W9-CFJ-959

A Digest of Medical Subjects

MEDICINE • SURGERY
NURSING • DIETETICS
PHYSICAL THERAPY
TREATMENT • DRUGS

TABER'S CYCLOPEDIC MEDICAL DICTIONARY

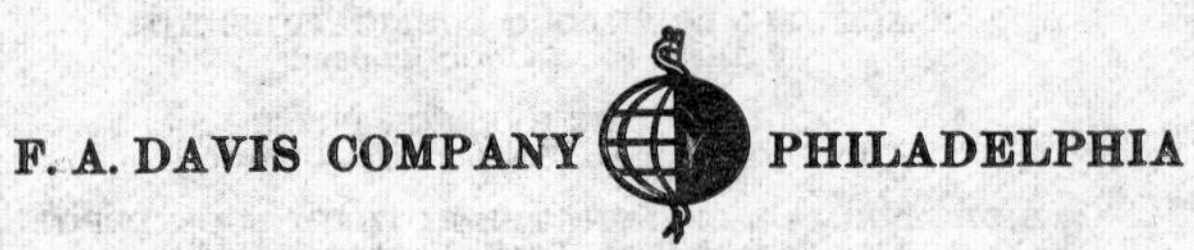

11TH EDITION • ILLUSTRATED

by Clarence Wilbur Taber

U.S.A.: F. A. DAVIS COMPANY
1915 Arch St., Philadelphia, Pa. 19103

GREAT BRITAIN, EUROPE & BRITISH COMMONWEALTH (except as noted):
BLACKWELL SCIENTIFIC PUBLICATIONS LTD.
5 Alfred St., Oxford, England

CANADA: THE RYERSON PRESS
330 Progress Ave., Scarborough, Ontario

INDIA, BURMA & CEYLON: THE KOTHARI BOOK DEPOT
King Edward Road, Parel, Bombay 12, India

Second Printing, January 1970
Third Printing, May 1970
Fourth Printing, January 1971
Fifth Printing, April 1971
Sixth Printing, November 1971

ISBN 0-8036-8300-6 (Thumb-indexed)
ISBN 0-8036-8301-4 (Plain)

PUBLISHER'S FOREWORD

WITH the publication of this Eleventh Edition we want to look both forward and to the past. Looking back, we find that during the past thirty years over 2,000,000 copies of *Taber's Cyclopedic Medical Dictionary* have been purchased by nurses, physicians and their professional colleagues throughout the world. We are pleased to have been part of this substantial effort to assist persons who by definition are dedicated to the service of mankind.

That we do not take this responsibility lightly is borne out by the improvement and changes included with this edition. Five hundred and fifty new entries have been added including Apgar Score, Indirect Measurement of Blood Pressure, Blood Components, Ponderal Index, and Thalidomide. Among the newly revised tables are Blood Components, Deciduous and Permanent Teeth, and Desirable Weights for Men and Women.

Literally thousands of changes have been made in areas which will not be immediately apparent. Some of these are Synonyms, Food Values, and those text changes necessitated by recent progress and developments in all branches of medicine, nursing, and related sciences. At the same time, entries which are no longer of value or in common usage have been removed.

There is no doubt that the quality of *Taber's Cyclopedic Medical Dictionary* has been enhanced by the many users who have taken the time to provide constructive criticism. To these we express our thanks and appreciation for being unofficial collaborators in the production of this edition.

F. A. DAVIS COMPANY

SOURCES CONSULTED

ALTHOUGH this dictionary is not a mere compilation, facts have been gathered from many sources. The author has personally scanned hundreds of medical and nursing textbooks and references for the latest information and procedures, and checked through countless numbers of medical, nursing, and biological journals. The information gleaned has been checked with many authorities, but the definitions are the author's own. To give individual credit to each book consulted and to each person written to would obviously be impossible.

The data on the content and chemical composition of foods have been largely based upon the findings of Sherman, although other eminent authorities in the field of food and nutrition have been drawn upon. It should, however, be understood that there can be no definite standard of values for any food, and that this accounts for the differences in the findings of various food specialists.

Much credit should be given to Edwin B. Steen, PH.D., Professor of Anatomy and Physiology, Western Michigan University, for his revisions and contributions pertaining to Bacteriology, Biology, and Parasitology in harmony with modern classifications of these subjects. New data have also been added to the subjects relating to the blood and to the endocrine glands with the help of well-known specialists.

C. W. TABER

FEATURES AND THEIR USE

ONLY a thoroughly trained mechanic would pretend to understand the workings of a complicated piece of machinery with its thousands of parts. Almost any one, however, feels competent to use successfully and to understand a dictionary that in reality represents hundreds of highly specialized subjects. To most persons, a dictionary is a dictionary. Nevertheless, *Taber's Cyclopedic Medical Dictionary* contains many subjects and features never before incorporated in such a reference work.

This work *is a medical dictionary,* but it is more than that. It is as much a dictionary of medical subject matter as it is a dictionary of medical terms. It is a source book of medical knowledge that will save much time in consulting a great many other works. A few of its more outstanding features are the following:

Pronunciations: Fully 99% of all words are respelled for pronunciation. Long and short vowels are marked diacritically, the primary accent is shown, and frequently the secondary accent. Latin rules cannot be depended upon for the pronunciation of medical words, and authorities do not agree upon any standardized pronunciations. Common usage, however, seems to prevail, and this has been followed as much as feasible in this book. Respellings for pronunciation are accurate and do not distort the actual spelling of the word any more than is necessary to indicate the proper phonetic sound.

Spellings: Diphthongs, for the most part, have been eliminated. Only proper nouns have been capitalized. Words formerly hyphenated, such as gastrointestinal, are now indicated as one word. Proper nouns used as adjectives do not take a capital initial. The letter "k" has been substituted for "c" in such words as leukocytes.

Vocabulary: This is sufficiently extensive to meet the daily needs of the practicing physician, the medical student, and the nurse. Highly specialized topics which belong in separate lexicons, such as botany, and obsolete words have been eliminated. Hundreds of drugs, for instance, that have not been in general use for ten or twenty years, have been weeded out of the vocabulary to make room for the inclusion of many new drugs. Medical literature has been combed to provide the very latest terms now in good medical standing.

Definitions: These stand out in a paragraph separate and apart from all collateral terms, and apart from additional supplementary matter, thus making it easy to read the definitions. The majority of synonyms have their own complete definitions, even at the risk of duplication. Words marked with an asterisk as they appear in a definition indicate that the word is defined in its proper place.

There probably is no profession in which there is less agreement regarding certain subjects than Medicine. The prevailing opinion of the profession, however, has been given in this dictionary, in so far as this has been available. Unfortunately, this may result in an adverse opinion in some instances, especially if the consultant is not familiar with opposing views, or unduly favorable to a definition other than the one expressed.

Subtopics: Many related words are listed and defined in most dictionaries in the same paragraph, such as the many *acids,* or different forms of the same disease. In this dictionary each of these words has its own vocabulary entrance with its definition separate and apart from other material. These topics are listed in alphabetical order, making access to them easy and quick.

Etymologies: This is the only abridged medical dictionary containing the derivations of words showing their Latin, Greek, and other sources with their meanings. These are not merely reproductions from other works, but the result of research which has made possible a great degree of accuracy. Prefixes and Suffixes also appear in alphabetical order the same as words.

Medical Synonyms: Medical synonyms are incorporated with the definition of a word; that is, when there *are* synonyms for a given term. This is a great aid to medical writers and speakers.

Words Pertaining To: Following important words will be found a list of other words pertaining to the one defined. In this way, a complete study or cycle of information pertaining to a given term may be acquired by reading the definitions of these words in the text. In many instances, following the definitions will be found a list of related subjects pertaining to the one defined.

First Aid: Practically every form of accident has been listed with first aid treatment. Included among these are poisons and their antidotes, bites and stings of all kinds, fractures, and other accidents, including different forms of unconsciousness.

Diseases: The principal diseases with their various forms are given, together with their diagnosis and symptoms, prognosis, treatment and nursing procedures, including diet.

Dietetics: Many foods and beverages are listed with all that is known about them. Also mineral content of the human body, and the physiology of digestion, assimilation, and elimination.

Drugs: Many of the terms for drugs have been given their trade-mark names, even though no references to the trade-mark or proprietary nature of the drug is made in the individual listing. These names are in common use by physicians and nurses who may be more familiar with them than with their scientific names.

Nursing Procedures: More of these are given than are usually found in the handbooks of nursing on the market.

Tabulations: Many important tabulations will be found in this text, but long tables which interfere with finding words in the dictionary have been grouped in the Appendix.

The Interpreter: This contains 373 questions and statements which are most often used during examination and taking the patient's history to aid in establishing diagnoses. Each item is in five languages: English, French, German, Italian and Spanish.

Only consistent use of this medical dictionary will prove its value and reveal much of its treasures.

FACT-FINDING INDEX

THE user of reference works seldom becomes aware of the many subjects they contain. The following index lists a few of the entries covering such important subjects as *Diagnosis, First Aid, Nursing Procedures,* and *Poisoning.* Many other subjects could be listed in the same manner. They, however, will be found in regular alphabetical order.

PRONUNCIATION

Diacritics: These are marks over or under vowels to indicate the pronunciations. In this dictionary, only two diacritics are used: The *macron*, showing the name sound or so-called long sound of vowels, as the *a* in rāte, *e* in ēat, *i* in īsle, *o* in ōver, and *u* in ūnite; also *e* as in ĕver, *i* as in ĭt, *o* as in nŏt, *u* as in cŭt.

Accents: These indicate the stress upon certain syllables. A single accent ′ is called a *primary* accent. A double accent ″ is called a *secondary* accent, indicating less stress upon a syllable than that given to a primary accent. Examples are "ob′ject," and "o″ar-i-al′ji-a."

Pronunciations only may be approximately indicated unless all the markings in Webster's New International Dictionary are used which is not practical in an abridged dictionary.

ABBREVIATIONS USED IN THE TEXT

abbr. abbreviation
adm. administration
anat. anatomy
ant. anterior
anti. antidote
app. appendix
art. artery
AS. Anglo-Saxon
at. no. atomic number
at. wt. atomic weight
bact. bacteriology
bet. between
biol. biology
BNA Basle Nomina Anatomica or Basel anatomical nomenclature
br. branch, branches
C. Centigrade
C carbon
Ca calcium
Cal. large Calorie or Calories
cal. small calorie or calories
carbo. carbohydrates
cc. cubic centimeter
cf. compare
chem. chemistry
Cl chlorine
CNS. Central nervous system
comp. composition
contra. contraindication
Cu copper, cuprum
der. derivative
dis. distribution
E. English
(e alternate word ending
e.g. for example
elect. electricity
esp. especially
etiol. etiology
ex. example
ext. exterior, external
F. Fahrenheit
F.A. first aid
Fr. French
Fe iron, ferrum
fem. female, feminine
ff. ind. fact-finding index
funct. function
G. Greek
Ger. German
Gm., gm. gram or grams
gr. grain or grains
gyn. gynecology
H hydrogen
I iodine
i.e. that is
ind. indication
inf. inferior
int. interior, internal
K potassium, kalium
L. Latin
lat. lateral
LL. Late Latin
m. male
ME. Middle English
med. medical
mg. milligram
Mg magnesium
N nitrogen
NA Nomina Anatomica (Parisiensia)
Na sodium, natrium
neur. neurology
NP. nursing procedure
NND. New and Nonofficial Drugs
nut. nutrients
O oxygen
OB. obstetrics
O. Fr. Old French
OPHTH. ophthalmology
opp. opposite
orig. origin
ORTH. orthopedics
OTO. otology
ONP operating nursing procedure
p page
P phosphorus
PATH. pathology
pert. pertaining
PHARM. pharmacy
PHYS. physiology
pl. plural
post. posterior
pre. prefix
pro. protein
prog. prognosis
PSY. psychiatry, psychoanalysis, psychology
PT. physical therapy
q.v. which see
rel. relating
RS. related subjects
S sulfur
sing. singular
sp. gr. specific gravity
sup. superior
SYM. symptoms
SYMB. symbol
SYN. synonym
USP United States Pharmacopoeia
viz. namely
***** denotes more information under the word indicated

A

A. Abbr. for *Angstrom unit;* chem. symbol formerly used for *argon.*

Å. Abbr. for *Angstrom unit.*

A_2. Abbr. for *aortic second sound.*

A.A. Abbr. for *achievement age, Alcoholics Anonymous.*

a. Abbr. for *accommodation, ampere, anode, anterior, area, artery.*

āa, āā [Abbr. G. *ana;* of each]. Prescription sign meaning *the stated amount of each of the substances is to be taken.*

aaa. Abbr. for *amalgam.*

a-, an- [G. *alpha*]. Prefix meaning *without, away from, not.*

A.A.A.S. American Association for the Advancement of Science.

A.A.G.P. American Academy of General Practice.

A.A.M.R.L. American Association of Medical Record Librarians.

A.A.P. American Academy of Pediatrics.

Aaron's sign [Charles D. Aaron, American physician, 1866-1951]. Distress in region of heart or stomach upon pressure over McBurney's point, *q.v.,* in appendicitis.

ab- [L.]. Prefix meaning *from, away from, negative, absent.*

abactus venter [L. *abactus,* driven away + L. *venter,* belly]. Induced abortion, *q.v.*

Abadie's sign (ă-bă-dēz'). 1. [C. Abadie, French ophthalmologist, 1842-1932]. In exophthalmic goiter, spasm of the levator palpebrae superioris. 2. [J. Abadie, French neurologist, 1873-]. In tabes dorsalis, insensibility to pressure over the Achilles tendon.

abaissement (ă-bās'mon) [Fr. a lowering]. 1. Depression. 2, In ophthalmology, a synonym for lenticular displacement (couching). 3. Falling.

abalienated (ăb-āl'yĕn-ā-tĕd) [L. *abalienare,* to separate from]. Insane.

abalienatio mentis (ab-al-yen-a'shĭ-o-men'tis). Insanity.

abalienation (ab-āl-yen-ā'shun) [L. *abalienāre,* to separate from]. Physical or mental decay; lunacy or derangement.

abaptiston (ă"bap-tis'ton) [G. *abaptistos, a-,* not + *baptistos,* dipped]. Trephine that cannot slip and injure the brain.

abarognosis (ăb-ar-og-nō'sĭs) [G. *a-,* priv. + *barys,* weight + *gnosis,* knowledge]. Without sense of weight.

abarthrosis (ab-ar-thrō'sis) [L. *ab,* from, + G. *arthron,* joint]. A movable joint or point upon which bones move freely upon each other. SYN: *diarthrosis.*

abartic'ular [" + *articulus,* joint]. At a distance from a joint.

abarticula'tion. 1. Dislocation of a joint. 2. Diarthrosis.

abasia (ă-bā'zĭ-ă) [G. *a-,* not, + *basis,* step]. Motor incoordination in walking. Inability to walk due to impairment of coordination.

a. -astasia. Lack of motor coordination with inability to stand or walk. Also called *astasia-abasia.*

a., atactic. Uncertain movements in walking. SYN: *ataxic abasia.*

a., choreic. That due to cramps in the limbs similar to movements of chorea.

a., paralytic. That in which the leg muscles are paralyzed.

a., paroxysmal trepidant. That caused by trembling and sudden stiffening of legs on standing, making walking impossible.

a., spastic. Paroxysmal trepidant abasia.

a., trembling, a. trepidans. That due to trembling of the legs.

abasic (ă-bā'sik). Pert. to abasia. SYN: *abatic.*

abate (ă-bāt') [L. *ab* from, + *battere,* to beat]. 1. To lessen or decrease. 2. To cease or cause to cease.

abatement (ă-bāt'mĕnt). Decrease in severity of pain or symptoms.

abatic (ab-at'ik). Pert. to abasia. SYN: *abasic.*

abaxial, abaxile (ab-ak'sĭ-al, ab-ak'sĭl) [L. *ab,* from + *axis*]. 1. Not in line of axis of the body or a part. 2. At opposite end of the axis of a part.

Abbe's catgut ring (ab'bē) [Robert Abbe, American surgeon, 1851-1928]. Ring of catgut for reinforcement of suture in intestinal anastomosis.

A.'s operation. 1. Resection of fifth nerve for tic douloureux. 2. Lateral anastomosis of the intestine.

Abbe's condenser (ab'bā) [Ernst Abbe, German physicist, 1840-1905]. Several achromatic lenses attached to a microscope to increase illumination.

Abbe-Zeiss apparatus. A device for counting blood cells in a specific quantity of blood. Called also *Thoma-Zeiss counting cell hemocytometer.*

Abbott's method [Edville G. Abbott, American orthopaedic surgeon, 1870-1938]. Treatment of scoliosis by a series of plaster jackets.

Abbott-Miller tube [W. Osler Abbott, Philadelphia physician, 1902-1943, and T. Grier Miller, Philadelphia physician, 1886-]. A double channel intestinal tube used to relieve intestinal distention. Commonly called Miller-Abbott tube.

Abbott-Rawson tube [W. Osler Abbott and Arthur J. Rawson, American scientist, 1896-]. Double barrelled gastroenterostomy tube.

A. B. C. method, process. The use of alum, blood, and charcoal in purification of water or sewage or deodorization.

Abderhalden's reaction, test (ăb'der-hăl-denz) [Emil Abderhalden, German physiologist, 1877-]. Creation of ferments in circulation as result of injection of foreign protein, fat, or carbohydrate. Has been used in testing for pregnancy, acute infections, malignancies, goiter. When used in dementia praecox, it is known as Abderhalden-Fauser reaction.

abdomen (ab-do'men, ab'do-men) [L. *abdomen,* of uncertain origin]. [NA]. That portion of the trunk located between the chest and the pelvis; the upper portion of the abdomino-pelvic cavity. SEE: *abdominal cavity; a. regions.*

Contains the stomach with lower part of esophagus, small and large intestines, liver, gallbladder, spleen, pancreas, and bladder. A serous membrane, the peritoneum, lines this cavity.

a., accordion. Swelling of the abdomen which comes and goes rapidly. Due to nervousness. SYN: *abdominal pseudotympany.*

a., acute. Medical jargon used to denote any acute abdominal condition demanding prompt operation.

a., boat-shaped. Scaphoid a.

a., carinate. Scaphoid a.

a., navicular. Scaphoid a.

a. obstipum. Congenital shortness of the rectus abdominis muscle.

a., pendulous. Condition in which the excessively relaxed anterior wall of the abdomen hangs down over the pubis.

a., scaphoid. One in which the anterior wall is hollowed, presenting a sunken appearance as in emaciation and some cerebral diseases.

a., surgical. Acute a.

abdominal (ab-dom'i-nal). Pert. to the abdomen, its function and disorders.

a. cavity. The cavity within the abdomen. It is lined with a serous membrane, the peritoneum, and contains the following organs: stomach with lower portion of esophagus, small and large intestines (except sigmoid colon and rectum), liver, gallbladder, spleen, pancreas, kidney and ureter. It is continuous with the pelvic cavity, the two comprising the abdomino-pelvic cavity.

a. crisis. Severe pain in the abdominal area. Usually refers to the pain which occurs during sickle cell anemia crisis or that due to syphilis.

a. examination. AUSCULTATION: Listening to sounds in the body. Of service in diagnosis of aneurysm, fetal heart sounds and uteroplacental murmur in pregnancy.

INSPECTION: Most satisfactorily performed with patient on back with thighs slightly flexed. In health, abdomen is of an oval form, marked by elevations and depressions corresponding to abdominal muscles, umbilicus, and in some degree by form of adjacent viscera. Is larger relatively, to size of chest, in children than in adults; more rotund and broader inferiorly in females than in males.

Alterations in shape due to disease are *first,* enlargement, which may be general and symmetrical, as in ascites; or partial and irregular, from tumors, hypertrophy of organs, as the liver and spleen, or from distention of portions of intestines by gas, as the colon in typhoid fever; *second,* retraction, as in extreme emaciation, and in several forms of cerebral disease, esp. noticeable in tuberculous meningitis of children.

The respiratory movements of abdominal walls bear a certain relation to movements of the thorax; are often increased when the latter are arrested and vice versa; thus abdominal movements are increased in pleurisy, pneumonia, pericarditis, etc., but decreased or wholly suspended when disease causes abdominal pain, or in peritonitis.

The superficial abdominal veins are also at times visibly enlarged, indicating an obstruction to the flow of blood, either in the portal system as in cirrhosis, or in the inferior vena cava.

PALPATION: May be performed with tips of fingers, whole hand, or both hands; pressure may be slight or forcible, continuous or intermittent. To obtain greatest amount of information, patient should be placed in horizontal position with head slightly raised and thighs flexed. Sometimes necessary to place in standing position or leaning forward.

INDICATIONS FURNISHED BY PALPATION: Size and position of viscera; existence of tumors and swellings, whether superficial or deep, large or small, hard or soft, smooth or nodulated, movable or fixed, solid or liquid, and whether they change position with respiration. Also ascertain whether tenderness exists in any portion of the abdominal cavity, and if pain is increased or relieved by firm pressure.

Impulse, if one exists, is systolic and expansive, though when situated high up there also may be a slight diastolic movement. A thrill is rarely perceptible. Surface of tumor, when not ruptured, is rounded and smooth. Effusion of blood into surrounding tissues may produce lobulations.

PERCUSSION: Patient should be placed in same position as for palpation, and percussion should be for most part mediate. In exploring abdomen by means of percussion, finger should first be placed immediately below the xiphoid cartilage, pressed firmly down, and carried along the median line toward the

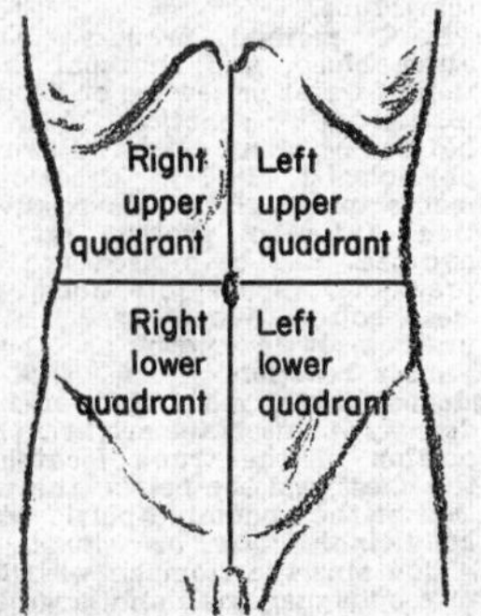

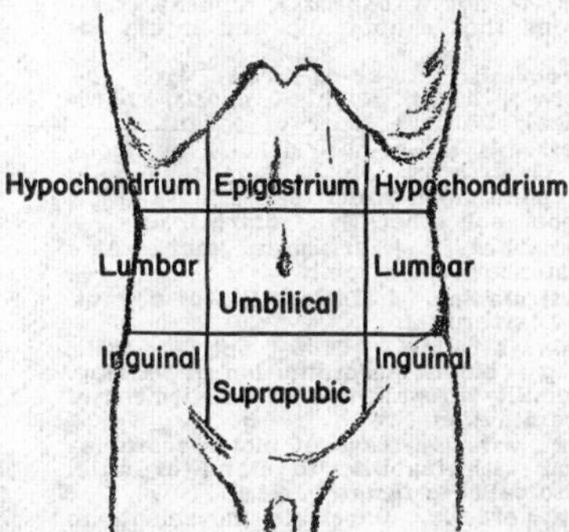

REGIONS OF ABDOMEN

pubes, striking it all the way, now forcibly, now gently. The *different tones* of stomach, colon, and small intestines will be distinctly heard. Percussion should then be made laterally, alternately to one side, then the other, till whole surface is percussed. *Abdominal aneurysm* gives dullness or flatness over it unless a distended intestine lies above it.

a. gestation. Abdominal pregnancy. Extrauterine pregnancy in belly cavity.

a. inguinal ring. The internal opening of the inguinal canal, bounded *inferiorly* by the inguinal ligament, *medially* by the inferior epigastric vessels, and *above* and *laterally* by the lower free border of the transversus abdominis muscle. SYN: *deep inguinal ring; int. abdominal ring.* SEE: *inguinal canal; inguinal ring.*

a. quadrants. Four parts or divisions of the abdomen determined by drawing a vertical and a horizontal line through the umbilicus. The quadrants and their contents are:

RIGHT UPPER Q.: Right lobe of liver, gallbladder, part of transverse colon, part of pylorus, hepatic flexure, right kidney, and duodenum.

RIGHT LOWER Q.: Cecum, ascending colon, small intestine, appendix, bladder if distended, right ureter, right spermatic duct in male, right ovary and right tube, and uterus, if enlarged, in female.

LEFT UPPER Q.: Left lobe of liver, stomach, transverse colon, splenic flexure, pancreas, left kidney, and spleen.

LEFT LOWER Q.: Small intestine, left ureter, sigmoid flexure, descending colon, bladder if distended, left spermatic duct in male, uterus, left ovary, and left tube in female.

a. reflexes. Contraction of the muscles of the abdominal wall upon stimulation of the overlying skin. Absence of these reflexes indicates damage to the pyramidal tract.

a. regions. The abdomen and its external surface are divided into nine regions by four imaginary planes: *two horizontal,* one at the level of the ninth costal cartilage (or the lowest point of the costal arch), and the other at the level of the highest point of the iliac crest; *two vertical,* through the centers of the inguinal ligaments (or through the nipples, or through the centers of the clavicles), or curved and coinciding with the lateral borders of the two abdominal rectus muscles.

a. rings. The apertures in the abdominal wall. *a.r., external:* An interval in aponeurosis of external oblique muscle, just above and to outer side of crest of the pubic bone. *a.r., triangular:* About one inch from base to apex, and half an inch transversely; gives passage to spermatic cord in male, round ligament in female. *a.r., internal or deep:* Situated in the transversalis fascia, midway between the ant. superior spine of ilium and symphysis pubis, half inch above Poupart's ligament; oval form, larger in male. Transmits spermatic cord in male, round ligament in female.

a. section. Abdominal incision for any operation on abdominal organs. SEE: *laparotomy.*

abdominalgia (ab-dom-ĭ-nal′jē-ă) [L. *abdomen* + G. *algos,* pain + ia]. Pain in the abdomen.

abdomino- (ab-dom′ĭ-nō). Combining form; relating to the stomach.

abdominoanterior (ab-dom″ĭ-nō-an-tē′rĭ-or). Position of fetus in uterus with belly facing anterior abdominal wall of mother.

abdom″inocar′diac re′flex. A change in heart rate, usually a slowing, resulting from mechanical stimulation of abdominal viscera.

abdom″inocentesis (ab-dom″ĭ-nō-sen-tē′sis) [L. *abdomen* + G. *kentēsis,* puncture]. Puncture of the abdomen with an instrument for withdrawal of fluid from the abdominal cavity. SYN: *paracentesis abdominis.*

abdom″inocys′tic [" + G. *kystis,* bladder]. Pertaining to abdomen and bladder.

abdom″inogen′ital [" + *genitalis*]. Pertaining to the abdomen and genital organs.

abdom″inohysterec′tomy [" + G. *ystera,* uterus, + *ektomē,* excision]. Removal of uterus through abdominal incision.

abdom″inohysterot′omy [" + " + *tome,* a cutting]. Incision of the uterus through a surgical opening in the abdomen.

abdom″inoposte′rior. Position of fetus in uterus with abdomen toward mother's back.

abdom″inos′copy [" + G. *skopein,* to view]. Examination, especially by instrument, of abdomen or its viscera.

abdom″inoscro′tal [" + *scrotum,* bag]. Pertaining to the abdomen and scrotum.

a. muscle. Cremaster muscle.

abdominothoracic (ab-dom″ĭ-nō-tho-ras′ik) [" + G. *thōrax,* breastplate]. Pertaining to the abdomen and thorax.

a. arch. The costal arch, a line dividing the thorax from the abdomen.

abdom′inous. Having a prominent abdomen.

abdom″inouterot′omy [" + *uterus,* womb, + G. *tomē,* incision]. Abdominohysterotomy.

abdom″inovag′inal [" + *vagina,* sheath]. Pertaining to the abdomen and vagina.

abdom″inoves′ical [" + *vesica,* bladder]. Pertaining to the abdomen and the urinary bladder.

a. pouch. Peritoneal fold which includes urachal folds.

abducens (ab-dū′senz) [L. drawing away from]. 1. Abducent nerve, *q.v.* 2. The rectus lateralis muscle of the eye, which moves the eyeball outward. 3. Pertaining to drawing away from the median line of the body.

a. labiorum. Elevates angle of mouth. SYN: *caninus muscle; levator anguli oris muscle, q.v. in Table of Muscles in Appendix.*

a. oculi. Rectus lateralis muscle of eye. SEE: *Table of Muscles in Appendix.*

a. oris. Elevates angle of mouth. SYN: *caninus muscle; levator anguli oris muscle, q.v. in Table of Muscles in Appendix.*

abdu′cent. 1. Abducting, leading away from. 2. Abducens.

a. nerve. Innervates rectus lateralis muscle of eye which rotates the eyeball outward. SYN: *6th cranial nerve.* SEE: *cranial nerves.*

abduct′ [L. *abductus,* past p. *abducere,* to lead away]. To draw away from the median plane of the body or one of its parts.

abduc′tion. 1. The lateral movement of the limbs away from the median plane of the body, or the lateral bending of the head or trunk. 2. The movement of the digits away from the axial line of a limb. 3. In ophthalmology, outward rotation of the eyes.

abduc′tor. A muscle which upon contraction draws a part away from median plane of body or axial line of an extremity. Opp. to *adductor*. SEE: *Table of Muscles in Appendix.*

Abel's bacillus [Rudolf Abel, German bacteriologist, 1868-1942]. *Klebsiella ozaenae;* found in ozena.

abenteric (ab-en-ter'ik) [L. *ab,* from + G. *enteron,* intestine]. Located in a part outside the intestines, as abenteric typhoid fever. SYN: *apenteric.*

abepithymia (ab-ep-ĭ-thī'mĭ-ă) [" + G. *epithymia,* desire]. 1. Paralysis of the celiac (solar) plexus. 2. This word is related to the Greek word *thymos,* meaning *soul.* The seat of the soul and desire was thought to be in the diaphragm. Thus the term has been used to describe unnatural or pathological desires.

Abernethy's fascia (ab'er-nē-thēz) [John Abernethy, British surgeon, 1764-1831]. A layer of areolar tissue separating the external iliac artery from the iliac fascia over the psoas muscle.

A.'s sarcoma. A circumscribed, usually malignant, fatty tumor occurring principally on the trunk.

aber'rant [L. *ab,* from, + *errare,* to wander]. Wandering from the normal or usual course.

a. pyramidal tract. Several groups of fibers from the midbrain to the cranial nerve motor nuclei and separating from the main fibers of the cortex.

aberratio (ab-er-ā'shĭ-o). Aberration.

a. lactis. Secretion of milk from a site other than the breast.

a. mensium. Vicarious menstruation.

a. testis. Location of a testis in a position away from the path of normal descent.

aberra'tion. 1. Deviation from a normal course. 2. Mental unsoundness, but not insanity. 3. Imperfect refraction.

a., chromatic. Unequal refraction of different wave lengths of light through a lens, producing a colored image.

a., chromosomal. Variations in chromosomes as to number (*aneurploidy, polyploidy*) or those involving alterations in chromosomal material (*translocation, deletion, duplication*).

a., diopteric. Spherical a.

a., distantial. Blurring of a distant object.

a., lateral. Deviation of a ray from the focus measured on a line perpendicular to the axis.

a., longitudinal. Deviation of a ray from the focus measured along the axis.

a., mental. Any deviation from normal mental functions.

a., spherical. Unequal refraction of different wave lengths of light through a lens, producing a blurred image.

aberrom'eter [L. *ab-,* from + *errare,* to wander + G. *metron,* measure]. An instrument for measuring errors in delicate observations or instruments.

abevacuation (ab-ē-vak-ū-ā'shun) [" + *evacuare,* to empty]. 1. Abnormal evacuation either in excess or in deficiency. 2. Metastases.

abeyance (a-bā'ăns) [Old French]. A temporary suspension of activity, sensation, or pain.

ab'ient. Tending to move away from the source of a stimulus. Opposite to *adient.*

abiochemistry (ab-ĭ-ō-kĕm'is-trĭ) [G. *a-,* priv. + *bios,* life, + *chēmeia,* chemistry]. Inorganic chemistry.

abiogenesis (ab-ĭ-ō-jĕn'ĕ-sis) [" + " + *genesis,* production]. Spontaneous generation of life; theoretical production of living from nonliving matter.

abiogenet'ic, abio'genous. Pertaining to spontaneous generation.

abiologic, abiological (ā-bī-ō-loj'ik, -al) Not related to biology or the science of life.

abiology (ā-bī-ol'ō-jī) [G. *a-,* priv. + *bios,* life, + *logos,* study of]. The study of inanimate things.

abionarce (ab"ĭ-o-nar'se) [" + G. *narke,* stupor]. Infirmity, especially of the aged, due to weakness of mind and body.

abionergy (ab-ĭ-on'ur-jĭ) [" + " + *energeia,* action, energy]. Premature degeneration. SYN: *abiotrophy.*

abiosis (ab-ĭ-ō'sis) [G. *a-,* priv. + *bios,* life]. Absence of life.

abiot'ic. Incompatible with life; not viable.

abiotro'phia. Abiotrophy.

abiotrophy (ab-ĭ-ot'rō-fĭ) [G. *a-,* priv. + *bios,* life + *trophē,* nourishment]. Premature loss of vitality or degeneration of tissues and cells with consequent loss of endurance and resistance.

abirritant (ab-ir'ĭ-tant) [L. *ab-,* from + *irritare,* to irritate]. Relieving irritation; soothing.

abirrita'tion. 1. Asthenia, or atony. 2. Lowered tissue irritability.

abiuret (a-bī'ū-ret) [G. *a-,* priv. + L. *bis,* double, + urea]. Nonbiuret; not giving the biuret reaction.

ablactation (ab-lak-tā'shun) [L. *ab,* from + *lac,* milk]. Free of, or cessation of, milk secretion; weaning.

ablastem'ic [G. *a-,* priv. + *blastos,* germ, seed]. Not germinal.

ablate (ab-lāt') [L. *ablatus,* taken away]. To remove, especially by excision.

ablatio (ab-lā'shĭ-ō) [L. *ablatio,* carrying away]. Ablation, removal, detachment.

a. placentae. Premature detachment of a normally situated placenta; apoplexy of placenta; abruptio placentae, *q.v.* SEE ALSO: *placenta.*

a. retinae. Detachment of retina. SEE: *retina.*

ablation (ab-lā'shun) [L. *ab,* from, + *latus,* carried]. Removal of a part, as by cutting.

ablepharia (ab-lĕ-fā-rē-a), [a- + G. *blepharon,* eyelid, + ia]. Congenital reduction in size or absence of the eyelids.

ablepharon (ă-bleph'ă-ron). Ablepharia.

ablepharous (ă-bleph'ă-rus). Without eyelids.

ablephary (ă-bleph'ă-rē). Ablepharia.

ablepsia (ă-blep'sĭ-ă) [G. *a-,* + *blepein,* to see]. Blindness.

ab'luent [L. *ab,* from, + *luens,* to wash]. An agent possessing cleansing qualities, as a detergent.

ablu'tion. A cleansing or washing.

ablutomania (ă-bloo"to-ma'nĭ-ă). Compulsion to wash or clean oneself.

abmor'tal [L. *ab,* from, + *mors,* death]. Passing from dead or dying to living fiber, as an electric current.

abner'val [L. *ab,* from, + *nervus,* nerve]. Away from a nerve, esp. with reference to the passage of an electric current through a muscle away from point where nerve enters the muscle. Opp. to *adnerval.*

abneural (ab-nū'ral) [L. *ab,* from, + G. *neuron,* nerve]. 1. Ventral. Remote from neural or dorsal aspect. 2. Abnerval.

abnor'mal [G. *anomalos*]. Not normal; deviating from the usual type in structure, form, or function; anomalous; irregular. SEE: *anomaly.*

ab"normal'ity. That which is not normal.

ab"norm'ity. 1. Deformity; abnormality. 2. A monstrosity.

abocclusion (ab″ŏ-klū′zhun). Dentition in which the teeth of the mandible and the maxilla are not in contact.

aborad (ab-ō′rad) [L. *ab,* from, + *oris,* mouth]. Away from the mouth.

aboral (ab-ō′ral). Opposite to, or away from, the mouth.

abort (ă-bort′) [L. *abortus* fr. *aboriri,* from being born, from rising]. 1. To cause expulsion of an embryo or of the fetus before time of viability. 2. To arrest progress of disease. 3. To arrest growth or development.

aborticide (a-bor′ti-sīd) [" + *caedere,* to kill]. Destruction of the fetus in the uterus.

abortient (ă-bor′shent). 1. Producing abortion. 2. Abortifacient.

abortifacient (ă-bor-tĭ-fā′shent) [L. *abortus,* abortion, + *facere,* to make]. A drug which causes an abortion.

abortion (ă-bor′shun). 1. The arrest of any physical action or disease. 2. The termination of pregnancy before the stage of viability, *i.e.,* sometime between the twentieth and twenty-eighth week of gestation, the fetus measuring less than 14 inches (20 cm.) and weighing less than 500 gm. Because laymen interpret the word *abortion* to mean criminal interruption of pregnancy, it is advisable to use the word *miscarriage* when discussing abortion with a patient or her family. 3. The immature product of conception which has been expelled prematurely.

Etiol: Among most common causes are: (a) faulty development of embryo; (b) abnormalities of the placenta; (c) endocrine disturbances; (d) acute infectious diseases; (e) severe trauma or shock.

Sym: Abdominal cramps and bleeding from vagina.

NP: Send for doctor. Keep patient quiet. Care as for uterine hemorrhage. Save discharges for doctor's inspection. Watch for shock and symptoms of sepsis.

a., accidental. That which occurs spontaneously and accidentally without criminal intent.

a., ampullar. Tubal abortion occurring from the ampulla of the oviduct.

a., artificial. When induced or performed purposely, as by a surgeon.

a., cervical. One in which the ovum is retained in the cervical canal.

a., complete. Abortion in which the complete product of conception has been expelled.

a., criminal. A. which is deliberately produced for other than medical purposes.

a., embryonic. One that occurs before the fifth month of pregnancy.

a., fetal. One that occurs after the fifth month of pregnancy.

a., habitual. A. in the course of three or more pregnancies, with no apparent cause.

a., imminent. That characterized by bleeding and colicky pains which progressively increase. Cervix usually effaced and patulous.

a., incomplete. Abortion in which part of the product of conception has been retained in the uterus.

a., induced. One brought on intentionally, as a criminal or therapeutic a. Abortions may be induced by use of drugs, instruments, or exposure to radiation. See: *curettage.*

a., inevitable. That which cannot be halted.

a., infected. When accompanied by infection of retained material with resultant febrile reaction.

a., justifiable. A. performed to save the mother's life. See: *abortion, therapeutic.*

a., missed. That in which a dead nonviable fetus and other products of conception are retained in the uterus for two months or longer.

a., ovular. That which occurs within first three weeks after conception.

a., partial. In multiple pregnancy, aborting of only one fetus, or less than the entire number.

a., psychiatric. A therapeutic abortion for the relief of symptoms of severe mental disease aggravated by or having its origin during pregnancy.

a., septic. That in which there is an infection of the product of conception and the endometrial lining of uterus usually resulting from attempted interference during early pregnancy.

a., spontaneous. Occurring naturally without interference.

a., therapeutic. A. performed legally before viability under certain conditions, as when the life of the mother is endangered by continuation of the pregnancy.

a., threatened. The appearance of signs and symptoms of possible loss of embryo. Vaginal bleeding with or without intermittent pain is usually the first sign. If embryo is still alive and attachment to uterus has not been interrupted, pregnancy may continue. Absolute bed rest essential with avoidance of coitus, douches, and strong cathartics.

a., tubal. 1. A tubal pregnancy in which the fetus has been expelled through the distal end of a uterine tube. 2. The escape of the product of conception into the peritoneal cavity by way of the uterine tube.

abortionist (ă-bor′shun-ist). One who performs a criminal abortion.

abortive (ă-bor′tiv). 1. Preventing the completion of. 2. Abortifacient; that which prevents a natural or regular course. 3. Rudimentary.

abortus (ă-bor′tus). An aborted fetus weighing less than 500 grams.

abouchement (ă-boosh-mon′) [Fr.]. The ending of a small vessel in a large one.

aboulia (ă-boo′lĭ-ă) [G. *a-,* + *boulē,* will]. Inability to exercise will power. Syn: *abulia, q.v.*

aboulomania (ă-boo′lō-mā′nĭ-ă) [" + " + *mania,* frenzy]. Mental disorder with loss of will power. Syn: *abulomania.*

abrachia (ă-brā′kē-ă) [G. *a-,* + *brachiōn,* arm]. The congenital anomaly of armlessness.

abrachiocephalia (ă-brā″kē-ō-sĕ-fā′lē-ă) [" + " + *kephalē,* head]. Congenital anomaly consisting of absence of arms and head.

abrachiocephalus (ă-brā″kē-ō-sĕf′ă-lus). A fetal monster without head or arms.

abrachius (ă_brā′kē-us). An individual without arms.

abradant (ă-brăd′ent). Abrasive.

abrade (ă-brăd′) [L. *ab,* from + *radere,* to scrape]. 1. To chafe. 2. To roughen or remove by friction.

Abrams' heart reflex [Albert Abrams, San Francisco physician, 1864-1924]. Reduction of area of cardiac dullness resulting from manual friction of precordial and epigastric areas.

abra′sio cor′neae [L. abrasion of cornea]. Removal of corneal excrescences by scraping.

abrasion (ab-rā'zhun) [L. *ab,* from, + *radere,* to scrape]. 1. A scraping away of a portion of skin or of a mucous membrane as a result of injury or mechanical means, as in dermabrasion for cosmetic purposes. A brush burn. 2. The wearing away of the substance of a tooth. Normally occurs from mastication; may be accomplished by mechanical or chemical means.

SEE: *avulsion; bruise.*

abra'sive. 1. Producing abrasion. 2. That which abrades.

abreaction (ăb-rē-ăk'shun) [L. *ab,* from, + *rē,* again, + *actus,* acting]. PSY: Reevaluation of an emotion-laden experience during its free discussion with an understanding psychotherapist. Freud called the process catharis, *q.v.*

abrosia (ab-rō'zĭ-ă) [" + *erodere,* to gnaw away]. 1. Fasting; abstaining from food. 2. A wasting away.

abruptio (ab-rup'shĭ-ō) [" + *ruptere,* a break]. A tearing away from.

a. placentae. Premature detachment of normally situated placenta; ablatio placenta. SEE ALSO: *placenta.*

ETIOL: Some causes are hypertensive disease, toxemia of pregnancy, chronic nephritis, violent labor of childbirth.

PATH: Extravasation of blood between placenta and uterine wall, occasionally between muscle fibers of the uterus. The peritoneal coat of the uterus may exhibit small linear fissures which allow free blood to enter the peritoneal cavity.

SYM: (a) Hemorrhage, concealed or evident, or a combination of both. (b) Pain, constant at point of separation of placenta due to blood extruding between muscle fibers. (c) Uterine contraction constant; occasionally tetanic in nature. (d) Evidences of fetal asphyxia and death, increased fetal movements, and changes in heart rate until final cessation of both. (e) Albumin in urine. (f) Anemia.

TREATMENT: (a) Mild cases: Rest in bed. (b) Severe cases: Shock must first be combated. A soft and partially dilated cervix is an indication for immediate artificial rupture of membranes followed by natural or artificial induction of labor. If the fetus is viable and alive, and if the mother's cervix is firm and not dilated, a cesarean section is the treatment of choice. If the uterus fails to contract after cesarean section, a rapid hysterectomy is usually necessary.

abscess (ăb'sĕs) [L. *abscessus,* a going away]. A localized collection of pus in any part of the body. SEE: *inflammation; pus.*

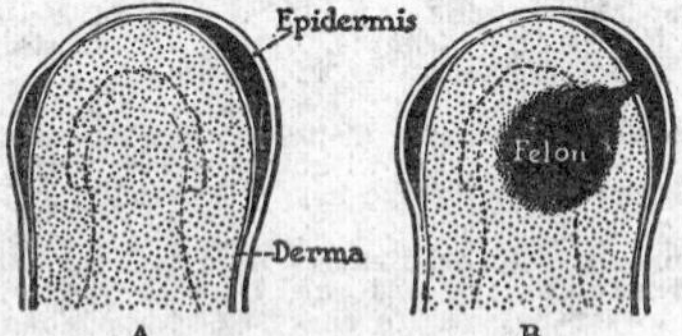

SUBEPITHELIAL ABSCESS

A, Abscesses located at tip of finger lie between dense epidermis and derma; B, Subepithelial abscess developed from felon which perforated derma and spread out beneath epiderma, which is lifted up in a manner similar to a blister.

a., acute, or warm. One with local symptoms of inflammation, with fluctuation, and pointing; also pressure and constitutional symptoms. Inflammation becomes intensified with increased heat, redness, swelling, and edema. Pain becomes throbbing and greater, with impaired loss of function of the part. An elevation appears, with fluctuation and softening as it reaches the surface, becoming necrotic and yellow, giving way with evacuation of pus. *Pressure symptoms,* according to size and depth. In floor of mouth or neck, swelling may cause dyspnea and dysphagia. *Constitutional symptoms* vary, from slight temperature (fever may be absent in a well walled-off abscess) to high temperature, with rigors and sweats if associated with pyemia and septicemia. Any or all general symptoms may be absent in deep-seated abscesses except loss of weight and strength.

TERMINATION: This may be by pointing, evacuation, and discharge of pus, which may become inspissated, encapsulated, and at times absorbed.

a., alveolar. Abscess about root of a tooth in alveolar cavity. Usually the result of necrosis and infection of dental pulp following dental caries.

a., amebic, of liver. Abscess occurring in the liver developing as a complication of amebic dysentery. Caused by *Entamoeba histolytica.*

a., anorectal. One in the tissue near the rectum. SYN: *ischiorectal a.; perirectal a.*

a., apical. One at the apex of lung or at extremity of root of a tooth.

a., appendiceal, appendicular. Pus formation around an inflamed vermiform appendix.

a., arthrifluent. A wandering abscess having origin in a diseased joint.

a., atheromatous. Softening in the wall of a blood vessel as the result of atherosclerosis.

a., axillary. One or multiple abscesses in axilla.

a., bartholin. A. of Bartholin's gland.

a., Bezold's. A deep abscess in the tissues of the neck resulting from osteomyelitis of sphenoid bone or nasopharyngeal infection.

a., bicameral. One with two pockets.

a., bile duct. A. of the bile duct. SYN: *cholangitic a.*

a., bilharziasis. One in an intestinal wall caused by *Schistosoma.*

a., blind. An abscess with no external opening such as a dental granuloma.

a., bone. Brodie's abscess, *q.v.*

a., brain. An intracranial abscess; one involving the brain or its membranes. They are seldom primary, usually occurring secondary to infections of middle ear, nasal sinuses, face, or skull, or from contamination from penetrating wounds or skull fractures. They may also have a metastatic origin arising from septic foci in the lungs (bronchiectasis, empyema, lung abscess), in bone (osteomyelitis), or in the heart (endocarditis). Infection of nervous tissue by the invading organism results in necrosis and liquefaction and edema of surrounding tissues.

Brain abscesses may be acute, subacute, or chronic. Their clinical manifestations depend on part of brain involved, size, virulence of infecting organisms, and other factors.

SYM: Severe and persistent headache usually localized over infected area; fever, vomiting, vertigo, malaise, sometimes irritability and other mental symptoms.

Treatment: Chemotherapy and antibiotic agents; sometimes puncture and aspiration or surgical extirpation is necessary.

a., breast. A. of breast marked by acute inflammation. Syn: *mammary a.*

a., Brodie's. Tuberculosis with suppuration of articular end of a bone, especially the tibia. Syn: *bone a.*

a., bursal. One in a bursa.

a., canalicular. An abscess of breast discharging into the milk ducts.

a., caseous. One in which the pus has a cheesy appearance.

a., cerebral. A brain abscess. Syn: *intracranial a.*

a., cheesy. Caseous abscess.

a., cholangitic. One of the bile duct.

a., chronic. One with pus but without signs of inflammation; usually of slow development. Formed by liquefaction of tuberculous tissue. May occur anywhere on the body but more frequently in the spine, hips, genitourinary tract, and lymph glands. Symptoms may be very mild, pain when present being due to pressure upon surrounding parts. Tenderness often absent. Chronic septic intoxication with hectic fever occurs when there is mixed infection. Amyloid disease may develop if the abscess persists for a prolonged period. Syn: *cold a.*

a., circumscribed. An abscess limited or confined by surrounding tissue.

a., circumtonsillar. An abscess around the tonsil. Syn: *quinsy; peritonsillar abscess.*

a., cold. Chronic abscess, *q.v.*

a., collar-button. Two cavities, one larger than the other, containing pus and connected by a narrow channel. Syn: *shirt-stud abscess.*

a., congestive. One that shows pus at a point distant from where formed.

a., deep. One arising from below the deep fascia.

a., Delpech's. A. without fever which develops rapidly, causing great prostration.

a., dental. An abscess about a tooth.

a., dentoalveolar. One in the alveolar process surrounding the root of a tooth.

a., diffuse. A collection of pus not circumscribed by a well-defined capsule.

a., dry. One that disappears without pointing or breaking.

a., Dubois'. One of the thymus formed in congenital syphilis.

a., embolic. One due to a septic embolus.

a., emphysematous. Tympanitic a., *q.v.*

a., encysted. One with pus circumscribed in a serous cavity.

a., endamebic; a., entamebic. Amebic a., *q.v.*

a., epidural. Extradural a., *q.v.*

a., epiploic. One in the omentum.

a., extradural. A. on the dura mater.

a., fecal. An abscess containing feces.

a., filarial. One caused by filaria.

a., fixation. One produced artificially by subcutaneous injection of an irritant.

a., Fochier's. Same as *fixation a.*

a., follicular. One forming in a follicle.

a., frontal. Abscess in the frontal lobe of the brain.

a., fungal. Abscess caused by a fungus.

a., gangrenous. One attended with gangrene of surrounding parts.

a., gas. A tympanitic abscess; one containing gas due to presence of gas-forming organisms such as ***Clostridium perfringens.***

a., gingival. An abscess of the gum.

a., glandular. One around a lymph node.

a., gravitation. An abscess in which the pus migrates, sinking to a lower part of the body.

a's., heart. In interstitial myocarditis, multiple small abscesses.

a., helminthic. One due to the presence of a parasitic worm.

a., hematic. One due to an extravasated blood clot.

a., hemorrhagic. One containing blood.

a., hepatic. Abscess of the liver, especially an amebic a.

a., hot. An acute abscess, *q.v.*

a., hypostatic. A wandering abscess, *q.v.*

a., idiopathic. One due to unknown causes.

a., iliac. One in the iliac region.

a., intracranial. A. of brain. Syn: *cerebral a.*

a., intradural. A. within the layers of the dura mater.

a., intramammary. An abscess of the mammary gland. Syn: *mammary a.; breast a.*

a., intramastoid. A mastoid process abscess of the temporal bone.

a., ischiorectal. One in the ischiorectal fossa.

a., kidney. One or multiple abscesses of renal cortex. Syn: *renal a.*

a., lacrimal. Suppuration of a lacrimal gland.

a., lacunar. One in the urethral lacunae.

a., lateral; a., lateral alveolar. A periodontal abscess.

a., lumbar. Abscess in the lumbar region.

a., lung. A. occurring in the lung.

a., lymphatic. An abscess of a lymph node.

a., mammary. One in the female breast, esp. an abscess involving the glandular tissue. Usually seen during lactation or at time of weaning. Syn: *breast a.; intramammary a.*

a., marginal. One near the orifice of the anus.

a., mastoid. Suppuration of the mastoid portion of the temporal bone.

a., mediastinal. Suppuration in the mediastinum.

a., metastatic. A secondary one at a distance from focus of infection.

a., migrating. A wandering abscess, *q.v.*

a., miliary. A small embolic abscess. One discharging numerous small collections of pus.

a., milk. A mammary abscess during lactation.

a., mother. A primary abscess giving rise to other abscesses.

a., multiple. A group of abscesses accompanying pyemia.

a., mural. One in tissues of the abdominal wall.

a., nocardial. One caused by *Nocardia.*

a., orbital. Suppuration in the orbit.

a., ossifluent. One dependent on degeneration of bone tissue.

a., Paget's. One recurring about the site of an earlier abscess. Same as *residual a.*

a., palatal. One in an upper lateral incisor, erupting toward the palate.

a., palmar. A purulent effusion into the tissues of the palm of the hand.

a., parafrenal. Abscess on the side of the frenulum of the penis. Usually involves Tyson's gland.

a., parametric; a., parametritic. One between the folds of the broad ligaments of the uterus.

a., paranephric, a., paranephritic. One in the tissues around the kidney.

a., parapancreatic. One in the tissues next to the pancreas.

a., parietal. A periodontal abscess arising in the periodontal tissue other than the orifice through which the vascular supply enters the dental pulp.

a., pelvic. Abscess of the pelvic peritoneum, especially Douglas' pouch.

a., pelvirectal. A deep rectal abscess.

a., periapical. A periodontal abscess at the root apex of a tooth.

a., peribronchitic. A. in inflamed tissue around the bronchi SYN: *Fauvel's granule.*

a., pericemental. An alveolar abscess not involving the apex of a tooth.

a., pericoronal. One around the crown of an unerupted molar tooth.

a., peridental. Periodontal abscess.

a., perinephric. One in tissue about the kidney. SYN: *perirenal a.*

a., periodontal. An abscess arising in the periodontal tissue (structures of support for teeth).

a., peripleuritic. In the tissue surrounding the parietal pleura.

a., periproctic. One in the areolar tissue about the anus. SYN: *perirectal a.*

a., perirenal. An a. in the tissue surrounding the kidney. SYN: *perinephric a.*

a., peritoneal. An abscess within the peritoneal cavity usually following peritonitis.

a., peritonsillar. Quinsy.

a., periurethral. One formed in tissue surrounding the urethra.

a., perivesical. One in the tissues around the urinary bladder.

a., phlegmonous. An acute abscess in the connective tissue.

a., pneumococcic. One due to infection with pneumococci

a., postcecal. One sometimes occurring in appendicitis.

a., postmammary. Retromammary abscess, *q.v.*

a., post-typhoid. A chronic abscess occurring as a complication of typhoid fever.

a., prelacrimal. One of the lacrimal bone producing a swelling at inner canthus.

a., premammary. A subcutaneous or subareolar abscess of the mammary gland.

a., primary. One originating at point of infection.

a., prostatic. A. within the prostate gland.

a., protozoal. One caused by a protozoan.

a., psoas. One with pus descending in sheath of psoas muscle due to vertebral disease, usually tuberculous in origin.

a., pulmonary. One of the lungs. Nontuberculous suppuration of lung tissue with one or more localized areas of necrosis resulting in pulmonary cavitation.

a., pulp. 1. A cavity discharging pus formed in the pulp of a tooth. 2. An a. of the tissues of the pulp of a finger.

a., pyemic. A metastatic one, usually multiple, due to pyogenic organisms.

a., rectal. One in the rectum.

a., renal. One or multiple abscesses of the renal cortex. SYN: *kidney a.*

a., residual. One occurring from old inflammatory products at the site of an earlier abscess. SYN: *Paget's a.*

a., retrocecal. Abscess situated behind the cecum.

a., retromammary. One between the mammary gland and the chest wall.

a., retroperitoneal. One located between the peritoneum and the posterior abdominal wall.

a., retropharyngeal. An a. of the lymph nodes in the walls of the pharynx. It sometimes simulates diphtheritic pharyngitis.

a., retrovesical. One behind the bladder.

a., root. An abscess of the root of a tooth. SYN: *apical a.*

a., sacrococcygeal. An a. over the sacrum and coccyx.

a., satellite. A secondary one arising from and located near the primary abscess.

a., scrofulous. One due to tuberculous degeneration of bone or lymph nodes.

a., secondary. Embolic abscess.

a., septicemic. An a. resulting from septicemia.

a's., shirt-stud. Two cavities, one larger than the other, containing pus and connected by a narrow channel. SYN: *collar-button abscess.*

a., spermatic. An a. of the seminiferous tubules.

a., spinal. One due to necrosis of a vertebra.

a., spirillary. One containing Spirilla.

a., splenic. One of the spleen.

a., stercoral; a., stercoralaceous. An abscess containing feces. SYN: *fecal abscess.*

a., stitch. One formed about a stitch or suture.

a., streptococcal. An abscess caused by streptococci.

a., subaponeurotic. One beneath an aponeurosis or fascia.

a., subarachnoid. A. of the midlayer of the covering of the brain and spinal cord.

a., subareolar. One underneath the areola of the mammary gland, sometimes draining through the nipple.

a., subdiaphragmatic. An a. beneath the diaphragm. SYN: *subphrenic a.*

a., subdural. One beneath the dura of brain or spinal cord.

a., subepidermal. One beneath the epidermis.

a., subfascial. One beneath a fascia.

a., submammary. An a. beneath the mammary gland.

a., subpectoral. One beneath the pectoral muscles.

a., subperiosteal. Bone abscess below the periosteum.

a., subperitoneal. One between the parietal peritoneum and the abdominal wall.

a., subphrenic. An a. beneath the diaphragm. SYN: *subdiaphragmatic a.*

a., subscapular. One between the serratus anterior and the posterior thoracic wall.

a., subungual. One beneath the distal portion of a finger nail. May follow injuries with pins, needles, or splinters.

a., sudoriparous. An a. of a sweat gland.

a., superficial. One occurring above the deep fascia.

a., suprahepatic. One in the suspensory ligament between the liver and the diaphragm.

a., sympathetic. One arising some distance from the primary cause.

a., syphilitic. One occurring in the final stage of syphilis.

a., thecal. One in a tendon sheath.

a., thymus. An a. of the thymus. SYN: *Dubois' a.*

a., tonsillar. Acute suppurative tonsillitis, or quinsy.

a., tooth. An alveolar abscess.

a., traumatic. One caused by injury.

a., tropical. Amebic a. of the liver.

a., tuberculous. Same as *chronic a.*

a., tympanitic. An abscess that contains air or gas.

a., tympanocervical. One arising in the tympanum and extending to the neck.

a., tympanomastoid. A combined abscess of the tympanum and mastoid.

a., urethral. One of the urethra.

a., urinary. One caused by escape of urine into the tissues.

a., urinous. One which contains pus with urine.

a., verminous. One which is caused by or contains insect larvae or other animal parasites.

a., wandering. One at a distance from focus of disease with pus along fascial sheaths of muscles. SYN: *migrating abscess.*

a., warm. An acute abscess, *q.v.*

a., worm. One caused by or containing worms.

abscission (ab-sĭ'zhun) [L. *abscindere,* to cut off]. The removal of a part by excision.

absence. Temporary mental inattention.

absentia epilep'tica (ab-sen'shĭ-ă ep-ĭ-lĕp'tĭk-ă). The loss of consciousness in the mild form of epilepsy.

abs. feb. Abbr. for *absente febre* (in the absence of fever).

Absidia (ab-sĭd'ē-ă). Genus of pathogenic fungi of the order Phycomycetes and the family Mucoraceae.

ab'sinthe, ab'sinth. A liquor containing oil of wormwood, anise, and other herbs. It is highly toxic, adversely affecting the nervous system.

ab'sinthism. Deterioration of the nerve centers following excessive use of absinthe.

ab'solute al'cohol. A. with not more than 1% of water.

a. temperature. Temperature reckoned from absolute zero.

a. zero. —273.16° C. The lowest possible temperature.

absorb [L. *absorbere,* to suck in]. To take in, suck up or imbibe. SEE: *absorption.*

absorbefacient (ab-sor-be-fā'shent) [" + *facere,* to make]. Causing or that which causes absorption.

absorbent. 1. A substance which absorbs, esp. a substance which brings about the absorption of diseased tissue. 2. Having the power to absorb.

absorptiometer (ab-sorp-shĭ-om'ĕ-ter) [L. *absorptio,* absorption + G. *metron,* measure]. 1. An instrument for measuring thickness of liquid, drawn by capillary attraction, between glass plates. 2. Instrument for measuring the absorption of gas by a liquid.

absorption (ab-sorp'shun) [L. *absorptio,* from *absorbere,* to suck in]. 1. The taking up of liquids by solids, or of gases by solids or liquids. 2. The taking up of light or of its rays by black or colored rays. 3. The taking up by the body of radiant heat, causing a rise in body temperature. 4. PHYS: The passage of a substance through some surface of the body into body fluids and tissues, as the passage of ether through the respiratory epithelium of lungs into the blood during anesthesia, or passage of oil of wintergreen through the skin, the result of several processes: diffusion, *q.v.,* filtration, *q.v.,* osmosis, *q.v.*

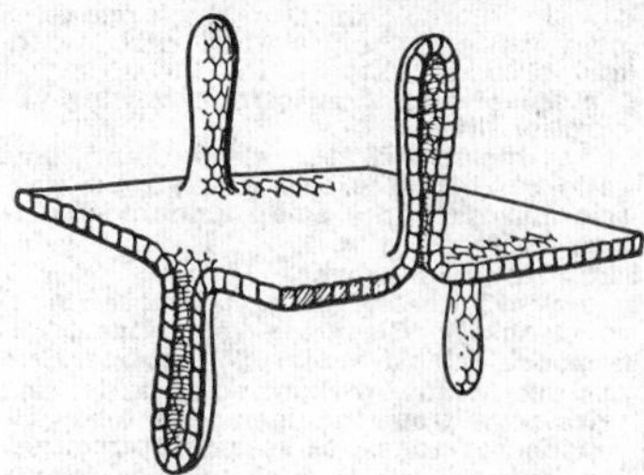

ABSORPTION—INTESTINAL SURFACE

Showing villi and crypts, which greatly increase the number of cells that have access to an epithelial surface and the contents of the lumen.

RS: *chondrolysis, imbibition, osmosis, resorption.*

a. coefficient. The ratio of the linear rate of change of intensity of roentgen rays in a given homogeneous material to the intensity at a given point within the same mass.

a., colon. Water (important in the conservation of body fluids) and products of bacterial action are normally absorbed esp. in the ascending colon. Some nutrients and drugs are absorbed by the lower bowel. Cellulose is not digested but passes from the body as residue.

a., cutaneous. A. through the skin.

a., disjunctive. Separation of a slough by absorption of a layer of adjacent healthy tissue.

a., external. Taking up of material by the skin and mucous membrane.

a., internal. Normal digestion.

a., interstitial. Removal of wastes by absorbent system.

a. lines. Dark lines of solar spectrum. SYN: *Fraunhofer's lines, q.v.*

a., mouth. Some substances, but no food nutrients, can be absorbed from the mouth; some drugs, esp. alkaloids, can pass through the oral mucosa.

a. of radiation. Grotthuss' law states that only rays which are absorbed are physiologically active. Sometimes called Draper's law.

a., pathologic. Absorption into the blood or lymph of substances normally excreted or of a product of disease processes, *e.g.,* pus.

a., protein. In the form of amino acids, produced by digestive hydrolysis, proteins enter the portal vein from the intestinal walls, and through the liver into the general circulation whence they are absorbed by the tissues. Each tissue synthesizes its own form of protein from the amino acids received from the blood.

a., small intestine. The most important absorption of products of digestion occurs in the small intestines, esp. the ileum. Products of digestion absorbed from the gastrointestinal tract pass into either blood or lymph. The mesenteric veins unite to form the portal vein and carry such blood to the liver; the mesenteric lymphatics are called *lacteals* because during absorption of a fatty meal the lymph which they contain looks milky and is called *chyle.* The lacteals empty into the *cisterna chyli* and are joined by lymphatics from other parts of the body; the mixed lymph travels, via the thoracic duct, to the large veins near the heart and is thus mixed with, and becomes part of, the blood.

a. spectrum. A spectrum showing absorption lines.

a., stomach. Water, alcohol, and some salts can be absorbed through the gastric mucosa and a small amount of glucose in food.

absorp'tive. Absorbent.

abstergent (ab-ster'jent) [L. *abstergere,* to cleanse]. Cleansing, purifying.

abstinence (ab'stĭ-nents) [L. *abstinere,* to abstain]. Going without voluntarily, esp. refraining from indulgence in food, alcoholic beverages, or sexual intercourse.

a. symptoms. Partial collapse resulting from withdrawal of alcohol, stimulants, and some opiates.

ab'stract [L. *abstrahere,* to draw away]. 1. A preparation containing the soluble principles of a drug evaporated and mixed with sugar of milk. 2. A summary or abridgment of an article, book, address, etc.

abstraction (ăb-străk'shŭn). 1. Removal or separation of a constituent from a mixture or compound. 2. Removal of blood; bloodletting. 3. Absorption of the mind; inattention or absent-mindedness.

abter'minal [L. *ab,* from, + *terminus,* end]. Away from an end and toward the center, said of electric currents in muscles.

abulia (a-boo'lĭ-ă) [G. *a-,* priv. + *boule,* will]. Absence of or inability to exercise will power; hesitation; indecision. Seen in schizophrenic reactions. SYN: *aboulia.*

abuse (a-būs). Misuse; excessive or improper use.

a., self. Masturbation.

abut'ment [Fr. *abouter,* to place end to end]. The tooth to which a partial denture is anchored.

A. C. Abbr. for *anodal closure, adrenal cortex, air conduction, alternating current, antiphlogistic corticoid, atriocarotid, auriculocarotid, axiocervical.*

a. c. Abbr. for L. *ante cibum,* before meals.

Ac. Chemical symbol for *actinium.*

acacia (ă-kā'shĭ-a). Gum arabic. USP. A dried, gummy exudation from the tree *Acacia senegal.* Used as a suspending agent or vehicle in pharmaceutical or other industrial products.

acalcicosis (ă-kăl"sĭ-kō'sĭs). Condition resulting from deficiency of calcium in diet. SYN: *acalcerosis.*

acalculia (ă-kal-kū'lĭ-ă) [G. *a-,* priv. + L. *calculare,* to reckon]. Inability to solve simple or complex mathematical problems.

acampsia (ă-kamp'sĭ-ă) [" + *kamptein,* to bend]. Inflexibility of a limb; rigidity, ankylosis.

acan'tha [G. *akantha,* thorn]. 1. The spine. 2. A vertebral spinous process.

acanthesthesia (a-kan-thes-thē'zi-ă) [" + *disthēsis,* sensation]. A sensation as of a pinprick; a form of paresthesia, *q.v.*

Acanthia lectularia (a-can'thĭ-a lĕc-tū-lā'rĭ-ă). The bedbug. SYN: *Cimex lectularis.*

acan'thion [G. *akanthion,* a thorn]. Tip of anterior nasal spine.

acan'tho-. Combining form meaning *thorn, spine.*

Acanthocephala (ă-kan-thō-sef'ă-lă) [" + *kephalē,* head]. A class of wormlike entozoa related to the Platyhelminthes, including a few species parasitic in man.

acanthocephaliasis (ă-kan"thō-sef-a-lī'ă-sis). Infestation with Acanthocephala.

acan'thoid [G. *akantha,* thorn, + *eidos,* form]. Thorny; spiny; of a spinous nature.

acanthokeratodermia (ă-kan"thō-ker"ă-tō-der'mĭ-ă) [" + *keras,* horn, + *derma,* skin]. Hypertrophy of the horny portion of the skin of the palms of hands and soles of feet, and thickening of the nails.

acantholysis (ă-kan-thol'ĭ-sĭs) [" + *lysis,* solution]. Any disease of the skin accompanied by degeneration of the cohesive elements of the cells of the outer or horny layer of the skin.

a. bullosa. A skin condition of large bullae produced by irritation or trauma. SYN: *Epidermolysis bullosa, q.v.*

acanthoma (ă-kan-thō'ma) [" + *-oma,* tumor]. 1. Papilloma. 2. Cancer of skin.

a. adenoides cysticum. A cystic tumor, often familial, occurring on chest, face and in axillary regions. Tumors contain tissues resembling sweat glands and hair follicles. SYN: *epithelioma adenoides cysticum.*

acanthopel'vis [" + *pelyx,* pelvis]. A prominent and sharp pubic spine on a rachitic pelvis.

acanthosis (ă-kan-thō'sĭs) [" + *-osis*]. Increased thickness of prickle cell layer of skin.

a. nigricans. Rare chronic inflammatory disease of skin in adult life sometimes associated with cancer of some internal organ. Characterized by symmetrically distributed hard and soft papillary growths accompanied by hyperpigmentation and hyperkeratosis. SYN: *keratosis nigricans.*

acanthot'ic. Pert. to acanthosis.

acap'nia [Gr. *akapnos,* smokeless]. The presence of less than normal amount of carbon dioxide in blood and tissues, *e.g.,* after voluntary overbreathing and the condition resulting therefrom.

SYM: Depressed respiration, giddiness, paresthesia, cramps, occasionally convulsions.

acap'nial. Showing or pert. to acapnia.

acar'bia [G. *a-,* priv. + L. *carbo,* coal]. Diminution of bicarbonate in the blood.

acardia (ă-car'dĭ-ă) [a-, + G. *kardia,* heart]. Congenital absence of the heart.

acar'diac. Having no heart.

acardiacus (ă-car-dī'ă-kus). A parasitic twin without a heart, therefore utilizing the circulation of its twin. SYN: *acardius.*

acardiohemia (ă-car-dĭ-ō-hē'mĭ-ă) [a-, + G. *kardia,* heart, + *haima,* blood, + ia]. Lack of blood in the heart.

acardioner'via. Lack of nerve stimulus to the heart.

acardiotro'pia. Atrophy of the heart.

acar'dius. Acardiacus, *q.v.*

acariasis (ak-ă-rī'ă-sis) [L. *acarus,* mite, + G. *-iasis,* condition]. Any disease caused by a mite or acarid. SYN: *acarinosis.*

acaricide (ă-kar'ĭ-sīd) [" + *caedere,* to kill]. An agent that destroys acarids. 2. Destroying a member of order *Acarina.*

acarid, acaridan (ăk'ă-rĭd, ă-kar'ĭ-dan). A tick or mite; member of the order Acarina.

acaridi'asis. Disease caused by a mite. SYN: *acariasis.*

Acarina (ăk"ă-rī'nă). An order of the class Arachnida which includes a large number of species of minute animals known as mites or ticks. Most are ectoparasites, infestation causing local dermatitis with pruritus and sometimes systemic reactions. They also are vectors of a number of diseases. SEE: *Dermocentor, Ixodidae, Sarcoptes, Sarcoptidea, scabies, tick.*

acarinosis (ă-kar-ĭ-nō'sis). Disease caused by a mite. SYN: *acariasis.*

acarodermatitis (ak-ă-rō-der-mă-tī'tis) [L. *acarus,* mite, + G. *derma,* skin, + *-itis,* inflammation]. The itch. Inflammation of skin caused by a mite.

ac'aroid [" + *eidos,* resemblance]. A mite, or resembling one.

acarophobia (a-kar-ō-fō'bĭ-ă) [" + *phobos,* fear]. PSY: Delusion that the skin is infested with mites or worms.

acarpia (ă-karp'i-ă) [G. *a-,* + *karpos,* fruit]. Barrenness; sterility.

Ac'arus [G. *akari,* a mite]. A genus of mites.

ac'arus. Any mite or tick.

acaryote (ă-kar'ĭ-ōt) [G. *a-,* + *karyon,* nucleus]. Without a nucleus.

acatalepsia, acatalepsy (ă-kat-ă-lep'sĭ-ă, ă-kat'ă-lep-sĭ) [" + *katalambanein,* to comprehend]. 1. Mental deficiency; inability to understand. 2. Diagnostic uncertainty.

acatalep'tic. 1. Deficient mentally. 2. Uncertain or doubtful.

acatamathesia (ă-kat-ă-mă-thē'zĭ-ă) [" + *katamathēsis,* understanding]. 1. Loss of ability to understand spoken words. 2. Inability to comprehend as a result of a brain or other lesion.

acataphasia (ă-kat-ă-fā'zĭ-ă) [" + *kataphasis,* affirmation]. Inability to express thoughts verbally. This condition is due to a cerebral lesion.

acataposis (ă-kat-ă-pō'sĭs) [" + *kataposis,* gulping down]. Dysphagia. Difficulty in swallowing.

acatastasia (ă-kat-ă-stā'zĭ-ă) [G. *akatastasis,* disorder]. Irregularity; deviation from normal.

acatharsia (ak-ă-thar'zĭ-ă) [G. *akatharsis,* uncleanness]. Foulness; impurity; lack of purging.

acathexia (ă-kă-theks'ĭ-ă). An inability to retain normal secretions.

acathexis (ă-că-theks'ĭs) [a-, + G. *kathexis,* retention]. PSY: Lack of emotion (affect) toward some thing or idea which is unconsciously important to the individual.

acathisia (ă-kă-thĭz'ĭ-ă) [G. *a-,* priv. + *kathisis,* sitting]. PSY: Fear of sitting down, hence the inability to remain seated. SYN: *akathisia.*

acaudal, acaudate (ā-kaw'dal, ă-kaw'-dāt). Having no tail.

ACC. Abbr. for *anodal closure contraction.*

acc. Abbr. for *accommodation.*

accelera'tion [L. *acceleratus,* past p. of *accelerare,* to hasten]. Increasing the speed of motion or rate, as pulse or respiration.

a., angular. A change in direction of motion, as when the body rotates about its own axis.

a., central. Centripetal acceleration, *q.v.*

a., centripetal. Movement of the body in a circular or curved course. SYN: *central acceleration.*

a., linear. A change in velocity either forward or backward.

a., negative. 1. SYMB: (−G). Acceleration which produces a force acting on the body in the long axis from seat to head, as when a pilot goes into a dive. 2. Retardation.

a., positive. SYMB: (+G). Acceleration which produces a force acting on the body in the long axis from head to seat, as when a pilot pulls out of a dive.

accelerator (ak-sel'ĕ-rā-tor). Anything that increases action or function. In chemistry, a catalyst.

a. nerves. Sympathetic nerves which contain fibers whose impulses increase rate and force of heart beat. Postganglionic fibers arise principally in cervical and thoracic ganglia.

a. reflexes. Statokinetic reflexes, *q.v.*

a. urinae. Obsolete term for *bulbocavernosus muscle.* SEE: *Table of Muscles in Appendix.*

accentua'tion [L. *ad,* to, + *cantus,* a singing]. Marked with a special stress; emphasis.

accept'or [L. *accipere,* to accept]. A substance absorbing nascent hydrogen or oxygen freed by a reducing enzyme.

a., hydrogen. Substance which receives hydrogen from a hydrogen donator.

accesso'rius [L. past p. *accedere,* move toward]. Accessory, supplementary, as certain muscles, glands, nerves.

a. Willis'ii. Accessory nerve, *q.v.;* 11th cranial nerve.

accessory. Auxiliary; assisting. Term applied to a lesser structure which resembles in structure and function a similar organ, as the accessory pancreatic duct (of Santorini) or accessory suprarenal glands. An organ or structure which assists other organs in performing their functions as accessory reproductive organs.

a. food substances. Substances necessary to maintain normal health but which are not sources of energy. Include water, inorganic salts, and vitamins.

a. nerve. 11th cranial nerve; spinal accessory nerve. Motor nerve made up of a cranial and a spinal part which supplies the trapezius and sternomastoid muscles and pharynx. Accessory portion joins the vagus, to which it supplies its motor and some of its cardio-inhibitory fibers.

a. sign. A nonpathognomonic sign.

ac'cident [L. *accidens,* happening]. 1. An unexpected event. 2. An unforeseen occurrence of an unfortunate nature; a mishap. 3. An unexpected complicating event in the course of a disease, or following surgery.

a., cerebrovascular. ABBR: CVA. A sudden, unexpected interference in brain function resulting from a vascular disturbance such as cerebral hemorrhage, occlusion of a vessel by a thrombus or embolus, vasospasm, or vasodilation. SYN: *apoplexy.*

a., serum. An allergic reaction following the therapeutic introduction of a foreign serum into a hypersensitive individual. SEE: *anaphylaxis.*

accident-prone. Said of persons having an unusually high rate of accidents.

accipiter (ak-sip'ĭ-tĕr) [L. a hawk]. A nose bandage with clawlike ends which spread over the face.

ACCl. Abbr. for *anodal closure clonus.*

acclimation, acclimatization (ak-lĭ-mā'-shun, a-klī-mă-tĭ-zā'shun) [F. *a,* to, + *climat,* climate]. The act of becoming accustomed to a new climate.

acclimatize (ak-klī'mă-tīz). To become accustomed to a different environment and climate.

accommodation [L. *accomodare,* to suit]. Adjustment or adaptation, esp. adjustment of the eye for seeing at different distance. ABBR: *a.; acc.* OPHTH: Term is applied to a phenomenon noted in receptors in which continued stimulation fails to elicit a sensation or response. SEE: *adaptation.*

The adjustment of the eye whereby it is able to focus the image of the object on the retina. In accommodation for *near vision*, the following changes occur: contraction of ciliary muscles which cause ciliary processes to approximate the lens, thus relaxing tension of the suspensory ligament on the capsule so that the anterior surface of the lens increases its curvature. In addition, the pupil contracts and the optic axes converge. These three actions, all reflex in nature, comprise the *accommodation reflex*. In accommodation for *far vision*, the reverse changes occur.

a., absolute. The amount of accommodation of one eye separately.

a., amplitude of. The difference between refracting power of the eye when accommodating for near and far vision. It is measured in diopters (D) and normally diminishes progressively from childhood to old age. It is approximately 16 D at age 12, 6.5 D at age 30, and 1 D at age 60.

a., binocular. Meeting of both eyes at a point in order to carry the object's image to the retina of both.

a., excessive. Greater-than-needed accommodation of the eye.

a., histologic. Change in cell form and function due to change in surrounding conditions.

a., mechanism. Method by which curvature of eye lens is changed in order to focus close objects on the retina.

a., negative. Relaxation by the eye to adjust itself for long distances.

a., positive. Contraction by the eye to adjust itself for short distances.

a., range of. Space of vision between its closest and most remote points.

a. reflex. A group of three reflexes closely associated with each other which facilitate the production of sharp images on corresponding points of the retinae. They are contraction of ciliary muscle resulting in rounding of lens, contraction of pupil, and convergence of eyes. Syn: *near reflex.*

a., relative. The extent to which accommodation is possible for any specific state of convergence of eyes.

a., spasm of. A spasm of the ciliary muscle usually resulting from excessive strain from over-use. Common in myopia in which accommodation is continually used in order to see anything, even distant objects, clearly.

a., subnormal. Insufficient accommodation of the eye.

a., synaptic. Condition in which nerve cells at synapses become less excitable to presynaptic impulses.

accom'modative iridoplegia. Noncontraction of pupils during accommodation.

accouchement (ă-koosh-mon'). The act of delivery in childbirth; parturition.

a. forcé. Forced delivery, especially by version, forceps or other means. Formerly denoted forcible hand delivery.

accoucheur (ă-koo-shur') An obstetrician.

accoucheuse (ă-koo-shuz'). A midwife.

accrementition (ak-rĕ-mĕn-tish'un) [L. *accrescere*, to increase]. Growth of tissues by addition of similar tissue.

accretio (ă-krē'shĭ-ō). Adhesion of parts normally separate from each other.

a. cordis. Condition in which fibrous bands extend from external pericardium to surrounding structures resulting in angulation and torsion of heart.

accretion (ă-krē'shun). 1. Increase by external addition; accumulation. 2. The growing together of parts naturally separate. 3. Accumulation of foreign matter in a cavity.

ACD. Abbr. for *absolute cardiac dullness.*

ACD sol. Citric acid, trisodium citrate, dextrose solution. The anticoagulant used when collecting blood for transfusions.

ACE. Abbr. for *adrenal cortical extract.*

acedia (ă-sē'dĭ-ă) [G. *a-*, + *kedos*, care]. Mental state of indifference, insensibility, lack of emotion. Syn: *apathy.*

acenesthesia (ă-sen-es-thē'zĭ-ă) [G. *a-*, + *koinos*, common, + *aisthēsis*, sensation]. Absence of a feeling of well-being, present in such disorders as hypochondriasis and neurasthenia.

acen'tric [G. *a-*, + L. *centrum*, center]. Not central; peripheral.

acephalia, acephalism (ă-sē-fā'lĭ-ă, ă-sĕf'ă-lĭzm) [*a*, + G. *kephalē*, head]. A developmental disorder in which the head is absent.

acephalo- (a-sĕf'a-lō-) [*a*, + G. *kephalē*, head]. Combined form meaning *without a head.*

acephalobrachia (ă-sĕf-ă-lō-brā'kĭ-ă) [" + " + *brachion*, arm + ia]. A developmental anomaly in which head and arms are absent.

acephalus (ă-sĕf'ă-lus). A malformed fetus.

acerate (ăs'er-āt). Sharp, pointed.

acerbity (ă-serb'ĭ-tĭ) [L. *acerbus*, sharp]. Astringency combined with acidity.

acervuline (ă-ser'vū-lĭn) [L. *acervulus*, a little heap]. Aggregated, occurring in clusters.

acervuloma (ă-ser-vū-lō'mă) [" + *-oma*, tumor]. Intracranial tumor containing psammoma bodies.

acer'vulus [L.]. Sandy, gritty, sabulous.

a. cer'ebri. Gritty matter filling the follicle of the pineal gland. Syn: *brain sand.*

acescence (ă-sĕs'ĕns) [L. *ascesere*, to become sour]. 1. Slight acidity. 2. Process of souring.

acescent (ă-sĕs'ĕnt). Slightly acid.

acesodyne (ă-sĕs'ō-dīn). An agent for relieving pain. Syn: *anodyne.*

acestoma (ă-sĕs-tō'mă) [G. *akestos*, curable, + *-oma*]. The fresh granulations which later form a cicatrix.

acetabular (as-ĕ-tab'ū-lar). Pert. to the acetabulum.

acetabulum (as-ĕ-tab'ū-lum) [L. a little saucer for vinegar]. 1. The rounded (cotyloid) cavity on the external surface of the innominate bone (*os coxae* or *os innominatum*) which receives head of femur. 2. The ventral sucker of the fluke.

acetanilid (as-ĕ-tan'ĭ-lĭd). A white powder or crystalline substance obtained by interaction of glacial acetic acid and aniline. Originally introduced as *antifebrin.*

Action and Uses: Analgesic, antipyretic, and anti-inflammatory. Acute or chronic poisoning may develop following prolonged administration or drug idiosyncrasy.

Poisoning: Sym: Cyanosis due to methemoglobin, cold sweat, irregular pulse, dyspnea, and unconsciousness. Sudden cardiac failure may occur.

F. A. Treatment: In *acute* poisoning, analeptics such as caffeine, pentylene tetrazol, external heat, inhalation of oxygen, gastric lavage or emetics, artificial respiration, blood transfusion. In *chronic* poisoning, stop use of drug; iron preparations for secondary anemia.

acetarsone (as-et-ar'sōn). An arsenical compound, acetylamino-hydroxy-phenylarsonic acid, contains 27% arsenic. Used in amebiasis and *trichomonas vaginalis* infections.

acetate (as'ĕ-tāt). A salt of acetic acid.

acetazolamide (ăs"ĕt-ăz"ol-am'īd). USP. A fine white powder, slightly soluble in alcohol or water. It is a sulfonamide compound used as a diuretic. It has been used also in glaucoma and in epilepsy.

acetic (a-sē'tĭk) [L. *acetum*, vinegar]. Pert. to vinegar; sour.

a. acid. CH_3COOH. The acid in vinegar. An aqueous solution containing not less than 36% or more than 37% by weight of CH_3COOH. Used as a reagent, a caustic; sometimes taken internally. SYN: *ethanoic acid.*

a. a., glacial. USP. A solution containing not less than 99.5% by weight of $C_2H_4O_2$.

acetify (ă-set'ĭ-fī) [L. *acetum*, vinegar, + *fieri*, to become]. To produce acetic fermentation or vinegar.

acetimeter (ă-sĕ-tim'ĕ-ter) [" + G. *metron*, measure]. An apparatus which determines the acetic acid in fluid.

acetoacetic acid (ăs'ĭ-tō-ă-sē'tĭk). A ketone body formed when fats are incompletely oxidized as in diabetes. Appears in the urine in abnormal amounts in starvation or diabetes. Also called *diacetic acid.*

Acetobacter (as-ĕ-tō-bak'tĕr). A genus of the family *Pseudomonadaceae.*

A. aceti. Produces vinegar from wine or cider. Also called *mother* of vinegar.

acetolase (a-set'o-lās). An enzyme which catalyzes conversion of alcohol into acetic acid.

acetonasthma (as"ĕ-tōn-as'ma). A form of asthma associated with acetonuria. Also called *uremic asthma.*

acetone (as'ĕ-tōn). Dimethyl ketone $(CH_3)_2CO$, a colorless, volatile, inflammable liquid, miscible with water, useful as a solvent, and having a characteristic sweet, fruity, ethereal odor. Found in the blood, and in urine in diabetes, faulty metabolism, and after lengthy fasting, produced when the fats are not properly oxidized, due to inability to oxidize glucose in the blood. SEE: *acetonuria, acidosis, ketone, ketosis,* and *tests.*

a. bodies. Certain substances related to acetone. An example is *acetoacetic acid, q.v.* SYN: *ketone bodies, q.v.*

a. in urine, test for. 1. Take 5 cc. of urine; add a few crystals of ammonium sulfate and dissolve; add a small crystal of sodium nitroprusside, and shake a little. Cover with a layer (about 2 cc.) of strong ammonia. The presence of acetone is indicated by the formation of a purple ring between the layers of liquid. 2. Test may also be done by wetting a specially treated paper with urine. If acetone is present, the paper will turn a certain color. These test papers or "sticks" are commercially available.

acetonemia (as-ĕ-tō-nē'mĭ-ă) [acetone + G. *aima*, blood]. Large amounts of acetone in blood. SYM: Abnormal excitement, gradual depression, acidosis.

acetonitrite (as"ĕ-to-ni'trīt). CH_3CN. Methyl cyanide. A substance which is found in an increased amount in the urine of persons who smoke three or more cigarettes a day.

acetonuria (as-ĕ-tō-nū'rĭ-ă) [" + G. *ouron*, urine]. The occurrence of acetone and diacetic bodies in the urine, as in the *ketosis* of diabetes, starvation, etc., which may be due to incomplete oxidation of fats. SEE: *acetone; acidosis; ests.*

acetophenetidin (as-ĕ-tō-fĕ-net'ĭ-dĭn). An odorless, white, crystalline substance derived from coal tar. An antipyretic and analgesic. Must be used cautiously as it is toxic and may cause hemolysis of red blood cells. SYN: *phenacetin.*

acetous (as'ĕ-tus) [L. *acetum*, vinegar]. 1. Pert. to vinegar. 2. Sour in taste.

acetum (a-se'tum) (pl. *aceta*) [L.]. Vinegar. The vinegars are solutions of medicinal substances in diluted acetic acid. They are seldom prescribed.

acetyl (ăs'ĕ-til). The univalent radical, CH_3CO.

acetylation (a-set-ĭ-lā'shun). The introduction of one or more acetyl groups into an organic compound.

acetylbetamethylcholine. A derivative of acetylcholine which is a strong stimulus to the parasympathetic nervous system.

ACTION: Lowers blood pressure, vasodilation, stimulates peristalsis, and increases sweating. Used in tachycardia.

acetylcholine (ă-sĕt-ĭl-kō'lēn). An ester of choline occurring in various organs and tissues of the body. It is thought to play an important role in the transmission of nerve impulses at synapses and myoneural junctions. It is quickly destroyed by an enzyme, cholinesterase. Either excessive or deficient action of acetylcholine at the motor endplates may result in neuromuscular block. ABBR: ACh. SEE: *cholinergic fibers.*

a. chloride. A salt of acetylcholine injected intramuscularly or subcutaneously as a parasympathetic stimulant. It lowers blood pressure by dilating peripheral vessels and relaxes smooth muscle spasms.

acetylene (a-sĕt'ĭ-lēn). C_2H_2. A colorless explosive gas with a garlic-like odor.

acetylsalicylic acid (as'et-il-sal-i-sil'ik). USP. A white crystalline solid formed by the action of acetic anhydride on salicylic acid. It is one of the most widely used analgesics and antipyretics. SYN: *aspirin.*

ACH. 1. An index of nutrition based on arm girth, chest depth, and hip width. 2. Abbr. for *adrenal cortical hormone.*

ACh. Abbr. for *acetylcholine.*

achalasia (ak-ă-lā'zĭ-ă) [G. *a-*, + *chalasis*, relaxation]. Failure to relax; said of muscles, such as sphincters, the normal function of which is a persistent contraction with periods of relaxation.

a. (of the) cardia. Failure of relaxation of lower segment of esophagus resulting in difficulty in passage of foods to the stomach. In advanced cases, dysphagia is marked and dilatation of the esophagus may occur. SYN: *cardiospasm.*

a., pelvirectal. Congenital dilatation of the colon.

a., sphincteral. Failure of intestinal sphincters to relax.

ache (āk). 1. A continued pain as distinguished from a sudden or spasmodic pain. May be dull or severe. 2. To suffer continued pain.

AChE. Abbr. for *acetylcholinesterase.*

acheilia (ă-kī'lē-ă) [*a-*, + G. *cheilos*, lip, + ia]. Developmental anomaly in which there is an absence of one or both lips.

acheiria (ă-kī'rĭ-ă) [*a-*, + G. *cheir*, hand, + ia]. 1. Congenital absence of one or both hands. 2. Loss of sensation in, with accompanying sense of loss of, one or both hands. May result from temporary or permanent injury or malfunction of sensory mechanism, or may occur in hysteria. 3. Inability to determine to which side of the body a stimulus has been applied. SYN: *achiria.*

acheiropodia (ă-kī″rō-pō′dĭ-ă) [" + " + *pous,* foot, + ia]. Developmental anomaly in which there is an absence of hands and feet.

achieve′ment age. Determined by test for proficiency in a subject. The result is compared with the score obtained by "average" children of that age group. ABBR: *A. A.* SEE: *age.*

a. quo′tient. A state of progress in learning ascertained by dividing the achievement age by the mental age. ABBR: *A. Q.*

Achilles jerk. The Achilles tendon reflex, *q.v.*

Achilles tendon. The tendon of the gastrocnemius and solens muscles of the leg. SYN: *tendo calcaneus.*

A. t. reflex. Plantar flexion extension of foot resulting from contraction of calf muscles following a sharp blow to the Achilles tendon. The variations and their significance correspond closely to to those of the knee jerk. It is exaggerated in upper motor neuron disease and diminished or absent in lower motor neuron disease. The character of the response is influenced by the metabolic rate. Thus attempts have been made to use this reflex as an index of thyroid function. The value of such use is questionable.

achillobursitis (ă-kil-ō-bur-sī′tis) [" + L. *bursa,* a pouch + G. *-itis,* inflammation]. Inflammation of the bursa lying over the tendo calcaneus.

achillodynia (ă-kil-ō-din′ĭ-ă) [" + *odyne,* pain]. Pain caused by inflammation between the tendo calcaneus and the bursa.

achillorrhaphy (ă-kil-or′ră-fĭ) [" + G. *raphē,* sewing]. Suture of tendo calcaneus.

achillotomy (ă-kil-ot′ō-mĭ) [" + *tomē,* incision]. A division of tendo calcaneus. SYN: *achillotenotomy.*

achiria (ă-kī′rĭ-ă) [" + *cheir,* hand]. 1. Congenital lack of hands. 2. Loss of sense of possession of one or both hands. 3. Inability to tell on which side of body a stimulus is applied. SYN: *acheiria.*

achlorhydria (ă-klor-hī′drĭ-ă) [" + *chlōros,* green, + *ydōr,* water]. Absence of free hydrochloric acid in the stomach.

ETIOL: May be due to gastric carcinoma, gastric ulcer, pernicious anemia, adrenal insufficiency, chronic gastritis. SEE: *achylia.*

a., histamine proved. Absence of free acid in gastric secretion even after subcutaneous injection of histamine hydrochloride.

achloride (ă-klō′rīd). A salt other than a chloride; nonchloride.

achloropsia (ă-klō-rop′sĭ-ă) [G. *a-,* priv. + *chloros,* green, + *opsis,* vision]. Color blindness in which green cannot be distinguished. SEE: *deuteranopsia.*

acholia (ă-kō′lĭ-ă) [G. *a-,* + *cholē,* bile]. An absence or want of bile or a condition which prevents bile from entering the duodenum.

a., pigmentary. Bile deficiency indicated by clay-colored feces in the absence of jaundice.

acholic (ă-kō′lĭk) [" + *cholē,* bile]. Pert. to acholia.

acholuria (ă-kō-lū′rĭ-ă) [" + " + *ouron,* urine]. In some forms of jaundice, absence of bile pigments in the urine.

achondroplasia (ă-kon-drō-plā′sĭ-ă) [" + *chondros,* cartilage, + *plasis,* a moulding]. Defect in the formation of cartilage at the epiphyses of long bones, producing a form of dwarfism; sometimes seen in rickets. SYN: *chondrodystrophy.*

achoresis (ă-kō-rē′sĭs) [G. *a-,* + *chōrein,* to make room]. A permanent reduction in size of the bladder, stomach, or other hollow viscus thus reducing its capacity.

Achorion (ă-kō′rĭ-on). Former name of a genus of fungi affecting skin, nails, and hair. Now called *Trichophyton, q.v.*

achreocythemia (a-krē-ō-sī-thē′mĭ-ă) [G. *achroios,* colorless, + *kytos,* cell, + *aima,* blood]. Absence of coloring in the red blood cells as a result of deficiency or lack of hemoglobin. SYN: *achroiocythemia.*

achroacyte (ă-krō′ă-sīt) [G. *a-,* + *chroa,* color, + *kytos,* cell]. A lymphocyte; a colorless cell.

achroacytosis (ă-krō″ă-sī-tō′sis) [" + " + " + *-osis,* condition]. Many lymphocytes in the peripheral circulation.

achroiocythemia (ă-kroy″ō-sī-thē′mĭ-ă) [G. *achroios,* colorless, + *kytos,* cell, + *aima,* blood]. Achreocythemia, *q.v.*

achroma (ă-krō′mă) [G. *a-,* + *chrōma,* color]. An absence of color or normal pigmentation as in leukoderma, albinism, etc. Hereditary, circumscribed skin areas deficient in pigmentation.

achromacyte (ă-krō′mă-sīt) [" + " + *kytos,* cell]. A decolorized erythrocyte; one in which hemoglobin is lacking or has been lost. SYN: *achromatocyte; ghost corpuscle; phantom corpuscle; Ponfick's shadow.*

achromasia (ak-rō-mā′zē-ă) [G. *achromatos,* without color]. 1. Absence of normal pigmentation of the skin as in albinism, vitiligo, leukoderma. 2. Pallor. 3. The lack of the ability to be stained, said of cells or tissues.

achromate (ă-krō′māt) [G. *a-,* + *chrōma,* color]. A person who is color blind.

achromatic (ak″rō-măt′ĭk) [G. *achrōmatos,* without color]. 1. Lacking in color. 2. Not dispersing light into its constituent components. 3 Not containing or composed of chromatin. 4. Staining with difficulty, with reference to cells and tissues.

a. lens. One correcting unequal refraction of different wave lengths of light.

achromatin (ă-krō′mă-tĭn). The weakly staining substance of a cell nucleus.

achro′matism. Colorlessness.

achromat′ocyte [" + " + *kytos,* cell]. A decolorized red blood cell. SYN: *achromacyte; ghost corpuscle; phantom corpuscle; Ponfick's shadow.*

achromatolysis (ă-krō-mă-tol′ĭ-sĭs) [" + " + *lysis,* loosing]. Dissolution of cell achromatin. SYN: *plasmolysis.*

achromatophil (ă-krō-mat′ō-fĭl) [" + " + *philos,* love]. A cell or tissue that is not stainable in the usual manner.

achromatopsia (ă-krō-mă-top′sĭ-ă) [G. *achrōmatos,* without color, + *opsis,* vision]. Color blindness.

achromatosis (ă-krō-mă-tō′sĭs) [" + *osis,* state]. Condition of being without natural pigmentation. SEE: *achroma.*

achromatous (ă-krō′mă-tus). Without color.

achromaturia (ă-krō″mă-tū′rĭ-ă) [G. *achrōmatos,* without color, + *-ouron,* urine]. Colorless or nearly colorless urine.

achromia [G. *a-,* + *chroma,* color]. 1. Absence of color; pallor. 2. Achromatosis. 3. Condition in which erythrocytes are pale and have large central pale areas; hypochromia.

a., congenital. Albinism, *q.v.*

achromic (ă-kro′mik). Lacking color.

achromoder'ma [G. *a-*, + *chroma*, color, + *derma*, skin]. Lack of color in skin. Leukoderma.

achro'mophil [" + " + *philos*, fond]. Achromatophil, *q.v.*

achromotrich'ia [" + " + *trichia*, condition of the hair]. Lack of color or graying of the hair. SYN: *canities*.

a., nutritional. Grayness of hair due to dietary deficiency.

achromycin (ăk-rō-mī'sĭn). Proprietary name for tetracycline, an antibiotic effective in treatment of many bacterial infections and, in topical form, of pyogenic infections of skin.

achroodextrin (ak"rō-ō-deks'trĭn) [G. *achroos*, colorless, + dextrin]. One of the varieties of dextrin resulting from hydrolysis of starch.

achylia (ă-kī'lĭ-ă) [G. *a-*, + *chylos*, chyle]. Absence of chyle or other digestive ferments.

a. gastrica. Complete absence or marked diminution in amount of gastric juice. SEE ALSO: *achlorhydria*.

a. pancreat'ica. Absence or deficiency of pancreatic secretion. Usually a manifestation of chronic pancreatitis.

achylosis (ă-kī-lō'sis). Achylia, *q.v.*

achylous (ă-kī'lus) [G. *achylos*, without chyle]. 1. Lacking in any kind of digestive secretion. 2. Without chyle.

achymia, achymosis (ă-kī'mĭ-ă, ak-ĭ-mō'-sis) [G. *a-*, priv. + *chymos*, juice]. Deficiency or absence of chyme.

acicular (ă-sĭk'ū-lar) [L. *aciculus*, little needle]. Needle-shaped.

a'cid [L. *acidus*, sour]. 1. Any substance of a group which characteristically is sour in taste, neutralizes basic substances, makes litmus paper red, and produces hydrogen ions (protons) when reacting with certain metals. SEE ALSO: *indicator*. 2. A sour substance.

a., acetic. $C_2H_4O_2$. USP. Gives sour taste to vinegar. Also used as a reagent, a caustic; sometimes taken internally. SYN: *ethanoic acid*.

a., a., dilute. Containing 6% pure acetic acid.

a., a., glacial. USP. Contains not less than 99.5% of acetic acid ($C_2H_4O_2$) by weight.

a., acetoacetic. CH_3COCH_2COOH. A ketone body formed when fats are incompletely oxidized. Appears in urine in abnormal amounts in starvation or diabetes. SYN: *diacetic acid; acetylacetic acid; 3-oxobutanoic acid*.

a., acetrizoic. $C_9H_6I_3NO_3$. USP. A white odorless powder used in solution as radiopaque medium.

a., acetylacetic. Acetoacetic acid, *q.v.*

a., acetylsalicylic. $CH_3COOC_6H_4COOH$. USP. Derivative of salicylic acid. It occurs as white crystals or powder and is odorless. Used extensively for analgesic and antipyretic actions. SYN: *aspirin; salicylic acid acetate; o-acetoxybenzoic acid*.

a., adenylic. A nucleotide; it occurs in muscle, blood corpuscles and yeast as well as other nuclear material. SYN: *adenosine monophosphate*.

a., amino. An organic acid containing one or more NH_2 (amino) groups and a COOH (carboxyl) group; these compounds are the basic building blocks for all of the body's protein elements. The end-products of digestion of proteins which are absorbed finally into the tissues. Certain of these acids are essential in the human body for growth and repair of tissues. Oral preparations of essential amino acids may be used as dietary supplements when necessary. SEE ALSO: *amino acid*.

a., aminoacetic. NH_2CH_2COOH. One of the simplest examples of an amino acid. Same as glycine.

a., aminosalicylic. Para-aminosalicylic acid, *q.v.*

a., ascorbic. $C_6H_8O_6$. Occurs naturally in fresh fruits, especially citrus fruits, and in fresh vegetables. Essential in maintenance of collagen formation, osteoid tissue of bones, and formation and maintenance of dentin. Produced synthetically (USP), it is used as a dietary supplement, and in the prevention and treatment of scurvy. SYN: *vitamin C; antiscorbutic vitamin*.

a., aspartic. $COOHCHNH_2CH_2COOH$. An amino acid; one of the products of pancreatic digestion.

a., barbituric. $C_4H_4O_3N_2$. A crystalline compound from which phenobarbital and other barbiturates are derived. SYN: *malonylurea*.

a., benzoic. $C_7H_6O_2$. USP. A white crystalline material having a slight odor. Used in keratolytic ointments, and as a food preservative. Saccharin is a derivative of this acid.

a., bile. Any substance occurring in the form of salt in the bile; *glycocholic acid* and *taurocholic acid*. On combination with a base they give rise to bile salts. They are formed by the reaction of *glycocoll* (glycine) or *taurin* with *cholic acid*.

a., boracic. Boric acid, *q.v.*

a., boric. H_3BO_3. USP. A white crystalline substance giving very weakly acid solutions, poisonous to plants and animals. Soluble in water, alcohol, or glycerin.

CAUTION: Because of its toxicity, the use of boric acid should be quite limited, particularly in areas where it could be accidentally swallowed by children. SEE ALSO: *boric*.

a., butyric. C_3H_7COOH. A liquid having a rancid odor; found in rancid butter, in cheese, perspiration, and cod liver oil.

a., butanedioic. Succinic acid, *q.v.*

a., carbolic. Obsolescent name for phenol.

a., carbonic. H_2CO_3. An acid formed from carbon dioxide dissolved in water.

a., carboxylic. Any one containing the group COOH. The simplest examples are *formic* and *acetic*.

a., cevitamic. Ascorbic acid, *q.v.*

a., chaulmoogric. A cyclic unsaturated fatty acid in chaulmoogra oil, formerly used in treatment of leprosy (Hansen's disease).

a., chromic. CrO_3. Escharotic sometimes used to remove warts. SYN: *chromic anhydride; chromium trioxide*.

a., citric. $C_6H_8O_7$. USP. Prepared from lemon or lime juice in form of colorless crystals or white crystalline powder. Soluble in water, ether or alcohol. Used as a preventive of scurvy. Hydrous form is used as a flavoring agent or vehicle.

a., deoxyribonucleic. The material of which chromosomes are primarily composed. It is believed to be the entire inheritable substance in living tissue. Sugar, phosphoric acid and a nitrogenous base are the essential components of this acid. ABBR: *DNA*.

a., desoxyribonucleic. Deoxyribonucleic acid, *q.v.*

a., diacetic. Same as *acetoacetic acid*.

a., ethanedioic. Oxalic acid, *q.v.*

a., ethanoic. Acetic acid, *q.v.*

a., ethylenediaminetetracetic. ABBR: EDTA. A compound which, in the form of its calcium or sodium salts, is useful in removing certain substances such as lead and digitalis from the body. This is done by *chelation, q.v.*

a., fatty. One of a series of carboxylic acids, with a general formula of RCOOH or $C_nH_{2n}O_2$, which can be combined with *glycerol* to form fats; the simplest members of the series are *formic* and *acetic;* most typical, *stearic* and *palmitic.*

a., folic. A member of the vitamin B complex. Used in control of pernicious anemia and in treatment of sprue. Found naturally in green plant tissue, liver and yeast. Produced synthetically, its formula is $C_{19}H_{19}N_7O_6$ and is identical with pteroylglutamic acid. USP. Also called *L. casei factor.*

a., formic. HCOOH. The first member of the monobasic fatty acid series, but is a much stronger acid than the others in the series. It occurs naturally in animal secretions and in muscle, but it may also be prepared synthetically. It is one of the irritants present in the sting of insects such as bees and ants. SYN: *methanoic acid.*

a., formiminoglutamic. ABBR: Figlu. $C_6N_2O_4H_{10}$. An intermediate product in the metabolism of histidine. Its increase in the urine after administration of histroline in patients with folic acid deficiency is the basis for the *Figlu excretion test.*

a., gallic. $C_6H_2(OH)_3COOH$. A colorless crystalline acid. It occurs naturally in plants such as nut galls and tea. It is used as a skin astringent, and in the manufacture of writing inks and dyes. SYN: *3,4,5-trihydroxybenzoic acid.*

a., glucuronic. $CHO(CHOH)_4COOH$. An oxidation product of glucose. Found in the urine. Toxic products (such as salicylic acid, menthol, and phenol) that have entered the body through the intestinal system are detoxified in the liver by conjugation with glucuronic acid. SYN: *glycuronic acid.*

a., glutamic. $COOH(CH_2)_2CH(NH_2)$-COOH. A non-essential amino acid formed during protein metabolism. Is used orally as an anticonvulsant. SYN: *glutaminic acid; aminoglutaric acid.*

a., glyceric. $CH_2OHCHOHCOOH$. An intermediate product of oxidation of fats. SYN: *2,3-dihydroxypropanoic acid.*

a., glycocholic. $C_{24}H_{39}O_4NHCH_2COOH$. A conjugate with glycine in the bile.

a., glycuronic. Glucuronic acid.

a., homogentisic. An acid found in the urine in alkaptonuria. SYN: *alkapton.*

a., hydriodic. HI. In solution, it is used in various forms of chemical analyses (quantitative, qualitative, etc.). A well-diluted solution is used orally in iodide treatment of thyroid gland disease. SYN: *hydrogen iodide.*

a., hydrochloric. HCl. USP. An inorganic acid. Occurs naturally in the gastric juice. Presence of this acid is essential to digestion. It also destroys fermenting bacteria which might cause intestinal tract disturbances. A further-diluted solution of 25% hydrochloric acid is used in hypoacidity or achlorhydria.

CAUTION: When so used, it must be accurately diluted and swallowed by using a drinking straw. This will prevent the acid from damaging the teeth. SYN: *muriatic acid.*

a., hydrocyanic. HCN. A colorless, extremely poisonous, highly volatile liquid. Occurs naturally in plants. It is obtained synthetically by several methods. Has many industrial uses: electroplating, fumigation, and production of dyes, pigments, synthetic fibers, and plastic. Exposure of man to 200-500 parts of acid per 1,000,000 parts of air for 30 minutes is fatal. It acts by preventing cellular respiration. SYN: *prussic acid; hydrogen cyanide.*

a., hydroxytoluic. Mandelic acid, *q.v.*

a., imino. An acid formed as a result of oxidation of amino acids in the body.

a., lactic. $C_3H_6O_3$. USP. Occurs in sour milk from fermentation of lactose present and is formed in muscles by exercise. Lactic acid milk (buttermilk or acidophilus milk) is administered to help prevent growth of putrefactive bacteria in the large intestine. SYN: *2-hydroxypropanoic acid; 2-hydroxypropionic acid.*

a., linoleic. $C_{18}H_{32}O_2$. An unsaturated fatty acid, a dietary essential. First isolated from linseed oil but is also found in corn oil. SYN: *linolic acid; 9,12-octadecadienoic acid.*

a., linolenic. $C_{18}H_{30}O_2$. An unsaturated fatty acid, a dietary essential.

a., linolic. Linoleic acid, *q.v.*

a., malic. $C_4H_6O_5$. Found in certain sour fruits as apples and apricots. Active in aerobic metabolism of carbohydrate.

a., malonic. $C_3H_4O_4$. A dibasic acid formed by oxidation of malic acid. Occurs in beets. Active in the tricarboxylic acid cycle in carbohydrate metabolism. Its inhibition of succinic dehydrogenase is the classic example of competitive inhibition.

a., mandelic. $C_8H_8O_3$. A colorless hydroxy acid. Its salt is used in urinary tract infections.

a., methanoic. Formic acid, *q.v.*

a., mineral. Acids prepared from inorganic materials, as sulfuric, hydrochloric, nitric, and phosphoric acids.

a., muriatic. Hydrochloric acid, *q.v.*

a., nicotinic. $C_6H_5NO_2$. USP. A member of the vitamin B complex. Occurs naturally in liver, yeast, milk, cheese, and cereals. Used for prevention and specific treatment of pellagra. SYN: *niacin; pellagra-preventive vitamin; 3-pyridinecarboxylic acid.*

a., nitric. HNO_3. A strong corrosive acid prepared from sulfuric acid and a nitrate. It is used in manufacture of explosives and dyes, and as a coagulant in testing urine for albumin (Heller's ring test).

a., nucleic. Combines with protein to form nucleoprotein, a substance in the nuclei of cells of all living things. SEE: *deoxyribonucleic a.*

a., octadecanoic. Name, approved by International Union of Chemistry, for stearic acid, *q.v.*

a., oleic. $C_{18}H_{34}O_2$. An unsaturated fatty acid that can be prepared from various fats and oils. SYN: *9-octadecenoic acid.*

a., organic. An acid containing the carboxyl radical COOH.

a., oxalic. $H_2C_2O_4$, or $(COOH)_2$. The simplest dibasic organic acid occurring as colorless monoclinic crystals. It occurs naturally in rhubarb, wood sorrel and many other plants. It is the strongest organic acid and is poisonous. It is effective in removing ink or rust stains from cloth. It is used also as a reagent. SYN: *ethanedioic acid.*

a., palmitic. $C_{15}H_{31}COOH$. A saturated fatty acid occurring as esters in most natural fats and oils. SYN: *hexadecanoic acid.*

acrochordon (ak-rō-kor'dŏn) [" + *chordē*, cord]. A soft pedunculated growth.

acrocinesia, acrocinesis (ăk-rō-sin-ē'sĭ-ă, -sis) [G. *akros*, extreme, + *kinesis*, movement]. Excessive motion.

acrocinetic (ak-rō-sin-et'ĭk). Showing excessive motion.

acrocontrac'ture [G. *akron*, extremity, + L. *contrahere*, to draw together]. Contracture of the hands or feet.

acrocyanosis (ak-rō-sī-ă-nō'sĭs) [" + *kyanōsis*, dark blue color]. Cyanosis of finger tips, and other extremities.

Etiol: Due to vasomotor disturbances. Seen in catatonia, hysteria, etc.

acrodermatitis (ak-rō-der-mă-tī'tis) [" + *derma*, skin, + *-itis*, inflammation]. Dermatitis of the extremities.

a. chronica atrophicans. Progressive dermatitis of hands and feet that moves slowly upward on the affected limbs.

a., continuous. An obstinate eczematous eruption confined to the extremities. See: *Hallopeau's disease*.

a. hiemalis. A form occurring in winter, affecting the extremities and tending to disappear spontaneously.

acrodynia (ak-rō-dĭn'ĭ-ă) [" + *odynē*, pain]. 1. Disorder of skin and limbs in children. See: *Swift's disease*. 2. Multiple neuritis of digits.

acroedema (ak"ro-ē-dē'mă) [" + *edema*]. Chronic edema of the hands or feet.

acroesthesia (ak-rō-es-thē'zĭ-ă) [" + *aisthēsis*, sensation]. 1. Marked hyperesthesia. 2. Pain in the extremities.

acrogeria (ak"ro-jĕr'ĭ-ă) [" + *geron*, old man]. A condtion wherein the skin of the hands and feet shows signs of premature aging.

acrogno'sis [" + *gnōsis*, knowledge]. Sensory perception of limbs.

acrohyperhidrosis (ăk-rō-hī-per-hī-drō'-sĭs). Excessive perspiration of hands and feet.

acrohy'pothermy [" + *hypo*, under, + *thermē*, heat]. Abnormal coldness of extremities.

acrokinesia (ak-ro-kin-e'sĭ-ă) [" + *kinesis*, movement]. Excessive motion. Syn: *acrocinesia*.

acrolein (ak-rō'lē-ĭn). A volatile liquid produced by dry distillation of glycerin. Irritating to the eyes. Used in chemical warfare. Syn: *acrylaldehyde*.

acromac'ria. Spider-fingers. Syn: *arachnodactyly*.

acromania (ak-rō-mā'nĭ-ă) [G. *akros*, extreme, + *mania*, frenzy]. Mania accompanied by great motor activity and sometimes by muteness.

acromasti'tis [" + *mastōs*, breast, + *-itis*, inflammation]. Inflammation of the nipple; thelitis.

acromegaly (ak-ro-meg'ă-lĭ), **acromegalia** ak-ro-me-ga'lĭ-ă) [" + *megas*, *megal-*, big]. A chronic disease characterized by elongation and enlargement of bones of the extremities and certain head bones, especially frontal bone and jaws, accompanied by enlargement of nose and lips and thickening of soft tissues of the face.

Etiol: Hyperfunction of the eosinophilic cells of the anterior lobe of the pituitary resulting in excess production of somatotrophic or growth hormone.

Sym: Facial features are enlarged, mandible and malar bones becoming prominent with protrusion of orbital ridge. Teeth become widely separated. Hands and feet become gradually enlarged. Early complaints include muscular pains, headache, sweating.

Treatment: X-ray therapy or surgery of pituitary gland.

acromelalgia (ak-rō-mel-al'jĭ-ă) [" + *melos*, limb, + *algos*, pain]. A disease of the extremities, especially the feet which are swollen and become painful upon walking. Syn: *erythromelalgia*.

Sym: Pain, redness, swelling of extremities, tachycardia, vertigo, and weakness.

acrometagenesis (ak"rō-mĕt"ă-jĕn'ē-sis) [" + *meta*, beyond, + *genesis*, origin]. Abnormal growth of extremities leading to deformity.

acromial (ak-rō'mĭ-al) [" + *ōmos*, shoulder]. Rel. to the acromion.

a. angle. The angle at edge of spine of the scapula where it ascends to become the acromion.

a. process. The acromion, *q.v.*

a. reflex. Flexion of forearm with internal rotation of hand resulting from quick blow upon acromion. Elicited in hyperkinetic states.

acromicria (ak-rō-mĭk'rĭ-ă) [" + *mikros*, small]. Congenital shortness or smallness of the extremities.

acromioclavicular joint (a-krō"mĭ-ō-klă-vik'ū-lar) [" + *ōmos*, shoulder, + L. *clavicula*, small key]. An arthrodial joint between the acromion and the acromial end of the clavicle.

acromiocoracoid (a-krō"mi-ō-kor'ă-koid) [" + " + *korax*, crow, + *eidos*, resemblance]. Pert. to the acromion and coracoid process.

acro'miohu"meral [" + " + L. *humerus*, shoulder]. Pert. to acromion and humerus.

acromion (ă-krō'mĭ-on) [G. *akron*, tip, + *ōmos*, shoulder]. The lateral, triangular projection of spine of scapula, forming point of the shoulder, and articulating with the clavicle. Syn: *acromial process*. See: *acromioclavicular*.

acromiothoracic (a-krō"mĭ-ō-thō-ras'ĭk) [" + " + *thorax*, breast plate]. Pert. to acromion and thorax.

a. artery. A branch of the axillary artery.

acromphalus (ak-rom'fal-us) [" + *omphalos*, umbilicus]. 1. Center of navel. 2. Beginning of umbilical hernia, marked by abnormal projection of umbilicus.

acromyotonia (ak"rō-mī-ō-tō'nĭ-ă) [" + *mys*, muscle, + *tonōs*, tension]. Myotonia of extremities causing spasmodic deformity.

acronarcotic (ak"rō-nar-kot'ĭk) [L. *acer*, *acris*, sharp, + G. *narcosis*, a benumbing]. Having the property of a narcotic and yet irritant in local effects.

ac"roneuro'sis [G. *akron*, extremity, + *neuron*, nerve]. Any neurosis, usually vasomotor, in extremities.

acronyx (ak'rō-nĭks) [L. *acer*, *acris*, sharp, + G. *onyx*, claw]. Ingrowing of a nail.

acroostolysis (ak"ro-os-tol'ĭ-sis) [G. *akron*, extremities, + *osteon*, bone, + *lysis*, dissolution]. An occupational disease seen in workers who come in contact with vinyl chloride polymerization processes. Characterized by Raynaud's phenomenon, *q.v.* Scleroderma-like skin changes and x-ray evidence of bone destruction of the distal phalanges of the hands. Recovery follows after removal from exposure.

acropachy (ak'rō-pak-ĭ) [G. *akron*, extremity, + *pachys*, thick]. Thickening of fingers or toes.

acroparal'ysis [" + *paralyein*, to disable at the side]. Paralysis of one or more extremities.

acroparesthesia (ak"rō-par-es-thē'zĭ-ă) [" + *para*, beside, + *aisthesis*, sensation]. Paresthesia (intense prickling, tingling or numbness) of fingers and hands occurring usually following sleep, more often in women than men. May be severe in some instances.

ac″ropathol′ogy [″ + *pathos*, suffering, + *logos*, science]. Pathology of disease of extremities.

acropathy (ak-rop′ă-thĭ). Any disease of extremities.

acrophobia (ak-rō-fō′bĭ-ă) [G. *akron*, top, + *phobos*, fear]. Morbid fear of high places.

acroposthitis (ak″rō-pos-thī′tis) [G. *akroposthis*, prepuce, + *-itis*, inflammation]. Inflammation of prepuce.

acroscleroderma (ak″rō-skler-ō-der′mă) [G. *akron*, extremity, + *sclēros*, hard, + *derma*, skin]. Hard, thickened skin condition of toes and fingers. Syn: *sclerodactylia*.

acrosclerosis (ăk-rō-skler-ō′sĭs). A scleroderma of the upper extremities, sometimes extending to neck and face. Usually follows Raynaud's disease.

ac′rose. A sugar prepared synthetically by formaldehyde or glucose condensation.

acrosome (ak′rō-sōm) [G. *akron*, extremity, + *soma*, body]. The ant. end of head of the spermatozoon.

acrosphacelus (ak-rō-sfas′ĕ-lus) [″ + *sphakelos*, gangrene]. Gangrene of digits. May be symptom of Raynaud's disease.

acroteric (ak-rō-tĕr′ĭk) [G. *akrōtērion*, summit]. Pertaining to the outermost parts of the extremities, as the tips of the fingers.

acrotic (a-krot′ĭk). 1. [G. *a-*, priv. + *krotos*, striking]. Pert. to failure of or defective beating of the pulse. 2. [G. *akrotēs*, an extreme]. Pert. to the surface or glands of the skin.

acrotism (ak′rō-tizm) [G. *a-*, priv. + *krotos*, a striking]. Apparent absence of the pulse.

acrotrophoneurosis (ak-ro-tro″fo-nu-ro′-sis) [G. *akron*, extremity, + *trophē*, nourishment, + *neuron*, nerve, + *-osis*, condition]. Trophoneurosis of extremities with trophic, neuritic, and vascular changes. Usually caused by prolonged immersion in water.

acrylaldehyde (ak-ril-al′dĕ-hīd). A volatile liquid from glycerin. Syn: *acrolein*.

acrylate (ak′ri-lāt). A salt of acrylic acid.

ACS. Abbr. for *American Cancer Society; American Chemical Society; American College of Surgeons; anodal closing sound; antireticular cytotoxic serum* (*Bogomolets serum*).

ACTH. Abbr. for *adrenocorticotropic hormone*, a pituitary hormone that stimulates the cortex of the adrenal glands. See also: *cortisone*.

actin (ak′tĭn). One of the proteins in muscle fiber, the other being myosin.

actinic (ak-tin′ĭk) [G. *aktis*, ray]. Pert. to radiant energy such as x-rays, ultraviolet light, sunlight, particularly the photochemical effects.

PT: Pert. to actinism, *q.v.* Capable of producing chemical changes as applied to radiant energy.

a. burns. Those caused by ultraviolet or sun rays. F. A. Treatment: As for dry heat burns. See: *burns*.

a. dermatitis. Inflammation and erythema of the skin due to exposure to actinic rays such as are present in x-rays, sunlight, ultraviolet light.

actinism (ak′tin-izm). That property of radiant energy which produces chemical changes, as in photography or heliotherapy.

actinium (ak-tin′ē-ŭm) [G. *aktis*, ray or beam]. A radioactive element. Symb: Ac. At. wt. 227; at. no. 89.

ac″tinochem′istry [G. *aktis*, ray, + *chēmeia*, chemistry]. Action of rays from a luminous source.

actinodermatitis (ak″tin-ō-der-mă-tī′tis) [″ + *derma*, skin, + *-itis*, inflammation]. Dermatitis caused by exposure to actinic rays.

actinogen (ak-tin′ō-jen). Any radioactive element.

actinogenesis (ak″tin-ō-jĕn′ĕ-sĭs) [G. *aktis*, ray, + *genesis*, source]. The source or production of actinic rays.

actinogenic (ak″tin-ō-jen′ik) [G. *aktis*, *aktin*, ray, + *gennan*, to produce]. Producing rays; radiogenic.

Actinomyces (ak-tin-ō-mī′sēz) [G. *aktis*, ray, + *mykes*, fungus]. A vegetable parasite (*Actinomycetaceae*) causing actinomycosis.

A. antibioticus. A species of fungus from which two antibiotics, actinomycins A and B, have been isolated.

A. bandetii. Similar to A. israelii. Cause of actinomycosis in dogs and cats.

A. bovis. The fungus causing lumpy jaw in cattle. Considered, by some authorities to be identical with *A. israelii*.

A. israelii. A nonmotile species. First isolated from human actinomycosis. Pathogenic for man.

actino″myce′tic. Pert. to Actinomyces.

actinomycetin (ak″tĭn-ō-mī-sĕt′ĭn). A substance that is antibacterial from *Actinomyces*, effective against some gram-positive and gram-negative organisms.

actinomycin A (ăk″tĭn-ō-mī′sĭn). An antibacterial substance from *Actinomyces antibioticus*, heat-stable and highly toxic, effective against gram-positive organisms. It is orange-colored, soluble in alcohol and ether.

a. B. Similar to actinomycin A but not soluble in alcohol and chemically unsuitable because of its great toxicity.

actino″myco′ma [G. *aktis*, ray, + *mykes*, fungus, + *-oma*, tumor]. A tumor produced by actinomycosis.

actinomycosis (ak″tin-ō-mī-kō′sis) [″ + ″ + *osis*, condition]. A noncontagious ray fungus disease in animals, sometimes communicated to man, invading the brain, lungs, gastrointestinal tract, or, most often, the jaw (lumpy jaw).

Etiol: *Actinomyces bovis* in cattle; *A. israelii* in man. This organism is normally present in the mouth.

Sym: Formation of slow growing granulomata, which later break down, discharging viscid pus containing minute yellowish ("sulfur") granules.

Treatment: The tetracyclines and penicillin are effective. Surgical incision and drainage of accessible lesions is helpful when combined with chemotherapy.

actinomycot′ic. Pert. to actinomycosis.

actinon (ak′tin-on) [G. *aktis*, *aktin*, ray]. Emanation from actinium, which is one of the radium, actinium, and thorium series. Syn: *radon*[219].

actinoneuri′tis [″ + *neuron*, nerve, + *-itis*, inflammation]. Neuritis due to exposure to radium or x-rays.

actinophytosis (ak″tin-ō-fī-tō′sis). Infection with organisms of genus Streptothrix, now classified as *Actinomyces*, *Streptomyces*, *Nocardia* and others. Syn: *streptothricosis*.

ac″tinoprax′is [″ + *praxis*, a doing]. Employment of light or radioactive rays in diagnosis and treatment.

actinos'copy [" + *skopein,* to write]. Examination of a body by x-rays.

actinostereos'copy [" + *stereos,* solid, + "]. Actinoscopy, *q.v.*

ac"tinother'apy [" + *therapeia,* healing]. Treatment of disease by rays of light, especially actinic or photochemically active rays, or by x-rays or radium.

ac"tinotoxe'mia [" + *toxikon,* poison, + *aima,* blood]. Blood-poisoning produced by x-ray or other radioactivity.

ac'tion [L. *actio,* from *agere,* to do]. Performance of a function, or process; in pathology, a morbid process.

a., antagonistic. The ability of a drug or a muscle to oppose or resist the action or effect of another drug or muscle. Opp. to *synergistic a.*

a., astringent. One in which the tissue cells are contracted by a chemical combination of drug and tissues, forming an albuminate. If this is not dissolved in fluids surrounding tissues, they are not acted upon further by the drug.

a., bacteriocidal. The lethal effect on bacteria.

a., bacteriostatic. The effect of stopping or preventing growth of bacteria without killing them.

a., ball-valve. Intermittent obstruction of a passageway or opening so that the flow of fluid or air is prevented from moving in the normal direction and at the usual rate.

a., cumulative. Sudden increased action of a drug after several doses have been given.

a. current. PT: Same as *action potential.*

a., drug. SEE: *drug action.*

a. of arrest. Inhibition.

a. potential. The momentary difference in electrical potential between active and resting parts of a nerve fiber found when the two parts are connected with a sensitive galvanometer.

a., reflex. Involuntary movement produced by a sensory nerve and carried to a center and returned by an efferent nerve to its origin or source of stimulus.

a., specific dynamic. Stimulation of metabolic rate by ingestion of certain foods, esp. proteins.

a., synergistic. The ability of a drug or muscle to aid or enhance the effect of another drug or muscle. Opp. to *antagonistic a.*

ac'tivate. 1. To make active. 2. To make radioactive.

ac'tivator. 1. A substance in the body which converts an inactive substance into an active agent, as the action of hydrogen ions on *pepsinogen* converting it to *pepsin.* 2. Any substance which specifically induces an activity such as an *inductor* or *organizer* in embryonic development, or a trophic hormone.

ac'tive prin'ciple. The chemical substance in a drug, without which the drug will have no therapeutic effect. Active principle is commonly a glycoside or an alkaloid. SEE: *drug action.*

actomyosin (ăk-tō-mī'ō-sĭn). The combination of actin and myosin in a muscle.

ACTP. Adrenocorticotropic polypeptide. Hydrolysate of ACTH.

actual (ak'chu-al) [L. *actus,* past p. of *agere,* to do]. Real, existent.

a. cautery. Cautery acting by virtue of its heat and not chemically.

acufilopressure (ak-ū-fī'lō-presh-ūr) [L. *acus,* needle, + *filum,* thread, + *pressura,* pressure]. Acupressure increased by a ligature.

acu'ity [L. *acuere,* to sharpen]. Clearness, sharpness.

a., visual. Acuteness or sharpness of vision.

acu'minate [L. *acuminatus,* sharpened]. Conical or pointed.

acupressure (ak'ū-presh"ur) [L. *acus,* needle, + *pressura,* pressure]. Compression of blood vessels by means of needles in surrounding tissue.

a. forceps. Spring-handled forceps for compressing blood vessels.

a. needles. Elastic needles for compressing blood vessels.

ac'upuncture [" + *punctura,* puncture]. Puncture with needles for diagnostic and therapeutic (counterirritation) purposes.

acus (ā'kus) [L. needle]. A surgical needle.

acusection (ak-ū-sek'shun) [" + *secare,* to cut]. Section by an electrosurgical needle.

acus'ticus [G. *akoustikos,* hearing]. The acoustic nerve, *q.v.*

acute (a-cūte') [L. *acutus,* sharp]. 1. Sharp, severe. 2. Having rapid onset, severe symptoms and a short course; not chronic.

acutenaculum (ak"ū-ten-ak'ū-lum) [L. *acus,* needle, + *tenaculum,* holder]. A needle holder.

acutor'sion [" + *torsio,* twisting]. Twisting of an artery with a needle to control hemorrhage.

acyanoblepsia (a"sī-ă-nō-blep'sĭ-ă) [G. *a-,* priv. + *kyanos,* blue, + *blepsis,* vision]. Inability to discern blue colors. SYN: *acyanopsia.*

acyanopsia (a-sī-ă-nop'sĭ-ă). Acyanoblepsia, *q.v.*

acyanotic (a-sī-ă-not'ik). Pert. to the absence of cyanosis.

acyclic (ă-sī'klĭk). 1. CHEM: Aliphatic; open chain compounds. 2. Without a cycle.

acyesis (ă-sī-ē'sis) [G. *a-,* priv, + *kyēsis,* pregnancy]. 1. Absence of pregnancy. 2. Sterility of the female.

acystia (ă-sis'tē-ă) [a-, + G. *kystis,* bladder]. Congenital absence of bladder.

acystineuria (ă-sĭs-tĭ-nū'rĭ-ă) [G. *a-,* priv. + *kystis,* bladder, + *neuron,* nerve]. Inability to control nervous mechanism of the bladder.

AD. Abbr. for *anodal duration; average deviation; diphenylchlorarsine.*

A. D. A. Abbreviation for *American Dental Association; American Dietetic Association.*

ad- [L.]. Prefix indicating adherence, increase, toward, as *adduct.*

-ad. [L.]. Suffix meaning toward; in direction of, as *cephalad.*

a. d. [L. *au'ris dex'tra*]. Abbr. for *right ear.*

adactylia (ă-dak-til'ē-ă) [a-, + G. *daktylos,* finger, + ia]. A congenital anomaly consisting of absence of digits of hands or foot.

adamantine (ăd-ă-măn'tin) [G. *adamantinos,* very hard]. Very hard, said of enamel of teeth.

ad"amantino'ma [" + *-oma,* tumor]. A tumor of the jaw, esp. the lower one, arising from the enamel organ. May be partly cystic, partly solid, and may reach a large size; of low-grade malignancy. SYN: *ameloblastoma.*

adamantoblast (ad-ă-măn'tō-blast) [" + *blastos,* germ]. An enamel cell from which tooth enamel is formed.

adamantoblastoma (ad-ă-man-tō-blas-tō'ma) [" + " + *-oma,* tumor]. Overgrowth of an adamantoblast.

adamanto'ma [" + *-oma,* tumor]. Adamantinoma, *q.v.*

Adam's apple [L. *pomum,* apple]. The laryngeal prominence. SYN: *prominentia laryngea* [NA]; *pomum Adami.*

Adams-Stokes syn'drome [Robert Adams, Dublin physician, 1791-1875, and William Stokes, Dublin physician, 1804-1878]. Sudden attacks of weakness, fainting, sweating, and sometimes convulsions. Caused by complete heart block or overdigitalization.

adaptation [L. *adaptare*, to adjust]. 1. In *biology*, the ability of an organism to adjust to a change in environment. 2. In *ophthalmology*, the ability of the eye to adjust to light of various intensities, accomplished by changing size of pupil accompanied by chemical changes occurring in the rods. 3. In *psychology*, a change in quality, intensity, or distinctness of a sensation which occurs after continuous stimulation of constant intensity. 4. In *dentistry*, the proper fitting of dentures, bands, etc. to the teeth, or closeness of a filling to walls of a cavity.

a., chromatic. A change in hue or saturation or both resulting from pre-exposure to light of other wave lengths.

a., dark. The adjustment of the eyes for vision in dim light. SYN: *scotopia.*

a., light. Adjustment of the eyes for vision in bright light. SYN: *photopia.*

adap'ter. A device for joining one part of an apparatus to another part.

adaxial (ăd-ăks'ĭ-ăl). Toward the main axis. Opposite to *abaxial.*

ADC. Abbr. for *anodal duration contraction; axiodistocervical.*

add. In prescription writing, abbr. for *adde* (*let there be added*).

ad'dict [L. *addictus*, past p. *addicere*, to consent]. One habituated to the use of a drug.

addiction (ă-dĭk'shun). Enslavement to some habit, esp. the drug habit.

Addis count or **method.** [Thomas Addis, American physician, 1881-1949]. Method for counting the sediment (casts and cells) in a 12-hour sample of urine.

addisonism (ad'ĭ-sŭn-izm). Symptom complex not due to disease of suprarenal glands but resembling Addison's disease. The presence of abnormal skin pigmentation with debility. Seen in pulmonary tuberculosis.

Addison's disease [Thomas Addison, English physician, 1793-1860]. Disease resulting from deficiency in the secretion of adrenocortical hormones. SYN: *adrenal cortical hypofunction; chronic hypoadrenocorticism.*

ETIOL: Progressive destruction of the adrenal cortex which is often invaded by chronic infectious diseases as tuberculosis, histoplasmosis, cryptococcosis and other fungus diseases. Commonly, idiopathic atrophy of the adrenal is the cause.

SYM AND SIGNS: Increased pigmentation of skin and mucous membranes, irregular milk-white patches (vitiligo) on skin, black freckles over head and neck, weakness, fatigability, hypotension, nausea, vomiting, anorexia, weight loss, and occasional hypoglycemia.

PROG: If untreated, the disease will continue a chronic course with progressive but relatively slow deterioration; in some patients the progression may be a rapid one of deterioration. Patients treated properly have an excellent prognosis.

NP: Freedom from anxiety, the prevention of fatigue. If confined to bed, as during an adrenal crisis, the patient should be kept warm and bedsores must be guarded against. Watch the pulse for sudden changes, as fainting and syncope may occur, and patient may die in such an attack. He never should be left alone if confined to the bed. Keep the patient as cheerful as possible.

TREATMENT: Adrenocortical hormone therapy is dramatic in its effect and in adrenal crisis must be given promptly in order to prevent death. SEE: *adrenal; adrenalin.*

addition. In chemistry, a reaction in which two substances unite without loss of atoms or valence.

ad'duct [L. *adductus*, past p. of *adducere*, to bring to]. 1. To draw towards the main axis of body or a limb. 2. In optics, to turn eye inwardly.

adduction (ăd-dŭk'shŭn). 1. Movement of a limb, or bending of trunk or head toward median plane of body or in case of digits, toward axial line of a limb. 2. In optics, inward rotation of the eye.

a.; convergent-stimulus. Convergence of eyes upon fixation of gaze on an object at the near point of vision.

adduc'tor [L. a drawer toward]. A muscle which draws toward the medial line of the body or to a common center.

a. reflex. Contraction of adductors of the thigh upon applying pressure to, or tapping, medial surface of thigh or knee.

adelomorphous (ad"el-ō-mor'fus) [G. *adelōs*, not seen, + *morphē*, shape]. Having undefined form. Word is applied to the central cells of the gastric glands.

adelphotaxis (ă-del'fō-tăk"sis) [G. *adelphos*, brother, + *taxis*, arrangement]. Grouping of cells in mutual relationships. SYN: *adelphotaxy.*

adenalgia (ad-en-al'jĭ-ă) [G. *aden*, gland, + *algos*, pain]. Pain in a gland. SYN: *adenodynia.*

ad'enase [" + *ase*, enzyme]. Enzyme secreted by the pancreas, spleen, and liver and which converts *adenine** into *hypoxanthine.** SEE: *enzymes.*

adenasthenia (ad"en-ăs-thē'nĭ-ă) [" + *astheneia*, weakness]. Deficient glandular functional activity.

adendrit'ic [G. *a-*, priv. + *dendritēs*, rel. to a tree]. Without dendrites, as certain cells in spinal ganglia. ALSO: *adendric.*

adenectomy (ad-en-ek'to-mĭ) [G. *aden*, gland, + *ek*, out, + *temnein*, to cut]. Excision of a gland.

ad"enecto'pia [" + " + *topos*, place]. A gland out of its normal place.

ad"enemphrax'is [" + *emphraxis*, stoppage]. Obstruction to discharge from a gland.

adenia (ad-e'nĭ-ă). Hypertrophy of lymphatic glands with hyperleukocytosis absent.

aden'iform [G. *adēn*, gland, + L. *forma*, shape]. Like a gland in form.

adenine (ad'ĕ-nēn). 6-aminopurine, $C_5H_5N_5$, a solid substance of the uric acid group, and derivable from the nucleic acids.

adeni'tis [G. *adēn*, gland, + *-itis*, inflammation]. Inflammation of lymph nodes or a gland.

adeniza'tion. Abnormal change into a glandlike structure.

adeno- (ad'ĕ-nō) [G. *aden*, gland]. A prefix denoting a gland.

adenoacanthoma (ad"ĕ-no-ak-an-thō'mă) [" + *akantha*, thorn, + *oma*, tumor]. Adenocarcinoma in which some cells have undergone squamous metaplasia.

adenocarcinoma (ad-ĕ-nō-kar-sin-ō'mă) [" + *karkinos*, cancer]. A malignant adenoma arising from epithelium of a glandular organ.

adenocele (ad'ĕ-nō-sēl) [" + *kēlē*, tumor]. A cystic tumor arising from a gland. A tumor of glandular structure.

adenocellulitis (ad″ĕ-nō-sel-ū-lī′tis) [" + L. *cella,* small chamber, + G. *-itis,* inflammation]. Inflammation of a gland and adjacent cellular tissue.

adenochondroma (ad″ĕ-nō-kon-drō′ma) [" + *chondros,* cartilage, + *-oma,* tumor]. Adenoma with added characteristics of chondroma.

adenocyst (ad′ĕ-nō-sist) [" + *kystis,* sac]. A cystic tumor arising from a gland.

adenocystoma (ad″ĕ-nō-sis-tō′mă) [" + " + *-oma,* tumor]. Cystic adenoma.

adenodynia (ad-ĕ-nō-din′ĭ-ă) [" + *odynē,* pain]. Pain in a gland. SYN: *adenalgia.*

adenoepithelioma (ad″ĕ-nō-ep″i-thēl-ē-ō′ma). Tumor consisting of glandular and epithelial elements.

adenofibro′ma [" + L. *fibra,* fiber, + G. *-oma,* tumor]. Fibrous and glandular tissue tumor frequently in uterus.

adenogenous (ad-ĕ-noj′ĕ-nus) [" + *gennan,* to produce]. Having origin in glandular tissue.

adenohypersthenia (ad″ĕ-nō-hī-per-sthē-nī-ă) [" + *yper,* excess, + *sthenos,* strength]. Excessive glandular activity.

adenohypophysis (ad″ĕ-no-hi-poph′i-sis). The anterior lobe or glandular portion of the hypophysis cerebri.

adenoid (ad′ĕ-noid) [G. *adēnoeides,* glandular]. Lymphoid; having the appearance of a gland.

a. hypertrophy. Enlargement of the pharyngeal tonsil occurring commonly in children. May result from infection of Waldeyer's ring or may be congenital.

a. tissue. The pharyngeal tonsil; adenoids, *q.v.*

adenoidectomy (ad-ĕ-noid-ek′tō-mĭ) [" + *ektomē,* excision]. Excision of adenoids.

NP: Watch color and pulse for signs of excessive bleeding; children often swallow blood, and signs are only as above. SEE: *tonsillectomy.*

adenoids (ăd′ĕ-noids) Lymphatic tissue forming a prominence on the wall of the pharyngeal recess of the nasopharynx. SYN: *pharyngeal tonsil.*

ad″enolipo′ma [G. *adēn,* gland, + *lipos,* fat, + *-oma,* tumor]. A benign tumor having glandular characteristics but composed of fat.

adenolymphitis (ad″ĕ-nō-lim-fī′tis) [" + L. *lympha,* lymph, + G. *-itis,* inflammation]. Inflammation of a lymph gland. SYN: *lymphadenitis.*

adenolymphocele (ad″ĕ-nō-lim′fō-sēl) [" + L. *lympha,* lymph, + G. *kēlē,* tumor]. Cystic dilatation of a lymph node from obstruction.

adenolymphoma (ad″ĕ-nō-lim-fō′ma) [" + " + *-oma,* tumor]. A lymph gland adenoma.

adenoma (ad-ĕ-nō′mă) (pl. *adenomata*) [" + *-oma,* tumor]. A neoplasm of glandular epithelium.

a., acidophil(ic. A tumor of the pituitary gland whose cells stain with acid dyes. Cause of acromegaly and gigantism. SYN: *eosinophil a.*

a., basophil(ic. A tumor of the pituitary gland whose cells stain with basic dyes. Cause of Cushing's syndrome.

a., chromophobe. Tumor of pituitary gland composed of cells that do not stain readily. May cause pituitary deficiency or diabetes insipidus.

a., eosinophil(ic. Same as acidophil(ic a., *q.v.*

a., fibroid. Fibroadenoma. SYN: *a. fibrosum.*

a., islet. Nonmalignant neoplasm of the pancreas sometimes containing beta cells. May be cause of hypoglycemia. SYN: *insuloma; langerhansian a.*

a., langerhansian. Islet a., *q.v.*

a., malignant. Adenocarcinoma, *q.v.*

a. sebaceum. Benign tumorlike growths on face developing from epithelium of sebaceous glands which undergo fatty but never colloid metamorphosis. Sometimes associated with mental deficiency.

a., tubular. An adenoma of the form of a tubular gland.

adenomalacia (ad″ĕ-nō-mă-lā′shĭ-ă) [" + *malakia,* softening]. Glandular softening.

adenomatome (ad″ĕ-nō′mă-tōm) [" + *tomē,* a cutting down]. Instrument for removing adenoids.

ad″enomato′sis [" + *-oma,* tumor, + *-osis,* increase]. The condition of multiple glandular tissue overgrowths.

adenomatous (ad-ĕ-no′mă-tus). Pert. to adenomas.

adenomere (ad′ĕ-nō-mēr) [G. *aden,* gland, + *mēros,* part]. The functional part of a gland.

adenomyoma (ad″ĕ-nō-mī-ō′mă) [" + *mys,* muscle, + *-oma,* tumor]. A tumor containing glandular and smooth muscular tissue.

adenomyometritis (ad″ĕ-nō-mī″ō-mē-trī′-tis) [" + " + *metra,* womb, + *-itis,* inflammation]. GYN: A hyperplastic condition of the uterus which is the result of pelvic inflammation and grossly resembles an adenomyoma.

adenomyosis (ad″ĕ-nō-mī-ō′sis) [" + *mys,* muscle, + *-osis,* increase]. Benign invasive growth of the endometrium into the muscular layer of the uterus.

ad″enomyxo′ma [" + *myxa,* mucus, + *-oma,* tumor]. A benign tumor with adenoma and myxoma characteristics.

ad″enomyx″osarco′ma [" + " + *sarx,* flesh, + *-oma,* tumor]. A malignant tumor with adenoma, myxoma, and sarcoma characteristics.

adenoncus (ad-ĕ-non′kus) [" + *onkos,* tumor]. A tumor of a gland or its enlargement.

adenopathy (ad-ĕ-nop′ă-thĭ) [" + *pathos,* suffering]. Swelling and morbid change in lymph nodes; glandular disease.

ad″enopharyngi′tis [" + *pharynx,* throat, + *-itis,* inflammation]. Inflammation of tonsils and pharyngeal mucous membrane.

ad″enophthal′mia [" + *ophthalmos,* eye]. Inflammation of the meibomian glands.

ad″enosarco′ma [" + *sarx,* flesh, + *-oma,* tumor]. A tumor with characteristics of adenoma and sarcoma.

adenosclerosis (ad″ĕ-nō-sklĕ-rō′sis) [" + *sclērōsis,* hardening]. Glandular hardening.

adenose (ad′ĕ-nōs). Glandlike.

adenosine (ad′ĕ-nō-sen). A nucleotide containing adenine and ribose.

a. diphosphate. A compound of adenosine containing two phosphoric acid groups. This enzyme is produced during muscle contraction. It is reformed when the muscle relaxes. ABBR: ADP.

a. triphosphate. A compound of adenosine containing three phosphoric acid groups. An enzyme found in all cells but particularly muscle cells. When this substance is split by enzyme action, energy is produced. The energy of the muscle is stored in this compound. ABBR: ATP.

adenosis (ad-ĕ-nō′sis) [G. *adēn,* gland, + *-osis,* increase]. Any disease of a gland, esp. of a lymphatic gland.

adenovirus. One of a group of closely related viruses which can cause infections of the upper respiratory tract. A large number have been isolated.

adeps (ad'eps) [L.]. Lard; omental hog-fat.

a. benzoina'tus. Benzoinated lard.

a. la'nae. USP. Wool fat. Purified anhydrous lanolin from sheep wool. Used as an ointment base.

a. lanae hydrosus. USP. Hydrous wool fat; lanolin.

ader'mia [G. *a-*, priv. + *derma*, skin]. Lack of skin, congenital or acquired.

ader"mogen'esis [" + " + *genesis*, production]. Imperfect growth or repair of skin.

A. D. H. Abbreviation for ***antidiuretic*** *hormone* (vasopressin).

adherent (ad-he'rent) [L. *ad*, to, + *haerere*, to stick]. Attached to, as of two surfaces.

adhe'sion. 1. A holding together by new tissue produced by inflammation or injury, of two structures which are normally separate. 2. A fibrous band which holds parts together which are normally separated. 3. An attraction to another substance; thus molecules or blood platelets adhere to each other or to dissimilar materials.

a., abdominal. Adhesion in the abdominal cavity, usually involving the intestines. Caused by inflammation or trauma. They are treated surgically if causing great pain or intestinal obstruction.

a., pericardial. Adhesion of the pericardial sac. If extensive enough may lead to restriction of the normal movement of the heart. SEE: *pericarditis.*

adhesiotomy (ad-hē-zĭ-ot'ō-mĭ). Surgical division of adhesions.

adhesive (ad-he'siv) [F. *adhésif*]. 1. Causing adhesion. 2. Sticky; adhering. 3. That which causes two bodies to adhere.

a. inflammation. A serous membrane inflammation exudating fibrinous matter making adhesions possible.

a. plaster, a. tape. A fabric or film, one side of which is coated with an adhesive substance, that remains in place after application by pressure.

adiadochokinesis (ă-dī"ă-dō-kō-kin-ē'sis) [G. *adiadochos*, perpetual, + *kinēsis*, movement]. 1. Inability to make rapid alternating movements. 2. Incessant movement. 3. NEUR: Rapid antagonistic movements which cannot be carried out with accuracy. Seen in cerebellar disease. SYN: *adiadochokinesia.* RS: *asynergia; dysmetria; gait.*

adiaphoresis (ă-dĭ-ă-fō-re'sis) [G. *a-*, priv. + *diaphoresis*, perspiration]. Deficiency or absence of sweat.

adiaphorous (ă"dĭ-af'o-rus) [G. *a-*, + *diaphoros*, different]. Neither harmful nor beneficial. Neutral.

adiapneustia (ă"di-ap-new'stĭ-ă) [G. *a-*, + *diaphnein*, to breathe through]. Anhidrous. Failure to, or lack of, sweat.

adiastole (ă-dĭ-as'tō-lē) [" + *diastolē*, dilatation]. Imperceptibility of diastole.

adiathermancy (ă-dĭ-ă-thur'măn-sĭ) [" + *dia*, through, + *thermē*, heat]. State of being impervious to heat.

adient (ad-ĭ'ent). Tending to move toward a stimulus. Opposite to *abient.*

adipectomy (ad"ĭ-pek'to-mĭ) [L. *adeps*, fat, + G. *ectome*, a cutting out]. Excision of fat or adipose tissue, usually a large quantity.

adipic (ă-dip'ik) [L. *adeps*, fat]. Relating to adipose tissues.

adipocele (ad'ĭ-pō-sēl) [" + G. *kēlē*, tumor]. A hernia which contains fat or fatty tissue. Lipocele.

adipocere (ad'ĭ-po-sēr) [L. *adeps*, fat, + *cera*, wax]. A brown waxlike substance composed of fatty acids and calcium soaps. It is formed in animal tissues which have been buried in a moist place. SYN: *grave wax.*

ad"ipofibro'ma [" + *fibra*, fiber, + G. *-oma*, tumor]. A fibroma and adipoma.

adipogenous (ad-ĭ-poj'en-us) [" + G. *gennan*, to produce]. Inducing the formation of fat.

adipoid (ad'ĭ-poid). Fatlike; lipoid.

adipolysis (ad-ĭ-pol'ĭ-sis) [" + *lysis*, setting free]. The hydrolysis of fat.

adipoma (ad-ĭ-po'mă) [L. *adeps*, fat, + *oma*, tumor]. Fatty tissue tumor. SYN: *lipoma.*

adipometer (ad-ĭ-pom'ĕ-ter). Instrument for measuring thickness of the skin.

adiponecrosis (ad"i-po-nĕ-kro'sis) [L. *adeps*, fat, + necrosis]. Necrosis affecting fatty tissue.

ad"ipopex'ia [" + G. *pēxis*, fixation]. The storing of fat. SYN: *lipopexia.*

ad'ipose. Fatty; pertaining to fat.

a. capsule. Renal fat.

a. fossae. Fatty accumulations on outer mammary surface.

a. tissue. Connective or areolar tissue containing masses of fat cells.

adiposis (ad-ĭ-po'sis) [L. *adeps*, fat, + G. *-ōsis*, increase]. Abnormal accumulation of fat in the body. SYN: ***corpulence;*** *liposis.*

a. cerebralis. Obesity due to intracranial disease especially of the hypophysis or pituitary.

a. doloro'sa. A disease, the symptoms of which are fatty painful formations, and nerve lesions. SYN: *Dercum's disease.*

a. hepat'ica. Fatty degeneration or infiltration of the liver.

a. tuberosa simplex. A disease resembling adiposis dolorosa in which the fat occurs in small circumscribed nodules sensitive or painful to touch. SYN: *Anders' disease.*

adipositis (ad-ĭ-pō-sī'tĭs) [L. *adiposa*, fatty tissue, + G. *-itis*, inflammation]. Infiltration of an inflammatory nature in and beneath subcutaneous adipose tissue.

adipos'ity. Excessive fat in the body. SYN: *adiposis; obesity.*

adipo"sogen'ital dystrophy. Combination of adiposity, impaired development of genital organs, and change in secondary sex characteristics. SYN: *Fröhlich's syndrome; sexual infantilism.*

ETIOL: A disturbance or tumor of the hypothalamus and pituitary gland.

adiposuria (ad-ĭ-pō-su'rĭ-ă). Fat in the urine. SYN: *lipuria.*

adip'sia, ad'ipsy [G. *a-*, priv. + *dipsa*, thirst]. Absence of thirst.

ad'itus [L.]. An approach; an entrance.

a. ad antrum tympanicum [NA]. The recess of the tympanic cavity which leads from epitympanic recess to the tympanic antrum.

a. ad aquaeductum cerebri. The entrance to the sylvian aqueduct, situated at lower posterior angle of third ventricle of brain.

a. ad infundibulum. A small canal leading from the third ventricle into the infundibulum.

a. glottidis inferior. Inferior entrance to the glottis.

a. glottidis superior. Superior entrance to the glottis.

a. laryngis [NA]. Upper aperture of larynx.

adjuster (ad-jus'ter). Device for holding together the ends of the wire forming a suture.

adjustment (ad-just'ment) [L. *adjuxtare,* to bring together]. 1. Biological adaptation to an altered or changing condition, particularly in the environment. 2. Mechanical change in a microscope so that the tube containing the lenses is moved up or down in order to bring the object into focus.

ad'juvant [L. *adjuvans,* from *adjuvare,* to aid]. That which assists, esp. a drug added to a prescription to hasten or increase the action of a principal ingredient; synergist.

Adler's organ-inferiority [Alfred Adler, Viennese psychiatrist, 1870-1937]. The theory that sexual or other organic inferiority is a cause of neuroses.

ad lib. Abbr. for L. *ad lib'itum,* at pleasure or as much as is wanted.

ad nauseum [L.]. Of such degree or extent as to produce nausea.

adner'val [L. *ad,* to, + *nervus,* nerve] Near or toward a nerve.

adneu'ral [" + G. *neuron,* nerve]. Adnerval.

adnex'a [L. *adnectere,* to tie or bind to]. Accessory parts of a structure.

a. oculi. Lacrimal glands.

a. uteri. Ovaries and oviducts.

adnex'al [L. *adnexus,* past p. *adnectere,* to tie to]. Adjacent or appending.

adnexi'tis [L. *adnexus* + G. *-itis,* inflammation]. Inflammation of the *adnexa uteri.*

adnexopexy (ad-neks'ō-peks-ē) [" + G. *pexis,* a putting together]. Fixing the fallopian tube and ovary to the abdominal wall.

adolescence (ad-o-les'ens) [L. *adolescens,* from *adolescere,* to grow up]. The period from the beginning of puberty until maturity. The onset of puberty and maturity is a gradual process and variable among individuals. Thus it is not practical to set exact age or chronological limits in defining the adolescent period.

ad"oles'cent. 1. Pert. to adolescence. 2. Young man or woman not fully grown.

adoral (ad-o'ral) [L. *ad,* to, + *os, oris,* mouth]. Toward or near the mouth.

A. D. P. Adenosine diphosphate.

adrenal (ăd-rē'năl) [L. *ad,* to, + *ren,* kidney]. 1. Near the kidney. 2. Pert. to or derived from the adrenal gland. 3. The adrenal gland, *q.v.*

a. gland. A triangular-shaped body adjacent to and covering the superior surface of each kidney. It is a gland of internal secretion producing hormones essential to life. Syn: *suprarenal gland.*

Embryology: The adrenal gland is essentially a double organ composed of an outer *cortex* and an inner *medulla.* The cortex arises in the embryo from a region of the mesoderm, which also gives rise to the gonads or sex organs. The medulla arises from ectoderm which also gives rise to the sympathetic nervous system.

Anat: The entire gland is enclosed in a tough connective tissue capsule from which *trabeculae* extend into the cortex. The cortex consists of cells arranged into three zones; the outer *zona glomerulosa,* the middle *zona fasciculata,* and the inner *zona reticularis.* The cells are arranged in a cordlike fashion. The medulla consists of chromaffin cells arranged in groups or anastomosing cords. The two adrenal glands are situated retroperitoneally, each embedded in perirenal fat above its respective kidney.

In the adult the average weight is 6 gm., and the range is 4 to 10 grams.

Phys: The Medulla. The medulla secretes two hormones, *epinephrine* and *norepinephrine,* the effects of which are similar but differ in degree. Both increase blood pressure, epinephrine acting through the heart by increasing heart rate and norepinephrine acting by increasing peripheral resistance through its vasoconstrictor effects. Epinephrine is a vasodilator and increases oxygen consumption by the tissues and glucose release by the liver. Both hormones inhibit gastrointestinal movements.

The adrenal medulla is under the control of the sympathetic nervous system and functions in conjunction with it. It is intimately related to adjustments of the body in response to emotional states. Anticipatory states tend to bring about the release of norepinephrine; the more intense emotional reactions, esp. those in response to extreme stress, tend to increase the secretion of both, epinephrine inducing reactions which adapt the organism to meet emergency situations. Norepinephrine is the neurohumor released at the ends of adrenergic nerve fibers.

The Cortex: Secretes a large number of substances, over forty steroids having been isolated from the adrenal cortex, including *glucocorticoids* which affect carbohydrate and protein metabolism, *mineralocorticoids* which affect water and electrolyte metabolism, and *sex hormones.* Cortical tissue is essential to life. Its removal or destruction results in disturbances in salt balance with loss of sodium and accumulation of potassium.

Cortical hormones include the following groups based on chemical structure and biologic activity: (a) the 11-oxygenated corticosteroids which primarily affect carbohydrate and protein metabolism. Ex: 17-*hydroxycorticosterone* (hydrocortisone, cortisol, or Compound F), *corticosterone* (Compound B) 11-*dehydrocorticosterone* (Compound A) and *cortisone* (Compound E). (b) Corticosteroids lacking oxygen at position 11, whose effects are principally on water and electrolyte metabolism. Ex: 11-*deoxycorticosterone* (DOC), 17-OH, 11-*deoxycorticosterone* (Compound S). (c) *Aldosterone,* of primary importance in electrolyte metabolism. (d) *Sex hormones* (androgens, estrogens, progesterone).

The secretion of cortical hormones is under the control of ACTH (adrenocorticotropic hormone) produced by the anterior lobe of the hypophysis.

Path: Medulla: *Hypersecretion* may result from tumors (*pheochromocytomas*) which involve chromaffin cells. Symptoms are paroxysmal attacks of hypertension, usually of sudden onset, with associated manifestations (viz. tachycardia, tremor of extremities, headache, weakness, sweating, dilatation of pupils and blurred vision).

Cortex: *Hypertension* may result from tumors involving cortical cells or from excessive production of ACTH by the ant. lobe of the hypophysis. The effects depend upon the kinds of hormones which are produced. If hydrocortisone and cortisone-like substances are secreted in excess, *Cushing's syndrome* results, characterized by obesity and weakness, protein loss, hypertension, and capillary fragility. If androgenic steroids predominate, the *adrenogenital syndrome* results, characterized by overmasculinization except for small testes in male adults and virilization in females, marked hirsutism, and pronounced muscular development. There are two types of this syndrome: prepubertal or congenital, and postpubertal or acquired. The signs and symptoms differ between these types. If aldosterone is secreted in excess, *primary aldosteronism* may result, characterized by edema, loss of potassium accompanied by intermittent paralysis, sodium retention, and hypertension.

Hyposecretion: Addison's disease. This disease is the result of chronic adrenal cortical insufficiency, brought about by invasion of the cortex by chronic infectious diseases as tuberculosis, histoplasmosis, and other fungus diseases. Commonly idiopathic atrophy of the adrenal is the cause. SEE: *Addison's disease* for symptoms, signs, etc.

RS: *Addison's disease, adrenalin, kidney.*

adrenalectomy (ad-rē-năl-ek'tō-mĭ) [" + G. *ektomē,* excision]. Excision of an adrenal body.

adrenalin (ă-dren'ă-lin). Proprietary name for epinephrine, *q.v.*

adrenaline (a-dren'ă-lēn). British designation for epinephrine, *q.v.*

adrenaline'mia [L. *ad,* to, + *rēn,* kidney, + G. *aima,* blood]. Epinephrine (adrenaline) in the blood.

adrenalinu'ria [" + G. *ouron,* urine]. Adrenalin (epinephrine) in the urine.

adren'alism. Illness caused by abnormal action of adrenal glands.

adrenalitis (ad-re"nal-i'tis). Inflammation of the adrenal glands; adrenitis.

adrenergic (ad-ren-er'jik) [L. *ad,* to, + *rēn,* kidney, + G. *ergon,* work]. Term applied to nerve fibers which when stimulated release epinephrine (adrenaline) at their endings. Includes nearly all sympathetic post-ganglionic fibers except those innervating sweat glands.

adreni'tis. Adrenalitis, *q.v.*

adrenochrome (ăd"rē'nō-krōm). A pigment obtained by oxidation of epinephrine. Its action is similar to that of epinephrine.

adrenocorticotrophic, adrenocorticotropic (ăd-rē-nō-kôr"tĭ-kō-trŏf'ĭk, -trŏp'ĭk). Having a stimulating effect on the adrenal cortex.

a. hormone. Abbr.: ACTH. A hormone secreted by ant. lobe of hypophysis which stimulates development of and secretion by the adrenal cortex. It also exerts extra-adrenal effects such as mobilizing depot fat and increasing liver fat. SYN: *corticotropin.*

adrenop'athy. Any disease of the adrenal glands.

adrenosterone (ăd"rēn-ŏs'tē-rōn). An androgenic hormone secreted by the adrenal cortex.

adrenotoxin (ad-rē"nō-toks'ĭn). A substance toxic to the adrenal glands.

adrenotrophic, adrenotropic (ad-rē"nō-trŏf'ĭk, -trŏp'ĭk). Nourishing or stimulating to the adrenal glands with reference especially to hormones which stimulate secretion by the adrenal glands.

adromia (ăd"rō'mĭ-ă). Failure of a muscle or nerve to conduct an impulse.

A. D. S. Antidiuretic substance; antidiuretic hormone (A.D.H.).

adsorb'ent. A substance which readily adsorbs, such as activated charcoal or magnesia.

adsorp'tion [L. *ad,* to, + *sorbere,* to suck in]. Adhesion by a gas or liquid to the surface of a solid.

adsternal (ad-ster'nal) [L. *ad,* toward + G. *sternon,* chest]. Near or toward the sternum.

A. D. T. *Adenosine triphosphate;* abbr. for a placebo, meaning *A* (*any*), *D* (*what you desire*), *T* (*thing*); *agar-gel diffusion test.*

adter'minal [L. *ad,* to, + *terminalis,* end]. Toward extremity of any structure, as end of nerve or muscle.

adtorsion [ad + L. *torsio,* **from** ***torguere,*** to twist]. Convergent squint; inward rotation of both eyes.

adultera'tion. The addition of an impure or weaker substance to another one.

advancement (ad-vans'ment) [Fr. *avancer,* to set forth]. Operation to remedy strabismus, by which the ocular muscle is severed and then attached at a point further removed from its origin.

a., capsular. Attachment of capsule of Tenon in front of its normal position.

adventitia (ad-ven-tish'ē-ă) [L. *adventitius,* coming from abroad]. The outermost covering of a structure or organ, such as the *tunica adventitia,* or outer coat of an artery.

adventitious (ad-ven-tish'us). 1. Acquired: accidental. 2. Arising sporadically. 3. Pert. to adventitia.

adynamia (ăd-ĭ-nā'mĭ-ă) [G. *a-,* priv. + *dynamis,* strength]. Weakness or loss of strength; asthenia, *q.v.*

adynamic (ad-ĭ-nam'ik, ā-dī-nam'ik). Pert. to adynamia.

a. ileus. Intestinal obstruction due to lack of intestinal motility. This causes abdominal distention and interferes with postsurgical recovery, particularly from abdominal surgery.

Aedes (ā-ē'dēs). A genus of mosquitoes belonging to the family Culicidae. Many species are troublesome pests and some are transmitters of disease.

A. aegypti. A species of A. which transmits yellow fever and dengue.

aeluropsis (ē"lū-rŏp'sĭs). Condition in which the eye or palpebral fissure is slanting.

aequum (ē'kwŭm). Basic amount of nutrients necessary for one to maintain body weight at a constant level while doing a specific amount of work.

aer- (air, a'er) [G. *aer,* air]. Combining form meaning relationship to gas or air.

aerated (ā'ĕr-ā-ted) [G. *aer,* air]. Containing air or gas.

aeration (ā-ĕr-a'shun). 1. Act of airing. 2. Change of venous into arterial blood in the lungs. 3. Saturation or charging of a fluid with gases.

aerendocardia (ā-ĕr-ĕn-dō-kar'dĭ-ă) [G. *aer,* air, + *kardia,* heart]. Bubble of air in the blood within the heart.

aerenterectasia (ā"er-en-ter-ek-tā'zĭ-ă) [" + *enteron,* intestine, + *ektasis.* stretching out]. Distention of intestine with gas.

aeriform (a-er'ĭ-form) [" + L. *forma,* shape]. Airlike; gaseous.

aero-, aer- (air'o, a'er-o). Combining form indicating relationship to air or gas.

Aerobacter (ā-ĕr-ō-bak'ter). A genus of aerobic, nonspore-bearing, gram-negative bacilli of the family Enterobacteriaceae.

A. aerogenes. A species of A. It occurs normally in the intestine of man and other animals and is found in decayed matter, on grains and plants..

a'erobe (pl. *aerobes*) [" + *bios,* life]. A microorganism which can live and grow only in the presence of free oxygen. SYN: *aerobion.*

a., facultative. A microorganism which prefers an environment that is devoid of free oxygen but which has adapted so that it can live and reproduce in the presence of free oxygen.

a., obligate. A microorganism which reproduces only when free oxygen is present.

aerobic (ā-er-ō'bik). 1. Living only in presence of oxygen. 2. Concerning an organism living only in oxygen.

aero'bion. Aerobe, *q.v.*

aerobiosis (ā-er-ō-bī-ō'sis). Living in an atmosphere containing oxygen.

aerocele (ā'er-ō-sēl) [G. *aer*, air, + *kēlē*, tumor]. Gas within and distending a cavity.

aerocolpos (ā"er-ō-kol'pos) [" + *kolpos*, vagina]. Distention of the vagina with air.

aerocoly (ā-ĕ-rok'ō-lī) [" + *kōlon*, colon]. Distention of colon with gas.

aerocystoscopy (ā-ĕr-ō-sis-tos'kō pī) [" + *kystis*, bladder, + *skopein*, to view]. Examination of the bladder, when distended by air, with a cystoscope.

aerodermectasia (ā-er-ō-der-mek-tā'zĭ-ă) [" + *derma*, skin, + *ektasis*, stretching out]. Subcutaneous emphysema.

aerodontalgia (ā"er-ō"dŏnt-ăl'gĭ-ă). Pain in the teeth resulting from reduction in atmospheric pressure, as at high altitudes.

aerodontia (ā-er-ō-dŏn'tĭ-ă). A branch of dentistry concerned with the effect of flying on the teeth.

aerodynam'ics [" + *dynamis*, force]. Science of air or gases in motion.

aeroembolism (ā-er-ō-em'bō-lizm) [G. *aer*, air, + *embolus*, blood]. A condition in which nitrogen bubbles form in fluids and tissues of body during rapid ascent to high altitudes.

SYM: Boring, gnawing pain in joints, itching of skin and eyelids, unconsciousness, convulsions and paralysis. Symptoms are relieved by recompression, *i.e.*, return to lower altitudes. Ascents above 30,000 feet should be avoided except in planes with pressurized cabins. SEE: *bends; caisson disease.*

aeroemphysema (a-er-ō-ĕm-fī-zē'ma). Aeroembolism, *q.v.*

aerogen (ā'er-ō-jen) [" + *gennan*, to produce]. A gas-forming microorganism.

aerogenesis (ā-er-ō-jĕn'ĕ-sis) [" + *genesis*, production]. Formation of gas.

aerogenic (ā-er-ō-jen'ik). Gas-forming.

aerogenous (ā-er-oj'en-us). Gas-forming.

aerogram (ā'er-ō-gram). Roentgenogram of an organ after it has been inflated or filled with air or gas.

aerohydrother'apy. Treatment by application of air and water. SYN: *aerohydropathy.*

aeroionotherapy (ā"er-ō-ī-on-ō-ther'ă-pī). Treatment of respiratory disorders by inhalation of air bearing electrically charged particles in a mist.

aeromed'icine. Aviation medicine.

aerometer (ā-er-om'ĕ-ter) [" + *metron*, measure]. Device for measuring density of gases.

aeroneurosis (ā-ĕr-ō-nū-rō'sĭs) [G. *aer*, air, + *neuron*, nerve]. A chronic functional nervous disorder affecting aviators.

ETIOL: Anoxia resulting from prolonged flights at high altitudes combined with intense emotional stress.

SYM: Acute exhaustion and fatigue, shallow irregular breathing, nervous irritability, emotional instability, anxiety, insomnia, gastric disorders, neurocirculatory failure, impaired functioning of higher nervous centers.

aeropathy (ā-er-op'ă-thĭ) [" + *pathos*, suffering]. Morbid condition caused by a marked change in atmospheric pressure, such as mountain sickness or caisson disease.

aeroperitoneum (ā-ĕr-ō-per"ĭ-tō-nē'um). Distention of peritoneal cavity with gas. SYN: *aeroperitonia.*

aerophagia (ā-er-ō-fā'jĭ-ă). Swallowing of air. SYN: *aerophagy.*

aerophilous (ā-ĕr-of'ĭ-lŭs) [" + *philos*, fond]. Requiring air for growth and development. SYN: *aerobic.*

aerophobia (ā-er-ō-fō'bĭ-ă) [" + *phobos*, fear]. Morbid fear of a draft or of fresh air.

aerophore (a'er-o-for, air'o-for) [" + *phoros*, breathing]. A portable apparatus for inflating the lungs of stillborn or asphyxiated infants.

aerophyte (a'er-o-fit, air'o-fit) [" + *phyton*, plant]. A plant or vegetative organism which derives its sustenance from air.

aeropiesotherapy (a"er-o-pi-e'so-ther'ă-pĭ, air'o-) [" + *piesis*, pressure, + therapy]. Therapeutic use of air at either increased or decreased barometric pressure. SEE: *hyperbaric; decompression chamber.*

aeroplethysmograph (ā-er-ō-plĕ-thiz'mō-graf) [" + *plethysmos*, enlargement, + *graphein*, to write]. Instrument for recording air respired.

aeropleura (ā-er-ō-plū'ră) [" + *pleura*, side]. Pneumothorax; air in pleural cavity.

aeroporotomy (ā-er-ō-pō-rot'ō-mĭ) [" + *poros*, passage, + *tomē*, cutting]. Operation, such as a tracheotomy, for admitting air into the air passages.

aeroscope (ā'er-ō-skōp) [" + *skopein*, to view]. Device for examining visible dust or other visible particles in the air.

aerosinusitis (ā-ĕr-ō-sī-nus-ī'tĭs). Chronic inflammation of nasal sinuses due to changes in atmospheric pressure.

aerosis (ā-er-ō'sĭs). Accumulation of gas in any of the tissues.

aerosol (air'o-sōl, air'o-sol). 1. Atomized particles of a substance suspended in air. 2. A solution of a bactericidal substance which can be atomized for sterilizing the air of a room. 3. A colloidal mixture in which gas is the continuous phase (dispersion medium).

a. therapy. The use of aerosolized medicines in the treatment of disease, especially pulmonary conditions such as asthma, bronchitis, and emphysema.

aerosolization. Producing an aerosol.

aerospace medicine (air'ō-spās). The branch of medicine which is concerned with the physiologic, pathologic, and psychologic problems man encounters in the environment of space.

aerosporin (ā"ĕr-ō-spor'ĭn). One of a group of antibiotics known as polymyxins and derived from *Bacillus polymyxa* (aerosporus), a soil organism. SEE: *polymyxin.*

aerotaxis (a"ĕr-o-tak'sis) [" + *taxis*, arrangement]. Movement of organisms away from or toward air, said of aerobic and anaerobic bacteria.

aerotherapy (ā-ĕr-ō-ther'ă-pĭ) [G. *aer*, air, + *therapeia*, treatment]. The use of air in the treatment of disease, utilizing changes in composition and density. SEE: *hyperbaric; decompression chamber; aeropiesotherapy.*

aerothermotherapy (ā-er-ō-ther-mō-ther'-ă-pĭ) [" + *thermos*, hot, + *therapeia*. treatment]. Therapeutic use of hot air.

aerothorax [G. " + thorax]. Presence of air in the intrapleural space. SYN: *pneumothorax.*

aerotonometer (ā-er-ō-tō-nom'ĕ-ter) [" + *tonos,* tension, + *metron,* measure]. Apparatus for measuring tension of gases of the blood.

aerotropism (ā-ĕr-ŏt'rō-pĭsm). The tendency of organisms, esp. bacteria and protozoa, to move toward a region where air is available as toward the surface of water or towards an air bubble.

aerourethroscope (a"er-o-u-rē'thrō-skōp) [" + *ourethra,* urethra, + *skopein,* to view]. An apparatus for examination of the urethra after dilatation by air.

aerourethroscopy (a"er-ō-ū-rē-thros'kō-pĭ). Examination of the urethra when distended with air.

Aesculapius (es-kū-lā'pē-us). The Latin name for the Greek god of medicine; son of Apollo and the nymph Coronis.

A., staff of. A staff or crude stick with a snake wound around it so that its head is at the top of the stick. This symbol is used to signify the art of healing and is used by many medical organizations.

aet. Abbr. for L. *aetatis,* of age.

afebrile (ă-fē'bril) [G. *a-,* priv. + L. *febris,* fever]. Without fever.

af'fect [L. *affectus,* from *afficere,* to apply oneself to]. PSY: The emotional reactions associated with an experience. SYN: *psychic trauma.*

affec'tion. 1. Love, feeling. 2. Disease, physical or mental.

affec'tive. Stimulating emotion.

a. insanity. Impulsive or emotional insanity.

a. memory. Memory of a psychic trauma causing recurrence of emotion.

a. psycho'sis. A psychotic reaction characterized by serious disorder of mood or emotional feeling. SYN: *manic-depressive reaction.*

a., spasms. Attacks of laughing, screaming, or weeping in hysteria.

af'ferent [L. *ad,* to, + *ferre.* to bear]. Carrying impulses toward a center, as when a sensory nerve carries a message toward the brain; also said of certain veins and lymphatics. Opp. to efferent, *q.v.*

affiliation (ă-fil-ĭ-a'shun). In nursing education, the administrative association of two hospitals or schools of nursing. This enables nurses to obtain specialized training and experience which might not otherwise be available to them.

affinity (ă-fin'ĭ-tĭ) [L. *affinis,* neighboring]. 1. Common relationship; attraction. 2. Chemical attraction bet. two substances, *i.e.,* oxygen and hemoglobin. SEE: *chemoreceptor.*

a., chemical. Force combining atoms of various substances.

a., elective. Force causing a substance to elect one substance rather than another with which to unite.

a., selective. Elective affinity, *q.v.*

af'flux [L. *ad,* to, + *fluere,* to flow]. Rush of blood to a part.

affu'sion [L. *affusus,* from *affundere,* to pour to]. The pouring of water upon, as on the body, for cooling, cleansing, or therapeutic purposes.

IND: Fever, agitation.

CONTRA: Typhoid accompanied by complications, or decompensating heart, or hemorrhagic cases.

NP: Patient may lie on a rubber sheet arranged to direct the water into a pail at bedside. A thin sheet may cover patient. Water can be poured on body through a watering can.

afibrinogenemia (ă-fī"brin-ō-jĕ-nē'mĭ-ă). In general, the term *hypofibrinogenemia* would more accurately describe the disease process. A rare blood disease characterized by the absence or decrease of fibrinogen in the blood plasma so that the blood is incoagulable; may be congenital or acquired. The acquired type is due to one of several causes which can reduce the plasma concentration of fibrinogen. This has been observed in severe trauma and burns, following extensive surgery, obstetric complications of abruptio placenta or retention of a dead fetus, neoplastic disease, hepatic cirrhosis, leukemia, sarcoidosis, and polycythemia vera.

TREATMENT: The clinical picture may develop suddenly. Administration of whole fresh blood and fibrinogen may prevent death from hemorrhage.

af'teraction. A term used particularly in connection with nerve centers to designate continued reaction for some time after the stimulus ceases. In the sensory centers this action gives rise to aftersensations.

af'terbirth. Placenta and membranes expelled after birth of child.

aftercare. Care of a convalescent after conclusion of treatment in a hospital or mental institution.

af'tercat"aract [*Cataracta secundaria*]. Retained portion of lens substance bet. agglutinated layers of capsule; seen after extracapsular cataract extraction.

TREATMENT: Discission or needling.

afterdischarge. The discharge of impulses from a reflex center after stimulation of the receptor has ceased. Results in prolongation of response.

aftereffect. A response occurring some time after the original stimulus or condition has produced its primary effect.

afterhearing. Persistence of sensation of sound after the stimulus causing the sound has ceased.

afterimage. Image which persists subjectively after the cessation of stimulus.

If colors are same as object it is called *positive; negative* if complementary colors are seen. In the former case, the image is seen in its natural bright colors without any alteration; in the latter, the bright parts become dark, while dark parts are light.

afterimpression. An aftersensation, *q.v.*

af'terpains. Uterine cramps due to contraction of uterus, occurring during first few days after childbirth (*puerperium*); commonly seen in multiparae.* Pains more severe during nursing. The pain rarely lasts for longer than 48 hours postpartum.

TREATMENT: Codeine, aspirin. The earlier given, the less needed.

afterperception. Perception of a sensation after cessation of stimulus.

af'tersensa'tion. Sensation persisting after stimulus causing it has ceased.

aftertaste. Persistence of gustatory sensations after cessation of stimulus.

aftertreatment. Secondary treatment; that following a primary treatment regimen. SEE: *aftercare.*

aftervision. SEE: *afterimage.*

Ag. [L. argentum]. Chem. symb. for *silver.*

agalactia (ag"ă-lak'shĭ-ă) [G. *a-,* priv. + *gala, galaktos,* milk]. Absence of milk secretion after childbirth.

agamic (ă-gam'ik) [G. *a-,* negate, + *gamos,* marriage]. 1. Reproducing asexually. 2. Asexual.

agalorrhea (ă-gal-ō-rē'ă) [" + " + *roia*, flow]. Arrest of milk flow.

agammaglobulinemia (ā-gam-ă-glŏb"ū-lĭn-ē'mĭ-ă). A rare disease characterized by the virtual absence of gamma globulin from the blood plasma with resulting loss of the ability to produce immune antibodies, and the absence of natural blood group isoantibodies from the serum; may be congenital or acquired. The sex-linked congenital form is inherited like hemophilia as a sex-linked recessive characteristic, and occurs only in male children. The non-sex-linked form occurs as an autosomal dominant characteristic. This latter form is quite rare.

agamogen'esis [G. *a-*, priv. + *gamos*, marriage, + *genesis*, development]. 1. Asexual reproduction. 2. Parthenogenesis.

agar (ă'gĕr, ăg'ĕr). 1. Sea weed (alga) belonging to the genus *Gelideum*. The source of agar-agar. 2. A dried mucilaginous product obtained from certain species of algae, especially Gelideum. It is unaffected by bacterial enzymes, hence widely used as a solidifying agent for bacterial culture media; also used as a laxative because of its great increase in bulk upon absorption of water. 3. A culture medium containing agar.

agar-agar. Agar, *q.v.*

agastria (ă-gas'trĭ-ă). Absence of the stomach.

agastric (ă-gast'rĭk). Lacking an alimentary canal as in certain animals such as tapeworms.

AgCl. Chem. symb. for *silver chloride.*

age [Fr. *age*, L. *aetas*]. 1. The time from birth to the present for a living individual as measured in units of time. 2. A particular period of life, as middle age or old age. 3. To grow old. 4. In psychology, the degree of development of an individual expressed in terms of the age of an average individual of comparable development or accomplishment.

a., achievement. One determined by a proficiency test, the results of which are measured with the mental ability of the average child of the same chronological age. ABBR: A. A.

a., chronological. Age as determined by years of existence. ABBR: C. A.

a., menarchial. Elapsed time expressed in years from menarche.

a., mental. The age of a person with regard to his mental development; this is determined by a series of mental tests as devised by Binet. Thus, if a woman of 30 can pass only the tests of a child of 12, she is said to have a mental age of 12. SEE: *Binet*. ABBR: M. A.

a., physiological. Age as determined by functional activity.

age, *words pert. to:* adolescence; Binet; climacteric; geriatrics; maturation; puberty; senility.

-age [L.]. Suffix: put in motion; to do; to move, as *manage.*

agenesia, agenesis (ă-jen-ē'sĭ-ă, ă-jen'ĕ-sĭs) [G. *a-*, priv. + *genesis*, production]. 1. Sterility; impotence. 2. Incomplete development.

agenitalism (ă-gen'ĭ-tal-ism) [" + L. *genitalis*, genital]. Symptoms resulting from absence of the testicles or ovaries.

agenosomia (ă-jen-ō-sō'mĭ-ă) [G. *a-*, priv. + *gennan*, to beget, + *soma*, body]. Imperfect development of genitals.

agent (a'jent) [L. *agere*, to do]. Something which causes an effect. Thus bacteria which cause disease are said to be agents of the specific diseases they cause.

agerasia (ă-jĕr-ā'sĭ-ă). Healthy, vigorous old age; youthful appearance of an old person.

ageusia (ă-gū'sĭ-ă) [" + *geusis*, taste]. Absence, a partial loss or an impairment of the sense of taste.

ETIOL: It may be due to disease of the chorda tympani on one side, or of the gustatory fibers, or to the excessive use of condiments, the effect of certain drugs, or lesions involving sensory pathways or taste centers in the brain.

a., central. That due to a cerebral lesion.

a., conduction. That due to a lesion involving sensory nerves of taste.

a., peripheral. That due to a disorder of taste buds of mucous membrane of tongue or pharynx.

agger (aj'ĕr). A small elevation or eminence; a mound.

a. nasi. A small elevation, the anterior part of the ethmoidal crest on medial surface of the frontal process of the upper jaw (maxilla), forming part of the nasal cavity.

agglomerate (ă-glom'ĕ-rāt) [L. *agglomeratus*, from *agglomerare*, to form into a ball]. To congregate; to form a mass.

agglu'tinable [L. *agglutinare*, to glue a thing]. Capable of agglutination.

agglutinant (a-glu'tĭ-nant). 1. Anything causing adhesion. 2. Causing to unite or adhere, as healing of a wound. 3. An antibody produced in the body in response to stimulation by an antigen (agglutinogen). SYN: *agglutinin.*

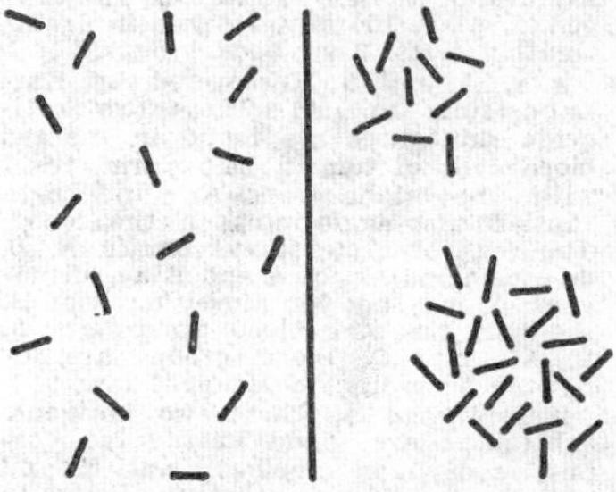

AGGLUTINATION REACTION
Left, negative, with uniform distribution of bacilli; right, positive, with the formation of clumps.

agglutination (ă-glū-tĭ-nā'shun). 1. Clumping of microorganisms when a specific immune serum is added to a bacterial culture. 2. Clumping of blood corpuscles when incompatible bloods are mixed. 3. Adhesion of surfaces of a wound.

agglu'tinative. Causing or capable of causing agglutination.

agglutinin (ă-glū'tĭ-nĭn). An antibody which causes agglutination; more specifically a substance present in normal or immune serum capable of causing agglutination or clumping of specific antigens (bacteria or cells). SEE: *agglutinogen; blood groups; blood typing; isoagglutinin.*

a., anti-Rh. A factor normally absent in human plasma but sometimes occurring in Rh-negative mothers, bearing an Rh-positive fetus or in Rh-negative individuals who have received multiple transfusions of Rh-positive blood.

a., chief. A specific one in the blood of a person who has been immunized against a specific disease or microorganism. It is active in higher dilutions than are the other agglutinins present.

a., cold. Agglutinins which act only at low temperatures. They are present in the serum of patients with atypical pneumonia and in certain blood diseases.

a., flagellar. One which agglutinates only the flagella of an organism.

a., group. A. acting as a specific on one species, but which will act on others.

a., haupt. SYN: *chief a.*

a., immune. A. causing immunity, found in the blood either because of recovery from the disease or of having been inoculated with the microorganism.

a., major. SEE: *chief a.*

a., minor. One acting on an organism related to the one utilized for immunization but in lower dilutions.

a., nonspecific. One found in individuals who have had a certain disease and which agglutinates organisms having no relation to the disease. Utilized in certain diagnostic tests.

a., O. One acting on the bodies of organisms, in contrast to flagellar or motile agglutinins. SYN: *somatic a.*

a., partial. Minor agglutinin, *q.v.*

a., somatic. O agglutinin, *q.v.*

agglutinogen (ă-glū-tĭn′ō-jĕn) [L. *agglutinare,* to glue a thing, + G. *gennan,* to produce]. 1. A substance which stimulates the development of a specific agglutinin, thereby acting as an antigen. 2. A specific antigen used in agglutination tests. SEE: *blood groups.*

a.'s, A and B. Discovered by Karl Landsteiner in 1901. These two antigenic substances are found in the red blood cells of human beings and react with the alpha (anti-A) and beta (anti-B) iso-agglutinins in the blood. The red corpuscles may contain A, B, or a combination of A and B agglutinogens, or may not contain either A or B; the four resulting blood groups are A, B, AB, and O. Blood groups are inherited according to Mendel's law.

a.'s, M and N. These two antigenic substances are found in the red corpuscles of human beings. Anti-M and anti-N agglutinins are rarely found in normal serum. The red blood cells may contain M, N, or M and N agglutinogens, resulting in blood types M, N, or MN, respectively.

a., Rh. A specific substance, called the Rh factor, present in red cells. It was discovered in 1940 by Landsteiner and Wiener who prepared anti-Rh serum by injecting red cells from Rhesus monkeys into rabbits or other animals. They found that the red cells of 85% of Caucasians will be agglutinated when in contact with anti-Rh. These persons are termed Rh-positive. The remaining 15% whose red cells are not agglutinated by anti-Rh are termed Rh-negative. More than 25 blood factors are known to belong to the Rh-Hr system. Their importance in blood typing and blood type incompatibility between mother and fetus makes this blood group system second in importance only to the ABO group.

agglutinoid (ă-glu′tin-oid) [L. *agglutinare,* to glue a thing, + G. *eidos,* resemblance]. An agglutinin that has lost its zymophore group as a result of the effect of heat, age, chemicals, etc., and, consequently, its ability to agglutinate its specific antigen although its ability to combine with its antigen remains.

agglutinophilic (ă-glū-tin-ō-fil′ik) [" + G. *philos,* fond]. Contributing to agglutination.

agglu′tinophore [" + G. *phorein,* to bear]. The active agent producing agglutination.

agglutogenic (ă-glū-tō-jen′ik) [" + G. *gennan,* to produce]. 1. Pert. to substances from which agglutinins originate. 2. Causing agglutinins.

agglutom′eter [" + G. *metron,* measure]. Device to simplify the agglutination or Widal test without the use of an ordinary microscope.

ag′gregate, ag′gregated [L. *aggregatus,* past p. of *aggregare,* to collect]. 1. Total substances making up a mass. 2. To cluster or come together.

a. glands. Lymphoid follicles found mainly in the ileum. SYN: *Peyer's patches.*

aggres′sin [L. *aggressus,* past p. *aggredi,* to approach]. A supposed substance which renders the action of bacteria more aggressive by lowering the activity of the phagocytes and weakening resisting power of the bacteria or organism.

aggression (ă-gresh′un) [L. *aggressio,* an attack]. PSY: A forceful attacking action, physical, verbal, or symbolic. May be justified and real or unrealistic and the result of disordered mental processes.

aging (a′jing). Growing old, maturing. Progressive changes related to the passage of time. There is no precise method for determining the rate or degree of aging.

agitated depression. PSY: A psychiatric depression characterized by continuous restlessness.

SYM: Patients are restless, depressed, and agitated, pacing up and down, wringing hands, crying, picking, and rubbing. They have feelings of guilt, unworthiness, and ideas of persecution, phobias, and obsessions.

NP: Similar to manic-depressive cases. Prevent patient from hurting self, as from pulling out hairs and tearing skin, etc. Divert patient but do not argue with him. Hydrotherapy may be indicated.

agitation (aj-ĭ-ta′shun) [L. *agitatio,* shaking]. 1. Excessive restlessness and increased mental and especially physical activity. 2. Tremor. 3. Shaking of a container so that the contents are rapidly moved and mixed.

agitographia (ăj-ĭ-tō-graf′ĭ-ă). Writing with excessive rapidity, with unconscious omission of word syllables, etc.

agitophasia (ăj-ĭ-tō-fā′zĭ-ă). Excessive rapidity of speech, with slurring, omission, and distortion of sounds. SYN: *agitolalia.*

aglaukopsia (ă-glaw-kop′sĭ-ă) [G. *a-,* priv. + *glaukos,* bluish-green, + *opsis,* vision]. Green blindness.

aglobu′lia [" + L. *globulus,* globule]. Marked decrease of red blood cells.

aglossia (ă-glos′ĭ-ă) [" + G. *glossa,* tongue, + ia]. Congenital absence of tongue.

aglossostomia (ă″glos-ō-sto′mĭ-ah) [" + G. *glossa,* tongue, + *stoma,* mouth, + ia]. Congenital absence of tongue and mouth opening.

aglutition (ag-lū-tish′un) [" + L. *glutire,* to swallow]. Difficulty in swallowing or inability to swallow.

aglycemia (ă-gli-se′mĭ-ă) [G. *a-*, + *glykis,* sweet, + *haima,* blood]. Lack of sugar in the blood.

aglycosu′ric [" + *glykus,* sweet, + *ouron,* urine]. Free from glycosuria.

agmatol′ogy [G. *agma,* fragment, + *logos,* study of]. The study of fractures.

agminate(d (ag′mĭ-nāt) [L. *agmen,* a crowd]. Aggregate; grouped in clusters.

a. follicles. Aggregations of solitary follicles or groups of lymph nodes, principally in lower portion of small intestine. SYN: *Peyer's patches.*

ag′nail [AS. *ang,* painful, + *naegel,* nail]. 1. Hangnail. 2. Whitlow, *q.v.*

agnathia (ag-nā′thĭ-a) [a + G. *gnathos,* jaw, + ia]. Condition in which the lower jaw is absent.

agne′a [G. *a-*, priv. + *gnosis,* knowledge]. A condition in which objects are not recognized; agnosis, *q.v.*

$AgNO_3$. Silver nitrate.

agnogenic (ag-no-jen′ik) [G. *a-*, + *gnosis,* knowledge, + *genein,* to produce]. Of unknown origin or etiology.

agno′sia [G. *ignorance*]. Los of comprehension of auditory, visual, or other sensations although the sensory sphere is intact; inability to recognize an object. SYN: *mind blindness.*

a., auditory. Mental inability to interpret sounds.

a., optic. Mental inability to interpret images that are seen.

a., tactile. Inability to distinguish objects by sense of touch.

-agogue (ă-gog) [G. *agogus,* leading, inducing]. Suffix meaning to produce or to lead.

agomphiasis (ag-ŏm-fī′ă-sĭs) [G. *agomphios,* toothless, + *iasis,* state]. 1. Looseness of the teeth. 2. Without teeth.

agonad (ă-gō′nad) [G. *a-*, priv. + *gonē,* seed]. A person without gonads.

agon′adal. Having no gonads.

ag′onal [G. *agōnia,* orig. a contest]. Rel. to death, or to agony.

ag′onist [G. *agōn,* a contest]. The muscle directly engaged in contraction as distinguished from muscles which have to relax at the same time.

Thus in bending the elbow, the *m. biceps brachii* is the agonist and the triceps the antagonist.

agony (ag′o-nĭ). 1. Extreme suffering, mental or physical. 2. Death struggle.

agoraphobia (ag-ō-ră-fō′bĭ-ă) [G. *agora,* market place, + *phobos,* fear]. Morbid dread of open spaces.

-agra [G. *seizure*]. Suffix: pertaining to a severe pain; seizure.

agraffe (ă-graf′) [F. *agrafer,* to hook, fasten]. An appliance for clamping together edges of a wound.

agramm′atism. Inability to form a grammatical or intelligible sentence or to arrange words in grammatical sequence.

ETIOL: Cerebral disease.

agranulocyte (ă-gran′ū-lō-sīt) [G. *a-*, priv. + L. *granulum,* granule, + G. *kytos,* cell]. A nongranular leukocyte.

agranulocytic (ă-gran-ū-lō-sĭt′ik). Pert. to agranulocytosis.

agranulocytosis (ă″gran-ū-lō-sī-tō′sĭs). An acute disease in which the white blood cell count drops to extremely low levels and neutropenia becomes pronounced. Characterized by high fever, prostration, necrotic ulcerations of the mouth, rectum, and vagina. Some cases idiopathic; others resulting from drugs or radiation. SYN: *granulocytopenia; agranulocytic angina.*

agranuloplas′tic [G. *a-*, priv. + L. *granulum,* granule, + G. *plastikos,* formative]. Capable of forming nongranular cells.

agranulo′sis. Same as agranulocytosis.

agraphia (ah-graf′ĭ-ă) [G. *a-*, priv. + *graphein,* to write]. A loss of ability to express oneself in writing due to a central lesion, or to muscular incoordination.

Copying or writing from dictation may still be possible. It is analogous to or associated with motor aphasia.* SYN: *logographia.* SEE: *anorthography.*

a., absolute. Complete inability to write.

a., acoustic. Inability to write words heard.

a., amnemonic. Inability to write a connected sentence expressing an idea, but letters or words may be written.

a., atactic. Absolute agraphia, *q.v.*

a., cerebral. Inability to express thoughts in writing.

a., mental. Cerebral a.

a., motor. A. due to inability to coordinate muscle movements.

a., optic. Inability to copy words.

a., verbal. Inability to write words although letters can be written.

agre′mia [G. *agra,* gout, + *aima,* blood]. Condition or state of the blood in gout.

agria (ag′rĭ-ă) [G. *agrios,* wild]. Malignant pustules; severe pustular eruption.

agroma′nia [G. *agros,* field, + *mania,* frenzy]. Unreasonable desire for solitude or solitudinous wandering. Morbid desire to live in solitude or in the country.

agrypnia (a-grip′nĭ-ă) [G. *agrypnos,* sleepless]. Inability to sleep. SYN: *insomnia; ahypnia; ahypnosis.*

agrypnot′ic. 1. Afflicted with insomnia. 2. That which causes wakefulness.

ague (ā′gū) [Fr. *aigu,* sharp, acute]. 1. Intermittent or malarial fever; typified by chills, fever, and sweating. 2. A chill.

ah. Abbr. for *hypermetropic astigmatism.*

Ahlfeld's sign (ahl′felts) [F. Ahlfeld, German obstetrician, 1843-1929]. OB: Uterine irregular contractions after the 3rd month of pregnancy.

ahypnia (ă-hip′nĭ-ă). [G. *a-*, priv. + *hypnos,* sleep]. Insomnia or sleeplessness. SYN: *agrypnia; ahypnosis.*

A. I. Abbr. for *aortic insufficiency; artificial insemination; axioincisal.*

aichmophobia (āk-mō-fō′bĭ-ă) [G. *aichmē,* point, + *phobos,* fear]. Morbid fear of pointed instruments or of being touched by them or with a finger.

A. I. D. Abbr. for *artificial insemination by donor* (heterologous insemination).

A. I. H. Abbr. for *artificial insemination by husband* (homologous insemination).

ailurophobia (ī″lū-rō-fō′bĭ-ă) [G. *ailuros,* cat, + *phobos,* fear]. PSY: Morbid fear of cats. A symbolism of psychoneurotic origin.

ainhum (ān′hum). A fissured constriction of unknown origin, causing eventual amputation of the digit. Affects usually the fourth or fifth toes and less commonly other digits of the feet or hands. It is predominately a disease of members of dark-skinned races; it apparently does not occur in Caucasians. There is no specific treatment.

air (ār) [G. *aer,* air]. The invisible, tasteless, odorless mixture of gases surrounding the earth.

The air, so-called "breath of life," is made up of approximately 21% oxygen, 0.8% argon, 78% nitrogen, aqueous vapor, carbon dioxide, and traces of ammonia, helium, neon, krypton, xenon, and other rare gases, but in mines, industrial communities and their environs it is polluted. The proportions, esp. of water vapor, are variable. The composition of dry atmospheric air is given approximately in the table below; in the column headed "inspired," the numbers are in volumes per cent.

a., alveolar. Air in the alveoli; that involved in the pulmonary exchange of gases between air and the blood. Its content is determined by sampling the last portion of a maximal expiration.

a., complemental (inspiratory reserve volume). The amount that may be breathed in over and above the tidal air, by deepest possible inspiration.

a., dead space. The volume of air that fills the respiratory passageways and not available for exchange of gases with the blood.

a., functional residual (functional residual capacity). The volume of air left in the lungs at the end of a natural unforced expiration. It is the sum of expiratory reserve volume (supplemental air) and residual air.

a., liquid. Air liquified by great pressure. It produces intense cold on evaporation.

a., minimal. The small amount of air left in the alveoli by collapse of small bronchi when the supplemental and residual air is driven out when the lungs collapse with the thorax open. This makes it possible for the excised lungs of animals to float, hence the term "lights."

a., reserve. Same as supplemental a.

a., residual (residual volume). The amount remaining in the lungs after the fullest possible expiration. About 1500 cc.

a., supplemental (expiratory reserve volume). Amount that may be forcibly expired after a quiet expiration. About 1600 cc.

a., tidal. The amount that flows in and out of the lungs with each quiet respiration; average of adult male about one pint (500 cc.).

air, *words pert. to:* "aer-" words, aspiration, atelectasis, expiration, inspiration, respiration, ventilation.

air bed. 1. Large inflated air cushion used as a mattress. SEE: *air cushion.* 2. A special bed which permits the patient actually to float on a cushion of air. The air which comes from the surface of the bed prevents the body from coming in contact with the surface. Especially useful in treating patients with burns or patients with bedsores.

air cell. An air vesicle.*

air conditioning. Adjustment of normal temperature and humidity while insuring adequate ventilation.

air cushion. An airtight inflatable cushion. To inflate, a pump, as a bicycle pump may be used.

NP: When inflating orally, place layer of gauze over opening and between lips.

air em'bolism. Obstruction of a blood vessel brought about by entrance of air into the blood stream.

ETIOL: A postoperative possibility, or air may enter during hypodermic injection, if syringe is not properly filled. Air should be excluded when giving an intravenous injection.

air hun'ger. Shortness of breath marked by rapid, labored breathing. SEE: *dyspnea.*

air sac. An air vesicle, *q.v.*

airsickness. Condition similar to seasickness occurring during airplane flight.

air swal'lowing. Oral intake of air either voluntarily or involuntarily. SYN: *aerophagia, q.v.*

Involuntarily, this condition mainly occurs in infants as a result of improper feeding; in adults it occurs in neurasthenia or hysteria or when on a fluid diet.

air vesicle. Pulmonary tissue saccule filling with air during breathing.

airway. 1. Any natural passageway for air in the body. 2. A device used to prevent or correct obstructed respiratory passage, especially during anesthesia.

akaryocyte (ă-kar'ē-ō-sīt). Erythrocyte; red blood cell; a non-nucleated cell.

akatamathesia (ă-kăt"ă-mă-thē'zĭ-ă) [G. *a-*, priv. + *katamathesis*, understanding]. The mental condition of being unable to understand.

akathisia (ăk-ă-thĭ'zĭ-ă) [G. *a-*, priv. + *kathisis*, a sitting]. PSY: Inability to remain seated. Seen in catatonia, *q.v.*, in agitated melancholia, and in some compulsive conditions. Also spelled *acathisia.*

akinesia (ă-kĭ-nē'zĭ-ă [G. *a-*, priv. + *kinēsis*, movement] . Complete or partial loss of muscle movement. Also spelled *acinesia.*

a. algera. Form with intense pain caused by any movement.

a. amnestica. Form marked by failure of muscular power due to lack of use.

akinet'ic. 1. Pertaining to akinesia. 2. Relating to or characterized by amitosis.

Al. Chemical symbol for *aluminum.*

-al [L.]. Suffix: Pert. to, as *abdominal.*

ala (ā'lă) (pl. *alae*) [L. wing]. 1. An expanded or winglike structure or appendage. 2. Axilla, *q.v.*

a. auris. The pinna of the ear.

a. cerebelli. A. of central lobule. SYN: *a. lobuli centralis.*

a. cinerea. Dark triangular area on the floor of the fourth ventricle. The autonomic fibers of the vagus nerve arise from the cells of the nucleus of this area. SYN: *triangle of the vagus nerve; trigonum nervi vagi.*

a. (of) ethmoid. Small projection on each side of the ethmoid bone.

a. (of) ilium. Broad, thin upper portion of the os ilium or iliac bone.

alae lateralis. 1. Greater wing of sphenoid bone. 2. Extended processes on each side of frontal bone.

a. major ossis sphenoidalis. Greater wing of the sphenoid bone.

a. minor ossis sphenoidalis. Lesser wing of the sphenoid bone.

a. nasi. Lower extended portion of lateral wall of nose.

a. (of) nose. A. nasi, *q.v.*

a. (of) sacrum. Large triangular surface on either side of the base of the sacrum.

a. vomeris. One of the two lateral extensions of bone on the superior border of the vomer.

alae (ā'lē). Plural of ala, *q.v.*

Composition of Dry Air	Inspired	Expired	Alveolar*
Oxygen	20.94	16.3	14.2
Nitrogen (including small amounts of argon and other inert gases)	79.02	79.7	80.3
Carbon Dioxide	0.04	4.0	5.5

ala'lia [G. *a-*, priv. + *lalia*, talking]. Loss of ability to speak due to defect or paralysis of the vocal organs. Aphasia.
ETIOL: Psychic or due to lesion.

alar (a'lar) [L. *ala*, wing]. 1. Pert. to or like a wing. 2. Axillary.
a. artery (of nose). Supplies tissues of ala of nose.
a. cartilage. One on each side of nose forming the tip.

alas'trim [Portuguese, *alastrar*, to spread]. A modified smallpox with sparse rash and low-grade fever. SYN: *variola minor.*

alate (ā'lāt) [L. *ala*, wing]. Winged.

al'ba [L. *albus*, white]. 1. White. 2. White substance of the brain.

albedo (al-bē'dō) [L. from *albus*, white]. Whiteness. Reflection of light from a surface.
a. ret'inae. Retinal edema.
a. unguium. White semilunar area at nail root. SYN: *lunula.*

Albee's operation (awl'bēz) [F. H. Albee. New York surgeon, 1876-1945]. Removal of upper end of head of femur and corresponding edges of the acetabulum with approximation; artificial ankylosis of the hip.

Albers-Schönberg disease (ăl-bārs-shĕn'-bārg) [H. E. Albers-Schönberg, German roentgenologist, 1865-1921]. Abnormal bone calcification giving bones spotted, marblelike appearance and causing them to fracture spontaneously. SYN: *marble bones; osteopetrosis.*

Al'bert's disease [Edward Albert, Viennese surgeon, 1841-1900]. Inflammation of the bursae lying over the Achilles tendon. SYN: *achillobursitis.*

al'bicans (pl. *albicantia*) [L. pres. p. *albicare*, to be white]. 1. White or whitish. 2. One of the *corpora albicantia.*
a., corpus. Whitish body in ovarian cortex.

albidum (ăl-bĭ-dum) [L.]. White.

albidu'ria [L. *albidus*, whitish, + G. *ouron*, urine]. 1. Passing of white or colorless urine and of low specific gravity. SYN: *albinuria.* 2. Chyluria, *q.v.*

albidus (al'bĭ-dus). Whitish.

Albini's nodules (ăl-bĭ'nĭ) [Giuseppe Albini, Italian physiologist, 1830-1911]. Minute nodules on margins of mitral and tricuspid valves of the heart; sometimes seen in newly born.

albinism (al'bin-ism) [Portuguese from L. *albus*, white]. Abnormal, nonpathological absence of pigment in skin, hair, and eyes, partial or total, frequently accompanied by astigmatism, photophobia, and nystagmus, because the choroid is not sufficiently protected from light because of lack of pigment.

albino (al-bī-nō). A person deficient in pigment; one afflicted with albinism.

albinu'ria [L. *albus*, white, + G. *ouron*, urine]. Passing of white or colorless urine of low specific gravity. SYN: *albiduria.*

albocinereous (al-bō-sĭn-ē'rē-ŭs) [" + *cinereus*, gray]. Pert. to both white and gray matter of brain and spinal cord.

Albright's disease. Same as Recklinghausen's disease and osteitis fibrosa cystica, *q.v.*

albuginea (al-bū-jĕn'ĭ-ă). A layer of firm, white, fibrous tissue forming the investment of an organ or part, as of the eye, testicle, ovary or spleen. SYN: *tunica albuginea.*
a. corporum cavernosorum. A strong, very elastic white fibrous coat, forming a sheath common to both corpora cavernosa of the penis.
a. oc'uli. Sclera, or tough white supporting covering of the eyeball.
a. ovarii. The layer of firm fibrous tissue lying beneath the epithelial ovarian covering.
a. testis. The thick, unyielding layer of white fibrous tissue lying under the tunica vaginalis.

albugineotomy (al-bū-jĕn"ē-ot'ō-mĭ) [L. *albus*, white, + G. *tomē*, cutting]. Incision of tunica albuginea of the testis.

albuginitis (al-bū-jĭn-ī'tis) [" + G. *-itis*, inflammation]. Inflammation of any tunica albuginea.

albu'go [L. whiteness from *albus*]. White opacity of the cornea.

albu'men [L. *albus*, white]. 1. White of an egg. 2. Former spelling for albumin, *q.v.*

albu'min [L. *albumen*, coagulated egg white]. One of a group of simple proteins.

Albumin is found in (a) the blood, as *serum albumin;* (b) in milk, as *lactalbumin*, and in (c) the white of egg, as *albumen.* It is soluble in cold water; coagulated on heating, then no longer dissolved by cold or hot water. In the stomach coagulated albumins are made soluble by *peptase*, being changed at the same time into albumoses* and peptones.*

In general, albumins from animal sources are of higher quality than those from vegetable sources, because animal proteins contain greater quantities of essential amino acids, *q.v.* SEE ALSO: *albumoses; peptones.*

a. test. The commonest type of albumin found in urine is serum albumin. Before testing, certain precautions must be observed: (a) The specimen of urine must be fresh. (b) The specimen must also be clear. To ensure this, the safest way is to filter it through special filter paper (blotting paper makes a good substitute). (c) The urine must be acid. (d) The specimen must be cold.

There are many tests for albumin, but the most usual are the following:

Acetic acid test: Over a Bunsen burner, heat the top inch or so of a test tube filled three parts full of urine. A cloudiness will form, which may be due to phosphate or albumin. Add 2 or 3 drops of acetic acid, and if the cloud disappears it is due to phosphates; if it becomes intensified, albumin is present.

Heller's cold test: Take about ½ in. of concentrated nitric acid in a test tube, and carefully overlay it with the urine, with a pipette. An opaque line appears at the junction of the fluids. This may take a few minutes to develop.

Sulfosalicylic acid test: To some urine in a test tube add 10 to 20 drops of sulfosalicylic acid. Albumin is shown as a white, cloudy precipitate. This may be carried out as a ring test, as in Heller's test.

Since albuminuria can be caused by many different conditions, the results require careful interpretation.

SEE: *Esbach's method; Esbach's quantitative estimation.*

a., acid. Compound resulting from action of acid on a.
a., alkali. Compound resulting from action of weak alkalies on a.
a., blood. Serum albumin, *q.v.*
a., circulating. A. present in the liquids of the body.
a., derived. A. changed by chemical action; albuminate.

a., egg. White of an egg; albumen; ovalbumin.

a., muscle. Form found in muscular tissue.

a., native. Any a. present in an organism normally, as serum a.

a., normal human serum. USP. Sterile solution of serum albumin from healthy donors. Administered intravenously to restore blood volume.

a., serum. The main proteins found in the blood. SYN: *blood a.*

a., urinary. Serum albumin, serum globulin, and any other proteins in urine.

a., vegetable. Any albumin in, or derived from, plant tissue.

albu'minate. Metaprotein, a product of hydrolysis of albumen and globulin.

albuminatu'ria [L. *albumen,* white of egg, + G. *ouron,* urine]. Albuminates in voided urine.

albuminiferous (ăl-bū-mĭn-ĭf'ĕ-rŭs) [" + *ferre,* to bear]. Producing albumin.

albuminimeter (ăl-bū-mĭn-ĭm'ĕ-ter) [" + G. *metron,* measure]. Instrument for measuring amount of albumin in urine.

albuminiparous (al-bū-mĭn-ĭp'ă-rŭs) [" + *parere,* to bear]. Yielding albumin.

albuminogenous (al-bū-mĭn-oj'ĕ-nus) [" + G. *gennan,* to produce]. Producing albumin.

albu'minoid [" + G. *eidos,* similarity]. 1. Resembling albumin. 2. A protein. 3. Scleroprotein.

albuminolysis (al-bū-mĭn-ŏl'ĭ-sĭs) [" + G. *lysis,* solution]. Proteolysis; decomposition of protein.

albu'minone. Noncoagulable protein in blood serum. SYN: *albumone.*

albuminoptysis (al-bū-mĭn-ŏp'tĭ-sĭs) [L. *albumen,* + G. *ptysis,* spitting]. Albumin in sputum.

albuminoreac'tion [" + *rē,* again, + *agere,* to act]. The presence or absence of albumin in the sputum. Positive reaction indicates inflammatory condition of lungs.

albuminorrhe'a [" + G. *roia,* flow]. Albumin in urine. SYN: *albuminuria, q.v.*

albuminose (al-bū'min-ōs). 1. Albumose. 2. Albuminous.

albumino'sis [L. *albumen,* + G. *-osis,* state of]. Abnormal increase of albuminous constituents in blood plasma.

albu'minous. Having the nature of or containing albumin.

albu"minuret'ic [L. *albumen,* + G. *ouretikos,* causing urine to flow]. Pert. to albuminuria.

albuminuria (al-bū-min-ū'rĭ-ă) [" + G. *ouron,* urine]. Presence of readily detectable amounts of serum protein, especially serum albumin but also serum globulin and others, in the urine. It is usually a sign of renal impairment; its presence, however, is not always a sign of disease because it may be found in normal persons following vigorous exercise. SYN: *proteinuria.*

It occurs in febrile states, malignant hypertension, congestive heart failure, nephrotic syndrome and other kidney disorders. SEE ALSO: *nephritis; nephrosis.*

a., cardiac. Caused by disease of the heart valves.

a., cyclic. Finding at regular diurnal intervals of small amounts of albumin in the urine, esp. in childhood and adolescence.

a., digestive. A. that occurs following the eating of certain foods. SYN: *dietetic a.*

a., extrarenal or accidental. Due to contamination of urine with pus, chyle, or blood.

a., functional or transient. One in which the only finding is occasional presence of albuminuria; not usually associated with kidney disease. Occurs in some after taking certain foods.

a., intrinsic. A. excreted in urine as a result of intrinsic renal disease. SYN: *true a.*

a., orthostatic. Postural albuminuria, *q.v.*

a., pathological. A. caused by a disease.

a., physiological. A., in a temporary form, existing without evidence of pathology.

a., postural. Albuminuria in normal individuals who have remained in an erect position for a considerable length of time. SYN: *orthostatic a.*

a., renal. Due to changes in epithelial cells of kidneys, making them pervious to proteins of the blood, as in all forms of nephritis.

a., toxic. Due to toxins generated within the body or by poison from outside source.

albuminu'ric retini'tis. inflammation of retina characterized by hazy retina, blurred disk margin, distention of retinal arteries, retinal hemorrhages, and white patches in the fundus, esp. the stellate figure at the macula. SEE: *retinitis.*

albumone (al-bū'mōn). A noncoagulable protein in blood serum. SYN: *albuminone.*

albu'moscope [L. *albumen,* + G. *skopein,* to view]. An instrument for determining the presence of albumin in the urine.

al'bumose. The intermediate product produced by enzymes in the splitting of proteins which, in the course of digestion, become peptones.

albumosemia (al-bū-mō-sē'mĭ-ă) [*albumose* + G. *aima,* blood]. Albumose in the blood.

albumosuria (al-bū-mō-sū'rĭ-ă) [" + G. *ouron,* urine]. The presence of Bence Jones protein in urine.

Alcaligenes (al-kă-lĭj'ĭ-nēz). Rod-shaped, gram-negative or gram-variable bacteria found in the intestinal tract of man, soil, and dairy utensils and products.

a. faecalis. Found normally in the intestinal tract of man. Rarely becomes pathogenic.

Alcock's canal [Benjamin Alcock, Irish anatomist, 1801-date of death unknown]. A space in the external fascia of the *ischiorectal fossa,* above the tuberosity of the ischium. It contains the internal pudendal artery, veins, and nerve.

al'cohol [Arabic *al,* the, + *koh'l,* fine antimonial powder]. 1. A class of organic compounds formed from hydrocarbons by substituting one or more hydroxyl (OH) group for a similar number of hydrogen atoms. 2. Ethyl alcohol, a colorless, volatile, flammable liquid of the formula C_2H_5-OH. Its molecular weight is 46.07; boiling point 78.5° C. It is a product of fermented or distilled liquors, and is obtained, in its pure form, from grain by fermentation and fractionation distillation. The USP standard is a liquid that contains not less than 92.3% by weight of C_2H_5OH. SYN: *ethanol; ethyl alcohol; grain alcohol; spirit of wine.*

ACTION AND USES: Used in preparing essences, tinctures, extracts; manufacturing of ether, ethylene and other industrial products; as a rubbing compound; as an antiseptic when in 70% solution. Arrests growth of putrefactive bacteria and is, therefore, used as a preservative of biological specimens and in certain patent medicines. Used in antifreeze products because of its low freezing point. Instruments may be sterilized by placing them in a 70% solution of alcohol for 30 minutes. Acts as a depressant to the nervous system when taken in excessive amounts.

a., absolute. Contains 99% alcohol and not more than 1% by weight of water.

a., dehydrated. Absolute a., *q.v.*

a., denatured. Alcohol rendered unfit for use as a beverage or medicine by adding toxic ingredients. Used commercially as a solvent.

a., diluted. USP. Alcohol containing not less than 41% and not more than 42% by weight of ethyl alcohol. Used as a solvent. SYN: *diluted ethanol; proof spirit.*

a., ethyl. Ordinary or grain alcohol. SEE: *alcohol* (def. 2).

a., grain. Same as *ethyl a.*

a., methyl. CH_3OH. A colorless, volatile, flammable liquid obtained from distillation of wood. Even though its physical properties are similar to those of ethyl alcohol, it is not fit for human consumption. Poisoning with methyl alcohol can lead to blindness and death. It is used as a solvent, for fuel, as an additive for denaturing ethyl alcohol, and in the preparation of formaldehyde. SYN: *carbanol; methanol; wood alcohol.*

a., wood. Same as methyl a., *q.v.*

alcoholase (al′ko-hŏl-ās). A ferment converting lactic acid into alcohol.

alcohol′ic. 1. Pertaining to alcohol. 2. One afflicted with alcoholism.

a. fermentation. That in which carbohydrates are converted to alcohol through action of yeast.

alcoholism (ăl′kō-hŏl-ĭzm) [Arabic *al,* the, + *koh′l,* fine antimonial powder]. An illness characterized by preoccupation with alcohol and loss of control over its consumption such as to lead to intoxication if drinking is begun; by chronicity; by progression; and by tendency toward relapse. It is typically associated with physical disability and impaired emotional, occupational, and/or social adjustments as a direct consequence of persistent and excessive use. (FROM: *Manual on Alcoholism of the American Medical Association,* Robert J. Shearer, coordinating ed., Chicago, 1967.)

ETIOL: Unknown. Psychological, physiological, and sociological factors play an important part. A deep-seated neurosis, subconscious feelings of insecurity and inadequacy, conflicts and frustrations are factors. The exhilaration factor is often the cause of intoxication in normal persons. Alcoholism is an illness and should be so treated.

a., acute. Acute intoxication with temporary mental disturbances and muscular incoordination.

CAUTION: When stupor or coma is observed in a patient who is suspected of being intoxicated by alcohol, other causes such as intracranial disease, insulin shock, etc., should also be considered. Acute alcoholism can cause death.

SYM AND SIGNS: There may be motor instability (staggered gait, blurred or double vision, impaired reflex action); reduced mental function; increased pulse rate; decreased blood pressure; dilated pupils; flushing of skin; drowsiness or stupor.

TREATMENT: When enough alcohol has been consumed to cause coma, vigorous therapeutic measures are indicated; thus insulin, dextrose, thiamine, chlorpromazine, and oxygen are used.

a., chronic. Pathologic state from habitual use of alcohol in toxic amounts.

SYM AND SIGNS: Malnutrition; vitamin deficiency; alcoholic cirrhosis of liver; gastritis; pancreatitis; and neurologic disorders such as tremulousness, hallucinosis, seizures, delirium tremens.

TREATMENT: Psychotherapy, tranquilizing drugs, withdrawal of alcohol, correction of vitamin deficiency. SEE: *delirium tremens; intoxication.*

a. psychoses. These include pathological intoxication, delirium tremens,* Korsakoff's psychosis,* acute hallucinosis.*

alcoholomania (al-kō-hol-ō-mā′nĭ-ă) [alcohol + G. *mania,* frenzy]. Abnormal craving for intoxicants.

alcoholometer (al-kō-hol-om′ĕ-ter) [" + G. *metron,* measure]. An instrument for measuring quantity of alcohol in a fluid.

alcoholophilia (al″ko-hol-o-fil′ĭ-ă) [" + G. *philos,* fond]. Morbid craving for alcohol.

alcoholu′ria [" + G. *ouron,* urine]. Alcohol in the urine.

aldehyde (al′dĕ-hīd) [*al.,* abbr. alcohol, + *dehyd,* abbr. dyhydrogenatum, alcohol deprived of hydrogen]. 1. Oxidation product of a primary alcohol; has the characteristic group —CHO. 2. Acetaldehyde. CH_3CHO. A colorless, fuming, flammable liquid. SYN: *acetic aldehyde; ethanol.*

aldolase (al′do-lās). An enzyme in muscle which is important in converting glycogen into lactic acid.

al′dose. A carbohydrate of the aldehyde group (—CHO).

aldosterone (al-dos′ter-ōn). The most biologically active mineralocorticoid secreted by the adrenal cortex. Functions in regulation of metabolism of sodium, chloride and potassium.

aldos′teronism. A condition in which the blood contains abnormally high levels of aldosterone. This causes retention of sodium, urinary loss of potassium, and alkalosis. The patient develops episodes of tetany, weakness, paralysis, hypertension, cardiac irregularity, polyuria, and polydipsia. SYN: *Conn's syndrome.*

alemmal (ă-lĕm′al) [G. *a-,* priv. + *lemma,* husk]. Without a neurilemma, as a nerve fiber.

Alep′po boil, button, evil or **sore.** Cutaneous leishmaniasis, caused by infection with the parasite Leishmania tropica. Characterized by one or multiple ulcerations of the skin. SYN: *Delhi boil; Oriental sore.*

alethia (ă-le′thĭ-ă) [G. *a-,* + *lethe,* forgetfulness]. Inability to forget.

aleukemia (ă-lū-kē′mĭ-ă) [" +" + G. *aima,* blood]. 1. Deficiency of white blood corpuscles. The existence of leukopenia or aleukocytosis. 2. Pseudoleukemia.

aleukemic (a-lū-kē′mik). Marked by aleukemia.

a. leukemia. Leukemia in which the total count of white blood corpuscles is normal or subnormal, regardless of quantitative changes of the blood or clinical changes consistent with leukemia.

aleukia (ă-lū'kĭ-ă) [G. *a-*, priv. + *leukos*, white]. 1.Absence or abnormal decrease in number of white blood cells. 2. Absence or abnormal decrease in number of blood platelets.

aleukocytosis (ă-lū-kō-sī-tō'sĭs) [" + " + G. *kytos*, cell]. A diminished production of white corpuscles in the blood.

aleuron, aleurone (al-u'ron) [G. flour]. The protein granules of seeds in which the vitamins are supposed to be stored.

aleuronate (al-ū'rō-nāt). Vegetable albumin flour used for bread for diabetics.

Alexand'er-Adam's operation. Shortening the round ligaments of the uterus and suturing their ends to the ext. abdominal ring, for uterine displacement.

alexeteric (ă-lĕk-sĕ-tĕr'ĭk) [G. *alexētērios*, fit to keep off]. Protective against infection, venom, and poison.

alex'ia [G. *a-*, priv. + *lexis*, speech]. Inability to read, due to a central lesion; word blindness. A form of sensory, optic, or visual aphasia.

a., cortical. That due to lesions involving the left angular gyrus.

a., motor. That in which printed or written words cannot be read aloud but are understood.

a., musical. Inability to read music. It may be sensory, optical or visual, but not motor. SEE: *anarthria; aphemia.*

alexic (a-lek'sik). Defensive, as an alexin.

alexin (a-lek'sin) [G. *alexein*, to ward off]. Defensive substance in normal serum which, in presence of a sensitizer, destroys bacteria and exerts a lytic action on cells. SYN: *complement, q.v.* RS: *immunity.*

alexin'ic un'it. The lowest amount of alexinic serum required to dissolve a measured quantity of red blood corpuscles in the presence of an excessive amount of hemolytic serum.

alexipharmic (ă-leks-ĭ-far'mik) [" + *pharmakon*, poison]. 1. An antidote. 2 Antidotal. Warding off the ill effects of a poison.

alexipyretic (ă-lĕk-sĭ-pī-ret'ĭk) [" + *pyretos*, fever]. That which lessens fever. SYN: *febrifuge.*

alexocyte (ă-lĕks'ō-sīt) [" + *kytos*, cell]. A leukocyte supposed to secrete alexin.

a-Leydigism (ă-lī'dĭg-ĭzm). Absence of Leydig cell function resulting in hypogonadism.

algae (al'je) [L. *pl. of alga*, seaweed). Plants belonging to the subphylum Algae of the phylum Thallophyta, the lowest division of the plant kingdom. They are independent plants without roots, stems or leaves but which contain chlorophyll, have a simple life history, and vary in size from microscopic forms to massive seaweeds. They live in fresh or salt water or in moist places. Some serve as food or as sources of medicinal products. Examples are rockweeds, kelps, and Irish moss.

algefacient (al-jē-fā'shent) [L. *algere*, to be cold, + *faciens*, making]. Cooling, or refrigerant.

algesia (al-jē'zĭ-ă) [G. *algēsis*, sense of pain]. Supersensitiveness to pain; hyperesthesia.

algesic (al-jē'sik). Hyperesthesic; painful.

algesichronometer (al-jē"sĭ-krō-nom'ĕ-tĕr) [G. *algēsis*, sense of pain, + *chronos*, time, + *metron*, measure]. An instrument for measuring time taken to feel pain.

algesimeter (al-jē-sĭm'ĕ-tĕr) [G. *algēsis*, sense of pain, + *metron*, measure]. An instrument for measuring skin sensitivity to pain. SYN: *algometer.*

algesthesia (al-jes-thē'zĭ-ă) [G. *algos*, pain, + *aisthesis*, sensation]. Unusual sensitivity to sensory stimuli, as pain or touch. SYN: *hyperesthesia.*

algetic (al-jet'ik). Painful.

-algia [G.]. Suffix signifying *pain*, as in neur*algia*.

algicide (al'jĭ-sīd) [L. *alga*, + *caedere*, to kill]. That which destroys algae.

algid (al'jid) [L. *algidus*, cold]. Cold; chilly.

a. pernicious fever. A form of malaria with symptoms of collapse.

a. stage. Cold and cyanotic skin occurring in cholera and some other diseases.

algiomotor (al"jĭ-ō-mō'tor) [G. *algos*, pain, + L. *motor*, a mover]. Causing painful contraction of muscles, particularly pain during peristalsis.

algiomus'cular [" + L. *musculus*, muscle]. Algiomotor, *q.v.*

algogenic (al-gō-jen-ik) [G. *algos*, pain, + *genesis*, production]. 1. Causing neuralgic pain. 2. Lowering body temperature below normal.

algolagnia (al-gō-lag'nĭ-ă) [G. *algos*, pain, + *lagneia*, lust]. A perversion whereby sexual satisfaction is derived by experiencing pain or by inflicting pain on others. SEE: *masochism; sadism.*

algolagnist (al-gō-lag'nist). One who practices algolagnia.

algomenorrhea (al"go-men"o-re'ă). Painful menstruation. SYN: *dysmenorrhea.*

algom'eter [G. *algos*, pain, + *metron*, measure]. Instrument for testing the sensitiveness to pain, as pinching the skin. SYN: *algesimeter.*

algophily (al-gŏf'ĭ-lĭ) [" + *philos*, fond]. Morbid love of pain. Algolagnia, *q.v.*

algophobia (al-gō-fō'bĭ-ă) [" + *phobos*, fear]. Morbid aversion to witnessing or experiencing pain.

algopsychalia (al-gō-sī-kā'lĭ-ă) [" + *psychē*, mind]. Mental distress of hysterical origin. SYN: *psychalgia.*

al'gor [L. cold]. 1. A chill. 2. The sensation of cold; cold.

a. mortis. The chill of death.

algos (al'gos) [G.]. Pain.

algospasm (al'gō-spăsm). A painful cramp or spasm.

alible (al'ĭ-ble) [L. *alibilis*, from *alere*, to nourish]. Absorbable; nutritive; assimilable.

alices (al'ĭ-sēz) [L.]. The red spots appearing before pustulation in smallpox, *q.v.*

alicyclic (ăl-ĭ-sī'klik). Having properties of both aliphatic (open-chain) and cyclic (closed-chain) compounds.

alienation (al-yen-ā'shun) [L. *alienare*, to make strange]. 1. Mental disorder; insanity. 2. Hostility or withdrawal.

a'lienism. Science of mental diseases.

a'lienist. One who studies mental disease; a psychiatrist.

aliform (al'ĭ-form) [L. *ala*, wing, + *forma*, shape]. Having form of a wing.

a. process. Wing of the sphenoid.

alignment. 1. Arranged in a straight line. 2. In orthopedics, the placing of portions of a fractured bone into correct anatomical position. SEE ALSO: *alinement.*

al'iment [L. *alere*, to nourish]. Nutriment, food.

alimen'tary [L. *alimentum*, nourishment]. Of or pertaining to nutrition.

a. canal or tract. The digestive tube from the mouth to anus, including mouth or buccal cavity, pharynx, esophagus, stomach, small and large intestine and rectum. Drugs administered orally (by mouth) are absorbed in the stomach or intestine by the portal vein and pass through the liver before entering the general circulation, or they may be absorbed into the lacteals and enter the blood stream by way of the thoracic duct.

a. duct. The thoracic duct.

alimenta'tion. The general process of nourishing the body; it includes mastication, swallowing, digestion, absorption, and assimilation.

RS: *anabolism, absorption, catabolism, digestion, metabolism, foods.*

a., artificial. Feeding, usually intravenous, of patient unable to take nourishment normally.

a., forced. 1. Feeding of a patient unwilling to eat. 2. Therapeutic feeding of more nourishment than necessary.

a., rectal. Injection, by enema, of food through the rectum.

alimentotherapy (al-i-men-tō-ther'a-pĭ) [L. *alimentum,* nourishment, + G. *therapeia,* healing]. Treatment employing dietetics. SYN: *dietotherapy.*

alina'sal [L. *ala,* wing, + *nasus,* nose]. Pert. to the *alae nasi* or wings of the nose.

alinement (ă-lĭn'ment) [Fr. *alignement*]. 1. Arranging in a line. 2. In dentistry, bringing artificial or natural teeth into normal articulation.

aliphatic (al-ĭ-fat'ik) [G. *aleiphar, aleiphatos,* fat, oil]. 1. Belonging to that series of carbon compounds characterized by open chains, including the fatty acids and the unsaturated compounds as the ethylenes. 2. Pertaining to a fat or oil.

aliquot (al'ĭ-kwot) [L. *alius,* other, + *quot,* how many]. A fractional part divisible into the whole without a remainder. A portion of a liquid or solid substance which represents a known quantitative relationship to the original amount.

alisphenoid (al-ĭ-sfe'noyd) [L. *ala,* wing, + G. *sphēn,* wedge, + *eidos,* resemblance]. Pert. to the greater wing of the sphenoid bone.

alizarin (ă-lĭz'ă-rĭn). A red dye obtained from coal tar or madder.

alkalemia (al-kă-lē'mĭ-ă) [Arabic *al-qili,* ashes of salt wort, + G. *aima,* blood]. An excessive alkalinity of the blood due to a decrease in the *hydrogen ion* concentration or an increase in hydroxyl ions. The blood is normally slightly alkaline (*p*H 7.35 to 7.45).

alkales'cence. 1. Slight alkalinity. 2. Process of becoming alkaline.

alkales'cent. Alkaline or becoming alkaline.

al'kali [Arabic *al-qili,* ashes of salt wort]. 1. A metallic hydroxide (except ammonia) that has the property of combining with an acid to form a salt, or with an oil to form soap. 2. Any substance which can neutralize acids and affect indicators in certain ways. Ex: *sodium hydroxide,* which turns litmus paper blue.

SEE: *"alkal-" words; corrosive alkali.*

a. poisoning (such as *lye, sodium* or *potassium hydroxide,* etc.). F. A. TREATMENT: Large amounts of water by mouth; diluted vinegar or lemon juice. Then olive oil or milk and egg whites by mouth. Mild stimulants to prevent shock. Tracheotomy if necessary.

FOLLOW-UP TREATMENT: Morphine is useful to allay the pain. Rest, heat, quiet, and adequate fluid intake are imperative. Bougies are used after about the 6th day to prevent esophageal strictures. Early use of adrenocortical steroids may help to prevent strictures.

CAUTION: Avoid emetics or lavage.

alkalimeter (al-kă-lĭm'ĕ-ter) [" + G. *metron,* measure]. Device for measuring strength of alkalies alone or in a mixture.

alkalim'etry. Measurement of degree of alkalinity in a mixture.

al'kaline. Pert. to an alkali or having the reactions of one.

al'kaline-ash diet. One consisting chiefly of milk, fruits and vegetables with very small amounts of protein foods such as meat, fish, cheese, poultry.

al'kaline effects of foods. Fruits and vegetables contain salts of alkaline metals, such as calcium, magnesium, potassium, and sodium and they exert an alkaline effect in the body. Original acid parts of the salts, and the free acids, such as citric, malic, tartaric, and lactic, are burned in the body to carbonic acid, eliminated by the breath. This makes possible the neutralization of the acidic products from proteins by the alkaline metals. The blood stream and tissues are protected against sudden changes in normal faintly alkaline reaction by the bicarbonates, phosphates, and proteins serving as buffer agents. The body never becomes actually acid in reaction although the alkaline reserve may become depleted. SEE: *acid effects.*

al'kaline reserve. The amount of base in the blood, principally bicarbonates, available for neutralization of fixed acids (hydrochloric, lactic, etc.). A fall in a. reserve is called acidosis; a rise, alkalosis.

Normally, the carbon dioxide-combining power of the serum is 24-35 mEq./L. and the carbon dioxide content is 24-33 mEq./L.

al'kaline tide. The increase in alkaline reserve and occasional occurrence of alkaline urine during gastric digestion.

alkalin'ity. State of being alkaline. SEE: *hydrogen ion.*

al'kalinize. To make alkaline; alkalize.

alkalinu'ria [*alkali* + G. *ouron,* urine]. An alkaline urine.

alkalipe'nia [" + G. *penia,* poor]. Low alkali reserve of the body.

alkalither'apy. Therapeutic use of alkalies.

alkaliza'tion. Process of making alkaline.

al'kalize. To make alkaline.

al'kaloid [*alkali* + G. *eidos,* resemblance]. 1. An active bitter principle obtained from plants that reacts with an acid to form a salt, the latter being used because of its solubility, rather than the alkaloid. 2. An alkaline principle of organic origin; any nitrogenous base, especially one of vegetable origin having a toxic effect. Ex: *Quinine, morphine, strychnine, nicotine.*

INCOMPATIBILITIES: *Tea (tannin), coffee (caffeine).*

alkalom'etry [" + G. *metron,* measure]. Dosimetry. A system of dosage in administration of alkaloids.

alkalo'sis [" + G. *-osis,* condition of]. A condition in which the alkalinity of the body tends to increase beyond normal due to excess of alkalies or withdrawal of acid or chlorides from the blood.

a., altitude. A condition due to exposure to high altitudes. This causes *respiratory alkalosis, q.v.*

a., metabolic. A condition characterized by a pH of blood and other body fluids that is higher than normal and a carbon dioxide content of the serum that is greater than 70 volumes per cent (30 mEq./L.). Commonly a result of loss of acid from excessive vomiting, but also of loss of potassium or ingestion of excessive amounts of sodium bicarbonate. Symptoms and signs are apathy, irritability, delirium, dehydration and occasionally tetany. TREATMENT: Correct primary disorder; administer sodium or potassium chloride, nonalkalinizing gels.

a., respiratory. A condition characterized by a pH of blood and other body fluids that is greater than normal but with a carbon dioxide content of the serum that is less than 21 mEq./L. Caused by hyperventilation of a neurotic or systemic source, as hysteria, salicylate poisoning, lesion of central nervous system, or decreased oxygen content of the air. Symptoms and signs are lightheadedness, fainting, tetany. TREATMENT: Discontinue use of salicylates (in salicylate poisoning), inhalation of expired CO_2 from paper bag (in neurosis), correction or alleviation of central nervous system disorder or lesion. SEE: *hyperventilation syndrome.*

alkalother'apy. Therapeutic use of alkalies.

alkalot'ic. Pert. to alkalosis.

alkaluria (al-kă-lū'rĭ-ă). The condition of alkali in the urine.

alkap'ton(e [" + G. *aptein,* to possess]. A yellowish-red substance sometimes occurring in urine, the result of incomplete oxidation of tyrosine and phenylalanine.

alkaptonuria (al-kap-tō-nū'rĭ-ă) [alkapton + G. *ouron,* urine]. A rare inherited disorder characterized by the excretion of large amounts of homogentisic acid in the urine, a result of incomplete metabolism of the amino acids tyrosine and phenylalanine. Presence of the acid is indicated by the darkening of urine when alkalinated and the dark staining of diapers or other linen.

alkyl (al'kil) [*al,* abbr. *alcohol,* + G. *yle,* stuff]. The univalent aliphatic or aromatic radical which results from removal of a hydrogen atom.

alkylating agent (al'kĕ-lāt-ing). 1. A substance which introduces an alkyl radical into a compound in place of a hydrogen atom. 2. One which adds a side chain to an aromatic compound.

alkylene (al'kĕ-lēn). A bivalent aliphatic compound formed by removal of two hydrogen atoms.

allachesthesia (al-ă-kes-thē'zĭ-ă) [G. *allachē,* elsewhere, + *aisthesis,* sensation]. Tactile sensation remote from point of stimulation.

allantiasis (al-an-tī'ă-sis) [G. *allanto,* sausage]. 1. Sausage poisoning. 2. Any poisoning caused by Clostridium botulinum. SEE: *botulism.*

allantochorion (al-lăn-tō-ko'rĭ-ŏn). Fusion of the allantois and chorion into one structure.

allanto'ic. Pert. to the allantois.

allan'toid [G. *allanto,* sausage, + *eidos,* resemblance]. 1. Sausage-shaped. 2. Pert. to the allantois.

allan'toin. A white crystalline substance derived from purine metabolism and also produced synthetically. Occurs in allantoic and amniotic fluids. At one time was used to promote wound healing.

allantoinu'ria [*allantoin* + G. *ouron,* urine]. Allantoin in the urine.

allantois (a-lan'tō-is) [G. *allanto,* sausage, + *eidos,* resemblance]. A kind of elongated bladder, between the chorion and amnion of the fetus, which grows out from the caudal extremity of the embryo, and communicates with the bladder of the urachus. It is very apparent in quadrupeds, but not in the human species. In primates, including man, the allantois has no function but its blood vessels function, being called the umbilical vessels. SEE: *chorion; urachus.*

allele (ă-lēl', ă-lĕl'). Allelomorph, *q.v.*

allelic genes (a-lel'ik). Genes which occupy the same locus on a specific pair of chromosomes and control the heredity of a particular characteristic. The heredity of eye color appears to depend on a series of allelic genes; the A-B-O blood groups are determined by allelic genes; the standard Rh-Hr types are transmitted by allelic genes. SYN: *allele; allelomorph, q.v.*

allelocatal'ysis [G. *allēlōn,* reciprocally, + *catalysis,* dissolution]. Stimulation of a bacterial culture by the addition of cells of same type.

allelomorph (ă-lē'lō-morph, ă-lĕl'ō-morph). One of two or more contrasted genetic forms occurring at the same locus (position) on homologous chromosomes, *e.g.,* the genes for A, B, and O blood types which are multiple alleles at the same locus. SYN: *allele; allelic gene(s.*

allel'otaxis [" + *taxis,* order]. Development of a part from different embryonic structures.

Allen-Doisy unit [Edgar V. Allen, American anatomist, and Edward A. Doisy, American biochemist and physiologist]. Injection in a spayed mouse of the smallest amount of estrus-producing hormone secreted during pregnancy, producing desquamation of vaginal epithelium in the mouse.

Allen's law. The more carbohydrate taken by a diabetic, the less he utilizes.

allen'thesis. Introduction of a foreign substance into the body.

allergen (al'er-jen) [G. *allos,* other, + *ergon,* work, + *gennan,* to produce]. Any substance which induces a state of, or brings on manifestations of allergy. It may or may not be a protein or an antigen. Among common allergens are: *inhalants*: dusts, pollens, fungi, smoke, perfumes, odors of plastics; *foods*: wheat, eggs, milk, chocolate, strawberries; *drugs*: aspirin, antibiotics, serums; *infectious agents*: bacteria, viruses, fungi, animal parasites; *contactants*: chemicals, animals, plants, metals; *physical agents*: heat, cold, light, pressure, radiations.

allergenic (ăl-ĕr-jĕn'ĭk). Producing or causing allergy.

aller'gic. Pertaining to, sensitive to or caused by an allergen.

allergization (ăl-lĕr-jĭ-zā'shŭn). Introduction of a foreign substance into the body in order to bring about a state of sensitivity.

al'lergy [G. *allos,* other, + *ergeia,* work]. An altered reaction of body tissues to a specific substance (allergen) which in nonsensitive persons will, in similar amounts, produce no effect.

It is essentially an antibody-antigen reaction but in some cases the antibody cannot be demonstrated. The reaction may be due to the release of histamine, or histamine-like substances from injured cells.

Ex: An infection of a common cold may render a patient more susceptible to future infection, while an attack of mumps or measles renders the patient less liable; hypersensitiveness of body cells due to proteins such as ferment in the protein molecules, and which causes hay fever or asthma through inhalation, resulting in lesions, or skin eruptions.

Allergic conditions include eczema; allergic rhinitis, or coryza; hay fever; bronchial asthma, and urticaria or hives. Gastrointestinal allergy may appear in children.

NP: *In children*: Avoid extremes of temperature and humidity. Skin must not be chilled and sweating must be kept to a minimum. Soap and water must not be used on eczematous parts of the skin. An ointment may be ordered which should be applied many times during the day in a thin layer, and as often as the child rubs it off.

Woolen clothing and blankets should not be used, or feather-stuffed pillows or mattresses. To prevent scratching, cuffs should be used so the child cannot bend the arm at the elbow. Other restraints of arms and legs may be necessary. Elimination diets are indicated.

ETIOL: Heredity, pollen, dust, hair, fur, feathers, scales, or dandruff; also specific foods, such as eggs, chocolate, milk, wheat, tomatoes, citrus fruits, oatmeal, and potatoes.

SYM: Eosinophilia frequently present; urticaria, eczema, rash, asthma, hay fever, migraine, or gastrointestinal disturbances.

RS: *anaphylaxis; atopy; hay fever; hypersensitiveness; immunity.*

a., food. Find the offending food by placing the patient on a diet consisting of commonly nonallergenic foods and suspected foods. Then add foods suspected to be allergenic to the diet one at a time. Skin tests are sometimes useful. Offending food should be eliminated. SEE: *anaphylaxis.*

a., heat and cold. Changes of temperature may cause cutaneous reactions such as urticaria and also internal reactions with sensitive persons. Itching, redness of skin, headache, asthmatic symptoms, dyspnea, and shock can follow exposure to cold water. Heat may produce same symptoms.

allesthesia (al-ĕs-thē'sĭ-ă) [G. *allos*, other, + *aisthesis*, sensation] A sensation in one limb which is referred to the other one; allochiria.

alliaceous (al-ĭ-ā'shus) [L. *allium*, garlic]. Tasting like garlic or onions.

allitera'tion [L. *ad*, to, + *littera*, letter]. Dysphrasia, in which words are spoken according to sound.

allo- [G. *allos*, other]. 1. A prefix meaning differentiation from the normal. 2. Indicating a body made stable by heat. 3. CHEM: An isomer, close relative or variety of a compound. Isomerism when there is relative asymmetry.

allochesthesia (al-ō-kĕs-thē'zĭ-ă) [G. *allachē*, elsewhere, + *aisthēsis*, sensation]. Tactile sensation remote from point of stimulation. SYN: *allochiria; allesthesia.*

allochezia, allochetia (al-ō-kē'zĭ-ă, al-ō-kē'shĭ-ă) [G. *allos*, other, + *chezein*, to defecate]. 1. Excretion of nonfecal matter from the bowels. 2. Excretion of feces through an abnormal opening.

allochiria (al-ō-kī'rĭ-ă), **allocheiria** [G. " + *cheir*, hand]. Sensation referred to side of body opposite its origin; allesthesia.

Observed in locomotor ataxia and in hysteria.

allochroism (al-ŏk'rō-izm) [" + *chroa*, color]. Change in color.

allochromasia (al-ō-krō-mā'sĭ-ă). Change in color of hair or skin.

allocinesia (al-ō-sĭn-ē'sĭ-ă) [G. *allos*, other, + *kinēsis*, movement]. Movement on side of body opposite to the one directed. SEE: *allokinesis.*

alloerot'icism. Alloerotism, *q.v.*

alloerotism (al-ō-er'ō-tism) [" + *Eros*, god of love]. Sexual urges stimulated by and directed toward another person. Opposite to *autoerotism.*

allokinesis (al-ō-kĭ-nē'sis) [G. *allos*, other, + *kinesis*, movement]. Movement on side of body opposite to the one directed.

allokinetic (al-ō-kĭ-net'ik) [" + *kinesis*, movement]. Movement caused by external forces.

allola'lia [" + *lalia*, talk]. Speech defect, esp. if due to disease of speech center.

allomorphic (al-lō-morph'ĭk). Assuming a different form but remaining unchanged in character.

al'lopath. A misnomer for a regular medical practitioner.

allopathy (al-op'a-thĭ). A misnomer for a system of therapeutics administering medicines which produce effects different from those of the disease treated; in principle, the opp. of homeopathy. A term erroneously used for the regular practice of medicine by physicians.

allophasis (al-off'ă-sis) [G. *allos*, other, + *phasis*, speech]. Incoherency, delirium.

alloplasia (al-ō-plā'zĭ-ă) [G. *allos*, other, + *plasis*, a molding]. Replacement of normal cell forms by other cell forms in the tissue. SEE: *heteroplasia.*

al'loplasty. Plastic surgery with nonhuman tissue.

allopolyploidy (al-ō-pol'ē-ploy-dē). Having more than two sets of chromosomes derived from different ancestral species.

allopsychic (al-ō-sī'kĭk) [" + *psychē*, mind]. Ideas not related to the patient's personality, but to the external environment.

allopsycho'sis [" + " + *-osis*, condition]. Derangement of perceptive powers.

allorhythmia (al-ō-rith'mĭ-ă) [" + *rythmos*, rhythm]. Irregular cardiac rhythm.

all-or-none law. That a stimulus to a nerve or muscle causes it to respond to its greatest extent or not at all. Applied specifically to a single striated muscle fiber, a single nerve fiber, or the heart as a whole.

allotherm (al'ō-therm) [" + *thermē*, heat]. An organism whose temperature is directly dependent on its environment. SEE: *homothermal; poikilthermal.*

allotox'in [" + *toxikon*, poison]. A substance within the body which protects by destroying toxins inimical to it.

allotransplantation (al"lo-trans-plan-ta'shun) [G. *allos*, other, + transplantation]. Grafting or transplanting tissue from one individual into another.

allotriogeustia (ă-lot-rĭ-ō-just'ĭ-ă) [G. *allotrios*, strange, + *geusis*, taste]. Perverted taste.

allotriophagy (ă-lot-rĭ-of'ă-jĭ) [" + *phagein*, to eat]. A perverted appetite for injurious, unusual, and nonedible substances. SEE: *pica.*

allotriuria (a-lot-rĭ-ū'rĭ-ă) [" + *ouron*, urine]. Abnormal urine.

allotropic (al-ō-trop'ik) [G. *allos*, other, + *tropos*, direction]. 1. CHEM: Pert. to different forms of the same element without change of chemical composition. 2. Altered by digestion so as to be changed in its nutritive value.

a. type. A person who is much concerned with what others think, say, or do.

allot'ropism, allot'ropy. Presence of an element in two or more distinct forms with unlike properties.

allox'an [L. *alloxanum*]. $C_4H_4N_2O_5$. A substance obtained as an oxidation product of uric acid. In experimental medicine, has caused diabetes in animals. It gives a red color to the skin, and has been used as a basis of cosmetic preparations.

allox'in. Any one of a series of *xanthin* bases derived from the splitting of *chromatin* which, on oxidation, produces uric acid.

allox'ur bases or bodies [*allox*(*an*) + *ur*(*ea*)]. Xanthine bases. Nitrogenous substances formed by splitting of nucleins.

alloxuremia (al-oks-ū-rē'mĭ-ă) [*alloxur* + G.*aima*, blood]. Xanthine bases in the blood.

alloxu'ria [" + G. *ouron*, urine]. Xanthine bases in the urine.

alloy (al'oi) [Fr. *aloi*, to combine]. A metallic substance (*e.g.*, brass) resulting from the fusion of two or more metals. Also, a substance (*e.g.*, steel) formed from the fusion of a metal and a nonmetal.

al'lyl [L. *allium*, garlic, + G. *ylē*, matter]. C_3H_5. A univalent radical. It is present in garlic and mustard CH_2CH-CH_2.

Almén's tests (ăl-māns'). Three tests of urine for blood, albumin, and sugar.

almond (ă'mond) [G. *amygdalē*]. Fruit of the almond tree. Highly nutritive and rich in nitrogenous components. High fat content. Heavy in cellulose. They contain considerable albumin. Source of thiamine, riboflavin and niacin. ROASTED, 100 gm. Calories: 627. Other values: 18.6 gm. protein; 54.2 gm. fat.

alochia (ă-lo'kĭ-ă) [G. *a*-, priv. + *lochios*, pert. to childbirth]. Absence of puerperal* vaginal discharge following childbirth.

aloe (al'ō). USP. The dried juice of several species of aloe. It is a necessary ingredient for compound benzoin tincture.

alo'gia [G. *a*-, priv. + *logos*, speech]. Inability to express oneself through speech. SYN: *aphasia*.

alopecia (al-ō-pe'shĭ-ă) [G. *alopēkia*, fox mange]. Natural or abnormal baldness or deficiency of hair, partial or complete, localized or generalized.

ETIOL: May result from: 1. Physiologic changes in senility. 2. Effects of serious illness, *e.g.*, typhoid fever. 3. Drugs, *e.g.*, arsenic, thallium. 4. Endocrine disorders, *e.g.*, hypothyroidism. 5. Certain forms of dermatitis. 6. Hereditary factors.

TREATMENT: Treatment of seborrheic dermatitis if present. There is no other effective therapy.

a. adnata. Congenital baldness.

a. areata. Baldness is sharply defined; circumscribed patches which leave the scalp smooth and white.

a., congenital. Form with absence of hair bulbs at birth.

a. follicularis. Inflammation of the hair follicles of the scalp causing loss of hair from affected areas.

a. furfuracea. Chronic in course and marked by dandruff and itching, and falling out of hair (exfoliation of scales). SYN: *a. pityroides*.

a. neurotica. Baldness following a nervous disease or injury to nervous system, and occurring at site of injury.

a. pityroides [G. *pityrōdes*, branny]. Falling of both scalp and body hair, together with abundant branlike desquamation.

a. prematura. Premature baldness.

a. senilis. Baldness of old age.

a. simplex. Baldness prematurely.

a. symptomatica. Loss of hair after prolonged fevers or during course of some disease; also may result from changes in internal secretions.

a. totalis. Complete loss of hair from the entire body.

a. toxica. Loss of hair thought to be due to toxins of infectious disease.

a. universalis. General loss of hair from all parts of body.

al'pha. First letter A or *α* of Greek alphabet. CHEM: Denotes first in a series of isomeric compounds.

a. leukocyte. One that disintegrates during blood coagulation.

a. rhythm. In electroencephalography, rhythmical oscillations in electric potential occurring at a rate of 8 to 13 per second. They are best recorded when the eyes are positioned in a particular way.

a. tocopherol (tō-kŏf'er-ŏl). One of a group of substances with vitamin E activity.

Therapeutic value has not been established.

a. wave. Alpha rhythm, *q.v.*

alphelasma (al-fel-as'ma). Leukoplakia.

alphus (al'fus) [L.], **al'phos** (G.]. 1. Psoriasis. 2. A pustular, scrofulous affection of the skin accompanied by white crusts.

al'ternate host [L. *alternare*, do by turns]. A carrier of disease germs, such as the louse, and other insects.

al'ternating cur'rent. PT: An electrical current the direction of which reverses constantly.

al'ternator. PT: So-called sinusoidal alternator; an electromagnetic device consisting of a revolving armature which cuts the lines of force in a magnetic field and which delivers a sinusoidal current from secondary coil of the apparatus.

al'therm, altherm pad. A device containing heat-producing chemicals for applying heat to the eye or a sinus.

alt. hor. Abbreviation for the Latin *alternis horis*, every other hour.

altricious (al-trish'us) [L. *altrix*, nourisher]. Slow in developing; requiring long nursing.

al'um [L. *alumen*] (ammonium alum, or potassium alum). USP. Large, colorless crystals, or white powder, with sweetish, strongly astringent taste. Used locally, in solution, as a mild astringent for mucous membranes.

Its manufacture (which is of great antiquity) is by subjecting alum stone to a roasting process, and treating with sulfuric acid.

alu'men [L.]. Alum.

a. exsiccatum. Alum that has been dried or burnt; used as a dusting powder.

aluminosis (al-ū-min-o'sis) [" + G. *-osis*, condition of]. Chronic catarrhal inflammation of the lungs in alum workers.

alu'minum. A silver-whitish metal. SYMB: Al. At. wt. 26.9815; at. no. 13.

a. acetate. A salt formed by the reaction between aluminum sulfate and lead acetate. Its aqueous solution, containing 4 to 5%, is known as Burow's solution.

USES: Regarded as a valuable local astringent.

a. hydroxide gel. USP. A white viscous suspension containing aluminum hydroxide and hydrated aluminum oxide; an antacid especially useful in treatment of peptic ulcer.

alusia (al-u'sĭ-ă) [G. *aluein*, to wander]. Morbidity; hallucination.

alveobronchioli'tis, alveobronchi'tis [L. *alveolus*, little tub, + G. *bronchos*, windpipe, + *-itis*, inflammation]. Inflammation of the bronchioles, and pulmonary alveoli; bronchopneumonia, *q.v.*

alve'olar [L. *alveolus*]. Pertaining to an alveolus, *q.v.*

a. air. That determined by sampling the last portion of a maximal expiration. SEE ALSO: *air; spirometry.*

a. bone. Bone of the alveolar processes of mandible and maxilla.

a. periosteum. The periodontal membrane.

a. process. One of four processes which make up each maxillary bone.

alveolar-capillary block. Impaired ability of gases to pass through the pulmonary alveolar-capillary membrane.

alve'olate [L. *alveola*]. Honeycombed; pitted.

alveoli (al-ve'ō-lī) [L.]. Pl. of alveolus, *q.v.*

a. dentales [NA]. Tooth sockets.

a. pulmonis [NA]. Air cells of the lungs.

alveoli'tis [L. *alveolus*, + G. *-itis*, inflammation]. Inflammation of the alveolar processes; pyorrhea.*

alveoloclasia (al-ve-o-lo-kla'zĭ-ă) [" + G. *klasis*, fracture]. Absorption of any part of the alveolar process.

alveolus (al-vē'ō-lus) (pl. *alve'oli*) [L. small hollow or cavity]. 1. A little hollow. 2. The socket of a tooth. 3. Air cell of the lungs. 4. A small depression such as those contained in the honeycomb cells of the gastric mucous membrane. 5. A follicle of a racemose gland.

a., mucous, of the salivary glands. Those that secrete the ropy material of the saliva, containing mucin.

a., parietal. An air space in the wall of an alveolar passage in the lung.

a. pulmoneus. A pulmonary air space.

a., serous, of the salivary glands. Those that secrete the serous albumin of the saliva, coagulating when heated.

a., terminal. An air space connected with a pulmonary infundibulum.

alveus (al'vē-us) [L. a hollow, a cavity]. A channel or groove.

a. ampullescens. Dilation of the receptaculum chyli.

a. hippocampi. A layer of white fibers covering ventricular surface of the hippocampal formation of the rhinencephalon.

alvine (al'vīn) [L. *alvus*, belly]. Pert. to the intestines or abdomen.

a. concretion. Intestinal stone.

a. discharge. Stools.

a. flux. Watery feces.

alvi'nolith [" + G. *lithos*, stone]. An intestinal mass formed from calcareous salts and other matter. SEE: *bezoar.*

al'vus. [L.]. Abdomen and viscera.

alymphopotent (a-lĭm'fō-pō"tĕnt) [G. *a-*, priv. + L. *lympha*, lymph, + *potens*, able]. Unable to develop lymphocytes or lymphoid cells.

Alzheimer's disease (ahlts'hī-merz) [Alois Alzheimer, German neurologist, 1864-1915]. NEUR: Presenile dementia with hyaline degeneration of the smaller blood vessels of the brain.

Am. Chemical symbol for *americium.* Abbr. for *mixed astigmatism; ametropia.*

ama (a'mă) [G. *amē*]. 1. Enlargement of a bony canal of labyrinth of the internal ear at the end opposite the ampulla. 2. An Oriental female diver.

A.M.A. Abbr. for *American Medical Association.*

amaas (ă'măhs). A mild form of smallpox; alastrim.

am'acrine cell [G. *a-*, priv. + *makros*, long, + *is, inos*, fiber]. Cell in inner nuclear layer of retina possessing only one branching process.

amal'gam [G. *malagma*, emollient]. Any alloy containing mercury.

amal'gamate. To make an amalgam.

Amantadine hydrochloride (ă-man'tă-dēn hi"dro-klor'īd). Proprietary name for an amine, 1-adamantanamine hydrochloride, used as a prophylaxis for influenza due to A-2 influenza virus.

amara (am-a'ră) [L. *amarus*, bitter]. Bitters.

amarthritis (am-ar-thri'tis) [G. *ama*, at same time, + *arthron*, joint, + *-itis*, inflammation]. Polyarthritis. Inflammation of more than one joint at the same time.

amasesis (ă-mas-ē'sis) [G. *a-*, priv. + *masesis*, chewing]. Inability to masticate food.

amas'tia [" + *mastos*, breast]. Lack of breast development. SYN: *amazia.*

am'ativeness [L. *amare*, to love]. 1. Sexual desire. 2. Propensity to love.

Amat'o bod'ies. Those seen in leukocytes in scarlet fever.

amaurosis (am-aw-ro'sus) [G. *amauros*, dark, dim, + *-osis*, condition]. Complete loss of vision, esp. that in which there is no evidence of pathologic condition of the eye.

a., albuminuric. A. caused by kidney affection.

a., amaurotic. A. caused by the atrophying of optic nerve or vision centers.

a., cerebral. A. caused by brain malady.

a., congenital. A. from birth on.

a., diabetic. A. in connection with diabetes.

a., epileptoid. Sudden seizure of blindness, considered to be similar to epilepsy.

a. fugax. Temporary loss of vision (blackout) from diminished blood supply to brain, as in acceleration.

a., lead. A. caused by lead poisoning.

a. partialis fugax. Sudden transitory blindness with symptoms similar to migraine: nausea, vomiting, dizziness, and disturbances of vision.

a., reflex. A. due to reflex action caused by irritation of a remote part.

a., saburral. A. in conjunction with acute gastritis.

a., tobacco. A. caused by tobacco poisoning.

a., toxic. Blindness from optic neuritis caused by poison.

a., uremic. A. caused by uremic condition.

amaurotic (am-ă-rot'ik). Pert. to one afflicted with amaurosis.

a. familial idiocy. Term for a group of related familial diseases marked by dementia, impaired vision, and lipid defect.

a.f.i., infantile. That occurring in infants between the ages of 1 and 12 months. Generally, the patients are members of Jewish families. It is marked by degeneration of the retina (cherry-red spot), progressive blindness, mental deterioration, loss of motor control, and death by age 3 years. SYN: *infantile cerebral lipoidosis; Tay-Sachs disease.*

a.f.i., juvenile. That form occurring between ages 5 and 10 years. Marked by deposits of pigment in retina, progressive blindness, progressive loss of motor control, mental deterioration, and death. SYN: *juvenile cerebral lipoidosis; Spielmeyer-Vogt disease.*

a.f.i., late infantile. That type occurring usually at the age of 3 or 4 years. Marked by optic atrophy, progressive blindness, spasticity and tremor, seizures, and death. SYN: *Bielschowsky disease; late infantile cerebral lipoidosis.*

a.f.i., late juvenile. (Also called *adult a.f.i.*) Similar to the juvenile form except for loss of vision which rarely occurs in the late juvenile type. Onset usually takes place between the ages of 15 and 25 years. Marked by tremors, muscle rigidity, dementia, convulsions, and death. SYN: *Kufs disease; late juvenile cerebral lipoidosis.*

amaxophobia (ă-maks-ō-fō'bĭ-ă) [G. *amaxa*, carriage, + *phobos*, fear]. Morbid dread of vehicles or riding in them.

amazia (ă-mā'zĭ-ă) [G. *a-*, priv. + *mazos*, breast]. Lack of development of the breasts. SYN: *amastia.*

ambi- [L.]. Prefix: both or both sides; around; about, as *ambidextrous.*

ambidex'trous [" + *dexter*, right]. Ability to work effectively with either hand.

ambilat'eral [" + *latus*, side]. Pert. to both sides.

ambilevous (am-bĭ-lē'vus) [" + *laevus*, left]. Awkward in use of either hand.

ambio'pia [" + G. *ops*, eye]. Double vision. SYN: *diplopia, q.v.*

ambisin'ister [" + *sinister*, left]. Awkward in use of either hand. SYN: *ambilevous.*

ambiten'dency [" + *tendere*, to stretch]. PSY: The association of a tendency with an opposite tendency—an essential mechanism in conflict.

ambivalence (am-biv'ă-lens) [" + *valere*, to be strong]. 1. Possessing ability of equal power or value in two directions. 2. PSY: Linking of opposite or contrary emotional values (love and hate) to the same idea, or toward the same person. The fluctuation from strong like to dislike found in schizophrenia.

ambiv'alency. The condition of being ambivalent.

ambiv'alent. Have equal power or value in both directions.

a. feelings. Two opposite emotions, such as love and hate, for the same person at same time. SEE: *ambivalence.*

ambivert (ăm'bĭ-vĕrt) [L. *ambo*, both, + L. *vertere*, to turn]. One intermediate between an extrovert and an introvert.

amblyacousia (am"blĭ-ă-koo'sĭ-ă) [G. *amblys*, dull, + *akousis*, hearing]. Dullness of hearing.

amblyaphia (am-blĭ-af'ĭ-ă) [" + *aphē*, touch]. Dull sense of touch.

amblychromasia (am"blĭ-kro-ma'sĭ-ă) [" + *chromatikos*, pert. to color]. The state in which the cell nucleus stains faintly.

amblychromat'ic. Staining faintly.

amblygeustia (am-blĭ-jūs'tĭ-ă) [G. *amblys*, dull, + *geusis*, taste]. Defective or blunted taste.

amblyphonia (ăm-blĭ-fō'nĭ-ă). Impaired hearing. SYN: *amblyacousia.*

amblyopia (ăm-blĭ-ō'pĭ-ă) [" + *ōps*, sight]. Reduced or dimness of vision, not dependent upon visible changes in the eye and not a refractive error (alcoholic, astigmatic, diabetic, *ex anopsia*, malarial, methyl alcohol, quinine, tobacco, toxic, uremic).

a., crossed. That of one eye with hemianesthesia of the opposite side of the face. SYN: *a. cruciata.*

a. ex anopsia. Dimness of vision resulting from disuse of the eyes. May be due to cataract, refractive errors.

a., reflex. A. due to irritation of peripheral area.

a., toxic. That due to effect of toxic substances such as alcohol or tobacco.

amblyoscope (am'blĭ-ō-skōp) [" + *skopein*, to view]. Instrument for training an amblyopic eye for better vision.

am'bo, ambon [G. *ambon*, edge of a dish]. Annular fibrocartilage producing an elevation about a joint cavity; also the elevation itself.

amboceptor (am-bō-sep'tor). So called by Ehrlich. An immune substance or antibody forming a union between an antigen and complement (agent that completes lytic action), as it is assumed it has one affinity for the antigen and one for the complement.

RS: *agglutinins, antibody, antigen, immune bodies, opsonin, precipitin, Ehrlich's theory.*

a. unit. Smallest amount of amboceptor required in the presence of which a given quantity of red blood corpuscles will be dissolved by an excess of complement.

am'bos. Incus or anvil bone of the middle ear.

am'bulance [L. *ambulare*, to move about]. A vehicle for transportation of the sick and wounded.

am'bulant, ambulatory. Able to walk, not confined to bed.

a. typhoid fever. A mild attack of typhoid fever, in which the patient is not confined to bed. SEE: *typhoid.*

ambustial (am-bus'shal) [L. *amburere*, to scorch]. Pert. to a burn or scald.

ambustion (am-bus'chun). A burn or scald.

Ameba. A genus of protozoa, class Sarcodina.

A. proteus. The common, large, fresh-water species.

ame'ba, amoeba (pl. *amebae, amoebae; amebas, amoebas*) [G. *amoibe*, change]. A one-celled protozoan minute animal form of life that constantly changes its shape by sending out processes of its protoplasm, by which it moves about and obtains its nourishment.

It is found in great numbers in pools, and in the green slime on the top of the water. It is also found in the mud at the bottom. It possesses an outer translucent substance called the *ectoplasm;* but the inner substance is denser, contains a nucleus, and is the *endoplasm.* It feeds by surrounding its victim and enclosing it in the so-called *food vacuole.* Oxygen is absorbed from the surrounding water, and CO_2 is eliminated through the plasma membrane. The organism moves by extending fingerlike protrusions of the protoplasm called pseudopodia. Reproduction is by binary fission in which the nucleus is divided by mitosis. One of the species found in the human colon, Entamoeba histolytica, may be pathogenic to man, causing amebic dysentery. In parasitic forms, encystment may occur.

amebiasis (am-ĕ-bī'ă-sis). An infectious disease from infestation by a species of ameba.

ETIOL: Entamoeba histolytica; acquired by ingesting food or drink containing encysted forms.

PATH: Small abscesses and, later, ulcers of mucous membrane of colon, sometimes resulting in perforation. Liver abscesses may result from amebas being carried to liver via portal vein.

SYM: Many patients are asymptomatic. Disease is generally characterized by dysentery with diarrhea, weakness and prostration. Nausea, vomiting and pain may be present and stools frequent. Complications may result in amebic hepatitis.

DIAG: Cysts or trophozoites of E. histolytica in stools.

TREATMENT: In acute amebiasis, antibiotics (as the tetracyclines), emetine and amebicidal agents as carbarsone or hydroxyquinolone. Chloroquine or emetine is useful in liver abscess.

a., hepatic. Infection of the liver by amebas, usually with abscess formation.

ame'bic. Pert. to or caused by amebas.

a. carrier state. That in which an individual harbors a form of pathogenic ameba.

a. dysentery. That caused by *Entamoeba histolytica.* SEE: *amebiasis.*

a. hepatitis. Amebic abscess of the liver.

ame'bicide [G. *amoibē,* change, + L. *caedere,* to kill]. Destructive to or any agent that kills amebas.

ame'biform [" + L. *forma,* shape]. Formed like an ameba.

amebocyte (ă-mē'bō-sīt) [" + G. *kytos,* cell]. A cell showing ameboid movements.

ame'boid [" + G. *eidos,* resemblance]. Having the appearance and characteristics of an ameba.

a. movements. Those possessed by leukocytes which "wander" through capillary walls into surrounding tissues; a process known as diapedesis.

ame'boidism. Ameba-like movements, noting a condition shown by certain nerve cells.

amebula (a-mē'bū-lă) [dim, *ameba*].The ameba-like spore of the malarial parasite.

amebu'ria [G. *amoibē,* change, + *ouron,* urine]. Amebas in the urine.

amelanotic (ă-mĕl-ă-not'ĭc). Without melanin; unpigmented.

amelia (ă-mē'lĭ-ă) [a, + G. *melos,* limb, + ia]. A congenital anomaly characterized by the absence of one or more limbs.

amelioration (ă-me-lĭ-or-a'shun) [L. *ad,* to, + *meliorare,* to make better]. Improvement; moderation of a condition.

ame'loblast [early English *amel,* enamel, + G. *blastos,* germ]. A cell from which tooth enamel is formed.

ameloblastoma (ă-mĕl-ō-blas-tō'mă). Highly destructive tumor of the jaw. SYN: *adamantinoma.*

ameloden'tinal [" + L. *dens, dent-,* tooth]. Pert. to both enamel and dentine.

ame'nia [G. *a-,* priv. + *mēn,* month]. Absence of the menses; amenorrhea.*

amenomania (ă-mē-nō-mā'nĭ-ă) [L. *amaenus,* pleasant, + G. *mania,* frenzy]. Manic phase of manic-depressive psychosis marked by excessive gaiety, lightheartedness, and morbidly cheerful disposition.

amenorrhea (a-men-ō-rē-ă) [G. *a-,* priv. + *mēn,* month, + *rein,* to flow]. Absence or suppression of menstruation; normal before puberty, after the menopause, during pregnancy and lactation.

ETIOL: Congenital abnormalities of the reproductive tract; metabolic disorders (obesity, malnutrition, diabetes); systemic diseases (syphilis, tuberculosis, nephritis); emotional disorders (excitement, anorexia nervosa); endocrine disorders, esp. those involving the ovaries, pituitary, thyroid, and adrenal glands; hormonal imbalance (excesses or inadequacies) of estrogen or progesterone, or of follicle-stimulating hormones. These are common causes.

TREATMENT: Underlying cause should be determined and corrected. If hormone deficiencies exist, substitutional therapy is recommended. If BMR is below normal, thyroid medication may be beneficial. Estrogen-progesterone therapy is effective in many cases.

a., emotional. That resulting from shock, fright, hysteria, etc.

a., functional. Condition with varying intervals of amenorrhea interspersed with normal menstrual periods.

a., partial. Appearing occasionally and at irregular intervals.

a., pathologic. That before the menarche, after menopause, and during pregnancy and lactation.

a., physiological. Periods when normally free from menstruation; prepuberty, pregnancy, lactation, postmenopause periods.

a., primary. *Emansio mensium.* That in which menses have never made their appearance.

a., secondary. *Suppressio mensium.* That in which, having appeared, the menses subsequently cease.

amenorrhe'ic. Pert. to amenorrhea.

ament (ă'ment) [L. *ab,* from, + *mens,* mind]. An idiot; one without evidence of mind.

amentia (a-men'shĭ-a). 1. Congenital mental deficiency; feeblemindedness. 2. PSY: Condition marked by subnormal intelligence; on the basis of intelligence tests, an I.Q. of 70 or below. Cf. *dementia.*

RS: *intelligence test; imbecile; idiot; moron.*

a., nevoid. Amentia with a nevoid condition, calcification of parts of the brain, glaucoma and epilepsy.

a., phenylpyruvic. A. with secretion of phenylpyruvic acid in urine.

americium (ăm-ĕr-ĭs'ē-um) [from the Americas]. A metallic element. SYMB: Am. At. wt. 243; at. no. 95.

ameristic (a-mer-is'tik) [G. *a-,* priv. + *meros,* part]. Not segmented.

ametria (ă-mē'trĭ-ă). Congenital absence of the uterus.

ametrohemia (ah-mĕt-rō-hē'mĭ-ă) [G. *a-,* priv. + *metra,* uterus, + *aima,* blood]. Lack of uterine blood supply.

ametrom'eter [G. *ametros,* disproportionate, + *ōps,* sight, + *metron,* measure]. Instrument for measuring ametropia.

ametropia (ă-mĕ-trō'pĭ-ă) [" + *ōps,* vision]. Imperfect refractive powers of eye (hyperopia, myopia, astigmatism), in which the principal focus does not lie on the retina.

amianthinopsy (ăm-ĭ-an'thin-op"sĭ) [G. *a-,* priv. + *ianthinos,* violet, + *opsis,* vision]. Violet blindness.

amicro'bic [G. *a-,* priv. + *mikros,* small, + *bios,* life] Lacking in microbes or microorganisms. Not due to microbes.

am'icron(e. A colloid particle unrecognizable through the ultramicroscope.

amicroscop'ic. Too small to be detected through the ultramicroscope.

am'idase. A deamidizing enzyme, one that catalyzes the hydrolysis of urea.

amide (am'ĭd). A chemical compound produced by the substitution of an acid radical for one of the hydrogen atoms of ammonia.

am'idin [F. *amidon*, starch]. 1. The part of starch soluble in water. 2. A monacid base. The group $C.NH.NH_2$.

amido-. A prefix signifying the presence of the radical $CO.NH_2$.

amid'ulin [Fr. *amidon*, starch]. Soluble starch.

am'igen. A proprietary name for a protein hydrolysate derived from casein; used to provide protein nutrients.

amimia (a-mim'ĭ-ă) [G. *a-*, priv. + *mimos*, mimic]. Loss of power to express ideas by signs or gestures.

a., amnesic. That in which signs and gestures can be made but their meaning is not remembered.

a., ataxic. That in which signs and gestures cannot be made because of nervous or muscular disorders.

amine (ă-mēn', am'ĭn). One of a group of nitrogen-containing organic compounds in which one or more of the hydrogens of ammonia have been replaced by one or more organic radicals.

amino- (ă-mē'nō, am'in-ō). Prefix denoting presence of the amino (NH_2) group combined with a radical, other than an acid radical.

amino acid. One of a large group of organic compounds marked by presence of both an amino (NH_2) and a carboxyl (COOH) radical. Their basic formula is NH_2-R-COOH in which R stands for any aliphatic or aromatic radical. They are amphoteric and exhibit properties marked by both the amino and carboxyl groups. They are the building blocks of which proteins are constructed, and they are the end-products of protein digestion or hydrolysis.

There are twenty or more amino acids of which ten are essential or indispensable for life. These are: histidine (may be essential for children but not for adults), isoleucine, leucine, lysine, methionine, phenylalanine, threonine, tryptophan, and valine. The nonessential amino acids are: alanine, aspartic acid, arginine, citrulline, cystine, glutamic acid, glycine, hydroxyglutamic acid, hydroxyproline, norleucine, proline, serine, and tyrosine. SEE ALSO: *deaminization; digestion; protein.*

All proteins do not contain all the essential amino acids as is the case with milk, cheese, eggs, and meat. Unused amino acids are converted into urea. They pass unchanged through the intestinal wall and portal vein into the blood, then through the liver into the general circulation from which they are absorbed by the tissues according to the specific protein for a specific tissue, each tissue making its own protein from the amino acid, and each deaminizing that which remains unused.

a. compound. Substance containing the group NH_2; same as amine, *q.v.*

a. group. The NH_2 group which characterizes the amines.

aminoacetic acid (am-in'o-ă-sē'tik). One of the simplest examples of an amino acid. A normal constituent of bile. Same as glycine.

a. acidemia. Amino acids in the blood.

aminophylline (am-ĭ-nof'ĭ-lĭn). USP. $C_{16}H_{24}N_{10}O_4.2H_2O$. A mixture of theophylline and ethylenediamine. Used esp. in acute asthma that has not responded to epinephrine. Used also as a stimulant to the respiratory center and heart muscle, and as a diuretic. SYN: *theophylline ethylenediamine.*

aminopterin (am-ĭ-nop'ter-ĭn). A proprietary name for 4-aminopteroylglutamic acid, a folic acid antagonist used in treatment of acute leukemia.

aminopyrine (am"in-ō-pī'rēn). An antipyretic and analgesic similar to antipyrine but with more lasting effects and effective in smaller doses. Same precautions should be used as in other antipyretics.

aminosis (am-ĭ-nō'sis) [*amino-* + G. *-osis*, state]. Excessive production of amino acids in the body.

aminuria (am-ĭ-nū'rē-ă) [" + G. *ouron*, urine]. Amines in voided urine.

amitosis (am-ĭ-tō'sis) [G. *a-*, priv. + G. *mitos*, a thread]. Simple or direct cell division without change in the nucleus.

amitotic (am-ĭ-tŏt'ik). Characterized by amitosis.

am'meter. PT: An instrument calibrated to measure in amperes the strength of a current flowing in a circuit. SEE ALSO: *milliammeter.*

ammone'mia. Ammonia in the blood due to urea decomposition. SYN: *ammoniemia.*

ammonia (ă-mō'nĭ-ă) [*Ammon*, Egyptian deity]. A gas formed by decomposition of nitrogen-containing substances such as proteins and amino acids. Ammonia is converted into urea in the liver. Its formula, NH_3, relates it to many poisonous substances but also to the proteins and to many useful chemicals. Dissolved in water, it neutralizes acids and turns litmus blue.

a., aromatic spirit of. A flavored solution of ammonia and ammonium carbonate in water and alcohol.

a., blood. Ammonia in the blood. Increased values are found in liver failure.

a. water. A solution of strong ammonia solution (USP). It has a very pungent odor. A necessary agent for aromatic ammonia spirit. SYN: *diluted ammonia solution; diluted ammonium hydroxide solution; hartshorn.*

a. water, stronger. A 28% solution of ammonia in water. SYN: *strong ammonia solution; stronger ammonium hydroxide solution.*

ammoni'acal. Having the characteristics of or pert. to ammonia.

ammo'niated. Containing ammonia.

ammoniemia (a-mō"nĭ-ē'mĭ-ă) [ammonia + G. *aima*, blood]. Ammonia in the blood due to decomposition of urea.

ammonium car'bonate (a-mō'nĭ-um). USP. Occurs as hard masses with strong odor of ammonia. On exposure to air, loses CO_2 and ammonia. It is a necessary agent in preparation of aromatic ammonia spirit.

a. chlor'ide. USP. White crystalline powder without odor. It is used as an expectorant, a diuretic, and as an aid in restoring acid-base balance.

a. hydrox'ide. This is a solution of ammonia gas in water, used about the house for cleaning purposes and as a refrigerant.

POISONING: See *Ammonia in Table of Poisons and Poisoning in Appendix.*

ammoniuria (ă-mō"nĭ-ū'rĭ-ă) [ammonia + G. *ouron*, urine]. An excessive amount of ammonia in the urine.

amnesia (am-nē'zĭ-ă) [G. forgetfulness]. A loss of memory.

This may be for recent experiences, those subsequent to the disease, and is then termed *anterograde.* When it involves more remote memory stores it is called *retrograde.* Amnesia is often applied to episodes during which the patient forgets his identity, though he may conduct himself properly enough, and following which no memory of the period persists. Such episodes are often hysterical, sometimes epileptic, while trauma, senility, alcoholism, and other organic reaction types account for a smaller number.

PSY: Partial a. is seen in confusional insanity, lack of retention in senility, and in hysteria there may be lack of recall.

a., auditory. Loss of memory for word meanings.

a., lacunar. Loss of memory for isolated events.

a., periodic. A. occurring in a period of double consciousness.

a., retroanterograde. A memory disorder in which present-day events are referred to the past and vice versa.

a., tactile. Inability to distinguish objects by sense of touch. SYN: *astereognosis.*

a. traumatica. A. caused by injuries.

a., visual. Inability to remember the appearance of objects that have been seen or to be cognizant of printed words.

amnesic (am-nē'sik). Pert. to amnesia.

a. aphasia. Loss of memory. SYN: *amnesia.*

amnestic (am-nes'tik). Amnesic, or causing amnesia.

amniochorial, amniochorionic (am"nĭ-ō-kō'rĭ-ăl, -kō-rĭ-on'ik). Relating to both amnion and chorion.

am"nioclep'sis [*amnion* + *kleptein,* to do secretly]. Gradual unperceived loss of amniotic fluid.

amniog'raphy [" + G. *graphein,* to write]. Radiography of amniotic sac.

am'nion [G. little lamb]. The inner of the fetal membranes, a thin, transparent sac which holds the fetus suspended in the *liquor amnii* or amniotic fluid, *q.v.* The amnion grows rapidly at the expense of the extra-embryonic coelom, and by the end of the second month it fuses with the chorion forming the amniochorionic sac. Commonly called the *bag of waters* or *caul.* SEE: *"amnio-" words; oligohydramnios.*

amniorrhea (am-ni-or-re'ă) [" + *roia,* flow]. Premature escape of the *liquor amnii.*

amniorrhexis (am-nĭ-o-rek'sis) [" + *rēxis,* rupture]. Rupture of the bag of waters, or amnion.

amnios (am'nĭ-os). The amnion, or the *liquor amnii.*

amniotic (am-nĭ-ot'ik). Pert. to the amnion.

a. cavity. 1. One that appears in the embryonic mass of the ovum. It is lined with a layer of cells called the embryonic ectoderm. The cavity enlarges rapidly as the embryo develops. 2. The fluid-filled cavity of the amnion.

a. fluid. *Liquor amnii.* The liquid or albuminous fluid contained in the amniotic sac, *q.v.* This fluid is transparent and almost colorless. The liquid protects the fetus from injury, helps maintain an even temperature, prevents formation of adhesions between the amnion and the skin of the fetus, and prevents conformity of the sac to the fetus (the last being an important consideration during labor). Premature rupture of the amniotic sac results in a so-called "dry labor." The amniotic fluid is continually being absorbed and renewed at a rapid rate. About one-third of the water in the amniotic fluid is replaced each hour.

a. sac. The bag or sac formed by the amnion, *q.v.*

amniotin. Proprietary name for a preparation of estrogenic substances used for atrophy of the genitalia.

amniotitis (am-nĭ-ō-tī'tis) [G. *amnion* + *-itis,* inflammation]. Inflammation of the amnion.

amniotome (am'nĭ-ō-tōm) [" + *tomē,* cutting]. Instrument for puncturing fetal membranes.

amnitis (am-nī'tis). Inflammation of the amnion. SYN: *amniotitis.*

amobarbital (am-ō-bar'bĭ-tal). USP. $C_{11}H_{18}N_2O_3$. An odorless, white, crystalline powder. Used as a sedative of intermediate action.

a. sodium. USP. $C_{11}H_{17}N_2NaO_3$. An odorless, white, granular powder. Following administration, it is absorbed rapidly, and is inactivated rapidly in the liver, Used as a sedative.

amodiaquine hydrochloride (am-ō-dī'ă-kwĭn). USP. $C_{20}H_{22}ClN_3O.2HCl.2H_2O$. Occurs as an odorless, yellow, crystalline powder. Used to control acute clinical attacks of falciparum or vivax malaria.

amoeba (ă-mē'ba). A one-celled protozoan animal form. SEE: *ameba.*

amok (ă-mok') [Malay *amoq,* furious]. A state of murderous frenzy. SYN: *amuck.*

amor (a'mor) [L.]. Love, esp. sexual love.

a. insanus [L. mad]. Unrestrained libido in the insane. SYN: *erotomania.**

a. lesbicus. Lesbianism, *q.v.*

a. sui [L. self]. Vanity; love of self.

amoralia (a-mō-rā'lĭ-ă) [G. *a-,* priv. + L. *moralis,* moral]. Moral imbecility.

amoralis (a-mō-rā'lis). A moral imbecile.

amorphia, amorphism (ă-mor'fĭ-ă, ă-mor'-fizm) [G. *a-,* priv. + *morphē,* form]. State of being without definite form.

amorphous (a-mor'fus). Without definite structure.

amotio (a-mō'shĭ-ō) [L. *amovere,* to move from]. A detachment.

a. retinae. Detached retina.

am"pelother'apy [G. *ampelos,* grape vine, + *therapeia,* treatment]. Grape cure.

amperage (ăm-pēr'āj). PT: Strength of the electrical current expressed in amperes or milliamperes.

ampere (ăm'pēr). PT: Practical unit of intensity of electric current, which is produced by 1 volt acting through resistance of 1 ohm.

The *international ampere* is practical equivalent of the unvarying current which deposits silver at the rate of 0.001118 gm. per second, when sent through a standard solution of nitrate of silver in water.

a. meter. Instrument denoting in amperes the strength of a current. SEE: *ammeter.*

amphetamine (am-fĕt'ă-mēn, -mĭn). A colorless liquid which volatilizes slowly at room temperature. It is a central nervous system stimulant. The preparation most commonly used is the sulfate, marketed in tablet or capsule form. Formerly used as an inhalant.

a. sulfate. USP. $(C_9H_{13}N)_2H_2SO_4$. A synthetic, white, crystalline substance which acts as a stimulant of the central nervous system. Used in treatment of narcolepsy, alcoholism, and certain types of mental depression; also for spasm of the gastrointestinal tract and in management of obesity. CAUTION: Large doses are toxic, and prolonged use may be habit-forming.

amphi- [G.]. Prefix. On both sides, as *amphibious.* CHEM: Denotes certain positions or configurations.

amphiarthrosis (am-fi-ar-thrō'sis) [*amphi-* + G. *arthrosis,* joint]. A form of articulation intermediate between diarthrosis and synarthrosis, in which the articulating bony surfaces are connected by an elastic cartilaginous substance; the mobility is slight, but may be exerted in all directions. The articulations of the bodies of the vertebrae are examples.

amphiaster (am'fĭ-ăs"ter) [" + *astēr* star]. Double star formed during mitosis, *q.v.*

Amphib'ia [G. *amphibios,* double life]. A class of animals which live on land and in water, as salamanders, frogs, etc.

amphiblas'tula [G. *amphi,* both, + *blastula,* little sprout]. A morula formed by unequal segmentation.

amphiblestri'tis [" + *blēstron,* fish net, + *-itis,* inflammation]. Inflammation of retina. SYN: *retinitis.*

amphibo'lia [G. *amphibolos,* doubtful]. The critical or uncertain period of a fever or disease when the outcome cannot be certain.

amphibolic (am-fi-bol'ik). Uncertain; ambiguous.

a. period, or stage. Amphibolia, *q.v.*

amphib'olous. Changeable; amphibolic.

amphicelous (am-fĭ-se'lus) [G. *amphi,* both, + *koilos,* hollow]. Concave on each end, as a vertebrae.

amphicentric (am-fĭ-sen'trik) [" + *kentron,* center]. Centering or converging at both ends.

amphichroic, amphichromatic (am-fĭ-krō'ik, -krō-mat'ik) [" + *chroma,* color]. 1. Turning red litmus paper blue, and blue, red. 2. Reacting both as an acid and an alkali.

amphicra'nia [" + *kranion,* skull]. Pain on both sides of head.

amphicre'atine, amphicreat'inine. A leukomaine formed in muscles.

amphicyte (am'fĭ-sīt) [G. *amphi,* both, + *kytos,* cell]. One of the capsule cells enveloping the bodies of cerebrospinal ganglionic neurons.

amphicyt'ula [" + L. *cytula,* little cell]. Impregnated ovum having unequal segmentation of the vitellus.

amphidiarthrosis (am-fĭ-dī-ar-thrō'sis) [" + *diarthrosis,* articulation]. An articulation with amphiarthrosis and diarthrosis, such as that of the lower jaw.

amphigas'trula [" + L. *gastrula,* little stomach]. The human ovum in advanced gastrula stage.

amphigony (am-fig'ō-nĭ) [" + *gonos,* begetting]. The sexual process of propagation.

amphimixis (am-fi-miks'is) [" + G. *mixis,* mingling]. 1. Mixing of maternal and paternal germ cells in reproduction. 2. PSY: Pregenital energies and mechanisms diverted to the urethra and anus during psychosexual maturity.

am"phimor'ula [" + L. *morula,* little mulberry]. The morula in ovum with unequal composing cells.

amphipyrenin (am"fĭ-pī'ren-in) [" + *pyrenos,* stone of a fruit]. The basophile substance of the nuclear membrane of a cell.

amphithe'atre [" + *theatron,* theater]. An operating room with rising tiers of seats arranged around it for students and other observers.

amphitrichate, amphitrichous (am-fit'rĭ-kāt, -kus) [" + *thrix,* hair]. Pert. to certain organisms having flagella, or a flagellum at both ends.

ampho- [G.]. Prefix: both.

am"phodiplo'pia [G. *amphō,* both, + *diploos,* double, + *ōps,* vision]. Double vision in each eye.

amphojel (am'fō-jĕl). A proprietary name for a suspension of aluminum hydroxide; aluminum hydroxide gel (USP.). Dried aluminum hydroxide gel tablets (USP.) is another dosage form. Used as an antacid.

am"phopep'tone. First peptone formed by tryptic digestion of protein.

amphophil, amphophilous (am'fo-fil, amfof'il-us) [G. *amphō,* both, + *philos,* fond]. Having affinity for acid and/or basic dyes.

amphor'ic [L. *amphora,* jar]. Pert. to a sound as that caused by blowing across the mouth of a bottle; a resonance; a cavernous sound heard on percussion of a pulmonary cavity.

amphoric'ity. Producing amphoric sounds.

amphoriloquy (am-fo-ril'ō-kwē) [L. *amphora,* jar, + *loqui,* to speak]. The presence of amphoric sounds in speaking.

amphoroph'ony [" + G. *phōnē,* voice]. Amphoric voice sound.

amphoter'ic, amphot'erous [G. *amphoteros,* both]. Having properties of both an acid and a base.

a. compounds. Those which may act as a base or an acid, *i. e., protein.*

a. reaction. A double reaction of certain liquids which turn red litmus paper blue, and blue, red.

amphotericin B (am-fō-tĕr'ĭ-sĭn). USP. An antibiotic agent obtained from a strain of *Streptomyces nodosus.* It is used in treatment of deep-seated mycotic infections, being especially effective in North American blastomycosis and histoplasmosis. It has been effective also in cryptococcosis and coccidioidomycosis. The drug is usually administered parenterally.

amphoterism (am-fo'ter-izm). Having both acid and basic properties.

amphot"erodiplo'pia [G. *amphoteros,* both, + *diploos,* double, + *ops,* vision]. Double vision in each eye. SYN: *amphodiplopia.*

amphoton'ic [G. *amphō,* both, + *tonos,* tone]. Pert. to both vagotony and sympathicotony.

amphot'ony [" + *tonos,* tone]. Tonicity of the sympathetic and parasympathetic nervous systems.

ampliation (am-plĭ-ā'shun) [L. *ampliare,* to make wider]. Distention of a part or cavity.

amplifica'tion [L. *amplificare*]. 1. Enlargement of visual area in microscopy. 2. Magnification of sound in telephony.

am'plifier. That which increases magnification of vision or sound.

am'plitude [L. *amplitudo*]. 1. Amount, extent, size, abundance or fullness. 2. PHYSICS: Extent of movement, as of a pendulum or sound wave. The maximum displacement of a particle, as that of a string vibrating as measured from the mean to the extreme.

ampule (am'pūl) [L. *ampulla*]. A small glass that can be sealed and its contents sterilized. This is a French invention for containing hypodermic solutions. SYN: *ampoule; ampul.*

ampul'la (pl. *ampullae*) [L. little jar]. 1. Sac-like dilatation of a canal or duct, as the semicircular canals or ductus deferens, *q.v.* 2. A small, hermetically sealed flask containing a solution for parenteral use; an ampule.

a. ductus deferens. An irregular and nodular dilatation of the vas deferens just before its junction with the excretory duct of the seminal vesicle.

a. of lacrimal duct. The slight dilatation of the lacrimal duct medial to the punctum.

a. of rectum. Slight dilatation of rectum proper just before continuing as anal canal. Also called infraperitoneal portion of rectum proper.

a. of semicircular canal. A dilatation at end of semicircular canal which houses an ampulla of a semicircular duct.

a. of semicircular ducts. Dilatation of semicircular ducts near their junction with the utricle. In their walls are the crista ampullares.

a. of uterine tube. The dilated distal end of a uterine tube terminating in a funnel-like infundibulum.

a. of vas deferens. A. ductus deferens.

a. of Vater. The duodenal end of the drainage systems of the pancreatic and common bile ducts. Although in common usage, the name is being discarded in favor of the more accurate *papilla of Vater.*

ampulli'tis [" + G. *-itis,* inflammation]. Inflammation of any ampulla, esp. of *ductus deferens.*

amputation (am-pū-tā'shun) [L. *ambi,* around, + *putāre,* to trim]. Surgical removal of a diseased member, part, or organ.

a., congenital. A. of parts of the fetus in utero, believed formerly to be caused by constricting bands but now believed to be a developmental defect.

a. in contiguity. A. at a joint.

a. in continuity. A. elsewhere than at a joint.

a., double flap. A. in which two flaps of soft tissue are formed.

a., primary. Before inflammation sets in.

a., secondary. During period of suppuration.

a., spontaneous. Nonsurgical separation of an extremity or digit. SEE: *ainhum.*

a., tertiary. A. performed following abatement of inflammatory reaction.

amuck' [Malay *amoq,* furious]. State of murderous frenzy. SYN: *amok.*

amusia (a-mu'sĭ-ă) [G. *amousos,* unmusical]. Music-deafness; inability to produce or comprehend music, as loss of the ability to play a musical instrument. ETIOL: Brain lesion, but cause not clearly understood.

a., motor. That in which music is understood, but without ability to produce by singing or otherwise.

a., sensory. Music deafness. Inability to understand the sounds of music.

Amussat's operation (am-ū-sāz'). Surgical formation of an artificial anus, by lumbar colotomy in ascending colon.

amychophobia (ă-mī-kō-fō'bĭ-ă) [G. *amychē,* scratch, + *phobos,* fear]. PSY: Morbid fear of being scratched; fear of the claws of any animal.

amyctic (a-mik'tik) [G. *amyktikos,* mangling]. 1. Irritating, caustic. 2. A caustic or corrosive agent.

amyelencephalia (ă-mī"ĕl-ĕn-sĕf-ā'lē-ă) [*a-,* + G. *myelos,* marrow, + *enkephalos,* brain, + *ia*]. Congenital malformation consisting of absence of brain and spinal cord.

amyelia (ă-mī-ĕ-lē'ă) [" + " + *ia*]. Absence of spinal cord.

amyeloneuria (ă-mī-el-ō-nū'rĭ-ă) [G. *a-,* priv. + *myelos,* marrow, + *neuron,* nerve]. Spinal cord paresis.

amyelotrophy (ă-mī-el-ot'rō-fĭ) [G. *a-,* priv. + *myelos,* marrow, + *atrophia,* atrophy]. Spinal cord atrophy.

amygdala (ă-mig'dă-lă) (pl. *amygdalae*) [L. from G. *amygdalē,* an almond]. 1. A mass of gray matter in the anterior portion of the temporal lobe. 2. Obsolete term for the tonsil.

amygdalectomy (ă-mig-dă-lek'tō-mĭ) [" + G. *ektomē,* excision]. Excision of a tonsil. NP: SEE: *tonsillectomy.*

amygdalin (a-mig'da-lĭn). A bitter tasting glucoside in bitter almonds and cherry laurel leaves. Used as a flavoring agent.

amygdaline (a-mĭg'dă-lĭn, -līn). 1. Pert. to a tonsil. 2. Pert. to or shaped like an almond. SYN: *amygdaloid.*

amygdalitis (a-mig-da-lī'tis) [L. *amygdala,* almond, + G. *-itis,* inflammation]. Inflammation of a tonsil; tonsillitis.

amygdaloid (a-mig'da-loid) [" + G. *eidos,* resemblance]. Resembling a tonsil or an almond.

a. fossa. A depression for the tonsil.

a. tubercle. A projection from the middle cornu of the lateral ventricle, marking area of the amygdaloid nucleus.

amygdalolith (a-mig'dă-lō-lith) [" + G. *lithos,* stone]. Stone in a distended crypt of a tonsil.

amygdalop'athy [" + G. *pathos,* suffering]. Any disease of a tonsil.

amygdalothrypsis (a-mig"dal-o-thrip'sis) [" + G. *thrypsis,* a crushing]. Crushing of a tonsil followed by excision.

amygdalotome (a-mig-dal'ō-tōm) [" + G. *tomē,* a cutting]. Instrument for excision of a tonsil.

amyl (am'il) [L. *amylum,* starch, + G. *ylē,* material]. A hypothetical univalent radical, C_5H_{11}, nonexistent in a free state.

a. nitrite. USP. $C_5H_{11}NO_2$. A volatile and highly flammable, clear liquid. Used as a vasodilator especially for anginal pain.

amyla'ceous. Starchy.

amylase (am'ĭ-lās) [L. *amylum,* starch, + G. *-asis,* pert. to a colloid enzyme]. A ferment or amylolytic enzyme of the saliva, pancreatic juice and intestinal juice that hydrolyzes starch, producing achroödextrin and maltose. These products are later acted upon by the maltase of the intestines and converted into dextrose before absorption.

Amylase is more powerful than ptyalin and it acts on uncooked as well as cooked starch. SEE: *antiamylase; enzymes.*

a., pancreatic. Amylopsin, *q.v.*

a., salivary. Ptyalin, *q.v.*

a., vegetable. Diastase, *q.v.*

amyle'mia [" + G. *aima,* blood]. Hypothetical presence of starch in the blood.

amylin (am'il-in). 1. Part of starch soluble in water. 2. A monacid base. The group C.NH.NH_2. SYN: *amidin*

amylodex'trin [L. *amylum,* starch, + dextrin]. Soluble substance produced during the change of starch into sugar.

amylodyspep'sia [" + G. *dys,* bad, + *pepsis,* digestion]. Inability to digest starchy foods.

amylogen (am-il'ō-jen) [" + G. *gennan,* to produce]. Soluble starch.

amylogenesis (am-i-lō-jen'ĕ-sis) [" + G. *genesis,* production]. The production of starch.

amylogenic (am-il-ō-jen'ik) [" + G. *gennan,* to produce]. Starch-producing.

am'yloid [" + G. *eidos,* resemblance]. 1. Resembling starch; starchlike. 2. A protein complex having starchlike characteristics produced and deposited in tissues during certain pathologic states.

It is a homogeneous, highly refractile substance staining readily with Congo red.

a. degeneration. That of organs or tissues from deposition of amyloid. Structures are waxy and translucent, having hyaline appearance. Liver, spleen and kidneys most involved but any tissue may be infiltrated.

a. disease. Amyloidosis.

a. kidney. Enlarged, firm, smooth kidney usually associated with amyloid diseases of spleen or liver.

ETIOL: Found in long continued bone suppuration or may be due to syphilis.

SYM: Face pale, waxy skin which may be edematous. Liver and spleen may also be enlarged. Not tender under pressure. Diarrhea if intestines are involved. Albumin, hyaline, and waxy casts in urine.

a. nephrosis. A nephrotic syndrome from myeloid degeneration of kidney.

amyloido'sis. A metabolic disorder marked by deposition of amyloid in organs and tissue. Thought to be the result of disturbed endogenous protein metabolism.

a., lichen. A form limited to the skin.

a., localized. That in which isolated amyloid tumors are formed.

a., secondary. That associated with chronic suppuration and tissue necrosis, as in tuberculosis, syphilis, Hodgkin's disease, rheumatoid arthritis, and in extensive tissue destruction. Spleen, liver, kidneys, and adrenal cortex most frequently involved.

amylolysis (am-il-ol'ĭ-sis) [" + G. *lysis*, solution]. Changing of starch into sugar in the process of digestion.

amylolytic (am-il-ō-lit'ik). Pertaining to the digestion of starches or their conversion into simple sugars (amylolysis, *q.v.*).

a. enzyme. A ferment that hydrolyzes starch, producing achroödextrin and maltose. SYN: *amylase.*

amylophagia (ăm-ĭ-lō-fā'jē-ă). Abnormal craving for starch.

amylop'sin [L. *amylum*, starch, + G. *opsis*, appearance]. Diastatic enzyme in pancreatic juice which changes starch into achroödextrin and maltose. SEE: *digestion; duodenum; enzymes.*

amylose (am'i-lōs). A group of carbohydrates containing starch, cellulose, and dextrin. SEE: *saccharose.*

amylosis (am-i-lō'sis) [G. *amylon*, starch]. Albuminoid degeneration of the cells.

amylosu'ria [*amylose* + G. *ouron*, urine]. Amylose in the urine.

amylum (am-i'lum) [L.]. USP. Starch; corn starch. Used as dusting powder.

amylu'ria [L. *amylum*, starch, + G. *ouron*, urine]. Starch in the urine.

amyocardia (ă-mī-ō-kar'dĭ-ă) [G. *a-*, priv. + *mys*, muscle, + *kardia*, heart]. Weakness of the heart muscle. SYN: *myasthenia cordis.*

amyostasia (a-mī-ō-stā'sĭ-ă) [" + " + *stasis*, standing]. Difficulty in standing because of lack of coordination or because of muscular tremors. SEE: *tremor.*

amyosthenia (a-mī-os-thē'nĭ-ă) [" + " + *sthenos*, strength]. Lack of muscular tone or power.

amyosthen'ic. Pert. to muscular weakness.

amyotaxy (a-mī-ō-taks'ĭ) [G. *a-*, priv. + *mys*, muscle, + *taxis*, order]. Muscular ataxia.

amyotonia (a-mī-ō-tō'nĭ-ă) [" + " + *tonos*, tone]. Deficiency or lack of muscular tone.

a. congenita. A non-inherited but sometimes familial disease characterized by absence of muscular development, with the lower extremities being the first involved. It is first seen at, or shortly after, birth. SYN: *Oppenheim's disease; myatonia congenita.*

amyotrophia (ă-mī-ō-trō'fĭ-a) [" + " + *trophē*, nourishment]. Muscular wasting.

a., progressive spinal. Progressive muscular atrophy.

amyotrophic (a-mī-ō-trof'ik). Pert. to atrophy.

a. lateral sclerosis. A syndrome marked by muscular weakness and atrophy with spasticity and hyperreflexia due to degeneration of motor neurons of spinal cord, medulla, and cortex. Prognosis is very poor. If only cells of motor cranial nuclei in the medulla are involved, condition is called progressive bulbar palsy.

amyotrophy (am-i-ot'rō-fĭ). Muscular wasting. SYN: *amyotrophia.*

amyous (am'ĭ-ŭs) [G. *a-*, priv. + *mys*, muscle]. 1. Congenitally lacking in muscular tissue. 2. Weak; deficient in muscular strength. 3. Without muscle; fleshless.

amytal (am'it-al). Proprietary name for amobarbital (USP.). It is used as an analgesic sedative, and as a hypnotic for preanesthetic medication.

amyxia (ă-miks'ĭ-a) [G. *a-*, priv. + *myxa*, mucus]. Deficient mucous secretion.

amyxorrhea (ă-miks-ō-rĭ'ă) [" + " + *roia*, flow]. Lack of normal secretion of mucus.

an- [G.]. Prefix: negative; without or not, as *anemia.*

An. Chem. symb. for *actinon;* abbr. for *anisometropia* and *anode.*

A. N. A. Abbr. *American Nurses Association.*

ana (an'ă) [G.]. Meaning "one of each"; used in writing prescriptions as āā. SEE: *prescription.*

anab'asis [G. *anabainein*, to go up]. Period of increased severity in a disease.

anabatic (an-ă-bat'ik). Increased severity; pert. to anabasis.

anabio'sis [G. *ana*, again, + *bios*, life]. Revival of a body which seemed lifeless. SYN: *resuscitation.*

anabiotic (an-ă-bi-ot'ik). Restorative. Any agent that resuscitates or restores.

anabol'ic. Promoting or pert. to anabolism.

a. nerve. Nerve controlling building processes.

anab'olin. A product of anabolism. SYN: *anabolite.*

anabolism (an-ab'ō-lizm) [G. *anabolē*, a building up]. The building up of the body substance; the constructive or synthetic chemical reactions included in metabolism; a process by which a cell takes from the blood the substance required for repair and growth, building it into a cytoplasm, thus converting a nonliving material into the living cytoplasm of the cell.

RS: *assimilation, catabolism, metabolism, nutrition, synthesis.*

anab'olite. Any product of anabolism. SYN: *anabolin.*

anabrosis (an-ă-brō'sis) [G. an eating up]. Superficial ulceration of soft tissue.

anacamp'tics [G. *anakamptein*, to bend back]. Study of reflection of light or sound.

anacamptometer (an-ă-camp-tom'ĕ-ter) [" + *metron*, measure]. Device for measuring reflexes.

anacatharsis (an-ă-kă-thar'sĭs) [G. *anakatharsis,* upward cleansing]. Vomiting; expectoration.

anacathar'tic. That which causes vomiting.

anachlorhydria (an-ă-klor-hīd'rĭ-ă). Decreased amount of free hydrochloric acid in the gastric juice.

anacidity (an-ă-sid'ĭ-tĭ). Abnormal lack or deficiency of acidity.

anaclasim'eter [G. *anaklasis,* refraction, + *metron,* measure]. Instrument for measuring refraction of eyes.

anaclisis (an-ak'lĭ-sis) [G. *anaklisis,* a lying back]. 1. Reclining. 2. State of being emotionally dependent upon another.

anaclit'ic choice. An early expression of psychosexual development, in which the object of one's love is influenced by dependence upon the mother or whoever is responsible for the child's early care, more or less inhibiting other expressions of the sex instinct. Opp. to narcissism, *q.v.*

anacroasia (an-ă-krō-ă'sĭ-ă) [G. *an-,* priv. + *akroasis,* hearing]. Inability to understand spoken words.

anacrotic (an-ă-krot'ik) [G. *ana,* up, + *krotos,* stroke]. 1. Pert. to a pulse with more than one expansion of the artery. 2. Pert. to two heartbeats traced on the ascending line of a sphygmogram. SYN: *anadicrotic.* SEE: *pulse.*

a. ***limb.*** Ascending or vertical upstroke of a sphygmogram.

a. ***pulse.*** One in which one or more small waves occur on ascending limb of tracing of pulse wave, as in aortic stenosis.

anac'rotism Existence of a double beat on ascending line of sphygmogram. SYN: *anadicrotism.*

anacusia, anacu'sis (an-ak-oo'sĭ-ă, -sis) [G. *an,* priv. + *kusis,* hearing]. Complete deafness.

anadenia (an-ă-dē'nĭ-ă) [" + *aden,* gland]. 1. Absence of glands. 2. Reduced glandular function.

anadicrot'ic. 1. Pert. to a pulse with more than one artery expansion. 2. Pert. to two heartbeats traced on the ascending line of a sphygmogram. SYN: *anacrotic.*

anadicrotism (an-ă-dik'ro-tizm) [G. *ana,* up, + *dikrotos,* double beating] Existence of a double beat on ascending line of the sphygmogram. SYN: *anacrotism.*

anadidymus (an-a-did'ĭ-mus) [G. *ana,* up, + *didymos,* twin]. A fetal monster divided above and united below.

anadipsia (an-ă-dip'sĭ-ă) [G. *ana,* intensive, + *dipsa,* thirst]. Intense thirst.

anadrenalism (an-ă-drē'nal-ism). Absence or failure of adrenal function. SYN: *hypodrenalism.*

anaerobe (an-ā'er-ōb) [G. *an,* priv. + *aer,* air, + *bios,* life]. A microorganism which thrives best or lives only without oxygen.

a., ***facultative.*** An organism showing preference for free oxygen yet capable of growing in its absence.

a., ***obligatory.*** Organism growing only in absence of free oxygen.

anaerob'ic. Having the power to use oxygen for metabolism from oxygen compounds; having the ability to live without air as some microbes.

anaerobiosis (an-a-er-ō-bī-ō'sis). 1. Life in an oxygen-free atmosphere. 2. Functioning of an organ or tissue in absence of free oxygen.

anaerobiotic (an-a-er-o-bi-ot'ik). Able to exist without free oxygen.

anagnosasthenia (an"ag-nōs-as-thē'nĭ-ă) [G. *anagnōsis,* reading, + *astheneia,* weakness]. Distressing symptoms when trying to read due to neurosis rather than organic disease of the eye.

anagoge, anagogy (an-ă-go'je) [G. *anagōgē,* a leading up]. PSY: Spiritual, moral or idealistic phases of thought.

anakatadidymus (an-ă-kat-ă-dĭd'ĭ-mus) [G. *ana,* up, + *kata,* down, + *didymos,* twin]. A fetal monster divided above and below but joined in the middle.

anakatesthe'sia [" + " + *aisthēsis,* sensation]. A sensation as of hovering or bearing down upon one.

anaku'sis. Complete deafness. SYN: *anacusia.*

anal (ā'nal) [L. *anus,* a ring]. Rel. to the anus or outer rectal opening.

a. ***canal.*** The terminal portion of the large intestine, its external aperture being the anus. This is protected by an internal and external sphincter muscle, and remains closed except during defecation. It is about 2.5 to 4 cm. (1½ inches) long.

a. ***character.*** PSY: A pattern of adult behavior characterized by excessive orderliness, stinginess, and obstinacy. If carried to an extreme, these qualities lead to the development of obsessive-compulsive type of behavior.

a. ***erotism.*** Stage in pregenital libido in which pleasurable sensations are experienced in the anal region.

a. ***reflex.*** Contraction of anal sphincter following irritation of skin about anus. Reflex is lost in lesions of posterior columns of cord and is exaggerated in anal fissures.

analepsis (an-ă-lĕp'sis) [G.*analēpsis,* a taking up]. Gaining strength after an illness. Restoration to health. 2. Epilepsy accompanied by gastric aura. 3. Suspension as in a swing.

analeptic (an-a-lep'tik) [G. *analēptikos,* restorative]. 1. A drug used to stimulate the central nervous system. Used especially in treatment of poisoning by drugs which depress the central nervous system, such as the barbiturates. 2. A restorative agent.

analgesia (an-al-jē'zĭ-ă) [G.*an-,* priv. + *algos,* pain]. Absence of normal sense of pain.

a. ***algera,*** *a.* ***dolorosa.*** Severe pain with loss of sensitivity in a part.

a., ***paretic.*** Complete a. of upper limb, in conjunction with partial paralysis.

analgesic (an-al-jē'sik). A medicine which relieves pain.

analgetic (an-al-jĕt'ik). Analgesic; producing freedom from pain, or an agent that lessens pain.

analgia (an-al'jĭ-ă) [G. *an-,* priv. + *algos,* pain]. State of being without pain.

analgic (an-al'jik). Without pain.

analogue (an'a-log) [G. *analogōs,* proportionate]. An organ or part similar in function, but differing in structure.

analogy (an-al'ō-jĭ). 1. Likeness or similarity between two things which otherwise are unlike. 2. In biology, similarity in function, but different in structure or embryonic origin. Opp. to homology.

analysand (an-al'ĭ-zand). PSY: A patient who is being psychoanalyzed.

analysis (ă-năl'ĭ-sĭs) [G. *analysis,* a dissolving]. 1. Separation of anything into its constituent parts. 2. CHEM: Determination of, or separation into, its constituent parts of a substance or compound. 3. PSY: Treatment by a physician trained as a psychoanalyst.

a., chromatographic. Separation of substances on the basis of color reaction of the constituents as they are differentially absorbed on one of a variety of materials, such as filter paper.

a., colorimetric. The separation, by adsorption, of a compound and the identification of its elements by color.

a., densimetric. A. by determination of the specific gravity (density) of a solution, and then estimation of the amount of solids.

a., gastric. A. of the stomach contents to determine the concentration of free hydrochloric acid and combined (total) acid, presence or absence of lactic acid, presence or absence of occult blood, presence of pus and excessive mucus, and amount and types of bacteria.

a., qual'itative. Determining the nature of the elements in a substance.

a., quantita'tive. Determining the nature and the quantity of elements in a substance.

a., spectrophotometric. Determination of the presence of materials in a compound by measuring amount of light they absorb in the infrared, visible, or ultraviolet regions of the spectrum.

a., spectrum. Analysis of substances by use of a spectroscope.

a., volumetric. Quantitative analysis performed by the measurement of the volume of solutions or liquids.

analyst (an'ă-list). 1. One who analyzes. 2. In psychiatry, a psychoanalyst.

analytic (an-ă-lit'ik). Pert. to any analysis.

analyze (an'a-līz). To make an analysis.

anamnesis (an-am-nē'sis) [G. *anamimnēskein*, to recall to memory]. 1. Recollection; faculty of remembering. 2. That which is remembered. 3. The personal and case history of a patient and his family history. SEE: *catamnesis*.

anamnes'tic. 1. Pert. to previous medical history of patient. 2. Assisting the memory.

anamniot'ic [G. *an-*, priv. + *amnion*]. Without an amnion.

ananabasia (an-an-a-bā'zĭ-ă) [G. *an-*, priv. + *anabasis*, an ascending]. An abulia (loss of will) in which the person seems unable to ascend heights.

ananaphylaxis (an-an-ă-fi-lak'sis) [G. *an*, priv. + *a-*, priv. + *phylaxis*, protection]. That which neutralizes anaphylaxis, *q.v.*

ananastasia (an-an-a-stā'zĭ-ă) [G. *an-*, priv. + *anastasis*, a rising up]. An abulia in which the person is unable to rise from a sitting position.

anandria (an-an'drĭ-ă) [" + *aner-*, *andr-*, man]. Impotence; lack in virility.

anangiopla'sia [" + *aggeion*, vessel, + *plassein*, to form]. Imperfect vascularization of a part.

anangioplas'tic. Pert. to imperfect development of the vascular system.

anapeiratic (an-ă-pī-rat'ik) [G. *anapeirasthai*, to try again]. Pert. to a nervous affection arising from excessive muscular activity, as an occupational neurosis.

a. cramp. One arising from excessive muscular activity.

a. c., cyclist's. Pain in scrotum, perineum, and thighs from excessive bicycling.

a. c., occupational. Writer's cramp.

a. c., professional. Spasmodic disorder affecting groups of muscles used in special work or movements.

anaphalantiasis (an"ă-phal-an-ti'ă-sis) [G. *ana*, up, + *phalanthos*, front baldness] Loss of hair of the eyebrow.

anaphase (an'a-fāz) [G. *ana*, up, + *phainein*, to appear]. Stage in mitosis between metaphase in which longitudinal halves of chromosomes (the chromatids) separate and move toward their respective poles.

anaphia (an-ă'fĭ-ă, an-ăf'ĭ-ă) [G. *an-*, priv. + *aphē*, touch]. 1. Abnormal sensitiveness to touch. 2. Loss or diminished sense of touch. 3. Palpation that reveals no diagnosis.

anaphoresis (an-ă-for-ē'sis) [" + *phoresis*, sweating]. 1. Insufficient activity of the sweat glands. 2. Transmission of electropositive bodies into tissues by passage of electric current, the flow toward the positive pole.

anaphoria (an-ă-for'ĭ-ă) [G. *ana*, up, + *phorein*, to carry]. Tendency of eyeballs to turn upward. SYN: *anatropia*.

anaphrodisia (an-af-rō-diz'ĭ-ă [G. *an-*, priv. + *Aphroditē*, goddess of love]. Diminished or absent sex desire.

anaphrodis'iac. An agent that will depress the sexual function.

anaphrodite (an-af'rō-dīt). One with an impairment of sexual desire or with an absence of it.

anaphylactia (an-ă-fĭ-lak-shĭ-ă) [G. *an*, again, + *a-*, priv. + *phylaxis*, protection]. Any anaphylactic condition.

anaphylactic (an-ă-fĭ-lak'tik). 1. Pertaining or relating to anaphylaxis. 2. Denoting increased activity to agents which are innocuous to others.

a. shock. State of collapse resulting from injection of a substance to which an animal has become sensitized. SEE: *anaphylaxis*.

anaphylactin (an-ă-fĭ-lak'tin). The substances supposed to produce hypersusceptibility following injection of a foreign protein.

anaphylac'togen [G. *an*, again, + *a*, priv. + *phylaxis*, protection, + *gennan*, to produce]. That which produces anaphylaxis or anaphylactin. SYN: *allergen*.

anaphylactogen'esis. The process of producing anaphylaxis.

anaphylactogenic (an-ă-fĭ-lak-tō-jen'ik). Producing anaphylaxis or the agent producing anaphylactic reactions.

anaphylatoxin (an-ă-fĭl-ă-toks'in) [*anaphylaxis* + G *toxikon*, poison]. The poisonous element in anaphylaxis.

anaphylatox'is. Anaphylatoxic reaction.

anaphylaxis (an-ă-fĭ-laks'is) [G. *an*, again, + *a-*, priv. + *phylaxis*, protection]. A condition produced artificially and experimentally in lower animals and dependent upon well defined antigen-antibody reaction.

A hypersensitive state of the body to a foreign protein or a drug, so that the injection of a second dose in 10 to 12 days brings about an acute reaction; known also as *protein sensitization* and *serum sickness*. The term implies symptoms severe enough to produce serious shock.

The reactions which constitute anaphylactic shock occur suddenly. They include increased irritability, dyspnea, cyanosis, sometimes convulsions, unconsciousness and death. Reactions primarily due to contraction of smooth muscle fibers and increased permeability of endothelia of capillaries. Death usually results from spasm of muscles of bronchioles.

Such diseases as asthma, hay fever, urticaria (hives) are thought to be of an anaphylactic nature, being caused by the irritation of a food or by the pollen of some plants and flowers, to which the individual may have become sensitized. Sometimes marked a. follows a blood transfusion. Serum sickness is an anaphylactic reaction which occasionally follows injection of foreign serums, especially horse serum.

SYM: (a).. *Mild a.*: Fever (slight), redness of skin, itching, urticaria. (b) *Severe a.*: Dyspnea, violent cough, chest constriction, cyanosis, fever, skin eruption, pulse variations, convulsions. collapse.

PROG: In mild cases, favorable; symptoms are self-limited. In severe cases, death may occur if emergency treatment is not given.

TREATMENT: Vasopressor agents, esp. epinephrine; corticosteroids; oxygen, artificial respiration.

NP: Oxygen inhalations, treatment for shock.

a., active. That resulting from injection of an antigen.

a., heterologous. Passive anaphylaxis by transfer of serum from an animal of a different species.

a., homologous. Passive anaphylaxis by transfer of serum from an animal of the same species.

a., local. Local inflammatory reaction following repeated injections of antigenic material. SYN: *Arthus phenomenon.*

a., passive. That induced by injection of serum from a sensitized animal into a normal one. After a few hours the latter becomes sensitized.

anaplasia (an-ă-plā'zĭ-ă) [G. *ana*, again, + *plasis*, a molding]. 1. Reversion of cells to a more embryonic type. 2. Alteration in cells which is believed, by some authorities, to produce malignancy.

anaplas'tic. Pert. to anaplasia or restoration of lost part.

anaplasty (an'a-plas-tĭ) [G. *ana*, again, + *plassein*, to form]. Grafting or restoring lost parts.

anaplero'sis [G. *anaplērōsis*, a filling up]. Surgical transplantation of tissue to fill a defect.

anapnea (an-ap-nē'ă) [G. *anapnein*, to breathe again]. 1. Respiration. 2. Regaining the breath.

anapneic (an-ap-nē'ik). Pert. to anapnea or relieving dyspnea.

anapnograph (an-ap'nō-graf). An instrument for measuring pressure and rate of respiration. SYN: *spirograph.*

anapnoic (an-ap-nō'ik). 1. Pert. to anapnea. 2. Relieving dyspnea.

anapnom'eter [G. *anapnoē*, respiration, + *metron*, measure]. Instrument for measuring respiratory movements. SYN: *spirometer, q.v.*

anapnother'apy [" + *therapeia*, treatment]. Inhalation therapy.

anapophysis (an-ă-pof'ĭ-sis) [G. *ana*, back, + *apophysis*, offshoot]. An accessory spinal process of a vertebra.

anap'tic [G. *an-*, priv. + *aptein*, to touch]. Pert. to anaphia or diminished or lost tactile sense.

anarithmia (an-ă-rith'mĭ-ă) [" + *arithmos*, enumeration]. Inability to count or to use numbers. ETIOL: Brain lesion.

anarthria (an-ar'thrĭ-ă) [" + *arthron*, joint]. Loss of motor power to speak distinctly. May be a result of a neural lesion or a muscular apparatus defect.

a. centralis. Partial aphasia caused by a lesion of the central nervous system.

a. literalis. Stammering.

anasarca (an-ă-sar'kă) [G. *ana*, throughout, + *sarx, sarkos*, flesh]. Severe generalized edema. SEE: *edema.*

anasarcous (an-ă-sar'kus). Dropsical; edematous.

anaspadias (an-ă-spa'dĭ-ăs) [G. *ana*, up, + *span*, to draw]. Epispadias, *q.v.*

anastal'tic [G. *anastaltikos*, checking]. 1. Very astringent. 2. Afferent.

anastasis (ă-nas'tă-sis) [G. a rising up]. 1. Return to health. 2. Resuscitation.

anastate (an'as-tāt). Anything characteristic of an anabolic process.

anastole (an-as'to-lē) [G. *anastolē*, laying bare a wound]. Shrinking away or retraction of the lips of a wound.

anastomose (a-nas'to-mōs) [G. *anastomōsis*, opening]. 1. Opening of one vessel into another, or the union of one nerve with another. 2. To make such a connection, surgically.

anastomosis (an-as-to-mo'sis) [G. opening]. 1. A communication between two vessels. 2. The surgical or pathologic formation of a passage between any two normally distinct spaces or organs. 3. An end-to-end union or joining together or intercommunication of parts of any network or set of fibers such as nerves, or connective tissue fibers.

a., antiperistaltic. Enterostomy in which the two parts are so joined that the peristaltic wave in one part proceeds in a direction opposite to the other.

a., arteriovenous. Anastomosis between an artery and a vein.

a., collateral. A natural one, as that of the arteries at knee joint.

a., crucial. An arterial anastomosis on the back of the thigh, formed by the medial femoral circumflex, inferior gluteal, lateral femoral circumflex, and first perforating arteries.

a., Galen's. The anastomosis between the sup. and inf. laryngeal nerves.

a., heterocladic. Anastomosis between branches of different arteries.

a., homocladic. Anastomosis between branches of the same artery.

a., Hyrtl's. An occasional looplike anastomosis bet. right and left hypoglossal nerves in geniohyoid muscle.

a., intestinal. The establishment of a communication between two portions of the intestines. SYN: *enterostomy.*

a., isoperistaltic. Intestinal anastomosis in which the two parts are so joined that the peristaltic wave in each part is in the same direction.

a., Jacobson's. The union of a nerve from the petrous ganglion with the Vidian nerve, or with the tympanic branch of the glossopharyngeal.

a., precapillary. Anastomosis between small arteries just before they become capillaries.

a., Schmidel's. Abnormal communications between the vena cava and the portal system.

a., terminoterminal. Anastomosis between the peripheral end of an artery and the central end of the corresponding vein, and between the central end of the artery and peripheral end of vein.

a., ureterotubal. An anastomosis between the ureter and the fallopian tube.

anastomot'ic. Pert. to, or marked by, anastomosis.

anatherapeusis (an-ă-ther"ă-pū'sis) [G. *ana*, up, + *therapeia*, treatment]. Treatment by steadily increasing doses.

anatomic (an-ă-tom'ik) [G. *anatomnein*, to cut up]. Of or rel. to the anatomy or structure of an organism.

anatomist (an-at'ō-mist). An individual skilled in anatomy.

anatomy (an-at'ō-mĭ) [G. *ana,* up, + *temnein,* to cut]. 1. The structure or study of structure of organisms or a treatise on same. 2. Dissection or cutting apart.

a., applied. That applied to diagnosis and treatment, esp. surgical treatment.

a., comparative. Comparison of structure of different animals.

a., descriptive. Study of individual parts of physical structure.

a., gross. Study of structures seen with the naked eye. SYN: *macroscopic anatomy.*

a., microscopic. Study of structure by use of a microscope. SYN: *histology.*

a., morbid or pathological. That of abnormal structure.

a., surface. Study of form and markings of the structure of the body, especially as they relate to underlying tissues and organs.

anat'opism [G. *ana,* without, + *topos,* place]. Inability to conform to social usage.

anatoxic (an-a-toks'ik) [G. *ana,* priv. + *toxikon,* poison]. 1. Pert. to anatoxin. 2. Anaphylactic.

anatoxin (an-a-toks'in) [G. *ana,* priv. + *toxikon,* poison]. A modified toxin retaining the antigenic properties with lessened toxic properties.

anatricrotic pulse (an-a-trī-krot'ik) [G. *ana,* up, + *treis,* three, + *krotos,* stroke]. Three beats on the ascending curve of a pulse wave.

anatripsis (an-a-trip'sis) [G. friction]. 1. A centripetal or upward movement in massage. 2. Inunction. Rubbing or removing by scraping. 3. Crushing as of a stone.

anatriptic (an-ă-trip'tik). An agent to be rubbed in.

anatro'pia [G. *ana,* up, + *tropē,* a turning]. Tendency of eyeballs to turn upward; anaphoria.

anaxon(e (an-aks'on) [G. *an-,* priv. + *axon,* axis]. A nerve cell, as of the retina, having no neuraxon.

anazoturia (an-az-ō-tu'rĭ-ă) [" + *a-,* priv. + *zōē,* life, + G. *ouron,* urine]. Without urea or nitrogenous substances in the urine.

ANC. Abbr. for *Army Nurse Corps.*

AnCC. Abbr. for *anodal closure contraction.*

anchone (ang-kō'nē) [G. *agchein,* to strangle]. Spasm of the throat in hysteria.

anchorage (ang'kĕr-ij). 1. Operative fixation of displaced viscus. 2. The part to which anything is fixed, as a tooth to which a bridge is fastened.

anconad (ang'ko-nad) [G. *ankōn,* elbow, + L. *ad,* to]. Toward the elbow.

anconagra (ang-ko-nag'ră) [" + *agra,* a seizure]. Gout of the elbow.

anconal, anconeal (ang'ko-nal, ang-kō'-nē-al). Pert. to the elbow.

a. fossa. Fossa olecrani.

anconeus (an-kō'nē-us) [G. *ankōn,* elbow]. Short extensor muscle of forearm located on the back of the elbow. It arises from the back portion of the lateral epicondyle of the humerus, and its fibers insert on side of the olecranon and upper fourth of shaft of ulna. Assists in extension of the elbow.

anconitis (ang-kō-nī'tis) [" + *-itis,* inflammation]. Inflammation of the elbow joint.

Ancylostoma (an-sil-os'tō-mă) [G. *agkylos,* crooked, + *stoma,* mouth]. A genus of nematodes of the family Ancylostomatidae including the hookworms. SEE ALSO: *Necator americanus.*

A. braziliense. Species of hookworm infesting dogs and cats, larvae of which may cause creeping eruption in man.

A. caninum. Species of hookworm infesting dogs and cats. Its larvae may cause creeping eruption in man.

A. duodenale. The Old World hookworm; commonly infests man causing ancylostomiasis, *q.v.* Primarily a parasite of southern Europe, North Africa and the Far East. Adult male hookworms average 8-11 mm. in length, and females 10-13 mm. Buccal capsule of the worm contains two pairs of teeth.

Ancylostomatidae (ăn-sĭ-lŏs"tō-măt'ĭ-dē). A family of nematodes belonging to the suborder Strongylata. It includes the genera *Ancylostoma* and *Necator,* common hookworms of man.

ancylostomiasis (ăn-kĭ-lŏs-tō-mī'ă-sĭs). Infestation by the hookworm, *Ancylostoma duodenale,* in the preintestinal phase. Infecting larvae enter through the skin of the bare foot of a person and cause ground itch or water sore characterized by inflammation, itching, and sometimes allergic reactions. Passing from the skin through the lungs, larvae may predispose to pulmonary infections, or if larvae are numerous, pneumonia or pneumonia-like symptoms may occur. In intestines, may cause nausea, colicky pains and diarrhea. Loss of blood leads to anemia; and, in children, normal mental and physical growth is retarded.

Ancyclostomiasis, known as hookworm disease, is common in tropical and semitropical areas where the climate, plus poor sanitation and damp earth, brings the larvae in contact with bare skin, usually of the foot.

ancyroid (an'sir-oid) [G. *ankyra,* anchor, + *eidos,* resemblance]. Shaped like fluke of an anchor.

Andernach's ossicles (ăn'der-năkh). Small bones found in cranial sutures. SYN: *Wormian bones.*

Anders' disease [James W. Anders, Philadelphia physician, 1854-1936]. One in which fat occurs in painful nodules. SYN: *adiposis tuberosa simplex.*

An'dersch's ganglion. Ganglion petrosum.

A.'s nerve. Tympanic nerve.

An'dral's decu'bitus [Gabriel Andral, French physician, 1797-1876]. Lying on sound side during beginning of pleurisy.

andrase (an'drāz) [G. *andrōs,* man, + *ase*]. The hypothetical substance determining male sex. Opp. of *gynase.*

andriat'rics [" + *iatreia,* medical treatment]. Study of diseases of male genitals.

andro- (an'drō) [G. *anēr,* man]. A prefix signifying man, male, or masculine.

androcyte (an'drō-sīt). A spherical cell produced by division of a secondary spermatocyte which develops into the spermatozoon.

androgalactozemia (an-dro-gal-ak-to-ze'-mĭ-ă) [" + *gala,* milk, + *zemia,* loss]. Oozing of milk from male breast.

androgen (ăn'drō-jĕn) [" + *gennan,* to produce]. Substance producing or stimulating male characteristics, as the male sex hormone, testosterone.

androgenesis (ăn-drō-jĕn'ĕ-sĭs). Development of an egg which has been fertilized by a spermatozoan but in which the egg nucleus has been experimentally removed or inactivated. Opp. of gynogenesis.

androgyne (an'dro-jīn) [" + *gynē,* woman]. Androgynus.

androgynoid (an-droj'ĭ-noyd) [" + " + *eidos*, resemblance]. A person possessing female gonads (ovaries) but secondary sex characteristics of a male; a female pseudohermaphrodite. Term is less commonly used for a person possessing male gonads (testes) but secondary sex characteristics of a female; a male pseudohermaphrodite.

androgynous (an-droj'in-us) [" + *gynē*, woman]. 1. Resembling or pert. to an androgynoid, *q.v.* 2. Without definite sexual characteristics.

androg'ynus [" + "]. A female pseudohermaphrodite.

android (ăn'droyd) [G. *aner, andr-*, man, + *eidos*, resemblance]. Shaped like that of a man, as an android pelvis in a female.

andrology (an-drol'ō-jĭ) [" + *logos*, study of]. Study of diseases of the male.

andromania (an-drō-mā'nĭ-ă) [" + *mania*, frenzy]. Abnormal sexual desire in the female. SYN: *nymphomania.**

andromimetic (ăn"drō-mĭm-ĕt'ĭk) [G. *aner, andr-*, man, + *mimētikos*, imitative]. Simulating human processes, as certain types of protozoa.

androp'athy [" + *pathos*, suffering]. Any disease peculiar to the male, as *prostatitis*.

an'drophile [" + *philos*, fond of]. Preferring man; said of certain parasitic organisms.

androphobia (an-dro-fo'bĭ-ă) [" + *phobos*, fear]. Abnormal fear of the male sex.

androphonomania (an-dro-fo-no-ma'nĭ-ă) [" + *phonos*, slaying, + *mania*, frenzy]. Psychotic homicidal trends, esp. when violent.

androstane (ăn'drō-stān). A steroid hydrocarbon $C_{19}H_{32}$, which is the precursor of androgenic hormones.

androsterone (ăn-drō-stēr'ōn, an-dros'tĕr-ōn). $C_{19}H_{30}O_2$. An androgenic steroid found in the urine and considered to be a metabolite of testosterone. It has been synthesized.

As one of the androgens (male sex hormones), androsterone contributes to the characteristic changes of growth and development of the genitals and axillary and pubic hair, deepening of the voice, and development of the sweat glands in the male.

-ane. Indicating a saturated hydrocarbon.

anebous (an-ē'bus) [G. *anebos*, immature]. Immature. Below the age of puberty.

anedeous (an-ē'dē-us) [G. *an-*, not, + *aidoia*, genitals]. Not possessing genitals.

anelectrotonus (an-el-ek-trot'ō-nus) [G. *ana*, up, + *elektrōn*, electric, + *tōnos*, tension]. The state of diminished irritability of a nerve or muscle produced in region near the anode during the passage of an electric current.

Anel's operation (ă-nel') [Dominique Anel, French surgeon, 1679-1730]. Ligation of an artery immediately above and on proximal side of an aneurysm.

A.'s probe. A probe for the lacrimal and nasal ducts.

anemato'sis [G. *an-*, priv. + *aima*, blood, + *-osis*, condition]. 1. General anemia. 2. Pernicious anemia.

anemia (an-e'mĭ-ă) [G. *an-*, priv. + *aima*, blood]. A condition in which there is a reduction in number of circulating red blood cells or in hemoglobin, or in the volume of packed red cells per 100 ml. of blood, or a combination of two or more of these factors. It exists when hemoglobin content is less than 13-14 gm. per 100 ml. for males or 11-12 gm. per 100 ml. for females.

If the onset of anemia is slow the body may adjust so well that there will be no functional impairment, even though the hemoglobin may be less than 6 gm. per 100 ml. of blood.

Classification: Anemias are classified on basis of (a) morphologic differentiation and mean corpuscular volume (MCV) as *normocytic, macrocytic* and *microcytic;* (b) mean corpuscular hemoglobin concentration (MCHC) as *normochromic, hypochromic,* and *hyperchromic;* and (c) etiology.

ETIOL: Anemia may result from (a) excessive blood loss or destruction, or (b) decreased blood cell formation. Anemia may follow acute or chronic hemorrhage or excessive blood cell destruction, as occurs in hemolytic diseases or hypersplenism. Anemias due to decreased blood formation may result from defective nucleoprotein synthesis (as in pernicious and other macrocytic anemias), iron deficiency, inhibition of bone marrow as occurs in certain toxic states, loss of bone marrow, or bone marrow failure.

SYM: Pallor of skin, fingernail beds, and mucous membranes, weakness, vertigo, headache, sore tongue, drowsiness, general malaise, dyspnea, tachycardia, palpitation, angina pectoris, gastrointestinal disturbances, amenorrhea, loss of libido, slight fever. In severe cases BMR may be increased.

NP: The nursing care of patients with anemia provides adequate rest, proper care of the skin, mouth, and teeth, proper elimination, a regulated diet, and antianemic medication prescribed by the physician.

Rest: Patients with mild and moderately severe anemias are usually ambulatory, but patients with very severe anemias must be kept in bed and spared all possible exertion. In acute anemia due to blood loss absolute rest is essential; the foot of the bed should be elevated, the patient kept comfortably warm but not hot. Warm, stimulating drinks may be given if the hemorrhage is not from the gastrointestinal tract.

Care of the skin: Daily warm baths and light massage are beneficial. In very severe anemias, special care of the buttocks and heels may be necessary to prevent the formation of pressure sores. Fresh air and sunshine are indicated, but chilling should be avoided.

Care of the mouth and teeth: Besides ordinary oral hygiene, special care of the mouth is indicated in anemic patients who have soreness of the tongue, mouth, and pharynx. Alkaline mouthwashes are beneficial; if the gums are very sore, pledgets of cotton or gauze may be substituted for a toothbrush for cleaning the teeth.

Elimination: This should be maintained through proper diet.

In severe anemias the function of the kidneys may be impaired; for this reason fluids should be given freely to insure an adequate output of urine.

Diet: The nurse's principal function in this regard is to see that the patient takes the diet which has been prescribed for him. This may be a difficult task, since he often has a poor appetite and his mouth and tongue may be sore. Tact and gentle persuasion often necessary.

Medicines: If the patient is taking iron or liver, it is most important that he does not miss a single dose. If he is given a transfusion, the nurse must watch carefully for reaction, and notify the doctor immediately if the patient complains of chilliness, pain in the chest or back, or shortness of breath, or if his temperature rises. Also if tenderness or swelling appears at the site of injection of liver extract.

Teaching the patient: Throughout the patient's illness the nurse should never lose the opportunity to impress the patient with the importance of his continuing proper treatment after he leaves the hospital. He should be made to understand that in order to get well and stay well he must continue to follow his diet and to take his medicine. He must also understand that he must revisit his doctor at frequent intervals for checkups and blood counts so that relapse may be prevented.

a., achlorhydric. Anemia in which there is an absence of free hydrochloric acid in gastric juice. SYN: *achylanemia.*

a., achrestic. A rare hyperchromic, macrocytic anemia resembling pernicious anemia yet gastric secretion is normal. Probably due to inability of bone marrow to utilize antianemic principle.

a., Addisonian. Pernicious anemia, *q.v.*

a., aplastic. A. caused by aplasia of bone marrow and destruction of same by chemical agents (benzene, arsenic, nitrogen mustards) or physical factors (x-rays, atomic explosions, radioactive phosphorus). An idiopathic form may occur.

a., blind loop. Megaloblastic anemia, *q.v.*, due to a blind loop or multiple diverticulosis of the jejunum which becomes infected with bacteria. These organisms destroy vitamin B_{12}, thus causing anemia. May be treated by removing blind loops or administering vitamin B_{12} and antibiotics.

a., chlorotic. Also called chloranemia, chlorosis and green sickness. Form of a. in adolescent girls and young women thought to be due to faulty diet. Same as iron-deficiency a., *q.v.*

a., congenital hemolytic. Inherited, chronic disease characterized by hemolysis of blood cells, jaundice, and splenomegaly. SYN: *congenital hemolytic icterus* or *jaundice.*

a., Cooley's. A. resulting from inheritance of a recessive trait responsible for interference with hemoglobin synthesis. SEE: *thalassemia.*

a., crescent cell. Sickle cell anemia, *q.v.*

a., deficiency. That resulting from lack of an essential ingredient such as iron or vitamins in the diet, or the inability of the intestine to absorb such. SYN: *nutritional a.*

a., drepanocytic. Sickle cell anemia, *q.v.*

a., erythroblastic. Thalassemia, *q.v.*

a., essential. Idiopathic anemia; pernicious anemia.

a., hemolytic. That resulting from hemolysis of red blood cells. Is either acquired as from the effects of toxic agents, or congenital (familial).

a., hyperchromic. Anemia in which mean corpuscular hemoglobin concentration (MCH) and color index (C.I.) are greater than normal (30% and 1.1 respectively). Term is actually a misnomer as red cells cannot contain an excess of hemoglobin.

a., hypersplenic. That resulting from excessive destruction of red blood cells in the spleen.

a., hypochromic. That in which there is a hemoglobin deficiency, and mean corpuscular hemoglobin concentration is below 30%.

a., idiopathic. That in which there is a lesion of the blood-forming tissue of unidentified cause.

a., iron-deficiency. A. resulting from a greater demand on the stored iron than can be supplied. Most commonly caused by a chronic loss of blood. Usually successfully treated with oral ferrous sulfate or ferrous gluconate and a well-balanced diet.

a., Jaksch's. Infantile pseudoleukemia, a painless, progressive enlargement of the lymphoid tissues, often beginning in the neck.

a., lymphatic. Anemia associated with tumors of the lymph nodes. SEE: *Hodgkin's disease.*

a., macrocytic. A. marked by abnormally large erythrocytes.

a., megaloblastic. A. in which megaloblasts are found in the blood.

a., microcytic. A. with abnormally small erythrocytes.

a., myelopathic, myelophthisic a. A. caused by disruption, usually by metastasis, in bone marrow function.

a., normocytic. Anemia in which size and hemoglobin content of red blood cells remain normal.

a., nutritional. Deficiency anemia, *q.v.*

a., pernicious. A chronic, macrocytic anemia characterized by achlorhydria. Occurs most commonly in the white race after fourth decade of life; occurs rarely before the age of 30 years. Also called *Addisonian a., Biermer's a., essential a., idiopathic a., primary a.*

ETIOL: Deficiency of an intrinsic factor, a thermolabile factor present in normal gastric juice, usually associated with atrophy of gastric mucosa and absence of hydrochloric acid. This factor is essential for absorption of vitamin B_{12}, the *extrinsic factor*, which is essential for normal bone marrow functioning. Vitamin B_{12} is stored in the liver and utilized in hematopoiesis as required. It constitutes the *antianemic* or *erythrocyte maturation factor (EMF)*.

SYM: Weakness, sore tongue, paresthesias (tingling and numbness) of extremities, and gastrointestinal symptoms as diarrhea, nausea, vomiting, pain; signs of cardiac failure may be present in severe anemia.

TREATMENT: Intramuscular injection of vitamin B_{12}.

a., physiologic. An anemia occurring sometimes in infants and disappearing at end of first year. Due to iron deficiency.

a., primary. Pernicious or idiopathic anemia.

a., secondary. A. which results from an injury or disease.

a., septic. A. due to septic condition in the body.

a., sickle cell. A hereditary, chronic, hemolytic anemia characterized by presence of large numbers of crescent or sickle-shaped red blood cells in the blood. Occurs almost exclusively in Negroes. Due to an abnormality in the hemoglobin molecule. SYN: *drepanocytic a.; meniscocytosis.*

a., splenic. Condition characterized by enlargement of the spleen (with accompanying anemia, leukopenia and sometimes thrombocytopenia), gastric hemorrhage, and usually cirrhosis of the liver. SYN: *Banti's syndrome; chronic congestive splenomegaly.*

anemia, words pert. to: anematosis, anemotrophy, antianemic, ischemia.

anemic (an-e'mik). Pert. to anemia; deficient in red blood cells, in hemoglobin, or in volume of blood.

a. factor. SEE: *vitamin B_{12}.* Also called hematinic principle.

a. hypoxia. Reduction in amount or capability of hemoglobin to transport oxygen.

anemophobia (an"ĕ-mō-fō'bĭ-ă) [G. from *anemos,* wind, + *phobos,* fear]. Abnormal fear of drafts, or of the wind.

anemot'rophy [G. *an-,* priv. + *aima,* blood, + *trophē,* nourishment]. Anemia from deficient formation of blood.

anempeiria (an-em-pi're-ă) [G. *an-,* + *empeiria,* experience]. Deficiency in practical knowledge or experience.

anencephalus (ăn-ĕn-sĕf'ăl-ŭs) [G. *an-,* priv. + *egkephalos,* the brain]. A monstrosity characterized by absence of brain and spinal cord, the cranium being open throughout its whole extent and the vertebral canal converted into a groove.

anephrogenesis (ā-nĕph-rō-jĕn'ĕ-sĭs) [G. *a-,* priv. + *nephros,* kidney, + genesis]. Congenital anomaly consisting of lack of kidney tissue.

anepia (an-ep'ĭ-ă) [" + *epos,* word]. Inability to speak.

anergasia (an-er-gā'sĭ-ă) [" + *ergon,* work]. Anergia; functional inactivity resulting from a structural lesion of the central nervous system.

anergastic reaction (an-er-gas'tik). Disorder involving cerebral lesions or organic psychoses.

SYM: *Physical.* Palsy, coma, fits or muscular contractions.

PSY: Loss of memory, impairment of judgment, etc.

anergia (an-er'jĭ-ă) [G. *an-,* priv. + *ergon,* work]. Inactivity; sluggishness.

anergic (an-er'jik). Sluggish; inactive. Deficient in energy; listless.

a. stupor. Acute phase of dementia.

anergy (an'er-jĭ) [G. *a-,* + *ergon,* work]. 1. Asthenia. 2. Impaired or absent ability to react to specific antigens.

aneroid (an'er-oid) [G. *an-,* priv. + *nēros,* wet, + *eidos,* form]. Operating without a fluid, as an aneroid barometer which utilizes atmospheric pressure instead of a liquid such as mercury.

anerythrocyte (an-ĕ-rith'rō-sīt) [" + *erythros,* red, + *kytos,* cell]. A red blood cell without hemoglobin.

anerythroplasia (an-ĕ-rith"rō-plā'zĭ-ă) [" + " + *plasis,* a molding]. Without formation of red blood cells.

anerythroplastic (an-ĕ-rith"rō-plas'tik). Marked by anerythroplasia.

anerythropsia (an-ĕ-rĭ-throp'sĭ-ă) [G. *an-,* priv. + *erythros,* red, + *opsis,* vision]. Inability to distinguish red clearly.

anesthecinesia, anesthekinesia (an"ĕs-thē"sĭn-ē'sĭ-ă, -kĭ-nē'sĭ-ă) [G. *an-,* priv. + *aisthesis,* sensation, + *kinesis,* movement]. Combined sensory and motor paralysis.

anesthesia (an-es-the'zĭ-ă). Partial or complete loss of sensation, with or without loss of consciousness, as result of disease, injury, or administration of a drug or gas.

STAGES OF ANESTHESIA: *First stage:* Preliminary excitement, until voluntary control is lost. Hearing is last sense to be lost. Avoid talking in presence of patient.

Second stage: Loss of voluntary control. Corneal reflex still present.

Third stage: Entire relaxation, no rigidity, deep regular breathing, sluggish corneal reflex, and conjunctival reflex lost.

TESTS FOR ANESTHESIA: *Reaction to light:* Exclude light by holding hand over eyes; withdraw hand quickly. Pupil will reduce in size if anesthesia is complete.

Conjunctival reflex: Place finger at corner of eye on conjunctiva when the eye will attempt to close. This reflex is lost during third stage.

Corneal reflex: If cornea is lightly touched with finger, the eyelid attempts to close. Reflex is brisk during first and second stages, sluggish during third stage and lost only in deep anesthesia.

Danger signals: If too deep, due to overdose, corneal reflex is lost, pupils widely dilate and cease to react to light. Cardiac and respiratory centers fail, patient ceases to breathe, and heart action stops.

EMERGENCY MEASURES: Artificial respiration by anesthetist; injection of cardiac stimulant, inhalation of oxygen, several seconds of brisk slapping over heart, injection of epinephrine into heart muscle. SEE: *resuscitation, cardiopulmonary.*

a., audio. A. produced by sound; used by dentists to kill pain.

a., block. That resulting from nerve blocking by injection of alcohol or other substance into or very near a nerve trunk. SYN: *conduction a.; nerve block a.*

a., bulbar. Pons lesion causing central a.

a., caudal. A form of epidural anesthesia in which needle is inserted into sacrococcygeal notch and local anesthetic injected into the epidural space. SYN: *sacral a.*

a. dolorosa. Painfulness of a part with anesthesia of that part, as in thalamic lesions.

a., general. One that is complete and affecting the entire body, with loss of consciousness, when the anesthetic acts upon the brain. This type of a. is usually accomplished following administration of inhalation or intravenous anesthetic. Commonly used for surgical procedures.

a., Gwathmey's. A. induced by injecting an olive oil and ether solution into the rectum.

a., hysterical. Bodily anesthesia occurring in hysteria.

a., infiltration. Local anesthesia achieved by injecting the local anesthetic solution directly into the tissues, such as injection of procaine solution into the gums for dental procedures.

a., inhalation. General anesthesia achieved by inhaling vapor or gas anesthetics such as ether, nitrous oxide, methoxyflurane, etc.

a., local. One affecting a local area only, the anesthetic acting upon nerves or nerve tracts. SEE: *block a.; infiltration a.*

a., mixed. Production of general anesthesia by more than one drug, as nitrous oxide gas for induction followed by ether for maintenance of a.

a., neural. Injection of an anesthetic into a nerve or immediately around it (*intraneural* and *paraneural*). Same as *block a.*

a., primary. First stage of anesthesia, *q.v.,* before unconsciousness.

a., rectal. General anesthesia produced by introduction of anesthetic agent into rectum.

a., refrigeration. Anesthesia induced by lowering temperature of a part to near freezing by topical ethyl chloride spray or by immersion of the body or a part in a container of finely cracked ice.

a., regional. Nerve or field blocking, causing insensibility over a particular area.

a. sexualis. Anaphrodisia or absence of sexual desire.

a., spinal. 1. Anesthesia resulting from injury to conduction pathways of the spinal cord. 2. Anesthesia produced by injection of anesthetic into subarachnoid space of spinal cord.

a., surgical. When depth of anesthesia produces relaxation of muscles and loss of sensation and/or consciousness.

a., tactile. Loss of sense of touch.

a., topical. Local anesthesia induced by application of an anesthetic directly to surface of body.

a., traumatic. Loss of sensation resulting from injury to nerve.

a., twilight. State of light anesthesia. SEE: *twilight sleep.*

anesthesia, *words pert. to:* a. c. e. mixture, words beginning anesthe-, avertin, barbotage, carbon dioxide, chloracetization, chloroform, cocaine, cyclopropane, ether, ethyl chloride, ethylene, halothane, labor, nitrous oxide, para-anesthesia, paraldehyde, procaine.

anesthesimeter (an-ĕs-thĕ-sim'e-ter) [G. *an-*, priv. + *aisthesis,* sensation, + *metron,* measure]. A device for measuring the amount of inhalation anesthetic administered.

anesthesin (ăn-es'thĕ-sĭn) [G. *an-*, priv. + *aesthēsis,* sensation]. Ethyl aminobenzoate, a local anesthetic. Same as *benzocaine.*

anesthesiology (an-es-thē-zĭ-ol'ō-jĭ) [G. *an-*, priv. + *aisthesis,* sensation, + *logos,* science]. Science of anesthesia.

anesthesiophore (an-es-thē'zĭ-ō-for) [" + " + *phoros,* bearer]. Carrying anesthetic action; the element of a chemical compound that carries the anesthetic action, as that in cocaine.

anesthetic (an-es-thet'ik). 1. An agent that produces insensibility to pain or touch. According to action, they are subdivided into general and local. 2. Causing or pert. to anesthesia. SEE: *anesthesia.*

anesthetist (an-es'thĕ-tist). One who administers anesthetics, esp. for general anesthesia.

a., nurse. A registered nurse who has had special training in anesthesia so that she is capable of administering anesthetic agents.

an"esthetiza'tion. Induction of anesthesia.

anesthetize (an-es'thĕ-tīz). To place under an anesthetic.

anetic (a-net'ik) [G. *anetikos,* relaxing]. 1. Relaxing, soothing. 2. Anodyne.

anetiologic (an-ē-tĭ-ō-loj'ik). Not etiologic; not according to the principles of etiology.

anetoderma (an-et-ō-der'mă [G. *anetos,* relaxed, + *derma,* skin]. Relaxation of the skin.

an'etus. Any intermittent fever.

aneuria (a-nu'rĭ-ă) [G. *a-*, priv. + *neuron,* nerve]. Defect in or deficiency of nervous energy.

aneur'ic. Pert. to aneuria.

aneurin (ă-nū'rĭn). Vitamin B_1; thiamine.

aneurysm (an'ū-rizm) [G. *aneurysma,* a widening]. Localized abnormal dilatation of a blood vessel. Due to congenital defect or weakness of the wall of the vessel.

ETIOL: Usually occurs secondary to syphilitic aortitis. Arteriosclerosis and atherosclerosis accompanied by hypertension are contributing causes. Bacterial or mycotic infection or trauma are common causes of aneurysms in peripheral arteries.

NP: No exertion permitted. Absolute rest in bed. Later, patient may get up, but warn against vigorous effort. General care in heart conditions should be observed. POSTOPERATIVE CARE: Observe circulation of the affected part. Keep limb warm with an electric pad or blanket, but, as sensation is impaired, apply heat with great care. Inspect affected part every 15 minutes, and adjust limb to aid circulation. SEE: *Berard's aneurysm; Cardarelli's sign.*

a., aortic. Affecting any part of the aorta; usually resulting from syphilitic infection, but may result also from necrosis of the structure of the aorta or from atherosclerosis. SEE ALSO: *a., dissecting.* PATH: Pressure on trachea, esophagus, veins, or nerves. SYM: Dyspnea, cough, sputum, dysphagia, congestion of head and neck. Inequality in the two radial pulses. TREATMENT: Surgery.

a., arteriovenous. One in which artery and vein become connected by a saccule. ETIOL: Trauma. Weak point, in walls of an artery, due to syphilis, sudden strain, or injury. SYM: Pain, expansile pulsation, bruit. NP: Avoid increasing heart action or raising blood pressure.

a., cirsoid. A dilatation of a network of vessels commonly occurring on the scalp. The mass may form a pulsating subcutaneous tumor. Also called *racemose aneurysm.*

a., dissecting. One in which the blood makes its way between the layers of a blood vessel wall, separating them; a result of necrosis of the arterial or aortic structure.

a., fusiform. All the walls of the blood vessels dilate more or less equally, creating a tubular swelling.

a., medical. A deeply located aneurysm inaccessible for surgery.

a., mycotic. One due to bacterial infection.

a., racemose. SYN: *cirsoid aneurysm, q.v.*

a., sacculated. One due to the yielding of a weak patch on one side of the vessel and which does not involve the entire circumference; usually due to an injury.

a., varicose. A. forming a blood-filled sac bet. an artery and a vein.

a., venous. Aneurysm of a vein.

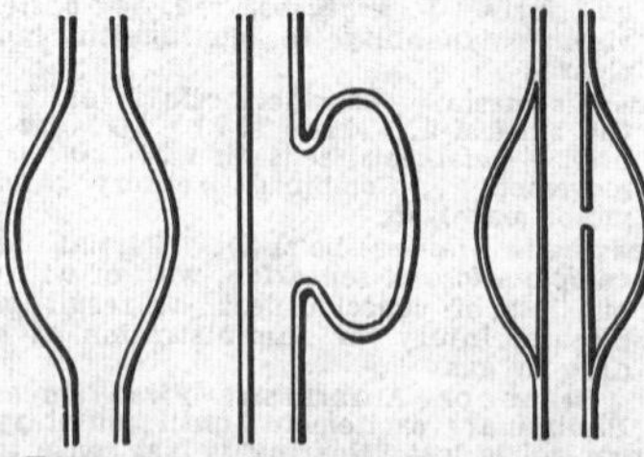

FUSIFORM ANEURYSM SACCULATED ANEURYSM DISSECTING ANEURYSM

aneurysmal (an-ū-riz'măl). Pert. to aneurysm.

aneurysmectomy (an-ū-riz-mek'tō-mĭ) [" + *ektomē*, a cutting out]. Extirpation of an aneurysm by removal of its sac.

aneurysmorrhaphy (an"ūr-iz-mor'ă-phe) [" + *rhaphe*, suture]. Surgical repair of an aneurysm.

aneurysmotomy (an-ū-riz-mot'ō-mĭ [" + *tomē*, cut]. Incision of the sac of an aneurysm, allowing it to heal by granulation.

anfractuosity (an-frak-tū-os'ĭ-tĭ) [L. *anfractus*, a winding]. A cerebral sulcus or fissure.

anfractuous (an-frak-tū'us). Bending; sinuous.

an'gel's wing. A condition usually caused by paralysis of the serratus anterior muscle and characterized by scapula projecting posteriorly. Syn: *winged scapula.*

Angelucci's syndrome (ăn-jĕ-loot'chē) [Arnaldo Angelucci, Italian ophthalmologist, 1854-1934]. Great excitability, palpitation, and vasomotor disturbance associated with vernal conjunctivitis.

angi (an'gĭ). Inguinal buboes.

angi-, angio- (an'jĭ, an'jĭ-ō) [G. *angeion*, vessel]. Prefix meaning a blood or lymph vessel.

angiasthe'nia [G. *angeion*, vessel, + *a-*, priv. + *sthenos*, strength]. Loss of vascular tone.

angiectasia, -sis (an-jĭ-ek-tā-zĭ-ă, -ek'tăsis) [" + *ektasis*, stretching]. Enlarged capillaries or abnormal dilation of a vessel.

angiec'tomy [" + *ektomē*, excision]. Excision or resection of a blood vessel.

angiectopia (an-jĭ-ek-tō'pĭ-ă) [" + *ektōpos*, out of place]. Displacement of a vessel.

angiemphraxis (an-jĭ-em-fraks'is) [" + *emphraxis*, stoppage]. Obstruction of any vessel.

angiitis (an-jĭ-ī'tis) [" + *-itis*, inflammation]. Inflammation of a blood or lymphatic vessel.

angina (ăn-jī'na, L. an'jĭ-na) [L. quinsy, from *angere*, to choke]. 1. A sense of suffocation. 2. Disease of the pharynx or fauces. 3. Any disease characterized by attacks of choking or suffocation.

a. abdominis. Severe abdominal pain resulting from sclerosis of abdominal blood vessels.

a., acute. Simple sore throat.

a. cruris. A. due to obstruction of an artery, causing pain and cyanosis of the affected part, with periodic lameness.

a. decubitus. Attacks of angina pectoris occurring during rest or sleep.

a., follicular. A. of the larynx and pharynx from public speaking, excessive drinking of alcoholic liquors.

a. laryngea. Inflammation of the larynx.

a. ludovici, a. ludwigii. Ludwig's a.

a., Ludwig's. Submaxillary cellulitis; a deep infection of tissues of the floor of the mouth.

a. maligna. Gangrenous inflammation of the throat; septic sore throat.

a., necrotic. Form with gangrenous patches in the mucosa of the air passages, seen in scarlet fever and occasionally in diphtheria.

a. parotidea. Inflammation of the parotid glands. Syn: *mumps.*

a. pectoris. Pain and oppression about the heart; a paroxysmal affection characterized by severe pain radiating from the heart to the shoulder, thence down the left arm, or, rarely, from the heart to the abdomen; apparently dependent upon some lesion of the coronary arteries of the heart, its walls, or valves. Attacks may occur in lesions of the aortic valves. Generally afflicts males of middle age.

Sym: Severe, steady pain and feeling of pressure in region of the heart; great anxiety, fear of approaching death (*angor animi*), and fixation of the body; face pale, ashen, or livid, brow bathed in sweat. Dyspnea often noted; pulse variable, usually tense and quick. Blood pressure is raised during an attack. Attack lasts from a few seconds to several minutes.

Prog: May be grave. Attacks may be intermittent, and with proper rest and care recovery is possible.

Treatment: During attack, inhalation of amyl nitrite or nitroglycerin sublingually. Avoidance of excitement; physical rest.

a. pectoris vasomotoria. Angina pectoris in which symptoms are relatively mild. Pallor, cyanosis, and coldness and numbness of the extremities are characteristic. Also called *mock, spurious,* or *false angina.*

a., phlegmonous. Inflammation of the deep tissues of the throat with edema and usually suppuration.

a., Plaut's. Same as *Vincent's a.*

a. simplex. Sore throat. See: *acute a.*

a. streptococcus. A. caused by the streptococcus.

a. tonsillaris. Quinsy.

a. trachealis. Croup.

a., Vincent's. A pseudomembranous affection of the mouth involving gingivae, oral mucosa, and sometimes pharynx and tonsils. Fusiform bacilli and a spirochete, *Borrelia vincenti,* are invariably associated with the disease but their relationship to it is not definitely established. Syn: *trench mouth.*

anginal (an'jĭ-nal). Pert. to angina.

anginoid (an'jĭ-noid) [L. *angina*, choking, + G. *eidos*, resemblance]. Resembling angina pectoris, or any angina.

anginophobia (an-jĭ-nō-fō'bĭ-ă) [" + G. *phobos*, fear]. Intense fear of an attack of angina pectoris.

anginose (an'jĭ-nōs). Pert. to or resembling angina.

an'ginous. Resembling angina. Syn: *anginose.*

angio- (an-gĭ-ō) [G. *angeion*, vessel]. A combining form denoting a seed, vessel, or something contained within a vessel.

an"gioatax'ia [" + G. *ataktōs*, out of order]. Variability in arterial tonus.

angioblast (an'jĭ-o-blast) [" + G. *blastos*, germ]. 1. The earliest tissue arising from mesenchyme cells of the embryo from which blood cells and blood vessels develop. 2. A cell which participates in vessel formation.

angiocardiography (an-jĭ-ō-car-dĭ-og'ră-phē) [" + G. *kardia*, heart, + *graphein*, to write]. Roentgenography of the heart and great vessels after intravenous injection of a radiopaque diagnostic solution.

angiocardiokinet'ic [" + G. *kardia*, heart, + *kinesis*, movement]. Stimulating or that which affects movements of heart and blood vessels.

angiocarditis (an-jĭ-ō-kar'dĭ-tis) [" + " *-itis*, inflammation]. Inflammation of the heart and large blood vessels.

angiocav'ernous [" + L. *caverna*, cavern]. Rel. to angioma cavernosum.

angiocholecystitis (an"jĭ-ō-kō-lĕ-sĭs-tī'tis) [" + *cholē*, bile, + *kystis*, bladder, + *-itis*, inflammation]. Inflammation of gallbladder and bile vessels.

angiocholitis (an-jĭ-ō-kō-lī'tis) [" + " + *-itis,* inflammation]. Inflammation of biliary vessels; cholangitis.
angiocrine (an'jĭ-ō-krĭn) [" + endocrine]. Marked by vasomotor disorders resulting from disturbances of the endocrine glands.
angiodermatitis (an"jĭ-ō-der-mă-tī'tis) [" + *derma,* skin, + *-itis,* inflammation]. Inflammation of cutaneous vessels.
angiodystrophia (an-jĭ-ō-dis-trō'fĭ-ă) [" + *dys,* bad, + *trophē,* nourishment]. Faulty nutrition of vessels.
angioedema. Angioneurotic edema, *q.v.*
angioendothelioma. A tumor consisting of endothelial cells, commonly occurring as single or multiple tumors of bone.
angiofibro'ma [" + L. *fibra,* fiber, + *-oma,* tumor]. An angioma having connective tissue overgrowth.
angiogenesis (an"jĭ-ō-jen'ĕ-sis) [" + *genesis,* origin]. Development of blood vessels.
angiogenic (an"jĭ-ō-jen'ik). Pert. to angiogenesis; of vascular origin.
an"giogIio'ma [G. *angeion,* vessel, + *glia,* glue, + *-ōma,* tumor]. A mixed angioma and glioma.
angiograph (an'jĭ-ō-graf) [" + *graphein,* to write]. A variety of sphygmograph.
angiography (an"jĭ-og'ră-fĭ). 1. A description of blood vessels and lymphatics. 2. Examination of blood vessels by roentgen rays. Vessels are made visible by injection of radiopaque substance.
a., cerebral. An x-ray of the vascular system.
angiohyalinosis (an"jĭ-ō-hī"ă-lin-ō'sis) [G. *angeion,* vessel, + *yalos,* glass, + *-ōsis,* production]. Hyaline or glassy degeneration of the muscular coat of blood vessels.
an"giohyperto'nia [" + *yper,* over, + *tonos,* tension]. Condition marked by spasm of blood vessels, esp. arteries. Syn: *vasospasm.* See: *hypertension.*
an"giohypoto'nia [" + *ypo,* under, + *tonos,* tension]. Angioparalysis; angioparesis; vascular dilatation. See: *hypotension.*
angioid (an'jĭ-oyd) [" + *eidos,* resemblance]. Resembling a blood vessel.
a. streaks. Dark, wavy, anastomosing striae lying beneath retinal vessels.
angiokeratoma (an"jĭ-ō-ker-ă-tō'mă) [" + *keras,* horn, + *-oma,* tumor]. A skin disorder occurring chiefly on feet and legs, and characterized by formation of telangiectases or warty growths (in groups), accompanied by thickening of the epidermis along the course of dilated capillaries.
angiokinet'ic [" + *kinesis,* movement]. Pert. to action of blood vessels.
angioleukasia (an-gĭ-ō-lū-kā'sĭ-ă) [" + *leukos,* white, + *asia,* condition]. Dilatation of lymphatics.
angioleukitis (an-jĭ-ō-lū-ki'tis) [" + *leukos,* white, + *-itis,* inflammation]. Inflammation of lymphatics.
angiolipo'ma [" + *lipos,* fat, + *-oma,* tumor]. A mixed angioma and lipoma.
angiolith (an'jĭ-o-lith) [" + *lithos,* stone]. Calcareous deposit in wall of a blood vessel.
angiology (an-jĭ-ol'o-jĭ) [" + *logos,* science]. The science of the blood vessels and lymphatics.
angiolu'poid. A tuberculous skin lesion consisting of small, oval, red plaques.
angiolymphitis (an"jĭ-ō-lim-fī'tis) [" + L. *lympha,* lymph, + *-itis,* inflammation]. Inflammation of the lymphatics. Syn: *lymphangitis.*
an"giolympho'ma [" + " + *-oma,* tumor]. Tumor of dilated lymphatics.
angiolysis (an-jĭ-ol'ĭ-sis) [" + *lysis,* destruction]. Obliteration of blood vessels in newly born infants after tying of the cord.
angioma (an-ji-o'mă) [" + *-oma,* tumor]. A form of tumor, usually benign, consisting principally of blood or lymph vessels. Considered to be remnants of fetal tissue misplaced or undergoing disordered development. Syn: *hemangioma; lymphangioma.* See also: *choristoma; epithelioma; hamartoma; nevus.*
a. cavernosum. Is congenital and appears as an elevated dark red tumor, ranging in size from a pea to that of the hand. It frequently has pulsation; commonly involves the subcutaneous or submucous tissue. They are nonmalignant and small ones may disappear without therapy. Syn: *strawberry mark.*
a., flat. A superficial angioma which may occur at any part of the body. Syn: *nevus flammeus; port-wine stain.*
a., senile. An angioma common in elderly persons and consisting of a compressible mass of blood vessels. Syn: *ruby spot.*
a., serpiginous. A skin disorder characterized by appearance of small, red vascular dots arranged in rings on the skin.
a. simplex. One that is congenital, made up of capillaries, nonelevated, bright red or purple-red in color; may cover a large surface; usually found on the face, commonly called "Mother's mark." No satisfactory treatment. Cosmetic creams are usually sufficient. Syn: *nevus flammeus; port-wine stain.*
a., stellate. An angioma in which numerous telangiectatic vessels radiate from a central point. They usually occur on the face and are commonly associated with hepatic disease, hypertension, and pregnancy. Syn: *spider nevus, spider hemangioma.*
a. venosum racemosum. Swelling associated with greatly enlarged superficial varicose veins.
angiomalacia (an-jĭ-ō-mă-lā'sĭ-ă) [" + *malakia,* softness]. Softening of blood vessel walls.
angiomatosis (an-jĭ-ō-mă-tō'sis) [" + *-oma,* tumor, + *-osis,* condition]. Condition of multiple angiomata.
a. retinae. Primary angioma of retina.
angiomatous (an-jĭ-ō'mă-tus). Resembling an angioma.
angiomeg'aly [G. *angeion,* vessel, + *megas,* large]. Enlargement of blood vessels, esp. in the eyelid.
angiometer (an-jĭ-om'ĕ-ter) [" + *metron,* measure]. Instrument for measuring tension and diameter of vessels.
angiomyocardiac (an-jĭ-ō-mī-ō-kar'dĭ-ak) [" + *mys,* muscle, + *kardia,* heart]. Pert. to blood vessels and cardiac muscle.
angiomyoma (an"jĭ-ō-mī-ō'mă) [" + " + *-oma,* tumor]. An angioma mixed with a myoma.
angiomyosarco'ma [" + " + *sarx,* flesh, + *-oma,* tumor]. Tumor containing elements of angioma, myoma, and sarcoma.
angioneurectomy (an-jĭ-ō-nū-rek'tō-mĭ) [" + *neuron,* nerve, + *ektomē,* excision]. Excision of vessels and nerves.
angioneurosis (an-jĭ-ō-nū-rō'sis) [" + " + *-osis,* condition]. Spasm or paralysis of blood vessels, resulting from a disturbance of vasomotor system.
angioneurotic (an-jĭ-ō-nū-rot'ik). Pert. to angioneurosis.
a. edema. A condition characterized by development of local allergic wheals accompanied by swelling of subcutane-

ous or submucous tissues. It is benign and thought to be an allergic disorder, usually a food allergy. SYN: *angioedema; hives; urticaria; giant urticaria; Quincke's disease.*

angioneurotomy (an-jĭ-o-nu-rot'o-mĭ) [G. *angeion*, vessel, + *neuron*, nerve, + *tomē*, cutting]. Cutting of vessels and nerves.

angionoma (an-jĭ-ō-nō'mă) [" + *nomē*, ulcer]. Ulceration of a vessel.

angioparal'ysis [" + *paralyein*, loosen, dissolve]. Vasomotor relaxation of blood vessel tone.

angioparesis (an-jĭ-ō-pă-rē'sis) [" + *paresis*, weakness]. Partial paralysis of the vasomotor system.

angiopathol'ogy [" + *pathos*, suffering, + *logos*, science]. Morbid changes of the blood vessels.

angiopathy (an-jĭ-op'a-thĭ) [" + *pathos*, disease]. Any disease of blood vessels or lymphatics.

angioplania (an"jĭ-o-plan'ĭ-ă) [" + *planē*, wandering]. Abnormality or irregularity in course of a blood vessel.

angioplas'ty [" + *plassein*, to form]. Plastic surgery upon blood vessels.

angiopoietic (an"jĭ-ō-poy-et'ik) [" + *poiein*, to make]. Pertaining to or causing the formation of blood vessels.

angiopres'sure. Control of hemorrhage by pressure.

angiopsathyrosis (an-jĭ-ō-sath-ĭ-rō'sĭs). Fragility of blood vessels.

angiorhigosis (an-jĭ-ō-rĭ-go'sis) [G. *angeion*, vessel, + *rigos*, cold]. Rigidity of vessels.

angiorrhaphy (an-jĭ-or'a-fĭ) [" + *raphē*, seam]. Suture of a vessel or vessels.

angiorrhea (an"jĭ-o-re'ă) [" + *rhoia*, flow]. Oozing of blood from vessels.

angiorrhexis (an-jĭ-or-eks'is) [" + *rēxis*, rupture]. Rupture of a blood vessel.

angiosarco'ma [" + *sarx*, flesh, + *-oma*, tumor]. Mixed sarcoma and angioma.

angiosclero'sis [" + *sklērōsis* hardening]. Hardening of the walls of the vascular system.

angioscope (an'jĭ-ō-skōp) [" + *skopein*, to view]. A microscope for studying capillary vessels.

angiosialitis (an"jĭ-ō-sĭ-ă-lĭ'tis) [" + *sialon*, saliva, + *-itis*, inflammation]. Inflammation of a salivary duct.

angiosis (an-jĭ-ō'sis) [" + *-osis*, condition]. Any disease of the lymphatics or blood vessels.

an'giospasm [" + *spasmos*, tension]. Spasmodic contraction of blood vessels. May cause cramping of muscles or intermittent claudication.

angiospas'tic. Pert. to angiospasm.

angiostaxis (an"jĭ-ō-stax'is) [G. *angeion*, vessel, + *staxis*, trickling]. 1. Hemophilia or hemorrhagic diathesis. 2. Oozing of blood.

angiosteno'sis [" + *stenoein*, to make narrow, + *-osis*, condition]. Narrowing of a tube or passage, especially a blood vessel.

angiosteosis (an"jĭ-os-tē-ō'sis) [" + *osteon*, bone]. Calcareous degeneration of walls of blood or lymph vessels.

angios'tomy [" + *stoma*, mouth]. Artificial fistulous opening into a blood vessel.

angiostrophy (an-jĭ-os'trō-fĭ) [" + *strophē*, twist]. Twisting cut end of a vessel.

angiosynizesis (an"jĭ-ō-sin-ĭ-zē'sis) [" + *synizesis*, contraction]. Collapse of walls of a vessel and their subsequent adhesion.

angiotelectasis (an"jĭ-ō-tel-ek'ta-sis) [" + *telos*, end, + *ektasis*, stretching out]. Dilatation of terminal arterioles.

angiotenic. Characterized by or caused by distention of blood vessels.

angiotensin (an-jĭ-ō-ten'sin). A pressor substance that is formed in the body by interaction of renin and a serum globulin fraction, and that increases arterial muscle tone. Formerly called angiotonin or hypertensin.

angiotitis (an-jĭ-ō-tĭ'tis [G. *angeion*, vessel, + *ous*, ear, + *-itis*, inflammation]. Inflammation of blood vessels of the ear.

angiotome (an'jĭ-ō-tōm) [" + *tomē*, cutting]. One of the segments of the vascular tissues of the embryo.

angiotomy (an-jĭ-ot'ō-mĭ) [" + *tomē*, a cutting]. Dissection of blood vessels.

angioton'ic [" + *tonos*, tension]. Pert. to increase of arterial tension.

angiotonin (an-jĭ-ō-tōn'in). Former name for angiotensin, *q.v.*

angiotribe (an'jĭ-ō-trīb) [" + *tribein*, to bruise]. Instrument for crushing the end of an artery to check hemorrhage.

angiotripsy (an'jĭ-ō-trip-sĭ) [" + *tripsis*, friction]. The use of an angiotribe to check hemorrhage.

angiotroph'ic [" + *trophē*, nourishment]. Pert. to nutrition of blood vessels.

angi'tis. Inflammation of the blood vessels or lymphatics. SYN: *angiitis.*

angle (ang'gl) [L. *angulus*]. 1. The space or area enclosed near the point or line where two lines or planes meet. 2. A projecting or sharp corner.

a., acromial. Point of junction of lateral and posterior borders of the acromion.

a., acute. An angle less than 90°.

a., alpha. One found by intersection of visual line with optic axis.

a., alveolar. Meeting point of the base of the nasal spine and the middle point of the alveolus of the upper jaw.

a., basilar. Formed by the intersection of a projection line from the nasal point to a line drawn at the base of the nasal spine.

a., biorbital. Formed by the meeting of the axes of the orbits.

a., carrying. Angle made at the elbow by extending the long axis of the forearm and the upper arm. This obtuse angle is more pronounced in the female than in the male.

a., cerebellopontine. Junction of the cerebellum and pons.

a. of convergence. Angle between the visual axis and the median line when an object is looked at.

a., costal. Meeting point of the lower border of the false ribs with the axis of the sternum.

a., craniofacial. The angle formed at the point where the basifacial and basicranial axes join at the midpoint of the sphenoethmoidal sutures.

a., facial. The angle made by lines from the nasal spine and external auditory meatus meeting between the upper middle incisor teeth.

a., gamma. Angle formed by line of fixation with optic axis.

a. of incidence. The angle between a ray incident on a surface and a line drawn perpendicular to the surface at the point of incidence.

a. of iris. Angle between the cornea and iris at the periphery of the ant. chamber of the eye.

a. of jaw. The angle at the point where the post. edge of the ramus of the mandible and the lower surface of the body of the mandible join.

a. of mandible. Angle of the jaw.

a., metafacial. Angle between the base of the skull and the pterygoid process.

a., obtuse. An angle greater than 90 degrees.

a., occipital. Formed by the intersection of lines from the basion and from the lower border of the orbit at the opisthion.

a., ophryospinal. Angle formed by the joining of lines drawn from the auricular point and the glabella at the ant. nasal spine.

a., optic. See: *visual angle.*

a., parietal. Formed by the meeting of the prolongation of the two lines tangent to the prominent portion of the zygomatic arch and the parietofrontal suture.

a., pontine. Same as cerebellopontine angle.

a., pubic. Junction of the rami of the pubes.

a., sphenoid. Formed by the intersection of lines coming from the nasal point and the tip of the rostrum of the sphenoid, at top of the sella turcica.

a., sternal. Angle between the manubrium and body of the sternum.

a., venous. Angle of the internal jugular and subclavian vein.

a., visual. The angle formed by drawing lines from the nodal point of the eye to the extreme edges of the visual object.

angophrasia (an-gō-frā'zĭ-ă) [G. *agchein,* to choke, + *phrasis,* utterance]. Drawling, choking speech in paralytic dementia.

angor (ang'gor) [L. quinsy, anguish]. Violent distress, as in angina pectoris.

angor animi (ang'or an'ĭ-me) [" + soul]. Overwhelming feeling of impending death or disaster.

angström unit (ōng'strum) [Anders J. Angstrom, Swedish physicist, 1814-1874]. PT: An internationally adopted unit of measurement of wave length: one ten-millionth of a millimeter, or one two hundred and fifty-four millionth inch. Abbr: *A°* or *A.*

Anguillula (an-gwil'ū-lă) [L. eel]. Genus of nematode worms.

A. aceti. Vinegar eel.

A. intestinalis. Parasitic form of nematode infesting intestine in tropics and near tropics. Syn: *Strongyloides intestinalis.*

A. stercoralis. Free stage of A. intestinalis. Syn: *Strongyloides stercoralis, q.v.*

anguilluliasis (an-gwil-ū-lī'ă-sĭs). Infestation with an anguillula.

angular [L.]. Having corners or angles.

a. artery. The artery at the inner canthus of the eye; facial artery.

angulation (ang-ū-lā'shun). Formation of angular loops in the intestine.

anhaphia (an-hā'fĭ-ă) [G. *an-,* priv. + *aphē,* touch]. Abnormal or defective sense of touch. Syn: *anaphia.*

anhedonia (an-hē-dō'nĭ-ă) [G. *an-,* priv. + *ēdonē,* pleasure]. Psy: Lacking in interest or pleasure; apathy.

anhedonic (an-hē-don'ik). Pert. to anhedonia.

anhelation (an-hel-ā'shun) [L. *anhelare,* to pant]. Dyspnea, shortness of breath.

anhematopoiesis (ăn-hē-mă-tō-poi-ē'sĭs). Defective blood formation. Syn: *anhematosis.*

anhemato'sis [G. *an,* priv. + *aimatoein,* to change into blood]. Defective or insufficient blood formation.

anhemolytic (an-hē-mō-lit'ik). Not destructive to the blood cells.

anhepatia (an-hē-pā'shĭ-ă) [G.*an-,* priv. +*ēpar,* liver]. Failure of or deficient liver function.

anhepat'ic. Not produced by the liver.

anhepatogenic (an-hep-ă-tō-jen'ik) [G. *an-,* priv. + *ēpar,* liver, + *gennan,* to produce]. Not produced by the liver. Syn: *anhepatic.*

anhidrosis (an-hī-drō'sis) [G. *an-,* priv. + *idros,* sweat]. Diminished or complete absence of secretion of sweat. May be generalized or localized, temporary or permanent, accompanying disease conditions or may be a congenital anomaly. Syn: *anidrosis.*

Treatment: Treatment of cause or accompanying conditions. Soft, nonirritating clothing; bland, soothing ointments and lubricants for skin. Air conditioning provides comfort in most instances.

anhidrotic (an-hī-drot'ik). Checking or anything that checks or prevents perspiration. Syn: *anidrotic.*

anhis'tic, anhis'tous [G. *an-,* priv. + *istos,* tissue]. Seemingly without structure.

anhydra'tion [" + *ydōr,* water]. The state of not being hydrated.

anhydremia (an-hī-drē'mĭ-ă) [" + " + *aima,* blood]. A lessening of the normal quantity of fluids in the blood.

anhydride (an-hī'drīd) [G. *anydros,* waterless]. A substance from which the hydrogen and oxygen, in the ratio in which they exist in water, have been removed.

anhydrochlo'ric [" + *chlōros,* green]. Lacking in hydrochloric acid.

anhydromyelia (an-hī-drō-mī-ē'lĭ-ă) [" + *myelos,* marrow]. Deficiency in spinal fluid.

anhy'drous. Containing no water.

anhypnia (an-hip'nĭ-ă) [G. *an-,* priv. + *ypnos,* sleep]. Insomnia; sleeplessness; anhypnosis.

anhypno'sis. Insomnia.

anianthinopsy (an-ĭ-an'thin-op"sĭ) [G. *an-,* priv. + *ianthinos,* violet, + *opsis,* vision]. Inability to recognize violet tints.

anidrosis (an-ĭ-drō'sis) [G. *an-,* priv. + *idrōs,* sweat]. Abnormal deficiency of sweat. Syn: *anhidrosis, q.v.*

anidrotic (an-ĭ-drot'ik). Pert. to anidrosis. Syn: *anhidrotic.*

anile (an'īl) [L. *anus,* an old woman]. 1. Infirm; as an old woman. 2. Senile.

aniline (an'ĭ-lĭn) [Ar. *an-nil,* the indigo plant]. The simplest aromatic amine, $C_6H_5NH_2$, an oily liquid derived from benzene. Used in manufacture of dyes for medical and industrial purposes. Syn: *aminobenzene; phenylamine.*

anilinophil, anilinophilous (an"ĭ-lin'ō-fil, -lin-oph'ĭ-lus) [" + G. *philos,* fond]. A structure staining readily with aniline dyes.

anilism (an'il-izm). Chronic aniline poisoning.

Sym: Cardiac block, weakness, intermittent pulse, vertigo, muscular depression, cyanosis. See: *Aniline in Table of Poisons and Poisoning in Appendix.*

anil'ity [L. *anus,* an old woman]. Old age in females.

anima (an'ĭ-mă) [L. soul]. An individual's true inner self as distinguished from the "image" or appearance or external character (*persona*) presented to the observer. Called *anima* in the male and *animas* in the female.

a. mundi. Paracelsus' term for the vital force essential to the continuity of life.

animal [L. literally *to breathe,* soul]. 1. A living organism, not a plant, which has certain features: mobility; a nervous system; nutritional requirements involving changing complex substances into simpler ones and then resynthesizing them. Animals usually do not store or manufacture chlorophyll. In some acellular organisms the distinction between plant and animal cannot be made. 2. Any animal, especially a four-footed one, other than man. 3. Pertaining to or from an animal. 4. A subhuman or inhuman person, one who is beastlike.

animalcule (an-ĭ-mal′kūl) [L. *animalculum,* little animal]. Unicellular animal organism; protozoan.

animation. State of being alive, or active.

a., suspended. Temporary cessation of vital activities such as respiration with loss of consciousness; state of apparent death.

anincretinosis (an-in-krē-tĭ-nō′sis) [G. *an-,* priv. + *incretus* + *-osis,* condition]. A disorder due to failure of some organ of internal secretion.

anion (an′ĭ-on) [G. *ana,* up, + *iōn,* going]. PT: An ion carrying a negative charge. Since unlike forms of electricity attract each other, the ion is attracted by, and travels to, the positive anode. Examples are acid radicals and corresponding radicals of their salts. SEE: *ion.*

anionic (an-i-on′ik). Containing or pertaining to anions.

a. detergent. A chemical substance with disinfectant properties due to the presence of an active negatively-charged chemical group. May be natural or synthetic.

anirid′ia [G. *an-,* priv. + *iris,* rainbows]. Congenital absence, complete or partial. of iris. SYN: *irideremia.*

anischuria (an-is-kū′rĭ-ă) [" + *ischouria,* retention of urine]. Incontinence of urine.

aniseikonia (an-is-ĭ-kō′nĭ-ă) [G. *anisos,* unequal, + *eikon,* image]. A condition in which the size and shape of the ocular image of one eye differs from that of the other.

anis′ergy [" + *ergon,* work]. Varying degrees of blood pressure in different parts of the system.

aniso- (an′is-ō) [G. *anisos*]. Prefix denoting unequal, unsymmetrical in combination.

anisochromatic (an-ĭ-sō-krō-mat′ik) [G. *anisos,* unequal, + *chrōma,* color]. Not of uniform color.

anisocoria (an-ĭ-sō-kō′rĭ-ă) [" + *korē,* pupil]. Inequality of the diameter of the pupils; may be normal or congenital.

Often seen in early stages of insanity, each pupil alternating in contraction and dilation. Found in *aneurysms, head trauma, diseases of the nervous system, sclerosis, brain lesion, paresis, and locomotor ataxia.*

anisocytosis (an-ĭ-sō-sī-tō′sis) [" + *kytos,* cell, + *-osis,* condition]. Inequality in size of cells, esp. erythrocytes. An abnormal condition.

anisog′amy [" + *gamos,* marriage]. Sexual fusion of two gametes of different form and size.

anisognathous (an-ĭ-sog′nă-thus) [" + *gnathos,* jaw]. Having upper jaw wider than lower one.

anisohypercytosis (an-ĭ-sō-hī-per-sī-tō′sis) [" + *yper,* above, + *kytos,* cell]. Increase in number of leukocytes with altered proportion of the different varieties. OPP: *anisohypocytosis.*

anisohypocytosis [" + *ypo,* below, + "]. Decrease in number of leukocytes with altered proportion of different varieties. OPP: *anisohypercytosis.*

anisoiconia (an-ĭ-so-ĭ-kō′nĭ-ă) [" + *eikon,* image]. Failure of retinal images to coalesce. SYN: *aniseikonia, q.v.*

an″isomas′tia [" + *mastos,* breast]. Breasts unequal in size.

an″isome′lia [" + *melos,* limb]. Inequality between two paired limbs.

anisometrope (an″ĭ-sō-met′rōp) [" + *metron,* measure, + *ops,* vision]. One afflicted with anisometropia.

anisometropia (an-i-sō-me-trō′pĭ-ă). Inequality in refractive power of the two eyes.

anisometrop′ic. Having unequal refractive power.

anisonormocyto′sis [G. *anisos,* unequal, + L. *norma,* rule, + G. *kytos,* cell]. Abnormal relation in numbers of different forms of leukocytes but with normal number of total leukocytes.

aniso′pia [" + *ops,* vision]. Inequality of visual power of both eyes.

anisopiesis (an-ĭ-sō-pī-ĕ′sis) [" + *piesis,* blood pressure]. Apparent inequality of blood pressure in different parts of the body.

anisorhythmia (an″ĭ-sō-rith′mĭ-ă) [" + *rythmos,* rhythm]. Absence of synchronism in rate of the atria and ventricles or irregular heart action.

anisospore (an′ĭ-sō-spōr) [" + *sporos,* seed]. A sexual cell. Opp. of *isospore.*

an″isosthen′ic [" + *sthenos,* strength]. Not of equal muscle strength.

anisotropal (an-is-ot′rō-pal) [" + *tropos,* a turning]. 1. Not equal in every direction. 2. Unequal in power of refraction.

anisotrop′ic. Having different optical properties in different directions, as have certain crystals; double polarizing.

anisotropous (an-ĭ-sot′ro-pus). 1. Not equal in every direction. 2. Unequal in refractive power. SYN: *anisotropal.*

anisuria (an-is-ū′rĭ-ă) [G. *anisos,* unequal, + *ouron,* urine]. Alternate polyuria and oliguria, *q.v.*

ankle (ăng′kl) [A. S. *anclēow*]. 1. The joint between the foot and lower end of leg. 2. In popular usage the region of this joint, including the tarsus and lower end of leg.

a. bone. The talus.

a. clonus. Repetitive extension-flexion movement of muscles of ankle, associated with increased muscle tonus. Commonly a symptom of corticospinal disease. NP: Keep patient's feet at right angles on a rectangular foot splint. When splint is removed for examination, etc., avoid dorsiflexion of foot to prevent movement of ankle, clonus or spasm.

a. c. reflex. Elicited by quick, vigorous dorsiflexion of the foot while the knee is held in a flexed position, resulting in repeated clonic movement of the foot so long as the foot is maintained in dorsiflexion.

a. jerk. Contraction of calf muscles resulting in extension of the foot following a blow upon the Achilles tendon.

a. joint. A hinge joint. Lower part of tibia, its medial malleolus and lateral malleolus of fibula, forming socket for the talus.

a., tailor's. An abnormal bursa over the head of the fibula in tailors from pressure caused by sitting cross-legged on the floor.

ankylo-. Combining form meaning crooked, bent, a fusion or growing together of parts.

ankyloblepharon (ang-kĭ-lo-blef'ar-on) [G. *ankylē*, a stiff joint, + *blepharon*, eyelid]. Adhesion of ciliary edges of lids to each other.

ankylochilia (ang-kĭ-lo-ki'lĭ-ă) [" + *cheilos*, lip]. Adhesion of lips to each other.

ankylocolpos (ang-kĭ-lo-kol'pos) [" + *kolpos*, vagina]. Imperforation or atresia of the vagina.

ankylodactylia (ang-kĭ-lo-dak-til'e-ah) [" + *daktylos*, finger]. Adhesion of two or more fingers or toes to one another.

ankyloglos'sia [" + *glōssa*, tongue]. Tongue-tie.

ankyloproctia (ang-kĭ-lo-prok'shĭ-ă) [" + *prōktos*, anus]. Stricture or imperforation of the anus.

ankylosed (ang'kĭ-lōst). Denoting fixation of a joint. Stiffened; held by adhesions.

ankylosis (an-kyl-o'sis) [G. *agkyle*, stiff joint]. Abnormal immobility and fixation of a joint due to pathological changes in the joint or its surrounding tissue.

Etiol: May be congenital, sometimes hereditary, or it may be result of disease. Seen in many joint conditions. May be performed surgically.

NP: If done surgically, maintain complete immobility of joint until bone has firmly united, which may be from 6 to 12 weeks. Keep joint in perfect position.

a., artificial. The surgical fixation of a joint.

a., bony. The abnormal union of the bones of a joint, also called true ankylosis.

a., extracapsular. That caused by rigidity of parts outside a joint.

a., false. Spurious ankylosis; that due to rigidity of the surrounding parts.

a., fibrous. That due to the formation of fibrous bands within a joint only.

a., intracapsular. That due to the undue rigidity of structure within a joint.

a., ligamentous. Ankylosis by ligaments or fibrous structures.

a., true. Same as bony ankylosis.

Ankylos'toma. Ancylostoma, *q.v.*

ankylos'toma [G. *agkylē*, stiff joint, + *stoma*, mouth]. Trismus, lockjaw.

ankylostomiasis. Ancylostomiasis, *q.v.*

ankylotia (ang-kĭ-lō'shĭ-ă) [G. *agkylos*, crooked, + *ot-*, ear]. Closure or imperforation of external auditory meatus of ear.

ankylotome (ang'kil-ō-tōm) [G. *agkylos*, bent, + *tomē*, a cutting]. An instrument for cutting the frenulum of the tongue in tongue-tie.

ankylurethria (ang-kĭl-ū-rē'thrĭ-ă) [" + *ourēthra*, urethra]. Stricture or imperforation of the urethra.

ankyroid (ang'kĭ-royd) [G. *agkyroeides*, anchor-shaped]. Hook-shaped.

a. cavity. The posterior or descending cornu of lateral ventricle of the brain.

anlage (ahn'lăg-ĕ). 1. A primordium. 2. The first accumulation of cells in an embryo which constitutes the beginning of a future tissue, organ, or part.

annatto (an-at'o). Reddish coloring matter obtained from the pulp of *Bixa orellana*, a tropical tree. Also spelled *annoto, arnotto.*

annec'tent [L. *annectens*, tying or binding to]. Linking together.

Annelida (ă-nel'ĭ-dă). The phylum which includes the segmented worms. Ex: *earthworm.* The only annelids of medical significance are *leeches*, belonging to the class Hirudinea, *q.v.* Some annelids serve as intermediate hosts for parasitic worms.

annex'a [L. *annectere*, to tie or bind to]. Accessory parts. Syn: *adnexa.*

annexi'tis [" + G. *-itis*, inflammation]. Inflammation of *adnexa uteri.* Syn: *adnexitis.*

annex'opexy [" + G. *pexis*, putting together]. Fixation of fallopian tubes and ovary to abdominal wall. Syn: *adnexopexy.*

annuens (an'ū-enz) [L. *annuens*, nodding]. *Rectus capitis anterior minor.*

ann'ular [L. *annulus*, ring]. Circular; ring-shaped.

annulorrhaphy (an-u-lor'ă-fĭ) [" + G. *raphē*, seam]. Closure of a hernial ring by suture.

ann'ulus [L.]. A ring-shaped structure; a ring. Syn: *anulus.*

a. abdominalis. The internal or deep inguinal ring.

a. ciliaris. Boundary between choroid and iris.

a. femoralis. The femoral ring.

a. inguinalis profundus. The abdominal inguinal ring.

a. inguinalis superficialis. Subcutaneous inguinal ring; superficial or external inguinal ring.

a. migrans. A disease of the tongue characterized by appearance of yellow-bordered red patches on dorsum and sides of tongue.

a. tympanicus. The tympanic ring.

a. umbilicalis. Fibrous ring which, in late fetal life, surrounds opening through which umbilical vessels enter and leave cord.

a. urethralis. Circular elevated ring in bladder surrounding internal orifice of urethra.

anoci-association (ă-nō-sĭ-ă-sō-sĭ-ā'shun). An anesthetic technique for helping to prevent shock from continuous preoperative apprehension. This is done by careful, prolonged use of preoperative sedation and narcotics, also local anesthesia used in conjunction with general anesthesia. This complex procedure is little used now.

anococcygeal (ā-nō-kok-sĭ'jē-al) [L. *anus*, + G. *kokkyx*]. Rel. to both anus and coccyx.

a. body. The muscle and fibrous tissue lying between the coccyx and anus.

a. ligament. A band of fibrous tissue joining the tip of the coccyx with the external sphincter ani.

anod'al [G. *ana*, up, + *odos*, way]. Pert. to the anode.

a. closure contraction. Contraction of muscles at anode on closure of circuit. Abbr: ACC.

anode (an'ōd) [G.]. The positive pole of an electrical source. Only galvanic (direct current) and static electricity have distinct polarity.

anodinia (an-ō-din'ĭ-ă) [G. *an-*, priv. + *dinos*, dizziness]. Absence of childbirth pains.

anodmia (an-od'mĭ-ă) [" + *odmē*, stench]. The want or absence of the sense of smell; anosmia, *q.v.*

anodontia (an"o-don'shĭ-ă) [G. *an-*, + *odous*, tooth]. Absence of teeth. Syn: *edentia.*

an'odyne [" + *odynē*, pain]. An agent that will relieve pain; milder in form than an analgesic, *q.v.* Ex: *morphine, codeine, acetylsalicylic acid.* Syn: *antalgesic; antalgic.*

anodyn'ia. 1. Cessation or absence of pain. 2. Loss of sensation.

anoesia (an-ō-ē'sĭ-ă) [G. *anoēsia*, want of understanding]. Without power of comprehension; anoia, imbecility, idiocy.

anoetic (an-ō-et'ik) [G. *anoētos*, unthinkable]. Rel. to the borderline of consciousness; not fully conscious.

anoia (an-oy'ă) [G. *a-*, priv. + *noos*, understanding]. Anoesia, *q.v.*

anomalous (ă-nom'ă-lus) [G. *anōmalos*, uneven]. Irregular. Contrary to the normal.

anom'aly [G. *anomalia*, irregularity]. 1. Anything contrary to general rule. 2. An organ or structure which is abnormal with reference to form, structure, or position; a malformation. SEE: *monster; teras; teratology.*

anomia (a-nō'mĭ-ă) [G. *a-*, priv. + *onoma*, name]. Inability to remember names of persons and objects.

anonychia (an-ō-nik'ĭ-ă) [" + *onyx*, nail]. Absence of the nails.

anoopsia (an-ō-op'sĭ-ă) [G. *anō*, upward, + *opsis*, vision]. Tendency of one eye to turn upward. SYN: *anopia; hyperphoria.*

anoperineal (a"no-per-ĭ-ne'al). Concerning the anus and perineum.

Anopheles (an-of'ĕ-lēz) [G. *anophelēs*, harmful, useless]. A genus of mosquitoes belonging to the family Culicidae, order Diptera. It is a vector of *Plasmodium*, the causative agent of malaria, and may be involved in the transmission of causative agent, of dengue, filariasis, and possibly other diseases.

anopho'ria [G. *ana*, up, + *phoros*, tending]. Tendency of one eye to turn upward. SYN: *anopia; hyperphoria.*

anophthal'mia [G. *an-*, priv. + *ophthalmos*, eye]. Congenital absence of eyes.

anopia (an-ō'pĭ-ă) [G. *an-*, priv. + *ops*, eye]. 1. Anophthalmos; lack of one eye or both. 2. Anopsia. 3. Tendency of one eye to turn upward; hyperphoria.

Anoplur'a. An order of the class insects which includes the sucking lice. SEE: *lice; pediculosis.*

anop'sia [G. *an-*, priv. + *opsis*, sight]. 1. Hyperphoria. 2. Inability to use the vision as in those confined in the dark, or from disuse of an eye in strabismus, or resulting from cataract, or in refractive errors.

anorchism (an-or'kĭzm). Congenital absence of one or both testes.

anorectal (an-ō-rek'tal) [L. *anus* + *rectum*]. Pert. to the anus and rectum.

anorectic, anorectous (an-ō-rek'tic, -tus). Having no appetite.

anorexia (an-ō-reks'ĭ-ă) [G. *an-*, priv. + *orexis*, appetite]. Loss of appetite.

Seen in malaise, commencement of all fevers and illnesses, also in disorders of alimentary tract, esp. of stomach, and as a result of alcoholic excesses and drug addiction, esp. cocaine. Also result of food fads and faulty feeding.

RS: *acoria, ageusia, bulimia, hyperorexia, nausea, parageusia, parorexia, pica, polyphagia, pyrosis, taste.*

a. nervo'sa. Loss of appetite for food not explainable by local disease. It is a mental illness.

anorexigenic (an"o-reks"ĭ-jen'ik). 1. A substance which produces loss of appetite. 2. Causing loss of appetite.

anorganic. Same as *inorganic.*

anor'mal [G. *a-*, priv. + L. *normalis*, according to pattern]. Abnormal.

anorrhorrhea (an-or-or-ē'ă) [G. *an-*, priv. + *orros*, serum, + *roia*, a flow]. Diminished or imperfect secretion of serous fluid.

anorthography (an-or-thog'ră-fĭ) [G. *an-*, priv. + *orthos*, straight, + *graphein*, to write]. Agraphia, esp. motor agraphia; loss of power to express oneself in writing. SEE: *agraphia.*

anorthopia (an-or-thō'pĭ-ă) [" + " + *ops*, eye]. 1. Vision in which straight lines do not appear straight; symmetry and parallelism not properly perceived. 2. Squinting.

anorthosis (an-or-thō'sis) [" + " + *osis*, condition]. Absence of, or diminished, erectility.

anoscope (a'no-skōp) [G. *anus* + *skopein*, to view]. Speculum for examining the anus and lower rectum.

anosmatic (an-oz-mat'ik) [" + *osmē*, smell]. Deficient sense of smell.

anosmia (an-oz'mĭ-ă). Absence of the sense of smell. Frequent in neurasthenia, hysteria, and sometimes in ataxia. SYN: *anodmia; anosphrasia.*

anosmic (an-oz'mik). Lacking in sense of smell.

anos'mous. Anosmic. Pert. to anosmia.

anosodiaphoria (an-ō-sō-dī-ă-for'ĭ-ă) [G. *a-*, priv. + *nosos*, disease, + *diaphoria*, difference]. Real or pretended indifference to presence of disease, esp. paralysis.

anosognosia (an-ō-sog-nō'zĭ-ă) [" + " + *gnosis*, knowledge]. Real or pretended ignorance of the presence of disease, esp. paralysis. OPP: *pathodixia, q.v.*

anosphrasia (an-os-frā'zĭ-ă) [" + G. *osphrēsis*, smell]. Absence or imperfect sense of smell.

anospi'nal [L. *anus* + *spina*, thorn]. Pert. to the anus and spinal cord, the center in the spinal cord which controls the contraction of the anal sphincter.

anostosis (an-os-tō'sis) [G. *an-*, priv. + *osteon*, bone]. A defective formation or development of bone; failure to ossify.

anotia (an-ō'shē-ă). Congenital malformation with absence of the ears.

anotro'pia [G. *ana*, up, + *tropē*, a turning]. Tendency of the eyes to turn upward and away from the visual axis.

anovaginal. Pertaining to the anus and vagina.

anovarism (an-ō'var-ĭzm). Absence of ovaries.

anoves'ical [L. *anus* + *vesica*, bladder]. Rel. in any way to both anus and urinary bladder.

anov'ular, anov'ulatory [G. *an-*, priv. + L. *ovarium*, ovary]. Pertaining to uterine hemorrhage not preceded by ovulation.

anoxemia (an-oks-ē'mĭ-ă) [" + *oxys*, sharp, + *gennan*, to produce, + *aima*, blood]. A diminution in the amount of oxygen in the blood. SEE: *hypoxia.*

anoxia (an-ox'ĭ-ă) [" + oxygen]. Deficiency of oxygen. SEE: *hypoxia.*

a., anemic. Deficiency in the oxygen-carrying power of the blood.

a., anoxic. Diminished oxygen in the arterial blood despite normal ability of the blood to contain and carry oxygen (oxygen capacity). May be due to reduced oxygen supply. respiratory obstruction, reduced surface area in lungs for exchange of gases (as in pneumonia) or inadequate respiratory movements.

a., hypokinetic. Stagnant anoxia, *q.v.*

a., stagnant. Generalized or localized oxygen lack due to deficiency in volume of blood as occurs in cardiac failure, shock, arterial spasm, thrombosis or other conditions which result in reduced circulation of blood.

anox'ic. Pert. to or caused by a general lack of oxygen, and characterized by a generally subnormal oxygen tension of the blood.

an'sa (pl. *ansae*) [L. a handle]. Any anatomical structure in the form of a loop.

a. capitis. The zygomatic arch.

a. cervicalis [NA]. Formerly called *a. hypoglossi.* A loop in the middle of the neck formed by the descending hypoglossal nerve and the descending cervical nerve.

a. hypoglos'si. A. cervicalis, *q.v.*

a. lenticula'ris. Fibers entering the lenticular nucleus from the thalamus by way of the thalamic radiation.

a. nervorum spinalium [NA]. A. of spinal nerves. Connecting loops of fibers between the anterior spinal nerves.

a. peduncularis. Fibers passing from the thalamus through the thalamic radiation, under the lenticular nucleus to the cortex of the temporal lobe and insula.

a. sacralis. Nerve cord connecting the sympathetic trunk with the ganglion impar.

a. subclavia. Loop of nerve fibers winding around the anterior aspect of the subclavian artery.

anselaphesia (an-sel-ă-fē-zĭ-ă). Absence of sense of touch or feeling or sensation, esp. of tactile sensibility.

anserine (an'ser-in) [L. *anser*, goose]. Pert. to a goose.

ansiform (an'sĭ-form). Shaped like a loop.

ant-, anti- [G.]. Prefix denoting opposed to, counteracting, against (as in antibiotic, *i.e.*, against life. Literally kills life).

antabuse (ăn-tĭ'būz). Proprietary name for disulfiram. Administered orally in alcoholism. Ingestion of alcohol following taking of drug causes unpleasant reaction including nausea and vomiting.

antacid (ant-as'id) [G. *anti*, against, + L. *acidum*, acid]. An agent that will neutralize acidity, esp. in digestive tract. Ex: *magnesium oxide, sodium bicarbonate.*

antag'onism [G. *antagōnizesthai*, to struggle against]. Opposition or contrary action, as bet. muscles or medicines.

a., bacterial. The inhibition of or killing of one bacterial organism by another.

antag'onist. That which counteracts the action of anything, as a muscle or drug.

antalge'sic [G. *anti*, against, + *algos*, pain]. Pain-relieving agent. Syn: *anodyne.*

antalgic (ant-al'jik). An anodyne or analgesic.

antalkaline (ant-al'ka-lĭn, -līn) [G. *anti*, against, + *alkaline*]. Neutralizing or reducing alkalinity.

antaphrodis'iac [" + *aphrodisiakos*, sexual]. Lessening sexual desire.

antarthritic (ant"ar-thrit'ik) [" + *arthritikos*, gouty]. Remedy for gout.

antasthenic (ant-as-then'ik) [" + *astheneia*, weakness]. 1. Strengthening, invigorating. 2. Agent which invigorates.

antasthmat'ic [" + *asthma*]. 1. An agent that prevents an asthmatic attack. 2. Relieving asthma.

antatrophic (ant-ă trō'fik) [" + *atrophia*, atrophy]. Preventing or curing atrophy.

ante- [L.]. Prefix meaning *before.*

antebrachium (an-tē-bra'kē-um) [L. *ante*, before, + *brachium*, arm]. The forearm.

antecornu (an-te-kor'nu). Anterior cornu or horn of the lateral ventricle of the brain.

antecurvature (an-tē-ker'va-tūr) [" + *curvatura*, bend]. Bending forward abnormally. Syn: *anteflexion.*

antefebrile (an-tē-fē'brĭl, -fē'brĭl, -fĕb'-rĭl) [" + *febris*, fever]. Pert. to the period before a fever.

anteflect (an'te-flekt). To bend or cause to bend forward.

anteflex'ion [" + *flectere*, to bend]. Abnormal bending forward, esp. bending forward of the uterus at its body and neck.

anteloca'tion [L. *ante*, before, + *locare*, to place]. Forward displacement of an organ or part of the human body.

antemetic (ant-ĕ-mĕt'ik) [G. *anti*, against, + *emetikos*, emetic]. 1. Arresting vomiting. 2. Remedy that controls vomiting and nausea. See: *antiemetic.*

ante mor'tem [L.]. Before death.

a.-m. statement. One made immediately preceding death. If made with belief that death is approaching, it is held in law as equally binding with a statement made on oath. Syn: *deathbed statement.*

antenatal (ăn"tē-nā'tal) [*ante-* + L. *natus*, birth]. Occurring before birth.

an'te par'tum [L.]. The time before the onset of labor.

antephialtic (ant-ĕ-fĭ-al'tik) [" + *ephialtēs*, nightmare]. Preventing nightmare.

anteposition. Anterior displacement of the uterus.

anteprostate (an-tē-pros'tāt). Cowper's gland.

anteprostati'tis [" + *prostata* + G. *-itis*, inflammation]. Inflammation of glands of Cowper.

antepyret'ic [" + G. *pyretos*, fever]. Before the development of fever; antefebrile. See: *antipyretic.*

ante'rior [L.]. Before, or in front of.

a. chamber. Aqueous chamber. Bounded in front by cornea, behind by iris and lens.

antero- [L.]. Prefix denoting anterior, front, before.

anterograde (an'ter-o-grād) [L. *antero*, anterior, + *gradior*, to step]. Extending frontward.

antero-infe'rior [" + *inferior*, below]. In front and below.

anterolat'eral [" + *latus*, side]. In front and to one side.

anterome'dian [" + *median*]. In front and toward the central line.

anteroposter'ior [" + *posterior*, rear]. Passing from front to rear.

anterosuper'ior [" + *superior*, above]. In front and above.

antever'sion [L. *ante*, before, + *vertere*, to turn]. 1. A tipping or bending forward of an organ. 2. A forward placement of the uterus.

a. uteri. A forward tipping of the uterus.

antevert'ed. Inclined or bent forward; said of uterus.

anthelix (ant-hē'liks, an-thē'liks) [G. *anti*, against, + *elix*, coil]. External ear's inner curved ridge. Syn: *antihelix.*

anthelmintic (an-thel-min'tik) [G. *anti*, against, + *elmins*, worm]. An agent used to expel intestinal worms. Ex: *diethylcarbamazine; piperazine; quinacrine hydrochloride.*

a. enema. One given to expel worms. See: *enema.*

Anthemis (an'them-is). Genus of plant, the flowers of which are used medicinally.

anthemis (an'them-is). Camomile; dried blossoms of A. nobilis. A bitter tonic; an antispasmodic.

anthemorrhagic (ant-hĕm-ō-raj'ik) [G. *anti*, against, + *aima*, blood, + *rēg-*

nunai, to discharge]. Agent for preventing or arresting hemorrhage.

anthocyanin (an-thō-sī'ă-nĭn). Any one of a group of pigments that cause flowers and plants to be reddish purple in color.

anthocyanine'mia [*anthocyanin* + G. *aima*, blood]. Anthocyanin in the blood.

anthocyaninu'ria [" + G. *ouron*, urine]. Anthocyanin in urine.

Anthomyia (an-thō-mī'ya) [G. *anthos*, flower, + *myia*, fly]. A genus of fly of the order Diptera, related to the housefly. Larvae sometimes infest man.

A. canalicularis. A small black horse fly, whose larvae may infest the human intestine, often resulting in alarming gastrointestinal symptoms.

anthopho'bia [G. *anthos*, flower, + *phobos*, fear]. Morbid dislike of flowers.

anthorism, anthorisma (an'thor-izm, -iz'-mă) [G. *anti*, against, + *orisma*, a boundary]. A diffuse swelling.

anthracemia (an"thra-sē'mĭ-ă) [G. *anthrax*, carbuncle, + *aima*, blood]. Presence in the blood of *B. anthracis*.

anthracia (an-thrā'sĭ-ă) [G. carbuncle]. Presence of carbuncles.

anthracoid (an'thra-koid). Resembling or pert. to anthrax.

anthracometer (an-thră-kom'ĕ-ter) [G. *anthrax*, coal, + *metron*, measure]. An instrument for measuring the carbon dioxide in the air.

an"thraconecro'sis [" + *nekrōsis*, deadness]. Necrosis of tissue into dry, black gangrene.

anthracosis [" + *-osis*, condition]. Miner's phthisis. A condition of the pulmonary organs due to coal dust inhalation; a pneumoconiosis probably caused by breathing coal dust and silica.

anthrax (ăn'thrăks) [G. coal, carbuncle]. 1. A carbuncle. 2. Acute, infectious disease caused by *Bacillus anthracis*, usually attacking cattle, sheep, horses and goats. Man contracts it from contact with animal hair, hides, or waste.

Etiol: B. anthracis. Workers in wools, hides, and brushes are commonly affected.

Sym: Disease may attack lungs (woolsorter's disease) or the loose cellular tissue, giving rise to malignant edema; more commonly it occurs in form of a pustule called anthrax boil or malignant pustule. Rarely, the disease may occur in intestinal tract. Anthrax often proves fatal if untreated.

Treatment: Antibiotics, especially penicillin.

NP: Isolation and complete bed rest of patient until lesions are healed. Daily cleansing baths and daily mouth and nose care. Diet—fluids when temperature is elevated, followed by progressive return to regular diet. Alcohol or tepid sponges for elevated temperature.

Medical aseptic technic. Dressings burned. Bed linen, gowns, instruments and gloves autoclaved. Fluid body wastes and bath water placed in cresol or solution of chloride of lime. Terminal disinfection of room and its contents after patient is discharged.

RS: *Ascoli's reaction*. Syn: *cacanthrax; charbon*.

an'thropo- [G.]. Prefix denoting relation to man.

anthropogeny (an-thrō-poj'ĕ-nĭ) [G. *anthrōpos*, man, + *gennan*, to produce] Origin and development of man

anthropoid (an'thrō-poid) [" + *eidos*, resemblance]. 1. Resembling a man. 2. An ape.

anthropol'ogy [" + *logos*, study of]. The science which treats of man in all aspects.

anthropometry (an-thro-pom'et-rĭ) [" + *metron*, measure]. Science of measuring the human body and its parts and functional capacities.

anthropophagy (an-thrō-pof'a-jĭ) [" + *phagein*, to eat]. The eating of human flesh; cannibalism.

anthropophile (an-thro'po-phĭl) [" + *philein*, to live]. One with a preference for man. Especially, an insect which chooses the blood of man rather than that of other mammals.

an"thropopho'bia [" + *phobos*, fear]. A morbid fear of society or of a particular man. An early symptom of mental disorder.

anthroposomatology (an"thrō-pō-sō-mă-tol'ō-jĭ) [" + *sōma*, body, + *logos*, study of]. Branch of anthropology dealing with human body.

anthropotomy (an-thrō-pot'ō-mĭ). Human anatomy.

an"thropotox'in [" + *toxikon*, poison]. Supposed poison exhaled by human lungs.

anthydropic (ant-hī-drop'ik) [G. *anti*, against, + *ydrops*, dropsy]. 1. Correcting dropsy. 2. Agent for relieving dropsy.

anthypnotic (ant-hip-not'ik) [" + *ypnos*, sleep]. 1. Preventing sleep. 2. Agent hindering sleep.

anthysteric (ant-his-ter'ik) [" + *ystera*, womb]. 1. Relieving hysteria. 2. Agent soothing hysteria.

anti- [G.]. Prefix meaning *against*.

antiagglu'tinin. A specific antibody opposing action of agglutinin.

antialbumate, antialbuminate (an-tĭ-al'bū-māt, -al-bū'mĭn-āt) [*anti-* + *albumin*]. A product resulting from incomplete proteolysis of albumin; parapeptone.

antialbu'min. An albumin constituent; supposed to be source of antialbumose.

antial'bumose. A product formed by peptic digestion of albumin; becomes antipeptone by further hydrolysis.

antialexin (an-tĭ-ă-lĕks'ĭn). Anticomplement.

antiamboceptor (an-tĭ-am'bō-sĕp-ter). Substance inhibiting action of an amboceptor.

antiamylase (an-tĭ-am'ĭ-lās). Substance neutralizing action of amylase.

antianaphylactin (an"tĭ-an-ă-fĭ-lak'tĭn). An antibody specific to anaphylactin.

antianaphylaxis (an"tĭ-an-ă-fĭ-laks'ĭs). A state of immunity.

antianemic (an-tĭ-ă-nē'mĭk). Curing or preventing anemia.

antiantibody (an-tĭ-an'tĭ-bod-ĭ). An antibody counteracting effect of antitoxin which produced it.

antiapoplectic (an-tĭ-ăp-ō-plek'tĭk). Relieving or preventing apoplexy.

antiarthritic (an-tĭ-ar-thrĭt'ik) [*anti-* + G. *arthritikos*, gouty]. Medicine given to relieve gout.

antibacte'rial. Destroying or stopping the growth of bacteria.

antibacterin (an-tĭ-bak'ter-in) [*anti-* + G. *baktērion*, little rod]. An antibody injected to prevent further germ growth in the body. See: *germ theory*.

antibechic (an-tĭ-bek'ik) [" + G. *bex*, cough]. 1. Relieving cough. 2. A cough remedy.

antibilious (an-tĭ-bil'yus). Relieving bilious conditions.

antibiosis (an-tĭ-bī-ō'sĭs) [" + G. *bios*, life]. An association of two organisms detrimental to one of them.

antibiotic (ăn-tĭ-bī-ŏt'ĭk). 1. Tending to destroy life. 2. A substance produced by a living organism which has power to inhibit the multiplication of, or to destroy, other organisms, especially bacteria. Some affect only gram-positive bacteria; others also the gram-negative forms. Some are effective against fungi and rickettsiae, and a few affect viruses. Antibiotics are produced by bacteria, molds and other fungi.

ANTIBIOTICS

SUBSTANCE	SOURCE*
amphotericin B	*Streptomyces nodosus*
ampicillin	*synthetic*
bacitracin	*Bacillus subtilis*
cephalothin	*semi-synthetic*
chloramphenicol	*Streptomyces venezuelae*
chlortetracycline	*Streptomyces aureofaciens*
cloxacillin	*synthetic*
colistin	*Bacillus colistinus*
cycloserine	*Streptomyces orchidaceus* or *Streptomyces garyphalus*
dapsone	*synthetic*
erythromycin	*Streptomyces erythreus*
ethionamide	*synthetic*
glucosulfone	*synthetic*
griseofulvin	*Penicillin griseofulvum*
kanamycin	*Streptomyces kanamyceticus*
lincomycin	*Streptomyces lincolnensis*
methenamine mandelate	*synthetic*
methicillin	*synthetic*
nafcillin	*synthetic*
neomycin	*Streptomyces fradiae*
nitrofurantoin	*synthetic*
novobiocin	*Streptomyces niveus* or *Streptomyces spheroides*
nystatin	*Streptomyces noursei*
oleandomycin	*Streptomyces antibioticus*
oxacillin	*synthetic*
oxytetracycline	*Streptomyces rimosus*
paromomycin	*Streptomyces rimosus*
penicillin	*Penicillium notatum* or *Penicillium chrysogenum*
phenethicillin	*synthetic*
phenoxymethyl penicillin	*synthetic*
polymyxin B	*Bacillus polymyxa*
pyrazinamide	*synthetic*
ristocetin	*Nocardia lurida*
streptomycin	*Streptomyces griseus*
subtilin	*Bacillus subtilis*
sulfonamides	*synthetic*
tetracycline	*Streptomyces* (unidentified strain)
tyrothricin	*Bacillus brevis*
vancomycin	*Streptomyces orientalis*
viomycin	*Streptomyces puniceus*

* Though originally isolated from sources listed, many of the substances are now produced synthetically.

This list of antibiotics (some of which are of historic interest and are not used clinically) can only be considered as being representative.

antiblennorrhagic (an-tĭ-blen-ō-raj'ik) [*anti-* + G. *blennos*, mucus, + *rēgnunai*, to burst forth]. 1. Preventing or curing gonorrhea or catarrh. 2. Remedy for these diseases.

antibody (an'tĭ-bod-ē). Protein substances developed by the body, usually in response to the presence of an antigen which has been administered parenterally or has otherwise gained access to the circulation. Normal antibodies are also present in the circulation, and may be transferred from the mother to the infant in utero or may be developed during life by subclinical contact with the disease-producing agent, thereby providing immunity to diseases.

Antibodies resemble enzymes in that they are associated with proteins of the serum. Most bacteria entering the body stimulate the production of antibodies. Antibodies do not seem to be activating agents except as they accelerate the action of other agents.

They consist of (a) *antitoxins*, which neutralize toxins; (b) *cytolysins* (bacteriolysins) which dissolve cells; (c) *agglutinins*, which cause cells to clump together; (d) *precipitins*, which bring about precipitation of substances; and (e) *opsonins*, which enhance the phagocytic activity of leukocytes by making bacteria more readily ingested. A substance which induces the production of antibodies is called an *antigen*. Antigen-antibody reaction is generally specific, *i.e.*, an antibody will act only against the antigen which induces its production.

The term antibody is not limited to substances which protect the body.

antibody, *words pert. to*: antianaphylactin, antiantibody, anticutin, anticytost, anticytotoxin, antiricin, antiserum, antitrypsin, autoantibody, autohemolysin, isoagglutinins, lysin, opsonin.

antibrachium (an-tĭ-brā'kĭ-um) [*anti-*, + G. *brachion*, arm]. The forearm.

antibro'mic [" + *brōmos*, smell]. 1. Deodorizing. 2. A deodorant.

antical'culous [" + L. *calculus*, a pebble]. Antilithic.

antican'crin [" + L. *cancrum*, cancer]. Cancroin. Supposed cancer antibody.

anticanitic (an-tĭ-kă-nĭt'ĭk), Counteracting graying of hair.

anticar'dium [" + *kardia*, heart]. Precordial depression.

anticarious (an-tĭ-kā'rĭ-us) [" + *caries*, decay]. Preventing decay of teeth.

anticatarrhal (an-tĭ-kă-tar'al). Counteracting catarrh.

anticathode (an-tĭ-kath'ōd). Portion of vacuum tube opposite cathode. SYN: *target*.

anticheirotonus (an-tĭ-kī-rot'ō-nus) [G. *anticheir*, thumb, + *tonos*, tension]. Spasmodic bending inward of thumb in epilepsy or before attack.

anticholagogue (an-tĭ-kō'lă-gog) [*anti-*, + G. *cholē*, bile, + *agōgos*, drawing forth]. Depressing hepatic function.

anticholerin (an-tĭ-kol'er-in) [" + *cholera*]. Substance from cultures of *Spirillum cholerae asiaticae:* employed as therapeutic agent in cholera.

anticholinergic (an-tĭ-kō"lĭn-ĕr'jĭk). 1. Impeding the impulses or action of the fibers of the parasympathetic nerves. 2. An agent that provides a cholinergic blocking action. SYN: *parasympatholytic*.

antic'ipating intermittent. Intermittent fever with paroxysms recurring earlier each day before the regular time.

anticlinal (an-tĭ-klī'nal) [G. *anti*, against, + *klinein*, to incline]. Leaning in opp. directions.

a. vertebra. Tenth thoracic vertebra.

anticoagulant (an-tĭ-kō-ag'ū-lant). 1. Preventing the process of clotting. 2. An agent which prevents or delays blood coagulation.

anticomplement (an-tĭ-kom'plē-ment). A substance combining with, and thus neutralizing, a complement.

anticonvul'sive [*anti-*, + L. *convulsio*, pulling together]. 1. Relieving convulsions. 2. Agent preventing convulsions.

anticreatinine (an-tĭ-krē-at'ĭ-nēn). A leukomaine from creatinine.

anticritical (an"tĭ-krit'ik-al). Preventing the crisis of a disease.

anticus (an-tī'kus) [L. foremost]. Anterior. That part nearest the ventral or front surface.

anticutin (an-tĭ-kū'tĭn). An antibody, in some individuals with tuberculosis, neutralizing tuberculin to prevent cutaneous tuberculin reaction.

anticyclic acid (an-tĭ-sĭ'klĭk). An antipyretic drug.

anticytol'ysin [*anti-*, + G. *kytos*, cell, + *lysis*, dissolution]. Antibody inhibiting cytotoxin. Syn: *anticytotoxin*.

anticy'tost. An antibody which gives immunity to cytost; named by Turck.

anticytotoxin (an-tĭ-sī-tō-toks'ĭn) [*anti-*, + G. *kytos*, cell, + *toxikon*, poison]. An antibody specifically inhibiting cytotoxin.

antidiabetic. 1. Preventing or alleviating diabetes. 2. Something which counteracts diabetes.

antidiarrhe'ic en'emas. These, which are rarely used, include the demulcents, astringents, antiseptics, carminative, or sedative enemas. See under: *enema*.

antidinic (an-tĭ-dĭn'ik) [*anti-*, + G. *dinos*, dizziness]. 1. Relieving giddiness. 2. Agent preventing vertigo.

antidiphtherin (an-tĭ-dif'thĕr-in). A substance taken from the culture of diphtheria bacillus and used to prevent the disease.

antidiuretic (an"tĭ-dī-ū-rĕt'ik) [*anti-*, + G. *dia*, intensive, + *ourēsis*, urination]. 1. Lessening urine secretion. 2. A drug having such an action.

antidotal (an-tĭ-dō'tal). Acting as or pert. to an antidote.

antidote (an'tĭ-dōt) [G. *antidotos*, given against]. A substance which neutralizes poisons or their effects.

a., chemical. These act chemically by reacting with the poison to produce an insoluble compound which is inert or less toxic. For example, table salt precipitates silver nitrate and forms an insoluble, harmless silver chloride. Chemical antidotes should be used sparingly and should be removed, as they may produce serious results if allowed to remain in the stomach.

a., mechanical. Those that envelop the poison inside the stomach or coat the mucous membrane of the stomach. These are fats, oils, milk (casein coagulum), whites of eggs, finely divided charcoal, fuller's earth, or mineral oil. (Fats and oils are not desirable in phosphorus, camphor, aspidium, and cantharides poisonings.)

a., physiologic. These produce physiological effects opposite to the effects of the poison, *e.g.*, sedatives are given for convulsives and hypnotics. These should not be given without physician's definite instructions.

a., universal. Two parts activated charcoal, one part tannic acid, and one part magnesium oxide. (The charcoal absorbs; the tannic acid precipitates metals, alkaloids, and some glucosides; and the magnesium oxide neutralizes acids). Give orally by dissolving 5 teaspoonsful of the mixture in ½ glass of warm water. After the patient has swallowed the antidote, the stomach contents should then be removed by gastric lavage.

antidromic (an-tĭ-drom'ik) [*anti-*, + G. *dromos*, running]. Running in a direction opposite the usual stream, as when a nervous impulse runs along a sensory fiber in the direction of the sense organ.

antidyscratic (an-tĭ-dis-krat'ik). Relieving dyscrasia.

antidysenteric (an-tĭ-dĭs-ĕn-ter'ik). 1. Relieving or preventing dysentery. 2. An agent curing dysentery.

antiemetic (an-tĭ-ē-mĕt'ik). An agent that will prevent or arrest vomiting. Ex: *dimenhydrinate, meclizine, promethazine.*

antienzyme (an-tĭ-ĕn'zīm). 1. Enzyme neutralizer. 2. An enzyme retarding the activity of another. Syn: *antiferment*.

antifebrile (an-tĭ-fē'brĭl, -fē'brĭl, -fĕb'rĭl). [*anti-*, + L. *febris*, fever]. 1. A medium reducing fever. 2. Reducing or relieving fever.

antifebrin (an-tĭ-feb'rin). Acetanilid, *q.v.*

antiferment (an-tĭ-fĕr'mĕnt) [*anti-*, + L. *fermentum*, leaven]. Hindering, or an agent which hinders, the action of an enzyme. Syn: *antienzyme*.

antifermen'tative. Preventing the fermentation process. Syn: *antizymotic*.

antifung'al. Checking the growth of fungus.

antigalactagogue (an-tĭ-gă-lak'tă-gog) [*anti-*, + G. *gala*, milk, + *agogos*, drawing forth]. An agent that lessens the secretion of milk. Ex: *estrogen*.

antigalactic (an-tĭ-ga-lak'tik). Diminishing or retarding the secretion of milk. Syn: *ischogalactic; lactifuge*.

antigen (an'tĭ-jĕn) [" + *gennan*, to produce]. A substance which induces the formation of antibodies. An antigen may be introduced into the body or it may be formed within the body. Examples are bacteria, bacterial toxins, foreign blood cells.

a. unit. Smallest quantity of antigen required to fix one unit of complement, preventing hemolysis.

antigenic (an-tĭ-jen'ik). Capable of causing the production of an antibody.

antigenophil (an-tĭ-jen'ō-fil) [" + " + *philos*, fond]. Having an affinity for the antigen. Syn: *antigentophil*.

antigenotherapy (an-tĭ-jĕn"ō-ther'ă-pĭ). Utilization of an antigen in treatment of a disease. Syn: *antigentotherapy*.

antiglobulin (an-tĭ-glob'ū-lĭn). A precipitin which precipitates globulin.

antigoitrogenic (an"tĭ-goy"tro-jen'ik) [" + goiter, + *gennan*, to produce]. Preventing the formation of a goiter.

antigonorrheic (an-tĭ-gon-ō-rē'ĭk). 1. Curing gonorrhea. 2. An agent relieving gonorrhea.

antihe'lix [G. *anti*, against, + *elix*, coil]. Inner curved ridge of external ear.

antihemol'ysin. A substance which neutralizes hemolysin.

antihemorrhagic (ăn-tĭ-hĕm-ō-răj'ĭk). Checking bleeding or hemorrhages.

a. vitamin. Vitamin K, *q.v.*

antihidrot'ic [G. *anti*, against, + *hidrotikos*, sweating]. Preventing or checking perspiration. Syn: *anhidrotic*.

antihistamine (an-tĭ-hĭs'tă-mēn, -mĭn). An agent, as chlorpheniramine maleate, which counteracts the effects of histamine. Used in treatment of allergies.

antihistaminic. 1. Inhibiting the production of or neutralizing the effect of histamine. 2. An agent used to counteract histamine.

antihormone (an-tĭ-hor'mōn). An inhibitory autacoid opposing hormone action.

antihydropic (an-tĭ-hī-drop'ĭk) [*anti-*, + G. *ydrops*, dropsy]. 1. Relieving dropsy. 2. Agent used to treat dropsy.

anti-icteric (an-tĭ-ĭk-tĕr'ĭk) [" + *ikteros*, jaundice]. 1. Relieving icterus. 2. Agent for treating jaundice.

anti-immune (an-tĭ-ĭ-mūn'). Preventing immunity.

anti-infectious. Counteracting infection.

anti-inflammatory. Counteracting or diminishing inflammation.

anti-isolysin (an-tĭ-ī-sol'ĭ-sĭn). A substance inhibiting action of an isolysin.

antikenotoxin (an-tĭ-kĕn-ō-toks'ĭn). A substance counteracting fatigue toxins.

antiketogenesis (an-tĭ-kē-tō-jĕn'ĕ-sis). [*anti-*, + G. *ketone* + *gennan*, to produce]. Lowering of acidosis through body oxidation of sugar, alcohol, glycerin, and allied substances.

antiketogenet'ic, antiketogen'ic. Pert. to antiketogenesis.

antilactase (an-tĭ-lak'tās) [*anti-*, + G. *lac*, milk]. An antibody counteracting lactase.

antilemic (an-tĭ-lē'mĭk) [" + *loimos*, plague]. 1. Preventing plague. 2. An agent curing the plague.

antilepsis (an-tĭ-lĕp'sis) [" + *lepsis*, a seizing]. 1. Application of a remedy to a healthy part; treatment by derivation or revulsion. 2. Support, as of a bandage.

antileptic (an-tĭ-lep'tĭk) [G. *antileptikos*, able to check]. 1. Assisting, supporting. 2. Revulsive.

antilethargic (an-tĭ-lĕ-thar'jik) [*anti-*, + G. *lethargos*, forgetfulness]. Preventing sleep.

antilithic (an-tĭ-lĭth'ĭk) [" + *lithos*, stone]. An agent that prevents the formation of, or favors the removal of stones or calculi in the urinary or biliary tracts.

antilobium (an-tĭ-lō'bĭ-ŭm) [" + *lobos*, ear lobe]. The tragus.

antilogia (an-tĭ-lō'jĭ-ă) [" + *logos*, science]. Contradictory symptoms which render diagnosis uncertain.

antiluetic (an-tĭ-lū-ĕt'ik) [" + L. *lues*, pestilence]. Antisyphilitic.

antilymphocytic serum (an"tĭ-lim"phosit'ik). ABBR: ALS. A substance used experimentally to reduce host rejection response to transplanted tissues. Produced by inoculating animals with certain tissues from other animals.

antilysin (an-tĭ-lī'sin). A substance neutralizing the lysins of a disease against which an animal has been immunized, thus preventing the lysis of cells.

antilysis (an-til'ĭ-sĭs). The result of the action of antilysin.

antilyssic (an-tĭ-lĭs'ĭk) [*anti-*, + G. *lyssa*, frenzy]. Preventing or checking rabies. SYN: *antirabic*.

antimalarial (an-tĭ-mă-lā'rĭ-al). An agent, such as quinine, that will prevent or relieve malaria.

antimere (an'tĭ-mēr) [*anti-*, + G. *meros*, a part]. Any body segment bounded by planes at right angles to the long axis of the body.

antimetabolite (an"tĭ-mĕ-tab'o-lĭt). A substance which, due to its similarity of structure, is utilized by an organism as if it were a preferred metabolic substance. The antimetabolite, once ingested, does not benefit the organism. It is believed that certain antibiotics are effective because they act as antimetabolites.

antimetropia (an-tĭ-mĕ-trō'pĭ-ă). An ocular disorder in which the eyes have different powers of refraction. Ex: one eye may be hypertropic; the other, myopic.

antimiasmatic (an-tĭ-mī-az-mat'ĭk). Antimalarial.

antimicrobic (an-tĭ-mī-krō'bĭk) [*anti-*, + G. *mikros*, small, + *bios*, life]. 1. Not believing in the pathogenicity of microorganisms. 2. Preventing the development or pathogenic action of microbes.

antimicro'bin. Antibody used to prevent further germ growth in the body. SEE: *germ theory*.

antimo'nial. Pert. to or containing antimony.

antimony (an'tĭ-mō"nĭ). SYMB: Sb. At. wt. 121.75, at. no. 51. An element of metallic appearance and crystalline structure. Its compounds are used in alloys and medicines, and may form poisons.

a. poisoning. SYM: Acrid metallic taste. Cardiac and arterial depressants with additional properties of inducing sweating and vomiting about 30 minutes after injection. In large doses they irritate lining of alimentary tract, resembling arsenic.

F. A. TREATMENT: Vomiting caused by the poison may be sufficient emesis. Wash stomach with strong tea or dilute tannic acid. Otherwise treat symptomatically. SEE: *tartar emetic*.

antimycotic (an-tĭ-mī-kot'ik) [*anti-*, + G. *mykēs*, fungus]. Checking or preventing the growth of fungi. SYN: *antibacterial*.

antinarcot'ic. Relieving stupor caused by a narcotic.

antinatriuresis (an"tĭ - na"trĭ - u - re'sis) Decreasing the excretion of sodium in the urine.

antinausea. Preventing or decreasing nausea.

antinephritic (an-tĭ-nĕ-frĭt'ik). Serviceable in renal inflammation.

antineuralgic (an-tĭ-nū-ral'jik). 1. Relieving neuralgic pain. 2. Agent curing neuralgia.

antineurit'ic. 1. Counteracting nerve inflammation. 2. An agent which relieves neuritis.

antineu'ritin. Antineuritic vitamin; vitamin B_1.

antin'ion [G. *anti*, against, + *inion*, nape of the neck]. Frontal pole of the skull.

antiop'sonin. A substance that retards opsonin action.

antioxida'tion. Prevention of oxidation.

antiox'ygen. A substance hindering oxidation.

antipaludian (an"ti-pă-loo'dĭ-an). Preventing malaria fever.

antiparalytic (an-ti-par-ă-lĭt'ik). Reputedly relieving paralysis.

antiparasitic (an-ti-par-ă-sĭt'ik). 1. Destructive to parasites. 2. Insecticide.

antiparastatitis (an-tĭ-păr"as-tă-tī'tĭs) [G. *anti*, against, + *parastates*, testicle, + *-itis*, inflammation]. Inflammation of Cowper's glands.

antipathic (an-tĭ-path'ĭk) [" + *pathein*, to feel]. Opposite; unlike.

antip'athy. 1. Aversion; disgust; or that which excites repugnance. 2. Chemical incompatibility.

antipepsin (an-tĭ-pĕp'sin). An antienzyme counteracting pepsin.

antipeptone (an-tĭ-pĕp'tōn). Peptone derived from antialbumose through hydrolysis.

antiperiod'ic [*anti-*, + G. *periodos*, a circle]. Antimalarial; preventing regular recurrences.

antiperistal'sis [" + *peri*, around, + *stalsis*, constriction]. A wave of contraction in the gastrointestinal tract moving towards the oral end.

In the duodenum it is associated with vomiting; in the ascending colon it occurs normally. SEE: *peristalsis*.

antiperistal'tic. 1. Pert. to antiperistalsis. 2. Impeding peristalsis.

antiperspirant. Inhibiting, or a substance which inhibits, perspiration.

antiphlogistic (an-tĭ-flō-jis'tik) [*anti-*, + G. *phlogistos*, on fire]. An agent that tends to relieve inflammation. Ex: *kaolin, ichthyol*.

antiphthisic (an-tĭ-tiz'ik) [" + *phthisis*, a wasting]. Checking or relieving phthisis.

antiphthi'sin. Modified tuberculin.

antiplas'tic. 1. An agent preventing granulation of tissue. 2. One which thins the blood.

antipneumotox'in [" + *pneumon*, lung, + *toxikon*, poison]. An antitoxin opposing pneumotoxin.

antipodal (an-tĭp'ō-dal) [G. *antipous*, with feet opposite]. Located at the opposite end or side.

a. cell. One of two nuclear cells at the base of embryo sac in a seed.

antipraxia (an-tĭ-praks'ĭ-ă). Functions or symptoms antagonistic to each other.

antiprostate (an-tĭ-pros'tāt). Anteprostate; Cowper's gland.

antiprostati'tis. Inflammation of Cowper's gland.

antiprothrom'bin [*anti-*, + G. *prō*, before, + *thrombos*, clot]. Agent preventing formation of thrombin; anticoagulant. SEE: *clotting.*

antiprotozo'al. Destructive to protozoa.

antipruritic (an-tĭ-prū-rĭt'ĭk). That which relieves itching.

antipsoric (an-tĭp-sō'rĭk) [*anti-*, + *psora*, the itch]. An agent used to prevent or arrest itching. It may be local or general.

antiputrefac'tive. Preventive of putrefaction.

antipyic (an-tĭ-pī'ĭk) [*anti-*, + G. *pyon*, pus]. Checking suppuration; antipyogenic.

antipyogenic (an-tĭ-pī-ō-jĕn'ĭk) [" + *pyon*, pus]. Preventing or checking pus formation.

antipyre'sis [" + *pyretos*, fever]. Use of antipyretics in fever.

antipyret'ic. An agent that reduces febrile temperatures. Ex: *quinine, antipyrine, acetylsalicylic acid.*

antipyrine (ăn"tĭ-pī'rēn) [*anti-*, + G. *pyr*, fire]. White crystalline powder, odorless and having a slightly bitter taste. An analgesic and antipyretic. Its pharmacologic actions are similar to those of phenacetin.

antipyrotic (an-tĭ-pī-rot'ĭk) [*anti-*, + G. *pyrōtikos*, burning]. Substance or technique used to treat, or effective in the treatment of, burns.

antirabic (an-tĭ-rā'bĭk). Preventive of, or curing rabies; antilyssic.

antirachit'ic [*anti-*, + G. *rachitis*]. 1. Helping to cure rickets. 2. Agent for treating rickets.

a. vitamin. Vitamin D, *q.v.*

antireticular cytotoxic serum. ABBR: ACS. First prepared by Alexander A. Bogomolets [Russian biologist, 1881-1946]. A serum obtained from horses which have been inoculated with certain human tissues. Believed, by some investigators, to stimulate the reticuloendothelial system when serum is given in small doses but to destroy the reticuloendothelial cells when given in large doses.

The developer of this serum allegedly believed that humans treated with it would live longer than their normal life spans. There is no evidence to support this. The serum is not available commercially.

antirheumat'ic. An agent that will combat rheumatism.

antiricin (an-tĭ-rī'sin). An antibody to ricin.

antiscabious (an-tĭ-skā'bĭ-us). Preventing or relieving scabies.

antiscorbutic (an-tĭ-skor-bū'tik). An agent effective against or a remedy for scurvy. Vitamin C is antiscorbutic.

antisep'sis [G. *anti*, against, + *sepsis*, putrefaction]. The prevention of sepsis by the exclusion, destruction, or inhibition of multiplication of microorganisms including viruses within body tissues.

antiseptic (an-tĭ-sep'tĭk). 1. Preventing decay, putrefaction, or sepsis. 2. An agent that will prevent the growth or arrest the development of microorganisms.

Chemically, antiseptics may be *inorganic*, such as the mercury preparations, or *organic*, such as carbolic acid (phenol). *Oxidizing* disinfectants liberate oxygen when in contact with pus or organic substances. When in use they should be washed away and replaced frequently to help remove pus, blood, and other substances. Different types of bacteria require different antiseptics. Antiseptics are more or less destructive to tissue. They should cause the serum to enter the wound rather than flow from it, and they should prevent absorption of infectious substances.

RS: *asepsis, disinfectant, deodorant, germicide, sterilization.*

antisep'ticism. Therapeutic employment of antiseptic measures.

antiserum (an-tĭ-sē'rum). A serum obtained from human donors (or an experimental animal, usually a goat or horse) who have been immunized against a specific bacterium or other antigenic agent. The serum contains antibodies specific for the antigen. SYN: *immune serum.*

antisialagogue (an-tĭ-si-al'ă-gog) [" + " + *agogos*, drawing forth]. An agent, as atropine, that lessens or checks the flow of saliva.

antisialic (an-tĭ-sī-al'ĭk) [*anti-*, + G. *sialon*, saliva]. Checking or that which checks the secretion of saliva.

antisocial. Pertaining to a person whose outlook or actions are socially negative, or to one who fails to obey the rules of society. SEE: *asocial.*

antispasmod'ic [" + *spasmos*, convulsion]. 1. Relieving or checking spasm. 2. An agent that will relieve spasm. SEE: *spasm.*

antispas'tic. Agent relieving muscular spasm. SYN: *antispasmodic.*

anti-stain formulary. An anti-stain formulary for removing stains from bed linens and other cotton fabrics is as follows:

BALSAM OF PERU: Use waste ether to dissolve it before laundering. CAUTION: Ether is explosive and toxic. It should not be used in closed areas. Use in open air or under a properly ventilated hood. Never use in presence of a flame or lighted cigarette.

BLOOD: Soak in cold water, then wash in lukewarm soap solution. For old stains, soak in 1% ammonia solution and then launder.

CHOCOLATE OR COCOA: Allow hot water to run through stained fabric; then wash in hot soap solution. Javelle water to bleach if necessary. Carbona for remaining grease stain.

COD LIVER OIL: Soak stained fabric in kerosene oil for 1 hour, rubbing lightly occasionally. Then boil for 10 minutes in water to which a naphtha soap product has been added. Rinse in clear water CAUTION: Kerosene is inflammable. Do not used in a closed area or near a flame.

COSMETICS: Nail polish, lipstick, or rouge — ordinary washing; stubborn stains remaining can be removed by acetone, followed by warm chlorine bleach.

FECES: Soak in cold water, rinse, then wash with soap and water (hot). Use a brush to scrub.

ANTISEPTICS

Used For	Chemicals	Uses
Hands	Bichloride of mercury (mercuric chloride)	One tablet (7½ grains) in one pint of water makes a 1:1000 solution, chiefly used to disinfect hands previous to an operation. Continued use irritates skin. Not used to disinfect instruments as it *corrodes the metal.* CAUTION: This solution is poisonous if ingested.
Skin	Alcohol (ethyl alcohol)	A 50 to 70 per cent solution will penetrate bacteria. but stronger solutions are not as active. Green soap owes its germicidal action to the alcohol (43 per cent) contained in it.
	Sulfur	Used as ointment to check growth of bacteria and destroy parasites, as in scabies.
	Ichthyol	An antiseptic in various skin diseases to relieve itching and soften skin.
Wounds and Ulcers	Hypochlorite solutions	Dakin's solution contains 45 to 50 per cent sodium hypochlorite. Free chlorine is liberated to combine with NH_2 radical of proteins in tissues to form chloramine; as an antiseptic about 15 times as effective as phenol, besides not being injurious to tissues.
	Potassium permanganate	An oxidizing disinfectant in 1 to 3 per cent solutions for wounds.
	Iodoform	Mostly used in gauze soaked with a 5 to 10 per cent solution of iodoform. Useful for slow-healing wounds.
Mucous Membranes	Silver nitrate	A 1 per cent solution, followed by physiologic saline solution, in eye of the newborn prevents gonorrheal infection. In strong solutions very destructive to tissues.
	Mild silver protein (Argyrol)	As a combination of silver and albumin it is used in 10 to 25 per cent solutions for antiseptic and astringent purposes.

FRUIT STAINS: Stretch stained article over a basin, pour boiling water directly over the spot until it disappears. If this fails, use Javelle water (a preparation of washing soda and chloride of lime), rinsing bet. each application.

GRASS STAINS: Use alcohol, afterwards washing soda and hot water. Put in the sun to bleach.

INK (Ordinary): If fresh, immerse in cold or tepid water, or skimmed milk. Old ink stains respond well to lemon juice, salt and sunlight. Whatever is used, the material should be rinsed thoroughly after using to remove all of the solution.

IODINE: Soapy water, ammonia solution and hot water rinse.

IRON RUST: Use lemon juice and salt; expose to the sunlight. For firm fabrics, use strong solution of oxalic acid. Rinse very thoroughly.

MEAT JUICES: Same as for blood.

MERCUROCHROME: Pour hot water through the material. Acid alcohol does very well, or Dakin's solution and 5% acetic acid (vinegar), equal parts of each. Then wash thoroughly.

MILDEW: If fresh, use strong soapsuds and hang in the sunlight. If an old stain, use Javelle water, rinse thoroughly and repeat the washing if indicated.

NAIL POLISH, LIPSTICK AND ROUGE: Ordinary washing or acetone, followed by a warm chlorine bleach.

PAINTS, VARNISHES: Turpentine or benzol applied in the open air. If old stain, soak well in grease to soften, then apply turpentine or the other solutions. Chloroform dissolves lacquer paint stains. Acetone sponged on fabric removes varnish. Shellac is soluble in 50% solution of alcohol. CAUTION: Chloroform is toxic and should be used only in a very well ventilated area.

PERSPIRATION: Wash in strong soap solution and hang in the sunlight.

PICRIC ACID: Boil fabric in dilute sodium hydroxide solution for ½ hr. and bleach in Javelle water.

SCORCH: Hydrogen peroxide applied to the area; then rub well with the material soaked in strong soap solution. Hang in the sunlight.

SILVER SALTS: If not too old, silver stains can be removed by sodium thiosulfate (hypo).

TEA OR COFFEE: If fresh, pour boiling water through it. If old, soak in borax before pouring boiling water over it.

URINE: Soak in boiling water, then pour 5% Lysol solution over it.

antistalsis (an-tĭ-stal'sis). Backward movement of bowel contents. Opp. to peristalsis, *q.v.*

antistaphylococ'cic. Destructive to staphylococcus.

antistaphylol'ysin. Blood serum substance counteracting staphylolysin.

antistreptococ'cic. Destructive to streptococcus.

antistreptococ'cin. The antitoxin of any type streptococcus.

antistreptolysin-O (ăn-tĭ-strĕp-tŏl'ĭ-sĭn). ABBR: *ASLO.* An antibody stimulated by infection with various streptococcus organisms and present in the serum of patients who have the infection.

antisu'doral. Checking perspiration. SYN: *anhidrotic; antihidrotic.*

antisudorific (ăn-tĭ-sūd-or-if'ik). 1. Checking perspiration. 2. An agent which reduces the secretion of sweat.

antisyphilit'ic. An agent that will cure or relieve syphilis.

antitabetic (an-tĭ-tă-bet'ĭk). 1. Preventing tabes dorsalis. 2. Agent which mitigates tabetic symptoms.

antithenar (an-tĭ-thē'nar). Placed opposite to the palm of hand or sole of foot.

antither'mic. 1. Reducing temperature. 2. Agent lowering temperature. SEE: *febrile; antipyretic.*

antithrombin (an-tĭ-throm'bin). A substance which inhibits coagulation of blood by preventing reaction between thrombin and fibrinogen.

antithromboplastin (an"tĭ-throm'bo-plastin). Substance which counteracts thromboplastin, thus interfering with normal blood coagulation.

antithyroi'din. A serum from sheep's blood after thyroid has been removed from animal.

USES: Exophthalmic goiter and other diseases due to hypersecretion of thyroid gland.

antiton'ic. Diminishing tone or tonicity.

antitoxic (an-tĭ-tok'sik) [*anti-*, + G. *toxikon*, poison]. Neutralizing a poison, especially a toxin such as bacterial toxin.

a. unit. Sufficient quantity of antitoxin to neutralize 100 toxic units. SYN: *immunizing unit.*

antitox'igen [" + " + *gennan*, to produce]. An antigen stimulating antitoxin production in the blood. SYN: *antitoxinogen.*

antitox'in. An antibody capable of neutralizing a specific toxin. It is produced by the body cells in response to the presence of a toxin. Examples are *diphtheria antitoxin, gas-gangrene antitoxin,* and *tetanus antitoxin* which counteract the toxins produced by the diphtheria, gas-gangrene and tetanus bacteria. Antitoxins are used for prophylactic and therapeutic purposes. SEE: *antivenin.*

a. serum. A serum which contains the antitoxin of a disease organism. The serum is obtained from the blood of an animal. It is given in toxic diseases, either subcutaneously, intramuscularly, intravenously.

antitoxin'ogen. An antigen promoting production of antitoxin in the blood. SYN: *antitoxigen.*

antitragicus (an-tĭ-traj'ik-us). A small muscle in the pinna of the ear.

antitragus (an-tĭ-trā'gus). A projection on the ear of the cartilage of the auricle in front of the tail of the helix, post. to the tragus.

antitrismus (an-tĭ-trĭs'mus). A condition in which the mouth cannot close because of tonic spasm.

antitrope (an'tĭ-trōp) [*anti-*, + G. *tropē*, a turn]. 1. A symmetrical pair of organs. 2. Antibody.

antitro'pin. An antibody, *q.v.*

antitryp'sin. An antibody or antiferment inhibiting tryptic action.

antitryp'tic. Counteracting trypsins.

antituberculot'ic. Inhibiting the spread or progress of tuberculosis in the body.

antitussive (an-tĭ-tus'iv). An agent which prevents or inhibits coughing.

a., centrally acting. An agent which depresses medullary centers thus suppressing the cough reflex.

antiuratic (an-tĭ-ū-rat'ik). Preventing the precipitation of urates.

antivaccina'tion. Opposition to vaccination.

antivaccina'tionist. One who is opposed to vaccination.

antiven'ene. Same as antivenin, *q.v.*

antivene'real. Preventing or curing venereal diseases.

antivenin (an-tĭ-ven'in). An antigenic substance prepared from immunized animal sera.

a., black widow spider. USP. An antitoxic serum obtained from horses immunized against venom of the black widow spider (*Latrodectus mactans*). Specific in treatment of bites of black widow spider.

a., crotaline, polyvalent. USP. Antisnakebite serum obtained from serum of horses immunized against venom of four types of pit vipers: *Crotalus atrox, C. adamanteus, C. terrificus,* and *Bothrops atrox* (Fam. Crotalidae). Specific in treatment of snakebites of these pit vipers.

antiven'om. A snake venom antitoxin.

antiven'omous. Inhibiting venom.

antivi'ral. Inhibiting a virus.

antivi'rus. A bacterial filtrate from a broth medium heated to reduce toxicity; used in the Besredka local immunity method.

antivitamin. A vitamin antagonist; one of a group of substances, natural or synthetic, which inhibits the normal functioning of certain vitamins. Ex: certain sulfonamides which are antagonistic to para-aminobenzoic acid.

antivivisection (an-tĭ-vĭv"ĭ-sek'shun). Opposition to the use of animals in experimentation.

antixenic (an-tĭ-zē'nĭk). Pert. to living tissue reaction to any foreign substance.

antizymot'ic. An agent that will prevent or arrest fermentation. Ex: *salicylic acid, alcohol.*

antodontalgic (an-tō-don-tal'jik) [G. *anti*, against, + *odont*, tooth, + *algos*, pain]. 1. Relieving toothache. 2. Remedy for toothache.

an'tra [L.]. Pl. of antrum.

antracele (an'tră-sēl) [L. *antrum*, cavity, + G. *kēlē*, tumor]. Accumulation of fluid in Highmore's antrum, *i.e.*, the maxillary sinus. SYN: *antrocele.*

antral (an'tral). Pert. to an antrum.

antrec'tomy [L. *antrum* + G. *ektomē*, excision]. Excision of the walls of an antrum.

antritis (an-trī'tis) [" + G. *-itis*, inflammation]. Inflammation of an antrum, especially that of the maxillary sinus.

antroatticotomy (an-trō-at-ĭ-kot'ō-mĭ) [" + *atticus*, + G. *tomē*, cutting]. Operation to open and remove contents of the antrum and the attic of the tympanum.

antrocele (an'trō-sēl) [" + G. *kēlē*, tumor]. Fluid accumulation in the maxillary sinus. SYN: *antracele.*

antrona'sal [" + *nasalis*]. Rel. to the maxillary sinus and nasal fossa.

antrophore (an'trō-for) [" + G. *phorein*, to carry]. A medicated bougie for local treatment of any accessible cavity or canal.

antroscope (an'trō-skōp) [" + G. *skopein*, to view]. An instrument for examining the maxillary sinus.

antros'copy. Examination of any cavity by the antroscope.

antros'tomy [L. *antrum,* cavity, + G. *stoma,* mouth]. Operation to open an antrum for drainage.

antrotome (an'trō-tōm) [" + G. *tomē,* incision]. An instrument for cutting open a cavity, esp. in bone.

antrot'omy. Opening an antral wall.

an"trotympan'ic [L. *antrum,* cavity, + G. *tympanon,* drum]. Rel. to the mastoid antrum and the tympanic cavity.

an"trotympani'tis. Chronic inflammation of tympanic cavity and mastoid antrum.

an'trum (pl. *antra*) [L. from G. *antron,* cavity]. Any nearly closed cavity or chamber, especially in a bone.

a. auris. External acoustic meatus.

a. cardiacum. The thoracic portion of the esophagus, functionally the superior portion of the stomach.

a., duodenal. The duodenal cap, a dilatation of duodenum near pylorus and seen during digestion.

a. mastoideum. Tympanic antrum.

a., maxillary. The maxillary sinus SEE: *sinus.*

a. of Highmore. The air sinus in the maxillary bone. Maxillary sinus.

a. puncture. Made near floor of nose 1½ inches from external opening. Pus is then drained. NP: Irrigate antrum 24 hours after puncture. May be necessary for first few days to cocainize nose before passing cannula. Attach syringe to cannula when placed. Teach patient to hold it and to treat self at home.

a. pyloricum. Bulge in the pyloric portion of the stomach along the greater curvature on distention.

a. tympanicum. The mastoid antrum.

ANTU. Alpha-naphthylthiourea, a powerful rat poison.

anuclear (a-nū'klē-ĕr). Without a nucleus, said of erythrocytes.

anulus. Spelling of *annulus,* according to Nomina Anatomica (Paris). SEE: *annulus.*

anure'sis [G. *an-,* priv. + *ouresis,* urination]. Failure of kidney to secrete sufficient urine, suppression or failure to reach bladder if secreted; found in acute nephritis, congestion, renal abscess, and last stages of chronic nephritis. SEE: *anuria.*

ETIOL: Inhalation of ether; lead, phosphorus, cantharides, or turpentine poisoning; Asiatic cholera; cholera infantum; cholera morbus; gastrointestinal perforation; shock; collapse; reaction to having been transfused with the incorrect type of blood; typhoid fever; yellow fever; pernicious anemia; hysteria; acute yellow atrophy of the liver. Obstructive suppression is the result of occlusion of one or both ureters.

NP: Aid action of skin and bowels. Care as in nephritis. Wash skin with hot water, 116° to 120° F., twice a day. Hot drinks. Cover patient well. Prevent chilling and keep out of drafts.

anuret'ic. Pert. to anuresis, *q.v.*

anuria (an-ū'rĭ-ă) [G. *an-,* priv. + *ouron,* urine]. Complete urinary suppression or failure of kidney function. SYN: *anuresis.*

ETIOL: Severe dehydration, shock, transfusion reactions, poisoning by metallic or industrial poisons, sulfonamide nephrosis, kidney disease, obstruction of ureters or renal pelves, obstruction of or reduction in blood flow to kidneys, severe hypotension.

a. postrenal. That due to obstruction of renal flow in renal pelvis or ureter. May result from stone, sulfonamide crystals, tumor, or spasm of ureter.

a., prerenal. That resulting from inadequate blood flow to kidney. May result from low blood pressure or low blood volume or both.

a., reflex. That which may follow trauma, stone, or instrumentation of the urinary tract.

a., renal. A. due to lesions involving kidney itself.

anus (ā'nŭs) [L.]. The outlet of the rectum lying in the fold between the nates or buttocks.

The end of the anal canal (2.5 to 3 cm.). Fissures of anus in newly born indicative of congenital syphilis.

a., artificial. Opening of the bowel usually by colostomy.

a., fissure in. A crack in mucosa of rectum.

a., fistula in. A fistulous connection bet. lumen of rectum and perianal skin. SYN: *fistula in ano.*

a., imperforated. Where the natural opening is closed.

a., vulvovaginal. An opening into the vulva from the anus.

anvil (an'vil) [A.S. *anfilt*]. Middle ossicle of ear. SYN: *incus.*

anxietas (ang-zi'ĕ-tăs) [L. *angere,* to vex, trouble]. Anxiety, apprehension, restlessness.

a. tibia'rum. Tiredness, twitching, and unrest in legs when in bed.

anxiety neuro'sis. Also called **anxiety reaction.** A functional disease in which fear (or the somatic evidences of fear) out of proportion to any apparent external cause is the essential part of the picture.

A symptomatic fear state can be differentiated by recognizing a justifiable organic cause such as thyrotoxicosis. Fear may exist consciously, or present a group of somatic symptoms not recognized for what they are; in fact, even denied as representing anxiety. Ordinarily, fear as a response to an environmental threat is quite conscious; it may be equally conscious without the patient having the slightest insight as to its causation.

Fear may be an emotional correlate of organic brain disease; it is outstanding in certain toxic states (notably delirium tremens), may coexist with depression, and occur as night waves.

Anxiety neurosis is manifested when an intact personality without organic disease, during clear consciousness, complains of palpitation; heart pain; dyspepsia; cold, sweaty, tremulous extremities; constriction of the throat; bandlike pressure about head, among other symptoms. Often these are interpreted as meaning regional disease.

The real significance is a feeling of inadequacy in meeting some situation, *e. g.,* a tempting situation which is so completely repressed as to be totally unacceptable to the patient as of significance. *Homosexuality* is such a frustrated impulse that may lead not only to an anxiety state but to the much more intense picture of panic—psychotic terror. It is always very important not to rationalize the symptoms as being due to some physical disease.

TREATMENT: The anxious patient needs therapy as much as if the disease were due to an organic illness. Comprehensive and understanding counseling may be provided by the family physician or by a psychiatrist. It is essential that the time required be made available if it is done by the family physician. The use of drugs, be they tranquilizers, sedatives, or antidepressants, may be indicated; this decision must be made for each patient individually.

anxious agitated depression. PSY: Depression accompanied by worry, uneasiness, and agitation, esp. rel. to poverty and want, or ruin.

SYM: Hallucinations may be present but generally they are absent. Delusions that a well-known phenomenon of nature has ceased to exist, such as the day or the night, the sun or the moon, aversion to eating, or the hearing of voices accusing the subject, are other symptoms.

anydremia (an-ĭ-drē'mĭ-ă) [G. *an-*, priv. + *ydōr*, water, + *aima*, blood]. Decrease in normal fluid content of the blood. SYN: *anhydremia, q.v.*

anypnia (an-ĭp'nĭ-ă) [" + G. *ypnos*, sleep]. Condition of sleeplessness.

A. O. A. 1. Abbr. for *Alpha Omega Alpha*, an honorary medical fraternity in the United States. 2 Abbr. for *American Osteopathic Association.*

A. O. C. Abbr. for *anodal opening contraction.*

aochlesia (ā-ok-lē'zĭ-ă) [G. *a-*, priv. + *ochlesis*, disturbance]. Tranquillity; rest; catalepsy.

aor'ta [G. *aortē*, aorta]. The main trunk of the arterial system of the body. It is about 3 cm. in diameter at its origin. It arises from the upper surface of the left ventricle, passes upward as the *ascending aorta*, turns backward and to the left (*arch of the aorta*) at about the level of the fourth thoracic vertebra and then passes downward as the *descending aorta*, which is divided into the *thoracic* and *abdominal aorta*. The latter terminates at its division into the two common iliac arteries. At its exit from the ventricle, the aortic orifice is guarded by three semilunar valves. The divisions and branches of the aorta are as follows:

The aorta, its three divisions, and numerous branches, and the areas they supply are:

I. **AORTIC ARCH** (5 branches)
- A. Two ***coronary arteries*** (right and left)—Provide blood supply to myocardium
- B. One ***innominate artery***—Divides into ***right subclavian artery*** which provides blood for the right arm and other areas and ***right common carotid artery*** which supplies the right side of the head and neck
- C. ***Left common carotid artery***—Supplies left side of head and neck
- D. ***Left subclavian artery***—Provides blood for left arm and portion of thoracic area

II. **THORACIC AORTA**
- A. Two or more ***bronchial arteries***—Provide blood for bronchi
- B. Four or five ***esophageal arteries***—Provide blood to esophagus
- C. ***Pericardial arteries***—Supply pericardium
- D. Nine pairs of ***intercostal arteries***—Supply blood for intercostal areas
- E. ***Mediastinal branches*** — Supply lymph glands and posterior mediastinum
- F. ***Superior phrenic arteries***—Supply diaphragm

III. **ABDOMINAL AORTA**
- A. ***Celiac artery***—Supplies stomach, liver, and spleen
- B. ***Superior mesenteric artery***—Supplies all of small intestine except superior portion of duodenum
- C. ***Inferior mesenteric artery***—Supplies all of colon and rectum except right half of the transverse colon
- D. ***Middle suprarenal branches***—Supply adrenal (suprarenal) glands
- E. ***Renal arteries***—Supply kidneys, ureters, and adrenals
- F. ***Testicular arteries***—Supply testicles and ureter
- G. ***Ovarian arteries***—Correspond to ***internal spermatic arteries*** of the male. Supply the ovaries, part of ureters, and uterine tubes
- H. ***Inferior phrenic arteries***—Supply diaphragm and esophagus
- I. ***Lumbar arteries***—Supply lumbar and psoas muscles and part of abdominal wall musculature
- J. ***Middle sacral artery***—Supplies sacrum, coccyx
- K. ***Right*** and ***left common iliac arteries***—Supply lower pelvic and abdominal areas and the lower extremities

aor'tal. Pert. to the aorta.

aortalgia (a-or-tal'jĭ-ă) [G. *aorte*, aorta, + G. *algos*, pain]. Pain in the aortic area.

aortarctia (a-or-tark'shĭ-ă) [" + L. *arctare*, to narrow]. Aortic narrowing.

aortectasia (a-or-tek-tā'zĭ-ă) [" + *ek*, out, + *tasis*, a stretching]. Dilatation of the aorta.

aor'tic. Pert. to aorta or its orifice in the left ventricle of the heart.

a. murmur. Symptom of a. valvular disease.

a. opening. 1. Path through diaphragm for aorta. 2. Post. opening in the diaphragm.

a. regurgita'tion. Leakage of the blood from the aorta back into the left ventricle at the recoil of the aorta's elastic walls. ETIOL: Diseases of the heart or aortic valves with defects or weakness of heart muscle. SYN: *aortic insufficiency.*

a. stenosis. Narrowing of aorta or its orifice due to lesions of the wall with scar formation, infection as in rheumatic fever, or embryonic anomalies. Hypertrophy of the heart is a common result.

a. valves. Three valves in left ventricle at the a. opening.

aortitis (ā-or-tī'tis) [G. *aortē*, aorta, + *-itis*, inflammation]. Inflammation of the aorta. Associated with syphilis in which vascular changes have taken place. A common cause of aortic aneurysm.

SYM: Possible cough, cyanosis, dyspnea, cardiac asthmatic attacks, hemoptysis.

aortoclasia (ā-or-tō-klā'zĭ-ă) [" + *klasis*, a breaking]. Aortic rupture.

aortog'raphy [" + G. *graphein*, to write]. Examination of abdominal aorta by x-ray after injection of contrast fluid.

aortolith (ā-or'tō-lith) [" + G. *lithos*, stone]. Calcareous deposit in the aortic wall.

aortomalacia (ā-or-tō-mă-lā'sĭ-ă) [" + G. *malakia*, softness]. Softening of the aorta's walls.

aortop'athy [" + G. *pathos*, disease]. Any aortic disease.

aortoptosia, aortoptosis (ā-or-top-tō'zĭ-ă, -sis) [" + G. *ptosis*, a falling]. Downward displacement of abdominal aorta.

aortorrhaphy (ā-or-tor'ă-fĭ) [" + *raphē*, suture]. Suture of the aorta.

aortosclero'sis [" + *skleros*, hard]. Aortic sclerosis.

aortostenosis (ā-or-tō-sten-ō'sis) [" + G. *stenōsis*, a narrowing]. Narrowing of the aorta.

aortot'omy [" + G. *tomē*, a cutting]. Incision of the aorta.

AOS. Abbr. for *anodal opening sound.*

aos'mic [G. *a-*, priv. + *osmē*, smell]. Without odor.

A. O. T. A. Abbr. for *American Occupational Therapy Association.*

A. P. A. Abbr. for *American Pharmaceutical Association; American Physiotherapy Association; American Psychiatric Association.*

apallesthesia (ă-pal"es-thē'zĭ-ă) [G. *a-*, priv. + *pallein*, to tremble, + *aisthēsis*, feeling]. Inability to detect vibrations of a tuning fork placed against the body.

apan'dria [G. *apo*, from, + *anēr* (*andr-*), man]. Aversion to males.

apanthropia, apanthropy (a-pan-thrō'pĭ-ă, a-pan'thrō-pĭ) [" + *anthrōpos*, man]. Morbid aversion to society or fear of human companionship.

aparalyt'ic [G. *a-*, priv. + *paralyein*, to loosen]. Marked by lack of paralysis.

aparathyrosis (ă-par-ă-thī-rō'sis) [" + *para*, near, + *thyreos*, an oblong shield, + *osis*, denoting increase]. Parathyroid deficiency.

apareunia (a-pă-rū'nĭ-ă) [" + *pareunos*, lying beside]. Impossibility or absence of coitus.

aparthrosis (ap-ar-thrō'sis) [G. *apo*, from, + *arthron*, joint, + *osis*, denoting increase]. 1. ANAT: A joint, such as the shoulder joint, which moves freely in any direction. SYN: *diarthrosis.* 2. Dislocation of a joint.

apastia (a-pas'tĭ-ă) [G. *apastia*, fasting]. Abnormal refusal to eat.

apathetic (ap-ă-thet'ik) [G. *a-*, priv. + *pathos*, disease]. Indifferent; without interest. SYN: *apathic.*

apath'ic. Indifferent. SYN: *apathetic.*

apathism (ap'ă-thĭzm) [G. *a-*, priv. + *pathos*, disease, + *ismos*, condition]. Slow to react; opp. to erethism, *q.v.*

ap'athy. Indifference; insensibility; without emotion, sluggish, opp. to erethism.

A. P. C. Abbr. for *acetylsalicylic acid, phenacetin,* and *caffeine*, common ingredients in various headache and cold tablets.

A-P-C virus. Adenoidal-pharyngeal-conjunctival v. A group of viruses. Some eight of the more than 30 types cause acute respiratory illness, especially at military camps where new recruits are brought together. Types 1, 2, 3, 4, 5, 7, 14, and 21 are most commonly involved. Type 8 is the principal cause of epidemic keratoconjunctivitis.

apectomy (a-pĕk'tō-mĭ) [L. *apex*, tip, + G. *ektomē*, incision]. Eradication of apex of a tooth root. SYN: *apicoectomy.*

ape hand. Nerve lesion in which the thumb remains extended at right angle from hand.

apeidosis (ap-ī-dō'sis) [G. *apo*, away, + *eidos*, form]. Slow disappearance of characteristic form in a disease.

apellous (ă-pel'us) [G. *a-*, priv. + L. *pellis*, skin]. 1. Without skin, or, in wounds, lack of formation of scar tissue. 2. Having a short prepuce, or circumcised.

apenteric (ap-en-ter'ik) [G. *apo*, from, + *enteron*, intestine]. Outside the intestine. SYN: *abenteric.*

apep'sia [G. *a-*, priv. + *pepsis*, a digesting]. 1. Absence of pepsin in the gastric juice. 2. Imperfect digestion or its cessation.

apepsin'ia. Absence of pepsin in the gastric juice.

aperient (a-pĕr'ĭ-ĕnt) [L. *aperire*, to open]. A very mild laxative. Ex: *magnesium oxide.*

NP: Usually given at night on an empty stomach if the drug acts slowly (10 to 12 hours). Saline a. and those having rapid action are given first thing in morning on an empty stomach, half-hour before first fluids are ingested.

Aperients should not be given in suspected appendicitis, in colic as a rule, in enteritis if diarrhea and vomiting are present.

aperistal'sis [G. *a-*, priv. + *peri*, around, + *stalsis*, constriction]. Absence of peristalsis.

aperitif [L. *aperire*, to open]. An alcoholic beverage such as wine taken before a meal to stimulate the appetite.

aper'itive [L. *aperire*, to open]. 1. An appetizer. 2. Mild purgative. SYN: *aperient, q.v.*

apertura (ap-er-tū'ră) (pl. *aperturae*) [L. *apertura*, opening]. An opening.

aperture (ap'er-tūr). An orifice or opening.

apex (ā'peks) (pl. *apices*) [L. apex, tip]. The summit or extremity of anything.

a. beat. The point of maximum impulse of the heart against the chest wall felt in the 5th left intercostal space, approximately 3½ inches from middle of sternum, about an inch within a line drawn from middle of clavicle parallel with sternum (the mammary line).

Generally may be detected by inspection or palpation; when these fail, may be localized by auscultation. In recumbent position apex beat may be elevated an inch or more. When body is inclined to left, beat may be detected in mammary line or even some distance outside. During forced inspiration, may become imperceptible or be found below its usual place. During forced expiration, beat becomes more forcible and position elevated. Patient as a rule should be examined in erect or sitting posture, while breathing quietly.

A weak apex beat may be noted in: Healthy persons at rest, degeneration or dilatation of heart, pericardial effusion, emphysema, shock or collapse.

CHANGES IN FORCE AND EXTENT: May be increased by hypertrophy of heart; excited action of heart from exercise, drugs, reflex irritation, excitement or disease (as exophthalmic goiter); shrinking of the lungs, as in phthisis.

DISPLACEMENT TO THE LEFT: May result from hypertrophy and dilatation of the heart (down and to the left); pneumothorax on the right; pericardial effusion (up and to left); chronic diseases of left lung and pleura, associated with retraction—as fibroid phthisis and pleural adhesions; abdominal tumors and effusions (up and to left); pressure of a pleural effusion on the right side (up and to left).

DISPLACEMENT TO RIGHT: May be caused by chronic disease of the right lung or pleura, associated with retraction; pneumothorax on the left; pressure of a pleural effusion on left side.

DISPLACEMENT DOWNWARD: May result from hypertrophy and dilatation of heart, chiefly the left ventricle; pressure of solid growths in upper mediastinum; aneurysm of aortic arch; enlargement of liver, causing traction through central tendon of diaphragm.

Deformity of chest may cause displacement in any direction.

PRECORDIAL PROMINENCE: May result from deformity, enlargement of heart, pericardial effusions.

a. murmur. One over the apex of the heart.

a. root. The end of the root of a tooth.

apex'igraph, apex'ograph [" + G. *graphein,* to write]. An instrument for determining location and size of apex of a tooth root.

Apgar score. System of scoring infant's condition one minute after birth. The heart rate, respiration, muscle tone, color, and response to stimuli are scored 0, 1, or 2. The maximum score for a normal baby is 10. Those with low scores require immediate attention if they are to survive. SEE: Table.

a., gibberish. Utterance of meaningless phrases.

a., motor. Patient knows what he wants to say but cannot say it. Muscles, controlling speech, unable to coordinate. May be complete or partial. Broca's area is disordered or diseased.

a., nominal. Inability to name objects.

a., optic. Inability to call name of an object recognized by sight without the aid of sound, taste, or touch; a form of agnosia, *q.v.*

a., semantic. Inability to understand meaning of words.

a., sensory. Inability to understand spoken words if word center is involved (auditory a.) or the written word if visual word center is affected (visual a.). If both centers are involved, will not understand spoken or written word.

a., syntactic. Loss of proper grammatical construction.

a., traumatic. A. caused by head injury.

a., Wernicke's. Sensory aphasia, *q.v.*

apha'sic, apha'siac. Pert. to aphasia.

aphelotic (af-el-ot'ĭk) [*aphelkein,* to draw away]. Absent minded; given to reverie.

aphemesthesia (ă-fem"es-thē'zĭ-ă) [G. *a-,* priv. + *phēmē,* speech, + *aisthesis,* sensation]. Word deafness, or word blindness.

APGAR SCORE TABLE

SIGN	SCORE 0	SCORE 1	SCORE 2
Heart rate	Absent	Slow or less than 100	Greater than 100
Respiratory effort	Absent	Slow, irregular	Good; crying
Muscle tone	Limp	Some flexion of extremities	Active motion
Reflex irritability	No response	Grimace	Cough or sneeze
Color	Blue, pale	Body pink; extremities blue	Completely pink

A.P.H.A. Abbr. for *American Public Health Association.*

aphacia (ă-fā'sĭ-ă). Aphakia, *q.v.*

aphacic (ă-fā'sĭk). Aphakic.

aphagia (a-fā'jĭ-ă) [G. *a-,* priv. + *phagein,* to eat]. Inability to swallow.

aphakia (ă-fā'kĭ-ă) [G. *a-,* priv. + *phakos,* lentil]. Absence of eye's crystalline lens.

aphakic (ă-fā'kĭk). Pert. to aphakia.

aphalangia (ă-fă-lan'jĭ-ă). Absence of fingers and toes.

aphanisis (ă-făn'ĭ-sĭs). Absence of sexuality in an individual.

aphasia (ă-fā'zĭ-ă) [" + *phasis,* speaking]. Inability to express oneself properly through speech, or loss of verbal comprehension.

It is considered to be complete or total when both sensory and motor areas are involved. SYN: *logagnosia.*

RS: *agraphia, alalia, anarthria, aphemia, atactic, mind blindness, mind deafness, paraphasia, word blindness.*

a., amnesic. Loss of memory for words.

a., ataxic. Inability to articulate. Similar to *motor a.*

a., auditory. Inability to understand meaning of spoken words; word deafness.

a., Broca's. Motor a., *q.v.*

a., conduction. ETIOL: Due to lesion of conduction path bet. motor and speech centers.

aphemia (ă-fē'mĭ-ă) [" + *phēmē,* speech]. Loss of speech due to impairment of the word memory center; ataxic aphasia.

aphephobia (af-ĕ-fō'bĭ-ă) [G. *aphē,* touch, + *phobos,* fear]. Abnormal aversion to being touched by anyone.

aphilopony (aph"ĭ-lop'o-nĭ) [G. *a-,* + *philein,* to love, + *ponos,* bodily exertion]. An abnormal dread of or dislike for work.

aphlogistic (ā"flō-jĭs'tik, af"lō-jĭs'tĭk) [G. *a-,* priv. + *phlogistos,* inflammable]. 1. Not inflammable. 2. Burning without flame.

aphonia (ă-fō'nĭ-ă) [" + *phonē,* voice]. Loss of voice with intact inner speech and not due to central lesion. May occur in chronic laryngitis.

ETIOL: Disease of vocal cords, paralysis of laryngeal nerves, pressure on recurrent laryngeal nerve, or it may be functional due to hysteria or psychiatric causes.

a. clericorum. Clergyman's sore throat.

a. paranoica. The silence of the mentally ill.

a., paralytic. A. resulting from paralysis of speech muscles.

a., spastic. A. resulting from spasm of vocal muscles, esp. that initiated by efforts to speak.

aphonogelia (ă-fo″no-je′lĭ-ă) [G. *a-*, + *phone*, voice, + *gelos*, laughter]. Inability to laugh out loud.

aphoresis (af-ō-rē′sis) [" + *phorēsis*, being transmitted]. 1. Lack of endurance, especially of pain. 2.Any separation or removal of a part.

aphoria (ă-fō′rĭ-ă) [" + *phoros*, carrier]. Sterility in the female.

aphose (af′ōz) [" + *phōs*, light]. A subjective visual perception of darkness, or of a shadow.

aphrasia (ă-frā′zĭ-ă) [" + *phrasis*, speech]. Inability in using connected phrases when speaking.

a., paralytic. Due to paralysis of the faculty of ideation.

a., superstitious. Avoidance of certain words because of scruples or aversion to their use.

aphrenia (a-frē′nĭ-ă) [" + *phrēn*, mind]. An apparent lack of intellect seen in some forms of dementia.

a. apoplexy. Unconsciousness.

aphrenic, aphrenous (ă-fren′ĭk, -′us). Pertaining to dementia.

aphrodisia (af-rō-dĭz′ĭ-ă) [G. *aphrodisios*, rel. to *Aphrodite*, goddess of love]. 1. Sexual passion, esp. when morbid, extreme or violent. 2. Sexual intercourse.

aphrodisiac (af-rō-diz′ĭ-ak). An agent which stimulates sexual desire.

aphronesia (ă-fro-ne′sĭ-ă) [G. *a-*, priv. + *phronēsis*, common sense]. 1. Silliness. 2. Dementia.

aphronia (ă-frō′nĭ-ă) [G. *aphrōn*, foolish]. Mental deficiency; defective functional activity of cerebrum.

aphtha (af′thă) (pl. *aphthae*) [G. small ulcer]. 1. Small ulcer on a mucous membrane of the mouth. 2. Thrush.

a., Bednar's. Whitish ulceration of hard palate in young children.

a., cachectic. Lesions formed beneath the tongue; accompanied by severe constitutional symptoms.

aphthenxia (af-thengks′ĭ-ă) [G. *a-*, priv. + *phthegxis*, utterance]. An aphasia with articulate sounds imperfectly expressed.

aphthongia (af-thon′jĭ-ă) [G. *a-*, priv. + *phthoggos*, voice]. Aphasia due to spasm of muscles controlling speech.

aphthous (af′thus) [G. *aphtha*, small ulcer]. Pert. to, or characterized by, ulcers.

a. fever. Foot and mouth disease, *q.v.*

aphylac′tic [G. *a-*, priv. + *phylaxis*, a protecting]. Having no immune power.

aphylaxis (ă-fi-laks′is). Without immunity against disease.

apical [L. *apex*, tip]. Pert. to the apex.

apicectomy (ap″is-ĕk′tō-mĭ) [L. *apex*, tip, + G. *tomē*, incision]. Eradication of apex of a tooth root. Syn: *apicoectomy; apicotomy.*

apices (a′pis-ez). Pl. of apex.

apicitis (ap-ĭ-sī′tis) [" + G. *-itis*, inflammation]. Inflammation of any apical structure, esp. apex of lung or tooth root.

apicoectomy (ap-ĭ-kō-ĕk′tō-mĭ) [" + G. *ektomē*, incision]. Amputation of apex of a tooth root. Syn: *apicectomy; apicotomy.*

apicoloca′tor [" + *locare*, to place]. Instrument for locating apex of a tooth root. Syn: *apexigraph; apexograph.*

apicolysis (ap-i-kol′ĭ-sis) [" + G. *lysis*, solution]. Artificial collapse of the apex of a lung by making an opening through the anterior chest wall.

NP: Keep patient on affected side and watch for shock and hemorrhage.

apicotomy (ap-ĭ-kot′ō-mĭ) [" + G. *tomē*, incision]. Removal of apex of a tooth root. Syn: *apicoectomy.*

apinealism (ă-pin′ē-al-izm) [G. *a-*, priv. + G. *pineus*, pert. to pine, + *ismos*, condition of]. Syndrome due to absence of pineal gland.

ap′inoid [" + *pinos*, filth, + *eidos*, appearance]. Free from dirt; clean.

a. cancer. Hard cancer.

apiphobia (ă-pĭ-fo′bĭ-ă) [L. *apis*, bee, + G. *phobos*, fear]. Abnormal fear of bees or of insects which buzz like a bee.

apisination (ă-pĭs-ĭ-nā′shun) [L. *apis*, bee]. Poisoning from bee stings.

apituitarism (ă-pĭ-tū′ĭ-tar-izm) [G. *a-*. priv. + L. *pituita*, phlegm, + *ismos*, condition of]. Condition due to total abeyance of function or removal of pituitary body. Leads to cachexia hypophyseopriva.

APL. 1. Abbr. for *anterior pituitary-like* (hormone), a substance with activity similar to chorionic gonadotropin. 2. Proprietary name for a preparation of chorionic gonadotropin.

aplanat′ic lens [" + *planētos*, wandering]. Free from spherical or chromatic aberration. Not wandering.

aplasia (ă-plā′zĭ-ă) [" + *plasis*, a developing]. Failure of an organ or part of the body to develop naturally.

a. axialis extracorticalis congenita. Congenital defect of the axon formation on the surface of the cerebral cortex.

aplas′tic [" + *plastikos*, shaped]. Having deficient or arrested development.

apnea (ap-nē′ă) [G. *a-*, priv. + *pnoē*, breath]. Cessation of breathing, usually of a temporary nature. May result from reduction in stimuli to the respiratory center as in overbreathing in which carbon dioxide content of the blood is reduced, or from failure of respiratory center to discharge impulses as occur when the breath is held voluntarily. It may also occur during Cheyne-Stokes respiration, *q.v.*

It is a serious symptom esp. in such conditions as arteriosclerosis, meningitis, coma, heart and kidney diseases, and also following an injury to the brain where concussion results. Sometimes this type of breathing is noticed in perfectly healthy children and in the aged during profound sleep.

Sym: It is characterized by a gradual increase in the rate until it ends in a gasp followed by a gradual decrease until the respiration ceases, then it begins again. Another form is sometimes noticed when the respirations gradually increase in force and frequency and then suddenly cease.

apneumatosis (ap-nū-mă-tō′sis). Noninflation of air cells; congenital atelectasis.

apneusis (ăp-nū′sĭs). A sustained respiratory inspiratory effort. Due to surgical removal of the upper portion of the pons.

apo- (ap′o) [G. *apo*, from]. Prefix denoting from, away, separation, as *apophysis.*

apobiosis (ap″o-bi-o′sis) [G. *apo-*, from or away, + *bios*, life]. Phys: Death of a part.

apocamnosis (ap-ō-kam-nō′sis) [G. *apokamnein*, to grow weary]. Weariness, easily induced fatigue.

apocenosis (ap-ō-sĕn-ō′sis) [G. *apokenoein*, to drain]. 1. Increased flow of blood or body fluids. 2. Partial evacuation.

apochromatic (ăp-ō-krō-măt′ĭk) [G. *apokenoein,* to drain, + *chrōmatikos,* colored]. Free from spherical and chromatic aberration, said of lenses.

apocope (ă-pok′ō-pē) [G. *apokopē,* a cutting off]. Amputation.

apocoptic (ap-ō-kop′tik) [G. *apokoptein,* to cut off]. The effect resulting from the removal of a part.

apocrine (ap′ō-krēn, -krĭn) [G. *apo,* from, + *krinein,* to separate]. 1. Pertaining to cells which lose part of their cytoplasm while functioning especially gland cells such as those of the mammary glands and certain sweat glands. 2. Describes sweat glands which differ from the usual (*eccrine*) in that they appear only in hairy areas such as axillae, groin, and mammary. They appear after puberty, are better developed in women than in men and in Negroes than in Caucasians. The characteristic odor of perspiration is produced by the action of bacteria on the material secreted by the apocrine sweat glands SEE: *holocrine; eccrine; merocrine.*

apocrustic (ap-ō-krus′tĭk) [G. *apokroustikos,* able to ward off]. 1. Astringent. 2. Repellent. 3. Defensive.

apodal (ă-pō′dal) [*a-,* + G. *pous,* foot, + al]. Having no feet.

apodemialgia (ap-ō-dē-mĭ-al′gĭ-ă) [G. *apodēmia,* away from home, + *algos,* pain]. 1. An abnormal desire to wander from one's abode or environment; wanderlust. 2. Morbid dislike of a home.

apodia (ă-pō′dē-ă). Developmental defect with absence of one or both feet.

apogee (ap′ō-gē) [G. *apo,* from, + *gē,* earth]. Most critical stage of a disease.

apokamnosis (ap-ō-kam-nō′sis) [G. *apokamnein,* to grow weary, + *osis,* denoting increase]. Abnormal tendency to fatigue, as in neurasthenia.

apolepsis (ap-ō-lep′sis) [G. *apolepsis,* a leaving off]. 1. Cessation of a function. 2. Retention or suppression of an excretion or secretion.

apolexis (ap-ō-leks′is) [G. *apolexis,* a declining]. 1. The catabolic condition or process. 2. Decline of life.

apomorphine (ap-ō-mor′fēn). A morphine derivative prepared from the alkaloid by removal of one molecule of water.

a. hydrochloride. USP. A grayish white powder which becomes green in color on exposure to water or air.

ACTION AND USES: 1. Emetic; sometimes valuable in cases of poisoning when stomach pump cannot be employed. 2. In small doses may be used as an expectorant.

apomyelin (ap-ō-mĭ′ĕ-lĭn) [G. *apo,* from, + *myelos,* marrow]. A brain substance containing no glycerol.

apomyttosis (ap″o-mĭ-to′sis) [G. *apomyssein,* to blow the nose]. Any disease in which stertorous breathing or sneezing is a characteristic sign.

apone (a′pōn) [G. *a-,* priv. + *ponos,* pain]. An anodyne.

ap″oneurol′ogy [" + *logos,* word]. The science of aponeuroses.

ap″oneuror′rhaphy [G. *apo,* from, + *neuron,* nerve, + *raphē,* suture]. Aponeurotic suture.

aponeurosis (ăp-ō-nū-rō′sĭs) (pl. *aponeuroses*) [G. *apo,* from, + *neuron,* sinew]. A flat fibrous sheet of connective tissue which serves to attach muscle to bone or other tissues at their origin or insertion.

a., epicranial. The *galea aponeurotica.* A fibrous membrane extending from occipital muscles anteriorly to frontal muscles.

a., lumbar. Superficial sheet of the a. of origin of the transversus abdominis muscle. With the lumbocostal a., encloses the sacrospinalis muscle.

a., lumbocostal. Deep sheet of the a. of origin of the transversus abdominis muscle. With the lumbar a., encloses the sacrospinalis muscle.

a., pharyngeal. Sheet of connective tissue lying just under the mucosa of pharynx.

aponeurositis (ap-ō-nū-rō-sī′tis) [" + *itis,* inflammation]. Aponeurotic inflammation.

aponeurot′ic. Pert. or rel. to an aponeurosis.

aponeurotome (ap-ō-nū′rō-tōm) [G. *apo,* from, + *neuron,* sinew, + *tomē,* cutting]. Knife for dividing an aponeurosis.

aponeurotomy ap-ō-nū-rot′ō-mĭ). Surgical cutting of an aponeurosis.

aponia (ă-pon′ĭ-ă) [G. *a-,* priv. + *ponos,* pain]. 1. Abstaining from labor. 2. Absence of pain.

aponic (a-pon′ik). Rel. to aponia.

aponoia, aponoea (ap-ō-noy′ă, ap-ō-nē′ă) [G. *apo,* from, + *nous,* mind]. Amentia.

apophlegmatic (ap-ō-fleg-mat′ik) [" + *phlegmatikos,* abounding in mucus]. Producing a mucous discharge; expectorant.

apophyseal (ap-ō-fĭz′ē-al) [" + *physis,* growth]. Rel. or pert. to an apophysis.

apophysis (ă-pof′ĭ-sĭs) (pl. *apophyses*) [from G. *apophysis,* offshoot]. 1. A projection esp. from a bone, an outgrowth without an independent center of ossification. Ex: a *tubercle* or *tuberosity.*

a. cerebri. The pineal body.

a. of Ingrassia. Smaller wing of sphenoid bone.

a. lenticularis. Temporal bone's orbicular process.

a. of Rau, a. raviana. Long process of malleus.

apophysitis (ă-pof-ĭ-sī′tis) [G. *apo,* from, + *physis,* growth, + *itis,* inflammation]. Inflammation of an apophysis, *q.v.*

apoplasmia (ap-ō-plaz′mĭ-ă) [" + *plasma,* formation]. Deficiency of blood plasma.

apoplectic (ap-ō-plek′tĭk) [G. *apoplēktikos,* crippled by stroke]. Pert. to apoplexy.

apoplec′tiform [G. *apoplexia,* stroke, + L. *forma,* appearance]. Like apoplexy. SYN: *apoplectoid.*

apoplectigenous (ap-ō-plĕk-tĭj′ĭ-nus) [" + *genos,* origin]. Causing apoplexy.

apoplec′toid [" + *eidos,* form]. Like apoplexy. SYN: *apoplectiform.*

apoplexia (ap-o-pex′ĭ-ă). Apoplexy, *q.v.*

a. uteri. Sudden hemorrhage from the uterus due to arterial degeneration or infarct.

apoplexy (ăp′ō-plĕk-sĭ) [G. *apoplēxia,* a stroke]. 1. Sudden loss of consciousness followed by paralysis due to hemorrhage into brain or spinal cord, or formation of an embolus or thrombus, which occludes an artery. SYN: *shock; stroke.** 2. Condition of an organ marked by a hemorrhage into its substance, as apoplexy of the lung.

SYM: Onset acute. Unconsciousness. Stertorous breathing due to paralysis of portion of the soft palate; expiration puffs out the cheeks and mouth. Pupils sometimes unequal, the larger one being on the side of the hemorrhage. Paralysis usually involves one side of the face, arm and leg of one side, with eyeballs turned away from the side of the body-paralysis, unequal pupils, skin covered clammy sweat, the surface tem-ure of which is often subnormal; disturbances, onset more gradual used by a thrombosis, *q.v.*

PROG: Depends upon symptoms. Often grave.

NP: As patient recovering from unconsciousness may hear all that is said in the room, care should be exercised about talking in presence of patient. Complete quiet. Guard against self-inflicted injuries to nonparalyzed side from movements due to irritation. Supine position: Head and body on same plane. Avoid pressure sores by moving patient frequently. Ease breathing by change of position once an hour, turning from paralyzed side to back and reverse. To lie on paralyzed side may require much effort to breathe. Turn body as a whole, not in part, flexing a paralyzed arm across chest, lower extremities flexed. Frequent cleansing of oropharyngeal passages.

Maintain body heat, but care must be exercised lest the unconscious patient be burned. Guard against sacral bed sores (not due to pressure; a cutaneous indication of lowered vitality). This is indicated by redness of skin which may be followed by superficial blisters, resulting in a gangrenous ulcer. Constant asepsis and antisepsis if break occurs in skin. Binders to hold dressings; no adhesive plasters.

A retention catheter may be used to avoid a wet bed. Use of a closed urinary drainage system is essential to prevent infection. Enemas instead of purgatives. Avoid pressure of bed clothes by using a bed cradle. Watch for contractures of muscles and avoid these by change of position and passive exercise.

Convalescence: Liquid or soft foods; solid ones as patient begins to masticate. Slight elevation of head when feeding which should be done from the paralyzed side unless patient exhibits imperfect sight, when position should be reversed to accommodate.

Feed slowly to avoid stoppage of windpipe. Loss of muscular power of pharynx, of tongue and cheeks must be considered. Frequent bathing; emollients or cocoa butter applied afterward. Watch for danger from heat or cold if loss of sensation is manifested in any part. Systematic massage. No strenuous rubbing. Passive exercises until active movements are possible.

Hemiplegic or chronic state: Careful training of muscles and organs of speech is necessary. Physical therapy, later followed perhaps by occupational therapy. Confidence must be inspired, memory trained and emotions controlled by patient. Nurse should teach patient how to sit and how to stand and walk.

F. A. TREATMENT: Keep patient quiet and sitting up or lying down with head and shoulders elevated. Do not give stimulants. Apply cooling applications to head and neck. Do not transport unless absolutely imperative—and then very carefully.

RS: *Aaron's sign, coma, hemiplegia.*

aporioneurosis (ap-or-ĭ-ō-nū-rō'sis) [G. *aporia*, doubt, + *neuron*, nerve, + *osis*, increased]. Anxiety neurosis, *q.v.*

aporrhegma (ap-ō-reg'mă) [G. *apo*, away, + *rēgma*, separation]. 1. A biological separation of one substance from another. 2. Any nitrogen-containing substance formed by the removal of carbon dioxide from protein-derivatives, as when histamine, $C_3H_3N_2(CH_2)_2NH_2$, is formed by putrefaction from histidine, $C_3H_3N_2CH_2CH(NH_2)COOH$.

aporrhipsis (ap-ō-rip'sis) [" + *riptein*, to throw]. Removal of clothing or bed clothes; seen in some psychotic conditions or in delirium.

aposia (a-pō'zĭ-ă) [G. *a-*, priv. + *posis*, drink]. Absence of thirst.

apositia (ap-ō-sit'ĭ-ă, -sish'ĭ-ă) [G. *apo*, away, + *sitos*, food]. Anorexia associated with disgust for food.

apospory (ă-pos'pō-rĭ) [" + *sporos*, seed]. In botany, absence of spore-producing ability.

apostasis (ă-pos'tă-sis) [G. *apostasis*, departure from]. 1. The crisis or end of a disease. 2. An abscess. 3. An exfoliation of bone.

apostaxis (ap-ō-staks'ĭs) [G. *apo*, from, + *stazein*, to drop]. 1. Epistaxis. 2. Discharge by drops.

apostem, apostema (ap'ō-stem, -stē'mă) [G. *apostēma*, abscess]. An abscess.

aposthia (ă-pos'thĭ-ă) [G. *a-*, priv. + *posthē*, foreskin]. Congenital absence of the prepuce.

apothanasia (ap-ō-thă-nā'zĭ-ă) [G. *apo*, away, + *thanatos*, death]. Prolongation of life.

apoth'ecaries' weights and measures. An outdated and obsolete system of weights and measures used by physicians and pharmacists. Has been replaced by the metric system, *q.v.*

The scruple and the pound are now seldom used. A portion of a grain is expressed fractionally, as gr. ½, not decimally. The quantity is written in Roman numerals, *q.v.*, with the symbol before it, as gr. v to indicate five grains, or ℥ $\frac{\cdot\cdot}{\text{xii}}$ for 12 ounces.

Weights

20 grains (gr.)	= 1 scruple	(℈)
60 grains (gr.) (3 ℈)	= 1 dram	(ʒ)
8 drams (ʒ)	= 1 ounce	(℥)
12 oz. (℥) (5760 gr.)	= 1 pound	(lb.)

Measures

60 minims	(♏)	= 1 fluidram	(f ʒ)
8 fluidrams	(f ʒ)	= 1 fluidounce	(f ℥)
16 fluidounces	(f ℥)	= 1 pint	(pt.)
2 pints	(pt.)	= 1 quart	(qt.)
4 quarts	(qt.)	= 1 gallon	(C)

Some points to remember are: The character ʒ represents 60 grains, while f ʒ represents 60 minims. ℥ represents 480 grains only, while f ℥ is necessary to express 480 minims. A minim is not the equivalent of a grain. 480 minims (1 f ℥) of water weighed at the standard temperature weigh 456.37 grains. This should be remembered for percentage solutions. Specific gravities of liquids vary; a pint of a liquid is not necessarily a pound.

apothecary (ă-poth'ĕ-kā-rĭ) [G. *apothēkē*, storing place]. A druggist or pharmacist. In England and Ireland one licensed by the Society of Apothecaries as an authorized physician and dispenser of drugs.

apothem, apotheme (ap'ō-thĕm, -thēm) [G. *apo*, away, + *thema*, deposit]. The brown precipitate which appears when vegetable decoctions or infusions are exposed to the air or are boiled a long time.

apothesis (ă-poth'ĕ-sĭs) [G. *apothesis*, a placing back]. Reduction of a fracture or dislocation.

apotheter (ă-poth'ĕ-ter) [G. *apothetein*, to stow away]. An instrument used during delivery to push up a prolapsed umbilical cord.

apotox'in [G. *apo*, away, + *toxikon*, poison]. The anaphylactic substance due to action of toxogenin on injected toxin.

apotrip'sis [G. *apotribein*, to abrade]. Removal of opacity in cornea.

apozem, apozeme (ap'ō-zĕm, -zēm) [G. *apo*, away, + *zein*, to boil]. A decoction.

apparatus (ap-ă-rā'tus) [L. *apparare*, to prepare]. 1. A number of parts acting together in the performance of some special function. 2. ANAT: A group of structures or organs which work together to perform a common function. 3. A mechanical appliance or appliances, used in operations and experiments.

a., acoustic. Auditory apparatus, the assemblage of parts essential for hearing.

a., biliary. The structures concerned with secretion and excretion of bile. Includes liver, gallbladder, and hepatic, cystic and common bile ducts.

a., Clover's. A device used in administering ether or chloroform.

a., Fell - O'Dwyer's. An instrument for performing artificial respiration, and for preventing collapse of the lung in chest operations.

a., Golgi. The internal reticular apparatus, *q.v.*

a., internal reticular. A cell organoid of variable shape—sometimes granular, reticular, or canalicular—present in most cells, esp. nerve and gland cells. It is rich in lipid materials and varies in size with functional activity of the cell. Its exact function is unknown but it is thought to be involved in secretory activity. Also called *Golgi complex, lipochondria, canalicular apparatus.*

a., juxtaglomerular. Thickened portion of an afferent arteriole in the cortex of a kidney. Consists of modified smooth muscles which acquire a clear swollen appearance. Considered to be the possible source of renin.

a., lacrimal. The tear-secreting gland and various structures by which tears are conveyed to the nasal cavity.

a. ligamentosus colli. The occipitoaxial ligament.

a., respiratory. The entire respiratory system.

a., sound conducting. Those parts of the acoustic apparatus that transmit sound.

a., sound perceiving. Those central parts of the acoustic apparatus that are essential for the perception of sounds.

a., vocal. The various organs collectively that subserve phonation.

appendage (ă-pĕn'dĭj). Anything attached or appended to a larger or major part, as a tail or a limb. SEE: *appendix.*

a., atrial. A small muscular pouch attached to each atrium of the heart.

a., auricular. Atrial a.

a., cutaneous. Appendages of the skin, as the nails, hair, sebaceous and sweat glands.

appendal'gia [L. *appendere*, hang to, + G. *algos*, pain]. Pain in lower right quadrant in region of vermiform appendix.

appendectomy (ap-en-dek'tō-mĭ) [L. *ad*, to, + *pendere*, hang, + G. *ektome*, cut out]. Surgical removal of the vermiform appendix.

appen'dical, appendiceal (ap-ĕn-dĭs'ē-al). Pert. to an appendix.

a. reflex. Tenderness at McBurney's point accompanied by rigidity considered a reflex expression by way of sympathetic cerebrospinal arc.

appendicectasis (a-pen-dis-ek'tă-sis) [L. *appendere*, hang to, + G. *ektasis*, a stretching]. Appendical dilatation.

appendicectomy (a-pen-dis-ek'tō-mĭ) [" + G. *ektome*, a cutting]. Surgical removal of the appendix.

appendices (a-pen'dĭ-sēz). Plural of appendix.

a. epiploicae. Pouches of peritoneum, filled with fat and attached to the colon.

appendicitis (a-pen-dĭ-sī'tis) [L. *appendere*, hang to, + G. *-itis*, inflammation]. Inflammation of the vermiform appendix.

It generally occurs in the young, very rarely before the fifth year or after the fiftieth. It is more common in male adults than in female adults. The disease may be acute, subacute, or chronic.

When this diagnosis is considered in the adult female, it must be differentiated from pain associated with ovulation ("mittelschmerz," *q.v.*), ruptured ectopic pregnancy, and pelvic inflammatory disease.

a., acute. SYM: (a) Abdominal pain, usually severe and generally throughout the abdomen followed by (b) nausea and vomiting, (c) localization of pain in the right lower quadrant of abdomen with tenderness and rigidity over right rectus muscle or McBurney's point, (d) fever usually rising within several hours, 99° F. to 101° F., (e) pulse increasing with temperature, (f) patient lying on back with right lower extremity frequently flexed to relieve muscle tension, (g) leukocytosis present shortly after onset; (h) in mild cases symptoms begin to subside on the second day, but in more severe cases there may be a cessation of pain indicating that the appendix has ruptured. After a few hours a well defined abscess may be felt in the right iliocecal region showing that nature has walled off the area.

TREATMENT: (1) Notify physician as soon as symptoms do not subside. (2) Refrain from giving foods, liquids, cathartics, enemas, and from applying heat. (3) Surgery within 24 hours of onset is safest procedure.

a., chronic. May follow an acute attack leaving a cicatricial narrowing of the lumen of the appendix, or adhesions. SYM: Gastric indigestion, frequently simulating a gastric ulcer, duodenal ulcer, or gallbladder disease. Tenderness manifested in the right lower abdomen. TREATMENT: Surgical.

a. obliterans, a., protective. A. with adhesions closing the appendiceal cavity.

appendico-enterostomy (a-pen-dik-o-en-ter-os'to-mĭ) [" + G. *enteron*, intestine, + *stoma*, mouth]. 1. Appendicostomy. 2. The establishment of an anastomosis between appendix and intestine.

appendicolithi'asis [" + G. *lithos*, stone]. Formation of calculi in the vermiform appendix.

appendicolysis (a-pen-dĭ-kol'ĭ-sis) [" + G. *lysis*, a loosening]. Operation which frees appendix from adhesions by a slit in the serosa at its base.

appendicopathy (a-pen-di-kop'ath-ĭ) [" + G. *pathos*, disease]. Any disease of the vermiform appendix.

a. oxyurica. Lesion of the appendical mucosa supposedly due to oxyurids (intestinal parasitic worms).

appendico'sis [" + G. *-osis,* increased]. Noninflammatory state of the appendix. SYM: Dull pain, local soreness, afebrile, but continual discomfort.

appendicostomy (a-pen-di-kos'tō-mĭ) [" + G. *stoma,* mouth]. Operation for irrigating cecum and colon.

appendic'ular. 1. Appendical. 2. Pert. to limbs or that appended to another part.

appen'dix (pl. *appendices*) [L.]. An appendage, esp. the vermiform appendix.

a., atrial. A small muscular pouch attached to each atrium of the heart.

a., auricular. Atrial a.

a., ensiform. The third or lowest portion of the sternum.

a. epididymidis. A cystic structure attached to epididymis, a vestigial remnant of cranial tip of mesonephric duct.

a., gangrenous. When inflammation is extreme, blood vessels are blocked in the mesentery, circulation to appendix cut off, and diffuse peritonitis ensues.

a. testis. A vestigial remnant of cranial portion of Müllerian duct forming a small bladderlike structure at cranial end of testis.

a., ventricular. SEE: *saccule of larynx.*

a. vermiformis [NA]. (*a., vermiform* or *processus vermiformis*). A worm-shaped process projecting from the cecum, whose mucous membrane also lines the appendix, which contains many solitary glands. Its average length is 8.3 cm.

a., vesicular. A cystic structure found in the broad ligament near the ovary attached to epoöphoron. It is a vestigial structure representing remains of cranial portion of mesonephric duct.

a., xiphoid. The xiphoid process, small terminal portion of sternum.

appen'dotome [L. *appendere,* hang to, + G. *tomē,* a cutting]. An instrument for excision of appendix.

apperception (ap-er-sep'shun) [L. *ad,* to, + *percipere,* to receive]. 1. The process of receiving (perceiving) and interpreting sensory stimuli. 2. Mental perception, consciousness, recognition.

appercep'tive. Pert. to apperception.

appestat (ap'ĕ-stat). An area of the hypothalamus which is supposed to control appetite for food.

ap'petence, ap'petency [L. *appetere,* to strive for]. An appetite or desire.

ap'petite [L. *appetitus,* longing for]. Desire, esp. for food; not necessarily hunger.

a. juice. Gastric secretion brought about by psychic causes such as sight or odor of food, and by tasting and chewing. It ceases 15 to 20 minutes after mastication is completed.

a., perverted. Desire to eat unnatural and indigestible substances such as paint or laundry starch.

appetite, *words pert. to:* Acoria, anorexia, apositia, bulimia, dysorexia, hyperorexia, malacia, parageusia, pica, polyphagia, taste.

appetition (ăp-ĕ-tĭsh'ŭn) [L. *ad,* toward, + *pe'tere,* to seek]. Desire for some object.

appeti'zer. That which promotes appetite.

applanation (ap-lă-nā'shun) [L. *applanatio*]. Abnormal flattening, as of the corneal surface.

apple (ap'l) [A. S. *aeppel*]. Most widely used of fleshy, many-celled fruits having a core. Fruit of tree of the genus *Malus.*

FRESH: Average serving 1 medium (2½ in. diam., 150 gm.). Calories: 85. Other values: 135 I.U. of vitamin A and small amounts of protein, fat, ascorbic acid and B complex.

a., Adam's. The laryngeal prominence formed by the two laminae of the thyroid cartilage.

ap'ple-head [" + *heāfod,* head]. Dwarf's broad, thick skull.

apple packer's diseases. Those which can afflict persons whose work involves the picking, sorting, or packing of apples.

a. p. epistaxis. Nosebleed due to handling packing trays containing certain dyes.

apple picker's disease. Bronchitis due to a fungicide used on apples.

apple sorter's disease. Contact dermatitis due to chemicals used in washing apples.

apple thinner's disease. Mild intoxication due to pesticide residues.

applicator (ăp'lĭ-kā-tĕr) [L. *applicāre,* to attach]. Device, usually a slender rod of glass or wood, used with a pledget of cotton on the end, to apply medicine to the nose, throat, uterus, or any other body cavity.

apposition (ap-ō-zĭ'shun) [L. *ad,* to, + *ponere,* to place]. 1. Development by accretion. 2. Addition of parts. 3. Fitting together, as the edges of two surfaces.

approximal (ă-proks'ĭ-mal) [L. *ad,* to, + *proximus,* nearest]. Contiguous; next to.

approximate (ă-prŏks'ĭ-māt) [L. from *ad,* toward, + *proximare,* to come near]. To bring a part toward another, as when bringing the fingers together or an arm toward the body.

apraxia (a-praks'ĭ-ă) [G. *apraxia,* inaction]. 1. Inability to perform certain purposive movements without loss of motor power, sensation, or coordination. 2. Ridiculous and out of the ordinary acts performed by the insane. Inability to understand the meaning of things.

a., akinetic. Inability to carry out spontaneous movements.

a., amnesic. Condition resulting from inability to remember orders or instructions.

a., ideational. Misuse of objects due to failure to identify them.

a., motor. Inability to willfully perform acts.

aprication (ap-rĭ-kā'shun) [L. *apricare,* expose to sun]. 1. Sunstroke. 2. Sunbath. Basking in the sun.

apricot (ā'prĭ-kot) [L. *praecoquum,* early ripe]. Fruit resembling small peach in appearance.

DRIED: 6 small uncooked halves (25 gm.). Calories: 65. Other values: 2225 I.U. of vitamin A; 17 mg. calcium; 27 mg. phosphorus; 1.4 mg. iron.

FRESH: 3 apricots (100 gm.). Calories: 51. Other values: 1.0 gm. protein; negligible amount of fat; 17 mg. calcium; 23 mg. phosphorus; 2700 I.U. vitamin A; 10 mg. ascorbic acid.

aproctia (ă-prok'shĭ-ă) [G. *a-,* priv. + *prōktos,* anus]. Imperforation or absence of anus.

a'pron [O. F. *naperon,* cloth]. Garment to cover front of the body, for protection of clothing during surgical operations, during certain nursing procedures, while working with plaster of Paris, etc.

a., Hottentot. Abnormally long labia minora. SYN: *velamen vulvae.*

aprosex'ia [G. *aprosexia,* want of attention]. Unintentional inattention, esp.

from defective hearing, sight, or mental weakness. Inability to concentrate on anything.

aprosopia (ap-rō-sō'pē-ă) [*a-*, + G. *prosopon*, face]. Congenital defect in which part or all of the face is absent.

apselaphesia (ap-sel-ă-fē'zĭ-ă) [G. *a-*, priv. + *pselaphēsis*, feeling]. Absence of tactile sense.

apsithyria (ap-sĭ-thĭ'rĭ-ă) [" + *psithyrizein*, to whisper]. Hysterical loss of voice with inability to whisper.

apsychia (ap-sĭk'ĭ-ă, -sĭ'kĭ-ă) [" + *psychē*, mind]. Unconsciousness; a faint.

apsychosis (ap-sī-kō'sis) [" + " + *-ōsis*, increased]. Inability to think.

A.P.T. Abbr. for *alum-precipitated toxoid.*

aptyalia (ap-tī-ā'lĭ-ă). Aptyalism, *q.v.*

aptyalism (ăp-tī'ă-lĭzm, ă-tī'a-lĭzm) [G. *a-*, priv. + *ptyalon*, saliva]. Lack of, or deficiency in, secretion of saliva. SYN: *oligosialia; xerostomia; dry mouth.*

ETIOL: Disease (mumps, typhoid fever), dehydration, effect of drugs, x-ray irradiation, old age, obstruction of salivary ducts. Sjogren's syndrome in which there is deficient secretion of lacrimal, salivary, and other glands.

apulmonism (ă-pul'mon-ĭzm) [*a-*, + L. *pulmo*, lung]. Defect in which a part of or the entire lung is absent.

apulosis (ap-ū-lō'sis) [G.*oulein*, to cicatrize]. A cicatrix.

apus (a'pus) [G. *a-*, + *pous*, foot]. A malformed fetus without feet.

apyetous (ă-pī'ĕ-tus) [G. *a-*, priv. + *pyēsis*, suppuration]. Nonsuppurative, nonpurulent.

apyknomorphous (ă-pik"nō-mor'fus) [" + *pyknos*, thick, + *morphē*, form]. Pert. to a cell which stains lightly as its stainable material is scattered.

apyogenous (ā-pi-oj'en-us) [" + *pyon*, pus, + *genos*, origin]. Not due to pus.

apyous (ă-pī'us). Without pus.

apyretic (ă-pī-ret'ik) [G. *a-*, priv. + *pyretos*, fever]. Without fever. SYN: *afebrile.*

apyrexia (ă-pī-reks'ĭ-ă) [" + *pyrexis*, feverishness]. 1. Absence of or intermission of fever. 2. Nonfebrile period of an intermittent fever.

apyrogenetic, apyrogenic (ā-pī-rō-jĕ-net'ĭk, -jen'ĭk) [" + " + *genos*, origin]. Not causing fever.

A.Q. Abbr. for *achievement quotient.*

aq. [L. *aqua*]. Water.

aqua (ak'wă) (pl. *aquae*) [L. *aqua*, water]. Water. ABBR: *a.; aq.*

a. ammoniae. Water charged with ammonia and stimulants.

a. astricta. Frozen water.

a. bulliens. Boiling water.

a. calcariae. Lime water.

a. camphorae. Camphor water.

a. chlori. Water charged with chlorine for antisepsis and cleaning.

a. chloroformil. Chloroform water.

a. cinnamomi. Cinnamon water.

a. communis. Faucet or common water.

a. destillata. A water obtained by distillation.

a. fervent. Hot water.

a. fluvialis. River water.

a. fontana. Spring water.

a. fortis. Weak nitric acid.

a. gaultheriae. Wintergreen water.

a. hamamelidis. Witch-hazel water.

a. labyrinthi. The fluid in the labyrinth of the ear.

a., medicated (water). An aqueous solution of a volatile substance. Usually contains only a comparatively small percentage of the active drug. Many of them are merely water saturated with a volatile oil. They are used more as vehicles and to give odor and taste to solutions.

a. menthae piperitae. USP. Peppermint water.

a. oculi. The fluid (aqueous humor) of the eye.

a. pura. Purified water.

a. purificata. Purified water.

a. re'gia. Nitrohydrochloric acid water (20% nitric acid and 80% hydrochloric acid).

a. rosae. Rosewater, used mainly as a perfuming agent. Obtained by diluting a. rosae fortior with an equal volume of purified water.

a. rosae fortior. USP. Stronger rose water; a perfuming agent. The water portion of distillate following distillation of water and fresh flowers of the family Rosaceae.

a. sedativa. Sedative lotion containing ammonia water and spirit of camphor.

a. tepida. Lukewarm water.

a. vitae. Brandy.

aquacapsuli'tis [" + *capsula*, a small box, + G. *-itis*, inflammation]. Serous iritis. SYN: *aquocapsulitis.*

aquaeductus (ak-we-duk'tus) [" + *ductus*, duct]. A channel or canal to convey fluids.

a. cerebri. Canal lined with ciliated epithelium and going from the posterior end of the third ventricle through the mesencephalon to the fourth ventricle.

a. cochleae. Canal connecting subarachnoid space and the perilymphatic space of the cochlea.

a. Fallopii. Canal for facial nerve in petrous part of temporal bone.

a. Sylvii. Aquaeductus cerebri.

a. vestibuli. Canal from vestibule of ear extending into temporal bone.

aquapuncture (ak'wă-pungh'chur) [L. *aqua*, water, + *punctura*, puncture]. 1. Injection of water hypodermically as a placebo. 2. A fine jet of water sprayed on the skin as a counterirritant.

aqueduct (ak'we-dukt) [" + *ductus*, duct]. Canal or passage. SYN: *aquaeductus.*

a., cerebral. Canal in midbrain connecting third and fourth ventricles. SYN: *a. cerebri.*

a., vestibular. Small passage reaching from the vestibule to the post. surface of the temporal bone's petrous section. SYN: *aquaeductus vestibuli.*

aqueous (ā'kwē-ŭs) [L. *aqua*, water]. Of the nature of water; watery.

a. chamber. Ant. chamber of the eye.

a. humor. Watery transparent liquid, containing trace of albumin and small amount of salts. Produced by the iris, ciliary body, and cornea. It circulates through the anterior and posterior chambers of the eye and leaves the eye through one of three routes: the posterior route through the zonula, the iris, and the canal of Schlemm. To enter the latter, it passes through the spaces of Fontana to the pectinate villi through which it is filtered.

aquiferous (ak-wif'er-us) [L. *aqua*, water, + *ferre*, to bear]. Carrying water or lymph.

aquiparous (ak-wĭp'ă-rus) [" + L. *parere*, to produce]. Producing water.

aquocapsuli'tis. Serous iritis.

A.R. Abbr. for *achievement ratio; alarm reaction.*

Ar. Symbol for *argon.*

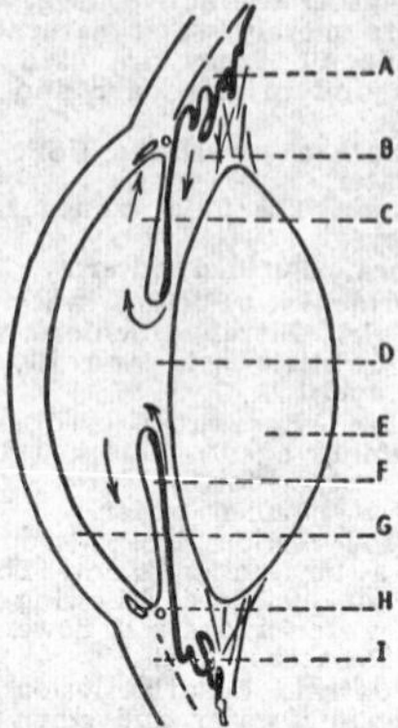

MOVEMENT OF AQUEOUS HUMOR IN THE EYE

Formed by the ciliary body in the posterior chamber, the aqueous humor streams out through the pupil into the anterior chamber and disappears into the sinus venosus sclerae. (Schematic). A, Ciliary body, with ciliary glands; B, posterior chamber; C, anterior chamber; D, pupil; E, lens; F, iris; G, cornea; H, sinus venosus sclerae (canal of Schlemm); I, sclera.

arabinose (ă-rab'ĭ-nōs, ar'ă-bĭ-nōs). Gum sugar, a pentose, obtained from boiling gum arabic and 0.5% sulfuric acid. Sometimes found in urine. SYN: *l-arabinose; pectinose.*

arabinosu'ria [*arabinose* + G. *ouron,* urine]. Arabinose in the urine.

arachnid (a-rak'nĭd). A member of the class Arachnida.

Arachnida (ă-rak'nĭ-dă) [G. *arachne,* spider]. A class of the Arthropoda, including the spiders, ticks, and mites.

arachnidism (ă-rak'nĭd-izm) [" + *eidos,* form, + *ismos,* condition of]. Systemic poisoning from spider bite. SYN: *arachnism.*

arachnitis (ă-rak-nī'tis) [" + *itis,* inflammation]. Inflammation of the arachnoid membrane. SYN: *arachnoiditis.*

arachnodactyly (a-rak-nō-dak'til-ĭ) [" + *dactylos,* finger]. Spider fingers; a state in which fingers and sometimes toes are abnormally long, slender, and curved. SYN: *acromacria, Marfan's syndrome.*

arachnoid (ă-rak'noid) [" + *eidos,* form]. 1. Resembling a web. 2. Arachnoid membrane; arachnoidea, *q.v.*

a. cavity. (a) The space between the arachnoid membrane and the dura mater (*cavum subdurale*); (b) the space between the arachnoid membrane and the pia mater (*cavum subarachnoidale* or *subarachnoid space*). The latter contains the cerebrospinal fluid.

a., cranial. SEE: *arachnoidea encephali.*

a. membrane. One (the middle) of the three membranes which cover the brain and spinal cord. SEE: *arachnoidea.*

a., spinal. SEE: *arachnoidea spinalis.*

arachnoidea (ă-rak-noid'ē-ă). A thin, delicate membrane, being the intermediate membrane which encloses the brain and spinal cord. It is located between the pia mater and dura mater, being separated from the pia by the subarachnoid space and from the dura by the subdural space.

a. encephali. The arachnoidea, the outer surface of which is separated from the dura over the brain by the subdural space. SYN: *cranial arachnoid.*

a. spinalis. The arachnoidea, the inner surface of which is separated from the pia mater by the subarachnoid space over the spinal cord. It is continuous with a. encephalis. SYN: *spinal arachnoid.*

arachnoidism (ă-răk-noid'ĭsm) [G. *arachnē,* spider]. The result produced by the bite of poisonous spiders.

arachnoiditis (ă-rak-noid-ī'tis) [" + *eidos,* form, + *itis,* inflammation]. Arachnitis; inflammation of the arachnoid membrane.

arachnolysin (ă-rack-nol'ĭ-sin) [" + lysin]. The hemolysin present in spider venom.

arachnopia (ă-rak-nō-pĭ'ă) [" + L. *pia,* protective membrane]. Pia and arachnoid considered as one membrane.

Aran-Duchenne disease (ar-ahn-du-shen). Muscular atrophy beginning in the extremities and progressing to other parts of the body. SYN: *progressive muscular atrophy.*

araneous (ă-rā'nē-us) [L. *aranea,* cobweb]. Arachnoid; resembling a cobweb.

Arantius's body, nodule (ar-an'shĭ-us). (pl. *Arantii*). Small nodule at center of each of the aortic valve cusps. SYN: *noduli valvularum aortae.*

arborescent (ar-bor-es'ent) [L. *arborescere,* to become a tree]. Branching; treelike.

arborization (ar-bor-ĭ-zā'shun) [L. *arbor,* a tree]. 1. Interlacing; ramification; applied to nerve process, terminations, fibers and arterioles. 2. A structure having the conformation of a tree. SEE: *nerve.*

a., terminal. The treelike termination of a nerve cell process, esp. the axis cylinder; the telodendria.

ar'bor vi'tae [L. *arbor,* tree, + *vita,* life]. ANAT: 1. A tree-like structure; a treelike outline seen in a section of the cerebellum. 2. A series of branching ridges within the cervix of the uterus. SYN: *plica palmatae.*

arc. A curved line; portion of the circumference of a circle.

a., reflex. The path followed by a nerve impulse in a reflex action. The impulse originates in a receptor at the point of stimulation, passes through an afferent neuron or neurons to a reflex center in the brain or spinal cord, and from the center out through efferent neurons to the effector organ, a muscle, or gland where the response occurs.

arcade (ar-kād'). Any anatomic structure composed of a series of arches.

a., Flint's. The arteriovenous anastomosis at the base of the pyramid of the kidney.

arcanum (ar-kā'num) (pl. *arcana*) [L. *arcanus,* a secret]. Secret remedy or nostrum; an elixir.

arcate (ar'kāt) [L. *arcatus,* bow shaped]. Arched, bow-shaped.

arch-, archi- [G. *archē,* primitive]. Prefix: First, principal, chief, beginning, as in *archetype.*

arch, arches [L. *arcus,* a bow]. Any structure or structures of a curved or bowlike outline.

a., abdominothoracic. The lower boundary of the front of the thorax.

a., alveolar. The arch of the alveolar process of either jaw.

a., aortic; a. of the aorta. Proximal curved part of the aorta, extending downward to the lower border of the fourth thoracic vertebra. The innominate, left common carotid, and left subclavian arteries arise from the aortic a.

a.'s, aortic. A series of six pairs of vessels which develop in the embryo and connect the aortic sac with the dorsal aortas. During the fifth to seventh weeks, the arches undergo transformation, some persisting as functional vessels, others persisting as rudimentary structures, and some disappearing entirely.

a.'s, branchial. Also called visceral or gill arches. A series of arches which support the gills of fishes. They occur in the human embryo and play an important role in the development of the head and neck. First is the *mandibular,* second, the *hyoid.* The third, fourth and fifth are transitory.

a., carotid. The third aortic arch which provides the common carotid artery.

a.'s of Corti. A series of arches made up of the rods of Corti.

a., costal. A. formed by the ribs.

a., crural. Femoral arch; Poupart's ligament.

a., deep crural. A band of fibers arching in front of sheath of femoral vessels; the downward extension of the transversalis fascia.

a., dental. An arch formed by the alveolar process on either jaw, containing teeth and covered by the gums.

a.'s, embryonic. Fetal arches, the aortic, branchial, mandibular, hyoid, pulmonary, and thyrohyoid arches.

a., femoral. Poupart's ligament.

a., glossopalatine. The anterior pillar of the fauces, *q.v.*

a., hemal. Arch formed by the body and processes of a vertebra, a pair of ribs and the sternum, or other like parts; also the sum of all such arches.

a., hyoid. The second branchial arch which persists in the styloid process, the stylohyoid ligament, and lesser cornu of the hyoid bone.

a., Langer's axillary. A thickened border of fascia forming a bridge across the occipital groove.

a., longitudinal. One of the two anteroposterior arches of the foot; the medial formed by calcaneus, talus, navicular, cuneiforms, and first three metatarsals; the lateral by the calcaneus, cuboid, and fourth and fifth metatarsals.

a., mandibular. The first branchial arch from which the upper and lower jawbones and associated structures develop. It also gives rise to the malleus and incus.

a., nasal. The arch formed by the nasal bones and by the nasal processes of the superior maxilla.

a., neural. The arch of a vertebra formed by its pedicles and laminae; also the sum of all such arches. SYN: *vertebral arch.*

a.'s of foot. The instep of the foot formed by longitudinal a. and transverse a.

a., palmar. *Deep,* an arch formed in the palm by the communicating branch of the ulnar and the radial artery. *Superficial,* an arch in the palm forming the termination of the ulnar artery.

a.'s, pharyngeal. The branchial arches of the fetus.

a., pharyngopalatine. The posterior pillar of the fauces, *q.v.*

a., plantar. The arch formed by the external plantar artery and deep branch of the dorsalis pedis artery.

a.'s, postaural. The branchial arches.

a., pubic. The portion of the pelvis formed by the rami of the ischia and the ossa pubis on either side.

a., pulmonary. The fifth of the aortic arches on the left side. It becomes the pulmonary artery.

a., stylohyoid. One of the embryonic arches made up of four segments, *viz*: the pharyngobranchial, which develops into the styloid process, the epibranchial, developing into the stylohyoid ligament, the ceratobranchial and hypobranchial which together develop into the lesser cornu of the hyoid bone.

a., superciliary. A curved process of the frontal bone lying just above the orbit and subjacent to the eyebrow.

a., supraorbital. A bony arch formed by the upper margin of the orbit.

a., tarsal. One of two branches, superior and inferior, of the median palpebral artery which supply the upper and lower eyelids, respectively.

a., thyroid. The third fetal arch; its cartilage is represented by the greater cornu of the hyoid bone.

a., transverse. An arch of the foot formed by the proximal portions of the metatarsal bones and anterior bones of the tarsus.

a., vertebral. The arched dorsal portion of a vertebra which, with the body, encloses the vertebral canal. SYN: *neural arch.*

a.'s, visceral. Branchial arches, *q.v.*

a., zygomatic. The arch formed by the malar and temporal bones.

archaic type of reaction. An inadequate immature reaction to reality; a reversion to a type once acceptable as normal (*e. g.,* in infancy).

archamphiaster (ark-am'fī-as"ter) [G. *archē,* origin, + *amphi,* around, + *astēr,* star]. Amphiaster formed when polar globules are extruded.

archegenesis (ar-kē-jen'ĕ-sis) [" + *genesis,* origin]. Generation spontaneously. SYN: *abiogenesis.*

archenteron (ark-ĕn'ter-ŏn) [G. *archē,* origin, + *enteron,* intestine]. The primitive digestive cavity of the gastrula which is lined with entoderm. Also called *primary gut* or *gastrocoele.* Its opening to the outside is the *blastopore.*

archeocyte (ar'kē-ō-sīt) [G. *archaios,* ancient, + *kytos,* a cell]. A wandering cell.

ar"cheokinet'ic [" + *kinētikos,* concerning movement]. Pert. to a low and primitive type of motor nerve mechanism as found in the peripheral and ganglionic nervous systems. SEE: *neokinetic; paleokinetic.*

archepyon (ar-ke-pī'on) [G. *archē,* a beginning, + *pyon,* pus]. Unusually thick pus.

archespore, archesporium (ar'kē-spor, -spō-ri-um) [" + *spora,* a seed]. Cells giving rise to mother cells of spores.

archetype (ar'kē-tīp) [" + *typos,* a variety]. 1. Primitive type, from which other forms have developed by differentiation. 2. An ideal or perfect anatomical type. Used as a standard in judging other individuals.

archiblast (ar'kĭ-blast) [" + *blastos,* a germ]. The outer layer which surrounds the germinal vesicle.

archiblas'tic. Derived from, or pert. to, the archiblast.

archiblastoma (ar-kĭ-blas-tō'ma) [G. *archē,* origin, + *blastos,* a germ, + *oma,* a tumor]. Tumor of archiblastic tissue.

archigaster (ar-kĭ-gas′ter) [" + *gastēr,* belly]. The primitive embryonic alimentary canal.

archinephron (ar-kĭ-nef′ron) [" + *nephros,* kidney]. Primordial kidney, an organ of the embryo. SYN: *mesonephros; wolffian body.*

archineuron (ar-kĭ-nū′ron) [" + *neuron,* sinew]. The central cell of the cerebral cortex, and all its processes.

archipallium (ar-kĭ-pal′ĭ-um) [" + L. *pallium,* a cloak]. Olfactory cortex, older than neopallium.

ar′chiplasm [" + *plasma,* a mold]. The substance of the attraction sphere.

archistome (ar′kĭ-stōm) [" + *stoma,* mouth]. Invagination of blastula making little opening into archenteron. SYN: *blastopore.*

architis (ar-kī′tis) [G. *archos,* anus, + *itis,* inflammation]. Inflammation of the anus; proctitis.

archocele (ar′kō-sēl) [" + *kēlē,* tumor]. Hernia of the rectum.

archocystocolposyrinx (ar-kō-sĭs-tō-kol-pō-sir′inks) [" + *kystis,* bladder, + *kolpos,* vagina, + *syrigx,* fistula]. Fistula of rectum, vagina, and bladder.

archocystosyrinx (ar-kō-sĭs-tō-sir′inks) [" + " + *syrigx,* fistula]. Anovesical fistula.

ar′chon. Poisonous radical of all proteins according to Vaughan.

archoptoma (ar-kop-to′mă) [G. *archos,* anus, + *ptōma,* a fall]. Prolapse of the rectum.

archoptosia, archoptosis (ar-kop-tō′sĭ-ă, -sis) [" + *ptōsis,* a falling]. Prolapse of rectum.

archorrhagia (ar-kō-ra′jĭ-ă) [G. *archos,* anus, + *rēgnunai,* to break out]. Hemorrhage from the rectum; archorrhea.

archorrhea (ar-kō-rē′ă) [" + *roia,* flow]. Rectal hemorrhage. SYN: *arcorrhagia.*

archostenosis (ar-kō-stĕ-nō′sis) [G. *archos,* anus, + *stenōsis,* a narrowing]. Stricture of the rectum.

arciform (ar′sif-orm) [" + *forma,* shape]. Bow-shaped. SYN: *arcuate.*

arc lamp [L. *arcus,* a bow]. Source of light consisting of gaseous particles from the electrodes of an electric arc which are raised to a temperature of incandescence by an electric current.

arctation (ark-tā′shun) [L. *arctatiō,* draw close together]. Stricture of any canal opening.

arcuate (ar′kū-āt) [L. *arcuatus,* bowed]. Bowed. SYN: *arciform.*

arcuation (ar-kū-ā′shun). A bending.

arculus (ar′kū-lŭs) [L. *arculus,* a small arch]. Support, in the form of an arch for bedclothes, to protect a part. SYN: *cradle.*

ar′cus (pl. *arcus*) [L. *arcus,* a bow]. An arc or arch.

a. alveolaris [NA]. Formerly called *limbus alveolaris.* The arch of the alveolar process of either jaw.

a. denta′lis [NA]. Dental arch.

a. juvenilis. Opaque ring about the corneal periphery similar to a. senilis; occurs in young individuals.

a. plantaris [NA]. The plantar arch.

a. seni′lis. Opaque white ring about corneal periphery, seen in aged persons. Due to deposit of fat granules in cornea or to hyaline degeneration.

ARD. Abbr. for *acute* undifferentiated *respiratory disease.*

ardanesthe′sia [L. *ardor,* heat, + G. *an-,* priv. + *aisthēsis,* feeling]. Inability to feel heat. SYN: *thermanesthesia.*

ardent (ar′dent) [L. *ardens,* burning]. Burning; feverish.

a. spirits. Distilled alcoholic liquors.

ar′dor [L. *ardor,* heat]. Burning; great heat.

a. urinae. A burning sensation during urination.

a. veneris. Sexual desire.

a. ventriculi. Heart burn; pyrosis.

area (a′rē-ă, ār′ē-ă) (pl. *areas, areae*) [L. *area,* an open space]. 1. A circumscribed space; one having definite boundaries. 2. A region of the cerebral cortex which differs in structure and function from other regions.

a. acustica. A. vestibularis, *q.v.*

a., association. Area of the cerebral cortex connected with other cortical areas through association and commissural fibers. Thought to be a region in which higher mental processes are mediated.

a., auditory. The hearing center of cerebral cortex located in floor of lateral fissure and coming to surface on dorsal surface of superior temporal gyrus. It receives auditory fibers from medial geniculate body.

a., Broca's. A. in the left hemisphere in post. portion of inferior frontal convolution. Controls speech. In left-handed persons it is in the right hemisphere. SYN: *motor speech a.*

a., Brodman's. Specific areas of the cerebral cortex, considered to be the seat of specific functions of the brain.

a. germinativa. A. of germination of the ovum.

a., Kiesselbach's. Area of anterior portion of nasal septum. Because of its abundant supply of capillaries it is a common site of nosebleed.

a., occipital. Portion of brain below the occipital bone.

a. pellucida. Clear central portion of *area germinativa.*

a., rolandic. A. situated in ant. central convolution in front of fissure of Rolando in each hemisphere. Governs motor acts of the body.

a. vestibularis [NA]. A rounded elevation in lateral portion of fourth ventricle above the vestibular nucleus. SYN: *a. acustica.*

areatus (a-re-a′tus). Occurring in circumscribed areas or patches.

areflex′ia [G. *a-,* priv. + L. *reflectere,* bend back]. State without reflexes.

arenaceous (ar-ĕ-na′se-us) [L. *arenaceus,* sandy]. Resembling sand or gravel.

arenation (ar-ĕ-na′shun) [L. *arena,* sand]. A sand bath or application of hot sand.

arenoid (ar′e-noid) [" + G. *eidos,* form]. Like sand.

areola (ă-rē′ō-lă) (pl. *areolae*) [L. *areola,* a small space]. 1. A small space or cavity in a tissue. 2. A form of macula* showing a hyperemic area about a skin lesion such as that about a boil. 3. A ringlike discoloration as that about the nipple. 4. The part of the iris enclosing the pupil.

a. mammae. The dark pigmented portion of the mammary gland which surrounds the nipple.

a. papilla′ris. The darkened ring about the female nipple. SYN: *a. mammae, q.v.*

a., primary. A space appearing in calcified cartilage which is undergoing degeneration in formation of endochondral bone.

a., secondary. An additional ring which during pregnancy is added around the *areola mammae.*

areolar (ă-rē′o-lar). Rel. to the areola.

a. glands. Large modified sweat glands lying beneath areola of the breast with ducts opening on its surface. They secrete a lipoid material which lubricates the breast and protects nipple during nursing. SYN: *glands of Montgomery.*

a. tissue. Connective tissue which occupies the interspaces of the body.

areoli'tis [L. *areola,* a small space, + G. *itis,* inflammation]. Inflammation of mammary areola.

areometer (a-re-om'ĕ-ter) [G. *araios,* thin, + *metron,* a measure]. Instrument for measuring sp. gr. of fluids.

areosis (ar-e-o'sis) [L. *area,* open place, + G. *osis,* increased]. Dilution; less compact.

arevareva (ar-e″va-rā'va) [Tahitian, skin rash]. Severe skin disease accompanied by general debility.

ETIOL: Excessive use of kava, an intoxicating beverage.

argamblyopia (ar-gam-bli-o'pi-ă) [G. *argos,* idle, + *amblus,* dulled, + *ops,* eye]. Amblyopia due to not using the eye.

Ar'gand burner. Gas or oil lamp having an inner tube by which air is supplied to the flame to increase combustion.

Argasidae [G. *argēēis,* shining]. Family of ticks usually infecting birds, but may attack man, causing severe pain, also fever.

argema (ar-jē'mă) [G. *argema,* ulcer]. White corneal ulcer.

argentaffin (ar-jent'ă-fin) [L. *argentum,* silver, + *affinis,* associated with]. Taking a silver stain. SYN: *argyrophil.*

argentaffino'ma [" + " + G. *ōma,* tumor]. Growth containing argentaffin elastic fibers. May be located in several body sites but usually in the ileum.

May be benign or malignant. When malignant will produce the carcinoid syndrome, *q.v.*

argen'tum. Silver. SYMB: Ag. At. wt. 107.870; at. no. 47.

argilla (ar-jĭl'ă) [G. *argillos,* white clay]. Clay or kaolin.

argillaceous (ar-jĭl-a'shus). Resembling or composed of clay.

ar'ginase. Enzyme of the liver that splits up arginine in hydrolysis, forming urea and ornithine.

arginine (ar'jĭ-nēn, -nĭn) [L. *argentum,* silver]. Crystalline basic amino acid, $C_6H_{14}N_4O_2$. Obtained from decomposition of vegetable tissues, protamines, proteins and also prepared synthetically.

It is a guanidine derivative, yielding urea and ornithine on hydrolysis. It is a hexone base.

ar'gol, ar'gal [G. *argos,* white]. Impure cream of tartar formed in wine casks.

ar'gon [G. *argos,* inactive]. An inert gas in the atmosphere. SYMB: Ar. At. wt. 39.948; at. no. 18.

Argyll Robertson pupil [Douglas Argyll Robertson, Scottish ophthalmologist, 1837-1909]. More properly the name of a symptom often present in paralysis and locomotor ataxia (due to syphilis), in which the light reflex is absent but there is no change in the power of contraction during accommodation. Usually bilateral.

argyria (ar-jir'ĭ-ă) [G. *argyros,* silver]. Bluish discoloration of skin and mucous membranes as a result of the administration of silver.

argyriasis (ar-jĭ-rī'ă-sĭs). Bluish discoloration of skin due to use of silver. SYN: *argyria.*

argyric (ar-jir'ik). Pert. to silver.

argyrism (ar'jir-izm). Bluish discoloration of skin due to use of silver. SYN: *argyria.*

argyrol (ar'jĭ-rol) (silver vitellin). Proprietary name for a dark brown, crystalline, protein substance, containing 20% silver.

USES: As an antiseptic in infections of the eye, nose and throat, and for urethral irrigations.

argyrophil (ar-ji'ro-fil) [G. *argyria,* silver, + *philos,* fond]. Staining readily or easily impregnated with silver. SYN: *argentaffin.*

argyrosis (ar-ji-ro'sis) [" + *osis,* increased]. Bluish discoloration of skin due to use of silver. SYN: *argyria.*

arhyth'mia. Arrhythmia, *q.v.*

ariboflavinosis (ă-rī-bō-flā″vĭn-ō'sĭs) [G. *a-,* priv. + riboflavin + G. *-ōsis,* disease]. Condition arising from a deficiency of riboflavin in the diet.

SYM: Lesions on the lips; stomatitis and, later, fissures in the angles of the mouth; seborrhea around the nose; vascularization of cornea.

TREATMENT: Riboflavin by mouth.

aridura (ar-ĭd-ū'ra) [L. *aridus,* parched]. Dryness, wasting, withering.

aristocar'dia [G. *aristos,* best, + *kardia,* heart]. Cardiac deviation to the right.

aristogen'ics [G. *aristos,* best, + *genea,* race]. Control of factors tending to improve the race. SYN: *eugenics.*

arithmomania (a-rĭth-mō-mā'nĭ-ă) [G. *arithmos,* a number, + *mania,* madness]. Repetition of consecutive numbers, unnecessary counting, and morbid interest in numbers.

arkyochrome (ar'kĭ-ō-krōm) [G. *arkus,* a net, + *chrōma,* a color]. A nerve cell in which the stainable substance is arranged in a network.

arkyostichochrome (ar″kĭ-ō-stik'ō-krōm) [" + *stichos,* a row, + *chrōma,* a color]. A nerve cell in which the stainable material is arranged both as a network and in parallel lines.

arm [L. *armus,* a shoulder]. 1. In *Anat.,* the upper extremity from shoulder to elbow. 2. In popular usage, the upper extremity from shoulder to hand or the entire upper extremity.

a., bird. Atrophy of the muscles of the forearm.

a. bone. The humerus.

a., brawny. Hard, swollen arm after removal of a breast.

a. center. Center in rolandic area controlling arm motion.

a., Saturday-night. A form of paralysis of the brachial plexus, sometimes seen in intoxicated persons. ETIOL: Sleeping in a chair, with the arm hanging over the back of the chair while the head rests on the shoulder or arm.

arm, *words pert. to:* axilla, "brachio" words, brachium, forearm, humerus, radius, ulna.

armamentarium (ar-mă-men-tā'rĭ-um) [L. *armamentum,* an implement]. All that a physician or surgeon uses in his practice such as instruments, drugs, books.

arm'ature [L. *armatura,* equipment]. A part of a dynamo consisting of a coil of insulated wire mounted around a soft iron core.

armil'la [L. *armilla,* bracelet]. The annular ligament of the wrist.

arm'pit [L. *armus,* shoulder, + *puteus,* a well]. Axilla.

arm-to-arm vaccination. Transferring vaccine virus from one patient to another.

ar'my itch. Chronic itch prevalent during U. S. Civil War.

Arneth's classification of neutrophils (ar'nāts) [Joseph Arneth, German physi-

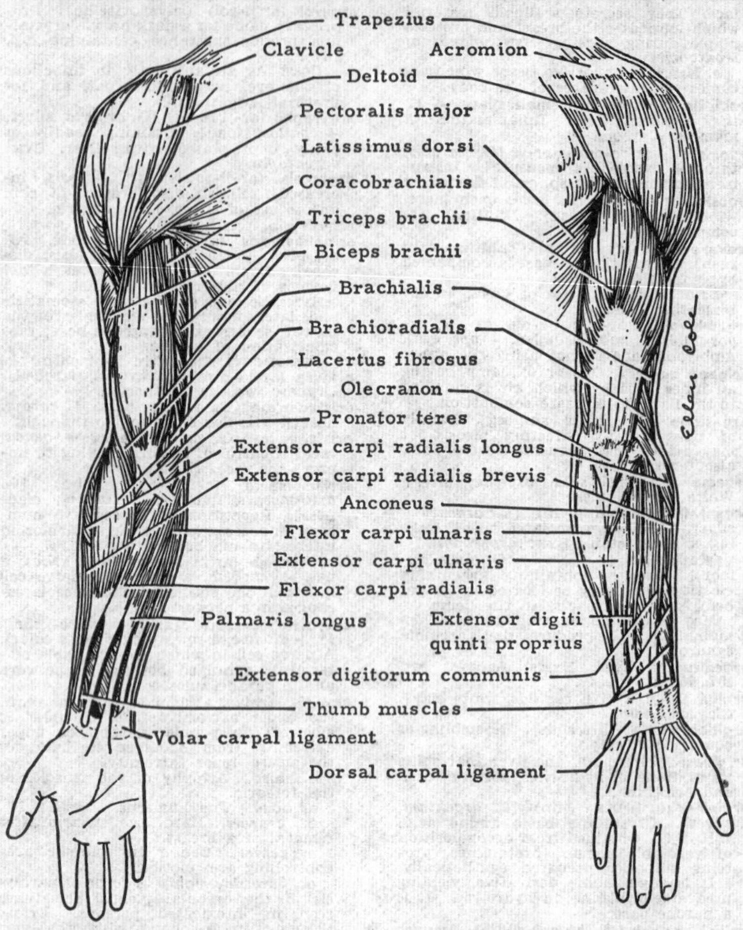

ARM'S ANTERIOR MUSCLES

ARM'S POSTERIOR MUSCLES

cian, 1873-]. Based on the number of nuclear lobes which polynuclear neutrophils contain. The normal are:

Lobes	1	2	3	4	5
%	5	35	41	17	2

A.'s formula. Method of procedure for elaborate differential blood count to estimate number of immature leukocytes.

Arnold-Chiari deformity, malformation [Julius Arnold, German pathologist, 1835-1915, and Hans Chiari, German pathologist, 1851-1916]. A condition in which there is displacement of the medulla and cerebellum into the opening in the basilar part of the occipital bone. It is one of the causes of hydrocephalus and is usually accompanied by spina bifida and meningomyelocele.

Ar'nold's canal [Friedrich Arnold, German anatomist, 1803-1890]. Passage in the temporal bone for small superficial petrosal nerve.

A.'s ganglion. Otic ganglion.

A.'s nerve. Auricular branch of vagus nerve. Stimulation of this nerve causes coughing.

aro'ma [G. *arōma,* spice]. An agreeable odor.

aromat'ic. 1. Having an agreeable odor. 2. Belonging to that series of carbon compounds in which the carbon atoms form closed rings (as in *benzene*) as distinguished from the *aliphatic* series in which the atoms form straight or branched chains.

a. compounds. Ring or cyclic compounds related to benzene, many having a fragrant odor.

a. ammonia spirit. USP. Contains 34 grams of ammonium carbonate in 1000 ml. of a solution containing diluted ammonia solution, fragrant oils, alcohol, and purified water.

Action and Uses: Antacid and carminative. Reflex stimulant when vapor is inhaled.

arrachment (ă-răsh-mon′) [Fr. *arrachement,* a tearing out]. Pulling out the capsule in a membranous cataract through a corneal incision.

arrectores pilorum (pl. *pili*) (ă-rek-tō-rēz pĭl-ō′rum) [L. *arrectores,* an erector, + from *pilus,* hair]. Involuntary muscle fibers inserted in the hair follicles on the side toward which the hair slopes. Under the influence of cold or terror they contract, straighten the follicles, and raise the hairs, resulting in "gooseflesh" or *cutis anserina.*

arrest (ă-rest′). Sudden stoppage.

a., cardiac. Sudden cessation of the heart.

a., epiphysial. Arrest of longitudinal growth of bone.

a., pelvic. In obstetrics, condition in which presenting part of fetus becomes fixed in maternal pelvis.

a., sinus. Condition in which sinus node does not initiate impulses for heart beat.

arrhea (ă-rē′ă) [G. *a-,* priv. + *roia,* a flow]. Suppression or cessation of a discharge.

arrhenoblastoma (ă-rē-nō-blas-tō′mă [G. *arrēn,* male, + *blastos,* germ, + *-oma,* tumor]. An ovarian tumor made up of masculine sex cells and producing secondary male sex characteristics (virilization) in the female.

arrhythmia (ă-rith′mĭ-ă) [G. *a-,* priv. + *rythmos,* rhythm]. Want of rhythm; irregularity.

a., cardiac. Irregular heart action caused by disturbances, either physiological or pathological, in discharge of cardiac impulses from SA node or their transmission through conductile tissue of the heart. SEE: *bradycardia* and *tachycardia.*

a., sinus. Irregular heart beat occurring commonly in children or in the aged in which the rate alternately increases and decreases.

arrhyth′mic. Signifying loss of rhythm.

arrosion (ă-rō′zhun) [L. *arrodere,* to gnaw at]. Ulcerous destruction of vessel walls.

ar′senfast. Resistant to the poisonous action of arsenic, esp. spirochetes which acquire immunity after repeated arsenic administration.

arseni′asis [L. *arsenium,* arsenic]. Chronic arsenical poisoning.

arsenic (ar′sen-ik) [L. *arsenium*]. A metallic element of grayish white color, very poisonous, used in the manufacture of dyes and medicines. SYMB: As. At. wt. 74.922; at. no. 33.

Minute traces of arsenic are found in vegetables and animal forms of life. It is a constant element of cell life and is present in eggs.

Many household and garden pesticides contain various forms of arsenic. All of these are toxic if ingested or inhaled in sufficient quantity.

CUMULATIVE EFFECT: Disorders of alimentary tract, nausea, vomiting, diarrhea, dehydration, neuritis, paralysis of wrist and ankle muscles.

a. triox′ide. As_2O_3. A white powder. Called also white arsenic or arsenous powder.

USES: Used internally in form of Fowler's solution (solution of potassium arsenite) 1%. Previously used for a variety of conditions but is little used now. More than a few grains may be fatal.

SYM: In acute poisoning, may appear in a few minutes or, when taken with solid food, may not appear for many hours. Metallic taste and odor of garlic on breath, burning pain throughout gastrointestinal tract, vomiting and purging, dehydration, shock syndrome, coma, convulsions, paralysis, death.

TREATMENT: F.A.: Lavage stomach with copious amounts of water. If this cannot be done, induce vomiting. Administer dimercaprol (British antilewisite). After first aid, maintain fluid and electrolyte balance. Morphine for pain. Treat for shock.

SEE ALSO: *Table of Poisons and Poisoning in Appendix.*

arsenic, words pert. to: acetarsone, arsphenamine, bismarsen, mapharsen, neoarsphenamine, neosilver arsphenamine, silver arsphenamine, sulfarsphenamine, tryparsamide.

arsenical (ăr-sĕn′ĭ-kăl) [L. *arsenica′lis*]. 1. Pertaining to or containing arsenic. 2. A drug containing arsenic.

arsenic-fast. Resistant to toxic action of arsenic. SYN: *arsenfast.*

arsenicism (ar-sen′ĭ-sĭzm) [L. *arsenicum,* arsenic, + G. *ismos,* condition of]. Chronic arsenic poisoning. SYN: *arseniasis.*

arsenicophagy (ar-sen-ĭ-kof′ă-jĭ) [G. *arsenikon,* arsenic, + *phagein,* to eat]. Habitual eating of arsenic. SYN: *arsenophagy.*

arsenionization (ar-sen-ī-on-ĭ-zā′shun). Electrolytic diffusion of arsenic ions in tissues.

arse′nium [L.]. Arsenic.

arsen′oblast [G. *arsēn,* male, + *blastos,* germ]. Male element in nucleus of impregnated ovum; a masculonucleus.

arsenoph′agy [L. *arsenium,* arsenic, + G. *phagein,* to eat]. Habitual eating of arsenic. SYN: *arsenicophagy.*

arsenorelap′sing [" + *re,* back, + *lapsus,* a slipping]. Pert. to syphilitic patient who relapses after apparent cure by arsenic.

arsenoresis′tant [" + *resistāre,* to withstand]. Resistant to arsenic compounds.

arsenother′apy [" + G. *therapeia,* treatment]. Treatment with arsenic and its compounds.

ar′senous. Of the nature of, or pert. to, arsenic or its compounds. SYN: *arsenical.*

ar′sin, arsine. A very poisonous gas used in chemical warfare. SYN: *arsenous hydride.*

arsphenamine (ars-fĕn′ă-mēn). A light yellow powder containing about 30% arsenic. Formerly used in treatment of syphilis. SYN: *606; salvarsan.*

ar′tefact [L. *ars,* art, + *factus,* made]. Artifact, *q.v.*

arterec′tomy [G. *artēria,* artery, + *ektomē,* excision]. Excision of an artery or arteries.

arte′ria (pl. *arteriae*) [G.]. Artery, *q.v.*

arteriag′ra [" + *agra,* a seizure]. Pain in an artery.

arte′rial. Pert. to one or more arteries.

a. bleeding. Blood is bright red and comes out in spurts. Arrest by pressure on proximal side of vessel (nearest heart).

a. circulation. It is maintained by the pumping of the heart, elasticity and extensibility of arterial walls, peripheral resistance in the areas of small arteries, and by the quantity of blood in the body. SEE: *circulation.*

a. varix. An enlarged and tortuous artery.

arterializa′tion. Aeration of the blood, changing it from venous to arterial.

arteriarctia (ar-tĕ-rĭ-ark'shĭ-ă) [G. *artēria,* artery, + L. *arctus,* bound]. Stenosis or constriction of an artery.

arteriasis (ar-tĕ-rī'ă-sis) [" + *iasis,* condition]. Degeneration of an artery.

arteriectasis, arteriectasia (ar-tĕ-rĭ-ek'tă-sis, -ek-tā'zĭ-ă) [G. *artēria,* artery, + *ektasis,* a stretching out]. Arterial dilatation.

arterio- [G. from *arteria,* artery]. Combining form indicating artery or arterial.

arterio-atony (ar-tē"rĭ-ō-at'ō-nĭ) [G. *artēria, artery,* + *atonia,* languor]. Lack of tone in arterial walls.

arteriocap'illary [" + L. *capillus,* like hair]. Pert. to arteries and capillaries.

a. fibrosis. Sclerosis of capillaries and arterioles.

arteriofibro'sis [" + L. *fibra,* fiber, + *osis,* increased. Arteriocapillary fibrosis.

arte'riogram [" + *gramma,* inscription]. 1. Recording of arterial pulse. SYN: *sphygmogram.* 2. X-ray picture of an artery which contains a radiopaque dye.

arteriog'raphy [" + *graphein,* to write]. 1. Description of arteries. 2. Sphygmography. 3. Roentgenography of arteries.

arterio'la (pl. *arteriolae*) [L. *arteriola,* small artery]. Small artery; an arteriole.

a. rec'ta. One of the small renal arteries going to the medullary pyramids.

arteriole (ar-tē'rĭ-ōl) (pl. *arterioles*). A minute artery, especially one which, at its distal end, leads into a capillary.

arte'riolith [G. *artēria,* artery, + *lithos,* stone]. An arterial calculus.

arteriol'ogy [" + *logos,* study]. Science of arteries, usually combined with study of other vessels, as in angiology.*

arteriolosclero'sis [L. *arteriola,* small artery, + G. *sklērōsis,* hardening]. Thickening of the walls of the arterioles with loss of elasticity and contractility. A type of arteriosclerosis.

arteriolosclerot'ic. Rel. to arteriolosclerosis.

arteriomala'cia [G. *artēria,* artery, + *malakia,* softening]. Softening of the arteries.

arteriom'eter [" + *metron,* measure]. Instrument measuring variations in the size of a beating artery.

arteriomo'tor [" + L. *movere,* to move]. Causing changes in size of arteries by dilatation and constriction.

arteriomyomatosis (ar-tē"rĭ-ō-mī-ō-mă-tō'sis) [" + *mys,* muscle, + *oma,* tumor, + *-osis,* increased]. Thickening of arterial walls due to overgrowth of muscle fibers.

arterio"necro'sis [" + *nekros,* dead, + *osis,* condition]. Arterial necrosis.

arteriopalmus (ar-tēr"ĭ-o-palm'us) [" + *palmus,* palpitation]. Pulsation of an artery or arteries.

arteriopathy (ar-tē"rĭ-op'ă-thĭ) [" + *pathos,* disease]. Any disease of the arteries.

arterio"pla'nia [" + *planasthai,* to wander]. The presence of an anomalous course of an artery.

arterioplasty (ar-tē'rĭ-ō-plăs-tĭ) [" + *plassein,* to form]. Repair of an aneurysm, restoring continuity of channel of the artery.

arteriopres'sor [" + L. *pressura,* force]. Causing increased arterial blood pressure.

arteriorrhaphy (ar-tē-rĭ-or'ă-fĭ) [" + *raphē,* suture]. Arterial suture.

arteriorrhexis (ar-tē-rĭ-ō-reks'ĭs) [" + *rēxis,* rupture]. Rupture of an artery.

arteriosclero'sis, arteriolosclero'sis [L. *arteriola,* small artery, + G. *sklērōsis,* hardening]. Term applied to a number of pathologic conditions in which there is thickening, hardening, and loss of elasticity of the walls of blood vessels, especially arteries. This results in altered function of tissues and organs. Changes may occur either in the intima or media. SEE: *atherosclerosis.*

ETIOL: Cause is unknown. Involutional changes associated with aging, altered lipoid metabolism and other factors are possibly involved.

TREATMENT: Moderate and regular exercise as walking; diet low in animal or hydrogenated vegetable fats; minimal use of tobacco; general moderation in all things to reduce or avoid stress; drugs for hypertension if present.

NP: Avoid all conditions which induce increase of blood pressure. Avoid either cooling or overheating of extremities. It is dangerous to apply intense local heat (hot water bottle or heating pad) to the arms or legs of an individual with inadequate blood supply due to arteriosclerosis. Massage of limbs to avoid cramps and start circulation. Moderation in food, drink and exercise. Avoid indigestion. It is not necessary to remain in bed unless heart is affected by strain, but rest is imperative. Anxiety should be eliminated. Avoid all strain upon the heart. Watch for signs of cerebral hemorrhage and guard against cerebral thrombosis by prevention of sudden or continued exertion by the patient.

a., medial. Arteriosclerosis involving the muscular arteries in which changes occur primarily in the media. SYN: *Monckeberg's a.*

a., Monckeberg's. Medial a.

a. of legs. A form due to failure of circulation in the legs.

arteriosclerot'ic. Pert. to arteriosclerosis.

arte'riospasm [G. *artēria,* artery, + *spasmos,* pain]. Arterial spasm.

arteriosteno'sis [" + *stenōsis,* a narrowing]. Narrowing of the lumen of an artery, either temporary or permanent.

arteriostosis (ar-tē"rĭ-os-tō'sĭs) [" + *osteon,* bone, + *osis,* increased]. Calcification of an artery.

arteriostrepsis (ar-tē"rĭ-ō-strep'sĭs) [" + *strepsis,* a twisting]. Twisting of divided end of an artery to arrest hemorrhage.

arteriosympathec'tomy [" + *sympatheia,* suffer with, + *ektomē,* excision]. Removal of arterial sheath containing fibers of sympathetic nerve.

arteriotome (ar-tē'rĭ-ō-tōm) [" + *tomē,* incision]. Knife for opening an artery.

arteriotomy (ar-tē-rĭ-ot'ō-mĭ). Surgical division or opening of an artery.

arteriotony (ar-tē-rĭ-ot'ō-nĭ) [G. *artēria,* artery, + *tonos,* tension]. Blood pressure; intra-arterial blood tension.

arteriovenous (ar-tē"rĭ-ō-vē'nus) [" + L.*vena,* a vein]. Rel. to both arteries and veins.

arteriover'sion [" + L. *versiō,* a twining]. Everting wall of artery to arrest hemorrhage from open end.

arterioverter (ar-tē-rĭ-ō-ver'ter). An instrument for everting cut end of an artery for arresting hemorrhage.

arteritis (ar-tē-rī'tis) [G. *artēria,* artery, + *-itis,* inflammation]. Inflammation of an artery. SEE: *polyarteritis.*

a. defor'mans. Inflammation of inner coat of an artery. SYN: *chronic endarteritis.*

a. oblit'erans. Inflammation of intima of artery causing closure of vessel's lumen. SYN: *endarteritis obliterans.*

artery (ar'ter-ĭ) (pl. *arteries*) [G. *artēria,* windpipe]. One of the vessels carrying blood from the heart to the tissues.

Frequently is nearly empty after death. The ancients supposed that air circulated through them; from which supposition the name, artery, was derived.

The arteries carry the blood from the right and left ventricles of the heart to all parts of the body. There are two sets, the *pulmonary* and the *systemic.* The pulmonary artery carries the venous blood from the right ventricle to the lungs. The systemic system begins as the *aorta* from the left ventricle.

ANAT: They have three coats: The inner, *tunica intima,* or serous; the outer, *tunica adventitia,* or white fibrous, and the middle, *tunica media,* or yellow fibrous. The blood they carry is red. SEE: *Tables in Appendix; Fig. A-88.*

a., coiled. SEE: *spiral artery.*

a., distributing. A muscular artery, *q.v.*

a., elastic. An artery in which elastic tissue is predominant in the tunica intima and tunica media. They include the aorta and its larger branches (innominate, common carotid, subclavian, and com. iliac), vessels which conduct blood to the muscular arteries.

a., end. An artery whose branches do not anastomose with those of other arteries, *e.g.,* arteries to brain and spinal cord.

a., muscular. An artery with smooth muscle tissue in its wall, esp. the tunica media, by means of which the flow of blood to tissues can be regulated through contraction and relaxation. These arteries also contract spastically when injured thus preventing excessive loss of blood.

a., sheathed. The terminal portion of a pulp artery in the spleen which has a peculiar thickened wall.

a., spiral. The coiled terminal branch of a uterine artery. They supply the superficial two-thirds of the endometrium and, in a pregnant uterus, they empty into intervillous spaces supplying blood which bathes the chorionic villi.

a., terminal. An end artery, *q.v.*

artery, words pert. to: adventitia, aneurysm, angina pectoris, circulation, endarteritis, hypertonia, hypotonia, lumen, media, mesarteritis, periarteritis, sclerosis.

arthragra (ar-thrag'ră) [G. *arthron,* joint, + *agra,* seizure]. Seizure in the joints. SYN: *gout.*

ar'thral. Pert. to a joint.

arthralgia (ar-thral'jĭ-ă) [G. *arthron,* joint, + *algos,* pain]. Pain in a joint.

a. saturnina. Joint pain resulting from lead poisoning.

arthrectomy (ar-threk'tō-mĭ) [" + *ektomē,* excision]. Excision of a joint.

arthredema (ar-thrĕ-dē'mă) [" + *oidema,* a swelling]. Edema of a joint.

arthrempyesis (ar-threm-pī-ē'sis) [" + *empyēsis,* suppuration]. Suppuration in a joint.

arthresthesia (ar-thres-thē'zĭ-ă) [" + *aisthēsis,* sensation]. Joint sensibility; the perception of articular motions.

arthric (ar'thrik). Pert. to a joint.

arthrifuge (ar'thrĭ-fūj) [G. *arthron,* joint, + L. *fugāre,* put to flight]. A remedy for gout.

arthritic (ar-thrĭt'ik). 1. Pert. to a joint. 2. Pertaining to arthritis. 3. A person afflicted with arthritis.

arthritides (ar-thrĭt'ĭ-dēz). 1. Collective term applied to various joint disorders. 2. Plural of *arthritis.*

arthritis (ar-thrī'tis) (pl. *arthritides*) [G. *arthron,* joint, + *-itis,* inflammation]. Inflammation of a joint, usually accompanied by pain and, frequently, changes in structure.

ETIOL: Arthritis may result from or be associated with a number of conditions including: Infection (gonococcal, tuberculous, pneumococcal); rheumatic fever; ulcerative colitis; trauma; neurogenic disturbances as tabes dorsalis; degenerative joint disease as osteoarthritis; metabolic disturbances as gout; neoplasms as synovioma; hydrarthrosis; para- or periarticular conditions as fibromyositis, myositis, or bursitis; various other conditions, as acromegaly, Raynaud's disease, etc.

a., acute secondary. One caused by osteitis. SYM: Severe pain, redness, and swelling.

a., acute suppurative. Purulent distention of synovial sac; a serious form.

a., allergic. That following ingestion of food allergens or occurring in serum sickness.

a., atrophic. Rheumatoid arthritis, *q.v.*

a. deformans. One with deformity. SYM: Begins in fingers; develops progressively. Deformity due to ankylosis, exostosis, and atrophy of soft parts. SYN: *rheumatoid a.*

a., degenerative. A chronic, usually progressive joint disease involving multiple joints, characterized by destruction of joint cartilage and other degenerative changes. SYN: *degenerative joint disease; hypertrophic arthritis; osteoarthritis.*

a. fungosa. Tuberculosis of a joint.

a., gonorrheal. One due to gonorrheal infection. SYM: Usually attacks knee joint; during acute stage several joints may be affected.

TREATMENT: Neoprontosil combined with typhoid vaccine relieves pain and effects speedy restoration of joint function.

a., gouty. That due to gout, *q.v.*

a., hypertrophic. Degenerative arthritis, *q.v.*

a., neurogenic. Neurotrophic arthritis, *q.v.*

a., neurotrophic. Neurogenic arthritis or that accompanying or following diseases of the nervous system. Occurs in tabes dorsalis and syringomyelia. SEE: *Charcot's arthropathy; Charcot's joint.*

a., osteo-. A form affecting the bones and joints.

a., palindromic. Recurrent arthritis characterized by fever, swelling of one or more joints. The attacks come on suddenly, last several days or less, and then go away without treatment leaving no evidence of injury to the joint. Most frequent in the hand joints.

a., pneumococcal. One sometimes appearing as a sequel to lobar pneumonia, affecting one or more joints, and the middle ear.

a., psoriatic. A form of arthritis which usually accompanies psoriasis, the exacerbations and remissions of arthritic symptoms paralleling those of psoriasis. May be a form of rheumatoid arthritis.

a., rheumatoid. A chronic systemic disease usually involving multiple joints characterized by inflammatory changes, atrophy and rarefaction of bones, transient swelling and stiffness, pain and tenderness, and structural changes usu-

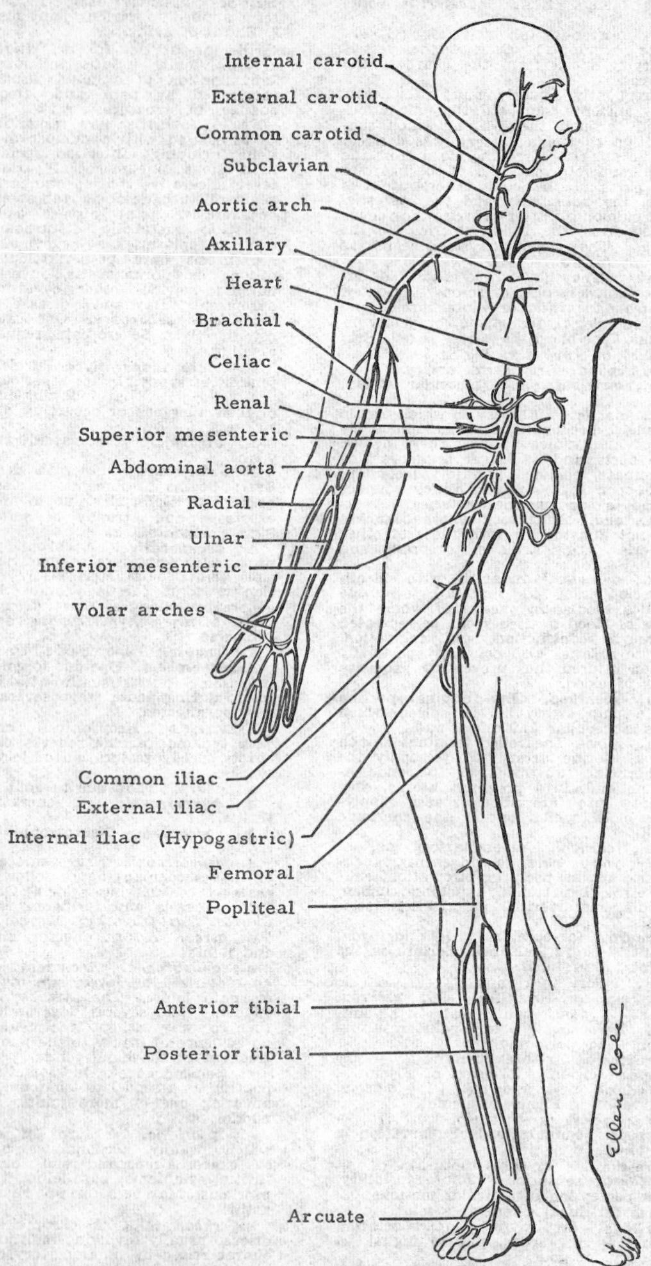

PRINCIPAL ARTERIES OF THE BODY

ally resulting, in later stages, in deformity and ankylosis of bones. Rheumatoid arthritis is considered to be one of the collagen diseases as it chiefly affects the collagen substance of connective tissue. SYN: *arthritis deformans; atrophic arthritis; chronic proliferative arthritis.*

ETIOL: The specific cause is unknown but certain precipitating factors may lead to its onset and development. These include emotional or physical shock, excessive physical or mental fatigue, trauma, infections, and sudden and repeated exposure to damp, cold weather. Heredity and constitutional factors are of importance.

TREATMENT: No specific cure; spontaneous remissions often occur. Physical therapy and orthopedic measures are utilized. Rest is essential for inflamed joints. Pain and muscle spasm can be relieved by local measures such as heat (hot baths, heat lamps, hot poultices). Aspirin is the most effective and safest analgesia for long-term use. Various special methods of treatment have been tried with diverse degrees of effectiveness. These methods include dietary and vitamin regimens, artificial hyperthermia, blood transfusions, use of gold salts and BAL, hormones (adrenal cortical steroids and ACTH), foreign proteins and vaccines. Hormone treatments often relieve acute symptoms but may produce undesirable side effects.

NP: Complete rest in bed imperative during acute stage when hands and feet and joints are swollen and painful. Usually, the patient is unable to use them. In order to protect them, complete rest is necessary. Splints may be applied for prevention of deformities but avoid pressure sores from rubbing. Due to poor circulation and limitation of motion, a daily bath necessary. Rub bony prominences with oily massaging solution. Position of patient should be changed frequently. A cradle may be used to avoid pressure from bedclothes. Apply heat over swollen joints. Maintain proper elimination by diet. An enema may be necessary. The mental condition needs special consideration. Strive to keep patient's mind occupied by some form of occupational therapy and if possible, a radio or television set placed in the room will aid in arousing interest.

a., suppurative. Arthritis occurring commonly in children; due to infection by pyogenic organisms usually *Streptococcus hemolyticus* and *Staphylococcus aureus.* Commonly referred to as a "surgical joint."

a., syphilitic. Arthritis occurring in secondary and tertiary stages of syphilis; characterized by tenderness, swelling, and limitation of motion.

a., tuberculous. A. involving epiphyseal cartilage, synovial membrane and joint.

arthritism (ar'thrĭ-tizm) [" + *ismos,* condition of]. A condition or tendency to inflammation and gouty conditions of the joints and their processes.

arthro- [G.]. Prefix: Pert. to joints.

arthrobacte'rium [G. *arthron,* joint, + *baktērion,* staff]. A bacterium which reproduces by segmentation or fission.

arthrocace (ar-throk'ă-se) [" + *kakē,* badness]. Caries of a joint.

arthrocele (ar'thro-sēl) [" + *kēlē,* tumor]. 1. Hernia of a synovial membrane, penetrating the capsule of a joint. 2. Any joint swelling.

arthrochondritis (ar-thrō-kon-drī'tĭs) [" + *chondros,* cartilage, + *-itis,* inflammation]. Inflammation of an articular cartilage.

arthroclasia (ar-thrō-klā'zĭ-ă) [" + *klasis,* a breaking]. Artificial breaking of an ankylosed joint to provide movement.

arthrodesis (ar-throd'ĕ-sis) [" + *desis,* binding]. The surgical fixation of a joint; artificial ankylosis.

arthrodia (ar-thrō'dĭ-ă) [G. *arthrōdia,* a gliding joint]. Gliding joints articulating by surfaces which glide upon each other.

arthrodynia (ar-thrō-dĭn'ĭ-ă) [G. *arthron,* joint, + *odynē,* pain]. Pain in a joint.

arthrodysplasia (ar"thrō-dĭs-plā'zĭ-ă). A familial disease characterized by abnormality of nails, dislocation of head of radius, and incomplete development of patella.

arthroempyesis (ar"thrō-em-pī-ē'sĭs) [" + *empyēsis,* suppuration]. Suppuration in a joint. SYN: *arthrempyesis.*

arthroendoscopy (ar"thrō-ĕn-dos'kō-pĭ) [" + *endon,* with, + *skopein,* to examine]. Inspection of interior of a joint by using an endoscope.

arthrog'raphy [" + *graphein,* to write]. 1. A description of the joints. 2. Roentgenography of a joint.

arthrogryposis (ar"thrō-grĭ-pō'sĭs) [" + *grypos,* curved, + *-osis,* increased]. 1. Persistent contracture of a joint. 2. Tetany.

arthrokleisis (ar-thrō-klī'sĭs) [" + *kleisis,* a closure]. Ankylosis, *q.v.,* both natural and surgical.

arthrolith (ar'thrō-lĭth) [" + *lithos,* stone]. Calculous deposit in a joint.

arthrology (ar-throl'ō-jĭ) [" + *logos,* study]. The science of joints.

arthrol'ysis [" + *lysis,* a loosening]. The operation of restoring mobility to an ankylosed joint.

arthromeningi'tis [" + *mēnigx,* membrane, + *-itis,* inflammation]. Inflammation of a synovial membrane. SYN: *synovitis.*

arthrometer (ar-throm'ĕ-ter) [" + *metron,* measure]. Instrument for measuring the degree of movement of a joint.

ar'thron. An articulation or joint.

arthron'cus [G. *arthron,* joint, + *ogkos,* tumor]. 1. Tumor of a joint. 2. Swelling of a joint.

arthroneural'gia [" + *neuron,* sinew, + *algos,* pain]. Pain in a joint.

arthrono'sos [" + *nosos,* disease]. Joint disease.

a. defor'mans. Arthritis causing deformity. SYN: *arthritis deformans.**

arthropathol'ogy [" + *pathos,* disease, + *logos,* study]. Joint disease pathology.

arthropathy (ar-throp'ă-thĭ) [" + *pathos,* disease]. Any joint disease.

a., Charcot's. Neurogenic arthropathy, *q.v.*

a., inflammatory. An inflammatory joint disease; arthritis.

a., neurogenic. A trophic joint disease with effusion of fluids into a joint, seen in locomotor ataxia due to syphilis, and in syringomyelia and sometimes in general paresis. SYN: *Charcot's disease; Charcot's joint, q.v.*

a., osteopulmonary. Enlargement and swelling of the ends of the long bones following pulmonary disease.

a., static. A disturbance in a joint of a given extremity secondary to a disturbance in some other joint of the same extremity, as one in the right knee joint secondary to one in the right hip joint.

a., tabetic. Same as neurogenic a.

arthrophlysis (ar-throf'lĭ-sĭs) [" + *phlysis,* eruption]. An eczematous eruption occurring in rheumatic subjects.

arthrophyma (ar-thrō-fī'mă) [" + *phyma,* swelling]. An articular swelling.

ar'throphyte [" + *phyton,* growth]. Abnormal growth in joint cavity.

arthroplasty (ar'thrō-plas-tĭ) [" + *plassein,* to form]. Surgical formation or reformation of a joint.

arthropod (ar'thrō-pod). A member of the phylum Arthropoda.

Arthropoda (ar-throp'ŏ-dă). A phylum of invertebrate animals characterized by bilateral symmetry, esp. chitinous skeleton, segmented bodies, and jointed paired appendages. Includes the crustaceans, insects, myriapods, arachnids, and similar forms. It is the largest animal phylum containing over 700,000 species. Many are of medical importance as causative agents of disease, as vectors, or as noxious pests.

arthropyosis (ar-thrō-pī-ō'sis) [" + *pyōsis,* suppuration]. Suppuration of a joint.

arthrorheu'matism [" + *rheumatismos,* flux]. Rheumatism of the joints.

arthrorrhagia (ar"thrō-rā'jĭ-ă). Hemorrhage into a joint.

arthrosclero'sis [" + *sklērōsis,* a hardening]. Stiffening or hardening of the joints, esp. in the aged.

ar'throscope [" + *skōpein,* to examine]. An endoscope for examining interior of a joint.

arthros'copy. Direct joint visualization by means of an arthroscope.

arthro'sis [G. *arthron,* joint, + *-osis,* increased]. 1. Joint. 2. Joint affection due to trophic degeneration.

ar'throspore [" + *sporos,* a seed]. A bacterial spore formed by segmentation.

arthrosteitis (ar-thros-tē-ī'tĭs) [" + *osteon,* bone, + *-itis,* inflammation]. Inflammation of the bony structures of a joint.

arthros'tomy [" + *stoma,* an opening]. The formation of a temporary opening into a joint for drainage purposes.

arthrosynovi'tis [" + G. *syn,* with, + *ōōn,* egg, + *-itis,* inflammation]. Inflammation of synovial membrane of a joint.

arthrotome (ar'thrō-tōm) [G. *arthron,* joint, + *temnein,* to cut]. Knife for making incisions into a joint.

arthrotomy (ar-throt'ō-mĭ) [" + *tomē,* incision]. Cutting into a joint.

arthrous (ar'thrus). Jointed or pert. to a joint.

arthroxesis (ar-throx-ē'sis) [" + *xesis,* scraping]. Scraping of diseased tissue from a joint.

Arthus reaction (ar'toos) [Maurice Arthus, French physiologist, 1862-1945]. A severe local inflammatory reaction which occurs at site of repeated injection of a nonirritating but antigenic substance such as egg albumin. SYN: *Arthus phenomenon.*

ar'tichoke [Italian *articioco*]. Perennial plant with edible flowery head. The globe artichoke is the edible variety cultivated for market in the United States. It is also known as the common, green, Italian, French or Paris artichoke.

Usually served with a thick, high-fat sauce. Value of 100 gm. boiled varies from 8 to 44 calories, a trace of fat, and 2.8 gm. protein. The carbohydrate present is in the form of inulin which is of doubtful availability.

artic'ular [L. *articularis,* joint]. Pert. to articulation.

artic'ulate [L. *articulatus,* jointed]. 1. To join together as a joint. 2. To adjust artificial teeth properly. 3. Clearly spoken. 4. To speak clearly.

artic'ulated. State of articulation or of being jointed.

articula'tion. 1. The connection of bones; a joint. It is classified as being immovable (*synarthrosis*), slightly movable (*amphiarthrosis*), or freely movable (*diarthrosis*). Cartilage, or fibrous or soft tissue lines the opposing surfaces of all joints. 2. The relative position of the tongue and palate necessary to produce a given sound. 3. Speech, clearly enunciated; enunciation.

a., confluent. Speech in which syllables are not clearly enunciated.

artic'ulo mor'tis [L. *articularis,* joint, + *mors,* death]. At the time of death.

articulus (ar-tik'ū-lus) [L.]. 1. A knuckle or a joint. 2. A segment.

ar'tifact [L. *ars,* craft, + *facere,* to make]. 1. Anything artificially produced. 2. An apparent structure produced in a cell or tissue by fixation, staining, or other manipulation.

artifi'cial [L. *ars,* art, + *facere,* to make]. Not natural; formed in imitation of nature. SEE: *feeding.*

a. hyperemia. Bringing blood to the superficial tissues by means of "cups," and elastic bandage, or unctions.

a. impregnation. Same as a. insemination, *q.v.*

a. insemination. Mechanical injection of semen into the vagina.

a. pneumothorax. Artificial introduction of air into pleural cavity. Oxygen or nitrogen, or filtered atmospheric air is used.

artifi'cial respira'tion. Maintenance of respiratory movements by artificial means.

Call a doctor at once. Laryngeal spasm often blocks air from lungs. Passage of catheter or airway tube may be necessary to convey air to lungs. Drugs may be needed to counteract spasm and promote circulation. Attempts at a. r., if such a spasm exists, may be useless.

METHODS: 1. *Manual methods.* In the past several relatively ineffective manual methods involving applying pressure to the chest and releasing it have been used. The most effective method is mouth-to-mouth breathing. SEE: illustration; ALSO SEE: *heart-lung resuscitation.* 2. *Mechanical methods.* These include Eve's rocking method and various pressure-cycling devices designed to alter pressure within the lungs and bring about the exchange of gases, for example, resuscitators, respirators (iron lungs), pulmotors, and lung motors. Devices with stimulation of phrenic nerves are also used.

TWO USES: (1) in which respiration needs only to be started and maintained artificially for a limited period. In asphyxia from such causes as gases, drowning, and electric shock, the mouth-to-mouth method is effective. If resuscitation apparatus is available, the use of O_2 and CO_2 is indicated. (2) cases where artificial respiration must be maintained for days, as in morphine poisoning and infantile paralysis. Apparatus such as a respirator is used.

SUPPLEMENTARY TREATMENT: Keep warm with blankets; massage with friction; hot water bottles, etc. If possible, head should be directed downhill to aid circulation to brain; it is desirable to turn the mouth toward the wind. Circulation must be maintained by massaging extremities toward the heart. Stimulants such as aromatic spirits of ammonia applied to nostrils intermittently, and injections of drugs, such as epinephrine (adrenalin), and ephedrine.

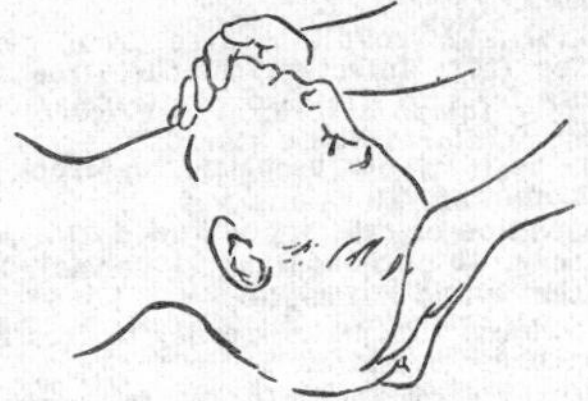

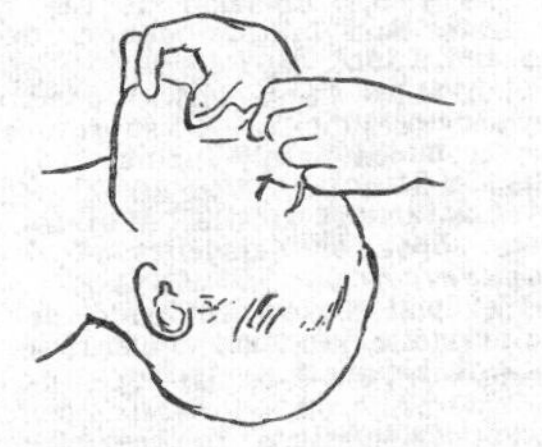

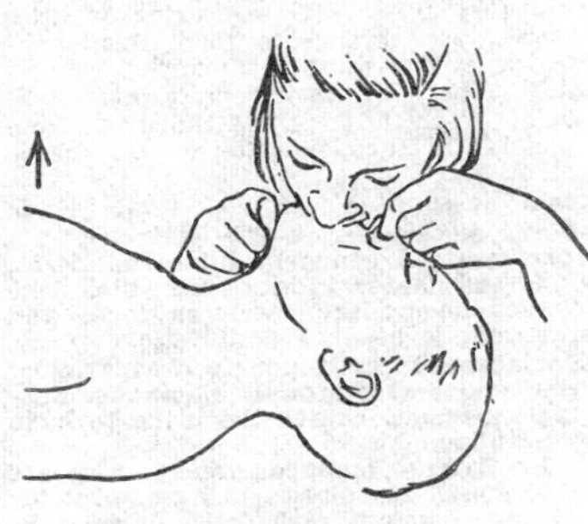

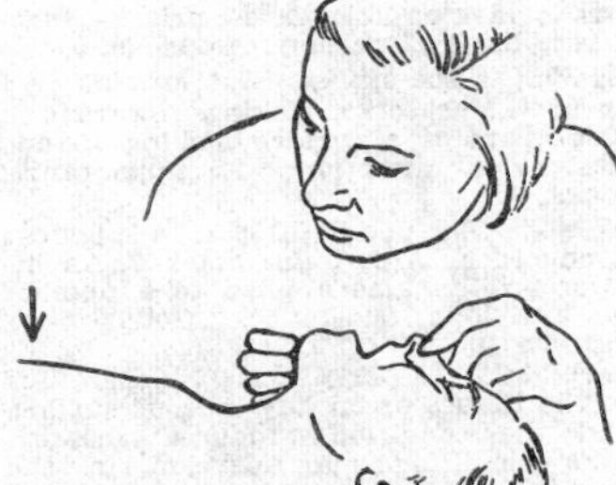

ARTIFICIAL RESPIRATION — MOUTH-TO-MOUTH BREATHING (RESCUE BREATHING) METHOD

Rectal instillations of hot, black coffee. This method should be continued for a prolonged period of time or until a physician pronounces patient dead. The use of oxygen or combination of oxygen and carbon dioxide mixtures is highly desirable if they can be obtained. Resuscitation has been necessary from several hours to many days. This method is more satisfactory than the ordinary mechanical device for inducing artificial respiration.

RS: *asphyxia; collapse; coma; drowning; respiration; syncope; shock; unconsciousness; Eve; Laborde; respirator.*

ar'tisan's cramp. A spasmodic affection of the muscles induced by prolonged work requiring delicate coordination and occurring only in performance of that particular work.

Occupations in which most apt to occur are writing, piano playing, sewing and telegraphing.

artus (ar'tus) [L. *artus,* joint]. A joint or joints; a limb.

aryepiglottic (ar-ĭ-ep-ĭ-glot'ik) [G. *arytaina,* pitcher, + *epi,* upon, + *glōttis,* glottis]. Pert. to the arytenoid cartilage and epiglottis.

ar'yl-. A prefix denoting a radical of the aromatic series.

a. group. In chemistry, a radical group of the aromatic or benzene series.

arylarsonate (ar-ĭl-ar'sō-nāt). Salt of arylarsonic acid.

arytenoid (ar-ĭ-tē'noyd) [G. *arytaina,* ladle, + *eidos,* form]. 1. Resembling a ladle or pitcher-mouth. 2. Relating to the a. cartilage, gland, ligament, or muscle.

arytenoidectomy (ar-ĭ-tē"noyd-ek'tō-mĭ) [" + " + *ektomē,* excision]. Excision of arytenoid cartilage.

arytenoid'itis. Inflammation of arytenoid cartilage.

Arzberger's pear. A hollow pear-shaped device used to pass cool water through after it has been inserted into the rectum. Used in treating rectal diseases such as hemorrhoids.

As. 1. Abbr. for *astigmatism.* 2. Symbol for *arsenic.*

a. s. [L. *auris sinistra*]. Abbr. *left ear.*

asafetida or **asafoetida** (as-ă-fet'id-ă [L. *asa,* gum, + *foetida,* fetid]. A gum resinous substance with characteristic strong odor and garlic taste. Even though this substance is no longer used in medicine, it is of historical interest. In the early part of the 20th century it was used as a carminative and also as an amulet, suspended in a small bag around the neck. When so used, asafetida was supposed to ward off disease.

asaphia (as-ă-fĭ'ă, ă-saf'ĭ-ă) [G. *asapheia,* uncertainty]. Inability to articulate properly due to cleft palate.

asbes'tiform [G. *asbestos,* quicklime, + L. *forma,* appearance]. Having structure similar to asbestos.

asbes'tos. Fibrous form of magnesium and calcium silicate.

asbesto'sis [G. *asbestos,* quicklime, + *osis,* increased]. Lung disease, a form of pneumonoconiosis, *q.v.,* due to protracted inhalation of asbestos particles.

ascariasis (as-kă-rī'ă-sĭs) [G. *askaris,* pinworm]. Condition resulting from infestation by *Ascaris lumbricoides,* the large roundworm. SEE: *Ascaris.*

ascar'ides. Pl. of Ascaris, *q.v.*

ascaridiasis (as-kar-ĭ-di'ă-sis). Ascarides in intestine and symptoms they cause.

Ascaris (as'ka-ris) (pl. *ascarides*). A genus of nematodes belonging to the superfamily Ascaridoidea which inhabits the intestine of vertebrates.

A. lumbricoides. A species of *Ascaris* which lives in the human intestine. Eggs are passed with the feces and are transmitted by contaminated water, food, or hands. After being swallowed, the eggs containing embryos hatch and the larvae enter the blood stream or lymph vessels, pass through the liver and heart to the lungs from which they migrate up the respiratory passages and are swallowed. A new cycle is then started.

Aschheim-Zondek test (ash'him-tson'dĕk). A test for pregnancy. SEE: *test.*

Asch'ner's phenomenon, reflex, sign. Slowing of the pulse caused by eyeball pressure. Sometimes used to slow the heart during attacks of supraventricular tachycardia. SYN: *oculocardiac reflex.*

Aschoff, Ludwig (ash'oph) [German pathologist, 1866-1942].

A.'s bodies. A.'s nodules, *q.v.*

A.'s cells. Large cells with basophilic cytoplasm and a large vesicular nucleus often multinucleated. Characteristic of Aschoff's nodules.

A.'s nodules. Small nodules found chiefly in association with small arteries in myocardium, a pathognomonic lesion of rheumatic fever. They may also occur in adventitia or aorta, pulmonary arteries and diaphragm.

asci (as'ī). Plural of ascus.

ascia (as'ĭ-ă, as'kĭ-ă) [L. *ascia,* ax]. Spinal bandage without reverse, each turn overlapping the previous one for a third of its width.

ascites (ă-sī'tez) [G. *askitēs,* bag]. The excessive accumulation of serous fluid in the peritoneal cavity. SEE: *edema.*

ETIOL: 1. Interference in venous return as occurs in cardiac disease, obstruction of flow in vena cava or portal vein. 2. Obstruction in lymphatic drainage. 3. Disturbance in electrolyte balance as occurs in sodium retention or in depletion of plasma proteins.

a. chylosus. Chyle in the ascetic fluid usually resulting from rupture of thoracic duct.

ascit'ic. Pert. to ascites.

a. fluid. Sp. gr. 1.005-1.015, clear and pale, straw-colored fluid occurring in ascites.

Ascoli's reaction (ahs-kō'lēz) [Alberto Ascoli, Italian serologist, 1877-]. Precipitation test for anthrax. Also called *Ascoli's test,* utilized for detection of anthrax bacilli in meat.

Ascomycetes (as-kō-mī-cē'tēz) [G. from *askos,* a bladder, + *mykes,* fungus]. The sac fungi; the largest class of Eumycetes, the true fungi (of the phylum Thallophyta). Organisms in this group are characterized by possession of a saclike sporangium (ascus, *q.v.*) in which ascospores are developed. Includes the yeasts, blue molds, mildews, and truffles.

ascorbic acid (ăs-kor'bĭk) [G. *a-,* priv. + *scorbutus*]. Vitamin C. It occurs naturally and can be synthesized. SEE: *acid, ascorbic; vitamin C.*

ascospore (as'kō-spor) [G. *askos,* bag, + *sporos,* seed]. A spore produced within an ascus or spore sac.

ascus (as'kus) (pl. *asci*). A saclike structure within which ascospores, typically eight, are formed; characteristic of the Ascomycetes, *q.v.*

-ase. A suffix used in forming the name of an enzyme. It is added to the name or a part of the name of the substance upon which it acts, as *lipase* which acts on fats (lipids).

asemia, asemasia (ă-sē'mĭ-ă, as"ĕ-mā'zĭ-ă) [G. *a-,* priv. + *sēmasia,* sign]. Inability to comprehend any type of symbol; a form of aphasia. SEE: *asymbolia.*

asep'sis. A condition free from germs; free from infection; sterile, free from any form of life. SEE: *antisepsis; sterilization.*

asep'tic. Rel. to asepsis; free from septic matter.

asep'tic-antisep'tic [G. *a-,* priv. + *sepsis,* decay, + *anti,* against, + *sepsis*]. Both aseptic and antiseptic.

asep'ticize. To make sterile; to free from pathogenic matter.

asexual (ā-sek'shoo-al) [G. *a-,* priv. + L. *sexualis,* having sex]. Without sex; nonsexual.

asexualiza'tion. Ablation of the ovaries or testes and in this manner desexing the individual.

ash (ăsh) [A.S. *asce,* ash]. Incombustible, powdery residue of a substance that has been completely incinerated.

asialia (as-ī-a'lĭ-ă, ă"sī-ā'lĭ-ă) [G. *a-,* priv. + *sialon,* spittle]. Failure to secrete saliva or deficiency of it. SYN: *aptylism.*

Asiat'ic cholera. An epidemic, acute infectious disease. SEE: *cholera.*

asiderosis (ă-sĭd-ĕ-rō'sĭs) [G. *a-,* priv. + *sidēros,* iron, + *-osis,* condition] Deficiency of iron in the circulating blood.

asitia (a-sish'ĭ-ă) [G. *a-,* priv. + *sitos,* food]. 1. Aversion to food. SEE: *anorexia.* 2. The want of food.

ASLO. Abbr. for *antistreptolysin-O.*

asocial (a-so'shil). 1. Withdrawn from society. 2. Inconsiderate of the needs of others.

asonia (ă-sō'nĭ-ă) [G. *a-,* priv. + L. *sonus,* sound]. Tone deafness.

Aspar'agus. A genus of liliaceous herbs.

A. officinalis. Plant of which the tender shoots are eaten as food, and the root is used as a diuretic.

aspar'agus. The common food asparagus; the tender shoots of *A. officinalis.* Eating asparagus causes the urine to have a peculiar odor.

AV. SERVING (canned, green): 6 spears (100 gm.). 21 calories; 2.3 gm. protein; 18 mg. calcium; 800 I.U. vitamin A; 15 mg. ascorbic acid.

aspastic (ă-spas'tik) [G. *a-,* priv. + *spastikos,* having spasms]. Nonspastic.

aspecific (a-spĕ-sif'ĭk). Not specific.

as'pect [L. *aspectus,* looking toward]. 1. That part of a surface looking in any designated direction. 2. Appearance, looks.

aspergillin (as"per-jĭl'ĭn). 1. A pigment produced by *Aspergillus niger.* 2. An inappropriate name applied to a number of antibiotic substances produced by various species of *Aspergillus.*

aspergillosis (ăs-pĕr-jĭl-ō'sĭs). Aspergillus in the tissues or on any mucous surface and the condition produced thereby. This condition may develop in the bronchi, lungs, mucous membranes of the eye, nose, or urethra, the aural canal, or the skin. It may even extend through the various viscera, producing mycotic nodules in the lungs, liver, kidney, and other organs.

a., aural. Otomycosis.

a., pulmonary. Disease of the lungs caused by *Aspergillus fumigatus.*

Aspergillus (ăs-pĕr-jĭl'ŭs) [L. *asper'gere,* to sprinkle]. A genus of Ascomycetes, including several species of the molds, some of which are pathogenic. The principal pathogenic species is *Aspergillus fumigatus,* although others (*A. flavus, A. nidulans* and *A. niger*) may be involved. SEE: *aspergillosis.*

A. auricula'ris. A species in the external auditory meatus.

A. bar'bae. A species found in mycosis of the head.

A. Bouffardi. Found in black mycetoma.

A. bronchialis. A species in the bronchi of a diabetic patient.

A. concen'tricus. A species once thought to be the cause of *Tinea imbricata* ringworm.

A. fla'vus. A mold found on corn and grain.

A. fumiga'tus. A species that has been found in the ear, nose, and lungs.

A. glau'cus. A bluish mold found on dried fruit, also in the human ear.

A. mucoroid'es. A form found in the lungs.

A. nid'ulans. A species causing one form of white mycetoma.

A. ni'ger. A pathogenic form with black spores, frequently present in the external auditory meatus.

A. ocra'ceus. The species which produces the characteristic and desirable odor of coffee.

A. pic'tor. A species found in the patches of pinta.

A. re'pens. A species found in the auditory canal.

aspermat'ic [G. *a-,* priv. + *sperma,* seed]. Pert. to aspermatism.

aspermatism (a-sper'mă-tizm) [" + " + *ismos,* condition of]. Absence or nonemission of semen. SYN: *aspermia.* SEE: *azoospermia.*

asper'mia. Lack of, or failure to ejaculate, semen.

asper'mous. Pert. to aspermia. SYN: *aspermatic.*

as'perous [L. *asper,* rough]. Uneven; having minute elevations.

asper'sion [L. *aspersio,* sprinkling]. Sprinkling an affected part with water; a form of hydrotherapy.*

asphalgesia (as-fal-jē'zĭ-ă) [G. *asphi,* own, + *algos,* pain]. A burning sensation and convulsions sometimes felt during hypnosis on touching certain articles.

asphyctic, asphyctous (as-fik'tik, -tus) [G. *a-,* priv. + *sphyxis,* pulse]. 1. Asphyxiated. 2. Without pulse.

asphyxia (ăs-fĭk'sĭ-ă) [" + *sphyxis,* pulse]. A decrease in the amount of oxygen and an increased amount of carbon dioxide in the body as a result of some interference with respiration.

ETIOL: *Extrinsic Causes:* Choking, gas (illuminating, sewer), exhaust gas (principally carbon monoxide), electric shock, drugs, anesthesia, traumatic asphyxia, crushing injuries of chest, also with compression of chest, injury of respiratory nerves or centers, diminution of oxygenation of environment, drowning. Tumors, such as goiter, pharyngeal and retropharyngeal abscesses. *Intrinsic Causes:* Hemorrhage into lungs or pleural cavity, drowning, foreign bodies in throat, swelling of air passages, diseases of air passages, ruptured aneurysm or abscess, edema of the lung, cardiac deficiency. *Other Causes:* Paralysis of the respiratory center, profound anesthesia, pneumothorax, narcotic drugs and electricity.

SYM: In general include dyspnea, cyanosis, rapid pulse, impairment of senses, mental disturbances, and in extreme cases convulsions, unconsciousness, and death.

F. A. TREATMENT: Artificial respiration, *q.v.*

a. carbonica. Suffocation from inhalation of coal or water gas.

a., fetal. That occurring in a fetus; results from interference in placental circulation or from premature separation of placenta as in placenta praevia.

a. livida. Asphyxia with cyanosis of the skin.

a., local. That in which a limited portion of the body is involved as the fingers, hands, toes, or feet.

a. neonatorum. Imperfect breathing in the newborn child.

a. pallida. When difficulty in breathing is accompanied by weak and thready pulse, pale skin, and absence of reflexes. This is the most serious type.

asphyx'ial. Pert. to asphyxia; asphyctic.

asphyx'iant. An agent, especially any gas, that will produce asphyxia.

asphyx'iate. To cause asphyxiation, or asphyxia.

asphyx''ia'tion [G. *a-,* priv. + *sphyxis,* pulse]. A state of asphyxia or suffocation. Act of producing asphyxia. SEE: *asphyxia.*

aspidium (as-pĭd'ĭ-um). USP. The root and stalk of *Dryopteris filix-mas* (male fern) or *Dryopteris marginalis* (marginal fern). Used medicinally in form of oleoresin. SYN: *male fern.*

a. oleoresin. USP. Extract of male fern; male fern oleoresin.

USE: As an anthelmintic in treatment of tapeworm infestations of intestines. Care should be taken that it is not administered with an oil, since absorption may occur.

as'pirate [L. *ad,* to, + *spirāre,* to breathe]. 1. Aspiration; to remove by suction. 2. A sound like that of the letter *h.*

aspiration (as-pĭ-rā'shun). 1. To draw in or out as by suction. Foreign bodies may be aspirated into the nose, throat, or lungs on inspiration. 2. The withdrawing of a fluid from a cavity by means of suction with an instrument called an aspirator.

Cavities most commonly aspirated are: (a) pericardial c., (b) pleural c., (c) theca (lumbar puncture), (d) abscess c.

OBJECT: (1) To remove fluid from an affected area such as pleural effusion, ascites. (2) To obtain specimens, as blood from a vein or serum from the spinal canal.

NECESSARY ARTICLES: (a) Disinfecting solution for the skin. (b) Local anesthetic. (c) Two aspirating needles with the aspirating apparatus as indicated. (d) Utensil for receiving the fluid, also a sterile receptacle for the specimen. (e) Sterile sponges, towels, basins, etc. (f) Sterile gloves, face masks, and gowns. (g) Sterile forceps. (h) Surgical dressings as the case may require. (i) Stimulant ordered if indication arises.

NP: (a) Place patient in a comfortable position. (b) Drape; be sure patient is warm. (c) Have all equipment in order and in readiness for the use of the physician. (d) Physician and nurse should wear face masks. If aspiration site is close to patient's face, patient should also wear a face mask. SEE: *foreign bodies; lumbar puncture.*

aspirator (as'pĭ-rā-tor). 1. Apparatus for evacuating fluid contents of a cavity.

VARIETIES: Piston pump, compressible rubber tube, rubber bulb, and siphon aspirators, a trocar and cannula, and hypodermic needle and syringe.

2. Instrument used in chemical analysis of gases.

aspirin (ăs'per-ĭn). Acetylsalicylic acid, *q.v.*

POISONING: See under *Salicylate in Table of Poisons and Poisoning in Appendix.*

asporogenic (as"pō-rō-jĕn'ik) [G. *a-*, priv. + *sporos,* seed, + *genos,* origin]. Not reproducing by spores.

asporous (ă-spō'rus). Having no spores.

assanation (as"ă-nā'shun) [L. *ad,* to, + *sanare,* heal]. Improvement of sanitary conditions.

assay (ă-sā', ăs'ā). The analysis of a substance to determine its constituents and the relative proportion of each. Physical, chemical, and biological methods are used.

assident (as'ĭ-dent) [L. *assidere,* to sit by]. Usually, though not always, associated with a disease, as *assident* symptoms.

assimilable (ă-sĭm'ĭ-lă-bl) [L. *assimilāre,* to make like]. Capable of assimilation.

assim'ilate. To absorb digested food.

assimila'tion. The processes whereby the products of digestion are changed to resemble the chemical substances of the body tissues, first passing through the lacteals and blood vessels; transformation of food into living tissue. The constructive phase of metabolism, *i.e.,* anabolism.

asso'ciated movements. Synchronous correlation of 2 or more muscles (or muscle groups) which, though apparently not essential for the performance of some function, normally accompany it, as the swinging of arms accompanies normal walking.

Associated movements are lost rather characteristically in cerebellar disease.

associa'tion. A joining or uniting together; coordination with another idea, structure, etc.

a. areas. Areas of the cerebral cortex which are connected to motor and sensory areas of the same side and to similar areas on the other side and to other regions of the brain as the thalamus. They serve to integrate the simpler motor and sensory functions.

a. center. One controlling associated movements.

a., controlled. An idea suggested by a word uttered by the physician.

a., free. In psychoanalysis, the uninhibited and uncensored oral expression of ideas as they arise in the mind.

a. of ideas. The linking together in a memory chain of two or more ideas, associated by some similarity, relationship, or by both having been experienced at the same time.

a. neuron. A neuron which transmits impulses from afferent to efferent neurons.

a. test. The patient is given a word (*stimulus word*) and he replies immediately with another word (*reaction word*) suggested to him by the first. The words chosen and the time taken in responding (*association time*) may be indicative of the patient's mental condition.

assonance (as'ō-nans) [L. *assonare,* to respond to]. Abnormal impulse to use alliteration.

assuetude (as'wē-tūd) [L. *assuetudō,* be persuaded to.] 1. Becoming habituated to conditions. 2. Acquiring tolerance to a drug until it loses its effect.

Ast. Abbr. for *astigmatism.*

astasia (ă-stā'zĭ-ă) [G. *a-*, priv. + *stasis,* stand]. Inability to stand or sit erect due to motor incoordination.

a. -abasia. Combined incoordination for standing or walking. PSY: A mental conflict making it difficult to stand or walk without swerving or swaying.

astatine (ăs'tă-tēn) [G. *astatos,* unstable]. An unstable element. At. wt. 210; at. no. 85. SYMB: At.

asteatosis (as"tē-ă-tō'sis) [G. *a-*, priv. + *stear,* tallow, + *-osis,* condition]. Any disease condition in which there is scantiness or absence of the sebaceous secretion.

a. cutis. A dry, fissured condition of the skin together with deficient secretion.

ETIOL: Symptomatic form due to senility, constitutional or local affections which give rise to trophic changes in the nervous system. Local form may be caused by frequent contact with irritants.

TREATMENT: Removal of underlying cause. Local application of oils and fats.

as'ter [G. *astēr,* star]. The stellate rays forming round the dividing centrosome during mitosis.

astereognosis (ă-ster-ē-og-nō'sis) [G. *a-*, priv. + *stereos,* solid, + *gnōsis,* recognition]. Inability to recognize objects or forms by touch.

aste'rion [G. *asterion,* starlike]. A craniometric point at junction of occipital, parietal, and temporal bones.

asterixis (as-ter-ix'is) [G. *a-*, + *sterixis,* fixed position]. Involuntary abnormal jerking muscular movements induced by dorsiflexion of the wrist and extension of fingers. May also be seen in other muscle groups such as those in the tongue and the feet. May be due to one of many illnesses which interfere with metabolism of the brain. When due to liver disease asterixis is called "liver flap" or liver tremor.

aster'nal [G. *a-*, priv. + *sternon,* chest]. 1. Not connected with the sternum. 2. Having no sternum.

asternia (ă-stĕr'nĭ-ă). Congenital anomaly with absence of the sternum.

asteroid (as'ter-oid) [G. *astēr,* star, + *eidos,* shape]. Star-shaped.

asthenia (as-thē'nĭ-ă) [G. *a-*, priv. + *sthenos,* strength]. Lack or loss of strength; debility. Any weakness, but one esp. originating in muscular or cerebellar disease.

a., neurocirculatory. A psychosomatic disorder characterized by mental and physical fatigue, dyspnea, giddiness, precordial pain and palpitation especially on exertion. SYN: *cardiac neurosis; effort syndrome; irritable heart; soldier's heart.*

ETIOL: Unknown but occurs in individuals who are under conditions of stress, either conscious or unconscious. It is common among soldiers.

TREATMENT: Removal from stress situation, and psychotherapy.

asthenic (as-then'ik). Weak; pert. to asthenia.

a. body type. PSY: A thin, more or less tall person with flat chest, accompanied by inferior muscular development, who centers his interest in his inner self. Usually an introvert. SEE: *pyknic type.*

asthenocoria (as-thē-nō-cō'rē-ă) [asthenia + G. *kore,* pupil, + *-ia*]. A sluggish pupillary light reflex.

asthenometer (as-the-nom'ĕ-ter) [G. *astheneia,* weakness, + *metron,* measure]. An instrument for determining loss of strength.

asthenope (as'thĕ-nōp) [G. *a-,* + *sthenos,* strength, + *opsis,* power of sight]. An individual who is affected with asthenopia, *q.v.*

asthenopia (as"thĕ-nō'pĭ-ă). Weakness or tiring of eyes due to fatigue of ciliary muscle or extraocular muscles. Painful vision.

SYM: Pain in or around eyes; headache, usually aggravated by use of eyes for close work; fatigue; vertigo; reflex symptoms, as nausea, twitching of facial muscles, migraine.

a., accommodative. Refractive errors such as hyperopia and astigmatism.

a., muscular. A. caused by weakness of extrinsic ocular muscles.

a., nervous. Hysteria and neurasthenia.

a., photogenous. Excessive or improper illumination.

a., reflex. Disease in other organs, as nose, sinuses, teeth.

asthenop'ic. Rel. to asthenopia.

asthenox'ia [G. *a-,* priv. + *sthenos,* strength, + *oxygen*]. Deficient oxygenation of waste products. Insufficient oxidation of fatty acids giving rise to ketosis.

asthma (az'mă) [G. *asthma,* panting]. Paroxysmal dyspnea accompanied by the adventitious sounds caused by a spasm of the bronchial tubes or due to swelling of their mucous membrane.

Status asthmaticus is a more or less continuous asthmatic state which may last for hours or days.

In all cases of asthma but particularly in the intrinsic group the importance of the emotions must be considered and the patient treated accordingly.

No age is exempt but occurs most frequently in childhood or early adulthood.

ETIOL: 1. *Extrinsic causes.* Allergens inhaled in the air (such as pollen, mold spores, animal dander, or dust), or infections of the respiratory tract. Occasionally foods (such as eggs, shellfish or chocolate), or drugs (such as aspirin) may precipitate an attack. 2. *Intrinsic causes.* In this situation asthma develops in persons who are found not to be allergic to specific antigens.

TREATMENT: Acute attacks may be relieved by a number of drugs such as epinephrine, ephedrine, or aminophylline. For persistent asthma (*status asthmaticus*), hormone injections are effective. Among hormones used are hydrocortisone, corticotropin, prednisone, and prednisolone. The use of sedatives and expectorants is sometimes necessary. In all cases effort should be made to control causative factors including the component of the disease due to emotional disturbance. Elimination of antigen or counteractivities such as immunization, desensitization, or hyposensitization is desirable. For asthma due to infections of respiratory tract, antibiotics should be used to control infection or prevent recurrence.

a., bronchial. Allergic asthma. Common form of asthma due to hypersensitivity to an allergen.

a., cardiac. Dyspnea due to heart disease.

TREATMENT: Upright position, morphine and venesection, if patient does not have anemia. When acute pulmonary edema sets in, strophanthin or digitalis.

a. convulsivum. Bronchial asthma, *q.v.*

a., extrinsic. Asthma due to dusts or other allergens inhaled in air or taken in with food.

a., hay. Hay fever, *q.v.*

a., intrinsic. Asthma resulting from allergens arising internally, usually the result of respiratory infections.

a., nonatopic. Intrinsic asthma, *q.v.*

a., renal. A. occurring in Bright's disease.

a., thymic. A. caused by a sudden closure of the larynx. Occurs in children, and it is believed to result from enlargement of the thymus.

asthmat'ic [L. *asthmaticus,* panting]. Pert. to or of the nature of asthma.

astigmatic (as-tig-mat'ik) [G. *a-,* priv. + *stigma,* point]. Pert. to or afflicted with astigmatism.

astigmatism (a-stig'mă-tizm) [" + " + *ismos,* condition of]. Form of ametropia in which refraction of several meridians of eyeball is different, usually due to change in curvature of cornea and lens. ABBR: As. SYN: *astigma.*

ETIOL: Congenital or acquired. Images do not properly focus on retina.

a., compound. Astigmatism in which both horizontal and vertical curvatures are involved.

a., index. Astigmatism resulting from inequalities in refractive indices of different parts of the lens.

a., mixed. Astigmatism when one meridian is myopic and the other hyperopic.

a., simple. Astigmatism along one meridian only.

astigmatometer, astigmometer (ă-stig-ma-tom'ĕ-ter, ă-stig-mom'ĕ-ter) [G. *a-,* priv. + *stigma,* point, + *metron,* measure]. An instrument for measuring astigmatism.

astigmat'oscope [" + " + *skopein,* to examine]. Instrument for detecting and measuring astigmatism.

astigmatos'copy. Use of the astigmatoscope.

astig'mia. Same as astigmatism, *q.v.*

astigmom'eter. Same as astigmatometer, *q.v.*

astigmoscope. Same as astigmatoscope, *q.v.*

asto'matous, as'tomous. Without mouth or oral aperture.

astomia (ă-stō'mē-ă) [G. *a-,* + *stoma,* mouth]. Congenital absence of the mouth.

astragalar (as-trag'ă-lar) [G. *astragalos.* ankle bone]. Pert. to the astragalus or talus.

astragalectomy (as-trag-ă-lek'tō-mĭ) [" + *ektomē,* excision]. Excision of astragalus or talus.

astragalus (as-trag'ă-lus). A bone of the foot which articulates with the tibia, fibula, calcaneus and navicular bone. SYN: *ankle bone; talus.*

astraphobia (as-tra-fō'bĭ-ă) [G. *astrapē,* lightning, + *phobos,* fear]. Anxiety and terror of thunderstorms.

astrict' [L. *astringere,* to contract]. 1. To contract or constrict, as the action of an astringent. To compress, as an artery in a hemorrhage. 2. To constipate.

astriction (a-strik'shun). Contraction; compression; constriction.

astringent (a-strĭn'jĕnt) [L. *astringere,* to contract]. 1. Drawing together, constricting, binding. 2. An agent that has a constricting or binding effect, *e.g.,* one which checks hemorrhages, secretion, etc. The principal astringents are salts of metals such as lead, iron, zinc (*e.g.*, ferric chloride, zinc oxide); permanganates; and tannic acid. SEE: *styptic.*

a. enema. One given to contract intestinal tissue and to provoke subsequent evacuation of worms. SEE: *enema.*

a., mineral. An agent that coagulates the albumins when applied to wounds or mucous surfaces, affording protection and healing, and halting bleeding.

astro- [G.]. Prefix: A star or star-shaped.

astroblast (as'trō-blast) [G. *astron*, star, + *blastos*, germ]. A cell which gives rise to an astrocyte. It develops from spongioblasts derived from embryonic neuroepithelium.

astroblasto'ma [" + " + *ōma*, tumor]. Tumor composed of astroblasts.

astrocyte (as'trō-sīt) [G. *astron*, star, + *blastos*, germ, + *kytos*, cell]. A star-shaped neuroglial cell possessing many branching processes.

astrocyto'ma [" + " + *ōma*, tumor]. Tumor formed from astrocytes.

astrog'lia [" + *glia*, glue]. Astrocytes making up neuroglial tissue.

astrokinet'ic motions [" + *kinesis*, motion]. Movements of centrosome.

astropho'bia [" + *phobos*, fear]. Morbid fear of stars and celestial space.

astrosphere (as'trō-sfēr) [" + *sphaira*, sphere]. A group of fibrils or fine rays which radiate from the centrosome (microcentrum) or the cell center. SYN: *aster.*

astrostat'ic [" + *statikos*, standing]. Pert. to astrosphere in its resting condition.

asurre'nalism [G. *a-*, priv. + L. *sur*, over, + *ren*, kidney, + G. *ismos*, condition of]. Deficient suprarenal function.

asyllabia (ă-sil-ā'bĭ-ă) [G. *a-*, priv. + *syllabos*, a collection]. Recognition of letters but not syllables or words.

asylum (ă-sī'lum) [L. from G. *asylos*, safe from violence]. An institution for the care of those unable to care for themselves, as the infirm, aged, insane, blind.

a. ear. Bloody tumor of ear found in the insane. SYN: *hematoma auris, q.v.*

asymbolia (ă-sim-bō'lĭ-ă, ā-) [G. *a-*, priv. + *symbolon*, a sign]. Inability to comprehend words, gestures, or any type of symbol; asemia. Sensory aphasia.

asymmetry (ă-sim'ĕ-trĭ) [" + *symmetria*, symmetry]. Lack of symmetry of parts or organs on opp. sides of body.

asymphytous (ă-sim'fĭ-tus) [" + *symphysis*, grow together]. Not grown together.

asymptomat'ic [" + *symptōmatikos*, symptom]. Without symptoms.

asynchronism (ă-sĭn'krō-nizm) [" + *syn*, together, + *chronos*, time, + *ismos*, condition of]. 1. The failure of events to occur in time with each other as they usually do. 2. Incoordination.

asynclitism (ă-sin'klĭ-tism) [" + *synklinein*, to lean together]. GYN: An oblique presentation of the fetal head.

a., anterior. Anterior parietal presentation. SYN: *Naegele's a.; obliquity, Naegele's, q.v.*

a., posterior. Posterior parietal presentation. SYN: *Litzmann's a.; obliquity, Litzmann's, q.v.*

asynechia (a-sin-e'kĭ-ă) [G. *a-*, + *synechia*, a holding together]. Lack of continuity of structure in an organ or tissue.

asynergia, asynergy (a-sin-er'jĭ-ă, ă-sin'-er-jĭ) [" + *syn*, together, + *ergon*, work]. Lack of coordination between muscle groups. Movements are in serial order instead of being made together. Seen in cerebellar diseases.

asynesia (ă-sĭn-ē'zĭ-ă) [G. *asynesia*, lack of intelligence]. Stupidness.

asynodia (ă-sĭn-ō'dĭ-ă) [G. *a-*, priv. + *syn*, with, + *odos*, way]. Failure of simultaneity of orgasm in male and female in coitus.

asynovia (ă-sin-ō'vĭ-ă) [" + *syn*, with, + L. *ovum*, egg]. Lack, or insufficient secretion, of synovial fluid of a joint.

systemat'ic [" + *systēma*, arrangement]. Diffuse; not limited to one system or set of organs.

asystole, asystolia (ă-sĭs'tō-lē, a"sis-to'-lĭ-ă) [G. *a-*, priv. + *systellein*, to draw together]. Faulty contraction of ventricles of the heart.

At. Symbol for *astatine.*

atabrine (at'ă-brin). Proprietary name for quinacrine hydrochloride. Used in treatment of malaria.

atactic (a-tak'tik) [G. *ataktos*, irregular]. Incoordinate, irregular, as muscular incoordination, esp. in aphasia. SYN: *ataxic.*

atactiform (ă-tak'tĭ-form) [" + L. *forma*, form]. Similar to ataxia.

atactilia (ă-tak-til'ĭ-ă) [G. *a-*, priv. + L. *tactilis*, pert. to touch]. Inability to recognize tactile impressions.

ataractic (at-ă-rak'tĭk). 1. Of or pertaining to ataraxia. 2. A drug that produces ataraxia.

atarax'ia, at'araxy [" + *taraktos*, disturbed]. A state of complete mental calm and tranquility. SYN: *imperturbability.*

atavism (ăt'ă-vĭzm) [" + G. *ismos*, condition of]. 1. Recurrence of characteristics of a remote ancestor, after remaining latent for one or more generations. 2. Reappearance, in a descendant, of a disease or abnormality experienced by a remote ancestor. A reversion to an original type.

atavis'tic. Pert. to atavism.

ataxaphasia (ă-taks-ă-fā'zĭ-ă) [G. *ataxia*, lack of order, + *phasis*, speech]. Inability to arrange words in sentences.

ataxaphemia (ă-taks-ă-fē'mĭ-ă) [" + *phēmē*, speech]. Lacking in lingual coordination.

ataxia (ă-taks'ĭ-ă). 1. Disorder or irregularity. 2. Muscular incoordination esp. that manifested when voluntary muscular movements are attempted. SYN: *ataxy.*

a., alcoholic. A. seen in drinkers, and caused by peripheral neuritis.

a., autonomic. Incoordination between sympathetic and parasympathetic nervous systems.

a., Briquet's. Hysteria accompanied by skin and leg muscle anesthesia.

a., Brun's frontal lobe. Condition resulting from lesions of the frontal lobes. Ability to perform skilled movements is lost but capacity for crude movements is retained.

a., bulbar. That due to a lesion in medulla oblongata or pons.

a., cerebellar. Muscular incoordination due to cerebellar disease.

a., choreic. Lack of muscular coordination seen in persons with chorea.

a., Friedreich's. Same as hereditary ataxia, *q.v.*

a., hereditary cerebellar. Disease of late adolescence. ETIOL: Atrophy of cerebellum. SYM: Ataxic gait, hesitating and explosive speech, nystagmus, and sometimes optic neuritis. SYN: *Marie's ataxia.*

a., hereditary. Hereditary degenerative disorder in which spinal pathways are involved. A cause of paraplegia in children and young adults. SYM: Ataxia in lower, and extending to upper, extremities; paralysis and contractures follow. SYN: *Friedreich's a.*

a., hysterical. Ataxia of leg muscles due to hysteria.

a., intrapsychic. A state in which emotional expressions appear to have no logical bases or relationship, other than those found in the unconscious. Thus a patient may cry when laughter would be appropriate.

a., locomotor. A sclerosis affecting the post. columns of spinal cord, most commonly due to syphilis. SYN: *tabes dorsalis.*

SYM: Characterized by incoordination, loss of deep reflexes, disturbances of nutrition, of sensation, and various ocular phenomena, with sometimes loss of sexual power, paralysis of sphincters, epileptiform seizures and dementia. Inability to control gait or to touch an article with the hand. SEE: *gait.*

TREATMENT: Penicillin. Response to treatment is often poor.

a., Marie's. Hereditary cerebellar ataxia, *q.v.*

a., motor. Lack of ability for proper coordination of muscles.

a., sensory. Ataxia resulting from interference in conduction of sensory responses esp. proprioceptive impulses from muscles; spinal ataxia, *q.v.*

a., spinal. Due to spinal cord disease, as in locomotor ataxia.

a., static. Loss of deep sensibility causing inability to preserve equilibrium in standing.

a., thermal. Condition in which body temperature changes irregularly.

a., vasomotor. Form of autonomic ataxia. ETIOL: Lack of coordination bet. sympathetic and parasympathetic nervous systems in connection with vasomotor phenomena. SYM: Irregularity in peripheral circulation, alternations of pallor and suffusion, due to spasm of smaller blood vessels.

ataxiadynamia (ă-taks"ĭ-ad-ĭ-nam'ĭ-ă) [G. *ataxia,* lack of order, + *a-,* priv. + *dynamis,* might]. Muscular weakness in combination with incoordination. SYN: *ataxoadynamia.*

atax'iagram [" + *gramma,* writing]. Ataxiagraph record or tracing.

ataxiagraph (ă-taks'ĭ-a-graf) [" + *graphein,* to write]. Instrument measuring swaying in ataxia.

ataxiam'eter [" + *metron,* measure]. Apparatus measuring ataxia.

ataxiamnesia (a-taks'ĭ-am-nē'zĭ-ă) [" + *amnēsia,* forgetfulness]. Suffering from muscular ataxia and amnesia.

atax'ic, atax'ial. Pert. to, or marked by, ataxia.

ataxoadynamia. Same as ataxiadynamia, *q.v.*

ataxophe'mia [" + *phēme,* speech]. Incoordination of speech muscles.

ataxopho'bia [" + *phobos,* fear]. Morbid dread of disorder or untidiness.

at'axy. Same as ataxia, *q.v.*

-ate. Word-ending noting a specific action of the affixed noun. For example: *hemolysate, activate, pulsate.*

atelectasis (at-ĕ-lek'tă-sis) [G. *atelēs,* imperfect, + *ektasis,* expansion]. 1. Condition in which lungs of a fetus remain unexpanded at birth. May be partial or total. 2. A collapsed or airless condition of the lung. May be caused by obstruction by foreign bodies, mucous plugs or excessive secretions, or by compression from without as by tumors, aneurysms, or enlarged lymph nodes. It sometimes is a complication following abdominal operations. A special chronic form, designated *middle lobe syndrome,* results from compression of a bronchus by surrounding lymph nodes.

atelencephalia (ăt-ĕl-ĕn-sĕ-fā'lē-ă) [G. *atelia,* incompleteness, + *enkephalos,* brain, + -ia]. Congenital anomaly with imperfect development of the brain.

atelia (a-tē'lĭ-ă) [G. *ateleia,* incompleteness]. The retention of childish characteristics in the adult. SYN: *ateliosis.*

ateliosis (ă-tē-lĭ-ō'sis) [G. *atelēs,* incomplete, + *-osis,* condition]. A form of infantilism due to pituitary causes in which growth may be arrested without deformity. The voice and face may resemble those of a child.

ateliot'ic. Infantile.

atelo- (at'ĕ-lō) [from G. *ateles,* imperfect]. Prefix denoting developmental or structural defect.

atelocardia (at-ĕ-lō-car'dĭ-ă) [" + G. *kardia,* heart]. Congenital anomaly with incomplete development of the heart.

atelocephalus (at-ĕ-lō-sef'ă-lus) [" + G. *kephale,* head]. Having an incomplete head.

atelocheilia (at-ĕ-lō-kĭ'lĭ-ă) [" + G. *cheilos,* lip, + ia]. Incomplete development of the lip.

atelocheiria (at-ĕ-lō-kĭ'rĭ-ă) [" + G. *cheir,* hand, + ia]. Incomplete development of the hand.

ateloencephalia (at-ĕ-lō-en"sĕ-fā'lĭ-ă). Same as atelencephalia, *q.v.*

ateloglossia (at-ĕ-lō-glos'ĭ-ă) [" + G. *glossa,* tongue, + ia]. Defective development of tongue.

atelognathia (at-ĕ-log-nā'thĭ-ă) [" + G. *gnathos,* jaw, + ia]. Incomplete development of jaw.

atelomyelia (at-ĕ-lō-mī-ē'lĭ-ă) [" + G. *myelos,* marrow, + ia]. Incomplete development of spinal cord.

atelopodia (at-ĕ-lō-pō'dĭ-ă) [" + G. *pous,* foot, + ia]. Developmental defect of foot.

ateloprosopia (at-ĕ-lō-prō-sō'pĭ-ă) [" + G. *prosopon,* face, + ia]. Defective development of face.

atelostomia (at-ĕ-lō-stō'mĭ-ă) [" + G. *stoma,* mouth, + ia]. Incomplete development of mouth.

athelia (ă-thē'lĭ-ă) [*a-,* + G. *thele,* nipple, + ia]. Absence of the nipples.

athermic, athermous (ă-ther'mĭk, -mus) [G. *a-,* priv. + *thermē,* heat]. Without fever.

athermosystaltic (ă-ther-mō-sis-tal'tĭk) [" + " + *systaltikos,* drawing together]. Not contracting or expanding due to action of heat or cold, said of striated muscle.

atheroma (ath-ĕr-ō'mă) [G. *athērē,* porridge, + *ōma,* tumor]. 1. A sebaceous cyst. SYN: *steatoma.* 2. Fatty degeneration or thickening of the wall of the larger arteries. SEE: *arteriosclerosis; atherosclerosis.*

atheromasia (ath-er-ō-mā'zĭ-ă). Atheromatous degeneration.

atheromatosis (ath-er-ō-mă-tō'sis). Generalized atheromatous condition.

atheromatous (ath-er-ō'mă-tus). Pert. to atheroma.

atheronecrosis (ath-er-ō-nĕ-crō'sĭs) [G. *athērē,* porridge, + *nekros,* dead, + *-osis,* condition]. Necrosis or degeneration accompanying arteriosclerosis.

atheroscleroʹsis [" + *sklērōsis*, hardness]. A form of arteriosclerosis in which there are localized accumulations of lipid-containing material (atheromas) within or beneath the intimal surfaces of blood vessels. It is thought to be due to a metabolic defect involving lipids and lipoproteins. It is one of the common causes of arterial occlusion.

atherosis (ath-er-ōʹsis) [" + *-osis*, condition]. Fatty degeneration of arterial walls. SYN: *arteriosclerosis.*

athetoid (athʹĕ-toid) [G. *athētos*, not fixed, + *eidos*, resemblance]. 1. Similar to athetosis. 2. Affected with athetosis.

athetosis (ath-ĕ-tōʹsis) [" + *-osis*, condition]. Slow, repeated, involuntary, purposeless, vermicular, muscular distortion involving part of a limb, toes, and fingers or almost the entire body. ETIOL: Brain lesion, chiefly in children.

athʹlete's foot. A fungus infection of the foot caused by various dermatophytes, esp. *Trichophyton rubrum, T. mentagrophytes,* and *Epidermphyton floccosum.* SYN: *dermatophytosis; ringworm of the foot; tinea pedis; trichophytosis pedis.*

TREATMENT: Various antifungal preparations are available, choice depending on seriousness of infection. Ointments, when used, should be applied at night and removed in the morning. Strong irritating medicaments should not be used. Soaking feet in 1:10,000 potassium permanganate solution and application of a drying lotion, such as calamine, or powder are usually effective.

athʹlete's heart. Incompetence of the aortic valves.

athrepsia, athrepsy (ă-threpʹsĭ-ă, -ĭ) [G. *a-*, priv. + *threpsis*, nourishment]. Malnutrition, marasmus.*

athreptic (ă-threpʹtĭk). Marasmic; pert. to or afflicted with athrepsia.

athromʹbia [G. *a-*, priv. + *thrombos*, a clot]. Defective blood clotting.

athymia (ă-thīʹmĭ-ă) [" + *thymos*, animation]. Without feeling or emotion, seen in certain mental disorders.

athymic (ă-thīʹmĭk). Pert. to athymia.

athyʹmism [G. *a-*, priv. + *thymos*, animation, + *ismos*, condition of]. Absence of thymus gland or its secretions. SYN: *athymia.*

athyrea (ă-thīʹrē-ă). Same as athyreosis, *q.v.*

athyreoʹsis [" + " + *-osis*, increased]. Hypothyroidism resulting from absence or malfunctioning of thyroid gland which may be due to maldevelopment, operative removal, or inactivation by irradiation or use of antithyroid agents. SYN: *athyrea; athyria.* SEE: *hypothyroidism.*

athyria (ă-thīʹrĭ-ă). Same as athyreosis, *q.v.*

athyʺroideʹmia [" + " + *eidos*, form, + *aima*, blood]. Morbid condition of blood due to absence of thyroid gland or its secretions.

athyroidism (ă-thīʹroy-dĭzm) [" + " + " + *ismos*, condition of]. Suppression of thyroid secretions, or absence of the thyroid gland; athyrea.

athyrosis (ă-thī-rōʹsis). Same as athyreosis, *q.v.*

atlanʹtad [G. *atlas*, a support]. Toward the atlas.

atlanʹtal. Pert. to the atlas.

atʹlas. The first cervical vertebra by which the head articulates with the occipital bone, so called because of Atlas who was supposed to support the world on his shoulders.

atloaxoid (at-lo-aksʹoid) [G. *atlas*, a support, + L. *axis*, a pivot, + G. *eidos*, form]. Pert. to atlas and axis.

atlodidymus (ăt-lō-dĭdʹĭ-mus) [atlas + G. *didymos*, twin]. A malformed fetus with one body and two heads.

atm. Abbr. for *atmosphere* or *atmospheric.*

atmiatrics, atmiatry (at-mĭ-atʹriks, at-mīʹă-trĭ) [G. *atmos*, vapor, + *iatreia*, art of healing]. Treatment of respiratory disease by medicated vapors.

atmic (atʹmik). Consisting of or pert. to vapor.

atmo- [G. *atmos*, vapor or steam]. Prefix: Vapor.

atmocauʹsis [G. *atmos*, steam, + *kausis*, burning]. Application of superheated steam; substitute for uterine curettage.

atmocautery (at-mō-kawʹter-ĭ) [G. *atmos*, steam, + *kausis*, burning]. Device for cauterization with steam.

atmograph (atʹmō-graf) [" + *graphein*, to write]. A spirograph. Device for tracing respiratory movements.

atmometer (at-momʹĕ-ter) [" + *metron*, measure]. Instrument for measuring exhalations.

atʹmos [G. *atmos*, air]. A unit of air pressure; one dyne per one sq. cc.

atʹmosphere [" + *sphaira*, sphere]. 1. The gases surrounding the earth. 2. Climatic condition of a locality. 3. PHYSICS: Pressure at sea level of the atmosphere—14.7 lbs. to the sq. in. 4. CHEM: Any gaseous medium around a body.

atmospherʹic. Pert. to the atmosphere.

atmospherizaʹtion. Process of transforming venous into arterial blood.

atmotherʹapy [G. *atmos*, air, + *therapeia*, treatment]. 1. Treatment of disease by medicated vapors. SYN: *atmiatrics.** 2. Treatment involving reduction of rate of respiration.

at. no. Abbr. for *atomic number.*

atocia (at-oʹsĭ-ă) [G. *a-*, priv. + *tokos*, birth]. Female sterility.

atʹom [G. *atomos*, indivisible]. The smallest particle of an element that can exist and take part in a chemical change, retaining its identity, and which cannot further be divided without change of its structure.

One hundred and three elements have been identified and named which in combination with one another or others like themselves make up all the various types of matter that we know. The elements are made up of atoms which are themselves composed of still smaller particles called *electrons, protons,* and *neutrons.* More than 30 particles in the atomic nucleus have been identified, and the search for other particles continues. Those identified include *positrons, mesons, neutrinos, pi-zero mesons.* Dimensions of atoms are of the order of 10^{-8} centimeters. SEE: *atomic theory; electron theory.*

a., tagged. An atom that has been made radioactive so that its course may be followed in the body. Also called radioactive tracer.

atomʹic. Pert. to an atom or atoms.

a. number. Number of protons in the nucleus of an atom. ABBR: *at. no.*

a. theory. Formulated by Dalton, who taught that all matter is composed ultimately of atoms.

a. weight. The ratio of weight of an atom of an element to one-twelfth the weight of the standard reference carbon atom. The carbon atom used as a standard is known as carbon-12 (C^{12}), with an assigned value of 12,000. For example, based on carbon-12, the atomic weight of hydrogen is 1.00797. ABBR: *at. wt.*

atomicity (at-om-is'ĭ-tĭ). 1. Chemical valence or combining power. 2. Number of hydroxyl groups in an alcohol, or in a base.

atomiza'tion. Converting a fluid into spray or vapor form.

at'omize. To reduce a liquid to the form of a spray or a vapor.

atomizer (at'om-ī-zer). Apparatus for changing jet of liquid to a spray.

atonic (a-ton'ik) [G. *a-*, priv. + *tonos*, strength]. Without tension or tone.

atonicity (at-ō-nis'ĭ-tĭ). State of being atonic, or without tone.

atony (at'ō-nĭ). Debility; or lack of normal tone.

a., gastric. Lack of muscle tone in stomach and failure to contract normally, causing slow movement of food out of stomach. Secondary to certain diseases. DIET: Small feedings at frequent intervals; soft foods; little fat. Avoid bulky foods and those requiring much mastication.

at'open [G. *a-*, priv. + *topos*, place]. An allergen, exciting cause of atopy, *q.v.*

atop'ic. Pert. to atopy. Displaced; misplaced.

atopognosis (at-ō-pog-nō'sis) [G. *a-*, priv. + *topos*, place, + *gnōsis*, knowledge]. An inhibited sense of touch or feeling, the victim not being able to know where one has touched his skin.

atopomenorrhea (at-ō-pō-men-ō-rē-'ă) [" + " + *mēn*, month, + *roia*, flow]. Periodic hemorrhage from any part of the female body other than the uterus; vicarious menstruation.

atopy (at'ō-pē). A term used clinically to apply to a group of diseases of an allergic nature. They differ from most allergies in that (1) they are inherited, (2) the antibody produced, called *atopic reagin* or *skin-sensitizing antibody* is deposited in cutaneous tissues and may enter the blood stream, and (3) the primary reaction which appears is edema as occurs in hay fever or rhinitis. The principal atopic manifestations are bronchial asthma, vasomotor rhinitis, and chronic urticaria.

atox'ic [G. *a-*, priv. + *toxikon*, poison]. Nonpoisonous.

ATP. Abbr. for *adenosine triphosphate.*

atremia (ă-trē'mĭ-ă) [G. *a-*, priv. + *tremein*, to tremble]. 1. Absence of trembling or tremor. 2. Hysterical condition characterized by inability to perform usual movements without discomfort and accompanied by paresthesia of back, neck, and head. Also called *Neftel's disease.*

atrepsy (ă-trep'sĭ) [" + *threpsis*, nutrition]. Infantile atrophy.

atre'sia [" + *trēsis*, a perforation] Pathological closure of a normal anatomical opening or congenital absence of the same, esp. that of the esophagus. Term also applied to the retrogression and disappearance of follicles in the mammalian ovary.

atre'sic. Imperforate; pert. to atresia.

atreto- (ă-trē'tō) [G. *atretos*, imperforate]. Prefix signifying absence of an opening.

atretogastria (ă-trēt-ō-gas'trĭ-a) [G. *atrētos*, imperforate, + *gaster*, stomach]. Imperforation of either the cardiac or pyloric orifice of the stomach or both.

atreturethria (ă-trēt-ū-rē'thrĭ-ă) [" + *ourēthra*, urethra]. Imperforation of the urethra.

atria (ā'trĭ-ă). Plural of atrium, *q.v.*

atrial (ā'trĭ-al). Pertaining to the atrium.

a. fibrillation. Irregular and rapid contractions of the atria working independently of the ventricles. Instead of the contraction beginning at the sinoatrial node and being conducted along the bundle of His to the ventricles, there is a rapid succession of beats at the atria. Contraction of the atrial muscle causes the waves to pass round and round the atrium. There is no atrial diastole or atrial heartbeat. SYN: *auricular fibrillation.*

ETIOL: Degeneration of cardiac muscle. Occurs in late stages of mitral disease of heart, after strain of the degenerated cardiac muscle; hyperthyroidism; infiltration of the atria by neoplastic tissue; and in acute rheumatism in children.

atrichia (ă-trik'ĭ-ă) [G. *a-*, priv. + *thrix*, hair]. Absence of hair.

atrichosis (ă-trĭ-ko'sis) [" + " + *-osis*, increased]. Having no hair, atrichia.*

atri'chous. Being without flagella.

atrionector (ā"trĭ-ō-nek'tor) [L. *atrium*, corridor, + *nector*, connector]. Sinoatrial node.

at'riotome [" + *tomē*, cutting]. Instrument which cuts connections between the cardiac atrium and ventricle.

atrioventric'ular [" + *ventriculus*, belly]. Pert. to both atrium and ventricle.

a. bundle. A bundle of modified cardiac muscle fibers which forms a part of the impulse-conducting system of the heart. It extends from the *atrioventricular (A-V) node* a short distance in the intraventricular septum, then divides into two branches which supply fibers to the two ventricles. SYN: *bundle of His.*

atriplicism (ă-trip'lĭ-sizm). Poisoning due to eating one form of spinach, *Atriplex littoralis.*

atrium (ā'trĭ-um) (pl. *atria*) [L. *atrium*, corridor]. A cavity or sinus.

a. (of) ear. Portion of the tympanic cavity lying below the malleus; the tympanic cavity proper.

a. (of) heart. The upper chamber of each half of the heart. The right atrium receives deoxygenated, dark red blood from the entire body (except lungs) through the sup. and inf. vena cavae and coronary sinus; the left atrium receives oxygenated red blood from the lungs through the pulmonary veins. Blood passes from the atria to the ventricles through the atrioventricular orifices. In the embryo the atrium is a single chamber which lies between the sinus venosus and the ventricle.

a., infection (of). Site of entrance of bacteria causing an infectious disease.

a. (of) lungs. The space at the end of an alveolar duct which opens into the alveoli or air sacs of the lungs.

atro'phia [G.]. Wasting of a part from lack of nutrition. SYN: *atrophy.*

atrophic (ă-tro'fik) [G. *a-*, priv. + *trophē*, nourishment]. Pert. to, or marked by, atrophy.

atrophied (ăt'rō-fēd). Wasted. Afflicted with atrophy.

atrophoderma (ăt-rō-fō-der'mă) [G. *a-*, priv. + *trophē*, nourishment, + *derma*, skin]. Atrophy of the skin.

a. pigmentosum. Rare skin disease characterized by ulcers, disseminated pigment discolorations, etc. SYN: *xeroderma pigmentosum, q.v.*

atrophodermato'sis [" + " + " + *-osis*, increased]. Any skin disease which has atrophied skin as a symptom.

at'rophy. 1. A wasting due to lack of nutrition of any part. 2. The reduction in size of a structure after having come to full functional maturity, as (a) atrophy of the ovary during menopause, or (b) the atrophy of an embryonic structure after having played its role in development, as the *ductus arteriosus.*

ETIOL: Disuse, disease, injury to trophic nerve centers in spinal cord, or interference with nerve or blood supply.

a., acute yellow. Extensive degeneration of liver cells with jaundice, mental disturbances, and cutaneous hemorrhages. Also called *acute necrosis; diffuse toxic necrosis; icterus gravis.*

SYM: Early nervous symptoms before jaundice sets in; slow onset; some fever with nausea and vomiting; black vomit; malaise.

a., Buchwald's. Progressive wasting of the skin.

a., compression. Compression of a part causing a.

a., correlated. Wasting of a part following destruction of another part.

a., Cruveilhier's. Progressive wasting of the muscles.

a. of disuse. A. from failure to normally use a part.

a., healed yellow. Postnecrotic cirrhosis of the liver.

a., Hoffman's. Progressive muscular wasting, in the legs, hands and forearms.

a., Landouzy-Dejerine. A form of progressive muscular dystrophy, *q.v.*, in which muscles of face, shoulders, and upper arms are the first involved. Called *facioscapulohumeral type.*

a., muscular. Atrophy of muscle tissue which may result from (a) interruption in nerve supply, or from a disorder involving motor centers of the brain, motor pathways of the spinal cord, motor neurons of the cord, or their endings in muscle; (b) disuse as may occur following immobilization of joints; or (c) pathological conditions involving muscles directly. Some conditions are hereditary and of unknown etiology.

a., myelopathic. Muscular atrophy resulting from degeneration of motor cells in anterior horns of gray matter of spinal cord.

a., myotonic. SEE: *myotonia congenita.*

a., optic. Atrophy of the second cranial (optic) nerve.

a., pathologic. That which results from the effects of disease processes.

a., peroneal muscular. A hereditary disease of unknown etiology in which peroneal nerves are primarily involved, the atrophy of muscles occurring secondary to nerve involvement. SYN: *Charcot-Marie-Tooth disease, q.v.*

a., physiologic. That which occurs as a result of the normal developmental and physiologic processes in the body (*e.g.*, atrophy of embryonic structures; atrophy of childhood structures upon reaching maturity, as the thymus; atrophy of structures in cyclic phases of activity, as the corpus luteum; atrophy of structures following cessation of functional activity, as the ovary and mammary glands; and, finally, atrophy of structures with aging).

a., progressive muscular. Chronic disease marked by progressive wasting of the muscles and paralysis, beginning with the extremities and ultimately causing death from paralysis of muscles of respiration. SEE: *dystrophy, progressive muscular; sclerosis, amyotrophic lateral.* SYN: *Aran-Duchenne disease.*

a., trophoneurotic. Wasting due to disease of the nerves or nerve centers.

a., unilateral facial. Progressive a. of the facial tissues on one side only.

a., white. Wasting of nerve, leaving only white connective tissue.

atropine sulfate (at'rō-pēn sul'fāt). USP. The salt of an alkaloid obtained from belladonna. It is a parasympatholytic agent; counteracts effects of parasympathetic stimulation.

ACTION AND USES: Respiratory and circulatory stimulant, also used to overcome spasm of involuntary muscles, to check secretion. When applied to the eye, it cause the pupil to dilate (mydriasis) and paralyzes the ciliary muscle (cycloplegia). This allows the eye to be easily examined for refractive errors.

Atropine is used to dilate pupils before testing eyes for glasses, to relieve muscle spasm, and for many other systemic effects.

POISONING: SYM: Dryness of mouth, thirst, burning pain in throat, skin is dry, hot and flushed, hyperpyrexia, palpitations, restlessness, excitement, delirium.

F. A. TREATMENT: Lavage with slurry of activated charcoal or 1% tannic acid. Pilocarpine will make patient more comfortable, but barbiturates must be used for controlling excitement.

For follow-up treatment, see *Table of Poisons and Poisoning in Appendix.*

at'ropinism, at'ropism. Atropine poisoning.

atropiniza'tion. Production of physiologic effect of atropine.

attack. The onset of an illness or symptom. One speaks of a *heart attack* or an *attack* of gout.

attendant. A nonprofessional paramedical hospital employee who assists in the care of patients.

atten'tion [L. *attendere,* wait upon]. Power to focus on some phase of consciousness including some aspect of the world of reality.

a. reflex. Change in size of pupil when attention is suddenly fixed. SYN: *Piltz's reflex.*

atten'uant [L. *attenuāre,* to thin]. 1. Diluting, making thin or weak. 2. An agent that thins the blood.

atten'uate. To render thin; or make less virulent.

atten'uated. 1. Diluted. 2. Pert. to reduced virulence of pathogenic microorganism.

a. virus. One made less virulent.

attenua'tion. 1. Dilution. 2. Lessening of virulence. This may be accomplished with bacteria and viruses by heating, drying, treating with chemicals, passing through another organism, or culturing under unfavorable conditions.

at'tic [G. *attikos,* upper part]. The upper portion of the middle ear or the portion lying above the tympanic cavity proper. SYN: *epitympanic recess.* SEE: *ear; tympanum.*

a. disease. Chronic suppurative inflammation of attic.

atticitis (at-ĭ-sī'tĭs) [" + *-itis,* inflammation]. Inflammation of the tympanic attic.

atticoantrotomy (at-ĭ-kō-an-trot'ō-mĭ) [" + *antron,* antrum, + *tomē,* cutting]. Operation to remove contents of the attic and mastoid antrum.

atticot'omy [" + *tomē*, a cutting]. Surgical opening of tympanic attic.

at'titude [L. *attitūdo*, posture]. Bodily posture or position assumed, esp. with reference to position of limbs. It is often a symptom of disease or abnormal mental state, *e.g.*, the stereotyped position assumed by catatonics or theatric expression seen in hysteria.

a. of combat. The rigid, defensile position a corpse assumes with flexion of legs, arms, and fingers; due to postmortem contraction of muscles.

a., crucifixion. Body rigid with arms at right angles.

a., defense. Position automatically assumed to avert pain.

a., forced. Abnormal position due to disease or contractures.

a., frozen. Stiffness of gait, seen in amyotrophic lateral sclerosis.

a., illogical. Peculiar attitudes caused by disease, esp. hysteroepilepsy.

a., passional, a., passionate. Theatric or dramatic gestures and expressions of face and figure assumed by hysteric patients.

a., stereotyped. Position taken and held for a long period, seen frequently in mental diseases.

attollens (a-tŏl'enz) [L. *attolere*, to lift up]. Raising or lifting up.

attrac'tion [L. *attractiō*, to draw toward]. Tendency of particles to approach each other.

a., capillary. The force by which liquids rise in fine tubes or through pores of loose material.

a., chemical. The tendency of atoms of one element to unite with those of another to form compounds.

a., molecular. The tendency of unlike molecules to attract each other. SEE: *cohesion; adhesion.*

attrahens (at-rā'henz) [L. *attrahere*, draw toward]. Drawing toward, as a muscle.

attrition (ă-trish'un) [L. *attritiō*, a rubbing against]. 1. A chafing or abrasion. 2. Any friction that breaks the skin.

at. wt. Abbr. for *atomic weight.*

atylosis (at-ĭ-lō'sĭs) [G. *a-*, priv. + *tylōsis*, a callus]. Nontypical tuberculosis.

atyp'ical [" + *typikos*, conformed to a type]. Deviating from the normal.

Au. Symb. for *gold* (*aurum*).

A.u. Abbr. for *Angstrom unit.*

auantic (aw-an'tik) [G. *auantikos*, wasted]. Wasted away. SYN: *atrophic.*

Aub-Dubois table (awb-du-bois'). Table of normal basal metabolic rates according to age.

audile (aw'dil). 1. Pert. to hearing. 2. Ear-minded. 3. PSY: One whose mental images are auditory. SEE: *visile; motile.*

audio-anesthesia. That produced by sound; used by dentists to kill pain.

audiogram (aw'dĭ-ō-gram) [L. *audire*, to hear, + G. *gramma*, drawing]. Record of the audiometer.

audiom'eter [" + G. *metron*, measure]. A delicate instrument for testing hearing.

audiom'etry. Testing of the hearing sense.

audiosound (aw'dē-ō-sound). Sound waves of frequencies perceptible to the human ear (12 to 20,000 cycles per second).

audiphone (aw'dĭ-fon) [L. *audire* + G. *phōnē*, voice]. Instrument for conveying sound to auditory nerve through the teeth or a bone.

audi'tion [L. *auditiō*, hearing]. Hearing.

a., chromatic. Condition in which certain color sensations are aroused by sound stimuli.

a., colored. Color sensation is perceived when certain sounds reach ear.

a., gustatory. Condition in which certain taste sensations are aroused by sound stimuli.

a., mental. The recollection of a sound based on previous auditory impressions.

auditive (aw'di-tiv). One who is auditory minded, depending upon hearing in learning, or recall.

auditognosis (aw-dĭt-og-nō'sĭs) [L. *auditiō*, hearing, + *gnōsis*, knowledge]. 1. Understanding and interpretation of sounds. 2. Diagnosis by percussion and auscultation.

auditooculogyric reflex (aw"dit-ō-ok"ū-lō-jī'rĭk). The sudden turning of the head and eyes in direction of an alarming sound.

aud'itory. Pert. to the sense of hearing.

a. canal. One of two canals leading to the ear. They are: the *external auditory meatus*, leading from concha to tympanic membrane, length 2.5 cm.; and the *internal auditory meatus*, located on post. surface of petrous portion of temporal bone and leads from cranial cavity to inner ear, transmitting the acoustic nerve.

a. muscles. The tensor tympani and stapedius muscles, *q.v.*

a. nerve (*n. acusticus*). The 8th cranial nerve; it is a sensory nerve with two sets of fibers: cochlear n. (of hearing), and vestibular n. (of equilibrium), the latter having three branches, the sup., inf., and middle br. SYN: *n. vestibulocochlearis* [NA]; *vestibulocochlear nerve.*

a. ossicles. The ear bones.

a. reflex. Blinking of the eyes upon the sudden unexpected production of a sound.

a. teeth. Toothlike projections in the cochlea.

a. tube. Eustachian tube, *q.v.*

aud'itus. The power or the sense of hearing.

Auenbrugger's sign (ow'en-broog-er's). Epigastric prominence due to marked pericardial effusion.

Auerbach's plexus. A plexus of sympathetic nerve fibers situated bet. the longitudinal and circular fibers of the muscular coat of the stomach and intestines. Also called the *plexus myentericus.*

Auer's bodies (ow'erz) [John Auer, American physician, 1875-1948]. Rod-shaped structures present in the cytoplasm of the cells in myeloid types of leukemia. The bodies may be found in myeloblasts, myelocytes and monocytes, and are peroxidase-positive.

Aufrecht's sign (owf'rekht's). Diminished breathing sound heard above the jugular notch in tracheal stenosis.

augment (aug'ment) [L. *augmentum*, increase]. 1. To add to or increase. 2. The increasing stage of a fever, or of an acute disease.

augmen'ter. Increasing.

a. nerves. Those increasing force and rapidity of the heartbeat.

augnathus (awg-nā'thŭs) [G. *au*, again, + *gnathos*, jaw]. Fetus with a double lower jaw.

aula (aw'lă) [G. *aulē*, hall]. 1. Anterior part of third ventricle. 2. Inflamed area around vaccination vesicle.

aulatela (aw-lă'tē-lă) [" + *tela*, web]. Membrane covering the aula.

auliplex'us [" + L. *plectere*, to twist]. Aulic part of choroid plexus.

aulix (aw'liks) [L. *aulix*, furrow]. Monro's sulcus or sulcus hypothalamicus.

au'ra [L. *aura*, breeze]. The preepileptic phenomenon.

Visual sensation of fire is rather characteristic, but sound, sense of movement of a part, or even dream states known as intellectual aurae, occur. A hysterical "attack" may present a similar phenomenon at its onset.

a., epileptic. A. preceding an attack of epilepsy.

aural (aw'ral) [L. *auris*, the ear]. 1. Pert. to the ear. 2. Pert. to an aura.

auranti'asis [L. *aurantium*, orange]. Yellowish skin color due to eating large quantities of oranges.

auran'tium [L.]. Orange.

aureomycin. A proprietary name for chlortetracycline, *q.v.*

auric (aw'rik) [L. *aurum*, gold]. Pert. to gold (*aurum*).

auricle (aw'rĭ-kl). Same as auricula, *q.v.*

auricula (pl. *auriculae*) (aw-rĭk'ū-lă) [L. *auricula*, the ear]. [NA]. 1. The external ear; pinna or flap. 2. The atrium, *q.v.* Upper chamber of heart.

(1) The protruding portion of the external ear which surrounds the opening of the external acoustic meatus; the pinna. (2) A small conical pouch forming a portion of the right and left atria of the heart. Each projects from the upper anterior portion of each atrium. (3) A term commonly used erroneously for the atrium.

auric'ular. 1. Rel. to the auricle of the ear. 2. Atrial.

auricula're (pl. *auricula'ria*). A craniometric point at center of opening of external auditory canal.

auric"ulocer'vical nerve reflex. Congestion of ear on same side resulting from stimulation of distal end of divided auriculocervical nerve. SYN: *Snellen's reflex.*

auric"ulopalpe'bral reflex. Closure of an eye resulting from stimulation by heat or some tactile irritant on the ext. auditory meatus or deeper portions of canal up to the tympanum. SYN: *Kisch's reflex.*

auriculoventricu'lar. Former term for *atrioventricular.*

a. bundle. Former name for *atrioventricular bundle, q.v.*

auriform (aw'rĭ-form) [L. *auris*, ear, + *forma*, shape]. Ear-shaped.

auriginous (aw-rij'ĭ-nus) [L. *auriginosis*, golden]. Pert. to jaundice.

aurilave (au'rĭ-lāv) [L. *auris*, ear, + *lavāre*, to wash]. An apparatus for cleansing the ear.

auripuncture (aw'rĭ-punk-tūr) [" + *punctura*, puncture]. Puncture of tympanic membrane.

auris (aw'ris) [L.]. The ear.

a. dextra. Right ear. ABBR: *a.d.*

a. externa. The external ear (pinna and ext. auditory meatus).

a. interna. The internal ear (semicircular canals, vestibule, cochlea).

a. media. The middle ear (tympanum).

a. sinistra. Left ear. ABBR: *a.s.*

au'riscalp, auriscal'pium [L. *auris*, ear, + *scalpere*, to scrape]. 1. Scraping instrument to remove foreign matter from ear. 2. Earpick.

auriscope (aw'rĭ-skōp) [" + G. *skopein*, to view]. Instrument for making an aural examination.

aurist (aw'rist). Ear specialist. SYN: *otologist.*

auris'tics. Art of treating ear diseases.

auristil'lae [L.]. Ear drops.

aurococcus (aw"ro-kok'us) [L. *aurum*, gold, + G. *kokkos*, berry]. Pyogenic microbe forming golden cultures found in boils, abscesses, carbuncles, pyemia, etc. SYN: *Staphylococcus pyogenes aureus.*

aurometer (aw-rom'ĕ-ter) [L. *auris*, ear, + G. *metron*, measure]. Instrument which measures hearing of each ear.

aurother'apy [L. *aurum*, gold, + G. *therapeia*, treatment]. Treatment of disease by adm. of gold salts; used in the treatment of rheumatoid arthritis. SYN: *chrysotherapy.*

aurum (aw'rum) [L.]. Gold.

auscult (aws-kult'). Auscultate, *q.v.*

auscultate (aws'kul-tāt) [L. *auscultāre*, listen to]. To examine by auscultation.

auscultation (aws-kul-tā'shun). Process of listening for sounds produced in some of the body cavities, esp. chest and abdomen, in order to detect or judge some abnormal condition.

INSTRUMENT: Stethoscope.

PROCEDURE: (Immediate a.): The chest should be draped with a loose-fitting garment which can easily be moved aside to allow the stethoscope to be placed directly against the skin. When chest is covered with hair moisten latter as otherwise it will produce friction sounds, resembling rales. Auscult all over chest anteriorly and posteriorly, on full inspiration, full expiration, and after coughing. In comparing the two sides auscult symmetrical parts. Parts should be in perfect repose. Position of examiner as unrestrained as possible, lest sounds of his own blood vessels be confused with sounds from within the subject.

a., immediate. When ear is applied directly to bared or thinly covered surface.

a., mediate. When sounds are conducted from the surface to ear through an instrument such as a stethoscope.

auscultation, words pert. to: abdominal a., bruit, cat's purr, egophony, percussion, râles, souffle, vocal resonance.

auscul'tatory. Pert. to auscultation.

a. percussion. Auscultation at the same time percussion is made.

auscultoplec'trum [L. *auscultāre*, listen to. + G. *plēktron*, hammer]. Instrument used for both auscultation and percussion.

autacoid (aw'ta-koyd) [G. *autos*, self, + *akos*, remedy]. A hormone which excites activity in the target organ or tissue. Opp. of *chalone* which inhibits activity. SEE: *hormone.*

autarcesiology (aw-tar-sē-sĭ-ol'ō-jĭ) [" + *arkein*, to protect, + *logos*, study]. Branch of immunology pert. to autarcesis.

autarcesis (aw-tar'sĕ-sis, aw-tar-sē'sis). Resistance to infection through natural immunity.

autarcetic (aw-tar-set'ik). Pert. to autarcesis.

autechoscope (aw-teck'ō-skōp) [G. *autos*, self, + *ēchos*, sound, + *skopein*, to inspect]. Instrument for self-auscultation.

autemesia (aw-tĕ-mē'zĭ-ă) [" + *emēsis*, vomiting]. Vomiting without apparent cause.

autism (aw'tizm) [" + *ismos*, condition of]. PSY: Mental introversion in which the attention or interest is fastened upon the victim's own ego. A self-centered mental state from which reality tends to be excluded.

autistic (aw-tĭst′ĭk). 1. Self-centered. 2. Daydreaming; phantasy of wish fulfillment.

auto- [G. *autos*, self]. Prefix meaning *self.*

autoactiva′tion [G. *autos*, self, + L. *activus*, acting]. Gland activation by its own secretion.

autoagglutina′tion [" + L. *agglutināre*, adhere to]. Blood corpuscle agglutination of an individual by his own serum.

autoanal′ysis [" + *analyein*, break down]. Patient's own analysis of mental state underlying his mental disorder.

autoanalyzer (aw″to-an′ă-līz-er). Apparatus for performing analytic tests on a large number of laboratory specimens. The testing is done automatically with each specimen being tested sequentially.

autoan′tibody [" + *anti*, against, + O. E. *bodig*, body]. Antibody acting against products of one in whom it is formed.

autoantitox′in [" + " + *toxikon*, poison]. Antitoxin produced by body itself.

autoau′dible [" + L. *audīre*, to hear]. Audible to oneself; pert. to sounds produced in one's own body.

au′toblast [" + *blastos*, germ]. Independent cell, as a bacterium.

autocatalysis (aw-tō-ka-tal′ĭ-sĭs) [" + *katalyein*, to dissolve]. Increase in the rate of a chemical reaction as result of products produced in the reaction which act as catalysts.

autocatharsis (aw-tō-kă-thar′sis). A form of psychotherapy in which the patient in discussing his own problems gains an insight into his mental difficulties.

autocath′eterism [" + *katheterismos*, a letting down into]. Passage of the catheter by oneself.

autochthonous (aw-tok′thō-nus) [" + *chthōn*, earth]. Found where developed as in the case of a blood clot or a calculus.

a. ideas. Ideas which compel attention, which are not in harmony with one's character, and which arise spontaneously, including auditory hallucinations.

autocinesia, autocinesis (aw-tō-sĭ-nē′sĭ-ă, -nē′sis) [" + *kinēsis*, motion]. Voluntary movement.

autoclasis (aw′tok′lă-sis) [" + *klasis*, a breaking]. Destruction of a part from internal causes.

autoclave (aw′tō-klāv) [" + L. *clavis*, a key]. Apparatus for sterilization by steam pressure, usually at 250° F. for a specified length of time.

autocondensa′tion [" + L. *con*, together, + *densāre*, to make thick]. A method of applying high frequency currents for therapeutic purposes.

autoconduc′tion [" + L. *con*, together, + *ductere*, lead]. A method, formerly much in vogue in France, of administering high frequency currents as therapy.

autocys′toplasty [" + *kystis*, bladder, + *plassein*, to mold]. Plastic repair of bladder with grafts from patient's own body.

autocytolysin (aw-tō-sī-tol′ĭ-sin) [" + *kytos*, cell, + *lysis*, dissolution]. Agent within patient's own blood plasma which destroys erythrocytes. SYN: *autolysin.*

autocytolysis (aw-tō-sī-tol′ĭ-sis) [" + " + *lyein*, break down]. Self-digestion or self-destruction of cells.

autoder′mic [" + *derma*, skin]. Pert. to one's own skin, esp. rel. to dermatoplasty with patient's own skin.

autodiagno′sis [" + *dia*, through, + *gignoskein*, to know]. Diagnosis of one's own disease.

autodiges′tion [" + L. *dis*, apart, + *gerere*, to carry]. Digestion of tissues by their own secretion as digestion of the stomach wall by gastric juice as occurs in certain stomach disorders.

autodrain′age [" + A. S. *drēhnigean*, strain]. Drainage of a cavity by sending the fluid through a channel made in patient's own tissues.

autoecholalia (aw″tō-ek-ō-lā′lĭ-ă) [" + *ēchō*, echo, + *lalia*, babble]. Repetition of words of one's own statements.

autoecic (aw-tē′sik) [" + *oikos*, house]. Pert. to parasite always infesting the same organism.

autoerotic (aw-tō-ē-rot′ĭk) [" + *erōtikos*, relating to love]. Attracted sexually to oneself.

autoeroticism (aw-tō-ē-rot′ĭ-sĭzm) [" + " + *ismos*, condition of]. Self-love sexually, apart from masturbation. SYN: *autoerotism.*

autoerotism (aw-tō-er′ō-tĭzm) [" + " + *ismos*, condition of]. The spontaneous generation of sexual emotion in the absence of an external stimulus, normally or abnormally, and apart from masturbation. SEE: *eroticism.*

autofundoscope (aw-tō-fun′dō-skōp) [" + L. *fundus*, bottom, + G. *skopein*, to examine]. Apparatus for autoexamination of eye vessels about macular region.

autogenesis (aw-tō-jen′ĕ-sis) [" + *genesis*, production]. Abiogenesis; self-production; spontaneous generation.

autogenetic (aw-tō-jĕ-net′ik). Pert. to self-production or autogenesis.

autogenic (aw-tō-jen′ik). Rel. to self-production. SYN: *autogenetic.*

autogenous (aw-toj′ĕ-nus). 1. Self-producing. 2. Originating within the body. 3. Denoting a vaccine from a culture of bacteria from the patient who is to be inoculated with it.

a. vaccine. A suspension of killed or attenuated bacteria prepared from bacteria obtained from the patient to whom the vaccine will be administered.

au′tograft [G. *autos*, self, + L. *graphium*, knife]. A graft taken from one part of a person's body to fill in another part.

autog′raphism [" + *graphein*, to write]. Condition in which tracings made upon the skin, with the edge of a tongue depressor or similar instrument, will be followed by appearance of wheals or elevated red areas. SYN: *dermographia.*

autohem′ic [" + *aima*, blood]. Done with one's own blood.

autohemol′ysin [" + *aima*, blood, + *lysis*, dissolution]. Antibody acting on corpuscles of individual in whose blood it is formed.

autohemol′ysis. Hemolysis of a person's blood corpuscles by his own serum.

autohemother′apy [G. *autos*, self, + *aima*, blood, + *therapeia*, treatment]. Treatment by withdrawal and injection of patient's own blood.

autohypnosis. Self-induced hypnosis.

autoimmuniza′tion [" + L. *immunis*, safe]. Immunization produced by an attack of the disease or by processes occurring within the body.

autoinfec′tion [" + L. *inficere*, to dye]. Infection by bacteria present within one's own body.

autoinfu′sion [" + L. *in*, into, + *fundere*, to pour]. Forcing blood from extremities to body by applying Esmarch bandages.

autoinocula′tion [" + L. *inoculāre*, to ingraft]. Inoculation by use of organisms obtained from another part of the body.

au"tointoxica'tion [" + L. *in*, into, + G. *toxikon*, poison]. A condition produced by poisonous products set free within the body. SEE: *autotyphization*.

Erroneously thought to be poisoning due to faulty digestive processes. SEE: *food poisoning; intoxication*.

autoisolysin (aw-tō-ī-sol'ī-sĭn). An antibody which causes dissolution of corpuscles of the individual from whom it was obtained. It also causes lysis of cells of other individuals of the same species.

autokeratoplasty (aw-tō-kĕr'ă-tō-plas-tē). Corneal grafting using tissue from the patient's other eye.

autokinesis (aw-tō-kī-nē'sis) [" + *kinesis*, motion]. Voluntary action.

autokinet'ic. Being able to move voluntarily.

autolesion (aw-tō-lē'shun) [G. *autos*, self, + L. *laedere*, to wound]. Injury self-inflicted.

autolysate (aw-tol'ī-sāt) [" + *lysis*, solution]. Specific product of autolysis.

autolysin (aw-tol'ī-sin). Agent in serum destroying erythrocytes.

autol'ysis. 1. The self-solution or self-digestion which occurs in tissues or cells by ferment in the cells themselves, even after death and in the absence of putrefactive bacteria. 2. Hemolysis of blood cells occurring as result of the action of an animal's own serum or plasma.

autolyt'ic. Rel. to autolysis. SEE: *enzymes*.

automat'ic [G. *automatos*, self acting]. Spontaneous; involuntary.

automatism (aw-tom'ă-tizm) [" + *ismos*, condition of]. 1. Automatic actions or behavior without conscious purpose or knowledge. The subject, though amnesic, appears normal to an observer but the "real" personality is "latent," during a secondary state or period of automatism, usually a hysterical trance. The patient is not responsible for his acts and must not be left for a second. He may carry out complicated acts without any idea of them and any after-memory. 2. The spontaneous activity of cilia or cells or tissues, as the movement of cilia or the contraction of smooth muscles in tissues or organs removed from the body.

automat'ograph [" + *graphein*, to write]. Instrument which records involuntary movements.

automysopho'bia [G. *autos*, self, + *mysos*, dirt, + *phobos*, fear]. Morbid dread of personal uncleanliness.

autonephrec'tomy [" + *nephros*, kidney, + *ektomē*, excision]. Ureteral stricture, completely closing it.

autonomic (aw-tō-nom'ik) [" + *nomos*, law]. Spontaneous, self-controlling.

a. nervous system. A part of the nervous system which is concerned with control of involuntary bodily functions. It controls function of glands, smooth muscle tissue and the heart. It is commonly defined so as to include the *sympathetic* or *thoracolumbar* division and the *parasympathetic* or *craniosacral* division.

THE SYMPATHETIC SYSTEM is made up of: The paired ganglionated sympathetic trunk, its connections (*rami communicantes*) with the thoracic and lumbar parts of the spinal nerve, the large and small splanchnic nerves, and certain ganglia in the abdomen (*e.g.*, the mesenteric ganglia).

THE PARASYMPATHETIC SYSTEM: Certain fibers of some cranial nerves such as the motor fibers of the vagus. Other fibers connected with the sacral part of the spinal cord.

It is best to use the word "autonomic" only in connection with efferent fibers; sensory fibers coming from the viscera and passing through the above named ganglia and trunks to reach the cord may be called "visceral afferents."

GENERAL FUNCTIONS OF THE AUTONOMIC SYSTEM: 1. Stimulating sympathetic fibers usually produces vasoconstriction in the part supplied, general rise in blood pressure, erection of the hairs, gooseflesh, pupillary dilation, secretion of small quantities of thick saliva, depression of gastrointestinal activity, and acceleration of the heart. In general these activities occur under emergencies such as fright and are associated or correlated with expenditure of energy. They are mediated through the release of a transmitter agent, norepinephrine. 2. Stimulating parasympathetic nerves generally produces vasodilation of the part supplied, general fall in blood pressure, contraction of the pupil, copious secretion of thin saliva, increased gastrointestinal activity, and slowing of the heart. SEE: *autonomotropic; nervous system*.

auton'omin. A hormone supposed to correlate endocrine gland activity, inhibiting or stimulating secretions of each according to systemic need.

autonomotrop'ic [G. *autos*, self, + *nomos*, law, + *tropēa*, turning]. Drawn to the autonomic nervous system.

auton'omous. Independent of external influences.

auton'omy. Functional independence.

autop'athy [G. *autos*, self, + *pathos*, disease]. A disease originating without apparent external cause. SYN: *ideopathy*.

autopep'sia [" + *peptein*, to digest]. Digestion by self, as of gastric wall by its own secretion.

autopha'gia, autoph'agy [" + *phagein*, to eat]. Biting oneself.

autophil (aw'tō-fil) [" + *philein*, to love]. Person having sensitive autonomic nervous system.

autophilia (aw-tō-fil'ī-ă). Narcissism, *q.v.* Self-love.

autophobia (aw-tō-fō'bī-ă) [G. *autos*, self, + *phobos*, fear]. 1. A psychoneurotic fear of being alone. 2. Abnormal fear of being egotistical.

autophonomania (aw-tō-phō-nō-mā'nī-ă) [" + *phonos*, murder]. Insanity with suicidal impulses.

autophony (aw-tof'ō-nī) [" + *phōnē*, voice]. The vibration and echolike reproduction of the patient's own voice, breath sounds, and murmurs; usually due to diseases of middle ear and auditory tube.

autoplasmother'apy [" + *plasma*, a thing formed, + *therapeia*, treatment]. Treatment through injecting patient's own blood plasma.

autoplas'tic [" + *plassein*, to form]. Pertaining to autoplasty, *q.v.*

autoplasty (aw'tō-plas-tī) [" + *plassein*, to form]. A grafting of fresh parts taken from the patient's body for the repair of wounds.

autoprecipitin (aw-tō-prē-sĭp'ī-tĭn) [" + L. *praecipitāre*, to cast down]. Precipitin active against serum of animal that was injected.

autopsia (aw-top'sī-ă) [" + *opsis*, view]. An exploratory incision to determine cause of a disorder or nature of a disease.

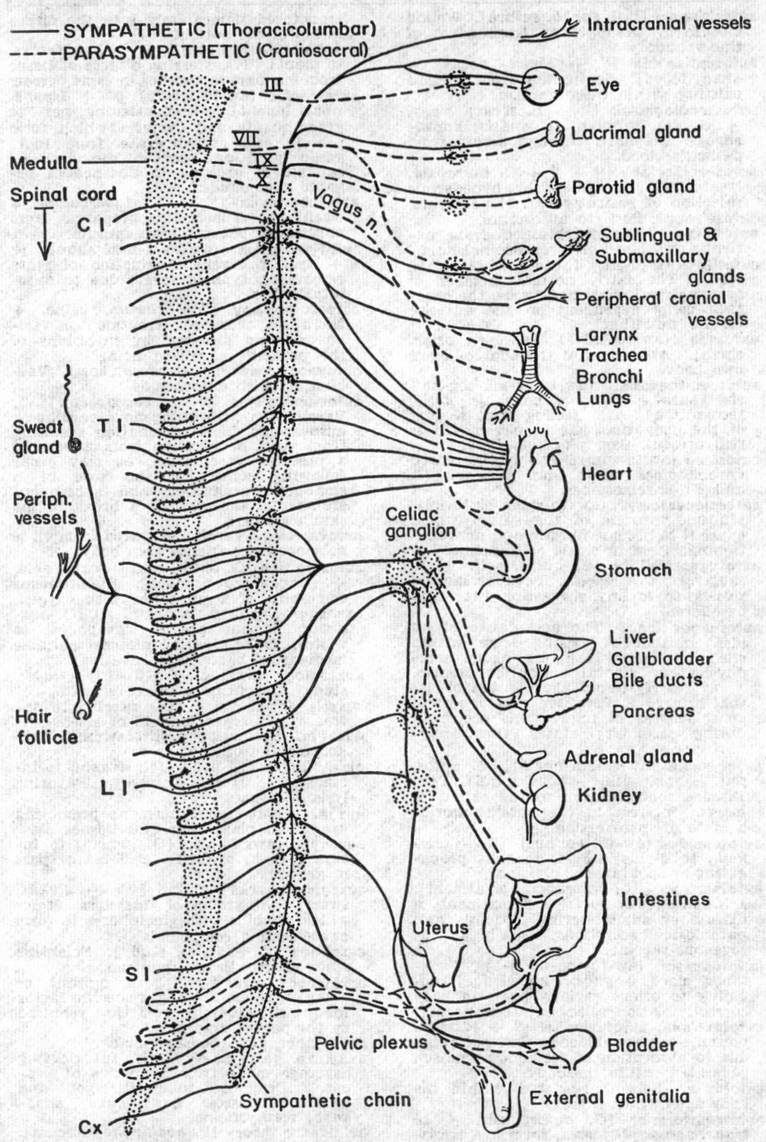

AUTONOMIC NERVOUS SYSTEM

autopsy (aw'top-sĭ). Examination of the organs of a dead body to determine cause of death, or pathological conditions. SYN: *post-mortem examination*.

autopsycho'sis [G. *autos*, self, + *psychē*, the soul]. Mental disease in which patient's ideas about himself are disordered.

autopyother'apy [" + *pyon*, pus, + *therapeia*, treatment]. Treatment of disease by adm. of patient's own pathological excretions.

autoreinfu'sion [" + L. *re*, back, + *in*-into, + *fundere*, to pour]. Intravenous injection of patient's blood which has been effused in his body cavities.

autor'rhaphy [" + *raphē*, suture]. Wound closure by tissue taken from edges of the wound.

autoseptice'mia [" + *sēpsis*, decay, + *aima*, blood]. Septicemia from poisons existing within the organism.

autoserodiagno'sis [" + L. *serum*, whey, + G. *dia*, through, + *gnōsis*, knowledge]. Diagnosis through serum from patient's blood.

autoserother'apy [" + " + G. *therapeia*, treatment]. Treatment by hypodermic injection of patient's own blood serum.

autose'rous. Pert. to autoserum.

autose'rum. Serum obtained from patient's own blood or cerebrospinal fluid.

autosite (aw'tō-sīt) [auto- + G. *sitos*, food]. The fairly normal member of asymmetrical conjoined twins, the other twin being dependent on the autosite for its nutrition.

autosmia (aw-toz'mĭ-ă) [G. + *osme*, smell]. Awareness of the odor of one's own body.

autosomatognosis (aw-tō-sō-mă-tog-nō'-sĭs) [auto- + G. *soma*, body, + *gnosis*, recognition]. The feeling that a part of the body that has been removed is still present. SEE: *phantom limb*.

autosome (aw'tō-sōm). Any of the paired chromosomes other than the sex (X and Y) chromosomes.

autosplenectomy (aw"to-splen-ek'to-mĭ). Multiple infarcts of the spleen which cause it to become fibrotic and nonfunctioning. Seen in sickle cell anemia.

autosuggestibil'ity [G. *autos*, self, + L. *suggerĕre*, to suggest]. Peculiar lack of resistance to any suggestion that may be offered.

autosugges'tion. The acceptance of an idea or thought arising from within one's own mind bringing about some physical or mental action or change.

PSY: 1. Hysteroid aggravation of actual injury. 2. Persistence into normal consciousness of impressions occurring during secondary states. SEE: *hypnotism*.

autosynnoia (aw-to-sĭn-noy'ă) [G. *autos*, self, + *syn*, with, + *nous*, mind]. PSY: Intense concentration to the extent of loss of interest in the outside world: a state of introversion.

autotemnous (aw-tō-tem'nus) [" + *temnein*, to divide]. Pert. to cells propagating by spontaneous division.

autother'apy [" + *therapeia*, treatment]. 1. Spontaneous cure. 2. Treatment of disease by administering patient's own pathological secretions, usually as autogenous vaccine.

autotopnosia (aw-tō-top-nō'zĭ-ă) [" + *topos*, place, + *gnōsis*, knowledge]. Inability to orient various parts of body correctly. Also called autotopagnosia.

autotoxe'mia, autotoxico'sis [" + *toxikon*, poison, + *aima*, blood]. Self-poisoning due to absorption of ferment or poison generated within the body.

autotox'in. Poison generated within the body upon which it acts.

autotransform'er [G. *autos*, self, + L. *trans*, across, + *forma*, form]. A transformer that has part of its turns common to both primary and secondary circuits. SEE: *transformer*.

autotransfusion (aw-tō-trans-fū'shun) [" + " + *fundere*, pour]. 1. Bandaging the limbs to force the blood to the vital centers. 2. A method of returning the patient's own extravasated blood to the circulation. Blood that is shed into the peritoneal cavity, particularly in a ruptured ectopic pregnancy or ruptured spleen, is collected during operation and transfused immediately into the circulation of the patient.

autotransplanta'tion [" + " + *plantāre*, to plant]. Transferring a piece of tissue from one part to another in same person.

autotrophic (aw-tō-trō'fik) [" + *trophē*, nourishment]. Self-nourishing; pert. to green plants and bacteria which form protein and carbohydrate from inorganic salts and carbon dioxide, *i.e.*, capable of growing in absence of organic compounds.

autotuber'culin [" + L. *tuberculum*, a swelling]. Tuberculin prepared from cultures of patient's own sputum.

autotyphization (aw-tō-tī-fi-ză'shun) [" + *typhos*, fever]. Production of state resembling typhoid fever; due to autointoxication.

autourother'apy [" + *ouron*, urine, + *therapeia*, therapy]. Treatment of various allergic diseases by injections of the patient's sterilized urine.

autovaccina'tion [" + *vacca*, cow]. Vaccination with autovaccine.*

autovaccina'tion [" + *vacca*, cow]. 1. Vaccination with autogenous vaccine or autovaccine. 2. A vaccination resulting from virus or bacteria from a sore of a previous vaccination, as may occur following scratching the sore of a smallpox vaccination and subsequent transfer of the virus to a break in the skin elsewhere.

autovac'cine. Vaccine prepared from virus developed in patient's own body.

autoxida'tion [G. *autos*, self, + *oxys*, acid, + *gennan*, to produce]. Spontaneous combining of a substance with oxygen.

auxanography (awks-an-og'ră-fĭ) [G. *auxanein*, to increase, + *graphein*, to write]. Determination of most suitable medium for bacterial cultivation.

auxanology (awks-an-ol'o-jĭ) [" + *logos*, study]. Scientific study of growth.

auxesis (awks-ē'sis) [G. *auxein*, to increase]. Enlarged in bulk or size.

auxet'ic. Promoting proliferation in leukocytes and other cells.

auxilytic (awks-ĭ-lit'ik) [G. *auxein*, to increase, + *lyein*, dissolve]. Favoring lysis (2), *q.v.*

aux'in. Plant-sprout hormone promoting growth in plant cells and tissues.

auxocyte (awks'ō-sīt) [G. *auxein*, to increase, + *kytos*, cell]. Cell taking part in growth.

auxogluc (awks'ō-glŭk) [" + *glukus*, sweet]. A group of tasteless atoms which combine with gluciphores to form sweet-tasting compounds.

auxol'ogy [" + *logos*, study]. Scientific study of growth of organisms.

auxotroph (awks'ō-trōf). A mutant or other organism needing a specific factor for growth different from that required by the parent organism.

A-V. Abbr. for *atrioventricular*.

ava-kava (a'va-kă-vă). 1. Intoxicating beverage made from a species of pepper. 2. Drug used in cystitis, gout and wasting illnesses. SYN: *kava; kavakava; methysticum*.

av'alanche theory [F. *avalanche*, descent]. Theory that nervous impulses increase in intensity in passing efferent nerves.

avascular (ă-văs'kū-lar). Lacking in blood vessels or having a poor blood supply, said of tissues such as cartilage.

avasculariza'tion [G. *a*-, priv. + L. *vasculāris*, having vessels]. Expulsion of blood, as by use of Esmarch bandage.

Avel'lis' syndrome, paralysis [George Avellis, German laryngologist, 1864-1916]. Paralysis of one-half of soft palate, the pharynx, larynx, and loss of pain and heat and cold sensation on opp. side.

aviation medicine. The branch of medicine concerned with diseases and pathologic conditions resulting from, or incident to air travel.

aviation physiology. The branch of physiology which deals with conditions encountered by man in high altitudes as in airplane flights, mountain climbing, or in space vehicles. The principal factors dealt with are hypoxia, physical factors such as extreme temperatures and radiation, effects of forces of acceleration and deceleration, weightlessness, enforced inactivity, and disturbance of biological rhythm.

avidin (av'ĭ-dĭn) [L. *avidus*, greedy]. A protein isolated from raw egg white. Said to be an inhibitor of biotin, thereby causing a deficiency in biotin. Formerly called vitamin H.

avirulent (ă-vir'ū-lent) [G. *a*-, priv. + L. *virus*, poison]. Without virulence.

avitaminosis (a-vī-tă-mĭ-nō'sis) [" + L. *vita*, life, + *amin*]. Disease due to lack of vitamins in the diet; a deficiency disease. SEE: *vitamin*.

avitaminotic (ă-vi-tam-in-ot'ĭk). Pert. to or affected with avitaminosis.

avivement (a-vēv-mon') [Fr. *avivement*, made alive again]. Refreshing of edges of a wound by operation to hasten healing.

avocado (ăv"o-kă'dō) [Portuguese *abacado*]. Pear-shaped, green fruit; alligator pear. Average serving (half of a peeled avocado), 100 gm. Calories: 167. Other values: 16.4 gm. fat; 6.3 gm. carbohydrate; 290 I.U. vitamin A; 14 mg. ascorbic acid.

Avocados contain a sugar, mannoneptose, which is excreted in the urine. This sugar will cause a positive test for reducing substances in the urine (*i.e.*, a false-positive reaction for excess sugar in the urine).

Avogad'ro's law [Amadeo Avogadro, Italian physicist, 1776-1856]. Equal volumes of gases contain equal numbers of molecules, pressure and temperature being same.

A.'s number. Number of molecules in one gram-molecular weight of a compound.

avoirdupois' meas'ure [Fr. *avoir*, to have, + *du*, of the, + *pois*, weight]. A system of weighing or measuring all coarse and heavy articles. 7000 grains equal one pound. Some medicines are bought and sold by avoirdupois weight.

Dry Measure

16 drams (dr.) equal ..	1 ounce (oz.)
16 ounces equal	1 pound (lb.)
25 pounds equal	1 quarter (qr.)
4 quarters equal	100 weight (cwt.)
20 cwts. equal	1 ton (T.)

Liquid Measure

2 pints equal	1 quart equals 57¾ cubic inches.
4 quarts equal	1 gallon equals 231 cubic inches.

To find the capacity of a vessel or space in gallons, divide the contents in cubic inches by 231 for liquid gallons, or by 268.8 for dry gallons.

To reduce gallons to inches, multiply the given number of liquid gallons by 231; then change to higher denominations if required. The dry gallon (half-peck) contains 268.8 cu. in. Six dry gallons are equal to nearly seven liquid gallons.

The bushel contains 2150.42 cu. in. and is a cylindrical measure 18½ in. in diameter and 8 in. deep. Measures of capacity are all cubic measures. The number of pounds in a bushel depends upon the article contained therein. SEE: *apothecaries' measure; household measures; metric system; Troy weight.*

avulsion (ă-vul'shun) [G. *a*-, priv. + L. *avulsio*, a turning away]. A tearing away forcibly of a part or structure. If surgical repair is necessary, merely apply a sterile dressing while waiting for surgery to be done. If fingers, toes, feet, or hands are completely avulsed, they may be successfully rejoined to the body if prompt and expert care is available.

axanthopsia (aks-an-thop'sĭ-ă) [G. *a*-, priv. + *xanthos*, yellow, + *opsis*, vision]. Yellow blindness.

axenic (ăks-ĕn'ĭk). Germ-free, as pertaining to animals, or pure, as pertaining to cultures or microorganisms.

axial (aks'ĭ-al) [L. *axis*, lever]. Situated in or pert. to an axis.

a. line. A line running in the main axis of the body or part of it. The *axial line of the hand* runs through the middle digit; the *axial line of the foot* runs through the second digit.

a. skeleton. Head and trunk.

axifugal (aks-if'u-gal) [" + *fugere*, to flee]. Receding from the axis. SYN: *centrifugal.*

axilem'ma [L. *axis*, pivot, + G. *lemma*, husk]. The plasma membrane of an axon.

axil'la (Pl. *axil'lae*) [L. *axilla*, little pivot]. The armpit.

axillary (aks'ĭ-lar-ĭ). Pert. to the axilla.

ax'ion [G. *axōn*, axis]. Brain and spinal cord. The cerebrospinal axis.

axioplasm (aks'ĭ-ō-plazm) [" + *plasma*, a thing formed]. Neuroplasm of an axis cylinder.

ax"ip'etal [L. *axis*, pivot, + *petere*, to seek]. Directed toward the axis. SYN: *axopetal; centripetal.*

ax'is (pl. *axes*). 1. A line, real or imaginary, which runs through the center of a body, or about which a part revolves. 2. [NA] The second cervical vertebra or *epistropheus* which bears the *odontoid process* (dens) about which the atlas rotates.

a., basicranial. A. connecting basion and gonion.

a., basifacial. A. from subnasal point to gonion.

a., binauricular. A. bet. the two auricular points.

a., celiac. Celiac artery from abdominal aorta.

a., cerebrospinal. Central nervous system.

a. cylinder. An axon (def. 2), *q.v.*

a., frontal. Imaginary line running transversely through the center of the eyeball.

a., neural. SEE: *cerebrospinal a.*

a., optic. A line which connects the anterior and posterior poles of the eye.

a., principal. In optics, a line which passes through the optical center or nodal point of a lens perpendicular to the surface of the lens.

a., sagittal. Imaginary line running through the eyeball anteroposteriorly.

a., visual. A line passing from object of vision directly through center of cornea and lens to the fovea.

axis traction (ak'sis trak'shun). Traction made on the fetus in the direction of the birth canal.

a. t. forceps. Device used to aid in traction made on the fetus.

axite (aks'īt). Any terminal filament of an axis cylinder.

axo- (aks'o) [G.]. Prefix: Axis.

axodendrite (aks-o-den'drīt) [G. *axōn*, axis, + *dendron*, tree]. Process given off from a nerve cell axon (not an axis cylinder).

axofugal (aks-of'u-gal) [" + L. *fugere*, to flee]. Axifugal, *q.v.*

axolem'ma [" + *lemma*, husk]. Axis cylinder sheath of a nerve fiber. SYN: *axilemma*.

axolysis (aks-ol'ĭ-sis) [" + *lyein*, to dissolve]. Destruction of the axis cylinder of a nerve.

ax'on, ax'one [G. *axōn*, axis]. 1. A process of a neuron which conducts impulses away from the cell body. Typically one arising from a portion of the cell devoid of Nissl granules, the *axon hillock*. Axons may possess either or both of two sheaths (myelin sheath and neurilemma) or neither. Axons are usually long and straight, and most end in synapses in the central nervous system or ganglia or in effector organs (*e.g.*, motor neurons). They may give off side branches or *collaterals*. An axon with its sheath(s) constitutes a nerve fiber. 2. A nerve cell process which resembles an axon in structure, specifically the peripheral process of a dorsal root ganglion cell (sensory neuron) which functionally and embryologically is a dendrite, but structurally is indistinguishable from an axon. SEE: *nerve; neuron*. SYN: *axis cylinder*.

axoneme (aks'o-nēm) [G. *axōn*, axis, + *nēma*, a thread]. Axial thread of a chromosome.

axoneuron (aks-ō-nū'ron) [" + *neuron*, sinew]. A nerve cell of the cerebrospinal system.

axonometer (aks-ō-nom'ĕ-ter) [" + *metron*, a measure]. Device for determining the axis of astigmatism.

axopetal (aks-op'ĕ-tal) [" + *petere*, to seek]. Conducted along an axon toward a cell body of a neuron.

axophage (aks'o-fāj) [" + *phagein*, to eat]. Glia cell found in myelin excavations in myelitis.

ax'oplasm [" + *plasma*, a thing formed]. The cytoplasm (neuroplasm) of an axon which encloses the neurofibrils.

axospongium (aks-ō-spon'jĭ-um) [" + *spoggos*, sponge]. The fine fibrillar network of axon of a nerve cell.

Ayerza's disease, syndrome (ā-yer'sa). One characterized by dyspnea, chronic cyanosis, erythemia, enlargement of spleen and liver, and hyperplasia of bone. Polycythemia usually results from pulmonary insufficiency.

Az. Abbr. for *azote*.

aza'lein [L. *azalea*, azalea]. A red dye. SYN: *fuchsin*.

azo-. Prefix indicating the presence of —N-N— group in a chemical. This group is usually connected at either end with carbon atoms. SEE: *azo compounds*.

azoamyly (az-ō-am'ĭ-lĭ) [G. *a-*, priv. + *zōon*, animal, + *amylon*, starch]. Diminution of amount of glycogen stored up in the liver.

azo compounds. Organic substance which contain the *azo* group. An example is azobenzene, $C_6H_5N:NC_6H_5$.

They are related to aniline, and include important dyes and indicators. The color changes shown by dimethylaminoazobenzene $C_6H_5N:NC_6H_4N(CH_3)_2$ are given under *"Indicators."*

azoic (ă-zō'ĭk) [G. *a-*, priv. + *zōē*, life]. Containing no living organisms.

azoospermia (ă-zo-o-sper'mĭ-ă) [" + *zōon*, animal, + *sperma*, seed]. Absence of spermatozoa from the semen.

azotation (az-ō-tā'shun) [*azote*, nitrogen]. Nitrogen absorption from the air.

az'ote [G. *a-*, priv. + *zōē*, life, so named by Lavoisier because it cannot support life]. Nitrogen.

azotemia (az-ō-tē'mĭ-ă) [" + *aima*, blood]. Presence of nitrogenous bodies, especially urea in increased amount, in the blood. SYN: *uremia, q.v.*

azotenesis (az-ō-tĕ-nē'sis) [" + *enesis*, injection]. Disease due to excess of nitrogen in system.

azotifica'tion. Atmospheric nitrogen fixation.

azotized (az'ot-īzd). 1. Containing nitrogen. 2. Converted into an azo compound.

Azotobacter (ă-zō'tō-bak-tĕr). Rod-shaped, gram-negative, nonpathogenic, soil and water bacteria that fix atmospheric nitrogen. The single genus of the family Azotobacteraceae.

azotom'eter [*azote*, nitrogen, + *metron*, measure]. Instrument measuring amount of uric acid and urea in urine.

azotorrhea (az-o-to-re'ă) [" + *roia*, flow]. Excess of nitrogenous matter in the feces or urine.

azotu'ria [" + *ouron*, urine]. An increase in nitrogenous compounds, esp. urea, in urine.

azurophil(e (azh-u'ro-fil) [M. E. *azure*, azure, + G. *philein*, to love]. Staining readily with azure dye.

azurophil'ia. Condition in which some blood cells have azurophil granules.

azygos (az'ĭ-gos) [G. *a-*, priv. + *zygos*, yoke]. Occurring singly, not in pairs.

azygous (az'ĭg-us). Single, not paired.

a. vein. A single vein arising in the abdomen as a branch of the ascending lumbar vein. It passes upward through the aortic hiatus of the diaphragm into the thorax, then along right side of vertebral column to level of fourth thoracic vertebra where it turns and enters sup. vena cava. In the thorax it receives the hemiazygous, accessory azygous and bronchial veins, as well as right intercostal and subcostal veins. In cases of obstruction to inf. vena cava, the azygous vein is the principal vein by which blood can return to the heart.

azymia (a-zi'mĭ-ă) [G. *a-*, priv. + *zymē*, ferment]. State of being without a ferment or enzyme.

azymic, azymous (ă-zi'mik, -mus). 1. Unfermented or unleavened. 2. Denoting the absence of a ferment.

Notes

Notes

B

B. Chemical symbol for *boron;* abbreviation for *Bacillus, balneum, barometric, base, bath, Baumé scale, behavior, Benoist scale, buccal.*

Ba. Chemical symbol for *barium.*

Bab'bitt metal. Antifriction alloy of copper, antimony, and tin used occasionally in dentistry.

Babcock-Levy test. PSY: The difference between a vocabulary and a nonvocabulary test indicating the degree of mental deterioration.

Babes-Ernst bodies (bă'bāz-ĕrnst) [Victor Babes, Roumanian bacteriologist, 1854-1926, and Paul Ernst, German pathologist, 1859-1937]. Metachromatic bodies, *q.v.*, seen in bacterial protoplasm.

Babesia (bă-bē'zĭ-ă) [named for Victor Babes]. A genus of Haemosporidia which are parasites in the blood of cattle, sheep, horses, dogs and other vertebrate animals. They infest red blood cells bringing about their destruction with resulting hemoglobinuria. They are transmitted by ticks.

B. bigemina. The causative organism of Texas fever in cattle.

B. bovis. Causes hemoglobinuria and jaundice (red water fever) in cattle.

babesiasis, babesiosis (bab"ĕ-zī'ă-sĭs, bă-bē"zĭ-ō'sĭs). Infection caused by a species of *Babesia.*

Babinski's reflex (bă-bĭn'skēz) [Joseph Babinski, Paris neurologist, 1857-1932]. Elicited by stroking of lateral aspect of sole of foot. Backward flexion of the great toe, sometimes accompanied by slight spreading of other toes, is indicative of pyramidal tract involvement, usually an upper motor neurone lesion on homolateral side. It is found in organic hemiplegia, *q.v.*, diseases of nervous system, but not in hysteria.

B.'s sign. A loss or diminished reflex contraction of the Achilles tendon. It is found in sciatica, not in hysteric sciatica.

baby. An infant.

b., blue. Infant born with cyanosis due to a congenital anomaly of the heart which permits venous blood to travel directly from the right to the left side of the heart without going through the lungs.

bacca (bak'ă) [L. berry]. A berry.

Baccelli's sign (bă-tchel'ēz). Whisper heard over the chest; an indication of pleural effusion.

bacciform (bak'sĭ-form) [L. *bacca*, berry, + *forma*, form]. Berry-shaped; coccal.

Bacillaceae (bas-ĭ-lā'sē-ē). A family (order *Eubacteriales*) of rod-shaped cells that can produce endospores. Usually gram-positive, commonly found in soil. Genera of family are *Bacillus* and *Clostridium.*

bacillaemia. Bacillemia, *q.v.*

bacillar, bacillary (bas'ĭ-ler, bas'ĭ-ler-ĭ). 1. Pert. to or caused by bacilli. 2. Rodlike.

b. layer. Rod and cone retinal layer.

bacillemia (bas-ĭ-lē'mĭ-ă [L. *bacillus*, rod, + G. *aima*, blood]. Presence of bacilli in the blood.

bacilli (bă-sĭl'ī). Plural of *bacillus.*

bacillicide (ba-sil'ĭ-sīd). An agent destructive to bacilli.

bacil'liculture [L. *bacillus*, rod, + *cultura* cultivation]. 1. Propagation of bacilli 2. Culture containing bacilli.

bacil'liform [" + *forma*, form]. Resembling a bacillus in shape.

bacilliparous (bas-ĭ-lip'a-rus) [" + *parere*, to produce]. Producing bacilli.

bacillogenic, bacillogenous (bas-ĭ-lō-jen'ĭk, bas-ĭ-loj'ĕ-nus) [" + G. *gennan*, to produce]. 1. Producing bacilli. 2. Originating in bacilli.

bacillophobia (bas-ĭ-lō-fō'bĭ-ă) [" + G. *phobos*, fear]. Morbid fear of bacilli.

bacillo'sis [" + G. *-osis*, infection]. Condition due to infection by bacilli.

bacilluria (bas-ĭ-lū'rĭ-ă) [L. *bacillus*, rod, + G. *ouron*, urine]. Bacilli in the urine. Most common infective organism is bacillus from the colon, usually *Escherichia coli.* SEE: *cystitis.*

Bacillus (ba-sil'us). A genus of bacteria belonging to the family Bacillaceae. All species are rod-shaped, sometimes occurring in chains. They are spore-bearing, aerobic, motile or nonmotile; most are gram-positive, and nonpathogenic. Only two species are pathogenic to man, the most important being *B. anthracis.*

B. an'thracis. An aerobic, spore-forming bacillus pathogenic to man and domestic animals, being the causative agent of anthrax, *q.v.* SYN: *Davaine's bacillus.*

B. subti'lis. The common hay bacillus but has a close resemblance to *B. anthracis.* It is considered to be nonpathogenic generally, but is believed by some occasionally to cause conjunctivitis in man. It is sometimes found as a contaminant of laboratory specimens. SYN: *hay bacillus.*

bacil'lus (pl. *bacilli*). 1. Any rod-shaped microorganism. 2. A rod-shaped microorganism belonging to the class Schizomycetes. See also the genus: *Bacillus.*

b., Abel's. *Klebsiella ozaenae.* Found in ozena.

b., abortus. *Brucella abortus.* Causes infectious abortion in cattle and other domestic animals. Causative agent of brucellosis (undulant fever) in man.

b., acid-fast. Bacillus not readily decolorized by acids or other means when stained.

b., Bang's. *Brucella abortus.* Abortus b., *q.v.*

b., Bordet-Gengou. *Bordetella pertussis*, formerly *Haemophilus pertussis.* Causative agent of whooping cough.

b., Boyd's. *Shigella boydii*, found in feces of patients with dysentery. Only a small number of bacilli found in feces of patients with bacillary dysentery.

b., butter. *Mycobacterium smegmatis.* Smegma b., *q.v.*

b., Calmette-Guerin. Attenuated *Mycobacterium bovis.* Used in BCG vaccine as a preventive of human tuberculosis.

b., cholera. *Vibrio comma.* Causative agent of cholera.

b., colon. *Escherichia coli.* A normal inhabitant of the intestinal tract; the cause of urinary tract infections. Certain types are responsible for enteritis in infants.

b., comma. *Vibrio comma.* Causative agent of cholera.

b., Davaine's. *Bacillus anthracis*, the cause of anthrax.

b., diphtheria. *Corynebacterium diphtheriae.* The causative agent of diphtheria.

***b.*, Döderlein's.** A large gram-positive bacillus usually present in the vagina. Considered identical with *Lactobacillus acidophilus.* Probably responsible for the acidity of the vagina.

***b.*, Ducrey's.** *Haemophilus ducreyi.* The cause of soft chancre or chancroid infection of the genitalia.

***b.*, Duval's.** *Shigella sonnei,* a cause of bacillary dysentery.

***b.*, dysentery.** A bacillus of the genus *Shigella* that causes bacillary dysentery.

***b.*, Eberth's.** *Salmonella typhosa,* the cause of typhoid fever.

***b.*, Flexner's.** *Shigella flexneri,* the most common cause of epidemic dysentery.

***b.*, Friedländer's.** *Klebsiella pneumoniae.* A cause of pneumonia.

***b.*, fusiform.** *Fusobacterium fusiforme.* The causative organism of Vincent's infection, is found also in the normal mouth.

***b.*, Gärtner's.** *Salmonella enteritidis.* The cause of Salmonella gastroenteritis and Salmonella food poisoning.

***b.*, gas.** *Clostridium perfringens.* A cause of gaseous gangrene.

***b.*, Ghon-Sachs.** *Clostridium septicum.* A causative agent of gaseous gangrene.

***b.*, Hansen's.** *Mycobacterium leprae.* Causative organism of Hansen's disease (leprosy).

***b.*, hay.** *Bacillus subtilis.* Nonpathogenic bacillus, sometimes found as a contaminant of laboratory specimens.

***b.*, Hofmann's.** *Corynebacterium pseudodiphtheriticum.* Causative agent of a type of diphtheria.

***b.*, influenza.** As *Haemophilus influenzae* type B, it is the cause of meningitis. Other types cause conjunctivitis, septicemia and respiratory infections. May cause complications, as a secondary invader, in influenza, pertussis, or other diseases.

***b.*, Johne's.** *Mycobacterium paratuberculosis.* Cause of chronic diarrhea in cattle.

***b.*, Klebs-Loeffler.** *Corynebacterium diphtheriae.* The cause of diphtheria.

***b.*, Koch-Weeks.** *Haemophilus aegyptius.* Cause of infectious conjunctivitis.

***b.*, leprosy.** *Mycobacterium leprae.* Cause of leprosy (Hansen's disease).

***b.*, Morax-Axenfeld.** *Moraxella lacunata,* a cause of conjunctivitis in man.

***b.*, Morgan's.** *Proteus morganii.* May cause abscesses and urinary tract infections. Usually a secondary invader. Isolated from patients with summer diarrhea.

***b.*, Nicolaier's.** *Clostridium tetani.* The cause of tetanus (lockjaw).

***b.*, Nocard's.** *Salmonella typhimurium.* One of the many types of Salmonellae.

***b.*, Novy's.** *Clostridium novyi,* a cause of gaseous gangrene.

***b.*, paracolon.** *Paracolobactrum.* Found in gastroenteritis.

***b.*, paratyphoid.** *Salmonella paratyphi.* One of the causes of paratyphoid fever.

***b.*, Pfeiffer's.** *Haemophilus influenzae.* SEE: *influenza bacillus.*

***b.*, plague.** *Pasteurella pestis.* The cause of bubonic plague.

***b.*, Schmitz.** *Shigella schmitzii,* a cause of bacillary dysentery.

***b.*, Shiga.** Name given to a representative dysentery bacillus first described in 1898 by Kiyoshi Shiga, a Japanese bacteriologist, for whom the genus *Shigella* was named.

***b.*, smegma.** *Mycobacterium smegmatis.* Found in smegma, and occasionally in feces and urine, of males and females.

***b.*, Sonne.** *Shigella sonnei,* a cause of bacillary dysentery in man.

***b.*, swine plague.** *Pasteurella multocida,* causing plague in swine.

***b.*, timothy.** *Mycobacterium phlei,* an organism found in timothy grass.

***b.*, tubercle.** *Mycobacterium tuberculosis,* the cause of tuberculosis in human beings.

***b.*, typhoid.** *Salmonella typhi,* the cause of typhoid fever.

***b.*, Vincent's.** *Fusobacterium fusiforme,* the cause of Vincent's infection, is found also in the normal mouth.

***b.*, Weichselbaum's.** *Neisseria meningitidis,* the causative agent of epidemic cerebral meningitis (cerebrospinal fever, spotted fever). SYN: *meningococcus.*

***b.*, Welch's.** *Clostridium perfringens.* A cause of gaseous gangrene.

***b.*, Whitmore.** *Pseudomonas pseudomallei,* an infection, similar to glanders, that is pathogenic in man in India and Indo-China.

bacitracin (băs-ĭ-trā′sĭn). USP. An antibiotic substance obtained from a strain of *Bacillus subtilis.* Its antibacterial actions are similar to those of penicillin, including gram-positive cocci and bacilli and some gram-negative organisms. Though available for intramuscular and for topical use, bacitracin is usually employed only topically in the form of ointment because of its toxicity when used parenterally.

back. 1. The dorsum or posterior surface of the body. 2. The posterior region of the body from neck to pelvis.

backache. A common syndrome characterized by pain and tenderness in the muscles or their attachments in the lower lumbar, lumbosacral, or sacroiliac regions. Pain is often referred to leg following distribution of sciatic nerve.

ETIOL: 1. Infection or abnormality in another part of the body, *e.g.*, uterine or prostatic disorders. 2. Disorders of vertebral column, such as intervertebral disk abnormality. 3. Local disturbances such as lumbar or sacral fractures, lumbosacral strain or sprain. 4. Structural inadequacies of supporting ligaments of the spinal column. 5. Muscle injury, spasm, myositis, or inflammation of fascial attachments. 6. Professional cramp. 7. Psychogenic factors.

TREATMENT: Treatment of specific primary cause. General treatment includes measures to allay pain and discomfort such as analgesics, preferably salicylates (codeine in severe cases), heat, and massage. Tender areas or "trigger points" may be anesthetized by local infiltration with 1% procaine or application of ethyl chloride spray. Special measures to relax tense muscles and improve blood flow are helpful. Orthopedic supports and strapping necessary in special cases. Muscle reeducation. Psychogenic treatment when necessary esp. in excessive muscle tension resulting from emotional maladjustments.

backbone. The vertebral column; spinal column.

backflow. Abnormal backward flow of fluids.

***b.*, pyelovenous.** Drainage from the renal pelvis into the venous system under some conditions of back pressure.

back-pressure arm-lift artificial respiration. Place the victim prone (face down) with elbows bent, one hand on the other, head to one side, cheek resting on folded hands. Kneel on one knee—or both, if you achieve better balance—at the victim's head. A. Place your hands on the flat of the victim's back, below the armpit, with your thumbs barely touching, fingers spread outward and downward. B. Rock forward slowly, keeping your elbows straight, until your arms are nearly vertical, thus exerting a steady downward pressure. C. Now rock backward, releasing pressure. Slide your hands outward to grasp the victim's arms just above the elbows. Continue to rock backward. D. As you rock backward, raise and pull the victim's arms toward you until you feel tension in his shoulders. Start over with step A. Repeat the full cycle about 12 times a minute. *Important:* When the victim begins to breathe on his own, synchronize your efforts with his breathing until he breathes strongly. Then stop.

bacteremia (băk-tĕr-ē'mĭ-ă) [G. *bakterion,* staff, + *aima,* blood]. Bacteria in the blood.

bacteria (pl. of *bacterium*). Unicellular, plant-like microorganisms, lacking chlorophyll.

Shape: There are three principal forms: (1) *Spherical or ovoid forms.* When appearing singly, they are called *micrococci;* when in pairs, *diplococci;* when in irregular clusters, *staphylococci;* when in chains, *streptococci;* when in regular groups of eight, *sarcinae.* (2) *Rod-shaped* forms known as *bacilli.* When the rods are somewhat oval, they are called *coccobacilli;* when attached end to end forming a chain, *streptobacilli.* (3) *Spiral forms.* When the spiral organisms are rigid they are called *spirilla;* when flexible, *spirochetes;* when forming curved rods, *vibrios.* (4) *Involution forms:* Most bacteria are relatively constant in form in growing cultures, but in old cultures or cultures grown under adverse environmental conditions, aberrant forms such as oversized and Y-shaped appear. These are considered by some to be involution or degenerating forms; by others to be stages in complex life cycles.

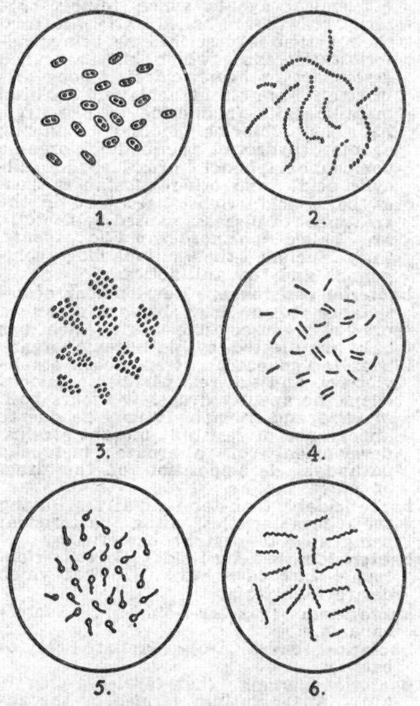

SHAPES OF BACTERIA

1. Diplococci. 2. Streptococci. 3. Staphylococci. 4. Bacilli. 5. Bacilli with spores. 6. Spirilla.

Characteristics

Size: An average rod-shaped bacterium measures about 1 micron in diameter by 4 microns in length. They vary considerably in size from 0.2 x 0.5 micron (influenza bacillus) to 2 x 20 microns (some of the longer spiral cells).

Motility: Some bacteria are incapable of movement (all cocci) but most bacilli and spiral forms exhibit independent movement. The power of locomotion depends on the possession of one or more flagella, slender whiplike appendages. Bacteria having no flagella are called *atrichous;* those having a flagellum at one end, *monotrichous;* those having flagella at each end, *amphitrichous;* those having a tuft at one end, *lophotrichous;* those having flagella protruding from all surfaces of the cell, *peritrichous.*

Capsules: Many bacteria possess a *capsule,* a layer of slimy mucoid substance which surrounds each cell. The presence of a capsule is associated with the virulence of certain pathogenic forms.

Spores: Certain species of the rod-shaped bacteria have the ability to develop an encysted or resting stage known as a *spore* or *endospore.* The size, shape, and position of the spore within the cell are characteristic of particular species. Spores are *terminal,* if formed at the end of a cell; *central,* if formed in the center; *subterminal,* if formed between the center and end. Spore formation is common among the bacilli but does not usually occur in the cocci or spiral forms. Bacterial spores are remarkably resistant to heat, drying, and the action of disinfectants. Few bacteria pathogenic to man form spores, *i.e.,* anthrax, botulinus, gas gangrene and tetanus bacilli. Unfavorable environmental conditions favor spore formation.

Reproduction: Binary fission is the usual mode of reproduction. Budding, branching, filamentous growth, and the development of conidia also occur.

Colony formation: A group of bacteria growing in one place is called a *colony.* A colony is usually composed of the descendants of a single cell. Colonies differ in shape, size, color, texture, type of margin, and in other characteristics. Each species of bacteria has a characteristic type of colony formation. Sometimes a single species may produce two types of colonies; one the *smooth or S-type,* the other the *rough* or *R-type.* Sometimes colonies contain clear spots and have a moth-eaten appearance. Such colonies are called *plaques* and are thought to be due to the lytic action of bacteriophage.

Food requirements: Bacteria possess no chlorophyll hence cannot carry on photosynthesis. A few can obtain their energy from inorganic substances. These are termed *autotrophic* and include many of the soil bacteria. The majority derive their nourishment from organic material and are termed *heterotrophic.* If they live on living organisms, they are called *parasites;* if their food is from nonliving organic matter, they are called *saprophytes.* If bacteria produce disease in their host, they are *pathogenic.*

Oxygen requirements: Most bacteria require free or atmospheric oxygen. These are called *aerobes.* Bacteria living in the absence of atmospheric oxygen are called *anaerobes.* Those showing a preference for free oxygen and yet are capable of living in its absence are called *facultative anerobes;* those which grow only in the absence of oxygen are called *obligate anaerobes.*

Temperature requirements: Most bacteria grow best at moderate temperatures. These are called *mesophilic.* Cold-living bacteria which thrive in temperatures between 0° and 30° C. (32° and 86° F.) are called *psychophilic;* those which thrive in high temperatures between 40° and 70° C. (104° and 158° F.) are called *thermophilic.* The optimum temperature for most saprophytes is around 25° C., for most pathogens, 37° C.

Activities of Bacteria

Enzyme production: Bacteria produce enzymes which act on complex food molecules breaking them down into simpler materials capable of assimilation. *Carbohydrases* act on sugars breaking them down to alcohol and carbon dioxide, a process called *fermentation. Proteolytic enzymes* bring about the decomposition of proteins with the formation of ill-smelling products, a process called *putrefaction.* The term *decay* is applied to the decomposition of organic substances in the presence of air without the formation of unpleasant odors. *Putrefaction* is the decomposition of organic substances, especially nitrogenous substances, in the absence of air and with resulting unpleasant odors. Bacteria are the principal agents of decay and putrefaction.

Toxin production: Many bacteria produce poisonous substances called *toxins,* which are of two types, (1) *exotoxins* which diffuse from the bacterial cell into the surrounding medium and (2) *endotoxins,* which are liberated only when the bacterial cell dies and disintegrates. Bacteria well known for their toxin production are the diphtheria, tetanus, and botulinus organisms.

Miscellaneous activities: Some bacteria produce *pigments;* some produce *light,* appearing *luminescent* at night. Many chemical substances are produced as a result of bacterial activity, among them acids, gases, alcohol, aldehydes, ammonia, indol. Pathogenic forms produce hemolysins, leukocidins, coagulases, and fibrolysins. Soil bacteria play an important role in various phases of the nitrogen cycle (nitrification, nitrogen fixation, and denitrification).

Methods of Studying Bacteria: The principal methods used in the study of bacteria are:

(1) Examination of unstained bacteria in a hanging-drop preparation. Dark-field illumination is necessary to see extremely small forms.

(2) *Staining methods.* General stains, differential stains, stains for special bacteria, and stains for specific parts are employed. Of the differential stains, Gram's method and staining for acid-fast bacteria are the most widely used. Bacteria fall into these groups: *Gram-positive bacteria:* Those which retain the stain. *Gram-negative bacteria:* Those which are decolorized by alcohol. *Acid-fast bacteria:* Those which, when stained with certain dyes, retain the stain even when treated with an acid.

(3) *Cultural methods.* The bacteria are grown on various culture media. Media may be *synthetic* or *nonsynthetic.* In the former, the exact composition of the medium is known; in the latter, the constituents are uncertain. Media, on the basis of consistency, may be *liquid* (nutrient broth, milk, blood serum); *liquefiable solid media* which consist of liquid media made solid by addition of gelatin or agar-agar; *nonliquefiable solid media* (potato, carrots, starch paste).

(4) *Animal inoculation.*

(5) *Immunological methods.*

(6) *Sterilization methods.*

Sterilization is the process of rendering any material free of living microorganisms. It may be accomplished by physical or chemical means. The use of chemical agents is usually designated *disinfection.* Physical agents employed are heat, light and filtration. Sterilization may be accomplished in a flame, in a hot-air oven (150° to 170° C. for one hour), in streaming steam (100° C. for 20 min. or longer) or by steam under pressure (10-15 lbs.) in an autoclave (121° C. for 20 min.). Ultraviolet light is destructive to bacteria as are certain gases such as ethylene oxide, methyl bromide, and hydrogen cyanide. Filtration is accomplished by the use of cotton or by special filters (Berkefeld, Pasteur, Chamberlain) of unglazed porcelain.

Chemical agents which inhibit bacterial growth are called *antiseptics* and their action is described as being *bacteriostatic;* those which kill are called *germicides* or *bactericides.* Among disinfectants are strong acids and alkalies, metallic salts (bichloride of mercury), halogens (chlorine, iodine), oxidizing agents (hydrogen peroxide), organic compounds (phenol, formaldehyde, salicylic acid), and other substances such as boric acid. Substances used in the treatment of diseases caused by bacteria are called *chemotherapeutic agents.* They include the sulfonamide compounds and the anitbiotics.

bacterial resistance. Development of resistance to a drug by an organism previously susceptible to it. Such has been manifested by pathogenic organisms (as gonococci, streptococci, staphylococci, and tubercle bacilli) to various chemotherapeutic drugs. It occurs both *in vitro* and *in vivo.* It may be due to appearance of resistant mutant strains, development of alternate metabolic pathways, decomposition of the drug, or *other* factors.

bactericidal (bak-ter-ĭ-sīd′al). Having the characteristics of a bactericide; being able to destroy bacteria.

bactericide (bak-ter′ĭ-sīd) [G. *baktērion,* rod, + L. *caedere,* to kill]. That which destroys bacteria.

bacteriemia (bak-ter-ĭ-ē′mĭ-ă). Bacteremia, *q.v.*

bacterio- (bak-tē′rĭ-ō). Prefix: Pert. to bacteria.

bacterioagglutinin (bak-tē″rĭ-ō-ă-gloo′tĭ-nĭn). An agglutinin formed by the action of bacteria.

bacteriocid′al. Bactericidal, *q.v.*

bacterioclasis (bak-tē-rĭ-ok′lă-sĭs). The break-up or fragmentation of bacteria.

bacteriogenic (bak-tē-rē-ō-jen'ĭk) [G. *baktērion,* rod, + *gennan,* to produce]. Caused by bacteria.

bacterioid (bak-tēr'ĭ-oyd). Resembling bacteria.

bacteriolog'ic, bacteriolog'ical [" + *logos,* study]. Pert. to bacteriology.

bacteriol'ogist. One versed in bacteriology.

bacteriol'ogy. Science of microorganisms.

bacteriolysin (bak-tē-rĭ-ol'ĭ-sĭn) [G. *baktērion,* rod, + *lysis,* solution]. A substance, especially an antibody produced within the body of an animal, which is capable of bringing about the dissolution or lysis of bacteria.

bacteriolysis (bak-tē-rē-ŏl'ĭ-sĭs). The disintegration of bacteria generally by a specific antibody.

bacteriolytic (bak-te"rĭ-ō-lit'ĭk). Pert. to bacteriolysis.

bacterioopsonin (bak-tē"rĭ-ō-op-sō'nĭn). Bacteriopsonin, *q.v.*

bacteriophage (băk-tē'rĭ-ō'fāj) [G. *baktērion,* rod, + *phagein,* to eat]. Term applied to a group of transmissible agents which are capable of inducing lysis or dissolution of certain bacterial cells. They are widely distributed in nature having been isolated from feces, sewage, and polluted surface waters. They are regarded as bacterial viruses, the phage particle consisting of a head composed of DNA and a tail by which it attaches to host cells. The clear zone formed by the lysis of bacteria is called a plaque. Syn: *phage.*

bacteriopha'gia. Destruction of bacteria by lytic agents.

bacterioprecip'itin. Precipitin occurring in bacteria-treated serum.

bacteriopro'tein. One of the proteins in bacteria bodies.

bacteriopsonin (bak-tē"rĭ-op'sō-nĭn). An opsonin acting on bacteria.

bacterios'copy. Microscopic examination of bacteria.

bacteriostasis (bak-tē-rĭ-ō-stā'sĭs) [" + *stasis,* a stopping]. The arrest of bacterial growth.

bacte'riostat. An agent inhibiting bacterial growth.

bacteriostatic (bak-tē-rĭ-ō-stat'ic). Inhibiting or retarding bacterial growth.

bacteriotox'ic. 1. Toxic to bacteria. 2. Due to bacterial toxins.

bacteriotox'in. Toxin specifically destructive to bacteria.

bacteriotropin (bak-tē-rĭ-ot'rō-pĭn). An opsonin or a substance which enhances the ability of phagocytes to engulf bacteria.

Bacterium (bak-tē'rĭ-ŭm). A former genus designation for rod-shaped bacteria without flagella. Term is no longer used in the taxonomic sense because of lack of an identified type species. The species formerly classified as Bacterium are now assigned to other genera such as *Aerobacter, Alcaligines, Mycobacterium, Pasteurella* and *Salmonella.*

B. aerogenes. *Aerobacter aerogenes.*

B. aertrycke. *Salmonella typhimurium.*

B. ambiguus. *Shigella ambigua.*

B. cholerae suis. *Salmonella choleraesuis.*

B. coli. *Escherichia coli.*

B. paratyphi (Type A). *Salmonella paratyphi.*

B. paratyphi (Type B). *Salmonella schottmuelleri.*

B. pneumonie crouposae. *Klebsiella pneumoniae.*

B. tularense. *Pasteurella tularensis.*

B. (Eberthella) typhi. *Salmonella typhosa.*

B. typhosum. *Salmonella typhosa.*

bacterium. Singular of *bacteria, q.v.*

bacteriuria (bak-tē"rĭ-ū'rĭ-ă) [G. *baktērion,* rod, + *ouron,* urine]. Presence of bacteria in the urine.

b., significant. Presence of more than 100,000 bacteria per ml. of urine. This is determined by culturing known dilutions of urine and counting the number of colonies.

bacteroid (bak'ter-oid) [" + *eidos,* appearance]. Resembling a bacterium.

Bacteroides (băk-ter-oyd'ēz). A genus of non-spore-forming anaerobic bacilli normally present in digestive, respiratory, and genital tracts, frequently found in abscesses, and oftentimes in the blood following infections. The species most commonly encountered is *B. funduliformis.*

baculiform (bak-ū'lĭ-form) [L. *baculum,* rod, + *forma,* shape]. Rod-shaped.

bag, hydrostatic [F. *bague,* sack]. Ob: Rubber or silk bag which is inserted into the uterine cavity and then distended with fluid in order to initiate labor and aid in dilatation of cervix.

The types of bags most frequently used are those of Barnes, Champetier de Ribes, and Voorhees.

b., Pol'itzer's. Soft rubber bag for middle ear inflation.

b. of waters. The amnion. The membrane enclosing the *liquor amnii* and the fetus.

It refers sometimes to that portion of the membrane protruding into the *os uteri.* It is the inner embryonic membrane, the *chorion* being the outer envelope.

bagassosis (bag-ă-sō'sĭs). Pulmonary disorder resulting from inhalation of bagasse dust, the dusty fibrous waste of sugar cane after removal of sugar-containing sap.

baker [A.S. *bacan,* cook by dry heat]. Two or more electric lamps mounted in semicircular containers, called electric light bakers. Used for applying heat to various parts of the body.

baker leg. Knock-knee; genu valgum.

Baker's cyst [William M. Baker, English surgeon, 1839-1896]. One containing synovial fluid communicating with synovial fluid of a joint.

baker's dermatitis. Eczematous affection of hand caused by yeast. Syn: *baker's itch.*

baker's itch. Manual eczema from irritation of yeast.

baker's stigmata. Manual callosities from kneading dough.

BAL [from *British anti-lewisite*]. Proprietary name for dimercaprol, a compound used as an antidote in poisoning from heavy metals. See: *dimercaprol.*

balance. 1. A device for weighing. 2. A state of equilibrium; condition in which the intake and output of substances such as water, nutrients, etc. are approximately equal. See: *homeostasis.*

b., acid-base. Condition in which the *p*H of the blood is maintained at a constant level (7.4). Accomplished by the action of buffers, respiration, and work of the kidney in formation of urine of varying degrees of acidity.

b., electrolyte. Condition in which electrolytes (Na^+, Ca^{++}, Cl^-, K^+, Mg^{++}, etc.) are maintained in suitable concentration for maintenance of fluid and osmotic environment proper for cellular and metabolic processes.

b., fluid. Condition in which the amount of water in the body and in various compartments (intracellular and extracellular) is maintained within certain optimal limits.

b., heat. Condition in which heat gain and heat loss are approximately equal thus maintaining a temperature of approximately 98.6° F. (37° C.).

b., nitrogen. Condition in which intake of nitrogen in protein foods is equal to nitrogen outgo, principally through loss of nitrogenous substances in the urine and feces.

balanic (ba-lan'ik) [G. *balanos,* glans]. Pert. to the glans clitoridis or glans penis.

balanism (bal'ă-nizm) [" + *ismos,* condition of]. Gynecological treatment by use of pessaries or suppositories.

balanitis (bal-ă-nī'tĭs) [" + *-itis,* inflammation]. Inflammation of the glans penis and of mucuous membrane beneath it with purulent discharge. The prepuce is often affected.

balano- (băl-ă-nō) [G.]. Prefix: Pert. to the *glans penis* or the *glans clitoridis.*

bal"anoblennorrhe'a [G. *balanos,* glans, + *blennos,* mucus, + *roia,* flow]. Gonorrheal inflammation of the external glans penis.

balanoplasty (bal'a-nō-plas-tĭ) [" + *plassein,* to form]. Plastic surgery of glans penis.

balanoposthitis (bal-ă-nō-pos-thī'tĭs) [" + *posthe,* prepuce, + *-itis,* inflammation]. Inflammation of the glans penis and prepuce; balanitis.

balanopreputial (bal-ă-nō-prē-pū'shĭ-al). Pert. to glans penis and prepuce.

balanorrhagia (bal"an-ŏ-ra'jĭ-ă) [G. *balanos,* glans, + *rēgnunai,* flow forth]. Hemorrhage from glans penis.

balanorrhea (bal-an-o-re'ă) [" + *roia,* flow]. Balanitis with purulent discharge.

balantidial (băl-ăn-tĭd'ĭ-ăl). Pert. to *Balantidium,* a genus of protozoans.

balantidiasis (băl-ăn-tĭ-dī'ă-sĭs). Disease caused by infestation with *Balantidium coli.*

Sym: Abdominal pain, diarrhea, vomiting, weakness, and loss of weight.

Treatment: Tetracyclines or diiodohydroxyquin.

Balantidium (băl-ăn-tĭd'ĭ-ŭm). A genus of ciliated protozoans belonging to the order Spirotrichida. It contains a number of species parasitic in the intestines of both vertebrates and invertebrates.

B. coli. A species of *Balantidium,* parasitic in man. It lives in the large intestine and is the cause of *balantidiasis.* It is a normal parasite of hogs.

balanus (bal'ă-nus). The glans penis or glans clitoridis.

baldness [M.E. *balled,* without hair]. Lack of hair on head. See: *alopecia.*

Balkan frame. A framework (usually wood) to fit over a bed so that weights may be suspended from it to produce the desired continuous traction and yet permit freedom of motion while maintaining immobilization of the desired part being treated.

ball-and-socket joint. Joint in which one rounded bone head fits into cavity of another bone. Syn: *enarthrosis.*

ball thrombus. A normal clot in the ante mortem heart. See: *thrombus.*

ballism (bal'izm) [G. *ballismos,* jumping about]. 1. Condition characterized by jerking, twisting movements. 2. Paralysis agitans.

ballis'tics [G. *ballein,* to throw]. Science of curves of projectiles.

ballistocardiograph (ba-lĭs"tō-kar'dĭ-ō-graf). Mechanism for measuring cardiac output.

ballistopho'bia [" + *phobos,* fear]. Morbid fear of missiles.

balloon'ing [It. *ballone,* great ball]. The distention of a cavity, as vagina, by air or otherwise for examination.

ballot'table [Fr. *balloter,* to toss about]. Capable of showing the ballottement* phenomenon.

ballottement (bal-ot-mon'). The rebound of a fetal part when lightly tapped when displaced by the examining finger either through abdominal wall or vagina. Technique may be used for examining the abdomen particularly when ascites is present.

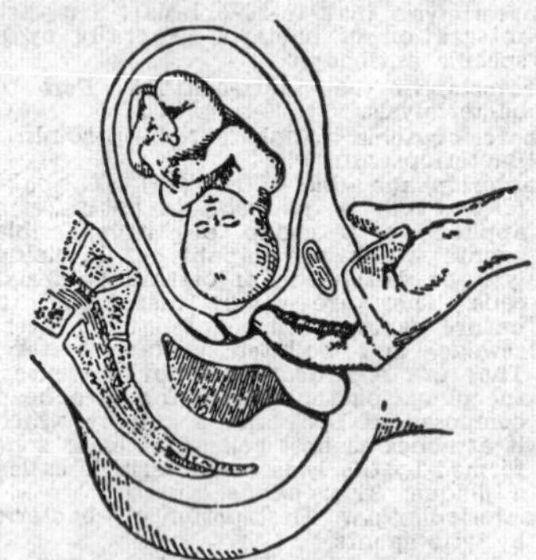

BALLOTTEMENT

balm [G. *balsamon,* balsam]. 1. A balsam. 2. A soothing or healing ointment.

b. of Gilead. 1. Mecca balsam from *Commiphora opobalsamum,* probably Biblical myrrh. 2. Balsam fir, source of Canadian balsam. 3. Poplar bud resin.

balneology (bal-ne-ol'o-jĭ) [L. *balneum,* bath, + G. *logos,* study]. The science of treating diseases by baths.

balneotherapy (bal-nē-ō-ther'ă-pĭ) [" + G. *therapeia,* treatment]. The treatment of disease by baths.

bal'neum (pl. *bal'nea*) [L. a bath]. A bath.

b. are'nae. A sand bath.

b. lu'teum. A mud bath.

balop'ticon [G. *ballein,* to throw, + *optikos,* pert. to sight]. Apparatus for projecting image of an opaque object on a screen.

bal'sam [G. *balsamon,* balsam]. Oleoresin or resin containing aromatic acids or essential oils.

b. of Peru. USP. A dark-brown, viscid, resinous liquid. Action and Uses: Locally for healing wounds; same as benzoin. It is used topically on the skin, usually in an alcohol solution or in ointment.

balsam'ic. 1. Pert. to balsam. 2. Aromatic.

b. tincture. Compound tincture of benzoin.

Balser's fatty necrosis (bahl'zerz) [W. Balser, German physician]. Gangrenous pancreatitis with fatty necrotic areas in interlobular tissue, and sometimes in pericardial fat and bone marrow.

banana. The edible fruit of the perennial herb *Musa sapientum.*

Raw: 1 banana (100 gm.). Calories: 85. Other main values: 190 I.U. vitamin A; 10 mg, ascorbic acid; 0.7 mg. iron,

b. oil. Amyl acetate, *q.v.*

GENERAL BANDAGING TECHNIQUES

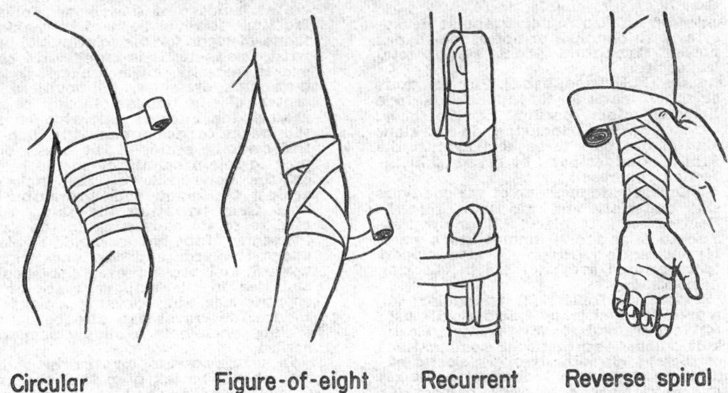

SPECIAL APPLICATIONS

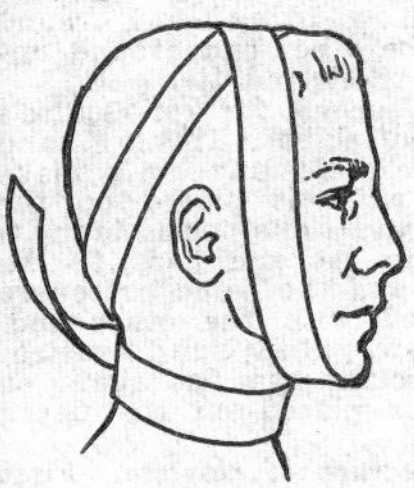

Barton

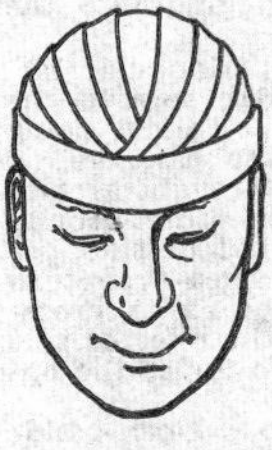

Recurrent of head

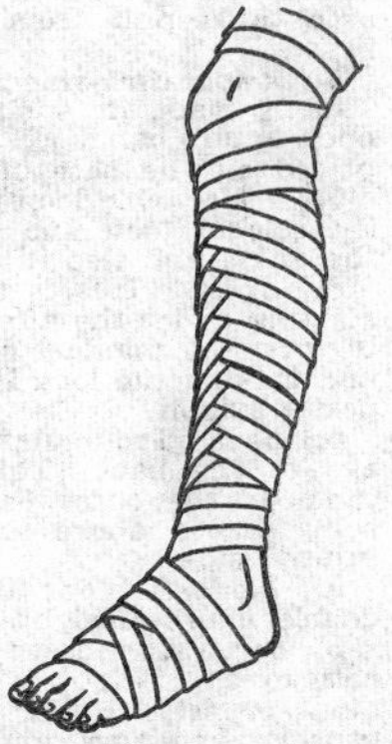

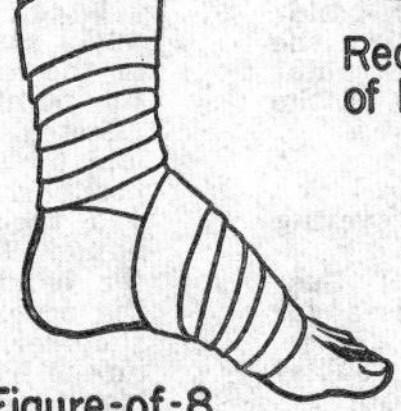

Figure-of-8 of ankle

Reverse spiral of leg

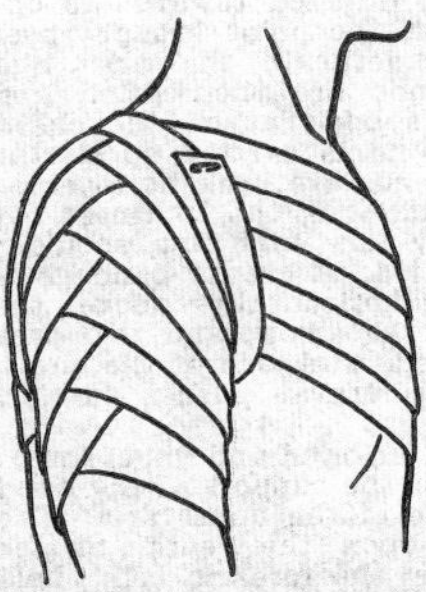

Spica of shoulder

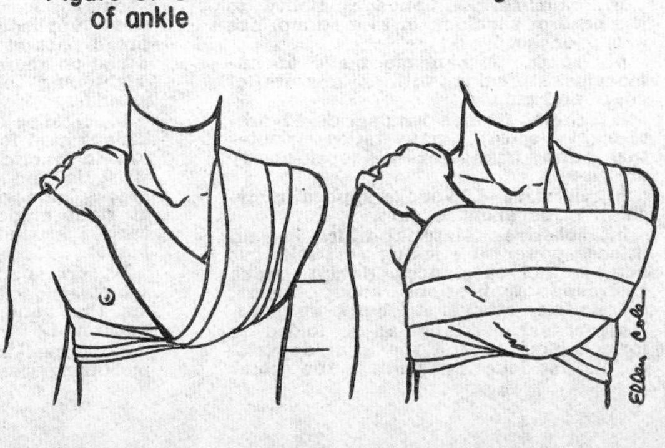

Velpeau ⟶

Ellen Cole

Bancroft's filariasis. A filarial infection caused by *Wuchereria bancrofti.* SEE: *elephantiasis.*

band. A cord or tapelike tissue which connects or holds structures together. SEE: *ligament; bundle; tract.*

band forms. Neutrophil granular leukocytes with bandlike or horseshoe-shaped nuclei. Consititute about 4% of total leukocytes.

band'age [M.E. *band,* band]. Piece of gauze or other material for application to a limb or other portion of the body. CAUTION: When bandaging, do not allow skin of one part to be held against the skin of another part, or severe skin infection can result.

Bandages are made up of various types and materials and are used to: (1) Hold dressing in place; (2) apply pressure to a part; (3) immobilize a part; (4) obliterate cavities; (5) give support to an injured area; (6) aid in checking hemorrhages.

TYPES: (1) Roller; (2) triangular; (3) four-tailed and many-tailed (scultetus); (4) quadrangular; (5) elastic (elastic knit, rubber, synthetic or combinations of these); (6) adhesive; (7) elastic adhesive; (8) newer cohesive bandages under various proprietary names; (9) impregnated bandages such as plaster of Paris, waterglass (silica), starch; (10) rubber; (11) stockinet.

b., abdomen (Triangular b.). A single wide cravat or several narrow ones may be used to hold dressing in place, or to exert a moderate pressure. A folded towel or handkerchief should be used to keep it from digging into the flesh.

b., amputation-stump (Triangular b.). This is made in a similar way to the open-hand bandage, the limb being placed on the base of the bandage.

b., ankle. One loop is brought around the sole of foot, and the other around the ankle and tied in front or side.

b., axilla. This is a spica-type turn starting under the affected axilla, crossing over the shoulder of the affected side and making the long loop under the opposite armpit.

b., back (Triangular b.). Open-bandage to the back: This is applied the same as the chest bandage, the point being placed above the scapula of the injured side.

b., Barton's. For the lower jaw. A double figure-of-eight b.

b., Borch's. An eye bandage covering both eyes.

b., breast. (Roller bandages.) Suspensory bandages and compresses for the breasts.

b., buttocks. Use (1) T or double-T bandage or (2) open triangle.

b., capeline. A bandage applied to the head or shoulder, or to a stump, like a cap or hood.

b., chalk. A bandage made of immovable stiffening with a mixture of chalk and gum.

b., chest. (Roller bandages.) Figure-of-eight (spica), many-tailed (scultetus), and triangular b. (open-chest) are used.

b., circular. A bandage applied in circular turns about a part.

b., cohesive. Material which has an intense power of sticking to itself, but not to other substances. Used to make encircling applications about fingers, extremities, etc., or to build up pads.

b., cravat. Triangular b. folded to form a band around the injured part.

This is done by pulling the point over towards the base, folding the base over the point and then folding again. This makes a bandage wide enough to cover a large knee. When folded a 2nd time, it is wide enough to make the cravat bandage of the elbow. Folded a 3rd time, it could be used in making a figure-of-eight for the foot, ankle, hand, wrist, head, etc. It is an effective bandage in arresting hemorrhages, retaining splints, dressings, and poultices. The center of the cravat should be laid against the affected part, the ends of the cravat carried around the limb and tied over the center of the base. When used to retain splints, it should be tied on the outer side of the limb and against the splint, thus preventing the knot from irritating the skin. When used to retain a dressing in the axilla, the center of the cravat should be placed under the arm and the ends carried upward and crossed over the shoulder and tied in the axillary space of the opposite side, thus forming a figure-of-eight. The cravat can also be used as a sling when only a simple support is needed.

In using cravats for ties or splints, care should be taken so that the knots do not pass over and press unduly on the surface of the limb. Knots should be placed where they are easily found and not subject to pressure, the ends should be neatly tucked in. All knots should be square or reef knots.

b., c., elbow. Bend the elbow about 45 degrees. Place center of bandage over point of elbow. Bring 1 end around forearm, and the other end around upper arm. Pull tight and tie.

b., c., for clenched fist (or Squire's diagonal figure-of-eight). This is a hand bandage to arrest bleeding or to make pressure. The wrist is placed on the center of the cravat, one end is brought around over the fist and back to the starting point, and the same procedure is then repeated with the other end. The two ends are pulled tight, twisted, and carried around the fist again so that pressure is placed on the flexed fingers.

b., c., for fracture of clavicle. First put a soft pad (2x4 in.) in the forepart of the axilla. A sling made by placing the point of the open bandage on the affected shoulder, the hand and wrist laid on it and directed toward the opposite shoulder, the point brought over and tucked underneath the wrist and hand. The ends are then lifted and the bandage is laid flat on the chest, the covered hand is carried up on the shoulder, the ends are brought together in the back and tied, the tightness being decided by how high the shoulder should be carried. A cravat bandage is then applied horizontally above the broad part of the elbow, and tied over a pad on the opposite side of the chest. Tightening this cravat pushes out the shoulder.

b., c., sling (for hand and upper arm). This is used for the support of the hand and in fracture of the upper arm. The wrist is laid upon the center of the cravat bandage, the forearm being held at right angle, and the two ends are carried around the neck and tied. SEE: *binder.*

b., crucial. Same as T bandage.

b., demigauntlet. A bandage that covers the hand, but leaves the fingers uncovered.

b., Desault's (de-sōz'). A special immobilizing bandage of the collarbone or

soluble salts in place of the insoluble sulfate. SEE: *Table of Poisons and Poisoning in Appendix.*

b. sulfate. A barium compound used in x-ray examination of the gastrointestinal tract.

bark [Dan. bark]. The outer cover of the woody parts of a plant. Ex: *cascara sagrada, cinchona, wild cherry.*

barley. The seed or grain of the cereal grass of the genus *Hordeum.*

Uncooked: 1 cup (203 gm.). Calories: 710. Other main values: 17 gm. protein; 32 mg. calcium; 4.1 mg. iron; 6.3 mg. niacin.

Barlow's disease [Sir Thomas Barlow, English physician, 1845-1945]. A deficiency disease due to lack of vitamin C (ascorbic acid). Occurs in both natural and bottle-fed babies who fail to receive adequate supplementary quantities of vitamin C. Occurs usually between 6 and 12 months of age. SYN: *Moeller-Barlow disease; infantile scurvy.*

TREATMENT: Supplemental vitamin C. Then adequate daily intake of fruit juices (orange, grapefruit, tomato).

Barnes' bag or **dilator** [Robert Barnes, English obstetrician, 1817-1907]. Rubber bag used to induce premature labor by dilating uterine cervix.

B.'s curve. The segment of a circle whose center is the sacral promontory.

baro- [G. *baros*, weight]. Prefix: Weight, heaviness.

barognosis (bar-og-nō'sis) [G. " + *gnōsis*, knowledge]. The ability to estimate weights. OPP: *baragnosis.*

barograph (bar'ō-graf) [" + *graphein*, to write]. Self-registering barometer.

bar'oscope [" + *skopein*, to examine]. Instrument which registers changes in the density of air.

bar'ospirator [" + *spirāre*, to breathe]. Apparatus producing artificial respiration by means of air pressure variations in a closed chamber.

barotax'is [" + *taxis*, turning]. Stimulation of cells by altering the pressure of the atmosphere.

barotitis (bar-o-ti'tis). Inflammation of the ear due to sudden changes in barometric pressure such as occur while flying. Closure of the eustachian tube due to upper respiratory infection prevents the middle ear from adjusting to pressure changes encountered during flight.

barot'ropism [" + *tropē*, turning]. Barotaxis.

Barr bodies. Sex chromatin. The deeply staining chromatin mass at the periphery of the cell nucleus. Found in normal females but not in males.

bar'rel chest. A chest that is rounded as in inspiration and has no apparent movement during respiration. Seen in emphysema.

bar'ren [M.E. *barain*, uncultivated land]. Sterile; incapable of producing offspring.

bar'rier. An obstacle or impediment.

b., blood-brain. A barrier which exists between circulating blood and the brain which prevents certain substances such as acid fat-soluble dyes from reaching brain tissue. It consists of either the perivascular glial membrane or the vascular endothelium or both. Also called *hematoencephalic barrier.*

b., hematoencephalic. The blood-brain barrier, *q.v.*

Bartholin's abscess (bar'to-linz) [Caspar Bartholin, Danish anatomist, 1655-1738]. This develops when B.'s glands become occluded in an acute inflammatory process.

B.'s cyst. In chronic inflammation of B.'s glands* cysts are commonly formed. Carcinoma is rare.

B.'s ducts. Large ducts of the sublingual salivary gland. They parallel Wharton's duct* and open with it.

B.'s glands. Two small compound, racemose, mucous glands, pea to bean size, situated beneath the vestibule, one on each side of the vaginal opening and at the base of the labia majora. SYN: *Duverney's g.; Tiedemann's g.; greater vestibular g.*

bartholinitis (bar-tō-lin-ī'tis) [Bartholin + G. *-itis*, inflammation]. Inflammation of a vulvovaginal gland.

Bartonella (bar-tō-nel'ă) [Named for A. L. Barton, S. American physician who first described it]. A genus of bacilli of the family Bartonellaceae.

B. bacilliformis. Motile gram-negative bacillus; the cause of bartonellosis.

bartonellosis (bar-tō-nel-ō'sĭs). A disease caused by infection with *Bartonella bacilliformis*, transmitted by female sandflies (Phlebotomus). The first clinical (noneruptive) stage is called Oroya fever, a severe anemia; the second (eruptive) stage is called verruga peruana, marked by appearance of small tumors on the skin and mucous membranes.

TREATMENT: Disease responds to several antibiotics, but chloramphenicol has the added advantage of being effective against *Salmonella* which may be present as a secondary infection.

Baruch's law. Water has a sedative effect when its temperature is the same as that of the skin, and a stimulating effect when it is below or above the skin temperature.

baruria (bar-u'rĭ-ă) [G. *baros*, weight, + *ouron*, urine]. Urine having a high specific gravity.

bary- [G.]. Prefix: Heavy, dull, hard.

baryecoia (bar"ĭ-ē-koy'ă) [G. *baryēkoia*, deafness]. Hardness of hearing; partial deafness.

baryglossia (bar-ĭ-glos'ĭ-ă) [" + *glōssa*, tongue]. Having a slow, thick utterance

barylalia (bar-ĭ-lā'lĭ-ă) [" + *lalia*, speech]. Indistinct, husky speech.

baryodmia (bar-ĭ-od'mĭ-ă) [" + *odmē*, stench]. Disagreeable, heavy odor.

baryodynia (bar-ĭ-ō-din'ĭ-ă) [" + *odynē*. pain]. Severe pain.

baryphonia (bar-ĭ-fo'nĭ-ă) [" + *phōnē*, voice]. Difficulty in speaking words.

barythymia (bar-ĭ-thī'mĭ-ă) [G. *barys*, heavy, + *thymos*, mind]. Sullen, gloomy, or melancholy state of mind.

basad (bā'sad) [G. *basis*, base]. Denoting the direction toward the base of anything.

ba'sal. 1. Pert. to the base of anything; the base. 2. Of primary importance.

b. ganglia. Four masses of gray matter located deep in the cerebral hemispheres, viz. *caudate, lentiform,* and *amygdaloid nuclei,* and the *claustrum.* The caudate and lentiform nuclei and the fibers of the internal capsule which separate them constitute the *corpus striatum.*

basal metab'olism [G. *basis*, base, + *metabolē*, change]. The amount of energy needed for maintenance of life when the subject is at digestive, physical and emotional rest.

basal metabolic rate. ABBR: BMR. The metabolic rate as measured under so-called *basal conditions:* (a) 12 hours after eating, (b) after a restful sleep, (c) no exercise or activity preceding test, (d) elimination of emotional excitement, and (e) in a comfortable temperature (between 62° and 87° F.).

It is usually expressed in terms of large calories per square meter of body surface per hour.

bascula'tion [Fr. *basculer*, to swing]. 1. Replacement of a retroverted uterus by swinging it into place. 2. Systolic recoil of the heart.

base [G. *basis*, base]. 1. The lower part of anything. 2. The principal substance in a mixture. 3. (Chem.) A compound containing a metal or the ammonium radical combined with the *hydroxyl* (OH) radical. In general, any substance which will neutralize an acid. SYN: *alkali*. Bases react with acids to form salts, turn red litmus blue, and have a bitter taste. Strong bases feel slippery and are corrosive to human tissues. Ex: Sodium hydroxide (NaOH) (lye or caustic soda); potassium hydroxide (KOH) (caustic potash).

This includes (a) compounds of metallic elements, as sodium hydroxide, and (b) various complex nonmetallic substances as ammonia, the amines, and the alkaloids. Such substances are detected in solution by the colors they give with indicators, *q.v.*

b. of heart. Heart surface back and upward, containing pulmonary vein and vena cavae openings.

baseball finger. Condition resulting from violent backward dislocation of the terminal phalanx onto the dorsum of the middle phalanx, as when a finger is struck on its tip when extended. SYN: *mallet finger; hammer finger.*

Basedow's disease (baz'e-dō) [Karl A. von Basedow, German physician, 1799-1854]. Grave's disease; exophthalmic goiter.

basement membrane [G. *basis* + L. *membrana*, membrane]. A thin layer of delicate noncellular material underlying the epithelium. Now called *basement lamina* or *basal lamina*.

base'plate. Plastic material for making dental trial plates.

basi-, basio- [G.]. Prefixes denoting *base* or *basion*.

ba'sial [G. *basis*, base]. Pert. to the basion.

basiarachnoiditis (ba-sĭ-a-rak-noy-dī'tis) [" + " + *eidos*, form, + *-itis*, inflammation]. Inflammation of the arachnoid membrane at base of brain. SYN: *basiarachnitis*.

basibregmat'ic axis [" + *bregmata*, pl. front of head, + *axis*, pivot]. Vertical line from the basion to junction of coronal and sagittal sutures.

ba'sic. 1. Possessing properties opposite to those of an acid. 2. Fundamental.

b. salt. A compound formed when only part of the hydroxide radicals of a base are replaced by the acid radical of an acid.

basicra'nial axis [G. *basis*, foundation, + *kranion*, skull, + *axis*, pivot]. Straight line from the basion to point of angle of mandible.

basifa'cial axis [" + L. *facies*, face, + G. *axis*, pivot]. Straight line from the point of angle of mandible to the subnasal point.

basihyal (ba-sĭ-hī'al) [G. *basis*, foundation, + *oeidēs*, hyoid]. The body of the hyoid bone.

bas'ilar. Basal; pert. to a base.

basilat'eral [G. *basis*, foundation, + L. *lateralis*, pert. to the side]. Both lateral and basilar.

basil'ic. Prominent, important.

b. vein. Large vein on inner side of biceps. Usually chosen for intravenous injection or for withdrawal of blood.

basiloma (bas-ĭ-lō'mă). Basal cell carcinoma.

basilysis (ba-sil'ĭ-sis) [G. *basis*, base, + *lysis*, loosening]. Crushing the fetal head in labor to aid delivery.

basilyst tractor (bas'ĭ-list). Instrument devised by Sir A. R. Simpson consisting of three blades for perforating the fetal head and obtaining a substantial grasp to facilitate delivery of the child.

basio- (bā'sĭ-ō). Prefix denoting *basion*.

basioccipital bone (bā-sĭ-ok-sip'ĭ-tal) [G. *basis*, base, + L. *occiput*, head, + A.S. *bān*, bone]. Basilar process of occipital bone.

ba'sion. Point at middle border of the foramen magnum.

basiotribe (ba'sĭ-ō-trīb) [" + *tribein*, to crush]. Instrument for crushing the fetal head.

basiotripsy (bā-sĭ-ō-trĭp'sĭ). Basilysis, *q.v.*

basiphobia (bā-sĭ-fo'bĭ-ă) [" + *phobos*, fear]. Fear of walking.

basirrhinal fissure (bā-sĭ-rī'nal) [G. *basis*, + *ris*, nose]. 1. Pert. to base of brain and to the nose. 2. A cerebral fissure at base of olfactory lobe.

basis (bā'sis). Base.

b. cranii. Base of skull.

basisphenoid (bā-sĭ-sfē'noid) [G. *basis*, base, + *sphēn*, wedge, + *eidos*, form]. Lower portion of sphenoid bone.

basisyl'vian fissure. Transverse basilar portion or stem of sylvian fissure.

basket. A netlike terminal arborization of an axon (or its collateral) of a basket cell which forms a network about the cell body of a Purkinje cell.

b. cell. Deep stellate cells (neurons) of the molecular layer of the cerebellum whose axons or collaterals terminate in baskets, *q.v.*

basocyte (ba'sō-sīt). A basophil cell or leukocyte.

basocytopenia (bā"so-sī"tō-pē'nĭ-ă) [basocyte + G. *penia*, poverty]. Reduced number of basophil leukocytes in the blood.

basocytosis (bā"sō-sī-tō'sis). Excess of basophilic leukocytes of the blood.

ba'sograph [G. *basis*, a walking, + *graphein*, to write]. Device for registering abnormalities of gait.

basophil(e (bā'sō-fil, -fīl) [G. *basis*, base, + *philein*, to love]. In histology, (a) applied to cells or parts of cells which are readily stained with basic dyes like methylene blue; (b) a type of white blood cell (leukocyte) characterized by possession of coarse granules which stain intensely with basic dyes. Constitute 0.5-1% of leukocytes. They are thought to bring anticoagulant substances to inflamed tissues. Increased numbers are found in myxedema, ulcerative colitis, smallpox, chickenpox and certain chronic diseases of the blood; (c) a type of cell found in the anterior lobe of the hypophysis.

b. degranulation response. A test for demonstration of sensitivity to penicillin.

basophilia (bā-sō-fil'ĭ-ă). 1. A pathological condition of the blood in which the erythrocytes develop basophil granules. 2. A condition in which many mast cells are present.

basophilic (bā-sō-fil'ik). Pert. to method of staining various cells.

basophilism (bā-sof'ĭ-lizm). Condition characterized by excessive numbers of basophils.

b., pituitary. A clinical syndrome (Cushing's disease) characterized by basophilic invasion or adenoma of the pituitary gland. SEE: *Cushing's disease.*

basophobia (bas-ō-fō'bĭ-ă) [G. *basis*, base, + *phobos*, fear]. 1. Abnormal fear of walking. 2. Emotional inability to stand or walk in the absence of muscle pathology.

bass deafness. Deafness to bass notes, the higher ones being heard.

Bassini's operation (bă-sē'nēz) [Edoardo Bassini, Italian surgeon, 1844-1924]. One for inguinal hernia.

bas'tard [O.Fr. *batard*, bastard]. 1. One born out of wedlock. 2. Not genuine.

bath [A.S. *baeth*, bath]. The medium and method of cleansing the body or any part of it, or to treat it therapeutically, as with air, light, steam, vapor, water, etc.

Room Temperature	*Water Temperature Should Be*
Below 76° F.	94-96° F.
Above 76° F.	92-94° F.
On hot summer days	90° F.

If Rectal Temperature Is	*Bath Water Should Be*
103° F.	90° F.
104° F.	86° F.
104.5° F.	82° F.
105° F.	76° F.
105.5° F.	70-60° F.

Baths May Be Indicated As:

Cold	45- 65° F.
Cool	65- 75° F.
Tepid	75- 85° F.
Warm	85- 95° F.
Hot	95-105° F.
Very Hot	105-110° F.

The general cleansing bath for a bed patient may be from 110°-115° F. with a room temperature of 75°-80° F.

THERAPEUTIC EFFECT OF: *Warm and Hot Baths and Applications*: They act to soothe both the *psyche* and the *soma.* Thus they calm and relax a nervous, agitated patient. *Gradually Elevated Hot Tub and Vapor Baths*: They relax all the muscles of the body. *Hot Baths*: They relax tissues, including the capillaries of the skin, drawing blood from the deeper tissues. They also relieve pain. They stimulate the nerves. *Cold Baths and Applications*: They abstract heat and stimulate reaction, especially if followed by brisk rubbing of the skin. They contract the small blood vessels when applied locally.

b., acid. 5 oz. hydrochloric acid or 1 gal. vinegar to 30 gal. water.

b., air. Therapeutic use of air warmed or vaporized, on the nude body.

b., alcohol. Use of alcohol on patient, as a stimulant and defervescent, in dilute form.

b., alkaline. 8 oz. of sodium bicarbonate or washing soda to 30 gal. of water.

b., alum. Use of alum in washing solution, as an astringent.

b., antipyretic. A bath in cool water (65° to 75° F.).

b., aromatic. One to which some volatile oil or perfume is added, or some herb.

b., astringent. Bathing in liquid containing an astringent.

b., bed. NP for giving bath to bed-patient. CAUTION: If patient is irrational or comatose, be certain to take precautions to prevent his falling from the bed. Also replace siderails if they were in place prior to beginning the bath.

1. Check temperature of room; clear bedside table for bath articles; tell patient about bath and desired results. Offer bedpan or urinal.
2. Remove top covers of bed, placing patient under cotton bath blanket; remove pillows if possible.
3. Bring clean linens and all necessary supplies to bedside, including bath basin of hot water (150° F.).
4. Place towel under area to be bathed; wash carefully, rinse, dry and cover immediately with bath blanket. The usual sequence is as follows: face, neck and ears, chest, abdomen, arms and hands, back, legs and feet, and genitalia. Change bath water as often as necessary but at least have fresh hot water to bathe back. Finish by rubbing back and buttocks with rubbing lotion. It is particularly important to use a lotion which does not dry the skin excessively. In order to reduce friction between skin and bedclothes, dust the skin with a bland powder at the completion of the bath.
5. Place clean gown on patient, comb hair, and clean finger and toe nails. Remake bed with clean linen. (SEE: *Bed*: *How to make an occupied bed.*).
6. Remove all bath articles, straighten and damp-dust room. Place call-bell, drinking water, etc. within easy reach of patient.
7. Clean up all used articles and restore to proper place.

b., bland. A bath containing substances such as starch, bran, or oatmeal for the relief of skin irritation; an emollient bath, *q.v.*

b., blanket. One in which wet pack and blankets are used.

b., borax. Glycerin and borax solution for bathing.

b., box. One in which patient is completely enclosed in box except for his head.

b., bran. Place bran (2 to 3 lb.) in a muslin bag and soak in hot water 15 min. Then add bag and hot water to bath water (30 gal., 95° F.), using bag as a washing-sponge.

b., brine. Saline bath, *q.v.*

b., bubble. A bath in which the water contains many small bubbles produced (a) mechanically as by an air pump or (b) chemically, by bubble-bath preparations.

b., cabinet. Exposure of the skin of the body except the head, to heat from electric lamps, live steam, steam radiators, or electric heaters.

b., carbon dioxide. An effervescent saline bath consisting of water, salts, and CO_2. The natural CO_2 baths are known as Nauheim baths, and approach closely CO_2 baths in their therapeutic effects.

b., cold. One in water at a temperature below 65° F.

b., colloid. An emollient bath, *q.v.*

b., continuous. One that is administered for hours, days, weeks, or months. It is a continuous, flowing bath if the prescribed temperature is maintained by keeping a stream of water flowing through the tub.

b., contrasted. Used for hands or feet. Two large basins or pails of sufficient depth, filled with water, one as hot as can be borne, the other as cold as can be borne. Change or add hot and cold water frequently to keep temperatures same as in beginning. Put part to be treated in hot water for 1 minute, then into cold for ½ minute, then again into hot water. Repeat for prescribed length of time, ending with cold water.

b., drip sheet. Modified sheet bath.

b., earth. Bathing in warmed earth or sand.

b., emollient. Used for irritation and inflammation of skin, and after erysipelas. SEE: *glycerin, oatmeal, powdered borax, starch baths.*

b., foam. Tub bath to which has been added an extract of a saponin containing vegetable fiber, and through this mixture, O or CO_2 is driven to form foam.

b., foot. Immersion of feet and legs to a depth of 4 inches above ankles in water at 98° F.

b., full. The whole body except the head is immersed in water.

b., galvanic. System using appropriate electrodes and direct current for stimulation of skin which acts as a transmitter for various physiologic effects, especially relief of pain. Effective in backaches, sciatica, various neuralgias, and subacute poliomyelitis.

b., glycerin. 10 oz. of glycerin added to 30 gal. water.

b., half. Tub bath with about 18 inches of water; the temperature depends on the case and the desired action.

b., herb. 1 to 2 lb. of herbs, such as chamomile, wild thyme, or spearmint, are tied in bag, boiled with 1 gal. of water, and the decoction added to the full bath.

b., hip. SEE: *sitz b.*

b., hot. Tub bath with the water covering the body to a little above the nipples and temperature gradually raised from 98° F. to desired degree, usually to 108° F.

b., hot air. Exposure of entire body except head to hot air contained in a bath cabinet.

b., hyperthermal. One in which the body except head is immersed in water from 105 to 120° F. for 1 to 2 minutes.

b., immersion. Free tub bath.

b., kinetotherapeutic. Bath given for underwater exercises of weak or partially paralyzed muscles.

b., lukewarm. Bath in which patient's body except head is immersed in water from 94 to 96° F. for 15 to 60 minutes.

b., medicated. Bath to which bran, oatmeal, starch, sodium bicarbonate, epsom salts, pine products, tar, sulfur, potassium permanganate, or salt is added.

b., milk. Bath taken in milk, as an emollient or cosmetic.

b., mud. Old form of applying moist heat which depends on availability of certain soils heated by thermal springs or artificially.

b., mustard. For stimulative hot foot bath, a mixture of 1 tablespoon of dry mustard in a quart of hot water which is then added to a pail or large basin filled with water of 100 to 104° F. Used in rheumatic conditions and in sprains or other muscular foot pains caused by trauma.

b., Nauheim (naw'him). A bath in which the human body is immersed in warm water through which carbon dioxide is bubbled.

b., neutral. One in which no circulatory or thermic reaction occurs, temperature 92 to 97° F.

b., neutral sitz. Same as hot sitz bath, except temperature between 92 to 97° F., and foot bath, 104 to 110° F., duration 15 to 60 minutes.

b., oatmeal. 2 to 3 lb. to 30 gal. water.

b., oxygen. Given by introducing O into the bath through a special device which is connected to an oxygen tank or by generating the O by chemicals.

b., paraffin. Member is immersed in warm paraffin, 140-150° F., quickly withdrawn, immersed again, withdrawn repeatedly until it is encased. For larger joints, may be applied with paint brush.

b., powdered borax. One-half lb. to 30 gal. water; 5 oz. glycerin may be added.

b., reducing. One given to reduce patient's temperature.

b., Russian. Warm vapor bath followed by rubbing and cold plunge.

b., saline. Given in artificial sea water made by dissolving 8 lb. of sea salt, or a mixture of 7 lb. of sodium chloride and ½ lb. of magnesium sulfate in 30 gal. of water.

b., sauna. A type of steam bath where the steam is produced by pouring water on heated rocks.

b., seawater or salt. Saline b.

b., sedative. A prolonged warm bath. Continuous flow of water may be used. Use air cushion and back rest.

b., sheet. Given by wrapping the patient in a sheet previously dipped in water 80 to 90° F., and rubbing the whole body with vigorous strokes on the sheet, until all parts of the sheet feel warm.

b., shower. Water sprayed down upon the body from an overhead source.

b., sitz. Immersion of thighs, buttocks, and abdomen below the umbilicus in water. In a hot sitz bath the water is first 92° F. and elevated to 106° F., duration 3 to 10 minutes.

b., sponge. One in which patient's body is washed by using a wash cloth and without immersing the body in a tub.

b., starch. 1 lb. mixed in cold water, pouring boiling water to make starch mucilage, which add to 30 gal. water.

b., steam. Given in a chamber into which steam under low pressure is allowed to escape. Best form of application is that in which subject sits in cabinet or lies in box with head outside. CAUTION: Temperature must be carefully controlled to avoid burning the patient.

b., stimulating. One which increases cutaneous effect; used for tonic purposes. SEE: *cold, mustard and saline baths.*

b., sulfur. A bath made by adding potassium sulfide (3 oz.) or zinc sulfate (8 tsp.), or sulfurated lime sol. N.F. (6 oz.) to 30 gal. water. Bath should be limited to 20 min.

b., sweat. One given to induce perspiration.

b., tonic. One which, through its stimulation of the cutaneous nerves and the response of the autonomic nervous system, quickens the circulation of the blood throughout the body.

b., towel. Given by applying towels dipped in water 70-60° F. to arms, legs, ant. and post. surfaces of trunk successively, removing towel, drying part.

b., vapor. Exposure of skin of body except head to vapor. Sometimes the vapor is impregnated with substances thought to possess therapeutic value, as sulfur, mercury, or camphor.

b., whirlpool. Continuous localized jets of water for the arm and leg. Water 105-120° F. from a thermostatic mixer is given a swirling motion in special reservoir as it mixes with air forced through an aerator.

bath'mism [" + *ismos,* condition of]. Force regulating nutrition and growth.

bathophobia [G. *bathos,* depth, + *phobos,* fear]. Abnormal fear of depths or of looking down from a high place.

bath"yanesthe'sia [G. *bathys,* deep, + *ana-,* priv. + *aisthēsis,* perception]. Loss of deep sensibility.

bathycar'dia [" + *kardia,* heart]. Abnormally low position of the heart in the thorax.

bathyesthesia (bath-ĭ-es-thē'zĭ-ă) [" + *aisthēsis,* sensation]. A consciousness of muscles, joints, and organs under skin.

bathygastry (bath-ĭ-gas'trĭ) [" + *gastēr,* stomach]. Abnormally low stomach. Syn: *gastroptosis.*

bathyhyperesthesia (bath-ĭ-hī"per-es-thē'zĭ-ă) [" + *yper,* above, + *aisthēsis,* sensation]. Excessive sensitiveness of muscular tissues and deep structures.

battarism (bat'ă-rizm). Stuttering.

bat'tery [Fr. *battre,* to beat]. Device for generating galvanic currents by chemical action.

Baudelocque's diameter (bō-dloks') [Jean Louis Baudelocque, Sr., French obstetrician, 1746-1810]. Distance bet. the depression just beneath the spine of the last lumbar vertebra and the ant. and upper margin of the *symphysis pubis.* The ext. conjugate diameter of the pelvis.

B.'s method. Manipulation to convert a face presentation into one of the vertex.

Baume scales (bō-māz') [Antoine Baumé, French chemist, 1728-1805]. Hydrometer scales for determination of the specific gravity of liquids, one being used for liquids heavier and one for liquids lighter than water.

bay'onet leg. Backward dislocation at knee joint of tibia and fibula.

Bazin's disease (bah-zanz'). Erythema induratum; tuberculosis of the skin.

B.C.G. Abbr. *Calmette-Guérin bacillus.*

B.C.G. vaccine. Tuberculosis vaccine. A freeze-dried preparation of an attenuated strain of *Mycobacterium tuberculosis* (bacillus Calmette-Guérin). Proposed for use in adults and children for immunization against tuberculosis. Also called *bacillus Calmette-Guérin vaccine.*

b. d. Abbr. L. *bis die,* twice a day.

bdellometer (del-om'ĕ-ter) [G. *bdella,* leech, + *metron,* measure]. Artificial substitute for a leech.

Be. Chemical symbol for *beryllium.*

beaded [A.S. *bed,* prayer]. Referring to disjointed colonies along the inoculation line in a streak or stab.

beads, rachitic. Visible swelling where the ribs join their cartilages, seen in rickets. Also called *rachitic rosary.*

beaker (bē'ker) [O.E. *becke,* beak]. Glass vessel with wide mouth for mixing or holding liquids.

beans [A.S.]. The seeds, and sometimes immature pods containing seeds, usually of the genus *Phaseolus* or *Vicia.*

Cooked (fresh green snap beans): 1 cup (100 gm.). Calories: 30. Other main values: 50 mg. calcium, 540 I.U. vitamin A, 0.06 mg. thiamine, 10 mg. ascorbic acid.

Canned (common varieties as navy beans): 1 cup (100 gm., white beans). Calories: 118. Other values: 7.8 gm. protein; 21.2 gm. carbohydrate; 148 mg. calcium; 7.0 mg. or less of iron depending on amount of water used in cooking.

bear'ing down. The expulsive effort of a parturient woman, in second stage of labor.

beat [A.S. *bēatan,* to strike]. A pulsation or throb resulting from contraction of the heart, or the passage of blood through a vessel.

b., apex. Impulse of the heart beat felt by the hand when held over the fifth intercostal space in left midclavicular line.

b., ectopic. One beginning at a place other than sinoatrial node.

b., forced. Extrasystole brought on by artificial heart stimulation.

b., premature. An extrasystole.

Bechterew's reflex (běk'tĕr-ĕv). 1. Contraction of facial muscles due to irritation of nasal mucosa. 2. Dilatation of pupil on exposure to light. 3. Plantar flexion of foot. 4. Flexion of foot in dorsal direction and flexive movement of knee and hip following passive flexion of toes and plantar extension of foot. 5. Contraction of lower abdominal muscles when skin of inner surface of thigh is stroked.

bed [A.S. *bedd,* bed]. A piece of furniture for resting of body.

How to Make an Occupied Bed:

Caution: Special drainage and irrigation tubes must be handled carefully in order not to disturb their function or to cause the patient great pain by tugging on them.

1. Assemble all necessary articles; place clean linens on back of chair at bedside.
2. Tell the patient what you are going to do; check temperature of room and adjust windows if necessary.
3. Loosen all bedclothes; remove and fold spread and all but one blanket. Hang on back of chair. Remove top sheet from under remaining blanket. Place in laundry bag or fold and place on seat of chair to form receiver for dirty linens.
4. Turn patient away from you, if possible, and insure safety by placing chair or bedrail for security.
5. Fold draw sheet to patient's back; straighten rubber draw sheet and fold likewise. Bottom sheet is also folded in neat, flat folds to center of bed.
6. Place clean bottom sheet on exposed half of mattress, folding neatly to center creases. Tuck top of sheet under head of mattress, miter corner and tuck under mattress to foot of bed. Sheet must cover mattress completely.
7. Pull rubber draw sheet out, straighten and place clean draw sheet with center crease to patient's back. Fold top of clean draw sheet over top edge of rubber sheet and tuck both securely under mattress.
8. Assist patient to roll toward you, under blanket, to clean side of bed. Again insure safety. Proceed to other side of bed. Remove soiled draw sheet and bottom

sheet and place in first piece of soiled linen on chair. Pull through clean bottom sheet, rubber sheet, and draw sheet. Proceed as for first side, tightening draw sheet to avoid any wrinkles. Ask patient to raise buttocks, if possible.

9. Remove pillows, remove pillow cases, and replace cases with clean ones. Pull mattress to head of bed; replace pillows and adjust to patient's comfort.
10. Place clean top sheet, wide hem to top, over blanket; draw blanket out from under sheet and replace with top of blanket well over patient's shoulders.
    Put on spread and turn top hem of sheet over spread at least 8 inches.
11. Remake foot of bed, allowing sufficient room for feet and toes of patient to move freely.

Remove soiled linens. Avoid shaking any bedclothes in order to prevent spreading dust which is a possible source of infection. Place signal light for patient, straighten room and evaluate comfort and appearance carefully.

b., air. One inflatable with air. Also, a special bed which literally floats the patient on a cushion of air which comes from holes in a special mattress. Used to prevent bed sores and in burn cases.

b., anesthetic. Same as recovery b., *q.v.*

b. blocking. Placing bedblocks under bed to raise it at head or foot.

Foot of b. raised: (a) In shock; (b) bleeding from lower limbs; (c) edema of lower limbs, vulva, or scrotum; (d) some cases of hemorrhoids; (e) to retain enema or aid high colonic irrigation; (f) when weight is used on lower limbs; (g) in reduction of inguinal hernia.

Head of b. raised: (a) To drain abdomen or pelvis; (b) to aid respiration; (c) in treatment for bleeding from head, neck, or upper chest.

b., capillary. A network of capillaries.

b., circular. Special bed which allows a patient to be turned end-over-end while held between two frames. This permits "turning" the patient without disturbing him, by turning the two frames inside a circular apparatus which holds the ends of the frames.

b., closed. One prepared to receive a new patient; an unoccupied bed.

b., ether. Same as recovery b., *q.v.*

b., "flotation." One in which the patient reclines in a hollow, flexible, mattress-shaped device which is filled with water. This enables equal distribution of pressure on the body. Used in treating and preventing decubiti.

b., fracture. One for patients with fracture.

b., Gatch. An adjustable bed which provides elevation of the back and knees.

b., hydrostatic. A water bed.

b., metabolic. One arranged to catch the feces and urine.

b., nail. The skin at tip of digit which lies beneath a nail.

b., open. One which is assigned to a patient who is not occupying it at the time it is made.

b., recovery. One prepared to receive a patient immediately following an operative procedure requiring anesthesia. SYN: ***anesthetic b.; ether b.***

b., surgical. One equipped with a mechanism by which the head or the foot of the bed can be raised or lowered independently of each other.

b., unoccupied. Same as closed b., *q.v.*

b., water. A rubber mattress filled with water. USES: Prevention of bedsores.

bedbug (*Cimex lectularius*). An insect, Cimex lectularius, the saliva of which contains an irritating substance causing a purpuric reaction, or an urticarial wheal.

TREATMENT: Antipruritic lotions containing phenol, camphor, and menthol.

CONTROL: Largely a matter of cleanliness. In heavy infestations use 5% DDT in kerosene, spraying furniture, mattresses, floors, baseboards, walls; 1% lindane is also effective.

bedfast. Unable or unwilling to leave the bed; bedridden.

Bed'nar's aph'thae. Two symmetrically placed, infected, traumatic ulcers appearing on hard palate of infants.

bedpan [A.S. *bedd,* bed, + *panna,* flat vessel]. Device for receiving fecal and urinal discharges from patient confined to the bed.

bedrest. 1. A device for propping up patients in bed. 2. The confining of a patient continuously to his bed for rest.

bedridden. Unable or unwilling to leave the bed; bedfast.

bedsore [" + O.E. *sāre,* open wound]. Pressure sore, especially over a bony prominence. SYN: *decubitus.*

Decubitus consists of ulceration and gangrene of a localized area, due to pressure from prolonged confinement in bed or from a cast or splint. Emaciated, weak, elderly patients and those who must remain in one position because of orthopedic or similar problems are especially likely to develop bedsores.

PREDISPOSING CAUSES: (1) Any factor which interferes with the circulation of the blood and mobility of the patient. (2) Prolonged fever. (3) Emaciation. (4) Obesity. (5) Paralysis. (6) Old age or senility. (7) Poorly made beds. (8) Lack of cleanliness. (9) Bruising. (10) Infrequent change of positions. (11) Cardiac diseases, nephritis, diabetes, anemia, etc.

LOCATION: The body prominences thinly covered with flesh, as: (1) The end of the spine. (2) The buttocks. (3) The heels. (4) Elbows. (5) Shoulder blades. (6) Back of the head and ears in children.

TREATMENT: (1) Best nursing care, as prevention is easier than a cure. (2) Prophylactic measures in keeping the bed dry and clean. (3) Relieving the pressure as soon as the first signs of redness appear. (4) Report to the nurse in charge or attending physician at once. (5) Use the prescribed medication as directed by the physician. (6) Thorough drying of skin after baths and gentle massage with alcohol to harden the skin and for stimulation of circulation. (7) Frequent change of position of patient if possible. (8) Exposure of area and protection of skin by silicone or similar preparation such as tincture of benzoin. (9) Maintenance of proper nutrition. (10) Chemical or surgical debridement of ulcers. (11) Use of sheepskin under vulnerable area. (12) Placing patient on special air bed, *q.v.*, or flotation bed, *q.v.*

bed'wetting. Enuresis, *q.v.*

beef [Fr. *boeuf*, flesh]. Meat from cattle that are one or more years old. COMP: *Protein:* Nitrogen is the essential characteristic of beef, it being richer in this element than any other food excepting cheese. The leaner the beef the greater the percentage of nitrogen.

OVEN-ROASTED (rib roast, 100 gm. of choice grade; 55% lean and 45% fat): Calories: 481. Other values: 18.3 gm. protein; 44.7 gm. fat; 80 I.U. vitamin A.

Poorer grade cuts of beef contain fewer calories than do the choice portions.

beer [A.S. *bēor*, fermented drink]. Fermented alcoholic beverage from a malt infusion of barley, malt or hops, with aid of brewer's yeast.

Contains about 4.5% alcohol by volume, 1% sugar, and approximately 42 calories per 100 gm. portion or 115 per 8 oz. glass.

Beer's operation [Georg Joseph Beer, German ophthalmologist, 1763-1821]. Flap operation for cataract or artificial pupil.

bee sting [A.S. *bēo*, bee, + *stingan*, to pierce]. The stinger, which is barbed, is usually left in the wound. Pain, mottled redness and edema result.

TREATMENT: Application of fairly strong household ammonia or baking soda paste. Remove stinger if present. If pain is severe, injection of 2% procaine solution. Antihistamines help to relieve discomfort. Some individuals are hypersensitive and may suffer severe anaphylactic reactions even leading to death. In such cases subcutaneous or intravenous administration of epinephrine is effective.

beeswax (bēēz'wax). Yellow wax obtained from honeycomb of bees. A purified form is used in ointments.

beets (red) [L. *beta*, beet]. A plant of the genus *Beta*, the common garden variety being *Beta vulgaris*. The root is most often eaten, but young plants (beet greens) are consumed also.

COOKED: 1 cup (100 gm.). Calories: 32. Other values: 23 mg. calcium; 0.5 mg. iron; 20 I.U. vitamin A; 6 mg. ascorbic acid.

beeturia (bēēt-ū'rĭ-ă). Pink to deep red color of urine which sometimes follows eating of beets.

behavior reflex. One acquired as result of training and repetition.

behav'iorism. A theory of conduct which regards normal and abnormal behavior as the result of conditioned reflexes quite apart from the concept of will. It does not apply to conditions resulting from structural disease.

bel (bĕl). A unit to measure the intensity of sound. A decibel, *q.v.* is one-tenth of a bel.

belch [A.S. *baelcian*, to eructate.] Escape of gas from the stomach through the mouth; to eructate.

belching. Raising of gas from the stomach. ETIOL: Gastric fermentation; air swallowing; gas-containing foods.

belemnoid (bĕ-lĕm'noyd) [G. *belemnon*, dart, + *eidos*, shape]. Dart-shaped; styloid.

Bell's disease [Luther Vose Bell, American physician, 1806-1862]. Acute delirious mania often terminating in death. Also called *Bell's mania*.

Bell's law [Sir Charles Bell, Scottish physiologist and surgeon, 1774-1842]. That anterior spinal nerve roots contain only motor fibers, and posterior roots only sensory fibers. SYN: *Bell-Magendie's law; Magendie's law*.

B.'s nerve. Long thoracic nerve; nervus thoracicus longus [NA].

B.'s palsy. Acute inflammatory reaction in or around the seventh, or facial, nerve at the stylomastoid foramen. Marked by pain and paralysis of muscles controlling facial expression, causing distortion of the face.

TREATMENT: Splint for prevention of drooping of lower face, massage of affected muscles, protection of eye during sleep to prevent ulceration of cornea, analgesics for pain.

Bell-Magendie's law. Bell's law, *q.v.*

bell-metal resonance. A metallic sound heard in pneumothorax.

bell sound. Bell-metal resonance.

belladonna (bel-ă-dŏn'ă) [It., fair lady]. *Atropa belladonna*, a poisonous plant with reddish flowers and shining black berries. Active principle of atropine. SYN: *deadly nightshade*.

ACTION AND USES: Mainly for sedative and spasmolytic effects on gastrointestinal tract.

b. leaf. USP. Powder from dried leaf and flowering top of *Atropa belladonna* Linné or *A. belladonna acuminata*. A parasympatholytic agent, it is used generally in tincture form though the dry extract in tablet form may be used. SYN: *deadly nightshade leaf*.

b. and atropine poisons. These include stramonium, hyoscyamus, scopolamine, belladonna, and atropine. SEE UNDER: *Atropine* in *Table of Poisons and Poisoning in Appendix*.

Bellini's ducts (bĕ-lē'nēz) [Lorenzo Bellini, Italian anatomist, 1643-1704]. Ducts in the kidney which open at tip of a renal pyramid after receiving several straight tubules. SYN: *papillary ducts*.

Belloc's cannula or **sound** (bel-oks'). An instrument for drawing in a plug through nostril and mouth to control epistaxis.

belly [A.S. *baelg*, bag]. 1. The abdomen or abdominal cavity. 2. The fleshy, central portion of a muscle.

b. ache. Colic, gastralgia.

b. button. Umbilicus.

belonephobia (bel-ō-nĕ-phō'bĭ-ă) [G. *belonē*, needle, + *phobos*, fear]. Morbid fear of sharp-pointed objects.

belonoid (bel'ō-noid) [" + *eidos*, shape]. Needle-shaped.

belonoskiascopy (bel-ō-nō-skī-as'kō-pĭ) [" + *skia*, shadow, + *skopein*, to examine]. Subjective retinoscopy by means of shadows and movements to determine refraction.

benadryl (ben'ă-drĭl). Proprietary name for diphenhydramine hydrochloride, an antihistaminic agent.

Bence Jones albumose [Henry Bence Jones, English physician, 1813-1873]. SEE: *protein, Bence Jones*.

bends. Painful condition caused by bubbles of nitrogen in blood and tissues as a result of too rapid decompression from greater-than-atmospheric pressure. SEE: *caisson disease*.

Benedict's solution [Stanley R. Benedict, American chemist, 1884-1936]. A solution used to test for presence of sugar. To 173 gm. sodium or potassium citrate and 100 gm. anhydrous sodium carbonate (dissolved in 700 ml. water) is added 17.3 gm. crystalline copper sulfate that has been dissolved in 100 ml. of water. Sufficient water is added to the mixture to make 1000 ml.

B.'s test (for sugar): Add 8 drops of clear urine (filtered if necessary) to a test tube containing 5 ml. of B.'s solution. Boil from 1 to 2 minutes, agitating the test tube during this time, and then allow it to cool undisturbed. Formation of red, yellow, olive green, or green precipitate indicates presence of sugar (2% or more [plus 4], 1% [plus 3], ¾% [plus 2], ½% [plus 1], respectively).

Ben'edikt's syndrome [Moritz Benedikt, Austrian physician, 1835-1920]. Hemiplegia with oculomotor paralysis and clonic spasm on opp. side.

benign (bē-nīn') [L. *benignus*, mild]. 1. Not recurrent. 2. Not malignant. 3. Mild.

b. stupor. A stupor sometimes seen in the depression of manic-depressive psychosis.

benzalkonium chloride (benz-al-kō'nĭ-um klō'rīd). USP. A bitter, aromatic, white powder. Used as a detergent and germicide.

benzedrine (bĕn'zĕ-drēn). Proprietary name for amphetamine, *q.v.*

b. sulfate. Proprietary name for amphetamine sulfate, *q.v.*

benzene [L. *benzinum*] C_6H_6. A volatile liquid, immiscible with water, able to dissolve fats.

Important theoretically because it is the simplest member of the *aromatic* series of hydrocarbons, and useful practically because, prepared in the distillation of coal tar, it serves in the synthesis of innumerable dyes, drugs, etc. The phenyl *radical*, C_6H_5, will be recognized in the formulae for *phenol*, dimethylaminoazobenzene (which see under *azo-compounds*), and *benzoic acid*. SYN: *benzol.*

POISONING (benzene or b. hydrochloride). SEE: *Table of Poisons and Poisoning in Appendix.*

benzestrol. A synthetic substance, which has an estrogenic effect when taken orally.

benzidine test. A test used to determine the presence of blood. Prepare benzidine sol. as follows: to a sat. solution of benzidine in glacial acetic acid, add equal volume of 3% hydrogen peroxide and about 1 ml. of the suspected fluid. Appearance of a blue color indicates presence of blood.

benzidine test diet. This consists of milk, crackers and rice.

An iron-free diet, its purpose being to free the alimentary tract of any iron; often the stool is tested for iron. Since no iron was in the food, if any is present in the food masses, it must come from the hemoglobin of the blood. Such a result is a positive test of bleeding into the intestinal tract, and an evidence of an ulcer. Patients should be watched to be sure that they eat nothing but those foods which are served at the prescribed times.

ben'zoate. Any salt of benzoic acid.

benzocaine (ben'zō-kān). Nontoxic local anesthetic.

benzo'ic acid. SEE: *acid, benzoic.*

benzoin (ben'zoin, -zō-in) [L. *benzoinum*]. USP. A balsamic resin obtained from various species of a tree, *Styrax*, especially *S. benzoin* or *S. paralleloneuris.* Used as a stimulant expectorant, as an inhalant in laryngitis and bronchitis, or as a protective coating for ulcers, etc.

ben'zol [L. *benzinum*]. Same as benzene, *q.v.*

benzyl benzoate (bĕn'zĭl ben'zō-āt). A sharp, colorless, oily liquid, used externally in scabies.

Berard's aneurysm [Auguste Berard, French surgeon, 1802-1846]. An arteriovenous aneurysm in the tissues surrounding the injured vein.

Beraud's valve (bā-rōz') [Bruno J. Beraud, French surgeon, 1823-1865]. Fold of mucous membrane at junction of lacrimal sac with lacrimal duct. SYN: *Krause's valve.*

beriberi (bĕr'ĭ-ber'ĭ) [Singhalese *beri*, weakness]. A deficiency disease associated with malnutrition. Endemic in the Orient, Philippines and other islands of the Pacific, and formerly in rice-growing sections of the United States (Louisiana).

ETIOLOGY: Deficiency of thiamine (vitamin B_1). Diet is usually a low-fat, low-protein, high-carbohydrate one, especially in which there is a high intake of rice highly milled.

SYM: Multiple neuritis, cardiovascular changes, and edema.

TREATMENT: Oral or parenteral administration of thiamine; establishment of a properly balanced diet.

berkelium (berk'lē-um) [from Univ. of California at *Berkeley*, where first produced]. SYMB: Bk. A transuranium element. At. wt. 247; at. no. 97.

Bernard's canal, duct (bĕr-narz') [Claude Bernard, French physiologist, 1813-1878]. An accessory pancreatic duct; ductus pancreaticus accessorius [NA]. SYN: *Santorini's duct.*

B.'s granular layer. Inner layer in cells lining acini of pancreas.

Bernreuter test (bern'rū-ter). A "yes" and "no" test of 125 questions, used to ascertain the attitudes and interest of a person.

Bertin, columns of (ber'tan) [Exupere Joseph Bertin, French anatomist, 1712-1781]. Renal cortical columns supporting the blood vessels in the kidneys. The part that separates the medullary pyramids.

B.'s ligament. Iliofemoral ligament.

beryllium (bĕ-rĭl'ĭ-um) [L. *beryl*]. SYMB: Be. A metallic element, also called glucinum. At. wt. 9.0122; at. no. 4.

besoin de respirer (ba-zwan dĕ res-pĭ-rā') [F. need to breathe]. Sensation inducing act of breathing.

bestiality (bes-tĭ-al'ĭ-tĭ) [L. *bestia*, beast]. Coition with an animal.

beta (bā'tă). 1. Second letter of Greek alphabet, written β. 2. Used as a prefix to chemical words to note isomeric variety or position in compounds of substituted groups.

b. cells. 1. Basophilic cells in the ant. lobe of hypophysis which give a positive periodic acid stain reaction. 2. Cells of the islets of Langerhans of the pancreas which secrete insulin.

b. rays. Negatively charged particles emitted by radium; more penetrating than alpha rays. Absorbed by 1 mm. lead or 0.6 mm. platinum.

betacism (bā'tă-sĭzm) [G. *bēta*, the letter *b*]. Speech defect giving the *b* sound to other consonants.

betaine hydrochloride (bē-tain'). A colorless crystalline substance, containing 23% hydrochloric acid, and obtained from an alkaloid found in the beet, and other plants. Used as a substitute for hydrochloric acid in hypochlorhydria.

betanaphthol (bā-tă-naf'thol). Occurs as a colorless or buff-colored crystalline powder, with faint odor of phenol $C_{10}H_7OH$.

ACTION AND USES: A parasiticide and fungicide. Ointment, 5-10%, used in the treatment of ringworm, psoriasis, and pediculosis. Formerly used in the treatment of hookworm infestation but has been replaced by safer drugs.

Betz cell. A form of giant pyramidal cell in the cortical motor area.

bezoar bē'zōr) [Persian]. A concretion from the stomachs and intestines of animals, and also in man as a hairball (*trichobezoar*), hair and vegetable fiberball (*trichophytobezoar*), and foodball (*phytobezoar*).

Bezold effect (be'zolt). Disturbances in respiration, *i.e.*, apnea followed by polypnea, resulting from the effect of veratrum alkaloids on pulmonary, cardiac, and carotid receptors. SYN: *Bezold reflexes.*

Bi. Chemical symbol for *bismuth.*

bi- (bī-) [L. *bis*, two]. Prefix: Two, double, twice.

biartic'ular [" + *articulus*, joint]. Pert. to two joints; diarthric.

bibasic (bī-bā'sik) [" + G. *basis*, foundation]. Pert. to an acid with two hydrogen atoms replaceable by bases to form salts.

bibulous (bĭb'ū-lus) [L. *bibere*, to drink]. Absorbent.

bicameral (bī-kam'ĕ-ral) [L. *bis*, two, + *camera*, a chamber]. Having two cavities or hollows, esp. an abscess divided by a septum.

bicap'sular [" + *capsula*, container]. Having a double capsule.

bicar'bonate [" + carbonate]. A salt resulting from the incomplete neutralization of carbonic *acid*, or from the passing of an excess of carbon dioxide into a solution of a *base*.

Sodium bicarbonate is $NaHCO_3$; calcium bicarbonate is $CaH_2(CO_3)_2$. A carbonate composed of two equivalents of carbonic acid and one of a base.

b., blood. That in the blood. An alkali reserve index.

bicar'diogram [" + G. *kardia*, heart, + *gramma*, a writing]. A cardiogram curve representing the combined effects of the right and left ventricles.

bicellular (bī-sĕl'ū-lar) [" + *cellulāris*, little cell]. 1. Composed of two cells. 2. Having two chambers or compartments.

biceps (bī'sĕps) [L. *bis*, two, + *caput*, head]. A muscle with two heads.

b. brachii. Muscle of the upper arm, having two heads. Flexes arm and forearm and supinates hand.

b. femoris. One of the hamstring muscles lying on posterior lateral side of thigh.

ACTION: Flexes knee and rotates it outward.

b. reflex. Biceps muscle contraction when tendon is percussed.

Bichat's canal (bĭ-shăs') [Marie Francois X. Bichat, French physiologist and anatomist, 1771-1802]. The subarachnoid canal extending from third ventricle to middle of B.'s fissure carrying the veins of Galen.

B.'s fat ball or ***pad.*** Mass of fat behind the buccinator muscle.

B.'s fissure. The horseshoe fissure separating cerebrum from cerebellum.

B.'s foramen. Same as B.'s canal.

B.'s ligament. Lower fasciculus of post. sacroiliac ligament.

B.'s membrane. *Lamina basalis.*

B.'s tunic. The tunica intima of the blood vessels.

bichloride of mercury (bī-klo'rīd) (corrosive mercuric chloride). A crystalline salt, $HgCl_2$. SEE: *mercuric chloride.*

POISONING: SEE: *Mercuric Chloride* in *Table of Poisons and Poisoning in Appendix.*

biciliate (bī-sil'ĭ-āt) [L. *bis*, two, + G. *kyla*, eyelids]. Having two cilia.

bicipital (bī-sĭp'ĭ-tal) [L. *biceps*, two heads]. 1. Pert. to a biceps muscle. 2. Having two heads.

$Bi_2(CO_3)_3$. Bismuth carbonate.

biconcave (bī-kon'kāv) [L. *bis*, two, + *concavus*, concave]. Concave on each side, as a lens.

bicon'vex [" + *convexus*, rounded raised surface]. Convex on two sides, as a lens.

bicornuate, bicornuous (bī-korn'ū-āt, -us) [" + *cornutus*, horned]. Having two processes or hornlike projections.

b. uterus. Anomalous uterus resulting from incomplete union of the mullerian ducts. May be double or single organ with two horns.

bicoro'nal [" + G. *korōnē*, crown]. Pert. to the two coronas.

bicor'porate [" + *corpus*, body]. Having two bodies.

bicuspid (bī-kus'pid) [" + *cuspis*, point]. Having two cusps or projections (*e.g.*, bicuspid tooth) or having two cusps or leaflets (*e.g.*, bicuspid valve).

b. tooth. SYN: premolar tooth.

b. valve. SYN: mitral valve. Valve between left atrium and left ventricle of the heart. SEE: *heart.*

bicuspid (bī-kus'pĭd). One of two teeth above and below on each side between the molars and canines.

b. i. d. Abbr. for *bis in die*, twice daily.

bidet (bĭ'det) [Fr. a small horse]. A receptacle with attachments for giving injections, for a hip bath or sitz bath, or for washing the genitals or for douching.

biduous (bid'u-us) [L. *bis*, two, + *diēs*, a day]. Continuing for two days.

Biederman's sign (be'der-mans) [Joseph B. Biederman, Cincinnati physician, 1907-]. Dusky redness of the lower ant. pillars of fauces in certain cases of syphilis.

Bielschowsky disease [Max Bielschowsky, German neuropathologist, 1869-1940]. SEE: *amaurotic familial idiocy, late infantile.*

Bier's cup (beers) [Karl G. A. Bier, Berlin surgeon, 1861-1949]. A clear glass cup provided with a pump and bulb named after the inventor. Its use is to induce hyperemia where there is pronounced external inflammation.

B.'s spots. White spots occurring in a congested extremity when arterial supply is occluded following venous obstruction.

bifa'cial ([L. *bis*, two, + *faciēs*, face]. Having similar opposite surfaces.

bi'fid [" + *findere*, to cleave]. Cleft or split into two parts.

b. spine. Congenital fissure of vertebral column.

b. tongue. Cleft tongue.

bifo'cal [" + *focus*, hearth]. Having two foci, as *b. eyeglasses.*

bifurcate (bī'fur-kāt, bī-fur'kāt) [" + *furca*, fork]. Having two branches or divisions; forked.

bifurcated (bī'fur-kāt"ĕd). Having two branches; forked.

bifurcation (bī-fŭr-kā'shŭn) [L. *bis*, two, + *furca*, fork]. A separation into two branches; the point of forking.

bigeminal (bī-jĕm'ĭ-nal) [L. *bigeminum*, twin]. Double, paired.

b. bodies. Either of the two anterior eminences of the corpora quadrigemina.

b. pulse. Pulse in which beats are in groups of two with pause in between groups. SEE: *pulse, b.*

bigem'inum. A bigeminal body.

bigeminy (bī-jĕm'ĭ-nĭ) [L. *bigeminum*, twin]. Pulse marked by occurrence of two beats close together followed by a pause before next pair of beats. SYN: *pulse, bigeminal.*

bilat'eral [" + *latus,* side]. Pert. to, affecting, or rel. to two sides of the body.

b. symmetry. Symmetry of paired organs. SYN: *bilateralism.*

bilateralism (bī-lat'ĕr-ăl-ĭzm) [" + " + G. *ismos,* condition]. Arrangement on two sides; symmetry.

bile (bīl) [L. *bilis,* bile]. A secretion of the liver.

It is a thick, viscid fluid with a bitter taste which passes from the bile duct of the liver into the common bile duct and then into the duodenum as needed. The bile from the liver is straw color, while that from the gallbladder varies from yellow to brown and green. There are more solids in green bile and it is mixed with mucus.

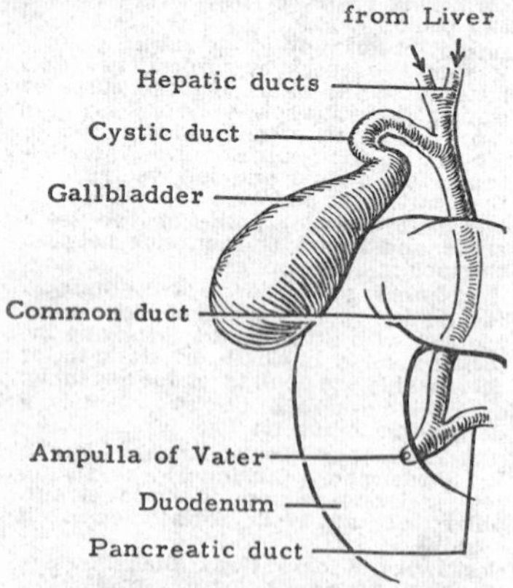

from Liver
Hepatic ducts
Cystic duct
Gallbladder
Common duct
Ampulla of Vater
Duodenum
Pancreatic duct

BILE AND PANCREATIC DUCTS

It is also stored in the gallbladder, drawn upon as needed, and discharged into the duodenum. Contraction of the gallbladder brought about by a hormone, cholecystokinin, produced by the duodenum, its secretion being brought about by the entrance of fatty foods (esp. egg yolk and cream) into the duodenum. Added to water, bile decreases surface tension, giving a foamy solution favoring the emulsification of fats and oils; this action is due to the bile salts, mainly sodium glycocholate and taurocholate.

COMP: The bile pigments (principally bilirubin* and biliverdin*) are responsible for the variety of the colors observed. In addition, bile contains cholesterol, lecithin, mucin, and other organic and inorganic substances.

FUNCT: Its importance as a digestive juice is due to its emulsifying action which facilitates the digestion of fats in the intestines by pancreatic steapsin, plus a further effect of the bile salts which form compounds with the fatty acids and are necessary for their absorption. Bile also stimulates peristalsis.

Normally the ejection of bile only occurs during duodenal digestion. Bile is both an antiseptic and a purgative. About 1800-2000 cc. are secreted per 24 hr. in the normal adult. SEE: *gallbladder.*

PATH: Interference with the flow of bile produces jaundice, resulting in unabsorbed fats being found in the feces. In such instances, fats should be restricted in the diet. Gallstones also may be produced in the gallbladder when the free flow of bile from the gallbladder is impeded, or when pathological conditions interfere with bile production.

TEST FOR IN URINE: There are several methods of testing for bile in the urine.

1. *Gmelin's Test:* 1 in. of concentrated nitric acid is carefully overlaid with the suspected urine. Bile is present when there is a play of colors at the junction of the fluids. This test can also be carried out by pouring some urine onto blotting or filter paper, and then placing a drop of concentrated nitric acid on the moist paper. From the spreading edge of the drop of acid will develop a ring of various colors in which green predominates and forms the outer band.

2. *Iodine Test:* Take an inch of the suspected urine in a test tube and carefully overlay it with dilute tincture of iodine. A bright green ring will appear at the junction of the fluids, if bile is present.

RS: *"bili-" words, "chol-" words, stercobilin, urobilin.*

b. acids. Complex acids, of which cholic, glycocholic, and taurocholic acids are examples, and which occur as salts (*e.g.,* sodium taurochlate) in bile. They give bile its foamy character, are important in the digestion of fats in the intestine, and are reabsorbed from the intestine to be used again by the liver; this circulation of the bile acids is called the enterohepatic circulation.

HAY'S TEST FOR: Some urine is placed in a watchglass, and a little powdered sulfur is thrown on the surface. If bile acids are present, the sulfur sinks due to the lowering of the surface tension by the bile salts.

b. ducts. Intercellular biliary passages conveying the bile from the liver to the hepatic duct which joins the duct from the gallbladder (cystic duct), to form the common bile duct (ductus choledochus), and which enters the duodenum about 3 inches (7.5 cm.) below the pylorus. SEE: *hepatic duct; cystic duct; common bile duct; gallbladder.*

b. pigments. Complex, highly colored substances found in bile, derived from the red pigment (hemoglobin) of the blood, and imparting the brown color to intestinal contents and feces. EX: *bilirubin, biliverdin.*

The van den Bergh test, *q.v.,* is used to detect the type of bilirubin in the blood serum.

b. salts. Alkali salts of bile. Sodium glycocholate and sodium taurocholate.

Bilharzia (bil-har'zĭ-ă). A term formerly used for *Schistosoma,* the human blood fluke. SEE: *Schistosoma.*

bilharzial, bilharzic. Pertaining to Bilharzia.

bilharziasis. Schistosomiasis.

bili- [L.]. Prefix: Pert. to bile.

biliary (bil'ĭ-ar-ĭ). Pert. to or conveying bile.

b. calculus. Cholelithiasis. Formation of stone in any of the biliary passages or in the gallbladder.

b. colic. Pain caused by the pressure or passing of gallstones.

b. ducts. Passages conveying bile from liver to hepatic duct. SEE: ***bile ducts.***

bilicy'anin. A blue or purple pigment, an oxidation product of biliverdin.

bilifaction. Bilification.

bilifica'tion [" + *fecere*, to make]. The formation of bile.

bilifla'vin [" + *flavus*, yellow]. A yellow pigment derived from biliverdin.

biliful'vin [" + *fulvus*, tawny]. Bilirubin mixed with other substances.

bilifuscin (bil-ĭ-fus'in) [L. *bilis*, bile, + *fuscus*, brown]. A dark brown pigment from bile and gallstones.

biligenesis (bil-ĭ-jen'ĕ-sis) [" + G. *genesis*, origin]. The formation of bile.

biligenet'ic, biligen'ic. Forming bile.

bilihu'min [L. *bilis*, bile, + *humus*, earth]. A dark insoluble residue after applying solvents to bile or gallstones.

bilineurine (bil"ĭ-nū'rin) [L. *bilis*, bile, + G. *neuron*, nerve]. Choline, *q.v.*

bil'ious. 1. Pert. to bile. 2. Afflicted with biliousness.

b. fever. Fever with vomiting of bile.

biliousness (bil'yus-nes). 1. A symptom due to disordered condition of the liver causing constipation, headache, loss of appetite, and vomiting of bile. 2. Excess of bile; bilious fever. Fever with vomiting of bile.

bilipra'sin [" + G. *prason*, leek-green]. Green pigment, similar to biliverdin and found in gallstones.

bilipur'pin, bilipurpu'rin [" + *purpur*, purple]. A purple pigment derived from biliverdin.

bilirachia (bil-ĭ-ra'kĭ-ă) [" + G. *rachis*, spine]. Bile in the spinal fluid.

bilirubin (bil-ĭ-ru'bin) [" + *ruber*, red] ($C_{33}H_{36}O_6N_4$). The orange-colored or yellowish pigment in bile.

It is carried to the liver by the blood, the product of degenerated hemoglobin in bone marrow, in the spleen, and elsewhere. It is chemically changed in the liver and excreted in the bile through the duodenum. As it passes through the intestines it is converted into urobilinogen by bacterial enzymes, most of it being excreted through the feces. If urobilinogen passes into the circulation it is excreted through the urine or re-excreted in the bile.

bilirub'inate. A salt of bilirubin.

bilirubinemia (bil-ĭ-roo-bin-ē'mĭ-ă) [" + " + G. *aima*, blood]. Bilirubin in blood. Bilirubin is normally present in the blood in small amounts. In certain pathologic conditions in which excessive destruction of red blood cells occurs, or in which there is interference with bile excretion, the amount is increased.

bilirubinu'ria [" + " + G. *ouron*, urine]. Bilirubin in urine.

biliuria (bil-ĭ-u'rĭ-ă) [" + G. *ouron*, urine]. Bile in the urine.

biliverdin (bil-ĭ-ver'dĭn) [" + G. *viridis*, green]. $C_{33}H_{34}O_6N_4$. A greenish pigment in bile formed by the oxidation of bilirubin.

bilobate (bĭ-lō'bāt). Having two lobes.

bilob'ular. Having two lobules.

biloc'ular [L. *bis*, two, + *loculus*, cell]. 1. Having two cells. 2. Divided into compartments.

biloc'ulate. Bilocular.

bilophodont (bĭ-loph'ō-dont) [L. *bis*, two, + G. *lophos*, ridge, + *odous* (odont), tooth]. Said of animals, such as the kangaroo, having teeth with two ridges.

biman'ual [L. *bis*, two, + *manus*, hand]. With both hands; with two hands, as *b. palpation.*

bimax'illary [G. *bios*, life, + L. *maxillaris*, pert. to the jaw]. Pert. to or afflicting both jaws.

binary (bī'nar-ĭ) [L. *binarius*, of two]. 1. Compounded of two elements. 2. Separating into two branches.

b. acid. One containing hydrogen and one other element.

b. digit. One of two digits, usually 0 or 1, used in a binary system of enumeration.

binau'ral [L. *bīni*, two, + *auris*, ear]. Pert. to or having two ears.

b. arc. The arc from one aural point to another across top of cranium.

binauric'ular. Binaural.

binder [A.S. *bindan*, to tie up]. A broad bandage, most commonly used as an encircling support of abdomen or chest. SEE ALSO: *bandage.*

b., abdominal. A wide band fastened snugly about the abdomen for support.

b., chest. A broad band used for encircling the chest to apply heat, dressings, or pressure, and supporting the breasts. Improved by using shoulder straps to keep from slipping.

b., double T. A horizontal band about the waist to which two vertical bands are attached in back, brought around leg and again fastened to horizontal band. Holds dressings about perineum or genitalia (esp. male).

b., obstetrical. A broad bandage encircling entire abdomen from ribs to pelvis, affording support.

b., T. Two strips of material fastened together, resembling a T, used as a bandage to hold a dressing on perineum of women; or vertex of head, etc.

b., towel. A towel encircling abdomen or chest with ends pinned or sewed together for support.

Binet age (bĭ-na') [Alford Binet, French physician, 1857-1911]. Intellect as measured by the Binet-Simon tests as compared with the age of a normal child. The Binet age of an idiot is 1-2 yr.; the imbecile, 3-9 yr.; the moron, 8-12 yr.

binoc'ular [L. *bini*, two, + *oculus*, eye]. Pert. to both eyes.

b. vision. Normal vision involving simultaneous use of both eyes.

binot'ic [" + G. *ous*, ear]. Pert. to or having two ears. SYN: *binaural.**

binov'ular [" + *ovum*, egg]. Derived from or pert. to two ova. SYN: *biovular.*

binuclear, binucleate (bī-nū'klē-er, -āt) [" + L. *nucleus*, kernel]. Having two nuclei.

bio- [G. *bios*, life]. Prefix: Life.

bio-assay (bī-ō-as-ā') [G. *bios*, life, + O.FR. *asaier*, to try]. Estimation of strength of a drug by noting its effect in a test animal and comparing such with effects of a standard preparation.

bioastronautics. Study of the effects of space travel on living plant and animal life.

bi'oblast [" + *blastos*, germ]. A corpuscle that has not yet become a cell; micella.

biocatalyst (bī-ō-kat'ă-list) [" + *katalyein*, to dissolve]. An enzyme; a biochemical catalyzer.

biochem'istry [" + *chēmeia*, chemistry]. The chemistry of living things; the science of the chemical changes accompanying the vital functions of plants and animals.

biochemorphic (bi"ō-kĕm-or'fik) [" + " + *morphē*, shape]. Pert. to the relation bet. biologic action of drugs and foods and their chemical constitution.

biochemorphology (bi"o-kĕ-mor-fol'o-jĭ) [" + " + " + *logos*, study]. Science of chemical structure of substances as related to their action on the body.

bioclimatology (bī"ō-klī-mă-tol'ō-jĭ) [" + *klima*, climate, + *logos*, study]. Relations of climate to life.

biocolloid (bi-o-kol'oyd) [" + *kollōdēs,* glutinous]. A colloid in animal or vegetable organism.

biocoenosis, biocenosis (bi"-o-se-no'sis) [G. *bios,* life, + *koines,* common]. The relationship between plants and animals sharing the same area and conditions. SEE: *ecology.*

biodynam'ics [" + *dynamis,* force]. The science of living force or energy; biophysiology.

bioenergetics. Science of energy transformation taking place within living tissues.

biogen'esis [" + *genesis,* origin]. Begetting living things from living things opp. to spontaneous generation.

biogenet'ic. Pert. to biogenesis.

biokinet'ics [G. *bios,* life, + *kinetikos,* moving]. The science of changes in developing organisms.

biolog'ic, biolog'ical [" + *logos,* study]. Pert. to biology.

biological false positive. A serological test for syphilis which is positive in the absence of infection with *Treponema.*

biological warfare. The use of biological agents such as viruses, bacteria, toxins, and molds to kill or injure enemy soldiers and civilians. SEE: *chemical warfare.*

biolog'icals. 1. Complex substances of organic origin, depending for their action on the processes effecting immunity, used esp. in diagnosis and treatment of disease, as vaccines, serums or antigens. 2. Complex products, of organic or synthetic origin, obtained or standardized by biological methods, as insulin

biol'ogist. A professional student of, or a specialist in biology.

biology (bī-ol'ō-jĭ) [G. *bios,* life, + *logos,* study]. Science of life and living things. It includes the study of plants (botany) and animals (zoology) and all their subdivisions.

biolysis (bi-ol'ĭs-ĭs) [G. *bios,* life, + *lysis,* dissolution]. Devitalization or destruction of living tissue by action of living organisms.

biolytic (bi-o-lit'ik). Capable of destroying life.

biomet'rics. Biometry.

biom'etry [G. *bios,* life, + *metron,* measure]. 1. Application of statistics to biological science. 2. Computation of life expectancy.

bion (bi'on) [G. *biōn,* living]. Any living organism.

bionergy (bi-on'er-jĭ) [G. *bios,* life, + *ergon,* work]. Vital energy or force.

bionics (bī-ŏn'ĭks). Study of how living organisms perform tasks and solve problems and the application of these findings to the design of machines, especially computers.

bion'omy. The science pertaining to life processes. SEE: *physiology; ecology.*

biono'sis [G. *bios,* life, + *nosos,* disease]. Any disease due to pathogenic organisms.

biophagism, biophagy (bi-of'ă-jizm, -ă-jĭ) [" + *phagein,* to eat]. Absorbing nourishment from living matter.

bioph'agous. Feeding on nonparasitic matter.

biophore (bi'o-fōr) [" + *phoros,* bearing]. The ultimate unit having vital energy.

biophylac'tic [" + *phylax,* a guard]. Tending to preserve life.

biophysics (bi-o-fiz'iks) [" + *physikos,* natural]. Application of physical laws to life processes and functions.

bi'oplasm [" + *plasma,* matter]. Protoplasm. Living substance.

bi'opsy [G. *bios,* life, + *opsis,* vision]. Excision of a small piece of tissue for microscopic examination.

bios (bi'os) [G. *bios,* life]. 1. Organic life. 2. A group of substances (including especially inositol, biotin and thiamine) necessary for the most favorable growth of some yeasts.

bios'copy [G. *bios,* life, + *skopein,* to examine]. Examination to determine life.

biospectrom'etry [G. *bios,* life, + L. *spectrum,* image, + G. *metron,* measure]. Use of a spectroscope to determine the amounts and kinds of substances in tissues.

biospectros'copy [" + ". + G. *skopein,* to examine]. Examination of tissue by use of a spectroscope.

biostat'ics [" + *statikos,* standing]. Science of the relation of structure to function.

biostatis'tics. 1. Application of statistical processes and methods to the analysis of biological data. 2. Vital statistics.

biota [G. *bios,* life]. Combined and total animal and plant life in an area.

biotax'is, bi'otaxy [G. *bios,* life, + *taxis,* arrangement]. 1. The selecting and arranging activity of living cells. 2. Systematic classification of living organisms.

biot'ics [G. *biōtikos,* living]. The sum of knowledge regarding life processes.

biotin (bī'ō-tin). Formerly designated as vitamin H, this substance is a component of the vitamin B complex. Though effects of deficiency of biotin have been determined in animals, such effects in man remain unconfirmed. Therapeutic value has not been proven.

biotomy (bi-ot'o-mĭ) [G. *bios,* life, + *tomē,* incision]. Operation on living animals for pathological or physiological study. SYN: *vivisection.*

biotox'in [" + *toxikon,* poison]. A toxin produced by or found in a living organism.

biotransformation. The biologic process of changing a substance so that it may be metabolized or excreted.

biotrip'sis [" + *tripsis,* rubbing]. A condition of the skin seen in old people in which skin wears away. May be smooth, pigmented, shiny, esp. on forehead, backs of hands, and shin.

Biot's breathing or **respiration** (bĭ-ōs'). Rapid breathing with rhythmical pauses. Unfavorable in meningitis.

biotype (bī'ō-tīp) [G. *bios,* life, + *typos,* mark]. 1. Fundamental constitution of an organism or those possessing it. 2. A genotype.

biov'ular twins [L. *bis,* two, + *ovulum,* ovum]. Twins from two separate ova.

bip'ara [" + *parēre,* to give birth]. Woman who has borne two children in separate labors.

biparasit'ic [" + G. *para,* beside, + *sitos,* food]. Pert. to parasite living upon another parasite.

biparen'tal [" + *parēre,* to bring forth]. Derived from both parents.

bip'arous. Giving birth to two at a time.

bipolar (bī-pōl'er) [" + *polus,* a pole]. 1. Having two poles or processes. 2. Pert. to the use of two poles in electrotherapeutic treatments.

When referring to an alternating current, biterminal should be used.

b. nerve cell. Cell with two processes.

biramous (bi-ra'mus) [L. *bi,* two, + *ramus,* a branch]. Possessing two branches.

birefrac'tive, birefrin'gent [L. *bis,* two, + *refrangere,* to break up]. Splitting a ray of light in two.

birhinia (bi-rĭn'ĭ-ă) [*bi* + G. *rhis*, nose]. Double nose.

birth [M.E. *byrthe*, birth]. Act of being born. Passage of a child from uterus.

b. canal. The uterus and vagina.

b. certificate. A legal form filled out by the physician or one in attendance at a birth and filed with the local health dept., giving pertinent information regarding the parents and child.

b., complete. The instant of complete separation of the body of the infant from that of the mother, regardless of cord or placenta detached.

b. control. Any method used to control the number of children conceived or born. This would include devices by either the male or the female, medicine, and abortion. Abstention from sexual intercourse is a form of birth control, as is surgical sterilization.

b., cross. With fetus across the uterus.

b., dry. Birth following premature rupture of the fetal membrane.

b., live. An infant showing one of the three evidences of life (breathing, heart action, movements of a voluntary muscle) after complete birth.

b. mark. Nevus; mark from birth injury.

b. palsy. Paraplegia or hemiplegia caused by birth injury. Injury to shoulder muscles may cause Erb's palsy.

b., premature. Birth of a fetus sometime after it is old enough to survive but before reaching 2500 gm. in weight. This weight limitation would not apply to races of small stature and weight.

b. rate. The number of live births in a given year per 1000 of total population.

b., still. An infant not exhibiting evidence of life after complete birth.

bisacro'mial [L. *bis*, two, + G. *akron*, point, + *ōmos*, shoulder]. Pert. to both acromial processes.

bisection (bī-sek'shŭn) [" + *sectiō*, a cutting]. Division into 2 parts.

bisex'ual [" + *sexus*, sex]. Hermaphroditic; having imperfect genitalia of both sexes in one person.

bisferious (bis-fer'ĭ-us) [" + *ferire*, to beat]. Having two beats; dicrotic.

bisiliac (bis-il'ĭ-ăk) [" + *ilium*, ilium]. Pert. to the two most distant points of the two iliac crests.

bis in d., bis in die [L.]. Twice a day.

bismuth (biz'muth) [Ger. *wismuth*, contraction of *weisse masse*, white mass]. A silvery metallic element. SYMB: Bi. At. wt. 208.980, at. no. 83. Its compounds are used as a protective for inflamed surfaces, and as an opaque medium for x-ray visualization. Its salts are used as an antiseptic, astringent, sedative, and in treatment of diarrhea.

POISONING: SYM: Metallic taste, foul breath, fever, gastrointestinal irritation. bluish line at gum margin, ulcerative process of gums and mouth, headache. Albuminuria; resembles lead poisoning with an absence of the blood changes and paralyses.

F. A. TREATMENT: Removal of source of bismuth; gastric lavage; high enemas; stimulants for respiration and heart if necessary; treat symptomatically.

b. subcarbonate. USP. USES: As an antacid, astringent, and protective. INCOMPATIBILITIES: Sulfides, acids, acid salts.

b. subgallate (Dermatol). A bright yellow powder without odor or taste. USES: First introduced for treatment of skin diseases. General use—same as bismuth subnitrate.

b. subnitrate. Occurs as heavy white odorless powder. INCOMPATIBILITIES: Acids, tannins, and sulfides. USES: Astringent, protective antiseptic.

bistoury (bis'to-rĭ) [Fr. *bistouri*, surgical knife]. Small surgical knife used in minor operations; special varieties are tenotomes, gum lancets, hernia knives, and lithotomy bistouries.

bite (bīt) [A.S. *bitan*, to bite]. 1. To cut with the teeth. 2. Puncture or tearing of the skin by the teeth as by an animal. SEE: *bites or stings.* 3. Occlusion of the teeth.

b., balanced. Balanced occlusion of the teeth.

b., close, closed. One in which lower incisors lie behind upper incisors.

b., end-to-end. One in which incisors of both jaws meet along cutting edge when jaw is closed.

b., open. One in which a space exists between the upper and lower incisors when the mouth is closed.

b., over. One in which upper incisors overlap lower ones when jaws are closed.

b., under (or ***underhung***). Lower incisors pass in front of upper incisors upon closing the mouth.

bitelock. Device for retaining position bite rims outside the mouth.

bitem'poral [L. *bis*, two, + *temporalis*, pert. to a temple]. Pert. to both temples or temporal bones.

bite rim. A rim of wax placed on base plate as a guide for inserting artificial teeth. SYN: *occlusion rim.*

bites or stings. Injuries in which body surfaces are torn by insects or animals, resulting in abrasions, punctured, or lacerated wounds. SEE: *dog bite; rabies; snake bite.*

SYM: May be evidence of a wound usually surrounded by a zone of redness and swelling, often accompanied by pain, itching, or throbbing. Often become infected and may contain specific noxious materials as bacteria or venom of rabies.

F. A. TREATMENT: If suspected of poison, apply tourniquet first. Wash wound with saline solution thoroughly, apply dry sterile dressing. Administer appropriate antitetanus therapy. Treatment for shock may be needed.

b. or stings, insect. They contain an acid substance resembling formic acid and consequently are relieved by alkalies, as ammonia water or baking soda paste. For intense local pain injection of local anesthetic may be required. Systemic medication may be needed for generalized pain.

Others, such as the bee, wasp, and hornet, contain unknown organic substances for which there is no specific antidote. (Remove the "stinger" if one is present.) At the site of bites or stings by poisonous spiders (especially the "black widow," *q.v.*), scorpions, *q.v.*, tarantulas, *q.v.*, poison fish, *q.v.*, etc., the tourniquet should be applied promptly.

Intravenous calcium gluconate given very slowly is specific for controlling muscle pain due to *black widow spider bite.*

Do not attempt to rub or pull off *jellyfish* (Portuguese man-of-war) sting tentacles because this will cause additional venom to be injected into area. Application of alcohol will cause tentacles to release. If this is not available, apply dry sand, salt or baking soda and allow to stand for 20 to 30 minutes. The tentacles can then be scraped off.

In *sting ray* injuries, first remove stinger, wash with water, and then immerse area in hot water for 30 to 90 minutes. If stinger has penetrated abdominal wall and entered perineal area, surgical exploration will be required.

Bitot's spots (bē'tōz) [Pierre A. Bitot, French physician, 1822-1888]. Triangular, shiny, gray spots on the conjunctiva seen in vitamin A deficiency.

bitter (bĭt'er) [A.S. *biter*, strong]. Having a disagreeable taste.

bitterling test (for pregnancy). A Japanese carplike fish is placed in a quart of fresh water with 2 teaspoonfuls of a woman's urine. A long tubular oviduct will protrude from the fish's belly if the woman is pregnant.

bituminosis (bĭ-tū-mĭ-nō'sĭs). Pneumoconiosis from dust of soft coal.

biuret (bī'ū-ret) [L. *bis*, two, + *urea*]. A crystalline decomposition derivative of urea.

b. reaction. Rose to violet coloring in an aqueous solution of protein, when dilute solution of copper sulfate and sodium hydroxide are added to it.

b. test. Use of above reaction to detect presence of urea or any soluble protein.

bivalent (bī-vā'lĕnt) [L. *bis*, two, + *valens*, powerful]. 1. Having a valence of 2 2. Biol: Double, as a chromosome consisting of two joined chromosomes. 3. A bivalent chromosome.

biven'ter [" + *venter*, belly]. A muscle with two bellies; pert. to several muscles.

biven'tral. Digastric; with two bellies.

Bjerrum screen. Tangent plane for mapping field of vision, esp. central and paracentral scotomata.

B. sign. One seen in glaucoma, a sickle-shaped blind spot usually found in central zone of the visual field. See: *sign*.

Bk. Symbol for *berkelium*.

B.L. Abbr. for *buccolingual*.

black (blăk) [A.S. *blaec*, dark]. 1. Devoid of color; reflecting no light. 2. Marked by dark pigmentation.

b. bone. Animal charcoal.

b. death. A contagious, malignant disease, as the bubonic plague.

b. eye. Subcutaneous extravasation of blood into the eye or orbit, usually the result of injury. Sym: Pain, swelling, discoloration. Treatment: Cold applications with pressure for 12 to 24 hr.—tends to prevent swelling.

b. fever. Kala-azar, *q.v.*

b. head. Comedo.*

b. measles. A severe type of measles in which the eruption is very dark due to hemorrhage under the skin.

b. vomit. The vomiting of black matter as in yellow fever.

blackberries. The dark fruit of a plant of the genus *Rubus*.

Canned, water packed without sugar added, 100 gm. Calories: 400. Protein and fat less than 1%. Other values: 22 mg. calcium; 0.6 mg. iron; 140 I.U. vitamin **A**; 7 mg. ascorbic acid.

blackhead. A plug of dried sebum in a sebaceous gland. Syn: *comedo*.

blackout. 1. Temporary loss of consciousness. 2. In aviators, temporary or transient loss of vision or consciousness due to a fall of blood pressure in the head. This is caused by the centrifugal force experienced in high-speed aircraft maneuvers.

blackwater fever [" + *waeter*, water]. Malarial hemoglobinuria, following chronic, falciparum malaria.

Symptoms and Signs: Sudden onset, fever, tender and enlarged liver and spleen, dark urine, epigastric pain, vomiting, jaundice, sudden shock.

black widow [" + A.S. *weoduwe*, widow]. *Lactrodec'tus mac'tans*. A poisonous spider.

bladder [A.S. *blaedre*, bladder]. 1. A membranous sac or receptacle for a secretion, as the *gallbladder, q.v.* 2. The vesicle which acts as a reservoir for urine. See: *urinary b.* and drawings under *genitourinary system*.

b., atony of. Inability to urinate, due to lack of muscular tone.

b., autonomous. One in which there is interruption in both afferent and efferent limbs of reflex arcs. Bladder sensations absent. Dribbling constant. Residual urine large in amount.

b., exstrophy of. The nonclosure of the bladder.

b., hypertonic. 1. One with excessive muscular tone. 2. Increased muscular activity of the bladder.

b., irritable. Marked by a constant desire to urinate.

b., nervous. Irritable b. with incomplete urination.

b., neurogenic. Dysfunction from lesion of central nervous system or nerves supplying the bladder.

b., spastic. An overactive bladder with reduced capacity and incontinence.

b., stammering of. Interruption of urination.

b., urinary (*vesica urinaria*). The muscular, membranous, distensible reservoir for the urine, which it receives from the kidneys through the ureters, and which it discharges from the body through the urethra. Its function is that of a reservoir for urine.

Anat: The lower portion continuous with the urethra, called the *neck;* its upper tip, connected with the umbilicus by median umbilical ligament, called the *apex*. The region between the two openings of the two ureters and the urethra is the *trigone*. The wall of the bladder consists of an inner mucous layer of transitional epithelium, a muscular coat of smooth muscle, the outer layer comprising the detrusor urinae, and a fibrous layer. On its free superior surface is a layer of peritoneum.

The bladder is supported by numerous ligaments, supplied by the sup., middle, and inf. vesical arteries, and numerous veins and lymphatics, and innervated with nerves derived from the third and fourth sacral by way of the hypogastric plexus.

It is situated in the ant. part of the pelvic cavity, in front of the ant. wall of the vagina and the uterus, and in the male it lies in front of the rectum. It has a storage capacity in health of one-half liter (500 ml.) or more. In disease states it may be greatly distended. A frequent cause of distention of the bladder in elderly males is hypertrophy of the prostate gland which surrounds the urethra and neck of the bladder.

Phys: An average of 40 to 50 oz. of urine are secreted within a 24-hr. period. This value is quite dependent upon amount of fluid ingested and loss of fluid through sweat and the bowels. Inability to empty the bladder is known as "retention" and may call for catheterization. Sphincter muscles are part of the mechanism which controls retention within the bladder.

The force of urination is much greater in the child than in the adult because the bladder is more nearly an abdominal than pelvic organ in the child. Thus the abdominal muscles help to expel the urine in the child.

Palpation of: The bladder cannot be palpated when empty. When full it appears as a tumor in the hypogastric region, which, on palpation, is smooth and oval.

Percussion of: When containing urine its rounded margin is easily made out by observing the tympanic sound of the intestines on one hand, and dull sound of the bladder on the other.

b. worm. A larval form of tapeworm with a rounded cyst or bladder into which a scolex is invaginated. The bladder worm of *Taenia solium* (pork tapeworm) encysts in muscles of pigs, that of *Taenia saginata* (beef tapeworm) in muscles of cattle. Syn: *cysticercus.*

bland [L. *blandus,* soft]. Soothing, mild.

b. diet. One soothing in flavor and texture; all food which causes chemical, mechanical, or thermal irritation is avoided.

Blandin's glands (blan-dăns') [Phillippe F. Blandin, French surgeon, 1798-1849]. Glandula lingualis ant. or Nuhn's glands. Glands near tip of tongue.

-blast. A suffix used to designate an immature cell or a structure which gives rise to a definitive structure. Ex: epiblast, erythroblast, fibroblast.

blast [G. *blastos,* germ]. 1. A nucleated erythrocyte; also called an *erythroblast.* 2. A violent movement of air such as accompanies the explosion of a shell or bomb; a violent sound as the blast of a horn.

b. injury. A clinical condition which follows severe nonpenetrating chest injuries due to explosions. Underwater explosions may cause this injury to swimmers.

blaste'ma [G. *blastēma,* sprout]. Immature or primitive material from which cells and tissues are formed.

blas'tid [G. *blastos,* germ]. The clear space marking site of the organizing nucleus in the impregnated ovum.

blasto- [G.]. Prefix: Germ or bud.

blastocele (blas'tō-sēl) [G. *blastos,* germ, + *koilos,* hollow]. The cavity of the blastula, an embryonic stage of development; the segmentation cavity.

blastochyle (blas'to-kīl) [G. *blastos,* germ, + *chylos,* juice]. Blastocelic fluid.

blastocyst (blas'tō-sist) [" + *kystis,* bag]. A stage in the development of a mammalian embryo which follows the morula. It consists of an outer layer or trophoblast to which is attached an *inner cell mass.* The enclosed cavity is the *blastocele.* The whole is called *blastodermic vesicle* or *blastocyst.*

blas'tocyte [" + *kytos,* cell]. The morula after change into a cyst.

blastocytoma (blas-tō-sī-tō'ma). Same as *blastoma.*

blas'toderm [" + *derma,* skin]. A disk of cells (*germinal disk* or *blastodisk*) which develops on the surface of the yolk in an avian or reptilian egg from which the embryo develops; also applied to the *embryonic disk* of mammalian embryos, a disk of cells lying between the yolk sac and the amniotic cavity from which the embryo develops. From the blastoderm, the three germ layers, *ectoderm, mesoderm,* and *endoderm* arise.

blastoderm'ic vesicle. A blastocyst.

blastogen'esis [G. *blastos,* germ, + *genesis,* generation]. 1. Multiplication by budding. 2. Transmission of characteristics from parents to offspring by the germ cells.

blastol'ysis [" + *lysis,* dissolution]. Lysis or destruction of a germ cell or a blastoderm.

blasto'ma (pl. *blastomata*) [" + *-ōma,* tumor]. A granular tumor formed by a single type of tissue, including *fibromas* and *chondromas.*

blastomere (blas'tō-mēr) [" + *meros,* a part]. One of the cells resulting from the cleavage or segmentation of a fertilized ovum.

blastomerot'omy [" + " + *tomē,* incision]. Destruction of blastomeres.

Blastomyces (blăst-ō-mī'sēz) (pl. *Blastomycetes*) [G. *blastos,* germ, + *mykes,* fungus]. A genus of pathogenic yeastlike organisms. They are dimorphic, occurring as budding yeastlike forms in tissues, but forming a mycelium in cultures.

B. brasiliensis. Fungus causing South American blastomycosis.

B. dermatitidis. The pathogen causing, in man, North American blastomycosis, a rare fungus infection.

blastomycetes (blas-to-mi-se'tēz) [" + *mykēs,* fungus]. Saccharomycetes; budding fungi; yeast fungi.

blastomyco'sis [" + *mykēs,* fungus]. A disease caused by budding yeastlike fungi in the tissues.

b., North American. A rare fungus infection caused by *Blastomyces dermatitidis.* Marked by inflammatory lesions of skin (cutaneous form) or lungs (pulmonary form); or a generalized invasion of skin, lungs, bones, central nervous system, kidneys, liver, and spleen (systemic form). Also called *Gilchrist's disease.*

b., South American. A serious infection caused by *Blastomyces brasiliensis.* Marked by inflammatory lesions of skin, mucous membranes and internal organs.

blastophore (blas'to-for). The part of the sperm cell which is not converted into the sperm.

blastopore (blas'to-pōr) [" + *poros,* passageway]. The small opening into the archenteron made by invagination of the blastula.

blas'tospore [" + *sporos,* seed]. A spore formed by budding from a hypha.

blastula (blas'tu-lă). An early stage in the development of an ovum consisting of a hollow sphere of cells enclosing a cavity, the *blastocele.* In large-yolked eggs, the blastocele is reduced to a narrow slit. In mammalian development, the blastocyst or blastodermic vesicle corresponds to the blastula of lower forms.

blas'tular. Pert. to a blastula.

Blatta. A genus of insects of the order Orthoptera which includes the cockroaches.

B. germanica. The German cockroach or croton bug.

B. orientalis. The oriental cockroach, a common house pest. Also called black beetle.

bleaching powder [A.S. *blaecan,* to pale]. Chlorinated lime.

blear-eye. Marginal blepharitis. Chronic inflammation of margins of eyelids.

bleb. Elevation of the epidermis, irregularly shaped. A blister or a bulla.

May vary in size from a bean to a goose egg and contain serous, seropurulent, or bloody fluid. A primary skin lesion. They occur in *dermatitis herpetiformis, pemphigus* and *syphilis*. SEE: *bulla*.

bleeder [A.S. *bledan*, to bleed]. One who lacks the facility to coagulate blood. Thus small cuts and injuries lead to profuse bleeding. Such a person may be treated with a blood fraction called *antihemophiliac factor*. SEE: *hemophilia*.

blee'der's disease. Hemophilia; a congenital blood condition marked by inability of blood to coagulate. SEE: *coagulation*.

bleeding (blēd'ing) [A.S. *bledan*, to bleed]. 1. Emitting blood. 2. Process of emitting blood, as a hemorrhage or operation of letting blood.

The plasma of the blood, when exposed to air, changes to allow fibrin to form. This entangles the corpuscles and forms a blood clot. SEE: *hemorrhage; blood clotting*.

b., arterial. This is indicated by bleeding in spurts. Color, bright red.

TREATMENT: Pressure with fingers above at nearest pressure point bet. it and heart. Locate artery and apply digital pressure above it until bleeding stops or until the artery is ligated.

b., breakthrough. Intermenstrual bleeding, especially that which occurs during use of progestational agents.

b., occult. Inapparent bleeding, especially that which occurs into the intestines and can be detected only by chemical tests of the feces.

b. time. Time required for blood to stop flowing from a small wound. This test is done by using one of several techniques. Depending on the method used, the time may vary from 1 to 3 (Duke method) or 1 to 9 minutes (Ivy method).

b., venous. Flow continuous. Color of blood, dark red.

TREATMENT: Patient recumbent. Pressure below wound with wound bet. heart and hand. Bandage over wound above and below.

blenn-, blenno- [G. *blennos*, mucus]. Combining form meaning mucus or pertaining to it.

blennadenitis (blen-ad-ĕ-nī'tis) [" + *adēn*, gland, + *-itis*, inflammation]. Inflammation of mucous glands.

blennemesis (blen-em'ĕ-sis [" + *emesis*, vomiting]. Vomiting of mucus.

blennogenic, blennogenous (blen-ō-jen'ik, blen-oj'ĕ-nus) [" + *gennan*, to produce]. Secreting mucus.

blennoid (blen'oid). Like mucus; mucoid.

blennometritis (blen-ō-mē-trī'tis) [G. *blennos*, mucus, + *mētra*, womb, + *-itis*, inflammation]. Inflammation of the uterus.

blennophthalmia (blen-off-thal'mĭ-ă) [" + *ophthalmos*, eye]. 1. Catarrhal conjunctivitis. 2. Gonorrheal ophthalmia.

blennorrhagia (blen-ō-rā'jĭ-ă) [" + *rēgnunai*, to break forth]. 1. A discharge from mucous membranes, esp. gonorrheal discharges from the genital or

BLEEDING: ARREST OF[1]

Artery	Bone Against Which Pressure Is Applied	Course	Spot to Apply Pressure
For Wounds of the Face			
Temporal	Temporal bone	Upwards of ½ in. in front of ear	Against bony prominence immediately in front of the ear or on temple
Facial	Low part of lower maxilla	Across the jaw diagonally upward from below	An inch in front of angle of lower jaw on the face
Carotid	Cervical vertebrae	From outer upper edge of sternum to angle of jaw	Deeply down and backwards an inch to the side of the prominence of the windpipe
For Wounds of the Upper Extremity			
Subclavian	First rib behind clavicle	Across middle of first rib to armpit	Deeply down and backwards over center of clavicle against first rib—(depress the shoulder first).
Axillary	Head of humerus	Descends across outer side of armpit to inside of humerus	High up in the armpit against upper part of humerus
Brachial	Shaft of humerus	Along inner side of humerus under edge of biceps muscle	Against shaft of humerus by pulling aside and gripping biceps, pressing deep down tips of fingers against the bone
For Wounds of the Lower Extremity			
(*a*) Femoral	Brim of pelvis	Down the thigh from the pelvis to the knee from a point midway bet. iliac spine and symphysis pubis to inner side of end of femur at knee joint	Against brim of pelvis, midway bet. iliac spine and symphysis pubis
(*b*) Femoral	Shaft of femur		High up on the inner side of the thigh, about 3 inches below brim of pelvis, over the line given in the direction of the knee
Posterior Tibial	Inner side of tibia, low down above ankle	Downwards to foot in hollow just behind the prominence of inner ankle	For wounds in the sole of the foot: against the tibia in center of the hollow behind the inner ankle

1. Hilda M. Gration, S.R.N.

urinary tract. 2. Gonorrhea. SEE: *blenorrhea.*

blennorrhagic (blen-ō-raj'ik). Pert. to blennorrhea; blennorrheal.

blennorrhea (blen-ō-rē'ă) [G. *blennos,* mucus, + *roia,* flow]. Discharge from mucous membranes, esp. gonorrheal discharge from genital or urinary tract. SYN: *blennorrhagia.*

b., inclusion. Inflammation of conjunctiva in newborn. Caused by a filtrable virus that forms cytoplasmic inclusion bodies in the epithelial cells.

b. neonatorum. Ophthalmia neonatorum caused by gonococci.

blennorrheal (blen-ō-re'ăl). Blennorrhagic; pert. to blennorrhea.

blennostasis (blen-os'tă-sĭs) [G. *blennos,* mucus, + *stasis,* a halt]. The checking of any mucous discharge.

blennostat'ic. Diminishing mucous secretion.

blennothorax (blen-ō-thō'raks) [" + *thōrax,* chest]. Accumulation of mucus in bronchial tubes or alveoli.

blennuria (blen-ū'rĭ-ă) [" + *ouron,* urine]. Excess of mucus in the urine.

blepharadenitis (blef-ar-ad-ĕ-nī'tis) [G. *blepharon,* eyelid, + *adēn,* gland, + *-itis,* inflammation]. Inflammation of the meibomian glands. SYN: *blepharoadenitis.*

blepharal (blef'ar-al). Pert. to an eyelid.

blepharectomy (blef"ă-rek'to-mĭ). Surgical excision of a lesion of the eyelid.

blepharedema (blef-ar-ĕ-dē'mă) [G. *blepharon,* eyelid, + *oidēma,* swelling]. Swelling of the eyelids.

blepharelosis (blef"ar-el-o'sis) [" + *eilein,* to roll]. Ingrowing eyelashes.

bleph'arism [" + *ismos,* condition of]. Twitching or blinking of the eyelids.

blepharitis (blef-ar-ī'tis) [" + *-itis,* inflammation]. Inflammation of the edges of the eyelids involving hair follicles and glands opening on surface; ulcerative and nonulcerative.

ETIOL: In ulcerative type, bacterial infection usually by staphylococci; in nonulcerative type, cause is often unknown. May be due to allergy, exposure to dust, smoke, or irritating chemicals.

SYM: Lids red, tender, and sore, with sticky exudate, ulcers on edges; lids may become inverted, lashes falling out, and epiphoria* occurring. Styes and meibomian cysts are associated with the condition.

NP: Bathe lids with warm saline solution to remove crusts. Ointment to edges.

b. angularis. B. in which medial angle of the eye is involved with blocking of openings of lacrimal ducts.

b. ciliaris. Inflammation affecting the ciliary margins of the eyelids.

b. marginalis. *B. ciliaris, q.v.*

b. parasitica. That caused by parasites such as mites or lice.

b. squamosa. B. with scaling.

b. ulcerosa. B. with ulceration.

blepharo- (blef-ar-o) [G.]. Prefix: Pert. to the eyelid.

blepharoadenitis (blef-ar-ō-ad-ĕ-nī'tis) [G *blepharon,* eyelid, + *adēn,* gland, + *-itis,* inflammation]. Inflammation of meibomian glands.

blepharoadenoma (blef-ar-ō-ad-ĕ-nō'mă) [" + " + *-ōma,* tumor]. Adenoma or glandular tumor of eyelid.

blepharoatheroma (blef"ar-ō-ath-ĕ-rō'mă) [" + *athērē,* thick fluid, + *-ōma,* tumor]. Sebaceous cyst of an eyelid.

blepharochalasis (blef-ar-ō-kal'ă-sis) [" + *chalasis,* relaxation]. Relaxation of skin of eyelid due to loss of elasticity following edematous swellings, such as in recurrent angioneurotic edema of lids. The redundant skin may droop over the edge of the eyelid when the eyes are open.

bleph"arochromidro'sis [" + *chrōma,* color, + *idrōs,* sweat]. Discolored sweat of the eyelid.

blepharoclonus (blĕf-ă-rok'lō-nus) [G. *blepharon,* eyelid, + *klonos,* tumult]. Clonic spasm of the muscles that close the eyelids (orbicularis oculi).

blepharoconjunctivitis (blef-ă-rō-con-junc-tĭ-vī-tis) [" + L. *conjunctiva,* + G. *-itis,* inflammation]. Inflammation of eyelids and conjunctiva.

blepharodiastasis (blef-ă-rō-dī-as'tă-sis) [" + *diastasis,* separation]. Excessive separation of eyelids.

blepharolithiasis (blef-ă-rō-lith-ī'ă-sĭs) [" + *lithos,* stone]. Concretions within the eyelid.

blepharon (blef'ă-ron). The eyelid; palpebra.

blepharoncus (blef-ă-ron'kus) [G. *blepharon,* eyelid, + *ogkos,* tumor]. Tumor of the eyelid.

blepharopachynsis (blef"ă-rō-pă-kin'sis) [" + *pachynsis,* thickening]. Thickening of the eyelid.

blepharophimosis (blef-ă-rō-fī-mō'sis) [" + *phimōsis,* narrowing]. Narrowing of slit between eyelids at external angle of eye due to angle being covered by vertical fold of skin.

blepharophryplasty (blef"ă-rof'rĭ-plas-tĭ) [" + *ophrys,* eyebrow, + *plassein,* to mold]. Plastic operation for restoration of eyelid and eyebrow.

bleph'aroplast [" + *plassein,* to form]. A minute mass of chromatin in a cell forming the base of a flagellum.

blepharoplasty (blef'ă-rō-plas-tĭ) [" + *plassein,* to form]. Plastic operation upon the eyelid.

blepharoplegia (blef-ă-rō-plē'jĭ-ă) [" + *plēgē,* a stroke]. Paralysis of an eyelid.

blepharoptosis (blef-ă-rop-tō'sis) [" + *ptōsis,* a falling]. Drooping of the upper eyelid.

blepharopyorrhea (blef-ă-rō-pī-or-ē'ă) [" + *pyon,* pus, + *roia,* flow]. Pus flowing from the eyelid.

blepharorrhaphy (blef"ă-ror'ă-fĭ) [" + *raphē,* seam]. Reducing length of or obliterating palpebral fissure by stitching margins of eyelids. May be required to prevent damage to the cornea. SYN: *tarsorraphy.*

blepharorrhea (blef-ă-rō-rē'ă) [" + *roia,* flow]. Discharge from the eyelid.

blepharospasm (blĕf'ă-rō-spăsm) [G. *blepharon,* eyelid, + *spasmos,* spasm]. A twitching or spasmodic contraction of the orbicularis oculi muscle due to habit spasm, eyestrain or nervous irritability.

blepharosphincterectomy (blef"ă-rō-sfink-ter-ĕk'tō-mĭ) [" + *sphigktēr,* a constrictor, + *ektomē,* excision]. Excision of part of the orbicularis palpebrarum to relieve pressure of eyelid on cornea.

blepharostat (blef'ă-rō-stat) [" + *istanai,* cause to stand]. Device for separating the eyelids during an operation.

blepharostenosis (blef"ă-rō-sten-ō'sis) [" + *stenōsis,* a narrowing]. Narrowing of the palpebral slit through inability to open the eye normally.

blepharosynechia (blef"ă-rō-sĭ-nĕk'ĭ-ă) [" + *synecheia,* a holding together]. Permanent adhesion of the eyelids.

blepharotomy (blef-ă-rot'ō-mĭ) [" + *tomē,* a cutting]. Cutting of eyelid.

blepsopathia (blep-sō-path'ī-ă) [G. *blepsis*, sight, + *pathos*, disease]. Neurasthenia caused by excessive eyestrain.

blind [A.S. *blind*, unable to see]. Without sight.

b. spot. Physiological scotoma situated 15° to outside of fixation point; corresponds to point where optic nerve enters the eye (optic disk), a region devoid of rods and cones. SYN: *optic disk.*

blindness [A.S. *blind*, unable to see]. Amaurosis; loss of sight.

b., color. Inability to distinguish one or more primary colors. SYN: *achromatopsia.*

b., c., amnesic. Inability to remember names of colors seen.

b., cortical. That resulting from a lesion of visual area of cerebral cortex.

b., day. Inability to see in daylight; hemeralopia.

b., eclipse. Blindness due to burning the macula while viewing an eclipse without using protective lenses.

b., flight. Blackout.

b., hysterical. Partial or total blindness associated with attacks of hysteria and occurring in absence of any organic defect.

b., letter. Inability to understand the meaning of letters; a form of aphasia.

b., night. Nyctalopia; inability to see at night.

b., psychic. Sight without recognition, due to brain lesion.

b., snow. Blindness resulting from glare of sunlight upon the snow. May result in photophobia and conjunctivitis, the latter resulting from effects of ultraviolet rays. Usually temporary.

b., word. Inability to understand written or printed words.

blindness, *words pert. to*: ablepsia, acatamathesia, achloropsia, "achro-" words, aglaukopsia, amianthinopsy, amaurosis, amaurotic, aphemesthesia, axanthopsia, acritochromacy, blind spot, blindness, chionblepsia, hemeralopia, hemiachromatopsia, hemianopia, meropia, nyctamblyopia, nyctophobia, nyctotyphlosis, tritanopia, typhlology, xanthocyanopia.

blister [M.E. *blester*, a swelling]. 1. A bleb or vesicle containing serum, sometimes caused by a pressure. 2. A collection of fluid below the epidermis, usually the result of a burn. 3. An agent producing a bleb.

TREATMENT: Mild antiseptic, protective dressing; if extremely painful due to pressure, may be aseptically punctured and then treated as a wound.

b., blood. Small subcutaneous or intracutaneous extravasation of blood due to rupture of blood vessels.

TREATMENT: Apply antiseptic and a firm dressing with moderate pressure to aid in stopping extravasation and hasten absorption. Sometimes desirable to puncture aseptically and aspirate.

b., fever. Herpes simplex of lip.

b., fly. Produced by application of *cantharides* to the skin.

b., flying. A therapeutic b. used long enough to produce redness but not actual blistering.

b., water. One containing water.

Blix's curve [Magnus G. Blix, Swedish physiologist, 1849-1904]. The curve demonstrated on a diagram of the tension produced against the length of a muscle when the muscle is detached from its insertion and made to contract isometrically at different lengths. SYN: *length-tension diagram.*

bloated (blōt'ĕd) [A.S. *blōtian*, to swell up]. Swollen or distended beyond normal size, as by serum, water, gas, etc.

block [O.Fr. *bloc*, a piece of wood, an obstruction]. 1. An obstruction or stoppage. 2. To stop the passage of sensory impulses in a nerve, nerve trunk, dorsal root of a spinal nerve, or spinal cord thus depriving a patient of sensation in the area involved. Accomplished by injection of a local anesthetic. SEE: *anesthesia.* 3. To obstruct any passageway or opening.

b., air. A leakage of air from the respiratory passageways and its accumulation in connective tissues of the lungs, there forming an obstruction to the normal flow of air.

b., atrioventricular. SYN: *A-V block.* SEE: *heart block.*

b., ear. Blockage of auditory tube to the middle ear. May result from trauma or from infection.

b., field. Regional anesthesia in which a limited operative area is walled off by an anesthetic.

b., heart. Interferences with the heart's contraction, causing dissociation of the atrial and ventricular rhythms. Due to failure of the contractile impulses to pass through the conductile tissue (atrioventricular node and bundle of His). SEE: *heart block.*

b., neuromuscular. A disturbance in transmission of impulses from motor endplate to a muscle. May be caused by an excess or deficiency of acetylcholine or by drugs which have an action simulating these effects.

b., paravertebral. Infiltration of stellate ganglion with a local anesthetic.

b., sinoatrial. SEE: *heart block, sinoatrial.*

b., spinal. Blockage in the flow of cerebrospinal fluid within spinal canal.

b., ventricular. Interference in the flow of cerebrospinal fluid between the ventricles or from the ventricles through the foramina to the subarachnoid space.

blocking. 1. Interruption in free association during psychoanalysis as a defense against unpleasant ideas. 2. PSY: A sudden, unaccountable stoppage of speech or thought. May be due to a conflict or painful thought. 3. Process of obstructing or deadening, as a nerve.

blood [A.S. *blōd*]. The fluid that circulates through the heart, arteries, veins, and capillaries carrying nourishment, electrolytes, hormones, vitamins, antibodies, heat, and oxygen to the tissues and taking away waste matter and carbon dioxide.

FUNCT: (a) Nutrition and respiration of tissues located far from the food and air supplies; (b) transportation of waste from the tissues to the excretory organs; (c) chemical and thermal coordination of the body; (d) defense against infection through the action of antibodies* and phagocytes.*

COMP: Human blood is composed of a fluid part (*plasma**) in which are suspended red and white corpuscles,* platelets* and fat globules. Blood consists of 22% solids and 78% water.

The amount of blood in man, measured in pints, can be computed approximately by dividing the weight in pounds by 14; using the metric system, an adult weighing 70 kg. has a blood volume of about 5.5 liters. Its *specific gravity* varies from 1.048 to 1.066, the corpuscles being heavier and plasma lighter than this. Blood is of slightly higher specific gravity in men than in women. Specific gravity is higher after exercise and at night.

In passing through the lungs the blood gives up carbon dioxide; after leaving the heart it is carried to the tissues as arterial blood, and then returned to the heart. It moves in the aorta at an average speed of 30 cm. per second and it makes the circuit of the vascular system in about 20 seconds. It constitutes approximately 7 to 8% of the body weight. SEE: *circulation.*

CHARACTERISTICS: It has a distinctive odor. Arterial blood is bright red or scarlet; the venous blood dark red or crimson.

b., clotting of. The process whereby blood changes into a jelly-like, nonfluid mass. Blood plasma normally contains fibrinogen, a protein. When blood is exposed to air, foreign substances, or juices from injured tissues, a new substance, thrombin, appears in it. Thrombin converts fibrinogen into the insoluble fibrin, a stringy, elastic substance that forms a meshwork in which the corpuscles are caught. Calcium deficiency causes tendency to slow clotting. SEE: *coagulation.*

b., components. Blood may be transfused in its whole state or one of its components may be administered. Some of these are:

Antihemophilic concentrates. Fractions of the blood rich in antihemophilic globulin. Prepared from quick-frozen plasma.

Immune and hyperimmune serum (gamma) globulin. Protein fractions used for persons who are deficient in gamma globulin or to produce passive immunity against certain diseases such as viral hepatitis.

Packed red cells. Blood from which the plasma has been removed. Used for patients who need red blood cells but do not need plasma. Use of this component reduces overload of the circulatory system and the risk of undesired antigenic response to the blood.

Packed frozen red cells. Type O, Rh-negative blood cells which have been separated from the plasma and frozen in a solution of glycerol, glucose, fructose and sodium ethylenediamine tetraacetic acid (Na_2 EDTA). The cells are thawed just before transfusion. The advantage of this technic is that the blood may be stored in a frozen state at —80° C. for as long as a year.

Plasma. Blood from which the cellular material has been removed. Though widely used in World War II and subsequently, the use of plasma has decreased. The risk of viral hepatitis when pooled plasma is used is considerable.

SEE ALSO: *table below.*

b., defibrinated. If whole blood is stirred in a dish (*e.g.*, with a stick of wood) the stringy, elastic *fibrin* comes out on the stirrer; it can be washed until white. The remaining thick, red blood can no longer clot, and is called defibrinated blood.

If it is centrifuged, the clear liquid which now appears in the upper half of the centrifuged tube is called *serum;* this differs from plasma chiefly in that it contains no more fibrinogen (the parent substance of fibrin). The corpuscles are in the lower half of the tube.

b., occult. Hidden blood; blood which has undergone changes, thereby preventing recognition of hemorrhaging.

b., sludged. Blood in which red corpuscles have massed together in the smaller blood vessels, and block or slow the blood flowing through the vessels.

RS: *erythrocytes; leukocytes.*

blood bank. Storing place for reserve blood kept for emergency transfusions.

Blood Components

Blood	Water 78%	Proteins	18.5%
		Glucose	0.1
		Lipids (fats)	1.4
	Solids 22%	Salts (inorganic)	1.5
		Waste products, etc.	0.5

Blood

- **Cells**
  - **Red blood cells (Erythrocytes)**
  - **White blood cells (Leukocytes)**
  - **Platelets**
- **Plasma**
  - **Water**
  - **Gases**
    - **Oxygen**
    - **Carbon dioxide**
    - **Nitrogen**
  - **Foods**
    - **Carbohydrate (Glucose)**
    - **Fat (fatty acids)**
    - **Protein (amino acids)**
  - **Blood proteins**
    - **Serum albumin**
    - **Serum globulin**
    - **Fibrinogen**
  - **Salts**
    - **Chlorides**, **Bicarbonates**, **Sulfates**, **Phosphates** —of— **Sodium**, **Calcium**, **Potassium**, **Magnesium**
  - **Protective substances:**
    - **Antitoxin**
    - **Opsonins**
    - **Agglutinin**
    - **Bacteriolysins**
  - **Autacoids (internal secretions from ductless glands)**
  - **Waste**
    - **Urea**
    - **Uric acid**
    - **Creatinine**
    - **Xanthine**
    - **Hypoxanthine**
    - **Guanine**
    - **Adenine**
    - **Carnine**

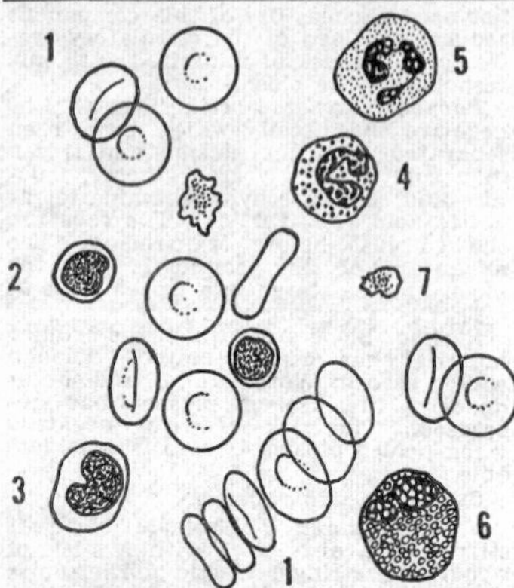

1. Red blood cells. 2. Immature (nucleated) red blood cell. 3. Lymphocyte. 4. Eosinophil. 5. Neutrophilic leukocyte. 6. Basophil. 7. Blood platelet.

Blood is mixed with sodium citrate, physiological saline solution and glucose (ACD solution), and is then stored at 4° C. (39° F.). Used up to 3 weeks after storage, but preferably should not be older than 5 days.

blood cell [A.S. *blōd*, blood, + L. *cella*, small chamber]. Minute body in the blood of two types: erythrocyte or red blood corpuscle, and leukocyte or white blood corpuscle. SYN: *b. corpuscle.*

b. c. casts. Masses of red cells molded by the renal tubules, the blood originating from the glomeruli. Abnormal microscopic body in the urine composed of coagulated serum covered with red blood cells.

blood clot. Coagulated mass of blood. SYN: *coagulum.* SEE: *b., clotting.*

blood corpuscles. The solid or cellular elements in the blood. SYN: *b. cell.* SEE: *erythrocytes; leukocytes.*

blood count. Enumeration of the red corpuscles and the leukocytes per cu. mm.

A blood count indicates the number of cells. The *differential blood count* tells the percentage of the various white cells in each 100 cells counted.

Normally in each cu. mm. of blood there are an average of five million erythrocytes in the male and four and a half million in the female. Prolonged exposure to altitude increases the number. The leukocytes average 5,000 to 10,000 per cu. mm. Platelets average 200,000 to 300,000 per cu. mm. by direct counting method.

A special chamber is filled with blood and the cells are counted using the microscope. The type of fluid used to dilute the blood depends upon whether the white or red cells are to be counted.

The differential count is done by counting at least 200 white cells in the stained smear of the blood which has been placed on a microscope slide. Pathologic cells are also looked for, and platelets, and hemoglobin and hematocrit tests are also made.

A DIFFERENTIAL BLOOD COUNT: This is an examination of the blood by stained specimens to ascertain the characteristic of the red blood cells and the variety of the white ones.

Some blood diseases, and inflammatory conditions may be recognized in this way. In a differential count, the varieties of the leukocytes and their percentages should be normally: Neutrophils (segmented), 40 to 60%; eosinophils, 1 to 3%; basophils, 0 to 1.0%; lymphocytes, 20 to 40%; monocytes, 4 to 8%.

blood crossmatching. The process of mixing a sample of the donor's red blood cells with the recipient's serum (major crossmatching), and mixing a sample of the recipient's blood with the donor's serum (minor crossmatching). This is used *before* transfusion to determine compatibility of blood.

blood donor. One who gives blood to be used for transfusion.

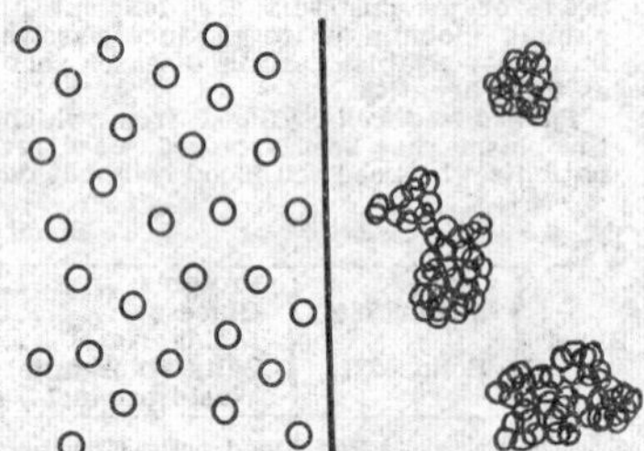

MAJOR CROSSMATCHING

The red blood cells of the donor are mixed with the serum of the recipient. **Left:** Compatibility; no agglutination. **Right:** Incompatibility with formation of clumps. This donor cannot be used.

Tabular Summary of Blood Corpuscles

Corpuscles (Cells)	Nucleus	Cytoplasm		Average diameter (Microns)	Number per cu. mm.
		Color	Granules		
Erythrocytes or red blood corpuscles	Absent	Red	None	5.5 to 8.8	4,300,000 to 6,000,000
Platelets (Not true cells)	?	None	None	2 to 4	200,000 to 500,000
Leukocytes or white blood corpuscles	Varies with different types	None	Varies with different types	7 to 20	5,000 to 10,000

blood dust. Minute colorless bodies in the blood, particles of the blood corpuscle. SYN: *hemoconia.*

blood examinations. They may be morphological, chemical, physical, bacteriological, and serological.

Blood is difficult to study because it so promptly clots unless anticoagulants are added to it. SEE: *table, Constituents in Blood, on B-29.*

WHAT THE EXAMINER LOOKS FOR: The number and character of the red blood cells, the percentage of hemoglobin, the coagulation time,* the number and character of white blood cells, the presence of parasites; also in chemical tests the amount of sugar, urea, urea-nitrogen, nonprotein nitrogen, creatinine, and uric acid. Complement fixation reactions, the basis of many tests, may be determined for infection, as syphilis, tuberculosis, etc. Culture should be made if bacteria are suspected.

CHEMICAL FINDINGS: Following amounts for some of the chemical constituents of blood are within so-called normal limits; deviations from these amounts, while not necessarily a sign of disease, indicate a need for further investigation:

calcium: 4.5-5.5 mEq./L. Serum (9.0 to 11 mg./100 ml.)
carbon dioxide combining power: 24-29 mEq./L., 53-64 vol.% (whole blood)
chloride: 100-106 mEq./L. serum
cholesterol, total: 150-250 mg./100 ml. serum
creatinine: 0.7-1.5 mg./100 ml. serum
glucose (fasting): 60-100 mg./100 ml. of blood
nonprotein nitrogen: 15-35 mg./100 ml. serum
sodium: 136-145 mEq./L. serum
urea nitrogen: 10-20 mg./100 ml. whole blood
uric acid: 3.0-6.0 mg./100 ml. serum

Whenever blood is to be collected from a vein the following points should be observed:

1. The syringe and needle should be not only sterile, but either dry or washed out with sterile normal saline solution. In particular the syringe should contain no trace of alcohol or ether, and preferably no distilled water.

2. The blood withdrawn is put into test tubes which are sterile and either (a) plain dry or (b) oxalated (*i. e.*, containing a small quantity of sodium or potassium oxalate powder). (a) Plain tubes are required for: Wassermann reaction, Widal and other agglutination reactions, van den Bergh reaction, blood calcium. (b) Oxalated tubes are required for: Blood sugar, blood urea, nonprotein nitrogen (N. P. N.), etc.

3. Immediately the blood has been expelled from the syringe, this and the needle should be washed out with normal saline or cold water. In this way "jamming" of the piston is avoided. This is of course unnecessary if disposable needles and syringes are used.

blood groups (or **types**). The separation of human bloods into four groups based on the presence or absence of *agglutinogens* in red cells and *agglutinins* in the plasma. When incompatible bloods are mixed, agglutination and hemolysis may occur followed by severe systemic reactions and possibly death. Blood groups have a hereditary basis and are dependent upon a series of alternative genes (triple alleles), a fact sometimes utilized in solving problems of disputed parentage. The groups are designated by the letters O, A, B, AB. SEE: *agglutinogens.*

bloodless. Without blood.

b. operation. One by which the blood is expelled by compresses from the part

Method of Testing Blood Groups

Serum of Group	Agglutinin in Serum	Recipient Red Blood Cells of Group				Remarks
		O	A	B	AB	
O	Anti-A and Anti-B	not agglutinated	agglutinated	agglutinated	agglutinated	Cells of Group O *not* agglutinated by any sera. Contains no agglutinable substances. *Universal Donors* (45% of adults).
A	Anti-B	not agglutinated	not agglutinated	agglutinated	agglutinated	Cells of Group A agglutinated by sera of Groups O and B (40% adults)
B	Anti-A	not agglutinated	agglutinated	not agglutinated	agglutinated	Cells of Group B agglutinated by sera of Groups O and A (10% adults).
AB	None	not agglutinated	not agglutinated	not agglutinated	not agglutinated	Cells of Group AB agglutinated by sera of Groups O, A, B. Serum of Group AB contains no isoagglutinins. *Universal recipient* (5% adults).

When recipient is Group O, select Donor from Group O
" " " " A, " " " " O or A
" " " " B, " " " " O or B
" " " " AB, " " " " O, A, B, AB

which is to be operated upon, or by electrocautery.

blood platelets. Small, colorless bodies in circulating blood, averaging about 3 microns in diameter which, in shed blood, tend to agglutinate into small clusters. They may originate from giant bone marrow cells (megakaryocytes). They play an important rôle in clotting through release of *thrombokinase* which, in the presence of calcium, reacts with prothrombin to form thrombin.

The normal number in circulating b., is about 200,000 to 500,000 per cu. mm. Reduction below normal is called *thrombocytopenia.* In certain forms of hemophilia, they are abnormally stable and fail to release thrombokinase, thus increasing coagulation time.

blood poisoning. A vague term usually used to indicate the presence of large numbers of bacteria in the circulating blood. SEE: *pyemia; septicemia; toxemia.*

blood pressure. As popularly used, the pressure existing in the large arteries at the height of the pulse wave; the systolic intra-arterial pressure.

More generally, the pressure exerted by the blood on the wall of any vessel. This pressure reaches its highest values in the left ventricle during systole, it is lower successively in the left arteries, capillaries, and veins, and sinks to subatmospheric values in the large veins during diastole.

The systolic arterial blood pressure itself rises during activity or excitement and falls during sleep. In the normal, relaxed, sitting adult, it is likely to be between 110 and 145 mm. of mercury.

The following findings are considered abnormal: (1) Systolic pressure persistently above 150; (2) diastolic pressure persistently above 100; (3) pulse pressure constantly greater than 50. Blood pressure varies with age, sex, altitude, muscular development, and according to states of worry and fatigue. It is usually lower in women than in men; low in childhood and high in advancing age as a rule. SEE: *Normal blood pressure.*

b. p., diastolic. That existing during relaxation phase between heart beats, normally about 80 mm. Hg. It is dependent primarily upon the elasticity of the arteries and peripheral resistance which in turn is dependent upon caliber of arterioles and capillaries.

b. p., indirect measurement of. The blood pressure may be measured by any intelligent person who will take the time to learn the procedure. The same arm, usually the right, should be used each time the pressure is measured. The arm should be at the level of the heart, and the patient should be sitting or recumbent. Either a mercury-gravity or aneroid manometer type of blood pressure apparatus may be used. The blood compression cuff should be of the width and length appropriate for the size of the subject's arm: narrow (2.5 to 6 cm.) for infants and children and wide (13 cm.) for adults.

The deflated cuff is placed evenly and snugly around the upper arm so that its lower edge is about one inch above the point on the brachial artery where the bell of the stethoscope will be applied.

While feeling the radial pulse, inflate the cuff until the pressure is about 30 mm. above the point where the radial pulse was no longer felt. Deflate the cuff slowly and record as accurately as possible the pressure at which the pulse returns to the radial artery. This is the *palpatory method* of obtaining the systolic blood pressure. Diastolic blood pressure cannot be determined by using this method.

To obtain the blood pressure using the *auscultatory method,* begin as above. After inflating the cuff until the pressure is about 30 mm. above the point where the radial pulse disappears, place the bell of the stethoscope over the brachial artery just below the blood pressure cuff. Then deflate the cuff slowly, about 2 to 3 mm. of mercury per heart beat. The first sound heard from the artery is recorded as the systolic pressure. The point at which sounds are no longer heard is recorded as the diastolic pressure. For convenience the blood pressure is recorded as figures separated by a slant. The systolic value is recorded first. For example, 120/80 indicates systolic pressure of 120 and diastolic of 80.

The experienced person will note the sounds heard over the brachial artery change in quality at some point prior to the point the sounds completely disappear. Some physicians consider this the diastolic pressure. This value should be noted when recording the blood pressure by placing it between the systolic pressure and the pressure noted when the sound disappears. Thus 120/90/80 would indicate a systolic pressure of 120, a *first diastolic pressure* of 90 and a *second diastolic pressure* of 80. The latter pressure would be the point of disappearance of all sounds from the artery. When the values are so recorded the physician may use either of the last two figures as the diastolic pressure. When the change in sound and the disappearance of all sound coincide, the result should be written as follows: 120/80/80.

b. p., mean. Half of the sum of systolic and diastolic values. For a normal person in good health, about 100 mm. Hg.

b. p., negative. That which is less than atmospheric pressure as in the great veins near the heart.

b. p., normal. In healthy young persons, 100 to 120 mm. of mercury systolic and 60 to 80 mm. diastolic. Upper limits of normal are 140/100, with systolic pressure greater than 140 mm. generally believed to be abnormal. Loss of resilience in the vascular tree and physiologic changes of age must be considered when levels above 140 mm. are obtained in apparently healthy, older persons.

b. p., systolic. The greatest force caused by the contraction of the left ventricle of the heart.

RS: *diastole; hypertension; hypotension; pulse pressure; systole.*

bloodshot. Locally congested with blood.

blood smear. Drop of blood spread on a slide for purpose of examination.

PROCEDURE: Clean glass with alcohol, rinse in warm water and wipe clean with lint-free towel or lens paper. Slide must be grease-free. Place a small drop of blood on the slide. Bring the end of another slide (spreader slide) against first slide at a 45° angle and pull it back against drop of blood so that the drop will spread between the two slides. Then push spreader slide forward against the first slide and the blood will follow forming an even smear. Smear must be thin. Dry slide by waving in air. Do not heat.

STAIN: A common method is as follows: Cover the blood smear with Wright's stain. Allow to stand 2 min. Add an equal amount of distilled water or buffer solution, mixing uniformly. Let stand 5 min. Gently wash off stain. Allow to dry. If permanent slide is desired, mount with balsam or methacrylate.

blood sugar. Sugar in the form of glucose, normally 60 to 100 mg. per 100 ml. of blood.

It rises after a meal to 150 mg. per 100 ml. of blood but this may vary. Above this amt. sugar enters the urine.

b. s. test. Increased glucose content of the blood, or presence of glucose in the urine indicates faulty metabolism and diabetes. The urine may be free of sugar but the blood sugar may have increased, which necessitates a glucose tolerance test being made.

blood test. To ascertain contents of the blood.

BLOOD UREA: For this test 10 cc. of blood are withdrawn into a sterile test tube containing a few crystals of calcium oxalate.

UREA CLEARANCE TEST: This test gives more accurate information as to the efficiency of the kidney than the above. It shows the amt. of blood cleared of urea in a given time. It is carried out bet. breakfast and lunch as follows:

The bladder is completely emptied. Exactly 1 hr. after, the bladder is again emptied. The specimen of urine obtained is kept. One hr. after, this is repeated. Blood, for blood urea, is withdrawn at the end of the first hr. No coffee is allowed for breakfast. Tea is sometimes allowed.

ORAL GLUCOSE TOLERANCE TEST: The fasting level of blood glucose is normally 60 to 100 mg. per 100 ml. whole blood. If large amounts of carbohydrate are taken, the glucose level may rise to as high as 150 mg. The level falls to fasting level within 3 hours.

TEST: No food or drink after 9 P. M. the evening before. In the morning blood is withdrawn and the amt. of glucose estimated. This represents the fasting level. The patient then empties the bladder completely and drinks a solution of 100 gm. of glucose in 500 ml. of water flavored with lemon juice. Samples of whole blood and urine are taken ½, 1, 2, and 3 hours after ingestion of glucose. The glucose level normally rises to about 150 mg. within 1 hour after ingestion of the glucose and then falls to the fasting level (60 to 100 mg. per 100 ml. whole blood) within 3 hours.

b., test for, in urine. Take 1 in. of urine in a test tube and add 1 or 2 drops of tincture of guaiacum. Carefully overlay this with ½ in. of ether. Hold the tube in the hand to warm it for a few minutes. Blood is indicated by the appearance of a blue line at the junction of the fluids.

blood transfusion. The transference of the blood of one person into the blood vessels of another. In direct or immediate transfusion, the blood is transferred without being exposed to air; in *indirect* or *mediate* transfusion, the blood is collected in a receptacle from the donor before transfusion.

blood typing. The method used to determine various factors when blood is tested according to blood group systems such as A-B-O, M-N, and Rh-Hr.

PROCEDURE: Place a drop of 2% saline suspension of patient's blood cells on each end of a slide labeling the drops A and B. Add a small drop of A typing serum to the A drop, of B typing serum to the B drop. Mix thoroughly. After 5 min. examine for agglutination. Type of blood can be determined by reactions as follows: No agglutination—Type O; Drop A only agglutinated—Type B; Drop B agglutinated only—Type A; Both drops agglutinated—Type AB. SEE: illustration page B-31.

bloody flux. Dysentery.

bloody sweat. Excretion of blood or blood pigment through the sweat glands. SYN: *hemathidrosis.*

bloody vomit. A result of rupture of the blood vessels of the upper alimentary tract due to injury, disease, or swallowing of blood.

TREATMENT: Do not give stimulants; nothing by mouth. Keep patient quiet and lying down. Cold applications to lower chest and upper abdomen.

bloody weeping. Hemorrhage from conjunctiva.

Blot's perforator (blōz) [Hippolyte Blot, French obstetrician, 1822-1888]. Instrument used to perforate the fetal skull to facilitate its delivery.

blotch. A blemish, spot, or area of discoloration on the skin.

blow'fly. One of a number of genera of flies belonging to the family Calliphoridae. Most are scavengers, their larvae living in decaying flesh or meat although occasionally they may live in decaying or suppurating tissue. One species, the screw-worm fly *Callitroga hominivorax,* however, attacks living tissue, laying its eggs in the nostrils or open wounds of the host domestic animals or man giving rise to *myiasis.*

blowing respiration. Bellows murmur of the heart.

blowpipe. A tube through which a gas is passed under pressure, the gas being directed upon a flame; it is employed to concentrate and intensify the heat of the flame.

blue [O.Fr. *bleu,* blue]. 1. A primary color of the spectrum; sky color; azure. 2. Cyanotic.

b. baby. A child born with a very blue color due to mixture of the venous and arterial blood through a defect in the heart.

b., brilliant cresyl. A dye used in staining blood.

b. drum. Bluish appearance of tympanic membrane.

b., Evans. A dye, injected intravenously, for determining blood volume.

b. mass. A compound pill of mercury.

b., methylene. A dye used for staining tissues; also used as an indicator.

b. ointment. Mercurial ointment.

b. stone. Copper sulfate, *q.v.*

b., toluidine. A metachromatic dye used as a stain for tissues.

b. vitriol. SEE: *copper sulfate.*

blueberries. The blue or blue-black fruit of several types of bush of the genus *Vaccinium.*

RAW: 100 gm. Calories: 62. Other values: 13 mg. calcium; 1.0 mg. iron; 100 I.U. vitamin A; 0.06 mg. riboflavin; 14 mg. ascorbic acid.

bluecomb (bloo'kōm). A disease of turkeys characterized by cyanosis. It is due to infection with *Erysipelothrix rhuziopathiae.*

Blumberg's sign. The occurrence of a sharp acute pain when the examiner presses his hand over McBurney's point and then releases the hand pressure suddenly. This sign is indicative of peritoneal inflammation.

Blu'menbach's clivus [Johann F. Blumenbach, German physiologist, 1752-1840]. Sloping part of sphenoid bone behind post. clinoid processses.

Blumenthal's disease. Leukemia in which there is an excessive amount of immature blood cells—both red and white—in the blood.

blush'ing [A.S. *blyscan,* to be red]. Rush of blood to the face caused by embarrassment or other emotion.

Blyth's test [Alexander W. Blyth, English physician, 1846-1921]. A test for the detection of lead in drinking water. In the presence of lead a white precipitate forms on the addition of a small amount of alcoholic tincture of cochineal to the water to be tested.

B.M.A. Abbr. for *British Medical Association.*

B.M.R. Abbr. for *basal metabolic rate.*

B.M.S. Abbr. for *Bachelor of Medical Science.*

BNA. Abbr. for *Basic Nomina Anatomica,* an anatomical nomenclature adopted by the German Anatomical Society in 1895, at Basle, Switzerland. It includes some 4500 terms.

Boas motor meal [Ismar I. Boas, German physician, 1858-1938]. Test for tonicity of bowels. If, the morning after an Ewald-Boas test meal was given, lavage shows the stomach to be empty, there is normal motility.

B. point. A tender spot left of the 12th dorsal vertebra in patients with gastric ulcer.

B. reagent. Formula for testing hydrochloric acid in gastric juice.

B. sign. The presence of lactic acid in the gastric contents.

Bochdalek's ganglion (bok'dal-ek) [Victor Bochdalek, Czechoslovakian anatomist, 1801-1883]. Ganglion of plexus of dental nerve in the maxilla above the canine tooth.

Bo'do. A genus of flagellate protozoa often found in stale feces or urine and sometimes in the urinary bladder. Nonpathogenic.

body [A.S. *bodig,* body]. Soma; corpus. 1. The physical man. 2. The trunk without the head and extremities. 3. The principal part of anything. 4. A small organ or a structure within an organ.

EXAMINATION: The nude body is examined and both sides compared. Physical examination is made by *inspection, palpation, manipulation, mensuration,* and *auscultation, q.v.* Chemical and microscopic examination may be made of the blood, sputum, feces, urine, cerebrospinal fluids, and other fluids of the body. X-ray, or roentgen ray, is also used, and checked with clinical findings. The electrocardiograph is used for determining heart rhythms.

b., acetone. One of a number of substances which increase in the blood as the result of faulty fat metabolism. SYN: *ketone b.'s.*

b., aortic. Two small bodies located in the arch of the aorta which contain the endings of the aortic nerve. They respond to oxygen concentration in the blood and to changes in blood pressure.

b., Aschoff. Microscopic foci of fibrinoid degeneration and granulomatous inflammation found in various tissues in rheumatic fever.

b., Barr. Sex chromatin present at the edge of the nucleus of cells from the female.

b., basal. A basal granule or blepharoblast. A small granule usually present at the base of a flagellum or a cilium in protozoa.

b., carotid. A flat structure at the bifurcation of the common carotid artery. Contains cells which respond to changes in concentration of oxygen in the blood and to changes in blood pressure.

b., cavernous. One of three cylindrical bodies of erectile tissue found in the penis. SEE: *corpora cavernosa.*

b. cavities. The thorax, abdomen, and pelvis.

b. cell. 1. The main portion of a cell, esp. a neuron; the portion that contains the nucleus. 2. Somatic cell. Any cell of the body excepting the reproductive or germinal cells.

b., chromaffin. A number of bodies composed principally of chromaffin cells, *q.v.* which lie serially arranged along both sides of the dorsal aorta. Also called *paraganglionic bodies.* They are ectodermal in origin, having the same origin as cells of the sympathetic ganglia.

b., chromatoid. Darkly staining bodies found in the encysted forms of parasitic amebae. Thought to serve as reserve food. They disappear as cysts grow older.

b., chromophilic. One of the granular bodies in cytoplasm of a nerve cell which stain readily with basic dyes.

b., ciliary. A structure in the eye consisting of the ciliary muscle and ciliary processes. Functions in accommodation.

b., coccygeal. A mass of tissue consisting of one or several small nodules located at tip of coccyx. It contains an arteriovenous anastomosis. Its function is unknown.

b., Donovan's. *Donovania granulomatis.* Organism causing granuloma inguinale.

b., geniculate, lateral. Two bodies forming elevations on the lateral portion of the posterior part of the thalamus. Each is the termination of afferent fibers from the retina which they receive through the optic nerves and tracts.

b., geniculate, medial. Two bodies lying in the posterior part of the dorsal thalamus, connected by the commissure of Gudden. Each receives fibers from the acoustic center of the medulla and from the inferior colliculus through the brachium.

b., Hassall's. Hassall's corpuscle, found in the medulla of the thymus.

b., Hensen's. A modified Golgi net found in the hair cells of the organ of Corti of the ear.

b., inclusion. Cell inclusions. Nonliving substances in the protoplasm of a cell. Seen in virus infections.

b.'s, ketone. One of a number of substances which increase in the blood as a result of faulty fat metabolism. Among them are B-hydroxybutyric acid, acetoacetic acid, and acetone. They increase in diabetes mellitus and are the primary cause of acidosis. They may also occur in other metabolic disturbances. SYN: *acetone b.'s.*

b.'s, Leishman-Donovan. Small bodies found in the spleen and liver of victims of kala-azar or dum-dum fever. Now known to be *Leishmania donovani,* causative organism of the disease. They are found both within and outside of living cells and in circulating blood.

b., Malpighian. (1) A renal corpuscle consisting of a glomerulus enclosed in Bowman's capsule; (2) a lymph nodule found in the spleen.

b., mammillary. A rounded body of gray matter found in the diencephalon. It forms a rounded eminence projecting into the anterior portion of the interpeduncular fossa. Their nuclei constitute an important relay station for olfactory impulses.

b., medullary. The deeper white matter of the cerebellum enclosed within the cortex.

b., metachromic. Metachromic granule, *q.v.*

b.'s, Negri. Inclusion bodies found in the cells of the central nervous system of animals infected with rabies. They are acidophilic masses appearing in large ganglion cells or in cells of the brain esp. those of the hippocampus and cerebellum.

b.'s, Nissl. Also called Nissl granules or chromophil substance. Conspicuous structures in nerve cells demonstrated by selective staining. They are absent in the axon and axon-hillock. They show changes under various physiological conditions and in pathological conditions may dissolve and disappear (chromatolysis). SYN: *tigroid b.*

b., Pacchionian. Arachnoid granulation. Numerous small ovoid or villuslike projections of the subarachnoid membrane of the brain. They may project into the superior sagittal sinus as arachnoid villi or they may press against the outer dura and grow into the inner plate of the cranium forming ovoid depressions.

b., perineal. The mass of tissue which separates the anus from the vestibule and the lower part of the vagina.

b., pineal. The epiphysis, a dorsal outgrowth of the diencephalon. Also called pineal gland.

b., pituitary. The hypophysis; pituitary gland, *q.v.*

b., polar. A small cell produced in oogenesis resulting from the divisions of the primary and secondary oocytes. It has no functional significance.

b., postbranchial. Ultimobranchial bodies. Two bodies which develop from the post. wall of the 4th pharyngeal pouch. They become incorporated into the thyroid gland.

b., psammoma. Laminated calcareous bodies seen in certain types of tumors. Term also applied to sandlike bodies (brain sand) found in the pineal body. Also seen in prostate gland.

b., restiform. The inferior cerebellar peduncles. Two bands of fibers which connect the medulla with the cerebellum.

b., tigroid. The chromophil substance of neurons; Nissl bodies.

b., vertebral. A short column of bone forming the weight-supporting portion of a vertebra. From its dorsolateral surfaces project the roots of the arch of a vertebra.

b., vitreous. A jelly-like body within the eye which fills the space between the lens and the retina. It is colorless, structureless, and transparent.

b., Wolffian. The mesonephros or middle kidney of the embryo.

body mechanics. Mechanical correlation of the various systems of the body.

body snatching. Robbing a grave of its body. Done in the past to obtain bodies for anatomical study in medical schools.

body type. Classification of the human body according to certain physical characteristics. SEE: *somatotype.*

Boeck's sarcoid (beks) [Caesar P. M. Boeck, Norwegian physician, 1845-1917]. Sarcoidosis, *q.v.*

boil [A.S. *byl*, a swelling]. A furuncle. An acute circumscribed inflammation of the subcutaneous layers of the skin, gland, or hair follicle.

The deeper tissue inflammation is so severe that blood clots in the vessels and the center dies. This is the cause of the acuteness of the pain; the dead core is ultimately expelled or reabsorbed. Contrary to general opinion, boils do not arise from "bad blood," but are the result of local infection due to an invasion of staphylococci.

TREATMENT: Protect from irritation; apply moist heat intermittently. Keep skin scrupulously clean and avoid injury or trauma to involved region. Bed rest may be necessary in severe cases. After lesions are fluctuant, surgical incision and debridement may be desirable. The area around draining abscesses should be protected by an antibiotic ointment to prevent new lesions on surrounding areas. If lesions are large and located on the face, penicillin or some other antibiotic should be used systemically to prevent possible complications such as meningitis or septicemia.

b., Aleppo. SEE: *leishmaniasis. cutaneous.*

b., oriental. SEE: *leishmaniasis, cutaneous.*

boiling. Vaporization of a liquid.

1. Boiling water destroys organic impurities. 2. Boiling toughens and hardens albumin in eggs. 3. Boiling toughens fibrin and dissolves tissues in meat. 4. Boiling bursts starch granules. 5. Boiling softens cellulose in cereals and vegetables.

b. point. The degree of heat required to bring a liquid to a boil. It depends upon the liquid. Water boils at 212° F. (100° C.) under ordinary conditions at sea level. To kill microorganisms, water should be boiled 3-15 minutes. Aeration (pouring from one vessel to another) will overcome the flat taste of boiled water.

bolom'eter [G. *bolē*, a throw, + *metron*, measure]. 1 Device for measuring the force of the heart beat apart from blood pressure. 2. An instrument for gauging minute degrees of radiant heat.

bo'lus [G. *bōlos*, a mass]. A pill-shaped mass.

b., alimentary. A mass of masticated food ready to swallow.

bond. A mark or short line bet. atoms to indicate the number and attachments of the valencies of an atom giving a graphic representation of arrangement of the atoms of elements in the molecules of compounds as H-Cl.

bone [A.S. *bān*, bone]. The hardest connective tissue that forms the framework of the body. (1) Osseous tissue. A specialized form of dense connective tissue consisting of bone cells (*osteocytes*) embedded in a *matrix* consisting of calcified intercellular substance. (2) An individual unit of the skeleton. Bones give shape to and support the body. They also serve as a storage place for mineral salts and play an important role in the formation of blood cells.

It consists of about 50% water, and 50% solid matter, the solids being chiefly

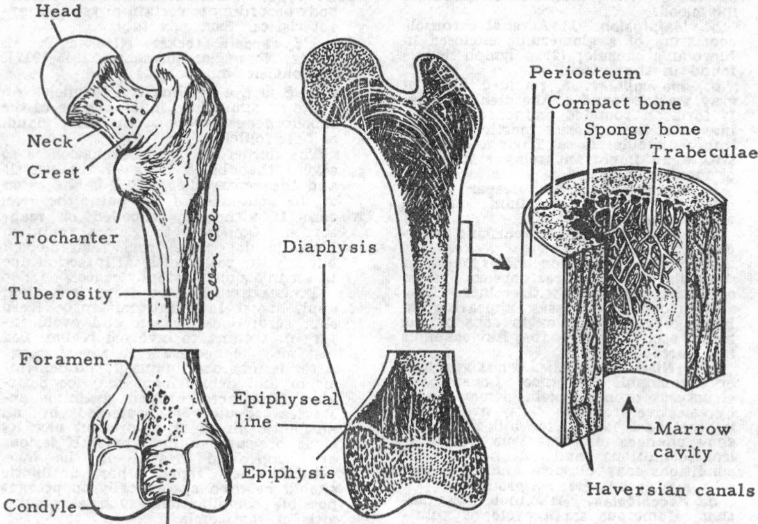

BONE — inner and outer structures

cartilage hardened by impregnation with inorganic salts, esp. carbonate and phosphate of lime. The proportion of lime in bone gradually increases and in old age there is such a large proportion that the bones are brittle and break easily.

They surround and protect some vital organs, and give points of attachment for the muscles, serving as levers and making movement possible.

The outer surface is less porous than the inner, and is called the compact tissue; the more porous portion is called cancellous tissue. The compact tissue is tunneled by a central canal containing marrow, and fine branching canals. In these canals run small blood vessels and lymphatics for the maintenance and repair of bone tissue. This is known as the Haversian system or canals. The exterior covering of the bone, or periosteum, serves to extend the blood supply to the bone. According to their shape, bones are classified as *flat, irregular, long,* and *short.*

CAVITIES: Depressions, openings, and cavities in bones consist of a *fissure,* a *foramen,* a *meatus* or *canal,* a *sinus* and *antrum, groove* or *sulcus,* and a *fossa.*

FORAMEN: Opening for blood vessels or nerves.

fossa. A concavity.

fissure. A slitlike opening.

meatus. A tubelike passage.

sinus. (a) Air cavity within a bone. (b) A groove lodging a blood sinus.

sulcus. A groove.

PROCESSES: Enlargements or protrusions.

crest. A ridge.

condyle. A rounded process for articulation.

head. Rounded end of a bone separated from the body by a constricted region: the neck.

spine. A pointed process.

trochanter. A very large process.

tubercle. A small rounded process.

tuberosity. A large rounded process.

b., ankle. The astragalus or talus.

b., breast. The sternum.

b., brittle. Abnormal brittleness of bones. SYN: *osteogenesis imperfecta.*

b., cancellous. A spongy bone in which the matrix forms connecting bars and plates partially enclosing many intercommunicating spaces filled with bone marrow.

b., cancer of. The red marrow becomes pale. Leukemic tissues tend to invade and destroy hard portions of the bone, anywhere in the body.

b., cartilage. Endochondral bone which develops from cartilage.

b., cavalry. Rider's b. Bony formation in adductor magnus femoris.

b., collar. The clavicle.

b., compact. Dense, hard bone with microscopic spaces.

b., cotyloid. One which during development forms a part of medial portion of the acetabulum. It fuses with the pubis.

b., cranial. A b. of the cranium or brain case.

b. cyst. B. tumor of cystic variety.

b., dermal. A membrane bone.

b., endochondral. Cartilaginous b.

b., Inca. An incarial b.

b., incarial. The interparietal b., part of the occipital b.

b., incisive. Part of maxilla bearing the incisor teeth.

b., innominate. Hip b., composed of the ilium, ischium, and pubis.

b., intracartilaginous. Cartilage or endochondral b.

b., ivory. Same as marble bone.

b., marble. Abnormally calcified bones with spotted appearance in a roentgenogram. SYN: *Albers-Schönberg disease; ivory bone; osteopetrosis.*

b., membrane. The intramembranous b.

b., perichondrial. One formed beneath the perichondrium.

b., periosteal. One formed by osteoblasts of the periosteum.

b., ping pong. The thin shell of osseous tissue covering a giant cell sarcoma in a bone.

b., replacement. Cartilage b., one which replaces cartilage.

b., sesamoid. One which develops in tendon, as the patella.

b., spongy. Cancellous bone.

b., sutural. A Wormian b.

b., thigh. The femur.

b., Wormian. A small irregularly shaped b., often found in the sutures of the cranium.

Names of principal bones: SEE: *skeleton.*

bone bank. Place for storage of bone to be used in bone grafts.

bone cell. One in osseous tissue or bone. It may be (a) an osteoblast or bone-forming cell; (b) an osteocyte which lies within a lacuna in bone matrix, or (c) an osteoclast, a giant, multinucleated cell occupying deep grooves (Howship's lacunae).

bone graft. A piece of bone taken either from some animal (foreign) or the body of the patient in which it is to be used (autogenous) and placed so as to encourage its growth and union with the bone it is being placed in contact with.

bone grafting. Transplanting a healthy bone to replace missing or defective bone.

bone'let. A small bone.

bone marrow. Medulla or soft tissues in the hollow of long bones and in the extremities of long bones. SEE: *marrow.*

bone reflex. A reflex action resulting from tapping or percussion; actually a tendon or muscle reflex.

bonine. Proprietary name for meclizine hydrochloride, an agent used for prevention and treatment of motion sickness and vomiting. Formerly marketed as *bonamine.*

bo'ny. Resembling or of the nature of bone. SYN: *osseous.*

boopia (bō-ŏp'ĭ-ă) [G. *bous,* ox, + *ōps,* eye]. The uninterested cowlike gaze seen in hysteria.

booster. An additional dose of an immunizing agent to increase the protection afforded by the original series of injections. The booster is given some months or years after the initial immunization.

bo'rate. A basic salt of boric acid.

bo'rated. That to which borax has been added.

borax [L.]. Sodium borate. It is found in some arid regions. Its chief use is as a detergent and water softener; also a weak antiseptic.

borborygmus (bor-bō-rig'mus) (pl. *borborygmi*) [G. *borborygmos,* rumbling in the bowels]. A gurgling, splashing sound heard over the large intestine; caused by passage of flatus through the intestine.

PATH: Its absence may denote such obstruction of the bowels as torsion, volvulus, or strangulated hernia.

border. The outer part or edge; boundary.

b., brush. A brushlike structure found on the free surface of epithelial cells in the proximal convoluted portion of a renal tubule. It consists of nonmotile hairs.

b., striated. A modified layer of the surface protoplasm of columnar epithelial cells lining the intestine. It consists of regular, perpendicular striations consisting of minute protoplasmic processes.

Bordet-Gengou bacillus (bor-dā'-zhon-goo') [Jules Bordet, Belgian physician, bacteriologist and physiologist, 1870-, and Octave Gengou, French bacteriologist]. *Bordetella pertussis,* the cause of whooping cough.

Bordetella [named for Jules Bordet]. A genus of Brucellaceae. Hemolytic gram-negative coccobacilli. The cause of whooping cough or an infection similar to whooping cough. SYN: *Bordet-Gengou bacillus.*

B. bronchiseptica. Cause of bronchopneumonia in rodents and dogs (as a complication of distemper in the latter), and of an infection resembling whooping cough in man.

B. pertussis. The cause of whooping cough. First isolated by Bordet and Gengou. Formerly called *Hemophilus pertussis.*

B. parapertussis. Cause of an infection similar to whooping cough.

boric acid. H_3BO_3. USP. An odorless, white, crystalline powder obtained by condensation and evaporation from certain mineral salts.

In solution it is used as mild antiseptic wash, esp. for the eyes, mouth, and bladder. As an ointment it is valuable in dressing burns, blisters, etc. When large doses are accidentally taken by mouth, as in children, it may be poisonous.

POISONING: SEE ALSO: *Table of Poisons and Poisoning in Appendix.*

SYM: Nausea, vomiting, diarrhea.

TREATMENT: Wash out stomach. Give saline cathartic and large volumes of water. Oxygen and plasma or blood transfusions as necessary.

bo'rism. Symptoms caused by internal use of borax or boron compounds include dry skin, eruptions, gastric disturbances.

boroglycerin (bor"ō-glis'ĕr-ĭn). A compound ($C_3H_5BO_3$) formed when boric acid and glycerin are heated together.

b. glycerite. A solution of boroglycerin (47-52%) in glycerin.

boroglycerol (bo-ro-glis'er-ŏl). Boroglycerin.

bo'ron [from Arabic *buroq*]. SYMB: B. A nonmetallic element, found only as a compound such as boric acid or borax. At. wt. 10.811; at. no. 5.

Borrelia (bor-rel'ĭ-ă). A genus of spirochetes including organisms responsible for relapsing fever.

B. duttonii. Causative agent for tick-borne relapsing fever.

B. recurrentis. Causative agent of louse-borne relapsing fever.

B. vincen'tii. A species found in Vincent's angina.

boss [O.Fr. *boce,* a swelling]. Any protuberance, esp. a round circumscribed swelling or growth such as occurs on a bone or tumor.

bos'selated. Marked by numerous bosses.

bossela'tion. One or more small bosses.

Bossi's dilator (bos'sēz). Metal instrument used to dilate the cervix by means of force.

botfly (pl. *botflies*). Insects belonging to the order Diptera of the family Oestridae. Parasitic on mammals, especially horses and sheep. Human infestation is rare.

botryoid (bot'rĭ-oid) [G. *botrys,* bunch of grapes, + *eidos,* appearance]. Resembling a bunch of grapes.

botryomycosis (bŏt-rĭ-ō-mī-kō'sĭs). Condition characterized by chronic granulomatous lesions caused by a fungus of the family Actinomycetaceae. SYN: *staphylococcal actinophytosis.*

bot'tle nose. Acne rosacea of the nose.

botuliform (bot-u'lĭ-form) [L. *botulus,* sausage, + *forma,* shape]. Shaped like a sausage.

botulin'ic acid. A toxin found in putrid sausage.

botulism (bŏt'ū-lĭzm). A severe form of food poisoning from food containing the botulinus toxin, produced by *Clostridium botulinum.* This organism is widely found in the soil and in the intestinal tract of domestic animals. Cases of human botulism are usually associated with development of the bacteria under anaerobic conditions in raw, improperly canned or otherwise preserved foods, esp. meats (as ham, sausage) and nonacid vegetables (as string beans). The toxin is a powerful exotoxin. It is very thermolabile losing its toxic properties when exposed to temperature of 80° C. for 30 min. or boiling for 10 min.

POISONING: The toxin has a selective action on the central nervous system. In fatal cases, cardiac and respiratory paralysis occur through involvement of the medullary centers.

SYM: Fatigue, weakness, dizziness, headache, and digestive complaints as nausea, vomiting, diarrhea and abdominal pain. Progresses to paralysis in the central nervous system, and of the cardiac and respiratory systems.

TREATMENT AND PROPHYLAXIS: Bivalent antitoxin for type A and B toxin should be administered to persons with clinical symptoms and to those persons who have eaten contaminated food but do not have symptoms. Type E antitoxin, which is available only from the Communicable Disease Center, Atlanta, Ga., should also be given. Careful and continuous nursing care is necessary. SEE: *Botulinus toxin* in *Table of Poisons and Poisoning in Appendix.*

bouba (boo-bah). Spanish-American term for *yaws.*

Bouchut's respiration (boo-shooz') [Jean A. E. Bouchut, French physician, 1818-1891]. Expiration longer than inspiration in children with bronchopneumonia and asthma.

B.'s tube. One used for intubation.

bougie (boo-zhē') [F. *bougie,* candle]. Instrument for exploring and dilating canals, esp. the male urethra.

b., armed. One with caustic attached.

bouillon (boo-yawn') [F. *bouillir,* to boil]. Clear beef broth.

b. culture. Bouillon used as a basis for a bacteriological culture.

boulimia (boo-lim'ĭ-ă) [G. *bous,* ox, + *limos,* hunger]. Abnormal hunger sensation a short time after a meal. SYN: *bulimia, q.v.*

bouquet (boo-kā') [F. nosegay]. 1. The aroma of a wine. 2. A cluster of anything, esp. of blood vessels or nerves.

bourdonnement (boor-dŏn-mon') [Fr. a droning]. A humming sound.

boutonnière operation (boo-tŏn-yār') [F. buttonhole]. 1. Incision through perineum behind an impervious stricture. 2. A buttonhole-like opening in a membrane.

boutons terminaux. Bulblike expansions at the tip of axons which come into synaptic contact with the cell bodies of other neurons.

bovine (bō'vīn) [L. *bovinus,* pert. to a cow]. Pert. to cattle.

b. lymph. Vaccine virus from a heifer.

bo'vinoid [" + *eidos,* resemblance]. Like that of cattle.

bow'el [O.Fr. *boel,* intestine, from L. *botellus,* little sausage]. The intestine.

b. movement. Evacuation of feces. SYN: *defecation.*

NUMBER OF: This varies in normal individuals, some having a movement after each meal, others one in the morning and one at night, and still others only one in several days. Thus to say that the healthy person must have at least one bowel movement a day in order to maintain health is unreasonable and not based on factual evidence. Also it is completely within the range of normal variation to have 2 to 3 bowel movements each day.

bowleg. A bending outward of the lower limb. Bandyleg, genu varum.

Bowman's capsule [Sir William Bowman, English physician, 1816-1892]. The expanded end of a renal tubule or nephron which invests a glomerulus, the two constituting the renal or Malpighian corpuscle. It consists of a visceral layer closely applied to the glomerulus and an outer parietal layer. It functions as a filter in the formation of urine.

B.'s glands. Branched tubulo-alveolar glands located in the lamina propria of the olfactory membrane which serves to keep the olfactory surface moist.

B.'s membrane. Thin homogeneous membrane separating corneal epithelium from corneal substance. SEE: *membrane.*

boxnote. A hollow sound heard on percussion in emphysema.

box splint. One for fractures below the knee.

Boyer's bursa (bwă-yāz') [Baron Alexis de Boyer, French surgeon, 1757-1833]. One ant. to the thyrohyoid membrane.

B.'s cyst. A subhyoid cyst.

Boyle's law. The volume of a given mass of gas, at any given temperature, varies inversely with the pressure put upon it.

Bozeman-Fritsch catheter (bōz'man-frĭtch) [Nathan Bozeman, American surgeon, 1825-1905, and Heinrich Fritsch, German gynecologist, 1844-1915]. Double-lumen uterine catheter with several openings at tip.

B. P., B. Ph. Abbr. for *British Pharmacopeia.*

Br. CHEM: Symbol for *bromine;* abbreviation for *Brucella.*

brachia (brā'kĭ-ă). Pl. of *brachium.*

brachial (brā'ki-al) [G. *brachiōn,* arm]. Pert. to the arm.

b. artery. Main artery of arm. Continuation of the axillary artery on the inside of the arm.

b. plexus. Network of lower cervical and upper dorsal spinal nerves supplying arm, forearm and hand. SEE: *nerve plexuses.*

b. veins. Those accompanying the brachial artery.

brachialgia (bra-kĭ-al'jĭ-ă) [" + *algos,* pain]. Intense pain in the arm.

brachialis (brā-kĭ-ăl'ĭs). A muscle of the arm lying immediately under the biceps brachii.

brachio- [G.]. Prefix: Pert. to the brachium.

brachiocephalic (brā-kĭ-ō-sĕ-fal'ĭk) [G. *brachiōn,* arm, + *kephalē,* head]. Pert. to arm and head.

brachiocrural (brā-kĭ-ō-kru'ral) [" + L. *cruralis,* pert. to the leg]. Pert. to arm and leg.

brachiocu'bital [" + L. *cubitus,* forearm]. Pert. to the arm and forearm.

brachiocyllosis (brā-kĭ-ō-sil-ō'sis) [" + *kyllōsis*, a bending]. Curvature of the arm.

brachiofa'cial [" + L. *facialis*, pert. to face]. Pert. to arm and face.

brachioncus (brā-kĭ-on'kus) [" + *ogkos*, a swelling]. A chronic, hard swelling of the arm.

brachioradialis (brā"kĭ-ō-rā"dĭ-ā'lĭs). A muscle lying on lateral side of the forearm. SEE: *Muscles of the Body*, in *Appendix*.

brachiotomy (brā-kĭ-ot'ō-mĭ) [" + *tomē*, a cutting]. Surgical removal or cutting of an arm of the fetus to facilitate delivery.

brachium (brā'kĭ-um) (pl. *brachia*) [L. from G. *brachiōn*, arm]. 1. The upper arm from shoulder to elbow. 2. One of the white tracts of the brain.

b. conjunctivum. The superior cerebellar peduncle, *q.v.*

b. pontis. The middle cerebellar peduncle, *q.v.*

brachy- [G. *brachys*, short]. Prefix: Short.

brachybasia (brăk-ĭ-bā'sĭ-ă) [" + *basis*, walking]. A slow, shuffling gait seen in partial paraplegia. SEE: *gait*.

brachycardia (brak-ĭ-kar'dĭ-ă) [" + *kardia*, heart]. Slowness of heart action. SYN: *bradycardia, q.v.*

brachycephalic, brachycephalous (brak-ĭ-sĕ-fal'ik, -sef'ă-lus) [" + *kephalē*, head]. Having a head disproportionately short.

brachyceph'alism, brachyceph'aly. Shortness of the head.

brachycheilia (brăk-e-ki'lĭ-ă) [" + *cheilos*, lip]. Condition of having abnormally short lip or lips.

brachydactylia (brak-ĭ-dak-til'ĭ-ă) [G. *brachys*, short, + *daktylos*, finger]. Shortness of the fingers.

brachygnathia (brak-ĭg-nā'thĭ-ă) [" + *gnathos*, jaw]. Abnormal shortness or recession of under jaw.

brachymetropia (brak-ĭ-mē-trōp'ĭ-ă) [" + *metron*, measure, + *opsis*, sight]. Myopia; nearsightedness.

brachymetropic (brak-ĭ-mē-trōp'ik). Nearsighted; myopic.

brachyphalan'gia. Shortness of phalanges.

brachypnea (brak-ĭp-nē'ă) [G. *brachys*, short, + *pnoē*, breathing]. Shortness of breath.

brachystasis (brăk-ĭs'tă-sĭs). Condition in which a muscle upon contracting does not relax but maintains its shortened state.

brachyuran'ic [" + *ouranos*, roof of mouth]. Having a short palate, or a palatomaxillary index over 115.

bradesthesia (brad-ĕs-thē'zĭ-ă) [G. *bradys*, slow, + *aisthēsis*, sensation]. Blunted perception. SYN: *bradyesthesia, q.v.*

Bradford frame [Edward H. Bradford, orthopedic surgeon, 1848-1926]. An oblong frame, about 7 x 3 feet, made of 1 in. pipe, covered with canvas strips, which run from one side of the frame to the other and which are movable, thus permitting the patient to urinate and defecate without moving the spine or changing position.

brady- [G. *bradys*, slow]. Prefix: Slow, as *bradycardia*.

bradyacusia (brad-ĭ-ă-koo'sĭ-ă) [" + *akouein*, to hear]. Hardness of hearing.

bradyarthria (brad-ĭ-ar'thrĭ-ă) [" + *arthron*, articulation]. Bradylalia; unusual slowness of articulation of words.

bradyauxesis (brăd-ĭ-awks-ē'sĭs). Term applied to the type of growth in which a part grows at a slower rate than that of the organism of which it is a part.

bradycardia (brad-ĭ-kar'dĭ-ă) [" + *kardia*, heart]. Slow heart action. SEE: *arrhythmia; tachycardia.*

b., sinus. A sinus rhythm with a rate below 60 in an adult, or below 70 in a child.

bradycar'dic. Pert. to bradycardia.

bradycinesia (brad-ĭ-sĭ-nē'sĭ-ă) [G. *bradys*, slow, + *kinēsis*, movement]. Extreme slowness of movement. SYN: *bradykinesia.*

bradycrotic (brad-ĭ-krot'ik). Pert. to slowness of pulse.

bradydiastole (brad-ĭ-dĭ-as'tō-lē) [G. *bradys*, slow, + *diastole*, dilatation]. Prolongation of the diastolic pause, as in myocardial lesions.

bradyecoia (brad-ĭ-ē-koy'ă) [G. *bradyēkoos*, hard of hearing]. Partial deafness.

bradyesthesia (brad-ĭ-ĕs-thē'zĭ-ă) [G. *bradys*, slow, + *aisthēsis*, perception]. Blunted perception.

bradyglossia (brad-ĭ-glos'ĭ-ă) [" + *glōssa*, tongue]. Unusual slowness of speech. SYN: *bradylalia, bradyarthria, bradylogia, bradyphasia, bradyphemia.*

bradykinesia (brad-ĭ-kĭ-nē'sĭ-ă) [" + *kinēsis*, motion]. Extreme slowness of movement. SYN: *bradycinesia.*

bradylalia (brad-ĭ-lā'lĭ-ă) [" + *lalein*, to talk]. Slowness of speech. SYN: *bradylogia; bradyphasia; bradyphemia.* SEE: *speech.*

bradylexia (brad-ĭ-lex'ĭ-ă) [" + *lexis*, word]. Slowness of reading not attributable to lack of intelligence. SEE: *dyslexia.*

bradypepsia (brad-ĭ-pep'sĭ-ă) [" + *pepsis*, digestion]. Slow digestion.

bradyphagia (brad-ĭ-fā'jĭ-ă) [" + *phagein*, to eat]. Slowness in eating.

bradyphrasia (brad-ĭ-frā'zĭ-ă) [" + *phrasis*, utterance]. Slowness of speech; seen in some types of mental disease.

bradyphre'nia [" + *phrēn*, mind]. Slowness of mental activity such as may result from epidemic encephalitis.

bradypnea (brad-ip-nē'ă) [" + *pnoē*, breathing]. Abnormally slow breathing.

bradyrhythmia (brad-ĭ-rĭth'mĭ-ă). 1. Slowness of heart or pulse rate. 2. In *electroencephalography*, slowness of brain waves (1 to 6 per sec.).

bradyspermatism (brad-ĭ-sper'mă-tizm) [" + *sperma*, semen]. Abnormally slow emission of semen.

bradysphygmia (brad-ĭ-sfig'mĭ-ă) [" + *sphygmos*, pulse]. Abnormally slow pulse.

bradystal'sis [" + *stalsis*, constriction]. Slow peristalsis.

bradytocia (brad-ĭ-to'sĭ-ă) [" + *tokos*, childbirth]. Slow parturition.

bradyuria (brad-ĭ-ū'rĭ-ă) [" + *ouron*, urine]. Slowness in passing urine.

braidism (bra'dizm). Hypnotism.

braille. Raised dots on paper used to communicate written language, signs, and symbols to the blind. The dots, which represent numerals and letters of the alphabet, are palpated by the fingers. Developed by Louis Braille (1809-1852), a French teacher of the blind.

brain [A.S. *braegen*]. A large, soft mass of nerve tissue contained within the cranium; the *encephalon*. Cranial portion of the central nervous system.

structure: It is composed of neurons which are nerve cells, and neurologia or supporting cells. The brain consists of gray and white matter. Gray matter is composed principally of nerve-cell bodies and is concentrated

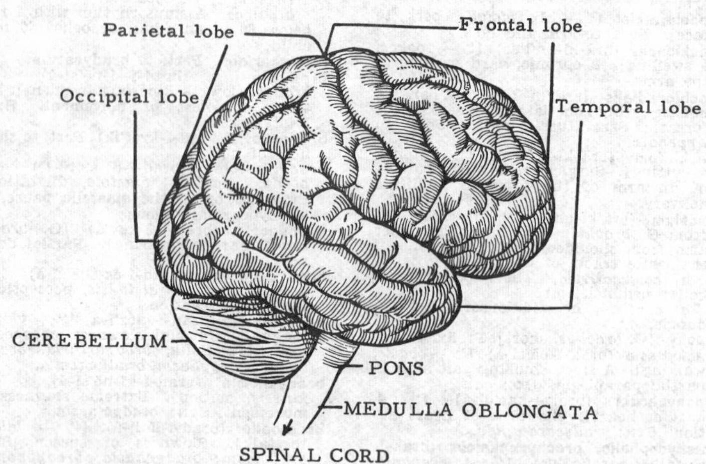

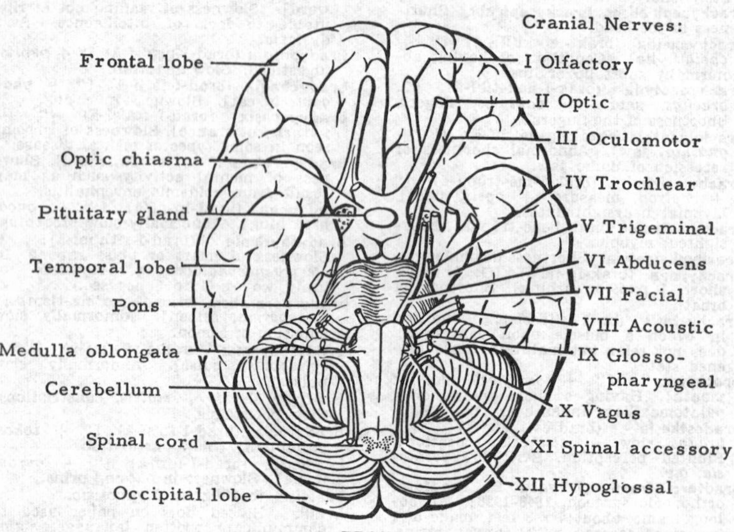

BRAIN
Above. Lateral exterior view. Below. Base of brain

in the cerebral cortex and the nuclei and basal ganglia. White matter is composed of nerve-cell processes which form tracts or commissures connecting various parts of the brain with each other.

It consists of 5 parts: the *cerebrum, cerebellum, pons Varolii, medulla oblongata,* and *midbrain.*

The cerebrum represents seven-eighths of the weight of the brain.

Lobes: 1. Frontal. 2. Parietal. 3. Occipital. 4. Temporal. 5. Insula.

Glands: Pituitary.

Membranes: Meninges, consisting of the dura mater (external), arachnoid (middle), and pia mater (internal).

Nerves: Cranial. See: *Nerves, cranial,* in *Appendix.*

The subdivisions of the brain are: *diencephalon.* This includes the epithalamus, thalamus, and hypothalamus (optic chiasma, hypophysis, tuber cinereum, and maxillary bodies).

myelencephalon. This includes the corpora quadrigemina, tegmentum, and crura cerebri.

metencephalon. This includes the cerebellum and pons.

myelencephalon. This includes the medulla oblongata.

telencephalon. This includes the rhinencephalon, corpora striata, and cerebrum (cerebral cortex).

ventricles: The cavities of the brain are (a) the *lateral* ventricles (1 and 2) which lie in the cerebral hemispheres; (b) the third ventricle of the diencephalon, and (c) the fourth ventricle of the medulla. The first and second communicate with the third by the interventricular foramina; the third with the fourth by the cerebral canal (aqueduct of Sylvius); the fourth with the subarachnoid spaces by the two *foramina of Luschka* and the *foramen of Magendie*. The ventricles are filled with cerebrospinal fluid which is formed by the choroid plexuses in the walls and roofs of the ventricles.

functions: The brain is the primary center for regulating and coordinating body activities. Sensory impulses are received through afferent nerves; these register as sensations which are the basis for perception. It is the seat of consciousness, thought, memory, reason, judgment, and emotion. Motor impulses are discharged through efferent nerves to muscles and glands initiating activities. Through reflex centers automatic control of body activities is maintained. The most important reflex centers are the *cardiac, vasomotor,* and *respiratory* centers which regulate circulation and respiration.

SEE: *illustration on B-39.*

The weight of brain and cord is about 1350-1400 gm., of which total the cord represents 2%. SEE: *spinal cord.*

b. fever. Meningitis.

b. stem. All the brain except the cerebellum and cerebrum.

b. sand. Laminated bodies consisting principally of phosphates, and carbonates of calcium, and magnesium found in the pineal body called *corpora arenacea.*

b. tumor. Usually used inexactly to describe any intracranial mass, neoplastic, cystic, inflammatory (abscess), or gummatous. Except the latter, treatment depends on surgery and thus on accurate diagnosis.

SYM: The general symptoms are those due to an increase in intracranial pressure such as headache, the change in the retina recognized by opthalmoscopic examination as "choked disk," and vomiting (without nausea).

Neoplasms of the brain do not metastasize to other parts of the body.

Malignancies of perineural nerves may appear as isolated lumps. They contain almost no blood vessels. May produce pain or other sensations. The most malignant ones in childhood are gliomas, *q.v.*

Mental changes (esp. dullness), epileptiform convulsions, giddiness, are often general but may be localized signs. In addition, history and cranial x-ray are of great value. The injection of air into the ventricles prior to x-ray is known as pneumoventriculography.

brain storm. Temporary outburst of mental excitement; often maniacal, esp. in paranoia.

Brain's reflex [W. Russell Brain, British physician, 1895-]. Extension of flexed arm on assuming quadripedal posture.

branchial (brang'kĭ-al) [G. *bragchia,* gills]. Pert. to gills.

b. arches. Five pairs of arched structures which form the lateral and ventral walls of the pharynx of the embryo. They are partially separated from each other externally by the branchial clefts; internally, by the pharyngeal pouches. The fifth arch is rudimentary. They play an important role in the formation of structures of the face and neck. The first is the *mandibular arch,* the second the *hyoid arch.* They are also called the visceral arches.

b. clefts. A series of openings between the branchial arches. They become functional gill slits in fishes.

b. grooves. A series of furrows separating the branchial arches. They are homologous to the branchial clefts of fishes and amphibians.

b. muscles. Those which develop from the mesoderm of the branchial arches. Include most of muscles of face and neck.

branchiogenic. Branchiogenous, *q.v.*

branchiogenous (brang-kĭ-oj'e-nus) [" + *gennan,* to generate]. Having origin in a branchial cleft.

branchioma (brang-kĭ-ō'mă). A tumor related to the branchial arches.

branchiomeric (brang-kĭ-ō-mĕr'ĭk). Of or pertaining to the branchial arches.

branchiomerism (brang-kĭ-om'er-izm) [" + *meros,* part]. Segmental division of the entoderm.

brandy. Spiritous liquor distilled from wine and containing about 50% alcohol by volume.

brash. A burning sensation in the stomach sometimes accompanied by belching of sour fluid. SYN: *heartburn; pyrosis; water b.*

brass founders' a'gue. Tremors due to zinc poison from inhalation of toxic fumes.

brass poisoning. Due to the inhalation of fumes of zinc and zinc oxide with destruction of tissue in respiratory passage.

SYM: Dryness and burning in respiratory tract; cough; headache; chills; rarely fatal.

TREATMENT: Entirely symptomatic; inhalations of humidified air make patient more comfortable.

Braun's hook (browns) [Gustave von Braun, Austrian gynecologist, 1829-1911]. Instrument for fracturing clavicle or to assist in decapitation of the fetal head.

Braune's canal (brow'nehs) [Christian Braune, German anatomist, 1831-1892]. The parturient canal formed by the uterus, dilated cervix and vulva.

braw'ny induration. Pathological hardening and thickening of tissues.

Braxton Hicks sign [John Braxton Hicks, English gynecologist, 1825-1897]. Intermittent painless uterine contractions which may occur every 10 to 20 minutes. They occur more frequently as pregnancy nears completion. These contractions do not represent true labor pains but are often so interpreted.

Brazil nut. An oily, three-sided nut from the tree *Bertholletia excelsa.*

RAW: 100 gm. Calories: 654. Other values: 14 gm. protein; 67 gm. fat; 186 mg. calcium; 3.4 mg. iron.

bread. A food made by baking a doughy mixture of flour (wheat, corn, rye, etc.), shortening, a leavening agent, and water. The dough may or may not contain yeast, which would cause air cells due to gas generated during its growth. Food value varies with type of bread.

break. 1. In orthopedics, a fracture. 2. To interrupt continuity in a tissue or electric circuit or channel of flow or communication.

b., chromatid. Fracture of the chromatid. This causes misalignment of the parts and leads to genetic abnormalities.

breakbone fever. Acute epidemic febrile disease. SEE: *dengue.*

breast [A.S. *breōst*]. 1. The upper ant. aspect of the chest. 2. Mammary gland, a compound alveolar gland consisting of 15-20 lobes of glandular tissue separated from each other by interlobular septa. Each lobe is drained by a *lactiferous duct* which opens on the tip of the nipple. The mammary gland secretes milk used for nourishment of young. SEE: *milk; lactiferous glands.*

DEVELOPMENT: Following puberty, *estrogens* from the ovary stimulate growth and development of the duct system; during pregnancy *progesterone* secreted by the corpus luteum and placenta acts synergistically with estrogens to bring the alveoli to complete development. Following parturition, *prolactin* (luteotrophin) in conjunction with adrenal corticoids initiate lactation and *oxytocin* from the post. pituitary induces ejection of milk. Suckling or milking reflexly stimulates both milk secretion and discharge of milk.

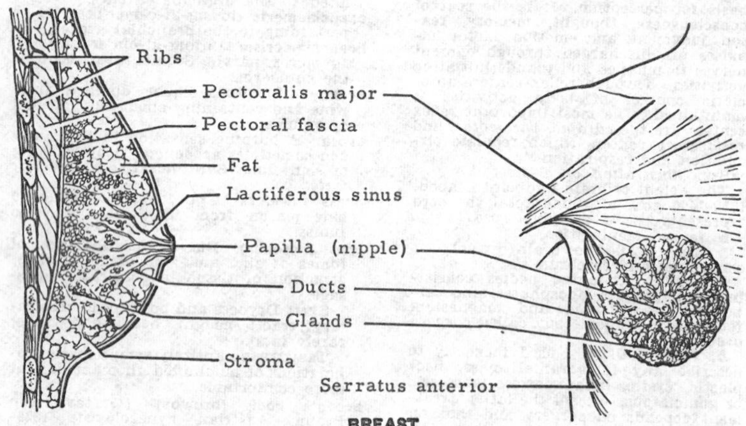

BREAST

CHANGES IN PREGNANCY: 6-12½ weeks, fullness and tenderness, erectile tissues in nipples, nodules felt, pigment deposited around nipple (primary areola), (in blondes the areolae and nipples become pinkish, in brunettes they become dark brown and in some cases even black), and few drops of fluid may be squeezed out. 16-20½ weeks (secondary areola), small, whitish spots in pigmentation. Due to hypertrophy of the sebaceous glands. These are the so-called *glands of Montgomery.*

NP: PREVENTIVE CARE: Most complications of the breast during the puerperal period will not occur if proper care is given.

POINTS TO OBSERVE: 1. Use aseptic technic in breast care to avoid infection of infant's mouth as well as mother's breasts. Clean nipples with sterile water before and after each nursing.

2. Early treatment of soreness, cracks and fissures: (a) By the use of sterile nipple shield while the baby nurses, (b) by taking the baby off the breast and pumping the breasts at the time the baby would be due to nurse. Pumping should be done under very low pressure and should be repeated until the nipple is well healed. This does away with the danger of infection from the infant's mouth and prevents him from making matters worse by his terrific nursing suction. Antiseptic oil, ointments, etc., may be used to favor the healing process.

3. Limit the nursing period during the first 3 days when no breast milk is available and during the engorgement period when the breasts are extremely sensitive from congestion and distention with milk. The use of the electric pump is stressed during this time.

4. Avoid bruising of the breasts. The use of the electric breast pump in place of excessively firm manual massage during the extreme sensitive period will prevent this.

5. Keep the nipples soft to avoid cracking. Applications which harden them predispose to cracking.

6. Avoid "caking" of the breasts by the use of the breast pump to remove any excess milk which may plug the ducts. In the home it will be necessary to resort to the hand breast pump or proper manual expression of the milk.

7. Proper support of the breast with a binder which pulls upward and inward. Do not bind so tightly that circulation is restricted.

8. Use ice bags during the engorgement period and when there is any tenderness. The ice bags are particularly soothing to cracked nipples as they relieve congestion.

CARE WHEN ABSCESS OCCURS: 1. When abscesses occur and drainage has been established, there is danger of carrying infection on your hands to other parts of the mother's body. The nurse must protect the mother, herself, and other patients by the use of proper technic. Gloves should be worn during the dressings. Dressings should be disposed of at once and before removing the gloves. Appropriate systemic antibiotic will be prescribed by the physician.

2. Remember the infant's milk supply is endangered. The infant is taken off the affected breast, but sometimes is permitted to nurse the normal breast. At other times pumping of the good breast is ordered during the height of the infection. Nursing orders will, of course, vary with the physician, but the infant's food intake must be kept up if necessary by artificial means.

3. Remember that an abscess may not only impair the function of the breast at this time but may also affect it in subsequent pregnancies.

b., chicken; b., pigeon. Deformity in which chest is protruding, caused by rickets or obstructed respiration in infancy.

b. milk. Mother's milk. SEE: *colostrum.*

b. pump. One to draw milk from the female breast. May be electric or hand-operated.

breath (brĕth) [A.S. *braeth,* odor]. The air inhaled and exhaled in act of respiration.

DIAG: Foul odor (*os fetor*) indicates neglect of mouth or teeth, improper diet, constipation, lack of exercise, use of drugs, alcohol or tobacco. It also depends upon the food ingested, and may indicate stomatitis, necrosis of jaw, caries of teeth, tonsillitis, diphtheria, gangrene and abscess of the lungs, fetid bronchitis, bronchiectasis, pyothorax, catarrh, diabetes, kidney disease, and other disorders.

If *os fetor* is due to systemic causes or ingestion of food such as garlic, mouth washes and gargles are ineffective in removing the odor.

Urinous odor: Indicates uremia.

Sweetish odor (that of ripe apples): Found in diabetes mellitus, esp. during coma. This sweet odor is due to the excretion of acetone in the breath. This condition develops quickly in infants and children who have gone several hours without food.

Odor of carnivorous animals: Noted in critical illness, in acidosis and alkalosis.

b., rattling and shortness of. Edema; presence of fluids in the air passages.

b., sighing. Air hunger. Occurs in internal hemorrhage.

NP: Watch for after abdominal operations and in typhoid fever.

breathing (brēth'ing) [A.S. *braeth,* odor]. Act of inhaling and exhaling air. SEE: *chest; respiration.*

b., asthmatic. Harsh breathing with a prolonged wheezing expiration. Is heard all over the chest.

b., bronchial or tubular. Harsh breathing with a prolonged high pitched expiration which has sometimes a tubular quality. Heard in consolidation of lung tissue.

b., cog-wheel or jerky. Respiratory murmur not continuous, but broken into waves, not indicative of any special disease, but frequently observed in bronchitis and in incipient phthisis.

b. of emphysema. Weak with prolonged, low pitched or inaudible expiration.

b., exaggerated. Almost same peculiarity as puerile b. Heard over lung that is doing extra work necessitated by some impairment of its fellow.

b., periodic. Cheyne-Stokes respiration, *q.v.*

b., puerile. Type heard normally over lungs of children, loud expiration, higher pitched than in vesicular breathing and almost as long as inspiration.

b., rapid. In pneumonia, high fevers, or interference with oxygenation.

b., slow. Found in narcotic poisoning, sleep, or rest, and in cases of increased intracranial pressure.

b., stertorous. Due to a relaxation of the palate and is characterized by a deep snoring sound on inspiration. It is most always present in apoplexy; the cheeks puff out with each breath on expiration. It is not regarded as a serious symptom, although it may indicate brain or nerve pressure. It is found in deep sleep and in coma.

b., weak or shallow. Noted: (a) When chest walls are thick; (b) in the old and feeble; (c) in emphysema; (d) in pleural effusion; (e) in incipient phthisis; (f) in painful affections of the chest, like pleurodynia and beginning pleurisy; (g) in pulmonary edema.

breath-o-lyzer (breth'o-lī-zer). Apparatus used to analyze the contents of expired air. One such device is used to test for presence of alcohol in expired air in order to determine whether or not a person is "legally" intoxicated.

bredouillement (brā-dwē-mon') [Fr.]. Pronunciation of only part of a word due to rapid utterance.

breech [A.S. *brēc,* buttocks]. The nates, or buttocks.

b. presentation. The presentation of the buttocks instead of the head in childbirth. Occurs in over 3% of all labors.

breeze [Fr. *brise,* wind]. A movement of air.

bregma (breg'mă) [G. front of head]. That point on the skull where the coronal and sagittal sutures join. The ant. fontanelle in the fetus and young infant.

bregmat'ic. Pert. to the bregma.

breg"mocard'iac reflex. Reduced heart rate following pressure on post. fontanel.

brei (bri). Tissue which has been finely divided; pulp.

Breisky's disease (bri'skēz) [August Breisky, German gynecologist, 1832-1889]. Atrophy of the vulva. Kraurosis vulvae.

Brenner's tumor [Fritz Brenner, German pathologist, 1877-]. A benign fibroepithelioma of the ovary.

brevilineal (brev-ĭ-lin'ē-al). Shorter and broader than usual, with reference to body type. SYN: *brachymorphic.*

bridge [A.S. *brycg*]. 1. Narrow band of tissue. 2. Dental plate fastened to a tooth at each end.

b. of nose. The ridge formed by the nasal bones.

bridgework (brij-werk). A partial plate held in place by permanent attachments to other teeth.

b., fixed. Partial plates held by crowns or inlays fastened to the natural teeth.

b., removable. Partial plates held by clasps which permit their removal.

Bright's disease [Richard Bright, English physician, 1789-1858]. A vague term for acute and chronic disease of the kidneys. It is usually associated with dropsy and albuminuria. SEE: *nephritis.*

brim [A.S. *seashore*]. 1. An edge or margin. 2. Brim of pelvis. Superior aperture of the lesser or true pelvis; the inlet. Formed by the iliopectineal line of the innominate bone and the sacral promontory. Oval-shaped in the female; heart-shaped in the male.

brisèment forcé (brēz-mon') [Fr. crushing]. Breaking, by forcible means, of adhesions.

Brissaud's reflex (brĭs-soz') [Edouard Brissaud, French physician, 1852-1909]. Contraction of fascial femoris muscle following tickling of sole of foot.

British Anti-Lewisite. Dimercaprol, *q.v.* ABBR: BAL.

British thermal unit. Amount of heat necessary to raise the temperature of one pound of water, at approximately 39°, 1 degree F. SEE: *calorie.*

broach [A.S. *broche*]. A dental instrument for enlarging a tooth canal or for removing the pulp.

broad ligament of uterus. A transverse fold of peritoneum arising from floor of the pelvic cavity between the bladder and rectum, dividing the minor pelvis into ant. and post. compartments. In its median portion lies the uterus to which it is attached on both sides. Its free superior border contains the uterine tube. A lateral portion of the upper border forms the suspensory ligament of the ovary.

Broadbent's sign [Sir William Henry Broadbent, English physician, 1835-1907]. A visible retraction of the left side and back in region of 11th and 12th ribs synchronous with the cardiac systole, in adhesive pericarditis.

Broca's area (brō'kăz) [Pierre Paul Broca, French surgeon, 1824-1880]. On left side of brain, controlling movements of tongue, lips, vocal cords, or motor speech area. Loss of speech may follow hemorrhage into this area. Area parolfactoria. SYN: *motor speech area.* SEE: *motor aphasia.*

broccoli (brok'ō-li). Green tops and stalks of a type of cauliflower.

COOKED: 100 gm. Calories: 26. Other values: 3 gm. protein; 88 mg. calcium; 1.1 mg. iron; 2500 I.U. vitamin A; 90 mg. ascorbic acid.

Brodie's abscess [Sir Benjamin Collins Brodie, English surgeon, 1783-1862]. An abscess of the head of the tibia, or it may be an abscess of any bone.

ETIOL: It is usually of tubercular origin or from subacute staphylococcal infection.

SYM: May be aching pains in area, followed by slight swelling and tenderness on movement. Symptoms less acute but similar to osteomyelitis.

Brokaw ring [Augustus V. L. Brokaw, American surgeon, 1853-1907]. Rubber tubing ring threaded with catgut for intestinal anastomosis.

brom-, bromo- [G. *brōmos*, stench]. Prefixes: Presence of bromine.

bromhidrosis (brom-hī-drō'sis). Bromidrosis, *q.v.*

bromide (bro'mīd) [G. *brōmos*, stench]. A binary compound of bromine combined with an element or a radical. It is a central nervous system depressant.

POISONING: SYM: Prompt vomiting, drowsiness, irritability, ataxia, vertigo, confusion, mania, hallucinations, coma. Also skin rashes (bromide acne) and neurological disturbances.

F. A. TREATMENT: Large doses of sodium or ammonium chloride by any route. Give saline cathartic. SEE ALSO: *Table of Poisons and Poisoning in Appendix.*

bromidrosiphobia (brō-mid-rō-sī-fō'bĭ-ă) [" + *idrōs*, sweat, + *phobos*, fear]. Abnormal fear of personal odors, accompanied by hallucinations.

bromidrosis (brom-ī-dro'sis) [" + *idrōs*, sweat]. Fetid or offensive sweat. It occurs mostly on *feet, groins,* and *axillae.*

NP: Cleanliness, use of an antiseptic, daily change of clothing, deodorant antiseptic powders.

RS: *anhidrosis; chromidrosis; uridrosis.*

bromine (bro'mēn, -min) [G. *bromos*, stench]. SYMB: Br. Liquid nonmetallic element. At. wt. 79.909; at. no. 35. It is obtained from natural brines from wells and sea water. Its compounds are used in medicine, photography and coal tar derivatives. SEE: *bromide.*

bromism, brominism (bro'mizm, bro'minizm) [" + *ismos*, state of]. Poisoning resulting from prolonged use of bromides, *q.v.* SEE: *Bromides* in *Table of Poisons and Poisoning in Appendix.*

bro"moder'ma [" + G. *derma*, skin]. Acne-like eruption due to chronic bromide poisoning.

bro"mohyperhidro'sis [" + *yper*, over, + *idrōsis*, perspiration]. Fetid and excessive sweat. SEE: *bromidrosis.*

bromoiodism (bro"mō-ī'ō-dizm) [" + iodine, + G. *ismos*, state of]. Poisoning from bromoiodides.

bromomania (brō-mō-mā'nĭ-ă) [" + G. *mania*, insanity]. Psychosis caused by use of bromides.

bromomenorrhea (brō-mō-men-o-rē'ă) [" + *mēnes*, menses, + *roia*, flow]. Foul odor to menstrual discharge.

bromopnea (brom-op-ne'ă) [" + *pnoē*, breath]. Offensive breath.

bronchadenitis (bronk"ad-ĕ-nī'tis) [G. *bronchia*, bronchia, + *adēn*, gland, + *-itis*, inflammation]. Inflammation of bronchial glands.

bronchi (bron'kī) (sing. *bronchus*). The primary divisions of the trachea; divides opp. 3rd dorsal vertebra. The right bronchus is shorter and more vertical than the left one.

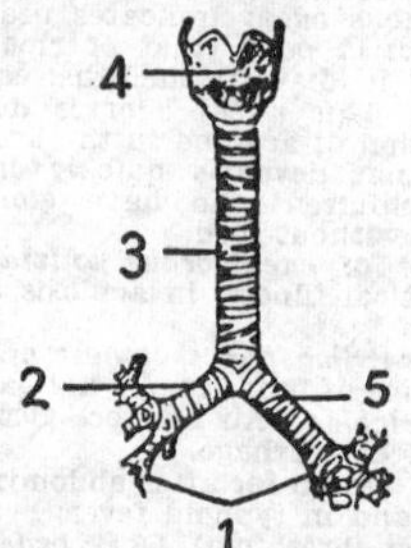

BRONCHI AND TRACHEA

1. Bronchioles. 2. Right bronchus. 3. Trachea. 4. Larynx. 5. Left bronchus.

They penetrate the lungs, one for the right and the other for the left lung, and terminate in the bronchioles or bronchial tubes.

b., foreign bodies in. May cause various diseases of bronchi, large objects leading to collapse of the lung. Metal bodies, if small, may produce no symptoms. Beans, nuts, seeds, etc., may cause pneumonia, bronchitis or lung abscess.

SYM: Choking and gagging immediately. Later, symptoms of bronchitis, atelectasis, pneumonia or lung abscess.

PROG: Good, if removed before complications. Better in case of metallic objects than in vegetable bodies.

TREATMENT: Removal through bronchoscope.

bronchi, words pert. to: alveobronchitis, "bronch-" words; mesobronchitis; rales.

bronchial (bron'kē-al). Pert. to the bronchi or bronchioles.

b. crises. Paroxysms of coughing in locomotor ataxia.

b. glands. Mucous or mixed glands in the bronchi or bronchioles.

b. tree. Bronchi and bronchial tubes.

b. tubes. The smaller divisions of the bronchi.

bronchiarctia (bron-kī-ark'shī-ă) [G. *bronchos,* windpipe, + L. *arctāre,* to compress]. Bronchial tube stenosis. SYN: *bronchiostenosis.*

bronchiectasis (bron-kī-ek'tă-sis) [" + *ektasis,* dilatation]. Dilatation of a bronchus or bronchi, usually secreting large amounts of offensive pus. Dilatation may be in an isolated segment or spread throughout the bronchi.

ETIOL: Acquired or congenital, on one or both sides of chest. Acquired b. usually secondary to obstruction or infections, as bronchopneumonia, chronic bronchitis, tuberculosis, whooping cough.

SYM: Cough, dyspnea, expectoration of foul secretion, esp. in the morning or when changing position. On standing, sputum separates into 3 layers: (a) bottom one that is thick and which contains pus cells; (b) a middle layer of greenish fluid; (c) an upper layer of froth.

TREATMENT: Antibiotics for treatment, and prophylaxis, and postural drainage. Resection of affected areas in selected patients. Aerosols for bronchodilation in bronchospasm.

NP: Position to assist drainage.

bronchiectatic (bron-kī-ĕk-tăt'ĭk) [" + *ektasis,* dilation]. Pert. to bronchiectasis.

bronchiloquy (bron-kil'ō-kwĭ) [" + L. *loqui,* to speak]. Unusual vocal resonance over a bronchus covered with consolidated lung tissue.

bronchiocele (bron'kĭ-ō-sēl) [" + *kēlē,* tumor]. Circumscribed dilatation of a bronchus.

bronchiogenic (bron-kĭ-ō-jen'ik) [" + *gennan,* to originate]. Having origin in the bronchi.

bronchiole (bron'kĭ-ōl) (pl. *bronchioles*) [L. *bronchiolus,* air passage]. One of the smaller subdivisions of the bronchi. They lack cartilage.

b., respiratory. The last division of the bronchial tree. They are branches of terminal bronchioles and lead to alveolar ducts leading to the alveoli.

b., terminal. Next to the last subdivision of a bronchiole, leading to the respiratory bronchioles.

bronchiolectasis (bron"kĭ-ō-lek'tă-sis) [" + G. *ektasis,* dilatation] Dilatation of the bronchioles; capillary bronchiectasis.

bronchiolitis (bron-kĭ-ō-lī'tis) [" + G. *-itis,* inflammation]. Inflammation of the bronchioles.

b., exudativa. A form with fibrinous exudation.

b., vesicular. Bronchopneumonia.

bronchiolus (bron-kī'ō-lus) (pl. *bronchioli*). Bronchiole, *q.v.*

bron'chiospasm [" + *spasmos,* fit]. Spasmodic narrowing of the lumen of the bronchial tubes.

bronchiosteno'sis [" + *stenōsis,* a narrowing]. Narrowing of the bronchial tubes. SYN: *bronchiarctia.*

bronchis'mus [" + *ismos,* state of]. Bronchiospasm, *q.v.*

bronchit'ic. Pert. to bronchitis.

bronchitis (bron-kī'tis) [G. *bronchos,* bronchos, + *itis,* inflammation]. Inflammation of bronchial mucous membrane.

ETIOL: Infectious agents such as viruses, esp. influenza virus or pyogenic organisms such as various species of *Streptococcus, Pneumococcus, Staphylococcus,* and *Hemophilus.* Infection often preceded by the common cold. Predisposing factors are exposure, chilling, fatigue and malnutrition. Acute bronchial irritation may also be caused by various physical and chemical agents such as dusts, fumes, etc. Allergic factors may be of importance.

b., acute. Chilliness, malaise. Soreness and constriction behind sternum, increased by coughing; slight fever, 100 to 102° F. Cough at first dry and painful, later mucopurulent expectoration which becomes free as inflammation subsides.

TREATMENT: Bed rest, increased intake of fluids, an antipyretic and analgesic, antibiotics, steam inhalations.

b., capillary. Inflammation of the secondary bronchi in children and debilitated persons.

SYM: Severe spells of coughing; rapid respiration—30 to 80 per minute; dyspnea, high fever—104°-105° F.; weak, rapid pulse. Later lips become blue, extremities cold, mind dull.

PROG: In young children very grave. May develop into bronchopneumonia.

TREATMENT: Absolute rest. Temp. of room kept uniformly at 70° or 75° F.—atmosphere kept moist by steam. Antibiotics.

b., chronic. A longstanding disease of the tracheobronchial tree characterized by chronic inflammation accompanied by fibrotic and atrophic changes in the mucous membrane.

SYM: Persistent cough, mucopurulent expectoration. Soreness behind sternum. Fever absent unless disease is severe; dyspnea on exertion.

NP: Whenever possible it is advisable for a person with chronic bronchitis to live in a mild stable climate, especially during the winter. The ward or room in the hospital should be kept warm. General health should be maintained. Diet should be nourishing. Anti-tussive agents, antibiotics, expectorants, steam or other inhalations.

b., plastic. Fibrinous bronchitis, *q.v.*

b., putrid. Chronic form with foul-smelling sputum.

b., vegetal. Bronchitis resulting from the lodgement of foods of vegetable origin such as a peanut in a bronchus.

bronchium (brong'kĭ-um) (pl. *bronchia*) [L. bronchus]. A bronchial tube.

broncho- [G. *bronchos,* windpipe]. Prefix: Rel. to the bronchi.

bronchoadeni'tis [" + *adēn,* gland, + *-itis,* inflammation]. Bronchadenitis, *q.v.*

broncho"blennorrhe'a [" + *blennos,* mucus, + *roia,* flow]. Copious, thick sputum accompanying chronic bronchitis.

bronchocele (brŏn'kō-sēl) G. *bronchos,* windpipe, + *kēlē,* tumor]. A dilatation of a bronchiole.

bronchoclysis (bron-kok'lĭ-sis) [" + *klysis,* washing]. Introduction of a medicated solution into the bronchi.

bron"choconstric'tion [" + L. *constringere,* to draw together]. Constriction of the lumen of the bronchi.

bron"chodilata'tion [" + L. *dilatāre,* to open]. Dilatation of a bronchus.

bronchoedema (brŏn-kō-ĕ-dē'mă). Edematous swelling of the mucosa of the bronchial tubes reducing size of air passageways and inducing dyspnea.

bronchoegophony (bron-kō-ĕ-gof'ō-nĭ) [" + *aig-*, goat, + *phōnē*, voice]. Egobronchophony; a goatlike sound.

bronchogenic (bron-ko-jen'ik) [" + *gennan*, to originate]. Having origin in the bronchi.

bron'chogram [" + *gramma*, a writing]. A roentgenogram of the lungs and bronchi.

bronchog'raphy [" + *graphein*, to write]. Radiography of the bronchi after a radiopaque substance has been injected into them, making a bronchogram.

broncholith (bron'kō-lith) [" + *lithos*, stone]. Calculus in the bronchus or bronchial tube.

broncholithiasis (bron-kō-lith-ī'ă-sis) [" + *lithos*, stone]. Calculi in the bronchi.

bronchomoniliasis (bron-kō-mon-ĭ-lī'ă-sis) [" + L. *monile*, necklace of chains]. Infection of the bronchial membrane with a species of Monilia.

bronchomo'tor [" + L. *motus*, moving]. Causing change of caliber of the bronchi.

bronchomycosis (brŏn-kō-mī-kō'sĭs) [G. *bronchos*, windpipe, + *mykēs*, fungus]. A fungus infection of the bronchi or bronchial tubes, usually caused by fungi of the genus *Candida*.

bronchopathy (brŏn-kŏp'ăth-ĭ) [" + *pathos*, disease]. Any pathological condition involving the bronchi or bronchioles.

bronchophony (bron-kof'ō-nĭ) [" + *phonē*, voice]. The voice as heard over a normal bronchus.

b., whispered. Bronchophony when patient whispers.

bronchoplasty (bron'kō-plăs-tĭ) [" + + *plasein*, to form]. Surgical repair of a bronchial defect.

bronchoplegia (bron-kō-plē'jĭ-ă) [" + *plēgē*, stroke]. Paralysis of the bronchial tubes.

bronchopleural (brŏn-kō-plūr'ăl). Pertaining to the bronchi and the pleural cavity.

bronchopneumonia (bron-ko-nu-mo'ne-a) [" + *pneumōnia*, lung inflammation]. Inflammation of the terminal bronchioles and alveoli. SEE ALSO: *pneumonia.*

ETIOL: It may be caused by various types of pneumococci; Group A hemolytic streptococcus; *Klebsiella pneumoniae* (Friedlander's bacillus) types A & B; various staphylococci; and *Pasteurella tularensis.* It may also be caused by other pathogenic bacteria as well as by viruses, rickettsias, and fungi.

SYM: Cough and expectoration; respiration short and shallow—from 50 to 75 per minute. Cyanosis may ensue. Nostrils dilate with each inspiration, and in children the temperature reaches 103° or 105° F.; before death, 108° F. Pulse, 140. Duration 2 to 3 weeks. Improvement may be followed by increased severity as new patches form. In the aged many of these symptoms are absent; slight cough and little sputum; temperature, 100 to 101° F. may or may not be in evidence. Weakness, sore throat, chills, chest pain. The elderly and bedridden are susceptible.

PROG: Depends principally upon time at which treatment is initiated, recovery generally occurring quicker in those treated during the first three days. Also prognosis more favorable for those under 50; unfavorable for the very young and very old. Mortality greatly reduced by use of antibiotics.

TREATMENT: Bed rest, increased intake of fluids, analgesics for pain, antibiotics, soft diet, oxygen for cyanosis, abdominal distention, and general comfort, treatment of shock if it occurs.

NP: Hygienic. Room, 65° to 70° F., humidified air. Cold sponge bath if necessary to control hyperpyrexia. Oxygen inhalations. Liquid or semiliquid food. Beware of relapse.

bron"chopul'monary [" + L. *pulmonarius*, pert. to lung]. Pert. to bronchi and lungs.

bron"chor'raphy [" + *raphē*, suture]. Suturing of a wound of the bronchus.

bronchorrhagia (bron-kor-ā'jĭ-ă) [" + *rēgnunai*, to break forth]. Bronchial hemorrhage.

bronchorrhea (bron-kō-rē'ă) [" + *roia*, flow]. Abnormal secretion from the bronchial mucous membrane, sometimes very offensive.

bronchorrhoncus (bron-kor-on'kus) [" + *rogchos*, snore]. A bronchial rale.

bronchoscope (bron'kō-skōp) [" + *skopein*, to examine]. An instrument for examining the interior of a bronchus.

bronchoscopy (bron-kos'kō-pĭ). Examination of the bronchi through a bronchoscope.

bronchosinusi'tis [G. *bronchos*, windpipe, + L. *sinus*, a hollow, + G. *-itis*, inflammation]. Infection of bronchi and sinuses at the same time.

bron'chospasm [" + *spasmos*, a spasm]. Spasm of the bronchus.

bronchospirochetosis (bron-kō-spī-rō-kē-tō'sis) [" + *speira*, coil, + *chaitē*, wavy hair]. Hemorrhagic bronchitis; bronchopulmonary spirochetosis resulting from spirochetes.

bronchospirometer (bronk"o-spī-rom'ĕ-ter). An instrument for determining the volume of air inspired from one lung and for collecting air for analysis.

bronchostaxis (bronk-o-stax'is). Hemorrhage from the walls of a bronchus.

bronchostenosis (bron-kō-sten-ō'sis) [" + *stenōsis*, a narrowing]. Narrowing of a bronchus.

bronchos'tomy [" + *stoma*, mouth]. Formation from without of an opening into a bronchus.

bron"chotet'any [" + *tetanos*, tetanus]. Extreme dyspnea due to spasm in the bronchi preventing access of air.

bronchotome (bron'kō-tom) [" + *tomē*, incision]. Instrument for making an incision of the trachea.

bronchotomy (bron-kot'o-mĭ). Surgical incision of a bronchus, the larynx, or trachea.

bron"chotra'cheal [G. *bronchos*, windpipe, + *tracheia*, trachea]. Pert. to both bronchi and trachea.

bron"choty'phoid [" + *typhos*, fever, + *eidos*, resemblance]. Typhoid fever marked by severe bronchitis in initial stage.

bronchovesic'ular [G. *bronchos*, windpipe, + L. *vesicula*, small bladder]. Pertaining to bronchial tubes and air vesicles with special reference to sounds intermediate between bronchial or tracheal sounds and vesicular sounds.

bronchus (bron'kus) (pl. *bronchi*) [G. *bronchos*]. One of the two large branches of the trachea. The trachea proper terminates at the level of the 4th dorsal vertebra. SEE: *bronchi.*

bronzed skin. A characteristic symptom of Addison's disease which is due to adrenal cortical insufficiency.

brood capsule or cyst. Cystlike bodies which develop within a hydatid cyst of *Echinococcus granulosus.*

brossage (brō-sazh′) [Fr. brushing]. Brushing the averted eyelids with stiff brush, to remove granulations, as in trachoma.

broth. 1. A nutrient drink such as bouillon usually served hot. 2. A liquid medium for culturing bacteria.

brow presentation. When the brow or face of the infant comes first on presentation in labor; makes birth almost impossible. Cesarean section is frequently needed if the presentation cannot be altered.

Brownian movement. Oscillatory movement of microscopic particles or particles of a colloidal system resulting from movement of the surrounding molecules. Based on the kinetic theory of matter, first described by Robt. Brown in 1827. This may be observed in bacteria but is distinguished from true motility resulting from activities initiated within the organism itself.

Brown-Séquard's paralysis (sa-kars′) [Charles E. Brown-Séquard, French physician, 1818-1894]. Reflex flaccid paraplegia occurring during some urinary tract affections.

B.-S.'s syndrome. Hemisection of the spinal cord with paralysis below the lesion on the affected side and with anesthesia and loss of tactile, pain, and temperature sensibility on the opposite side below the lesion.

Brucella (bru-sel′ă). A genus of bacteria, nonmotile. Aerobic, gram negative, and pathogenic to man causing undulant fever, and contagions and abortion in cattle, hogs, and goats.

brucel′lar. Pert. to Brucella.

brucellosis (brū-sĕl-ō′sĭs) [brucella, + *osis*]. A widespread infectious, febrile disease affecting principally cattle, swine, and goats, but sometimes affecting other animals including man. It is caused by bacteria of the genus *Brucella,* three species being involved: *B. melitensis* and *B. suis* the cause of brucellosis in goats and swine, respectively, and *B. abortus,* the cause of contagious abortion in cattle and other domestic animals. In man it is called *undulant fever* or *Malta fever* and is caused by any of the three species.

Bruch's membrane. A glassy membrane of the uvea of the eye lying between the chorioid membrane and the pigmented epithelium of the retina.

brucine (bru′sin). A poisonous alkaloid from *Strychnos nux vomica* and other *Strychnos* species. Similar to but less powerful than strychnine, *q.v.*

Bruck's disease (brooks) [Alfred Bruck, German physician, 1865-]. A rare disease characterized by muscle atrophy and skeletal disorders such as multiple fractures, ankyloses, etc.

bruise [Fr. *bruiser,* to break]. An injury with diffuse effusion into subcutaneous tissue, and in which skin is discolored but not broken. A contusion, *q.v.*

b. of head, chest, and abdomen. May be associated with internal injuries.

Sʏᴍ: Pain, swelling, tenderness, discoloration. NP: Mild antiseptic if skin is scratched. Cold applications with pressure.

b. or contusion of breast. Sʏᴍ: Pain, swelling, discoloration. NP: Apply cold applications and snug bandage with pressure and elevation. Sᴇᴇ: *contusion.*

bruissement (bru-ēs-mon′) [Fr. droning noise]. A purring sound heard by auscultation.

bruit (broo′ē) [Fr. noise]. An adventitious sound of venous or arterial origin heard on auscultation.

b. de craquement. Crackling.

b. de diable. 1. The venous hum of anemia. 2. Subjective tinnitus of chlorotic patients and a humming hallucination of hearing in the insane.

b. de frottement. Friction-like sound.

b., placental. A purring or blowing noise heard in the pregnant uterus due to fetal circulation of blood, and synchronous with the maternal pulse.

b. de pot fêlé. Cracked pot sound.

b. de râpe. Rasping.

b. de soufflet. Bellows sound.

Brunner's glands. Compound glands of the duodenum and upper jejunum. Also known as duodenal glands.

They are embedded in the submucous tissue and lined with columnar epithelium. They are similar to the pyloric glands of stomach. They secrete intestinal juice.

Brussels sprouts. The small, green, cabbage-like heads of the plant *Brassica oleracea gemmiferma.*

Cᴏᴏᴋᴇᴅ: 100 gm. Calories: 36. Other values: 4.9 gm. protein; 8.3 gm. carbohydrate; 4.9 mg. iron; 520 I.U. vitamin A; 0.14 mg. riboflavin; 87 mg. ascorbic acid.

bruxism (brŭks′izm). Grinding of the teeth, especially during sleep.

BSR. Abbr. for *basal skin resistance.*

bubo (bū′bō) (pl. *buboes*) [G. *boubōn,* groin]. An inflamed, swollen or enlarged lymph node often exhibiting suppuration, occurring commonly after chancroid, gonorrhea, or lymphogranuloma venereum. Nodes most commonly affected are those of the groin and axilla. Buboes may also develop after other infectious diseases, especially bubonic plague.

b., axillary. One in the axilla or armpit.

b., indolent. One in which suppuration does not occur.

b., inguinal. One in the region of the groin.

b., pestilential. One occurring in bubonic plague.

b., venereal. One resulting from a venereal disease.

bubonadenitis (bu-bon-ad-en-i′tis) [" + *adēn,* gland, + *-itis,* inflammation]. Inflammation of an inguinal gland.

bubonal′gia [" + *algos,* pain]. Pain in the groin.

bubon d'emblée (bu-boh″ dăhm-blā′) [Fr.]. Venereal bubo appearing without previous lesion.

bubon′ic plague [" + L. *plāgā,* epidemic]. An acute, infectious disease, common in the Orient, esp. India. The Black Death of the Middle Ages. It is frequently fatal.

Eᴛɪᴏʟ: Caused by *Pasteurella pestis,* usually from infected rats and ground squirrels, which is imparted to human beings by bite of the rat-flea. It is characterized by enlargement of lymphatic glands, severe toxic symptoms, accompanied by intense adenitis or pneumonia. Sᴇᴇ: *plague.*

bubonocele (bu-bon′o-sēl) [" + *kēlē,* tumor]. Inguinal hernia.

bubononcus (bu-bon-on′kus) [" + *ogchos,* tumor]. A swelling in the inguinal region.

bucar′dia [G. *bous,* ox, + *kardia,* heart]. Severe hypertrophy of the heart.

bucca (buk′a) [L. mouth, cheek]. 1. The mouth. 2. Hollow part of the cheek.

buc'cal. Pert. to the cheek or mouth.

b. cavity. The mouth.

b. fat pad. The corpus adiposum or suctorial pad, an encapsulated mass of fat lying superficial to the buccinator muscle. It is well developed in infants and is thought to aid in the act of sucking.

b. glands. Small glands situated in the mucous membranes of the mouth which secrete saliva.

buccella'tion [L. *buccella,* morsel]. Hemostasis by use of a lint pad or compress.

buccinatolabialis (buk-sin-at-o-lā-bĭ-a'lis) [L. *buccinator,* trumpeter, + *labialis,* pert. to the lips]. The buccinator and orbicularis oris as one.

buccinator (buk'sin-a-tor) [L. *buccinator,* trumpeter]. The muscle of the cheek. SEE: *muscles.*

buccoversion (buk-o-ver'shun) [L. *bucca,* mouth, + *versiō,* a turning]. Position of part buccal to line of occlusion; said of a tooth.

buccula (buk'ū-lă) [L. a little cheek]. A double chin.

Buck's extension [Gurdon Buck, American surgeon, 1807-1877]. An apparatus consisting of a weight and pulley for applying extension to a limb.

buclamase (buck'lă-mās). Proprietary name for alpha amylase, a starch-splitting enzyme. Used orally as an adjunct in management of inflammation, edema and pain of traumatic injuries, postoperative tissue reactions, allergic reactions, infection, and connective tissue disorders.

bucnemia (buk-ne'mĭ-ă) [G. *bous,* ox, + *knēmē,* leg].Tense inflammatory swelling of the leg; elephantiasis.

bud. 1. In *Anat.,* a small structure resembling a bud of a plant as a taste bud. 2. In *Embryol.,* a small protuberance or outgrowth which is the anlage or primordium of an organ or structure, as a *limb bud.*

b., taste. An ovoid body embedded in the stratified epithelium of the tongue and also found sparingly on the epiglottis and soft palate. Buds contain the sensory receptors for taste.

bud'ding [M.E. *budde,* to swell]. A method of asexual reproduction in which a budlike process grows from the side or end of the parent and develops into a new organism which in some cases remains attached, in others separates and lives an independent existence. It is common in lower animals (sponges, coelenterates) and plants (yeasts, molds).

Buerger's disease (bur'gers) [Leo Buerger, New York physician, 1879-1943]. A chronic recurring inflammatory occlusive disease, chiefly of the peripheral arteries and veins of a limb, with an extraordinary affinity for males between the ages of 15 and 50 years. It is fairly rare in occurrence. SYN: *thromboangiitis obliterans.*

SYM: Paresthesia of the foot, or pain confined to one toe. Easy fatigue. Cramps in legs but not to be confused with those occurring in the aged. Legs give out, esp. when walking. Ulceration or moist gangrene may set in; amputation may be necessary.

TREATMENT: Absolute and continued abstinence from tobacco in all forms is extremely important. AVOID: excessive use of affected limb; exposure to temperature extremes; trauma; use of drugs which diminish blood supply to extremities; fungus infections. If gangrene, rest pain, or ulceration are present, however, complete bed rest is advised. For arterial spasm, blocking of the sympathetic nervous system by injection of various drugs or by sympathectomy may be done. SEE: *thromboangiitis obliterans.*

buffer (bŭf'ĕr) [Fr. *buffe,* blow]. 1. A substance, esp. a salt of the blood, tending to preserve original hydrogen-ion concentration of its solution, upon adding an acid or base. 2. A substance tending to offset reaction of an agent administered in conjunction with it.

b. action. Ability of chemical solutions to neutralize excess acid or base and thus prevent change in the pH of the solution.

b., blood. One present in the blood. The principal buffers are: carbonic acid, carbonates and bicarbonates, monobasic and dibasic phosphates, and proteins. Hemoglobin is an important protein buffer.

b. salts. Substances in the blood which act as a buffer.

buf'fy coat [Fr. *buffe,* buffalo]. Light stratum of a blood clot seen when the blood is allowed to stand in a test tube. The red blood cells settle to the bottom, then between the plasma and the red blood cells there is a light-colored layer which contains mostly white blood cells.

bug (M.E. *bugge,* swollen). A term applied loosely to any small insect or arthropod; more specifically a member of the order Hemiptera which includes the squash bug, chinch bug, and bedbug. They have sucking mouth parts, incomplete metamorphosis, and two pairs of wings, the fore pair being half membranous. The following bugs are of medical importance:

b., assassin. One belonging to the family Reduviidae. Many are predaceous; others are blood-sucking. *Pantastrongulus, Triatoma,* and *Rhodnius* are vectors of trypanosome diseases (Chagas' disease) in man.

b., bed. A member of the family Cimicidae, esp. of the genus *Cimex.*

b., kissing. Several species of the family Reduviidae. *Melanolestes picipes* is the common kissing bug, or black corsair.

b., red. The larvae of mites of the family Trombiculidae, commonly called "chiggers".

buggery (bug'er-ĭ) [Fr. *bougrerie,* heresy]. Unnatural sexual relations through the anus. SYN: *sodomy.*

bulb [G. *bolbos,* a bulbous root]. 1. An expansion of a canal vessel or organ. 2. Obsolete term for the medulla oblongata.

b., aortic. Dilated portion of the truncus arteriosus in the embryo which gives rise to the roots of the aorta and pulmonary arteries.

b., duodenal. Upper duodenal area just beyond pylorus.

b. of the eye. The eyeball.

b., hair. The expanded portion at the lower end of the hair root.

b., olfactory. The ant. enlargement of the olfactory tract.

b., terminal, of Krause. An encapsulated sensory nerve-ending similar in structure to the corpuscles of Pacini. Also called corpuscle of Golgi-Manzoni.

b. of the urethra. The post. portion of the spongy body.

b. of the vestibule. The vaginal bulb or *bulbus vestibuli, q.v.*

bul'bar. 1. Pert. to a bulb. 2. Shaped like a bulb. 3. Pert. to the medulla oblongata.

b. paralysis. Paralysis due to changes in motor centers of the oblongata. SEE: *paralysis.*

bul'biform [G. *bolbos*, bulbous root, + L. *forma*, shape]. Shaped like a bulb.

bulbitis (bul-bī'tis) [" + *-itis*, inflammation]. Inflammation of the urethra in its bulbous portion.

bul'bi vestib'uli vaginae. Two elongated masses of erectile tissue on either side of the vaginal orifice. They are united in front by a narrow band.

bulbocaverno'sus [G. *bolbos*, + L. *cavernosus*, hollow]. A muscle ensheathing the bulb of the penis in the male or covering the bulbus vestibuli in the female. Also called in the male *ejaculator urinae, accelerator urinae;* in the female *sphincter vaginae.*

bulbocav'ernous reflex. Contraction of bulbocavernous muscle on percussing dorsum of penis.

bulbomim'ic reflex. Contraction of facial muscles following pressure on eyeball.

bulbonu'clear [" + L. *nucleus*, kernel]. Pert. to the nuclei in the medulla oblongata.

bulbourethral glands (bul"bō-ū-rē'thral) [" + *ourēthra*, urethra]. Cowper's glands.

Two small glands about the size of a pea, one on each side of the prostate gland, each with a duct about 1 inch (2.5 cm.) long, terminating in the wall of the urethra. They secrete a viscid fluid forming part of the seminal fluid.

RS: *prostate gland; urethra.*

bulbous. Bulb-shaped; swollen; terminating in an enlargement.

bul'bus [G. *bolbos*, bulbous root]. Bulb, *q.v.*

b. corpus cavernosum. Bulb of the urethra. A bulbous swelling of the corpus cavernosum at base of the penis.

b. vestibuli. Two oval masses of erectile tissue lying beneath the vestibule and resting on the urogenital diaphragm. They are homologous to the bulbus cavernosum urethra of the male.

bulesis (bu-lē'sis) [G. *boulēsis*, a willing]. An act of the will; the will.

bulimia (bu-lim'ĭ-ă) [G. *bous*, ox, + *limos*, hunger]. Hunger experienced a short time after a meal; morbid hunger.

bulim'ic. Pert. to bulimia.

bulla (bul'la) (pl. *bullae*) [L. a bubble]. A large blister or skin vesicle filled with fluid; a bleb, *q.v.* SEE: *pompholyx.*

b. ethmoidal'is. A rounded projection into the middle meatus of the nose underneath the middle turbinated bone, formed by an ant. ethmoid cell.

b. ossea. The dilated portion of the bony external meatus of the ear. SEE: *pompholyx.*

bullate (bul'āt). Said of a surface growth which appears blistered because of convex prominences.

bullation (bul-a'shun) [L. *bulla*, a bubble]. 1. Division into small compartments. 2. Inflation.

bullet wound. Puncture wound from a bullet. SEE: *wounds.*

bullous (bul'us) [L. *bulla*, bubble]. Having the nature of a bulla.

BUN. Abbr. for *blood urea nitrogen.*

bun'dle. A group of fibers; a fasciculus.

b., Arnold's. The frontopontile tract. It passes from the cerebral cortex of frontal lobe through the internal capsule and cerebral peduncle to the pons.

b., atrioventricular. A bundle of fibers of the impulse-conducting system of the heart. From its origin in the A-V node it enters the interventricular septum where it divides into two branches whose fibers pass to the right and left ventricles respectively, the fibers of each trunk becoming continuous with the Purkinje fibers of the ventricles. SEE: *heart block.* SYN: *A-V bundle; bundle of His.*

b., Bechterew's. The spino-olivary fasciculus or Helweg's bundle.

b. of His. Atrioventricular b., *q.v.*

b., Schultze's. Comma-shaped path of fibers in middle of spinal cord's fasciculus cuneatus.

b. of Turck. The temporopontile tract. Fibers pass from the cerebral cortex of temporal lobe and terminate in the pons.

bundle branch block. A defect in the heart's construction system wherein there is failure of conduction down one of the main branches of the *bundle of His.* SEE: *heart block.*

bunion (bun'yun) [G. *bounion*, turnip]. Inflammation and thickening of the bursa of the joint of the great toe, usually associated with marked enlargement of the joint and displacement of the toe, laterally. SEE: *hallux valgus.*

bunodont (bū-nō'dŏnt). Having round or conical cusps, said of molar teeth, in contrast to *lophodont* in which crowns bear ridges or crests.

bunogaster (bu-nō-gas'ter) [G. *bounos*, mound, + *gastēr*, belly]. Protrusion of the abdomen.

Bunsen burner [Robert W. E. von Bunsen, German chemist, 1811-1899]. A gas burner named after its inventor.

It has an adjustment by which the air holes at the bottom of the tube can be closed or open and the flame made either yellow or blue. If the holes are closed, the flame burns yellow, *i.e.*, it will give light but a relatively small amount of heat. Its action may be reversed by the opening of the holes.

buphthalmia, buphthalmos (buf-thal'mĭ-ă, -mos) [G. *bous*, ox, + *ophthalmos*, eye]. Condition of infantile glaucoma resulting in uniform enlargement of eye, particularly the cornea.

Disease may stop spontaneously or continue until it produces blindness.

TREATMENT: Iridectomy, sclerotomy, miotics. SEE: *hydrophthalmos.*

Burdach's tracts. Continuation of dorsolateral column of spinal cord into medulla oblongata. SYN: *cuneate fasciculus*

buret, burette (bû-ret') [Fr. small holder for fluid]. A graduated tube for measuring a reagent.

burn (bern) [A.S. *brinnan*, to burn]. Tissue injury resulting from excessive exposure to thermal, chemical, electrical, or radioactive agents. The effects vary according to the type, duration, and intensity of the agent and part of body involved. The effects may be *local* resulting in cell injury or death, or *systemic* involving primary shock (that occurring immediately after the injury and rarely fatal) or secondary shock (that developing insidiously following severe burns and often fatal).

Burns are usually classified as:

(a) *First degree burns.* Superficial burns, damage being limited to outer layer of the epidermis. Characterized by erythema, hyperemia, tenderness and pain. No vesiculation.

(b) *Second degree burns.* Burns in which damage extends through the epidermis and into the dermis but not of sufficient extent to interfere with regeneration of epidermis. Vesicles usually present.

(c) *Third degree burns.* Burns in which both epidermis and dermis are destroyed with damage extending into underlying tissues. Vesiculation often absent. Tissues may be charred or coagulated.

TREATMENT: Emergency treatment of burns which cover less than ½ of the body should be cooling of the burned portion by immersion in water of approximately 50° F. temperature. This will bring about almost immediate relief of pain and will aid subsequent healing of the wound. If facilities for immersion are not available, cold compresses may be used. Treatment varies with type of burn and extent of body involved. Therapy for all burns involves asepsis and proper care of wounds, relief from pain, prevention or control of infection if it occurs, prevention or relief of shock, maintenance of water and electrolyte balance, and proper nutrition esp. to correct hypoproteinemia which usually accompanies burns.

In severe burns shock is always present and may cause death. Morphine is administered immediately, followed by intravenous injections of whole blood and of salt solutions to prevent shock. When pain has eased, charred clothing is removed and burned area is gently washed with a sterile normal saline solution.

Treatment may be by use of pressure dressings or by open technic. Experimentation with technics such as an air bed, which keeps the body suspended on a layer of air, and use of topical silver nitrate are in progress and show promise. Also, the use of split-thickness skin grafts from the patient are being used much sooner after the burn than formerly.

The use of appropriate antibiotics, blood protein and fluid replacement have made possible the salvage with full recovery of extensively burned patients who were formerly almost certain to die.

PRECAUTIONS: 1. Never allow a person whose clothing is burning to run. Make him lie down and roll. Wrap him in a rug, blanket, or anything within reach and smother the flames. Be careful not to allow him to inhale the smoke. Cut away the clothing, taking care not to pull any portion of the skin away. 2. Do not open any blisters, as this increases the chance for infections.

COMPLICATIONS (in burns and scalds): Sloughing, gangrene, erysipelas, nephritis, pneumonia, or intestinal disturbances; sudden attacks of rigor, vomiting, rise of temperature or convulsions are all suspicious symptoms. A superficial burn covering a large part of the body is more serious than a small, deep one, unless important nerves and blood vessels are involved. If two-thirds of the skin are destroyed, death may be expected, even in a burn of the first degree. Shock must always be anticipated regardless of degree of burn.

Forms

b., acid. Due to exposure to corrosive acids, as sulfuric, hydrochloric, nitric, etc. F. A. TREATMENT: Wash with large volumes of water; apply dilute alkalies, as baking soda (sodium bicarbonate) paste, soap solution dressing, chalk paste, etc. Follow with a bland oil or ointment.

b., alkali. Due to caustic alkalies, as lye, caustic potash (potassium hydroxide), caustic soda (sodium hydroxide), etc. SYM: Painful lesion of skin often associated with gelatinization of tissue. F. A. TREATMENT: Wash with large volumes of water. Follow by wet dressings of dilute acid, as citrus fruit juices, weak vinegar, dilute acetic acid, etc. Later dress with bland ointments or oils, or irrigate with boric acid solution. Follow by instillation of liquid paraffin or other bland oil.

b., brush. A combined burn and abrasion resulting from friction. TREATMENT: Like abrasion, *q.v.*

b., chemical. Injuries due to the action of corrosive or irritating chemicals, as acid burns, *q.v.*, alkali burns, *q.v.*

Burns from chemical acids or alkalies should be treated by flushing the surface with water, thereby removing all traces of the drug. Remember that usually an acid counteracts an alkali, so that weak vinegar, weak ammonia, or a solution of sodium bicarbonate is always safe. A carbolic acid burn is almost always counteracted by alcohol. Never use oil as it helps in the absorption of acid. If lime gets into the eye, flush the eye with water and follow with a solution of weak vinegar.

b., electric. A result of exposure to electricity. The extent of destruction is much greater than that evidenced by initial inspection. TREATMENT: SEE: *electric injuries.*

b. of eye. F. A. TREATMENT: Wash well with warm water and instill bland oil, as sweet oil or paraffin oil. SEE: *lye.*

b., fireworks. Such injuries are usually burns, often with embedded foreign bodies and a high incidence of infection and tetanus which should be prevented by meticulous care of injury and use of antitetanus serum.

b., flash. A burn resulting from an explosive blast as occurs from ignition of highly inflammable fluids, or in war, from a high-explosive shell or a nuclear blast.

b., gunpowder. Often followed by tetanus which should be prevented by administration of antitetanus serum and meticulous care of injury.

b., radiation. One resulting from overexposure to radiant energy as from roentgen rays, radium emanations, sunlight, or nuclear blast.

b., respiratory. One in which the respiratory tract is injured, as from inhalation of hot gases.

b., thermal. One resulting from contact with fire, hot objects, or fluids.

b., x-ray. SEE: *radiation burn.*

Burns' amauro'sis [G. *amauroein,* to darken] [John Burns, Scotch obstetrician, 1774-1850]. Dimness of sight or blindness following sexual excesses.

burrow. A tunnel made in the skin by the itch mite, *Sarcoptes scabei.*

bur'rowing. The formation of: (1) A subcutaneous tunnel made by a parasite, or (2) a fistula or sinus containing pus.

bur'sa [G. a leather sac]. 1. A padlike sac or cavity found in connecting tissue usually in the vicinity of joints. They are lined with synovial membrane and contain a fluid synovia which acts to reduce friction between tendon and bone, tendon and ligament, or between other structures where friction is likely to occur. 2. A blind sac or cavity.

b., Achilles. One located between the tendon of Achilles and the calcaneus.

b., adventitious. One not usually present but which develops in response to friction or pressure.

b., olecranon. One at the elbow joint lying between olecranon process and the skin.

b., omental. The lesser peritoneal cavity; the cavity of the great omentum. It communicates with the greater or true peritoneal cavity via the vestibule and epiploic foramen.

b., patellar. One of several bursae located in region of the patella. Includes the suprapatellar, infrapatellar, and prepatellar bursae. Some communicate with the cavity of the knee joint.

b., pharyngeal. A small, median, blind sac found in lower portion of the pharyngeal tonsil.

b., subacromial. A large bursa lying between the acromium and coracoacromial ligament above, and the insertion of the supraspinatus below.

bursae. Plural of bursa, *q.v.*

bur'sal. Pert. to a bursa.

bursa'lis [L. *bursalis*, pert. to a bursa]. Obturator internus muscle.

bursalogy (ber-sal'ō-jĭ) [G. *bursa*, leather sac, + *logos*, study]. Anatomy, pathology, and physiology of bursae.

bursectomy (ber-sek'tō-mĭ) [" + *ektomē*, excision]. Excision of a bursa.

bursitis (ber-sī'tĭs) [" + *-itis*, inflammation]. Inflammation of a bursa, especially those located between bony prominences and muscle or tendon, as the shoulder, knee, etc.

Common forms include painful shoulder (subacromial bursa, *q.v.*) miner's or tennis elbow (olecranon bursa, *q.v.*), housemaid's knee (prepatellar bursa, *q.v.*), and bunion, *q.v.*

TREATMENT: Rest, immobilization of affected part during acute stage. Active mobilization as soon as acute symptoms subside will help to prevent adhesions. Analgesics, heat, and diathermy are helpful. Injection of local anesthetics or cortisone into bursa may be required. In chronic bursitis surgical removal of calcification may be necessary.

bur'solith [" + *lithos*, stone]. A calculus formed in a bursa.

bursop'athy [" + *pathos*, disease]. Any pathological condition of a bursa.

bursula (bur'sū-la) [L. *bursula*, little sac]. A small bursa.

b. testium. The scrotum.

Burton's line [Henry Burton, British physician, 1799-1849]. A blue line along the margin of the gums visible in chronic lead poisoning.

butacaine sulfate (bū'tă-kān). A topical local anesthetic.

butane (bu'tān). C_4H_{10}. A gaseous, inflammable hydrocarbon from petroleum.

butazolidin. Proprietary name for phenylbutazone, used in treatment of acute rheumatic disease. It has a potent anti-inflammatory action.

butisol sodium. Proprietary name for butabarbital sodium, a sedative and hypnotic.

butter [G. *bouturon*]. COMP: It consists largely of butter fat which is made up of stearin. Butyric, palmitic, and oleic acid are the acids found in butter fat. 100 gm. salted (approximately 10 "pats" or 7 tablespoons). Calories: 720. Other values: 81 gm. fat; 20 mg. calcium; 3300 I.U. vitamin A; 23 mg. sodium.

buttermilk. Cultured from skim milk. Av. SERVING: 100 gm. Calories: 36. Other values: 3.6 gm. protein; 5.1 gm. carbohydrate; 121 mg. calcium; 0.10 mg. thiamine; 0.18 mg. riboflavin; 0.1 mg. niacin; 1.0 mg. ascorbic acid.

buttocks (but'uks) [M.E. *butte*, thick end]. The gluteal prominence, commonly called the "seat" or "rump."

button anastomosis. One made to unite severed portions of the hollow viscera without suture. Devised by Murphy.

button forceps. Those for holding parts of an anastomosis button while it is being adjusted and placed.

buttonhole. A straight cut through the wall of a cavity.

b. fracture. Perforation of a bone by a missile.

b., mitral. Contraction of any orifice to a slit, as that of the heart.

b. operation. Boutonnière's operation. An artificial slit in a membrane.

button suture. One for preventing a suture from cutting through or into underlying tissue. VARIETIES: *Getchell's, lead, Powell's and silver wire.* Also perforated shot.

butylchloral hydrate (bu'til-klo'ral hi'drāt). A preparation similar in action to chloral, but said to be less depressant and more analgesic.

USES: Recommended for relief of facial neuralgia.

butyn (bu'tin). Proprietary name for butacaine sulfate, *q.v.*

butyraceous (bu-ti-rā'shus) [G. *bouturon*, butter]. Containing or resembling butter.

butyrate (bu'tĭ-rāt). A salt of butyric acid.

butyr'ic acid. A fatty acid (C_3H_7COOH); about 5% butter but rare in most fats. It is a viscid liquid with a rancid odor.

butyrin (bū'tir-in). A soft, yellowish, semiliquid fat which is present in butter.

butyroid (bu'tĭ-roid) [G. *bouturon*, butter, + *eidos*, appearance]. Having the appearance or consistency of butter.

butyrometer (bu-tĭ-rom'ĕ-ter) [" + *metron*, measure]. Device for estimating amt. of butter fat of milk.

butyrous (but'ĭ-rus). Of butter-like consistency.

Byrd-Dew method [Harvey L. Byrd, American physician, 1820-1884, and James H. Dew, American physician, 1843-1914]. One for resuscitating newborn child suffering from asphyxia. Operator supports supine child on palms of his hands, allowing head to fall backward. By supination of forearms, operator flexes child's body and effects expiration. By pronation of arms, body is again extended, causing inspiration.

bysma (bĭs'mă) [G. plug]. A plug or tampon.

byssinosis (bĭs-ĭ-nō'sĭs) [G. *byssos*, cotton, + *-osis*]. Pulmonary disease caused by the inhalation of cotton dust and the foreign materials contained therein, including bacteria, mold, and fungi.

byssocausis (bis-ō-kaw'sis) [" + *kausis*, burning]. Cauterization by moxa; moxibustion.

bys'soid [" + *eidos*, form]. Consisting of a filamentous fringe, the filaments being of unequal length.

byssophthisis (bis-o-this'is) [" + *phthisis*, a wasting away]. Byssinosis, *q.v.*

byssus (bis'us) [G. *byssos*, cotton]. The growth of hair on the pubic region.

Notes

Notes

Notes

C

C. Symb. for *carbon.* Abbr. for *congius* (gallon) *compound, centigrade, Celsius* (scale or thermometer), *clonus, closure,* L. *centum* (one hundred), L. *cum* (with).

C_3 population. Those who have imperfect mental or physical development.

C^{14}. Radioactive carbon.

Ca. Symb. for *calcium.*

Ca. Abbr. for *cathode.*

cabagin. Vitamin U.

cabbage [Fr. *cabocher,* to make a swelling]. A leafy vegetable, growing in a head. A base-forming food.

RAW (shredded): 1 cup (100 gm.). Calories: 24. Other main values: 1.3 gm. protein; 5.4 gm. carbohydrate; 49 mg. calcium; 47 mg. ascorbic acid.

Cabot's ring bodies [Richard C. Cabot, Boston physician, 1868-1939]. Ring shaped bodies sometimes seen in red blood cells in pernicious anemia, lymphatic leukemia, and lead poisoning.

cac-, caco- [G. from *kakos,* bad]. Prefix denoting *bad,* or *diseased.*

CaC_2. Calcium carbide.

cacan'thrax [" + *anthrax,* carbuncle]. Cutaneous form of anthrax.

cacao (kă-kā'ō, kă-kă'ō) [Mexican from Spanish *cacahuatl,* seed]. 1. Seed of *Theobroma cacao* used to prepare cacao butter (theobroma oil), chocolate, and cocoa. 2. USP. A reddish to brown powder prepared from the roasted ripe seeds of *Theobroma cacao* Linné (family Sterculiaceae) and having a chocolate odor and taste. Used in a syrup base, as a flavoring vehicle for certain medications. SEE ALSO: *cocoa, q.v.*

cacatory (kak'ă-tor-ĭ). Accompanied by diarrhea or excessive bowel movements.

cacemia (kas-ē'mĭ-ă) [G. *kakos,* bad, + *aima,* blood]. A poor condition of the blood.

cacesthesia (kak-es-thē'zĭ-ă) [" + *aisthē*-work]. Defective functioning, mentally or physically.

cacesthesia (kak-es-thē'zĭ-ă) [" + *aisthēsis,* sensation]. 1. Disorder of sensibility, morbid or otherwise. 2. Malaise.

caché (kash-ā') [Fr. covered]. A lead cone covered with paper layers, with mica bottom, used for applying radiotherapy, radium or any radioactive substance.

cachectic (kă-kek'tĭk) [G. *kakos,* ill, + *exis,* habit]. Pert. to cachexia.

cachet (kă-shā') [Fr. a seal]. Two concave pieces of wafer (rice paper) bet. which is placed medicine to be administered, the margins being pressed together so they will adhere.

cachexia (ka-keks'ĭ-ă) [G. *kakos,* ill, + *exis,* habit]. A state of ill health, malnutrition and wasting. It may occur in many chronic diseases as certain malignancies, advanced pulmonary tuberculosis, etc.

c., cancerous. C. caused by cancerous condition.

c., hypophyseal. Pituitary c., *q.v.*

c. hypophysiopri'va. Symptoms resulting from removal of the hypophysis cerebri.

c., lymphatic. C. caused by Hodgkin's disease of the lymph nodes.

c., malarial. C. due to chronic malaria.

c., pachydermic. C. due to myxedemic condition.

c., pituitary. Group of symptoms caused by atrophy of pituitary gland, including emaciation, premature aging, atrophy of genitals with loss of secondary sex characteristics and lowering of basal metabolic rate. SYN: *Simmond's disease.*

c. splenetica. C. caused by disease of the spleen. SYN: *pseudoleukocythemia.*

c. strumipri'va. Myxedema due to removal of the thyroid gland.

c., thyreopriva. Strumipriva c., *q.v.*

cachinna'tion (kak-ĭ-nā'shun) [L. *cachinnāre,* to laugh aloud]. Hysterical laughter.

$CaCl_2$. Calcium chloride; a bleaching powder.

$Ca(ClO_3)_2$. Calcium chlorate.

caco-, cac- [G. from *kakos,* bad]. Prefix denoting *bad* or *diseased.*

$CaCO_3$. Calcium carbonate; chalk.

CaC_2O_4. Calcium oxalate.

cacochylia (kak-o-ki'lĭ-ă) [" + *chylos,* chyle]. Impaired digestion.

cacochy'mia [" + *chymos,* chyme]. 1. Disordered metabolism. 2. Cacochylia.

cacodontia (kak-o-don'tĭ-ă) [" + *odous, odont-,* tooth]. Bad teeth.

cacodyl (kak'o-dil). Poisonous arsenical compound, $As(CH_3)_2$.

cacodylate. A salt of cacodylic acid, used in skin diseases or where arsenic is indicated.

cacoethes (kak-o-e'thes) [" + *ēthos,* character]. Any bad habit, propensity, or disorder.

cacogenesis (kak-o-jen'ĕ-sis) [G. *kakos,* bad, + *genesis,* development]. Any abnormal development or growth.

cacogen'ic. Pert. to race degeneration.

cacogen'ics [G. *kakos,* bad, + *gennan,* to produce]. Race degeneration resulting from reproduction of inferior persons.

cacomelia (kak-ō-me'lĭ-ă). Congenital deformity of a limb.

cacomorphia (kak-ō-mor'fĭ-ă) [" + *morphē,* form]. Malformation; deformity.

cacop'athy [" + *pathos,* disease]. Malignant disease; a severe disorder.

cacoplas'tic [" + *plastikos,* formed]. 1. Pert. to or causing morbid growth. 2. Incapable of normal development or formation.

cacorhythmic (kak-o-rith'mĭk) [" + *rythmos,* rhythm]. Showing irregularity of rhythm.

cacosmia (kă-kos'mĭ-ă) [" + *osmē,* smell]. 1. An unpleasant odor. 2. A form of parosmia. Imaginary foul odors which do not exist.

cacothenics (kak-ō-then'ĭks) [" + *thēnia,* state of being]. Racial degeneration from hostile environment.

cacothymia (kak-o-thi'mĭ-ă) [" + *thymos,* spirit]. A disorder of the mind; moral depravity; insane morbidity of temper.

cacot'rophy [" + *trophē,* nourishment]. Malnutrition.

cacumen (kak-ū'mĕn) (pl. *cacumina*) [L. *cacumina,* summit]. 1. Part of cerebellum below the declivis. 2.The top of anything.

cadaver (kă-dav′er) (pl. *cadav′era*) [L. corpse, from *cadere*, to fall]. A dead body; a corpse.

cadaveric (kă-dav′er-ĭk). Pert. to a dead body.

cadaverous (kă-dav′er-us). Resembling, esp. having the color or appearance of, a corpse.

cadmium (kad′mĭ-ŭm) [G. *cadmia*, earth]. A metallic element occurring in zinc. It is a soft, bluish white metal and is used industrially in electroplating and in atomic fission. SYMB: Cd. At. wt. 112.40; at. no. 48.

caduca (kă-dū′kă) [L. *caducus*, falling off]. Thickened membrane of the uterus; the decidua of the uterus.

caduceus (kă-dū′shus) [L. a herald's wand]. The wand of Hermes or Mercury; used as a symbol of the medical profession.

caffeine (kaf′ēn) [L.]. USP. $C_8H_{10}N_4O_2$. An alkaloid of coffee and tea that is a stimulant and a diuretic.

About 100 mg. are found in a strong cup of coffee.

ACTION AND USES: Diuretic, cardiac, and respiratory stimulant, and as a headache remedy.

INCOMPATIBILITIES: Alkalies, tannic acid, quinine sulfate.

c., citrated. A mixture of caffeine and citric acid, containing about 52% caffeine. Possesses same properties as caffeine, but more likely to disagree with the digestive functions.

c. and sodium benzoate. USP. A mixture of equal parts of caffeine and sodium benzoate.

ACTION AND USES: Same as caffeine.

c. and sodium salicylate. NF. A mixture of caffeine with sodium salicylate, containing about 52% caffeine.

USES: Same as caffeine.

caffeinism (kaf′ēn-ĭzm) [L. *caffeina*]. Chronic effects of excessive use of coffee.

SYM: Sudden flushing of the face, palpitation of the heart, trembling, general depression, anxiety, insomnia, and nervousness.

cainotophobia (ki-no-to-fo′bĭ-ă) [G. *kainotēs*, novelty, + *phobos*, fear]. Fear of novelty. Cenotophobia, *q.v.*

caisson disease (kā′son) [Fr. *caisse*, a box, from L. *capsa*, box]. A condition induced in divers subject to too rapid reduction of air pressure after coming to the surface and after breathing compressed air in caissons. SYN: *decompression sickness; bends, q.v.*

caked breast. A stagnation of milk in the secreting ducts.

Cal. Abbr. of *large calorie*.

cal. Abbr. of *small calorie*.

calage (kal-azh′) [Fr. wedging]. Fixation of body in a berth by means of pillows to prevent movement and so to relieve seasickness.

calamine (kal′ă-mīn). USP. A pink powder, containing zinc oxide with small amt. of ferric oxide.

USES: Externally in various skin conditions, as a protective and astringent, as an ointment, or as a lotion.

calcaneal, calcanean (kal-kā′nē-ăl, -an) [L. *calcaneus*, heel bone]. Pert. to the calcaneus, the heel bone.

calcaneodynia (kal-kā″nē-ō-din′ĭ-ă) [" + G. *odynē*, pain]. Pain in the heel.

calcaneum (kal-kā′nē-ŭm) (pl. *calcanea*) [L. *calcaneus*, heel bone]. Same as calcaneus, *q.v.*

calcaneus (kal-kā′nē-us) (pl. *calcanei*) [L. *calcaneus*, heel bone]. 1. [NA] The heel bone, or *os calcis*. It articulates anteriorly with the cuboid bone, and with the astragalus above. 2. Talipes calcaneus, *q.v.*

calcanodynia (kal-kan-o-din′ĭ-ă) [" + *odynē*, pain]. Pain in the heel when standing or walking.

cal′car [L. a spur]. A spurlike process.

c. avis. Hippocampus minor, lower of two elevations on inner wall of post horn of lateral ventricle of brain.

c. femorale. A bony spur that strengthens the femoral neck.

c. pedis. The heel.

calcareous (kal-ka′re-us) [L. *calcarius*, pert. to lime]. Of the nature of lime; chalky.

calcarine (kal′kar-ĭn) [L. *calcar*, spur]. Spur-shaped.

calcariuria (kal-kar-ĭ-ū′rĭ-ă) [L. *calcarius*, pert. to lime, + G. *ouron*, urine]. Calcium salts in the urine.

calcaroid (kal′kar-oid) [" + G. *eidos*, appearance]. Calciumlike deposit in brain tissue.

calcemia (kal-sē′mĭ-ă) [" + G. *aima*, blood]. Excess of calcium in the blood.

calcic (kal′sĭk). Pert. to calcium or lime.

calcicosis (kal-sĭ-ko′sis) [L. *calx*, lime, + G. *-ōsis*, infection]. Pneumoconiosis caused by inhaling dust from limestone, esp. by marblecutters.

calcidin (kal′sĭ-dĭn). Proprietary name for an available iodine combination with lime and starch plus calcium iodate. Used for dry cough due to simple colds.

calciferol (cal-sĭf′ĕr-ol). Vitamin D_2. A synthetic vitamin D; it has the most vitamin D activity of those substances derived from ergosterol. It is used for prophylaxis and treatment of vitamin D deficiency, rickets and in hypocalcemic tetany.

calciferous (kal-sif′er-us) [" + *ferre*, to carry]. Containing calcium, chalk, or lime.

calcific (kal-sif′ĭk) [" + *facere*, to make] Forming lime.

calcification [" + *facere*, to make]. Deposit of lime salts in the tissues, and commonly in bone.

c., arterial. Deposition of calcium in walls of arteries.

c., metastatic. That of soft tissue with transference of calcium from bone, as in osteomalacia and disease of the parathyroid glands.

calcigerous (kal-sij′er-us) [" + *gerere*, to bear]. Containing lime or lime salts.

c. tubes. Dentinal tubules of dentin

calcim′eter [L. *calx*, lime, + G. *metron*, measure]. Device for measuring the calcium in the blood.

calcina′tion [L. *calcindre*, to char]. Drying by roasting to produce a powder.

calcinorrhachia (kal-sin-o-ra′kĭ-ă) [L. *calx*, lime, + *rachis*, spine]. Calcium in the spinal fluid.

calcino′sis [" + G. *-ōsis*, infection]. Deposit of lime salts in tissues.

calcipectic (kal-sĭ-pek′tik) [" + G. *pēgnunai*, to fix]. Pert. to calcipexis, *q.v.*

calcipenia (kal-sĭ-pē′nĭ-ă) [" + G. *penia*, poverty]. Calcium deficiency in body tissues and fluids.

calcipexic (kal-sĭ-pĕx′ĭc). Pertaining to calcipexis.

calcipexis, calcipexy (kal-sĭ-pĕk′sis, -pĕks′ĭ) [" + *pēgnunai*, to fix]. The fixation of calcium in body tissues.

calciphilia (kal-sĭ-fĭl′ĭ-ă) [" + *philein*, to love]. Tendency to calcification.

calciphylaxis (kal″sĭ-fĭ-laks′is). A state of induced tissue sensitivity characterized by calcification of tissue when challenged by an appropriate stimulus.

calciprivia (kal-sĭ-priv'ĭ-ă) [" + *privus,* without]. Deficiency or absence of calcium.

calciprivic (kal-sĭ-priv'ĭk). Pert. to deficiency or absence of calcium in the body.

cal'cium [L. *calx,* lime]. SYMB: Ca. Silver-white metallic element, the basis of limestone. At. wt. 40.08; at. no. 20.

Lime is its oxide. Calcium phosphate constitutes 75% of the body ash, and about 85% of mineral matter in bones.

FUNCTION: Calcium must be carried by the blood in solution before being available for bone growth. Unless certain activating substances, such as vitamin D, are present, increased calcium intake does not affect the tissues or blood calcium. The secretions of the parathyroid glands are a factor in the utilization of calcium, making it possible for the blood to carry dissolved calcium.

Quantities of bread, rice, oatmeal, and corn in the diet decrease absorption of calcium and phosphorus, and the alkalinity of the small intestines promotes the formation of insoluble salts.

Calcium is of great importance: (a) for coagulation of the blood, (b) to give firmness and rigidity to bones and teeth, (c) as a preventive of rickets, (d) as an ion balance, (e) as essential to lactation, (f) for activating enzymes, (g) for the functions of the muscles, nerves, and heart, (h) for maintaining the permeability of membranes.

Calcium is taken into the body as a constituent of various foods. While much of it may prove insoluble and escape absorption, some of it passes through the intestine into the blood, where it can be found by chemical tests. Its level in the serum is normally 10.5 to 11.0 mg. per 100 ml. Low blood calcium causes tetany with muscular twitching, spasms and convulsions. Blood deprived of its calcium will not clot, and milk without calcium will not curdle.

Calcium is deposited in the bones, but can be mobilized again to keep the blood level constant when there is a period of insufficient intake. At any given time the body of an adult contains about 700 Gm. of calcium phosphate; of this, 120 Gm. are the element calcium. Ordinarily an adult takes in 0.8 Gm. of calcium per day. During pregnancy 1.3 Gm. of calcium a day will be required.

SOURCES: *Excellent*: Cheese, cream, milk, chard, cauliflower, egg yolk, kale, molasses, beans, rhubarb. *Good:* Almonds, beets, bran, cabbage, celery, carrots, chocolate, dates, figs, kohl-rabi, lettuce, lemons, oatmeal, oranges, pineapples, parsnips, raspberries, spinach, shell fish, turnips, rutabagas, oysters, water cress, walnuts.

SEE: *acalcerosis, "calci-" words.*

c. carbonate. $CaCO_3$ (precipitated chalk). USP. A fine, white, tasteless and odorless powder.

ACTION AND USES: An antacid, also antidote to corrosive acid poisoning.

c. chloride ($CaCl_2$). USP. A very deliquescent salt occurring as translucent crystals having a sharp saline taste.

ACTION AND USES: To raise the calcium content of the blood in disorders resulting from lack of sufficient calcium, such as in hypocalcemic tetany. Used in solution and administered intravenously.

INCOMPATIBILITIES: Ephedrine.

c. deficiency. SYM: Brittle bones, poor development of bones and teeth, dental caries, rickets, tetany, heart atony, hyperirritability, excessive bleeding.

DIAG: Normal content in blood serum is 9 to 10.5 mg. per 100 ml. of blood. In evaluating the calcium level, laboratory error and variation may be the causes of inaccurate or inconsistent values.

c. gluconate. A granular or white powder without odor or taste.

ACTION AND USES: Same as calcium chloride; more pleasant to taste, and nonirritating when administered orally, or intramuscularly in a 10% solution.

c., high, in diet. A normal adequate diet including 1½ qt. milk, cheese, eggs, clams, and vegetables especially broccoli, cauliflower, beans, and beet nd other greens.

c. lactate. USP. A white, odorless and nearly tasteless powder, less irritating than the chloride.

USES: Orally or parenterally as an alternative to calcium gluconate.

c. levulinate. Soluble white powder used when intravenous administration of calcium is required.

c., low, in diet. Milk, cheese. and other foods high in calcium are avoided.

c. oxide. USP. Occurs as white or grayish-white hard mass.

ACTION AND USES: Germicide and disinfectant.

calcium phosphate precipitated. A white, amorphous powder.

USES: As an antacid in treatment of gastric hyperacidity.

calciuria (kal-sĭ-ū'rĭ-ă). Calcium in the urine.

calcopherous (kal-kof'er-us) [" + G. *phoros,* bearing]. Containing or producing lime or any salts of calcium.

calcospherite (kal-kos-fe'rīt) [" + G. *sphaira,* a sphere]. One of many small calcareous bodies found in tumors, nervous tissue, the thyroid, and prostate.

calcreose (kal'kre-oze). A chemical combination of creosote and lime containing approximately 50% creosote.

calculary (kal'ku-la-rĭ) [L. *calculus,* pebble]. Pert. to calculus.

cal'culi. Pl. of calculus, *q.v.*

calculif'ragous [L. *calculus,* pebble, + *frangere,* to break]. Breaking or reducing a stone in the bladder.

calculo'sis [" + G. *-ōsis,* infection]. Having a calculus.

calculous (kal'kū-lus). Like a calculus.

calculus (kal'kū-lus) (pl. *calculi*) [L. pebble]. Commonly called "stone"; any abnormal concretion within the animal body, and usually composed of mineral salts.

These pathological concretions occur in kidneys, ureter, bladder, urethra, usually formed of crystalline, urinary salts held together by viscid organic matter.

ETIOL: Abnormal function of the parathyroid glands, disordered uric acid metabolism as in gout, excess intake of milk and alkali, all can cause urinary calculi. However, most kidney stones form from a cause which is unexplainable.

c., biliary. Cholelithiasis*; gallstones. SEE: *gallbladder.*

c., hemic. One formed of coagulated blood.

c., pancreatic. Calculus in the pancreas, *q.v.*

c., renal. Calculus in the kidney. SYN: *nephrolithiasis.*

SYM: Urinary retention, sudden and paroxysmal renal colic, ulceration with possibly perforation, ureteral stricture, inflammation of various degrees.

PROG: Serious in uremic stage.

TREATMENT: Relief of pain, force fluids unless passage is completely blocked by the calculus. Medicines to relax smooth muscle help to allow the stone to pass and to relieve pain. If the stone is preventing urine flow or if the stone continues to grow and cause infection, surgery must be performed.

c., salivary. Calculus in salivary duct. Usually affects duct of submaxillary gland.

SYM: Obstructs flow of saliva, causing severe pain and swelling of gland, esp. when eating.

TREATMENT: Removal of stone by surgery.

c., urinary. Calculus in any part of the urinary system.

SYM: Sudden stoppage of flow of urine with sharp pain in obstruction, and, if firmly impacted, complete retention or dysuria.*

TREATMENT: Extraction of calculus.

c., vesical. Calculus in the bladder.

SYM: Frequency of urination, pain, diurnal hematuria increased by exercise are suggestive.

PROG: Stone is usually small enough to pass through urethra.

TREATMENT: The use of a non-addicting analgesic such as pentazocine and an antispasmodic if necessary, adequate fluid. Special urologic or surgical procedure if stone is large or impacted.

calculus, *words pert. to:* "calcu-" words; "chol-" words; gravel; "lith-" words.

calefacient (kal-ĕ-fa'shent) [L. *calere,* to be warm, + *facere,* to make]. Conveying or that which conveys a sense of warmth when applied to a part of the body.

calf [A.S. cealf]. The swelling on back part of the leg below the knee formed by the gastrocnemius and soleus muscles.

cal'iber [Fr. *calibre,* diameter of bore of gun]. The diameter of any orifice or opening.

calibration (kal-ĭ-brā'shun) [Fr. *calibre,* diameter of bore of gun]. Estimation of the caliber of an opening.

cal'ibrator. 1. Instrument for measuring the size of tubes or orifices. 2. Device for dilating tubes such as the esophagus or ureter.

c., anastomosis. One for determining size of opening to be united by anastomosis.

c., vaginal. One for determining degree of vaginal relaxation.

calic'ulus [L. *calyculus,* small cup]. A cup-shaped structure.

c. gustato'rius [NA]. A taste bud.

c. ophthal'micus [NA]. The optic cup.

caliectasis (kal-ĭ-ek'tas-is) [G. *kalix,* cup, + *ektasis,* dilatation]. Dilatation of the renal calyx.

californium (kal-ĭ-for'nĭ-ŭm) [Named for the state and the university of California where it was first discovered in 1950.]. A chemical element prepared by bombardment of curium with alpha particles. It has properties similar to dysproprium. SYMB: Cf. At. wt. 251; at. no. 98.

caliga'tion. Caligo, *q.v.*

cali'go [L. darkness]. Dimness of vision. SYN: *caligation.*

caliper(s (kal'ip-er) [corruption from caliber]. Instrument for measuring diameters, as those of chest or pelvis.

calix. Calyx, *q.v.*

Calliphora vomitoria (kă-lĭf'ĕr-ă). Common blowfly sometimes causing myiasis disorders.

callisec'tion [L. *callus,* insensitive, + *sectio,* a cutting]. Vivisection under anesthesia.

callomania (kal-o-ma'nĭ-ă) [G. *kalos,* beautiful, + *mania,* madness]. Belief in one's own beauty; a delusion of the insane.

callosal (kă-lō'sal) [L. *callus,* tough substance]. Pert. to the *corpus callosum.*

callosity, callositas (kal-os'ĭ-tĭ, -tas) [L. *callōsus,* thick-skinned]. Circumscribed thickening and hypertrophy of the horny layer of the skin. SYN: *callus.*

ETIOL: Friction, pressure, or other irritation, oval or elongated, on flexor surfaces of hands and feet, grayish or brownish and slightly elevated, with smooth, burnished surfaces.

TREATMENT: Temporary removal by salicylic acid or careful shaving. Permanent removal only by removal of cause. SEE: *porosis.*

callosomar'ginal [L. *callus,* tough, + *margo,* margin]. Pert. to the corpus callosum and marginal gyrus, marking sulcus bet. them.

callosum (kal-o'sum) [L. *callōsus,* hard]. The great commissure of the brain bet. the cerebral hemispheres. SYN: *corpus callosum.*

callous (kal'us) [L. *callus,* hard]. Hard; like a callus.

cal'lus. 1. Hypertrophied thickening of circumscribed area of horny layer of skin; callosity, *q.v.* 2. The osseous material thrown out bet. ends of a fractured bone.

c., definitive. Cartilage found bet. two ends of a fractured bone.

c., provisional. Temporary deposit bet. ends of a fractured bone.

calm'ative. 1. Sedative; soothing. 2. An agent that acts as a sedative.

Calmette's reaction (kal-mets') [Leon Charles A. Calmette, French bacteriologist, 1863-1933]. Slight injection of conjunctiva in one with an infective disease upon introduction of toxins of same disease. SYN: *ophthalmoreaction.*

calomel (kal'o-mel) [G. *kalos,* beautiful, + *melas,* black]. Mercurous chloride, *q.v.*

calor (ka'lor) [L. heat]. 1. Heat. 2. Moderate heat of fever; with *rubor, tumor, dolor* (*i.e.,* redness, swelling, pain), it represents the four classical signs of inflammation.

calora'diance [L. *calor,* heat, + *radiāre,* to shine]. Giving out heat rays.

calorescence (kal-or-es'ens). Producing by means of a lens incandescence of a body.

Calori's bursa (kal-ō'rez) [Luigi Calori, Italian anatomist, 1807-1896]. One sometimes found between arch of aorta and trachea.

caloric (kă-lor'ĭk) [L. *calor,* heat]. Relating to heat or to a calorie.

caloricity (kal-or-is'ĭ-tĭ). Heating power of the body.

calorie (kăl′ŏ-rē) [L. *calor*, heat]. A unit of heat. Also spelled *calory.*

c., *gram.* Small calorie, *q.v.*

c., *kilogram.* Large calorie, *q.v.*

c., *large.* The amount of heat needed to change temperature of one kilogram of water from 14.5° C to 15.5° C. Commonly employed in metabolic studies. When writing of human nutrition the large or kilogram calorie is used. Calorie is always capitalized in order to distinguish it from a small calorie. ABBR: Cal., or KCAL in British literature. SYN: *kilogram calorie.*

c., *small.* The amount of heat needed to change temperature of one gram of water one degree centigrade. SYN: *gram calorie; microcalorie.* ABBR: cal.

CALORIE EQUIVALENTS

	Ergs	Gm.-cm.	Ft.-lb.	Cal.	Kw.-hr.
1 erg	= 1.000	$= 1.02 \times 10^{-3}$	$= 7.37 \times 10^{-8}$	$= 2.39 \times 10^{-11}$	$= 2.77 \times 10^{-14}$
1 gm.-cm.	$= 9.81 \times 10^{2}$	= 1.000	$= 7.23 \times 10^{-5}$	$= 2.34 \times 10^{-8}$	$= 2.73 \times 10^{-11}$
1 ft.-lb.	$= 1.36 \times 10^{7}$	$= 1.38 \times 10^{4}$	= 1.000	$= 3.23 \times 10^{-4}$	$= 3.76 \times 10^{-7}$
1 calorie	$= 4.18 \times 10^{10}$	$= 4.26 \times 10^{7}$	$= 3.08 \times 10^{3}$	= 1.000	$= 1.17 \times 10^{-3}$
1 kw.-hr.	$= 3.61 \times 10^{13}$	$= 3.66 \times 10^{10}$	$= 2.66 \times 10^{6}$	$= 8.58 \times 10^{2}$	= 1.000

Calorie Allowances for Adult Individuals of Various Body Weights and Ages*

(At a mean environmental temperature of 20° C. (68° F.) assuming average physical activity)

Desirable Weight		*Calorie Allowance*†		
kgs.	*pounds*	*25 years*	*45 years*	*65 years*
MEN:				
50	110	2300	2050	1750
55	121	2450	2200	1850
60	132	2600	2350	1950
65	143	2750	2500	2100
70	154	2900	2600	2200
75	165	3050	2750	2300
80	176	3200	2900	2450
85	187	3350	3050	2550
WOMEN:				
40	88	1600	1450	1200
45	99	1750	1600	1300
50	110	1900	1700	1450
55	121	2000	1800	1550
58	128	2100	1900	1600
60	132	2150	1950	1650
65	143	2300	2050	1750
70	154	2400	2200	1850

* Adapted from a report of the Food and Nutrition Board, National Academy of Sciences, National Research Council: Recommended Dietary Allowances, 6th revised ed., National Academy of Sciences, Washington, D. C., 1964.

† Values have been rounded to nearest 50 Calories.

calorific (kal-ō-rif′ĭk). Producing heat; calorifacient.

calorigen′ic. Pert. to heat production or its increase.

calorimeter (kal-ō-rĭm′ĕ-ter) [L. *calor*, heat, + G. *metron*, measure]. Instrument for determining heat of bodies.

c., *bomb.* Apparatus for determination of potential energy of foods by measuring heat in combustion.

c., *respiratory.* Apparatus for determination of heat production calculated from exchange of respiratory gases.

calorimetry (kal-ō-rim′ĕ-trĭ). Determination of heat loss or gain.

c., *indirect.* Determination of heat production from amt. of oxygen used and carbon dioxide eliminated.

caloripuncture (kal-ō″rĭ-punk′tur). Use of heated needles in cauterization by puncture. SYN: *ignipuncture.*

cal′ory. Calorie, *q.v.*

calva′ria [L. human skull]. Skull cap; cranium, skull.

calvities (kal-vish′ĭ-ēz) [L. *calvus*, bald]. Baldness, alopecia.*

calx (kalks) [L. lime]. 1. Lime. 2. The heel.

c. *chlorinata.* Chlorinated lime. Used as a deodorant and disinfectant.

c. *sulfurata.* Sulfurated lime. Used as a depilatory.

c. *usta*, c. *viva*. Burnt lime; quicklime.

calyciform (ka-lis′ĭ-form) [G. *kalix*, cup. + L. *forma*, shape]. Cup-shaped.

calyx (kā′lix) (pl. *calyces*) [G. *kalix*, cup]. Any cuplike division of the kidney pelvis. The minor calyces enclose the tips of the renal pyramids, receiving the urine from the papillary ducts which open at their tips.

c. *major.* One of the major subdivisions of the renal pelvis, two or three in number.

c. *minor.* A subdivision of a major calyx, each terminating in relation to one to three papillae.

camera (kam′er-ă) [L. vault]. 1. A chamber or compartment. 2. In anatomy, any open space, chamber, or cavity.

c. *aqueosa.* Anterior aqueous chamber of the eye.

c. *pulpi.* The pulp cavity of a tooth.

camisole (kam′ĭ-sōl) [Fr. little shirt, from Italian, *camisa*, shirt]. A straitjacket used for restraining violent mental patients.

Cammidge reaction (kam'ĭj) [Percy J. Cammidge, English physician, 1872-]. Urinal reaction in pancreatic disease.

The result is a light yellow flocculent precipitation in a few hours following test.

cam'omile. SEE: *chamomile.*

cam'phor [G. *kamphora*]. USP. A gum obtained from an evergreen tree native to China and Japan.

ACTION AND USES: Topically, as 0.1% preparation, as an antipruritic.

cam'phorated. Combined with or containing camphor.

c. oil. Liniment containing camphor.

camphoromania (kam-for-ō-mā'nĭ-ă) [G. *kamphora,* camphor, + *mania,* madness]. Abnormal craving for camphor.

campimeter (kamp-im'ĕ-ter) [L. *campus,* field, + G. *metron,* measure]. Device for measuring field of vision.

campimetry (kamp-im'ĕ-trĭ). Measurement of field of vision. SYN: *perimetry.*

cam'pospasm. Camptocormia, *q.v.*

camptocor'mia [G. *kamptos,* bent, + *kormos,* body]. Abnormal flexing of body.

camptodactylia (kamp-to-dak-til'ĭ-ă) [" + *dactylos,* finger]. Permanent flexion of fingers or toes.

camp'tospasm [" + *spasmos,* spasm]. Camptocormia, *q.v.*

canal (pl. *canals*). A narrow tube, channel, or passageway. SEE ALSO: *duct; groove; space; foramen.*

c., adductor. Hunter's canal; a triangular space lying beneath the sartorius muscle and between the adductor longus and the vastus medialis muscles. It extends from the apex of the femoral triangle to the popliteal space and transmits the femoral vessels and the saphenous nerve.

c., Alcock's. A canal on the pelvic surface of the obturator internus muscle formed by the obturator fascia. It transmits the pudendal vessels and nerve. SYN: *canalis pudendalis* [NA]; *pudendal canal.*

c., alimentary. The digestive tract from mouth through the intestine.

c., alveolar, inferior. Mandibular c., *q.v.*

c.'s, alveolar. Canals in the maxilla for transmitting the posterior superior alveolar blood vessels and nerves to the upper teeth. SYN: *dental c.'s; canales alveolares* [NA].

c., anal. The terminal portion of the rectum opening at the anus. SYN: *canalis analis* [NA].

c., auditory, external. The external auditory meatus; transmits sound waves.

c., auditory, internal. A canal in the petrous portion of the temporal bone which transmits the acoustic and facial nerves and the acoustic artery.

c., birth. Parturient canal; passageway through which the fetus passes in parturition, specifically the uterus and vagina.

c., carotid. A canal in the petrous portion of the temporal bone which transmits int. carotid artery and the int. carotid plexus of sympathetic nerves. SYN: *canalis caroticus* [NA].

c., central. A small canal lying in the center of the spinal cord extending from the fourth ventricle to the conus medullaris. Contains cerebrospinal fluid. SYN: *canalis centralis* [NA].

c., cervical. Canal in cervix of uterus extending from internal to external os. SYN: *canalis cervicis uteri* [NA].

c., cochlear, spiral. A part of the bony labyrinth of the ear. A spiral tube about 30 mm. long making two and three-quarters turns about a central bony axis, the modiolus. Contains the scala tympani, scala vestibuli, and cochlear duct. SYN: *canalis spiralis cochleae* [NA].

c., condylar. A canal in the occipital bone which transmits emissary vein from the transverse sinus. Opens anterior to the occipital condyle. SYN: *condyloid c.; canalis condylaris* [NA].

c., craniopharyngeal. A canal in the sphenoid bone of a fetus which contains the stalk of Rathke's pouch.

c.'s, dental. Alveolar c.'s, *q.v.*

c., ethmoidal. Two grooves running transversely across the lateral mass of the ethmoid bone to the cribiform plate. Lie between ethmoid and frontal bones. The *anterior ethmoidal canal* transmits the anterior ethmoidal vessels and the nasociliary nerve; the *posterior ethmoidal canal* transmits the posterior ethmoidal vessels and nerve.

c., facial. A canal in the internal acoustic meatus of the temporal bone which transmits the facial nerve. SYN: *canalis facialis* [NA].

c., femoral. The medial division of the femoral sheath. It is a short compartment about 1.5 cm. long lying behind the inguinal ligament. Contains some lymphatic vessels and a lymph node. SYN: *canalis femoralis* [NA].

c., gastric. A longitudinal groove on the inner surface of the stomach following the lesser curvature. Extends from esophagus to pylorus.

c., Haversian. Minute canals found in compact bone which contain blood and lymph vessels, nerves, and sometimes marrow. Each is surrounded by lamellae of bone comprising a Haversian system. SEE: *bone.*

c., hyaloid. A canal in the vitreous body of the eye extending from the optic papilla to the post. surface of lens. It serves as a lymph channel. In the fetus it transmits the hyaline artery to the lens. SYN: *canalis hyaloideus* [NA].

c., hypoglossal. A canal in the occipital bone which transmits the hypoglossal nerve and a branch of the post. meningeal artery. SYN: *canalis hypoglossi* [NA].

c., incisive. A short canal in the maxillary bone leading from incisive fossa in roof of mouth to the floor of nasal cavity. Transmits nasopalatine nerve and branches of the greater palatine arteries to the nasal fossa. SYN: *canalis incisivus* [NA].

c., infraorbital. A canal in the maxilla lying in the floor of the orbit which transmits the infraorbital nerve and artery. It terminates anteriorly at the infraorbital foramen. SYN: *canalis infraorbitalis* [NA].

c., inguinal. A slit in the lower lateral portion of the abdominal wall, extending from the abdominal inguinal ring to the subcutaneous inguinal ring. It is an oblique passageway about 1½ inches long and serves in the male to transmit the spermatic cord and the ilioinguinal nerve and in the female the round ligament of the uterus and the ilioinguinal nerve. It forms a channel through which an inguinal hernia descends. SYN: *canalis inguinalis* [NA].

c., intestinal. The alimentary canal from stomach to anus.

c., lacrimal. The lacrimal duct, *q.v.*

c., mandibular. C. in the mandible that transmits the inferior alveolar blood vessels and nerve to the teeth. SYN: *canalis mandibularis* [NA].

c., maxillary. Alevolar c.'s, *q.v.*

c., nasolacrimal. A canal lying between the lacrimal bone and the inf. nasal conchae. Contains the nasolacrimal duct.

c., Nuck's. In the female, a persistent peritoneal pouch corresponding to the saccus vaginalis of the male.

c., nutritive. An opening on the surface of compact bone through which blood vessels gain access to the medullary cavity of long bones. Also transmits veins.

c., obturator. An opening in the obturator membrane of the hip-bone which transmits the obturator vessels and nerve.

c., pharyngeal. A canal between sphenoid and palatine bones for transmission of branches of sphenopalatine vessels.

c., portal. The connective tissue (continuation of Glisson's capsule) and its contained vessels (interlobular branches of hepatic artery, portal vein, and bile duct and lymphatic vessel) located between adjoining liver lobules.

c., pterygoid. A canal of the sphenoid bone transmitting pterygoid vessels, artery, and nerve. Also called canal of Vidian. SYN: *canalis pterygoideus* [NA].

c., pterygopalatine. A canal lying between maxillary and palatine bones which transmits descending palatine nerves and artery. SYN: *canalis palatinus major* [NA].

c., pudendal. Alcock's c., *q.v.*

c., pulp. The central cavity of a tooth filled with pulp. Contains blood vessels and sensory nerve endings.

c., sacral. Cavity within the sacrum, a continuation of the vertebral canal. SYN: *canalis sacralis* [NA].

c., Schlemm's. A space or series of spaces at the junction of the sclera and the cornea of the eye into which aqueous humor is drained from the anterior chamber through the pectinate villi.

c.'s, semicircular, bony. Located in the bony labyrinth of the internal ear and enclose the three semicircular ducts: the superior, posterior, and lateral which open into the vestibule. They are enclosed within the petrous portion of the temporal bone.

c.'s, semicircular, membranous. Semicircular ducts. SEE UNDER: *duct.*

c., spinal. The vertebral c., *q.v.*

c., spiral, cochlear. SEE: *cochlear c., spiral.*

c., spiral [of the modiolus]. A series of irregular spaces which follow the course of the attached margin of the osseous spiral lamina to the modiolus. They serve for the transmission of filaments of the cochlear nerve and blood vessels. The spiral ganglion lies in the spiral canal. SYN: *canalis spiralis modioli* [NA].

c., uterine. The cavity of the uterus.

c., uterocervical. The cavity of the cervix of the uterus.

c., uterovaginal. The combined cavity of the uterus and vagina.

c., vaginal. The cavity of the vagina.

c., vertebral. The cavity formed by the foramina of the vertebral column. Also called spinal canal, neural canal. It contains the spinal cord and its meninges. SYN: *canalis vertebralis* [NA].

c., Volkmann's. Small canals found in bone through which blood vessels pass from the periosteum. They connect with the blood vessels of Haversian canals or the marrow cavity.

canales (kă-nā'lēz). Plural of *canalis.*

canalicular (kan-ă-lik'ū-lar) [L. *canaliculаris,* pert. to a small canal]. Pert. to a canaliculus.

canaliculi (kan-a-lik'ū-lī). Plural of *canaliculus.*

canaliculus (kan-ă-lĭk'ū-lus) (pl. *canaliculi*). A small channel or canal.

canalis (kă-nā'lĭs) (pl. *canales*) [L.]. Canal, *q.v.*

canalization (ka-nal-ĭ-za'shun). Formation of channels in tissue.

can'cellated [L. *cancellus,* lattice]. Reticulated; latticelike.

cancelli (kan-sel'ī) (pl. of *cancellus*) [L. *cancellus,* lattice]. Reticulations forming spongy tissue of bones.

can'cellous [L. *cancellus,* a grating]. Having a reticular or latticework structure, as the spongy tissue of bone.

cancellus (kăn-sĕl'us) (pl. *cancelli*) [L. a lattice]. An osseous plate of which cancellous bone is composed.

cancer (kan'ser) [L. a crab; ulcer]. A malignant tumor or neoplasm; a sarcoma or carcinoma.

ETIOL: Origin unknown. May be caused by various forms of chronic irritation. Some forms in animals at least are apparently caused by viruses.

SYM: The important warning signals of cancer are: Unusual bleeding or discharge from any body site internal or external; a lump or thickening in any area but especially the breast; a sore that does not heal; a change in bowel or bladder habits; hoarseness or persistent cough; indigestion or difficulty in swallowing; change in size or shape or appearance of a wart or mole; unexplained loss of weight. These are the major signs of cancer and once any one of them is observed in oneself or in a patient it should be brought to a physician's attention without delay.

TREATMENT: Surgery, cytotoxic agents, radium and x-rays are the only recognized effective methods of treatment for cancer.

Early diagnosis and application of proper method or combination of methods are necessary for complete cure.

NP: Small pillows and sandbags to relieve strained muscles. Cradles to hold bedclothes away from painful parts. Light bedclothes; 1 wool blanket instead of several cotton ones. Olive oil added to rubbing alcohol prevents chafing and rawness. Bland, neutral soap should be used for bathing.

Cater to individual idiosyncrasies. Do not deny particular foods unless there is a good reason for it. Serve 4 to 6 small meals. Attractively decorated trays stimulate appetite in patient. Diet with minimum of 2000 calories per day.

Keep patient cheerful. Talk and soothe patient out of complaint when possible. Censor literature and talk of visitors so that cheerful attitude will be maintained.

c., black. Cancer with dark pigmentation.

c. cell. A cell found in neoplasm which possesses characteristics which differentiate them from normal tissue cells. Among such are degree of anaplasia, irregularity in shape, indistinctness of cell outline, nuclear size, changes in structure of nucleus and cytoplasm, increased number of mitoses and ability to metastasize.

c., hard. C. composed of fibrous tissue.

c., lip. Epithelioma, usually in men, smokers and on lower lip.

c., scirrhous. SEE: *hard c.*

cancer, words pert. to: adenocarcinoma; carcinoma; epithelioma; sarcoma; scirrhus.

cancerogenic (kan″ser-o-jen′ĭk). Carcinogenic.

cancerology (kan-ser-ol′o-jĭ) [" + G. *logos*, study]. The science of cancer. SYN: *cancrology*.

cancerophoʹbia [" + G. *phobos*, fear]. Morbid fear of cancer.

canʹcerous. Pert. to malignant growth.

cancra (kang′kră). Plural of *cancrum*.

cancriform (kang′krĭ-form) [L. *cancer*, ulcer, + *forma*, appearance]. Having the appearance of cancer.

cancroid (kan′kroid) [" + G. *eidos*, appearance]. 1. Like a cancer. 2. A type of keloid.* 3. Epithelioma.*

cancrology (kang-krol′o-jĭ). Cancerology, *q.v.*

cancrum (kang′krum) (pl. *cancra*) [L. *cancer*, ulcer]. A rapidly spreading ulcer.

c. na′si. Gangrenous inflammation of nasal membranes.

c. o′ris. Gangrenous stomatitis, noma.

TREATMENT: Good oral hygiene and massive doses of appropriate antibiotic.

c. puden′di. Ulceration of vulva.

Candida (kan′dĭ-dă). A genus of yeast-like fungi which develop a pseudomycelium and reproduce by budding. They are the primary etiologic agents for many mycotic infections in man. Formerly called *Monilia*.

C. albicans. A small oval, budding fungus which is the primary etiologic organism of moniliasis (candidiasis). Formerly called *Monilia albicans*.

candidiasis. Infection with any species of *Candida*. SEE: *moniliasis*.

candle, international. A unit of luminosity.

c. power. Amt. of light thrown out by a lighted candle, measured in international candles. SEE: *unit; light unit; lux*.

cane. A slender stick held in the hand and used for support during walking.

cane sugar. Sucrose. Table sugar obtained from sugar cane. SEE: *saccharose*.

canescent (kan-es′ent) [L. *canus*, gray]. Grayish in color.

ca′nine [L. *caninus*, pert. to a dog]. 1. Pert. to a dog. 2. Pert. to the canine teeth or the 4 teeth known as the eyeteeth (upper and lower) bet. the incisors and molars. 3. A canine tooth.

c. appetite. Abnormal hunger a short time after eating. SYN: *bulimia.**

c. eminence. Ridge on ant. surface of sup. maxilla.

c. fossa. Depression on sup. maxilla external to the c. eminence.

c. tooth. Tooth situated bet. incisors and 1st premolar tooth. SEE: *dentition; tooth*.

canities (kan-ish′ĭ-ēz) [L. gray hair]. Congenital (rare) or acquired whiteness of the hair.

Acquired form may develop rapidly or slowly, partial or complete.

ETIOL: Hereditary tendency, prolonged fevers, wasting diseases, worry, overwork, grief, anxiety, nervous shock. In localized type, nerve injury.

c. unguium. Gray or white streaks in nails.

canker (kang′ker) [L. *cancer*, ulcer]. Thrush; white spots on mucous membrane of the mouth, aphthae, noma, gangrenous stomatitis.

cannabis [G. *kannabis*, hemp]. Marihuana, *q.v.*

cannula (kan′u-lă) [L. a small reed]. A tube or sheath enclosing a trocar, the tube allowing the escape of fluid after withdrawal of the trocar from the body.

cantaloupe, cantaloup [I. *cantalupo*]. A type of muskmelon.

RAW: 100 gm. Calories: 30. Other main values: 0.7 gm. protein; trace of fat; 7.5 gm. carbohydrate; 14 mg. calcium; 3400 I.U. vitamin A; 33 mg. ascorbic acid.

can′thal [G. *kanthos*, angle]. Pert. to a canthus.

canthar′idal [G. *kantharos*, beetle, + *eidos*, form]. Pert. to or containing cantharides.

cantharides (kan-thar′ĭ-dēz) (pl. of *Cantharis*) [" + *eidos*, form]. Dried insects of the species Cantharis vesicatoria obtained from Spain or Russia. SYN: *Spanish fly*.

ACTION AND USES: Locally, a counterirritant and vesicant. Its use has been almost entirely discontinued. Poisonous if taken internally in large doses.

Cantharis (kan-thar′ĭs) (pl. *cantharides*). A genus of beetles, C. vesicatoria being used for Spanish fly. SEE: *cantharides*.

canthectomy (kan-thek′tō-mĭ) [G. *kanthos*, canthus, + *ektomē*, excision]. Excision of a canthus.

can′thi. Plural of *canthus*.

canthitis (kan-thī′tis) [" + *-itis*, inflammation]. Inflammation of a canthus.

cantholysis (kan-thol′ĭ-sĭs) [" + *lysis*, a loosening]. Incision of a canthus to widen palpebral slit.

canthoplasty (kan′thō-plas-tĭ) [" + *plassein*, to form]. Plastic surgery of canthus of the eye. Enlargement of palpebral fissure by division of the external canthus.

canthorraphy (kan-thor′ă-fĭ) [" + *raphē*, suture]. Suturing of a canthus.

canthotomy (kan-thot′ō-mĭ) [" + *tomē*, a cutting]. Division of a canthus.

can′thus (pl. *canthi*) [G. *kanthos*, angle]. The angle at either end of the slit bet. the eyelids; the external canthus or *commissura palpebrarum lateralis* [NA], and the internal canthus or *commissura palpebrarum medialis* [NA].

CaO. Calcium oxide, quicklime, calx.

CaOC. Abbr. for *cathodal* or *negative opening contracture*.

$Ca(OH)_2$. Calcium hydroxide; slaked lime.

cap (kăp) [A.S. *caeppe*, hood]. 1. A covering. SYN: *tegmentum*. 2. First part of the duodenum. SYN: *pyloric cap*.

c., cradle. Seborrhea, oily crusts on the head, seen in infants.

c., knee-. Bone in front of the knee. SYN: *patella, q.v.*

capac′itance [L. *capacitās*, the taking]. That property of a system of conductors and dielectrics which permits the storage of electric charges. SEE: *farad*.

capac′ity. 1. Capability. 2. Cubic content. 3. Holding power. SEE: *capacitance*.

c., cranial. Volume of the cranial cavity.

c., unit of. Unit of electrical capacity. SEE: *farad*.

c., vital. Volume of air that can be forcibly exhaled after a full inspiration.

capeline (kap′ĕ-lĭn) [Fr. a hat]. A bandage used for the head, or the stump of an amputated limb.

capiat (ka′pĭ-at) [L. "let it take"]. An instrument for removing foreign substances or bodies esp. from the uterus.

capillarectasia (kap″ĭ-lar-ek-tā′sĭ-ă) [L. *capillaris*, hairlike, + G. *ektasis*, dilatation]. Dilatation of capillary vessels.

capillaries (kap'ĭ-lā-rēz). 1. Minute blood vessels. 2. Small lymphatic ducts. Plural of *capillary, q.v.*

capillari'tis [" + G. *-itis,* inflammation]. Inflammation of the capillaries; telangiitis.

capillar'ity. Process by which a liquid's surface, at the point of contact with a solid, is elevated or lowered. SYN: *capillary attraction.*

capillarop'athy [L. *capillaris,* hairlike, + G. *pathos,* disease]. Capillary disorders or disease.

capillaros'copy [" + G. *skopein,* to examine]. Examination of capillaries for diagnostic purposes.

cap'illary (pl. *capillaries*) [L. *capillaris,* hairlike]. 1. Minute blood vessel, 0.008 mm. in diameter, carrying blood and forming the capillary system. Capillaries connect the smallest arteries (arterioles) with the smallest veins (venules). 2. One of the small lymphatic ducts which allow passage of nutrient matter and oxygen from the blood to the tissues, and of waste matter from the tissues into the blood. 3. Pert. to a hair; hairlike.

c., *arterial.* The very small vessels which are the terminal branches of the arterioles or metarterioles.

c. *attraction.* Capillarity, *q.v.*

c., *bile.* Intercellular biliary passageways which convey bile from liver cells to the interlobular bile ducts.

c.'s, *blood.* Minute blood vessels which convey blood from the arterioles to the venules. They form an anastomosing network which brings the blood into intimate relationship to the tissue cells. Their wall consists of a single layer of squamous cells called *endothelium* through which blood and oxygen diffuse to the tissue and products of metabolic activity enter the blood stream. They average about 8 microns in diameter, but are capable of being constricted so as to have almost no lumen at all.

c.'s, *lymphatic.* The smallest lymphatic vessels. They are thin-walled tubes forming a dense network in most tissues of the body. They differ from blood capillaries in that they are generally slightly larger in diameter and end blindly. They collect tissue fluid from the tissues. Lymph capillaries unite to form larger lymphatic vessels.

c. *permeability.* The ability of substances to diffuse through capillary walls into the tissue spaces. It is influenced by anoxia, adrenal cortical hormone and the concentration of calcium ions in the blood.

c.'s, *venous.* The minute vessels which convey blood from a capillary network into the small veins or venules.

capillus (kă-pĭl'us) (pl. *capilli*) [L.]. 1. A hair, esp. of the head. 2. A filament. 3. A hair's breadth.

cap'ital [L. *capitalis,* pert. to the head]. 1. Pert. to the head. 2. Of great importance to life.

cap'itate [L. *caput,* head]. Headshaped; having a rounded extremity.

c. *bone.* Capitatum, *q.v.*

capitatum (kap-ĭ-tā'tum). Third bone in distal row of carpus. SYN: *capitate; os magnum; os capitatum* [NA].

capitel'lum [L. dim. of *caput,* head]. The round eminence at lower end of the humerus articulating with radius; its radial head. SYN: *capitulum humeri* [NA].

capitular (kă-pit'ū-lar) [L. dim. of *caput,* head]. Pert. to a capitulum.

capit'ulum. A small, rounded articular end of a bone.

c. *fibulae.* The proximal extremity or head of the fibula; articulates with tibia.

c. *humeri* [NA]. Rounded prominence at distal end of humerus. Articulates with the radius. SYN: *capitellum.*

c. *mallei.* The head or large rounded extremity of the malleus; bears facet for the incus.

c. *stapedis.* The head of the stapes; articulated with lenticular process of incus.

capotement (kă-pōt-mon') [Fr.]. A splashing sound in the stomach.

capsicum (kap'sĭ-kum). Cayenne pepper; dried, ripe fruit of capsicum.

ACTION AND USES: Carminative, stimulant and rubefacient.

capsitis (kap-sī'tis) [L. *capsa,* small box]. Capsulitis of crystalline lens.

cap'sula (pl. *capsulae*) [L. a little box]. In anatomy a sheath or continuous enclosure around an organ or structure.

c. *articula'ris.* Capsule of a joint.

c. *bul'bi.* Tenon's capsule.

c. *fibro'sa perivascularis hep'atis* [NA]. Glisson's capsule.

c. *glomer'uli* [NA]. Bowman's capsule; malpighian capsule.

c. *len'tis* [NA]. Crystalline lens capsule.

cap'sular. Pert. to a capsule.

c. *ligament.* A ligament which surrounds a movable joint.

capsula'tion. Enclosure in a capsule.

cap'sule [L. *capsula,* small box]. 1. Capsula, *q.v.* 2. A special container made of gelatin for a single dose of a drug; the enclosure prevents the patient from tasting the drug.

c., *auditory.* Embryonic cartilaginous capsule enclosing the developing ear.

c., *Bowman's.* The glomerular capsule of the kidneys.

c., *brain (external of).* A thin layer of white matter which separates the claustrum from the putamen.

c., *brain (internal of).* A broad band of white matter which separates the lentiform nucleus on lateral side from the caudate nucleus and thalamus on the medial side.

c., *cartilage.* The layer of matrix which forms the innermost portion of the wall of a lacuna enclosing a single cell or a group of cartilage cells. It is basophilic.

c., *Glisson's.* An outer capsule of fibrous tissue in which is invested the liver, its ducts and vessels. SYN: *capsula fibrosa perivascularis hepatis* [NA].

c., *joint.* The fibrous tissues enclosing a joint.

c. *of the kidney.* Fat-containing connective tissue surrounding the kidney.

c., *lens.* A transparent structureless membrane which surrounds and encloses the lens of the eye.

c., *nasal;* c., *optic;* c., *otic.* Cartilaginous capsules which develop in embryonic skull enclosing each of the paired sense organs, as nasal cavity, eyes, and ears, respectively.

c., *suprarenal or adrenal.* A tough connective tissue capsule which encloses the adrenal gland.

c. *of Tenon.* A thin fibrous sac enveloping the eyeball, forming a socket in which it rotates. SYN: *fascia bulbi.*

capsuli'tis [L. *capsula,* a little box, + G. *-itis,* inflammation]. Inflammation of a capsule.

capsulocil'iary [" + *ciliāris,* pert. to the

eyelashes]. Pert. to capsule of lens and ciliary structures.

cap″suloplas′ty [" + G. *plassein,* to mold]. Plastic surgery of a capsule, esp. one of a joint.

capsulorrhaphy(kap-sū-lor′ă-fĭ) [" + G. *raphē,* suture]. Suture of a joint capsule or of a tear in a capsule.

capsulotome (kap′sū-lō-tōm) [" + G. *temnein,* to cut]. Instrument for incising into capsule of crystalline lens.

capsulotomy (kap-sū-lot′ō-mĭ) [" + G. *temnein,* to cut]. Cutting of capsule of crystalline lens.

captation (kap-tā′shun) [L. *captātiō,* seizure]. The first stage of hypnosis.

caput (ka′put, kap′ut) (pl. *cap′ita*) [L.]. 1. The head. 2. The upper part of an organ.

c. gallinaginis. Round protuberance on urethral floor. SYN: *colliculus seminalis* [NA].

c. medusae. Plexus of veins about the umbilicus in one form of cirrhosis of the liver (Cruveilhier-Baumgarten syndrome) indicating portal vein obstruction.

c. obstipum. Wryneck; torticollis.

c. succedaneum. Swelling produced on the presenting part of the fetal head during labor. It may be mistaken for the bag-of-waters.

ETIOL: Effusion of serum into cellular tissue of exposed scalp through venous interference from pressure.

carbacrylamine resins (kar″ba-krĭl′ă-mine res′ins). Combined carbacrylic resin, potassium carbacrylic resin, polyamine-methylene resin, which is used to increase removal of sodium via fecal excretion by processes of ion exchange. Proprietary name is Carbo-resin.

carbamide (kär′bă-mīd). Urea, $CO(NH)_2$.

carbarsone (kar′bar-sōn). USP. A white, crystalline, odorless powder; contains about 28% arsenic, having a chemical structure resembling tryparsamide.

USES: An antiamebic agent, it is also used in treatment of Trichomonas vaginitis.

carbohydrase (kar-bō-hī′drās). One of a group of enzymes (such as amylase and lactase) that hydrolyze carbohydrates.

carbohyd′rates [L. *carbo,* carbon, + G. *ydōr,* water]. The monosaccharoses, disaccharoses, and polysaccharoses. A class of organic compounds so called because in them the hydrogen and oxygen are in the same ratio as they are in water, so that the group can be represented by the formula $Cx(H_2O)y$.

Glucose, $C_6H_{12}O_6$, and sucrose, $C_{12}H_{22}O_{11}$ are typical carbohydrates, but the group also includes the noncrystalline dextrins and starches.

c. foods. These contain only carbon combined with hydrogen and oxygen, such as sugars, starch, and cellulose. Carbohydrates, principally starches, provide a major source of calories in an average diet.

CLASSIFICATION: SEE: tables below.

carbohydratu′ria [" + " + *ouron,* urine]. Sugar in the urine. SYN: *glycosuria.*

carbolic acid [L. *carbo,* coal, + *oleum,* oil]. Obsolete name for phenol, *q.v.*

carbolism (kar′bo-lizm). Poisoning by carbolic acid. SEE: *phenol.*

car′bolize [" + *oleum,* oil]. To add or mix with carbolic acid.

carbolu′ria [" + " + G. *ouron,* urine]. Phenol in the urine.

carbomycin (kar-bō-mī′sĭn). An antibiotic obtained from *Streptomyces halstedii* and effective against gram-positive bacteria.

car′bon [L. *carbo,* carbon or coal]. SYMB: C. This nonmetallic element is the characteristic constituent of organic compounds. At. wt. 12.0111; at. no. 6.

A common form is coal. Carbon is found in all living things in its various forms and combinations. It is the basis of all organic matter and makes life

Classification of Important Carbohydrates

Classification	Examples	Some Properties
Monosaccharides (monoses) $(C_6H_{10}O_5)_1 \cdot H_2O$ or $C_6H_{12}O_6$	Glucose Fructose	Crystalline, sweet, very soluble. Readily absorbed.
Disaccharides (dioses) $(C_6H_{10}O_5)_2 \cdot H_2O$ or $C_{12}H_{22}O_{11}$ hydrolyzed to simple sugars.	Sucrose Lactose Maltose	Crystalline, sweet, soluble, digestible.
Polysaccharides (polyoses) $(C_6H_{10}O_5)\,n$ composed of many molecules of simple sugars. (Since the molecular weight is unknown, *n* refers to an unknown number of these groups, the exact molecular weight being undetermined.)	Starch Dextrin Cellulose Glycogen	Amorphous, with little or no flavor, less soluble. Vary in solubility and digestibility. Form colloidal solutions which cannot be dialyzed.

Digestion of Carbohydrates

Enzyme	Found in	Carbohydrates	End-product
Sucrase (invertase) Maltase Lactase	Intestine Intestine Intestine	Sucrose Maltose Lactose	Glucose and fructose Glucose Glucose and galactose
Salivary amylase (ptyalin) Pancreatic amylase (amylopsin)	Saliva (mouth) Pancreas	Starch Starch	Dextrin to maltose Dextrin to maltose

possible through a number of combinations with hydrogen, nitrogen, and oxygen. In foods it is a fuel creating heat. The diamond is crystallized carbon.

car'bon diox'ide. CO_2. USP. A colorless gas, heavier than air, generally produced in the combustion, decomposition, or fermentation of carbon or its compounds, and found in the air and exhaled by all animals.

The final product of combustion of carbon in food, which the body exhales through the lungs, or eliminates through the kidneys in urine, or in perspiration through the skin.

It is also given off by decomposition of vegetable or animal matter, or formed by alcoholic fermentation, as in rising bread. It is necessary to all plant life and it is absorbed directly from the air.

Although a waste product, in small quantities (up to about 5%) in inspired air, it stimulates respiration; in greater quantities, it produces an uncomfortable degree of hyperpnea with mental confusion.

Although not supposed to be poisonous, it will cause death by suffocation. Over 500,000,000 tons are passed into the air per year, but as it is used by green plants, the air content is kept down to about 0.03%. One sq. yd. of leaf surface can absorb the carbon dioxide from 2500 liters of air in 1 hour. An acre of trees uses 4½ tons a year.

c. d. combining power test. This test, done on blood serum, is a determination of the amount of carbon dioxide which the blood serum can hold in chemical combination.

The blood serum is saturated with carbon dioxide by blowing one's breath into it, removing the carbon dioxide by producing a vacuum, and measuring its volume directly. It is used to detect acidosis or alkalosis and to determine their degree. Carbon dioxide in solution forms a weak acid (H_2CO_3), and the amount of this acid which the blood serum can take up is a measure of its reserve power to prevent the occurrence of acidosis. The normal amount is from 50 to 70 ml. for each 100 ml. of blood (usually expressed as 50-70 volumes %). Values below 50 indicate *acidosis*, above 70 *alkalosis*.

c. d., inhalation. Carbon dioxide, (5 to 7½%), mixed with oxygen for inhalation stimulates breathing the same way as increased carbon dioxide production from exercise. Inhalation of oxygen and carbon dioxide is used as an accessory during artificial respiration and as a continuation of resuscitation after spontaneous breathing has returned. Also used to stimulate respiration in patients with pulmonary diseases such as pneumonia.

c. d. poisoning. C. d. gas is most commonly used in carbonated drinks and commercially used in dry ice; of itself, it is rarely fatal, unless the patient is in a closed space. It is a profound respiratory stimulant.

SYM: Violent increased breathing; sensation of pressure in the head; ringing in ears, acid taste in mouth; slight burning in nose. Within a short time, respiration almost ceases and patient becomes unconscious.

TREATMENT: Remove to fresh air, administer artificial respiration, inhalation of oxygen.

c. d. test. The alkalinity reserve in the plasma is indicated by the volume percentage of carbon dioxide in the blood. Acidosis shows a percentage below 50, while in coma it is as low as 20. Acidosis indicates faulty metabolism. Diacetic acid is produced as the result of accumulated fatty acids, the product of incomplete oxidation of fats. A test is often made before an operation and the patient treated if acidosis is present, as a mild acidosis might develop into a very acute one from the effect of the ether.

c. d. (solid) therapy. Solid carbon dioxide (CO_2 snow) is used for therapeutic refrigeration. Solid CO_2 has a temperature of —80° C. Application to skin 1-2 seconds causes superficial frostbite, 4-5 seconds a blister, 10-15 seconds superficial necrosis, 15-45 seconds ulceration. Now used mostly for certain nevi and warts, occasionally for telangiectasia.

car'bonate [L. *carbo,* carbon]. A salt of carbonic acid.

c. of soda. Sodium carbonate commercially in crude form, as washing soda. The free alkali present is irritating and in larger concentrations has the effect of sodium hydroxide, *q.v.*

carbonemia (kar-bo-ne'mĭ-ă) [L. *carbo,* carbon, + G. *aima,* blood]. Excess accumulation of carbonic acid in the blood.

carbon'ic. Pert. to carbon.

c. acid. H_2CO_3. Acid resulting from mixture of carbon dioxide and water.

c. anhydrase. An enzyme which catalyzes union of H_2O and CO_2 to form carbonic acid or reverse action. Present in red blood cells.

c. a. gas. Carbon dioxide, *q.v.*

car'bonize. To char or convert into charcoal.

car'bon monox'ide. CO. An insidious poisonous gas. It is a colorless, tasteless, odorless gas, gives no warning of its presence, and it is widely distributed as the result of imperfect combustion and oxidation.

It is found in the exhaust gas from all internal combustion engines, such as are used in most motor-powered vehicles. It is likewise present in illuminating gas and it results from the inefficient and incomplete combustion of coal. It is found in sewers, cellars, and mines.

POISONING: May take place even from small amounts inhaled over a long period of time, or from large amounts inhaled over a short time. For example, riding in a closed automobile or parking in an automobile with motor running may result fatally from the inhalation of these noxious fumes, from leaking exhausts and exhaust heaters, or from operating a gasoline motor in an enclosed area, such as a closed garage or basement.

Poisoning from carbon monoxide is produced as a result of a chemical combination of this gas with the hemoglobin of the blood, thus preventing the blood from carrying oxygen to the tissues, and since this combination is a relatively stable one, such a patient may need oxygen administration for prolonged periods in addition to artificial respiration.

SYM: The symptoms of carbon monoxide poisoning are somewhat variable. Respiration is deep and difficult. There may be reddish patches of color about the face and chest. The mucous membrane may have a brighter red hue than normal. The pulse initially may be slowed but it soon becomes increased.

There may be pounding of the heart; dizziness is frequent, although the muscular system is often affected so that the extremities may fail. There may be ringing in the ear, throbbing in the temples, headache, faintness and nausea, dilated pupils. If the patient is still breathing when found, he usually recovers when brought into the fresh air and given stimulants.

TREATMENT: Oxygen with 5% CO_2, preferably with a face mask; artificial respiration if necessary. Keep patient warm. Give antibiotics at first sign of infection. Give whole blood transfusions and 50% dextrose I.V.

COMPLICATIONS: When such patients recover, they often have some nervous system involvement, including various types of paralysis, blindness, or interference with sensation, or muscular spasms, or twitchings, for an indefinite period of time. Most of these complications disappear in time, but occasionally they remain permanently.

carbonom'etry [L. *carbo,* carbon, + G. *metron,* measure]. Determination of presence and amt. of carbon dioxide exhaled.

car'bon tetrachloride (tet-ră-klō'rīd). CCl_4. A clear, colorless liquid, with ethereal odor resembling chloroform; not inflammable.

USES: Although having narcotic and anesthetic properties resembling chloroform, it is too toxic to be suitable as an anesthetic. In general this substance is too toxic for use. Inhalation of a small quantity has been known to produce death. The mechanism of injury is acute atrophy of the liver and kidney.

POISONING: Toxic effects due to prolonged inhalation.

SYM: Irritation of eyes, nose, and throat, headache, nausea, anorexia, weakness.

F. A. TREATMENT: Oxygen inhalation, and artificial respiration. Lavage with saline solution. Leave saline cathartic in stomach.

SEE ALSO: *Table of Poisons and Poisoning in Appendix.*

carbonu'ria [L. *carbo,* carbon, + G. *ouron,* urine]. The presence or excretion of carbon compounds in the urine.

carbonyl (kar'bon-īl) [" + G. *ylē,* matter]. The divalent radical CO, characteristic of aldehydes and ketones.

carbo-resin. Proprietary name for carbacrylamine resins, *q.v.*

carboxyhemoglobin (kar-bok"sī-hē"mō-glō'bin) [L. *carbo,* carbon, + G. *oxys,* acid, + *aima,* blood, + L. *globus,* sphere]. Compound formed by carbon monoxide and hemoglobin in poisoning by carbon monoxide.

carboxyl (kar-box'īl). The characteristic group (COOH) of organic carboxylic acids, *e.g.,* formic acid (H-COOH), acetic acid (CH_2COOH).

carboxylase (kar-boks'ĭ-lās). An enzyme which brings about the removal of the carboxyl group (COOH) from amino acids; an enzyme found in brewer's yeast which catalizes the decarboxylation of pyruvic acid with the production of acetaldehyde and carbon dioxide. In the body this requires the presence of vitamin B_1 (thiamine) which acts as a coenzyme.

carbuncle, carbunculus (kar'bun-kl, kar-bunk'ū-lus) [L. *carbunculus,* little coal]. A circumscribed inflammation of the skin and deeper tissues which terminates in a slough and suppuration and is accompanied by marked constitutional symptoms.

ETIOL: Staphylococci. Predisposing factors the same as in furuncle.* Occurs more frequently in men, and in adults than children. Diabetics are particularly susceptible.

SYM: It is characterized by a painful node at first covered by a tight, reddened skin which later becomes thin and perforates, discharging pus through several openings. Also fever, leukocytosis and sometimes prostration. Most commonly found on nape of neck, on upper back, or on buttocks.

TREATMENT: Antibiotics given systemically are usually effective. Incision and drainage when lesion is about to point. Keep covered with warm compresses to promote blood supply to the area.

NP: Use sterile technic when dressing area. Disinfect all contaminated equipment and destroy soiled dressings.

carbun'cular. Pert. to a carbuncle.

carbunculosis (kar-bunk-ū-lō'sis). Appearance of several carbuncles in succession.

carcinectomy (kar-sĭ-nek'tō-mĭ) [G. *karkinos,* crab cancer, + *ektomē,* excision]. The excision of a cancerous growth.

carcinelcosis (kar-sĭ-nĕl-kō'sis) [" + *elkōsis,* ulceration]. An ulcer of a cancerous nature.

carcinogenesis (kar"sĭ-nō-jen'ĕ-sis) [" + *genesis,* production]. The production or origin of cancer.

carcinogenic (kar"sĭ-nō-jen'ik). Causing cancer.

carcinoid (kar'sĭ-noid) [G. *karkinos,* cancer, + *eidos,* resemblance]. An argentaffin cell tumor which may arise in the intestinal tract, bile ducts, pancreas, bronchus or ovary. These tumors secrete serotonin (5-hydroxytryptamine).

c. *syndrome.* A group of symptoms which develop when a carcinoid tumor, by metastasis or on its own, produces excess amounts of serotonin. Symptoms include one or more of the following: brief episodes of flushing, especially of the face and neck; tachycardia; facial and periorbital edema; hypotension; intermittent abdominal pain with diarrhea; valvular lesions of the heart; loss of weight; hypoproteinemia; signs of pellagra. The latter symptom is due to the body's available tryptophan, which is the precursor of serotonin, being used for serotonin production instead of for manufacture of niacin and protein.

TREATMENT: Symptoms usually develop only after the tumor has metastasized. Nevertheless surgical removal of accessible tumors is indicated. High protein diet with niacin supplement. Serotonin antagonist for control of diarrhea and malabsorption. Cortisone may be helpful in controlling inanition.

carcinolysis (kar-sĭ-nol'ĭ-sis) [" + *lysis,* destruction]. Destruction of carcinoma cells.

carcinolytic (kar-sĭ-nō-lit'ik). Destructive to cancer cells.

carcinoma (kar-sĭ-nō'mă) [" + *-ōma, tumor*]. An epithelial cell new growth or malignant tumor, enclosed in connective tissue, and tending to infiltrate and give rise to metastases. SYN: *cancer.*

It may affect almost any organ or part of the body and spread through the blood stream. Etiology is unknown.

c., *basal cell.* An epidermoid carcinoma common on face of elderly. It has a low degree of malignancy. It gives rise to the typical rodent ulcer.

c., chorionic. A tumor containing cells characteristic of the chorion of the embryo. It occurs in the testis, ovary, and other parts of the body. SYN: *choriocarcinoma.*

c., cylindrical-cell. A carcinoma of glands usually of entodermal origin including adenocarcinoma and carcinoma simplex.

c., epidermoid. A tumor on a surface such as the skin which is covered with stratified epithelium; usually of two types, one a wartlike growth, slow-growing, mildly malignant; the other a flat and rapidly infiltrating neoplasm.

c., glandular. C. with cells of the secreting variety. SEE: *adenocarcinoma.*

c., lipomatous. C. with fatty tissue.

c., melanotic. C. containing melanin.

c., scirrhous. A form of cylindrical-cell c., with a firm, hard structure.

c., squamous-cell. A form of epidermoid carcinoma principally of squamous cells.

carcinomatophobia (kar-sĭ-nō″mă-tō-fō′-bĭ-ă) [G. *karkinos,* cancer, +-*ōma,* tumor, + *phobos,* fear]. Morbid fear of carcinoma.

carcinomatosis (kar-sĭ-nō-mă-tō′sĭs) [" + " + -*ōsis,* infection]. The condition of having a carcinoma anywhere in the body. SYN: *carcinosis.*

carcinomatous (kar-sĭ-nō′mă-tus). Pert. to or affected with cancer.

carcinomec′tomy [G. *karkinos,* cancer, + -*ōma,* tumor, + *ektomē,* excision]. Excision of a cancer.

carcinomelcosis (kar-sĭ-nō-mel-kō′sis) [" + " + *elkōsis,* ulceration]. An ulcerating cancer.

carcinopho′bia [" + " + *phobos,* fear]. Morbid fear of cancer.

carcinosarco′ma [" + " + *sarx,* flesh, + -*ōma,* tumor]. A mixed tumor of carcinoma and sarcoma.

carcinosectomy (kar-sĭ-nō-sĕk′tō-mĭ) [" + " + *ektomē,* excision]. Excision of a cancer.

carcinosis (kar-sĭ-nō′sis) [" + " + -*ōsis,* infection]. Carcinomatosis, *q.v.*

car′damom, car′damon [G. *kardamōmon*]. Dried ripe fruit of an herb *Elettaria repens* or *E. cardomomum,* used as an aromatic and carminative.

Cardarelli's sign (kar-dă-rel′lēz). Tracheal tugging significant of aneurysm of aorta.

cardia (kar′dĭ-ă) [G.]. 1. Upper orifice (esophageal) of stomach connecting with the esophagus. 2. The heart.

cardiac (kar′dĭ-ak). 1. Pertaining to the heart or to the cardiac orifice into the stomach. 2. Having heart disease. 3. A heart tonic.

c. arrhythmia. SEE: *arrhythmia.*

c. atrophy. Fatty degeneration of the heart.

c. compensation. The ability of the heart through its reserve power to compensate for impaired functioning of its valves.

c. cycle. The period from the beginning of one beat of the heart to the beginning of the next succeeding beat, including the *systole,* or contraction of the atria and ventricles propelling the blood onward, and the *diastole,* the period during which the cavities are being refilled with blood.

The atria contract immediately before the ventricles. The ordinary cycle lasts 8/10 of a second with the heart beating at 72 times per minute. The *atrial systole* lasts 0.1 second; the *ventricular systole,* 0.3 second, and the *diastole,* 0.4 second, thus even though the heart seems to be "working" continuously it rests for a good portion of each cardiac cycle.

RS: *circulation; diastole; heart; systole.*

c. diet. Variable. Maintenance without labor upon heart.

Avoid gas-producing foods, such as cabbage, onions, turnips, beans, and bulky foods causing distention and pressure upon heart. Fluid intake restricted to 1500 cc. or less. Eliminate salt if edema is present. Small quantities of food at a time. Karrell diet, *q.v.*

c. diet, Smith. A variation of the Karrell diet, *q.v.* Maintenance protein (⅔ to 1 gm. per kg.) mostly milk or eggs. The calories made adequate by addition of some cream by the liberal use of carbohydrates. Fluids limited, salt restricted in cases complicated with edema. For the first few days diet is liquid, milk and cream, orange juice and added sugars. After that soft foods are added, pureed vegetables, fruits, toast, cereal, carbohydrate pushed by use of sugars, jelly, honey or sugar candy.

Advantages: An adequate diet; foods may be varied so diet is not so monotonous. The emphasis on carbohydrates is beneficial.

c. failure. Condition resulting from inability of the heart to pump sufficient blood to meet the needs of the body. SEE: *heart failure.*

c. hypertrophy. Enlargement of the heart. SEE: *heart, hypertrophy of.*

c. insufficiency. Inadequate cardiac output due to failure of the heart to function properly, as in valvular deficiency.

c. output. The amount of blood discharged from the left (or right) ventricle per minute. Also called *minute volume.* For an average adult cardiac output is approximately 3.0 liters per square meter of body surface area each minute.

c. plexus. *Plexus cardiacus.* SEE: *plexuses in Appendix.*

c. reflex. A reflex in which the response is a change in cardiac rate. Stimulation of sensory nerve endings in the wall of the carotid sinus by increased arterial blood pressure reflexly slows the heart (Marey's law); stimulation of vagus fibers in the right side of the heart by increased venous return reflexly increases heart rate (Bainbridge's reflex).

c. reserve. The capacity of the heart to increase cardiac output and raise blood pressure above basal pressure to meet body requirements.

cardiactia (kar-dĭ-ak′tĭ-ă) [G. *kardia,* heart, + L. *actio,* function]. Cardiac stenosis.

cardiagra (kar-dĭ-ag′ră) [" + *agra,* seizure]. Serious pains in the chest of a constricting nature. SEE: *angina pectoris.*

cardialgia (kar-dĭ-al′jĭ-ă) [" + *algos,* pain]. Pain at the pit of the stomach or region of the heart, usually occurring in paroxysms.

cardiam′eter [" + *metron,* measure]. Device for marking position of the cardia.

cardianastrophe (kar-dĭ-an-as′trō-fĭ) [" + *anastrophē,* reversal of position]. Congenital transposition of the heart to the right side. SYN: *dextrocardia.*

cardianesthe′sia [" + *anaisthēsia,* lack of sensation]. Lack of sensation in the heart.

cardiant (kar'dĭ-ant). 1. Affecting, or that which affects the heart. 2. A cardiac stimulant.

cardiaortic (kar-dĭ-ā-or'tĭk) [G. *kardia*, heart, + *aortē*, aorta]. Pert. to the heart and the aorta.

cardiasthenia (kar-dĭ-as-thē'nĭ-ă) [" + *astheneia*, weakness]. Type of neurasthenia with predominance of cardiac symptoms.

cardiasthma (kar-dĭ-az'mă) [" + *asthma*, panting]. Dyspnea due to heart disease.

cardiataxia (kar-dĭ-ă-taks'ĭ-ă) [" + *ataxia*, lack of order]. Incoordination of the heart contractions; very irregular heart action.

cardiectasia, cardiectasis (kar-dĭ-ek-ta'-sĭ-ă, kar-dĭ-ek'tă-sis) [" + *ektasis*, dilatation]. Dilatation of the heart.

cardiectomy (kar-dĭ-ek'tō-mĭ) [" + *ektomē*, excision]. Excision of the cardiac end of the stomach.

cardinal [L. *cardinalis*, important]. Of primary importance such as the cardinal symptoms: temperature, pulse, respiration.

cardio- [G. *kardia*, heart]. Prefix: Pert. to the cardia or heart.

cardioaccel'erator [" + L. *accelerāre*, to hasten]. That which increases the rate of the heart beat.

cardioangiology (kar"dĭ-ō-an-jĭ-ol'ō-jĭ) [" + *aggeion*, vessel, + *logos*, study]. The science of the heart and blood vessels.

cardioaortic (kar"dĭ-ō-ā-or'tĭk) [" + *aortē*, aorta]. Pert. to the heart and the aortic artery.

cardiocele (kar'dĭ-ō-sēl) [" + *kēlē*, tumor]. Hernia of the heart.

cardiocentesis (kar-dĭ-ō-sen-tē'sis) [" + *kentesis*, puncture]. Surgical incision or puncture of the heart.

cardiocinetic (kar"dĭ-ō-sĭ-net'ĭk) [" + *kinesis*, motion]. Cardiokinetic, *q.v.*

cardiocirrhosis (kar-dĭ-ō-sĭ-rō'sĭs). Cirrhosis of the liver associated with or occurring secondary to heart failure.

cardioclasia, cardioclasis (kar-dĭ-ō-klā'-zĭ-ă, kar-dĭ-ok'lă-sĭs) [" + *klasis*, break]. Rupture of the heart.

cardiodi'lator [" + L. *dilatāre*, to enlarge]. Device for dilating the cardia of the esophagus.

cardiodynamics (kar-dĭ-ō'dĭ-năm-ĭks). Science of forces involved in propulsion of blood from heart to tissues and back to heart.

cardiodynia (kar-dĭ-ō-din'ĭ-ă) [" + *odynē*, pain]. Pain in the region of the heart.

cardiogen'ic [" + *gennan*, to produce]. Having origin in the heart itself.

car'diogram [" + *gramma*, mark]. A graph, on special paper, of the electrical activity of the heart muscle. Made with an electrocardiograph machine. Syn: *electrocardiograph.*

cardiograph (kar'dĭ-ō-graf) [" + *graphein*, to write]. A device for registering the electrical activity of the heart muscle.

cardiograph'ic. Pert. to cardiography.

cardiog'raphy. The recording and study of the electrical activity of the heart.

cardiohepat'ic [G. *kardia*, heart, + *epar*, liver]. Pert. to heart and liver.

car"dioinhib'itory [" + L. *inhibere*, to check]. Slowing action of the heart.

cardiokinet'ic [" + *kinēsis*, motion]. Pert. to that which excites heart action.

car'diolith [" + *lithos*, stone]. A concretion or calculus in the heart.

cardiol'ogist [" + *logos*, study]. A specialist in treatment of heart disease.

cardiol'ogy. The study of the heart.

cardiol'ysin [G. *kardia*, heart, + *lysis*, loosening]. A lysin acting on heart muscle.

cardiolysis (kar-dĭ-ol'ĭ-sĭs) [" + *lysis*, loosening]. Freeing pericardial adhesions to surrounding tissues, involving resection of the ribs and sternum.

cardiomalacia (kar-dĭ-o-mă-lā'sĭ-ă) [" + *malakia*, softening]. Softening of the heart walls.

cardiomegaly (kar-dĭ-ō-meg'ă-lĭ) [" + *megas*, large]. Hypertrophy of the heart.

cardiometer (kar-dĭ-om'ĕ-ter) [" + *metron*, measure]. Device for locating impulse or apex of the heart's beat.

cardiomotil'ity [" + L. *motilis*, moving]. The ability of the heart to function.

cardiomyoliposis (kar"dĭ-o-mi"ō-lĭ-pō'sis) [" + *mys*, muscle, + *lipos*, fat]. Fatty degeneration of the heart.

cardionecro'sis [" + *nekros*, dead]. Necrosis of the heart.

cardionephric (kar-dĭ-ō-nef'rĭk) [" + *nephros*, kidney]. Pert. to heart and kidney.

cardioneu'ral [" + *neuron*, nerve]. Pert. to nervous control of the heart.

cardioneuro'sis [" + *neuron*, nerve]. Functional neurosis with cardiac symptoms.

cardiopalmus (kar-dĭ-ō-păl'mus) [" + *palmos*, palpitation]. Palpitation of the heart.

cardiopal'udism [" + L. *palus*, marsh, + G. *ismos*]. Irregularity of heart action resulting from malaria.

car'diopath [" + *pathos*, disease]. A person with heart disease.

cardiopathy (kar-dĭ-op'ă-thĭ). Any disease of the heart.

cardiopericardi'tis [" + *peri*, around, + *kardia*, heart, + *-itis*, inflammation]. Inflammation of myocardium and pericardium.

cardiophobia (kar"dĭ-ō-fō'bĭ-ă) [" + *phobos*, fear]. Morbid fear of heart disease.

cardiophone (kar'dĭ-ō-fōn) [" + *phonē*, voice]. Device, esp. a stethoscope, for listening to sound of the heart.

cardioplasty (kar-dĭ-ō-plas'tĭ) [" + *plassein*, to form]. Operation on the cardia to relieve cardiospasm.

cardioplegia (kar-dĭ-ō-plē'jĭ-ă) [" + *plēgē*, stroke]. Paralysis of the heart.

cardiopneumat'ic [" + *pneuma*, breath]. Pert. to the heart and the lungs.

cardiopneumograph (kar-dĭ-ō-nū'mō-graf) [" + " + *graphein*, to write]. Device for recording motion of heart and lungs.

cardioptosis (kăr-dĭ-ŏp-tō'sĭs) [" + *ptōsis*, falling]. Prolapse of the heart.

cardiopul'monary [" + L. *pulmō*, lung]. Pert. to both heart and lungs.

car'diopuncture [" + L. *punctura*, piercing]. Surgical puncture of the heart. Syn: *cardiocentesis.*

cardiopylor'ic [" + *pyloros*, gatekeeper]. Pert. to the cardiac and pyloric ends of the stomach.

cardiore'nal [" + L. *rēnalis*, pert. to kidney]. Pert. to both heart and kidneys.

cardiorrhaphy (kar-dĭ-or'af-ĭ) [" + *raphē*, a suture]. Suturing of the heart muscle.

cardiorrhexis (kar-dĭ-or-reks'is) [" + *rēxis*, rupture]. Heart rupture.

cardiosclerosis (kar-dĭ-o-sklĕ-ro'sis) [" + *sklērōsis*, hardening]. Hardening of the cardiac tissues and arteries.

car'dioscope [" + *skopein*, to examine]. Instrument for examining the interior of the heart.

cardioscopy (kar-dĭ-ŏs'kō-pĭ). Examination of the interior of the heart, without opening the chest, by using a cardioscope.

cardiospasm (kar'dĭ-ō-spazm) [" + *spasmos*, spasm]. Disordered motor function of the distal end of the esophagus and failure of the esophageal orifice (cardia) of the stomach to relax. Thus the word is a misnomer in that failure of relaxation (achalasia) and absence of esophageal motility (aperistalsis) are the disease processes involved.

Etiol: Due to absence or injury of ganglion cells in Auerbach's plexus.

Sym: Substernal fullness, dysphagia, regurgitation, esp. at night.

Treatment: Bland semi-solid foods warmed to body temperature are of some help, but dilatation of the esophageal sphincter will allow the esophagus to drain by force of gravity. It may be possible to do this mechanically, but if not surgical myotomy may be required.

cardiosphyg'mograph [" + *sphygmos*, throb, + *graphein*, to write]. Instrument for graphically recording movements of the heart and pulse.

cardiostenosis (kar-dĭ-o-sten-o'sis) [" + *stenōsis*, narrowing]. Heart constriction and its development.

cardiosym'physis [G. *kardia*, heart, + *symphysis*, growing together]. Mediastinopericarditis, *q.v.*

cardiotachometer (kar"dĭ-ō-tak-om'ĕ-ter) [" + *takos*, speed, + *metron*, measure]. An instrument for measuring the total number of heart beats over a long period of time.

cardiother'apy [" + *therapeia*, treatment]. The treatment of cardiac diseases.

cardiotomy (kar-dĭ-ot'ō-mĭ) [" + *temnein*, to cut]. Incision of the heart.

cardioton'ic [" + *tonos*, tone]. Increasing tonicity of the heart.

cardiotoxic (kar-dĭ-ō-toks'ik) [" + *toxikon*, poisoning]. Exercising a poisonous effect upon the heart.

cardiovalvuli'tis [" + L. *valvula*, valve, + G. *-itis*, inflammation]. Inflammation of valves of the heart. Valvular endocarditis.

cardiovalvulotome (kar-dĭ-ō-val'vū-lō-tōm) [" + " + G. *tomē*, cut]. An instrument for excising part of a valve, esp. the mitral valve.

cardiovas'cular [" + L. *vasculum*, small vessel]. Pert. to the heart and blood vessels.

c. reflex. 1. Sympathetic increase in heart rate when increased pressure in, or distention of, great veins occurs. Syn: *Bainbridge reflex.* 2. Reflex vasoconstriction resulting from reduced venous pressure.

cardiovasology (kar"dĭ-ō-vas-ol'ō-jĭ) [" + L. *vas*, vessel, + G. *logos*, study]. Science of the heart and blood vessels. Syn: *cardioangiology.*

carditis (kar-dī'tĭs) [" + *-itis*, inflammation]. Inflammation of the heart muscles. Usually involves two of the following: pericardium, myocardium, or endocardium.

caries (ka'rēz, ka'rĭ-ēz) [L. rottenness]. Gradual decay and disintegration of a bone or tooth associated with inflammation and the formation of abscesses in the periosteum and surrounding tissues.

c., dental. Decay of the teeth. A progressive decalcification of the enamel and dentine of a tooth. The etiology is not fully known. Early detection and dental fillings offer the best form of control. Topical application of fluorine promotes resistance to dental caries if applied during the stage of tooth formation.

Chronic abscess, tuberculosis, and bacterial invasion of teeth are examples. In caries the bone disintegrates by pieces, while in necrosis large masses of bone are discharged. Deficiency of vitamins C and D has a direct influence upon caries of the teeth.

c. fungo'sa. A type of tuberculosis of bone.

c., necrotic. Caries with masses of bone in a suppurative cavity.

c. sic'ca. Dry tuberculosis of ends of bones and joints unaccompanied by fluid or swelling.

c., spinal. Pott's disease. Caries of the vertebrae, usually tuberculous.

carina (kă-rī'nă) (pl. *carinae*) [L. keel of a boat]. A keel-like structure.

c. nasi. A cleftlike space between the agger nasi and roof of nasal cavity. Syn: *olfactory sulcus.*

c. tracheae [NA]. A ridge at lower end of trachea separating openings of the two bronchi.

c. urethralis. Ridge extending posteriorly from urethral orifice and continuous with anterior column of the vagina.

carinate (kar'ĭ-nāt). Keel-shaped; possessing a keel or keel-shaped process.

cariogenic (ka"rĭ-o-jen'ik) [" + G. *gennan*, to produce]. Conducive to caries formation.

carious (ka'rĭ-us) [L. *cariēs*, rottenness]. 1. Affected with or relating to caries. 2. Having pits or perforations. See: *caries.*

carmin'ative [L. *carmināre*, to cleanse]. An agent that will remove gases from the gastrointestinal tract.

c. enema. Given to relieve distention caused by flatulence and also to stimulate peristalsis.

carnal (kar'nal) [L. *carō, carnis*, flesh]. Relating to the flesh.

c. knowledge. A phrase used in medicolegal cases to denote sexual intercourse especially with a minor female child.

carneous (kar'nē-us) [L. *carneus*, fleshy]. Fleshy.

carnification (kar-nĭ-fĭ-kā'shun) [L. *carō*, cornis, flesh, + *facere*, to make]. Alteration of tissues, esp. the change of pulmonary tissue to a form resembling skeletal muscle.

carnitine (kar'nĭ-tĭn). A base derived from betaine.

carnivorous (kar-niv'o-rus) [" + *vorāre*, to devour]. Flesh eating.

carnopho'bia [" + G. *phobos*, fear]. Abnormal aversion to meat.

carnose (kar'nōs). Having the consistency of or resembling flesh.

carnosity (kar-nos'ĭ-tĭ) [L. *carnōsitās*, fleshiness]. An excrescence resembling flesh; a fleshy growth.

carot'enase [G. *karōton*, carrot]. An enzyme that converts carotene into vitamin A. Also *carotinase.*

carotene (car'ō-tēn). A yellow crystalline pigment present in various plant and animal tissues. It is abundant in yellow vegetables (carrots, squash, corn). Carotene, which exists in several forms, is the precursor of vitamin A. Carotene is stored in the liver and converted to vitamin A in the liver.

carotenemia, carotinemia (kar"ō-tē-nē'mĭ-ă) [G. *karōton*, carrot, + *aima*, blood]. Carotene in the blood characterized by yellowing of the skin (pseudojaundice). Carotenemia can be distinguished from true jaundice by the lack of yellow discoloration of the conjunctivae in carotenemia. Syn: *carotenosis.*

carotenoid (kă-rot'ĕ'-noid). 1. One of a group of pigments (as carotene, *q.v.*) ranging in color from light yellow to purple, widely distributed in plants and animals. 2. Resembling carotene.

caroteno'sis. Carotenemia, *q.v.*

carotic (kă-rot'ik) [G. *karoun*, to stupefy]. 1. Carotid. 2. Resembling stupor; stupefying. 3. A sleep-producing drug.

carotid (kă-rot'ĭd) [G. *karōtides*, from *karos*, heavy with sleep, because ancient Greeks believed the carotid arteries caused sleep]. 1. The right and left common carotid arteries, both of which arise from the aorta, are the principal blood supply to the head and neck. Each of these two arteries divides to form external and internal carotid arteries. 2. Pertaining to any carotid part, as c. sinus.

c. body. SEE: *body, carotid.*

c. sinus. A dilated area at the bifurcation of the common carotid artery which is richly supplied with sensory nerve endings of the sinus branch of the vagus nerve. These when stimulated by distention of the vessel wall brought about by a rise in blood pressure, bring about reflex vasodilation and a slowing of the heart rate.

carotidynia (kar-ot-ĭ-din'ĭ-ă) [" + *odynē*, pain]. Pain elicited by pressure on the common carotid artery. Also spelled *carotodynia.*

car'otin [G. *karōton*, carrot]. Carotene, *q.v.*

car'otinase. Carotenase, *q.v.*

carotine'mia. Carotenemia, *q.v.*

car'pal [G. *karpos*, wrist]. Pertaining to the carpus or wrist.

c. articulation. Wrist joint.

c. tunnel syndrome. Pressure on the median nerve at the point it goes through the carpal tunnel of the wrist. Causes soreness, tenderness, and weakness of the muscles of the thumb.

TREATMENT: Surgical relief of tension if conservative therapy fails.

carpale (kar-pā'lĕ). Any wrist bone.

carpec'tomy [G. *karpos*, wrist, + *ektomē*, excision]. Excision of the carpus or portion of it.

carphologia, carphology (kar-fo-lo'jĭ-ă, -fol'ō-ji) [G. *karphos*, chaff, + *legein*, to pluck]. Involuntary picking at bed clothes, seen esp. in febrile or exhaustive delirium, of the low muttering type. A grave symptom in cases of extreme exhaustion or approaching death. SYN: *floccilation.*

carpo- [G.]. Prefix: Pert. to the carpus.

car"pometacar'pal [G. *karpos*, wrist, + *meta*, beyond, + *karpos*]. Pert. to both carpus and metacarpus.

carpoped'al [" + L. *pēs, ped*, foot]. Pertaining to both the wrist and the foot.

c. spasm. Spasm of the hands and feet, sometimes seen in laryngismus stridulus, *q.v.*

carpoptosis (kar-pop-tō'sis) [" + *ptōsis*, a falling]. Wrist drop.

carpus (kar'pus) [G. *karpos*]. The 8 bones of the wrist. SEE: *wrist.*

Carrel-Dakin treatment [Alexis Carrel, French American surgeon, 1873-1944, and Henry D. Dakin, American chemist, 1880-1952]. Method of wound irrigation first utilized in 1915.

Most suitable for deep septic wounds. A special apparatus is necessary: A glass receptacle for the solution constructed on the principle of a vacuum flask for maintaining a constant temperature. From this leads a rubber tube, attached to a glass connection piece, from which are suspended several perforated fine gauge rubber tubes. Each is tied at the lower end, and perforated for about half its length. Any number of tubes can be used, depending on size of wound. The flow is regulated so that a slow dropping occurs continually, thus keeping the wound constantly bathed. A Dakin's special solution of sodium hypochlorite (0.45-0.50%) is used. It decomposes under light. Must be kept in dark bottle and not be older than 36-72 hours.

carrier [Fr. *carier*, to bear]. 1. A person who harbors a specific pathogenic organism in the absence of discernible symptoms or signs of the disease and who is potentially capable of spreading the organism to others. 2. That which carries anything as (a) an insect such as a fly which passively carries infectious organisms; (b) a substance which, when combined with another substance (transport substance), is capable of passing through cell membranes as occurs in active transport mechanisms. SEE: *vector; microorganisms.*

CLASSIFICATION: *Infection by Animal Carriers:* Some microorganisms may be carried from an animal to man by *direct contact, indirect transfer*, or *by intermediary hosts.*

Air-borne Infection: Pathogenic organisms in the respiratory tract, discharged from the mouth or nose, may be borne on the air and settle on food, clothing, walls and floors, and if they are of the type which resists drying for a long period they may remain virulent until transmitted to another person. Coughing, sneezing, and expectorating may be responsible for "droplet infection."

Contact Infection: This is the result of transmission from person to person, as in kissing, coming in contact with those afflicted with communicable diseases, or with utensils handled by one with an infection.

Food-borne Infection: Bacteria may be communicated through food. Root and salad vegetables may carry bacteria from the soil or from manure. Cooking safeguards by destroying microorganisms on food.

Human Carriers: Some parasites may live in or upon the body of those who themselves do not suffer from them, but may be carried by them to others. Carriers may be: (*a*) *Contact* carriers, or those who never show symptoms; (*b*) *incubationary* carriers, or those in whom the infection is starting but has not completed the incubation period, and (*c*) *convalescent* carriers, or those who have recovered but who still harbor tne organism causing their disease

Insect Vectors: An insect may act as a physical carrier, as the tick. which may transmit the organism causing Rocky Mountain spotted fever, or one that acts as an active intermediate host such as the Anopheles mosquito which transmits malaria.

Prenatal Infection: This is the result of the fetus being infected from the mother's blood stream, or from contiguity with the maternal membranes.

Soil-borne Infection: Soil-borne, spore-forming organisms commonly enter the body through wounds, as in tetanus and gas gangrene.

Water - borne Infection: Organisms producing typhoid, dysentery, cholera, and amebic infections may be carried through a water supply, or water in public pools used for bathing. These organisms may pass into the water from the feces of an infected person and be communicated to others.

c., active. One who harbors a pathogenic organism for a considerable period following recovery from disease due to the organism. A chronic carrier.

c., chain saw. Instrument for carrying one end of a thread around a bone to be cut.

c., chronic. Active c., *q.v.*

c., convalescent. One who harbors the organism during recovery from the disease caused by the organism.

c., drainage tube. Instrument for placing drainage tubes in narrow or deep seated tracts.

c., healthy. One who harbors an infectious organism but infection is inapparent throughout entire course.

c., incubatory. One who harbors and spreads an infectious organism during the incubation period of a disease.

c., intermittent. One who is capable of spreading infectious organisms at intervals.

c., ligament. Flat needlelike instrument for drawing ligament through perforations made in the fascia.

c., ligature. An instrument for carrying ligatures through tissue.

c., passive. A healthy carrier, *q.v.*

c., renal. An instrument for introduction into kidneys. Flexible ones, about 20 in. long.

c., suppository bladder. C. for depositing suppositories, etc., in the bladder.

c., temporary. Healthy c., *q.v.*

c., urethral. C. for introduction into ureters. Flexible ones, about 12 in. long.

Carrion's disease [named for Daniel A. Carrion, 1850-1885, a Peruvian student who lost his life after voluntarily taking an injection]. Bartonellosis, *q.v.*

Carron oil (kar'on) [From Carron Iron Works, England]. A mixture of linseed oil and lime water used as a dressing in treatment of burns. SYN: *lime liniment.*

car'rots [G. *karōton*, carrot]. The orange root of a plant *Daucus carota.*

RAW: 100 gm. Calories: 42. Other main values: 1.1 gm. protein; trace of fat; 9.7 gm. carbohydrates; 37 mg. calcium; 11,000 I.U. vitamin A; 8 mg. ascorbic acid.

car sickness. Sickness induced by riding in cars. A form of motion sickness, *q.v.*

cartilage (kar'til-ăj) [L. *cartilagō*, gristle], A type of dense connective tissue consisting of cells embedded in a ground substance or matrix. The matrix is firm and compact rendering it capable of withstanding considerable pressure or tension. Cartilage has a bluish white or gray color and is semiopaque; it has no nerve or blood supply of its own. The cells lie in cavities called lacunae. They may be single or in groups of two, three, or four.

Cartilage constitutes a part of the skeleton occurring in the costal cartilages of the ribs, the nasal septum, in the external ear and lining the eustachian tube, in the wall of the larynx, in the trachea and bronchi, between bodies of the vertebrae, and covering the articular surfaces of bones. It forms the major portion of the embryonic skeleton.

c., articular. Hyaline cartilage covering the articular surfaces of bones.

c., costal. Cartilage connecting the true ribs and the sternum.

CARTILAGE

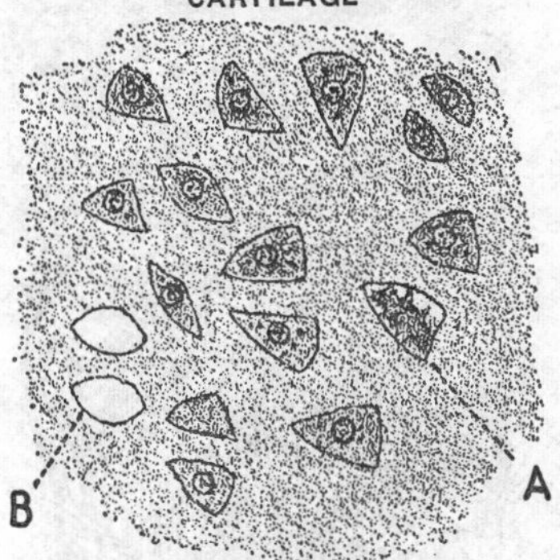

HYALINE CARTILAGE

Section of articular cartilage of the frog. A, Shrunken cartilage cells. B, Lacuna.

c. hyaline. A bluish-white glassy translucent cartilage. The matrix appears homogeneous although it contains collagenous fibers forming a finelike network. The walls of the lacunae stain intensely with basic dyes. Hyaline cartilage is flexible and slightly elastic. Its surface is covered by the *perichondrium* except on articular surfaces. Found in articular cartilage, in costal cartilages, in septum of nose, in larynx and trachea.

c., semilunar. One of the interarticular cartilages of the knee joint.

c., thyroid. Shield-shaped cartilage of the larynx, forming the prominence known as the Adam's apple.

c., yellow or elastic. A network of yellow elastic fibers, holding cartilage cells, and pervading intercellular substance. Found in the epiglottis, the external ear, the auditory tube, strengthening them and maintaining their shape.

cartilage, words pert. to: "cartilag-" words; "chondr-" words; cricoid.

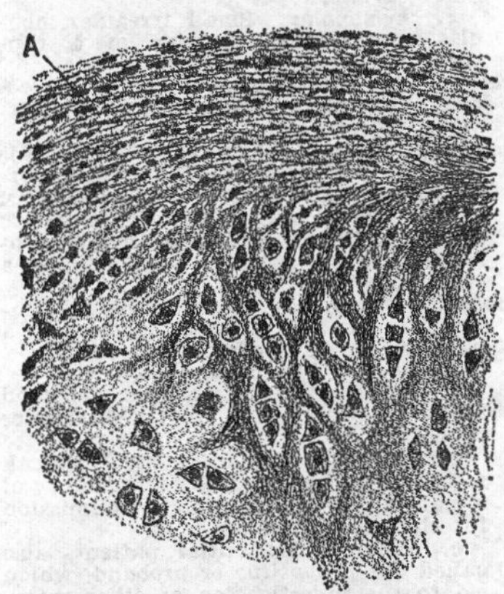

FIBROUS CARTILAGE

Section of intervertebral cartilage, calf's tail. A, Perichondrium.

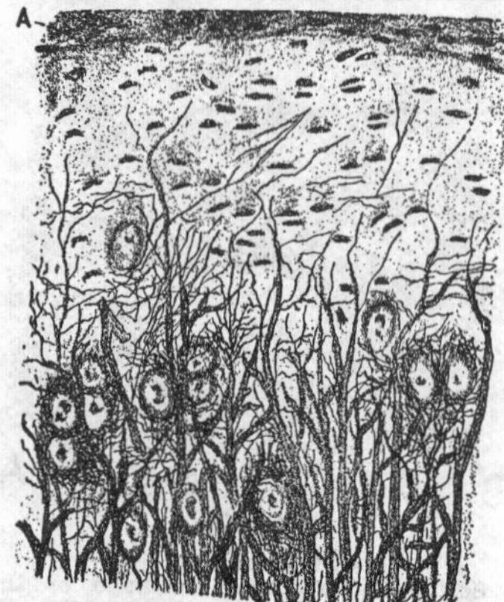

ELASTIC CARTILAGE
External ear, calf. A, Perichondrium.

cartilaginification (kar-tĭ-lă-jĭn″ĭ-fĭ-kā′-shun) [L. *cartilagō*, + *facere*, to make]. Cartilage formation or chondrification; the development of cartilage from undifferentiated tissue.

cartilaginoid (kar-tĭ-laj′ĭ-noid) [" + G. *eidos*, form]. Resembling cartilage.

cartilaginous (kar-tĭ-laj′ĭ-nus). Pert. to or consisting of cartilage.

cartilago (kar-tĭ-lā′gō) (pl. *cartilagines*). Cartilage, *q.v.*

car′uncle [L. *caruncula*, dim. *carō*, flesh]. A small fleshy growth.

c., *lacrimal*. One found on the conjunctiva near the inner canthus. A small, reddish elevation of modified skin. SYN: *caruncula lacrimalis* [NA].

c., *urethral*. A small, red, papillary growth, highly vascular, sometimes found in the urinary meatus in females. It is characterized by pain on urination and is very sensitive to friction.

caruncula (kar-ung′kū-lă) (pl. *carunculae*) [L.]. A tiny, fleshy protuberance. SYN: *caruncle.*

c., *hymenales*. Small irregular nodules representing remains of a ruptured hymen. SYN: *c. myrtiformes.*

cary-, caryo- [G. *karyon*, nucleus]. A combining form meaning nucleus. SEE: *kary-, karyo-*.

cascara sagrada (kas-kar′ă să-grā′dă). USP. The dried bark of *Rhamnus purshiana*, a small tree grown on western U. S. coast, and in parts of South America. The main ingredient in aromatic cascara sagrada fluid extract, a cathartic.

case [L. *casus*, happening]. 1. A particular example of a disease; incorrectly a patient. 2. An enclosing structure.

c., *brain*. The cranium, *q.v.*

c. *fatality rate*. Number per thousand of fatal terminations from a disease or operation.

c. *history*. The complete medical, family, social, and psychiatric history of a patient up to the time of admission for the present illness.

c., *index*. The initial patient, also called the *propositus* or *proband*, which led to the investigation of other members of a family for presence of genetic factors in the disease the original (index) case has.

caseate (kā′sē-āt) [L. *caseus*, cheese]. 1. To undergo cheesy degeneration. 2. A lactate.

caseation (kā-sē-ā′shun) [L. *caseus*, cheese]. 1. Process of conversion of necrotic tissue into a granular amorphous mass resembling cheese. 2. Precipitation of casein during coagulation of milk.

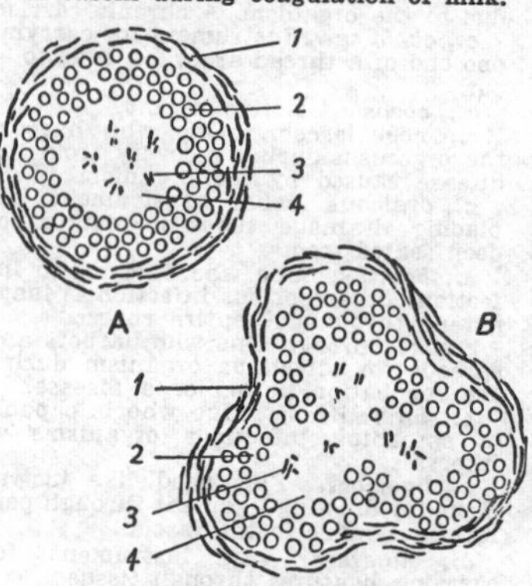

CASEATION
Diagram illustrating: A, Single tubercle; B, Three tubercles running together to produce a large central area of caseation. 1. Fibrous tissue. 2. Inflammatory cells (lymphocytes). 3. Tubercle bacilli. 4. Caseous material.

casein (ka′se-in) [L. *caseus*, cheese]. The principal protein in milk, seen in milk curds.

It supplies all of the amino acids necessary for body tissue. It is a derived protein. When coagulated by rennin or acid it becomes one of the principal ingredients of cheese. SEE: *caseinogen.*

caseinogen (ka-sē-in′ō-jen) [L. *caseus*, cheese, + G. *gennan*, to produce]. The principal protein in milk from which casein is derived.

It is the substance in solution, and casein is the result of its precipitation. Its conversion into casein is the essential process in the curdling of milk.

caseous (ka′sē-us). Resembling cheese; pert. to transformation of tissues into a cheesy mass.

$CaSO_4$. Calcium sulfate.

Casoni's reaction (ka-so′nĭz) [Tomaso Casoni, Italian physician, 1880-1933]. Appearance of a wheal surrounded by an erythematous zone following intradermal injection of sterile hydatid fluid. A test for presence of hydatid cysts resulting from infection with *Echinococcus granulosus.*

cassava (kă-să′vă) [Sp. *cazabe*, starch]. A tropical plant, the starch of which is used to make tapioca and bread. The rootstocks, from which the starch is obtained, are used also as a vegetable in tropical countries.

cassete (kă-set′) [F. little box]. A flat light-tight box, with an intensifying screen in it, for holding x-ray film.

cast [M.E. *casten*, to carry]. 1. A solid mold of a part, usually applied *in situ* for immobilization, as in fractures, dislocations and other severe injuries. Most often made of plaster of Paris, sodium silicate, starch, or dextrin which is rubbed into crinoline, then soaked in water, carefully applied to the part and allowed to harden.

2. Plastic or fibrous material thrown off in various pathological conditions, the product of effusion. It is molded to the shape of the part in which it has been accumulated. According to source, casts are classified as bronchial, intestinal, nasal, esophageal, renal, tracheal, urethral and vaginal; as to constituents, classified as bloody, fatty, fibrinous, granular, hyaline, mucous and waxy.

HOW TO RECOGNIZE: They have a limiting membrane enclosing a matrix or substance in which are epithelial cells, pus cells, red blood cells, granules, and fat globules. From these latter characters they take their name as epithelial casts, red blood casts, etc. Casts usually have square ends, their diameter is the same throughout, and usually they do not bend or twist.

c., *blood*. A cast composed principally of red blood cells.

c., *bronchial*. Seen in sputum of patients with asthma and some with bronchitis.

c., *epithelial*. Contain cells from inner lining of uriniferous tubules. Seen in acute nephritis.

c., *fatty*. Those containing epithelium that has undergone degenerative changes, found in very advanced cases of renal degeneration.

c., *fibrinous*. Yellowish-brown, sometimes with ragged fractures and highly refractile.

c., *granular*. Of varying sizes and made up of albumin and white blood cells, and of serious import in nephritis in its acute and chronic forms.

c., *hyaline*. Pale cylinders with rounded edges and variable size. Found in irritating conditions of the kidneys, nephritis, and its varying forms.

c., *pseudo-*. These are epithelial cells swollen and held in groups, resembling casts. Alkaline urine has a tendency to dissolve casts.

c., *pus*. Found in urine in suppuration of kidney.

c., *urinary*. Those found in the urine.

c., *uterine*. Those from the uterus passed in exfoliative endometritis or membranous dysmenorrhea.

c., *waxy*. Light yellowish, well defined, with tendency to split transversely, found in some cases of amyloid degeneration, and advanced nephritis.

Castle's intrinsic factor [William Bosworth Castle, American physician and university professor, Harvard University. Born 1897.]. A substance secreted by the stomach which is essential for the absorption of cyanocobalamin (vitamin B_{12}; *extrinsic factor*). Absence of intrinsic factor causes pernicious anemia.

cas'tor oil. USP. A fixed oil expressed from the seed of the plant *Ricinus communis*.

USES: Externally as an *emollient;* internally as a *cathartic.* In the digestive tract it is hydrolyzed to ricinoleic acid which acts as an irritant type of laxative.

cas'trate [L. *castrāre,* to prune]. 1. To remove the testicles or ovaries. 2. One who has been castrated. SEE: *spay.*

cas'trated. Desexed; emasculated.

castration (kăs-trā'shun) [L. *castrāre,* to prune]. 1. Emasculation; excision of the testicles or ovaries. 2. Destruction or inactivation of the gonad.

c. *complex*. Morbid fear of castration.

c., *female*. Removal of the ovaries. SYN: *oophorectomy; spaying.*

c., *male*. Removal of the testes. SYN: *orchiectomy; orchotomy.*

c., *parasitic*. Destruction of the gonads by parasitic organisms. It may result from direct infestation of the gonad or indirectly from effects of infestation in other parts of the body.

casualty (kaz'ū-al-tĭ) [L. *casualis,* accidental]. 1. Accident causing injury or death. 2. One so disabled, as a soldier.

casuistics (kaz-ū-is'tiks) [L. *casus,* a case]. Study of pathological cases.

cata- [G.]. Prefix: Down or downward; against, or according to, as *catabolism.*

catabasis (kă-tab'ă-sĭs) [G. *kata,* down, + *basis,* going]. The decline of a disease.

catabat'ic. Pert. to catabasis.*

catabolic (kat-a-bol'ik). Pert. to catabolism.

catab'olin. Catabolite, *q.v.*

catabolism (kă-tab'ō-lizm) [G. *katabolē,* a casting down]. 1. The destructive phase of metabolism, the opposite of *anabolism,* the constructive phase. 2. Catabolism includes all the processes in which complex substances are converted into simpler substances, usually with the release of energy. SEE: *anabolism; metabolism.*

catabolite (kă-tab'o-līt). Any catabolism product. SYN: *catabolin.*

catacrotic [G. *kata,* down, + *krotos,* beat]. Manifesting the downstroke of a pulse tracing interrupted by an upstroke.

catacrotism (kă-tak'rō-tizm) [" + " + *ismos*]. A pulse with one or more secondary expansions of artery following main beat.

catadicrotic (kat-ă-dī-krot'ik) [" + *dis,* twice, + *krotos,* beat] Manifesting one or more secondary expansions of a pulse on the descending limb of the tracing.

catadi'crotism [" + " + " + *ismos*]. Two minor expansions following the main beat of an artery.

catadioptric (kat"ă-dī-op'trik) [" + *diopsesthai,* to see through]. Pert. to refraction and reflection of light simultaneously.

catagenesis (kat-ă-jen'ĕ-sis) [" + *genesis,* production]. Retrogression or involution.

catalase (kat'a-lās). An enzyme present in cells esp. anaerobic bacteria which catalyzes the decomposition of hydrogen peroxide to water and oxygen.

catalepsy (kat'ă-lep-sĭ) [G. *kata,* down, + *lēpsis,* seizure]. A condition seen in psychotic patients wherein there is generalized diminished responsiveness usually characterized by a trance-like state. Doctors and nurses should keep in mind that even though the patient is in a trance, conversations may be heard. Therefore one's actions toward and talk about the patient should be no different than if he were not in a cataleptic state.

catalep'tic. Pert. to catalepsy.

cataleptiform (kat-ă-lep'tĭ-form) [G. *kata,* down, + *lēpsis,* seizure, + L. *forma,* shape]. Having the form of catalepsy.

catalep'toid [" + " + *eidos,* resemblance]. Resembling or simulating catalepsy.

catalysis (kă-tal'ĭ-sĭs) [G. *katalysis,* dissolution]. The speeding up of the rate of a chemical reaction by a catalyst, *q.v.*

catalyst (kat'ă-list) [G. *katalysis,* dissolution]. 1. An agent producing catalysis. A substance which speeds up the rate of a chemical reaction without itself being permanently altered in the reaction. Catalysts are effective in small quantities and are not used up in the reaction, *i.e.*, they can be recovered unchanged. Ex: hydrochloric acid which catalyzes the hydrolysis of sucrose; ptyalin which catalyzes the hydrolysis of starch. SYN: *catalyzer; catalytic agent.*

catalytic (kat-al-it'ik) [G. *katalysis*, dissolution]. Pert. to catalysis.*

c. agent. A catalyst, *q.v.*

catalyzer (kăt'ă-lī-zer) [G. *kata*, down, + *lysis*, loosening]. A catalyst, *q.v.*

catamenia (kat-ă-mē'nĭ-ă) [" + *mēn*, month]. The menses. Periodic menstrual discharge of blood from the uterus.

catame'nial. Pert. to the menses or catamenia.

c. device. That which collects or absorbs the menstrual flow. SEE: *perineal pad; vaginal tampon.*

catamnesis (kat-am-nē'sis) [G. *kata*, down, + *mnēmē*, memory]. A patient's history, after first being seen by physician, including all subsequent examinations. SEE ALSO: *anamnesis.*

cataphasia (kat-ă-fā'zĭ-ă) [" + *phasis*, speech]. A speech disorder causing an involuntary repetition of the same word.

cataphora (kă-taf'ō-ră) [G. *kataphora*, lethargy]. Lethargy with short remissions.

cataphoresis (kat-ă-fō-rē'sis) [G. *kata*, down, + *phorēsis*, being carried]. The transmission of electronegative ions or drugs into the body tissues or through a membrane by use of an electric current.

cataphoria (kat-ă-fō'rĭ-ă) [" + *pherein*, to bear]. Tendency of visual axes to incline below the horizontal plane.

cataphor'ic. Pert. to cataphora or cataphoresis.

cataphre'nia [G. *kata*, down, + *phrēn*, mind]. A dementia type tending to recovery but which shows mental debility.

cataphylaxis (kat-ă-fī-laks'is) [" + *phylaxis*, guard]. 1. The process of carrying antibodies, leukocytes, etc., to the site of an infection. 2. The breaking down of the body's natural defenses against infection.

cataplasia (kat-ă-plā'zĭ-ă) [" + *plassein*, to form]. Degenerative change in tissues or cells. SYN: *cataplasis.*

cataplasis (ka-tap'lă-sis). Cataplasia, *q.v.*

cat'aplasm [G. *kataplassein*, to spread over]. A poultice, *q.v.*

cataplectic (kat-ă-plek'tĭk) [G. *kata*, down, + *plēxis*, stroke]. Pert. to cataplexy.

cataplexy, cataplexia (kat'ă-pleks-ī, kat-ă-pleks'ĭ-ă) [" + *plēxis*, stroke]. A form of sudden shock, accompanied by loss of muscular tone, without loss of consciousness, the patient falling to the floor.

ETIOL: May be the result of intense emotion or the sudden onset of a disease or rarely a part of a narcoleptic attack.

cat'aract [G. *katarraktēs*, a rushing down]. Opacity of lens of eye or its capsule or both.

VARIETIES: Capsular, polar, lamellar, nuclear, cortical, morgagnian (fluid cataract with hard nucleus). Also, congenital, infantile, traumatic, diabetic, and senile, occurring bet. 50-60 years.

STAGES: (a) Incipient stage (spoke-shaped opacities, cloudlike opacities, opacity of cortex or nucleus. (b) Stage of swelling, or immature stage (swollen lens, shallow ant. chamber). (c) Mature stage (lens shrinks due to loss of fluid and becomes opaque, ant. chamber regains its normal depth, no shadow thrown by iris or lens with focal illumination). (d) Hypermature stage (lens becomes either solid and shrunken or soft and liquid).

ETIOL: Common form is result of senility; other forms may be congenital or caused by infection or injury.

TREATMENT: Surgical removal of lens except in presence of associated inflammation. Application of glasses.

c., operation for. NP: *Preoperative*: Explain to patient the need for postoperative restriction of movement. Cathartic and/or enema; sedative if ordered. *Postoperative:* Avoid turning, jarring, or startling patient. Always announce your approach to the patient in a calm, unhurried tone. If medicines are to be instilled into the eyes, be certain to warn the patient several times. Sand bags at sides of head to prevent turning until permitted. Knee roll and small pillow under small of back to relieve strain. Liquid diet for first few days with gradual return to regular diet. Bowel movement not encouraged for first 48 hours to prevent straining which could exert pressure on eye. Dressing changed after first 48 hours unless otherwise ordered; patient's unoperated eye then uncovered and he is permitted to turn to that side. He is allowed up in chair by end of week. Dark glasses for patient as ordered.

Use skill in feeding patient in *calm*, quiet atmosphere.

c., capsular. Cataract from opacity of the capsule.

c., lenticular. Occurring in the lens.

c., Morgagnian. A fluid cataract with a hard nucleus.

c., overripe. Stage following a mature cataract in which lens solidifies and shrinks or becomes soft. Also called *hypermature cataract.*

c., senile. Cataract of old persons.

cataractous (kat-a-rak'tus). Affected with or of the nature of a cataract.

catarrh (kă-tar') [G. *katarrein*, to flow down]. Term formerly applied to inflammation of mucous membranes.

c., dry. Severe spells of coughing with little or no expectoration. Generally seen in the old in association with emphysema or asthma.

SEQUELAE: Emphysema, bronchiectasis, and dilation of right ventricle.

PROG: Perfect recovery rarely attainable, but not incompatible with long life.

TREATMENT: Careful regulation of the hygiene. Constitutional.

catarrhal (kă-tar'al). Of the nature of or pert. to catarrh.

catastalsis (kat-ăs-tăl'sĭs) [G. *kata*, down, + *stalsis*, contraction]. Movement of a contraction-wave of the stomach downward, not preceded by a wave of inhibition.

catato'nia [G. *kata*, down, + *tonos*, tension]. 1. A phase of schizophrenia in which the patient is unresponsive. The tendency to assume and remain in a fixed posture, refusal to move or talk are characteristic of this phase. 2. Stupor.

cataton'ic. Stuporous; pert. to catatonia.

catatricrotic (kat-ă-trī-krot'ik) [G. *kata*, down, + *treis*, three, + *krotos*, beat]. Manifesting a third impulse in the descending stroke of the sphygmogram.

catatricrotism (kat-ă-trī'krō-tĭzm) [" + " + *krotos*, beat]. State in which the pulse is catatricrotic.

catatropia (kat-ă-trō'pĭ-ă) [" + *trepein*, to turn]. Having both eyes turned downward.

cat bite. Usually a punctured or lacerated wound, potentially infected.

Frequently infected wounds follow even under careful management. If animals are rabid, may lead to hydrophobia.

TREATMENT: Generously applied antiseptic to all parts of bite. Consider cautery and debridement. Antirabies treatment when indicated. Sterile dressings. SEE ALSO: *bites*.

cat scratch disease. A benign, self-limited disease lasting from two weeks to several months following a cat scratch or other skin injury. Etiology unknown but thought to be caused by a virus. SYN: *nonbacterial regional lymphadenitis; benign lymphoreticulosis of inoculation.*

cat unit. Amount of a drug (*i.e.*, digitalis) per Kg. of cat's weight, required to kill it when injected intravenously.

catecholamines (kat"ĕ-kōl-am'ēnz). Biologically active amines, epinephrine and norepinephrine, derived from the amino acid tyrosine. They have marked effect on the nervous system, cardiovascular system, metabolic rate, temperature, and smooth muscle.

cat"electrot'onus [G. *kata*, down, + *ēlektron*, amber, + *tonos*, tension]. The state of increased excitability produced in a nerve or muscle in the region near the cathode during the passage of an electric current.

catenoid (kat'ĕ-noid) [" + G. *eidos*, resemblance]. Chainlike; pert to protozoan colonies whose individuals are joined end-to-end.

cat'gut [A.S. *catta*, to whelp, + *guttas*, to pour]. Sheep's intestine twisted for use as an absorbable ligature.

cathar'sis [G. *katharsis*, purification]. 1. Purgative action of the bowels. 2. The freudian method of freeing the mind by recalling the patient's memory of an event or experience that was the exciting cause of a psychoneurosis; abreaction, *q.v.*

cathar'tic [G. *kathartikos*, purging]. An active purgative, usually producing several evacuations which may or may not be accompanied by pain or tenesmus.

EX: *Castor oil; cascara sagrada.* SEE: *purgative.*

catheresis (kath-ĕ-rē'sĭs) [G. *kathairesis*, destruction]. 1. Weakness resulting from medication. 2. Caustic or feebly caustic action.

catheter (kath'ĕ-ter) [G. *katheter*, a tube placed down into]. A tube for evacuating or injecting fluids. Made of elastic, elastic web, rubber, glass, or metal,

c., cardiac. A long, fine catheter especially designed for passage through a blood vessel into the chambers of the heart. SYN: *intracardiac c.* SEE: *catheterization, cardiac.*

c., double channel. One providing for inflow and outflow. SYN: *two-way channel c.*

c., elbowed. One which has an acute bend near the beak. USES: Cases of enlarged prostate. SYN: *prostatic c.*

c., eustachian. One for injection into eustachian tube through nasal passages.

c., female. A short c., about 5 inches in length, used to pass into bladder of the female.

c., indwelling. One which keeps its position in the ureter.

c., male. One used to pass into the bladder of the male. C. is 12-13 inches long.

c., prostatic. One designed to pass prostatic obstruction. 15-16 inches long. SYN: *elbowed c.*

c., self-retaining. One which can be retained at will, effecting bladder drainage.

c., vertebrated. One in sections to be fitted together, so that it is flexible.

c., winged. One with little flaps at each side of beak to aid in retaining it in the bladder.

catheter fever. Reactionary rise in temperature caused by a urinary tract infection following passage of a catheter or urethral bougie.

catheterization (kath"ĕ-ter-ĭ-zā'shun) [G. *katheterismos*, an inserting of a catheter]. Use or passage of a catheter.

c., cardiac. The passage of a catheter into the heart through an arm vein and blood vessels leading into the heart for the purpose of obtaining cardiac blood samples, detection of abnormalities, and determination of intracardiac pressure.

c., urinary bladder. Introduction of a catheter through the urethra into the bladder for withdrawal of urine.

NP (for female patient): Treatment should be explained to patient who lies on back with knees drawn up, slightly separated; pillows under head and shoulders to relax abdominal muscles; feet flat on bed. Place screen around bed, tray at right side within reach. Arrange top covers so they may be separated with elbow. This is an aseptic procedure; scrub hands and place sterile towels, one above and one below vulva of female patient. Separate labia with first and second finger of left hand and pick up sterile cotton balls dipped in soap solution with right hand. Use downward stroke on one side of vulva, discard cotton ball and proceed to cleanse area, swabbing orifice of meatus *last.*

Sterile receiver is placed bet. patient's legs. Nurse holds catheter about inch from open end, inspects for flaws, and inserts it into meatus of urethra, being careful not to touch any other part of vulval surface. Insert gently until urine begins to flow, holding it steadily until flow ceases. By withdrawing it slowly more urine may flow. Repeat unitl catheter is withdrawn.

Place finger over open end of c., invert over receiver and empty. Dry patient and cover. Report findings and condition of patient, also time. Place urine in appropriately labelled container and send to laboratory for whatever tests have been ordered. SEE: *autocatheterism.*

catheterize (kath'e-ter-īz). To pass or introduce a catheter into a part.

cathexis (kă-thĕk'sĭs) [G. *kathexis*, retention]. The emotional or mental energy imparted to an idea.

cath'odal [G. *kathodos*, downward path]. Pert. to the cathode.

cath'ode [G. *kathodos*, from *kata*, down, + *odos*, way]. ABBR: *ca.* 1. The negative pole, as opposed to the anode or positive pole. 2. In a vacuum tube, the electrode which serves as the source of the electron stream.

c. stream. Negatively charged electrons, sent out as particles from the cathode in discharges through the vacuum. SEE: *rays, cathode.*

cathod'ic. 1. Pertaining to a cathode. 2. Proceeding outwardly or efferently as applied to a nerve impulse.

cation (kat'ī-on) [G. *kation*, descending]. The name given by Faraday to the element or elements of an electrolyte in electrochemical decomposition appearing as a positive ion at the negative pole, or cathode.

catlin (kat'lin). Surgical knife with double edges.

catoptric (kat-op'trik) [G. *katoptrikos*, reflecting]. Pert. to reflected light or mirrors.

catoptrophobia (kat-op-trō-fo'bī-ă) [G. *katoptron*, mirror, + *phobos*, fear]. Morbid fear of mirrors or of breaking them.

cat's-eye pupil. A slitlike pupil.

cauda (kaw'dă) [L. tail]. A tail or tail-like structure.

c. *epididymidis* [NA]. The inferior portion of the epididymis which is continuous with the ductus deferens.

c. *equina* [NA]. The terminal portion of the spinal cord and the roots of the spinal nerves below the first lumbar nerve.

c. *helicis* [NA]. A pointed process extending inferiorly from the helix of the auricular cartilage of the ear.

c. *pancreatis.* The tail of the pancreas.

c. *striati.* Tail-like posterior extremity of the corpus striatum.

caudad (kaw'dad) [" + *ad*, toward] Toward the tail; in a post. direction.

caudal (kawd'al) [L. *caudalis*, pert. to a tail]. 1. Pert. to any tail-like structure. 2. Inferior in position.

caudate (kaw'dāt) [L. *caudātus*, having a tail]. Possessing a tail.

caudation (kaw-dā'shun) [L. *cauda*, tail]. 1. A lengthened or elongated clitoris. 2. Having a tail or tails.

caul (kawl) [Fr. *cale*, a small cap]. 1. The great omentum. 2. Membranes or portions of the amnion covering head of fetus at birth.

caul'iflower [L. *caulis*, cabbage, + *flos, floris*, flower]. The edible thickened flower head of the plant *Brassica oleracea botrytis*, a member of the cabbage family.

COOKED: 100 gm. Calories: 27. Other main values: 2.7 gm. protein; trace of fat; 5.2 gm. carbohydrates; 25 mg. calcium; 55 mg. ascorbic acid.

cauli'flower ear. Malformation of cartilage of ear due to injury, as seen in boxers.

caumesthesia (kaw-mes-the'zī-ă) [" + *aisthēsis*, sensation]. A sense of heat when surrounding temperature is normal.

causalgia (kaw-sal'jī-ă) [G. *kausis*, heat, + *algos*, pain]. Intense burning pain.

cause. That which induces or brings about a particular condition, result, or effect.

c., *constitutional.* One that is inherent within the body.

c., *predisposing.* One which favors but does not directly induce an effect.

c., *primary.* The immediate or precipitating cause.

caustic (kaw'stik) [G. *kaustikos*, capable of burning]. 1. Corrosive and burning. 2. An agent that will destroy living tissue. Ex: *silver nitrate, potassium hydroxide, nitric acid.*

c. *Lugol's.* One part iodine, one part potassium iodide, and two parts water.

c., *lunar.* Toughened silver nitrate, USP.

c. *potash.* Potassium hydroxide, *q.v.*

c. *soda.* Sodium hydroxide, *q.v.*

cauterant (kaw'ter-ant) [G. *kautēr*, a burner]. 1. Escharotic; caustic. 2. A caustic agent.

cauterization (kaw-ter-i-za'shun) [G. *kautēriazein*, to burn]. Burning a part; cautery.

RS: *byssocausis, chemicocautery, electrocautery, galvanocautery, moxibustion, ustion, zestocausis.*

c., *actual.* By hot iron. Atmocausis. By steam.

c., *chemical.* Cauterization by the use of chemical agents, especially caustic substances.

c., *electrical.* By platinum wires heated to incandescence by an electric current. SYN: *electrocautery, q.v.; galvanocautery.*

cauterize (kaw'ter-īz) [G. *kautēriazein*, to burn]. To burn with a cautery, or to apply one.

cautery (kaw'ter-ī) [G. *kautēr*, a burner]. A means of destroying tissue by electricity, heat, or corrosive chemicals.

Used in potentially infected wounds; to destroy exuberant granulations (proud flesh) or some neoplasms. Thermocautery consists of red hot or white hot object, usually piece of wire or pointed metallic instrument, heated in a flame or with electricity (electrocautery, galvanocautery).

ca'val. Pert. to the vena cava.

cav'alry bone. Rider's bone; bony deposit in the adductor muscles of the thigh.

cavascope (kav'ă-skōp) [L. *cavum*, hollow, + G. *skopein*, to examine]. Instrument for examining cavities.

caverni'tis [L. *caverna*, hollow, + G. *-itis*, inflammation]. Inflammation of the *corpus cavernosum penis.*

caverno'ma [" + G. *-ōma*, tumor]. A cavernous angioma.

cavernosi'tis [L. *cavernosus*, having hollows, + G. *-ītis*, inflammation]. Inflammation of the *corpora cavernosa.*

cavernosum (kăv-ĕr-nō'sŭm). One of two erectile columns of the dorsum of the penis or clitoris. SYN: *corpus cavernosum.*

cavernous (kăv'ĕr-nŭs) [L. *caverna*, a hollow]. Containing hollow spaces.

c. *angioma.* A vascular tumor with many large spaces.

c. *body.* Corpus cavernosum.

c. *râle.* Bubbling hollow sound.

c. *resonance.* Amphoric resonance.

c. *respiration.* Hollow sound heard when there is a lung cavity.

c. *rhoncus.* A cavernous râle.

c. *sinus.* A venous space in the dura mater on either side of the sphenoid bone.

c. *tumor.* An angioma.

cavita'tion [L. *cavitas*, a cavity]. Formation of a cavity. May occur as a normal process as in the formation of the amnion in human development or pathologically as in the development of cavities in lung tissue in pulmonary tuberculosis.

cavitis (ka-vi'tis) [L. *cavum*, hollow, + G. *-itis*, inflammation]. Inflammation of a vena cava.

cavity (kav'ī-tī) [L. *cavitas*, hollow]. A hollow space, such as a body organ or the hole in a carious tooth.

c., *abdominal.* The cavity of the peritoneum bet. the diaphragm and pelvis.

c., *alveolar.* A tooth socket.

c., *amniotic.* That within the amnion.

c., *articular*. The synovial cavity of a joint.

c., *body*. In vertebrates the space between the body wall and the visceral organs; the coelum, *q.v.*

c., *buccal*. The mouth.

c., *cotyloid*. The acetabulum.

c., *cranial*. The cavity of the skull which contains the brain.

c., *glenoid*. A shallow concavity on lateral surface of the head of the scapula which receives the head of the humerus.

c., *oral*. The mouth or buccal cavity. Includes the vestibule and the oral cavity proper.

c., *pelvic*. The cavity of the pelvis. Includes the *major pelvic cavity* which lies between the iliac fossa and above the iliopectineal lines and the *minor pelvic cavity* which lies below the iliopectineal lines or the inlet of the pelvis.

c., *pericardial*. The space between the epicardium (visceral pericardium) and the parietal pericardium.

c., *peritoneal*. The potential space between the parietal peritoneum lining the body-wall and the visceral peritoneum forming surface layer of visceral organs.

c., *peritoneal, lesser*. The omental bursa; also called lesser peritoneal sac.

c., *pleural*. The potential space between the parietal pleura and visceral pleura.

c., *pulp*. One in a tooth containing the dental pulp and nerve termination.

c., *Rosenmüller's*. One on either side of openings of eustachian tube.

c., *serous*. A space between two layers of serous membrane. Ex: pleural pericardial, and peritoneal cavities.

c., *splanchnic*. One of three, the cranial, thoracic, and abdominal, including the pelvic cavity.

c., *tympanic*. The cavity of the middle ear. Syn: *tympanum; ear drum.*

cavum (kā'vŭm) [L. *cavus*, a hollow]. A cavity or space.

c. *abdominis* [NA]. The abdominal cavity.

c. *conchae* [NA]. The inferior portion of the cavity of the auricle of the ear. It leads to the ext. acoustic meatus.

c. *mediastinale*. The mediastinum, *q.v.*

c. *medullare*. The medullary cavity of a long bone.

c. *oris* [NA]. The oral cavity.

c. *pelvis* [NA]. The pelvic cavity.

c. *tympani* [NA]. Middle ear cavity.

c. *uteri* [NA]. The cavity of the uterus.

ca'vus [L. hollow]. Condition of exaggerated height of arch of foot. Syn: *talipes cavus.*

Cayenne pepper (kī-ĕn', kā-ĕn'). Capsicum, *q.v.*

Cazenave's lupus (khaz-năv'). Pemphigus foliaceus.

C.B.C. Abbr. for *complete blood count.*

C.C. 1. Abbr. for *Commission Certified*, with reference to certification of stains by the Biological Stain Commission. 2. Abbr. for *chief complaint.*

cc. Abbr. for *cubic centimeter.*

CCl_3.CHO. Chloral.

CCl_4. Abbr. for *carbon tetrachloride.*

Cd. Symb. of *cadmium.*

Ce. Symb. of *cerium.*

ceasmic (se-as'mĭk) [G. *keasma*, chip]. Pert. to an abnormal cleavage of parts or to a fissure.

cebione (sē'bī-ōn). Proprietary name for an antiscorbutic preparation of ascorbic acid.

cecal (se'kal) [L. *caecalis*, pert. to blindness]. 1. Pert. to cecum. 2. Blind, terminating in a closed extremity.

cecectomy (sē-sĕk'tō-mĭ) [L. *caecum*, blindness, caecum, + G. *ektomē*, excision]. Removing part of or incision into the cecum.

NP: Preparation for appendectomy slightly modified.

cecitis (sē-sī'tĭs) [" + G. *-ītis*, inflammation]. Inflammation of the cecum.

cecoileostomy (sē-kō-il-ē-os'tō-mĭ) [" + *ileum*, ileum, + G. *stoma*, opening]. Making an opening through the abdominal wall into the ileum at the ileocecal valve.

cecopexy (sē'kō-pĕks-ĭ) [" + G. *pēxis*, fixation]. Surgical fixation of the cecum to the abdominal wall.

cecoplica'tion [" + *plica*, fold]. Reduction of a dilated cecum by making a fold in its wall.

cecoptosis (sē-kop-tō'sĭs) [" + G. *ptōsis*, a dropping]. Falling displacement of the cecum.

cecosigmoidostomy (sē-kō-sĭg-moid-os'tō-mĭ) [" + G. *sigmoeidēs*, shaped like letter S, + *stoma*, opening]. Formation of a communication bet. the cecum and sigmoid.

cecos'tomy [" + G. *stoma*, opening]. Surgical formation of a cecal fistula or artificial anus.

cecot'omy [" + G. *tomē*, a cutting]. Cutting into the cecum.

cecum (sē'kŭm) [L. *caecum*]. A blind pouch or cul-de-sac which forms the first portion of the large intestine, located below the entrance of the ileum at the ileocecal valve. It averages about 6 cm. in length and 7.5 cm. in width and bears at its lower end the vermiform process or appendix.

-cele [G. hernia, tumor]. Suffix: A swelling.

celectome (sē-lĕk'tōm) [G. *kēlē*, tumor, + *tomē*, a cutting]. Instrument for obtaining a piece of tissue from a tumor for examination.

celery [Fr. *celeri*, from G. *selinon*, parsley]. The edible stalks and leaves of the plant *Apium graveolens.*

Raw: 100 gm. Calories: 17. Other main values: 0.9 gm. protein; trace of fat; 3.9 gm. carbohydrates; 39 mg. calcium; 9 mg. ascorbic acid.

celiac (se'lĭ-ak) [G. *koilia*, belly]. Rel. to the abdominal regions.

c. *artery*. The first branch of the abdominal aorta. Branches supply the stomach, liver, spleen, duodenum, and pancreas.

c. *axis*. Same as *celiac artery.*

c. *disease*. Intestinal malabsorption characterized by diarrhea, malnutrition, bleeding tendency, and hypocalcemia.

Treatment: Gluten-free diet which may have to be continued for months before it is completely effective.

c. *plexus*. Sympathetic plexus lying near the origin of celiac artery. See: *plexuses.*

celiagra (sē-lĭ-ag'ră) [G. *koilia*, belly, + *agra*, seizure]. Gouty affection of any abdominal organ.

celial'gia [" + *algos*, pain]. Abdominal pain.

celiectasia (sē-lĭ-ĕk-tā'sĭ-ă) [" + *ektasis*, extension]. Distention of the abdomen.

celiectomy (se-lĭ-ek'to-mĭ) [" + *ektomē*, excision]. Complete or partial removal of an abdominal organ.

celiocentesis (sē-lĭ-ō-sĕn-tē'sĭs) [" + *kentēsis*, puncture]. Puncture of the abdomen.

celiocolpotomy (se"lĭ-o-kol-pot'o-mĭ) [" + *kolpos*, vagina, + *tomē*, incision]. Surgical incision of the vagina through the abdominal wall.

celioenterotomy (se-lĭ-ō-en-ter-ot′o-mĭ) [" + *enteron*, intestine, + *tomē*, incision]. Incision in the abdominal wall to gain access to the intestines.

celiogastrostomy (se-lĭ-ō-gas-tros′to-mĭ) [" + *gastēr*, stomach, + *stoma*, opening]. Incision in the abdominal wall for making a gastric fistula.

celiogastrotomy (sel-ĭ-o-gas-trot′o-mĭ) [" + " + *tomē*, incision]. Incision into the stomach through the abdominal wall.

celiohysterectomy (se″lĭ-o-his-ter-ek′to-mĭ) [" + *ystera*, uterus, + *ektomē*, excision]. Removal of uterus through the abdomen.

ce″liohysterot′omy [" + " + *tomē*, incision]. Opening into the uterus through an abdominal incision.

celioma (se-lĭ-o′mă) [" + *-ōma*, tumor]. An abdominal tumor.

celiomyal′gia [" + *mys*, muscle, + *algos*, pain]. Rheumatic pain in muscles of the abdomen.

celiomyomotomy (sē-lĭ-ō-mī-ō-mot′ō-mĭ) [" + " + " + *tomē*, incision]. Incision of muscles of abdomen.

celiomyositis (sē-lĭ-ō-mī-ō-sī′tĭs) [" + " + *-itis*, inflammation]. Inflammation of muscles of the abdomen.

celioncus (se-lĭ-on′kus) [" + *ogkos*, tumor]. An abdominal tumor.

celioparacentesis (se-lĭ-o-par-ă-sen-te′sis) [" + *para*, beside, + *kentēsis*, puncture]. Puncture of the abdomen for purposes of tapping or drainage.

celiopathy (se-lĭ-op′ă-thĭ) [" + *pathos*, disease]. Any disease of the abdomen.

celiopyosis (se-lĭ-ō-pī-ō′sĭs) [" + *pyōsis*, suppuration]. Purulent peritonitis.

celiorrhaphy (se-lĭ-or′ă-fĭ) [" + *raphē*, suture]. Suture of wound in the abdominal wall.

celiosalpingectomy (se-lĭ-o-sal-pin-jek′to-mĭ) [" + *salpigx*, tube, + *ektomē*, excision]. Removal of the fallopian tubes through an abdominal incision.

celiosalpingotomy (se-lĭ-o-sal-pin-got′o-mĭ) [" + " + *tomē*, incision]. Opening of the fallopian tube through an abdominal incision.

celioscope (se′lĭ-ō-skōp) [" + *skopein*, to examine]. Device for illumination of abdominal cavity.

celioscopy (se-lĭ-os′ko-pĭ) [" + *skopein*, to examine]. Use of the celioscope.

celiotomy (se-lĭ-ot′o-mĭ) [" + *tomē*, incision]. Surgical incision into the abdominal cavity.

c., vaginal. Entering the abdomen through the vagina.

celitis (se-li′tis) [" + *-itis*- inflammation]. Peritonitis; abdominal inflammation.

cell [L. *cella*, a small chamber]. 1. A small, enclosed or partly enclosed cavity, such as an air cell. 2. A mass of protoplasm containing a nucleus or nuclear material. It is the unit of structure of all

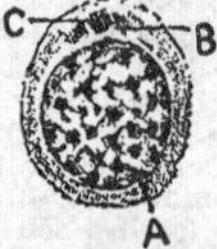

CELL

From testicle of salamander showing: A, Nucleus with chromatin network. B, Centrosome. C, Centriole.

animals and plants and is the physical basis of all life processes.

Cells and the products of cells comprise all the tissues of the body. All functional activities of the body are carried on by cells. The structure and form of a cell is closely correlated with its functioning. Cells arise only from preexisting cells, new cells arising by cell division. Growth and development result from the increase in numbers of cells and the differentiation of cells into different types of tissues. Reproduction is accomplished by specialized germ cells, the spermatozoa and ova, which contain in their nuclei the genes or determiners for hereditary characteristics.

Cell inclusions or paraplastic bodies include (1) *food substances:* fat droplets, glycogen and protein granules; (2) *chromophilic substance* (Nissl bodies); (3) *pigment granules* (melanin); (4) *crystals* of various substances; (5) secretory granules.

Also present in the cytoplasm are submicroscopic bodies once called *microsomes*, demonstrated by differential centrifugation. They are small fragments of the endoplasmic reticulum and contain particles of ribonucleoprotein (ribosomes). Thus microsomes should be called ribosomes. Ribosomes are important in protein synthesis within the cell.

Structure. A typical cell, when killed, fixed and stained, exhibits a centrally located *nucleus* surrounded by *cytoplasm.* (a) *Nucleus.* The nucleus possesses a *nuclear membrane* which encloses a clear *nuclear sap* or *karyoplasm.* Usually present are one or more densely staining bodies, the nucleoli. (b) *Cytoplasm.* This includes the cell protoplasm lying outside the nucleus. Its outermost layer constitutes the *cell membrane* which forms the limiting membrane of the cell. Within the ground substance of the cytoplasm is the *ergastoplasm* (granular endoplasmic reticulum) which contains ribonucleoprotein, a substance which can be identified only by use of the electron microscope. Ribonucleoprotein is important in protein synthesis.

A cell may produce other cells, and it has the power of exercising the vital processes of life. Cells of one tissue differ from those of other tissues, depending upon the function they perform. Those of one tissue in man are very similar to those of corresponding tissues in other vertebrates.

c., acidophil. One which stains with eosin or other acid dyes.

c., acinar. A cell present in the acinus of an acinar gland, as those of the pancreas.

c.'s, adelomorphous. Transparent columnar cells lining the glands of the stomach, believed to secrete pepsinogen.

c., adipose. A fat cell.

c., adventitial. A macrophage along a blood vessel, together with perivascular undifferentiated cells associated with it.

c., air. A small cavity in one of the bones of the skull containing air (*e.g.*, mastoid air cells, air cells comprising the ethmoid sinus).

c.'s, alpha. Acidophil cells of (a) the hypophysis (ant. lobe) and (b) the pancreas. In the latter they are the source of glucagon.

c.'s, argentaffin. Cells found in the epithelium of the digestive tract (stomach, intestine, appendix). Cytoplasm of the c.'s contains granules which stain selectively with silver.

c., basal. (a) A basket c., *q.v.* (b) A type of cell in the olfactory epithelium lying between bases of the supporting cells.

c., basket. (a) A branching basal or myoepithelial cell of the salivary and other glands. (b) Certain cells of the molecular layer of the cerebellar cortex.

c.'s, beta. (a) Insulin-secreting cells of the pancreatic islets of Langerhans. (b) Basophil cells of the ant. lobe of the hypophysis.

c.'s, Betz. Large pyramidal cells of the motor area of cerebral cortex.

c., bipolar. A neuron with two processes, an axon and dendrite. Found in retina of eye and in cochlear and vestibular ganglia of the acoustic nerve.

c., blood. Erythrocyte or leukocyte.

c. body. Part of the nerve cell or neuron which contains the cell nucleus and cytoplasm. SEE: *nerve.*

c.'s, capsule. Cells forming a single layer about the cell bodies of sensory neurons of spinal ganglia. SYN: *satellite cells; amphicytes.*

c., castration. An enlarged and vacuolated basophil cell of the hypophysis in gonadal insufficiency or following castration.

c., centro-acinar. Duct cells of the pancreas more or less invaginated into the lumen of an acinus.

c., chief. (a) The cells of the parathyroid gland which secrete the hormone. (b) Zymogenic cells of gastric glands which secrete pepsin or its precursor. (c) Chromophobe cells of the hypophysis.

c., columnar. An epithelial cell with height greater than width.

c., cone. A cell in the retina whose scleral end forms a cone which serves as a light receptor. Vision in bright light, color vision, and acute vision depend upon functioning of the cones.

c., cuboidal. A cell with height about equal to width and depth.

c., daughter. One from a mother cell.

c., delomorphous. Large cells in the glands of the stomach, believed to secrete the acid of gastric juice.

c., endothelial. A flat c. making up the lining membranes of vessels.

c., epithelial. One forming epithelial surfaces of membranes and skin.

c., ethmoidal. One of several cavities which honeycomb the lateral masses of the ethmoid bone, forming a part of the paranasal air sinuses. SYN: *ethmoid sinus.*

c., ganglion. (a) Any neuron whose cell body is located within a ganglion. (b) A neuron of the retina of the eye whose cell body lies in the ganglion cell layer. The axons of ganglion cells form the fibers of the optic nerve.

c., giant. Large multinucleated cells found in bone marrow; a megakaryocyte. They are thought to give rise to blood platelets.

c., glia. A neuroglia cell, *q.v.*

c., goblet. Epithelial c. distended with mucus.

c., granule. Certain small neurons of the cerebrum and cerebellum.

c., gustatory. A neuroepithelial cell or taste cell of a taste bud.

c., horizontal. A neuron of the inner nuclear layer of the retina. The axons of these cells run horizontally and serve to connect various parts of the retina.

c., interstitial. One of the many found in connective tissue of the seminiferous tubules of the testes, and such tissues of the ovary which account for their internal secretion.

c., Kupffer. A fixed phagocytic cell found in the sinusoids of the liver.

c., L.E. A lupus erythematosus cell.

c., Leydig's. Interstitial c., *q.v.*

c., littoral. A macrophage found in the sinuses of lymphatic tissue.

c., lupus erythematosus. Cells characteristic of lupus erythematosus disseminatus in which denaturation of nuclear material of leukocytes occurs. Such cells are highly chemotactic causing phagocytic leukocytes to congregate about them in a rosette fashion.

c., lutein. A cell of the corpus luteum of the ovary which contains lutein. *Granulose lutein cells* are hypertrophied follicle cells; these *lutein (paralutein) cells* develop from the theca interna.

c., mast. A cell found in connective tissue of vertebrates. Contains heparin and histamine.

c., microglia. Neuroglial cells of mesodermal origin present in the brain and spinal cord.

c., mother. Any type of cell which divides and gives rise to two or more cells. The latter are called daughter c.'s.

c., mucous. (a) A cell which secretes mucus found in mucus secreting glands. (b) A goblet cell.

c., neuroglia. Non-nerve cells found in the central nervous system and the retina of the eye. Includes astrocytes, oligodendrocytes, and microglia.

c., parent. Mother c., *q.v.*

c.'s, phalangeal. Cells which support the hair cells of the organ of Corti. They form several rows of outer phalangeal cells (Deiter's cells) and a single row of inner phalangeal cells.

c., plasma. Cells derived from lymphoid elements. They are found in lymphoid tissue and the cellular connective tissue of the intestinal tract. They are important in antibody production. Patients with hyperglobulinemia have a great number of mast cells in their tissues.

c., prickle. A cell possessing spine-like protoplasmic processes which connect with similar processes of adjoining cells. Found in the stratum germinativum of the epidermis.

c., pus. A leukocyte present in pus. They are often degenerated or necrotic.

c., pyramidal. A nerve cell of the cerebral cortex.

c., Reider. A cell present in certain leukemias possessing a lobulated or double nucleus.

c., rod. A cell in the retina of the eye whose scleral end is long and narrow forming a *rod,* a sensory element of the eye. Rods are stimulated by dim light.

c., Rouget. Cells with branching processes which, in a frog, surround the walls of a capillary. They are capable of contracting upon stimulation.

c., satellite. A neuroglia cell lying adjacent to the cell body of a sensory neuron in cranial or spinal ganglia.

c., segmented. A segmented neutrophil, *i.e.,* one with a nucleus of two or more lobes connected together by slender filaments.

c., sensory. A sensory neuron; a cell which when stimulated gives rise to nerve impulses which are conveyed to the central nervous system.

c.'s, septal. Cells attached to or in the septa of the lungs. They function in some animals as macrophages.

c., sickle. An abnormal erythrocyte shaped like a sickle. SEE: *anemia, sickle-cell.*

c., spider. An astrocyte.

c., squamous. Flat, scalelike, epithelial cell.

c., sympathicotrophic. Large epithelial cells occurring in groups in the hilus of the ovary. Thought to be chromaffin cells.

c., sympathochromaffin. Chromaffin cells of ectodermal origin present in fetal adrenal from which sympathetic and medullary cells arise.

c., target. An erythrocyte with a rounded, central area surrounded by a clear ring lightly stained, and this in turn surrounded by a dense ring of peripheral protoplasm. Present in certain blood disorders.

c., Türck's irritation. A cell found in plasma cell leukemia, multiple myeloma, and rubella. SYN: *proplasmocyte.*

c., visual. A rod or cone cell of the retina.

c.'s, zymogenic. Chief cells or enzyme producing cells of the gastric glands.

cell center. Centrosome, *q.v.*

cell-division. Mitosis, *q.v.* SEE ALSO: *amitosis.*

cell mass. In *embryology,* a mass of cells which is the anlage or primordium of an organ or structure.

c. m., inner. A mass of cells attached eccentrically to the inner surface of the wall of the blastocyst of mammals. From it develops the embryo proper and certain related structures as the amnion and yolk sac.

c. m., intermediate. A nephrotome, *q.v.*

cell membrane. A thin membrane (*plasmalemma*) which encloses a cell. It is too thin to be seen with the light microscope.

cell organelle. A specific structure in the cytoplasm of a cell consisting of organized living substance, in contrast to *inclusions* which are lifeless constituents. Cell organelles include the cell membrane (plasma membrane), mitochondria, endoplasmic reticulum (ergastroplasm), Golgi complex or apparatus, ribosomes, agranular reticulum, lysosomes, cell center and centriole.

cell wall. Cell membrane, *q.v.* Plant cells are enclosed by a wall which contains cellulose. Some animal cells have a thin coat outside the cell membrane. It is not known whether or not this should be regarded as part of the cell.

Cellano factor (sĕl'ăn-ō făk'tôr). One rarely found lacking in the blood; 99.8% have it. Named for woman by that name who did not have this blood factor, but who did possess the antibody. SYN: *k factor.*

cellobi'ose. A disaccharide resulting from the hydrolysis of cellulose.

cellophane (sĕl'ō-fān). Thin, transparent, waterproof sheet of viscose.

Used as a wound dressing because it does not crack, is singularly free of infection, and wound can be seen without its removal.

cell'ula (pl. *cellulae*) [L. little cell]. 1. A minute cell. 2. A small compartment.

cell'ular. Pert. to, composed of, or derived from cells.

cell'ulase. An enzyme which converts cellulose to cellobiose. Present in some microorganisms and marine life.

cellulicidal (sel-ū-lĭ-si'dal) [" + *caedere,* to kill]. Destructive to cells.

cellulif'ugal [" + *fugere,* to flee]. Extending or moving away from a cell.

cellulipetal (sel-ū-lip'ĭ-tal) [L. *cellula,* little cell, + *petere,* to seek]. Extending or moving toward a cell.

cellulitis (sel-ū-lī'tis) [" + G. *-itis,* inflammation]. Inflammation of cellular or connective tissue, spreading as in erysipelas.

An infection in or close to the skin is usually localized by the body defense mechanisms. If this does not happen and the inflammation spreads through the tissue, then the process is called *cellulitis.*

c., pelvic. Parametritis; inflammation of the parametrium.* May occur in puerperal fever, or septic conditions of the uterus and appendages.

cellulofi'brous [" + *fibra,* fiber]. Both cellular and fibrous.

celluloneuritis (sel"u-lo-nū-rī'tis) [" + G. *neuron,* nerve, + *-itis,* inflammation]. Inflammation of nerve cells.

c., acute anterior. Acute anterior poliomyelitis.

cellulose (sĕl'ū-lōs) [L. *cellula,* little cell]. A fibrous form of carbohydrate constituting the supporting framework of plants; plant fiber. It is composed of a great number of glucose units.

It stimulates peristalsis and aids in intestinal elimination. It is not ordinarily chemically changed or absorbed in digestion, remaining a polysaccharide.*

c. or fiber-containing foods. Apples, apricots, asparagus, beans, beets, bran flakes, broccoli, cabbage, celery, mushrooms, oatmeal, onions, oranges, parsnips, prunes, spinach, turnips, wheat flakes, whole grains, whole wheat bread.

c. high diet. High residue diet, *q.v.*

c., oxidized. Cellulose which has been oxidized by nitrogen dioxide and is made in the form of cotton or gauze. Used as surgical packing.

cellulotox'ic [" + G. *toxikon,* poison]. 1. Poisonous to cells. 2. Caused by cell toxins.

celology (sē-lol'ō-jĭ) [G. *kēlē,* hernia, + *logos,* study]. The surgical study of hernias.

celom, celoma (sē'lom, sē-lō'mă) [G. *koilōma,* a hollow]. The coelom, *q.v.*

celonychia (sē-lō-nik'ĭ-ă) [G. *koilos,* hollow, + *onyx, onych-,* nail]. Koilonychia, *q.v.*

celoschisis (se-los'kĭ-sis) [G. *koilia,* belly, + *schisis,* fissure]. Congenital fissure of the abdominal wall.

celoscope (se'lō-skōp) [G. *koilos,* hollow, + *skopein,* to examine]. Device for throwing light into a cavity.

celosomia (sē-lō-sō'mĭ-ă) [G. *kēlē,* hernia, + *sōma,* body]. Congenital protrusion of viscera.

celotomy (se-lot'o-mĭ) [" + *tomē,* incision]. Kelotomy, *q.v.*

celozo'ic [G. *koilia,* belly, + *zōon,* animal]. Inhabiting any cavity of the body, such as parasitic protozoa.

Celsius scale (sĕl′sĭ-us) [Anders Celsius, Swedish astronomer, 1701-1744]. A temperature scale on which the boiling point of water is 100° and the melting point of ice is 0°.

cementi′tis [L. *caementum*, cement, + G. *-itis*, inflammation]. Inflammation of the dental cementum.

cementoblast (se-men′to-blast) [" + G. *blastos*, germ]. A cell of the inner layer of the dental sac of a developing tooth. They deposit cementum, *q.v.*, upon the dentine of the root.

cementocla′sia [" + G. *klasis*, breaking]. Decay of the cementum of a tooth root.

cemento′ma [" + G. *-ōma*, tumor]. A tumor having its origin in the substantia ossea.

cementum. Thin layer of modified bone formed by cementoblasts and deposited upon the dentine of the root of a tooth; the substantia ossea. To it is attached the alveolar periosteum or peridental membrane which binds the tooth to its socket.

cenesthesia ***(coenesthesia)*** (sen-es-the′zĭ-a) [G. *koinos*, common, + *aisthēsis*, feeling]. The normal feeling of being alive and aware.

cenesthe′sic, cenesthet′ic [" + *aisthēsis*, feeling]. Pert. to cenesthesia.

cenesthopathia, cenesthopathy (sen-es-tho-path′ĭ-ă, sen-es-thop′a-thĭ) [" + " + *pathos*, disease]. Malaise or a general feeling of lack of well-being in illness.

cenogen′esis. The development of characters in an individual which are absent in ancestors and which do not have a phylogenetic significance.

cenopsychic (sen-ō-si′kik) [G. *kainos*, new, + *psychē*, mind]. Only recently appearing in mental development.

cenosis (se-no′sis) [G. *kenos*, empty, + *-ōsis*, infection]. 1. A morbid discharge. 2. Inanition.

cenosite (se′no-sīt) [G. *koinos*, common, + *sitos*, food]. A microorganism not depending for life upon its host, but parasitic in character.

cenotic (se-not′ik) [G. *kenos*, empty]. 1. Purgative; drastic. 2. Pert. to cenosis.

cenotophobia (sē-nō-tō-fō′bĭ-ă) [G. *kainotes*, novelty, + *phobos*, fear]. Morbid aversion to new things and new ideas. SYN: *cainotophobia.*

cenotype (sĕn′ō-tīp) [G. *koinos*, common, + *typos*, a type]. An original type.

cen′sor [L. *censere*, to judge]. PSY: A psychic inhibition that prevents abhorrent unconscious thoughts or impulses from seeking objective expression unless in a form unrecognized by consciousness.

center (sen′ter) [G. *kentron*, middle]. 1. Middle point of a body. 2. A group of nerve cells within the central nervous system which control a specific activity or function.

c., auditory. One for hearing, in the gyri in sylvian fissure. SEE: *area, auditory.*

c., autonomic. A center in the brain or spinal cord which regulates any of the activities under the control of the autonomic nervous system. There are a few cortical centers but most are located in the hypothalamus, medulla oblongata, and spinal cord.

c., Broca's. Speech center.

c., cardioaccelerator. A center in the medulla oblongata which gives rise to impulses which speed up the heart rate. They reach the heart by way of sympathetic fibers.

c., cardioinhibitory. A center in the medulla oblongata containing neurons whose axons, parasympathetic fibers, pass by way of the vagus nerves to the heart. Impulses slow down heart rate.

c., chondrification. A center of cartilage formation.

c., ciliospinal. A center in the spinal cord from which arise sympathetic impulses which dilate the pupils of the eyes.

c.'s, defecation. Two centers, a *medullary center* located in the medulla oblongata and a *spinal center* located in second to fourth sacral segments of the spinal cord. The anospinal centers controlling the sphincter reflexes for the process of defecation.

c., deglutition. A center in the medulla oblongata on the floor of the fourth ventricle which controls swallowing.

c., epiotic. Ossification center of mastoid process.

c., gustatory. Little is known about it but it is thought to be in the hypothalamus. SYN: *gustatory area; taste center.*

c.'s, heat-regulating. Two centers, a heat loss center and a heat-production center located in the hypothalamus. They regulate body temperature.

c., higher. 1. A center in the cerebrum from which impulses based on conscious sensations, wishes, or desires are initiated. 2. A center in any portion of the brain in contrast to one in the cord.

c., lower. One in the brain stem or spinal cord.

c., micturition. C. controlling reflexes of urinary bladder. Located in second to fourth and fourth to sixth sacral segments of the cord; higher centers are present in medulla oblongata, hypothalamus, and cerebrum.

c., motor cortical. The area in the frontal lobe, the origin of impulses for voluntary movements.

c., nerve. One of many in cerebrospinal or ganglionic systems originating or controlling vital function.

c., ossification. Spot where ossification begins in bones.

c., pneumotaxic. SEE: respiratory c.

c.'s, psychocortical. Centers of cerebral cortex concerned with mental operations.

c., reflex. A region within the brain or spinal cord where connections (synapses) are made between afferent and efferent neurons of a reflex arc.

c., respiratory. A region in the medulla oblongata which controls respiratory movements. It consists of inspiratory, expiratory, and pneumotaxic centers.

c., speech. SEE: *area, Broca's.*

c., taste. A gustatory c., *q.v.*

c., temperature. A thermoregulatory c., *q.v.*

c., thermoregulatory. Temperature-regulating centers in the hypothalamus.

c., trophic. One of many located in cerebrospinal and sympathetic systems presiding over nutrition.

c., vasoconstrictor. A center in the medulla which brings about the constriction of blood vessels.

c., vasodilator. A center located in the medulla oblongata which brings about vasodilation of blood vessels.

c., vasomotor. A center through which the diameter of blood vessels is controlled; the vasoconstrictor and vasodilator centers.

c., visual. In occipital lobe. Controls sight.

c., vomiting. A center in the medulla oblongata.

centesis (sĕn-tē'sĭs) [G. *kentēsis*, puncture]. Puncture of a cavity.

centigrade (sen'ti-grād) [L. *centum*, a hundred, + *gradus*, a step]. 1. Having 100 degrees. 2. Pert. to a thermometer divided into 100°. The boiling point is 100° and the freezing point is 0°. ABBR: C. SEE: *thermometer*.

cen'tigram [" + G. *gramma*, a small weight]. A measure of weight; the hundredth part of a gram; 0.15432 gr. SEE: *metric measures*.

centiliter (sen'tĭ-lē-ter) [" + G. *lĭtra*, measure of wt.]. One-hundredth part of a liter; 10 cc.

centimeter (sen'tĭ-mē-ter) [" + G. *metron*, measure]. One-hundredth part of a meter; 2/5 of a linear inch (0.3937 in.).

centinormal (sen-tĭ-nor'măl) [" + *norma*, rule]. One-hundredth part of the normal, as the strength of a solution.

centipede. An arthropod of the subclass Chilopoda characterized by an elongated, flattened body of many segments each with a pair of jointed legs. The first pair of appendages are hooklike claws bearing openings of ducts from poison glands. The bites of large tropical centipedes may cause severe local and sometimes general symptoms but they are rarely fatal.

centrad (sen'trad) [G. *kentron*, center, + L. *ad*, toward]. Toward the center.

central (sen'tral). Situated at, or rel. to, a center.

c. bodies. Attraction center of a cell. SYN: *centrosome, q.v.*

c. nervous system. Brain and spinal cord, including their nerves and end organs, controlling voluntary acts. Also called cerebrospinal system, and voluntary nervous system.

Composed of nerve tissue which forms the brain, spinal cord and the nerves from both. Tissue is made up of gray and white matter. Gray matter is composed of cells of nervous tissue, while the white matter is composed of nerve fibers from the cells. White matter in the brain and cord carries messages or impulses from the body, or outside world, to the cells or gray matter.

GENERAL FUNCTION OF CENTRAL NERVOUS SYSTEM: Includes: (1) Parts of the brain governing consciousness and mental activities; (2) parts of brain, spinal cord and their sensory and motor nerve fibers controlling skeletal muscles, and (3) end-organs of the body-wall. SEE: *autonomic, parasympathetic, and sympathetic nervous systems*.

centraphose (sen'tră-fōz) [G. *kentron*, center, + *a-*, priv. + *phōs*, light]. A subjective sensation of darkness originating in the optic brain centers. SEE: *centrophose; chromophose*.

cen'tre. Center.

centriciput (sen-tris'ĭ-put) [G. *kentron*, center, + L. *caput*, head]. The central part of upper surface of skull, bet. the occiput and sinciput.

centrifugal (sen-trif'u-gal) [" + L. *fugere*, to flee]. Receding from the center. SEE: *axifugal; centrifuge*.

c. force. The force which impels a thing, or parts of it, outward from the center of rotation.

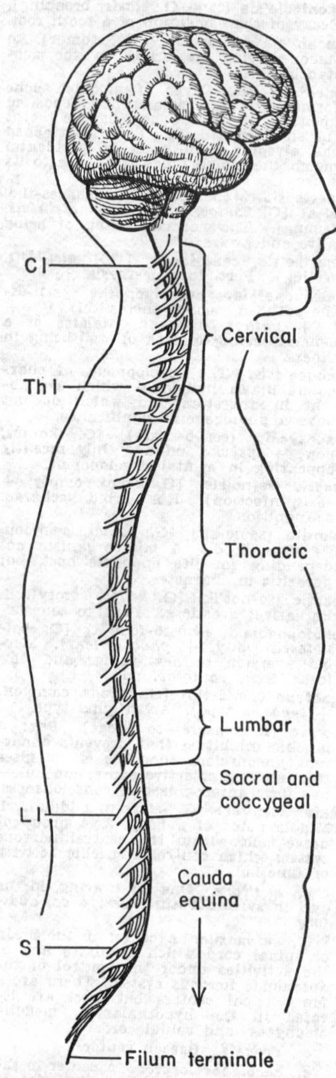

THE CENTRAL NERVOUS SYSTEM

centrifuge (sen'trĭ-fūj). 1. A machine for the separation of heavier materials from lighter ones, through the employment of centrifugal force. 2. To subject to centrifugation.

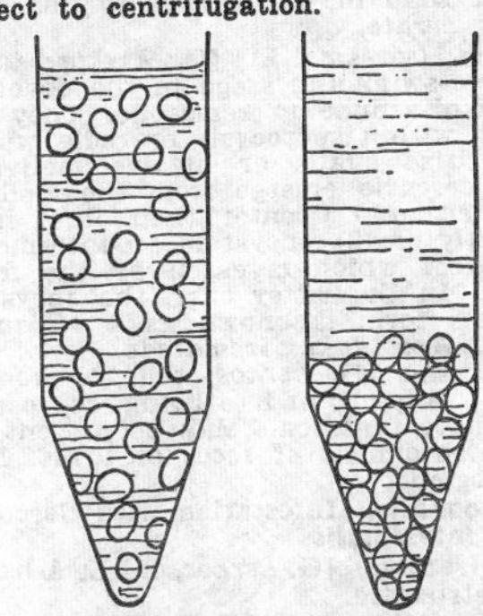

EFFECT OF CENTRIFUGING

Rapidly whirling a tube of blood in a centrifuge hastens sedimentation, and separates corpuscles from plasma. Generally 12 cc. of blood yield 6 cc. of packed corpuscles and 6 cc. of supernatant plasma. (Highly schematic.)

centriole (sĕn'trĭ-ōl). A minute body found in the cell center or attraction sphere of a cell. Preceding mitosis it divides, forming two daughter centrioles (diplosomes). During mitosis the centrioles migrate to opposite poles of the cell and each form the center of the aster to which the spindle fibers are attached. SEE: *mitosis.*

centripetal (sen-trip'ĕ-tal) [G. *kentron,* center, + L. *petere,* to seek]. Toward the center.

centrocyte (sen'trō-sīt) [G. *kentron,* center, + *kytos,* cell]. A cell having single and double, hematoxylin stainable granules of varying size in its protoplasm.

centrodesmus (sen-trō-dez'mus) [" + *desmos,* a band]. The matter connecting the two centrosomes in a nucleus during mitosis.

centrolecithal (sen-tro-les'ĭ-thal) [" + *lekithos,* yoke]. Pertaining to an egg, especially an ova, with the yolk centrally located.

centromere (sen'trō-mēr). A clear region on a chromosome which marks the junction of its two arms.

centrophose (sĕn'trō-fōz) [" + *phōs,* light]. A subjective sensation of a light spot having its origin in the optic brain centers. SEE: *centraphose; chromophose.*

centrosome (sen'trō-sōm) [G. *kentron,* center, + *soma,* body]. A region of the cytoplasm of a cell usually lying near the nucleus, containing in its center one or two *centrioles,* the *diplosome.* The cell spare center is active during cell division. SYN: *cell center.*

centrosphere (sen'tro-sfēr) [" + *sphaira,* sphere]. The envelope encasing two centrosomes.

centrostaltic (sen-tro-stal'tĭk) [" + *stalsis,* contraction]. Pert. to a center of motion.

centrother'apy [" + *therapeia,* therapy]. Any local application that acts upon nerve centers.

centrum (sen'trum) [L. from G. *kentron.* center]. 1. Any center, esp. an anatomical one. 2. Body of a vertebra.

c. semiova'le. A mass of white matter at center of each cerebral hemisphere.

c. tendin'eum. Central tendon of the diaphragm.

cephalad (sef'ă-lad) [G. *kephalē,* head, + L. *ad,* toward]. Toward the head.

cephalalgia (sef-ă-lal'jĭ-ă) [" + *algos,* pain]. Headache, pain in the head.

A symptom of numerous diseases and disorders. Commonly due to eyestrain and to gastrointestinal upset. SEE: *headache.*

cephalalgic (sef-al-al'jik). Of the nature of cephalalgia.

cephalea (sef-ă-lē'ă) [G. *kephalē,* head]. Cephalalgia, *q.v.*

cephaledema (sef-ăl-ĕ-dē'mă) [" + *oidēma,* swelling]. Edema of the head.

cephalhematocele (sef"ăl-hem-at'o-sēl) [" + *aima,* blood, + *kēlē,* tumor]. A bloody tumor communicating with the dural sinuses.

cephalhematoma (sef-al-hē-mă-tō'mă) [" + *aima,* blood, + *-ōma,* swelling]. A subcutaneous swelling containing blood, often found on the head of a baby several days after birth, when delivery was accompanied by use of forceps. The swelling disappears within two to three months. RS: *caput succedaneum.*

cephal'ic. 1. Cranial; pert. to the head. 2. Superior in position.

c. version. Turning the fetus during labor so head will present.

cephalin (sĕf'ă-lĭn). A phospholipid, resembling lecithin, present in the brain of mammals.

cephalin-cholesterol test. A test for liver function.

cephalitis (sef-al-i'tis) [G. *kephalē,* head, + *-itis,* inflammation]. Same as *encephalitis, q.v.*

cephalocele (sĕf'ă-lō-sēl) [G. *kephalē,* head, + *kēlē,* hernia]. Protrusion of the brain from the cranial cavity.

cephalocentesis (sef-ă-lō-sen-tē'sis) [" + *kentēsis,* puncture]. Surgical puncture of cranium.

cephalodynia (sef-ă-lō-din'ĭ-ă) [" + *odynē,* pain]. Pain in the head; headache, cephalalgia.

cephalogyric (sĕf-ă-lō-jī'rĭk). Of or pertaining to rotation of the head.

cephalohemometer (sef-ă-lō-hē-mom'ĕ-ter) [" + *aima,* blood, + *metron,* measure]. Instrument for determining changes in intracranial blood pressure.

cephalo'ma [" + *-ōma,* tumor]. A soft carcinoma.

cephalomenia (sef-ă-lō-mē'nĭ-ă) [" + *mēn,* month]. Vicarious menstruation from the nose or head.

cephalomeningitis (sef-ă-lō-mĕn-ĭn-jī'tis) [" + *menigx,* membrane, + *-itis,* inflammation]. Inflammation of the cerebral meninges.

cephalometer (sef-ă-lom'ĕ-ter) [" + *metron,* measure]. Device for measuring the head.

cephalometry (sef-ă-lom'ĕ-trĭ). Measurement of the head.

cephalomo'tor [G. *kephalē,* head, + L. *motus,* motion]. Pert. to movements of the head.

cephalone (sef'a-lōn) [" + It. *-one,* augmentative particle]. An idiot with a large head and sclerotic enlargement of the brain.

cephalonia (sef-a-lo'ni-a). A condition marked by idiocy, enlarged head, and sclerotic enlargement of the brain.

cephalopathy (sef-ă-lop'ă-thĭ) [G. *kephalē,* head, + *pathos,* pain]. Any disease of the head or brain.

cephaloplegia (sef-ă-lō-plē'jĭ-ă) [" + *plēgē*, stroke]. Paralysis of muscles about head or, less accurately, face.

cephalorhachidian (sef"ă-lō-ră-kid'ĭ-an) [" + *rachis*, spine]. Pert. to the head and spine.

cephaloscope (sef'ă-lō-skōp) [" + *skopein*, to examine]. Device for auscultation of the head.

cephalothoracopagus (sef-ă-lō-thō-ră-kop'ă-gus). A double fetus joined at head and thorax.

cephalotome (sef'ă-lō-tōm) [" + *tomē*, incision]. Instrument for cutting the head of the fetus.

cephalotomy (sef-ă-lot'ō-mĭ) [" + *tomē*, cutting]. Cutting the fetal head to facilitate delivery.

cephalotractor (sef-ă-lō-trak'tor) [" + L. *tractus*, drawing along]. Obstetrical forceps.

cephalotribe (sef'ă-lō-trīb) [" + *tribein*, to crush]. Instrument for crushing head of fetus.

cephalotripsy (sef'ă-lō-trĭp-sĭ) [" + *tribein*, to crush]. Crushing of fetal head in dystocia.

cephalotrypesis (sef-ă-lō-trip-ē'sis) [" + *trypesis*, a boring]. Removing a bone disk from the skull. Syn: *trephination*.

cephaloxia (sĕf-ă-lŏks'ĭ-ă). Torticollis or wryneck, *q.v.*

ceptor (sep'tor). [L. *capere*, to take]. General term for a nerve ending which upon being stimulated passes the stimulus on to the cell to which the ceptor is attached.

c., chemical. One which initiates chemical reactions in the body.

c., contact. One which apprehends stimuli contributed by direct physical contact.

c., distance. One which perceives stimuli at a distance, by aerial or ethereal forces.

cera (sē'ră) [L. from G. *kēros*]. Wax.

c. alba. White wax.

c. flava. Yellow wax.

ceratotome or keratotome (se-rat'o-tōm) [" + *tomē*, incision]. A knife for division of the cornea.

ceratum (se-ra'tum) [L. waxed]. An unctuous solid for application to the skin. Syn: *cerate, q.v.*

cercaria (sĕr-ka'rĭ-ă) [G. *kerkos*, tail]. A free-swimming stage in the development of a fluke or trematode. They develop within sporocysts or redia which parasitize snails or bivalve molluscs. The cercaria emerge from the mollusc and either (1) enter their final host directly or (2) encyst in an intermediate host which is eaten by the final host. In the latter case, the encysted tailless form is known as a *metacercaria*. See: *fluke; trematode*.

Cercom'onas [G. *kerkos*, tail, + *monas*. unit.] A genus of free-living, coprozoic, flagellate protozoa. May be present in stale specimens of feces or urine. Not pathogenic.

cercomoni'asis. Infestation with *Cercomonas intestinalis*.

cercus (ser'kus) [G. *kerkos*, tail]. A hairlike structure.

cerea flexibilitas (sē'rē-ă fleks-ĭ-bil'ĭ-tas) [L. *cera*, wax, + *flexibilitas*, flexibility]. Psy: A condition in which the limbs can be molded into any desired position.

ce'reals [L. *Cerealis*, pert. to Ceres, goddess of agriculture]. Edible grains.

Comp: The composition of all cereals is of a similar character. The carbohydrates are in greater proportion than are the other properties. They are mostly in the form of starch (70-80%, oatmeal 67%), and about 10-15% protein.

Vitamin B complex abundant in wheat germ. Sodium chloride small, potash and phosphorus predominate. Magnesium abundant. Iron found in the germ and outer layer. Water low. Some of the cellulose is lost in milling. The whole grain contains about 1% fat.

Absorption of Cereals: Proteins, 85%; carbohydrates, 98%; fats, 90%.

Comparison of Food Value of Principal Cereals*
(Source: USDA Handbook #8, 1963.)

	Calories mg.	*Protein* gm.	*Starch* gm.	*Fat* gm.	*Fiber* gm.	*Calcium* mg.	*Phosphorus* mg.	*Magnesium* mg.	*Potassium* mg.
Barley	16	8.2	78.8	1.0	0.5	16	2	37	160
Corn	6	7.8	76.8	2.6	0.7	6	164	47	–
Oatmeal	53	14.2	68.2	7.4	1.2	53	405	110	352
Rice	24	6.7	80.4	0.4	0.3	24	94	28	92
Rye	22	9.4	77.9	1.0	0.4	22	185	115	156
Wheat	16	11.8	74.7	1.1	0.3	16	95	25	95

* In their raw, uncooked, unenriched flour form.

ceram'ics, dental [G. *keramos*, potters' clay]. The use of porcelain or porcelain-type materials in dental work.

ceramodon'tia [" + *odous*, tooth]. Dental ceramics.

ceramuria (ser-am-u'rĭ-ă) [" + *ouron*, urine]. Excessive phosphate excretion in urine. Syn: *phosphaturia*.

cerate (se'rat) [L. *ceratum*, from *cera*, wax]. Unctuous substance containing wax and of such consistency that it may be spread easily, at ordinary temperature, upon muslin or similar material, with a spatula, and yet not so soft as to liquefy and run when applied to the skin. Rarely prescribed.

ceratocele or keratocele (ser'ă-to-sēl) [G. *keras*, horn, + *kēlē*, hernia]. Hernia of Descemet's membrane through outer layer of the cornea.

cerebellar (ser-ē-bel'ar) [L. dim. *cerebrum*, brain]. Pert. to the cerebellum.

cerebellif'ugal [" + *fugere*, to flee]. Extending or proceeding from the cerebellum.

cerebellip'etal [" + *petere*, to seek]. Extending toward the cerebellum.

cerebellitis (ser-ĕ-bel-ī-tis) [" + G. *-itis*, inflammation]. Inflammation of the cerebellum.

cerebellospinal (ser-ĕ-bel-ō-spī'nal) [" + *spina*, a thorn]. Pert. to cerebellum and spinal cord.

cerebellum (ser-ĕ-bel'um) [L.]. A portion of the brain forming the largest portion of the rhombencephalon. It lies dorsal to the pons and medulla oblongata, overhanging the latter. It consists of two lateral *cerebellar hemispheres* and a narrow medial portion, the *vermis*. It is connected to the brain stem by three pairs of fiber bundles, the inferior, middle, and superior peduncles. The cerebellum is involved in synergic control of skeletal muscles and plays an important role in the coordination of voluntary muscular movements. It receives afferent impulse and discharges efferent impulse but does not serve as a reflex center in the usual sense; however it may intensify some reflexes and depress others.

cerebral (ser'ĕ-bral, sĕ-rē'bral) [L. *cerebrum*, brain]. Pert. to the cerebrum.

c. hemorrhage. The result of rupture of a sclerosed or diseased blood vessel in brain. Often associated with high blood pressure. RS: *apoplexy; hemiplegia.*

c. infantile lipoidosis. SEE: *amaurotic familial idiocy, infantile.*

cerebration (ser-ĕ-brā'shun) [L. *cerebratiō*, brain activity]. Mental action of the brain.

cerebrifugal (ser-ĕ-brif'u-gal) [L. *cerebrum*, brain, + *fugere*, to flee]. Away from the brain; pert. to efferent nerve fibers.

cerebrin (ser'ĕ-brin). One of a number of fatty nitrogenous principles from nerve tissue, containing phosphorus.

cerebrip'etal [L. *cerebrum*, brain, + *petere*, to seek]. Proceeding toward the cerebrum, as nerve fibers or impulses.

cerebri'tis [" + G. *-ītis*, inflammation]. Inflammation of the brain, esp. the cerebrum.

cerebromalacia (ser-ĕ-bro-mă-lā'sĭ-ă) [" + G. *malakia*, softening]. Softening of the brain, esp. of the cerebrum.

cerebromedullary (ser"ĕ-brō-med'ū-lā-rē). Pertaining to the brain and spinal cord; cerebrospinal.

cerebromeningitis (ser-ĕ-brō"men-in-jī'tis) [" + G. *menigx*, membrane, + *-itis*, inflammation]. Inflammation of the cerebrum and its membranes.

cerebrometer (ser-ĕ-brom'ĕ-ter) [" + G. *metron*, measure]. Device for registering pulsations of the brain.

cerebropathy (ser-ĕ-brop'ă-thĭ) [" + G. *pathos*, disease]. Any disease of the brain, esp. cerebrum.

cerebrophysiology (ser"ĕ-brō-fiz-ĭ-ol'ō-jĭ) [" + G. *physis*, nature, + *logos*, study]. Physiology of the brain.

cerebropontile (ser-ĕ-brō-pon'tĭl) [" + *pons, pont-*, bridge]. Pert. to the cerebrum and pons varolii.

cerebropsychosis (ser-ĕ-brō-sī-kō'sis) [" + *psychōsis*, life]. Any mental disorder due to cerebral lesion.

cer"ebrosclero'sis [" + G. *sklērōsis*, hardening]. Hardening of the brain, esp. of the cerebrum.

cerebroscope (ser-ĕ'brō-skōp) [" + G. *skopein*, to examine]. Instrument for brain diagnosis.

cerebroscopic (ser-ĕ-brō-skŏp'ĭk). Pert. to cerebroscopy.

cerebroscopy (ser-ĕ-brŏs'kō-pĭ) [" + G. *skopein*, to examine]. Diagnostic use of the ophthalmoscope as applied to the brain.

cerebrose (ser'ĕ-brōs). $C_6H_{12}O_6$, a compound (brain sugar) derived from brain tissue.

cerebroside (sĕr'ĕ-brō-sīd). One of a class of substances present in brain tissue which upon hydrolysis yield galactose, a nitrogenous base, and a fatty acid, *e.g.*, kerasin, phrenosin, nervone. SYN: *galactolipids.*

cerebrosis (ser-ĕ-brō'sis) [L. *cerebrum*, brain, + G. *-ōsis*, infection]. Any brain disease. SYN: *encephalosis.*

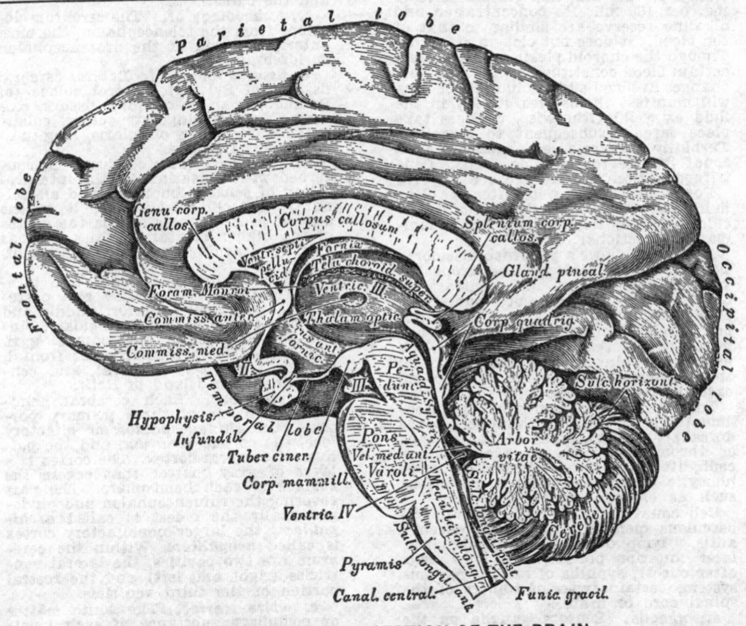

MEDIAN SAGITTAL SECTION OF THE BRAIN.

cerebrospinal (ser″ĕ-brō-spī′nal) [" + *spina*, thorn]. Referring to the brain and spinal cord, as the cerebrospinal axis.

c. axis. The central nervous system (brain and spinal cord).

c. fever. Cerebrospinal meningitis. Inflammation of the meninges of the brain and spinal cord; sometimes called "spotted fever" because of rash on the body.

c. fluid. A water cushion protecting the brain and spinal cord from shock.

Shrinking or expanding of the cranial contents is usually quickly balanced by increase or decrease of this fluid. Possibly cell nourishment and the removal of waste are minor functions.

FORMATION OF: The fluid is formed by the choroid plexuses of the lateral and third ventricles, that of the lateral ventricles passing through the foramen of Monro to the third, and through the aqueduct of Sylvius to the fourth ventricle. Here it may escape through the central foramen of Magendie, or the lateral foramen of Luschke into the *cisterna magna*, and so over the brain and cord surfaces, occupying the subarachnoid spaces. It is absorbed by the arachnoid villi and through the perineural lymph spaces of both brain and cord.

CHARACTERISTICS: The fluid is watery, clear and colorless. Normally, the initial pressure of spinal fluid in a recumbent man (as determined by spinal puncture) is equivalent to 70 to 180 mm. of water. Amt. in normal adult is 100 to 140 ml. Sp. Gr.: 1.003 to 1.008.

Total cell count in adults is 0 to 10 cu. ml.; in children 0 to 20 cu. ml. (they should be counted at once and not remain in the fluid); total protein 20 to 45 mg. per 100 ml.; and glucose 50 to 75 mg. per 100 ml. Its concentration and alkaline reserve are similar to that of the blood. It does not clot on standing. Though the choroid plexuses can express certain blood constituents (*e.g.*, iodides), changes in blood sugar, chloride, or urea will manifest themselves quickly in the fluid as well. Otherwise, changes take place largely subsequent to secretion. Turbidity suggests an excessive cell count, if due to red blood cells. Centrifugalization will show a red deposit.

Formation of a web after a clear fluid has stood is characteristic of tuberculous meningitis (rarely other inflammatory reactions).

It usually shows a yellowish discoloration when containing blood from the subarachnoid spaces (in contrast to blood from trauma of puncture), though for a few days the cells may not be entirely disintegrated. A similar appearance may result from a spinal block above the point of puncture; the fluid spontaneously coagulating due to an excessive albumen content.

Total protein is increased in infections (as meningitis, brain abscess, tabes dorsalis), various types of hemorrhage or thrombosis, virus diseases (as encephalitis, anterior poliomyelitis, lymphocytic meningitis), and conditions such as chronic alcoholism.

Cell count increases especially in tuberculous meningitis, epidemic encephalitis, lymphocytic choriomeningitis, later anterior poliomyelitis (few days after onset), syphilis of central nervous system, certain types of tumors of the spinal cord or brain.

c., ganglia. Sensory ganglia on the roots of cranial and spinal nerves.

c. nerves. The cranial and spinal nerves, *q.v.*

c. puncture. A puncture for the collection of cerebrospinal fluid. It may be collected from spaces around the spinal cord (*lumbar puncture*), from the cisterna magna (*cisternal puncture*), or in infants with open fontanelles (by *ventricular puncture*).

cerebrosuria (ser″ĕ-brō-sū′rĭ-ă) [L. *cerebrum*, brain, + G. *ouron*, urine]. Cerebrose in the urine.

cer″ebrot′omy [" + G. *tomē*, incision]. 1. Incision of the brain to evacuate an abscess. 2. Dissection of the brain.

cerebrum (ser′ĕ-brum, ser-ē′brum) [L.]. The largest part of the brain consisting of two hemispheres separated by a deep longitudinal fissure. They are united by three *commissures*, the corpus callosum and the anterior and posterior hippocampal commissures. The surface of each hemisphere is thrown into numerous folds or convolutions called *gyri* separated by furrows called *fissures* or *sulci*.

c. areas. On the basis of function, several areas have been identified and located. Among them are (a) *Motor projection areas* which give rise to fibers carrying efferent impulses to effector organs, the skeletal muscles. (b) *Sensory projection areas* which receive impulses from sense organs or sensory receptors by way of the brain stem. These include the somesthetic (visual, auditory, gustatory, and olfactory) areas. (c) *Association areas*, which are concerned with the higher mental faculties.

c. basal ganglia. These are masses of gray matter deeply embedded within each hemisphere. They are the *caudate*, *lentiform*, and *amygdaloid nuclei* and the *claustrum*.

c., embryology of. The cerebrum develops from the telencephalon, the most anterior portion of the prosencephalon or forebrain.

c. fissures and sulci. Lateral cerebral fissure (of Sylvius), central sulcus (of Rolando), parieto-occipital fissure, calcarine fissure, cingulate sulcus, collateral fissure, sulcus circularis, longitudinal cerebral fissure.

c. functions. The cerebrum is concerned with sensations or the interpretation of sensory impulses, and all voluntary muscular activities; it is the seat of consciousness and is the center of the higher mental faculties such as memory, learning, reasoning, judgment, intelligence, and the emotions.

c. gyri. Superior, middle, and inferior frontal gyri; anterior and posterior central gyri; superior, middle and inferior temporal gyri; cingulate, lingual, fusiform, and hippocampal gyri.

c. lobes. The principal lobes: frontal, parietal, occipital, temporal, and central (insula or island of Reil).

c. structure. Each cerebral hemisphere consists of three primary portions, the *rhinencephalon* or olfactory lobe, the *corpus striatum*, and the *pallium* or cerebral cortex. The cortex is a layer of gray matter that covers the surface of each hemisphere. The part covering the rhinencephalon and phylogenetically the oldest is called *archipallium;* the larger nonolfactory cortex is called *neopallium*. Within the cerebrum are two cavities, the lateral ventricles (right and left) and the rostral portion of the third ventricle.

c. white matter. The white matter or medullary substance of each hemisphere consists of three kinds of fibers

(1) *commissural fibers* which pass from one hemisphere to the other, (2) *projection fibers* which convey impulses to and from the cortex, and (3) *association fibers* which connect various parts of the cortex within one hemisphere.

cerium (sē'rĭ-um). A metallic element obtained from the rare earths. It is used as a sulfate, in quantitative analysis. SYMB: Ce. At. wt. 140.12; at. no. 58.

ceroma (se-ro'mă) [L. *cera*, wax, + -*ōma*, mass]. A waxy tumor that has undergone amyloid degeneration.

ce'roplasty [" + *plassein*, to mold]. Manufacture of anatomical models and pathological specimens in wax.

cerosis (se-ro'sis) [" + -*ōsis*, infection]. Morbid condition of membranes resembling waxlike scales.

cer'tifiable. Pert. to infectious diseases which must be reported to the health authorities.

cerumen (se-rū'men) [L. *cera*, wax]. The waxlike, soft brown secretion found in the external canal of the ear; inspissated, dried earwax.

ceru'minal. Pert. to the cerumen.

cerumino'sis [L. *cera*, wax, + G. -*ōsis*, infection]. Excessive wax formation.

ceru'minous. Pert. to cerumen.

c. glands. Modified sweat glands in the skin lining the external auditory canal, which secrete cerumen.

ceruse (se'rūs) [L. *cerussa*]. White lead paint.

cervical (ser'vĭ-kal) [L. *cervicalis*, pert. to neck]. 1. Of, pertaining to, or in the region of the neck. 2. Pertaining to the cervix of an organ, as the *cervix uteri*.

c. nerves. The first eight spinal nerves.

c. plexus. That formed by loops joining the ant. rami of first four cervical nerves; it receives communicating rami from the sympathetic ganglia. SEE: *Nerve plexuses in Appendix*.

c. vertebrae. First seven bones of the spinal column. SEE: *skeleton*.

cervicectomy (ser-vĭ-sek'tō-mĭ) [L. *cervix*, neck, + G. *ektomē*, excision]. Removal of the cervix uteri.

cervicitis (ser-vĭ-sī'tĭs) [" + G. -*ītis*, inflammation]. Inflammation of the cervix uteri.

cervico- (ser'vĭ-kō) [L.]. Prefix: Pert. to the neck.

cervicobra'chial [" + G. *brachion*, arm]. Pert. to the neck and arm.

cervicobuc'cal [" + *bucca*, cheek]. Pert. to the buccal surface of neck of a molar or premolar tooth.

cervicodynia (ser-vĭ-kō-dĭn-ĭ-ă). A pain or cramp of the neck; cervical neuralgia.

cervicofa'cial [" + *faciēs*, face]. Pert. to the neck and face.

cervicovagini'tis. Inflammation of the cervix of the uterus and the vagina.

cervicoves'ical [" + *vesica*, bladder]. Pert. to the cervix uteri and bladder.

cervix (sĕr'vĭks) [L.]. The neck or a part of an organ resembling a neck. SEE: *"cervico-" words*.

c. uteri. Neck of the uterus. The lower part from the internal os, outward to the external os.

It is rounded and conical in shape, and a portion protrudes into the vagina. It is about 1 in. long, penetrated by the cervical canal through which the fetus and menstrual flow escape. It is apt to be torn in childbirth, in which case it must be sutured. SEE: *cauliflower excrescence*.

c. uteri, laceration of. There may be slight tearing in most primipara. Deeper tears in manual dilatation and use of forceps; breech presentation also may be a cause. Laceration may be post., ant., single and bilateral, stellate and incomplete. Tears are repaired by suturing in order to prevent hemorrhage and later complications.

c. vesicae, c., vesical. Neck of the bladder.

c.e.s. Abbr. for *central excitatory state*.

cesarean section (sē-zar'ē-ăn) [L. Caesar, because he was supposed to have been born in this manner; this derivation is probably inaccurate.]. Removal of the fetus by means of an incision into uterus, usually by way of abdominal wall.

May be performed by extraperitoneal or intraperitoneal abdominal route.

CONSERVATIVE: One in which the uterus is not removed. *Classical*: The incision is made across the fundus of the uterus. *Low Fundal*: The incision is made through the contractile portion of the uterus from a point just above the reflection of the bladder upward for a space of 2 to 3 inches. *Laparotrachelotomy*: Low cervical cesarean section. The incision is made in the noncontractile lower uterine segment after stripping back the bladder flap. After removal of the fetus and placenta the uterus is sutured and the bladder flap is sewed up over the uterine scar, thus peritonealizing the scar. *Extraperitoneal*: An abdominal incision is made parallel to Poupart's ligament. The incision in the uterus is made extraperitoneally by pushing the bladder to the side.

RADICAL: *Porro*: Cesarean section with removal of the uterus after the fetus has been taken out. This is a supracervical hysterectomy. *Total*: This is a total hysterectomy after the removal of the fetus, used in cases of badly lacerated cervices or in cases of early carcinoma of the cervix.

c. s., absolute. Where the child cannot be delivered through the natural passages under any circumstances.

IND: (1) Contraction of the bony pelvis with a conjugata vera diameter of less than 5.5 cm. (2) Exostoses of the bony pelvis completely obstructing the birth canal. (3) Tumor masses of the soft parts which hinder the passage of the fetus (fibroid tumors, ovarian cysts). (4) Placenta previa and premature separation of the placenta. (5) Previous cesarean section without an absolute indication but where the postoperative course was stormy and a weakened uterine scar is suspected.

In general terms: The most frequent cause for cesarean section is dystocia due to fetopelvic (also called cephalopelvic) disproportion, *i.e.*, for some reason the fetus is too large to be delivered through the pelvic outlet or the pelvis is abnormally small or there is a combination of these factors.

c. s., relative. Where the child could be delivered through the natural passages, but where the danger of such a delivery might be greater by way of the vaginal route.

IND: (1) Moderate degrees of contraction of the bony pelvis with a conjugata vera diameter of about 9.5 cm. (2) Prolapsed cord in some instances. (3) Transverse presentation of the fetus. (4) Oblique presentation of the fetus. (5) A large baby with a moderate degree of disproportion. (6) Habitual death of the fetus during the course of labor. (7) Impacted brow or face presentation where the fetus is alive. (8) Preeclamptic toxemia in patients where a difficult labor is anticipated. (9) Carcinoma of the cervix with rigidity. (10) In cases where hysterectomy is indicated and is to be done in conjunction with the cesarean section. (11) In cases where oophorectomy is indicated. (12) In cases where sterilization is desired, although to allow that patient to deliver normally and sterilize through the vaginal route at a later time is more satisfactory. There are several varieties of cesarean section differing mainly in the technic employed.

cesarotomy (sez-ă-rot'o-mĭ) [Caesar, + G. *tomē,* incision]. Cesarean* section.

cesium (sē'zĭ-ŭm) [L. *caesius,* sky blue]. A metallic element. It has a number of isotopes, radioactive isotopes, Cs^{137} being used therapeutically for irradiation of cancerous tissue. SYMB: Cs. At. wt. 132.905; at. no. 55.

Cestoda (ses-tōd'ă). A subclass of the class Cestoidea, phylum Platyhelminthes, which includes the tapeworms. Have a scolex and a chain of segments (proglottids). Ex. *Taenia.* They are intestinal parasites of man and other vertebrates.

cestode (ses'tōd) [G. *kestos,* girdle, + *eidos,* form]. A tapeworm; one of the Cestoda.

cestodiasis (sĕs-tō-dī'ă-sĭs). Infestation with tapeworms, *q.v.* SEE: *Cestoda.*

ces'toid. Like a tapeworm.

Cestoidea (ses-toi'de-ă). A class of flatworms of the phylum Platyhelminthes. Includes the tapeworms.

Cetraria (sē-trā'rĭ-ă). 1. A genus of lichens, chiefly found in northern latitudes. 2. *C. islandica,* or Iceland moss, a lichen used in treating lung and bowel disorders.

cetylpyridinium chloride. USP. A quaternary ammonium compound, soluble in water. Used as an antiseptic.

cevitamic acid (sev-i-tam'ik). Crystalline vitamin C. SEE: *acid, ascorbic.*

CF. Abbr. for *citrovorum factor.*

Cf. Symbol for *californium.*

C.F.T. Abbr. for *complement fixation test.*

C. G. S. Abbr. for *centimeter-gram-second,* a name given to a system of units for distance, weight and time.

C_2H_4. Ethylene.

CH_4. Methane; marsh gas.

C_2H_2. Acetylene.

C_6H_6. Benzene.

Chaddock's reflexes (chad'dok) [Charles G. Chaddock, American neurologist, 1861-1936]. 1. Extension of great toe resulting from irritation around ext. malleolus. 2. Flexion of wrist and fanning of fingers when forearm is irritated above and near wrist.

chaeromania (ke-ro-ma'nĭ-ă) [G. *chairein,* to rejoice, + *mania,* madness]. Mania characterized by exaltation and cheerfulness. SYN: *amenomania.*

chafe. To injure by rubbing or friction.

chaf'ing. A superficial inflammation which develops when skin is subjected to friction from clothing or adjacent skin as may occur at the axilla, groin, anal region, or between digits of hands and feet or at the neck or wrists. Erythema, maceration, and sometimes fissuring occur. Bacterial or mycotic infection may result secondarily. SYN: *erythema intertrigo.*

Chagas' disease. South American trypanosomiasis. Caused by *Trypanosoma cruzi* and transmitted by the biting reduviid bug. Also sometimes called *Chagas-Cruz disease.*

chain [Fr. *chaine,* from L. *catēna,* chain]. In bacteriology, 3 or more cells attached end to end. In chemistry, a series of atoms held together by valence bonds.

c. reflex. One in a consecutive series.

chalarosis (kal-ă-rō'sis). Infection with *Chalara,* a fungus producing subcutaneous nodules which break down, forming ulcers.

chalazion (ka-la'zĭ-on) (pl. *chalazia, chalazions*) [G. dim. of *chalaza,* sty]. Small, hard tumor analogous to sebaceous cyst developing on the eyelids, formed by distention of a meibomian gland with secretion. A meibomian cyst. SEE: *steatoma.*

chalcosis (kal-ko'sis) [G. *chalkos,* copper, + *-ōsis,* infection]. 1. Chronic poisoning from copper. 2. Copper deposits in lungs and tissues.

chalice cell (tshal'is) [G. *kalix,* cup]. Crateriform shell remaining after mucus has been discharged from an epithelial cell. SYN: *goblet cell, q.v.*

chalicosis (kal-ĭ-ko'sis) [G. *chalix,* limestone, + *-ōsis,* infection]. Lung disorder due to inhalation of stone particles. SYN: *pneumoconiosis, q.v.*

chalinoplasty (kal-in'o-plas-tĭ) [G. *chalinos,* corner of mouth, + *plassein,* to mold]. Plastic surgery of the mouth and lips, esp. of corners of mouth.

chalone (kal'ōn) [G. *chaloun,* to relax]. A substance carried through the blood which has an inhibitory effect on the tissue or organ which responds to its action. SEE: *autacoid; hormone.*

chalybeate (kă-lĭb'ē-āt) [L. *chalybs,* from G. *chalyps,* steel]. 1. Pert. to or composed of iron; ferruginous. 2. Agent containing iron.

chamber (chām'ber) [G. *kamara,* vault]. Compartment or closed space.

c., anterior. The space bet. the cornea and iris.

c., aqueous. Ant. and post. chambers of the eye, containing the aqueous humor.

c., hyperbaric. An airtight enclosure strong enough to withstand high internal pressure. Used to expose animals or an entire surgical team to increased air pressure. Used to treat gas gangrene, bends, and for certain surgical procedures.

c., low pressure. One designed to simulate high altitudes by exposing men or animals to low atmospheric pressure. Such studies are essential to provide background for human flights into the atmosphere and space.

c., posterior. Space behind the iris, ant. to the lens.

c., vitreous. Cavity behind the lens in the eye containing the vitreous humor.

Chamberland filter (sham-ber-län) [Charles E. Chamberland, French bacteriologist, 1851-1908]. An unglazed porcelain filter through which water can be forced under pressure. Intercepts all but ultramicroscopic microorganisms.

chamomile, camomile (kam'o-mīl) [G. *chamaimelon,* earth apple, so called from smell of its flowers]. Flowers of the *Anthemis* yielding a bluish volatile oil and a bitter infusion.

chancre (shang'ker) [Fr. anything that consumes, from L. *cancer,* ulcer]. A hard, syphilitic, primary ulcer. The first sign of syphilis, approximately two to three weeks after infection. SEE ALSO: *syphilis.*

CAUTION: During the chancre stage, the patient is highly contagious and the chancre itself contains many spirochetes. Discovery of these organisms in the chancre is the basis for the positive darkfield test for syphilis. Syphilis may occur, however, without a chancre developing.

SYM: Begins as erosion or papule which ulcerates superficially. Generally single; sometimes multiple. Has a scooped out appearance due to level or sloping edges which are adherent. It has a shining red or raw floor with some deposit. Induration constant. No pain. Slightly purulent secretion. Heals without leaving scar. May appear at almost any site including mouth, penis, urethra, eyelid, conjunctiva.

c., hard; c., hunterian. Primary lesion of syphilis. SEE: *chancre.*

c., simple; c., soft. A nonsyphilitic venereal ulcer. SYN: *chancroid.*

c., true. The primary lesion of syphilis. SEE: *chancre.*

chancroid (shang'kroyd) [" + G. *eidos*, form]. A nonsyphilitic venereal ulcer, highly infectious; a simple or soft chancre. It is caused by *Hemophilus ducreyi* (also called Ducrey's bacillus), a gram-negative bacillus.

INCUBATION: Approximately three to five days.

SYM: Begins with pustule or ulcer; multiple; abrupt edges; rough floor; yellow exudate; purulent secretion; sensitive and inflamed. Scar remains. Rapid progress. May affect the penis, urethra, vulva, or anus. Multiple lesions may develop by autoinoculation. Types include *transient, phagedenic, giant,* and *serpiginous.*

TREATMENT: Sulfonamides, tetracyclines, chloramphenicol.

chancrous (shang'krus). Pert. to or of the nature of chancre.

change of life. The menopause;* climacteric.*

chapped (chapt). Inflamed, roughened, fissured, as from exposure to cold.

charbon (shar-bon') [Fr. coal]. Infection with *B. anthracis.* SYN: *anthrax.*

charcoal (shăr'kōl) [M.E. *charken*, to creak, + *coal*]. Wood charcoal. USP. Very fine powder prepared from soft charred wood.

ACTION AND USES: Internally for adsorption of gastrointestinal gas. Also for adsorption of poisonous alkaloids which have been swallowed.

c. fumes. SEE: *carbon monoxide.*

Charcot's joint (shar-kōz) [Jean M. Charcot, French neurologist, 1825-1893]. A type of joint associated with tabes dorsalis, syringomyelia, or other conditions involving disease or injury to the spinal cord, characterized by hypermobility. Decalcification of bone on joint surfaces occurs accompanied by overgrowth of bone about margins. Pain is usually absent although there are exceptions. Deformity and instability of the joint are characteristic. SYN: *neurogenic arthropathy.*

Charcot-Leyden crystals (shar-kō'lī'den) [Charcot, and Ernest V. von Leyden, German physician, 1832-1910]. Colorless, hexagonal, double-pointed and often needle-like crystals found (a) in the sputum in asthma, bronchial bronchitis and (b) in the feces, in ulcerative cases of the intestine especially amebiasis.

Charcot-Marie-Tooth disease [Charcot; Pierre Marie, French neurologist, 1853-1940; and Howard Tooth, English physician, 1856-1926]. A form of progressive neural muscular atrophy, a disease with hereditary tendencies, characterized by progressive weakness of distal muscles of the arms and feet. The muscles atrophy, reflexes are lost, foot drop develops, and there is loss of cutaneous sensations. Usually develops in childhood but may occur in adults; more commonly in males. Its cause is unknown. SYN: *peroneal muscular atrophy.*

charlatan (shar'lă-tăn) [Italian *ciarratano*, seller of papal indulgences]. A boasting pretender to special knowledge or ability, as in medicine. SYN: *quack.*

charlatanry (shar'lă-tăn-rĭ) [Italian *ciarlataneria*]. Undue pretension to knowledge or skill or an instance of it. SYN: *quackery.*

Charles' law [Jacques A. C. Charles, French physicist, 1746-1823]. At constant pressure a given amount of gas will expand its volume in direct proportion to the absolute temperature. SYN: *Gay-Lussac's law.*

charleyhorse. A pulled muscle, intramuscular bleeding; torn muscle fibers commonly of the quadriceps muscle or the hamstrings, associated with soreness and stiffness. Often occurs as an athletic injury.

F. A. TREATMENT: Cold applications.

charpie (shar'pĭ) [Fr.]. Shreds of linen for dressing wounds.

chart [L. *charta*, paper]. 1. A simple form or sheet of paper for recording the course of a patient's illness. Includes records of temperature, pulse, respiratory rate, blood pressure, urinary and fecal output, and doctors' and nurses' notes. 2. To record on a graph the sequence of events such as vital signs. SEE: *charting.*

charta (kar'ta) [G. *chartēs*, piece of paper]. Preparation intended principally for external application, made either by saturating paper with medicinal substances or by applying the latter to the surface of the paper by the addition of some adhesive liquid.

chart'ing. The making of a tabulated record of the progress of a disease; a clinical record.

ITEMS TO RECORD: Information about the patient and his treatment that may be gathered only by the nurse who is in constant attendance. The doctor needs detailed information which the nurse may contribute through her observation of and contact with the patient. These notes then aid the doctor in making his diagnosis, and upon the details of the patient's reactions and progress he bases his treatment. The nurse's responsibility for supplying this information is very great. Verbal reports are not sufficient; they take time, and make mistakes possible.

Record the following:

General: BATHS: Record an accurate description of medicinal baths and also reaction to same.

BLOOD PRESSURE: Record under "Remarks."

DIET: If patient is on regular diet, it is sufficient to chart *Breakfast, Dinner, and Supper,* but when on any other diet, chart exactly what the patient takes. The *amount* of liquids taken should be charted, not "Water P. R. N." 1. Hours of giving. 2. Kind: full, light, soft, liquid, special. 3. Appetite: good, poor, special likes and dislikes.

Discharge or Death: Chart discharge or death of patient, with *hour* and *date* of same.

Dressings: Chart the *change* of dressings on wounds and the *amount* and *character of drainage;* remark "Specimen Saved" if this has been done. 1. Hour. 2. By whom done. 3. Stitches or drains removed. 4. Patient's reaction if pained or shocked by dressing.

Drugs: Any unfavorable reaction from drugs or treatments should be charted. Chart *time* when drugs or treatments are administered. All medicines, treatments, preparation, etc., are to be charted by the nurse who administers same, whether she has charge of the patient or not. Confine name of medicine and dose to the prescribed column. When administering soluble salts, dispensed in solution, state dose actually administered, *not the amount of solution.* The administration of medicines other than by mouth should be indicated, as *per hypodermic, per injection, per inunction,* or *per rectum.* Any prominent or unusual therapeutic action or idiosyncrasy resulting from a drug should be recorded as a "Remark." A special prescription is written in full in the medication column the first time it is given. After that, chart ℞ Medicine or ℞ Capsule, as the case may be. After first charting, chart the name of principal ingredient, adding the word "Compound." Note discontinuance of medicine or treatment as a "Remark."

Fluids: 1. Hours of giving. 2. Kind. 3. Amount. The amount should be totaled and the total charted every 12 hours.

Heat: Chart by *whose* order heat is applied to an unconscious patient, and *who executed* the order.

Infant Feeding: The *formula* should be charted the *first time;* afterwards, *amount* given, and if regurgitated, approximate the *amount.*

Laboratory: 1. Hour. 2. Kind of specimen. 3. By whom taken. 4. By whom ordered (not necessary in case of routine urine specimen on admission).

Medications: 1. Hour of giving. 2. Kind; name of drug and preparation. 3. Amount. 4. By whom given. 5. Manner of giving: mouth, hypo, rectum, intravenous, etc. 6. Patient's reaction.

Nursing Care: 1. Hour. 2. Baths: shampoos. 3. Alcohol rubs; decubitus dressing. 4. Special mouth care. 5. Sitting up for first time. 6. Out of bed for first time. 7. Walking for first time. 8. Narcotics. (Treatments are also charted, but as treatments.)

Operations: 1. Name of operation. 2. Preparation for operation. 3. Preliminary anesthetic if given by nurse or on ward. 4. Hour of going to O. R. 5. Hour of going to and leaving recovery room. 6. Hour of return to room. 7. Condition on return to room. 8. Hour of recovery from anesthetic. 9. Condition every half hour for next 3 or 4 hours, depending on state patient is in and severity of operation. Recovery room staff members will record treatment and condition while patient is in their care.

Physician: Record his visit. Doctor's orders must be recorded and time when they are carried out.

Physiotherapy: Occupational Therapy: 1. Hour of going for treatment. 2. Hour of return. 3. Condition of patient.

Postoperative: *Changing position* of postoperative patients should be recorded under "Remarks." Record passive and active exercise of patient.

Specimens: Record the taking of *specimens* of blood, exudates, transudates, etc., for examination. The result will be shown by the report of the pathologist.

Surgical Preparations: The nurse who does surgical preparations will sign her name after "Preliminary preparation of field of operation." Also observe the same rule for narcotics.

Symptoms: Record accurate descriptions of all symptoms, such as *character of pulse* and *respiration, psychic condition, description of pain,* and *nature of any discharge,* etc. The remarks should be appropriate and well chosen. *Subjective* as well as *objective symptoms* should be recorded.

Time: Everything relating to the patient's progress should be charted as it occurs. Record the *hour* with all statements on charts. Record on the first line of the sheet the *day* and *date of admission,* whether the patient *walked in,* or was admitted *per ambulance,* and *condition* of patient. Four-hour graphic charts are kept for all surgical and obstetrical cases the first 3 days (time 8-12-4); and for all patients whose temperature is above normal. The T. P. R. of all other patients are charted at 6 A. M. and 4 P. M.

Treatments: 1. Hour of giving. 2. Nature of treatment. 3. By whom given. 4. Patient's reaction.

Visits of Clergyman (specially important in case of Roman Catholic patients): 1. Hour. 2. Name of clergyman. 3. Rite performed.

X-ray: 1. Hour. 2. To x-ray room, or portable at bedside. 3. Return from x-ray room. 4. Condition of patient.

Miscellaneous: Any sudden or marked change in patient's condition. Notification of patient's relatives and clergyman. Special charts are also provided for certain purposes, such as the temperature, pulse and respiration chart; an anesthesia chart, generally kept by the anesthetist; blood-pressure chart, used in conditions apt to affect the blood pressure; intake and output charts used in nephritis, and laboratory records usually filed with the patient's chart. If any laboratory records have been made and not filed with the chart, their existence should be noted on the clinical chart at the time made and also upon the final page of the chart.

Physical Symptoms: 1. Appetite: Good. Poor. Special likes or dislikes.

2. Convulsions: Type. Duration. Consciousness lost. Note fecal or urinary incontinence. Was patient injured during convulsion or in fall which came with convulsion. Aura.

3. Defecation: See: *Excretions; Feces; Urine.*

4. Diaphoresis (perspiration): State whether slight, moderate, or profuse.

5. Emesis: State the *amount, color, odor, consistency* of the vomitus, and *manner of ejecting.* (See: Nausea.)

6. Enemas: Results and *unusual appearances,* distention before or after; describe *results* fully. Note whether or not flatus was expelled with the return of the enema. Chart the *solution,* the

Charting: Abbreviations and Their Meanings*

Abbr.	Latin Phrase	Meaning
a or āā	ana	of each
abs. feb.	absente febre	when there is no fever
a.c.	ante cibum	before eating
ad	ad	to, up to
ad effect.	ad effectum	until effectual
ad grat. acid.	ad gratum aciditatem	to an agreeable acidity
ad grat. gust.	ad gratum gustum	to an agreeable taste
adhib.	adhibendus	to be administered
ad lib.	ad libitum	at pleasure; as much as is needed
ad neut.	ad neutralizandum	to neutralization
ad part. dolent.	ad partes dolentes	to the painful parts
ad sat.	ad saturandum	to saturation
adst. feb.	adstante febre	when fever is present
ad us.	ad usum	according to custom
ad us. ext.	ad usum externum	for external use
aeq.	aequales	equal
ag. feb.	aggrediente febre	when the fever increases
agit. ante sum.	agita ante sumendum	shake before taking
alt. dieb.	alternis diebus	every other day
alt. hor.	alternis horis	every other hour
alt. noc.	alternis nocte	every other night
aq.	aqua	water
aq. bull.	aqua bulliens	boiling water
aq. cal.	aqua calida	warm water
aq. dest.	aqua destillata	distilled water
aq. ferv.	aqua fervens	hot water
aq. frig.	aqua frigida	cold water
aq. menth. pip.	aqua menthae piperitae	peppermint water
aq. pur.	aqua pura	pure water
arg.	argentum	silver
bal.	balneum	bath
bal. sin.	balneum sinapis	mustard bath
bib.	bibe	drink
b. i. d.	bis in die	twice daily
bis.	bis	twice
bis in 7d.	bis in septem diebus	twice a week
b.p.		blood pressure; boiling point
bull.	bulliat	let it boil
C.		Centigrade carbon calorie (large)
c.	cum	with
cap.	capsula	a capsule
cat.	cataplasma	a poultice
cc.		cubic centimeter
chart.	charta	paper
cito disp.	cito dispensetur	let it be dispensed quickly
c.m.	cras mane	tomorrow morning
c.m.s.	cras mane sumendus	to be taken tomorrow morning
c.n.	cras nocte	tomorrow night
cochl. amp.	cochleare amplum	heaping spoonful
cochl. mag.	cochleare magnum	a tablespoonful
cochl. med.	cochleare medium	a dessertspoonful
cochl. parv.	cochleare parvum	a teaspoonful
comp.	compositus	compounded of
cong.	congius	a gallon
contra	contra	against
cont. rem.	continuetur remedia	let the medicines be continued
c.v.	cras vespere	tomorrow night
cyath.	cyathus	glassful
cyath. vinos.	cyathus vinosus	wineglassful
D.	dosis	dose
d.	da	give
d. d. in d.	de die in diem	from day to day
decub.	decubitus	lying down
det.	detur	let it be given
dieb. alt.	diebus alternis	on alternate days
dil.	dilue	dilute
dim.	dimidius	half
div.	divide	divide
div. in p. aeq.	divide in partes aequales	divide into equal parts
don.	donec	until
emp.	emplastrum	a plaster
en., enem.		enema
exhib.	exhibeatur	let it be given
ext.	extractum	extract
ext. liq.	extractum liquidum	liquid extract
F., Fahr.		Fahrenheit (temperature scale)

* NOTE: A considerable number of these abbreviations are used rarely if at all. They are recorded for historical purposes.

Charting: Abbreviations and Their Meanings (*Continued*)

Abbr.	Latin Phrase	Meaning
Fe.	ferrum	iron
f.h.	fiat haustus	let a draught be made
f.m.	fiat mistura	let a mixture be made
f.p.	fiat potio	let a potion be made
f. pil.	fiat pilula	let a pill be made
ft.	fiat	let it be made
Gm., gm.		gram
gr.	granum	grain
gt.	gutta	a drop
gtt.	guttae	drops
h. n.	hoc noc'te	tonight
hor. som, h. s.	hora somni	at bedtime
in d.	in dies	daily
inf.	infusum	an infusion
inj.	injectio	an injection
liq.	liquor	a liquor or liquid
m.	misce	mix
mod. praesc.	modo praescripto	as prescribed
mor. dict.	more dicto	in the manner directed
mor. sol.	more solito	in the usual manner
n. b.	no'ta be'ne	note well
noct.	noc'te	night
non rep.	non repetatur	do not repeat
O.	octarius	a pint
o. d.	oculus dexter	right eye
ol.	oleum	oil
o.m.	omni mane	every morning
omn. bid.	omnibus bidendis	every 2 days
omn. bih.	omni bihoris	every 2 hours
omn. hor.	omni hora	every hour
omn. noct.	omni nocte	every night
o. s.	oculus sinister	left eye
p.a.a.	parti affectae applicetur	let it be applied to the affected region
part aeq.	partes aequales	equal parts
post. cib. or p. c.	post cibum	after meals
p.r.	per rectum	through the rectum
p. r. n.	pro re nata	as needed
pulv.	pulvis	a powder
p.v.	per vaginam	through the vagina
q. i. d.	qua'ter in di'e	four times a day
q.l.	quantum libet	as much as is wanted
q. p.	quantum placeat	at will
q. s.	quantum sufficiat	a sufficient quantity, as much as may be needed
℞	recipe	take (thou)
rep.	repetatur	let it be repeated
s.a.	secundum artem	by skill
sig.	signetur	let it be labeled
sing.	singulorum	of each
s. o. s.	si o'pus sit	if necessary
ss.	semis	one-half
stat.	statim	at once
sum.	sumat, sumendum	let him take, to be taken
s.v.	spiritus vini	alcoholic spirit
s. v. v.	spiritus vini vitis	brandy
T.		temperature
tab.	tabella, tabellae	a tablet, tablets
t. i. d.	ter in die	thrice daily
tinct. or tr.	tinctura	tincture
ung.	unguentum	ointment
ur.		urine

strength, and *amount* used. Also for douches and irrigations.

7. Excretions: Chart *time, character,* and *other facts.*

8. Feces: Enema or natural movement. Amount. Consistency. Abnormal constituents. Defecation accompanied by pain or tenesmus.

9. General Appearance: Color. Posture. Rash. Mood. Mental State.

10. Hemorrhages, Discharges, etc.: Chart a *description,* etc. When unusual, *save specimens* for examination.

11. Nausea: Accompanied by vomiting. Following certain foods, drugs or treatments.

12. Nerves: All nervous symptoms, excitability, etc.

13. Pain: Location. Time of onset. Character: Sharp, dull, burning, grinding, throbbing. Duration: Constant, for how long. Intermittent, intervals.

14. Pathological Conditions: *Vomiting, convulsions,* etc. Record *time, duration, severity, general appearance* of patient before, during, and after the attack. *T. P. R.* immediately after, and *what was done* to relieve condition. Chart explanation as to the cause if known.

15. Pulse: Rate: beats per minute. Character: full, bounding, weak, thready,

faint. Rhythm: regular, irregular, intermittent.

16. RESPIRATION: Rate per minute. Character: deep, shallow, difficult, easy, labored, quiet, stertorous, Cheyne-Stokes. Rhythm: regular, irregular, gasping.

17. SLEEP: Record should be made of the *hours of sleeping* during the day, as well as at night. If impossible to estimate same accurately, approximate it. *Time* and *amount* of sleep obtained by the patient should be noted, if possible. Sleepwalking, nightmares, or talking in sleep should be recorded.

18. TEMPERATURE: If for some legitimate reason temperature is omitted, write *hour* in designated space, leave temperature space unmarked. When recording next temperature, bring line across this space to the adjoining and record the next temperature. By mouth, rectum or axilla. Degree. Following chill, or treatment. If temperature is quite high and patient does not appear to have fever of that extent, take temperature again but remain at bedside to be sure patient is not placing thermometer against some hot object.

19. T. P. R.: Temperature, pulse and respiration taken as ordered. The nurse charts the T. P. R. and general condition of the patient before going to the operating room, and the pulse and respiration with general condition upon return from the operating room.

20. UNCONSCIOUSNESS OR COMA: Time of onset. Conditions associated with or which caused onset. Appearance of patient while in coma. Medicines or treatment given while in coma. Duration.

21. UNUSUAL CONDITIONS: Chart these, such as appearance of blood, twitching, convulsions, coma, drowsiness, lethargy, unconsciousness.

22. URINE: State *time* of voiding, the *amount, color* and *appearance,* whether voided or per catheter. Note time of beginning 24-hour specimen; when bladder is emptied for the purpose, this specimen is sent to laboratory for qualitative test. Remark the *ending* of 24-hour specimen. Note *amount* on chart and on laboratory label. Send specimen to the laboratory for all patients remaining in the hospital over night. At 7 P.M. and 7 A.M., day and night nurses remark whether or not very ill patients voided during the day or night. Immediately upon admission begin 24-hour specimen of urine for all diabetic patients. Check may be used in the urine column: (*a*) When patient uses lavatory. (*b*) When he voids with defecation. At all other times the amount of urine is to be charted (totaled every 12 hours and *total* charted also). Accompanied by pain or burning. Any abnormal appearance. Specimen to laboratory.

23. VISITORS: Reaction to visitors and mood change after visitors depart. Especially important in depressed and psychiatric patients.

24. VOMITING: Cause. Forcible or projectile. Vomitus: Amount. Color. Odor. Consistency. Any unusual constituents.

Mental Symptoms: 1. Calmness. 2. Cheerfulness. 3. Delirium: Kind. 4. Depression: Degree. Apparent effect of visitors, etc. 5. Delusions, on what special subjects. 6. Hallucinations. 7. Illusions, on what special subjects. 8. Temper fits. 9. Willingness to cooperate. 10. Worry.

chartula (kar′tu-lă) [L. dim. of *charta,* piece of paper]. A paper folded to form a receptacle containing a dose of medicinal substance.

chaude-pisse (shōd-pēs′). A burning sensation during urination esp. in acute gonorrhea.

chauffage (sho-fazh′) [Fr. *chauffer,* to heat]. A heated cautery at low temperature applied over a part about ¼ in. from it.

chaulmoogra oil, chaulmugra, chaulmaugra (chawl-moo′gră, chawl-mū′gră, chawl-maw′gră). A vegetable oil used in treatment of leprosy and some dermatoses. Though generally replaced by sulfones in treatment of leprosy, c. is still used in endemic areas where it is readily available and has a low cost.

Chaussier's areola (sho-sĭ-ās′) [Francois Chaussier, Paris physician, 1746-1828]. Indurated tissue around the lesion of a malignant pustule.

check. 1. To slow down or arrest the course of. 2. To verify.

c. *bite*. Impression of teeth on plastic material to check articulation.

c. *experiment*. Control experiment, or one checked against another.

cheek [A.S. *ceáce,* check]. Side of face forming lateral wall of mouth below eye. SYN: *bucca.*

c. *bone*. The malar bone; os zygomaticum [NA]; zygomatic bone.

c. *retractor*. Device for enclosing cheek at the mouth's angle for properly exposing operating field.

cheese [A.S. *cēse,* from L. *caseus,* cheese]. The compressed casein of milk, flavored and altered by bacterial action.

COMP. (Domestic cheddar often called *American*): 100 gm. Calories: 398. Other main values: 25 gm. protein; 32 gm. fat; 2 gm. carbohydrates; 750 mg. calcium; 1310 I.U. vitamin A.

cheilitis (ki-li′tis) [G. *cheilos,* lip, + *-ītis,* inflammation]. Inflammation of the lip.

c. *actinica*. Irritation of lips resulting from exposure to sunlight.

c. *exfoliativa*. Seborrheic dermatitis of the lips.

c. *glandularis*. Disorder of the lips resulting from hypertrophy of mucous glands and their ducts.

c. *venenata*. Dermatitis of the lips resulting from chemicals present in lipsticks, lip cream, and other cosmetics.

cheilognathopalatoschisis (kī-lōg″năth-ō-păl-ă-tōs′kĭ-sĭs) [" + *gnathos,* jaw, + L. *palatum,* palate, + G. *schisis,* cleft]. Malformation in which there is a cleft in the hard and soft palate, upper jaw and in the lip. SYN: *cheilognathouranoschisis.*

cheiloplasty (kī′lō-plas-tĭ) [" + *plassein,* to form]. Plastic operation upon the lips.

cheiloschisis (kī-los′kĭ-sis). Harelip.

cheilosis (kī-lō′sĭs) [G. *cheilos,* lip, + *-ōsis,* disease]. Morbid condition of lips with reddened appearance and fissures at the angles, seen frequently in deficiency of vitamin B complex, especially riboflavin.

cheilostomatoplasty (kil-os-to′mat-o-plas-tĭ) [" + *stoma,* mouth, + *plassein,* to form]. Plastic surgery of and restoration of mouth.

cheilotomy, chilotomy (ki-lot′o-mĭ) [" + *tomē,* incision]. Excision of part of the lip.

cheirognostic (ki″rog-nos′tik) [G. *cheir,* hand, + *gnostikos,* knowing]. 1. Able to distinguish left from right side of body. 2. Able to perceive which side of the body is being stimulated.

cheiropompholyx (kī"rō-pom'fō-liks) [G. *cheiro,* hand, + *pompholyx,* bubble]. A skin disease with groups of blebs or vesicles on the palms of hands, soles of feet.

cheirospasm (ki'ro-spasm) [" + G. *spasmos,* spasm]. Writer's cramp.

chelation (kē-lā'shun). Combination of a group or compound with a central metallic atom, thereby forming a heterocyclic ring.

cheloid (ke'loid) [G. *chēlē,* claw, + *eidos,* form]. Keloid, *q.v.*

chem'ical [G. *chēmeia,* chemistry]. Pert. to chemistry.

c. change. A change in which a substance breaks up or combines with other substances to make new substances with new properties or characteristics. Ex: Oxygen and hydrogen combine together to form *water.* Sodium (a metal) and chlorine (a gas) combine together to form *sodium chloride,* or common salt. Oxygen combines with hemoglobin when the hemoglobin in the blood comes into contact with the oxygen in the air in the alveoli of the lungs to form *oxyhemoglobin.* The difference can be seen by comparing the bright scarlet of the arterial blood containing oxyhemoglobin with the bluish color of the venous blood containing hemoglobin.

c. compound. (1) A substance consisting of two or more chemical elements in definite proportions and in chemical combination and for which a chemical formula can be written. Ex: *water* H_2O), *salt* (NaCl). (2) A substance which can be separated by chemical means into simpler substances.

c. element. 1. Element, *q.v.* 2. Of the nature of, caused by, or performed by the use of chemicals. 3. Any chemical compound or substance composed of chemical elements.

c. reflex. Any reflex action initiated by a chemical stimulus.

c. warfare. The use in wars of chemicals such as gases, or irritants to kill or disable human beings or animals or both.

chemicocautery (kem-ĭ-kō-kaw'ter-ĭ) [G. *chēmeia,* chemistry, + *kautērion,* branding iron]. Cauterization by chemical agents.

chemilumines'cence. Cold light or light produced as a result of a chemical reaction and without the production of heat, *e.g.,* the light produced by certain bacteria, fungi, or fireflies.

cheminosis (kem-in-o'sis) [" + *-ōsis,* infection]. Any disease caused by chemical agents.

chemiotaxis (kem-ĭ-o-taks'is) [" + *taxis,* arrangement]. Chemotaxis, *q.v.*

chemise (she-mēz') [Fr. shirt]. Surgical dressing consisting of a square bandage tied around a catheter passing through the center of the bandage.

chemist (kem'ist). One trained in chemistry.

chem'istry [G. *chēmeia,* chemistry]. The science that treats of the molecular and atomic structure of matter and the composition of substances, their formation, decomposition, and various transformations which they may undergo.

c., analytical. That concerned with the detection of the presence of chemical substances (*qualitative analysis*) or the determination of the amounts of substances present (*quantitative analysis*).

c., biological. The chemistry of living things, involving all the chemical processes which take place within an organism such as the digestion of food, anabolism, and catabolism. SEE: *biochemistry.*

c., general. The study of the entire field of chemistry with emphasis on fundamental concepts and laws.

c., inorganic. The chemistry of compounds not containing carbon.

c., nuclear. Radiochemistry or the study of changes which take place within the nucleus of an atom especially when the nucleus is bombarded by electrons, neutrons, or other subatomic particles.

c., organic. The chemistry of carbon compounds.

c., pathological. The study of chemical changes induced by disease processes, *e.g.,* changes in the chemistry of organs and tissues, blood, secretions, excretions, etc.

c., physical. Theoretical chemistry or that concerned with fundamental laws underlying chemical changes and the expression of these laws mathematically.

c., physiological. The study of the chemical nature of living matter and the changes occurring in the metabolic activities of plants and animals.

chemoceptor (kem'ō-sep-ter). A chemoreceptor, *q.v.*

chem'ocoagulation. Coagulation brought about by chemical agents.

chem'oreceptor. A sense organ or sensory nerve ending (as a taste bud) which is stimulated by a chemical substance.

chemore'flex [" + L. *reflectere,* to bend back]. Reflex resulting from chemical stimulus.

chemosis (ke-mo'sis) [G. *chēmē,* cockleshell, + *-ōsis,* infection]. Swelling of conjunctiva about the cornea.

chemotactic (kem-o-tak'tĭk) [G. *chēmeia,* chemistry, + *taxikos,* arranging]. Pert. to chemotaxis.

chemotaxis (kem-o-tak'sis) [" + *taxis,* arrangement]. Attraction and repulsion of living protoplasm to a chemical stimulus.

chemotherapy (kem-o-ther'a-pĭ) [" + *therapeia,* treatment]. Application of chemical reagents in treatment of disease, that have a specific and toxic effect on microorganism causing the disease, without harming the patient.

chemotic (kē-mot'ĭk). Pert. to chemosis.

chemotropism (kē-mot'ro-pizm) [" + *tropos,* direction]. Ability of impulse to progress or turn in a certain direction due to the influence of certain chemical stimuli, as the root of a plant toward its food supply.

chenopodium oil (ken-o-po'dĭ-um). USP. Oil of American wormseed. Colorless, a pale yellow volatile oil with pungent, irritating odor.

ACTION AND USES: Anthelmintic against hookworm.

cherophobia (ker-o-fo'bĭ-ă) [G. *chairein,* to rejoice, + *phobos,* fear]. Morbid fear of and aversion to gaiety.

cherries [G. *kerasion,* the fruit]. The fruit of the tree of the genus *Prunus, P. cerasus* bearing the sour variety of cherry and *P. avium* bearing the sweet fruit.

RAW: 100 gm. Calories: 58. Other main values: 1.2 gm. protein; 1 gm. fat; 14.3 gm. carbohydrates; 22 mg. calcium; 1000 I.U. vitamin A.

chest [A.S. *cest*, a box]. The thorax.

MENSURATION: *Object*: First, to ascertain the comparative bulk of the two sides; second, to ascertain amt. of expansion and retraction accompanying inspiration and expiration of the two sides.

The points of measurement are the spinous processes behind and the median line in front on the level of the 6th costosternal articulation. The right side is from half an inch to an inch larger than the left.

When a pleural cavity is distended with air or fluid the measurement of the affected side may exceed that of the healthy side by 2 or 3 inches; after removal of the fluid there may be an equal diminution in the measurement of the affected side, as compared with the healthy one. In emphysema the total difference bet. the fullest inspiration and fullest expiration on the affected side will scarcely exceed 1/16 of an inch, while on the other side there may be a difference of 2 or 3 inches.

PALPATION: Serves to detect any thoracic tenderness, edema, friction fremitus or râles, and to determine the vocal fremitus and amt. of expansion. Edema of chest walls is recognized by "pitting" when pressure is made with finger. It may be observed in empyema and in various types of dropsy.

The friction sound of pleurisy and harsh, sonorous râles can sometimes be detected by palpation. Thoracic tenderness is observed in pleurisy; pneumonia from being associated with pleurisy; in pleurodynia, in intercostal neuralgia (confined to certain spots); in surgical affections like caries, and fracture of the ribs; and in contusion and inflammation of the parietes.

PERCUSSION: *Precautions*: Place finger being used as a pleximeter firmly against chest and preferably parallel to ribs. Make finger which is used as plexor strike the one on chest perpendicularly, fix forearm, and use no more force than can be obtained from a gentle swing of the wrist. Percuss all parts of chest anteriorly and posteriorly, both in inspiration and expiration. In comparing sides be sure to percuss corresponding parts.

Normal Resonance: On the right side pulmonary resonance extends from half an inch to an inch above the clavicle, downward to upper border of 6th rib in front, and to a line drawn through the 10th spinous process posteriorly. On left side pulmonary resonance extends from a half inch to an inch above the clavicle downward, within the mammary line to the 10th rib and posteriorly to a line drawn through the 10th spinous process.

Cracked Pot Sound: Modified tympany, can be simulated by percussing over the cheek when mouth is partially open. May be normally heard over the chest of a crying infant. In the adult it usually indicates a cavity which has a free communication with a bronchus. Best detected by keeping ear near open mouth of patient while percussing.

Dullness or flatness is recognized in: (1) Tuberculous condition; (2) pneumonic consolidation; (3) pleural effusions of all kinds, except air; (4) collapse of lung; (5) congestion and edema of lung; (6) enlargement of liver or spleen (at base); (7) morbid growths in the lung.

It is important to determine the extent of movement of the diaphragms. To do this have the patient, while in a sitting position, hold his breath in deep inspiration. Then quickly percuss the chest on both sides posteriorly to find and mark the lowest point of pulmonary resonance. Repeat this while the patient holds his breath following complete expiration. On both sides of the chest the top and bottom marks should be from 2 to 6 cm. apart. The top line on the right is usually a cm. or two higher than the left due to the presence of the liver below the right diaphragm. Diseases which interfere with aeration of the lungs or which paralyze the diaphragms will cause the normal movement of the diaphragms to be altered.

Hyperresonance is observed in: (1) Pneumothorax; (2) cavities, tuberculous or bronchiectatic; (3) emphysema; (4) lowered pulmonary tension in the initial stage of pneumonia, and above a pleural effusion (Skoda's resonance); (5) flatulent distention of the stomach or colon frequently observed over the left base. A *tympanitic note* is a hollow, drumlike sound, like that which is normally obtained by percussing the larynx or empty stomach. The above conditions are also capable of producing tympany.

Pitch: Depends largely upon the volume of air, tension of walls of cavity, and upon size of opening that communicates with the cavity. The less the air the greater the tension, and the smaller the opening the higher will be the pitch of the note. In beginning tuberculous consolidation, the note over the affected apex is higher pitched. It must be remembered that normally the note over the right apex is higher pitched than that over the left.

Resistance: The greater the dullness the greater will be the resistance; therefore, there is always more resistance over a large pleural effusion than over a pneumonic or tuberculous consolidation.

RS: *breathing; fremitus; resonance; respiration; "thoraco-" words.*

c., emphysematous. In advanced emphysema thorax is short and round; anterior-posterior diameter is often as long as the transverse diameter; ribs are horizontal; angle formed by divergence of the costal margin from the sternum is very obtuse or quite obliterated. Often termed "barrel shaped."

c. prominences and depressions. An unnatural prominence or depression is often observed over the lower part of the sternum and is generally congenital. The term "funnel" breast or "shoemaker's" breast (because it may result from pressure of tools) has been applied to the sternal depression. The correct term is pectus excavatum.

A unilateral or local depression may be due to: (a) consolidation; (b) cavity; (c) pleurisy with fibrous adhesions.

A unilateral or local prominence may be due to: (a) Pleurisy with effusion; (b) pneumothorax, hydrothorax, hemothorax; (c) aneurysm or tumor; (d) compensatory emphysema, resulting from impairment of the opposite lung; (e) cardiac enlargements (left side); (f) enlargements of abdominal organs, esp. liver and spleen.

c., phthinoid. Ant. post. diameter is short, thorax long and flat, ribs oblique. Scapula prominent; spaces above and below clavicles are depressed. Angle formed by divergence of the costal margins from the sternum is very acute.

c., rachitic. May resemble phthinoid, but usually sides are considerably flattened and sternum prominent, so term pigeon breast has been applied. The sternal ends of the ribs are enlarged or "beaded" and this characteristic has given rise to the term "rachitic rosary." Is often a circular construction of the thorax at level of the xiphoid cartilage.

c. regions. Ant., post., and lateral. *Ant. Divisions* (R. and L.): Clavicular, infra- and supraclavicular, mammary and inframammary, upper and lower sternal. *Post. Divisions* (R. and L.): Scapular, infrascapular, interscapular and suprascapular. *Lateral Divisions*: Axillary and infra-axillary. C. symptoms, *q.v.*

chest expansion, normal. In the male, 2 in.; in the female, 2½ in. *Capacity*: Normal male, 22 yr. old, 5.8 ft., 230 to 240 cu. in. Normal female, 19 yr. old, 5.25 ft., 145 to 150 cu. in. Expansion denotes capacity of air taken into lungs. This varies with age, the young adult having a greater capacity than the aged. Those given to exercise or physical work have a greater lung capacity than others.

Cheyne-Stokes respiration [John Cheyne, Scottish physician, 1777-1836, and William Stokes, Irish physician, 1804-1878]. An irregular or cyclic type of arrhythmic breathing occurring in certain acute diseases of the central nervous system, heart, lungs, and in intoxications.

At first it is slow and shallow, then it increases in rapidity and depth until it

APNEA

Diagram illustrating the respiratory movements in Cheyne-Stokes breathing.

reaches a maximum. Then it decreases gradually until it stops for 10 to 20 seconds, then repeating in the same manner. It may occur in heart failure, intracranial pressure, cerebral disease, or drug sensitivity; all of which interfere with the blood-oxygen supply to the centers in the brain which control respiration.

Chiari's deformity (kē-ar'ēz). SEE: *Arnold-Chiari deformity.*

chiasm, chiasma (ki'azm, ki-az'ma) [G. from *chiazen,* to mark with letter X]. A crossing or decussation.

c., optic. An incomplete crossing of the optic fibers (the outer fibers not crossing each other); the point of crossing of the fibers of the optic nerves.

chicken [A.S. *cicen*]. Dark meat without skin, fried: 100 gm. Calories: 220. Protein 30.4 gm.; fat 9.3 gm.; carbohydrate 1.5 gm.; calcium 14 mg.; 130 I.U. vitamin A.

Light meat fried without skin has almost the same food value as dark meat. It contains about 10% fewer Calories, 7% more protein, two-thirds as much fat and less than half as much vitamin A.

c. breast. Abnormal prominence of the sternum. SYN: *pectus carinatum; pigeon b.*

c. fat clot. A yellowish blood clot after death.

chickenpox. Varicella; a mild, highly contagious disease, marked by an eruption of vesicles on skin and mucous membranes. SEE: *varicella.*

chig'gers. Redbugs. The six-legged larvae of mites of the family Trombiculidae, order Acarina of the class Arachnida. Also called rougets, harvest mites, scrub mites. They are parasitic on insects, various vertebrates, and man. Eggs are laid on the ground and hatch in about 12 days, after which they attach to host at first opportunity. The redbugs attach themselves to the surface of the skin and inject a salivary secretion which dissolves the surrounding tissues. A tubular structure, a *stylostome,* is developed which is used in ingesting the semidigested tissue debris. The mites do not feed on blood. The most common species attacking humans in N. America is *Trombicula alfreddugesi.* The irritation is the result of sensitization to the injected saliva. To prevent being infested when exposed, wear clothes which are tight at the neck and arms and stuff pant legs into shoe with high tops. DDT powder or diethyltoluamide (Off) will repel chiggers.

TREATMENT: Commercial preparations are available which, when applied to the affected area, asphyxiate the mite. One of these, Kwell, contains hexachlorohexane. Benzyl benzoate ointment is also effective.

chigo, chigre (chē'go, chē'grā) [Sp.]. A jigger or sand flea.

chilblain (chil'blān) [A.S. *cele,* cold, + *blegen,* to boil]. Inflammation and swelling of the feet, toes, or fingers caused by cold, damp atmosphere. Also called *frostbite; pernio.*

SYM: Reddish, violaceous plaques or patches on hands and feet, occasionally the ears. Persistent, giving rise to smarting, burning, itching, esp. when parts become warm. In severe types frostbite corresponds to second degree burns, showing vesicles, bullae, ulcer, and necrosis.

NP: If circulation is not restored, warm gradually by placing parts in lukewarm water or with warm hands. Do *not* rub. Place patient in warm but not hot room; give warm nutritious drinks (no alcohol). Protect the part from abrasion of bed clothes by using a cradle.

TREATMENT: Analgesics, antibiotics, anticoagulants, and vasodilators are used to attempt to prevent loss of blood supply to the affected area.

SEE: *windchill; windchill factor.*

child [A.S. *cild*]. A young person of either sex, bet. infancy and puberty. SEE: *pediatrics.*

child'bed. Puerperium. Period during and immediately subsequent to parturition.

c. b. fever. Puerperal sepsis, *q.v.*

childbirth. The process of bringing forth a child; parturition. SEE: *labor.*

child crowing. Spasmodic closure of glottis, of brief duration, and succeeded by noisy inspiration. SYN: *laryngismus stridulus.*

chilectro'pion [G. *cheilos,* lip, + *ektropos,* turning out]. Eversion of the lip or cheilectropion.

chilitis (ki-li'tis) [" + *-itis,* inflammation]. Inflammation of the lips. SEE: *cheilitis.*

chill (chĭl) [A.S. *cele,* cold]. An attack of shivering accompanied by the sensation of coldness and pallor of the skin. It is due to a disturbance in the temperature-regulating centers of the hypothalamus.

Chills accompany various diseases, esp. malaria and pneumococcal pneumonia, and are coarse or fine, diffuse, trembling, etc. SEE: *windchill.*

ETIOL: Infections or diseases (as malaria, pneumococcal pneumonia, bacteremia), parasites in blood, bacterial vaccines, and transfusion reactions. Postoperative chills or chills in puerperium indicative of infection.

SYM: A real chill is ushered in by extreme sensation of cold, shivering, chattering of the teeth and, in extreme cases, a marked tremor of the entire body followed by a rapidly rising temperature.

NP: (a) Make patient comfortable by supplying external heat and extra blanket. (b) Give hot drink when permitted or tolerated. (c) Give patient moral support. (d) Take temperature as soon as possible, then again about 20 minutes after chill subsides. (e) Chart a report to attending physician, duration and degree of severity of chills, and temperature. SEE: *ague.*

c., nervous. Accompanied by a chilly sensation but not with fever. It may follow severe pain or extreme nervousness. It usually passes quickly and is seldom serious.

chilo-, cheilo- [G. *cheilos,* lip]. Prefix denoting relationship to the lip.

chiloangioscopy (kī-lō-an-jĭ-os′kō-pĭ) [G. *cheilos,* lip, + *aggeion,* vessel, + *skopein,* to examine]. Microscopic examination of the circulation in the lip.

chilognathopalatoschisis (kī-log″nath-o-pal-ă-tos′kis-is) [" + *gnathos,* jaw, + L. *palatum,* palate, + G. *schisis,* fissure]. Fissure of the lip, palate, and alveolar process.

Chilomas′tix mesnil′i. A species of Mastigophora. A nonpathogenic protozoa which is parasitic in the intestines.

chiloschisis (ki-los′kis-is) [G. *cheilos,* lip, + *schisis,* fissure]. Harelip.

chilostomatoplasty (kī-los-to′mă-to-plas″-tĭ) [" + *stoma,* mouth, + *plassein,* to form]. Plastic operation for harelip.

chim′ney-sweeps′ cancer. Epithelioma of the scrotum. Due to chronic irritation by coal soot.

chin [AS. *cin,* chin]. Point of the lower jaw; mentum; region below lower lip.

c. cough. Pertussis, *q.v.*

c. jerk. Reflex contraction of muscles of mastication on suddenly depressing the jaw.

c. reflex. Clonic movement resulting from percussing or stroking lower jaw.

chionablepsia (kī-on-ab-lep′sĭ-ă) [G. *chiōn,* snow, + *ablepsia,* blindness]. Snow blindness.

chiragra (kī-răg-ră). Pain in the hand.

chiralgia (kī-răl′jĭ-ă). Pain in the hand of nontraumatic or neuralgic origin.

c. paresthetica. Numbness and pain in the hand esp. in the region supplied by the radial nerve.

chirapsia (kī-răp′sĭ-ă) [G. *cheirapsia,* a touching with the hands]. Friction; massage.

chirismus (kī-rĭs′mŭs). Spasm of hand muscles.

chirognostic (kī-rog-nos′tĭk) [G. *cheir,* hand, + *gnōstikos,* knowing]. Having the ability to distinguish the right from the left, or the side of body being stimulated.

chirokinesthesia (kī-rō-kin-ĕs-thē′sĭ-ă) [" + *kinēsis,* movement, + *aisthēsis,* sensation]. Subjective perception of motions of the hand.

chiromeg′aly [" + *megas,* large]. Enlargement of the hands, wrists, or ankles.

chi′roplasty [" + *plassein,* to form]. A plastic operation on the hand.

chiropodist (kī-rop′o-dist, kī-) [" + *pous,* foot]. One who practices chiropody.

chiropody (kī-rop′ō-dĭ) [" + *pous,* foot]. Treatment of minor disorders of the feet.

chiropompholyx (kī-rō-pom′fō-liks) [" + *pompholyx,* a bubble]. Inflammatory disease of skin confined to hands and feet. SYN: *pompholyx, q.v.*

chiropractic (kī-rō-prak′tik) [" + L. *practos,* done with the hand]. A system of manipulative treatment which teaches that all diseases are caused by impingement on spinal nerves and can be corrected by spinal adjustments.

chi′ropractor. One who practices chiropractic methods.

chirospasm (ki′ro-spazm) [" + *spasmos,* spasm]. Spasmodic affection of muscles of hand, or writers′ cramp.

chirurgery (ki-rur′jer-ĭ) [" + *ergon,* work]. Surgery.

chirurgia (ki-rur′jĭ-ă). Surgery.

chirurgical (ki-rur′jĭk-al). Surgical.

chitin (kī′tin). A white horny substance in outer covering of body of invertebrates such as crabs. Also occurs in some fungi.

chitinous (ki′tin-us) [G. *chitōn,* a tunic]. Pertaining to or composed of chitin.

c. degeneration. Amyloid degeneration.

chloasma (klo-az′mă) [G. *chloazein,* to be green]. Pigmentary skin discolorations, usually those occurring in yellowish brown patches or spots.

SYM: Areas rounded or oval with ill-defined margins, light yellow to black. In those due to external factors pigmentation develops only at sight of irritation or beyond. In symptomatic forms constitutional cause underlies.

TREATMENT: Constitutional when indicated.

c. gravida′rum. Brownish pigmentation of the face, often occurring in pregnancy. It usually disappears after delivery. Also seen in some persons who take progestational agents. SYN: *Mask of pregnancy.*

c. hepaticum. So-called "liver spot" following dyspepsia.

c., idiopathic. C. caused by external agents, such as sun, heat, mechanical means, x-rays, etc.

c., symptomatic. C. caused by various diseases, as syphilis or cancer.

c. traumaticum. Skin discolorations from traumatic agencies.

c. uteri′num. Chloasma of pregnancy and seen in other uterine conditions.

chloral (klo′ral). 1. An oily liquid having a bitter taste. 2. Chloral hydrate.

c. hydrate. USP. Colorless, transparent crystals having aromatic, slightly acrid odor, and caustic, faintly bitter taste; soluble in alcohol and water.

ACTION AND USES: As a sedative and hypnotic.

POISONING: *Sym:* Depresses and eventually paralyzes the central nervous system. Can be toxic to the liver. There may be nausea and vomiting due to gastric irritation. Pulse is feeble, respirations are shallow and irregular, lassitude, weakness, dizziness, sleep.

F. A. TREATMENT: Gastric lavage with coffee or tea. Central nervous system stimulants by mouth, injection, or rectum. Artificial respiration, Trendelenburg position, I.V. glucose. SEE: *Table of Poisons and Poisoning in Appendix.*

chloramines (klō'ră-mĭns). Organic chlorine compounds which decompose slowly liberating chlorine. Used extensively in dairies, food manufacturing establishments, etc., as a germicide. Ex: *chloramine-T; dichloramine-T.*

chloramphenicol (klor-ăm-phĕn'i-cŏl). USP. An antibiotic originally isolated from *Streptomyces venezuelae.* It is now made synthetically. It is a broad-spectrum agent and is especially useful in typhoid fever (in which it is the antibiotic of choice) and other infections caused by Salmonellae, and in rickettsial infections.

CAUTION: Certain blood dyscrasias may follow the use of chloramphenicol, consequently it should *not* be used indiscriminately or for minor infections. If used for prolonged periods, careful blood checks should be made. Be sure to read the literature which comes with each package of this medicine prior to deciding to use it rather than another antibiotic.

chloranemia (klor-a-ne'mĭ-ă) [G. *chlōros,* green, + *a-,* priv. + *aima,* blood]. A form of iron-deficiency anemia, *q.v.* SEE UNDER: *anemia.*

chlorate (klo'rāt). A salt of chloric acid. SEE: *potassium chlorate.*

chlorbu'tanol. Chlorobutanol, *q.v.*

chlorcosane (klor-co-sān') (chlorinated paraffin). Used as a solvent for dichloramine T, *q.v.*

chlorcy'clizine hydrochloride. USP. Official name for 1-(p-chlorobenzhydryl)-4-methylpiperazine hydrochloride, an antihistaminic drug.

chloremia (klo-re'mĭ-ă) [G. *chlōros,* green, + *aima,* blood]. 1. Anemia with diminution of hemoglobin and decrease in number of red corpuscles. SEE: *chlorosis* under *anemia.* 2. Excess chloride in the blood.

chlorephidrosis (klor-ef-ĭ-dro'sis) [" + *ephidrōsis,* perspiration]. Greenish perspiration.

chloretone (klō'rĕ-tōn). Proprietary name for chlorobutanol, *q.v.*

chlorhydria (klor-hi'drĭ-ă) [" + *ydōr,* water]. Excess of hydrochloric acid in stomach.

chloride (klō'rĭd) [G. *chlōros,* green]. A binary compound of chlorine; a salt of hydrochloric acid. Blood serum contains 100-110 mEq./L. (350-390 mg./100 ml.) principally as sodium chloride. Chlorides are increased in nephritis, eclampsia, anemia, and cardiac disease; decreased in fevers, diabetes, and pneumonia.

c., test for in urine. To a test tube half filled with urine is added a drop or 2 of nitric acid, which holds the phosphates in solution. Then a 3% solution of silver nitrate is added to the specimen, drop by drop, till about 6 drops have passed. This forms a white, curdled precipitate at once. The test should be compared with a known normal specimen of urine. *Diminished chlorides* are found in chronic nephritis, early stages of pneumonia, malignant disease, and in gastritis. Chlorides are increased in a diet rich in salt, in rickets, and hepatic cirrhosis.

chloridemia (klor-ĭ-de'mĭ-ă) [" + *aima,* blood]. Chlorides in the blood.

chloridim'eter [" + *metron,* measure]. An instrument for estimating amt. of chlorides in a fluid. SYN: *chloridometer.*

chloridimetry (klor-ĭ-dim'e-trĭ). Determination of amt. of chlorides in the body fluids.

chloridom'eter. Same as chloridimeter, *q.v.*

chloriduria (klor-ĭ-dū'rĭ-ă) [G. *chlōros,* green, + *ouron,* urine]. Presence or excess of chlorides in urine.

chlorinated (klor'in-ā-ted) [G. *chlōros,* green]. Impregnated with chlorine.

c. lime. Calcium hypochlorite widely used in solution as a bleach and as an antiseptic.

chlorina'tion. Treatment of water by addition of chlorine and its compounds for the killing of bacteria. For effective disinfection, a concentration of 0.5 to 1 part of chlorine per million parts of water is necessary.

chlorine (klo'rēn) [G. *chlōros,* green]. SYMB: Cl. A highly irritating gas and destructive to the mucous membranes of the respiratory passages. It is very poisonous and excessive inhalation may cause death. Carefully inhaling ammonia or alcohol will counteract the effects of chlorine inhalation. Chlorine is an active bleaching agent and germicide. Both of these effects are due to its oxidizing powers. It is used extensively in the disinfection of water supplies and in treatment of sewage. It is a chemical element. At. wt. 35.453; at. no. 17.

FUNCTIONS: Chlorine is found combined with sodium in the blood and exercises some influence upon metabolism, helps to maintain osmotic pressure, and aids in the regulation and stimulation of muscular action. The body fluids contain 0.85% salt solution. The inorganic salts keep in solution the proteins of the blood, milk, and other secretions. Chlorine is present in the hydrochloric acid of the gastric juice. It aids digestion, activates enzymes, and is essential to normal gastric secretion.

EXCRETION: The excretion of chlorine during a 31-day fast measured from 3.77 gm. on the first day to 0.13 gm. on the last day of the fast. It leaves the body in the form of chloride ions.

c. preparations. Those used for disinfecting.

Compounds (hypochlorites), as Dakin's solution or Javelle water, are very effective in their germicidal power. As a disinfecting agent in washing dishes and utensils used by infected patients, 1/10 of 1% solution should be used; the dishes should then be washed well in soap and hot water and rinsed well, or boiled and then washed well after the boiling.

STOOLS: For disinfection of the stools of patients, 5% or even stronger solutions may be used for one-half hour or longer. The utensil is set aside and covered while the solution functions. Dakin's solution is nonirritating and is used as a wound disinfectant, but it must be carefully prepared daily by the laboratory and used only when fresh.

chlorite (klo'rīt). A salt of chlorous acid; used as a disinfectant and bleaching agent.

chlormerodrin (klor-mer'o-drin). Generic name, [3-(chloromercuri-2-methoxy-propylurea)], an orally effective mercurial diuretic.

chloroanemia (klor-o-ă-ne'mĭ-ă) [G. *chlōros,* green, + *a-,* priv. + *aima,* blood]. A type of iron-deficiency anemia, *q.v.* SEE UNDER: *anemia.*

chloroazodin (klŏr-ō-ăz'ō-dĭn). a, a, Azobis-(chloroformamidine), a germicidal preparation of chlorine.

chlorobutanol (klō-ro-bū'tă-nol). USP. Colorless crystals, with camphor odor and taste. SYN: *chlorbutanol; chlorbutol.*

USES: Antiseptic and local anesthetic, and as a preservative in many pharmaceuticals.

INCOMPATIBILITIES: Decomposed by alkalies, and should not be mixed with borax, carbonates, etc. Soluble in ether, chloroform, and volatile oils.

chlor'oform [L. *chloroformum*]. $CHCl_3$. USP. A heavy, clear, colorless liquid with strong ethereal odor, formed by the action of chlorinated lime on methyl alcohol.

ACTION AND USES: A general anesthetic, having a small margin of safety. Locally an irritant used in liniments. Internally a carminative and sedative.

c. anesthesia. For some time chloroform anesthesia was more popular than ether. It is 6 times as strong, but it was found to be more harmful.

When employed, the chloroform is well diluted with air. It is not flammable except when mixed with alcohol, although volatile at low temperatures. It tends to decompose and to form hydrochloric acid and carbonyl chloride. Chloroform should be kept in tightly closed, dark containers in a cool place with temperature not exceeding 85° F.

ADVANTAGES: The period of excitement following anesthesia is relatively short. It does not irritate the mucous membranes and it produces excellent muscular relaxation. Neither does it cause excessive secretion of the respiratory mucous membrane. It has a pleasant odor and it acts more agreeably than some other anesthetics.

PHYSIOLOGICAL ACTION: When inhaled it is promptly absorbed through the mucous membranes of the respiratory tract. After being eliminated by the lungs it seems to remain unchanged.

DANGERS: Dangerous symptoms may develop very suddenly. Circulatory depression may develop with cardiac arrest. It is a severe cardiac and respiratory depressant. It lowers body temperature and blood pressure. It produces toxic changes in body chemistry, and is very detrimental to the bladder and kidney functioning. It should never be given without plenty of oxygen. This form of anesthesia should not be used for a patient with disease of the heart, liver, or kidneys. Because it is not flammable it may be used when work is to be done with a cautery, diathermy, or when the x-ray is used around the head or mouth. It also may be used in acute pulmonary pathology.

chloroformism (klo'ro-form-izm). The habit of inhaling chloroform and the resulting symptoms.

chloroguanide hydrochloride (klor"ō-gwan'id). An antimalarial compound.

chloroleukemia (klo-ro-lū-ke'mĭ-ă) [G. *chlōros*, green, + *leukos*, white, + *aima*, blood]. Leukemia with chlorosis.

chloroma (klo-ro'mă) [" + *-ōma*, growth]. A greenish sarcoma of the periosteum of cranial bones; "green cancer."

chloromycetin (klor-ō-mī-sē'tĭn). Proprietary name for chloramphenicol, *q.v.*

chloromyeloma (klo-ro-mī-ĕ-lō'mă) [" + *myelos*, marrow, + *-ōma*, growth]. Chloroma accompanied by multiple growths in bone marrow.

chloropenia (klo-ro-pe'nĭ-ă) [" + *penēs*, poor]. Deficiency in chlorine; hypochloremia.

chloropenic (klo-ro-pēn'ik). Deficient in chlorine.

chlorophane (klo'ro-fān) [G. *chlōros*, green, + *phainein*, to show]. A green-yellow pigment in the retina.

chlorophenothane (klo"rō-phĕn'o-thān). USP. An insecticide, used especially to prevent helminthic, malarial and other infestations of man. SYN: *DDT*.

chlorophyll, chlorophyl (klo'ro-fĭl) [" + *phyllon*, leaf]. The green coloring matter in plants consisting of chlorophyll *a* and chlorophyll *b*. It acts as a catalytic agent in the process of photosynthesis in which carbon dioxide from the air reacts with water from the soil to form simple carbohydrates, which are used for energy or converted into more complex substances and stored.

Chemically it is quite similar to hemoglobin except the element in chlorophyll which corresponds to iron in hemoglobin is magnesium.

chloro'pia [" + *opsis*, vision]. Vision in which all things appear green.

chloroplast. Small round green bodies found in the cells of leaves and stem of plants which are important in the process of photosynthesis. They possess a stroma and contain four pigments: chlorophyll *a*, chlorophyll *b*, carotene, and xanthophyll.

chloroplas'tid [G. *chlōros*, green, + *plastos*, form]. A chloroplast, *q.v.*

chloroprivic (klor-o-priv'ĭk) [" + L. *privāre*, to deprive of]. Lack of, or due to loss of, chlorides.

chlorop'sia [" + *opsis*, vision]. Vision in which all things seem green. SYN: *chloropia*.

chloroquine phosphate. USP. $C_{18}H_{26}ClN_3 \cdot 2H_3PO_4$. A white crystalline powder used for its antimicrobial action, especially in the treatment of malaria. It is useful also in amebic dysentery complicated by liver abscess.

chlorosarco'ma [" + *sarx*, flesh, + *-ōma*, tumor]. Sarcomatous form of chloroma.

chloro'sis [" + *-ōsis*, infection]. A form of iron-deficiency anemia, *q.v.* SEE UNDER: *anemia*.

chlorotic (klo-rot'ĭk). Of the nature of or afflicted with chlorosis.

chloroxyl (klō-roks'il). Cinchophen hydrochloride.

chlorpromazine (klor-prō'mă-zēn). A tranquilizing agent, it is used, primarily in its hydrochloride form, in major and minor psychotic states. Also used for the prevention of motion sickness. Proprietary name is thorazine.

chlortetracycline (klor-tĕt-ră-sī'klēn). A golden colored antibiotic isolated from a strain of *Streptomyces aureofaciens*. It is a broad-spectrum antibiotic, inhibiting growth of or destroying some strains of streptococci, staphylococci, pneumococci, rickettsiae, and viruses. Proprietary name is Aureomycin.

Ch.M. Abbr. for *Chirur'giae magis'ter*, Master of Surgery.

choana (kō'ă-nă) (pl. *choanae*). A funnel-shaped opening, especially one of the posterior nares, the communicating passageways between the nasal fossae and the pharynx.

choanoid (ko'an-oyd) [" + *eidos*, shape]. Shaped like a funnel.

chocolate [Sp. from Mexican *choco*, cacao, + *latl*, water]. 1. Preparation made by grinding roasted cacao or theobroma seeds. 2. Beverage prepared by dissolving chocolate in water or milk. SEE: *cocoa*.

choke. 1. To strangle or suffocate. 2. To check progress, growth, or an action.

choked disk. Inflammation of the optic disk. Also called papillitis or optic neuritis. SEE: *disk*.

chokes. Respiratory symptoms such as substernal distress, paroxysmal cough, tachypnea, or asphyxia which may occur in decompression illness especially in cases of aeroembolism resulting from exposure to pressure lower than atmospheric.

choking [A.S. *aceocian*, to suffocate]. Obstruction within respiratory passage or constriction about the neck, interfering with breathing and circulation of brain. May also result from spasm of the larynx induced by an irritating gas.

Sym: Face purple, eyes protrude, arms thrown about, coughing. Constriction and injury about neck, cyanosis, dizziness, unconsciousness.

Treatment: Remove constriction. Artificial respiration. Slap violently on back. Severe blow bet. shoulders. With children, compress chest with the hands squeezing suddenly and vigorously. If foreign body in throat, such as meat, insert thumb and forefinger and try to grasp it. If child, grasp by legs and hold upside down for a moment. If the article is swallowed, do not give purgative. If lodged in throat and breathing is possible, interference should be limited until professional aid is at hand. Tracheotomy may be needed.

cholago'gia [G. *cholē*, bile, + *agein*, to lead forth]. Excretion of bile from gallbladder.

cholagogue (kō'lă-gŏg) [G. *cholē*, bile, + *agein*, to lead forth]. An agent which increases the flow of bile into the intestine, *i.e.*, a choleretic, or cholecystagogue.

cholangiogastrostomy (ko-lan"jĭ-o-gas-tros'to-mĭ) [" + *aggeion*, vessel, + *gastēr*, stomach, + *stoma*, mouth]. Formation of a communication bet. bile duct and the stomach.

cholangiography (ko-lan-jĭ-og'ră-fĭ) [" + " + *graphein*, to write]. X-ray or skiagraphic examination of the bile ducts.

cholangioma (ko-lan-jĭ-o'mă) [" + " + *-ōma*, tumor]. A tumor of the biliary ducts.

cholangiostomy (kō-lan-jĭ-ŏs'tō-mĭ) [" + " + *stoma*, mouth]. The surgical formation of a fistula into the gallbladder.

cholangiotomy (kō-lan-jĭ-ŏt'ō-mĭ) [" + " + *tomē*, incision]. Incision of an intrahepatic bile duct for removal of gallstones.

cholangitis (kō-lăn-jĭ'tĭs) [G. *cholē*, bile, + *aggeion*, vessel, + *-itis*, inflammation]. Inflammation of the bile ducts.

cholascos (ko-las'kos) [" + *askos*, bag]. Escape of bile into the peritoneal cavity.

cholecyst (kō'lē-sĭst) [G. *cholē*, bile, + *kystis*, cyst]. The gallbladder, *q.v.*

cholecystalgia (ko-lē-sis-tal'jĭ-ă) [" + " + *algos*, pain]. Biliary colic.

cholecystectasia (ko-lē-sis-tĕk-tā'zĭ-ă) [" + " + *ektasis*, dilatation]. Dilatation of the gallbladder.

cholecystectomy (ko-lē-sis-tĕk'tō-mĭ) [" + " + *ektomē*, excision]. Excision of a gallbladder.

cholecystendysis (ko-lē-sis-tĕn'dĭ-sis) [" + " + *endysis*, entrance]. Removal of a gallstone by incision, suturing wound in gallbladder and abdominal wall.

cholecystenterorrhaphy (ko-le-sis-ten-ter-or'ă-fĭ) [" + " + *enteron*, intestine, + *raphē*, suture]. Suture of gallbladder to intestinal wall.

cholecystenterostomy (kō-lē-sĭs-tĕn-ter-ŏs'tō-mĭ) [G. *cholē*, bile, + *kystis*, cyst, + *enteron*, intestine, + *stoma*, opening]. The establishment of a connection between the gallbladder and the small intestine.

cholecystic (ko-le-sis'tĭk) [" + *kystis*, cyst]. Pert. to the gallbladder.

cholecystitis (ko-lē-sis-tī'tis) [" + " + *-itis*, inflammation]. Inflammation of the gallbladder. It may be acute or chronic.

Etiol: *Acute c.* nearly always caused by gallstones. Other causes may be bacteria or chemical irritants. *Chronic c.* may be with or without stones.

Sym: *Acute c.*—Fever, gradually developing or sudden pain in upper abdomen, nausea and vomiting. Visible jaundice in about 25% of patients. Approximately 10% of patients do not have pain. *Chronic c.*—Less severe than in acute c., but recurring. May be with or without stones.

Treatment: *Acute c.*—Cholecystectomy; if this is not possible, draining of gallbladder (cholecystostomy) followed by cholecystectomy at a later date. *Chronic c.*—If stones are present, cholecystectomy is treatment. If there are no stones, antispasmodics, laxatives, rest, and sedation if necessary, and further study to determine cause.

NP: *Postoperative*—Patient in bed in semi-Fowler position to aid drainage. Inspect dressing for bleeding and drainage tube. If tube is present, check to be sure it is fastened securely to dressing. Inspect dressings, check pulse rate and blood pressure frequently during first 24 hours. Observe color of skin, sclera, urine, stools, for evidence of jaundice. Encourage patient to move from side to side and to take deep breaths. This is essential to help prevent postoperative complications. Be alert for complications as shock or hemorrhage. Maintain drainage, check for obstruction of drainage tube by patient's position, chart amount of drainage every 24 hours. Low-fat diet.

cholecystnephrostomy (ko"le-sist-nĕ-fros'-tō-mi) [" + " + *nephros*, kidney, + *stoma*, mouth]. Making an anastomosis of gallbladder into renal pelvis.

cholecystocolostomy (ko-le-sis-to-ko-los'-to-mĭ) [" + " + *kolon*, colon, + *stoma*, mouth]. Making a passage from gallbladder to colon.

cholecystocolotomy (ko-le-sis-to-ko-lot'-o-mi) [" + " + *tomē*, incision]. Incision into gallbladder and colon.

cholecystoduodenostomy (kol-e-sis-to-du-o-dē-nos'to-mĭ) [" + " + L. *duodeni*, twelve, + G. *stoma*, mouth]. Surgical formation of a passage from gallbladder to duodenum.

cholecystogastrostomy (ko-le-sis-to-gas-tros'to-mĭ) [" + " + *gastēr*, belly, + *stoma*, mouth]. Surgical formation of a passage from the gallbladder to the stomach.

cholecys'togram [" + " + *gramma*, mark]. An x-ray picture of the gallbladder.

cholecystography (ko-le-sis-tog'ră-fĭ) [" + " + *graphein*, to write]. Examination of the gallbladder by x-ray.

cholecystoileostomy (ko-le-sis-to-ĭl-e-os'-to-mĭ) [" + " + L. *ileum* + G. *stoma*, mouth]. Forming a communication bet. the gallbladder and ileum.

cholecystojejunostomy (ko-le-sis-to-je-ju-nos'to-mĭ) [" + " + L. *jejunum*, empty, + *stoma*, mouth]. Forming a communication bet. the gallbladder and jejunum.

cholecystokinin (ko"le-sĭs"tō-kĭ'nĭn) [" + " + *kinein*, to move]. A hormone secreted by the mucosa of the duodenum which induces contraction of the gallbladder.

cholecystolithiasis (ko-le-sis-to-lĭ-thī'ă-sis) [" + " + *lithos*, stone]. Gallstones in the gallbladder.

cholecystolithotripsy (ko-le-sis-to-lith'o-trip-sĭ) [" + " + " + *tripsis*, a crushing]. Crushing of a gallstone in the unopened gallbladder.

cholecys'tomy [" + " + *tomē*, incision]. Cholecystotomy, *q.v.*

cholecystopathy (ko-le-sis-top'ă-thĭ) [" + " + *pathos*, disease]. Any gallbladder affection.

cholecystopexy (ko-le-sis'to-pek-sĭ) [" + " + *pēxis*, fixation]. Suturing the gallbladder to the abdominal wall.

cholecystoptosis (ko-le-sis-top-to'sis) [" + " + *ptōsis*, fall]. Displacement of the gallbladder downward.

cholecystorrhaphy (kō-lē-sis-tor'ă-fĭ) [" + " + *raphē*, suture]. Suturing of the gallbladder.

cholecystostomy (kol-e-sis-tos'to-mĭ) [" + " + *stoma*, opening]. Surgical formation of an opening into gallbladder through abdominal wall.

cholecystotomy (ko-le-sis-tot'o-mĭ) [" + " + *tomē*, incision]. Incision of gallbladder through the abdominal walls for removal of gallstones.

choledochal (kō-lē-dŏk'ăl). Relating or pertaining to the common bile duct.

choledochectasia (ko-led"-o-kek-ta'zĭ-ă) [G. *choledochos*, common bile duct, + *ektasis*, distention]. Distention of the common bile duct.

choledochectomy (kŏ-led"ō-kek'tō-mĭ). Excision of a portion of the common bile duct.

choledochitis (ko-led"o-ki'tis) [" + *-itis*, inflammation]. Inflammation of common bile duct.

choledochoduodenostomy (ko-led"o-ko-du-o-dē-nos'to-mĭ) [" + L. *duodeni*, twelve, + G. *stoma*, opening]. Surgical communication bet. the common bile duct and duodenum.

choledochoenterostomy (ko-led"o-ko-en-ter-os'to-mĭ) [" + *enteron*, intestine, + *stoma*, opening]. Surgical passage bet. common bile duct and intestine.

choledochography (kō-lĕd"ō-kog'ră-phē). The photographing by x-ray of the bile duct following administration of a radiopaque substance.

choledocholithiasis (ko-led"o-ko-lĭ-thī'ă-sis) [" + *lithos*, stone]. Calculi in the common bile duct.

choledocholithotomy (ko-led"o-ko-lith-ot'-o-mĭ) [" + " + *tomē*, incision]. Removal of a gallstone through an incision of the bile duct.

choledocholithotripsy (ko-led-o-ko-lith'o-trip-sĭ) [" + " + *tripsis*, a crushing]. Crushing of a gallstone in the common bile duct.

choledochoplasty (ko-led'o-ko-plas"tĭ) [" + *plassein*, to form]. Operation for repair of common bile duct.

choledochorrhaphy (ko-led-o-kor'ă-fĭ) [" + *raphē*, suture]. Suturing the severed ends of the common bile duct.

choledochostomy (ko-led"o-kos'to-mĭ) [" + *stoma*, mouth]. Surgical formation of an opening into common bile duct through abdominal wall.

choledochotomy (ko-led"o-kot'o-mĭ) [" + *tomē*, incision]. Surgical incision of the common bile duct.

choledochus (ko-led'o-kus) [G. *cholē*, bile, + *dechesthai*, to receive]. The common bile duct. SYN: *ductus choledochus.*

cholehemia (ko-le-he'mĭ-ă) [" + *aima*, blood]. Cholemia, *q.v.*

choleic (ko-le'ĭk). Cholic; pert. to the bile.

chol'elith [G. *cholē*, bile, + *lithos*, stone]. A biliary concretion or gallstone.

cholelithiasis (kol-e-lĭ-thī'as-is) [" + *lithos*, stone]. Formation or presence of calculi or bilestones in the gallbladder or common duct.

They may remain dormant or be responsible for few symptoms.

SYM: Digestive disturbances; heaviness in right hypochondrium, tenderness on pressure over gallbladder. Gallstone colic when passing through bile duct if obstructed. Pain may radiate to back and right shoulder. Colic usually manifest when stomach is empty. Jaundice if flow of bile is obstructed. Pain may be associated with vomiting and sweating. Gallbladder may be palpated if distended.

TREATMENT: Cholecystectomy; in very poor-risk patients, cholecystostomy.

cholelithic (ko-le-lith'ĭk). Pert. to or caused by biliary calculus.

cholelithotomy (ko-le-lĭ-thot'o-mĭ) [G. *cholē*, bile, + *lithos*, stone, + *tomē*, incision]. Removal of gallstones through a surgical incision.

cholelithotripsy (kō-lē-lith'ō-trĭp-sē). Same as cholelithotrity, *q.v.*

cholelithotrity (ko-le-lĭ-thot'rĭ-tĭ) [" + " + L. *tritus*, crushing]. Crushing of a biliary calculus.

cholemesis (kol-em'e-sis) [" + *emein*, to vomit]. Bile in the vomitus.

cholemia (ko-le'mĭ-ă) [" + *aima*, blood]. Bile or its pigments in the blood.

cholemic state (kō-lē'mĭk). A condition of stupor and delirium which progress into somnambulence and coma, accompanied by intense jaundice, seen in final stages of Laennec's cirrhosis or in carcinoma of the liver.

cholepathia (ko-le-path'ĭ-ă) [" + *pathos*, disease]. Faulty contractions of bile ducts.

c. spas'tica. Spasmodic contraction of biliary ducts.

choleperitoneum (ko-le-per-ĭ-to-ne'um) [" + *peri*, around, + *teinein*, to stretch]. Bile in the peritoneum.

cholepoiesis (ko-le-poy-ē'sis). The formation of bile.

cholepyrrhin (ko-le-pir'ĭn) [" + *pyrros*, flame colored]. Impure bilirubin. SYN: *biliphein.*

chol'era [" + *rein*, to flow]. An acute, specific, infectious disease characterized by diarrhea with severe loss of fluids and electrolytes, painful cramps of muscles, and tendency to collapse. Also called *Asiatic c.*, *Indian c.*, *algid c.*, *asphyctic c.*, *epidemic c.*, *malignant c.*, and *pestilential c.*

ETIOL: Causative organism, *Vibrio comma* (also called *Vibrio cholerae*, cholera bacillus, comma bacillus, Koch's bacillus), a short, curved, motile, gram-negative rod which produces a potent endotoxin which interferes with cellular metabolism, and a mucolytic enzyme. Transmission is through water, milk, or other foods contaminated with excreta of patients or carriers.

INCUBATION: A few hours to 4 to 5 days.

SYM: Four stages are usually described as follows:

Invasion: At the conclusion of the incubation period there is malaise, headache, diarrhea, and anorexia. Headache and slight fever are present. May last a few days, and then subside. Under such circumstances, may be termed cholerine. Sometimes this stage is lacking entirely.

Evacuation: Purging, violent vomiting, and muscular cramps. Stools loose, copious, and watery, and present a typical rice water appearance. Sometimes there are particles of blood, as well as mucus. Vomiting severe and persistent; material expelled may also resemble rice water. Muscular cramps commonly start in extremities, involve calves of legs, and later even arms, hands, feet, and trunk. Thirst unquenchable and hiccough sometimes develops. Signs of depression soon terminate in collapse. Duration of stage, 2 to 12 hours; seldom more.

Stage of Collapse: Almost complete arrest of circulation, eyes sunken, cheeks hollow, nose pinched, skin dry and wrinkled, body surface cold, covered with clammy sweat, breath cool, temperature in axilla 85-95° F., while in the rectum it may be 103° F. or more. Respirations quickened, pulse weak, systolic blood pressure from 50 to 60, urine suppressed; evacuation and cramps may continue. Mind usually clear until toward the close when coma develops. Stage lasts from few hours to 1 or 2 days, and generally ends in death.

Stage of Reaction: Sometimes, even when death seems imminent, surface temperature begins to rise, vomiting ceases, bowel evacuations become less frequent, more feculent* and convalescence is established. Complete recovery may ensue in from 1 to 2 weeks. Occasionally, typhoid symptoms set in, temperature goes from 106-107° F. and outcome is fatal. Sometimes in this stage, an erythemal eruption or one of the urticarial type appears, particularly on extremities. Such eruptions have no special significance.

TREATMENT: Vigorous replacement of fluid and electrolytes by intravenous administration of saline solution. Sodium lactate or sodium bicarbonate intravenously for acidosis. Tetracycline therapy is effective in limiting the diarrhea.

PROPHYLAXIS: Proper sanitation. Cholera vaccine: Following the initial two or three injections, booster doses should be administered every six months if the person remains in an endemic area.

c. infantum. An acute disease of childhood, usually occurring in summer months, accompanied by vomiting, purging, and collapse. An obsolete term.

c. morbus. Old term formerly applied to an inflammatory intestinal disease resembling cholera, characterized by intense cramps and purging.

c. sicca. A term sometimes applied to a fulminating variety of cholera which occurs without vomiting or purging.

cholerase (kol'er-ās). The special bacteriolytic enzyme of cholera vibrio.

choleresis (kol-ĕr-ē'sis) [G. *cholē*, bile, + *erēsis*, removal]. The secretion and excretion of bile by the liver.

choleretic (kol-er-et'ĭk). Pert. to choleresis, or any agent that increases excretion of bile by the liver.

choleric (kol'er-ik). Irritable; quick-tempered without apparent cause.

choleriform (kol-er'ĭ-form) [G. *cholē*, bile, + *rein*, to flow, + L. *forma*, shape]. Appearing like cholera.

cholerigenous (kol-er-ij'en-us) [" + " + *gennan*, to produce]. Giving rise to cholera.

cholerine (kol'er-ēn). A mild form or initial stages of Asiatic cholera.

cholerization (kol-er-i-za'shun) [G. *cholē*, bile, + *rein*, to flow]. Inoculation against cholera.

choleroid (kol'ĕr-oid). Having a resemblance to cholera.

choleromania (kol-ĕr-ō-mā'nĭ-ă). Morbid fear of contracting cholera.

cholerophobia (kol-er-o-fo'be-a) [" + " + *phobos*, fear]. Morbid fear of acquiring cholera.

cholerrhagia (kol-er-ra'jĭ-ă) [" + *rēgnunai*, to burst forth]. A flow of bile.

cholerythrin (kol-er'ĭ-thrin) [" + *erythros*, red]. 1. Cholera-red. 2. Pigment in urine of tropical residents.

cholesta'sia [" + *stasis*, stoppage]. Arrest of the bile excretion.

chol"estat'ic. Caused by arrest of biliary excretion.

cholesteatoma (kol-es-te-ă-to'ma) [G. *cholē*, bile, + *stear*, fat, + *-ōma*, tumor]. 1. (Primary.) A pearl tumor or pearly nodules in brain. 2. (Secondary.) One of suppurative otitic origin in presence of marginal perforations. Fatty degeneration of epithelium containing cholesterin crystals caused by nature's effort to arrest suppuration. Chloroform test to determine green ring.

cholesteremia (ko-les-ter-e'mĭ-ă) [" + " + *aima*, blood]. Excess cholesterol in the blood.

cholesterin (ko-les'ter-in) [" + *stereos*, solid]. Cholesterol, *q.v.*

cholesterinemia (ko-les-ter-in-e'mĭ-ă) [" + " + *aima* blood]. Cholesteremia, *q.v.*

cholesterinuria (ko-les-ter-ĭn-u'rĭ-ă) [" + " + *ouron*, urine]. Presence of cholesterin in the urine.

cholesterol (ko-les'ter-ol) [" + *stereos*, solid]. A monohydric alcohol ($C_{27}H_{45}$-OH). A sterol, widely distributed in animals, tissues, occurring in the yolk of eggs, various oils, fats, and nervous tissue (brain and spinal cord). It can be synthesized in the liver and is a normal constituent of bile. It is the principal constituent of gallstones. It is important in bodily metabolism serving as a precursor of various steroid hormones, *e.g.*, sex hormones, adrenal corticoids, etc. SYNS *cholesterin.*

cholesterolemia (ko-les-ter-ol-e'mĭ-ă) [" + " + *aima*, blood]. Cholesteremia, *q.v.*

cholesteroluria (ko-les-ter-ol-u'rĭ-ă) [" + " + *ouron*, urine]. Cholesterol in voided urine.

cholesterosis (ko-les-ter-o'sis) [" + " + *-ōsis*, infection]. Cholesterol deposition, esp. in excessive amounts, as in the gallbladder.

choletelin (ko-let'el-ĭn) [" + *telos*, end]. Yellow coloring derived from bilirubin.

cholestyramine (ko"lē-stī'ră-mēn). A resin used to treat itching associated with jaundice. It acts by lowering the level of bile acids in the serum.

choleuria (ko-le-u'rĭ-ă) [" + *ouron*, urine]. Bile in urine.

choleverdin (ko-le-ver'din) [" + L. *viridis*, green]. Green pigment appearing in gallstones and in urine in jaundice. SYN: *biliverdin.**

choline (kō'lēn) [G. *cholē*, bile]. C_5H_{15}-NO_2. An amine, widely distributed in plant and animal tissues, a constituent of lecithin and other phospholipids. It is essential in normal fat and carbohydrate metabolism, a deficiency resulting in lipoidosis of the liver. It is also involved in protein metabolism serving as a methylating agent, and is a precursor of acetylcholine.

cholinergic. Term applied to nerve endings which liberate acetylcholine.

c. fibers. They include all preganglionic fibers, (2) all postganglionic parasympathetic fibers, (3) postganglionic sympathetic fibers to sweat glands, (4) efferent fibers to skeletal muscle.

cholinesterase (kō-lĭn-ĕs'ter-ās). Any enzyme which catalyzes the hydrolysis of choline esters, *e.g., acetylcholinesterase* which catalyzes the breakdown of acetylcholine to acetic acid and choline. Cholinesterases are inhibited by physostigmine (eserine).

cholochrome (ko'lo-krōm) [" + *chrōma,* color]. Any bile pigment.

cholohemothorax (ko-lo-hĕm-o-tho'raks) [" + *aima,* blood, + *thōrax,* chest]. Bile and blood in the thorax.

chololith (kol'o-lith) [" + *lithos,* stone]. A gallstone; biliary calculus.

chololithiasis (kol"o-lith-i'ăs-is). Presence of concretions in the gallbladder. SYN: *cholelithiasis.*

cholorrhea (kol-or-re'ă) [G. *cholē,* bile, + *roia,* flow]. Excessive secretion of bile.

choloscopy (ko-los'ko-pĭ) [" + *skopein,* to examine]. Testing the biliary function.

choluria (ko-lu'rĭ-a) [" + *ouron,* urine]. Bile salts in the urine.

chondral (kon'dral) [G. *chondros,* cartilage]. Pert. to cartilage.

chondralgia (kon-dral'jĭ-ă) [" + *algos,* pain]. Pain in or around a cartilage.

chondralloplasia (kon"dral-o-pla'zĭ-ă) [" + *allos,* other, + *plassein,* to form]. Presence of cartilage in abnormal places.

chondrectomy (kon-drek'to-mĭ) [" + *ektomē,* excision]. Surgical excision of a cartilage.

chondric (kon'drik) [G. *chondros,* cartilage]. Pert. to cartilage.

chondrification (kon-drĭ-fi-ka'shun) [" + L. *facere,* to make]. Conversion into cartilage.

chon'drigen [" + *gennan,* to produce]. Basal substance of cartilage, which turns into chondrin on boiling. SYN: *chondrogen.*

chondrin (kon'drĭn) [G. *chondros,* cartilage]. Gelatinlike matter obtained by boiling cartilage.

chondriosome (kon'drĭ-o-sōm) [" + *sōma,* body]. Any of the organelles of a cell comprising the chondriome. Includes the *mitochondria* (granules) and *chondrioconts* (rods or filaments).

chondritis (kon-dri'tis) [" + *-itis,* inflammation]. Inflammation of cartilage.

chon"droadeno'ma [" + *adēn,* gland, + *-ōma,* tumor]. Cartilaginous tissue in an adenoma.

chon"droangio'ma [" + *aggeion,* vessel, + *-ōma,* tumor]. Cartilaginous elements in an angioma.

chondroblast (kŏn'drō-blăst) [G. *chondros,* cartilage, + *blastos,* germ]. A cell which forms cartilage.

chondroclast (kon'dro-klast) [" + *klastos,* broken into bits]. A cell concerned in the absorption of cartilage.

chondrocostal (kon-dro-kos'tal) [" + L. *costa,* rib]. Pert. to costal cartilages.

chondrocranium (kon-dro-kra'nĭ-um) [" + *kranion,* head]. The cartilaginous embryonic cranium before ossification.

chondrocyte (kon'dro-sīt) [" + *kytos,* cell]. A cartilage cell.

chondrodynia (kon-dro-din'ĭ-ă) [" + *odynē,* pain]. Pain in or about a cartilage.

chondrodysplasia (kon"dro-dis-pla'zĭ-ă) [" + *dys,* bad, + *plassein,* to form]. Chondrodystrophy.

chondrodystrophy (kon-dro-dis'tro-fĭ) [" + *dys,* difficult, + *trophē,* nourishment]. Defect in cartilage formation at epiphyses of long bones. SYN: *dyschondroplasia, q.v.*

c., hypoplastic. Achondroplasia, *q.v.*

chondrofibroma (kon-dro-fi-bro'mă) [" + L. *fibra,* fiber, + G. *-ōma,* tumor]. A mixed tumor with elements of chondroma and fibroma.

chondrogen (kon'dro-jen) [" + *gennan,* to produce]. Chondrigen, *q.v.*

chondrogenesis (kon-dro-jen'es-is) [" + *genesis,* production]. Formation of cartilage.

chondroid (kon'droid) [" + *eidos,* resemblance]. Resembling cartilage; cartilaginous.

chondroituria (kon-dro-ĭ-tu'rĭ-ă) [" + *ouron,* urine]. Chondroitic acid in urine.

chondrolipoma (kon-dro-lip-o'mă) [" + *lipos,* fat, + *-ōma,* tumor]. Cartilaginous and fatty tissue tumor.

chondrology (kon-drol'o-jĭ) [" + *logos,* study]. The science of cartilages.

chondrolysis (kon-drol'ĭ-sis) [" + *lysis,* dissolution]. The breaking down and absorption of cartilage.

chondro'ma [" + *-ōma,* tumor]. A cartilaginous tumor of slow growth.

It may occur any place where there is cartilage. It causes no pain.

chondromalacia (kon-drō-mal-a'sĭ-ă) [" + *malakia,* softening]. Softness of any cartilage.

chondromatous (kon-dro'mă-tus) [" + *-ōma,* tumor]. Pert. to chondroma, or tumor of a cartilage.

chondromucoid (kon-drō-mū'koid) [G. *chondros,* cartilage, + L. mucus, *mucus,* + G. *eidos,* form]. A basophilic glycoprotein present in interstitial substance of cartilage.

chondromyoma (kon-dro-mi-o'mă) [" + *mys,* muscle, + *-ōma,* tumor]. Myoma and cartilaginous neoplasm combined.

chondromyxoma (kon-dro-mĭk-sō'mă) [" + *myxa,* mucus, + *-ōma,* tumor]. Chondroma with myxomatous elements.

chondromyxosarcoma (kon-dro-mĭk"sō-sar-kō'mă) [" + " + *sarx,* flesh, + *-ōma*-tumor]. A cartilaginous and sarcomatous tumor.

chondropathology (kon-dro-path'ol-o-jĭ) [" + *pathos,* disease, + *logos,* study of]. Pathology of cartilages.

chondropathy (kon-drop'ath-ĭ) [" + *pathos,* disease]. Any disease of cartilage.

chondroplast (kon'drō-plast). Chondroblast, *q.v.*

chondroplasty (kon'dro-plas-tĭ) [G. *chondros,* cartilage, + *plassein,* to mold]. Plastic or reparative surgery on cartilage.

chondroporosis (kon-dro-po-ro'sis) [" + *poros,* passage]. The porous condition of cartilage, pathological or normal, during ossification.

chondroproteins (kon-dro-pro'te-ins) [" + *prōtos,* first]. A group of glucoproteins found in cartilage, tendons, and connective tissue.

chondrosarcoma (kon-dro-sar-ko'mă) [" + *sarx,* flesh, + *-ōma,* tumor]. Cartilaginous sarcoma.

chondro'sis [" + *-ōsis,* infection]. The development of cartilage.

chon"droster'nal [" + *sternon,* chest]. Pert. to sternal cartilage.

chondrotome (kon'dro-tōm) [" + *tomē,* a cutting]. Device for cutting cartilage.

chondrotomy (kon-drot'o-mĭ) [" + *tomē,* incision]. Dissection or surgical division of cartilage.

Chondrus. A genus of red algae which includes *Chondrus crispus* the source of *carrageenin,* a mucilaginous substance used as an emulsifying agent. Commonly called *Irish moss* or *carrageen.*

Chopart's amputation (sho-pars') [Francois Chopart, French surgeon, 1743-1795]. Disarticulation at the midtarsal joint.

chorda (kor'da) (pl. *chordae*) [G. *chordē,* cord]. A string or tendon.

c. dorsalis. The notochord.

c. gubernaculi. An embryonic structure forming a part of the gubernaculum testis in the male and the round ligament in the female.

c. obliqua [NA]. The oblique ligament, an oblique cord which connects the shafts of the radius and ulna. Extends from lateral side of tubercle of ulna to a point just below radial tuberosity.

chordae tendinea [NA]. A small tendinous cord which connects the free edge of an atrioventricular valve to a papillary muscle.

c. tympani [NA]. A branch of the facial nerve which leaves the cranium through the stylomastoid foramen, transverses the tympanic cavity and joins a branch of the lingual nerve. Efferent fibers innervate the submaxillary and sublingual glands; afferent fibers convey taste impulses from ant. two thirds of the tongue.

c. umbilicalis. Umbilical cord connecting fetus and placenta.

c. Willisii. One of several fibrous cords across the superior longitudinal sinus.

chordal (kor'dal). Pert. to a chorda, esp. the notochord.

Chord'ata. A phylum of the animal kingdom which includes all vertebrates.

chordée (kor-de') [Fr. corded]. Downward, painful curvature of the penis on erection in gonorrhea caused by inflammatory infiltration of the corpus spongiosum which interferes with its distensibility.

chorditis (kor-di'tis) [G. *chordē,* cord, + *-ītis,* inflammation]. Inflammation of a cord, esp. the spermatic or a vocal cord.

c. nodo'sa. Formation of small, whitish nodules on one or both vocal cords.

SYM: Hoarseness, inability of singers to register tones properly.

TREATMENT: Vocal hygiene. Surgical removal of nodules if they do not respond to conservative therapy.

chordot'omy [" + *tomē,* dissection]. Division of any cord to relieve pain.

chorea (ko-re'ă) [G. *choreia,* dance]. A nervous affection marked by muscular twitching. SEE: *Sydenham's c.*

c., electric. A myoclonic form of epidemic encephalitis, *q.v.* SYN: *Dubini's disease.*

c., epidemic. Religious emotional neurosis, manifest in the 14th century in Europe, exhibited in form of dancing mania. SYN: *dancing mania.*

c. gravidarum. A form of Sydenham's c. seen in some pregnant women, usually in those who have had chorea before, esp. in their first pregnancy.

c., Huntington's. A hereditary and chronic form manifested in adult life.

c., hyoscine. Movements simulating chorea, and sometimes accompanied by delirium, seen in acute hyoscine intoxication.

c., insaniens. Movements so violent patient is unable to walk, eat or even lie down.

SYM: Fever develops, mind becomes delirious. Death frequently results from exhaustion. This form usually observed in adults, and esp. in primipara.

PROG: Frequently terminates fatally through exhaustion.

TREATMENT: Quiet, hygienic life. Forced feeding. Severe cases complicating pregnancy will call for induction of premature labor. Constitutional remedies.

NP: Rest in bed. Protect from injury by use of siderails. Light bed clothes, soft and free from wrinkles to avoid dermatitis. Isolation necessary. Visitors restricted; esp. no children. If possible tub baths prolonged as sedative; warm water and hot sponging. Rhythmic breathing and rhythmic exercises as improvement sets in. Quietness. If violent, make bed on floor surrounded by bolsters. Rubber under sheets, soft blanket. Nourishing diet. Food in small pieces, as patient may not masticate. No glass utensils. Feed slowly. Precautions against bed sores. Mouth hygiene. Water bet. meals. Measure and test urine for albumin. No exertion. Sedatives or tranquilizers as indicated.

c., major. C. with violent hysterical muscular action.

c., mimetic. C. due to imitative movements.

c. minor. Sydenham's c., *q.v.*

c., posthemiplegic; c., postparalytic. Involuntary movements of patients subsequent to a hemiplegic attack.

c., rheumatic. Sydenham's c., *q.v.*

c., rhythmic. C. with movements at regulated times.

c., senile. C. developing in senility.

c., Sydenham's. A disease of childhood commonly occurring between 5 and 15 years of age; more females than males are affected. Usually associated with rheumatic fever. Characterized by involuntary, purposeless contractions of the muscles of the trunk and extremities; anxiety; impairment of memory and sometimes of speech.

SYN: *chorea minor; infectious chorea; rheumatic chorea; St. Vitus' dance.*

PROG: Usually recover in course of 6 to 10 weeks. Relapses not infrequent especially in pregnancy. Rare complication is death from heart disease. Among possible sequelae are imbecility and chronic chorea.

TREATMENT: Rest of body and mind, remove child from school; place under most favorable hygienic conditions. Protection against injury in severe cases. Sedation in most cases.

choreal (ko-re'al). Pert. to chorea.

choreic (ko-re'ik). Pert. to or of nature of chorea.

choreiform (ko-re'ĭ-form) [G. *choreia,* dance, + L. *forma,* form]. Of the nature of chorea.

choreomania (ko-re-o-ma'nĭ-ă) [" + *mania,* madness]. Epidemic chorea, as the dancing mania of the middle ages.

chorioadenoma (ko-rĭ-o-ad-en-o'mă) [G. *chorion,* skin, + *adēn,* gland, + *-ōma,* tumor]. Adenoma of the chorion.

chorioangioma (ko-rĭ-o-an-jĭ-o'mă) [" + *aggeion,* vessel, + *-ōma,* tumor]. A vascular tumor of the chorion.

choriocapillaris (ko-rĭ″o-kap-il-la′ris) [″ + L. *capillaris*, hairlike]. Capillary layer of choroid.

choriocarcinoma (ko‴rĭ-ō-kar″sĭ-nō′mă). An extremely rare, very malignant neoplasm usually of the uterus but sometimes at site of ectopic pregnancy. Though actual cause is unknown, it occurs following hydatid mole, pregnancy, abortion.

choriocele (ko′rĭ-o-sēl) [″ + *kēlē*, hernia]. A protrusion of the chorioid coat of the eye through a defective sclera.

chorioepithelioma (ko-ri-o-ep-ĭ-thē-lĭ-o′mă). Choriocarcinoma, *q.v.*

chorioid (ko′rĭ-oid). Choroid, *q.v.*

chorioma (ko-rĭ-o′mă) (pl. *chorio′mata*) [″ + *-ōma*, tumor]. A tumor of the chorion. There are a number of types including chorioadenoma, choriocarcinoma, and syncytioma, *q.v.*

choriomeningitis (ko-rĭ-o-men-in-ji′tis) [″ + *menigx*, membrane, + *-ītis*, inflammation]. Cerebral meningitis with cellular infiltration of the meninges.

c., *lymphocytic*. An acute central nervous system disease probably of viral origin characterized by grippelike symptoms (fever, malaise, headache, etc.) sometimes followed by acute septic meningitis.

chorion (kō′rĭ-ŏn) [G.]. An extraembryonic membrane which, in early development, forms the outer wall of the blastocyst. It is formed from the trophoblast and its inner lining of mesoderm. From it chorionic *villi* develop which establish an intimate connection with the endometrium giving rise to the placenta. SEE: *trophoblast*.

chorionepithelioma. Choriocarcinoma, *q.v.*

chorionic (ko-rĭ-on′ik). Pert. to the chorion.

c. *villi*. The vascular projections from the chorion.

chorionitis (ko-rĭ-on-i′tis) [G. *chorion*, skin, + *-ītis*, inflammation]. 1. Inflammation of the chorion. 2. Scleroderma, *q.v.*

chorioretinitis (ko-rĭ-o-ret″in-i′tis) [″ + L. *rete*, network, + G. *-ītis*, inflammation]. Inflammation of choroid and retina.

chorista (ko-ris′tă) [G. *chōristos*, separated]. An error of development showing separation from the rudiments in a developing embryo.

choristoma (ko-ris-to′mă) [″ + *-ōma*, tumor]. A neoplasm due to overdevelopment of embryonic rudiments.

choroid (ko′roid) [G. *chorioeidēs*, skinlike]. Dark brown, vascular coat of eye bet. sclera and retina, extending from *ora serrata* to optic nerve.

Consists of blood vessels, united by connective tissue containing pigmented cells, and is made up of 5 layers: (1) suprachoroid; (2) layer of large vessels; (3) layer of medium sized vessels; (4) layer of capillaries; (5) *lamina vitrea* (homogeneous membrane placed next to pigmentary layer of retina).

It is a part of the uvea or vascular tunic of the eye.

choroideremia (ko-roy-der-e′mĭ-ă) [G. *chorioeidēs*, skinlike, + *erēmia*, destitution]. Absence of the choroid coat of the eye.

choroiditis (ko-roid-i′tis) [″ + *-itis*, inflammation]. Inflammation of choroid.

c., *anterior*. When outlets of exudation are at the choroidal periphery.

c., *areolar*. In which inflammation spreads from around the macula lutea.

c., *central*. Exudation is limited to the macula.

c., *diffuse or disseminated*. When the fundus is covered with spots.

c., *exudative*. When covered with patches of inflammation.

c., *guttata*. Tay's c., *q.v.*

c., *metastatic*. When due to embolism.

c., *suppurative*. When suppuration occurs.

c., *Tay's*. A familial condition characterized by degeneration of the choroid esp. in the region about the macula lutea. Occurs in aged persons.

choroidocycli′tis [″ + *kyklos*, a circle, + *-ītis*, inflammation]. Inflammation of the choroid coat and ciliary processes.

choroidoiritis (ko-royd-o-i-ri′tis) [″ + *iris*, iris, + *-ītis*, inflammation]. Inflammation of the choroid coat and iris.

choroidoretinitis (ko-royd-o-ret-in-i′tis) (″ + L. *rete*, network, + G. *-ītis*, inflammation]. Inflammation of choroid and retina.

choromania (ko-ro-mā′nĭ-ă) [G. *choros*, dance, + *mania*, madness]. Epidemic chorea, *q.v.*

Christian Science. A religion that derives its teachings from the Scriptures as understood by its adherents, and that includes a practice of spiritual healing based upon the teaching that cause and effect are mental and that sin, sickness, and death will be destroyed by a full understanding of the divine principle of Jesus' teaching and healing. (Webster's *Third New Int. Dictionary*.)

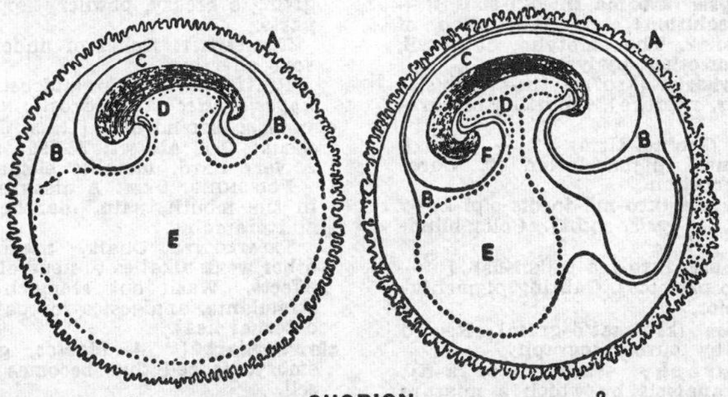

CHORION

A, Chorion with villi. The villi are shown to be best developed in the part of the chorion to which the allantois is extending; this portion ultimately becomes the placenta. B, Extraembryonic coelom. C, Amniotic cavity. D, Primitive gut or embryonic intestine. E, Yolk sac or umbilical vesicle.

Christmas disease [Named for person in whom the disease was discovered]. A form of hemophilia in males resulting from plasma thromboplastin component (PTC or Factor IX) deficiency.

C. factor. A thromboplastin activator present in blood plasma, *viz.* plasma thromboplastin component (PTC).

chromaffin (krō-măf'ĭn) [G. *chrōma*, color, + L. *affinis*, having affinity for]. 1. Staining readily with chromium salts. 2. Noting pigmented cells forming medulla of the adrenal glands and the paraganglia.

c. cells. Cells such as those of the adrenal medulla which contain granules which stain brown when cells are stained with a fluid containing potassium bichromate. SEE ALSO: *c. reaction.*

c. reaction. The turning brown of cytoplasmic granules containing epinephrine when subjected to stains containing chromium salts. Such granules stain green with ferric chloride, yellow with iodine, and brown with osmic acid. SEE ALSO: *c. cells.*

c. system, c. tissue. The mass of tissue forming paraganglia and medulla of suprarenal glands, which secretes adrenalin and stains readily with chromium salts. Similar tissue is found in the organs of Zuckerkandl, and in the liver, testes, ovary, and heart. SEE: *adrenal gland.*

chromaffino'ma [" + " + G. *-ōma*, tumor]. A chromaffin cell tumor. SYN: *paraganglioma.*

chromaffinopathy (kro-maf-in-op'ă-thĭ) [" + " + G. *pathos*, disease]. Any disease of chromaffin tissue.

chromaphil (kro'maf-ĭl) [" + *philein*, to love]. Pert. to a histological element or cell which stains readily with chromium salts. SYN: *chromaffin, q.v.*

chromate (kro'māt) [G. *chrōmatos*, color]. A salt of chromic acid. SEE: *potassium c.*

chromatelopsia (kro"mat-ĕ-lop'sĭ-ă) [G. *chrōma*, color, + *atelēs*, imperfect, + *opsis*, sight]. Color blindness.

chromat'ic. Pert. to color.

chromatid (kro'mă-tĭd). Either of the two bodies resulting from longitudinal splitting of a chromosome.

chromatin (krō'mă-tĭn) [G. *chrōma*, color]. A deeply staining substance present in the nucleus of a cell, and considered to be the physical basis of heredity. In a cell in interphase, it is in the form of a fine network bearing coarse granules.

chromatinolysis (kro"mă-tin-ol'ĭ-sis) [" + *lysis*, dissolution]. 1. Destruction of chromatin. 2. The emptying of a cell, bacterial or other, by lysis.

chromatinorrhexis (kro"mă-tin-or-rek'sis) [" + *rēxis*, rupture]. Splitting of chromatin.

chromatism (kro'mă-tĭzm) [" + *ismos*]. 1. Unnatural pigmentation. 2. Chromatic aberration.

chromatodysopia (kro-mă-to-dis-o'pĭ-ă) [" + *dys*, ill, + *opsis*, sight]. Color blindness.

chromatogenous (kro-mă-toj'en-us) [" + *gennan*, to produce]. Causing pigmentation or color.

chromatogram (krō-mat'ō-gram). Record produced by chromatography.

chromatography (krō-mă-tog'ră-fĭ). Chemical analysis by which a mixture of substances is separated by fractional extraction or adsorption on a porous solid (column of aluminum oxide or filter paper) by means of flowing solvents.

c., paper. C. in which paper strips are used as the porous solid medium.

chromatolysis (kro-mă-tol'ĭ-sis) [" + *lysis*, dissolution]. Dissolution of chromophil substance (Nissl's bodies) in neurons in certain pathological conditions, or following injury to the cell body or axon.

chromatometer (kro-ma-tom'et-er) [" + *metron*, measure]. A scale of colors for testing color perception.

chromatopathy (kro-ma-top'ă-thĭ) [" + *pathos*, disease]. Any skin disease that is marked by pigmentation.

chromat'ophil, chromatophil'ic [" + *philein*, to love]. Staining easily.

chromatophore (kro-mat'o-fōr) [" + *pherein*, to bear]. A pigment-bearing cell.

chromatopsia (kro-mă-top'sĭ-ă) [" + *opsis*, vision]. Abnormally colored vision.

chromatoptometry (kro-mat-op-tom'e-trĭ) [" + *optein*, to see, + *metron*, measure]. Measurement of color perception.

chromatosis (kro-mă-to'sis). 1. Pigmentation. 2. The pathological deposition of pigment in any part of the body where it is not normally present or excessive deposition where it is present.

chromaturia (kro-mă-tu'rĭ-ă) [" + *ouron*, urine]. Abnormal color of the urine.

chromesthe'sia. The association of color sensations with words, taste, smell or sounds.

chro'micized. Mixed with a chromium salt.

chromidiosis (kro-mid-ĭ-o'sis) [G. *chrōma*, color]. Overflow of chromatin and nuclear substance into cell protoplasm.

chromid'ium (pl. *chromidia*) [" + *-idion*, a dim. termination]. An extranuclear granule seen in the cytoplasm of a cell.

chromidrosis (kro-mid-ro'sis) [" + *idrōs*, sweat]. Excretion of colored sweat.

(a) It may be *black*. This may be present in hysteria due to indican in the sweat, and associated with constipation. (b) *Red sweat.* It may be due to an exudation of blood into the sweat glands, or to microorganisms in those glands.

ETIOL: May be due to ingestion or absorption of certain substances, as pigment-producing bacteria. May be caused by certain disorders of metabolism.

SYM: Localized in eyelids, breasts, axillae, genitocrural regions, occasionally hands and limbs, grayish, bluish, violaceous, brownish, collecting on skin, giving a greasy, powdery appearance to parts.

TREATMENT: Relief of underlying nervous affection.

RS: *anhidrosis; bromidrosis; hidrosis; hyperidrosis; chromidrosis; uridrosis.*

chromium (kro'mĭ-um) [G. *chrōma*, color]. SYMB: Cr. At. wt. 51.996; at. no. 24. A very hard, metallic element.

POISONING: SYM: A disagreeable taste in the mouth, pain, diarrhea, collapse and cramping.

TREATMENT: Chalk, magnesia, and other weak alkalies to neutralize its acid effects. Wash out stomach and give stimulants, analgesics for pain. Provide external heat.

chro'moblast [" + *blastos*, germ]. An embryonic cell that becomes a pigment cell.

chromoblastomycosis (kro"mo-blas"tō-mĭ-kō'sĭs). One of a group of diseases marked by itching and warty plaques on the skin and subcutaneous swellings of feet, legs and other exposed areas.

Caused by fungi, *Phialophora verrucosa* and *Hormodendrum pedrosoi*.

chromocholoscopy (kro-mo-ko-los'ko-pĭ) [" + *cholē*, bile, + *skopein*, to examine]. Examination of the biliary function by a pigment extraction test.

chromocrinia (kro-mo-krin'ĭ-ă) [" + *krinein*, to separate]. The secretion or excretion of pigmented matter.

chromocystoscopy (kro-mo-sis-tos'ko-pĭ) [" + *kystis*, cyst, + *skopein*, to examine]. Determination of functional activity of kidneys by use of dyes.

chromocyte (kro'mo-sīt) [" + *kytos*, cell]. Any colored cell.

chromocytometer (kro-mo-sī-tom'et-er) [" + " + *metron*, measure]. Instrument for determining the hemoglobin in red blood corpuscles.

chromodermatosis (kro-mo-der-mă-to'sis) [" + *derma*, skin, + *-ōsis*, infection]. Any pigmented skin disease.

chromogen (kro'mo-jen) [" + *gennan*, to produce]. Any principle that may be changed into coloring matter.

chromogen'esis [" + *genesis*, production]. Production of pigment.

chromogen'ic. Pigment producing.

chromolipoid (kro-mo-lip'oid) [G. *chrōma*, color, + *lipos*, fat, + *eidos*, appearance]. Any lipoid, such as carotin, that is pigmented. Syn: *lipochrome*.

chromolume (kro'mo-lūm) [" + L. *lumen*, light]. Device for producing colored light rays.

chromolysis (kro-mol'ĭ-sĭs) [" + *lysis*, dissolution]. Chromatolysis, *q.v.*

chromomere (kro'mo-mēr) [" + *meros*, part]. 1. One of a series of chromatin granules found in a chromosome. 2. A highly refractile purple granule which forms the central portion of a blood platelet.

chromometer (kro-mom'ĕ-ter) [" + *metron*, measure]. Device for determining the pigment in a substance. Syn: *colorimeter*.

chromometry (kro-mom'et-rĭ). The estimation of coloring matter.

chromopar'ic [G. *chrōma*, color, + L. *parēre*, produce]. Producing color; chromogenic.

chromopex'ic [" + *pēxis*, fixation]. Fixing coloring matter, as the liver.

chromophage (kro'mo-fāj) [" + *phagein*, to eat]. A phagocyte that destroys pigment believed to be present in the blanching of hair. Syn: *pigmentophage*.

chromophane (kro'mo-fān) [" + *phainein*, to show]. Retinal pigment.

chromophil(e (kro'mo-fil) [" + *philein*, to love]. 1. Any structure that stains easily. 2. Staining readily. 3. One of two types of cells present in *pars distalis* of the pituitary gland. It is considered a secretory cell.

chromophilic (kro-mo-fil'ik). Staining readily; chromophilous.

chromophilous (kro-mof'il-us). Chromophilic.

chromophobe (krō'mō-fōb) [G. *chrōma*, color, + *phobos*, fear]. A type of cell found in *pars distalis* of the pituitary gland. Also called *chief* or *C cells*.

chromophobic (krō-mō-fō'bĭk). Resistant to staining.

chromophor'ic [G. *chrōma*, color, + *pherein*, to bear]. Pert. to or bearing color.

chromophose (kro'mo-fōz) [" + *phōs*, light]. A subjective sensation of a spot of color in the eye. See: *centraphose; centrophose*.

chromophytosis (kro-mo-fi-to'sis) [" + *phyton*, plant, + *-ōsis*, infection]. Pigmentation of skin due to a vegetable parasite. Tinea, or pityriasis versicolor.

chro'moplasm [" + *plasma*, matter]. The network of a cell nucleus.

chromoplas'tid [" + *plastos*, formed]. Colored plastids other than chloroplasts present in plant cells.

chromoprotein (kro-mo-pro'te-in) [" + *prōtos*, first]. One of a group of conjugated proteins consisting of a protein combined with hematin or another colored, metal-containing, prosthetic group. Ex: *hemoglobin; hemocyanin; chlorophyll; flavoproteins; cytochromes*.

chromop'sia [" + *opsis*, vision]. Chromatopsia; colored vision.

chromoptometer (kro-mop-tom'ĕ-ter) [" + *optein*, to see, + *metron*, measure]. Instrument for determining keenness of color vision.

chro"moradiom'eter [" + L. *radius*, ray, + G. *metron*, measure]. An instrument for measuring penetrative power of roentgen rays.

chromoscope (krō-mō-skōp) [" + *skopein*, to examine]. Instrument for determining color perception.

chromoscopy (krō-mos'kō-pĭ) [" + *skopein*, to examine]. Examination for color vision.

chromosome (kro'mō-sōm) [G. *chrōma*, color, + *sōma*, body]. A microscopic rod-shaped (J- or V-shaped) body which develops from the nuclear material of a cell and is especially conspicuous during mitosis. They stain deeply with basic dyes. They contain the genes or hereditary determiners.

The number of chromosomes is constant for each species being 46 in man (*i.e.*, 23 pairs in all somatic cells) which constitutes the diploid number. In the formation of the gametes the number is reduced to one-half (haploid number), *i.e.*, the ovum and sperm each contain 23 or one of each of the 23 pairs. Of these, 22 are autosomes and one is the sex chromosome (X or Y).

At time of fertilization the chromosomes from the sperm unite with the chromosomes from the ovum. At that time the sex of the embryo is determined. The female sex chromosome from the ovum may contribute *only* an *X* to the embryo. The sperm or male sex chromosome may contribute an *X* or a *Y* as its half to join with the chromosome derived from the ovum. Thus the embryo may have *XX* in its sex chromosome in which case a female would develop, or *XY* in which case a male would develop.

2. The unit of chromatin in the nucleus of a cell.

See: *heredity*.

c., accessory. An unpaired monosome, a sex c., *q.v.*

c., bivalent. A double chromosome resulting from the conjugation of two homologous chromosomes in synapsis which occurs during the first meiotic division.

c., giant. Extremely large chromosomes seen in the salivary glands and in other organs and tissues of insects. Also called polytenic chromosomes.

c., sex. One of two chromosomes, the X- and Y-chromosomes, which are concerned with the determination of sex and carry the genes for sex-linked characters. In birds, they are designated the Z- and W-chromosomes.

c., somatic. An autosome, *i.e.*, any chromosome except a sex chromosome.

c., X-. One of a pair of female-determining chromosomes (XX) present in the somatic cells of all human females.

c., Y-. The male-determining member of a pair of chromosomes (XY) present in the somatic cells of all human males. It is usually devoid of genes and in certain lower animals may be absent.

chro"mother'apy [" + *therapeia,* treatment]. The use of colored light in the treatment of disease.

chromotox'ic [" + *toxikon,* poison]. Caused by toxic action on the hemoglobin.

chromoureteroscopy (kro-mo-ū-ret-er-os'-ko-pĭ) [" + *ourētēr,* ureter, + *skopein,* to examine]. Inspecting orifices of ureters after giving a substance to dye the urine.

chronaxia (kron-ak'sĭ-ă). Chronaxie, *q.v.*

chronaxie (kro'nak-sĭ) [" + *axia,* value]. A number expressing the sensitiveness of a nerve to electrical stimulation.

It is the minimum duration, measured in seconds, during which a current of prescribed strength must pass through a motor nerve in order to cause contraction in the associated muscle; the strength of direct current (the rheobasic voltage) which will just suffice if given an indefinite time is first determined, and exactly double this strength is taken for the final determinations.

chronaximeter (kron-aks-im'et-er) [" + " + *metron,* measure]. Device for measuring chronaxia.

chron'ic [G. *chronos,* duration]. Long drawn out; applied to a disease that is not acute.

chronicity (kro-nis'it-ĭ). State of being chronic.

chronobiol'ogy [G. *chronos,* time, + *bios,* life, + *logos,* study of]. Science of duration of life, and methods of prolonging it.

chronograph (kron'o-graf) [" + *graphein,* to write]. Device for recording short intervals of time.

chronological (krŏn"ō-lŏj'ĭ-kăl) [G. *chronos,* time, + *logos,* understanding]. Occurring in natural sequence according to time.

c. age. The number of years of one's life.

chron'oscope [G. *chronos,* time, + *skopein,* to examine]. Device for measuring extremely short intervals of time.

chronot'ropism [" + " + *ismos,* condition of]. Modification of periodic events such as the heart beat through external causes.

chrysarobin (kris-ă-rō'bin). USP. A mixture of neutral principles obtained from goa powder, which is deposited in the wood of Araroba, a leguminous tree of South America. It is used topically, as an ointment, for treatment of psoriasis.

chthonophagia (thon-o-fa'jĭ-ă) [G. *chthōn,* earth, + *phagein,* to eat]. Eating clay or dirt; geophagy.

Chvostek's sign (shvos'teks) [Franz Chvostek, Austrian surgeon, 1835-1884]. Local spasm following a tap on one side of face.

chylangioma (ki-lan-jĭ-o'mă) [G. *chylos,* chyle, + *aggeion,* vessel, + *-ōma,* tumor]. 1. Tumor of intestinal lymph vessels containing chyle. 2. Retention of chyle in lymphatic vessels with dilatation.

chyle (kīl) [G. *chylos*]. The milklike contents of the lacteals and lymphatic vessels of the intestine consisting of the products of digestion and principally absorbed fats. It is carried by the lymphatic vessels to the cisterna chyli and then by way of the thoracic duct to the left subclavian vein where it enters the blood stream. A large quantity is formed in 24 hours. Reaction is alkaline.

RS: *achylia; cisterna chyli; oligochylia; recepaculum chyli; secretion.*

chylemia (ki-le'mĭ-ă) [" + *aima,* blood]. Chyle in the peripheral circulation.

chylidrosis (ki-lĭ-dro'sis) [" + *idrōs,* sweat]. A milklike sweat resembling chyle.

chylifacient (ki-lĭ-fa'shent) [" + L. *facere,* to make]. Forming chyle.

chylifaction (ki-lĭ-fak'shun) [" + L. *facere,* to make]. The formation of chyle. Syn: *chylification.*

chylifactive (ki-lĭ-fak'tiv). Forming chyle; chilifacient.

chyliferous (ki-lif'er-us) [G. *chylos,* chyle, + L. *ferre,* to carry]. Carrying chyle.

chylification (ki-lĭ-fĭ-kā'shun). Chylifaction, *q.v.*

chylocele (ki'lo-sēl) [" + *kēlē,* tumor]. Infused chyle in *tunica vaginalis testis.*

chyloderma (ki-lo-der'mă) [" + *derma,* skin]. Lymph accumulated in the enlarged lymphatic vessels and thickened skin of the scrotum; lymph scrotum; scrotal elephantiasis.

chylology (ki-lol'o-jĭ) [" + *logos,* study of]. The study of chyle.

chylomediastinum (kī-lo"me-dĭ-as-tī'num) [" + L. *mediastinum,* being in the middle]. Chyle in the mediastinum.

chylomicron (ki-lo-mi'kron) [" + *mikros,* small]. Small particle of fat in the blood after digestion and absorption of fat in the food, and perceptible under a microscope.

chylopericardium (ki-lo-per-ĭ-kar'dĭ-um) [" + *peri,* around, + *kardia,* heart]. Chyle in the pericardium.

chyloperitone'um [" + " + *teinein,* to stretch]. Effused chyle in peritoneal cavity.

chylophoric (ki-lo-for'ĭk) [" + *phoros,* bearing]. Conveying chyle; chyliferous.

chylopoiesis (ki-lo-poi-e'sis) [" + *poiēsis,* production]. Formation of chyle and absorption by lacteals in the intestines. Syn: *chylification.*

chylotho'rax [" + *thōrax,* chest]. Chyle in pleural cavities.

chylous (kī'lus) [G. *chylos*]. Pert. to or of the nature of chyle.

chyluria (ki-lu'rĭ-ă) [" + *ouron,* urine]. Chyle or fat globules in the urine.

chyme (kīm) [G. *chymos,* juice]. The mixture of partly digested food and digestive secretions found in the stomach and small intestine during digestion of a meal; it is a varicolored, thick, but nearly liquid mass. See: *enchyma; oligochymia.*

chymosin (kī'mō-sin) [G. *chymos,* juice]. The enzyme in gastric juice which converts the milk protein caseinogen into casein. Calcium ions are necessary for this reaction. Syn: *rennin; chymase.*

chymosinogen (kī-mo-sin'o-jen) [" + *gennan,* to produce]. A substance from which chymosin is formed.

chymotrypsin (kī'mo-trip'sin). A proteolytic enzyme present in the intestine which, with trypsin, hydrolyzes proteins to peptones or further. It is secreted by the pancreas.

C. I. Abbr. for *color index;* also *chemotherapeutic index* (parasitology).

cibisitome (si-bis'it-ōm) [G. *kibisis,* pouch, + *tomē,* a cut]. Instrument for incision of capsule of the lens.

cibophobia (sī-bō-fō'bĭ-ă). A morbid aversion to or fear of food.

cicatricial (sik-ă-trish'al) [L. *cicatrix*, scar]. Pert. to a cicatrix, *q.v.*

cicatricotomy (sik-ă-trik-ot'o-mĭ) [" + G. *tomē*, incision]. Incision of a cicatrix or scar.

cicatrix (sik'ă-triks, sik-a'triks) [L.]. A scar left by a healed wound.

Lack of color is due to absence of pigmentation. Cicatricial tissue is less elastic than normal tissue, hence it usually presents a contracted appearance. SEE: *keloid.*

cicatrizant (sĭk-at'rĭ-zant) [L. *cicatrix*, scar]. Favoring or causing, or an agent that aids in, cicatrization.

cicatrization (sik-ă-trĭ-za'shun) [L. *cicatrix*, scar]. Healing by scar formation. SEE: *intention.*

cicatrize (sik'ă-trīz) [L. *cicatrix*, scar]. To heal by scar tissue.

cicutism (sĭk'ū-tizm). Poisoning resulting from ingestion of *Cicuta maculata* or *C. virosa*, water hemlock.

cilia (sil'ĭ-ă) (sing. *cilium*) [L. pl.]. 1. Eyelashes. 2. Hairlike processes projecting from epithelial cells, as in the bronchi, which wave mucus, pus, and dust particles upward. SEE: *biciliate.*

ciliariscope (sil-ĭ-a'rĭ-skōp) [L. *ciliaris*, pert. to eyelash, + G. *skopein*, to examine]. Instrument for examination of the ciliary region of the eye.

ciliarotomy (sil-ĭ-ă-rot'o-mĭ) [" + G. *tomē*, incision]. Surgical section of the ciliary zone in glaucoma.

cil'iary [L. *ciliaris*, pert. to eyelash]. Pert. to any hairlike processes, especially the eyelashes, and to eye structures as the ciliary body.

c. arteries. Branches of the ophthalmic artery which supply the choroid layer.

c. body. Extends from base of iris to ant. part of choroid; consists of ciliary processes and ciliary muscle.

c. ganglion. A ganglion lying in the posterior part of the orbit. Receives preganglionic fibers through the oculomotor nerve from the nucleus of Edinger-Westphal of the midbrain. From it six short ciliary nerves pass to the eyeball. Postganglionic fibers innervate the ciliary muscle, sphincter of the iris, and the smooth muscles of blood vessels of these structures and the cornea.

c. glands. Glands of Moll, a form of sweat glands of the eyelid.

c. muscle. Smooth muscle forming a part of the ciliary body of the eye. Contraction pulls the choroid forward, lessening tension on fibers of the zonula (suspensory ligament) thereby allowing the lens, which is elastic, to assume a more spherical shape; thus accommodation for near vision is accomplished.

c. processes. Consist of about 70 folds arranged meridionally so as to form a circle, have same structure as rest of choroid and secrete nutrient fluids which nourish neighboring parts, as cornea, lens, vitreous body. They also serve as points of attachment for the suspensory ligament of the lens. SYN: *processus ciliaris* [NA].

c. reflex. Normal contraction of pupil in accommodation of vision from distant to near.

cil'iate [L. *cilia*, eyelashes]. Ciliated.

ciliated (sil'ĭ-a-ted). Possessing cilia.

c. epithelium. Epithelium with hairlike processes on surface. They waft only in one direction and line the respiratory tract and fallopian tubes.

ciliectomy (sil-ĭ-ek'to-mĭ) [L. *cilium*, eyelash, + G. *ektomē*, excision]. Excision of portion of ciliary body or ciliary border of eyelid.

ciliospinal (sil-ĭ-o-spi'nal) [" + *spina*, thorn]. Pert. to the ciliary body and spinal cord.

c. center. Spinal cord center which controls dilatation of the pupil.

c. reflex. Dilation of pupil following stimulation of the skin of the neck by pinching or scratching the skin.

ciliostatic (sil"ĭ-o-stat'ik). Interfering with or preventing movement of the cilia.

cilium (sĭl'ĭ-um). Singular of cilia, *q.v.*

cillosis (sil-o'sis) [L.]. Spasmodic twitching of the eyelid.

cimbia (sim'be-ă) [L.]. Slender band of white fibers crossing the ventral surface of a cerebral peduncle.

Cimex lectularius (sī'mĕks lĕk-tū-lā'rĭ-ŭs). The bedbug. An insect belonging to the order Hemiptera.

cinchona (sin-ko'nă) [Sp. *cinchon*, from Countess of Cinchon who was erroneously credited with having introduced it into Europe]. The dried bark of the tree cinchona, the source of quinine. SYN: *Peruvian bark.* SEE: *quinine.*

cinchonism (sin'kon-izm) [" + G. *ismos*, condition of]. Poisoning from cinchona or its alkaloids.

cinchophen (sin'ko-fen) (atophan). Light yellow powder with slightly bitter taste. It frequently produces serious side effects, *e.g.*, a fatal form of hepatitis; consequently it is seldom used in present-day medical therapy.

c. poisoning. SYM: Gastric irritation, nausea, vomiting, belching, heartburn, vertigo, weakness, diarrhea, itching, rash, jaundice, stupor. When chronic it is often associated with profound liver damage. Those with gallbladder disease, inflammation, or cirrhosis of liver, the undernourished and those suffering from alcoholism are esp. susceptible.

F. A. TREATMENT: Largely symptomatic. Wash out stomach; give large quantities of fluids and saline catharsis. Sugars, glucose, intravenously. Insulin if sugar appears in the urine.

cincture sensation (sink'tūr) [L. *cinctura*, from *cingere, cinctum*, to gird]. Sensation of a tight girdle about the waist. SYN: *zonesthesia.*

cinemat'ics [G. *kinema*, motion]. Science of motion; kinematics.

cinematoradiography (sin-e-mat"o-rā-dĭ-og'ra-fĭ) [" + L. *radius*, ray, + G. *graphein*, to write]. Radiography of an organ in motion.

cineplas'tics [G. *kinein*, to move, + *plastikos*, formed]. Formation after amputation of muscles of a stump, so that it is possible to impart motion and direction to an artificial limb.

cineraceous (sin-e-ra'shus) [L. *cinis, ciner-*, ash]. Like ashes.

cinerea (sin-ē'rē-ă) [L. *cinerius*, ashenhued]. Gray matter of the brain or spinal cord.

c., ala. An area at the post. end of the fourth ventricle. Called the triangle of the vagus nerve.

cine'real. Pert. to the cinerea.

cineritious (sin-er-ish'us) [L. *cineritius*, ashen]. Ashen, as the gray matter.

cinesi- [G. *kinēsis*, motion]. Prefix: Motion. See also *kinesi-*.

cingulum (sin'gu-lum) (pl. *cin'gula*) [L. girdle]. 1. A band of association fibers in the cingulate gyrus extending from anterior perforated substance posteriorly to the hippocampal gyrus. 2. An eminence on the lingual surface of the incisor teeth especially the upper ones. It is situated near the gum. Also called *basal ridge*.

cion (sī′ŏn) [G. *kiōn*, uvula]. The uvula, *q.v.*

circa (sir′kă) [L.]. Prefix: About.

circadian (sir-kā′dĭ-en) [L. *circa*, about, + *dies*, day]. Pertaining to events which occur at approximately 24-hour intervals, such as certain biological rhythms. SEE: *clock, biological*.

circinate (sur′sĭ-nāt) [L. *circinatus*, made round]. Circular.

cir′cle [L. *circulus*, dim. of *circus*, a ring]. Any ringshaped structure.

c. of diffusion. One or more on projection plane of an image not in focus of the lens.

c. of Willis. Union of the ant. and post. cerebral arteries (branches of the carotid) forming an anastomosis at base of the brain.

cir′cuit [L. *circuire*, to go around]. 1. Course or path of an electric current. 2. The path followed by a fluid circulating in a system or tubes or cavities. 3. The path followed by nerve impulses in a reflex arc from sensory receptor to effector organ.

cir′cular [L. *circularis*, pert. to a ring]. 1. Shaped like a circle. 2. Recurrent.

c. insanity. That in which manic and depressive attacks follow one another without intervals of lucidity.

circulation [L. *circulatio*, movement in a circle]. Movement in a circular course.

c. of the aqueous humor of the eye. SEE: *aqueous*.

c. of bile salts. The sodium glycocholate and taurocholate found in hepatic bile pass with it into the duodenum and then into the intestine, where they are absorbed along with the fats.

c. of the blood. The blood leaving the left ventricle enters the aorta, from which it escapes into the various large arteries. It thus reaches the coronary arteries of the heart itself and the arteries of the head, body wall, abdominal viscera, and extremities. Passing through the various capillary systems, it is gathered into veins, of which there are two systems. (1) Most veins empty their blood into the *venae cavae superior* and *inferior*. (2) The veins from the stomach, pancreas, spleen, and intestine unite to form the portal vein, which runs to the liver. Here it breaks up into a new capillary system, which drains through the hepatic veins into the *vena cava inferior*. The combined blood of the *venae cavae* and the coronary veins enters the right atrium, passes through the right ventricle, and is forced out into the pulmonary artery. The pulmonary capillary system drains by way of the pulmonary veins into the left atrium and thence into the left ventricle.

c. of the cerebrospinal fluid. SEE: *cerebrospinal*.

c., collateral. Circulation which is established through an anastomosis between two vessels supplying or draining two adjacent vascular areas. Such enables the blood to bypass an obstruction in the larger vessel supplying or draining the two areas or will enable blood to flow to or from a tissue although the principal vessel involved may be obstructed.

c., coronary. Circulation through the muscular tissue of the heart. Blood leaves the aorta through the r. and l. coronary arteries which supply the myocardium. Blood passes through capillaries and is collected in veins most of which empty into the coronary sinus which opens into the right atrium. A few of the small veins open directly into the atria and ventricles.

c., fetal. Circulation through the fetus. Blood, oxygenated in the placenta passes through the umbilical vein and ductus venosus to the inferior vena cava and thence to the right atrium from which it may follow one of two courses (1) through the *foramen ovale* to the left atrium and thence through the aorta to the tissues or (2) through the right ventricle, pulmonary artery, and ductus arteriosus to the aorta, and thence to the tissues. In either case the blood bypasses the lungs which are not functioning before birth. Blood is

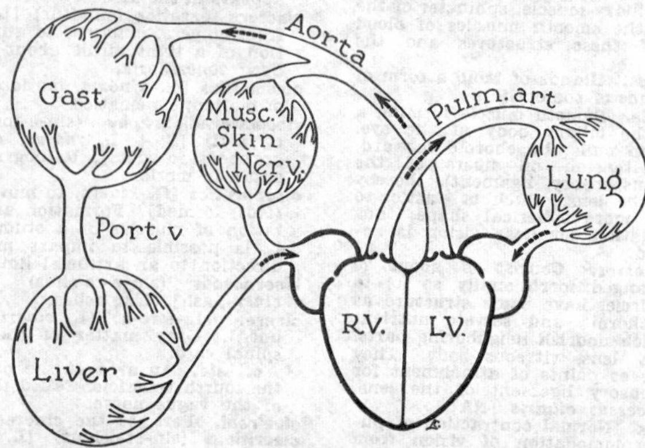

CIRCULATION

General scheme of the circulation of blood in man. Beginning with the lung, the abbreviations follow in this order: LV, left ventricle; Gast, gastrointestinal organs; Port. v., portal vein; Musc., System of voluntary muscles; Nerv., Nervous system; RV., right ventricle; Pulm. art., pulmonary artery.

returned to the placenta through the umbilical arteries which are continuations of the hypogastric arteries. At birth or shortly after, the ductus arteriosus and the foramen ovale close, establishing normal circulation. Failure of either to occur gives rise to a "blue baby."

c. of the lymph. Lymph is formed from the tissue fluid which fills the tissue spaces of the body. It is collected into lymph capillaries which carry the lymph to the larger lymph vessels. These converge to form one of two main trunks, the right lymphatic duct and the thoracic duct. The rt. lymphatic duct drains the right side of the head, neck, and trunk and right upper extremity; the thoracic duct drains all the remaining portion of the body. The latter has its origin at the cisterna chyli which receives the lymphatics from the abdominal organs. It courses upward through the diaphragm and thorax and empties into the left subclavian artery near its junction with the l. int. jugular vein. The rt. lymphatic duct empties into the rt. subclavian vein. Lymph vessels have along their course lymph nodes which function as filtering structures filtering out bacteria and particulate substances preventing their entrance into the blood stream. Lymph flow is maintained by difference in pressure at the two ends of the system. Important accessory factors aiding the flow of lymph are breathing movements and muscular activities.

c., portal. Blood from the systemic arteries is supplied to the abdominal organs and is collected into the portal vein through which the blood enters the liver. It passes into sinusoids which lead to central veins of the lobules and eventually to the hepatic veins which empty into the inf. vena cava.

c., pulmonary. The venous blood which is received into the right atrium passes through the tricuspid valve into the right ventricle. From there into the pulmonary artery, which divides into two branches, one going to each lung. (This is the only instance when an artery contains venous or dark blood deficient in oxygen.) The artery breaks up in the lung into capillaries, and here, by means of the hemoglobin in the red corpuscles, takes up oxygen from the inspired air. Red arterial blood returns to the heart by the four pulmonary veins, two from each lung entering the left atrium. (This is the only instance where veins contain oxygenated blood.)

c. rate. The minute volume or output of the heart per minute. In an average size adult with a pulse rate of 70, the amount is about 3 liters per square meter of body surface each minute.

c., systemic. General circulation through the whole body except the lungs.

c., venous. C. of the blood via the veins.

circulation time. The time required by a particle of blood to make the complete circuit of both the systemic and pulmonary systems. Circulation time is determined by injecting a substance into a vein and timing its reappearance in arteries at the point of injection or some other point in the body. Such would necessitate the blood with the contained substance passing through veins to the heart and through the right atrium and ventricle, through the pulmonary circuit to the lungs and back through the left atrium and ventricle, and then out through the aorta and arteries to the place where detected. Dyes such as florescein, methylene blue or substances such as potassium ferrocyanide or histamine have been used as tracers. Average circulation time is 18 to 24 seconds. Circulation time is reduced in anemia and hyperthyroidism; increased in hypertension, myxedema, and cardiac failure.

May also be measured by injecting in a vein a substance which can be detected by the sense of taste when it is transported to the tongue. The normal circulation time from an arm vein to the tongue is 10 to 16 seconds.

c. time, pulmonary. The time required for blood to pass through the lungs. Average time 11 seconds.

cir'culatory. Pert. to circulation.

c. failure. Failure of the cardiovascular system to provide bodily tissues with an adequate amount of blood for proper functioning. It may be due to heart (cardiac) failure or peripheral circulatory failure, as occurs in shock in which there is loss of blood plasma into the tissues with resulting decreased venous return.

c. system. The cardiovascular system consisting of the heart and blood vessels (arteries, arterioles, capillaries, venules, veins, and sinuses) and the lymphatic system.

c. system, inspection of. Inspection detects any abnormal centers of pulsation,* the apex* beat and its position, force, and extent, and any unnatural prominence over the precordial region. SEE: *abdomen; apex beat; chest; heart; lungs; pulsation.*

circum- [L.]. Prefix: Around, as *circumduction.*

circumarticular (sĭr″kŭm-ar-tĭk′ū-lar) [L. *circum,* around, + *articulus,* a joint]. Surrounding a joint. SYN: *periarthric.*

circumcision (sir-kum-sĭ′shun) [L. *circumcisio,* a cutting around]. Surgical removal of the end of the prepuce. Done for hygienic reasons. Rate of occurrence of carcinoma of the penis is much less in persons who were circumcised at birth compared to those who were not. SYN: *posthetomy.*

NP: The foreskin is often tight after birth. It should be pulled back gently at the first bath to see that the meatus is clear, and then left alone for 8 days. After this, if still tight, it should be picked up in the thumb and finger and gently coaxed backwards twice a day. If it is inclined to bleed, smear it with an antiseptic ointment. Care must be taken not to strip it backwards too far or constriction of the glans (paraphimosis) may occur. If tightness still persists or there is any difficulty in passing urine, a doctor should be consulted. Often the gentle passage of a probe by the doctor, underneath the skin of the prepuce, will obviate any need to circumcise. Strict asepsis must be maintained in the dressing of a circumcision.

c., ritual. The religious rite performed by the Jews and Muslims of removal of the prepuce.

circumclusion (sir-kum-klu′zhun) [L. *circumcludere,* to shut in]. Acupressure by use of a pin under an artery and a wire loop over it, attached to each end of the pin.

circumcor'neal [L. *circum,* around, + *corneus,* horny]. Around the cornea.

circumduction (sir-kum-duk′shun) [" + *ducere,* to lead]. 1. The action or swing of a limb, such as the arm, in such a manner that it describes a coneshaped figure, the apex of the cone being formed by the joint at the proximal end, while the complete circle is formed by the free distal end of the limb. 2. Circular movement of the eye.

circumflex (sir'kum-fleks) [" + *flectere,* to bend]. Winding around, as a vessel.

c. nerve. A motor and sensory nerve. SYN: *axillary nerve; nervus axillaris* [NA]. SEE: *Table of Nerves in Appendix.*

circumin'sular [" + *insula,* island]. Surrounding the island of Reil.

circumlen'tal [" + *lens,* lens]. Situated around the lens.

circumnu'clear [" + *nucleus,* kernel]. Surrounding the nucleus.

circumoc'ular [" + *oculus,* eye]. Surrounding the eye.

circumor'al [" + *os, or-,* mouth]. Encircling the mouth.

c. pallor. White area around the mouth contrasting vividly with color of face, esp. seen in scarlet fever.

circumorbital (sĕr"kŭm-or'bĭt-ăl) [" + *orbita,* orbit]. Around an orbit.

circumpolariza'tion [" + *polaris,* polar]. The rotation of a ray of polarized light.

circumre'nal [" + *rēnalis,* pert. to kidney]. Around or about the kidney.

cir'cumscribed [" + *scrībere,* to write]. Limited in space.

cir"cumstantial'ity [L. *circumstantia,* a standing around]. The mention of irrelevant facts and details in conversation. Usually a symptom of mental disorder.

circumval'late [L. *circum,* around, + *vallāre,* to wall]. Surrounded by a wall or raised structure.

c. papillae. V-shaped row of papillae at base of tongue.

circumvascular. Perivascular; around a blood vessel.

cirrhosis (sĭ-rō'sĭs) [G. *kirros,* yellow, + *-ōsis,* infection]. A chronic disease of the liver characterized by formation of dense perilobular connective tissue, degenerative changes in parenchymal cells, alteration in structure of the cords of liver lobules, fatty and cellular infiltration, and sometimes development of areas of regeneration.

ETIOL: May be due to various factors as nutritional deficiency (lack of proteins, choline or methionine), or poisons (carbon tetrachloride, phosphorus), or may be due to previous inflammation caused by a virus or bacteria.

c., alcoholic. That occurring commonly in alcoholics. SYN: *portal c., q.v.*

c., atrophic. Portal c., *q.v.*

c., biliary. That marked by prolonged jaundice due to chronic retention of bile and inflammation of bile ducts. SEE ALSO: *obstructive biliary c.; primary biliary c.*

c., cardiac. Congestive cirrhosis resulting from passive congestion of the liver due to cardiac disorders.

c., cholangiolitic. Primary biliary cirrhosis, *q.v.*

c., coarse nodular. Postnecrotic cirrhosis, *q.v.*

c., fatty. C. with fatty infiltration of the liver cells.

c., hypertrophic. In which the connective tissue hyperplasia causes the liver to be greatly enlarged.

c., infantile. Cirrhosis occurring in childhood, resulting from protein malnutrition. Also called *kwashiorkor.*

c., Laennec's. Portal cirrhosis, *q.v.*

c., obstructive biliary. Cirrhosis resulting from obstruction of the common duct by a stone, tumor, etc.

c., portal. Cirrhosis of the liver occurring chiefly in males following middle age and formerly thought to be caused by excessive use of alcohol but now attributed to faulty nutrition. SYN: *alcoholic c.; atrophic c.; hobnail c.; Laennec's c.*

c., postnecrotic. Form characterized by extensive destruction of liver cells as occurs in poisoning or following infections. Massive scarring occurs with areas of regeneration. SYN: *coarse nodular c.; healed yellow atrophy; toxic c.*

c., primary biliary. A rare, progressive form of cirrhosis characterized by enlargement of the liver, jaundice, and pruritus. SYN: *cholangiolitic c.*

c., syphilitic. Form occurring in tertiary syphilis in which gummas form in the liver and, on healing, cause coarse lobulation. SYN: *hepar lobatum.*

c., toxic. That resulting from toxic substances as in poisoning by carbon tetrachloride or phosphorus. SEE: *postnecrotic c.*

c., zooparasitic. Cirrhosis resulting from infestation with animal parasites especially blood flukes of the genus *Schistosoma* or liver flukes, *Clonorchis sinensis.*

cirrhotic (sĭ-rot'ĭk). Pert. to or affected with cirrhosis.

cirsectomy (sir-sek'to-mĭ) [G. *kirsos,* varix, + *ektomē,* excision]. Excision of a portion of a varicose vein.

cirsenchysis (sir-sen'kĭ-sis) [" + *enchysis,* a pouring in]. Injection of varicose veins with a sclerosing substance.

cirsocele (sir'so-sēl) [" + *kēlē,* hernia]. Dilation of veins of spermatic cord. SYN: *variocele, q.v.*

cirsodesis (sir-sod'ĕ-sis) [" + *desis,* ligation]. Ligation of varicose veins.

cirsoid (sir'soid) [" + *eidos,* resemblance]. Resembling a varix. SYN: *varicose.*

cirsomphalos (sir-som'fă-los) [" + *omphalos,* navel]. Varicose veins around the navel.

cirsotome (sir'so-tōm) [" + *tomē,* incision]. Instrument for cutting varicose veins.

cirsotomy (sir-sot'o-mĭ) [" + *tomē,* incision]. Treatment of a varicosity by multiple incisions.

C.I.S. Abbr. for *central inhibitory state.*

cis'tern [L.]. Cisterna, *q.v.*

c. of Pecquet. Cisterna chyli, *q.v.*

c., subarachnoid. Cisterna subarachnoidalis, *q.v.*

cister'na [L. a vessel]. A reservoir or cavity.

c. chy'li [NA]. *Receptaculum chyli.* A dilated sac into which is emptied the intestinal, two lumbar, and two descending lymphatic trunks; the origin of the thoracic duct.

c., subarachnoidalis [NA]. Wide spaces in the cranial cavity between the arachnoid and the pia mater. They contain cerebrospinal fluid.

cisternal (sĭs-ter'năl). Concerning a cavity filled with fluid.

c. puncture. A spinal puncture with a hollow needle bet. the cervical vertebrae, through the dura mater into the cisterna at base of brain.

PURPOSE: (a) To inject a drug or a serum as in cerebral meningitis or cerebral syphilis, or (b) to remove excess spinal fluid and consequent pressure which inhibits the flow of spinal fluid to the lumbar region, esp. when the fluid cannot be obtained by lumbar puncture. SEE: *cerebrospinal fluid; spinal puncture.*

Citel'li's syndrome. Poor memory, mental backwardness, insomnia or drowsiness, and lack of concentration in those with adenoids or sphenoid sinusitis.

citochol reaction (sī'to-kol). The use of concentrated cholesterolized extract of heart muscle as the antigen for a rapid flocculation test. SYN: *flocculation test; Sachs-Georgi test; Sachs-Witebsky test.*

citrate (sit'rāt, sī'trāt). Compound of citric acid and a base.

c. solution. One used to prevent clotting of the blood. Its use permits blood to be stored in a refrigerator until it is needed for transfusion.

citric acid. $C_6H_8O_7.H_2O$. A tribasic acid present in the juice of many fruits, esp. citrus fruits. Sometimes present in urine, esp. in alkalosis. SEE ALSO UNDER: *acid.*

citric acid cycle. A complicated series of reactions in the body involving the oxidative metabolism of pyruvic acid and liberation of energy. It is the main pathway of terminal oxidation in the process of which not only carbohydrates but proteins and fats are utilized. SYN: *Kreb's cycle; tricarboxylic acid cycle.*

citrin (sit'rin). Vitamin P. Antiscorbutic in action and found in lemon juice.

Cl. Chem. symbol for *chlorine.* Abbr. for *chloride; clavicle; Clostridium.*

cladosporiosis (klad″o-spo-rī-o'sis) [G. *klados,* branch, + *sporos,* seed, + *-ōsis,* infection]. Infection with *Cladospo'rium,* a fungus, marked by appearance of gummatous nodules.

cladothricosis (klad-o-thrī-ko'sis) [" + *thrix,* hair, + *-ōsis,* infection]. Infection with *Cladothrix.* Former name for *Nocardia asteroides.*

clam. A bivalve belonging to the phylum Mollusca. RAW (meat only): 100 gm. Calories: 82. Other main values: 14 gm. protein; 1.9 gm. fat; 1.3 gm. carbohydrates.

clamp (klamp) [Danish, *klamp,* hook]. Device for compression of vessels.

clang [L. *clangere,* to peal]. A loud, metallic sound.

c. tint. A delicate tone.

clap. Colloquial term for gonorrhea.

clapotage, clapotement (klă-po-tazh', klă-pot-mon') [Fr.]. Any splashing sound in succussion of a dilated stomach.

Clap'ton's lines. Green lines on dental margin of gums in copper poisoning.

clar'et stain or **cheek** [L. *clarētum,* light red]. Capillary nevus of cheek. SYN: *nevus flammeus.*

clarificant (klar-if'ik-ant) [L. *clarus,* clear, + *facere,* to make]. Any agent that clears the turbidity of a liquid.

Clarke's bodies [Jacob A. Clarke, English physician, 1817-1880]. Alveolar sarcomatous intranuclear bodies of breast.

C.'s column. The dorsal nucleus of the spinal cord.

clasmatoblast (klaz-mat'o-blast) [G. *klasma,* fragment, + *blastos,* germ]. A mast cell.

clasmatocyte (klaz-mat'o-sīt) [" + *kytos,* cell]. A large, wandering, uninucleated cell, with many branches.

A fixed macrophage of loose connective tissue. They are capable of ingesting particulate material and have the property of electively storing certain dyes in colloidal solution. In inflammatory conditions they become actively ameboid and are important in providing protection against local invasion by bacteria which they ingest. SYN: *histiocyte* or *tissue, macrophage.*

clasmatodendro'sis [" + *dendron,* tree, + *-ōsis,* infection]. A breaking up of astrocytic protoplasmic expansions.

clasmato'sis [" + *-ōsis,* infection]. Crumbling into small bits; fragmentation, as of cells.

clasp-knife rigidity. Spastic action in a joint in cerebral palsies.

clastic (klas'tik) [G. *klastos,* broken, from *klaein,* to break]. Causing division into parts.

clastothrix (klas'to-thriks) [" + *thrix,* hair]. Brittleness of the hair. SYN: *trichorrhexis.*

claudication (klaw-dī-ka'shun) [L. *claudicāre,* to limp]. Lameness; limping.

c., intermittent. A severe pain in calf muscles occurring during walking but which subsides with rest. It results from inadequate blood supply which may be due to arterial spasm, atherosclerosis, arteriosclerosis, or an occlusion.

c., venous. That resulting from inadequate venous drainage.

Claudius' cells (klaw'dī-us) [Friedrich Claudius, Austrian anatomist, 1822-1869]. Large columnar cells external to the organ of Corti.

C.'s fossa. Small depression in post. part of pelvis, on either side, in which lies the ovary.

claustrophilia (klaws-tro-fil'ī-ă) [L. *claustrum,* a closed space, + G. *philein,* to love]. Dread of being in an open space; a morbid desire to be shut in with doors and windows closed.

claustrophobia (klaws-tro-fo'bī-ă) [" + *phobos,* fear]. PSY: Fear of being confined in any space, as in a locked room. Opp. of *agoraphobia.**

claustrum (klaws'trum) [L. a closed space]. 1. A barrier. 2. Thin layer of gray matter separating the ext. capsule from the island of Reil.

clausura (klaws-su'ră) [L. closure]. Atresia of a passage, closure.

clava (kla'vă) (pl. *clavae*) [L. club]. An elevation on dorsal surface of the medulla oblongata caused by the underlying *nucleus gracilis,* the superior extremity of the *fasciculus gracilis.*

cla'vate [L. *clavatus,* pert. to a club]. Clubshaped.

clav'icle [L. *clavicula,* dim. of *clavis,* key]. The collarbone; a bone curved like the letter f, which articulates with the sternum and the scapula.

c., dislocation of. *Forward. Sternal end.* TREATMENT: (a) Knee placed against spine. (b) Draw shoulders back. (c) Apply clavicle bandage with pad on dislocated end of bone.

Outer Extremity: Bone upon upper surface of acromion, or upon ant. part of spine of the scapula. SYM: (a) Prominence upon surface of acromion which disappears when arm is raised. (b) Shoulders flattened, arm hanging close to trunk. TREATMENT: (a) Raise shoulder, draw backward. (b) Place pad in axilla, bringing elbow close to side. (c) Secure arm and forearm to chest with pad in axilla. (d) Pressure by pad and gutta percha plate on projecting clavicle strapped in place. SEE: *jugulum.*

c., fracture of. SYM: (1) Swelling, pain, protuberance with sharp depression over the injured bone. (2) Patient supports arm at the elbow, arm useless.

F. A. TREATMENT: (a) Place ball of cloth, 1 or 2 handkerchiefs, tightly rolled, under armpit. (b) Apply arm sling. Bandage elbow to side, hand and forearm extending across the chest. (c) Or, lay patient on back, on the floor, with rolled-up blanket under shoulders until medical aid arrives. This position keeps shoulders back and prevents broken ends of bone from rubbing.

TREATMENT (medical): (a) Have assistant draw arms and shoulders backward. (b) Raise shoulders and support in upward, backward, and outward direction. (c) Cover parts with adhesive plaster and bandage.

clavicular (kla-vik'u-lar). Pert. to the clavicle.

cla'vus [L. nail]. 1. A corn or callosity. 2. A sharp head pain like the driving of a nail into the head.

clawfoot (klaw'fut). A deformity of the foot characterized by excessively high longitudinal arch usually accompanied by dorsal contracture of toes. SYN: *pes cavus; hollow foot; contracted foot.*

clawhand. A hand characterized by hyperextension of the proximal phalanges of the digits and extreme flexion of middle and distal phalanges. Usually the result of injury to ulnar and median nerves. SYN: *main en griffe.*

claw toe. A hammer toe; extreme flexion of a toe.

Clayton gas. Sulfur dioxide.

clear'ance. The elimination of a substance from the blood plasma by the kidneys. SEE: *renal clearance.*

clear'ing agent. One that makes tissues prepared for microscopic examination more transparent.

cleavage (kle'vej) [A.S. *cleoflan,* to adhere]. 1. Splitting a complex molecule into two or more simpler ones. 2. Cell division following the fertilization of an egg. SYN: *segmentation.*

c. cell. The blastomere.

c., hydrolytic. Hydrolysis.

c. lines. Lines indicating the prevailing direction of fibers in the corium of the skin. In a living subject or fresh cadaver, a puncture wound does not remain round but becomes elliptical in the direction of the fibers. Lines in general run obliquely. This is important to the surgeon because an incision parallel to these lines will heal with much less scarring than one across the lines. SYN: *Langer's lines; tension lines.*

cleft [M.E. *clyft,* crevice]. 1. A fissure. 2. Divided or split.

c., branchial. An opening between the branchial arches of an embryo. In lower vertebrates it becomes a gill cleft.

c. cheek. Macrostomia; transverse facial cleft.

c., facial. An anomaly resulting from failure of facial processes of embryo to fuse. Common ones are *oblique facial cleft,* an open nasolacrimal furrow extending from eye to lower portion of nose which is sometimes continuous with a cleft in upper lip. *Transverse facial cleft* extends laterally from the angle of the mouth.

c., foot. A bipartite foot resulting from failure of a digit and its corresponding metatarsal to develop.

c. hand. A bipartite hand resulting from failure of a digit and its corresponding metacarpal to develop.

c. palate. A congenital fissure in the palate (roof of mouth) forming a communicating passageway between mouth and nasal cavities. May be *unilateral* or *bilateral, complete* or *incomplete.*

c. sternum. A congenital fissure of the breastbone.

c. tongue. A bifid tongue; one with a separated tip.

cleido- (kli'do) [G. *kleis,* clavicle]. Prefix: Pert. to the clavicle.

cleidorrhexis (kli-do-rek'sis) [G. *kleis,* clavicle, + *rēxis,* rupture]. Fracture or bending the clavicles of the fetus for delivery.

cleidotomy (kli-dot'o-mĭ) [" + *tomē,* a cutting]. Dividing a fetal clavicle to facilitate delivery.

cleptoma'nia [G. *kleptein,* to steal, + *mania,* madness]. Impulsive stealing, the intrinsic value of the article not being the motive. SYN: *kleptomania, q.v.*

clergyman's sore throat. A form of granular pharyngitis.

climacteric (kli-mak'ter-ĭk, kli-mak-ter'-ĭk) [G. *klimaktēr,* a round of a ladder]. That period that marks the cessation of a woman's reproductive period (female climacteric); a corresponding period of lessening of sexual activity in the male (male climacteric).

c., grand. The 63rd year.

climatol'ogy [G. *klima,* climate, + *logos,* study of]. Branch of meteorology which is the study of climate and its relation to disease. SEE: *bioclimatology.*

climatotherapy (kli-mat-ō-ther'ap-ĭ) [" + *therapeia,* treatment]. Treatment of disease by having patient move to a more favorable climate.

cli'max [G. *klimax,* ladder]. 1. Period of greatest intensity. 2. The orgasm, *q.v.*

cli'mograph [G. *klima,* climate, + *graphein,* to write]. A graph of the effect of climate on health.

clinic (klin'ĭk) [G. *klinikos,* pert. to a bed]. 1.Medical instruction in which patients are observed directly, symptoms noted, treatment discussed, etc. 2. A center for physical examination and treatment of ambulant patients who are not hospitalized. 3. A place where individuals gather together with patients for the study of disease. 4. A place where preliminary diagnosis is made and treatment given, as an *X-ray clinic* or *child-guidance clinic.*

clin'ical. 1. Founded on actual observation and treatment of patients as distinguished from data or facts obtained by experimentation or pathology. 2. Pert. to a clinic.

c. analysis. The chemical analysis and study of body fluids, excreta, and tissues in the diagnosis and treatment of disease.

c. pathology. That division of pathology which utilizes clinical analysis and other laboratory procedures in the diagnosis and treatment of disease.

c. procedures. Procedures usually carried out by a physician or under his immediate supervision, and usually at the patient's bedside in contrast to *bedside procedures* (those carried on by nurses) or *office procedures.* Such involves route of medication, local anesthesia, aspiration of fluids, administration of oxygen, etc.

c. thermometer. One which measures body temperature.

They may be disinfected by first cleansing with cotton and soap solution, using a rotary motion downward to bulb end. This removes adherent mucus which coagulates in some disinfectants, thereby retaining organisms. Rinse thoroughly in water and submerge in 70% alcohol for 10 minutes. Rinse before use. SEE: *thermometer.*

clinician (klin-ish'an) [G. *klinikos*, pert. to a bed]. A practicing physician.

clinodactylism (kli'no-dak'tĭ-lizm). Clinodactyly.

clinodactyly (kli'no-dak'tĭ-le) [G. *klinein*, to bend + *daktylos*, finger]. Permanent deflection, either medial or lateral, of one or more fingers.

clinoid (kli'noid) [G. *klinē*, bed, + *eidos*, appearance]. Resembling a bed in shape.

c. processes. Three pairs of prominences on upper surface of sphenoid bone.

clinom'eter [G. *klinein*, to decline, + *metron*, measure]. Instrument for estimation of torsional deviation of eyes. This is used to measure ocular muscle paralysis. SYN: *clinoscope.*

cli'noscope [" + *skopein*, to examine]. Instrument for measuring the weakness of ocular muscles.

clinostat'ic [G. *klinē*, bed, + *stasis*, position]. Caused by assuming a recumbent position.

clinostat'ism. The recumbent position.

clip. Instrument for holding tissue or other material together.

cliseometer (klis-e-om'et-er) [G. *klisis*, inclination, + *metron*, measure]. Device for measuring the inclination which the female pelvis makes with the spinal column.

clithrophobia (klith-ro-fo'bĭ-ă) [G. *kleithria*, keyhole, + *phobos*, fear]. Morbid fear of being locked in.

clition (klit'ĭ-on) [G. *klitus*, slope]. A craniometric point in center of highest part of the clivus on the sphenoid bone.

clitoridauxe (klit-or-id-awk'sĕ) [G. *kleitoris*, clitoris, + *auxē*, increase]. Hypertrophy of the clitoris.

clitoridectomy (klit-or-ĭ-dek'to-mĭ) [" + *ektomē*, excision]. Excision of clitoris.

clitoriditis (klit-or-id-i'tis) [" + *-itis*, inflammation]. Inflammation of the clitoris.

clitoridotomy (klit-or-ĭ-dot'ō-mĭ) [" + *tomē*, incision]. Incision of the clitoris.

clitoris (klĭ'to-rĭs, klit'ō-rĭs) [G. *kleitoris*]. One of the organs of the female genitalia. It is an erectile structure located beneath the anterior labial commissure and partially hidden by the anterior ends of the labia minora. It is homologous to the penis of the male.

Structure. It consists of three parts: a body, two crura, and a glans. (a) The body, about an inch in length, consists of two fused corpora cavernosa. It extends from the pubic arch above to the glans below. (b) The two *crura* are continuations of the corpora cavernosa and serve to attach them to the inferior rami of the pubic bones. They are covered by the ischiocavernosus muscles. (c) The *glans* which forms the free distal end is a small rounded tubercle composed of erectile tissue. It is highly sensitive. The glans is usually covered by a hood-like prepuce and its ventral surface is attached to the frenulum of the labia.

c. crises. Recurring involuntary crises of excess of sexual excitement in women. Occurs in tabes dorsalis.

clitorism (klit'or-izm) [G. *kleitoris*, + *ismos*]. 1. The counterpart of priapism. A long continued, painful condition in the female with recurring erection of the clitoris. 2. Enlargement of the clitoris.

clitoritis (klit-o-ri'tis) [" + *-itis*, inflammation]. Inflammation of the clitoris. SYN: *clitoriditis.*

clivus (klĭ'vus) [L. a slope]. A surface that slopes, as the sphenoid bone.

c. blumenbach'ii. The slope at base of skull.

clo. A unit of thermal insulation.

cloaca (klo-ā'kă) [L. a sewer]. 1. Cavity lined with endoderm at the posterior end of the body which serves as a common passageway for urinary, digestive and reproductive ducts. Present in adults of birds, reptiles and amphibia and in the embryos of all vertebrates. 2. An opening in the sheath covering necrosed bone.

clock. Device for measuring time.

c., biological. An internal mechanism which apparently regulates cyclic phenomena such as the wake–sleep cycle, menstrual cycle, and hourly variations in the level of hormones such as those from the adrenal cortex. SEE ALSO: *circadian.*

clone (klōn) [G. *klon*, a cutting used for propagation]. In tissue culture, a group of cells descended from a single cell.

clonic (klon'ik) [G. *klonos*, turmoil]. Pert. to alternate contraction and relaxation of muscles.

c. spasm. One marked by muscular rigidity and then relaxation.

clonicity (klon-is'ĭ-tĭ) [G. *klonos*, turmoil]. Being clonic.

clonicotonic (klon-ĭ-ko-ton'ĭk) [" + *tonikos*, tone]. Both clonic and tonic, as some forms of muscular spasm.

clon'ism, clonis'mus [" + *ismos*, condition of]. Condition of being affected with clonic spasms, or a succession of them.

clon'ograph [" + *graphein*, to write]. An instrument for registering spasmodic movements.

clon'ospasm [" + *spasmos*, spasm]. Rapid alternation of muscular contraction and relaxation.

The rate is much slower than a tremor. In upper motor neurone paralysis, sharp flexion of ankle often produces ankle clonus.

clon'us [G. *klonos*, turmoil]. Spasmodic alternation of contraction and relaxation; opposite of *tonus*. SEE: *wrist clonus.*

Cloquet's canal (klo-kās'). An irregular passage (hyaloid) through center of the vitreous body in the fetus.

Clostrid'ium. A genus of bacteria belonging to the family Bacillaceae. They are anaerobic, spore-forming rods and are widely distributed in nature. They are common in the soil and in the intestinal tract of man and animals and are frequently found in wound infections. Several are pathogenic in man, being the primary causative agents for gas gangrene.

Cl. botulinum. Grows in improperly processed food. Produces a powerful toxin, the cause of botulism, *q.v.*

Cl. chauvoei. Cause of blackleg, or symptomatic anthrax, in cattle.

Cl. histolyticum. A proteolytic organism found in gas gangrene.

Cl. novyi. Found in cases of gas gangrene. SYN: *Novy's bacillus.*

Cl. perfringens. A cause of gas gangrene. SYN: *gas bacillus; Cl. welchii.*

Cl. septicum. Found in cases of gangrene in man, cattle, hogs, and other domestic animals. SYN: *Ghon-Sachs bacillus.*

Cl. sporogenes. Frequently associated with other organisms in mixed gangrenous infections.

Cl. tetani. The causative organism of tetanus or lockjaw. Produces a powerful exotoxin, a portion of which affects nerve tissue, another portion is hemolytic. SYN: *Nicolaier's bacillus.*

Cl. welchii. Cl. perfringens, *q.v.*

clot (klŏt) [A.S. *clott*]. 1. To coagulate. 2. A thrombus; a coagulum, as of blood or lymph.

SEE: *blood, clotting of; thrombosis.*

c., agony. One formed in the heart when death ensues from prolonged heart failure.

c., antemortem. One formed in the heart or its cavities before death.

c., blood. A coagulum formed of blood. SEE: *blood, clotting of; thrombosis.*

c., chicken fat. A yellow-colored blood clot having no erythrocytes.

c., currant jelly. A clot of fibrin of reddish color and jellylike consistency.

c., distal. One formed in a vessel on distal side of a ligature.

c., external. One formed outside a blood vessel.

c., heart. A thrombus within the heart.

c., internal. One formed by solidification of blood.

c., laminated. One formed in a succession of layers filling an aneurysm.

c., muscle. One formed in coagulation of muscle plasma.

c., passive. One formed in the sac of an aneurysm.

c., plastic. One formed from the intima of an artery at the point of ligation.

c., postmortem. One formed in the heart or blood vessel after death.

c., proximal. One formed on the proximal side of a ligature.

c., stratified. Thrombus consisting of layers of different colors.

clothes louse. *Pediculus corporis;* a body louse.

cloth'ing [A.S. *clāthian,* to clothe]. Clothes conserve heat energy. A greater amount of energy is required to heat the body in cold weather if insufficient clothing is worn.

Air spaces in a fabric conserve heat. It is texture, not the material alone, that makes for warmth. Woolen fabrics lose in warmth when the material is matted down and the air spaces are destroyed. Wool and silk absorb more moisture than other fabrics but silk loses it more readily. Cotton and linen come next but linen loses moisture quicker than cotton. Open mesh is necessary to prevent chill from evaporation. Knitted fabrics absorb and dry more readily than woven fabrics of the same material. Temperature inside a hat worn by a man varies from 13° to 20° hotter than outside temperature. Body heat increased when moisture from wet garments cannot escape.

clot'ting. Coagulation, *q.v.*

c. time. Coagulation time, *q.v.*

clouding of consciousness. PSY: A state of mental confusion characterized by insufficiency of perception and impaired attention, and resulting in loss of orientation of time and place. amnesia and ill-adjusted reactions. Occurs in toxic, febrile, and other deliria as well as in cases where insufficient oxygen is being supplied to the brain. SEE: *consciousness.*

clou'dy swelling. Degeneration in which the tissues swell and become turbid.

clove, oil of. USP. A volatile oil distilled from the dried flower buds of the clove tree. SYN: *Caryophyllus.*

ACTION AND USES: Antiseptic and aromatic. Useful also as an anodyne in dental practice.

clo'ven spine. Spina bifida. Congenital defect of spinal canal walls caused by lack of union bet. laminae of the vertebrae.

clown'ism. Grotesque actions and attitudes, esp. that in certain hysterical states or in epilepsy.

clubbed fingers. Rounding of ends and swelling of fingers in children with congenital heart disease and in older children and adults with long standing pulmonary disease.

clubfoot. Nontraumatic congenital foot deformity. SEE: *talipes.*

clubhand. Deformity of the hand resembling clubfoot. SYN: *talipomanus, q.v.*

clumping [A.S. *clympre,* a lump]. Clumping of microorganisms in a culture when specific immune serum is added. SYN: *agglutination.*

clu'nes [L. pl. of *clunis,* buttock]. The buttocks; nates.

cluttering. A speech defect characterized by omission of letters or syllables.

Clutton's synovitis [Henry H. Clutton, English surgeon, 1850-1909]. Hydroarthrosis of the knee joint often associated with interstital keratitis, seen in congenital syphilis. SYN: *Clutton's joint.*

clysis (kli'sis) [G. *klyzein,* to cleanse]. Injection of fluid for washing out the blood in a cavity.

clysma (klis'mă) [G.]. An enema.*

clys'ter [G. *klystēr,* enema]. An enema; a clysma.

C. M. Abbr. for *chirurgiae magister,* Master in Surgery.

C/M. Abbr. for *counts per minute.*

cm. Abbr. for *centimeter.*

CN. Abbr. for *cyanogen radical.*

cnemial (ne'mĭ-al) [G. *knēmis,* leg]. Pert. to the leg, esp. the shin.

cnemis (ne'mis) [G. *knēmis,* leg]. Shin, lower leg, tibia.

cnemitis (ne-mi'tis) [" + *-itis,* inflammation]. Inflammation of the tibia.

CNS. Abbr. for *central nervous system.*

CO. Symb. for *carbon monoxide.*

CO_2. Symb. for *carbon dioxide.*

CO_2 therapy. Therapeutic application of low temperatures with solid carbon dioxide. Also inhalation of carbon dioxide to stimulate breathing. SEE: *refrigeration.*

Co. Chem. symb. for *cobalt.*

co"activ'ity [L. *coactāre,* to force]. Action that aids an enzyme to function, as the action of bile salts upon lipase, but not the same as that incited by an activator.

Dialysis will remove the bile salts, whereas an active enzyme cannot be transformed back to an inactive zymogen, proving the difference bet. coactivity and *activation.*

coadunation (ko-ad-u-na'shun) [L. *co,* together, + *ad,* to, + *unus,* one]. Union or junction of dissimilar substances in one mass.

coagglutina'tion [" + *agglutinans,* gluing]. Clumping by an antigen and the homologous antibody of the corpuscles of another organism.

coagglu'tinin. An antibody that is effective on two or more organisms.

coag'ula [L. pl. a blood clot]. Plural of *coagulum.*

coagulable (ko-ag'u-lă-bl) [L. *coagulum,* blood clot]. Capable of clotting; apt to clot.

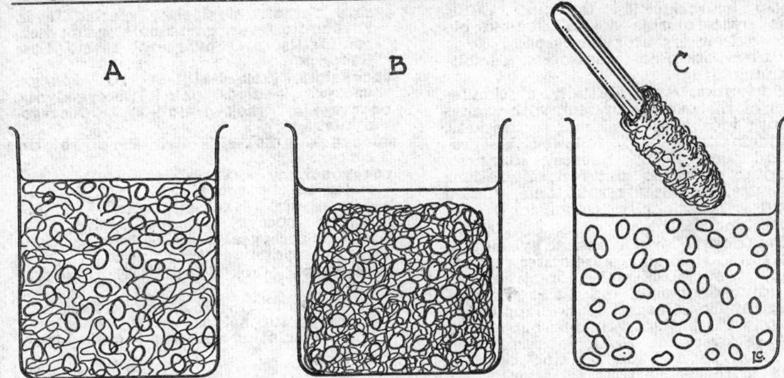

COAGULATION AND DEFIBRINATION
A, A fresh clot contains fibrin threads, corpuscles, and serum. B, On standing, the fibrin contracts, retaining most of the corpuscles, but releasing some of the serum. C, If blood is stirred before and during the process of coagulation, the fibrin clings to the stirring rod and leaves the mixture of corpuscles and serum called defibrinated blood.

coagulant (ko-ag'u-lant) [L. *coagulans*, congealing]. 1. That which causes a fluid to coagulate. 2. Causing coagulation.

coagulase (ko-ag'u-lāz) [L. *coagulum*, blood clot]. Any enzyme, such as thrombin, which causes coagulation.

coagulate (kō-ăg'ū-lāt) [L. *coagulāre*, to congeal]. To solidify or to change from a fluid state to a semisolid mass.

coag'ulated. Clotted or curdled.

c. proteins. Derived proteins (insoluble), resulting from the action of alcohol on protein, or heat on protein solutions.

coagula'tion [L. *coagulatiō*]. The process of clotting.

Coagulation depends upon the presence of several substances. Some of the most important are: (1) prothrombin, (2) thrombin, (3) thromboplastin (thrombokinase), (4) calcium in ionic form, and (5) fibrinogen. Prothrombin is converted to thrombin by the action of thromboplastin in the presence of calcium ions. Thrombin then acts on the soluble fibrinogen of the plasma converting it to insoluble fibrin. The fibrin forms a meshwork of fibers in which the corpuscles of the blood become entangled thus forming a clot. Shrinkage of the fibrin causes the exudation of plasma minus fibrinogen which constitutes blood serum. When blood is shed through an injured vessel, thromboplastin is liberated from the injured tissues and from degenerating blood platelets. This initiates the clotting mechanism.

In schematic form, the clotting process is as follows: *prothrombin* + *thromboplastin* + *calcium ions* → *thrombin*

Thrombin + fibrinogen → fibrin.

Clotting is retarded by (1) cold, (2) smooth surfaces, (3) substances which combine with calcium, such as EDTA (ethylenediamine tetraacetic acid), (4) neutral salts such as magnesium or sodium sulfate, (5) certain substances of biological origin such as hirudin, heparin, snake venoms, cysteine, and dicoumarol.

Clotting is hastened by (1) warming, (2) providing a rough surface, (3) use of chemical substance such as adrenalin, thrombin, thromboplastin.

coagulation time. The time required for a small amount of blood to coagulate. This can be determined by (1) collecting blood in a small test tube and noting elapsed time from moment blood is shed to time it coagulates or (2) collecting blood in a small capillary tube and breaking off small pieces of the tube at 30 sec. intervals. Coagulation is indicated by the appearance of fine threads of fibrin between the broken ends of the tube. Normal time, using the capillary tube method is 6 to 17 minutes. SYN: *clotting time.*

coag'ulative. Causing coagulation.

coagulometer (ko-ag-u-lom'et-er) [" + G. *metron*, measure]. Device for measuring the blood's coagulation time.

coag'ulum [L.]. 1. A blood clot. 2. A curd.

coalesce (ko-al-es') [L. *coalēscere*, to grow together]. To fuse; run or grow together.

coales'cence [L. *coalēscere*, to grow together]. Fusion or growing together of two or more parts of bodies.

coal tar. A tar that is produced in the destructive distillation of bituminous coal, as crude creosol.

coapta'tion [L. *coaptāre*, to fit together]. The adjustment of separate parts to each other, as the edges of fractures.

coarctate (ko-ark'tāt) [L. *coarctāre*, to tighten]. To press or pressed together.

c. retina. Funnelshaped retina.

coarcta'tion [L. *coarctatio*, a tightening]. 1. Compression of the walls of a vessel. 2. Shriveling. 3. A stricture.

c. of aorta. Narrowing of the aorta.

coarctotomy (ko-ark-tot'o-mĭ) [" + G. *tomē*, incision]. Cutting or division of a stricture.

coat. A covering or a layer in the wall of a tubular structure as the inner coat (tunica intima), middle coat (tunica media), and outer coat (tunica adventitia) of an artery.

cobalt (kō'balt). A chemical element, a gray, hard, ductile metal. In experimental animals it stimulates erythropoiesis. SYMB: Co. At. wt. 59.933; at. no. 27.

cobra venom solution (kō'bră vĕn'ŭm). Minute quantities of the secretion of the cobra in sterile physiological salt solution.

cocaine hydrochlor'ide (ko-kān'). USP. The hydrochloride of an alkaloid obtained from erythroxylin cocoa.

CHIEF USES: Local anesthetic. A habit-forming drug.

POISONING: SYM: Initially, a stimulation of the nervous system, with excitement, incoherent talking, restlessness, hallucinations, etc., followed by profound depression, nausea, dizziness, tingling of hands and feet, alterations of pulse, increased respirations, dilated pupils; occasionally convulsions, collapse, and death.

TREATMENT: When taken by mouth, evacuate stomach. Administer tannic acid, strong black coffee, or strong tea to dilute the poison and act as a stimulant. Apply external heat. Slapping or moving the patient valuable, but should not be overdone. Artificial respiration and oxygen and short-acting barbiturate to relieve nervous agitation.

CAUTION: Do not administer morphine or opium derivatives.

cocainism (ko-kān'izm) [L. *cocaina,* + G. *ismos,* condition of]. The habitual use of cocaine; more rare than morphinism. Cocaine is often used with morphine, or as a substitute. SEE: *cocaine hydrachloride.*

cocainization (ko-kān-ĭ-za'shun). Inducing analgesia by use of cocaine.

cocainomania (ko-kān-o-ma'ne-ă) [L. *cocaina,* + G. *mania,* madness]. Intense desire for cocaine and its results.

Coccidia (kok-sĭd'ĭ-ă). An order of protozoa belonging to the class Sporozoa. All are intracellular parasites usually infecting epithelial cells of the intestine and associated glands. They are principally parasites of lower animals causing great economic loss among domestic and game animals. Practically all domestic animals suffer from coccidial disease. Only one species, *Isospora hominis* infects humans. The geographic area of infestation is largely confined to the Far East.

coccidioidomycosis (kŏk-sĭd-ĭ-oyd-ō-mī-kō'sĭs). A coccidioidal granuloma. SYN: *valley fever; desert rheumatism; San Joaquin Valley fever.*

Exists in two forms (1) *primary coccidioidomycosis* which is an acute, self-limiting disease involving only the respiratory organs and (2) *progressive coccidioidomycosis,* a chronic, diffuse, malignant disease that may involve almost any part of the body.

ETIOL: Caused by a pathogenic fungus, *Coccidioides immitis.*

PROG: For the primary type, favorable; for the progressive type, grave, often fatal.

coccidiosis (kok-sid-ĭ-o'sis) [G. dim. of *kokkos,* berry, + *-ōsis,* infection]. Pathogenic condition resulting from infestation with coccidia. SEE: *Coccidia.*

coccobacilli (kŏk-ō-bă-sĭl'ī). Bacilli which are short and thick and somewhat ovoid in form.

coccogenous (kok-oj'en-us) [" + *gennan,* to produce]. Produced by cocci.

coccoid (kok'oid) [" + *eidos,* appearance]. Resembling a micrococcus.

coccus (kok'us) (pl. *cocci*) [G. *kokkos,* berry]. A type of bacteria which is spherical or ovoid in form. When they appear singly they are designated *micrococci;* in pairs, *diplococci;* in clusters like bunches of grapes, *staphylococci;* in chains, *streptococci;* in cubical packets of eight, *sarcinae.* Many are pathogenic causing such diseases as septic sore throat, erysipelas, scarlet fever, rheumatic fever, pneumonia, gonorrhea, meningitis, and puerperal fever. SEE: *Bacteria.*

coccyalgia (kok-sĭ-al'jĭ-ă) [G. *kokkyx,* coccyx, + *algos,* pain]. Coccygodynia.

coccydynia (kok-sĭ-din'ĭ-ă). Coccygodynia.

coccygeal (kok-sij'ē-al). Pert. to the coccyx.

coccygectomy (kok-sĭ-jek'to-mĭ). Excision of the coccyx.

coccygodynia (kok-sĭ-go-din'ĭ-ă) [G. *kokkyx,* coccyx, + *odynē,* pain]. Pain in the coccygeal region. SYN: *coccyalgia; coccydynia; coccyodynia.*

coccyodynia (kok-sĭ-o-din'ĭ-ă). Coccygodynia.

coccyx (kok'siks) [G. *kokkyx*]. Last four bones of the spine. Usually ankylosed and articulating with the sacrum above.

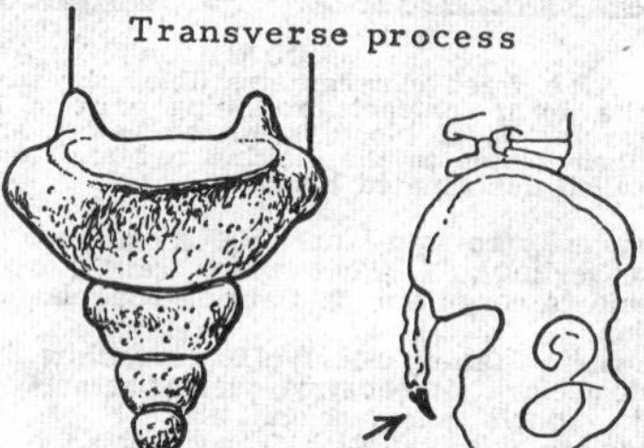

COCCYX, Anterior and lateral views.

cochineal (koch'in-ēl) [L. *coccinella*]. Dried female insect, used as a dye in laboratory work.

cochlea (kok'lē-ă) [G. *kochliās,* a spiral]. A winding cone-shaped tube forming a portion of the inner ear. It contains the *organ of Corti,* the receptor for hearing.

The cochlea is coiled resembling a snail shell, winding two and three-quarters turns about a central bony axis, the *modiolus.* Projecting outward from the modiolus is a thin bony plate, the *spiral lamina* which partially divides the cochlear canal into an upper passageway, the *scala vestibuli* and a lower one, the *scala tympani.* Lying between the two scalae is the *cochlear duct,* in the floor of which lies the *spiral organ* (of Corti). The base of the cochlea adjoins the vestibule; at the cupola or tip, the two scalae are joined at the *helicotrema.*

cochlear (kok'le-ar). Pert. to the cochlea.

c. nerve. The division of the stato-acoustic nerve (8th cranial nerve) which supplies the cochlea. SEE ALSO: *vestibulocochlear nerve.*

cochleare (kok-le-a're) [G. *kochliarion*]. Spoonful.

cochleariform (kok-le-ar'ĭ-form) [" + L. *forma,* shape]. Spoonshaped.

cochleitis (kok-le-ī'tis) [G. *kochliās,* spiral, + *-ītis,* inflammation]. Inflammation of the cochlea. SYN: *cochlitis.*

cochleo-orbicular reflex (kok-le-o-or-bik'u-lar). Contraction of orbicularis palpebrarum muscle resulting from sudden noise being produced near ear. SYN: *cochleopalpebral reflex.*

cochleopalpebral reflex (kok-lē-ō-pal'pē-bral). Contraction of orbicularis palpebrarum muscle resulting from sudden noise being produced near ear. SYN: *cochleo-orbicular reflex.*

cochleovestibular (kok-le-o-ves-tib'u-lar) [G. *kochliās*, spiral, + L. *vestibulum*, from *vestis*, garment]. Pert. to the cochlea and vestibule of the ear.

cochlitis (kok-li'tis) [" + *-itis*, inflammation]. Cochleitis, *q.v.*

cock'roach [Sp. *cucaracha*]. *Blatta orientalis.* A common insect belonging to the order Orthoptera, which infests homes and eating places. They are swift-running omnivorous insects averaging about 2 cm. in length. Through their dual contact with filth and food, they may mechanically transmit bacteria, protozoan cysts, and helminth ova. Common genera are *Blatta, Blatella* and *Periplaneta.*

COCL. Abbr. for *cathodal opening clonus.*

co'coa [Sp. *coco*, from G. *kokkos*, berry]. 1. A food substance obtained from the ripe seed of the cacao or cocoa tree. *Theobroma cacao.* It is prepared by pulverizing the residue after most of the fat has been removed from plain chocolate. 2. A beverage prepared from the powder.

Cocoa (mix for hot chocolate beverage): 100 gm. Calories: 392. Other main values: 9.4 gm. protein; 10.6 gm. fat; 74 gm. carbohydrates; 275 mg. calcium.

cocoa butter (theobroma oil). USP. The fat obtained from the roasted seed of cacao. Uses: Suppositories and in toilet preparations as a lubricant.

cocon'sciousness [L. *co*, together, + *conscius*, aware]. A conscious objective state in which subconscious impressions rise to the surface.

cocontraction (kō-kon-trak'shun) [" + *contractio*, a drawing together]. Adjustment of two muscles during contraction, said of antagonist muscles in coordination.

co'conut [fruit of *Cocos nucifera*]. The edible fruit of the coconut palm.

Dried (shredded and sweetened): 100 gm. Calories: 548. Other main values: 3.6 gm. protein; 39 gm. fat; 53 gm. carbohydrates; 16 mg. calcium; 2 mg. iron.

c. water (liquid from coconuts). 100 gm. Calories: 22. Trace of fat and protein. 4.7 gm. carbohydrates.

coctolabile (kok-to-la'bĭl) [L. *coctus*, cooked, + *labilis* perishable]. Unaltered when subjected to boiling water.

coctoprecipitin (kok-to-pre-sip'it-in) [" + *praecipitāre*, to cast down]. A precipitin produced by injecting a serum that has been boiled.

coctostabile (kok-to-sta'bĭl) [" + *stabilis*, resisting]. Incapbale of being altered or destroyed by boiling water.

codeine (ko'de-ĭn) [L. *codina*, from G. *kōdeia*, poppyhead]. An alkaloid obtained from opium, or synthetically from morphine as methylmorphine.

Action and Uses: Analgesic, hypnotic sedative with effects resembling morphine. Used commonly for its effectiveness in suppressing coughs.

Poisoning: Sym: Depression of central nervous system to the point of sleep.

Treatment: Similar to morphine.

Incompatibilities: Ferrous iodide, Lugol's solution.

c. phosphate. USP. Phosphate of the alkaloid codeine with a preference because of its free solubility in water. Much weaker than morphine. Used as codeine.

c. sulfate. The sulfate of the alkaloid codeine. Action and Uses: Same as codeine.

Codivilla's extension (ko-di-vil'lă). One for fractures made by weight pulling on a nail passed through the lower end of the bone.

cod liver oil (oleum morrhuae). USP. A fixed oil obtained from the fresh livers of the cod fish. The official oil is standardized for its vitamin A and D content.

Action and Uses: Used in cases of nutritional deficiency to supply vitamins A and D. Especially used for prophylaxis of rickets in infants.

Incompatibilities: Light and air, both being contributing factors toward rancidity.

coefficient (ko-ef-fish'ent) [L. *con*, together, + *efficere*, to produce]. A figure put before a chemical formula to express amt. or degree of normal change in a substance under stated conditions.

c. of absorption. Volume of gas absorbed by a unit volume of a liquid at 0° C. and a pressure of 760 mm.

c., isotonic. Number showing the amt. of salt to be added to distilled water to prevent the destruction of erythrocytes when it is added to blood.

c., lethal. Concentration of disinfectant that will kill bacteria in the shortest length of time at 20-25° C.

coelom (sē'lom). The cavity in an embryo between the split layers of lateral mesoderm. In mammals it develops into the pleural, peritoneal, and pericardial cavities.

c. extraembryonic. In man, the cavity in the developing blastocyst which lies between the mesoderm of the chorion and the mesoderm covering the amniotic cavity and yolk sac.

coenocyte (sē'nō-sīt, sĕn'ō-sīt). A multinucleated mass of protoplasm; a mass of protoplasm in which cell membranes are lacking between the nuclei, as in striated muscle cells; a syncytium.

coen'zyme [L. *co*, together, + G. *en*, with, + *zymē*, leaven]. Enzyme activators. A diffusible, heat stable substance of low molecular weight which when combined with an inactive protein called *apoenzyme*, forms an active compound or a complete enzyme called *holoenzyme*. Examples are adenylic acid, riboflavin, and coenzymes I and II. See: *coactivity.*

coetaneous (ko-e-ta'ne-us) [" + *aetās*, age]. Having the same age or date.

coexcitation (ko-ek-sī-ta'shun) [" + *excitāre*, to arouse]. Simultaneous excitation of two parts or bodies.

coferment (ko-fer'ment) [" + *fermentātiō*, ferment]. A coenzyme.

cof'fee [L. *caffea*]. Seed of the berry of *Coffea arabica.*

Comp: Coffee has no nutritive value. Caffeine is its essential principle and this is combined with caffeotannic acid, making it slightly antiseptic.

A cup of coffee contains 90 mg. of caffeine. This principle is a trimethyl xanthine and its use promotes excretion of uric acid in the urine.

Action: *Stomach*: Action is light and aids digestion. Cold coffee with plenty of water does not fatigue the stomach. Even with dyspepsia strong coffee does not always prove baneful.

Circulation: Raises the tension of the vascular and nervous systems. Raises the temperature, modifies the heart beats. Relieves fatigue, stimulates activity, esp. cerebral and muscular activity. Prevents sleep in some individuals through increased cerebral stimulation. Whether it diminishes the consumption of albumin is a debatable question.

Kidneys: It is a diuretic, producing uric acid and taxing the suprarenal capsules. Overdoses are toxic, causing caffeinism, *q.v.*

IND: Use where a quick stimulation is necessary. As an antidote for morphine and opium, in acute alcoholism, and where it is necessary to keep one awake.

CONTRA: Do not use in affections of the heart; in angina; hypertension; scleroma; neurasthenia; dyspepsia; acne rosacea; psoriasis; uremia; gout; arthritis; liver complaints, and congestion of the visual organs, or when alkaloids or quinine sulfate are being administered. SEE: *chocolate, cocoa, tea.*

c.-ground vomitus. Vomit similar to coffee-grounds in pigment and consistency, occurring as a result of blood mixed in the vomitus.

Cogan's syndrome (ko'ganz). Interstitial keratitis, associated with tinnitus, vertigo, and usually deafness.

cogni'tion [L. *cognōscere,* to know]. Awareness, having perception and memory.

cog'wheel respira'tion. A sudden, brief halt in inspiration and expiration.

cohabita'tion [L. *cohabitāre,* to dwell together]. 1. Sexual intercourse. 2. State of monogamy.

coherent (kō-hēr'ĕnt). 1. Sticking together, as parts of bodies or fluids. 2 Consistent; making a logical whole.

cohe'sion [L. *cohaerere,* to adhere]. The property of adhering.

cohe'sive. Adhesive; sticky.

Cohnheim's areas (kōn'hīmz) [Julius Friedrich Cohnheim, German pathologist, 1839-1884]. Irregular groups of fibrils seen in a cross section of a striated muscle fiber. Also called *Cohnheim's fields.*

C.'s theory. Theory that tumors result from embryonal cells not utilized for fetal development.

coiled posture. A natural position with some, but esp. assumed in cerebral diseases, in hepatic, intestinal, or renal colic. SEE: *posture; illustration C-66.*

coilonychia (koy-lo-nik'ĭ-ă). Koilonychia, *q.v.*

coin counting. A sliding movement of tips of thumb and index finger over each other in paralysis agitans. SYN: *pill rolling tremor.*

c. test. A metallic sound heard in pneumothorax. SYN: *bell metal resonance, q.v.*

coital (ko'ĭ-tal). Pert. to sexual intercourse.

coition (ko-ish'un) [L. *coitus,* a uniting]. Coitus, sexual intercourse.

coitophobia (ko-i-to-fo'bĭ-ă) [" + G. *phobos,* fear]. Morbid fear of sexual intercourse.

coitus (ko'i-tus) [L. a uniting]. Coition, copulation, *q.v.* Sexual intercourse bet. man and woman.

c. à la vache. Coitus from behind with the female in the knee-chest position.

c. interrup'tus. Withdrawal of the penis from the vagina before the seminal emission occurs.

c. reservatus. Coitus with intentional suppression of ejaculation.

cola (kō'lă). Also spelled kola. A genus of tropical trees which produce the kola nut. An extract of the kola nut is used in pharmaceutical preparations and as a main ingredient in some carbonated beverages.

colal'gia [G. *kōlon,* + *algos,* pain]. Pain in the colon.

colation (ko-la'shun) [L. *colatiō,* from *colāre,* to strain]. Straining, filtering.

colauxe (kol-awks'e) [G. *kōlon,* + *auxē,* increase]. Distention of the colon.

cold [A.S. *cold, ceald*]. 1. A catarrhal affection of the respiratory mucous membranes known as the common cold. 2. The opposite of heat, *q.v.*

c., common. An acute catarrhal inflammation of the upper respiratory tract. It is highly contagious. Incubation period is from 18 to 48 hours. Lasting immunity does not develop. Also called *coryza; rhinitis.*

ETIOLOGY: May be due to one of a considerable number of viruses.

SYMPTOMS: Congestion of nasal mucosa with partial or complete occlusion of nostrils; continuous watery discharge with more or less continuous sniffing and blowing of nose. Headaches and dull pains in the face and head are common. Constitutional symptoms may appear, such as fever, body aches, easy fatigability and sensations of chilliness. Symptoms are usually resolved within 5 to 10 days.

TREATMENT: Treatment is mainly for the relief of symptoms. Spraying with ephedrine hydrochloride or inhalation of benzedrine or menthol relieves nasal congestion. Analgesics are useful to relieve aching. Preparations containing codeine will usually relieve a cough but should not be used when the cough is productive. Antihistamines sometimes are effective in controlling the nasal secretions. Bed rest is recommended for febrile patients.

c., asphyxia from. Place patient in cold room, rub with snow or ice water, use artificial respiration. SEE: *artificial respiration; respiration.*

c., chest. Bronchitis.* Inflammation of the bronchial mucous membranes.

c. cream. USP. White perfumed ointment used mainly as a cosmetic and for chapped skin, minor excoriations of the face, and herpes labialis.

c., head. A common cold, *q.v.*

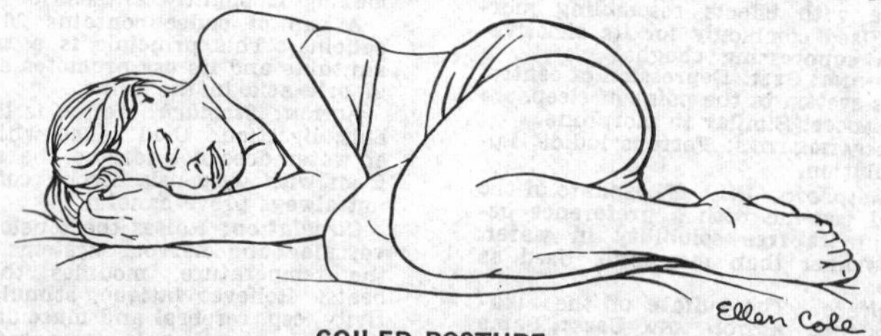

COILED POSTURE.

c. pack. Used to apply cold to an area, usually for pain, swelling or inflammation.

c. pressor test. A rise in blood pressure after immersion of hand in cold water for 1 min.

c. sore. Fever blister. Eruption of vesicles on an inflammatory base. SEE: *herpes simplex.*

colectomy (ko-lek'to-mĭ) [G. *kōlon,* + *ektomē,* excision]. Excision of part of the colon.

coleitis (kol-ē-ī'tĭs) [G. *koleos,* sheath]. Same as vaginitis, *q.v.*

coleocele (ko'le-o-sēl) [G. *koleos,* sheath, vagina, + *kēlē,* hernia]. A vaginal hernia.

coleocystitis (ko-le-o-sĭs-ti'tĭs) [" + *kystis,* bladder, + *-ītis,* inflammation]. Inflammation of the vagina and bladder.

coleoptosis (kō-lē-op-tō'sĭs). Prolapse of the wall of the vagina.

coleot'omy [" + *tomē,* incision]. Incision into the pericardium or into the vagina. SYN: *colpotomy.*

colibacellemia (ko-lĭ-bas-ĭl-le'mĭ-ă) [G. *kōlon,* colon, + L. *bacillus,* little rod, + G. *aima,* blood]. Colon bacillus in the blood.

colibacillo'sis [" + " + G. *-ōsis,* infection]. Infection with the colon bacillus.

colibacilluria (ko-lĭ-bas-ĭl-u'rĭ-ă) [" + " + G. *ouron,* urine]. Colon bacillus in the urine.

colibacil'lus [" + L. *bacillus,* little rod]. The colon bacillus, *Escherichia coli.*

colic (kol'ik) [G. *kōlikos,* pert. to the colon]. 1. Spasm in any hollow or tubular soft organ accompanied by pain. 2. Pert. to the colon. SEE: *cholecystalgia; tormina.*

c., biliary. In bile ducts usually associated with a gallstone.

c., infantile. Occurring in infants, principally first few months.

c., intestinal. Pain may occur throughout the abdomen.

c., lead. Associated with lead poisoning, occupational, painters, etc. Severe abdominal colic. Lead line may be found on gums and basic stippling in red blood cells. SYN: *Devonshire c.*

c., menstrual. Abdominal pain during menses. SYN: *dysmenorrhea.*

c., renal. In region of one of the kidneys and toward the thigh. Pain radiates from kidney region around over abdomen into the groin. It accompanies the passage of calculus. Rigors pronounced.

c., uterine. Painful menstruation. SYN: *dysmenorrhea.*

col'ica [L.]. 1. Abdominal colic; colic. 2. Colic artery.

colicoli'tis [G. *kōlon,* colon, + *-ītis,* inflammation]. Colon inflammation due to *Escherichia coli.*

colicople'gia [" + *plēgē,* stroke]. Lead poisoning with colic and lead paralysis.

colicystitis (ko"lĭ-sis-ti'tis) [G. *kōlon,* colon bacillus, + *kystis,* bladder, + *-ītis,* inflammation]. Inflammation of bladder resulting from infection with *Escherichia coli.*

colicystopyelitis (ko"lĭ-sis"to-pi-ĕ-li'tis) [" + " + *pyelos,* pus, + *-ītis,* inflammation]. Inflammation of bladder and pelvis of kidney caused by *Escherichia coli.*

col'iform [L. *colum,* sieve, + *forma,* form]. 1. Sieve form; cribriform. 2. Pertaining to a group of bacteria which includes *Aerobacter aerogenes* and *Escherichia coli.* Their presence in water, esp. the *E. coli.,* is presumptive evidence of fecal contamination.

colilysin (ko-lil'ĭ-sin) [G. *kōlon,* colon bacillus, + *lysis,* dissolution]. A hemolysin formed by *Escherichia coli.*

colinephri'tis [" + *nephros,* kidney, + *-ītis,* inflammation]. Nephritis caused by the colon bacillus, *Escherichia coli.*

coliplication (ko-lĭ-pli-ka'shun) [G. *kōlon,* colon, + L. *plica,* fold]. Operation for correcting a dilated colon.

colipuncture (ko-lĭ-punk'tūr) [" + L. *punctura,* a piercing]. Puncture of the colon to relieve distention. SYN: *colocentesis.*

colipyuria (ko-lĭ-pĭ-u'rĭ-ă) [" + *pyon,* pus, + *ouron,* urine]. Pus in urine due to *Escherichia coli.*

colisep'sis [" + *sepsis,* putrefaction]. Infection caused by the colon bacillus.

coli'tis [" + *-ītis,* inflammation]. Inflammation of the colon.

c., mucous. Colitis accompanied by large quantities of mucus.

SYM: Attacks occur paroxysmally sometimes followed by constipation. Spastic, colicky pain in midabdomen. Tenacious, gelatinous mucus and shreds of mucous membrane may be passed.

c., ulcerative. Ulceration of mucosa of colon.

SYM: Passage of watery, offensive stools with mucus and pus. Abdominal pain, tenderness, or colic. Intermittent or irregular fever. Hemorrhage and perforation may occur.

colitoxemia (ko-lĭ-toks-e'mĭ-ă) [" + *toxikon,* poison, + *aima,* blood]. Toxemia caused by the colon bacillus, *Escherichia coli.*

colitoxico'sis [" + " + *-ōsis,* infection]. Systemic poisoning caused by the colon bacillus, *Escherichia coli.*

colitox'in [" + *toxikon,* poison]. A toxin generated by the colon bacillus.

coliuria (ko-lĭ-u'rĭ-ă) [" + *ouron,* urine]. Presence of *Escherichia coli* in the urine. SYN: *colibaciluria.*

collagen (kol'ă-jen) [G. *kolla,* glue, + *gennan,* to produce]. A fibrous insoluble protein found in the connective tissue including skin, bone, ligaments and cartilage. Collagen represents about 30% of the total body protein.

c. diseases. A group of clinical syndromes which cause similar cellular changes. That is, they affect the body's connective tissue. The joints, blood vessels, heart, skin and supporting tissue of various organs contain lesions. How these lesions are spread throughout the body determines the clinical picture in the various diseases. Collagen diseases include systemic lupus erythematosus (SLE) dermatomyositis, polyarteritis, rheumatoid arthritis, progressive systemic sclerosis, and others.

collapse' [L. *collapsus,* fallen to pieces]. 1. An abnormal retraction of the walls of an organ. 2. A sudden failure of vital power due to reflex inhibition of the heart and respiratory system, or to loss of blood, low metabolism, or undue lowering of the blood pressure.

The term *collapse* designates a profound degree of shock, *q.v.,* induced by functional inhibition of the vasomotor center, to distinguish it from the shock of exhaustion of the same center resulting from physical violence or impressions of fear. Intense fear may induce a complete collapse, as is sometimes seen in a victim about to be executed.

SYM: Similar to those of hemorrhage. The peripheral arteries are depleted of blood, and the veins, esp. in the splanchnic region, are congested; apathy; extreme pallor; cold, clammy perspiration; thin, rapid pulse; fall of blood pressure; unconsciousness.

NP: The head of bed, or head and shoulders of patient should be lowered. Hot blankets and hot water bottles may be placed about the patient's body. SEE ALSO: *shock*.

c. of lung. Artificially induced by: (a) Artificial pneumothorax; (b) thoracoplasty, or (c) avulsion of phrenic nerve.

collap'sing. Falling into extreme and sudden prostration resembling shock.

c. pulse. Pulse of aortic insufficiency or regurgitation; water-hammer pulse. SYN: *Corrigan's pulse.*

collapsother'apy [L. *collapsus*, fallen to pieces, + G. *therapeia*, treatment]. Treatment of pulmonary affections by unilateral pneumothorax and immobilization of affected lung. SYN: *collapse therapy.*

collar (kol'ar) [L. *collum*, neck]. 1. A band worn round the neck. 2. Structure or marking formed like a neckband.

c. of Venus, c., venereal. Mottled appearance of the skin of the neck occasionally seen in syphilis. SYN: *melanoleukoderma colli.*

col'larbone. The clavicle, *q.v.*

collat'eral [L. *con*, together, + *lateralis*, pert. to a side]. 1. Accompanying, as side by side. 2. Subordinate or secondary. 3. Not related lineally. 4. An accessory nerve or blood vessel. 5. A minute side branch of the axon or axis cylinder of a neuron which passes outward at right angles to the axon.

c. circulation. That of small anastomosing vessels, esp. when a main artery is obstructed.

c. eminence. An elevation in the floor of the lateral ventricle.

c. fissure. A fissure on the median surface of the cerebral hemisphere.

c. ganglia. Ganglia of the sympathetic division of the autonomic nervous system, located near origins of the celiac and mesenteric arteries. Include the celiac and mesenteric ganglia. Also called *prevertebral ganglia.*

c. trigone. The angle between the diverging inferior and posterior horns of the lateral ventricle.

collat'erals [L. *con*, together, + *lateralis*, pert. to a side]. Plural of *collateral* (def. 5), *q.v.*

collecting tubules. Small ducts which receive urine from several renal tubules and discharge it into papillary ducts which open into a renal calyx at the tip of a papilla.

collemia (kol-e'mĭ-ă) [G. *kolla*, glue, + *aima*, blood]. A colloidal form of matter in the blood causing capillary obstruction.

Colles' fascia (kol'ēz) [Abraham Colles, Irish surgeon, 1773-1843]. Inner layer of superficial fascia of perineum.

C.'s fracture. The transverse fracture of the distal end of radius (just above wrist) with displacement of hand backward and outward.

C.'s law. A theory, long accepted but now obsolete, that a child affected with congenital syphilis, its mother showing no signs of the disease, will not infect its mother.

colliculectomy (kol-lik"u-lek'to-mĭ) [L. *colliculus*, mound, + G. *ektomē*, excision]. Removal of the *colliculus seminalis.*

colliculi'tis [" + G. *-itis*, inflammation]. Inflammation of the *colliculus seminalis.*

collic'ulus [L. mound]. A little eminence.

c. bulbi, c. bulbi intermedius. Erectile tissue encircling the male urethra at the entrance to the bulb.

c. cervicalis (*urethrae muliebris*). The crest on the posterior wall of the female urethra.

c. inferior. One of two elevations forming the lower portion of the corpora quadrigemina of the midbrain.

c. seminalis. An oval enlargement on the crista urethralis, an elevation in the floor of the prostatic portion of the urethra. On its sides are the openings of the ejaculatory ducts and numerous ducts of the prostate gland.

c. superior. One of two elevations forming the upper portion of the corpora quadrigemina of the midbrain.

c. urethralis. C. seminalis.

collimation (kol"ĭ-ma'shun) [L. *collineare*, to align]. The process of making parallel. Thus x-ray machines are fitted with a collimator to insure that the rays are parallel and not diffuse.

Collip unit [James B. Collip, Canadian biochemist, 1892-]. Dosage unit of parathyroid extract. One-one hundredth of the quantity necessary to increase by 5 mg. the amount of calcium in 100 cc. of blood after 15 hours in a dog weighing 20 kg.

colliquation (kol-ĭ-kwa'shun) [L. *con*, together, + *liquāre*, to melt]. 1. Abnormal discharge of a body fluid. 2. Softening of tissues to liquefaction. 3. A wasting.

colliquative (ko-lik'wă-tiv). Pert. to a liquid and excessive discharge, as a *c. diarrhea.*

collodion (ko-lo'di-on) [G. *kollodes*, resembling glue]. USP. A preparation containing pyroxylin dissolved thoroughly in ether and alcohol. It is a viscous liquid having an odor of ether and is highly flammable. When applied, it dries to form a strong, thin transparent film and is useful in sealing the edge of a dressing, especially on the scalp.

c., flexible. USP. A preparation of collodion containing camphor and castor oil. It is more elastic than collodion in ether and alcohol.

c., salicylic acid. USP. Flexible c. with salicylic acid. Used as a keratolytic agent, commonly for corns.

colloid (kol'oid) [G. *kollōdēs*, glutinous]. 1. A colloidal system. A gluelike substance such as a protein or starch whose particles (molecules or aggregates of molecules) when dispersed in a solvent to the greatest possible degree remain uniformly distributed and fail to form a true solution. The size of colloid particles ranges from 1 to 100 millimicrons. 2. A homogeneous gelatinous substance found within the follicles of the thyroid gland and containing the thyroid secretion.

c. chemistry. This deals with such systems and substances, and with the problems of emulsions, mists, foams, and suspensions.

c. cyst. A sac containing a jellylike liquid.

c. degeneration. A mucoid degeneration seen in the protoplasm of epithelial cells.

c. suspension. A mixture holding particles in suspension, the forms of which change with the forces acting upon them, such as milk, fat, etc.

c. thyroid. Semi-fluid, jelly-like substance filling the follicles of the thyroid gland. It contains the thyroid hormone.

colloidal (kol-loyd'ăl). Pert. to a colloid.

colloidal dispersion. A mixture containing colloid particles which fail to settle out and are held in suspension. They are common in animal and plant tissues, the protoplasm of cells being a colloidal mixture. Particles of colloidal dispersions are too large to pass through cell membranes and such dispersions usually appear cloudy.

colloidin (kol-loi'din). A jellylike substance seen in colloid degeneration.

colloidoclasia (kol-oid-o-kla'sĭ-ă) [G. *kollōdēs,* glutinous, + *klasis,* fracture]. An alteration in the equilibrium of body colloids resulting from entrance into the blood stream of unaltered colloids such as proteins with an end result of anaphylactic shock.

colloidopexy (kol-oid'o-pek-sĭ) [" + *pēxis,* fixation]. Fixation of colloids during metabolism.

collo'ma [G. *kolla,* glue, + *-ōma,* tumor]. A colloid degeneration of a cancer.

collonema (kol-o-ne'mă) [" + *nēma,* yarn]. A tumor, esp. a lipoma, which has undergone mucoid degeneration.

collopexia (kol-o-peks'ĭ-ă) [L. *collum,* neck, + G. *pēxis,* fixation]. Fixation of the *cervix uteri.*

col'lum (pl. *colla*) [L. neck]. 1. The necklike part of an organ. 2. The neck.

collutory (kol'lu-to-rĭ) [L. *colluĕre,* to rinse]. A gargle or mouth wash.

collyrium (kol-lir'ĭ-um). An eyewash.

colobo'ma [G. *kolobōma,* a mutilation]. A lesion or defect of the eye, usually a fissure or cleft of the iris, ciliary body or choroid. May be congenital, pathological or surgical. Sometimes the eyelid is involved.

colocentesis (ko-lo-sen-te'sis) [G. *kōlon,* colon, + *kentēsis,* puncture]. Surgical puncture of the colon to relieve distention.

colocholecystostomy (ko-lo-kol-e-sis-tos'to-mĭ) [" + *cholē,* bile, + *kystis,* bladder, + *stoma,* opening]. Surgical formation of a communication bet. colon and gallbladder. Syn: *cholecystocolostomy.*

colocleisis (ko-lo-kli'sis) [" + *kleisis,* closure]. Occlusion of the colon.

coloclysis (ko-lok'li-sis) [" + *klysis,* washing]. A colonic enema.

coloclyster (ko-lo-klis'ter) [" + *klyzein,* to cleanse]. A colonic enema.

colocolostomy (ko-lo-kol-os'to-mĭ) [" + *kōlon,* colon, + *stoma,* mouth]. Formation of a connection bet. two portions of the colon.

colocynth (kol'o-sinth) [G. *kolokynthē,* fruit of *Citrullus colocynthis*]. Dried pulp of unripe colocynth fruit.

Action and Uses: A drastic hydragogue cathartic.

coloenteritis (ko-lo-en-ter-i'tis) [G. *kōlon,* colon, + *enteron,* intestine, + *-ītis,* inflammation]. Inflammation of mucous membrane of small and large intestines.

colofixa'tion [" + L. *fixātiō,* fixation]. Suspension of the colon in ptosis.

co'lon [G. *kōlon*]. The large intestine from the end of the ileum and beginning with the cecum to the anus, about 1.5 meters (4.5 feet) long, and divided into the ascending, transverse, descending, and the sigmoid or pelvic colon.

Beginning at the cecum, the first part of the large intestine, the ascending colon, passes upward to the right colic or hepatic flexure, where it turns as the transverse colon passing ventral to the liver and stomach. On reaching the spleen, it turns downward (left colic or splenic flexure) and continues as the descending colon to the brim of the pelvis where it is continuous with the sigmoid colon.

c. bacteria. *Escherichia coli* is the most common one found. Whatever digestion takes place in the colon is due to bacteria. A large number of fermentative bacteria are found in the middle portion of the colon. They change carbohydrates into carbon dioxide, alcohol, and lactic acid. This is the only way cellulose may be acted upon in the body. Putrefying bacteria are found in the lower part of the colon. These may produce toxic products, *e.g.,* indol, skatol; however, if absorbed such products undergo detoxification in the liver.

c. functions. *Mechanical:* Mixing the contents of the intestines.

Chemical: No digestive enzymes are secreted in the colon, but an alkaline fluid aids in the completion of digestion begun in the small intestines. Those products of bacterial action which are absorbed into the blood stream are carried by the portal circulation to the liver before they get into the general circulation. There is also a great deal of water absorbed in the colon rather than in the small intestines. The fluids of the body are conserved in this way, and in spite of the large volumes of secretions (saliva, etc.) added to the food during its progress through the alimentary canal, the contents of the colon are gradually dehydrated until they assume the consistency of normal feces or even become quite hard.

See: *absorption; defecation.*

colon, words pert. to: anus, appendices, epiploicae, cecum, cholecystocolostomy, colalgia, colitis, "colo-" words, diverticulitis, jejunum, peristalsis, rectum, small intestines.

colonalgia (ko-lon-al'ji-a) [G. *kōlon,* colon, + *algos,* pain]. Pain in the colon.

colonic (ko-lon'ik). Pert. to the colon.

c. irrigation. Injection into the colon of a large amt. of fluid which is intended to fill colon and flush it.

Administered not to induce defecation but to wash out material situated above the defecation area and to wash the wall of the bowel as high as the water can be made to reach. Two primary methods: 1-tube, involving filling colon to capacity through a single tube and allowing liquid to run out through the same tube, and, 2-tube method, employing separate inflow and outflow tubes.

colonitis (ko-lon-i'tis) [G. *kōlon,* colon, + *-ītis,* inflammation]. Colitis, *q.v.*

colonom'eter [L. *colonia,* colony, + G. *metron,* measure]. Device for estimating colonies of bacteria on a culture plate.

colonopexy (ko'lon-o-pek-sĭ) [G. *kōlon,* colon, + *pēxis,* fixation]. Process of attaching part of colon to abdominal wall.

colonorrhagia (ko"lon-o-ra'jĭ-ă) [" + *regnunai,* to burst forth]. Hemorrhage from the colon.

colonorrhea (ko"lon-o-re'ă) [" + *roia,* flow]. Mucous colitis.

colonoscope (ko-lon'o-skōp) [" + *skopein,* to examine]. Instrument for examination of the colon. See: *sigmoidoscope.*

colonos'copy. Examination of upper portion of rectum with an elongated speculum.

col'ony [L. *colonia*]. A collection of microorganisms in a culture.

colopexos'tomy [G. *kōlon,* colon, + *pēxis,* fixation, + *stoma,* mouth]. Resection of the colon and fixation to abdominal wall to establish an artificial anus.

colopexotomy (ko-lo-peks-ot'o-mĭ) [" + " + *tomē,* incision]. Incision and fixation of colon.

colopexy, colopexia (ko'lo-pek-sĭ, ko-lo-peks'ĭ-ă) [" + *pēxis,* fixation]. Fixation of the sigmoid or cecum to the abdominal wall by suture.

coloplication (ko-lo-pli-ka'shun) [" + L. *plica,* fold]. Making a fold in the colon to reduce its lumen.

coloprocti'tis [" + *prōktos,* anus, + *-itis,* inflammation]. Colonic and rectal inflammation. SYN: *colorectitis.*

coloproctostomy (ko-lo-prok-tos'to-mĭ) [" + " + *stoma,* opening]. Making a communication bet. a segment of colon and the rectum.

coloptosia (ko-lop-to'sĭ-ă) [" + *ptōsis,* dropping]. Prolapse of the colon, esp. of the transverse c.

coloptosis (ko-lop-to'sis) [" + *ptōsis,* dropping]. A downward displacement of the colon.

colopuncture (ko'lo-punk-chur) [" + L. *punctura,* piercing]. Puncturing the colon.

col'or [L.]. A visible quality, distinct from form, and light and shade.

c. *blindness.* Inability to identify one or more of the primary colors. SYN: *daltonism.*

c. *gustation.* A sense of color aroused by stimulation of taste receptors.

c. *hearing.* A sense of color caused by a sound.

c. *index.* An outmoded method of expressing the amount of hemoglobin present in each red cell.

color, *words pert. to:* achromate, achromodermia, "acro-" words, alba, albedo, albicans, allochroism, allochromasia, anerythropsia, anisochromatic, aurantiasis, auric, canescent, carotene, "chrom-" words, flavescent, isochromatic, melanin, nigrescent, pigmentation, rubescent, rubiginous, rubor, vermilion, versicolor, xanthic.

colorectitis (ko-lo-rek-ti'tis) [G. *kōlon,* colon, + L. *rectum,* + G. *-itis,* inflammation]. Inflammation of colon and rectum. SYN: *coloproctitis.*

colorectostomy (ko-lo-rek-tos'to-mĭ) [" + " + G. *stoma,* opening]. Formation of passage bet. colon and rectum.

colorim'eter [L. *color,* color, + G. *metron,* measure]. Instrument for measuring intensity of color in a substance or fluid, especially one for determining the amt. of hemoglobin in the blood.

colostomy (ko-los'to-mĭ) [G. *kōlon,* colon, + *stoma,* mouth]. Incision of the colon for purpose of making a more or less permanent fistula between the bowel and the abdominal wall. The location is usually indicated in the description as *inguinal colostomy, lumbar colostomy,* etc.

c. *diet.* A low residue diet.*

c., *inguinal.* Incision of colon to form artificial anus.

NP: Change dressings *p.r.n.* Protect skin around opening from discharge by covering with sterile zinc oxide ointment. Remove ointment when cleaning with sterile sweet oil. Chart amt. and nature of discharge. Prevent impaction, watch diet orders, irrigate through upper or lower loop *as ordered.* Special colostomy bags which cover the opening and greatly facilitate colostomy care are available.

colostra'tion [L. *colostrum*]. Infant diarrhea assumed to be caused by colostrum.

colostrorrhea (ko-los-tro-re'ă) [" + G. *roia,* flow]. Abnormal secretion of colostrum.

colos'trum [L.]. Secretion from the breast before the onset of true lactation 2 or 3 days after delivery.

The secretion contains, mainly, serum and white blood corpuscles. So-called "first milk."

colotomy (ko-lot'o-mĭ) [G. *kōlon,* colon, + *tomē,* incision]. Incision of colon. SEE: *Callisen's operation.*

colotyphoid (kol-ō-tī'foid) [" + *typhos,* fever, + *eidos,* resemblance]. Typhoid fever with ulceration of colon.

colpalgia (kol-pal'jĭ-ă) [G. *kolpos,* vagina, + *algos,* pain]. Vaginal pain.

colpatresia (kol-pă-trē'zĭ-ă) [" + *a-,* priv. + *trēsis,* a perforation]. Occlusion or pathological closure of the vagina; vaginal atresia.

colpectasia (kol-pek-ta'sĭ-ă) [" + *ektasis,* distention]. Dilatation of the vagina.

colpec'tomy [" + *ektomē,* excision]. Surgical removal of the vagina.

colpeurynter (kol-pu-rin'ter) [" + *eurynein,* to dilate]. A bag for dilatation of the vagina.

colpeurysis (kol-pu'ris-is) [" + *eurynein,* to widen]. Dilatation of the vagina by surgery.

colpitis (kol-pi'tis) [" + *-itis,* inflammation]. Inflammation of the vagina. SEE: *vaginitis.*

colpocele (kol'po-sēl) [" + *kēlē,* hernia] Hernia into the vagina.

colpoceliotomy (kol'po-se-lĭ-ot'o-mĭ) [" + *koilia,* belly, + *tomē,* a cut]. Entering the abdomen surgically through the vagina.

colpocleisis (kol-po-klī'sis) [" + *kleisis,* a closure]. Operation of occluding the vagina.

colpocystitis (kol-po-sis-ti'tis) [" + *kystis,* bladder, + *-itis,* inflammation]. Inflammation of vagina and bladder.

colpocystocele (kol-po-sis'to-sēl) [" + " + *kēlē,* hernia]. Prolapse of the bladder into the vagina.

colpocys'toplasty [" + " + *plassein,* to form]. Treatment of vesicovaginal fistula.

colpocystosyrinx (kol"po-sis-to-sir'inks) [" + " + *syrigx,* fistula]. Fistula bet. bladder and vagina.

colpocystotomy (kol-po-sis-tot'o-mĭ) [" + " + *tomē,* incision]. Cutting into the bladder through the vagina.

NP: Prevent bladder distention. Record intake and output. If retention catheter is present, irrigate twice daily with solution ordered and be sure catheter is kept draining. Keep patient clean and comfortable with external irrigations over the vulva. Dry skin thoroughly after each irrigation.

colpocystoureterocystotomy (kol"po-sis"-to-u-re"ter-o-sis-tot'o-mĭ) [" + " + *ourētēr,* ureter, + *kystis,* bladder, + *tomē,* incision]. Incision into the ureter through the walls of the bladder and vagina.

colpodesmorrhaphy (kol-po-des-mor'ă-fĭ) [" + *desmos,* band, + *raphē,* suture]. Repair of the vaginal sphincter.

colpodynia (kol-po-din'ĭ-ă) [" + *odynē,* pain]. Pain in the vagina. SYN: *colpalgia.*

colpohyperplasia (kol-po-hi-per-pla'zĭ-ă) [" + *yper,* over, + *plasis,* a forming].

Excessive growth of mucous membrane of the vagina.

c. cystica. Infectious inflammation of the vaginal walls which is characterized by the production of small blebs.

colpo″hysterec′tomy [" + *ystera,* uterus, + *ektomē,* excision]. Removal of the uterus through the vagina.

NP: Watch for vaginal packs and remove as ordered. Watch for retention catheters and care for per routine orders.

colpohysteropexy (kol-po-his′ter-o-pek-sĭ) [" + " + *pēxis,* fixation]. Fixation of uterus through the vagina.

colpohysterot′omy [" + " + *tomē,* incision]. Incision through the vagina into the uterus, as for excision of a fibroma.

colpomyomectomy (kol-po-mi-o-mek′to-mĭ) [" + *mys,* muscle, + *-ōma,* tumor, + *ektomē,* excision]. Removal of a fibroid tumor of the uterus through the vagina.

colpomyomotomy (-mot′o-mĭ) [" + " + " + *tomē,* incision]. Incision of uterus through the vagina for removal of tumor.

colpopathy (kol-pop′ă-thĭ) [" + *pathos,* disease]. Any pathology of the vagina.

colpoperineoplasty (kol-po-per-in-ē′o-plas-tĭ) [" + *perinaion,* perineum, + *plassein,* to form]. Plastic operation on vagina and perineum.

colpoperineorrhaphy (kol-po-per-in″e-or′ră-fĭ) [" + " + *raphē,* suture]. Operation for mending perineal tears in vagina. Syn: *colpoperineoplasty.*

col′popexy [" + *pēxis,* fixation]. Suture of a relaxed and prolapsed vagina to the abdominal wall.

colpoplasty (kol′po-plas-tĭ) [" + *plassein,* to form]. Plastic operation upon vagina.

colpoptosis (kol-pop-to′sis) [" + *ptōsis,* a falling]. Prolapse of the vagina.

colporrhagia (kol-po-ra′ji-ă) [" + *rēgnunai,* to burst forth]. Excessive vaginal discharge. Vaginal hemorrhage.

colporrhaphy (kol-por′ă-fĭ) [" + *raphē,* suture]. Suture of vagina.

colporrhexis (kol-po-reks′is) [" + *rēxis,* rupture]. Laceration or rupture of the vaginal walls.

colposcope (kol′po-skōp) [" + *skopein,* to examine]. An instrument for examining the fornices of the vagina and *cervix uteri.*

col′pospasm, colpospas′mus [" + *spasmos,* spasm]. Spasm of the vagina. Syn: *vaginismus.*

col′postat [" + L. *stāre,* to stand]. Device for holding an instrument such as a radium applicator in place in the vagina.

colpostenosis (kol-po-sten-o′sis) [" + *stenōsis,* narrowing]. Stenosis or narrowing of the vagina.

colpostenotomy (kol-po-sten-ot′o-mĭ) [" + " + *tomē,* incision]. A cutting operation for dilating the lumen in stricture of the vagina.

colpotherm (kol′po-thurm) [" + *thermē,* heat]. Electrical device introduced into the vagina to convey heat.

colpotomy (kŏl-pŏt′ō-mĭ) [G. *kolpos,* vagina, + *tomē,* incision]. Incision into the wall of the vagina.

colpoureterocystotomy (kol-po-u-re″ter-o-sis-tot′o-mĭ) [" + *ourētēr,* ureter, + *kystis,* + *tomē,* incision]. Exposure of the ureteral orifices by incision through the walls of the vagina and bladder.

colpoureterot′omy [" + " + *tomē,* incision]. Incision of the ureter through the vagina.

colpoxerosis (kol-po-zē-rō′sis) [" + *xērōsis,* dryness]. Abnormal dryness of the vulva and vagina.

columbium. See: *niobium.*

columella (kol-ū-mel′lă) [L. dim. of *columna,* column]. 1. A column. 2. Bact: Portion of the sporangiophore upon which are borne the spores.

c. cochleae. The modiolus of the cochlea.

c. na′si. The ant. part of the septum of nose; a turbinate bone.

column (kŏl′ŭm) [L. *columna,* pillar]. A cylindrical supporting structure.

c., anterior. (a) The ant. portion of the gray matter on each side of the spinal cord. Also called *anterior horn.* (b) With ref. to white matter, the *post. funiculus.*

c. of Burdach. The fasciculus cuneatus, *q.v.*

c., Clarke's. A group of large cells in medial portion of the base of the posterior gray column of the spinal cord.

c., fornicis. A column of the fornix, two arched bands of fibers which form the anterior portion of the fornix. Fibers lead to mammillary body.

c. of Goll. The fasciculus gracilis, *q.v.*

c. of Gowers. Tract of ascending fibers ant. to the direct cerebellar column, and on the lateral surface of the spinal cord.

c., lateral. (a) A column in lateral portion of gray matter of spinal cord. Contains cell bodies of preganglionic neurons of sympathetic nervous system. (b) The lateral funiculus or the white matter between roots of spinal nerves.

c. of Morgagni. One of several vertical ridges in mucous membrane at junction of anus and rectum.

c., posterior. (a) The post. horn of the gray matter of the spinal cord. It consists of an expanded portion or *caput* connected by a narrower *cervix* to the main portion of gray matter. (b) The post. funiculus of the white matter.

c., renal. A column of Bertin, cortical material of the kidney which extends centrally, separating the pyramids.

c., spinal. The line of vertebrae from the head to the pelvis, making up the bony flexible case for the spinal cord. The vertebral column, *q.v.*

c., vertebral. The spinal column; the portion of the axial skeleton consisting of vertebrae (7 cervical, 12 thoracic, 5 lumbar, a sacrum and coccyx) joined together by intervertebral disks. It forms the main supporting axis of the body, encloses and protects the spinal cord, and serves for attachment of the appendicular skeleton and muscles for moving the various bodily parts.

c., vesicular. Line of ganglion cells on inner side of post. column.

columna (ko-lum′na) (pl. *columnae*) [L.]. A column or pillar.

c. bertini. Interpyramidal extension or renal column supporting renal blood vessels.

c. carnea. A muscular projection within the cardiac ventricles. Syn: *trabecula carnea* [NA].

c. nasi. Nasal septum.

c. rugarum vaginae. Fold of mucous membrane of the vagina which is arranged in a columnar fashion.

colum'nar layer. Retinal rod-and-cone layer.

columning (kol'um-ing). Introduction of tampons in vagina to support the prolapsed uterus.

co'ma [G. *kōma,* a deep sleep]. An abnormal deep stupor occurring in illness, or as a result of it, or it may be due to an injury. The patient cannot be aroused by external stimuli.

ETIOL: May be due to alcoholism, to hysteria, epilepsy, narcotics, poisons, gases, sunstroke, heat exhaustion, uremia, or injury. More than 50% of cases are due to trauma to the head or circulatory accidents in the brain due to hypertension, sclerosis, thrombosis, tumor or abscess formation. The chief causes of coma are: (a) Trauma, as in accidents, hemorrhage, and shock; (b) vascular disease; (c) organic disease of the central nervous system; (d) metabolic disorders; (e) acute infections of the brain or meninges; (f) acute infections and bacterial intoxications, as in fevers, botulism, and other diseases; (g) parasites; (h) the effects of drugs; alcohol, atropine, barbiturates, chloral, chloroform, cyanides, carbon dioxide, carbon monoxide, hyoscine, phenols, paraldehyde, ether, gases and various fumes; (i) extreme temperatures; (j) excessive loss of blood; (k) neurotic causes, as in malingering.

GENERAL TREATMENT: First aid treatment should be strictly limited; patient should not be moved other than to slightly raise the head. Movement without aid of a physician is dangerous. The collar should be loosened. Cold compresses to head and hot ones to the spine and abdomen may be indicated. Stomach pump in case of poisoning indicated. Insulin injection for diabetic coma may be given unless the coma is due to too much insulin.

CAUTION: If there is a question of whether the coma is due to an overdose of insulin or is a diabetic coma, it is safe to give glucose intravenously; insulin might be disastrous.

Urine should be examined for albumin and sugar.

In uremic coma, stimulate elimination. In coma due to hysteria, the patient requires careful nursing care and observation but no specific therapy is indicated.

NP: Test urine for cause, and for retention. Clean mouth. Keep water out of trachea. Keep eyes cleansed. Apply an ointment to prevent lids from sticking together. Guard against bed sores. May have to be fed artificially.

c., *alcoholic*. Due to alcohol.

c., *apoplectic*. Due to cerebral hemorrhage or apoplexy; one side of body, or the extremities, one or more, will be paralyzed. No fever at first but one pupil may be larger than the other. Coma usually indicates increased cranial pressure. SEE: *apoplexy.*

c., *diabetic*. Occurring in diabetes, due to lack of insulin which causes metabolic changes with excess production of *acetone bodies, q.v.,* and metabolic acidosis. Paralysis not present. SYM: Sweet breath. Hyperglycemia is present, and softening of eyeballs may occur.

TREATMENT: Insulin has prevented diabetic coma to a large extent but an overdose may induce hypoglycemic coma. Thus do not give insulin until the diagnosis of diabetic coma is made. Examine urine hourly for dextrose; if urine is sugar-free, more dextrose must be given.

c., *uremic*. The result of disturbed kidney metabolism, causing autointoxication through the retention of metabolic end products which would normally be excreted by the kidneys. Interference with the acid-base balance develops.

SYM: In general, respiration stertorous, face livid, skin dry and may be covered with "uremic frost" which is a collection of urea excreted in the sweat, hard and rapid pulse, blood pressure elevated, sphincters relaxed according to cause; urinous odor on breath, urine scanty and containing many casts and albumin. Complete retention may occur.

c. *vigil*. Delirious lethargy with open eyes and partial consciousness.

co'matose. In a condition of coma.

comedo (kom'e-do) (pl. *comedon'es, com'edos*) [L. a glutton]. Blackhead. Discolored dried sebum plugging an excretory duct of the skin.

ETIOL: Either increased activity of sebaceous glands or material secreted is unable to escape through a too-narrow opening.

SYM: Commonly affects the face, back, and ears; chronic, frequently associated with seborrheic dermatitis, or acne, usually during adolescence.

Diagnosis of Diabetic and Hypoglycemic Coma[1]

	Diabetic Coma	Hypoglycemic Coma
Onset	Gradual.	Often sudden.
History	Often of acute infection in a diabetic or no previous history of diabetes.	Recent insulin injection, or inadequate meal or excessive exercise after insulin.
Skin	Flushed, dry.	Pale, sweating.
Tongue	Dry.	Moist.
Breath	Smell of acetone.	No acetone.
Respiration	Deep (air hunger).	Shallow.
Pulse	Rapid, feeble.	Normal or bounding.
Eyeball Tension	Low.	Normal or raised.
Urine	Sugar and acetone.	None, unless bladder has not been emptied for some hours.
Blood Sugar	Raised [over 200].	Subnormal [40-70].
Blood Pressure	Low.	Normal.
Abdominal Pain	Common and often acute.	Sometimes sense of constriction.

[1] Sears. *Medicine for Nurses.*

PROG: Obstinate and persistent, but amenable to treatment.

TREATMENT: Aside from careful and gentle removal of plugs, treatment is essentially that of acne, *q.v.*

comes (ko'mēz) (pl. *com'ites*) [L. *companion*]. A blood vessel which accompanies a nerve or another blood vessel.

comma bacillus (named from shape). *Vibrio comma*, the causative organism of cholera.

comma tract of Schultz. The fasciculus interfascicularis, a tract of descending fibers located between the fasciculus cuneatus and fasciculus gracilis in the post. funiculus of the spinal cord.

commen'sal [L. *com*, together, + *mensa*, table]. One of two organisms which live in an intimate, nonparasitic relationship, one to the other.

commensalism. The symbiotic relationship of two organisms of different species in which neither is harmful to the other and one gains some benefit such as protection or nourishment. Ex: Nonpathogenic bacteria in human intestine.

comminute (kom'in-ūt) [" + *minuēre*, to crumble]. To break into pieces.

com'minuted fracture. A crushed bone.

comminution (kom-in-u'shun) [L. *comminutiō*, crumbling]. Reducing a solid body to varying sizes by grating, pulverizing, slicing, granulating, and by other processes. SEE: *attenuation; dynamization.*

commissu'ra (pl. *commissurae*) [L. a joining together]. A commissure.

commissu'ral. Pert. to a commissure.

commissure (kŏm'ĭ-shūr) [L. *commissura*, a joining together]. 1. A transverse band of nerve fibers passing over the midline in the central nervous system. 2. The coming together of two structures, as the lips, eyelids, or nymphae.

c., *anterior cerebral*. A band of white fibers which passes through lamina terminalis connecting the two cerebral hemispheres.

c., *anterior gray*. One in spinal cord lying anterior to central canal.

c., *anterior white*. One in spinal cord lying anterior to central canal and anterior to the ant. gray commissure.

c. *of fornix*. A band of fibers connecting the two crura.

c., *middle*. The mass intermedia, *q.v.*

c., *posterior* (of brain). One just above the midbrain containing fibers which connect the superior colliculi.

c., *posterior* (of spinal cord). A gray commissure connecting two halves of spinal cord. It lies post. to central canal.

common bile duct. Duct carrying bile to the duodenum and receiving it from the cystic and hepatic ducts. SYN: *common duct; ductus choledochus.* SEE: *bile.*

commu'nicable disease. 1. A disease which may be transmitted directly or indirectly from one individual to another. 2. One due to an infectious agent or toxic products produced by it.

communicable disease, *words pert. to*: alternate host, carriers, contagion, endemic, epidemic, immunity, incubation, infection, isolation, microbe, micrococcus, microorganism, quarantine, transmissible, vector.

commu'nicans [L. *communicare*, to connect with]. One of a number of communicating nerves or arteries.

Comolli's sign (ko-mol'lĭs). A triangular swelling corresponding to the outline of the scapula when fractured.

compact' [L. *compactus*, joined together]. Dense, packed, solid.

c. *bone*. Hard or dense bone which forms the superficial layer of all bones, in contrast to spongy or cancellous bone found chiefly in the ends of long bones.

compar'ative anat'omy. Human anatomy compared with that of animals.

compatibil'ity [L. *con*, with, + *pati*, to suffer, + *habilis*, to fit]. 1. State of suitability to be mixed or taken together without unfavorable results, as drugs. 2. The ability of two individuals or groups to live together without undue strife or tension.

compat'ible. Not opposed to; able to mix with another substance without destructive changes.

com'pensating. Making up for a deficiency.

c. *operation*. Tenotomy of the associated antagonists in diplopia.

compensa'tion [L. *cum*, with, + *pensāre*, to weigh]. Making up for a defect, as cardiac circulation competent to meet demands made upon it, regardless of valvular defect.

PSY: A far reaching psychic mechanism, best described by an example. The individual handicapped by a physical deformity or variation, or by a character defect, may escape the consciousness or revelation of the inferiority, by accomplishment resulting from compensatory ambition. More simply, the short man struts or the incompetent brags.

Sublimation* is often similar, but varies in the sense that the substitution of a higher social goal gratifies the infrasocial drive by replacement—rather than going to the opposite extreme in a merely camouflaging manner.

c., *failure of*. Inability of heart muscle to cope with cardiac output required. It indicates a diseased heart muscle.

ETIOL: Diseased myocardium; back pressure, due to mitral regurgitation, mitral or aortic stenosis, or aortic regurgitation.

comp'lement [L. *complēre*, to complete]. A substance or body producing bacteriolysis or hemolysis which, by means of an amboceptor, is connected with a bacterial or animal cell.

It is present in all sera. Strictly speaking, c. is not an antibody, but a natural property of blood.

RS: *albumin, antialbumin, anticomplement, Ehrlich's theory.*

c. *fixation*. SEE: *fixation of complement.*

complement'al, complement'ary. Supplying something that is lacking.

c. *air*. Amount of air that can be inspired over and above the tidal air by the deepest inspiration. SEE: *air.*

c. *colors*. Any two primary colors which, when blended, produce white light.

complemen'toid [L. *complēre*, to complete, + G. *eidos*, form]. A complement, the lysis-causing power of which has been destroyed.

complementophil (kom-ple-ment'o-fil) [" + G. *philein*, to love]. Having the power to combine with a complement.

com'plex [L. *complexus*, woven together]. 1. PSY: A subconscious idea (or group of ideas) which has become associated with a repressed wish or emotional ex-

(Cont. p. C-75)

Method of Transfer of Some Common Communicable Diseases

Disease	How Agent Leaves the Bodies of the Sick	How Organisms May Be Transferred	Method of Entry Into the Body
Typhoid.	Feces and urine.	Direct contact. Hands of nurse or attendant. Linen and all articles used by and about patient. Hands of "carriers" soiled by their own feces. Water polluted by excreta. Food grown in or washed with such water. Milk diluted or milk cans washed with such water. Flies.	Through mouth in infected food or water and thence to intestinal tract.
Diphtheria.	Sputum and discharges from nose and throat.	Direct contact. "Droplet infection" from patient coughing. Hands of nurse. Articles used by and about patient.	Through mouth to throat or nose to throat.
Scarlet fever.	Discharges from nose and throat.	Direct contact. Hands of nurse. Articles used by and about patient.	Through mouth and nose.
Pneumonia.	Sputum and discharges from nose and throat.	Direct contact. Hands of nurse. Articles used by and about patient.	Through mouth and nose to lungs.
Influenza.	As in pneumonia.	As in pneumonia.	As in pneumonia.
Smallpox.	Discharges from nose and throat. Skin lesions.	Direct contact. Hands of nurse. Articles used by and about patient.	Thought to be through mucous membrane of respiratory tract.
Syphilis.	Infected tissues. Lesions. Blood.	Direct contact. May be by kissing or by sexual intercourse. Needles and syringes.	Directly into blood and tissues through breaks in skin or membrane. Needles and syringes.
Tetanus.	Excreta from infected herbivorous animals and man.	Soil, especially that with manure or feces in it. Dust, etc. Articles used about stables.	Directly into blood stream through wounds. (Is anaerobe and prefers deep, incised wound.)
Tuberculosis, Human.	Sputum. Lesions. Feces.	Direct contact, such as kissing. "Droplet infection" from person coughing with mouth uncovered. Sputum from mouth to fingers, thence to food and other things. Soiled dressings.	Through mouth to lungs and intestines. From intestines *via* lymph channels to lymph vessels and to tissues.
Tuberculosis, Bovine.		Milk.	Same as Tuberculosis, Human.
Cholera.	Excreta from intestinal tract.	As in typhoid, through feces.	As in typhoid, through mouth to intestinal tract.

Method of Transfer of Some Common Communicable Diseases (*Continued*)

Disease	How Agent Leaves the Bodies of the Sick	How Organisms May Be Transferred	Method of Entry Into the Body
Dysentery.	As in cholera.	As in cholera.	As in cholera.
Hookworm.	Feces.	Direct contact with soil polluted with feces. Eggs in feces hatch in sandy soil. Feces may also contaminate food.	Larvae enter through breaks in skin, specially skin of feet, and, after devious passage through the body, settle in the intestine.
Meningitis.	Discharges from nose and throat.	Direct contact. Hands of nurse or attendant. Articles used by and about patient. Flies.	Mouth and nose.
Infantile paralysis.	Discharges from nose and throat, and via feces.	Direct contact. Hands of nurse or attendant.	Through mouth and nose.
Gonorrhea.	Lesions. Discharges from infected mucous membranes.	Direct contact, as in sexual intercourse. Towels, bathtubs, toilets, etc. Hands of infected persons soiled with their own discharges. Hands of attendant.	Directly onto mucous membrane. Through breaks in membrane.
Ophthalmia neonatorum (gonorrheal infection of eyes of newborn).	Pus discharges from eye.	Direct contact with infected areas, as vagina of infected mother during birth. Other infected babies. Hands of doctor or nurse. Linens, etc.	Directly on the conjunctiva.
Whooping cough.	Discharges from respiratory tract.	Direct contact with persons affected.	Mouth and nose.
Mumps.	Discharges from infected glands and mouth.	Direct contact with persons affected.	Mouth and nose.
Measles.	As in scarlet fever.	As in scarlet fever.	As in scarlet fever.
Trachoma.	Discharges from infected eyes.	Direct contact. Hands, towels, handkerchiefs, possibly clothing.	Directly on conjunctiva.
Leprosy.	Uncertain, may be from lesions. Bacilli found in nodules which may break down, forming lesions.	Uncertain.	Uncertain.

perience and which may influence behavior although the person may not have any appreciation of the connection between the repressed desire and his thoughts or actions. 2. All the ideas, feelings, and sensations connected with a subject. 3. Intricate. 4. An atrial or ventricular systole as it appears on an electrocardiograph tracing.

In Freudian psychology a grouping of ideas with an emotional background. These may be harmless, and the individual fully aware of them, *e. g.*, an artist sees every object with a view to a possible picture, and is said to have established a complex for art. Often, however, the complex is aroused by some painful emotional reaction, such as fright or excessive grief, which, instead of being allowed a natural outlet, becomes unconsciously repressed, and later manifests itself in some abnormality of mind or behavior. According to Freud, the best method of determining the complex is through the medium of psychoanalysis. SEE: *Oedipus c.; Electra c.*

c., castration. Morbid fear of being castrated.

c., Electra. Excessive love of the father by an adult female.

c., inferiority. A repressed state of mind in which one feels himself inferior to others.

c., Oedipus. Excessive mother-love manifested by an adult male, usually accompanied by hostility toward father.

c., superiority. Exaggerated conviction of one's own superiority; also pretense of being superior to compensate for a supposed inferiority.

complex'us [L.]. 1. The total indications or phenomena of a morbid state. 2. Semispinalis capitis muscle.

complica'tion [L. *cum,* with, + *plicāre,* to fold]. An added difficulty; a complex state. A disease or accident superimposed upon another without being specially related, yet affecting or modifying the prognosis of the original disease, *e. g.,* pneumonia is a complication of measles, and is the cause of many deaths from that disease.

component. A constituent part.

component blood therapy. Use of a specific blood component, such as plasma, or washed red cells, instead of an entire unit of whole blood. This practice reduces the chances for adverse reaction to blood therapy without interfering with treatment.

com'pos men'tis [L.]. Of sound mind; sane.

com'pound [L. *componere,* to place together]. 1. A substance composed of two or more units or parts combined in definite proportions by weight and having specific properties of its own. Compounds are formed in plants and animals and are of two types, *organic* and *inorganic.* 2. Made up of more than one part.

c. astigmatism. Myopia of both vertical and horizontal meridians.

c. fracture. Fracture of bone where broken end of bone has penetrated the skin.

c., inorganic. One of many compounds which, in general, contain no carbon.

c. microscope. One consisting of two or more lenses.

c., organic. A compound containing carbon. Examples are carbohydrates, proteins, and fats.

compress (kom'pres) [L. *compressus,* squeezed together]. 1.Cloth, wet or dry, folded and applied firmly to a part. 2. (kŏm-prĕs'). To press together into smaller space. 3. To close by squeezing together, as a wound.

c., abdominal. Three folds of linen reaching from sternum to pubis, overlapping sides of abdomen, wrung out of the water at 70° F., held in place by flannel binder little wider than linen, long enough to reach around the body.

c., chest. Application of 2 pieces of old linen of sufficient size to fit the entire chest from the clavicles down to the umbilicus, wrung out of water at 60° F., and covered with flannel.

c., cold. Soft, absorbent cloth, several layers thick, dipped in cold water, slightly wrung out, applied to given part. To maintain constant temperature, compress is frequently renewed, ice bag or rubber coil through which ice water is circulating is placed on it. Duration, 30-60 minutes.

c., cribriform. A compress with holes for drainage from a wound.

c., forehead. A soft towel wrung out of water below 60° F. renewed at least every 2 minutes.

c., hot. Soft, absorbent cloth folded into several layers, dipped in hot water (107-115° F.) slightly wrung out and placed on part to be treated, covered with a piece of flannel large enough to overlap the linen slightly. Temperature is maintained at constant level by renewing compress or by rubber coil through which hot water (107-115° F.) is circulated.

c., neck. Application of a soft towel wrung out of water bet. 42-60° F.

c., precordial. Pad of four layers of cloth, moistened in water 60-65° F., is applied over the heart region. On this is placed a coil through which water at 60-65° F. is circulating. This water temperature is reduced until ice water is used. Duration, 10-45 minutes. Twice daily.

c., spinal. Usually the application of a soft cloth wrung out of ice water, renewed every 2-3 minutes. Applied to cervical region for meningitis, cerebral congestion and nervous asthenia; dorsal region for hysterical vomiting and to lumbar region for renal and uterine hemorrhage.

c., throat. Application of two strips of absorbent cloth 3 inches wide and long enough to reach from beneath one ear under the chin to the opposite ear, wrung out of water at 60° F.; a piece of flannel ¼ inch wider covers it and overlaps at top of head.

c., trunk. Consists of three folds of linen from axilla to pubis and reaching around the trunk, wrung out of water 60-75° F., covering with flannel bandage secured by pins. Changed every hour.

c., wet. Application of two or more folds of soft cloth wrung out of water at prescribed temperatures and covered with flannel.

compression [L. *compressio,* a compression]. A squeezing together; state of being pressed together.

c. atrophy. That in a part due to steady compression.

c. of the brain. Same as cerebral compression, *q.v.*

c., cerebral. Pressure on the brain produced by increased intercranial fluids, embolism, thrombosis, tumors, and skull fractures. More serious than concussion.*

SYM: Deep unconsciousness; full, bounding pulse; deep, stertorous, slow respiration; flushed face; high blood pressure; pupils varying in size. Temperature may rise and there may be retention or incontinence of urine and feces. *Danger Signals:* Coma, Cheyne-Stokes respiration, rise in temperature, quickening of pulse.

NP: Watch for change of symptoms; pulse, respiration, color, urine, and bed sores; also convulsions, bleeding from ears and nose, and oozing at back of throat, or for cerebrospinal fluid from ears, which may indicate fracture. Constant care of mouth and eyes.

c., digital. Arterial compression by means of the fingers.

c., myelitis. That caused by pressure on the spinal cord, often due to a tumor.

compres'sor. 1. Instrument for making pressure on a part. 2. A muscle which compresses a part as the *compressor hemispherium bulbi* which compresses the bulb of the urethra.

compul'sion [L. *compulsiō*, an urging]. Act performed to relieve fear connected with obsession; dictation by the patient's subconscious, arising against the subject's wishes and, if denied, causing uneasiness. Impulsive actions, on the contrary, often seem to express the personality.

c. neurosis. Obsession or psychoneurosis urging one to perform an absurd act or to say something silly.

compul'sive. Exercising or applying compulsion.

c. ideas. Psy: An idea that continues to suggest against one's will the commitment of an overt act which would normally be against one's better judgment.

compul'sory. Compelling action against one's will.

c. movements. Movements caused by injury to a nerve center.

con- [L.]. Prefix: Together with, as *congenital.*

conarium (ko-na'rĭ-um) [G. *konarion*, a little cone]. The pineal gland. Syn: *corpus pineale* [NA].

conation (ko-na'shun) [L. *conatio*, an attempt]. The desire or impulse, arising from inside one, to act.

concassation (kon-kas-a'shun) [L. *con*, with, + *quassere*, to crush]. 1. Shaking of a precipitate in a bottle or pulverizing by beating. 2. Mental distress.

concatenation (kon-kat"ĕ-na'shun) [L. *con*, together, + *catena*, chain]. A group of events or effects acting in concert or occurring at the same time.

Concato's disease (kon-kă'tōz) [Luigi M. Concato, Italian physician, 1825-1882]. Progressive inflammation of serous membranes. Etiol: Tuberculosis.

concave (kon'kāv) [L. *con*, with, + *cavus*, hollow]. Having a spherically depressed or hollow surface.

concav'ity [" + *cavitas*, a hollow]. A hollowed surface, with curved, bowl-like sides.

conca"vocon'cave [" + *cavus*, hollow, + *con*, with, + *cavus*, hollow]. Concave on opposing sides.

concavocon'vex [" + " + *convexus*, vaulted]. Concave on one side and convex on opp. surface. See: *convex.*

conceive (kŏn-sēv'). 1. To become pregnant. 2. To form a mental image or to bring into mind; to form an idea.

concentration (kon-sen-tra'shun) [L. *concentratiō*, in the center]. 1. Increase in strength of a fluid by evaporation. 2. Medicine strengthened by evaporation. 3. Fixation of mind on one subject to exclusion of all other thoughts.

c., hydrogen ion. Concentration of hydrogen ions in a solution; the symbol is pH.

con'cept [L. *conceptum*, something devised]. An idea.

concep'tion [L. *conceptiō*, a conceiving]. 1. The mental process of forming an idea. 2. The union of the male sperm and the ovum of the female; fertilization.

With a cycle of 28 days, menstruation normally lasts 5 days followed by a period of repair and proliferation of about a week. Until ovulation occurs the female is sterile. In general, ovulation occurs about 12 to 14 days *prior to the beginning of the next menstrual period.* Thus sexual intercourse during the middle of the menstrual cycle is most likely to result in conception. During this period, the ovum is discharged from the follicle and makes its way through the Fallopian tube to the uterus. If fertilization does not occur during this time the ovum disintegrates and for the remaining portion of the menstrual cycle (the 10 days preceding menstruation) conception is very unlikely to occur.

Caution: One of the most variable events known in human biology is the menstrual cycle. It is therefore quite difficult, and in many cases impossible, to predict optimum time of conception or the reverse by attempting to calculate ovulation time from the time the last menstrual period occurred. Also sperm survival time in the female reproductive tract is variable.

concep'tus. The products of conception.

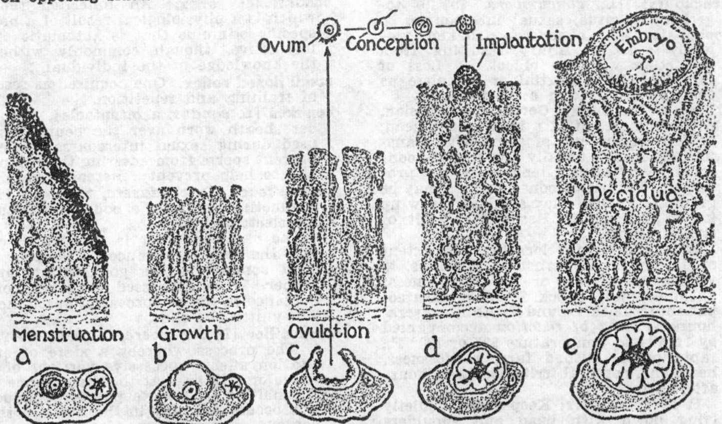

MENSTRUATION, CONCEPTION, AND IMPLANTATION

(a) Menstruation. (b) Growth. (c) Ovulation, ovum becomes impregnated. (d) Ovum in morula stage becomes implanted. Endometrium in pregravid stage, corpus luteum of pregnancy developing. (e) Endometrium has become decidua and ovum is growing in it.

concha (kong'kă) (pl. *conchae*) [G. *kogchē*, shell]. 1. The outer ear or the pinna. 2. One of the three nasal conchae, *q.v.* 3. Patella. 4. Vulva.

c. auriculae. A concavity on the median surface of the auricle of the ear, divided by a ridge into the upper *cymba conchae* and a lower *cavum conchae*. The latter leads to the ext. auditory meatus.

c. bullosa. Turbinated bone expansion, during chronic rhinitis.

c. nasal. One of the three scroll-like bones which project medially from the lateral wall of the nasal cavity; a turbinate bone. The superior and middle conchae are processes of lateral mass of the ethmoid bone; the inferior concha is a face bone. Each overlies a meatus.

c. Santorini. C. nasalis suprema.

c. sphenoidalis. In a fetal skull, one of two curved plates located on anterior portion of body of sphenoid bone. Forms part of roof of nasal cavity.

conchitis (kong-ki'tis) [" + *-itis*, inflammation]. Inflammation of any concha.

conchoidal (kong-koi'dal) [" + *eidos*, shape]. Having the shape of a shell.

conchoscope (kong'ko-scōp) [" + *skopein*, to examine]. Instrument for examination of the nasal cavity.

conchotome (kong'ko-tōm) [" + *tomē*, incision]. Device for excision of middle turbinated bone.

concoc'tion [L. *con*, with, + *coquere*, to cook]. Mixture of two medicinal substances usually done with the aid of heat.

concom'itant [L. *cum*, together, + *comēs*, companion]. Accessory; taking place at the same time.

concrement. A concretion as of protein and other substances. If infiltrated with calcium salts, such is termed a calculus.

concrescence (kon-kres'ens) [L. *con*, together, + *crescere*, to grow]. The union of separate parts; coalescence.

concrete (kon'krēt) [L. *concretus*, solid]. Condensed, hardened, or solidified.

concre'tion [L. *con*, with, + *crescere*, to grow]. A calculus.

concub'itus [L. *concumbere*, to lie together]. Coitus, sexual intercourse.

concus'sion [L. *concussus*, shaken violently]. 1. An injury resulting from impaction with an object. 2. Loss of function either partial or complete as that resulting from a blow or fall.

c. of the brain. Cerebral concussion. A common result of a blow to the head, or fall on the end of spine with transmitted force, usually causing unconsciousness, either temporary or prolonged. Return of consciousness may be gradual. Patient may suddenly draw up knees and vomit. Resembles result of skull fracture.

Sym: Vary with location and extent of injury from transient dizziness to various paralyses, or unconsciousness; unequal pupils, shock. If uncomplicated, patient comes round within several hours. *Period of reaction* accompanied by vomiting, temperature 99° or 100° F., rapid pulse, flushed face, restlessness, headache, cerebral irritation 12-24 hours afterwards.

F. A. Treatment: Keep patient quietly lying down with head and shoulders slightly elevated. *Do not* give stimulants. Transportation should be delayed if possible. Sedatives only if patient is hyperexcited. Caution: Do not give morphine. Cool applications to head and neck are soothing. Reassure patient if conscious. Heat to extremities if cold. Report any adverse symptoms, such as bleeding, at once. Darkened room best. See: *contusion; transportation of injured.*

c. of labyrinth. Deafness resulting from a blow to the head or ear.

c., spinal. Loss of function in spinal cord resulting from a blow or severe jarring. May be with or without lesion.

condensa'tion [L. *con*, with, + *densāre*, to make thick]. 1. Making more dense or compact. 2. Changing a liquid to a solid or a gas to a liquid. 3. Psy: The union of ideas to form a new mental pattern.

Chem: A type of reaction in which two or more molecules of the same substance react with each other and form a new substance with higher molecular weight and different chemical properties.

conden'ser [" + *densāre*, to make thick]. Device for solidifying vapors and liquids. See: *capacitor.*

c., electrical. Device for storing of electricity by using two conducting surfaces and a nonconductor.

con'diment [L. *condere*, to pickle]. Appetizing ingredient added to food.

Classification: 1. *Aromatic*: Vanilla, cinnamon, cloves, chervil, parsley, bay leaf, etc. 2. *Acrid or Peppery*: Pepper, ginger, allspice, etc. 3. *Alliaceous or Allylic*: Onion, mustard, horseradish. 4. *Acid*: Vinegar, capers, gherkins, citron. 5. *Animal Origin*: Caviar, anchovies.

In general, condiments have little Caloric value. Sugar is an exception. They are extremely useful in making food more appetizing.

Action: They seem to stimulate the stomach and intestines, perhaps by chemical action although this is questioned. They do irritate, esp. if taken in too large quantities. They are appetizers and stimulate the secretion of saliva and intestinal juices.

Sugar is a food producing muscular energy; salt is a chemical substance maintaining the mineral equilibrium.

condi'tional reflex. An inherited reflex which is a physiological result of a nonspecific stimulus that is automatic and instinctive, though commonly without the knowledge of the individual.

condi'tioned reflex. One acquired as result of training and repetition.

con'dom [L. *condus*, a receptacle]. A rubber sheath worn over the penis. It is used during sexual intercourse to help prevent sperm from entering the vagina, and to help prevent venereal disease.

conduc'tance [L. *conducere*, to lead]. The conducting ability of a body or a circuit for electricity.

The best conductor is that which offers the least resistance. Examples of good conductors are gold, silver, and copper. When expressed in figures, conductance is the reciprocal of resistance. The unit is the ohm.

conduc'tion [L. *conducerè*, to read]. Phys: 1. The process whereby a state of excitation affects successive portions of a tissue or cell, so that the disturbance is transmitted to remote points. Conduction occurs not only in the fibers of the nervous system, but also in muscle fibers. 2. The transfer of electrons, ions, heat, or sound waves through a conductor or conducting medium.

c., bone. Sound conduction through cranial bones.

conductiv'ity. The specific electric conducting ability of a substance.

Numerically, conductivity is the reciprocal of unit resistance, or resistivity. The unit is the ohm per cm. Specific conductivity is sometimes expressed as a percentage. In such cases the conductivity is given as a percentage of the conductivity of pure copper under certain standard conditions.

conductor (kon-duk'tor) [L. *conducere,* to lead]. 1. Medium transmitting a force. 2. A guide directing a surgical knife or probe.

condylar (kon'dĭ-lăr) [G. *kondylos,* knuckle]. Pert. to a condyle.

condylarthrosis (kon-dil-ar-thro'sis) [" + *arthrōsis,* a joint]. A form of diarthrosis;* an ovoid head in an elliptical cavity.

condyle (kon'dīl) (pl. *condyles*) [G. *kondylos,* knuckle]. A rounded protuberance at the end of a bone forming an articulation.

condylectomy (kon-dĭ-lek'to-mĭ) [" + *ektomē,* excision]. Excision of a condyle.

condylion (kon-dĭl'ĭ-on) [G. *kondylion,* knob]. A point on either the lateral or medial surface of the mandibular condyle.

condyloid (kon'dĭ-loid) [G. *kondylos,* knuckle, + *eidos,* appearance]. Pert. to or resembling a condyle.

c. process. Articular process on ramus of mandible consisting of a capitulum and neck. Articulates with mandibular fossa of temporal bone.

c. tubercle. A tubercle on capitulum of condyloid process of the mandible for attachment of temporomandibular ligament.

condyloma (kŏn-dĭ-lō'mă) [" + *-ōma,* tumor]. A wartlike growth of the skin, usually seen on the external genitalia or near the anus.

There are two types, a pointed variety, and a broad, flat form which is usually of syphilitic origin.

c. latum. A mucous patch on the vulva or anus, coated with gray exudate, flattened in form, with delimited area, characteristic of syphilis.

condylomatous (kon-dĭ-lo'mă-tus) [" + *-ōma,* tumor]. Pert. to a condyloma.

condylotomy (kon-dĭ-lot'o-mĭ) [" + *tomē,* incision]. Division without removal of a condyle.

condylus (kon'dĭ-lus) (pl. *condyli*). Condyle.

cone (kōn) [G. *kōnos,* cone]. 1. A three-dimensional figure with circular base with sides sloping to a point above. May be solid or hollow. 2. Retinal flask-shaped figure in layer of rods and cones. 3. A receptor cell concerned with color vision.

c. of light. Triangular light areas on the membrana tympani extending downward from the umbo.

c., ocular. Cone of light in eye with tip on the retina.

confabula'tion [L. *confabulārī,* to talk together]. PSY: The relation of imaginary experiences to fill in gaps in the memory.

confec'tio, confec'tion [L. *con,* with, + *facere,* to make]. Sugarlike soft solids in which one or more medicinal substances are incorporated with the object of affording an agreeable form for their administration and a convenient method for their preservation. Not often prescribed, and not official.

confinement (kon-fīn'ment) [Fr. *confiner,* to restrain in a place]. The puerperal state or period of childbirth.

con'flict [L. *con,* with, + *fligere,* to strike]. 1. Opposing action of incompatibles. 2. PSY: The conscious or unconscious struggle bet. two opposing desires or courses of action. A technical term applied to a state in which social goals dictate behavior contrary to more primitive (often subconscious) desires.

confluence of sinuses. The union of the sagittal sinus with the transverse sinuses. SYN: *Confluens sinuum* [NA]; *torcular Herophili.*

con'fluent [L. *confluere,* to run together]. Running together, as when the pustules in smallpox merge.

confrontation (kon-frun-ta'shun) [" + *frons,* face]. 1. The examination of two patients together, one with a disease and the other from whom the disease was supposed to be contracted. 2. A method employed in determining extent of visual fields in which that of the patient is compared with that of the examiner.

congelation (kon-je-la'shun) [L. *congelāre,* to freeze]. Freezing, or a frostbite.

congenerous (kon-jen'er-us) [L. *con,* with, + *genus,* race]. Possessing the same function, as synergistic muscles.

congen'ital [L. *congenitus,* born together]. Present at birth.

congested (kon-jes'ted) [L. *congerere,* to heap together]. Hyperemic; containing an abnormal amt. of blood.

conges'tion [L. *congerere,* to heap together]. The presence of an excessive amount of blood or tissue fluid in an organ or in tissue.

c., active. Congestion resulting from increased flow of blood to a part or dilatation of blood vessels.

c., passive. Hyperemia resulting from interference with flow of blood from capillaries into venules. May also result from myocardial insufficiency.

congestive (kon-jes'tiv). Pertaining to congestion.

congius (kon'jĭ-us) (pl. *con'gii*) [L.]. A gallon.

conglo'bate [L. *con,* with + *glōbāre,* to make round]. In one mass, as lymph glands.

congloba'tion [" + *globus,* a ball]. Aggregation of particles in a mass.

conglom'erate [" + *glomerāre,* to heap]. 1. An aggregation in one mass. 2. Clustered; heaped together.

conglutin (kon-glu'tin) [L. *conglutināre,* to glue together]. A protein resembling casein found in peas, beans, and almonds.

conglu'tinant. Promoting adhesion, as of the edges of a wound.

conglu'tinate [L. *conglutinātiō,* an adhering]. Having the quality of adhesiveness.

conglutination (kon-glu-tin-a'shun) [L. *conglutinātiō,* an adhering]. 1. Coalescence, adhesion. 2. Reaction, such as agglutination.

coniasis (kon-i'ă-sis) [G. *konis,* dust]. Dustlike calculi in gallbladder and bile ducts.

conidia (ko-nid'ĭ-ă) (pl. of *conidium*) [G. *konidion,* a particle of dust]. Asexual spores of fungi.

conidiophore (kon-id'ĭ-o-for) [" + *phoros,* bearing]. The stalk supporting conidia.

coniol'ogy [G. *konis,* dust, + *logos,* study of]. The study of dust and its effects.

conio'sis [" + *-ōsis,* infection]. Any condition caused by inhalation of dust.

coniza'tion [G. *kōnos,* cone]. Excision of a cone of tissue, as of the mucous membrane of the cervix.

conjugata (kon-ju-gā'tă) [L.]. Diameter of pelvis, measured from center of the promontory of the sacrum to the back of the symphysis pubis. SYN: *conjugate.*

c. vera. Sometimes written *c.v.* Same as conjugata.

conjugate (kon'jū-gāt) [L. *con,* with, + *jugum,* yoke]. 1. Paired or joined. 2. An important diameter of the pelvis, measured from the center of the promontory of the sacrum to the back of the symphysis pubis. In obstetrics the diagonal conjugate is measured and the true conjugate is estimated. SEE: *c., diagonal; c., external.*

c. deviation. Deviation of both eyes to either side.

c., diagonal. Measured from the lower edge of the symphysis to the sac and can be determined during life, whereas the true conjugate cannot be measured. The true conjugate is estimated by deducting 1.5 to 2.0 cm. from the length of the diagonal conjugate. It is about ½-¾ in. longer than the true conjugate, or about 5 in.

c. diameter. Same as conjugate (def. 2).

c., external. Measured from the spine of the last lumbar vertebra to the front of the pubes (this is done by using calipers), and is normally about 8 in.

c., true. Same as conjugate (2). SYN: *conjugata vera.*

conjuga'tion [" + *jugum,* yoke]. A coupling together. In biology, the union of two unicellular organisms accompanied by an interchange of nuclear material as in *Paramecium.*

conjunctiva (con-junk-tī'vă) [" + *jungere,* to join]. Mucous membrane which lines eyelids and is reflected onto eyeball.

DIVISIONS: (1) Palpebral, covering under surface of lids; (2) bulbar, coating ant. portion of eyeball; (3) fornix, transition portion forming fold bet. lid and globe.

INSPECTION: Palpebral and ocular portions should be examined. Color and degree of moisture and presence of foreign bodies should be observed; also petechial hemorrhages and inflammation.

PATH. CONDITIONS: Trachoma and pannus as well as discoloration. *Yellowish discoloration*: Seen in jaundice, certain fevers, and hemolysis. May be due to fatty deposits. *Bluish-white or pearly discoloration*: Seen in anemia, nephritis, and phthisis. Sky-blue coloring is noted in whooping cough. *Pale conjunctivae*: Observed in anemias.

conjunctival reflex (kon-junk-ti'val). Closure of eyelids when conjunctiva is touched or threatened.

conjunctivitis (kon-junk-tī-vi'tis) [L. *con,* with, + *jungere,* to join, + G. *-itis,* inflammation]. Inflammation of conjunctiva.

TREATMENT: Directed against the specific type of infection.

c., actinic. Conjunctivitis resulting from exposure to ultraviolet (actinic) rays.

c., acute contagious. Pink eye. ETIOL: Koch-Weeks bacillus.

c., angular (of Morax-Axenfeld). Chronic catarrhal conjunctivitis.

c., catarrhal. One due to irritation or cold.

c., follicular. Type characterized by pinkish round bodies in retrotarsal fold.

c., gonorrheal. A severe, acute form of purulent conjunctivitis caused by the gonococcus, *Neisseria gonorrhea.*

c., granular. Acute, contagious, inflammatory c. with granular elevations on the lids which ulcerate and cicatrize. SYN: *trachoma.*

c., membranous. Acute conjunctivitis characterized by a false membrane; with or without infiltration.

c. of newborn. Ophthalmia neonatorum, *q.v.*

c., phlyctenular. Circumscribed type characterized by lymphoid tissue in small red nodules.

c., purulent. SEE: *c., gonorrheal.*

c., vernal. One beginning in the spring.

conjunctivo'ma [" + " + G. *-ōma,* tumor]. A tumor of the conjunctiva.

conjunctivoplasty (kon-junk-tī'vo-plas-tī) [" + " + G. *plassein,* to form]. Removal of part of cornea, but replacing with flaps from the conjunctiva.

connec'tive [L. *connectere,* to bind]. That which connects or binds together.

c. tissue. One of the four main tissues of the body. It includes an embryonic connective tissue (mesenchyme and mucous) and adult connective tissue. The latter is subdivided into four general groups (1) vascular tissues (blood, lymph), (2) connective tissue proper (areolar, white fibrous, yellow fibrous, reticular, adipose), (3) cartilage and (4) bone. Connective tissues are concerned primarily with supporting bodily structures and binding parts together. They also are involved in other functions such as food storage, blood formation, and defensive mechanisms of the body.

co'noid [G. *kōnos,* cone, + *eidos,* shape]. Resembling a cone; conical.

c. ligament. Lower and inner portion of coracoclavicular ligament.

c. tubercle. Eminence on inf. surface of clavicle to which is attached the conoid ligament.

consanguinity (kon-san-gwin'ī-tī) [L. *consanguinitās,* kinship]. Relationship by blood.

conscious (kon'shus) [L. *conscius,* aware]. Being aware and having perception.

con'sciousness [L. *conscius,* aware]. PSY: A state of awareness.

It implies an orientation to time, place, and person; *i. e.,* the individual knows approximately the date, the nature of his environment, his name and other pertinent personal data.

The content of consciousness is a composite of memories and the comprehension of external reality; the emotional status and the individual's goals also enter. It is then a large part of that described as "personality" in its largest sense.

Consciousness varies its intensity and extent from minute to minute. In crises, vivid ideational association may lead to an exaggerated state of awareness. In states of relaxed contentment, it lessens, to disappear completely in sleep. This differs from the pathologic condition of coma in which the patient cannot be aroused.

In so-called pathologic sleep (*e. g.,* encephalitis lethargica) and in stupor, though aroused, the patient is unable to postpone again lapsing into dullness; normal sleep can be adequately combated by the demands of reality. Stupor is produced largely by the factors resulting in coma; the personality is relatively intact but "hazy." In contrast there are conditions in which a real personality change manifests itself. Clouding of consciousness may simulate the dullness but usually not the other characteristics of stupor. On the contrary, such patients may impress one as relatively alert.

The loss of orientation to time and place but not to person constitutes delirium. A quiet delirium may not easily reveal itself even in certain states of automatism in which one finds evidence of the "real personality"; there may appear on casual examination little to arouse suspicion, yet brutal acts, total absence of memory, reveal these as major abnormalities. The "clouded" patient with obvious emotionalism (fear) and violent hallucinations is obviously psychotic.

Clouding of consciousness may be diagnosed from the appearance of the patient in catatonic stupor and it may be difficult to realize the patient is quite lucid and that experiences are being registered accurately and can be later recalled. In true clouding, stimuli usually fail to register.

Again, in some ambulistic states, experiences may register but cannot be recalled after return to a normal state. During a later secondary state, it is apparent that the failure of memory is only a repression and not truly absent. Consciousness, on the other hand, may erroneously appear to be present in so-called "coma vigil" because the eyes are open and expression may be alert.

c., *clouding of.* A phase of delirium in which the patient's consciousness is cloudy or not clear.

c., *cosmic.* The inner reaches of consciousness in which there is recognition of knowledge or facts independent of physical influence.

c., *levels of.* Altered consciousness from any cause may be classified as follows:

Somnolence. Patient may be delirious and restless, or still, and fall asleep when left alone. Even though he can answer questions he may be confused.

Stupor. Patient may be restless or combative, and may make twitching or picking motions. He should be protected from injuring himself. Responds to sensory stimuli including bright lights and loud sounds.

Semicoma. Spontaneous movement is absent unless the patient is roused. Even then, the response may be only a groan or a mutter. Withdraws from painful stimuli and is usually incontinent.

Deep coma. If patient responds at all, it is only to very painful stimuli. Spontaneous movements and resistance to passive movement are absent.

consen'sual [L. *con,* with, + *sentire,* to feel]. Reflex stimulation from another part.

c. *light index.* When one eye is exposed to an intensity of light different from that to which the other is exposed, both pupils will react.

c. *reflex.* Any reflex occurring on opposite side of body from point of stimulation.

consolidation (kon-sol-ĭ-dā'shun) [L. *consolidāre,* to make firm]. The act of becoming solid. Esp. used in connection with the solidification of the lungs due to engorgement of the lung tissues, as occurs in acute pneumonia.

constella'tion [L. *con,* with, + *stella,* star]. Ideas arising from unrepressed emotions.

constipation (kŏn-stĭ-pā'shun) [L. *constipāre,* to press together]. Difficult defecation; often infrequent passage of feces with passage of unduly hard and dry fecal material; sluggish action of the bowels.

Predisposing Causes: No habitual bowel movement from childhood; worry, anxiety, fear, sedentary life.

Direct Causes: Failure to establish definite and regular times for bowel movements; improper diet; intestinal obstruction; tumors; excessive use of laxatives; weakness of intestinal musculature (atony) or excessive tonicity (spasticity); use of certain drugs; presence of anal lesions.

General Corrective Measures: Plenty of fresh vegetables, fruits, milk, and an abundance of water. Cut down starches. Plenty of physical exercise, avoid all that worries, establish regular habit time for bowel movement, and do not eat when under the influence of strong emotion.

c., *atonic.* That due to weakness of muscles of colon and rectum.

c., *obstructive.* Due to an obstruction in the intestines. Surgical aid needed. Preoperative diet should contain low residue and no gas forming foods.

c., *spastic.* That due to excessive tonicity of the intestinal wall, esp. the colon.

constitu'tion [L. *constituere,* to establish]. The physical makeup and functional habits of the body.

constitu'tional. Pert. to the body as a whole.

c. *disease.* One that affects the entire body rather than a specific part. 2. One that is dependent upon an individual's hereditary makeup, *e.g.,* hemophilia.

c. *psychosis.* Functional psychosis; not of organic origin.

constric'tion [L. *con,* with, + *stringere,* to draw]. 1. A binding or squeezing of a part. 2. The narrowing of a vessel or opening as constriction of blood vessels or the pupil of the eye.

constric'tor [" + *stringere,* to draw]. 1. That which binds or restricts a part. 2. A muscle which contricts a vessel, opening, or passageway, as the *constrictors* of the faucial isthmus and pharynx, the circular fibers of the iris, intestine, and blood vessels.

construct'ive metabolism. The binding up or anabolic process.

consult'ant [L. *consultāre,* to counsel]. A consulting physician or surgeon who acts in an advisory capacity.

consulta'tion [L. *consultātiō*]. Diagnosis and proposed treatment by two or more physicians at one time.

consumption (kon-sump'shun) [L. *consumere,* to waste away]. 1. Tuberculosis.* 2. Wasting. 3. The using up of anything.

consump'tive. Pert. to or afflicted with tuberculosis.

con'tact [L. *con,* with, + *tangere,* to touch]. 1. Mutual touching or apposition of two bodies. 2. One who has been exposed to contagion.

c., *complete.* When entire surface of a tooth touches entire surface of an adjoining tooth, proximally.

c., *direct.* Communication of a contagious disease through a healthy person touching an infected body.

c., immediate. Same as direct contact.

c., indirect. The spread of a contagious disease by some medium other than direct touch of the sick person.

c., lens. A thin bowl-shaped shell of glass made to fit over the cornea.

c., mediate. Same as indirect contact.

c., proximal or **proximate.** Touching of teeth on their adjacent surfaces.

c. surface. Proximal surface of a tooth.

conta'gion [L. *contangere,* to touch]. The process of transferring a specific disease either by direct or indirect contact. SEE: *virulent; virus.*

conta'gious. Communicable; transmitted readily from one person to another either directly or indirectly, with reference to the organism which causes a disease.

contagium (kon-ta'jĭ-um) [L.]. The agent causing infection or contagion.

containers, care and handling of. As contamination of the container in which a specimen is to be placed may render the results of the examination futile, and so interfere with the doctor's diagnosis based upon it, the nurse must avoid contamination of any container used for the collection of specimens.

1. See that the containers are perfectly clean, inside and outside, and that the surfaces are intact. Cracked or broken containers must not be used. The containers must never be completely filled.

2. If the presence of bacteria is suspected, the container must first be sterilized, unless this has already been done by the laboratory.

To clean glassware: (a) Using very little soap-powder, boil in water. (b) Brush well under running water. (c) Rinse well in running water. (d) Place in potassium bichromate solution for 20 minutes. (e) Rinse well in running water. (f) Rinse in distilled water. (g) Rinse again in distilled water. (h) Invert in basket and drain dry or dry in a hot-air oven.

Sterilization of glassware: This is accomplished by hot air or dry heat, boiling water, flowing steam, steam under pressure, certain gases, and the use of germicidal chemicals.

3. *Labels*: All containers should be labeled, when used, with the name of the patient and his room number; also the name of the attending physician. "Request forms," sometimes used as labels, are made up to suit the individual laboratory or hospital. Provision is made for recording necessary data as indicated, including date when specimen was taken, and under what circumstances, and for what substances the examination is to be done, together with other information desired.

4. *Time*: If the required specimen cannot be furnished at once, make a note of what is needed, inform the patient, the supervisor, and any other nurse who may attend to the patient in your absence.

5. *Charting*: Note on the chart all specimens sent to the laboratory, when sent, and any other data that seem pertinent such as the appearance of the specimen or unusual occurrences while obtaining it.

6. *Care of specimen*: Cover immediately after depositing in the container; check label or "request form," and see that the container is intact, and that there is no danger of spilling while in transit.

contam'inate. 1. To soil, stain, or pollute. 2. To render unfit for use through introduction of a substance which is harmful or injurious. 3. To make impure or unclean.

contamina'tion. 1. The act of contaminating, esp. introduction of disease germs or infectious material into or on normally sterile objects. 2. In psychiatry, the fusion and condensation of words.

content. That which is contained in something.

c., dream. What one dreams.

contiguity (kon-tĭ-gū'ĭ-tĭ) [L. *contiguus,* touching]. Contact or closely associated.

c., amputation in. Amputation through a joint.

c., law of. If two ideas occur in association they are apt to be repeated.

c., solution of. Dislocation or displacement of two normally contiguous parts.

con'tinence [L. *continere,* to hold back]. Self-restraint, used esp. in connection with refraining from sexual indulgence. Also used in reference to the ability to control urination and defecation.

continent (kon'tĭ-nent). Capable of controlling urination and defecation. SEE ALSO: *continence.*

continuity (kon-tĭ-nū'ĭ-tĭ) [L. *continuus,* continued]. The state of being continuous or intimately united.

c., amputation in. Amputation through a long bone.

c., solution of. Division of normally continuous parts by fracture, rupture, laceration, incision.

contin'uous [L. *continere,* to hold together]. Without break, cessation, or interruption.

c. spec'trum. An unbroken series of wave lengths, either visible or invisible. Such a spectrum is produced by light from incandescent solids, liquids, or gases under high pressure passed through a prism. Also an unbroken range of radiations of different wave lengths in any portion of the invisible spectrum.

contor'tion. A twisting into an unusual shape.

contour (kon'toor) [L. *con,* with, + *tornāre,* to turn around]. Outline or surface configuration of a part.

contoured (kon'toord). Having an irregular, smooth, undulating surface resembling a relief map.

contra- [L.]. Prefix: Opposite; against, as *contraindication.*

contra-ap'erture [L. *contra,* against, + *apertura, opening*]. A second opening made in an abscess.

contraception (kon-tra-sep'shun) [" + *conceptiō,* a conceiving]. The prevention of conception.

contracep'tive. Any agent or device used to prevent conception.

contract' [L. *contrahere,* to draw together]. 1. To draw together, reduce in size, or shorten. 2. To acquire through infection, as to contract a disease.

contrac'tile. Able to contract or shorten.

contractil'ity [L. *contrahere,* to draw together]. Having the ability to contract or shorten.

contrac'tion [L. *contractio,* a drawing up]. A shortening or tightening, as that of a muscle, or a reduction in size; a shrinking. SEE: *cholepathia spastica.*

c., isometric. Muscular contraction in which the muscle does not change its length.

c., isotonic. Muscular contraction in which the muscle maintains constant tension by changing its length during the action.

contracture (kon-trak'chur) [L. *contractura*]. 1. Permanent contraction of a muscle due to spasm or paralysis. 2. A condition of fixed high resistance to the passive stretch of a muscle, as may result from fibrosis of tissues surrounding a joint.

c., Dupuytren's. Flexion deformity of hands and fingers due to contraction of the palmar fascia.

c., functional. Decrease of a contracture during anesthesia or sleep.

c., physiological. A temporary condition in which tension and shortening of a muscle are maintained for a considerable time although there is no tetanus. May be induced by heat, action of drugs, acids, etc.

c., Volkmann's. Pronation and flexion of the hand, with shrinking and hardening of the muscles of the forearm.

contrafissura (kon"tră-fī-shu'ră) [L. *contra*, against, + *fissura*, fissure]. A skull fracture at a point opp. from where the blow was received.

contraindication (kŏn"tră-ĭn-dĭ-kā'shŭn) [" + *indicāre*, to point out]. Any symptom or circumstance indicating the inappropriateness of a form of treatment, otherwise advisable.

contralat'eral [" + *latus*, side]. Originating in, or affecting, the opposite side of the body. Antonym: *ipsilateral.*

c. reflexes. 1. Passive flexion of one part following flexion of another. 2. Passive flexion of one leg causing similar movement of opposite leg.

con'trast sprays. Those administered by sitting on side of bathtub, spraying feet and legs with warm water for 1 minute and cold water for 1 minute. Alternate for 10 minutes twice daily.

contravolitional (kon"tră-vō-lĭ'shun-al) [L. *contra*, against, + *velle*, to wish]. In opposition to or without the will; involuntary.

contrecoup (kaun"tră-koo) [Fr. counter-blow.] Occurring on the opposite side.

c. injury. An injury to parts of the brain located on the side opposite that of the primary injury, as when the frontal and temporal lobes of the brain are forced against the irregular bones of the anterior portion of the cranial vault as a result of a blow on the back of the head.

contrectation (kon-trek-ta'shun) [L. *contrectāre*, to handle]. 1. Touch with the hands. 2. Caressing or sexually fondling one of the opposite sex.

control (kon-trōl') [L. *contra*, against, + *rotulus*, catalogue]. 1. To regulate or maintain. 2. A standard against which observations or conclusions may be checked in order to establish their validity, as a control animal, one which has not been exposed to the treatment or condition being studied in the other animals.

c. animal. An animal subjected to the same conditions as the experimental animal except for the specific factor being tested.

c., birth. Practice of contraception.

contrude (kon-trūd') [L. *con*, with, + *trūdere*, to thrust]. 1. Abnormal lingual curve or line of dental arch. 2. To crowd together, as the teeth.

contru'sion. Having the teeth crowded.

contuse (kon-tuz') [L. *contundere*, to bruise]. To bruise.

contusion (kon-tu'zhun) [L. *contusiō*, a bruise]. An injury in which the skin is not broken.

Sym: Pain, swelling and discoloration.

F. A. Treatment: Apply cold applications. Follow with firm bandage to prevent swelling. Twenty-four to 48 hours later, heat is desirable followed by gentle massage. See: *concussion.*

co'nus [G. *kōnos*]. 1. A cone. 2. Post. staphyloma of myopic eye.

c. arteriosus. Right cardiac ventricle's upper rounded ant. angle, where pulmonary artery arises.

c. medullaris. Conical portion of lower spinal cord.

convalescence (kon-val-es'ens) [L. *convalescere*, to become strong]. The period of recovery after the termination of a disease or an operation.

convales'cent. 1. Getting well. 2. One who is recovering from a disease or operation.

c. diet. A diet suitable for the condition from which the patient is recovering.

convection (kon-vek'shun) [L. *convehere*, to convey]. The transference of heat by means of currents in liquids or gases which result from changes in density.

convergence (kon-ver'jens) [L. *con*, with. + *vergere*, to incline]. 1. Visual lines directed to a nearby point. 2. The moving of two or more objects toward the same point. 3. In reflex activity, the coming together of several axons or afferent fibers upon one or a few motor neurons; the condition whereby impulses from several sensory receptors converge upon the same motor center resulting in a limited and specific response.

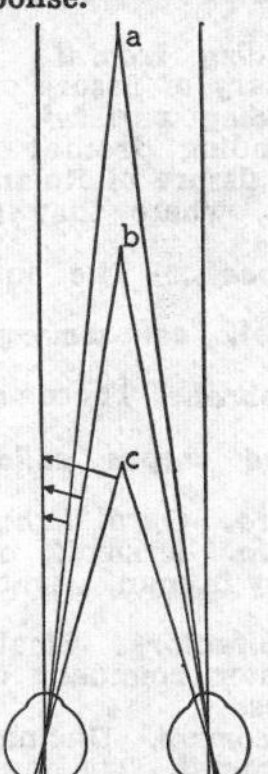

CONVERGENCE

When an object is brought from a distant position (a) to a near position (b), the eyes are rotated medially to make the lines of vision meet at the object. The closer the object, the greater the degree of convergence as measured by the angles indicated by arrows.

convergent (kon-ver'jent). Tending toward a common point.

conver'sion [L. *convertere*, to turn round]. Change from one state to another. In obstet., the change in position of a fetus in order to facilitate delivery. See: *version.*

c. symptom. Psy: A term for a repressed emotion that becomes manifested through a physical symptom; seen in hysteria.

con'vex [L. *convexus,* vaulted, arched]. Curved evenly; resembling the segment of a sphere.

convex"ocon'cave [" + *con,* with, + *cavus,* hollow]. Concave on one side and convex on opp. surface. Syn: *concavoconvex.*

convexocon'vex [L. *convexus,* arched]. Convex on two opp. faces.

convolute (kon'vo-lūt) [L. *convolvere,* to roll together]. Rolled, as a scroll.

con'voluted. Convolute, rolled.

c. tubule. In the kidney the proximal convoluted tubule lies between Bowman's capsule and the loop of Henle; the distal convoluted tubule lies between the loop of Henle and the collecting duct.

convolution (kŏn"vō-lū'shŭn) [L. *convolvere,* to roll together]. 1. A turn, fold, or coil of anything which is convoluted. 2. In *anat.*, a gyrus, one of the many folds on the surface of the cerebral hemispheres. They are separated by grooves (sulci or fissures). See: *gyrus.*

c., angular. A gyrus forming post. portion of inf. parietal lobule.

c.'s, annectant. The four gyri connecting the c.'s on upper surface of occipital lobe with parietal and temporophenoidal lobes.

c., ant. central. Ascending frontal c., *q.v.*

c., ant. choroid. *Gyrus choroides.*

c., anteroparietal. Ascending frontal c., *q.v.*

c., ant. orbital. One which lies in front of the orbital sulcus.

c., Arnold's. *Gyri posteriores inferiores.*

c., ascending frontal. One forming ant. boundary of fissure of Rolando.

c., ascending parietal. One parallel with ascending frontal c. separated from it by fissure of Rolando, except at extremities, where they are generally united.

c.'s, Broca's. The inf., or third, frontal c.

c., callosal, callosomarginal. *Gyrus fornicatus.*

c.'s, cerebral. Those of the cerebrum.

c. of the corpus callosum. *Gyrus fornicatus.*

c., cuneate. *Gyral isthmus.*

c., dentate. A small, notched gyrus rudimentary in man, situated in dentate fissure.

c., ext. olfactory. Small projections forming outer boundary of the olfactory grooves.

c., hippocompal. Uncinate gyrus.

c., inf. frontal. The lower and outer part of frontal lobe.

c., inf. occipital. A small one lying bet. middle and inf. occipital fissures.

c., inframarginal. Superior temporosphenoidal c.

c., insular. One of a group of small c.'s forming the island of Reil, entirely concealed by the operculum.

c., int. orbital. The gyrus next outside of the gyrus rectus.

c.'s, intestinal. The coils of the intestines.

c., marginal. One beginning in front of locus perforatus anterior and bounding longitudinal fissure on mesial aspect of the hemisphere.

c., middle frontal. One continuous post. with ascending frontal c. and extending forward over ant. end of hemisphere to its orbital surface.

c., middle occipital. One between the first and third occipital c.'s.

c., middle temporosphenoidal. A small gyrus continuous with the middle occipital or angular gyrus.

c., occipitotemporal. Two small c.'s on lower surface of temporosphenoidal lobe.

c., olfactory. Olfactory lobe.

c.'s, orbital. Small gyri on orbital surface of frontal lobe.

c.'s, parietal. Ascending parietal c. and superior parietal c.

c., post. orbital. A small one on post. and outer side of orbital sulcus, and continuous with inf. frontal c.

c., second (or middle) frontal. One continuous post. with ascending frontal c.

c., sup. frontal. One which bounds great longitudinal fissure, arising post. from upper end of ascending frontal c.

c., sup. occipital. Upper of the three c.'s on sup. surface of occipital lobe.

c., sup. parietal. Portion of parietal lobe limited ant. by upper part of the fissure of Rolando, post. by ext. parieto-occipital fissure, and inf. by intraparietal sulcus.

c., sup. temporosphenoidal. Upper of three c's forming temporosphenoidal lobe. It lies just below and is parallel with sylvian fissure.

c., supramarginal. The ant. portion of inf. parietal lobule behind inf. extremity of intraparietal fissure (sulcus), below which it joins the ascending parietal c.

c. of the sylvian fissure. The c. that bounds the fissure of Sylvius.

c., transverse orbital. The gyrus occupying post. portion of inf. surface of frontal lobe, at ant. extremity of fissure of Sylvius.

c., uncinate. One extending from near post. extremity of occipital lobe to apex of temporosphenoidal.

convul'sant [L. *convulsio,* a pulling together]. 1. An agent which produces a convulsion. 2. Causing onset of a convulsion.

c. poisons. The common ones are strychnine and other drugs of the nux vomica groups, and various infrequently used drugs, such as picrotoxin.

Sym: These produce a sense of suffocation, dyspnea, and then muscular rigidity; there are powerful tetanic contractions which may be very painful. These spasms may be brought on by trivial stimuli, such as touching the patient or they may come on at varying intervals of from 3 to 30 minutes and may last from 1 to 5 minutes. Trismus, cyanosis, and tachycardia are frequent accompaniments. Death results from asphyxia or exhaustion.

Treatment: Appropriate therapy will depend upon substance which caused the convulsion. General measures for emptying the stomach or attempting to neutralize the drug may be indicated. Sedatives may be ordered by the physician. Oxygen and artificial respiration may be indicated.

convul'sion [L. *convulsio,* a pulling together]. Paroxysms of involuntary muscular contractions and relaxations generally in children.

Convulsions due to tetanus and rabies are easily distinguished and for the most part involve a small portion of the voluntary musculature. On the contrary, strychnine poisoning convulsions involve the entire body. The word is accurately applied to unilateral attacks as seen in jacksonian epilepsy and, less likely, in hysteria. They are usually accompanied by unconsciousness. This is not the case in strychnine poisoning, hysteria, or in jacksonian epileptic attacks until the second side is involved.

NOTE: It is important for the person who observes the convulsion to later record on the chart the following: time of onset; duration; whether or not convulsion started in a certain area of the body and became generalized from the start; type of contractions; whether or not the patient became incontinent; was there an abnormal odor to the patient's breath; did the convulsion cause the patient to be injured or strike his head during the convulsion. This information will be quite valuable in diagnosing the patient's illness and caring for him.

ETIOL: *In General*: Epilepsy, eclampsia, meningitis, tetanus, uremia. Poisoning from aspidium, brucine, camphor, cyanides, strychnine, santonin. In *children* the cause is often dietary; other causes: rickets, neuropathic tendency, spasmophilia, syphilis, malnutrition, malaria, acute infectious disease, cervical disease, toxemias, or unknown. Calcium is low. Guanidine should be considered. In *adults*, due to epilepsy, heat cramps, strychnine, brain lesions, or food poisoning.

TREATMENT: If an infant, put him in a bath of 95° F. or mustard and water at 85° F. Cold applied to head. Cause must first be found or injury may result from bath. If cause is undetermined, keep patient from injuring self. Soft pad bet. teeth to avoid biting tongue or cheeks. Warm bath, with cold to head; if fever is present, tepid or cool bath. Sedatives or anesthesia may be advised by physician. *After Care*: Rest in bed, absolute quiet, careful diagnosis without unduly disturbing patient.

c., clonic. One having intermittent contractions, muscles being alternately contracted and relaxed.

c., epileptiform. One accompanied by unconsciousness.

c., hysterical. C. caused by hysteria.

c., mimetic. A spasm of facial muscles.

c., oscillating. One involving separate bundles of muscle fibers which contract alternately.

c., puerperal. Eclamptic c. in pregnant or puerperal woman.

c., salaam. Nodding spasm. SEE: *eclampsia nutans.*

c., tonic. One in which the contractions are maintained for a time, as in tetany.

c., toxic. C. caused by action of a toxin on nervous system.

c., uremic. C. caused by uremic condition.

convulsion, words pert. to: anticonvulsive, athetosis, chill, chorea, epilepsy, hysteria, ictus, jactitation, mimetic, paroxysm, rabies, spasm center, spasmophilia, strychnine poisoning, tetanus, tic, tremor.

convul'sive. Pert. to convulsions.

c. reflex. Incoördinate contraction of muscles in a convulsive manner.

c. tic. Spasm of face.

cook'ing [L. *coquere, coctum,* to cook]. The process of preparing foods for eating. *Purpose* . . . cooking makes most foods more palatable, easier to masticate, improves their digestibility, and destroys or inactivates harmful organisms or toxins which may be present.

Action on Protein: Soluble proteins become coagulated.

Action on Soluble Substances: These are often lost in boiling, and even sugars, mineral substances and starches, though insoluble to a certain extent, suffer a certain loss in this process.

Action on Starch: The starch granules now swell and are changed from insoluble (raw) starch to soluble starch capable of being converted into sugar in the process of digestion and of being assimilated in the system.

Cooking releases the aromatic substances and extractives that contribute odors and taste to foods. These odors help to stimulate the appetite.

Most microorganisms are destroyed in the ordinary processes of cooking, but some require a higher degree of heat and longer cooking to effect this result, as pork.

Cooley's anemia [Thomas Cooley, American pediatrician, 1871-1945]. Anemia resulting from inheritance of a recessive trait responsible for interference with hemoglobin synthesis. SYN: *thalassemia, q.v.*

Coo'lidge tube. An x-ray tube whose cathode consists of a spiral tungsten wire surrounded by a molybdenum tube.

Coombs' test [R. R. A. Coombs, British immunologist, 20th century]. A test for antiglobulins in the red cell; used in diagnosing various hemolytic anemias.

coordination (ko-or-din-a'shun) [L. *con,* with, + *ordināre,* to arrange]. The working together of various muscles for the production of a certain movement.

More generally, the working together of different systems of the body in a given process as the coordination bet. the system of glands and involuntary muscles in digestion.

cope (kōp). The ability to effectively deal with and handle the stresses to which one is subjected.

copiopia (ko-pĭ-o'pĭ-ă) [G. *kopos,* fatigue, + *opsis,* sight]. Eyestrain causing eye fatigue.

copodyskinesia (ko-po-dis-kın-e'sĭ-ă) [" + *dys,* difficult, + *kinēsis,* motion]. Fatigue of or difficulty in moving a group of muscles used in working. May be out of proportion to that which would be expected from the amount of work done, in which case it is called occupational neurosis.

cop'per (cuprum) [G. *kupros*]. SYMB: *Cu.* A metal, small quantities of which are utilized by the body. Its salts are an irritant poison. At. wt. 63.54; at. no. 29.

FUNCTION AND USES: It functions with iron in its transformation into such substances as hemoglobin, and it seems to be an activating principle when used in the treatment of blood dyscrasias. It aids tissue respiration and the synthesis of cytochrome. It is present in the liver at all times and is excreted by the kidneys.

DEFICIENCY SYM: Anemia, weakness, impaired respiration and growth, and poor utilization of iron.

SOURCES: Found in many vegetable and animal tissues. SEE: *chalcosis; Clapton's lines; names of foods.*

cop'per sul'fate (blue vitriol). $CuSO_4$ USP. Deep blue, shiny crystals or granular powder.

ACTION AND USES: Stimulant, astringent, and powerful emetic.

POISONING: SYM: A disagreeable, coppery, metallic taste, with tightness in the throat, nausea and vomiting, thirst; abdominal pains, cramps, and suppression of urine.

F. A. TREATMENT: Wash out stomach, give egg whites raw or beaten. Give demulcent drinks.

copperas (kop'er-ăs). Green vitriol. Pale bluish-green crystals. SEE: *ferrous sulfate.*

copperhead. A poisonous snake, *Agkistrodon mokassen,* common in the southern United States.

copremesis (kop-rĕm'ĕ-sĭs). The vomiting of fecal material.

coprolagnia (kop-ro-lag'nĭ-ă) [" + *lagneia,* lust]. An erotic satisfaction at the sight or odor of excreta.

coprolalia (kop-ro-la'lĭ-ă) [" + *lalia,* babble]. PSY: A morbid desire to use sacrilegious or obscene words in ordinary conversation. Seen in obsessional neurosis or dementia precox.

coprolith (kop'ro-lith) [" + *lithos,* stone]. Hard, inspissated feces.

coprology (kop-rol'o-jĭ) [" + *logos,* study of]. Examination of the feces. SYN: *scatology.*

coprophagy (ko-prof'ă-jĭ) [" + *phagein,* to eat]. The eating of excrement.

coprophilia (kop-ro-fil'ĭ-ă) [" + *philein,* to love]. Abnormal interest in feces; a perversion in adults.

coprophil'ic. Term applied to organisms which normally live in fecal material.

coprophobia (kop-ro-fo'bĭ-ă) [" + *phobos,* fear]. A morbid disgust at the sight of filth of any kind.

copropor'phyrin. A porphyrin present in feces. Coproporphyrins I and II are normally present in minute and equal amounts, but quantities are altered in certain diseases as poliomyelitis, infectious hepatitis and in lead poisoning.

copros'tanol. A derivative of cholesterol present in feces, usually the result of bacterial action in the large intestine.

coprozo'a [" + *zōon,* animal]. Protozoa in fecal matter outside of the intestine.

coprozo'ic. Pert. to coprozoa; found in feces or fecal matter.

copula (kŏp'ū-lă) [L. *copulāre,* to bind together]. A median elevation on floor of embryonic pharynx representing future root of the tongue.

copulation (kop-u-la'shun) [L. *copulātiō*]. Sexual intercourse. SYN: *coition; coitus; cohabitation; concubitus.*

cor, cordis (kor) [L.]. The heart.

c. pulmonale. Hypertrophy or failure of right ventricle resulting from disorders of the lungs, pulmonary vessels, or chest wall.

coracoacromial (kor"ă-ko-ă-kro'mĭ-ăl) [G. *korax,* raven, + *akron,* point, + *ōmos,* shoulder]. Pert. to acromial and coracoid processes.

cor'acoid [G. *korax,* raven, + *eidos,* appearance]. Resembling, in shape, a crow's beak.

c. process. Process on upper anterior surface of scapula.

coramine (cō'ra-mēn). Proprietary name for nikethamide, a respiratory stimulant.

cord [G. *chordē*]. 1. A stringlike structure. 2. The umbilical cord.

c. bladder. Distention of the bladder without discomfort. Tending to void frequently and dribbling after urination.

ETIOL: Lesion affecting the posterior roots of the spinal column at the level of bladder innervation.

c., spermatic. Cord by which the testis is connected to the abdominal inguinal ring. It consists of the ductus deferens, blood vessels, lymphatics, and nerves supplying the testis and epididymis. These are enclosed in the cremasteric fascia which forms an investing sheath. SYN: *funiculus spermaticus* [NA].

c., spinal. That portion of the central nervous system contained in the spinal canal. The center of the cord consists of gray matter, which is composed of nerve cells, dendrites, and their processes. The white matter is arranged in tracts outside the gray matter. It consists of medullated nerve fibers which are (a) going to and from the brain, (b) connecting various layers of gray matter in the cord, (c) leaving and entering the spinal column. The cord serves as a conducting pathway for sensory impulses to the brain and motor impulses from the brain. It also serves as a reflex center for many reflex acts. SYN: *medulla spinalis* [NA].

c., umbilical. One which connects the umbilicus of the fetus to the placenta.

cor'date. Shaped like a heart.

cor'diform [L. *cor,* heart, + *forma,* shape]. Shaped like a heart.

cordi'tis [" + G. *-ītis,* inflammation]. Inflammation of a spermatic cord; funiculitis.

cor'dopexy [G. *chordē,* cord, + *pēxis,* fixation]. Operative fixation of an anatomical cord, esp. the vocal cords.

cordot'omy [" + *tomē,* incision]. Spinal cord section of lateral pathways to relieve pain. SYN: *chordotomy.*

core (kor). The center of a structure.

c. temperature. The body's temperature in deep structures such as the liver or heart.

coreclisis (kor-e-kli'sis) [G. *korē,* pupil, + *kleisis,* closure]. Occlusion of the pupil.

corectasia, corectasis (kor-ek-ta'zĭ-ă, ek'ta-sis) [" + *ektasis,* dilatation]. Dilatation of the pupil of the eye; corediastasis.

corectome (ko-rek'tōm) [" + *ektomē,* excision]. Instrument used for cutting or removing the iris. SYN: *iridectome.*

corectomedialysis (kor-ek"to-me-dĭ-al'ĭ-sis). Coredialysis, *q.v.*

corectomy (ko-rek'to-mĭ) [" + *ektomē,* excision]. Surgical removal of the iris. SYN: *iridectomy.*

corectopia (kor-ek-to'pĭ-ă) [" + *ek,* out of, + *topos,* place]. Having the pupil to one side of center of iris.

coredialysis (ko-re-di-al'ĭ-sis) [G. *korē,* pupil, + *dialysis,* separation]. Separation of iris' outer border from its ciliary attachment. SYN: *corectomedialysis.*

corediastasis (kor-e-dĭ-as'ta-sis) [" + *diastasis,* a standing apart]. Dilatation of pupil. SYN: *corectasia.*

corelysis (kor-el'ĭ-sis) [" + *lysis,* destruction]. Obliteration of pupil because of adhesions of iris to cornea.

coremorphosis (kor-e-mor-fo'sis) [" + *morphē,* form, + *-ōsis,* infection]. Establishment of an artificial pupil.

corenclesis (kor-en-kli'sis). Iridencleisis, *q.v.*

coreometer (ko-re-om'ĕ-ter) [" + *metron*, measure]. Instrument for measurement of the pupil.

coreom'etry [" + *metron*, measure] Measurement of the pupil of the eye.

coreoplasty (ko're-o-plas-tĭ) [" + *plassein*, to form]. Any operation for forming an artificial pupil.

corestenoma (kor-e-sten-o'mă) [" + *stenōma*, contraction]. Narrowing of pupil.

c. congen'itum. Partial congenital obliteration of pupil by excrescences.

coretomedialysis (kor-et-o-mē-dĭ-al'ĭ-sis). [" + *temnein*, to cut, + *dialysis*, division]. Making of an artificial pupil through the iris. SYN: *iridodialysis.*

coretomy (ko-ret'o-mĭ) [" + *tomē*, incision]. Any cutting of the iris. SYN: *iridotomy, q.v.*

Cori cycle [Carl F. Cori, American pharmacologist and biochemist, 1896-; and Gerty T. Cori, American biochemist, 1896-1957]. In carbohydrate metabolism, the breakdown of muscle glycogen, with formation of lactic acid which enters the blood stream, is converted to liver glycogen which in turn breaks down into glucose which is carried to muscles where it is reconverted to muscle glycogen.

corium (ko'rĭ-um) [G. *chorion*, skin]. [NA, BNA]. The layer of the skin lying immediately under the epidermis, the dermis, or true skin. Consists of two layers, papillary and reticular. It is composed of loose connective tissue in which are numerous capillaries, lymphatics, and nerve endings. In it lie hair follicles, sebaceous glands, sweat glands and their ducts and smooth muscle fibers. SYN: *cutis vera; dermis.*

corm [G. *kormos*, a stem]. A short bulb-shaped, underground stem of a plant. Ex: *Colchicum.*

corn [A.S.]. Indian corn or maize. Fresh (cooked): 1 ear (5" x 1¾", 140 gm.). Calories: 65. Other main values: 2 gm. protein; 1 gm. fat; 16 gm. carbohydrates; 4 mg. calcium; 300 I. U. vitamin A (yellow corn).

corn [L. *cornu*, horn]. Horny induration and thickening of the skin, hard or soft, according to location. SYN: *clavus.*

ETIOL: Pressure or friction or both from ill-fitting shoes.

SYM: Hard corns on exposed surfaces have a horny core of conical shape extending down into the derma, causing pain and irritation. Soft corns occur bet. the toes, kept soft by moisture and maceration, and may lead to inflammation beneath the corn. Infection with pyogenic organisms results in suppuration.

TREATMENT: Remove cause. Properly fitting shoes of soft leather and proper shape. New materials for absorbing energy and thus preventing friction are available for lining shoes or bandaging the area of the foot being abraded. Local application of a keratolytic agent for removal of corn. Corn pads to relieve pressure. Services of a chiropodist may be necessary. Special care to patients with diabetes or a circulatory condition. Soft corns dissected similarly with cotton pad protection to prevent maceration.

cor'nea [L. *corneus*, horny]. The clear, transparent anterior portion of the fibrous coat of the eye comprising about one-sixth of its surface. Its curvature being greater than that of the remainder of the bulb enables it to function as an important refractive medium. It is continuous at its periphery with the sclera.

Composed of 5 layers: (1) Layer of epithelium; (2) Bowman's membrane (ant. limiting membrane); (3) substantia propria; (4) Descemets' membrane; (5) layer of endothelium.

cornea, words pert. to: abrasio corneae, albugo, anterior chamber, applanatio c., arcus senilis, argema, "cera-" words, chemosis, circumcorneal, "kerat-" words, leukoma, macula corneae, megalocornea, microcornea, nebula, obfuscation, pannus, peritomy, phlyctenula, rhytidosis, rutidosus, staphyloma, synechia.

cor'neal. Pert. to the cornea.

c. reflex. Closure of eyelids resulting from direct corneal irritation.

corneitis (kor-ne-i'tis) [L. *corneus*, horny, + G. *-ītis*, inflammation]. Inflammation of the cornea. SYN: *keratitis.*

corneoiri'tis [" + G. *iris*, iris, + *-ītis*, inflammation]. Inflammation of iris and cornea.

corneomandibular reflex (kor-ne-o-man-dĭb'u-lar). Deflexion of mandible toward opposite side when cornea is irritated while mouth is open and relaxed.

corneosclera (kor-ne-o-skle'ră) [" + *sklēros*, hard]. The cornea and sclera considered together comprising the *tunica fibrosa* or fibrous coat of the eye.

corneous (kor'ne-us) [L. *corneus*]. Horny; hornlike.

c. layer. Horny outer layer of the epidermis. SYN: *stratum corneum.*

cornic'ulum [L. *cornu*, horn]. A small, hornlike process.

cornifica'tion (L. *cornu*, horn, + *facere*, to make). The process by which squamous epithelial cells are converted into hard, horny material as in the corneum of the skin or in structures such as horns, hair, and feathers which are derived from epithelium.

cor'nu (pl. *cornua*) [L. horn]. Any excrescence like a horn.

c. ammo'nis. Hippocampus major of brain.

c. anterius [NA]. The anterior horn of the lateral ventricle.

c. coccy'geum [NA]. Two upward projecting processes which articulate with the sacrum.

c. cuta'neum, c. huma'num. Hornlike excrescence on skin.

c. inferius [NA]. The inferior horn of the lateral ventricle.

c. of the hyoid. The greater and lesser horns of the hyoid bones, *q.v.*

c. of the sacrum. Two small processes projecting inferiorly on either side of the sacral hiatus leading into the sacral canal.

c. posterius [NA]. The posterior horn of the lateral ventricle.

cor'nua. Plural of cornu.

cor'nual. Pert. to a cornu.

coro'na [G. *korōnē*, crown]. Any structure resembling a crown.

c. capitis. Crown of head.

c. ciliaris [NA]. Circular figure on inner surface of ciliary body.

c., dentis [NA]. Crown of a tooth.

c. glandis [NA]. Post, border of glans penis.

c. radiata. 1. Ascending and descending fibers of the internal capsule which, above the corpus callosum, extend in all directions to the cerebral cortex. Many of the fibers arise in the thalamus. 2. A thin mass of follicle cells which adhere firmly to the zona pellucida of the human ovum following ovulation.

c. veneris. Syphilitic blotches on forehead parallel to hairline.

co'ronal. Pert. to a corona.

c. suture. One which joins the parietal and frontal bones of the cranium.

coronary (kor'o-na-rĭ) [L. *coronarius,* pert. to a crown or circle]. A term applied to blood vessels of the heart which supply blood to its walls. Coronary pain is usually dull and heavy, as a vise.

c. arteries. 1. One of a pair of arteries which supply blood to the myocardium of the heart. They arise within the right and left aortic sinuses at base of the aorta. Decreased flow of blood through these arteries induces attacks of angina pectoris. 2. The cervical branch of the uterine artery.

c. plexus. A network of autonomic nerve fibers which lies close to base of heart.

c. sinus. The vessel cavity or passage which receives the cardiac veins from the heart. It opens into rt. atrium.

c. thrombosis. Occlusion of one or more of the coronary arteries of the heart.

coronary care unit. A specially equipped area of a hospital for providing intensive nursing and medical care for patients who have acute coronary thrombosis.

cor'oner [L. *corōnātor,* crown officer]. An official who investigates and holds inquests over those dead from unknown or violent causes. He may or may not be a physician, depending upon the law in each state.

cor'onoid [G. *korōnē,* crow or crown, + *eidos,* appearance]. Shaped like a crow's beak or crown.

c. fossa. An oval depression on ant. surface of distal end of humerus. Receives coronoid process of ulna.

c. process. 1. A process on proximal end of ulna. Forms ant. portion of semilunar notch. 2. A process on the ramus of the mandible which serves for attachment of the temporalis muscle.

coroparelcysis (kor"o-par-el'si-sis) [G. *korē,* pupil, + *parelkein,* to draw aside]. Surgically bringing the pupil to one side in central corneal opacity so that it lies under a transparent area.

coroscopy (ko-ros'ko-pĭ) [" + *skopein,* to examine]. Shadow test to determine refractive error of an eye. SYN: *skiascopy.*

corot'omy [" + *tomē,* incision]. Surgical incision of the iris. Iridotomy, *q.v.*

cor'pora. Plural of corpus, *q.v.*

c. aranacea. Brain sand; psammoma bodies found in the pineal body.

c. Arantii. Tubercle found in center of semilunar valves of heart.

c. cavernosa penis. Two columns of erectile tissue on dorsum of the penis.

c. olivaria. Two oval masses behind pyramids of the oblongata.

c. quadrigemina. The superior portion of the midbrain consisting of two pairs of rounded bodies, the superior and inferior colliculi.

corpulence (kor'pū-lĕns) [L. *corpulentia*]. Fatness of the body. SYN: *obesity.*

corpulent (kor'pū-lĕnt) [L. *corpulentus*]. Fat; obese.

cor'pus (pl. *corpora*) [L. body]. The principal part of any organ; any mass or body.

c. albicans. A mass of fibrous tissue which replaces the regressing corpus luteum following rupture of the graafian follicle. It forms a white scar which gradually decreases in size and eventually disappears.

c. amylaceum. Mass having an irregular, laminated structure like a starch grain, found in the prostate, meninges, lungs and other organs in various pathological conditions.

c. annulare. Pons varolii.

c. callosum. The great commissure of the brain bet. the cerebral hemispheres.

c. cavernosum. Any erectile tissue, esp. the erectile bodies of the penis, clitoris, male or female urethra, bulb of the vestibule, or the nasal conchae.

c. cerebellum. The two lateral portions of the cerebellum exclusive of the central flocculonodular node.

c. ciliare. Ciliary body.

c. dentale, c. dentatum. Gray layer in white substance of the cerebellum.

c. fimbriatum. White layer edging the lower cornu of the lateral ventricle.

c. fornicis. The body of the fornix.

c. flavum. A waxy body seen in the central nervous system.

c. geniculatum. The medial or lateral geniculate body, *q.v.*; a mass of gray matter lying in the thalamus.

c. hemorrhagicum. Blood clot formed in the cavity left by rupture of the graafian follicle.

c. highmorianum. Mediastinum testis.

c. interpedunculare. Gray matter bet. peduncles before the pons Varolii.

c. luteum. A small yellow body which develops within a ruptured ovarian follicle. It is an endocrine structure secreting progesterone.

c. mammillare. A mammillary body; a rounded body in the anterior part of the interpeduncular fossa.

c. pampiniforme. Parovarium, or the remnant of the wolffian body of the female.

c. pineale. The pineal body or pineal gland.

c. pyramidale. 1. Pyramid of the oblongata. 2. A lobe of the epididymus.

c. restiforme. The restiform body or inferior cerebellar peduncle. A band of fibers, principally ascending, in the medulla oblongata which connects the spinal cord below with the cerebellum.

c. rhomboidale. SEE: *c. dentatum.*

c. spongiosum. Erectile tissue surrounding the urethra.

c. striatum. A structure in the cerebral hemispheres consisting of two basal ganglia (the caudate and lentiform nuclei), and the fibers of the internal capsule which separate them.

c. subthalamicum. The subthalamic nucleus (corpus Luysii), lying in the ventral thalamus.

c., trapezoideum. The trapezoid body, *q.v.*

c. vitreum. Vitreous portion of eye.

c. wolffianum. Wolffian body.

cor'puscle [L. *corpusculum,* little body]. 1. Any small rounded body. 2. An encapsulated sensory nerve ending. 3. Old term for a blood cell. SEE: *erythrocyte; leukocyte.*

c., amniotic; c., amylaceous. Corpus amylaceum, *q.v.*

c., axile; c., axis. The center of a tactile c.

c., blood. An erythrocyte or leukocyte.

c., bone. A bone cell.

c., Burckhardt's. Yellowish particles found in secretion of trachoma.

c., *cancroid.* Characteristic nodule in cutaneous epithelioma.

c., *cartilage.* A cell characteristic of cartilage.

c., *chromophil.* Tiny body found in cytoplasm of a nerve cell. SYN: *Nissl's body.*

c.'s, *chyle.* C. seen in chyle.

c., *colloid.* Corpus amylaceum, *q.v.*

c., *colostrum.* A cell containing phagocytosed fat globules present in milk secreted the first few days after parturition. Also called *colostrum body.*

c., *compound granular.* Gitter cells. Microglia cells when functioning as phagocytes.

c.'s, *corneal.* Connective tissue c's. found in fibrous tissue of cornea.

c's, *Drysdale's.* Elements found in the fluid of certain ovarian cysts.

c., *genital.* Encapsulated sensory nerve endings resembling pacinian corpuscles present in skin of external genitalia and nipple.

c., *ghost.* A decolorized red blood cell. SYN: achromatocyte; phantom c.; Ponfick's shadow.

c.'s, *Gierke's.* Particles seen in the thymus gland. SYN: *Hassall's c.'s.*

c.'s, *Gluge's.* Particles seen in diseased nervous tissue.

c., *Golgi-Mazzoni.* Terminal corpuscle of Krause.

c.'s, *Hassall's.* C's. found in the thymus gland. SYN: *Gierke's c.'s.*

c.'s, *Krause's.* Sensory encapsulated nerve endings in mucosa of genitalia, mouth, nose and eyes.

c., *lymph.* A lymphocyte, *q.v.*

c., *malpighian.* 1. A renal corpuscle consisting of a glomerulus and Bowman's capsule which encloses it. 2. A malpighian body of the spleen.

c's., *Mazzoni's.* Nerve endings resembling Krause's c.'s.

c., *Meissner's.* A tactile corpuscle; an encapsulated touch receptor found in connective tissue immediately underlying the epidermis of the skin, esp. on palmar and volar surfaces of hands and feet.

c., *milk.* Fat-filled globules present in milk. They represent the distal ends of mammary gland cells which are broken off in apocrine secretion.

c., *pacinian.* A large, ovoid, sensory end organ consisting of concentric layers or lamella of connective tissue surrounding a nerve ending. They are present in tendons, intermuscular septa, connective tissue membranes, and sometimes internal organs, and function as proprioceptive receptors and as receptors of deep pressure.

c., *phantom.* Ghost c.

c., *red.* An erythrocyte, *q.v.*

c., *renal.* A glomerulus and the capsule (Bowman's capsule) which surrounds it. It is located at proximal end of a renal tubule. SYN: *malpighian c.*

c., *reticulated.* Erythrocytes which when properly stained show filamentous reticulations.

c., *splenic.* A nodule of lymphatic tissue present in the spleen.

c., *tactile.* A sensory end-organ which responds to touch, as Meissner's c., *q.v.*

c., *terminal.* A nerve ending. SEE: *nerve.*

c., *thymic.* Hassall's c.

c., *touch.* Tactile c.

c., *Wagner's.* Tactile c.

c., *white.* A leukocyte, *q.v.*

corpus'cular. Pert. to corpuscles.

corpus'culum [L. little body]. Corpuscle.

c. *renis.* A renal corpuscle, *q.v.*

correc'tive [L. *corrigere,* to correct]. 1. A drug that modifies action of another. 2. Pert. to such a drug.

correla'tion. The processes by which the various activities of the body, especially nervous impulses, occur in proper relation to each other.

correspondence. The act or state of corresponding, i.e. occurring in proper relationship to other phenomena.

c., *retinal.* Condition occurring in normal vision in which images formed on the maculae or other points of the retinas of the two eyes are mentally blended and seen as a single image.

corresponding. Agreeing with, matching, or fitting.

c. *points* (of retina). Identical points; points on the retinas of the two eyes which when stimulated give rise to a single image.

Corrigan's pulse. [Sir Dominic J. Corrigan, Dublin physician, 1802-1880]. A full bounding pulse, which appears to be completely empty bet. beats; is associated with aortic insufficiency. SYN: waterhammer pulse.

corro'sion [L. *con,* with, + *rodere,* to gnaw]. Disintegration, esp. carious disintegration of a tooth.

corro'sive. Disintegrating, as eating away.

c. *alkalies.* These are corrosive hydroxides most commonly of sodium, ammonium, and potassium, as well as carbonates.

Because of their great combining power with water, and their action on the fatty tissues they cause rapid deep destruction. They have a tendency to gelatinize tissue with a somewhat grayish color forming a soapy, slippery surface, accompanied by pain and burning.

c. *poisons.* These include (a) strong acids, alkalies, strong antiseptics, including bichloride of mercury, carbolic acid (phenol), lysol, cresol compounds, tincture of iodine, and arsenic compounds. They are destructive and have a disintegrating effect upon tissues similar to burns, and may result in death. If swallowed, any part of alimentary canal may be affected. Tissues involved are altered, easily perforated, or destroyed. Death comes very shortly from shock, or swelling of throat and pharynx, which causes choking; or by closure of esophagus, causing slow starvation.

SYM: Intense burning about mouth, throat, pharynx, and abdomen; abdominal cramping, retching, nausea, vomiting, and often collapse. There may be bloody vomitus (hematemesis) and diarrhea, the stools being watery, mucoid, bloody, and possibly stained with the poison or its products, resulting from its action on the contents of the alimentary tract. Stains about the lips, cheeks, tongue, mouth, or pharynx are often characteristic brown; violaceous or black stain on mucous membranes, which appear dry or parched. Carbolic acid or phenol leaves a white or gray stain resembling boiled meat; hydrochloric acid stains are grayish; nitric acid leaves a yellow stain; sulfuric acid leaves tan or dark burns.

TREATMENT: First, dilute the poison before giving any emetic and apply weak acids for prolonged periods.

Such dilution always delays absorption somewhat and makes it easier to induce vomiting. Second, remove the poison; this is best done by making the patient vomit. Emesis is more easily produced in a distended stomach. Titillate the uvula or pharynx with the finger, and again give the patient more fluid, repeating the process until the fluid returns clear. Among the most useful diluents and emetics for this purpose are (a) tepid water, (b) soapy water, (c) salty water, (d) baking soda (sodium bicarbonate) water (*do not use washing soda*), (e) milk. A useful and widely available first aid emetic of this type is warm, soapy, greasy dish water. Any of these emetics should be used in generous amounts in all ordinary cases. (About 4 to 7 glassfuls may be used).

Where the corrosives, such as lye or mineral acids, have been in the stomach for some time, there may be danger of perforating the stomach. In such cases there is excruciating abdominal pain, muscular rigidity, and often collapse. Following the washing of the stomach, the appropriate antidote may be administered if it is available.

In addition to the therapy directed toward removing the corrosive substance from the gastrointestinal tract, analgesic drugs and intravenous fluids may be required.

cor'rugator. A muscle which lies above the orbit arising medially from frontal bone and having its insertion on skin of medial half of the eyebrows. It draws the brow medially and inferiorly.

cor'tex [L. rind]. (*Pl. cortices.*) 1. The outer layer of an organ as distinguished from the inner medulla as in the adrenal gland, kidney, ovary, lymph node, thymus, and cerebrum and cerebellum of the brain. 2. The outer layer of a structure as a hair, or the lens of the eye. 3. The outer superficial portion of the stem or root of a plant.

c., *cerebellar.* The surface layer of the cerebellum consisting of three layers: outer or molecular, middle, and inner or granular layer. Puukinje cells are present in the middle layer.

c., *cerebral.* The thin, convoluted surface layer of gray matter of the cerebral hemispheres, consisting principally of cell bodies of neurons arranged in five layers. There are also numerous fibers.

c., *fetal.* SYN: *X-zone.* A thick boundary zone which lies between the definitive cortex and medulla of the adrenal gland in early development. It is capable of secreting adrenal steroids. It undergoes involution in early post-natal life.

c., *interpretive.* The temporal c. where memories of the past may be evoked by electric stimulation.

c., *renal.* SEE: kidney.

c., *temporal.* Outer layer of brain behind the temples.

Corti, canal of [Alfonso Corti, Italian anatomist, 1822-1888]. Tunnel of Corti, *q.v.*

C., *organ of.* An elongated spiral structure running the entire length of cochlea in the floor of the cochlear duct and resting on the basilar membrane. It is the end organ of hearing containing *hair cells, supporting cells,* and neuroepithelial receptors stimulated by sound waves. SYN: *papilla basilaris.*

C., *tunnel of.* A triangular shaped canal extending the entire length of the organ of Corti. Its walls are formed by the external and internal pillar cells.

cortiadrenal (kor-tĭ-ad-re'nal) [" + *ad,* toward, + *rēn,* kidney]. Pert. to cortex of adrenal gland.

cor'tical. Pert. to the cortex.

cortices. Plural of cortex.

corticifugal (kor-tĭ-sif'u-gal) [L. *cortex,* rind, + *fugere,* to flee]. Conducting away from the cortex, *e.g.,* axons of pyramidal cells of the cerebral cortex. SYN: *corticoefferent.*

corticipetal (kor-tĭ-sĭp'e-tal) [" + *petere,* to seek]. Conducting towards the cortex, e.g. fibers of the thalamic radiation conveying impulses to sensory areas of cerebral cortex. SYN: *corticoafferent.*

corticoadre'nal [" + *ad,* toward, + *rēn,* kidney]. Pert. to cortex of adrenal gland.

corticoaf'ferent [" + *afferre,* to bear to]. Corticipetal, *q.v.*

corticobul'bar. Pertaining to the cerebral cortex and upper portion of the brain stem, as corticobulbar tract.

corticoef'ferent [" + *efferre,* to bring out of]. Corticifugal, *q.v.*

cor'ticoid. Any of a number of steroid substances obtained from the cortex of the adrenal gland. SYN: corticosteroid.

corticopedun'cular [" + *pedunculus,* little foot]. Pert. to cortex and cerebral peduncles.

corticopleuritis (kor-tĭ-ko-plū-ri'tis) [" + G. *pleura,* rib, + *-itis,* inflammation]. Inflammation of the outer parts of the pleura.

corticospi'nal [" + *spīna,* thorn]. Pert. to cerebral cortex and spinal cord.

corticosteroid (kor"ti-ko-stēr'oid). Same as corticoid.

corticosterone (kor"tĭ-kos'tĕ-rōn). A hormone of the adrenal cortex. Corticosterone influences carbohydrate metabolism and metabolism of potassium and sodium. It is essential for normal absorption of glucose, the formation of glycogen in the liver and tissues, and the normal utilization of carbohydrates by the tissues.

corticotrophic (kor"tĭ-ko-tro'fik). Pertaining to corticotrophin.

corticotrophin (kor"tĭ-ko-tro'fin). Pertaining to the adrenocorticotrophic factor or principle in the ant. lobe of the pituitary gland. Stimulates adrenal cortex in secreting steroid hormones. SYN: *ACTH, q.v.*

c. *releasing factor.* A substance found in the hypothalamus which controls secretion of adrenocorticotrophin.

cor'tin [L. *cortex,* rind]. An extract of the cortex of the adrenal gland; contains the active steroid agents such as corticosterone, etc.

cortisone (kor'tĭ-sōn). A hormone isolated from the cortex of the adrenal gland and also prepared synthetically. It is closely related to hydrocortisone. It is important for its regulatory action in metabolism of fats, carbohydrates, sodium, potassium, and proteins. It is used principally in treatment of adrenal insufficiency. SYN: *compound E; ACTH.*

coruscation (ko-rus-kā'shun). The subjective sensation of flashes of light.

Corynebacterium (kō-rī"nē-bak-tē'rĭ-um) [G. *coryne,* a club, + *bacterium,* a small rod]. A genus of the family Corynebacteriaceae. The bacteria are rod-shaped, gram-positive, and non-motile. Though many of the species are pathogens in domestic animals, birds, reptiles and plants, the most important is the species, C. diphtheriae, pathogenic in man.

C. diphtheriae. The cause of diphtheria in man. SYN: *diphtheria bacillus; Klebs-Loeffler bacillus.*

coryza (ko-ri'ză). [G. *koryza*]. Cold in the head; an acute catarrhal inflammation of the nasal mucous membrane.

c. spasmod'ica. Hay fever.

cosen'sitize [L. *con,* with, + *sensitīvus,* sensitive]. To sensitize to more than one infection.

cosmesis (kŏs-mē'sĭs). A regard for the appearance of a patient with special reference to surgical operations.

cosmetic (koz-met'ik) [G. *kosmētikos,* pert. to adornment]. 1. Powder or cream for improving complexion. 2. To preserve or promote beauty.

c. surgery. Surgical procedures, usually plastic surgery, directed towards preserving beauty or correcting ugly scars or burns.

cos'mic. Pertaining to the universe as a whole.

cos'ta (pl. *costae*) [L.]. Rib.

c. fluctuans. A floating rib.

c. spuria. A false rib.

c. vera. A true rib.

cos'tal. Pert. to a rib.

c. cartilage. A cartilage which connects the end of a true rib with the sternum or the end of a rib with the costal cartilage above.

c. pit. Cup-shaped depression at distal end of transverse process of a thoracic vertebra for articulation with tubercle of rib.

costal'gia [L. *costa,* rib, + G. *algos,* pain). Pain in a rib or in the intercostal spaces, *e.g.,* intercostal neuralgia.

cos'tive [L. contraction, from *constipāre,* to press together]. Constipated.

cos'tiveness [L. contraction, from *constipāre,* to press together]. Constipation.

costochon'dral [L. *costa,* rib, + G. *chondros,* cartilage]. Pert. to a rib and its cartilage.

costoclavic'ular [L. *costa,* rib, + *clavicula,* a little key]. Pert. to ribs and clavicle.

costocor'acoid [" + G. *korax,* crow, + *eidos,* form]. Pert. to ribs and coracoid process of scapula.

costopneumopexy (kos"to-nu'mo-pek-sĭ) [" + G. *pneumōn,* lung, + *pēxis,* fixation]. Anchoring a lung to a rib.

costoster'nal [" + G. *sternon,* chest]. Pert. to a rib and the sternum.

costotome (kos'to-tōm) [" + G. *tomē,* incision]. Knife or shears for cutting through a rib or cartilage.

costotomy (kos-tot'o-mĭ) [" + *tomē,* incision]. Excision of a rib or part of one. SYN: *costectomy.*

costo"transverse' [" + *transvertere,* to turn aside]. Pert. to the ribs and transverse processes of articulating vertebrae.

costover'tebral [" + *vertebra,* joint]. Pert. to a rib and a vertebra.

cot'ton [M.E. *coton,* from Ar. *qutun,* cotton]. A soft, white, fibrous material obtained from the fibers enclosing the seeds of various plants of the Malvaceae, esp. those of the genus *Gossypium.*

c., absorbent. Cotton fibers from which the oil has been completely removed enhancing ability to absorb liquids.

c., styptic. Cotton impregnated with an astringent.

c. wool sandwiches. These are used when a sharp pointed foreign body, such as a pin, has been swallowed, and when it has been determined by examination that the foreign body is not lodged in the esophagus, lung, etc.

Wisps of finely separated cotton wool are placed bet. bread. Bread and butter may be used, but cotton wool is rather apt to collect into a pasty mass in the mouth with butter; therefore it is better to use only bread or bread and jam, or any jam containing pips which, mingling with the cotton wool, prevent its rolling up into a ball.

To *prepare,* cut thin pieces of bread, spread fine wisps of cotton wool onto it, and smear a little jam over it to make it stick to the bread. Care should be taken to arrange the cotton wool so that pieces will not be pulled out when the sandwich is bitten.

Several small sandwiches should be given at each meal until the pin has been passed in the feces.

cotyledon (kot-ĭ-le'don) [G. *kotylēdōn,* hollow of a cup]. 1. Mass of villi on chorionic surface of the placenta. 2. Any of rounded portions into which the placenta's uterine surface is divided. 3. Seed leaf of a plant embryo.

cotyloid (kot'ĭ-loid) [G. *kotyloeidēs,* cup shaped]. Shaped like a cup.

c. cavity. The acetabulum or socket receiving the head of the femur.

couching (kow'ching) [Fr. *coucher,* to lay down]. Displacement of the lens downward in cataract.

cough [M.E. *coughen*]. A forceful and sometimes violent expiratory effort preceded by a preliminary inspiration. The glottis is partially closed, the accessory muscles of expiration are brought into action, and the air is noisily expelled.

c., aneurysmal. Brassy and clanging, heard in patients suffering from aneurysm.

c., asthmatic. More like an attack of dyspnea than a cough.

c., brassy. Heard in patients in whom there is pressure on the left recurrent laryngeal nerve, as in aortic aneurysm.

c., bronchial. Heard in patients with bronchiectasis.* May be provoked by change of posture, as in getting up in morning. SPUTUM: Fetid odor and copious. Dirty gray. That heard in bronchitis,* in earlier stages, is hacking and irritating; in later stages, looser and easier. SPUTUM: Thin, frothy mucus.

c., diphtherial. Heard in laryngeal diphtheria; noisy and brassy, with stridulous breathing.

c., dry. One unaccompanied by moisture.

c., ear. A reflex cough induced by irritation in the ear which stimulates Arnold's nerve (*ramus auricularis nervi vagi*).

c., effective. When sputum or an exudate is expectorated. SYN: *productive c.*

c., hacking. A series of repeated efforts, as occurs in the early stages of pulmonary tuberculosis.

c., harsh. A metallic cough occurring in laryngitis.

c., moist. A loose cough accompanied by moisture.

c., paroxysmal. That occurring in whooping cough and bronchiectasis. Also described as spasmodic.

c., productive. That in which mucus or an exudate is expectorated.

c., pulmonary. Hard and painful in pneumonia. SPUTUM: 1. *Scanty,* very tenacious, rusty colored from being tinged with blood. In early stages of tuberculosis, hacking and irritating; in later stages, frequent and paroxysmal. 2. *Purulent,* greenish-yellow; may be streaked with blood. In later stages, nummular or coinshaped.

c., reflex. Due to irritation from the middle ear, pharynx, stomach, or intestine. It may occur singly or coupled, or it may be hacking in character.

c., uterine. A reflex cough resulting from irritation of female organs, esp. the uterus.

c., whooping. 1. A paroxysmal cough ending in a whooping inspiration. Occurs in pertussis, *q.v.* 2. Synonym for *pertussis.*

coulomb (koo-lom'). Unit of electrical quantity. It is the quantity of electricity transferred by 1 ampere in 1 second.

count. The number obtained by determining the number of units of the object being counted per unit of volume, as bacteria count, red cell count, platelet count, reticulocyte count, differential count, parasite count, etc.

counter'act. To act against or in opposition to.

counterac'tion. That action or a drug or chemical agent having an action opposing that of another agent.

counterextension (kown-ter-eks-ten'shun) [L. *contra,* against, + *extendere,* to extend]. Back pull or resistance to extension on a limb.

counterir'ritant [" + *irritāre,* to excite]. An agent that is applied locally to produce inflammatory reaction with the object of affecting some other part, usually adjacent to or underlying the surface irritated. Ex: *mustard.*

There are three degrees of irritation produced by the following classes of agents: *rubefacients,* which redden the skin, the 1st degree; *vesicants,** which produce a blister or vesicle, the 2nd degree; and *escharotics,** which form an eschar or slough or death of tissue, the 3rd degree. SEE: *aquapuncture* (2); *seton.*

counterirrita'tion [" + *irritāre,* to excite]. Superficial irritation which relieves some other irritation of deeper structures.

countero'pening [" + A.S. *open*]. A second opening, as in an abscess, not draining satisfactorily from first incision.

coun'terpressure instrument. To provide counter-retraction to offset that exerted by exit of needle.

coun'terpuncture [L. *contra,* against, + *punctura,* puncture]. Counteropening. An additional opening made to help drainage, as an abscess.

coup de soleil (koo-da-sō-lay') [Fr.]. Sunstroke.

courses (kōr'siz) [L. *cursus,* a flowing]. Menses; catamenia.

Courvoisier's law (koor-vwă'ze-āz) [named from Dr. Ludwig Courvoisier, a French surgeon who died in 1918]. Disease processes which cause sudden blockage of the common bile duct such as a stone do not usually cause dilatation of the gallbladder. When the duct is obstructed slowly, as would be the case in infiltration of tissue around the duct (as in cancer), dilatation of the gallbladder is usually present.

couvade (koo-văd') [Fr. to brood upon]. A custom among some primitive peoples which entails the father going to bed when his child is born. He stays there until his wife has recovered.

cover cell (kŭv'ĕr). A cell which serves to protect another cell of specialized function. SEE: *cell.*

cov'erglass. Thin glass disk to cover a tissue or bacterial specimen to be examined microscopically.

cowperi'tis [Cowper + G. *-ītis,* inflammation]. Inflammation of Cowper's glands.

Cowper's glands. The bulbourethral glands. A pair of compound tubular glands about the size of a pea beneath the bulb of the male urethra, and emptying a mucous secretion into it.

Discovered by Wm. Cowper, an English anatomist (1666-1709). They are small round bodies, yellow in color. They correspond to the Bartholin* glands in the female.

cowpox (kow'pox). Vaccinia; pustular eruption on teats and bag of a cow in form of bluish vesicles, similar to smallpox. When given to humans, usually by vaccination, some degree of immunity against smallpox is obtained.

cox'a [L. haunch]. 1. The *os innominatum.* 2. The hip joint or hip bone.

c. valga. Opp. of *c. vara.* Deformity produced when angle of head of femur with the shaft is increased above 120°.

c. vara. A deformity produced by decrease in angle made by head of femur with the shaft. Normally it should be 120°; but in c. vara it may be 80-90°. It occurs in rickets or may be due to bone injury.

coxal'gia [" + G. *algos,* pain]. 1. Pain in the hip. SYN: *coxodynia.* 2. Hip joint disease. SYN: *coxitis.*

coxi'tis [" + G. *-ītis,* inflammation]. Hip joint disease. SYN: *coxalgia* (def. 2)

coxodyn'ia [" + G. *odynē,* pain]. Pain in the hip joint. SYN: *coxalgia* (def. 1).

coxofem'oral [" + *femur,* thigh]. Pert. to the hip and femur.

coxo"tuberculo'sis [" + *tuberculum,* a little swelling]. Tuberculous condition of the hip joint.

C.P. Abbr. for *candle power; cerebral palsy; chemically pure.*

Cr. Symb. for *chromium.*

crab louse. *Phthirius inguinalis* and *Phthirius pubis.* One that infests the pubic region and other hairy areas of the body. SEE: *pediculosis.*

crachotement (kră-shōt-mon) [Fr.]. Inability to spit, even when the patient has a strong desire to do so; usually accompanied by syncope following utero-ovarian operation.

cracked pot sound. Percussion sound resembling that heard when striking a cracked pot, indicative of a pulmonary cavity.

cra'dle [A.S. *cradel*]. Frame for keeping bedclothes from pressing on a wound or fractured part. SYN: *arculus.*

craigiasis (kră-gī'ă-sis). Infection with Craigia microorganism causing symptoms peculiar to dysentery.

cramp [M.E. *crampe*]. A spasmodic, esp. a tonic, contraction of one or many muscles, usually painful.

In certain occupations, the attempted use of muscle groups habitually employed may lead to a so-called "professional cramp," though other motor formulae are easily executed by the affected muscles. In writer's cramp, the attempt to write induces painful spasm of the hand muscles (similarly telegrapher's, watchmaker's, seamstress' cramp, etc.).

SYM: Excruciating pain, hard and contracted lumps of muscle.

TREATMENT: Depends upon cause and location. In muscular cramps try to extend muscle, compress it and apply heat and massage.

SEE: *bricklayer's cramp; heat cramp; systremma; writer's cramp.*

c., clonic. Wryneck caused by rheumatism. SYN: *rheumatic torticollis.**

c., heat. SEE: *heat cramps.*

cran'berries. A bright red, acid berry of the plant *Oxycoccus.*

COOKED: 1 cup (sauce, sweetened, 100 gm.). Calories: 146. Other main values: trace of protein; 0.2 gm. fat; 37.5 gm. carbohydrates; 6 mg. calcium.

cra'nial [G. *kranion,* skull]. Pert. to the cranium.

c. bones. Those that comprise the cranium or brain case.

c. nerves. Twelve pairs of nerves which have their origin in the brain. In addition to the 12 pairs of cranial nerves, there is a small combined efferent and afferent nerve which goes from the olfactory area of the brain to the nasal septum. This nerve, which is thought by some anatomists to be the first cranial nerve, is called *terminal nerve.*

The twelve cranial nerves are listed in the table.

LESIONS OF THE CRANIAL NERVES GIVE RISE TO THE FOLLOWING MANIFESTATIONS:

The lesions are described as if one of each pair of nerves were diseased.

First (Olfactory): Loss or disturbance of the sense of smell.

Second (Optic): Blindness, of various types depending upon the exact location of the lesion.

Third (Oculomotor): Ptosis (drooping) of the eyelid, deviation of the eyeball outward, dilatation of the pupil, double vision.

Fourth (Trochlear): Rotation of the eyeball upward and outward, double vision.

Fifth (Trigeminal): *Sensory root:* Pain or loss of sensation in face, forehead, temple and eye. *Motor root:* Deviation of the jaw toward paralyzed side, difficulty in chewing.

Sixth (Abducens): Deviation of the eye outward, double vision.

Seventh (Facial): Paralysis of all the muscles on one side of the face; inability to wrinkle the forehead, to close the eye, to whistle; deviation of the mouth toward the sound side.

Eighth (Vestibulocochlear): Deafness or ringing in the ears; dizziness; nausea and vomiting; reeling.

Ninth (Glossopharyngeal): Disturbance of taste; difficulty in swallowing.

Tenth (Vagus): Disease of the vagus nerve is usually limited to one or more of its divisions. Paralysis of the main trunk on one side causes difficulty in swallowing and talking, and hoarseness. The commonest disease of the vagus is of its left recurrent branch (see above) which causes hoarseness as its principal manifestation.

Eleventh (Spinal Accessory): Drooping of the shoulder; inability to rotate the head away from affected side.

Twelfth (Hypoglossal): Paralysis of one side of the tongue; deviation of tongue toward paralyzed side; "thick" speech.

craniectomy (kra-nĭ-ek'to-mĭ) [" + *ektomē,* excision]. Opening of skull and removal of a portion of the skull.

NP: Take blood pressure every 15 minutes for first 12 hours, every half hour for second 12 hours, and then as ordered until discontinued. Do not leave patient alone for first 24 hours. Watch for and report at once any changes in blood pressure, pulse, respiration, temperature, and any evidence of paralysis.

cranio (krā'nĭ-ō) [G. *kranion,* skull]. Prefix; pertaining to the skull or cranium.

cranioacromial (krā-nĭ-ō-ă-krō'mĭ-al) [" + *akron,* extremity]. Relating to the cranium and the acromion.

craniocele (kra'nĭ-o-sēl) [" + *kēlē,* hernia]. Protrusion of the brain from the skull. SEE: *encephalocele.*

craniocer'ebral [" + L. *cerebrum,* brain]. Rel. to skull and brain.

cranioclast (kra'nĭ-o-klast) [" + *klastos,* broken]. Instrument for crushing fetal skull in delivery.

cra'nioclasty [" + *klastos,* broken]. Crushing of fetal head in dystocia.

craniocleidodysostosis (kra"nĭ-o-kli"do-dis-os-to'sis) [" + *kleis,* clavicle, + *dys,* bad, + *osteon,* bone, + *-ōsis,* infection]. Defective ossification of bones of head, face and clavicles; a congenital condition.

cra'niograph [" + *graphein,* to write]. Device for making graphs of the skull.

craniol'ogy [" + *logos,* study of]. The study of the skull, its size, and shape, esp. in reference to different races.

craniomalacia (kra-nĭ-o-mă-la'sĭ-ă) [" + *malakia,* softening]. Softening of the skull bones.

craniometer (kra-nĭ-om'ĕ-ter) [" + *metron,* measure]. Instrument for making cranial measurements.

craniomet'ric points. Any prominences or marks on skull for defining the configuration of the cranium; for use in craniometry.

craniom'etry [G. *kranion,* skull, + *metron,* measure]. Study of the skull and measurement of its bones.

craniopagus (krā-nĭ-op'ă-gus) [" + *pagos,* a fixed or solid thing]. Twins joined at the skulls.

craniopharyngeal (kra"nĭ-o-far-in'je-al) [" + *pharygx,* the pharynx]. Pert. to cranium and pharynx.

craniopharyngioma (kra-nĭ-o-far-in-jĭ-o'-mă) [" + " + *-ōma,* tumor]. Tumor of portion of the *hypophysis cerebri.*

cranioplasty (kra'ne-o-plas-tĭ) [" + *plassein,* to form]. Plastic operation on skull.

cra'niopuncture [" + L. *punctura,* puncture]. Puncture of the skull.

craniorhachischisis (kra-nĭ-o-ră-kis'kĭ-sis) [" + *rachis,* spine, + *schizein,* to split]. Congenital fissure of skull and spine.

craniostosis (kra-nĭ-os-to'sis) [" + *osteon,* bone]. Congenital ossification of cranial sutures.

craniotabes (kra-nĭ-o-ta'bēz) [" + L. *tabes,* a wasting]. Atrophy in infancy of cranial bones.

ETIOL: Marasmus, rickets, or syphilis.

craniotome (kra'nĭ-o-tōm) [" + *tomē,* incision]. Device for forcible reduction of fetal skull in labor.

craniotomy (kra-nĭ-ot'o-mĭ) [" + *tomē,* incision]. 1. Breaking up fetal skull to facilitate delivery in difficult parturition. 2. Incision through the cranium

TABLE OF CRANIAL NERVES

NERVES	COMPOSITION	FUNCTION	ORIGIN OF DISTAL FIBERS
I Olfactory	Afferent	Smell	Olfactory nerves
II Optic	Afferent	Vision	Rods and cones of retina
III Oculomotor	Efferent	Movement of eyes	Four of the six extraocular eye muscles
	Efferent	Contracts pupil and controls accommodation	Ciliaris and sphincter pupillae muscles
	Afferent	Sensory endings in eye muscles	Proprioceptive endings in ocular muscles
IV Trochlear	Efferent	Movement of eyes	Superior oblique muscle of eye
	Afferent	Sensory endings in eye muscles	Proprioceptive endings in eye muscles
V Trigeminal	Afferent	Receives sensory impulses	Sensory nerve endings in area of eye, skin, and mucous membranes of face and head
	Afferent	Sensory endings in chewing muscles	Proprioceptive endings in chewing muscles
	Efferent	Chewing	Muscles of chewing
VI Abducent	Efferent	Eye movement	Rectus lateralis muscle of each eye
	Afferent	Sensory endings in eye muscles	Proprioceptive endings in rectus lateralis
VII Facial	Efferent	Muscles of expression of face. Muscles which assist in swallowing. Muscle which moves one of the bones of the middle ear.	Facial muscles and stapedius; stylohyoid and digastricus muscle
	Efferent	Salivary gland secretion	Salivary glands
	Afferent	Taste	Tongue
	Afferent	Deep sensory endings	Soft palate, inner ear
	Afferent	Sensory endings in skin	External ear and mastoid area
VIII Acoustic	Afferent	Hearing	Organ of Corti in inner ear
	Afferent	Sense of balance	Semicircular canals of inner ear
IX Glossopharyngeal	Afferent	Taste	Taste buds of posterior tongue
	Afferent	Sensory impulses from tongue, ear, and carotid sinus	Tympanic nerve to middle ear; tongue and pharynx; carotid sinus nerve
	Efferent	Glandular secretions	Parotid gland
	Efferent	Swallowing	Stylopharyngeus muscle
X Vagus	Efferent	Control of involuntary muscle and glands	Heart, pulmonary area, esophagus, digestive tract down as far as the transverse colon
	Efferent	Swallowing and speech muscles	Muscles of pharynx and larynx
	Afferent	Sensory impulses from viscera	Thoracic and abdominal viscera and carotid and aortic bodies
	Afferent	Taste	Epiglottis and tongue
	Afferent	Sensory impulse from skin	Skin of ear
XI Accessory	Efferent	Swallowing and speech muscles	Muscles of pharynx and larynx
	Efferent	Movement of head and shoulder	Muscles of neck and shoulder
XII Hypoglossal	Efferent	Movement of tongue	Tongue

craniotonos'copy [" + *tonos*, tone, + *skopein*, to examine]. Auscultatory percussion of cranium.

craniotympan'ic [" + *tympanon*, kettledrum]. Pert. to skull and middle ear.

cra'nium [L. from G. *kranion*]. That portion of the skull which encloses the brain; consists of single frontal, occipital, sphenoid, and ethmoid bones and the paired temporal and parietal bones. SEE: *skeleton*.

c., metabolic. Hyperostosis frontalis interna, a condition occurring in women in which bone is deposited on inner surface of the frontal bone. Also called *calvarial hyperostosis* and *Stewart-Morel syndrome*.

crap'ulent, crap'ulous [L. *crapula*, excessive drinking]. Related to, or excessive, drinking and eating. Intoxicated.

crassamen'tum [L. *crassare*, to make thick]. Coagulum, blood clot.

crater'iform [G. *kratēr*, bowl, + L. *forma*, shape]. BACT: Saucer-shaped, craterlike, or goblet-shaped.

cravat' ban'dage [Fr. *cravate*, a Croatian]. Triangular b. folded to form a band around the injured part. SEE: *bandage*.

cream [L. *cremor*, thick juice]. The rich, yellowish part of milk.

LIGHT (table or coffee): 1 tablespoon (15 gm.). Calories: 30. Other main values: 3 gm. fat; 0.4 gm. protein; 15 mg. calcium; 120 I.U. vitamin A; 0.02 mg. riboflavin, 0.6 gm. carbohydrate.

creamalin (krēm'ă-lĭn). Proprietary name for an antacid preparation.

cream of tartar. Potassium bitartrate, $KHC_4H_4O_6$. An aperient and diuretic. SEE: *argol*.

crease (krēs) [L. *crista*, tuft]. A line produced by a fold.

c., gluteofemoral, c., ileofemoral. The crease that bounds the buttocks below.

creatinase (kre-at'in-ās) [G. *kreas*, flesh, + *ase*, enzyme]. An enzyme that decomposes creatinine.

creatine (kre'ă-tĭn) [G. *kreas*, flesh]. Methylglycocyamine, $NH:C(NH_2)N(CH_3).CH_2.COOH + H_2O$, a colorless, crystalline substance that can be isolated from various animal organs and body fluids.

It combines readily with phosphate to form phosphocreatine (creatine phosphate) which serves as a source of high energy phosphate released in the anaerobic phase of muscle contraction. Found esp. in muscle juice and in blood. Creatine may be present in a greater quantity in the urine of women than men. Creatine excretion is increased in pregnancy and decreased in hypothyroidism.

creatinemia (krē-ă-tĭn-ē'mē-ă) [" + *aima*, blood]. Excess of creatine in circulating blood.

creatinine (kre-at'in-in) [G. *kreas*, flesh]. Methylglycocyamidine, $C_4H_7ON_3$. It is the end product of creatine metabolism.

It can also be isolated as colorless crystals from animal material. It is one of the nonprotein constituents of blood, and increased quantities of it are found in advanced stages of renal disease. It is a normal and an alkaline constituent of urine and blood. About 0.02 gm. per kg. of body weight is excreted by the kidneys per day.

creatinuria (kre-ă-tin-u'rĭ-ă) [" + *ouron*, urine]. Creatinine in urine.

creatorrhea (kre-ă-to-re'ă) [" + *roia*, flow]. The presence of undigested muscle fibers in the feces, seen in some cases of pancreatic disease.

crèche (krăsh) [Fr.]. A day nursery for children.

Credé's method (krē-dā') [Karl S. F. Credé, German gynecologist and obstetrician, 1819-1892]. 1. The means whereby the placenta is expelled by downward pressure on the uterus through the abdominal wall with the thumb on the post. surface of the fundus uteri and the flat of the hand on the ant. surface, the pressure being applied in the direction of the birth canal. 2. For treatment of the eyes of the newborn, the use of 1% silver nitrate solution instilled into the eyes immediately after birth for the prevention of *ophthalmia neonatorum* (gonorrheal ophthalmia).

creek dots. Small shining dots sometimes present in the retina. Their nature or cause is unknown. Sometimes familial.

creeping eruption. Larva migrans, *q.v.*

cremaster (krē-mas'ter) [G. *kreman*, to suspend]. One of the fascialike muscles suspending and enveloping the testicles and spermatic cord.

cremaster'ic [G. *kremastos*, hanging]. Pert. to the cremaster muscle.

c. fascia. One of the coverings of the spermatic cord.

c. reflex. Retraction of testis when skin is stroked on front inner side of thigh.

cremate (kre'māt) [L. *cremātus*, burned to ashes]. Dispose by burning the body of a dead person. The ashes may or may not be buried.

crenate (kre'nāt) [L. *crena*, a notch]. Notched or scalloped, as crenated condition of blood corpuscles.

crenation (krē-nā'shun) [L. *crena*, a notch]. The conversion of normally round red corpuscles into shrunken, knobbed, starry forms, as when blood is mixed with salt solution of, say, 5% strength. SEE: *plasmolysis*.

creosote (kre'o-sōt) [G. *kreas*, flesh, + *sōzein*, to preserve]. A mixture of phenols obtained from wood tar. Used as a disinfectant and as a preserver of wood.

crepitant (krĕp'ĭ-tănt) [L. *crepitāre*, to crackle]. Crackling; having or making a crackling sound.

crepitation (krĕp-ĭ-tā'shŭn) [L. *crepitāre*, to crackle]. 1. A crackling sound heard in certain diseases, as the râle heard in pneumonia. 2. A grating sound heard on movement of ends of a broken bone.

crep'itus [L. *crepitāre*, to crackle]. 1. The noise of gas discharged from the intestines. 2. Crepitation.

c. redux. Râle indicating approaching recovery in pneumonia.

crepuscular (kre-pus'kū-lar) [L. *crepusculum*, twilight]. Pert. to twilight.

cres'cent [L. *crescere*, to grow]. Shaped like a sickle or the new moon.

c., articular. A crescent-shaped cartilage present in certain joints as the menisci of the knee joint.

c. of Gianuzzi (jăn-noot'tse). A crescent-shaped group of serous cells lying at the base of or along the side of a mucous alveolus of a salivary gland, also called demilune of Heidenhein.

c., myopic. Grayish patch in fundus of eye due to atrophy of choroid.

crescentic (kres-en'tik). Sickle-shaped.

cresol (kre'sol). USP. Yellowish brown liquid obtained from coal tar and containing not more than 5% of phenol.

USE: A disinfectant, in a 1 to 5% solution, for inanimate objects such as dishes.

cresomania (kres-o-ma'nĭ-ă) [*Croesus,* wealthy king of Lydia, 6th Century B. C., + G. *mania,* madness]. Hallucination of possessing great wealth.

crest [L. *crista,* tuft]. A ridge or an elongated prominence, esp. one on a bone.

cretin (krē'tin) [Fr.]. One afflicted with congenital myxedema; a mentally retarded dwarf. SEE: *cretinism.*

A cretin is characterized by lack of growth and mental development; rarely if ever exceeds the mental age of 10.

The skin is rough and dry, and the hair coarse, dry, and brittle. Teeth erupt slowly and are of poor quality and irregularly placed. The tongue is large and apt to protrude from a mouth which constantly drools saliva. A cretin child is potbellied, swaybacked, and prone to umbilical hernia. Adult cretin is myxedematous.

cretinism (kre'tin-izm) [" + G. *ismos,* condition]. Congenital affection, characterized by a lack of physical and mental development.

ETIOL: A congenital deficiency in secretion of the thyroid hormones.

SYM: An abnormal condition of the thyroid gland, myxedema and impaired mental ability.

TREATMENT: Dessicated thyroid orally.

c., endemic. C. resulting from iodine deficiency of mother during pregnancy or genetic factors.

c., sporadic. C. resulting from congenital absence of, or lack of normal development of, the thyroid gland.

cretinoid (cre'tĭ-noid) [" + G. *eidos,* resemblance]. Having the symptoms of cretinism, or resembling a cretin, due to a congenital condition.

cre'tinous. Pert. to a cretin or to cretinism.

crevice (krev'is) [Fr. *crever,* to break from L. *crepāre,* to break]. A small fissure, or crack.

c., gin'gival. The fissure produced by the marginal gingiva with the tooth surface.

crevicular (krev-ik'u-lar). Pert. to the gingival crevice.

CRF. Abbr. for *corticotrophin-releasing factor,* esp., the substance present in extract of the hypothalamus which brings about the release of ACTH from the anterior pituitary.

crib. Bassinette for newborn to lie in.

c. death. Sudden unexplained death of an infant. Cause is unknown but viral origin is suspected. Most cases occur between one month and four months of age in fall of year, during normal sleep.

cribbing. Aerophagia; swallowing air.

crib'rate [L. *cribrum,* a sieve]. Profusely pitted or perforated like a sieve.

cribra'tion [L. *cribrum,* a sieve]. The state of being perforated.

crib'riform [" + *forma,* form]. Sievelike.

c. fascia. The portion of deep fascia which covers the fossa ovalis of the thigh.

c. plate. The thin, perforated, medial portion of the horizontal plate of the ethmoid bone.

cricoarytenoid (krĭ-ko-ă-rit'en-oid) [G. *krikos,* ring, + *arytaina,* pitcher, + *eidos,* form]. Extending bet. the cricoid and arytenoid cartilages.

cricoderma (kri-ko-der'mă) [" + *derma,* skin]. Ringshaped infiltrations in center of indurations on the skin.

cricoid (krī'koid) [G. *krikos,* ring, + *eidos,* form]. Shaped like a signet ring.

c. cartilage. The lowermost cartilage of the larynx. It is shaped like a signet ring, the broad portion or lamina being posterior, the anterior portion forming the arch.

cricoidectomy (kri-koid-ek'to-mĭ) [" + " + *ektomē,* excision]. Excision of cricoid cartilage.

cricoidynia (kri-koi-dĭn'ĭ-ă) [" + " + *odynē,* pain]. Pain in cricoid cartilage.

cricopharyn'geal [" + *pharygx,* gullet]. Pert. to the cricoid cartilage and pharynx.

cricothyreotomy (kri-ko-thi-re-ot'o-mĭ) [" + *thyreos,* shield, + *tomē,* a cut]. Division of the cricoid and thyroid cartilage.

cricothyroid (kri-ko-thi'roid) [" + " + *eidos,* form]. Pert. to the thyroid and cricoid cartilages.

cricot'omy [" + *tomē,* incision]. Division of the cricoid cartilage.

cricotracheot'omy [" + *tracheia,* windpipe, + *tomē,* incision]. Division of the cricoid cartilage and upper trachea in closure of the glottis.

Crigler-Najjar syndrome. A rare congenital disease characterized by nonhemolytic jaundice. SYN: *congenital familial nonhemolytic jaundice.*

crinogenic (krin-o-jen'ik) [G. *krinein,* to secrete, + *gennan,* to produce]. Producing or stimulating secretion.

crisis (kri'sis) (pl. *crises*) [G. *krisis*]. 1. The turning point of a disease; a very critical period often marked by a long sleep and profuse perspiration. 2. The term used for the sudden descent of a high temperature to normal or below; generally occurs within 24 hours. 3. Sharp paroxysms of pain occurring over the course of a few days in certain diseases, *e.g.,* Dietl's c.

c., abdominal. Severe abdominal pain due to one of several causes. SEE: *c., tabetic; c., sickle cell.*

c., blood. The appearance in the blood of large numbers of nucleated erythrocytes over the course of a few days.

c., Dietl's. In cases of floating kidney, the ureter becomes kinked and

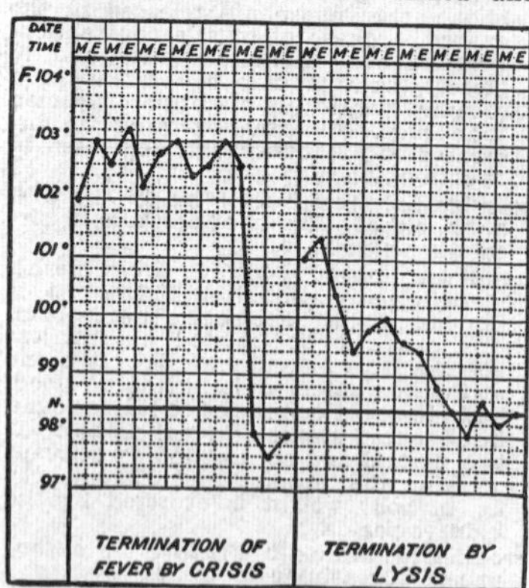

CRISIS LYSIS
After Sears.

urine is obstructed, producing symptoms of renal colic.

c., *false*. When temperature falls and the pulse rate remains high, suggesting that later on the temperature may rise again.

c., *sickle cell*. Severe abdominal pain due to sickle cell anemia.

c., *tabetic*. Abdominal pain due to syphilis.

c., *thyroid*. Sudden increase in severity of symptoms of thyrotoxicosis; marked by fever and extreme tachycardia. Outcome occasionally fatal. SYN: *thyroid storm.*

c., *true*. One accompanied by a fall in the pulse rate.

crista (kris'tă) (pl. *cristae*) [L.]. 1. A crest or ridge. 2. A projection, sometimes branched, of the inner wall of a mitochondrion into its fluid-filled cavity.

c. *ampullaris* [NA]. A localized thickening of the membrane lining the ampullae of the semicircular canals; it is covered with neuroepithelium containing auditory cells.

c. *galli* [NA]. A ridge on the ethmoid bone to which the *falx cerebri* is attached.

c. *lacrimalis posterior*. A vertical ridge on the lateral surface of the lacrimal bone.

c. *spiralis*. A ridge on the spiral lamina of the cochlea.*

criterion (Pl. *criteria*) [G. *krites*, judge]. Standard or attribute for judging a condition or establishing a diagnosis.

critical (krit'ik-al) [G. *krinein*, to judge]. 1. Pert. to a crisis. 2. Dangerous.

c. *reflex*. Abnormal tension of an area resulting from direct stimulation of that area.

Crohn's disease [Burrill B. Crohn, American gastroenterologist, 1884-]. Regional ileitis; regional enteritis.

Crookes' dark space. Nonluminous region enveloping outline of the cathode in a discharge tube. SEE: *cathode, dark space.*

C. *tube*. An early form of vacuum discharge tube devised by Sir William Crookes and used by him for the study of cathode rays.

cross. In genetics, the mating, or the offspring of the mating, of two individuals of different strains, races, or species.

cross birth. Presentation of the fetus where the long axis of the fetus is at right angles to that of the mother and requiring version.

cross eye. Manifest inward deviation of one eye when looking at an object. SYN: *strabismus; squint; esotropia.*

cross fertilization. The combining of gametes of two different individuals of the same species.

crossed. Passing from one side to the other, as crossed pyramidal tract in which nerve fibers cross from one side of the medulla to the other.

c., *reflexes*. 1. Passive flexion of one part following flexion of another. 2. Passive flexion of one leg causing similar movement of opposite leg.

crossing over. In genetics the mutual interchange of blocks of genes between two homologous chromosomes. It occurs during synapsis in miosis.

crossmatching. Test to establish blood compatibility before transfusion. SEE: *blood crossmatching.*

crossover. Abbr: CO. An individual which results from a new combination of linked genes.

crotaphion (kro-ta'fī-on) [G. *krotaphos*, the temple]. Tip of greater wing of sphenoid bone.

crotchet (krotch'et) [Fr. *crochet*, small hook]. Sharp hook for extracting fetus after craniotomy.

cro'tonism. Poisoning from croton oil.

croton oil (kro'ton) [G. *krotōn*, shrub]. (*oleum tiglii*). USP. A fixed oil expressed from the seed of the croton plant *croton tiglium.*

ACTION: Drastic cathartic, externally as a rubefacient. Rarely used in modern medical therapy.

POISONING: SYM: Severe abdominal pains, vomiting, marked diarrhea, and shock. Skin cold and clammy; face pinched; pulse rapid and small; collapse follows.

TREATMENT: Stomach pump or an emetic. Give soothing drinks, such as milk, barley water, or whites of eggs. Stimulate; apply external heat. Atropine, belladonna, or morphine to relieve cramping.

crounotherapy (kroo"no-ther'ă-pī) [G. *krounos*, spring, + *therapeia*, treatment]. Use of mineral waters for therapeutic purposes. SYN: *crenotherapy.*

croup (crōōp) [Fr. *croupe*]. Disease characterized by suffocative and difficult breathing, laryngeal spasm, and sometimes by the formation of a membrane.

c., *catarrhal*. Acute catarrhal laryngitis.

c., *diphtheritic*. Diphtheria of the larynx.

c., *false*. SEE: *spasmodic croup.*

c., *membranous*. Croupous laryngitis or true croup. Inflammation of larynx with exudation forming a false membrane. SYM: Those of laryngitis; loss of voice; noisy, difficult, and stridulous breathing; weak, rapid pulse; livid surface, fever moderate. PROG: Grave, unless tracheostomy has been performed. TREATMENT: Similar to that for diphtheria, *q.v.* Hot fomentations to throat, emetics, and medicated steam inhalations. SEE: *carpopedal spasm; steam tent.*

c., *spasmodic* or *false*. Catarrhal laryngitis without formation of false membrane, but with spasm of the glottis. Occurs in children. SYM: Difficult breathing, metallic cough, swollen membrane with tenacious mucus. PROG: Favorable. TREATMENT: Hot fomentations to throat, inhalation of steam.

croupous (kroo'pus). Pert. to croup or having a fibrinous exudation.

crown'ing [L. *corōna*, crown]. Stage in delivery when fetal head presents at the vulva.

crownwork [L. *corōna*, crown]. Artificial crown for a tooth.

crucial (krōō'shal) [L. *crucialis*, from *crux*, cross]. 1. Cross-shaped. 2. Decisive.

cruciate (krōō'shĭ-āt) [L. *crux*, cross]. Cross shaped as in the cruciate ligaments of the knee.

cru'cible [L. *crucibulum*]. A vessel for melting substances with great heat.

cruciform (krōō'sĭ-form) [L. *crux*, cross, + *forma*, shape]. Shaped like a cross.

crude (krōōd) [L. *crudus*, unripe; raw]. Raw, unrefined, or in a natural state. When used to describe a person, indicates one who is unrefined or uncouth.

crura (krōō'ră) (plural of *crus*) [L. legs]. A pair of elongated masses or diverging bands, resembling legs.

c. *cerebel'li*. Cerebellar peduncles.

c. cer'ebri. Pair of bands joining cerebellum to medulla and pons.

c. of diaphragm. Two pillars connecting spinal column and diaphragm.

c. of the fornix. Arches made by division of the fornicate extremities.

crural (krōō'ral) [L. *cruralis*, pert. to the leg]. Pert. to the leg or thigh; femoral.

c. arch. Femoral arch.

c. hernia. Femoral hernia.

c. nerve. SEE: *femoral nerve.*

c. palsies. Those of the nerves to the legs (*e.g.*, 12th thoracic, 1st to 5th lumbar, and 1st to 3rd sacral spinal nerves).

crus (pl. *cru'ra*) [L.]. 1. The leg. 2. Any structure resembling the leg.

c. cerebri. Either of the 2 peduncles connecting the cerebrum with the pons.

crush syndrome. Renal failure following severe local injuries, esp. those involving crushing of the lower extremities.

crust, crust'a [L. *crusta*]. 1. A scab. A secondary lesion; dry serous or seropurulent, brown, yellow, red or green exudations on a free surface. 2. An outer covering or coat.

Seen in eczema, seborrhea, syphilis, impetigo, favus and ringworm of the scalp.

c. lactea. Seborrhea of scalp in nursing infants. SEE: *galactophlysis.*

crutch. 1. A device for aiding a lame or weak person in walking. Usually a long staff with padded crescent-shaped portion at the top for placing under the armpit. 2. PSY: The use of some affliction which may be real or imaginary to explain personal inadequacy or failure.

Cruveilheir-Baumgarten syndrome (krōō-vāl-yā' bowm'gar-ten). Thrombosis of the portal vein.

cryalgesia (krī-al-je'zĭ-ă) [G. *kryos*, cold, + *algos*, pain]. Pain from the cold. SYN: *crymodynia.*

cryanesthesia (krī-an-es-the'zĭ-ă) [G. *krymos*, cold, + *an-*, priv. + *aisthēsis*, sensation]. Loss of sense of cold.

cryesthesia (krī-es-the'zĭ-ă) [" + *aisthēsis*, sensation]. Sensitiveness to the cold.

crymodynia (krī-mo-din'ĭ-ă) [G. *krymos*, cold, + *odynē*, pain]. Pain from cold esp. rheumatic pain aggravated by cold. SYN: *cryalgesia.*

crymophilic (krī-mo-fil'ĭk) [" + *philein*, to love]. Showing preference for cold. as certain microorganisms. SYN: *cryophilic.*

crymophylactic (krī-mo-fī-lak'tĭk) [" + *phylaxis*, guarding against]. Resistant to cold.

crymother'apy [" + *therapeia*, treatment]. The use of cold in treating disease. SYN: *cryotherapy.*

cryo-aerotherapy (krī-o-a-er-o-ther'ă-pĭ) [G. *kryos*, cold, + *aēr*, air, + *therapeia*, treatment]. Cold air bath in which, by degrees, the patient is accustomed to freezing temperature.

cryobiology (krī"o-bi-ol'o-jĭ) [" + biology]. Study of effect of cold on biological systems.

cryocautery (krī-o-kaw'ter-ĭ) [" + *kauter*, a burner]. Device for collection and application of solid carbon dioxide.

cry'ogen [" + *gennan*, to produce]. Substances which produce low temperatures.

cryogenic (krī-o-jen'ĭk). Producing or pert. to low temperatures.

cryoglobulinemia (krī'o-glob'u-lin-e'me-ah) [" + L. *globulus*, globule + G. *haima*, blood]. Presence in the blood of an abnormal protein which forms gels at low temperatures. Found in association with pathologic conditions such as multiple myeloma, leukemia, and certain forms of pneumonia.

cryom'eter [G. *kryos*, cold, + *metron*, measure]. A thermometer for measuring very low temperature.

cryophil'ic [" + *philein*, to love]. Preferring low temperatures.

cryothalamotomy (krī"o-thal"ă-mot'o-mĭ) [" + thalamotomy]. Destruction of a portion of the brain by cooling the end of a slender probe placed in the thalamus. This is usually done by circulating liquid nitrogen through the hollow stylus. Used in treating parkinsonism.

cryotherapy (krī-o-ther'ă-pĭ) [G. *kryos*, cold, + *therapeia*, treatment]. The therapeutic use of cold.

cryotol'erant [" + L. *tolerāre*, to bear]. Able to tolerate very low temperatures.

crypt (kript) [G. *kryptein*, to hide]. 1. A small sac or cavity extending into an epithelial surface. 2. A tubular gland, esp. one of the intestine.

c., anal. One of a number of small indentations lying immediately behind junction of anal skin and rectal mucosa.

c., of the iris. An irregular excavation on ant., surface of the iris near pupillary and ciliary margins.

c. of Lieberkuhn. A tubular gland of the intestine which secretes intestinal juice. Its wall is composed of columnar epithelium containing *argentaffin cells* and, at the base of the gland, *cells of Paneth.* They open between bases of the villi.

c., synoviparous. A saclike extension of the synovial cavity into capsule of a joint. Sometimes they become blind sacs.

c., tonsillar. A deep invagination of the surface stratified epithelium into substance of the lingual or palatine tonsils. It is surrounded by lymph nodules and may be branched.

cryptanamnesia (kript-an-am-ne'zĭ-ă) [" + *an-*, priv. + *amnēsia*, forgetfulness]. Subconscious memory.

cryptectomy (krip-tek'to-mĭ) [" + *ektomē*, excision]. Excision of a crypt.

cryptesthesia (krip-tes-the'zĭ-ă) [" + *aisthesis*, perception]. Intuition.

cryptic (krip'tĭk) [G. *kryptikos*, hidden]. Having a hidden meaning; occult.

cryptitis (krip-ti'tis) [G. *kryptein*, to hide, + *-itis*, inflammation]. Inflammation of a crypt or follicle, esp. an anal crypt.

cryptococcosis (krip-to-kok-o'sĭs). A systemic fungus infection which may involve any organ of the body, lungs, skin, but having a marked predilection for the brain and its meninges. SYN: *torulosis.*

ETIOL: *Cryptococcus neoformans* (*Torula histolytica*), a fungus.

SYMPTOMS: Development of single or multiple abscesses. In the cerebral type, headache, dizziness, vertigo, stiffness of neck muscles; in final stages coma and respiratory failure. Often mistaken for brain tumor.

PROG: Poor; in cerebral and meningeal forms usually fatal.

TREATMENT: Amphotericin B is somewhat beneficial in certain cases.

Cryptococcus (krip-to-kok'us). SYN: *Torula.* A genus of pathogenic yeastlike fungi which is the causative agent of cryptococcosis.

cryptodidymus (krip-to-did'ĭ-mus) [" + *didymos*, twin]. One fetus concealed within another.

cryptogenetic (krĭp-to-jen-et'ĭk) [" + *gennan,* to produce]. Of unknown or indeterminate origin.

c. infection. The invasion of bacteria without outward evidence of entry into the body. SEE: *infection.*

cryptolith (krip'to-lith) [" + *lithos,* stone]. A concretion in a glandular follicle.

cryptomenorrhea (krip-to-men-o-re'ă) [" + *mēn,* month, + *roia,* flow]. Monthly subjective symptoms of menses without flow of blood. May be due to imperforate hymen.

cryptomerorachischisis (krip"to-mer"o-ră-kis'kĭ-sis) [" + *meros,* part, + *rachis,* spine, + *schisis,* cleavage]. *Spina bifida occulta* without a tumor but with bony deficiency.

cryptomnesia (krip-tom-ne'zĭ-ă) [" + *mnēsis,* memory]. Subconscious memory.

cryptophthal'mus [" + *ophthalmos,* eye]. Complete congenital adhesion of eyelids to globe of eye.

cryptoplas'mic [" + *plasma,* matter]. Having existence in a concealed form.

cryptopodia (krip-to-po'dĭ-ă) [" + *pous,* foot]. Fibromata of feet so diffuse as to resemble pads.

cryptopyic (krip-to-pi'ĭk) [" + *pyon,* pus]. Having concealed suppuration, as a pyemia without apparent etiology.

cryptorchid (kript-or'kid) [" + *orchis,* testis]. An individual with testicles which have not descended into the scrotum.

cryptorchidectomy (kript-or-kĭ-dek'to-mĭ) [" + " + *ektomē,* excision]. Operation for an undescended testicle.

cryptorchidism (kript-or'kid-izm) [G. *kryptos,* hidden, + " + *ismos,* condition of]. Failure of testicles to descend into scrotum.

cryptor'chis. Cryptorchid.

cryptor'chism. Cryptorchidism.

cryptorrhea (krip-to-re'ă) [" + *roia,* flow]. Excessive secretion of a ductless gland.

cryptorrhet'ic [" + *roia,* flow]. Pert. to the internal secretions. SYN: *cryptorrheic.*

cryptoscope (krip'to-skōp) [" + *skopein,* to examine]. Fluoroscope.

cryptotox'ic [" + *toxikon,* poison]. Having unknown toxic properties.

cry reflex. 1. Normal ability of an infant to cry. Not present in premature infants. 2. Spontaneous crying by infants during sleep. Due to some painful disease such as tuberculosis of the joints.

crystal [G. *krystallos,* clear ice]. A solid body in which the atoms are arranged in a definite symmetrical pattern and having faces lying at definite angles to each other, as crystals formed from salts, water, etc.

c., Böttcher's. SEE: *c., spermin.*

c., Charcot-Leyden. Found in sputum from patients with asthma, leukemic blood, etc. Octahedral and composed of a phosphate.

c., Charcot-Neumann. Spermin crystals found in semen and some animal tissues.

c., Charcot-Robin. A type formed in blood in leukemia.

c. hemin. Yellowish or brown crystals which appear when dried blood or hemoglobin is heated with a few drops of acetic acid and salt. They are crystals of hemin, the hydrochloride of heme. Their presence constitutes a delicate and reliable test for blood. SYN: *Teichmann's c.*

c., spermin. Composed of spermine phosphate and seen in prostatic fluid on addition of a drop of ammonium phosphate solution.

crystallin (krĭs'tăl-ĭn). Globulin of the crystalline lens.

crys'talline. Resembling crystal.

c. deposits (in urine). ACID GROUP: Includes the urates, oxalates, carbonates, and sulfates. ALKALINE GROUP: Includes the phosphates, cholesterin ammonium urate.

c. lens. The lens of the eye in the capsule behind the pupil. It separates the *aqueous* from the *vitreous* humor. It is transparent and refracts the rays of light, impinging them upon the surface to bring them to a focus on the retina.

crystalliza'tion [G. *krystallos,* clear ice]. The formation of crystals.

crys'talloid [" + *eidos,* form]. 1. Like a crystal. 2. Opposite of *colloid;* a substance capable of crystallization, which in solution can be diffused through animal membranes.

crystalloiditis (kris-tal-oid-i'tis) [" + " + *-itis,* inflammation]. Inflammation of crystalline lens.

crystallopho'bia [" + *phobos,* fear]. Abnormal fear of glass or objects made of glass.

crystallu'ria. The appearance of crystals in the urine. May occur following the administration of sulfonamides. Their formation can be prevented by administration of adequate amounts of alkali.

crystalluridrosis (krist-al-ū-rĭd-ro'sis) [G. *krystallos,* clear ice, + *ouron,* urine, + *idrōs,* sweat]. Crystallization of urinary elements on the skin.

Cs. Symb. for *cesium.*

Ctenocephalides (tĕn-ō-sĕf'ă-lĭds). A genus of fleas belonging to the order Siphonaptera. Common species are *Ct. canis* and *Ct. felis,* the dog flea and cat flea. The adults feed on their hosts while larvae live on dried blood and feces of adult fleas. Adults may attack man and other animals. They serve as intermediate host of the dog tapeworm, *Dipylidium caninum,* and may transmit other helminth and protozoan infections.

Cu. Symb. for *copper* (*cuprum*).

cubic measure. SEE: *Appendix.*

cu'bital [G. *kubiton,* the elbow]. Pert. to the ulna, or to the forearm.

c. fossa. Triangular area lying anterior to and below the elbow, bounded medially by the pronator teres and laterally by the brachioradialis muscle.

cu'bitus [L. from G. *kubiton*]. Elbow; forearm; ulna.

c. valgus. A deformity of the arm in which the forearm deviates laterally. May be congenital or due to injury or disease. In females, slight cubitus valgus is normal and is one of the secondary sex characteristics.

c. varus. A deformity of the arm in which the forearm deviates medially.

cu'boid [G. *kubos,* cube, + *eidos,* resemblance]. Like a cube.

c. bone. Outer bone of tarsal or instep bones articulating posteriorly with the 4th and 5th metatarsus. SYN: *os cuboideum* [NA].

cucumbers. Fruit of *Cucumis saturis* vine. RAW (unpared): 100 gm. Calories: 15. Other main values: 0.9 gm. protein; 3.4 gm. carbohydrates; 46 mg. calcium; 1.1

mg. iron; 250 I.U. vitamin A; 11 mg. ascorbic acid.

cucurbit (ku-ker'bit) [L. *cucurbita,* gourd]. Cupping glass.

cuff (kuf). Anatomical structure encircling a part.

cul-de-sac [Fr. *cul,* bottom, + *de,* of, + *sac,* bag]. 1. A blind pouch or cavity. 2. The rectouterine pouch or pouch of Douglas, an extension of the peritoneal cavity which lies between rectum and posterior wall of uterus.

cul'doscope. An endoscope used in performing a culdoscopic examination.

culdos'copy. Examination of the viscera of the pelvic cavity of the female after introduction of an endoscope in the vagina.

-cule, -cle [L.]. Suffix: Little, as *molecule, corpuscle.*

Culex (kū'leks). A genus of small to medium sized mosquitoes of cosmopolitan distribution. Some species are vectors of disease organisms.

C. pipiens. The common house mosquito. Serves as a vector of *Wuchereria bancrofti,* the causative agent of filariasis.

C. quinquefasciatus. Common in the tropics and subtropics; the most important intermediate host of *Wuchereria bancrofti.*

Culicidae (kū-lĭs'ĭ-dē). A family of insects belonging to the order Diptera. Includes the mosquitoes.

culicifuge (ku-lis'ĭ-fūj) [L. *culex,* gnat, + *fugere,* to flee]. An agent to repel mosquito attacks.

cul'men [L. summit]. Top or summit of a thing.

c. cerebelli. Most prominent part of the vermis sup. near its ant. extremity.

cultiva'tion [L. *cultivāre,* to cultivate]. Growing microorganisms in an artificial medium.

cultural (kul'tu-ral) [L. *cultura,* tillage]. Pert. to cultures of microorganisms.

cul'ture [L. *cultura*]. 1. Psy: The total pattern or life style of an individual or a group as judged by speech, intellectual attainment, and degree of realization of potential. 2. Bact: A mass of microorganisms growing in laboratory culture media.

c., blood. Used in the diagnosis of specific infectious diseases. Test consists of withdrawing blood from a vein, under sterile precautions, placing it in or upon suitable culture media, and determining whether or not bacteria grow in the media. If organisms do grow, they are identified by bacteriologic methods.

c., gelatin. A c. of bacteria on gelatin.

c., hanging block. A thin slice of agar seeded on its surface with bacteria, and then inverted on a cover slip and sealed in the concavity of a hollow glass slide.

c., hanging drop. A c. accomplished by inoculating the bacterium into a drop on a cover glass, and mounting it in the depression on a concave slide.

c. medium. A substance on which microorganisms may grow. Those most commonly used are broths, gelatin, and agar, which contain the same basic ingredients.

c., negative. A c. made from suspected matter which fails to reveal the suspected organism.

c., physical. The training of the body by means of gymnastics.

c., positive. A c. which reveals the suspected organism.

c., pure. The c. of a single form of microorganism uncontaminated by other organisms.

c., stab. A bacterial c. made by thrusting into the c. medium a point inoculated with the matter under examination.

c., stock. A permanent c. from which transfers may be made.

c., tissue. The growing of tissue cells in artificial nutrient media.

cu.mm. Abbr. for cubic millimeter.

cumulative (ku'mu-la-tiv) [L. *cumulus,* a heap]. Increasing in effect.

c. drugs. Those which, after being received into the body in small doses, often repeated, are not immediately eliminated, but tend to accumulate in the system and eventually produce symptoms of poisoning. Carbolic acid, lead, silver, and mercurial preparations are examples of drugs which act in this way.

cu'mulus. A raised place; a heap of cells.

c. oophorus. A mass of follicle cells which surrounds the ovum. It projects into the antrum of the graafian follicle. Also called *discus proligerus.*

cuneate (ku'ne-āt) [L. *cuneus,* wedge]. Wedge-shaped.

c. fasciculus, c. funiculus. Continuation of posteroexternal column of cord into the medulla.

c. nucleus. Gray matter at end of cuneate fasciculus.

cuneiform (ku-ne'ĭ-form) [L. *cuneus,* wedge, + *forma,* shape]. Wedge-shaped.

c. bones. Those of the tarsus, internal, middle, and external.

c. cartilage. One of two small pieces of yellow elastic cartilage which lies in the aryepiglottic fold of the larynx immediately anterior to the arytenoid cartilage.

cuneo- (ku'ne-o) [L.]. Prefix: A wedge.

cu"neocu'boid [L. *cuneus,* wedge, + G. *kubos,* cube, + *eidos,* shape]. Pert. to cuboid and cuneiform bones.

cuneohysterectomy (ku-ne-o-his-ter-ek'-to-mĭ) [" + *ystera,* uterus, + *ektomē,* excision]. Excision of a wedge of tissue from the post. surface of the *cervix uteri* to correct abnormal anteflexion.

cu'neus [L.]. Wedge-shaped lobule of brain on mesial surface of occipital lobe.

cuniculus (ku-nik'u-lus) (pl. *cuniculi*) [L. an underground passage]. Burrow in epidermis made by the itch mite.

cunnilinguist (kun-ĭ-lin'gwist). One who practices cunnilingus, *q.v.*

cunnilingus (kun-nĭ-lin'gus) [L. *cunnus,* vulva, + *lingua,* tongue]. Sexual activity in which the mouth and tongue are used to stimulate the female genitalia.

cun'nus [L.]. The vulva,* pudenda.

cup [G. *kupe,* hollow]. 1. Small drinking vessel. 2. A cupping glass. 3. An athletic supporter (jockey strap) reinforced with a piece of firm material to cover the genitalia. Worn to protect the penis and testicles during vigorous and contact sports. 4. Either of the two cup-shaped halves of a brassiere which fits over a breast. 5. A method of producing counterirritation. See: *cupping.*

c., favus. A cup-shaped crust which develops in certain fungus infections. See: *favus.*

c., glaucomatous. A depression in the optic disk occurring in late stages of glaucoma.

c., optic. In the embryo a double layered cuplike structure connected to the diencephalon by a tubular optic stalk. It gives rise to the sensory and pigmented layers of the retina.

c., physiologic. A slight concavity in the center of the optic disk.

Cupid's bow. The normal shape of the upper lip is that of a bow.

cu'pola [L. *cūpula,* little tub]. 1. The little dome at apex of cochlea and of spiral canal. 2. The portion of costal pleura which extends superiorly into the root of the neck. It is dome-shaped and accommodates the apex of the lung.

cupping. Application of glass vessel from which the air has been exhausted by heat or a special suction apparatus to the skin in order to draw blood to the surface. SEE: *leech.*

cu'prum [L.]. Abbr. Cu. Copper, *q.v.*

curare, curari (kū-ră'rē) [Spanish *curaré,* he, to whom it comes, falls]. An extract of the bark and other parts of the plants of various species of *Chondrodendron* and *Strychnos* used as an arrow poison by South American Indians. It contains alkaloids which induce paralysis by selective action on the myoneural junction inhibiting the action of acetylcholine. It is used in the control of convulsions and spasms, and for relaxation of skeletal muscles in anesthesia.

curarization (kū"ră-rī-ză'shun) [Spanish *curaré,* he, to whom it comes, falls]. Condition following introduction of curare: eyelids heavy, nystagmus, husky voice, weak jaw and throat muscles, inability to raise head, arms and legs.

Employed to lessen severity of convulsions produced by pentylenetetrazol and electric shock therapy and relaxation of muscles as in tetanus, etc.

cur'ative. Having healing or remedial properties.

curd [M.E.]. Milk coagulum. Milk coagulated in the stomach forming what is known as a "curd."

cure [L. *cura,* care]. 1. Course of treatment of patients. 2. Restoration to health.

curet, curette (ku-ret') [Fr. *curette,* a cleanser]. A spoon-shaped scraping instrument for removing foreign matter from a cavity.

curettage (ku-ret'aj) [Fr.]. Scraping of a cavity.

c., uterine. Scraping with a curette to remove contents of uterus (as is done following inevitable or incomplete abortion). Done to obtain specimens for use in diagnosis and to remove growths (as polyps).

NP: 1. It is essential that the patient's buttocks are not pulled down below edge of table. If this is done when legs are elevated in leg rests or stirrups, an undue strain is placed on the sacroiliac structures. Prolonged pressure on the leg muscles by stirrups is to be avoided, if possible, to prevent muscular soreness, paralysis of muscles, or thrombosis of a varicose vein.

2. The exterior surfaces are either scrubbed and irrigated with sterile water or painted using an antiseptic. The vaginal surfaces are included, as is also the cervix. The patient has already been placed on a Kelly pad, on which a sterile towel has been placed. A sterile towel is now placed across the pubes. Another is now placed crosswise across the buttocks. The "floating" nurse takes a strip of narrow adhesive plaster, about 18 in. long, holding it by the ends, well away from her. The "sterile" nurse then throws over the middle of the tape a sterile towel so that tape holds towel in middle fold. The "floating" nurse places edges of tape around patient's hips so that sterile towel is stretched tightly across rectum. Sterile leggings are now pulled over patient's legs and a lithotomy sheet draped down on the perineum.

3. Sterile packing for the uterus should be ready. This form of packing is usually of gauze 1½ in. wide and 18 in. long.

curettement (ku-ret'ment) [Fr.]. Curettage, *q.v.*

curie (ku-re'). The standard unit of quantity of radon, being the amt. in equilibrium with 1 gm. of radium element. This quantity decays at the rate of 3.7×10^{10} disintegrations per second.

cu'riegram [Curie + G. *gramma,* writing]. A photogram made by radium rays.

curietherapy (kū-rī-ther'ă-pī) [" + G. *therapeia,* treatment]. Radium therapy.

curium (kū'rī-ŭm). A transuranium element, named after Pierre and Marie Curie. SYMB: Cm. At. wt. 247; at. no. 96.

curled. BACT: Said of parallel chains in wavy strands, such as in anthrax colonies.

Curling's ulcer (kurl'ingz) [after a British physician, Thomas Curling, 1811-1888]. Acute peptic ulcer which sometimes occurs following a severe burn. A form of stress ulcer, *q.v.*

cur'rant jelly clot. Postmortem, soft, red clot in heart and vessels.

cur'rent [L. *currere,* to run]. A flow, as of water, or the transference of electrical impulses.

c., alternating. A current which periodically flows in opposite directions. Alternating current waves may be either sinusoidal or nonsinusoidal. The alternating current wave used most commonly therapeutically is the sinusoidal.

c., direct. A current that flows in one direction only. When used medically it is called the "galvanic" current.

curriculum (kur-rik'u-lum) [L. a course]. A course of study covering a specific time.

Curschmann's spirals (koorsh'mahnz). Coiled spirals of mucus occasionally seen in sputum of asthma patients, etc. SEE: *sputum.*

curvature (kŭr'vă-chŭr) [L. *curvatura,* a slope]. A bending or sloping away either normal or abnormal; a curve.

c., angular. A sharp bending of the vertebral column. Also called *Pott's curvature.*

c. of the spine. One of four normal curves or flexures of the vertebral column as seen in profile, *viz.* cervical, thoracic, lumbar, and sacral. Abnormal curvatures may occur as a result of maldevelopment or disease processes. SEE: *kyphosis; lordosis; scoliosis.*

curve [L. *curvus*]. A bend.

c. of Carus. An arc corresponding with the pelvic axis.

c., probability. Frequency curve in statistics.

c., temperature. Line representing changes of temperature during a given period.

c., Wunderlich's. Typical temperature curve of typhoid fever.

curvi- [L.]. Combining form, meaning curved.

Cus'co's spec'ulum. A duckbill vaginal speculum manipulated by a screw.

Cushing's syndrome. A syndrome resulting from hypersecretion of the adrenal cortex in which there is excessive production of glucocorticoids. May be due to a tumor of the adrenal gland or to excess stimulation of that gland as a result of hyperfunction of the anterior pituitary. Symptoms are protein loss, adiposity, fatigue and weakness, osteoporosis, amenorrhea, impotence, capillary fragility, edema, excess hair growth, diabetes mellitus, skin discoloration and turgidity (plethora), and purplish striae of skin.

cushion. In *Anat.*, a mass of connective tissue, usually adipose, which acts to prevent undue pressure upon underlying tissues or structures.

cusp (kusp) [L. *cuspis*, a point]. 1. Point of the crown of a tooth. 2. One of the leaflike divisions or parts of the valves of the heart. SEE: *bicuspid valve; tricuspid valve; semilunar valve.*

cuspid (kus'pid) [L. *cuspis*, a point]. The 4 teeth with conic crowns (canine).

cuspidate (kus'pĭ-dāt) [L. *cuspis*, point]. Having cusps.

cuta'neous [L. *cutis*, skin]. Pert. to the skin.

c. nerves. Sensory nerves of the skin of the arms and legs.

c. respiration. The transpiration of gases through the skin.

cu'ticle [L. *cuticula*, dim. of *cutis*, skin]. 1. A layer of solid or semisolid substance which covers the free surface of a layer of epithelial cells. It may be of a horny or chitinous consistency; sometimes it is calcified. Examples are enamel of a tooth, capsule of lens of eye. 2. The epidermis of the skin.

c. of hair. A single layer of clear cells which forms the outer layer of a hair.

c. of inner root sheath. A layer of scalelike cells which forms innermost layer of the root sheath. Lies next to the cuticle of the hair.

cuticula (ku-tĭk'u-lă) [L.]. Cuticle.

cuticulariza'tion. Growth of epidermis over a sore or wound.

cutireaction. Reaction appearing on the skin; skin reaction.

c., von Pirquet's. Reaction of skin after inoculation with tuberculosis toxins.

cutis (ku'tis) [L). The skin.

c. anserina. "Gooseflesh" caused by erection of skin papillae, as from cold, shock, fright, or fear.

c., aurantiasis. Yellow discoloration of the skin resulting from ingesting excessive quantities of vegetables, such as carrots, containing carotenoid pigments.

c., hyperelastica. A congenital or familial condition characterized by excessive elasticity of the skin, loose-jointedness, easy bruisability, and development of pseudotumors at joints. SYN: *Ehlers-Danlos syndrome.*

c. laxa. Dermatolysis, or hypertrophy of the skin and subcutaneous tissue.

c. marmorata. Purplish discoloration of skin on exposure to cold.

c. pendula. Condition in which the skin hangs in flabby folds or wrinkles.

c. testacea. Condition characterized by formation of plates of greasy material on trunk and extremities. SYN: *seborrhea.*

c. unctosa. Excessive secretion of sebaceous glands. SEE: *seborrhea.*

c. vera. The corium*; deep layer of skin, the dermis, *q.v.*

c. verticis gyrata. Looseness and hypertrophy of the scalp skin which may hang in folds.

cutitis (ku-ti'tis) [" + G. *-itis*, inflammation]. Inflammation of skin. SYN: *dermatitis.*

cutization (kū-tĭ-za'shun) [L. *cutis*, skin]. Skinlike condition of a mucous membrane as result of continued exposure.

cut throat. Injury depends upon position in which it was caused.

NP: *First Aid*: Send for doctor. Have subject lying down, head and shoulders raised. Press head on chest. If trachea is severed, keep open and free from clot. Compress bleeding points with clean, wet cloths. Reassure patient, keep his lips moist, do not leave him for an instant. Artificial respiration if necessary.

cyanemia (sī-an-e'mĭ-ă) [G. *kyanos*, dark blue, + *aima*, blood]. Blue color of blood.

cyanephidrosis (sī-ăn-ef-ĭ-dro'sis) [" + *ephidrōsis*, sweating]. Bluish sweat.

cyanhidrosis (sī-ăn-hĭ-dro'sis) [" + *idrōsis*, sweat]. Exuding bluish sweat.

cyanide (sī'ă-nīd). A compound containing the radical —CN, as potassium cyanide (KCN) sodium cyanide (NaCN).

c. poisoning. Cyanides are among the most common and most deadly poisons known. They stop cellular respiration by inhibiting the action of cytochrome oxidase, carbonic anhydrase, and other enzyme systems.

SYM: Start within a few seconds, rarely longer than 2 minutes. The patient utters a cry and falls insensible. Respiration is first rapid and convulsive, later slow and gasping. Death usually comes within 5 minutes. When smaller doses are taken, there is an acrid taste, a choking feeling, anxiety, dizziness, confusion, and headache. Convulsions with frothing of the mouth. Often incontinence. Pulse rapid, feeble, and irregular.

F. A. TREATMENT: Must be very prompt. Have victim inhale amyl nitrite immediately for 15 to 30 seconds. Do this every 2 to 3 minutes. While this is being done, give I.V. sodium nitrite 0.3 gm. in 10 ml. of water at rate of 2.5 to 5 ml. per minute. As soon as this is completed, through the same needle give 25 to 50 ml. of 50% solution of sodium thiosulfate.

Immediate artificial respiration is also required.

In one hour repeat half doses of medicines above.

Wash out the stomach with 3% hydrogen peroxide or 1:5000 potassium permanganate solution.

External heat, epinephrine for collapse and having the patient lying flat are also indicated.

cyano- [G.]. Combining form, meaning *dark blue.*

cyanochroia (sī-an-o-kroi'ă) [G. *kyanos*, dark blue, + *chroia*, color]. Cyanosis.

cyanocobalamin (sī"an-o-co-bal'ă-min). USP. A component of the vitamin B complex. Also called vitamin B_{12}. It has blood-forming action and is used in treatment of certain anemias and sprue.

cyanoder'ma [" + *derma*, skin]. Blue discoloration of skin. SYN: *cyanosis.*

cyan'ogen. (1) The radical CN; (2) A poisonous gas, CN-CN.

cyanomycosis (sī"an-o-mī-ko'sis) [G. *kyanos*, dark blue, + *mykēs*, fungus]. Development of blue pus due to *Micrococcus pyocyaneus.*

cyanopathy (sī-an-op'ă-thĭ) [" + *pathos*, disease]. Blue discoloration of skin. SYN: *cyanosis.*

cyanophil (si-an'o-fil) [" + *philein*, to love]. Blue staining substance of plants and animals.

cyanophilous (si-an-of'il-us). Having an affinity for a blue dye or stain.

cyanopia, cyanopsia (si-an-op'ī-ă, -si-a) [G. *kyanos*, dark blue, + *opsis*, vision]. Vision in which all objects appear to be blue.

cy'anosed. Affected with cyanosis.

cyanosis (si-an-o'sis) [G. *kyanos*, dark blue, + *-ōsis*, infection]. Slightly bluish, grayish, slatelike, or dark purple discoloration of the skin due to presence of abnormal amounts of reduced hemoglobin in the blood. May not appear in patients with severe anemia even though their blood is poorly oxygenated because there is not enough reduced hemoglobin present to cause the blue color to be visible.

When entire body is affected the color is dusky leaden.

Etiol: Deficiency of oxygen and excess of carbon dioxide in blood caused by gas or any condition interfering with entrance of air in the respiratory tract; also by overdoses of certain drugs, or any form of asphyxiation.

Treatment: Remove cause. Artificial respiration together with oxygen inhalation or oxygen plus carbon dioxide. Stimulants; heat and massage are valuable adjuncts. See: *asphyxia, unconsciousness.*

c., congenital. Usually associated with stenosis of the pulmonary orifice, an imperfect ventricular septum, or a patulous foramen ovale or ductus arteriosus. See: *tetralogy of Fallot.*

c., delayed. Tardive cyanosis, *q.v.*

c., enterogenous. Induced by intestinal absorption of toxins. See: *methemoglobinemia.*

c., hereditary methemoglobinemic. Presence of methemoglobin in the blood; present at birth, and occurring generally in males.

c. retinae. Bluish appearance of retina seen in congenital heart disease, polycythemia, and in certain poisonings, as dinitrobenzol.

c., tardive. That resulting from an interatrial or interventricular septal defect. Also called *delayed cyanosis.*

cyanotic (si-an-ot'ik). Of the nature of, affected with, or pert. to, cyanosis.

cyasma (si-az'mă) [G. *kyēsis*, pregnancy]. Lenticular pigmentation of skin of pregnant women.

cyclarthrosis (si-klar-thro'sis) [G. *kyklos*, circle, + *arthron*, joint, + *-ōsis*, infection]. A lateral ginglymus or pivot joint which makes possible rotation.

cycle (sī'kl) [G. *kyklos*, circle]. A series of movements or events; a sequence.

c., cardiac. The series of consecutive movements through which the heart passes in performing one heart beat; it includes contraction or *systole*, relaxation or *diastole*, and a short rest pause, the *diastasis cordis;* a complete cycle corresponds to one pulse beat, which requires a variable length of time depending upon the heart rate.

c., Cori. A series of reactions which accounts for the disposal of lactate formed during muscular activity, *viz.*, muscle glycogen to lactic acid to liver glycogen to blood glucose to muscle glycogen.

c. gastric. Progression of peristaltic waves over the stomach.

c., genesial. The period from puberty to menopause.

c. glycolytic. The successive steps by which glucose is broken down in living tissue.

c., Krebs'. A series of reactions occurring in muscle cells and possibly all tissues in which pyruvic acid (or two-carbon derivatives of carbohydrate, fat, or protein) formed anaerobically are converted, through a series of interrelated oxidation-reduction and other reactions to carbon dioxide and water with the release of energy principally utilized in the formation of adenosinetriphosphate (ATP). It is considered to be the final common pathway for the oxidation of and interconversions between the three primary classes of foods. Syn: *tricarboxylic acid cycle* (TCA); *citric acid cycle.*

c., menstrual. A series of periodically recurring changes in endometrium of the uterus culminating in menstruation, *q.v.*

c., ornithine. A cycle which takes place in the liver in which products of the citric acid cycle (glutamic acid, aspartic acid) are converted into ornithine and arginine, an amino acid which if not used for protein synthesis forms urea and ornithine. Syn: *urea cycle.*

cyclectomy (si-klek'to-mī) [" + *ektomē*, excision]. Excision of a portion of the ciliary body or muscle or ciliary border of eyelids.

cy'clic. Periodic; occurring in cycles.

c. insanity. Manic depressive psychosis; a form in which mania, melancholia, and sanity succeed each other at intervals; circular insanity.

c. vomiting. Periodic and recurring attacks of vomiting occurring in persons of a nervous temperament. The condition is usually associated with acidosis.

Sym: Dizziness, loss of appetite, headache, nausea may occur. Patient then vomits about every ½ hr. for 1-2 days. Great thirst, slight rise of temperature, rapid pulse, prostration.

NP: At first, glucose, barley sugar, or easily assimilated carbohydrate. Nothing during attacks. Keep warm in bed; mouth washes.

See: *nausea; vomiting.*

cyclicot'omy [G. *kyklikos*, circular, + *tomē*, incision]. Cutting of the ciliary muscle.

cycli'tis [G. *kyklos*, circle, + *-itis*, inflammation]. Inflammation of ciliary body.

Sym: Tenderness in ciliary region, swelling of upper lid, circumcorneal injection, deposits on Descemet's membrane, reduced or hazy vision, increased or decreased tension. Pain in or about the eye, worse at night, and on pressure. Its course is rapid, progressively unfavorable.

Complications: Iritis, choroiditis, scleritis, glaucoma.

Treatment: Local (atropine, heat, protection from light); general (salicylates, diaphoresis, rest; treat underlying cause if possible).

c., plastic. Ciliary body inflammation accompanied by that of entire uveal tract, giving rise to a fibrinous exudate in ant. chamber and vitreous.

c., purulent. Suppurative inflammation of ciliary body and iris.

c., serous. Simple inflammation without iritis.

cyclo- [G.]. A combining form meaning (1) circular or pertaining to a cycle;

(2) pertaining to the ciliary body of the eye.

cycloceratitis (si-klo-ser-ă-ti'tis). Cyclokeratitis, *q.v.*

cyclochoroiditis (si-klo-ko-roid-i'tis) [G. *kyklos*, circle, + *chorioeidēs*, skinlike, + *-itis*, inflammation]. Inflammation of ciliary body and choroid coat of eye.

cyclodial'ysis [" + *dialysis*, dissolution]. Operation performed in certain types of glaucoma to produce communication bet. ant. chamber and suprachoroidal space for the escape of aqueous humor.

cycloid (sī'kloid) [" + *eidos*, form]. 1. Denoting a ring of atoms. 2. Extreme variations of mood from elation to melancholia.

cyclokerati'tis [" + *keras*, cornea, + *-itis*, inflammation]. Inflammation of cornea and ciliary body.

cyclophoria (si-klo-fo'rĭ-ă) [" + *phoros*, bearing]. Rotation of eyeball due to insufficiency of oblique muscles.

cyclople'gia [" + *plēgē*, a stroke]. Paralysis of ciliary muscle.

cycloplegic (si-klo-ple'jik). Producing cycloplegia.

cyclopro'pane (C_3H_6). A gaseous anesthetic agent, colorless, slightly heavier than air, with a not unpleasant odor. Administered with 70 to 95% oxygen it produces unconsciousness in 1 to 2 minutes. Fire and explosion must be guarded against.

cyclops (sī'klops) [G. *kyklos*, circle + *ōps*, eye]. A fetal monster with one eye.

cyclo'sis [G. *kyklōsis*, circulation]. A streaming movement of protoplasm such as is seen in certain plant and animal cells.

cyclothymia (si-klo-thi'mĭ-ă) [G. *kyklos*, circle, + *thymos*, mind]. Psy: Cyclic insanity.

cyclothy'mic. Pert. to cyclothymia.

c. personality. Psy: One in which periods of elation and sadness alternate.

cyesedema (si-e-se-de'mă) [G. *kyēsis*, pregnancy, + *oidēma*, swelling]. Thickening of cutis; bloating in pregnancy.

cyesiology (si-e-si-ol'o-jĭ) [" + *logos*, study of]. The study of pregnancy.

cyesis (si-e'sis) [G. *kyēsis*]. Pregnancy.

cyetic (si-et'ĭk). Pert. to pregnancy.

cylicotomy (sil-ik-ot'o-mĭ) [G. *kylix*, cup, + *tomē*, incision]. To cut ciliary muscle. Syn: *cyclotomy*.

cylin"droadeno'ma [G. *kylindros*, cylinder, + *adēn*, gland, + *-ōma*, tumor]. An adenoma containing cylindrical masses of hyaline material.

cylindroid (sil-in'droid) [" + *eidos*, shape]. 1. Cylinder shaped. 2. A mucous, spurious cast in urine. How to Recognize: They have twists and turns, varying markedly in diameter in different places, most frequently pointed at the ends and frequently crossing an entire field. They do not usually have cellular intrusions.

cylindro'ma [" + *-ōma*, tumor]. Malignant tumor containing a collection of cells forming cylinders.

cylindrosarco'ma [" + *sarx*, flesh, + *-ōma*, tumor]. A tumor containing properties of a cylindroma and sarcoma.

cylindruria (sil-in-dru'rĭ-ă) [" + *ouron*, urine]. Cylindroids in the urine.

cyllosis (sil-o'sis) [G. *kyllōsis*]. Clubfoot.

cymbocephalic (sim-bo-sef-al'ik) [G. *kymbē*, boat, + *kephalē*, head]. Having a boatshaped head.

cynanthropy (sin-an'thrō-pē) [G. *kyon*, dog, + *anthrōpos*, man]. Insanity in which the patient behaves like a dog.

cyn'ic spasm [G. *kynikos*, doglike]. Spasm of face muscles causing a grin or snarl like a dog. Syn: *risus sardonicus*.

cynobex (sin'o-beks) [G. *kyōn*, dog, + *bēx*, cough]. Dry, barking cough.

cynophobia (sin-o-fo'bĭ-ă) [" + *phobos*, fear]. Unreasonable fear of dogs. Syn: *lyssophobia*.

cynorex'ia [" + *orexis*, appetite]. Morbid appetite, bulimia.*

cyotrophy (si-ot'ro-fĭ) [G. *kyos*, fetus, + *trophē*, nutrition]. Nourishment of the fetus.

cypridopathy (sip"rĭ-dop'ă-thĭ) [G. *Kypris*, Venus, + *pathos*, disease]. Any venereal disease.

cypridophobia (sip"rĭ-do-fo'bĭ-ă) [" + *phobos*, fear]. 1. Morbid fear of venereal disease. 2. Abnormal fear of the sexual act. 3. False belief of having a venereal disease.

cypriphobia (sip-rĭ-fo'bĭ-ă) [" + *phobos*, fear]. Morbid aversion to and fear of coitus.

cyrtometer (sir-tom'ĕ-ter) [G. *kyrtos*, bent, + *metron*, measure]. Instrument for measuring circumference of chest and comparison of chest curves. Also used to measure other curved portions of the body.

cyrtosis (sir-to'sis) [" + *-ōsis*, infection]. Having any abnormal curvature of the spine. See: *kyphosis*.

cyst (sĭst) [G. *kystis*, bladder, sac]. 1. A closed sac or pouch with a definite wall which contains fluid, semifluid or solid material. It is usually an abnormal structure resulting from developmental anomalies, obstruction of ducts, or from parasitic infection. 2. In *Biol.* a structure formed by, and enclosing, certain organisms in which they become inactive, as the cyst of certain protozoans or of the metacercariae of flukes. It may serve as a reproductive structure or in hydatid cysts.

c., adventitious. One formed about a foreign body.

c., blood. Bloody tumor. Syn: *hematoma*.

c., branchial. A cervical cyst, *q.v.*

c., cervical. A closed epithelial sac derived from a branchial groove or its corresponding pharyngeal pouch.

c., chocolate. Ovarian c. with darkly pigmented gelatinous content.

c., colloid. C. with gelatinous contents.

c., congenital. One present at birth resulting from (a) abnormal development, as a dermoid cyst; (b) imperfect closure of a structure, *e.g.*, spina bifida, or (c) nonclosure of embryonic clefts, ducts, or tubules, *e.g.*, cervical cysts, *q.v.*

c., daughter. C. growing out of the walls of another cyst.

c., dentigerous. One containing teeth. Syn: *follicular odontoma*. See: *dermoid cyst*.

c., dermoid. One containing elements of hair, teeth, or skin. They occur commonly in the ovary and contain derivatives of all three germ layers.

c., distention. One formed in a natural enclosed cavity as a follicular cyst of the ovary.

c., extravasation. C. arising from hemorrhage into tissues.

c., follicular. One arising from a follicle, as a follicular cyst of the thyroid gland or ovary.

c., Gartner's. One developing from a vestigial mesonephric duct (Gartner's duct) in a female.

c., hydatid. A cyst formed by the growth of the larval form of the Echinococcus granulosus, usually in the liver.

c., implantation. One resulting from displacement of portions of the epidermis as may occur in injuries.

c., intraligamentary. Cystic formation between the layers of the broad ligament.

c., involutional. One occurring in the normal involution of an organ or structure as in the mammary gland.

c., meibomian. Tumor or cyst produced by inflammation of a meibomian gland. SYN: *chalazion.*

c., mucous. Retention cyst composed of mucus.

c., nabothian. Cystic formation caused by closure of the ducts of the nabothian glands in the cervix uteri as a result of healing of an erosion.

c., odontogenic. One associated with the teeth as a *dentigerous* or *radicular* cyst, *q.v.*

c., ovarian. Cystic formation in the ovary. SEE: *ovary.*

c., parasitic. A cyst enclosing the larval form of certain parasites as the cysticercus or hydatid of tapeworms or the larva of certain nematodes, *e.g., Trichinella.*

c., parovarian. Cystic formation of the parovarium.

c., pilonidal. An elongated closed sac lined with stratified epithelium and usually containing hair, usually occurs in midline over sacral area of back. SYN: *pilonidal sinus.*

c., porencephalic. An anomalous cavity of the brain which communicates with the ventricular system.

c., proliferative. One lined with epithelium which proliferates, forming projections which extend into the cavity of the cyst.

c., radicular. A granulomatous cyst located alongside the root of a tooth.

c., retention. One retaining the secretion of a gland, as in a mucous or sebaceous cyst.

c., sebaceous. One of a sebaceous gland.

c., seminal. A cyst of the epididymis, ductus deferens, or other sperm-carrying ducts which contains semen.

c., suprasellar. A cyst of the hypophyseal stalk just above the floor of the sella turcica. Its wall is frequently calcified or ossified.

c., tubo-ovarian. An ovarian cyst which ruptures into the lumen of an adherent uterine tube.

c., unilocular. C. containing only one cavity.

c., vaginal. Cystic formation in the vagina.

cyst, words pert. to: atheroma, encysted, endocyst, hydrocyst, hydroma, steatoma.

cystadenoma (sist-ad-en-o'mă) [G. *kystis,* bladder, + *adēn,* gland, + *-ōma,* tumor]. An adenoma containing cysts. Cystoma blended with adenoma.

c., pseudomucinous. One filled with a thick, viscid fluid and lined with tall epithelial cells.

c., serous. One filled with a clear, serous fluid and lined with cuboidal epithelial cells.

cystalgia (sis-tal'jĭ-ă) [" + *algos,* pain]. Paroxysms of pain in the bladder.

cystauxe (sist-awk'sē) [" + *auxe,* increase]. Enlargement or thickening of the urinary bladder.

cystectasy (sis-tek'tă-sĭ) [" + *ektasis,* dilatation]. 1. An operation for extracting calculus from the bladder by dividing the membranous portion of the urethra, and then dilating neck of bladder. 2. Dilatation of bladder.

cystectomy (sis-tek'to-mĭ) [G. *kystis,* bladder, + *ektomē,* excision]. 1. Removal of a cyst. 2. Excision of a cystic duct. 3. Excision of the gallbladder. 4. Excision of the urinary bladder or a part of it.

cysteine (sist'e-in). A sulfur-containing amino acid, $C_3H\text{-}NSO_2$, found among the decomposition products of proteins.

cys'tic. 1. Of or pertaining to a cyst. 2. Pertaining to the gallbladder. 3. Pertaining to the urinary bladder.

c. duct. The duct of the gallbladder which unites with the hepatic duct from the liver to form the common bile duct.

c. fibrosis. SYN: *fibrocystic disease of the pancreas; mucoviscidosis.* A disease of infants, children, adolescents, and young adults involving the exocrine glands, especially those secreting mucus, and resulting in pancreatic insufficiency, chronic pulmonary disease, abnormally high sweat electrolyte levels, and, in some cases, cirrhosis of the liver. Incomplete forms lead to variations in the manifestations. It has become apparent that cystic fibrosis is a disease which affects all of the exocrine glands including in most cases the pancreas and sweat glands. The affection is believed to be genetically transmitted. Although prognosis is poor, with the advent of effective antibiotics the life span of many of these patients has been prolonged.

c. tumor. Tumor composed of cysts.

cysticercoid (sĭs-tĭ-sĕr'koid). The larval encysted form of a tapeworm. It differs from a cysticercus in having a much reduced bladder.

cysticercosis (sis-tĭ-ser-ko'sis) [G. *kystis,* bladder, + *kerkos,* tail, + *-ōsis,* infection]. Infestation by larva *Taenia solium.*

cysticercus (sĭs-tĭ-sĕr'kŭs). The encysted larval form of a tapeworm consisting of a rounded cyst or bladder into which the scolex is invaginated. SYN: *bladderworm.*

c. cellulosae. Infestation by bladderworms (cysticerci) of the pork tapeworm, *Taenia solium.*

cysticotomy (sis-tĭ-kot'o-mĭ) [" + *tomē,* incision]. Incision of cystic bile duct. SYN: *choledochotomy.*

cys'tiform [" + L. *forma,* form]. Having the form of a cyst.

cystigerous (sis-tij'er-us) [" + L. *gerere,* to bear]. Containing cysts.

cystine [G. *kystis,* bladder]. $C_6H_{12}N_2S_2O_4$. A sulfur-containing amino acid, which can be obtained by oxidation from cysteine and which is likewise obtained from proteins.

cystinemia. The presence of cystine in blood.

cystinuria (sĭs-tĭn-ū'rĭ-ă) [G. *kystis,* bladder, + *ouron,* urine]. 1. The presence of cystine in urine. 2. A hereditary, metabolic disorder characterized by excretion of large amounts of cystine, lysine, arginine, and ornithine in the urine. Results in the development of recurrent urinary calculi.

cystistax'ia [" + *staxis,* dripping]. Blood oozing from the mucous membrane of the bladder.

cystitis (sis-tĭ'tis) [G. *kystis,* bladder, + *-ītis,* inflammation]. Inflammation of the bladder usually occurring secondarily to infections of associated organs (kidney, prostate, urethra). May be acute or chronic.

SYM: *Acute*: Frequent and painful urination. *Chronic:* Secondary to some other lesion with possibly pyuria as only symptom.

c. cystica and **granulosa.** *Chronic*: Slight frequency of urination. Chronic pyuria and painful irritation, perhaps hematuria. TREATMENT: Appropriate therapy for the underlying cause.

cystitome (sis′tĭ-tōm) [" + *tomē*, incision]. Instrument for incision into sac of crystalline lens.

cystit′omy [" + *tomē*, incision]. 1. Incision of capsule of crystalline lens. 2 Incision into the gallbladder. SYN: *cholecystotomy.*

cysto- [G.]. Prefix: Pert. to the urinary bladder or a cyst.

cystoadenoma (sis″to-ad-ĕ-no′mă) [G. *kystis*, bladder, + *adēn*, gland, + *-ōma*, tumor]. A tumor containing cystic and adenomatous elements.

cystocarcino′ma [" + *karkinos*, ulcer, + *-ōma*, tumor]. Glandular tumor distended with fluid secretion of the gland.

cystocele (sis′to-sēl) [" + *kēlē*, hernia] A bladder hernia.

Injury to the vesicovaginal fascia during delivery may allow the bladder to pouch into the vagina causing a cystocele.

cystocolos′tomy [" + *kōlon*, colon, + *stoma*, mouth]. Formation of communication bet. the gallbladder and colon.

cystodiaphanoscopy (sis″to-di-ă-fan-os′ko-pĭ) [" + *dia*, through, + *phanein*, to shine, + *skopein*, to examine]. Transillumination of abdomen by an electric light in bladder.

cystodyn′ia [" + *odynē*, pain]. Paroxysmal pains in the bladder. SYN: *cystalgia.*

cystoelytroplasty (sis″to-el′ĭ-tro-plas-tĭ) [" + *elytron*, vagina, + *plassein*, to form]. Repair of a vesicovaginal fistula

cystoepiplocele (sis″to-ĕ-pip′lo-sēl) [" + *epiploon*, omentum, + *kēlē*, hernia] Herniation of a portion of the bladder and the omentum.

cystoepithelio′ma [" + *epi*, upon, + *thēlē* nipple, + *-ōma*, tumor]. Epithelioma in stage of cystic degeneration.

cystofibro′ma [" + L. *fibra*, fiber, + G *-ōma*, tumor]. Fibrous tumor containing cysts.

cystogram (sis′to-gram) [" + *gramma* mark]. A roentgenogram of the bladder.

cystography (sis-tog′ră-fĭ) [" + *graphein* to write]. Taking roentgenograms of the bladder by using a radiopaque dye injected into the bladder.

cys′toid [" + *eidos*, appearance]. Bladderlike.

cystolith (sis′to-lith) [" + *lithos*, stone] A vesical calculus.

cystolithectomy (sis-to-lĭ-thek′to-mĭ) [" + " + *ektomē*, excision]. Excision of a stone from the bladder.

cystolithiasis (sis-to-lĭ-thi′ă-sis) [" + *lithos*, stone]. Calculi in the bladder.

cystolith′ic. Pert. to a vesical calculus.

cystolutein (sis-to-lu′te-in) [G. *kystis*, cyst, + L. *luteus*, yellow]. Yellow coloring matter in cysts.

cysto′ma (pl. *cysto′mata, cysto′mas*) [" + *-ōma*, tumor]. A cystic tumor; a growth containing cysts.

cystometer [" + *metron*, measure]. Device for estimating the capacity of the bladder and its changes in the bladder pressure.

cystomor′phous [" + *morphē*, form]. Cystlike; cystoid.

cystomyxoadenoma (sis″to-mik″so-ad-en-o′mă) [" + *myxa*, mucus, + *adēn*, gland, + *-ōma*, tumor]. Myxoma and adenoma with cystic degeneration.

cystomyxo′ma [" + " + *-ōma*, tumor] Myxoma with cystic formation.

cys′topexy [" + *pēxis*, fixation]. Surgical fixation of bladder to wall of abdomen.

cystoplasty (sis′to-plas-tĭ) [" + *plassein* to form]. Plastic operation upon the bladder.

cystoplegia (sis-to-ple′jĭ-ă) [" + *plēgē* stroke]. Paralysis of the bladder.

cystopto′sia, cystopto′sis [" + *ptōsis*, a dropping]. Prolapse into the urethra of the vesical mucous membrane.

cystopyelitis (sis-to-pi-ĕ-li′tis) [" + *pyelos*, pelvis, + *-itis*, inflammation]. Cystitis with pyelitis.

cystopyelonephritis (sis-to-pi-ĕ-lo-nef-ri′-tis) [" + " + *nephros*, kidney, + *-itis*, inflammation]. Inflammation of urinary bladder, kidney, and pelvis of kidney.

cystoradiog′raphy [" + L. *radius*, ray, + G. *graphein*, to write]. Radiography of the gallbladder or urinary bladder.

cystorectostomy (sis-to-rek-tos′to-mĭ) [" + L. *rectum*, + G. *stoma*, opening]. Establishment of a surgical communication bet. the bladder and rectum.

cystorrha′gia [" + *rēgnunai*, to burst forth]. Hemorrhage from the urinary bladder.

cystorrhaphy (sist-or′ă-fĭ) [" + *raphē*, suture]. Suture of bladder.

cystorrhe′a [" + *roia*, flow]. A discharge of mucus from the urinary bladder.

cystosarco′ma [" + *sarx*, flesh, + *-ōma*, tumor]. Sarcoma containing cysts or cystic formations.

cystoscope (sist′o-skōp) [" + *skopein*, to examine]. Instrument for interior examination of bladder.

cystoscopy (sis-tos′ko-pĭ) [" + *skopein*, to examine]. Examination of the bladder with the cystoscope.

cys′tospasm [" + *spasmos*, spasm]. Spasmodic contractions of the urinary bladder.

cystos′tomy [" + *stoma*, opening]. Surgical incision into the bladder to establish a temporary opening.

cystotome (sis′to-tōm) [" + *tomē*, incision]. Knife for incision of bladder.

cystotomy (sis-tot′o-mĭ) [" + *tomē*, incision]. Incision of bladder.

cystotrachelotomy (sis-to-tra-ke-lot′o-mĭ) [" + *trachelos*, neck, + *tomē*, incision]. Incision into neck of bladder. SYN: *cystauchenotomy.*

cystoureteritis (sis-to-u-re″ter-i′tis) [" + *ourētēr*, ureter, + *-itis*, inflammation]. Inflammation of ureter and urinary bladder.

cystoureterogram (sis″to-ū-rē′tĕr-ō-grăm] [" + " + *gramma*, mark]. Roentgenographic study of the bladder and ureter.

cystoure′throscope [" + *ourēthra*, urethra, + *skopein*, to examine]. Device for examining the post. urethra and urinary bladder.

cystovesiculography (sis″to-vĕ-sik-u-log′-ră-fē). Roentgenographic examination of the bladder and seminal vesicles.

cytase (si′tās) [" + *ase*, enzyme]. A ferment in phagocytes.

-cyte (sīt) [G. *kytos*, cell]. Suffix denoting cell.

cyto- [G.]. Indicating the cell.

cytoarchitectonic (si″to-ark-ĭ-tek-ton′ĭk) [G. *kytos*, cell, + *architektonikē*, architecture]. Pert. to structure and arrangement of cells.

cytobiology (si-to-bi-ol′o-jĭ) [″ + *bios*, life, + *logos*, study of]. Biology of cells.

cytobiotax′is [″ + ″ + *taxis*, arrangement]. The influence of cells upon other living cells. SYN: *cytoclesis.*

cy′toblast [″ + *blastos*, germ]. A cell nucleus. SEE: *cyton.*

cytocentrum (si-to-sen′trum) [″ + *kentron*, center]. Sphere of attraction.

cytoceras′tic [″ + *kerastos*, mixed]. Pert. to cells changing to a higher form. SYN: *cytokerastic.*

cytochemism (si-to-kem′izm) [″ + *chemeia*, chemistry, + *ismos*, condition of]. Reaction of body cells to chemical agents or the injections of antitoxin.

cytochem′istry [″ + *chemeia*, chemistry]. The chemistry of the living cell.

cytochrome (si′to-krōm) [″ + *chrōma*, color]. A pigment widely distributed in animals and plants. It plays an important role in cellular respiration. It is a mixture of three hemochromogens, designated cytochromes A, B and C.

c. oxidase. An enzyme of importance in biological oxidations functioning in the transfer of electrons from cytochromes to oxygen, thus activating oxygen which unites with hydrogen to form water.

cytochylema (si-to-ki-le′mă) [″ + *chylos*, juice]. The more fluid constituent of cell protoplasm. SYN: *hyaloplasm, q.v.*

cytoci′dal. Lethal to cells.

cytocide (si′to-sīd) [G. *kytos*, cell, + L. *caedere*, to kill]. That which causes the death of cells.

cytoclas′tic [″ + *klasis*, destruction]. Destructive to cells.

cytoclesis (si-to-kle′sis) [″ + *klēsis*, a call]. The influence of living cells upon other cells. SYN: *cytobiotaxis.*

cytocyst (si′to-sist) [″ + *kystis*, a cyst]. The remains of a cell enclosing a mature schizont.

cytoden′drite [″ + *dendron*, tree]. A dendrite given off from the body of a nerve cell.

cytodiagno′sis [″ + *dia*, through, + *gignoskein*, to know]. Diagnosis of pathogenic conditions by the study of cells present in exudates, fluids, etc.

cytodieresis (si-to-di-er′ĕ-sis) [″ + *diairesis*, division]. Cytokinesis, *q.v.*

cytodistal (si-to-dis′tal) [″ + *distāre*, to be distant]. Pert. to a neoplasm remote from the cell of origin.

cytofin (si′to-fin) [G. *kytos*, cell]. An alloxur body allied to a purine formed by thymic acid.

cy′togene. A plasmagene or cytoplasmic body responsible for extrachromosomal transmission of hereditary traits.

cytogenesis (si-to-jen′es-is) [″ + *genesis*, origin]. Origin and development of the cell.

cytogenet′ics. The study of cytology in relation to genetics, esp. the study of chromosomal behavior in mitosis and meiosis. Modern cytogenetics has led to the identification of chromosomes as bearers of the genes and deoxyribonucleic acid (DNA) as the key molecule of the gene.

cytogenous (si-toj′en-us) [″ + *gennan*, to produce]. Pertaining to the origin of cells.

cytogeny (si-toj′ĕ-nĭ) [″ + *gonē*, seed]. The formation of the cell.

cytoglobin (si-to-glo′bĭn) [″ + L. *globus*, sphere]. A globin from lymphocytes and leukocytes. SYN: *cytoglobulin.*

cytoglycopenia (si-to-gli-ko-pe′nĭ-ă) [″ + *glukos*, sweet, + *penia*, poverty]. Deficient glucose of blood cells. Also spelled *cytoglucopenia.*

cytohistogen′esis [″ + *istos*, web, + *genesis*, origin]. The structural development of cells.

cytohyaloplasm (si-to-hi′al-o-plazm) [″ + *yalos*, transparent, + *plasma*, matter]. Reticular network of protoplasm.

cytoid (si′toid) [″ + *eidos*, form]. Resembling a cell.

cytoinhibition (si″to-in-hĭ-bish′un) [″ + L. *inhibere*, to restrain]. Phagocytic cell action in preventing the destruction of ingested bacteria.

cytokalipenia (si″to-kal-ĭ-pē′nĭ-ă) [″ + L. *kalium*, potassium + G. *penia*, poverty]. A potassium deficiency in body or blood cells.

cytokeras′tic [″ + *kerastos*, mixed]. Pert. to cellular development from a lower to a higher form.

cytokine′sis [″ + *kinēsis*, movement]. The separation of the cytoplasm into two parts which occurs in the latter stages of mitosis or cell division. SYN: *cytodieresis.*

cytology (si-tol′o-jĭ) [″ + *logos*, study of]. The science which deals with the structure and function of cells.

cytolymph (si′to-limf) [″ + L. *lympha*]. Matrix of cytoplasm of cells.

cytolysin (si-tol′ĭ-sin) [″ + *lysis*, dissolution]. An antibody which causes disintegration of cells.

cytol′ysis [″ + *lysis*, destruction]. Dissolution or destruction of living cells. *Hemolysis* is the term used in case of red blood corpuscles, and *bacteriolysis* for bacteria.

cytomachia (si-to-mak′ĭ-ă) [″ + *machē*, fight]. Cellular activities and resistance during infection by microorganisms.

cytometaplasia (si″to-met-ă-pla′zĭ-ă) [″ + *metaplasis*, change]. Change of form or function of cells.

cytometer (si-tom′ĕ-ter) [″ + *metron*, measure]. Instrument for counting and measuring cells.

cytom′etry [″ + *metron*, measure]. The counting and measuring of cells.

cytomicrosome (si-to-mi′kro-sōm) [″ + *mikros*, small, + *sōma*, body]. Minute granules in the protoplasm (cytoplasm) of the cell.

cytom′itome [″ + *mitos*, thread]. Any part of the network of the cytoplasm.

cytomorphol′ogy [″ + *morphē*, form, + *logos*, study of]. The study of the structure of cells.

cytomorphosis (si-to-mor′fo-sis, - mor-fo′sis) [″ + ″ + *-ōsis*, infection]. The cellular transformations which a cell undergoes during its life.

cyton (si′ton) [G. *kytos*]. 1. A cell. 2. The body of a nerve cell; also called perikaryon.

cytopathogenic effect. In tissue culture, the morphologic changes seen in the cultured cells due to the effect of some pathogenic agent such as a virus.

cytopathology (sī″tō-păth-ŏl′ō-jĭ) [″ + *pathos*, disease, + *logos*, study]. Study of the cellular changes in disease.

cytope′nia [″ + *penia*, lack]. Diminution of cellular elements in blood or other tissues.

cytophagocyto′sis [″ + *phagein*, to eat, + *kytos* + *-ōsis*, infection]. Destruction of other cells by phagocytes. SYN: *cytophagy.*

cytophagous (si-tof'ă-gus) Devouring or destructive of cells.

cytophagy (si-tof'ăjĭ) [G. *kytos,* cell, + *phagein,* to eat]. Cell destruction by phagocytes. SYN: *cytophagocytosis.*

cytophilic (si-to-fil'ik) [" + *philein,* to love]. Having an affinity for or attracted by cells, *e.g.,* antibodies.

cytophylaxis (si-to-fi-lak'sis) [" + *phylaxis,* guarding against]. The protection of cells against lysis.

cytophylet'ic [" + *phylē,* tribe]. Pert. to genealogy of cells.

cytophys'ics [" + *physikē,* study of nature]. The physics of cellular activity.

cytophysiol'ogy [" + *physis,* nature, + *logos,* study]. Physiology of the cell.

cytoplasm (si'to-plazm) [" + *plasma,* matter]. 1. The protoplasm of a cell which envelops the nucleus. 2. Cell plasm not including the nucleus. SYN: *cytosome.*

cytoplas'tin [G. *kytos,* cell]. The plastin substance of the cytoplasm.

cytoproximal (si-to-proks'ĭ-mal) [" + L. *proximus,* nearest]. Pertaining to the portion of an axon nearest to the cell body from which it originates.

cytopyge (si-to-pī'jē). The cell anus or anal spot from which waste material is discharged from a cell as in certain protozoans.

cytoreticulum (si-to-ret-ik'u-lum) [" + L. *reticulum,* network]. The fibrillar network supporting fluid of protoplasm.

cytoscopy (si-tos'ko-pĭ) [" + *skopein,* to examine]. Microscopic examination of cells for purposes of diagnosis.

cytosome (si'to-sōm) [G. *kytos,* cell, + *sōma,* body]. The cytoplasm or the portion of the protoplasm of a cell exclusive of the nucleus.

cytospongium (si-to-spun'jĭ-um) [G. *kytos,* cell, + *spoggos,* sponge]. The fibrillar network of the cytoplasm of a cell.

cytost (si'tost) [G. *kytos,* cell]. A specific toxin given off by an injured or destroyed cell.

cytostasis (si-tos'tă-sis) [" + *stasis,* stoppage]. Stasis of white blood corpuscles, as in incipient stage of inflammation.

cytostatic (si"to-stat'ik) [" + *stasis,* standing still]. Preventing the growth and proliferation of cells.

cytotactic (si-to-tak'tik). Pert. to cytotaxia.

cytotax'ia, cytotax'is [G. *kytos,* cell, + *taxis,* arrangement]. Attraction or repulsion of cells for each other.

cytother'apy [" + *therapeia,* treatment]. 1. Treatment by use of glandular extracts; organotherapy. 2. Use of cytotoxic or cytolytic substances or serums in treating disease.

cytothesis (si-toth'ĕ-sis) [" + *thesis,* a placing]. Restoration or repair of injured cells.

cytotoxin (si-to-toks'in) [" + *toxikon,* poison]. An exotoxin that attacks different organs and tissues.

SEE: *endotoxin; erythrotoxin; exotoxin; leukocidin; lysis; neurotoxin.*

cytotrophoblast (si-to-tro'fo-blast) [" + *trophē,* nourishment, + *blastos,* germ]. The thin inner layer of the trophoblast composed of cuboidal cells, the outer layer being the syntrophoblast; also called layer of Langhans.

cytotropic (si-to-trop'ik, - trōp'ik) [" + *tropē,* a turn]. Having an affinity for cells.

cytozoon (sī-tō-zō'on). A protozoon which lives as an intracellular parasite.

cytozo'ic [" + *zōon,* animal]. Living within or attached to a cell, as certain protozoa.

cytula (si'tū-lă) [L. dim. of G. *kytos,* cell]. The impregnated ovum.

cyturia (si-tu'rĭ-ă) [G. *kytos,* cell, + *ouron,* urine]. Presence of any kind of cells in the urine.

Czermak's spaces (chār'māks). The interglobular spaces in dentine because of failure of calcification.

Notes

Notes

D

D. 1. Abbreviation for *da* (L. give); *detur* (L. let it be given); *dexter* (L. right); *deciduous; diopter; distal; divorced; dorsal; duration.* 2. Chem. symbol for *deuterium.*

D. and C. Abbreviation for the surgical procedure of dilatation of the cervix and curettage of the uterus.

dacnomania (dak"no-ma'nĭ-ă) [G. *daknein,* to bite + *mania,* insanity]. An irrational impulse to kill.

dacrocystitis (dak"ro-sis-ti'tis [G. *dakyron,* tear, + *kystis,* cyst, + *itis,* inflammation]. Inflammation of the lacrimal (tear) sac. SYN: *dacryocystitis, q.v.*

dacryadenal'gia [" + *adēn,* gland, + *algos,* pain]. Pain in a lacrimal gland.

dacryadeni'tis [" + " + *-ītis,* inflammation]. Inflammation of a lacrimal gland.

dacryadenoscirrhus (dak-rĭ-ad-ĕ-no-skir'-us) [" + " + *skirros,* hardening]. Induration of a lacrimal gland.

dacryagogatresia (dak'rĭ-ă-gog-ă-tre'sĭ-ă) [" + *agōgos,* leading, + *a-,* priv. + *trēsis,* perforate]. Occlusion of a tear duct.

dacryagogue (dak'rĭ-ă-gog) [" + *agōgos,* leading]. That which stimulates the secretion of tears.

dacrycystal'gia [" + *kystis,* cyst, + *algos.* pain]. Pain in a lacrimal gland; dacryocystalgia.

dacryelcosis (dak-rĭ-el-ko'sis) [" + *elkōsis,* ulceration]. Ulceration of the lacrimal apparatus.

dacryoadenal'gia [G. *dakryon,* tear, + *adēn,* gland, + *algos,* pain]. Dacryadenalgia; pain in a lacrimal gland.

dacryoadenitis (dak-rĭ-o-ad-ĕ-ni'tis) [" + " + *-ītis,* inflammation]. Inflammation of lacrimal gland.

Rare; seen as complication in epidemic parotitis (mumps of lacrimal gland); also present in Mikulicz's disease; may be acute or chronic. Neoplasms.

dacryoblennorrhe'a [" + *blenna,* mucus, + *roia,* flow]. Discharge of mucus from a lacrimal sac, and chronic inflammation of the sac.

dacryocele (dak'rĭ-o-sēl) [" + *kēlē,* hernia]. Protrusion of a lacrimal sac.

dacryocyst (dak'rĭ-o-sist) [" + *kystis,* cyst]. The lacrimal (tear) sac.

dacryocystalgia (dak-rĭ-o-sis-tal'jĭ-ă) [" + " + *algos,* pain]. Pain in the lacrimal sac.

dacryocystec'tomy [" + " + *ektomē,* excision]. The excision of membranes of the lacrimal sac.

dacryocystitis (dak-rĭ-o-sis-ti'tis) [" + " + *-ītis,* inflammation]. Inflammation of the tear sac involving mucous membrane of the lacrimal sac, together with submucous membrane, which later extends to connective tissue surrounding it, terminating in phlegmonous inflammation. Usually secondary to prolonged obstruction of the nasolacrimal duct.

SYM: Epiphora, redness and swelling in area of sac which may also extend to lids and conjunctiva; pain, esp. on pressure over the lacrimal sac; overflow of tears.

TREATMENT: Hot compresses; oral and ophthalmic antibiotic preparations; incision and drainage if fluctuant; attempt to restore permeability of duct with probe when acute symptoms have subsided; in chronic cases extirpate sac or do intranasal operation (dacryocystorrhinostomy).

dacryocystoblennorrhea (dak-rĭ-o-sis"to-blen-o-re'ă) [" + " + *blenna,* mucus, + *roia,* flow]. Chronic inflammation of and discharge from the lacrimal sac.

dacryocystocele (dak-rĭ-o-sis'to-sēl) [" + " + *kēlē,* hernia]. Protrusion of lacrimal sac.

dacryocystopto'sis [" + " + *ptōsis,* a falling]. Prolapse of the lacrimal (tear) sac.

dacryocystorrhinostomy (dak-rĭ-o-sis-to-rĭ-nos'to-mĭ) [" + " + *ris,* nose, + *stoma,* opening]. Lumen of tear sac brought into direct communication with nasal cavity.

dacryocystosyringotomy (dak"rĭ-o-sis"to-sĭr-in-got'o-mĭ) [" + " + *syrigx,* tube, + *tomē,* incision]. Making an opening bet. the lacrimal sac and the nasal cavity.

dacryocystotome (dak-rĭ-o-sis'to-tōm) [" + " + *tomē,* incision]. Device for incision of lacrimal sac.

dacryocystot'omy [" + " + *tomē,* incision]. Incision of the lacrimal sac.

dacryohemorrhea (dak"rĭ-o-hem-o-re'ă) [" + *aima,* blood, + *roia,* flow]. Shedding of bloody tears.

dac'ryolin [G. *dakryon,* tear]. An albuminous matter in tears.

dac'ryolith [" + *lithos,* stone]. Concretion in lacrimal passages. SYN: *dacryolite.*

dacryoma (dak-rĭ-o'mă) [" + *-ōma,* tumor]. 1. A lacrimal tumor. 2. Obstruction of lacrimal puncta producing epiphora.

dacryon (dak'rĭ-on) [G. *dakryon*]. The lacrimal point of juncture of the lacrimal, frontal, and upper maxillary bones.

dacryops (dak'rĭ-ops) [G. *dakry,* tear, + *ops,* eye]. Constant flow of tears; dacryorrhea.

dacryopyorrhea (dak"rĭ-o-pi-o-re'ă) [" + *pyon,* pus, + *roia,* discharge]. Discharge of pus from lacrimal duct.

dacryopyo'sis [" + *pyōsis,* suppuration]. Suppuration in the lacrimal sac or duct.

dacryorrhe'a [" + *roia,* flow]. Excessive flow of tears.

dacryosolenitis (dak"-rĭ-o-so-len-i'tĭs) [" + *sōlēn,* duct, + *-ītis,* inflammation]. Inflammation of a lacrimal or nasal duct.

dacryosteno'sis [" + *stenōsis,* narrowing]. Stricture of a lacrimal or nasal duct.

dacryosyr'inx [" + *syrigx,* tube]. A lacrimal fistula.

dactyl (dak'til) [G. *daktylos,* finger]. A finger or toe; a digit of the hand or foot.

dactyl'ion [G. *daktylos,* finger]. Adhesions bet. or union of fingers or toes.

dactyli'tis [" + *-ītis,* inflammation]. Chronic inflammation of bones of fingers and toes in very young children.

ETIOL: Usually tuberculous or syphilitic.

d., sickle cell. Painful swelling of the feet and hands during the first several years of life of children with sickle cell anemia. SYN: *hand and foot syndrome.*

dactylocampsodynia (dak"tĭ-lo-kamp"so-din'ĭ-ă) [" + *kampsis,* bend, + *odynē,* pain]. Painful contraction of one or more fingers.

dactyl'ogram [" + *gramma,* a mark]. A fingerprint.

dactylog'raphy [" + *graphein,* to write]. 1. The study of fingerprints. 2. The act of using a machine for blind deaf mutes to convey by touch the signs of speech.

dactylogryposis (dak-tĭ-lo-grĭ-po'sis) [" + *gryposis,* curve]. Permanent contraction of the fingers.

dactylology (dak-til-ol'o-jĭ) [" + *logos,* study]. Representing words by signs made with the fingers. SYN: *sign language.*

dactylomeg'aly [" + *megas,* large]. Abnormal size of fingers and toes.

dactylos'copy [" + *skopein,* to examine]. Examination of fingerprints for purpose of identification.

dactylospasm (dak'til-o-spazm) [" + *spasmos,* spasm]. Cramp of a finger or toe.

dactylus (dak'ti-lus) [G. *daktylos*]. A toe or finger.

Dakin's solution [Henry D. Dakin, American chemist, 1880-1952]. A solution for cleansing wounds; developed during World War I.

A very dilute neutral solution (0.45 to 0.5%) of sodium hypochlorite and 0.4% boric acid.

SEE: *chlorine preparations.*

daltonism (dawl'ton-izm). Color blindness.

dam. A thin sheet of rubber to protect cavities or the field of dental operation from fluids.

damp (damp). 1. Moist, humid. 2. A noxious gas.

d., after-. Air containing large percentage of carbon dioxide.

d., black, choke. A gas formed by oxygen and the giving off of carbon dioxide by the coal.

d., cold. Vapor charged with carbon dioxide.

d., fire. Methane, CH_4, found in coal mines.

d., stink. Hydrogen sulfide.

d., white. Carbon monoxide.

damping. The steady diminution of the amplitude of successive vibrations, as of an electric wave or current.

dance, St. Vitus'. A disease characterized by involuntary and irregular jerkings and movements in diverse groups of muscles. SEE: *chorea.*

Dan'ce's sign [Jean B. H. Dance, French physician, 1797-1832]. Slight retraction in the right iliac region in some cases of intussusception.

dan'cing disease. Epidemic dancing mania of Europe during the Middle Ages, supposed to have been caused by the bite of the tarantula. SEE: *tarantism.*

d. mania. Epidemic chorea.

dandelion greens. Those of a well-known plant which grows both as a weed and cultivated. They are bitter and tonic, and are eaten like spinach.

COOKED: 100 gm. Calories: 35. Other main values: 2 gm. protein; 0.6 gm. fat; 6.4 gm. carbohydrate; 140 mg. calcium; 11,700 I.U. vitamin A; 18 mg. ascorbic acid.

dan'druff. Exfoliation of the epidermis of the scalp in the form of dry, white scales. Sometimes due to seborrhea.*

dandy fever (dan'dĭ). Dengue, *q.v.* An acute, epidemic, febrile disease occurring in tropical areas.

Danielssen's disease [Daniel C. Danielssen, Norwegian physician, 1815-1894]. Anesthetic leprosy.

d'Arsonvalism (ar-son-val'izm). Obsolete term indicating the employment of d'Arsonval current therapeutically.

d'Arsonvalization (ar-son-val-iz-a'shun). The employment of the d'Arsonval current in the form of autocondensation, autoconduction, or the direct biterminal method. SEE: *diathermy.*

dartoid (dar'toid) [G. *dartos,* skinned, + *eidos,* form]. Resembling the *tunica dartos* in its slow, involuntary contractions.

dar'tos [G.]. The muscular, contractile tissue beneath the skin of the scrotum. SYN: *tunica dartos* [NA].

d. muscle reflex. Wormlike contraction of dartos muscle following sudden cold application to perineum.

dartre (dar'tr) [Fr.]. Any chronic skin disease.

dar'trous [G. *dartos,* skinned]. Of the nature of herpes; herpetic.

darwin'ian ear. An exaggeration of darwinian tubercle, *q.v.*

d. tubercle. A blunt point projecting from upper part of the helix.

dasetherapy (das-e-ther'ă-pĭ) [G. *dasos,* forest, + *therapeia,* treatment]. Treatment of disease by residence in a region of pine and spruce trees.

dasym'eter [" + *metron,* measure]. Device for estimating density of gases.

date. The fruit of the palm; an oblong berry with a grooved seed.

NATURAL, DRY: 100 gm. Calories: 275. Other main values: 2.2 gm. protein; 0.5 gm. fat; 73 gm. carbohydrate; 59 mg. calcium; 50 I.U. vitamin A.

daturine (da-tu'rin). The active principle of stramonium. A poisonous alkaloid. USES: Manias, epilepsy, as a hypnotic in insanity, etc. Action resembles atropine, *q.v.*

daughter cell. One formed by the division of a mother cell.

d. cyst. A small c. growing out of the walls of a large c.

d. nucleus. Formation of a new n. by a diaster.

Davidsohn's sign [Hermann Davidsohn, Prussian physician, 1842-1911]. The lessening or absence of pupillary light reflex when an electric light is held in the closed mouth. Indicates presence of a tumor or fluid in the maxillary sinus.

day blind'ness. Inability to see well in a bright light.

DDT. Abbreviation for dichloro-diphenyl-trichloroethane now called chlorophenothane. A powerful insecticide effective against a wide variety of insects, esp. the flea, fly, louse, mosquito, bedbug, cockroach, Japanese beetle and European corn borer.

Toxicity. When ingested orally may cause acute poisoning. Symptoms are vomiting, numbness and partial paralysis of limbs, anorexia, tremors, depression and death.

de- [L.]. Prefix: Down or from.

deacidifica'tion [L. *de,* from, + *acidus,* sour, + *facere,* to make]. Neutralization of acidity.

deactivation [" + *activus,* acting]. The process of becoming inactive.

dead [A.S. *dēad*]. Cessation of life or life processes.

When death has occurred in a hospital or other institution for care of the sick, the patient's name, hour of death, and name of the ward should be written on a piece of paper and pinned to the front of the nightdress, or identified according to the custom of the institution. It is important that the "laying out" be completed before the commencement of rigor mortis. If the doctor is not present at the time of death immediate steps must be taken to inform him, since no preparation of the body may be begun until the doctor has officially pronounced the patient dead. It will sometimes happen that the private duty nurse will be asked to continue on duty for several hours, but, in any case, she will not hurry away until assured everything in the room is in order, and that she can be of no further service. SEE: *death.*

deaf mute. A person who is unable to hear or speak.

deaf-mut'ism. The state of being both deaf and dumb.

deafness [A.S.]. Loss of ability to hear, complete or partial.

ETIOL: May occur from several causes, such as (1) injury or disease of that part of the *cortex* controlling the center for hearing; (2) hysteria, without any abnormality of the ear or brain; (3) injury of the ear from loud noises such as the firing of a gun at close range; (4) disease of the labyrinth of the internal ear; (5) an abnormal mental state may produce auditory aphasia or psychic d., *q.v.* (6) Congenital defects.

Some forms of conduction deafness may be remedied by a fenestration operation or stapes mobilization. SEE: *otosclerosis.*

d., aviator's. A nerve deafness temporary or permanent, found in a moderate percentage of aviators. This form of deafness is due to prolonged exposure to loud noise levels.

d., bass. Inability to hear some of the low tones.

d. central. Deafness resulting from lesions of auditory tracts of the brain or auditory centers of the cerebral cortex.

d., cerebral. Due to brain lesion.

d., ceruminous. Deafness due to plugs of cerumen (ear wax).

d. conduction. Deafness resulting from any condition which prevents sound waves from being transmitted to the auditory receptors. May be due to (a) wax obstructing ext. auditory meatus; (b) inflammation of the middle ear; (c) ankylosis of ear bones; (d) fixation of footplate of stirrup. SEE: *otosclerosis.*

d., cortical. D. due to disease of the cortical centers.

d., mind. SEE: *psychic d.*

d., nerve. Perception d.

d., occupational. That which is caused by working in places where noise levels are quite high. Persons working in such an environment should wear devices to protect the hearing sense from the noise.

d. perception or nerve deafness. Deafness resulting from lesions involving sensory receptors of cochlea or fibers of the acoustic nerve.

d., psychic. Condition in which auditory sensations are perceived, but the sounds are not comprehended.

d., simulated. Malingering.

d., tone. Inability to distinguish musical sounds.

d., word. Ability to hear sounds but interpretation of the meaning of words is not possible.

dealbation (de-al-ba'shun) [L. *dē,* from, + *albāre,* to whiten]. Bleaching.

deam'inase. An enzyme which causes deaminization.

de"amina'tion. Deaminization, *q.v.*

deaminization (de-am-in-i-za'shun). A chemical decomposition whereby substances like the amino acids and alkaloids lose their amino groups and form ammonia.

Alanine can be deaminized to give ammonia and pyruvic acid: $CH_3CH(NH_2)$-$COOH + O = CH_3.CO.COOH + NH_3$. Each tissue is supposed to deaminize its amino acids. Deaminization may be simple, oxidative, or hydrolytic. Oxidizing enzymes are called deaminizing enzymes, when the oxidation is accompanied by splitting off of amino groups.

deanesthe'siant [L. *dē,* from, + G. *an-,* priv. + *aisthēsis,* sensation]. That which will overcome anesthesia.

deaquation (de-ă-kwa'shun) [" + *aqua.* water]. Dehydration, *q.v.*

dearterializa'tion [" + G. *artēria,* artery]. Changing character of arterial into venous blood; deoxygenation.

death (dĕth) [A.S. *death*]. Permanent cessation of all vital functions.

The following definitions of death have also been considered: 1. Total irreversible cessation of cerebral function, spontaneous function of the respiratory system, spontaneous function of the circulatory system. 2. The final and irreversible cessation of perceptible heart beat and respiration. Conversely, as long as any heart beat or respiration can be perceived, either with or without mechanical or electrical aids and regardless of how the heart beat and respiration were maintained, death has not occurred.

NOTE: Defining death is complicated. Conditions such as cardiac standstill or complete lack of renal function would have meant certain death at one time. The use of cardiac pacemakers, artificial hearts and kidneys, heart transplants, and kidney transplants have made delaying death possible.

d., black. Plague, *q.v.*

d., causes. (1) *Gradual wearing out of tissue and loss of energy with cessation of function without disease* as in old age. (2) Result of *disease represented by the culmination of its ravages* in the ordinary progress of the affection or as sudden death. (3) Result of *injury from accidents.* Injury is considered the major cause of death, although there is scarcely a disease known that may not be a cause of sudden death. (4) *Sudden death* may be result of circulatory failure, cerebral causes, respiratory causes, neuroendocrinohumeral causes, shock, intoxications, obstetrical causes, infantile causes. (5) *Loss of will to live.* In some cases persons who would be expected to recover from their illness die despite extreme effort being made to keep them alive. For want of a better explanation, these persons are said to have lost their will to live. They have in fact willed to die.

d., local. Gangrene or necrosis of a part.

d., molar. SEE: *local d.*

d., molecular. That of cell life.

d. rate. This is the number of deaths occurring per 1000 of the population in a given area within a specified time.

d. rattle. Sound heard in the throat of the dying.

d., signs of. NURSES'S OBSERVATIONS: The principal one is (a) cessation of the heart's action. Other indications are (b) opaqueness of the cornea; (c) the absence of reflexes; (d) manifestations of *rigor mortis;* (e) a mottled discoloration of the body, esp. over all parts where there is pressure. Many cases of death have been reported only to find after 24 hours that the person was not dead. For such reasons more or less elaborate tests have sometimes been used to determine without doubt whether life is or is not extinct. The signs mentioned usually are sufficient to confirm one's opinion that death has taken place. Call doctor.

d., somatic. That of the entire organism.

d. tests. Both the electrocardiogram and electroencephalogram have been used to determine death but neither test is infallible. Other tests are: (a) A drop of ether is instilled into the conjunctival sac of one eye, the other being used as control. A reddening of the conjunctiva proves that life is present. (b) Sometimes the physician may pass a stylet through a small incision in the first intercostal spaces to the heart. Any movement of the heart will be communicated through the stylet. Removing the stylet may induce cardiac movement which may be augmented by artificial respiration. (c) A piece of litmus paper has been used under the eyelid, an acid reaction being shown by contact with the tears, the blood, or the organ in contact with the paper if death has taken place. (d) Moisture appearing upon the face of a mirror held over the mouth and nostrils is indicative that life is not extinct.

d., to determine how long since it occurred. Take the rectal temperature. In general the body loses one degree of Fahrenheit temperature each hour following death. The rate of heat loss would, of course, vary with the temperature of the surrounding air, water or snow.

In an emergency, the usual symptoms of death are often found to be unreliable. Attempts at resuscitation should continue to be made indefinitely. No harm can be done in attempting to resuscitate one who seems to be deceased. Successes are numerous.

d., voodoo. In studying certain primitive societies it has been established that the witch doctor or *shaman* may at least appear to cause death in persons who he has caused to believe are under his "spell" or control.

death, *words pert. to:* agonal, agonia ante mortem, autophonia, autopsy, demise, euthanasia, in articulo mortis, in extremis, lethal, "necr-" words, posthumous, post mortem, putrefaction, rigor mortis, suicide.

death-bed state'ment. A declaration made at the time immediately preceding death.

Such a statement, if made with the consciousness and belief that death is impending, is held in law as equally binding with a statement made under oath. SYN: *ante-mortem statement.*

debil'itant [L. *debilis,* weak]. 1. A remedy used to reduce excitement. 2. That which weakens.

debil'itate [L. *debilis,* weak]. To produce weakness or debility.

debil'ity [L. *debilis,* weak]. Weakness of tonicity in functions or organs of the body.

debouchement (da-boosh-mon') [Fr.]. Opening or emptying into another part.

Debove's membrane (de-bovz') [George Maurice Débove, French physician, 1845-1920]. Layer of connective tissue cells bet. the epithelium and basement tissue of mucous membranes of air passages and intestinal mucosa.

débridement (da-bred-mon') [Fr.]. In surgery, the removal of foreign material, dead or damaged tissue especially in a wound.

debris (dĕ-brē') [F. remains]. The remains of broken down or damaged cells or tissue.

deca-, dec- [G. *deka*]. Prefix: Ten.

decagram (dek'a-gram) [G. *deka,* ten, + *gramma,* weight]. A weight of 10 gm. or 154.323 gr.

decalcification (dē-kăl-sĭ-fĭ-kā'shŭn) [L. *dē,* down, + *calx,* lime, + *facere,* to make]. The removal of or the withdrawal of lime salts from bone.

decal'cify [" + *calx,* lime]. To soften bone by removal of calcium or its salts by acids.

decaliter (dek'ă-le-ter([G. *deka,* ten, + Fr. *litre*]. A measure of 10 liters; 610.28 cu. in.

decalvant (de-kal'vant) [L. *dēcalvāre,* to make bald]. Destroying hair or making bald.

decameter (dek'ă-mē-ter) [G. *deka,* ten, + *metron,* measure]. A measure of 10 meters; 393.71 in.

decanormal (dek-ă-nor'mal) [" + L. *norma,* rule]. Pert. to a solution 10 times as strong as a normal one.

decant (dē-kant') [L. *dē,* from, + *canthus,* corner]. To pour off liquid so the sediment remains in the bottom of the container.

de"canta'tion [" + *canthus,* corner]. The gentle pouring off of a liquid from its sediment.

decapita'tion (dē-kăp-ĭ-tā'shŭn) [" + *caput, head*]. SYN: *decollation.* (1) The separation of the head from the body; beheading. (2) In obstetrics, the separation of the head of the fetus from the body to facilitate delivery. (3) Separating the head from the shaft of a bone.

decapryn succinate. Proprietary name for doxylamine succinate, an antihistaminic agent.

decapsula'tion [" + *capsula,* little box] Removal of a capsule of an organ.

decarboxylation, decarboxylization (de-kar-boks-ĭ-la'shun, i-za'shun). A chemical decomposition whereby substances like the amino acids lose their carboxyl (COOH) groups. SEE: *aporrhegma* (def. 2).

decay' [L. *dē,* down, + *cadere,* to fall]. 1. Gradual loss of vigor with physical and mental deterioration as in aging. SEE: *senility.* 2. To waste away. 3. Decomposition of organic matter by the action of microorganisms in the presence of air. SEE: *cementoclasia.* 4. Disintegration of radioactive substances.

deceleration (de-sel"ĕ-ra'shun). To decrease in speed or rate.

decerebrate (de-ser'ĕ-brāt). A person or animal who has been subjected to decerebration.

decerebration (de-ser-ĕ-bra'shun) [" + *cerebrum,* brain]. Removal of the brain or cutting the spinal cord at the level of the brain stem.

dechlorina'tion [" + G. *chloros,* green]. Reduction in the amount of chlorides in the body by reduction of or withdrawal of salt in the diet. SYN: *dechloridation.*

deci- [L.]. Prefix: *Decimus,* tenth.

decibel (des'ĭ-bel) [L. *deci,* + *bel,* unit of sound]. The unit of intensity and volume of sound.

decidua (de-sid'u-ă) [L. *deciduus,* falling off]. The name given to the endometrium or mucous membrane when conception occurs and which envelops the impregnated ovum.

This may be seen in both the uterine and ectopic pregnancies. The gland structures of the endometrium and the interstitial cells undergo marked hypertrophy. The decidua divides itself into an outer, or compact layer, and an inner spongy layer.

d. basalis [NA]. That part of the decidua which unites with the chorion to form the placenta. SYN: *d. serotina.*

d. capsularis [NA]. That part of the decidua which surrounds the chorionic sac. SYN: *d. reflexa.*

d. graviditatis. The pregnancy decidua.

d. menstrualis. The layer of the uterine endometrium that is shed during menstruation.

d. parietalis [NA]. The nonplacental lining of the uterus; the decidua. SYN: *d. vera.*

d., reflexa. Decidua capsularis.

d. serotina. Decidua basalis.

d. vera. Decidua parietalis.

decidual (de-sid'u-al). Pert. to or resembling the decidua.

decidualitis (de-sid-u-al-i'tis) [L. *deciduus,* falling off, + G. *-ītis,* inflammation]. A bacterial infection of the decidua.

deciduation (de-sid-u-a'shun) [L. *deciduus,* falling off]. The loss of the decidua during menstruation.

deciduitis (de-sid-u-i'tis) [" + G. *-ītis,* inflammation]. Inflammation of the decidua.

deciduoma (de-sid-u-o'ma) [" + G. *-ōma,* tumor.] A uterine tumor containing decidual tissue. Thought to arise from portions of decidua retained within the uterus following an abortion.

d., benign. The more or less normal invasion of the uterine musculature by the syncytium which disappears after the gestation is completed.

d., Loeb's. Decidual tissue produced within the uterus of experimental animals as a result of mechanical or hormonal stimulation.

d., malignant. A tumor consisting of syncytial and Langhans cells which have a tendency to invade the general system by means of the blood stream, and having a high mortality. SYN: *choriocarcinoma; chorionepithelioma.*

ETIOL: This tumor arises following a full term pregnancy, an ectopic pregnancy, an abortion, a miscarriage, and particularly a vesicular mole.

DIAG: May be made by histologic study, aided by the symptoms and the Aschheim-Zondek test which remains strongly positive during the presence of this type of tumor.

TREATMENT: The treatment is the surgical removal of the uterus, and adnexae, and any local growths that may be accessible. This should be followed by deep x-ray therapy over the pelvis and the secondary growths.

deciduomatosis (de-sid-u-o-mă-to'sis) [" + " + *-ōsis,* infection]. Excessive and irregular formation of decidual tissue in the nonpregnant state.

deciduosarco'ma [" + G. *sarx,* flesh, + *-ōma,* tumor]. A tumor of the chorion. SYN: *choriocarcinoma; chorionepithelioma.*

deciduous (de-sid'u-us) [L. *deciduus,* falling off]. Falling off.

d. teeth. The milk teeth or temporary teeth, 10 in each jaw: 4 incisors, 2 canines, and 4 molars. They usually appear at 6 months and are lost by the end of 6 years. Those of the lower jaw appear before the upper ones, as follows: *Lower central incisors,* at 5-9 months. *Upper incisors,* at 8-12 months. *Lower lateral incisors and first molars,* at 12-15 months. *Canines,* at 18-24 months. *Second molars,* at 24-30 months. SEE: *dentition.*

decigram (des'ĭ-gram) [L. *deci,* ten, + G. *gramma,* weight]. One-tenth of a gram, about 1.54 gr.

deciliter (des'ĭ-lī-ter) [" + Fr. *litre*]. One-tenth of a liter; 6.1 cu. in.

decimeter (des'ĭ-me-ter) [" + G. *metron,* measure]. One-tenth of a meter; 3.93 in.

decinor'mal (des-ĭ-nor'mal) [" + *norma,* rule]. Having one-tenth the standard strength.

declinator (dek'lin-a-tor) [L. *declināre,* to turn aside]. Instrument used during trephining for holding apart the dura mater.

decline (de-klīn') [L. *declināre,* to turn aside]. 1. Progressive decrease. 2. Declining period of a disease.

declivis cerebel'li (de-klīv'is). Sloping post. portion of the monticulus of the sup. vermis of the cerebellum.

decoction (de-kok'shun) [L. *dē,* down, + *coquere,* to boil]. A liquid preparation made by boiling vegetable substances with water.

When the strength and method of preparation are not otherwise specified, it is made by boiling 5 parts of the coarsely comminuted drug for 15 minutes with enough water to make 100 parts. There are no official decoctions. SEE: *apothem, apozeme.*

decollation (de"kol-a'shun) [" + *collum,* neck]. Fetal decapitation. SYN: *detruncation.*

decollator (de'kol-ă-ter). Device for decapitation of the fetus.

décollement (de-kol-mon') [Fr. ungluing]. Separation of 2 normally adherent structures.

decompensa'tion [L. *dē* + *compensāre,* to make good again]. Failure of compensation, as in circulation of the heart.

decom'plementize. To take away the complement from.

decomposition (de-com-po-zish'un) [" + *componere,* to put together]. 1. The putrefactive process; decay. 2. Reducing a compound body to its simpler constituents. SEE: *fermentation, resolution.*

d., double. A chemical change in which the molecules of 2 interacting compounds exchange a portion of their constituents.

d., hydrolytic. 1. Chemical change in substances due to addition of a molecule of water.

d., simple. A chemical change by which a molecule of a single compound breaks into its simpler constituents or substitutes the entire molecule of another body for 1 of these constituents.

decompres'sion [" + *compressio*, a squeezing together. 1. The removal of pressure, as from gas in the intestinal tract. SEE: *Wangensteen's method.* 2. The slow reduction or removal of pressure on deep-sea divers and caisson workers to prevent development of bends, *q.v.*

d. chamber. A tank in which patients suffering from decompression sickness are placed. After entry into the chamber, the barometric pressure is increased and then very slowly decreased until pressure is equal to outside pressure.

d., explosive. In aviators or divers, decompression resulting from an extremely rapid rate of change from one pressure to a much less pressure. This may occur if a high altitude aircraft suddenly loses its cabin pressurization or if a diver ascends quite rapidly. Causes violent expansion of involved gases.

d. illness or sickness. Caisson disease, or bends, q. v., compressed air illness.

de"contamina'tion. The process of rendering an object, person, or area free of a contaminating substance such as a poison-gas or radioactive substance.

de"cortica'tion [" + *cortex*, bark]. The removal of the surface layer of an organ or structure, as the removal of a portion of the cortex of the brain from the underlying white portion.

d. pulmonary. Removal of the pleura of the lung, or a portion of the surface lung-tissue.

d. renal. Removal of capsule of the kidney.

dec'rement [L. *decrementum*, decrease]. Declining period of a disease.

decrep'itate [L. *decrepitāre*, to crackle]. To cause decrepitation or a crackling noise.

decrepita'tion [L. *decrepitāre*, to crackle]. A crackling noise.

decrepitude (de-krep'ĭ-tud) [L. *decrepitāre*, to rattle]. Senile breaking down.

decubation (de-ku-ba'shun) [L. *dē*, down, + *cumbere*, to lie]. 1. The act of lying down. 2. The recovery stage of an infectious disease.

decu'bital [" + *cumbere*, to lie]. Pert. to a bed sore.

decubitus (de-ku'bi-tus) [L. a lying down]. 1. A bedsore.* 2. A patient's position in bed.

d., acute. Bedsore on one side due to hemiplegia.

decussate (de-kus'at) [L. *decussāre*, to cross, as an x]. To cross, or crossed, as in the form of the letter *x*. Interlacing or crossing of parts.

decussa'tion. 1. A crossing of structures in form of an x. 2. The place of crossing; chiasma.

d. of the pyramids. Crossing of fibers of pyramids of the medulla oblongata from 1 pyramid to the other.

d. optic. The crossing of the fibers of the optic nerves; the optic chiasma.

decussorium (de-kus-o'rĭ-um) [L. *decussāre*, to cross, as an x]. Instrument for depression of the dura following trephining.

deep reflexes (dēp). Opposite of superficial or skin reflexes; reflexes within, or fractional stretch reflexes.

Deer fly. A biting fly, *Chrysops discalis*, which transmits the causative organism of deerfly fever, a form of tularemia.

d.f. fever. Tularemia, *q.v.*

defat'ted [" + A.S. *fǣlt*, to fatten]. Deprived of fat.

defecalgesiophobia (def"ĕ-kal-je-sĭ-o-fo'-bĭ-ă) [L. *defaecāre*, to remove dregs, + G. *algēsis*, pain, + *phobos*, fear]. Fear of defecating because of pain.

defecation (def-ĕ-ka'shun) [L. *defaecāre*, to remove the dregs]. Evacuation of the bowels.

The bulk of the feces depends upon the amount and composition of food ingested. One does not, however, have to eat in order to have bowel movements. A large quantity of cellular material is desquamated from the epithelial lining of the intestinal tract each day.

The food residues, reaching the rectum, cause a sensation referred to as a "call to stool," or the urge to defecate. The sensation is related to periodic increase of pressure within the rectum and contracture of its musculature.

The expulsion of a fecal mass is accompanied by coordinated action of the following mechanisms: (1) Involuntary contraction of the circular muscle of the rectum behind the mass, followed by contraction of the longitudinal muscle; (2) relaxation of the internal (involuntary) and external (voluntary) sphincter ani; (3) voluntary closure of the glottis, fixation of the chest, and contraction of the abdominal muscles, causing an increase in intra-abdominal pressure. SEE: *cacatory; constipation; feces; stool.*

de'fect. A flaw or imperfection.

d., congenital. Imperfection present at birth.

d., filling. Interruption in the contour of the inner surface of the stomach or intestine revealed by roentgenography.

defec'tive [L. *defectus*, a failure]. 1. Not perfect. 2. A person deficient in one or more physical, mental, or moral powers.

defensive protein. An antibody, *q.v.*

d. reflex. Retraction or tension in defense against an action or threatened action.

deferens (def'er-enz) [L. carrying away]. Ductus or *vās deferens.*

deferent (def'er-ent) [L. *deferre*, to carry away]. Away from or downward. SEE: *afferent; efferent.*

d. duct. Ductus deferens.

deferentectomy (def-er-en-tek'to-mĭ) [" + G. *ektomē*, excision]. Cutting of the ductus deferens. SYN: *vasectomy.*

deferential (def-er-en'shal) [L. *deferre*, to carry away]. Pert. to or accompanying the ductus deferens.

deferentitis (def-er-en-ti'tis) [" + G. *-ītis*, inflammation]. Inflammation of the ductus deferens.

deferred' shock. Delayed onset of symptoms of shock.

deferves'cence [L. *defervescere*, to become calm]. The period that marks the subsidence of fever to normal temperature.

defibrina'tion, defibriniza'tion [L. *dē*, from, + *fibra*, fiber]. Process of being deprived of fibrin. SEE: *coagulation.*

defi'ciency [L. *deficere*, to lack]. A lack, something missing.

d. disease. One due to a deficiency of a substance essential in body metabolism.

The deficiency may be due to inadequate intake, inadequate digestion, inadequate absorption, inadequate utilization, or excessive loss through excretory channels, or excess loss to a parasite such as a hookworm or tapeworm.

EXAMPLES: Night blindness and keratomalacia due to lack of vitamin A; beriberi, polyneuritis, due to lack of thiamine; pellagra due to lack of niacin; ariboflavinosis due to lack of riboflavin; scurvy due to lack of vitamin C; rickets and osteomalacia due to lack of vitamin D; pernicious anemia due to lack of folic acid and vitamin B_{12}.

d., mental. Feeblemindedness.

definition [L. *definire*, to limit]. The precise determination of the limits of anything, esp. a disease process.

defin'itive. Clear and final; without question.

deflagra'tion [L. *deflagrāre*, to burn furiously]. Sudden, sharp combustion usually with a crackling sound.

defloration (def-lo-ra'shun) [L. *dē*, from, + *flos, flor-*, flower]. Rupture of the hymen, either during coitus, by accident, or vaginal examination. As a rule the tear is in the posterior edge. NOTE: Not many females have a hymen which is of such size or consistency as to require its rupture. SEE: *virginity; hymen.*

deflores'cence. Disappearance of an eruption of the skin.

defluvium (dē-flu'vĭ-um) [L. *defluere*, to flow down]. Falling out or sudden loss of the hair.

defluxio (de-fluk'she-o) [L.]. A flowing down.

d. capillorum. A falling out of hair.

d. ciliorum. A falling out of eyelashes.

defluxion (de-fluk'shun) [L. *defluxio*, a down flowing]. A flowing down; copious discharge or loss of any kind.

deforma'tion [L. *dē*, from, + *forma*, form]. The act of deforming; a disfiguration.

deform'ities. If present after injury, usually imply presence of fracture or dislocation, or both. May be due to extensive swelling, extravasation of blood, rupture of muscles, etc.

deform'ity. An unnatural alteration in the form of a part or organ. Distortion of any part or general disfigurement of the body. It may be acquired or congenital.

d., anterior. Abnormal ant. convexity of the spine. SYN: *lordosis.**

d., gunstock. One in which the forearm when extended makes an angle with the arm, because of displacement of axis of the extended arm. ETIOL: Condylar fracture at elbow.

d., Madelung's. Distortion of the radius at its lower end, with ulnar displacement backward.

d., seal fin. Outward deflection of the fingers in rheumatoid arthritis.

d., silverfork. The peculiar deformity seen in Colles' fracture of the forearm.

d., Sprengel's. Congenital upward displacement of the scapula.

d., Velpeau's. Silverfork deformity.

d., Volkmann's. Congenital tibiotarsal dislocation.

defunda'tion [L. *dē*, from, + *fundus*]. Excision of the uterine fundus.

defurfura'tion [" + *furfur*, bran]. Shedding of epidermis in scales; branny desquamation.

Deg. Abbr. for *degeneration* or *degree.*

degan'glionate [L. *dē*, from, + G. *gagglion*, tumor]. To deprive of ganglia.

degen'erate [" + *genus*, race]. 1. A sexual pervert; loosely applied to a low mental or moral type. 2. To deteriorate.

degen'erates [L. *degenerāre*, to degenerate]. A term used to include all cellular masses whose staining reactions, form, size, etc., do not admit of classification. Although the number of these cells is determined in each differential they do not enter into the per cents of the differential.

degenera'tion. Deterioration or impairment of an organ or part in structure of cells and the substances of which they are a part.

ETIOL: Due to changes in size (decrease or increase) and other changes.

d., Abercrombie's. SEE: *amyloid d.*

d., adipose. SEE: *fatty d.*

d., albuminoid. SEE: *amyloid d.*

d., amyloid. Degeneration resulting from deposition of amyloid between cells in various organs and tissues. It especially affects blood vessels in the parts affected.

d., ascending. Nerve fiber d. progressing to the center from the periphery.

d., bacony. SEE: *amyloid d.*

d., calcareous. Deposits of lime salts in tissues and parts.

d., caseous. Cheesy alteration in tissues seen in tuberculosis of same.

d., cloudy swelling. A condition in which protein substances in cells become cloudy, the cells increasing in size, with minute droplets of protein substances. Occurs in infectious diseases, and in those of the kidneys, liver, the heart and its muscles, and in the glands.

d., colloid. Jellylike disorganization of a part.

d., cystic. Cyst formation accompanying degeneration.

d., descending. Nerve fiber d. progressing toward the periphery from the original lesion.

d., fatty. Disturbance of fat metabolism changing a part into an oily substance.

d., fibroid. Change of membranous tissue into that of a fibrous nature.

d., gray. Gray d. in nerve tissue due to chronic inflammation.

d. hepatolenticular. Degeneration of the liver and of the lenticular nucleus. SEE: *Wilson's disease.*

d., hyaline. A form in which the tissues assume a homogeneous and glassy appearance. Caused by hyaline deposits, replacing musculoelastic elements of blood vessels with a firm, transparent substance which causes loss of elasticity. It is responsible for hardening of the arteries and is often followed by calcification or deposit of lime salts in dead tissue. Calcification also may result in concretions.

d., lardaceous. SEE: *amyloid d.*

d., mucoid. Disorganization of mucous cells.

d., myxomatous. SEE: *mucoid d.*

d., Nissl. Nerve cell degeneration after division of the axon.

d., parenchymatous. SEE: *cloudy swelling d.*

d., polypoid. Formation of polyp-like growths on mucous membrane.

d., secondary. SEE: *wallerian d.*

d., senile. Bodily and mental changes of the aged.

d., vitreous. SEE: *hyaline d.*

d., wallerian. Nerve fiber d. after separation from its nutritive center.

d., waxy. Amyloid or lardaceous degeneration.

d., Zenker's. Amyloid d. in muscular tissue.

degeneration, *words pert. to:* amylosis, "ather-" words, athetoid, atrophic, cacogenic, cardiomyoliposis, caseation, catalysis, colloid, sarcomatosis, steatosis.

degen'erative. Pert. to or accompanied by degeneration.

deglutible (de-glū'tĭ-bl). [L. *deglutire,* to swallow]. Capable of being swallowed.

deglutition (deg-lu-tish'un) [L. *deglutire,* to swallow]. The act of swallowing.

deglu'titive. Pert. to deglutition.

degusta'tion [L. *degustāre,* to taste]. The sense of taste.

dehiscence (de-his'ens) [L. *dehiscere,* to gape]. A bursting open, as of a graafian follicle or a wound, especially an abdominal wound.

dehy'drate [L. *dē,* from, + G. *ydōr,* water]. CHEM. to deprive of or lose, or to become free of water.

MED. To deprive the body or tissues of water.

dehydration (dē-hī-drā'shŭn) [" + G. *ydōr,* water]. The process of dehydrating. Occurs when output of water exceeds water intake. May result from deprivation of water, excessive loss of water, reduction in total quantity of electrolytes, or injection of hypertonic solutions.

dehydroandrosterone (dē-hī-drō-an-drō-stēr'ōn, dros'ter-ōn). An androgenic substance $C_{19}H_{28}O_2$ present in urine with about one-fifth the potency of androsterone. SYN: *dehydroisonandrosterone.*

dehydrocholesterol (dē-hī-drō-kō-lĕs'tĕr-ol). A sterol (found in the skin and other tissues) which after activation by radiation then forms vitamin D.

dehydrocorticosterone (dē-hī-drō-kôrt-ĭ-kō-stēr'ōn, -kos'ter-ōn). 11-dehydrocorticosterone (Kendall's compound A). $C_{21}H_{28}O_4$. A physiologically active steroid isolated from the adrenal cortex. It is important in water and salt metabolism.

dehydrogenase (dē-hī-droj'ĕ-nās). An enzyme which catalyzes the oxidation of a specific substance causing it to give up its hydrogen.

dehydroisoandrosterone (dē''hī'drō-ī-sō-an-dro-stēr'ōn, -drŏs''ter-ōn). A 17-ketosteroid excreted in normal male urine. It possesses androgenic activity.

Deiters's cells (dī'terz) [Otto F. C. Deiters, German anatomist, 1834-1863]. 1. Supporting cells in organ of Corti. 2. Spider cells of the neuroglia. 3. Neuro cells, the neuraxons of which become the axis cylinders of nerve fibers. SEE: *cell.*

D.'s nucleus. Collection of cells back of the acoustic nucleus.

D.'s process. Axis cylinder process or neuraxon.

déjà vu (da-zhă vĭ) [F. already seen]. The impression that something seen or some situation being experienced for the first time has been previously seen or experienced.

dejecta (de-jek'tă) [L. *dejicere,* to cast down]. Feces; intestinal waste.

dejection, dejecture (de-jek'shun, -tūr) [L. *deficere,* to cast down]. 1. A cast down feeling, or mental depression. 2. Defecation or act of defecation.

Dejerine's disease (da-zhĕ-rēns') [Joseph J. Dejerine, Paris neurologist, 1849-1917]. Interstitial neuritis of infants.

D.'s syndrome. S. with deep sensitivity repressed but with normal tactile sense, caused by lesion of long root fibers of post. column.

dekanormal (dek-ă-nor'mal) [G. *deka,* ten, + L. *norma,* rule]. Having 10 times the strength of normal, as a solution.

delacrimation (de-lak-rī-ma'shun) [" + *lacrimāre,* to shed tears]. More or less constant overflow of tears. SEE: *epiphora.*

delactation (de-lak-ta'shun) [" + *lactāre,* to suckle]. Weaning or cessation of lactation.

delamina'tion [" + *lamina,* plate]. The division into laminae, esp. that of a blastoderm into two layers: epiblast and hypoblast.

delayed reflex (dē-lād'). Any in which the response is abnormally delayed.

d. symptoms. Delayed onset of symptoms, as of shock.

delectatio morosa [L.]. Dallying with voluptuous thoughts.

deligation (del-ĭ-ga'shun) [L. *deligāre,* to tie up]. The application of ligatures or binder.

delimita'tion [L. *dē,* down, + *limitāre,* to limit]. Determination of limits of an area or organ in diagnosis.

deliquesce (del-ĭ-qwes'). To cause liquefication.

deliquescence (del-ĭ-kwes'ens) [L. *deliquescere,* to grow moist]. The process of becoming liquefied as result of absorption of water from the air. Ordinary table salt has this property.

deliquescent (del-i-kwes'ent). Pert. to a substance which absorbs water from the atmosphere.

delire de toucher (de-lĭr dĕ too-shā') [Fr.]. An abnormal desire to touch things.

delir'iant [L. *delirāre,* to be out of one's head]. An agent that will produce delirium. EX: *atropine, hyoscine.*

delirifacient (de-lir'i-fa'shĭ-ent) [" + *facere,* to make]. A drug causing delirium. SYN: *deliriant.*

delirium (de-lĭr'ĭ-um) [L.]. Disorientation for time and place, usually with illusions and hallucinations. A state of mental confusion and excitement.

The mind wanders and speech is incoherent, and the patient is in a state of continual, aimless physical activity. There are many forms of delirium, depending mainly upon the cause.

RS: *alcoholism; carphologia; consciousness, clouding of; dipsomania; mussitation; potomania; restraints.*

d., acute. One developing suddenly and speedily, resulting in recovery or death.

d., alcoholic. SEE: *delirium tremens.*

d., chronic. D. of chronic psychoses, without febrile characteristics.

d. constantium. D. of patients with reiteration of same fixed idea.

d. cordis. Violent heart beat. Atrial fibrillation.

d. epilepticum. D. either following an epileptic attack or appearing instead of an attack.

d., febrile. D. occurring with fever.

d. hystericum. Delirium of hysteria.

d., lingual. Form where meaningless sounds are muttered constantly.

d. mussitans. Excitement causing lingual d.

d. of negation. Form in which patient thinks parts of his body are missing.

d., partial. D. reacting on only a portion of the mental faculties, causing only some of the patient's actions to be unreasonable.

d. of persecution. D. in which patient feels he is being persecuted by those about him.

d., toxic. D. produced by presence of toxins in the body.

d., traumatic. D. following injury or shock.

d. tremens. A psychic disorder involving hallucinations, both visual and auditory, found in habitual and excessive users of alcoholic beverages.

SYM: Hallucinations, as seeing snakes or monsters, hearing noises. Patient is excited and usually talking or yelling incoherently.

F. A. TREATMENT: Sedatives, esp. paraldehyde and bromides. Treat for shock if present. Glucose and fluids in large quantities. Induce free perspiration. Restraints may be necessary. Hypodermics of apomorphine hydrochloride may be sedative in the maniacal individual.

NP: The patient must never be left alone for an instant, since attempts at suicide are frequent in such cases. The nursing of delirium needs endless patience, tact, and understanding. Restraint should be avoided if possible.

d., violent. Feverish d. with exaltation and great strength.

delitescence (del-ĭ-tes'ens) [L. *delitescere,* to be hidden]. An unusually complete and speedy resolution of an inflammation.

deliv'er [Fr. *delivrer,* to free]. To aid in childbirth by removal of a fetus or placenta.

deliv'ery [Fr. *delivrer,* to free]. Expulsion of the child at birth with placenta and membranes from the mother. SEE: *labor.*

d., abdominal. Removal of the child by Cesarean section.

d., forceps. Delivery of the child by the use of tractor instruments.

d., postmortem. Delivery of the child after death of the mother either by the abdominal or vaginal route.

d., precipitate. A precipitate delivery is one that occurs under nonaseptic conditions and when the physician is not present. In the true sense it is one which follows a precipitate labor regardless of who is present.

TO PREVENT A PRECIPITATE DELIVERY: *Watch the patient carefully.*

A multipara needs more careful watching against this predicament than a primipara. However, this should not be taken as an excuse because it is possible for it to occur in a primipara.

Do not wait for the head to be visible in a multipara if she is having frequent hard pains, particularly if they are bearing down in type, but have her seen by the physician immediately. In a primipara it is fairly safe to wait, in the majority of cases, until a small portion of the head is seen at the vaginal orifice during a pain before putting the patient up for delivery.

Remember to watch the primipara or multipara who has received an analgesic, since precipitation can occur with little or no warning. This means watching for bulging of the perineum during the pains by viewing the vulva and not taking it for granted that because the patient is fairly quiet no progress is being made.

d., premature. Delivery of a fetus after the twenty-eighth week but before full term.

d., spontaneous. Delivery of the child without external aid.

delomorphous (del-o-mor'fus) [G. *dēlos,* evident, + *morphē,* form]. Having definite form and shape.

d. cells. Granular cells which stain easily; found next to basement membrane in stomach; glands in cardiac region.

delousing (de-lows'ing) [L. *dē,* from, + A.S. *lūs*]. Ridding of lice by their destruction.

del'ta for'nicis [L.]. A triangular surface on lower side of fornix; *commissura hippocampi.*

del'toid [G. *delta,* letter d, + *eidos,* resemblance]. Shaped like the Greek letter Δ.

d. ligament. Internal lateral ligament of ankle joint.

d. muscle. The *musculus deltoideus,* which covers the shoulder prominence.

d. ridge. Ridge on humerus where deltoid muscle is attached.

de lunat'ico inquiren'do [L.]. Legal process to determine alleged incompetence of a person.

delusion (de-lu'zhun) [L. *deludere,* to cheat]. A false belief, as that the individual is Napoleon. Differs from hallucination which involves the false excitation of one or more of the senses.

MOST IMPORTANT DELUSIONS: Those which cause the patient to harm others, or himself, such as: (a) Fear of being poisoned, causing the patient to refuse food; (b) those leading to suicide, or inflicting injury upon self; (c) false beliefs, such as having been guilty of an unpardonable sin; (d) those of persecution.

d., depressive. One causing a saddened state.

d., expansive. Conviction of one's own fineness, power or importance.

d., fixed. One that remains unaltered.

d., fleeting. A type that comes and goes.

d. of grandeur. A false sense of possessing wealth or power.

d. of negation. SEE: *nihilistic d.*

d., nihilistic (ni-hil-is'tik). One that causes the victim to believe that everything has ceased to exist.

d. of persecution. D. in which patient feels everyone about him is against him.

d., reference. One that causes the victim to read a meaning not intended in the acts or words of others, usually an interpretation of slight or ridicule.

d., systematized. Logical correlation with false reasoning and deduction.

d., unsystematized. D. without any correlation between ideas and surroundings.

delu'sional [L. *deludere,* to cheat]. Pert. to a delusion.

dement' [L. *de,* from, + *mens,* mind]. One who has lost his sanity.

demented (de-men'ted). Of unsound mind.

dementia (de-men'shi-ă) [L. *de,* from, + *mens,* mind]. Irrecoverable deteriorative mental state, the common end result of many entities.

SEE: *cataphrenia.*

d., alcoholic. D. in terminal portion of chronic alcoholic state.

d., apathetic. D. with diminished sensitivity, occurring usually in the last stages of disease.

d., apoplectic. Form following cerebral hemorrhage or tumors.

d., catatonic. A form of d. praecox.

d., chronic. An incurable form occurring at any time of life.

d., epileptic. That accompanied by mental deterioration, and due to long continued epilepsy.

d. naturalis. Congenital form; idiocy.

d., organic. D. caused by lesions of nerve centers.

d. paralytica. Paresis or general paralysis of the insane. A paretic form of neurosyphilis characterized by progressive dementia and a diffuse generalized paralysis. Generally terminates in death if untreated. ETIOL: Antecedent syphilitic infection. DURATION: Several months to 3 or 4 years.

IN GENERAL: (1) Often seen in the young who have inherited syphilis, usually 10 or 20 years later. (2) If not treated, leads to physical and mental deterioration. May eventually be fatal. (3) Sometimes classified into 3 common types, spoken of as the *deluded*, the *depressed*, and the *demented*. (4) Without treatment, the disease may pass through 3 stages of development.

THE DELUDED TYPE: *The First Stage*: (1) Memory defective. (2) Very excitable. (3) Hallucinations of hearing. (4) Judgment defect. (5) Weaken self control. (6) Acute excitement may occur. (7) Peculiar "in and out" movement of tongue. "Trombone tremor." (8) Slurred, hesitating speech with drawling. (9) Ankle and knee jerks absent, increased, or floppy. (10) Restlessness and irritability. (11) Pleased with self. (12) Delusions of grandeur. (13) Feels unusually well. (14) Feels able to work when not fit. (15) Mental weakness steadily progresses. (16) Tremors of tongue, face, and hands. (17) Unsteady gait. (18) Loss of facial expression due to muscular weakness. (19) Irregular, unequal pupils without reflex to light. (20) Difficult urination.

The Second Stage: (1) About beginning of 2nd year. (2) Delusions may be repeated but gradually forgotten. (3) Dull, stupid; shows no emotion. (4) Seizures occur. (5) Patient becomes dull and flushed, then unconscious. (6) Unconsciousness may last few minutes to an hour. (7) Seizures resemble epilepsy but less severe. (8) Seizures followed by hemiplegia or monoplegia. (9) Congestive attacks. (10) Rise of temperature before seizure. (11) Physical signs more marked. (12) Muscular weakness shown in gait, handwriting and in speech. (13) Often becomes fat.

The Third Stage: (1) Little interest shown except in food. (2) Evidence of mind disappears. (3) Grinding of teeth. (4) Becomes wasted. (5) Unable to control excretions. (6) Becomes bedridden. (7) Seizures may continue.

THE DEPRESSED TYPE: (1) Remissions not so common. (2) Depression. (3) Physical signs same as the deluded type. (4) Runs longer course. (5) Delusions of unworthiness or persecution. (6) Delusions are of much greater magnitude.

THE DEMENTED TYPE: (1) All become demented but not noticeable from the start. (2) Run a prolonged course. (3) Delusions do not occur. (4) Dull, forgetful, unable to work. (5) Commonest type in females.

TREATMENT: Penicillin therapy.

NURSING OF GENERAL PARALYTICS: (1) Patient must be under constant observation. (2) Their bones are fragile, hence they should be handled carefully. (3) Prevent decubitus. (4) Artificial fever is sometimes induced. (5) Must be kept warm during rigors. (6) If patient has convulsions, he must be watched carefully to prevent him from injuring himself. (7) Watch for distended bladder. (8) Check on elimination. (9) Avoid all quarreling. (10) Patients have a tendency to eat greedily and may have difficulty in swallowing. Care must be exercised to prevent choking. (11) Watch for possible collapse. (12) Death may occur during a seizure.

d. paranoides. D. praecox with paranoid tendencies.

d., paretic. Paralytic dementia, *q.v.*

d., postfebrile. D. following severe cases of infectious diseases.

d. praecox. Though a disease entity, it is best replaced by the term "schizophrenia,"* since it is not always associated with dementia nor always occurring in the young. It has been characterized as a "dream state," a psychosis represented by a dreaming mind in a sleeping body, the latter being easily aroused but not the former.

d., presenile. One beginning in middle age, usually resulting from cerebral arteriosclerosis. SYM: Apathy, loss of memory, disturbances of speech and gait.

d., primary. Dementia occurring by itself, without relation to another form of psychosis.

d., secondary. D. occurring after a primary mental disease, such as mania.

d., senile. That occurring in the aged. SYM: Progressive mental deterioration with loss of memory, esp. for recent events, with occasional intercurrent attacks of excitement.

d., syphilitic. D. caused by lesion of syphilis.

d., tabetic. Dementia that may occur following tabes dorsalis.

d., terminal. D. following another form of mental disease. SEE: *secondary d.*

d., toxic. That due to the excessive use of some drug.

demerol (dĕm'er-ŏl). Proprietary name for meperidine hydrochloride, a white, colorless, crystalline compound, soluble in water, having a neutral reaction and an analgesic effect similar to morphine. It may be habit forming.

demi- [L.]. Prefix: Half.

demibain (dem'ĭ-ban) [F. half bath]. Half a bath, sitz bath.

demic (dem'ik) [G. *demos*, people]. Concerning the living body of man.

demilune (dĕm'ĭ-lūn) [L. *demi*, half, + *luna*, moon]. A crescent-shaped group of serous cells which forms a cap-like structure over a mucous alveolus. They are present in mixed glands, esp. the submandibular gland.

demineraliza'tion [L. *de*, from, + *minare*, to mine]. Loss of mineral salts esp. from the bones.

demise (de-mīz') [L. *demittere*, to send from]. Death.

Dem'odex. Genus of mites and ticks of the class *Arachnida* and order *Acarina*.

D. folliculorum. The hair follicle or face mite, an elongated wormlike organism which infests the hair follicles and sebaceous glands of various mammals including man.

demog'raphy [G. *demos*, the people, + *graphein*, to write]. Statistical study of births, marriages, and deaths, and physical, moral, and intellectual development.

demonoma'nia [G. *daimon*, devil, + *mania*, madness]. Obsolete term for psychotic belief that one is possessed by demons.

Demours' membrane (de-moorz') [Pierre Demours, French ophthalmologist, 1702-1795]. A fine membrane bet. the endothelial layer of the cornea and the substantia propria. SYN: *Descemet's membrane; lamina elastica posterior.*

demucosa'tion [L. *dē,* from, + *mucus*]. Excision of mucosa of any part of body.

demul'cent [L. *demulcere,* to stroke softly]. An agent that will soothe the part or soften the skin to which applied. The term is usually restricted to agents acting on mucous membrane. Ex: *Glycerin, honey, lanolin, olive oil.*

demutiza'tion [L. *dē,* down, + *mutus,* mute]. Overcoming mutism by teaching the patient to speak or to use the sign language.

demyelinate (de-my'ĕ-lin-āt) [" + G. *myelos,* marrow]. Destruction or removal of the myelin sheath of nerve tissue.

dena'tured [" + *natura,* nature]. Subject to having the nature of a substance changed, or to render unfit for consumption, as alcohol, *q.v.*

d. protein. A protein which has been treated in some manner that caused it to lose some of its physical and chemical properties. Cooking egg white denatures the albumen present.

dendraxon (den-drak'son) [G. *dendron,* tree, + *axōn,* axle]. The terminal filaments of the neuraxon of a nerve cell.

den'dric. Pert. to or possessing a dendron.

dendriform (den'drĭ-form) [G. *dendron,* tree, + L. *forma,* shape]. Branching or like a tree in shape.

den'drite [G. *dendritēs,* pert. to a tree]. A branched protoplasmic process of a neuron which conducts impulses to the cell body. There are usually several to a cell. They form synaptic connections with other neurons.

d., extracapsular. Dendrites of neurons of autonomic ganglia which pierce the capsule surrounding the cell and which extend for considerable distances from the cell body.

d., intracapsular. Dendrites of neurons of autonomic ganglia which ramify beneath the capsule forming a network about the cell body.

dendrit'ic. Treelike in form.

d. calculus. A renal stone molded in the form of the pelvis and calyces.

dendroid (den'droid) [G. *dendron,* tree, + *eidos,* form]. 1. Dendriform, pert. to dendrites. 2. Arborescent, treelike.

dendron (den'dron) [G. tree]. A dendrite. A protoplasmic branch from a nerve cell.

dendrophagocytosis (den"dro-fag-o-sī-to'-sis) [" + *phagein,* to eat, + *kytos,* cell, + *-ōsis,* infection]. The absorption of portions of astrocytes by microglia cells.

dener'vated [L. *dē,* from, + G. *neuron,* nerve]. 1. Excision, incision, or blocking of a nerve supply. 2. A condition in which the nerve supply is blocked or cut off.

dengue (deng'gā, -ge) [Sp.]. Acute, epidemic, febrile disease lasting 5 to 7 days, seldom fatal. SYN: *breakbone fever; dandy fever.*

ETIOL: A virus transmitted by the mosquito, *Aedes aegypti,* and other species of *Aedes.*

INCUBATION PERIOD: 3 to 15 days, usually 5 to 6 days.

SYM: Two fever periods with intermissions; eruptions similar to measles; severe pain in muscles and joints.

TREATMENT: No specific treatment. Analgesic and sedative agents. Mosquito control for prophylaxis.

denidation (de-ni-da'shun) [L. *dē,* from, + *nidus,* nest]. Removal during menstruation of the superficial mucosal surface of the uterus.

dens (denz) (pl. *dentes*) [L.]. 1. A tooth. 2. The odontoid process of the axis. A process on the body of the axis which serves as a pivot for the rotation of the atlas. SEE: *illustration under dentition.*

d. bicuspidus. Same as *d. premolaris.*

d. caninus (pl. *dentes canini* [NA]). The canine tooth.

d. deciduus (pl. *dentes decidui* [NA]). Milk tooth, first tooth.

d. incisivus (pl. *dentes incisivi* [NA]). Incisor tooth.

d. moliris (pl. *dentes molares* [NA]). Molar tooth, grinder.

d. permanens (pl. *dentes permanentes* [NA]). One of the 32 teeth making up the so-called permanent teeth.

d. premolaris (pl. *dentes premolares* [NA]). One of the premolar teeth.

d. sapientiae. A wisdom tooth; late tooth; third molar; *d. serotinus.*

d. serotinus [NA]. A wisdom tooth; third molar.

densimeter (den-sim'ĕ-ter) [L. *densus,* thick, + G. *metron,* measure]. Instrument for measuring densities.

densitom'eter [" + G. *metron,* measure]. A special densimeter for measuring bacterial growth and effect upon it of antiseptics and bacteriophages.

den'sity [L. *densitās,* thickness]. 1. Relative weight of a substance compared with some other substance of equal bulk. SEE: *specific gravity.* 2. The quality of being dense.

dentag'ra [L. *dens,* tooth, + G. *agra,* seizure]. 1. Toothache. 2. Forceps for removing teeth.

den'tal. Pert. to the teeth.

d. abscess. SEE: *abscess, dental.*

d. arch. The arch formed by the cutting and chewing surfaces of the teeth.

d. caries. Decay of the teeth. SEE: *caries.*

d. consonant. A consonant pronounced with the tongue at or near the front upper teeth. Term used in speech therapy.

d. curve. The curve or bow of the line of the teeth in the jaw. The different portions of the curve are described as follows: *Alignment c.* The line passing through the center of the teeth from the middle line through the last molar. *Buccal c.* The curve extending from the cuspid to the 3rd molar. *Compensating c.* The occlusal line of bicuspids and molars. *Labial c.* The curve extending from cuspid to cuspid.

d. disk. A thin, circular piece of paper, cloth, or other substance charged with abrasive powder for cutting or polishing teeth and fillings.

d. dysfunction. Malfunctioning of the parts of the dental structure.

d. engine. A machine operated with foot power, or by an electric or a water motor, to give a swift rotary motion to drills, burs, and burnishers.

d. engineering. Use of the principles of engineering in dentistry.

d. floss. Waxed silk thread used for cleaning between the teeth and testing for defects in the teeth.

d. formula. A method of expressing briefly the dentition of mammals in which the numbers of the teeth are given in the form of a fraction, the numbers of the upper teeth forming the numerator, those of the lower teeth the denominator.

The dental formula of man is: Abbreviations used are *i* for incisors, *c* for canine, *b* for bicuspid, *pm* for premolar, and *m* for molar.

$$\text{i. } \frac{2\text{-}2}{2\text{-}2} \text{ c. } \frac{1\text{-}1}{1\text{-}1} \text{ b. or pm. } \frac{2\text{-}2}{2\text{-}2} \text{ m } \frac{3\text{-}3}{3\text{-}3} \text{ 32.}$$

d. geriatrics. The scientific study and treatment of dental conditions of the aged.

d. hygienist. A trained person who professionally cleans teeth and, usually in schools or institutions, offers instruction on general care of the teeth.

d. index. A system of numbers for indicating comparative size of the teeth.

d. prosthesis. An artificial part used in the mouth to replace missing structural tissue or teeth. Also called a denture.

dentalgia (den-tal'jĭ-ă) [L. *dens,* tooth, + G. *algos,* pain]. Toothache.

dentaphone (den'tă-fōn) [" + G. *phōnē,* sound]. Device for conveying sound through the teeth.

dentate (den'tāt) [L. *dentātus,* toothed]. Notched; having short triangular divisions of the margin; toothed.

den'tes [L.]. Teeth; plural of *dens, q.v.*

dentibuc'cal [L. *dens,* tooth, + *bucca,* cheek]. Pert. to both the cheek and teeth.

dent'icle. 1. A small toothlike projection. 2. A small tooth.

dentic'ulate [L. *denticulatus,* small toothed]. Finely toothed or serrated.

d. body. Corpus dentatum.

dentifica'tion [L. *dens,* tooth, + *facere,* to make]. Conversion into dental structure.

den'tiform. Toothlike.

dentifrice (den'ti-fris) [" + *fricāre,* to rub]. A powder or other substance for cleaning teeth.

dentigerous (den-tij'er-us) [" + *gerere,* to bear]. Having or containing teeth.

dentila'bial [" + *labium,* lip]. Pert. to both teeth and lips.

dentilin'gual [" + *lingua,* tongue]. Pert. to both teeth and tongue.

dentim'eter [" + G. *metron,* measure]. Device for measuring teeth.

dentin (den'tin). The main, or osseous, tissues of a tooth, surrounding the pulp cavity. SYN: *dentine.*

den'tinal. Pert. to dentin.

dentinalgia (den-tin-al'jē-ă). Pain in dentin.

dentine (den'tēn) [L. *dens,* tooth]. Dentin, *q.v.*

dentinifica'tion [" + *facere,* to make]. Formation of dentin.

dentini'tis [" + G. *-itis,* inflammation]. Inflammation of dentin.

dentinoblast (den'tin-ō-blast) [L. *dens,* tooth, + G. *blastos,* germ]. A dentin-forming cell.

dentinogenesis (dĕn-tĭn-ō-jĕn'ĕ-sis). Formation of dentin in development of a tooth.

d. imperfecta. Aplasia or hypoplasia of the enamel and dentin of a tooth.

d. nucleus. A mass of gray matter in the medulla of each cerebellar hemisphere.

den'tinoid [" + G. *eidos,* form]. 1. Resembling dentin. 2. A tumor arising from dentin; a dentinoma.

dentino'ma [" + G. *ōma,* tumor]. A dentin tumor.

dentinos'teoid ["+ G. *osteon,* bone, + *eidos,* form]. Dentinoid (def. 2).

dentiparous (den-tip'ă-rus). Pert. to development and formation of teeth.

den'tist [L. *dens,* tooth]. A practitioner of dentistry.

dent'istry. 1. That branch of medicine which deals with the care of the teeth and associated structures. It is concerned with the prevention, diagnosis, and treatment of diseases of the teeth, and gums. 2. The art or profession of a dentist.

d., esthetic. Repair and restoration or replacement of carious or broken teeth.

d., operative. Phase dealing with dental operations on mouth as contrasted with dental laboratory work.

d., prosthetic. Pertaining to prosthodontia.

d., prosthodontic. The art of replacing defective or missing teeth through the use of artificial appliances such as bridges, crowns, artificial dentures, etc.

denti'tion [L. *dentitiō*]. The process and time of teething. SEE: *illustration.*

d., primary. Eruption of 20 deciduous, or milk teeth. ORDER OF ERUPTION: Two lower central incisors, 5-9 months. Two upper central incisors, 8-12 months. Two upper lateral incisors, 10-12 months. Two lower lateral incisors, 12-15 months. Four anterior molars, 12-15 months. Four canines, 18-24 months. Four posterior molars, 24-30 months.

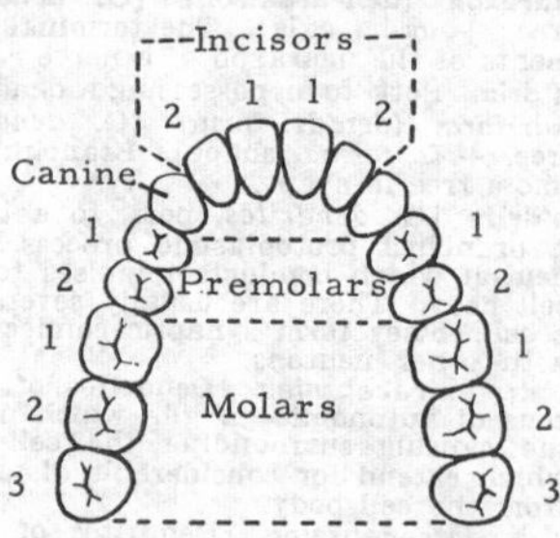

DENTITION—TEETH IN SITU

d., secondary (32 teeth). The eruption of the permanent teeth, beginning at about the age of six years. Completed by the 15th year with the exception of the "wisdom" teeth, which appear between the 17th and 25th years. ORDER OF ERUPTION: The incisors and canines are followed by the same teeth. The frontal molars are followed by 1st bicuspids. The posterior molars are followed by 2nd bicuspids, then the 1st, 2nd and 3rd molars follow. SEE: *teeth.*

dentoalve'olar [L. *dens,* tooth, + *alveolus,* small hollow]. Pert. to alveolus of a tooth.

dentoalveoli'tis [" + " + G. *-itis,* inflammation]. A purulent inflammation of the tooth socket linings, characterized by looseness of the teeth and gum shrinkage. SYN: *pyorrhea alveolaris.*

den'toid [" + G. *eidos,* form]. Dentiform; odontoid; tooth-shaped.

dentoid'in. Organic substance of a tooth.

dentoliva (den-to-lē'vă) [" + *oliva,* olive]. Olivary body.

denture (den'chur) [L. *dens,* tooth]. A set of teeth either natural or artificial.

d., artificial. A dental appliance for support of one or more artificial teeth. Used in the mouth to replace missing natural teeth. Dentures are usually made of a combination of synthetic plastic and metal.

NP: Dentures should be cleaned after each meal. When patient's condition prevents his doing this for himself it will need to be done by the nursing staff. The simplest method of cleaning dentures is to use a soft brush and either plain soap or tooth paste, with lukewarm water (hot water may damage dentures). They should be thoroughly rinsed after each washing.

Instruct patient to store dentures in opaque covered jar. If wrapped in tissue paper they are easily lost or thrown away.

Dentures are removed from comatose or moribund patients and prior to any surgical procedure.

The following solutions and mixtures are accepted by the Am. Dental Assn. for cleaning dentures: 1. Ammonia water 28%. Dilute 2 ml. in 2 ounces of water. 2. Trisodium phosphate. 600 mg. in 2 ounces of water. 3. Sodium hypochlorite (bleach). Two ml. in 4 ounces of water.

d., full. Complete set of artificial teeth.

d., immediate. A complete set of artificial teeth to be inserted immediately after removal (extraction) of natural teeth.

d., partial. An appliance with one or more artificial teeth but less in number than that in a full denture.

denucleated (de-nu′kle-āt-ed) [L. *dē,* from, + *nucleus,* kernel]. Deprived of a nucleus.

denuda′tion [L. *denudāre,* to lay bare]. Removal of a protecting layer or covering.

denutrition (de-nu-trish′un) [L. *dē,* from, + *nutrīre,* to nourish]. Malnutrition.

deob′struent [" + *obstruere,* to block up]. Having the property of removing obstructions.

deodorant (de-ō′dor-ant) [" + *odorāre,* to perfume]. An agent which destroys or neutralizes foul odors. Those in common use are: Chloride of lime, creolin, iodoform, permanganate of potash, chlorine and hydrogen peroxide. SEE: *odor.*

deodorize (de-o′dor-īz) [" + *odor,* odor]. To remove foul odor.

deodorizer (de-o′dor-ī-zer) [" + *odor,* odor]. That which deodorizes.

deontology (de-on-tol′o-jĭ) [G. *deonta,* things to be done, + *logos,* study of]. Medical ethics.

deoppila′tion [L. *dē,* from, + *oppilāre,* to stop up]. The doing away with obstructions.

deor′sum [L.]. Downward or turning downward.

d. ver′gens. Turning downward.

deorsumduction (de-or″sum-duk′shun) [" + *ducere,* to lead]. Bending downward.

deos′sification (dē-ŏs-ĭ-fĭ-kā′shŭn) [L. *dē,* from, + *os,* bone, + *facere,* to make]. Loss of or the removal of mineral matter from bone or osseous tissue.

deox′idate [" + G. *oxys,* sharp]. To deprive a chemical of oxygen.

deoxida′tion [" + *oxys,* sharp]. Process of depriving of oxygen.

deoxidizer (de-ok′sĭ-di-zer) [" + *oxys,* sharp]. A deoxidizing substance.

deoxycholic acid (de-ok″sĭ-ko′lik). $C_{24}H_{40}O_4$, a crystalline acid found in bile.

deoxyribonuclease (de-ok″sĭ-ri-bo-nu′kle-ās). An enzyme, produced by certain streptococci, which hydrolyzes deoxyribonucleoprotein of cells.

deoxyribonucleic acid (de-ok″sĭ-ri″bo-nu′klē-ik). ABBR: DNA. A complex protein of high molecular weight consisting of deoxyribose, phosphoric acid, and four bases (two purines, *adenine* and *guanine,* and two pyrimadines, *thymine* and *cystosine*). It is a nucleic acid present in chromosomes of the nuclei of cells and is considered the chemical basis of heredity and the carrier of genetic information. Formerly spelled desoxyribonucleic acid.

deoxyribose (de-ok″sĭ-ri′bōs). A phosphoric ester of a pentose present in nucleic acid.

depancreatize (de-pan′kre-ă-tīz). To remove the pancreas surgically.

dependence (de-pen′dents). In narcotic addicts, the mental and physical state of being dependent upon narcotics in order to achieve a feeling of well being. The nature of most narcotics is such that an increasingly larger dose is required to obtain that feeling. Decreasing the dose causes wihdrawal signs and symptoms. SEE: *habituation.*

depersonaliza′tion [" + L. *persona,* person]. A sense of being someone else; a lessened sense of one's own identity.

depilate (dep′il-ate) [L. *depilāre,* to pluck out hair]. To remove hair.

depilation (dep-il-a′shun) [L. *de* + *pilus,* hair]. The process of hair removal. SEE: *epilation.*

depil′atory [" + *pilus,* hair]. An agent used for the removal of hair.

deplete (de-plēt′) [" + *plēre,* to fill]. To empty, as in blood letting; to produce depletion.

depletion (de-ple′shun) [" + *plēre,* to fill]. Removal of substances from the body such as blood, fluids, iron, fat, protein.

deplumation (de-plu-ma′shun) [" + *pluma,* down]. Falling of eyelashes as result of disease.

depolarization (dē-pō″lăr-ĭ-zā′shŭn) [" + *polus,* pole]. The process of reducing to a nonpolarized condition; destruction of polarity.

deposit (de-poz′it) [" + *ponere,* to place]. 1. Sediment. 2. Matter collected in any part of an organism, normal or otherwise.

deprava′tion [L. *depravāre,* to impair]. 1. Deterioration, esp. of secretions. 2. Perversion.

depraved (de-prāvd′). 1. Perverted; abnormal. 2. Deteriorated.

depress′ant [L. *depressus,* pressed down]. An agent that will depress a body function or nerve activity. Ex: *Bromides, aconite, chloral hydrate.*

d., cardiac. One which lessens heart action, so that it beats slower and weaker.

d., cerebral. One lessening brain activity, making patient dull and less active. Large doses may produce sleep.

d., motor. One which lessens contractions of involuntary muscles.

d., respiratory. A drug lessening frequency and depth of breathing.

d., secretory. One making gland secretions less.

depressed (de-prest′). 1. Hollowed. 2. Low in spirits.

depression (de-presh′un) [L. *depressiō,* a pressing down]. 1. A hollow or lowered region. 2. The lowering of a part as the mandible. 3. The lowering of a vital function such as respiration. 4. A mental state characterized by dejection, lack of hope, and absence of cheerfulness. Observed in manic depressive psychoses. Depression is to be differentiated from grief which is realistic and is proportionate to that which has been lost.

d., averse. Melancholia.

d., cardiac. Notch in ant. margin of left lung for the cardiac apex.

d., pacchionian. Depressions in the skull which contain the pacchionian bodies.

depres'somotor [" + *motor,* mover]. A drug which diminishes muscular movements by lessening the impulses for motion sent from the brain or spinal cord.

depressor (de-pres'or) [L.]. Instrument for depressing a part.

d. nerve. A nerve, the stimulation of which brings about a fall in blood pressure through reflex vasodilation and slowing of heart beat.

d. reflex. More or less transient stimulation of depressor fibers.

d., tongue. Device used to flatten tongue for throat examinations.

dep'rimens oc'uli [L.]. *Musculus rectus inferior.*

depri'val [L. *dē,* from, + *privāre,* to remove]. Deprived of or without organs, parts, or functions.

depriva'tion [" + *privāre,* to remove]. Deprival.

d., sensory. A situation or environment wherein the usual sensory stimuli, such as noise and light, as well as human contact are absent or, in the case of noise, masked by a continuous dull noise. Persons exposed partially or completely to such an environment include astronauts, patients in artificial respirators, and patients with both eyes bandaged. Prolonged exposure to lack of sensory stimuli may cause hallucinations and other signs and symptoms of mental disorder.

deprive'ment [" + *privāre,* to remove]. Being without function, parts or organs. Syn: *deprival.*

depuliza'tion [" + *pulex,* flea]. Destruction of fleas which carry the plague bacillus.

dep'urant [L. *depurāre,* to purify]. A medicine that purifies through the removal of *excreta.*

depura'tion [L. *depurāre,* to purify]. Process of freeing from impurities.

dep'urative. Cleansing.

depura'tor [L. *dē* + *purus,* pure]. 1. That which purifies. 2. An emunctory.

deradelphus (der-ă-del'fus) [G. *derē,* neck + *adelphos,* brother]. Twin monster fused above the thorax and having one head, but separated below the chest as two bodies.

deradenitis (der-ad-ĕ-ni'tis) [G. *derē,* neck, + *adēn,* gland]. Inflammation of a lymph gland of the neck.

deradenoncus (der-ad"e-non'kus) [" + *ogkos,* tumor]. Swelling or tumor of a neck gland.

derangement (de-rānj'ment) [Fr. disorder]. Disorder of the mental functions, especially those involving the intellect.

Dercum's disease (der'kŭm) [Francis X. Dercum, American neurologist, 1856-1931]. Dystrophy of subcutaneous connective tissue; painful. Syn: *adiposis dolorosa; paratrophy.*

dereistic (de-re-is'tik). Pert. to overexercise of the imagination to the extent of ignoring reality, as seen in day dreaming. See: *autism.*

der'ic (der'ik) [G. *deros,* skin]. Pertaining to the skin or surface of the body as distinguished from enteric.

derivation (der-ĭ-va'shun) [L. *derivāre,* to draw off]. 1. Diversion of fluids from one part to another. 2. The formation of a substance from its source.

deriv'ative [L. *derivāre,* to draw off]. 1. That which is not original or fundamental. 2. Anything derived from another body or substance. 3. That which produces derivation. 4. In embryology that which develops from a preceding structure as the derivatives of the germ layers.

derm, derma [G. *derma,* skin]. The *cutis vera,* or true skin.

dermabrasion (derm'ă-bra-zhun). A procedure for removal of acne scars or nevi on the skin by utilization of sandpaper or other abrasive. Procedure is dangerous and should not be used indiscriminately.

Dermacentor (der-mă-sent'or). A genus of ticks belonging to the order Acarina, family Ixodidae.

D. andersoni. The wood tick, a species of ticks which is parasitic on man or other mammals during some part of their life cycle. May transmit causative agents of Rocky Mountain spotted fever, typhus fever, scrub typhus, tularemia, anaplasmosis. brucellosis, Q fever, and several forms of virus encephalomyelitis, also causes tick paralysis.

D. variabilis. A species of ticks similar to *D. andersoni.* On east coast of United States, it is the common dog tick, and transmits especially Rocky Mountain spotted fever.

der'mad [G. *derma,* skin, + L. *ad,* toward]. Toward the skin; externally.

dermal. Relating to the skin or derma.

dermalax'ia [G. *derma,* skin, + *malaxis,* softening]. Morbid relaxation or softness of the skin.

dermalgia (der-mal'jĭ-ă) [" + *algos,* pain]. Pain in the skin.

dermametropathism (der"mă-mĕ-trŏp'ă-thizm) [" + *metron,* measure, + *pathos,* disease]. Diagnosis of skin disease by observing the markings made by drawing a blunt pencil across the skin.

dermamyiasis (der-mă-mī-ī'ă-sis) [" + *myia,* fly]. Skin disease caused by invasion of larva of dipterous insects.

dermanaplasty (der-man'ă-plas-tĭ) [" + *anaplassein,* to reform]. Skin grafting.

dermapos'tasis [" + *apostasis,* a falling away]. Abscess formation accompanying a disease of the skin.

dermat-, dermato- [G.]. Prefixes: Skin.

dermatalgia (der-mă-tal'jĭ-ă) [" + *algos,* pain]. Paresthesia with localized pain in the skin. Syn: *dermalgia.*

dermatatrophia (derm-at-ă-tro'fĭ-ă) [" + *atrophia,* atrophy]. Atrophy of the skin.

dermatauxe (der-mă-tawk'sē) [" + *auxē,* increase]. Hypertrophy of the skin.

dermatitis (der-mă-ti'tis) [" + *-itis,* inflammation]. Inflammation of skin evidenced by itching, redness and various skin lesions.

Etiol: Skin irritants, as poison ivy, corrosives, acids, alkalies; or hypersusceptibility on part of patient to conditions which would not cause skin irritation in persons who were not hypersusceptible.

Treatment: Remove irritant by washing with soap and water. Dress with calamine lotion or bland oils or ointment.

d. aestivalis [L. *aestiva,* summer]. Hot weather dermatitis.

d., allergic. Inflammation supposed to be due to an allergy.

d. calorica [L. *calor,* heat]. That due to heat or cold, as sunburn, etc.

d., cercarial. Dermatitis resulting from infestation with the cercaria of blood flukes belonging to the genus *Schistosoma.* Schistosome dermatitis or swimmer's itch.

d. congelationis [L. *congelatio,* cold] Frostbite, chilblain. SEE: *chilblain.*

d., contact. Inflammation and irritation of the skin due to contact with an irritating substance. Usually due to a combination of reduced ability of the skin to resist injury and exposure to a material in strong concentration such as soap or chemical. Some individuals are sensitive to such apparently innocuous compounds as perfumes and deodorants.

TREATMENT: Remove patient from offending material and treat skin as indicated. SYN: *dermatitis venenata.*

d. exfoliativa. Chronic inflammation of the skin commonly involving whole surface and characterized by redness and abundant flaky desquamation.

ETIOL: Unknown.

SYM: May be primary with constitutional symptoms (fever, debility, and gastrointestinal upset), with sudden eruption, pink turning dark red, followed by thin, flaky, loosely adherent, grayish or brownish scales, tender skin, tension and stiffness. In secondary type it follows certain scaly diseases of the skin (eczema, seborrheic dermatitis, psoriasis); pigmentation (slate or mahogany color) is frequent.

TREATMENT: Attention to general health. Locally, soothing oily applications. Corticosteroid and antibiotic therapy.

d. gangraenosa. Skin inflammation of gangrenous form.

d. herpetiformis. Chronic, inflammatory disease characterized by erythematous, papular, vesicular, bullous, or pustular lesions with tendency to grouping and with itching and burning.

ETIOL: Direct cause unknown. Occurs mostly in adult males though no age is exempt.

SYM: Slight; constitutional. Lesions develop suddenly and spread peripherally. Disease is variable and erratic and attack may be prolonged for weeks or months. Secondary infection may follow from trauma.

PROG: Amelioration of attack, but permanent relief cannot be promised.

TREATMENT: Removal of sources of reflex irritation. Soothing mixtures externally. Excoriated areas to be protected by mild antiseptics.

d. hiemalis [L. *hiems,* winter]. Dermatitis occurring in cold weather.

d. infectiosa eczematoides. Pustular eruption during or following a pyogenic disease. SYN: *Engman's disease.*

d. medicamentosa. Drug eruption.

ETIOL: Idiosyncrasy or sensitization to the drug in question. Most probably anaphylactoid, not true anaphylactic reaction. Cosmetics, arsenic (wallpaper, etc.), iodides, bromides, butyn, phenobarbital, etc., are some of the offending drugs.

SYM: With exception of bromine and iodine, the eruption is not characteristic and may resemble almost any condition or disease.

TREATMENT: Removal of cause.

d. multiformis. Form with lesions of a pustular nature.

d. papillaris capillitii. Formation on scalp and neck of surface elevations interspersed with pustules and ending in scarlike elevations resembling keloids.

d., poison ivy. D. resulting from ivy poisoning, *q.v.* SYN: *rhus dermatitis.*

d., rhus. A contact dermatitis caused by substances present in certain plants. SEE: *poison ivy.*

d. seborrheica. Acute or subacute inflammatory skin disease beginning on the scalp, characterized by rounded, irregular, or circinate lesions covered with yellowish or brownish-gray greasy scales.

ETIOL: Unknown.

SYM: On the scalp it may be dry with abundant grayish branny scales, or oozing and crusted, constituting eczema capitis,* and may spread to forehead and postauricular regions. On the forehead it shows scaly and infiltrated lesions with dark red bases, some itching, localized loss of hair; on eyebrows and eyelashes dry, dirty white scales, itching; on nasolabial folds or vermilion border of lips (SEE: *Cheilitis exfoliativa*); on sternal region, greasy and unctuous to the touch; in interscapular, axillary, and genitocrural regions.

TREATMENT: When limited to scalp, frequent shampooing and use of mild keratolytic agents. Selenium-containing shampoos have been helpful. Generalized seborrheic dermatitis requires careful attention including scrupulous skin hygiene, keep skin as dry as possible, dusting powders. Topical and systemic cortisone preparations may be required.

SYN: *alopecia furfuracea, pityriasis capitis, seborrhea corporis, seborrhea sicca.*

d. venenata. Any inflammation caused by local action of various animal, vegetable, or mineral substances on the surface of the skin. Commonly called ivy poisoning.

ETIOL: Drugs, acids, alkalies, plants (poison ivy, oak, or sumac). Runs an acute course with recurrence on reexposure to the sensitizing agent.

SYM: Vary from simple hyperemia to gangrene and sloughing. Majority are erythematous, limited to part touched by irritant, becoming papular, vesicular, or pustular with burning or itching.

TREATMENT: Incision and drainage of bullae followed by alcohol sponge and preceded by soap and water to remove toxicodendron (poison ivy) oil. Locally drying solutions such as aluminum acetate. Calamine lotion is helpful in drying the lesions and for control of itching. In ivy poisoning desensitization with poison ivy extract injections may be effective. SEE: *skin.*

In severe cases, the use of topical and systemic cortisone may be needed.

d. verrucosa. SYN: *Chromoblastomycosis q. v.* A dermatitis characterized by the formation of wartlike nodules on the skin. These may enlarge and form papillomatous structures which sometimes ulcerate.

ETIOL: May be due to one of several fungi including *Hormodendrum pedrusoi* or *Phialophora verrucosa.*

d., x-ray. Skin inflammation due to overdose of x-ray.

dermatoautoplasty (der"mă-to-aw'to-plas-tĭ) [" + *autos,* self, + *plassein,* to form]. Grafting of skin taken from some portion of the patient's own body.

Dermatobia (dĕr-mă-tō'bĭ-a). A genus of botflies belonging to the order Diptera of the family Oestridae.

D. hominis. A species of botflies found in parts of tropical America whose larvae infest man and cattle. The eggs are transported by mosquitoes.

dermatobiasis (der-mă-to-bi'ă-sis) [" + *bios,* life]. Infestation by the larvae of *Dermatobia hominis,* the eggs of which are carried to the skin by mosquitoes. The larvae then hatch and bore into the skin while the mosquito feeds. Marble-like boils form at the site of infestation.

dermatocele (der'mă-to-sēl) [" + *kēlē,* hernia]. Tendency of hypertrophied skin and subcutaneous tissue to hang loosely in folds. SYN: *dermatolysis.*

d. lipomato'sis. A pedunculated lipoma with cystic degeneration.

dermatocelidosis (der-mă-to-sel"ĭ-do'sis) [G. *derma,* skin, + *kēlis,* spot, + *-ōsis*]. Freckles; a macular eruption. SYN: *dermatokelidosis.*

dermatocellulitis (der-mă-to-sel-u-li'tis) [" + L. *cellula,* little cell, + G. *-itis,* inflammation]. Inflammation of subcutaneous connective tissue.

dermatoconiosis (der-mă-to-ko-nĭ-o'sis) [" + *konia,* dust]. Any irritation of the skin caused by dust, esp. one due to occupational exposure.

dermatocyst (der'mă-to-sist) [" + *kystis,* cyst]. A skin cyst.

dermatodyn'ia [" + *odynē,* pain]. Pain in the skin; dermatalgia.*

dermatofibro'ma [" + L. *fibra,* fiber, + G. *-ōma,* tumor]. A skin fibroma.

dermatogen (der-mat'o-jen) [" + *gennan,* to form]. Antigen from a skin disease.

dermatogenous (der-mă-toj'ĕ-nus) [" + *gennan,* to produce]. Of the nature of or producing skin or disease of skin.

dermatoglyphics (der-mă-to-glif'ĭks) [" + *glyphē,* a carving]. Study of surface markings of the skin, esp. those of hands and feet. May be very useful in genetic studies.

dermat'ograph [" + *graphein,* to write]. 1. A device for marking the body for diagnosis. 2. A wheal made on the skin in dermatography. SYN: *dermographia.*

dermatograph'ia, dermatog'raphy [" + *graphein,* to write]. 1. A treatise on the skin. 2. A form of urticaria in which wheals are made by pressure. SYN: *dermographia.*

der"matohet'eroplasty [" + *eteros,* other, + *plassein,* to mold]. Skin grafting with grafts from another's skin.

dermatoid (der'mă-toid) [" + *eidos,* form]. Resembling skin.

dermatokelidosis (der-mă-to-kel-ĭ-do'sis) [" + *kēlidoun,* to stain]. A macular eruption; freckle.

dermatol'ogist [" + *logos,* understanding]. A skin specialist.

dermatol'ogy [" + *logos,* understanding]. The science of the skin and its diseases.

dermatolysis (der-mă-tol'ĭ-sis) [" + *lysis,* a loosening]. Tendency of hypertrophied skin and subcutaneous tissue to hang in folds. Loose skin. SYN: *cutis laxa; cutis pendula.*

dermato'ma [G. *derma,* skin, + *-ōma,* growth]. Circumscribed thickening of skin.

dermatome (der'mă-tōm) [" + *tomē,* incision]. 1. Instrument for incising the skin or for cutting thin transplants of skin. 2. A segmental skin area innervated by various spinal cord segments. 3. The lateral portion of the somite of an embryo which gives rise to the dermis of the skin; the cutis plate.

dermatomere (der'mă-to-mēr) [" + *meros,* part]. A segment of embryonic integument.

dermatomucosomyositis (der"mă-to-mū-ko"so-mi-o-si'tis) [" + L. *mucosa,* mucous membrane, + G. *mys,* muscle, + *-itis,* inflammation]. Inflammation of the skin, involving mucosa and muscles.

dermatomycosis (der"mă-to-mi-ko'sis) (pl. *dermatomycoses*) [" + *mykes,* fungus, + *-ōsis*]. A skin infection caused by certain fungi of the genera *Trichophyton, Epidermophyton,* and *Microsporum.*

dermatomyo'ma [" + *mys,* muscle, + *-ōma,* tumor]. Myoma of the skin.

dermatomyositis (der"mă-to"mi-o-si'tis) [" + " + *-itis,* inflammation]. One of the so-called collagen diseases, *q.v.* An acute, subacute, or chronic disease of unknown etiology. Characterized by edema, dermatitis, and inflammation of the muscles. Fever, malaise, and weakness may be the presenting symptoms along with weakness of the pelvic and shoulder girdle muscles. Skin and mucosal lesions are often present.

TREATMENT: Symptomatic: bed rest, physiotherapy, salicylates. Adrenal cortical steroids are helpful in most cases.

NP: Rest in bed with skillful turning is essential. Mouth lesions should be irrigated frequently with saline solution. Hot baths and hot fomentations help stiffness. Avoid fatigue and chilling. Massage, graduated exercise and electrotherapy are helpful in preventing or treating muscular atrophy and contractures.

dermatoneuro'sis [" + *neuron,* nerve, + *-ōsis*]. Skin disease of nervous origin. SEE: *neurodermatitis.*

dermatopath'ia [" + *pathos,* disease]. Any disease of the skin.

dermatopathol'ogy [" + " + *logos,* study of]. Study of diseases of the skin.

dermatop'athy [" + *pathos,* disease]. Any skin disease. SYN: *dermatopathia.*

dermatopho'bia [" + *phobos,* fear]. Abnormal fear of having a skin disease.

dermatophyte (dĕr'măt-ō-fīt) [" + *phyton,* plant]. A plant parasite which grows in or on the skin. They rarely penetrate deeper than the epidermis or its derivatives, hair, and nails. They cause such skin diseases as favus, tinea, or ringworm, eczema, erythrasma. Important dermatophytes include the genera *Microsporum, Trichophyton,* and *Epidermophyton.* All are fungi.

dermatophytid (der-mă-tof'ĭ-tid) [" + *phyton,* plant]. A toxic rash or eruption occurring in dermatomycosis.

dermatophytosis (der"mă-to-fi-to'sis). A fungus infection of the skin of the hands and feet, especially between the toes. SYN: *tinea pedis; athlete's foot; ringworm of feet.*

dermatoplas'tic [" + *plassein,* to form]. Pert. to skin grafting.

dermatoplasty (der'mat-o-plas-tĭ). Transplanting living skin to cover cutaneous defects caused by injury, operation, or disease. Any restoring operation on the skin.

NP: DRESSING: Safety pins. Gauze, cotton, roller bandage. Great care must be taken in adjusting bandage. If too much pressure is put on grafts they will die because of lack of vascularity. These wounds are sometimes dressed with a light compress of sterilized gauze, saturated with a warm physiologic saline solution.

dermatorrhagia (der"mă-to-ra'jĭ-ă) [G. *derma,* skin, + *rēgnunai,* to burst forth]. Hemorrhage into or from the skin.

dermatorrhea (der"mă-to-re'ă) [" + *roia*, flow]. Excessive secretion of sebaceous glands.

dermatosclerosis (dĕr-mă-tō-sklĕ-rō'sis). Scleroderma, *q.v.*

dermatoscopy (der-mă-tos'ko-pĭ) [" + *skopein*, to examine]. Examination of the skin with a high powered lens.

dermatosiophobe (der-mă-to'sĭ-o-fōb) [" + *-ōsis* + *phobos*, fear]. One having a morbid fear of acquiring a skin disease.

dermatosiophobia (der-mă-to"sĭ-o-fō'bĭ-ă). Dread of skin disease.

dermatosis (der-mă-to'sis) (pl. *dermatoses*) [G. *derma*, skin, + *-ōsis*]. Any disease of the skin in which inflammation is not necessarily a feature. Not a synonym for dermatitis.

d., actinic. Dermatosis due to exposure to sunlight.

d., papulosa nigra. Eruption consisting of many tiny tumors on skin of face.

d., progressive pigmentary. Reddish papules principally on legs; eruption is progressive. Syn: *Schamberg's disease.*

dermatosome (der'ma-to-sōm) [" + *sōma*, body]. Section of equatorial plate in mitosis.

der"matother'apy [" + *therapeia*, treatment]. Treatment of skin diseases.

dermatothlasia (der"mă-to-thla'zĭ-ă) [" + *thlasis*, a bruising]. An uncontrollable tic or impetus to bruise, rub, or pinch the skin.

dermatotome (der'mă-to-tōm) [" + *tomē*, incision]. 1. One of the fetal skin segments. 2. A knife for incising the skin or small lesions.

dermatotropic (der-mă-to-trop'ĭk) [" + *tropē*, a turning]. Acting esp. on the skin.

dermatoxerasia (der"mă-to-ze-ra'sĭ-ă) [" + *xērasia*, dryness]. Roughening of skin. Syn: *xeroderma.*

dermatozo'on [" + *zōon*, animal]. Animal parasite of the skin.

dermatrophia (der-ma-tro'fĭ-ă) [" + *atrophia*, atrophy]. Atrophy of the skin.

dermic (der'mik) [G. *derma*, skin]. Pert. to the skin.

dermis (der'mis) [L.]. The skin; *cutis vera* or true skin. Syn: *corium* [NA, BNA].

dermi'tis [G. *derma*, skin, + *-ītis*, inflammation]. Inflammation of skin. Syn: *dermatitis.*

der'moblast [" + *blastos*, germ]. Part of mesoblastic layer, developing into the corium.

dermographia, dermography (der-mo-graf'ĭ-ă, -mog'ră-fĭ) [" + *graphein*, to write]. The appearance of elevated red marks on the skin as the result of pressure or stroking its surface.

der'moid [" + *eidos*, form]. 1. Resembling the skin. 2. A dermoid cyst.

d. cyst. A nonmalignant cystic tumor in which are found elements derived from the ectoderm, such as hair, teeth, or skin. They occur frequently in the ovary but may develop in other organs such as the lungs. 2. An ovarian teratoma.

dermoidec'tomy [" + " + *ektomē*, excision]. Excision of a dermoid cyst.

dermolysin (der-mol'ĭ-sin) [" + *lysis*, loosening]. A substance in the blood supposed to be capable of dissolving the skin.

dermol'ysis [" + *lysis*, loosening]. A rare destructive disease of the skin.

dermomycosis (der-mo-mi-ko'sis) [" + *mykēs*, fungus, + *-ōsis*]. A skin disease produced by a vegetable parasite. Syn: *dermatomycosis.*

dermonosology (der"mo-no-sol'o-jĭ) [" + *nosos*, disease, + *logos*, study of]. The classification of skin affections.

dermopathy (der-mop'ă-thĭ) [" + *pathos*, disease]. Any skin disease.

dermophlebitis (der-mo-fle-bi'tis) [" + *phleps*, vein, + *-ītis*, inflammation]. Inflammation of superficial veins and surrounding skin.

dermophylax'is [" + *phylax*, a guard]. The protective function of the skin in warding off infections.

dermophyte (der'mo-fīt) [" + *phyton*, plant]. A vegetable skin parasite. Syn: *dermatophyte.*

dermoskel'eton [" + *skeleton*, skeleton]. The exoskeleton. The remnants in man are seen in the hair, nails, and teeth.

dermostenosis (der-mo-sten-o-'sis) [" + *stenōsis*, narrowing]. A tightening of the skin. See: *scleroderma.*

dermosynovitis (dĕr-mō-sĭn-ō-vī'tĭs) [" + *syn*, with, + L. *ovum*, egg, + G. *-ītis*, inflammation]. Inflammation of the synovial sheaths and the adjacent skin.

dermosyphilopathy (der"mo-sif"ĭ-lop'ă-thĭ) [" + *syn*, together, + *philein*, to love, + *pathos*, disease]. Any syphilitic disease of the skin.

dermotrop'ic [" + *tropē*, a turning]. Acting esp. on the skin.

dermovac'cine [" + L. *vaccinus*, pert. to a cow]. A vaccine for skin inoculation.

derodidymus (der"o-did'ĭ-mus) [*derē* + G. *didymos*, double]. A malformed fetus with a single body, two necks and heads, and two upper and lower limbs. Syn: *dicephalus.*

desatura'tion [L. *dē*, from, + *saturāre*, to fill]. A process whereby a saturated organic compound is converted into an unsaturated one, as when stearic acid, $CH_3.(CH_2)_{16}.COOH$, is changed into oleic acid, $C_{17}H_{33}.COOH$. The product has different physical and chemical properties after this transformation.

Desault's appara'tus or **ban'dage** (de-sōz') [Pierre J. Desault, French surgeon, 1744-1795]. Bandage used for fracture of clavicle. See: *bandage.*

descemetitis (des-em-et-i'tis) [G. *-ītis*, inflammation]. Inflammation of Descemet's membrane on the corneal post. surface; serous cyclitis.

Descemet's membrane. (des'māz) [Jean Descemet, French anatomist, 1732-1810]. A fine membrane bet. the endothelial layer of the cornea and the substantia propia; *lamina elastica posterior.* See: *Demours' membrane.*

descemetocele (des-se-met'o-sēl) [G. *kēlē*, hernia]. Protrusion of Descemet's membrane.

descendens (de-sen'dens) [L. *dē*, from, + *scandere*, to climb]. Descending; a descending structure.

d. hypoglossi, d. noni. A branch of the hypoglossal nerve given off at the point where it curves around the occipital artery, which passes down obliquely across the sheath of the carotid vessels (sometimes within it) to form a loop just below the middle of the neck with branches of the 2d and 3rd cervical nerves.

descensus (de-sen'sus) [L. a falling]. Falling, descent. Syn: *ptosis.*

d. testis. Passage of the testicle down into the scrotum. Syn: *migration of testicle.*

d. uteri. Defective pelvic floor allowing the uterus or part of the uterus to protrude out of the vagina. Syn: *pro-*

lapse of uterus; prolapsus uteri; procidentia.

VARIETIES: *First Degree*: Where the cervix uteri reaches down to the vaginal introitus. *Second Degree*: Where the cervix uteri protrudes out of the vagina. *Third Degree*: Where the entire uterus lies outside of the vagina. This is the condition known as procidentia uteri.

ETIOL: This condition may be congenital or acquired, although it is most usually acquired. The etiological factors are congenital weakness of the uterine supports; injury to the pelvic floor or uterine supports during childbirth.

SYM: The condition is most often seen following instrumental deliveries, or where the patient has been allowed to bear down before the cervix is fully dilated. With it there is frequently associated a prolapsus of the ant. and post. vaginal walls, as seen in cystocele and rectocele. In the early stages there are dragging sensations in the lower abdomen, backache while standing and on exertion, sensation of weight and bearing down in the perineum, frequency of urination and incontinence of urine in cases associated with cystocele. In the later stages a protrusion or a swelling at the vulva is noticed on standing or straining, and leukorrhea. In procidentia there is frequently pain on walking, inability to urinate unless the mass is reduced, and quite commonly cystitis.

TREATMENT: The treatment depends upon the age of the patient, the degree of prolapsus, and the associated pathology. Where conservation is desired the use of the pessary is clearly indicated, or conservative surgery (round ligament shortening and pelvic floor repair) may be practiced. In the elderly patient where the uterus is pathological, a hysterectomy (abdominal or vaginal) accompanied by vaginal plastic work is indicated.

d. ventriculi. Downward displacement of the stomach. SYN: *gastroptosis.*

desensitiza'tion. 1. Term applied to the condition when sensitized animals on recovering from an anaphylactic shock do not react to a subsequent injection of the antigen within a reasonable period. 2. Loss of sensitivity.

desen'sitize [L. *dē,* from, + *sentire,* to perceive]. 1. To deprive of or lessen sensitivity by nerve section or blocking. 2. To abate anaphylactic sensitiveness by administration of the specific antigen in low dosage.

desex'ualize [" + *sexus,* sex]. To castrate, to remove testicles or ovaries.

deshydremia (des-hi-dre'mĭ-ă) [" + *ydōr,* water, + *aima,* blood]. Lack of fluid elements of the blood.

desiccant (des'ĭk-ant). Causing desiccation or dryness.

des'iccate [L. *desiccāre,* to dry up]. To dry.

desicca'tion [L. *desiccāre,* to dry up]. The process of drying up. SEE: *electrodesiccation.*

d., electric. Electric therapy to cure a lesion.

desiccative (des'ĭ-ka-tiv). Causing to dry up.

desmalgia (dez-mal'jĭ-ă) [G. *desmos,* band, + *algos,* pain]. Pain in a ligament.

desmectasia, desmectasis (des-mek-ta'zĭ-ă, -tă-sis) [" + *ektasis,* dilatation]. The stretching of a tendon.

desmepithelium (des-mep-ĭ-the'lĭ-um) [" + *epi,* upon, + *thēlē,* nipple]. The epithelial lining of vessels and synovial cavities.

desmitis (des-mi'tis) [" + *-ītis,* inflammation]. Inflammation of a ligament.

desmo- [G. *desmos*]. Prefix: A bond, a ligature.

desmocyte (des'mo-sīt) [" + *kytos,* cell]. A supporting tissue cell. SYN: *fibroblast, fibrocyte.*

desmocytoma (des-mo-sī-to'ma) [" + " + *ōma,* tumor]. A tumor formed of desmocytes; a sarcoma.

desmodyn'ia [" + *odynē,* pain]. Pain in a ligament.

desmo'enzyme. An enzyme which is bound to the protoplasm of cells and difficult to extract, in contrast to *lyoenzymes* which can be readily extracted.

desmogenous (des-moj'ĕ-nus) [" + *gennan,* to produce]. Of connective tissue origin.

desmog'raphy [" + *graphein,* to write]. A description of or treatise on ligaments.

des'moid [" + *eidos,* form]. 1. Tendonlike; fibroid. 2. A very tough and firm fibroma.

desmology (des-mol'o-jĭ) [" + *logos,* science]. Science of tendons and ligaments.

desmo'ma [" + *-ōma,* tumor]. A tumor of the connective tissue.

desmoneoplasm (dez-mo-ne'o-plazm) [" + *neos,* new, + *plasma,* matter]. A connective tissue tumor.

desmopathy (des-mop'ă-thĭ) [" + *pathos,* disease]. Any disease affecting ligaments.

desmopexia (des-mo-peks'ĭ-ă) [" + *pēxis,* fixation]. Fixation of round ligaments to the abdominal wall for the correction of uterine displacement.

desmoplas'tic [" + *plassein,* to form]. Causing or forming adhesions.

desmopyknosis (dez-mo-pik-no'sis) [" + *pyknōsis,* a condensation]. Dudley's operation. Shortening of round ligaments by attaching them by loops to the ant. uterine wall.

desmorrhexis (des-mo-reks'is) [" + *rēxis,* rupture]. Rupture of a ligament.

desmosis (des-mo'sis) [" + *-ōsis*]. Any disease of the connective tissue.

desmosome (des'mo-sōm) [" + *sōma,* body]. A small thickening in an intercellular bridge.

desmotomy (des-mot'o-mĭ) [" + *tomē,* incision]. Dissection of ligament.

desoxy. Prefix meaning *deoxidized* or *a reduced form of.* SEE ALSO: *deoxy-,* words.

desoxycorticosterone (dĕs-ok"sĭ-kôr-tĭ-kŏs'tĕr-ōn). An active steroid hormone produced by the adrenal cortex. It plays an important role in the regulation of water and salt metabolism.

d. acetate. USP. An acetate ester of desoxycorticosterone and the form in which the hormone is usually administered in its therapeutic use. It may be injected intramuscularly or used buccally.

desoxyephedrine (dĕs-ok"sĭ-ĕf'ĕd-rĭn). A synthetic compound, related to amphetamine and ephedrine, which acts as a cerebral stimulant and vasoconstrictor. Usually used in the form of dextrodesoxyephedrine hydrochloride for the relief of fatigue, to overcome sleepiness or drowsiness, and to counteract a depressed mood.

desoxyribonucleic acid. Former spelling for deoxyribonucleic acid, *q.v.*

despumation (de-spu-ma'shun) [L. *dē,* from, + *spuma,* froth]. Separation of froth or scum from a liquid.

des'quamate [" + *squamāre,* to scale off]. To shred or scale off the surface epithelium.

desquamation (des-kwă-ma'shun) [" + *squama,* scale]. Shedding of the epidermis.

d., furfuraceous. Shedding of branlike scales.

desquamative (des-kwam'ă-tiv) [" + *squamāre,* to scale off]. Of the nature of desquamation or pert. to, or causing it.

desudation (de-su-da'shun) [L. *dē,* from, + *sudāre,* to perspire]. Excessive sweating often followed by slight pustular eruption.

desynchronosis (de"sin-kro-no'sis). The time difference between that of a person's present location and that to which he is accustomed. This causes an upset of the individual's internal *biological clock.*

det. Abbr. for [L.] *detur,* let it b given.

detachment [F. *detacher,* to unfasten]. To become separate.

d., retinal. The pathological condition where the retina or a part of it becomes separated from the choroid.

detector. Device for determining the presence of something.

d., lie. A device which, by indicating changes in pulse rate and force, and electrical property of the skin, may be useful in indicating when a person is telling a lie.

detelec'tasis [" + *ektasis,* dilatation]. Lack of normal inflation; collapse of an organ.

deter'gent [L. *detergere,* to cleanse]. 1. A medicine that purges or cleanses; cleansing. 2. A cleaning or wetting agent prepared synthetically from higher alcohols, sulfuric acid and caustic soda.

deteriora'tion [L. *deteriorāre,* to deteriorate]. Retrogression; said of impairment of mental or physical functions.

determina'tion [L. *determināre,* to limit]. 1. A tendency in a definite direction, as of blood, to a part. 2. A quantitative analysis.

determinism (de-term'in-izm) [" + G. *ismos,* condition of]. The theory that all human action is the result of innate urges although they may not be conscious ones.

deter'sive [L. *detergere,* to cleanse]. Detergent; cleansing or purging.

dethyroidism (de-thi'roid-izm) [L. *dē,* away + G. *thyreoeides,* like a shield]. Condition resulting from removal of the thyroid.

dethy'roidized [" + G. *thyreoeides,* like a shield]. Without a thyroid gland.

detonation (det-o-na'shun) [L. *detonāre,* to thunder loudly]. A violent noise caused by an explosive combustion.

detoxicate (de-tok'sĭ-kāt) [L. *dē,* from + G. *toxikon,* poison]. To remove the toxic principle of a substance. Syn: *detoxify.*

detoxify (de-toks'ĭ-fi) [" + " + L. *facere,* to make]. To remove the toxic quality of a substance. Syn: *detoxicate.*

detrition (de-trish'un) [" + *terere,* to wear]. The wearing away of a part, esp. through friction, as that of the teeth.

detritus (de-tri'tus) [" + *terere,* to wear]. Any broken down or degenerative tissue or carious matter.

detruncation (de-trun-ka'shun) [" + *truncus,* trunk]. Decapitation, esp. of a fetus. Syn: *decollation.*

detrusor urinae (de-tru'sor u-ri'ne) [L.]. Ext. longitudinal layer of muscular coat of bladder.

detumescence (de-tu-mes'ens) [L. *dē,* down, + *tumescere,* to swell]. 1. Subsidence of a swelling. 2. Subsidence of erectile tissue of genital organs (penis and clitoris) following erection.

deutencephalon (dūt-en-sef'ă-lon) [G. *deuteros,* second, + *egkephalos,* brain]. The interbrain. Syn: *thalamencephalon; diencephalon.*

deuteranopia, deuteranopsia (du-ter-an-o'pĭ-a, -op'sĭ-ă) [" + *anopia,* blindness]. Green blindness, so named because green is the 2nd of the primary colors. See: *protanopia, tritanopia.*

deuterium (dū-te'rĭ-um) [G. *deuteros,* second]. Heavy hydrogen; the mass 2 isotope of hydrogen, symbol H^2 or D.

d. oxide. Heavy water.

deuteroal'bumose [" + L. *albumen,* white of egg]. An albumose formed in peptic digestion of proteins.

deuteroelas'tose [" + L. *elasticus,* elastic]. A deuteroalbumose formed in the peptic digestion of elastin.

deuteromyosinose (du-ter-o-mī-o'sĭn-ōz) [" + G. *mys,* muscle]. A product of myosin digestion.

deuteron (du'ter-on). The nucleus of deuterium or heavy hydrogen. Syn: *deuton.*

deuteropathi'a, deuterop'athy [" + *pathos,* disease]. A disease associated with or secondary to another disease.

deu'teroplasm [" + *plasma,* matter]. Inclusion bodies. Syn: *paraplasm.*

deutoscolex (du-to-sko'lex) [" + *skolex,* intestinal worm]. Secondary daughter cysts which develop on the inner wall of a hydatid cyst.

devasation (de-vas-a'shun) [L. *dē,* away, + *vasa,* vessel]. Destruction of blood vessels.

devascularization (de-vas"ku-lar-ĭ-za'-shun) [" + *vascularis,* pert. to a vessel]. 1. Loss or draining of blood from a part. 2. To decrease the blood supply to a part of the body.

devel'opment [Fr. *de'velopper,* to unwrap]. Growth to full size or maturity. Progress of an egg to the adult state. Evolution.

development, words pert. to: anoria, aplasia, apposition, ateliosis, auxology, cacogenesis, caryogenesis, cavalry bone, cenopsychic, chondrosis, chorista.

developmental (de-vel-op-men'tal) [Fr. *développer,* to unwrap]. Pert. to development.

deviation (de-vĭ-a'shun) [L. *dē,* from, + *via,* way]. Going out of the way; departure from normal.

d., axis. A change in the direction of the major electrical axis of the heart as determined by the electrocardiogram.

d., conjugate. Deviation of face and eyes to the same side in paralytics.

d., minimum. The smallest deviation that a prism can produce.

d. of complement. Incapable of hemolysis.

d., standard. Measure of variability of any frequency curve.

deviom'eter [" + " + G. *metron,* measure]. Device for estimating degree of strabismus.

devisceration (de-vis-er-a'shun) [" + *viscus, viscer-,* internal organ]. Removal of viscera. Syn: *evisceration.*

devitaliza'tion [" + *vita,* life]. 1. Destruction or loss of vitality. 2. Anesthetizing sensitive pulp of a tooth; known as "killing the nerve."

devolution (dev-o-lu'shun) [L. *devolvere*, to roll down]. Catabolism; degeneration.

dew cure. Walking with bare feet in grass wet with dew. SYN: *kneippism.*

dew point. Temperature at which dew begins to form.

dexter (deks'ter) [L. *dexter*, right]. On the right side.

dextrad (dex'trad) [L. *dexter*, right, + *ad*, toward]. Toward the right side.

dextral (dex'tral). Pert. to the right side.

dex'tran [L. *dexter*, right]. $C_6H_{10}O_5$. A monodextrin, it is used as a substitute for blood plasma in severe burns and shock.

dex'trase [L. *dexter*, right]. An enzyme that splits dextrose and converts it into lactic acid.

dex'trin [L. *dexter*, right]. A yellowish-white powder which forms mucilaginous solutions in water and can be prepared by the action of heat or acid on starch.

It is a *carbohydrate* of the formula $(C_6H_{10}O_5)n$. In digestion it is soluble or gummy matter into which starch is converted by diastase and is the result of the first chemical change in the digestion of starch.

dextrinuria (deks-trin-u'rĭ-ă) [" + G. *ouron*, urine]. Dextrin in the urine.

dextro- [L. *dexter*, *dextr-*]. Prefix: To the right.

dextroamphetamine sulfate (deks'tro-am-fet'ă-mēn sul'fāt). USP. A compound related to amphetamine sulfate (*i.e.*, an isomer of amphetamine). Used as a central nervous system stimulant in treatment of mild depression; used also for control of appetite in obesity. Sometimes written *d-amphetamine sulfate* or *dextro-amphetamine sulfate.*

dextrocardia (deks-tro-kar'dĭ-ă) [" + G. *kardia*, heart]. Having the heart on the right side of body.

dextrocar'diogram [" + " + *gramma*, a writing]. A cardiogram representing action of the right ventricle.

dextroc'ular [" + *oculus*, eye]. Having a stronger right eye than the left one.

dextrocularity (deks-trok-ū-lar'ĭ-tĭ) [" + *oculus*, eye]. The condition of having the right eye stronger than the left.

dextroduc'tion [" + *ducere*, to lead]. The movement of visual axis to the right.

dextrogas'tria [" + G. *gastēr*, belly]. Having the stomach on right side of body.

dextrogyrate (deks-tro-ji'rāt). To turn to the right. Bending of light rays to the right.

dextrogyre (deks'tro-jīr) [" + *gyrāre*, to turn]. A substance turning to the right.

dextroman'ual [" + *manus*, hand]. Right-handed.

dextropedal (deks-trop'ĕ-dal) [" + *pēs*, *ped-*, foot]. Having greater dexterity in using the right leg than the left one.

dextropho'bia [" + G. *phobos*, fear]. Abnormal aversion to objects on right side of body.

dextrorotatory (deks-tro-ro'tă-tor-ĭ) [" + *rotāre*, to turn]. Turning rays of light to the right.

dextrose (deks'trōs) [" + *ose*, chemical name for sugar]. A simple sugar of the monosaccharose* group; also known as glucose, or grape sugar. $C_6H_{12}O_6$, a crystalline solid which can be made by the action of acids on starches (USP.) and occurs naturally in the juices of plants and the body fluids of animals.

It is very soluble in water, is an important constituent of corn syrup and honey, and is an example of one kind of carbohydrate, *q.v.* The most important of the monosaccharide group. It is usually associated with levulose. Its presence in the urine in large amounts is symptomatic of diabetes. This may also obtain in brain injuries, cirrhosis of the liver, in normal pregnancies, and as a result of the administration of epinephrine or thyroxin. It is formed in the digestive tract by the action of enzymes on carbohydrates. It occurs naturally.

NP: For rectal, intravenous, or subcutaneous injection, a 5% glucose in sterile pyrogen-free water solution is used.

USP: SEE: *disaccharose, glucose.*

RS: *diabetes, glycosuria, hyperglycemia, hypoglycemia.*

dextrosinistral (deks-tro-sin-is'trăl) [" + *sinister*, left]. From right to left.

dextrosuria (deks-trōs-ū'rĭ-ă) [*dextrose* + G. *ouron*, urine]. Dextrose in the urine.

dextrotropic, dextrotropous (deks-tro-trop'ik, trot'ro-pus) [L. *dexter*, right, + G. *tropos*, a turning]. Turning to the right.

dextrover'sion [" + *vertere*, to turn]. Turned toward the right.

dezymotize (de-zi'mo-tīz) [L. *dē*, from, + G. *zymē*, leaven]. To free of ferments or germs.

dg. Abbreviation for *decigram.*

dhobie itch (do'be). Tropical name for form of *Tinea cruris* that is more intense than that of temperate zone.

di- [G.]. Prefix: Twice.

diabetes (di-ă-be'tēz) [G. *dia*, through, + *bainein*, to go].

d., brittle. About 15% of patients with diabetes mellitus have an unstable form of the disease which is difficult to regulate. Many of these patients developed their disease prior to the age of 15 years. Diabetics who are extremely difficult to regulate are said to have "brittle" or unstable diabetes.

d., bronze. Hemochromatosis. A disease of metabolism characterized by deposition of pigment in various organs of the body, cirrhosis of the liver and pancreas, and diabetes.

d., hysterical. Polyuria induced by a hysterical attack or state.

d. insipidus. Polyuria* due to vasopressin deficiency. SYM: Enormous amounts of urine, pale and watery. Sp. gr. 1.002-5. No sugar or albumin. More common in the young. Thirst, weakness, dry skin. ETIOL: In almost half of all cases, the cause is unknown. Trauma to the head which causes damage to the pituitary or a tumor in that area causes the remainder of cases. PROG: Essentially chronic. TREATMENT: Eradication of causative factor (as tumors) if determined. When not due to specific injury of the pituitary, the disease is easily controlled by use of vasopressin replacement therapy. This may be given by injection or nasal spray.

d., juvenile-onset. Diabetes which has its onset prior to the age of 15 years. This form is usually quite difficult to regulate.

d. melli'tus. A disorder of carbohydrate metabolism characterized by hyperglycemia, and glycosuria, resulting from inadequate production or utilization of insulin.

ETIOL: Basic cause is still unknown but direct cause is failure of beta cells of the pancreas to secrete an adequate amount of insulin. In the absence of insulin, glycogenesis and glycolysis are adversely affected. It is currently thought that insulin acts primarily at the cell membrane facilitating transport of glucose into cells.

SYM: Principal symtoms are: elevated blood sugar (hyperglycemia), sugar in urine (glycosuria), excessive urine production (polyuria), excessive thirst (polydipsia), and increase in food intake (polyphagia).

Urine sp. gr. 1.020-40; sugar excessive; urine shows diacetic acid, betaoxybutyric acid, acetone when disease process is in advanced stage. More common in women and after the age of 40. Increased thirst; frequent urination, 3 to 10 qt. a day; itching, frequently about the genitals. Fasting blood sugar raised above normal range of 90 to 120 mg. per 100 cc. (ml.) of blood; boils and carbuncles; loss of weight, emaciation, weakness, and debility. When severe diabetes is allowed to progress without proper treatment, coma ensues with weakness, and sweet odor of breath; nausea, headache, vomiting, dyspnea, sense of intoxication, delirium, deep coma, and death. The isolation and eventual production of insulin in 1921 by Doctors Banting and Best made it possible to allow persons with this disease to lead a normal life.

COMPLICATIONS: Diabetic acidosis due to excessive production of ketone bodies; low resistance to infections especially those involving extremities; increase in incidence of toxemia in pregnancy and cardiovascular disorders; disturbances in electrolyte balance; eye disorders.

PROG: Diabetes is a chronic, incurable disease but symptoms can be ameliorated and life prolonged by modern treatment.

TREATMENT: Consists of diet, insulin and exercise. When first discovered, the patient should be placed on well-balanced diet adequate in all basic essentials: carbohydrates, proteins, fats, vitamins, minerals, and fluids. In many patients this may be all that is required. It is important that obese persons with this disease be placed on a diet which will enable them to lose weight. Control of diabetes is much more difficult in an obese person. Blood sugar determinations should be made at frequent intervals. NOTE: Blood sugar and glucose are considered to be the same.

When a patient is given an adequate diet and the glucose still appears in the urine, insulin may be necessary. Its use is not required in every case and may be dangerous if not properly given. In the last several years certain drugs have been given by mouth for the control of mild cases of diabetes. These have been used with success mostly in middle-aged and older patients.

DIET: Standardization of patients—a balanced diet of approximately 1000-1200 calories may be prescribed. This should be increased promptly if levels of glucose in the blood are brought within normal limits. In planning a diet, the age, weight and type of work or physical activity in which the patient is engaged is important. Standardized diets have been worked out in which the necessary proportions of carbohydrates, proteins, and fats are standardized. The diets vary from 1200 to 3000 calories. Frequent feedings (five or six in 24 hours) rather than the standard three meals is preferred. The older the patient, as a rule, the smaller the proportion of fat in the diet.

NP: The nursing care of the patient with diabetes includes general hygienic care, giving insulin, collecting specimens, preventing and treating complications, serving the prescribed diet, and teaching how to take care of himself.

General hygienic care: Care of the skin and feet. The skin must be kept scrupulously clean. Daily warm baths are essential. Irritation or bruises should be promptly attended to, as any break in the skin heals with difficulty, and diabetics are susceptible to bedsores, infection and gangrene. Because of the poor circulation in the feet they should have special care, being kept clean and dry, especially between the toes. Care should be taken in trimming the toenails, as the slightest abrasion of the skin may become infected. Olive oil or lanolin to keep the feet soft and smooth. Tight shoes must be avoided. The care of the mouth and teeth is most important. The teeth should be brushed well at least three times a day and a mouthwash should be used before and after eating. The patient should be encouraged to see his dentist regularly. The bowels should be kept open by regulation of the diet, if possible, or by laxatives or enemas. Constipation should be guarded against as it predisposes to coma.

Administration of Insulin: The dosage and frequency in which insulin is given will depend on the individual patient and the physician prescribing it. In administering the drug, precautions necessary in giving hypodermic injections should be observed. Care taken not to inject the drug repeatedly in the same area and trauma should be avoided. Every diabetic patient should be taught to give himself insulin or if he is unable to give it to himself, some member of the family should be instructed.

Collecting Specimens: Both single and 24-hour urine specimens may be collected. They are usually examined daily. It is especially important that the specimens are accurately collected, labeled, and sent to the laboratory on time. The diagnosis and treatment are based mostly upon the results of the urine examination. Specimens of blood may be collected by the physician for blood chemistry. The specimen is taken early in the morning before the patient has his breakfast.

Prevention of Complications: Close observation of the patient is necessary. Shock may be avoided if the patient is closely watched or if the patient has been taught that when he has the slightest symptom of insulin reaction to call the nurse. He may be instructed to eat a lump or two of sugar or to keep a piece of hard candy within his reach.

Acidosis and coma may also be prevented by the recognition of first symptoms and prompt treatment. The chief symptoms of acidosis are pain in the abdomen, nausea, vomiting, drowsiness, and difficult breathing. The doctor should be notified when the first symptoms appear. The patient kept warm with blankets and hot water bottles. He should not be left alone. His pulse should be closely watched.

Teaching the Patient: There is perhaps no other disease in which it is as important that the patient is taught all the factors involved in the management and treatment. The patient should understand that he will have to continue treatment all his life and that he must abide strictly by everything taught him in the hospital. His mouth and teeth should be kept in good condition. It is necessary to pay particular attention to his feet (see above). His diet must be followed. He should also understand the complications that may arise and the measures he may take to prevent them. He is taught to take his insulin and examine his urine. He should be taught importance of reporting to physician for frequent check-ups. SEE ALSO: *coma, diabetic.*

d., pancreatic. D. associated with disease of the pancreas.

d., phlorizin. Glycosuria caused by administration of phlorizin.

d., renal. Renal glycosuria. Condition characterized by a low renal threshold for sugar. Glucose tolerance is normal and diabetic symptoms are lacking.

d., true. SEE: *d. mellitus.*

diabetic di-ă-bet'ik). Pert. to diabetes.

d. center. Area in the floor of the fourth ventricle.

d. coma. Loss of consciousness due to severe diabetes mellitus which has not been treated or treatment has not been adequately regulated.

d. ear. Otitis media diabetica.

d. neuritis. Multiple neuritis of diabetes.

d. sugar. Glucose in the sugar of the urine of diabetics.

d. tabes. Diabetes with neuritic pains in leg and loss of knee jerk.

diabetide (di-ă-be'tid). A cutaneous form of diabetes.

diabetin (di-ă-be'tin) [G. *dia,* through, + *bainein,* to go]. Pure crystallized levulose used as a substitute for cane sugar in diabetes.

diabetogenic (di-ă-bet-o-jen'ik) [" + " + *gennan,* to produce]. Causing diabetes.

diabetogenous (di-ă-bĕ-toj'ĕ-nus) [" + " + *gennan,* to produce]. Diabetogenic*; caused by diabetes.

diabetometer (di-ă-bĕ-tom'ĕ-ter) [" + " + *metron,* a measure]. A device for measuring sugar in diabetic urine.

diaboleptic (di-ab-o-lep'tik) [G. *diabolos,* devil, + *lepsis,* a seizure]. One professing to have supernatural communication, esp. with the devil.

diabrosis (di-ă-brō'sis) [G. *diabrōsis,* an eating through]. A corrosion causing perforation.

diabrot'ic [G. *diabrōsis,* an eating through]. 1. Corrosive. 2. An escharotic or corrosive.

diacele (di'ă-sēl) [G. *dia,* between, + *koilia,* a hollow]. The 3rd ventricle of the brain. SYN: *diacoele.*

diacetate (di-as'et-āt). A salt of diacetic acid.

diacetemia (di-as-ĕ-te'mĭ-ă) [diacetic acid + G. *aima,* blood]. Diacetic acid in the blood.

diacetic acid (di-ă-set'ik). Acetoacetic acid, found in acidosis and in the urine of the diabetic.

It is similar to acetone and is found in serious diabetes and in any condition which produces starvation, such as persistent vomiting.

d. a. test (in urine). Half fill a test tube with freshly voided urine. Then add, drop by drop, some ferric chloride solution, which will cause a deposit of iron phosphate to form. Now filter the mixture and add a few more drops of ferric chloride. If diacetic acid is present a port wine color develops. The specimen is now divided into two parts, one being used as a control. One part is boiled, when the color will quickly disappear if it is due to diacetic acid.

diacetonu'ria [diacetic acid + G. *ouron,* urine]. Diacetic acid in urine; diaceturia.

diaceturia (di-as-ĕ-tu'rĭ-ă) [" + G. *ouron,* urine]. Diacetonuria; diacetic acid in urine.

diacid (di-as'id) [G. *dis,* twice, + L. *acidus,* soured]. Having 2 atoms of hydrogen replaceable with a base.

diaclasia (di-ă-kla'zĭ-ă) [G. *dia,* through, + *klan,* to break]. A fracture, esp. breaking a bone before surgery.

diaclast (di'ă-klăst) [" + *klan,* to break]. Device for perforating the fetal skull.

diacoele (di'ă-sēl). The third ventricle of brain. SYN: *diacele.*

diacrinous (di-ăk'rin-us) [G. *diakrinein,* to separate]. Pert. to cells which secrete outwardly; exocrine.*

diacrisis (di-ăk'rĭ-sis) [G. *diakrisis,* separation]. 1. A change in the character of a secretion. 2. Any disease having an altered secretion. 3. A critical discharge.

diacrit'ic, diacrit'ical [G. *dia,* apart, + *krinein,* to judge]. Diagnostic; said of symptoms.

diad (di'ad) [G. *dis,* twice]. An element or radical having an atomicity of 2; a bivalent element.

di'aderm. Blastoderm composed of ectoderm and entoderm, and containing bet. them the segmentation cavity.

diadochokinesia (di-ad"ō-ko-kĭ-ne'zĭ-ă) [G. *diadokos,* succeeding, + *kinesis,* motion]. Ability to make antagonistic movements, as pronation and supination, in quick succession. SEE: *disdiadochokinesia.*

diagnose (di'ag-nōs) [G. *dia,* through + *gignoskein,* to know]. To determine the cause and nature of a pathological condition; to recognize a disease.

diagnosis (di-ag-no'sis) (pl. *diagnoses*) [" + *gnōsis,* knowledge]. 1. The term denoting name of the disease a person has or is believed to have. For example, one is found to have pneumonia. Thus the *diagnosis* is pneumonia. 2. The use of scientific and skillful methods to establish the cause and nature of a sick person's disease. This is done by evaluating (a) the history of the disease process (b) the signs and symptoms present (c) laboratory data (d) special tests such as x-ray and electrocardiograms.

The value of establishing a diagnosis is to provide a logical basis for treatment and prognosis.

d., clinical. One determined by symptoms alone; they may be *objective* (visible symptoms); *subjective* (those of internal or mental origin), and *cardinal* (those pert. to respiration, pulse, and temperature). Symptoms may be *local* or conditions may be pathological. Most diseases have a symptom or symptoms in common with some other disease.

d., cytological. D. based on cells present in body tissues or exudates.

d., differential. Comparison of symptoms of two similar diseases to determine from which the patient is suffering. SEE: *differential diagnosis.*

d. by exclusion. Establishing a diagnosis by eliminating other possibilities.

d., pathological. D. based on structural lesions present.

d., physical. D. by external examination only.

d., roentgen. D. based on roentgenograms.

d., serum. D. by means of serum and its effects.

diagnosis, *words pert. to:* abdomen; auscultation; blood; breathing; chest; colic; coma; constipation; convulsion; cough; diffusion, ear; examination, physical; eye; face; fatigue; feces; fever; gait; gums; head, examination of; headache; infection; inflammation; inspection; nail; nausea; organ, see name of; pain; pallor; palpation; palpitation; percussion; perspiration; position; pulse; pus; reflexes; respiration; skin; sputum; syncope; teeth; temperature; tongue; unconsciousness; urine; vertigo; vomiting.

diagnos′tic. Pert. to a diagnosis.

diagnostician (di-ag-nos-tish′un) [G. *dia,* through, + *gignoskein,* to know]. One skilled in diagnosis.

diagraph (di′ă-graf) [" + *graphein,* to write]. Device for recording outlines, esp. of the cranium.

Dialister (di-ă-lis′ter). A genus of bacteria of the family Bacteroidaceae found in the respiratory tract during influenza.

D. pneumosin′tes. A bacterium found in the nasal secretions at beginning of influenza.

dialy- [G.]. Prefix: To separate.

dialysate (di-al′ĭ-sāt) [G. *dia,* through, + *lyein,* to loosen]. A liquid that has been dialyzed.

dialysis (di-al′ĭ-sis) [" + *lysis,* loosening]. 1. The passage of a solute through a membrane. 2. A process in which a liquid to be purified or studied is enclosed in a thin, membranous sack and exposed to water or any other solvent which continually circulates or changes outside the sack.

Diffusible substances pass through the membrane, but colloidal material does not. SEE: *absorption; diffusion; osmosis.*

dialyt′ic. Belonging to or resembling the process of dialysis.

di′alyze [G. *dia,* through, + *lyein,* to loosen]. To make a dialysis or to have made one.

dialyzable (di-ă-liz′ă-bl). Capable of dialysis.

dialyzer (di-ă-liz-er) [G. *dia,* through, + *lyein,* to loosen]. Membrane used in performing dialysis.

diamagnet′ic [" + *magnēs,* magnet]. Repulsion by the magnet.

diameter (di-am′ĕ-ter) [" + *metron,* a measure]. The distance from any point on the periphery of a surface, body, or space to the opposite point.

d., anterior transverse, of the fetal head. SEE: *temporal d.*

d., anteroposterior, of the pelvic cavity. The distance bet. middle of symphysis pubis and upper border of 3rd sacral vertebra.

d., a., of pelvic inlet. The distance from upper part of symphysis pubis to promontory of sacrum (about 11 cm. in female). SYN: *true conjugate d. of pelvic inlet.*

d., anteroposterior, of pelvic outlet. Distance between tip of coccyx and lower edge of symphysis pubis (from 9 to 11.5 cm. in female).

d., a., of skull. The distance in a straight line bet. the metopic point and the most remote point upon the external surface of the tabular portion of the occipital bone, or bet. most prominent point of the glabella and the most prominent point upon the external surface of the occipital bone.

d., basilobregmatic. Distance in a straight line bet. basilon and bregma.

d., biauricular. 1. Distance in a straight line bet. two points on a line passing over the vertex and uniting the two auricular points, each immediately above the ridge which continues the zygomatic arch backward. 2. Transverse distance bet. the centers of external auditory meatuses, or bet. middle point of the upper margins of each external auditory meatus.

d., biglenoid. Distance bet. the center of one glenoid cavity of the temporal bone and that of the other.

d., biischial. D. between the ischial spines.

d., bijugal. Horizontal distance bet. two malar points.

d., bijugular. Transverse distance bet. two jugular points.

d., bimalar. The transverse distance bet. two malar points.

d., bimandibular. Transverse distance bet. tubercles on the inferior borders of the inferior maxilla.

d., bimastoid. Transverse distance bet. two mastoid processes of the temporal bone.

d., biparietal. Transverse distance bet. parietal eminences on each side (about 9.25 cm.).

d., bisacromial. Transverse distance bet. two acromial processes.

d., bisiliac. Transverse distance bet. most distant points of the iliac crests. SYN: *intercristal d.*

d., bisischiadic. SEE: *transverse d. of pelvis.*

d., bitemporal. Distance between the temporal bones (about 8 cm.).

d., bitrochanteric. Distance bet. the highest point of one of the greater trochanters and that of the other. SYN: *intertrochanteric d.*

d., bizygomatic. Greatest transverse distance bet. most prominent points of the zygomatic arches.

d., cervicobregmatic. Distance bet. anterior fontanel and junction of the neck with floor of the mouth.

d., diagonal conjugate, of the pelvis. The distance from the upper part of the symphysis pubis to the most distant part of the brim of the pelvis.

d., external biorbital. Greatest transverse distance bet. outer borders of external orbital apophyses of the frontal bone.

d., external conjugate, of the pelvis. Anteroposterior d. of the pelvic inlet measured externally; distance from the skin over the upper part of symphysis pubis to the skin over a point corresponding to the sacral promontory.

d. of fetal skull. Important diameters at full term are: Suboccipitobregmatic, 3¾ in.; cervicobregmatic, 3¾ in.; frontomental, 3 1/5 in.; occipitomental, 5 in.; supraoccipitomental, 5½ in.; occipitofrontal, 4½ in.; suboccipitofrontal, 4 in.; biparietal, 3¾ in.; bitemporal, 3 1/5 in.

d., frontomental. Distance from top of forehead to point of chin.

d., inial. Distance in a straight line, in median line of skull, bet. most prominent points of the inion and the glabella.

d., internal biorbital. Greatest transverse distance bet. inner borders of the external orbital apophyses of the frontal bone.

d., interspinous. Distance bet. the two anterior superior spines of the ilia.

d., maximum anteroposterior, of the skull. Distance, in the median line. bet. the most prominent part of the glabella and the most prominent point in the middle line upon the tabular portion of the occipital bone.

d., m. frontal. Distance bet. two stephanions.

d., m. occipital. Distance in a straight line bet. two asterions.

d., m. transverse, of the skull. Longest horizontal transverse line that can be drawn within the cranium.

d., mentobregmatic. Distance from chin to middle of anterior fontanel.

d., minimum frontal. Distance bet. two extremities of supraorbital line.

d., oblique, of pelvic inlet. Distance from iliopectineal eminence of one side to sacroiliac articulation on opposite side (about 12.5 cm. in female).

d., obstetric, of pelvic inlet. Shortest distance between sacrum and symphysis. This d. is shorter than the true conjugate.

d., occipitofrontal. That extending from the most prominent parts of the frontal and occipital bones (about 12 cm.).

d., occipitomental. Greatest distance bet. occiput and point of chin (about 13 cm.).

d. of pelvis. OBST: *Anteroposterior*: the distance bet. the sacrovertebral angle and the symphysis pubis. *Bi-ischial*: Bet. the ischial spines. *Conjugata diagonalis:* Bet. the sacrovertebral angle and the symphysis pubis. *Conjugata vera*: The true conjugate. Bet. the sacrovertebral angle and the middle of the post. aspect of the symphysis pubis (about 1.5 cm. less than the diagonal conjugate). *Deventer's Oblique*: Bet. the sacroiliac synchondrosis on one side and the ileopectineal eminence on the other side. *Intercristus*: Bet. the crests of the ilium. *Interspinous*: Bet. the spines of the ilium. *Intertrochanteric*: Bet. the greater trochanters when the hips are extended and the legs are held together. *Internal conjugate*: Bet. the promontory of the sacrum and the upper edge of the symphysis pubis. *Pelvic*: Any diameter of the pelvis found by measuring a straight line bet. any two points. *Transverse d. of the inlet*: Distance from the middle of brim, across greatest width of pelvic inlet, to same point of opposite side (about 13.5 cm. in female). *Transverse d. of the pelvic outlet*: Bet. the tuberosities of the ischium. SEE: *pelvis.*

d., posterior sagittal, of midpelvis. Distance between midpoint of interspinous diameter and sacrum (about 5.0 cm.).

d., sacrosubpubic. Distance bet. middle of promontory of sacrum and middle of lower border of the triangular ligament of pubic symphysis.

d., sagittal. SEE: *basilobregmatic d.*

d., sternovertebral. Distance from sternum to vertebral column, measured externally.

d., suboccipitobregmatic. That extending from the bregma to the undersurface of the occiput (about 9.5 cm.).

d., suboccipitofrontal. Greatest distance bet. forehead and junction of occiput with the neck.

d., subtemporal. Distance bet. point upon sphenotemporal suture which is crossed by the ridge upon the inferior surface on the greater wing of the sphenoid bone of one side and a similar point on the other side.

d., temporal. Greatest horizontal distance bet. two opposite points upon the line passing over the vertex and uniting the two auricular points, on surface of the temporal bones.

d., trachelobregmatic. D. bet. ant. fontanel and meeting point of neck with floor of mouth.

d., transverse, of pelvic inlet. Distance from middle of brim, across greatest width of pelvic inlet, to same point on opposite side (about 13.5 cm. in female).

d., transverse, of pelvic outlet. Distance between posterior portions of ischial tuberosities (about 11 cm. in female).

d., true conjugate, of pelvic inlet. Distance between sacrovertebral angle and symphysis pubis (about 11 cm. in female). SYN: *anteroposterior d. of pelvic inlet.*

d., vertical, of fetal head. That extending from highest point of head to ant. margin of foramen magnum.

diamid(e (di-am'ĭd, -īd) [L. *di,* two, + *amide*]. A double amide. SEE: *hydrazine.*

diamine (di-am'ĭn, ēn) [" + *amine*]. A chemical compound with two NH_2 radicals.

diaminu'ria [" + " + " G. *ouron,* urine]. Diamines in the urine.

dianoetic (di"ă-no-et'ik) [G. *dia,* through, + *nous,* mind]. Pertaining to intellectual function, particularly logic and orderly analysis.

diapason (dī-ă-pa'sun) [G. *dia,* through, + *pasōn,* all]. A diagnostic tuning fork used to determine the degree of deafness.

diapedesis (di-ă-ped-e'sis) [" + *pēdan,* to leap]. Passage of blood cells, esp. leukocytes by ameboid movements through the unruptured wall of a capillary vessel.

diaphane (di'ă-fān) [" + *phainein,* to appear]. 1. The investing membrane of a cell. 2. A very small electric light utilized in transillumination.

diaphanometer (di"ă-fan-om'ĕ-ter) [" + " + *metron,* a measure]. A device for estimating the amount of solids in a fluid by its transparency.

diaphanom'etry [" + " + *metron,* measure]. Determination of translucency of a fluid, as the urine.

diaphanoscope (di-ă-fan'o-skōp) [" + " + *skopein,* to examine]. Device for electric examination of body cavities.

diaphanoscopy (di"ă-fan-os'ko-pē). Examination of fluids by the diaphanoscope.

diaphemetric (di"ă-fē-met'rĭk) [" + *aphē,* touch, + *metron,* measure]. Pert. to degree of tactile sensibility.

diaphoresis (di-ă-fo-re'sis) [" + *pherein,* to carry]. Profuse sweating.

diaphoretic (di-ă-fo-ret'ik) [" + *pherein,* to carry]. A sudorific or an agent which increases perspiration. The term sudorific is usually confined to those active agents that cause drops of perspiration to collect on the skin. Ex: *camphor, opium, pilocarpine.* Heat may also be included as such an agent.

d. drugs. These produce their effects either by stimulation, or general applications, or both.

d., refrigerant. One that acts on sweat centers in the spinal cord and medulla, and reduces circulation, *i. e.,* lobelia, tobacco.

d., sedative. One, such as warm drinks or sweat baths, which dilates superficial capillaries and causes relaxation.

d., simple. One that stimulates sudoriferous glands, such as sulfur.

diaphragm (dī'ă-fram) [" + *phragma*, wall]. 1. Thin membrane such as one used for dialysis; 2. In microscopy, an apparatus located beneath the opening in the stage by means of which the amount of light passing through the object can be regulated; 3. A rubber or plastic cup which fits over the cervix uteri and used for contraceptive purposes; 4. A musculomembranous wall separating the abdomen from the thoracic cavity with its convexity upward. It contracts with each inspiration, flattening out downward, permitting the descent of the bases of the lungs. It relaxes with each expiration, elevating it and restoring its inverted basin shape. The deeper the inspiration, the lower the descent of the diaphragm; the greater the expiration, the higher does it rise.

Its origin is at a level with the 6th ribs or intercostal spaces ant., and the 11th or 12th ribs post. The right half rises higher than the left. The lower surface is in relation to the suprarenal bodies of the kidney, the liver, spleen, and cardiac end of the stomach. It aids in defecation and parturition by its ability to cause an increase in intra-abdominal pressure while the person attempts to exhale with the glottis closed. SEE: *straining; Valsalva maneuver.* It becomes spasmodic in hiccoughs and sneezing.

SEE: *midriff, phrenic, "phren-" words.*

d., Bucky. A grid, suspended immediately beneath the x-ray table and above the film tray, so constructed that the effects of backscatter and secondary radiation are eliminated when x-ray photographs of dense structures are taken. Also called Potter-Bucky d.

d., hernia of. Protrusion of abdominal contents through the diaphragm. ETIOL: Congenital or through injury.

d., pelvic. The musculofascial layer forming the lower boundary of the abdominopelvic cavity.

It is funnelshaped, and is pierced in the midline by the urethra, vagina, and rectum. Consists of a muscular layer made up of the paired levator ani and coccygeus muscles. The fascial layer consists of 2 portions, the parietal and visceral layers, the former being made up of the peritoneum continuous with the connective tissue sheaths of the psoas and iliac muscles; the visceral layer is split from the parietal layer at the white line passing downwards and inwards to form the upper sheath of the levator ani muscles; the ant. part of this layer unites the bladder to the post. wall of the pubes.

The middle portion splits into 3 parts: (a) The vesical layer investing bladder and urethra; (b) rectovaginal layer forming the rectovaginal septum; (c) the rectal layer investing the rectum; the post. part is the base of the broad ligament where it sheaths the uterine arteries and supports the cervix.

d., urogenital. Urogenital trigone, or triangular ligament. A musculofascial sheath which lies between the ischiopubic rami. It lies superficial to the pelvic diaphragm and in the male

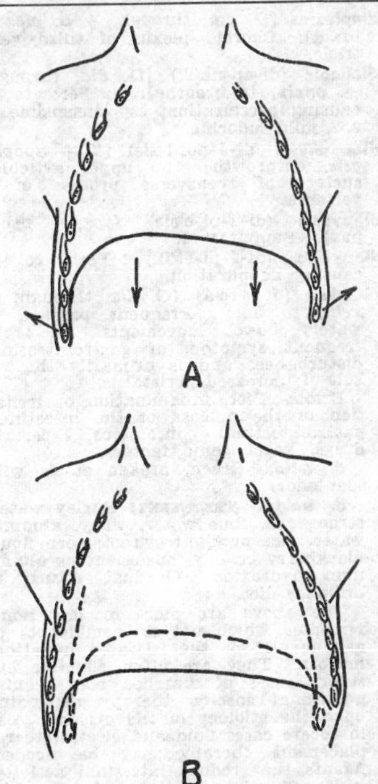

ACTION OF THE DIAPHRAGM

A. Expiration
B. Inspiration

surrounds the membranous urethra, in the female it surrounds the vagina.

diaphragmalgia (dī"ă-frag-mal'jĭ-ă) [G. *dia*, through, + *phragma*, wall, + *algos*, pain]. Pain in the diaphragm.

diaphragmat'ic. Pert. to the diaphragm.

diaphragmatitis. Diaphragmitis, *q.v.*

diaphragmatocele (dī"ă-frag-mat'o-sēl) [" + " + *kēlē*, hernia]. Hernia of the diaphragm.

diaphragmitis (dī"ă-frag-mī'tis) [" + " + *-ītis*, inflammation]. Inflammation of the diaphragm. SYN: *diaphragmatitis.*

di"aphragmodyn'ia [" + " + *odynē*, pain]. Pain in the diaphragm.

diaphysary (dī-af'ĭ-sa-re) [" + *phyein*, to grow]. Pert. to or affecting the shaft of a bone. SEE: *diaphysis.*

diaphysec'tomy [" + " + *ektomē*, excision]. Removal of part of the shaft of a long bone.

diaphysis (dī-af'ĭ-sis) [" + *plassein*, to grow]. The shaft or middle part of a long cylindrical bone. SEE: *apophysis; epiphysis.*

diaphysitis (dī-ă-fī-sī'tis) [" + " + *-ītis*, inflammation]. Inflammation of shaft of a long bone.

diaplasis (dī-ap'lă-sis) [" + *plassein*, to form]. Reduction of a fracture or dislocation. SYN: *diorthosis.*

di'aplex [" + L. *plexus*]. Choroid plexus of third ventricle.

diaplex'al. Pert. to the diaplex.

diaplex'us [G. *dia*, through, + L. *plexus*, braid]. Choroid plexus of third ventricle.

diapnoic (di-ap-no'ik) [G. *dia*, through, + *pnein*, to breathe]. 1. Pert. to or causing perspiration, esp. insensible p. 2. A mild sudorific.

diapophysis (di-ă-pof'ĭ-sis) [" + *apophysis*, outgrowth]. An upper articular surface of transverse process of a vertebra.

diapyesis (di-ă-pi-e'sis) [" + *pyon*, pus]. Suppuration.

diapyetic (di-ă-pi-et'ik). Pert. to or causing suppuration.

diarrhea (di-ă-re'ă) [G. *dia*, through, + *rein*, to flow]. Frequent passage of watery bowel movements. It is a frequent symptom of gastrointestinal disturbances and is primarily the result of increased peristalsis.

Etiol: Diet, inflammation or irritation of the mucosa of the intestines, gastrointestinal infections, certain drugs, psychogenic factors.

d., acid. Green, broken stools with sour odor.

d., acute. Treatment: Barley water, strong tea, lime water, whey, albumin water, rice milk, arrowroot, corn flour, blackberry brandy, adsorbent as aluminum hydroxide. Gradual return to ordinary diet.

The above are more or less home remedies which act as demulcents or astringents for the irritated intestinal mucosa. They are often effective but severe cases of diarrhea may require additional specific therapy depending upon the etiology of the disease. Also in severe cases fluid and electrolyte replacement therapy may be needed. Agents that reduce intestinal activity, such as antispasmodics and paregoric, may provide distinct relief.

d., bilious. Bile in the stools.

d., catarrhal. D. caused by degeneration in the intestines.

d., choleraic. D. accompanying cholera in severe form with vomiting and collapse.

d., chronic. Treatment: (a) Light food; lean meat, white fish, white of eggs, tongue, scraped meat, potted meat, poultry; spinach, vegetable marrow, puree of potato; milk puddings, arrowroot, corn flour; jelly; cooked apples; toast, cereals, but not whole wheat; cake; dry toast, rusk; whey, buttermilk, sour milk; tea, coffee, or cocoa (in moderation); red wine, whortleberry or blackberry wine. Avoid oatmeal, all fibrous foods and causes of intestinal fermentation, meat extracts, strong soups, much sugar, and fat.

(b) Pure milk diet; fresh milk, sour milk.

(c) If very persistent, try protein diet: Raw meat, sandwiches, eggs on toast, chicken, fish, sweetbread, custard, junket, jelly; with small allowance of zwieback, rusk, or toast; butter, sour milk, alum, whey; red wines.

(d) Any food which has been passed through a fine sieve.

d., colliquative. Variety causing collapse, due to frequency of evacuation.

d., congestive. Form caused by congestion of alimentary tract.

d., critical. D. causing a crisis, or occurring at the time of a crisis.

d., emotional. Form caused by emotional stress.

d., epidemic, in newborn. Diarrhea in newborn, caused by Escherichia coli infection and occurring in epidemics in hospitals.

d., fatty. D. with stools containing undigested fat particles.

d., infantile. In children under 2 years. Dysentery, *q.v.* Sym: Skin dry, temperature, high; thirst, pains, increase of stools with change of color and consistency.

d., lienteric. Watery stools with undigested food particles.

d., membranous. D. with passage of pieces of intestinal mucosa.

d., nervous. Increase of peristalsis due to nervousness of patient.

d., mucous. D. with mucus in stools.

d., purulent. Presence of pus in stools, a result of intestinal ulceration.

d., serous. Watery stools.

d., simple. Variety in which stools contain only normal excreta.

d., summer. D. occurring in children during summer heat.

d., ulcerative. Severe d. with ulceration of mucosa of intestines.

diarthric (di-ar'thrik). Pert. to two or more joints.

diarthrosis (di-ar-thro'sis) [G. *dia*, through, + *arthrōsis*, a joining]. An articulation in which opposing bones move freely; a hinge joint.

diartic'ular [G. *dis*, two, + L. *articulus*, joint]. Pert. to two joints.

diaschisis (di-as'kĭ-sis) [G. *dia*, apart, + *schizein*, to split]. Disturbance or injury to one part of central nervous system may cause alteration in function of some distant part.

diascope (di'ă-skōp) [" + *skopein*, to examine]. A glass plate held against the skin for ascertaining noncongestive changes.

diastalsis (di-ă-stal'sis) [" + *stalsis*, contraction]. A wave of inhibition before a downward contraction in the intestine. Similar to peristalsis.

diastal'tic. Denoting reflex action.

diastase (di'as-tās) [G. *diastanai*, to separate]. A specific enzyme or ferment in plant cells, such as in sprouting grains and malt, and in the digestive juice which converts starch into sugar.

diastasis (di-as'tă-sis) [G. a separation]. 1. In surgery, injury to a bone involving separation of an epiphysis. 2. In cardiac physiology, the last part of diastole.

It follows the period of most rapid diastolic filling of the ventricles, consists of a period of retarded inflow of blood from atria into ventricles, lasts (in man under average conditions) about 0.2 seconds, and is immediately followed by atrial systole.

d. recti. A separation lateralward of the two halves of the *m. rectus abdominis.*

diastema (di-ă-ste'mă) (pl. *diaste'mata*) [G. an interval or space]. 1. A fissure. 2. A space bet. two teeth.

diastematocrania (di-ă-stem"ă-to-kra'nĭ-ă) [" + *kranion*, cranium]. Congenital sagittal fissure of the skull.

diastematomyelia (di-ă-stem"ă-to-mi-e'lĭ-ă) [" + *myelos*, marrow]. Congenital fissure of the spinal cord.

diastematopyelia (di-ă-stem"ă-to-pi-e'lĭ-ă) [" + *pyelos*, pelvis]. Median slit of the pelvis; congenital.

dias'ter [G. *dis*, twice, + *astēr*, star]. In mitosis the achromatic figure consisting of a double star. See also: *mitosis.* Syn: *amphiaster.*

diastole (di-as'to-le) [G. *diastellein*, to expand]. PHYS: The normal period in the heart cycle during which the muscle fibers lengthen, the heart dilates, and the cavities fill with blood, the atria before the ventricles; roughly, the period of relaxation alternating with systole or contraction. SEE: *heart; murmurs; pulse; systole.*

diastolic (di-as-tol'ik). Pert. to diastole.
d. pressure. This is the point of least pressure in the arterial vascular system.
If the diastolic pressure does not drop in proportion to the systolic pressure this is known as a sign of danger.
RS: *blood pressure; pulse p.; systolic p.*

diatax'ia [G. *dis*, two, + *ataxia*, lack of order]. Ataxia of both sides of body.
d. cerebra'lis infanti'lis. Birth palsy.

diatela, diatele (di-ă-te'lă, -lē) [G. *dia*, between, + L. *tela*, web]. Membranous roof of third ventricle.

diater'ma [" + *terma*, end]. Portion of the floor of third ventricle.

diathermal (di-ă-ther'mal) [" + *thermē*, heat]. Permeable by radiant heat.

diather'manous. Diathermal, *q.v.*

diather'mia [" + *thermē*, heat]. Diathermy, *q.v.*

diather'mic. Of the nature of diathermy or of its results.

diathermy (di'ă-ther"mĭ) [G. *dia*, through, + *thermē*, heat]. The therapeutic use of a high frequency current to generate heat within some part of the body.
The frequency is greater than the maximum frequency for neuromuscular response, and ranges from several hundred thousand to millions of cycles per second.
d., medical. The generation of heat within the body by the application of high frequency oscillatory current for warming, but not damaging, tissues.
d., short wave. Treatment by use of wave lengths of 3 to 30 meters.
d., surgical. D. of high frequency for electrocoagulation, cauterization, etc.

diathesis (di-ath'ĕ-sis) [G. *diathenai*, to dispose]. Constitutional predisposition to a certain disease, conditions, or group of diseases. For example: *allergic d., hemorrhagic d., or rheumatic d.*

diathet'ic. Pert. to diathesis, or predisposition.

diatom (di'ă-tom) [G. *dis*, twice, + *atomos*, atom]. One of a group of unicellular microscopic algae. They possess a siliceous cell wall.

diatom'ic. 1. Containing two atoms; said of molecules. 2. Bivalent.

diato'ric [G. *diatoros*, bored through]. Artificial teeth attached with vulcanized rubber to their bases.

diax'on, diax'one [G. *dis*, twice, + *axōn*, axis]. A neuron having two axons.

diazo-. Prefix used in chemistry to note that a compound contains the N_2 radical.
d. reaction. A deep red color in urine.

dibasic (di-ba'sik) [G. *dis*, twice, + *basis*, base]. Containing in each molecule two atoms of hydrogen replaceable by a base; said of acids.

diblastula (di-blas'tu-lă) [" + *blastos*, sprout]. A blastule containing the ectoderm and entoderm.

Dibothriocephalus (di-both"rĭ-o-sef'al-us). Diphyllobothrium, *q.v.*

dicalcic (di-kal'sik) [" + *calx*, lime]. Containing two atoms of calcium in a molecule.
d. orthophosphate. $CaHPO_4$. A salt, often found in the urine.

dicalcium phosphate (di-kal'sĭ-um fos'fāt). Dibasic calcium phosphate, USP. Used as a calcium supplement.

dichloramine-T (di-klor'a-mēn). White powder containing about 28% chlorine.
ACTION AND USES: Germicide and disinfectant.

dichloro-diphenyl-trichloroethane. Former chemical name for an insecticide, commonly abbreviated DDT, *q.v.* Accepted chemical name is chlorophenothane.

dichotomy, dichotomization (di-kot'o-mĭ, di-kot"o-mi-za'shun) [G. *dicha*, twofold, + *tomē*, a cut]. 1. Division into two parts, as bifurcation of the embryo. 2. Sharing of fees between practitioner and consultant.

dichroic (di-kro'ĭk). Pert. to dichroism.

dichroism (di'kro-izm) [G. *dis*, twice, + *chroa*, color]. Property of a substance appearing to be one color by direct light and another by transmitted light.

dichromasy (di-kro'-mă-sĭ) [" + *chrōma*, color]. Able to see only two colors. Partial colorblindness. SYN: *dichromatism.*

dichromat'ic. Being able to see only two colors.

dichromatopsia (di-kro-mă-top'sĭ-ă) [G. *dis*, twice, + *chrōma*, color, + *opsis*, sight]. Ability to distinguish only two primary colors.

dichro'mic. 1. Containing two atoms of chromium. 2. Seeing only two colors.

dichro'mophil [G. *dis*, twice, + *chrōma*, color, + *philein*, to love]. Double staining with both acid and basic dyes.

dichromophilism (di-kro-mof'il-izm) [" + " + " + *ismos*, condition of]. Having the capacity for double staining.

dick. A gas, ethyldichlorarsine, used in chemical warfare.

Dick method [George F. and Gladys H. Dick, American physicians, 1881-]. A toxin-antitoxin injection for the prevention of scarlet fever.
D. test. *Negative Reaction*: Some slight inflammatory changes due to irritation by proteins in fluid administered. SEE: *Schick method; Schick test.*
In a manner somewhat similar to the Schick testing for diphtheria, a person's susceptibility to scarlet fever may be ascertained by the injection of a standardized toxin of the *Streptococcus hemolyticus.* A positive reaction in the shape of erythema appears in about 12 to 24 hours. Patients convalescent from scarlet fever invariably give a negative reaction. Susceptible persons can subsequently be actively immunized by graded doses of a specific toxin, or passively immunized by the administration of scarlet fever antitoxic serum.

dicliditis (dik-lĭ-di'tis) [G. *diklides*, valve, + *-itis*, inflammation]. Inflammation of heart valve. SYN: *valvulitis.*

diclidostosis (di-klid-os-to'sis) [" + *osteon*, bone]. Ossification of the venous valves.

diclidot'omy [" + *tomē*, incision]. Cutting a valve, esp. a rectal or heart valve. SYN: *valvotomy.*

dicoria (di-ko'rĭ-ă) [G. *dis*, double, + *korē*, pupil]. Double pupil in each eye.

dicrotic (di-krot'ik) [G. *dikrotos*, beating double]. One heartbeat for two arterial pulsations; rel. to a double pulse.
d. notch. In a pulse tracing, a notch on the descending limb.
d. wave. A positive wave following the dicrotic notch.

dicrotism (di'krot-izm) [" + *ismos,* condition of]. The state of being dicrotic.

dictyoma (dik-tĭ-o'ma) [G. *diktyon,* net, + *-ōma,* tumor]. A retinal tumor. Also spelled diktyoma.

dicumarol (di-koo'mă-rol). Proprietary name for bishydroxycoumarin, USP., an anticoagulant that decreases activity of prothrombin in the blood plasma and hence increases prothrombin time.

Uses: In prophylaxis and treatment of intravascular clotting, in postoperative thrombophlebitis, pulmonary embolism, acute peripheral embolism and thrombosis, and recurrent idiopathic thrombophlebitis. Used also in management of acute coronary thrombosis. Frequently an adjunct to *heparin, q.v.* RS: *heparin, menadione sodium bisulfite, vitamin K.*

Contraindications: Subacute bacterial endocarditis, recent brain and spinal surgery, purpura and blood dyscrasias, and in absence of prothrombin determination.

didactylism (di-dak'tĭ-lizm) [G. *dis,* twice, + *daktylos,* finger]. The congenital condition of having only two digits on a hand or foot.

didelphic (di-del'fik) [" + *delphys,* uterus]. Having or pertaining to a doubled uterus.

didymalgia (did-ĭ-mal'jĭ-ă) [G. *didymos,* testis, + *algos,* pain]. Pain in a testicle. Syn: *didymodynia.*

didymitis (did-ĭ-mi'tis) [" + *-itis,* inflammation]. Inflammation of a testicle. Syn: *orchitis.*

didymodynia (did"ĭ-mo-din'ĭ-ă) [" + *odynē,* pain]. Pain in a testicle. Syn: *didymalgia.*

didymus (did'ĭ-mus) [G. *didymos,* twin, testis]. 1. A twin. 2. A double monstrosity. 3. A testicle.

diechoscope (di-ek'o-skōp) [G. *dis,* twice, + *ēcho,* echo, + *skopein,* to examine]. A stethoscope for simultaneous auscultation from two different sites.

di"elec'tric [G. *dia,* through, + *elektron,* amber]. An insulating substance offering great resistance to passage of electricity by conduction through which electric force may act by induction.

dielectrolysis (di"e-lek-trol'i-sis) [" + " + *lysis,* loosening]. The forcing of a drug or medicinal compound to a particular part of the body by osmosis brought about or accelerated with an electric current.

diencephalon (di-en-sef'ă-lon) [" + *egkephalos,* brain]. Second portion of the brain or that lying between the telencephalon and mesencephalon. It includes the epithalamus, thalamus, metathalamus, and hypothalamus. Syn: *thalamencephalon; between brain; 'tween-brain.*

dienestrol (di"ēn-es'trol). A nonsteroid, synthetic estrogen used for estrogen therapy.

Dientamoeba (dī-ĕn-tă-mē'bă). A genus of parasitic protozoa characterized by possession of two similar nuclei. They belong to the class *Sarcodina.*

D. fragilis. A species of parasitic amebae inhabiting the intestine of man. There is strong evidence that it may sometimes be pathogenic producing symptoms such as intestinal colic, diarrhea, and lowered vitality.

dieresis (di-er'ĕ-sis) [G. *dia,* apart, + *airein,* to take]. 1. Breaking up or dispersion of things normally joined, as by an ulcer. 2. Mechanical separation of parts by surgical means.

dieret'ic. Pertaining to dieresis; dissolvable or separable.

diet [G. *diaita*]. 1. Food substances, liquid and solid, regularly consumed in the course of normal living. 2. A prescribed allowance of food adapted for a particular state of health or disease, as a diabetic diet. 3. To cause to eat or drink sparingly in accordance with prescribed rules.

d., balanced. One adequate in energy-providing substances (carbohydrates and fats), tissue-building substances (proteins), inorganic substances (water and mineral salts), regulating substances (vitamins), substances for certain physiological processes such as bulk for promoting peristaltic movements of the digestive tract.

diet, *words pert. to:* alkaline ash d.; basic d.; bland d.; calcium high and low d.; carbohydrate high d.; cardiac d.; cardiac d., Smith; cellulose high d.; colostomy d.; elimination d.; fat low d.; feeding; fluid d.; iron high d.; ketogenic d.; light d.; liquid full d.; liquid high caloric d.; liquid or fluid d. without milk; liquid restricted d; liquid surgical d.; residue d. high and low; roughage d.; saltfree d.; salt low d.; salt poor d.; Sippy d.; soft d.; water balance d.

dietary (dī'ĕ-ta-rĭ). A regulated diet.

dietetic (dī-ĕ-tet'ik). Pert. to diet.

dietet'ics [G. *diaitētikos*]. The science of the use of foods in health and disease. Some fundamental principles and facts of this science will be summarized here.

Conservation of Energy: In order to obtain metabolic balance, there must be as much chemical energy in the food as will equal the amt. of work done by the subject or patient plus the heat which he constantly loses. The number of calories in his daily food must in the long run equal his *basal metabolic rate* plus his additional metabolism due to muscular work and added heat losses. Thus a subject whose basal rate is 1700 calories per 24 hours may, during the day, do work and lose heat adding, say, 2000 calories to his output; he must, therefore, obtain 3700 calories in his diet.

1 gm. of fat gives about	9.3 cal.
1 gm. of carbohydrate	4.0 cal.
1 gm. of protein	4.0 cal.

Conservation of Matter: Everything that leaves the body, whether exhaled as carbon dioxide and water, or excreted as urea and minerals, must be replaced in the food and can be accounted for by chemical analysis. Thus if a man excretes 10 gm. of nitrogen daily he must receive 10 gm. of it in his diet, for the element can neither be created nor destroyed.

Difficulty of Some Organic Syntheses: The power of the body to build tissue is limited, and for a given purpose only certain raw materials can be used. Thus proteins are "made up" of carbon, hydrogen, oxygen, and nitrogen; but eating charcoal and inhaling the gases would not enable one to make tissue protein. For instance, hemoglobin cannot be synthesized unless the body is supplied with proteins containing the pyrrole ring. This group occurs in the amino acids: tryptophan, proline, and hydroxyproline; proteins which do not contain these amino acids therefore are insufficient for needs of the body.

Summary: A diet should contain: (a) Water, (b) carbohydrates, (c) fats, (d) proteins, (e) minerals, (f) roughage (indigestible residue), (g) vitamins and other accessories.

diethylstilbestrol (dī"eth"ĭl-stĭl"bĕs'trōl). USP. A synthetic preparation possessing estrogenic properties. It is several times more effective than natural estrogens and may be given orally. It is used therapeutically in the treatment of menopausal disturbances and other disorders due to estrogen deficiencies. SYN: *stilbestrol.*

dietitian (dī-ĕ-tish'an) [G. *diaita,* diet]. One scientifically trained in dietetics (which includes nutrition).

Dietl's crisis (de'tlz). Renal colic; accompanied by scanty, bloodstained urine.

Dieulafoy's triad. Tenderness, muscular contraction, and skin hyperesthesia in acute appendicitis at McBurney's point.

differential (dif-er-en'shal) [L. *dis,* apart, + *ferre,* to bear]. Marked by differences.

d. blood count. Determination of the number of each variety of leukocytes in a cubic millimeter of blood. SEE: *blood count.*

d. diagnosis. Diagnosis based on comparison of symptoms of two or more similar diseases to determine which the patient is suffering from. SEE: *diagnosis.*

differentia'tion [" + *ferre,* to bear]. Acquirement of functions different from those of the original type.

diffraction (dĭ-frak'shun). The change which occurs in light when it passes through crystals, prisms, or parallel bars in a grating in which the rays appear to be turned aside producing dark or colored bands or lines, or other phenomena. Term is also applied to similar phenomena in sound and electricity.

diffusate (dĭ-fu'zāt) [" + *fundere,* to pour]. In the process of dialysis, that portion of a liquid which passes through a membrane and which contains crystalloid matter in solution. SYN: *dialysate.*

diffuse (dĭ-fūs') [" + *fundere,* to pour]. Spreading, scattered, spread.

d. inflammation. One not localized.

diffusible (dĭ-fuz'ĭ-bl). Capable of being diffused.

diffusion (dĭ-fu'zhun) [L. *dis,* apart, + *fundere,* to pour]. 1. Absorption of a liquid such as the absorption, by cells, of water from lymph when the percentage of salt is less in lymph than in the cells. *See illustration this page.*

When the percentage is greater in the lymph than in the cells water is withdrawn from the latter. SEE: *osmosis.*

2. A process whereby different gases interpenetrate and become mixed, due to the incessant motion of their molecules. Similarly, if aqueous solutions of different materials stand in contact, mixing occurs on standing, even if the solutions be separated by thin membranes.

3. The tendency of molecules of a substance (gaseous, liquid, or solid) to move from a region of high concentration to one of lower concentration.

digastric (di-gas'trĭk) [G. *dis,* double, + *gastēr,* belly]. Having two bellies; said of certain muscles.

digen'esis [" + *genesis,* production]. Reproduction in which alternate generations are asexual.

Digenetica (di-jĕ-net'ĭ-kă). An order of parasitic flatworms belonging to the class Trematoda and characterized by having an asexual generation, living

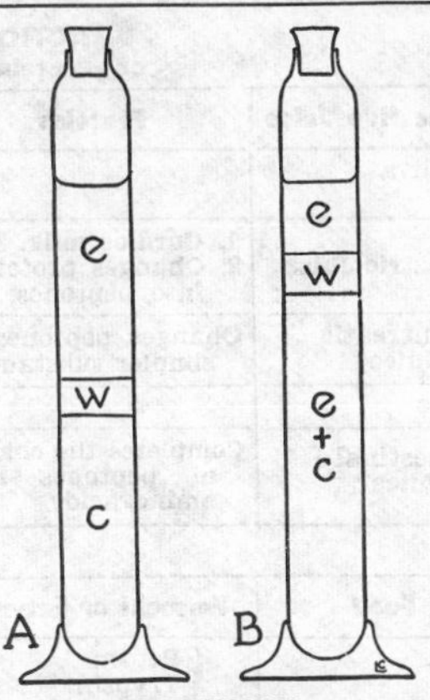

DIFFUSION

The experiment begins in A with a thin layer of water, w, separating a large volume of ether, e, above from an equal volume of the much heavier carbon tetrachloride, c, below. B. Three weeks later the layers are still distinct, but the lowest layer has visibly increased in volume at the expense of the uppermost layer. Ether has passed through the water into the carbon tetrachloride.

usually in molluscs, alternating with a sexual generation living in vertebrates as their final host. It includes all the flukes parasitic in man. These include four groups of flukes, *q.v.*

digest' [L. *dis,* apart, + *gerere,* to carry]. 1. To undergo digestion. 2. To make a condensation of a subject.

diges'tant [" + *gerere,* to carry]. 1. An agent that will digest food or aid in digestion. Ex: *pepsin, pancreatin.* 2. A preparation made from the digestive glands or lining membrane of the stomach, classified according to the foods it digests, such as *carbohydrate* or *protein.*

diges'tible. Pert. to that which may be digested.

diges'tion [L. *digestio,* a taking apart]. The process by which food is broken down, mechanically and chemically, in the gastrointestinal tract and is converted into absorbable forms.

Salt, the simplest sugars (such as glucose), crystalloids in general, and water can be absorbed unchanged; but starches, fats, and proteins for the most part are not absorbable until disintegrated by the digestive fluids, and even the sugar, sucrose (a disaccharose*), must first undergo inversion.

The chemical actions are chiefly hydrolytic; they are brought about by a variety of enzymes, each of which acts in an acid or alkaline or neutral juice according to its peculiar properties.

The higher carbohydrates are converted into monosaccharoses*; proteins (through successive stages of peptones and polypeptides) ultimately into amino acids, and fats into fatty acids and glycerine. In the stomach the soluble casein of milk is converted into insoluble paracasein resulting in its coagulation or clotting. This is brought about by the enzyme, pepsin. The *rennin* and *acid* are responsible for the clotting (curdling) of milk, which nor-

ACTION OF DIGESTIVE JUICES
on Proteins, Fats, and Carbohydrates

Digestive Juice	Proteins	Fats	Carbohydrates
Saliva			Changes cooked starch into maltose.
Gastric Juice	1. Curdles milk. 2. Changes proteins into peptones.		
Pancreatic Juice	Changes peptones to simpler substances.	Changes fats to fatty acids and glycerol	Changes sugars into simpler forms.
Bile		Emulsifies fats.	
Intestinal Juice	Completes the change of peptones into amino acids.		Completes the change of all sugars into the simplest form, glucose.

On Foods

Food	Ferment or Enzyme	Digestive Juice	Where Juice Acts
Protein	Pepsin.	Gastric juice, acid.	Stomach.
	Trypsin.	Pancreatic juice, alkaline.	Small intestine.
	Erepsin.	Succus Entericus, alkaline.	Small intestine.
Fats	Lipase.	Pancreatic juice.	Small intestine.
Carbohydrates	Ptyalin.	Saliva, alkaline.	Mouth and in stomach.
	Amylopsin.	Pancreatic juice, alkaline.	Small intestine.
	Invertase.	Succus Entericus.	Small intestine.

mally occurs in the stomach. An enzyme, lipase, is able to attack fats in emulsified form. It liberates, for instance, butyric acid from the fats in milk, and thus causes the characteristic odor of vomitus. The chemical actions are facilitated by the churning, wavelike motions of the stomach walls. When the chyme is ready to leave the stomach, the pylorus opens from time to time and the chyme is spurted into the duodenum.

d., artificial. D. outside the living organism by a ferment.

d., duodenal. The acid, chyme, is made alkaline, and the fats it contains are emulsified by the action of bile. A fresh set of enzymes adapted to these new conditions are supplied by the pancreatic juice which enters by two ducts and by the intestinal juice which comes from small glands in the wall of the intestine itself. The hydrolysis of starches, fats, and proteins is carried to its physiological completion here, and in the remainder of the small intestine.

d., extracellular. That occurring outside the body of the cell.

d., gastric. Portion of the digestive process taking place in the stomach.

d., intestinal. Hydrolytic processes continue here, and absorption of the products is active. SEE: *absorption.* From the ileum the food residues pass in a nearly liquid state through a small opening into the ascending colon. A sphincter muscle prevents backflow. True digestive processes in the colon are slight, but there is normally much bacterial action (the products of which are mostly absorbed) and reabsorption of water. The remaining substances, now colored by pigments which entered with bile and changed to a firm consistency by the loss of water, pass on through the transverse colon, the descending colon, and the sigmoid flexure into the rectum. They are retained in the rectum by the action of sphincters until defecation occurs.

d., intracellular. Digestion within the cell body.

d., oral. Portion of the digestive process taking place in the mouth.

d., pancreatic. Portion of digestive process influenced by pancreatic juice.

d., peptic. Gastric d.

d., primary. Portion of digestive process taking place in the gastrointestinal tract.

d., salivary. Digestive action by the saliva. SEE: *salivary digestion.*

d., secondary. Cellular assimilation of nutritive material.

digestive (di-jes'tiv). Pert. to digestion.

d. juice. One of several secretions which aid in processes of digestion.

digit (dij'it) (pl. *digits*) [L. *digitus,* finger]. A finger or toe.

digital (dij'ĭ-tal) [L. *digitus,* finger]. Pert. to or resembling a finger or toe.

d. reflex. Sudden flexion of terminal phalanx of a finger or thumb when nail is suddenly tapped.

digitalis (dij-ĭ-tal'is) [L. *digitus,* finger, because of its finger-shaped corolla]. USP. Foxglove. The dried leaves of *Digitalis purpurea* used in powdered form as tablets or capsules. Cardiotonic glycosides, especially digitoxin and digoxin, are obtained from various species of the Digitalis plant.

ACTION AND USES: Heart stimulant, indirectly diuretic.

POISONING: A valuable drug widely used in treatment of cardiac diseases, but toxicity may develop acutely or chronically from its cumulative effect.

SYM: Digestive disturbances, as nausea, and vomiting. Frequently distressing headache. Cardiac irregularities are common, esp. slowing of heart with ventricular extrasystoles or partial heart block.

F. A. TREATMENT: Evacuate stomach, administer diffusible stimulants; cathartics and sedatives are desirable. Because these patients are usually chron-

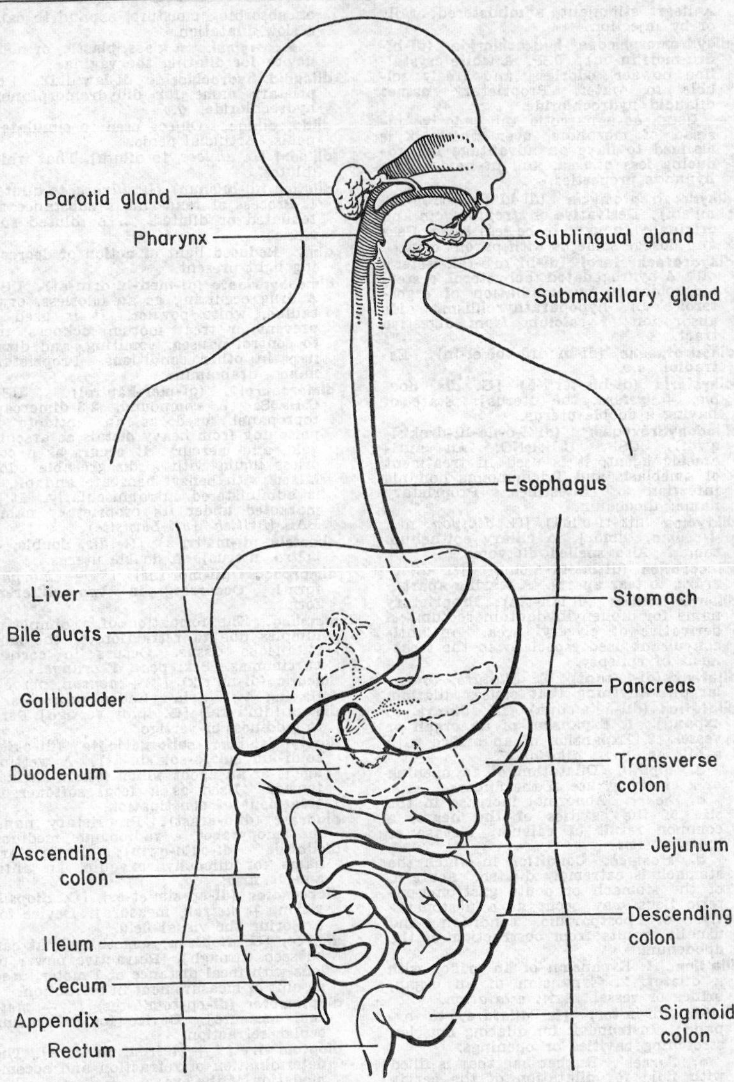

THE DIGESTIVE SYSTEM

ically ill special care is necessary in their management.

digitalism (dij'ĭ-tal-izm) [" + G. *ismos*, condition of]. The poisonous effects produced by digitalis.

digitalization (dij-ĭ-tal-ĭ-za'shun). Subjection of an organism to the action of digitalis.

dig'itate [L. *digitus*, finger]. Having fingerlike impressions or processes.

digitation (dij-ĭ-ta'shun) [L. *digitus*, finger]. A fingerlike process.

digiti (dij'ĭ-ti). Plural of *digitus;* toes or fingers.

digitoxin dij-ĭ-tok'sin). USP. A cardiotoxic glycoside obtained from various species of the Digitalis plant. A heart stimulant, administered orally or by injection. SEE: *digitalis.*

dig'itus (pl. *digiti*) [L.]. A finger or toe.

diglossia (dī-glos'ĭ-ă) [G. *dis*, double, + *glōssa*, tongue]. Having a double tongue.

digoxin (dī-jok'sin). USP. A cardiotonic glycoside obtained from Digitalis lanata.

A heart stimulant, administered orally or by injection.

dihydromorphinone hydrochloride (dī-hī-drō-morf'ĭn-ōn). USP. A white crystalline powder, odorless, and freely soluble in water. Proprietary name: dilaudid hydrochloride.

USES: As a narcotic and sedative instead of morphine, over which it is claimed to have an advantage in producing less nausea, and in having less hypnotic properties.

dihydrostreptomycin (dī-hī"drō-strĕp-tō-mī'sĭn). Derivative of *streptomycin* and originally thought to be less toxic. Uses and dosage same as with parent drug.

dihydrotachysterol (dī-hī"drō-tăk-ĭ-ster'-ol). A hydrogenated tachysterol, a steroid, obtained by irradiation of ergosterol. In hypoparathyroidism, aids absorption of calcium from digestive tract.

dihydrotheelin (dī-hī"drō-thē'ĕl-ĭn). Estradiol, *q.v.*

dihysteria (di-his-ter'ĭ-ă) [G. *dis,* double, + *ystera,* the uterus]. State of having a double uterus.

diiodohydroxyquin (di"i-o-do-hi-drok'sĭ-qwin). USP. $C_9H_5I_2NO$. An antiamebic agent, it is used in treatment of amebiasis and Trichomonas hominis infection of intestines. Proprietary name: diodoquin.

diktyoma (dik-tĭ-o'mă) [G. *diktyon,* net, + *-ōma,* tumor]. A ciliary epithelium tumor. Also spelled dictyoma.

dilaceration (dī"las-er-a'shun) [L. *dilacerāre,* to tear apart]. A tearing apart.

dilantin sodium (dī'lăn-tĭn). Proprietary name for diphenylhydantoin sodium. A derivative of glyceryl urea. An anticonvulsant used especially in the treatment of epilepsy.

dilatant (di-la'tant) [L. *dilatāre,* to enlarge]. Anything that causes dilation.

dilatation (dil-ă-ta'shun) [L. *dīlatāre,* to expand]. 1. Expansion of an organ or vessel. 2. Expansion of an orifice with a dilator. SYN: *dilation.*

d., digital. Dilatation of an opening or a cavity by use of the fingers.

d., heart. Abnormal increase in the size of the cavities of the heart, a common result of valvular disease or hypertension.

d., stomach. Condition in which the stomach is extremely dilated. Acute d. of the stomach or acute gastromesenteric ileus may occur as a postoperative or postpartum condition and usually results from obstruction of the duodenum.

dila'tion. 1. Expansion of an orifice with a dilator. 2. Expansion of an organ, orifice or vessel. SYN: *dilatation.*

dilator (dī-lā'tor) [L. *dilatāre,* to expand]. Instrument for dilating muscles, stretching cavities or openings.

d., Barnes'. Rubber bag that is filled with fluid for dilatation of the cervix uteri.

d., Bossi's. A multiple pronged instrument that dilates by separation of the prongs. Used for dilatation of the cervix uteri.

d., Goodell's. Similar to the Bossi except that it has but three prongs.

d., gyn. An instrument for dilating the cervix uteri.

d., Hegar's. Graduated metal sounds that are inserted into the cervical canal and cause a graded dilatation.

d.'s, tent. Small cones made of seaweed, sponge, or tree roots which are inserted into the uterine canal dry and, on absorbing moisture, expand to cause a slow dilatation.

d., vaginal. A glass, plastic, or metal device for dilating the vagina.

dilaudid hydrochloride dī-law'did). Proprietary name for dihydromorphinone hydrochloride, *q.v.*

dildo, dildoe. Object used to simulate a penis. Artificial penis.

dil'uent [L. *diluere,* to dilute]. That which dilutes.

dilution (di-lu'shun) [L. *diluere,* to dilute]. 1. Process of rendering a substance attenuated or diluted. 2. A diluted substance.

dim. Reduced light or action of decreasing light present.

dimenhydrinate (di-men-hi'drin-āt). USP. A drug occurring as an odorless, crystalline, white powder. It is used to prevent or treat motion sickness and to control nausea, vomiting, and dizziness in other conditions. Proprietary name: dramamine.

dimercaprol (dī-mer-kăp'rōl). USP. $C_3H_8OS_2$. A compound, 2,3-dimercaptopropanol, used as an antidote in poisoning from heavy metals as arsenic, gold, and mercury. It occurs as a colorless liquid with a disagreeable odor. Mixed with benzyl benzoate and oil, it is administered intramuscularly. It is marketed under its proprietary name, BAL (*British Anti-Lewisite*).

dimetria (di-me'trĭ-ă) [G. *dis,* double, + *mētra,* uterus]. A double uterus.

dimorphous (di-mor'fus) [" + *morphē,* form]. Occurring in two different forms.

dimpling. The formation of a dimple or dimples due to retraction of the subcutaneous tissue. Occurs in certain carcinomas. SEE: *peau d' orange.*

dineuric (di-nu'rik) [" + *neuron,* nerve]. Having two axis-cylinder processes.

dinical (din'ĭ-kal) [G. *dinos,* vertigo]. Pert. to giddiness or vertigo.

dioctyl sodium sulfosuccinate (dī-ok'til so'dĭ-um sul"fo-suk'sin-āt). A wetting agent or an agent which lowers surface tension. Used as a fecal softener in treatment of constipation.

diodrast (dī'o-drast). Proprietary name for iodopyracet, a radiopaque medium.

diodoquin (di-od'o-qwin). Proprietary name for diiodohydroxyquin, an antiamebic drug.

diopsimeter (dī-op-sim'et-er) [G. *diopsis,* vision, + *metron,* measure]. Device for exploring the visual field.

diop'ter [G. *dioptron,* something that can be seen through]. Refractive power of lens with focal distance of 1 meter, used as unit of measurement in refraction.

dioptometer (di-op-tom'ĕ-ter) [" + *metron,* measure]. Device for measuring ocular refraction.

dioptom'etry [" + *metron,* measure]. The determination of refraction and accommodation of the eye.

dioptral (di-op'tral) [G. *dioptron,* something that can be seen through]. Pert. to a diopter.

dioptre (di-op'ter). Diopter, *q.v.*

dioptric (di-op'trik). Dioptral; pert. to refraction of light.

diop'trics [G. *dioptron,* something that can be seen through]. The science of refraction of light.

diorthosis (di-or-tho'sis) [G. *dia,* through, + *orthos,* straight]. Reduction of a fracture or dislocation. SYN: *diaplasis.*

diosmosis (di-oz-mo'sis) [" + *ōsmos,* a pushing]. Passage of a fluid through a membrane. SEE: *dialysis; osmosis.*

dioxide (di-oks'īd) [G. *dis*, twice, + *oxys*, sharp]. A compound having two oxygen atoms to one of another element.

dipeptid(e) (di-pep'tid, -tīd) [" + *peptein*, to digest]. A derived protein obtained by hydrolysis of proteins or condensation of amino acids.

dipeptidase (dī-pĕp'tĭ-dās). An enzyme that hydrolyzes dipeptids to amino acids.

diphallus (dī-făl'ŭs). A condition in which there is either a complete or incomplete doubling of the penis or clitoris.

diphasic (di-fa'zik) [" + *phasis*, a phase]. Having two phases.

diphenhydramine hydrochloride (di-fen-hi'dră-min hi-dro-klo'rīd). USP. An antihistaminic agent, occurring as an odorless, white, crystalline powder.

diphenylhydantoin sodium (di-fen"il-hi-dan'to-in). USP. A white odorless powder, freely soluble in water. An anticonvulsant used especially in the treatment of epilepsy.

diphonia (di-fō'nĭ-ă) [" + *phōnē*, voice]. Simultaneous production of two different voice tones.

diphtheria (dif-the'ri-ă) [G. *diphthera*, a skin]. An acute infectious disease characterized by the formation of a false membrane on any mucous surface and occasionally the skin. Usually accompanied by great prostration.

Etiol: Causative organism, *Corynebacterium diphtheriae*, a gram-positive nonmotile, non-spore-forming, club-shaped bacillus. In stained smears the bacilli are usually arranged at sharp angles with each other. This gives the characteristic Chinese letter appearance. The disease is rare under 1 year of age. The vast majority of cases occur before the age of 10, but older children and adults are not exempt. Both sexes equally susceptible. Esp. prevalent in fall and winter months. Transmission through direct contact with a human carrier, or as a result of exposure through contact with articles that have been contaminated by the diphtheria patient. Incubation: 2 to 5 days, occasionally longer.

Sym: Onset gradual. Usually slight headache and malaise. Temperature 100° F. to 101° F., and sore throat with presence of yellowish-white membrane adherent to tonsils or pharyngeal walls. Cervical adenitis may develop early in severe types. In nasal diphtheria, fever is a much more evident symptom. Adenitis often severe, serous discharge from nostrils which may be blood tinged; strong fetid odor of breath common.

d. antitoxin. The antibody which counteracts the diphtheria toxin; the blood serum of a horse or some other animal which has been immunized against diphtheria toxin.

d. carrier. A person harboring in his body the causative organism without manifest symptoms, thus acting as a potential distributor of the infection.

The bacillus usually disappears from the throat of carrier within 4 weeks even without treatment. However, administration of penicillin or erythromycin is the most effective treatment for acute or chronic carrier.

d., laryngeal. Considered to be a complication of diphtheria. Results from extension of the membrane from the pharynx with gradual occlusion of the airway. Signs are restlessness, use of accessory respiration muscles, and development of cyanosis. If this is not remedied effectively, death results.

d. toxin. An exotoxin produced by the diphtheria bacillus. A thermolabile substance capable of producing in susceptible animals the same symptoms brought about by inoculation with the living organism.

d. toxin-antitoxin. A mixture of diphtheria toxin and antitoxin. Formerly used in the treatment of diphtheria to produce active immunity. It has been replaced by d. toxoid, *q.v.*, or d. antitoxin; the latter is administered to patients exposed to the disease but who have not been immunized previously.

d. toxoid. Diphtheria toxin which has been detoxified. Used to produce active immunity against diphtheria.

Differential Diagnosis: Tonsillitis, scarlet fever, acute pharyngitis, streptococcus sore throat, peritonsillar abscess, infectious mononucleosis, Vincent's angina, acute moniliasis, and staphylococcous infections in the respiratory tract following chemotherapy may frequently require consideration. Examination of a smear from infected area is advisable, but cultures should be obtained in every instance for the purpose of confirming the diagnosis. In the laryngeal type, edema of the glottis, foreign bodies, and retropharyngeal abscess may require consideration.

Prog: Favorable when antitoxin in sufficient amounts is administered within 3 days from time of onset. If given on 1st day, death should hardly ever occur. In laryngeal diphtheria, intubation or, rarely, tracheotomy, is usually necessary, as well as an adequate dose of diphtheria antitoxin. Age is important factor, with death more frequent in very young or very old patients than in intermediate age groups.

When therapy is not given promptly the incidence of nerve damage is quite high.

Active Immunization: Since all individuals are not susceptible to diphtheria, and because this doubtful factor may be determined by means of the Schick test, it is usually advisable to make use of this test in adults before administering either toxin-antitoxin or toxoid. Routine immunization should begin at age 3 months, d. toxoid being administered in combination with pertussis vaccine and tetanus toxoid; this is then followed by booster doses. Diphtheria toxoid, following a subcutaneous test for hypersensitivity, is used for immunization of adults.

General Measures: Strict bed rest during acute and convalescent stages of disease. In cases with myocardial involvement, prolonged rest in bed may be as important as the early administration of diphtheria antitoxin.

Treatment: Specific treatment consists of diphtheria antitoxin after determination of sensitivity to horse serum. No interference with the diphtheria membrane is advisable. Gargles should not be used, although cleansing mouthwashes are permissible. On the other hand, the use of suction in nasal cases is sometimes of distinct advantage. A liquid diet (consisting of plenty of water, fruit juices, and nourishing broths) or a soft diet is recommended. In the acute stage, stimulants of any description are rarely necessary. In fact, they are more likely to do harm than good.

In laryngeal diphtheria, surgical interference is sometimes a necessity. Intubation is always to be preferred to tracheotomy, provided an experienced operator is available, and furthermore that the patient is safeguarded by hospitalization which will make possible any attention required within a moment's notice.

SEE: *anatoxin, antitoxin, diphtheria carrier, Klebs-Loeffler bacillus, Schick test.*

d., surgical or **wound.** Diphtheric membrane formation on wounds.

diphthe'rial. Pert. to diphtheria.

diphtheriaphor (dif-the'rĭ-ă-for) [G. *diphthera,* a skin, + *phorein,* to carry]. A diphtheria carrier or vector.

diphtheric (dif-the'rik). Pert. to diphtheria. SYN: *diphtheritic.*

diphtherin (dif'the-rin) [G. *diphthera,* a skin]. The toxin of diphtheria, from *Corynebacterium diphtheriae.*

diphtheritic (dif-ther-it'ĭk). Pert. to diphtheria.

diph'theroid (dif'the-roid) [" + *eidos,* appearance]. 1. Resembling diphtheria or the bacteria which cause diphtheria. 2. The formation of a false or pseudomembrane not due to the diphtheria bacillus.

diphtherotox'in [" + *toxikon,* poison]. The specific toxin of the diphtheria bacillus.

diphthongia (dif-thon'jĭ-ă) [G. *dis,* double, + *phthoggos,* voice]. The simultaneous utterance of two vocal sounds of different pitch in pathological conditions of the larynx.

Diphyllobothrium (di-fil"o-both'rĭ-um) [" +*phyllon,* leaf, + *bothrion,* pit]. A genus of tapeworms belonging to the order Pseudophyllidea and characterized by possession of a scolex possessing two slit-like grooves or bothria. Formerly called *Dibothriocephalus.*

D. cordatum. The heart-headed tapeworm, a small species infesting carnivores in Greenland, formerly known as *D. mansoni.* The plerocercoids are occasionally found in man.

D. erinacei. A species infesting dogs, cats, and other carnivores. Larval stages are occasionally found in man.

D. latum. The broad or "fish" tapeworm. The adult lives in the intestine of fish-eating mammals and man. It is the largest human tapeworm and may reach a length of 50 to 60 feet (ave. 20 ft.). The eggs develop into ciliated larvae called *coracidia* which are eaten by certain species of copepods in which each becomes an *onchosphere* which develops into a *procercoid.* Further development occurs in a fish where it develops into a worm-like *plerocercoid* or *sparganum* larva. Infection of the final host occurs following eating improperly cooked fish. Pathological effects are abdominal pain, loss of weight, digestive disorders, progressive weakness, and a severe type of anemia which is clinically identical with pernicious anemia.

diphyodont (dif'ĭ-o-dont) [" + *phyein,* to produce, + *odous,* tooth]. Having two sets of teeth; as man.

diplacusis (dip-lă-ku'sis) [G. *diploos,* double, + *akousis,* hearing]. Variety of disturbed perception of pitch characterized by hearing two tones for every sound produced.

diplegia (di-ple'jĭ-ă) [G. *dis,* twice, + *plēgē,* a stroke]. Paralysis of similar parts on both sides of the body. SYN: *double hemiplegia.*

d., infantile. Birth palsy.

d., spastic. Congenital spastic stiffness of the limbs. SYN: *Little's disease.*

diplegic (di-ple'jik). Pert. to diplegia.

diploalbuminuria (dip"lo-al-bu"min-u'rĭ-ă) [G. *diploos,* double, + L. *albumen,* white of egg, + G. *ouron,* urine]. Coexistence of physiologic and pathologic albuminuria.

diplobacil'lus [" + L. *bacillus,* a little stick]. A double bacillus, two being linked end to end.

diplobacte'rium [" + *baktērion,* little rod]. An organism made up of two adherent bacteria.

diploblastic (dip-lo-blas'tĭk) [" + *blastos,* germ]. The ectoderm and endoderm having two germ layers.

diplocar'dia [" + *kardia,* heart]. Having a double heart.

diplocephaly (dip"lo-sef'ă-lĭ). State of having two heads.

diplococcemia (dip"lo-kok-se'mĭ-ă) [" + *kokkos,* berry, + *aima,* blood]. Diplococci in the blood.

Diplococcus (dĭp-lō-kok'us) [" + *kokkus,* berry]. A genus of bacteria belonging to the family Lactobacillaceae. They are gram positive organisms occurring in pairs.

D. pneumoniae. SYN: *pneumococcus, D. lanceolatus, Micrococcus pneumoniae, Micrococcus lanceolatus, Streptococcus pneumoniae.* A species of bacteria, oval or spherical in shape, gram-positive, nonmotile. They possess a capsule. The species is made up of a number of distinct strains of which more than 80 serological types have been isolated. It is the causative agent of certain types of pneumonia esp. lobar pneumonia and is associated with other infectious diseases such as cerebrospinal meningitis, otitis media, and septicemia.

diplocoria (dĭp"lo-ko'rĭ-ă) [G. *diploos,* double, + *korē,* pupil]. Double pupil in the eye.

diploe (dip'lo-e) [G. *diploē,* fold]. Cancellated tissue bet. the tables of the skull.

diploet'ic, diplo'ic [G. *diploē,* fold]. Pert. to the diploe or cancellated tissue bet. cranial tables.

diplogen'esis [G. *diploos,* double, + *genesis,* production]. Having two parts or producing two substances.

diploid (dĭp'loyd). Having double the haploid number of chromosomes. Said of somatic cells which contain twice the number of chromosomes present in the egg or sperm.

diplokaryon (dĭp-lō-kar'ĭ-ŏn). A nucleus containing twice the diploid number of chromosomes.

diplomellituria (dĭp-lō-mĕl'ĭ-tur'ĭ-ă) [" + *meli,* honey, + *ouron,* urine]. Condition in which diabetic and nondiabetic glycosuria occur either simultaneously or alternately in the same individual.

diplomyelia (dip-lo-mi-e'lĭ-ă) [" + *myelos,* marrow]. Condition in certain types of spina bifida in which the spinal cord is doubled.

diploneu'ral [" + *neuron,* nerve]. Having two nerves from different origins, as certain muscles.

diplopagus (dip-lop'ă-gus) [" + G. *pagos,* a thing fixed]. Conjoined twins which share some organs.

diplophonia (dip-lo-fo'nĭ-ă) [" + *phōnē,* voice]. Having two different voice tones at the same time. SYN: *diphonia.*

diplopia (dip-lo'pĭ-ă) [" + *opsis,* sight]. Double vision; monocular (astigmatism, subluxated lens, incipient cataract); binocular (due to derangement of extraocular muscles).

d., binocular. Double vision occurs when both eyes are used but not in focus. Seen in disease of the eyeballs, cranial-nerve affections, disease of the cerebellum, cerebrum, and meninges.

d., crossed. Binocular vision in which the images are reversed.

d., direct. SEE: *homonymous d.*

d., heteronymous. SEE: *crossed d.*

d., homonymous. Double vision in which right-hand image appears on right side and left-hand image on left side. OPP: *crossed d.*

d., monocular. Double vision with one eye.

d., unocular. SEE: *monocular d.*

d., vertical. D. with one of two images higher than the other.

diplopiometer (dip-lo-pĭ-om'ĕ-ter) [" + " + *metron*, measure]. Device for estimating double vision.

dip'loscope [" + *skopein*, to examine]. Device for study of binocular vision.

diplosoma'tia [" + *sōma*, body]. Twins joined at one or more points. SYN: *diplosomia.*

diploso'mia [" + *sōma*, body]. Twins joined together. SYN: *diplosomatia.**

dipping (dip'ing). 1. Palpation of the liver by a quick depression of the abdomen. 2. The act of immersing an object in a solution, esp. applied to the dipping of cattle for the control of cattle ticks.

diprosopus (dĭp-rō-sōp'ŭs). A malformed fetus characterized by possession of a double face.

dipsesis (dip-se'sis) [G. *dipsa*, thirst]. Extreme thirst or craving for abnormal liquids.

dipsomania (dip-so-ma'nĭ-ă) [G. *dipsa*, thirst, + *mania*, mania]. PSY: A morbid and uncontrollable craving for alcoholic beverages. SEE: *alcoholism.*

dipsopathy (dip-sop'ă-thĭ) [" + *pathos*, disease]. Dipsomania.

dipsophobia (dĭp-so-fo'bĭ-ă). Morbid fear of drinking.

dipsosis (dip-so'sis) [" + *-ōsis*]. Abnormal thirst.

dipsotherapy (dip-so-ther'ă-pĭ) [" + *therapeia*, treatment]. Limitation of water to be drunk as a cure.

Diptera (dĭp'ter-ă). An order of insects characterized by having sucking or piercing mouth parts, one pair of wings, and complete metamorphosis. It includes the flies, gnats, midges, and mosquitoes. It contains many species involved in the transmission of pathogenic organisms.

dipterous (dĭp'ter-ŭs). Having two wings; characteristic of the order Diptera.

dipylidiasis (dip"ĭ-lĭ-di'ă-sis). Infestation with the tapeworm, *Dipylidium caninum.*

Dipylidium (dip"ĭ-lĭd'e-um). A genus of tapeworms belonging to the family *Dipyliidae* which infests dogs and cats.

D. caninum. A species of *Dipylidium*, a common parasite of dogs and cats. Occasionally human infestation may occur through the accidental ingestion of lice or fleas which serve as the intermediate host.

direct'. Immediate, uninterrupted.

d. current. One flowing in one direction only.

d. light reflex. One in which response occurs in same side as the stimulus.

d. murmur. That due to stenosis of cardiac orifices.

d. reflex. Prompt contraction of sphincter of iris when light entering through pupil strikes retina of eye.

director (dĭ-rek'tor) [L. *dirigere*, to lay straight]. Grooved device for guiding a knife.

dirigomotor (dir"ĭ-go-mo'tor) [" + *motor*, mover]. Controlling or directing muscular activity.

dis- [L.]. Prefix: Free of, undo, as *disable.*

disaccharide (di-sak'ĭ-rĭd) [G. *dis*, two, + *sakcharon*, sugar]. A member of the disaccharose* group of carbohydrates. SEE: *carbohydrates.*

disaccharose (di-sak'ă-rōs) [" + G. *sakcharon*, sugar]. A *complex* sugar that may be split into two molecules of monosaccharides. The two monosaccharoses resulting from the decomposition may be different or identical. Thus the disaccharose *maltose*, $C_{12}H_{22}O_{11}$, for each molecule yields two molecules of glucose, $C_6H_{12}O_6$, while the disaccharose sucrose, $C_{12}H_{22}O_{11}$, yields a molecule each of glucose and fructose.

The disaccharoses consist of the following:

LEVULOSE: The same as *fructose.* In the body this is formed in the digestion of sucrose. It is found in fruits, plants, and in honey.

MALTOSE: This is found in malt and malt products, and in germinating seeds. It is acted upon in the intestines by maltase, resulting in production of 2 molecules of glucose. It is a reducing sugar. Commercial maltose is a mixture of maltose and dextrins.

SUCROSE: Cane sugar or table sugar. A nonreducing sugar. It comes from sugar cane, sorghum, maple sugar, sugar beets, and honey. An increase in temperature while heating sucrose results in caramel. It is acted upon in the intestines by *sucrase*, an enzyme converting it into one molecule each of glucose and fructose.

Some sugars undergo fermentation by yeasts, or decomposition is brought about by bacteria or molds. They oxidize sugars into carbon dioxide and water. Alcohol is produced when dextrose ferments.

Most of the sugar on the market consists of beet and cane sugar. Ripe fruits, and vegetables contain sucrose. The starch of green fruits is changed to a mixture of sucrose, glucose, and levulose. Sucrose gives the sweet flavor to ripe fruits. It has the following chemical characteristics:

1. Extremely soluble. Cold water will hold in solution almost twice its weight of sucrose. Hot water will dissolve even more.
2. It crystallizes very easily.
3. It melts at about 160° C., changing to an amber hue and growing darker, becoming less sweet and when heated to about 200° C. becomes a brown, syrupy mass, with a distinctive flavor, called caramel.

SEE: *carbohydrates; monosaccharide; polysaccharide.*

disarticula'tion [L. *dis*, apart, + *articulus*, joint]. Amputation through a joint.

disassimila'tion [" + *ad*, to, + *similāre*, to make like]. Changing assimilated material into less complex compounds for the production of energy.

disc [G. *diskos*, a flat dish]. A round, flat, platelike structure. SEE: *disk.*

discharge (dis-charj', dis'charj) [M.E. *dischargen*, an oozing out]. 1. The escape (especially by violence) of pent up or accumulated energy or of explosive material. 2. The flowing away of a secretion or excretion of pus, feces, urine, etc. 3. The material ejected by discharge (2nd def.).

d., cerebral cortical. The violent action of a diseased portion of the cerebral cortex that gives rise to an epileptic paroxysm.

d., convective. One from a high potential source in the form of electrical energy passing through the air to the patient.

d., disruptive. A passage of current through an insulating medium due to the breakdown of the medium under electrostatic stress.

d., electric. A slow or instantaneous bringing back to a neutral electric condition, by which every highly electrified body loses its surplus electricity, giving it up to surrounding bodies less highly electrified.

d., lochial. Uterine excretion following childbirth. SEE: *lochia.*

discharg'ing. The emission of or the flowing out of material as the discharge of pus from a lesion. Excreting.

d. lesion. A lesion of nerve center in brain suddenly discharging motor impulses.

dischrona'tion [L. *dis,* apart, + G. *chronos,* time]. Failure of relativity in the consciousness of time.

discission (dĭ-sizh'un) [" + *scindere,* to cut]. Rupture of the capsule of the crystalline lens in operation for cataract.

discitis (dis-ki'tis) [G. *diskos,* disk, + *-ītis,* inflammation]. Diskitis, *q.v.*

discoblas'tic [" + *blastos,* germ]. Pert. to discoid segmentation of yolk in an impregnated ovum.

discoblastula (dĭs-kō-blăst-ŭl'ă). A modified blastula found in highly telolecithal eggs as in birds in which the blastomeres form a cellular cap (germinal disc or blastoderm) which is separated from the yolk by a space, the blastocoele.

dis'coid [" + *eidos,* form]. Like a disc.

discoplacen'ta [" + *plakous,* a flat cake]. A disklike placenta.

discrete (dis-krēt') [L. *discretus,* separated]. Separate; opposed to *confluent.** Said of certain eruptions on the skin.

discrimi'nation. The process of distinguishing or differentiating.

d., one-point. The ability to locate specifically a point of pressure on the surface of the skin.

d., tonal. The ability to distinguish one tone from another. This is dependent upon the integrity of the transverse fibers of the basilar membrane of the organ of Corti.

d., two-point. The ability to localize two points of pressure on the surface of the skin, and to identify them as discrete sensations. Also called tactile discrimination.

dis'cus (pl. *discuses*). A disk.

d. articularis [NA]. An interarticular fibrocartilage; an articular disk.

d. proligerus. The cumulus oophorus, *q.v.*

discuss' [L. *discutere,* to dissipate]. To disperse, scatter, or cause to disappear.

discussion (dis-kush'un) [L. *discutere,* to dissipate]. Dispersal of a tumor or swelling.

discussive (dis-kus'iv) [L. *discutere,* to strike asunder]. An agent which causes a disease process to disperse or undergo resolution.

discutient (dis-ku'shent) [L. *discutere,* to dissipate]. Agent which disperses a lesion or tumor.

disdiaclast (dis-di'ă-klast) [G. *dis,* two, + *diaklan,* to break through]. A doubly refracting element in the tissues of striated muscles.

disdiadochokinesia (dis-di″ă-do″ko-kĭ-ne'zĭ-ă) [L. *dis,* apart, + G. *diadochos,* succeeding, + *kinesis,* motion]. Inability to make finely coordinated movements of a part in opposite directions. For example, quickly supinating and pronating the hand. SEE: *diadochokinesia.*

disease (di-zēz') [L. *dis,* apart, + Fr. *aise,* ease]. Literally the lack of ease; a pathological condition of the body that presents a group of symptoms peculiar to it and which sets the condition apart as an abnormal entity differing from other normal or pathological body states.

d., acute. D. having a rapid onset and of relatively short duration.

d., bridegroom's. Thrombosis of the pampiniform plexus of the penis.

d., chronic. One having a slow onset and lasting for a long period of time.

d., communicable. D. the causative organism of which is transmissible from one person to another, either directly or indirectly through a carrier or vector.

d., congenital. D. which is present at birth. May be due to hereditary factors, or prenatal infection.

d., constitutional. (1) D. due to an individual's hereditary make-up. (2) A disease involving the body as a whole in contrast to one involving specific organs. SEE: *diathesis.*

d., contagious. An infectious disease readily transmitted from one person to another.

d., deficiency. A disease resulting from inadequate intake or absorption of essential dietary factors such as vitamins or minerals.

d., degenerative. A disease resulting from degenerative changes that occur in tissues and organs, characteristic of old age.

e., endemic. A disease which is present more or less continuously or recurs in a community.

d., epidemic. D. which attacks a large number of individuals in a community at the same time.

d., familial. A d. which occurs in several individuals of the same family.

d., functional. A d. in which no anatomical changes can be observed to account for the symptoms present.

d., hereditary. D. due to hereditary factors transmitted from parent to offspring.

d., hypokinetic [G. insufficient motion]. Physical and mental illness produced by lack of or insufficient exercise.

d., idiopathic. D. for which no causative factor can be recognized.

d., infectious. D. resulting from the presence in the body of a pathogenic organism.

d., malignant. (1) Cancer, *q.v.* (2) D. including cancer but not limited to that in which the progress is extremely rapid, generally threatening or resulting in death within a short time.

d., molecular. A heredity disease that may be caused by a defective molecule.

d., occupational. D. resulting from factors associated with the occupation engaged in by the patient.

d., organic. D. resulting from recognizable anatomical changes in an organ, or tissue of the body.

d., pandemic. An epidemic disease which is extremely widespread involving an entire country, continent, or possibly the entire world.

d., parasitic. D. resulting from the growth and development of parasitic organisms (plants or animals) in or upon the body.

d., periodic. Disease that occurs at more or less regular intervals or at the same time each year.

d., psychosomatic. D. in which structural changes in or malfunctioning of organs are due to the mind, esp. the emotions. NOTE: It is not possible for a human being to be consciously sick without there being some interplay between the emotions and the bodily functions.

d., sporadic. D. in which only occasional cases occur; not epidemic or endemic.

d., subacute. D. in which symptoms are less pronounced but more prolonged than in an acute disease; intermediate between acute and chronic disease.

d., venereal. ABBR: V. D. Includes syphilis, gonorrhea, and chancroid. Disease usually acquired through sexual relations.

disengage'ment [Fr. désengagement]. GYN: The displacement of the fetal head from within the maternal pelvis.

disequilib'rium [L. *dis*, apart, + *aequus*, equal, + *libra*, balance]. On unequal and unstable equilibrium.

disinfect (dis-in-fekt') [" + *inficere*, to corrupt]. To free from infection by physical or chemical means.

disinfec'tant [" + *inficere*, to corrupt]. A chemical which kills bacteria. SYN: *germicide, bactericide.* Common disinfectants are (1) the halogens: chlorine, fluorine, iodine; (2) salts of heavy metals: mercuric chloride (bichloride of mercury), silver nitrate; (3) acids: sulphurous acid; (4) alkalies: chloride of lime; (5) organic compounds: formaldahyde, alcohol 70%, iodoform, organic acids, phenol (carbolic acid), cresols, benzoic and salicylic acids and their sodium salts; (6) misc. substances: thymol, hydrogen peroxide, potassium permanganate, boric acid.

An agent that frees from infection. Term is usually applied to a chemical or physical agent which kills vegetative forms of microorganisms.

disinfecting agents. SEE: *alcohol, borax, boric acid, chlorine preparations, cresols, formaldehyde, hydrogen dioxide, kreseptol, mercuric chloride, nitric acid, phenol, potassium permanganate, sulfur, urotropin.*

disinfec'tion [L. *dis*, apart, + *inficere*, to corrupt]. The application of disinfectants. It is not possible to insure a 100% disinfection of a room unless the entire room and its contents are treated with a gaseous agent such as ethylene oxide. Disinfestation, or the killing of vermin by chemicals and their vapors, however, is possible.

d. of blankets and woolens. May be steam disinfected, or soaked for 2 hours in 5% carbolic acid solution and then washed. Cotton goods may also be so treated, or boiled before washing. Materials which might be harmed by conventional methods of disinfection may be treated in a chamber with ethylene oxide gas.

d. of excreta. Should be soaked in 5% carbolic acid solution for 1 hour before disposal. All infected excreta should be burned, but sputum may be treated as excreta if impossible to burn.

d. of field of operation. A safe rule is to make the disinfection, if anything,

DISINFECTANTS

Used For	Chemicals	Uses
Purifying air in rooms Preserving tissues	Formaldehyde (gas)	A 40% solution of formaldehyde gas is called by the trade name "formalin." A 4% solution preserves tissues, a 1 to 2% solution disinfects instruments.
	Sulfur dioxide	Formed by burning sulfur. Disinfects but will bleach colored fabrics.
Purifying the air and certain solutions	Chlorine	This gas in the presence of moisture is a powerful disinfectant. It is used mostly as chlorinated lime to disinfect stools and urine, and also to remove odors. Used commercially to purify drinking water. Oxidizes bacteria directly, or combines with the amino group (—NH_2) of bacterial cell to form chloramine (NH_2Cl) which kills the bacteria by oxidation.
Sinks, etc.	Phenol (carbolic acid)	Two to 5% solutions are fatal to all bacteria. Concentrated solutions are corrosive.
	Cresols	Generally prepared as emulsions or soapy solutions (common trade name of Lysol). They are more powerful than phenol.
Skin	Iodine 70% Ethyl alcohol	A 2½ to 3½% solution of iodine in alcohol (or in water +KI) is used to disinfect the skin before an operation. Disinfection is due to oxidation and precipitation of protein. This is followed by thorough washing of the area with the alcohol solution.
Wounds	Plain soap and water	For cleaning and irrigating dirty wounds. Followed by thorough rinsing with sterile isotonic saline solution.

too extensive. Thus, in operations of any magnitude upon scalp and large wounds of this structure, and all operations on the skull and its contents the entire scalp must be shaved and disinfected.

In operations upon the breast, the axilla and half of the chest must be prepared, and if glands of neck are involved the entire neck must be included in field of operation.

In amputation of foot and lower third of leg the disinfection must extend as far as knee, and in all higher amputations it should include the whole limb and corresponding side of pelvis.

In all abdominal operations below the umbilicus the pubic area must be shaved, and the surface disinfection must include the whole ant. surface and both sides as far as the breasts.

In operations on the stomach, liver, and bile ducts the field extends from the pubic area to the breasts. A general warm bath, liberal use of tincture of green soap should precede disinfection of the field of operation in all abdominal and pelvic operations, including hernia and varicocele.

In operations upon parts of the body difficult to disinfect, as scalp, palm of hand, and sole of foot, it is advisable to scrub with hot water and tincture of green soap, then rinse; then use 70 per cent solution of alcohol, benzalkonium chloride, hexachlorophene, or other disinfectant. Alcohol is universally useful in hand and surface disinfection.

The mucous membranes are active, absorbing surfaces so that the use of solutions of carbolic acid, mercuric bichloride, and other potent antiseptics is not advisable. The free use of any of these agents in the vagina, uterus, or rectum has frequently resulted in serious poisoning, and in some instances death.

Disinfection of the mouth should invariably precede the use of a general anesthetic, as in doing so the danger of inflammatory complications of the air passages following anesthetization is greatly diminished. For this purpose and to prepare the mouth for operation, cetyl pyridinium or benzalkonium chloride mouthwashes are especially effective.

In grave operations, such as excision of superior or inferior maxilla, and amputation of tongue, the employment of a disinfecting solution is preceded by thorough cleansing of the teeth and the mucous membrane is swabbed with hydrogen peroxide.

In operations upon the rectum the procedure in common use is made up of shaving perianal area, and enemas.

Vaginal disinfection is more satisfactory. After a thorough cleansing with warm water and tincture of green soap, a douche of warm water with a suitable disinfectant is recommended. The vaginal disinfection is preceded by shaving and disinfection of the external genitals.

Catheterization should always be preceded by disinfection of the meatus with green soap and rinsing thoroughly with sterile water.

The ear should be mechanically cleansed of wax, dirt, blood clot, etc., and then be carefully disinfected by a low-pressure stream of warm hydrogen peroxide, till it is absolutely clean.

disinfestation (dis-in-fes-ta'shun) [" + *infestāre,* to strike at]. The process of killing infesting insects or parasites.

disinsected. Freed of insects.

disintegra'tion [" + *integer,* entire]. The product of catabolism; the falling apart of the constituents of a substance.

disjoint'. To disarticulate or to separate bones from their natural positions in a joint.

disk [G. *diskos,* a disk]. A round, flat, platelike structure.

d., anisotropic. A dark, shining, highly refractile disk forming a part of the striation of the myofibril of a striated muscle fiber. Also called A or Q stripe.

d., articular. A disk of dense fibrous tissue or fibrocartilage found in the structure of certain joints, esp. the temporomandibular joint.

d., blood. A red blood corpuscle.

d., Bowman's. Segment of a muscle fiber.

d., choked. A swollen optic disk due to inflammation or edema. SYN: *papilledema.*

d. diameter. Optic disk diameter.

d., embryonic. An oval disk of cells in the blastocyst of a mammal from which the embryo proper develops. Its lower layer, the endoderm, forms the roof of the yolk sac; its upper layer, the ectoderm, forms the floor of the amniotic cavity. The primitive streak develops on the upper surface of the disk.

d., epiphyseal. Disklike epiphysis at vertebral centrum's ends.

d., germinal. A disk of cells on the surface of the yolk of the eggs of reptiles and birds from which the embryo develops; the blastoderm.

d., Hensen's. A pale disk occurring in the middle of a muscle fiber.

d., herniated. Rupture or herniation of the intervertebral disk, esp. between the 4th and 5th lumbar vertebrae. This usually causes pain in the affected side. SYN: *herniated nucleus pulposus.*

d. holder. Microscope joint to enable mobility in every direction.

d., intercalated. A highly refractive band which extends transversely across the fiber of cardiac muscle. It is bounded on each side by Z lines.

d., intermediate. Myofibrils. Also called Z line or Krause's membrane.

d., interpubic. Disk of cartilage bet. the pubic bones at their symphysis.

d., intervertebral. A fibrocartilage substance bet. vertebral surfaces.

It may rupture but it does not slip. It serves as a shock absorber. The gelatinous mass in the center is called the *nucleus pulposus.* When the disk material protrudes into the neural canal, pressure on the adjacent nerve root is manifested by pain. This is called herniation of an intervertebral disk. Symptoms will depend upon the location of the herniation. Those in the cervical area produce distinctive signs and symptoms in the cervical area. Those in the lumbar area cause symptoms of lumbar nerve root pressure.

d., isotropic. A disk lying between the A disk of a striated muscle myofibril. Also called I or J disk. It extends across the entire muscle fiber.

d., M. A thin line lying in the center of Hensen's disk.

d., Merkel's. A disklike expansion found at the end of sensory nerve fibers in the epidermis. It is a touch receptor. Also called *tactile disk.*

d., optic. Area of the retina where optic nerve enters it.

d., proligerous. SEE: *germinal d.*

d., Q. The anistropic or A disk of a striated muscle myofibril.

d., tactile. Merkel's disk, *q.v.*

d., Z. The intermediate disk of a striated muscle fiber, *q.v.*

diskitis (disk-i'tis). Inflammation of a disk, esp. an interarticular cartilage. SYN: *meniscitis.*

dis"loca'tion [L. *dis,* apart, + *locāre,* to place]. The displacement of any part, esp. the removal temporarily of a bone from its normal position in a joint.

d., closed. Simple dislocation, *q.v.*

d., complete. One which completely separates the surfaces of a joint.

d., complicated. One which is associated with other important injuries.

d., compound. One in which the joint communicates with the external air.

d., congenital. One which exists from or before birth.

d., consecutive. One in which the luxated bone has changed its position since its first displacement.

d., divergent. One in which the ulna and radius are dislocated separately.

d., habitual. One which often recurs after replacement.

d., incomplete. A subluxation; a slight displacement.

d., intrauterine. One which occurs to the fetus in utero.

d., metacarpophalangeal joint. D. of finger.

This is usually complicated by an interposition of tendons or other structures, and if reduced tends to slip out immediately. In many instances manipulating of this region only tends to make it more difficult for a subsequent reduction; therefore, immobilize* the disturbed area with well placed and padded splints of hand and wrist. Send patient to doctor, promptly.

d., Monteggia's. Dislocation of hip joint in which head of femur is near anterosuperior spine of the ilium.

d., Nelaton's. Dislocation of the ankle in which the astragalus is forced up bet. the end of the tibia and the fibula.

d., old. A dislocation in which no reduction has been accomplished, even after many days, weeks, or months.

d., partial. Same as incomplete.

d., pathologic. One which results from paralysis or disease of joint or supporting tissues.

d., primitive. One in which the bones remain as originally displaced.

d., recent. One seen shortly after it occurred.

d., simple. One in which the joint is not penetrated by a wound.

d., subastragalar. Separation of the calcaneum and the scaphoid from the astragalus.

d., thyroid. Displacement of the head of the femur into the thyroid foramen.

d., traumatic. One due to injury or violence.

dismemb'er. To remove an extremity or a portion of it.

disorganiza'tion [" + G. *organon,* a unified organ]. Alteration in an organic part, causing it to lose most or all of its distinctive characteristics.

disomus (di-so'mus). A malformed fetus with a double trunk.

disorientation (dis-o-ri-en-ta'shun) [" + Fr. *orienter,* to face the east]. Inability to estimate direction or location, or to be cognizant of time or of persons.

disparate points (dis'par-at) [L. *disparare,* to separate]. Points on the 2 retinas which are not corresponding or identical, causing objects to appear double.

dispen'sary [L. *dispensare,* to give out]. Place or clinic for dispensation of medicines and treatment.

dispense (dis-pens') [L. *dis,* out, + *pensare,* to weigh]. To prepare or deliver medicines.

dispireme (di-spi'rēm) [G. *dis,* two, + *speirēma,* coil]. Stage that succeeds the diaster and precedes division of cell body, when threads of daughter cell are convoluted.

disperse (dis-pers') [" + *spergere,* to scatter]. To scatter, esp. applied to the scattering of light rays.

dispersion (dis-per'zhun). 1. Act of dispersing. 2. That which is dispersed.

d., coarse. Mechanical suspension.

d., colloidal. Colloid solution.

d. medium. Liquid in which a colloid is dispersed.

d., molecular. A true solution.

d. particles. Colloid particles in a colloid system.

d. system. A colloid solution.

dispersonalization (dis"per-son-al-ī-za'shun). Mental state in which the individual denies the existence of his personality or parts of the body.

displace'ment [Fr. *déplacer,* to lay aside]. 1. Removal from the normal or usual position or place. 2. Adding to a fluid one of greater density causing the first fluid to be dispersed. 3. Attachment of emotion from repressed conflict to some apparently indifferent idea.

PSY: The transfer of an emotion pert. to one set of ideas to an inappropriate idea; although properly thus associated in the unconscious.

disposi'tion. A natural tendency or aptitude exhibited by an individual or group of individuals. This may be manifested toward acquiring a certain disease, presumably due to hereditary factors. SEE: *diathesis.*

dissect (dis-sekt') [L. *dissecāre,* to cut up]. To separate tissues and parts of a cadaver for anatomical study.

dissection (dis-sek'shun) [L. *dissecāre,* to cut up]. The cutting of parts for purpose of separation and studying of the same.

dissem'inated. Scattered or disturbed over a considerable area, esp. applied to disease organisms; scattered throughout an organ or the body.

d. sclerosis. A degenerative disease of the nervous system.

dissipa'tion (dis-ĭ-pa'shun) [L. *dissipāre,* to scatter]. Dispersion of matter. Act of being wasteful and living a dissolute life, esp. drinking to excess.

dissociation (dis-so-sĭ-a'shun) [L. *dis,* apart, + *sociatiō,* union]. Separation, as the separation by heat of a complex compound into simpler molecules.

d., microbic. Substrains arising from pure strains.

d. of personality. Split in consciousness resulting in two different phases of personality, neither being aware of the words, acts, and feelings of the other. SEE: *dual personality, multiple personality.*

d., psychological. Disunion of mind of which the person is not aware. Dual personalities, fugues, somnambulism, selective amnesia, are so classified.

d. symptoms. Anesthesia to heat, cold, and pain, without loss of muscular sense or tactile sensibility.

dissolu'tion [L. *dissolvere,* to dissolve]. Death; pathological resolution or breaking up of the integrity of an anatomical element.

dissolve (dĭ-zolv') [L. *dissolvere,* to dissolve]. To cause absorption of a solid in and by a liquid.

dissolvent (diz-ol'vent) [L. *dissolvens,* dissolving]. 1. Having the power to dissolve. 2. That which is capable of disintegrating.

dissol'ving. To cause to enter into a solution.

distad (dis'tad) [L. *distāre,* to be distant + *ad,* toward]. Away from the center.

distal (dis'tal) [L. *distāre,* to be distant]. Farthest from the center, from a medial line, or from the trunk. Opposite of *proximal.*

distend' [L. *distendere,* to stretch out]. 1. To stretch out. 2. To become inflated.

disten'tion [L. *distendere,* to stretch out]. The state of being distended. SEE: *goblet cell, Wangensteen's method.*

distichiasis (dis-tĭ-ki'a-sis) [G. *dis,* two, + *stichos,* row]. Two rows of eyelashes, one or both of which are directed inward toward the eye.

distill [L. *destillāre,* to drop from]. To vaporize by heat, condensing and collecting the volatilized products.

distillate (dis'til-āt) [L. *destillāre,* to drop from]. The portion of a substance subject to distillation which passes off in the form of a vapor and condenses.

distilla'tion [L. *destillāre,* to drop from]. Condensation of a liquid, heated to a volatilization point, as the condensation of steam from boiling water.

It is used for the purification of water, and other purposes. Distilled water should not be exposed as it readily takes up impurities from the atmosphere.

d., destructive. The process of decomposing complex organic compounds by heat in the absence of air, and condensing the vapor of the liquid products.

d., dry. D. of solids without liquids.

d., fractional. Separation of liquids based upon the difference in their boiling points.

distinctometer (dis-tink-tom'ĕ-ter) [L. *distinguere,* to mark out, + G. *metron,* measure]. Device for palpation of abdomen along its borders.

distobuccal (dis-to-buk'al [L. *distāre,* to be distant, + *bucca,* cheek]. Pert. to the distal and buccal walls of bicuspid and molar teeth.

Dis'toma, Dis'tomum (dis'to-ma, -mum) [G. *distomios,* double mouthed]. Former name of genus of trematode worms. Its members have been placed in many new genera.

dis'tome. A fluke with two suckers; an oral and a ventral sucker or *acetabulum.*

distomiasis (dĭs-tō-mī-ās'ĭs). Infestation with flukes, which flukes may infest the intestine, liver, bile ducts, gallbladder, blood vessels, or lungs.

distor'tion. 1. A twisting or bending out of regular shape. 2. A writhing or twisting movement as of the muscles of the face. 3. A deformity in which the part or structure is altered in shape. 4. In ophthalmology, visual perception of an image which does not provide a true picture. This is due to astigmatism or to retinal abnormalities. 5. In psychiatry, adapting an idea to conform with a patient's wishes.

distractibil'ity [L. *dis,* apart, + *tractio,* a drawing]. PSY: A condition of mental wandering in which the thoughts are attracted by extraneous conditions or influenced by a dissociation of consciousness.

distraction (dis-trak'shun). 1. State of mental confusion or derangement. 2. Separation of the surfaces of a joint by extension without injury or dislocation of the parts.

distraught (dis-trawt'). The mental state of being in doubt, deeply troubled, and having conflicting thoughts. Patient may be frantic and have need to be continuously occupied.

distress (dis-tres') [L. *distringere,* to hinder or molest]. Physical or mental trouble or suffering.

distribution [L. *distribuere,* to allot]. 1. The dividing and spreading of anything, esp. blood vessels and nerves, to tissues. 2. The presence of entities at various sites or in particular patterns throughout the body such as hair, fat, nutrients, etc.

districhiasis (dis-trik-i'ă-sis) [G. *dis,* double, + *thrix,* hair]. Two hairs growing from the same hair follicle.

distrix (dis'triks). The splitting of ends of the hairs.

disulfiram (di-sul'fĭ-ram). A drug administered orally to deter ingestion of alcohol as an intoxicant. If alcohol is ingested following taking of drug, there occurs an unpleasant reaction including nausea and vomiting. SYN: *tetraethylthiuram disulfide.* Proprietary name: Antabuse.

Dittrich's plugs (dit'ricks) [Franz Dittrich, German pathologist, 1815-1859]. Small particles in fetid sputum composed of pus, detritus, bacteria, and fat crystals.

diuresis (di-u-re'sis) [G. *dia,* through, + *ourein,* to urinate]. Secretion and passage of abnormally large amounts of urine.

This occurs in diabetes mellitus. It is an early sign of chronic interstitial nephritis. May also be due to: (a) hysteria or as a result of fear and anxiety, (b) ingestion of large quantities of liquids, (c) diabetes insipidus, (d) the action of drugs which have the ability to cause diuresis.

diuretic (di-u-ret'ik). Increasing or an agent which increases the secretion of urine.

Diuretics act in two ways (1) by increasing glomerular filtration or (2) by decreasing reabsorption from the tubules. An increase in blood flow in the renal vessels increases urine formation by increasing glomerular filtration-pressure and by increasing the number of glomeruli functioning.

Diuretics act on the kidney cells, increasing permeability, and also on the circulation to the kidneys. Alcohol dilates the blood vessels of the kidneys and thus increases circulation to them.

Cold applications have a diuretic action by contracting superficial vessels and raising blood pressure. SEE: *diuresis.*

d., alterative. One eliminated by the kidney which aids diseased urinary tract surfaces.

d., hydragogue. One increasing renal flow.

d., refrigerant. One which makes the urine less irritating.

diuril (dĭ'ū-rĭl). Proprietary name for chlorothiazide, a diuretic agent.

diur'nal [L. *diēs,* day]. 1. Daily. 2. Happening in the daytime, or pert. to it; opposed to *nocturnal.*

divagation (di-vă-ga'shun) [L. *divagari*, to wander about]. Disconnected and incoherent speech.

divergence (di-ver'jens) [L. *divergere*, to tend apart]. Separation from a common center, esp. that of the eyes.

diver'gent [L. *divergere*, to tend apart]. Radiating in different directions.

diver's paralysis. Occupational disease due to returning too suddenly to normal atmosphere after working under high air pressure. SYN: *bends, caisson disease, tunnel disease.*

divertic'ula [L. *diverticulāre*, to turn aside]. Plural of *diverticulum, q.v.*

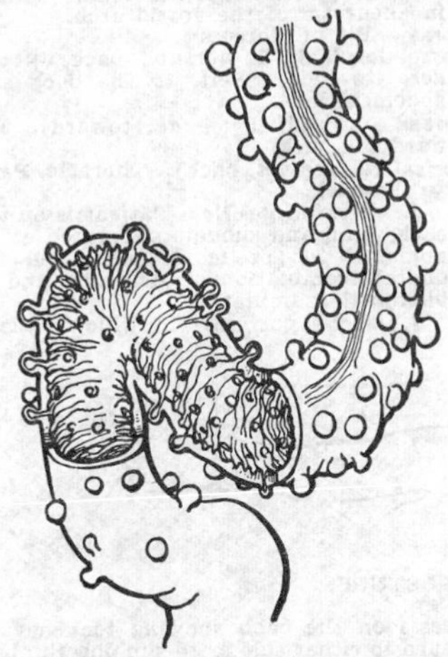

MULTIPLE DIVERTICULA OF THE COLON

diverticulec'tomy [" + G. *ektomē*, excision]. Surgical removal of a diverticulum.

diverticuli'tis [" + G. *-itis*, inflammation]. Inflammation of a diverticulum or of diverticula in the intestinal tract esp. the colon, causing stagnation of feces in little distended sacs of the colon (diverticula).

d., acute. SYM: Similar to appendicitis; inflammation of peritoneum, formation of an abscess, and finally gangrene accompanied by perforation may ensue. Symptoms are felt on left side.

d., chronic. SYM: Constipation growing worse, mucus in stools, griping abdominal pains at intervals. Wall of bowels may thicken, which may produce chronic intestinal obstruction.

diverticulo'sis [" + G. *-ōsis*]. Diverticula of the colon without inflammation or symptoms. Only a small per cent of persons with diverticulosis go on to develop diverticulitis.

diverticulum (di-ver-tik'u-lum) (pl. *diverticula*) [L. *diverticulāre*, to turn aside]. A sac or pouch in the walls of a canal or organ.

d., false. D. without muscular coats in wall of pouch. This type of d. is acquired.

d., Meckel's. Caused by continued existence of the omphalomesenteric duct. Its occurrence is fairly common. Usually located on ileum close to ileocecal valve.

d. of duodenum. D. commonly located near entrance of common and pancreatic ducts.

d. of jejunum. D. marked usually by severe pain in upper abdomen, followed occasionally by massive hemorrhage from intestine.

d. of stomach. D. of wall of stomach.

d., true. D. consisting of all the coats of muscle in the pouch wall. Usually congenital.

division [L. *dividere*, divide]. 1. A separation into parts. 2. That which separates as anatomical boundary, partition, or wall.

d., cell. The formation of two daughter cells from the original cell.

divulsor (di-vul'sor) [L. *dis*, apart, + *vellere*, to pluck]. Device for dilatation of a part.

d., pterygium. Instrument for separating corneal portion of the pterygium.

d., tendon. Device for separating tendon from surrounding tissue.

dizygotic twins (di-zi-got'ik) [G. *dis*, two, + *zygon*, yoke]. Twins who are the product of two ova. Fraternal twins. SEE: *twin, monozygotic.*

diz'ziness [A.S. *dyzig*, foolish]. Giddiness, vertigo.

DNA. ABBR. for *deoxyribonucleic acid, q.v.*

Dobell's solution (do'belz) [Horace B. Dobell, English physician, 1828-1917]. Carbolic acid, borax, sodium bicarbonate, glycerine, and water in solution.

Dobie's globule (dō'bē's) [William M. Dobie, English physician, 1828-1915]. A very tiny spherical body in a striated muscle fiber's light band.

DOCA. *Desoxycorticosterone.* SEE: *STH.*

dochmiasis, dochmiosis (dok-mi'as-is, -mī-o'sis) [*Dochmius*, a nematode parasite]. Hookworm disease. SYN: *ankylostomiasis, uncinariasis.*

Dochmius (dok'mī-us). A species of parasite. SYN: *ankylostoma.*

Dock's test meal [George Dock, American physician, 1860-]. Shredded wheat biscuit and 9-12 oz. water. SEE: *Ewald's t. m.*

doctor [L. teacher]. 1. A teacher, a learned person. 2. The recipient of an advanced degree, *i.e.*, doctor of medicine (M.D.); doctor of philosophy (Ph.D.); doctor of science (D.Sc.); doctor, of divinity (D.D.); etc. 3. One who, after being licensed to do so, practices medicine.

The use of the word *doctor* is sometimes confusing. This may be remedied when writing or speaking of those who possess an M.D. degree by using the word *physician.*

In some countries persons are, after college, awarded the degree of *Doctor of Jurisprudence* and are referred to thereafter as *doctor.*

dog bite. Lacerated wound by a dog. SEE: *rabies.*

Preserve the dog alive if possible. Animal should be observed for 10 days to determine the presence of rabies.

TREATMENT: Thorough cleansing of bite wounds with strong soap or detergent solutions (as 1:1000 solution of benzalkonium hydrochloride), followed by infiltration of the wound areas with antirabies serum. For rabies vaccine, see under: *Rabies.*

dol. Symbol for degree of pain registered on the dolorimeter.

dolichocephalic (dol''ī-ko-se-fal'ik) [G. *dolichos*, long, + *kephalē*, head]. Having a skull with a long ant. post. diameter.

dolichohieric (dol-ĭ-ko-hi-er′ĭk) [" + *ieros,* sacred]. Having a long, slender sacrum.

dolichopellic, dolichopelvic (dol-ĭ-ko-pel′-ĭk, -pel′vĭk) [" + *pellis,* pelvis]. Having an abnormally long or narrow pelvis.

dolichosigmoid (dol-ĭ-ko-sig′moid) [" + *sigma,* the letter S, + *eidos,* form]. Having an abnormally long sigmoid flexure.

dolor (do′lor) [L.]. Pain. SEE: *calor, rubor, tumor.*

d. cap′itis. Headache.

dolorific (dol-or-if′ik). [L. *dolor,* pain]. Causing pain.

dolorimeter (dŏl-ŏr-ĭm′ĕ-ter) ′L. *dolor,* pain, + *meter,* measure]. SYMB: *dol.* Device for measuring degree of pain.

dolorogen′ic [" + G. *gennan,* to produce]. Causing pain.

domatophobia (do-mat-o-fo′bĭ-ă) [G. *dōma,* house, + *phobos,* fear]. A form of claustrophobia; abnormal aversion to being in a house.

domicil′iary [L. *domis,* house]. Pert. to a house.

dom′inant [L. *dominans,* ruling]. That which is inherited from 1 parent developing to the exclusion of a contrasting character from the opp. parent. One who, or that which, gives something.

born 1863]. *Leishmania donovani,* a small protozoan parasite occurring as a small oval or round body in bone marrow or in spleen or liver. The causative agent in kala-azar.

DOPA. A chemical substance, 3,4-dihydroxyphenylalanine, produced by the oxidation of tyrosine to typosinase.

doraphobia (do-ră-fo′bĭ-ă) [G. *dora,* hide, + *phobos,* fear]. Abnormal aversion to touching the hair or fur of animals.

Dorel′lo's canal. A bony canal in tip of temporal bone enclosing abducens nerve.

Dorendorf's sign [Hans Dorendorf, German physician, 1866-]. A filling up or fullness of the supraclavicular groove in aneurysm of the aortic arch.

dorsa. Pl. of dorsum.

dorsabdom′inal [L. *dorsum,* back, + *abdere,* to hide]. Pert. to the back and abdomen.

dorsad (dor′sad) [" + *ad,* toward]. Toward the back.

dor′sal [L. *dorsum,* back]. Thoracic. Pert. to the back.

d. elevated position. Patient is on the back, head and shoulders elevated at an angle of 30° or more. Employed for digital examination of genitalia, and in bimanual examination.

d. inertia posture. In which patient rests on the back showing tendency to turn to either side or to slip down in bed if head of bed is elevated.

This may be seen in great weakness, in acute infectious diseases such as typhoid, mental apathy, and in muscular weakness.

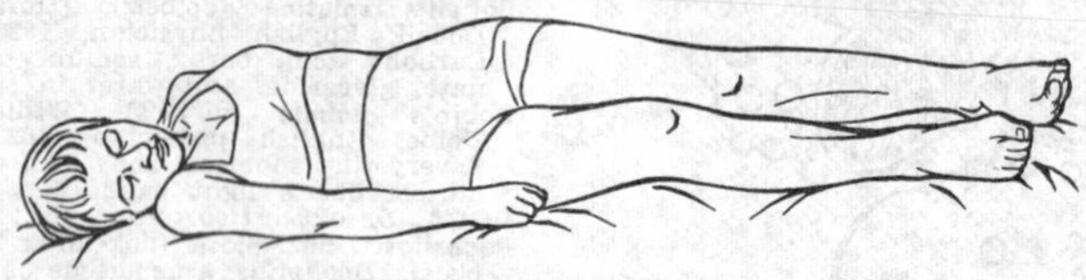

DORSAL INERTIA POSTURE.

d. nerves. Nerves emerging from the dorsal vertebrae.*

d. recumbent position. Same as dorsal elevated, except extremities are moderately flexed and rotated outward, the soles of the feet resting upon bed or table, or legs may be extended. With legs not flexed it is used for examination of chest, abdomen, and lower limbs. With legs flexed, it is used in giving douches, for bathing, for catheterizing.

d., hydrogen. A substance which gives up hydrogen to another substance. SEE: *hydrogen acceptor.*

donee (dō-nē′) [L. *donāre,* to give]. One who receives something such as a blood transfusion from a donor.

do′nor [L. *donāre,* to give]. One who furnishes blood, tissue, or an organ to be used in another person.

d., universal. One whose blood is of Group O, and whose blood is usually compatible with most other blood types. In actual practice this rarely occurs because of the many factors other than the major blood antigens (A, B, AB) which determine blood compatibility.

Don′ovan body [Charles Donovan, Irish physician in Sanitary Service of India,

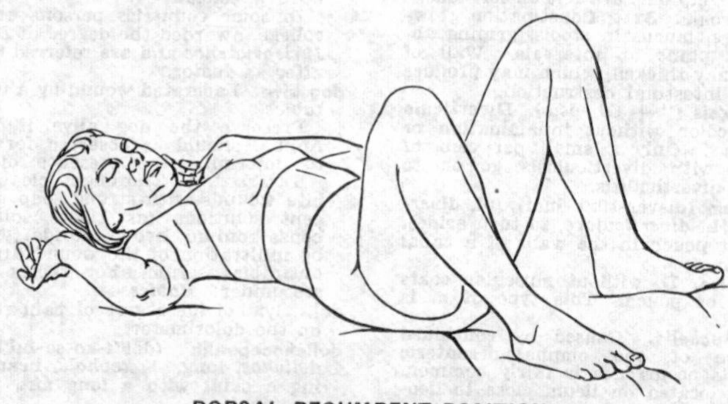

DORSAL RECUMBENT POSITION.

and for applying abdominal compresses. The patient may be placed in this position for bimanual palpation, or for vaginal examinations and repair of lesions following parturition.

d. reflex. Irritation of the skin over the erector spinal muscles, causing contraction of muscles of the back.

d. rigid posture. One in which both legs (or the right one) are drawn up; observed in peritonitis, meningitis, ascites, and tympanites. The right leg is drawn up in appendicitis, in pelvic inflammation, renal calculus in right ureter, in psoas abscess or in peritonitis on the right side.

d. vertebrae. Twelve bones of the spinal column bet. the cervical and lumbar vertebrae. SEE: *position; posture.*

dorsalgia (dor-sal'jĭ-ă) [" + G. *algos*, pain]. Pain in the back. SYN: *nostalgia; rachialgia.*

dorsi-, dorso-, dors- [L.]. Combining form for *dorsum*, back.

dorsiduct (dor'si-dukt) [L. *dorsum*, back, + *ducere*, to lead]. To draw toward the back or backward.

dorsiduc'tion [" + *ducere*, to lead]. Drawing toward the back.

dorsiflect (dor'sĭ-flekt) [" + *flectere*, to bend]. Bending backward.

dorsiflex'ion [" + *flectere*, to bend]. The act of bending or flexion toward the dorsum or rear; opposite of plantarflexion. Also applied to straightening or extending the toes.

dorsimesad (dor-sĭ-mes'ad) [" + G. *mesos*, middle, + L. *ad-*, toward]. In the direction of the dorsimeson.

dos'age [G. *dosis*, dose]. The amt. of medicine to be administered to a patient at one time.

d., calculation of, for children. There is no absolutely reliable formula for calculating the dose of a medicine an infant or child should receive. Several rules for calculating a child's dose are given below.

Young's rule for children:

FOR CHILDREN FROM 1-12 YEARS

Formula:

$$\frac{\text{Age in yr.}}{\text{Age} + 12} \times \text{Adult dose} = \text{child's dose.}$$

Example: The adult dose of a substance is 500 mg. How much should a 4-year-old child receive?

$$\frac{4}{4+12} \times 500 = 125$$

The child should receive 125 mg.

Body surface area: The surface area in square meters is divided by 1.7 and multiplied by the adult dose. Example: A child of 0.4 sq. meters of surface who needs a drug for which the adult dose is 500 mg.:

$$\frac{0.4}{1.7} \times 500 = 117$$

Thus the dose would be 117 mg. Obviously medicines are not packaged in 117 mg. doses; so either 100 mg. or 125 mg. could be safely given. If the medicine were in liquid form, the dose could be easily determined by using the same formula.

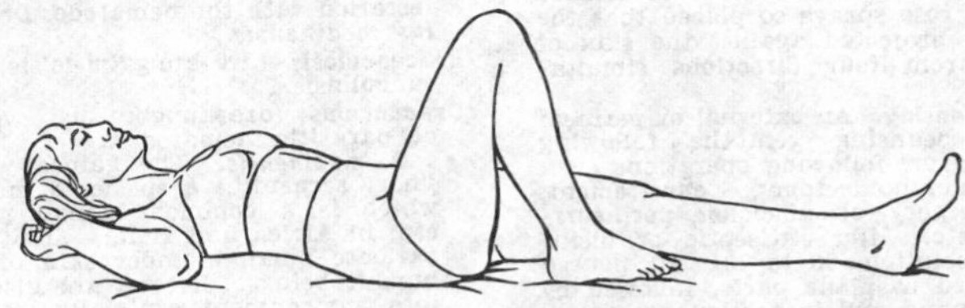

DORSAL RIGID POSTURE.
With right leg drawn up.

dorsimeson (dor-sĭ-mes'on) [" + G. *mesos*, middle]. The median plane of the back.

dorsispinal (dor"sĭ-spi'nal) [" + *spina*, thorn]. Pert. to the back and spine.

d. veins. Veins around the vertebrae.

dorsocephalad (dor-so-sef'ă-lad) [" + G. *kephalē*, head, + L. *ad*, toward]. Situated toward the back of the head.

dorsodynia (dor-so-din'ĭ-ă) [" + G. *odynē*, pain]. Pain in the muscles of upper part of back.

dorsosa'cral [" + *sacrum*, sacred, "sacred bone"]. Pert. to lower back.

d. position. Patient lies upon the back, same as in the dorsal recumbent position,* excepting that thighs are flexed upon abdomen and legs upon thighs which are abducted. Leg holders are used to support legs in position.

Used for gynecological examinations and treatments, in plastic operations on genital tract, in vaginal hysterectomy, and in diagnosis and treatment of diseases of urethra and bladder. SYN: *lithotomy position* (illus., p. L-34).

dor'sum (pl. *dorsa*) [L.]. The back or post. surface of a part.

d. meter. An instrument designed to estimate the quantity of radiation, so as to determine the duration of exposure when using roentgen rays. SYN: *dosimeter.*

dose (dōs) [G. *dosis*]. Amt. of a medicinal preparation to be taken at one time.

d., divided. Fractional portions adm. at short intervals.

d., erythema. Smallest amount of x-rays that will produce erythema within two weeks following treatment.

d., lethal. A fatal dose.

d., maximum. Largest dose it is safe to administer.

d., minimum. Smallest dose that will be effective.

dosimeter (do-sim'ĕ-ter) [" + *metron*, measure]. Device for measuring doses, especially of x-rays.

dosimetric (do-sĭ-met'rik). Pert. to dosage.

d. system. One of regular or determinate dosage.

dosimetry (do-sim'et-rĭ) [G. *dosis*, dose, + *metron*, measure]. Measurement of doses.

do'tage [M.E. *doten*, to doze]. Senility; feeblemindedness of very old age.

dothienenteria, dothienenteritis (do"the-en-en-te'rĭ-ă, -en-ter-i'tis) [G. *dothien*, a boil, + *enteron*, intestine, + *-ītis*, inflammation]. Typhoid fever.

double (dŭb'l) [L. *duplus*, twofold]. Combining two things or qualities.

d. consciousness. Expression of two phases of personality.

d. personality. A split in consciousness, neither personality being aware of acts and words of other. SEE: *dual personality; multiple personality.*

d. touch. Exploration with a finger in one cavity and thumb in another.

d. uterus. State of having a double uterus. SYN: *dihysteria.*

d. vision. Seeing two images of an object at the same time. SYN: *diplopia.*

douche (doosh) [Fr. *doucher*, to pour]. A current of vapor or stream of water, hot or cold, directed against a part.

Douches may be made up of plain water or water that is medicated. The douche may be for the purpose of personal hygiene or for the treatment of a local condition.

d., air. Air current directed on body for therapeutic purposes.

d., alternating. SEE: *Scotch d.*

d., astringent. One containing substances for shrinking the mucous membrane, such as alum or zinc sulfate.

d., circular. Needle spray or application of water to body through horizontal jets size of a needle from number of small rose sprays so placed that the water is projected against the skin of bather from four directions simultaneously.

d., cleansing. An external or perineal d. for cleansing genitalia following defecation or following operations such as hemorrhoidectomy, curettement, rectal surgery, circumcision, perineorrhaphy, etc. Mild antiseptic or disinfectant solution, 98 to 104° F., poured or sprayed over the parts, followed by gentle drying and inspection for cleanliness. SYN: *external d.; perineal d.*

d., deodorizing. One to deodorize the vagina and vaginal secretions when they have an offensive odor.

d., high. One where the bag is at least four feet above the hips of the patient.

d., jet. A solid stream from the douche hose.

d., low. One where the bag is 1-1½ feet above the hips of the patient.

d., medicated. One containing a medicinal substance for the treatment of local conditions.

d., neutral. Douche given at average surface temperature of body—90°-97° F.

d., perineal. One projected upward from a bidet* placed just above floor; patient sits in armchair, crescent-shaped seat, and receives douche upon perineum. SYN: *cleansing d., q.v.*

d., rain. Overhead shower.

d., Scotch. Alternating of hot and cold jets of water against local area of skin.

d. solutions. *Alum:* ½ to 1%. *Green Soap:* 1%. *Sodium Bicarbonate:* 2%.

d., vaginal. D. of vagina ordered for deodorant, antiseptic, stimulating or hemostatic purposes. Temperature of solutions: antiseptic or deodorant d., 105 to 112° F.; stimulating or hemostatic d., 118 to 120° F. Solution should flow slowly with little pressure, the douche can being elevated up to two feet above patient's pelvis. Quantity generally two to three quarts of solution unless otherwise ordered.

Douglas' cul-de-sac [James Douglas, Scottish anatomist, 1675-1742]. Peritoneal sac which lies behind uterus and in front of rectum.

D.'s pouch. Same as D.'s *cul-de-sac.*

douglasitis (dug-las-i'tis) [G. *-ītis*, inflammation]. Inflammation of the *cul-de-sac* of Douglas.

dow'el [Fr. *douille*, socket, from L. *ductus*, leading]. Metal pin for fastening an artificial crown to a tooth root.

Down's syndrome [J. Langdon Down, English physician, 1828-1896]. Mongolism, a variety of congenital, moderate to severe mental retardation. Marked by sloping forehead, presence of epicanthal folds causing an Oriental appearance of eyes, bridge of nose flat or sometimes absent, low-set ears, and generally dwarfed physique.

Doyère's eminence (dwah-yair') [Louis Doyère, French physiologist, 1811-1863]. Elevation where a nerve filament enters a muscle.

D. P. Abbr. for *Doctor of Pharmacy.*

dr. Abbr. for *dram* or *drachm.*

D. R. Abbr. for *reaction of degeneration.*

drachm (dram) [G. *drachmē*, a weight]. A unit of weight in apothecaries' system. SYMB: ʒ. ABBR: *dm.* SEE: *dram.*

dracontiasis (drā-kŏn-ti'ă-sis) [G. *drakontian*, little dragon]. Dracunculiasis.

dracunculiasis (dra-kung"ku-li'ă-sis). Infestation with the nematode, *Dracunculus medinensis.*

dracunculosis (drā-kung"ku-lo'sis). Dracunculiasis.

Dracunculus (dra-kung'ku-lus) A genus of parasitic nematodes.

D. medinensis. The guinea worm or "fiery serpent". A species of nematode which is a common human parasite, esp. in Africa and India. Adult female parasite burrows under skin of leg of human beings. Larvae are discharged into environment especially when legs are in water. Fleas in water swallow larvae and become infective. Man becomes infected after drinking contaminated water.

drain (drān) [A.S. *drehnigean*, to draw off]. 1. Exit or tube for discharge of morbid matter. 2. To draw off a fluid.

d., capillary. Drawing off by capillary attraction.

d., cigarette. Drain made by covering a small strip of gauze with rubber covering.

d., Mikulicz'. Single layer of gauze pushed into the wound cavity, to which is added thick gauze wicks that project from the cavity.

d., nonabsorbable. One made from horsehair, gauze, rubber, glass, or metal. TYPES: *abdominal, antrum, perineal, suprapubic,* etc.

d., Penrose. A cigarette d. made with a piece of small rubber tubing through which gauze has been pulled.

drainage (drān'ij) [A.S. *drehnigean*, to draw off]. The free flow or withdrawal of fluids, as pus from a cavity or wound. SEE: *autodrainage; drain.*

d., capillary. D. by method of capillary attraction.

d., funnel. D. with glass funnels.

d., postural. D. for draining nasal area, bronchi, and the sinuses.

The patient lies on his back on a bed with shoulders over the side and head hanging down.

d., tidal. A method, controlled mechanically, of filling the bladder with solution by gravity, and periodically emptying the vesicle by siphonage. Usually used when the patient lacks control of the bladder, as in injuries or lesions of the spinal cord.

d. tube. Device for allowing escape of pus, serum, blood, or other fluids from a wound, abscess, etc.

d. t. carrier. Device for placing drainage tube in position.

d. t. trocar. Device to introduce drainage tube without making a large incision.

dram [G. *drachmē,* a weight]. A unit of weight in apothecaries' system. Sixty gr. or ⅛ oz. apothecary weight; 3.888 gm., 27.34 gr. or 1/16 oz., avoirdupois.

d., fluid. A teaspoonful or ⅛ of a fluid ounce or 57.1 gr. of distilled water, the equivalent of 3.70 cc. or ml. In Great Britain 54.8 gr. of distilled water or 3.50 cc.

dramamine (dram'ă-mēn). Proprietary name for dimenhydrinate.

dram'atism [G. *drama,* acting, + *ismos,* state of]. Dramatic behavior and lofty speech in insanity.

drapetomania (drap-et-o-ma'nĭ-ă) [G. *drapetēs,* runaway, + *mania,* madness]. Insane impulse to wander from home.

dras'tic [G. *drastikos,* effective]. 1. Acting strongly. 2. A very active purgative, usually producing many evacuations, and accompanied by pain and tenesmus. Ex: *croton oil, elaterin.*

draught (draft) [A.S. *dragan,* to draw]. 1. A drink. 2. Drawing liquid into the mouth. 3. Breeze produced by wind or fan.

draw sheet. Historically, the term "draw sheet" was given to a long roll or bolt of muslin with the free end placed under the patient's buttocks. When this became soiled, it was drawn from under the patient and rolled up on the opposite side of the cot or bed, allowing the patient to lie on a clean section of the roll of muslin.

The draw sheet is now used to cover a rubber sheet which protects the mattress from soiling and drainage. A crib sheet or one-half a regular sheet is the usual size but it must be wide enough to extend from the patient's shoulders to below the knees and long enough to tuck under both sides of mattress. (See *Bed, Making an Occupied,* for method of changing.)

drepanocyte (drep'ă-no-sīt) [G. *drepanē,* sickle, + *kytos,* cell]. Sickle or crescent cell.

drepanocytemia (drep"ă-no-si-te'mĭ-ă) [" + " + *aima,* blood]. Sickle cell anemia.

drepanocytic (drep"ă-no-sit'ik) [" + *kytos,* cell]. Pert. to or resembling a sickle cell.

dressing [Fr. *dresser,* to treat a wound]. Covering, protective, or support for diseased or injured parts.

NP: These rules should be followed when preparing to dress any type of wound:

1. Assemble all necessary articles either on a tray or surgical dressing cart.
2. Scrub hands thoroughly with soap under hot running water. Use sterile rubber gloves for procedure, if doctor so advises. Also the nurse, physician, and patient may be required to wear surgical-type masks.
3. Tell the patient what is going to be done; then drape with a sheet or bath blanket, exposing only the area necessary to be dressed.
4. Place sterile towel beside the wound and, using sterile forceps, place upon it the sterile instruments, gauze, etc., from their sterile containers immediately.
5. Using clean forceps, remove soiled dressings and place in paper bag for burning. Follow doctor's instructions as to use of antiseptics, powders, petroleum gauze, etc.
6. If drainage is profuse, reinforce the dressing with absorbent cellulose pads.
7. Make the patient comfortable; remove all articles from room; take tray or cart to area for cleaning and replenishing supplies.

RS: *bandages; compresses.*

d., absorbent. Gauze, sterilized gauze, absorbent cotton.

d., antiseptic. Dressing consisting of gauze permeated with an antiseptic solution.

d., dry. Dressing consisting of dry gauze, absorbent cotton, or other dry material.

d., fixed. Dressing permeated with starch, silicate of soda, or plaster of Paris. When this dressing dries it provides fixation of the part so treated.

d., hot moist. Most common form is hot normal saline solution, heated to as hot as can be borne by bare forearm of nurse. Sterile towel unfolded, gauze dressings dropped into it, immersed in solution at middle, wrung out by turning dry ends in opposite directions. Dressing is then applied, with sterile forceps, directly to the wound and a dry, sterile towel is sometimes used over it, to keep dressing in place. Heat is best maintained by infrared lamp. CAUTION: Do not burn patient.

d., occlusive. Dressing that seals a wound completely to prevent infection from without and to prevent moisture from escaping from the dressing.

d., pressure. One applies pressure to the wound. May be used following skin grafting.

d., protective. Dressing applied for purpose of preventing injury or infection to the part so treated.

d., water. Dressing consisting of gauze, cotton, or similar dressing material which is kept wet by the application of sterilized water.

Drinker respirator [Philip Drinker, American engineer in industrial hygiene, 1894-]. Apparatus in which alternating positive and negative air pressure upon the patient creates artificial respiration. Commonly called the "iron lung."

drip [A.S. *dryppan,* to drip]. 1. To fall in drops. 2. To instill drop by drop.

d., intravenous. Slow injection of a solution (glucose, saline, etc.), a drop at a time, intravenously.

d., Murphy. Slow rectal instillation of a fluid drop by drop. SEE: *Murphy's drip or method.*

d., nasal. Method of administering fluid slowly to dehydrated babies by means of a catheter placed through the nose with one end in the esophagus.

d., postnasal. A condition due to chronic sinusitis in which a discharge drips from the postnasal region into the pharynx.

drip sheet. Modified sheet bath.

drive (drīv). The force or impulse to act.

dromomania (dro-mo-ma'nĭ-ă) [G. *dromos,* a running, + *mania,* madness]. Insane impulse to wander.

dromotrop'ic [" + *trepein,* to turn]. Pert. to supposed fibers in cardiac nerves which influence conductivity of muscles.

drop [A.S. *dropa*] [L. *gutta*]. 1. A minute spherical mass of liquid. 2. Falling of a part from paralysis or injury.

d., culture. A bacterial culture in a drop of culture media.

d.'s, ear. Medication administered by drops placed in the external canal of the ear.

d. finger. Baseball finger.

d. foot. Toes dragging in walking with falling of foot due to paralysis of dorsal flexor muscles.

d., hanging. Application of a drop of solution to a small glass cover-slip. This is then inverted over a glass slide with a depression in it. The contents of the suspended solution can then be examined microscopically.

d.'s, knockout. A drug to cause unconsciousness; usually adm. for criminal purposes, as robbery.

d. wrist. Paralysis of extensor muscles causing hand to hang down from forearm.

droplet. Very small drop.

d. infection. That conveyed by means of infective particles, as when carried in a spray from the nose or mouth. Usual mode of infection from common cold.

dropsy (drop'sĭ) [contraction L. *hydrops,* dropsy, from G. *ydōr,* water]. A condition rather than a disease. Morbid accumulation of water in the tissues and cavities; hydrops.

ETIOL: Heart disease, kidney disease, cirrhosis of the liver, and other causes such as excess sodium retention. SEE ALSO: *nephritis.*

DIET: Sufficient proteins, carbohydrates, fats, vitamins, and iron, reducing the sodium intake: a salt free diet with an acid base. Salt substitutes may be used.

d. of amnion. OB: Abnormal increase in amt. of amniotic fluid. SYN: *polyhydramnios.*

d. of the belly. Ascites.

d. of brain. Hydrocephalus.

d., cardiac. That due to cardiac disease.

d. of chest. Hydrothorax.

d. of peritoneum. Hydroperitoneum.

d., tubal. A collection of fluid in the fallopian tube. SYN: *hydrosalpinx.*

d., uterine. A collection of fluid in the uterine cavity. SYN: *hydrometra.*

Drosophila (dro-sof'ĭ-lă). A genus of flies belonging to the order Diptera. Includes the common fruit flies.

D. melanogaster. A genus of fruit flies used extensively in the study of genetics. The development of the chromosome theory of heredity was largely the outcome of research on this species.

drowning [A.S. *druncnian,* to drown]. A special type of asphyxia resulting from the body being submerged in water. External respiration is blocked by a spasm of the larynx or the filling of the lungs with fluid.

SYM: Unconsciousness, cessation of respiration, cyanosis, etc., depending upon duration of submersion. Due to action of the epiglottis, there is very little, if any, water in the lung.

F. A. TREATMENT: Artificial respiration at once. Do not waste time trying to get water out of lungs. Use oxygen or oxygen-carbon dioxide mixtures with resuscitation. May have to be kept up for several hours.

RS: *artificial respiration; asphyxia, shock; syncope; unconsciousness.*

drownproofing. A method of staying afloat by using a minimum amount of energy. May be kept up for hours even by nonswimmers, whereas only the most fit and expert of swimmers could stay afloat for more than 30 minutes. Details of the drownproofing technique may be obtained from local chapters of the American Red Cross.

drug [Fr. *drogue*]. A medicinal substance, used in the treatment of disease.

drug action. LOCAL: When the drug is applied locally or direct to a tissue or organ it combines to form an albuminate with the cells' albumins. This action may be: 1. *Astringent a.*: When the drug cannot act because the albuminate does not dissolve. 2. *Corrosive a.*: When the drug is strong enough to destroy cells. 3. *Irritating a.*: When too much of the drug combines with cells to impair them.

GENERAL OR SYSTEMIC ACTION: When the drug enters the blood stream by absorption or direct injection affecting tissues and organs not near the site of entry. Systemic action may be: 1. *Specific*: When specific in the cure of a certain disease. 2. *Substitutive*: When it supplies substances deficient in the body. 3. *Physical*: When some of the constituents of a cell are dissolved by the action of the drug in the blood stream. 4. *Chemical*: When the drug or some of its principles combine with the constituents of cells or organs to form a new chemical combination. 5. *Salt Action*: Osmosis* caused by dilution of salt (also acids, sugars, and alkalies) in the stomach or intestines by fluid withdrawn from the blood and tissues, or diffusion* when water is absorbed by cells from the lymph. 6. *Selective*: Action produced by drugs which only affect certain tissues or organs. 7. *Synergistic*: The stimulating of the action of one drug by another drug. 8. *Antagonistic*: Counteraction of one drug by another one. 9. *Physiological*: The effect of a drug on a normal animal body. 10. *Therapeutic*: The effect upon diseased organs or tissues. 11. *Side Action*: Creating an effect not desired. 12. *Empiric*: An effect produced but not proved by laboratory experiment. 13. *Toxicological*: A poisonous effect generally from result of an overdose.

CUMULATIVE: The effect of drugs too slowly excreted or absorbed so that with repeated doses an accumulation of the drug in the body produces a poisonous effect. Such drugs should not be administered continuously.

d. a., incompatible. Ill effects produced by two or more drugs antagonistic to each other.

Drugs and Their Common Names

Chemical Names	Common Names
Nitric Acid	Aqua Fortis
Nitrohydrochloric Acid	Aqua Regia
Copper Sulfate	Blue Vitriol
Potassium Bitartrate	Cream of Tartar
Calcium Carbonate	Chalk
Potassium Carbonate	Salt of Tartar
Potassium Hydroxide	Caustic Potash
Sodium Chloride	Common Salt
Ferrous Sulfate	Copperas, or Green Vitriol
Aluminum and Potassium Sulfate	Dry Alum
Magnesium Sulfate	Epsom Salts
Sodium Sulfate	Glauber's Salts
Glucose	Grape Sugar
Nitrous Oxide	Laughing Gas
Calcium Oxide	Lime
Silver Nitrate	Lunar Caustic
Calcium Chloride	Muriate of Lime
Potassium Nitrate	Niter or Saltpeter
Sulfuric Acid	Oil of Vitriol
Iron Oxide	Rust of Iron
Ammonium Chloride	Sal Ammoniac
Calcium Hydroxide	Slaked Lime
Sodium Carbonate	Soda
Ammonia	Spirits of Hartshorn
Hydrochloric Acid	Spirits of Salt
Calcium Sulfate	Stucco, or Plaster of Paris
Basic Copper Acetate	Verdigris
Acetic Acid (Diluted)	Vinegar
Ammonia	Volatile Alkali
Hydrogen Oxide	Water
Ammoniated Mercury	White Precipitate
Zinc Sulfate	White Vitriol

drug action, *words pert. to*: active principles, alkaloids, antidotes, dosage, medical preparations, names of individual drugs, names of poisons, names of preparations, preparations usually given by rectum, prescription writing.

drug addiction. A condition caused by excessive or continued use of habit-forming drugs. SYM: The symptom-pattern may be changed according to the drug used. In general there may be a change in personality, loss of appetite, or the appetite is dulled; disturbance in normal sleep-rhythm; generally a weight loss. The addict may be dull, sleepy, and incoordinated in movement having the appearance of intoxication. The eyes often tearing, and bloodshot; a watery fluid at times dripping from the nose. When intramuscular or intravenous injection is used there may be scars, hardening and swelling of the arm tissues. Serum hepatitis may occur when narcotic addicts use dirty needles and syringes for administering drugs to themselves or fellow addicts. SEE: *hepatitis, homologous*.

drug-fast. Resistance, as of bacteria, to action of a drug or drugs.

drug rashes: Rashes produced in some patients by application or ingestion of drugs.

Antipyrin: Papular, erythematous rash, sometimes accompanied by edema and much irritation.

Arsenic: Papular or erythematous rash, sometimes urticarial. Prolonged use may produce pigmentation of skin.

Belladonna: Erythematous rash, usually accompanied by intense itching.

Bromides: Usually like acne vulgaris. Sometimes erythema.

Chloral: Papular erythema.

Iodides: Usually papular erythema, sometimes with acnelike pustules.

Phenolphthalein: Macular rash, sometimes purpuric.

Quinine: Very irritable erythema or urticaria.

Salicylate: Erythematous rash, possibly morbilliform.

Serum: Usually urticaria.

Sulfonal: Erythematous or urticarial rash.

drugs (special) **and their administration.** ACIDS: When acids are administered orally they should be given well diluted through a glass tube or by stomach tube because they are corrosive to the enamel and the dentine of the teeth. They should be given with much water and the drinking tube should be placed well back in the mouth to prevent the fluid coming in contact with the teeth before passing into the throat. Hydrochloric acid is one preparation that should always be given with the above thought in mind.

ARTIFICIAL TEETH: SEE: *dentures*.

BARBITAL DERIVATIVES: All such preparations should be given from one-half to one hour before sleep is desired. All procedures should be taken care of before the medicament is given in order that nothing shall disturb the patient after the drug is administered.

ELIXIR OF IRON, QUININE AND STRYCHNINE: When administering these drugs they should be given well diluted with much water, through a glass tube. A bitter effect will be produced if given before meals.

HABIT-FORMING DRUGS: These should be given as ordered by the physician.

INSULIN: When this is administered, it should be given hypodermically according to the instructions of the attending physician. The type of insulin, dosage, and frequency of dosage vary greatly with each patient.

LAXATIVES: These are best given in the evening, because it usually takes 6 or 8 hours for them to produce an effect. The saline purgatives are usually given well diluted on an empty stomach, in the morning. The other purgatives are usually given as ordered and needed.

MOUTHWASH: Stock solutions used for mouthwash should be diluted one-half or more before being given to the patient. The special solutions, such as S.T. 37, or Dobell's solution, should be diluted according to instructions from the attending physician. Only enough for the immediate mouth washing should be used at a particular time. To take into the patient's room a glass or cupful, when the patient will only use about one-half of the amt., is not an economic procedure.

HORSE SERUM: When injections containing it are administered, information should be obtained as to whether the patient has ever received horse serum and what his reaction to it was, as a reaction is liable to occur. If the patient is allergic to horse serum, a test for sensitivity should always be done by injecting a few drops of the greatly diluted material containing horse serum hypodermically, and within a short time a reaction will occur. A small spot appears at the site of the injection if the patient has a tendency toward an unfavorable reaction. If the person is allergic to horse serum the physician will provide instructions for desensitizing him.

OXYGEN: The most commonly used method for the administration of oxygen consists of inserting a catheter into a nostril, or into each nostril. Oxygen may also be given from a tank by means of a mask over the patient's nose and mouth, or the patient may be placed in an oxygen tent, or an oxygen chamber or room. The last two methods are not only expensive but also extremely dangerous and must be used cautiously, as the danger from fire hazard is very great.

SALINE PURGATIVES: Should always be given to the patient when the stomach is empty, preferably in the morning.

SEIDLITZ POWDERS: These should be mixed or dissolved in about one-fourth glass of water; a separate glass for each powder, the white and the blue. At the bedside, the mixture in one glass is poured into the other and the patient drinks this mixture before it effervesces.

VACCINES: Most of these are administered subcutaneously. Pertussis vaccine, USP., may be given subcutaneously or intramuscularly, while adsorbed pertussis vaccine, USP., is given via the intramuscular route.

drugs, handling of. Read the label or other printed instruction issued with medicine carefully; measure out accurately the doses (quantities) ordered, and never guess.

A measuring glass or spoon should be employed, marked either in drams and ounces only, or with the words teaspoon and tablespoon also.

One drop equals 1 minim. Symbol, ♏. One teaspoonful equals 1 dram. Symbol, ʒ. Two teaspoonfuls equal 2 drams. Four teaspoonfuls equal ½ ounce or 1 tablespoonful. Two tablespoonfuls equal 1 ounce. Symbol, ℥.

Important Points: (1) The cork must never be left out of the bottle, as a necessary property may evaporate or the drug may become dangerously concentrated. (2) The drug compartment must be kept locked.

To Give a Dose of Medicine: Make quite sure: (a) To whom it has to be given; (b) what has to be given; (c) when it has to be given; (d) the amt. to be given. If an oral preparation is ordered, the nurse should not leave the bedside until she sees the patient actually swallow the medicine.

drugs, words pert. to: absorbent, action, alkaloids, alterative, ampule, analeptic, analgesic, anesthetic, anodyne, antacid, anthelmintic, antiarthritic, antidiuretic, antiemetic, antilithic, antiperiodic, antipyretic, antiseptic, antisialagogue, antispasmodic, antizymotic, aperient, aromatic, balsam, biochemorphic, bitters, cachet, calmant, capsule, carminative, cathartic, caustic, cerate, cholagogue, confection, convulsant, correctant, corrosive, counterirritant, decoction, delirifacient, demulcent, deodorant, depilatory, depressant, detergent, diaphoretic, digestant, disinfectant, diuretic, ecbolic, elixir, emetic, emmenagogue, emollient, emulsion, enzyme, epispastic, errhines, escharotic, evacuant, expectorant, extract, febrifuge, ferment, fluidextract, galactagogue, glucoside, glycerite, hematinic, hemostatic, hormone, hydragogue, hypnotic, idiosyncrasy, infusion, irritation, lamella, laxative, liniment, lozenge, mixture, mucilage, mydriatic, myotic, oil, ointment, oleate, oleoresin, oxytocics, paper, pharmacognosy, pharmacology, pill, plaster, powder, prophylactic, purgative, refrigerant, resins, revulsant, rubefacient, saline purgative, saponins, sedative, sensitization, serum therapy, sialagogue, solution, somnifacient, soporific, specific, spirit, stimulant, stomachic, styptic, sudorific, suppository, synergism, tablet, tincture, tonic, vaccine, vasoconstrictor, vasodilator, vermicide, vermifuge, vesicant, vinegar, vulnerary, water, wine.

drum [A.S. *drumme*]. The ear drum or tympanic cavity; the tympanum or cavity of the middle ear.

drunkenness [A.S. *drincan*, to drink]. Alcoholic intoxication. NOTE: In legal medicine, intoxication or being "under-the-influence" of alcohol is defined according to the concentration of alcohol in the blood or exhaled air.

drusen (dru'zen) [Ger. *Druse* "a rock cavity lined with crystals"]. Small, hyaline, globular pathological growths formed on optic papilla or on Descemet's membrane.

dry diet. A temporary high carbohydrate diet with measured liquid given bet. meals only.

dry ice. Proprietary name for solidified carbon dioxide used for commercial refrigeration. The temperature of solid carbon dioxide is —78.5° C. SYN: *carbon dioxide snow.*

dry measure. A measure of volume for dry commodities, as follows:

2 pints (pt.)	=	1 quart (qt.)
8 quarts	=	1 peck (pk.)
4 pecks	=	1 bushel (bu.)

Drys'dale's corpuscles [Thomas M. Drysdale, American gynecologist, 1831-1904]. Non-nucleated, granular cells present in the fluid of certain ovarian cysts.

dualism (du'ă-lizm) [L. *dualis*, pert. to two]. 1. The condition of being double or two-fold. 2. The theory that the human body consists of two entities, mind and matter, which are independent of each other. 3. The theory that blood corpuscles arise from two types of stem cells; myeloblasts giving rise to the myeloid elements and lymphoblasts giving rise to the lymphoid elements.

dual personality. A split in consciousness which results in the expression of two different phases of personality at various intervals, neither personality, as a rule, being aware of the words, acts, and feelings of the other. When this does rarely occur it has been called coconsciousness.

SEE: *coconsciousness; dissociation of personality; multiple personality; vigilambulism.*

Dubini's disease (doo-be'nēz) [Angelo Dubini, Italian physician, 1813-1902]. Rhythmic, rapid contractions of a group or groups of muscles. SYN: *electric chorea; spasmus Dubini.*

duboisine (du-boi'sin). Alkaloid derivative of plant *Duboisea myoporoides.* It is a form of hyoscyamine.

d., poisoning from. Resembles atropine, *q.v.*

Duchenne's disease (du-shen') [Guillaume B. A. Duchenne, French neurologist, 1806-1875]. 1. Bulbar paralysis. 2. Tabes dorsalis.

Ducrey's bacillus (du-kray') [Augusto Ducrey, Italian physician, 1860-1940]. *Hemophilus ducreyi.* The cause of chancroid or soft chancre; small, rod-shaped organism found in pairs.

duct [L. *ducere,* to lead]. 1. A narrow tubular vessel or channel, especially one serving to convey secretions from a gland. 2. A narrow enclosed channel containing a fluid, as the semicircular duct of the ear.

d. accessory pancreatic. D. of the pancreas, leading into the pancreatic d. or the duodenum near the mouth of the common bile duct. SYN: *ductus pancreaticus accessorius* [NA].

d., alveolar. A branch of a respiratory bronchiole which leads to the alveolar sacs of the lungs. SYN: *ductulus alveolaris* [NA].

d., Bartholin's. The major duct of the sublingual gland. SYN: *ductus sublingualis major* [NA].

d.'s, biliary. The canals which carry bile. The intrahepatic ducts include the bile canaliculi and interlobular ducts; the extrahepatic ducts include the hepatic duct, cystic duct, and common bile duct. SYN: *bile ducts.*

d., cochlear. Canal of the cochlea. SYN: *ductus cochlearis* [NA].

d., common bile. Duct formed by the confluence of the hepatic and cystic ducts. Conveys bile to the duodenum opening at the papilla of Vater. SYN: *ductus choledochus* [NA].

d., cystic. Excretory duct of the gallbladder. SEE: *gallduct.* SYN: *ductus cysticus* [NA].

d., efferent. Any duct conveying secretion from a gland.

d., ejaculatory. Conveys semen into urethra. SYN: *ductus ejaculatorius* [NA].

d., endolymphatic. In the embryo, a tubular projection of the otocyst ending in a blind extremity, the endolymph sac. In the adult, it connects the endolymphatic sac with the utricle and saccule. SYN: *ductus endolymphaticus* [NA].

d., excretory. Any duct which conveys a product from an organ, as the excretory duct of a salivary gland.

d., galactophorous. Duct carrying milk in lobes of mammary glands. SYN: *ductus lactiferi* [NA].

d., Gartner's. A remnant of the wolffian duct extending from the parovarium through the broad ligament into the vagina. SYN: *ductus epoophori longitudinalis* [NA].

d.'s, hepatic. Right and left ducts receive bile from right and left lobes of liver and carry bile to common bile duct. SYN: *ductus hepaticus dexter* [NA] and *ductus hepaticus sinister* [NA].

d.'s, interlobular. One of the d.'s carrying bile. SEE: *biliary duct.*

d., lacrimal. One of two short ducts, inferior and superior, which conveys tears from the lacrimal lake to the lacrimal sac. Their openings are on the margins of the upper and lower eyelids. SYN: *canaliculus lacrimalis* [NA].

d.'s, lactiferous. A group of 15 to 20 ducts which drain the lobes of the mammary gland. Each opens in a slight depression on the tip of the nipple. SYN: *ductus lactiferi* [NA].

d., Leydig's. Mesonephric duct, *q.v.*

d., lymphatic. One of two main ducts conveying lymph to the blood stream: the left lymphatic duct (thoracic duct) and the right lymphatic duct.

d., lymphatic, left. Thoracic duct.

d., lymphatic, right. A duct, smaller than the left lymphatic duct, draining the right side of the body above the diaphragm. Discharges into the right innominate vein. SYN: *ductus lymphaticus dexter* [NA].

d., mammary. Lactiferous duct.

d., mesonephric. The duct which, in the embryo, connects the mesonephros with the cloaca. In the male it develops into the ductus deferens. SYN: *ductus mesonephricus* [NA]; *wolffian d.*

d., metanephric. Ureter.

d., milk. Lactiferous ducts.

d., Muller's; mullerian d. Bilateral ducts in the embryo that form the uterus, vagina, and fallopian tubes. SYN: *ductus paramesonephricus* [NA].

d., nasolacrimal. The duct which conveys tears from the lacrimal sac to the nasal cavity. It opens beneath the inferior nasal concha. SYN: *ductus nasolacrimalis* [NA].

d., omphalomesenteric. The vitelline duct.

d., pancreatic. Conveys pancreatic juice to the duodenum. SYN: *d. of Wirsung; ductus pancreaticus* [NA].

d.'s, paraurethral. Skene's ducts.

d., parotid. Discharges secretions from the parotid gland into mouth. SYN: *ductus parotideus* [NA].

d.'s, prostatic. About 20 ducts which discharge prostatic secretion into the urethra. SYN: *ductus prostatici* [NA].

d.'s of Rivinus. Five to fifteen ducts (the minor sublingual ducts) which drain the posterior portion of the sublingual gland. SYN: *ductus sublinguales minores* [NA].

d., salivary. Any of the ducts which drain a salivary gland. SYN: *ductus pancreaticus accessorius* [NA].

d. of Santorini. Accessory pancreatic duct. SYN: *ductus pancreaticus accessorius* [NA].

d., secretory. The smaller canals of a gland.

d., segmental. A pair of embryonic tubes located between visceral and parietal layers of mesoblast on each side of the body.

d.'s, semicircular. Three membranous tubes forming a part of the membranous labyrinth of the inner ear. They lie within the semicircular canals and bear corresponding names, anterior, posterior and lateral. SYN: *ductus semicirculares* [NA].

d., seminal. Any of the ducts which convey semen, specifically the ductus deferens and the ejaculatory duct.

d.'s, Skene's. Paraurethral ducts. Two slender ducts of Skene's glands which open on either side of the urethral orifice in the female. SYN: *ductus paraurethrales* [NA].

d., spermatic. Excretory duct of the testicle which later joins the duct of the seminal vesicle to become the ejaculatory duct. SYN: *vas deferens; ductus deferens* [NA].

d., Stensen's; Steno's duct. Parotid duct.

d.'s, sublingual. The excretory ducts of the sublingual gland. SEE: *d.'s of Rivinus; Bartholin's d.*

d., submandibular. Duct of the submandibular gland. It opens on a papilla at the side of the frenulum linguae. SYN: *submaxillary d.; Wharton's d.; ductus submandibularis* [NA].

d., submaxillary. Submandibular duct.

d., sudoriferous. Sweat duct.

d., tear. A duct that conveys tears including excretory ducts of lacrimal glands, lacrimal and nasolacrimal ducts.

d., testicular. Spermatic duct.

d., thoracic. The left lymphatic duct. Drains the left side of the body above the diaphragm and all of the body below the diaphragm. Discharges into the left innominate vein. SYN: *ductus thoracicus* [NA].

d., umbilical. The vitelline duct.

d., utriculosaccular. A narrow tube emanating from the utricle and opening into the endolymphatic duct. SYN: *ductus utriculosaccularis* [NA].

d., vitelline. The narrow duct which, in the embryo, connects the yolk sac (umbilica vesicle) with the intestine. SYN: *umbilical d.; yolk stalk.*

d., (of) Wirsung. Pancreatic duct.

duct'less [" + A.S. *læssa*]. Having no duct, secreting only internally.

d. glands. Ductless glands secrete internally one or more hormones which have a specific action upon the body. SEE: *endocrine; exocrine.*

ductule (duk'tūl) [L. *ducere,* to lead]. A very small duct.

d., aberrant. One of a group of small tubules associated with the epididymis. They are blindly ending, representing the vestigial remains of the caudal group of mesonephric tubules.

ductus (duk'tus) (pl. *ductus*) [L.] [NA]. Duct. SEE ALSO: *duct.*

d. arteriosus. A channel of communication bet. main pulmonary artery of the fetus and aorta.

d. arteriosus, patent. Persistence after birth of the foramen ovale. A treatable form of congenital heart defect.

d. choledochus. The common bile duct, *q.v.*

d. cochlearis. The cochlear duct, *q.v.* Also called *scala media.*

d. communis. One about 3 in. long formed by union of cystic and hepatic d.'s; carries the bile to the intestine.

d. deferens. Excretory duct of the testicle. Conveys sperm from the epididymis to the ejaculatory duct. SYN: *vas deferens.*

d. efferent. One of a group of 12-14 small tubes which constitute the efferent ducts of the testis. They lie within the epididymis and connect the rete testis with the ductus epididymis. Their coiled portions constitute the lobulus epididymis.

d. hemithoracicus. Ascending branch of thoracic opening either into right lymphatic duct or close to angle of union of right subclavian and right internal jugular veins.

d. hepaticus dexter. One issuing from the right lobe of the liver, uniting with the d. hepaticus sinister and forming the hepatic duct.

d. hepaticus sinister. One issuing with d. hepaticus dexter to form hepatic duct.

d. prostatici. Ducts for secretion of prostate into the urethra.

d. sacculo-utricularis. Small tube connecting saccule of internal ear with utricle.

d. venosus. Smaller, shorter, and post. of 2 branches into which umbilical vein divides after entering the abdomen; empties into the inf. vena cava.

duipara (dū-ip'ă-ră) [L. *duo,* two, + *parēre,* to bear]. A female pregnant for the second time. SYN: *secundipara.*

dulcite. A sugar ($C_6H_{14}O_6$) found in certain plants. Also called *dulcin, dulcitol* or *dulcose.*

dull [A.S. *dol*]. 1. Not resonant on percussion. 2. Not mentally alert.

dullness, dulness (dul'nes) [A.S. *dol*]. 1 Lack of normal resonance on percussion 2. State of being dull.

dumb [A.S.]. Mute. Unable to speak.

d. ague. Latent malaria not expressed by ordinary signs.

dumb'ness [A.S.]. Muteness.

dumping syndrome. A syndrome characterized by sweating and weakness after eating. Occurs in patients who have had gastric resections. Exact cause is unknown but rapid emptying (*i.e.,* dumping of the stomach contents) into the small intestine is associated with the symptoms.

duodenal (du-o-de'nal) [L. *duodeni,* twelve]. Pert. to the duodenum.

d. activities. The entry of acid chyme into the duodenum brings about discharge of bile from the gallbladder and the secretion of pancreatic juice by the pancreas. These enter through the common bile duct. Bile salts alkalinize the chyme and emulsify the fats. Through the action of pancreatic enzymes, the following changes occur: steapsin (pancreatic lipase), hydrolyzes neutral fats to fatty acids and glycerol; *amylopsin* (pancreatic amylase) hydrolyzes starch to maltose; *maltase* hydrolyzes maltose to glucose. Three proteolytic enzymes: *trypsin, chymotrypsin,* and *peptidase* act on proteins hydrolyzing them to *proteoses,* peptones, and amino acids.

d. bulb. Area of duodenum just beyond the pylorus.

SECRETORY PHENOMENA: Two substances are secreted by the duodenum. One of these, secretin, *q.v.,* excites the pancreas to increased production of its juice; the other, cholecystokinin, causes the gallbladder to contract and force its contents through the ductus choledochus into the duodenum. In addition, nervous mechanisms contribute to the coordination which exists here, regulating the rate of discharge of chyme from the stomach, varying both quality and quantity of the various secretions, and determining the rate of passage through the duodenum. For the action of particular juices: SEE: *bile; digestion; enzyme; functions of pancreas; juice, gastric; juice, pancreatic; succus entericus.*

MOTOR PHENOMENA: (a) First part of duodenum (*pars superior, duodenal cap, d. bulb*) is the small portion immediately following the pylorus. It is regularly full of material and consequently visible in roentgenograms as a spade-shaped shadow. (b) The next part (*pars descendens*) is that into which the common bile duct (*ductus choledochus*) and pancreatic ducts open. Movement through it and through (c) the pars inferior and (d) the pars ascendens is rapid, so that they are normally inconspicuous by x-ray. Throughout the duodenum the mucosa is thrown into folds (*plicae circulares*) and shows the active projections called villi. The folds are permanent and inactive. The villi, which stud the surface of the folds as well as the spaces bet. them, exhibit waving and thrusting movements.

d. delay. Delay in the movement of food through the duodenum due to conditions such as inflammation of lower portion on the intestine which reflexly inhibits duodenal movements.

d. papilla. Raised surface near entrance of ductus choledochus communis into duodenum.

d. p. major. Slight elevation in descending portion of the duodenum bearing openings of the common bile duct and main pancreatic duct.

d. p. minor. Slight elevation about 2 cm. above the p. major bearing opening of the accessory pancreatic duct.

d. ulcer. Broken mucous membrane, usually accompanied by suppuration and perhaps a sore is present which bleeds with more or less danger of perforation.

It heals slowly due to constant passage of irritating fluids and food over it.

DIET: Same as for peptic ulcer. SEE: *peptic ulcer*.

duodenectasis (dū-ō-děn-ěk′tă-sĭs). Chronic dilatation of the duodenum.

duodenectomy (du-o-den-ek′to-mĭ) [" + G. *ektomē*, excision]. Excision of part or all of the duodenum.

duodenitis (du-od-ĕ-ni′tis) [L. *duodeni*, twelve, + G. *-ītis*, inflammation]. Inflammation of the duodenum.

duodenocholecystostomy (du-o-de″no-ko-le-sis-tos′to-mĭ) [" + G. *cholē*, bile, + *kystis*, bladder, + *stōma*, mouth]. Formation by surgical means of a fistula bet. duodenum and gallbladder.

duodenocholedochotomy (du-o-de″-no-ko-led-o-kot′o-mĭ) [" + G. *choledochos*, bile duct, + *tome*, incision]. Surgical incision of the duodenum to reach the gallbladder.

duodenocystostomy (du-od-en″o-sist-os′to-mĭ). Duodenocholecystostomy.

duodenoenterostomy (du-ō-de″no-en-ter-os′to-mĭ) [" + G. *enteron*, intestine, + *stōma*, opening]. Formation of passage bet. the duodenum and intestine.

duodenogram (du-o-de′no-gram) [" + G. *gramma*, a writing]. A roentgenogram of the duodenum.

duodenohepatic (du-o-de″no-he-pat′ik) [" + G. *ēpar, epat-*, liver]. Pert. to duodenum and liver.

duodenojejunostomy (du-o-de″no-jĕ-joo-nos′to-mĭ) [" + *jejunum*, empty, + G. *stōma*, opening]. Making a passage bet. the duodenum and jejunum.

duodenoscopy (du-od″ĕ-nos′ko-pĭ) [" + G. *skopein*, to examine]. Inspection of the duodenum with an endoscope.

duodenostomy (du-od″ĕ-nos′to-mĭ) [" + G. *stoma*, opening]. Operation of making a permanent opening into the duodenum through the wall of the abdomen.

duodenotomy (du-od″ĕ-not′o-mĭ) [" + G. *tomē*, incision]. An incision into the duodenum.

duodenum (du-o-de′num) [L. *duodeni*, twelve, from twelve fingerbreadths in length]. The first part of the small intestines connecting with the pylorus of the stomach and extending to the jejunum.

It receives the hepatic and pancreatic secretions through the same duct. It is 8 to 11 inches long, the average length being 10 inches (25 cm.). Brunner's glands are found in the duodenum, and the chyle is formed here. Lieberkühn's glands are also found here.

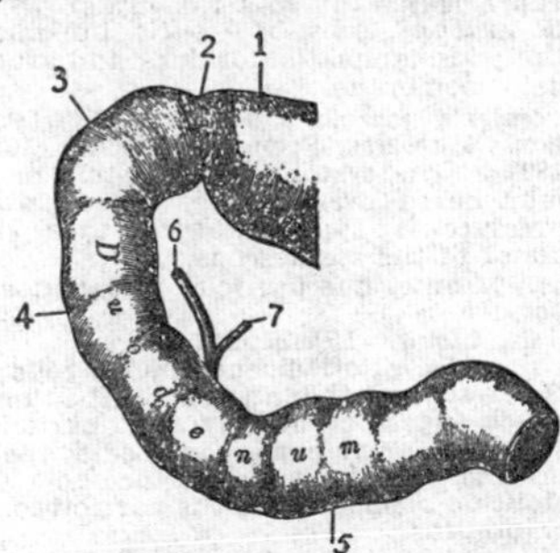

THE DUODENUM

1. Pyloric end of the stomach. 2. Pyloric valvule. 3. Upper transverse part. 4. Descending part. 5. Lower transverse part. 6. Choledochus duct. 7. Pancreatic duct.

It is a crucial section of the alimentary canal, since in it occurs the mixing of (1) the acid chyme from the stomach, (2) the bile from the liver and gallbladder, (3) the pancreatic juice entering by way of two ducts, and (4) the intestinal juices secreted by the glands of Brunner and the crypts of Lieberkühn.

NERVE SUPPLY: From the celiac plexus.

BLOOD SUPPLY: Pancreaticoduodenal branches of hepatic and sup. mesenteric arteries and the right gastric artery.

RS: *Brunner's glands; choledochoduodenostomy; duodenal digestion; duodenal ulcer; gallbladder; intestines; Lieberkühn's glands; liver; pancreas.*

duplica′tion, du′plicature [L. *duplicāre*, to double]. A doubling or folding, or state of being folded.

duplicitas (du-plis′ĭ-tas). Fetal abnormality in which the cephalic and/or the pelvic end is doubled.

dupp (dŭp) [imitative origin]. Part of the word *lubb-dupp*, denoting 2nd sound at cardiac apex heard in auscultation. It is due to the closing of the pulmonary and aortic semilunar valves.

The 1st sound is longer and pitched lower. SEE: *heart, auscultation of; lubb; lubb-dupp.*

Dupuytren's contracture (du-pwē-trănz′) [Baron G. Dupuytren, French surgeon, 1778-1835]. Contracture of palmar fascia causing ring and little fingers to bend into palm so that they cannot be extended.

dura (du′ră) [L. *durus*, hard]. Dura mater.

d. mater [L. hard mother]. The outer membrane covering the spinal cord (*d. m. spina'lis* [NA]) and brain (*d. m. cer'ebri or enceph'ali* [NA]). SEE: *pia mater, tentorium.*

dural (du'ral) [L. *durus,* hard]. Pert. to the dura.

durama'tral [" + *mater,* mother]. Pert. to the dura. SYN: *dural.*

du'raplasty [" + G. *plassein,* to form]. Plastic repair of the dura mater.

durematoma (dū-rem-ă-to'mă) [" + G. *aima,* blood, + *-ōma,* tumor]. Accumulation of blood bet. arachnoid and dura.

duritis (du-ri'tis) [" + G. *-itis,* inflammation]. Inflammation of the dura. SYN: *pachymeningitis.*

duroarachnitis (dū-ro-ă-rak-ni'tis) [" + G. *arachnē,* cobweb, + *-itis,* inflammation]. Inflammation of dura and arachnoid membrane.

Durorziez's murmur (du-ro-zĭ-ez') [Paul Louis Duroziez, French physician, 1826-1897]. The systolic and diastolic murmur heard over a large artery when pressure is applied to the area just distal to the stethoscope.

dust. Minute, fine particles of earth; any powder.

d., blood. Hemoconia.

d. cells. Reticuloendothelial cells in the walls of the alveoli of the lungs which ingest or destroy dust particles.

d., ear. Fine calcareous bodies found in the gelatinous substance of the otolithic membrane of the ear; otoconia or otoliths.

dust'ing powder. Any fine powder for dusting on skin.

Duverney's gland (doo-ver-nās') [Joseph G. Duverney, French anatomist, 1648-1730]. The vulvovaginal gland.

dwarf. An abnormally short or undersized person; a pygmy.

d., achondroplastic. One with normal trunk but possessing shortened extremities, with a large head, and protruding buttocks.

d., asexual. One with deficient sexual development.

d., diabetic. One due to diabetes.

d., hypophyseal. One due to hypofunction of ant. lobe of the hypophysis.

d., infantile. One showing marked physical, mental and sexual underdevelopment.

d., Levi-Lorain. An hypophyseal or pituitary dwarf.

d., micromelic. One with very small limbs.

d., ovarian. An undersized female due to absence or underdevelopment of the ovaries.

d., phocomelic. One with abnormally short diaphyses of either pair of extremities or all four.

d., physiologic. A normal dwarf.

d., pituitary. A hypophyseal one.

d., primordial. One in whom there is a selective deficiency of growth hormone but with otherwise normal endocrine function.

d., rachitic. One due to rickets.

d., renal. One due to renal osteodystrophy.

d., sexual. One showing normal sexual development.

dwarfism. Condition of being abnormally small. May be hereditary, or a result of endocrine dysfunction, deficiency diseases, renal insufficiency, diseases of the skeleton or other causes.

dy'ad. 1. A pair. 2. A pair of chromosomes formed by the division of a tetrad in miosis. A dyad represents a single chromosome split precociously for a subsequent division. 3. In *Chem.* A bivalent element or radical.

dynamia (di-nam'ĭ-ă) [G. *dynamis,* power]. Vital energy or ability to combat disease.

dynamic (di-nam'ik) [G. *dynamis,* power]. Pert. to vital force or inherent power, opp. of *static.*

d. psychology. A theory that energy is inherent in mind.

dynam'ics [G. *dynamis,* power]. The science of bodies in motion and their forces.

dynamization (di-nam-iz-a'shun) [G. *dynamis,* power]. The attempt to add to the potency of medicine by agitation or comminution.* SEE: *attenuation.*

dynamogenesis (di"nă-mo-jen'ĕ-sis) [" + *genesis,* growth]. The capacity to call forth increased energy.

dynamogen'ic [" + *gennan,* to produce]. Pert. to, or caused by, an increase of energy.

dynamograph (di-nam'o-graf) [" + *graphein,* to write]. Device for recording muscular strength.

dynamometer (di"nă-mom'ĕ-ter) [" + *metron,* measure]. 1. A device for measuring muscular strength. Simple dynamometer is spring scales bet. segment to be examined and examiner's hand. 2. A device for giving the magnifying power of a lens.

dynamoneure (di-nam'o-nūr) [" + *neuron,* nerve]. A motor, spinal nerve cell.

dynamoscope (di-nam'o-skōp) [" + *skopein,* to examine]. Instrument for auscultation of muscles.

dynamoscopy (di-nam-os'ko-pĭ) [" + *skopein,* to examine]. Auscultation of muscles.

dyne (dīn) [G. *dynamis,* power]. A unit of force which would accelerate a mass of weight of 1 gram with a velocity of 1 cm. in a second.

dys- [G.]. Prefix meaning bad, difficult, painful.

dysacousia, dysacousma (dis"ă-koo'zĭ-ă, -kooz'mă) [G. *dys,* bad, + *akousis,* hearing]. 1. Discomfort caused by loud noises. 2. Difficulty in hearing.

dysadrenia (dis-ă-dre'nĭ-ă) [" + L. *ad-* toward, + *rēn,* kidney]. Functional disorder of the kidneys.

dysalbumose (dis-al'bū-mōs) [" + L. *albumen,* white of egg]. A variety of albumose insoluble in water or hydrochloric acid.

dysantigraphia (dis-an-tĭ-graf'ĭ-ă) [" + *anti,* against, + *graphein,* to write]. Inability to copy writing or printed letters.

dysaphia (dis-af'ĭ-ă) [" + *aphē,* touch]. Dullness of the sense of touch.

dysarteriotony (dis"ar-te-rĭ-ot'o-nĭ) [" + *artēria,* artery, + *tonos,* tension]. Abnormal blood pressure, either too low or too high.

dysarthria (dis-ar'thrĭ-ă) [" + *arthron,* articulation]. 1. Difficulty in articulation of joints, as in amyostasia. 2. Incorrectly applied to imperfect speech; stammering.

dysarthro'sis [" + *arthrōsis,* joint]. Joint malformation.

dysautonomia (dis"aw-to-no'mĭ-ă) [" + *autonomia,* freedom to use own laws]. A rare hereditary disease involving the autonomic nervous system with mental retardation, motor incoordination, vomiting, frequent infections, and convulsions.

dysbarism (dis-bar'izm) [" + G. *barys,* heavy, + *-ism,* condition]. Symptom complex following exposure of body to less-than-atmospheric pressure in air flight or altitude chamber. When occurring in severe form, sometimes called decompression sickness or bends.

dysbasia (dis-ba'zĭ-ă) [" + *basis,* a step]. Difficulty in walking, esp. when due to disease of the brain or spinal cord.

dysbolism (dis'bo-lizm) [" + *bolē,* a throwing]. Disordered metabolism.

dysbulia (dis-bu'lĭ-ă) [" + *boulē,* will]. 1. Inability to fix the attention; difficulty experienced in thinking; mind weariness. 2. Weak and uncertain willpower.

dyschezia (dis-ke'zĭ-ă) [" + *chezein,* go to defecate]. Constipation due to habitual neglect to respond to stimulus to defecate.

dyschiria (dis-ki'rĭ-ă) [" + *cheir,* hand]. Inability to tell which side of the body has been touched.

If referred to the wrong side it is called *allochiria;** to both sides, *synchiria.** Syn: *achiria.*

dyscholia (dis-ko'lĭ-ă) [G. *dys,* bad, + *cholē,* bile]. Morbid condition of the bile.

dyschondroplasia (dĭs-kŏn-drō-plā'zĭ-a). Disease, usually hereditary, resulting in disordered growth. Characterized by multiple exostoses of growth of the epiphyses, esp. of the long bones, metacarpals, and phalanges. Also called multiple cartilaginous exostoses, dyschondroplasia, Ollier's disease; diaphyseal aclasia.

dyschroa, dyschroia (dĭs-krō-ă, dis-kroy'ă). Discolored skin, esp. of the face; poor or bad complexion.

dyschromatopsia (dis-kro-mă-top'sĭ-ă) [" + *chrōma,* color, + *opsis,* vision]. Imperfect color vision.

dyschro'mia [" + *chrōma,* color]. Discoloration, as of the skin.

dyschronism (dis-chron'izm) [" + *chronos,* time]. 1. Disturbed time relation esp. that which occurs when one is transported from one time zone to one that is 5 to 10 hours ahead of or behind the original. This leads to disturbances of biological rhythms. 2. Separate as to time.

dyscinesia (dis-sin-e'zĭ-ă). Dyskinesia.

dyscoimesis (dis-koy-me'sis). Dyskoimesis.

dyscoria (dis-ko'rĭ-ă) [" + *korē,* pupil]. Abnormal form of the pupil.

dyscrasia (dis-kra'sĭ-ă) [" + *krasis,* mixture]. Disease, particularly one due to developmental or metabolic, but not usually infectious, causes.

d. blood. A general nonspecific term for blood disease.

dyscrasic (dis-kra'sik) [" + *krasis,* mixture]. Pert. to dyscrasia.

dyscrinism (dis-kri'nizm) [" + *krinein,* to secrete, + *ismos,* condition of]. Any disorder of secretions, esp. of an endocrine gland.

dysdiadochokinesia (dis"di-ad'o-ko-kĭ-ne'sĭ-ă) [" + *diadochos,* succeeding, + *kinesis,* movement]. Inability to quickly substitute antagonistic motor impulses.

dysdiemorrhysis (dis-di-em-or'ĭ-sis) [" + *dia,* through, + *aima,* blood, + *rysis,* a flowing]. Sluggish circulation of capillaries.

dyse'mia [" + *aima,* blood]. Any blood disease.

dysendocriniasis (dis-en-do-krin-i'ă-sis) [" + *endon,* within, + *krinein,* to secrete]. Faulty function of the endocrine glands.

dysendocrinism (dis - en - dok'rĭ - nizm). Faulty function of the endocrine glands; dysendocriniasis.

dysendocrisi'asis [" + " + *krinein,* to secrete]. Dysendocriniasis.

dysenteric (dis-en-ter'ĭk) [" + *enteron,* intestine]. Pert. to dysentery.

dysentery (dis'en-ter-e) [" + *enteron,* intestine]. A term applied to a number of intestinal disorders, esp. of the colon, characterized by inflammation of the mucous membrane.

Etiol: Bacterial or viral infection, infestation by protozoa or parasitic worms, or chemical irritants.

Sym: Abdominal pain, tenesmus, diarrhea with passage of mucus or blood.

d., amebic. Due to amebas. Sym: Similar to catarrhal d. with intermissions.

d., bacillary. An acute infectious disease caused by bacteria of the genus *Shigella,* esp. *Sh. dysenteriae, Sh. boydii, Sh. flexneri,* and *Sh. sonnei.* It may occur sporadically or in epidemics. In addition to intestinal symptoms, a severe toxemia may occur due to exo- and endotoxins produced by the organisms.

d., balantidial. B. caused by ciliate protozoan, Balantidium coli.

d., malignant. A form in which symptoms are very pronounced and progress rapidly, usually terminating fatally.

d., viral. D. caused by virus.

dysepulotic (dis"ep-u-lot'ik) [" + *epulotikos,* to scar over]. Slow formation of a scar.

dysergasia (dis-er-ga'sĭ-ă) [" + *ergon,* work]. Inability to function properly. Syn: *neurasthenia.* In Psy., a behavior disorder characterized by disorientation, hallucinations, dreamstates, and delirium. Possibly due to toxic conditions such as uremia, or alcohol intoxication.

dysergastic (dis-er-gas'tik). Pert. to dysergasia.

d. reaction. Hallucinations, fears, disorientation, dream states, and other mental disorders resulting from poor circulation and nutrition of the brain.

dysergia (dis-er'jĭ-ă) [G. *dys,* bad, + *ergon,* work]. Lack of coordination in muscular voluntary movements.

dysesthesia (dis-es-the'zĭ-ă) [" + *aisthesis,* sensation]. 1. Sensations, as of the pricks of pins and needles, or of crawling. Syn: *formication.* 2. Failing sensitivity, esp. of touch. 3. Painfulness of any sensation which is not normally painful.

d., auditory. Abnormal discomfort from loud noises. Syn: *dysacusia.*

dysfunction (dis-funk'shun) [" + L. *fungi,* to be busy]. Absence of complete normal function.

dysgalac'tia [" + *gala,* milk]. Defective milk secretion.

dysgenesia, dysgenesis (dis-jen-e'sĭ-ă, -jen'ĕ-sis) [" + *genesis,* procreation]. Impairment or loss of procreative powers.

dysgen'ic [" + *gennan,* to produce]. Causing racial deterioration.

dysgen'italism [" + L. *genitalis,* pert. to genitals, + G. *ismos,* state of]. Condition caused by abnormal genital development.

dysgerminoma (dis-jer-min-o'mă) [" + L. *germen,* a sprout, + G. *-ōma,* tumor]. A malignant neoplasm of the ovary.

dysgeusia (dis-gu'sĭ-ă) [" + *geusis,* taste]. Perversion or impairment of sense of taste.

dysglan'dular [" + L. *glans, gland-,* acorn]. Abnormal functioning of glands, esp. those of internal secretion.

dysglycemia (dis-gli-se'mĭ-ă) [" + *glykus*, sweet, + *aima*, blood]. Faulty blood sugar metabolism.

dysgnosia (dis-no'sĭ-ă) [" + *gnōsis*, knowledge]. Any anomaly of intellect. SYN: *dysthymia*.

dysgonesis (dis-go-ne'sis) [" + *gonē*, seed). 1. Functional disorder of the genital organs. 2. Poor growth of bacterial culture.

dysgon'ic [" + *gonē*, seed]. Bacterial cultures of sparse growth.

dysgraph'ia (dĭs-grăf'ĭ-ă) [" + *graphein*, to write]. 1. Inability to write properly. Usually the result of a brain lesion. 2. Writer's cramp.

dyshematopoiesis (dis-hem"ă-to-poy-e'-sĭ-ă) [" + *aima*, blood, + *poiēsis*, making]. Imperfect blood formation.

dyshidria (dis-hi'drĭ-ă) [" + *idrōs*, sweat]. Dyshidrosis.

dyshidrosis (dis-hi-dro'sis). 1. Disorder of the sweating apparatus. 2. A recurrent vesicular eruption on skin of hands and feet; marked by intense itching. SYN: *pompholyx*.

dyshor'monal [" + *orman*, to excite]. Caused by endocrine disturbance.

dyshor'monism [" + " + *ismos*, state of]. Deficiency or excessive production of hormones or any internal secretions.

dysidrosis (dis-i-dro'sis) [" + *idrōs*, sweat, + *-ōsis*]. Dyshidrosis.

d., trichophytic. Athlete's foot.

dysin'sulinism [" + L. *insula*, island, + G. *ismos*, state of]. Imperfect secretion of insulin.

dyskerato'sis [" + *keras*, horn, + *-ōsis*]. Epithelial alterations in which a certain number of isolated malpighian cells become differentiated. Any alteration in the keratinization of the epithelial cells of the epidermis. Characteristic of many skin disorders.

dyskine'sia [" + *kinēsis*, movement]. Defect in voluntary movement.

d. al'gera. Condition in which active movement is painful.

d. intermit'tens. Limb disability occurring intermittently.

d., uterine. Pain in the uterus on movement.

dyskinet'ic [G. *dys*, bad, + *kinēsis*, movement]. Having disordered normal movement.

dyskoimesis (dis-koy-me'sis) [" + *koimēsis*, sleeping]. Difficulty in going to sleep.

dyslalia (dis-lal'ĭ-ă) [" + *lalein*, to talk]. Impairment of speech due to defect of speech organs.

dyslexia (dis-leks'ĭ-ă) [" + *lexis*, diction]. 1. Difficulty in reading as result of brain lesion. 2. Visual confusion by which similarly shaped letters, such as o, e, c, b, p, h, or n, cause the victim to transpose letters in reading, seeing such a word as "pot" for "top."

dyslochia (dis-lo'kĭ-ă) [" + *lochia*, lochia]. Disordered lochial discharge, or premature cessation.

dyslogia (dis-lo'jĭ-ă) [" + *logos*, understanding]. Difficulty in expression of ideas.

dysmasesis (dis-mă-se'sis) [" + *masēsis*, mastication]. Difficulty in masticating. SYN: *dysmastesis*.

dysmegalop'sia [" + *megas*, size, + *opsis*, vision]. Inability to visualize correctly the size and shape of things.

dysmenorrhea (dis-men-o-re'ă) [" + *mēn*, month, + *rein*, to flow]. Painful or difficult menstruation, either primary or secondary.

d., congestive. Condition caused by pelvic congestion.

d., inflammatory. Condition caused by pelvic inflammation.

d., membranous. A severe spasmodic dysmenorrhea which is accompanied by the passage of a cast of the uterine cavity. Treated by curettage, and if not relieved, hysterectomy.

d., neurotic. Form caused by neurosis.

d., primary. Difficult menstruation starting from the first period and for which there is no known etiology.

d., secondary. When periods were, at the outset, normal, but, because of the development of some pathological state in the pelvis, there is a disturbance of menstruation.

ETIOL: *Cervix:* Diseases of the cervix; lacerations with scar formation; acute, subacute, and chronic endocervicitis. *Body of the Uterus:* Chronic endometritis; hyperplastic endometrium; fibroids, particularly the submucous and intramural types of fibroids; chronic metritis; acquired malposition of the uterus. *Tubal Conditions*: Acute, subacute, and chronic salpingitis. *Ovarian Conditions:* Cystic oöphoritis, endometrial cysts of the ovary, ovarian tumors of marked size. *Parametrium*: Uterosacral and broad ligament parametritis.

d., spasmodic. D. caused by uterine contractions of spasmodic form.

dysmetria (dis-me'trĭ-ă) [" + *metron*, measure]. An inability to fix the range of a movement.

Rapid and brusk movements made with more force than necessary. Seen in cerebellar affections. RS: *adiadochokinesis, asynergia, gait.*

dysmetrop'sia [" + " + *opsis*, vision]. Inability to visualize correctly the size and shape of things. SYN: *dysmegalopsia*.

dysmimia (dis-mim'ĭ-ă) [" + *mimeisthai*, to imitate]. 1. Inability to express oneself by gestures or signs. 2. Inability to imitate.

dysmnesia (dis-ne'zĭ-ă) [G. *dys*, bad, + *mnēmē*, memory]. Any impairment of memory.

dysmorphophobia (dis-mor-fo-fo'bĭ-ă) [" + *morphē*, form, + *phobos*, fear]. Morbid fear of deformity.

dysmorphosis (dis-mor-fo'sis) [" + " + *-ōsis*]. Not normal in form.

dysmyoto'nia [" + *mys*. muscle, + *tonos*, tone]. 1. Muscle atony. 2. Abnormal muscle tonicity.

dysneuria (dis-nu'rĭ-ă) [" + *neuron*, nerve]. Impairment of the nervous function.

dysodontiasis (dis-o-don-ti'ă-sis) [" + *odous*, tooth]. Painful or difficult dentition.

dysontogenesis (dis-ŏn-to-jĕn'ĕ-sis) [" + *ōn*, being, + *genesis*, development]. Defective development of an organism.

dysontogenet'ic [" + " + *gennan*, to produce]. Pert. to defective development.

dysopia, dysopsia (dis-o'pĭ-ă, -op'si-ă) [" + *opsis*, vision]. Defective or painful vision.

dysorexia (dis-o-rek'sĭ-ă) [" + *orēxis*, appetite]. Perverted or lessened appetite

dysosmia (dis-oz'mĭ-ă) [" + *osmē*, smell]. Impairment of the sense of smell.

dysostosis (dis-os-to'sis) [" + *osteon*, bone]. Defective bone formation.

d., cleidocranial. A congenital ossification of the skull with partial atrophy of clavicles.

d., mandibulofacial. Hypoplasia of the facial bones, downward sloping of the palbebral tissues, defects of the ear, macrostomia, and a fish-face appearance. It is supposed to be a sex-linked recessive trait. SYN: *Treacher-Collins syndrome.*

dysovarism (dis-o'var-izm) [" + L. *ovarium,* ovary, + G. *ismos,* condition]. Defective ovarian internal secretion.

dysox'idizable [" + *oxys,* sour]. Not easy to oxidize.

dyspan'creatism [" + *pagkreas,* pancreas, + *ismos,* condition of]. Impaired pancreatic function.

dyspareunia (dis-pă-ru'nĭ-ă) [G. *dyspareunos,* unhappily mated as bedfellows]. Painful coitus experienced by women.

ETIOL: May be due to physical or mental causes.

dyspepsia (dis-pep'sĭ-ă) [G. *dys,* bad, + *peptein,* to digest]. Imperfect digestion. Not a disease in itself, but symptomatic of other diseases or disorders.

d., acid. With excessive acid.

d., alcoholic. Caused by excessive use of alcoholic beverages.

d., atonic. Due to lack of muscular tone in the digestive organs.

d., biliary, bilious. Form in which there is insufficient quantity or quality of bile secretion.

d., cardiac. Form occurring during heart disease.

d., catarrhal. Due to inflammation of the stomach.

d., fermentative. D. caused by excessive fermentation of food and characterized by frequent eructation of gas; also called "gaseous" or "flatulent" d.

d., gastric. D. caused by faulty stomach function.

d., gastrointestinal. D. caused by faulty function of stomach and intestines.

d., hepatic. D. caused by liver disease.

d., hysterical. D. present during hysterical attacks.

d., intestinal. Due to abnormal state of pancreatic, biliary, and intestinal secretions.

d., nervous. Indicated by gastric pain and palpitation due to a lesion of nerves innervating the digestive tract, or to emotional states.

dyspeptic (dis-pep'tik) [" + *peptein,* to digest]. 1. Affected with or pert. to dyspepsia. 2. One afflicted with dyspepsia.

dyspeptone (dis-pep'tōn) [" + *peptein,* to digest]. An insoluble product of gastric digestion.

dysperma'sia [" + *sperma,* seed]. Dysspermia, *q.v.*

dysper'matism [" + " + *ismos,* condition]. Dysspermia, *q.v.*

dysper'mia [" + *sperma,* seed]. Dysspermia, *q.v.*

dysphagia (dis-fa'jĭ-ă) [" + *phagein,* to eat]. Inability or diffculty in swallowing.

d. constricta. D. due to narrowing of the pharynx or esophagus.

d. lusoria. D. caused by pressure exerted on the esophagus by anomalous origin of the right subclavian artery.

d. paralytica. D. due to paralysis of muscles of deglutition.

d. spastica. D. resulting from a spasm of pharyngeal or esophageal muscles.

dysphagy (dis'fă-jĭ). Dysphagia, *q.v.*

dysphasia (dis-fa'zĭ-ă) [" + *phasis,* speech]. Impairment of speech resulting from a brain lesion.

dysphemia (dis-fe'mĭ-ă) [" + *phēmē,* speech]. Stammering of psychoneurotic origin.

dysphonia (dis-fo'nĭ-ă) [" + *phōnē,* voice]. Difficulty in speaking; hoarseness.

d. clerico'rum. Clergyman's sore throat.

d. pu'berum. Change of voice in boys during puberty.

dysphoria (dis-fo'rĭ-ă) [" + *pherein,* to bear]. Exaggerated feeling of depression and unrest without apparent cause.

dysphrasia (dis-fra'zĭ-ă) [" + *phrasis,* a speech]. Impairment of speech due to a brain lesion. SYN: *dysphasia.*

dysphrenia (dis-fre'nĭ-ă) [" + *phrēn,* mind]. Functional or constitutional psychosis; the opp. of the organic type.

dysphylaxia (dis-fi-laks'ĭ-ă) [" + *phylaxis,* watching]. Waking too early from sleep.

dyspinealism (dis-pin'e-al-ism) [" + L. *pinealis,* pert. to a pine cone, + G. *ismos,* condition of]. Functional impairment of pineal gland.

dyspitu'itarism [" + L. *pituita,* mucus]. Condition due to disorder of the pituitary body.

dyspla'sia [" + *plassein,* to form]. Abnormal development of tissue. SYN: *alloplasia; heteroplasia.*

d., anhidrotic. A congenital condition marked by a few, absent or deficient sweat glands; intolerance of heat; and abnormal development of teeth and nails.

d., chondroectodermal. Condition marked by defective development of bones, nails, teeth and hair, and by congenital heart disease. SYN: *complete achondroplasia; Ellis-Van Creveld syndrome.*

d., hereditary ectodermal. Hereditary defect marked by few or absence of sweat glands and hair follicles, smooth shiny skin, abnormalities or absence of teeth, nail deformities, cataracts or alterations of cornea, absence of mammary glands, concave face, prominent eyebrows, conjunctivitis, deficient hair growth, and mental retardation. SYN: *anhidrotic ectodermal dysplasia; congenital ectodermal defect; Siemen syndrome.*

d., monostotic fibrous. Replacement of bone by fibrous tissue. Marked by pain usually in tibia or femur. Cause is unknown.

d., polyostotic fibrous. Replacement of bone by avascular fibrous tissue. Marked by difficulty in walking, and multiple bone deformities and fractures. Usually commences in childhood. Cause is unknown.

dyspnea (disp-ne'a) [" + *pnoē,* breathing]. Air hunger resulting in labored or difficult breathing usually accompanied by pain. Is normal when due to vigorous work or athletic activity.

ETIOL: Insufficient oxygenation of the blood resulting from disturbances in the lungs, low oxygen pressure of air, circulatory disturbances, hemoglobin deficiency; other causes may be: acidosis, excessive CO_2 content of blood, lesions of the respiratory center, emotional excitation, hyperexcitability of Hering-Breuer reflex, cardiac asthma, and orthopnea. It may be a subjective feeling.

SYM: Audible, labored breathing, distressed, anxious expression, dilated nostrils, protrusion of abdomen and expanded chest; gasping; marked cyanosis.

d., cardiac. D. due to cardiac insufficiency.

d., expiratory. As in asthma and bronchitis; wheezing and painful expiration. Secretions in respiratory tract cause of sound.

POISONS: May be induced by cyanides, carbon monoxide, strychnine during convulsions.

d., inspiratory. D. due to interference in passage of air to the lungs.

d., renal. D. due to kidney disorder.

dyspneic (disp-ne'ik) [G. *dys*, bad, + *pnoē*, breathing]. Affected with or due to dyspnea.

dyspragia (dis-pra'jĭ-ă) [" + G. *pragein*, to do]. Dyspraxia.

dyspraxia (dis-prax'ĭ-ă) [" + G. *prassein*, to perform]. Difficulty or pain in performing any function. SYN: *dyspragia*.

dysprosium (dis-pro'sĭ-um). ABBR: Dy. A metallic element of the yttrium group of rare earths. At. wt. 162.50; At. no. 66.

dysraphia, dysraphism (dis-raf'ĭ-ă, -izm) [" + *rhaphē*, a seam]. In the embryo, failure of raphe-formation, or failure of fusion of parts which normally fuse.

d. spinal. A general term applied to failure of fusion of parts along the dorsal midline. May involve any of the following structures: skin, vertebrae, skull, meninges, brain and spinal cord.

dysspermatism (dis-sper'mă-tizm). Dysspermia.

dysspermia (dis-sper'mĭ-ă). Difficult or painful emission of sperm during coitus.

dyssta'sia [" + *stasis*, standing]. Difficulty in standing.

dysstat'ic [" + *stasis*, standing]. Showing difficulty in standing.

dyssyner'gia [" + *syn*, with, + *ergon*, work]. Failure of muscular co-ordination. SYN: *ataxia*.

dyssystole (dis-sis'to-lē) [" + *systolē*, contraction]. Dilatation with cardiac insufficiency. Asystole; incomplete systole.

dystaxia (dis-tax'ĭ-ă) [" + *taxis*, arrangement]. Partial ataxia.

dystectia (dis-tek'shĭ-ă) [" + L. *tectum*, roof]. In the embryo, failure of closure of the neural tube. Thus deformities such as spina bifida or meningocele are produced.

dysteleology (dis-te-le-ol'o-jĭ) [" + *teleos*, complete, + *logos*, knowledge]. A theory, esp. in biology, that rudimentary organs have no useful purpose to life of organism.

dysthymia (dis-thi'mĭ-ă) [" + *thymos*, mind]. 1. Mental perversion; melancholia. 2. Condition resulting from malfunctioning of the thymus gland during childhood.

dysthyreosis (dis-thi-re-o'sis) [" + *thyreos*, shield, + *-ōsis*]. Impaired functional activity of thyroid gland. SYN: *dysthyroidism*.

dysthyroidism (dis-thi'roi-dizm) [" + " + *eidos*, form, + *ismos*, state of]. Imperfect development and function of the thyroid gland.

dystith'ia [" + *tithēnia*, nursing]. Difficulty or inability to nurse at breast.

dystocia (dis-to'sĭ-ă) [" + *tokos*, birth]. Difficult labor. May be produced by either the passenger (the fetus) or the passage (the pelvis of the mother).

FETAL CAUSES: (a) Usually large babies; (b) malpositions of the fetus (transverse presentation, face, brow, breech, or compound presentations); (c) abnormalities of the fetus (hydrocephalus, tumors of the neck or abdomen, hydrops; (d) multiple pregnancy (interlocked twins).

MATERNAL CAUSES: *Uterus*: (a) Primary and secondary uterine inertia; (b) congenital anomalies of the uterus (bicornuate uterus); (c) tumors of the uterus (fibroids, carcinoma of the cervix); (d) abnormal fixation of the uterus by previous operation.

Bony Pelvis: Contracted pelves, the commoner clinical types of which are (a) flat pelvis, rachitic and nonrachitic; (b) generally contracted pelvis; (c) flat and generally contracted pelvis; (d) funnel pelvis; (e) exostoses of the pelvic bones; (f) tumors of the pelvic bones.

Cervix Uteri: (a) Bandl's contraction ring; (b) rigid cervix that will not dilate; (c) stenosis and stricture preventing dilatation.

Ovary: Ovarian cysts that block the pelvis.

Vagina and Vulva: (a) Cysts; (b) tumors; (c) atresias and stenoses.

DIAG: Can generally be made by vaginal examination and external pelvimetry before the patient goes into labor.

TREATMENT: Varies according to the condition present that causes the dystocia. In general it aims toward the correction of the abnormality in order to allow the fetus to pass. If this is not possible, operative delivery must be resorted to. SEE: *cephalotripsy*.

dystonia (dis-to'nĭ-ă) [G. *dys*, bad, + *tonos*, tone]. Impairment of tonicity.

dyston'ic [" + *tonos*, tone]. Pert. to distonia or hyper- or hypotonicity of tissues.

dysto'pia [" + *topos*, place]. Malposition; displacement of any organ.

dystopic (dis-top'ik) [" + *topos*, place]. Not in place.

dys'topy [" + *topos*, place]. Dystopia, *q.v.*

dystro'phia [" + *trephein*, to nourish]. Progressive weakening of a muscle. SYN: *dystrophy*.

d., progressive muscular. Progressive atrophy of muscles beginning in terminals of motor nerves.

d., pseudohypertrophic muscular. An hereditary disease usually beginning in childhood in which muscular ability is lost. At first certain muscles atrophy followed by atrophy. Also called Erb's paralysis.

dystrophic (dis-trof'ik) [" + *trephein*, to nourish]. Pert. to dystrophia.

dystrophoneurosis (dis-trof"o-nu-ro'sis) [" + " + *neuron*, nerve, + *-ōsis*]. Defective nutrition accompanied by a nervous disease.

dystrophy (dis'tro-fĭ) [" + G. *trephein*, to nourish]. 1. Imperfect or defective nutrition. 2. Degeneration of an organ or structure resulting from defective nutrition, abnormal development, infection or unknown causes. SYN: *dystrophia*.

d., adiposogenital. A condition characterized by a peculiar type of obesity and hypogenitalism due to a disturbance in the hypothalamus which controls food intake and of the pituitary which controls gonadal development. SYN: *Fröhlich's syndrome; sexual infantilism*.

d., Landouzy-Dejerine. A form of d., in which there is marked atrophy of facial muscles, shoulder girdle and arm. Facial atrophy produces a peculiar expression called *myopathic facies*.

d., progressive muscular. A familial disease characterized by progressive atrophy and wasting of muscles. Onset is usually at an early age and it occurs more frequently in males than females. Its cause is thought to be a genetic defect in muscle metabolism.

d., pseudohypertrophic muscular. An hereditary disease usually beginning in childhood in which muscular ability is lost. At first there is muscular pseudohypertrophy followed by atrophy.

dystrypsia (dis-trip'sĭ-ă) [" + *tripsis*, digestion]. Impaired secretion of pancreas.

dysuria (dis-u'rĭ-ă) [" + *ouron*, urine]. Painful or difficult urination, symptomatic of numerous conditions.

There is usually frequent urination. This may be indicative of cystitis, neuralgia of the bladder, urethritis; urethral stricture; hypertrophied, cancerous, or ulcerated prostate in the male; prolapsus of uterus in the female; pelvic peritonitis and abscess; metritis; cancer of the cervix, or dysmenorrhea. Pain and burning may also be caused by concentrated acid urine.

dysu'riac [" + *ouron*, urine]. One affected with dysuria.

dyszooamylia (dis-zo"o-am-il'ĭ-ă) [" + *zōon*, animal, + *amylon*, starch]. Failure to transform dextrose into glycogen.

dyszoospermia (dis"zo-o-sperm'ĭ-ă) [" + " + *sperma*, seed]. Imperfect formation of spermatozoa.

Notes

E

E. Abbr. for *electromotive force, emmetropia, energy, Escherichia, experimenter,* and *eye;* chemical symbol for *einsteinium.*

e. Abbr. for *electric charge, electron, ex* (L. *from*).

ea. Abbr. for *each.*

ead. Abbr. for *eadem* (L. *the same*).

EAHF. Abbr. for *eczema, asthma, hay fever complex.*

Eales' disease (ēlz). Repeated hemorrhages into the retina and vitreous.

ear [A.S. *eáre*]. Organ of hearing. Consisting of external, middle, and internal ear.

e., Blainville's. Congenital asymmetry of the two ears.

e. bones. Ossicles of tympanic cavity: malleus, incus, and stapes.

e., Cagot. An ear without a lower lobe.

e., cauliflower. A deformity consisting of a thickening of the external ear resulting from repeated blows. Commonly seen in prize fighters.

e. drum. The tympanum, or cavity in middle ear.

e. dust. Calcareous concretions in membranous labyrinth. Syn: *otoconia; otolith.*

e., examination of. Watch test for hearing, color, size, and shape, discharge from middle or inner ear, tenderness upon pressure in front or back of ear; inflammation or bulging, perforations, or scars of drum.

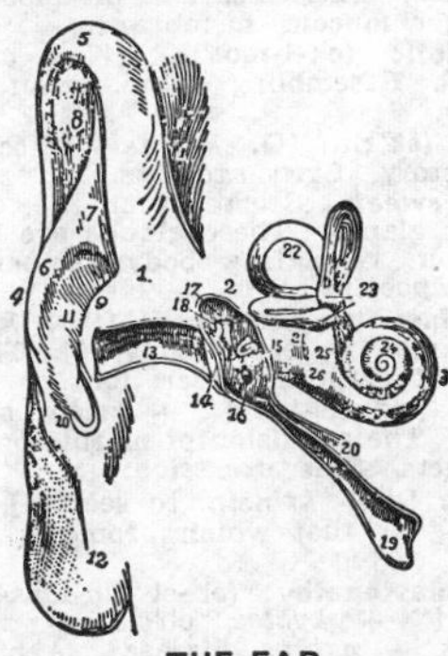

THE EAR

1. External ear; 2. Middle ear; 3. Internal ear; 4. Pinna; 5. Helix; 6. Antihelix; 7. & 8. Scapha (scaphoid fossa; fossa helicis); 9. Tragus; 10. Antitragus; 11. Concha; 12. Lobe; 13. External acoustic (auditory) meatus; 14. Tympanic membrane; 15. Tympanic promontory; 16. Fenestra cochleae; 17. Posterior wall of the tympanum; 18. Auditory ossicles; 19. Auditory or eustachian tube; 20. Facial canal; 21. Vestibule; 22. Semicircular canals (superior, posterior, lateral); 23. Ampulla; 24. Cochlea; 25. Prominentia spiralis; 26. Scala tympani.

Acute hearing sometimes precedes delirium. *Deafness* may indicate want of attention, wax in external ear passage, paralysis of auditory nerve or effect of quinine or other drugs. *Pallor of ears, tongue, and gums* indicates shock or anemia. *Ringing in ears* is noted in nervous debility, cerebral hyperemia and anemia, in disease of ear. Ménière's disease, and after use of certain drugs like quinine and salicylic acid.

e., external. Comprises auricle and external auditory canal; is separated from middle ear by tympanic membrane or eardrum.

e., foreign bodies in. These are usually insects, pebbles, beans, or peas. Insects in the ear cannot be attracted from the ear by a bright light inasmuch as they crawl in head first and usually do not see the light, or they may be stimulated to crawl in deeper by the bright light.

Sym: Pain, ringing or buzzing in the ear, and, if an insect, there is a great noise.

Treatment: Drop in bland oil and so float insect out of ear. In case of a solid foreign body, oil or water should not be used, inasmuch as it may cause the body to be pushed further in the ear or may cause it to swell and become firmly embedded. Such foreign bodies in the ear do not constitute an emergency and should be left untreated until seen by a physician.

Swimmers sometimes find that water enters the ear and will not flow out spontaneously. This may occasionally be dislodged by a sudden tap on the side of the head above the ear, or by introducing a long wisp of cotton which will draw out the water by capillarity. Also a few drops of 70% alcohol instilled in the canal will hasten evaporation of the so-called trapped water. Occasionally this sensation of water in the ear is not due to water but to swelling of the cerumen* that is usually present. In such instances a physician should be consulted.

e., internal. Consists of the cochlea containing the sensory receptors for hearing and the vestibule and semicircular canals which contain the receptors for equilibrium and the sense of position. Innervated by the vestibulocochlear nerve.

e., middle. An irregular cavity in temporal bone. In front it communicates with eustachian tube which forms an open channel bet. middle ear and cavity of nasopharynx. Behind, middle ear opens into mastoid antrum, and this in turn communicates with the mastoid cells. There are two openings into the inner ear, both of which are covered with membrane. Three ossicles (small bones), joined together, extend from the tympanic membrane to the *fenestra vestibuli;* these are the malleus, incus, and stapes.

e., nerve supply of. *External:* branches of facial, vagus, and mandibular nerves and from cervical plexus.

Middle: tympanic plexus and branches of mandibular, vagus, and facial nerves. *Internal:* vestibulocochlear nerve.

e. oximeter. A device which determines the oxygen content of the blood flowing through the ear.

e. plug. A device for helping to prevent sound from entering the ear by occluding the external auditory canal. Should not be used while swimming because the device may interfere with pressure equalization.

e., swelling in front or behind. ETIOL: Mumps, mastoid disease, scurvy, anthrax, or gangrenous stomatitis.

e. wax. Wax in the ear. SYN: *cerumen.*

ear, *words pert. to:* acoustic meatus, aditus, angiotitis, annulus, antihelix, antitragus, antrotympanitis, auricle, "auris-" words, binaural, blennotorrhea, bulla ossea, cavum tympani, cerumen, cochlea, concha, crista ampullaris, cupola, deafness, endolymph, epitympanum, eustachian, foreign bodies, helix, hydrotis, incus, labyrinth, labyrinthitis, malleus, ossicles, "ot-" or "oto-" words, pinna, scala tympani, tinnitus aurium, tympanum, "utri-" words, vestibule, vitreous.

earache. Aural pain. SYN: *otalgia.*

earth eating. Eating clay or dirt. Sometimes done by children who lack lime; also by the insane. SYN: *chthonophagia; geophagism; geotragia.*

ear trumpet. A tubular device to aid the deaf in hearing.

eat [A.S. *etan*]. 1. To devour as food. 2. To take solid food. 3. To corrode.

eating, *words pert. to:* abrosia, acataposis, acoria, allotriophagy, amasesis, apastia, appetite, bradyphagia, bulimia, chthonophagia, dysphagia, esculent, fastidium, fasting, geophagia, hunger, hyperorexia, mastication, parorexia, pica, polyphagia.

Eberthella (e-ber-thel'ă) [K. J. Eberth, German pathologist, 1835-1926]. Formerly a genus of bacteria. Now classified under *Salmonella.*

E. typhosa. *Salmonella typhosa.*

eberthian (e-ber'thĭ-en). Pert. to or caused by Eberth's bacillus. (*Salmonella*).

Eb'ner's glands. [A. G. Victor von Ebner, Austrian histologist, 1842-1925]. Serous glands of the tongue usually found in the vicinity of the circumvallate papillae.

ebonation (e-bo-na'shun) [L. *ē,* out, + A.S. *ban,* bone]. Removal of bony fragments from a wound.

Ebstein's anomaly of tricuspid valve. [Wilhelm Ebstein, German physician, 1836-1912]. A congenital condition of the heart, symptoms of which are fatigue, palpitation and dyspnea, resulting from downward displacement of the tricuspid valve from the annulus fibrosus. SYN: *downward displacement of tricuspid valve.*

ebullism (eb'u-lizm) [L. *ebullire,* to boil]. Spontaneous boiling of body fluids which occurs when the body is exposed to atmospheric pressure below that of the boiling point of the fluids.

ebullition (eb-u-lish'un) [L. *ebullīre,* to boil]. 1. Boiling. 2. Effervescence.

eburnation (e-bur-nā'shun) [L. *eburnus,* made of ivory]. Changes in bone causing them to become dense like ivory and hardened.

eburneous (e-bur'ne-us) [L. *eburnus,* made of ivory]. Resembling ivory; ivory-colored.

ecaudate (e-kaw'dāt) [L. *ē,* without, + *cauda,* tail]. Without a tail.

ecbolic (ek-bol'ik) [G. *ekbolikos,* throwing out]. 1. Hastening labor by causing contractions of the uterine muscles. 2. Causing abortion. 3. Any agent producing or hastening labor or abortion. Ex: *ergot; oxytocin.* SYN: *abortifacient.*

eccentric (ek-sen'trik) [G. *ekkentros,* from the center]. 1. Peculiar, abnormal in action or ideas. 2. Proceeding away from a center. 3. Peripheral.

e. atrophy. Atrophy with dilatation.

e. convulsion. One caused by peripheral irritation.

e. hypertrophy. Hypertrophy of a hollow organ with dilatation.

e. limitation. Having smaller visual field than normal.

eccentro-osteochondrodysplasia. A pathological condition of bones due to imperfect bone formation. Ossification occurs in eccentric centers instead of one common center.

eccentropiesis (ek-sen"tro-pi-e'sis) [" + *piēsis,* pressure]. Pressure from within exerted outward.

ecchondroma, ecchondrosis (ek-on-dro'mă, -dro'sis) [G. *ek,* out, + *chondros,* cartilage, + *-ōma,* tumor]. A chondroma or cartilaginous tumor.

ecchondrotome (ek-on'dro-tōm) [" + " + *tomē,* incision]. Knife for excision of cartilage.

ecchymoma (ek-ĭ-mo'mă) [" + *chymos,* juice, + *ōma,* tumor]. An extravasated blood tumor. A swelling due to the accumulation of blood in subcutaneous tissues such as occurs following a bruise.

ecchymosis (ek-ĭ-mo'sis) (pl. *ecchymoses*) [" + " + *ōsis*]. A form of macula appearing in large irregularly-formed hemorrhagic areas of the skin. The color is blue-black, changing to greenish brown or yellow.

ETIOL: Extravasation of blood into skin or mucous membrane.

ecchymotic (ek-i-mot'ĭk) [" + *chymos,* juice]. Resembling or rel. to an ecchymosis.

eccrine (ek'rin) [G. *ekkrinein,* to secrete]. Excretory. SYN: *exocrine.*

e. sweat. Sweat from the eccrine sweat glands. These glands are important in regulating body temperature. SEE: *apocrine.*

eccrinology (ek-rin-ol'o-jĭ) [" + *krinein,* to secrete, + *logos,* study of]. The science of glandular secretions.

eccrisis (ek'kris-is) [" + *krisis,* separation]. The expulsion of morbid or waste products. SYN: *excretion.*

eccrit'ic [" + *krinein,* to secrete]. Promoting or that which promotes excretion.

eccyclomastopathy (ek-si"klo-mas-top'ă-thĭ) [" + *kyklos,* circle, + *mastos,* breast, + *pathos,* disease]. A mass of lesions of the breast made up of connective tissue and/or epithelial cells. SYN: *cyclomastopathy.*

eccyesis (ek-si-e'sis) [" + *kyēsis,* pregnancy]. Extrauterine or ectopic pregnancy.

ecdem'ic [G. *ekdēmos,* foreign]. Neither endemic nor epidemic, as a disease carried to a region from without.

ecdemomania (ek"de-mo-mo-ma'nĭ-ă) [" + *mania,* madness]. Wanderlust; abnormal desire to wander. SYN: *drapetomania; dromomania; vagabondage.*

ecderon (ek'dĕ-ron) [G. *ek,* out, + *deros,* skin]. Epidermis, or outer portion of skin, as distinguished from *enderon,** or inner portion.

ecdysis (ek'dĭ-sis) (pl. *ecdyses*). 1. The shedding or sloughing off of the epidermis of the skin; desquamation. 2. The shedding of the outer covering of the body as occurs in certain animals such as insects, crustaceans, and snakes; molting.

ECG., ecg. Abbr. for *electrocardiogram.*

echidnase (ĕ-kid'nās). An enzyme present in snake venom which produces inflammation.

echidnin (ĕ-kĭd'nĭn). 1. The venom of poisonous snakes. 2. The active principle present in snake venom.

Echidnophaga (ĕ"kid-nof'ă-gă). A genus of fleas belonging to the family Pulicidae.

E. gallinacea. The sticktight flea which is the most important flea pest of poultry. It collects in clusters on the heads of poultry and in the ears of mammals. It may infest humans, esp. children.

echinate (ek'ĭ-nāt) [G. *echinos,* hedgehog]. 1. Spiny.. 2. In agar streak, a growth with pitted or toothed margins along the inoculation line; in stab cultures, coiled growth with pointed outgrowths. SYN: *echinulate.*

echinococcosis (e-ki"no-kok-o'sis, ek"ĭ-no-kok-o'sis) [" + *kokkos,* berry]. Infestation with echinococcus.

echinococcotomy (e-ki"no-kok-ot'o-mĭ) [" + " + *tomē,* incision]. Operation for evacuation of an echinococcus cyst.

Echinococcus (e-ki"no-kok'us) (pl. *Echinococci*) [" + *kokkos,* berry]. A genus of tapeworms. They are minute forms consisting of a scolex and three or four proglottids.

e. cyst. A cyst resulting from the development of the larva of the dog tapeworm.

e. cysticus. Disease resulting from a single hydatid cyst occurring in the liver.

e. disease. Infestation with the larva of Echinococcus which causes the formation of hydatid cysts.

e. granulosus. A species of tapeworms which infests dogs and other carnivors. Its larva called a hydatid develops in other mammals including man and causes the formation of hydatid cysts in the liver and/or lungs.

e. hydatidosus. Variety of E. characterized by development of daughter cysts from the mother cyst.

Echinorhynchus (e-ki"no-rin'kus) [" + *rygchos,* beak]. Formerly considered a genus of parasitic worms belonging to the Acanthocephala. It has been divided into many sub-groups.

E. gigas. Macracanthorhynchus hirudinaceus, a worm commonly parasitic in pigs, but occasionally found in man.

echinosis (ek"i-no'sis) ["+ *-ōsis*]. Blood corpuscles appearing like a sea urchin, having lost their smooth outlines. Crenation of red blood cells.

Echinostoma (ek"ĭ-nos'tō-mă). A genus of flukes characterized by a spiny body and the presence of a collar of spines near the anterior end. They are found in the intestines of many vertebrates, esp. aquatic birds. They occasionally occur as accidental parasites in man.

echinulate (ĕ-kin'u-lāt) [G. *echinos,* hedgehog]. A bacterial growth having lateral spines. Seen along line of inoculation. SYN: *echinate.*

echo (ĕk'ō) [G. *ēchō,* echo]. A reverberating sound.

e. acou'sia. Subjective echoes of sounds just normally heard.

e., amphor'ic. Amphoric sound sometimes heard in auscultation of chest. SEE: *chest, percussion of.*

e. sign. Repetition of closing word of a sentence, a sign of epilepsy or other brain conditions.

e. speech. Echolalia.

ECHO virus. A virus belonging to the group known as Enteric Cytopathogenic Human Orphan group. Cause of nonbacterial viral meningitis, enteritis, and various infections with or without fever and rash.

echokinesia (ek-o-kin-e'sĭ-ă) [" + *kinēsis,* movement]. Involuntary repetition of another's gestures.

echolalia (ek-o-la'lĭ-ă) [" + *lalia,* babble]. An involuntary, parrotlike repetition of words spoken by others, often accompanied by twitching of muscles. Frequently seen in catatonic schizophrenia.

echomatism (ĕ-ko'mă-tizm) [" + *ismos,* condition of]. Automatic repetition of another's actions.

echomimia (ek"o-mim'ĭ-a) [" + *mimēsis,* imitation]. The imitation of the actions of others without meaning as seen in dementia precox.

echomotism (ek"o-mo'tizm) [" + L. *motus,* moving]. Imitation of movements. SYN: *echomatism.*

echopathy (ĕ-kop'ă-thĭ) [" + *pathos,* disease]. Imitation of another's actions and repetitions of his words; a neurosis.

echophotony (ek"o-fot'o-nĭ) [" + *phos,* light, + *tonos,* tone]. Production of color sensations by stimulus of sounds heard.

echophra'sia [" + *phrasis,* speech]. Echolalia, *q.v.*

echopraxia (ek"o-praks'ĭ-ă) [" + *prassein,* to perform]. Imitation, without meaning, of motions made by others. SYN: *echomatism.*

echoprax'is [" + *prassein,* to perform]. Echopraxia, *q.v.*

eclabium (ek-la'bĭ-um) [G. *ek,* out, + L. *labium,* lip]. Eversion of a lip.

eclampsia (ĕ-klamp'sĭ-ă) [" + *lampein,* to flash]. A major toxemia of pregnancy accompanied by high blood pressure, albuminuria, oliguria, tonic and clonic convulsions, and coma. May occur during pregnancy or shortly after delivery. SEE ALSO: *preeclampsia.*

ETIOL: Unknown. Occurs more often in primiparae. Hypertension and glomerulonephritis contribute to cause.

PATH: Seen most frequently in the kidney, liver, brain, and placenta. The kidney shows degenerated tubal nephritis, the tubal epithelium showing cloudy swelling, fatty degeneration, and coagulation necrosis. The liver is enlarged and mottled, there are portal vein thrombosis and degeneration of the periphery of the lobules with subcapsular hemorrhages. The brain shows edema, hyperemia, thrombosis, and hemorrhages. The placenta shows infarcts, thromboses, and hemorrhages. There is also retinal edema.

SYM. AND SIGNS: Edema of the legs and feet, puffiness of the face, hyperpiesis,* and albuminuria.* Severe headaches, dizziness, spots before the eyes, epigastric pain and nausea, convulsions (beginning with fixation of the eyeballs, rolling of the eyes, twitchings of the face, arms, and hands; the paroxysms then involve the entire body), and coma. There may be one or many convulsions. The pulse is rapid and bounding, the temperature usually rises to 103° or 104° F., and the blood pressure varies bet. 140 and

200 mm. Hg systolic. The patient may continue in coma until death.

TREATMENT: *Prophylactic*: The most important. Good prenatal care, with careful watching of the patient's blood pressure, urine, and weight; instituting medical management as soon as any abnormal findings are presented, and terminating pregnancy if unsuccessful in reducing the signs of danger.

The Attack: Prevent the patient from doing herself bodily harm (tie her in bed, protect the tongue by keeping the teeth separated). Relieve vasoconstriction; promote diuresis. Sedatives only on order by physician. Tracheostomy may be performed to aid oxygenation.

Delivery: This should not be instituted until the general condition of the patient has improved unless the patient is in active labor, in which case the labor should be conducted by most conservative methods. Cesarean section should not be done unless there is some other obstetrical reason. If medical management effects no improvement, then labor must be instituted by one of the recognized methods, but local rather than general anesthesia is preferred.

NP (during a convulsion): (a) The patient *must not* be left alone. (b) Restrain only enough to keep her in bed. Side boards or some type of restraint must be used after the convulsion to make certain the patient will not fall out of bed during the coma, delirium, and restless stage. (c) Use mouth gag to keep patient from biting her tongue. (d) See that the physician is notified immediately. (e) Have the fetal heart checked frequently, in cases of convulsion before delivery, because the fetal circulation is interfered with and the infant may register signs of distress.

e., infantile. A convulsion occurring in children. It is of reflex origin being associated with teething, acute digestive disorders, worm infestation, or cerebral congestion.

e. nutans. SYN: *nodding spasm, salaam convulsion.* E. characterized by nodding movements.

e., puerperal. A convulsion occurring near the end of pregnancy, during labor, or immediately following labor.

e., uremic. E. resulting from uremia due to suppressed urine formation.

eclampsism (e-klamp'sizm) [" + " + *ismos,* state of]. Puerperal eclampsia without convulsive seizures.

eclamp'tic [" + *lampein,* to flash]. Rel. to, or of the nature of, eclampsia.

eclamptism (ĕ-klamp'tizm) [" + " + *ismos,* state of]. Condition due to autointoxication incident to pregnancy.

eclamptogen'ic [" + " + *gennan,* to produce]. Causing convulsions.

eclamptogenous (ek-lamp-toj'en-us) [" + " + *gennan,* to produce]. Producing convulsions. SYN: *eclamptogenic.*

eclectic (ek-lek'tik) [G. *eklektikos,* selecting]. Selecting from various sources what seems to be the best.

e. school of medicine. One employing a selected method, as indigenous plants or "specifics" according to patient's symptoms.

eclecticism (ek-lek'tĭ-sizm) [" + *ismos,* state of]. A system of medicine treating disease through specific remedies for individual pathological conditions, rather than by treating body as a whole. Remedies, principally botanical.

eclysis (ĕk-lĭ'sĭs). A mild syncope.

ecmnesia (ek-ne'zĭ-ă) [G. *ek,* out, + *mnēsis,* memory]. Inability to remember recent events as seen in senility. The memory of before and after events not affected.

ecoid (e'koyd) [G. *oikos,* house, + *eidos,* resemblance]. The framework of a red blood corpuscle.

ecology (e-kol'o-jĭ) [" + *logos,* study of]. The physiology of organisms as affected by their environment. SYN: *bionomics.*

ecomania (e-ko-ma'nĭ-ă) [" + *mania,* madness]. An extreme humbleness manifested before those in authority but a dominating, irritable attitude towards members of the family. Manifested in chronic alcoholism.

ecostate (e-kos'tāt) [L. *e-,* without, + *costa,* rib]. Without ribs.

ecosystem (ek'o-sis"tem). The smallest ecology unit. The living organisms and plants and their environment in a defined area.

écouvillonage (a-koo-vĭ-yon-ahzh') [Fr.]. The cleansing and application of remedies to a cavity by means of a brush or swab.

ecphoria (ĕk-fôr'ĭ-ă). An engram, or the reestablishment of a memory trace or engram.

ecphyadectomy (ek-fĭ-ă-dek'to-mĭ) [G. *ekphyas,* appendix, + *ektomē,* excision]. Removal of vermiform appendix. SEE: *appendectomy.*

ecphyaditis (ek-fĭ-ă-di'tis) [" + *-ītis,* inflammation]. Inflammation of vermiform appendix. SYN: *appendicitis.*

ecphylactic (ek-fĭ-lak'tĭk) [G. *ek,* out, + *phylaxis,* guarding]. Pert. to ecphylaxis.

ecphylax'is [" + *phylaxis,* protection]. Impotent antibodies or phylactic agents in the blood.

ecphyma (ek-fĭ'mă) [" + *phyma,* growth]. An outgrowth or excrescence, as a wart.

écrasement (ā-krăz-mon') [Fr. *ecraser,* to crush]. Excision by means of an écraseur.

écraseur (ā-kră-zer') [Fr. *ecraser,* to crush]. A wire loop used for excisions.

ecstasy (ek'sta-sĭ) [G. *ekstasis,* a standing out]. An exhilarated, trancelike, or exalted state.

ecstrophy (ek'stro-fĭ) [G. *ekstrophe,* a turning out]. Turning an organ inside out. SYN: *exstrophy.*

ECT. Abbreviation for *electroconvulsive therapy.*

ec'tad [G. *ektos,* without]. Toward the surface; outward; externally.

ec'tal [G. *ektos,* without]. External, outer, on the surface.

ectasia, ectasis (ek-ta'sĭ-ă, ek'tă-sis) [G. *ek,* out, + *teinein,* to stretch]. Dilatation of any tubular vessel.

e., hypostatic. Dilatation of a blood vessel from the settling of blood in dependent parts, especially the legs.

e. iridis. Smallness of the pupil of the eye caused by displacement of the iris.

e. ventriculi paradoxa. Hourglass stomach.

ectasin (ek'tas-in) [" + *teinein,* to stretch]. A tuberculin-derived substance causing vasomotor dilation.

ectat'ic [" + *teinein,* to stretch]. Distensible or capable of being stretched.

ecten'tal [G. *ektos,* without, + *entos,* within]. Pert. to entoderm and ectoderm.

e. line. Point of entodermal and ectodermal junction in the gastrula.

ectethmoid (ek-teth'moyd) [" + *ēthmos*, sieve, + *eidos*, form]. Lateral mass of the ethmoid bone.

ecthyma (ek-thi'mă) [G. *ek*, out, + *thyein*, to rush]. An infection of the skin. Usually a result of neglected treatment of impetigo, *q.v.* It is marked by shallow lesions containing pus and may be followed by pigmentation and scarring. Treatment is the same as that for impetigo. SYN: *ulcerative impetigo*.

e. scrofulosum. Form seen in scrofula.

e. syphiliticum. Pustular eruption occurring in tertiary syphilis.

ecthyreosis (ek-thī-rē-o'sis) [" + *thyreos*, shield, + *-ōsis*]. Loss of thyroid gland or its function.

ectiris (ek-ti'ris) [G. *ektos*, without, + *iris*, iris]. The external portion of the iris.

ecto- [G. *ekto*]. Prefix: Outside.

ectoan'tigen [G. *ektos*, out, + *anti*, against, + *gennan*, to produce]. 1. Any toxin or stimulator of antibody formation. 2. An antigen assumed to have its origin in ectoplasm of bacterial cells or one loosely attached to the surface of bacteria and capable of being separated from the bacterial cell.

ec'toblast [" + *blastos*, germ]. 1. Wall of a cell. 2. Ectoderm. 3. Any outer membrane.

ectocardia (ek-to-kar'dĭ-ă) [" + *kardia*, heart]. Having the heart out of normal position.

ectochoroidea (ek"to-ko-roy'de-ă) [" + *chorioidēs*, choroid]. Outer layer of choroid coat of the eye.

ectocinerea (ek-to-sin-e're-ă) [" + L. *cinereus*, ashen]. The outer gray matter of the brain.

ectocolos'tomy [G. *ektos*, outside, + *kōlon*, colon, + *stōma*, opening]. Formation through the abdominal wall of an opening into the colon.

ectocondyle (ek-to-kon'dĭl) [" + *kondylos*, knuckle]. The outer condyle of the bone.

ectocornea (ek-to-kor'ne-ă) [" + L. *corneus*, horny]. External layer of the cornea.

ectocuneiform (ek-to-ku'ne-ĭ-form) [" + L. *cuneus*, wedge, + *forma*, form]. External cuneiform bone.

ectocytic (ek-to-si'tĭk) [" + *kytos*, cell]. Outside of the cell.

ectodactylism (ek-to-dak'til-izm) [" + *daktylos*, finger, + *ismos*, state of]. Lack of a digit or digits.

ectoderm (ek'to-derm) [" + *derma*, skin]. The outer layer of cells in a developing embryo.

From it are developed skin structures, the nervous system, organs of special sense, the pineal and part of pituitary and suprarenal glands. SYN: *epiblast*. SEE: *entoderm*.

ectoder'mal [" + *derma*, skin]. Rel. to the ectoderm.

ectodermatosis (ek-to-der-mă-to'sis) [" + " + *-ōsis*]. Disorder due to faulty development of the ectoderm. SYN: *ectodermosis*.

ectoder'mic [" + *derma*, skin]. Pert. to the ectoderm. SYN: *ectodermal*.

ectodermoi'dal [" + " + *eidos*, resemblance]. Pert. to or resembling the ectoderm.

ectodermo'sis [" + " + *-ōsis*]. Illness resulting from congenital maldevelopment of ectodermal structures. SYN: *ectodermatosis*.

e. pluriorificialis. A form of erythema multiforme characterized by fever, chills, profuse salivation, small blisters on tongue, lips and cheeks, and erythematous lesions on the hands. The disease is rare, occurring in children and young persons. SYN: *dermatostomatitis*.

ectoen'tad [" + *entos*, within]. From without inward.

ectoen'zyme [" + *en*, in, + *zymē*, leaven]. An extracellular enzyme or one that acts outside of the cell that secretes it.

ectogenous (ek-toj'ĕ-nus) [" + *gennan*, to produce]. Having its origin outside of a body or structure, as infection.

ectoglia (ek-tog'lĭ-ă) [G. *ektos*, outside, + *glia*, glue]. Superficial embryonic layer in beginning of stratification of the medullary tube.

ectoglob'ular [" + L. *globulus*, globule]. Not within blood cells or globular bodies.

ectog'ony [" + *gonos*, seed]. Influences on the mother's body and metabolism from the developing zygote.

ectokelostomy (ek-to-ke-los'to-mĭ) [" + *kēlē*, hernia, + *stōma*, opening]. Making an external opening into a hernial sac to prepare for a radical operation.

ectolecithal (ek-to-les'ĭ-thal) [" + *lekithos*, yolk]. Pert. to ovum having food yolk placed near the surface.

ectol'ysis [" + *lysis*, dissolution]. Ectoplasmic lysis.

ectomere (ek'to-mēr) [" + *meros*, part]. One of the blastomeres forming the ectoderm.

ectomesoblast (ek-to-me'so-blast) [" + " + *blastos*, germ]. Cells from which will be developed the ectoblast and mesoblast.

ectomorphy (ek'to-mor-fe) [" + *morphe*, form]. Body build characterized by predominance of tissues derived from the ectoderm. SEE: *endomorphy; mesomorphy; somatotype*.

ectomy (ek'to-mĭ) [G. *ektomē*]. Excision of any organ or gland.

ectonuclear (ek-to-nu'kle-er) [G. *ektos*, outside, + L. *nucleus*, kernel]. Occurring outside a cell nucleus.

ectopagus (ek-top'ă-gus). An abnormal fetus consisting of twins fused at the thorax.

ectopar'asite. A parasite that lives on the outer surface of the body.

ectoperitoni'tis [" + *peritonaion*, peritoneum, + *-itis*, inflammation]. Inflammation of the parietal layer of peritoneum (layer lining the abdominal wall).

ectopia (ek-to'pĭ-ă) [G. *ek*, out, + *topos*, place]. Malposition or displacement, especially congenital, of an organ or structure.

e. cordis. Malposition of the heart in which heart lies outside the thoracic cavity.

e. lentis. Displacement of the crystalline lens of the eye.

e., pupillae. Displacement of the pupil. SYN: *corectopia*.

e. renis. Displacement of the kidney.

e. testis. Displacement of the testis.

e. vesicae. Displacement of the bladder, esp. exstrophy of the bladder.

e., visceral. An umbilical hernia.

ectopic (ek-top'ik) [" + *topos*, place]. In an abnormal position; said of a fetus.

e. beat. Cardiac beat beginning at a point other than sinoatrial node.

e. gestation or **pregnancy.** Implantation of the fertilized ovum outside of the uterine cavity. There is usually a decidual reaction in the uterus, but the decidua is poorly developed and the decidua reflex is absent. The tubal decidual reaction is meager.

Locations: *Abdominal*: In the free abdominal cavity and attached to one of the abdominal viscera, usually secondary to tubal. *Interstitial*: In the interstitial portion of the tube. *Ovarian*: In the ovary. The ovarian and primary abdominal types are very rare. *Tubal*: In the fallopian tube, the most frequently encountered. The pregnancy may be situated in the interstitial, ampullar, or isthmic portion of the tube, the isthmic type being the most common.

Etiol: Most commonly associated with inflammatory conditions of the tube and other conditions which mechanically interfere with the downward passage of the ovum, such as diverticula, polypi in the tubal lumen, peritoneal adhesions, and a large migrating ovum. Any variety of pregnancy or any combination of varieties may occur (uterine plus ectopic, bilateral ectopic, etc.).

Sym: (a) Missed menstruation; (b) tenderness, soreness, pain on affected side; (c) pallor, weak pulse, signs of shock or hemorrhage; (d) pain may be reflected to shoulder; (e) perhaps bluish discoloration of umbilicus.

Unruptured: Amenorrhea may or may not be present; vague pains in the abdomen usually on one side; irregular hemorrhage. The diagnosis at this stage can be made only by the absence of definite signs of uterine pregnancy, and colpotomy incision with an inspection of the internal genitalia.

Ruptured: *Without a severe hemorrhage*: Severe pain in the lower abdomen with fainting spells which occur repeatedly. Diagnosis made by puncture which reveals the free blood in the abdominal cavity.

Tragic, with overwhelming hemorrhage: Sudden collapse with cold, clammy sweat, rapid pulse, Cullen's sign in women with thin abdominal walls, lowering blood pressure, gaseous distention of the abdomen, desire to defecate with no relief of the pressure on defecation (due to bloody distention of the *cul-de-sac*), shock, air hunger, and other signs of severe hemorrhage. Diagnosis is confirmed by the return of free blood on post. puncture. After several attacks there is a leukocytosis of 12,000 to 15,000, and the hemoglobin is lowered.

Differential Diagnosis: Ectopic must be differentiated from uterine pregnancy, acute salpingitis, twisting of the pedicle of an ovarian cyst or pedunculated fibroid tumor, and hemorrhage from a ruptured graafian follicle or corpus luteum cyst.

Treatment: Once the diagnosis of ectopic pregnancy is made, operative treatment is indicated. In those cases where there is profound shock from hemorrhage, the patient should be supported by blood transfusion and saline infusions before major surgery is attempted. See: *celiocolpotomy*.

e. rhythm. Any cardiac rhythm that is abnormal or irregular.

ec'toplasm [G. *ektos*, outer, + *plasma*, a thing formed]. The outermost layer of cell protoplasm.

ec"toplas'mic [" + *plasma*, a thing formed]. Pert. to ectoplasm.

ectoplas'tic [" + *plassein*, to form]. Formed at the periphery; ectoplasmic.

ectopotomy (ek-to-pot'o-mĭ) [G. *ek*, out, + *topos*, place, + *tomē*, incision]. Removal of the fetus in ectopic pregnancy.

ectopterygoid (ek"to-ter'ĭ-goyd) [G. *ektos*, outside, + *pteryx*, wing, + *eidos*, form]. External or lateral pterygoid muscle. Acts to bring jaw forward. Syn: *musculus pterygoideus lateralis* [NA].

ectopy (ek'to-pĭ) [G. *ek*, out, + *topos*, place]. Displacement. Syn: *ectopia*.

ectoret'ina [G. *ektos*, outside, + L. *rete*, net]. Outer layer of retina.

ectos'copy [" + *skopein*, to examine]. Diagnosis by study of thoracic movements when patient speaks, or by abdominal movements.

ectostosis (ek-tos-to'sis) [" + *osteon*, bone, + *-ōsis*]. Formation of bone beneath the periosteum.

ectotoxe'mia [" + *toxikon*, poison, + *aima*, blood]. Toxemia from introduction of a toxin into the body.

Ectotrichophyton (ĕk-tō-trī-kŏf'ĭ-tŏn). Term applied to *Trichophyton megalosporon ectothrix*, a genus of parasitic fungi, causing tinea or ringworm of the hair.

ectozoon (ek-to-zo'on) [" + *zōon*, animal]. Parasitic animal that infests the outer integument of the body.

ectrodactylism (ek-tro-dak'til-izm) [G. *ektrōma*, abortion, + *daktylos*, finger, + *ismos*, state of]. Congenital absence of 1 or more fingers or toes.

ectromelia (ek"tro-me'li-ă). Congenital absence of one or more limbs.

ectropic (ek-tro'pĭk) [G. *ek*, out, + *trepein*, to turn]. Pert. to complete or partial eversion of a part, generally the eyelid.

ectropion (ek-tro'pĭ-on) [" + *trepein*, to turn]. Ophth: Eversion, as the edge of an eyelid.

Etiol: Old age; relaxation of skin; cicatrix following trauma; infection; palsy of facial nerve.

e. of the cervix uteri. Gyn: A turning out of the edges of the cervix following laceration.

ectro'pionize [" + *trepein*, to turn]. To evert, or cause an eversion.

eczema (ek'zĕ-mă) [G. *ekzein*, to boil out]. This word has become synonymous with chronic dermatitis. It has therefore no specific connotation, particularly with respect to etiology. Cutaneous inflammatory condition, acute or chronic, with erythema, papules, vesicles, pustules, scales, crusts, or scabs alone or in combination, dry, or with watery discharge, and with thickening or infiltration and more or less itching or burning. More a symptom than a disease.

Etiol: Essential cause unknown. No class, age, or sex is exempt, but those with thin, dry skins are more susceptible. Not infectious. Two classes of causes: (1) External or exciting (parasitic, irritation, occupational and nonoccupational, chemicals, etc.). (2) Constitutional or predisposing (nerve strain and reflex irritation, anaphylactic reactions, hyperglycemia, etc.).

Sym: Primary type characterized by erythematous, papular, vesicular, or pustular lesions. In secondary type, the lesions evolve from primary variety. Invasion by pathogenic organisms may cause suppuration.

e. capitis. That on the head. Oozing dermatitis seborrheica.*

e., erythematous. Dry, pinkish, ill-defined patches with itching and burning, slight swelling with tendency to spread and coalesce, branny scaling, roughness and dryness of skin. May become generalized.

e. fissum. Form of e. with painful fissures.

e. hypertrophicum. E. with a permanent enlargement of papillae of the skin, or skin growths.

e., lichenoid. E. with a thickened condition of the skin.

e. madidans. Variety with raw, erythematous points exuding moisture.

e. marginatum. E. caused by ringworm. SYN: *tinea cruris.*

e., papular. Pin-point to pinhead-sized reddish, pinkish, or violaceous papules with rounded or acuminate thin-walled vesicles which, when ruptured, become covered with thin yellowish crust of dried sebum or inspissated pus interspersed with raw areas of denuded epithelium. Skin as a result of irritation and chronic congestion becomes thick and infiltrated and dark red.

e., pustular. Includes many forms: Follicular, impetiginous or consecutive types, including *eczema rubrum* (red, glazed surface with little oozing); *eczema madidans* (raw, red, and covered with moisture); *eczema crustosum* (more or less crusting with exudate); *eczema fissum* (thick, dry, inelastic skin with cracks and fissures); *squamous eczema* (chronic, on soles, legs, scalp; multiple, circumscribed infiltrated patches with thin, dry scales); *eczema sclerosum* (marked thickening, elephantiasis-like papillary hypertrophy resulting in rough, horny, verrucose patches on legs, soles, and palms with fissuring); *furrowed eczema* (slightly erythematous skin, harsh and dry, with innumerable cracks on outer epidermal layer).

PROG: Chronic, amenable to treatment but prone to relapse and recurrence.

TREATMENT: Depends upon the etiology and will therefore be highly individualized according to the causive agent, organism, or condition. SEE: *allergy; dermatitis, contact.*

e. rubrum. SEE: *e. madidans.*

e., seborrheic. Form marked by excessive secretion from the sebaceous glands. SYN: *seborrhea.*

e. squamosum. E. with scaly formation.

e. vaccinatum. Generalized vaccinial lesions or local lesions elsewhere than at vaccination site in persons who have eczema and have been vaccinated.

e., vesicular. Formation of vesicles on the scalp in eczema.

eczem'atous [G. *ekzein,* to boil out]. Marked by or resembling eczema.

ED. Abbr. for *effective dose, erythema dose.*

Edebohls' position (ed'e-bols) [George M. Edebohls, American surgeon, 1853-1908]. The dorsal recumbent position with the buttocks resting upon end of table, the lower limbs flexed backward toward the abdomen sufficiently to permit holding the position with legs supported from ankles in a support attached to two straight uprights extending one on each side at end of table.

edema (e-de'mă, ĕ-de'mă) [G. *oidēma,* swelling]. In England, spelled *oedema.* A condition in which the body tissues contain an excessive amount of tissue fluid. It may be local or general. Generalized edema is sometimes called dropsy, or anasarca.

ETIOL: Edema may result from increased permeability of the capillary walls; increased capillary pressure due to venous obstruction or heart failure; lymphatic obstruction; disturbances in renal functioning; reduction of plasma proteins; inflammatory conditions; fluid and electrolyte disturbances, particularly those causing sodium retention; malnutrition; starvation; chemical substances such as bacterial toxins, venoms, caustic substances, and histamine.

May occur by diffusion,* osmosis,* or dialysis.* Acid in the tissue, such as resulting from a sting, produces absorption of water which causes local edema.

TREATMENT OF GENERAL EDEMA: Bed rest desirable. Salt intake restricted. This may be moderate or severe restriction, depending upon degree of edema. Fluid intake restricted; may be as low as 600 cc. in 24 hours. This proscription may be relaxed when free diuresis has been attained. Diuretics are effective when renal function is good, edema mild, and when underlying abnormality of cardiac function, capillary pressure, or colloid osmotic pressure is being corrected, simultaneously. Diuretics contraindicated in the true nephritic edema of acute diffuse glomerulonephritis. They are often useless in cardiac edema associated with advanced renal insufficiency. Useful diuretics are acetazolamide, aminophylline ammonium chloride, cation exchange resins, dextran, potassium salts, theobromine, theophylline, thiazide derivatives, urea, and mercurial diuretics. The diet in edema should be adequate in protein, high in calories, rich in vitamins, and low in salt. When diuresis appears, the patient may resume a normal diet.

e., acute circumscribed. Form with separated swellings on the body, but usually on the face.

e., angioneurotic. Also called *angioedema.* Large areas of swelling of subcutaneous tissues, mucous membranes, and occasionally the viscera. May be due to allergic sensitivity to drugs, food, or physical agents such as cold or wind.

e., blue. Hysteric paralysis inducing a swollen, bluish condition of a limb.

e. bullosum vesicae. Form affecting the bladder.

e. of glottis. An infiltration of the submucosa of the larynx, with cough, loss of voice and feeling of suffocation.

e., inflammatory. E. of inflamed tissues.

e., malignant. E. characterized by a rapid course, and speedy destruction of tissue.

e. neonatorum. Edema in newborn, especially premature infants. Condition is usually transitory, involving hands, face, feet and genitalia, and it rarely becomes generalized.

e., purulent. E. caused by purulent infiltration.

e., salt. Form caused by increase of salt in the diet.

edema, words pert. to: angioneuroedema, cephaledema, chemosis, lung, nephritis, phlegmasia alba dolens, hives, giant urticaria, angioedema.

edematous (e-dem'at-us) [G. *oidēma,* swelling]. Pert. to, or affected with, edema.

edentia (e-den'she-ă) [L. *e,* without, + *dens,* tooth]. Absence of teeth.

edentulous (e-dent'u-lus). Without teeth.

edible (ĕd'ĭ-bl) [L. *edere,* to eat]. Suitable for food.

edul'corant [L. *ē,* out, + *dulcorāre,* to sweeten]. Sweetening.

edulcorate (e-dul'ko-rāt) [" + *dulcorāre,* to sweeten]. 1. To sweeten. 2. To wash out salts or acids.

EEE. Abbr. for *Eastern equine encephalitis.*

EEG. Abbr. for *electroencephalogram.*

effect. Result of an action or force.

e., additive. A therapeutic effect of a combination of two or more drugs which is greater than the sum of the individual drug effects.

e., cumulative. A sudden increased e. following a number of doses of a drug; caused by excretion or metabolic degradation of only a fraction of the active principles of a substance. Though this type of effect is usually avoided, it is sometimes therapeutically desirable.

effect'or [L. *effectus,* accomplishing, from *efficere*]. One of the nerve endings having the efferent process end in a gland or muscle cell. The terminal arborizations of efferent or motor nerves. Also applied to effector organs (muscles and glands).

e. organ. A structure which when stimulated produces an effect, specifically muscles and glands.

effemination (ĕ-fem-ĭ-na'shun) [L. *effeminare,* to make feminine]. The state or condition of a male having the mental and physical characteristics of a female.

ef'ferent [L. *ex,* out, + *ferre,* to carry]. Carrying away from as efferent nerves which conduct impulses from the brain or spinal cord to the periphery, efferent lymph vessels which convey lymph from lymph nodes, and efferent arterioles which carry blood from glomeruli of the kidney.

e. nerves. Motor nerves. They can carry impulses having the following effects: (1) Motor, causing contraction of muscles; (2) secretory, causing glands to secrete, and (3) inhibitory, causing some organ to become quiescent.

effervesce (ef-er-ves') [L. *effervescere,* to boil up]. To boil, or form bubbles on the surface of a liquid.

effervescence (ef-er-ves'ents) [L. *effervēscere,* to boil up]. Formation of bubbles of gas coming up to surface of fluid.

efferves'cent. Bubbling. Rising in little bubbles of gas.

effleurage (ef-flūr-ahzh') [Fr. *effleurer,* to touch lightly]. In massage, deep or gentle stroking.

efflorescence (ef-flor-es'ents) [L. *efflorescere,* to bloom]. A rash; a redness of the skin. SYN: *exanthem.**

efflorescent (ef-flor-es'ent) [L. *efflorescere,* to bloom]. Becoming powdery or drying from loss of water of crystallization.

effluent (ef'lu-ent) [L. *effluere,* to flow out]. 1. A flowing out. 2. Fluid material discharged from a sewage treatment plant or an industrial plant.

effluvium (ef-lu'vĭ-um) (pl. *effluvia*) [L. a flowing out]. A malodorous exhalation, particularly one that is toxic. SYN: *odor; vapor.*

effuse' [L. *ex,* out, + *fundere,* to pour]. Thin, widely spreading. Applied to a bacterial growth which forms a very delicate film over a surface.

effu'sion [" + *fundere,* to pour]. Escape of fluid into a part, as the pleural cavity, such as pyothorax (pus), hydrothorax (serum), hemothorax (blood), chylothorax (lymph), pneumothorax (air), hydropneumothorax (serum and air), and pyopneumothorax (pus and air).

e., pleural. Fluid in the pleural space.

egersis (ē-ger'sĭs). Extreme or abnormal wakefulness; extremely alert.

egesta (e-jes'tă) [" + *gerere,* to bear]. Waste matter eliminated from the body.

egg [A.S. *aeg*]. 1. The female sex cell or ovum applied especially to an ovum which after fertilization is passed from the body and develops outside as in fowls. 2. The mammalian ovum.

e. albumen. The white of an egg. SEE: *vitellin; vitellus; yellow sac.*

e., nutritive values of. RAW: two large eggs (100 gm.). Calories: 163. Other values: 12.9 gm. protein; 11.5 gm. fat; 0.9 gm. carbohydrate; 54 mg. calcium; 2.3 mg. iron; 1180 I.U. vitamin A; 0.11 mg. thiamine; 0.15 mg. riboflavin; trace, niacin.

ego (e'go) [G. *egō,* I]. PSY: One of the three major divisions in the model of the psychic apparatus. The others are *id* and *superego.* The ego possesses consciousness and memory and serves to mediate beween the primitive instinctual or animal drives (*i.e.,* the *id*), internal social (the *superego*) prohibitions and reality. Thus the ego allows one to adapt to what might otherwise be a very unpleasant situation. The psychiatric use of the term should not be confused with its common usage in the sense of "self-love" or "selfishness."

e. ideal. The unconscious perfection of an individual's pattern or standard of character, usually identified with one greatly admired.

The social standards of the individual in contrast to his instinctive unsocial desires. While undoubtedly there is an inherent difference in the child's capacity to attain an ego ideal as definitely as to attain mature intelligence, much of its formulation depends upon teaching and example in the early years.

Organic disease modifies its evolution, and even more definitely may effect its involution. The later experiences of life, each in turn, add some little modification. It constitutes one phase of "conflict." Overdevelopment or compensatory overemphasis may lead to manifestations neither desirable from the social nor personal viewpoints.

e. instincts. All instincts not of a sexual nature.

e. libido. One concentrated in and upon the ego and not manifested toward external objects. Manifested in narcissistic disorders.

e., super. An inner censor (outside of the field of consciousness) of the ego.

egobronchophony (e"go-bron-kof'o-nĭ) [G. *aix, aig-,* goat, + *brogchos,* + *phōnē,* voice]. A bleating sound with bronchophony. SEE: *egophony.*

egocen'tric [G. *ego,* I, + *kentron,* center]. Pert. to a withdrawal from external world with concentration upon inner self.

egoma'nia [" + *mania,* madness]. Abnormal self-esteem and self-interest.

egophony (e-gof'o-nĭ) [G. *aix, aig-,* goat, + *phōnē,* voice]. A nasal sound somewhat like the bleat of a goat heard in auscultation of the chest when the subject speaks in a normal tone. Heard in pleural effusion.

egotrop'ic [G. *ego,* I, + *tropos,* a turning]. Interested chiefly in oneself; self-centered.

Eh'renritter's ganglion. The jugular ganglion.

Ehrlich's side-chain theory (air'lik) [Paul Ehrlich, German bacteriologist, 1854-1915]. So named because the protoplasmic cell is said to possess the certain receptors or "side-chains" which are capable of becoming fixed to certain protein groups with which they have a chemical affinity. This "fixation" is of value to the cell in that it enables it to attach the various food substances which it needs for nourishment. The molecules of a toxin, according to this theory, contain two groups for attachment to the cell.

HAPTOPHORE GROUP: It becomes fixed to a suitable cell receptor. When this happens, the receptor detaches from the cell and floats off in the blood stream. The cell responds to this loss by producing more effectors, which are again liberated into the blood, where they combine with toxins and thereby render them inert, and so form free antitoxin.

TOXOPHORE GROUP: Toxicity results when this becomes attached to certain receptors of the cell called toxiphiles, and this union is prevented by rendering the haptophore group inert. SEE: *immunity.*

E.'s theory of immunity. A theory which attempts to explain the formation of antitoxin in the blood. Also known as E.'s side-chain theory, *q.v.*

Ehrlich-Hata preparation or treatment, "606" [Paul Ehrlich; S. Hata, Japanese physician]. A specific for syphilis. SYN: *arsphenamine.*

Eichhorst's corpuscles (īk'horst) [Hermann Ludwig Eichhorst, Swiss physician, 1849-1921]. Spherical, small blood corpuscles found in pernicious anemia.

E.'s neuritis. Neuritis involving nerve sheath and interstitial muscular tissues.

eidetic (i-det'ik) [G. *eidos,* form]. Relating to or having the ability of total visual recall of anything previously seen.

eidoptometry (i-dop-tom'ĕ-trĭ) [G. *eidos,* form, + *optein,* to see, + *metron,* measure]. Determination of visual acuteness.

eighth cranial nerve. Acoustic nerve, *q.v.*

eikonom'etry [G. *eikon,* image, + *metron,* measure]. Determination of distance of an object by measuring the image produced by a lens of known focus.

eiloid (i'loid) [G. *eilein,* to coil, + *eidos,* appearance]. Having a coil-like structure.

Eimeria (i-me'rĭ-ă). A genus of sporozoan parasites belonging to the class Telosporidea, subclass Coccidiida. They are intracellular parasites living in the epithelial cells of vertebrates and invertebrates. They rarely are parasitic to man.

E. hominis. A species in the pleural exudate of man.

einsteinium (īn-stīn'ĭ-um) [Named for Albert Einstein, American physicist, 1879-1955]. A radioactive element. SYMB: Es. At. no. 99.

eisodic (i-sod'ik) [G. *eis,* into, + *odos,* way]. Centripetal or afferent, as nerve fibers of a reflex arc.

ejaculatio (e-jak-u-la'she-o) [L.]. Sudden expelling, as of semen.

e. precox (pre'kox) [L.]. Premature ejaculation. Inability to prevent ejaculation of semen at the beginning of copulation, or prior to it.

ejaculation (e-jak-u-la'shun) [L. *ejaculārī,* to throw out]. Ejection of the seminal fluids from the male urethra, or of the secretions of the vaginal glands, esp. Bartholin's glands, in the female.

e. mechanism of. Ejaculation consists of two phases, (1) the passage of semen and the secretions of the accessory organs (bulbourethral and prostate glands and seminal vesicles) into the urethra and (2) the expulsion of the seminal fluid from the urethra. The former is brought about by contraction of the smooth muscle of the ductus deferens, and the increased secretory activity of the glands; the latter by the rhythmical contractions of the bulbocavernosus and ischiocavernosus muscles and the levator ani.

The prostate discharges its secretions before those of the seminal vesicle. The sensations associated with ejaculation constitute the male orgasm.

Ejaculation is a reflex phenomenon. Afferent impulses arising principally from stimulation of the glans penis pass to the spinal cord by way of the internal pudendal nerves. Efferent impulses arising from a reflex center located in the upper lumbar region of the cord pass through sympathetic fibers in the hypogastric nerves and plexus to the ductus deferens and seminal vesicles. Other impulses arising from the 3rd and 4th sacral segments pass through the internal pudendal nerves to the ischiocavernous and bulbocavernous muscles.

Erection of the penis usually precedes ejaculation. Ejaculation occurs normally during copulation or it may occur as a nocturnal emission. The amount of seminal fluid discharged contains up to 300,000,000 spermatozoa.

RS: *coitus; excitation; orgasm; semen.*

ejac'ulatory. Pert. to ejaculation.

e. duct. The terminal portion of the seminal duct formed by the union of the ductus deferens and the excretory duct of the seminal vesicle.

ejecta (e-jek'tă) [L. *ejaculāri,* to throw out]. Matter thrown off by the body. SYN: *dejecta, egesta.*

EKG. Abbr. for *electrocardiogram.* SEE ALSO: *ECG.*

ekphorize (ek'fo-rīz) [G. *ek,* out, + *phorein,* to bear]. PSY: A bringing back of the effect of a psychic experience in an attempt to experience it again in memory. SEE: *engram.*

elaiopathy (e"la-op'ă-thĭ) [G. *elaion,* oil, + *pathos,* disease]. Swelling of joints due to contusion, followed by fatty deposits. SYN: *eleopathy.*

elastic (e-las'tik) [G. *elastikos,* elastic]. Capable of being stretched and returning to its original state; having elasticity.

e. bandage. One which can be stretched.

e. cartilage. Yellow cartilage such as is found in the epiglottis, pharynx, external ears, and auditory tube.

e. lamina. Descemet's membrane.

e. skin. Rare condition in which there is unusual elastic state of the skin.

e. stocking. One worn to place pressure on surface of the foot, or portion of the leg.

e. tissue. Connective tissue supplied with elastic fibers as found in the middle coat of arteries.

elasticity (e-las-tis'ĭ-tĭ) [G. *elastikos,* elastic]. The quality of returning to original size and shape after compression or stretching.

elastin (e-las'tin) [G. *elastikos,* elastic]. 1. An albuminoid substance forming the principal constituent of yellow elastic tissue, comprising about 30% of this tissue. 2. A protein which can be prepared from various connective tissues. SEE: *albumoid.*

elas'tinase [G. *elastikos,* elastic]. A ferment that dissolves elastin.

elas'toid [G. *elastikos,* elastic, + *eidos,* form]. Pert. to a substance formed by hyaline degeneration.

e. degeneration. Hyaline degeneration of elastic fibers of an artery.

elasto'ma [" + -*ōma*, tumor]. A chronic disease of the skin; pseudoxanthoma.

elastometer (e-las-tŏm'ĕ-ter) [" + *metron*, measure]. Device for measuring elasticity.

elastom'etry [" + *metron*, measure]. The measurement of elasticity of tissues.

elas'tose. A peptone resulting from gastric digestion of elastin.

elaterin (e-lăt'er-in) [G. *elatērios*, driving]. The neutral principle obtained from *elaterium*, a plant grown in the Mediterranean region. A cathartic.

ela'tion [L. *elatus*, borne out of]. PSY: Joyful emotion. It is pathologic when out of accord with patient's actual circumstances.

elbow (el'bō) [A.S. *eln*, forearm + *boga*, bend]. Joint of arm and forearm.

e. jerk. Striking tendon of biceps or triceps muscle causes involuntary bending or jerk of elbow.

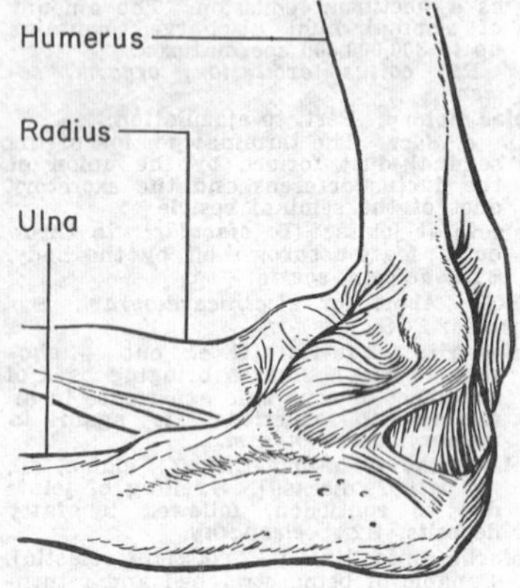

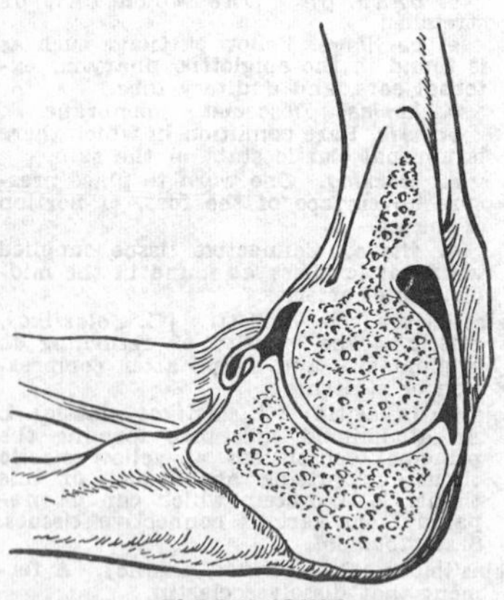

ELBOW JOINT
Upper, external view.
Lower, internal view.

e. joint. Joint between arm and the forearm. Includes the humeroulnar, humeroradial, and proximal radioulnar articulations.

e. reflex. Sharp extension of forearm resulting from tapping of triceps tendon while arm is held loosely in bent position.

elbow, words pert. to: anconad, anconeus, anconitis, tennis elbow.

elcosis (el-ko'sis) [G. *elkōsis*, ulceration]. Fetid ulceration.

Electra complex [G. *Elektra*, Agamemnon's daughter, who helped assassinate her mother, because of love for her father, whom the former had slain]. PSY: A group of symptoms due to suppressed sexual love of daughter for father. OPP: *Oedipus complex, q.v.*

elec'tric [G. *ēlektron*, amber]. Pert. to, caused by, or resembling electricity.

e. baker. Device for placing intense heat on a part, as in arthritis. SEE: *baker.*

e. contacts and injuries. Injuries from electricity vary with type and strength of current, length of contact, location of contact, such as legs, arms, etc., and hence vary from trivial burns to complete charring; or unconsciousness from either paralysis of the respiratory center, fibrillation of the heart, or both.

Direct currents of less than 300 volts are seldom fatal, but alternating currents of 15 to 60 cycles may be fatal, even when below 100 volts. Ordinary household or office currents vary from 30 to 220 volts.

INSULATION: Protection against such currents may be made with dry nonconductors, such as folded newspapers, magazines, cardboard, wood, rubber, clothing, etc. These may be used to move patient from the contact or to remove wire from patient. It is always preferable to turn off the current if possible. If patient is in water, remember that it is electrically charged and special precautions must be taken. On a humid or rainy day ordinary insulators may contain sufficient moisture to conduct electricity. Make sure insulators are dry.

High tension currents, such as those used about the x-ray or in conducting currents for long distances or for special industrial locations cannot be insulated by such means. Such currents may jump through rubber, paper, or strips of wood. A safe procedure is to ascertain the source of current and have it shut off, otherwise multiple tragedies result.

TREATMENT: SEE: *electric shock.*

e. field. Field exerting force of one dyne on unit positive charge.

e. shock. SYM: Burns, with loss of consciousness; contact or proximity to source of current are principal symptoms.

F. A. TREATMENT: Carefully free victim from source of current with nonconductors such as dry wood, paper, rubber, etc., or shut off current. Prolonged artificial respiration may be necessary. SEE: *resuscitation; shock.*

electri'city [G. *ēlektron*, amber]. "A form of energy which exhibits magnetic, chemical, mechanical, and thermal effects. Composed of two parts: positive which is protons and negative which is electrons.

e., frictional. Generation of static e. by rubbing two articles together.

e., galvanic. E. generated by chemical action.

e., induced. E. generated in a body from another body close by, without contact.

e., magnetic. E. induced by means of a magnetic device.

e., negative. Electric charge caused by an excess of electrons negatively charged.

e., positive. Electric charge caused by loss of negative electrons.

e., static. E. generated by friction.

e., unit of. SEE: *ampere; coulomb; farad; ohm; volt; watt.*

elec'trify [" + L. *facere,* to make]. To charge a body with electricity.

electriza'tion [G. *ēlektron,* amber]. The act of charging the body with electricity.

electroanesthesia [" + *a-,* priv. + *aisthēsis,* sensation]. 1. Local anesthesia induced by an anesthetizing substance injected into tissues by electricity. 2. General anesthesia produced by a device which passes electricity of a certain frequency, amplitude, and wave form through the brain. Has been used experimentally in both the U.S.S.R. and U.S.A.

electrobiol'ogy [" + *bios,* life, + *logos,* study of]. Science of electric phenomena in the living body.

electrobios'copy [" + " + *skopein,* to examine]. Electric test to determine if life is extinct.

electro"car'diogram [" + *kardia,* heart, + *gramma,* writing]. A record of the electrical activity of the heart; shows certain waves called P, Q. R, S, and T waves. Sometimes a U wave is seen. The first or P wave is caused by contraction of the atria. During this time the heart muscle is electrically polarized and then depolarized. The Q, R, S, and T waves are related to contraction of the ventricles. The cause of the U wave is unknown. The electrocardiogram gives important information concerning the spread of excitation to the different chambers of the heart and it is of value in the diagnosis of cases of abnormal cardiac rhythm and myocardial damage. ABBR: *ECG; EKG.*

electrocar'diograph [" + " + *graphein,* to write]. Device for recording electrical variations in action of heart muscles.

electrocardiog'raphy [" + " + *graphein,* to write]. The making and study of graphic records (electrocardiograms) produced by electrical currents originating in the heart.

elec"trocar"diopho'nograph [" + " + *phone,* voice, + *graphein,* to write]. Device for recording heart sounds.

elec"trocatal'ysis [" + *kata,* down, + *lysis,* loosening]. Chemical decomposition produced by electricity.

electro"cau'tery [" + *kauter,* burner]. Cauterization by means of an apparatus consisting of a holder containing a wire, which may be heated to a red or white heat by a current of electricity, either direct or alternating.

electrochem'istry [" + *chēmeia,* chemistry]. Science of chemical changes produced by electricity.

elec'trochemy [" + *chēmeia,* chemistry]. Therapy concerned with physical applications, such as electricity, which produce chemical effects in the tissues.

electrocis'ion [" + L. *caedare,* to cut]. Excision by electric current.

elec"trocoagula'tion [" + L. *coagulare,* to thicken]. Coagulation of tissue by means of a high frequency electric current. The heat producing the coagulation is generated within the tissue to be destroyed.

electrocontractility (e-lek"tro-kon-trak-tĭl'ĭ-tĭ) [" + L. *contrahere,* to contract]. Contraction of muscular tissue by electrical stimulation.

electrocryptectomy (e-lek"tro-krip-tek'to-mĭ) [" + *kryptos,* concealed, + *ektomē,* excision]. Destruction of tonsillar crypts by diathermy.

electrocu'tion [G. *ēlektron,* amber, + L. *secutus,* following]. The destruction of life by means of electric current.

electrocystoscopy (e-lek"tro-sis-tos'ko-pĭ) [" + *kystis,* bladder, + *skopein,* to examine]. The use of electric light to see the interior of the bladder.

elec'trode [" + *odos,* way]. A medium intervening bet. an electric conductor and the object to which the current is to be applied. In electrotherapy an electrode is an instrument with a point or a surface from which to discharge current to the body of a patient.

e., active. SEE: *therapeutic e.*

e., brush. A wire brush used to apply electricity to a part of the body.

e., depolarizing. E. with greater resistance than the part of the body in the circuit.

e., disper'sive. When electrodes may be applied in pairs dissimilar in size and shape, then the smaller electrode is called the active, and the larger, the dispersive, indifferent, or inactive electrode.

e., exciting. SEE: *therapeutic e.*

e., hydrogen. Form absorbing hydrogen gas.

e., impregnated. SEE: *therapeutic e.*

e., indifferent. SEE: *e., dispersive.*

e., multiple point. Several sets of terminals providing for the use of several electrodes. SEE: *multiterminal.*

e., negative. Cathode.

e., point. An electrode with an insulating handle at one end and a metallic point at the other for use in applying static sparks.

e., positive. Anode.

e., prescription. Therapeutic e. made according to a physician's prescription.

e., silent. SEE: *dispersive e.*

e., spark ball or point. An insulating handle having on one end a metallic ball or point. Used in giving static sparks.

e., therapeutic. E. devised so the carbon is impregnated with medicinal preparations.

elec"trodesicca'tion [" + L. *desiccāre,* to dry up]. The destructive drying of cells and tissue by means of short high frequency electric sparks, in contradistinction to fulguration, which is the destruction of tissue by means of long high-frequency electric sparks.

electro"dial'ysis. A method of separating electrolytes from colloids by passing a current through a solution containing both.

electrodynamometer (e-lek-tro-di-nă-mom'ĕ-ter) [" + *dynamis,* power, + *metron,* measure]. An instrument to measure the strength of an electric current.

electroencephalogram (ē-lek-trō-en-sef'ă-lō-gram) [G. *ēlektron,* amber, + *egkephalos,* brain, + *gramma,* a writing]. A tracing on an electroencephalograph.

electroencephalograph (ē-lĕk-trō-ĕn-sĕf'ă-lō-grăf) [" + " + *graphein,* to write]. An instrument for recording electrical activity of the brain.

electro"hemos'tasis. The arrest of bleeding by means of a high-frequency current.

electrol'ogy [" + *logos,* science]. The branch of science that deals with the phenomena and properties of electricity.

electrolysis (e-lek-trol'ĭ-sis) [" + *lysis,* a dissolution]. The decomposition of a substance by passage of an electrical current through it. Hair follicles may be destroyed by use of this method.

electrolyte (e-lek'tro-līt) [" + *lytos,* solution]. 1. A solution which is a conductor of electricity. 2. A substance which, in solution, conducts an electric current and is decomposed by the passage of an electric current.

Ex: Acids, bases, and salts are common electrolytes.

e., amphoteric. One which produces both hydrogen (H^-) and hydroxyl (OH^-) ions.

electrolytic (e-lek-tro-lit'ĭk) [" + *lytos,* solution]. Caused by or rel. to electrolysis.

e. conduction. In metals the electrical charges are carried by the electrons of inappreciable mass.

In solutions the electrical charges are carried by electrolytic ions, each one of a mass several thousand times as great as the electron. When a direct current passes through an electrolytic solution bet. metallic electrodes immersed in it, the positive ions move to the cathode, the negative ions to the anode.

electromag'net [" + *magnes,* magnet]. A magnet consisting of a length of insulated wire wound around soft iron core.

electromagnet'ic [" + *magnes,* magnet]. Pert. to an electromagnet.

e. induc'tion. Generation of an electromotive force in an insulated conductor moving in an electromagnetic field, or in a fixed conductor in a moving magnetic field.

electromag'netism [" + " + *ismos,* state of]. Magnetism produced by an electrical current.

electromassage [" + *massein,* to knead]. Massage combined with application of electrization.

electrom'eter [" + *metron,* measure]. An instrument for measuring pressure quantity and intensity of electricity, *i. e.,* differences in electric potential.

electromo'tive [" + L. *motor,* motion]. Pert. to passage of electricity in a current, or motion produced by it.

e. force. ABBR: EMF. That effect of differences of potential which, on the closing of a circuit, causes a flow of electricity from one place to another, giving rise to an electric current. The strength of an electric current is directly proportional to the impressed electromotive force, and inversely proportional to the resistance in the case of direct current and to the impedance in the case of alternating current. Electromotive force is measured in volts or in some convenient multiple or fraction of a volt. Microvolt, millivolt and kilovolt are, respectively, one-millionth volt, one-thousandth volt and 1000 volts.

electro"my'ogram. A graphic record of the contraction of a muscle as a result of electrical stimulation.

electro"myog'raphy. The preparation, study of, and interpretation of electromyograms.

elec'tron [G. *elektron,* amber]. An extremely minute corpuscle or charge of negative electricity which revolves about the central core or nucleus of an atom. They are the smallest known particles that exist, their mass being 1/1845 that of a hydrogen atom. When emitted from radioactive substances, they are known as *beta particles* or rays.

electro"narco'sis. The induction of narcosis by the application of electricity to the body. Used in the treatment of schizophrenia.

electro"neg'ative [" + L. *negāre,* to deny]. Condition of being charged with negative electricity which results in the attraction of bodies positively charged and the repulsion of bodies negatively charged.

electron'ic [G. *ēlektron,* amber]. Pert. to electrons.

electroniza'tion [G. *ēlektron,* amber]. The use of radiation to restore electrical equilibrium to diseased cells.

electropathol'ogy [" + " + *logos,* study of]. Determining electrical reaction of muscles and nerves as means of diagnosis.

electro"phore'sis (e-lek-tro-for-e'sis [" + *phorein,* to bear]. Diathermy or iontophoresis. SEE: *phoresis.* The movement of charged colloidal particles through the medium in which they are dispersed as a result of changes in electrical potential. Electrophoretic methods are useful in the analysis of protein mixtures as protein particles move with different velocities dependent principally on the number of charges carried by the particle.

electrophorus (e-lek-trŏf'o-rus) [" + *phorein,* to bear]. An instrument for obtaining static electricity by means of induction. SYN: *electrophore.*

electrophotother'apy [" + *phōs,* light, + *therapeia,* treatment]. Treatment by means of electric light.

electro"phre'nic. Pertaining to stimulation of the phrenic nerve by electricity.

electropos'itive [" + L. *positivus,* emphatic]. The condition of being subject to repulsion by bodies positively electrified, and to attraction by bodies negatively electrified.

electro"physiol'ogy [" + *physis,* nature, + *logos,* study of]. A branch of physiology which deals with the relations of body functions to electrical phenomena such as the effects of electrical stimulation upon the tissues, the production of electrical currents by organs and tissues, the therapeutic use of electric currents, etc.

elec'tropuncture [" + L. *punctura,* a piercing]. Piercing tissues with an electric needle.

electropyrexia (e-lek"tro-pi-REKS'ĭ-ă) [" + *pyressein,* to be feverish]. Elevation of temperature by electricity.

electroradiometer (e-lek"tro-ra-dĭ-om'ĕ-ter) [" + L. *radius,* ray, + G. *metron,* measure]. An electroscope for differentiation of radiant energy.

electro'retin'ogram. A record of the action currents of the retina made by placing one electrode upon the cornea and the other on the optic nerve or the posterior pole of the darkened eyeball.

electroscission (e-lek"tro-sĭ'zhun) [G. *ēlektron,* amber, + L. *scindere,* to cut]. Division of tissues by electrocautery.

electroscope (e-lek'tro-skōp) [" + *skopein,* to see]. An instrument which detects positive or negative static electricity.

elec'troshock. Shock produced by an electric current.

e. therapy. The induction of convulsive seizures by the passing of an electric current through the brain.

Used in the treatment of certain types of psychoses.

electrostat'ic [" + *statikos,* causing to stand]. Pert. to static electricity.

e. generator. A device that generates static electricity. SEE: *influence machine.*

e. unit. Any unit of electrical measurement based on the attraction or repulsion of a static charge, as distinguished from an electromagnetic unit, which is defined in terms of the attraction or repulsion of magnetic poles.

electrosur'gery [" + *cheir,* hand, + *ergon,* work]. Surgery accomplished by means of an electrical knife.

elec"trotax'is [" + *taxis,* arrangement]. The movement of a cell or an organism toward or away from an electrical stimulus.

elec"trothana'sia. Death resulting from electric shock; electrocution.

electrotherapeutics (e-lek"tro-ther-ă-pu'-tiks) [" + *therapeutikē,* treatment]. The use of electricity in the treatment of disease.

electrotherapist (e-lek"tro-ther'a-pist) [" + *therapeia,* treatment]. A physician who has had special training and has acquired skill in the therapeutic use of electricity. The term is sometimes used incorrectly to designate anyone who administers electrical treatments.

elec"trother'apy [" + *therapeia,* treatment]. Use of electricity in treating disease. SYN: *electrotherapeutics.*

elec'trotherm. An electrical apparatus for the therapeutic application of heat to the surface of the body. Used for relief of pain.

electrothermotherapy (e-lek"tro-ther"mo-ther'a-pĭ) [" + *thermē,* heat, + *therapeia,* treatment]. The production of heat within the living tissues for therapeutic purposes by means of bodily resistance to the passing of an electric current.

elec'trotome. An electrocautery device used for surgical procedures.

electroton'ic [" + *tonos,* tone]. Of or pert. to electrotonus.

electrotonus (e-lek-trot'o-nus) [" + *tonos,* tone]. The change in the irritability of a nerve or muscle during the passage of an electric current.

electrotropism (e-lek-trot'ro-pizm) [" + *tropē,* a turning, + *ismos,* condition of]. Reaction of cells to an electrical current.

electuary (e-lek'tu-a-rĭ) [G. *ekleichein,* to lick up]. Medicinal substance mixed with saccharine matter to form pasty mass.

eleidin (ĕ-lē'ĭ-din) [G. *elaion,* oil]. An acidophil substance present in the stratum lucidum of the epidermis.

el'ement [L. *elementum,* a rudiment]. In modern chemistry, a substance which cannot be separated into substances different from itself by ordinary chemical processes. They exist in a free and in a combined state. More than 100 have been identified. SEE: *Appendix for table of Chemical Elements.*

The e.'s of which the human body is composed are: oxygen, silicon, aluminum, carbon, hydrogen, nitrogen, calcium, phosphorus, potassium, sulfur, sodium, chlorine, magnesium, iron, fluorine, iodine, copper, manganese, and zinc.

e.'s, formed, of the blood. Erythrocytes, thrombocytes and leukocytes.

e.'s, trace. Chemical elements, extremely small amounts of which are present in the body or in the diet. Some are necessary in metabolism.

element, words pert. to: atom, body, chemical e., mineral e., monad, name of each element, oxidation, oxide, radical.

eleoma (el-e-o'mă) [G. *elaion,* oil, + *ōma,* tumor]. A neoplasm sometimes following injection of oil into the tissues.

eleometer (el-e-om'ĕ-ter) [" + *metron,* measure]. Instrument for determining quality and specific gravity of oils.

eleomyenchysis (el"e-o-mi-en'kis-is) [" + *mys,* muscle, + *egchysis,* infusion]. 1. The intramuscular injection of oils for chronic local spasms. 2. Prosthesis* by paraffin injection.

eleop'athy [" + *pathos,* disease]. Swelling of joints due to fatty deposits. SYN: *elaiopathy.*

eleoptene (el-e-op'tēn) [" + *ptēnos,* fleeting]. The fluid part of a volatile oil.

eleosaccharum (el"e-o-sak'ă-rum) [" + *sakcharon,* sugar]. A mixture of powdered sugar with a volatile oil.

eleotherapy (el-e-o-ther'ă-pĭ) [" + *therapeia,* treatment]. The use of oil for therapeutic purposes.

eleotho'rax [" + *thōrax,* chest]. The injection of oil into the pleural cavity to compress a tuberculous lung.

elephantiasis (el-ĕ-fan-ti'ă-sis) [G. *elephas,* elephant]. A chronic condition characterized by pronounced hypertrophy of the skin and subcutaneous tissues resulting from obstruction of the lymphatic vessels. The lower extremities and the scrotum are parts most frequently involved.

ETIOL: E. may be congenital (Milroy's disease), or the result of metastatic invasion of the lymph nodes by tumor cells; inflammatory e. results from filariasis or local infection of the lymph nodes. Elephantiasis is most common in tropical countries and is caused by infestation by *Wuchereria bancrofti,* a filarial worm; this type is called Bancroft's filariasis.

e. arabum. SYN: *elephantiasis.*

e. graecorum. Leprosy.

e. telangiectodes. E. which affects only a limited area of skin.

el'evator [L. *elevāre,* to lift]. 1. Curved retractor for holding lid away from the globe of the eye. 2. One for raising depressed bones by levers or screws.

eleventh cranial nerve. Accessory nerve, *q.v.*

eliminant (e-lim'ĭ-nant) [L. *ē,* out, + *līmen,* threshold]. 1. Effecting evacuation. 2. Agent aiding in elimination.

eliminate (e-lim'ĭ-nāte) [" + *līmen,* threshold]. To expel; to rid the body of waste material.

elimina'tion [" + *līmen,* threshold]. Excretion of waste body products by the skin, kidneys, and intestines.

e. diet. Based on patient's history of food sensitiveness and results of skin tests. The "elimination diet" found to relieve the patient's symptoms is increased by gradual addition of foods to which patient has been found to be nonsensitive, until insofar as possible all the essentials of an adequate diet are included.

elimination, words pert. to: constipation, defecation, dejecta, ejecta, evacuate, feces, names of excretions, nisus.

elinguation (e-lin-gwa'shun) [L. *ē,* out, + *lingua,* tongue]. The operation of removing the tongue from the oral cavity.

elixir [Arabic *alexir,* philosopher's stone]. A sweetened, aromatic, hydro-alcoholic liquid used in the compounding of oral medicines. Elixirs constitute one of the most commonly used classes of

Elements Having Medicinal Uses

Element	Compound Form	Some Medicinal Uses
Aluminum (Al)	Alum	Astringent to contract mucous membranes; as a gargle and a douche.
	Aluminum acetate	Astringent and antiseptic in surgical dressings.
	Aluminum hydroxide Aluminum phosphate	Antacids for gastric hyperchlorhydria.
Barium (Ba)	Barium sulfate	Coats the stomach and intestines for taking x-ray pictures.
Bismuth (Bi)	Bismuth subnitrate	Insoluble compounds used as dusting powders on the skin.
	Bismuth subcarbonate	Astringent, antacid and coating in diarrhea and gastroenteritis.
Bromine (Br)	Sodium and Potassium Bromide	Nerve sedatives.
Calcium (Ca)	Calcium carbonate (chalk)	Antacid.
	Calcium chloride Calcium gluconate Calcium phosphate	Replenish electrolytes.
	Calcium cyclamate	Noncaloric sweetening agent.
	Calcium hydroxide (lime water)	Antacid; calcium replacement; antidote in acid poisonings.
Chlorine (Cl)	Sodium chloride	Common salt.
	Chlorinated lime	Disinfectant for urinals and excreta. A deodorant.
Copper (Cu)	Copper sulfate (blue vitriol)	Removes granulations on the eyelids in trachoma. Produces vomiting. Used as an astringent.
Hydrogen (H)	All acids, *e. g.*, hydrochloric	Dilute solutions extract water from the tissues, and in the stomach aid digestion.
	Hydrogen peroxide	Antiseptic.
Iodine (I)	Iodine tincture Potassium iodide	Antiseptic.
Iron (Fe)	Ferrous salts	Hematinic as in cases of anemia. Astringent.
Magnesium (Mg)	Magnesium carbonate	Antacid.
	Magnesium hydroxide suspension (milk of magnesia)	Antacid and laxative.
	Magnesium oxide	Antacid.
	Magnesium silicate, hydrous (talc)	Dusting powder.
	Magnesium sulfate (Epsom salt)	Cathartic; local anti-inflammatory agent.
	Magnesium trisilicate	Antacid.
Nitrogen (N)	Nitrous oxide (laughing gas)	General anesthetic.
	Ammonia water	Cleanser; reflex stimulant by inhalation.
Oxygen (O)		Used in resuscitation in anoxemia and in determination of basal metabolic rate.
Phosphorus (P)	Sodium phosphate	Saline purgative. Reduces accumulation of fluid in the tissues, as in edema.
Potassium (K)	Potassium acetate	Diuretic.
	Potassium bicarbonate	Electrolyte replenisher.
	Potassium chloride	Electrolyte replenisher.
	Potassium iodide	Expectorant. Also source of iodine.
	Potassium permanganate	In solution, as a topical anti-infective agent in various skin affections, or for gastric lavage in certain poisonings.
	Potassium sodium tartrate (Rochelle salts)	Mild cathartic.

Elements Having Medicinal Uses

Element	Compound Form	Some Medicinal Uses
Radium (Ra)	Radium salts	Treatment for neoplasms.
Silver (Ag)	Silver nitrate	Antiseptic to contract mucous membranes of eye, to cauterize, and for nose and throat inflammations.
Sodium (Na)	Sodium bicarbonate (baking soda)	In intravenous fluids.
Sulfur (S)		Used in ointments for skin diseases. May be used as a laxative.
Zinc (Zn)	Zinc oxide	Astringent and protective for skin conditions.
	Zinc peroxide	Anti-infective and deodorant for skin diseases.
	Zinc stearate	Dusting powder (irritating if inhaled).
	Zinc sulfate	Ophthalmic astringent.

preparations, and contribute largely toward the possibility of pleasant medication.

El'liott treatment [Charles R. Elliott, American gynecologist]. Treatment given by means of rubber bag that distends vagina when attached to machine delivering water at temperature of 115° to 128° F. maintained for 45 to 60 minutes; used in pelvic inflammatory disease.

Ellis-Van Creveld syndrome. SEE: *dysplasia, chondroectodermal.*

elutriation (e-lū-trĭ-a'shun) [L. *elutriāre,* to cleanse]. The separation of insoluble particles from finer ones by decanting the fluid.

elytritis (el-ĭ-tri'tis) [G. *elytron,* vagina, + *itis,* inflammation]. Inflammation of the vagina. SYN: *colpitis.*

elytrocele (el'ĭ-tro-sēl) [" + *kēlē,* hernia]. Hernia into the vagina. SYN: *colpocele.*

elytroclasia (el"ĭ-tro-kla'sĭ-a) [" + *klasis,* rupture]. Rupture of the vagina.

elytrocleisis (el"ĭ-tro-kli'sis) [" + *kleisis,* closure]. Surgical closure of the vagina. SYN: *colpocleisis.*

elytroplasty (el'ĭ-tro-plas"tĭ) [" + *plassein,* to form]. Plastic operation upon the vagina. SYN: *colpoplasty.*

elytroptosis (ĕl"ĭ-trŏp-tō'sĭs) [" + *ptōsis,* a dropping]. Prolapse of the vagina. SYN: *colpoptosis.*

elytrorrhaphy (el-ĭ-tror'ră-fĭ) [" + *raphē,* suture]. Suture of vaginal wall. SYN: *colporrhaphy.*

elytrostenosis (el"i-tro-sten-o'sis) [" + *stenōsis,* narrowing]. Narrowing of the vagina. SYN: *colpostenosis.*

elytrotomy (el-ĭ-trot'o-mĭ) [" + *tomē,* incision]. Incision into vaginal wall. SYN: *colpotomy.*

emaciate (e-mā-sĭ-āt) [L. *ēmaciāre,* to grow thin]. To cause to become excessively lean.

ema'ciated. Excessively lean.

emacia'tion [L. *ēmaciāre,* to grow thin]. Wasting of the flesh; state of being extremely lean.

ETIOL: Malnutrition; diseases of gastrointestinal canal. If rapid: Marasmus, Addison's d., tuberculosis, cancer, diabetes, suppuration, hyperthyroidism, chronic diarrhea, stricture of esophagus, pyloric obstruction; parasites; loss of sleep, exophthalmic goiter, starvation. SEE: *lean, tabes, wasting.*

emaculation (em-ak-u-la'shun) [L. *ēmaculāre,* to remove spots]. Removal of spots from the skin.

emailloid (em-a'loid) [Fr. *ēmail,* enamel, + G. *eidos,* form]. Tumor having its origin in tooth enamel.

emana'tion [L. *ē,* out, + *manāre,* to flow]. 1. Something given off; radiation; emission. 2. A disintegration product.

e., actinium. One given off by actinium. SYN: *actinon.*

e., radium. A radioactive gas given off by radium. SYN: *niton.*

e., thorium. One given off by thorium. SYN: *thoron.*

emansio mensium (em-an'sĭ-o men'sĭ-um) [L.]. Amenorrhea in which menstruation has never occurred.

emasculation (e-mas-ku-la'shun) [L. *ēmasculāre,* to castrate]. 1. Castration. 2. Excision of the entire male genitalia.

embalming (em-bahm'ing) [L. *in,* in, + *balsămum,* balsam] Preservation of a dead body against putrefaction.

embed'ding [" + A.S. *bedd,* to bed]. In histology, the process by which a piece of tissue is placed in a firm medium such as paraffin or celloidin in order to support it and keep it intact during the subsequent cutting into thin sections for microscopic examination.

embola'lia [G. *embolos,* thrown in, + *lalia,* babble]. Meaningless language of the insane. SYN: *embolophrasia.*

embole (em'bo-lĕ) [G. a throwing in]. 1. Reduction of a dislocation. 2. Formation of the gastrula by invagination. 3. Enarthrosis. SYN: *emboly.*

embol'ic. Pert. to or caused by embolism.

embol'iform [G. *embolos,* thrown in, + L. *forma,* form]. 1. Resembling a nucleus. 2. Wedge-shaped, as the *nucleus emboliformis.*

embolism (em'bo-lizm) [G. *embolē,* a throwing in, + *ismos,* condition]. Obstruction of a blood vessel by foreign substance or a blood clot. RS: *embolus, thrombosis, thrombus.*

Diagnosis depends upon the factors predisposing. Arteriosclerosis favors a diagnosis of thrombosis, while atrial fibrillation, bacterial endocarditis, or thrombophlebitis points to embolism. Nearly always embolism is due to blood clots.

NP: Postoperative cases must be handled with great care. Sudden sitting up or turning over may displace an embolus into the circulation and cause sudden death. Fat embolism is not uncommon in bone injuries and fractures, and bacterial emboli may be present in so-called blood poisoning.

e., air. One caused by air bubble. SEE: *air embolism.*

e., fat. Globules of fat obstructing blood vessels.

e., pulmonary. Obstruction of the pulmonary artery or one of its branches. Usually caused by an embolus from thrombosis in lower extremities.

e., pyemic. E. caused by purulent matter.

embolophrasia (em"bol-o-fra'zĭ-ă) [" + *phrasis*, utterance]. Meaningless speech. SYN: *embolalia.*

em'bolus (pl. *emboli*) [G. *embolos*, plug]. A mass of undissolved matter present in a blood or lymphatic vessel brought there by the blood or lymph current. Emboli may be solid, liquid, or gaseous. Other emboli may consist of bits of tissue, tumor cells, globules of fat, air bubbles, clumps of bacteria, and foreign bodies such as bullets. Emboli may arise within the body or they may gain entrance from without. Occlusion of vessels from emboli usually results in the development of infarcts, *q.v.* SEE: *thrombus, thrombosis.*

e., air. An air bubble in the veins, the right atrium, or ventricle, or in the capillaries. SEE: *air embolism.*

e., coronary. May be complication of arteriosclerosis and cause angina pectoris. SYM: Similar to pulmonary e.

e., pulmonary. E. in pulmonary artery or one of its branches.

em'boly [G. *embolē*, a throwing in]. Formation of the gastrula from invagination. SYN: *embole.*

embrace reflex (em-brās') [L. *brachium*, arm]. A variety of defensive reflex. The throwing out of the arms in an attitude of embrace, in fearful response. SYN: *Moro's reflex.*

embrasure (em-bra'shur) [Fr. *embrasér*, to widen an opening]. An opening widening outwardly or inwardly.

e., buccal. Opening spreading toward the buccal aspect.

e., labial. Embrasure opening toward the labial aspect.

e., lingual. One spreading to the lingual aspect.

e., occlusal. Space mesially and distally bet. marginal ridges of approximating teeth.

embroca'tion [G. *embrochē*, fomentation]. 1. Application of a liniment to the skin, esp. one that acts as a counterirritant to the skin. For example: turpentine; methyl salicylate. 2. A drug rubbed into the skin.

embryectomy (em-brĭ-ek'to-mĭ) [G. *embryon*, embryo, + *ektomē*, excision]. Removal of an extrauterine embryo.

embryo (em'brĭ-o) (G. *embryon*]. 1. The young of any organism in an early stage of development. 2. Stage in prenatal development of a mammal between the ovum and the fetus. In humans, stage of development between the second and eight weeks, inclusive.

STAGES OF DEVELOPMENT: Following fertilization, cells multiply (cleavage) resulting in formation of a *morula* which develops into a *blastocyst*, consisting of a trophoblast and inner cell mass. Two cavities (amniotic cavity and yolk sac) arise within the *inner cell mass.* These are separated by the *embryonic disk* which gives rise to the three germ layers (*ectoderm, mesoderm,* and *endoderm*) which develop into the *embryo proper;* the blastocyst wall or *trophoblast* gives rise to auxiliary structures.

During the period of the embryo (3rd to 8th weeks) the germ layers of the embryonic disk give rise to the principal organ systems and the body acquires a somewhat human form. After the second month, the developing young is called a *fetus.*

e., development of. 1. *Period of the ovum;* (first two weeks) Blastocyst forms. Embryo enters uterus and implantation occurs. 2. *Period of the embryo* (3rd to 8th weeks). Embryo increases in length from about 1.5 mm. to 23 mm. Organ systems arise and embryo acquires human form. 3. *Period of the fetus* (3rd to 9th month) (a) 3rd month, 4 in. long.

The alimentary canal, liver, pancreas, and lungs develop from *endoderm;* muscle, all connective tissues, blood, lymphatic tissue and the epithelium of blood vessels, body cavities, kidney, gonads, and suprarenal cortex develop from *mesoderm;* the epidermis nervous tissue, hypophysis, and the epithelium of the organs, nasal cavity, mouth, salivary glands, bladder, and urethra develop from *ectoderm.*

embryocardia (em-brĭ-o-kar'dĭ-ă) [G. *embryon*, embryo, + *kardia*, heart]. Heart action in which first and second sounds are equal, and resemble the fetal heart sounds. A sign of cardiac distress. SYN: *tic-tac rhythm.*

embryoctony (em-brĭ-ok'to-nĭ) [" + *kteinein*, to kill]. Destroying the fetus in utero, as in cases where delivery is impossible, or for abortion. SEE: *craniotomy.*

embryogenet'ic, embryogen'ic [" + *gennan*, to originate]. Pert. to or giving rise to an embryo.

embryogeny (em-brĭ-oj'ĕ-nĭ) [" + *gennan*, to develop]. The growth and development of an embryo.

embryog'raphy [" + *graphein*, to write]. A treatise on the embryo.

embryol'ogy [" + *logos*, study]. The science which deals with the origin and development of an individual organism.

embryo'ma (em-brĭ-o'mă) [" + *ōma*, tumor]. A tumor consisting of derivatives of the embryonic germ layers but lacking in organization; a dermoid cyst.

em'bryonal [G. *embryon*, embryo]. Pert. to or resembling an embryo.

embryonic (em-brĭ-on'ĭk) [G. *embryon*, embryo]. Pert. to or in condition of an embryo.

embryoniza'tion [G. *embryon*, embryo]. Reversion of a cell or tissue to an embryonic structure.

embryonoid (em'brĭ-o-noyd) [" + *eidos*, form]. Having the appearance of an embryo.

embryoplas'tic [" + *plassein*, to form]. Having a part in the formation of an embryo; said of cells.

embryotocia (em"brĭ-o-to'sĭ-ă) [" + *tokos*, birth]. An abortion; delivery of an embryo.

embryotome (em'brĭ-o-tōm) [" + *tomē* incision]. Instrument used in dismemberment of fetus in utero.

embryotomy (em-brĭ-ot'o-mĭ) [" + *tomē*, incision]. The dissection of a fetus to aid its delivery.

embryotoxon (em-brĭ-o-tox'on) [" + *toxon*, bow]. Congenital marginal opacity of the cornea. SYN: *arcus juvenilis.*

embryotroph (em′bri-o-trof) [" + *trophē*, nourishment]. A fluid resulting from the enzyme action of the trophoblasts upon the neighboring maternal tissue and which nourishes the embryo from the time of implantation into the uterus.

embryotrophy (em-brĭ-ot′ro-fĭ) [" + *trophē*, nourishment]. Nutrition of the fetus.

embryulcia (em-brĭ-ul′sĭ-ă) [" + *elkein*, to draw]. Forcible removal of the fetus as by embryotomy or taking a dead fetus with instruments.

embryulcus (em-brĭ-ul′kus) [G. *embryoulkos*]. Instrument for extracting a fetus.

emedullate (e-med′u-lāt) [L. *ē*, out, + *medulla*, marrow]. To remove the marrow from a bone.

emer′gency [L. *emergere*, to raise up]. An unexpected serious happening, demanding immediate action.

e. *light reflex.* Marked pupillary contraction, frowning, and closure of eyelids, resulting from sudden powerful light stimulus of retina.

e. *theory.* Formulated by Cannon: Adrenal secretion is stimulated by sympathetic nervous system activity to meet bodily emergencies, as emotional excitement, pain, etc.

emergency, *words pert. to:* asphyxia, asphyxiation, bites, choking, convulsion, dislocation, drowning, fainting, fire emergencies, foreign bodies, fumes, gases, poisoning, shock, stings, unconsciousness.

emer′gent [L. *emergere*, to raise up]. 1. Growing from a cavity or other part. 2. Sudden, unforeseen.

emesis (em′ĕ-sis) [G. *emein*, to vomit]. Vomiting.

May be gastric, systemic, nervous, reflex, or irritation of vomiting center.

NP: The relation of vomiting to eating is important, and the nurse should determine how it is affected by pain, by soft or solid foods, by liquids, by odors before or after eating or drinking. Note the type, character, and color of vomitus.

If patient is extremely weak, barely conscious, or comatose while vomiting, then great care must be exercised to prevent aspiration of food into the lungs. Elevate foot of bed and have suction apparatus available for removing vomitus from hypopharynx if necessary. Tracheotomy may be required. SEE: *anacathartic, antemetic, emetic, vomit, vomitus.*

e., *gastric.* In gastric ulcer, gastric carcinoma, acute gastritis, chronic gastritis, gastrectasis, gastric hyperesthesia, hyperacidity and hypersecretion, Asiatic cholera, pressure upon stomach.

e. *gravidarum.* Vomiting of pregnancy.

e., *irritation.* Drugs, uremia, nephritis, some brain tumors, chloroform, ether.

e., *nervous.* Tumor or abscess of brain, sea sickness, acute myelitis, meningitis, anemia and hyperemia of brain, concussion and contusion of brain, fracture of skull, Ménière's disease, migraine, paresis, sclerosis.

e., *reflex.* Irritation of fauces and pharynx; coughing, removal of viscous secretion from nasopharynx, eyestrain, unpleasant odors and sights, shock, nervousness, anticipation, anxiety, hysteria, morning sickness, gastric crisis of tabes, various heart troubles, hiccough.

e., *systemic.* Pulmonary tuberculosis, whooping cough, peritonitis, irritations of bowels, acute obstruction of bowels, renal or biliary colic, Addison's disease.

emetic (e-met′ik) [G. *emein*, to vomit]. Medicine that produces vomiting. Ex: *apomorphine, a. hydrochloride, ipecac, mustard, sodium chloride.*

e., *direct.* Those acting directly on gastric nerves, *e.g.*, mustard.

e., *indirect.* Those acting on vomiting center of brain, as apomorphine.

e., *local.* Those which act through nerve irritation, such as salt.

e., *systemic.* Those acting through the circulation, irritating vomiting centers by stimulation, such as mustard, soapy water, syrup of ipecac.

One tablespoonful of mustard in ½ pint of water; or 2 tablespoons of common salt with sufficient water to be swallowed.

PROCEDURE TO INDUCE VOMITING: Dilute contents of stomach before giving any emetic. Emetics may be dangerous because of their own toxic effect, as in severe heart or blood vessel diseases, tuberculosis, advanced pregnancy, rupture, ulcers of the stomach, or corrosive poisoning. For these reasons chemical emetics are omitted from the nurse's treatment of poisoning.

Vomiting may be induced by generous amounts of warm water, preferably warm soapy water and by titillating the uvula or posterior pharynx. Gastric lavage is preferable to emetics in poisoning. Emetics may induce vomiting by their local effect, as copper sulfate or zinc sulfate, mustard, ipecac, etc., in small doses diluted in water; or by their effect on the central nervous system, such as apomorphine hydrochloride which works by hypodermic injection. Emesis is much more likely to take place when the stomach is distended.

emetine (em′ĕ-tēn, -tin) [G. *emein*, to vomit]. Powdered, white alkaloid obtained from ipecac, *q.v.*

e. *bismuth iodide.* A combination of emetine and bismuth containing about 20% emetine and 20% bismuth.

ACTION AND USES: Same as emetine.

e. *hydrochloride.* USP. The hydrated hydrochloride of an alkaloid obtained from ipecac. It has an antiamebic action.

em′etism [G. *emein*, to vomit, + *ismos*, condition of]. Poisoning from overdose of ipecac.

SYM: Acute inflammation of pylorus, hyperemesis, diarrhea, and perhaps coughing and suffocation.

emetocathar′tic [" + *katharsis*, a purging]. Producing both emesis and catharsis.

emetol′ogy [" + *logos*, understanding]. Study of emetics and their action.

E. M. F. Abbr. for *electromotive force; erythrocyte maturation factor.*

emiction (e-mik′shun) [L. *ē* + *mingere*, to urinate]. The act of urination.

emigra′tion [" + *migrāre*, to move]. Passage of white blood corpuscles through the walls of capillaries and veins during inflammation.

em′inence [" + *minere*, to hang on]. A prominence or projection, esp. of a bone.

e., *arcuate.* A rounded eminence on upper surface of petrous portion of temporal bone. SYN: *eminentia arcuata* [NA].

e., *articular, of the temporal bone.* A rounded e. forming ant. boundary of the glenoid fossa. SYN: *tuberculum articulare* [NA].

e., auditory. A collection of gray matter on floor of 4th ventricle of brain at its lower part, forming the deep origin of the auditory nerve.

e., bicipital. A tuberosity for insertion of biceps muscle on radius.

e., blastodermic. An elevated mass of cells of a developing ovum forming the blastoderm.

e., canine. A vertical ridge on the external surface of the superior maxilla.

e., collateral. One bet. middle and post. horns in lat. ventricle of brain. SYN: *eminentia collateralis* [NA].

e. of Doyère. Slight elevation of muscular fiber corresponding to entrance of a nerve fiber.

e., frontal. A rounded prominence on either side of median line, a little below center of frontal bone. SYN: *tuber frontale* [NA].

e., germinal. Cumulus oophorus, *q.v.*

e., hypothenar. One on ulnar side of palm, formed by muscles of little finger.

e., iliopectineal; e., iliopubic. E. on upper aspect of pubic bone above the acetabulum, marking the junction of bone with the ilium. SYN: *eminentia iliopectinea* [NA].

e., intercondyloid. A process on the head of the tibia lying between the two condyles. SYN: *intercondylar e.; eminentia condyloidea; eminentia intercondylaris* [NA].

e., mamillary. Projection of inner pillars of fornix. SYN: *mammillary body; corpora mammillares* [NA].

e., median. Ant. bodies of medulla oblongata separated by ant. median fissure. SYN: *eminentia medialis* [NA].

e., nasal. A prominence on vertical portion of frontal bone above the nasal notch and bet. the two superciliary ridges.

e., occipital. Protuberance on occipital bone.

e., olivary. Oval projection at upper part of medulla oblongata above extremity of lateral column. SYN: *olivary body; oliva* [NA].

e., parietal. The marked convexity on outer surface of parietal bone. SYN: *parietal tuber; tuber parietale* [NA].

e.'s, portal. The small median lobes on lower surface of liver.

e., pyramidal. An elevation on the mastoid wall of the tympanic cavity. It contains a cavity in which lies the stapedius muscle. SYN: *pyramid of tympanum; eminentia pyramidalis* [NA].

e., thenar. E. formed by muscles, below the thumb on the palm of the hand.

eminentia (em-in-en'shĭ-ă) [L.]. An eminence, *q.v.*

emissary (em'ĭ-sa-rĭ) [L. *ē*, out, + *mittere*, to send]. 1. Providing an outlet. 2. An outlet.

e. veins. Small veins piercing the skull, carrying blood from the sinuses within the skull to the veins without.

emissio (e-mis'sĭ-o) [L.]. A discharge; emission.*

e. seminis. Discharge of semen.

emission (e-mish'un) [L. *ē*, out, + *mittere*, to send]. The sending forth or discharge of a portion of that which remained as an atomic particle, exhalation, or a light or heat wave.

e., nocturnal. Involuntary discharge of semen during sleep.

emmenagogue (em-en'ă-gog) [G. *emmēna*, menses, + *agein*, to lead]. A substance which assists the menstrual function.

e., direct. That which has a direct effect on the reproductive tract such as a hormone.

e., indirect. An agent which alters the menstrual function by changing the general state of health.

emmenia (em-me'nĭ-ă) [G. *emmēna*]. The menstrual flow.

emmen'ic. Pert. to the menses.

emmeniopathy (em-me-nĭ-op'ă-thĭ) [" + *pathos*, disease]. Any disorder of menstruation.

emmenology (em"en-ol'o-jĭ) [" + *logos*, science]. Science of menstruation.

emmetrope (em'mĕ-trōp) [G. *emmetros*, in due measure, + *opsis*, sight]. One endowed with normal vision.

emmetropia (em-me-tro'pĭ-ă) [" + *opsis*, sight]. Normal condition of eye in refraction; with eye at rest parallel rays are focused on retina; ability to focus on the retina a luminous point from 3.9 to 4.7 in. from the eye. SEE: *astigmatism; myopia*.

emmetrop'ic. Normal in vision. SEE: *hypermetropic; myopic*.

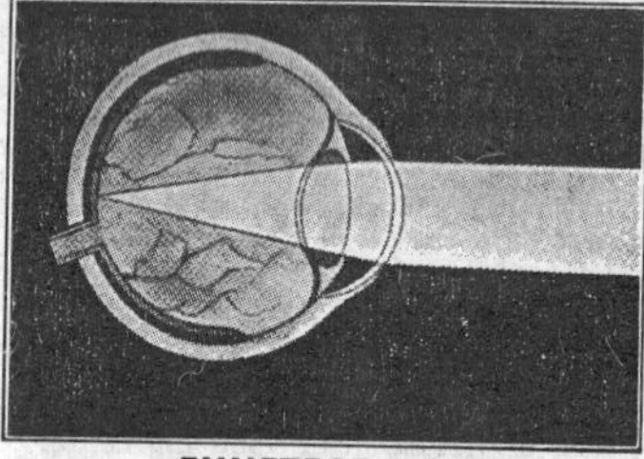

EMMETROPIC EYE

Parallel light rays brought to a focus upon retina, with lens at rest.

Em'met's operation [Thomas A. Emmet, American gynecologist, 1828-1919]. 1. Uterine trachelorrhaphy. 2. Suturing of a lacerated perineum. 3. Converting a sessile submucous tumor of the uterus into a pedunculated one. 4. Operation for prolapse of uterus.

emollient (e-mol'yent) [L. *ē*, out, + *mollīre*, to soften]. An agent that will soften and soothe the part when applied locally. The term is usually confined to agents affecting the surface of the body. Ex: *ointment of rose water, olive oil, petrolatum*. SEE: *demulcent*.

e. enema. One for the purpose of coating membranes and allaying local pain and irritation, in order to soften and protect tissues. SEE ALSO UNDER: *enema*.

emotion (e-mo'shun) [L. *ēmovēre*, to disturb]. 1. A mental state or strong feeling affect usually accompanied by physical changes in the body such as alteration in heart rate and respiratory activity, vasomotor reactions, and changes in muscle tone. 2. A mental state or feeling such as fear, hate, love, anger, grief, joy. These constitute the "drive" which brings about the motor adjustment necessary to satisfy instinctive needs.

Frustration is normally associated with displeasure and the intensifying of need; the process of gratification is accompanied by pleasurable feeling tone which persists for a variable period in less intense form. Physiologic changes invariably accompany the emotion but such change may not be apparent to either the person experiencing the emotion or an observer.

Anxiety, or fear, arises when one doubts his ability adequately to meet a situation; neutralization consists of "flight" from the danger, and a struggle (fight) to remove the threat. The physical changes are those favorable to success and phylogenetically may well have antedated the psychic phase of the fear. Often a partial syndrome of fear may exist with this latter phase apparently absent (and denied), and then the condition may be considered heart disease, stomach trouble, toxic goiter, etc. Other physical affect reactions may be similarly confusing. Civilized man may find an instinctive goal unattainable because his conditioned (moral) reactions regard the goal as socially objectionable (or even deny the goal entirely). Here arise the conflict and the starting point of psychogenic disease.

e., disorders of. An emotion is not felt in the same way by healthy persons as by one suffering from schizophrenia. In the latter, there is a decrease of pleasure, hate, love, and other emotions. There is loss of ability to feel and express emotions such as love or hate. The patient is said to be *blunted*. The emotions he does show are not in harmony with his ideas; for example, he may smile while describing tortures and terrors.

Unhappiness is marked in manic depressive psychosis. It varies in degree and may lead to suicide. In the excited stage undue happiness is marked. Depressions and elations have no apparent cause.

Emotions are easily aroused in aged persons and in alcoholics.

Depressed patients are so wrapped up in their own misery they take no notice of anything else. Excited patients cannot concentrate their attention. Confused ones may not realize they are not in the proper place for their actions. Hallucinating patients are influenced by imaginary voices, visions, places and persons. Deluded ones have unreasonable fears.

emotion, words pert. to: affective, alusia, amor, athymia, cathexis, manias, parapathia, psychiatry, sex.

emo'tional [L. *ēmovere*, to disturb]. Relating to any of the emotions.

e. attitudes. Those which express any of the emotions, such as joy, sorrow, etc. Seen in hysteroepilepsy.

e. disturbance. Mental illness.

e. instability. Psy: Given to easy rage, brooding, and vastly fluctuating moods.

emotivity (e-mo-tiv'ĭ-tĭ) [L. *ē*, out, + *motus*, moving]. One's capability for emotional response.

em'pasm. A powder, usually perfumed, for external application to the body.

empath'ic. Pert. to, or characterized by, empathy.

empathy (em'pă-thĭ) [G. *en*, in, + *pathos*, feeling]. Objective awareness of and insight into the feelings, emotions, and behavior of another person; and their meaning and significance. Not the same as sympathy which is usually nonobjective and noncritical.

emphlysis (em'flis-is) (pl. *emphlyses*) [" + *phlysis*, an eruption]. Any vesicular or exanthematous eruption.

emphractic (em-frak'tik) [G. *emphraxis*, an obstruction]. 1. Obstructive, as clogging of pores of skin. 2. Anything that obstructs a function.

emphraxis (em-frak'sis). A stoppage, or obstruction; an infarction.

emphysatherapy (em-fiz-ă-ther'ă-pĭ) [G. *emphysan*, to inflate, + *therapeia*, treatment]. Injection of gas into a cavity for therapeutic purposes.

emphysema (em-fi-se'mă) [G. *emphysan*, to inflate]. 1. Distention of tissues by gas or air in the interstices. 2. A condition in which the alveoli of the lungs become distended or ruptured. Usually the result of an interference with expiration, or loss of elasticity of the lung. Syn: *pulmonary emphysema*.

e., atrophic. Senile e.

e., chronic hypertrophic. E. accompanied with bony changes resulting in the so-called barrel chest.

e., compensatory. E. which results from overstretching of a functional part of the lung when another portion fails to function. A secondary condition seen in tuberculosis or pneumonia. Also called *complemental e.*

e., interstitial. Rupture of air cells from overdistention, and escape of air into interlobular tissue.

e., subcutaneous. Presence of air or gas in subcutaneous tissues, with consequent distention. Often caused by infection by gas-producing organisms, esp. *Clostridium perfringens*.

e., surgical. Subcutaneous emphysema due to operation, esp. after wounds of respiratory tract.

e., vesicular. Overdistention of alveoli and smaller bronchial tubes with air. Sym: Dyspnea upon exertion; accelerated pulse, cough, and expectoration of whitish mucus. Short inspiration, prolonged expiration.

emphysematous (em-fi-sem'ă-tus) [G. *emphysan*, to inflate]. Affected with or pert. to emphysema.

empir'ic [G. *empeirikos*, experimental]. 1. Based on experience. See: *empirical*. 2. A physician whose skill or art is based upon what has been learned through experience.

empirical (em-pir'ik-al) [G. *empeirikos*, skilled]. Based on experience and usually without respect to scientific principles.

empiricism (em-pir'is-izm) [" + *ismos*, condition of]. 1. Experience, not theory, as basis of medical science. 2. Quackery.

empirin compound. Proprietary name for an analgesic and antipyretic compound for oral administration. Each tablet contains acetylsalicylic acid, acetophenitidin, and caffeine.

emplastic (em-plas'tik) [G. *emplastikos*, clogging]. 1. A constipating medicine. 2. Adhesive or able to be used as a plaster or in one.

emplas'trum (pl. *emplastra*) [G. *emplastron*, a plaster]. Preparation for external application; adheres to the skin when applied. See: *plaster*.

emprosthotonos (em-pros-thot'o-nos) [G. *emprosthen*, forward, + *tonos*, tension]. Lying with body incurved and resting upon forehead and feet with face downward. See: *Illustration*, p. E-19.

Sometimes seen in tetanus and strychnine poisoning. The reverse of *opisthotonos*. See: *posture*.

emptysis (ĕmp'tĭ-sĭs) [G. a spitting]. Expectoration of blood or blood-stained mucus; hemoptysis.

empyema (em-pī-e'ma) [G. *en*, within, + *pyon*, pus]. Pus in a body cavity, esp. in the pleural cavity (pyothorax). Usually result of a primary infection in the lungs.

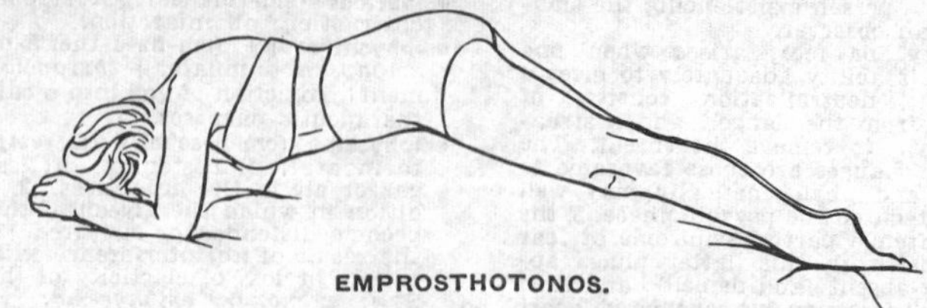

EMPROSTHOTONOS.

SYM: Chills, fever, and sweating. Skin is gray, malar flush, appetite poor, marked malaise, pain in chest, cough, emaciation. Dyspnea may ensue.

TREATMENT: Antibiotic therapy, aspiration of pleural fluid. Treatment of primary condition. Surgical drainage may be necessary.

NP: *Postoperative*: Patient should sit up inclined to affected side to facilitate drainage, then to opp. side to aid expansion of lung; high protein, high vitamin diet; breathing exercises. SEE: *resection.*

e., interlobular. Form with pus bet. lobes of lung.

e. necessitatis. Form in which pus can escape spontaneously.

e., pulsating. Form with cardiac beats causing pulsation of chest wall.

empyesis (em-pī-e'sis) [G. *empyein,* to suppurate]. A pustular eruption on the skin.

empyocele (ĕm'pī-ō-sēl) [" + *kēlē,* tumor]. A collection of pus in a sacculated cavity, especially in the scrotum; a suppurating hydrocele.

emul'gent [L. *ēmulgere,* to drain out]. Extracting or draining.

e. vessel. Blood vessel of the kidney.

emulsifica'tion [L. *emulsio,* emulsion, + *facere,* to make]. 1. Process of making an emulsion. 2. The breaking down of large fat globules in the intestine to smaller, uniformly distributed particles, accomplished largely through the action of bile acids which lower surface tension.

emul'sifier [" + *facere,* to make]. Anything used to make an emulsion.

emulsify (e-mul'sĭ-fī) [" + *facere,* to make]. To form into an emulsion.

emul'sion [L. *emulsiō*]. A mixture of two liquids not mutually soluble.

If they are thoroughly shaken, one will divide into globules and is called the *discontinuous* or *dispersed* phase; the other is then the *continuous* phase. Milk is an emulsion in which butter fat is the discontinuous and water the continuous phase.

emul'soid (ē-mŭl'soyd) [" + G. *eidos.* form]. A colloid in an aqueous solution in which the colloid has a marked attraction for water to the extent that the dispersoid contains large quantities of water. Also called hydrophilic or lyophilic colloids. Protoplasm, starch, soap, gelatin, and egg white are common examples.

emulsum (e-mul'sum) [L.]. A fluid in which oil or resin is suspended by means of a mucilaginous substance.

emunctory (e-munk'to-rĭ) [L. *ēmungere,* to cleanse]. 1. Pert. to organ or duct having an excretory function. 2. An excretory duct, *i. e.,* pores of skin.

enamel (en-am'el) [A.S. *en,* on, + *amaile,* ivory]. It is the hardest substance in the body. The hard, white, dense substance forming a covering for the crown of the teeth. SYN: *enamelum* [NA]; *substantia adamantina.*

e., mottled. Condition in which the enamel acquires a mottled appearance as a result of the ingestion of excessive amounts of fluorides in water or foods.

e. organ. A cup-shaped structure which forms on the dental lamina of an embryo. It produces the enamel and serves as a mold for the remainder of the tooth.

enam'elum [NA]. Enamel, *q.v.,* of teeth.

enanthem, enanthema (en-an'them, -an-the'ma) [G. *en,* in, + *anthēma,* blossoming]. Eruption of mucous membrane. Ex: Koplik's spots. SEE: *rash.* OPP: *exanthem.*

enanthematous (en-an-them'ă-tus) [G. *en.* + *anthēma,* a blossoming]. Of the nature of an enanthema.

enanthesis (en-an-the'sis) [" + *anthein,* to bloom]. A skin eruption due to internal disease.

enanthrope (en'an-thrōp) [" + *anthrōpos,* man]. Any disease originating within the body.

enantiobiosis (en-an"tĭ-o-bi-o'sis) [G. *enantios,* opposite, + *bios,* life]. The condition in which associated organisms are antagonistic to each other. SEE: *symbiosis.*

enantiopathy (en-an-tĭ-op'ă-thĭ) [" + *pathos,* disease]. Treatment of one disease by another disease antagonistic to it, as malaria in general paresis.

enarkyochrome (en-ar'kĭ-o-krōm) [G. *en,* in, + *arkus,* network, + *chrōma,* color]. A nerve cell arranged like a network, taking a stain best in the cell body.

enarthri'tis [" + *arthron,* joint, + *itis,* inflammation]. Inflammation of a ball-and-socket joint.

enarthrosis (en-ar-thro'sis) (Pl. *enarthroses*) [" + *arthrōsis,* joint]. A ball-and-socket joint; a form of diarthrosis.

RS: *amphiarthrosis, condylarthrosis, diarthrosis, synarthrosis, synchondrosis.*

encan'this [G. *en,* in. + *kanthos,* angle of the eye]. An excrescence or new growth at the inner angle of the eye.

encapsula'tion [L. *en,* in, + *capsula,* a little box]. 1. Enclosure in a sheath not normal to the part. 2. The process of the formation of a capsule or a sheath about a structure.

encatarrhaphy (en-kat-ar'ă-fĭ) [G. *egkatarraptein,* to sew in]. Insertion of an organ or tissue into a part where it is not normally found.

enceinte (on-sant') [Fr.]. Pregnant.

encelial'gia [G. *en,* in, + *koilia,* belly, + *algos,* pain]. Abdominal pain.

encephalalgia (en-sef-al-al'jĭ-ă) [G. *egkephalos,* brain, + *algos,* pain]. Deep-seated head pain. SYN: *cephalalgia.*

encephalasthenia (en-sef"al-as-the'nĭ-ă) [" + *asthenia,* weakness]. Deficiency in brain power.

encephalatrophy (en-sef-al-at'ro-fĭ) [" + *a-,* priv. + *trophē,* nourishment]. Cerebral atrophy.

encephalic (en-sef-al'ĭk) [G. *egkephalos,* brain]. Pert. to the brain or its cavity.

encephalitis (en-sef-ă-li'tis) [" + *ītis,* inflammation]. Inflammation of the brain.

ETIOL: It may be a specific disease entity due to an arthropod-borne (arbor) virus, or it may occur as a sequela of influenza, measles, German measles, chickenpox, smallpox, vaccinia, or other diseases.

e., *cat-scratch.* Results from contact with a cat, a rare form of cat-scratch disease.

e., *cortical.* E. of brain cortex only.

e., *epidemic.* Any form of e. which occurs as an epidemic.

e., *equine.* Originally isolated as an e. affecting horses, it has been found to be transmitted to man by vectors also.

e., e., *Eastern.* Primarily a disease of birds and wild animals, transmitted to horses and man by mosquitoes. More severe than other types of e. Outbreaks have occurred in the Eastern and Gulf Coast states.

e., e., *Western.* A mild type of e., having occurred in Western United States and Canada.

e., *hemorrhagic.* Hemorrhage in brain inflammation.

e. *hyperplastica.* Acute encephalitis without suppuration.

e., *infantile.* Brain inflammation in the young causing cerebral palsy.

e., *Japanese B.* Similar to St. Louis e., it is caused by a different strain of virus. Occurs in summer and fall.

e., *lead.* Encephalitis due to lead poisoning.

e. *lethargica* (leth-ar'jĭ-ka). Epidemic neurotaxis, epidemic stupor. An infective disease believed to be of viral origin which first appeared pandemically in 1916-1917. It appeared epidemically in various regions of the world up to 1925 usually following epidemics of influenza. Since that time, it has occurred sporadically. Occurs usually in winter months. SYN: *Economo's disease; sleeping sickness.*

e., *meningo-.* E. combined with meningitis.

e. *neonato'rum.* A form occurring within the first several weeks of life.

e. *periaxialis.* Inflammation of the white matter of the cerebrum, occurring mainly in the young.

e., *postinfection.* E. occurring following a smallpox vaccination or one of the common communicable diseases, as chickenpox.

e., *purulent.* E. characterized by abscesses in the brain.

e., *St. Louis.* A virus disease which first occurred epidemically in the summer of 1933 in and around St. Louis. Now endemic in America. Occurs most frequently during summer and early fall.

e., *toxic.* That resulting from metal poisonings, as lead poisoning.

encephalocele (en-sef'ă-lo-sēl) [L. *en,* in + *kēlē,* hernia]. Protrusion of the brain through a cranial fissure. SYN: *hydrencephalocele.*

encephalocystocele (en-sef-ă-lo-sis'to-sēl) [" + *kystis,* a bladder, + *kēlē,* hernia]. Protrusion of brain distended by hernial sac containing fluid.

encephalodialysis (en-sef"ă-lo-di-al'ĭ-sis) [" + *dialysis,* loosening]. Softening of the brain.

encephalogram (en-sef'ă-lo-gram) [" + *gramma,* a writing]. A roentgen ray picture of the brain.

encephalography (en-sef-ă-log'ră-fĭ) [" + *graphein,* to write]. X-ray examination of head, esp. one obtained following the introduction of air into the ventricles through a lumbar or cisternal puncture.

encephaloid (en-sef'ă-loyd) [" + *eidos,* form]. 1. Resembling the cerebral substance. 2. A malignant neoplasm of brainlike texture.

e. *cancer.* Malignant tumor of the brain. SYN: *encephaloma.*

encephalolith (en-sef'ă-lo-lith) [L. *en,* in, + G. *egkephalos,* brain, + *lithos,* stone]. A calculus of the brain.

encephalology (en-sef-ă-lol'o-jĭ) [" + " + *logos,* study of]. That division of medical science which deals with the structure, function, and pathology of the brain.

encephalo'ma [" + *ōma,* tumor]. Tumor of the brain.

encephalomalacia (en-sef"ă-lo-mă-la'sĭ-ă) [" + *malakia,* softening]. Brain softening.

encephalomeningi'tis [" + *mēnigx,* membrane, + *ītis,* inflammation]. Inflammation of the brain and its membranes.

encephalomeningocele (en-sef"ă-lo-men-in'jo-sēl) [" + " + *kēlē,* hernia]. Protrusion through the cranium of membranes and brain substance.

encephalomere (en-sef'-ă-lo-mēr) [L. *en,* in + *meros,* part]. A primitive segment of the embryonic brain; a neuromere.

encephalometer (en-sef-ă-lom'ĕ-ter) [" + *metron,* measure]. An instrument for measuring the cranium and locating brain regions.

encephalomyelitis (en-sef"ă-lo-mi-el-i'-tis) [" + *myelos,* marrow, + *ītis,* inflammation]. An acute inflammation of the brain and spinal cord.

e., *acute disseminated.* Acute disorder of the brain and spinal cord due to causes such as vaccination or acute exanthema. SYN: *postinfection encephalomyelitis.*

e., *equine.* Virus disease of horses that may be communicated to man. Includes Eastern and Western equine encephalitis.

encephalomyelopathy (en-sef"ă-lo-mi"el-op'ă-thĭ) [" + " + *pathos,* disease]. Any disease of brain and spinal cord.

encephalon (en-sef'ă-lon) [G. *egkephalos,* brain]. The brain, including the cerebrum, cerebellum, medulla oblongata, and pons, diencephalon and mid-brain.

encephalop'athy [" + *pathos,* disease]. Any dysfunction of the brain.

e. *lead.* Neuronal degeneration and cerebral edema, apparently due to presence of lead in the brain.

enceph'alopuncture [" + L. *punctura,* a piercing]. Puncture into the brain substance.

encephalopyosis (en-sef"ă-lo-pi-o'sis) [" + *pyōsis,* suppuration]. Abscess of the brain.

encephalorrhagia (en-sef"ă-lo-ra'jĭ-a) [" + *rēgnunai,* to burst forth]. Hemorrhage of the brain.

encephalosclerosis (en-sef"ă-lo-skle-ro'-sis) [" + *sklērōsis,* hardening]. Brain hardening.

encephalo'sis [" + *osis*]. A degenerative process of the brain.

encephalospi'nal [" + L. *spina,* thorn]. Pert. to brain and spinal cord.

e. *axis.* Cerebrospinal axis.

encephalothlipsis (en-sef"ă-lo-thlip'sis). Compression of the brain.

encephalotome (en-sef'ă-lo-tōm) [" + *tomē*, incision]. Instrument for incising brain tissue.

encephalotomy (en-sef"ă-lot'o-mĭ) [" + *tomē*, a cutting]. 1. Brain dissection. 2. Surgical destruction of the brain of a fetus to facilitate delivery.

enchondroma (en-kon-dro'mă) [G. *en*, in, + *chondros*, cartilage, + *ōma*, tumor]. A cartilaginous tumor occurring generally where cartilage is absent or within a bone where it expands the diaphysis.

enchondrosarcoma (en-kon"dro-sar-ko'mă) [" + " + *sarx*, flesh, + *ōma*, tumor]. Sarcoma made up of cartilaginous tissue.

enchondrosis (en-kon-dro'sis). A cartilaginous outgrowth from bone or cartilaginous tissue; an enchondroma.

enchylema (en-ki-le'mă) [" + *chylos*, juice]. Fluid granular matter in interstices of cell body and nucleus. SYN: *cytochylema*.

enchyma (en'kĭ-mă) [" + *chymos*, juice]. A fluid formed from chyme which elaborates and repairs tissues and cells.

enclave (ĕn-klāv') [Fr. *enclavér*, to surround]. A mass of tissue which becomes enclosed by a tissue of another kind.

enclavement (en-klāv'ment) [Fr.]. GYN: An impaction of the fetus in the pelvic strait.

enclitic (en-klit'ik) [G. *egklinein*, to incline]. Having the planes of the fetal head inclined to those of the maternal pelvis.

encolpism (en-kol'pizm) [G. *en*, in, + *kolpos*, vagina, + *ismos*, condition]. Medication by vaginal suppositories and injections.

encolpitis (en-kol-pi'tis) [" + *kolpos*, vagina, + *itis*, inflammation]. Inflamed condition of the vaginal mucosa. SYN: *endocolpitis*.

encopresis (en-kop-re'sis). Fecal incontinence not due to illness or organic defect.

encra'nial [" + *kranion*, cranium]. Intracranial or within the cranium.

encyesis (en-si-e'sis) [" + *kyēsis*, pregnancy]. Normal uterine pregnancy.

encysted (en-sist'ed) [" + *kystis*, cyst]. Surrounded by membrane; encapsulated.

end [A.S. *ende*]. A termination; extremity.

e. *artery*. An artery which does not anastomose directly or indirectly with other arteries, *e.g.*, in kidney and spleen, etc.

e. *body*. Substance that kills bacteria in immunity to typhoid. SYN: *complement*.

e. *brain*. The telencephalon.

e. *bud*, e. *bulb*, e. *capsule*. The terminal of a sensory nerve.

e. *bulb of Krause*. An encapsulated nerve ending found in the skin and mucous membranes.

e. *organ*. An encapsulated sensory nerve ending.

e. o., *neuromuscular*. Spindle-shaped bundle of specialized muscle fibers in which sensory nerve fibers terminate in muscles; muscle spindle.

e. o., *neurotendinous*. Specialized tendon fasciculi in which sensory nerve fibers terminate in tendons; a tendon spindle.

e. *plate*. The special area in which motor axons terminate in the skeletal muscle.

e. *result*. The ultimate or final result.

Endamoeba (en"dă-me'bă). *Entamoeba, q.v.*

endangeitis, endangiitis (end-an-je-i'tis) [G. *endon*, within, + *aggeion*, vessel, + *itis*, inflammation]. Inflammation of the endangium.

endangium (en-dan'jĭ-um) [" + *aggeion*, vessel]. Innermost coat or intima of blood vessels.

endaortitis (end"a-or-ti'tis) [" + *aortē*, aorta, + *itis*, inflammation]. Inflammation of inner coat of the aorta.

endarterial (end-ar-te'rĭ-al) [" + *artēria*, artery]. 1. Pert. to the inner portion of an artery. 2. Within an artery.

endarteritis (end-ar-ter-i'tis) [" + " + *itis*, inflammation]. Inflammation of innermost coat or intima of an artery resulting from syphilis, trauma, pyogenic bacteria, or infective thrombi.

e., *acute*. Of large arteries. Rare.

e., *chronic*. Degeneration of arterial coats in the aged. SYN: *atheroma*.

e. *deformans*. Thickening of intima or replacement with atheromatous or calcareous deposits.

e. *obliterans*. Chronic progressive thickening of intima leading to stenosis or obstruction of lumen.

e., *syphilitic*. E. caused by syphilis. SYN: *syphilitic vasculitis*.

endeictic (en-dīk'tĭk). Symptomatic.

endem'ic [G. *en*, in, + *dēmos*, people].

e. *disease*. A disease which is present more or less continuously in a community. Used in contrast to sporadic or epidemic.

e. *neuritis*. A form of polyneuritis. SYN: *beriberi*.

endemoepidemic (en-de"mo-ep-ĭ-dem'ik) [" + " + *epi*, on, + *dēmos*, people]. Endemic, but becoming epidemic periodically.

endermat'ic, enderm'ic [" + *derma*, skin]. Administering medicine through the skin.

endermo'sis [" + " + *ōsis*]. 1. Administration of medicines through the skin. 2. Herpetic affection of any mucous membrane.

en'deron [" + *deros*, skin]. The dermis or corium; the portion of a mucous membrane underlying the epithelial layer.

en'dive. Fresh (curly including escarole): 100 gm. Calories: 20. Other main values: 1.7 gm. protein; trace of fat; 4.1 gm. carbohydrates; 81 mg. calcium; 3300 I.U. vitamin A.

endoaneurysmorrhaphy (en"do-an-ū-ris-mor'af-ĭ) [G. *endon*, within, + *aneurysma*, aneurysm, + *raphē*, suture]. Opening an aneurysmal sac and suturing its orifice.

endoangiitis (en"do-an-jĭ-i'tis) [" + *aggeion*, vessel, + *itis*, inflammation]. Inflammation of the coat of blood vessels. SYN: *endangiitis; endoarteritis; endophlebitis*.

en"doantitox'in [" + *anti*, against, + *toxikon*, poison]. An antitoxin within a cell.

en"doappendici'tis [" + L. *appendere*, to hang, + G. *itis*, inflammation]. Inflammation of mucosa of the vermiform appendix.

endoarteritis (en"do-ar-ter-i'tis) [G. *endon*, with, + *arteria*, artery, + *-itis*, inflammation]. Endarteritis, *q.v.*

en"doausculta'tion [" + L. *auscultāre*, to listen to]. Auscultation by esophageal tube passed into the stomach.

endobiotic (en"do-bi-ot'ik) [" + *bios*, life]. Pertaining to an organism living parasitically in the host.

endoblast (en'do-blast) [" + *blastos,* germ]. 1. The nucleus cell. 2. Inner layer of the blastoderm. SYN: *endoderm; hypoblast.*

endobronchi'tis [" + *brogchos,* windpipe, + *itis,* inflammation]. Inflammation of bronchial mucosa.

endocar'diac, endocar'dial [" + *kardia,* heart]. Within the heart or arising from the endocardium.

endocarditis (en-do-kar-di'tis) [" + " + *itis,* inflammation]. Inflammation of the lining membrane of the heart or *endocardium.*

It is usually confined to the external lining of the valve, sometimes to the lining membrane of its chambers. Generally of bacterial origin.

NP: Practically the same as that for pericarditis and other heart conditions. Rest in bed essential, but during symptoms of dyspnea patient should be propped up in bed and supported by pillows with arms resting on pillows. All bodily activities should be kept at a minimum. Patient should not reach for anything. Pulse should be taken before and after any exertion and if it does not return to original pulse within two minutes after the effort it indicates strain as a result. Maintain proper elimination.

TREATMENT: Antibiotic therapy for at least one month. Procaine penicillin in large doses is usually employed, although other antibiotics may be required.

e., acute bacterial. One that progresses rapidly; usually caused by staphylococci or the pneumococcus.

e., chronic. SEE: *ulcerative endocarditis.*

e., exudative. Begins as an acute affection. Rheumatism chief cause. SYM: Auscultation may give only indication—a prolongation of heart sound. PROG: Guarded. TREATMENT: Absolute rest.

e., malignant. Usually secondary to suppurative inflammation elsewhere. SEE: *ulcerative endocarditis.*

e., subacute bacterial. A condition caused by lodgment of the *Streptococcus viridans* group (mainly *S. salivarius, S. mitis, S. bovis, S. fecalis, S. sanguis*) in an abnormal heart or in valves damaged previously by rheumatic fever.

e., ulcerative. A rapidly destructive form of acute bacterial e., characterized by necrosis or ulceration of the valves and the deposition of colonies of micrococci. Usually fatal.

e., vegetative. Fibrinous clots on ulcerated valvular surfaces. SEE: *exudative endocarditis.*

e. verrucous. Nonbacterial e. occurring frequently in lupus erythematosus. SYN: *Libman-Sacks disease; nonbacterial verrucous e.*

e. viridans. Subacute bacterial endocarditis.

endocar'dium [" + *kardia,* heart]. Lining (serous) membrane of inner surface and cavities of the heart.

It is continuous with the intima or int. coat of arteries.

endocervical (en-do-ser'vĭ-kal) [" + L. *cervix,* neck]. Pert. to the endocervix.

endocervicitis (en-dō-ser-vĭ-si'tis) [" + " + G. *itis,* inflammation]. Inflammation of mucous lining of the cervix uteri. Usually chronic and due to infection, and accompanied by cervical erosion.

SYM: White or yellow mucoid discharge.

TREATMENT: Electrocauterization of cervical lesion; warm douches daily for two to three weeks following electrocautery. An antibiotic for local application may be prescribed.

endocervix (en-do-ser'viks) [G. *endon,* within, + L. *cervix,* neck]. The lining of the canal of the cervix uteri.

endochondral (en-do-kon'dral) [" + *chondros,* cartilage]. Within a cartilage.

endochorion (en-do-ko'rĭ-on) [" + *chorion,* chorion]. The inner chorion; vascular layer of allantois.

endochrome (en'do-krōm) [" + *chrōma,* color]. The coloring matter (not green) of a cell's endoplasm.

endocoli'tis [" + *kōlon,* colon, + *itis,* inflammation]. Inflammation of the mucosa of colon. SEE: *colitis.*

endocolpitis (en-do-kol-pi'tis) [" + *colpos,* vagina, + *itis,* inflammation]. Inflammation of the vaginal mucosa. SYN. *encolpitis.*

endocom'plement [" + L. *complēre,* to fill]. An intracellular complement or one contained within the erythrocyte.

endocorpus'cular [" + L. *corpusculum,* corpuscle]. Within a corpuscle.

endocra'nial [" + *kranion,* cranium]. 1 Intracranial or within the cranium. 2 Pert. to the endocranium.

endocrani'tis [" + " + *itis,* inflammation]. Inflammation of endocranium. SYN: *pachymeningitis, external.*

endocra'nium [" + *kranion,* cranium]. The dura mater of the brain which forms the lining membrane of the cranium.

endocrinasthenia (en"do-krin-as-the'nĭ-ă) [" + *krinein,* to secrete, + *astheneia,* weakness]. Neurasthenia due to dysfunction of the endocrines.

endocrine (ĕn'dō-krĭn, -krīn) [" + *krinein* to secrete]. 1. An internal secretion. 2. Endocrinous. 3. Pertaining to a gland that produces an internal secretion.

e. gland. A ductless gland; a gland which produces an internal secretion discharged into the blood or lymph and circulated to all parts of the body. The active principles of the glands, hormones, produce effects on tissues more or less remote from their place of origin. In addition to their endocrine function, some glands also produce an external secretion (Ex: pancreas, testes).

The endocrine glands include: hypophysis (pituitary gland), thyroid gland (the thymus and pineal body have not been shown to produce any hormones), parathyroid glands, adrenal (suprarenal) glands, islands of Langerhans of the pancreas, and the gonads (ovaries and testes). Other structures such as the gastrointestinal mucosa and the placenta have an endocrine function.

The hormones secreted by the ductless glands may have a specific effect on an organ or tissue, or in some cases the effect is general affecting the entire body as in the case of the thyroid hormone which affects the rate of metabolism. Among the physiological processes affected by hormones are: rate of metabolism and the metabolism of specific substances such as carbohydrates and calcium; growth and developmental processes; the secretory activity of other endocrine glands; the development and functioning of the reproductive organs; sexual characteristics and libido; the development of personality and higher nervous functions; the ability of the body to meet conditions of stress; resistance to disease.

PRINCIPAL ENDOCRINE GLANDS

Name	Position	Function	Endocrine Disorders
Thyroid	Two lobes in neck	Influences basal metabolic rate. Indirectly influences growth and nutrition	Hypofunction—Cretinism in young; myxedema in adult Goiter in hyperfunction and hypofunction
Parathyroid	Four or more small glands near thyroid	Calcium and phosphorus metabolism. Indirectly affect muscular irritability	Hypofunction—Tetany Hyperfunction—Resorption of bone. Renal calculi
Suprarenal Cortex (Adrenal Cortex)	One above each kidney	Steroid hormones regulating carbohydrate metabolism and salt and water balance. Some effects on sexual characteristics	Hypofunction – Addison's disease Hyperfunction – Adrenogenital syndrome
Adrenal Medulla	Embedded in adrenal surrounded by cortex	Effects on sympathetic nervous system and carbohydrate metabolism	Hypofunction – Almost unknown Hyperfunction – Phenochromocytoma
Anterior Pituitary (Adenohypophysis	Small gland at base of brain	Influences growth, sexual development, skin pigmentation, thyroid function, adrenal cortical function through effects on other endocrine glands (except for growth factor which acts directly on cells)	Hypofunction—Dwarf in child. Decrease in all other endocrine gland functions except parathyroids Hyperfunction – Acromegaly in adult; diabetes, gigantism in child
Posterior Pituitary (Neurohypophysis)	Attached to anterior pituitary	Oxytocic factor influencing some aspects of uterine contraction. Antidiuretic factor influencing absorption of water by kidney tubule	Unknown Hypofunction—Diabetes insipidus
Testes and Ovaries	Testes—in the scrotum Ovaries—in the pelvic cavity	Development of secondary sex characteristics; some effect on metabolism	Hypofunction—Lack of sex development or regression in adult. Hyperfunction – Abnormal sex development

Endocrine dysfunction may result from (a) *hyposecretion* in which an inadequate amount of the hormone(s) is secreted or (b) *hypersecretion* in which excessive amounts of hormones are produced. Secretion of endocrine glands may be under nervous control, or it may be controlled by chemical substances in the blood; in some cases, other hormones. Many pathological conditions are the result of, or associated with, the malfunctioning of the endocrine glands.

endocrinic (en-do-krin'ik). Same as endocrinous.

endoc'rinism [" + " + *ismos*, condition]. Disease due to malfunction of one or more of the endocrine glands. SYN: *endocrinopathy.*

endocrino-. Combining form for endocrine.

endocrinology (en-do-krin-ol'o-jĭ) [" + " + *logos*, science]. The science of the endocrines, or ductless glands, and their functions.

endocrinopath (en"do-krin'o-path) [" + " + *pathos*, disease]. One affected by a disorder of one or more glands of internal secretion.

endocrinopathic (en"do-krin-o-path'ĭk) [" + " + *pathos*, disease]. Of the nature of endocrinopathy.

endocrinopathy (en"do-krin-op'ă-thĭ) [" + " + *pathos*, disease]. A disease due to disorder of an endocrine gland or glands.

endocrinosis (en"do-krin-o'sis) [" + " + *ōsis*]. Condition resulting from dysfunction of an endocrine gland.

endocrinotherapy (en"do-krin-o-ther'ă-pĭ) [" + " + *therapeia*, treatment]. Treatment with endocrine preparations.

endocrinous (en-dok'rin-us) [" + *krinein*, to secrete]. Pert. to internal secretions or endocrine glands.

endocrit'ic [G. *endon*, within + *krinein*, to secrete]. Referring to internal secretions.

en'docyst [" + *kystis*, cyst]. The innermost layer of any hydatid cyst.

endocystitis (en-do-sis-ti'tis) [" + " + *itis*, inflammation]. Inflammation of mucous membrane of bladder. SEE ALSO: *cystitis.*

endoderm (en'do-derm) [" + *derma*, skin]. Inner layer of cells of an embryo. SYN: *entoderm, q.v.; hypoblast.*

endoderm'al. Pertaining to the entoderm. SYN: *entodermal.*

Endodermophyton (en"do-derm"o-fi'ton). Former name of a genus of parasitic fungi growing in the epidermis of the skin. Now included in the genus *Trichophyton, q.v.*

endodiascope (en-do-di'ă-skōp). X-ray tube that may be placed within the body for radiologic examination and radiation therapy.

endodiascopy (en-do-di-as'kō-pĭ) [" + *dia*, through, + *skopein*, to examine]. X-ray examination with an endodiascope of a body cavity.

endodontia (en-do-don'shĭ-ă). Endodontics.
endodontics (en-do-don'tiks). A branch of dentistry concerned with diagnosis, treatment and prevention of diseases of the dental pulp and its surrounding tissues.
endodon'tist. A specialist in the practice of endodontics.
endodontitis (en"do-don-ti'tis) [" + *odous, odont-*, tooth, + *ītis*, inflammation]. Inflammation of the dental pulp. Syn: *pulpitis.*
endodon'tium. Obsolete term for pulp of a tooth. See: *dental pulp.*
endodontol'ogist. An endodontist.
endodontol'ogy. Endodontics, *q.v.*
endoectothrix (en"do-ek'to-thrix) [" + *ektos*, outside, + *thrix*, hair]. Any fungus growth on and in the hair.
en"doenteri'tis [" + *enteron*, intestine, + *ītis*, inflammation]. Inflammation of lining membrane of intestines.
endoen'zyme [" + *en*, in, + *zymē*, leaven]. An intracellular enzyme.
endogamy (en-dog'ă-mĭ). 1. Inbreeding; the custom or tribal requirement of marriage within a tribe or group. 2. In biology, reproduction by joining together gametes descended from the same ancestral cell.
endogastrectomy (en-do-gas-trek'to-mĭ) [" + *gastēr*, belly, + *ektome*, excision]. Excision of the gastric mucosa.
endogastric (en-do-gas'trik) [" + *gastēr*, stomach]. Pert. to the stomach's interior.
endogastritis (en-do-gas-tri'tis) [" + " + *itis*, inflammation]. Inflammation of the lining membrane of the stomach.
endogenic (en-do-jen'ik) [" + *gennan*, to produce]. Having origin within the organism. Syn: *endogenous.*
endogenous (en-doj'ĕ-nus) [" + *gennan*, to produce]. 1. Produced or arising from within a cell or organism. 2. Concerning spore formation within the bacterial cell. Syn: *endogenic.*
endogeny (en-doj'ĕ-nĭ). Formation or growth within the cell.
endoglobar (en-do-glōb'ar). Endoglobular, *q.v.*
endoglob'ular [" + L. *globulus*, a globule]. Within the blood corpuscles, as malarial germs.
endointoxica'tion [" + L. *in*, into, + G. *toxikon*, poison]. Poisoning due to an endogenous toxin.
endolabyrinthitis (en"do-lab-ĭ-rin-thi'tis) [" + *labyrinthos*, labyrinth, + *ītis*, inflammation]. Inflamed condition of the membranous labyrinth.
endolaryn'geal [" + *larygx*, larynx]. Within the larynx.
endolemma (en-do-lem'ă). Neurilemma, *q.v.* Syn: *sheath of Schwann.*
Endolimax na'na (en-do-li'maks) [" + *leimax*, meadow]. A minute species of ameba inhabiting the intestine of man, monkeys, and other mammals. It is nonpathogenic in man and is found in the intestines of healthy persons.
endolum'bar [" + L. *lumbus*, loin]. In the lumbar portion of the spinal cord.
endolymph (en'do-limf) [" + L. *lympha*]. Pale, limpid fluid within the labyrinth of the ear.
endolymphat'ic [" + L. *lympha*]. Rel. to the endolymph.
  e. duct. A slender duct extending from posterior surface of the saccule of the inner ear. It ends blindly in the petrous portion of temporal bone as a dilated pouch, the endolymphatic sac.
endolysin (en-dol'ĭ-sin) [" + *lysis*, a loosening]. Bacterial substance within a leukocyte which destroys bacteria.
endol'ysis [G. *endon*, within, + *lysis*, a dissolution]. Disintegration of cell cytoplasm.
endomastoiditis (en"do-mas-toy-di'tis) [" + *mastos*, breast, + *eidos*, form, + *ītis*, inflammation]. Inflammation of mucosa lining the mastoid cavity and cells.
endometrectomy (en"do-me-trek'to-mĭ) [" + *mētra*, uterus, + *ektomē*, excision]. Excision of uterine mucosa. See: *curettage.*
endometrial (en-do-me'trĭ-al) [" + *mētra*, uterus]. Pert. to the lining mucosa of the uterus.
  e. cyst. An ovarian cyst or tumor that bleeds. Usually seen in ovarian endometriosis. Syn: ***chocolate cyst of ovary.***
endometrioma (en-do-me-trĭ-o'mă) [" + " + *ōma*, tumor]. A tumor containing shreds of ectopic endometrium; found most frequently in the ovary, *cul-de-sac*, rectovaginal septum, and the peritoneal surface of the post. portion of the uterus.
endometriosis (en-do-me-trĭ-o'sis) [" + " + *ōsis*]. Ectopic endometrium located in various sites throughout the pelvis or in the abdominal wall.
  e., direct. Invasion, by the mucous membrane lining the uterus, of the myometrium. Syn: *adenomyoma of the wall of the uterus.*
  e., implantation. Same as peritoneal endometriosis, *q.v.*
  e., internal. Same as direct endometriosis, *q.v.*
  e., metastatic. Extraperitoneal lesions in circumstances resembling metastatic pelvic carcinoma.
  e., peritoneal. Endometrial tissue found throughout the pelvis.
  e., primary. Same as direct endometriosis, *q.v.*
  e., transplantation. Endometriosis taking place within abdominal incision scar following pelvic surgery.
endometritis (en-do-me-tri'tis) [" + " + *itis*, inflammation]. Inflammation of the endometrium, the inner mucous lining of the uterus.
  Etiol: Produced by bacterial invasion. May be acute, subacute, or chronic, the acute cases most commonly resulting from infection by staphylococci, colon bacilli, or gonococci; trauma; septic abortion. The subacute type is the result of repeated acute attacks as is the chronic type. Occasionally the chronic type may be a tuberculous infection. There are many other conditions which are labeled as endometritis but which are of either vascular or endocrine origin. Some of these conditions are senile endometritis, hyperplastic endometritis, hypertrophic endometritis, etc.
  Sym: In acute cases the symptoms are usually low back and low abdominal pain, dysmenorrhea, menorrhagia, sterility, constipation. In chronic e., there is scant serosanguineous vaginal discharge. A positive diagnosis cannot be made without a curettage and a histological study of the recovered material. See: *cervix uteri; endometrium; uterus.*
  e., cervical. Inflammation of the inner portion of the cervix uteri.
  e., decidual. Inflammation of the mucous membrane of a gravid uterus.
  e. dissecans. E. accompanied by development of ulcers and shedding of the mucous membrane.

e., septic. Form caused by septic poisoning.

endometrium (en-do-me'trĭ-um) [" + *mētra,* uterus]. The mucous membrane lining the inner surface of the uterus. Histologically, it consists of a surface epithelium made up of a single layer of columnar cells, a few of which bear cilia. Invaginations of the epithelium form simple, branched tubular glands which extend to the myometrium. The glands are separated by connective tissue resembling mesenchyme which forms the *stroma.* There is no submucosa; the mucosa lying closely attached to the myometrium.

The endometrium is supplied by two types of arteries; *straight arteries* which supply the deeper third or basal layer of the endometrium and *spiral arteries* which supply the spongy and compact layers. They penetrate between the glands and form a subepithelial capillary plexus. These arteries show marked changes in response to hormonal stimulation during the menstrual cycle.

Between puberty and the menopause, the uterine endometrium passes through cyclic changes which constitute the menstrual cycle, *q.v.* These changes are related to the development and maturation of the graafian follicle, the discharge of the ovum, and the subsequent development of the corpus luteum in the ovary.

Following fertilization of the ovum, the endometrium serves as nesting place and implantation occurs. The endometrium fuses with the developing chorion of the embryo and at birth there is a splitting off and shedding of the uterine lining or *decidua.* During pregnancy, the *decidua basalis,* the endometrium lying between the chorionic vesicle and the myometrium, develops into the maternal portion of the placenta, *q.v.*

endom'etry [" + *metron,* measure]. Measurement of the interior of a cavity or organ.

endomorphy (en"do-mor'fe) [" + *morphe,* form]. Body build characterized by predominance of tissues derived from the endoderm. SEE: *ectomorphy; mesomorphy; somatotype.*

endomyocarditis (en"do-mī-o-kar-dī'tis) [" + *mys,* muscle, + *kardia,* heart, + *ītis,* inflammation]. Inflammation of the endocardium and myocardium.

endomysium (en-do-miz'ĭ-um). A thin sheath of connective tissue consisting principally of reticular fibers which invests each striated muscle fiber and binds the fibers together within a fasciculus.

endoneuri'tis [" + *neuron,* nerve, + *ītis,* inflammation]. Inflammation of the endoneurium.*

endoneurium (en-do-nu'rĭ-um) [" + *neuron,* nerve]. Henle's sheath. A delicate connective tissue sheath which surrounds nerve fibers within a fasciculus.

endoparasite (en-do-par'ă-sīt) [" + *parasitos,* parasite]. Any parasite living within its host.

endopathy (en-dop'ă-thĭ) [" + *pathos,* disease]. Any endogenous disease.

endopelvic (en-do-pel'vic) [" + L. *pelvis,* basin]. Within the pelvis.

e. fasciae. The downward continuation of the parietal peritoneum of the abdomen to form the pelvic fasciae which have a very important part in the support of the pelvic viscera.

endopericarditis (en"do-per"ĭ-kar-dī'tis) [" + *peri,* around, + *kardia,* heart, + *ītis,* inflammation]. Endocarditis complicated by pericarditis.

endoperimyocarditis (en"do-per-ĭ-mi"o-kar-dī'tis) [" + " + *mys,* muscle, + *kardia,* heart, + *ītis,* inflammation]. Inflammation of the pericardium, myocardium, and endocardium.

endoperitonitis (en"do-per-ĭ-to-nī'tis) [" + *peritonaion,* peritoneum, + *ītis,* inflammation]. Superficial inflammation of the peritoneum.

endophlebitis (en"do-fle-bī'tis) [" + *phleps,* vein, + *ītis,* inflammation]. Inflammation of inner coat of a vein.

e. obliterans. E. causing obliteration of a vein.

e. portalis. Inflammation of the portal vein.

en'doplasm [" + *plasma,* matter formed]. The internal, more fluid protoplasm of a cell which lies within the ectoplasm which forms the peripheral layer.

end organ. The expanded end of a nerve fiber in a peripheral structure.

e. o., sensory. An encapsulated termination of a nerve fiber which serves as a receptor.

endorrhachis (en-do-rā'kis) [G. *endon,* within, + *rachis,* spine]. Membrane lining; the spinal dura mater.

endorrhinitis (en-do-ri-nī'tis) [" + *ris, rin-,* nose, + *ītis,* inflammation]. Inflammation of the mucous membranes of the nose. SYN: *coryza.*

endosalpingitis (en"do-sal-pin-jī'tis) [" + *salpigx,* tube, + *ītis,* inflammation]. Inflammation of lining of fallopian tubes.

endoscope (en'do-skōp) [" + *skopein,* to examine]. A device consisting of a tube and optical system for observing the inside of an organ or cavity. This may be done through a natural body opening or through a small incision.

endoscopy (en-dos'ko-pĭ) [" + *skopein,* to examine]. Inspection of body organs or cavities by use of the endoscope.

endosep'sis [" + *sēpsis,* decay]. Septicemia having its origin within the body.

endoskel'eton [" + *skeleton,* skeleton]. Internal bony framework of the body. SEE: *exoskeleton.*

endosmometer (en-dos-mom'ĕ-ter) [" + *ōsmos,* a thrusting, + *metron,* measure]. Device for estimating passage by osmosis of a substance through a membrane or tissue.

endosmose, endosmosis (en'dŏs-mōs", en-dos-mō'sis) [" + *ōsmos,* a thrusting, + *ōsis*]. Osmosis in which flow of water is from the outside liquid to the solution within a membranous cell.

en'dospore [" + *sporos,* a seed]. BIOL: Thick walled spore within the bacterium.

endosteitis (en"dos-te-i'tis) [" + *osteon,* bone, + *ītis,* inflammation]. Inflammation of the endosteum or of medullary cavity of a bone.

endosteo'ma [" + " + *ōma,* tumor]. A tumor in the medullary cavity of a bone.

endos'teum [" + *osteon,* bone]. Membrane lining bone in the medullary cavity.

endostitis (en"dos-tī'tis) [" + " + *ītis,* inflammation]. Inflammation of the endosteum or the medullary cavity of a bone.

endostoma (en-dos-to'mă) [" + " + *ōma,* tumor]. Osseous tumor within a bone.

endostosis (en-dos-to'sis) [" + " + *ōsis*]. The development of an endostoma.

endothelial (en-do-the'lĭ-al) [" + *thēlē,* nipple]. Pert. to or consisting of endothelium.

endotheliocyte (en"do-the'lĭ-o-sīt) [" + *kytos,* cell]. Large, phagocytic, wandering cell found in circulating blood and in tissue.

endotheliocytosis (en″do-the″lĭ-o-si-to′sis) [" + " + *kytos,* cell, + *ōsis*]. Abnormal increase in endothelial cells.

endothelioinoma (en″do-the″lĭ-o-ĭ-no′mă) [" + " + *is, in-,* fiber, + *ōma,* tumor]. Tumorous growth arising from endothelium containing fibrous substance.

endotheliolysin (en″do-the-lĭ-ol′ĭ-sin) [" + " + *lysis,* dissolution]. An antibody found in snake venom which dissolves endothelial cells.

endotheliolytic (en″do-thē-lĭ-o-lit′ĭk) [" + " + *lysis,* dissolution]. Capable of destroying endothelial tissue.

endothelioma (en″do-the-lĭ-o′mă) [" + " + *ōma,* tumor]. Malignant growth of lining cells of the blood vessels.

endotheliomyoma (en″do-the″lĭ-o-mi-o′-ma) [" + " + *mys,* muscle, + *ōma,* tumor]. Muscular tumor with elements of endothelium.

endotheliomyxoma (en″do-the″lĭ-o-miks-o′-mă) [" + " + *myxa,* mucus, + *ōma,* tumor]. Myxoma with element from endothelium.

endotheliotoxin (en″do-the-lĭ-o-toks′in) [" + " + *toxikon,* poison]. A specific toxin which acts on endothelial capillary cells, causing hemorrhages.

endothe′lium [" + "+ *thēlē,* nipple]. A form of squamous epithelium consisting of flat cells which line the blood and lymphatic vessels, the heart, and various other body cavities. It is derived from mesoderm.

end′otherm knife. A knife devised for using a high frequency current.

endother′mal [G. *endon,* within, + *thermē,* heat]. 1. Pert. to production of heat within an organism. 2. Pert. to absorption of heat during formation of chemical compounds. SYN: *endothermic.*

endother′mic [" + *thermē,* heat]. 1. Storing up potential energy or heat. 2. Absorbing heat. 3. Accompanied by heat absorption.

endothermy (en′do-ther″mĭ) [" + *thermē,* heat]. A term used as a synonym for surgical diathermy.

en′dothrix [" + *thrix,* hair]. Any fungus growing inside the hair.

endothyreopexy (en-do-thi′re-o-peks″ĭ) [" + *thyreos,* shield, + *pēxis,* fixation]. Displacing the thyroid gland and fixing it to the side of the neck.

endothyroidopexy (en″do-thi″royd-o-peks′ĭ) [" + " + *eidos,* form, + *pēxis,* fixation]. Operative displacement of the thyroid gland and fixing it to the side of the neck. SYN: *endothyreopexy.*

endotoscope (end-o′to-skōp) [" + *ous, ot-,* ear, + *skopein,* to examine]. An ear speculum. SYN: *otoscope.*

en″dotoxico′sis [" + *toxikon,* poison, + *-ōsis*]. Poisoning due to an endotoxin.

en′dotoxin [" + *toxikon,* poison]. Bacterial toxin confined within the body of a bacterium, freed only when the bacterium is broken down.

SEE: *cytotoxin; erythrotoxin; exotoxin; leukotoxin; neurotoxin.*

endotracheitis (en-do-tra-ke-i′tis) [" + *tracheia,* trachea, + *ītis,* inflammation]. Inflammation of the tracheal mucosa.

endotrachelitis (en″do-tra-kel-i′tis) [" + *trachēlos,* neck, + *ītis,* inflammation]. Inflammation of the endocervical tissues. SYN: *endocervicitis.*

en″dovasculi′tis [" + L. *vasculum,* vessel, + G. *ītis,* inflammation]. Inflammation of the endangium or inner coat of a blood vessel. SYN: *endangeitis.*

endove′nous [" + L. *vēna,* vein]. Within a vein. SYN: *intravenous.*

end plate. The terminal mass of a nerve fiber ending on a muscle cell.

e. p., motor. An ending in a striated muscle fiber; a myoneural junction.

end product. The final waste or excretory product of digestion that passes from the system.

endyma (en′dĭm-ă). Membranous lining of cerebral ventricles. SYN: *ependyma.*

en′ema (pl. *enemas* or *enem′ata*) [G.]. Injection of water, either plain or containing various drugs, etc., into the rectum and colon to empty the lower intestine or to introduce food or medicine for therapeutic purposes.

e., analeptic. One with ½ teaspoonful of salt to a pint of tepid water; a "thirst" enema.

e., anthelmintic. One given to expel worms if oral anthelmintics are not available. Use of enema for this purpose is of doubtful value.

e., antidiarrheic. One given for diarrhea.

e., antiseptic. One for the destruction of microorganisms.

e., antispasmodic. One to counteract spasms.

e., astringent. One given to contract intestinal tissue and to provoke subsequent evacuation of worms. Those given for anthelmintic* purposes are also useful when an astringent is needed. The following astringents are credited with inhibiting worms by dehydration, and with reducing the intestinal mucosa which harbors them:

Alum in a 1 to a 250 parts solution, mixed with water.

Calumba as ordered by the physician.

Limewater in a saturated strength solution.

Phenol (carbolic acid) in a one-fourth of 1% solution, to a one-half of a 1% solution.

Quinine bisulfate in a 1 to 2000 parts solution, or a 1 to 500 solution. Also used in amebic colitis for an irrigation

Sodium chloride in a hypertonic solution. This in double strength or 1 tablespoonful to the quart.

Tannic acid solution, 1 to 2500 parts of water.

Vinegar in a one-half dilution.

e., barium. Administration of barium sulfate in solution as a diagnostic aid in x-ray examination of colon.

e., blind. The insertion of a rubber tube to cause expulsion of gas or flatus. SEE: *carminative enema.*

e., carminative. One given to relieve distention caused by flatus and to stimulate peristalsis.

It calls for an examination of the patient's abdomen both before and after administering the enema. Special attention must be paid to the exclusion of flatus and of fecal matter. Often there is a high degree of distention, and it is vastly important to know of the relief from flatulence and accumulated feces. A very detailed description must be given after a careful examination has been made of the returns.

The carminative enema should be sufficiently warm, as it is to reach more of the intestinal tissues than the general cleansing enema, and as it also causes a greater hyperemia. It should penetrate farther than most enemas. An effective solution is 8 ounces of milk and 8 ounces of molasses.

e., cleansing. One to empty the lower intestine or the colon.

PROCEDURE: 1. Bring all equipment to bedside. 2. Screen bed and explain to patient what is to be done and why it is being done. Take time to gain patient's cooperation. 3. Turn patient on left side, with right leg flexed, in as comfortable a position as possible. 4. Place small rubber sheet covered with large towel under buttocks. 5. Cover patient with bath blanket while fan-folding top covers. Drape to expose required area. 6. Hang enema can on stand, having it about 2 feet above patient (not more), and see that stopcock is working properly. 7. See that solution is the proper temperature. 8. Lubricate rectal or enema tube for about 2 inches at end. 9. Run a little of the solution through tube into bedpan to warm tube. Close stopcock. 10. Insert tube into rectum. If you meet with resistance wait a few seconds, then proceed. 11. Open stopcock and let fluid run in. If it seems to be flowing too fast pinch the tube with your finger and thumb. 12. If patient complains of sharp pain, or is unable to retain fluid, stop flow for a minute. 13. When all fluid has been run in slowly remove tube and place bedpan. 14. Detach enema or rectal tube and place it in emesis basin. *Do not put it into the can.* 15. See that patient is comfortable on pan, covered with the bath blankets and the signal within reach. 16. Remove and care for enema tray. 17. When patient has finished expelling enema remove pan and do perineal toilet as usual. 18. Remove bath blankets and replace upper bedding. 19. If patient has used toilet paper himself provide soap and water for his hands. 20. Chart enema as directed.

e., demulcent. SEE: *emollient enema.*

e., Dobell's. One for nutritive purposes.

e., double-contrast. An enema of barium or other radiopaque material is injected and evacuated. This is followed by injection of air. X-rays of the lower intestinal tract are then taken.

e., egg and ether. Used as a last resort in the relief of distention. CAUTION: Ether should be handled with great care because it is inflammable.

It consists of magnesium sulfate, 1 ounce of ether, and the whites of 2 eggs. Water enough is added to make 1 pint of fluid. Mix the egg whites with the ether and beat until the mixture bubbles, then add the magnesium sulfate which has been dissolved in hot water; lastly, add the remaining warm water. All should be ready before the final water is added.

CHARTING: The results of a carminative enema for flatulence should be noted and charted. The abdomen should be examined both before and afterward to be sure of the results obtained. If hard and distended before giving the enema, and soft and flat afterwards it is evident good results have been obtained. Do not rely entirely upon the patient's word. If there should be any amt. of foam in the bedpan this indicates relief from the flatulence has been obtained.

e., emollient. One given to soothe and protect the intestinal mucosa by making a coating over membranes, allaying local pain and irritation, and to act as a vehicle for the rectal administration of drugs.

It should be given at a temperature of about 105° F., or in a severe case at about 100° F. After giving, the record must show if the patient felt relieved, and to what extent; also if the solution was retained in its entirety.

1. Mix *amylum* 2 drams with 1 ounce of cold water, then add 5 ounces of boiling water. Boil mixture 1 or 2 minutes to the consistency of mucilage. Now cool to about 105° F., and give slowly with a large catheter. If too small a catheter is used the solution will not pass through, if of a pastelike constituency. A bulb or piston syringe attached to a rectal tube may be used. From 10 to 30 minims of laudanum are often used in this enema as prescribed by the attending physician. It is best given by means of a small hand syringe, the solution being injected rather than flowing by gravity. The results are also better given in this manner.

2. *Olive oil or cottonseed oil* will also act as an emollient when injected. The tissues in this way are prevented from coming in contact with irritating substances, thus relieving the pain of inflammations through protecting the delicate membrane.

3. *Mucilage of acacia* is used as an emollient, 1 ounce to 5 ounces of water, or a thin, strained tea from boiled flaxseed, 4 or 5 ounces, also acts as a good emollient. This, of course, is only used on a doctor's order.

4. *The bismuth enema* may be given for its emollient effect. This also must be prescribed by the physician. Four or 5 ounces of water are used in which to dissolve the bismuth. Too large an amt. of enema may not be retained, in which case the effect desired is lost; the water will be absorbed and the bismuth will form a coating over the intestinal mucosa.

5. *Thin, strained gruel,* 4 ounces, may be given for emollient effect, and it may be absorbed as a nutrient.

e., evacuating. SEE: *cleansing enema.*

e., Ewald's. A nutritive enema containing red wine, 20% grape sugar solution with wheat flour boiled in it, mixed with eggs.

e., flatus. One to relieve gas pressure. Contains 1 dram of glycerine and ½ ounce of magnesium sulfate in 4 ounces of water.

e., high. One to reach the colon. Insertion of rubber tube into rectum to carry water as far as possible. Too frequent irrigation, esp. with hot water, may cause diverticula.

e., lubricating. Administered after an operation for hemorrhoids, and in order to soften the feces and lubricate the passage or anal canal to the external orifice or anus. When there is an impaction of feces, a lubricating enema may be given, followed in 2 hours by a cleansing enema.

OLIVE OIL, 4 to 6 ounces, warmed, may be given, or cottonseed oil warmed in quantities of from 4 to 6 ounces in the evening. The patient should remain in a prone position with hips elevated for half an hour following the enema in order to help retain the oil and thus aiding it in passing higher in the colon.

WARM SWEET OIL, 4 ounces, injected into the rectum with a bulb or piston syringe, will serve the purpose better than the usual enema apparatus. The hips should be elevated, and a cotton pad held against the anal region for a few minutes in order to help retention.

e., m. and m. Eight ounces of milk, and 8 ounces of molasses. The mixture may also be in proportions of 6 to 6. This is esp. efficient, as the sugar of the molasses with the milk forms gases which distend the bowels, causing frequent copious bowel movements. Starch water may be added to a 6 to 6 mixture to the extent of 4 ounces.

e., Mayo. Granulated sugar, 2 ounces, 1 ounce of sodium bicarbonate, and 8 ounces of water.

The sodium bicarbonate is added to the sugar and water mixture at the bedside, just before the solution is ready to be given. The combination of the sugar with the acid content of the intestine coming in contact with the bicarbonate causes a fermentation and production of gases. The bowels thus become inflated, causing a hyperdistention which produces bowel action.

e., medicinal. An enema to which some drug or medication has been added on order of attending physician. It is necessary that this enema be retained and absorbed. It may be given to medicate diseased conditions of the rectum, sigmoid, or colon, or for absorption for its general effects. Although substances (other than fluids) are not absorbed in the large intestine as extensively as in the small intestine, the chemical changes that may occur must be very simple if any absorption may be expected. SEE: *preparations usually given by rectum.*

e., nutrient or nutritive. One to give sustenance to a patient unable to be fed otherwise.

It may consist of peptonized milk, glucose, and other solutions. The temperature must be about body heat, and whatever food material is used should never be boiled.

The various prescriptions usually ordered are: (1) Foods most apt to be absorbed; (2) concentrated, easily digested and assimilable substances; (3) predigested foods; those that have been peptonized, such as milk, eggs, and meat broth.

Dilute alcohol, brandy, and whisky produce energy but they do not feed the tissues. The energy produced reduces the tax upon the body's tissues for energy, and conserves the proteins as nourishing factors. Alcohol, however, should be restricted as too much is destructive to the tissues. Dextrose is irritating although otherwise nutritive and absorbable.

TEMPERATURE OF SOLUTION: This should be 105° F. The attending physician prescribes the diet and the time of feeding. Much depends upon the condition of the patient and the diet prescribed.

GLUCOSE: If glucose is prescribed, 3 ounces of a 5-10% solution may be used. A very good nutritive enema is prepared by peptonized milk, 4 ounces, liquid beef preparation, ½ ounce, the white of 1 egg stirred into the mixture, and about 15 grains of salt. To this 15 cc. of *spiritus frumenti, i.e.,* ethyl alcohol U.S.P., may be added. This serves a double purpose because it is both nutritive as well as stimulating. Another formula is malted milk, 15 grams; Somatose, 4 grams; water, 4 ounces; sodium chloride, 15 grains; white of egg and peptonized milk, 1 ounce. Another is peptonized milk, 5 ounces, with white of 1 egg, alcohol, 1 dram, and 15 grains of salt. These solutions are best heated by setting in a pan of hot water.

NP: An evacuating enema of normal saline solution is usually given every 24 hours as an aid to absorption and to remove any mucus. The feedings may be given at 4 A. M. and at 8 A. M., followed at 12 noon with the cleansing enema, and a feeding at 4 P. M. and 8 P. M. The feedings should not consist of more than 4 to 8 ounces. The cleansing enema, however, is preferably given in the morning at about 6 o'clock, then the feeding may be given at 7 o'clock. This interval gives time to recover from any peristaltic irritation.

Not too much should be given at one time, and not at too frequent intervals. Every 2 hours should be sufficient *if only 2 or 3 ounces are given* at a time. The nurse should endeavor to estimate the amt. absorbed in a given time. Some feedings are ordered every 3 hours during the day, or every hour to 6 hours. If given every 4 hours during the day, the feeding at 4 or 6 o'clock in the morning may be omitted because the cleansing enema is usually given early in the morning to prepare the intestinal tract for the day's feedings.

The injections are given with a catheter which should be lubricated. Glycerine should not be used, as it activates peristalsis. At least 15 to 20 or 30 minutes should be taken for giving a nutritive enema, as the slower the feeding is given, the better are the chances of retention.

If patient cannot lie on left side for injection, hips should be elevated on a pillow (rubber covered). No air should be introduced through the rectal tube while giving the enema, as there may be a tendency to expel the solution.

PRECAUTION: Avoid anything that incites peristalsis. Be sure that the cleansing enema is administered before beginning a series of feedings as indicated. Every precaution should be taken to prevent the expulsion of the feeding, as the patient depends on this feeding for sustenance. Any expulsion of the feeding would defeat the purpose of the treatment.

e., olive oil. Mix 4 ounces of olive oil with 1 dram of turpentine, beating the mixture well so as to break the oil globules. This will cause sufficient peristalsis to move the bowels.

e., one-two-three. Magnesium sulfate, 1 ounce; glycerine, 2 ounces, and hot water, 3 ounces (115° F.).

This mixture must be given with a small tube because of the small quantity, and the action desired. The results following the injection are more satisfactory if given very carefully with assistance to help the patient retain it.

e., pancreatic. One containing pancreatin.

e., physiological salt solution. One teaspoonful of salt to a pint of water is a normal salt solution. It may be abbreviated as N. S. Sol. The distention made by this enema excites peristalsis and evacuation. There is no harm in retaining this enema. Often ordered when there is dehydration.

e., quantity of. For retention, 3 to 8 ounces. Cleansing: For a child: ½-1½ pints; infants: ½-2 ounces; adults: 2-4 pints.

e., retention. This is one to retain. It may be used to provide nourishment, to medicate a diseased mucous membrane, or for absorption purposes, or for general, local, or systemic action. This enema must be of constituents which will not stimulate the nerve endings and reflexly promote peristalsis. It necessarily must consist of a small amt. of solution. The rectum and lower bowel must first be well cleansed, and all irritation resulting from evacuation must subside before giving, or the purpose will be defeated. The patient should be placed on left side with knees flexed, and the rectal tube inserted high; 6 inches or more. Allow the fluid to flow through the tube before inserting to expel air. Pressure on tube should be made with fingers to prevent loss of liquid. Lubricate tube before inserting, and introduce with a twisting motion, slowly pushing it in so as not to bring discomfort to the patient. Unless absolutely necessary, the tube should not be slipped forward or backward to make the solution flow. Pushing may stimulate peristalsis. If the fluid does not readily flow, grasp tube in one hand, squeezing, compressing, and relaxing, so that suction will cause solution to flow. Allow fluid to run very slowly, stopping occasionally to aid retention. If the least desire to expel is manifested fluid should be stopped until the desire to evacuate has passed. Upon withdrawal of tube, which should be done quickly, pressure with a pad of cotton should be made over anus for a minute or two to prevent evacuation. The patient should be informed of the purpose of this enema so that cooperation may be secured. Enemas classed in the retention group may include the following: *emollient, lubricating, medicinal, nutritive, sedative, stimulating, q.v.*

e., Rosenheim's. A nutrient one, containing cod liver oil, sugar, and peptone in a 3% soda solution.

e., saline. One with solution of magnesium sulfate in warm water.

e., sedative. Retention enema given for its soothing action and to allay irritability. The temperature should be about 100°-105° F. Before and after it has been administered, the condition of the patient must be noted and recorded. Watch for untoward effects.

Paraldehyde may be ordered in delirium tremens, and this should be dissolved in thin, boiled starch solution. In water it dissolves in the proportion of 1 to 8. It must be injected with a small catheter. Paraldehyde is also sometimes ordered in epilepsy, manias, and various nervous irritations. The dosage varies in different institutions and among different physicians.

Chloral Hydrate: This may be administered as a sedative but only on a doctor's order. There are dangers attendant upon the administration of the drug in almost any form. The drug is dissolved in olive oil, hot milk, or boiled cornstarch. It should be given at a temperature of 105° F. and administered with a small catheter as a *high* enema. The higher, the better the absorption.

Paregoric: The tincture may be given per rectum if added to at least 2 ounces of thin starch water. The mixture should contain at least 2 ounces but not more than 4 ounces. It is prescribed for some specific result desired and given only on a physician's order.

e., simple mixed. A soapsuds enema to which is added 1 dram of salt and ½ ounce of molasses.

e., soapsuds. The soapsuds are either ready prepared, or may be made by placing soap particles in a shaker and agitating the water until the right consistency is obtained. If liquid soap is used, 1 ounce to 1 quart of water is the right proportion. A milky solution is of sufficient strength. Strong soapsuds should not be used, as there is danger of injuring the intestinal mucosa. The mild white soaps, such as castile, are best for suds.

INCOMPATIBILITIES: *Magnesium sulfate.*

e., s. s. & p. A mixture of 1 dram of peppermint added to a soapsuds solution. The peppermint may be added to a plain water solution, 1 dram to 16 ounces; a good enema to relieve flatulence.

e., s. s. & t. A mixture of thick liquid soap; green soap is best. Add ¼ ounce or 1 dram of turpentine and beat the 2 ingredients thoroughly together. The emulsion of this mixture is stirred into 1 quart of water at 115° F.

e., stimulating. This may be grouped with the medicated and the retention enemas. It is supposed to cause irritation. Should be given at 115° F. It is intended to excite activity and ordered when the patient is in shock, or in some unconscious state, as from narcotic poisoning. The patient's condition must be compared both before and after giving. Ingredients used are the following:

COFFEE: Eight ounces black coffee with 1 of *spiritus frumenti* given in 4-ounce doses and repeated in 2 hours if absorption has taken place. Otherwise, 4 ounces every 4 to 6 hours. Black coffee and warm saline solution, the coffee being cooked in the solution. A cup of coffee made from 1 tablespoonful of ground coffee to 1 cup of water gives the equivalent of 0.1 to 0.2 gram or 1½ to 3 grains of caffeine.

SALINE SOLUTION: Hot normal saline solution, 4 ounces, with ½ to 1 ounce of *spiritus frumenti.*

LUGOL'S SOLUTION: This solution with normal saline solution may be given per rectum as ordered.

e., temperature of. Carminative, stimulating, and for inflammations, 115° F. For hemorrhage, 120° F. For others, 105° F.

e., thirst. Analeptic enema, *q.v.*

e., yeast. One quart of warm water and ½ cake of yeast, thoroughly mixed and given very warm.

enema, *words pert. to:* coloclyster, colonic irrigation, clyster, enteroclysis, medication (rectal).

enepidermic (en-ep-ĭ-der′mĭk) [G. *en,* in, + *epi,* upon, + *derma,* skin]. Pert. to drugs applied without friction. SEE: *inunction.* Applied to or placed upon the surface of the skin. A term used in connection with application of medicinal agents to the skin without friction.

energometer (en-er-gom′ĕ-ter) [" + *ergon,* work, + *metron,* measure]. An instrument for measuring blood pressure. Especially one used in studying pulse pressure.

energy (en′er-jĭ) [" + *ergon,* work]. The capacity of a system for doing work or its equivalent in the strict physical sense.

Energy is manifested in various forms: Motion (kinetic e.), position (potential e.), light, heat, sound, and so on. These forms are mutually interchangeable according to certain laws. Thus, the chemical energy residing in 1 gram of glucose can be liberated in the form of heat, so that if complete oxidation (to carbon dioxide and water) is carried out at 20° C. and atmospheric pressure, one obtains 3.74 calories of heat. This fact is fundamental in the science of *dietetics.* SEE: *calorie.*

e. changes. These may be physical or chemical, or both. Movement of a part of the body, as the arm, shortens and thickens the muscles involved and changes the position and size of cells, temporarily, but the intake of oxygen in the blood, combining with sugar and fat, creates a chemical change, producing heat and waste products within the cells, which in turn produce fatigue if not eliminated.

e., conservation of. The theory that no energy in the universe can be lost, but that it may be transformed into other forms.

e., latent. That which exists but which is not being used.

e., potential. SEE: *latent e.*

e., radiant. That form of energy which is transmitted through space without the support of a sensible medium. Radio waves, infrared waves, visible rays, ultraviolet rays, x-rays, gamma rays and cosmic rays are energy in this form.

e., static. SEE: *latent e.*

energy, words pert. to: chemism, chemokinesis, dietetics, kinetic, metabolism, physical agents, radiant, synergic, unit, vril.

enerva'tion [L. *enervatio,* to weaken, + *nervus,* nerve]. Weakness; failure of nerve energy.

engagement. In obs. the entrance of the fetal head or the part being presented into the superior pelvic strait.

En'gelmann's disk [Theodor W. Engelmann, German physiologist, 1843-1909]. A narrow zone of transparent material lying on each side of the intermediate disk in the isotropic or I disk of a striated muscle fiber.

englobe' [G. *en,* in, + L. *globus,* a ball]. To absorb within a spherical body, as the ingestion of bacteria by the phagocytes.

Engman's disease [Martin F. Engman, American dermatologist, 1869-1953]. Pustular eruption resembling eczema, which often occurs simultaneously with a pyogenic process. SYN: *dermatitis infectiosa eczematoides.*

engorged (en-gorjd') [Fr. *engorger,* to obstruct, to devour]. Distended, as with blood.

engorge'ment [Fr. *engórger,* to obstruct, to devour]. Vascular congestion; distention.

engram (en'gram) [G. *en,* in, + *gramma,* mark]. 1. A memory trace. A theory that traces on protoplasm made by irritants or stimuli which, when repeated, form a habit after the stimulus ceases; the mnemic hypothesis. 2. The result of a psychic experience supposed to have established a pattern in memory. SEE: *ekphorize; mnemic theory.*

engraphia (en-graf'ĭ-ă) [" + *graphein,* to write]. The process of making engrams, *q.v.*

enhem'atospore [" + *aima,* blood, + *sporos,* spore]. A spore of the malarial parasite. SYN: *enhemospore; merozoite, q.v.*

enhemospore (en-hem'o-spōr) [" + " + *sporos,* spore]. A spore of the malarial parasite. SYN: *enhematospore; merozoite, q.v.*

enkatarrhaphy (en-kat-ar'af-ĭ) [G. *egkatarrhaptein,* to sew in]. Artificial implantation of a structure where it does not normally occur.

enolase (e'no-lās). An enzyme present in muscle tissue which converts phosphoglyceric acid to phosphopyruvic acid.

enomania (e"no-ma'nĭ-ă) [G. *oinos,* wine, + *mania,* madness]. Craving for alcoholic beverages; delirium tremens.

enophthalmus (en-of-thal'mus) [G. *en,* in, + *ophthalmos,* eye]. Recession of eyeball into orbit.

enosimania (en-os-ĭ-ma'nĭ-ă). A mental state characterized by excessive and irrational terror.

enostosis (en-os-to'sis) [" + *osteon,* bone, + *ōsis*]. An osseous tumor within the cavity of a bone.

ensiform (en'sĭ-form) [L. *ensis,* sword, + *forma,* form]. Swordlike structure.

e. cartilage. Lower part of sternum, below the gladiolus. SYN: *xiphoid cartilage or process.* SEE: *chondroxiphoid; xiphodynia.*

ensisternum (en-sĭ-ster'num) [" + G. *sternon,* sternum]. The tip of the sternum; ensiform or xiphoid appendix. SYN: *metasternum.*

enstrophe (en'stro-fe) [G. *en,* in, + *strephein,* to turn]. Inversion; a turning inward, esp. of eyelids.

en'tad [" + L. *ad,* toward]. Toward the inside; inwardly.

en'tal [G. *entos,* within]. Pert. to the interior; inside, central.

entamebiasis (ent-ă-me-bi'ă-sis) [" + *amoibē,* change]. Infestation with *Entamoeba.*

Entamoeba (ent-ă-me'bă) [" + *amoibē,* change]. A genus of ameba several of which live in the intestine of man. Some are parasitic. Characterized by the presence of 4 or 8 nuclei in their cysts.

E. buccalis. *E. gingivalis, q.v.*

E. coli. Found normally in the upper intestinal tract. Nonpathogenic to man.

E. gingivalis. Nonpathogenic species which inhabits the mouth.

E. histolytica. A pathogenic form of ameba, the cause of amebic dysentery and tropical abscess.

E. kartul'isi. Found in the pus of necrotic bone abscesses.

E. tetrage'na. Now considered identical with *E. histolytica.*

E. un'dulans. A species found in the intestine.

entasia (en-ta'sĭ-ă) [G. *entasis,* a straining]. Spasmodic muscular contraction.

entelechy (en-tel'ĕ-kĭ) [G. *entelecheia,* actuality]. 1. Complete development. 2. The activating cause of everything.

enteradeni'tis [G. *enteron,* intestine, + *adēn,* gland, + *-itis,* inflammation]. Inflammation of intestinal glands.

en'teral [G. *enteron,* intestine]. Within the intestine as distinguished from *parenteral.*

enteralgia (en-ter-al'jĭ-ă) [" + *algos,* pain]. Neuralgia or pain in the intestines. Intestinal cramps or colic.

enterectasia (en-ter-ek-tā'sĭ-ă) [" + *ektasis,* dilatation]. Dilatation of the small intestines.

enterectomy (en-ter-ek'to-mĭ) [" + *ek-tomē,* excision]. Excision of a portion of the intestines.

enterelcosis (en-ter-el-ko'sis) [" + *el-kōsis,* ulceration]. Intestinal ulceration.

enterepiplocele (en-ter-ep-ip'lo-sēl) [" + *epiploon,* omentum, + *kēlē,* hernia]. Hernia involving the bowel and omentum.

enteric (en-ter'ik) [G. *enteron,* intestine]. Pert. to the intestinal tract.

e. -coated tablets. Tablets which are coated with a substance that does not dissolve until reaching the intestine where the drug is then released.

e. fever. Typhoid fever.

enter'icoid [" + *eidos,* resemblance]. Resembling typhoid fever.

enteritis (en-ter-i'tis) [" + *-ītis,* inflammation]. Inflammation of the intestines, more particularly of the mucous and submucous tissues usually of the small intestines.

e., acute catarrhal. Acute inflammation of ileum and colon with diarrhea and intestinal catarrh. SYM: Frequent, watery, light colored stools, abdominal colic, flatus. Attack short. TREATMENT: Liquid diet, laxatives, milk purgatives; complete rest.

e., chronic catarrhal. Chronic inflammation of intestines and colon with chronic diarrhea. SYM: Less severe than acute catarrhal enteritis. TREATMENT: Diet restricted to milk, soups, cooked fruits, and vegetables. Rest.

e., croupous. Diphtheritic. A sequel of typhoid fever and other diseases. Often characterized by formation of false membrane. TREATMENT: SEE: *chronic c. e.*

e., mucous. A condition involving the intestinal mucosa characterized by excessive secretion of mucus and passage in the stools of shreds of pseudomembranous material. Usually accompanied by constipation or diarrhea or both alternating; intestinal myxoneurosis.

entero- [G. *enteron,* intestine]. Prefix: Noting some relation to the intestines.

enteroanastomosis (en"ter-o-an-as"to-mo'sĭs) [" + *ana,* up, + *stomōsis,* a mouth]. Intestinal anastomosis.

enteroan'tigen [" + *anti,* against, + *gennan,* to form]. An antigen derived from the feces.

enteroapokleisis (en"ter-o-ap-o-klī'sis) [" + *apokleisis,* a shutting out]. Operation for exclusion of a part of the intestine.

enterobacteriotherapy (en"ter-o-bak-te"rĭ-o-ther'ă-pĭ) [" + *bakterion,* little rod, + *therapeia,* treatment]. Use of vaccines containing intestinal bacteria.

enterobi'asis [" + *bios,* life]. Infestation with pinworms (*Enterobius vermicularis*).

enterobil'iary [" + L. *bilis,* bile]. Pert. to the intestines and the bile passages.

Enterobius (en-ter-o'bĭ-us). A genus of parasitic nematode worms, formerly *Oxyuris vermicularis.*

E. vermicularis. A species of nematode worms which inhabits the cecum, appendix, and neighboring regions of the intestine. In females, the genital organs and bladder may become infected. Female worms average 8 to 13 mm. in length, male worms, 2 to 5 mm. Distribution is world wide. Infestations characterized by irritation of the anal region and allergic reaction of the neighboring skin, accompanied by intense itching which may result in loss of sleep, excessive irritability, and a secondary infection of the area around the anus as a result of the scratching. SYN: *pinworm.*

enterobro'sia [" + *brōsis,* an eating]. Perforation of the intestine.

enterocele (en'ter-o-sēl) [" + *kēlē,* hernia]. 1. A hernia of the intestine. 2. Post. vaginal hernia.

enterocentesis (en"ter-o-sen-te'sis) [" + *kentēsis,* puncture]. Puncture of intestine to withdraw gas or fluids.

enterochirurgia (en"ter-o-ki-rur'jĭ-ă) [" + *cheir,* hand, + *ergon,* work]. Intestinal surgery.

enterocholecystostomy (en"ter-o-ko"le-sis-tos'to-mĭ) [" + *cholē,* bile, + *kystis,* a bladder, + *stōma,* opening]. Making an opening bet. the gallbladder and small intestine. SYN: *cholecystenterostomy.*

enterocholecystotomy (en"ter-o-ko"le-sis-tot'o-mĭ) [" + " + " + *tomē,* incision]. Incision of both gallbladder and intestine.

enterocinesia (en"ter-o-sin-e'sĭ-ă) [" + *kinēsis,* movement]. Intestinal movement. SYN: *peristalsis.*

enterocinetic (en"ter-o-sin-et'ik) [" + *kinēsis,* movement]. Pert. to or promoting peristalsis.

enteroclysis (en-ter-ok'lĭ-sis) [" + *klysis,* injection]. 1. Injection of a nutrient or medicinal liquid into bowel. 2. Irrigation of colon with large amt. of fluid intended to fill the colon completely and flush it. SEE: *proctoclysis.* SYN: *enteroclysm; high enema.*

PREPARATIONS USED: 1. Bicarbonate of soda, 1 teaspoonful of soda to a pint or quart of normal saline solution. 2. Powdered alum, 1 teaspoonful to a quart of water, may be used. 3. Flaxseed-tea, made very thin. 4. Normal salt solution, 1 teaspoonful of salt to 1 pint of water. This need not be sterile, unless indicated by rectal operation or condition. 5. Oil of peppermint or cinnamon, 5 to 15 drops to a pint of saline solution or plain water. 6. Potassium permanganate, 3 to 10 grains to 2 quarts of water.

NP: After a cleansing enema, administer the solution, and note and chart the following: All symptoms of the patient; the amount of the solution given; its nature; time of administering; length of treatment; results obtained and the reaction of the patient as to relief, discomfort, or untoward symptoms.

en'teroclysm [G. *enteron,* intestine, + *klysmos,* an injection]. A high enema. SYN: *enteroclysis.*

enterococcus. Any species of streptococcus inhabiting the intestine.

enterocoele (en'ter-o-sēl) [" + *koilia,* hollow]. The abdominal cavity.

enterocolitis (en"ter-o-ko-li'tis) [" + *kōlon,* colon, + *ītis,* inflammation]. Inflammation of intestines and colon. The more common types are acute pseudomembranous e. and tuberculous e. Necrosis of mucosa of large and small bowel takes place. This serious condition requires immediate treatment of shock, regulation of electrolyte balance, antibiotics if ordered by physician.

enterocrinin (en-ter-ok'rĭ-nin) [G. *enteron,* intestine, + *krinein,* to separate]. Hormone from animal intestines which aids digestion by stimulating the secretion of intestinal juice by the intestinal glands.

enterocyst (en'ter-o-sist) [" + *kystis,* cyst]. A cyst of the intestinal wall.

enterocystocele (en"ter-o-sis'to-sēl) [" + " + *kēlē,* hernia]. Hernia of the bladder wall and intestine.

enterocysto'ma [" + " + *ōma,* tumor]. Cystic tumor of the intestinal wall. SYN: *enterocyst.*

enterodyn'ia [" + *odynē,* pain]. Pain in the intestine. SYN: *enteralgia.*

en"teroenteros'tomy [" + *enteron* + *stōma,* opening]. Formation of a communication bet. two segments (not continuous) of the intestine.

enteroepiplocele (en"ter-o-e-pip'lo-sēl) [" + *epiplōon,* omentum, + *kēlē,* hernia]. Hernia of small intestine and omentum.

en"terogastri'tis [" + *gastēr,* belly, + *ītis,* inflammation]. Inflammation of stomach (gastritis) and of the intestines (enteritis).

enterogastrone (en"ter-o-gas'trōn) [" + *gastēr,* belly]. A hormone secreted by the intestinal mucosa which, by depressing gastric motility and secretion, controls the release of food from the stomach into the duodenum.

enterogenous (en-ter-oj'ĕ-nus) [" + *gennan,* to produce]. Originating in the intestines.

en'terogram [" + *gramma,* mark]. Tracing or graph of intestinal movements.

enterog'raphy [" + *graphein,* to write]. 1. A description of the intestines. 2. Making of an enterogram.

en"terohepat'ic [" + *ēpar, ēpat-,* liver]. Pert. to intestines and the liver.

en"terohepati'tis [" + " + *ītis,* inflammation]. Inflamed condition of both intestine and liver.

enterohydrocele (en"ter-o-hi'dro-sēl) [" + *ydōr,* water, + *kēlē,* hernia]. Hydrocele with loop of intestine in the sac.

enteroidea (en-ter-oyd'e-ă) [" + *eidos,* form]. The intestinal fevers; those caused by intestinal bacilli including typhoid fever.

enterokinase (en-ter-o-ki'nās) [" + *kinēsis,* movement]. A substance or hormone occurring in the mucosa of the duodenum, necessary for the activation of the trypsinogen of the pancreatic juice which is converted into trypsin. One of the enzymes of the *succus entericus.* It has no fat-splitting properties.

RS: *enzyme, prosecretin, trypsin, trypsinogen.*

enterolith (en'ter-o-lith) [" + *lithos,* stone]. An intestinal concretion.

enterolithiasis (en"ter-o-lĭ-thi'ă-sis) [" + *lithos,* stone]. The formation or existence of intestinal calculi.

enterol'ogy [" + *logos,* study]. The study of the intestinal tract.

en"teromega'lia, en"teromeg'aly [" + *megas,* large]. Abnormal enlargement of the intestines. SYN: *megacolon; megaloenteron.*

Enteromonas hominis (ĕn-tĕr-ŏm'ō-nās). A minute flagellated, protozoan parasite which lives in the intestine of man. It is rare and considered nonpathogenic.

enteromyco'sis [" + *mykēs,* fungus, + *ōsis*]. Disease of intestine due to bacteria. May include bacterial diseases.

enteromyiasis (ĕn-tĕr-ō-mī-ă'sĭs). Disease due to the presence of maggots (the larvae of flies) in the intestines.

enteron (en'ter-on) [G.]. The intestine.

enteroneuri'tis [G. *enteron,* intestine, + *neuron,* nerve, + *ītis,* inflammation]. Neuritis of the intestine.

enteronitis (en-ter-on-i'tis) [" + *ītis,* inflammation]. Inflammation of the small intestine. SYN: *enteritis.*

enteropareis (en-ter-o-par'ĕ-sis) [" + *paresis,* relaxation]. Flaccidity of the intestinal walls with diminished peristalsis.

enteropathy (en-ter-op'ă-thĭ) [" + *pathos,* disease]. Any intestinal disease.

enteropexy (en'ter-o-peks-ĭ) [" + *pēxis,* fixation]. Fixation of the intestine to the abdominal wall.

enteroplasty (en'ter-o-plas-tĭ) [" + *plassein,* to form]. Plastic operation on intestines. NP: Watch diet and fluid orders. Care of mouth. SEE: *laparotomy.*

enteroplegia (en"ter-o-ple'jĭ-ă) [" + *plēgē,* stroke]. Paralysis of the bowels.

enteroplex (en'ter-o-pleks) [" + *plexis,* a weaving]. Instrument for joining cut edges of intestines.

en'teroplexy [" + *plexis,* a weaving]. Union of divided parts of the intestine.

enteroproctia (en-ter-o-prok'shĭ-ă) [" + *proktos,* anus]. The condition of having an artificial anus.

enteroptosis (en-ter-op-to'sis) [" + *ptōsis,* a dropping]. Prolapse of the intestine or abdominal organs.

enterorrhagia (en"ter-o-ra'jĭ-ă) [" + *rēgnunai,* to burst forth]. Hemorrhage from the intestines.

enterorrhaphy (en-ter-or'ă-fĭ) [" + *raphē,* suture]. The stitching of the lips of an intestinal wound, or of the intestines to some other structure.

enterorrhexis (en-ter-o-reks'is) [" + *rēxis,* rupture]. Rupture of the intestine.

enteroscope (en'ter-o-skōp) [" + *skopein,* to examine]. Device for examination of intestines.

enterosep'sis [" + *sēpsis,* decay]. Intestinal toxemia; sepsis developed from the intestinal contents.

enterosite (en'ter-o-sīt) [" + parasite]. Any parasite which inhabits the intestinal tract.

enterospasm (en'ter-o-spazm) [" + *spasmos,* spasm]. Painful peristalsis.

enterosta'sis [" + *stasis,* a standing]. Intestinal stasis. Cessation of or delay in the passage of food through the intestine.

enterosteno'sis [" + *stēnōsis,* a narrowing]. Narrowing or stricture of the intestine.

enterostomy (en-ter-os'to-mĭ) [" + *stoma,* opening]. Surgical formation of a permanent opening into the intestine through the abdominal wall.

enterotome (en'ter-o-tōm) [" + *tomē,* incision]. Instrument for incision of intestines.

enterotomy (en-ter-ot'o-mĭ) [" + *tomē,* a cutting]. Incision or dissection of the intestines.

en"terotox'in. 1. A toxin produced in or originating in the intestinal contents. 2. A toxin specific for the cells of the mucosa. 3. A toxin produced by certain species of bacteria which produces symptoms characteristic of food poisoning.

enterotox'ism [" + *toxikon,* poison, + *ismos,* condition]. Absorption of intestinal toxins. SYN: *enterosepsis.*

enterotrop'ic [" + *tropē,* a turning]. Affecting or attracted by the intestines.

enterovac'cine [" + L. *vacca,* a cow]. A vaccine composed of fecal bacteria.

enterovi'rus. A member of a group of human viruses including the three polioviruses, the Coxsackie viruses, and the ECHO viruses.

enterozo'ic [" + *zōon,* animal]. Pert. to parasites inhabiting the intestines.

enterozo'on [" + *zōon,* animal]. Any intestinal animal parasite.

entheomania (en-the-o-ma'nĭ-ă) [G. *entheos,* inspired, + *mania,* madness]. Religious insanity.

enthesis (en'thĕ-sis) [G. a putting in]. The use of metallic or other inorganic substances to substitute for or replace lost tissue.

enthetic (en-thet'ik) [" + *tithenai,* to place]. Introduced from outside. SYN: *exogenous.*

enthlasis (en'thlă-sis) [" + *thlan,* to dent]. Depressed fracture of the skull.

ento- [G.]. Prefix, *entos,* within, inside.

en'toblast [G. *entos,* within, + *blastos,* germ]. The entoderm, *q.v.,* or hypoblast.

entocele (en'to-sēl) [" + *kēlē,* hernia]. 1. Internal hernia. 2. Displacement of a part, inward.

entochondrostosis (en"to-kon-dros-to'sis) [" + *chondros,* cartilage, + *ōsis*]. The development of bone within cartilage.

entochoroidea (en"to-ko-roy'de-ă) [" + *chorioeidēs,* choroid]. The inner layer of the choroid; coat of the eye.

entocineria (en-to-sin-e'rĭ-ă) [" + L. *cinereus,* ashen]. The internal gray matter of nerve centers, esp. of the brain.

entocone (en'to-kōn) [" + *kōnos,* cone]. The inner post. cusp of an upper molar tooth.

entocor'nea [" + L. *corneus,* horny]. Post. or inner lining membrane of cornea. SYN: *Descemet's membrane.*

entocyte (en'to-sīt) [" + *kytos,* cell]. Int. part of a cell within the ectoplasm. SYN: *endoplasm.*

entoderm (en'to-derm) [" + *derma,* skin]. SYN: *endoderm; hypoblast.* Inner layer of cells in the blastoderm.* Innermost of the three primary germ layers of a developing embryo. It gives rise to the epithelium of the digestive tract and its associated glands, the respiratory organs, bladder, vagina and urethra.

entoectad (en-to-ek'tad) [" + *ektos,* without, + L. *ad,* toward]. From within outward.

entome (en'tōm) [G. *en,* in, + *tomē,* a cut]. Knife for division of urethral stricture.

entomion (en-to'mĭ-on) [G. *entomē,* notch]. The tip of mastoid angle of the parietal bone.

entomol'ogy [G. *entomon,* insect, + *logos,* science]. The study of insects.

e., medical. That branch of entomology which deals with insects and their relationship to disease.

entophyte (en'to-fīt) [G. *entos,* within, + *phyton,* plant]. Any vegetable parasite living within the body.

entopic (en-top'ik) [G. *en,* in, + *topos,* place]. Normally situated; in a normal place.

entoptic (en-top'tĭk) [G. *entos,* within, + *optikos,* seeing]. Situated in the eyeball.

entoptoscopy (en"top-tos'ko-pĭ) [" + *ōps,* eye, + *skopein,* to examine]. Inspection of intraocular shadows.

entoral (en-to'răl) [" + L. *os, or-,* mouth]. Proprietary name for an oral cold vaccine.

entoret'ina [" + L. *rete,* a net]. Internal layer of the retina.

entorrhagia (en-tor-a'jĭ-ă) [" + *rēgnunai,* to burst forth]. Enterorrhagia.

entos'thoblast [G. *entosthe,* from within, + *blastos,* germ]. Hypothetical nucleus of the nucleolus.

entotic (ent-o'tik, ent-ot'ik) [G. *entos,* within, + *ous, ot-,* ear] Pert. to int. of ear or to perception of sound due to condition of the auditory apparatus.

entozoon (en-to-zo'on) (pl. *entozo'a*) [" + *zōon,* animal]. Any animal parasite in any internal organ.

entrophia (en-tro'fĭ-ă) [G. *en,* in, + *trophē,* nourishment]. Normal growth and nourishment.

entro'pion [" + *trepein,* to turn]. Inward curling of eyelid, esp. lower lid, with lashes.

e., cicatricial. An e. resulting from scar tissue on the inner surface of the lid.

e., spastic. An e. resulting from a spasm of the orbicularis oculi muscles.

entro'pionize [" + *trepein,* to turn]. To invert or correct by turning in.

entro'pium [" + *trepein,* to turn]. Entropion, *q.v.*

entropy (en'tro-pĭ). That portion of energy within a system which cannot be utilized for mechanical work but is available for internal use.

enucleate (e-nu'kle-āt) [L. *enucleāre,* to remove the kernel of]. 1. To remove a tumor or a structure from the body without rupturing; to remove a part entire. 2. To destroy or take out the nucleus of a cell.

enucleation (e-nu-kle-a'shun) [L. *enucleāre,* to remove the kernel of]. 1. Removal of a tumor or structure from its capsule. 2. Act of unfolding.

enu'cleator [L. *enucleāre,* to remove the kernel of]. Instrument for separating a tumor mass, as a myoma.

enuresis (en-u-re'sis) [G. *enourein,* to void urine]. Incontinence. Involuntary discharge of urine, complete or partial, diurnal or nocturnal, dependent upon pathologic or functional causes, although it may be voluntary as representative of a behavior pattern.

A child, for instance, may feel neglected, or feel a desire for attention, and attempt to center attention upon himself by deliberately wetting his bed. Urinary control, however, is generally established after the second year, although incontinence may be reestablished as a pathological manifestation.

Condition in adults is called incontinence, *q.v.*

e., diurnal. Urinary incontinence during the day and its etiology is of a pathological nature. It may be caused by muscular contractions brought about by laughing, coughing, or crying, and it often persists for long periods of time, esp. after protracted illness, but more frequently in the female.

ETIOL: Enuresis may result from urethral irritation, and fecal incontinence is sometimes associated with it. Excessive water drinking. There may be deficiency of the cord due to injury, cystitis may be present, and it may be associated with various diseases, such as diabetes insipidus and mellitus, epilepsy, or mental deficiency.

Children suffering from enuresis may be shy and sensitive; sometimes gloomy. These nervous manifestations may result from the reaction to the condition, or they may be a part of the behavior pattern of which the enuresis is a symptom.

NP: Examine the urine as soon as possible, esp. to ascertain the presence of white cells which are indicative of abnormality of the urinary tract. Great concern or censure should be avoided as it adds to apprehensiveness on part of child. If the result of a behavior pattern, the condition should be ignored as much as possible, but the cause of the behavior difficulty needs to be found and corrected.

Fluid should be restricted late in day,

and diurnal voidings should be spaced at more than ordinary intervals. The child may be awakened once or twice in the night and when fully awake, robed and walked to the bathroom. As improvement is noticed the number of awakenings may be lessened. The foot of the bed may also be elevated.

e., nocturnal. Urinary incontinence during the night. Wetting is irregular, and unaccompanied by urgency or frequency. Incontinence may cease for several weeks only to return. This type is more common in boys than in girls.

envi'ronment [L. *in,* in, + *virer,* to turn]. The surroundings, conditions, or influences which affect an organism, or the cells within an organism.

e., external. Those influences which are outside the body.

e., internal. Those influences within the body. Specifically, the tissue fluid constitutes the internal environment.

enzygotic (en-zi-got'ik) [G. *en,* in, + *zygon,* yoke]. Developed from the same ovum.

e. twins. Identical twins; those developed from one ovum. SEE: *dizygotic.*

enzyme (en'zīm) [" + *zymē,* leaven]. An organic catalyst produced by living cells but capable of acting independently of the cells producing them. They are complex colloidal substances which are capable of inducing chemical changes in other substances without themselves being changed in the process.

Enzymes are found particularly in digestive juices, acting upon food substances causing them to break down into simpler compounds. They are capable of accelerating greatly the speed of chemical reactions.

The reactions affected by the digestive enzymes are chiefly decompositions of a hydrolytic nature, but enzymes are equally important in the synthetic reactions of assimilation.

Each hydrolytic enzyme has been given a name which indicates the substance upon which it acts with the addition of the suffix *-ase.* As an example, *lipases* indicate fat-splitting enzymes; *amylases,* starch-splitting ones, and *proteases,* protein-splitting enzymes. Some of them take a qualifying adjective, as salivary or pancreatic enzymes. Exceptions are the enzymes rennin, pepsin, and trypsin.

The substance acted upon by an enzyme is called the *substrate.* Zymogen is the name given to the precursor of an enzyme. The more common groups of enzymes are: (a) Hydrolytic e., fat, protein, starch, and sugar-splitting e.'s. (b) Coagulating e.'s or those which cause clotting. (c) Oxidases or oxydizing e.'s, deaminizing e.'s. Those destroying amines or amino groups during oxidation. (d) Reductases or reducing e.'s. (e) Those producing carbon dioxide without the use of free oxygen. (f) Those which produce the breakdown of a larger molecule into a smaller one without change of composition. (g) Mutases, those which bring about chemical rearrangement without change of the molecules in size.

Enzymes are specific in their action,

Summary of the Main Enzymatic Processes in Digestion*

Site	Secretion	Enzyme	Substrate	Degree of Digestion	Products of Digestion
Mouth.	Saliva.	Ptyalin.	Starch.	Slight.	Dextrins, maltose.
		Maltase.	Maltose.	Very slight.	Glucose.
Stomach.	Gastric juice.	Pepsin.	Protein.	Incomplete.	Proteoses, peptones.
		Rennin.	Casein.	Nearly complete.	Paracasein.
		Lipase.	Emulsified fats.	Very slight.	Fatty acids, glycerol.
Intestine.	Pancreatic juice.	Trypsin. Chymotrypsin. Carboxypeptidase.	Proteins. Proteoses. Peptones. Peptides.	Nearly complete.	Amino acids.
		Steapsin.	Fats.	Nearly complete.	Insoluble fatty acids, glycerol.
		Amylopsin.	Starch.	Nearly complete.	Dextrins, maltose.
Intestine.	Intestinal juice and intestinal mucosa.	Erepsin.	Ordinary peptides.	Nearly complete.	Amino acids.
		Amylase.	Starch.	Nearly complete.	Dextrins, maltose.
		Enterokinase.	Trypsinogen.		Trypsin.
		Maltase.	Maltose.	Complete.	Glucose.
		Lactase.	Lactose.	Complete.	Glucose, galactose.
		Sucrase.	Sucrose.	Usually complete.	Glucose, fructose.
		Nucleosidases (in mucosa).	Nucleosides.	Usually complete.	Purine bases, carbohydrates.

*Adapted from Biddle, H. C., and Floutz, V. W.: Chemistry in Health and Disease, 6th ed. F. A. Davis Company, Philadelphia. 1965.

i. e., they will act only upon a certain substance or a group of chemically closely related substances and no other; each enzyme has an optimum temperature at which it acts with greatest efficiency; each enzyme is influenced by the reaction of the medium in which it acts, there being an optimum degree of acidity or alkalinity.

Enzyme activity can be retarded or inhibited by (a) low temperatures, (b) high temperatures, (c) presence of salts of heavy metals (copper, mercury), (d) dehydration, (e) ultraviolet radiation.

Enzymes sometimes require the presence of additional substances in order to make them active. Nonspecific substances which activate enzymes are called *activators* (Ex: HCI for pepsin); specific substances which act selectively with certain enzymes only are called *coenzymes* (Ex: enterokinase for trypsinogen). More than 650 enzymes are known.

e., amylolytic. E. changing starch to sugar.

e., autolytic. E. producing autolysis, or cell digestion.

e., bacterial. E. developed by bacteria.

e., coagulating. E. converting soluble proteins into insoluble ones. Ex: *rennin.* A coagulase.

e., deamidizing. E. dividing amino acids into ammonia compounds.

e., decarboxylating. E. which separates CO_2 from organic acids. (Ex: *carboxylase*).

e., digestive. E. which is involved in digestive processes in the alimentary canal.

e., extracellular. E. which produces its effects outside the cell that produces it.

e., fermenting. E. produced by bacteria or yeasts which bring about the fermentation of substances, esp. carbohydrates.

e., glycolytic. E. oxidizing sugar.

e., hydrolytic. E. which reacts on a substance to form smaller molecules by the addition of water.

e., inorganic. A metallic colloidal solution, acting somewhat like an e.

e., intracellular. An enzyme that acts within the cell which produces it.

e., inverting. E. that converts a double sugar (sucrose) into simple sugars.

e., lipolytic. E. that acts on fats hydrolyzing them to glycerol and fatty acids; a lipase.

e., oxidation. SEE: *deamidizing e.*

e., oxidizing. E. that catalyzes oxidative reactions; an oxidase or dehydrogenase.

e., polypeptolytic. E. having a hydrolytic action on the polypeptides.

e., proteolytic. E. changing proteins into peptones.

e., reducing. Reductase. One that withdraws oxygen.

e., respiratory. E. that acts within tissue cells catalyzing oxidative reactions with the release of energy. Ex: *flavoproteins, cytochromes.*

e., steatolytic. SEE: *lipolytic e.*

e., sucrolastic. E. dividing or decomposing sugar.

e., uricolytic. E. converting uric acid into urea.

e., yellow. A flavoprotein. One of a group of enzymes involved in cellular oxidations.

enzymolysis (en-zim-ol'ĭ-sis) [G. *en,* in, + *zymē,* leaven, + *lysis,* dissolution]. Chemical change caused by an enzyme. SYN: *enzymosis.*

enzymo'sis [" + " + *ōsis*]. Enzymolysis.

enzymuria (en-zīm-u'rĭ-ă) [" + " + *ouron,* urine]. Enzymes in the urine.

eonism (e'on-izm). Desire to dress in the clothing of the opposite sex; a sexual perversion. SYN: *transvestism.**

eosin (e'o-sin) [G. *ēōs,* dawn (rose colored)]. ($C_{20}H_8Br_4O_5$.) 1. A dye derived from action of bromine on fluorescein. An acid dye much used for staining tissues for microscopic examination. Brownish-red crystals used in microscopy as a stain. SYN: *tetrabromfluorescein.* 2. Any of several similar dyes. 3. Rosy-red; dawn colored.

eosin'oblast [G. *eōs,* dawn, + *blastos,* germ]. A bone marrow cell which develops into a myelocyte. SYN: *myeloblast.*

eosinopenia (e"o-sin-o-pe'nĭ-ă) [" + *penia,* poverty]. Abnormally small number of eosinophil cells in the peripheral blood.

eosinophil (e-o-sin'o-fĭl) [" + *philein,* to love]. A cell or cellular structure that stains readily with the acid stain, *eosin;* specifically an eosinophil leukocyte.

e. leukocytes. Spherical cells found in blood and sometimes in connective tissues having a diameter of 9 to 14 microns. The nucleus is polymorphic usually having two lobes connected by a thin strand. The cytoplasm contains numerous coarse, highly refractile granules which stain intensely with eosin or other acid stains. They constitute 2% to 4% of the white cell count.

Eosinophil leukocytes originate in the red bone marrow. Their function is not well established. They are ameboid but do not exhibit phagocytic activity. They increase in number in certain diseases such as asthma and in certain infestations with animal parasites. They decrease in number in circulating blood following the administration of ACTH or cortisone.

eosinophile (e-o-sin'o-fĭl). 1. Eosinophilic. 2. Eosinophil, *q.v.*

eosinophilia (e"o-sin-o-fil'ĭ-ă) [" + *philein,* to love]. 1. Accumulation of ununusual number of eosinophils in the blood. 2. Condition of being eosinophilic.

eosinophilic (e"o-sin-o-fil'ik) [" + *philein,* to love]. Readily stainable with eosin.

eosinophilous (e"o-sin-of'ĭ-lus) [" + *philein,* to love]. 1. Easily stainable with eosin. 2. Having eosinophilia.

eosinotactic (e-o-sin-o-tak'tik) [" + *taktikos,* arranged]. Attraction or repulsion of eosinophil cells.

epacmastic (ep-ak-mas'tĭk) [G. *epi,* upon, + *akmē,* prime]. Denoting increase of symptoms. RS: *acmastic, paracmastic.*

epac'tal [G. *epaktos,* added to]. Supernumerary.

e. bone. Wormian bone.

eparsalgia (ep-ar-sal'jĭ-ă) [G. *epairein,* to lift, + *algos,* pain]. Any disorder due to overstrain of a part. SYN: *epersalgia.*

eparterial (ep-ar-te'rĭ-al). Located over or above an artery.

epaxial (ep-ak'sĭ-al) [G. *epi,* upon, + L. *axis,* axis]. Situated above or behind any axis.

epencephalon (ep-en-sef'ă-lon) [" + *egkephalos,* brain]. The metencephalon; the anterior portion of the embryonic hindbrain (rhombencephalon) from which arise the pons and cerebellum.

ependyma (ep-en'dĭ-mă) [G. *ependyma,* wrap]. Membrane lining the cerebral ventricles and central canal of spinal cord.

e. *medullae spinalis.* The spinal portion of the e.

e. *ventriculorum cerebri.* The ventricular portion of the e.

epen'dymal. Pertaining to the ependyma.

e. *cells.* Cells of the developing neural tube which give rise to the ependyma. They arise from spongioblasts derived from the neural epithelium.

e. *layer.* The innermost of three layers which form the neural tube of an embryo.

ependymitis (ep"en-dĭ-mī'tis) [" + *-itis,* inflammation]. Inflammation of the ependyma.

ependymoblast (ep-en'dĭ-mo-blast [" + *blastos,* germ]. An embryonic ependymal cell or ependymocyte.

ependymocyte (ep-en'dĭ-mo-sīt) [" + *kytos,* cell]. A cell of the ependymal region.

ependymo'ma [" + *ōma,* tumor]. A tumor arising from fetal inclusion of ependymal elements.

EPF. Exophthalmos-producing factor.

ephebiatrics (ĕ-fe-bĭ-at'riks). A branch of medicine dealing with adolescents.

ephebic (ĕ-fe'bik) [G. *ephēbikos,* pert. to puberty]. Pert. to adolescence.

ephebology (ĕ-fe-bol'o-jĭ) [G. *ephēbos,* puberty]. The study of puberty and its changes.

ephedrine (ĕ-fed'rin, ef'ĕ-drin). An alkaloid originally obtained from species of *Ephedra;* first isolated by Nagai in 1887. In ancient Chinese medicine it was used as a diaphoretic and antipyretic. It was not until recent times, however, that its action was studied and its valuable therapeutic properties made known. It is a sympathomimetic drug, and is usually produced synthetically.

Action: Similar to that of adrenalin. Its effects, although less powerful, are more prolonged, and it exerts an action when given orally, whereas adrenalin is effective only by injection. Ephedrine orally (or by injection) dilates the bronchial muscles, contracts the nasal mucosa, and raises the blood pressure. Chiefly used for its bronchodilator effect in asthma, and for its constricting effects on the nasal mucosa in hay fever.

Incompatibilities: *Calcium chloride, iodine, tannic acid.*

e. *hydrochloride.* A more soluble salt of the alkaloid, having the same action and uses as e.

e. *sulfate.* USP. The sulfate of ephedrine. It occurs as fine white crystals or as a powder. Its action and uses are the same as those for e.

ephelis (ef-e'lis) (pl. *ephelides*) [G. *ephēlis,* freckle]. Freckle, lentigo.*

ephemeral (e-fem'er-al) [G. *epi,* upon, + *ēmera,* day]. Of brief duration.

ephidrosis (ef-i-dro'sis) [G. *ephidrōsis,* a sweating]. Abnormal amt. of sweating.

e. *cruenta.* Sweat containing blood.

e. *saccharata.* Diabetic condition in which sugar is present in sweat.

e. *tincta.* Colored sweat. Syn: *chromidrosis.*

epi-, ep- [G.]. Prefix meaning upon, at, in addition to.

epiallopregnanolone (ep"ĭ-al"o-preg-nan'-o-lōn). Male sex hormone in urine of pregnant women, which helps to form male sex characteristics.

epiblast [G. *epi,* upon, + *blastos,* germ]. Outer layer of cells of the blastoderm. Syn: *ectoderm, q.v.*

epiblastic (ep-ĭ-blas'tik) [" + *blastos,* germ]. Pert. to the epiblast.

epibole, epiboly (ĕ-pib'o-lĭ) [G. *epibolē,* cover]. Inclusion of the hypoblast within the epiblast, due to swifter growth of the latter. See: *emboly.*

epibulbar (ep-ĭ-bul'bar). Lying upon the bulb of any structure; more specifically, located upon the eyeball.

epican'thus [G. *epi,* upon, + *kanthos,* canthus]. A fold of skin extending from the root of the nose to the median end of the eyebrow, covering the inner canthus and caruncle. It is a characteristic of certain races and may occur as a congenital anomaly in Caucasians.

epicardia (ep-ĭ-kard'ĭ-ă) [" + *kardia,* heart]. The abdominal portion of the esophagus extending from the diaphragm to the stomach, about 2 cm. in length.

epicar'dium [" + *kardia,* heart]. The inner or visceral layer of the pericardium,* which forms a serous membrane forming the outermost layer of the wall of the heart.

epichordal (ep-ĭ-kord'al). Located dorsad to the notochord.

epicomus (ĕ-pik'o-mus). A congenital malformation consisting of a parasitic twin, or head attached to the summit or vertex of the skull.

epicondylalgia (ep"ĭ-kon-dĭ-lal'jĭ-ă) [" + *kondylos,* condyle, + *algos,* pain]. pain]. Pain in the elbow joint in the region of the epicondyles.

epicondyle (ep-ĭ-kon'dīl) [" + *kondylos,* condyle]. The eminence at the articular end of a bone above a condyle.

epicra'nium [" + *kranion,* cranium]. Soft parts covering the cranium.

epicranius (ep-ĭ-kra'nĭ-us) [" + *kranion,* cranium]. Occipitofrontal muscle and scalp.

epicri'sis [" + *krisis,* crisis]. A supplementary or secondary crisis following a return of morbid symptoms.

epicritic (ep-ĭ-krit'ik) [G. *epikritikos,* judging]. 1. Pertaining to extreme sensibility, such as that of the skin when it discriminates between degrees of sensation caused by touch or temperature. 2. Pertaining to an epicrisis, *q.v.*

epicysti'tis [G. *epi,* upon, + *kystis,* bladder, + *itis,* inflammation]. Inflammation of cellular tissue above the bladder.

epicystot'omy [" + " + *tomē,* incision]. Opening above the symphysis pubis into the bladder.

epicyte (ep'ĭ-sīt) [" + *kytos,* cell]. 1. An epithelial cell. 2. A cell membrane.

epidem'ic [" + *dēmos,* people]. Appearance of an infectious disease or condition which attacks many people at the same time in the same area.

e. *jaundice.* Infectious or spirochetal jaundice; Weil's disease. An infectious disease caused by a spirochete, *Leptospira icterohaemorrhagiae.* Sym: Onset of sudden fever, in a few days followed by jaundice, hemorrhage into skin, and anemia. See: *caribi; endemic; pandemic.*

epidemiography (ep"ĭ-de-mĭ-og'ră-fĭ) [" + " + *graphein,* to write]. Study of epidemic diseases.

epidemiologic (ep"ĭ-de-mĭ-o-loj'ik) [" + " + *logos,* study]. Pert. to the study of epidemics.

epidemiologist (ep″ĭ-de-mĭ-ol′o-jist) [" + " + *logos*, study]. One who specializes in epidemic diseases.

epidemiology (ep-ĭ-de-mĭ-ol′o-jĭ) [" + " + *logos*, study]. The division of medical science concerned with defining and explaining the interrelationships of the host, agent, and environment in causing disease.

epider′mal, epider′mic [" + *derma*, skin]. Pert. to the epidermis.

epidermatoplasty (ep-ĭ-der-mat′o-plas-tĭ) [" + " + *plassein*, to mould]. Grafting with pieces of epidermis with the underlying layer of the corium.

epidermic (ep-ĭ-der′mik) [" + *derma*, skin]. Pert. to the external layer of the skin or epidermis.

epidermidol′ysis [" + " + *lysis*, loosening]. Epidermolysis, *q.v.*

epidermidosis [" + " + *ōsis*]. Epidermosis, *q.v.*

epider′mis [" + *derma*, skin]. Cuticle, or outer layer of skin; scarf skin. It is nonvascular and is formed from within outward.

It consists of four layers or strata: (1) *stratum germinativum* (*s. mucosum;* malpighian layer), the innermost layer; (2) *s. granulosum* (*epidermis*), located immediately above the *s. germinativum;* (3) *s. lucidum*, the clear layer; (4) *s. corneum*, the outermost layer of the e.

epidermi′tis [" + " + *ītis*, inflammation]. Inflammation of the superficial layers of the skin.

epidermization (ep-ĭ-der-mĭ-za′shun) [" + *derma*, skin]. 1. Skin grafting. 2. Conversion of deeper germinative layer of cells into outer layer of epidermis.

epidermoid (ep-ĭ-der′moyd) [" + " + *eidos*, form]. 1. Resembling or pert. to the epidermis. 2. A tumor arising from aberrant epidermal cells. SYN: *cholesteatoma.*

epidermolysis (ep-ĭ-der-mol′ĭ-sis) [" + " + *lysis*, loosening]. Loosening of the epidermis.

e. bullosa. A form characterized by formation of deep-seated bullae appearing after irritation or rubbing of a part.

epidermo′ma [" + " + *ōma*, growth]. An excrescence on the skin.

epidermomycosis (ep-ĭ-der″mo-mi-ko′sis) [" + " + *mykēs*, fungus, + *ōsis*]. Skin disease caused by a fungus.

Epidermophyton (ep-ĭ-der-mof′ĭ-ton) [" + " + *phyton*, plant]. A genus of fungi, similar to Trichophyton but affecting the skin and nails, instead of the hair.

E. floccosum. The causative agent of certain types of tinea, esp. tinea pedis (athlete's foot), tinea cruris, tinea unguium, and tinea corporis.

epidermophytosis (ep-ĭ-der-mo-fi-to′sis) [" + " + " + *ōsis*]. Infection by a species of *Epidermophyton.*

epidermo′sis [" + " + *ōsis*]. Any disease affecting the skin, esp. the epidermis.

epidi′ascope [" + *dia*, through, + *skopein*, to examine]. Lantern used for projection of images on a screen. SYN: *episcope.*

epididymectomy (ep-ĭ-did-ĭ-mek′to-mĭ) [G. *epi;* upon, + *didymos;* testis, + *ektomē*, excision]. Removal of the epididymis.

epididymis (ep-ĭ-did′ĭ-mis) (Pl. *epididymides*) [" + *didymos*, testis]. A small, oblong body resting upon and beside the post. surface of the testes, consisting of a convoluted tube 13 to 20 ft. long, enveloped in the tunica vaginalis, ending in the ductus deferens.

It consists of (1) the *head* (caput or globus major) which contains 12 to 14 efferent ducts of the testis, (2) the *body*, and (3) the *tail* (cauda or globus minor). It constitutes the first part of the excretory duct of each testis. The epididymis is supplied by the internal spermatic, deferential, and external spermatic arteries; it is drained by corresponding veins.

epididymitis (ep-ĭ-did-ĭ-mi′tis) [" + " + *ītis*, inflammation]. Inflammation of the epididymis.

ETIOL: May be complication of gonorrhea, syphilis, tuberculosis, mumps, prostatitis, urethritis, prostatectomy, or following prolonged use of indwelling catheter.

SYM AND SIGNS: Fever and chills, pain in inguinal region, swollen epididymis.

TREATMENT: Bed rest, support of scrotum, and antibiotics or other drug therapy for primary infection (as penicillin for gonorrhea, streptomycin for tuberculosis, etc.).

epididymodeferentectomy (ep-ĭ-did-ĭ-mo-def′er-en-tek′to-mĭ) [" + " + L. *deferens*, carrying away, + G. *ektomē*, excision]. Excision of epididymis and ductus deferens.

epididymodeferen′tial [" + " + L. *deferens*, carrying away]. Concerning both the epididymis and ductus deferens.

epididymoorchitis (ep-ĭ-did-im-o-or-ki′-tis) [" + " + *orchis*, testis, + *ītis*, inflammation]. Epididymitis with orchitis.*

epididymot′omy [" + " + *tomē*, incision]. Incision into the epididymis.

epididymovasostomy (ep-ĭ-did″ĭ-mo-vas-os′to-mĭ) [" + " + L. *vas*, vessel, + *tomē*, incision]. Making an anastomosis bet. the epididymis and the vas.

epidu′ral [" + L. *durus*, hard]. Located over or upon the dura.

e. space. Space outside of dura mater of brain and spinal cord.

epifascial (ep-ĭ-fash′ĭ-al). On or upon a fascia.

epifolliculitis (ep-i-fol-lik-u-li′tis) [" + L. *folliculus*, follicle, + G. *ītis*, inflammation]. Inflammation of hair follicles of the scalp.

epigas′ter [" + *gastēr*, belly]. Embryonic structure which develops into the large intestine. SYN: *hindgut.*

ep″igastral′gia [" + " + *algos*, pain]. Pain in the epigastrium.

epigas′tric [" + *gastēr*, belly]. Pert. to the epigastrium. SEE: *precordia.*

e. reflex. Contraction of the upper portion of the rectus abdominis muscle when skin of the epigastric region is scratched.

epigastrium (ep-i-gas′trĭ-um) [" + *gastēr*, belly]. Region over the pit of the stomach. SEE: *Auenbrugger's sign.*

epigastrocele (ep-ĭ-gas′tro-sēl) [" + " + *kēlē*, hernia]. Hernia in the epigastrium.

epigastrorrhaphy (ep-i-gas-tror′ă-fĭ) [" + " + *raphē*, suture]. Suture of an abdominal wound in the epigastric area.

epigenesis (ep-ĭ-jen′ĕ-sis) [" + *genesis*, formation]. In embryology, the theory that parts of an organism arise by a process of progressive development from simple to complex structures through the utilization of cells as building units; in contrast to preformation which holds that parts exist in the ovum preformed.

epiglottid′ean [" + *glōttis*, glottis]. Pert. to the epiglottis.

epiglottidectomy (ep″i-glot-id-ek′to-mī) [" + " + *ektomē*, excision]. Excision of the epiglottis.

epiglottiditis (ep″ĭ-glot-tid-i′tis) [" + " + *itis*, inflammation]. Inflammation of the epiglottis. SYN: *epiglottitis*.

epiglot′tis (pl. *epiglottidēs*) [" + *glōttis*, glottis]. A thin leaf-shaped structure located immediately posterior to the root of the tongue which covers the entrance of the larynx when swallowing. It consists of the epiglottic cartilage, an impaired laryngeal cartilage, and is covered with mucous membrane.

epiglottitis (ep″ĭ-glot-i′tis) [" + " + -*itis*, inflammation]. A disease caused by *Hemophilus influenzae*. Death results, usually from respiratory obstruction, in nearly all untreated patients. Appears most commonly in young children.

SYM: Sore throat, fever, croupy cough, drooling, cyanosis, and even coma.

TREATMENT: Establishment of airway by tracheostomy if necessary. Administration of tetracyclines.

epihy′al [" + *uoeidēs*, U-shaped]. Pert. to the arch of the hyoid.

e. bone. Ossified stylohyoid ligament.

epilate (ep′ĭ-lāt) [L. *ē*, out, + *pilus*, hair]. To extract the hair by the roots.

ep′ilating [" + *pilus*, hair]. Depilating; extracting a hair.

e. dose. The quantity of roentgen rays or radium necessary to cause temporary loss of hair.

e. forceps. Tweezers for pulling out hairs.

epilation (ep-ĭ-la′shun) [" + *pilus*, hair]. Extraction of hair. SYN: *depilation*.

epilatory (e-pil′ă-tor-ĭ) [" + *pilus*, hair]. Pert. to removal of hairs, or that which removes them. SYN: *depilatory*.

epilemma (ep-ĭ-lem′ă) [G. *epi*, upon, + *lemma*, husk]. Neurilemma of small branches of nerve filaments.

ep″ilep′sy [G. *epilēpsia*, seizure]. An episodic disturbance of consciousness during which generalized convulsions may occur.

ETIOL: May be due to one of many causes; electroencephalographic studies reveal a direct relationship between changes in electrical brain potentials and the occurrence of seizures. Heredity plays an important role.

SYM: Often a peculiar sensation or feeling (the aura) precedes loss of consciousness. The patient falls during the attack, often injuring himself; he may bite his tongue, pass urine, and awake to realize something has happened because of muscular soreness.

There is a tendency to sleep following the attack; indeed attacks may occur only during sleep. The convulsion may be replaced by a so-called equivalent—during the unconsciousness, violent, antisocial or unnatural conduct may occur (automatism), which may have vast medicolegal significance.

On recovery, amnesia is complete and so no precautions to hide the antisocial acts are taken; this in itself is significant, esp. if associated with postautomatism, sleep, and a particularly vicious type of crime. The epileptic may gradually deteriorate, and in some cases finally become completely demented.

NP: Do not attempt to stop attack. During attack arrange head so as to facilitate breathing. Prevent tongue from being bitten, or from obstructing windpipe. Place pad between teeth during attack. Afterward allow patient to sleep. Dilantin is used as an anticonvulsant without depressive action, but toxicity must be guarded against.

GENERAL TREATMENT: Remove causative or precipitating factors (as operable brain tumors, endocrine disturbances, etc.). Regular well-balanced diet; no alcoholic beverages. Regular bowel habits. Regular amounts of sleep. Anticonvulsant drugs.

GRAND MAL: Often preceded by a peculiar sensation known as an aura, beginning in finger or toe and rising until head is involved, when patient gives shrill cry and falls unconscious; tonic spasm followed by clonic movements; face cyanosed; frothing at mouth; coma.

PROG: Unfavorable, although not fatal.

PETIT MAL: Seizure consists of momentary unconsciousness.

e., cortical. SEE: Jacksonian e.

e., focal. Jacksonian e., *q.v.*

e., hemiplegic. Jacksonian e., *q.v.*

e., idiopathic. Presence of epilepsy without known cause.

e., Jacksonian. E. in which convulsions tend to be restricted to certain groups of muscles, or limited to one side of the body, due to disease involving the cortex. Also called cortical, focal, hemiplegic, partial, or symptomatic e.

e., menstrual. Form in which attacks coincide with menstruation.

e., myoclonic. E. in which clonic contractions of muscles, esp. those of the extremities, occur between seizures. SEE: *myoclinia*.

e., nocturnal. Occurs only during sleep. Symptoms similar to grand mal. PROG: Favorable.

e., partial. Jacksonian e., *q.v.*

e., reflex. E. in which attacks are induced by peripheral irritation.

e., sleep. Spasmodic uncontrollable desire to sleep. SYN: *narcolepsy*.

e., spinal. E. due to lateral sclerosis of the spinal cord.

e., symptomatic. Jacksonian e., *q.v.*

e., thalamic. Form with lesion of the thalamus, causing hallucinations.

e., toxemic. E. due to presence of toxic substances in the blood.

e., traumatic. E. caused by trauma, particularly of the cranial vertex.

e., uncinate. E. due to a lesion of the uncinate gyrus of the temporal lobe.

epilepsy, *words pert. to:* absentia epileptica, analepsis, aura, cataptosis, fit, furor epilepticus, haut mal, ictus, status epilepticus.

epilep′tic [G. *epilēptikos*, pert. to a seizure]. 1. Concerning epilepsy. 2. Individual suffering from epileptic attacks.

epilep′tiform [G. *epilēpsia*, seizure, + L. *forma*, form]. Having the form of epilepsy.

epileptogenic, epileptogenous (ep″ĭ-lep-to-jen′ik, -toj′ĕ-nus) [" + *gennan*, to produce]. Giving rise to epileptoid convulsions.

e. zone. Certain motor areas in cerebral cortex, irritation of which gives rise to an epileptic seizure.

epilep′toid [" + *eidos*, resemblance]. Resembling epilepsy. SYN: *epileptiform*.

epileptol′ogy [" + *logos*, study]. Study of epilepsy.

epileptosis (ep-ĭ-lep-to′sis) [" + *ōsis*]. Any mental disease due to epilepsy.

epiloia (ep-ĭ-loy′ă). A syndrome consisting of mental deficiency, adenoma sebaceum, epileptic fits, hypertrophic sclerosis of the brain, tumors in the kidneys, and nodules on floor of lateral ventricle. SYN: *tuberous sclerosis.*

epilose (ep'ĭ-lōs) [L. *e,* without, + *pilus,* hair]. Bald, without hair.

epimandibular (ep"ĭ-man-dib'u-lar) [G. *epi,* upon, + L. *mandibulum,* jaw]. Above or upon the lower jaw.

epimenorrhagia (ep-ĭ-men-o-ra'jĭ-ă) [" + *mēn,* month, + *rēgnunai,* to burst forth]. Too much and too frequent menstruation.

epimenorrhea (ep-ĭ-men-o-re'ă) [" + " + *roia,* flow]. Menstruation occurring too frequently.

epimerite (ep-ĭ-mer'īt) [" + *meros,* part]. An organ of certain protozoa by which they attach themselves to epithelial cells.

epimysium (ep-ĭ-mis'ĭ-um) [" + *mys,* muscle]. Outermost sheath of connective tissue which surrounds a skeletal muscle. Consists of irregularly distributed collagenous, reticular, and elastic fibers, connective tissue cells, and fat cells.

ep'inasty [" + *nastos,* pressed close]. More vigorous growth on the upper than on the under surface, leading to a downward curvature of an organ.

epinephrectomy (ep-ĭ-ne-frek'to-mĭ) [" + *nephros,* kidney, + *ektomē,* excision]. Excision of the suprarenal gland. SYN: *adrenalectomy.*

epinephrine (ep-ĭ-nef'rĭn) [G. *epi,* upon, + *nephros,* kidney]. ($C_9H_{13}NO_3$). USP. This substance along with norepinephrine are the two active hormones produced by the adrenal medulla. Epinephrine which has been synthesized is also produced by tissues other than the adrenal. It is employed therapeutically as a vasoconstrictor, cardiac stimulant, to induce uterine contractions and to relax bronchioles. Its effects are similar to those brought about by stimulation of the sympathetic division of the autonomic nervous system. SYN: *adrenaline; adrenin; suprarenin.*

USES: To check local hemorrhage, to relieve asthmatic paroxysms, shock, etc. Also to prolong action of local anesthetics by constricting blood vessels, which prevents rapid absorption.

INCOMPATIBILITIES: Light, heat, and air, iron salts, and alkalies.

e. bitartrate. USP. A white or grayish white crystalline powder ($C_9H_{13}NO_3C_4H_6O_6$). It is a sympathomimetic agent used as a topical ophthalmic ointment.

epinephrinemia (ep"ĭ-nef"rĭ-ne'mĭ-ă) [" + " + *aima,* blood]. Epinephrine in the blood.

epinephritis (ep"ĭ-nef-ri'tis) [G. *epi,* upon, + *nephros,* kidney, + *-itis,* inflammation]. Inflammation of an adrenal gland.

epinephro'ma [" + " + *ōma,* tumor]. A lipomatoid tumor of the kidney. SYN: *Grawitz's tumor; hypernephroma.*

epineural (ep-ĭ-nu'ral) [" + *neuron,* nerve]. Located upon a neural arch.

epineurium (ep"ĭ-nu'rĭ-um) [" + *neuron,* nerve]. The general connective tissue sheath of a nerve. SEE: *nerve.*

ep"iot'ic [" + *ous, ot-,* ear]. Located above the ear.

e. center. Ossification center of temporal bone forming upper and post. part of the auditory capsule.

epipas'tic [" + *passein,* to sprinkle]. Resembling a dusting powder.

epipharynx (ep-ĭ-far'inks) [" + *pharygx,* pharynx]. Nasal portion of pharynx. SYN: *rhinopharynx.*

epiphenom'enon [" + *phainomenon,* phenomenon]. An exceptional and extraneous phenomenon in a disease.

epiphora (ĕ-pif'o-ră) [G. downpour]. Abnormal overflow of tears down the cheek due to excess secretion of tears or to obstruction of the lacrimal duct.

epiphylac'tic [G. *epi,* upon, + *phylaxis,* protection]. Pert. to epiphylaxis.

epiphylax'is [" + *phylaxis,* protection]. Increase of defensive powers of the body.

epiphyseal (ep-ĭ-fiz'e-al) [G. *epiphysis,* a growing upon]. Pert. to or of the nature of an epiphysis. Also spelled epiphysial.

epiphyseolysis (ep"ĭ-fiz-e-ol'ĭ-sis) [" + *lysis,* loosening]. Separation of an epiphysis.

epiphyseopathy (ep"ĭ-fiz-e-op'ă-thĭ) [" + *pathos,* disease]. Any disease of an epiphysis or of the pineal gland.

epiphysial (ep-ĭ-fiz'-ĭ-al) [G. *epiphysis,* a growing upon]. Of the nature of or concerning an epiphysis. Also spelled epiphyseal.

epiphysis (ĕ-pif'ĭ-sis) (pl. *epiphysēs*) [G. a growing upon]. 1. In the developing infant and child, a secondary bone-forming (ossification) center separated from a parent bone in early life by cartilage. As growth proceeds and at a different time for each epiphysis, it becomes a part of the larger (or parent) bone. By use of x-ray studies, it is possible to judge the age of a child from the development of these ossification centers. 2. A center for ossification at each extremity of long bones. SEE: *diaphysis.*

e. cerebri. The pineal body.

epiphysitis (ĕ-pif"ĭ-si'tis) [" + *-ītis,* inflammation]. Inflammation of an epiphysis, esp. that at the hip, knee, and shoulder in infants.

epipial (ep-ĭ-pi'al) [G. *epi,* upon, + L. *pia,* tender]. Situated above or upon the pia mater.

epiplocele (ĕ-pip'lo-sēl) [G. *epiploon,* omentum, + *kēlē,* hernia]. Hernia containing omentum.

epiploenterocele (e-pip"lo-en'ter-o-sēl) [" + *enteron,* intestine, + *kēlē,* hernia]. Hernia consisting of omentum and intestine.

epiploic (ep-ĭ-plo'ik) [G. *epiploon,* omentum]. Pert. to the omentum.

e. foramen. The opening between the greater and lesser peritoneal cavities.

epiploitis (ĕ-pip"lo-i'tis) [" + *-ītis,* inflammation]. Inflammation of the omentum.

epiplomerocele (ĕ-pip"lo-me'ro-sēl) [" + *mēros,* thigh, + *kēlē,* hernia]. Femoral hernia containing omentum.

epiplomphalocele (ĕ-pip"lom-fal'o-sēl) [" + *omphalos,* navel, + *kēlē,* hernia]. Umbilical hernia with omentum protruding.

epiploon (ĕ-pip'lo-on) [G. omentum]. The omentum, esp. the greater omentum. SEE: *omentum.*

epiplopexy (ĕ-pip'lo-peks-ĭ) [" + *pēxis,* fixation]. Suturing of omentum to the ant. abdominal wall.

epiplosarcomphalocele (ĕ-pip"lo-sar"kom-fal'o-sēl) [" + *sarx,* flesh, + *omphalos,* navel, + *kēlē,* hernia]. An umbilical hernia with protruding omentum. SYN: *epiplomphalocele.*

epiploscheocele (ĕ-pip"los-ke'o-sēl) [" + *oscheon,* scrotum, + *kēlē,* hernia]. Omental hernia into the scrotum.

epipygus (ep-ĭ-pi'gus). A developmental anomaly in which an accessory limb is attached to the buttocks.

episclera (ep-ĭ-skle'ră) [G. *epi*, upon, + *sklēros*, hard]. Loose connective tissue between sclera and conjunctiva.

episcleral (ep-ĭ-skle'ral) [" + *sklēros*, hard]. 1. Pertaining to the episclera. 2. Overlying the sclera of the eye.

episcleritis (ep-ĭ-skle-ri'tis) [" + " + *-itis*, inflammation]. Inflammation of the subconjunctival layers of the sclera.

ep'iscope [" + *skopein*, to examine]. Projection lantern for examination of an object on a screen. SYN: *epidiascope*.

episioclisia (ĕ-pis"ĭ-o-klis'ĭ-ă) [G. *episeion*, pudenda, + *kleisis*, closure]. Surgical closure of the vulva.

episioelytrorrhaphy (ĕ-pis"ĭ-o-el-ĭ-tror'ră-fĭ) [" + *elytron*, vagina, + *raphē*, suture]. Narrowing of vagina and vulva.

episioperineorrhaphy (ĕ-pis"ĭ-o-per-ĭ-ne-or'ă-fĭ) [" + *perinaion*, perineum, + *raphē*, suture]. Suturing the vulva and perineum for the support of a prolapse of the uterus.

NP: Prevent necessity for straining on defecation, routine perineal care.

episioplasty (ĕ-pis"ĭ-o-plas'tĭ) [" + *plassein*, to form]. Plastic surgery on the vulva.

episiorrhaphy (e-pis"ĭ-or'a-fĭ) [" + *raphē*, suture]. Sewing of a lacerated perineum.

episiostenosis (ĕ-pis"ĭ-o-stĕ-no'sis) [" + *stenōsis*, narrowing]. Narrowing of the vulvar slit.

episiotomy (ĕ-pis"ĭ-ot'o-mĭ) [" + *tomē*, incision]. Incision of perineum at end of second stage of labor to avoid laceration of perineum.

epispadias (ep-ĭ-spa'dĭ-as) [G. *epi*, upon, + *span*, to tear away]. Congenital opening of urethra on dorsum of penis; in the female, opening by separation of the labia minora and a fissure of the clitoris.

epispas'tic [" + *span*, to draw]. An agent that, applied locally, will produce a serous or puriform discharge by exciting inflammation.

episplenitis (ep"ĭ-sple-ni'tis) [" + *splēn*, spleen, + *-ītis*, inflammation]. Inflammation of the splenic capsule.

epistasis (ĕ-pis'ta-sis) [" + *stasis*, standing]. 1. A substance rising to the surface instead of sinking; scum, as on the urine. 2. In heredity a condition in which the presence of a gene or determiner prevents another gene not allelomorphic to it from expressing itself. 3. The checking of any discharge. SEE: *hypostasis*.

epistax'is [G. *epistaxein*, to bleed from nose]. Hemorrhage from nose.

ETIOL: Trauma, picking the nose with finger, direct blow, postoperative, foreign bodies; diseases (local and general), violent exertion, basilar skull fracture, vicarious menstruation, and high altitudes.

TREATMENT: Lie quietly propped up in bed, cold compresses, epinephrine locally, followed by cautery of bleeding vessel, packing.

NP: Simple nose bleed may be stopped ordinarily by elevating head of patient and pinching nostrils. Refrain from breathing through or blowing nose. Pressure across upper lip or cold cloths placed over nose and on back of neck are beneficial.

In severe nose bleeding, if necessary, pack entire nose or upper pharynx (retrograde packing). Occasionally epinephrine, styptics, or astringents may be used. However, for most first-aid purposes, these are unsatisfactory.

episternal (ep-ĭ-ster'nal) [G. *epi*, upon, + *sternon*, chest]. Situated above the sternum.

epister'num [" + *sternon*, chest]. Upper portion of the sternum. SYN: *manubrium*.

epistropheus (ep-ĭ-stro'fe-us) (pl. *epistrophei*) [" + *strephein*, to turn]. Second cervical vertebra. SYN: *axis*.

epitendineum (ep-ĭ-ten-din'e-um) [" + *tenōn*, tendon]. The fibrous sheath enveloping a tendon.

epitenon (ep-ĭ-ten'on) [" + *tenōn*, tendon]. The connective tissue holding a tendon within its sheaths. SYN: *epitendineum*.

epithalamus (ep-ĭ-thal'ă-mus) [" + *thalamos*, chamber]. The uppermost portion of the diencephalon. It includes the pineal body, trigonum habenulae, striae medullares thalami, and the posterior commissure.

epithalaxia (ep-ĭ-thă-lak'sĭ-ă) [" + *thēlē*, nipple, + *allaxis*, falling]. Desquamation of epithelial cells, esp. of lining of the intestine.

epithe'lia [" + *thēlē*, nipple]. Epithelial layer or cells.

epithelial (ep-ĭ-the'lĭ-al) [" + *thēlē*, nipple]. Pert. to or composed of epithelium.

e. cancer. Carcinoma composed of epithelial cells. SYN: *epithelioma*.

e. casts. Aggregations of renal epithelium, with cells filled with granules or fat droplets. They often preserve their original form in the epithelial tubes.

e. cells. Cells which are irregular in shape, having a single nucleus. Frequently 2 or 3 are joined together.

e. tissue. Those cells which form the outer surface of the body, and line the body cavities and the principal tubes and passageways leading to the exterior. They form the secreting portions of glands and their ducts, and important parts of certain sense organs. The cells of epithelial tissues lies closely approximated to each other and contain very little intercellular substance. They are arranged in one or a few layers and are devoid of blood vessels. SEE ALSO: under *tissue*.

epithe"lioblasto'ma [" + " + *blastos*, germ, + *ōma*, tumor]. Epithelial cell tumor.

epitheliogenic, epitheliogenetic (ep-ĭ-the"lĭ-o-jen'ik, -jĕ-net'ik) [" + " + *gennan*, to produce]. Caused by epithelial proliferation.

epithelioid (ep-ĭ-the'lĭ-oyd) [" + " + *eidos*, form]. Resembling epithelium.

epitheliolysis (ep-ĭ-the-lĭ-ol'ĭ-sis) [" + " + *lysis*, dissolution]. Death of epithelial tissue. The destruction or dissolving of epithelial cells by an epitheliolysin.

epithelioma (ep-ĭ-the-lĭ-o'mă) [" + " + *ōma*, tumor]. A malignant tumor consisting principally of epithelial cells; a carcinoma. A tumor originating in the epidermis of the skin or in a mucous membrane.

e. adamantinum. An adamantinoma, *q.v.*

e. adenoides cysticum. A basal cell carcinoma of low malignancy, occurring on the surface of the body, esp. the face. Characterized by formation of cysts.

e., basal cell. One derived from cells in the basal layer of the epidermis (stratum germinativum). SYN: *e. adenoides cysticum; rodent ulcer*.

e., deep seated. Involving lymphatic glands; irregular rounded ulcers, occurring after several months.

e. molluscum. Molluscum contagiosum, *q.v.*

e., papillary. Malignant, more often occurring in men and after middle life. Attacks genitals, nose, eyelids, or lower lip, etc.

e., superficial. Papules, yellowish or brownish, degenerating and forming ulcers, secreting a yellowish fluid.

epitheliomatous (ep″ĭ-thē-lĭ-o′mă-tus) [" + " + *ōma,* tumor]. Pert. to epithelioma.

epitheliosis (ep-ĭ-thē-lĭ-o′sis) [" + " + *ōsis*]. Trachomatous proliferation of the conjunctival epithelium.

epithelium (ep-ĭ-the′lĭ-um) (pl. *epithelia*) [" + *thēlē,* nipple]. The layer of cells forming the epidermis of the skin and the surface layer of mucous and serous membranes. The cells rest on a basement membrane and lie closely approximated to each other with little intercellular material between them. Epithelium may be *simple,* consisting of a single layer, or *stratified,* consisting of several layers. Cells comprising epithelium may be flat (squamous), cube-shaped (cuboidal) or cylindrical (columnar). Modified forms of epithelium include: ciliated, pseudostratified, glandular, and neuroepithelium. Epithelium may include *goblet cells,* which secrete mucus. Squamous epithelium is classified as *endothelium,* which lines the blood vessels and the heart, and *mesothelium,* which lines the serous cavities. Epithelium serves the general functions of protection, absorption, secretion, and specialized functions such as movement of substances through ducts, production of germ cells, and reception of stimuli. Its ability to regenerate is high.

e., ciliated. Epithelial cells with fine hair-like protuberances, called cilia, on their free border. These cells are able to sweep particles in a certain direction.

e., columnar. E. composed of cells shaped like pillars.

e., cuboidal. E. consisting of cube-shaped or prismatic cells with height approximately equal to width.

e., cylindrical. SEE: *columnar e.*

e., germinal. The e. which covers the surface of the genital ridge of the urogenital folds of an embryo. It gives rise to seminiferous tubules of the testes and the surface layer of the ovary. It is thought to give rise to the germ cells (spermatozoa and ova).

e., glandular. E. consisting of cells which secrete.

e., laminated. Stratified epithelium.

e., maternal. Uterine e. contrasted with that of the embryo.

e., mesenchymal. E. of the squamous type which lines the subarachnoid and subdural cavities, the chambers of the eye, and the perilymphatic spaces of the ear.

e., neuro-. E. terminating the nerves of special sense.

e., pavement. E. of flat, platelike cells.

e., pigmented. E. consisting of cells containing pigment granules.

e., pseudostratified. E. in which the bases of cells rest on the basement membrane but the distal ends of some do not reach the surface. Nuclei of the cells lies at different levels giving the appearance of stratification.

e., squamous. SEE: *pavement e.*

e., stratified. E. with the cells in layers.

e., transitional. A form of stratified epithelium in which the cells have the ability of adjusting themselves to mechanical changes such as stretching and contracting. Found only in the urinary system (pelvis of kidney, ureter, bladder, and a part of the urethra).

epithem (ep′ĭ-them) [G. *epithēma,* a cover]. Any external application, as a poultice.

epitonic (ep-ĭ-ton′ik) [G. *epitonos* strained]. Increased tonus.

epitox′oid [G. *epi,* upon, + *toxikon,* poison, + *eidos,* form]. Any toxoid which has less affinity for an antitoxin than is possessed by the toxin. SYN: *toxon.*

epitrichium (ep-ĭ-trik′ĭ-um) [" + *trichion,* hair]. Superficial layer of the epidermis of the fetus.

epitrochlea (ep-ĭ-trok′le-ă) [" + *trochalia,* pulley]. The inner condyle of the humerus.

epitrochlear (ep-i-trok′le-ar) [" + *trochalia,* pulley]. Pert. to the inner condyle of the humerus.

epituberculo′sis [" + L. *tuberculum,* tubercle, + G. *ōsis*]. Resembling tuberculosis but without tubercle bacilli. SYN: *paratuberculosis.*

epitur′binate [" + L. *turbo,* top]. The tissue upon or covering the turbinate bone.

epitympanum (ep-ĭ-tim′pă-num) [" + *tympanon,* drum]. The attic of middle ear; area above the drum membrane.

epityphlitis (ep″ĭ-tif-li′tis) [" + *typhlon,* cecum, + *-itis,* inflammation]. Appendicitis.

epizoic (ep-ĭ-zo′ik) [" + *zōon,* animal]. Parasitic on the epidermis.

epizoicide (ep-ĭ-zo′ĭ-sīd) [" + " + L. *caedere,* to kill]. That which destroys epizoa. SEE: *epizoon.*

epizoon (ep-ĭ-zo′on) (pl. *epizoa*) [" + *zōon,* animal]. An animal organism externally parasitic.

épluchage (ā-plū-shazh′) [Fr. cleaning]. Wound excision for removing contaminated tissues.

eponychium (ep-o-nik′ĭ-um) [G. *epi,* upon, + *onyx, onych-,* nail]. The horny embryonic structure from which the nail develops.

eponym (ep′o-nim) [G. *epōnymos,* named after]. A name for anything (diseases, organs, functions, places) adapted from the name of a particular person.

eponym′ic [G. *epōnymos,* named after]. Pert. to eponym. SYN: *eponymous.*

epon′ymous [G. *epōnymos,* named after]. Named after a person.

epoophorectomy (ep″o-o-fo-rek′to-mĭ) [G. *epi,* upon, + *ōophoron,* ovary, + *ektomē,* excision]. Removal of the parovarium.

epoophoron (ĕp″ō-ŏf′o-ron) [G. *epi,* upon, + *oophoron,* ovary]. A rudimentary structure located in the mesosalpinx consisting of a longitudinal duct (duct of Gartner) and ten to fifteen transverse ducts. It is the remains of the upper portion of the mesonephros and is the homolog of the head of the epididymis in the male. SYN: *parovarium; organ of Rosenmuller.*

epsom salt (ep′sŭm). Magnesium sulfate, *q.v.*

epulis (ep-u′lis) [G. *epoulis,* a gumboil]. A fibrous, sarcomatous tumor having its origin in the periosteum of the lower jaw.

e., malignant. Jaw sarcoma made up of giant cells.

epuloid (ep′u-loyd) [" + *eidos,* form]. 1.

Like an epulis. 2. Tumor of the jaw or gum appearing like an epulis.

epulosis (ep-u-lo'sis) [" + *-ōsis*]. Cicatrization; a cicatrix.

epulot'ic [G. *epoulis*, gumboil]. Promoting cicatrization.

equa'tion [L. *aequāre*, to make equal]. 1. State of being equal. 2. In chem. a symbolic representation of a chemical reaction.

e., personal. The difference between the results of observations as influenced by the personal qualities of the observers.

equa'tor. Line encircling a round body and equidistant from both poles.

e. of a cell. The boundary of a plane through which the division of a cell occurs.

e. of crystalline lens. Line which marks the junction of the anterior and posterior surfaces; the aequator lentis. To it are attached the fibers of the suspensory ligament.

e. oculi. An imaginary line encircling the bulb of the eye midway between ant, and post poles.

equato'rial [L. *aequāre*, to make equal]. Pert. to an equator.

e. plate. Mass of chromosomes at equator of the nuclear spindle during karyokinesis.

equi- [L.]. Prefix meaning *equal*.

equilibrating (e-kwil'ĭ-brāt-ing). Maintaining equilibrium.

e. operation. Section of the antagonist of a paralyzed ocular muscle. SEE: *tenotomy*.

equilib'rium [L. *aequus*, equal, + *libra*, balance]. State of balance or rest. Condition in which contending forces are equal.

e., nitrogenous. Having amt. of nitrogen in egesta equal to that of ingesta.

e., physiological. Having egesta equal to the ingesta.

equilin (ek'wĭl-ĭn) [L. *equus*, horse]. Crystalline estrogenic hormone derived from pregnant mares' urine, which affects growth of female sex organs. SYN: *theelin*.

equinia (e-kwin'ĭ-ă) [L. *equus*, horse]. Infectious disease of horses which can also affect man. SYN: *glanders*.

equinovarus (e-kwi"no-va'rus) [L. *equinus*, equine, + *varus*, bent inward]. A form of clubfoot with a combination pes equinus and pes varus.

equivalence (e-kwiv'ă-lents) [L. *aequis*, equal, + *valere*, to be worth]. 1. Quality of being equivalent. 2. Condition in which two radicals reacting are of the same valence and one displaces the other in a compound.

equivalent (e-kwĭv'a-lent) [" + *valere*, to be worth]. 1. Equal in power, force, or value. 2. Amount of weight of any element needed to replace a fixed weight of another body.

e., epilepsy. Any mental or physical disturbance, which may take the place of an epileptic seizure.

e., Joule's. Energy expended in raising the temperature of one unit of water one degree.

Er. Symbol for *erbium*.

E.R. Symbol for external resistance.

erasion (e-ra'zhun) [L. *ē*, out, + *radere*, to scrape]. 1. Laying open a diseased part and scraping away diseased tissue. 2. Scraping away morbid products.

Erb's paralysis or palsy [Wilhelm H. Erb, Heidelberg neurologist, 1840-1921]. Paralysis of group of muscles of shoulder and upper arm involving cervical roots of 5th and 6th spinal nerves.

The arm hangs limp, the hand rotates inward and normal movements are lost. SEE: *paralysis*.

Erben's reflex (erb'ens) [Siegmund Erben, Vienna physician, 1863-]. Retardation of pulse when head and trunk are forcibly bent forward.

er'bium. A rare metallic element. SYMB: Er. At. wt. 167.26; at. no. 68.

erectile (e-rek'tĭl) [L. *erigere*, to erect]. Able to become erect.

e. tissue. Vascular tissue which, when filled with blood, becomes erect or rigid, as the clitoris or penis.

erec'tion [L. *erigere*, to erect]. The state of swelling, hardness, and stiffness observed in the penis and to a lesser extent in the clitoris of the female, generally during sexual excitement.

Due to engorgement with blood of the *corpora cavernosa* and the *corpus spongiosum* of the penis and the *c. cavernosa clitoridis* of the female.

It is necessary in the male for the intromission of the penis into the vagina of the female and for the emission of semen. After ejaculation the blood withdraws from the penis and the erection is reduced. Erection of the penis also occurs normally under other special conditions. Abnormal, persistent erection of the penis is called priapism.*

e. center. This is in lumbar and sacral region; responds to organic and psychic stimuli and with the genitalia responding to peripheral irritation of the sensory nerves. This center is not directly under control of the will. The *nervi erigentes* in the first 3 sacral nerves under excitation convey their impulse to the *corpora cavernosa*. Reflex stimuli also affect it.

erec'tor [L. *erigere*, to erect]. A muscle that raises a part.

e. spinae reflex. Irritation of the skin over the erector spinae muscles causing contraction of muscles of the back. SYN: *dorsal r.; lumbar r.*

erect posi'tion. One having the occiput and heels in line, with nose, groin, and great toes in same relative plane.

eremacausis (er"em-ă-kaw'sis) [G. *ērema*, slowly, + *kausis*, burning]. Slow oxidation of organic matter exposed to heat.

eremophobia (er-em-o-fo'bĭ-ă) [G. *erēmos*, solitude, + *phobos*, fear]. Dread of being alone.

erep'sin. Term applied to a peptide-splitting enzyme found in the succus entericus (intestinal juice). The peptide-splitting action is due to the action of several peptidases which act on peptides which have escaped pancreatic digestion transforming them to amino acids.

erethin (er'ĕ-thin) [G. *erethizein*, to irritate]. The principle of tuberculin which causes fevers.

erethism (er'ĕ-thizm) [G. *erethisma*, stimulation]. Abnormal excitement or irritation which may be combined with collapse.

erethis'mic [G. *erethisma*, stimulation]. Pert. to or causing erethism. SYN: *erethitic*.

erethisophrenia (er-ĕ-thĭ-so-fre'nĭ-ă) [G. *erethizein*, to irritate, + *phrēn*, mind]. Unusual mental excitability.

erethistic (er-ĕ-this'tik) [G. *erethisma*, stimulation]. Erethismic, exciting.

erethitic (er-ĕ-thit'ĭk) [G. *erethisma*, stimulation]. Causing erethism; irritable, excited.

ereuthrophobia (er"u-thro-fo'bĭ-ă) [G. *erythros*, red, + *phobos*, fear]. Pathological fear of blushing. SYN: *erythrophobia.*

erg [G. *ergon,* work]. In physics, the amount of work done when a force of 1 dyne acts through a distance of 1 centimeter.

One erg is roughly 1/980 gram-centimeter; that is, to raise a load of 1 gram against gravity the distance of 1 centimeter requires that a force of 980 dynes operate through a distance of 1 centimeter and hence that 980 ergs of work be done. SEE: *unit, work.*

ergasia (er-ga'sĭ-ă) [G. *ergasia,* work]. Functions of the mind and behavior resulting therefrom in contrast to those depending upon physiological functions.

ergasiodermatosis (er-ga"sĭ-o-der-mă-to'-sis) [" + *derma,* skin, + *-ōsis*]. Dermatosis due to occupational cause.

ergasiomania (er-ga"sĭ-o-ma'nĭ-ă) [" + *mania,* madness]. Active interest in a task without completing it, seen in certain phases of manic excitement.

ergasiophobia (er-ga"sĭ-o-fo'bĭ-ă) [" + *phobos,* fear]. Abnormal dislike for assuming responsibility or for work of any kind.

ergasthenia (er-gas-the'nĭ-ă) [G. *ergon,* work, + *astheneia,* weakness]. Overwork and debility caused therefrom.

ergas'tic [G. *ergon,* work]. Possessing potential energy.

ergograph (er'go-graf) [" + *graphein,* to write]. An apparatus for recording the contractions of muscles and measuring the amount of work done.

ergom'eter [" + *metron,* measure]. An apparatus for measuring the amount of work done by a human or animal subject.

ergopho'bia [" + *phobos,* fear]. Morbid dread of working.

ergophore (er'go-for) [" + *pherein,* to bear]. That part of an antigen on which the specific properties of the substance depend. SYN: *toxophore.*

er'goplasm [G. *ergon,* work, + *plasma,* a thing formed]. Protoplasm peculiar to the centrosome, and composing the attraction sphere. SYN: *kinoplasm; archoplasm.*

er'gostat [" + *statos,* standing]. A machine for measuring work done by a contracting muscle.

ergos'terol. A substance derived from yeast, ergot, and other fungi, and resembling cholesterol in composition.

e., irradiated. E. subjected to ultraviolet radiation, vitamin D_2. A remedy for rickets. SYN: *viosterol.*

ergot (er'got) [L. *ergota*]. A drug obtained from *Claviceps purpurea,* a fungus which grows parasitically on rye. Several valuable alkaloids, as ergotamine, *q.v.,* are obtained from ergot.

e. poisoning. May come from eating bread made with diseased grain or by taking overdoses of the drug.

SYM: Appear several hours after administration. Vomiting, burning, and cramping in abdomen, great thirst, profound weakness, diarrhea; slow, weak pulse; anesthesia, tingling and twitching in extremities; dilated pupils; occasionally convulsions, anuria; if patient survives may develop gangrene of fingers, toes or limited areas of skin, and cataracts.

F. A. TREATMENT: Slurry of activated charcoal by mouth, followed by emesis or gastric lavage, and instillation of a saline cathartic, external heat. For supportive and follow-up treatment, see: *Table of Poisons and Poisoning in Appendix.*

ergotamine (er-got'ă-mēn). A crystalline alkaloid ($C_{33}H_{35}O_5N_5$) derived from ergot.

e. tartrate. A white crystalline substance which stimulates smooth muscle of blood vessels and the uterus inducing vasoconstriction and uterine contractions. Used in the treatment of migraine.

ergotherapy (er-go-ther'ă-pĭ) [G. *ergon,* work, + *therapeia,* treatment]. Work used as a treatment of disease.

e., passive. Generalized muscular exercise excited by faradic current.

ergotism (er'go-tizm) [L. *ergota,* ergot, + G. *ismos,* condition]. Poisoning resulting from excessive use of ergot or from eating food made from rye or wheat infected with the fungus *Claviceps purpurea.* May be acute or chronic. SEE: *ergot poisoning.*

ergotrate (er'go-trāt). An active principle isolated from ergot.

USES: Same as ergot.

ergotrop'ic [G. *ergon,* work, + *tropos,* a turning]. Pert. to ergotropy.*

ergotropy (er-got'ro-pĭ) [" + *tropos,* a turning]. Injection of nonspecific proteins to increase body resistance.

eriom'eter [G. *erion,* wool, + *metron,* measure]. Device for measuring size of minute particles.

Eristalis. A genus of flies belonging to the family Syrphidae. The larva, called rat-tailed maggot (*E. tenax*) may cause intestinal myiasis in man.

erode (e-rōd') [L. *erodere,* to gnaw away]. 1. To wear away. 2. To eat away by ulceration.

erogenous (e-roj'ĕ-nus) [G. *erōs,* love, + *gennan,* to produce]. Causing sexual excitement. SYN: *erotogenic.**

e. zone. Any part of the body which, by touching or stroking, causes sexual excitement.

erosion (e-ro'zhun) [L. *erodere,* to gnaw away]. An eating away of tissue; destruction of a surface layer, either external or internal, by physical or inflammatory processes.

e. of the cervix uteri. The alteration of the epithelium on a portion of the cervix as a result of irritation by infection.

SYM: In the early stages, the epithelium shows necrosis which nature tries to heal by a downgrowth of epithelium from the endocervical canal. If this is accomplished by a single layer of tissue, having a grossly granular appearance, it is called a simple granular erosion. If the downgrowth is excessive and shows papillary tufts, it is called a papillary erosion.

Histologically, the papillary erosion shows many glands of the branching racemose type whose epithelium is the mucus-bearing cell with the nucleus at the base. In the healing process, squamous epithelium grows over the eroded area with the following results: the squamous cells take the place of the tissue beneath it completely, giving a complete healing, or the glands fill with squamous plugs and remain in that state, or the mouths of the glands are occluded by the squamous cells and cysts are formed (nabothian cysts). In the congenital type of erosion the portio is covered by high columnar epithelium.

TREATMENT: Prophylaxis, proper care of the cervix following delivery, proper hygiene by means of douches, and cauterization of the early erosion with the electrocautery is usually curative.

e., dental. The wearing away of the surface layer (enamel) of a tooth.

erosive (e-ro'siv) [G. *erodere*, to gnaw away]. 1. Able to produce erosion. 2. An agent that erodes anything.

erotic (e-rot'ĭk) [G. *erōtikos*, pert. to love]. Pert. to sexual passion. SYN: *lustful*.

erot'icism [" + *ismos*, condition of]. Excessive or morbid libido; also intense sex desire.

e., allo-. Eroticism directed to an external object rather than to self. SEE: *eroticism; erotomania*.

e., anal. Sensations of pleasure experienced by the child through defecation.

e., auto-. 1. Self-gratification of the sexual instinct. 2. Self-admiration combined with sexual emotion, such as that obtained from viewing one's naked body, or one's genitals. SEE: *erotomania*.

e., oral. Sensation of pleasure experienced when nursing at the breast, modified and sublimated but continuing into adult life through normal contacts of the lips, mouth, and throat.

er'otism [" + *ismos*, condition of]. PSY: eroticism.

erotogenic (e-ro-to-jen'ĭk) [G. *erōs*, love, + *gennan*, to produce]. Producing sexual excitement. SEE: *zones, erotic*.

erotology (er-o-tol'o-jĭ) [" + *logos*, study]. The study of love and its manifestations.

erotomania (e-ro"to-, e-rot"o-ma'nĭ-ă) [" + *mania*, madness]. Pathological exaggeration of sexual behavior. SEE: *eroticism*.

erotopathia (e-ro"to-, e-rot"o-path'ĭ-ă) [" + *pathos*, disease]. Any abnormal or perverted sex impulse.

erotophobia (e-ro"to-, e-rot"o-fo'bĭ-ă) [" + *phobos*, fear]. Aversion to sexual love or its manifestations.

erotopsychic (e-ro"to-, e-rot"o-si'kik) [" + *psychē*, mind]. Mental perversion of the sexual impulse.

errat'ic [L. *errāre*, to wander]. Wandering, having an unpredictable or fluctuating course or pattern. SYN: *eccentric*.

errhine (er'in) [G. *en*, in, + *ris, rin-*, nose]. An agent that will increase the secretion of the mucous membrane lining the nose. SYN: *sternutatory*. EX: *quillaja, salicylic acid*.

erubes'cence [L. *erubēscere*, to grow red]. Reddening of the skin; a blush.

eructa'tion [L. *eructāre*, to belch]. Raising of gas or acid fluid from the stomach; belching. SEE: *oxyrygmia*.

eruption (e-rup'shun) [L. *eruptio*, a breaking out]. 1. A breaking out and becoming visible, esp. applied to the appearance of a skin lesion or rash accompanying a disease such as measles or scarlet fever. 2. The appearance of a lesion such as redness or spotting on the skin or mucous membrane. 3. The breaking through of a tooth through the gum; the cutting of a tooth.

e., creeping. A skin lesion characterized by a tortuous elevated red line which progresses at one end while fading out at the other. It is caused by the migration of the larvae of certain nematodes, esp. *Ancylostoma braziliense* and other cat and dog nematodes which occur as accidental invaders of man. SYN: *larva migrans*.

e., drug. Dermatitis medicamentosa; skin reaction resulting from the ingestion of certain drugs, such as iodides.

Eruptive, Infective, and Contagious Diseases

Name	Period of Incubation	Time of Eruption	Duration of Eruption	Period of Quarantine
Scarlet Fever	1- 7 days	12-24 hr. after onset	7-10 days	10 days
Smallpox	8-21 days	3rd or 4th day of fever	14-21 days	21 days or until all scabs disappear
Measles (Rubeola)	7-18 days	4th day of fever	4-8 days	7 days past onset of catarrhal symptoms
Rubella	5-21 days	2nd day of fever	1-3 days	Until rash disappears
Mumps	4-26 days			Until all swellings have subsided
Whooping Cough	7-14 days			4-6 weeks
Chickenpox	14-21 days	2nd day of fever	7-21 days	7 days
Diphtheria	2-5 days			7 days, and until 2 successive nose and throat cultures, 24 hr. apart, are negative
Typhus Fever	7-14 days	3rd to 8th day of fever	14 days	15 days, but not required if person and area are completely rid of lice
Typhoid Fever	1-21 days	4th day of fever	3-5 days for each crop of spots	Release after 2 successive negative cultures of urine and feces not less than 24 hr. apart
Erysipelas	Acute onset	2nd day of fever	5-7 days	

e., primary. Blebs, macules, papules, pustules, tubercles, tumors, vesicles, wheals or pomphus, *q.v.*

e., secondary. Crusts, excoriations, fissures, pigmentations, scales, scars, ulcers, *q.v.*

e., serum. E. caused by the injection of a serum.

erup'tive [L. *eruptio,* a breaking out]. Breaking out, as with a rash.

erysipelas (er-ĭ-sip'ĭ-las) [G. *erythros,* red, + *pella,* skin]. Acute, febrile disease with localized inflammation and swelling of skin and subcutaneous tissue accompanied by systemic disturbance of variable degree. SYN: *St. Anthony's fire.*

ETIOL: *Streptococcus pyogenes.*

SYM AND SIGNS: Fever, chills, nausea, vomiting, painful and warm skin; face and head lesions that are hot and red usually seen within 24-48 hours. Bullae may develop.

TREATMENT: Penicillin or erythromycin. Cool magnesium sulfate solution compresses for skin. Aspirin for pain.

PROG: Excellent with treatment.

e., ambulant. E. which disappears from one part of the body and reappears in another.

e., erythematous. E. in a mild form.

e., facial. Form found mainly on the face.

e., idiopathic. E. which does not develop subsequent to trauma or injury.

e. migrans. Widely spread form of e.

e., phlegmonous. Purulent form of e.

e., surgical. E. developing in a wound.

e., traumatic. SEE: *surgical e.*

erysipelatous (er"ĭ-sĭ-pel'ă-tus) [" + *pella,* skin]. Of the nature of or pert. to erysipelas.

erysipeloid (er-ĭ-sip'ĭ-loyd) [" + " + *eidos,* form]. An infective dermatitis resembling erysipelas usually limited to the hands and characterized by hyperemia, edema, and occasionally systemic complications.

ETIOL: It is caused by *Erysipelothrix rhusiopathiae,* usually acquired by handling of fish products.

Erysipelothrix (er-ĭ-sĭ-pel'o-thriks). A genus of bacteria belonging to the family Corynebacteriaceae. They are branching filamentous, rod-shaped, nonmotile organisms.

E. rhusiopathiae. The causative agent of swine erysipelas and erysipeloid in man.

erysip'elotox'in. The toxin produced by *Streptococcus pyogenes,* the causative agent of erysipelas.

erythema (er-ĭ-the'mă) [G. redness]. A form of macula showing diffused redness over the skin.

ETIOL: Caused by capillary congestion, usually due to dilatation of the superficial capillaries as a result of (1) some nervous mechanism within the body, (2) inflammation, (3) as a result of some external influence, such as heat, sunburn, etc.

e. annulare. E. with rounded, raised marginal lesions.

e. circinatum. In red circles.

e. congestivum. E. with congestive state of skin.

e., diffuse. Widely spread over body.

e. dose. The amount of radiant energy sufficient to evoke perceptible redness of the skin.

e. hyperaemicum. Caused by heat or cold (erythema caloricum, chilblain), sun (erythema solare), artificial heat as from hot water bottle or electric pad (erythema ab igne).

e. infectiosum. Contagious form with rose-colored eruption.

e. intertrigo. Chafing of opposing surfaces, with erythema and often with maceration and abrasion.

e. multiforme. A macular eruption with dark red papules or tubercles. Usually on extremities appearing in successive eruptions of short duration. No itching, burning or rheumatic pains. May appear in separate rings, concentric rings, disk-shaped patches, distributed elevations, and figured arrangements.

e. nodosum. Red and painful nodules on legs associated with rheumatism. Also caused by certain drugs and food poisoning.

e., punctate. In minute points, as scarlet fever rash.

e. symptomaticum. Hyperemia of the skin with level patches.

e. venenatum. Form caused by contact with an irritating substance.

erythemat'ic, erythem'atous [G. *erythēma,* redness]. Pert. to or marked by erythema.

erythemogen'ic [" + *gennan,* to produce]. Pert. to erythema.

erythemomegalalgia (er-ĭ-the'mo-mĕg-al-al'jĭ-ă) [" + *megas,* great, + *algos,* pain]. Painful redness of skin. SYN: *erythromelalgia.*

erythralgia (er-ĭ-thral'jĭ-ă) [G. *erythros,* red, + *algos,* pain]. A condition of painful redness of the skin. SYN: *erythromelalgia.*

erythrasma (er-ĭ-thraz'mă) [G. *erythros,* red]. Reddish-brown eruption in patches in the axillae and groins formerly thought to be due to a fungus, but now considered to be bacterial in origin.

erythredema (ĕ-rĭth"rĕ-de'mă) [" + *oidēma,* swelling]. A disease occurring in infants characterized by lesions of the skin on the hands and feet, swelling of the extremities, digestive disturbances. It is frequently followed by multiple arthritis. Its cause is unknown. SYN: *acrodynia; pink disease.*

erythre'mia [" + *aima,* blood]. Excessive increase of red blood corpuscles with cyanosis. SYN: *polycythemia rubra.*

erythrism (er'ĭ-thrizm) [" + *ismos,* condition of]. Redness of the hair and beard with ruddy complexion.

erythristic (er-ĭ-thris'tik) [G. *erythros,* red]. Ruddy complexion. Having reddish hair.

erythro-. Prefix meaning red.

erythroblast (ĕ-rith'ro-blast) [" + *blastos,* germ]. The youngest erythroblasts are called basophilic erythroblasts or proerythroblasts. Successive stages are polychromatophile erythroblasts and normoblasts. Erythroblasts possess hemoglobin. In the embryo they are found in blood islands of the yolk sac, body mesenchyma, liver, spleen, and lymph nodes; after the third month they are restricted to the bone marrow.

erythroblaste'mia [" + " + *aima,* blood]. An excessive number of erythroblasts in the blood.

erythroblas'tic [" + *blastos,* germ]. Pert. to erythroblasts.

erythroblasto'ma [" + " + *ōma,* tumor]. A tumor (myeloma) with cells resembling megaloblasts.

erythroblasto'sis [" + " + *ōsis*]. A condition marked by many erythroblasts in the blood.

e. fetalis. A hemolytic disease of the newborn characterized by anemia, jaundice, and enlargement of the liver and spleen, generalized edema (hydrops fetalis). ETIOL: It is due to the development in an Rh negative mother of antibodies against an Rh positive fetus. This occurs following a preceding pregnancy in which the fetus was Rh positive or following transfusion of Rh positive blood.

erythrochloropia (ĕ-rith″ro-klor-o′pĭ-ă) [" + *chlōros*, green, + *ōps*, eye]. Partial color blindness with ability to see only red and green.

erythrochromia (ĕ-rith″ro-kro′mĭ-ă) [" + *chroma*, color]. Hemorrhagic red pigmentation of the spinal fluid.

erythroclas′tic [" + *klan*, to break]. Destructive to red blood cells.

eryth′roconte [G. *erythros*, red]. An abnormal rod-shaped structure found in erythrocytes in cases of pernicious anemia.

erythrocyano′sis [" + *kyanos*, blue, + *ōsis*]. Red or bluish discoloration on the skin with swelling, itching, and burning.

erythrocyte (ĕ-rith′ro-sĭt) [" + *kytos*, cell]. Red blood corpuscle.

Each is a non-nucleated, biconcave disk averaging 7.7 microns in diameter. The body of the cell consists of a spongelike *stroma* containing a respiratory pigment, *hemoglobin*, enclosed in a cell membrane of proteins in combination with lipoid substances. Hemoglobin is a conjugated protein consisting of a colored iron-containing portion, *hematin*, and a simple protein, *globin*. It combines readily with oxygen to form an unstable compound, *oxyhemoglobin*.

The total surface area of the red cells of an average man is 3820 square meters or about 2000 times greater than his total body surface area.

NUMBER. In a normal person, the number of erythrocytes average about 5,000,000 per cu. millimeter (5,500,000 for males, 4,500,000 for females). The total number in an average-sized person is about 35 trillion. The number per cubic millimeter varies with (1) *age*, being higher in infants, (2) *time of day*, being lower during sleep, (3) *activity* and *environmental temperature*, increasing in both conditions, and (4) *altitude*. Persons living at altitudes of 10,000 ft. or more may have a red cell count of 8,000,000 or more.

FUNCTIONS: The primary function of the red blood cells is to carry oxygen and carbon dioxide. They also play a role in the regulation of the acid-base balance of the blood and in the formation of bile pigments which are derived from decomposition products of hemoglobin.

ORIGIN: Red cell formation (*erythropoiesis*) in the adult takes place in the red bone marrow, principally in the vertebrae, ribs, sternum, diploe of cranial bones, and proximal ends of the humerus and femur. They arise from large nucleated stem-cells (*proerythroblasts*) which give rise to *erythroblasts* in which hemoglobin appears. These give rise to *normoblasts* which extrude their nuclei. Red cells at this stage possess a fine reticular network and are known as *reticulocytes*. This reticular structure is lost before the cells enter circulation as *mature erythrocytes*.

The proper formation of erythrocytes depends upon several factors among them: (a) healthy condition of the bone marrow; (b) dietary substances such as iron, cobalt, and copper, all essential for the formation of hemoglobin; essential amino acids, and certain vitamins, esp. B_{12} and folic acid (pteroylglutamic acid); (c) an *antianemic factor* stored in the liver.

LIFE HISTORY AND FATE: The average length of life of a red blood cell is estimated to be about 120 days. Cells are continuously dying and disintegrating. The cellular debris is picked up by the cells of the reticuloendothelial system, esp. those of the spleen, liver, and bone marrow. Hemoglobin is broken down, and proteins and iron are stored and utilized in the formation of new erythrocytes. The iron-containing portion, *hematin*, gives rise to *bilirubin*, which is excreted in the bile as one of the bile pigments.

VARIATIONS: On microscopic examination, erythrocytes may reveal variations in the following respects (1) *Size* (anisocytosis), (2) *Shape* (poikilocytosis), (3) *Staining reaction* (achromia, hypochromia, hyperchromia, polychromatophilia), (4) *Structure* (possession of bodies such as Cabot's rings, Howell-Jolly bodies, Heinz bodies, parasites such as malaria, a reticular network, or nuclei), (5) *Number* (anemia, polycythemia).

e., achromatic. A phantom corpuscle or one from which the hemoglobin has been dissolved; a colorless corpuscle.

e., basophilic. E. in which cytoplasm stains blue indicating the presence of basophilic material. May be diffuse (basophilic material uniformly distributed) or punctate (material appearing as pin point dots).

e., crenated. E. with a serrated or indented edge usually the result of withdrawal of water from the cell as occurs when cells are placed in hypertonic solutions.

e., immature. An erythroblast.

e., orthrochromatic. E. that stains with acid stains only, cytoplasm appearing pink.

e., polychromatic. E. that does not stain uniformly.

erythrocythemia (ĕ-rith″ro-si-the′mĭ-ă) [" + " + *aima*, blood]. Enormous increase in red blood cells. SYN: *erythremia; polycythemia*.

erythrocytolysis (ĕ-rith″ro-si-tol′ĭ-sis) [" + " + *lysis*, dissolution]. Dissolution of red blood corpuscles with the escape of hemoglobin; hemolysis.

erythrocytom′eter [" + " + *metron*, measure]. Instrument for counting red blood corpuscles.

erythrocytoopso′nin [" + " + *opsōnein*, to prepare food for]. A substance opsonic for red corpuscles.

erythrocytorrhexis (ĕ-rith″ro-si″to-reks′-is) [" + " + *rēxis*, rupture]. The breaking up of red blood cells with particles or fragments of the cell escaping into the plasma; plasmorrhexis.

erythrocytoschisis (ĕ-rith″ro-si-tos′kĭ-sis) [" + " + *schisis*, division]. The breaking up of red blood cells into small disk-like particles resembling blood platelets.

erythrocytosis (ĕ-rith″ro-si-to′sis). Abnormal increase in the number of red blood cells in circulation; polycythemia, erythemia, erythrocytothemia.

erythroderma (ĕ-rith″ro-der′mă). Erythema, erythrodermia, *q.v.*

e. desquamativum. A disease, resembling seborrhea, of breast-fed infants characterized by redness of skin and development of scales; Leiner's disease.

e. ichthyosiforme congenitum. A congenital condition characterized by thickening and redness of the skin; may resemble ichthyosis or lichen.

e., maculopapular. A condition of the skin characterized by redness and eruption of macules and papules.

e. squamosum. An eruption of the skin consisting of groups of papules covered by scales; parapsoriasis.

erythrodermia (ĕ-rith″ro-der′mĭ-ă) [" + *derma*, skin]. Abnormal redness in the skin. SYN: *erythema.*

erythrodextrin (ĕ-rith″ro-dex′trin) [" + L. *dexter*, right]. Form of dextrin from splitting of a polysaccharide molecule. SEE: *achroodextrin.*

erythrogen′esis [" + *genesis*, development]. The development of red blood corpuscles.

erythroleukemia (ĕ-rith″ro-lu-ke′mĭ-ă) [G. *erythros*, red, + *leukos*, white, + *aima*, blood]. Many immature cells in the blood causing anemia.

erythroleukosis (ĕ-rith″ro-lu-ko′sis) [" + " + *ōsis*]. Abnormal increase of red cells and granulocytes.

erythrolysin (er″ĭ-throl′ĭ-sin) [" + *lysis*, dissolution]. An agent causing erythrolysis. SYN: *hemolysin; erythrocytolysin.* SEE: *lysin.*

erythrol′ysis [" + *lysis*, dissolution]. Dissolution of red blood corpuscles. SYN: *erythrocytolysis.*

erythromelalgia (ĕ-rith″ro-mel-al′jĭ-ă) [" + *melos*, limb, + *algos*, pain]. A skin neurosis accompanied by burning and throbbing which come and go, affecting any one of the extremities, esp. the feet.

erythrome′lia [" + *melos*, limb]. Erythema of extensor surfaces of extremities but without pain.

erythromycin (e-rith″ro-mi′sin). An antibiotic from Streptomyces erythreus. It is effective orally against many gram positive and some gram negative organisms.

erythron (er′ĭ-thron). The concept of blood as a body system including the circulating red cells and the organ from which they arise, *i.e.*, the bone marrow.

erythroneocytosis (ĕ-rith″ro-ne″o-si-to′sis) [" + *neos*, new, + *kytos*, cell, + *ōsis*]. Regenerative forms of red blood cells in the blood.

erythronoclastic (er-ĭ-thron-o-klas′tĭk) [" + *klan*, to break]. Destructive to the erythron.

erythropar′asite [" + *parasitos*, parasite]. A red blood corpuscle parasite.

erythrop′athy [" + *pathos*, disease]. Disease of the red blood corpuscles.

erythropenia (e-rith″ro-pe′nĭ-ă) [" + *penia*, poverty]. Deficiency of red blood corpuscles.

erythrophage (ĕ-rith″ro-fāj) [" + *phagein*, to eat]. A phagocyte which destroys red corpuscles.

erythropha′gia [" + *phagein*, to eat]. Destruction of red blood cells by phagocytes.

erythrophile, erythrophilous (ĕ-rith′ro-fil, er-ĭ-throf′ĭ-lus) [" + *philein*, to love]. Readily staining red.

erythrophobia (ĕ-rith″ro-fo′bĭ-ă) [" + *phobos*, fear]. 1. Abnormal dread of blushing or fear of being diffident or of being embarrassed. 2. A morbid fear of, or aversion to, anything colored red.

erythrophose (ĕ-rith′ro-fōs) [" + *phōs*, light]. Any red subjective perception of a bright spot. SEE: *phose.*

erythrophthisis (ĕ-rith″ro-thi′sis) [" + *phthisis*, wasting]. Serious damage to the restorative power of the red corpuscles.

erythrophthoric (ĕ-rith″rof-thor′ik) [" + *phtheirein*, to destroy]. 1. Rapid destruction of erythrocytes. 2. By any means other than hemolysis.

erythropia, erythropsia (er″ĭ-thro′pĭ-ă, -throp′sĭ-ă) [" + *opsis*, vision]. Condition in which objects appear to be red.

erythroplasia (ĕ-rith″ro-pla′sĭ-ă). A condition considered to be precancerous characterized by the appearance of erythematous lesions involving the junctions of the epithelium of the skin and mucous membranes at the mouth, anus, penis, and vulva.

erythropoiesis (ĕ-rith″ro-poy-e′sis) [" + *poiēsis*, making]. The formation of red blood corpuscles.

erythropoietic (ĕ-rith″ro-poy-et′ik) [" + *poiēsis*, making]. Pert. to red blood cells.

erythroprosopalgia (ĕ-rith″ro-pro-so-pal′-jĭ-ă) [" + *prosōpon*, face, + *algos*, pain]. A neuropathy characterized by redness and pain in the face.

erythropsia (er-ĭ-throp′sĭ-ă) [" + *opsis*, vision]. Perversion of color vision in which all objects look red.

erythrop′sin [" + *opsis*, vision]. Pigment in the external portion of the rods of the retina. SYN: *rhodopsin; visual purple.*

erythrorrhexis (ĕ-rith″ro-reks′is) [" + *rexis*, rupture]. Rupture of a red cell and escape of its plasma. SYN: *erythrocytorrhexis; plasmorrhexis.*

erythrosis (er-ĭ-thro′sis) [" + *ōsis*]. A reddish-purple discoloration of the skin and mucous membranes in polycythemia.

erythrothrombomonoblastosis (ĕ-rith″ro-throm″bo-mo″no-blas-to′sis). A disorder characterized by appearance in the blood of excessive numbers of erythroblasts, thrombocytes, and immature monocytes. Other symptoms include enlargement of the spleen, increase in basal metabolism, and bone atrophy.

erythrotoxin (ĕ-rith″ro-toks′in) [" + *toxikon*, poison]. An exotoxin that attacks red blood cells. SEE: *leukotoxin.*

erythruria (er-ĭ-thru′rĭ-ă) [" + *ouron*, urine]. Red color of the urine.

Esbach's method (es′baks) [Georges H. Esbach, Paris physician, 1843-1890]. A method of estimating quantity of albumin in urine. The urine is collected for 24 hours, and after stirring well, a specimen is taken.

The specific gravity is read and, if necessary, urine is diluted until it shows a reading of 1.010 or below. It should be slightly acid. It is poured into a special Esbach's test tube, which is marked off in grams, until the letter U (urine) is reached. Then Esbach's reagent is poured in up to the mark R. The tube is tightly corked and gently inverted once or twice, care being taken to prevent bubbles forming.

The tube is now set aside, upright, for 12 hours. It must not be disturbed, and the temperature of the room should be kept constant. The albumin is seen as a precipitate at the bottom of the tube, and is read off in grams per liter. If grains per ounce are required, multiply the result by 0.4. Esbach's reagent contains picric acid and citric acid. RS: *albumin.*

E.'s quantitative estimation of albumin. Apparatus required:

(*a*) An Esbach's albuminometer. This is a large test tube marked with a scale for reading off the precipitate in grams per liter. Above this is the letter U, and about 2 in. higher is the letter R.

(*b*) Esbach's reagent. Consists of:

Picric acid, 10 gm.; citric acid, 20 gm.; water, 1 liter.

The following points should be noted before carrying out the test:

1. The urine must be acid.
2. Its specific gravity must be 1.010 or below. If above this the urine must be diluted with an equal quantity of water, the final result being multiplied by 2.
3. The urine should be cold.
4. Keep the specimen in a room with a constant temperature.

Technic: Same as E.'s method, *q.v.*

escape mechanism. In psychiatry, the reaction of a person in adjusting temporarily to difficult, unpleasant, or intolerable situations by unconsciously employing another means which is less difficult or more pleasant.

e., vagal. Occurrence of a ventricular contraction when the normal rhythmical beat of the heart has been stopped or inhibited by stimulation of the vagus nerve. Also called "escape from inhibition", "escape of the heart", or "vagus escape."

e., ventricular. Occurrence of single or repeated ventricular contractions from impulses arising in the atrioventricular node. Also called nodal extrasystole.

eschar (es'kar) [G. *eschara*, scab]. A slough, esp. one following a cauterization or burn. SEE: *escharotic*.

escharotic (es-kar-ot'ik) [G. *eschara*, scab]. Agent used to destroy tissue and to cause sloughing which produces what is known as an *eschar*. The third degree of counterirritation.

They are caustics, the mild ones being used in the treatment of skin diseases; the stronger being employed to destroy infected tissue, and to counteract the bites of animals and insects; caustic soda and antimonial ointment being applied for this purpose. They may be acids, alkalies, metallic salts, phenol or carbolic acid, carbon dioxide, or the cautery; epispastics, *q.v.*

Escherich's reflex (esh'er-ik) [Theodor Escherich, German physician, 1857-1911]. Pursing or muscular contraction of lips resulting from irritation of mucosa of lips.

Escherichia (esh-er-ik'ĭ-ă) [Named for Theodor Escherich who first isolated the type species, E. coli, of the genus]. A genus of bacteria belonging to the family Enterobacteriaceae, tribe Eschericheae. They are common inhabitants of the alimentary canal of man and other animals.

E. coli. The colon bacillus. A short, plump, gram-negative, nonsporeforming motile bacillus almost constantly present in the alimentary canal of humans and some animals. They are normally nonpathogenic. Outside the body and under certain conditions, E. coli is responsible for infections of the urinary tract and other systems and for enteritis in infants. The presence of the bacilli in milk or water is an indicator of fecal contamination.

eschrolalia (es-kro-lal'ĭ-ă) [G. *aischros*, indecent, + *lalia*, babble]. Utterance, without meaning, of obscene words. SYN: *coprolalia*.

Escudero's test [Pedro Escudero, Buenos Aires physician, 1877-]. A test for gout.

es'culent [L. *esculentus*, eatable]. Suitable to be eaten.

escutcheon (es-kutch'un) [Fr. *escuchon*, shield, from L. *scutum*, shield]. The coarse pubic hair in the adult.

eserine (es'er-ĭn). SEE: *physostigmine salicylate*.

ESF. Abbr. for *erythropoietic stimulating factor*.

Es'march's bandage [Johannes F. A. von Esmarch, German surgeon, 1823-1908]. A rubber bandage for controlling bleeding. Before operation commences, bandage is applied tightly to limb, commencing at distal end and reaching above site of operation, where a rubber tourniquet is firmly applied. The bandage is then removed. This renders operative area virtually bloodless. CAUTION: Tourniquet must not be applied so tightly as to cause nerve damage. Also it must be removed in time to prevent injury due to lack of blood flow to the distal tissues. SEE: *bandage*.

esodic (e-sod'ik) [G. *esō*, within, + *odos*, way]. Centripetal or afferent; pert. to sensory nerves conducting impulses toward the brain and spinal cord.

esoethmoiditis (es-o-eth-moy-di'tis) [" + *ēthmos*, sieve, + *eidos*, form, + *-ītis*, inflammation]. Inflammation of membrane of ethmoid cells.

esogastri'tis [" + *gastēr*, belly, + *-ītis*, inflammation]. Catarrhal inflammation of the gastric mucous membranes.

esophagalgia (e-sof-ă-gal'jĭ-ă). Pain in the esophagus.

esophageal (e-sof"ă-je'al) [G. *oisophagos*, esophagus]. Pert. to the esophagus.

esophagectasia, esophagectasis (e-sof"ă-jek-ta'sĭ-ă, -jek'ta-sis). Dilatation of the esophagus.

esophagec'tomy [" + *ektomē*, excision]. Excision of a part of the esophagus.

esophagismus (e-sof-ă-jis'mus) [" + *ismos*, condition of]. Esophageal spasm.

esophagitis (e-sof-ă-ji'tis) [" + *-ītis*, inflammation]. Inflammation of the esophagus.

esophagocele (e-sof'ă-go-sēl) [" + *kēlē*, hernia]. Hernia of the esophagus.

esophagodyn'ia [" + *odynē*, pain]. Pain in the esophagus.

esophagoenterostomy (e-sof"ă-go-en-ter-os'to-mĭ) [" + *enteron*, intestine, + *stoma*, mouth]. Formation of communication bet. the esophagus and intestine following excision of stomach.

esophagogastros'copy [" + *gastēr*, belly, + *skopein*, to examine]. Inspection of esophagus and stomach through an illuminated instrument.

esophagogastrostomy (e-sof"ă-go-gas-tros'to-mĭ) [" + " + *stoma*, mouth]. Formation of a communication bet. the esophagus and stomach.

esophagomalacia (e-sof"ă-go-mă-la'sĭ-ă) [" + *malakia*, softness]. Softening of the esophageal walls.

esophagomycosis (e-sof"ă-go-mi-ko'sis) [" + *mykēs*, fungus, + *ōsis*]. Bacterial or fungus disease of esophagus.

esophagoplasty (e-sof'ă-go-plas"tĭ) [" + *plassein*, to form]. Repair of the esophagus by a plastic operation.

esophagoplication (e-sof"ă-go-pli-ka'shun) [" + L. *plicāre*, to fold]. Reduction of dilation of the esophagus by taking tucks in its walls.

esophagopto'sia, esophagopto'sis [" + *ptōsis*, a falling]. Relaxation and prolapse of the esophagus.

esophagoscope (e-sof'ă-go-skōp) [" + *skopein*, to examine]. Device for examination of esophagus.

esoph'agospasm [" + *spasmos*, spasm]. Spasm of walls of the esophagus.

esophagostenosis (e-sof"ă-go-stĕ-no'sis) [" + *stenōsis*, contraction]. Stricture or narrowing of the esophagus.

esophagostomy (e-sof-ă-gos'to-mĭ) [" + *stoma,* opening]. Formation of esophageal fistula.

esophagotome (e-sof'ă-go-tōm) [" + *tomē,* incision]. Instrument for forming an esophageal fistula.

esophagotomy (e-sof-ă-got'o-mĭ) [" + *tomē,* incision]. Making of an incision in esophagus, so as to remove foreign substance.

esophagus (e-sof'ă-gus) (pl. *esophagi*) [G. *oisophagos*]. A musculomembranous canal extending from the pharynx to the stomach. Length about 9 inches. RS: *epicardium, gullet.*

e., foreign bodies in the. F. A. TREATMENT: The patient may complain of pain or an uncomfortable feeling deep in the chest. The article often can be dislodged by making the patient vomit by wiggling the finger in the back part of the throat.

A physician should always be called. Foreign bodies in the stomach are ordinarily not dangerous and usually pass through the alimentary tract in a few days without danger. However, it may be dangerous to give cathartics or enemas. These patients should always be under the care of a physician.

esophoria (es-o-fo'rĭ-ă) [G. *esō,* inward, + *pherein,* to bear]. OPTH: Tendency of visual lines to converge. SEE: *exophoria.*

esophylac'tic [" + *phylaxis,* protection]. That which is phylactic or protective.

esophylaxis (es"o-fi-laks'is) [" + *phylaxis,* protection]. The protective biological action against disease exercised by the fluids and cells of the body. SEE: *exophylaxis.*

esosphenoiditis (es"o-sfe-noy-di'tis) [" + *sphēn,* wedge, + *eidos,* form, + *itis,* inflammation]. Osteomyelitis of the sphenoid bone.

esoteric (es-o-ter'ik) [G. *esōteros,* within]. Coming from within the organism.

esotropia (es-o-tro'pĭ-ă) [G. *esō,* inward, + *trepein,* to turn]. Marked turning inward of eye, crossed eyes.

ESP. Abbr. for *extrasensory perception.*

ESR. Abbr. for *electron spin resistance; erythrocyte sedimentation rate.*

-ess [Fr.]. Suffix noting female sex.

es'sence [L. *essentia,* being or quality]. 1. The spirit or principle of anything. 2. An alcoholic solution of volatile oil.

essen'tial [L. *essentia,* being or quality]. 1. Pert. to an essence. 2. Indispensable. 3. Specific; independent of a local morbid condition. SYN: *idiopathic.*

e. oil. Any volatile oil of vegetable or animal origin.

es'ter. In organic chemistry, a compound formed by the combination of an organic acid with an alcohol.

Ex: Ethyl acetate is an ester formed by combining acetic acid with ethyl alcohol. Esters are commonly liquids with characteristic fruity or flowery odors.

esterase (es'ter-ās). Generic term for an enzyme that catalyzes the hydrolysis of esters.

e. acetylcholine. Cholinesterase, an enzyme that quickly hydrolyzes acetylcholine to acetic acid and choline.

es'terize. To convert into an ester.

es"thematol'ogy [G. *aisthēma,* sensation, + *logos,* science]. Science of the sense organs and their function.

esthesia (es-the'zĭ-ă) [G. *aisthēsis,* sensation]. 1. Perception, feeling, sensation. 2. Any disease that affects the senses or perceptions. It forms the termination of many medical words.

esthe'sioblast [" + *blastos,* germ]. An embryonic ganglion cell. SYN: *ganglioblast.*

esthesiol'ogy [" + *logos,* science]. Science of sensory phenomena. SYN: *esthematology.*

esthesiomania (es-the"zĭ-o-ma'nĭ-ă) [" + *mania,* madness]. Insanity with sensory hallucinations and perverted moral sensibilities.

esthesiometer (es-the-zĭ-om'ĕ-ter) [" + *metron,* measure]. Device for measuring tactile sensibility.

esthesioneurosis (es-the'zĭ-o-nu-ro'sis) [" + *neuron,* nerve, + *ōsis*]. A loss of feeling without any apparent organic lesion.

esthe"siophysiol'ogy [" + *physis,* nature, + *logos,* study]. Physiology of the sense organs.

esthesioscopy (es-the'zĭ-os'ko-pĭ) [" + *skopein,* to examine]. Testing tactile and other forms of sensibility.

estheticokinetic (es-thet"ĭ-ko-kin-et'ik) [" + *kinēsis,* motion]. Being both sensory and motor.

esthiomene (es-thĭ-om'en-e) [G. *esthiomenos,* eating]. A chronic hypertrophic ulcerative vulvovaginitis. A complication of lymphogranuloma venereum. SYN: *esthiomenus.*

es'tival [L. *aestivus,* pert. to summer]. Relating to or occurring in summer.

estivoautumnal [" + *autumnalis,* pert. to autumn]. 1. Pert. to summer and autumn. 2. A term applied to form of malaria.

estradiol (es-tră-di'ol). $C_{18}H_{24}O_2$, a crystalline steroid possessing estrogenic properties found in the ovary, the follicular fluid, corpus luteum, placenta, and adrenal gland. Large quantities are found in the urine of pregnant women and mares and in the urine of stallions; the latter two serving as sources of the commercial product. In the body it is converted to estrone and estriol. It is believed to be the true ovarian hormone. SYN: *dihydrotheelin; dihydroxyestrin.*

e. dipropionate. An ester of estradiol. Exerts a more sustained effect than e.

es'triol. Hormone found in urine of pregnancy. SYN: *theelol.*

es'trogen. Any substance, natural or artificial, which induces estrogenic activity; more specifically the estrogenic hormone produced by the ovarian follicle and other structures; the female sex hormone. Estrogens are responsible for the development of secondary sexual characteristics, cyclic changes in the vaginal epithelium (and the endothelium) of the uterus. They are used in the treatment of menopausal symptoms. Natural estrogens include estradiol, estrone, and estriol.

estrogenic (es-tro-jen'ĭk) [G. *oistros,* mad desire, + *gennan,* to produce]. Causing estrus.

es'trone. Theelin, $C_{18}H_{22}O_2$; an estrogenic hormone found in the urine of pregnant women and mares. It is also prepared synthetically. Used in the treatment of estrogen deficiencies. It is less active than estradiol, but more active than estriol. Also called folliculin, follicular hormone.

es'trual [G. *oistros,* mad desire]. Pert. to the rutting of animals.

estrua'tion [G. *oistros,* mad desire]. Rutting of animals during heat period.

es'trum, es'trus [G. *oistros,* mad desire]. In mammals other than primates, the recurrent period of sexual activity called "heat", characterized by congestion of and secretion by the uterine mucosa, proliferation of vaginal epithelium, swelling of the vulva, ovulation, and acceptance of the male by the female.

e. cycle. The cycle from the beginning of one estrus period to the beginning of the next. Includes proestrus, estrus, and metestrus followed by a short period of quiescence called *diestrus.*

estua'rium [L. *aistus,* heat]. Vapor bath.

état mamelonné (ā-tă' mă-mĕ-lon-nă') [Fr. knobby state]. Condition of gastric mucosa in chronic inflammation with nodular projections.

ethanol (eth'ă-nol). Ethyl alcohol. SEE: *alcohol.*

e'ther [G. *aithēr,* air]. 1. Hypothetic substance once regarded as permeating all space and capable of transmitting electromagnetic vibrations. 2. Any organic compound in which an oxygen atom links together two carbon chains.

The general formula is R'OR". The ether used for anesthesia is diethyl ether. $C_4H_{10}O$. As an anesthetic it causes postoperative nausea and profuse salivation.

CAUTION: Ether is highly flammable and should be handled with great care. Also it should not be stored once the can is opened, because toxic products form when ether is exposed to light.

e. anesthetic. Ethyl oxide, or diethyl ether $C_4H_{10}O$, the common ether used in anesthesia. It is a thin, colorless, highly volatile, and highly inflammable liquid with a specific gravity at 25° of 0.713-0.716. It was formerly called sulfuric ether because it was prepared from ethyl alcohol and sulfuric acid. It is widely used for general anesthesia. The action of ether is slower than other general anesthetics and the margin of safety is greater.

PHYS. ACTION: Ether stimulates the respiratory mucous membranes and the respiratory center in the medulla oblongata. It stimulates and accelerates the action of the heart. It lowers body temperature and raises blood pressure unless given in large doses or continued over a long period, when it lowers blood pressure. It produces fair muscular relaxation and increases mucus and other secretions. It produces slight changes in body chemistry. It is usually chosen for most brain surgery.

CONTRA: Its use is contraindicated in diabetes, liver damage, kidney disease, chronic pulmonary conditions (especially tuberculosis), surgical shock, or following recent severe blood loss.

AFTER EFFECTS: Excitement with desire to talk follows ether anesthesia, the patient perspires freely, and exhibits signs of nausea and begins to vomit, all before the return to consciousness which may not be regained for several hours. Upon awakening he feels dizzy, complains of headache and thirst. These effects may last for hours. The flow of saliva and the secretion of mucus may be increased. It is usually excreted from the body within 24 hr. Pneumonia is the most common complication following ether anesthesia. Gas pains may give trouble.

NP: Warm or cold water; the quantity permitted to relieve thirst depends upon the surgeon. Foot of bed elevated and the head should be turned to one side when vomiting, to prevent vomitus from passing into the trachea. Cold compresses may be placed to head and a rectal irrigation may be given to relieve gas pressure, or a rectal tube may be inserted for the purpose. SEE: *chloroform a.; ethylene a.*

e. asphyxia. Suffocation during ether anesthetization. SEE: *e. anesthesia; gases; resuscitation.*

e. bed. One prepared to receive patient immediately following an operative procedure requiring anesthesia.

ARTICLES NECESSARY: Bedding for making an ordinary closed bed. Two small rubber sheets. Two draw sheets (or special "ether sheets"). Two bath blankets. Two pieces of bandage about 3 in. wide. Two towels. Two emesis basins. Pad and pencil. Small pieces of gauze or paper wipes. Paper bags. Safety pins. Shock blocks. Rubber pillow case. Hot water bottles filled and covered (if they are to be used).

PROCEDURE: 1. Make up bottom part of bed as usual. 2. Place 1 small rubber sheet where region of operation will come. 3. Place another across head of mattress where patient's head will lie. 4. Cover each with a draw sheet, tucking it firmly under mattress. 5. Spread the two bath blankets one over the other, with tops 6 in. from top of mattress. Hot water bottles to be placed between these. Tuck lower blanket in at sides. 6. Place top bedding as usual but do not tuck in. 7. Fan-fold top sheet over bed blanket to protect it. Fold all top bedding together, including the top bath blanket, even with mattress edge all around, then fold toward side of bed away from the door, or where the stretcher will be placed, until it lies in a neat fold. 8. Tie one pillow upright on its side against bars at top of bed with bandage. 9. Put rubber pillow case on other pillow and have it ready to put under patient's knees if needed. 10. Place shock blocks at foot of bed on each side ready for instant pushing into position. 11. Place pad, pencil, emesis basin, wipes and one towel on bedside table, other towels over headbar of bed. 12. Place chairs and table out of way of the stretcher.

e. drunkenness. Intoxication produced by imbibing ether.

ethereal (e-the're-al) [G. *aithēr,* air]. Pert. to or made with ether.

e. oil. A volatile oil.

etherin (e'ther-in) [G. *aithēr,* air]. A tuberculous toxin extracted by ether. SYN: *etherobacillin.*

etherization (e"ther-ī-za'shun) [G. *aithēr,* air]. Administering ether to induce anesthesia.

e'therize [G. *aithēr,* air]. To anesthetize by use of ether.

e"therobacil'lin [" + L. *bacillus,* rod]. Etherin, *q.v.*

etheromania (e"ther-o-ma'nĭ-ă) [" + *mania,* madness]. Addiction to use of ether.

ethics. A system of moral principles or standards governing conduct.

e., medical. A system of principles governing medical conduct. It deals with the relationship of a physician to the patient, the patient's family, his fellow physicians, and society at large.

e., nursing. A system of principles governing conduct of a nurse. It deals with the relationship of a nurse to the patient, the patient's family, her associates and fellow nurses, and society at large.

ethiopifica'tion [G. *Aithiops,* an Ethiopian, + L. *facere,* to make]. Pathological blackening of the skin from use of silver or other metals.

ethmocardi'tis [G. *ēthmos,* sieve, + *kardia,* heart]. Chronic inflammation and proliferation of cardiac connective tissue. SYN: *cardiosclerosis.*

eth'moid [G. *ethmos,* sieve, + *eidos,* form]. Sievelike; cribiform.

e. bone. Sievelike spongy bone which forms a roof for the nasal fossae and part of floor of ant. fossa of skull, and containing air sinuses.

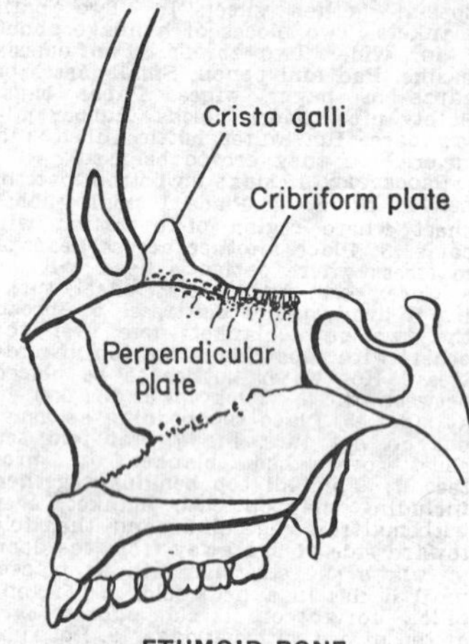

ETHMOID BONE

e. sinus. Air cells or space inside ethmoid bone.

ethmoi'dal [" + *eidos,* form]. Pert. to the ethmoid bone or sinuses.

ethmoidectomy (eth-moy-dek'to-mĭ) [" + " + *ektomē,* excision]. Excision of ethmoid cells.

NP: Patient in sitting position, ice packs to nose often ordered.

ethmoidi'tis [" + " + *-ĭtis,* inflammation]. Inflammation of ethmoidal cells. May be acute or chronic. SYM: Headache, acute pain bet. eyes, nasal discharge.

ethmyphitis (eth-mif-i'tis) [" + *yphē,* tissue, + *-ĭtis,* inflammation]. Diffuse inflammation of cellular tissue. SYN: *cellulitis.*

ethnog'raphy [G. *ethnos,* race, + *graphein,* to write]. The description of the human race.

ethnol'ogy [" + *logos,* science]. The science of human races.

ethyl (eth'il) [G. *aithēr,* air, + *ylē,* matter]. In organic chemistry, the radical C_2H_5 which enters into the constitution of many compounds such as ethyl ether, ethyl alcohol, and ethyl acetate.

e. acetate. $CH_3COOC_2H_5$. A colorless flammable liquid used as a solvent. SYN: *acetic ether.*

e. alcohol. C_2H_5OH. Grain alcohol. SEE: *alcohol, ethyl.*

e. aminobenzoate. Same as benzocaine, a topical anesthetic.

e. bromide. CH_3CH_2Br, hydrobromic ether. Used for local anesthesia as a topical spray, and as inhalation anesthetic.

e. carbamate. $NH_2COOC_2H_5$. Used in the treatment of myeloid and lymphatic leukemia. SYN: *urethan.*

e. chaulmoograte. The ethyl esters of the fatty acids of chaulmoogra oil. Used in the treatment of leprosy.

e. chloride. CH_3CH_2OH, hydrochloric ether. USP. A very volatile liquid with a pleasant odor. When sprayed on the skin, it evaporates so quickly that the tissue is cooled immediately. Because of this property the skin is anesthetized. USES: Local anesthetic in minor surgery. It is a topical anesthetic and is used only for a very short anesthesia.

e. formate. $HCOOC_2H_5$, formic ether; a volatile antispasmodic and anesthetic.

e. iodide. C_2H_5I, hydriodic ether; used by inhalation in treatment of asthma.

e. nitrite, spirit of. Commonly known as sweet spirit of niter. Alcoholic solution of an oily liquid. ACTION AND USES: Diuretic and for relief of arterial spasm.

e. salicylate. A volatile liquid, characteristic odor, same effects but less irritant than methyl salicylate.

ethylamine. $CH_3CH_2NH_2$. An amine formed in the decomposition of certain proteins.

ethylene (eth'il-ēn). A colorless gas (CH_2CH_2) prepared from alcohol by dehydration and found in illuminating gas to the extent of 4%. It is colorless, and has a sweetish taste but a pungent, foul odor. It is lighter than air and diffusable when liberated. It is inflammable and explosive.

e. anesthesia. Since ethylene is a rather weak anesthetic, it usually is given in a combination of oxygen 20%, cyclopropane 10%, and ethylene 70%.

PHYS. EFFECTS: It causes less alteration in the blood gases than does nitrous oxide. The CO_2 content is not altered. Full muscular relaxation and slight irregularity in heart action, respiration, and blood pressure. Analgesia results before loss of hearing or before complete unconsciousness. Nausea and vomiting seldom persist as long as 24 hr., but it generally disappears before consciousness has returned.

ADVANTAGES: Slightly stimulating to cardiac and respiratory systems. It lowers body temperature; less toxic than any known anesthetics. It is not irritating to mucous glands and kidneys. It has a short period of induction and makes possible a very rapid recovery. There is an absence of cyanosis, and a minimum of emesis. The difference between ethylene and any other anesthetic known today is that there is a less marked effect on all the systems of the body. It is the choice anesthetic for old patients and for poor surgical risks, and when moderate anesthesia is desired or where complete relaxation is not required.

DISADVANTAGES: Has an objectionable smell; is highly inflammable and explosive; increases capillary bleeding; the relaxation is not so complete or as perfect as from the use of ether anesthetics.

PRECAUTIONS: *Many lives have been lost because someone was careless and a spark was emitted from some immediate source. Ethylene should be stored where there is plenty of air. The administration must be done away from fire or electric appliances or x-ray apparatus. All lights should be turned on before bringing the tanks into the room to prevent sparking from the plug or lighting fixture. Furniture should never be dragged into the room or rolled into the room while the anesthetic is being given. The humidity of the room should be checked during the administration of this anesthetic.* Nylon clothing or undergarments should not be worn by anyone in the room. Friction from the material may generate static electricity.

Ethylene does not combine with air as do other anesthetics but floats around as clouds; as the vapor rises in a cloud-like form any gust of air may carry it out of the room and should someone be on the outside smoking or the elevator cause a sparking, an explosion would result with the destruction of life in a most devastating manner. Ethylene always comes in red tanks. Oxygen is stored in green tanks. Nitrous oxide is stored in blue tanks. Carbon dioxide is stored in gray tanks. SEE: *chloroform a.; ether a.*

etiolate (e'tĭ-o-lāt) [Fr. *étioler,* to blanch]. Pale or sickly from lack of light or long continued illness.

etiologic, etiological (e"tĭ-o-loj'ik, e-tĭ-o-loj'ik-ăl) [G. *aitia,* cause, + *logos,* study]. Pert. to causes.

etiology (e-tĭ-ol'o-jĭ) [" + *logos,* study]. The study of the causes of disease which result from an abnormal state producing pathological conditions.

CONGENITAL: Embryonic malformations and conditions occurring during fetal life, such as abnormalities, anomalies, and monstrosities.

e"tiotrop'ic. Directed toward the cause of a disease, said of a drug or treatment which destroys or inactivates the causal agent of a disease; opposite of nosotropic, *q.v.*

etrohysterectomy (e"tro-his-ter-ek'to-mĭ). Excision of the uterus through the abdominal wall in the hypogastric region.

etymology (et-ĭ-mol'o-jĭ) [G. *etymon,* true meaning of a word, + *logos,* science]. The science of the derivation of words.

Most medical words are derived from the Latin and Greek, but many of those from the Greek have reached us through the Latin, being modified by that language. When two Greek words are used to form one word, they generally are connected by the letter "o."

Many medical words have been formed from one or more *roots,* forms used or adapted from the Latin or Greek, and many of them are modified either by a *prefix* or a *suffix,* or both. A knowledge of important Latin or Greek roots, and of prefixes will reveal the meaning of a great many other words. SEE: Prefixes and Suffixes, App. 30-31.

eu- (ū) [G. *eu,* well]. Prefix meaning healthy, normal, good, well.

Eubacteriales (u"bak-te-rĭ-a'lēz) [G. *eu,* well, + *baktērion,* little rod]. The true bacteria. Includes the simplest and least differentiated forms. SEE: *bacteria, classification of.*

eubiotics (u-bi-ot'iks) [G. *eu,* well, + *bios,* life]. The science of healthy and hygienic living.

eu'bolism [" + (*meta*)*bolē,* change, + *ismos,* condition]. Normal metabolism.

eucaine hydrochloride (u'kān-hi-dro-klo'-rīd). USP. White, crystalline powder. Used as a local anesthetic.

eucalyptol. USP. A substance obtained from oil of eucalyptus.

eucalyptus, oil of (u-kă-lip'tus) [G. *eu,* well, + *kalyptein,* to cover]. USP. Oil distilled from fresh leaves of the plant.

ACTION AND USES: As an expectorant and antiseptic.

eucapnia (u-kap'nĭ-ă). Presence of normal amounts of carbon dioxide in the blood.

euchlorhydria (u"klor-hi'drĭ-ă). Presence of the normal amount of free hydrochloric acid in the gastric juice.

eucholia (u-ko'lĭ-ă). Normal condition of bile regarding its constituents and amount secreted.

euchylia (u-ki'lĭ-ă) [" + *chylos, chyle*]. Normal condition of the chyle.

eucrasia (u-kra'sĭ-ă). Condition of normal health; state of the body in which all activities are in normal balance.

eudiaphoresis (u"di-ă-fo-re'sis) [" + *dia,* through, + *pherein,* to carry]. Normal secretion of perspiration.

eudiemorrhysis (u"di-ĕ-mor'ĭ-sis) [" + " + *aima,* blood, + *rysis,* flow]. The normal blood flow through the capillaries.

eudiom'eter [G. *eudia,* good weather, + *metron,* measure]. An instrument for testing purity of air and analysis of gases.

euesthesia (u-es-the'sĭ-ă) [G. *eu,* well, + *aisthēsis,* sensation]. Having normal senses.

eugenics (u-jen'iks) [" + *gennan,* to produce]. The science which deals with the physical, moral, and intellectual improvement of the human race by careful and judicious mating. It is also concerned with (1) the sterilization of mental defectives; (2) intermarriages; (3) restriction of marriage bet. persons physically unfit; (4) birth control and allied problems. SEE: *aristogenics.*

e., negative. Those measures which seek to restrict the numbers of offspring with genetically undesirable traits.

e., positive. Those measures which seek to bring about an increase in the numbers of offspring of families with genetically desirable traits.

eugenism (u'jen-izm) [" + " + *ismos,* condition]. The circumstances of environment and heredity which tend to bring about happy and healthy existence.

euglobulin (u-glob'u-lin). A true globulin, or one soluble in distilled water and dilute salt solution. SEE: *pseudoglobulin.*

eugonic (u-gon'ik) [" + *gonē,* seed]. Pertaining to a luxuriant growth of bacteria.

eukinesia (u-kin-e'sĭ-ă) [" + *kinēsis,* motion]. Normal power of movement.

Eulenburg's disease [Albert Eulenburg, German neurologist, 1840-1917]. Paramyotonia congenita.

eumenorrhea (u"men-o-re'ă). Normal menstruation.

eunoia (u-noy'ă) [" + *nous,* mind]. Soundness of mind.

eunuch (u'nuk) [G. *eunē,* bed, + *echein,* to guard]. Castrated male; one who has had his testicles removed.

The absence of the testicular secretions produce certain symptoms, such as a female type of voice and loss of hair on the face.

In some countries eunuchs were employed to guard the women of a harem.

eunuchism (u'nuk-izm). Condition resulting from complete androgen deficiency, as occurs following castration.

eunuchoid. Having the characteristics of a eunuch, such as retarded development of external and accessory sex organs, absence of beard and bodily hair, high-pitched voice, and striking lack of muscular development.

e., pituitary. E. due to failure of the ant. lobe of the pituitary to secrete gonadotrophic hormones; secondary hypogonadism.

eunuchoidism (u-nuk'oyd-ism). Condition resulting from androgen deficiency of the testes regardless of etiology.

eupancreatism (u-pan'kre-ă-tizm) [G. *eu*, well, + *pagkreas*, pancreas, + *ismos* condition]. Normal condition of the pancreas.

eupep'sia [" + *pepsis*, digestion]. Normal digestion, as distinguished from dyspepsia.

eupep'tic [" + *pepsis*, digestion]. Possessed of a good digestion.

euphonia (u-fōn'ĭ-ă). Having a normal clear voice.

euphoria (u-fo'rĭ-ă) [" + *pherein*, to bear]. 1. A condition of good health. 2. PSY: An exaggerated feeling of well-being; mild elation.

euplas'tic [" + *plassein*, to form]. Healing quickly and well.

eupnea (ūp-ne'ă) [" + *pnein*, to breathe]. Normal breathing, as distinguished from dyspnea and apnea.

eupraxia (u-prak'sĭ-ă) [" + *prassein*, to do]. Normal capacity to execute a motor pattern. SEE: *paralysis*.

eupraxic (u-prak'sik) [" + *prassein*, to do]. Contributing to proper functioning.

europium (u-ro'pi-um). An element of the lanthanide series. SYMB: Eu. At. no. 63; at. wt. 151.96.

Eurotium (u-ro'shĭ-um). A genus of molds.

E. malig'num. A species causing inflammation in ext. auditory meatus.

euryon (u're-on) [G. *eurys*, broad]. Either end of bilateral diameter of head.

euryosomic, eurysomatic (u"rĭ-o-so'mik, u"rĭ-so-mat'ik) [" + *sōma*, body]. Having a thick, squat body.

eustachian (u-sta'kĭ-an). [After Eustachio, an Italian anatomist]. Pert. to the auditory tube.

RS: *salpingemphraxis, syringitis, syrinx.*

e. catheter. Instrument for insertion into eustachian tube.

e. tube. The auditory tube (from the middle ear to the pharynx, 3-4 cm. long and lined with mucous membrane).

e. valve. At the entrance of the inf. vena cava. SYN: *valvula venae cavae inferioris.*

eustachitis (u-sta-ki'tis). Inflammation of the eustachian tube.

eusystole (u-sis'to-lē) [G. *eu*, well, + *systellein*, to draw together]. A state of the systole of the heart that is normal in time and force.

eutectic (u-tek'tik) [" + *tēktos*, melting]. Easily melted.

e. mixture. A mixture of two or more substances which has a melting point lower than that of any of its constituents.

euthanasia (u-thă-na'zĭ-ă) [" + *thanatos*, death]. 1. An easy death. 2. The proposed practice of ending of life in case of incurable disease.

euthenics (u-then'iks) [G. *euthēnia*, well-being]. The science of improvement of the race through modification of the environment; in contrast to eugenics. *q.v.*

euthyroid (ū-thi'royd) [" + thyroid]. Normal thyroid gland function.

eutocia (u-to'sĭ-ă) [G. *eu*, well, + *tokos*, birth]. Normal or natural labor and childbirth.

evacuant (e-vak'u-ant) [L. *evacuans*, making empty]. Drug which moves the bowels.

evac'uate [L. *evacuāre*, to empty]. 1. To discharge, esp. from the bowels; to empty the uterus. 2. To move patients from place or site of accident to a hospital.

evacuation (e-vak-u-a'shun) [L. *evacuāre*, to empty]. 1. Emptying, esp. the bowels. 2. The material discharged from the bowels; stool. 3. Removal of air from a closed container; the production of a vacuum. RS: *absorption, feces, stool.*

evacuator (e-vak'u-a-tor) [L. *evacuāre*, to empty]. Device for emptying, as of the bowels or for irrigating the bladder and removing calculi.

evaginate (e-vaj'ĭ-nat) [L. *ē*, out, + *vagina*, sheath]. Pert. to protrusion of some part or organ from its normal place.

evagination (e-vaj-ĭ-na'-shun) [" + *vagina*, sheath]. 1. Emergence from a sheath. 2. Protrusion of an organ or part. SEE: *invagination.*

evanes'cent [L. *evanescere*, to vanish]. Not permanent; of brief duration; passing gradually.

Evans blue [Herbert M. Evans, California anatomist, 1882-]. A diazo dye occurring as a bluish-green powder, very soluble in water. It is used intravenously as a diagnostic agent.

evapora'tion [L. *ē*, out, + *vaporāre*, to steam]. 1. Change from liquid form to vapor. 2. Loss in volume due to conversion of a liquid into a vapor.

Eve's method (F. C. Eve, physician, Hull, England) (resuscitation in drowning). NOTE: This method of artificial respiration is presented mostly for historical reasons. *Mouth-to-mouth* method of artificial respiration is much more effective. Place the victim downward on a stretcher with ankles and wrists tied to handles, arms extending away from the body beyond the head. Support stretcher on a trestle about 34 inches high. Hold head of stretcher down to a tilt of about 45 degrees, and keep it there until no more water drains from the mouth. Then start rocking for a few minutes; then reduce tilt about 30 degrees each way with ten double rockings a minute. Remove wet clothing as the rocking proceeds, rub the body, and place hot-water bottle at back of neck, adding warm blankets about the patient. Paralysis of the diaphragm is thus prevented. SEE: *resuscitation; artificial respiration.*

evec'tics [L. *evehere*, to carry up]. Acquiring good body vigor and habits.

eventra'tion [L. *ē*, out, + *venter*, belly]. 1. Partial protrusion of the abdominal contents through an opening in the abdominal wall. 2. Removal of contents of the abdominal cavity.

e. of the diaphragm. Elevation of the diaphragmatic dome into the thoracic cavity.

eversion (e-ver'zhun) [" + *vertere*, to turn]. Turning outward. SEE: *chilectropion.*

e. of the cervix. A turning out of the cervical edges subsequent to laceration. SYN: *ectropion of cervix.*

évidement (ā-vēd-mòn') [Fr. a scooping out]. Scraping away diseased tissue.

evil. Disease or illness.

eviration (e-vi-ra'shun) [L. *ē*, out, + *vir*, man]. 1. Castration. 2. Effemination or defemination, or transformations of psychical personality due to the development of contrary sexual instincts.

evisceration (e-vis-er-a'shun) [" + *viscera*, viscera]. 1. Removal of the viscera. 2. Removal of the contents of a cavity. 3. Protrusion of the viscera.

e., obstetrical. Removal of the thoracic and abdominal contents of a fetus to facilitate delivery.

evisceroneurotomy (e-vis"er-o-nu-rot'o-mĭ) [" + " + G. *neuron*, nerve, + *tomē*, incision]. Scleral evisceration of the eye with division of optic nerve.

evolu'tion [" + *volvere*, to roll]. A process of orderly and gradual change or development.

More generally, any orderly and gradual process of modification whereby a system, whether physical, chemical, social, or even intellectual, becomes more highly organized.

e., doctrine of. The view that all present-day species of plants and animals, including man, have come into existence by gradual, continuous change from earlier pre-existing forms. It considers that life first came into existence as a simple primordial mass of protoplasm from which, through a series of progressive changes, the highly complex, specialized forms of today arose.

e., spontaneous. Spontaneous birth of a child in transverse presentation.

evul'sion [" + *vellere*, to pluck]. 1. Tearing away of a part or new growth. 2. Forcible extraction, as of teeth.

ex- [L.]. Prefix: *Out, away from, completely.*

exacerbation (eks"as-er-ba'shun) [L. *ex*, completely, + *acerbus*, harsh]. Aggravation of symptoms or increase in the severity of a disease.

exacrinous (eks-ak'rin-us) [G. *ex*, outside, + *krinein*, to secrete]. Concerning a gland's external secretion.

exaltation. A mental state characterized by feelings of grandeur, excessive joy, elation, and optimism; an abnormal feeling of personal well-being or self-importance.

examina'tion, phys'ical [L. *examināre*, to examine]. The act or process of examining the body and its products as to fitness or for symptoms of a disease.

Local examination includes specific parts and organs. Four procedures utilized are *inspection, palpation, percussion*, and *auscultation*. Laboratory examination includes urinalysis, tests, cultures, basal metabolism, etc.

Terms employed indicating type of examination are: physical, bimanual, digital, oral, rectal, O.B. (obstetrical), roentgenological, cystoscopic.

exangia (eks-an'jĭ-ă) [G. *ex*, out, + *aggeion*, vessel]. Any dilatation of a blood vessel. Ex: *aneurysm, varix.*

exanthem (eks-an'them) (pl. *exanthems*) [G. *exanthēma*, eruption]. Any eruption of the skin, accompanied by inflammation, *e.g.*, measles, scarlatina, erysipelas, *q.v.*

e. subitum. An acute virus disease of infants. Marked by high fever for 3 or 4 days and convulsions. Treatment is symptomatic. SEE ALSO: *convulsion.* SYN: *pseudorubella; roseola infantum; sixth disease.*

exanthema (eks-an-the'mă) (pl. *exanthemas, exanthemata*). Exanthem.

exanthematous (eks-an-them'ă-tus) [G. *exanthēma*, eruption]. Pert. to an exanthem, eruption or rash.

exanthrope (eks'an-thrōp) [G. *ex*, out, + *anthrōpos*, man]. A cause or source of a disease originating outside the body.

exarteritis (eks-ar-ter-i'tis) [" + *artēria*, artery, + *ītis*, inflammation]. Inflammation of the outer coat of an artery.

exarticula'tion [L. *ex*, out, + *articulus*, joint]. 1. Amputation of a limb through a joint. 2. Excision of a part of a joint.

excava'tion [" + *cavus*, hollow]. 1. A hollow or depression. 2. Formation of a cavity.

e., dental. The preparation of a cavity in a tooth prior to filling.

e. of the optic nerve. A slight depression in the center of the optic papilla or disk from which retinal vessels emerge. Depression is total in glaucoma as a result of high intraocular pressure.

e., rectouterine. The rectouterine pouch or pouch of Douglas.

excen'tric [G. *ex*, out, + *kentron*, center]. Eccentric.

excerebration (eks-ser-e-bra'shun) [L. *ex*, out, + *cerebrum*, brain]. Removal of brain.

excernant (ek-ser'nant) [L. *excernere*, to excrete]. Bringing about an evacuation or excretion. SYN: *excretory.*

excip'ient [L. *excipiens*, from *ex*, out, + *capere*, to take]. Any substance added to a medicine to permit it to be formed into the proper shape and consistency. The excipient should have no action of its own and should not interfere with the solubility of the medicine.

excise (ex'sīsz) [" + *caedere*, to cut]. To cut out or remove surgically.

excis'ion [L. *excisiō*, from *ex*, out, + *caedere*, to cut]. An act of cutting away or taking out.

excitabil'ity [L. *excitāre*, to rouse]. Sensitiveness to being stimulated.

e., independent. Power of a muscle to respond to a stimulus without intervention of motor nerves.

e., reflex. Sensitiveness to reflex irritation.

excitant (ek-sīt'ant) [L. *excitāre*, to rouse]. An agent that will excite a special function of the body; subdivided, according to action, as *motor, cerebral*, etc. Ex: *alcohol, cocaine, strychnine.*

excita'tion [L. *excitāre*, to rouse]. 1. The act of exciting. 2. Condition of being stimulated or excited.

e., direct. Stimulation of a muscle by placing an electrode in it or physically stimulating it.

e., indirect. Stimulation of a muscle *via* its nerve.

e. wave. The wave of irritability originating in the atrioventricular node which sweeps over the conductile tissue of the heart and induces contraction of the atria and ventricles.

excit'ing [L. *excitāre*, to rouse]. Causing excitement.

e. cause. Acting immediately as a cause of disease.

excitoglan'dular [" + *glans, gland-*, kernel]. Increasing glandular function.

excitometabol'ic [" + G. *metabolē*, change]. Inducing metabolic changes.

excitomo'tor [" + *motor*, moving]. Increasing rapidity of muscular activity.

excitomus'cular [" + G. *mys*, muscle]. Causing muscular activity.

excitonu'trient [" + *nutrire*, to nourish]. Stimulating nutrition.

exci'tor [L. *excitāre*, to rouse]. That which incites to greater activity. SYN: *stimulant.*

excitosecre'tory [" + *secretiō*, a hiding]. Tending to bring about secretion.

excitovas'cular [" + *vasculāris,* pert. to a vessel]. Increasing circulation.

exclave (eks'klāv) [L. *ex,* out, + *clavis,* key]. Detached part of an organ.

excochleation (eks-kok-le-a'shun) [" + *cochlea,* spoon]. Curettage of a cavity.

excoriation (eks-ko-rĭ-a'shun) [" + *corium,* skin]. Abrasion of the epidermis or of the coating of any organ of the body by trauma, chemicals, burns, or other causes.

excrement (eks'krĕ-ment) [L. *excernere,* to take away]. The feces, excreta, dejecta. SEE: *excretion.*

e., menstruum. Menstrual discharge

excrementitious (eks-krĕ-men-tish'us) [L. *excernere,* to take away]. Of the nature of excrement.

excrescence (eks-kres'ens) [L. *ex,* out, + *crescere,* to grow]. 1. Normal outgrowth from the surface of a part such as hair. 2. Diseased or useless growth on the surface of a part as a wart or mole.

excreta (eks-kre'tă) [L. from *excernere,* to take away]. Waste intestinal matter; dejecta; feces. Waste material cast off by the body.

CAUTION: When using the disinfecting materials listed below, be certain they do not come in contact with skin or eyes.

e., disinfection of. CARBOLIC ACID: A 5% solution to be used in quantity at least equal to the amount of the material to be disinfected.

CAUSTIC LIME: In the form of freshly prepared milk lime—this should contain about 1 part by weight of hydrate of lime mixed with 8 parts of water, to be used in an amount equal to that of the excreta to be disinfected.

CHLORIDE OF LIME: Dissolve in the proportion of 4 ounces to 1 gallon of water. One quart of this solution for disinfection of each liquid discharge. For solid fecal matter a stronger solution or a larger quantity of above solution will be required.

It will be prudent to use a large quantity of the standard solution recommended for a copious liquid discharge. With a spatula the formed material should be broken up and covered with chlorinated lime. The container should be set aside and the feces or urine, with the coating of lime, covered with a lid or newspapers. Let the mixture stand for 1 hour, stirring the lime into the contents from time to time, then it may be emptied into the sewer.

CUPRIC SULFATE: Is used as chloride of lime but in a 4% solution.

INVOLUNTARY DISCHARGES: These should be cared for by placing cellulose pads under the patient. The pads should be thoroughly wrapped in strong paper after being soiled to prevent scattering of the feces. In handling all infected discharges, the nurse should wear rubber gloves.

e., kinds of. (1) Carbon and oxygen. Both given off as carbon dioxide from the lungs. (2) Hydrogen and oxygen. Both forming water and given off as: (a) Vapor from the lungs; (b) perspiration from the skin; (c) in urine from the kidneys. (3) Nitrogen: Given off in urine from the kidneys. (4) Intestinal excreta: (a) Waste mineral matter; (b) foreign matter; (c) unassimilated food material; (d) water and liquids.

excrete (eks-krēt') [L. *excernere,* to separate]. To separate and expel useless matter not utilized by the body.

excre'tin. A crystalline substance found in the feces. A fraction of the hormone, secretin, which stimulates pancreatic secretion.

excre'tion [L. *excernere,* to separate]. 1. Waste matter, excreta. 2. The elimination of waste products from the body.

e., organs of. INTESTINES: Indigestible residue, water and bacteria.

KIDNEYS: Filter from the blood water, nitrogenous substances (urea, uric acid, creatin, creatinine) mineral salts.

RESPIRATORY SYSTEM: Carbon dioxide, water vapor, and other gases.

SKIN: Small amt. through perspiration of water, salts, minute quantities of urea. Its excretory function is stimulated by kidney inactivity. Diaphoretics, hot packs, and warm blankets stimulate skin and aid kidneys, thus helping to avoid uremic coma.

excretion, *words pert. to:* defecation, dejecta, elimination, excrement, excreta, expectoration, feces, hydragogue, incontinence, lung, perspiration, pore, respiration, semen, skin, sputum, sweat, urine, void.

ex'cretory [L. *excernere,* to separate]. Pert. to or bringing about excretion.

excur'sion [L. *ex,* out, + *currere,* to run]. 1. Wandering from the usual course. 2. Extent of movement of the eyes from a central position.

excurva'tion [" + *curvus,* bend]. A curvature outward. SYN: *kyphosis.*

excystation (eks"sis-ta'shun) [G. *ex,* out, + *kystis,* cyst]. Pertaining esp. to the escape of certain organisms (parasitic worms, protozoa) from an enclosing cyst wall or envelope. Process which occurs in the life cycle of an intestinal parasite after encysted form is ingested.

exemia (eks-e'mĭ-ă) [" + *aima,* blood]. Loss of blood from circulation, though accumulation in a part.

exencephalia (eks-en-sef-a'lĭ-ă). Condition in which the brain is located outside the skull. A congenital anomaly. A term for *encephalocele, hydrencephalocele, meningocele,* and *synencephalocele.*

exenteration (eks-en-ter-a'shun) [" + *enteron,* intestine]. 1. Evisceration. 2. Removal of viscera of fetus in embryotomy.

exercise [L. *exercitātiō,* training the body]. Functional activity of the muscles, voluntary or otherwise.

e., active. A form of bodily movement which the patient performs with or without the personal supervision of the operator.

e., assistive. A form of bodily movement which the patient performs assisted by the operator or some mechanical means such as a pulley or weight.

e., blowing. One in which water is blown from one bottle to another, thus increasing intrabronchial pressure which tends to aid in expansion of the lung. It is by this means that obliteration of an empyema cavity is facilitated. SEE ALSO: *empyema.*

e., Buerger's postural (bur'gers). Used for circulatory disturbances of the extremities.

e., corrective. Use of specific exercises to correct deficiencies caused by trauma or inactivity.

e., crawling. Devised for treatment of scoliosis,* essentially for children.

e., free. Form of bodily movement which is carried through by patient against least possible resistance.

e., Frenkel's. Used to teach tabetics to walk.

e., Krida knee. In intertrochanteric fractures of femur, remove post. half of plaster cast from the knee to the toes: anterior portion of leg cast remains attached to spica, and maintains position of hip. When patient is face down, this permits knee to be flexed and extended and ankle exercised.

e., Lewin circulatory. Passive exercise for leg for circulatory disturbance of extremity. (1) Patient lying supine, limb is elevated 60°, allowed to rest on support 30 seconds to 3 minutes. (2) Leg is then lowered to hang over side of bed 2-5 minutes. (3) Limb is then placed horizontal and heat applied 3-5 minutes.

e., Master's. Ascending and descending 2 steps a variable number of times. Used as a tolerance test for circulatory efficiency and as an exercise in heart disease. SYN: *Master two-step test.*

e., Mosher's. For dysmenorrhea. Lie on back on floor with knees bent, feet on floor. Raise abdomen, relax it, contract it forcibly and relax. Repeat 10 times.

e., muscle-setting. Contracting and relaxing a muscle or group of muscles without moving the part or changing the muscle length. SYN: *isotonic contraction; static exercise.*

e., passive. Form of bodily movement which is carried through by the operator without the assistance or resistance of the patient. Same as relaxed movement.

e., resistive. Form of supervised bodily movement, with or without apparatus, which offers resistance to muscle action.

e., rhythm. Used in obstetrical paralysis. Exercise to song or music.

e., Schott's. Named after the Dr. Schott of Nauheim, who first scientifically administered Nauheim baths. It consists of slowly and evenly executed exercises with slight resistance, for cardiac diseases.

e., sling suspension. Method of supporting arm or leg to be exercised in a sling suspended from overhead, thus eliminating the weight of the extremity as a hindrance during movement.

e., static. Alternate contraction and relaxation of a muscle or group of muscles without movement of the joint. Also known as muscle setting. SEE: *muscle-setting exercise.*

e., therapeutic. Scientific supervision of bodily movement, with or without apparatus, for purpose of restoring normal function to diseased or injured tissues.

e., water. Hydrogymnastics.

ex'ercise bone. Bony growth developing in a muscle due to overexercise.

exeresis (eks-er'ĕ-sis) [G. *ex*, out, + *eiresis*, taking]. Excision of any part.

exfetation (eks-fe-ta'shun) [L. *ex*, out, + *foetus*, fetus]. Ectopic gestation.

exflagellation (eks"flaj-ĕ-la'shun) [" + *flagellum*, a switch]. The formation of microgametes (flagellated bodies) from the microgametocytes. Occurs in the malarial organism (Plasmodium) in the stomach of a mosquito.

exfolia'tion [" + *folium*, leaf]. The scaling off of dead tissue. RS: *apostasis.*

exhala'tion [" + *halāre*, to breathe]. The process of breathing outward; the opposite of inhalation; emanation of a gas or vapor.

exhaus'ter [" + *haurīre*, to drain]. A cataract evacuator for removal of loosened or fluid matter by vacuum pressure through a hollow needle.

exhaus'tion [" + *haurīre*, to drain]. 1. State of being exhausted, extreme fatigue, or weariness; loss of vital powers; inability to respond to stimuli; 2. Process of removing the contents of or using up a supply of anything; 3. To draw or let out.

e., heat. Heat prostration; a condition resulting from exposure to high temperatures. Characterized by drowsy state of mind, rapid breathing, paleness, cold and sweaty skin, and normal or below normal temperature. May be due to salt deficiency, failure of the sweating mechanism, deficient water intake, or a combination of these factors.

exhib'it [L. *exhibere*, to display]. 1. To show. 2. To administer a drug. 3. Collection of objects for public inspection.

exhibi'tionism [L. *exhibere*, to display, + G. *ismos*, condition]. 1. An abnormal impulse that causes one to expose the genitals to one of the opposite sex. A psychoneurosis. 2. Tendency to attract attention in other ways.

exhibitionist (ek-sĭ-bish'un-ist) [L. *exhibere*, to display]. 1. One with an abnormal desire to attract attention. 2. One who yields to an impulse to expose the genitals to the view of one of the opposite sex.

exhilarant (eks-ĭl'ă-rant) [L. *exhilāre*, to gladden]. That which is mentally stimulating.

exhuma'tion [L. *ex*, out, + *humus*, earth]. Removal of the dead body from the grave after it has been buried.

exitus (ex'ĭ-tus) [L. exit]. Death.

Ex'ner's nerve [Sigmund Exner, Austrian physiologist, 1846-1926]. One from the pharyngeal plexus to the cricothyroid membranes.

E. plexus. A plexus of nerve fibers forming a layer near the surface of the cerebral cortex.

exo- [G.]. Prefix: Without; outside of.

exocar'dia [G. *exō*, out, + *kardia*, heart]. Congenitally abnormal position of the heart.

exocar'dial [" + *kardia*, heart]. Occurring outside of the heart.

exocataphoria (eks-o-kat-ă-for'ĭ-ă) [" + *kata*, down, + *pherein*, to bear]. A downward and outward turning of the visual axes.

exocoli'tis [" + *kōlon*, colon, + *ītis*, inflammation]. Inflammation of the peritoneal coat of the colon.

exocrine (eks'o-krēn, -krin) [" + *krinein*, to separate]. 1. The external secretion of a gland, opp. of endocrine. 2. Term applied to glands whose secretion reaches an epithelial surface either directly or through a duct.

exodic (eks-od'ik) [" + *odos*, way]. Efferent, centrifugal. Transmitting impressions outward from the central nervous system.

exodontia (eks-o-don'shĭ-ă) [" + *odous*, *odont-*, tooth]. 1. Extraction of a tooth. 2. Protrusion of teeth forward.

exodontol'ogy [" + " + *logos*, science]. Branch of dentistry concerned with extraction of teeth.

exoen'zyme [" + *en*, in, + *zymē*, leaven]. One that does not function within the cells from which it is secreted.

exogamy (eks-og'ă-mĭ) [" + *gamos*, marriage]. 1. Marriage outside of same family; outbreeding. 2. BIOL: Conjugation bet. gametes of different ancestry, as in some protozoans. SEE: *heterosexuality.*

exogastri'tis [" + *gastēr*, belly, + *ītis*, inflammation]. Inflammation of the peritoneal coat of stomach.

exogenous (eks-oj'ĕ-nus) [" + *gennan*, to produce]. Originating outside an organ or part.

exohemophylaxis (eks"o-hem"o-fi-laks'is) [" + *aima*, blood, + *phylaxis*, protection]. Injection of one's own blood mingled with arsphenamine.

exohysteropexy (eks-o-his-ter-o-peks'sĭ) [" + *ystera*, uterus, + *pēxis*, fixation]. Fixation of the uterus by implanting the fundus into the abdominal wall.

exometritis (eks-o-me-tri'tis) [" + *mētra*, womb, + *ītis*, inflammation]. Inflammation of the peritoneal coat of the uterus.

exomphalos (eks-om'fă-lus) [G. *ex*, out, + *omphalos*, navel]. 1. Umbilical protrusion. 2. Umbilical hernia. Syn: *exumbilication*.

exopath'ic [G. *exō*, out, + *pathos*, disease]. Pert. to a disease originating outside of the body.

exophoria (eks-o-fo'rĭ-ă) [" + *pherein*, to bear]. Ophth: Tendency of visual axes to diverge outward. See: *esophoria*.

exophthalmia (eks"of-thal'mĭ-ă) [G. *ex*, out, + *ophthalmos*, eye]. Abnormal protrusion of the eyeball. Syn: *exophthalmos*.

e. cachectica. Exophthalmic goiter.

e. fungosa. Late stage of glioma retinae.

exophthalmic (eks-of-thal'mik) [" + *ophthalmos*, eye]. Pert. to protrusion of the eyeball.

e. goiter. A condition marked by protrusion of the eyeballs, increased heart action, enlargement of the thyroid gland, weight loss, nervousness. Syn: *Graves' disease; Parry's disease; Basedow's disease.*

exophthal'mos, exophthal'mus [" + *ophthalmos*, eye]. Abnormal protrusion of eyeball. May be due to thyrotoxicosis, tumor of the orbit, orbital cellulitis, leukemia, or aneurysm.

e., pulsating. E. accompanied by pulsation and bruit due to an aneurysm behind the eye.

exophylac'tic [G. *exō*, out, + *phylaxis*, guarding]. Pert. to exophylaxis.

ex"ophylax'is [" + *phylaxis*, guarding]. Protection from disease originating outside the body, as by the skin.

ex'oplasm [" + *plasma*, matter]. Outer protoplasm of a cell. Syn: *ectoplasm.*

exorbitism (eks-or'bĭ-tizm) [L. *ex*, out, + *orbita*, eye]. Protrusion of eyeball. Syn: *exophthalmos.*

exormia (eks-or'mĭ-ă) [G. *ex*, out, + *ormē*, rash]. Any papular skin disease.

exosep'sis [G. *exō*, out, + *sēpsis*, decay]. Septic poison of external origin.

exoserosis (eks-o-ser-o'sis) [L. *ex*, out, + *serum*, whey, + G. *ōsis*]. An oozing of serum or discharging of an exudate.

exoskel'eton [G. *exō*, out, + *skeleton*, skeleton]. 1. The hard outer covering of certain invertebrates such as the molluscs and arthropods. Composed of chitin or calcareous material or both. 2. In vertebrates, the hard outer covering such as the shell of a turtle, or more specifically, the hard parts of the body surface derived principally from the ectoderm. These include such structures as hair, hooves, horns, nails, feathers, scales, etc.

exosmo'sis [G. *ex*, out, + *ōsmos*, a thrusting, + *ōsis*]. Diffusion of a fluid from within outward, as from a blood vessel.

exosplenopexy (eks-o-sple'no-peks-ĭ) [G. *exō*, out, + *splēn*, spleen, + *pēxis*, fixation]. Suturing the spleen to opening in the abdominal wall.

exostosis (eks-os-tō'sis) [G. *ex*, out, + *osteon*, bone]. A bony growth which arises from the surface of a bone, often involving the ossification of muscular attachments.

e. bursata. An e. arising from the epiphysis of a bone and covered with cartilage and a synovial sac.

e. cartilaginea. E. consisting of cartilage underlying the periosteum.

e., dental. E. on the root of a tooth.

e., multiple osteocartilaginous. A disorder of growth characterized by the development of multiple exostoses, usually located on the diaphyses of long bones near the epiphyseal lines. Results in irregularities of growth of the epiphyses and often times secondary deformities. Syn: *dyschondroplasia, q.v.*

Etiol: Unknown; tends to be hereditary occurring more frequently in males than females.

exoter'ic [G. *exōterikos*, outer]. Pert. to causes developing outside the body. Syn: *exopathic.*

exother'mal, exother'mic [G. *exō*, out, + *thermē*, heat]. Chemical reaction with production of heat.

exothy'mopexy [" + *thymos*, thymus, + *pēxis*, fixation]. Suturing of an enlarged thymus gland to the sternum.

exothyreopexy (eks-o-thi're-o-peks-ĭ) [" + *thyreos*, shield, + *pēxis*, fixation]. Exothyropexy.

exothy'ropexy [" + " + *pēxis*, fixation]. Suture of the thyroid and external fixation to induce atrophy. Syn: *exothyreopexy.*

exotic (ex-ot'ik) [G. *exotikos*, foreign]. Originating in a foreign country.

exotoxin (eks-o-toks'ĭn) [" + *toxikon*, poison]. A toxin produced by a microorganism and excreted into its surrounding medium. It can usually be recovered from the liquid medium in which the toxin-producing organisms have developed. Exotoxins are usually unstable being sensitive to the effects of chemicals, light, and heat. Exotoxins are produced by the diphtheria and tetanus organisms.

The exotoxins differ with regard to the particular tissues of the host that may be affected.

RS: *cytotoxin, endotoxin, erythrotoxin, leukocidin, leukotoxin, neurotoxin.*

exotro'pia [" + *tropē*, a turning]. Divergent strabismus; abnormal turning of one or both eyes outward.

expansion (eks-pan'shun) [L. *expandere*, to spread out]. Increase of volume; spreading out.

e., coefficient of. Increase in length or in volume when temperature is raised 1° C. from zero.

e., muscle. Degree a muscle may be stretched by an attached weight.

expansive delusion. Belief in one's power and wealth, accompanied by a feeling of well-being. See: *megalomania.*

expec'tant [L. *ex*, out, + *spectāre*, to watch]. Waiting.

e. treatment. Treatment of symptoms as they arise.

expecta'tion. Hoping, anticipation.

e. of life. Probable duration of life after a given age.

expec'torant [L. *ex*, out, + *pectus, pector-*, breast]. An agent that facilitates the removal of the secretions of the bronchopulmonary mucous membrane.

Expectorants are sometimes classed as *sedative* expectorants and *stimulating* expectorants.

Ex: *Ammonium carbonate, ammonium chloride, ipecac.*

expectoration (eks-pek'to-ra'shun) [" + *pectus, pector-*, breast]. Expulsion of mucus or phlegm from the throat or lungs.

May be mucous, mucopurulent, serous, or frothy.

It is viscid and tenacious in *pneumonia,* sticks to anything, and is rusty in appearance. It is frothy, often streaked with blood, and greenish-yellow in character from pus in *bronchitis.* In *tuberculosis* it varies from small amt. of frothy fluid to abundant greenish-yellow, offensive sputum often streaked with blood.

SEE: *anabole, anacatharsis, apophlegmatic, sputum, vomica.*

expel' [L. *expellere,* to drive out]. To drive out.

experiment (ex-per'ĭ-ment). The scientific procedure used to test the validity of a hypothesis; or to gain further evidence or knowledge.

e., controlled. One wherein part of a group of similar entities, animals, or human beings is tested or treated; the others do not receive the test or treatment.

expira'tion [L. *ex,* out, + *spirāre,* to breathe]. The expulsion of air from the lungs in breathing. Its sound is the shortest breath sound heard.

Any longer sound will be pathological. In emphysema it is longer than the inspiration.

Muscles used in expiration are the *int. intercostal muscles, m. rectus abdominis, m. transversus abdominis,* the *triangularis sterni* and possibly the *iliocostalis, serratus post. inf.,* and *quadratus lumborum.* SEE: *inspiration; respiration.*

e., active. Expiration accomplished as a result of muscular activity, as in forced respiration. The muscles used in respiration are: the muscles of the abdominal wall (ext. and int. oblique, rectus, and transverse abdominus); the internal intercostals, serratus posticus inferior, and quadratus lumborum.

e., passive. E. during quiet respiration in which no muscular effort is required. It is brought about by the elasticity of the lung, recoil of the elastic tissues of the chest, such as the costal cartilages, and the weight of the thoracic wall.

expiratory (eks-pi'ră-tor-ĭ) [" + *spirāre,* to breathe]. Pert. to expiration.

e. center. The part of the respiratory center in the medulla controlling e. movements.

expire. 1. To breathe out or exhale. 2. To die.

explant' [" + *planta,* sprout]. To remove a piece of living tissue from the body and transfer to an artificial culture medium for growth as in tissue culture. Opp. of implantation, *q.v.*

explora'tion [L. *explorāre,* to search out]. Examination by various means of an organ or part.

explo'ratory [L. *explorāre,* to search out]. Pert. to an exploration.

explorer. An instrument used in diagnosis.

explo'sive speech. Sudden and explosive utterance. SEE: *speech.*

express' [L. *expressus,* from *expremere,* to press out]. To squeeze out.

expres'sion [L. *expressus,* from *expremere,* to press out]. 1. Expelling anything by pressure. 2. Facial disclosure of feeling or emotion. SYN: *facies.* SEE: *face.*

expul'sive [L. *ex,* out, + *pellere,* to drive]. Having a tendency to expel.

e. pains. Labor pains which are effective, contracting the uterine muscle.

exsanguinate (eks-san'gwin-āt) [" + *sanguis,* blood]. 1. To deprive of blood. 2. Bloodless.

exsanguination (eks-san-gwin-a'shun) [" + *sanguis,* blood]. The process of expressing blood from a part.

exsanguine (ek-san'gwin) [" + *sanguis,* blood]. Anemic; bloodless.

exsec'tion [" + *secāre,* to cut]. Excision.

exsiccant (ek-sik'ant) [" + *siccāre,* to dry]. 1. Absorbing or drying up a discharge. 2. An agent that absorbs moisture. 3. A dusting or drying powder.

exsicca'tion [" + *siccāre,* to dry]. The act of drying by heat. SYN: *desiccation.*

exsic'cative [" + *siccāre,* to dry]. Causing to dry up or that which dries. SYN: *desiccative.*

exso'matize [G. *ex,* out, + *sōma,* body]. To remove from the body.

exstrophy (eks'trof-ĭ) [" + *strephein,* to turn]. Eversion; turning inside out of a part.

e. of the bladder. A congenital malformation in which the lower portion of the abdominal wall and anterior wall of the bladder are lacking and the bladder is everted through the opening; *ectopia vesicae.*

exsufflation (ex"sŭ-fla'shun) [" + *sufflare,* to blow]. Forceful expulsion of air from the lungs either by natural means or by use of a mechanical exsufflator.

ext. Abbr. of L. *extractum,* extract.

extempora'neous [L. *extemporaneus,* without time]. Not prepared according to formula but devised for the occasion.

e. mixture. A preparation to be taken at once because of tendency to deteriorate.

extension (eks-ten'shun) [L. *extendere,* to stretch out]. 1. The movement by which both ends of any part are pulled asunder. A movement which brings the members of a limb into or toward a straight condition. 2. The opposite of flexion. 3. The application of a pull (traction) to a fractured or dislocated limb.

e., Buck's. A method of producing traction by applying adhesive tape or moleskin to the skin and keeping it in smooth close contact by means of circular bandaging of the part to which it is applied. The adhesive strips are placed longitudinal to the member, the superior ends being about 1 in. from fracture site. Weights sufficient to produce the required extension are fastened to the inferior end of the adhesive strips, by means of a rope which is run over a pulley to permit of free motion.

exten'sor [L. *extendere,* to stretch out] A muscle that extends a part.

exte'rior [L.]. Outside of; external.

exte'riorize. 1. In surg. to temporarily expose a part; marsupialization, *q.v.* 2. In psych. the process of turning one's interests outward.

extern(e (ek'sturn) [L. *externus,* outside] A medical student living outside of a hospital who assists in the medical and surgical care of patients. SEE: *intern.*

external [L. *externus,* outside]. Exterior; lateral; opp. of medial or internal.

externa'lia [L. *externus,* outside]. External genitalia.

exteroceptive (eks″ter-o-sep′tiv) [″ + *ceptus,* from *capere,* to take]. Pert. to end organs receiving impressions from without.

exteroceptor (eks-ter-o-sep′tor) [″ + *ceptus,* from *capere,* to take]. A sense organ, as the eye, adapted for the reception of stimuli from outside the body.

exterofec′tive [″ + *facere,* to make]. Pertaining to responses to stimuli mediated by the central nervous system and somatic nerves in contrast to those mediated through the autonomic nervous system.

ex′tima [L. outermost]. The outer layer of a blood vessel; the tunica adventitia.

extinction. 1. The process of extinguishing or putting out. 2. The complete inhibition of a conditioned reflex as a result of failure to reinforce it.

e. of mercury. Causing the disappearance of mercury by rubbing with lard or some other agent.

extirpation (eks-tir-pa′shun) [L. *extirpāre,* to root out]. Excision of a part; taking out by the roots.

extor′sion [L. *ex,* out, + *torquire,* to twist]. Rotation of an organ or limb outward.

extra- [L.]. Prefix: Outside of, in addition to.

extra-artic′ular [L. *extra,* outside, + *articulus,* joint]. Outside a joint.

ex′tract [L. *extractum,* from *extrahere,* to draw out]. 1. A solid or semisolid preparation made by extracting the soluble portion of a compound by using water or alcohol and evaporating the solution. 2. Active principle of a drug obtained by distillation or chemical processes.

e., alcoholic. One in which alcohol acts as the solvent.

e., aqueous. One in which water is the solvent.

e., aromatic fluid. E. made from an aromatic powder.

e., compound. E. prepared from more than one drug or substance.

e., ethereal. E. using ether as the vehicle.

e., fluid. One made into a solution from a vegetable drug, which contains medicinal components.

e., powdered. A crushed, dried extract.

e., soft. E. of the consistency of honey.

e., solid. E. made by evaporating the fluid part of a solution.

extrac′tion [L. *extractum,* a drawing out]. 1. Pulling out, as a tooth. 2. The removing of the active portion of a drug.

extract′or [L. *extractum,* a drawing out]. Instrument for removing foreign bodies. VARIETIES: Esophageal, throat, shot, tympanum, tissue, etc.

e., tissue. Needles, trocars or pointed instruments with a form of barb for extracting soft tissue for examination.

e., tube. Device for removing an intubation tube from trachea.

extrac′tum (ext.) [L. a drawing out]. Solid or semi-solid preparations produced by evaporating solutions of vegetable principles.

The official extracts are either powders or soft solids. The majority can be obtained in powdered form and many prefer them that way. Extracts are usually about five times the strength of the crude drug. SEE ALSO: *fluidextract.*

extracys′tic [L. *extra,* beyond, + G. *kystis,* bladder]. Outside of or unrelated to a bladder or cystic tumor.

extradu′ral [″ + *durus,* hard]. 1. On outer side of the dura mater. 2. Unconnected with the dura mater.

extragenital (eks-trā-jen′ĭ-tal) [″ + *genitalis,* genital]. Outside of or unrelated to the genital organs.

extrahep′atic [″ + G. *ēpar, ēpat-,* liver]. Outside of or unrelated to the liver.

extraligamen′tous [″ + *ligāre,* to bind]. Outside of or unrelated to a ligament.

extramalle′olus [″ + *malleōlus,* little hammer]. The external or lateral malleolus.

extramar′ginal [″ + *margō,* margin]. Pert. to subliminal consciousness.

extramastoiditis (eks-trā-mas-toy-dī′tis) [″ + G. *mastos,* breast, + *eidos,* form, + *-ītis,* inflammation]. Inflammation of outside tissues contiguous to the mastoid process.

extramedullary (eks″trā-med′u-la-rĭ) [″ + *medulla,* marrow]. Outside or unrelated to any medulla, esp. the m. oblongata.

extraneous (eks-tra′ne-us) [L. *extraneus,* external]. Outside and unrelated to an organism.

extranu′clear [L. *extra,* beyond, + *nucleus,* kernel]. Outside of a nucleus.

extrapo′lar [″ + *polus,* pole]. Outside instead of bet. poles, as the electrodes of a battery.

extrasensory. Pertaining to forms of perception not dependent upon the five primary senses; *e. g.,* thought transference.

e. perception. Perception, esp. of another person's thoughts or actions not received by use of the senses.

extrasys′tole [″ + G. *systellein,* to contract]. Premature contraction of the heart, which may be induced experimentally by stimulating the heart at any time except during the absolute refractory period. In humans it is the result of some factor that initiates an impulse in the impulse–conducting system. It may occur either in the presence or absence of organic heart disease. It may be of reflex origin being initiated by stimuli from almost any part of the body or it may be of central origin.

e., atrial. Premature contraction of the atrium at some point outside the S-A. node.

e., nodal. E. occurring as a result of the origin of an impulse in the A-V node.

e., ventricular. E. which occurs after the normal contraction of the ventricle has ceased. Usually followed by a long compensary pause.

extrau′terine [″ + *uterus,* womb]. Outside the uterus.

extravag′inal [″ + *vagina,* vagina]. Outside the vagina.

extravasate (eks-trav′ă-sāt) [″ + *vas,* vessel]. 1. To escape from a vessel into the tissues, said of serum, blood, or lymph. 2. Exudate so escaping.

extravasation (eks-trav″ă-sa′shun) [″ + *vas,* vessel]. The escape of fluids into the surrounding tissue.

extravas′cular [″ + *vasculum,* vessel]. Outside a vessel.

extraventric′ular [″ + *ventriculus,* little belly]. Outside of any ventricle, esp. one of the heart.

extrem′ital [L. *extrēmus,* last]. Pert. to an extremity. SYN: *distal.*

extrem′ity [L. *extrēmus,* last]. 1. The terminal part of anything. 2. An arm or leg. RS: *acanthokeratodermia, "acro-" words, dactyl, dactylus.*

e., lower. The lower limb, including the hip, thigh, leg, ankle, and foot.

e., upper. The upper limb, including the shoulder, arm, forearm, wrist and hand.

extrin'sic [L. *extrinsecus*, from *extra*, outside, + *secus*, otherwise]. From or coming from without.

e. muscles. Those partly attached to the trunk and partly to a limb.

extrospection (ex"tro-spek'shun) [L. *extra*, + *spectare*, to look]. Continual inspection by the patient of his skin for evidence of dirt. Caused by mysophobia, compulsive fear of dirt.

extroversion (eks-tro-ver'shun) [L. *extra*, out, + *vertere*, to turn]. 1. Eversion; turning inside out. 2. Psy: The direction of attention and energy outward from the self. See: *introversion*.

ex'trovert [" + *vertere*, to turn]. A personality-reaction type; one who is interested mainly in ext. objects and actions.

The extreme pathologic extrovert reaction is seen in manic depressive insanity. Opp: *introvert, q.v.*

extrude (eks-trūd') [L. *extrudere*, to squeeze out]. To push out of a normal position or situation.

extru'sion [L. *extrudere*, to squeeze out]. 1. Occupying an abnormal external position. 2. Position of a tooth pushed forward from line of occlusion.

extubation (eks-tu-ba'shun) [L. *ex*, out, + *tuba*, tube]. Removal of a tube, as the laryngeal tube.

exudate (eks'u-dāt) [" + *sudāre*, to sweat]. 1. Accumulation of a fluid in a cavity, or matter that penetrates through vessel walls into adjoining tissue, or the passing out of pus or serum, or the matter so passed.

They may be classified as *catarrhal, fibrinous, hemorrhagic, diphtheritic, purulent*, and *serous*, the fluids being different in various affections. A fibrinous exudate may wall off a cavity, resulting in adhesions following an operation, as in empyema* and appendicitis. Inflammatory processes tend to wall off the injured area to localize the inflammation and to prevent its spread. 2. An inflammatory product withdrawn through a membrane for exploratory purposes. See: *exudation, infection, inflammation, pus, resorption*.

exuda'tion [" + *sudāre*, to sweat]. Morbid oozing of fluids, usually the result of inflammatory conditions. See: *choroiditis; exudate*.

ex'udative [" + *sudāre*, to sweat]. Having the property of exudation.

exude' [" + *sudāre*, to sweat]. To pass off slowly through the tissues; said of a semisolid or fluid.

exumbilica'tion [" + *umbilicus*, navel]. Protrusion of navel. Syn: *exomphalos*.

exuviae (eks-u'vĭ-e) [L. *exuere*, to strip]. Cast-off parts, as desquamated epidermis; a slough.

eye [A.S. *ēáge*]. Organ of vision; composed of 3 coats: (a) *Retina*, sensory for light; (b) *uvea* (choroid, ciliary body, and iris), nutritional; (c) *sclera* and *cornea*, serve to protect delicate retina.

These layers enclose two cavities, the more anterior or *ocular chamber* being the space lying in front of the lens. It is divided by the *iris* into an *anterior chamber* and a *posterior chamber*, both of which are filled with a watery *aqueous humor*. The cavity behind the lens is much larger and filled with a jelly-like *vitreous body*. The lens is suspended behind the iris by the ciliary zonule. Anteriorly, the cornea is covered by the *conjunctiva* which con-

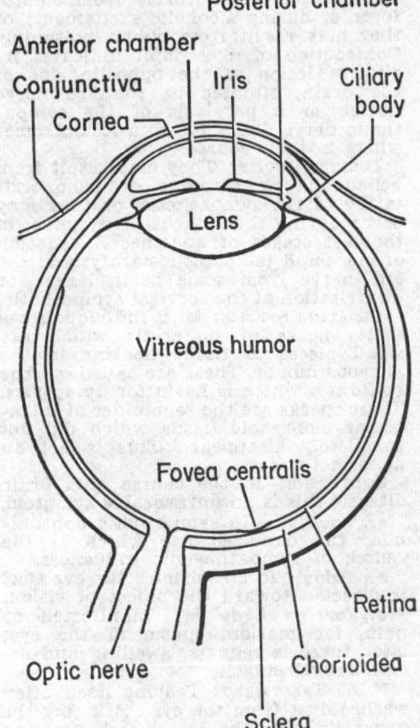

THE EYE

tinues and forms the inner layer of the eyelids.

e., aphakic. An eye from which the crystalline lens has been removed.

e., black. Ecchymosis of the tissues surrounding the eye.

e. closure reflex. Contraction of orbicularis palpebrarum with closure of lids resulting from percussion above supraorbital nerve. Syn: *McCarthy's reflex; supraorbital reflex*.

e., cold compresses: Purpose: (a) To relieve congestion of eyelids; (b) to control intraocular hemorrhage; (c) occasionally for conjunctivitis and early lid injuries to prevent hemorrhage into tissues.

Procedures: Scrub hands: (a) Wring compresses out of boric acid solution with forceps and place on ice to chill; (b) place over lids and extend over cheek; (c) change every 30 seconds. Each compress may be used over and over if there is no pus. When pus is present, may be used only once.

e., cross. Strabismus, *q.v.*

e., dark adapted. An eye which has become adjusted for viewing objects in dim light; one adapted for scotopic or rod vision. Depends upon the regeneration of a light sensitive substance, visual purple.

e., dominant. The eye which a person unconsciously gives preference to as a source of stimuli for visual sensations.

e., examinations and diagnosis. The diagnosis of disease which the physician makes from an examination depends largely upon symptoms manifested by the pupils of the eyes.

Contracted Pupils: They may denote irritative lesions of the 3rd nerve (in early stages of anesthesia from chloroform, or during alcoholic excitement) or they may result from opium poisoning. Contraction of *one* pupil indicates irritative lesion of the opposite side of the brain, situated at the 3rd nerve nuclei, or a paralysis of the sympathetic nerve fibers due to a lesion somewhere in their course.

DILATED PUPILS: They may result from belladonna or atropine or from irritating of the sympathetic, or they may occur during the attacks of dyspnea, in the last stages of anesthesia. Dilation of one pupil indicates a paralysis of the 3rd nerve from some brain lesion, or an irritation of the cervical sympathetic.

FLOATING SPECKS: Most individuals see little specks of materials which are small pieces of tissue floating in the vitreous humor. These are called *muscae volitantes* which is Latin for *flying flies.* These specks are the remainder of intraocular embryonic tissue which did not completely disappear. This is not an abnormal condition.

SQUINTING: In the course of a brain disease, this is an unfavorable symptom.

e., exciting. In sympathetic ophthalmia, the damaged eye which is the source of sympathogenic influences.

e., fixing. In strabismus, the eye that is directed toward the object of vision.

e., foreign body in. Manifested by pain, lacrimation, spasm of the eye; later there is redness, swelling and occasionally headache.

F. A. TREATMENT: Tearing itself often washes dust from the eye. Bringing the upper lid over the lower and directing patient to roll eye, often deposits dust on the margin of the lower lid.

Great care is necessary in removing larger particles, and should be done in a quiet place with excellent illumination and by using clean, preferably sterile, materials. Follow by instillation of 1 or 2 drops of a bland oil into the eye. A mild antiseptic, as 5%-10% mild silver proteinate, is desirable. If inflamed, use repeated hot compresses.

If for any reason patient cannot be taken care of at once, the eye should be bandaged to keep it closed and thus avoid scratching the lid. There should be no delay in having the speck removed, as serious injury to the eyeball or to the vision may result. The longer the foreign body remains in the eye the deeper it becomes embedded.

Infection may be carried into the eye, resulting in an ulcer of the cornea. Metal produces a chemical effect, as it disintegrates, which affects the eyeball. The x-ray is sometimes used to detect any tiny particles of metal, and the electromagnet to remove them. Sympathetic ophthalmia,* the transference of inflammation from an injury to the normal eye, may be produced by wounds which pierce the eyeball. Loss of vision in both eyes may result.

e., hare's. Lagophthalmos; condition in which the eye cannot be completely closed.

e., hot compresses: PURPOSE: (a) To increase the blood supply to the eyelids and eyeballs; (b) to relieve pain.

PROCEDURES: Scrub hands: (a) Apply petroleum jelly with clean swab to area to which compresses are to be applied; (b) wring compresses dry with forceps and test on wrist and apply as hot as patient can tolerate; (c) to increase blood supply to eyelids, place compresses over lids and extend over cheek; to increase blood supply to eyeballs, place compresses over lids and extend over brow; (d) use new compresses for each application if pus is present; (e) when last compress is removed, dry the eyelid.

e., light adapted. An eye that has become adjusted to viewing objects in bright light; one adapted for photopic or cone vision. One in which visual purple has been bleached.

e. muscles. Movements of the eye ball are brought about by six muscles: the superior, inferior, medial and external rectus muscles and the superior and inferior oblique muscles.

e., nerve supply of. 2nd. or optic nerve; *eye muscles,* 3rd. or oculomotor, 4th. or trochlear, and 6th. or abducens; *lid muscles,* facial to orbicularis oculi and oculomotor to levator palpebrae. Sensory fibers to orbit furnished by ophthalmic and maxillary fibers of the 5th or trigeminal. Sympathetic postganglionic fibers are derived from the carotid plexus, their cell bodies lying in the superior cervical ganglion. They supply the dilator muscle of the iris, lacrimal gland, and smooth muscle fibers in the eyelid; parasympathetic, fibers from the ciliary ganglion pass to the ciliary muscle and constrictor muscles of the iris.

e., pink. Acute epidemic conjunctivitis.

e., refracting media of. Aqueous humor, lens, and vitreous body.

e., refracting surfaces of. Cornea and anterior and post. surfaces of the lens.

e., squint. Strabismus, *q.v.*

e., squinting. The eye affected in strabismus.

e., sympathizing. In sympathetic ophthalmia, the uninjured eye which responds to sympathogenic influences.

e. vision. Light entering the eye passes through the cornea, then through the *pupil,* an opening in the iris, and on through the crystalline lens and the vitreous body to the retina. The aqueous humor, lens and vitreous body constitute the refracting media of the eye. Through changes in the curvature of the lens brought about by its elasticity and contraction of the ciliary muscles, light rays are focused on the retina where they stimulate the rods and cones, the sensory receptors. The cones are concerned with color vision; rods with vision in dim light. Sensory impulses are conveyed over the optic nerve to the brain where, in the visual area of the cerebral cortex located in the occipital lobe, they register as visual sensations. The amount of light entering the eye is regulated by the pupil, its size being controlled by the dilator and constrictor muscles of the iris.

e., watery. Epiphora; abnormal secretion of tears.

eyeball [A.S. *ēage* + M. E. *bal*]. The body of the eye.

It has 3 humors: Aqueous, lens or crystalline, and vitreous. Tension and position in relation to orbit should be noted.

PATH: *Exophthalmos,* or protrusion. If bilateral may be due to goiter. Eyeball may appear to protrude in fright, asthma, and spasmodic croup. It is noted in thrombosis of sup. longitudinal sinus, cardiac atrophy, laryngeal stenosis and paralysis of ocular movements. One or both may be affected due to hemorrhage in orbit, to aneurysm, exostosis, or tumor of orbit, or enlarged lacrimal glands. *Enophthalmos*: Bilateral or unilateral recession of eyeball.

eye'brow [A.S. *ēáge*, eye, + *braew*, brow]. The arch over the eye; also its covering, esp. the hairs.

eye'cup. 1. The optic vesicle, evagination of the embryonic brain from which the retina develops. 2. A small cup which fits over the eye and used for bathing the surface of the eye.

eye'glass. A glass lens used to aid the defective eye in seeing.

eye'ground [A.S. *ēáge* + *grund*, earth]. Fundus of eye, seen with ophthalmoscope.

eye'lash [" + *lasche*, a thin whip]. Cilium.* A stiff hair on the margin of the eyelid. SEE: *capsulociliary; "cili-" words; phalangosis; trichiasis.*

eye'lid (*palpebra*) [" + *hlīdan*, to cover]. One of two movable protective folds which when closed, cover the anterior surface of the eyeball. They are separated by the *palpebral fissure.* The upper (palpebrae superior) is the larger and more movable. It is raised by contraction of the levator palpebral superioris muscle. Angles formed by the lids at inner and outer ends are known as the *canthi.* The *cilia*, or eyelashes, are attached. The post, surface is lined by the *conjunctiva*, a mucous membrane.

e. *dropping*. Ptosis.

e., *fused*. A congenital anomaly resulting from failure of the fetal eyelids to separate.

eyestrain. Tiredness of the eye due to overuse or uncorrected defect. SYN: *asthenopia.*

eyetooth. A cuspid or upper canine tooth.

eye worm, African. *Loa Loa*, a genus of nematode which frequently infests the eye.

Notes

F

F. 1. Abbr. for *Fahrenheit, field of vision, formula, Fusiformis.* 2. Chem. symbol for *fluorine.*

F₁. In genetics the first filial generation, the offspring of a cross between two unlike individuals.

F₂. The second filial generation or the offspring of a cross between two individuals of the F₁ generation.

FA.; F.A. Abbr. for *fatty acid; filterable agent; first aid; fluorescent antibody; fortified aqueous.*

fabel'la [L. little bean]. Fibrocartilages or bones which sometimes develop in the head of the gastrocnemius muscle.

fabrication (fab-rĭ-kā'shun) [L. *fabricāre,* to forge]. Stating that which is not true, seen in Korsakow's syndrome.

F. A. C. D. Abbr. for *Fellow of the American College of Dentists.*

face [L. *facies*]. Anterior part of the head from forehead to chin and extending laterally to but not including the ears; the visage or countenance.

Anat: *Arteries of Face and Head:* Left common carotid with ext. and int. branches. Right common carotid with ext. and int. branches and circle of Willis. *Bones of:* The face has 14 bones. See: *skeleton. Veins of Face and Neck:* Ext. and int. jugular.

Coloring: *Brownish-yellow spots:* Liver spots. Seen in pregnancy, malignancies of liver or uterus, and in exophthalmic goiter. Cosmetics and facial irritants, sunburn and exposure to weather also factors. Occur in many diseases including Addison's disease, diabetes, hemochromatosis, pellagra, acanthosis nigricans, and others. Also occurs in arsenic poisoning.

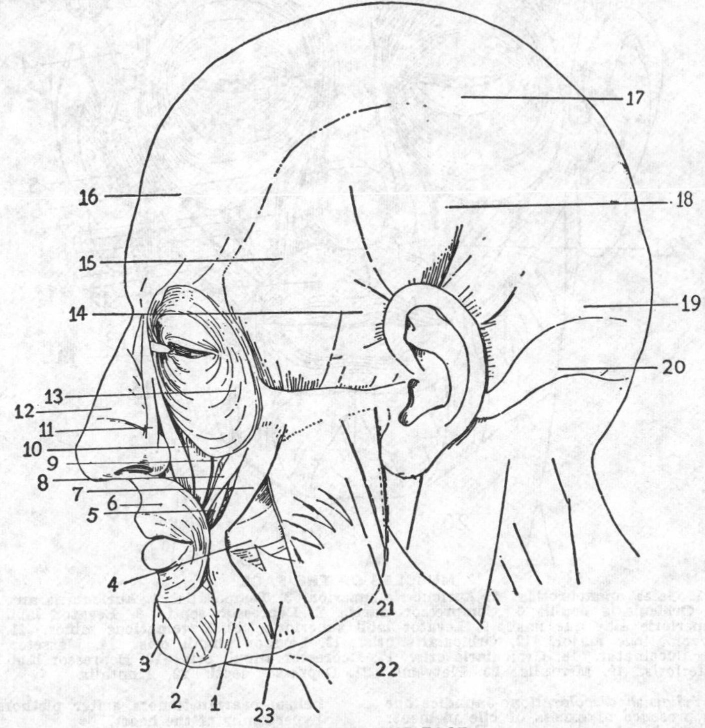

MUSCLES OF THE FACE

1. Depressor anguli oris. 2. Depressor labii inferioris. 3. Mentalis. 4. Buccinator. 5. Levator anguli oris. 6. Orbicularis oris. 7. Zygomaticus major. 8. Zygomaticus minor. 9. Depressor septi. 10. Levator labii superioris. 11. Levator labii superioris alae que nasi. 12. Compressor naris. 13. Orbicularis oculi. 14. Auricularis anterior. 15. Temporalis. 16. Frontalis. 17. Galea aponeurotica. 18. Auricularis superior. 19. Auricularis posterior. 20. Occipitalis. 21. Masseter. 22. Platysma. 23. Risorius.

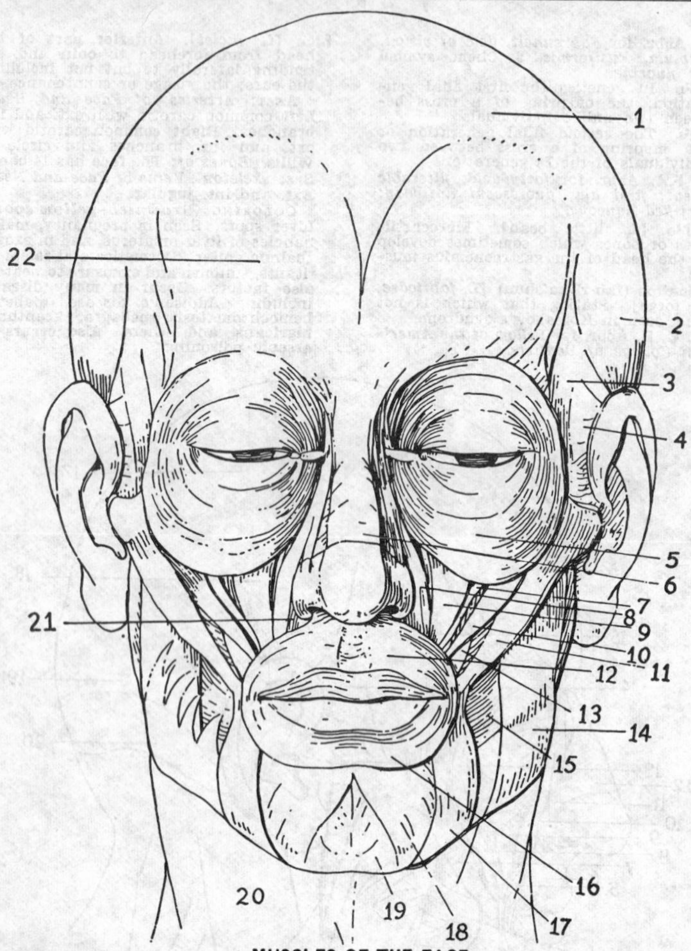

MUSCLES OF THE FACE

1. Galea aponeurotica. 2. Auricularis superior. 3. Temporalis. 4. Auricularis ant. 5. Orbicularis oculi. 6. Compressor naris. 7. Depressor septi. 8. Levator labii superioris alae que nasi. 9. Levator labii superioris. 10. Zygomaticus minor. 11. Zygomaticus major. 12. Orbicularis oris. 13. Levator anguli oris. 14. Masseter. 15. Buccinator. 16. Orbicularis oris. 17. Depressor anguli oris. 18. Depressor labii inferioris. 19. Mentalis. 20. Platysma. 21. Depressor septi. 22. Frontalis.

Yellowish discoloration: Jaundice due to presence of excess of bile pigments in the blood.

Cyanosis: Deficient oxygenation of the blood which may be due to acquired or congenital malformations of the heart, to asthma, whooping cough, pulmonary tuberculosis, croup, obstruction of trachea, aneurysm, tumor, asphyxia, drug poisoning, emphysema, dilation of right side of the heart. SEE: *cyanosis.*

Flushing (hyperemia): May be permanent or evanescent. Produced by the emotions if temporary. Permanent flushing may be due to febrile diseases, pulmonary tuberculosis, convulsions, alcoholism, ovarian tumors, goiter, plethora, hypertrophy of the heart.

Pallor: Absence of color. May be due to excessive confinement indoors, malnourishment, anemia, hemorrhage, shock, fright.

Redness, alternating with pallor: Emotion such as anger, cerebrospinal meningitis, typhoid, menopause, and general vasomotor disturbances.

Sallowness: Cachexia, cancer, lead poisoning, chronic gallbladder disease, some anemias, Addison's disease, arthritis deformans, constipation, hepatic, pancreatic, and enteric diseases.

DIAGNOSIS BY: The following conditions affect the features: Mouth breathing, chronic alcoholism, drug habits, abdominal diseases, facial hemiplegia, cretinism, myxedema, congenital syphilis, exophthalmic goiter, myopathic and myasthenic conditions, paralysis agitans, encephalitis lethargica, locomotor ataxia, acromegaly, mongolian idiocy, acute diffuse peritonitis, dyspnea, hysteria, late stages of pulmonary tuberculosis, lobar pneumonia, renal diseases, typhoid fever, hippocratic facies.

EDEMA: Swelling of the face from edema is noted in cardiac, renal, and blood diseases, pneumothorax, mediastinal tumors, and aneurysm. It may be localized and evanescent due to urticaria, angioneurotic edema, or anaphylaxis. Seen in thrombosis of sup. longitudinal sinus.

EXPRESSION: *Absence of expression from half the face downward, drawn and distorted*: Indicates facial paralysis of opposite side. *Anxious or pinched look*: Forerunner of unfavorable conditions. *Hippocratic facies*: A cadaverous appearance seen in cholera and acute general peritonitis. *Risus sardonicus*: A sardonic smile caused by contraction of mouth muscles which indicates abdominal affections, such as spasms and peritonitis. *Sudden lack of expression*: Apathy and immobility, generally bad symptoms, except in mental weakness and hysteria.

f., moon. Full, round face, seen in Cushing's syndrome. May also be a side effect of corticosteroid therapy.

f. presentation. Fetal face presentation in childbirth.

f., spasms of. May be intermittent, continuous, bilateral or unilateral.

May be due to teeth, disorders of skin, nose, eyes, or constitutional nervous disorders. May be *mimic* or *habit* spasms; choreic, winking spasms, convulsive tic, blepharospasm. Closure of eyelids caused by spasm of orbicular muscles, due to affection of the nerve supply, the eye muscles, or to eye diseases. Clonic unilateral spasm due to epilepsy. Spasm of eyelids, chin, upper lips, or muscles of face seen in early stages of meningitis. Tonic spasms due to tetanus, spasms following paralysis, hysteria, and tic douloureux.

facet, facette (fas'et) [Fr. *facette*, small face]. A small, smooth area on a bone or other hard surface.

fa'cial [L. *facies*, face]. Pert. to the face.

f. center. Brain center causing facial movements.

f. nerve. Seventh cranial nerve, a mixed nerve consisting of efferent fibers supplying the facial muscles, the platysma muscle, the submaxillary and sublingual glands; afferent fibers from taste buds of the ant. two thirds of the tongue and from the muscles. *Orig.* afferent fibers from geniculate ganglion; motor and secretory fibers from nuclei in pons. DIS: Ear, face, palate, tongue. BR: Tympanic, chorda tympani, post. auricular, digastric, stylohyoid, temporal, malar, infraorbital, buccal, supramaxillary, inframaxillary. SYN: *nervus facialis* [NA]. SEE: *cranial nerves.*

f. paralysis. Affecting the muscles of the face. The 7th cranial nerve is involved.

f. reflex. Contraction of facial muscles following pressure on eyeball.

f. spasm. Tic. SEE: *cranial nerves; face, spasms of.*

facies (fa'shĭ-ēz) (pl. *facies*) [L.]. 1. Face. 2. [NA] Surface.

f. abdomina'lis. Pinched, anxious, shrunken and drawn expression seen in abdominal troubles.

f., adenoid. Stupid appearance with open mouth.

f. aor'tica. Expression seen in aortic valve insufficiency, bluish sclera, cheeks sunken, face sallow.

f. hepat'ica. Seen in liver affections: Skin sallow, conjunctivae yellow, and eyeballs sunken.

f. hippocrat'ica. Seen in those dying from long continued illness or from cholera; cheeks and temples hollow, eyes sunken, complexion leaden, and lips relaxed.

f. leontina. Lion-like face seen in certain forms of leprosy.

f., mask-like. Expressionless face with little or no animation. Seen in parkinsonism.

f. mitra'lis. Seen in mitral insufficiency. Capillaries more or less visible, cheeks pink, more or less cyanosis.

f., myopath'ic. Due to muscular weakness, esp. that of the face, lids drop and lips protrude.

f. ovari'na. Seen in women with ovarian tumor; face drawn and pinched.

f., typhoid. Dusky complexion, injected conjunctivae and dull expression.

facilitation (fă-sil"ĭ-ta'shun) [L. *facilis*, easy]. Making an action or process easier, the energy of an impulse being added to that of other impulses activated at the same time.

fa'cing [L. *faciēs*, face]. An inlay to form the outer surface of a tooth.

faciobrachial (fa-shĭ-o-bra'kĭ-al) [" + G. *brachion*, arm]. Pert. to the face and arm, esp. to juvenile muscular dystrophy.

faciocephalalgia (fa"shĭ-o-sef"ă-lal'jĭ-ă) [" + *kephalē*, head, + *algia*]. Neuralgia of the face and head.

faciocer'vical [" + *cervix*, neck]. Pert. to the face and neck, esp. to progressive dystrophy of facial muscles.

faciolin'gual [" + *lingua*, tongue]. Pert. to the face and the tongue, esp. a paralysis of them.

fa'cioplasty [" + G. *plassein*, to form]. Plastic surgery of the face.

facioplegia (fa"sĭ-o-ple'jĭ-ă) [" + G. *plēgē*, stroke]. Facial paralysis. SYN: *prosopoplegia.*

facioscapulohumeral (fa"shĭ-o-skap"u-lo-hu'mer-al) [" + *scapula*, shoulder blade, + *humerus*, shoulder]. Pert. to the face, the scapula, and the upper arm.

F. A. C. P. Abbr. for *Fellow of the American College of Physicians.*

F. A. C. S. Abbr. for *Fellow of the American College of Surgeons.*

factitious (fak-tish'us) [L. *factitius*, made by art]. Something produced artificially.

f. fever. Fever produced artificially, usually by the patient in order to feign illness.

factor. A condition, element, influence, or circumstance that contributes to a result.

f., accessory food. A substance in food which does not serve as a source of energy but is essential for normal growth and development or normal metabolic activities; a vitamin, *q.v.*

f., antianemic. A substance stored in the liver, essential for the normal development of red blood cells in the bone marrow. It is formed in the stomach and intestine by the interaction of an *extrinsic factor,* vitamin B_{12}, and an *intrinsic factor* present in gastric juice. Also called *antianemic principle, hematinic principle, erythrocyte maturation factor (EMF).* It is used in the treatment of pernicious anemia.

f., hereditary. A gene.

f., lethal. A gene which, when homozygous, causes the death of an individual before development is complete.

f., milk. A substance present in certain strains of mice which is transferred to offspring through milk from the mammary glands, and is capable of inducing the development of mammary cancer.

f., Rh. SEE: *Rh blood factor.*

fac'ulta"tive [L. *facere,* to do]. BIOL: 1. Able to live under conditions of temperature or oxygen supply which vary 2. Able to do something not compulsory voluntary.

fac'ulty [L. *facultās,* function]. 1. A mental attribute or sense. 2. Ability to function.

f., affective. Capacity for expressing emotions.

f., germinative. Power of a germ to develop.

fagopyrism (fag-ō-pīr'izm, fag-op'ĭ-rizm) [L. *fagopyrum,* buckwheat]. Buckwheat poisoning.

Fahrenheit scale [Gabriel D. Fahrenheit, German physicist, 1686-1736]. The temperature scale used in the U.S.A. and England. The freezing point of water is 32° and the boiling point 212°. Indicated by F.

SEE: *thermometer.*

Fahrenheit and Centigrade Scales

F.	C.	F.	C.	F.	C.
500°	260°	248°	120°	95°	35°
401	205	239	115	86	30
392	200	230	110	77	25
383	195	212	100	68	20
374	190	203	95	50	10
356	180	194	90	41	5
347	175	176	80	32	0
338	170	167	75	23	—5
329	165	140	60	14	—10
320	160	122	50	+5	—15
311	155	113	45	—4	—20
302	150	105	40.54	—13	—25
284	140	104	40	—22	—30
275	135	100	37.8	—40	—40
266	130	98.5	36.9	—76	—60

1 deg. F. = .54° C.
1.8 " = 1° C.
3.6 " = 2° C.
4.5 " = 2.5° C.
5.4 " = 3° C.

faint [O.F. *faindre,* to feign]. 1. To feel weak, as though about to lose consciousness. 2. Weak. 3. Syncope. SEE: *fainting.*

fainting (fānt'ing) [O.F. *faindre,* to feign]. Loss of consciousness due to cerebral anemia or insufficient blood to the brain.

SYM: Prior to onset, patient may be pale, weak, dizzy, have cold perspiration, uncomfortable abdominal sensation, and may fall on the ground unconscious. Pulse is usually weak, rapid, often irregular.

F. A. TREATMENT: If patient is sitting, lower head between the knees, or preferably have patient lie down with the head lower than the body. Elevate lower extremities. Rub extremities toward the heart. Stimulate by administering spirits of ammonia to the nostrils at intervals. When able to swallow, give hot black coffee, strong tea, or other hot drinks.

Twenty drops of aromatic spirits of ammonia in hot water may be given by mouth.

RS: *apoplexy, asphyxia, coma, shock, swoon, syncope, unconsciousness.*

faint'ness [O.F. *faindre,* to feign]. 1. A sensation of impending loss of consciousness. 2. A sensation due to lack of food. SEE: *lipothymia.*

falcate (fal'kāt) [L. *falx,* sickle]. Sickle-shaped.

falcial (fal'shal) [L. *falx,* sickle]. Pert. to the falx.

falciform (fal'sĭ-form) [" + *forma,* form]. Sickle-shaped.

f. ligament. The triangular ligament attached to sides of the sacrum and coccyx by its base. SYN: *sacrotuberous ligament.*

f. l. of liver. That portion of the peritoneum reflected around the ligamentum teres, and attaching the upper surfaces of the liver to the diaphragm and abdominal wall. SYN: *ligamentum falciforme hepatis* [NA].

f. process. That portion of the f. ligament along the inner margin of the ramus of the ischium.

fal'cula [L. little sickle]. The falx cerebelli.

fal'cular [L. *falcula,* little sickle]. 1. Sickle-shaped. 2. Pertaining to the *falx cerebelli.*

fallec'tomy [G. *ektomē,* excision]. Cutting away part of the fallopian tube.

falling drop. 1. A metallic tinkle heard over the normal stomach and bowel when inflated. 2. The same sound heard over large cavities containing fluid and air, as observed in hydropneumothorax.

f. sickness. Epileptic condition.

f. of the womb. Dropping of the uterus, so that it protrudes into vagina. SYN: *descensus uteri.*

fallo'pian. Pert. to parts named for the Italian anatomist Fallopius.

f. canal. C. in petrous bone for *nervus facialis.*

f. ligament. Round ligament of the uterus.

f. tube. The tube or duct which extends laterally from the lateral angle of the uterus, terminating near the ovary. It serves to convey the ovum from the ovary to the uterus and spermatozoa from the uterus towards the ovary. Medially each tube opens into the uterus; distally each opens into the peritoneal cavity. Each lies in the superior border of the broad ligament. SYN: *oviduct; tuba uterina* [NA]; *uterine tube.*

BLOOD SUPPLY: Derived from branches of the uterine and ovarian arteries.

NERVE SUPPLY: Pelvic, ovarian, and uterine nerve plexuses send fibers to the tubes.

ANAT: The narrow region near the uterus, the isthmus, continues laterally as a wider *ampulla.* The latter expands to form the terminal funnel-shaped *infundibulum,* at the bottom of which lies a small opening, the *ostium,* through which the ovum enters the oviduct. Surrounding each ostium are a number of fingerlike processes called *fimbria,* one of which the *fimbria ovarica* is considerably longer than the others, extending towards and may be connected to the ovary. Each tube averages about 4½ in. in length and ¼ in. in diameter. Its wall consists of three layers: mucosa, muscular layer, and serosa. The epithelium of the mucosa consists of ciliated and non-ciliated cells. Ciliary action aids in the movement of the ovum towards the uterus. The muscular layer consists of an inner circular and an outer longitudinal layer of smooth muscle. The serosa consists of connective tissue underlying the outermost layer of peritoneum.

fallostomy (fal-os'to-mĭ) [G. *stoma,* opening]. Surgical opening of the fallopian tube. SYN: *salpingostomy.*

Fallot, tetralogy of [Etienne L. A. Fallot, French physician, 1850-1911]. A congenital condition characterized by defect in the interventricular septum, stenosis of the pulmonary artery, dextroposition of the aorta, and hypertrophy of the right ventricle. The defects are sometimes carried into adult life.

fallot'omy. Division of the fallopian tubes. SYN: *salpingotomy.**

fallout. Settling of radioactive fission products from the atmosphere after explosion of an atomic bomb.

false ribs. The lower 5 pairs of ribs. SEE: *ribs, vertebrae.*

falx [L.]. Any sickle-shaped structure.

f. cerebelli [NA]. A fold of the dura mater which forms a vertical partition between the hemispheres of the cerebellum.

f. cerebri [NA]. A fold of the dura mater which lies in the longitudinal fissure and separates the two cerebral hemispheres.

f. inguinalis [NA]. The conjoined or conjoint tendon which forms the origin of the transversus abdominis and internal oblique muscles.

f. ligamento'sa. The broad ligament of the liver. SYN: *falciform ligament of liver.*

famil'ial [L. *familiā,* family]. Pert. to or common to the same family, as *f. symptoms.*

family (fam'il-e) [L. *familiā,* family]. 1. A group consisting of parents and their children. 2. In biological classification, the division bet. the *order* and *genus.*

f., degenerate. One that produces offspring of low or subnormal mentality.

f., Jukes. A family whose history covers 5 generations of degeneracy.

f., Kallikak. An American family with one branch mentally unfit and another of average intelligence.

fam'ine fever. Relapsing fever.

F. and R., F & R. Abbr. for *force and rhythm* (of pulse).

fang [A.S. *fōn,* to seize]. 1. A sharp-pointed tooth. 2. The root of a tooth.

f.'s, poison. Two teeth in upper jaw of poisonous reptiles adjacent to their poison glands.

far'ad. A unit of electrical capacity. The capacity of a condenser which, charged with 1 coulomb, gives a difference of potential of 1 volt.

This unit is so large that one-millionth part of it has been adopted as a practical unit called a microfarad.

farad'ic. Pert. to induced electricity.

f. contrac'tion, graduated. Produced by Smart or Bristow coils.

far'adism. The therapeutic use of an interrupted current to stimulate muscles and nerves. Such a current is derived from the secondary or induction coil.

faradiza'tion. The treatment of nerves or muscles with the faradic current; the condition of nerves or muscles so treated.

faradother'apy [G. *therapeia,* treatment]. Treatment of disease by the faradic current.

far'cy [L. *farcire,* to stuff]. A form of glanders.

f. bud. A glanderous tumor.

f., button. Farcy marked by dermal tubercular nodules.

farina (fă-rī'nă) [L.]. Finely ground meal commonly made from wheat or other grain. Used as cereal and flour.

farina'ceous [L. *farina,* flour]. 1. Starchy. 2. Pert. to flour.

far-point. The farthest point of vision at which objects can be distinctly seen with eyes in complete relaxation.

Farre's tubercles (fars) [John R. Farre, British physician, 1775-1862]. Carcinomatous masses on surface of the liver.

far-sight'ed. Pert. to far-sightedness. SYN: *hypermetropic; hyperopic.*

far-sight'edness. An error of refraction in which, with accommodation completely relaxed, parallel rays come to a focus behind the retina. SYN: *hypermetropia; hyperopia.*

fascia (fash'ĭ-ă) (pl. *fasciae*) [L. a band]. 1. [NA]. A fibrous membrane covering, supporting, and separating muscles. It also unites the skin with underlying tissue. Fascia may be *superficial,* a nearly subcutaneous covering permitting free movement of the skin, or *deep,* enveloping and binding muscles. 2. A bandage.

f., Abernethy's. SEE: *Abernethy's fascia.*

f., anal. F. of connective tissue covering levator ani muscle from the perineal aspect.

f., Buck's. A fascial covering of the penis, derived from Colles' fascia.

f., cervical, deep. Fascia of the neck covering the muscles, vessels and nerves.

f., c., superficial. Fascia of the neck just inside the skin.

f., Cloquet's. Femoral fascia.

f., Colles'. Inner layer of the perineal fascia.

f., cremasteric. F. covering the cremaster muscle of the spermatic cord. SYN: *f. cremasterica* [NA].

f., cribriform. The fascia of the thigh covering the saphenous opening. SYN: *f. cribrosa* [NA].

f., dentate. Gray matter in the cerebral dentate convolution. SYN: *gyrus dentatus* [NA].

f., infundibuliform. Funnel-shaped f., derived from interior abdominal wall, encasing the spermatic cord and testis. SYN: *f. spermatica interna* [NA].

f., intercolumnar. F. derived from external abdominal ring sheathing the spermatic cord and testis.

f., ischiorectal. SEE: *anal f.*

f. lata [NA]. Wide covering encasing thigh muscles.

f., lumbodorsal. Deep investing membrane covering deep muscles of the trunk and back.

f., pectineal. Pubic section of f. lata.

f., pelvic. Fascial tissues of extreme importance in the maintenance of normal strength in the pelvic floor. SEE: *pelvic diaphragm under "diaphragm."*

f., thyrolaryngeal. F. covering thyroid gland.

f., transversalis. F. located between perineum and transversalis muscle; lines the abdominal cavity.

fasciae (fash'ĭ-ē). Plural of fascia.

fascial (fash'ĭ-al) [L. *fascia,* band]. Pert. to or of the nature of fascia.

f. reflex. Muscular contraction resulting from percussing facial fascia.

fasciaplasty (fash'ĭ-ă-plas"tĭ) [" + G. *plassein,* to form]. Plastic surgery of fascia.

fascicle (fas'ik-'l). A fasciculus.

fascicular (fas-sik'u-lar) [L. *fasciculus,* little bundle]. 1. Arranged like a bundle of rods. 2. Pert. to a fasciculus.

fasciculus (fa-sik'u-lus) (pl. *fasciculi*) [L. a little bundle]. A bundle of nerve or muscle fibers. More specifically a division of a funiculus of the spinal cord consisting of fibers of one or more tracts. Sometimes the term is used as a synonym for "tract." SYN: *fasciola.*

f. cuneatus [NA]. A triangular shaped bundle of nerve fibers lying in the dorsal funiculus of the spinal cord. Its fibers enter the cord through the dorsal roots of spinal nerves and terminate in the medulla. Also called tract of Burdach.

f., fundamental. Portion of ant. column of spinal cord continuing into medulla oblongata.

f. gracilis [NA]. A bundle of nerve fibers lying in the dorsal funiculus of the spinal cord medial to the f. cuneatus. Conducts sensory impulses from the periphery to the medulla.

f. longitudinal. *Inferior longitudinal fasciculus.* A bundle of association fibers connecting the occipital and temporal lobes of the brain; *medial longitudinal fasciculus,* a bundle of fibers running from the spinal cord to the upper portion of the midbrain; *dorsal longitudinal fasciculus,* a bundle of association fibers connecting the frontal lobe with the occipital and temporal lobes.

f., posterior longitudinal. Nerve fiber bundle running bet. corpora quadrigemina and nuclei of 4th and 6th nerves.

f. teres. Column on both sides of median furrow in floor of fourth ventricle.

f., unciform. Fibers within sylvian fissure connecting frontal and temporosphenoid lobes. SYN: *f. uncinatus* [NA]; *uncinate f.*

fasciectomy (fash"ĭ-ek'to-mĭ) [L. *fascia,* band, + G. *ektomē,* excision]. Excision of strips of fascia.

fasciod'esis [" + G. *desis,* binding]. Operation of attaching a fascia to a tendon or another fascia.

fasciola (fă-si'o-la) (pl. *fasciolae*) [L. little band]. A bundle of nerve or muscle fibers. SYN: *fasciculus, q.v.*

f. cinerea. Upper portion of dentate fascia.

Fasci'ola [L. *fascia,* band]. A genus of flukes belonging to the class Trematoda.

F. hepatica. A species of flukes infesting the liver and bile ducts of cattle, sheep, and other herbivores; the common liver fluke. An occasional parasite of man. Intermediate hosts are snails belonging to the genus *Limmeus.* Formerly called *Distomum hepaticum.*

fasci'olar [L. *fasciola,* little band]. Pert. to the fasciola cinerea.

fascioliasis (fash"ĭ-o-li'ă-sis) [L. *fascia,* band]. Infection of the body with a genus of trematode worms. SYN: *distomiasis.*

fas'cioplasty [" + G. *plassein,* to form]. Plastic operation on a fascia.

fasciorrhaphy (fash-ĭ-or'ă-fĭ) [" + *raphē,* suture]. Suturing a fascia.

fasciotomy (fash-ĭ-ot'o-mĭ) [" + G. *tomē,* incision]. Surgical incision and division of a fascia.

fascitis (fă-si'tis) [" + G. *itis,* inflammation]. Inflamed condition of a fascia.

fast [A.S. *faest,* fixed]. 1. Resistant to the effects or action of a chemical substance. 2. Fasting.

f., acid. Term applied to bacteria esp. the tuberculosis group which after staining are not decolorized when treated with acid.

f., drug. Term applied to bacteria or other organisms which become resistant to drugs such as penicillin.

fastidium (fas-tid'ĭ-um) [L. aversion]. Aversion to food or to eating.

Sometimes seen in hysteria but not as the result of delusions.

fastigatum (fas-tig-a'tum) [L. pointed]. The gray matter on both sides of the inf. vermiform process of the cerebellum. SYN: *nucleus fastigii.*

fastigium (fas-tij'ĭ-um) [L. ridge]. 1. The highest point. The full period of development of acute, infectious diseases when the temperature reaches the maximum or *stadium* and all symptoms have developed. 2. The most posterior portion of the 4th ventricle formed by the junction of the ant. and post. medullary vela projecting into the medullary substance of the cerebellum.

fast'ing [A.S. *faest,* firm]. Going without food for a stated period.

Energy requirements of body metabolism during fasting are supplied by the oxidization of fats which, if glucose is not supplied, results in the products of incomplete fat combustion, such as fatty acids, diacetic acid, and acetone, producing ketosis or a mild acidosis. This condition occurs quickly in children as they have little glycogen reserve.

fast'ness [A.S. *faest,* firm]. Resistance to stains or destructive agents.

fat. 1. Adipose, obese, corpulent. 2. Greasy, oily. 3. CHEM. A triglyceride ester of fatty acids; one of a group of organic compounds closely associated in nature with the phosphatides, cerebrosides, sterols. The term *lipids* or *lipides, q.v.,* is applied in general to fats or fatlike substances. Fats are insoluble in water but soluble in ether, chloroform, benzene and other fat solvents. Upon hydrolysis, fats break down into fatty acids and glycerol (an alcohol). Fats are hydrolyzed by the action of acids, alkalies, lipases (fat-splitting enzymes) and superheated steam.

Chem. structure. In the fat molecule, one molecule of glycerol is combined with three of fatty acids. Three fatty acids, oleic acid ($C_{18}H_{34}O_2$), stearic acid ($C_{18}H_{36}O_2$), and palmitic acid ($C_{18}H_{32}O_2$) comprise the bulk of the fatty acids present in the neutral fats found in body tissues. According to the fatty acid with which the glycerol is combined, corresponding fats are *triolein, tristearin,* and *tripalmitin.* These three fats are the principal fats present in foods.

Physiologic functions of: 1. Fats serve as a source of energy. 2. Subcutaneous fats form an insulating layer which prevents loss of heat. 3. Fat acts to support and protect certain organs such as the eye and kidney. 4. It provides a concentrated reserve of food. 5. It provides essential fatty acids necessary for normal growth and well-being. 6. It is a vehicle for natural fat-soluble vitamins. 7. In conjunction with carbohydrates, fats serve as protein sparers. 8. They are an important constituent of cell structure forming an integral part of the cell membrane. 9. When properly distributed, fat gives a pleasing contour to the body.

Digestion and absorption of fats. In the stomach, emulsified fats such as cream or egg yolk are acted on by gastric lipase; however, most fats undergo digestion in the intestine where they are acted on by a pancreatic lipase, *steapsin,* which hydrolyzes them to fatty acids and glycerol. Although containing no lipolytic enzymes bile is essential for the digestion of fats. Bile aids in the emulsification of fats and also has a hydrotropic action, *i. e.,* renders substances such as fatty acids, which are normally insoluble in water, readily soluble in the fluids of the intestine. Bile salts also act as specific activators of the pancreatic lipase. Bile salts react with fatty acids forming water-soluble, diffusible soaps which facilitate the emulsification of fats. Glycerol and fatty acids enter the epithelial cells where they recombine to form neutral fats most of which enter the lacteals. The fats are carried by the lymph through lymph vessels to the thoracic duct from which they enter the blood stream. After a meal rich in fats the mesenteric lymph vessels are filled with a milklike fluid, the *chyle,* containing finely emulsified fat particles, called *chylomicrons.*

Metabolism of fats. Absorbed fats are utilized in the following ways: (a) oxidized with the release of energy, (b) deposited in adipose tissue as storage fat, (c) incorporated in the cells of tissues as an integral part of the protoplasm, (d) desaturated and stored in the liver, (e) excreted in the secretions of the mammary and sweat glands, and in the feces.

Sources of body fats. In addition to fat being absorbed from the intestine, body fat may arise from the conversion of carbohydrates (glucose) or proteins into fat. Fat may possibly be converted into carbohydrates but this occurs only to a limited extent.

Intermediary metabolism of fats. In the oxidation of fat to carbon dioxide and water, several intermediary substances (ketones) are formed. The principal ones are acetoacetic acid, beta-hydroxybutyric acid, and acetone. Excessive production of ketone bodies which occurs when fats are incompletely oxidized is called ketosis. This especially occurs when there is an interference in carbohydrate metabolism, as in diabetes. Ketosis also occurs in certain fevers, in toxemias of pregnancy, and hyperthyroidism. Ketosis results in acidosis.

Fat nutrition. Fats have a high caloric value yielding 9.3 Cal. per gram. as compared with 4.0 and 4.1 Cal. for carbohydrates and proteins respectively. The average diet of 3000 Cal. should contain 30 to 40 per cent of its caloric value in fats. The average diet contains from 50 to 130 grams of fat. Quantities in excess of 150 grams are repulsive and difficult to digest. In addition to their nutritive values, fats improve the taste and odor of foods, provide a feeling of satiety, are absorbed slowly prolonging their nutritive effects, and because of their high caloric content, are of especial importance in high-caloric diets.

Contra. Fat intake should be reduced in diseases of the gallbladder and liver.

RS: *bile, gallbladder, liver, fatty acids, lipases, ketones, glycerol.*

f. depot. Accumulations of fat in certain regions of the body such as the buttocks or abdominal wall.

f., low-, diet. Approximately 40 to 50 gm. fat daily. SEE: *reduction diet.*

f., neutral. Compounds of the higher fatty acids (palmitic, stearic, and oleic) with glycerol. They are the common fats of animal and plant tissues.

f.- and protein-free diet. 1. Carbohydrates. 2. Honey. 3. Fruit juices. 4. Juicy fruits. 5. Melons. 6. Cucumbers. 7. Marmalades and jellies. 8. Rhubarb. 9. Fresh tomatoes.

f.-pad. The buccal pad of fat seen in cheeks of nursing infants.

f.-soluble. Soluble in fat as in the case of certain vitamins.

fat, *words pert. to:* absorption, acid, "adip-" words, calorie, chondrolipoma, chromolipoid, digestion, fatty acids, fuel value, hydrogenation, ketogenic diet, "lip-" words, obesity, palmitic acid, palmitin, stearin.

fatal (fa'tʹl) [L. *fatalis,* pre-ordained]. Inevitable. Causing death.

fatigue (fă-tēg') [L. *fatigare,* to tire]. 1. A feeling of tiredness or weariness resulting from continued activity. 2. The state or condition of an organ or tissue in which its response to stimulation is reduced or lost as a result of overactivity. 3. To bring about a condition of fatigue.

Fatigue may be the result of: (a) excessive activity which results in the accumulation of metabolic waste products such as lactic acid, (b) malnutrition (deficiency of carbohydrates, proteins, minerals, or vitamins), (c) circulatory disturbances such as heart disease or anemia which interfere with the supply of oxygen and energy materials to tissues, (d) respiratory disturbances which interfere with the supply of oxygen to tissues, (e) infectious diseases in which toxic products are produced or body metabolism altered, (f) endocrine disturbances such as occur in diabetes, hyperinsulinism, and menopause, (g) psychogenic factors such as emotional conflicts, frustration, worry, boredom, (h) physical factors such as incorrect posture, flat feet, (i) miscellaneous factors such as eye strain.

f., acute. Fatigue with sudden onset such as occurs following excessive exertion; relieved by rest.

f., chronic. Long-continued fatigue not relieved by rest. Indicative of disease such as tuberculosis or diabetes or other conditions of altered body metabolism.

f., muscular. The reduced capacity of a muscle to perform work as a result of repeated contractions. Fatigue may be partial or complete.

f. reaction. In tuberculosis, an elevation of temperature following exertion.

f. stance. Fatigue resulting from standing for long periods of time.

f. syndrome. Neurasthenia, *q.v.*

fatty. Of or pertaining to fats or fatty substances; adipose.

SEE: *fat; heart.*

f. acid. A hydrocarbon in which one of the hydrogen atoms has been replaced by a carboxyl (COCH) group; a monobasic aliphatic acid made up of an alkyl radical attached to a carboxyl group.

The saturated fatty acids include: acetic, butyric, caproic, caprylic, capric, lauric, formic, myristic, palmitic, and stearic acids all of which contain an even number of carbon atoms. All are homologues of formic acid.

The unsaturated fatty acids include: Those of (a) the *oleic series:* oleic, tiglic, hypogeic, palmitoleic, and physetoleic acids and (b) the *linoleic* or *linolic series:* linoleic, linolenic, clupanodonic, arachidonic, hydrocarpic, and chaulmoogric acids.

f. a., essential. The unsaturated fatty acids, *q.v.* In certain animals, the absence of these fatty acids in their diet leads to loss of weight, eczematous condition of the skin, and kidney disorders.

By boiling with alkalies, esp. in alcoholic solutions, also by the action of many ferments, as the steapsin of the pancreatic juice, fats are split up into glycerine and free fatty acids.

The fatty acids unite with the alkalies present, forming salts of fatty acids, the soaps (sodium soap, or hard soap, and potassium soap, or soft soap). If fats contain free fatty acid (rancid fats) they can, on melting, form an emulsion with water and a little soda; in this process of emulsion the fats are finely divided, forming a milky fluid.

As emulsification is dependent upon the presence of soap, formed by the union of fatty acid and alkali, a purely neutral fat cannot be emulsified. Emulsification is an important process in the absorption of fats in foods. SEE: *digestion.*

f. casts. Casts seen in the urine sediments. They are usually abnormal. Consist of a mass of fat globules.

f. degeneration. A change involving the deposition of fat in the cytoplasm.

fauces (faw'sēz) [L. the throat]. [NA]. The aperture leading from the mouth into the pharynx, or cavity of the throat.

The ant. pillars of the fauces are known as the *glossopalatine arch,* and the post. pillars, as the *pharyngopalatine arch.* SEE: *fossa.*

fau'cial [L. fauces, the throat]. Pert. to the fauces.

f. reflex. Gagging or vomiting resulting from irritation of fauces.

faucitis (faw-si'tis) [" + G. *-itis,* inflammation]. Inflammation of the fauces.

faveolate (fav-e'o-lāt) [L. *faveŏlus,* little honeycomb]. Honeycombed. SYN: *alveolate.*

fave'olus [L. little honeycomb]. A depression or small pit, esp. on the skin.

favism (fa'vizm). A condition common in Sicily and Sardinia resulting from sensitivity to a species of bean, *Vicia faba.* It is characterized by fever, anemia, abdominal pain, and may lead to prostration and coma. It is caused by ingestion of the beans, or inhalation of the pollen.

favus (fa'vus) [L. honeycomb]. Contagious skin disease characterized by pinhead to pea-sized, saucer-shaped, yellowish crust usually over hair follicles and accompanied by musty odor and itching. It may spread all over the body.

ETIOL: Fungus, *Trichophyton schoenleini schönleinlii.*

SYM: As stated.

PATH: Invasion of hair shafts and epidermis.

PROG: Good.

TREATMENT: Griseofulvin or ointments containing salicylanilide or copper undecylenate.

SYN: *crusted or honeycomb ringworm; tinea favosa.*

F.D. Abbr. for *fatal dose; focal distance.*

Fe. Chem. symb. for iron (*ferrum*).

fear [A.S. *faer*]. PSY: Primitively, the emotional reaction to an environmental threat, it now also presents itself frequently as an indicator of inner problems; fright, dread.

A partial fear reaction may be considered the expression of somatic disease. Fear is met with clinically, esp. in anxiety neuroses, anxious psychotic pictures (*e. g.,* depression), and in toxic deliria (*e. g.,* delirium tremens). At the somatic level, hyperthyroidism and hyperadrenalism may strongly simulate the fear state. SEE: *emotion.*

febricide (feb'-rĭ-sīd) [L. *febris,* fever, + *caedere,* to kill]. Destructive to fever. SYN: *antipyretic.*

febric'ula [L. little fever]. Mild fever of short duration without other pathology.

febrifacient (feb-rĭ-fa'sĭ-ent) [L. *febris,* fever, + *facere,* to make]. Producing fever.

febrific (fē-brif'ĭk) [" + *facere,* to make]. Producing or conveying fever.

febrifugal (feb-rif'u-gal) [" + *fugarē,* to put to flight]. Reducing fever.

febrifuge (feb'rĭ-fūj) [" + *fugāre,* to put to flight]. That which lessens fever. SYN: *antipyretic.*

febrile (fe'bril, fe'brīl, feb'ril) [L. *febris,* fever]. Feverish; pert. to a fever. SEE: *fever.*

f. convulsions. A convulsion occurring during fever but not due to an infection in the brain. Occurs almost exclusively between the ages of six months and five years and more commonly in boys. Children with high fever should be sedated in order to attempt to prevent convulsions.

f. state. A term used to describe constitutional symptoms which accompany a rise in temperature. Pulse and respiration usually rise with headache, pains, malaise, loss of appetite, concentrated and diminished urine, constipation, restlessness, hot dry skin, insomnia, irritability.

febripho'bia [" + G. *phobos,* fear]. Anxiety or fear induced by a rise in body temperature.

febris (fe'bris) [L.]. Fever.

f. acmastica. Continued fever.

f. castrensis. Typhus and remittent fever.

f. enterica. Typhoid fever.

f. flava. Yellow fever.

f. lactea. Milk fever.

f. remittens. Remittent fever.

f. undulans. Brucellosis.

f. variolosa. A form of smallpox.

fe'cal [L. *faeces,* feces]. Pert. to, or of the nature of, feces.

f. vomit. Feces in vomitus.

ETIOL: Strangulated hernia or intestinal obstruction preventing anal outlet.

fecalith (fe'kal-ith) [" + G. *lithos,* stone]. A fecal concretion. SYN: *coprolith.*

fecaloid (fe'kal-oid) [" + G. *eidos,* form]. Resembling feces.

fecaloma (fe-kal-o'mă) [" + G. *ōma,* tumor]. [L. *faeces, feces*]. SYN: *Coproma, scatoma, stercoroma.* A large mass of accumulated feces in the rectum resembling a tumor. SYN: *Coproma; scatoma; stercoroma.*

fecalu'ria [" + G. *ouron,* urine]. Fecal matter in the urine.

feces (fe'sez) [L. *faeces*]. Stools; excreta; dejecta; excrement. Body waste, such as food residue, bacteria, epithelium, and mucus, discharged from the bowels by way of the anus. SYN: *Stool.*

AMOUNT OF: Twenty-five to fifty gm. of solid, or 100-200 gm. of moist substance on a mixed diet, per day. From 0.5-0.9 gm. per day of nitrogen is excreted on a non-nitrogenous diet.

COLOR OF: The color of the feces may be indicative of various disorders as shown by the following: *Black*: May follow intestinal hemorrhage, or the use of drugs such as bismuth, iron, tannin, manganese, or charcoal. *Bloody*: May indicate hemorrhoids, cancer of the rectum, ulcers, fissures, abraded rectal membrane from dry feces, eroded rectal polypus, acute proctitis, foreign bodies, colitis, and intussusception or strangulated hernia in children. May also result from cancer of the colon, rupture of abdominal aneurysm, typhoid fever, phosphorus poisoning, jaundice, yellow fever, dengue, septicemia and yellow atrophy of the liver. *Clay-colored*: May denote impaired bile formation or obstruction, phosphorus poisoning or yellow atrophy of the liver. *Green:* Seen as the result of increased flow of bile, the use of calomel, and, commonly, diarrheas in young children. In the latter cases, may be due to bacterial growth.

COMPOSITION: Residue of food, water, products of secretions, of bacterial decomposition, indole, skatole, cholesterol, mucous and epithelial cells, purine bases, pigment, microorganisms, inorganic salts, and sometimes foreign substances.

DIAGNOSIS BY: The reducing effect of the intestinal flora upon the feces is considered an index of intestinal conditions, the less reduction indicating the best condition. Low reduction may be caused by green vegetables, fruits, and milk, while meat and egg protein result in the opposite condition.

FORM AND CONSISTENCY: (a) Normally, soft and formed; (b) hard, nodular, or scybalous in constipation; (c) fluid or mushy in diarrhea; (d) flattened or ribbonlike in rectal obstruction or spastic colitis; (e) frothy in fermentative conditions; (f) greasy in jaundice, etc.

INSPECTION OF: This should include the *color,* the *formation,* their *odor,* and the presence of any observable *foreign substances,* including *calculi.*

MUCUS: Amount should be noted. Present in both abnormal as well as normal circumstances. May occur: (a) As superficial gelatinous streaks or blobs; (b) mixed with the stool, and only apparent on making a thin paste with water; (c) mixed with blood, as in dysentery; (d) composing almost the entire stool, sometimes as firm bands or cords.

ODOR: This varies much with disease and dietary differences. It is most marked on a meat diet, and almost absent on a milk diet. Variations, such as sour, pungent, putrid, etc., occur in different diseases. *Offensive*: Obtain in jaundice, acute indigestion, enteritis, erysipelas, typhoid fever, rachitis, and occasionally in constipation. *Putrid*: May be the result of syphilitic or carcinomatous ulceration of the rectum or gangrenous dysentery. *Sour*: Normal stools of infants.

PARASITES: The presence of various intestinal parasites can be determined by examination of the feces. Gross examination may reveal the presence of nematodes or tapeworms; however, microscopic examination is necessary to determine the presence of protozoa, helminth ova, or larvae. In examination of feces, stools are collected in clean, dry, containers. For microscopic examination, representative bits of feces, or mucus are emulsified in saline solution on a clean slide, then spread evenly, and covered with a coverglass. Enterobiasis is best diagnosed by examination of scrapings from the anal and perianal regions.

REACTION: The normal reaction is neutral or slightly alkaline. An acid reaction usually indicates some fermentation in the gut or an excess of vegetables in the diet. The stools of infants are usually acid.

f., sheep. Small masses broken off from stonelike feces remaining in colon too long.

feces, *words pert. to:* acoprosis, acoprous, anus, bilifecia, colon, constipation, defecation, dejecta, elimination, excreta, excretion, hypostasis, impaction, intestine, meconium, melanorrhea, melena, rectum, scatology, scybalum, sigmoid, steatorrhea, stercoremia, stool.

$Fe(C_3H_5O_3)_2$. Ferrous lactate; lactate of iron.

$Fe(C_6H_5O_7)$. Citrate of iron.

Fechner's law (fek'nerz) [Gustav T. Fechner, Prussian philosopher, 1801-1887]. The magnitudes of sensation produced by given stimuli form an arithmetical progression, the stimuli forming a geometrical progression. SYN: *psychophysical law.*

$FeCl_2$. Ferrous chloride.

$FeCl_3$. Ferric chloride.

$FeCO_3$. Ferrous carbonate; c. of iron.

fec'ula [L. *faecula,* dregs]. 1. Sediment. 2. Starch.

feculent (fek'u-lent) [L. *faecula,* dregs]. Having sediment.

fecundate (fe'kun-dāt) [L. *fecundāre,* to bear fruit]. To fertilize or impregnate or render fertile.

fecundation (fe-kun-da'shun) [L. *fecundāre,* to bear fruit]. Impregnation; fertilization.

f., artificial. Impregnation by injecting the seminal fluid into the uterus by mechanical means. SYN: *artificial insemination.*

fecundity (fe-kun'dĭ-tĭ) [L. *fecundāre,* to bear fruit]. Ability to produce offspring; fertility.

feeblemind'edness [L. *flebilis,* tearful, + A.S. *gemynd,* to think]. Arrested mental development as distinguished from temperamental abnormality. Mental deficiency, *q.v.*

feedback. In medical electronics or in biology, the automatic perception of information which is under control by the system that receives the information. To a certain degree, blood pressure and blood sugar are regulated by feedback mechanisms. Feedback may be negative or positive.

feed'ing [A.S. *fedan,* to give food to]. Taking or giving nourishment, esp. extra-orally.

The latter is sometimes necessary because the patient either refuses or is unable to eat.

f., artificial. 1. This is accomplished through the *nostrils,* the *esophagus,* and the *rectum;* also through *gastrostomy* or *duodenostomy.* 2. Feeding of a baby with food other than mother's milk.

f., breast. Feeding of an infant at the breast.

f., colonic. Less useful with psychotic than with physically sick patients but at times it can be utilized. The limited ability for absorption in the colon limits the usefulness of this method of feeding.

f., esophageal. Used after operations on tongue or jaw, diseases of mouth, in mental cases, and forcible feedings. Also used for test meals.

f., forcible. This is by way of esophagus or rectum.

f., nasal. Largely used for children, and when unable to take nourishment normally, such as in delirium, coma, and stupor, diseases of mouth and pharynx. Any strained liquid food that will pass through catheter can be used. Temperature of feeding, 100° F. Olive oil and swabs needed for cleaning nostrils.

f., rectal. Commonest form used although it is admitted that little nourishment can be absorbed through colon. Normal saline often used with glucose, making a 5-10% solution by adding ½ to 1 oz. of glucose to 10 oz. of normal saline. Rectal washout should be given once in 24 hr., preferably in the morning.

f., tube. Done through the mouth or nostril, the latter requiring a much smaller tube and a little more dexterity, but less likely to be successfully resisted. If the patient is delirious or insane the procedure is best done with patient lying, arms bound to body by encircling sheets, the lubricated (glycerine) tube is gently passed into pharynx and, avoiding the larynx, it is projected into the stomach. Entry into the larynx may produce struggling and cyanosis. CAUTION: Be certain tube is in stomach and not in the bronchus prior to feedings. This can be determined by aspirating the tube and observing for gastric contents; or by listening to the end of the tube. If air comes out of the tube with each expiration, the tube is not in the stomach. Foods or nutritional substances as ordered by the physician are then fed slowly.

feel'ing [A.S. *fēlan,* to feel]. The conscious phase of nervous activity. The (a) emotions or centrally stimulated f.'s and (b) those sensations peripherally produced by excitation of peripheral nerves including those of the special senses.

feet (pl. of *foot*) [A.S. *fēt*]. The pedal extremities of the legs.

SEE ALSO: *foot.*

Fehl'ings solution [Hermann von Fehling, German chemist, 1812-1885]. A solution used for detecting the presence of sugar in urine. It consists of equal parts of Solutions A and B prepared as follows: Solution A (copper solution): dissolve 34.66 gm. of copper sulfate crystals in an amount of water to make 500 cc. (ml.). Solution B (alkaline tartrate solution): dissolve 173 gm. of crystallized potassium sodium tartrate and 50 gm. of sodium hydroxide in an amount of water to make 500 cc. Mix equal portions of Solutions A and B immediately before using.

fel [L.]. Bile.

f. bo'vis. Ox gall. USP. Dried fresh bile of the ox, used principally in form of an extract. SYN: *bilis bovina.*

ACTION AND USES: A laxative, intestinal antiseptic, chologogue.

fellatorism (fel-a'tor-izm). A form of sex perversion in which gratification is accomplished by buccal intromission of the penis; buccal coitus. SYN: *irrumation.*

Fell-O'Dwyer's method (George E. Fell, Buffalo physician, 1850-1918; Joseph O'Dwyer, New York physician, 1841-1898). Artificial respiration by means of a bellows, forcing air through an intubation tube into the lungs.

fel'on [A.S. *feloun,* malignant]. Suppuration of terminal joint of a finger. SYN: *paronychia*; runaround; whitlow.*

felt'work [Ger. *falzen,* to join, + A.S. *worc,* to make]. 1. Fibrous network. 2. A plexus of nerve fibrils. SYN: *neuropilem.*

fe'male [L. *femella,* little woman]. 1. A woman or girl-child. 2. Pert. to a woman. SEE: *genitalia, female.*

f. sex hormone. H. secreted by the ovaries which cause development of the uterus, vagina, and breasts at puberty, aids in regeneration of mucosa following menstruation, stimulates uterine contraction. SYN: *estrin; estrogen.*

fem'inism [L. *femina,* woman]. 1. The female character. 2. Possession of female characteristics by the male. 3. Social movement for female independence.

feminiza'tion [L. *femina,* woman]. Acquiring or adoption of female characteristics.

fem'oral [L. *femur, femor-,* thigh]. Pert. to the thigh bone or femur.

f. artery. One beginning at *ext. iliac a.,* terminating behind the knee as the popliteal a., on inner side of femur. SYN: *arteria femoralis* [NA].

f. reflex. Extension of knee and flexion of foot resulting from irritation of skin over upper ant. third of thigh.

f. vein. Continuation of the popliteal vein upward toward the *ext. iliac vein.* SYN: *vena femoralis* [NA].

fem'orocele [L. *femur,* thigh, + G. *kēlē,* hernia]. Femoral hernia.

femorotib'ial [" + *tibia,* pipe]. Rel. to the femur and tibia.

fe'mur [L.]. [NA]. The thigh bone. It extends from the hip to the knee and is the longest and strongest bone in the skeleton.

RS: *calcar femorale, cavalry bone, cotyloid cavity, femoral, trochanter.*

fenes'tra (pl. *fenestrae*) [L. window]. 1. An aperture frequently closed by a membrane. 2. An open area, as in the blade of a forceps.

f. cochleae [NA]. Leading into the cochlea. It is closed by a membrane, the secondary tympanic membrane. SYN: *f. rotunda.*

f. vestibuli [NA]. An oval opening on the inner wall of the middle ear or tympanum leading to the vestibule, into which the base of the stapes fits. SYN: *f. ovalis.*

fen'estrated [L. *fenestra,* window]. Having openings.

f. membrane of Henle. Elastic tissue layer in intima of larger arteries.

fenestra'tion [L. *fenestra,* window]. 1. Condition of having a fenestra. 2. An operation in which an artificial opening is made into the labyrinth of the ear. Performed in cases of otosclerosis.

ferment' [L. *fermentum,* from *fervere,* to ferment]. 1. To decompose. 2. (fer'ment). A substance capable of producing fermentation in other substances. 3. A catalytic agent which is capable of inducing fermentation in substances

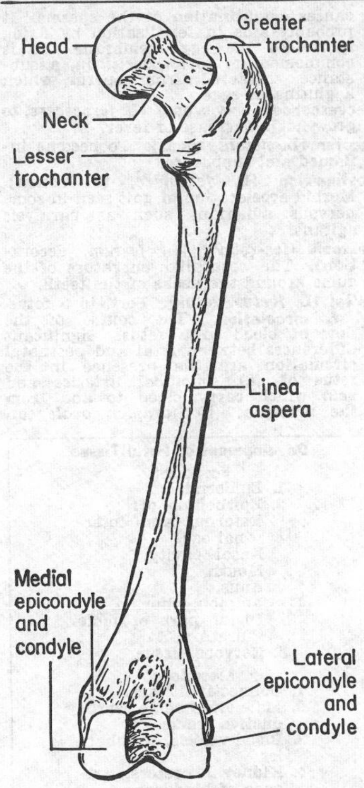

THE FEMUR

with which it comes in contact. SYN: *enzyme, q.v.*

RS: *bromelin, cacozyme, chymase, cholesterase, enzyme, hydrolyst, myopsin, pancreatin, papain, steapsin, trypsin, trypsinogen, tyrosinase, yeast.*

fermenta'tion [L. *fermentum,* leaven]. The oxidative decomposition of complex substances through the action of enzymes or ferments, produced by microorganisms. Bacteria, molds, and yeasts are the principal groups of organisms involved in fermentation. Fermentations of economic importance are those involved in the production of alcohol, lactic and butyric acids, and the baking of bread.

f., acetic. The production of acetic acid by the bacterial oxidation of ethyl alcohol under aerobic conditions.

f., alcoholic. The production of ethyl alcohol from carbohydrates usually through the action of yeasts.

f., amylolyt'ic. The process of hydrolyzation of starch with the formation of sugar.

f., autolyt'ic. Disintegration of tissues after death due to enzymes present in the tissues.

f., butyric. Formation of butyric acid from bacterial action on carbohydrates under anaerobic conditions.

f., citric acid. Formation of citric acid from action of molds on carbohydrates.

f., invertin. One that converts cane sugar into dextrose and levulose.

f., lactic. That which sours milk.

f., lactic acid. Formation of lactic acid from carbohydrates by action of lactic acid bacteria. The genera *Streptococcus* and *Lactobacillus* are the forms usually involved. Lactic acid is responsible for the souring of milk.

f., oxalic acid. Formation of oxalic acid from carbohydrates from the action of certain molds, esp. *Aspergillus.*

f., propionic acid. Formation of propionic acid from carbohydrates from action of certain bacteria.

f. test. A confirmation test for sugar in the urine. Gas forms in the fermentation tube if sugar is present.

f., viscous. Production of gelatinous material by different forms of bacilli.

fermen'toid [" + G. *eidos,* form]. A ferment without fermentive power.

fermentum (fer-men'tum) [L.]. Yeast; a ferment.

fermium (fer'mĭ-um) [Named for Enrico Fermi, winner of the Nobel Prize in physics in 1938]. Radioactive element. SYMB: Fm. At. no. 100.

fern. A flowerless plant belonging to the class Filicinae, of the division Tracheophyta (formerly phylum Pteridophyta).

f., male. *Dryopteris filix-mas* or *D. marginalis,* from the rhizomes and stipes of which is obtained oleoresin, a polyhydric phenol, the most commonly used anthelmintic for all species of tapeworms.

-ferous [L.]. Suffix meaning producing.

ferrated. Combined with iron or containing iron.

ferri-, ferro- [L. *ferrum,* iron]. Prefix used to indicate *presence of iron.*

fer'ric [L. *ferrum,* iron]. SYN: *ferruginous.* 1. Pertaining to or containing iron. 2. Denoting a compound containing iron in its trivalent form.

f. ammo'nium cit'rate. Thin, garnet-red crystals, containing about 17% of iron. Used in hypochromic anemia.

f. chlo'ride ($FeCl_3$). Used principally in form of tincture.

ACTION AND USES: An astringent, used in application to throat, also as a hematinic.

ferricyanide. A salt of hydroferricyanic acid.

ferrihemoglobin. Methemoglobin, a reduced form of hemoglobin.

fer'rin. An iron-containing compound isolated from liver tissue.

ferrit'in. An iron-phosphorus-protein complex containing about 23% iron. It is formed in the intestinal mucosa by the union of ferric iron with a protein, *apoferritin.* Ferritin is the form in which iron is stored in the tissues, principally in the reticuloendothelial cells of the liver, spleen and bone marrow.

ferrom'eter [L. *ferrum,* iron, + G. *metron,* measure]. Device for estimating proportion of iron in the blood.

ferropectic (fer-o-pek'tik) [" + G. *pēxis* fixation]. Pert. to fixing iron.

ferropexia (fer-o-pek'sĭ-ă) [" + G. *pēxis,* fixation]. Iron fixation.

ferroprotein. A protein combined with an iron-containing radical. Ferroproteins are important oxygen-transferring enzymes (*e.g.,* Warburg's enzyme, cytochrome, oxidase) *q.v.*

ferrous (fer'us) [L. *ferrum,* iron]. 1. Pertaining to iron. 2. Denoting a compound containing iron of a lower valence than three. SYN: *ferruginous.*

f. car'bonate ($FeCO_3$). Iron carbonate, used chiefly in form of Blaud's pills.

ACTION AND USES: To increase number of red blood cells, indicated in anemia.

f. gluconate. USP. Occurs as a yellowish powder or granules. Used as a hematinic.

f. i'odide (FeI_2). An unstable preparation of iron used in form of syrup. Should be transparent, pale or yellowish-green liquid.

ACTION AND USES: Same properties as iron and iodide.

INCOMPATIBILITIES: Codeine, quinine.

f. sulfate ($FeSO_4$). USP. Iron sulfate. Pale, bluish-green crystals.

ACTION AND USES: Internally, same as other preparations of iron.

INCOMPATIBILITIES: Alkalies, chlorides, tannic acid, and oxidizing agents.

ferruginous (fĕr-rū'jĭn-ŭs) [L. *ferrugo*, iron rust]. 1. Pertaining to or containing iron. 2. Of the color of iron rust. SYN: *chalybeate*.

fer'rule [L. *viriola*, little bracelet]. A band or ring of metal applied to the end of root or crown of a tooth to strengthen it.

fer'rum [L. iron]. SYMB: Fe. Iron.

fer'tile [L. *fertilis*, from *ferre*, to bear]. Capable of reproduction.

fertility (fer-til'ĭ-tĭ) [L. *fertilis*, from *ferre*, to bear]. Quality of being productive or fertile.

fertiliza'tion [L. *fertilis*, from *ferre*, to bear]. 1. Fecundation; impregnation of an ovum with the spermatozoon of the male, the male sex cell being carried in the seminal discharge.

This usually takes place in the fallopian tube. Spermatozoa have been found in the tube alive 48 hours after the last coitus. On meeting the ovum the head of the spermatozoon penetrates it and its tail drops off. Cell division begins and the fertilized ovum enters the uterus.

2. BOT: The union of the male and female gametes. In higher plants, when the pollen tube enters the ovule, two gametes emerge, one uniting with the egg to form the zygote, from which the embryo develops; the other uniting with two endosperm nuclei to form a primary endosperm cell from which the endosperm (reserve food) develops.

RS: *chemicogenesis, coitus, conception, impregnation, ovum, spermatozoa, sterile, sterility.*

fertilizin. A substance, possibly a glycoprotein, extracted from eggs which when added to a suspension of sperms causes agglutination of the sperms. It probably aids in fertilization by fixing sperm to the egg membrane. It is complementary to *antifertilizin*, a substance extracted from sperm which agglutinates eggs.

fervescence (fer-ves'ens) [L. *fervescere*, to grow hot]. Increase of fever.

fes'ter [L. *fistula*, ulcer]. To become inflamed and suppurate.

festina'tion [L. *festināre*, to hasten]. Morbid acceleration of gait seen in some nervous afflictions such as paralysis agitans.

festoon (fes-tōōn') [L. *festum*, decoration]. The wreathlike curvature of the gums around the necks of the teeth.

fe'tal [L. *foetus*, fetus]. Pert. to a fetus.

f. circulation. The course of the flow of blood in a fetus. Significant differences between fetal and postnatal circulation are the presence in the fetus of (a) *umbilical arteries* and *vein* which carry blood to and from the placenta. (b) *foramen ovale*, an

Development of Fetal Tissue

Ectoderm

1. Epidermis.
2. Epithelium of:
   External and internal ear.
   Nasal cavity.
   Mouth.
   Anus.
   Amnion, chorion.
   Distal part of male urethra.
3. Nervous tissue.

Mesoderm

1. Connective tissues.
2. Male and female reproductive tracts.
3. Blood vessels, lymphatics.
4. Kidneys, ureters, trigone of bladder.
5. Pleura, peritoneum, pericardium.
6. Muscles.

Entoderm

1. Respiratory tract except nose.
2. Digestive tract except mouth and anus.
3. Bladder except trigone.
4. Male urethra, proximal portion.
5. Female urethra.

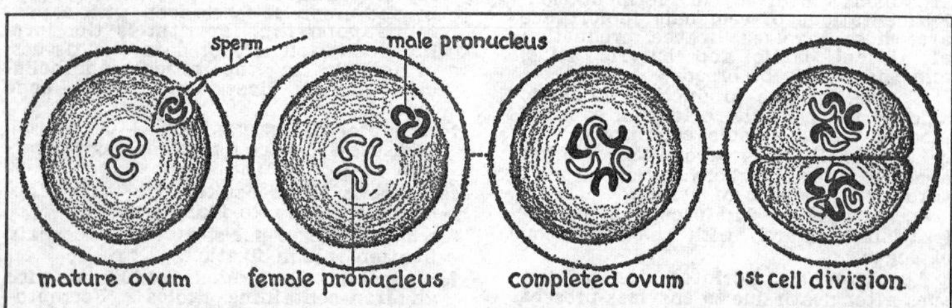

FERTILIZATION

(Diagrammatic): a. Sperm enters mature ovum. b. Sperm loses its tail and becomes male pronucleus. c. Male and female pronuclei fuse to form complete nucleus containing half male and half female chromosomes. d. Complete nucleus divides, each new nucleus containing half male and half female chromosomes.

opening in the interatrial septum, and (c) *ductus arteriosus*, a vessel connecting the pulmonary artery with the aorta. The latter two enable the blood to by-pass the lungs which are nonfunctional in the fetus. SEE: Fig. of fetal circulation p. F-13.

fetalism (fe'tal-izm) [" + G. *ismos*, condition]. Retention of fetal structures after birth.

feta'tion [L. *foetus*, fetus]. Pregnancy.

feticide (fe'tĭ-sīd) [" + *caedere*, to kill]. Intentional destruction of fetal life. SEE: *infanticide*.

fet'id [L. *fetere*, to stink]. Rank or foul in odor.

fetish, fetich (fe'tish) [Portug. *feitico*, from L. *factitius*, artificial]. That which attracts one of the opposite sex to another, or which excites the libido.

It may be the hair, the lips, or the dress. Undue value set upon such a fetish is called fetishism, *q.v.* Religious fetishism sees divine attributes in its idols and holy images. The fetish becomes a symbol. SEE: *libido*.

fe'tishism [" + G. *ismos*, state]. 1. Belief in some object as possessing power, or being capable of inspiring a stimulus. 2. Substitution for a normal love object (a person) of parts or possessions of such a one. Libido gratification from contact with articles of dress, braid of hair, etc.

A form of mental illness which finds a sex stimulus at the sight of a woman's

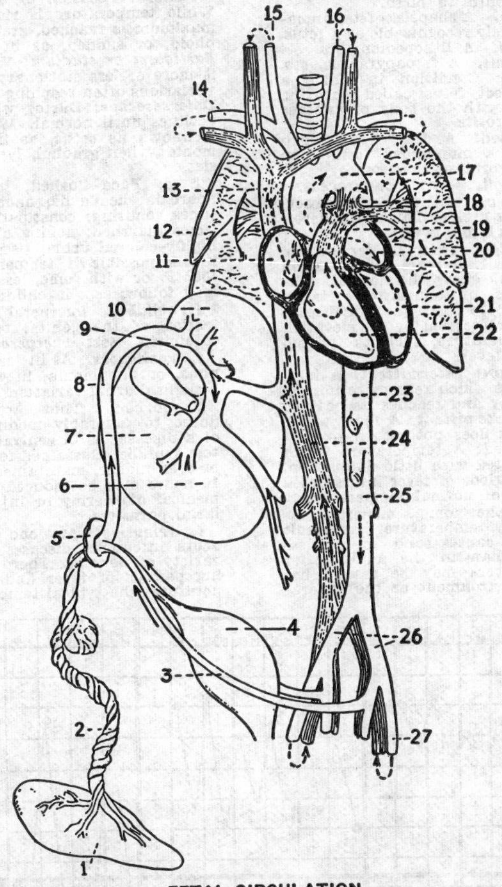

FETAL CIRCULATION

1. Placenta. 2. Umbilical cord. 3. Left hypogastric artery. 4. Bladder. 5. Umbilicus. 6. Right lobe of liver. 7. Liver. 8. Umbilical vein. 9. Ductus venosus. 10. Left lobe of liver. 11. Right atrium. 12. Right lung. 13. Superior vena cava. 14. Right subclavian artery. 15. Right common carotid. 16. Left common carotid. 17. Arch of the aorta. 18. Aorta. 19. Pulmonary artery. 20. Left atrium. 21. Left ventricle. 22. Right ventricle. 23. Aorta. 24. Inferior vena cava. 25. Aorta. 26. Common iliac arteries. 27. External iliac artery.

shoe or glove, or other article of apparel, or of some part of the body such as the hair, esp. the pubic hair. To the masochist,* all such symbols are indicative of the woman's domination.

fetom'etry [L. *foetus*, fetus, + G. *metron*, measure]. Estimation of size of the fetus or its head before delivery.

fetoplacen'tal [" + *placenta*, a flat cake, from G. *plakous*]. Pert. to the fetus and its placenta.

fe'tor [L. *fetere*, to stink]. Stench; an offensive odor.

f. ex ore. Offensive breath, halitosis.

f. oris. Halitosis.

fe'tus [L. *foetus*]. 1. The latter stages of the developing young of an animal within the uterus or within an egg. 2. In humans, the child in utero from the third month to birth.

f. amorphus. A shapeless fetal anomaly, one scarcely recognizable as a fetus.

f., calcified. A lithopedion, *q.v.*

f. compressus. A f. papyraceus, *q.v.*

f. in fetu. Condition in which a small imperfect fetus called *parasite*, is contained with the body of another fetus, the *autosite*.

f., mummified. A dead fetus which has assumed a mummified form upon failure of resorption to occur.

f., paper doll. SEE: *f. papyraceus.*

f. papyraceus. In twin pregnancy, the dead fetus pressed flat by the development of the living twin.

fe'ver [A.S. *fēfer*, from L. *fervere*, to grow warm]. 1. Pyrexia, or elevation of temperature above the normal. The normal range of temperature taken orally is 96.8° to 99.5° F. 2. A disease which is characterized by an elevation of body temperature, such as typhoid fever, yellow fever.

CLASSIFICATION: *Intermittent:* A temperature curve which returns to normal during the day and reaches its peak in the evening. *Remittent:* A fever which fluctuates but does not return to normal. *Sustained:* A temperature which remains elevated with little fluctuation. *Relapsing:* Periods of fever interspersed with periods of normal temperature.

ETIOL: In the young, moderate increase in body temperature may result from minor causes and is of less significance than in the adult. After childhood, fevers may be caused by: (a) a hot environment or the generation of body heat by physical means such as exercise, (b) neurogenic factors such as injury to the diencephalon or midbrain (the diencephalon contains reflex centers regulating heat loss), (c) dehydration such as occurs after excessive diuresis, (d) chemical substances such as caffeine or cocaine when injected into the blood stream, (d) the injection of proteins or their products, or the breakdown of necrotic tissue (these are the *aseptic fevers* such as follow surgery or coronary occlusion), (e) infectious diseases or inflammation (fever is the result of the breakdown of bacterial proteins or toxins liberated by the disease organisms which affect the heat-regulating centers), (f) severe hemorrhage.

PERIODS: *Invasion or onset of fever:* While temperature is rising and until maximum is reached, gradual, as in typhoid, or sudden, as in scarlet fever. *Fastigium or stadium*: When the fever is more or less stationary with possible variations often reaching the maximum. *Defervescence*: During which the fever declines until normal. When sudden it is known as *crisis*, as in lobar pneumonia; when gradual, *lysis*, as in measles.

SYM: Face flushed; hot, dry skin; anorexia; headache; nausea and sometimes vomiting; constipation and sometimes diarrhea; aching all over; scant, highly-colored urine; tissue waste. Delirium possible if temperature is over 105° F. or with some, less. Convulsions may follow, esp. in children; coma.

f., childbed. Puerperal sepsis. An infection of the genital tract following childbirth. SEE: *puerperal sepsis.*

f., continuous. As in scarlet fever, typhus, or pneumonia, in which there is a slight diurnal variation.

f., induced. That artificially produced to favorably modify the course of a disease, as in central nervous system syphilis. Sustained fever of 105° F., or even higher, maintained for 6 to 8 or 10 hours may be induced by the use of medical diathermy or injection of malarial parasites.

f., relapsing. Any one of a group of acute infectious diseases caused by a variety of *Borrelia*. There are alternating periods of fever and normal temperature; the typical temperature curve

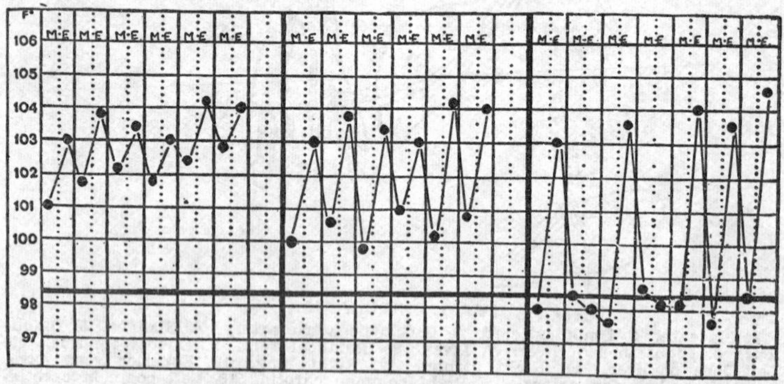

FEVER

being a characteristic of the disease. SEE UNDER: *relapsing*.

f., remittent. As in typhoid fever, septic fever, or remittent fever, with minimum temperature above normal, and with marked diurnal variation.

f., septic. One due to septic matter in the body.

fever, words pert. to: ague, antifebrile, apyrexia, crisis, dengue, febrifacient, febrifuge, food f., gastric f., hectic flush, lysis, name of fever, pulse, "pyr-" words, quartan, quintan, quotidian, respiration, temperature.

fi'at (pl. *fi'ant*) [L.]. "Let there be made," a term used in writing prescriptions.

fi'ber [L. *fibra*]. Threadlike or filmlike element, as a nerve fiber. A neuron or the axonal portion of a neuron.

RS: *chondrofibroma, cilia, cimbria, cingula, "fibr-" words, filament, filum.*

f., accelerator. One causing increased heart pulsations.

f., afferent. One carrying incoming impulses to nerve cells.

f., efferent. One carrying outgoing impulses.

f., inhibitory. One causing slower heart action.

f., medullated; f., myelinated. Nerve fiber in which axis cylinder is sheathed in myelin.

f., nonmedullated; f., unmyelinated. Nerve fiber in which there is no myelin sheath bet. axis cylinder and neurilemma.

f., nerve. The part of a nerve cell which carries impulses. SEE: *nerve*.

f.'s, Purkinje. SEE UNDER: *Purkinje*.

fi'bra (pl. *fibrae*) [L.]. A fiber.

fibralbu'min [" + *albumen*, white of egg]. Globulin.

fibremia (fi-bre'mĭ-ă) [" + G. *aima*, blood]. Fibrin formed in the blood, causing embolism or thrombosis. SYN: *inosemia*.

fi'bril [L. *fibrilla*, little fiber]. A small fiber. A very small filamentous structure, oftentimes the component of a cell or a fiber.

f., muscle. A myofibril; an extremely minute fibril found within the cytoplasm of smooth muscle cells and in the sarcoplasm of striated and cardiac muscle fibers.

f., nerve. A neurofibril; delicate fibrils found in the cell body and processes of a neuron.

fibril'la (pl. *fibrillae*) [L.]. A fibril or small fiber.

fibril'lar, fib'rillary [L. *fibrilla*, little fiber]. Pert. to, or consisting of, fibrils.

fib'rillated [L. *fibrilla*, little fiber]. Composed of minute fibers. SYN: *fibrillar; fibrous*.

fibrillation (fi-bril-a'shun) [L. *fibrilla*, little fiber]. 1. The formation of fibrils. 2. Quivering of muscular fibers. 3. Tremor or rapid action of the heart.

f., atrial. Extremely rapid, incomplete, contractions of the atria resulting in fine, rapid, irregular, and uncoordinated movements. Also called *auricular f.*

f. ventricular. A condition similar to atrial fibrillation resulting in rapid, tremulous, and ineffectual contractions of the ventricles. May result from (a) mechanical injury to the heart, (b) occlusion of coronary vessels, (c) effects of certain drugs such as excess of digitalis or chloroform, and (d) electrical stimuli.

fibrillolysis (fi-bril-ol'ĭ-sis) [" + G. *lysis*, dissolution]. Dissolution of fibrils.

fibrillolyt'ic [" + *lysis*, dissolution]. Dissolving fibrils.

fibrin [L. *fibra*, fiber]. A whitish, filamentous protein formed by the action of thrombin on fibrinogen. The conversion of fibrinogen, a hydrosol, into fibrin, a hydrogel, is the basis for the clotting of the blood. The fibrin is deposited as fine interlacing filaments in which are entangled red and white blood cells and platelets, the whole forming a coagulum or clot.

RS: *blood clot, clotting, fibrinogen, prothrombin, thrombin.*

f. foam. A spongelike substance prepared from human fibrin. When impregnated with thrombin it is used in surgery as a hemostatic agent. It is especially useful in neurosurgery and in injuries to parenchymatous organs. It is slowly absorbed.

fibrination (fi-brĭ-na'shun) [L. *fibra*, fiber]. Abnormal amt. of fibrin in the blood.

fibrinemia (fi-brĭ-ne'mĭ-ă) [" + G. *aima*, blood]. Presence of fibrin in the blood. SYN: *fibremia*.

fibrinogen (fi-brin'o-jen) [" + G. *gennan*, to produce]. A protein present in the blood plasma which through the action of thrombin in the presence of calcium ions is converted into fibrin; this brings about the clotting of the blood. SEE: *blood, clotting of; coagulation*.

fibrinogen'ic, fibrinog'enus [" + G. *gennan*, to produce]. Producing fibrin.

fibrin"ogenopen'ia. Reduction in the amount of fibrinogen in the blood usually the result of a liver disorder.

fi'brinoid [" + G. *eidos*, form]. Resembling fibrin.

f. material. A fibrinous substance which develops in the placenta, increasing in quantity as the placenta becomes older. Its origin is attributed to the degenerating decidua and trophoblast. Its forms an incomplete layer in the chorion and decidua basalis and also occurs in the form of small irregular patches on the surface of the chorionic villi. In late pregnancy, the material may have a striated or canalized appearance to which the term *canalized fibrinoid* is applied.

fibrinolysin (fi-brin-ol'ĭ-sin) [" + G. *lysis*, dissolution]. The substance, also called *plasmin*, formed from plasminogen. Its function is to dissolve fibrin. SEE: *fibrinolysis*.

fibrinol'ysis [" + *lysis*, dissolution]. Dissolution of fibrin by fibrinolysin. Caused by the action of a proteolytic enzyme system. This system is continually active in the body, but its action is greatly increased by various stress stimuli such as intense exercise, anoxia, hypoglycemia, or bacterial infections.

fibrinolyt'ic [" + *lysis*, dissolution]. Pert. to the splitting up of fibrin.

fibrinope'nia [" + G. *penia*, poverty]. Fibrin and fibrinogen deficiency in the blood.

fibrinoplas'tic [" + G. *plassein*, to form]. Of the nature of fibrinoplastin.

fibrinopu'rulent [" + *purulentus*, festering]. Consisting of pus and fibrin.

fibrinos'copy [" + G. *skopein*, to examine]. Physical and chemical examination of the fibrin of blood clots and exudates. SYN: *inoscopy*.

fibrino'sis [" + G. *ōsis*]. Excess of fibrin in the blood.

fibrinous (fi'brin-us) [L. *fibra*, fiber]. Pert. to, of the nature of, or containing, fibrin.

fibrinuria (fi-brin-u'rĭ-ă) [" + G. *ouron,* urine]. Passage of fibrin in the urine.

fibro- [L.]. Prefix: Relation to fibers or fibrous tissues.

fibroadenia (fi-bro-ă-de'nĭ-ă) [L. *fibra,* fiber, + G *adēn,* gland]. Fibrous degeneration of glandular tissue.

fibroadenoma (fi-bro-ad-ĕ-no'mă) [" + " + *ōma,* tumor]. Adenoma with fibrous tissue forming a dense stroma.

fibroad'ipose [" + *adeps, adip-,* fat]. Being fibrous and fatty.

fibroangio'ma [" + G. *aggeion,* vessel, + *ōma,* tumor]. A fibrous tissue angioma.

fibroareolar (fi-bro-ă-re'o-lar) [" + *areola,* little space]. With fibrous tissue and areolar arrangement.

fi'broblast [" + G. *blastos,* germ]. Any cell or corpuscle from which connective tissue is developed. Syn: *desmocyte; fibrocyte.*

fibroblastoma (fi-bro-blas-to'mă) [" + " + *ōma,* tumor]. Tumor of connective tissue or fibroplastic cells.

fibrobronchi'tis [" + G. *brogchia,* air tubes, + *itis,* inflammation]. Croupous or fibrinous bronchitis.

fibrocarcino'ma [" + G. *karkinos,* cancer, + *ōma,* tumor]. A carcinoma in which the trabeculae are resistant and thickened with granular degeneration of the cells.

f. cysticum. A f. with enclosed cysts

fibrocar'tilage [" + *cartilagō,* gristle]. A type of cartilage in which the matrix contains thick bundles of white or collagenous fibers. Found in the intervertebral disks.

fibrocell'ular [" + *cellula,* little cell]. Both fibrous and cellular. Syn: *fibroareolar.*

fibrochondritis (fi"bro-kon-dri'tis) [" + G *chondros,* cartilage, + *-itis,* inflammation]. Inflammation of fibrocartilage.

fibrochondro'ma [" + " + *ōma,* tumor] Tumor of fibrous tissue and cartilage.

fi'brocyst [" + G. *kystis,* cyst]. A fibrous tumor that has undergone cystic degeneration or one which has accumulated fluid in the interspaces.

fibrocystic (fi-bro-sis'tik) [" + G. *kystis,* cyst]. 1. Consisting of fibrocysts. 2. Fibrous with cystic degeneration.

f. disease of pancreas. See: *cystic fibrosis.*

fibrocysto'ma [" + " + *ōma,* tumor] Fibroma combined with cystoma.

fibrocyte (fi'bro-sīt) [" + *kytos,* cell]. A fibroblast.

fibroelas'tic [" + G. *elastikos,* elastic]. Pertaining to connective tissue containing both white, nonelastic, collagenous fibers and yellow elastic fibers.

fibroelastosis. Overgrowth of fibroelastic tissue.

f. endocardial. Fibroelastosis of the endocardium, leading to cardiac failure.

fibroenchondroma (fi-bro-en-kon-dro'mă) (pl. *fibroenchondromata*) [" + G. *en,* in + *chondros,* cartilage, + *ōma,* tumor]. An enchondroma containing fibrous elements.

fibroglio'ma [" + " + *ōma,* tumor]. A fibroma partly glioma.

fi'broid [" + G. *eidos,* form]. 1. Containing or resembling fibers. See: *degeneration.* 2. A colloquial term for fibroma, esp. fibroma of the uterus. Syn: *fibroma, q.v.*

f., interstitial. Tumor in muscular wall of uterus which may grow inward and form a *polypoid fibroid,* or outward and become a *subperitoneal fibroid.*

f., uterine. F. in uterus. See: *fibroma, uterine.*

fibroidectomy (fi-broyd-ek'to-mĭ) [" + " + *ektomē,* excision]. Surgical removal of a fibroid tumor.

fibrolipo'ma [" + G. *lipos,* fat, + *ōma,* tumor]. A lipoma having much fibrous tissue.

fibro'ma (pl. *fibromata*) [" + G. *ōma,* tumor]. A fibrous, encapsulated, connective tissue tumor.

A fibroma is irregular in shape and slow in growth. Consistency, firm. Painless except by pressure or cystic degeneration. May be found in the periosteum. May affect the jaws, the occiput, pelvis, vertebrae, ribs, long bones and sternum.

f. of breast. A benign tumor, nonulcerative and painless.

f., intramural. Located in muscle tissue of uterus bet. peritoneal coat and endometrium.

f. molluscum pedunculum of vulva. A pedunculated fibroid tumor of the vulva.

f., submucous. Encroaching upon endometrial cavity; sessile or pedunculated.

f., subserous. Lying beneath peritoneal coat of uterus, often pedunculated.

f., uterine. A fibroid tumor of the uterus.

Path: A benign tumor varying in size from a millet seed to a size large enough to fill the entire abdominal cavity. May be single or multiple. These tumors are completely encapsulated by a fibrous connective tissue capsule in which the blood vessels that supply the tumor are found. They are subjected to numerous benign degenerations, such as necrobiotic changes (red and gray degeneration), hyaline changes, telangiectatic and lymphangiectatic changes, calcareous degeneration, fatty degeneration, and infection. Occasionally, a fibroid will show sarcomatous degeneration.

Sym: Fibromata rarely cause symptoms before the age of 30. The occurrence is common after the age of 30, especially in the Negro race. Although the cardinal symptoms of fibromata are supposed to be dysmenorrhea, menorrhagia, and leukorrhea, these symptoms are found only infrequently and the symptomatology is directly related to the location of the tumors in the uterus. Following this contention, tumors that encroach upon the bladder region cause frequency and dysuria;* those pressing on the rectum cause a rectal tenesmus;* those that encroach upon the endometrium cause menorrhagia* and dysmenorrhea,* and very large subserous growths may be absolutely symptomless.

Treatment: Fibromata producing no symptoms should be left in place and the patient kept under observation. If unusually rapid growth is evidenced, they should be removed. Tumors that produce symptoms need intervention. The type of treatment depends upon age of patient, location, and size of tumor, and symptoms present. In general, wherever possible, conservation of the menstrual function should be considered. Tumors larger than a fetal head are best treated by surgical removal. Fibromectomy is clearly indicated in patients who hope subsequently to become pregnant.

See: *fibrosis uteri.*

fibromatosis (fi"bro-mă-to'sis) [L. *fibra,* fiber, + G. *ōma,* tumor, + *ōsis*]. The development simultaneously of many fibromas. Syn: *fibrosis.*

fibromatous (fi-bro′mă-tus) [" + G. *ōma*, tumor]. Pert. to, or of the nature of, a fibroma.

fibromectomy (fi-bro-mek′to-mĭ) [" + " + *ektomē*, excision]. Removal of a fibroid tumor.

fibromem′branous [" + *membrana*, web]. Having both fibrous and membranous tissue.

fibromus′cular [" + *musculus*, muscle]. Consisting of muscle and connective tissue.

fibromyi′tis [" + G. *mys, my-*, muscle, + *-itis*, inflammation]. Inflammation of the muscular system followed by fibrous degeneration of muscular fibers and atrophy.

fibromyoma (fi-bro-mi-o′mă) [" + " + *ōma*, tumor]. 1. Fibrous tissue myoma. 2. SYN: A fibroid tumor of the uterus that contains more fibrous than muscle tissue.

fibromyomectomy (fi-bro-mi-o-mek′to-mĭ) [" + " + *ektomē*, excision]. Removal of a fibromyoma from the uterus, leaving that organ in place.

fibromyosi′tis [" + " + *-ītis*, inflammation]. Chronic muscular inflammation with hyperplasia of connective tissue. SYN: *inomyositis*.

fibromyotomy (fi-bro-mi-ot′o-mĭ) [" + " + *tomē*, incision]. Opening of a fibroid tumor.

fibromyxoma (fi-bro-miks-o′mă) [" + G. *myxa*, mucus, + *-ōma*, tumor]. A fibroma that has partially undergone myxomatous degeneration.

fibromyxosarco′ma [" + " + *sarx*, flesh, + *ōma*, tumor]. 1. A sarcoma containing fibrous and myxoid tissue. 2. A mucoid degenerated sarcoma.

fibroneuroma (fi″bro-nu-ro′mă) [" + G. *neuron*, nerve, + *ōma*, tumor]. A mixed neuroma and fibroma. SYN: *inoneuroma*.

fibroosteoma (fi″bro-os-te-o′mă) [" + G. *osteon*, bone, + *ōma*, tumor]. Tumor containing bony and fibrous elements.

fibropapilloma (fi″bro-pap-ĭ-lo′mă) [" + *papilla*, nipple, + G. *ōma*, tumor]. A mixed fibroma and papilloma sometimes occurring in the bladder.

fibropericardi′tis [" + G. *peri*, around, + *kardia*, heart, + *-ītis*, inflammation]. Fibrinous pericarditis.

fibropla′sia [L. *fibra*, fiber, + G. *plasis*, a molding]. The development of fibrous tissue, as in wounds.

f., retrolental. Fibrous overgrowth of the vascular tissue of the eye. Occurs in some premature infants who have been exposed to excess oxygen concentration while in an incubator.

fibroplas′tic [" + G. *plassein*, to form]. Giving formation to fibrous tissue.

f. tumor. Small spindle-celled sarcoma.

fibroplastin (fi-bro-plas′tin) [" + G. *plassein*, to form]. A globulin in blood serum and other body fluids. SYN: *fibrinoplastin; paraglobulin*.

fibropsammoma (fi-bro-sam-o′mă) [" + G. *psammos*, sand, + *oma*, tumor]. A tumor containing fibromatous and psammomatous tissue.

fibropu′rulent [" + *purulentus*, festering]. Pus containing flakes of fibrous tissue.

fibrosarco′ma [" + G. *sarx*, flesh, + *ōma*, tumor]. A spindle-celled sarcoma containing much connective tissue.

fibrosis (fi-bro′sis) [" + G. *ōsis*]. Abnormal formation of fibrous tissue.

f., arteriocapillary. Arteriolar and capillary fibroid degeneration.

f. of lungs. Formation of scar tissue in connective tissue framework of lungs following inflammation, pneumonia, and in pulmonary tuberculosis.

f. uteri. A condition of the uterus manifested by excess of fibrous tissue, predominating symptom being menorrhagia.*

The uterus may be large or small. The endometrium* may be normal, atrophic, or in the larger number show hyperplastic and hypertrophic glandular and interstitial endometritis of vascular origin.

ETIOL: Not definitely known, but it is seen in patients with syphilis, those who have had a number of pregnancies, and in conditions where venous stasis has been present over a long period, such as in chronic retroversion with or without infection and procidentia.

fibrositis (fi-bro-si′tis) [" + G. *itis*, inflammation]. Nonsuppurative inflammation of white fibrous connective tissue anywhere in the body. SYN: *muscular rheumatism*.

f., bursal. F. of a bursa; bursitis.

f., intramuscular. F. of fibrous sheaths of muscles; muscular rheumatism; interstitial myositis.

f., periarticular. F. of the fibrous tissue of the articular capsule.

f., perineural. F. of the fibrous sheath surrounding nerves, esp. the sciatic nerve; sciatica.

f., subcutaneous. F. of the subcutaneous tissue; panniculitis.

fibrous (fi′brus) [L. *fibra*, fiber]. Composed of or containing fibers; as in contradistinction to (osseous) bony composition.

fibrot′ic [L. *fibra*, fiber]. Marked by or pert. to fibrosis.

fib′ula [L. pin]. [NA]. Calf bone (*peroneal bone*). One of the longest and thinnest bones of the body. The outer and smaller bone of the leg from the ankle to the knee, articulating above with the tibia, and below with the tibia, and talus (astragalus). SEE: *peroneal, peroneus, tibia*.

fib′ular [L. *fibula*, pin]. Rel. to the fibula.

fibulocalcaneal (fib″u-lo-kal-ka′ne-al) [" + *calcaneus*, pert. to the heel]. Pert. to the fibula and calcaneus, or *os calcis*.

field [A.S. *feld*]. A specific area in relation to an object.

f., au′ditory. The space or distance within the limit of hearing.

f. of vision. That portion of space which the fixed eye can see.

fifth cranial nerve. Trigeminal or trifacial n., *q.v.*

f. ventricle. Space separating layers of septum lucidum.

fig [L. *ficus*, fig]. A fruit of *Ficus carica*.

RAW: 100 gm. Calories: 80. Other main values: 1.2 gm. protein; trace of fat; 20 gm. carbohydrates; 35 mg. calcium; 80 I.U. vitamin A. SEE: *dates; fruit*.

fig′ure. A body; form, shape, or outline.

f., achromatic. In mitosis or meiosis, the spindle fibers and the asters.

f., chromatic. The chromosomes or the chromatin material.

fila (fi′lă) [L. *filum*, thread]. Plural of filum, *q.v.*

filaceous (fil-a′she-us) [L. *filum*, thread]. Composed of filaments. SYN: *filamentous*.

fil′ament [L. *filum*, thread].

f., axial. A fine filament forming the central axis of the tail of a spermatozoan.

filamen'tous [L. *filum,* thread]. BIOL: Made up of long, interwoven or irregularly placed filaments.

Filaria (fil-a'rĭ-ă) [L. *filum,* thread]. Term formerly applied to a genus of nematodes belonging to the superfamily Filarioidea.

F. bancrofti. *Wuchereria bancrofti, q.v.*

F. loa. Loa loa, *q.v.*

F. medinensis. *Dracunculus medinensis, q.v.*

F. sanguinis hominis. *Wuchereria bancrofti, q.v.*

filaria. A long filiform nematode belonging to the superfamily Filarioidea. The adults live in vertebrates including man, inhabiting man, being found in the lymphatic vessels and lymphatic organs, circulatory system, connective tissues, esp., subcutaneous tissues, and serous cavities. Typically, the female produces larvae called *microfilariae* which may be sheathed or sheathless. These reach the peripheral blood or lymphatic vessels where they may be ingested by a blood sucking arthropod (mosquitos, gnats, flies). In the intermediate host, they transform into *rhabditoid larvae,* which metamorphose into infective filariform larvae. These migrate to the proboscis and are deposited in or on the skin of the vertebrate host.

fila'rial [L. *filum,* thread]. Pert. to or caused by filariae.

filariasis (fil-ă-ri'ă-sis) [L. *filum,* thread]. A chronic disease due to one of the filariae.

filarici'dal [" + *caedere,* to kill]. Pert. to that which is destructive to Filaria.

fil'iform [L. *filum,* thread, + *forma,* form]. 1. BIOL: Pert. to a growth that is uniform along the inoculation line in stab or streak cultures. 2. Hairlike, filamentous.

f. papillae. Smallest tongue papillae.

fil'ipuncture [" + *punctura,* a piercing]. Insertion of a slender wire or thread in an aneurysm to induce coagulation.

fil'let [L. *filum,* thread]. 1. A bandage shaped like a loop. 2. Two bundles of sensory fibers in the medulla, pons, and brain. SYN: *lemniscus.*

f. of corpus callosum. Fibers forming white substance of the gyrus fornicatus.

f., olivary. Nerve fasciculus surrounding olivary body.

filling (fil'ing) [A.S. *fyllan,* to fill]. 1. The material for insertion in a tooth cavity; usually gold, amalgam, or cement. 2. The operation of filling tooth cavities.

film. 1. A thin skin, membrane, or covering. 2. A thin sheet of material, usually cellulose, coated with a light-sensitive emulsion used in taking photographs. 3. In microscopy, a thin layer of blood or other material spread on a slide or cover slip.

fil'opressure [L. *filum,* thread, + *pressura,* pressure]. Pressure on a blood vessel caused by a ligature.

filovaricosis (fi"lo-var-ĭ-ko'sis) [" + *varix,* a dilated vein, + G. *ōsis*]. Dilatation or thickening of the axis cylinder of a nerve fiber.

filter [L. *filtrāre,* to strain through]. 1. To pass a liquid through any porous substance which prevents particles larger than a certain size to pass through. 2. Device for filtering liquids, light rays, or radiations. SEE: *absorption; osmosis.*

f. bed. Large-scale filter to purify the water supply.

f., Berkefeld. One of diatomaceous earth which will not allow bacteria to pass through.

f., infrared. Cell of water and red glass which confines radiation to spectral region from 600 to 1400 mu, red glass alone from 600 to 4000 mu.

f., Kitasato's. Suction variety of filter, using porcelain dilator.

f., Pasteur-Chamberlain. Filters of unglazed porcelain capable of retaining bacteria and some viruses; either pressure or suction is required to force or draw the liquid through the filter.

f. paper. Coarse form of paper used in filtering solutions.

f., Wood's A glass screen allowing passage of ultraviolet rays and absorbing rays of visual light. Used in diagnosing certain dermatologic conditions, especially tinea capitis.

filterable [L. *filtrāre,* to strain through]. Capable of passing through the pores of a porcelain filter, through which bacteria cannot pass.

fil'trate [L. *filtrāre,* to strain through]. The fluid which has been passed through a filter. The residue is the *precipitate.*

f., glomerular. The fluid which passes from the blood through the capillary walls of the glomeruli of the kidney. It is a protein-free plasma from which urine is formed.

filtra'tion [L. *filtrāre,* to strain through]. Passage of a fluid through a semipermeable membrane as a result of a difference in hydrostatic pressures. SEE: *filter.*

f. of roentgen rays. The absorption of some of the relatively longer wave lengths of roentgen radiation by placing in the path of the rays some absorbing medium, such as aluminum, copper, or zinc.

filtratometer (fi-tra-tom'ĕ-ter) [" + G. *metron,* measure]. Device for measuring gastric filtrates.

fil'trum [L.]. A filter.

filum (fi'lum) (pl. *fila*) [L.]. A threadlike structure.

f. coronaria. A fibrous band extending from the base of the medial cusp of the tricuspid valve to the aortic annulus.

f. olfactoria. Groups of fibers consisting of the axons of olfactory cells which form the olfactory nerves. These pass from the olfactory epithelium through the cribriform plate and terminate in the olfactory bulb.

f. terminale. A long, slender filament forming end of spinal cord.

fimbria (fim'brĭ-ă) (pl. *fimbriae*) [L. fringe]. Any structure resembling fringe.

f. ova'rica. The longest fringelike extremity of the fallopian tubes; extending from the infundibulum close to the ovary.

f. tubae. Fringelike portion at abdominal end of the fallopian tubes.

fimbriate (fim'brĭ-āt) [L. *fimbria,* fringe]. 1. BIOL: Having fingerlike projections. 2 Fringed.

f. body. Corpus fimbriatum.

fim'briated [L. *fimbria,* fringe.]. Fringed.

fimbriocele (fim'brĭ-o-sēl) [L. *fimbria,* fringe, + G. *kēlē,* hernia]. Hernia including the fimbriated portion of the oviduct.

fin'ger [A.S.]. A digit of the hand.

f., dislocation of the. First, be certain that there is no fracture. Dislocations occur only at a joint. If there has been a crushing injury, assume that a fracture is present until an x-ray has been made. Dislocations of a finger are usually easily diagnosed and quite easily reduced. They may be caused by blows, falls, and similar causes.

If there is no fracture, it may be treated by asking the patient to steady and support his own wrist (or getting somebody else to do so) for countertraction. Then take hold of the finger beyond the dislocated muscles and tendons, and with the other (free) hand slip the dislocated bone into place.

This is to be followed by an application of a splint from the tip of the finger well into the palm of the hand. This may be made of cigar box wood, wire, tongue depressors, heavy cardboard, etc.

Do not under any circumstances attempt to reduce a dislocation of the thumb joint nearest to the palm of the hand.

f. print. An imprint made by the cutaneous ridges of the fleshy portion of the distal end of a finger. Finger prints are used for purposes of identification.

f. stall. A finger cot.

finger, *words pert. to:* acroataxia, acrodynia, arachnodactyly, baseball f., camptodactylia, dactyl, dactylus, digit, nail, phalanx.

Finsen light [Niels R. Finsen, Danish physician, 1860-1904]. Blue and violet light with heat waves excluded. Formerly used in the treatment of lupus.

fire [A.S. *fyr*]. Flame producing heat.

f. emergencies. If a person's clothing catches fire, he should be rolled in a rug or blanket to smother flames. It may be necessary to trip him to prevent his running about, as this only fans the flames.

If patient is trapped in a burning building, this particular room should have doors closed to prevent cross breezes from increasing the fire. The window should be opened if patient is to be rescued by lowering him, using any appropriate carry. Do not open any door more than a few inches to ascertain possibility of escape. A burst of flame or hot air may push door in and asphyxiate anyone in the room. Wet cloths or towels should be held over mouth and nostrils to keep out smoke and gases. SEE: *burn, flame, gases, transportation.*

f., St. Anthony's. Erysipelas. Also called *St. Francis' fire.*

first aid. The administration of emergency assistance to individuals who have been injured or otherwise disabled, prior to the arrival of a doctor, or transportation to a hospital or doctor's office. In no sense assume to be the substitution for definitive medical care.

first aid, *words pert. to:* antidote, apoplexy, artificial respiration, asphyxia, bites, burn, coma, dislocation, drowning, emetic, fainting, flames, food poisoning, foreign bodies, fracture, freezing, frost bite, fumes, gases, insect bites, laceration, name of poison, poison, shock, snake bite, triage, unconsciousness. SEE ALSO: First Aid, in Fact-Finding Index (page viii).

first cranial nerve. Olfactory nerve, *q.v.*

fish poisoning. A form of food poisoning caused by eating poisonous fish. Some fish are inherently poisonous, others become poisonous through decomposition, infection, by feeding on other poisonous forms, or by poisonous metabolic substances produced during the spawning season.

The symptoms are very similar to those of meat poisoning, but perhaps more intense. Headache, vertigo, thirst, indigestion, vomiting, cramps, diarrhea and skin eruptions. Convulsions may occur.

SHELL FISH: The onset is very rapid, but seldom are there gastrointestinal symptoms. Collapse may ensue and death occur in a few hours. Other fish poisonings only differ in degree in gastrointestinal symptoms from meat poisoning.

TREATMENT: Emetics, purgatives, and stimulants. Medical treatment for convulsions. Follow treatment with oatmeal or barley water, esp. if nauseated; later, water with a pinch of salt. SEE: *food poisoning; meat poisoning.*

fish skin disease. A disease of the skin characterized by increase of the horny layer and deficiency of the skin secretions. SYN: *ichthyosis, q.v.*

fission (fish'un) [L. *fissiō*, from *findere*, to cleave]. 1. Splitting into two or more parts. 2. A method of asexual reproduction seen in bacteria, protozoa, and other lower forms of life in which the cell or the body divides into two or more parts each of which develops into a complete individual. 3. Splitting of the nucleus of an atom into smaller nuclei. SYN: *nuclear fission.*

fissip'arous [L. *fissiō-*, *findere*, to cleave, + *parere*, to bring forth]. Reproducing by fission.

fissura (fis-u'ră) (pl. *fissurae*) [L.]. Fissure. SYN: *cleft, sulcus.*

fis'sural [L. *fissura*, fissure]. Pertaining to a fissure.

fissure (fish'ur) [L. *fissura*]. 1. A groove or natural division, cleft or slit, deep furrow in the brain, liver, spinal cord, and other organs. 2. Ulcer or crack-like sore. 3. A break in the enamel of a tooth.

f., anal. A linear ulcer on the margin of the anus.

f., auricular. F. of petrous portion of the temporal bone.

f. of Bichat. A fissure below the corpus callosum in the cerebellum.

f., Broca's. Fissure encircling the third left frontal convolution of the brain.

f., Burdach's. F. connecting lateral surface of insula and inner surface of operculum of the brain.

f., calcarine. F. extending from the cerebrum's occipital end to the occipital f.

f., callosomarginal. A conspicuous sulcus in mesial surface of cerebral hemisphere running above and concentric with the curved upper surface of the corpus callosum.

f., central. SEE: *Rolando's f.*

f., Clevenger's. Inferior temporal sulcus.

f., collateral. F. on inferior surface of cerebral hemisphere separating subcalcarine and subcollateral gyri.

f.'s, Henle's. Connective tissue areas bet. the muscular fibers of heart.

f., hippocampal. F. of brain extending from post. part of corpus callosum to the tip of temporal lobe.

f., inferior orbital. A fissure at the apex of the orbit through which pass the infraorbital blood vessels and maxillary branch of the trigeminal nerve; the sphenomaxillary fissure.

f., interparietal. Intraparietal sulcus.

f., longitudinal. A fissure on the lower surface of the liver.

f., occipitoparietal. The fissure bet. the occipital and parietal lobes of the brain.

f., palpebral. Opening separating the upper and lower eyelids.

f., portal. The opening into the liver on its under surface: continues into the liver as the portal canal.

f., Rolando's. F. separating frontal and parietal lobes.

f., sphenoidal. F. separating the wings and body of the sphenoid.

f. of Sylvius. The lateral cerebral fissure. A f. separating the frontal and parietal lobes from the temporal lobe of the brain.

f., transverse. 1. The fissure bet. the cerebellum and cerebrum of the brain. 2. A f. on lower surface of the liver which serves as the hilum transmitting vessels and ducts to the liver.

f., umbilical. Ant. portion of liver's longitudinal fissure which contains the round ligament, the obliterated umbilical vein.

f., Wernicke's. F. dividing the temporal and parietal lobes from the occipital lobe.

fistula (fis'tu-la) [L. a pipe]. An abnormal tubelike passage from a normal cavity or tube to a free surface or to another cavity. May be congenital due to incomplete closure of parts or may result from abscesses, injuries, or inflammatory processes.

f., anal. F. near the anus.

f., biliary. One through which bile is discharged after a biliary operation.

f., blind. One open at only one end.

f., branchial. An open branchial cleft.

f., cervical. 1. An abnormal opening into the cervix uteri. 2. An opening in the neck leading to the pharynx, resulting from incomplete closure of the brachial clefts.

f., cervicovaginalis laqueatica. Fistula in the vaginal portion of the cervix uteri bet. the uterine canal and the vagina.

f., complete. F. with both external and internal opening.

f., enterovaginal. One bet. the bowel and vagina.

f., fecal. One in which there is a discharge of feces through the opening.

f., metroperitoneal. F. between uterine and peritoneal cavities.

f., parotid. One through which there is an abnormal leakage of saliva onto ext. surface of cheek.

f., perineovaginal. Opening from vagina through the perineum.

f., rectovaginal. Opening bet. rectum and vagina.

f., ureterovaginal. Opening bet. ureter and vagina.

f., vesicouterine. Opening bet. uterus and bladder.

f., vesicovaginal. Opening from bladder into the vagina.

fistulatome (fis'tu-lă-tōm) [" + G. *tomē*, incision]. Instrument for incising a fistula.

fistulectomy (fis-tu-lek'to-mĭ) [" + G. *ektomē*, excision]. Excision of a fistula.

fistulization (fis"tu-li-za'shun) [L. *fistula*, pipe]. Becoming fistulous.

fistuloenterostomy (fis"tu-lo-en-ter-os'to-mĭ) [" + G. *enteron*, intestine, + *stoma*, opening]. Operative closure of a biliary fistula and formation of new passage of bile into the intestine.

fistulous (fis'tu-lus) [L. *fistula*, pipe]. Pert. to, or containing, a fistula.

fit (fĭt) [A.S. *fitt*]. A sudden attack, convulsion or paroxysm. SEE: *convulsion.*

F. A. TREATMENT: Do not try to stop attack. Prevent patient from hurting or injuring self. Place a pad between teeth to prevent biting tongue or cheeks. Allow patient to sleep.

fixa'tion [L. *fixus*, from *figere*, to fasten]. 1. The act of holding or fastening in a fixed position. The condition of being fixed. Immobilizing, making rigid. 2. PSYCH: A phase of psychosexual development in which the libido is arrested at an inferior or presexual level. For example, father or mother fixation.

f., complement. The action of a complement, a constituent of fresh blood serum, on an antigen, which, in turn, has been acted on by its antibody. During the uniting of antigen, antibody, and complement, the complement is rendered inactive or destroyed, and this process is known as f. of complement. The basis of the Wassermann and Kolmer tests for syphilis and other tests for infectious diseases.

f., field of. The widest limits of vision in all directions within which the eyes can fixate.

f. forceps. Forceps for holding a part.

f. of eyes. The movement of the eyes for the most acute vision in which they are directed toward an object so that the visual axes meet and the image of the object falls on corresponding points of each retina.

f. point. The fovea or the point on the retina where the visual axes (fixation lines) meet the point of clearest vision.

fix'ative [L. *fixus*, from *figere*, to fasten]. 1. A substance that serves to make firm or fixed. 2. One used to harden and preserve pathological specimens.

fix'ing [L. *fixus*, from *figere*, to fasten]. Rapid killing of tissue elements so that their normal living form is preserved.

Fl. Abbr. for fluid; symb. for fluorine.

flabel'lum [L. fan]. White fibers in form of a fan-shaped bundle in corpus striatum.

flaccid (flak'sid) [L. *flaccidus*, flabby]. Relaxed, flabby, having defective or absent muscular tone.

flagella (flă-jel'ă). Plural of flagellum, *q.v.*

flagellant (flaj'ĕ-lant) [L. *flagellum*, whip]. 1. Pert. to flagella. 2. Pert. to stroking in massage. 3. One who practices flagellation.

flagellate (flaj'ĕ-lāt) [L. *flagellum*, whip]. 1. With one or more flagella. 2. A protozoon with one or more flagella.

f. cell. One with long cilia for propulsion.

flagella'tion [L. *flagellum*, whip]. 1. Flogging. 2. Massage by strokes. 3. Applying electricity by tapping the body. 4. A form of sexual perversion through which the libido is stimulated by striking the gluteal region with a whip or lashes.

It was practiced during the 13th and 15th centuries as an atonement, and to kill the desires of the flesh, but instead it stimulated sensuality and so it was discontinued.

It is practiced by masochists on the opposite sex. The pervert sometimes subjects himself to this form of castigation to stimulate the libido.

flagellum (flă-jel'um) (pl. *flagella*) [L. whip]. A hairlike, motile process on the extremity of a bacterium or protozoon.

flail joint. A joint with excessive mobility after resection.

flames, inhalation of. SYM: Intense irritation of nose, throat, pharynx, windpipe and lungs; with choking, coughing, interference with respiration; intense swelling of throat; breathing is markedly limited. Shock.

TREATMENT: Administration of oxygen; occasionally tracheotomy necessary. Pain relieved by spraying nose and throat with a local anesthetic of low toxicity. Follow with oil sprays. Steam inhalations are very soothing, and may have to be kept up for long periods of time. SEE: *burn; fire; gases.*

flank [Fr. *flanc,* side]. The part bet. ribs and upper border of ilium. SEE: *latus.* Also loosely used to refer to the outer side of the thigh, hip, and buttock.

flap [Dutch *flappen,* to strike]. A mass of partly detached tissue attached at the base after resection.

f., amputation. A flap covering the end of a part left after an amputation.

f., extraction. Removal of cataract so as to make a flap in the cornea.

flare. A flush or spreading area of redness which surrounds a line made by drawing a pointed instrument across the skin. It is the second reaction in the "triple response" *q.v.* and due to dilatation of the arterioles.

flarim'eter. A modified spirometer for estimating vital capacity, blood pressure, heart rate, etc.

flash method. Means of pasteurizing milk by rapidly raising temperature of milk to 178° F., maintaining it there for a few minutes and letting it fall to 40° F.

f. point. The temperature at which a substance will burst into flame.

flatfoot. Abnormal flatness of sole and arch of foot. This condition may exist without causing symptoms or interfering with normal function of the foot.

The inner longitudinal and ant. transverse metatarsal arches are those that may be depressed. It may be *acute, subacute, or chronic.* SYN: *pes planus; splayfoot.*

f., spasmodic. The foot is held everted by spasmodic contraction of the peroneal muscle.

flat'ness. Resonance heard on percussing over solid organs, or fluid in the thoracic cavity.

flatulence (flat'u-lens) [L. *flatulentiā,* a blowing]. Excesive gas in the stomach and intestines.

NP: *If of the stomach,* seat patient upright, apply heat to epigastrium or a counterirritant. Give sodium bicarbonate in water or give an effervescent beverage.

If in intestines, have patient lying down for ½ hr. before and after meals. No fluids with meals but hot water may be sipped afterwards. Give carminatives, carminative enema if needed, or pass a flatus tube. SEE: *distention; gastrointestinal decompression; Wangensteen method.*

flatulent (flat'u-lent) [L. *flatulentiā,* a blowing]. Affected with or caused by gas in the alimentary tract.

fla'tus [L. a blowing]. 1. Gas in digestive tract. 2. Expiration of air; eructation. SEE: *borborygmus.*

f. tube. A rectal tube to procure expulsion of flatus in distention and before a saline enema.

NP: It may be passed 6-8 inches. It may be left in position for 20-30 minutes. Patient on back or side. Lubricate tube and insert gently. Lower end of tube is placed in a deodorant solution in vessel beside the bed.

f. vaginalis. GYN: Expulsion of air from vagina.

flatworm. A worm belonging to the phylum Platyhelminthes, *q.v.*

flavedo (flă-ve'do) [L. *flavus,* yellow]. Yellowness, as of the skin; sallowness; jaundice.

flavescent (flă-ves'ent) [L. *flavus,* yellow]. Yellowish.

flav'icin. An antibiotic substance obtained from certain fungi, especially *Aspergillus flavus.*

flavin (fla'vin). One of a group of natural water-soluble pigments occurring in milk, yeasts, bacteria, and some plants. All contain the flavin or isoalloxazine nucleus and are yellow in color. Present in riboflavin and in Warburg's yellow enzyme.

fla'vism [" + G. *ismos,* condition]. Having a yellow tinge to the hair.

flavo- [L. *flavus,* yellow]. Prefix: yellow.

Flavo"bacter'ium. A genus of rod-shaped bacteria belonging to the Achromobacteriaceae. They are found in soil and water and produce an orange-yellow pigment in cultures.

flavo"pro'tein. One of a group of conjugated proteins which constitute the yellow enzymes essential in cellular respiration.

flax'seed. Seed of *Linum usitatis simum.* SYN: *linseed.*

f. poultice. A soft, usually hot and moist paste for external application, such as a flaxseed poultice, linseed meal, bran, flour, or hops boiled with water and wrapped in cheesecloth or other fabrics.

PURPOSE: (a) Action is mainly through heat; (b) counterirritant effect is slight; (c) used for inflammations, abscesses, relief of pain, and pulmonary congestion.

PROPORTIONS: One part flaxseed meal and 1½ parts boiling water. One cup of meal and 1½ cups of water make a poultice approximately 6 x 4 x 1.

ARTICLES NEEDED: (a) Flaxseed meal; (b) boiling water; (c) saucepan; (d) large spoon; (e) one teaspoonful of soda bicarbonate powder; (f) old muslin, size in proportion to that of affected area; (g) bandage or binder; (h) hot water bottle and cover or flannel protector; (i) cup for measuring.

PROCEDURE: (a) Put the required amount of water on to boil. (b) Collect the necessary articles. Fill the hot water bottle, 125° F. (c) Spread the muslin on the table. (d) When the water is boiling briskly, add flaxseed gradually and stir vigorously. Cook until it drops from the spoon. When removed from the stove, add one teaspoonful of soda bicarbonate powder. (e) Beat well to incorporate air. (f) Spread it on the old muslin about 1 inch thick and fold the muslin in envelope fashion. Fill the saucepan with water. (g) Obtain the hot water bottle and carry the poultice to the patient between the folds of the hot water bottle. (h) Test the temperature of the poulice by applying it to the back of the wrist. Apply the poultice to the area slowly and lay the hot water bottle over it. (i) Secure poultice with binder or bandage. If previous poultices have been applied and the hot water bottle is over the area, remove it, place the poultice, and refill and replace the bottle.

When the treatment is discontinued,

remove the poultice, dry the part, and place the hot water bottle or flannel over the area for 2 or 3 hours.

fl. dr. Abbr. of *fluidram.*

flea (flē) [A.S. *flēa*]. Fleas of the genus *Xenopsylla* transmit the bacillus of plague *(Pasteurella pestis)* from rats to humans. Fleas may transmit other diseases such as tularemia, endemic typhus, and brucellosis, and they serve as intermediate hosts for the cat and dog tapeworms.

f. bites. Hemorrhagic puncta* surrounded by erythematous* and urticarial patches, as the result of the injection of their saliva.

PREVENTION: Treat the skin with an insect repellent available in form of a powder, spray or oil for topical use.

f., cat. *Ctenophalides felis.*

f., chigger. *Tungra penetrans.* Also called chigger, jigger, and sand fleas.

f., dog. *Ctenophalides canis.*

f., human. *Pulex irritans.*

f., rat. *Xenopsylla cheopis.*

fleam (flēm) [Fr. *flieme,* from G. *phleps,* vein]. Lancet used in venesection.

Flechsig's areas (flekh'zig) [Paul E. Flechsig, Leipzig neurologist, 1847-1929]. Ant., lateral, and post. areas of each lateral half of the medulla.

fleece of Stilling. Meshwork of white fibers that surrounds the dentate nucleus of the cerebellum.

flesh [A.S. *flaesc*]. The soft tissues of the animal body, esp. the muscles. SEE: *carnivorous, carnophobia, meat, meat poisoning.*

f., examination of animal. *General rule*: Examine for (1) Color; (2) consistency; (3) proportion of fat; (4) odor; (5) taste.

COLOR: *Yellow*—May be produced by food. In disease due to biliary compounds. *Brown*—Rare, except in old meat undergoing decomposition. *Dark Purple*—May indicate animal has died a natural death, suffered from acute fever, tuberculosis, or rinderpest. Avoid. *Dark Reddish-Brown*—May indicate animal has been hunted or overdriven, poisoned, drowned or suffocated. Avoid. *Scarlet*—Rare. Indicates arsenic or monoxide poisoning. *Diffused redness*—Indicates that animal may have been poisoned, or the meat frozen. *Green or Violet*—Indicates the beginning of putrefaction. Dangerous. *Saffron*—Indicates artificial coloring of smoked pork. *Briliant Red*—Due to poisonous bacteria. *Gray*—Usually in sausages. Due to bacteria. *Phosphorescent Flesh*—Not due to putrefaction. Usually found in fish and shellfish. Sometimes in meat, esp. veal. Due to bacteria and generally transmitted from fish kept in the same place with meat. Increased by warmth. *White*—Rare, except in calves. Found in certain diseases. Avoid.

GENERAL TEST: *Color* — Neither very pale nor dark purple. *Appearance*—Marbled. *Consistency* — Firm and elastic. Not flabby or sodden. Should hardly moisten the finger. *Odor*—Free from odors.

f., goose. Cutis anserina, *q.v.*

f., proud. 1. Fungus growth. 2. Excessive granular tissue in a wound or ulcer.

fletch'erism. Taking small amounts of food at a time with excessive mastication.

flex [L. *flexus,* from *flectere,* to bend]. To bend upon itself, as a muscle; flexion, bending.

flexibilitas cerea (fleks-ĭ-bil'ĭ-tas se're-ă) [L.]. A cataleptic state in which a subject maintains the limbs in the position in which they are placed. Characteristic of catatonic patients.

flexibil'ity [L. *flexus,* from *flectere,* to bend]. Quality of being bent without breaking; adaptability. SYN: *pliability.*

flex'ible [L. *flexus,* from *flectere,* to bend]. Capable of being bent without breaking.

flexile (fleks'il) [L. *flexus,* bent]. Pliant; flexible.

flexion (flek'shun) [L. *flexus,* bent]. The act of bending or condition of being bent, in contrast to extending. SEE: *antecurvature; clawfoot; clawhand.*

flex'or [L. *flectere,* to bend]. A muscle that bends a part, in a generally proximal direction; as opposed to an extensor.

flexure, flexura (flek'sher, flek-shu'ra) [L. *flexura,* a bending]. A bend.

f., duodenojejunal. Curve at meeting point of jejunum and duodenum.

f., hepatic. The bend on right side forming junction of the ascending with the transverse colon.

f., sigmoid. The s-like loop (in *left iliac fossa*) of the descending colon as it meets the rectum. SEE: *colon.*

f., splenic. Bend at junction of transverse with descending colon.

flick'er. The sensation of alternating intervals of brightness caused by interruptions in light stimuli.

flight of ideas. PSY: Continuous but fragmentary stream of talk.

Connection can be followed but direction is frequently changed, often by chance stimuli from the environment.

flint disease. Deposit of fine particles in the lungs. SYN: *chalicosis.*

floating [A.S. *flota,* a raft]. Moving about. Out of normal location.

f. kidney. One movable from its normal bed of fat.

ETIOL: A blow, a sudden movement, laxity of the peritoneum complicated by inflammation, kinking of ureter and damming of urine.

SYM: Dragging pain in loin, chronic indigestion, albuminuria, painful urination, urine scanty and frequent. Neurasthenic complaints.

TREATMENT: Rest in bed. Diet to increase weight. A kidney pad may be ordered. If so, adjust before getting out of bed. Patient should not be told nature of condition. *Nephropexy* may be indicated if kidney is healthy; otherwise, possible *nephrectomy.*

f. ribs. The 11th and 12th ribs which do not articulate with the sternum.

floats [A.S. *flota,* a raft]. Glass capsules containing labels to float in an exposed liquid to designate its nature.

floccillation, floccitation (flok-sĭ-la'shun, -ta'shun) [L. *flocculus,* little tuft]. Semiconscious picking at bedclothes in fevers and stupors. SYN: *carphologia, carphology.*

floccose (flok'ōs) [L. *floccōsus,* full of wool tufts]. BIOL: Pert. to a growth made up of short and densely but irregularly interwoven filaments.

floccular (flok'u-lar) [L. *flocculus,* little tuft]. Pert. to the flocculus of the cerebellum.

floc'culence [L. *flocculus,* little tuft]. State of being flocculent or resembling shreds or tufts of cotton.

flocculent (flok'u-lent) [L. *flocculus,* little tuft]. Resembling the white portion of "floating island" or a fluid or culture containing whitish shreds of mucus.

flocculoreac'tion [" + *rē*, again, + *agere*, to act]. Flocculation of a serum reaction.

floc'culus (pl. *flocculi*) [L. tuft]. 1. A lobe below and behind the middle peduncle of the cerebrum on each side of the median fissure. 2. A small tuft of wool-like fibers.

f. retinae. Ciliary process of retina.

flooding (flŭd'ing) [A.S. *flōd*]. Profuse uterine bleeding.

Flood's ligament [Valentine Flood, Irish surgeon, 1800-1847]. A band of ligaments attached to lower part of lesser tuberosity of the humerus.

floor. The surface which forms the lower limit of a cavity or space, as the floor of the cranial cavity, fourth ventricle, mouth, nasal fossa, or pelvis.

flora (flō'ra) [L. *flos, flor-*, flower]. 1. Plant life as distinguished from animal life. 2. Plant life occurring or adapted for living in a specific environment, as flora in the intestines.

florid (flor'id) [L. *flos*, flower]. Having a bright deep red color. Used to describe skin coloration.

floss, dental. Fibers used in dentistry to clean between the teeth.

flour [A.S. flower of meal, from L. *flos, flor-*, flower]. Finely ground meal obtained from wheat, or other grain; any soft fine powder. SEE: *bread; cereal.*

Flourens' theory (floo-ronz') [Marie J. P. Flourens, French physiologist, 1794-1867]. That thought is a process dependent upon the entire cerebrum.

flow [A.S. *flōwan*, to flow]. 1. Action of flowing; said of liquids. 2. The menstrual discharge. Bleeding from the uterus, but not as profusely as in flooding.

flower [L. *flōs, flor-*, flower]. That part of a plant which comprises the organs of reproduction. Ex: *anthemis, arnica, matricaria.* A complete flower includes a calyx, corolla, stamens which produce pollen, and a pistil which produces the ovule.

flowmeter. Device for measuring the flow of a gas. Used esp. in monitoring flow of anesthetic gases.

flucticuli (fluk-tik'ū-lī) (sing. *flucticulus*) [L. "little waves"]. Wavelike markings on lateral wall of 3rd ventricle.

fluctua'tion [L. *fluctuāre*, to flow in waves]. A wavy impulse felt in palpation and produced by vibration of body fluid.

DIAG: If felt over lower bowel ascites usually is present. May be caused by peritoneal hemorrhage. If confined to limited portion of abdomen, tuberculous peritonitis may be indicated; over central portion, bladder distention. In lower abdomen in women, an ovarian cyst or pregnancy. In right hypochondria, a hydatid cyst; abscess of liver, distended gallbladder; over left hypochondria, cysts or abscess. Above umbilicus, dilated colon or stomach partly filled with fluid and gas.

flu'id [L. *fluidus*]. A nonsolid, liquid, or gaseous substance. SEE ALSO: *secretion.*

f., amniotic. GYN: The fluid that fills the fetal membranes in pregnancy. A clear, yellowish fluid. Spec. grav. approximately 1.006. It is composed of albumin, salts (chiefly urea), and water, and suspended in it are lanugo, epidermal cells, *vernix caseosa*, and meconium.* It is derived from the cells of the amnion, although some claim it comes from the fetal urine and others that it is derived from the maternal circulation. Its chief function is protection for the fetus. SEE: *amnion.*

f. balance. Regulation of amount of water in the body by its controlling mechanism. The balance is upset when fluids are lost by vomiting, bleeding, or when dehydration occurs. When vital reflexes are disorganized, as in shock, collapse, septicemia, and toxemias, dehydration ensues. Increased fluid intake is indicated, but vitality may be so low fluid may pool in stomach, or if given rectally may lie in colon and not be absorbed. Intravenous, subcutaneous, and intraperitoneal injections may then be indicated.

f., cerebrospinal. That found in central canal of spinal cord and in the ventricles of the brain, also in the subarachnoid space about the brain and spinal cord. It is formed by the choroid plexuses of the ventricles.

f. diet. One for postoperative cases: carbonated water, ginger ale, tea, albumin, water, beef tea, broth, coffee. Raw fruit juices and milk should not be given unless ordered. SEE: *liquid diet.*

f., extracellular. The tissue fluid or the fluid occupying spaces between the tissue cells; interstitial fluid.

f., extravascular. All the body fluids outside the blood vessels; includes tissue fluid, fluids within the serous and synovial cavities, the cerebrospinal fluid, and lymph.

f., interstitial. The tissue fluid.

f., intracellular. The fluid contained within cells, and comprising about 50% of body weight.

f., intraocular. The fluid within the ant. and post. chambers of the eye.

f. retention. Failure to expel fluids of the body normally. OPP: *fluid balance.*

It occurs in nephritis with massive albuminuria. When protein content of plasma falls below 4% fluid cannot be attracted back into the blood stream and edema occurs. Fluid is retained in congestive heart failure. It should be detected by decreased urinary output. Retention of salt is another cause of fluid retention. Salt retention attracts fluid to maintain the isotonic concentration. A salt-free diet is indicated in fluid retention.

f., serous. A fluid in the serous cavities.

f., synovial. The fluid contained within synovial cavities, bursae, and tendon sheaths. SYN: *synovia.*

f., tissue. The interstitial or extracellular fluid.

fluidextract, fluidextractum (flext.) [L. *fluidus* + *extractum*, extract]. Solution of the soluble constituents of vegetable drugs of such strength that each cc. or ml. represents 1 gm. of the drug.

Fluidextracts contain alcohol as a solvent and/or preservative, and many of these give precipitates with water.

f., aromatic cascara sagrada. USP. Liquid preparation of cascara sagrada, the dried bark of *Rhamnus purshiana.* It is used as a cathartic.

f., glycyrrhiza. USP. A liquid preparation of glycyrrhiza (licorice root). It is a flavoring and a necessary ingredient for aromatic cascara sagrada f.

f., ipecac. USP. A fluid preparation of the powdered rhizome and roots of *Cephaelis ipecacuana* or *C. acuminata.* It is used as an emetic and expectorant.

flu'idounce. Eight fluidrams. SYMB: f ℥.

flu'idram. Measure of capacity equal to 57.1 gr. of distilled water; equal to 3.697 ml. SYMB: f ʒ.

fluke (flook) [A.S. *flōc*, flatfish]. A parasitic worm belonging to the class Trematoda, phylum Platyhelminthes. Those parasitic in man belong to the order Digenea. Most flukes have complex life cycles which include asexual generations that live in a mollusc (snail or bivalve). Stages of a typical fluke include adult, egg, miracidium, sporocyst, redia, cercaria, and metacercaria.

f., blood. A schistosome. Flukes of the genus *Schistosome, S. haematobium, S. mansoni,* and *S. japonicum.* Adults live principally in the mesenteric and pelvic veins. They cause schistosomiasis and schistosome dermatitis (swimmer's itch).

f., intestinal. Species of intestinal flukes infesting man include: *Gastrodiscoides hominis, Fasciolopsis buski, Heterophyes heterophyes, Metagonimus yokogawai.*

f., liver. Flukes which live in the liver and bile ducts. Species infesting man include: *Clonorchis sinensis, Fasciola hepatica, Dicrocoelium dendriticum,* and *Opisthrochis felineus.*

f., lung. Only one species is common in man, namely *Paragonimus westermani.*

flu'mina pilo'rum [L. rivers of hair]. The curved lines along which the hairs of the body are arranged, esp. in the fetus.

flu'or al'bus [L. white flow]. White discharge from the uterus or vagina. Syn: *leukorrhea.*

fluorescein (flu-o-res'e-in) A red crystalline powder.

Uses: Chiefly in diagnostic purposes, detecting foreign bodies in the eye, or corneal lesions.

fluorescence (flu-o-res'ents) [L. *fluere,* to flow]. Luminescence of a substance when acted on by short wave radiation.

Usually ultraviolet, first noted in fluorspar; caused by absorption of certain wave lengths and simultaneous emission of a longer wave length, which terminates simultaneously with the cessation of the incident exciting radiation.

fluorescent (flu-o-res'ent) [L. *fluere,* to flow]. 1. Biol: Having one color by transmitted light and another by reflected light. 2. Luminous when exposed to other rays.

f. antibody. Abbr: FA. An antibody which has been stained or marked by a fluorescent material. Use of the FA technique permits rapid diagnosis of various kinds of infections.

f. screen. 1. A sheet of cardboard, paper, or glass coated with a material which fluoresces visibly, such as calcium tungstate, used as the chief part of a fluoroscope when roentgen rays, radium rays, or electrons impinge upon it; a substitute for a fluoroscope in a darkened room. 2. A sheet of cardboard, paper, or glass, coated with anthracene or other fluorescing materials, to observe ultraviolet radiations.

fluoridation (flu-o-rĭ-da'shun). The addition of fluorides to a water supply as a means of preventing dental caries.

fluoride (flu-o-rīd) [L. *fluere,* to flow]. A compound of fluorine with a radicle; a salt of hydrofluoric acid.

fluorine (flu'o-rēn) [L. *fluere,* to flow]. Gaseous, chemical element. Symb: F. At. wt. 18.9984; at. no. 9.

This is found in the soil in combination with calcium. It seems absolutely necessary to plant life and in animal life it helps to form the bones and teeth. Insoluble mineral elements must be absorbed by plant life and taken into the animal body as food before they can be assimilated, but f. was liquefied by Moissan and Dewar in 1897. It is found in cow's milk, yolk of egg, and brain.

fluorometer (flu-o-rom'ĕ-ter) [" + G. *metron,* to measure]. Device for adjusting the shadow in skiagraphy.

fluoroscope (flu'o-ro-skōp or flu-or'o-skōp) [" + G. *skopein,* to examine]. A device consisting of a fluorescent screen suitably mounted, either separately or in conjunction with a roentgen tube, by means of which the shadows of objects interposed between the tube and the screen are made visible.

fluoros'copy [" + G. *skopein,* to examine]. The use of a fluoroscope for medical diagnosis or for testing various materials by roentgen rays.

fluorosis (flu-or-o'sis) [" + G. *ōsis*]. Chronic fluorine poisoning, sometimes marked by mottling of tooth enamel. Often results from too much fluoride in drinking water.

flush [A.S. *fluschen,* to fly up]. 1. Sudden redness of the skin. 2. Flushing of a cavity with water.

f., Harris. (Def. 2.) A technic used to relieve flatulence and distention of abdomen, esp. following abdominal surgery. About 200 cc. of water from an enema can (containing 500 cc.) is allowed to flow into the rectum. The enema can is then lowered so that the fluid from the rectum can return to the enema can. Bubbles seen in the fluid in the enema can indicate expulsion of gas.

f., hec'tic. Redness of the cheeks seen in some chronic affections, such as pulmonary tuberculosis, and due to rise of temperature.

f., hot. One accompanied with sensation of heat; common in neuroses and psychoneuroses and during menopause.

flut'ter [A.S. *floterian,* to fly about]. A tremulous movement, esp. of the heart as atrial and ventricular flutter.

f., atrial. Condition in which contractions of the atrium become extremely rapid (200-400 per min.). In *pure flutter,* a regular rhythm is maintained, in *impure flutter,* the rhythm is irregular. Syn: auricular f.

flux [L. *fluxus,* a flow]. 1. An excessive flow or discharge from an organ or cavity of the body; diarrhea. 2. Discharge from the bowels.

f., bloody. Dysentery.

f., menstrual. Menstrual flow.

fly [A.S. *flēoge*]. An insect belonging to the order Diptera, characterized by possessing sucking mouth parts, one pair of wings, and incomplete metamorphosis. Term is sometimes applied to insects belonging to other orders (ex. May fly, dragon fly). See: *Diptera.*

f., black. *Simulium, q.v.*

f., blow. Flies of the family *Calliphoridae.* They breed in dung or the flesh of dead animals. Also called *bluebottle flies.* See: *Calliphora vomitoria.*

f., bot. Botfly, *q.v.*

f., flesh. The *Sarcophagidae, q.v.*

f., house. *Musca domestica, q.v.*

f., sand. *Phlebotomus, q.v.*

f. screwworm. A fly belonging to the families *Calliphoridae* and *Sarcophagidae, q.v.*

f., Spanish. Cantharides, *q.v.*

f., tsetse. *Glossina palpalis.* One which transmits African sleeping sickness or trypanosomiasis.

f., warble. The *Dermatobia q.v.*

FM., FMN. Abbr. for *flavin mononucleotide.*

f.m. [L.]. Abbr. for *fiat mistura* (make a mixture).

foam. A mixture of finely divided gas bubbles interspersed in a liquid.

fo'cal [L. *focus,* hearth]. Pert. to a focus.

f. infection. One occurring near a focus, such as the cavity of a tooth.

f. lesion. A limited central lesion.

foci (fo'si) [L.]. Plural of focus, *q.v.*

fo'cus (pl. *foci*) [L. the hearth]. The point of convergence of light rays or waves of sound.

f., real. Point at which convergent rays intersect.

f., virtual. The point at which divergent rays would intersect if prolonged backward.

fog'ging, fog'ging sys'tem. A method of testing vision, used particularly in testing astigmatism, and in postcycloplegic examination.

fold [A.S. *foltan,* to fold]. A ridge; a doubling back. Syn: *plica.*

f., amniotic. Folded edge of the amniotic membrane where it rises over and finally encloses the embryo of birds, reptiles and some mammals.

f., genital. Fold of skin in the embryo on each side of the genital tubercle which develops into the labia minora in the female.

f., mesouterine. Fold of peritoneum supporting the uterus.

fo'lia. Plural of folium, *q.v.*

foliaceous (fo-lĭ-a'she-us) [L. *folia,* leaves]. Resembling or pert. to a leaf.

folic acid (fō'lik'. Pteroylglutamic acid. Found in liver, yeast, and green leaves. Used in treating macrocytic anemia due to folic acid deficiency, cliac syndrome, and sprue. Caution: Pernicious anemia should not be treated with folic acid but with vitamin B_{12}.

folie (fol-e') [Fr. foolish, mad]. Mania; psychosis.

f. à deux (ah-du'). Occurrence of psychosis at the same time in two closely associated persons.

f. circulaire. Frequent repetition of excited and depressed phases of manic-depressive psychosis. Syn: *circular insanity.*

f. du doute (du doot). Abnormal doubts about ordinary acts and beliefs; inability to decide upon definite standards of conduct.

folium (pl. *folia*) [L. leaf]. Thin, broad, leaflike structure.

f. vermis, f. cacuminis. A fold on the posterior part of the upper surface of the vermis of the cerebellum.

foll'icle [L. *folliculus,* little bag]. 1. A small secretory sac or cavity. 2. A lymphatic nodule (obs.).

f., aggregated. Peyer's patch, *q.v.*

f., atretic. An ovarian follicle that has undergone degeneration or involution.

f., graafian. Gyn: The complete development of the primary oocyte in the cortex of the ovary to the stage where the ovum is fully developed. See: *ovary.*

f., growing. A developing follicle of the ovary.

f., hair. An invagination of the epidermis from which a hair develops.

f., nabothian. Dilated cyst of the glands of the cervix uteri.

f., ovarian. A spherical structure in the cortex of the ovary consisting of an oogonium, or an oocyte and its surrounding epithelial (follicular) cells. Follicles are of three types: 1. *Primary,* consisting of an oogonium and a single layer of follicular cells. 2. *Growing,* in which the follicle cells proliferate forming several layers and the first maturation division occurs. 3. *Vesicular,* or *graafiian* follicle which possesses a cavity *(antrum)* containing the follicular fluid *(liquor folliculi).* The oocyte lies in the *cumulus oophorus,* a mass of cells on the inner surface. The cells lining the follicle constitute the *stratum granulosum.* The follicle is a secretory structure producing estrogens.

f., sebaceous. Oil gland of the skin.

f., solitary. A single lymph nodule of the intestine.

f., thyroid. Spherical or ovoid structure found in the thyroid gland lined with a single layer of cuboidal epithelial cells which secrete the thyroid hormone. The follicles are filled with *colloid,* a viscid substance rich in iodine.

f., vesicular. One containing a cavity; a mature ovarian or graafian follicle.

folliclis (fol'ik-lis) [L. *folliculus,* little bag]. Indolent papulonecrotic lesion, esp. on the extremities and possibly the face due to tuberculosis.

follic'ular [L. *folliculus,* little bag]. Pert. to a follicle or follicles.

f. tonsillitis. Inflammation of follicles on surface of the tonsil which become filled with pus.

f. tumor. A sebaceous cyst.

follic'ulin [L. *folliculus,* little bag]. An internal secretion of the ovary which, with lutein and ovulin, forms the oophorin hormone. See: *estrin.*

folliculitis (fol-ik-u-li'tis) [" + G. *-itis,* inflammation]. Inflammation of a follicle or follicles.

f. barbae. *Tinea barbae, q.v.*

f. decalvans. Purulent follicular inflammation of the scalp resulting in irregular alopecia and scarring. Syn: *acne decalvans, Quinquad's disease.*

Etiol: Essential cause unknown. Believed to be caused by staphylococci. Affects mostly males between 2nd and 4th decades.

Sym: Initial inflammatory papule or pustule at mouth of follicle pierced by a hair is followed by crusting and desiccation, when it drops off along with loosened hair. Bald patches, with slight depressed whitish center surrounded by inflamed margin. Extends peripherally.

Path: Perivascular, particularly lower half of follicle sheaths; sebaceous gland atrophy and flattened papillae.

Prog: Baldness is permanent, though extension may be arrested.

Treatment: Externally, topical antibiotics or corticosteroids, frequent shampoos, and daily antiseptic.

f. sebacea. Inflammation of the sebaceous glands, with accumulation of secretion. Syn: *acne.*

folliculoma (fol-ik-u-lo'mă) [" + G. *ōma,* tumor]. A tumor of the ovary originating in a graafian follicle, in which the cells resemble the cells of the *stratum granulosum.*

folliculose (fol-ik'u-lōs) [L. *folliculus,* little bag]. Composed of follicles.

folliculo'sis [" + G. *-ōsis*]. Presence of an abnormal quantity of lymph follicles.

folliculus (fŏ-lik'u-lus) (pl. *fol'liculi*) [L. little bag]. A follicle.

f. oophorus vesiculosus. A graafian follicle, *q.v.*

fomentation (fo-men-ta'shun) [L. *fomentāre,* to apply a poultice]. A hot, wet application for the relief of pain or inflammation. SEE: *stupe.*

f., boracic. This may be prepared with boracic lint, which is already impregnated with boracic acid, and is colored pink as a distinguishing mark; or boracic acid may be added to lint, either in form of powder or crystals, and then wrung out of boiling water as before.

f., medical. Instead of lint, 2 or 3 thicknesses of flannel are used, and the fomentation is applied to unbroken skin, otherwise procedure is same as for a surgical fomentation; it is unnecessary to boil it; flannel is used because it retains the heat better than lint. This fomentation is also called a *stupe, q.v.*

f., surgical. SEE: *hot moist dressing.*

fomes (fo'mēz) (pl. *fomites*) [L. tinder]. Any substance that absorbs and transmits infectious material.

fomites (fo'mĭ-tēz). Plural of fomes, *q.v.*

Fontan'a's spaces [Felice Fontana, Italian scientist, 1730-1805]. Spaces bet. the processes of ligamentum pectinatum of the iris. These convey the aqueous humor.

fontanel, fontanelle (fon-tan-el') [Fr. *fontanelle,* little fountain]. An unossified space or "soft spot" lying between the cranial bones of the skull of a fetus.

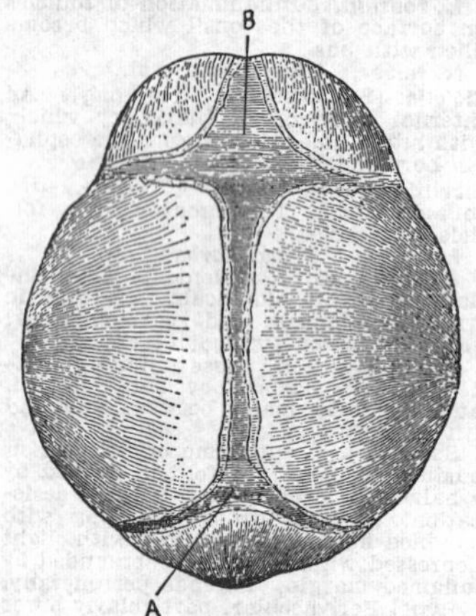

THE FONTANELS
A. Posterior fontanel.
B. Anterior fontanel.

f., anterior. At the junction of the coronal, frontal, and sagittal sutures.

f., posterior. At the junction of the sagittal and lambdoid sutures.

fonticulus (fon-tik'u-lus) [L. little fountain]. SYN: *fontanel.*

food (pl. *foods*). Nutritive substance which provides heat and energy, etc. for maintenance of well-being of the body. SEE ALSO: specific names of food items in alphabetical order.

f. accessories. Nutrient substances which do not provide energy but furnish substances essential for the growth and well-being of the body. Includes water, mineral salts, and vitamins.

f. allergies. Allergic reactions resulting from ingestion of foods to which a person has become sensitized. One may become sensitive to almost any food; shellfish, pork, eggs, milk, spinach, lettuce, strawberries and tomatoes are the most common offenders.

SYM: Urticaria (hives), certain eczemas, nausea, vomiting, diarrhea, and intestinal cramps. A syndrome (angioneurotic edema) characterized by a transient swelling of various parts of the body and spasm of the intestine may result.

f. ball. Gastric stone made up of fruit and vegetable skins, seeds and fibers. SYN: *phytobezoar.*

f., course of (through the alimentary canal). Foods enter the mouth and in the buccal area are reduced to a pulp or semifluid mass through the processes of mastication and insalivation (the mixing of food with saliva). Swallowing or deglutition then occurs. In swallowing, the food mass or *bolus* passes into the *pharynx* and then through the *esophagus* to the *stomach,* the entrance to which is controlled by the cardiac sphincter.

Stomach. In the stomach the food is stored and mixed with gastric juice. After it attains a certain fluid consistency, it passes through the *pyloric* sphincter into the small intestine.

Small intestine. In the first portion or *duodenum* the intestinal contents, now called *chyme,* are mixed with bile, secreted by the liver, and the pancreatic juice, both of which enter through the opening of the common bile duct. In the next two portions, the *jejunum* and *ileum,* the chyme is mixed with the intestinal juice secreted by the intestinal glands or crypts of Lieberkuhn. In the small intestine, digestion is completed and the end products of digestion (simple sugars, amino acids, fatty acids and glycerol) are absorbed into the capillaries and lacteals of the intestinal mucosa.

Large intestine. Undigestible material passes from the small intestine into the large intestine (colon) through the *ileocecal valve* located at the junction of the ascending colon and the cecum, a blind pouch which terminates in the vermiform appendix. The material continues through the colon (ascending, transverse, descending and sigmoid) to the *rectum* from which it is discharged through the *anal canal* as the feces, at the anus or anal orifice. In the large intestine, the major portion of the water of the intestinal contents is absorbed. Digestive changes are limited to the action of bacteria which bring about putrefaction and fermentation of incompletely digested foods. No enzymes are secreted by the glands of the large intestine.

f., enriched. F. to which have been added vitamins or minerals removed in refining and processing; foods in which the vitamin and (or) mineral content has been increased either by addition or by irradiation.

f. fever. Sudden rise in temperature accompanying digestive disturbances in children, supposed to be result of intestinal autointoxication.

f. infections. Illness resulting from infectious organisms which enter the body in food or drink. Among the organisms which may be ingested are (1) bacteria, esp. those of the salmonella group and certain staphylococci and streptococci, typhoid, paratyphoid, and dysentery bacilli, (2) the eggs, encysted forms or larvae of

ORGANIC

Proteins

Elements	Symbol	Per Cent
1. Carbon	C	53 %
2. Hydrogen	H	7 %
3. Oxygen	O	22 %
4. Nitrogen	N	16 %
5. Sulfur	S	1½%
6. Phosphorous	P	½%
7. Other Minerals		trace
		100%

End Products

Urea, uric acid, H_2SO_4, CO_2, H_2O.
Salts set free.
Proteins are tissue, including muscle and nerve, builders and also furnish heat and energy.

Classification of Proteins

Albumen	Casein	Gluten	Myosin
Eggs	Milk	Cereals	Fowls
Meat	Cheese	Beans	
		Peas	
		Lentils	
		Nuts	

Carbohydrates (Cx(H_2O)y)

Elements	Symbol	Per Cent
1. Carbon	C	76%
2. Hydrogen	H	12%
3. Oxygen	O	12%
		100%

End Products

Salts set free

CO_2 and H_2O

Classification of Carbohydrates

Glucose	Cane Sugar	Cellulose
$C_6H_{12}O_6$	$C_{12}H_{22}O_{11}$	$C_6H_{10}O_5$

Carbohydrates as well as fats are heat and energy producers, but neither can take the place of proteins, as they contain no nitrogen. They consist principally of the sugars, starch, cellulose and fibers.

Fats

Elements	Symbol	Per Cent
1. Carbon	C	45%
2. Hydrogen	H	06%
3. Oxygen	O	49%
		100%

End Products

CO_2 and H_2O

Fats are heat and energy producers and not tissue or cell builders.

Origin of Fats

Animal	Oils	Nuts	Fruits
Butter, Lard, Meat	Cottonseed, Corn, Sunflower	Peanuts	Palm, Olive

Food Accessories
Water, Minerals, Vitamins

TEMPERATURE BEST SUITED FOR STORAGE OF FOODS

Fruits

	Degrees F.
Apples	31-32
Bananas	34-36
Berries	34-36
Cantaloupe	32
Cranberries	33-34
Dried Fruits	35-40
Fresh Fruits	33-40
Lemons	36
Oranges	36
Watermelons	32

Vegetables

	Degrees F.
Fresh	33-35

Meats and Fish

	Degrees F.
Brined Meats	35-40
Beef, Fresh	37-39
Fish, Fresh	25-30
Fish, Frozen	25
Fish, Dried	25
Ham	30-35
Lard	34-35
Mutton	32-36
Oysters	33-40
Oysters in Shell	40
Oysters in Tubs	35
Pork	30-33
Poultry	29
Poultry, Frozen	5-10
Veal	32-36
Milk	50-60

animal parasites such as *Trichinella*, tapeworms, and other parasitic worms.

f., nutrient substances of. Substances which in the body serve as a source of energy or provide materials for the growth and repair of tissue. Foods are organic substances (proteins, carbohydrates, fats) present in animal and plant tissues. Nutrient substances which do not provide energy are called *food accessories, q.v.* The term "food" is commonly used to refer to any substance taken into the body which serves a nutrient function.

f. poisoning. An attack of illness or a digestive disorder resulting from the ingestion of foods containing poisonous substances. True food poisoning includes mushroom poisoning, shellfish poisoning, poisoning resulting from foods contaminated with poisonous insecticides or other poisons, milk sickness (due to milk from cows that have fed on certain poisonous plants); and occasionally poisoning resulting from eating foods that have undergone putrefaction or decomposition. It may also be due to bacteria, especially paratyphoid bacilli and staphylococci ingested in food.

f., protective. Foods which are the richest sources of basic nutritional needs (water, proteins, vitamins, essential fatty acids, inorganic salts). These include milk, milk products, eggs, fruits, and leafy vegetables.

f. rashes. In those with an idiosyncrasy to some protein certain rashes may be the only symptom of toxemia. They may be in form of *urticaria, erythema,* or *papules,* or a combination of these.

f. requirements. "It is ordinarily assumed that an average man in health performing light to moderate muscular work requires per day about 0.25 pound protein and 3050 calories of energy, the latter being supplied in part by protein, but mostly by fat and carbohydrates. Persons in sedentary occupations require smaller amounts.

"A diet made up of ordinary foods and supplying the necessary amounts of protein and energy would undoubtedly supply an abundance of mineral matter. It has been found that women and children consume somewhat less food than men. The assumption is usually made that, provided a woman is engaged in some moderately active occupation, she requires about eight-tenths as much as a man with a similar amount of work.

"In calculating the results of dietary studies (which may be most conveniently expressed in amounts for 1 man for 1 day), it is further assumed that a boy 13-14 years old and a girl 15-16 years old also require about eight-tenths as much food as a man at moderately active muscular labor; a boy of 12 and a girl 13-14 years old, about seven-tenths; a boy 10-11 and a girl 10-12 years old, about six-tenths; a child 6-9 years old, about five-tenths; one 2-5, about four-tenths, and an infant under 2 years, about three-tenths."—*U. S. Dept. Agriculture.*

(Daily quantities of the principal foods for a patient weighing about 132 lb.):

Salad and Vegetable	200 gm.
Raw Vegetable	100 gm.
Fruit	375 gm.
Fat (butter, oil, etc.)	100 gm.
Milk	1250 gm.
Cream	100 gm.
Egg	One to one-and-a-half
Meat, Viscera, Fish	70 gm.
Potatoes	125 gm.
Bread	60 gm.
Zwieback or Cookie	20 gm.
Starch (flour, rice, farina, oatmeal, etc.)	30 gm.
Sugar or Honey	30 gm.

Contain about 90 gm. protein, 164 gm. fat, 244 gm. carbohydrate, with total calories 2886 and about 3.4 gm. sodium chloride.

By the Average Healthy Adult Man at Moderate Work

Proteins	100 gm.	12-15% caloric value
Fats	100 gm.	20-30% caloric value
Carb.	500 gm.	50-70% caloric value
Water	3000 cc.	

Minerals as follows: calcium 0.8 gm., phosphorus 1.5 gm., sodium 3 to 6 gm., potassium 2 to 4 gm., sodium chloride 5 to 15 gm. and vitamins, *q.v.*

Seven Basic Food Groups as recommended by the U. S. Dept. of Agriculture are: 1. Leafy Green and Yellow Vegetables, 2. Citrus fruit, tomatoes, raw cabbage, 3. Potatoes and other vegetables and fruits, 4. Milk, cheese, ice cream, 5. Meat, poultry, fish, eggs, dried peas, beans, 6. Bread, flour, cereals, whole grain or enriched, 7. Butter and fortified margarine.

SEE: *names of condiments, drinks, and foods, according to alphabetical order.*

foot [A.S. *fōt*]. (*pes*). 1. The terminal portion of the lower extremity. The bones of the foot include the *tarsus, metatarsus,* and *phalanges.* SEE: *skeleton.* 2. A unit of measurement.

f. arches. Four arches: (a) Int. longitudinal; (b) outer l., and (c) 2 transverse ones.

f., athlete's. SEE: ***athlete's foot.***

f. bath, mustard. AIM: To aid action of hot water in relieving congestion in some distant part of the body.

ARTICLES NEEDED: Bath blanket. Small rubber sheet and large bath towel. Foot tub with water at 110° F. and bath thermometer which is left in tub during treatment. Mustard. Old muslin about 6 in. square. Tablespoon. Hot water bottle filled and covered. Pitcher of very hot water.

PROCEDURE: 1. Measure mustard in the proportion of 1 tablespoonful to 1 gallon of water and tie in the square of muslin. 2. Put in tub and add water. Rub mustard bag between fingers to dissolve mustard and allow it to diffuse through the water. 3. Loosen upper bedding at foot of bed and turn back to patient's knees. 4. Flex knees. 5. Place rubber sheet covered with bath towel across bed under patient's feet. 6. Put tub on towel and place feet in tub, arranging patient as comfortably as possible. 7. Cover knees, feet and tub with bath blanket, tucking under tub so it does not drop into water. 8. Lay upper bedding down over blanket and tub but do not tuck in. 9. Continue treatment 20 minutes unless patient complains of burning sensation. In that case stop it at once. 10. As bath cools add hot water from pitcher. Lift feet out before doing this. Check temperature with thermometer. 11. Watch patient and if she feels faint stop treatment at once. The swift withdrawal of blood from head to feet may cause syncope. 12. At end of treatment lift feet, draw tub toward you and put feet down on towel. Remove tub. Dry feet well. 13. Put hot water bottle at foot of bed if desired and permitted. Arrange bedding and make patient comfortable. 14. Clean and replace equipment. 15. Record treatment.

f. and mouth disease. Aphthous fever, *q.v.*

f. candle. (Def. 2.) Amt. of light radiated 1 ft. from a standard candle. SYN: *light u.*

f., cleft. Condition in which a cleft extends between the digits to the metatarsal region, usually due to a missing digit.

f., contracted. Clawfoot or *pes cavus, q.v.*

f., flat. Flatfoot, *q.v.;* pes planus.

f., immersion. Condition resulting from prolonged immersion of the feet in water.

f., Madura. Bone hypertrophy and degeneration, frequently followed by suppuration or gangrene.

f. plate. Base of the stapes; an ossicle of the tympanum. It fits into, and closes, the *fenestra vestibuli* (oval window).

f. pound. (Def. 2.) Amt. of energy required to raise 1 pound 1 foot from a level.

f. print. An impression of the foot, esp., an ink impression used for identification of infants.

f., splay. Flatfoot accompanied by extreme eversion of the foot.

f., weak. Condition resulting from weakened muscles, or from faulty walking habits. Results in chronic eversion of the foot.

footdrop. A falling or dragging of the foot from paralysis of the flexors of the ankle.

foot'ling presentation. Presentation of feet foremost in labor.

forage (for-azh') [Fr. boring]. Cutting

FOOT

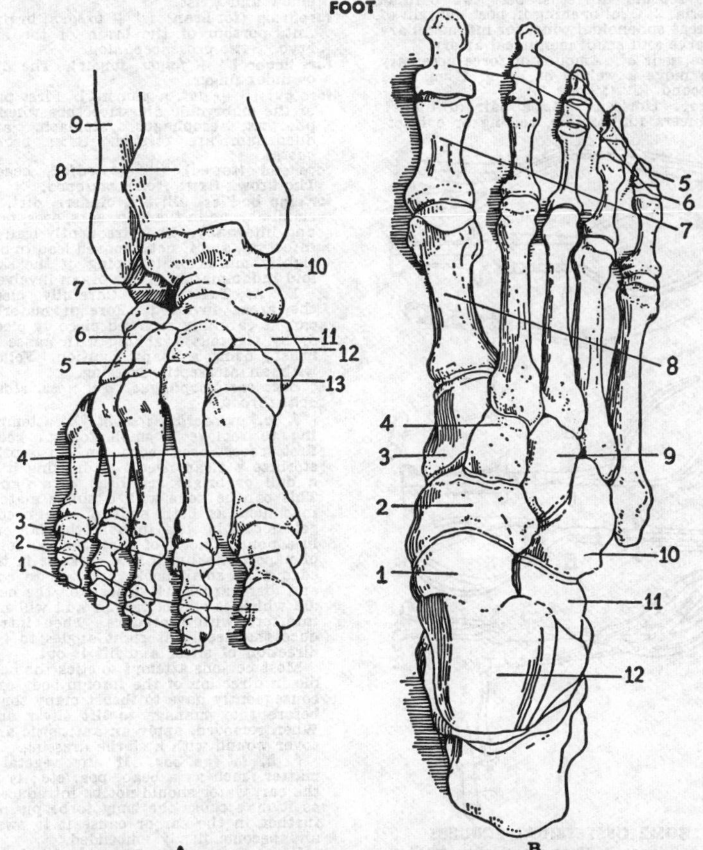

TARSAL AND METATARSAL BONES AND PHALANGES

A 1. 3rd Phalanges. 2. 2nd Phalanges. 3. 1st Phalanges. 4. Metatarsals. 5. External Cuneiform. 6. Cuboid. 7. Os Calcis. 8. Tibia. 9. Fibula. 10. Astragalus. 11. Scaphoid. 12. Middle Cuneiform. 13. Internal Cuneiform.

B 1. Astragalus. 2. Scaphoid. 3. Internal Cuneiform. 4. Middle Cuneiform. 5. 3rd Phalanges. 6. 2nd Phalanges. 7. 1st Phalanges. 8. Metatarsals. 9. External Cuneiform. 10. Cuboid. 11. Os Calcis. 12. Astragalus (talus).

a channel by diathermy through an enlarged prostate or other tissue.

foramen (for-a'men) (pl. *foram ina*) [L. an opening]. A passage or opening; an orifice, a communication between two cavities of an organ, or a hole in a bone for passage of vessels or nerves.

f., intervertebral. Opening between every two articulated vertebrae for passage of nerves to and from spinal cord.

f. magnum. It pierces the occipital bone through which passes the spinal cord from the brain.

f. of Monro. Opening bet. third and lateral ventricles of the brain.

f., obturator. Large oval f. below acetabulum bounded by the pubis and ischium. SEE: *Magendie's f.*

f., olfactory. An opening in the ethmoid bone for passage of the olfactory nerves.

f. ova'le. 1. Opening at lower post. of septum in fetus, bet. two cardiac atria. 2. Oval opening in post. margin of great sphenoidal wing, for inf. maxillary nerve and small meningeal artery.

force, unit of. Amount of force necessary to move a weight of 1 gm. 1 cm. in 1 second. SYN: *dyne.*

forceps (for'seps) [L. a pair of tongs]. Pincers for holding, seizing or extracting. There are many distinct types of forceps, varying according to the operation for which they are intended.

f., artery. F. for holding ends of an artery in order to perform ligation.

f., bone. F. used for cutting bone and removal of bone fragments.

f., dressing. F. for general use in dressing wounds—removing dead tissue, drainage tubes, etc.

f., needle. F. for grasping and holding a needle.

f., ronguer. F. used for cutting bone.

forcipate (for'sip-āt) [L. *forceps, forcip-*, tongs]. Forceps shaped.

for'cipressure [" + *pressura,* pressure]. Arresting hemorrhage by pressure on an artery with forceps.

fore- [O.Eng.]. Prefix meaning *before* or *in front of.*

forearm (fōr'arm) [A.S. *fore,* in front, + *arm,* arm]. The part of arm between elbow and wrist.

forebrain (fōr'brān) [" + *bregen,* brain]. Ant. portion of the brain of the embryo. SYN: *prosencephalon.*

fore'finger [" + *finger,* finger]. The first or index finger.

fore'gut [" + *gut,* a pouring]. First part of the embryonic digestive tube whence pharynx, esophagus, stomach, and duodenum are formed. SYN: *protogaster.*

forehead (for'ed) [" + *heāfod,* head]. The brow. SYN: *frons, metopon.*

for'eign bod'ies. Slivers, cinders, dirt, or small objects in the skin, ears, eyes, nose and internally. They frequently lead to infection, and if not removed lead to unsightly marks or tattooing of the skin and inflammation of the organ involved.

F. A. TREATMENT: Carefully clean the areas involved. Foreign material can be carefully removed piece by piece, or by vigorous swabbing with gauze or brush, using a soapy solution. Follow with an antiseptic dressing.

SEE: *ear, esophagus, eye, nose, stomach, throat.*

f. b., extracting a small. In attempting to remove a small foreign body, first cover area with an antiseptic; sterilize a clean needle by heating it to a dull or bright red heat in a flame. This can be done with a single match; inasmuch as both ends of the needle get hot it is wise to hold the far end in a nonconductor of heat, such as folds of paper, sticking it in a cork, or in the edge of a small book; allow it to cool and disregard black deposit on the needle which is sterile carbon and will not interfere with procedure. Then introduce the needle at right angles to the direction of sliver and lift it out.

Most persons attempt to stick the needle in direction of the foreign body and consequently have to thrust many times before they manage to lift sliver out. When removed, apply an antiseptic and cover wound with a sterile dressing.

f. b. in the ear. If any vegetable matter, such as a bean, pea, etc., is in the ear, water should not be introduced, as it may cause the body to be pushed further in the ear or cause it to swell and become firmly embedded.

F. A. TREATMENT: Place a globule of glue on the end of a match stick or an applicator; gently introduce it until it touches the foreign body and then remove gently.

If an insect is in the ear, the patient may experience loud buzzing, pain and dizziness. TREATMENT: Flood ear with

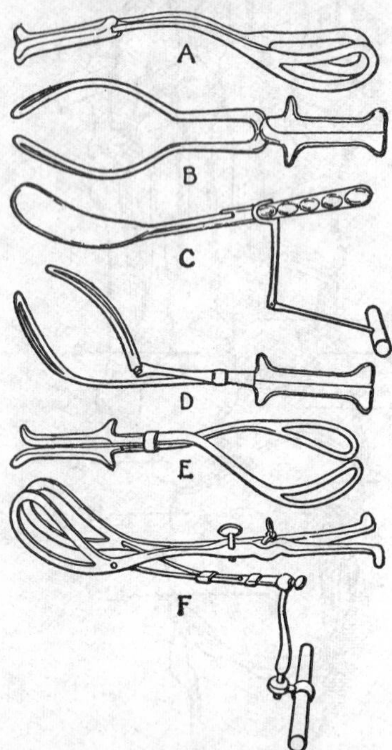

SOME OBSTETRICAL FORCEPS

A, Piper; B, Simpson (DeLee modification); C, Tucker-McLean with Bill's axis traction handle; D, Barton; E, Kielland; F, Tarnier axis traction. (From Bryant and Overland: Woodward & Gardner's Obstetric Management and Nursing, 7th ed., 1964.)

warm oil or water, letting insect float out.

f. b. in wounds. They are often present in wounds and generally should be left undisturbed if a surgeon is available within a short time. If small, as a sliver, it may be desirable to remove it. If large, it may be very dangerous to try any method of removing, inasmuch as it might be embedded in large blood vessels, muscles, etc., and removing it might result in much loss of blood or might cause breaking off of splinters, particles of rust, dirt, etc.; within a very few moments tissue juices, blood, and the natural reaction of swelling would tend to fill in the wounds and cover this foreign material, making it exceedingly difficult for the doctor to care for the patient.

In such instances, it is much wiser when possible, to leave the large foreign body in position, and obtain the services of a doctor promptly.

forensic (for-en'sik) [L. *forensis,* pert. to a forum]. Pert. to the law; legal.

f. medicine. Legal medicine or medicine in relation to the law.

fore'pleasure [A.S. *fore,* before, + L. *placere,* to please]. Any action that induces or intensifies sexual desire before orgasm.

fore'skin [" + *skinn,* skin]. Prepuce* or loose skin at and covering the end of the penis.

Excision of the prepuce constitutes circumcision. *Smegma* praeputii* is secreted by Tyson's glands and collects under the foreskin. SEE: *circumcision.*

NP: In infant cases the nurse must see that the prepuce is not adherent or interfering with urination. Abnormalities must be reported to the doctor.

-form [L. *forma*]. Suffix meaning *having the form of.*

formaldehyde (for-mal'de-hīd). USP. CH_2O. A colorless, pungent, irritant gas commonly made by oxidation of methyl alcohol; the simplest member of the group of aldehydes.* It is used in medicinal form as *formaldehyde solution* which contains 37% of f. with methanol added.

ACTION AND USES: A disinfectant; also a preservative and fumigant. A 10% solution is useful as an astringent.

A 1% or 2% solution used for cleansing dishes, instruments, or fabrics. Formaldehyde is a powerful disinfectant, esp. in the form of gas, because of its penetrating power, but it is active only in the presence of an abundance of moisture. The solution is germicidal in the strength of from 1% to 2%, but the action may be delayed from 20-30 minutes. It hardens tissues and is often used in histology for this purpose. It has a similar hardening effect on the living skin; it is very irritating to mucous membranes and produces reddening, inflammation, and necrosis, if applied repeatedly or continuously. It is sometimes used in soap for disinfection of the hands. A 10% solution is used for sterilizing feces, urine, and sputum; 5% to 10% for clothing and towels. SEE: *fumigation.*

POISONING: SYM: Local irritation of eyes, nose, mouth, throat; respiratory and gastrointestinal tracts and central nervous system; causing vertigo, stupor, abdominal pain, convulsions, unconsciousness, renal damage.

F. A. TREATMENT: Administration of dilute aromatic spirits of ammonia, very dilute ammonia water, as ammonium acetate which seems to combine with the formaldehyde, forming nonpoisonous methenamine. Otherwise symptomatic treatment.

for'malin. Aqueous solution of 37% of formaldehyde with methanol added. SEE: *aldehyde.*

formate (for'māt). A salt of formic acid.

formatio (for-ma'shĭ-ō [L. formation]. A structure with definite arrangement and shape.

f. reticula'ris [NA]. Dorsal part of of the medulla oblongata.

forma'tion. 1. A structure, shape, or figure. 2. The giving of form or shape to, or the development of a structure.

f. reaction. Development of attributes that hold in check and repress the components of infantile sexuality.

f., reticular. A reticular structure formed of gray matter and interlacing fibers of white matter found in the medulla oblongata between the pyramids and the floor of the 4th ventricle. It is also present in the spinal cord, midbrain, and pons. SYN: *formatio reticularis.*

forme fruste (form früst) [Fr. from L. *forma,* form, + *frustra,* without effect]. An aborted form of disease arrested before running its course.

for'mic [L. *formica,* ant]. Pert. to ants or to formic acid.

for'mic acid. H.COOH, a clear, pungent, liquid obtained from the oxidation of formaldehyde or wood alcohol. It was originally obtained from the distillation of the bodies of red ants, and is probably the cause of the pain and swelling resulting from the bites or stings of certain insects or the irritation from nettles.

f. aldehyde. Formaldehyde.

f. ether. Volatile anesthetic liquid ethyl formate.

formica'tion [L. *formica,* ant]. A sensation as of ants creeping upon the body; a form of paresthesia.

formiciasis (for-mis-i'ă-sis) [L. *formica,* ant]. Symptoms caused by ant bites.

formilase (for'mĭ-lās). A ferment which converts acetic acid into formic acid.

formin (for'mĭn). SEE: *methenamine.*

for'mula [L. a little form]. 1. A rule prescribing ingredients with proportions for the preparation of a compound. 2. CHEM: An expression by symbols of the constitution of a molecule consisting of letters, each denoting 1 atom of 1 elementary substance, with figures denoting the number of atoms present.

Collections of atoms which constitute a group by themselves (radical) are often separated by periods or parentheses, and in this case figures prefixed or appended to the parentheses or placed before an expression contained within periods apply to all the symbols embraced by the parentheses or periods.

In all other cases, a figure prefixed to a symbolical expression for a molecule, like a coefficient in an algebraical f., is understood to be a multiplier of all the symbols following.

f., Arneth's. Method of estimating number of immature leukocytes by means of an elaborate differential blood count.

f., dental. F. showing the number and arrangement of the teeth. For the permanent teeth,

$$i\frac{2}{2},\ c\frac{1}{1},\ pm\frac{2}{2},\ m\frac{3}{3} = \frac{8}{8} \times 2\ 32.$$

f., empirical. The f. of a compound which shows the atoms and their numbers in a molecule, as H_2O.

f., official. One in a pharmacopeia.

f., structural. The formula of a compound which shows the relations of the atoms to each other in a molecule. The atoms are shown joined by valence bonds, for example: H-O-H.

form'ulary [L. *formula,* a little form]. A book of formulas.

f., national. One issued by the *American Pharmaceutical Association.*

formyl. The radical of formic acid, HCO.

for'nicate [L. *fornix,* arch; brothel]. 1. Arched or vaultlike. 2. To indulge in illicit sexual intercourse.

fornica'tion [L. *fornix,* brothel]. The act of illicit sexual intercourse.

fornices (for'nĭ-sēz). Plural of fornix, *q.v.*

for'nicolumn [L. *fornix,* arch, + *columna,* column]. The ant. pillar of the fornix.

fornicommissure (for-nĭ-kom'is-ūr) [" + *commissura,* a joining together]. The commissure or body of the fornix uteri.

for'nix (pl. *fornices*) [L. arch]. 1. A fibrous vaulted band connecting the cerebral lobes. 2. Any body with vaultlike or arched shape.

f. conjunctivae [NA]. Ophth: Loose fold connecting palpebral and bulbar conjunctivae.

f. uteri. Ant. and post. spaces into which the upper vagina is divided. These recesses are formed by protrusion of the cervix uteri into the vagina.

f. vaginae. The f. uteri, *q.v.*

f. supratonsillaris [NA]. Space bet. anterior and posterior pillars of the fauces above the tonsil.

fossae (fos'e). Plural of fossa, *q.v.*

fossette (fos-et') [Fr. a little ditch]. 1. A small depression or fossa. 2. A small but deep corneal ulcer.

foulage (foo-lazh') [Fr. impression]. Kneading with pressure of the muscles.

fourchet, fourchette (foor-shet') [Fr. *fourchette,* a fork]. A tense band or transverse fold of mucous membrane at the post. commissure of the vagina, connecting the post. ends of the labia minora.

The *fossa navicularis,* a more or less deep *cul-de-sac* anterior to the fourchette, separates it from the hymen. It disappears after defloration or parturition, leaving a more open vulva below and behind. Syn: *frenulum labiorum pudendi.*

fourth cranial nerve. Trochlear nerve, *q.v.*

fovea (fo've-ă) [L. pit]. A pit or cuplike depression. See: *fossa.*

f. centralis retinea [NA]. Pit in the middle of macula lutea.

foveate (fo've-āt) [L. *fovea,* pit]. Pitted; having depressions.

foveation (fo-ve-a'shun) [L. *fovea,* pit]. Pitting, as in smallpox.

foveola (fo-ve'o-lă) [L. little pit]. A minute pit or depression.

Fow'ler's position [George R. Fowler, American surgeon, 1848-1906]. This places the patient in a semi-sitting position.

The head of bed may be raised on blocks, pins, or other support, or the back rest may be elevated, or patient may rest upon 4 or 5 pillows. It is more easily maintained if the patient sits in a swing or hammock, made by folding a bedsheet lengthwise, placing center of sheet tightly across the buttocks, with one end on each side. The ends are fastened securely at head of the bed, or as high as ends will reach.

This position may be ordered if patient is suffering from dyspnea,* after a thyroid or an abdominal operation and where there is drainage expected. Some pneumonia patients are placed in this position. In many instances it is contraindicated.

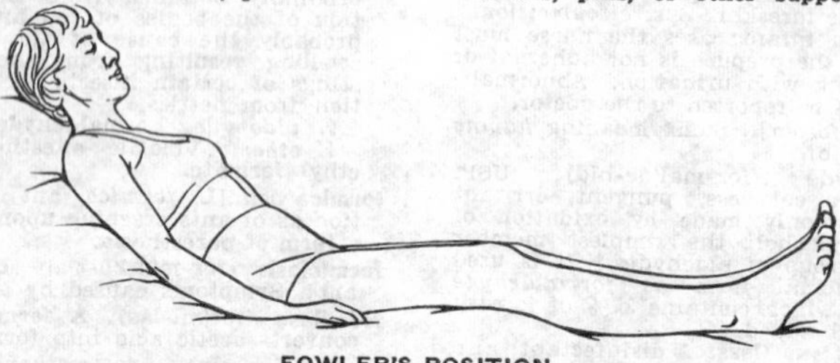

FOWLER'S POSITION.

fortifica'tion spectrum. Appearance of dark patch with zigzag outline in visual field. Syn: *scintillating scotoma; teichopsia.*

Foshay's serum [Lee Foshay, American physician, 1896-]. One used in the treatment of tularemia.

fossa (fos'ă) (pl. *fossae*) [L. ditch]. A furrow or shallow depression.

f., amygdaloid. Depression containing the tonsil.

f., axillary. The armpit.

f., Claudius'. Triangular area harboring the ovary.

f., iliac. One of the concavities of the iliac bones of pelvis. The right one contains the apepndix. Syn: *f. iliaca* [NA].

f. lacrimalis. Hollow of frontal bone holding the lacrimal gland.

f. navicularis. One bet. the vulva and fourchette. Syn: *f. vestibuli vaginae* [NA].

f. ovalis. 1. Opening in thigh for large saphenous vein. 2. [NA] Remnant of embryonic foramen ovale in right cardiac atrium.

f., Rosenmuller's. Depression in pharynx posterior to opening of eustachian tube.

Fowler-Murphy method [George R. Fowler; John B. Murphy, American surgeon, 1857-1916]. Elevation of head of bed with tube through an incision in right iliac fossa for drainage in diffuse suppurative peritonitis. Continuous rectal irrigation with a physiological salt solution accompanies the treatment.

Fowler's solution [Thomas Fowler, English physician, 1736-1801]. An arsenical solution containing 0.95 to 1.5 gm. of arsenic trioxide for each 100 cc. of solution. Syn: *potassium arsenite solution.*

Fr. Chem. symb. for *francium.*

fraction. One or more of the separable parts of a substance.

fractional. Pertaining to a fraction or a portion of a whole.

fractional test meal. *Fractional examination of stomach contents.* A method for the collection and examination of stomach contents as follows. First the residual contents are removed and then the test meal given. After the meal, samples are removed every 15 min. for two hours, examined and submitted to chemical tests.

Free hydrochloric acid, bile, blood, starch, mucus, and the total of acids are looked for. Free hydrochloric and total acids are normally small in amt.

In peptic ulcers there is a high acid curve, and a low one in carcinoma, and an absence of acid in pernicious anemia.

fracture (frak'tūr) [L. *fractura, frangere,* to break]. 1. A sudden breaking of a bone. 2. A broken bone.

RS: *buttonhole f., cerclage, extension, green stick f., Lucas-Championnière's method, malunion, name of bone fractured, splint, thrypsis.*

f., cause of:

1. *By direct violence,* when the bone is broken directly at the spot where the force was applied, as in fracture of the tibia by being run over.

2. *By indirect violence,* where the bone is fractured by a force applied at a distance from the site of fracture and transmitted to the fractured bone, as in a clavicle fractured by falling on the outstretched hand.

3. *By muscular contraction,* when the bone is broken by a sudden violent contraction of the muscles. The patella is the bone most frequently fractured in this way.

In certain diseases and conditions bones break easily with scarcely any violence, *e. g.,* osteomalacia, syphilis, osteomyelitis, etc.

f., varieties of:

1. *Simple*: The bone is broken, but there is no external wound.

2. *Compound*: The bone is broken, and there is an external wound leading down to the site of fracture.

3. *Complicated*: The bone is broken, and has injured some internal organ, *e. g.,* a broken rib piercing a lung.

4. *Comminuted*: The bone is broken or splintered into pieces.

5. *Impacted*: The bone is broken, and one end is wedged into the interior of the other.

6. *Incomplete*: The line of fracture does not include the whole bone.

7. *Green Stick*: The bone is partially bent and partially broken, as when a green stick breaks. It occurs in children, especially in those with rickets.

8. *Depressed*: When a piece of the skull is broken and driven inwards.

9. *Separation of an epiphysis* takes place between the shaft of a bone and its growing end, and occurs only in young patients.

f., signs of:

(a) Loss of power of movement.

(b) Pain with acute tenderness over the site of fracture.

(c) Swelling and bruising.

(d) Deformity and possible shortening.

(e) Unnatural mobility. The nurse should never try to obtain this sign.

(f) Crepitus or grating which is heard when the ends of the bone rub together. The nurse should never try to obtain this sign.

To find out the kind of fracture and its exact position, x-rays are used.

f., treatment of:

1. First Aid Treatment: In simple fractures the limb or part must be kept immovable by means of splints, such as folded newspapers or umbrellas, or proper wooden splints if they are at hand. The clothing should not be removed unless there is dangerous hemorrhage. If it is necessary to remove clothing, do so by cutting the cloth away so as to cause a minimum of motion of the affected part.

If it is an upper extremity it should be supported in a sling, and the patient may then walk. If a lower limb is injured the patient should remain lying, and no attempt to walk should be made.

2. Later Treatment:

(a) Reducing the fracture, *i. e.,* placing the fragments in proper position.

(b) Keeping the bone in position by means of splints until union has taken place.

(c) Restoring the limb's former functions under instruction.

In compound fractures, before treating the fracture any bleeding must be arrested, the wound is then washed and cleaned with some antiseptic lotion, and when quite clean a sterilized dressing is put on and secured by a bandage. Splints are then applied as in simple fractures.

fragilitas (fra-jil'ĭ-tas) [L. brittleness]. Fragility.

f. crin'ium. Brittleness, as of the hair, showing splitting and breaking of the shaft. Cause unknown.

Treatment: Scalp cleanliness with occasional petrolatum rub. Clipping may retard splitting of distal ends. Singeing is harmful.

f. oss'ium. Brittleness of bones. Syn: *osteopsathyrosis.*

f. sanguinas. Red blood cell fragility.

fragil'ity [L. *fragilitās,* brittleness]. State of brittleness.

f., capillary. Breaking down of capillaries with oozing of blood beneath skin surface.

f. of the blood. Tendency of blood corpuscles to divide up or dissolve; due to changes in saline content of the blood.

f. test. If red blood cells are placed in distilled water, they rapidly swell and burst, since they normally are suspended in a solution of much greater osmotic pressure. This phenomenon is called *hemolysis.* If they are suspended in a solution of normal saline, the cells retain their normal shape and do not burst. If they are placed in successively weaker solutions of saline, a point is reached at which some of the cells burst and liberate their hemoglobin within a given length of time, while others do not (*partial hemolysis*). Finally, at a given dilution, all of the cells have burst within the allotted time, which is usually 2 hours. The cells of normal blood begin to hemolyze in about 0.44%, and complete hemolysis occurs in about 0.35% saline. If the cells are abnormally "fragile," hemolysis occurs in stronger solutions of saline.

fragmenta'tion [L. *fragmentum, frangere,* to break]. Breaking up into fragments.

frambe'sia [L. *framboesia,* raspberry]. Infectious tropical disease. Syn: *yaws.*

frambesioma (fram-be-zĭ-o′mă) [" + G. *ōma,* swelling]. Primary lesion of yaws.

Francisella tularensis (fran″cis-el′lă tu-lă-ren′sis) [named in honor of Edward *Francis,* pioneer investigator of tularemia, and *Tulare,* a California county in which tularemia was first observed and investigated]. The microorganism is a very small, nonmotile, gram-negative rod or coccus and is found in animals such as wild rabbits, flies and ticks, but it may be transmitted to man by flies and ticks and contact with infected animals. Formerly referred to as Pasteurella tularensis.

francium (fran′sē-ūm) [Named for France, the country in which it was discovered]. A metallic element occurring as a natural isotope. SYMB: Fr. At. wt. 223; at. no. 87.

Frankenhäuser's ganglion (frang′ken-hoy-zerz). A nerve ganglion sometimes found in lateral walls of the cervix uteri.

Frank′lin glasses [Benjamin Franklin, American statesman and inventor, 1706-1790]. Bifocal spectacles.

franklin′ic electric′ity. Electricity produced by friction. SEE: *electricity, static.*

Fraunhofer's lines (frown′hō-fer). Absorption bands or lines seen in a spectrum, caused by the absorption of groups of light rays in their passage through solids, liquids, or gases.

freckle (frek′l) [Old Norse *frecken,* a freckle]. Small local pigmentation, brownish or yellowish, of the skin.

ETIOL: Exposure to sun in majority. Universal types are probably symptomatic (anemia, abdominal disorders etc.).

SYM: Minute circumscribed brownish pigmentary macules appearing chiefly on face and dorsal surfaces of hands, more marked in spring and summer. In *lentigo senilis* the forearms are affected in individuals showing other senile skin changes.

TREATMENT: Protection from the sun. Locally, mercuric chloride-alcohol-water with circumspection, symptoms of dermatitis to be controlled by calamine lotion or cold cream. SYN: *lentigines; lentigo; ephalis.*

free associa′tion. 1. Uncontrolled ideas when not under mental restraint or direction. 2. PSY: The procedure which requires the patient to speak aloud his thought flow, word for word, without censorship.

freez′ing [A.S. *frēosan,* to freeze]. Frigidity of a limb due to cold.

Most common in the debilitated, the exhausted, and those accustomed to alcoholic beverages.

SYM: Paleness, cyanosis, coldness. Unconsciousness usually develops.

F. A. TREATMENT: Protect part with a cradle and apply dry heat at room temperature. Sudden applications of heat undesirable. SEE: *frostbite.*

f. microtome. One for cutting frozen objects.

f. mixtures (for ice bags). 5 oz. sal ammoniac, 5 oz. niter and 1 part of water.

Equal parts of sal ammoniac, salt, and niter.

f. point. Temperature at which liquids freeze.

Frei's disease [William S. Frei, German dermatologist, 1885-1943]. Venereal disease affecting the inguinal area, chiefly, with formation of buboes. SYN: *lymphogranuloma inguinale* or *venerea; Nicolas-Favre disease.*

F.'s test. Test given to confirm diagnosis of lymphogranuloma inguinale.

Consists of injecting an extract from the lymph nodes of a patient with lymphogranuloma into the skin. Positive reaction is evidenced by marked reddening and thickening of the skin about the site of the injection.

fremitus (frem′ĭ-tus) [L. a clashing]. Vibratory tremors felt by palpation through the chest wall.

VARIETIES: Vocal or tactile, friction, hydatid, rhonchal or bronchial, cavernous or succussion, pleural, pericardial, tussive, thrills. SEE: *palpation.*

f., vocal. Vibrations of the voice transmitted to the ear on auscultation of the chest of a person speaking. In determining the vocal fremitus observe following precautions: Palpate symmetrical parts of chest; make firm pressure; when comparing use the same pressure on both sides; apply hands as nearly parallel to ribs as possible; remember the fremitus is normally increased over the right apex. Is decreased in: (1) Pleural effusions—air, pus, blood, serum, or lymph; (2) emphysema; (3) pulmonary collapse from an obstructed bronchus; (4) pulmonary edema; (5) morbid growths of the lung.

fre′nal [L. *fraenum,* bridle]. Pert. to the frenum.

frenosecretory (fre-no-se′krē-to-rĭ) [" + *secernere,* to secrete]. Exercising an inhibitory power over the secretions.

frenotomy (fre-not′o-mĭ) [" + G. *tomē,* incision]. Division of any frenum, esp. for tongue-tie.

frenulum (pl. *frenula*). [L. a little bridle.] 1. A small frenum. SYN: *vinculum.* 2. A small fold of white matter on the upper surface of the anterior medullary velum extending to the corpora quadrigemina.

f. clitoridis [NA]. The union of inner parts of the labia minora on undersurface of the clitoris, *q.v.*

f. labiorum pudendi [NA]. Fold of membrane connecting post. ends of labia minora.

f. linguae [NA]. A fold of mucous membrane which extends from the floor of the mouth to the inferior surface of the tongue along its midline.

f. prepu′tii [NA]. One that unites the foreskin (prepuce) to the glans penis.

f. of tongue. One attaching lower side of tongue to the gum.

frenum (fre′num) (pl. *frena*) [L. *fraenum,* bridle]. A fold of mucous membrane which connects two parts, one more or less movable and which serves to check the movement of this part. SEE: *frenulum.*

frenzy. A state of violent mental agitation; maniacal excitement.

fre′quency [L. *frequens,* often, constant]. 1. The number of repetitions of a phenomenon in a certain period of time as the f. of heart beat, f. of sound vibrations. 2. In biometry, the ratio of the number of individuals falling into a single group (having a certain characteristic, disease, or condition) to the total number of individuals in the population being studied. This is usually expressed for a definite period of time. SEE: *incidence.* 3. The rate of oscillation or alternation in an alternating current circuit, in contradistinction to periodicity in the interruptions or regular variations of current in a direct current circuit.

The frequency is computed on the basis of a complete cycle, a complete cycle being one in which the current rises from zero to a maximum, returns to zero, and rises to an opposite maximum and returns to zero.

Freud, Sigmund (froyd) [Neurologist in Vienna, 1856-1939]. A famous Austrian psychoanalyst, whose teachings stress the theory:

1. Of the existence of a subconscious mind.

2. That psychical processes are never accidental or due to chance, but are determined by laws, as are physical events.

3. That emotional processes have the attributes of quantity, and can be displaced from one idea to another.

4. That the sex instinct does not develop at puberty, but that the child experiences a rich sexual life, and from this is derived the later stages of *narcissism* or self-love, *homosexuality* or attraction to the same sex, *heterosexuality,* which is the normal attraction to the opposite sex. SEE: *Œdipus complex.*

5. That dreams are fulfillments of wishes which find no realization in waking hours; theories are also formulated with regard to the importance of sex in dreams.

6. Freud also suggests that forgetting, misplacing articles, and slips of the tongue or pen are the outward manifestation of repression. SEE: *abreaction, psychoanalysis, etc.*

freudian (froy'di-an). Pert. to Sigmund Freud or his theories of unconscious or repressed libido or past sex experiences or desires as the cause of various neuroses, the cure for which is the restoration of such conditions to consciousness through psychoanalysis.

fri'able [L. *friāre,* to crumble]. Easily broken or pulverized.

fric'tion (in massage) [L. *fricare,* to rub]. In massage, strong, circular manipulations always followed by centripetal stroking.

In hydrotherapy, friction is used in drying patients after tonic baths, shampoos, salt glows, wet mitten friction and drip sheet rubs.

f., dry. F. using no liquid.

f., moist. F. using a liquid or oil.

f. murmur, f. sound. A frictional sound heard in pleurisy.

fric'tional electric'ity. Electricity produced by friction. SEE: *electricity, static.*

Friedländer's bacillus frēd'len-derz) [Karl Friedländer, German physician, 1847-1887]. *Klebsiella pneumoniae.*

F.'s disease. Extreme degree of fibrous tissue in the intima closing the lumen. SYN: *endarteritis obliterans.*

Fried'man's test [Maurice H. Friedman, American physiologist, 1903-]. The injection, in 4 cc. doses twice a day for 2 days, of the urine of a woman suspected of pregnancy into an unmated female rabbit will cause the formation of corpora lutea and corpora hemorrhagica in the rabbit at the end of 2 days if the woman is pregnant.

Fried'mann's disease [Max Friedmann, German physician, 1858-1925]. Relapsing infantile spastic spinal paralysis.

Fried'reich's ataxia (freed'rix) [Nikolaus Friedreich, German neurologist, 1825-1882]. Rare disease resembling locomotor ataxia occurring in the children, esp. girls, of the same family. SYN: *hereditary ataxia.*

F.'s disease. SEE: *F.'s ataxia.*

F.'s sign. Sudden collapse of the cervical veins previously distended, at each diastole, caused by an adherent pericardium. The lowering of the pitch of the percussion note during inspiration which occurs over an area of cavitation.

fright [A.S. *fryhto,* fear]. Extreme sudden fear.

f. neuroses. Traumatic hysteria.

f., precordial. Anxiety felt before melancholic frenzy.

frigid (frij'id) [L. *frigor,* cold]. 1. Cold. 2. Irresponsive to emotion, applied esp. to the inability to feel sex desire on the part of a woman.

frigid'ity [L. *frigor,* cold]. In the female, absence of sexual desire. Inability to have an orgasm.

frigolabile (frig-o-la'bl) [L. *frigor,* cold, + *labilis,* unstable]. Capable of being destroyed by low temperature.

frigorific (frig-o-rif'ik) [" + *facere,* to make]. Generating cold.

frig'orism [" + G. *ismos,* condition]. A condition due to long exposure to cold.

frigostabile (frig-o-sta'bl) [" + *stabilis.* firm]. Incapable of being destroyed by low temperature.

frigotherapy (frig-o-ther'ă-pĭ) [" + G. *therapeia,* treatment]. The use of cold in treatment of disease.

Frisch's bacillus. *Klebsiella rhinoscleromatis,* a gram-negative encapsulated bacillus found in the lesions of rhinoscleroma.

frit [Fr. *fritte, frire,* to fry]. 1. The material from which glass or the glazed portion of pottery is made. 2. A similar material for making the glaze of artificial teeth.

frog belly. Flaccid abdomen in children afflicted by rickets, and atony of abdominal cells resulting from dyspepsia, accompanied by flatulence.

f. face. Flatness of face resulting from intranasal disease.

Fröhde's reagent (freh'dez). A test for alkaloids; 1 part of sodium molybdate in 1000 parts of strong sulfuric acid.

Fröhlich's syndrome (frā'liks) [Alfred Fröhlich, Austrian neurologist, 1871-]. A condition characterized by adiposity of the female type, atrophy or hypoplasia of the gonads, and altered secondary sex characteristics. Due to disturbance of the hypothalamus and hypophysis. SYN: *adiposogenital dystrophy; sexual infantilism.*

Froin's syndrome (fro-wans') [Georges Froin, French physician, 1874-]. Yellow cerebrospinal fluid which rapidly coagulates. It contains an excess of lymphocytes, and also globulin.

frolement (frol-mon') [Fr.]. 1. Very light friction with the hand in massage.* 2. A sound resembling rustling heard in auscultation.

Frommann's lines (from'mahnz) [Carl Frommann, German anatomist, 1851-1892]. Transverse lines in the axis cylinder of medullated nerve fibers after being stained by silver nitrate.

frons (fronz) [L.]. The forehead.

fron'tad [L. *frons, front-,* brow, + *ad,* toward]. Toward the frontal aspect.

frontal (fron'tal) [L. *frons, front-,* brow]. 1. Anterior. 2. Pertaining to the forehead bone.

f. bone. Forehead bone.

f. lobe (of the cerebrum). Four main convolutions in front of the central *sulcus.*

f. plane. A plane parallel with the long axis of the body and at right angles to the median sagittal plane.

f. sinuses. A pair of hollow spaces in the frontal bone lying above the orbits. They are lined with mucous membrane, contain air, and communicate with the middle nasal meatus by means of the nasofrontal duct.

fronto- [L. *frons, front-,* brow]. Prefix: Ant. position, or relationship with the forehead.

frontoma'lar [" + *mala,* cheek]. Rel. to the frontal and malar bones.

frontomax'illary [" + *maxilla,* jaw]. Rel. to the frontal bone and maxillary bones.

frontoparietal (fron"to-pă-ri'ĕ-tal) [" + *parietalis,* pert. to a wall]. Pert. to the frontal and parietal bones.

frontotem'poral [" + *tempora,* the temples]. Pert. to frontal and temporal bones.

front-tap reflex. Contraction of gastrocnemius muscles resulting from percussing stretched muscles of extended leg.

frost. A vapor deposit similar to frozen dew.

f., urea. Deposit of crystals on the skin in a patient whose kidneys are severely impaired such as in uremia.

frost'bite. Freezing or effect of freezing of a part of the body.

The nose, fingers, and toes are usually the parts affected.

SYM: Tingling, redness, followed by paleness and numbness of affected area. It is of three degrees: (a) Transitory hyperemia following numbness; (b) formation of vesicles, and (c) gangrene.

F. A. TREATMENT: Slow rewarming or rapid rewarming (bath water at 114° F.); the latter to be used if it is certain that the vascular tissues are not injured. Stimulate with tea, coffee, beef tea. Artificial respiration if unconscious. Patients have been known to recover when parts were black and all hope had been given up, except amputation.

f.-itch. Itching skin disease in cold climates. SYN: *pruritus hiemalis.*

frottage (fro-tazh') [Fr. rubbing]. 1. A condition of *hyperesthesia sexualis* often associated with lowered virility inducing an irresistible impulse of pressing up behind women in crowds, thus producing an orgasm. 2. Massage technic using rubbing.

frotteur (fro-ter') [Fr. *frottage,* rubbing]. One who practices frottage.

frozen sleep. Hypothermia, *q.v.*

fruc'tose [L. *fructus,* fruit]. Levulose. Fruit sugar.

A monosaccharose and a hexose, having the same empirical formula as glucose, $C_6H_{12}O_6$, and found in corn syrup, honey, fruit juices, and in the syrup resulting from the inversion of sucrose; an invert sugar. It produces glycogen and maintains normal content of glucose in the blood. In the liver, it may be converted into glycogen which, in turn, may be converted into glucose. SEE: *disaccharose.*

fructosuria (fruk"to-sū'rĭ-ă) [" + G. *ouron,* urine]. Fructose in the urine.

fruit [L. *fructus,* fruit]. BOT: A ripened ovary consisting of a seed or seeds and the surrounding tissue. Ex: *pod of a bean, nut, grain, pome, or berry.* The edible product of a plant consisting of ripened seeds and the enveloping tissue.

Fruits in general tend to add bulk to the diet. This quality, as well as in some cases their containing specific laxative substances, makes fruits quite helpful in treating constipation.

COMP: Carbohydrates in the form of fruit sugar form the chief nutritive value of fruits. Seventy-five per cent of it is a mixture of dextrose and levulose. Proteins and energy factors are variable. Good source of vitamins and mineral elements. Iodine content, 6 to 120 parts per billion. *Pectose bodies*: The principle in fruits that causes them to jelly *Pectose,* found in unripe fruit. *Pectin,* found in ripe fruit. *Pectosic acid,* from pectose, in cooked fruit. *Pectic acid,* from pectin, in fruit cooked a long time.

PRINCIPAL ACIDS IN FRUITS AND OTHER FOODS: 1. Acetic, in wine and vinegar. 2. Citric, in lemons, oranges, limes, citron, etc. 3. Malic, in apples, pears, apricots, peaches, currants, gooseberries, etc. 4. Tannic, in gallnuts. 5. Oxalic, in rhubarb, sorrel, cranberries, etc. 6. Tartaric, in grapes, pineapples and tamarinds. 7. Salicylic, in currants, cranberries, cherries, plums, grapes, crabapples and berries. *Combined acids*: (a) Citric; (b) malic, in raspberries, strawberries, gooseberries, cherries, etc. (a) Citric, (b) malic, (c) oxalic in cranberries. They contain iron and other mineral substances.

fruit sugar. Fructose, levulose, *q.v.*

frumentaceous (fru-men-ta'she-us) [L. *frumentum,* grain]. Resembling or belonging to grain.

frumenti, spiritus [L. essence of grain] Whisky.

frumentum (fru-men'tum) [L. grain]. Wheat or other grain.

frustration [L. *frustrā,* in vain]. 1. The failure of libido to find adequate outlet. 2. The condition which results from the thwarting or prevention of acts which if performed would bring satisfaction or gratification of physical or personality needs.

FSH. The follicle stimulating hormone secreted by the ant. lobe of the hypophysis.

Ft. Abbr. of L. *fiat,* or *fiant,* let there be made. Also for *florentium,* former name for *promethium.*

fuadin (fu'ah-din) [Fuad I, King of Egypt]. Proprietary brand of stibophen. Used in the treatment of granuloma inguinale and schistosomiasis.

fuel value. Energy to be produced by oxidation of edible foods after eating. SEE: *calory, energy, food requirements.*

-fuge [L.]. Suffix meaning *to expel.*

fugitive (fu'jit-iv) [L. *fugitivus,* wandering]. 1. Temporary, transient. 2. Wandering; pert. to inconstant symptoms.

fugue (fŭg) [L. *fuga,* flight]. Serious personality dissociation. Leaving home or surroundings on a hysterical impulse generally with loss of memory as to identity and the past.

Fuld's test [Ernst Fuld, German internist, 1873-]. A test for the antipyretic power of the blood serum.

fulgurant (ful'gu-rant) [L. *fulgurāre,* to lighten]. Severe and sudden, as a *f. pain.*

ful'gurating [L. *fulgurāre,* to lighten]. Pert. to fulguration. SYN: *fulgurant.*

fulguration (ful-gu-ra'shun) [L. *fulgurāre,* to lighten]. Destruction of tissue by means of long high frequency electric sparks. SEE: *electrodesiccation.*

fuliginous (fu-lij'in-us) [L. *fuligō,* spot]. Resembling soot, esp. in color.

full'ing [A.S. *fullian,* to fill]. A movement in massage; kneading.

Palms hold a limb bet. them, the fingers extended, the limb being rolled backward and forward.

full term. Normal end of pregnancy, when the fetus is 20-21 in. long, has well-developed finger- and toenails, and, if a boy, with both testicles descended. It should weigh from 7 lb. upward and have been nourished in the womb for not less than 40 weeks.

ful'minant [L. *fulmināre,* to lighten]. Fulgurant. Coming in lightninglike flashes of pain, as in tabes dorsalis.

ful'minating [L. *fulmināre,* to lighten]. Fulgurant; occurring with very great rapidity, said of certain pains.

fumes [L. *fumus,* smoke]. Vapors, esp. those having irritating qualities.

f., nitric acid. Used in various chemical processes.

SYM: Choking, gasping, swelling of mucous membranes, tightness in chest, cough and shock. Symptoms may last for 1 week or more.

TREATMENT: Allow patient to inhale aromatic spirits of ammonia, followed by steam inhalations at intervals and oily spray repeatedly. Oxygen may be necessary because of limited space for air exchange.

fu'migant. An agent used in fumigation. Common fumigants are hydrocyanic acid, calcium cyanids, methyl bromide, sulfur dioxide, naphthalene, and ortho- and paradichlorobenzene.

fumiga'tion [L. *fumigāre,* to fumigate]. 1. The use of poisonous fumes or gases to destroy living organisms, esp., rats, mice, insects, and other vermin. Fumigants are relatively ineffective against bacteria and viruses, consequently the practice of terminal disinfection of the sick room, formerly a common practice, has been discontinued. 2. The disinfecting of rooms by gases.

fu'ming [L. *fumus,* smoke]. Having a visible vapor.

function (fŭng'shŭn) [L. *functia, fungi,* to perform]. 1. The action performed by any structure. In a living organism this may pertain to a cell or a part of a cell, tissue, organ, or system of organs. 2. The act of carrying on or performing a special activity. Normal function is the normal action of an organ. Abnormal functioning or the failure of an organ to perform its function are the bases of disease or disease processes. Structural changes in an organ constitute pathological changes and are common cause of malfunctioning although an organ may function abnormally in the absence of observable structural changes.

function, *words pert. to:* absorption, anabolism, analogue, assimilation, atelic, cacergasia, catabolism, catabiotic, choloscopy, digestion, excretion, metabolism, secretion, syzygiology.

func'tional [L. *functio, fungi,* to perform]. 1. Pertaining to function. 2. A word applied to disturbances of function in a variety of ways.

The disturbance of function of one organ by structural change in another is at times termed functional, but incorrectly, as it represents organic change. Disturbances of function resulting from unfortunate conditioning of the organism to an external situation may more suitably be called functional, though this "conditioning" may be purely structural.

f. disease. One not organic, or in which changes of an organ are not in evidence; a disturbance of any organ's functions.

f. psychosis. One exhibited in psychosis, in which no pathology of the central nervous system is apparent.

funda (fun'dă) [L. a sling]. A four-tailed bandage.

fundal (fun'dal) [L. *fundus,* base]. Pert. to a fundus.

fund'ament [L. *fundamentum,* foundation]. 1. A foundation. 2. The anus.

fund'ic. Pertaining to a fundus.

fun'diform [L. *fundus,* sling, + *forma,* shape]. Sling-shaped or looped.

fun'dus (pl. *fundi*) [L. base]. 1. The larger part, base, or body of a hollow organ. 2. The portion of an organ most remote from its opening.

f. glands. Minute tubelike glands of the gastric mucosa in the cardiac section.

f. oculi. Post. inner part of eye as seen with ophthalmoscope.

f. uteri. The body of the uterus from the internal os of the cervix upward above the fallopian tubes.

fundusectomy (fun-dus-ek'to-mĭ) [" + G. *ektomē,* excision]. Excision of the fundus of the stomach. SYN: *cardiectomy.*

fun'gate [L. *fungus,* mushroom]. To grow like a fungus.

fungating (fun'gāt-ing) [L. *fungus,* mushroom]. Growing rapidly like a fungus, applied to certain tumors.

fungemia (fun-je'mĭ-ă). Presence of fungi in the blood.

fungi (fun'jī) [L. *fungus,* mushroom]. 1. Plural of fungus. 2. A division of plants which includes slime molds, sac fungi, club fungi, and imperfect fungi. They were formerly considered as a subdivision of the Thallophytes. Fungi are simple dependent plants lacking chlorophyll. Their bodies show little differentiation and they have relatively simple life cycles. They include the molds, rusts, mushrooms, toadstools, lichens, and yeasts. Many forms are pathogenic to plants and animals.

f., fission. The bacteria or Schizomycetes.

f., imperfect. The Fungi Imperfecti, or Deuteromycetes, a class of fungi so-called because their life cycles are only partly known, the sexual stage being absent. Many species are parasitic, causing disease.

f., slime. The slime molds (*Myxomycetes*).

f., true. Fungi with a plant body composed of hyphae. Include the algal fungi (*Phycomycetes*), sac fungi (*Ascomycetes*), club fungi (*Basidiomycetes*) and imperfect fungi (*Fungi Imperfecti*).

fungicide (fun'jĭ-sīd) [" + *caedere,* to kill]. Bactericide; that which destroys bacteria or fungi.

fungicidin (fun-jĭ-si'din). An antibiotic obtained from *Streptomycetes griseus* which possesses fungistatic and fungicidal properties. It is not antibacterial.

fungiform (fun'jĭ-form) [" + *forma,* shape]. Fungus-shaped.

f. papillae. Small, rounded eminences on middle and ant. parts of dorsum and esp. along sides of tongue.

fungista'sis [" + G. *stasis,* a halting]. A condition in which the growth of fungi is inhibited. SEE: *fungicide.*

fun'gistat [" + G. *statikos,* standing]. That which inhibits the growth of fungi.

fungistat'ic [" + G. *statikos,* standing]. Inhibiting the growth of fungi.

fungoid (fun'goid) [" + G. *eidos,* form]. Having the appearance of a fungus.

f., chignon. Bacterial growth of the hair. SEE: *chignon f.*

fungosity (fun-gos'ĭ-tĭ) [L. *fungus,* mushroom]. A soft excrescence.

fungous (fun'gus). Fungus, *q.v.*

fungus (fun'gus) (pl. *fungi*) [L. *mushroom*]. 1. A vegetable cellular organism that subsists on organic matter. 2. A plant belonging to the division Fungi. 3. A sponge-like morbid excrescence on the body resembling fungus. SEE: *actinomycosis; cladosporiosis.*

f. haematodes. Malignant bleeding growth.

fu'nic [L. *funis,* cord]. Pert. to the umbilical cord.

f. souffle. The purring sound heard over the pregnant uterus, and having the same rate at the fetal heart beat.

fu'nicle [L. *funiculus,* little cord]. A small, threadlike structure. SYN: *funiculus.*

funicular (fu-nik'u-lar) [L. *funiculus,* little cord]. Pert. to the spermatic, or umbilical cord.

f. process. That part of the tunica vaginalis that covers the spermatic cord.

funiculitis (fu-nik-u-li'tis) [" + G. *-ītis,* inflammation]. Inflammation of the spermatic cord.

funiculopexy (fu-nik'u-lo-peks-ĭ) [" + G. *pēxis,* fixation]. Suturing the spermatic cord to the tissues in cases of undescended testicle.

funiculus (fu-nik'u-lus) (pl. *funiculi*) [L. little cord]. 1. Any small structure resembling a cord. 2. A division of the white matter of the spinal cord consisting of fasculi or fiber tracts lying peripherally to the gray matter. Differentiated into dorsal, lateral, and ventral funiculi. 3. Old term for the umbilical cord or the spermatic cord. 4. Formerly a synonym for *fasciculus, q.v.*

fu'niform [L. *funis,* cord, + *forma,* shape]. Cordlike.

fu'nis [L. cord]. 1. A cordlike structure. 2. The umbilical cord.

fun'nel [L. *fundere,* to pour]. Conical, wide, open-mouthed device for pouring through its open tube at end into another vessel.

f. breast. Sternal depression of chest walls resembling a funnel.

f. drainage. Drainage by funnels.

funny bone. The internal condyle of the humerus.

F.U.O. Abbr. for *fever of unknown origin.*

furacin. Trade name for *nitrofurazone, q.v.*

fur'cal [L. *furca,* fork]. Forked.

furcula. The hypobranchial eminence, an elevation in the floor of the embryonic pharynx at the level of the 3rd and 4th branchial arches. It gives rise to the epiglottis and the aryepiglottic folds.

furfur (fur'fur) [L. bran]. Scurf; dandruff.

furfuraceous (fur-fu-ra'shus) [L. *furfur,* bran]. Scaly, or resembling scales.

furibund (fu'rĭ-bund) [L. *furibundus, furere,* to rage]. Maniacal; raging, as in certain types of insanity.

fu'ror [L. rage]. PSY: Extremely violent outbursts or anger, often without provocation.

f. amatorius. Insatiable sexual desire.

f. epilepticus. Epileptic insanity, or sudden anger as expressed by epileptics.

f. femininus. Nymphomania.*

f. genitalis. Erotomania.*

f. uterinus. Nymphomania.

furred (ferd). Said of the tongue on which a deposit has formed.

furrow. A groove.

furuncle (fu'rung-kl) [L. *furunculus,* a boil]. A boil. SYN: *furunculus.*

furunc'ular [L. *furunculus,* a boil]. Pert. to a boil.

furunculoid (fu-rung'ku-loid) [" + G. *eidos,* form]. Resembling a furuncle or boil. SYN: *furunculous.*

furunculosis (fu-rung-ku-lo'sis) [" + G. *ōsis*]. A condition resulting from boils.

furunc'ulous [L. *furunculus,* boil]. Pert. to or of the nature of a boil or boils.

furunculus (fu-rung'ku-lus) [L. a boil]. Boil, furuncle. Acute, deep-seated phlegmonous inflammation formed in the skin usually ending in suppuration and necrosis.

ETIOL: Staphylococcal infection of follicular or sebaceous glands.

SYM: Neck, axillae, face, buttocks and breasts are common sites of predilection, beginning in hair follicle or sudoriparous gland as subcutaneous swelling or acuminate pustule around hair shaft, skin smooth and shining, with pain and tenderness. Lesion may come to head, or become boggy and fluctuant, or regression may take place before suppuration, resulting in disappearance by absorption (blind boil). Lesion ruptures spontaneously or following incision, discharging core, necrotic tissue, and pus; healing follows.

TREATMENT: Moist heat, incision on pointing of lesion, systemic antibiotic.

Fusarium (fū-za'rĭ-um) [L. *fusus,* a spindle]. A genus of fungi.

fuscin. A brown pigment, a melanin, present in the outermost layer (pigmented epithelium) of the retina.

fuse [L. *fusus, fundere,* to pour]. A safety device comprising a strip of wire of easily fusible metal, the conductance of which is predetermined. The metal fuses and breaks circuit when excess of current passes through. Convenient forms mounted in plugs, bet. hard metal ends under screwheads.

fu'sible [L. *fusus,* a thing poured]. Capable of being melted.

fu'siform [L. *fusus,* spindle, + *forma,* shape]. 1. Tapering at both ends. Spindle-shaped. 2. BIOL: Pert. to gelatin which liquefies in parsnip form.

Fusifor'mis [" + *forma,* shape]. Old term for *Fusobacterium.*

F. ac'nes. *Corynebacterium acnes.*

F. den'tium. *Fusobacterium fusiforme.*

fusion (fu'shun) [L. *fundere,* to pour]. Meeting and joining together through liquefaction by heat. The process of fusing of uniting.

f. faculty. Blending of the images of binocular vision into a single perception having the quality of depth.

f., spinal. The fusion of two or more vertebrae, an operation resorted to in the treatment of certain deformities of the spine.

Fus"obacter'ium. A genus of nonspore forming, nonencapsulated, nonmotile, gram-negative bacteria usually found in necrotic lesions, associated with spirochaetes.

F. fusiforme. The causative organism of Vincent's infection. It is found also in the normal mouth. SYN: *fusiform bacillus.*

F. plauti-vincenti. F. fusiforme.

fusocel'lular [L. *fusus*, spindle, + *cellulus*, little cell]. Spindle celled.

fusospirillosis (fū"so-spir-il-o'sis) [" + *spirillum*, coil, + G. *-ōsis*]. Vincent's angina.

fusospirochetal (fū"so-spi-ro-ke'tăl) [" + G. *speira*, coil, + *chaitē*, hair]. Pert. to fusiform bacilli and spirochetes such as found in Vincent's angina.

fusospirocheto'sis [" + " + " + *-ōsis*]. Infection with fusiform bacilli and spirochetes.

fusostreptococcosis (fū"so-strep"to-kok-ko'sis) [" + G. *streptos*, twisted, + *kokkos*, berry, + *-ōsis*]. Infection with fusiform bacteria and streptococcus.

fustiga'tion [L. *fustigare*, to beat with a rod]. In massage, beating with light rods.

fututrix (fu-tu'triks). A girl or woman who practices tribadism, *q.v.*

Notes

G

G. 1. A constant in Newton's law of gravitation. 2. In aviation physiology, G. is a unit of force resulting from acceleration or centrifugal motion. 3. Abbreviation for *gingival; gram(s)*.

G-6-PD. Glucose-6-phosphate dehydrogenase. An enzyme of the red blood cells. A deficiency of the enzyme may cause the red cells to hemolyze more rapidly than normal following administration of certain drugs to, or ingestion of fava beans by patients. There are several variants of this disease.

Ga. Chemical symb. for *gallium*.

GABA. Abbreviation for *gamma-aminobutyric acid*.

gad'fly. An insect which lays eggs under the skin of its victim, which cause swellings simulating a boil. Multiple furuncles appear with hatching of larva. A fly belonging to the family Tabanidae, *q.v.* Includes horseflies, deerflies, and other bloodsucking flies. SEE: *botfly*.

gadolinium (gad-o-lin'ĭ-um). SYMB: Gd. A very rare element. At. wt. 157.25; at. no. 64.

Gaffkya (gaf'kĭ-ă) [Georg T. A. Gaffky, German bacteriologist, 1850-1918]. A genus of bacteria of the family *Micrococcaceae*.

G. tetrag'ena. Found associated with the tubercle bacillus and present in lesions of the respiratory passageways, in the blood, and spinal fluid. Of low pathogenicity. SYN: *Micrococcus tetragenus*.

gag [imitative]. 1. Device for keeping the jaws open or forcibly opening the mouth. 2. To retch or cause to retch.

g. reflex. Gagging and vomiting resulting from irritation of fauces.

Gaisböck's disease (gīs'beks) [Felix Gaisböck, German physician]. Abnormal number of red corpuscles in blood with cardiac hypertrophy and elevated blood pressure, without splenic enlargement. SYN: *polycythemia hypertonica*.

gait (gāt) [A.S. *geat*, gate, door]. Manner of walking.

CHARACTERISTIC: 1. Body leans backward and feet are widely separated in pregnancy, obesity, ascites, and large abdominal tumors. 2. Limping or hobbling gait is seen in rheumatism, sciatica, hip or knee joint disease or injury, metatarsal neuralgia, and affections of lower extremities such as poliomyelitis. 3. When standing with feet close together in locomotor ataxia, aural vertigo, disease of middle cerebellar lobe, patient sways and may fall. 4. Gait is slovenly in the weak, anemic, and apathetic, and in chronic mental or physical defects.

SEE: *asynergia; adiadochokinesis; dysmetria; walking*.

g., ataxic. Raising foot high, striking ground suddenly with entire sole.

g., brachybasic. Shuffling gait of partial paraplegia.

g., cerebellar. A staggering movement.

g., cow. Swaying due to knock-knees.

g., equine. Raising foot by flexing thigh on abdomen. Characteristic of peroneal paralysis. Slow, awkward.

g., festinating. Body bent forward and rigid. Walks on toes as though pushed. Starts slowly, increases and does not stop until patient meets an obstruction. Seen in paralysis agitans.

g., flat-footed. Toes everted, legs often bowed.

g., frog. That of infantile paralysis: hopping.

g., hemiplegic. Patient abducts paralyzed limb, swings it around and brings it forward so foot comes to ground in front of him.

g., Huntington's chorea. A few normal paces, a long slow one, and then one or two hops.

g., multiple neuritis. That of a high-stepping horse. Steppage gait, *q.v.*

g., paralysis agitans. Tendency to begin slowly, then rapidly, falling forward. SYN: *festinating g.*

g., paralytic. Feet dragged with slow movements. Stumbles easily. Seen in chronic myelitis.

g., scissor. One in which legs cross in walking.

g., spastic. A stiff movement, toes seeming to catch and drag, legs held together, hips and knee joints slightly flexed. Seen in spastic paraplegia, sclerosis of lateral pyramidal columns of cord. Also in tumor of spinal cord and arachnoiditis.

g., steppage. Foot and toes lifted high, heel brought down first. Seen in peripheral neuritis, late stages of diabetes, alcoholism, chronic arsenical poisoning.

g., waddling. Feet wide apart and walk resembling that of a duck. Seen in coxa vara and double congenital displacement of hip when lordosis is present.

galact-, galacto- [G.]. Combining forms, pert. to *milk*.

galactacrasia (gă-lak"tă-kra'zĭ-ă) [G. *gala*, milk, + *krasis*, mixture]. An abnormal composition of milk from the breast.

galactagogue (gă-lak'tă-gog) [" + *agōgos*, leading]. Agent that promotes the flow of milk.

galactan (gă-lak'tan) [G. *gala*, milk]. A complex carbohydrate forming galactose upon hydrolysis.

galac'tase [G. *gala*, milk]. An enzyme or proteolytic ferment of milk.

galactemia (gă-lak-te'mĭ-ă) [" + *aima*, blood]. Milky condition of the blood.

galactic (gă-lak'tik) [G. *gala*, milk]. Pert. to flow of milk.

galactidrosis (gă-lak"tĭ-dro'sis) [" + *idrōs*, sweat]. A milklike sweat.

galactin (gă-lak'tin) [G. *gala*, milk]. A basic amorphous substance in milk. SYN: *prolactin*.

galactischia (gă-lak'tis-kĭ-ă). Suppression of the secretion and flow of milk. SYN: *galactoschesia*.

galactoblast (gă-lak'to-blast) [" + *blastos*, germ]. Body found in mammary acini; contains fat globules.

galactocele (gă-lak'to-sēl) [" + *kēlē*, hernia]. 1. A tumor caused by occlusion of a milk duct. 2. Hydrocele containing a milklike liquid.

galac'toid. Resembling milk.

galactolip'in. A phosphorus-free lipid combined with galactose; a cerebroside.

galactoma (gal-ak-to'ma) [" + *ōma*, tumor]. Cystic tumor of female breast. SYN: *galactocele*, 1.

galactom'eter [" + *metron*, measure]. Device for measuring amt. of cream in milk by its specific gravity. SYN: *lactometer*.

galactop'athy [" + *pathos*, disease]. 1. Treatment of nursing infants by drugs administered to the mother. 2. Therapeutic use of milk. SYN: *galactotherapy*.

galactopex'ic [G. *gala*, milk, + *pēxis*, fixation]. Holding galactose. SEE: *galactopexy*.

galac'topexy [" + *pēxis*, fixation]. The fixation of galactose by the liver.

galactophagous (gal-ak-tof'ă-gus) [" + *phagein*, to eat]. Feeding upon milk.

galactophlysis (gal-ak-tof'lĭ-sis) [" + *phlysis*, eruption]. 1. Eruption of vesicles containing milklike contents. 2. Infantile seborrhea of scalp.

galac'tophore [" + *pherein*, to bear]. A milk duct.

galactophoritis (gal-ak-tof-o-ri'tis) [" + " + *-itis*, inflammation]. Inflammation of a milk duct.

galactophorous (gal-ak-tof'or-us) [" + *pherein*, to bear]. Giving milk.

g. ducts. Excretory ducts of the mammae.

galactophthisis (gal-ak-tof'this-is) [" + *phthisis*, wasting]. Debility and emaciation as result of excessive milk secretion.

galactophygous (gal-ak-tof'ĭ-gus) [" + *phygē*, flight]. Arresting flow of milk.

galactoplania (gă-lak"to-pla'nĭ-ă) [" + *planē*, wandering]. Secretion of milk in some abnormal part due to suppression of normal lactation.

galactopoietic (gă-lak"to-poy-et'ik) [" + *poiein*, to make]. Having to do with the production of milk.

galactopyra (gă-lak"to-pi'ră) [" + *pyr*, fire]. Milk fever.

galactorrhea (gă-lak"to-re'ă) [" + *roia*, flow]. 1. Continuation of lactation, or flow of milk at intervals after cessation of nursing. 2. Excessive flow of milk.

galactoschesia, galactoschesis (gal-ak-tos-ke'sĭ-ă, -tos'kĭ-sis) [" + *schesis*, suppression]. A stopping of the milk secretion.

galactoscope (gă-lak'to-skōp) [" + *skopein*, to examine]. Device for measuring quality of milk. SYN: *galactometer*.

galactose (gă-lak'tōs) [G. *gala*, milk]. $C_6H_{12}O_6$ a monosaccharide or simple hexose sugar.

Galactose is an isomer of glucose and is formed along with glucose, in the hydrolysis of lactose. It is dextrorotatory and reduces alkaline copper solutions such as Fehling's solution. It is a component of cerebrosides. In the digestive tract, galactose is readily absorbed; in the liver it is converted into glycogen.

g. tolerance test. Patient fasts overnight and then empties bladder. 40 gm. of galactose in 500 cc. of water are taken orally, then specimens of urine are collected hourly for five hours and the amount of galactose excreted determined. A normal person will excrete up to 3 gm. in this period. Amounts esp. above 6 gm. in excess of this indicate impairment of liver function.

galactosemia (gă-lak"to-se'mĭ-ă). Galactose in the blood.

galactosis (gal-ak-to'sis) [" + *ōsis*]. The secretion of milk.

galactostasis (gal-ak-tos'tă-sis) [" + *stasis*, a stopping]. Cessation or checking of milk secretion. SYN: *galactoschesia*.

galactosu'ria [" + *ouron*, urine]. Galactose in the urine.

galactotherapy (gă-lak"to-ther'ă-pĭ) [" + *therapeia*, treatment]. 1. Treatment of a nursing infant by drugs administered to the mother. 2. Therapeutic use of milk, as a milk diet. SYN: *galactopathy*.

galactotoxin (gă-lak"to-toks'in) [" + *toxikon*, poison]. A poison in milk produced by bacteria.

galactotox'ism [" + " + *ismos*, state of] Milk poisoning.

galactotrophy (gal-ak-tot'ro-fĭ) [" + *trophē*, nourishment]. Feeding with nothing but milk.

galactoxism (gal-ak-toks'izm) [" + *toxikon*, poison, + *ismos*, state of]. Poisoning by milk. SYN: *galactotoxism*.

galactozymase (gă-lak"to-zi'mās) [" + *zymē*, leaven]. A starch-hydrolyzing ferment in milk.

galactu'ria [" + *ouron*, urine]. The passing of milky urine. SYN: *chyluria*.*

galea (ga'le-ă) [L. helmet]. 1. The epicranial aponeurosis which connects the bellies of the occipitofrontal muscle. 2. A type of head bandage.

galeanthropy (ga-le-an'thro-pĭ) [G. *galē*, cat, + *anthrōpos*, man]. A delusion that one has become transformed into a cat.

Ga'len, Claudius. (130-200?) A noted Greek physician and medical writer, born in Mysia and later residing in Rome. Recognized as the "authority" on medicine until the Middle Ages. Called the father of experimental physiology.

G.'s veins. The veins running through the tela chorioidea formed by the joining of the terminal and choroid veins, and forming the v. cerebri magna which empties into the straight sinus.

galena (gă-le'nă). Lead sulfide ore.

galen'ic. Pertaining to Galen or his teachings.

galenicals, galenics (gă-lĕn'ĭ-kăls, -ĭks). 1. Herb and vegetable medicines. 2. Crude drugs and medicinals as distinguished from pure active principles contained in them. 3. A medicine prepared according to an official formula.

galeophilia (gal-e-o-fil'ĭ-ă) [G. *galē*, cat, + *philein*, to love]. Fondness for cats.

galeophobia (gal-e-o-fo'bĭ-ă) [" + *phobos*, fear]. Abnormal aversion to cats.

galeropia, galeropsia (gal-er-o'pĭ-ă, -op'-sĭ-ă) [G. *galeros*, cheerful, + *opsis*, vision]. Unusual clearness of vision.

gall [A.S. *galla*]. 1. An excoriation. 2. The bitter secretion of the liver stored in the gallbladder bile.

It has no ferments and it assists in the emulsifying of fats. It also stimulates intestinal action and multiplies the action of the pancreatic juice threefold. It is discharged through the cystic duct into the duodenum.

RS: *bile duct; calculus; "chol-" words; colic, biliary; cystic duct; vesica fellea.*

gallate (gal'lāt). A salt of gallic acid.

gall'bladder [A.S. *galla* + *blaeddre*, bladder, blister]. Pear-shaped sac on undersurface of right lobe of liver holding bile from the liver until discharged through cystic duct; 3–4 in. long, 1 in. greatest diameter; capacity 50-75 cc. concentrated bile equivalent to 1½ pt. liver bile. See illustration of gallbladder on page B-20.

SYN: *vesica fellea.*

gall'duct [" + L. *ductus,* a passage]. Tube carrying bile from the liver and gallbladder.

gallium (gal'ĭ-um). A rare metal, small amounts of which are found in bauxite and zinc blende. SYMB: Ga. At. wt. 69.72; at. no. 31.

gal'lon. Four quarts; 231 cubic inches or 3785 ml.

gall'stone [A.S. *galla,* bile, + *stān,* stone]. Concretion formed in the gallbladder or bile ducts.

Gallstones may be classified as (1) *pure,* consisting of either cholesterol, calcium bilirubin, or calcium carbonate, or (2) *mixed,* consisting of cholesterol in combination with one or more of the other constituents. In addition to the substances named, gallstones may contain albuminates, cellular debris, or foreign substances such as bacteria, esp. typhoid bacilli. So called "soft" stones (those consisting principally of cholesterol) can be visualized by x-ray only under optimal conditions by cholecystography.

SYM: Stone may remain dormant and give little distress unless inflammation and distention of the gallbladder take place or unless it enters and is unable to pass through the biliary ducts, when colic ensues. The pain may radiate to the back and right shoulder, usually several hours after eating and when the stomach is empty; flatulence, jaundice usually absent.

TREATMENT: Morphine under physician's directions; surgical aid. Surgery.

NP (postoperative): Position, propped up in bed to prevent pneumonia, to permit free drainage, and relieve pressure on diaphragm. Lavage if vomiting is persistent. Only liquids in small amt. given. Note character of drainage and stools for color and nature of contents, and for proper discharge of bile. Protect drainage from all areas. Use cradle if no dressing is permitted, and absorbent pad at side for discharge. SYN: *biliary calculus.*

RS: *bilifuscin, biliphein, biliprasin, calculus, cholelithiasis.*

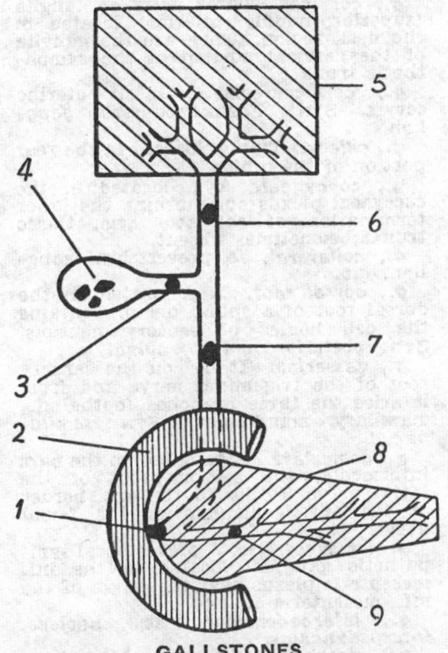

GALLSTONES
(After Sears)

Diagram showing the positions in which gallstones may be found. 1. Gallstone impacted at entrance of bile duct into duodenum. 2. Duodenum. 3. Cystic duct. 4. Gallbladder with stones. 5. Liver. 6. Hepatic duct. 7. Common bile duct. 8. Pancreas. 9. Pancreatic duct with pancreatic calculus.

Gal'ton's whistle [Sir Francis Galton, English scientist, 1822-1911]. A whistle with which a note may be changed, used to test the hearing.

galvan'ic. Pert. to galvanism.

g. battery. A series of cells, giving a combined effect of all the units, and generating electricity by chemical reaction.

g. cell. One of a series of cells generating electricity through chemical reaction.

gal'vanism. Therapeutic use of direct current of electricity.

galvanization (gal-van-i-za'shun). Employment of a galvanic current.

galvanocau'tery. Cauterization of tissue by means of an electric current. SEE: *electrocautery.*

galvanocontractil'ity. Capability of a muscle of contracting under a galvanic stimulation.

galvanofaradiza'tion. Combined use of galvanic and faradic current made possible by use of a De Watteville switch.

galvanom'eter. An instrument that measures current by electromagnetic action.

galvanopalpa'tion. A method of measuring tactile sensibility of the nerves of the skin by the electric current.

galvanopunc'ture. Introduction of needles to complete a galvanic current.

galvanoscope (gal-van'o-skōp). Instrument which shows the presence and direction of a galvanic current.

galvanosur'gery. Use of galvanism in surgery.

galvanotax'is. The tendency of a living organism to arrange itself in a medium so that its axis bears a certain relation to the direction of the current in the medium.

galvanotherapeu'tics, galvanother'apy. Treatment by means of electricity. SYN: *electrotherapy.*

gal'vanotherm"y. Treatment by the heat from a galvanic battery.

galvanot'onus. Tonic contractions caused by a galvanic current.

galvanot'ropism. The tendency of an organism to grow, turn, or move into a certain relation with an electric current.

gamete (gam'ēt) [G. *gametēs,* spouse]. A male or female reproductive cell; the spermatozoon or ovum, *q.v.*

RS: *chromosome, conception, embryo, fertilization, gene, maturation, ovum, spermatozoon.*

The ovum (1/125 in. in diameter) and the spermatozoon (1/500 in. in length). Each mature human germ cell has 46 chromosomes or 23 pairs which are reduced to one-half the number during maturation.

gamet'ic [G. *gametēs,* spouse]. Pert. to gametes.

gametocide (gam'ĕ-to-sīd) [" + L. *caedere,* to kill]. An agent destructive to gametocytes, particularly those of malaria.

gametocyte (gă-me'to-sīt) [" + *kytos,* cell]. The sexual cell forming the gamete. An oocyte or spermatocyte.

gametogen'esis. For formation of gametes: oogenesis or spermatogenesis. SEE: *maturation.*

gametog'ony. The phase in the life cycle of the malarial parasite (*Plasmodium*) in which male and female gametocytes, which infect the mosquito, are formed.

gamet'ophyte. In plants, the sexual or gamete-producing generation which alternates with the asexual or spore-producing generation.

Gam'gee tissue [Sampson Gamgee, British surgeon, 1826-1886]. A dressing made of a thick layer of absorbent cotton between two layers of absorbent gauze; used for surgical dressing.

gam'ic. Sexual, esp. as applied to eggs which develop only after fertilization in contrast to those which develop parthenogenetically.

gam'ma (G. letter g.). 1. Third letter of the Greek alphabet, γ. 2. In Chem., used to designate the third of a series, as the third carbon atom in an aliphatic chain. 3. One microgram; or one thousandth of a milligram (0.001 mg.); one millionth of a gram.

g. globulin. A protein formed in the blood. Ability to resist infection is related to concentration of such proteins.

g. rays. Electromagnetic waves of extremely short wave length emitted by radioactive substances. They are thought to be of the same nature as x-rays. They have greater penetrating power than alpha or beta rays, and, when passing through a magnetic field, are not deflected. SEE: *rays.*

gam'macism [G. *gamma,* g, + *ismos,* state of]. Inability to pronounce correctly *g* and *k* sounds.

Gamna's disease. Splenomegaly with slow, progressive enlargement of the spleen.

G.'s nodules. Nodules stained yellow or brown in certain varieties of splenic enlargement. SEE: *G.'s disease.*

gamo- [G.]. Combining form from *gamos,* sexual union.

gam'ont [" + *ontos,* being]. A sexual form of certain protozoons.

gamophobia (gam-o-fo'bĭ-ă) [" + *phobos,* fear]. Psychoneurotic aversion to the marriage relationship.

gampsodactylia (gamp"so-dak-til'ĭ-ă) [G. *gampsos,* curved, + *daktylos,* finger]. Deformity of the toes resembling claws. SYN: *clawfoot.*

ganglial (gang'lĭ-ăl) [G. *gagglion,* ganglion]. Pert. to a ganglion. SYN: *ganglionic.*

gangliated (gang'lĭ-at-ed) [G. *gagglion,* ganglion]. 1. Having ganglia. 2. Intermixed.

g. cord. Main trunk of sympathetic nervous system.

gangliec'tomy [" + *ektomē,* excision]. Excision of a ganglion.

gangliform (gang'lĭ-form) [" + L. *forma,* shape]. Formed like a ganglion.

ganglioform (gang'lĭ-o-form). Same as gangliform, *q.v.*

ganglioglio'ma [" + *glia,* glue, + *ōma,* tumor]. A ganglion cell glioma.

ganglioglioneuroma (gang"glĭ-o-glĭ"o-nu-ro'mă) [" + " + *neuron,* nerve, + *ōma,* tumor]. Ganglion cells, glia cells, and nerve fibers in a nerve tumor.

ganglioma (gang-lĭ-o'mă) [" + *ōma,* tumor]. 1. Tumor of a lymphatic gland. 2. A swelling of lymphoid tissue.

ganglion (gang'lĭ-ŏn) (pl. *ganglia*) (G. *gagglion,* ganglion). 1. A mass of nervous tissue composed principally of nerve-cell bodies and lying outside the brain or spinal cord: e.g. the chain of ganglia which form the main sympathetic trunks; the dorsal root ganglion of a spinal nerve. 2. Cystic tumors developing on a tendon or aponeurosis; sometimes occur on the back of the wrist.

g., abdominal. Any one of the abdominal ganglia.

g., ant. cerebral. Corpus striatum. Corpus striatum and corpus lenticulare considered together.

g., aorticore'nal. A g. lying near to the lower border of the celiac g. It is located near the origin of the renal artery.

g., Arnold's auricular. Tiny g. located beneath foramen ovale. SYN: *otic g.; otoganglion.*

g., auricular. SEE: *Arnold's auricular g.*

g., autonomic. A ganglion of the autonomic division of the nervous system.

g., basal. Mass of gray matter beneath 3rd ventricle. Consisting of the caudate, lentiform, and amygdaloid nuclei and the claustrum.

g., basal optic. Mass of gray matter beneath 3rd ventricle.

g., cardiac. Tiny g. toward which converge the fibers of superficial cardiac plexus. It lies on the right side of the ligamentum arteriosus. SYN: *ganglion of Wrisberg.*

g., carotid. G. formed by filamentous threads from the carotid plexus beneath the carotid artery.

g., celiac. One of a pair of prevertebral or collateral ganglia located near the origin of the celiac artery. They form a part of the celiac plexus. SYN: *semilunar g.*

g., cerebral. Main cerebral nerve centers.

g., cervical. Three pairs of ganglia (superior, middle, inferior) located in the neck region. They are the ganglia of the cervical portion of the sympathetic trunk.

g., cervicouterine. G. of uterine cervix. SYN: *Frankenhauser's ganglion.*

g., ciliary. Tiny g. located in the rear portion of the orbit.

g., coccygeal. A g. located in the coccygeal plexus and forming the lower termination of the two sympathetic trunks; sometimes absent.

g., collateral. A prevertebral ganglion, *q.v.*

g., dorsal root. A g. located on the dorsal root of a spinal nerve. Contains the cell bodies of sensory neurons. SYN: *posterior root g.; spinal g.*

g., gasserian. It lies on the sensory root of the trigeminal nerve and from it arise the three branches (opthalmic, maxillary, mandibular). SYN: *semilunar g.*

g., geniculate. A ganglion on the pars intermedia, the sensory root of the facial nerve. It lies in the ant. border of the ant. geniculum of the facial nerve.

g., inf. mesentric. A prevertebral sympathetic ganglion located in the inf. mesenteric plexus near the origin of the inf. mesenteric artery.

g., interpeduncular. SEE: *nucleus, interpeduncular.*

g., intervertebral. A spinal ganglion, *q.v.*

g., jugular. A g. located on the root of the vagus nerve and lying in upper portion of jugular foramen.

g., lateral. One of a chain of ganglia forming the main sympathetic trunk; also called vertebral ganglion.

g., lenticular. SEE: *ciliary g.*

g., lumbar. G. usually four in number in the lumbar portion of the sympathetic trunk.

g., Meckel's. SEE: *sphenopalatine ganglion.*

g., nodose. G. of the trunk of the vagus nerve. Located immediately below jugular ganglion. It makes connections with the spinal accessory nerve, hypoglossal nerve, and the sup. cervical ganglion of the sympathetic trunk.

g., ophthalmic, g., optic. SEE: *ciliary g.*

g., otic. A small ganglion located deep in the zygomatic fossa immediately below the foramen ovale. It lies medial to the mandibular nerve. It supplies postganglionic parasympathetic fibers to the parotid gland. SYN: *Arnold's g.*

g., petrous. G. located on lower margin of temporal bone's petrous portion.

g., pharyngeal. G. in contact with the glossopharyngeal nerve.

g., phrenic. One of a group of ganglia joining the phrenic plexus.

g., renal. One of a group of ganglia joining the renal plexus.

g., sacral. Four small ganglia located in the sacral portion of the sympathetic trunk. They lie on the anterior surface of the sacrum and are connected to the spinal nerves by gray rami.

g., semilunar. 1. The gasserian g. *q.v.* 2. The celiac g., *q.v.*

g., sphenopalatine. A g. associated with the great superficial petrosal nerve (branch of facial) and the maxillary nerve. It transmits both sympathetic and parasympathetic fibers to the nasal mucosa, palate, pharynx and orbit.

g., spinal. Ganglionic enlargement of spinal nerves' dorsal roots. SYN: *dorsal root g.; post. root g.*

g., spiral. A long coiled ganglion in the cochlea of the ear. It contains bipolar cells, the peripheral processes of which terminate in the organ of Corti. The central processes form the cochlear portion of the acoustic nerve and terminate in the cochlear nuclei of the medulla.

g., submaxillary. A g. lying between the mylohyoideus and hyoglossus muscles and suspended from the lingual nerve by two small branches. Peripheral fibers pass to the submandibular, sublingual, lingual, and adjacent salivary glands. SYN: *submandibular g.*

g., superior mesenteric. A prevertebral ganglion of the sympathetic nervous system which lies close to the celiac ganglion and with it forms a part of the celiac (solar) plexus. It lies close to the base of the sup. mesenteric artery.

g., suprarenal. G. situated in the suprarenal plexus.

g., sympathetic. Those of the thoracolumbar (sympathetic) division of the autonomic nervous system. Include vertebral or lateral ganglia (those forming the sympathetic trunk) and prevertebral or collateral ganglia, more peripherally located.

g., temporal. Tiny g. joining the ant. branches of sup. cervical g.

g., terminal. A ganglion of the autonomic division of the nervous system which lies close to or within the organ innervated.

g., thoracic. One of 12 ganglia of thoracic area of sympathetic nerve.

g., tympanic. On tympanic portion of the glossopharyngeal nerve.

g., vestibular. A bilobed g. located on the vestibular branch of the acoustic nerve at the bottom of the int. acoustic meatus. Its peripheral fibers arise in the maculae of the sacculus and utriculus and the cristae of the ampullae of the semicircular ducts. SYN: *g. of Scarpa.*

gang'lionated (G. *gagglion,* ganglion). Having or consisting of ganglia.

ganglionectomy (gang-lĭ-o-nek'to-mĭ) [" + *ektomē,* excision]. Excision of a ganglion.

ganglioneuroma (gang"lĭ-o-nū-ro'mă) [" + " + *ōma,* tumor]. A neuroma containing ganglion cells.

ganglionic (gang-lĭ-on'ik) [G. *gagglion,* ganglion]. Pert. to or of the nature of a ganglion.

ganglionitis (gang-lĭ-on-i'tis) [" + *-itis,* inflammation]. Inflamed condition of a ganglion.

gang'lioside. A cerebroside present in the brain and containing neuraminic acid, a particular type of fatty acid.

gangosa. A lesion of the nose and hard palate, regarded as a late stage of yaws: rhinopharyngitis mutilans.

gangrene (gan'grēn) [G. *gaggraina,* an eating sore]. The putrefaction of soft tissue; a form of necrosis. SYN: *mortification.*

ETIOL: Usually results from cutting off of blood supply to an organ or tissue, which may result from inflammatory processes, injury, or degenerative changes such as arteriosclerosis. It is commonly a sequela of boils, frostbite, crushing injuries, or diseases such as diabetes, tuberculosis, syphilis, and Raynaud's disease. The part that dies is known as a *slough* if the soft tissues are involved, or a *sequestrum* if it is a bone that dies. It must be removed before healing can take place.

g., anemic. G. resulting from an obstructed circulation in the part.

g., angioneurotic. State resulting from thrombotic arteries and veins.

g., diabetic. Moist gangrenous condition arising in some diabetics.

g., dry. This results when the part that dies has little blood and when it remains aseptic. The arteries but not the veins are obstructed. The tissues dry and drop off, the process continuing for weeks or months. SYM: Pain in early stages. The part is cold and black and begins to wither. The toes are generally first affected spreading to the knee. Usually seen in advanced diabetes and arteriosclerosis.

g., embolic. Gangrenous condition arising subsequent to an embolic obstruction.

g., gas. This is gangrene in a wound infected by a gas bacillus, the most common etiologic agent being *Clostridium perfringens.*

TREATMENT: Surgical intervention, antibiotics, clostridial antitoxin.

g., hospital. Moist gangrene due to wound contamination by putrefactive bacteria. It was common in hospitals in the days when overcrowding and lack of cleanliness were the rule.

g., humid. SEE: *moist g.*

g., idiopathic. When the cause is unknown.

g., infective. Due to infection, as in carbuncle necrosis, cancrum oris and cancrum noma.

g., moist. This occurs after a crushing injury, usually at distal part of an extremity, or when dry gangrene is infected with putrefactive bacteria, and when the part is full of blood. SYM: The part is hot, red, later cold and bluish, commencing to slough. It spreads rapidly and there is an offensive odor. The process is known to the layman as "mortification." Death may result in a few days.

g., primary. G. developing in a part without previous inflammation.

g., secondary. G. developing subsequent to local inflammation.

g., senile. G. developing in the limbs of the senile. Believed to be due to arteriosclerosis.

g., symmetric. G. on opposite sides of the body in corresponding parts. Usually the result of vasomotor disturbances. Characteristic of Raynaud's and Buerger's disease.

g., traumatic. Result of extensive injuries.

gangrenosis (gang-gren-o'sis) [" + *-ōsis*]. Condition of mortification or gangrene.

gan'grenous [G. *gaggraina,* an eating sore]. Of the nature of gangrene.

gan'oblast [G. *ganos,* brightness, + *blastos,* cell]. The cell which forms enamel of a tooth. SYN: *ameloblast.*

Ganser's syndrome (gan'zerz sin'drōm) [Sigbert J. M. Ganser, German psychiatrist, 1853-1931]. "Nonsense syndrome." Absurd acts and speech seen in prison psychosis, hysteria, and other states.

gap. An opening or a break; an interruption in continuity.

g., auscultatory. A period of silence which occurs in the determination of blood pressure by the auscultatory method. Exact cause unknown. May cause a false reading of the blood pressure. SEE: *blood pressure.*

g., cranial. A congenital fissure in the skull.

gargarism (gar'gar-izm) [G. *gargarisma,* a gargle]. A gargle or throat wash.

gargle (gar'gl) [L. *gurguliō,* windpipe]. 1. A wash for the throat. 2. To wash out the mouth and throat by tipping the head back so that the fluid runs to the tonsils and is there agitated by expired air that is forced out of the lungs.

gargoylism. A condition usually congenital characterized by dwarfism, kyphosis, and other skeletal abnormalities, disturbances in lipoid metabolism, and usually mental deficiency. SYN: *lipochondrodystrophy; Hurler's disease.*

garlic [A.S. *gar,* spear, + *leak,* the leek]. An edible, strongly flavored bulb of *Allium sativum* used mainly for seasoning. COMP: The active principle of garlic is sulfide of allyl.

ACTION: It is a gastric stimulant and an intestinal antiseptic.

gar'rot [Fr. *garroter,* to tie fast]. A form of tourniquet.

Gart'ner's duct [Hermann T. Gartner, Danish surgeon and anatomist, 1785-1827]. A small duct, the mesosalpinx lying parallel to the uterine tube. It is a vestigial structure representing the persistent mesonephric duct. Also called duct of the epoophoron; ductus epoophori longitudinalis.

G.A.S. Abbreviation for *general adaptation syndrome.*

gas. 1. One of the basic forms of matter. The molecules are free and move swiftly in all directions. Thus a gas not only takes the shape of the containing vessel but expands and fills the vessel no matter what its volume. 2. An airlike fluid subject to expansion and convertible into a liquid by cooling or compression.

Among the common important gases are oxygen; illuminating gas; exhaust gas; sewer gas, which contains carbon monoxide (*q.v.*), carbon dioxide (*q.v.*); the anesthetic gases (SEE: *anesthesia*); ammonia (*q.v.*); the poison war gases, etc. Liquids and solids when heated often give off fumes which may be poisonous; among the more common are the mineral acids, ammonia water, mercury and its compounds, cyanides, zinc-containing metals, etc. SEE: *gases.*

g. bacillus. SEE: *gangrene.*

g. (in the) blood. The principal gases found in the blood are oxygen, nitrogen, and carbon dioxide. They may be dissolved in the plasma or they may exist in loose chemical combination with other compounds, as oxygen combined with hemoglobin.

g., digestive tract. Among the gases in the digestive tract are: oxygen, nitrogen, hydrogen, carbon dioxide, methane, and in decomposition of proteins, hydrogen sulfide, indole, skatole, ammonia, etc.

g., distention. Abdominal distention is result of abnormal gaseous, fluid, or solid accumulation in abdominal cavity. It may be: (a) acute; (b) chronic; (c) local, or (d) general. The abdominal wall, the cavity, or the intra-abdominal viscera may be involved. *Postoperative*: Result of complication following an operation. Limited to lower part of small, and all of large intestines. Careless administration of anesthesia may be a cause, as is degree of peritonitis. *Preoperative*: Enema is a preventive. TREATMENT: No cold fluids, change of posture, insertion of rectal tube, enemata only as advised by surgeon.

g. excretions. Oxidation produces carbon dioxide or carbonic acid gas, from one-half to two-thirds of a cubic ft. per hr. being produced by an adult male of average weight. Activity increases the amount. Ordinarily only water vapor and carbon dioxide are given off.

g. gangrene. That caused by the gas bacillus. SEE: *gangrene.*

g., illuminating. This is a mixture of various combustible gases including hydrogen and carbon monoxide. Its poisonous effects are largely due to carbon monoxide, *q.v.* TREATMENT: Resuscitation, *q.v.*

g. in the blood. Dissolved gases are found in the blood in the form of oxygen, nitrogen, and a small portion of carbon dioxide, with carbonic acid from the tissues.

g., laughing. Nitrous oxide.

g., marsh. Methane.

g., mustard. Poisonous gas used in warfare (dichlorethyl sulfide).

g., refrigerant. A number of these gases are used in ordinary household mechanical refrigerators. Poisoning may be caused by leaks, faulty connections or breakage, and gas dissipated into the atmosphere. Among these gases are methyl chloride, ammonia, sulfur dioxide and more than 20 other gases. Most of these are toxic. Careful researches are now being carried on to develop nontoxic gases. Warning agents mixed with these gases are not a guarantee of protection to infants, children, hospital patients, firemen and refrigerator workers; therefore, instead of merely adding a protective agent, it would be wiser to have a nontoxic refrigerant. *Methyl chloride* is responsible for more poisoning than other refrigerant gases. *Sulfur dioxide*: As this is a respiratory irritant it is easily detected, so serious poisoning is not likely to occur.

g., tear. A gas that irritates the conjunctiva and which produces a flow of tears.

gaseous (gas'e-us). Of the nature or form of gas.

gases, war. Any chemical substances whether solid, liquid, or vapor, used to produce poisonous gases with irritant effects. They can be classified as *lacrimators, sternutators, lung irritants, vesicants,* and those that act as a systemic poison. Some gases have multiple effects.

They are known as persistent or nonpersistent, *i. e.,* those which diffuse and are dispersed fairly rapidly, and those which linger and evaporate slowly.

It is of the greatest importance that persons rendering first aid should avoid becoming casualties; precautions must be taken, masks worn, as well as being applied to the patients. Strict discipline must be maintained during gas raids in order to avoid panic. If gas training has been thorough and if organization is good, much may be done to lessen the effect, and maintain a good morale.

Decontamination centers are essential and nurses must understand that thorough decontamination of clothing, boots, ambulances, etc., is vitally necessary, and they should make themselves familiar with the necessary procedures.

g., lewisite. Contains arsenic and smells of geraniums.

SYM: Similar to those of vesicant gas, *q.v.,* but come on at once and as a rule are not so severe. Arsenic can be recovered from the serum of the blisters and symptoms of arsenic poisoning may occur.

TREATMENT: Similar to that for vesicant gas, *q.v.*

g., lung irritant. Ex: *Chlorine and phosgene.*

SYM: Burning sensation of the eyes, nose, and throat, bronchitis and pneumonia, sometimes followed by edema of the lungs and probably death.

TREATMENT: Remove patient from exposure, apply respirator; if there has been exposure to phosgene (smells like musty hay) the symptoms may be delayed and the patient may collapse later. It is important, therefore, to provide complete rest, remove patient on a stretcher, and provide warmth; oxygen may be required in large quantities over a fairly long period.

g., mustard. Dichlorethyl sulfide. SEE: *g., vesicant.*

g., nose irritant. Diphenylchloroarsine. An irritant smoke.

SYM: Intense pain in the nose, throat, and air passages and sneezing followed by headache and aching in teeth and jaws, acute mental depression, and sometimes vomiting.

TREATMENT: Casualties must be reassured that no permanent harm is done and should be warned against removing respirator in spite of the fact the symptoms may get worse after donning it. This is a gas likely to lead to "panic." Nasal douching with warm sodium bicarbonate is helpful.

g., suffocating. Made from chlorine compounds.

g., tear. Substance which, when dispersed into the air, causes the eyes to be blinded by tears. Ex: *bromoacetone.*

SYM: Causes much inconvenience. Irritation of the nose and eyes, and free lacrimation so that it is impossible to see.

TREATMENT: As a rule, none is necessary, for upon removal from the contaminated area, the symptoms tend gradually to subside.

g., toxic. Hydrocyanic acid type.

g., vesicant. Attack every part of body; clothing and boots are infected and a source of danger. Ex: *mustard g., lewisite.*

SYM: Do not appear at once; may be 6 hr. or longer before the patient is aware of anything wrong. Pain in the eyes, lacrimation, and discharge may be the first evidence, the eyelids swelling and the patient being unable to see; there is a diffuse redness of the skin, followed by blistering and ulceration.

PROG: Healing is very slow, but generally follows if treatment is prompt and efficient.

TREATMENT: Decontamination is essential and must be thorough. Bathe eyes freely with normal saline or plain water; a drop or 2 of castor oil will prevent lids sticking; no bandage should be worn. The patient should be scrubbed, if possible, under a hot or warm shower for 10 minutes. Bleach cream or powder, if ordered, should be applied first, and left in contact with the skin for 5 minutes. If, in spite of these precautionary measures, blisters arise, they may be successfully treated with tannic acid.

g., vomiting. That induces emesis, specifically chloropicrin.

gas'oline. A product of the destructive distillation of petroleum.

Most motor fuel contains ethyl lead, ethyl antimony or ethyl arsenic combinations which increase the toxicity markedly. Slightly antiseptic if free from these compounds, and may be used to wash grease out of wounds, although ether is better.

SYM. OF POISONING: Giddiness, headache, intoxication, nervous disturbance, muscular tremors, difficulty in respiration, paralyses, convulsions, cyanosis, unconsciousness, pulmonary hemorrhage. Usually no local disturbance of stomach.

F. A. TREATMENT: Fresh air, inhalation of oxygen and carbon dioxide; artificial respiration when necessary. Otherwise treat symptoms.

gasomet'ric. Pert. to measurement of gases.

gasometry (gas-om'ĕ-trĭ) [G. *metron,* measure]. Estimation of amount of gas present in a mixture.

gasp. To catch the breath; to inhale and exhale with quick, difficult breaths; the act of gasping.

gasserectomy (gas-er-ek'to-mĭ) [G. *ektome,* excision]. Excision of the gasserian ganglion.

gasse'rian arteries. A branch from the int. carotid a. and one of the middle meningeal a. to the gasserian ganglion. SEE: *ganglion.*

gas'sing. The use of war gases, *q.v.*

gaster-, gastero-, gastro-. Combining forms meaning "pertaining to the stomach or the region of the stomach."

gasteral'gia [G. *gastēr,* belly, + *algos,* pain]. Gastralgia, *q.v.*

gasterangiemphraxis (gas"ter-an"jĭ-em-fraks'is) [" + *aggeion,* vessel, + *emphraxis,* obstruction]. 1. Congestion of blood vessels of stomach. 2. Pyloric obstruction.

gasterasthenia (gas-ter-as-the'nĭ-ă) [" + *asthĕneia,* weakness]. Gastrasthenia, *q.v.*

gasterhysterotomy (gas"ter-his-ter-ot'o-mĭ) [" + *ystera,* uterus, + *tomē,* incision]. Incision of uterus through abdomen. SEE: *cesarean operation.*

gastorrhagia (gas-tor-a'jĭ-ă) [" + *rēgnunai,* a bursting forth]. Gastorrhagia, *q.v.*

gastradenitis (gas-trad-en-i'tis) [" + *adēn,* gland, + *-itis,* inflammation]. Inflammation of the stomach glands.

gastralgia (gas-tral'jĭ-ă) [" + *algos,* pain]. Pain in the stomach from any cause.

gastralgocenosis (gas-tral"go-sen-o'sis). Gastralgokenosis, *q.v.*

gastralgokenosis (gas-tral-go-ken-o'sis) [" + " + *kenōsis,* emptiness]. Gastric pain due to emptiness of stomach; hunger pangs due to hunger contractions, powerful peristalic contractions which sweep over the stomach.

gastraneuria (gas-tra-nu'rĭ-ă) [" + *neuron,* nerve]. Defective action of nerves of the stomach.

gastrasthe'nia [" + *asthĕneia,* weakness]. Debility of the stomach. SYN: *gasterasthenia.*

gastratrophia (gas-tră-tro'fĭ-ă) [" + *atropheia,* atrophy]. Atrophy of the stomach.

gastrecta'sia, gastrec'tasis [" + *ektasis,* dilatation]. Dilatation of the stomach. May be acute or chronic.

ETIOL: Obstruction of pylorus; atony, overeating, congenital weakness, imperfect peristalsis, omental hernia, periduodenal adhesions, gastroptosis.

SYM: *Chronic*: Vomiting of food taken several days before, vomitus sour, contains fatty acids, mucus, bacteria. *Acute*: Severe, sudden pain accompanied by collapse. Small, rapid pulse, temperature subnormal, upper abdominal pain resembling angina pectoris. Distended and tympanic abdomen. Vomiting of fluids and eructation of gas.

gastrectomy (gas-trek'to-mĭ) [G. *gaster,* belly, + *ek-tomē,* excision]. Surgical removal of a part or the whole of the stomach.

gas'tric [G. *gaster,* stomach]. Pert. to the stomach.

g. analysis. Determines quality of secretion, amount of free and combined hydrochloric acid, absence or presence of blood, bile, bacteria, fatty acids. Esp. necessary if gastric ulcer or carcinoma is suspected.

g. digestion. 1. As food passes through the cardiac orifice into the stomach, it tends to accumulate in the lowest part of the major curvature. 2. Successive portions of food are added to this, tending to accumulate in the innermost portion of the mass. The walls of the stomach gradually relax adapting themselves to the amount of the contents. This is the result of a *gastric feeding reflex* which also inhibits peristalsis in the remaining portion of the stomach. 3. Within the mass, salivary digestion continues for a short time, but in those portions touching the stomach wall, the salivary ptyalin is destroyed by the acid.

CHEMICAL ASPECTS: During the meal, nervous impulses from the brain are carried to the stomach by way of the vagi; they result from the sensations of sight, smell, and taste. In addition, the stretching of the stomach wall excites the gastric glands by local nervous mechanisms, and chemical substances initially present in the food (preformed secretagogues) or produced during the digestion of the food (derived secretagogues) are absorbed and further stimulate the gastric glands.

The following changes occur in the food while in the stomach. Pepsin acts on proteins of high molecular weight hydrolyzing them to proteoses and peptones. Pepsin also coagulates milk. Hydrochloric acid is essential for the activity of pepsin. It also dissolves collagen, disintegrates nucleoproteins, hydrolyzes double sugars, and is responsible for the antiseptic action of the gastric juice. Gastric lipase acts on emulsified fats reducing them to fatty acids and glycerol but its action is limited.

MOTOR ASPECTS: After the initial relaxation, the stomach increases its pressure upon its contents. The cardiac sphincter closes firmly to prevent regurgitation into the esophagus. The pyloric part of the stomach begins to exhibit wavelets of contraction which run toward the pylorus. They become deeper, and their focus of origin shifts in the direction of the cardia.

At first the pylorus, like the cardia, remains firmly closed, and the wavelets result only in mixing and in facilitating the chemical comminution and solution. Now the pylorus begins to open occasionally, allowing the acid chyme to spurt at intervals into the duodenum. The further course of the chyme is described under *duodenal digestion.*

g. fever. Fever accompanied by gastric disturbances.

g. glands. Cardiac, fundic or oxyntic, and pyloric glands of the stomach.

These are tubular glands lying in the mucosa of the wall, and the gastric juice exudes from them just as sweat drips from one's forehead. The general result of gastric digestion is the reduction of the ingested mass to a mushy, gray mixture called "acid chyme."

They contain (a) chief, zymogenic, or peptic cells which secrete pepsinogen, the inactive form of pepsin; (b) parietal border, or oxyntic cells which secrete hydrochloric acid, and (c) mucous cells found in the neck of the gland, which secrete mucin.

g. juice. The digestive juice of the gastric glands of the stomach. It contains pepsin, hydrochloric acid, mucin, small quantities of inorganic salts, and the "intrinsic factor" of the antianemic principle. It is strongly acid having a pH of 0.9 to 1.5. It is a thin colorless fluid, its total acidity being equivalent to 10 to 50 ml. of tenth normal (10%) hydrochloric acid; free HCl from 0 to 30 ml. of tenth normal HCl. The amount secreted in 24 hours varies greatly.

The mixture of acid and pepsin has effects which neither substance has alone, and dissolves some proteins with remarkable speed. Rennin is the cause of the normal clotting or curdling of milk in the stomach. There is also a lipase which can release butyric fat from butter fat and this gives the characteristic odor to vomitus.

DIAG. (findings): *Carcinoma*: Lactic acid, blood, Boas-Oppler bacilli, sarcinae, and sometimes tumor cells are present; frequently no hydrochloric acid is found. *Hyperacidity*: May indicate gastric ulcer. *Lactic Acid*: Present in carcinoma. *Pus Cells*: Indicate severe damage to stomach. *Red Cells*: Same significance as pus cells.

RS: *gastric analysis, hydrochloric acid, hyper- and hypochlorhydria, stomach (digestion in).*

g. lavage. Washing out of the stomach.

USES: 1. To empty stomach when contents are irritating, as in prolonged postanesthetic vomiting, and in some cases of regurgitant vomiting in acute intestinal obstruction. 2. To clean cavity before an operation is performed upon it. 3. To remove poison in cases in which this method of treatment is indicated. 4. For removal of a test meal.

METHOD: If possible patient is propped up in bed; a rubber sheet and towel are placed around neck and arranged to protect clothing in front. The apparatus required is: An esophageal tube, with plastic or glass connection; a length of rubber tubing and a funnel; several pints of solution and a solution thermometer; glycerine to lubricate tube; a towel and receiver for vomit, which patient may be allowed to hold; a pint measure and pail for returned fluid; a receiver for stomach contents, and sodium bicarbonate solution, a dram to the pint. Should be prepared at a temperature of 100° F.

The procedure is explained to the patient if he is capable of understanding. His mouth is cleaned and he is asked to swallow the lubricated tube which is placed in his mouth. He is encouraged to try and control the desire to retch. As the tube is swallowed the nurse will gently help to pass it along. When a special mark on the tube is on a level with the patient's lips the tube may be expected to be in the stomach, and the funnel is attached to glass connection by short length of rubber tubing and is then inverted to empty the stomach of its contents; if nothing is seen, the tube should be passed farther in until it is found to be in the stomach.

If possible collect stomach contents in receiver provided. Then pinch the tube below funnel and fill the funnel with solution, expel air from the tube by pinching and rubbing it upwards towards the funnel. Let fluid run in very slowly, using from ½ to 1 pint at a time; invert funnel and let this run out, repeat until all fluid has been used or until it returns clear. When the treatment is finished, pinch tube and withdraw it quickly, giving patient a mouthwash immediately, and then place soiled tube in a basin of tepid water.

The siphoned gastric contents should be examined, and the amount of returned solution measured and inspected for blood, bile, and mucus. If necessary, it should be saved for the doctor's inspection or labeled and specimen sent to laboratory if so ordered.

g. motor meals. These meals are used to test the motor activity of the stomach and intestines. SEE: *Boas motor m.; Von Leube m.*

g. mucin (mu'sin). A fine, straw-colored powder, prepared from hog stomach. Used as a protective in peptic ulcer.

g. ulcer. An ulcer of the stomach. SYN: *peptic ulcer, q.v.*

gastricism (gas'trĭ-sizm) [G. *gastēr*, belly, + *ismos*, state]. Any gastric disorder.

gas'trin [G. *gastēr*, belly]. A hormone that stimulates secretion of the glands in the cardiac end of the stomach. It is formed at the pyloric end of the stomach.

gastritis (gas-tri'tis) [" + *-ītis*, inflammation]. Inflammation of the stomach.

Characterized by epigastric pain or tenderness, thirst, nausea, vomiting, and diarrhea. The mucosa may be atrophic or hypertrophic.

ETIOL: Generally unknown. May result from infection, excessive indulgence in alcoholic beverages, dietary indiscretions. Pain in the region of the stomach may be due to causes other than gastritis, such as cancer. Gastritis may be due to an excess or a deficiency of hydrochloric acid, and a remedy suitable for one would not be proper for the other condition. The type must first be determined before medication.

g., acute. SYM: Moderate fever; anorexia, coated tongue; intense pain in epigastrium, persistent vomiting, thirst; prostration. PROG: Good. TREATMENT: Absolute rest. In severe cases no food by mouth till stomach becomes retentive. Thirst allayed with cracked ice.

g., atrophic. Chronic g. with atrophied mucosa and glands.

g., chronic. SYM: Weight and distress after eating; often tenderness on palpation. Eructations of gas and some liquid, nausea and vomiting frequently, constipation. PROG: Good. TREATMENT: Hygienic conditions, regulated diet.

g., excess acid (hyperchlorhydria). SYM: Pain more intense than in acid deficiency. Good appetite.

g., hypertrophic. G. combined with glandular hypertrophy and infiltration.

g., phlegmonous. Acute g. with suppuration of the mucosa and submucosa.

g., polypous. G. characterized by knoblike projections on the surface.

g., pseudomembranous. G. marked by membranous patch formation.

gastro- [G. *gastēr*, stomach]. Used as a combining form to denote the *stomach.*

gastroanastomosis (gas"tro-an-as"to-mo'sis) [" + *ana*, up, + *stoma*, mouth, + *-ōsis*]. Formation of passage bet. two pouches of stomach for relief of hour-glass contraction.

gastroblennorrhea (gas-tro-blen-o-re'ă) [" + *blennos*, mucus, + *roia*, flow]. Excessive secretion of gastric mucus.

gastrobrosis (gas-tro-bro'sis) [" + *brōsis*, eating]. Perforating ulcer of the stomach.

gastrocamera (gas"tro-kam'ĕ-ră). A camera small enough to be swallowed. Used to photograph inside of stomach.

gastrocele (gas'tro-sēl) [" + *kēlē*, hernia]. Hernia of the stomach.

gastrochronorrhea (gas-tro-kron-o-re'ă) [" + *chronos*, time, + *roia*, flow]. Chronic gastric disease marked by permanent hypersecretion with dilatation and thickening of stomach walls and hypertrophy of glands. SYN: *Reichmann's disease.*

gastrocnemius (gas-trok-ne'mĭ-us) [" + *knēmē*, leg]. The large muscle of the leg. Extends foot and helps to flex knee upon thigh.

gastrocol'ic [" + *kōlon*, colon]. Pert. to stomach and colon.

g. omentum. The great omentum. SYN: *epiploon.*

g. reflex. Peristaltic wave in colon induced by entrance of food into fasting stomach.

gastrocoli'tis [" + " + *-ītis*, inflammation]. Inflammation of stomach and colon.

gastrocoloptosis (gas-tro-kol-op-to'sis) [" + " + *ptōsis,* dropping]. Downward prolapse of stomach and colon.

gastrocolostomy (gas-tro-kol-os'to-mĭ) [" + " + *stoma,* opening]. Establishment of permanent passage bet. stomach and colon.

gastrocolotomy (gas-tro-ko-lot'o-mĭ) [" + " + *tomē,* incision]. Incision into stomach and colon.

gastrocolpotomy (gas-tro-kol-pot'o-mĭ) [G. *gastēr,* belly, + *kolpos,* vagina, + *tomē,* incision]. An incision through the abdominal wall into upper part of vagina.

gastrodiaphane (gas-tro-di'ă-fān) [" + *dia,* through, + *phainein,* to show]. Device for electrically illuminating stomach interior, making visible its outlines through the abdomen.

gastrodiaphanos'copy, gastrodiaph'any [" + " + " + *skopein,* to examine]. Examination of interior of the stomach by rendering its walls translucent by an electric light introduced through the esophagus into the stomach.

gastrodisciasis (gas-tro-dis-kĭ-a'sis). Infestation by a fluke, *Gastrodiscoides hominis.*

Gastrodiscoides (gas"tro-dis-koy'dēz). A genus of flukes belonging to family Gastrodiscidae, suborder Amphistomata.

G. hominis. A species of flukes commonly infesting hogs but occasionally found in man.

gastroduodenal (gas"tra-du-o-dēn'al). Related to the stomach and duodenum.

gastroduodenitis (gas"tro-dū-od-en-i'tis) [" + L. *duodenum,* duodenum, + G. *-ītis,* inflammation]. Inflammation of stomach and duodenum.

gastroduodenostomy (gas"tro-du-o-den-os'to-mĭ) [" + " + G. *stoma,* mouth]. Formation of an artificial opening between the stomach and duodenum.

gastrodynia (gas-tro-din'ĭ-ă) [" + *odynē,* pain]. Pain in the stomach. Syn: *gastralgia.**

gastroelytrotomy (gas-tro-el-ĭ-trot'o-mĭ) [" + *elytron,* vagina, + *tomē,* incision]. Cesarean section through linea alba into upper portion of vagina. Syn: *gastrocolpotomy.*

gastroenteralgia (gas"tro-en-ter-al'jĭ-ă) [" + *enteron,* intestine, + *algos,* pain]. Pain in stomach and intestines.

gastroenter'ic [" + *enteron,* intestine]. Pert. to stomach and intestines or to a condition involving them both.

gastroenteritis (gas-tro-en-ter-i'tis) [" + " + *-ītis,* inflammation]. Inflammation of the stomach and intestinal tract.

gastroenterocolitis (gas"tro-en"ter-o-kol-i'tis) [" + " + *kōlon,* colon, + *-ītis,* inflammation]. Inflammation of stomach, small intestine, and colon.

gastroenterocolostomy (gas-tro-en-ter-o-ko-los'to-mĭ) [" + " + " + *stoma,* opening]. Creation of a passage bet. the stomach, small intestine, and colon.

gastroenterol'ogy [" + " + *logos,* study]. The branch of medical science concerned with study of the physiology and pathology of the stomach, intestines, and related structures such as the esophagus, liver, gallbladder, and pancreas.

gastroenteroptosis (gas"tro-en-ter-op-to'sis) [" + " + *ptōsis,* a dropping]. Prolapse of stomach and intestines.

gastroenterostomy (gas-tro-en-ter-os'to-mĭ) [" + " + *stoma,* opening]. Surgical anastomosis between the stomach and small bowel.

This operation is required for patients who are suffering from carcinoma or cicatricial stricture of pyloric orifice of the stomach.

gas"troenterot'omy [" + " + *tomē,* incision]. Incision of stomach and intestine through abdominal wall.

gas"troepiplo'ic [G. *gastēr,* belly, + *epiplōon,* omentum]. Pert. to stomach and great omentum.

gastroesophagitis (gas-tro-e-sof-ă-ji'tis) [" + *oisophagos,* gullet, + *-ītis,* inflammation]. Inflammation of stomach and esophagus.

gastroesophagostomy (gas"tro-e-sof-ă-gos'to-mĭ) [" + " + *tomē,* incision]. Formation of passage from the esophagus into the stomach.

gastrogastrostomy (gas-tro-gas-tros'to-mĭ) [" + *gastēr,* belly, + *stoma,* opening]. Formation of passage in hourglass contraction bet. the two gastric pouches. Syn: *gastroanastomosis.*

gastrogavage (gas-tro-gă-vazh') [" + Fr. *gaver,* to gorge fowls]. Artificial feeding through an opening into the stomach.

gastrogen'ic [" + *gennan,* to produce] Having its origin in the stomach.

gastrohelcosis (gas"tro-hel-ko'sis) [" + *elkōsis,* ulceration]. Ulcer of the stomach.

gas"trohepat'ic [" + *ēpar, ēpat-,* liver]. Pert. to stomach and liver.

gastrohepatitis (gas-tro-hep-ă-ti'tis) [" + " + *-ītis,* inflammation]. Combination of gastritis and hepatitis at same time.

gastrohydrorrhea (gas-tro-hi-dro-re'ă) [" + *ydōr,* water, + *roia,* flow]. Excretion of much watery fluid, other than gastric juice, into the stomach.

gastrohysterectomy (gas-tro-his-ter-ek'-to-mĭ) [" + *ystera,* uterus, + *ektomē,* excision]. Removal of the uterus through an abdominal incision.

gastrohysteropexy (gas"tro-his"ter-o-peks'ĭ) [" + " + *pēxis,* fixation]. Ventrofixation of the uterus.

gastrohysterorrhaphy (gas-tro-his-ter-or'-ă-fĭ) [" + " + *raphē,* suture]. Fixation of uterus to the abdominal wall. Syn: *gastrohysteropexy.*

gastrohysterotomy (gas-tro-his-ter-ot'o-mĭ) [" + " + *tomē,* incision]. Incision of uterus through abdomen. Syn: *gasterhysterotomy.*

gastroiliac (gas-trō-ĭl'ĭ-ak) [" + L. *iliacus*]. Pert. to stomach and ileum.

g. reflex. Physiologic relaxation of ileocecal valve resulting from food in stomach.

gastrointes'tinal [" + L. *intestinum,* intestine]. Pert. to stomach and intestine.

g. decompression. Drainage of gases from the body cavities and tissues by use of suction through a tube inserted through the nostrils and into the digestive tract. See: *Wangensteen method.*

gastrojejunostomy (gas-tro-je-ju-nos'to-mĭ) [" + L. *jejunus,* empty, + G. *stoma,* opening]. Surgical anastomosis between the stomach and jejunum.

gastrolith (gas'tro-lith) [G. *gastēr,* belly, + *lithos,* stone]. A concretion in the stomach.

gastrolithiasis (gas"tro-lith-i'ă-sis) [" + *lithos,* stone]. Formation of calculi in the stomach.

gastrology (gas-trol'o-jĭ) [" + *logos,* study]. Study of function and diseases of the stomach.

gastrol'ysis [" + *lysis,* loosening]. Breaking adhesions bet. stomach and adjoining structures.

gastromalacia (gas-tro-ma-la'sĭ-ă) [" + *malakia*, softening]. Softening of the stomach walls.

gastromegaly (gas-tro-meg'ă-lĭ) [" + *megas, megal-*, large]. Enlargement of the stomach.

gastromenia (gas-tro-me'nĭ-ă) [" + *mēn*, month]. A form of vicarious menstruation through the stomach.

gastromycosis (gas-tro-mi-ko'sis) [" + *mykēs*, fungus, + *-ōsis*]. Disease of the stomach due to fungi.

gastromyotomy (gas-tro-mi-ot'o-mĭ) [" + *mys*, muscle, + *tomē*, incision]. Incision of circular muscular fibers of stomach.

gastromyxorrhea (gas-tro-miks-o-re'ă) [" + *myxa*, mucus, + *roia*, flow]. Excessive secretion of gastric mucus.

gastronephritis (gas-tro-nĕ-fri'tis) [" + *nephros*, kidney, + *-itis*, inflammation]. Inflammation of the stomach and kidney at same time.

gastronesteostomy (gas-tro-nes-te-os'to-mĭ) [" + *nēstis*, jejunum, + *stoma*, opening]. Formation of communication bet. jejunum and stomach. Syn: *gastrojejunostomy.*

gastropancreatitis (gas″tro-pan″kre-ă-ti'-tis) [" + *pagkreas*, pancreas, + *-itis*, inflammation]. Inflammation of the stomach and pancreas at same time.

gastroparalysis (gas″tro-par-al'ĭ-sis) [" + *paralyein*, to loose from sides]. Paralysis of the stomach.

gastroparesis (gas″tro-par'ĕ-sis) [" + *paresis*, paralysis]. Mild form of gastroparalysis.

gastropathy (gas-trop'ă-thĭ) [G. *gastēr*, belly, + *pathos*, disease]. Any disorder of the stomach.

gastroperiodynia (gas″tro-per″ĭ-o-din'ĭ-ă) [" + *periodos*, period, + *odynē*, pain]. Periodic pain in the stomach. Syn: *gastralgia.*

gastropexy, gastropexis (gas-tro-peks'e, -is) [" + *pēxis*, fixation]. Suture of the stomach to the abdominal walls for correction of displacement.

Gastrophilus (găs-trŏf'ĭ-lus). A genus of botflies belonging to the family Oestridae, order of Diptera. The larvae infest horses.

G. *hemorrhoidalis.* A species which infests horses.

G. *intestinalis.* Infest stomach of horses.

G. *nasalis.* The chin fly. Eggs are laid on shafts of hairs on lower lip and jaw of horses.

gastrophrenic (gas-tro-fren'ĭk) [" + *phrēn*, diaphragm]. Rel. to the stomach and diaphragm.

gastroplasty (gas'tro-plas″tĭ) [" + *plassein*, to form]. Plastic operation on the stomach.

gastroplegia (gas-tro-ple'jĭ-ă) [" + *plēgē*, stroke]. Paralysis of the stomach.

gastroplication (gas-tro-pli-ka'shun) [" + L. *plicāre*, to fold]. Stitching the walls of the stomach to reduce dilatation.

gastroptosia, gastroptosis (gas-trop-to'-sĭ-ă, -sis) [" + *ptōsis*, a dropping]. Abnormal falling of the stomach, Glénard's disease.

Usually accompanied by the displacement of other organs, the abdomen being pendulous. See: *bathygastry.*

gastroptyxis, gastroptyxy (gas-trop-tiks'-is, -ĭ) [" + *ptyxis*, a folding]. Reduction of a dilated stomach by surgery. Syn: *gastroplication.*

gastropylorectomy (gas-tro-pi-lor-ek'to-mĭ) [" + *pylōros*, pylorus, + *ektomē*, excision]. Excision of stomach at pyloric end.

gastropylor'ic [" + *pylōros*, pylorus]. Rel. to stomach and pylorus.

gastroradiculitis (gas-tro-ră-dik″u-li'tis) [" + L. *radix*, root, + G. *-itis*, inflammation]. Inflammation of the post. spinal nerve roots, the sensory fibers of which supply the stomach.

gastrorrhagia (gas-tro-ra'jĭ-ă) [" + *rēgnunai*, to burst forth]. Hemorrhage from stomach.

gastrorrhaphy (gas-tror'ă-fĭ) [G. *gastēr*, belly, + *raphē*, suture]. Suture of a stomach wall.

gastrorrhea (gas-tror-re'ă) [" + *roia*, flow]. An excessive secretion of gastric juice.

gastrosalpingotomy (gas-tro-sal-pin-got'o-mĭ) [" + *salpigx*, tube, + *tomē*, incision]. Incision of the oviduct by abdominal section.

gastroschisis (gas-tros'kĭ-sis) [" + *schisis*, cleft]. A congenital fissure in wall of abdomen which remains open.

gastroscope (gas'tro-skōp) [" + *skopein*, to examine]. Device for inspecting stomach's interior.

gastros'copy [" + *skopein*, to examine]. Examination of the stomach and abdominal cavity.

gastro'sis [" + *-ōsis*, disease]. Any disease of the stomach.

gas'trospasm [" + *spasmos*, spasm]. A spasm of the stomach.

gastrosplen'ic [" + *splēn*, spleen]. Of or pert. to stomach and spleen.

gastrostaxis (gas-tro-stak'sis) [" + *staxis*, trickling]. Hemorrhage of blood from membrane of the stomach.

gastrostenosis (gas-tro-sten-o'sis) [" + *stēnōsis*, narrowing]. Contracted state of the stomach.

g. *cardiaca.* Stenosis of cardiac orifice.

g. *pylorica.* Stenosis of pylorus.

gastrostogavage (gas-tros″to-gă-vazh') [" + *stoma*, opening, + Fr. *gaver*, to gorge fowls]. Injection of food through a gastric fistula.

Peptonized milk, albumen water, or eggnog during first week, soft diet the second week with more liberal diet with improvement. Temperature: 100° F. See: *gavage.*

gastros'toma [G. *gastēr*, belly, + *stoma*, opening]. A fistula of the stomach.

gastros'tomize [" + *stoma*, opening]. To perform a gastrostomy.

gastrostomy (gas-tros'to-mĭ) [" + *stoma*, opening]. Surgical creation of a gastric fistula through the abdominal wall.

It is necessary in carcinoma, and in some cases of cicatricial stricture of the esophagus; made for purpose of introducing food into stomach.

NP: Teach patient to care for self after hospitalization. Help patient to make mental adjustment. Mouth should receive special care because it is not being used to help process food prior to swallowing.

gastrosuccorrhea (gas-tro-suk-or-e'ă) [" + L. *succus*, juice, + G. *roia*, flow]. An excessive secretion of gastric juice with increased acidity; hypersecretion.

gastrother'apy [" + *therapeia*, treatment]. 1. Treatment of gastric diseases. 2. Treatment with extract of gastric mucosa; used esp. in pernicious anemia.

gastrotome (gas'tro-tōm) [" + *tomē*, incision]. Instrument for incising stomach or abdomen.

gastrotomy (gas-trot'o-mĭ) [" + *tomē*, incision]. Gastric or abdominal incision.

gastrotonometer (gas-tro-to-nom'ĕ-ter) [" + *tonos*, tension, + *metron*, measure].

Instrument for measuring intragastric pressure by insufflation of air or carbonic acid gas.

gastrotrachelotomy (gas-tro-tra-kel-ot′o-mĭ) [" + *trachelos*, neck, + *tomē*, incision]. Cesarean section in which the uterus is opened by a transverse incision across the cervix.

gastrotrop′ic [" + *tropikos*, turning]. Attracted to or affecting the stomach.

gastrotubotomy (gas-tro-tu-bot′o-mĭ) [" + L. *tuba*, tube, + G. *tomē*, incision]. Incision into fallopian tube through abdomen. SYN: *gastrosalpingotomy.*

gastrotympanites (gas″tro-tim-pan-i′tēz) [" + *tympanon*, drum]. Gaseous distention of the stomach.

gastroxynsis (gas-troks-in′sis) [" + *oxynein*, to sharpen]. Excessive hydrochloric acid secretion by stomach. SYN: *hyperchlorhydria.*

gastrula (gas′tru-lă) [L. dim. G. *gastēr*, belly]. Stage in embryonic development following the blastula in which the embryo assumes a two-layered condition. The outer layer being the *ectoderm* or *epiblast;* the inner layer, the *endoderm* or *hypoblast.* The latter lines a cavity, the *gastrocoele* or *archenteron* which opens to the outside through an opening, the *blastopore.*

gastrula′tion [L. *gastrula*, little belly]. The development of the gastrula.

Gatch bed [Willis D. Gatch, American surgeon, 1878-]. A bed in which the patient can be raised and held in a half-sitting position.

gath′ering [A.S. *gaderian*, to collect]. An abscess or swelling.

ga′tism [Fr. *gater*, to spoil]. Vesical or rectal incontinence.

gatophilia (gat-o-fil′ĭ-ă) [G. *gatos*, cat, + *philein*, to love]. Abnormal love for cats. SYN: *ailurophilia.*

gatophobia (gat-o-fo′bĭ-ă) [" + *phobos*, fear]. Aversion to cats. SYN: *ailurophobia; galeophobia.*

Gaucher's disease (go-shāz′) [Philippe C. E. Gaucher, French physician, 1854-1918]. A rare chronic congenital disorder of lipid metabolism. Associated with enlarged spleen, increased skin pigmentation, and bone lesions.

gauge (gāj) [Fr. a measuring rod]. Device for measuring size, capacity, amount or power of an object or substance; a standard of measurement.

Gault's reflex (galt). Contraction of orbicularis palpebrarum muscle resulting from sudden noise being produced near ear.

gauntlet (gawnt′let). A glovelike bandage which fits the hand and fingers.

gauss (gows). The unit of intensity of a magnetic flux.

Gauss' sign (gows) [Carl J. Gauss, German gynecologist, 1875-]. Unusual mobility of the uterus in the early weeks of pregnancy.

gauze (gawz) [Fr. *gaze*, gauze]. Thin, transparent fabric used in surgery.

g., absorbent. G. from which oily matter and sizing has been removed.

g., antiseptic. G. containing antiseptic material.

g., aseptic. 1. A gauze sterilized and packaged in an aseptic container and ready for surgical use. 2. A gauze rendered free of microorganisms.

gavage (gă-vazh′) [Fr. *gaver*, to gorge fowls]. Feeding with a stomach tube, or with a tube passed through the nares, pharynx, and esophagus into the stomach; the food is in liquid or semiliquid form at a temperature of about 100° F. SEE: *gastrostogavage.*

Gavard's muscle (ga-varz′) [Hyacinthe Gavard, French anatomist, 1753-1802]. The oblique muscular fibers of the stomach's coat.

Gawalowski's test (gav-al-ov′skĭ). Test for sugar made by use of ammonium molybdate and indicated by a blue color.

Gayet's disease (ga-yas′) [Prudent Gayet, French surgeon]. A lethargic sleep resembling sleeping sickness. It is rare and fatal.

Gay-Lussac's′ law [Joseph L. Gay-Lussac, French naturalist, 1778-1850]. All gases on heating expand equally and on cooling contract equally, according to temperature relation. SEE: *Charles' law.*

Geigel's reflex (gī′gel) [Richard Geigel, German physician, 1859-1930]. Reflex in females resembling cremasteric reflex* in males.

Geiger counter (gī′ger cown′ter) [Hans Geiger, German physicist, 1882-1945]. An instrument for detecting ionizing radiation.

gel (jel) [L. *gelāre*, to congeal]. 1. A semisolid condition of a precipitated or coagulated colloid. Jelly. A jellylike colloid. 2. Coagulum of a sol.

g., aluminum hydroxide. A white, viscous suspension; antacid.

gelatin (jel′ă-tin) [L. *gelatina*, gelatin]. A derived protein obtained by the hydrolysis of collagen present in the connective tissues of the skin, bones, and joints of animals.

USES: As a food, in preparation of pharmaceuticals, as a medium for culture of bacteria.

g. culture. Gelatinous base for bacterial growth.

g. peptone. Digestive product of gelatin.

g. sponge. A spongy sheet of gelatin prepared for use as a hemostatic.

g., nutrient. SEE: *g. culture.*

gelat′inase [L. *gelatina*, gelatin]. An enzyme that liquefies gelatin.

gelatiniferous (jel-at-in-if′er-us) [" + *ferre*, to bear]. Producing gelatin.

gelatinize (jel-at′in-īz) [L. *gelatina*, gelatin]. To convert into gelatin.

gelatinoid (jel-at′in-oyd) [" + G. *eidos*, resemblance). Resembling gelatin.

gelatinolytic (jel-at″in-o-lit′ĭk) [" + G. *lysis*, dissolution]. Dissolution or splitting up of gelatin.

gelat″inotho′rax [" + G. *thōrax*, chest]. Injection of gelatin solution intrapleurally.

gelatinous (jel-at′in-us) [L. *gelatina*, gelatin]. Containing or of the consistency of gelatin.

gelation (jel-a′shun) [L. *gelāre*, to congeal]. The transformation of a colloid from a sol into a gel.

gelfoam. Proprietary name for absorbable gelatin sponge. It is used as a surgical sponge in operative wounds.

Gellé's test (zhel-ā′) [Marie Ernst Gellé, French physician, 1834-1923]. A tuning fork is connected with a rubber tube inserted in the ear. Pressure is produced by an attached bulb and, if ear is normal, vibrations are felt. SEE: *test.*

gelodiagno′sis [L. *gelāre*, to congeal, + G. *dia*, through, + *gnōsis*, knowledge]. Identification of bacteria by means of a gelose culture medium.

gelose (jĕ′lōs) [L. *gelāre*, to congeal]. 1. Gelatinous element of agar, $C_6H_{10}O_5$. 2. Bacterial culture medium.

gelosis (jel-o′sis) [" + G. *ōsis*]. A hard lump appearing to be frozen.

gelotherapy (jel-o-ther′ă-pĭ) [G. *gelōs*, laughter, + *therapeia*, treatment]. Inducing hilarity in treatment of certain morbid states of the mind.

gelotripsy (jel′o-trip-sĭ) [L. *gelāre*, to congeal, + G. *tripsis*, a rubbing]. The massaging away of indurated swellings.

-gels. A termination to indicate colloids in a solid state.

Gély's suture (zhā-lē′) [Jules A Gély, French surgeon, 1806-1861]. One for closing intestinal wounds employing cross stitches. SYN: *cobbler's suture.*

gemellus (jem-el′us) [L. twin]. Either of two muscles inserted in the obturator internus tendon.

geminate (jem′ĭ-nāt) [L. *geminātus*, paired]. In pairs.

gemination. 1. Development of two teeth within a single alveolus. 2. To produce twins.

gem′ma. 1. A small budlike, reproductive structure, produced by lower forms of life. 2. Any small budlike structure such as a tastebud or end-bulb.

gemmation (jem-ma′shun) [L. *gemmāre*, to bud]. Fission by budding.

Budlike processes or daughter cells, each containing chromatin, separate from the mother cell from which the bud is projected.

gemmule (jem′ūl) [L. *gemmula*, little bud]. 1. A gemma, *q.v.* 2. One of numerous minute processes present on the dendrites of a neuron.

gena (je′na) [L. *gena*, cheek]. The side of the face or cheek.

genal (je′nal) [L. *gena*, cheek] Pert. to the cheek. SYN: *buccal.*

gene (jēn) [G. *gennan*, to produce]. 1.An hereditary determiner. 2. A factor present in the gametes which is responsible for the transmission of hereditary characteristics to the offspring. Genes are self-reproducing ultramicroscopic particles found within cells and located at definite points on chromosomes. They are capable under certain circumstances of giving rise to a new character, such a change being called a mutation.

g., epistatic. One of a pair of factors which masks the expression of another pair.

g., holandric. A gene located in the nonhomologous portion of the Y-chromosome.

g., inhibiting. A gene which prevents the expression of another gene.

g., lethal. A gene which when in a homozygous condition brings about an effect which results in the death of an individual.

g., modifying. A gene which influences or alters the effect of another gene.

g., multiple. A group of genes which have more or less equal and cumulative effects upon the same character.

g., sex-linked. A gene contained within the X or sex chromosome.

gen′era. Plural of genus.

gen′eralize [L. *genus*, race]. 1. To become or render general. 2. To become systemic, as a local disease.

generation (jen-er-a′shun) [L. *generāre*, to beget]. 1. An act of forming a new organism. 2. A group of animals or plants the same distance removed from an ancestor, as the first filial (F_1) generation. 3. The average span between one generation and the next, for humans, approximately thirty-three years. 4. The production of an electric current.

g's., alternation of. A mode of reproduction in which a sexual generation alternates with an asexual generation, characteristic of all plants above the Thallophytes. It also occurs in some of the lower animals.

g., asexual. Reproduction which occurs without the union of sexual elements or gametes, such as reproduction by fission, or spore production.

g., F_1. The first filial generation; the offspring of a given mating or cross.

g., sexual. Reproduction by the union of male and female cells.

g., spontaneous. The theory that living things can originate from nonliving matter. SYN: *abiogenesis.*

g., viviparous. Normal method of g. among higher animals.

generative (jen′er-a-tiv). Concerned in reproduction of or affecting the species.

generic (jen-er′ik) [L. *genus*, *gener-*, kind]. 1. General. 2. Pert. to a genus. 3. Distinctive.

g. name. The nonproprietary name of a drug or pharmaceutical preparation.

genes (sing. *gene*) (jēnz) [G. *gennan*, to produce]. The units controlling heredity which are believed to be situated in the chromosomes. There are specific points on the chromosomes for genes governing each characteristic. Genes on different chromosomes are transmitted independently; genes on the same chromosome are said to be linked. The genes occur in pairs, corresponding to the pairing of the chromosomes, one derived from each parent, and each pair of genes determines the individual's genotype for the trait in question. SEE: *chromosome; heredity.*

genesiology (jen-e-sĭ-ol′o-jĭ) [" + *logos*, science]. The science of reproduction.

genesis (jen′ĕ-sis) [G. origin]. 1. Act of reproducing; generation. 2. The origin of anything.

genetic (jen-et′ik) [G. *genesis*, origin]. Pert. to generation.

geneticist (jen-et′ĭ-sist) [G. *gennan*, to produce]. One who specializes in genetics.

genet′ics [G. *gennan*, to produce]. The science that accounts for natural differences and resemblances among organisms related by descent. 2. The study of heredity and its variation.

genetopathy (jen-ĕ-top′ă-thĭ) [G. *genesis*, origin, + *pathos*, disease]. Disease affecting the generative function.

genetous (jen′ĕ-tus) [G. *genesis*, origin]. From birth. SYN: *congenital, q.v.*

genial (je′nĭ-al) [G. *geneion*, chin]. Rel. to the chin.

g. tubercle. A nodule on the lower jawbone on either side of the symphysis.

geniculate (jen-ik′u-lāt) [G. *geniculāre*, to bend the knee]. 1. Kneed. 2. Bent as a knee. 3. Pert. to the ganglion or geniculum of the facial nerve.

g. otalgia. Pain transmitted from the facial nerve to the ear.

geniculum (jen-ik′u-lum) [L. little knee]. A structure resembling a knot, or a knee. Indicates an abrupt bend or angle in a small structure.

genion (je′nĭ-on) [G. *geneion*, chin]. Apex of the spina mentalis.

genioplasty (je′nĭ-o-plas″tĭ) [" + *plassein*, to form]. Plastic surgery of the chin or cheek.

genital (jen′ĭ-tal) [L. *genitalis*, genital]. Pert. to the genitals.

genitalia, geni′tals (jen-ĭ-tal′ĭ-ă) [L. *genitalis*, genital]. Organs of generation; reproductive organs.

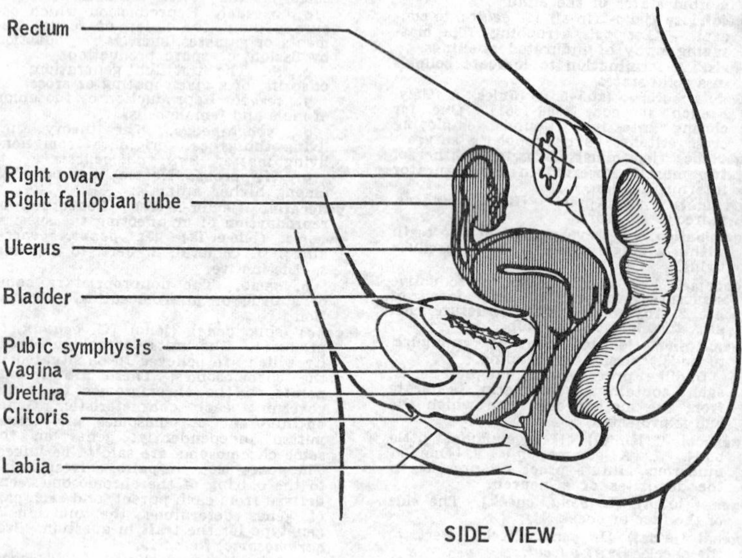

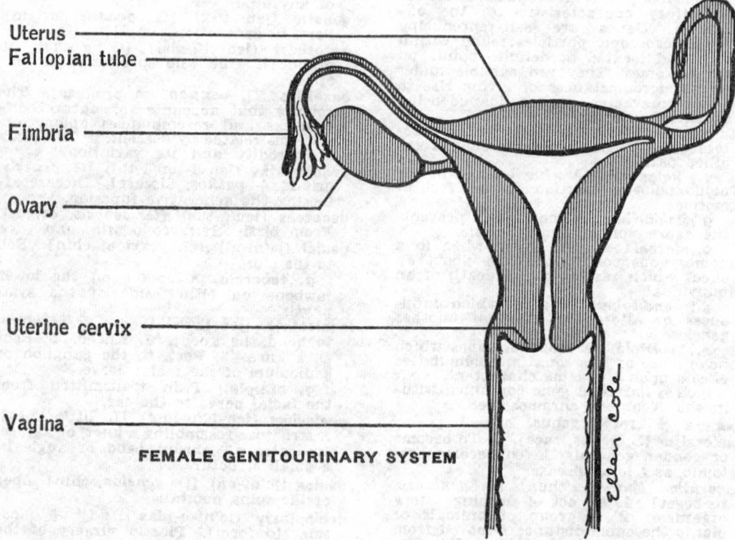

FEMALE GENITOURINARY SYSTEM

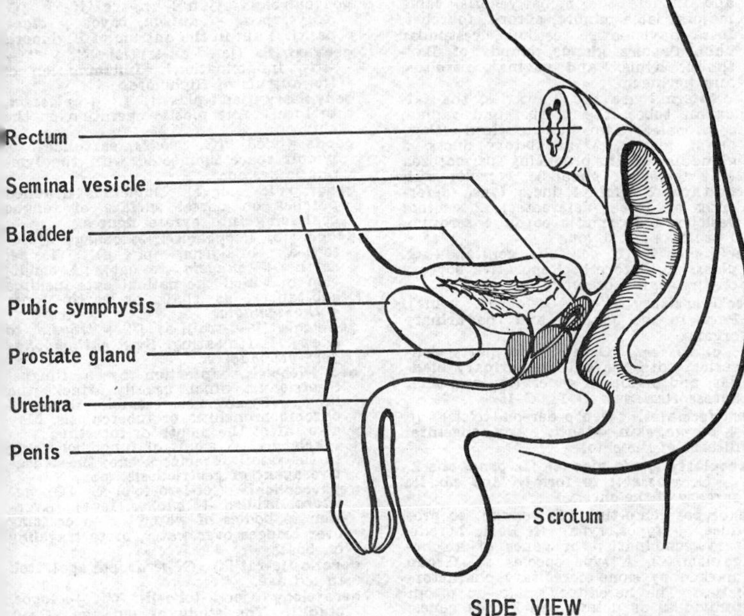

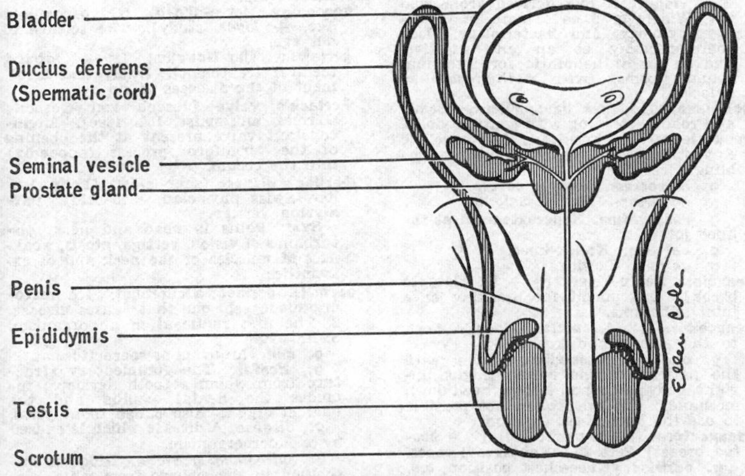

MALE GENITOURINARY SYSTEM

g., female. Those concerned with reproduction.

The *external* genitalia collectively are termed the vulva or *pudendum* and include the mons veneris, labia majora, labia minora, clitoris, fourchet, fossa navicularis, vestibule, vestibular bulb, Skene's glands, glands of Bartholin, hymen and vaginal introitus, and perineum.

Internal are the 2 ovaries, the fallopian tubes, the uterus, and vagina.

g., male. Two bulbourethral (Cowper's) glands, 2 ejaculatory ducts, 2 glandular organs producing spermatozoa (the testes or gonads), 1 penis with urethra, 2 seminal ducts (vasa deferentes or ductus deferentes), 2 seminal vesicles, 2 spermatic cords, 1 scrotum, 1 prostate gland, *q.v.*

gen'itoplas"ty [L. *genitalis,* genital, + G. *plassein,* to form]. Reparative surgery on the genital organs.

gen"itou'rinary [" + G. *ouron,* urine]. Pert. to the genitals and the urinary organs.

g. system. Organs and parts concerned with the kidneys, urinary bladder, and organs of generation and their accessories. SEE: G-14, G-15.

genodermatosis (jen"o-der-mă-to'sis) [" + *derma,* skin, + *-ōsis*]. Any congenital disease of the skin.

genoplasty (jen'o-plas-tĭ) [L. *gena,* cheek, + G. *plassein,* to form]. Any plastic surgery of the cheek.

genotype (jen'o-tīp) [G. *gennan,* to produce, + *typos,* type]. 1. Basic hereditary combination of genes of an organism. 2. A type species. 3. Group marked by same hereditary characteristics. The hereditary make-up of an individual as determined by his genes. Each pair of genes determines the genotype for a different characteristic. SEE: *phenotype.*

gentian (jĕn'shĭ-ăn). USP. Dried rhizome roots of the plant *Gentiana lutea.*

g. violet. A dye derived from coal tar. Widely used as a stain in histology, cytology, and bacteriology. Used therapeutically as an anti-infective, and as an anthelmintic for intestinal round worms. SYN: *methylrosaniline chloride.*

gen'tianophil(e, gen"tianoph'ilous. Easily and readily staining with gentian violet.

genu (je'nu) [L. knee]. 1. The knee. 2. Any structure of angular form resembling a bent knee.

g. extrorsum. SEE: *g. varum.*

g. introrsum. SEE: *g. valgum.*

g. recurvatum. Hyperextension at the knee joint.

g. val'gum. Knock-knee.

g. va'rum. Bowleg.

genuclast (jen'u-klăst) [" + G. *klan,* to break]. Instrument for breaking knee joint adhesions.

genucu'bital [" + *cubitus,* elbow]. Pert. to the elbows and knees.

g. position (knee-elbow). One with the patient on the knees, thighs upright, body resting on elbows, head down on hands; employed when not possible to use the knee-chest position.

genupectoral (jen"u-pek'to-ral) [" + *pectus,* breast]. Pert. to the chest and knees.

g. position. Knee-chest position, *q.v. for illustration.*

A position assumed by the female patient in which the patient is supported upon her knees and chest, and when the vaginal lips are open the vagina fills with air. This position is used for purposes of examination and treatment.

ge'nus [G. *genos,* race]. BIOL: The division between the species and the family.

genyantralgia (jen"ĭ-an-tral'jĭ-ă) [G. *genys,* jaw, + *antron,* cave, + *algos* pain]. Pain in the antrum of Highmore.

genyantritis (jen"ĭ-an-tri'tis) [" + " + *-itis,* inflammation]. Inflammation of the antrum of Highmore.

genyplasty (jen'ĭ-plas-tĭ) [" + *plassein,* to form]. Any plastic operation on the chin.

geode (je'ōd) [G. *geōdēs,* earthlike]. A lymph space connected with the lymphatic system.

geograph'ic tongue. Numerous denuded patches on dorsal surface of tongue coalescing into gyrate figures.

geophagia, geophagism, geophagy (je-o-fa'jĭ-ă, -of'ă-jĭzm, -of'ă-jĭ) [G. *gē,* earth, + *phagein,* to eat]. A condition in which the patient eats inedible substances, as chalk or earth. SYN: *chthonophagia.*

geotragia (je-o-tra'jĭ-ă) [" + *trōgein,* to chew]. Earth eating. SYN: *chthonophagia; geophagism.*

geo"tricho'sis. Infection by a fungus, *Geotrichum* which usually attacks the lungs. Symptoms resemble those of chronic bronchitis or tuberculosis. May also infect the mouth or intestine.

Geot'richum. A genus of fungi belonging to the family Eremascaceae; the causative agent of geotrichosis, *q.v.*

gephyrophobia (jef-ĭ-ro-fo'bĭ-ă) [G. *gephyra,* bridge, + *phobos,* fear]. Aversion to bodies of water, or to crossing over bridges over water, or to traveling on boats.

geratic (je-rat'ik) [G. *gēras,* old age]. Rel. to old age.

geratology (jer-ă-tol'o-jĭ) [" + *logos,* study]. The study of old age. SYN: *gereology.*

Gerdy's fibers (zher'dēz) [Pierre N. Gerdy, French physician, 1797-1856]. The superficial transverse ligament of the fingers.

gereology (jer-e-ol'o-jĭ) [G. *gēras,* old age, + *logos,* study]. The science of old age.

geriatrics (jer-ĭ-at'riks) [" + *iatrikē,* medical treatment]. Study and treatment of the diseases of old age.

Gerlach's valve [Joseph von Gerlach, German anatomist, 1820-1896]. An inconstant valve present at the opening of the vermiform process (appendix) into the cecum.

Gerlier's disease (zher-le-āz') [Felix Gerlier, Swiss physician, 1840-1914]. Paralyzing vertigo.

SYM: Pains in head and neck, disturbance of vision, vertigo, ptosis, weakness of muscles of the neck and of extremities.

germ [L. *germen,* a microbe]. 1.A microorganism, esp. one that causes disease. 2. The first rudiment of an organism. 3. An ovum.

g. cell. An ovum or spermatozoon.

g., dental. The rudimentary structure from which a tooth develops; includes the dental papilla and the enamel organ. Also called *tooth germ.*

g., disease. A disease which is caused by a microorganism.

g. epithelium, g. ridge. Ridge of epithelium in the embryo from which develops the sexual portions of the body.

g., hair. The rudimentary structure from which a hair develops. Consists of an ingrowth of epidermal cells called *hair peg* which pushes into the corium.

g. layers. Three primary layers of cells in an embryo from which the organs and tissues develop. They are the *ectoderm, mesoderm,* and *entoderm, q.v.*

g. plasm. The reproductive tissues in contrast to the non-reproductive tissues which constitute the *soma.*

g. theory. The hypothesis that disease is the result of the presence of microorganisms or their products in the body.

German measles. Acute contagious disease with rash of short duration, resembling measles and scarlet fever. SYN: *rötheln; rubella.*

germanium (jer-ma'nĭ-um). A grayish white metallic element of the silicon group. SYMB: Ge. At. wt. 72.59; at. no. 32.

germicidal (jerm-ĭ-si'dal) [L. *germen,* microbe, + *caedere,* to kill]. 1. Destructive to germs. 2. Pert. to an agent destructive to germs.

germicide (jer'mis-īd) [" + *caedere,* to kill]. A substance that destroys germs. SEE: *disinfectant; bactericide.*

Bacteria and spores may be killed by boiling for 30 minutes, by dry heat at 160° to 170° C. for an hour, by steam at 121° C. for 20 minutes.

germ'inal [L. *germen,* microbe]. Pertaining to a germ or reproductive cells, egg or sperm, or to germination.

g. center. A light area of lymphocytopoietic cells which occupies the center of lymphatic nodules of the spleen, tonsils, and lymph nodes.

g. disk. A disk of cells on the surface of the yolk of a teloblastic egg from which the embryo develops; the blastoderm.

g. epithelium. 1. The epithelium which covers the surface of the genital ridge of an embryo. 2. The epithelium which covers the surface of a mature mammalian ovary.

g. vesicle. Nucleus of oocyte, *q.v.*

germina'tion [L. *germināre,* to sprout] 1. Development of an impregnated ovum into an embryo. 2. The sprouting of the spore or seed of a plant.

gerocomia (jer-o-ko'mĭ-ă) [G. *gerōn,* old man, + *komein,* to care for]. The hygiene of old age, or old men.

geroder'ma, gerodermia (jer-o-der'mĭ-ă) [" + *derma,* skin]. An appearance of senility brought about by premature loss of hair, wrinkling of the skin, and general atrophy.

geromaras'mus. Emaciation which accompanies extreme old age.

geromorphism (jer-o-mor'fizm) [" + *morphē,* form, + *ismos,* state of]. Appearance of age in youth.

gerontal (jĕ-ron'tal) [G. *gerōn,* old man]. Pert. to an old man or to the aged. SYN: *senile.*

gerontology (je-ron-tol'o-jĭ) [" + *logos,* study of]. The study of the phenomena of old age. SYN: *geriatrics.*

gerontophil'ia. Fondness or love for old people.

gerontopia (jĕ-ron-to'pĭ-ă) [" + *ops,* vision]. Second sight due to change in the refractive power of the lens. SYN: *senopia.*

gerontoxon (jĕ-ron-toks'on) [" + *toxon,* bow]. Degenerative circle about corneal ext. surface seen in the aged. SYN: *arcus senilis.*

Gerota's capsule [Dumitru Gerota, Roumanian anatomist, 1867-1939]. The perirenal fascia.

gestal'tism. The theory that the objects of mind come as wholes which cannot be split up into parts and which are unanalyzable.

gestation (jes-ta'shun) [L. *gestāre,* to bear]. Period of intrauterine fetal development.

g., abdominal. Ectopic g. in which the product of conception is lodged in the peritoneal cavity.

g., cornual. G. in an ill-developed cornu of a bicornuate uterus.

g., ectopic. Conception outside the uterus.

g., interstitial. Tubal g. in which the ovum is developed in that portion of oviduct that traverses wall of uterus.

g., ovarian. A form of ectopic g. in the ovary.

g., plural. G. with more than one embryo.

g., prolonged, g., protracted. G. prolonged beyond the usual period.

g. sac. The amnion and its contents.

g., secondary. The ovum becomes dislodged from original seat of implantation, and continues to develop in a new situation.

g., secondary abdominal. Extrauterine g. in which the fetus, originally situated in oviduct or elsewhere, has become lodged in abdominal cavity because of the rupture of the fetal sac

g., tubal, g., tubarian. Ectopic g. in which the product of conception is lodged in the oviduct.

g., tuboabdominal. Extrauterine g. in which fetal sac is formed partly of the abdominal extremity of the oviduct and partly of plastic exudation in the area.

g., tubo-ovarian. Extrauterine g. in which the fetal sac is made up of the ovary and the abdominal end of the oviduct.

g., uterotubal. G. in which the ovum is developed partly in uterine portion of oviduct and partly within cavity of uterus.

gestosis (jes-to'sis) [L. *gestāre,* to bear, + G. *ōsis*]. Any disorder of pregnancy.

geumophobia (gu"mo-fo'bĭ-ă) [G. *geume,* taste, + phobia]. Abnormal dislike or fear of tastes.

GH. Growth hormone.

gher'kin. A form of pickle. COMP: It is more of a condiment than a vegetable or a food.

ACTION: An appetizer and probably a gastric stimulant to a small degree.

Ghon's primary lesion, tubercle [Anton Ghon, Czechoslovakian pathologist, 1866-1936]. A bean-shaped shadow in the x-ray of the lung seen in certain cases of pulmonary tuberculosis in children. It is the primary lesion of tuberculosis in children.

ghost corpuscle. Depigmented red blood corpuscle. SYN: *phantom corpuscle.*

giant cell. One of large size with several nuclei, appearing to be made up of many cells, but not clearly outlined, found in both kinds of marrow, esp. in red marrow and spleen; a megakaryocyte.

g. c. tumor. Rare, benign, encapsulated tumor in lower jaw or on alveolar process of upper jaw in the young.

giantism (ji'an-tizm) [G. *gigas, gigant-,* giant]. Abnormal development of the body or its parts. SYN: *gigantism.*

Gianuzzi's cells or crescents (jan-oot'sez). Crescent-shaped groups of serous cells found in the mixed salivary glands. They appear as darkly-staining cells forming a caplike structure on the alveoli. Also called *demilunes of Heidenhain.*

Giardia (gĭ-ar'dĭ-ă) [Alfred Giard, Paris biologist, 1846-1908]. A genus of protozoa possessing flagella which inhabit the small intestine of man and other animals. They are pear-shaped, possess two nuclei and four pairs of flagella. They attach themselves to the cells of the intestinal mucosa, from which they absorb their nourishment.

G. lamblia. Species of Giardia found in man. They were formerly considered nonpathogenic but evidence indicates that they interfere with the absorption of fats, their presence being connected with recurring attacks of diarrhea and the passage of stools containing large amounts of unabsorbed fats and quantities of yellow mucus. They form cysts intermittently.

giardiasis (gĭ-ar-di'ă-sis). Infection with *Giardia lamblia.* SYN: *lambliasis.*

Gibbon's hydrocele (gĭb'ŏn) [Q. V. Gibbon, American surgeon, 1813-1894]. A hydrocele and large hernia combined.

gibbos'ity [L. *gibbōsus,* humped]. 1. Condition of having a humpback. 2. A hump or gibbus, as the deformity of Pott's disease.

gibbous (gib'bus) [L. *gibbus,* humped]. Humped; protuberant or humpbacked.

gid'diness. State of dizziness. SYN: *vertigo.*

Giemsa's stain (gēm'zah) [Gustav Giemsa, Hamburg chemist, 1867-1948]. A stain for staining blood smears. Used for differential leukocyte counts and for the detection of parasitic microorganisms.

Gifford's reflex (gĭf'ford) [Harold Gifford, American oculist, 1858-1929]. Pupillary contraction resulting from endeavoring forcibly to close eyelids which are held apart.

gigan'tism [G. *gigas, gigant-,* giant, + *ismos,* state of]. Abnormal development of the body or of a part. SYN: *giantism.*

g., acromegalic. G. in which acromegalic features (overgrowth of the bones of the hands, feet, and face) are present. Due to excessive production of the growth hormone after full skeletal growth has been attained.

g., eunuchoid. G. accompanied by eunuchoid features and sexual insufficiency.

g., normal. G. of the body in which the bodily proportions and functional activities are normal. Usually the result of hypersecretion of the growth hormone.

gigan'toblast [" + *blastos,* germ]. A very large nucleated red corpuscle.

gigantocyte (ji-gan'to-sīt) [" + *kytos,* cell]. 1. A giant cell. 2. A very large erythroblast.

gigantosoma (ji-gan-to-so'mă) [" + *sōma,* body]. Abnormal size of the body. SYN: *giantism; gigantism.*

Gigli's saw (gēl'yēz) [Leonardo Gigli, Italian gynecologist, 1863-1908]. A wire saw originally used to cut the pubis. Now used in removing the scalp in craniotomy.

Gimbernat's ligament (zham-bār-nahz') [Antonio de Gimbernat, Spanish surgeon, 1734-1790]. Ligamentum lacunare.

gin'ger. Dried rhizome of the plant *Zingiber officinale.*

ACTION AND USES: A carminative, aromatic and stimulant. Chiefly in form of tincture.

gingiva (jin-ji'vă) [L. gum]. The gum; the tissues which surrounds the necks of the teeth and covers the alveolar processes of the maxilla and mandible.

g., labial. G. covering labial surfaces of the teeth.

g., lingual. G. covering lingual surface of the teeth.

gingival (jin'jiv-al) [L. *gingiva,* gum]. Rel. to the gums.

gingival'gia [" + G. *algos,* pain]. Pain in the gums.

gingivally (jin-ji'val-e) [L. *gingiva,* gum]. Toward the gums.

gingivectomy (jin"jĭ-vek'to-mĭ) [" + G. *ektomē,* excision]. Excision of gum tissue in pyorrhea. SYN: *ulectomy.*

gingivitis (jin-jĭ-vi'tis) [L. *gingiva,* gum, + G. *-itis,* inflammation]. Inflammation of the gums, characterized by redness, swelling, and tendency to bleed. SYN: *ulitis.*

ETIOL: May be local due to improper dental hygiene, poorly fitting dentures, or appliances, poor occlusion, or it may accompany generalized stomatitis associated with mouth and upper respiratory infections. May also occur in deficiency diseases such as scurvy, blood dyscrasias, or metallic poisoning.

g., expulsive. Osteoperiostitis of a tooth in which the tooth is expelled from its socket.

g. gravidum. Gingivitis of pregnancy. Characterized by generalized hypertrophy of the gums which may progress to the state of tumor formation.

g., interstitial. Inflammation of the gums and alveolar processes which precede pyorrhea.

g., phagedenic. A rapidly spreading ulceration of the gums accompanied by extensive ulceration and sloughing of tissue.

g., Vincent's. An ulcerative necrotizing inflammation. An associated spirillum and a fusiform bacillus have been recovered in this condition. SYN: *Vincent's angina; Vincent's stomatitis.*

gingivoglossitis (jin"jĭ-vo-glos-si'tis) [" + G. *glōssa,* tongue, + *-itis,* inflammation]. Inflammation of the gums and tongue. SYN: *stomatitis.*

ginglyform (jing'lĭ-form) [G. *gigglymos,* hinge, + L. *forma,* shape]. In the form of a hinge. SYN: *ginglymoid.*

ginglymoarthrodial (jing"lĭ-mo-ar-thro'dĭ-al) [" + *arthrōdia,* gliding joint]. Pert. to a joint that is both hinged and arthrodial. SEE: *arthrodia.*

ginglymoid (jing'lĭ-moyd) [" + *eidos,* form]. Pert. to or shaped like a hinged joint.

ginglymus (jing'lĭ-mus) [G. *gigglymos,* hinge]. A hinge joint; diarthrosis.* SEE: *joint.*

Giraldès' organ (zhir-al-dās') [Joachim A. C. C. Giraldès, Portuguese surgeon in Paris, 1808-1875]. A vestige of the wolffian body at post. side of the testicle. SYN: *paradidymis.*

girdle (gir'del) [A.S. *gyrdel*]. 1. A zone or belt; cingulum, the waist. 2. A structure which resembles a circular belt or band.

g. anesthesia. A portion around the body without sensation.

g., Neptune. Stimulating or heating compress of linen covered by flannel encircling trunk from lower end of sternum to pubes.

g. pain. Painful sensation around the body.

g., pelvic. The portion of the lower extremities to which the lower limbs are attached. Composed of the two innominate or hip bones.

g. sensation. Same as g. pain.

g., shoulder. The portion of the upper extremities to which the upper limbs are attached. Composed of the two clavicles and two scapulae.

g. symptom. A symptom in tabes as of a tight girdle, such as a feeling of constriction about the chest; also found in compression of the cord due to collapse of the vertebrae as in Pott's disease. SYN: *Hitzig's g.*

gitalin (jit'ă-lin). A cardiac glycoside from digitalis.

glabel'la [L. *glaber*, smooth]. The smooth surface of the frontal bone lying between the superciliary arches; the portion directly above the root of the nose.

gla'brate [L. *glaber*, smooth]. 1. Bald. 2. Smooth

glabrificin (glab-rif'ĭ-sin) [" + *facere*, to make]. A variety of antibody which exposes a capsulated bacterium to the action of lysin.

gla'brous [L. *glaber*, smooth]. 1. Bald. 2. Smooth. SYN: *glabrate.*

glacial (gla'shal) [L. *glacialis*, icy]. Glassy; resembling ice.

glad'iate [L. *gladius*, sword]. Sword-shaped. SYN: *ensiform; xiphoid.*

gladi'oline. An alkaloid from tissue of the brain.

gladiolus (glă-di'o-lus) [L. *gladiolus*, little sword]. The intermediate and principal segment of the sternum, *q.v.*

glairin (glār'in) [L. *glair*, mucus]. Gelatinous substance in water of some sulfur springs.

glair'y [L. *glair*, mucus]. Viscous; albuminous; mucoid.

gland [L. *glans, gland-*, kernel]. 1. A secretory organ or structure. 2. A cell or a group of cells which has the ability to manufacture a substance (secretion) which is discharged and used in some other part of the body or is excreted.

On the basis of complexity of structure, glands may be *simple* (consisting of one or a few secreting units) or *compound* (consisting of many secreting units whose secretions leave the gland by a common duct). Simple tubular glands may be *straight, coiled,* or *branched.*

Glands consisting of one cell are called *unicellular;* those of more than one cell, *multicellular.*

On the basis of their secretion, glands are *mucous* (those producing a viscous, slimy secretion), *serous* (those producing a clear watery secretion) or *mixed* (those producing both).

On the basis of the presence or absence of ducts, glands are *exocrine* (those which possess ducts which carry the secretions to an epithelial surface) and *endocrine* (those without ducts and whose secretions enter the blood or lymph).

On the basis of the shape of the secreting units, glands are *tubular* (secreting portion elongated with a narrow lumen) or *saccular* (secreting portion in the form of a sac or flask). If the lumen of the secreting portion is wide, it is termed an *alveolus,* if narrow, an *acinus.* Glands composed of these types of units are termed *alveolar* and *acinar,* respectively.

On the basis of the manner by which secretion is accomplished, glands are *merocrine* (secretion forms within cells and is passed through cell membranes into excretory ducts); *apocrine* (secretion forms in apical ends of cells which break off and form a part of the secretion), *e.g.,* mammary gland; and *holocrine* (entire cell with its contents is extruded as the secretion), *e.g.,* sebaceous glands.

Glands may be *simple* (tubular or saccular), opening by a single duct upon a surface, or *compound,* consisting of many tubular or saccular cavities. The secretory glands are of two kinds: (a) ductless or endocrine; (b) having ducts. In those without a duct, the secretion leaves the duct by way of the lymph or blood. They are: The *gonads* or sex glands, the *pineal, pituitary, thyroid, parathyroid, thymus,* and *adrenal glands.*

GLANDS PECULIAR TO THE FEMALE: Bartholin's g., Duverney's g., nabothian g., ovaries, Skene's g., uterine g., glans clitoridis, mammary g.

GLANDS PECULIAR TO THE MALE: Cowper's g., seminal g., prostate g., Tyson's g.

g., absorbent. Any one of the lymphatic glands.

g., accessory. Gland functioning as an accesory to another gland of similar structure some distance removed.

g., acinotubular. A gland structurally midway bet. an acinous and a tubular g.

g., acinous. A g. whose secreting units are composed of saclike structures each possessing a narrow lumen.

g., adrenal. An endocrine gland lying above each kidney. SEE: *adrenal glands.*

g.'s, aggregate. Lymphatic glands in patch formation found mainly in ileum. SYN: *Peyer's patches.*

g.'s, agminated. SEE: *aggregate g.'s.*

g.'s, albuminous. Digestive tract glands secreting a fluid containing albumin.

g., anal. Glands in the region of the anus.

g., apocrine. A gland whose cells lose some of their cytoplasmic contents in the formation of the secretion. Ex: *mammary gland, some sweat glands.*

g.'s, areolar. Large sebaceous and rudimentary milk glands present in the areola surrounding the nipple of the female breast. SYN: *Montgomery's g.'s.*

g.'s, auricular. External otic lymph nodes.

g.'s, axillary. Axillary lymph nodes.

g.'s, Bartholin's. Numerous glands which open into the vestibule of the female. Homologous to bulbourethral glands of the male. SYN: *major vestibular g.'s.*

g.'s, Blandin's; g.'s, Blandin-Nuhn's. Tiny racemose g.'s secreting mucus and saliva, near the tip of the tongue on the undersurface.

g.'s, Bowman's. Simple, branched, tubular glands present in the olfactory mucosa of the nasal cavity.

g.'s, brachial. Lymph glands in the arm and forearm.

g.'s, bronchial. Mixed glands lying in the submucosa of the bronchi and bronchial tubes.

g.'s, Bruch's. Conjunctival lymph nodes in lower lids.

g.'s, Brunner's. Glands in the duodenal submucosa secreting intestinal juice.

g.'s, buccal. Acinous glands in the cheek tissue.

g., bulbourethral. Cowper's gland. Two small glands above the bulb of corpus spongiosum, whose secretion forms part of seminal fluid.

g.'s, cardiac. Glands of the stomach near the cardiac orifice of the esophagus.

g., carotid. Tiny gland at bifurcation of the common carotid artery. SYN: *carotid body.*

g.'s, cecal. Cecal lymph nodes.

g.'s, ceruminous. Glands in auditory canal excreting cerumen.

g.'s, cervical. Lymph glands situated in the neck.

g.'s, ciliary. SEE: *Moll's g.'s.*

g.'s, circumanal. The anal glands, *q.v.*

g.'s, Cobelli's. Glands in the esophageal mucosa.

g.'s, coccygeal. SEE: *Luschka's g.'s.*

g., compound. A g. consisting of a number of branching duct systems which open into the main excretory duct.

g., compound tubular. G. composed of numerous minute tubules leading to a lone duct.

g., conglobate. Lymphatic gland.

g., conglomerate. SEE: *acinous gland.*

g., Cowper's. SEE: *bulbourethral g.*

g.'s, cutaneous. Glands of the skin, esp. the sebaceous and sudoriferous glands. Also includes modified forms such as the ciliary, ceruminous, anal, preputial, areolar, meibomian glands.

g., cytogenic. A gland whose product is living cells, such as the testis or ovary.

g.'s, decidual. Glands possessing no secretory duct.

g., ductless. A gland which lacks an excretory duct; an endocrine gland, *q.v.*

g.'s, duodenal. SEE: *Brunner's g.'s.*

g.'s, Duverney's. SEE: *Bartholin's g.'s.*

g., Ebner's (g. of von Ebner). Serous glands of the tongue located in the region of the vallate papillae, their ducts opening into the furrows surrounding the papillae.

g., endocrine. An organ or structure which secretes a hormone that is absorbed into the blood or lymph; a ductless gland. The principal endocrine glands are the hypophysis, thyroid, and testes, *q.v.* SEE: *endocrine glands.*

g.'s, Frankel's. Tiny glands located below the margin of the vocal cords.

g., fundic. Glands of the body and fundus of the stomach; gastric glands which secrete gastric juice.

g.'s, Gay's. Multiple sweat glands developed to a great extent in the perianal area.

g., genal. Gland in buccal submucosa.

g.'s, genital. Ovaries (in female) and testes (in male).

g.'s, gingival. Glands at gum margins.

g.'s, hair. Sebaceous glands opening into each hair follicle.

g.'s, haversian. Glands secreting synovial fluid.

g.'s, hematopoietic. Glands participating in blood production.

g.'s. hemolymph. Modified glands containing blood and lymph sinuses, which probably participate in the formation of the leukocytes and the destruction of red blood corpuscles.

g.'s, hepatic. Lymph nodes located in front of the portal vein.

g.'s, inguinal. Lymph nodes in the inguinal region.

g., interscapular. Embryonic lymphatic tissue.

g., interstitial. G. in connective tissue of seminiferous tubules of testes and which produce internal secretions. SYN: *interstitial or Leydig's cells.*

g.'s, intestinal. Simple or branched tubular glands of the intestine which secrete the succus entericus. Include Brunner's glands, and crypts of Lieberkühn.

g.'s, jugular. SEE: *cervical g.*

g.'s, Krause's. Small glands in the conjunctiva of the eyelids, also called accessory lacrimal glands.

g.'s, labial. Multiple acinous glands bet. the mucosa of the lips and the opening on the inner lip.

g., lacrimal. A compound tubuloalveolar gland, located in the roof of the orbit which secretes tears.

g.'s, lactiferous. SEE: *mammary g.'s.*

g.'s, Lieberkühn's. Tiny tubular glands on the intestinal mucosa. SYN: *intestinal g.'s.*

g., lingual. Glands of the tongue, includes the ant. lingual glands (g.'s of Nuhn), post. lingual glands (g.'s of von Ebner) and mucous glands at the root of the tongue.

g.'s, Littre's. Tiny mucous glands in the urethral mucosa in the cavernous portion.

g.'s, lumbar. Lymphatics located behind the peritoneal region and the lower section of the diaphragmatic post. part.

g., Luschka's. G. located near the coccygeal tip.

g., lymph, g., lymphatic. Nodule of lymphatic tissue, found along the path of a lymphatic vessel.

g., mammary. A compound alveolar gland which secretes milk.

g., mandibular. The submaxillary gland, *q.v.*

g.'s, meibomian. Tarsal g.'s, *q.v.*

g., merocrine. A gland in which the cells remain intact in the process of the elaboration and discharge of their secretion.

g.'s, Mery's. Bulbourethral g.'s, *q.v.*

g.'s, Moll's. Modified sweat glands in the eyelid.

g.'s, Montgomery's. Areolar glands, *q.v.*

g.'s, Morgagni's. SEE: *Littré's g.'s.*

g.'s, muciparous; g.'s, mucous. G.'s secreting mucus.

g.'s, nabothian. Dilated mucous g.'s in the uterine cervix.

g.'s, odoriferous. G.'s exuding odoriferous materials, as those around the prepuce or anus.

g.'s, oxyntic. Gastric glands usually found in the abdominal cardiac region.

g.'s, pacchionian. Small masses along the surface of the dura mater in the cranium.

g.'s, palatine. Mucous glands in the tissue of the palate.

g., palpebral. Tarsal g.'s, *q.v.*

g., parathyroid. SEE: *parathyroid.*

g.'s, paraurethral. Small rudimentary glands which open on either side of the posterior portion of the urethral orifice in the female; Skene's glands.

g., parotid. Largest salivary gland located in front of the ear. It is a compound tubuloacinous, serous gland.

g.'s, Peyer's. SEE: *aggregate glands.*

g., pineal. Tiny glandular body of conical shape located bet. 2 sup. quadrigeminal bodies, connected with the thalamus, but not a part of the brain.

g., pituitary. The hypophysis cerebri, *q.v.* ALSO SEE *pituitary.*

g.'s, preputial. SEE: *Tyson's glands.*

g., prostate. G. surrounding male bladder neck and urethra. SEE: *prostate.*

g.'s, pulmonary. Glands in lung tissue.

g.'s, pyloric. Gastric glands near the pylorus secreting gastric juice.

g., racemose. SEE: *acinous g.*

g.'s, Rivini's. SEE: *sublingual g.'s.*

g., saccular. An alveolar gland.

g., salivary. Any gland secreting saliva, as parotid, sublingual and submaxillary. SEE ALSO under *salivary.*

g., sebaceous. A simple or branched alveolar gland which secretes sebum. They are found in the skin. Their ducts usually opening into hair follicles.

g.'s, serous. SEE: *albuminous g.'s.*

g., sex. Old term for the ovary or testis.

g.'s, Skene's. The paraurethral glands, *q.v.*

g.'s, solitary. SEE: *intestinal g.'s.*

g.'s, sublingual. Tiny salivary glands situated on either side of the tongue.

g.'s, submaxillary. Tiny salivary glands on either side of the tongue in the submaxillary triangles.

g.'s, sudoriferous. Glands secreting perspiration situated in the skin. SEE ALSO under *sweat.* SYN: *sudoriparous g.'s; sweat g.'s.*

g., suprarenal. The adrenal gland, *q.v.*

g.'s, sweat. SEE: *sudoriferous, q.v.*

g.'s, synovial. Glands secreting synovial fluid. SYN: *haversian g.'s.*

g.'s, tarsal. G.'s situated in the eyelid secreting sebaceous substance which keeps the lids from adhering to each other. SYN: *meibomian g.'s.*

g., thymus. The thymus body or thymus, *q.v.*

g., thyroid. Ductless g. situated in the neck in front of the trachea. SEE ALSO under *thyroid.*

g.'s, tracheal. Acinous g.'s of the tracheal mucosa.

g., tubular. A g. whose terminal secreting portions are narrow tubes.

g.'s, Tyson's. Tiny sebaceous glands found on the inner surface of the prepuce and on the glans of the penis.

g.'s, urethral. SEE: *Littre's g.'s.*

g.'s, vaginal. Acinous g.'s in the vaginal mucosa. These are found only in uppermost portion near the cervix. The major portion of the vaginal mucosa is devoid of glands.

g.'s, vestibular. G.'s of the vaginal vestibule. They include the *minor vestibular glands* and the *major vestibular glands* (glands of Bartholin).

g.'s, vulvovaginal. SEE: *Bartholin's g's.*

g.'s, Waldeyer's. G.'s in the eyelid.

g.'s, Weber's. G.'s in the tongue mucosa.

g.'s of Zeis. Large sebaceous glands found in the eyelids. They are associated with the follicles of the eyelashes.

g., Zuckerkandl's. Tiny tawny lobe occasionally seen bet. geniohyoid muscles.

gland, words pert. to: "aden-" words, "adreno-" words, bulbourethral, endocrine, gastric, holocrine, name of each gland, seborrhea, "sial-" words.

glanders (glan'derz) [L. *glans, gland-*, kernel]. Contagious infection by *Malleomyces mallei* in horses and mules, communicable to man.

SYM: Fever, inflammation of the skin and mucous membranes esp. those of the nasal cavity, with formation of ulcers and abscesses. Small subcutaneous nodules (farcy buds) develop which break down giving rise to ulcers. Beginning as small areas, these tend to spread and coalesce involving large areas and giving rise to a viscid, mucopurulent discharge with a foul odor. May occur in acute or chronic form. In the acute form, prognosis is grave, the disease often ending fatally.

glandula (glan'du-la) (pl. *glandulae*) [L. little kernel]. A small gland. SYN: *glandule.*

glan'dular [L. *glandula*, little kernel]. Pert. to or of nature of a gland.

g. therapy. Treatment of disease with endocrine glands or their extracts. SYN: *organotherapy.*

glandule (glan'dūl) [L. *glandula*, little kernel]. A small gland. SYN: *glandula.*

glans (pl. *glandes*) [L. kernel]. 1. A gland. 2. Goiter. 3. A nut.

g. clitoridis [NA]. The head of the clitoris. SEE: *clitoris.*

g. penis [NA], **g. phalli.** Bulbous end of the penis. SEE: *penis.*

glare [M.E. *glaren*, to glow]. Temporary blurring of vision, with possible permanent injury to retina from intense light (visible radiation) emanating from highly reflecting objects, such as sunlight reflected from water or snow, or projected by automobile headlight, or by a therapeutic lamp.

glase'rian artery [Johann Heinrich Glaser, Swiss anatomist, 1629-1675]. A branch of internal maxillary artery; goes to tympanum. SYN: *tympanic artery.*

g. fissure. A fissure in the temporal bone. SYN: *petrotympanic fissure.*

glass, polarized. A medium that permits the exiting light waves to vibrate in only one direction.

g., ultraviolet transmitting. Glass designed to admit ultraviolet radiation through it.

The best transmits from 50 to 60% of the solar radiation, between 290 and 320 millimicrons. With age the transparency to these rays drops off 50%.

glass'es [A.S. *glaes*, glass]. 1. Transparent refractive device worn to correct eye defects. 2. Device worn to protect eyes from glare or particles in the air.

g., bifocal. Those in which the refracting power of the lower portion differs from that in the upper portion, the lower portion being used for viewing near objects or reading, the upper portion for distant objects. SYN: *Franklin g.'s.*

glas'sy [A.S. *glaes*, glass]. Hyaline; vitreous; like glass, smooth and shiny.

Glau'ber's salt [Johann R. Glauber, German physician, 1604-1668]. Sodium sulfate used as a hydragogue purgative.

glaucoma (glaw-ko'mă) [G. *glaukos*, green, + *oma*, swelling]. Disease of eye characterized by increase in intraocular pressure which results in atrophy of optic nerve and blindness of two general types, *primary* which sets in without known cause, and *secondary* in which there is an increase in intraocular pressure due to other eye disease. The acute type often attended by acute pain. The chronic type has an insidious onset. Normal tonometer reading is 13 to 22.

An early sign of glaucoma is a subjective complaint that lights appear to have halos around them.

ETIOL: Closing of the canal of Schlemm due to a variety of conditions.

TREATMENT: *Nonoperative*: Miotics (eserine, pilocarpine), phospholine iodide. Control of associated disorders, as diabetes.

Operative: Paracentesis of cornea, iridectomy (broad peripheral), cyclodialysis, ant. sclerotomy, sclerotomy with inclusion of iris as iridotasis or iridocleisis, sclerectomy.

SEE: *ciliarotomy.*

g. absolutum. Eye completely blind, cornea insensitive, ant. chamber shallow, excavated optic disk, eye as hard as stone, extremely painful.

g., chronic. Pressure up to 45-50, enlargement of ant. ciliary veins, cornea clear, dilated pupil, pain, poor vision during attacks, field may be normal, no cupping early.

g., infantile. Buphthalmos resulting in uniform enlargement of eye with increased pressure.

g. simplex. Pressure not high, contracted field, glaucomatous cupping, blindness, no acute attacks. TREATMENT: Neostigmine.

glaucomatous (glaw-ko′mă-tus) [" + *ōma,* swelling]. Pert. to glaucoma.

gleet [Fr. *glette,* slime]. A mucous discharge from the urethra in chronic gonorrhea.

Glénard's disease (gla-narz′) [Frantz Glenard, French physician, 1848-1920]. Prolapse of one or more of the internal organs. SYN: *enteroptosis; splanchnoptosis.*

glenohumeral (gle-no-hu′mer-al). Pert. to the humerus and the glenoid cavity.

g. ligaments. Three ligaments in shoulder.

gle′noid [G. *glēnē,* cavity, + *eidos,* form]. Having the appearance of a socket.

g. cavity. The socket which receives the head of the humerus, below the acromium at the junction of the superior and axillary borders.

g. fossa. The mandibular fossa, which receives the capitulum of the mandible.

gli′a [G. glue]. The neuroglia, *q.v.;* the non-nervous or supporting tissue of the brain and spinal cord.

g. cells. Neuroglia cells, includes astrocytes, oligodendroglia (oligoglia), and microglia. SEE: *cell; neuroglia.*

gliacyte (gli′ă-sīt) [" + *kytos,* cell]. A neuroglia cell.

gli′adin [G. *glia,* glue]. A protein separable from the gluten of wheat.

It is deficient in lysine. It contains 94.11% amino acid.

glial (gli′al) [G. *glia,* glue]. Concerning glia or neuroglia.

gliarase (gli′ă-rās) [G. *glia,* glue]. Astrocytic mass with fission of cytoplasm.

gliobacte′ria [" + *baktērion,* little rod]. A zoogleal mass containing bacilli.

glioblasto′ma [" + *blastos,* germ, + *ōma,* tumor]. A neuroglia cell tumor. SYN: *glioma.*

g. multiforme. A neoplasm of the central nervous system, esp. the cerebrum, consisting of a variety of cellular types.

gliococ′cus [" + *kokkos,* berry]. A micrococcus in a mass of zooglea.

gliocyte (gli′o-sīt) [" + *kytos,* cell]. A neuroglia cell. SYN: *gliacyte.*

gliocyto′ma [" + " + *ōma,* tumor]. A neuroglia cell tumor.

gliogenous (gli-oj′ĕ-nus) [" + *gennan,* to produce]. Of the nature of neuroglia.

glio′ma (pl. *glio′mata*) [" + *ōma,* tumor]. 1. A sarcoma of neuroglial origin. 2. Neoplasm or a tumor composed of neuroglia cells.

g. retinae. Malignant tumor of retina; occurs in children; metastasizes late. SEE: *pseudoglioma.*

gliomatosis (gli-o-mă-to′sis) [" + " + *ōsis*]. Formation of a glioma.

gliomatous (gli-o′mă-tus) [G. *glia,* glue, + *ōma,* tumor]. Affected with or of the nature of a glioma.

gliomyoma (gli-o-mi-o′mă) [" + *mys, myo-,* muscle, + *ōma,* tumor]. A mixed glioma and myoma.

glioneuroma (gli-o-nū-ro′mă) [" + *neuron,* nerve, + *ōma,* tumor]. A tumor having the characteristics of glioma and neuroma.

gliosarco′ma [" + *sarx,* flesh, + *ōma,* tumor]. Glioma combined with fusiform cells of sarcoma.

gliosis (G. *glia,* glue, + *-osis*). Proliferation of neuroglial tissue in the central nervous system.

gliosome (gli′o-sōm) [" + *sōma,* body]. One of the rounded bodies seen in neuroglia cells.

gliotoxin. An antibiotic obtained from several different fungi, esp. *Trichoderma.*

glischrin (glis′krin) [G. *glischros,* gluey]. Mucinous substance produced in urine by bacterial activity.

glischruria (glis-kru′rĭ-ă) [" + *ouron,* urine]. Glischrin in the urine.

glisso′nian cirrhosis. Inflammation of peritoneal coat of the liver. SYN: *perihepatitis.*

glissoni′tis [G. *-ītis,* inflammation]. Inflammation of Glisson's capsule.

Glisson's capsule (glis′uns) [Francis Glisson, English physician, 1597-1677]. The outer capsule of fibrous tissue investing the liver. SYN: *capsula fibrosa hepatis.*

glo′bin [L. *globus,* globe]. 1. A protein constituent of hemoglobin. 2. One of a particular group of proteins.

g. insulin. SEE: *insulin, globin.*

globinom′eter [" + G. *metron,* measure]. Device for determining the number of red blood cells in a certain volume of blood.

glo′boid [" + G. *eidos,* form]. Spheroid; resembling a globe.

g. bodies. Minute ultramicroscopical microorganisms such as pathogens of poliomyelitis.

globular (glob′u-lar) [L. *globus,* a globe]. Resembling a globe or globule; spherical.

globule (glob′ūl) [L. *globulus,* globule]. Any small rounded body.

globulicidal (glob″u-lĭ-si′dal) [" + *caedere,* to kill]. Destructive to red blood corpuscles.

globulim′eter [" + G. *metron,* measure]. Device for determining the per cent of oxyhemoglobin in the blood. SYN: *cytometer.*

globulin (glob′u-lin) [L. *globulus,* globule]. One of a group of simple proteins insoluble in pure water but soluble in neutral solutions of salts of strong acids with strong bases.

Ex: *serum, globulin, fibrinogen, myosinogen, lactoglobulin.*

g., Ac. Accelerator globulin; a globulin present in blood serum which speeds up the conversion of prothrombin to thrombin in the presence of thromboplastin and calcium ions.

g., antihemophiliac. A clotting component present in the plasma which is essential for the normal agglutination and disintegration of blood platelets. It is deficient in the blood of hemophiliacs. SYN: *thromboplastinogen; thrombocytolytic factor.*

g., gamma. That fraction of serum globulin with which most of the immune antibodies are associated. Most of the antibodies to viruses, bacterial agglutinogens, exotoxins, and injected foreign proteins are contained in the gamma globulin fraction. They are thought to arise from plasma cells.

g., placental. A preparation of globulins, antibodies obtained from the human placenta. It contains the antibodies or immune factors against measles and is used in the prevention, modification, and treatment of measles.

g., serum. Globulins present in blood plasma or serum; the fraction of the blood serum with which antibodies are associated. By electrophoresis, they can be separated into alpha-, beta-, and gamma-globulins, which differ in their isoelectric points.

glob'ulism [" + G. *ismos*, state]. 1. Abnormal amt. of red corpuscles in the blood. 2. Administration of medicine in globules.

globulolysis (glob-u-lol'ĭ-sis) [" + G. *lysis*, dissolution]. Red blood corpuscle destruction. SYN: *hematolysis.*

globulolytic (glob-u-lo-lit'ik) [" + G. *lysis*, dissolution]. Capable of destroying red blood corpuscles.

globulose (glob'u-lōs) [L. *globulus*, globule]. Albumose or protein produced by the digestion of globulins.

globu'lysis [L. *globus*, globe, + G. *lysis*, destruction]. Destruction of red blood corpuscles. SYN: *globulolysis; hemolysis.*

globus [L.]. A globe or sphere.

g. hystericus. A lump in the throat in hysteria and other neuroses.

g. major. Head of epididymus.

g. minor. Lower end of epididymus.

g. pallidus. Pale section within the lenticular nucleus of the brain. SEE: *paleostriatum.*

glomangioma (glo"man-jĭ-o'mă). A benign tumor which develops from an arteriovenous glomus of the skin.

glom'erate [L. *glomerāre*, to wind into a ball]. Conglomerate, clustered, grouped.

glomer'ular [L. *glomerulus*, little skein]. Clustered. Pert. to a glomerulus.

glomerule (glom'er-ūl) [L. *glomerulus*, little skein]. A glomerulus.

glomer'uli (sing. *glomerulus*) [L. *glomerulus*, little skein]. 1. Small structures in the malpighian body of the kidney made up of capillary blood vessels in a cluster and enveloped in a thin wall, giving off uriniferous tubules. 2. Plexuses of capillaries. Twisted secretory parts of sweat glands.

glomerulitis (glo-mer"u-li'tis) [" + G. *-ītis*, inflammation]. Inflammation of glomeruli, esp. of the renal glomeruli. SYN: *glomerulonephritis.*

glomerulonephritis (glo-mer"u-lo-ne-fri'-tis) [L. *glomerulus*, little skein, + G. *nephros*, kidney, + *-ītis*, inflammation]. A form of nephritis in which the lesions involve primarily the glomeruli. May be acute, subacute, or chronic. Etiology is unknown but it frequently follows other infections, esp. those of the upper respiratory tract. Characterized by hematuria, edema, hypertension, and in severe cases, dyspnea, delirium, convulsions, and coma. SYN: *glomerulitis.*

glomerulus (glo-mer'u-lus) (pl. *glomeruli*) [L. little skein]. 1. A small rounded mass or spherical structure. 2. A small tuft of capillary loops enclosed within Bowman's capsule, the expanded end of a renal tubule, and two comprising a malpighian body or renal corpuscle. It serves as a filtering structure in the formation of urine.

g., olfactory. A rounded body found in the olfactory bulb formed by the numerous terminal branches of the dendrites of a mitral cell intertwining with the terminal fibers of several olfactory receptor cells.

glomus (glo'mus) [L.]. A small, round swelling made up of tiny blood vessels and found in a stroma containing many nerve fibers.

g. caroticum [NA]. The carotid body, *q.v.*

g. choroideum [NA]. An enlargement of the choroid plexus at its entrance into the inferior corum of the lateral ventricle.

g. coccygeum. The coccygeal body, *q.v.*

glos'sa [G. tongue]. The tongue.

glos'sal [G. *glōssa*, tongue]. Rel. to the tongue.

glossalgia (glos-sal'jĭ-ă) [" + *algos*, pain]. Pain in the tongue. SYN: *glossodynia.*

glossectomy (glos"ek'to-mĭ) [" + *ektome*, excision]. Partial or complete excision of tongue. SYN: *elinguation; Kocher's operation.*

Glossina (glos-si'nă). A genus of flies called tsetse flies. Includes about 20 species of bloodsucking flies which are confined principally to central and southern Africa. They transmit the trypanosomes (*Trypanosoma gambiense, T. rhodesiense*) the causative agents of sleeping sickness in man and other trypanosomes which infect wild and domestic animals. Important species are *Glossina palpalis, G. morsitans, G. tachinoides,* and *G. swynnertoni.* SEE: *Trypanosoma; sleeping sickness.*

glossi'tis [" + *-ītis*, inflammation]. Inflammation of the tongue.

g., acute. Associated with stomatitis, *q.v.* The tongue is covered with ulcers and is tender and painful. Another form affects the parenchyma of tongue and is characterized by edema, which may spread to surrounding structures, producing asphyxia and necessitating tracheotomy operation.

SYM: Tongue is painful; saliva thick and viscid, rendering swallowing difficult. Marked malaise, and often a rise in temperature.

TREATMENT: Oral cleanliness by frequent use of antiseptic mouthwashes. Anesthetic solution as oral rinse for pain. Corticosteroid dental ointment. Bland or liquid diet.

g. areata exfoliativa. Geographic tongue.

g., chronic. Sometimes while suffering from chronic ill health, chronic dyspepsia, and septic teeth, this condition arises.

SYM: Tongue is large, pale, and flabby, and shows indentation marks from teeth pressure. Mouth is uncomfortable and there may be an unpleasant taste or foul odor.

TREATMENT: Improvement of the general health, relief of constipation, careful attention to oral hygiene.

g. desic'cans. A painful, raw, and fissured tongue.

g., median rhomboidal. An inflammatory area, somewhat diamond shaped, found on the dorsum of the tongue anterior to the vallate papillae.

g., Moeller's. Glossodynia exfoliativa, *q.v.*

g. parasit'ica. Black tongue. SYN: *glossophytia.*

glosso- [G. *glōssa*, tongue]. Prefix: Signifies *pert. to the tongue.*

glossocele (glos'so-sēl) [G. *glōssa*, tongue, + *kēlē*, swelling]. Swelling and protrusion of the tongue due to disease or malformation.

glossodynamometer (glos"so-di"nă-mom'-ĕ-ter) [" + *dynamis*, power, + *metron*, measure]. Device for measuring contractile power of the tongue muscles.

glossodynia (glos-o-din'ĭ-ă) [" + *odynē*, pain]. Pain in the tongue. SYN: *glossalgia.*

g. exfoliativa. Moeller's glossitis. A chronic superficial inflammation of the tongue characterized by burning or pain and increased sensitivity to hot and spicy foods.

glos"soepiglot'tic [" + *epi*, upon, + *glōttis*, back of tongue]. Pert. to the ligament bet. base of tongue and epiglottis.

glossoepiglottidean (glos"o-ep-ĭ-glŏ-tid'e-an) [" + " + *glōttis*, back of tongue]. Rel. to the tongue and epiglottis.

g. folds. Three mucous membrane folds from base of tongue to the epiglottis. SYN: *plicae epiglotticae.*

g. ligament. Elastic band from base of tongue to the epiglottis in middle g. fold.

glossograph (glos'o-graf) [" + *graphein*, to write]. A graph for showing the tongue's movements in speaking.

glossohyal (glos-o-hi'al) [" + *yoeidēs*, U-shaped]. Rel. to tongue and hyoid bone. SYN: *hyoglossal.*

gloss"okin"esthet'ic. Pertaining to movements of the tongue, esp. those in speech.

glosso"la'bial. Pertaining to the tongue and lips.

glossolalia (glos-so-lal'ĭ-ă) [" + *lalia*, babble]. Repetition of senseless remarks not related to the subject or situation involved.

glossology (glos-sol'o-jĭ) [" + *logos*, study]. 1. Study of the tongue and its diseases. SYN: *glottology.* 2. Science of nomenclature. SYN: *onomatology.*

glossolysis (glos-sol'ĭ-sis) [G. *glōssa*, tongue, + *lysis*, loosening]. Paralysis of tongue. SYN: *glossoplegia.*

glosso"pal'atine. Pertaining to the tongue and the palate.

glossopathy (glos-sop'ă-thĭ) [" + *pathos*, disease]. Disease of the tongue.

glossopharyngeal (glos"o-far-in'je-ăl) [" + *pharygx*, pharynx]. Rel. to tongue and pharynx.

g. nerve. Ninth cranial n. FUNCT: Special sensory (taste), visceral sensory, motor. ORIG: by several roots from the medulla oblongata. DIST: Pharynx, ear, meninges, tongue, tonsils. BRS: Carotid, tympanic, pharyngeal, lingual, tonsillar, and sinus nerve of Hering.

glossophytia (glos"so-fi'tĭ-ă). Black or hairy tongue, characterized by the appearance on the dorsum of the tongue of a dark furlike patch consisting of hypertrophied filiform papillae, pigment, and shed epithelial cells. SYN: *hyperkeratosis linguae.*

glossoplasty (glos-so-plas'tĭ) [" + *plassein*, to form]. Reparative surgery of the tongue.

glossoplegia (glŏs-sō-ple'jĭ-ă). Paralysis of tongue, usually unilateral. ETIOL: Cerebral hemorrhage, disease, or injury which involves the hypoglossal nerve. SYN: *glossolysis.*

glossopto'sis [" + *ptōsis*, a dropping]. A dropping of the tongue downward out of normal position.

glosso"pyros'is. A burning sensation of the tongue.

glossorrhaphy (glos-sor'ă-fĭ) [" + *raphē*, suture]. Suture of wound of the tongue.

glossos'copy [" + *skopein*, to examine]. Inspection of the tongue.

glossospasm (glos'so-spazm) [" + *spasmos*, spasm]. Spasmodic contraction of muscles of the tongue.

glossotomy (glos-ot'o-mĭ) [" + *tomē*, incision]. Incision of tongue.

glosso"trich'ia. Hairy tongue, due to greatly elongated filiform papillae which gives the tongue a hairy appearance.

gloss'y [M.E. *glōse*]. Smooth and shining.

g. skin. Shiny appearance of the skin due to atrophy or injury to nerves.

glot'tic [G. *glōttis*, back of tongue]. Of or pert. to the tongue, or the glottis.

glottis (glŏt'is) [G. *glottis*, back of tongue]. The sound-producing apparatus of the larynx consisting of the two *vocal folds* and the intervening space, the *rima glottidis.* A leaf-shaped lid of fibrocartilage (the epiglottis) protects this opening.

g., edema. The accumulation of fluid in the tissues lining the larynx. It may result from irritation of the larynx from improper use of the voice, excessive use of tobacco or alcohol, chemical fumes, acute infections, or more serious conditions such as tuberculous or syphilitic laryngitis.

SYM: Hoarseness, and later complete aphonia, extreme dyspnea at first on inspiration, but later on expiration also. Stridulous respiration, barking cough when epiglottis is involved.

g. spuria. Space situated bet. the false vocal cords.

glotti'tis [" + *-itis*, inflammation]. Inflammation of the tongue. SYN: *glossitis.*

glottol'ogy [" + *logos*, study]. The study of the tongue and its diseases. SYN: *glossology.*

glucagon (glu'kă-gon). ABBR: HGF. A hyperglycemic glycogenolytic factor secreted by the alpha cells of the pancreas. It stimulates the breakdown of glycogen and the release of glucose by the liver.

glucase (glu'kās) [G. *glukus*, sweet]. An old term for a ferment converting starch into glucose.

glucatonia (glu-ka-to'nĭ-ă) [" + *a-*, priv. + *tonos*, tone]. Reduction of blood sugar brought about by insulin therapy. Insulin shock.

glucinum. Former name for *beryllium.*

gluciphore (glu'sĭ-fōr) [" + *phorein*, to carry]. An atomic group which, when combined with other tasteless atoms called auxoglucs, forms sweet compounds. SEE: *auxogluc.*

glucocorticoid (gloo"ko-kort'ĭ-koyd). A general classification of adrenal cortical hormones which are primarily active in protecting against stress and in affecting protein and carbohydrate metabolism. SEE: *mineralocorticoid.*

glucohe'mia [" + *aima*, blood]. Sugar in the blood. SYN: *glycosemia.*

gluco'neogenesis [G. *glukus*, *sweet*, + *neos*, new, + *genesis*, origin]. The formation of glucose from noncarbohydrate sources such as proteins, and possibly fats. It occurs in the liver under such conditions as low carbohydrate intake or starvation. SYN: *glyconeogenesis.*

glu'cose [L. *glucosum* from G. *glukus*, sweet]. 1. USP. Dextrose ($C_6H_{12}O_6$), a crystalline monosaccharide, more specifically dextro- or d-glucose. 2. An intermediate in metabolism of carbohydrates in the body. Formed during digestion.

Glucose is the most important carbohydrate in body metabolism. It is formed during digestion from the hydrolysis of di- and polysaccharides, esp. starch, and absorbed from the intestines into the blood of the portal vein. In its passage through the liver excess glucose is converted into glycogen (*glycogenesis*). The concentration of sugar in the blood is approximately 0.1 per cent (100 mg.) the amount being maintained at a fairly constant level (80 to 120 mg.) through the action of insulin produced by the islets of Langerhans of the pancreas. Failure of the pancreas to produce adequate insulin results in *hyperglycemia* in which the blood sugar (glucose) level may rise to 200 mg. or higher. When above the renal threshold (about 180 mg.), glucose appears in the urine (glycosuria), a symptom of diabetes. Overproduction of insulin or injection of insulin as in insulin shock treatment, reduces the blood sugar below normal, a condition known as *hypoglycemia, q.v.*

In the tissue glucose may be (a) converted into glycogen, (b) converted into fat, or (c) oxidized to carbon dioxide and water. Free glucose is not used in the tissues until phosphorlyated by ATP (adenosinetriphosphate). This occurs through the action of an enzyme, hexokinase, with the resultant production of glucose-6-phosphate. Through a complex series of reactions involving several enzymes, the action of certain hormones, and the formation of several intermediate products including lactic and pyruvic acids, oxidation to carbon and water is brought about. Hormones of the anterior lobe of the hypophysis, the adrenal gland (cortex and medulla), thyroid and the gonads play a role in carbohydrate metabolism.

When the blood sugar is below normal, fats are consumed. Incomplete combustion leads to the formation of ketone bodies, also a symptom of diabetes. Blood sugar acts as a protein sparer, *q.v.* Nervous tissue is especially dependent upon glucose as its source of energy, the brain being able to oxidize glucose directly.

g., conditions which change blood. The glucose found in the blood stream has a dual origin. First, glucose is present normally in both the whole blood and plasma; secondly, the greater percentage of the normal glucose concentration has an exogenous origin—that is, from the food intake. ***A. Normal:*** 80 to 120 mg. per 100 cc. ***B. Increased:*** (1) Acromegaly, (2) Adrenal tumors, (3) Cortical or medullary, (4) Diabetes mellitus, (5) Hemochromatosis, (6) Hyperthyroidism, (7) Hyperpituitarism, (8) Hyperadrenalism, (9) Intracranial pressure, (10) Severe exercise. ***C. Decreased:*** (1) Addison's disease, (2) Adenoma or carcinoma of islets of Langerhans, (3) Cretinism, (4) Hyperinsulinism, (5) Hypopituitarism, (6) Hypothyroidism, (7) Insulin shock, (8) Muscular dystrophy, (9) Myxedema.

g., liquid. A liquid obtained from the incomplete hydrolysis of starch. It is a thick syrupy liquid, sweet in taste, containing d-glucose (dextrose), dextrins, and other carbohydrates. It is used for nutritive purposes and in various pharmaceutical and food preparations.

glucose tolerance test. A test done by giving a certain amount of glucose to the patient orally or intravenously. Blood samples are drawn at specified intervals and the blood glucose determined in each sample. By this means, the ability of the patient to metabolize glucose can be determined. In suspected cases of hyperinsulinism, the test is prolonged to six hours with samples of blood being drawn hourly and analyzed for sugar content. If the blood-sugar level continues to drop after 3 hours, falling below 80 mg. per 100 cc., hyperinsulinism is indicated although other conditions may produce a deficiency in blood sugar (hypoglycemia).

glucosidase (glu'ko-sĭ-dās). An enzyme which catalyzes the hydrolysis of a glucoside.

glucoside (glu'ko-sīd) [G. *glukus,* sweet]. A substance glycoside, which upon hydrolysis, yields a sugar, glucose, and one or two additional products. They are numerous and widely distributed in plants. Many glucosides have medicinal properties, for example digitalin and strophanthin, present in digitalis and strophanthus respectively, which have a specific effect upon the heart. SEE: *glycoside.*

glucosin (glu'ko-sin) [G. *glukus,* sweet]. Any one of a series of bases derived by action of ammonia on glucose.

glucosu'ria [" + *ouron,* urine]. Abnormal amt. of sugar in the urine. SYN: *glycosuria.*

gluelike tumor. Glioma. Also a colloid degenerative cancer or colloma.

Glu'ge's corpuscles [Gottlieb Gluge, German pathologist, 1812-1898]. Granular cells containing fat droplets, usually found in degenerating nervous tissue.

glu'side. USP. White crystals or powder, about 500 times sweeter than sugar but with no caloric value. Used as a sweetening agent in some pharmaceuticals, and as a sugar substitute where sugar is forbidden in diet. SYN: *saccharin.*

glutam'ic acid. An amino acid (COOH $(CH_2)_2CHNH_2COOH$) formed in the

glutam'inase. An enzyme which catalyzes the breakdown of glutamine into glutamic acid and ammonia.

glutam'ine. The mono-amide of aminoglutaric acid. It is present in the juices of many plants and is essential in the hydrolysis of proteins.
metabolism of certain bacteria. It is also present in animal tissues such as the brain, liver and kidney.

glutathione (glū-tă-thi'ōn) [G. *theion,* sulfur]. A tripeptide of glutamic acid, cysteine, and glycine.

Found in small quantities in active animal tissues; takes up and gives off hydrogen; fundamentally important in cellular respiration.

gluteal (glu'te-al) [G. *gloutos,* buttock]. Pertaining to the buttocks.

g. fold. Crease between the thigh and the buttocks. SEE: *rump.*

g. reflex. Contraction of gluteal muscles from stimulation of their skin.

glutelin (glu'tĕ-lin). A simple protein found in grain seeds, soluble in alkalies and dilute acids, but not in neutral solutions. SEE: *protein.*

glu'ten [L. glue]. Vegetable albumin, a protein which can be prepared from wheat and other grain.

g. enteropathy. Adult celiac disease. A condition associated with malabsorption of food from the intestinal tract. The symptoms of diarrhea and malnutrition are usually controlled by eliminating gluten from the diet. SEE: *gluten-free diet.*

g.-free diet. Elimination of gluten from the diet by avoiding all products containing wheat, rye, oats, or barley and vegetables such as beans, cabbage, turnips, dried peas, and cucumbers. Rice, potatoes, corn, and cornmeal are allowed.

glu'tin [L. glue]. The viscid portion of wheat gluten. SYN: *gliadin.*

glutinous (glū'tin-us) [L. *glutinōsus, gluey*]. Adhesive; sticky.

gluti'tis [G. *gloutos,* buttock, + *-ītis,* inflammation]. Inflammation of muscles of buttocks.

glu'tolin. An albumoid substance found in small amts. in paraglobulin.

glycase (gli'kās) [G. *glykus*, sweet]. The enzyme that converts maltose into dextrose. SEE: *enzyme; ferment.*

glycemia (gli-se'mĭ-ă) [" + *aima*, blood] Sugar or glucose in the blood. SYN. *glycosemia.**

glyceride (glis'er-id, -īd) [G. *glykus*, sweet]. An ester of glycerin compounded with an acid.

glycerin (glis'er-in) [G. *glykus*, sweet]. USP. $C_3H_8O_3$. A trihydric alcohol, trihydroxy-propane present in chemical combination in all fats. It is a syrupy, colorless liquid, soluble in all proportions in water and alcohol. It is made commercially by the hydrolysis of fats, esp. during the manufacture of soap. SYN: *glycerol.*

USES: Extensively as a solvent, as a preservative, as an emollient in various skin diseases, and in form of suppositories as an evacuant.

glycerite (glis'er-īt) [G. *glykus*, sweet]. Drug dissolved in glycerin.

glyceri'tum (pl. *glycerita*) [L glycerite]. Medicinal substance mixed or dissolved in glycerin.

glycerol (glis'er-ol) [G. *glykus*, sweet]. Clear, colorless, syrupy liquid formed by hydrolysis of fat. SYN: *glycerin, q.v.*

g. trinitrate. Nitroglycerin, USP. Made by the action of nitric acid on glycerin in presence of sulfuric acid. Commonly in tablet form for sublingual use.

ACTION AND USES: To dilate blood vessels in some cases of angina pectoris.

glyc'eryl. The trivalent radical C_3H_5 of glycerol.

glycine (gli'sēn, gli-sēn') [G. *glykus*, sweet]. Aminoacetic acid derived from gelatin and from many proteins. SYN: *glycocin; glycocoll.*

glyco- (gli'ko). Prefix from G. *glykus*, sweet. Used in chemical compounds to indicate presence of glycerol or similar substance.

gly'cocin. Glycine, *q.v.*

glycoclas'tic [G. *glykus*, sweet, + *klassein*, to break]. Pert. to the hydrolysis and digestion of sugars.

glycogen (gli'ko-jen) [G. *glykus*, sweet, + *gennan*, to produce]. It is a polysaccharide $(C_6H_{10}O_5)x$ and is commonly called "animal starch", a whitish powder which can be prepared from mammalian liver and muscle, and other animal tissues.

Formation of glycogen from carbohydrate sources is called *glycogenesis;* from noncarbohydrate sources, *glyconeogenesis.* The conversion of glycogen to glucose is called *glycogenolysis.*

It is the form in which carbohydrate is stored in the animal body for future conversion into sugar, and for subsequent use in performing muscular work or for liberating heat.

It is formed from sugar and a part of the fat and protein in the blood. It is converted when needed by the tissues into glucose. It is a muscle food, and with the contraction of the muscles it breaks down into lactic acid, causing fatigue. Oxygen is then needed to convert lactic acid back into glycogen, at which time some of the lactic acid is burned, producing carbonic acid and heat. Sugar from the blood takes the place of the lactic acid consumed.

Oxygen and sugar are necessary to prevent fatigue from muscular exertion long continued. SEE: *azoamyly.*

glycogenase (gli'ko-jen-ās) [" + *gennan*, to produce]. An enzyme in the liver which hydrolyzes glycogen. Its end product is dextrose.

glycogenesis (gli-ko-jen'ĕ-sis) [" + *genesis*, formation]. The formation of glycogen, as occurs in man after the eating of a carbohydrate meal.

glycogenet'ic [" + *gennan*, to produce]. Pert. to the formation of glycogen.

glycogen'ic [" + *gennan*, to produce]. Rel. to glycogen.

glycogenolysis (gli"ko-jen-ol'ĭ-sis) [" + " + *lysis*, dissolution]. Conversion of glycogen into dextrose in the liver.

glycogenolytic (gli-ko-jen-o-lit'ik) [" + " + *lysis*, dissolution]. Pert. to the hydrolysis of glycogen.

glycogenosis (gli-ko-jen-o'sis) [" + " + *ōsis*]. Abnormal amt. of glycogen in children resulting in an enlarged liver. SYN: *glycogen disease; von Gierke's disease; glycogenic hepatonephromegaly.*

glycogeusia (gli-ko-ju'sĭ-ă) [" + *geusis*, taste]. A sweet taste.

glycohemia (gli-ko-he'mĭ-ă) [" + *aima*, blood]. Abnormal amt. of sugar in the blood. SYN: *glycosemia.*

glycol (gli'kol) [G. *glykus*, sweet]. Any one of the dihydric alcohols related to ethylene glycol, $C_2H_4(OH)_2$. The general formula is $C_2H_{2}n(OH)_2$.

The glycols are thick, colorless, water-soluble liquids similar to glycerol.

glycolipid(e (gli"ko-lip'id) [" + *lipos*, fat]. Compound of fatty acids with a carbohydrate, containing nitrogen, but no phosphoric acid. Found in myelin sheath of nerves. Also spelled glycolipide. SYN: *cerebroside.*

glycolysis (gli-kol'ĭ-sis) [" + *lysis*, dissolution]. Hydrolysis of sugar by a ferment in the body.

glycolyt'ic [" + *lysis*, dissolution]. Pert. to hydrolyzing sugar.

g. enzyme. An enzyme which catalyzes the hydrolysis of sugars.

glycometabol'ic [" + *metabolē*, change]. Rel. to the metabolism of sugar.

glycometabolism (gli"ko-mĕ-tab'o-lizm) [" + " + *-ismos*, process]. Utilization of sugar* by the body. SYN: *saccharometabolism.* SEE: *metabolism.*

glyconeogenesis (gli"ko-ne-o-jen'ĕ-sis) [" + *neos*, new, + *genesis*, formation]. The formation of carbohydrates from noncarbohydrates, such as fat or protein. SYN: *gluconeogenesis.*

glyconucleopro'tein [" + L. *nucleus*, kernel, + G. *prōtos*, first]. A carbohydrate group unduly developed in a nucleoprotein.

glycopenia (gli-ko-pe'nĭ-ă) [" + *penia*, poverty]. Having a tendency to hypoglycemia.

glycopex'ic [" + *pēxis*, fixation]. Pert. to the fixing or storing of sugar.

glycopex'is [" + *pēxis*, fixation]. The storing of glycogen in the liver.

glycophilia (gli-ko-fil'ĭ-ă) [" + *philein*, to love]. A condition in which there is a marked tendency to hyperglycemia.

glycopolyuria (gli"ko-pol-ĭ-ū'rĭ-ă) [" + *polys*, much, + *ouron*, urine]. Diabetes mellitus with *polyuria* greater than *glycosuria.*

glycopri'val, glycopri'vous [" + L. *privus*, deprived of]. Lacking in or without carbohydrates.

glycoprotein (gli-ko-pro'te-in) [" + *prōtos*, first]. A compound or conjugated protein such as mucin. SEE: *protein.*

glycoptyalism (gli-ko-ti'al-izm) [" + *ptyalon*, saliva, + *ismos*, state of]. Excretion of glucose in the saliva.

glycoregula'tion [" + L. *regula*, rule]. The dietary and insulin control of sugar metabolism.

glycoreg'ulatory [" + L. *regula*, rule]. Rel. to glycoregulation.

glycorrhachia (gli-ko-rak'ĭ-ă) [" + *rachis*, spine]. Sugar in the cerebrospinal fluid.

glycorrhea (gli-ko-re'ă) [" + *roia*, flow]. Discharge of sugar from the body as in urine.

glycosecretory (gli"ko-se'krĕ-to-rĭ) [" + L. *secretus*, from *secernere*, to separate]. Pert. to or determining the secretion of glycogen.

glycose'mia [" + *aima*, blood]. Abnormal amount of sugar in the blood.

glycosialia (gli-ko-si-al'ĭ-ă) [" + *sialon*, saliva]. Sugar in the saliva.

glycosialorrhea (gli"ko-si"al-o-re'ă) [" + " + *roia*, flow]. Excessive secretion of saliva containing sugar.

gly'coside. A substance derived from plants which upon hydrolysis yields a sugar and one or more additional products. Depending on the sugar formed, glycosides are designated *glucosides, galactosides*, etc. SEE: *glucoside*.

glycosom'eter [" + *metron*, measure]. Device for determining proportion of sugar in urine in glycosuria.

glycosuria (gli-ko-su'rĭ-ă) [" + *ouron*, urine]. The presence of sugar (glucose) in the urine.

Traces of sugar, particularly glucose, may occur in normal urine, but are not detected by ordinary qualitative methods. In routine urinalyses the presence of a reducing substance is suspicious of diabetes mellitus. It is found when the blood sugar level exceeds the renal threshold (about 170 mg. per cent). Fasting level of blood glucose is usually between 80 and 120 mg. per 100 ml. of blood. SYN: *glycosuria*.

Glycosuria may result from (a) pancreatic (insulin) insufficiency, (b) disorders of the endocrine glands esp. hypophysis, adrenals, thyroid, or ovaries, (c) excessive carbohydrate intake, (d) excessive glycogenolysis, (e) reduction of renal threshold.

g., alimentary. Following ingestion of large amounts of starches or sugars.

g., diabetic. G. resulting from hyposecretion of insulin.

g., emotional. G. resulting from emotional states such as worry or anxiety.

g., pituitary. G. resulting from dysfunction of the ant. pituitary.

g., phloridzin. G. resulting from the injection of phloridzin which reduces the renal threshold for glucose.

g., renal. When glucose is persistent and not accompanied by hyperglycemia.

glycuresis (gli-ku-re'sis) [" + *ourēsis*, urination]. Presence of sugar (glucose) in the urine. SYN: *glycosuria*.*

glycuronuria (gli-kū-ro-nu'rĭ-ă) [*glycuronic acid* + G. *ouron*, urine]. Glycuronic acid in the urine.

glycylglycine (glis-il-glis'in). The simplest form of a polypeptide.

glycyltryptophan (glis"il-trip'to-fan). A dipeptide of glycine and tryptophan.

glycyrrhiza (glis-ĭ-ri'ză). The licorice root. SEE: *licorice*.

glyoxalase. An enzyme which catalyzes the conversion of methylglyoxal to lactic acid by the addition of water.

gm., Gm. Abbr. for *gram*.

gnat (nat). Any of a number of small insects belonging to the order Diptera, suborder Orthorrhapha. Term applied generally to insects smaller than mosquitoes. Includes black flies, midges, and sand flies.

g., buffalo. A small dipterous insect belonging to the family Simuliidae, *q.v.*

gnathalgia (nath-al'jĭ-ă) [G. *gnathos*, jaw, + *algos*, pain]. Pain in the jaw. SYN: *gnathodynia*.

gnathic (nath'ĭk) [G. *gnathos*, jaw]. Pert. to an alveolar process or to the jaw.

gnathion (nath'ĭ-on) [G. *gnathos*, jaw]. Lowest point of middle line of lower jaw; a craniometric point.

gnathitis (nath-i'tis) [" + *-itis*, inflammation]. Inflammation of the jaw or adjacent soft parts.

gnatho- (nath'o) [G.]. Prefix: Pert. to jaw or cheek.

gnathocephalus (nath-o-sef'ă-lus). A malformed fetus in which the head consists principally of the jaws.

gnathodynia (nath-o-din'ĭ-ă) [G. *gnathos*, jaw, + *odynē*, pain]. Pain in the jaw. SYN: *gnathalgia*.

gnathoplasty (nath'o-plas-tĭ) [" + *plassein*, to form]. Reparative surgery of jaws or cheek.

gnathoschisis (nath-os'kĭ-sis) [" + *schizein*, to split]. Congenital jaw cleft.

Gnathostoma (nath-os'to-mă). A genus of nematode worms which infest the stomach walls of domestic and wild animals. They occasionally accidentally infest man.

gnathostomiasis (nath-o-sto-mi'ă-sis). Infestation with *Gnathostoma*, *q.v.*

gnosia (no'sĭ-ă) [G. *gnōsis*, knowledge]. The perceptive faculty of recognizing persons, things and forms.

gnotobiotics (no-to-bi-ot'iks). Study of animals that have been raised in germ-controlled or germ-free surroundings.

goat-leap pulse. Term applied to an irregular and bounding pulse. SEE: *pulse*.

goat milk. Fluid (whole): 100 gm. Calories: 77. Other main values: 1.1 gm. protein; 4 gm. fat; 4.6 gm. carbohydrate; 129 mg. calcium; 160 I.U. vitamin A.

goblet cell. A type of secretory cell found in the epithelium of the intestinal and respiratory tracts; a unicellular gland which secretes mucus. Mucin droplets accumulate in the distal end of the cell, forming a large ovoid mass which causes the cell to become swollen and distorted in shape. The free surface of the cell finally ruptures liberating the mucus. SEE: *cell; gland; secretion; mucus*. SYN: *mucous cell*.

gog'gle eyed. Having an abnormally protruding eye. SYN: *exophthalmic*.

goiter (goi'ter) [L. *guttur*, throat]. An enlargement of the thyroid gland.

ETIOL: It may be due to lack of iodine in diet, thyroiditis, or inflammation from infection, to tumors, or hyper- or hypofunction of the thyroid gland. SYN: *Derbyshire neck; struma*.

g., aberrant. Supernumerary thyroid enlargement.

g., acute. G. growing rapidly.

g., adenomatous. Thyroid enlargement due to growth of encapsulated adenomata. Nodular goiter.

g., basedowified. SEE: *toxic g.*

g., colloid. One in which there is a great increase of follicular contents.

g., congenital. One present at birth.

g., cystic. A g. in which a cyst or a number of cysts are formed. May result from the degeneration of tissue or liquification within an adenoma.

g., diffuse. G. in which the thyroid tissue is diffuse in contrast to its nodular form as in adenomatous goiter.

g., diver, g., diving. Movable g.

g., endemic. G. development in certain geographic localities, especially those in which iodine is deficient in food and water.

g., exophthalmic. G. with exophthalmos. Syn: *Graves', Parry's or Basedow's disease; hyperthyroidism; thyrotoxicosis.*

Etiol: Unknown. Occurs in constitutionally predisposed individuals. Incidence higher in females.

Sym: Bulging eyeballs generally present. Many eye signs, enlarged thyroid, delayed coagulation time, tremor of fingers and muscles of hands, tachycardia, increased metabolism, vomiting and diarrhea, profuse perspiration, nervous irritability, skin eruptions, emaciation, anemia, hyperglycemia. Goiters are more prevalent in fresh water and lake countries, and less so on the sea coast, due to the lack of iodine in fresh water. Iodine and iodized salt are used as remedies and preventives.

g., fibrous. G. with hyperplastic capsule and stroma of the thyroid gland.

g., follicular. See: *parenchymatous g.*

g., hyperplastic. Parenchymatous g., *q.v.*

g., intrathoracic. G. in which a portion of the thyroid tissue lies within the thoracic cavity.

g., lingual. Hypertrophied mass forming a tumor at post. portion of dorsum of tongue.

g., parenchymatous. G. characterized by multiplication of cells lining the follicles or alveoli. There is usually a reduction in colloid and the follicular cavities assume various sizes and are often obliterated by infoldings of their walls. Fibrous tissue may increase markedly. Iodine content of gland is low. Goiter usually of a diffuse nature.

g., perivascular. G. surrounding a large blood vessel.

g., retrovascular. G. development behind a large blood vessel.

g., simple. Thyroid gland hyperplasia unaccompanied by constitutional symptoms.

g., substernal. Enlargement of lower part of thyroid isthmus.

g., suffocative. G. causing shortness of breath due to pressure.

g., toxic. Exopthalmic goiter or goiter in which there is an excessive production of the thyroid hormone.

g., vascular. G. due to distention of blood vessels.

gold. A metallic element, yellow in color. Symb: Au. [from L. *aurum,* shining dawn]. At. no. 79; at. wt. 196.967. Its salts are used in early rheumatoid arthritis and in nondisseminated lupus erythematosus. Radioactive gold is used in treatment of certain types of cancer.

gold-beaters' skin. A membrane from the cecum of the ox for surgical use.

Gold'berger's diet [Joseph Goldberger, American physician, 1874-1929]. One for pellagra. Eggs, lean meat, and brewer's yeast.

Gold'flam's disease [Samuel V. Goldflam, Polish physician, 1852-1932]. Excessive tiring of voluntary muscles and rapid decrease of contractility. Syn: *myasthenia gravis pseudoparalytica.*

gold seed. Thin capillary glass tube covered with gold containing some form of radium.

Golgi's apparatus [Camillo Golgi, Italian histologist, 1843-1926]. The internal reticular apparatus of Golgi. A network of irregular wavy threads present in the cytoplasm of all nerve cells, and many other cells, esp. secretory cells.

G.'s cells. Multipolar nerve cells in the cerebral cortex and post. horns, of spinal cord. There are two types: Type I, those that possess long axons and Type II, those that possess short axons.

G.'s corpuscle. A sensory nerve ending or receptor found in tendons, or aponeuroses; an end organ of muscle sense. Also called *organ of Golgi.*

Goll's tract (golz) [Friedrich Goll, Swiss anatomist, 1829-1904]. One in post. white column of spinal cord. Syn: *fasciculus gracilis.*

gomphi'asis [G. *gomphios,* molar tooth]. Loosening of the teeth.

gomphosis (gom-fo'sis) [G. *gomphos,* nail, + *ōsis*]. A conical process fitting into a socket in immovable (synarthrosis*) joint. See: *joint.*

gon'ad [G. *gonē,* semen]. A generic term referring to both the female sex glands, or ovaries, and the male sex glands, or testes. The embryonic sex gland before differentiation into definitive testis or ovary.

Each forms the cells necessary for human reproduction, *spermatozoa* from the testes, *ova from* the ovaries.

Internal Secretions: *Female*: The vesicular follicles of the ovaries secrete estrogen, which maintains the nutrition and mature size of the female generative organs; also the *corpus luteum,* producing the luteal secretion (progesterone) which sensitizes the interior membrane of the uterus to contact with the ovum to assist in the implantation of the fertilized ovum.

Male: The interstitial cells of the testes secrete an internal secretion containing androgens which stimulates metabolism, increases muscular strength, and develops secondary sex characteristics.

Hormones from both sexes have been isolated and standardized, and are used in the treatment of conditions arising from an insufficiency of these hormones. See: *ovary; testicle.*

gonadal (gon'ă-dal) [G. *gonē,* seed]. Pert. to a gonad. Syn: *gonadial.*

gonadectomy (gon-ă-dek'to-mĭ) [" + *ektomē,* excision]. Excision of a testis or ovary.

gonad'ial [G. *gonē,* semen]. Pert. to a reproductive gland. Syn: *gonadal.*

gonadogen (gon-ad'o-jen) [" + *gennan,* to produce]. Commercial gonadotropic substance from pregnant mare's serum.

Induces ovulation, and, in male, growth of genitalia and secondary sex characteristics..

gonadop'athy [" + *pathos,* disease]. Any disease of the sexual glands.

gonadother'apy [" + *therapeia,* treatment]. Treatment by injection of extracts containing testicular or ovarian hormones.

gonadotrope (gon-ad'o-trōp) [" + *tropē,* turning]. One dominated by the sex instinct.

gonadotrophic (go-nad-o-trŏf'ĭk) [G. *gonē,* semen]. Relating to stimulation of the gonads.

g. hormones. Gonadotrophins, *q.v* or gonad-stimulating hormones.

gonadotrophin [G. *gonē,* semen, + trope, a turning]. A gonad-stimulating hormone.

g.'s, ant. pituitary. Those produced by the anterior lobe of the hypophysis. Include (a) follicle-stimulating hormone (FSH), (b) leuteinizing hormone (LH). In the male this is called the interstitial cell stimulating hormone (ICSH), (c) luteotrophic hormone (LTH).

g., chorionic. G.'s produced by the chorionic villi of the placenta. They are present in the blood and urine of pregnant women and in the blood of pregnant mares. Their presence in urine is the basis of the Ascheim-Zondeck, Friedman, and other pregnancy tests. Also called ant. pituitary-like hormone, pregnancy hormone.

gonadotropism (go-nad-ot'ro-pizm) [" + " + *ismos,* state of]. Domination by the sex impulse.

gon'aduct [" + L. *ductus,* canal]. The seminal duct or the oviduct.

gonagra (gon-ag'ră) [G. *gonu,* knee, + *agra,* seizure]. Gout in the knee.

gonal'gia [" + *algos,* pain]. Pain in the knee.

gonangiectomy (gon-an-jĭ-ek'to-mĭ) [G. *gonē,* seed, + *aggeion,* vessel, + *ektomē,* excision]. Excision of the vas deferens or a part of it. SYN: *vasectomy.*

gonarthritis (gon-ar-thri'tis) [G. *gonu,* knee, + *arthron,* joint, + *-itis,* inflammation]. Inflammation of knee joint.

gonarthrocace (gon-ar-throk'ă-se) [" + " + *kakē,* evil]. White swelling of knee joint.

gonarthromeningitis (gon-ar"thro-men-in-ji'tis) [" + " + *mēnigx,* membrane, + *-itis,* inflammation]. Synovitis of the knee joint.

gonarthrotomy (gon-ar-throt'o-mĭ) [" + " + *tomē,* incision]. Incision of knee joint.

gonatag'ra [" + *agra,* seizure]. Gout in the knee.

gonatocele (gon-at'o-sēl) [" + *kēlē,* swelling]. White swelling; tumor of the knee.

gonecyst, gonecystis (gon'e-sist, gon-e-sis'tis) [G. *gonē,* semen, + *kystis,* a bladder]. A seminal vesicle.

gonecystitis (gon-e-sis-ti'tis) [" + " + *-itis,* inflammation]. Inflammation of seminal vesicles.

gonecystolith (gon-e-sis'to-lith) [" + " + *lithos,* stone]. A concretion or calculus in a seminal vesicle.

gonecystopyosis (gon-e-sist"o-pi-o'sis) [" + " + *pyōsis,* suppuration]. Suppuration in a seminal vesicle or gonecyst.

goneitis (go-ne-i'tis) [G. *gonu,* knee, + *-itis,* inflammation]. Inflammation of the knee.

gonepoiesis (gon-e-poy-e'sis) [G. *gonē,* semen, + *poiein,* to make]. The secretion of the semen.

Gonglyonema (gon"jĭ-lo-ne'mă). A genus of nematode worms belonging to the suborder Spirurata. They are parasitic in wall of the esophagus and stomach of domestic animals. Occasionally, they are accidental parasites in man. *G. pulchrum* is the species most frequently involved.

goniometer (gon-ĭ-om'ĕ-ter) [G. *gōnia,* angle, + *metron,* measure]. Apparatus to measure joint movements and angles.

gonion (go'nĭ-on) [G. *gōnia,* angle]. Point of angle of the mandible or lower jaw.

gonioscope (go'nĭ-o-skōp) [" + *skopein,* to examine]. An instrument for inspecting angle of ant. chamber of eye and for determining ocular motility and rotation.

gono-, gon- (gon'o) [G.]. Prefix meaning *generation, offspring, semen.*

gonoblast (gon'o-blast). SEE: *ganoblast.*

gonocide (gon'o-sīd) [G. *gonē,* semen, + L. *caedere,* to kill]. Destructive to the gonococcus.

gonococ'cal [" + *kokkos,* berry]. Rel. to or caused by gonococci.

gonococcemia (gon-o-kok-se'mĭ-ă) [" + " + *aima,* blood]. Gonococci in the blood.

gonococ'ci. Pl. of gonococcus.

gonococcic (gon-o-kok'sik) [" + *kokkos,* berry]. Pert. to the gonococcus.

g. smears. Gonococci are in pairs and tetrads, never in chains. They are biscuit-shaped with concave adjacent surfaces, Gram negative and intracellular. *Stains*: Gram's method, methylene blue.

gonococcide (gon-o-kok'sīd) [" + " + L. *caedere,* to kill]. Destructive to or that which kills gonococci.

gonococ'cocide [" + *kokkos,* berry, + L. *caedere,* to kill]. Gonococcide.

gonococcus (gon-o-kok'us) (pl. *gonococci*) [" + *kokkos,* berry]. The organism causing gonorrhea. *Neisseria gonorrhoeae.*

It is an intracellular biscuit-shaped diplococcus and tends to occur in pairs. It is classified as a Gram negative bacterium and may be found in or on the genitalia, in the blood, the eye, urine, feces, and in boils.

gon'ocyte [G. *gonos,* seed, + *kytos,* cell]. The primitive reproductive cell.

gonohemia (gon-o-he'mĭ-ă) [G. *gonē,* semen, + *aima,* blood]. General gonorrhea infection. SYN: *gonococcemia.*

gonophage (gon'o-fāj) [" + *phagein,* to eat]. The bacteriophage produced by the gonococcus.

gon'ophore [" + *phorein,* to carry]. Any body that stores up or activates sex cells, as the spermatic duct, seminal vesicle, oviduct, or uterus.

gonorrhea (gon-o-re'ă) [" + *roia,* flow]. A specific, contagious, catarrhal inflammation of the genital mucous membrane of either sex.

ETIOL: Infection by the gonococcus, *Neisseria gonorrhoeae.*

The disease also may affect other structures of the body, such as the conjunctiva, the oral mucosa, the rectum, or the joints. In the female the parts involved may be the urethra, vulva, vulvovaginal glands, vagina, endocervix, Skene's glands, Bartholin's glands, or fallopian tubes.

SYM: *Male*: Yellow mucopurulent discharge from the penis. Inception in the urethra. May become deep-seated and affect the prostate. Slow, difficult and painful urination, and sometimes rigidity of the penis with great pain.

Female: The labia may become red, hot, tender, and inflamed. A sticky, serous exudate may cover the surfaces. Labia may become so swollen as to prevent inspection. Two strawberry points may show just beneath the external meatus, the latter being red and tender. The urethral canal is inflamed, painful micturition and frequency of urination may occur. Thick, creamy or greenish mucopurulent discharge develops shortly after invasion. Later it subsides and if the cervix is involved, becomes mucopurulent, and in final stages, whitish. The positive diagnosis is made by finding the organism on smear. Very commonly the disease is subacute or chronic from its inception, in the female.

PROG: It may clear up without serious results, or become chronic (involving deeper tissues and producing urethral stricture), or produce complications (prostatitis, epididymitis, orchitis, cystitis, etc., arthritis and endocarditis). No case of acute gonorrhea should be considered as cured until 3 successive negative smears from the cervix, Bartholin's and Skene's glands are obtained, at least 2 of which should be examined immediately after a menstrual period. Even then the patient must be regarded with suspicion.

NP: Every precaution for self-protection. Always wash hands after tending patient. Rubber gloves and a gown should be worn. The latter should not be worn in caring for another patient, and gloves should be sterilized after treatment. All linens and equipment should be sterilized after using and dressings immediately disposed of. The danger of an infected eye on part of the nurse is very considerable.

PROPHYLAXIS: Avoidance of contact with infected persons; immediate penicillin as a preventive following contact. In newborn, instillation of silver nitrate or penicillin solution in both eyes.

TREATMENT: Local measures, including urethral instillations, have largely given way to penicillin therapy. Penicillin is specific, and is regarded as superior to sulfadiazine and other sulfonamides. Strains of gonococcus resistant to penicillin are known but, in general, penicillin is the drug of choice. Local therapy may be required for eradication of foci of infection in the female, involving such structures as Skene's duct, Bartholin's glands, and the cervix.

gonorrhe'al [G. *gonē*, seed, + *roia*, flow]. Of the nature of or pert. to gonorrhea.

g. arthritis, g. rheumatism. Arthritis. or rheumatism resulting from gonorrheal infection.

gonycamp'sis [G. *gonu*, knee, + *kampsis*, bending]. Abnormal curvature of the knee or ankylosis.

gonycrote'sis [" + *krotēsis*, knocking]. Knock-knee.

gonyectyposis (gon"ĭ-ek-tĭ-po'sis) [" + *ektypōsis*, displacement]. Bowlegs. SYN: *genu varum*.

gonyocele (gon'e-o-sēl) [" + *kēlē*, swelling]. Tuberculous synovitis of the knee. SYN: *white swelling*.

gonyoncus (gon"ĭ-on'kus) [" + *ogkos*, tumor]. Tumor of the knee. SYN: *white swelling*.

goose flesh. A skin reaction caused by erection of skin papillae from cold or shock due to contraction of the arrector pili muscles. SYN: *cutis anserina*.

Gordon's reflex (gord'on) [Afford Gordon, American neurologist, 1874-1929]. Extension of great toe when sudden pressure is made on deep flexor muscles of calf of leg.

gorget (gor'jet) [Fr. *gorge*, throat, because of shape of instrument]. A grooved instrument to protect soft tissues from injury from point of knife.

gouge (gowj). Instrument for cutting away hard tissue of bone.

Goulard's extract (goo'lars) [Thomas Goulard, French surgeon, 1724-1784]. USP. An aqueous solution of lead subacetate, containing 18% lead.

ACTION AND USES: Diluted from 15 to 39 volumes of distilled water, as an astringent in inflammatory conditions of skin, for sprains and bruises.

INCOMPATIBILITIES: Exposure to air, acacia, albumen.

gout (gowt) [L. *gutta*, drop]. Paroxysmal metabolic disease marked by acute arthritis and inflammation of the joints. Joints affected may be at any location but gout usually begins in the knee or foot.

ETIOL: Excessive uric acid in blood and deposits of urates of sodium in and around joints.

SYM: Nocturnally painful with swelling and pain around joints.

NP: The painful joints may be wrapped in cotton. They should be elevated and supported on a pillow. The weight of the bedclothes should be carried on a cradle. Hot fomentations may afford some relief. Massage and radiant energy may be employed. Watch for vomiting and purgation resulting from the use of colchicum. Plentiful liquids should be given and proper elimination maintained.

DIET: Milk, diluted fruit juices, and farinaceous foods may be given. The diet, however, should be a light one. Meat should not be given more than once a day. Rich game, kidneys, liver, sweetbreads, and duck are prohibited.

g., abarticular. G. which involves structures other than the joints.

g., chronic. Persistent form of g.

g., latent, g., masked. Lithemia without regular symptoms of gout.

g., misplaced, g., retrocedent. Subsidence of joint symptoms followed by severe constitutional upsets.

g., tophaceous. G. marked by the development of tophi (deposits of sodium urate) in the joints, the external ear, and about the fingernails.

gout'y [L. *gutta*, drop]. Of the nature of, or rel. to, gout.

g. diathesis. Predisposition to gout.

Gowers' tract (gow'erz) [Sir William R. Gowers, English neurologist, 1845-1915]. One formed of fibers from post. roots of lateral tract of the spinal cord reaching the cerebellum by way of the sup. peduncle. The anterior spinocerebellar tract, *q.v.*

gr. Abbr. for *grain*.

graaf'ian fol'licle. A mature, vesicular follicle of the ovary.

Beginning with puberty and continuing until the menopause, except during pregnancy, a graafian follicle develops each four weeks. Each follicle contains a nearly mature ovum (an oocyte) which, upon rupture of the follicle, is discharged from the ovary, a process called *ovulation*. Ovulation occurs usually about the 13th day of the menstrual cycle, dated from the first day of the next menstrual period. Within the ruptured graafian follicle, the corpus luteum develops. Both the follicle and the corpus luteum are glands of internal secretion, the former secreting estrogens, the latter, progesterone.

gracile (gras'il) [L. *gracilis*, delicate]. Slender; slight.

g. nucleus. Mass of medullary gray matter terminating the funiculus gracilis.

gracilus (gras'ĭ-lus). A long slender muscle on the medial aspect of the thigh.

grada'tim [L.]. Gradually or by degrees.

Gradenigo's syndrome (grä-den-e'gōz) [Giuseppe Gradenigo, Italian physician, 1859-1926]. Suppurative otitis media with abducens paralysis and pain in temporal region.

gradient (gra'dĭ-ent). A slope or grade; an increase or decrease of varying degrees; or the curve which represents such.

g., axial. A gradient of physiological or metabolic activity exhibited by embryos and many adult animals, the principal one of which follows the main axis of the body, being highest at the anterior end and lowest at the posterior end.

graduate (grad'u-āt) [L. *gradus*, a step]. 1. A vessel marked by lines for measuring liquids. 2. One who has been awarded an academic or professional degree from a college or university.

grad'uated. Marked by a series of lines indicating degrees of measurement, weight, or volume.

g. tenotomy. Partial surgical division of tendon of an eye muscle.

Graefe's, von, sign [Albrecht von Graefe, German ophthalmologist, 1828-1870]. Failure of the upper lid to follow a downward movement of the eyeball when the patient changes his vision from upward, downward. Seen in Graves' disease with exophthalmos.

graft [L. *graphium*, grafting knife]. Skin or other living substance inserted into a similar substance to supply an absence or defect by attachment and growth into an integral part of the original substances.

RS: *autograft, skin grafting, transplantation, zoografting.*

g., autoplastic. One taken from another part of the patient.

g., bone. A piece of bone generally taken from the tibia and inserted elsewhere in the body to replace another osseous structure.

Bones for grafting can be kept in icebox until needed.

g., heteroplas'tic. One taken from another person.

g., nerve. Healthy nerve, usually from an animal, implanted to join a degenerated nerve in a human being.

g., ovarian. Implantation of a section of an ovary into the muscles of the abdominal wall.

g., pinch. A graft consisting of small bits of skin.

g., postmortem. Tissue taken from body after death and stored under proper conditions to be used later on a patient requiring a graft of such tissue.

g., skin. Removal of small sections of skin to a raw, clean surface such as a large superficial burn.

g., sponge. Small piece of sponge placed over an ulcerating part to stimulate epidermal growth.

g., Thiersch's. One in which only epidermis and small amt. of dermis are used.

g., Wolfe's. One in which the whole thickness of the skin is used.

g., zooplas'tic. One taken from an animal.

grain [L. *granum*]. 1. The seed or seedlike fruit of many members of the grass family, esp. corn, wheat, oats, and other cereals. 2. A weight; 0.065 of a gram. 3. Direction of fibers or layers.

g. poisoning. Poisoning due to a fungus which develops on grain, as ergot. *Gangrenous*: Tingling, pain, spasmodic muscular contractions, blood stasis and gangrene, fingers, toes, nose or ears. *Convulsive*: May be similar to gangrenous form followed by nervous disturbance. Headache, slight fever, spasm and cramps of muscles, delirium, epilepsy, dementia.

TREATMENT: Provoke vomiting; wash out stomach; give a purgative; give an enema; give powdered charcoal freely; give peroxide of hydrogen. Collapse should be fought with external heat; whiskey, strychnine, atropine, etc.

gram. ABBR: gm., Gm., g. A unit of weight (mass) of the metric system. It equals approximately the weight of a cubic centimeter or one milliliter of water. It is equal to 15.437 grain (Troy).

gram-meter. A unit of work energy equivalent to that expended in raising

Gram Conversion into Ounces

Gm.	Oz.	Gm.	Oz.	Gm.	Oz.	Gm.	Oz.
1	0.03	30	1.06	59	2.08	88	3.10
2	0.07	31	1.09	60	2.11	89	3.14
3	0.11	32	1.13	61	2.15	90	3.17
4	0.14	33	1.16	62	2.18	91	3.21
5	0.18	34	1.20	63	2.22	92	3.24
6	0.21	35	1.23	64	2.26	93	3.28
7	0.25	36	1.27	65	2.29	94	3.31
8	0.28	37	1.30	66	2.33	95	3.35
9	0.32	38	1.34	67	2.36	96	3.38
10	0.35	39	1.37	68	2.40	97	3.42
11	0.39	40	1.41	69	2.43	98	3.46
12	0.42	41	1.44	70	2.47	99	3.49
13	0.45	42	1.48	71	2.50	100	3.53
14	0.49	43	1.51	72	2.54	125	4.41
15	0.53	44	1.55	73	2.57	150	5.30
16	0.56	45	1.59	74	2.61	175	6.18
17	0.60	46	1.62	75	2.64	200	7.05
18	0.63	47	1.65	76	2.68	250	8.82
19	0.67	48	1.69	77	2.71	300	10.58
20	0.70	49	1.73	78	2.75	350	12.34
21	0.74	50	1.75	79	2.79	400	14.11
22	0.77	51	1.80	80	2.82	450	15.87
23	0.81	52	1.83	81	2.85	453.6	16.00
24	0.84	53	1.87	82	2.89	500	17.64
25	0.88	54	1.90	83	2.93	600	21.16
26	0.91	55	1.94	84	2.96	700	24.69
27	0.95	56	1.97	85	3.00	800	28.22
28	0.99	57	2.01	86	3.03	900	30.75
29	1.02	58	2.04	87	3.07	1000	35.33

a weight of 1 gram vertically a height of 1 meter.

gram mol′ecule. The weight in grams of a substance equal to its molecular weight.

gram negative organisms will lose the stain and take the color of the counterstain.

gram positive organisms will retain the color of the gentian violet stain.

Gram's method [Hans C. J. Gram, Danish physician, 1853-1938]. A method

The Chief Gram Negative Bacteria

Genus	Species	Colloquial or Old Names	Disease Caused in Man
Actinobacillus	*P. mallei.*	Bacillus mallei, or the glanders bacillus.	Glanders.
Pseudomonas	*P. aeruginosa.*	Bacillus pyocyaneus.	Suppuration ("blue pus").
Vibrio	*N. meningitidis.*	Comma bacillus.	Cholera.
Neisseria	*V. comma.*	Meningococcus.	Cerebrospinal meningitis.
	N. gonorrhoeae.	Gonococcus.	Gonorrhea.
	N. catarrhalis.	Micrococcus catarrhalis.	Nasopharyngeal catarrh.
Proteus	*P. vulgaris.*	Bacillus proteus.	Suppuration.
Escherichia	*E. coli.*	Bacillus coli.	Occasionally suppuration, cystitis and pyelitis.
Klebsiella	*K. pneumoniae.*	Pneumobacillus or Bacillus mucosus capsulatus.	Occasionally pneumonia.
Salmonella	*S. typhosa.*	Typhoid bacillus.	Typhoid fever.
	S. paratyphi (A&B). *S. enteritidis.* *S. typhimurium.*	Bacillus paratyphosus, etc. (Salmonella group).	Paratyphoid fever, gastroenteritis (food poisoning).
Shigella	*S. dysenteriae.*	The dysentery bacilli.	Bacillary dysentery.
Pasteurella	*Past. pestis.*	Bacillus pestis; plague bacillus.	Plague.
Hemophilus	*H. influenzae.*	Pfeiffer's bacillus.	Meningitis conjunctivitis, and influenza.
Bordetella	*B. pertussis.*	Bordet-Gengou bacillus.	Whooping cough.
Brucella	*Br. melitensis.*	Micrococcus melitensis.	Undulant fever.
	Br. abortus.	Bang's bacillus.	
	Br. suis.		
Borrelia	13 species		Relapsing fever.
	B. vincentii.	Vincent's bacillus.	Vincent's angina (trench mouth).
Leptospira	*L. icterohaemorrhagiae.*		Weil's disease (infectious jaundice).
Treponema	*T. pallidum.*		Syphilis.
	T. pertenue.		Yaws.

The Chief Gram Positive Bacteria

Genus	Species	Colloquial or Old Names	Disease Caused in Man
Actinomyces	*A. bovis.* *A. israelii.*	Nocardia actinomyces; ray fungus.	Actinomycosis.
Mycobacterium	*Myco. tuberculosis.*	Tubercle bacillus.	Tuberculosis.
	Myco. leprae.	Leprosy bacillus.	Leprosy (Hansen's disease).
Corynebacterium	*C. diphtheriae.*	Diphtheria bacillus; Klebs-Löffler bacillus.	Diphtheria.
Streptococcus	*Str. pyogenes.*		Suppuration, scarlet fever, septicemia.
	Str. viridans.	*Str. mitis.*	Subacute bacterial endocarditis.
Staphylococcus	*Staph. aureus, albus, etc.*		Suppuration, pyemia, osteomyelitis.
Sarcina	*Sarcina lutea.*		Rarely suppuration.
Bacillus	*B. anthracis.*	Anthrax bacillus.	Anthrax.
	B. subtilis.	Hay bacillus.	Nonpathogenic.
Clostridium	*Cl. tetani.*	Tetanus bacillus.	Tetanus.
	Cl. botulinum.	Bacillus botulinus.	Botulism.
	Cl. perfringens.	Cl. welchii.	Gas gangrene.
Diplococcus	*D. pneumoniae.*	Streptococcus pneumoniae.	Lobar and bronchopneumonia; other infections.

for staining bacteria of importance in the identification of bacteria. 1. Prepare a film on a slide, dry and fix with heat. 2. Stain with aniline gentian violet or ammonium oxalate crystal violet 1 min. 3. Rinse in water, then immerse in Gram's iodine solution for 1 min. 4. Rinse off iodine solution then decolorize in 95% ethyl alcohol or acetone. 5. Counterstain with dilute carbolfuchsin or safranine, 30 sec. 6. Rinse with water, blot dry, and examine.

Gran'cher's disease [Jacques J. Grancher, French physician, 1843-1907]. Massive pneumonia. SYN: *splenopneumonia.*

G.'s sign. Raised pitch of expiratory murmur in pulmonary consolidation.

grand mal (grahn mal) [Fr. great evil]. The typical epileptic attack with or without coma.

gran'ular [L. *granulum,* little grain]. Of the nature of granules. Roughened by prominences like those of seeds.

g. cast. Coarse or fine granule, short and plump, sometimes yellowish, similar to hyaline cast.

Soluble in acetic acid. Seen in inflammatory and degenerative nephropathies. SEE: *cast.*

granula'tion [L. *granulum,* little grain]. 1. Formation of granules, or state or condition of being granular. 2. Fleshy projections formed on the surface of a gaping wound that is not healing by first intention* or indirect union.

Each granulation represents the outgrowth of new capillaries by budding from the existing capillaries and then joining up into capillary loops supported by cells which will later become fibrous scar tissue. Granulations bring a rich blood supply to the healing surface.

OB: When the umbilical cord separates by wet gangrene there is left a raw area and granulation tissue is formed to heal it. If these granulations are left unchecked they will grow beyond the edge of the navel and form an umbilical polypus which is really an exuberant mass of granulation tissue.

g., arachnoidal. Villus-like projections of the subarachnoid layer of the meninges which project into the superior sagittal sinus and other venous sinuses of the brain. Through them cerebrospinal fluid reenters the blood stream. SYN: *pacchionian bodies; arachnoid villi.*

g., exuberant. An excessive mass of granulation tissue formed in the healing of a wound or ulcer; proud flesh.

gran'ule [L. *granulum,* little grain]. 1. A small, grainlike body. 2. In histology: (a) A minute mass in a cell, which has an outline, but no apparent structure; (b) any minute mass; (c) the crossing points of an intracellular reticulum endwise. 3. In pharmacy, a small globule of sugar and gum tragacanth, combined with a medicinal substance. SEE: *chromomere.*

g., acidophil. Alpha g., *q.v.*

g., agminated. Small round or angular particle of disintegrated red blood corpuscle in the blood.

g., albuminous. Cytoplasmic granule in many normal cells, not affected by ether or chloroform, but disappears from view when acetic acid is added.

g., aleuronoid. Pigment cell g.; colorless, myeloid, and colloidal.

g., alpha. Albuminous g. in leukocytes. Coarse, eosinophil, and highly refractive. SYN: *acidophil g.; eosinophil g.; oxyphil g.*

g., Altmann's. Mitochondria, *q.v.*

g., amphophil. One which stains with both acid and basic dyes; beta granule, *q.v.*

g., azurophil. One which takes a stain with azure dyes easily. Found in lymphocytes and monocytes; small and red or reddish-purple in color; they are inconstant in number being present in about 30% of the cells.

g., basal. A small deeply staining granule found in certain protozoa from which the flagellum arises. SYN: *blepharoplast, q.v.*

g., beta. An azurophil granule found in beta cells of the hypophysis or islets of Langerhans of the pancreas. SYN: *amphophil g.*

g., chromatin. Small masses of deeply staining substance suspended within the meshes of the linin network of the nucleus of a cell.

g., chromophil. A granule of chromophil substance present in the cytoplasm of neurons; Nissl granules.

g.'s, cone. The nuclei of the cones, sensory cells of the retina. They form the outer zone of the outer nuclear layer of the retina.

g., delta. Small granules in the delta cells of the pancreas.

g., eosinophil. Alpha g., *q.v.*

g., Fauvel's. Peribronchitic abscess, *q.v.*

g., glycogen. Minute particles of glycogen seen in liver cells following fixation.

g., Grawitz's. Found in lead poisoning basophilia, in the red blood corpuscles.

g., iodophil. Found in polymorphonuclear leukocytes and staining easily with iodine. Seen in various acute infectious diseases.

g., Kölliker's interstitial. Appears in various sizes in muscle fiber sarcoplasm.

g., metachromatic. Found in protoplasm of numerous bacteria. Stains deeply; irregular in size. SYN: *Babes-Ernst body; metachromatic body.*

g., Much's. Rod found in sputum of tuberculosis which stains with Gram's stain; considered to be a modified tubercle bacillus.

g., neutrophil. Granules such as those found in neutrophil leukocytes which stain with both basic and acid dyes, assuming a neutral tint.

g., Nissl. Chromophil granules found in the cell bodies of neurons; Nissl bodies.

g., oxyphil. SEE: *alpha g.*

g., pigment. Particle of coloring matter seen esp. in pigment cells.

g., Plehn's. Basophilic and seen in conjugating form of *Plasmodium vivax.*

g., protein. Protein particles of minute size in cells.

g., rod. Nucleus of the rod visual cell found in the external nuclear layer of the retina; connected with the rods.

g., Schüffner's. Polychrome methylene blue-staining g. found in parasitized erythrocytes of tertian malaria; coarse and red.

g., secretory. Zymogen granules, *q.v.*

g., seminal. Minute particles in semen, supposed to derive from disintegrated nuclei in nutritive cells from seminiferous tubules.

g., vitelline. SEE: *yolk g.*

g., yolk. Minute particles of fatty and albuminous nutritive substances present in the yolk (deutoplasm) of ova.

g., zymogen. Granules present in gland cells esp. secretory cells of pancreas, chief cells of the gastric glands, and serous cells of the salivary glands. They are the precursors of the enzymes secreted.

granulitis (gran-u-li'tis) [L. *granulum*, little grain, + G. *-itis*, inflammation]. Acute miliary tuberculosis.

gran'uloblast [L. *granulum*, + G. *blastos*, germ]. Mother cell of a granulocyte. A myeloblast, found in bone marrow.

granulocyte (gran-u-lo-sīt) [L. *granulum*, little grain, G. *kytos*, cell]. A granular leukocyte. A polymorphonuclear leukocyte (neutrophil, eosinophil, or basophil).

granulocytopenia (gran"u-lo-si"to-pe'nĭ-ă) [" + " + *penia*, poverty]. Abnormal reduction of granulocytes in the blood. Syn: *granulopenia*.

granulocytopoiesis (gran"u-lo-si"to-poy-e'sis) [" + " + *poiein*, to form]. The formation of granulocytes.

granulo'ma [L. *granulum*, + G. *oma*, tumor]. A granular tumor or growth, usually of lymphoid and epitheloid cells. They occur in various diseases such as leprosy, cutaneous leishmaniasis, yaws, and syphilis.

g., annulare. A condition of the skin characterized by development of reddish nodules arranged in the form of a circle.

g., apical. Dental granuloma, *q.v.*

g., coccidioidal. A chronic, generalized granulomatous disease caused by *Coccidioides immitis*. See: *Coccidioidomycosis*.

g., dental. G. developing at the root of a tooth. May contain epithelial rests or colonies of bacteria.

g., eosinophilic. G. containing eosinophils and usually accompanied by eosinophilia.

g., fungoides. Mycosis fungoides, *q.v.*

g., infectious. Any infectious disease in which granulomas are formed, such as tuberculosis or syphilis. Granulomas are also formed in mycoses, protozoan infections, and in certain metazoal diseases.

g. inguinale. A granulomatous disease common in the tropics caused by Donovan bodies (*Leishmania donovani*). Characterized by purulent lesions of the skin in region of the groin and often involving external genitalia.

g. iridis. G. which develops on the iris.

g., malignant. Lymphogranulomatosis; Hodgkin's disease.

g. pyogenicum. G. containing pyogenic organisms, which develop at the site of a wound. They may also occur at the tip of the fingers along the sides of the nails or beneath the free edge of the nail. They bleed easily and are usually painful to touch. Also called *septic granuloma*.

g., venereal. Lymphogranuloma venereum, *q.v.*

granulomato'sis [L. *granulum*, little grain, + G. *ōma*, tumor, + *-ōsis*]. The development of multiple granulomas.

g. infantiseptica. Listeriosis, *q.v.*, of the newborn.

g., lipoid. Xanthomatosis, *q.v.*

g. siderot'ica. Brownish (Gamna) nodules in the enlarged spleen.

granulope'nia [" + G. *penia*, poverty]. Abnormal decrease of granulocytes in the blood. Syn: *granulocytopenia*.

granuloplastic (gran"u-lo-plas'tik) [" + G. *plassein*, to form]. Developing granules.

granulopoiesis (gran"u-lo-poy-e'sis) [" + G. *poiein*, to make]. The formation of granulocytes.

granulopo'tent [" + *potentia*, power]. Potentially capable of forming granules.

granulosa. The membrana granulosa, *q.v.*

gran'ulose [" + G. *ōsis*]. The soluble portion of starch.

It is converted into sugar by hydrolysis.

granulo'sis [" + G. *ōsis*]. A mass of minute granules.

g. ru'bia na'si. Disease of the skin of the nose.

Etiol: Inflammatory infiltration about nose with slightly elevated papules, and dilated sweat glands.

Sym: Moist erythematous patch on numerous macules.

grape'fruit. A citrus fruit. Fresh (pink or red): 100 gm. Calories: 41. Other main values: 0.5 gm. protein; trace of fat; 10.6 gm. carbohydrate; 16 mg. calcium; 80 to 440 I.U. vitamin A depending upon kind.

Juice (canned, sweetened): 100 gm. Calories: 39. Other main values: 0.5 gm. protein; trace of fat; 10 gm. carbohydrate; 9 mg. calcium; 38 mg. ascorbic acid; 80 to 440 I.U. vitamin A depending upon kind.

grapes [Fr. *grappe*, a cluster]. Comp: Contain acid potassium tartrate. Acidity decreases with the age of the grape and sugar increases. The sugar is nearly all glucose and is more abundant than in any other fruit. Mannite, dulcite, and saccharose also represented. Raisins contain more sugar and less water.

Fresh (American type): 100 gm. Calories: 69. Other main values: 1.3 gm. protein; 1 gm. fat; 16 gm. carbohydrate; 16 mg. calcium; 100 I.U. vitamin A.

grape sugar. Dextrose.

-graph [G.]. Suffix: Pert. to *a writing* or *treatise*.

graph [G.]. A presentation of statistical, clinical, or experimental data by dots and lines.

graphesthe'sia. The sense by which outlines, numbers, words, or symbols traced or written upon the skin are recognized.

graphite (graf'īt) [G. *graphein*, to write]. A soft form of carbon. Syn: *plumbago*.

grapho- [G.]. Prefix: To write.

graphology (graf-ol'o-jĭ) [G. *graphein*, to write, + *logos*, study]. Examination of handwriting in diseases of the nerves as a means of diagnosis.

graphomotor. Pertaining to movements involved in writing.

graphophobia. Abnormal fear of writing.

graphorrhea (graf-o-re'ă) [" + *roia*, flow]. Writing of many meaningless words and phrases; manifested in dementia praecox.

graphospasm (graf'o-spazm) [" + *spasmos*, spasm]. Writer's cramp.

grattage (grat-ahzh') [Fr. a scraping]. Removal of morbid growths by rubbing with a brush or harsh sponge.

grave [L. *gravis*, heavy]. Serious; dangerous; severe.

g. wax. Waxlike matter on flesh caused by exposure to moisture with exclusion of air, as a body in the water or underground. Syn: *adipocere*.

grav'el [Fr. *gravelle*, coarse sand]. Crystalline dust, or concretions of crystals from the kidneys.

Generally made up of phosphates, calcium, oxalate, and uric acid.

Graves' disease [Robert J. Graves, Irish physician, 1797-1853]. Exophthalmic goiter.

gravid (grav'id) [L. *gravida*, pregnant]. Pregnant; heavy with child.

gravida (grav′id-ă) [L.]. A pregnant woman.

grav′idism [" + G. *ismos,* state of]. State of being pregnant.

gravidity (gră-vid′ĭ-tĭ) [L. *gravida,* pregnant]. Pregnancy.

gravidocardiac (grav″id-o-kar′dĭ-ak) [" + G. *kardia,* heart]. Pert. to cardiac disorders resulting from pregnancy.

gravimet′ric [L. *gravis,* weight, + G. *metron,* measure]. Determined by weight.

g. method. Examination of blood by weighing.

gravistatic (grav-ĭ-stat′ik) [" + G. *statikos,* standing]. Resulting from gravitation, as in a form of congestion.

gravita′tion [L. *gravitas,* weight]. Force and movement tending to draw every particle of matter together, esp. the attraction of the earth for bodies at a distance from its center.

grav′ity [L. *gravitās,* weight]. Property of possessing weight. The force of the earth's gravitational attraction.

g., specific. Weight of a substance compared with a known standard such as that of water, air, or hydrogen.

gray [A.S. *graey*]. Black or brown mixed with white.

g. matter. Nervous tissue of a grayish color, in which myelinated nerve fibers *do not* predominate. It contains large numbers of cell-bodies of neurons; also called *substantia grisea.*

The term is generally applied to gray portions of the central nervous system, which include the cerebral cortex, basal ganglia, and nuclei of the brain and the gray columns of the spinal cord which form an H-shaped region surrounded by white matter. Sympathetic ganglia and nerves may also be gray.

green. A color intermediate bet. blue and yellow, afforded by rays of wave length between 4920 and 5750 Angstrom units. SEE: *"chloro-" words.*

g. blindness. *Aglaucopsia;* a type of color-blindness in which green colors cannot be distinguished.

g., malachite. A dye used as a stain and antiseptic.

g. sickness. A form of anemia in adolescent girls, perhaps due to faulty diet during puberty. SYN: *chlorosis.*

g. soap. A solution of soft soap in alcohol, molded and dried.

g. soft′ening. Cranial abscess with pus of a greenish hue.

g. vit′riol. Ferrous sulfate. SYN: *copperas.*

green′stick fracture. One involving only part of the thickness of a bone. SEE: *incomplete fracture.*

greffotome (gref′o-tōm) [Fr. *greffe,* graft, + G. *tomē,* incision]. Instrument for making tissue grafts.

grenz rays. Roentgen rays with an average wave length of 2 angstroms. SEE: *ray.*

griffe des orteils (grēf daz or-ta′) [Fr.]. Muscular atrophy of foot with contraction. SYN: *clawfoot.*

grinder (grin′der) [A.S. *grindan,* to gnash]. A molar tooth. SYN: *dens molaris.*

grind′ers' disease. Chronic lung disease due to dust inhalation. SYN: *siderosis; pneumoconiosis.*

grip, grippe (grĭp) [Fr. *gripper,* to seize]. Acute, infectious disease marked by fever, prostration, pains in head and back, and by catarrh of respiratory tract. SYN: *influenza, q.v.*

gripes (grīps) [A.S. *grīpan,* to grasp]. Intermittent severe pains in bowels. SYN: *colic; tormina, q.v.*

griseofulvin. An antifungal antibiotic for oral administration. Especially effective in ringworm.

gris′tle [A.S.]. Cartilage.

gro′cers' itch. Eczema or psoriasis of the hands due to irritation from handling flour, sugar, etc.

Groff electrosurgical knife. Device for use of cutting current.

groin [A.S. *grynde,* abyss]. The depression between the thigh and trunk. The inguinal region. SEE: *bubonalgia, venereal bubo.*

groove [Danish *groeve,* to dig]. A furrow or elongated channel. SYN: *sulcus.*

g., biciptal. Depression for long tendon of the triceps located on ant. surface of humerus. SYN: *intertubercular groove.*

g., branchial. In the embryo, a groove lined with ectoderm which lies between two branchial arches. SEE: *branchial groove* and *branchial arches.*

g., carotid. A broad groove on the inner surface of the sphenoid bone lateral to the body. It lodges the carotid artery and the cavernous sinus. SYN: *cavernous g.*

g., costal. A groove on the lower internal border of a rib. It lodges the intercostal vessels and nerve. SYN: *subcostal groove.*

g., costovertebral. A broad groove extending along each side of the vertebrae. It lodges the sacrospinalis muscle and its subdivisions. SYN: *vertebral g.*

g., infraorbital. A groove on the orbital surface of the maxilla which transmits the infraorbital vessels and nerve.

g., intertubercular. The bicipital groove, *q.v.*

g., labial. A groove which develops in each of the primitive jaws. It gives rise to the vestibule separating the lips from the gums.

g., lacrimal. 1. A groove on post. surface of frontal process of the maxilla. 2. A groove on ant. surface of the post. lacrimal crest of the lacrimal bone. The two grooves serve to lodge the lacrimal sac.

g., laryngotracheal. A groove along the ventral surface of the ant. portion of the embryonic gut which gives rise to the respiratory organs.

g., malleolar. G. on ant.. surface of distal end of tibia which lodges tendons of the tibilalis posterior and flexor digitorum longus muscles.

g., medullary. Neural groove, *q.v.*

g., musculospiral. The radial groove, *q.v.*

g., mylohyoid. G. on inner surface of the mandible which runs obliquely forward and downward lodging the mylohyoid nerve and artery. In the embryo it lodges Meckel's cartilage.

g., nasolacrimal. In the embryo, a g. extending from inner angle of the eye to the primitive olfactory sac. It separates the maxillary and lateral nasal processes and its epithelial lining gives rise to the nasolacrimal duct.

g., nasopalatine. G. on vomer lodging nasopalatine nerve and vessels.

g., neural. A longitudinal g. on dorsal surface of the embryo lying between the neural folds. Upon closure of the folds to form the neural tube, the groove becomes the cavity of the neural tube eventually giving rise to the ventricles of the brain and the central canal of the spinal cord.

g., obturator. A g. at the sup. and post. angle of the obturator foramen through which pass the obturator vessels and nerve.

g., *olfactory.* A shallow g. on sup. surface of cribriform plate of the ethmoid on each side of the crista galli. It lodges the olfactory bulb.

g., *palatine.* One of a number of grooves on the inferior surface of the palatine process of the maxilla. They lodge the palatine vessels and nerves.

g., *peroneal.* 1. A shallow groove on lateral aspect of the calcaneus. 2. A deep groove on inferior surface of the cuboid bone. Each transmits the tendon of the peroneus longus muscle.

g., *pharyngeal.* A branchial groove, *q.v.*

g., *primitive.* In the embryo, a shallow groove in the primitive streak of the blastoderm and bordered by the primitive folds.

g., *pterygopalatine.* The pterygopalatine sulcus. A groove on the maxillary surface of the perpendicular portion of the palatine bone which, with corresponding grooves on the maxilla and pterygoid process of the sphenoid, transmits the palatine nerve and descending palatine artery.

g., *radial.* The musculospiral groove; a broad shallow groove running in a spiral direction on post. surface of the humerus. It transmits radial nerve and the profunda brachi artery.

g., *rhombic.* One of seven transverse grooves in the floor of the developing rhombencephalon. They separate the neuromeres.

g., *sagittal.* The sagittal sulcus; a shallow groove on inner surface of the parietal bones which lodges the sup. sagittal sinus.

g., *sigmoid.* G. on inner surface of the mastoid portion of temporal bone. It transmits the transverse sinus.

g., *subcostal.* SEE: *costal groove.*

g., *tympanic.* A. g. at the bottom of the ext. auditory meatus which receives the inferior portion of the tympanic membrane.

g., *urethral.* A g. on caudal surface of the genital tubercle or phallus bordered by the urethral folds. The latter close, transforming the groove into the cavernous urethra.

g., *vertebral.* SEE: *costovertebral groove.*

g., *visceral.* A branchial groove, *q.v.*

gross [L. *grossus,* thick]. Not minute; in mass.

g. *anatomy.* That of organs and parts seen without the aid of a microscope.

g. *lesion.* One visible to the eye without the aid of a microscope.

Grotthuss, law of. Only those light rays which are absorbed are biologically active.

ground. Basic substance or foundation; reduced to a powder; pulverized.

g. *bundle.* Fasciculus proprius, a bundle of nerve fibers which immediately surrounds the gray matter of the spinal cord. It is divided into three regions, the anterior, lateral, and posterior bundles which lie in the corresponding funiculi. These consist principally of short descending fibers.

g. *itch.* Ancylostomiasis cutis. Inflammation of the skin resulting from the invasion of the larvae of hookworms (*Ancylostoma* or *Necator*).

g. *substance.* The material, fluid, semifluid, or solid which occupies the intercellular spaces in fibrous connective tissue, cartilage, or bone. SYN: *matrix; interstitial substance.*

group'ing [It. *gruppo,* bunch]. Classification.

g., *blood.* Classifying blood of different individuals according to agglutinating and hemolyzing qualities before making a blood transfusion. SEE: *blood groups; blood transfusion.*

g. *serum.* A serum used for determining the blood group to which unknown cells belong. The grouping serums commonly used are human serums secured from donors and rabbit antiserums prepared commercially.

grow'ing pains. Pains, probably rheumatic, in the limbs of young persons.

growth [A.S. *grōwan,* to grow]. The progressive development or increase in size of a living thing, as cyst, excrescence, tumor, benign or malignant.

Methods of growth. 1. By the synthesis of new protoplasm and multiplication of cells. 2. By the intake of water. 3. By the manufacture and deposition of nonliving substances either within or outside of cells.

There are four main types of growth:

1. Organs of the *lymphoid* type, such as the thymus and the lymph nodes, grow fastest early in life, reach their peak of development at the age of about 12, and then regress.

2. The *neural* type of organ, such as the brain, cord, eye, and meninges, grows definitely in childhood, but is close to its adult size by the age of 8 years. This size is maintained without regression.

3. The *general* type of growth is seen in the weight of the body, the height of the body, and lengths of various bones, the total weight of the muscles, and various internal organs. It is a slower and steadier growth than the first two, but has a marked acceleration at the time of puberty.

4. The *genital* type of growth is seen in the testes, ovaries, and other genitourinary structures. Their growth is the slowest of these four types in infancy, but at puberty they grow faster than the others and cause the striking changes in appearance noted in the reproductive organs.

Not all of the organs of the body are included in the above four types. Some structures, such as the mammary glands, have several cycles of growth and regression in a lifetime, and many other peculiarities of particular organs might be mentioned.

g. *hormone.* Hormone liberated by the anterior pituitary which is important in regulating growth.

g., *new.* A neoplasm or tumor.

g., *postnatal.* Growth subsequent to birth.

g. *prenatal.* Growth occurring before birth.

gru'el [L. *grutum,* meal]. Any cereal boiled in water.

gru'mose, gru'mous [L. *grumus,* heap]. 1. BACT: Made up of coarse granular bodies in the center. 2. Lumpy, clotted.

Grünfelder's reflex (grün'feld-ĕr). Fanlike spreading of toes with upward flexion of great toe resulting from pressure over post. fontanel.

grutum (gru'tum) [L. meal]. 1. Small pink and white patches most frequently on skin of face and scrotum caused by inspissated sebum beneath the horny epidermis. SYN: *milium.* 2. Oaten grits.

GSH. Abbr. for *glomerular stimulating hormone.*

GSR. Abbr. for *galvanic skin response.*

gtt. Abbr. of *guttae,* drops.

guaiacol (gwi'ak-ol). A phenol obtained from wood creosote.

ACTION AND USES: Antiseptic and germicide, intestinal antiseptic and expectorant.

g. carbonate. USP. A white crystalline powder used internally as a tasteless, nonpoisonous substitute for guaiacol.

guanase (gwan'ās). An enzyme in a number of glands; it converts guanine into xanthine.

guanidine (gwan'ĭ-din). A crystalline organic compound, NH: $C(NH_2)_2$, found among the decomposition products of proteins.

guanidinemia (gwan'id-ĕn-e'mĭ-ă) [*guanidine* + G. *aima*, blood]. Guanidine in the blood.

guanine (gwah'nin). An organic compound, $C_5H_5N_5O$, which can be extracted from guano and is related to guanidine and xanthine. It is also found in the liver, pancreas, and muscle.

gubernaculum (gu-ber-nak'u-lum) [L. helm). A structure which guides; a cordlike structure uniting two structures.

g. dentis. A connective tissue band which connects the tooth sac of an unerupted tooth with the overlying gum.

g. testis. A fibrous cord in the fetus which extends from the caudal end of the testis through the inguinal canal to the scrotal swelling. It plays a role in the descent of the testis into the scrotum.

Gubler's line (goob'lerz) [Adolphe Gubler, French physician, 1821-1879]. The level of superficial origin of the trigeminus or 5th nerve.

G.'s paralysis. Hemiplegia affecting parts on opposite sides of the body. SYN: *alternate* or *crossed hemiplegia.*

G.'s tumor. A fusiform swelling on wrist in lead palsy.

Gudden's inferior commissure (good'enz in-fe'ri-or com'mis-sure) [Bernard A. von Gudden, German neurologist, 1824-1886]. Fibers of optic tract. SYN: *arcuate c.*

G.'s law. When a nerve is divided, degeneration in the proximal portion is toward the nerve cell.

guillotine (gil'o-tēn) [Fr. instrument for beheading]. Instrument for excising tonsils and laryngeal growths.

Guinea worm. *Dracunculus medinensis, q.v.*

gul'let [L. *gula*, throat]. The esophagus. *q.v.*

Gull's disease [Sir William W. Gull, English physician, 1816-1890]. Atrophy of the thyroid gland and resulting myxedema.

gum (L. *gummi*). 1. The fleshy substance or tissue covering the alveolar processes of the jaws. SYN: *gingiva.* 2. A substance which is given out or extracted from certain plants which is sticky when moist but hardens upon drying. Roughly any resinlike substance given out by plants.

DIAG: *Bleeding Easily*: Indicates scurvy, or inflammation as in trench mouth or pyorrhea, etc.

Bluish Red: Indicates mercurial stomatitis or lead poisoning, if bluish line is at edge of teeth.

Greenish Line: At edge of teeth, may indicate copper poisoning.

Purplish Line or Color: Scurvy.

Red Line: In youth, indicates gingivitis, pyorrhea, scurvy.

Spongy g., and Ulceration: Gingivitis, scurvy, stomatitis, leukemia, tuberculosis, diabetes, and digestive disturbances.

RS: ***diagnosis, gingiva, oulorrhagia, ulatropia, ulemorrhagia, uletic, ulitis, uloglossitis, uloncus, ulorrhea.***

gumboil. (gum'boyl). Gum abscess. SYN: *parulis.*

ETIOL: Subperiosteal infection associated with a carious tooth, irritation or injury by a denture.

SYM: Gum is red, swollen, tender, and very painful. A fluctuating swelling may appear containing pus. It may point and break or require incision.

TREATMENT: Hot mouthwashes and applications over gum or externally. Warn patient not to swallow pus. Frequent mouthwashes after being evacuated. SEE: *gum.*

gumma (gum'mă) [L. *gummi*, gum]. A soft tumor of the tissues characteristic of the tertiary stage of syphilis. It is a granuloma varying in size from a millimeter to a centimeter or more in diameter. They may be single or multiple, and tend to be encapsulated. Each consists of a central necrotic mass surrounded by an inflammatory zone and fibrosis. The necrotic portion may be firm or elastic, gelatinous or hyalinized. Infectious organisms may be present. They occur most frequently in the liver but may occur in other organs such as the brain, testis, heart, bone, and skin.

SYM: Depend upon location. Bursting of a gumma leads to a gummatous ulcer, painless, but slow to heal. The base is formed by a "wash-leather" slough but surrounding tissues are healthy. SEE: *syphilis.*

gummose (gum'ōs). A sugar from animal gum. $C_6H_{12}O_6$.

gum'my [L. *gummi*, gum]. Sticky, swollen, puffy.

gun'shot wound. Penetrating or perforating wound which may contain a foreign body, as a bullet. SEE: *wound.*

gun'stock deform'ity. Deformity in which the long axis of the extended forearm turns outwardly from the arm, caused by fracture at the elbow.

gustation (gus-ta'shun) [L. *gustāre*, to taste]. Sense of taste.

gustatory (gus'tă-to-rĭ) [L. *gustāre*, to taste]. Pert. to sense of taste.

gustom'etry [" + G. *metron*, measure]. Measurement of the degree of the sense of taste.

gut (A.S.). 1. The bowel or intestine. 2. The primitive gut or embryonic digestive tube which includes the foregut, midgut, and hindgut. 3. Short term for catgut.

g., blind. Cecum.

gut'ta (pl. *guttae*) [L. a drop]. A drop. The amount in a drop varies with the nature of the liquid, being about a minim of water.

g. rosacea. Acne rosacea, *q.v.*

g. serena. Blindness. SEE: *amaurosis.*

guttadiophot test (gut-ă-di'ă-fŏt) [L. a drop]. A test for detecting pathological conditions of the blood. Consists of examining by transmitted light strips of red, green, and blue absorbent paper upon which two drops of blood have been placed.

gutt'ate [L. *gutta*, drop]. Resembling a drop, said of certain cutaneous lesions.

gutta'tim [L.]. Drop by drop.

gut'tur [L.]. The throat.

guttural (gut'u-ral) [L. *guttur*, throat]. Pert. to the throat.

gutturotet'any [" + G. *tetanos*, tension]. Laryngeal spasm of throat with temporary stutter.

Guyon's sign (gwy-onz') [Felix J. C. Guyon, Paris surgeon, 1831-1920]. Ballottement of kidney.

Gwath'mey's meth'od or technic [James T. Gwathmey, American surgeon, 1863-1944]. Adm. of rectal anesthetic of ether and olive oil solution in labor. SEE: *anesthesia.*

gymnas'tics [G. *gymnastikos,* pert. to nakedness]. Systematic bodily exercise, with or without special apparatus.

g., ocular. Systematic exercise of the eye muscles to improve muscular coordination and efficiency.

g., Swedish. A system of movements made by a patient against a resistance provided by the attendant.

gymnophobia (jim-no-fo'bĭ-ă) [" + *phobos,* fear]. Abnormal aversion to viewing a naked body.

gynander (guy-nan'der) [G. *gynē,* woman, — *anēr, andr-* man]. A gynandromorph, *q.v.* A pseudohermaphrodite; an individual possessing both male and female characteristics.

gynandroid (guy-nan'droyd) [" + " + *eidos,* form]. An individual having sufficient hermaphroditic sexual characteristics to be mistaken for a person of the opposite sex.

gynandromorph (guy-nan'dro-morf). An individual in which certain parts of the organism are male and certain parts female. SYN: *gynander.*

gynandromorphous (guy-nan-dro-morf'us) [" + " + *morphē,* form]. Having the characteristics of both the male and female.

gynandry (guy-nan'drĭ) [G. *gynē,* woman, + *anēr, andr-* man]. Condition of pseudohermaphroditism.

gynatresia (guy-nă-tre'zĭ-ă) [" + *a-,* priv. + *trēsis,* perforation]. Atresia* of the vagina.

gynecic (guy-ne'sik) [G. *gynē,* woman]. Pert. to women.

gyneco-, gyno- [G.]. Prefix meaning *woman, female.*

gynecologic, gynecological (guy-nĕ-ko-loj'ik, -ĭ-kal) [G. *gynē,* woman, + *logos,* study]. Pert. to gynecology, or study of women's diseases.

gynecologist (guy-nĕ-kol'o-jist) [" + *logos,* study]. Physician who specializes in the diseases of women.

gynecology (guy-nĕ-kol'o-jĭ) [" + *logos,* study]. The study of the diseases of the female, particularly of the genital, urinary or rectal organs.

NP: *Preoperative*: Empty bladder. Local preparation from nipple to anus. *Postoperative*: Count and chart pulse every 15 minutes for first few hours. Report immediately any change in rate or volume. Watch for shock or internal hemorrhage. Keep warm and quiet; no visitors. Fluids when tolerated, tap water being best. Hypodermoclysis or infusions in excessive vomiting instead of fluids by mouth.

Care must be taken to prevent retention of urine. Sterile, closed, continuous drainage of the bladder may be preferable to repeated catheterization.

Patient catheterized every 12 hours after operation, then every 8 hours until able to void. Catheterization after voiding to prevent retention, until less than ½ oz. urine is thus obtained after 2 successive voidings. A solution of silver nitrate, as ordered, instilled after each catheterization. Thrombophlebitis with embolism is a dreaded complication.

gynecomania (guy-nĕ-ko-ma'nĭ-ă) [" + *mania,* madness]. Abnormal sex desire in the male. SYN: *satyriasis, q.v.*

gynecomastia, gynecomasty, gynecomazia (guy-nĕ-ko-mas'tĭ-ă, -tĭ, -ma'zĭ-ă) [" + *mastos, mazos,* breast]. Abnormally large mammary glands in the male; sometimes may secrete milk.

gynecopathy (guy-nĕ-kop'ă-thĭ) [G. *gynē,* woman, + *pathos,* disease]. Diseases peculiar to women.

gynecophonus (guy-nĕ-kof'on-us) [" + *phōnē,* voice]. Having an effeminate voice.

gynephobia (guy-nĕ-fo'bĭ-ă) [" + *phobos,* fear]. Abnormal aversion to the company of women, or fear of them.

gynergen (guy'nĕr-jĕn). Proprietary name for a preparation of ergotamine tartrate. Used as an oxytocic and sympatholytic agent.

gynesic (guy-nē'sik) [G. *gynē,* woman]. Pert. to the diseases of women.

gyniatrics (guy-nĭ-at'riks) [" + *iatreia,* treatment]. Treatment of diseases of women.

gynopath'ic [" + *pathos,* disease]. Pert. to disease of women.

gynoplastic [G. *gynē,* woman, + *plassein,* to form]. Pertaining to gynoplasty.

gynoplastics (guy-no-plas'tiks) [" + *plassein,* to form]. Reparative surgery of female genitalia.

gynoplasty (guy-no-plas'tĭ) [" + *plassein,* to form]. Plastic surgery of the female reproductive organs.

gyrate (jī'rāt) [G. *gyros,* circle]. 1. Ring-shaped, convoluted. 2. To revolve.

gyration (ji-ra'shun) [G. *gyros,* circle]. A rotary movement.

gyre (jīr) [G. *gyros,* circle]. Convolution. SYN: *gyrus.*

gyrencephalic (ji-ren-sef-al'ik) [" + *egkephalē,* head]. Having a brain marked by numerous convolutions.

gyri (ji'ri). Plural of gyrus, *q.v.*

gyro- [G.]. Combining form meaning a *circle, spiral, ring.*

gyrochrome (ji'ro-krōm) [G. *gyros,* circle, + *chrōma,* color]. A nerve cell in which the stainable substance occurs in rings.

gyroma (ji-ro'mă) [" + *ōma,* tumor]. Ovarian tumor consisting of a convoluted mass.

gyromele (ji'ro-mēl) [" + *mēlē,* a probe]. Revolving stomach tube for massage and cleansing of stomach, determining its location, size and condition.

gyrometer (ji-rom'ĕ-ter) [" + *metron,* measure]. A device for measuring the cerebral gyri.

gyrosa (ji-ro'să) [" + *ōsis*]. Gastric vertigo causing one to close one's eyes to prevent falling, as everything turns round when standing.

gyrose (ji'rōs) [" + *ōsis*]. BACT: Marked by wavy lines or circles applied to bacterial colonies.

gyrospasm (ji'ro-spasm) [" + *spasmos,* spasm]. Spasmodic rotary head movement.

gyrotrope (ji'ro-trōp) [" + *tropē,* a turning]. Cord connecting an electrode with source of an electric current. SYN: *rheotrope.*

gyrous (ji'rus) [G. *gyros,* circle]. Marked by circular lines. SYN: *gyrose.*

gyrus (ji'rus) (pl. *gyri*) [G. *gyros,* circle]. A convolution of the cerebral hemisphere of the brain. They are separated by shallow grooves (sulci) or deeper grooves (fissures).

g., angular. G. of the parietal lobe embracing post. end of the superior temporal sulcus.

g., annectent. Any of many short folds of gray matter which are formed as a result of short branches or twigs of sulci extending into adjacent gyri. They are inconstant.

g., ant. central. G. of the frontal lobe extending vertically between precentral and central sulci.

gyri breves insulae. Preinsular g.

g., Broca's. Inf. frontal g.

g., callosal. A large g. on medial surface of cerebral hemisphere which lies directly above the corpus callosum, and arches over its anterior end.

g. cerebelli. Layer of the cerebellum.

g., dentate. A g. marked by indentations which lie on the upper surface of the hippocampal gyrus.

g. fornicatus. G. on medial surface of cerebrum which includes the g. cinguli, the isthmus, the hippocampus, hippocampal gyrus and uncus.

g., frontal, inferior. Convolution on external surface of frontal lobe of cerebrum located bet. the sylvian fissure and the inferior frontal sulcus.

g., frontal, middle. G. bet. the superior and inferior frontal sulci.

g., frontal, superior. Convolution of cerebral frontal lobe situated above the superfrontal fissure.

g., fusiform. G. beneath the collateral fissure joining the occipital and temporal lobes.

g., Heschl's. Transverse temporal g.

g., hippocampal. G. situated bet. the hippocampal and collateral fissures.

g., lingual. G. bet. the calcarine and collateral fissures.

g. longus insulae. Lengthy g. composing the postinsula.

g., marginal. SEE: *frontal superior g.*

g., middle temporal. G. located between middle temporal sulcus and superior temporal sulcus.

g., occipital. Any of the gyri on the lateral surface of the occipital lobe. They are inconstant but grouped roughly into two groups, the *inferior* or *lateral occipital gyri* and the *superior occipital gyri.*

g., occipitotemporal. SEE: *fusiform g.*

g., orbital. One of four g. (ant., post., lat., and med.), forming inf. surface of the frontal lobe.

g., paracentral. Area on mesial aspect of the cerebrum; the paracentral lobule. Lies above cingulate sulcus.

g., parietal. G. on lateral aspect of parietal lobe. Include post. central gyrus, sup. and inf. parietal gyri.

g., postcentral. G. situated bet. the central and postcentral fissures.

g., primary. Fetal cerebral regions marked by the primary fissures.

g. profundi cerebri. Very deep gyri of the cerebrum.

g., rectus. G. on the orbital aspect of the frontal lobe, located bet. the mesial margin and the olfactory sulcus.

g., Retzii, g., sagittal. The supra- and subcallosal gyri.

g., subcallosal. A narrow band of gray matter on median surface of hemisphere below the rostrum of the corpus callosum.

g., subcollateral. SEE: *fusiform g.*

g., supracallosal. A rudimentary gyrus on the upper surface of the corpus callosum.

g., supracallosus. Gray matter layer covering the corpus callosum.

g., supramarginal. G. in the inferior parietal lobule twisting about the upper terminus of the sylvian fissure.

g., temporal. Three gyri (sup., middle, inf.) on lateral surface of temporal lobe.

g., transitivus. SEE: *annectent g.*

g., uncinate. Ant. hooked portion of the hippocampal g.

Notes

H

H. or **h.** Abbr. for *haustus* (a draught), *height; henry; Holznecht unit; hora* or *hour; horizontal; hypermetropia.* Symb. for *hydrogen.*

H+. Symb. for *hydrogen ion.*

H1. Symb. for *protium.*

H2. Symb. for *deuterium,* an isotope of hydrogen.

H & E. Hematoxylin and eosin, a staining method much used in histology.

Haab's reflex [O. Haab, professor of ophthalmology in Zurich, 1850-1931]. Contraction of pupils without alteration of accommodation or convergence when gazing at a bright object. A sign of a cortical lesion.

habena (hă-be'nă) [L. rein]. 1. A frenum. 2. Bandage for a wound. 3. Pineal gland peduncle. SYN: *habenula, 2.*

habe'nal, habe'nar [L. *habena,* rein]. Pert. to the habena or habenula.

habenula (hă-ben'u-lă) [L. strap]. 1. A frenum, or any rein- or whip-like structure. 2. [NA]. A peduncle of the pineal gland. 3. A narrow bandlike stricture.

h. urethra'lis. One of two whitish bands between the clitoris and meatus urethra in young females.

habenul'ar. Pertaining to the habenula, esp. the stalk of the pineal body.

h. trigone. A depressed triangular area located on the lateral aspect of the post. portion of the third ventricle. Each contains a *medial* and *lateral habernacular nucleus.*

h. commissure. A band of transverse fibers connecting the two habenular areas.

habit [L. *habitus, habēre,* to hold]. SYN: *habitus, q.v.* 1. A motor pattern executed with facility following constant or frequent repetition; an act at first performed in a typical voluntary manner but which after sufficient repetition is performed as a reflex action. Habits result from the passing of impulses through a particular set of neurons and synapses many times. 2. A particular type of dress or garb. 3. Mental or moral constitution or disposition. 4. Bodily appearance or constitution, esp. as related to a disease or predisposition to a disease, as the *apoplectic habit.* 5. Addiction to the use of drug or beverage as the *opium habit, alcoholic habit.*

h., chorea. SEE: *h. spasm.*

h., full. Full bloodedness, as in a disease.

h. spasm. A spasmodic voluntary movement that has become involuntary. Often due to something irritating; sometimes from mimicry. SYN: *tic.**

h. training. Schedule for 24 hr., adapted and rigidly enforced to train mentally ill patients in habits of cleanliness and to stimulate mental activity.

habitua'tion [L. *habitus,* habit]. Act of becoming accustomed to anything from frequent use.

hab'itus [L. habit]. Indications in appearance of tendency to disease or abnormal conditions.

h. apoplecticus. The supposed body build and appearance of one predisposed to develop apoplexy: short, thicknecked with flushed face and prominent temporal arteries.

h. enteroptoticus. Physical state marking enteroptosis.

h. phthisicus. Predisposition to pulmonary tuberculosis characterized by poor bone development, pallor, thin chest and dry skin.

habromania (hab-ro-ma'nĭ-ă) [G. *abros,* cheerful, + *mania,* madness]. A psychosis accompanied by pleasant delusions.

hachement (hash-mon') [Fr. chopping]. Strokes with edge of hand in massage. SYN: *hacking.*

hack'ing [A.S. *haccian,* to chop]. Strokes with edge of hand in massage. SYN: *hachement.*

h. cough. A frequent, short cough.

haem. Heme, *q.v.*

Haemadipsa (hē″mă-dĭp'să). A genus of terrestrial leeches found in Asia which attack man and animals.

H. ceylonica and ***H. japonica*** are species found in Ceylon and Japan, respectively.

Haemagogus (he″mă-gog'us). A genus of mosquitoes. Includes the species *H. capricorni* which serves as a vector of yellow fever.

Haemophilus (hem-of'ĭl-us) [G. *aima,* blood, + *philein,* to love]. A genus of Bacteriaceae growing best in hemoglobin. SEE: *Hemophilus.*

Haemosporidia (he″mo-spo-rid'ĭ-ă). An order of sporozoa which live in the blood cells of vertebrates and reproduce sexually in invertebrates; includes the genus *Plasmodium,* four species of which cause malaria in man.

haf'nium. A rare chemical element of at. wt. 178.49; at. no. 72. SYMB: Hf.

Hagedorn needle (hā'gĕ-dorn) [Werner Hagedorn, German surgeon, 1831-1894]. A curved surgical needle with flattened sides.

Haines formula [Walter S. Haines, American chemist, 1850-1923]. The number of grains of solid in a fluidounce of urine determined approximately by multiplying the last two figures of the sp. gr. of a specimen by 1.1.

hair [A.S. *haer*]. 1. A keratinized, threadlike outgrowth from the skin of mammals. 2. Collectively, the threadlike outgrowths which form the fur of animals, or which grow on the human head.

A hair is a thin flexible shaft of cornified cells which develops from a cylindrical invagination of the epidermis, the *hair follicle.* Each consists of a free portion or *shaft* (scapus pili) and a *root* (radix pili) embedded within the follicle. The shaft consists of three layers of cells: the *cuticle* or outermost layer, the *cortex,* forming the main horny portion of the hair, and the *medulla,* the central axis. Hair color is due to pigment in the cortex.

Hairs in each part of the body have a definite period of growth after which they are shed. In man there is a constant gradual loss and replacement of hairs. Hairs of the eyebrows last only three to five months; those of the scalp two to five years. Baldness or *alopecia* results when replacement fails to keep up with hair loss. It may be due to hereditary factors or pathological con-

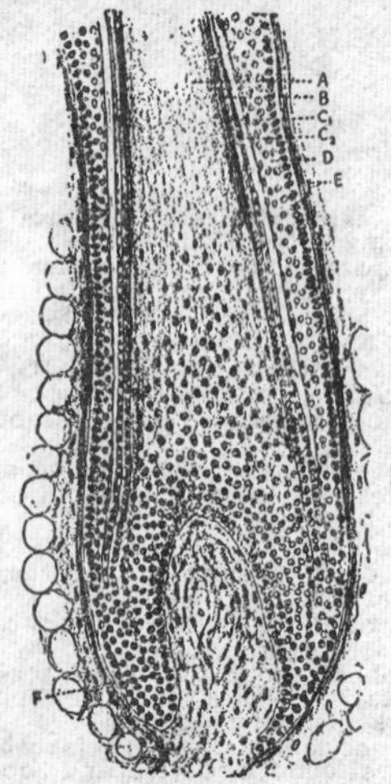

HAIR

Root of hair, longitudinal section. A. Hair. B. Cuticle of hair. C. Internal root sheath: C1. Cuticle of root sheath. C2. Huxley's layer of internal root sheath. D. External root sheath. E. Hair follicle. F. Hair papilla.

ditions such as infections or injury from irradiation.

h. bulb (bulbus pili). Lower expanded portion of a hair root. Growth of a hair results from the proliferation of cells of the hair bulb.

h. cell. An epithelial cell possessing fine nonmotile cilia found in the maculae and the organ of Corti of the membranous labyrinth of the inner ear. They are receptors for the senses of position and hearing.

h. dye. May contain silver nitrate or aniline dyes which are often irritating to skin or eyes, causing severe dermatitis or conjunctivitis. Occasionally results in blindness.

F. A. TREATMENT: Wash with sterile salt solution, followed by soap and water, followed by sponging with alcohol; cover with bland ointment, as cold cream or lanolin. The eye should be washed with normal saline and then instill paraffin oil, sweet oil or other bland oil.

h. follicle. An invagination of the epidermis which forms a cylindrical depression, penetrating the corium into the connective tissue which holds the hair root.

Sebaceous glands which secrete an oily fluid, and tiny muscles which cause the hair to stand (*arrectores pili*), are attached to these follicles.

h., gustatory. A taste-hair. One of several fine hairlike process extending from the ends of gustatory cells in a taste bud. They project through the inner pore of a taste bud.

h. papilla. A projection of the corium which extends into the hair bulb at the bottom of a hair follicle. It contains capillaries through which a hair receives nourishment.

h., pubic. That over the pubes. SYN: *escutcheon.* SEE: *pubic.*

hairball. A mass in the stomach consisting of hair. SYN: *trichobezoar.*

hair'y heart. A heart covered with a rough exudation.

h. tongue. One covered with hairlike papillae.

hala'tion [G. *alōs,* a halo]. Blurring of vision due to light from a wrong direction.

half-life. The time required for a radioactive substance to lose one half of its energy.

half-value layer. SEE: half-value thickness.

h.-v. thickness. The thickness of a substance which, when placed in the path of a given beam of rays, will lower its intensity to ½ of the initial value.

halisteresis (hă-lis"ter-e'sis) [hali- from G. *halos,* salt + *sterēsis,* deprivation]. Lack of calcium (lime salt) in bone. SYN: *osteomalacia.*

halistere'tic [" + *sterēsis,* privation]. Rel. to or affected with halisteresis, *q.v.*

halitosis (hal-ĭ-to'sis) [L. *halitus,* breath, + G. *-ōsis*]. Offensive breath.

halituous (hal-it'u-us) [L. *halitus,* breath]. Covered with moisture. SYN: *vaporous.*

hal'itus [L. breath]. 1. The breath. 2. Warm vapor.

Hal'ler's cir'cles [Albrecht von Haller, Swiss physiologist, 1708-1777]. Circles of veins and arteries in the eye.

hal'lex (pl. *hal'lices*) [L.]. The great toe. SYN: *hallus, hallux.*

hallucination (hă-lu-sĭ-na'shun) [L. *alucinari,* to wander in mind]. PSY: False perception having no relation to reality and not accounted fro by any ext. stimuli. May be *visual, auditory, olfactory, etc.*

Commonly, the patient is unable to consider it as not constituting reality, but judgment may at times recognize discrepancies, and even at times deny the hallucination entirely. Usually, then, the patient reacts emotionally and behaves as one would to a real situation. An indifferent attitude strongly suggests deterioration. Any sense may be involved, or elaborate combinations may occur. As in dreams, here the patient might be terrified at seeing an approaching assaulter, hear his threats, and feel his blows, and struggle in desperate defense. Emotional tone, delusions, and hallucinations tend to harmonize and this may be ascribed to the last, reflecting rather than determining the others.

Structural disease of the sensory organ and conducting mechanism may favor the formation of hallucinations, *e. g.,* the deafness of an old otitis media often is associated with tinnitus, and at times the paresthesia is associated with phonemes. An irritative lesion of the visual cortex may produce more directly the hallucination, but even here an intact mind probably quickly would recognize the perception as unreal.

Hallucinations must then be considered the product of mental distortion, and the recognition of cause must be based on associated symptoms. It follows that hallucinations with few exceptions are presumptive evidence of a psychosis (insanity). Those experienced during sleep are notable exceptions.

RS: *acousma, delusion, hallucinosis, hypnagogic, illusion.*

h., extracampine. H. of hearing words spoken at a great distance.

h., haptic. One pert. to touching the skin, or to sensations of temperature or pain.

h., hypnagogic. Pre-sleep phenomena having the same practical significance as a dream but experienced while consciousness persists. Includes sense of falling, sinking, or of the ceiling moving.

h., kinetic. Sensation of flying or moving the body or a part of it.

h., microptic. One in which things seem reduced in size. SYN: *lilliputian h.*

h., motor. Imaginary perceptions of movement.

h., somatic. Sensation of pain attributed to visceral injury.

h., teleologic. One which advises or guides the subject, such as those of Jeanne d'Arc.

hallucinogen (hă-lu-sin-o'jen). An intoxicant and narcotic, according to the additives used. It produces telepathy, fantastic visions, hallucinations, and other psychic effects. It is precognitive and psychic in its results.

hallucinosis (hal-lu"sin-o'sis) [" + G. *ōsis*]. The state of having hallucinations more or less persistently. SEE: *hallucination.*

h., acute. PSY: Alcoholic psychosis. SYM: Fear or anxiety and auditory hallucinations.

hallus, hallux (hal'us, -uks) (pl. *hal'luces*) [L.]. The great toe.

h. doloro'sus. Pain in the metatarsophalangeal joint of the great toe due to flat foot.

h. flexus. Hammer toe.

h. valgus. Displacement of great toe toward other toes.

h. varus. Displacement of great toe away from other toes.

halmatogenesis (hal"ma-to-jen'ĕ-sis) [G. *alma,* jump, + *genesis,* development]. A sudden deviation of type from one generation to the other one. SYN: *saltatory variation.*

ha'lo [G. *alōs,* a halo]. 1. The areola, esp. of the nipple. 2. A ring surrounding the macula lutea in ophthalmoscopic images. 3. A circle of light surrounding a shining body.

h. glaumato'sus. A whitish ring surrounding the optic disk; seen in glaucoma.

h. symptom. Colored circle around lights in glaucoma.

halogen (hal'o-jen) [G. *als,* salt, + *gennan,* to form]. A salt former; one of a group of elements (chlorine, Cl; bromine, Br; iodine I; and fluorine, F), having very similar chemical properties.

They combine with hydrogen to form acids and with metal to form salts.

haloid (hal'oid) [" + *eidos,* form]. Resembling salt.

h. salt. A salt made up of a base and a halogen, resembling common salt.

halometer (ha-lom'ĕ-ter) [G. *alōs,* a halo, + *metron,* measure]. 1. Device for measuring diffraction halo of a red blood cell. 2. Device for measuring the halo around optic disk.

halosteresis (ha-lo-ster-e'sis) [G. *als,* salt, + *sterēsis,* privation]. Deficiency of lime salts in the bones. SYN: *halisteresis.*

halothane (hal'o-thān). A fluorinated hydrocarbon used as a general anesthetic.

Hal'sted's opera'tion [William Stewart Halsted, Baltimore surgeon, 1852-1922]. Operation for inguinal hernia and one for amputation of breast with carcinoma.

H.'s suture. An interrupted one for intestinal wounds.

ham [A.S. *haum,* haunch]. 1. The popliteal space or region behind the knee. 2. Common name for the thigh, hip, and buttock. 3. The thigh of an animal, esp. the hog, prepared for food.

hamartia (ham-ar'shĭ-ă) [G. *amartia,* defect]. Error in development due to imperfect tissue combination.

hamartoma (ham-ar-to'mă) [" + *ōma,* tumor]. 1. A tumor due to new growth of blood vessels; opp. to dilatation of pre-existing vessels. 2. A tumor due to failure of development.

hamartomatosis (ham-ar-to-mă-to'sis) [" + *ōma,* tumor + *-ōsis*]. Existence of multiple hamartomas.

hamatum (hă-ma'tum) [L. *hamatus,* hooked]. The unciform bone, *os hamatum.*

hammer. 1. An instrument with a head attached crosswise to the handle for striking blows. 2. Common name for the malleus, the middle ear bone.

h., percussion. A h. with a rubber head used for tapping surfaces of the body in order to produce sounds for diagnostic purposes. SEE: *plexor.*

h., reflex. A h. used for tapping parts of the body such as a muscle, tendon, or nerve in order to initiate certain reflex responses.

ham'mer toe. A toe with dorsal flexion of 1st phalanx and plantar flexion of 2nd and 3rd phalanges.

hamster. A rodent *Cricetus cricetus* belonging to the family Cricetidae, common in Europe and W. Asia. It is extensively used as a laboratory animal.

ham'string [A.S. *haum,* haunch]. One of the tendons which form the medial and lateral boundaries of the popliteal space.

h.'s, inner. Tendons of the semimembranosus, semitendinosus, and gracilis muscles.

h.'s, outer. The tendon of the biceps femoris.

hamstrings. Three muscles on the posterior aspect of the thigh, the semitendinosus, semimembranosus, and biceps femoris. They flex the leg and adduct and extend the thigh.

ham'ular [L. *hamulus,* a small hook]. Unciform; hook-shaped.

hamulus [L. a small hook]. 1. Any hook-shaped structure. 2. Hooklike process on the hamate bone.

h. cochleae. A hooklike process at the tip of the osseous spiral lamina of the cochlea.

h. lacrimalis [NA]. Hooklike process on the lacrimal bone.

h. pterygoideus [NA]. Hooklike process at tip of medial pterygoid process of the sphenoid bone.

hand [A.S. hand]. That part of the body attached to the forearm at the wrist.

It includes the wrist (*carpus*) with its 8 bones, the metacarpus, or body of the hand (*ossa metacarpalia*) having 5 bones, and the phalanges (fingers) with their 14 bones.

h., ape. Deformity of hand in which thumb is permanently extended.

h., claw. SEE: *clawhand.*

h., cleft. Deformity of hand in which the division between the fingers, particularly between the third and fourth, extends into the carpus.

h., opera-glass. Deformity of hand due to chronic absorptive arthritis. The phalanges appear to be telescoped into one another like an opera glass.

hand'edness. The tendency to use one hand in preference to the other.

h., left. Sinistrality; preferential use of the left hand.

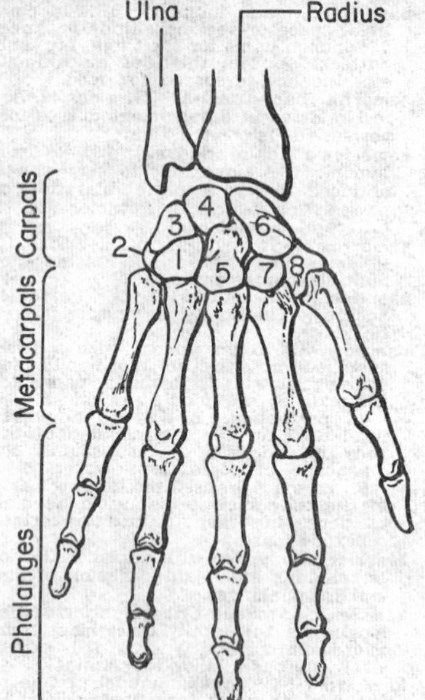

BONES OF THE HAND AND WRIST

h., right. Dextrality; preferential use of the right hand.

hands and skin. Disinfection of hands commonly consists of thorough scrubbing with a bristle brush in hot water and soap for 5 minutes. Mechanical cleansing alone removes a major part of the organisms. The hands may be immersed in a germicidal solution such as 70% alcohol for 1 minute. After drying with sterile towel, sterile rubber gloves are worn.

Hand-Schüller-Christian syndrome or disease [Alfred Hand, Jr., American pediatrician, 1868-1949; Artur Schüller, Austrian neurologist, 1874-; Henry A. Christian, American pathologist, 1876-1951]. A condition of unknown cause. Pathological lesion is that of reticuloendothelial cell proliferation with granuloma formation. SYN: *histiocytosis X; Schuller-Christian disease; xanthoma disseminatum.*

hang'ing drop culture. A method of culturing microorganisms by placing a drop of the culture medium containing organisms on a coverslip, then inverting the coverslip over a concavity of a hanging drop slide.

hang'nail [A.S. *hangian* to hang, + *naegel,* nail]. Partly detached piece of skin at root of fingernail. SYN: *agnail.*

Hanot's disease (han'os) [Victor C. Hanot, French physician, 1844-1896]. Hypertrophic cirrhosis of liver with jaundice.

Hansen's bacillus [Gerhard H. A. Hansen, Norwegian physician, 1841-1912]. *Mycobacterium leprae,* which he discovered in 1871.

H.'s disease. Leprosy.

Han'son unit [Adolph M. Hanson, American surgeon, 1888-]. One one-hundredth of the quantity of parathyroid extract solution necessary to elevate by 1 mg. the concentration of calcium in blood serum of a parathyroidectomized dog whose weight is 15 Kg.

hapalonychia (hap-al-o-nik'ĭ-ă) [G. *apalos,* soft, + *onyx, onych-,* nail]. Lack of rigidity of the nails. SYN: *onychomalacia.*

haphalgesia (haf-al-ge'zĭ-ă) [G. *aphē,* touch, + *algēsis,* pain]. A sensation of pain upon touching the skin with an object which is not an irritant.

haphephobia (haf-e-fo'bĭ-ă) [" + *phobos,* fear]. Aversion to being touched by another person.

haplodermatitis (hap"lo-der-mă-ti'tis) [G. *aploos,* simple, + *derma,* skin, + *-itis,* inflammation]. Simple inflammation of the skin. SYN: *haplodermitis.*

hap"lodermi'tis [" + " + *-ītis,* inflammation]. Uncomplicated inflammation of the skin.

hap'loid. Possessing half the diploid or normal number of chromosomes found in somatic or body cells. Such is the case of the germ cells, ova or sperm, following the reduction divisions in gametogenesis, the haploid number being 23 in man.

haplop'ia. Single vision; condition in which an object viewed by two eyes appears as a single object in contrast to *diplopia,* in which it appears as two objects.

hap'ten(e [G. *aptein,* to seize]. The portion of an antigen containing the grouping on which the specificity depends.

haptic (hap'tik) [G. *aptein,* to touch]. Pert. to touch. SYN: *tactile.*

hap'tics [G. *aptein,* to touch]. The science of the touch sense.

haptin (hap'tin) [G. *aptein,* to seize]. Haptene, *q.v.*

haptophil(e (hap'to-fil, -fīl) [" + *philein,* to love]. That portion of a receptor that unites with the haptophore group of a toxin.

haptophore (hap'to-for) [" + *pherein,* to bring]. The atom group of an antigen causing a combination with its corresponding antibody. SEE: *Ehrlich's sidechain theory.*

haptophor'ic, haptoph'orous [" + *pherein,* to bring]. Pert. to the action of a haptophore.

har'dening [A.S. heardian, to harden]. 1. Rendering a pathological or histological specimen firm or compact for making thin sections for microscopic study.

2. Increased resistance to changes in temperature of the atmosphere.

If the body is exposed to low temperatures, a contraction of skin vessels takes place, with a corresponding dilatation of the capillaries of the mucous membranes.

Hardening is induced by bathing to cause a prompt skin vascular reaction.

hard'ness [A.S. *heardness*]. 1. Quality of water containing certain substances, esp. soluble salts of calcium and magnesium. These react with soaps forming insoluble compounds which are precipitated out of solution, thus interfering with their cleansing action. 2. That quality of x-rays determining their penetrating power. Hardness lessens as wave lengths become longer.

h. of a gas tube. A term used to qualify the condition of a tube according to the degree of rarefaction of the residual gas.

The higher the vacuum, the harder the tube and the rays emitted, the higher the voltage required to cause a discharge with a cold cathode, and hence the shorter the wave length of the resulting roentgen rays.

hare'lip [A.S. *hara*, hare, + *lippa*, lip]. A vertical cleft or clefts in the upper lip. It is congenital resulting from the faulty fusion of the median nasal process and the lateral maxillary processes. It is usually unilateral and on the left side although it may be bilateral. It may involve the lip or the upper jaw alone or both together, and often occurs with cleft palate. SYN: *cheiloschisis.*

h. suture. A twisted figure-of-eight suture.

harlequin fetus (har'lĕ-kwin). A newlyborn infant with *ichthyosis congenita.* SYN: *hyperkeratosis congenitalis.*

Harris flush. A therapeutic procedure, similar to an enema, used to relieve flatus and abdominal distention, esp. following abdominal surgery.

Har'rison's groove [Edwin Harrison, London physician, 1779-1847]. Depression on lower edge of the thorax caused by tug of the diaphragm; seen in adenoids and rickets.

Has'ner's valve or fold [Joseph R. Hasner, Prague ophthalmologist, 1819-1892]. A fold of the mucous membrane at the opening of the nasolacrimal duct in the inf. meatus of the nasal cavity. SYN: *plica lacrimalis.*

Has'sall's corpuscles or bodies [Arthur H. Hassall, English chemist and physician, 1817-1894]. SYN: *thymic corpuscle.* Spherical or oval bodies present in the medulla of the thymus. Each consists of central area of degenerated cells surrounded by concentrically arranged flattened or polygonal cells. They are characteristic of the thymus.

Hatchcock's sign. Tenderness just beyond the angle of the jaws when the finger follows on the under surface of the mandible towards the angle. Found in mumps before any swelling can be detected.

haunch (hawnsh) [Fr. *hanche*]. The hips and buttocks.

h. bone. The ilium. SYN: *os coxae.*

haustra (haws'tra) (sing. *haustrum*) [L. *haurire,* to draw, drink]. The sacculated elevations of the colon.

h. coli. Sacculations of the colon resembling tucks caused by the fact that the gut is longer than the longitudinal bands or taeniae.

haustral (haw'stral) [L. *haurire,* to draw, drink]. Pert. to the colonic haustra.

h. churning. Agitation of the intestinal contents.

haustrum (haw'strum) (pl. *haus'tra*) [L. *haurire,* to draw, drink]. One of the sacculations of the colon caused by longitudinal bands shorter than the gut which causes formation of pouches in the colon. SYN: *haustra coli.*

haus'tus [L. a drink]. A draught of medicine.

haut-mal (o'mahl) [Fr. high evil]. Grand mal when at its height.

haver'sian canal. Minute vascular canals found in osseous tissue.

h. canaliculi. Delicate canals extending from the lacunae into the matrix of bone. They anastomose with canaliculi of adjacent lacunae forming a network of fine channels which communicate with Haversian and Volkmann's canals. They transmit nutrient materials.

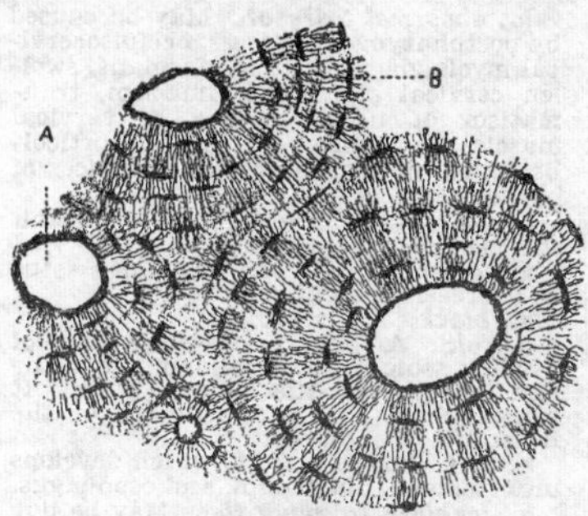

HAVERSIAN SYSTEM OF BONE, MAGNIFIED

Cross section femur, dog. A. Haversian canal. B. Lacunae and canaliculi.

h. gland. A mass of fatty tissue lodged in the acetabular fossa of the innominate bone. Also called *synovial gland.*

h. system. Architectural unit of bone consisting of a central tube (*h. canal*) with alternate layers of intercellular material (*matrix*) surrounding it in concentric cylinders. Alternating layers of matrix and cells are called *haversian lamellae.* SEE: *bone.*

hay fever. SYN: *allergic coryza; rose cold; vasomotor rhinitis; pollinosis.* An allergic disease of mucous passages of nose and upper air passages induced by external irritation.

SYM: Inflammation, catarrh, watery discharges from the eyes, cold in the head, coryza, headache, asthmatic symptoms.

ETIOL: Air-borne pollens. *Spring type* due to pollens of trees such as oak, elm, hickory, ash; *Summer type* due to pollens of plants such as grasses, plantain, and sorrel; *Fall type* due principally to the pollen of ragweeds. Nonseasonal hay fever may result from (a) inhalation of irritating substances such as the danders of animals, or dust such as hay, straw, or house dust. (b) Ingestion of substances such as drugs or foods to which the subject is allergic.

TREATMENT: 1. Change of climate, sea voyage. 2. Filtration of air by air conditioning, masks, and nasal filters. 3. Drug therapy in which epinephrine, antihistamines, or other drugs are given orally or used as nose drops, or nasal sprays. 4. Prophylactic treatment consisting of injection of pollen extracts made from pollen to which the subject is sensitive.

Hay'garth's deformities, nodes or nodosities [John Haygarth, English physician, 1740-1827]. Exostoses or bony tumors on joints in arthritis deformans.

hb. Abbr. for *hemoglobin.*

HCG. Abbr. for *human chorionic gonadotrophin.*

H. D. Abbr. for *hearing distance.*

h.d. Abbr. for *hora decubitus* (the hour of going to bed).

He. Symb. for *helium.*

head [A.S. *heafod*]. 1. Caput. That part of the animal body containing the brain and organs of sight, hearing, smell, and taste. It includes the facial bones. 2. The proximal end of a bone. 3. The larger extremity of any structure or body.

h., abnormal fixity of. May be caused by postpharyngeal abscess, occipitocervical myelalgia, arthritis deformans, swollen cervical glands, rheumatism, traumatism of neck, sprains of cervical muscles, congenital spasmodic torticollis, caries of a molar tooth, cicatrices of burns.

h., abnormal movement of. Habit spasms, such as nodding.

h., aftercoming. The head of a fetus in a breech presentation.

h., black. A comedo, *q.v.*

h. fold. A fold of the blastoderm of a chick which grows caudad under the ant. portion of the neural plate. It brings about the establishment of the head and the foregut.

h. gut. Part of embryo which develops into stomach, duodenum, and esophagus.

h., inability to move the. May be due to caries of cervical vertebrae and diseases of articulation bet. occiput and atlas or paralysis of neck muscles.

h. kidney. Embryonic kidney.

h. lock. Interlocking of chins in twin birth.

h., nerve. The optic disk.

h. process. A strand of cells in the embryo extending forward from the primitive knot. Also called *notochordal plate.*

h., retracted. Seen in acute meningitis, cerebral abscess, tumor, thrombosis of sup. longitudinal sinus, acute encephalitis, laryngeal obstruction, tetanus, hydrophobia, epilepsy, spasmodic torticollis, strychnine poisoning, hysteria, and rachitic conditions. Also in painful neck lesions at the back.

h., rhythmical nodding of. Seen in aortic regurgitation, chorea, torticollis, *q.v.*

h. scald. Affection of scalp accompanied by crusts or scales.

head, *words pert. to:* acromegaly, caput, "ceph-" words, coryza, face, gyrospasm, macrocephalous, nutation, occipital, sinciput, skeleton, temple, vertex.

head'ache [A.S. *heafod* + *acan,* to ache]. A diffuse pain in different portions of the head and not confined to any nerve distribution area.

It may be *frontal, temporal* or *occipital;* confined to one side of head or to region immediately over one eye. The character of pain may vary; may be dull ache; acute, almost unbearable pain; intermittent, intense pain; throbbing pain; pressure pain when head feels as if it will burst, or penetrating pain driving through head.

Etiol: (a) Associated with disorders of alimentary tract, probably due to absorption of toxins, as in indigestion or constipation. (b) Due to toxemia. A constant symptom in nephritis and jaundice; also occurs in septic absorption from foci present in body, as in septic teeth, septic tonsils, infected cranial sinuses. (c) Frequently a symptom at onset of febrile diseases, esp. pneumonia, typhoid fever, scarlet fever, smallpox, erysipelas, tetanus, and influenza. (d) Defective sight and, less commonly, defective hearing are causes. With defective sight, pain may occur over eyes, also at occiput owing to fatigue of visual area, situated in the occipital lobe of the brain. (e) Mental strain, worry, and anxiety will cause headache; this may be associated with eyestrain or be independent of it. (f) Abnormalities in blood pressure give rise to headache. In some cases due to low blood pressure, in which anemia of brain occurs; in other cases blood pressure is high. Sudden changes in blood pressure also cause headache. (g) Changes in intracranial pressure give rise to headache. The acutely painful headache following intrathecal anesthesia is an example, as is the headache associated with meningitis. (h) Diseases of central nervous system are characterized by headache. (i) Any injury resulting in concussion or compression of brain or cord.

Summary:

1. Toxic Factors—

(a) *Of exogenous origin*—Foul air, from poor ventilation, etc.; poisonous gases, including fumes from furnaces or gas fires; drugs (quinine, morphine, etc.); alcohol, tobacco, etc.

(b) *Of endogenous origin* (any absorption of the toxins of bacterial infection will cause headache).

Chronic infections—Nose and sinuses, teeth, middle ear, pharynx, tonsils, appendix, gallbladder, pelvic viscera.

Fever in general.

Bacteremias—Typhoid fever, malaria, smallpox, tuberculosis, grippe and influenza, puerperal fever, etc.

Systemic diseases—Nephritis with uremia, biliary tract disease (including acute yellow atrophy of the liver), rheumatism, diabetes, anemia, polycythemia, eclampsia, syphilis.

2. Gastrointestinal Disturbances—Dyspepsia, gastric hyper- and hypoacidity, intestinal stasis and constipation.

3. Physicochemical Disturbances — Acidosis, alkalosis.

4. Cardiovascular Disturbances—High blood pressure, low blood pressure, myocardial and valvular insufficiency causing either congestion or anemia.

5. Endocrine Disorders — Pituitary, thyroid, suprarenals, ovaries.

6. Gynecological Factors (due to functional disturbances of one or more of the above glands)—Puberty, menstruation, pregnancy, menopause.

7. Neurological Factors — Nervous shock; nervous exhaustion; worry, excitement, anger, or nervous tension; migraine; hysteria; epilepsy; psychoneuroses; headache which may be psychic with reflex symptoms to various regions or which may be, itself, a reflex pain secondary to organic disease.

8. Diseases of Special Sense Organs —Iritis, glaucoma, etc.; adenoids, deviated septum, etc.; middle ear affections.

9. Organic Disease of Brain—Causing pressure: Tumor, abscess, gumma, cyst, hydrocephaly, intracranial hemorrhage. Intracranial vascular disease; arteriosclerosis; embolism, thrombosis or aneurysm; encephalitis.

10. Various Forms of Meningitis, including meningismus.

11. Functional Causes (almost any disturbance of body function may cause headache)—External pressure and constriction of head; trauma to head; sunstroke; persistent noises; persistent motion (seasickness, train sickness, etc.); irritation of mucous membrane of nose and sinuses by dust, pollen, etc.; fatigue (physical mental); insomnia; eyestrain (uncorrected defects, overwork); spinal puncture usually followed by headache.

Treatment: Depends entirely on cause, and there is great danger of headache, which is probably only a symptom, being treated without regard to cause. Provided that due consideration has been given to this, the following points may receive general attention: (a) The diet; (b) adequate rest; (c) possible constipation; (d) the amount of urine being passed. Applications of cold to head may relieve, esp. if evaporating lotion is used. A hot bath may help, by stimulating circulation generally. Heat applied to back of neck may relieve by reflex effect. A stimulant, such as tea, coffee, or sal volatile (effervescent salt), may relieve when headache is due to fatigue or overstrain. Drugs for the relief of headache should be given with care. SYN: *cephalgia*.

h., histamine. H. resulting from injection of histamine or excessive histamine in circulating blood. Due to dilatation of branches of the carotid artery.

h., sick. A nervous headache occurring periodically, usually on one side of the head, accompanied by nausea and vomiting.

SEE: *migraine*.

heal (hēl) [A.S. *hael*, whole]. To cure; to make whole or healthy.

heal'ing [A.S. *hael*, whole]. The restoration to a normal condition, esp. of an inflammation or a wound.

HEALING BY FIRST INTENTION: This process closes the edge of a wound with little or no inflammatory reaction, and in such a manner that no scar is left to reveal the site of the injury. The free bleeding of the cut edges and the intact living cells not affected by the injury make this possible. New cells are formed to take the place of dead ones, and the capillary walls stretch across the wound to join themselves to each other in a smooth surface. New connective tissue may form an almost imperceptible scar which proves temporary.

HEALING BY SECOND INTENTION: This is healing by granulation or indirect union. Granulation tissue is formed to fill the gap between the edges of the wound with a thin layer of fibrinous exudate. It bars out bacteria and aids in checking bleeding by the coagulation of the blood. Connective tissue cells support the new capillaries. This form of healing is slower than that by first intention and its grayish-red surface may become pale and flabby if the healing is too long delayed. If the granulations show above the surface they may have to be removed with caustics. If the granulations first form at the top instead of the bottom of the wound, it may have to be kept open by drainage.

HEALING BY THIRD INTENTION: Of an ulcer, wound, or cavity by filling with granulations. It generally results in the formation of a scar.

COMPLICATIONS IN HEALING: These may result from: (a) The formation of a scar interfering with functioning of the part, and possible deformity; (b) the formation of a *keloid*,* the result of overgrowth of connective tissue forming a tumor in the surface of a scar; (c) necrosis of the skin and mucous membrane producing a raw surface that results in an ulcer; (d) a sinus or fistula which may be due to bacteria, or some foreign substance remaining in the wound; (e) proud flesh. This represents excessive granulations, the result of a fungus growth.

health (helth) [A.S. *hǣlth*, wholeness]. A condition in which all functions of body and mind are normally active.

h., bill of. Public health certificate certifying that passengers on a public conveyance or ship are free of infectious disease.

h., board of. A public body in charge of the health of a community.

h. certificate. An official statement signed by a physician which attests to the state of health of a particular individual.

h., department of. Branch of a government (city, county, or nation) for regulation and protection of the people's health.

h., industrial. The health of employees of industrial firms.

h., public. The state of health of the population of a particular community, such as a city, county, state, or nation, as opposed to individual or personal health; community health.

h. nurse, public. One employed by a board or dept. of health to serve the public.

health'y [A.S. *hǣlth*, wholeness]. Being in a state of health or enjoying it.

h. ulcer. Ulcer which heals easily.

hear'ing [A.S. *hēran*, to hear]. The act or power of perceiving sound.

h., after. Perception of sound after the stimulus producing it has ceased to act.

h. aid. An apparatus used by those with impaired hearing for amplifying sound waves.

h. distance. That at which a given sound can be heard. On the prairies a voice may be heard for 2 miles or more.

h., functional tests for. Hearing acuity can be determined by: (1) Determining the distance at which a person can hear a certain sound, such as a watch tick. (2) By the use of *audiometers*, in which electrically produced sounds are conveyed by wires to a receiver applied to the subject's ear. Intensity and pitch of sound can be altered and is indicated on dials. Results are plotted on a graph known as an *audiogram*. (3) By bone conduction tests in which a device such as tuning fork or an apparatus which converts an electrical current into mechanical vibrations is applied to the skull. This is of value in distinguishing between perceptive and transmission deafness.

h. hallucinations. Subjective sensations of sound such as "hearing voices" when none actually exists.

heart (hart) [A.S. *heorte*]. A hollow, muscular, contractile organ, the center of the circulatory system. Its wall possesses three layers, the outer *epicardium*, a serous layer, the middle *myocardium*, composed of cardiac muscle, and the inner *endocardium*, a layer which lines the chambers of the heart and covers the valves. The heart is enclosed in a fibroserous sac, the *pericardium*, the space between the pericardium and the epicardium forming the *pericardial cavity*.

CHAMBERS: Each lower cavity is the *ventriculum*, or ventricle; each upper one the *atrium*, or auricle. The right auricle is called the *atrium dexter*, and the left one the *atrium sinistrum*, the two ventricles being known as *ventriculus dexter* (right) and *v. sinister* (left) respectively.

Contraction of the heart chambers is called *systole;* relaxation with accompanying dilation, *diastole*. The complete series of events which occurs in a single heart beat is known as the *cardiac cycle*. In a heart beating at the rate of 72 per minute, each cycle lasts about 0.85 sec. The heart is divided perpendicularly from base to apex by the *interatrial* and *interventricular septa,* the right side having no communication with the left. The right side receives *deoxygenated* blood from the tissues and pumps it to the lungs; the left side receives *oxygenated* blood from the lungs and pumps it to the tissues.

The atria, serving as receiving chambers, are thin walled; the ventricles, serving as pumping chambers, are thick walled.

Accelerator impulses are conveyed over nerves and ganglia of the sympathetic division. Preganglionic neurons which lie in the thoracic portion of the spinal cord synapse with postganglionic neurons located in the cervical ganglia of sympathetic trunk whose axons pass to the heart. Impulses over these nerves known as *augmentor nerves* increase rate and force of heart beat. Impulses regulating the heart arise in the cardiac center in the medulla oblongata.

Afferent fibers: these pass through the vagus trunks to the medulla. Some are *depressor* fibers originating in receptors in the base of the aorta. Impulses over these fibers reflexly slow the heart rate. Others are *pressor fibers* originating in receptors in the vena cavae and rt. atrium. These reflexly increase heart beat. Fibers conveying pain impulses are also present.

VALVES: The atrioventricular orifice bet. each atrium and ventricle. 1. *Valvula tricuspidalis* (tricuspid) guards the opening bet. the *atrium dexter* and the *ventriculus dexter.* 2. *Valvula bicuspidalis* (bicuspid or mitral valve), bet. the *atrium sinistrum* (left atrium) and the *ventriculus sinister* (left ventricle). 3. *Valvulae semilunares* (semilunar valves) guard the orifice bet. the *ventriculus dexter* and the pulmonary artery. 4. *Valvulae semilunares aortae* (aortic valves) guard the orifice bet. the *ventriculus sinister* and the aorta.

NERVE SUPPLY: *Inhibitory*: Vagus or pneumogastric, acceleratory: By way of the sympathetic ganglia of the autonomic system and phrenic nerve. *Afferent*: A depressor nerve running from the heart to a cardioinhibitory center in the medulla, through the sheath of the vagi nerves, causing reflex inhibition of the heart. Efferent fibers: *Inhibitory impulses* are conveyed by preganglionic fibers of the vagus nerve, which synapse with postganglionic neurons located in terminal ganglia in the wall of the heart. They are distributed to the S-A node and other conductile tissue of the heart.

WORK OF HEART. Two to 3 oz. of blood are driven into the arteries by each heartbeat. The power exerted by the heart is said to equal that necessary to lift 80 lb. 1 ft. each minute. At the rate of 72 times each minute, the human heart beats 104,000 times a day, 38,000,000 times during a year. At every stroke 5 cu. in. of blood are forced out into the body, or 500,000 cu. in. a day. In terms of work this is the equivalent of raising 1 ton to a height of 41 ft. every 24 hr.

h., abdominal. **A heart that is displaced into the abdominal cavity.**

h., armoured. Condition characterized by deposit of calcareous matter in the pericardium.

h., athletic. Supposed hypertrophy of the heart as a result of strenuous physical activity. Of little or no significance in the absence of diseased valves.

h., auscultation of. Shows intensity, quality, and rhythm of heart sounds and

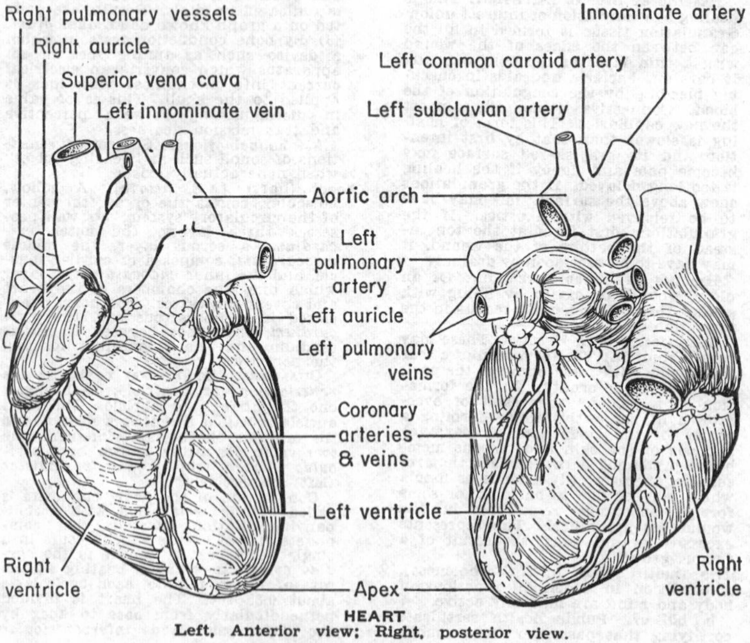

HEART
Left, Anterior view; Right, posterior view.

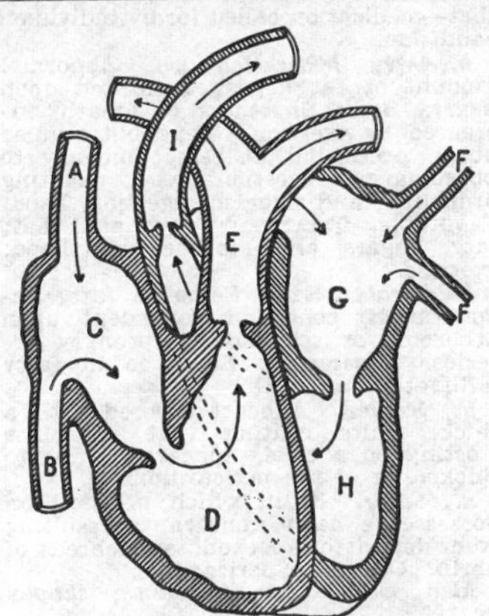

CIRCULATION OF THE BLOOD THROUGH THE HEART

A. Superior vena cava. B. Inferior vena cava. C. Right atrium. D. Right ventricle. E. Pulmonary artery. F. Pulmonary veins. G. Left atrium. H. Left ventricle. I. Aorta.

detects the presence of any adventitious sounds, as murmurs. Both sounds over the heart have been represented by the syllables "lubb," "dupp." The first sound (systolic) results from the contraction of the ventricle, tension of the atrioventricular valves, and the impact of the heart against the chest wall, and is synchronous with the apex beat and carotid pulse. This sound is prolonged and dull; after the first sound is a short pause, then the second sound (diastolic), which results from the closure of the aortic and pulmonary valves. This sound is short and high pitched. After the second sound a longer pause follows before the first is heard again.

INTENSITY: Both sounds are accentuated in: (1) Excitement of heart from any cause; (2) anemia; (3) cardiac hypertrophy; (4) subjects with thin chest walls; (5) consolidation of the lung, as in phthisis and pneumonia. *Accentuation of the aortic second sound results from*: (a) Hypertrophy of the left ventricle; (b) high arterial tension, as in arteriosclerosis with hypertension; (c) aortic aneurysm. *Accentuation of the pulmonary second sound results from*: (a) Pulmonary obstruction, as in emphysema, pneumonia and congestion of the lungs following mitral disease; (b) hypertrophy of the right ventricle. *Weakness of both sounds is noted in*: (a) General obesity; (b) general debility; (c) degeneration or dilatation of the heart; (d) pericardial or pleural effusion; (e) emphysema.

REDUPLICATION — HEART SOUNDS: Probably due to a lack of synchronous action in the valves of both sides of the heart, and results from many conditions, but notably from increased resistance in the systemic or the pulmonary circulation, as in arteriosclerosis of chronic nephritis and in emphysema. Frequently noted in mitral stenosis and pericarditis.

ADVENTITIOUS SOUNDS: *Murmurs*: A murmur is an abnormal sound heard over the heart or blood vessels and may result from: (1) Obstruction or regurgitation at the valves following endocarditis; (2) dilatation of the ventricle or relaxation of its walls rendering the valves relatively insufficient; (3) aneurysm; (4) a change in the blood constituents, as in anemia; (5) roughening of the pericardial surfaces, as in pericarditis; (6) irregular action of the heart.

Murmurs produced within the heart are termed endocardial, those outside exocardial; those produced in aneurysms, bruits; those produced by anemia, hemic murmurs.

Hemic murmurs. They are soft and blowing in character, usually systolic in time, heard best over pulmonary valves. Associated with symptoms of anemia, and disappear with the latter.

Aneurysmal murmur or bruit. Usually loud, booming in character, systolic in time, heard best over the aorta or base of heart and is often associated with an abnormal area of dullness and pulsation, and with symptoms resulting from pressure on neighboring structures.

Pericardial friction sounds. Pericardial murmurs or friction sounds are superficial, rough, and creaking in quality, to and fro in time, not transmitted beyond the precordium and may be modified by pressure of the stethoscope.

PROCEDURE: Patient should be recumbent when beginning examination; then, having elicited all the signs possible, repeat with patient sitting or standing and note any variations from change of position. First listen while patient is breathing naturally, then while holding breath, and finally have patient take 3 or 4 forced inspirations. Explore whole thoracic cavity and endeavor to localize the points at which heart sounds, both normal and abnormal, are heard with the greatest intensity. Proceed from below upward, from left to right.

VALVES: *Location for auscultation*: *Aortic,* 3rd intercostal space; close to left side of sternum. *Pulmonary,* in front of aorta, behind junction of 3rd costal cartilage with sternum, left side. *Tricuspid,* behind middle of sternum about level of 4th of costal cartilage. *Mitral,* behind 3rd intercostal space about 1 in. to the left of sternum.

h., beriberi. **Heart failure due to vitamin deficiency.**

h. block. Condition in which the conductile tissue of the heart (S-A node, A-V node, bundle of His, Purkinje fibers) fails to conduct impulses normally from the atrium to the ventricles. Such results in altered rhythm of heart beat with loss of every other, or of every 3rd beat, the atrial systole not always being followed by the ventricular systole, the bundle of His failing to transmit the regular systolic impulse. The ventricle contracts regularly at a much slower rate than the atrium. The contractions begin at the sinoatrial node, or normal point, but they are interrupted before they reach their destination. The pulse is very slow, usually under 30.

ETIOL: (a) Structural changes as from tumor or degeneration or embryonic maldevelopment. (b) Toxic effects of drugs or the toxins of infections. (c) Nutritional or functional factors.

h. b., arborization. B. in which there is interference in terminal fibers of the Purkinje system.

h. b., atrioventricular. B. in which impulses are impeded at the A-V node.

h. b., bundle branch. B. in which impulses are blocked in one of the branches of the bundle of His, resulting in ventricles beating independently of each other.

h. b., complete. Condition in which there is a complete dissociation between atrial and ventricular systoles. Ventricles may beat at a rate of 30 to 40 per min. while atria are beating the normal 70 beats per min.

h. b., congenital. H. b. present at birth due to improper development of the impulse-conducting system.

h. b., incomplete. H. b. in which conduction time of impulses is prolonged; usually recognized only by electrocardiograph; partial h.b.

h. b., interventricular. Bundle branch block, *q.v.*

h. b., partial. One of 2 or 3 impulses passes to ventricle; pulse is thus 40-50.

h. b., sinoatrial. H. b. in which there is interference in the passage of impulses from the S-A node. May be partial or complete.

h., boatshaped. H. in which one ventricle is dilated and hypertrophied as a result of aortic regurgitation.

h., bony. A heart having calcareous patches in its walls and pericardium.

h., cervical. A heart that is located in the neck.

h., dilatation of. Enlargement of heart due to stretching of its walls. VARIETIES: 1. Dilatation with thickening of walls. 2. Dilatation with thinning of walls. SYM: So long as the associated hypertrophy keeps pace with the dilatation no symptoms result, but otherwise dyspnea, cough, dyspepsia, scanty urine, dropsy, feeble pulse. TREATMENT: Rest, light, nutritious diet—improve general condition.

h. disease. Any pathological disorder of the heart.

h., encased. State resulting from chronic constrictive pericarditis.

h. failure. 1. Cessation of the beat of the heart. 2. A syndrome or clinical condition resulting from failure of the heart to maintain adequate circulation of blood. May result from failure of the right or left ventricle or both.

ETIOL: Hypertension, infections, valvular insufficiency, coronary disease, congenital malformations, arteriosclerosis, atherosclerosis.

SYM: Dyspnea, cardiac asthma, stasis in systemic or portal circulation, edema, cyanosis, hypertrophy of heart. Symptoms vary depending on which side of the heart is affected.

h. f., backward. H. f. in which venous return to the heart is reduced with resulting venous stasis and congestion. Due principally to failure of the right ventricle.

h. f., congestive. Condition characterized by weakness, breathlessness, abdominal discomfort, edema in lower portions of body resulting from venous stasis and reduced outflow of blood. Also called *myocardial insufficiency; cardiac decompensation.*

h. f., forward. H. f. in which forward flow of blood to the tissues is inadequate due to failure of the left ventricle.

h., fatty degeneration of. Cardiac muscle has been metamorphosed into fat. SYM: All signs of heart failure, *viz.*: dyspnea; asthma; cough; weak, irregular pulse; poor digestion; attacks of syncope. PROG: Unfavorable. Death may occur on slight exertion. TREATMENT: Rest of body and mind—light, nutritious diet—medication called for by individual condition.

h., fatty infiltration of. Abnormal amount of fat deposited in and upon heart. SYM: Shortness of breath, increased by exertion. Weak but regular pulse, precordial distress, tendency to pulmonary congestion, with resulting bronchitis and sluggish digestion. PROG: Favorable. TREATMENT: Regulated diet: fats, sugars and starches restricted; exercise.

h., fibroid. SYM: Same as fatty degeneration, condition dependent upon atheroma or sclerosis of coronary arteries. TREATMENT: Same as in fatty infiltration of h.

h., frosted. A heart covered with a thick, white coating that resembles frosting on a cake. Appearance due to thickening of the pericardium.

h., hairy. H. in which pericardium possesses a hairy appearance resulting from deposit of an exudate or shreds of fibrin. Occurs in pericarditis.

Also called *cor villosum; shaggy heart.*

h., hypertrophy of. Enlargement due to overgrowth of its muscle. VARIETIES: 1. *Simple h.* Thickened muscle and cavities normal size. 2. *Eccentric h.* Thickened muscle and cavities dilated. 3. *Concentric h.* Thickened muscle and cavities diminished in size. Always congenital. SYM: Unless advanced, no symptoms. Extreme hypertrophy, precordial distress, palpitation. Strong pulse. Sometimes flushed face, ringing in ears, flashes of light, headache, and disturbed sleep. TREATMENT: Graduated exercise, light diet, sedatives.

h., icing. **Frosted heart, *q.v.***

h., irritable. Neurocirculatory asthenia, or effort syndrome. Syndrome characterized by breathlessness, palpitation, weakness and exhaustion. Also called *soldier's heart.*

h., left. Medical jargon for left side of the heart—the left atrium and ventricle. This is the portion of the heart that receives the aerated blood from the lungs and propels it into the systemic circulation.

h., palpation of. Not only determines position, force, extent, and rhythm of apex beat, but also detects existence of any fremitus or thrill. A thrill is a vibratory sensation likened to that received when the hand is placed on the back of a purring cat. Thrills at base of heart may result from valvular lesions, atheroma of aorta, aneurysm, and from roughened pericardial surfaces, as in pericarditis. A presystolic thrill at apex is almost pathognomonic of mitral stenosis.

h., palpitation of. May result from dyspepsia; excitement, mental or physical; organic heart disease; exophthalmic goiter; overwork, as the "irritable heart" of untrained recruits; anemia; hysteria; or an independent neurosis. Also: *endocarditis, myocarditis, pericarditis* due to infection, to trauma, circulatory disturbances, disorders of metabolism, nutrition, and growth.

h., percussion of. Determines shape and extent of cardiac dullness. The normal area of superficial or absolute percussion—dullness (part uncovered by lung) is detected by light percussion and extends from the 4th left costosternal junction to the apex beat; from the apex beat to the juncture of the xiphoid cartilage, with the sternum, and thence up left border of the sternum. The normal area of deep percussion dullness (the heart projected on the chest wall) is detected by firm percussion and extends from 3rd left costosternal articulation to the apex beat; from apex beat to junction of the xiphoid cartilage with the sternum; and hence up right border of sternum to the 3rd rib. The lower level of the cardiac dullness fuses with the liver dullness and can rarely be determined. The area of cardiac dullness is increased in: (1) Hypertrophy and dilation of the heart; (2) pericardial effusion. It is apparently increased in shrinking of the lungs, as in phthisis. The area of detectable cardiac dullness is diminished in: (1) Emphysema; (2) pneumothorax; (3) pneumocardium (rare); (4) gaseous distention of stomach.

h., pulmonary. Right heart, *q.v.*

h. reflex. A cardiac reflex; any reflex in which the stimulation of a sensory nerve brings about an increase or decrease in heart rate. Ex.: Bainbridge's reflex in which stimulation of sensory receptors in rt. atrium by increased venous return results in increase of heart rate.

h., right. Medical jargon for right side of the heart—the right atrium and ventricle. This portion of the heart receives the venous blood and propels it to the lungs.

h. sounds. SEE: *h., auscultation of.*

h., systemic. Left heart, *q.v.*

h. test. Various methods of testing the heart clinically have been devised. These are usually based upon the ability of the healthy heart to return to a normal rate within a specified time following exertion. The amount of exercise is usually precisely measured.

heart'burn. Acid liquid raised from the stomach, causing sensation of burning in the esophagus. SYN: *pyrosis.* SEE: *ardor ventriculi.*

heat [G. *heito*, fever]. 1. Condition of being hot; warmth. 2. High temperature. 3. A form of energy manifested to the senses, as in the effects of fire, sun's rays, etc. 4. Sexual excitement in lower mammals; period of such excitement. SYN: *estrus.* 5. To make hot. 6. To become warm.

Heat is constantly being produced within the body as a result of exothermic chemical processes occurring in metabolic activities. Ultimately all heat produced in the body results from oxidative processes. Body temperature (normally 98.6° F. or 37° C.) is the result of a balance between heat produced (*thermogenesis*) and heat loss (*thermolysis*).

The temperature of the body is not uniform. Oral temperatures range from 96.6° F. to 100° F. (average 98.6° F.). Axillary temperature averages 0.5° F. lower; rectal temperature averages 0.6° higher. SEE: *fever.*

Reducing the temperature of the skin reflexly brings about a constriction of the blood vessels, thus reducing heat loss and conserving heat within the body. The application of heat reflexly induces the dilation of blood vessels thus increasing blood flow to the skin with consequent increase in heat loss.

The application of heat to the skin reflexly produces effects in the deeper portions of the body. In general, internal organs are reflexly related to the region of the skin lying directly over them, and the effects are the same as those produced in the cutaneous area stimulated. Heat application induces muscle relaxation, increased blood supply and stimulates metabolic activity. Physiological effects resulting are hyperemia, sedation of sensory or motor activity. Application of cold tends to produce the opposite effects.

Relaxation of muscular tissue results in relief of pain, which may be due to rigidity and tension in tissues. Local hot applications may have some reflex effect on deep organs, as in cases of lobar pneumonia, when the lung is known to be in a state of congestion; local heat is applied in order to relieve, probably, the congestion of the lung by inducing a superficial hyperemia.

H., APPLICATION OF, GENERAL. May be dry, as in the form of electric and radiant heat and hot air baths, or moist, when water or water vapor is used. The *effect* is first to produce a slight contraction of vessels in skin, thus increasing blood pressure and driving blood into the internal organs; this makes patient feel that his head is full and bursting. This effect is, however, only of very short duration, and discomfort can be avoided by application of cold compress or ice bag to head.

The true effect follows immediately, when blood vessels in skin are dilated, due to relaxation of involuntary muscle contained in their walls; the skin is reddened, increased blood supply to the sweat glands causes them to act freely, and waste products are better eliminated and heat is lost to the body. For this reason applications of heat are most often used to increase sweating and so relieve work of kidneys in cases of renal disease.

NP: During a general application of heat it is necessary to watch the patient carefully, noting any apparent discomfort caused, also state of pulse and respiration and color.

H., APPLICATION OF LOCAL. May be dry or moist. Dry applications include hot absorbent wool, rubber hot-water bottles, bags of hot salt or bran previously heated in an oven, radiant heat, electric pads, and diathermy.

The mode of elimination of body heat and the per cent of heat lost through each of the following is:

Mode	Per cent	Total
Radiation	55%	94%
Convection and Conduction	15%	
Evaporation through skin and lungs	24%	
Warming inspired air	2%	6%
Elimination of CO_2 from lungs	3%	
Warming ingested food and water and loss through feces and urine	1%	

Figures are approximate and vary with physiological activity of the body.

H., APPLICATION OF MOIST. Considered more penetrating than dry heat, thus more readily relaxing muscular spasm and relieving pain due to this. Hot compresses of hypertonic saline will relieve edema and tension in tissues which may be causing great pain.

Ex: Fomentations or stupes, either simple or medicated; poultices such as bread, linseed, linseed and mustard, linseed and charcoal. A starch poultice may also be applied hot.

h., atomic. That amount which will raise an atom from 0° to 1° C.

h., body, loss of. The skin loses approximately 87.5 cal., the lungs 10.7 cal., and through excreta, 1.8 cal. In a healthy adult man weighing about 154 lb., loss in elimination has been estimated in the table above.

h., conductive. A term applied to heat transferred by conduction from poultices, bags, etc.

h., convective. That supplied from heated particles of gases or liquids, such as superheated air, melted paraffin, incandescent light apparatus, or the whirlpool bath.

h., conversive. A term used to designate heat generated in the tissues by a current of electricity or by some form of radiant energy.

h. cramps. Severe, intermittent, spasmodic cramping of muscles in abdomen and extremities.

ETIOL: Profuse sweating due to deficiency of salt in the tissues. Often found in individuals who have been drinking large volumes of water and perspire profusely for long period of time; not fatal.

SYM: Hypochloremia. In addition to free sweating, cramps are felt in the legs and in other regions accompanied by fever, rapid pulse, pains, increased blood pressure, and loss of weight.

F. A. TREATMENT: Adm. ¼ teaspoonful of ordinary table salt (sodium chloride) in glass of water. Repeat at 5- to 30-minute intervals until cramping ceases. May be prevented by adding salt to drinking water on hot days, particularly for hard working individuals.

As a *preventive,* 100–300 gr. of salt per day is necessary to compensate for each 2 quarts of sweat excreted. The salt aids in holding the water in the tissues. If the supply of salt is lowered, thirst calls for more water, but the intake of water is dependent upon the increase of the salt. Local applications of heat to reduce pain and salt solution by mouth or injection. SEE: *cramps; salt.*

h., diathermy. Electrical energy is converted into heat by the use of diathermy and short wave.

h., dry. May be adm. in form of hot, dry pack; hot water bottle; electric light bath; heliotherapy; hot bricks; resistance coil; electric pad or blanket; hot air bath, or therapeutic lamp.

h. exhaustion. Must not be mistaken for heatstroke, *q.v.* Usually affects adults, esp. the debilitated and fatigued.

SYM: Dizziness, nausea, faintness, weakness. Unconsciousness often follows. Skin pale, cool, moist; pulse rapid; respiration shallow and hurried.

PROG: Favorable under proper treatment.

F. A. TREATMENT: Lower head and shoulders; elevate lower extremities. Stimulate with aromatic spirits of ammonia to nostrils. Hot, black coffee or tea. External heat and massage. No cold drinks.

h., initial. Muscular heat produced (a) during contraction when tension is increasing, (b) during maintenance of tension, and (c) during relaxation when tension is diminishing.

h., latent. The heat which is required to convert a solid into a liquid or a liquid into a gas at the same temperature.

h., latent, of fusion. That which is required to convert 1 gm. of a solid into liquid at the same temperature, *e.g.,* when 1 gm. of ice at 0° C. is converted into water at 0° C.; this process requires 80 calories, and until it is completed there will be no rise of temperature.

h., latent, of vaporization. That required to change 1 gm. of a liquid at its boiling point to vapor at the same temperature. The latent heat of steam is 540 calories; therefore, when steam cools to liquid, each gm. gives out 540 calories. This explains why it is that a scald from steam is much more severe than one caused by boiling water.

h., luminous. That derived from light. This may be borne better than other forms of radiation. Light may be converted into heat. Short infrared rays penetrate subcutaneous tissues to a greater extent than long, invisible rays.

h., mechanical equivalent of. The value of heat units in terms of work units. One calorie equals 426.5 grammeters or 3.085 foot-pounds.

h., moist. May be applied as hot bath pack, hot wet pack, hot foot bath, fomentations, poultices or vapor bath. WARNINGS: Watch for chill, fainting, dizziness, headache, collapse, faintness, increased pulse, weakness. Cold applications to head should be used during and after treatment. Opinion regarding therapeutic use of heat or cold differs.

h., molecular. Result of multiplying a substance's molecular weight by its specific heat.

h., prickly. Vesicles due to obstruction or acute inflammation of sweat glands. SYN: *miliaria.*

h., radiant. Heat given off from a heated body and which passes through the air in form of waves.

h. rays. Visible rays from 4000-7000 A. U. and infrared rays from 6000-14,000 A. U.

h. recovery. Muscular heat produced after relaxation is complete.

h., sensible. Heat producing a temperature rise when absorbed by a body.

h., specific. The heat or number of calories needed to raise the temperature of 1 gram of a substance 1° C.

h. therapy. Use of heat in treatment of the body.

h. therapy, wet. Application of heat by hot water, steam and mud baths, and the hot pack, etc.

h. unit. A calorie, *q.v.*

heat'stroke. Result of direct exposure to high temperatures or to sun, usually in adults; esp. those who have been taking alcoholic beverages or who are debilitated or fatigued. This disease is the direct result of excess storage of heat in the body.

SYM: Early symptoms are dizziness, weakness, nausea, spots before the eyes and ringing in the ears. Bright red, dry skin; rapid, strong pulse, later becoming weak. Unconsciousness usually follows. Temperature may reach 108°; occasionally 112°. Latter patients usually do not recover.

F. A. TREATMENT: Patient should be cooled off in any conceivable manner. Remove clothing. Apply cold cloths, or pour cold water over person. Gently massage to help circulate blood. Cold water irrigations of the bowel are of value. Do not give stimulants of any sort. Heatstroke is a grave emergency, and must be treated promptly.

hebeosteotomy (he″be-os-te-ot′o-mĭ) [G. *ēbē*, pubes, + *osteon*, bone, + *tomē*, incision]. Section of the pubic bone in order to enlarge the pelvic opening for facilitation of delivery. SYN: *pubiotomy*.

hebephrenia (hē-bē-frē′nĭ-ă) [G. *ēbē*, puberty, + *phrēn*, mind]. A type of schizophrenic reaction characterized by infantile behavior, regression and deterioration, shallow emotional responses, illogical and senseless thought processes and actions, delusions and hallucinations. Patient may laugh often without cause, talk incoherently and excessively, undergo rapid mood change. Occurs often at age of or following puberty.

hebosteotomy (he-bos-te-ot′o-mĭ) [G. *ēbē*, pubes, + *osteon*, bone, + *tomē*, incision]. Enlargement of pelvic diameter by section of the pelvis to aid delivery. SYN: *hebotomy; pubiotomy*.

hebot′omy [" + *tomē*, incision]. Section through the pubis to facilitate labor. SYN: *hebosteotomy; pubiotomy*.

hecateromeric (hek-ă-ter″o-mer′ik) [G. *ekateros*, each of two, + *meros*, part]. Having processes on a spinal neuron, one supplying each side of the spinal cord.

hecatomeric (hek-ă-to-mer′ik) [G. *ekateros*, each of two, + *meros*, part]. Having a process which divides into two parts, as that of a spinal sensory neuron, one passing to each side of the spinal cord.

hectic (hek′tik) [G. *ektikos*, habitual]. Habitual or constitutional.

h. fever. A form of fever that occurs in connection with an organic disease, that is attended by some continuous and exhausting drain upon the system, as in pulmonary tuberculosis or abscess of liver or kidney.

Heatstroke *versus* Heat Exhaustion

Heat or Sunstroke	Heat Exhaustion
Definition: A condition or derangement of the heat-control centers due to exposure to the rays of the sun or very high temperatures	**Definition:** A state of very definite weakness produced by the loss of the normal fluids and sodium chloride of the body
History: Exposure to sun's rays or extreme heat.	**History:** Exposure to heat, usually indoors
Differential Symptoms:	**Differential Symptoms:**
Face: Red, dry, and hot	*Face:* Pale, cool, and moist
Skin: Hot, dry, and no diaphoresis	*Skin:* Cool, clammy, with profuse diaphoresis
Temperature: High, 106° to 110° F.	*Temperature:* Slight elevation to subnormal
Pulse: Full, strong, bounding	*Pulse:* Weak, thready, and rapid
Respirations: Dyspneic and sonorous	*Respirations:* Shallow and quiet
Muscles: Tense and possible convulsions	*Muscles:* Tense and contracted
Eyes: Pupils are dilated but equal	*Eyes:* Pupils are normal, eyeballs may be soft
Treatment: Absolute rest with head elevated. Cold packs to promote heat loss.	**Treatment:** Keep patient quiet; head should be lowered. Keep body warm to prevent shock symptoms
Drugs: Allow no stimulants; give infusions of normal saline (to force fluids)	*Drugs:* Aromatic spirits of ammonia. Salt tablets and fruit juices in abundant amounts. Intravenous isotonic saline will be required if patient is unconscious.

hebephrenic (he-be-fren′ik) [" + *phrēn*, mind]. Pert. to hebephrenia.

Heb′erden's asthma [William Heberden, English physician, 1710-1801]. Paroxysms of severe pain about heart and down left arm, with sense of oppression. SYN: *angina pectoris, q.v.*

H.'s disease. Arthritis deformans.

H.'s nodes. Hard nodules or enlargements of tubercles of last phalanges of fingers; seen in osteoarthritis.

hebetic (he-bet′ik) [G. *ēbē*, puberty]. Pert. to or occurring at the time of puberty.

hebet′omy [G. *ēbē*, pubes, + *tomē*, incision]. Section through pelvis to aid obstructed delivery. SYN: *pubiotomy*.

hebetude (heb′ĕ-tūd) [L. *hebetūdō; hebere*, to be dull]. Mental dullness, as seen in exhaustive conditions.

There may be latent conditions suddenly manifesting themselves during the course of a disease not concerned with such a condition but aggravated by the sickness, such as a sudden appearance of hysteria, or the development of a phobia, hallucinations, or delusions.

h. flush. The bright pink-red spot that appears on the cheek during a paroxysm of hectic fever.

hec′togram [G. *ekaton*, hundred, + *gramma*, weight]. One hundred grams, or 1543.7 grains.

hec′toliter [" + *litra*, a pound]. One hundred liters.

hec′tometer [" + *metron*, measure]. One hundred meters.

hedge′hog crys′tals. Globular crystals of ammonium urate with spines found in urine.

hedonia. Excessive cheerfulness; amenomania.

hedonism (he′don-izm) [G. *ēdonē*, pleasure, + *ismos*, state]. A theory or standard of conduct in which the principal object of life is pleasure.

hedrocele (hed′ro-sēl) [G. *edra*, anus, + *kēlē*, hernia]. Hernia; prolapse through the anus. SYN: *proctocele*.

heel [A.S. *huela*, heel]. Post. extremity of foot. SYN: *calx*.

h. bone. Bone at back of tarsus. SYN: *os calcis; calcaneum; calcaneus*.

Hegar's sign (hay'garz) [Alford Hegar, Freiburg gynecologist, 1830-1914]. Sign present during 2nd and 3rd month of pregnancy, due to: (1) Softening of lower segments of uterus; (2) at this stage, the ovum does not fill the uterine cavity, so there is an empty space in its lower part. On bimanual examination the lower part of uterus is easily compressed bet. fingers in the vagina and those of the other hand.

Heidenhain's demilunes (hi'den-hinz) [Rudolph P. Heidenhain, German physiologist, 1834-1897]. Crescent-shaped groups of serous cells at the base of or along the sides of the mucous alveoli of the salivary glands, esp. sublingual and submaxillary; also called *crescents of Gianuzzi.*

height (hīt) [A.S. *hiehthu*]. Distance to which anything rises above that surface on which it rests.

Heine-Medin disease (hi'ne-ma'dĭn) [Jacob Heine, German physician, 1800-1879; Karl O. Medin, Swedish physician, 1847-1928]. Acute infectious disease accompanied by motor paralysis and muscular atrophy, frequently with permanent deformity. SYN: *acute anterior poliomyelitis.**

Heinz bodies. Degenerated red blood cells due to damaged hemoglobin. The altered hemoglobin appears as a granule in the red cell. The bodies are seen easily when the blood is stained with a special stain. Condition is usually associated with hemolytic anemia due to drug sensitivity. May also be seen in premature infants.

Heinz body anemia. Hemolytic anemia of infancy associated with the finding of Heinz bodies in the red cells.

Heister, spiral valve of [Lorenz Heister, German anatomist, 1683-1758]. A spiral fold of the mucous membrane lining the cystic duct. It serves to keep the lumen open.

helcoid (hel'koid) [G. *elkos*, ulcer, + *eidos*, form]. Resembling an ulcer.

helcology (hel-kol'o-jĭ) [" + *logos*, study]. The study of ulcers.

helcoplasty (hel'ko-plas-tĭ) [" + *plassein*, to form]. Grafting healthy skin on ulcers. SEE: *dermatoplasty.*

helco'sis [" + *ōsis*]. The development of an ulcer. SYN: *ulceration.*

helicine (hel'ĭ-sin) [G. *elix*, coil]. Pert. to a helix or coil; spiral.

h. arteries. Term applied to tortuous arteries in cavernous tissue of the penis and clitoris, and in the uterus.

helicoid (hel'ĭ-koyd) [" + *eidos*, resemblance]. Resembling a helix or spiral.

helicopodia (hel''ĭ-ko-po'dĭ-ă) [G. *elix*, coil, + *pous, pod-*, foot]. A peculiar movement in which the foot, when brought forward, drags and describes a partial arc. Results in a gait such as seen in spastic hemiplegia.

helicotrema (hel-ĭ-ko-tre'mă) [G. *elix*, coil, + *trema*, a hole]. The opening at the tip of the cochlear canal where the scala tympani and scala vestibuli unite.

heliencephalitis (he''lĭ-en-sef-ă-li'tis) [G. *elios*, sun, + *egkephalos*, brain, + *-itis*, inflammation]. Inflammation of the brain as the result of sunstroke.

heliopho'bia [" + *phobos*, fear]. Abnormal fear of the sun's rays esp. by one who has suffered a sunstroke.

helio'sis [" + *-ōsis*]. Sunstroke.

heliotherapy (he-lĭ-o-ther'ă-pĭ) [" + *therapeia*, treatment]. The therapeutic application of radiation from the sun which includes infrared, ultraviolet and visible radiation. SEE: *solarium.*

heliotropism (he-lĭ-ot'ro-pizm) [" + *trepein*, to turn, + *ismos*, state of]. Chemotropism induced by the action of

HEIGHT AND WEIGHT TABLE

Person	Age	Height (in.) Without shoes	Weight (lb.)		
	Months:				
Infants	2-6	24	13		
	7-12	28	20		
	Years:				
Children	1-3	34	27		
	4-6	43	40		
	7-9	51	60		
	10-12	57	79		
Boys	13-15	64	108		
	16-19	69	139		
Girls	13-15	63	108		
	16-19	64	120		
			Frame		
			Small	Medium	Large
Women	25 and over	62	108-116	113-126	121-138
		64	114-123	120-135	129-146
		66	122-131	128-143	137-154
Men	25 and over	66	128-137	134-147	142-161
		69	140-150	146-160	155-174
		72	152-162	158-175	168-189

sunlight; the tendency of an organism to turn toward or grow toward sunlight.

he'lium [G. *elios*, sun]. SYMB: He. A gaseous element. It is given off by radium and other radioactive elements as charged helium ions known as alpha rays. At. wt. 4.0026; at. no. 2.

Because of its low density, it being next to the lightest element known, it is mixed with air or oxygen and used in the treatment of various respiratory disorders. Because of its low solubility, it is mixed with air supplied to workers laboring under high atmospheric pressure, as in caissons. When so used, it reduces time required in adjustment to increasing or decreasing air pressure and reduces the danger of "bends."

helix (he'lix) [G. coil]. 1. Margin of the external ear. 2. A coil or spiral.

h., Watson-Crick. A double helix named after the two scientists who established its existence. Each half of the helix contains chemical compounds arranged in a specific sequence. Variation in the sequence of these compounds enables genetic information to be transmitted. The double helix is DNA or deoxyribonucleic acid.

Hel'ler's test [Johann F. Heller, Austrian pathologist, 1813-1871]. A test for the presence of albumin in urine.

Pour ½ in. of pure nitric acid into a clean test tube, and carefully overlay it with an equal quantity of urine. The presence of albumin is indicated by the appearance of an opaque white ring at the junction of the fluids; also known as the "cold" test. RS: *albumin, urine.*

Hel'lin's law [Dyonizy Hellin, Polish pathologist, 1867-1935]. Occurrence of twins once in 80 pregnancies, triplets once in 6400 pregnancies, quadruplets once in 512,000 pregnancies.

hel'minth [G. *elmins, elminth-*, worm]. 1. A worm-like animal. 2. More specifically any animal, either free-living or parasitic, belonging to the phyla Platyhelminthes (flatworms), Acanthocephala (spiney-headed worms), nemathelminthes (threadworms or roundworms) or Annelida (segmented worms).

helminthagogue (hel-minth'ă-gog) [" + *agōgos*, leading]. A remedy that expels worms. SYN: *vermifuge.*

helminthemesis (hel-min-them'ĕ-sis) [" + *emesis*, vomiting]. The vomiting of intestinal worms.

helminthiasis (hel-min-thi'ă-sis) [G. *elmins, elminth-*, worm]. Having intestinal parasites or worms.

helmin'thic [G. *elmins, elminth-*, worm]. 1. Pertaining to worms. 2. Pert. to that which expels worms. SYN: *anthelmintic; vermifugal.*

helminthicide (hel-min'thĭ-sīd) [" + L. *caedere*, to kill]. A worm-expelling drug. SYN: *vermicide.*

helminthoid. Wormlike or resembling a worm.

helminthol'ogy [" + *logos*, study]. The study of intestinal vermiform parasites.

helmintho'ma [" + *ōma*, tumor]. A parasitic worm tumor.

helminthophobia (hel-min-tho-fo'bĭ-ă) [" + *phobos*, fear]. Morbid dread of worms or delusion of being infested by them.

helmitol (hel'mi-tol). Proprietary name for a methenamine compound. Used as a urinary antiseptic.

heloma (he-lo'mă) [G. *ēlos*, nail, + *ōma*, tumor]. A callosity or corn. SYN: *clavus.*

helosis (he-lo'sis) [" + *-ōsis*]. The state of having corns.

helotomeia (he-lo-to-mi'ă) [" + *tomē*, incision]. Helotomy.

helot'omon [" + *tomē*, incision]. Surgical knife for cutting corns.

helotomy (he-lot'o-mĭ) [" + *tomē*, incision]. Surgical treatment of corns.

Helweg's bundle [Hans K. S. Helweg, Danish physician, 1847-1901]. A tract in cervical region of spinal cord. Fibers arise from cell bodies in olive of the medulla and upper region of cord. SYN: *Helweg's tract; Bechterew's bundle.*

hemabarometer (hem"ă-bă-rom'ĕ-ter) [G. *aima*, blood, + *baros*, weight, + *metron*, measure]. Device for determining sp. gr. of blood.

hemachrome (hem'a-krōm) [" + *chrōma*, color]. The red coloring substance of blood. SEE: *hemoglobin.*

hemachro'sis [" + *chrōsis*, coloring]. Abnormal redness of blood.

hemacytom'eter [" + *kytos*, cell, + *metron*, measure]. Apparatus for counting blood corpuscles.

hemacytozoon (hem-ă-si-to-zo'on) [" + " + *zōon*, animal]. A protozoan parasite infesting red blood corpuscles.

hemad (he'mad) [A.S. *hem*, border, + L. *ad*, toward]. Toward the ventral or hemal aspect of the body. Opp. to neural or dorsal.

hemadostenosis (hem"ă-do-sten-o'sis) [G. *aimas, aimad-*, blood stream, + *stenōsis*, narrowing]. Contraction of blood vessels.

hemadromom'eter [G. *aima*, blood, + *dromos*, course, + *metron*, measure]. Device for recording rapidity of flow of blood. SYN: *hemodromometer.*

hemadynamometer (hem"ă-di"nă-mom'ĕ-ter) [" + *dynamis*, power, + *metron*, measure]. Device for determining blood pressure.

hemadynamometry (hem"ă-di-nă-mom'ĕ-trĭ) [" + " + *metron*, measure]. Measurement of blood pressure.

hemafa'cient [" + L. *facere*, to make]. A blood producing agent. SYN: *hematopoietic; sanguifacient.*

hemafecia (hem-ă-fe'sĭ-ă) [" + L. *faex, faec-*, dregs]. Feces containing blood.

hemagglutination (hem"ă-glu-tin-a'shun) [" + L. *agglutināre*, to paste to]. The clumping of red blood corpuscles.

hem"agglu'tinin [" + L. *agglutināre*, to paste to]. An antibody that induces clumping of red blood corpuscles.

h., cold. Agglutination of erythrocytes (usually sheep) at low temperatures by the serum of patients with certain diseases.

hemagogue (hem'ă-gog) [" + *agōgos*, leading]. An agent that favors the flow of blood or of the menses. SYN: *emmenagogue.*

he'mal [G. *aima*, blood]. 1. Pert. to the blood or blood vessels. 2. Pert. to side of the body in which the heart is located.

h. arch. The ribs, breastbone, and that part of the vertebrae which, together, enclose the heart and viscera.

h. gland. A hemal or hemolymph node.

h. node. A body resembling a lymph node in structure but associated with blood vessels instead of lymph vessels. Present in certain ungulates. SYN: *hemal gland; hemolymph gland or node.*

hemanal'ysis [" + *analysis*, a dissolving]. A blood analysis. SEE: *blood.*

hemangiectasis (hem"an-jĭ-ek'tă-sis) [" + *aggeion*, vessel, + *ektasis*, dilatation]. Dilatation of blood vessels.

hemangioblastoma (hem-an"ji-o-blas-to'mă) [" + " + *blastos*, germ, + *ōma*, tumor]. Hemangioma of the brain of a capillary nature.

hemangioendothelioma (hem"an-jĭ-o-en"-do-the-lĭ-o'mă) [" + " + *endon,* within, + *thēlē,* nipple, + *ōma,* tumor]. An overgrowth of the endothelium of the minute capillary vessels frequently on the cerebral meninges.

hemangioma (hem-an-jĭ-o'mă) (pl. *hemangiomata*) [" + " + *ōma,* tumor]. An angioma consisting of blood vessels.

hemangiomatosis (hem"an-jĭ-o-ma-to'sis) [" + " + " + *-ōsis*]. Multiple angiomata of blood vessels.

hemangiosarcoma (hem"an-jĭ-o-sar-ko'mă) [" + " + *sarx,* flesh, + *ōma,* tumor]. A mixed sarcoma and hemangioma. Syn: *angiosarcoma.*

hemaphein (hem-af-e'in) [G. *aima,* blood, + *phaios,* tawny]. Brown coloring matter in the blood; a decomposition product of hematin.

hemapoiesis (hem-ă-poy-e'sis) [" + *poiein,* to form]. Blood formation. Syn: *hematopoiesis.*

hemapoietic (hem-ă-poy-et'ik) [" + *poiein,* to form]. Pert. to hemapoiesis. Syn: *hematogenic; hematoplastic.*

hemapophysis (hem-ă-pof'ĭ-sis) [G. *aima,* blood, + *apo,* from, + *physis,* growth]. Portion of a developing vertebra which forms a rib and costal cartilage.

hemarthros (hem-ar'thros) [" + *arthron,* joint]. Bloody effusion into cavity of a joint. Syn: *hemarthrosis.*

hemarthrosis (hem-ar-thro'sis) [" + " + *-ōsis*]. Effusion of blood in a joint cavity.

hematachometer (hem-ă-tă-kom'ĕ-ter) [" + *tachus,* swift, + *metron,* measure]. Device for determining rapidity of the circulation.

hematapostema (hem"at-ap-os-te'mă) (pl. *hematapostemata*) [" + *apostēma,* abscess]. Abscess containing extravasated blood.

hemateikon (hem-at-i'kon) [G. *aima,* blood, + *eikon,* image]. A microscopic picture of the blood.

hematemesis (hem-at-em'ĕ-sis) [" + *emesis,* vomiting]. Vomiting of blood.

Sym: Blood often clotted and mixed with food, acid in reaction. Subsequent stools may be tarry; associated symptoms point to stomach. If of gastric origin, the blood is generally dark and acid. If of pharyngeal origin, it is bright red and alkaline in reaction. If loss of blood is severe enough, shock and collapse may occur.

Treatment: Absolute rest, nothing by mouth, nourishment through rectal enemas. No stimulants. May take broth. Have patient lie down; cold applications—ice bag to abdominal region. Keep quiet. Surgery may be necessary. See: *hemoptysis; hemorrhage.*

hematencephalon (hem-at-en-sef'ă-lon) [" + *egkephalos,* brain]. Cerebral hemorrhage.

hematherapy (hem-ă-ther'ă-pĭ) [" + *therapeia,* treatment]. Adm. of fresh blood in treatment of disease.

hemathermal [G. *aima,* blood, + *thermē,* heat]. Warm blooded, applied to animals whose blood remains at a fairly constant temperature. Syn: *hematothermal.*

hemather'mous [" + *thermē,* heat]. Warm blooded. Syn: *hemathermal; hematothermal.*

hemathidrosis, hematidrosis (he-mat-hi-dro'sis) [" + *idrōs,* sweat, + *-ōsis*]. Condition of sweating blood.

hematic (he-mat'ik) [G. *aima,* blood]. 1. Rel. to the blood. 2. A remedy for anemia.

hematimeter (hem-ă-tim'ĕ-ter) [" + *metron,* measure]. Apparatus for counting blood corpuscles in a cu.mm. of blood. Syn: *hematometer; hemocytometer.*

hem'atin [G. *aima,* blood]. An acid radicle or brown amorphous substance that unites with globin in the formation of hemoglobin.

It can be prepared from hemoglobin by the action of acids, alkalies, or enzymes. It is the iron-containing pigment of hemoglobin.

h. hydrochloride. The hydrochloric acid ester of hematin, crystalline in form.

Crystals dark brown and often seen in groups. Syn: *Teichmann's crystals.*

hematinemia (hem-ă-tin-e'mĭ-ă) [hematin + G. *aima,* blood]. Hematin in the circulating blood.

hematinic (hem-ă-tin'ĭk) [G. *aima,* blood]. 1. Pert. to blood. Syn: *hematic.* 2. An agent which increases the amount of hemoglobin in the blood.

hematinometer (hem-ă-tin-om'ĕ-ter) [" + *metron,* measure]. Device for determining quantity of hemoglobin in blood.

hematinu'ria [" + *ouron,* urine]. Hematin in the urine. Syn: *hemoglobinuria.*

hematischesis (hem-ă-tis'kĭ-sis) [" + *schesis,* checking]. Arrest of bleeding or hemorrhage.

hemato'bium [" + *bios,* life]. A parasite that lives in the blood. Syn: *hematozoon.*

hematoblast (hem'ă-to-blast) [G. *aima,* blood, + *blastos,* germ]. 1. A hemocytoblast, *q.v.* 2. Old term for blood platelet.

hematocele (hem'ă-to-sēl) [" + *kēlē,* hernia]. 1. A blood cyst. 2. Effusion of blood into a cavity. 3. Swelling due to effusion of blood into the *tunica vaginalis testis.*

h., parametric, pelvic, retrouterine. Tumor formed by blood effusion in the *cul-de-sac* of Douglas walled off by adhesions.

Etiol: Usually leakage from a fallopian tube, the seat of ectopic gestation.

Treatment: Rest, applications of cold and pressure to limit increase of size. Aspiration may be needed or incision if there are clots.

h., pudendal. A bloody tumor of the labium.

hematocelia (hem"ă-to-se'lĭ-ă) [" + *koilia,* cavity]. Hemorrhage into the peritoneal cavity.

hematoceph'alus [G. *aima,* blood, + *kephalē,* head]. Fetus born with infusion of blood in the head.

hematochezia (hem"ă-to-ke'zĭ-ă) [" + *chezein,* to go to stool]. Passage of stools containing blood.

hematochromato'sis [" + *chrōma,* color, + *-ōsis*]. A condition showing staining of tissues with blood pigment due to abnormal and excessive deposition of iron from hemoglobin or excessive ingestion of iron. Syn: *hemochromatosis.*

hematochyluria (hem"ă-to-ki-lu'rĭ-ă) [" + *chylos,* juice, + *ouron,* urine]. Blood and chyle in the urine.

hematocolpometra (hem"ă-to-kol"po-me'-tra) [" + *kolpos,* vagina, + *mētra,* uterus]. Retention of menstrual blood in the vagina and uterus.

hematocolpos (hem-ă-to-kol'pos) [" + *kolpos,* vagina]. Retained menstrual blood in the vagina from an imperforate hymen.

hematocrit (he-mat′o-krit) [" + *krinein*, to separate]. 1. Centrifuge for separating solids from plasma in the blood. 2. The volume of erythrocytes packed by centrifugation in a given volume of blood. The hematocrit is expressed as the percentage of total blood volume which consists of erythrocytes or as the volume in cubic centimeters of erythrocytes packed by centrifugation of blood. Normal values, at sea level, men: average 47%, range 40% to 54%; women: average 42%, range 37% to 47%.

hematocryal (hem-ă-to-kri′al) [" + *kryos*, cold]. Possessing cold blood.

hematocrystallin (hem-ă-to-kris′tal-in) [" + *krystallos*, crystal]. The coloring matter of the blood. SYN: *hemoglobin*.

hematocyst (hem′ă-to-sist) [" + *kystis*, a bladder]. A blood cyst.

hematocyte (hem′ă-to-sīt) [G. *aima*, blood, + *kytos*, cell]. A blood corpuscle.

hematocytoblast (hem″ă-to-si′to-blast) [" + " + *blastos*, germ]. A cell in bone marrow.

Granular leukocytes of myeloid origin are assumed to be derived from it. SYN: *leukoblast; lymphoidocyte; myeloblast*.

hematocytolysis (hem″ă-to-si-tol′ĭ-sis) [" + " + *lysis*, dissolution]. Dissolution of blood corpuscles freeing hemoglobin. SYN: *hemolysis*.

hematocytometer (hem″ă-to-si-tom′ĕ-ter) [" + " + *metron*, measure]. Device for determining number of corpuscles in given quantity of blood.

hematocytozoon (hem″ă-to-si-to-zo′on) [" + " + *zōon*, animal]. A parasite which lives in red blood corpuscles.

hematocyturia (hem″ă-to-si-tu′rĭ-ă) [" + " + *ouron*, urine]. Red blood corpuscles in urine; hematuria* as differentiated from hemoglobinuria.*

hematodyscrasia (hem″ă-to-dis-kra′zĭ-ă). A pathological condition of the blood.

hematodystrophy (hem″ă-to-dis′tro-fĭ) [" + *dys*, bad, + *trophē*, nutrition]. Any disorder of blood, such as anemia.*

hematogenesis (hem″ă-to-jen′ĕ-sis) [" + *genesis*, formation]. The development of blood corpuscles. SYN: *hematopoiesis*.

hematogenic, hematogenous (hem-ă-to-jen′ik, -toj′ĕ-nus) [" + *gennan*, to produce]. 1. Pert. to formation of blood. 2. Pert. to or originating in the blood. SYN: *hematopoietic*.

hematoglob′ulin [" + L. *globus*, globe]. Coloring matter of blood. SYN: *hemoglobin; oxyhemoglobin*.

hematohidrosis (hem″ă-to-hī-dro′sis) [" + *idrōs*, sweat, + *-ōsis*]. Excretion of bloody sweat. SYN: *hemathidrosis*.

hematohistioblast (hem″ă-to-his′tĭ-o-blast) [" + *istos*, tissue, + *blastos*, germ]. A polymorphous white blood cell of large size forming connective tissue.

hematoid (hem′ă-toyd) [G. *aima*, blood, + *eidos*, resemblance]. Resembling blood.

hematoidin (hem-ă-toy′din) [" + *eidos*, resemblance]. An iron-free principle in remains of old blood clots.

hematokolpos. Hematocolpos.

hematokrit. Hematocrit.

hem′atolith [" + *lithos*, stone]. Concretion in a blood vessel wall. SYN: *hemolith*.

hematologist (he″mă-tol′o-jist). One who specializes in the study of the blood.

hematology (he″mă-tol′o-jĭ) [" + *logos*, science]. The science of the blood.

hematolymphangioma (hem″ă-to-limf-an″-jĭ-o′mă) [" + L. *lympha*, lymph, + G. *aggeion*, vessel, + *ōma*, tumor]. A tumor consisting of dilated blood vessels and lymphatics.

hematolysis (hem-ă-tol′ĭ-sis) [" + *lysis*, dissolution]. A term applied to (a) diminished coagulability, or (b) to the destruction or disorganization of the blood and its corpuscles. SEE: *hemolysis*.

hematolytic (hem-ă-to-lit′ik) [" + *lysis*, dissolution]. Pert. to hematolysis. SYN: *hemolytic*.

hematoma (hem-ă-to′mă) [G. *aima*, blood, + *ōma*, tumor]. A blood tumor.

h. auris. One beneath perichondrium of ear cartilage.

h., pelvic. One affecting cellular tissue of pelvis. TREATMENT: Cold applications, rest, compression, massage.

h., subdural. H. located beneath the dura, usually the result of head injuries.

h., vulvar. H. occurring on the vulva. SYM: Distention and purplish swelling. TREATMENT: Surgical; light pack which is removed in approximately 24 hours.

hematomediastinum (hem″ă-to-me″dĭ-ă-sti′num) [" + L. *mediastinus*, in the middle]. Blood effusion into the mediastinum.

hematometer (he-mă-tom′ĕ-ter) [" + *metron*, measure]. Device for determining the properties of blood.

hematometra (he″mă-to-me′tră) [" + *mētra*, uterus]. 1. Hemorrhage in the uterus. 2. Accumulation of menstrual blood in the womb. SEE: *hematocolpos; hydrometra; pyometra*.

hematom′etry [" + *metron*, measure]. Determination of varieties and number of blood cells and percentage of hemoglobin in the blood.

hematomphalocele (hem″at-om-fal′o-sēl) [" + *omphalos*, navel, + *kēlē*, hernia]. Effusion of blood into an umbilical hernia.

hematomyelia (he-mă-to-mi-e′lĭ-ă) [" + *myelos*, marrow]. Hemorrhage of blood into the spinal cord.

hematomyelitis (hem″ă-to-mi-el-i′tis) [" + " + *-itis*, inflammation]. Inflammation of spinal cord with bloody effusion.

hematomyelopore (hem-at-o-mi′el-o-pōr) [" + " + *poros*, opening]. Porous condition of the spinal cord resulting from hemorrhages.

hematonephrosis (hem-ă-to-ne-fro′sis) [" + *nephros*, kidney, + *ōsis*]. Blood distending the pelvis of the kidney.

hematopathol′ogy [" + *pathos*, disease, + *logos*, study]. The study of morbid conditions of the blood.

hematopericar′dium [" + *peri*, around, + *kardia*, heart]. Bloody effusion into the pericardial sac.

hematoperitone′um [" + *peritonaion*, peritoneum]. Bloody effusion into the peritoneal cavity. SYN: *hemoperitoneum*.

hematopex′in [" + *pēxis*, fixation]. That which coagulates blood. SYN: *hemopexin*.

hematopex′is [" + *pēxis*, fixation]. Coagulation of the blood. SYN: *hemopexia*.

hem′atophage [" + *phagein*, to eat]. A phagocytic cell which destroys red blood corpuscles.

hematophagia (hem-ă-to-fa′jĭ-ă) [" + *phagein*, to eat]. 1. Subsistence on blood. 2. Adm. of blood as a treatment.

hematophagous (hem-ă-tof′ă-gus) [" + *phagein*, to eat]. Living on blood.

hematophilia (hem-ă-to-fil′ĭ-ă) [G. *aima*, blood, + *philein*, to love]. Congenital condition characterized by defective blood coagulation causing copious hemorrhages. SYN: *hemophilia.*

hematophobia (hem"ă-to-fō'bĭ-ă) [G. *aima, aimat-,* blood, + *phobos,* fear]. Abnormal aversion to the sight of blood.

hematophyte (hem'ă-to-fīt) [" + *phyton,* plant]. Plant organism or bacteria in the blood.

hematopla'nia [" + *planē,* wandering]. Condition of vicarious menstruation.

hematoplas'tic [" + *plassein,* to form]. Pert. to formation of blood. SYN: *hematopoietic.*

hematopneic (hem-ă-top-ne'ĭk) [" + *pnein,* to breathe]. Rel. to oxygenation of the blood.

hematopoiesis (he"mă-to-poy-e'sis) [" + *poiein,* to form]. The formation of red blood corpuscles.

Tissues which can produce red corpuscles are said to be *hematopoietic,* as, for instance, the red bone marrow.

h., extramedullary. Normally the blood cells are formed exclusively in the bone marrow. In severe anemia and in other diseases affecting the blood, blood cell formation takes place in tissues other than bone marrow (extramedullary hematopoiesis).

hematopoietic (hem"ă-to-poy-et'ik) [" + *poiein,* to make]. Rel. to blood-making processes. SYN: *hematogenic; hematoplastic.*

hematoporphyrin (hem"ă-to-por'fĭ-rin) [" + *porphyra,* purple]. Iron-free hematin; a decomposition product of hemoglobin in the urine in certain conditions.

hematoporphyrinuria (hem"ă-to-por"fĭ-rin-u'rĭ-ă) [" + " + *ouron,* urine]. Hematoporphyrin in urine.

hematorrhachis (he-mă-tor'ră-kis) [" + *rachis,* spine]. Hemorrhage into the spinal cord.

hematorrhea (he-mă-to-re'ă) [" + *roia,* flow]. Profuse hemorrhage.

hematosalpinx (he-mă-to-sal'pinks) [" + *salpigx,* tube]. Retained menstrual fluid in the fallopian tube.

hematoscheocele (hem-ă-tos'ke-o-sēl) [" + *oscheon,* scrotum, + *kēlē,* hernia]. Blood accumulated in the scrotum.

hematoscope (hem'ă-to-skōp) [" + *skopein,* to examine]. Device for examining the blood.

hematoscopy (hem-ă-tos'ko-pĭ) [" + *skopein,* to examine]. Examination of the blood.

hematose (hem'ă-tōs) [" + *-ōsis*]. Full of blood.

hematosepsis (hem-ă-to-sep'sis) [" + *sēpsis,* putrefaction]. Blood toxemia. SYN: *septicemia.*

hematospec'troscope [" + L. *spectrum,* image, + G. *skopein,* to examine]. Spectroscope for inspecting the blood.

hematospectros'copy [" + " + G. *skopein,* to examine]. Examination of the blood with the hematospectroscope.

hematospermatocele (hem"ă-to-sper-mat'-o-sēl) [" + *sperma,* seed, + *kēlē,* tumor]. A blood-filled spermatocele.

hematospermia (hem-ă-to-sper'mĭ-ă) [" + *sperma,* seed]. Bloody semen.

h. spuria. When coming from the prostatic urethra.

h. vera. When coming from the seminal vessels.

hematostatic (hem"ă-to-stat'ik) [G. *aima,* blood, + *stasis,* a standing]. 1. Retaining blood in a part. 2. Pertaining to the arrest of blood flow in a hemorrhage. SYN: *hemostatic.*

hematosteon (hem-ă-tos'te-on) [" + *osteon,* bone]. Bleeding into the medullary cavity of a bone.

hematother'mal [" + *thermē,* heat]. Warm blooded. SYN: *hemathermal; hemathermous.*

hematothorax (hem-ă-to-tho'raks) [" + *thōrax,* chest]. Blood in the chest. SYN: *hemothorax.*

hematotox'ic [" + *toxikon,* poison]. Pert. to toxemia.

hematotrachelos (hem"ă-to-tră-ke'los) [" + *trachēlos,* neck]. Retained menstrual blood in cervix uteri causing distention.

hematotympanum (hem-ă-to-tĭm'pan-um) [" + *tympanon,* drum]. Blood in the middle ear.

hematoxylin. A colorless crystalline compound, $C_{16}H_{14}O_6$. obtained by extraction with ether from logwood. Upon oxidation it is converted into hematein, an oxidation product of hematoxylin, which stains certain structures a deep blue color. It is an excellent nuclear stain, and widely used in histological work.

hematozoon (hem"ă-to-zo'on) [" + *zōon,* animal]. Any living organism in the blood.

hematozymosis (hem-ă-to-zi-mo'sis) [" + *zymōsis,* fermentation]. Blood fermentation.

hematuria (hem"ă-tu'rĭ-ă) [G. *aima,* blood, + *ouron,* urine]. Blood in the urine. NOTE: The occurrence of bright red blood in the urine and its appearance in the toilet bowl is quite frightening to the patient. Both the patient and the nurse should realize that a very small amount of blood may cause the entire toilet bowl contents to appear to be full of pure blood.

SYM: Urine may be slightly smoky, reddish, or very red.

ETIOL: Lesion of urinary tract, or blood dyscrasia, contamination during menstruation or puerperium, prostatic disease, tumors, poisoning esp. carbolic acid and cantharides, malaria and toxemias and calculus.

DIAG: If well mixed with urine, probably from kidneys. If clotted in tubular casts of ureters, from kidneys or ureters. If passed at beginning of urination, from the urethra; if at the end, from bladder.

h., renal. Urine smoky, sometimes bright red.

h., urethral. Always bright red. Precedes urination.

h., vesical. Urine bright red, not uniform.

hemaurochrome (hem"ă-u'ro-krōm) [" + *ouron,* urine, + *chrōma,* color]. A hematin derivative found in the urine in sarcoma and carcinoma, malaria, anemias and other disorders. Supposed to result from dissolution of red blood corpuscles.

heme (hēm). An iron-containing protoporphyrin derived from hemin when hemin is treated with sodium hydroxide. Heme can combine with a large number of organic nitrogenous substances to form *hemochromogens.* Formerly called *hematin.*

hemeralopia (hem-er-al-o'pĭ-ă) [G. *ēmera,* day, + *alaos,* blind, + *ōps,* eye]. Day blindness or night blindness, found particularly in macular lesions. Term formerly erroneously applied to night blindness or *nyctalopia* (inability to see in dim light).

The latter, *nyctalopia,* indicates inability to see in dim light though otherwise vision is normal.

In day blindness, the sight is poor in sunlight and in good illumination; it is good at dusk, at twilight, and in poor illumination. This is noted in albinism, retinitis with central scotoma, toxic amblyopia, coloboma of the iris and choroid, opacity of the crystalline lens or cornea, and in conjunctivitis with photophobia.

hemi- [G.]. Prefix meaning *half*.

hemiacephalus. A malformed fetus with a markedly defective head. SEE: *anencephalus*.

hemiachromatopsia (hem-ĭ-ă-kro-mă-top′-sĭ-ă) [G. *ēmi*, half, + *a-*, priv. + *chrōma*, color, + *opsis*, vision]. Color blindness in one-half, or in corresponding halves, of the visual field.

hemialbumin (hem-ĭ-al-bu′min) [" + L. *albumen*, white of egg]. A product resulting from the digestion of albumin. SYN: *antialbumin*.

hemialbumose (hem-ĭ-al′bu-mōs) [" + L. *albumen*, white of egg]. An albumoid product from the digestion of certain proteins. It occurs in bone marrow.

hemialbumosu′ria [" + " + G. *ouron*, urine]. Hemialbumose in the urine.

hemialgia (hem-ĭ-al′jĭ-ă) [" + *algos*, pain]. Pain in one-half of the body.

hemiamaurosis (hem″ĭ-am-aw-ro′sis) [" + *amaurosis*, darkness]. Blindness in one-half the visual field. SYN: *hemianopsia*.

hemiamblyopia (hem″ĭ-am-blĭ-o′pĭ-ă) [" + *amblys*, dim, + *ōps*, sight]. Blindness in half the visual field. SYN: *hemianopsia*.

hemiamyosthenia (hem″ĭ-a″mi-os-the′nĭ-ă) [" + *a-*, priv. + *mys*, *myo-*, muscle, + *sthenos*, strength]. Absence of normal muscular power on one side of the body. SYN: *hemiparesis*.

hemianacusia (hem″ĭ-an-ă-ku′zĭ-ă) [G. *ēmi*, half, + *an-*, priv. + *akousis*, hearing]. Deafness in one ear.

hemianalgesia (hem″ĭ-an-al-je′zĭ-ă) [" + " + *algos*, pain]. Lack of sensibility to pain (analgesia) on one side of the body.

hemianesthesia (hem″ĭ-an-es-the′zĭ-ă) [" + " + *aisthēsis*, sensation]. Anesthesia of one-half of the body.

hemianopia, hemianopsia (hem-ĭ-ă-no′pĭ-ă, -nop′sĭ-ă) [" + " + *ōps*, eye]. Blindness for one-half field of vision in one or both eyes.

h., altitudinal. Blindness in upper or lower half in each eye.

h., binasal. Affection of nasal half of visual field in each eye.

h., bitemporal. Affection of temporal half of visual field in each eye.

h., complete. H. of half of each eye.

h., crossed. Bitemporal or binasal hemianopsia.

h., heteronymous. SEE: *crossed h.*

h., homonymous. Blindness of nasal half of one eye and temporal half of the other or right-sided or left-sided h. of corresponding sides in both eyes.

h., incomplete. H. of less than half of each eye.

h., quadrant. Affection of symmetrical quadrant of the field in each eye.

h., unilateral, uniocular. Hemianopsia affecting only one eye.

hemianosmia (hem″ĭ-an-os′mĭ-ă) [G. *ēmi*, half, + *an-*, priv. + *osmē*, smell]. Loss of smell in one nostril.

hemiapraxia (hem″ĭ-ă-prak′sĭ-ă) [" + *a-*, priv. + *prassein*, to do]. Incapacity to exercise purposeful movements on one side of the body.

hemiarthrosis (hem-ĭ-ar-thro′sis) [" + *arthron*, joint, + *ōsis*]. A false articulation bet. two bones. SYN: *synchondrosis*.

hemiasynergia (hem″ĭ-as-in-er′jĭ-ă) [" + *a-*, priv. + *syn*, with, + *ergon*, work]. Lack of coordination of parts affecting one side of the body.

hemiataxia (hem-ĭ-ă-taks′ĭ-ă) [" + *ataxia*, lack of order]. Impaired muscular coordination causing awkward movements of the affected side of the body.

hemiathetosis (hem″ĭ-ath-ĕ-to′sis) [" + *athetos*, without fixed position, + *-ōsis*]. Slow change of position; athetosis of one side of the body.

hemiatrophy (hem-ĭ-at′ro-fĭ) [" + *atrophia*, atrophy]. Impaired nutrition resulting in atrophy of one side of the face or other part; marked by white or yellow macules on affected side.

hemiballism (hem-ĭ-bal′izm) [" + *ballismos*, jumping]. Jerking and twitching movements of one side of the body. SYN: *hemichorea*.

he′mic [G. *aima*, blood]. Pert. to blood. SYN: *hemal*.

hemicanities (hem″ĭ-kan-ish′ĭ-ēz) [G. *ēmi*, half, + L. *canitiēs*, gray hair]. Grayness (*canities*) of hair on one side only.

hemicardia (hem-ĭ-kar′dĭ-ă) [" + *kardia*, heart]. Half of a four-chambered heart.

hemicellulose (hem-ĭ-sel′u-lōs) [G. *aima*, blood, + L. *cellula*, little cell]. One of a group of polysaccharides which differ from cellulose in that they may be hydrolyzed by dilute mineral acids and from other polysaccharides in that they are not readily digested by amylases. Includes pentosans, galactosans (agar agar), and pectins.

hemicentrum (hem-ĭ-sen′trum) [" + *kentron*, center]. Either lateral half of the centrum of a vertebra.

hemichorea (hem-ĭ-ko-re′ă) [" + *choreia*, a dancing]. Convulsive movements (*chorea*) of but one side of the body.

hemichromatopsia (hem″ĭ-kro-mă-top′-sĭ-ă) [" + *chrōma*, color, + *opsis*, vision]. Blindness to color in one-half of the visual field. SYN: *hemiachromatopsia*.

hemicrania (hem-ĭ-kra′nĭ-ă) [" + *kranion*, skull]. 1. Unilateral head pain, usually migraine. 2. Malformed fetus having only one-half of the skull developed.

hemicraniectomy (hem″ĭ-kra-nĭ-ek′to-mĭ) [" + " + *ektomē*, excision]. Surgical division of cranial vault from before backward, exposing half of the brain.

hemicraniosis (hem″ĭ-kra-nĭ-o′sis) [" + " + *ōsis*]. Enlargement of half of cranium or face.

hemidiaphoresis (hem″ĭ-di″ă-fo-re′sis) [" + *dia*, through, + *pherein*, to carry]. Sweating on one side of the body.

hemidi′aphragm [" + " + *phragma*, wall]. Paralysis affecting only one-half of the diaphragm.

hemidro′sis [" + *idrōsis*, sweat]. Bloody sweating. SYN: *hemathidrosis*.

hemidyser′gia [" + *dys*, bad, + *ergon*, work]. Lack of coordination of muscles (*dysergia*) on one side of the body.

hemidysesthesia (hem″ĭ-dis-es-the′zĭ-ă) [" + " + *aisthēsis*, sensation]. Impaired sensation (*dysesthesia*) of one-half of the body.

hemidystrophy (hem″ĭ-dis′tro-fĭ) [" + " + *trophē*, nourishment]. Inequality in development of the two sides of the body.

hemiep′ilepsy [" + *epilēpsia*, seizure]. Epilepsy with convulsions confined to lateral half of the body.

hemifa′cial [G. *ēmi*, half, + L. *faciēs*, face]. Pert. to one side of the face.

hemigastrectomy (hem″ĭ-gas-trek′to-mĭ) [" + *gastēr*, belly, + *ektomē*, excision].

Excision of pyloric end of the stomach for hourglass contraction.

hemigeusia (hem-ĭ-gu'sĭ-ă) [" + *geusis,* taste]. Loss of sense of taste on one side of the tongue.

hemiglossi'tis [" + *glōssa,* tongue, + *-ītis,* inflammation]. Vesicular eruption on one-half of the tongue and inner surface of cheek. Herpetic in character.

hemihidro'sis [" + *idrōsis,* perspiration]. Sweating on only one side of the body. SYN: *hemidiaphoresis.*

hemihyperesthesia (hem"ĭ-hi-per-es-the'-zĭ-ă) [" + *yper,* over, + *aisthēsis,* sensation]. Abnormal tactile and painful sensitiveness of one side of the body.

hemihyperidrosis (hem"ĭ-hi-per-ĭ-dro'sis) [" + " + *idrosis,* sweating]. Excessive perspiration confined to one side of the body.

hemihyperto'nia [" + " + *tonos,* tone]. Exaggerated tonicity of muscles on lateral half of the body.

hemihyper'trophy [" + " + *trophē,* nourishment]. Hypertrophy of muscles of one-half of the body or face.

hemihypesthesia (hem"ĭ-hi-pes-the'zĭ-ă) [" + *ypo,* under, + *aisthēsis,* sensation]. Diminished sensibility on one side of the body.

hemihypotonia (hem"ĭ-hi-po-to'nĭ-ă) [" + " + *tonos,* tone]. Partial loss of tonicity of muscles on one side of the body.

hemilat'eral [" + L. *latus,* side]. Rel. to one side only.

hemimelia (hem"ĭ-me'lĭ-ă) [G. " + *melos,* limb]. A malformed fetus with defective development of the extremities esp. the distal portion.

hemin (he'min) [G. *aima,* blood]. SYN: *heme hydrochloride.* A brownish red crystalline salt of heme formed when hemoglobin is heated with glacial acetic acid and sodium chloride. Used in testing for presence of blood.

h. crystals. Teichmann's crystals, formed when the above test is made.

heminephrectomy. Excision or removal of a portion of a kidney.

hemineurasthenia (hem"ĭ-nu-ras-the'nĭ-ă) [G. *ēmi,* half, + *neuron,* nerve, + *astheneia,* weakness]. Neurasthenia affecting one side of the body only.

hemiopia (hem-ĭ-o'pĭ-ă) [" + *ōps,* eye]. Blindness in half of the visual field. SYN: *hemianopia.*

hemiopic (hem-ĭ-op'ik) [" + *ōps,* eye]. Pert. to hemiopia.

hemiparal'ysis [" + *paralyein,* to loosen from the sides]. Paralysis of one side of the body only.

hemiparanesthesia (hem"ĭ-par-an-es-the'-zĭ-ă) [" + *para,* beyond, + *an-,* priv. + *aisthēsis,* sensation]. Anesthesia of one lower extremity or lower half of one side.

hemiparaplegia (hem"ĭ-par-ă-ple'jĭ-ă) [" + " + *plēgē,* stroke]. Paralysis of the lower half of one side or of one leg.

hemipar'esis [" + *paresis,* paralysis]. Slight paralysis of one side of the body.

hem"iparesthe'sia [" + *para,* beyond, + *aisthēsis,* sensation]. Numbness of one side of body.

hemipeptone (hem-ĭ-pep'tōn) [" + *peptein,* to digest]. One of the two compounds of peptone in pepsin digestion which later forms leucin, tyrosin, and amino acids.

hemiplegia (hem-ĭ-ple'jĭ-ă) [" + *plēgē,* a stroke]. Paralysis of only one-half of the body.

ETIOL: A brain lesion involving upper motor neurons and resulting in paralysis of the opposite side of the body. May result from cerebral apoplexy, softening or tumors of the cerebrum.

NP: Elevate head and shoulders. See that tongue does not obstruct breathing. Avoid stimulants. Do not move patient until arrival of doctor.

Chart nursing care and observations every 4 hours for the first 2 days. Turn patient frequently to avoid hypostatic pneumonia. Watch for bedsores, retention of urine, which should be measured and tested for albumin and sugar. Avoid burning with hot water bottles. Do not discuss patient when apparently unconscious.

SEE: *Benedict's syndrome; paralysis; thalamic syndrome.*

h., alternate. Affecting one side of face and trunk and opposite of extremities.

h., capsular. H. resulting from a lesion of the internal capsule.

h., cerebral. Due to brain lesion.

h., crossed. Alternate h.

h., facial. Paralysis of muscles of one side of face.

h., spastic. H. accompanied by spasms, usually occurring in infants.

h., spinal. H. resulting from a lesion of the spinal cord. SEE: *Brown-Sequard's paralysis.*

hemiplegic (hem-ĭ-ple'jik) [G. *ēmi,* half, + *plēgē,* stroke]. Pert. to hemiplegia.

Hemiptera (hem-ip'ter-ă). The true bugs; an order of insects characterized by piercing and sucking mouth parts; 1st pr. of wings leathery at base and membranous at tip, 2nd pair of wings membranous; incomplete metamorphosis. Includes bedbugs, kissing bugs, and several other species which are pests or transmitters of pathogenic organisms.

hemirachischisis (hem-ĭ-ră-kis'kis-is). Rachischisis in which protrusion of the spinal meninges does not occur; *spina bifida occulta, q.v.*

hemisec'tion [G. *ēmi,* half, + L. *sectio,* a cutting] The act of dividing a part or an organ into two halves; bisection. SYN: *bisection.*

hemisomus (hem"ĭ-so'mus) [G. " + *soma,* body]. Fetus with lateral half of body missing or malformed.

hemispasm (hem'ĭ-spazm) [" + *spasmos,* spasm]. Spasm of only one side of the body or face.

hemisphere (hem'ĭ-sfēr) [" + *sphaira,* sphere]. Either half of the cerebrum or cerebellum.

h., dominant. The cerebral hemisphere in which the higher cortical functions, esp. those relating to speech and certain motor activities, are associated; the left one in right-handed individuals. Results in phenomenon known as "cerebral dominance."

Hemis'pora stella'ta. A variety of fungus causing mycosis.

hemispore (hem'ĭ-spōr) [G. *ēmi,* half, + *sporos,* seed]. A spore which reproduces by division of terminal part of a hyphus.*

hemisporosis (hem-ĭ-spo-ro'sis) [" + *sporos,* seed, + *ōsis*]. Infection with a fungus (*Hemispora stellata*) resulting in swellings of bone and other tissue of a gummatous nature. They may later ulcerate.

hemistrumectomy (hem"ĭ-stru-mek'to-mĭ) [" + L. *struma,* goiter, + G. *ektomē,* excision]. Excision of about one-half of a goiter.

hemisyndrome (hem-ĭ-sin′drōm) [" + *syndromē*, a running with]. One indicating a unilateral lesion of the spinal cord.

hemisystole (hem-ĭ-sis′to-le) [G. *ēmi*, half, + *systole*, a contracting]. One pulse beat to every two heart beats. Results from failure of the ventricle to contract every other time.

hem″iterat′a. Individuals possessing congenital malformations but not to such a degree as to be designated a monster.

hemiteric, hemiteratic (hem-ĭ-ter′ĭk, -ter-at′ik) [" + *teras*. monster]. Congenitally deformed, but not severely so.

hemivertebra (hem″ĭ-ver′te-bră). Congenital absence of one-half of a vertebra.

hem′lock [A.S. *hemléac*]. 1. A species of fir tree. 2. Volatile oil extracted from hemlock tree.

Poisoning: Sym: Nausea, vomiting, diarrhea, salivation, pupils dilated.

Treatment: Empty stomach by means of a stomach pump or an emetic. Give a teaspoonful of tannic acid in glass of water. Stimulate.

he′mo-. Prefix meaning pertaining to the blood. See also *haemo- haem- hem- hema-* and *hemato-*.

he″moagglutina′tion [G. *aima*, blood, + L. *agglutināre*, to paste to]. The clumping of red blood corpuscles.

he″moagglu′tinin [" + L. *agglutināre*, to paste to]. An agglutinin which clumps the red blood corpuscles.

he″moalkalim′eter [" + Arab. *alkali*, the kali plant, + G. *metron*, measure]. A device for estimating degree of alkalinity of blood.

hemobilinuria (he″mo-bil-in-u′rĭ-ă) [" + L. *bilis*, bile, + G. *ouron*, urine]. Urobilin in the blood and urine.

he′moblast [" + *blastos*, germ]. Immature red blood corpuscles; a blood platelet. Syn: *hematoblast; hematocytoblast.*

hemoblastosis (he″mo-blas-to′sis) [" + " + *-ōsis*]. Changes occurring in or increase in amount of the blood-forming tissues.

hemocatheresis (he″mo-kath-er-e′sis) [" + *kathairesis*, destruction]. Dissolution of red blood corpuscles as in the spleen.

hemocatheretic (he″mo-kath-er-et′ik) [" + *kathairetikos*, destructive]. Destructive to blood corpuscles.

hemochorial (he″mo-kor′ĭ-al). Pertaining to the relationship between blood of the mother and the chorionic ectoderm. See: *placenta.*

hemochromatosis (he″mo-kro″mă-to′sis) [" + *chrōma*, color, + *-ōsis*]. A disease characterized by deposits of hemosiderin throughout the body. Occurs mostly in males. The majority of patients have bronzing of the skin, cirrhosis of the liver, and diabetes. Syn: *bronzed diabetes.*

he′mochrome [" + *chrōma*, color]. The red pigment of the blood.

he″mochro′mogen [G. *aima*, blood + *gennan*, to produce). General term applied to compounds of heme with nitrogen-containing substances such as a protein.

hemochromometer (he″mo-kro-mom′ĕ-ter) [G. *aima*, blood, + *chroma*, color, + *metron*, measure). A colorimeter used for estimating the amount of hemoglobin in the blood.

hemocla′sia, hemoc′lasis [" + *klasis*, destruction]. Disintegration of red blood corpuscles. Syn: *hemolysis.*

hemoclas′tic [" + *klasis*, destruction]. Destructive of erythrocytes. Syn: *hemolytic.*

he″moconcentra′tion. An increase in the number of red blood cells resulting from a decrease in the volume of plasma. Syn: *anhydremia.*

hemoco′nia [G. *aima*, blood, + *konis*, dust]. Minute colorless bodies in blood thought to be the products of disintegration of red blood cells. Also called *blood dust.* Syn: *hemokonia.*

hemoconio′sis [" + " + *-ōsis*]. Having an abnormal amt. of hemoconia in the blood.

he′moculture [" + L. *cultura*, development]. A bacteriological blood culture.

hemocyte (he′mo-sīt) [" + *kytos*, cell]. Blood corpuscle.

he″mocy′toblast [G. *aima*, blood, + L. *cultura*, + *blastos*, germ). The common lymphoid stem cell found in bone marrow from which all blood cells are thought to arise.

hemocytoblastoma (he″mo-si″to-blas-to′mă) [" + " + " + *ōma*, tumor]. A tumor containing embryonic blood cells.

hemocytocatheresis (he″mo-si″to-kath-er-e′sis) [" + " + *kathairesis*, destruction]. The dissolution of blood corpuscles.

hemocytogenesis (he″mo-si″to-jen′ĕ-sis) [G. *aima*, blood + *kytos*, cell, + *genesis*, development]. The formation of blood cells. Syn: *hematopoiesis.*

hemocytology (he″mo-si-tol′o-jĭ) [" + " + *logos*, study]. The science of blood cells.

hemocytolysis (he″mo-si-tol′ĭ-sis) [" + " + *lysis*, dissolution]. Dissolution of the blood corpuscles. Syn: *hematocytolysis; hemolysis.*

hemocytometer (he″mo-si-tom′ĕ-ter) [" + " + *metron*, measure]. Device for determining relative number of corpuscles in the blood.

hemocytopoiesis (he″mo-si″to-poy-e′sis) [" + " + *poiein*, to form]. The development of blood cells.

hemocytotripsis (he″mo-si″to-trip′sis) [" + " + *tripsis*, a crushing]. Fragmentation of the red blood corpuscles.

hemocytozoon (he″mo-si″to-zo′on) [" + " + *zōon*, animal]. An animal microparasite of the blood cells. Syn: *hematobium.*

hemo′dia. Extreme sensitivity of the teeth.

hemodiagno′sis [G. *aima*, blood, + *dia*, through, + *gnōsis*, knowledge]. Examination of the blood for diagnostic purpose.

hemodialysis (he″mo-di-al′ĭ-sis) [" + *dia*, through, + *lysis*, dissolve]. Removal of chemical substances from the blood by passing it through tubes made of semipermeable membranes. The tubes are being continually bathed by solutions which selectively remove the unwanted material from the blood.

Used to cleanse the blood of patients in whom one or both kidneys are defective or absent and to remove excess accumulation of drugs or toxic chemicals in the blood. See: *kidney, artificial.*

hemodi′astase [" + *diastasis*, separation]. An amylolytic ferment in the blood.

he″modilu′tion. An increase in the volume of blood plasma resulting in reduced concentration of red blood cells.

hemodromometer (he″mo-dro-mom′ĕ-ter) [" + *dromos*, course, + *metron*, measure]. Device for determining the blood's velocity.

hemodynam′ics [" + *dynamis*, power]. The study of circulation of the blood.

hemodynamometer (he″mo-di″nă-mom′ĕ-ter) [" + " + *metron*, measure]. Device for measuring blood pressure.

hemodystrophy (he″mo-dis′tro-fī) [" + *dys*, bad, + *trophē*, nutrition]. Imperfect nutrition of the blood. SYN: *hematodystrophy*.

hemoendothelial (he″mo-en″do-the′lĭ-al). Pertaining to the relationship between blood of the mother and the endothelium of chorionic vessels. SEE: *placenta*.

hemoferrum (he″mo-fer′um) [" + L. *ferrum*, iron]. The iron element of hemoglobin. SYN: *oxyhemoglobin*.

he″moflag′ellate. Any flagellate protozoan parasite of the blood. Includes trypanosomes and leishmanias.

hemofuscin (he″mo-fu′sin) [" + L. *fuscus*, brown]. Brown coloring matter derived from hemoglobin.

hemogenesis (he″mo-jen′ĕ-sis) [" + *genesis*, formation]. Blood formation. SYN: *hematogenesis*.

hemoge′nia [" + *gennan*, to produce]. A hemorrhagic condition of the blood-forming apparatus.

hemogen′ic [" + *gennan*, to produce]. Rel. to the production of blood.

hemoglobin (he-mo-glo′bin) [G. *aima*, blood, + L. *globus*, globe]. The iron-containing pigment of the red blood cells. Its function is to carry oxygen from the lungs to the tissues.

The amount of hemoglobin in the blood averages 14 to 16 grams per 100 ml. One gram of hemoglobin can combine with 1.34 ml. of oxygen, the resulting compound being oxyhemoglobin.

Hemoglobin is a crystallizable, conjugated protein consisting of an iron-containing pigment called *heme* or *hematin*, and a simple protein, *globin*. In the lungs it combines readily with oxygen to form a loose, unstable compound called *oxyhemoglobin*, a process called *oxygenation*. In the tissues where oxygen tension is low, oxyhemoglobin decomposes and oxygen is liberated. The resulting compound is *reduced hemoglobin*. Hemoglobin is a weak acid and in the red corpuscles is combined with potassium, an alkali, to form potassium hemoglobinate (an alkali), which acts to buffer carbonic acid formed from carbon dioxide entering the blood from the tissues. The buffering action is accomplished by a mechanism known as the *chloride shift*.

Hemoglobin liberated from disintegrating red blood cells is removed from circulation by the cells of the reticuloendothelial system, esp. those of the liver and spleen. The globin is converted to amino acids and reutilized. Iron from the iron-containing portion is stored in the liver and spleen and reutilized; the noniron containing pigment is converted to *bilirubin* which is excreted as one of the bile pigments.

Hemoglobin combines with carbon monoxide to form the stable compound carboxyhemoglobin. Oxidation of the ferrous iron of hemoglobin to the ferric state produces methemoglobin.

A large number of different types of hemoglobin have been discovered. Study of these has facilitated investigating human genetics. Hemoglobin is named according to the way the amino acid components of the globin move when studied by electrophoresis. There are more than a hundred different types of abnormal hemoglobin. Hemoglobin S is the abnormal form of hemoglobin found in persons with *sickle-cell disease*.

h., fetal. Hemoglobin found in the erythrocytes of the fetus which is capable of taking up and giving off oxygen at lower oxygen tensions than that in the erythrocytes of the adult.

hemoglobinemia (he″mo-glo-bin-e′mĭ-ă) [" + " + G. *aima*, blood]. Presence of hemoglobin in the blood plasma.

hemoglobinocholia (he″mo-glo″bin-o-ko′lĭ-ă) [" + " + G. *cholē*, bile]. Hemoglobin in the bile.

hemoglobinolysis (he″mo-glo-bin-ol′ĭ-sis) [" + " + G. *lysis*, dissolution]. Dissolution of hemoglobin.

hemoglobinometer (he″mo-glo-bin-om′ĕ-ter) [" + " + G. *metron*, measure]. Device for determining the hemoglobin in the blood.

hemoglobinopepsia (he″mo-glo″bin-o-pep′sĭ-ă) [" + " + G. *pepsis*, digestion]. Destruction of hemoglobin. SYN: *hemoglobinolysis*.

hemoglobinophilic (he″mo-glo-bin-o-fil′ik) [G. *aima*, blood, + L. *globus*, globe, + G. *philein*, to love]. Pert. to organisms which grow better in presence of hemoglobin.

hemoglo′binous [" + L. *globus*, globe]. Pert. to or containing hemoglobin.

hemoglobinuria (he″mo-glo-bin-u′rĭ-ă) [G. *aima*, blood, + L. *globus*, globe, + G. *ouron*, urine]. The presence of hemoglobin in the urine, but free from red blood corpuscles.

Occurs when hemoglobin from disintegrating red blood cells or from rapid hemolysis of red cells exceeds the ability of the blood proteins to combine with the hemoglobin.

ETIOL: Hemolytic anemia, scurvy, purpura, or certain drugs, such as arsenic, phosphorus, or typhus fever, or pyemia.

SEE: *Buhl's disease; Winckel's disease.*

h., cold. H. following local or general exposure to cold. SYN: *paroxysmal cold h.*

h., epidemic. H. of the newborn characterized by jaundice, cyanosis, and fatty degeneration of heart and liver. SYN: *Winckel's disease*.

h., malarial. Blackwater fever.

h., march. H. occurring esp. in young soldiers following strenuous exercise.

h., paroxysmal. Intermittent, recurring attacks of h. following exposure to cold (cold h.) or strenuous exercise (march h.). Results from increased fragility of red blood cells, or presence of a thermolabile autohemolysin.

h., toxic. H. resulting from: toxic substances such as muscarine, or snake venom; toxic products of infectious diseases, such as yellow fever, typhoid fever, syphilis and certain forms of hemolytic jaundice; organisms such as *Plasmodium* which destroy red blood cells; foreign proteins in blood as may follow blood transfusion or serum therapy.

he″moglobinu′ric [" + " + G. *ouron*, urine]. Rel. to or marked by hemoglobinuria.

h. fever. Malarial hemoglobinuria.

he′mogram [" + *gramma*, a writing]. A graph of the differential blood count. SEE: *Schilling's h.*

hemohistioblast (he″mo-his′tĭ-o-blast) [G. *aima*, blood, + *istos*, tissue, + *blastos*, germ]. Free macrophages which sometimes appear in the blood in certain diseases, esp. those of a septic nature. SYN: *hematohistioblast*.

he′moid [" + *eidos*, resemblance]. Having the appearance of blood.

hemoko'nia (pl. *hemokoniae*) [" + *konis*, dust]. Minute, highly refractive body in the blood, said to be disintegrated particle of blood corpuscle. SYN: *hemoconia; blood dust; blood mote.*

hemokoniosis (he"mo-ko-nī-o'sis) [" + " + -*ōsis*]. Abnormal amount of hemokoniae in the blood. SYN: *hemoconiosis.*

he'molith [" + *lithos*, stone]. A calculus in the wall of a blood vessel.

he'molymph [" + L. *lympha*, lymph]. Blood and lymph.

hemol'ysin [" + *lysis*, dissolution]. An agent in a serum destructive of erythrocytes.*

hemolysis (he-mol'ĭ-sis) [G. *aima*, blood, + *lysis*, dissolution]. The destruction of red blood cells with the liberation of hemoglobin which diffuses into the fluid surrounding them. Also called "laking" of the blood. May occur as a result of the effects of bacterial toxins, snake venoms, immune bodies (hemolysins), and hypotonic saline solutions.

Their stroma is ruptured or dissolved, and the hemoglobin is liberated into the plasma. As a result, the blood, examined grossly, appears to be more transparent and to have a richer, red color; under the microscope the dissolution of the red corpuscles can be observed.

When the hemolysis occurs within the blood vessels, the body is unable to retain the hemoglobin, which is lost through the kidneys and imparts a red color to the urine, a condition called *hemoglobinuria, q.v.*

Injection of a hypotonic saline solution or distilled water into the blood stream induces hemolysis and may result in death. The red blood cells swell, and become globular; their membranes stretch and hemoglobin is liberated. All solutions injected intravenously must be isotonic to the blood. Hemolysis may result from infection by certain disease organisms, e.g. certain streptococci, staphylococci, the tetanus bacillus, and the scarlet fever organism. Hemolysis also occurs in smallpox, diphtheria, and following severe burns. SEE: *fragility test; laked.*

hemolytic (he"mo-lit'ik) [G. *aima*, blood, + *lysis*, dissolution]. Pert. to the breaking down of red blood corpuscles.

h. unit. The amount of inactivated immune serum which causes complete hemolysis of 1 cc. of a 5% emulsion of washed red blood corpuscles in the presence of complement.

hemolytopoietic (he-mol"ĭ-to-poy-et'ik) [" + " + *poiein*, to form]. Rel. to processes of production and destruction of blood cells.

he'molyze. To produce hemolysis.

hemomediastinum (he"mo-me"dĭ-ă-stī'-num) [" + L. *mediastinus*, in the middle]. Effusion of blood into mediastinal spaces. SYN: *hematomediastinum.*

hemometra (he-mo-me'tră) [" + *mētra*, uterus]. Retention of blood within the uterus. SYN: *hematometra.*

hemonephro'sis [" + *nephros*, kidney, + *ōsis*]. Blood in pelvis of the kidney. SYN: *hematonephrosis.*

hemopath'ic [" + *pathos*, blood]. Rel. or due to disease of the blood.

hemopathol'ogy [" + " + *logos*, study]. The science of blood disorders.

hemop'athy [" + *pathos*, disease]. A disease of the blood.

hemoperitone'um [" + *peritonaion*, peritoneum]. Effusion of blood into the peritoneal cavity.

hemopex'in [" + *pēxis*, fixation]. A protein of high carbohydrate content which combines with heme. It is normally present in the blood.

hemopex'is [" + *pēxis*, fixation]. Blood coagulation.

he'mophage [" + *phagein*, to eat]. A cell destroying red blood corpuscles by phagocytosis.

hemophagocyte (he-mo-fag'o-sīt) [" + " + *kytos*, cell]. A white blood corpuscle which ingests other blood corpuscles, esp. red.

RS: *anemia, blood, leukocyte.*

hemophilia (he-mo-fil'ĭ-ă) [G. *aima*, blood, + *philein*, to love]. A hereditary blood disease characterized by greatly prolonged coagulation time. The blood fails to clot and abnormal bleeding occurs. It is a sex-linked hereditary trait, being transmitted by normal heterozygous females who carry the recessive gene. It occurs almost exclusively in males.

The term *hemophilia* has been used to designate a variety of coagulation disorders of blood. This has led to confusion which can be prevented by using the word *hemophilia* to mean what it originally meant and to designate conditions resembling it by the name of the specific coagulation factor which is lacking.

ETIOL: The cause of true hemophilia is deficiency of a factor in plasma necessary for coagulation of blood. This factor is called by several names including *factor VIII, antihemophilic globulin,* and *antihemophilic factor.*

SYM: Abnormal tendency to bleed. May cause swelling of the joints.

PROG: Unfavorable; depends upon severity of the disease. In about one-third of cases, death may occur in the first year of life and 57% during the first 5 years.

TREATMENT: There is no cure for hemophilia. In an emergency, transfusion of fresh whole blood or plasma is required. This provides factor VIII. Hemophiliacs should avoid trauma. Excellent pamphlets concerning home care of the hemophiliac child are available from the National Hemophilia Foundation, 25 West 39th Street, New York, N. Y., U.S.A.

Subject should carry notice on person that he or she is a *hemophiliac* so that in case of accident requiring an operation the surgeon may be forewarned and take necessary precautions. SEE: *angiostaxis; blood.*

h. B. This term refers to Christmas disease which is a hemophilia-like disease, caused by a lack of factor IX which is the plasma thromboplastin component. The surname of one of the first families in which the disease was recognized was *Christmas.*

hemophiliac (he-mo-fil'ĭ-ak) [" + *philein*, to love]. One afflicted with hemophilia.

he"mophil'ic. 1. Fond of blood, said of bacteria which grow well in culture media containing hemoglobin. 2. Pertaining to hemophilia or hemophiliacs.

Hemophilus (hē-mŏf'ĭl-us) [G. *aima*, blood, + *philein*, to love]. A genus of bacteria belonging to the family Brucellaceae. Small, pleomorphic, nonmotile and motile gram negative, rod-shaped hemophilic organisms.

H. aegyptius. A cause of conjunctivitis. SYN: *Koch-Weeks bacillus.*

H. ducreyi. The causative organism of chancroid or soft chancre. Also called Ducrey's bacillus.

H. duplex. Former name for *Moraxella lacunata* or Morax-Axenfeld bacillus, the causative organism of angular conjunctivitis.

H. influenzae. An organism found in respiratory infections and formerly thought to be the cause of influenza, but now considered to be a primary and a secondary invader. It is the causative organism of influenzal meningitis, conjunctivitis, septicemia, respiratory infections. Also called Pfeiffer's bacillus.

H. pertussis. Former name for *Bordetella pertussis,* the causative organism of whooping cough.

hemophobia (he-mo-fo'bĭ-ă) [" + *phobos,* fear]. Aversion to seeing blood or to bleeding.

hemophor'ic [" + *pherein,* to carry]. Conveying blood.

hemophthal'mia, hemophthal'mus [" + *ophthalmos,* eye]. Effusion of blood into eyeball.

hemoplas'tic [" + *plassein,* to form]. Blood-forming. SYN: *hematoplastic; hematopoietic.*

hemopneumothorax (he"mo-nu-mo-tho'raks) [" + *pneuma,* air, + *thōrax,* chest]. Blood and air in the pleural cavity.

hemopoie'sis [" + *poiein,* to make]. Formation of red blood corpuscles. SYN: *hematopoiesis.*

hemoptysis (he-mop'tĭ-sis) [G. *aima,* blood, + *ptyein,* to spit]. Expectoration of blood arising from hemorrhage of the larynx, trachea, bronchi, or lungs.

SYM: Attack sudden. Salty taste. Blood frothy, bright red.

TREATMENT: Cold applications over chest.

Hemoptysis	Hematemesis
1. Probable previous history of tuberculosis.	1. Probable previous history of gastric or duodenal trouble.
2. Blood is coughed up.	2. Blood is vomited.
3. Blood is frothy, bright red, and alkaline in reaction.	3. Blood is usually (not always) dark, usually not frothy, and acid in reaction. Often clotted.
4. Blood may be mixed with sputum.	4. Blood may be mixed with food.
5. There is some dyspnea, pain, and a tickling sensation in the chest.	5. There is often nausea and pain referred to stomach.

NP: Patient must be kept perfectly quiet in bed in a semirecumbent position with head of bed slightly elevated. No movement or excitement permitted and no visitors. No talking by patient, who should be reassured. No hot drinks. Light diet.

In tuberculosis, in absence of doctor in case of hemorrhage, follow these rules:

1. Support the patient's head and shoulders with pillows. Patient in a semirecumbent position. If the bleeding side is known, incline him towards that side, and, if any feeling of suffocation, loosen clothing about throat and chest.

2. If there be thirst, give chipped ice in small amounts.

3. Open the window. Keep patient warm but not hot.

4. Keep patient calm and comforted.

5. Do not adm. any drugs until doctor comes, and on no account give stimulants. An injection of morphine may be prescribed. Should patient faint, hemorrhage may cease. This is often nature's means of cure.

SEE: *bleeding; hemorrhage; hematemesis.*

The table below gives the more important distinguishing features between hemoptysis and hematemesis, *q.v.*

h., endemic. Paragonimiasis. SEE: *h., parasitic.*

h., parasitic. Spitting of blood resulting from infection of the lungs by *Paragonimus westermanii, q.v.,* a parasitic fluke.

hemorrhage (hem'o-rij) [G. *aima,* blood, + *rēgnunai,* to burst forth]. Abnormal discharge of blood, either external or internal; venous, arterial, or capillary from blood vessels into tissues, into or from the body.

Venous blood is dark red; flow is continuous. Arterial blood is bright red; flows in jets. Capillary blood is of a reddish color; exudes from tissue.

SYM: When visible, diagnosis is obvious. When internal, diagnosis may be made from the general condition. Patient is in shock; pulse weak, rapid and irregular; face pale; skin cold and moist.

NP: Depends upon location. Remove all dirt with absorbent cotton, using moisture of the blood, not water; apply sterilized gauze sponge; bandage firmly; elevate limb. Patient should recline. Very cold water contracts vessels. Warm water increases bleeding. Do not use alum, iron solutions, etc., if avoidable. If an open wound, apply sterile dressing and a firm bandage. In an emergency, when bleeding is from a small vessel, firm pressure over the actual site of bleeding may be sufficient to stop the bleeding. Continue to apply pressure until definitive treatment can be provided. In the case of a ruptured varicose vein, pressure may be best applied with a flat firm object such as a coin of suitable size.

h., accidental. OB. AND GYN: H. caused by premature rupture of the placenta. SEE: *ablatio placentae.*

h., antepartum. Hemorrhage appearing before the onset of labor.

h., armpit. Place sterile gauze sponge into wound; apply pressure over pad and bandage over shoulder and under armpit. Also bandage under opposite armpit over shoulder already bandaged.

h., armpit and elbow (between). Insert sterile gauze sponge into wound and apply pressure over pad; or tourniquet.

h., arterial. In arterial bleeding (red) the blood ordinarily comes through in waves or spurts, unless the torn artery is deep or buried, when the flow may be steady. SEE: *tourniquet.*

F. A. TREATMENT: It is usually necessary: (1) To make pressure along the course of artery, somewhere between heart and bleeding point, by means of

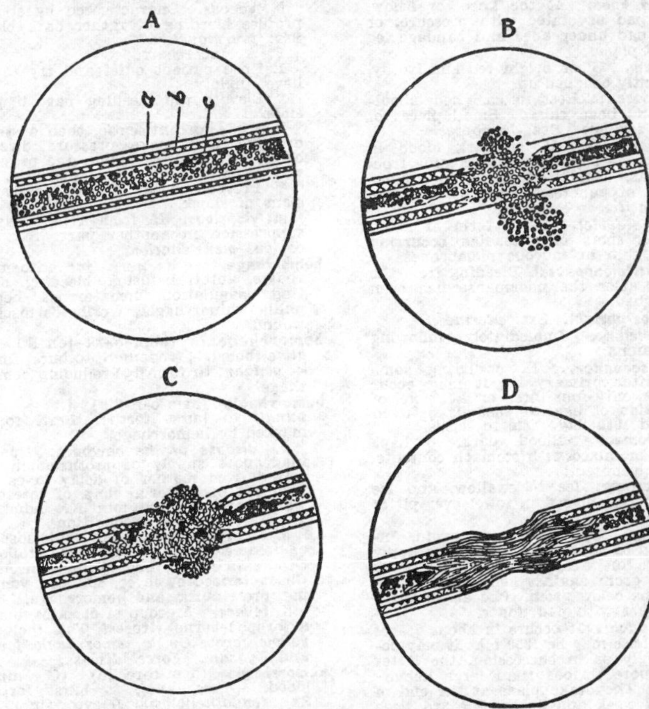

ARREST OF HEMORRHAGE

Temporary and permanent, diagrammatic. A, Normal small artery: a, outer coat, adventitia; b, middle coat, muscular; c, inner coat, intima. B, Artery torn across. Retraction of middle and inner coats; contraction of muscular coat. C, Clotting of blood outside and inside the vessel; temporary arrest. D, Obliteration of the lumen of the vessel with fibrous tissue; permanent arrest.

fingers (digital pressure) on the pressure points. (2) Then by a tourniquet above the point of injury. NOTE: Tourniquet should be used only if absolutely required after other means failed to stop the bleeding. When used, apply only the pressure required to stop the bleeding. Improperly applied, a tourniquet may cause permanent damage to nerves. (3) Elevate the part. (4) A sterile dressing. (5) A *firm* bandage. (6) Gradually release tourniquet after 12 to 15 minutes; if bleeding, retighten. *Do not give* stimulants until bleeding is controlled.

h., capillary. Bleeding from minute blood vessels, present in all bleeding; when large vessels are not injured they may be controlled by simple elevation and pressure as with sterile compress.

TREATMENT: Astringents, styptic. Best is simply dry compress applied with pressure.

h., carotid artery. Usually accompanied by bleeding from the jugular veins and may be fatal in a short time.

F. A. TREATMENT: Compression with the thumbs transversely across the neck, both above and below the wound, the fingers directed around the back of the neck to aid in compression. It may be more desirable to pack the wound with sterile gauze and compress it with the closed fist. Wounds of the jugular vein are sometimes the cause of air embolism.

h., cerebral. Escape of blood into tissues of brain.

ETIOL: hypertension, arteriosclerosis, or atherosclerosis, infections.

SYM: Unconsciousness, slow pulse, stertorous breathing; hemiplegia, death. May be speech disturbance, incontinence of bladder and rectum, or constipation according to location of damaged brain tissue.

TREATMENT: Ice bag over head and heat at feet.

h., consecutive. Some time after an injury, 20 to 24 hours after an operation.

TREATMENT: Compress applied to main artery and wound. Elevate parts. Reopen and tie bleeding vessels.

h., contact. Hemorrhage from the cervix uteri coming on as a result of exertion, or contact during coitus, douching, or instrumentation.

h., elbow and hand (bet.). Put pad in elbow, apply bandage over it as a tourniquet.

h. of foot. Apply pad and pressure and bandage.

h. of hand. If from palmar area, fill hand with sterile gauze sponge, clasp fingers around it and bandage.

h. of knee. At the knee, or below, apply pad as stated with pressure, or put a pad under knee and bandage leg at that place.

h., lung. Blood bright red and frothy, frequently coughed up.

TREATMENT: Rest in cool bed, shoulders and head raised. Small pieces of ice to swallow. SEE: *hemoptysis.*

h., pancreas. H. of dark blood in vomitus with slimy mucus, coming from pancreas, usually occurring in inflammation of pancreas. SEE: *hemorrhagic pancreatitis.*

h., petechial. H. in form of small rounded spots or petechiae occurring in the skin or mucous membranes.

h., postmenopausal. Bleeding from the vagina after the menopause has been established.

h., postpartum. SEE: *uterine h.*

h., primary. Immediately following any trauma.

h., secondary. H. occurring some time after primary h. It may occur after twenty-four hrs. or at time of separation of ligature, usually between 7th and 10th day. Due to sepsis.

h., stomach. Blood dark, perhaps clotted or mixed with stomach contents, usually vomited.

TREATMENT: Ice to swallow, and ice cracked and placed in towel over pit of stomach.

h., thigh. Upper part near groin. Insert pad of gauze into wound and apply pressure or press thumb in center of fold of groin against bone until bleeding stops below groin. Pad as above or tourniquet with pad under.

h., typhoid. It occurs in about 7% of cases. Loss may be 1000 ml. It may occur singly or in succession, the latter being more serious than large hemorrhages. They take place at the end of the 2nd week and during the 3rd week of the disease.

h., unavoidable. Ceaseless, painless bleeding from placenta previa, *q.v.*

h., uterine. One into cavity of uterus.

ETIOL: Common causes are (1) trauma, (2) congenital abnormalities, (3) pathological processes such as tumors, (4) infections esp. of alimentary, respiratory, and genitourinary tracts, (5) generalized vascular disorders such as various purpuras, (6) coagulation defects, and (7) retained products of conception following criminal or therapeutic abortion.

TREATMENT: A wet, sterile packing is used by some but condemned by others. A retained placenta, when present and causing hemorrhage, should be removed with uterine forceps. A relaxed uterus may need a hypodermic injection of posterior pituitary extract. The patient may need transfusion and, in some cases, surgery will be required to prevent fatal hemorrhage.

There are three types of uterine h.: *Essential uterine h.*: H. occurring in connection with pelvic, uterine, or cervical diseases. SYN: *metropathia haemorrhagica.* SEE: *fibrosis uteri.*

Intrapartum h.: Hemorrhage coming on during labor.

Postpartum h.: Occurring after 3rd stage of labor. Due to inversion, rupture, lacerations, relaxation of the uterus and hematoma.

NP: Lower head, elevate hips, grasp uterus with hand and make firm compression.

h., venous. Characterized by steady, profuse bleeding of rather dark blood. SEE: *tourniquet.*

F. A. TREATMENT:

1. Keep patient quiet and try to relieve anxiety.

2. Elevate the bleeding part if possible.

3. Apply an antiseptic, then a sterile dressing and make pressure directly over the wound. Elevation and pressure will control most venous bleeding.

4. Prevent shock; observe closely for signs of shock.

h., vicarious. H. from a part due to suppression in another part. SEE: *vicarious menstruation.*

hemorrhage, *words pert. to:* anthemorrhagic, autotransfusion, bleeding, clotting, coagulation, hematorrhea, hemophilia, rhinorrhagia, Werlhoff's disease, wound.

hemorrhagenic (hem-o-ră-jen′ik) [G. *aima,* blood, + *rēgnunai,* to burst forth, + *gennan,* to form]. Producing hemorrhage.

hemorrhagic (hem-o-raj′ik) [" + *rēgnunai,* to burst forth]. Pert. to or marked by hemorrhage.

h. disease of the newborn. Due to inadequate supply of prothrombin received from mother or delay in establishment of bacterial flora of intestine which produces vitamin K. Adm. of vit. K. corrects the condition.

h. fever, epidemic. An acute disease of unknown but probably viral etiology. Occurs in spring and autumn in Asia. Characterized by fever, collapse, vomiting, proteinuria, and hemorrhage.

h. fevers. A group of diseases due to arthropod-borne viruses. This includes *yellow fever, Omsk hemorrhagic fever,* and *Kyasanur Forest disease.*

hemorrhagin (hem-o-raj′in) [G. *aima,* blood, + *regnunai,* to burst forth]. SYN: *endotheliolysin.* A cytolysin present in venom of snakes and other toxins responsible for hemorrhages and effusion of blood by destroying capillary endothelium.

h. unit. Quantity of venom needed to produce vascular hemorrhage in 3-day-old chick embryos.

hemorrhagiparous (hem-o-răj-ip′ă-rus) [" + " + L. *parēre,* to produce]. Producing hemorrhage. SYN: *hemorrhagenic.*

hemorrhea (hem-o-re′ă) [" + *roia,* flow]. Hemorrhage.

hemorrhoid (hem′o-royd) [G. *aimorrois,* vein liable to discharge blood]. A tumor in form of dilated blood vessels in the anal region. SEE: *hemorrhoidectomy; piles.*

h., external. Cutaneous and thrombotic, outside the sphincter.

TREATMENT: Sitz baths; hot or cold applications; petrolatum; or surgical treatment.

h., internal. Venous, arterial and capillary, within the sphincter but beneath the mucous membrane.

TREATMENT: Local applications of heat or cold. Laxatives. Rest in bed. Operation and excision.

hemorrhoidal (hem-o-roy′dal) [G. *aimorrois,* veins liable to discharge blood]. 1. Rel. to hemorrhoids. 2. Pert. to certain anal arteries, *arteria hemorrhoidalis.*

hemorrhoidectomy (hem-o-royd-ek′to-mĭ) [" + *ektomē,* excision]. Surgical excision of hemorrhoids.*

DRESSING, etc.: Petrolatum, gauze, sponges, gauze strips 3 and 8 in. wide, cotton and T bandages, 6 towels, leg holders, solution for irrigation, Dudley or Kelly pad.

NP: *Preoperative*: The patient is placed in lithotomy position. A towel, wet with antiseptic solution, is placed over external genitalia. The operating field is thoroughly scrubbed with soap and water and flushed with an iodine solution of 3% strength. The patient is draped with leggings; lithotomy sheet.

Postoperative: Knees tied together until anesthetic is worn off. Head and shoulders elevated on pillows. Keep weight off buttocks. Retard bowel action 3-5 days. Cool fluids; avoid foods stimulating peristalsis. Swab margin of anus with a local anesthetic before stool. Bathe after with an antiseptic and renew dressing. After a week give daily bath. Inspect dressing carefully. Repack as necessary. Re-dress 2nd day with petrolatum gauze or dry dressing. Watch for retention of urine and possibility of hemorrhage.

hemosal'pinx [G. *aima*, blood, + *salpigx*, tube]. Blood accumulated in an oviduct. SYN: *hematosalpinx.*

he"mosid'erin. An iron-containing pigment derived from hemoglobin from disintegration of red blood cells.

he"mosidero'sis. Condition characterized by the deposition, esp. in liver and spleen, of hemosiderin. Occurs in diseases in which there is marked red cell destruction such as hemolytic anemia and malaria. Hemosiderin may be deposited in pulmonary lymphatics in congenital and rheumatic heart disease.

hemosozic (hem-o-so'zik) [" + *sozein*, to save]. 1. Protective of blood corpuscles. 2. Rel. to an antiserum (*antihemolysin*) that prevents hemolysis.

hemospasia (hem-o-spa'zĭ-ă) [" + *spaein*, to draw]. Withdrawal of blood by cupping or leeching.

hemosper'mia [" + *sperma*, seed]. Bloody semen. SYN: *hematospermia.*

hemostasis (he-mos'tă-sis) [" + *stasis*, a stopping]. SYN: *hemostasia.* 1. Arrest of bleeding or of circulation. 2. Stagnation of blood.

he'mostat [" + *statikos*, standing]. 1. Device or medicine which arrests the flow of blood. 2. Compressor for controlling hemorrhage of the tonsils.

hemostatic (he-mo-stat'ik) [" + *statikos*, standing]. 1. Checking hemorrhage. 2. Any substance which checks bleeding without being directly applied to the bleeding areas. Ex: *calcium lactate; ergot; whole blood.*

hemostyp'tic [" + *styptikos*, astringent]. An astringent that stops bleeding; chemically hemostatic.

hemotachometer (he"mo-tak-om'ĕ-ter) [" + *tachos*, swiftness, + *metron*, measure]. Device for measuring velocity of the blood.

hemotherapeu'tics [" + *therapeutikē*, medical practice]. The use of blood, by transfusion or otherwise, in treatment of disease.

hemother'apy [" + *therapeia*, treatment]. Blood transfusion as a therapeutic measure. SYN: *hematotherapeutics.*

hemothorax (he-mo-tho'raks) [" + *thōrax*, chest]. Bloody fluid in the pleural cavity caused by rupture of small blood vessels, due to inflammation of the lungs in pneumonia, or to pulmonary tuberculosis, or to a malignant growth.

hemothy'mia [" + *thymos*, anger]. An irresistible impulse to murder.

hemoto'nia [" + *tonos*, tension]. The tension of the solid elements of the blood.

hemotox'in [" + *toxikon*, poison]. A toxin destructive of red blood cells. SYN: *hemolysin.*

hemotrip'sia [" + *tripsis*, a rubbing]. Hemorrhage in one part that induces hemorrhage in another part.

hemotrophic (he-mo-trof'ik). Pertaining to nutrient substances carried in the blood.

h. nutrition. Nutrition of the fetus by substances in the maternal blood which pass to the blood of the fetus through vessels within the villi.

hemotropic (he-mo-trop'ik). Attracted to or having an affinity for blood or blood cells.

hemotym'panum [" + *tympanon*, drum]. Blood in the middle ear.

hemozoin (he"mo-zo'in). A dark pigment found within malarial organisms (plasmodia). It is derived from the disintegration of hemoglobin.

he'mozoon. A hematozoon, *q.v.*

henbane (hen'bān). SYN: *Hyoscyamus, q.v.*

Henle's ampul'la [Friedrich G. J. Henle, German anatomist, 1809-1885]. A ductus deferens dilatation just above the ejaculatory duct.

H.'s layer. Outer layer of cells of inner root sheath of hair follicle.

H.'s loop. A U-shaped portion of a renal tubule lying between the proximal and distal convoluted portions. Consists of a thin descending limb and a thicker ascending limb.

H.'s membrane. Bruch's layer forming inner boundary of the choroid.

H.'s sheath. Connective tissue support of individual nerve fibers in a funiculus. SYN: *endoneurium.*

He'noch's angina [Edouard H. Henoch, German pediatrician, 1820-1910]. Form of angina with gangrenous patches found in mucosa of air passages in scarlet fever and diphtheria. SYN: *necrotic angina.*

H.'s purpura. Purpura with intestinal disturbances. Infectious disease of children.

SYM: Erythema, urticaria, purpura, gastroenteric disorders, and perhaps arthritis.

henry (hen're). Unit designating electrical inductance.

Hensen's cells [Victor Hensen, German anatomist and physiologist, 1835-1924]. Tall columnar cells which form the outer border cells of the organ of Corti of the cochlea.

H.'s disk. Band in center of the A disk of a sarcomere of striated muscle. During contraction it appears lighter than the remaining portion and in its center, a dark stripe, the M stripe, is seen.

H.'s stripe. A dark band on the under surface of the tectorial membrane.

he'par [G. *ēpar*, liver]. The liver, *q.v.*

heparin (hep'ă-rin) [G. *ēpar*, liver]. A mucoitin polysulfuric acid which has been isolated from the liver, lung, and other tissues. It is produced by the mast cells of the liver and by basophil leukocytes. It inhibits coagulation by preventing conversion of prothrombin to thrombin by forming an antithrombin, and by preventing liberation of thromboplastin from blood platelets. The action of heparin requires the presence of a co-factor found in serum albumin of the plasma. SYN: *heparin sodium.*

USES: An anticoagulant; used in prevention and treatment of thrombosis and embolism. Sometimes employed concurrently with *dicumarol, q.v.*

hep'arinize [G. *ēpar,* liver]. To inhibit coagulation of blood with heparin.

hepatalgia (hep-ă-tal'jĭ-ă) [G. *ēpar, ēpat-,* liver, + *algos,* pain]. Pain in the liver. SYN: *hepatodynia.*

hepatal'gic [" + *algos,* pain]. Pert. to hepatalgia.

hepatatrophia (hep-at-ă-tro'fĭ-ă) [" + *atrophia,* atrophy]. Atrophied condition of the liver.

hepatauxe (hep"at-awk'se) [" + *auxē,* increase]. Enlargement or hypertrophy of the liver.

hepatectomy (hep-ă-tek'to-mĭ) [" + *ektomē,* excision]. Excision of part or all of liver.

hepat'ic [G. *ēpar, ēpat-,* liver]. Pertaining to the liver.

h. amebiasis. Infection of the liver by *Entamoeba histolytica* resulting in hepatitis and abscess formation. Usually a sequel to amebic dysentery. SEE ALSO: *amebiasis.*

h. duct. The canal that receives bile from the liver. It unites with cystic duct to form the common bile duct.

h. flexure. The right bend of colon under the liver. The junction of the ascending and transverse colon.

h. lobes. Divisions of the liver.

h. veins. The three vessels returning blood from the liver and discharging into the inferior vena cava.

h. zones. Venous, arterial, and portal hepatic regions.

hepaticoduodenostomy (hĕ-pat"ĭ-ko-du"-o-dĕ-nos'to-mĭ) [" + L. *duodenum,* duodenum, + G. *stoma,* opening]. Making an artificial opening bet. hepatic duct and duodenum.

hepaticoenterostomy (hĕ-pat"ĭ-ko-en-ter-os'to-mĭ) [" + *enteron,* intestine, + *stoma,* opening]. Operation for artificial opening bet. hepatic duct and intestine.

hepaticogastrostomy (hĕ-pat-ĭ-ko-gas-tros'to-mĭ) [" + *gastēr,* stomach, + *stoma,* opening]. The operation for a passage bet. the hepatic duct and the stomach.

hepaticolithotripsy (hĕ-pat-ĭ-ko-lith'o-trip-sĭ) [" + *lithos,* stone, + *tripsis,* a crushing]. The crushing of a biliary calculus in the hepatic duct.

hepaticos'tomy [" + *stoma,* opening]. Establishment of permanent fistula into hepatic duct.

hepaticot'omy [" + *tomē,* incision]. Incision into the hepatic duct.

hepatin (hep'ă-tin) [G. *ēpar, ēpat-,* liver]. Carbohydrate formed in the liver, which is changed to dextrose to meet body requirements. SYN: *glycogen.*

hepatitis (hep-ă-ti'tis) [G. *ēpar, ēpat-,* liver, + *-itis,* inflammation]. Inflammation of the liver of virus or toxic origin. It is usually manifest by jaundice and, in some instances, liver enlargement. Fever and other systemic disorders are usually present.

h., acute anicteric. H. marked by slight fever, gastrointestinal upset and anorexia, but no jaundice.

h., cholangiolitic. H. characterized by jaundice, tiredness, pruritus, vomiting of bile, and hepatomegaly. SYN: *cholestatic h.*

h., fulminant. H. marked by sudden onset of nausea and vomiting, chills, high fever, severe and early jaundice, convulsions, shock, deep coma, and death usually within 10 days. SYN: *massive necrosis of liver.*

h., homologous serum. H. in which the virus is transmitted parenterally by blood transfusion, plasma, needles or other parenteral instruments. Incubation period varies from 6 weeks to 6 months. Marked by sudden onset of headache, fever, chills, general weakness, nausea, vomiting, abdominal pain, prostration, jaundice, pruritus, enlarged and tender liver. SYN: *serum h.; inoculation h.; homologous serum jaundice; transfusion jaundice.*

h., infectious. H. occurring sporadically and in epidemics. Transmitted by oral or parenteral route. Incubation period is 2 to 6 weeks. Gastrointestinal and respiratory disturbances followed by sudden onset of jaundice, enlarged and tender liver, pruritus, muscle pain, splenomegaly, loss of weight. SYN: *epidemic h.; epidemic jaundice.*

h., toxic. H. caused by exposure to certain poisons (as carbon tetrachloride) or drugs (as sulfonamides), the latter causing hypersensitivity in some patients.

hepatization (hep"ă-tĭ-za'shun) [G. *ēpar, ēpat-,* liver]. The second and third stages in consolidation in lobar pneumonia, the surface of the lung has the appearance of liver tissue.

hepato- [G.]. Prefix: The liver.

hepatocele (hep'ă-to-sēl) [G. *ēpar, ēpat-,* liver, + *kēlē,* hernia]. Hernia of the liver.

hepatocholangiocystoduodenostomy (hep"-ă-to-ko-lan" jĭ-o-sis" to-du-o-dĕ-nos'to-mĭ) [" + *cholē,* bile, + *aggeion,* vessel, + *kystis,* bladder, + L. *duodenum* + G. *stoma,* opening]. Establishment of drainage of bile ducts into the duodenum through the gallbladder.

hepatocholangioduodenostomy (hep"ă-to-ko-lan"jĭ-o-du-o-dĕ-nos'to-mĭ) [" + " + " + L. *duodenum* + G. *stoma,* opening]. Establishment of drainage of bile ducts into the duodenum.

hepatocholangioenterostomy (hep"ă-to-ko-lan"jĭ-o-en-ter-os'to-mĭ) [" + " + " + *enteron,* intestine, + *stoma,* opening]. Establishment of a passage bet. the liver and intestine.

hepatocholangiogastrostomy (hep"ă-to-ko-lan"jĭ-o-gas-tros'to-mĭ) [" + " + " + *gastēr,* belly, + *stoma,* opening]. Establishment of drainage of bile ducts into the stomach.

hepatocholangiostomy (hep"ă-to-ko-lan-jĭ-os'to-mĭ) [" + " + " + *stoma,* opening]. Establishment of free drainage by opening into the gall duct.

hepatocirrhosis (hep-ă-to-sĭ-ro'sis) [" + *kirros,* tawny, + *ōsis*]. Cirrhosis of liver.

hepatocol'ic [" + *kōlon,* colon]. Rel. to both liver and colon.

hepatocys'tic [" + *kystis,* bladder]. Rel. to the liver and gallbladder, or the gallbladder.

hepatoduodenos'tomy [" + L. *duodenum* + G. *stoma,* opening]. Establishment of an opening from the liver into the duodenum. SYN: *hepaticoduodenostomy.*

hepatodynia (hep-ă-to-din'ĭ-ă) [" + *odynē,* pain]. Pain in the liver.

hepatodys'entery [" + *dys,* painful, + *enteron,* intestine]. Inflammation of the liver causing dysentery.

hepatoenter'ic [" + *enteron,* intestine]. Rel. to the liver and intestines.

hepatogas'tric [" + *gastēr,* belly]. Rel. to the liver and stomach.

hepatogenic (hep-ă-to-jen'ik) [" + *gennan,* to produce]. Having its origin in the liver.

hepatogenous (hep-ă-toj'ĕ-nus) [" + *gennan,* to produce]. Originating in the liver.

hepatog'raphy [G. *ēpar, ēpat-,* liver, + *graphein,* to write). 1. Treatise on human liver. 2. Roentgenography of the liver.

hepatohemia (hep"ă-to-he'mĭ-ă) [" + *aima,* blood]. Liver congestion.

hep'atoid [G. *ēpar, ēpat-,* liver, + *eidos,* form]. Having the structural form of the liver.

hepatolentic'ular [" + L. *lenticula,* lentil, lens]. Rel. to lenticular nucleus and the liver.

h. degeneration. Progressive lenticular degeneration in cirrhosis of the liver. SYN: *Wilson's disease.*

hepatolith (hep'ă-to-lith) [" + *lithos,* stone]. A biliary concretion in the liver.

hepatolithiasis (hep-ă-to-lĭ-thi'ă-sis) [" + *lithos,* stone]. Calculi or concretions in the liver.

hepatol'ogist [" + *logos,* study]. A specialist in diseases of the liver.

hepatolysin (hep-ă-tol'ĭ-sin) [" + *lysis,* dissolution]. A cytolysin destructive to hepatic cells.

hepatol'ysis [" + *lysis,* dissolution]. Liver cell destruction.

hepatolyt'ic [" + *lysis,* dissolution]. Destructive to tissues of the liver.

hepatoma (hep-ă-to'mă) [" + *ōma,* tumor]. A tumor of the liver.

hepatomalacia (hep"ă-to-mă-la'sĭ-ă) [" + *malakia,* softening]. Softening of the liver.

hepatomegaly (hep"ă-to-meg'ă-lĭ) [" + *megas,* large]. Enlargement of the liver.

hepatomelanosis (hep"ă-to-mel"ă-no'sis) [" + *melas,* black, + *-ōsis*]. Pigmented deposits or melanosis in the liver.

hepatonephri'tis [" + *nephros,* kidney, + *-ītis,* inflammation]. Inflammation of both liver and kidneys.

hepatonephromegaly (hep"ă-to-nef"ro-meg'ă-lĭ) [" + " + *megas,* large]. Hypertrophy of both liver and kidney or kidneys.

h. glycogenica. Von Gierke's disease, characterized by hypertrophy of liver and excess accumulation of glycogen resulting from failure of glycogenolysis to occur.

hepatopathy (hep-ă-top'ă-thĭ) [" + *pathos,* disease]. Disease of the liver.

hepatoperitonitis (hep"ă-to-per"ĭ-to-ni'tis, [" + *peritonaion,* peritoneum, + *-ītis,* inflammation]. Inflammation of the peritoneal covering of the liver. SYN: *perihepatitis.*

hep'atopexy [G. *ēpar, ēpat-,* liver, + *pēxis,* fixation]. Fixation of a movable liver to abdominal wall.

hepatophage (hep'ă-to-fāj) [" + *phagein,* to eat]. A phagocyte that attacks liver cells.

hepatoptosia, hepatoptosis (hep"ă-top-to'sĭ-ă, -to'sis) [" + *ptōsis,* a dropping]. Downward displacement of the liver.

hep"atopul'monary [" + L. *pulmō,* lung]. Rel. to both liver and lungs.

hepatore'nal [" + L. *rēn,* kidney]. Pert. to both liver and kidneys.

hepatorrhaphy (hep-ă-tor'ă-fĭ) [" + *raphē,* suture]. The suturing of a wound of the liver.

hepatorrhea (hep-ă-to-re'ă) [" + *roia,* flow]. 1. Bilious diarrhea. 2. Morbid flow from the liver.

hepatorrhexis (hep"ă-to-reks'is) [" + *rēxis,* rupture]. Rupture of the liver.

hepatos'copy [" + *skopein,* to examine]. Inspection of the liver.

hepatosplenitis (hep"ă-to-sple-ni'tis) [" + *splēn,* spleen, + *-ītis,* inflammation]. Inflamed condition of both liver and spleen.

hepatosplenomegaly (hep"ă-to-sple"no-meg'ă-lĭ) [" + " + *megas,* large]. Enlargement of both liver and spleen.

hepatostomy (hep-ă-tos'to-mĭ) [" + *stoma,* opening]. The making of an artificial fissure into the liver.

hep"atother'apy [" + *therapeia,* treatment]. 1. Treatment of liver disease. 2. The use of liver or liver extract.

hepatotomy (hep-ă-tot'o-mĭ) [" + *tomē,* incision]. Incision into the liver.

hepatotoxemia (hep"ă-to-toks-e'mĭ-ă) [" + *toxikon,* poison, + *aima,* blood]. Autointoxication due to malfunctioning of the liver.

hepatotox'in [" + *toxikon,* poison]. A cytotoxin specific for liver cells.

heptachromic (hep"tă-kro'mik) [G. *epta,* seven, + *chrōma,* color]. Possessing normal color vision.

hep'tad [" + L. *ad,* to]. Any element with a valence of seven.

heptose (hep'tōs). Any sugar containing seven carbon atoms in its molecule.

heptosuria (hep"to-su'rĭ-ă) [G. *epta,* seven, + *ouron,* urine]. Heptose in the urine.

herb (erb) [L. *herba,* grass]. A plant with a soft stem containing little wood.

herbivorous (her-biv'o-rus) [" + *vorāre,* to eat]. Vegetarian living on grasses and herbs.

herd [A.S. *heord*]. Any large aggregation of people or animals.

h. instinct. The urge to remain one of the social group and to conform to social patterns and general opinions. An aversion to excessive individualism.

hered'itary [L. *hereditarius,* an heir]. Transmitted from one's ancestry.

h. ataxia. Hereditary spinal ataxia.* SYN: *Friedreich's ataxia.*

heredity (hĕ-red'ĭ-tĭ) [L. *hereditas,* heir]. Innate capacity of an individual to develop traits and characteristics (body size and form, skin and hair color, intellectual capacity, tendency to certain diseases) possessed by its ancestors. Such is dependent upon the presence of genes (hereditary factors or determiners) in the chromosomes of the fertilized ovum from which the individual develops.

RS: *chromosome, gene, genetics, linkage, sex.*

heredo- [L.]. Prefix: *heredity.*

heredoataxia (her"ĕ-do-ă-taks'ĭ-ă) [L. *heres, hered-,* heir, + G. *ataxia,* lack of order]. Hereditary spinal ataxia. SYN: *Friedreich's ataxia.*

Hering-Breuer reflex. Reflex inhibition of inspiration resulting from stimulation of pressoreceptors by inflation of the lungs.

Hering's nerves [Heinrich Ewald Hering, Austrian physician, 1866-]. Afferent nerve fibers leading from carotid sinus via glossopharyngeal nerve to the brain. They are pressoreceptor nerves responding to changes in blood pressure which reflexly control heart rate. An increase in pressure diminishes heart rate.

Her'ing's theory [Carl Ewald K. Hering, Leipzig physiologist, 1834-1918]. A theory of color vision in which it is assumed that the retina possesses three photochemical substances which, depending on their decomposition or resynthesis, produce different color sensations by their stimulation of different nerve endings.

heritage (her'ĭ-tij) [L. *heres,* heir]. All the characteristics transmitted by parents to their children.

hermaphrodism (her-maf'ro-dizm). Hermaphroditism, *q.v.*

hermaphrodite (her-maf′ro-dīt) [G. *Hermaphroditos,* son of Hermes and Aphrodite, who was man and woman combined]. One possessing genital and sexual characteristics of both sexes. SYN: *androgyne.*

The clitoris is usually enlarged, resembling the penis of the male.

RS: *gynandry.*

hermaphroditism (her-maf′ro-dīt-izm) [G. *Hermaphroditos,* son of Hermes and Aphrodite, who was man and woman combined, + *ismos,* state of]. Condition in which both ovarian and testicular tissue exist in the same individual. Occurs rarely in humans. SYN: *hermaphrodism.*

h., complex. Having internal and external organs of both sexes.

h., dimidiate. Lateral h., *q.v.*

h., false. Pseudohermaphroditism; possession of the sex glands of one sex (ovary or testis) but accompanied by secondary sexual characteristics and external genitalia of the opposite sex.

h., lateral. Possession of a testis on one side and an ovary on the other.

h., spurious. False hermaphroditism.

h., transverse. Having the outward organs indicating one sex, and the internal ones the other.

h., true. Double sex.

h., unilateral. H. in which an ovary and a testis or an ovotestis are present on one side and either an ovary or testis present on the other side.

hermet′ic [G. *ermēs,* Hermes]. Airtight.

hermetical (her-met′ik-al) [G. *ērmes,* Hermes]. Airtight.

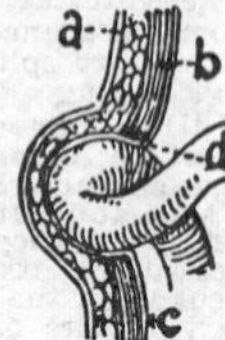

DIAGRAM OF HERNIA

a. Skin and superficial fascia; b. muscular and aponeurotic layer; c, peritoneum; d, neck of the sac.

hernia (her′nĭ-ă) [G. *ernos,* a young shoot]. The protrusion or projection of an organ or a part of an organ through the wall of the cavity which normally contains it. SYN: *rupture.*

ETIOL: Failure of certain normal openings to close during development; weakness resulting from debilitating illness, old age, or injury, prolonged distention as from tumors, pregnancy, or corpulence; increased intraabdominal pressure resulting from lifting heavy loads, or coughing.

TREATMENT: 1. Surgery. 2. Mechanical reduction; taxis. 3. In very large hernias, mechanical devices or trusses may be used.

h., abdominal. H. through the abdominal wall.

h., acquired. H. which develops any time after birth in contrast to one present at birth (congenital hernia). Usually the result of excessive strain on the muscular wall. Frequently occurs following injuries or operations.

h., bladder. Protrusion of the bladder or a part of bladder through normal or abnormal orifice.

h., cerebral. H. of the brain through the cranial wall.

h., Cloquet's. A type of femoral hernia.

h., complete. H. in which sac and its contents have passed through the aperture.

h., concealed. H. that is imperceptible when palpated.

h., congenital. H. existing from birth.

h., crural. SEE: *femoral h.*

h., cystic. Bladder hernia. SYN: *cystocele.*

h. of diaphragm. There are three groups: congenital, acquired or traumatic, and esophageal. In the latter, a portion of the diaphragm is pushed through the esophageal hiatus into the stomach; or h. protruding through the diaphragm.

h., direct. SEE: *inguinal hernia.*

h., diverticular. Protrusion of intestinal congenital diverticulum.

h., encysted. Scrotal protrusion which, enveloped in its own sac, passes into the tunica vaginalis.

h., epigastric. H. of the intestine through an opening in the midline above the umbilicus.

h., fascial. Protrusion of muscular tissue through its fascial covering.

h., femoral. Descending of intestines besides femoral vessels and through femoral ring.

h., funicular. H. into the umbilical or spermatic cord.

h., hiatus. Protrusion of the stomach upward into the mediastinal cavity through the esophageal hiatus of the diaphragm.

h., Holthouse's. SEE: *inguinocrural h.*

h., incarcerated. H. completely obstructing the bowels.

h., incomplete. H. which has not gone completely through the aperture.

h., indirect. SEE: *inguinal hernia.*

h., inguinal. Protrusion of the hernial sac containing the intestine at the inguinal opening. In *indirect lateral* or *oblique inguinal hernia,* the sac protrudes through the internal inguinal ring into the inguinal canal often descending into the scrotum; in *direct medial inguinal hernia* the hernial sac protrudes through the abdominal wall in the region of Hesselbach's triangle, a region bounded by the rectus abdominus muscle, inguinal ligament, and inf. epigastric vessels. Inguinal hernia accounts for about 80% of all hernias.

h., inguinocrural. H. which is femoral and inguinal.

h., internal. H. which occurs within the abdominal cavity. May be intraperitoneal or retroperitoneal.

h., interstitial. Form of inguinal hernia in which the hernial sac lies between layers of the abdominal muscles. SYN: *intermuscular hernia.*

h., irreducible. H. which cannot be returned to its original position out of its sac by manual methods.

h., labial. Protrusion of a loop of bowel into the labium majus.

h., lateral. SEE: *inguinal hernia.*

h., lumbar. In lumbar regions or loins.

h., medial. SEE: *inguinal hernia.*

h., mesocolic. H. bet. the layers of the mesocolon.

h., nuckian. H. into canal of Nuck.

h., oblique. SEE: *inguinal hernia.*

h., obturator. H. through the obturator foramen.

h., omental. H. containing a portion of the omentum.

h., ovarian. Presence of an ovary in a hernial sac.

h., phrenic. Projecting through the diaphragm into one of the pleural cavities.

h., posterior vaginal. H. of Douglas' sac downward bet. rectum and post. vaginal wall. SYN: *enterocele, q.v.*

h., properitoneal. Protrusion through the peritoneum and into the abdominal wall.

h., reducible. H. which can be replaced by manipulation.

h., retroperitoneal. H. into peritoneal sac extending behind the peritoneum into the iliac fossa.

h., Richter's. H. in which only a portion of wall of intestine protrudes, the main portion of the intestine being excluded from the hernial sac and the lumen remaining open.

h., scrotal. One that descends into the scrotum.

h., strangulated. One so tightly constricted that gangrene results if operation does not relieve. Not reducible by ordinary means.

h., umbilical. Occurring at the navel. More frequent in women than men. TREATMENT: Surgical.

h., uterine. Presence of the uterus in the hernial sac.

h., vaginal. Hernial protrusion of the vagina.

h., vaginolabial. Hernia of a viscus into the posterior end of the labium majus.

h., ventral. If stretching and thinning of an abdominal scar occur, pressure from the abdomen may cause protrusion of part of the gut. It is then protected only by a layer of thin scar tissue.

hernia, words pert. to: archocele, Bassini's operation, Beclard's h., bubonocele, cardioclasia, caryorrhexis, cephalocele, ceratocele, cerebroma, herniotomy, liparocele, rupture.

her'nial [G. *ernos,* a young shoot]. Pert. to a hernia.

h. sac. The pouch of peritoneum pushed before a hernia and into which it descends.

her'niated [G. *ernos,* a young shoot]. Having a hernia.

h. disk. Rupture or herniation of the intervertebral disk, esp. between the 4th and 5th lumbar vertebrae. This usually causes pain in the affected side. SYN: *herniated nucleus pulposus.*

herniation (her-nĭ-a'shun) [G. *ernos,* a young shoot]. Development of a hernia.

hernioenterotomy (her"nĭ-o-en"ter-ot'o-mĭ) [" + *enteron,* intestine, + *tome,* incision]. Herniotomy at same time as enterotomy.

her'nioid [" + *eidos,* resemblance]. Resembling a hernia.

herniolaparotomy (her"nĭ-o-lap-ă-rot'o-mĭ) [" + *lapara,* loin, + *tomē,* incision]. Abdominal section for the cure of hernia.

herniol'ogy [" + *logos,* study]. The science of hernia.

her'nioplasty [" + *plassein,* to form]. Surgical operation for hernia.

her"niopunc'ture [" + L. *punctura,* puncture]. Puncture of a hernia with hollow needle for withdrawal of fluid or gas.

herniorrhaphy (her-nĭ-or'ă-fĭ) [" + *raphē,* a suture]. Surgical operation for hernia.

herniotomy (her-nĭ-ot'o-mĭ) [G. *ernos,* a young shoot, + *tomē,* incision]. Surgery for the relief of hernia; an operation for the correction of irreducible hernia, esp. strangulated hernia.

NP: Paint area with iodine, 3½ or 7% as ordered. Place sterile towel over chest and abdomen, place lap ring (small sheet about a yard square, with opening in center) over area of incision. Place an open regular lap sheet on abdomen. Place 4 towels around area of incision, 2 lengthwise and 2 crosswise.

When the operator is finished with an instrument, discard it into a basin of Lysol solution (it may then be removed for resterilization and meanwhile has not contaminated anything). While the skin is being sutured prepare final dressing. The operating nurse washes off her gloves thoroughly before removing them. She then assists in replacing the dressing. In bilateral hernias, each side should be draped and treated as a separate operation.

DRESSING: Towels, gauze sponges, gauze compresses, safety pins, bandages, and cotton. One pillow under head until otherwise ordered, knee roll under knees, prevent strain on abdominal muscles—assist in turning, etc. The surgeon's requisites vary with the operator.

heroin (her'o-in). A narcotic derived from morphine, commonly used by addicts. Formerly used for treatment of asthma and cough. Importation of this drug is illegal in the United States. SYN: *diacetylmorphine.*

heroinism (her'o-in-izm) [*heroin* + G. *ismos,* condition]. Addiction to habitual use of heroin.

herpangina (herp-an-ji'nă, herp-an'jĭ-nă) [G. *erpēs,* herpes, + L. *angina,* a choking]. A disease of children marked by fever and small ulcers in the throat.

ETIOL: One of several strains of Coxsackie virus.

herpes (her'pēz) [G. *erpēs,* herpes]. 1. A form of vesicles appearing in clusters on inflammatory base but with no tendency to rupture; in *herpes zoster* they are distributed along the nerve trunks. 2. Inflammatory skin disease characterized by formation of groups of vesicles.

h. circinatus. Dermatitis herpetiformis, an inflammatory skin disease of a herpetic nature.

h. desquamans. Tinea imbricata, *q.v.*

h. facialis. A form of herpes simplex which occurs on the face.

h. febrilis. Herpes simplex accompanying a febrile disease.

h. genitalis. Herpetic lesions on the male or female genitalia.

h. iris. Erythema multiforme, *q.v.*

h. labialis. Herpes simplex occurring on the lips. SYN: *cold sore; fever blister.*

h. menstrualis. Herpetic lesions appearing at the time of the menstrual period.

h., mouth. H. marked by appearance of multiple whitish areas on soft palate and mucosa of mouth. SYN: *gingivostomatitis, q.v.*

h. praeputialis. Herpes of the male genitals.

h. progenitalis. Herpes simplex of vulva.

h. simplex. So-called fever blisters.

SYM: Occurrence of clusters of vesicles on erythematous edematous base on face or genital regions marked by itching and localized hyperemia, the lesions drying up and shedding yellowish crusts in 10-14 days if unmolested.

ETIOL: A medium-sized virus which is found in early vesicles but usually absent in later pus-filled vesicles. Indigestion, febrile and toxic states, physical fatigue, and emotional disturbances are precipitating factors. The virus apparently lives within the body cells between recurrent manifestations.

h. zoster. SYN: *shingles, zona.* An acute, infectious, inflammatory disease of the skin.

SYM: Usually unilateral.

ETIOL: A large filtrable virus related to that causing chickenpox.

PATH: The skin vesicles are usually confined to the epidermis accompanied by inflammation of the underlying corium. The nerve, its sensory ganglion and post. horn of the gray matter may show inflammatory reaction.

PROG: Acute course conferring immunity. Hemorrhagic, gangrenous and supraorbital cases are serious.

TREATMENT: Aspirin and codeine and mild sedation for pain. Gauze pad with petroleum jelly applied locally to prevent pain from irritation by clothing. Calamine lotion for skin lesions.

herpet'ic [G. *erpēs,* herpes]. Pert. to herpes.

h. neuralgia. Neural pain with herpes zoster.

h. sore throat. Herpetic tonsillitis.

herpet'iform [" + L. *forma,* form]. Resembling herpes.

her'petism [" + *ismos,* state of]. Predisposition to herpetic eruption.

hersage (ār-sazh') [Fr. a harrowing]. Splitting of a nerve trunk into separate fibers.

Herter's infantilism [Christian A. Herter, American physician, 1865-1910]. Celiac disease; a form of infantilism resulting from defective fat and calcium absorption. Resembles sprue in adults.

hertz'ian waves. Electromagnetic vibrations that have wave lengths of a centimeter or longer.

hes'peridin. A derivative of a white glycoside found in ripe and unripe citrus fruits. Decreases capillary fragility and prevents localized hemorrhage.

Hesselbach's hernia (hes'el-bakhs) [Franz K. Hesselbach, German surgeon, 1759-1816]. A lobated hernia which passes through the cribiform fascia.

H.'s triangle. The triangular space bounded by Poupart's ligament below, ext. border of rectus muscle internally, and epigastric artery ext.

heteradenia (het-er-ă-de'nĭ-ă) [G. *eteros,* other, + *adēn,* gland]. 1. Glandular substance in a part not provided with glands. 2. Abnormal glandular tissue.

heteradenic (het-er-ă-den'ik) [" + *adēn,* gland]. Pert. to heteradenia.

heteradenoma (het"er-ad-ĕ-no'mă) (pl. *heteradenomata*) [" + " + *ōma,* tumor]. A heteradenic tissue tumor; any hyaline cylindroma.

heterecious (het-er-e'shus) [" + *oikos,* house]. Living upon different hosts at different stages of development.

heterecism (het"er-ē'sizm) [" + *oikos,* house]. Development of different cycles of existence on different hosts, said of certain parasites.

heteresthesia (het-er-es-the'zĭ-ă) [" + *aisthēsis,* sensation]. Variation in degree (plus or minus) of sensory response to cutaneous stimuli.

heteroagglutinin. An agglutinin formed as result of injection of an antigen from an animal of a different species; an agglutinin capable of agglutinating blood cells of other species of animals.

heteroal'bumose [" + L. *albumen,* white of egg]. Albumose insoluble in water but soluble in saline solutions, in acid or alkaline solutions. SYN: *hemialbumose.*

heteroautoplasty (het"er-o-aw'to-plas-tĭ) [" + *autos,* self, + *plassein,* to form]. Grafting skin from one person to another.

heteroblas'tic [" + *blastos,* germ]. Having origin in tissue of another kind. Opp. of homoblastic.

heterocel'lular. Composed of different kinds of cells.

heterochiral (het-er-o-ki'ral). Pertaining to the other hand.

het"erochro'matin. A type of chromatin that stains less distinctly than the *euchromatin,* forming clear disks interposed between dark bands on chromosomes. In interphasic nuclei it constitutes the chromocenters. It is thought that it controls certain metabolic activities of cells. It contains no genes. SEE: *euchromatin.*

heterochromatosis (het"er-o-kro-mă-to'sis) [" + *chrōma,* color, + *ōsis*]. 1. Pigmentation of skin from foreign substances. 2. Difference in color. SYN: *heterochromia.*

heterochromia (het-er-o-kro'mĭ-ă) [" + *chrōma,* color]. A difference in color.

h. iridis. Different color of iris in the two eyes; the lighter colored iris is atrophic due to previous iridocyclitis, congenital or otherwise.

heterochromosome (het-er-o-kro'mo-sōm). An allosome; a chromosome which differs from the ordinary chromosomes or autosomes; the X and Y or sex chromosomes. Also called *accessory chromosome.*

heterochromous (het-er-o-kro'mus) [G. *eteros,* other, + *chrōma,* color]. With abnormal difference in coloration.

heterochro'nia [" + *chronos,* time]. Denoting an abnormal time for the occurrence of a phenomenon or production of a structure.

heterochron'ic [" + *chronos,* time]. Occurring at different or at abnormal times.

heterochylia (het-er-o-ki'lĭ-ă) [" + *chylos,* juice]. A change in character of the gastric juice without apparent cause.

heterocinesia (het-er-o-sĭ-ne'sĭ-ă) [" + *kinēsis,* movement]. Movements different from those the patient is instructed to make.

heterocladic (het"er-o-klad'ik). Pertaining to an anastomosis between branches of two different arteries, in contrast to *homocladic, q.v.*

heterocri'sis [" + *krisis,* division]. Irregular crisis with abnormal symptoms.

heterocyclic (het"er-o-si'klik) [" + *kyklos,* circle]. Pert. to ring compounds which contain other atoms in addition to carbon atoms as part of the ring.

heteroder'mic [" + *derma,* skin]. Pert. to a method of skin grafting when grafts are taken from another person. SEE: *dermatoheteroplasty.*

het'erodont [" + *odous, odont-,* tooth]. Having teeth of various shapes.

heteroecious. Heterecious, *q.v.*

heteroecism. Heterecism, *q.v.*

heteroerotism (het"er-o-er'o-tizm) [" + *erōs,* love, + *ismos,* state of]. Sexual desire for another person.

heterogametic (het"er-o-gă-met'ik). Pertaining to the production of unlike gametes, applied esp. to a male which produces two types of sperm, one containing the X chromosome, the other the Y chromosome.

heterogamy (het"er-og'ă-mĭ). The union of gametes which are dissimilar in size and structure. Occurs in higher plants and animals. SEE: *isogamy.*

heterogeneous (het-er-o-je'ne-us) [G. *eteros,* other, + *gennos,* type]. Of unlike natures composed of unlike substances. In contrast to homogeneous, *q.v.*

h. vaccine. That made from some source other than patient's own organism. Opp. of *autogenous.*

heterogen'esis [G. *eteros,* other, + *genesis,* production]. Alternation of generations; mode of reproduction in which an asexual generation alternates with a sexual generation, or a dioecious generation alternates with a parthenogenetic generation. Occurs in lower forms such as coelenterates and trematodes.

heterogenet'ic [" + *gennan,* to produce]. Rel. to heterogenesis.

het'erograft [" + L. *graphium,* grafting knife]. A graft taken from another individual or an animal of a different species from the one for whom it is intended. SEE: *autograft; isograft.*

heterog'raphy [" + *graphein,* to write]. Writing different words from those the writer intended.

heteroinfec'tion [G. *eteros,* other, + L. *in,* in, + *facere,* to make]. Infection by virus originating outside of the body. SYN: *exogenous infection.*

het"eroinocula'tion [" + " + *oculus,* bud]. Inoculation from other organisms.

heterola'lia [" + *lalia,* babbling]. The use of meaningless words instead of those intended.

heterol'ogous [" + *logos,* relation]. Made up of cell tissue not normal to the part, as certain new growths.

heterol'ogy [G. *eteros,* other, + *logos,* relation]. Different from the normal in structure or method of growth.

heterolysin (het-er-ol'ĭ-sin) [" + *lysis,* solution]. Lysins formed from an antigen from an animal of a different species. SEE: *autolysin; hemolysin.*

heterolysis (het-er-ol'ĭ-sis) [" + *lysis,* solution]. Hemolytic action of blood serum of an animal upon corpuscles of another species. SEE: *isolysis.*

heteromeric (het-er-o-mer'ik) [" + *meros,* part]. 1. Pert. to spinal neurons with processes to opposite side of cord. 2. Possessing a different chemical composition.

heterometaplasia (het"er-o-met-ă-pla'zĭ-ă) [" + *meta,* beyond, + *plassein,* to form]. Transformation of tissue to a tissue foreign to the part where produced.

heteromorphous (het-er-o-mor'fus) [" + *morphē,* form]. Deviating from the normal type.

heteronomous (het-er-on'o-mus) [" + *nomos,* law]. Abnormal; differing from type.

heteronymous (het-er-on'ĭ-mus) [" + *onyma,* name]. 1. Expressed in or having different names. 2. On opposite sides.

h. diplopia. Having a false image on same side as the sound eye.

hetero-os'teoplasty [" + *osteon,* bone, + *plassein,* to form]. Grafting of bone, esp. with a graft from an animal.

heteropathy (het-er-op'ă-thĭ) [" + *pathos,* disease]. 1. Abnormal reaction to irritation or to stimuli. 2. Creation of a morbid condition to neutralize another disorder.

heterophany (het-er-of'ă-nĭ) [" + *phainein,* to appear]. Having different expressions of the same disorder.

heterophasia (het-er-o-fa'zĭ-ă) [" + *phasis,* speech]. Expression of meaningless words instead of those intended. SYN: *heterolalia; heterophemy.*

heterophe'mia, heteroph'emy [" + *phēmē,* speech]. Expressing one thing when another is intended. SYN: *heterolalia; heterophasia.*

heterophil(e (het'er-o-fĭl) [" + *philein,* to love]. 1. Pert. to an antibody reacting with other than the specific antigen. 2. Pert. to a tissue or microorganism that takes a stain other than the ordinary one.

heterophonia (het-er-o-fo'nĭ-ă) [G. *eteros,* other, + *phōnē,* voice]. Change of voice.

heterophoralgia (het-er-o-for-al'jĭ-ă) [" + *phoros,* bearing, + *algos,* pain]. Deviation of one eye accompanied by pain.

heteropho'ria [G. *eteros,* other, + *phoros,* bearing]. The tendency of the eyes to deviate from their normal position, esp. when one eye is covered; latent deviation or squint.

ETIOL: Imbalance or insufficiency of ocular muscles.

heterophthalmos (het-er-of-thal'mus) [" + *ophthalmos,* eye]. Difference in appearance of the eyes due to the irides differing in color. SEE: *heterochromia.*

Heterophyes (het-er-oph'ĭ-ēz). A genus of flukes belonging to the family Heterophyidae, *q.v.*

H. heterophyes. A species of intestinal fluke commonly infesting man. In heavy infestations may cause diarrhea, nausea, and abdominal discomfort.

heterophyiasis (het"er-o-fi-i'ă-sis). Infestation by any fluke belonging to the family *Heterophyidae, q.v.*

Heterophyidae. A family of Trematoda (flukes) which infests the intestines of dogs, cats and other mammals including humans. Infestations are common in Egypt and in the Far East. Includes the genera Heterophyes, Haplorchis, Diorchitrema and Metagonimus. Intermediate hosts are snails, the cercaria encysting in fishes, esp. mullets, or frogs. The eggs of foreign species may cause serious damage to organs, esp. the heart.

heteroplasia (het-er-o-pla'zĭ-ă) [" + *plassein,* to mold]. Production of a part where it does not belong.

heteroplastic (het-er-o-plas'tĭk) [" + *plassein,* to form]. Rel. to heteroplasia.

het'eroplasty [" + *plassein,* to form]. Grafting with tissue from another person or an animal.

heteroploid. Possessing a chromosome number that is a multiple of the haploid number common for the species.

heteroproteose (het"er-o-pro'te-ōs). An intermediate product formed in the hydrolysis of proteins to peptones.

heteropsia (het-er-op'sĭ-ă) [" + *opsis,* vision]. Inequality of vision in the two eyes.

heteroptics. Perversion of vision such as seeing objects that do not exist or misinterpreting what is seen.

heteropyknosis (het"er-o-pik-no'sis). The property whereby various parts of a chromosome stain with varying degrees of intensity; thought to be due to variations in concentration of nucleic acid.

heteros'copy [" + *skopein,* to examine]. Finding range of vision in strabismus.

heteroserotherapy (het"er-o-se"ro-ther'ă-pĭ) [" + L. *serum,* whey, + G. *therapeia,* treatment]. Treatment by serum from another person.

heterosex'ual [" + L. *sexus,* sex]. Having normal attraction for the opposite sex.

het"erosexual'ity [" + L. *sexus,* sex]. The normal state of love for one of the opposite sex.

heterosis (het-er-o'sis). Hybrid vigor; condition in which the offspring of individuals belonging to different races or species possess greater vitality, sturdiness, and resistance to disease or unfavorable environmental conditions.

heterotax'ia [G. *eteros*, other, + *taxis*, arrangement]. Abnormal position of organs or parts. SEE: *dextrocardia; situs inversum viscerus.*

heteroto'pia [" + *topos*, place]. Displacement of an organ or part.

heterotop'ic [" + *topos*, place]. Misplaced; pert. to heterotopia.

heterotopous (het-er-ot'o-pus) [" + *topos*, place]. Pert. esp. to teratomata consisting of tissues out of normal placement.

heterotopy (het-er-ot'o-pĭ) [" + *topos*, place]. Displacement of an organ or a portion of the body.

heterotox'in [" + *toxikon*, poison]. A toxin introduced from without the patient's body.

heterotrans'plant [G. *eteros*, other, + L. *trans*, across, + *plantare*, to plant]. An organ tissue, or structure taken from an animal and grafted into, or on, another animal of a different species. Such transplants usually atrophy.

heterotrichosis (het"er-o-trĭ-ko'sis) [" + *trichōsis*, growth of hair]. Growth of different kinds or color of hairs on the scalp or body.

heterotroph (het"er-o-trŏf). An organism which obtains its energy by the oxidation of organic compounds, such as *heterotrophic bacteria*. SEE: *autotrophic.*

heterotro'pia [" + *tropos*, a turn]. Manifest deviation of the eyes due to absence of binocular equilibrium. SEE: *strabismus.*

heterovac'cine [" + L. *vaccinus*, pert. to a cow]. A vaccine from a source other than that of the disease for which it is intended.

heteroxanthine (het"er-o-zan'thin) [" + *xanthos*, yellow]. Methyl xanthine found in the urine.

heterozygosis (het"er-o-zi-go'sis). Condition in which the two members of a pair of genes in the zygote differ from each other; the result of cross breeding. SEE: *homozygosis.*

heterozygote (het"er-o-zi'gōt). An individual in which the members of one or more pairs of genes are unlike.

heterozygous (het-er-o-zi'gus). Genetically impure, not breeding true. Having one or many pairs of genes in the phase of heterozygosis resulting from cross breeding. Having unlike genes. SEE: *homozygous.*

hettocyrtosis (het-o-sir-to'sis) [G. *ēttōn*, less, + *kyrtōsis*, curvature]. A slight curvature of the spine.

Heublein method (hoyb'līn) [Arthur C. Heublein, American radiologist, 1879-1932]. Low voltage doses of x-ray given over the entire body for cancer.

Heubner's disease (hoib'ners) [Johann Otto L. Heubner, Berlin pediatrician, 1843-1926]. Syphilitic endarteritis of the brain.

heurteloup (hert-loo'). An artificial leech; a cupping apparatus.

hexa- [G.]. Prefix: *Six.*

hexaba'sic [G. *ex*, six, + *basis*, base]. Having six replaceable hydrogen atoms.

hexachlorophene (heks"ă-klo'ro-fēn). USP. A bactericidal and bacteriostatic compound, used in emulsions and soaps for preoperative cleansing of skin and mucous membranes and for hand scrubs.

hexachro'mic [" + *chrōma*, color]. Not being able to distinguish more than six of the seven colors of the spectrum or to distinguish violet from indigo.

hexad (heks'ad) [G. *ex*, six]. The atom of an element having a valence of 6.

hexadactylism (heks"ă-dak'til-izm). Possession of six fingers or six toes.

hexamethonium (heks"ă-me-tho'nĭ-um). A compound which acts as a ganglionic blocking agent. Used in the treatment of hypertension.

Hexapoda (heks-ă-po'dă). The insects or six-legged arthropods.

hexatomic (heks-ă-tom'ik) [G. *ex*, six, + *atomos*, indivisible]. Pertaining to a compound consisting of six atoms, or a compound having six replaceable hydrogen or univalent atoms.

hexavac'cine [" + L. *vaccinus*, pert. to a cow]. A vaccine made from six different microorganisms.

hexavalent (heks"ă-va'lent) [G. *ex*, six, + L. *valere*, to have power]. Having a valence of 6. SYN: *sexivalent.*

hexestrol. A synthetic estrogen said to be more active than diethylstilbestrol.

hexokinase (heks"o-ki'nās). An enzyme present in muscle tissue which catalyzes the phosphorylation of glucose. It has also been isolated from yeast.

hex'one, or **hex'one base** [G. *ex*, six]. One of the amino acids, as histidine, arginine and lysine, so called because they contain chains of 6 carbon atoms.

hexon'ic [G. ex, six]. Rel. to hexone bases.

hexosephosphate (heks"ōs-fos'fāt) [G. *ex*, six, + *phosphas*, phosphate]. A phosphoric acid ester of glucose. One of several esters (Cori, Robison, *et al.*) formed in the muscles and other tissues in the metabolism of carbohydrates.

hex'oses [G. *ex*, six]. Monosaccharides of the general formula $C_6H_{12}O_6$; the group includes particularly dextrose and levulose, *q.v.*

hexylresorcinol (heks"il-re-sor'sĭ-nol). USP. $C_{12}H_{18}O_2$. White needle-shaped crystals. Used as an anthelmintic.

Hey's lig'ament [William Hey, English surgeon, 1736-1819]. The semilunar lateral margin (falciform margin) of the fossa ovalis which lies between iliac and pubic portions of the fascia lata.

Hg. Symb. for *mercury* (*hydrargyrum*).

$HgCl_2$. Mercuric chloride; corrosive sublimate.

Hg_2Cl_2. Mercurous chloride; calomel.

HgI_2. Mercuric iodide.

HgO. Mercuric oxide.

HgS. Mercuric sulfide.

$HgSO_4$. Mercuric sulfate.

hiatus (hi-a'tus) [L. an opening]. 1. An opening, a foramen. 2. The vulva. 3. An aperture.

h. aorticus [NA]. Opening in diaphragm through which pass the aorta and the thoracic duct.

h. canalis facialis [NA]. Opening on superior (ant.) portion of petrous portion of temporal bone. It transmits the great superficial petrosal nerve and branch of facial and petrosal branch of middle meningeal artery.

h. fallopii. H. canalis facialis, *q.v.*

h. maxillaris [NA]. Opening of maxillary sinus into the nasal cavity, located on nasal surface of maxillary bone.

h. oesophageus [NA]. Opening in diaphragm through which the esophagus passes.

h. semilunaris [NA]. The groove in the external wall of middle meatus of nasal fossa into which the antrum of

Highmore, frontal series, and ant. ethmoid cells open.

hiccough, hiccup (hik'up) [probably of imitative origin]. Spasmodic periodic closure of the glottis following spasmodic lowering of the diaphragm, causing a short, sharp, inspiratory cough. SYN: *singultus*.

ETIOL: It may be caused by indigestion, an overloaded stomach, irritation under surface of diaphragm, alcoholism, new growths of the pleura, or certain cerebral lesions, or hysteria, or influenza. May be due to a disturbance of the phrenic nerve and diaphragm and if prolonged it has serious significance. The time of occurrence and whether accompanied by a burning sensation in the throat or by an unpleasant sensation, should be noted.

TREATMENT: Antiemetic drugs, rebreathing in a paper bag, carbon dioxide breathing, gastric suction. Stimulation of the pharynx with a soft rubber tube should also be tried. If these are not effective, anesthetization of the phrenic nerve may be helpful.

Hicks' (Braxton) sign [John B. Hicks, English gynecologist, 1825-1897]. Uterine intermittent contractions at end of 3rd mo. of pregnancy, or in presence of tumor.

hide'bound disease' [A.S. *hyd*, a skin, + *bindan*, to tie up]. Hardening and thickening of the skin with loss of elasticity. SYN: *scleroderma*.

hidradenitis (hi-drad-ĕ-ni'tis) [G. *idrōs*, sweat, + *adēn*, gland, + *-ītis*, inflammation]. Inflammation of sweat glands by staphylococcus, usually in the axillae.

hidradenoma (hi-drad-ĕ-no'mă) [G. *idros*, sweat, + *aden*, gland, + *oma*, tumor]. Adenoma of the sweat glands. SYN: *syringocystadenoma*.

hidroa (hi-dro'ă) [G. *idrōs*, sweat]. 1. Vesicles due to retention of sweat. SYN: *sudamina*. 2. Any bullous eruption. SYN: *hydroa*.

hidrocystoma (hi-dro-sis-to'mă) [" + *kystis*, cyst, + *ōma*, tumor]. A cystic tumor of a sweat gland.

hidropoiesis (hi-dro-poy-e'sis) [G. *idrōs*, sweat, + *poiēsis*, formation]. The formation of sweat.

hidropoiet'ic [" + *poiēsis*, formation]. Pert. to hydropoiesis. SYN: *sudorific*.

hidrorrhea (hi-dro-re'ă) [" + *roia*, flow]. Abnormal sweating.

hidrosadenitis (hi-drōs-ad-ĕ-ni'tis) [" + *adēn*, gland, + *-ītis*, inflammation]. Inflammation of sweat glands. SYN: *hidradenitis*.

hidroschesis (hi-dros'kĕ-sis) [" + *schesis*, a holding]. Retention of perspiration.

hidrosis (hi-dro'sis) [G. *idrōs*, sweat, + *ōsis*]. 1. Formation and excretion of sweat. 2. Excessive sweating.

hidrot'ic. 1. Causing the secretion and excretion of sweat. SYN: *diaphoretic; sudorific*. 2. Any drug or medicine that induces sweating.

hieralgia (hi-er-al'jĭ-ă) [G. *ieron*, sacrum, + *algos*, pain]. Pain in the region of the sacrum.

hierophobia (hi"er-o-fo-bĭ'ă). Abnormal fear of sacred things, or persons connected with religion.

high blood pressure. Abnormal pressure in arteries at height of pulse wave.

TREATMENT: Many drugs and some surgical procedures are used to bring blood pressure to normal.

RS: *blood, blood pressure, hypertension, hypotension, pulse pressure*.

high calorie diet. One that provides maintenance and extra heat and energy. *Indicated*: 1. To prevent loss of weight. 2. In wasting diseases. 3. In high basal metabolism. 4. After long illness. 5. In deficiency caused by anorexia, poverty, poor dietary habits. 6. During lactation when 1000 to 1200 extra calories are indicated.

Three meals plus between-meal feedings. Milk, eggs, as under normal conditions, a slight excess of proteins and fats. Fermentable and bulky foods to be avoided.

Breakfast: Three oz. cream, extra butter. *Dinner*: Salad with mayonnaise, extra butter, 3 oz. cream. *Supper*: Same as for dinner. Each in addition to the general diet, with a 10 A. M. and 2:30 P. M. high caloric lunch, and a glass of milk at 8 P. M.

high cellulose diet. The general diet plus the following: *Breakfast*: Bran muffin or a tablespoon of bran added to a cereal, and extra large serving of fruit. *10 A. M.*: Fruit juice. *Dinner*: Salad, extra serving of vegetables, fruit. *Supper*: Salad, extra serving of vegetables and fruits.

high frequency treatment. High frequency current passed through the body to produce heat in the tissues. RS: *circuit, current, diathermy*.

High'more, antrum of [Nathaniel Highmore, English surgeon, 1613-1685]. The air sinus in the maxillary bone. SEE: *antracele; antrum*.

H.'s body. Fibrous tissue mass, a prolongation of albuginea testis, projecting forward along posterior border of testis. SYN: *mediastinum testis*.

highmori'tis. Inflammation of the maxillary sinus or antrum of Highmore. SYN: *antritis; sinusitis maxillaris*.

hill'ock. A small eminence or projection.

h., anal. One of two small eminences which lie lateral and posterior to the cloacal membrane, and later, the anal fissure in the embryo.

h., axon. A small conical elevation on the cell body of a neuron from which the axon arises. It is devoid of Nissl bodies. SYN: *implantation cone*.

h., seminal. The *colliculus seminalis*, *q.v.*

Hil'ton's law [John Hilton, English surgeon, 1804-1878]. The trunk of a nerve, which sends branches to a particular muscle, also sends branches to the joint moved by that muscle and to the skin overlying the insertion of the muscle.

H.'s line. A white one at junction of skin of perineum and anal mucosa.

H.'s muscle. The aryepiglottic muscle.

H.'s sac. Pit along external portion of false vocal cords. SYN: *sacculus laryngis*.

hi'lum, hi'lus (pl. *hila, hili*) [L. a trifle]. 1. Depression or recess at exit or entrance of duct into a gland, or of nerves and vessels into an organ. 2. The root of the lungs at level of 4th and 5th dorsal vertebrae.

himantosis (hi-man-to'sis) [G. *imantōsis*, a long strap]. Abnormal lengthening of the uvula.

hind'brain [A.S. *hindan*, behind, + *bragen*, brain]. The most caudal of the three divisions of the embryonic brain; the *rhombencephalon*. It differentiates into the *metencephalon* which gives rise to the cerebellum and pons, and the *myelencephalon* which gives rise to the medulla oblongata.

hindgut. The caudal portion of the entodermal tube which develops into the alimentary canal. It gives rise to the ileum, colon, and rectum.

hind kidney. The metanephros, the most caudal of three embryonic kidneys. It persists and develops into the permanent kidney. SEE: *metanephros.*

hinge joint. An articulation which permits flexion and extension about a single axis; *ginglymus.*

Hin'ton's test [William A. Hinton, American bacteriologist, 1883-1959]. Agglutination test for syphilis.

hip [A.S. *hype*]. 1. Upper part of thigh, formed by the femur and innominate bones. 2. The region on each side of the pelvis.

***h.* bone.** *Os coxae.* Its three portions are: (a) The ilium (pl. *ilia*); (b) ischium (pl. *ischia*), and (c) pubis (pl. *pubes*).

***h.*, dislocation of.** Dislocations of the hip are very often accompanied by a fracture and it is extremely difficult even for a well-trained surgeon to distinguish a pure dislocation from a fracture dislocation without an x-ray.

DIAG: If person has great difficulty in straightening the hip following an accident. It is always accompanied by pain. The knee on the injured side resistantly points inwardly toward the other knee and it is difficult to straighten the leg.

SYM: Pain, rigidity, loss of function, and the dislocation may be obvious by the abnormal position in which the leg is held, or by seeing or feeling the head of the femur in an abnormal position.

F. A. TREATMENT: Place the patient on a large splint as in a fractured back. In addition, place a large pad, such as a pillow, under the knee of the affected side. Treat for shock.

***h.*, dislocation of, backward.** Onto the dorsum ilii or sciatic notch. SYM: 1. Inward rotation of thigh, with flexion, inversion, adduction, shortening. 2. Pain, tenderness. 3. Loss of function and immobility. TREATMENT: (a) Patient anesthetized. (b) Dorsal position, leg flexed on thigh, latter upon abdomen. (c) Adduct thigh, rotate outward; circumduction outwardly across abdomen, back to straight position. (d) Possibly traction, even incision and direct replacement.

***h.*, dislocation of, downward.** Rare. TREATMENT: (a) Traction in flexed position. (b) Outward rotation and extension.

***h.*, dislocation of, forward.** Through obturator foramen, on pubis, in perineum, or through fractured acetabulum. SYM: 1. Pain, tenderness, and immobility. 2. In pubic and suprapubic forms, shortening; lengthening in obturator and perineal forms. TREATMENT: (a) Hyperextension and direct traction. (b) Flexion, abduction with inward rotations, adduction.

hip joint. Articulation bet. femur and innominate bone. A ball and socket (enarthrosis) formed by the head of the femur fitting into a concavity, the acetabulum. SYN: *articulatio coxae* [NA].

***h. j.*, arthritis of.** Usually occurring before age of 14 years. VARIETIES: Arthritic, acetabulum, femoral. SYM: cardinal symptoms, wasting, spasm, lameness, pain, swelling, deformity. PROG: Influenced by circumstances. Tendency toward recovery. TREATMENT: Maintain general state of good health, mechanical and surgical treatment.

***h. j.* disease.** May be: 1. Tubercular. 2. Pustular (pyogenic). 3. Fracture. 4. Congenital deformities. 5. Dislocation of. 6. Dystrophies of (internal glandular). 7. Legg's disease. SYM: *General:* 1. Early—pain, limp, muscle spasm. 2. Later—muscle wasting, swelling, deformity. TREATMENT: *General:* Build up patient's general health by: 1. Diets. 2. Fresh air and sunshine. 3. Tonics. *Specific:* Varies with disease. *General to all:* Put on spica plaster cast, surgery or mechanical manipulation.

***h. j.*, snapping.** A slipping around of the hip joint, sometimes producing an audible snapping sound.

hip lift (artificial respiration). Following application of the prone-pressure or Schafer method, operator leans forward and inserts his clenched fist under one hip, elevating it about 2 inches; then with the other fist under the other hip, it is lifted 4 to 6 inches, producing a rotary motion on the stationary hip. This is alternated with the back-pressure method. This procedure provides more than twice the amount of air in respiration than the prone-pressure method. SEE ALSO: *artificial respiration; resuscitation.*

hip lift–back pressure (artificial respiration). This method combines alternate lifting of the hips with pressure on the midback (just below the scapulas), with the fingers spread and the thumbs about an inch from the spine. As the operator lifts the hips, he rocks backward; and as he exerts back pressure, he rocks forward. In each phase, he keeps the arms straight, so that the work of lifting and pressing is distributed over the shoulders and back, rather than being imposed primarily on the arms. Active inspiration results from lifting the hips and active expiration from pressure on the midback. SEE ALSO: *artificial respiration; resuscitation.*

hip roll–back pressure (artificial respiration). This is a modification of the hip lift–back pressure method in which a roll is substituted for the lift in order to increase the ease of performance. The operator kneels astride the prone subject as described for the hip lift; instead of lifting both hips, he uses the knee on which he is kneeling as a fulcrum on which to roll the victim. The operator keeps his arm straight and rolls himself in the same direction in which he rolls the victim. Great care must be exercised to insure that the victim is rolled up onto the operator's knee or thigh so that both hips are raised from the ground. SEE ALSO: *artificial respiration; resuscitation.*

hippocam'pal [G. *ippokampos,* seahorse]. Pert. to the hippocampus.

***h.* commissure.** A thin sheet of fibers passing transversely under post. portion of the corpus callosum. They connect the medial margins of the crura of the fornix. SYN: *commissure of the fornix; commissura fornicis* [NA]; *lyra; psalterium.*

***h.* fissure.** Fissure above the temporal lobe on mesial surface of cerebrum. SYN: *sulcus hippocampi* [NA].

***h.* formation.** Olfactory structures lying along the medial margin of the pallium. It includes the hippocampus, dentate gyrus, supracallosal gyrus, longitudinal striae, subcallosal gyrus, diagonal band of Broca, and hippocampal commissure. SYN: *formatio hippocampalis.*

hippocam'pus ma'jor [G. *ippokampos,* seahorse]. Elevation of floor of inf. horn of lat. ventricle of the brain, occupying nearly all of it.

h., digitations of. Three or four shallow grooves on ant. portion of hippocampus.

h. minor. A small elevation on mesial wall of lat. ventricle formed by end of the calcarine fissure. SYN: *calcar avis* [NA].

Hippocrates (hĭ-pok'ră-tēz) [B.C. 460-359 or 377). Greek physician who is referred to as the "father of medicine."

hippocrat'ic fa'cies. The appearance of the face at the time of impending death.

SYM: Dark brown, livid, or lead colored skin; hollow appearance of eyes, collapse of temples, sharpness of nose, lobes of ears contracting and turning outward. SEE: *facial.*

h. oath. Oath exacted of his students by Hippocrates: "I swear by Apollo the physician, and Aesculapius, and Hygeia, and Panacea, and all the gods and goddesses, that according to my ability and judgment, I will keep this oath and its stipulation—to reckon him who taught me this art equally dear to me as my parents, to share my substance with him, and to relieve his necessities if required; to look upon his offspring in the same footing as my own brothers, and to teach them this art if they shall wish to learn it, without fee or stipulation, and that by precept, lecture, and every other mode of instruction, I will impart a knowledge of the art to my own sons, and those of my teachers, and to disciples bound by a stipulation and oath according to the law of medicine, but to none other.

"I will follow that system of regimen which, according to my ability and judgment, I consider for the benefit of my patients, and abstain from whatever is deleterious and mischievous. I will give no deadly medicine to anyone if asked, nor suggest any such counsel; and in like manner I will not give to a woman a pessary to produce abortion. With purity and with holiness I will pass my life and practice my art. I will not cut persons laboring under the stone, but will leave this to be done by men who are practitioners of this work. Into whatever houses I enter, I will go into them for the benefit of the sick, and I will abstain from every voluntary act of mischief and corruption; and, further, from the seduction of females or males, of freemen and slaves. Whatever, in connection with my professional practice, or not in connection with it, I see or hear, in the life of men, which ought not to be spoken of abroad, I will not divulge, as reckoning that all such should be kept secret.

"While I continue to keep this Oath unviolated, may it be granted to me to enjoy life and the practice of this art, respected by all men, in all times. But should I trespass and violate this Oath, may the reverse be my lot."

In part, some of these points are still the accepted standard for the ethical physician today.

hip'pulin(e [G. *ippos,* horse]. An estrogenic substance, obtained from urine of pregnant mares.

hippu'ria [G. *ippos,* horse, + *ouron,* urine]. Large quantities of hippuric acid in the urine.

hippu'ric acid. An acid formed and excreted by the kidneys. It is formed in the human body from the combination of benzoic acid and glycine, the synthesis taking place in the liver and to a limited extent by the kidney.

Seven to 15 gr. (0.5 to 1.0 gm.) is eliminated every 24 hr. It is increased by eating prunes, greengage plums, cranberries, and some vegetables. They increase acidity of the urine, as the hippuric acid is not metabolized.

hippur'icase. An enzyme found in the liver, kidney, and other tissues which catalyzes the synthesis of hippuric acid from benzoic acid and glycine. SYN: *hippurase; histozyme.*

hippus (hip'us) [G. *ippos,* horse]. Rhythmical and rapid dilatation and contraction of the pupils. Tremor of iris, spasmodic in character.

h., respiratory. Dilatation during inspiration, and contraction of pupil during expiration.

Hirschberg's reflex (hirsh'berg). Adduction of foot when sole at base of great toe is irritated.

Hirschsprung's disease (hirsh'sprungs) [Harold Hirschsprung, Danish physician, 1830-1916]. Congenital hypertrophic dilatation of the colon.

hirsute (hur'sūt) [L. *hirsutus,* shaggy]. Hairy.

hirsuties (hur-su'shĭ-ēz) [L. *hirsutus,* shaggy]. Hirsutism.

hirsutism (hur'sūt-izm). Condition characterized by the excessive growth of hair or the presence of hair in unusual places.

hirudicide (hĭ-ru'dĭ-sīd) [L. *hirūdō,* a leech, + *caedere,* to kill]. Any substance that destroys leeches.

hir'udin. A substance present in the secretion of the buccal glands of the leech which prevents coagulation of the blood. It inactivates thrombin.

Hir''udin'ea. A class of annelida. They are hermaphroditic, lack setae or appendages, and usually possess two suckers. Includes the blood-sucking leeches. A number of species, including *H. medicinalis,* were formerly used extensively for blood-letting.

hir''udini'asis. Infestation by leeches. In *external h.,* leeches attach themselves to the skin and suck blood. After the leeches drop off, bleeding may continue as a result of the action of hirudin. Bites may become infected or ulcerate.

h., internal. Results from accidental ingestion of leeches in drinking water, which may attach to wall of pharynx, nasal cavity, or larynx.

Hiru'do. A genus of leeches belonging to the family Gnathobdellidae.

His, bundle of [Wilhelm His, Jr., German physician, 1863-1934]. The *atrioventricular bundle,* A-V bundle, a group of modified muscle fibers, Purkinje fibers forming a part of the impulse conducting system of the heart. It arises in the atrioventricular node and continues in the interventricular septum as a single bundle, the *crus commune* which divides into two trunks which pass respectively to the right and left ventricles, fine branches passing to all parts of the ventricles. It conducts impulses from the atria to the ventricles which initiate ventricular contraction.

histaffine (his'tă-fēn) [G. *istos,* tissue, + L. *affinis,* having affinity for]. 1. Having affinity for tissues. 2. A hypothetical substance in the blood serum assumed to fix certain constituents of normal and esp. pathological tissues.

histaminase (hĭs-tăm'ĭ-nās). An enzyme widely distributed in the body which inactivates histamine. It is used in the treatment of certain allergies and other conditions resulting from release of excessive quantities of histamine.

histamine (his'tă-min, -mēn). 1. A substance in the body found wherever tissues are damaged. Red flush of a burn is due to the local production of histamine; product of histidine catabolism.

2. An amine found in almost all animal tissues, and produced by the action of putrefactive bacteria.

Injected under the skin, if the circulation is normal, it produces a wheal surrounded by a flare, suggesting a mosquito bite. Given intravenously, causes gastric secretion, flushing of skin, lowered blood pressure, and headache.

h. cataphoresis. Method of treating rheumatic afflictions in which histamine solution is applied to the skin by the positive pole of the galvanic current.

h. phosphate. USP. A chemically made product, which may be produced from citric acid by a lengthy process.

Uses: Most frequently as a diagnostic agent in determining the acid secreting power of the stomach.

histamine'mia [*histamine* + G. *aima*, blood]. Histamine in the blood.

histamin'ia. Shock induced by histamine in the body.

his'tase [G. *istos*, tissue, + *ase*, enzyme]. An enzyme which digests tissue.

histen'zyme [" + *en*, in, + *zymē*, leaven]. An enzyme in renal tissues which splits up hippuric acid into benzoic acid and glycocol. Syn: *histozyme.*

his'tidase. An enzyme present in the liver which acts on l-histidine. It splits the imidazole ring with the resultant formation of glutamic and formic acids and ammonia.

histidine (his'tĭ-din, -dēn). An amino acid, $C_6H_9N_3O_2$, obtained by hydrolysis from tissue proteins and necessary for tissue repair and growth.

histiocyte (his'tĭ-o-sīt) [G. *histos*, web, + *kytos*, cell]. A cell present in all loose connective tissues. It may exhibit active ameboid movement and show marked phagocytic activity. These cells take up readily substances such as trypan blue, colloidal carbon, and other foreign substances of a particulate nature. Histiocytes belong to the reticuloendothelial system. Syn: *macrophage; clasmatocyte; pyrrhol cells; adventitial cells; resting wandering cells.*

histiocytoma. A tumor containing histiocytes.

histiocytosis (his"tĭ-o-si-to'sis) [G. *histion* dim. of *histos*, web, + *kytos*, cell, + *ōsis*]. Histocytes in the blood in unusual numbers.

h., lipoid. Niemann-Pick disease, *q.v.*

histiogenic (his-tĭ-o-jen'ĭk) [" + *gennan*, to form]. Formed by the tissues. Syn: *histogenous.*

his'tioid [" + *eidos*, form]. Resembling or composed of one of the body tissues. Syn: *histoid.*

his"tioir'ritative [" + L. *irritāre*, to excite]. Irritative to connective tissue.

histio'ma [" + *ōma*, tumor]. A tissue tumor.

histo- [G.]. Prefix: *Relation to tissue.*

his'toblast [G. *istos*, tissue, + *blastos*, germ]. A tissue cell.

histochemistry (his"to-kem'is-trĭ). Study of chemistry of tissue by use of microscopes and stained or otherwise prepared tissue.

histochromatosis (his"to-kro-mă-to'sis) [" + *chrōma*, color, + *ōsis*]. Name of disorders of reticuloendothelial system.

histoclas'tic [" + *klastos*, breaking]. Decomposing tissue.

histocyte (his'to-sīt) [" + *kytos*, cell]. A tissue cell. Syn: *histoblast.*

his"todiagno'sis [" + *dia*, through, + *gnōsis*, knowledge]. Diagnosis made from examination of the tissues.

histodial'ysis [" + *dialysis*, a loosening]. Disintegration of tissue. Syn: *histolysis.*

histogenesis (his-to-jen'ĕ-sis) [" + *genesis*, formation]. Development into differentiated tissues of the germ layer; origin and development of tissue.

histogenetic (his-to-jĕ-net'ik) [" + *genesis*, formation]. Pert. to histogenesis.

histogenous (his-toj'ĕ-nus) [" + *gennan*, to form]. Made by the tissues.

histogram (his'to-gram) [" + *gramma*, a writing]. A graph showing frequency distributions.

histog'raphy [" + *graphein*, to write]. A written description of the tissues.

histohem'atin [" + *aima*, blood]. A hemoglobin pigment in various tissues.

histohematogenous (his"to-hem-ă-toj'ĕ-nus) [" + " + *gennan*, to form]. Arising from both the tissues and the blood.

histoid (his'toyd) [" + *eidos*, form]. 1. Resembling one of the tissues. 2. Developed from a single tissue, as *fibroma.*

histokinesis (his-to-kĭ-ne'sis) [" + *kinēsis*, movement]. Movement in the tissues of the body.

histolog'ical [" + *logos*, knowledge]. Pert. to microscopic tissue anatomy.

histol'ogy [" + *logos*, study]. Study of the microscopic structure of tissue.

h., normal. Study of healthy tissue.

h., pathologic. Study of diseased tissue.

histolysis (his-tol'ĭ-sis) [" + *lysis*, dissolution]. Disintegration of tissues.

histolyt'ic [" + *lysis*, dissolution]. Pert. to histolysis.

histo'ma [" + *ōma*, tumor]. A tumor composed of tissue. Syn: *histioma.*

his'ton(e [G. *istos*, web]. A class of simple proteins derived from cell nuclei which interferes with coagulation, yielding certain amino acids (the histone or hexone bases) as a result of hydrolysis.

Histones are found in the thymus, sperm, and blood cells.

histonec'tomy [G. *istos*, tissue, + *ektomē*, excision]. Periarterial excision of parts of the sympathetic nerve.

histon'omy [" + *nomos*, law]. The law governing development and structure of tissues.

histonu'ria [" + *ouros*, urine]. Excretion of histon in the urine.

histopathol'ogy [" + *pathos*, disease, + *logos*, study]. Histology of diseased tissues.

histophysiol'ogy [" + *physis*, nature, + *logos*, study]. Study of functions of cells and tissues.

Histoplas'ma. A genus of parasitic fungi.

H. capsulatum. The causative agent of histoplasmosis, *q.v.*

histoplas'min. An antigen prepared from cultures of *Histoplasma capsulatum* and used as a skin test for the diagnosis of histoplasmosis.

histoplasmo'sis [" + *plasma*, plasma, + *ōsis*]. A systemic, fungal, respiratory disease due to *Histoplasma capsulatum.* It spreads from the lungs throughout all parts of the body.

h. organs. Structures which are morphological equivalents as the arm of man and forelimb of quadrupeds; penis of male and clitoris of female. Homologous organs indicate relationship, or descent from a common ancestor.

h. series. Compounds with a similar chemical structure and properties, arranged in order of their molecular complexity, such as *methane* and *ethane*.

h. tissues. Those identical in structure.

h. vaccine. One from the microorganism infecting the patient. SYN: *autogenous vaccine.*

homology (ho-mol'o-jĭ) [G. *omos*, same, + *logos*, relation]). Similarity in structure and in origin.

h., serial. Anterior-posterior correspondence of parts of an organism which occur in a serial fashion, as the appendage of a crayfish, or the fore- and hind limbs of quadrupeds.

homolysin (ho-mol'ĭ-sin) [G. *omos*, same, + *lysis*, solution]. SYN: *isolysin.* An agent in a serum destructive of erythrocytes.

homonomous (ho-mon'o-mus) [G. *omos*, same, + *nomos*, law]. Pertaining to parts arranged in a series which are similar in form and structure as metameres of a segmented animal or the fingers and toes.

homonymous (ho-mon'ĭ-mus) [" + *onyma*, name]. Having the same name.

h. diplopia. D. in which the image seen by the right eye is on the right side and *vice versa.*

homophil (ho'mo-fĭl) [" + *philein*, to love]. Pert. to an antibody reacting only with a specific antigen.

homoplas'tic [" + *plassein*, to form]. Having similar form and structure.

ho'moplasty [" + *plassein*, to form]. Repair by tissue similar to the one replaced.

Homo sapiens. The species to which all races of modern man belong.

homosex'ual [" + L. *sexus*, sex]. 1. An invert, one sexually attracted to another of the same sex. 2. Pert. to attraction to another of same sex.

ho"mosexual'ity [" + L. *sexus*, sex]. A condition in which the libido is directed toward one of the same sex.

homostim'ulant [" + L. *stimulāre*, to arouse]. Stimulating the organ from which an extract is derived.

homotherm'al [G. *omos*, same, + *therma*, heat]. Condition in which the body temperature is maintained at a fairly constant level regardless of the temperature of the environment. SYN: *warm-blooded.*

homotonic (ho-mo-ton'ik) [" + *tonos*, tension]. Of uniform tension.

homotype (ho'mo-tīp) [" + *typos*, type] One organ or part similar in form and function to another, as one of two paired parts or organs.

homotypic (ho-mo-tip'ik) [" + *typos*, type]. Of the same form and type.

homozygote (ho-mo-zi'gōt). A homozygous individual; an individual developing from like gametes and thus possessing like pairs of genes for any hereditary characteristic.

homozygous (ho-mo-zi'gus). 1. Produced by similar gametes. 2. Pure bred. 3. Said of an organism when all germ cells transmit identical genes resulting from inbreeding.

homunculus (ho-mun'ku-lus). A dwarf in which the parts of the body develop in their normal proportions.

honey. A sweet thick liquid substance made by bees from the nectar of flowers and stored in their hive. An excellent source of carbohydrate. The earliest known fermented alcoholic beverage, now called *mead*, was made from honey. Calories: 304 per 100 grams. Other main values: 3 gm. protein; 82 gm. carbohydrate; 5 mg. calcium; 1 mg. ascorbic acid.

hook [A.S. *hōk*, an angle]. A curved instrument.

h., blunt. One used in extraction of fetus or in embryotomy.

hook-up. Term used in speaking of the method of arranging circuits, appliances and electrodes in the giving of any particular treatment; as, for instance, the hook-up for direct sparks.

hook'worm. A parasitic nematode belonging to the superfamily Strongyloidea, esp. *Ancylostoma duodenale* and *Necator americanus, q.v.*

hook'worm disease. A condition brought about by the presence of the hookworm in the intestinal tract. SYN: *Ancylostomiasis; uncinariasis.*

hordeolum (hor-de'o-lum) [L. barleycorn]. Inflammation of a sebaceous gland of the eyelid. SYN: *sty, q.v.*

h. internum. Suppuration of Zeiss or meibomian glands.

horismascope (hor-is'mă-skōp) [G. *orizma*, a boundary, + *skopein*, to examine]. A U-shaped tube for an acid test for albumin in the urine.

horizocardia (ho-ri"zo-kar'dĭ-ă) [G. *orizōn*, horizon, + *kardia*, heart]. Horizontal position of the heart.

horizon'tal posi'tion [G. *orizōn*, horizon]. Lying supine with feet extended. Employed in palpitation and auscultation of fetal heart beat and in operative procedures.

h. p., abdominal. The patient lies flat on the abdomen with feet extended. Employed in examination of back and spinal column.

hormion (hor'mĭ-on) [G. *ormion*, a little chain]. Junction of post. border of the vomer with the sphenoid bone.

hormone (hor'mōn) [G. *ormanein*, to excite]. 1. A chemical substance originating in an organ, gland, or part, which is conveyed through the blood to another part of the body, stimulating it to increased functional activity and increased secretion.

Contains amino acids which may be the precursors of hormones.

2. The secretion of the ductless glands, such as insulin, by the pancreas.

They are active in minute quantities and do not supply energy. A hormone

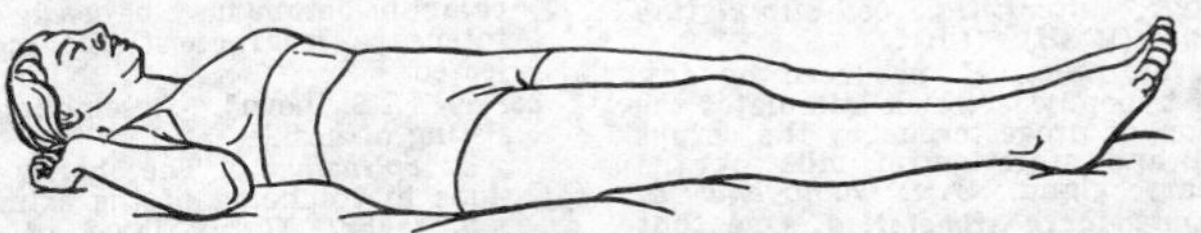

HORIZONTAL POSITION.

that induces an excitatory effect is called an *autacoid;* an inhibitory effect, a *chalone.*

h., adrenocortical. H. secreted by the cortex of the adrenal gland. SEE: the cortex, under *adrenal.*

h., adrenocorticotropic. A hormone secreted by the ant. lobe of the hypophysis (pituitary gland) which stimulates the adrenal cortex. SYN: *corticotropin; ACTH.*

h., androgenic. Includes *testosterone, androsterone,* and *dehydroandrosterone.* H. which regulates the development and maintenance of the male secondary sexual characteristics; an androgen, *q.v.* Androgens are secreted by the interstitial tissue of the testis and by the adrenal cortex of both sexes. SYN: *male sex hormones.*

h., anterior pituitary. H. secreted by ant. lobe of the hypophysis. Includes the somatotropic (SH), thyrotropic (TH), gonadotropic, follicle-stimulating (FSH), interstitial-cell stimulating (ICSH), luteotropic (LH), lactogenic, and adrenocorticotropic (ACTH) hormones.

h., A.P.L. Anterior pituitary-like hormone. A chorionic gonadotropin secreted by the placenta and found in the urine of pregnant women and serum of pregnant mares. Used in pregnancy tests, *q.v.*

h., basal. One that reduces urine excretion to normal levels.

h., chromatophorotrophic. Melanocyte stimulating h.

h., corpus luteum. Progesterone, *q.v.*

h., corticoadrenal. Adrenocortical hormones, *q.v.*

h., diabetogenic. H. antagonistic to insulin.

h., estrogenic. A hormone, as estrogen, which stimulates the development and maintenance of female sexual characteristics. Estrogens are secreted by the ovary, the placenta, and the adrenal cortex in both sexes. *Female hormones.* Include estradiol, estrone, estriol.

h., follicle, h., follicular. H. secreted by the ovarian follicles; an estrogen.

h., follicle-stimulating (FSH). H. secreted by the ant. lobe of hypophysis which stimulates development of the ovarian follicles.

h., gastric. Gastrin, *q.v.*

h., gonadotropic. Ant. pituitary h affecting the gonads. SEE: *follicle-stimulating h.; luteinizing h.; luteotropic h.*

h., growth. Ant. pituitary h. promoting normal growth.

h., interstitial cell-stimulating (ICSH). SEE: *luteinizing hormone.*

h., intestinal. A hormone produced by the mucosa of the intestine. SEE: *secretin; cholecystokinin.*

h., lactogenic. Luteotropic hormone, *q.v.*

h., luteal. H. produced by the corpus luteum. SYN: *progesterone, q.v.*

h., luteinizing. H. produced by the ant. lobe of hyphophysis which induces ovulation and the formation of the corpus luteum. Also stimulates development of interstitial cells of the testes. SYN: *interstitial cell-stimulating hormone* (ICSH) (LH).

h., luteotropic. H. produced by ant. lobe of hypophysis which stimulates the secretion of progesterone by the corpus luteum and secretion of milk by the mammary gland. SYN: *lactogenic h.*

h., melanocyte stimulating. One that darkens the skin in man.

h., ovarian. A h. produced by the ovary. SEE: *estradiol; estrone; estriol; progesterone.*

h., pancreatic. H. produced by the islets of Langerhans of the pancreas. SEE: *insulin; lipocaic.*

h., parathyroid. H. secreted by the parathyroid glands which regulates calcium and phosphorus metabolism. Deficiency results in tetany. SEE: *parathyrin; parathormone.*

h., placental. H. secreted by the placenta. Includes estrogens and chorionic gonadotropin.

h., post. pituitary. H. secreted by post. lobe of hypophysis. Includes *pitressin,* which produces vasopressor and antidiuretic effects and *ditocin* (oxytocin) which causes contraction of smooth muscles of the uterus.

h.'s, sex, female. Estrogenic hormones, *q.v.*

h.'s, sex, male. Androgenic hormones, *q.v.*

h., testicular. H. produced by the interstitial tissue of the testis, *e. g.. testosterone, androsterone,* and *dehydroandrosterone, q.v.*

h., thyroid. Thyroxine, the h. secreted by follicles of the thyroid gland.

h., thyrotropic. H. produced by ant. lobe of hypophysis which regulates development and functioning of the thyroid gland.

h., wound. Traumatin.

hormon'ic [G. *ormanein,* to excite]. Rel. to or acting as a hormone. SYN: *hormonal.*

hormonogenesis (hor"mo-no-jen'ĕ-sis) [" + *genesis,* production]. Production of an internal secretion. SYN: *hormonopoiesis.*

hormonogenic (hor"mo-no-jen'ik) [" + *gennan,* to produce]. Producing hormones. SYN: *hormonopoietic.*

hormonol'ogy [" + *logos,* study]. The study of hormones. SYN: *clinical endocrinology.*

hormopoiesis (hor-mo-poy-e'sis) [" + *poiēsis,* formation]. The production of hormones. SYN: *hormonopoiesis.*

hormopoietic (hor-mo-poy-et'ik) [" + *poiēsis,* formation]. Rel. to hormones and their formation. SYN: *hormonopoietic.*

horn. A cutaneous outgrowth composed chiefly of keratin. A horn-like projection. SYN: *cornu.*

h. (of) Ammon. Hippocampus, *q.v.*

h., dorsal. Post. projection of gray matter of the spinal cord. SYN: *posterior column.*

h., ventral. Anterior projection of gray matter of the spinal cord. SYN: *anterior column.*

Hor'ner's syndrome [Johann F. Horner, Swiss ophthalmologist, 1831-1886]. Anidrosis, enophthalmos, miosis, and ptosis from paralysis of cervical sympathetic nerves.

hor'net sting. Sting by a hornet.

A general urticaria may result from the sting of this insect.

TREATMENT: Remove the stinger; apply tincture of iodine and cold compresses. Household ammonia in 10% solution applied to the area is beneficial and subsequent soothing lotions such as calamine lotion may be used. If pain is intense a local anesthetic may be injected.

hor'ny [A.S. horn]. Resembling or consisting of horn.

h. epithelium. The horny granulations in trachoma of the skin.

h. layer. Horny layer of the skin. SYN: *stratum corneum.*

horopter (hor-op'ter) [G. *oros,* limit, + *optēr,* observer]. Sum of all points in the binocular vision.

horripilation (hor-ĭ-pĭ-la'shun) [L. *horrēre,* to bristle, + *pilus,* hair]. Goose flesh. SYN: *cutis anserina.*

horse'shoe fis'tula. A fistulous tract in a semicircle in front or behind the anus.

h. kidney. A congenital abnormality. Both kidneys are united at their lower poles forming a horseshoe mass generally at a lower level than normal.

hos'pital [L. *hospitalis,* pert. to a guest]. Institution for treatment of the sick and wounded.

h., base. A hospital unit within the lines of an army for reception of wounded and patients from the front, as well as for those within the line itself.

h., camp. An immobile military unit for care of sick and wounded in camp.

h., cottage. A collection of detached cottages for care of the sick.

h., evacuation. A mobile advance hospital unit to take the place of field hospitals and to supplement base hospitals.

h., field. A portable military hospital beyond the zone of conflict and beyond the dressing stations.

hos'pitalism [L. *hospitalis,* pert. to a guest, + G. *ismos,* state]. 1. The air of depression and apathy which often surrounds a group of seriously ill patients esp. if they are in the same ward and overcrowded. 2. A neurotic tendency to seek hospitalization and, once hospitalized, to resist being discharged.

hospitalization. Removal of a patient to and confinement in a hospital.

host [L. *hostis,* a stranger]. 1. The organism from which a parasite obtains its nourishment. 2. In embryology, the larger and relatively normal of conjoined twins. 3. In transplantation of tissue, the individual who receives the graft.

h., accidental. A host other than the usual or normal host.

h., alternate. Intermediate host, *q.v.*

h., definitive. The final host or host in which the parasite reaches sexual maturity. 2. The vertebrate, when the intermediate host is an invertebrate.

h., final. The definitive host, *q.v.*

h., intermediate. H. in which a parasite passes through its larval or asexual stages of development. The invertebrate host, when final host is a vertebrate.

h., primary. The final host, *q.v.*

h., reservoir. A host other than the usual or normal one in which a parasite is capable of living and serving as a source of infestation.

h., secondary. The intermediate host, *q.v.*

hot. 1. Possessing a high temperature. 2. Actively conducting an electrical current. 3. Contaminated with dangerous radioactive material.

h. flashes. Crises of vasodilation in skin of head, neck, and chest accompanied by sensation of suffocation and sweating. Occurs commonly during menopause.

Hot'tentot ap'ron. Excessive elongation of the labia minora seen in Hottentot women. SYN: *velamen vulvae.*

H. deformity. Abnormal fatness of the buttocks. SYN: *steatopygia.*

hot'tentotism. Abnormal form of stuttering.

hot water bag. Rubber or plastic bag of various shapes and sizes for applying dry heat to circumscribed areas and for keeping moist applications warm.

hourglass contrac'tion. Excessive, irregular contraction of an organ at its center, as the pregnant uterus during 3rd stage of labor.

The placenta is held in upper part of uterus by a tightly constricting band bet. lower and upper uterine segments. SYN: *ectasia.*

h. stomach. Division of stomach (in form of an hourglass) by a muscular constriction; often associated with gastric ulcer.

house fly. *Musca domestica,* a fly belonging to the order Diptera. Serves as a transmitter of organisms of many infectious diseases.

house'maid's knee. A traumatism resulting from kneeling which produces a swelling of the bursa, ant. to the patella.

house physician. A physician, especially an intern or resident, who is responsible for caring for patients under the direction of the medical and surgical staff.

house staff. The interns and externs of a hospital acting under direction of the general staff.

house surgeon. The senior surgical member of the hospital staff who acts for the attending surgeon in his absence.

Houston's muscle (hūs'tonz) [John Houston, Irish surgeon, 1802-1845]. The ant. part of the *musculus bulbo-cavernosus.*

H.'s valves. The folds of mucous membrane or valves formed by them in rectum; supposed to keep feces from entering the anus too rapidly. SYN: *plica transversalis recti.*

Howell-Jolly bodies [William H. Howell, American physiologist, 1860-1945; Justin Jolly, French histologist, 1870-1953]. Spherical granules seen in erythrocytes in slides of stained blood. They are thought to be nuclear particles.

Howship's lacunae [John Howship, English surgeon, 1781-1841]. Small pits, grooves or depressions found where resorption of bone is occurring. They are usually occupied by *osteoclasts, q.v.*

H.'s symptom. Paresthesia, or pain in obturator hernia, on inner side of thigh.

HPO_3. Metaphosphoric acid.

H_3PO_2. Hypophosphorous acid.

H_3PO_3. Phosphorous acid.

H_3PO_4. Orthophosphoric acid.

$H_4P_2O_6$. Hypophosphoric acid.

Hr factors. Structures including *Hr agglutinogens* and *Hr antigens,* on surface of the red blood cells responsible for reactions with *Hr antiserums.* A number of related factors of human blood, so named because of their reciprocal relationship to the Rh factors. The factors, Hr', Hr'', and Hr_0 have been identified. These blood factors are important because sensitization may give rise to dangerous blood transfusion reactions. The baby of a sensitized Hr-negative pregnant woman may develop the blood disease, erythroblastosis fetalis, just as with sensitized Rh-negative mothers.

h.s. Hora somni, bedtime.

H. S. Abbr. for *house surgeon.*

H_2S. Hydrogen sulfide.

H_2SO_3. Sulfurous acid.

H_2SO_4. Sulfuric acid.

H-substance. A substance similar to or identical with histamine, *q.v.*

Ht. Abbr. for *total hypermetropia.*

Hub'bard tank. One used for underwater exercises.

Húguier's canal (ü-ge-a') [Pierre C. Huguier, French surgeon, 1804-1873]. A canal through which the chorda tympani nerve exits from the cranium.

H.'s circle. Anastomosis around the isthmus of the uterus.

H.'s diseases. Lupus of vulva, and uterine fibroma.

H.'s glands. Two tiny vaginal glands

Huhner test [Max Huhner, American urologist, 1873-1947]. One for sterility in the male. SEE: *test.*

hum [of imitative origin]. A soft continuous sound.

h., venous. Sound from large veins in certain anemias. SYN: *bruit de diable.*

hu'man [L. *humanus,* pert. to man]. Pert. to or characterizing man or mankind.

h. bite. Wound caused by human teeth.

SYM: Intense swelling, edema, and foul discharge may develop. The organisms most frequently found in wounds from such bites are a fusiform bacillus, and a spirillum of streptococcus.

TREATMENT: If lymphangitis, moderate fever, and leukocytosis occur, a wide incision may be necessary with hot wet pack applied to the whole arm or hand that has been injured. Smears should be taken from the drainage. Induration in the palm of the hand may occur. All such victims need the immediate attention of a physician.

humectant (hu-mek'tant). A moistening or diluent agent.

humeral (hu'mer-al) [L. *humerus,* shoulder]. Pert. to the humerus.

humeroradial (hū"mer-o-ra'dĭ-ăl) [" + *radius,* wheel spoke, ray]. Pert. to humerus and radius, esp. in comparison of their length.

humeroulnar (hu"mer-o-ul'ner) [" + *ulna,* forearm]. Pert. to the humerus and ulna, esp. in comparison to their length.

hu'merus [L. shoulder]. Upper bone of arm from the elbow (articulating with the ulna and radius) to the shoulder joint, where it articulates with the scapula.

h., fracture of. 1. If the fracture is of the upper end the arm is abducted on a wire splint for about 4 weeks. Movements of the elbow and wrist are started early and movements (active) of shoulder in about 3 weeks.

2. Fracture of shaft and lower end. The limb is put in plaster in a position midway between pronation and supination with the humerus at right angles to the forearm. Movement of the shoulder, wrist, and finger is allowed at once.

RS: *acromiohumeral, capitellum, cubitus, glenoid cavity.*

hu'mid [L. *humidus,* moist]. Moist, damp.

h. gangrene. G. with serous exudation and rapid decomposition. SEE: *gangrene.*

humidifier (hu-mid'ĭ-fi-er) [L. *humidus,* moist]. Apparatus to increase moisture content of the air in a room.

humid'ity [L. *humiditās,* moisture]. Moisture in the atmosphere.

If air was saturated at a temperature of 70° F., water would condense on all objects if the temperature fell to 68° F.

THE SATURATION OF THE AIR OCCURS AT:

If It Contains

50°	4.2 grains of water per cu. ft.
60°	5.8 grains of water per cu. ft.
70°	7.9 grains of water per cu. ft.
90°	14.3 grains of water per cu. ft.

The air can contain at 90° almost twice as much as at 70° F. The relative humidity at 70° F. would be 50% if the air held 3.88 grains of water per cu. ft. A room with a humidity of from 40-50° F. means the presence of 1½ gal. of water every 24 hours if it represents a content of 10 cu. ft., or 8 or more gal. for a 6-room house. SEE: *relative humidity.*

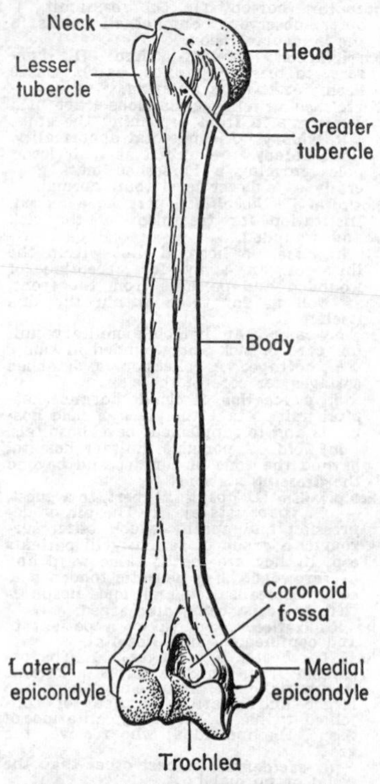

RIGHT HUMERUS, ANTERIOR VIEW

humor [L. fluid]. 1. Any fluid or semifluid substance in the body. 2. In ancient medicine, the four "juices" or fluids (blood, phlegm, black bile, yellow bile) of which the body was thought to be composed.

h., aqueous. A watery fluid in the anterior and posterior chambers of the eye.

h., crystalline. The fluidlike substance of the crystalline lens of the eye.

h., vitreous. The vitreous body, *q.v.* A semifluid, transparent substance occupying the space between the lens and retina of the eye.

hu'moral [L. *humor,* fluid]. Pertaining to body fluids or substances contained in them.

h. control or ***correlation.*** The control of various bodily activities by chemical substances, esp. hormones transported by the blood or lymph. In contrast to *nervous control* brought about through nerve impulses.

humpback [origin uncertain]. Curvature of the spine. SYN: *kyphosis.*

hung'er [A.S. *hungur*]. 1. A sensation resulting from lack of food, characterized by dull or acute pain referred to the epigastrium or lower part of chest. Usually accompanied by weakness and an overwhelming desire to eat. Hunger pains coincide with powerful contractions of the stomach. Distinguished from *appetite* in that the latter is a pleasant sensation based on previous experience which causes one to seek food for the purpose of tasting and enjoying. 2. To have a strong desire.

h., air. Dyspnea, breathlessness.

h. contractions. Those observed, and often felt, in the normal empty stomach. They may be painful. A series of such contractions is followed by a period of rest, after which they may return with greater intensity unless food is taken. Digestion may be activated under such conditions.

h. cure. Restricted diet or fasting for cure of disease. SYN: *nestiatria, nestitherapy.*

h., hormone. Deficiency of special hormone in an organ.

hungry. Craving food.

hunte'rian chancre. Indurated, syphilitic chancre. SEE: *chancre.*

Hun'ter's canal [John Hunter, English anatomist and surgeon, 1728-1793]. *Canalis adductorius.*

Hurler's syndrome. Lipochondrodystrophy, *q.v.*

Huschke's canal (hoosh'kēz) [Emil Huschke, German anatomist, 1797-1858]. One formed by juncture of the *annulus tympanicus* tubercules. Usually present only during early childhood.

H.'s foramen. Perforation found in arrested development near inner extremity of tympanic plate.

H.'s teeth. Tiny, toothlike protuberances at edge of cochlear labium vestibulare.

H.'s valve. Plica lacrimalis, *q.v.*

Hutchinson's patch (hŭtsh'ĭn-sŏn) [Sir Jonathan Hutchinson, English surgeon, 1828-1913]. Salmon-colored area in the cornea seen in syphilitic keratitis. SYN: *salmon patch.*

H.'s teeth. A congenital condition; pegged, lateral incisors and notched central incisors along the cutting edge. A sign of congenital syphilis.

Hux'ley's layer [Thomas H. Huxley, English physiologist and naturalist, 1825-1895]. Inner layer of nucleated cells forming the inner root sheath of a hair follicle.

hyalin (hi'ă-lin) [G. *yalos*, glass]. 1. A substance obtainable from the products of amyloid, colloid, or hyaloid degeneration. 2. Basement substance of hyaline cartilage.

hyaline (hi'ă-lin) [G. *yalos*, glass] Crystalline, glassy, translucent. SEE: *casts; degeneration.*

h. bodies. Homogeneous substance; the result of colloid degeneration and found in degenerated cells.

h. cartilage. The true cartilage. Smooth and pearly. It covers the articular surfaces of bones.

h. casts. The commonest form of cast. They are transparent, pale, and homogeneous with rounded ends, and they indicate nephropathy.

h. membrane disease. A respiratory disease of the newborn infant. A formation inside the lung of a thin membrane interfering with the normal flow of oxygen.

hyalino'sis [" + *ōsis*]. Waxy or hyaline degeneration.

hyalinu'ria [" + *ouron*, urine]. Hyalin present in the urine.

hyalitis (hi-ă-li'tis) [" + *-ītis*, inflammation]. Inflammation of the vitreous humor.

h., asteroid. Spherical bodies in the vitreous.

h. puncta'ta. A form marked by minute opacities in the vitreous humor.

h. suppurati'va. A purulent inflammation of the vitreous humor.

hyalo- [G.]. Prefix: Transparent.

hyaloenchondroma (hi"a-lo-en-kon-dro'-mă) [G. *yalos*, glass, + *en*, in, + *chondros*, cartilage, + *ōma*, tumor]. A chondroma composed of hyaline cartilage.

hyalogen (hi-al'o-jen) [" + *gennan*, to produce]. A protein substance in cartilage and the vitreous humor.

hyaloid (hi'ă-loyd) [" + *eidos*, form]. Hyaline, glassy.

h. artery. Present in the fetus. Supplies nutrition to lens. Disappears in later months of gestation.

h. canal. Lymph channel in vitreous extending from optic disk to post. capsule of lens; contains hyaloid artery in fetus.

h. membrane. That which envelops the vitreous humor.

hyaloiditis (hi"ă-loyd-i'tis) [" + " + *-ītis*, inflammation]. Inflammation of the hyaloid membrane of the vitreous humor. SYN: *hyalitis.*

hyaloma (hi-ă-lo'mă) [G. *yalos*, glass, + *ōma*, tumor]. A small yellow papule which develops in the corium of the skin as a result of colloid degeneration. SYN: *colloid milium.*

hyalomere (hi'ă-lo-mēr) [" + *meros*, part]. Homogeneous part of a blood platelet, pale in color, as contrasted with the chromomere.

hyalomu'coid [" + L. *mucus*, mucus, + G. *eidos*, form]. Mucoid in vitreous body.

hyalonyxis (hi"ă-lo-nik'sis) [" + *nyxis*, puncture]. Puncture of vitreous body.

hyalophagia (hi"ă-lo-fa'jĭ-ă) [" + *phagein*, to eat]. The eating of glass by the demented.

hyalophagy (hi-ă-lof'ă-jĭ) [" + *phagein*, to eat]. Eating of glass by the demented. SYN: *hyalophagia.*

hyalopho'bia [" + *phobos*, fear]. Fear of touching glass.

hyaloplasm (hi'ă-lo-plazm) [G. *yalos*, glass, + *plasma*, a thing formed]. The fluid portion of protoplasm. The basic ground substance; also called basic or fundamental protoplasm. SYN: *hyalomitome.*

h., nuclear. Clear substance filling the meshes of the nuclear reticulum. SYN: *karyolymph; nuclear sap.*

hyaloserositis (hi"ă-lo-se-ro-si'tis) [" + L. *serōsus*, serous, + G. *-ītis*, inflammation]. Inflammation of a serous membrane with fibrinous exudate undergoing hyaline transformation.

h., progressive multiple. Phthisis of serous membranes.

hyalotome (hi-al'o-tōm) [G. *yalos*, glass]. Fluid portion of protoplasm. SYN: *hyaloplasm.*

hyaluron'ic acid. An acid mucopolysaccharide found in the ground substance of connective tissue which acts as a binding and protective agent. Also found in the synovial fluid, vitreous and aqueous humors.

hyaluronidase (hi"ă-lur-on'ĭ-dās) An enzyme found in the testes and other tissues and present in semen. It depolymerizes hyaluronic acid thus increasing the permeability of connective tissues by dissolving the substances that hold body cells together. It acts to disperse the cells of the corona radiata about the newly ovulated ovum. SYN: *Duran-Reynals spreading factor.*

hybrid. The offspring of unlike parents; a heterozygous individual.

hybridization. The mating of individuals which differ in one or more pairs of genes; cross breeding.

hydan'toin. A colorless base, glycolyl urea, $C_3H_4N_2O_2$, from urea or allantoin.

hydatid (hi'dă-tid) [G. *ydatis*, a drop of water]. 1. A cyst formed in the tissues, esp. liver, resulting from the development of the larval stage of the dog tapeworm, *Echinococcus granulosus.* The cysts develop slowly forming a hollow bladder from the inner surface of which hollow brood capsules are formed. These are attached by slender stalks or they may fall free into the fluid-filled cavity of the mother cyst. Scolices form on the inner surface of the older brood capsules. In older cysts there is a granular deposit of brood capsules and scoleces called *hydatid sand.* Hydatids may grow for years sometimes attaining an enormous size. SEE: *Echinococcus granulosus.* 2. A small cystic remnant of an embryonic structure.

TREATMENT: Surgical.

h. fremi'tus. A tremulous sensation felt on palpating a hydatid tumor.

h. mole. Degenerative process in chorionic villi, which gives rise to multiple cysts and rapid growth of uterus with hemorrhage. DIAG: Indicated by the latter and expulsion of some of the cysts.

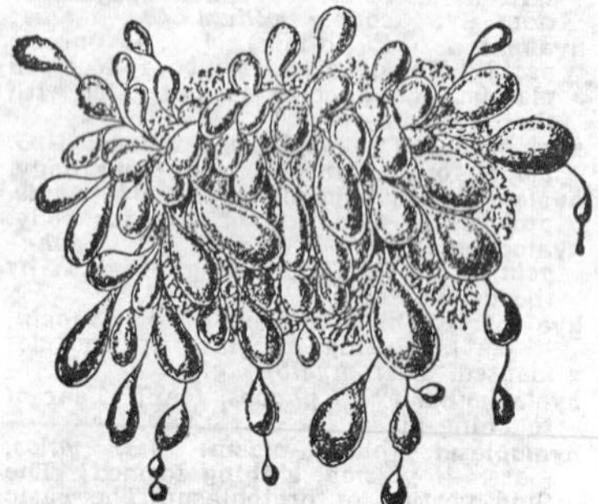

HYDATID MOLE

The entire placenta is transformed into a large number of edematous vesicles which resemble a bunch of grapes. Only a small part of the placenta is represented in this picture.

h. of Morgagni. Cystlike remnant of the mullerian duct which is attached to the fallopian tube.

h., sessile. Morgagnian h. connected with a testicle.

h., stalked. Morgagnian hydatid connected with a fallopian tube.

hydatidiform (hi"dă-tid'ĭ-form) [" + L. *forma*, shape]. Having the form of a hydatid.

hydatidocele (hi"dă-tid'o-sēl) [" + *kēlē*, tumor]. Hydatid cyst of scrotum or testicle.

hydatido'ma [" + *ōma*, tumor]. A tumor consisting of hydatids.

hydatidosis (hi"dă-tid-o'sis) [" + *ōsis*]. Condition caused by infestation with hydatids.

hydatidostomy (hi"dă-tid-os'to-mĭ) [" + *stoma*, opening]. Evacuation of a hydatid cyst.

hydat'iform [" + L. *forma*, form]. Having the form of a hydatid.

hy'datism [" + *ismos*, state of]. The sound produced by fluid in a cavity.

hydradenitis (hi-drad-ĕ-ni'tis) [G. *idrōs*, sweat, + *adēn*, gland, + *-ītis*, inflammation]. Inflammation of a sweat gland.

hydradeno'ma [" + " + *ōma*, tumor]. Tumor of a sweat gland.

hydraeroperitoneum (hi-dra-er-o-per-ĭ-to-ne'um) [G. *ydōr*, water, + *aēr*, air, + *peritonaion*, peritoneum]. Collection of fluid and gas in the peritoneal cavity.

hydragogue (hi'dră-gog) [" + *agōgos*, leading]. Drug promoting watery evacuation of the bowels.

EX: *magnesium sulfate, sodium phosphate, solution of magnesium citrate.*

hydramnion, hydramnios (hi-dram'nĭ-on, -os) [" + *amnion*, a caul on a lamb]. An excess of liquor amnii which leads to overdistention of the uterus and the possibility of malpresentations.

The normal amount is 500 to 1,000 ml. It may increase to 2,500 ml. and not be regarded as abnormal.

Liquor amnii is secreted by the fetus, and abnormal amounts are probably due to some abnormality of the fetus. Nearly half the cases occur in twin pregnancies. Hydramnios begins about 5th month of pregnancy and the pressure of the enlarged uterus gives rise to breathlessness, edema, cyanosis, and varicose veins in the mother. The uterus is large for the date given and the fetus may be felt bobbing about in the liquor and the fetal heart is not easily heard.

hydrargyrum (hi-drar'jir-um) [" + *argyros*, silver]. Mercury or quicksilver. SEE: *mercury.*

hydrarthrosis (hi-drar-thro'sis) [" + *arthron*, joint, + *ōsis*]. Serous effusion in a joint cavity; white swelling.

hydrase. An enzyme which catalyzes the addition of or the withdrawal of water from a compound without hydrolysis occurring.

hydrate (hi'drāt) [G. *ydōr*, water]. A crystalline substance formed by water combining with various compounds.

hydrated (hi'dra-ted) [G. *ydōr*, water]. Combined chemically with water.

hydration. The chemical combination of a substance with water.

hydrazine (hi'dră-zin). 1. A colorless gas, H_4N_2, with peculiar odor; soluble in water. 2. One of a class derived from hydrazine.

hydre'mia [G. *ydōr*, water, + *aima*, blood]. Excess of watery fluid in the blood.

hydrencephalocele (hi-dren-sef'ă-lo-sēl) [" + *egkephalos*, brain, + *kēlē*, tumor]. A hernia through a cranial defect of brain substance and meninges, in which fluid occupies the space between the two.

hydrencephalus (hi-dren-sef'ă-lus) [" + *egkephalos*, brain]. Accumulation of fluid in the cerebral ventricles or outside of the brain. SYN: *hydrocephalus.*

hydrepigastrium (hi-drep-ĭ-gas'trĭ-um) [" + *epi*, upon, + *gastēr*, belly]. Accumulation of fluid bet. the peritoneum and the abdominal muscles.

hydriatics (hi-drĭ-at'iks) [" + *iatikos*, healing]. Application of water in treatment of disease. SYN: *hydrotherapeutics.*

hydriatric (hi-drĭ-at'rik) [" + *iatrikos*, healing]. Pert. to treatment of disease with water, as hydriatric procedures or hydriatric institutions.

hydriat'rist [" + *iatrikos*, healing]. One who practices hydrotherapy.

hydride [G. *ydōr*, water]. Chemical compound containing hydrogen and an element or radical.

hy'drion. The hydrogen ion (H^+).

hydro- [G.]. Prefix: Water; also hydrogen.

hydro'a [G. *ydōr*, water]. Chronic inflammatory skin disease.

SYM: Bullae, erythema, itching, papules, pustules, and vesicles.

SYN: *dermatitis herpetiformis; pemphigus pruriginosus.*

hydroappen'dix [" + L. *appendere*, to hang]. Watery fluid distending the vermiform appendix.

hydrobilirubin (hi"dro-bil-ĭ-ru'bin) [" + L. *bilis*, bile, + *ruber*, red]. A brownish red bile pigment perhaps identical with stercobilin and urobilin.

hydrobromate (hi-dro-bro'māt) [" + *bromos*, stench]. A salt of hydrobromic acid.

hydrocarbon [G. *ydōr*, water, + L. *carbo*, carbon]. A compound made up only of hydrogen and carbon.

Hydrocarbons may exist as aliphatic chain compounds in which the carbon atoms are arranged in the form of a chain, or as aromatic or cyclic compounds in which the carbon atoms form one or more rings.

h., saturated. H. in which the carbon atoms are linked by a single electron pair and in which all valences are satisfied.

h., unsaturated. H. in which carbon atoms share two or three pairs of electrons.

hydrocele (hi'dro-sēl) [G. *ydōr*, water, + *kēlē*, hernia]. The accumulation of serous fluid in a saclike cavity, esp. the tunica vaginalis testis; serous tumors of the testes or associated parts.

h., acute. Most common, majority of cases bet. 2nd and 5th years. H. occurring suddenly, usually the result of inflammation of the epididymis or testis.

h., cervical. H. in the neck resulting from accumulation of serous fluid in persistent cervical duct or cleft.

h., chronic. H. usually seen in men of middle age. May result from filariasis.

h., congenital. That present at birth, resulting from failure of closure of the vaginal process.

h., encysted. H. in the vaginal process in which openings to the scrotal and peritoneal cavities are closed.

h. feminae. H. in labium majus or canal of Nuck.

h. hernialis. When hernia accompanies infantile or congenital h. and there is an accumulation of peritoneal fluid in a hernia sac.

h., infantile. Peritoneal fluid in the tunica vaginalis and vaginal process with the latter closed at the abdominal ring.

h. muliebris. H. feminae, *q.v.*

h., spermatic. Spermatic fluid in the tunica vaginalis of the testes.

h. spinalis. Spina bifida.

hydrocenosis (hi-dro-sen-o'sis) [" + *kenōsis*, an emptying]. Evacuation of a dropsical fluid by tapping or by a hydragogue. SYN: *paracentesis.*

hydrocephal'ic [G. *ydōr*, water, + *kephalē*, head]. Pert. to hydrocephalus.

hydrocephalocele (hi-dro-sef'ă-lo-sēl) [" + " + *kēlē*, hernia]. Watery hernia of the brain. SYN: *hydrencephalocele.*

hydroceph'aloid [" + " + *eidos*, resemblance]. Resembling or pert. to hydrocephalus.

h. disease. One of infants similar to hydrocephalus.

SYM: Depressed fontanels, pulse irregular, tendency to vomit.

hydrocephalus (hi-dro-sef'ă-lus) [G. *ydōr*, water, + *kephalē*, head]. The increased accumulation of cerebrospinal fluid within the ventricles of the brain. Results from interference with normal circulation and absorption of the fluid, esp. destruction of the foramina of Magendie and Lushka. This may result from developmental anomalies, infection, injury, or brain tumors.

In children, in severe cases, the head is usually globular or pyramidal in shape. Face disproportionately small. Eyes hidden in sockets and turned upward. Sutures separated, with bulging fontanels and thin cranial bones.

In older individuals after skull has formed there are headache, vomiting, choked disks, atrophy of optic nerve, mental disturbances.

h., communicating. H. in which normal communication between fourth ventricle and subarachnoid space is maintained.

h., congenital. Chronic type occurring in infancy. Also called *infantile h.*

h., external. Accumulation of fluid in subdural spaces.

h., internal. Accumulation of fluid within ventricles of the brain.

h., secondary. H. following injury or infections such as meningitis or syphilis.

hydrochlorate (hi-dro-klo'rāt) [" + *chlōros*, green]. Any salt of hydrochloric acid.

hy"drochlo'ric acid (HCl) [G. *ydōr*, water, + *chlōros*, green). An aqueous solution of hydrogen chloride, containing 35 to 38% (HCl). Crude commercial hydrochloric acid is known as *muriatic acid.*

It is a normal constituent of gastric juice amounting to 0.4 to 0.5% and is produced by the parietal cells of gastric glands. It serves the following functions: 1. Converts pepsinogen into pepsin and produces an acid medium favorable for the activity of pepsin. 2. Dissolves and disintegrates nucleoproteins and collagen. 3. Hydrolyzes sucrose. 4. Precipitates caseinogen. 5. Inhibits multiplication of bacteria, esp. putrefactive lactic acid fermentation, and certain pathogenic forms. 6. Stimulates secretion of secretin by the duodenum. It inhibits the action of ptyalin and thus stops salivary digestion in the stomach.

Average amount found in the food content of stomach is about 0.2% due to dilution and neutralization by alkaline contents. In pernicious anemia there is an absence of this acid (achlorhydria).

h. a., dilute. Aqueous solution of 10% HCl.

hydrocholecystis (hi-dro-ko-le-sis'tis) [G. *ydōr*, water, + *cholē*, bile, + *kystis*, bladder]. Dropsy of gallbladder.

hydrocholeresis (hi"dro-ko"ler-e'sis). Choleresis in which water content of the bile is increased resulting in production of bile with reduced specific gravity, viscosity, and total solid contents.

hydrocirsocele (hi-dro-sir'so-sēl) [" + *kirsos*, varix, + *kēlē*, tumor]. Hydrocele with varicose veins of spermatic cord.

hydrocollidine (hi-dro-kol'ĭ-din) [" + *kolla*, glue]. A poisonous ptomaine from putrefying fish or animal flesh.

hydrocolpos (hi-dro-kol'pos) [" + *kolpos*, vagina]. Retention cyst of the vagina containing watery, nonsanguineous fluid, or mucus.

hydroconion (hi-dro-ko'nĭ-on) [" + *konis,* dust]. An atomizer.

hy'drocyst [" + *kystis,* a bladder]. A cyst containing watery fluid.

hydrocysto'ma [" + " + *ōma,* tumor]. Disease marked by small hydrocysts. Sudamina on the face, esp. in women after middle age. SYN: *hidrocystoma.*

hydrodiascope (hi-dro-di'ă-skōp) [" + *dia,* through, + *skopein,* to examine]. Device to correct astigmatism.

hydrodictiotomy (hi"dro-dik-ti-ot'o-mĭ) [" + *dictyon,* retina, + *tomē,* incision]. Incision of retina for edema.

hydroelec'tric bath. Administration of an electrically charged bath.

hydroencephalocele (hi"dro-en-sef'ă-lo-sēl) [G. *ydōr,* water, + *egkephalos,* brain, + *kēlē,* hernia]. Brain substance expanded into a watery sac protruding through a cleft in the cranium. SYN: *hydrencephalocele.*

hydrogel (hi'dro-jel) [" + L. *gelāre,* to congeal]. A colloid containing water that solidifies in gelatinous form.

hy'drogen [G. *ydōr,* water, + *gennan,* to produce]. An element existing as a colorless, odorless, tasteless gas. SYMB: H. At. no. 1; at. wt. 1.00797. It possesses one valence electron. Three isotopes of hydrogen (*protium, deuterium,* and *tritium*) exist having atomic weight of 1, 2, and 3, respectively.

OCCURRENCE: H. occurs in its free state in natural gases and volcanic eruptions only in minute quantities. It is present in the sun and stars and on the earth it comprises about 1% of all known terrestrial matter. It occurs principally as hydrogen oxide (water, H_2O) and is a constituent of all hydrocarbons. It is present in all acids and in ionic form is responsible for the properties characteristic of acids. It is present in nearly all organic compounds and is a component of all carbohydrates, proteins, and fats.

USES: It is highly inflammable and used in the oxyhydrogen flame in welding, in hydrogenation of oils for solidifying purposes, as a reducing agent, and in many syntheses.

h. acceptor. In oxidation reduction reactions a substance which receives hydrogen atoms from another substance. SEE: *coenzyme.*

h. donator. In oxidation-reduction reactions a substance which gives up hydrogen atoms to another substance, the acceptor.

hy'drogenate [" + *gennan,* to produce]. To bring about a combination with hydrogen.

hydrogenation (hi-dro-jen-a'shun) [" + *gennan,* to produce]. A process of changing an unsaturated fat to a solid saturated fat by the addition of hydrogen in the presence of a catalyst, as olein and stearin.

hydrogen dioxide (di-oks'ĭd) [" + " + *di,* two, + *oxys,* acid]. Hydrogen peroxide (H_2O_2), *q.v.*

hydrogen ion. The positively charged nucleus of a hydrogen atom.

h. ion concentration. The relative proportion of hydrogen ions in a solution, the factor responsible for the acidic properties of a solution.

h. ion or pH scale. A scale used to express the degree of acidity or alkalinity of a solution. It extends from 0.00 (total acidity) to 14 (total alkalinity), the numbers running in reverse order of H-ion concentration. The *p*H value is the negative logarithm of the H-ion concentration of a solution, expressed in gram ions (moles) per liter.

As the hydrogen ion concentration decreases, a change of 1 *p*H unit means a ten-fold increase in hydrogen-ion concentration or true acidity. Thus a solution with a *p*H of 1.0 is ten times more acid than one with a *pH* of 2.0 and 100 times more acid than one with a *p*H of 3.0. A *p*H of 7.0 indicates neutrality.

As the hydrogen-ion concentration varies in a definite reciprocal manner with the hydroxyl ion (OH—) concentration, a *p*H reading above 7.0 indicates alkalinity. The blood and body fluids are slightly alkaline having a *p*H of 7.35 to 7.45.

hydrogen peroxide [G. *ydōr,* water, + *gennan,* to form, + L. *per,* through, + G. *oxys,* acid]. H_2O_2, a colorless, syrupy, liquid with an irritating odor and acrid taste. It decomposes readily, liberating oxygen.

USES: As a commercial bleaching agent, as an oxidizing and reducing agent. In a 3% solution, as a mild antiseptic, germicide, and cleansing agent.

h. p., solution of. The action kills bacteria because of its oxidizing power. The most important use is as an antibacterial agent, although its germicidal activity is generally greatly overestimated. In the presence of organic matter (pus, blood, etc.) this compound is so rapidly broken down that it has little efficiency. In contact with tissues its germicidal power is very limited, owing to the fact that organic matter decomposes it. As long as there is effervescence caused by its application to a wound there is no great destruction of bacteria.

It is of value chiefly as a cleansing agent for suppurating wounds and inflamed mucous membranes. It is esp. useful for this purpose because of the development of gas, which tends to loosen adherent deposits. Its value in cleansing infected wounds and freely suppurating ulcers is probably due more to removal of organic detritus* which forms a breeding place for the microorganisms rather than to its antibacterial action.

Its styptic action—probably due to activation of the fibrin ferment of the blood and consequent more rapid coagulation—as well as its harmless nature, make it a very popular antiseptic for household use. It is sometimes injected into deep cavities to determine the presence of pus, which will be indicated by effervescence. Because of its lack of toxicity it is a favored disinfectant for application to various mucous membranes, esp. those of the nose and throat. Diluted with equal parts of water used as a gargle in pharyngitis, or mouthwash in stomatitis.

hydroglossa (hi-dro-glos'ă) [" + *glōssa,* tongue]. Cystic tumor beneath the tongue. SYN: *ranula.*

hydrogymna'sium [" + *gymnasion,* exercising]. Pool for underwater exercises.

hydrogymnas'tics [" + *gymnastikos,* pert. to nakedness]. Underwater exercises.

hydrohematonephrosis (hi"dro-hem"ă-to-nef-ro'sis) [" + *aima,* blood, + *nephros,* kidney, + *ōsis*]. Blood and urine in pelvis of the kidney.

hydrohepatosis (hi"dro-hep-ă-to'sis) [" + *ēpar, ēpat-,* liver, + *ōsis*]. Accumulation of fluid in the liver.

hydrohymenitis (hi"dro-hi-men-i'tis) [" + *ymēn,* membrane, + *-itis,* inflammation]. Any inflammation of a serous membrane.

hydrokinet'ics [G. *ydōr,* water, + *kinēsis,* motion]. Science of fluids in motion.

hydrolase (hi'dro-lās) [" + *ase,* enzyme]. An enzyme that causes hydrolysis. SYN: *hydrolyst.*

hydrology (hi-drol'o-jĭ) [G. *ydōr,* water, + *logos,* science]. The science of water in all its aspects.

hydrolysis hi-drol'ĭ-sis) [G. *ydōr,* water, + *lysis,* solution]. Any reaction in which water is one of the reactants, more specifically the combination of water with a salt to produce an acid and a base, one of which is more dissociated than the other. The reverse of neutralization. A chemical decomposition in which a substance is split into simpler compounds by the addition of and the taking up of the elements of water.

Reactions of this kind are extremely frequent in life processes. The conversion of starch to maltose, of fat to glycerol and fatty acid, and of protein to amino acids, are examples of hydrolysis, as are more of the other reactions involved in digestion. A simple example is the reaction in which the hydrolysis of ethyl acetate yields acetic acid and ethyl alcohol: $C_2H_5C_2H_3O_2 + H_2O = HC_2H_3O_2 + C_2H_5OH$. Such reactions can be reversed, usually; the reversed reaction is called neutralization, esterification, or condensation. SEE: *assimilation; enzyme.*

hydrolyst (hi'dro-list) [" + *lysis,* solution]. A ferment that produces hydrolysis.

hydrolyt'ic [" + *lysis,* solution]. Rel. to hydrolysis.

hydrolyze. To cause to undergo hydrolysis.

hydroma (hi-dro'mă) [" + *ōma,* tumor]. A collection of serous fluid in a cyst.

hydromel (hi'dro-mel) [" + *meli,* honey]. Mixture of honey and water.

hydromeningitis (hi-dro-men-in-ji'tis) [" + *mēnigx,* membrane, + *itis,* inflammation]. 1. Inflammation of membranes of brain with serous effusion. 2. Inflammation of Descemet's membrane.

hydromeningocele (hi"dro-men-in'go-sēl) [" + " + *kēlē,* hernia]. Protrusion of meninges or spinal cord in a sac of fluid.

hydrom'eter [" + *metron,* measure]. An instrument which measures the density of a liquid by the depth to which a graduated scale sinks into the liquid.

hydrometra (hi-dro-me'tră) [" + *mētra,* uterus]. Collection of watery fluid or mucus in the uterus.

hydromphalus (hi-drom'fă-lus) [" + *omphalos,* navel]. Watery tumor at the umbilicus.

hydromyelia (hi"dro-mi-e'lĭ-ă) [G. *ydōr,* water, + *myelos,* marrow]. Increased fluid in central canal of spinal cord. SYN: *hydrorrhachis.*

hydromyelocele (hi-dro-mi'ĕ-lo-sēl) [" + " + *kēlē,* hernia]. Protrusion of sac with cerebrospinal fluid through a spina bifida.

hydromyoma (hi-dro-mi-o'mă) [" + *mys, myo-,* muscle, + *ōma,* tumor]. Cystic fibroid, usually uterine, filled with fluid.

hydronephrosis (hi"dro-nef-ro'sis) [" + *nephros,* kidney, + *ōsis*]. Collection of urine in the kidney pelvis due to obstructed outflow, forming a cyst by production of distention and atrophy of organ.

DIAG: Large, fluctuating, soft mass in region of kidney, appearing and disappearing as retained urine passes into the ureters and bladder.

TREATMENT: Aspiration, nephrectomy, or nephrotomy.

hydroparasalpinx (hi"dro-par-ă-sal'pinks) [" + *para,* beside, + *salpigx,* tube]. Accumulation of serous fluid in the accessory tubes of the fallopian tube.

hydroparoti'tis [" + *para,* near, + *ous, ot-,* ear, + *itis,* inflammation]. Accumulation of fluid in the parotid gland.

hydropath'ic [" + *pathos,* disease]. Rel. to hydropathy.

hydropathy (hi-drop'ă-thĭ) [" + *pathos,* disease]. A treatment regimen involving the use of large amounts of water internally and externally. It is falsely claimed that such treatment will cure a great variety of diseases. SEE: *hydrotherapy.*

hydropenia (hi"dro-pe'nĭ-ă) [" + *penia,* poverty]. Deficiency in body water.

hydropericardi'tis [" + *peri,* around, + *kardia,* heart, + *itis,* inflammation]. Serous effusion accompanying pericarditis.

hydropericardium (hi"dro-per-ĭ-kar'dĭ-um) [" + " + *kardia,* heart]. Pericardial dropsy. Accumulation of water in pericardial sac without inflammation.

SYM: Distress in region of heart; dysphagia, disturbed cardiac action and dyspnea.

TREATMENT: Paracentesis. Governed by cause of attack.

hydroperinephrosis (hi"dro-per-ĭ-ne-fro'sis) [" + " + *nephros,* kidney, + *ōsis*]. Accumulation of serum of connective tissue surrounding the kidney.

hydroperion (hi-dro-per'ĭ-on) [G. *ydōr,* water, + *peri,* around, + *ōon,* egg]. Fluid supposedly present between decidua capsularis and decidua parietalis.

hydroperitone'um [" + *peritonaion,* peritoneum]. Accumulation of fluid in peritoneal cavity. SYN: *ascites.*

hydropexis (hi"dro-pex'is) [" + *pexis,* fixation]. The holding or fixing of water.

hydroph'ilism. Tendency of tissues to attract and hold water.

hydrophilous (hi-drof'ĭ-lus) [" + *philein,* to love]. Taking up moisture. SYN: *bibulous.*

hydrophobia (hi-dro-fo'bĭ-ă) [G. *ydōr,* water, + *phobos,* fear]. SYN: *lyssa.* 1. Morbid fear of water. 2. Common name for rabies, *q.v.,* resulting from bite of a rabid animal.

hydrophobophobia. Morbid fear of contracting hydrophobia, sometimes resulting in a hysterical condition resembling hydrophobia.

hydrophthalmos (hi-drof-thal'mos) [G. *ydōr,* water, + *ophthalmos,* eye]. Distention of the eyeball due to accumulation of fluid within it. SYN: *ouphthalmia; infantile glaucoma.*

hydrophysometra (hi"dro-fi-so-me'tră) [" + *physa,* gas, + *mētra,* uterus]. Presence of water and gas in the uterus.

hydrop'ic [G. *ydrōpikos,* pert. to dropsy]. Dropsical or pert. to dropsy.

hydropigenous (hi-dro-pij'ĕ-nus) [G. *ydrōps,* dropsy, + *gennan,* to produce]. Producing dropsy.

hydropneumatosis (hi"dro-nu-mă-to'sis) [" + *pneuma,* air, + *ōsis*]. Liquid and gas in the tissues producing combined edema and emphysema.

hydropneumogony (hi-dro-nu-mog'ō-nĭ) [" + " + *gonu,* knee]. Diagnosis of joint effusion by injecting air in joint.

hydropneumopericardium (hī-dro-nu″mo-per-ĭ-kar′dĭ-um) [" + " + *peri*, around, + *kardia*, heart]. Serous effusion with gas in the pericardium.

hydropneumoperitoneum (hī″dro-nu″mo-per-ĭ-to-ne′um) [" + " + *peritonaion*, peritoneum]. Gas and serous fluid in the peritoneal cavity.

hydropneumothorax (hī″dro-nu″mo-tho′-raks) [" + " + *thōrax*, chest]. Gas and serous effusion in pleural cavity. SYN: *pneumohydrothorax*.

hy′drops, hydrop′sy [G. *ydrōps*, dropsy]. Dropsy or edema.

h. **abdominis.** Dropsy of the abdominal cavity; ascites.

h., **endolymphatic.** H. labyrinthine, *q.v.*

h. **fetalis.** Erythroblastosis fetalis, *q.v.*

h. **folliculi.** Accumulation of fluid in graafian follicle of ovary.

h. **gravidarum.** Edema accompanying pregnancy.

h., **labyrinthine.** Dilatation due to an accumulation of fluid in the endolymphatic space of the ear. A characteristic of Meniere's disease, *q.v.*

h. **tubae.** Collection of fluid in an oviduct. Hydrosalpinx.

h. t. **profluens.** A hydrops of the tube in which the distention becomes so great that the tube is forced to empty itself by the pressure, the emptying taking place via the uterine cavity. SYN: *intermittent hydrosalpinx*.

h. **vesi′cae fel′leae.** Fluid in the gallbladder causing distention.

hydropyonephrosis (hī″dro-pī″o-nef-ro′sis) [G. *ydōr*, water, + *pyon*, pus, + *nephros*, kidney, + *ōsis*]. Dilatation of kidney pelvis with pus and urine.

hydrorheostat (hī-dro-re′o-stat) [" + *reos*, current, + *istanai*, to place]. A device used to control the flow of electrical current by changes in water resistance.

hydrorrhachis (hī-dro′ră-kis) [" + *rachis*, spine]. Condition of increased cerebrospinal fluid bet. membranes and spinal cord or its central canal or cavities.

hydrorhachitis (hī-dro-ră-kī′tis) [" + " + *itis*, inflammation]. Serous effusion from the spinal cord or its membranes with inflammation of the cord.

hydrorrhea (hī-dro-re′ă) [" + *roia*, flow]. Copious watery discharge from any part, as from the nose.

h. **gravidarum.** Discharge of a watery fluid from the vagina during pregnancy, sometimes mistaken for amniotic fluid.

hydrosalpinx (hī-dro-sal′pinks) [" + *salpigx*, tube]. Distention of fallopian tube by clear fluid.

h., **intermittent.** A discharge of watery fluid from the oviduct. SYN: *hydrops tubae profluens*.

hydrosarcocele (hī-dro-sar′ko-sēl) [" + *sarx*, flesh, + *kēlē*, hernia]. Hydrocele with chronic swelling of testis.

hydro′sis [" + *-ōsis*]. Hidrosis.

hydrosol. The fluid state of a colloidal solution; a sol. State of a colloidal solution in which the colloid particles, separated by water in a continuous phase, are free to move about. SEE: *hydrogel*.

hydrosphygmograph (hī-dro-sfig′mo-graf) [" + *sphygmos*, pulse, + *graphein*, to write]. A sphygmograph with indicator consisting of a column of water.

hydrostat′ic [" + *statikos*, standing]. Pert. to the pressure of liquids in equilibrium and that exerted on liquids.

h. **test.** Putting lungs of a dead infant in water. If they float, the infant was born alive.

hydrostat′ics [G. *ydōr*, water, + *statikos*, standing]. Science of properties of fluids in equilibrium.

hydrosudotherapy (hī″dro-su″do-ther′ă-pĭ) [" + L. *sudor*, sweat, + G. *therapeia*, treatment]. Treatment of disease by sweating and hydrotherapy.

hydrosyringomyelia (hī″dro-sir-in″go-mī-e′lĭ-ă) [" + *syrigx*, tube, + *myelos*, marrow]. Distention of central canal of spinal cord with effusion of fluid and formation of cavities.

hydrotaxis. The response of an animal toward or away from moisture. SEE: *hydrotropism*.

hydrotherapeu′tics [" + *therapeutikè*, treatment]. Treatment of disease with water. SYN: *hydrotherapy*.

hydrotherapist (hī-dro-ther′ă-pist) [" + *therapeia*, treatment]. One who practices hydrotherapy.

hydrotherapy (hī-dro-ther′ă-pĭ) [" + *therapeia*, treatment]. Scientific application of water in treatment of disease.

The therapeutic effects of hydrotherapy are as follows:

Brief Hot Tub and Shower Baths: Relieve fatigue but may cause cerebral congestion and wakefulness unless cold compresses are used on the head.

Cold Baths and Applications: Abstract heat and stimulate reaction, esp. if followed by friction and percussion. They contract the small blood vessels when applied locally.

Cold and Hot Applications: One followed by the other stimulates the cardiovascular system.

Gradually Elevated Temperature of Hot Tub and Vapor Baths: Relax all muscles of the body.

Hot Baths: Relax tissues including capillaries of skin, drawing blood from deeper tissues; also relieve pain.

Warm and Hot Baths and Applications: They soothe cutaneous nerves, and nerves of internal organs in reflex relation with skin areas to which heat is applied.

SEE: *Kneipp cure*.

hydrothionammonemia (hī″dro-thī″on-am-o-ne′mĭ-ă) [" + *theion*, sulfur, + L. *ammonia*, ammonium, + G. *aima*, blood]. Ammonium sulfide in the blood.

hydrothionemia (hī″dro-thī-on-e′mĭ-ă) [" + " + *aima*, blood]. Condition caused by hydrogen sulfide in the blood.

hydrothionuria (hī-dro-thī-on-u′rĭ-ă) [" + " + *ouron*, urine]. Condition caused by hydrogen sulfide in the urine.

hydrothorax (hī-dro-tho′raks) [G. *ydōr*, water, + *thōrax*, chest]. Dropsy of the chest, or effused fluid in pleural cavity.

SYM: Dyspnea, absence of vesicular breath sounds, murmur, flatness over location of fluid.

TREATMENT: According to cause. Aspiration.

hydro′tis [" + *ous*, *ot-*, ear]. Serous effusion in the internal ear or tympanum.

hydrotomy (hī-drot′o-mĭ) [" + *tomē*, dissection]. Dissection of tissue by forcible injection of water into the vessels.

hydrotropism. Response of plants toward (positive h.) or away (negative h.) from moisture.

hydrotym′panum [" + *tympanon*, drum]. Dropsy of the middle ear.

hydroure′ter [" + *ourētēr*, ureter]. Dropsy of the ureter.

hydrovarium (hī-dro-va′rĭ-um) [" + L. *ovarium*, ovary]. Dropsy or cyst of the ovary.

hydroxide (hi-droks'īd) [G. *ydōr*, water, + *oxys*, acid]. A compound which contains the hydroxyl (OH) group. Ex: NaOH (sodium hydroxide, or caustic soda).

hydroxy acids (hi-droks'ĭ). Acids containing one or more hydroxyl groups in addition to the carboxyl group, as *lactic acid.*

hydrox'yl. The univalent radical OH which, when combined with a metallic ion or a radical which acts as a metal (*e. g.*, NH_4), forms a hydroxide. Commonly called a base or alkali.

hydrozone (hi'dro-zōn) [G. *ydōr*, water, + *ozein*, to smell]. A bactericide of an aqueous solution of pure hydrogen dioxide.

hydruria (hi-dru'rĭ-ă) [" + *ouron*, urine]. Increase of watery constituents of the urine with diminished solids in proportion. Syn: *polyuria.*

hygiene (hi'jēn) [G. *ygiēinos*, healthful]. The study of health and observance of health rules.

***h.*, community.** That branch of hygiene which deals with the health of a large group of individuals such as a city, state, or nation, and esp. the control of communicable diseases.

***h.*, industrial.** That branch of hygiene which deals primarily with health of industrial workers, esp. prevention of occupational diseases.

***h.*, mental.** Science of developing and maintaining mental health, preventing neurosis and mental unsoundness.

***h.*, military.** That branch of hygiene that deals with the health of men in military service.

***h.*, oral.** Scientific care of teeth and mouth.

hygienic (hi-jĭ-en'ik) [G. *ygiēinos*, healthful]. 1. Pert. to health or its preservation. 2. In a healthy condition.

hygien'ics [G. *ygiēinos*, healthful]. A system for promoting health.

hygienist (hi'jĭ-en-ist) [G. *ygiēinos*, healthful]. A specialist in hygiene.

***h.*, dental.** One trained in dental prophylaxis.

hygienization (hi"jēn-ĭ-za'shun) [G. *ygiēinos*, healthful]. The establishment of sanitary conditions and rules of hygiene.

hy'gric [G. *ygros*, moisture]. Pert. to moisture.

hygro- [G.]. Prefix: Rel. to moisture.

hygroma (hi-gro'mă) (pl. *hygromata*) [" + *ōma*, tumor]. A sac or bursa containing fluid.

***h.*, cystic.** A rapidly growing hygroma in the maxillary region of infants.

hygrometer (hi-grom'ĕ-ter) [" + meter]. An instrument for measuring the amount of moisture in the air.

hygroscopic (hi-gro-skop'ik) [" + *skopein*, to examine]. 1. Pert. to hygroscopy. 2. Absorbing moisture readily. Syn: *bibulous; hydrophilous.*

hygros'copy [" + *skopein*, to examine]. Estimation of the quantity of moisture in the atmosphere.

hygrostomia (hi-gro-sto'mĭ-ă) [" + *stoma* mouth]. Excess flow of saliva. Syn: *ptyalism; salivation.*

hyla (hi'lă) [G. *ylē*, matter]. A lateral extension of the *aquaeductus cerebri.* Syn: *paraqueduct.*

hylo'ma [" + *ōma*, tumor]. A tumor composed of or in the hylic tissues, such as *hypohyloma*, and *mesohyloma.*

hymen (hi'men) [G. *ymēn*, membrane]. A fold of mucous membrane which normally partially covers the entrance to the vagina. Contrary to folklore, presence or absence of the hymen cannot be used to prove or disprove virginity or history of sexual intercourse.

Its rupture is no longer considered as a loss of virginity.

RS: *carunculae myrtiformes, defloration, hymenorrhaphy, hymenotomy.*

***h.* annularis.** Hymen with a ring-shaped opening in the center.

***h.* biforis.** One with two parallel openings with a thick septum between.

***h.* cribriformis.** One with many small perforations.

***h.* denticulatis.** One with an opening with serrated edges.

***h.*, fenestrated.** Same as cribriform.

***h.* imperforatus.** A hymen with no opening in it.

***h.*, lunar.** H. shaped like the moon.

***h.*, ruptured.** Hymen that has been torn by coitus, injury or operation.

***h.* septus or *h.*, septate.** Hymen in which the opening is separated by a thin septum.

***h.*, unruptured.** Imperforate hymen.

hymenal (hi'men-al) [G. *ymēn*, membrane]. Pert. to the hymen.

hymenectomy (hi-men-ek'to-mĭ) [" + *ektomē*, excision]. 1. Removal of a membrane. 2. Removal of the hymen.

hymenitis (hi-men-i'tis) [" + *-itis*, inflammation]. Inflammation of the hymen or a membrane.

Hymenolepis (hi-men-ol'ĕ-pis) [G. *ymēn*, membrane, + *lepis*, rind]. A genus of tapeworm. Parasitic in birds and mammals.

***H.* nana.** The dwarf tapeworm, a parasite in the intestine of rats and mice and commonly found in man. It averages about 1 in. (2.5 cm.) in length and differs from other tapeworms in that it is capable of completing its life cycle within a single host. It causes severe toxic symptoms, esp. in children.

hymenology (hi-men-ol'o-jĭ) [" + *logos*, science]. Science of the membranes and their diseases.

hymenorrhaphy (hi-men-or'ă-fĭ) [" + *raphē*, suture]. Plastic operation on the hymen, occluding the vagina.

hymenotome (hi-men'o-tōm) [" + *tomē*, incision]. Knife used to divide membranes.

hymenotomy (hi-men-ot'o-mĭ) [" + *tomē*, incision]. 1. Incision of the hymen. 2. Dissection of a membrane.

hyo- [G.]. Prefix: Connection with hyoid bone.

hyobasioglossus (hi"o-ba"sĭ-o-glos'us) [G. *yoeidēs*, shape like letter U, + *basis*, base, + *glōssa*, tongue]. The part of hyoglossal muscle attached to the hyoid bone. Syn: *basioglossus.*

hyoepiglottic (hi"o-ep-ĭ-glot'ik) [" + *epiglōttis*, epiglottis]. Rel. to hyoid bone and epiglottis.

hyoepiglottidean (hi"o-ep-ĭ-glot-id'e-an) [" + *epiglōttis*, epiglottis]. Rel. to hyoid bone and epiglottis. Syn: *hyoepiglottic.*

hyoglos'sal [" + *glōssa*, tongue]. 1. Pert. to the hyoglossus. 2. Extending to the tongue from the hyoid bone.

hyoglossus. A muscle arising from body and greater cornu of hyoid bone and inserted into dorsum of tongue.

Action: Draws down sides and retracts tongue.

hy'oid [G. *yoeidēs*, U-shaped]. Bone at ant. surface of neck at root of the tongue, suspended from styloid processes by the stylohyoid ligament.

It is shaped like the Greek letter U.

***h.* arch.** Second branchial arch.

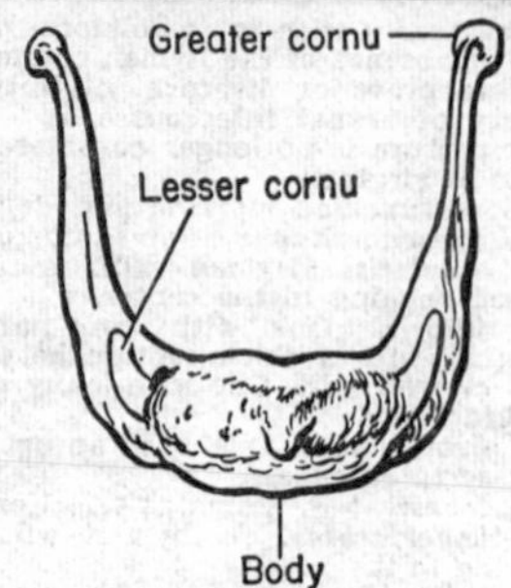

HYOID BONE

hyopharyngeus (hi-o-far-in'je-us) [" + *pharygx,* gullet]. Middle pharyngeal constrictor.

hyoscine (hi'o-sin) Scopolamine.

h. hydrobromide. Scopolamine hydrobromide.

Hyoscyamus (hi-o-si'ă-mus) [G. *ys,* a pig, + *kyamos,* bean]. USP. Dried leaves of the plant *Hyoscyamus niger.* A narcotic. SYN: *henbane.*

POISONING: Related to atropine, *q.v.*

hypacousia, hypacusia, hypacusis (hi"pă-koo'sĭ-ă, -ku'sĭ-ă, -sis) [G. *ypo,* under, + *akousis,* hearing]. Impaired hearing.

hypalbuminosis (hi"pal-bu-min-o'sis) [" + L. *albumen,* white of egg, + G. *ōsis*]. Deficiency in proportion of albumin in blood.

hypalgesia (hi-pal-je'zĭ-ă) [" + *algēsis,* pain]. Lessened sensitivity to pain. SEE: *hyperalgesia.*

hypalgia (hi-pal'jĭ-ă) [" + *algos,* pain]. Lessened sensitivity to pain. SYN: *hypalgesia.*

hypamnios (hi-pam'nĭ-os) [" + *amnion,* caul of a lamb]. Deficiency in amt. of amniotic fluid.

hypanakinesis (hi-pan-ă-kin-e'sis) [" + *anakinēsis,* exercise]. Lowered rate of movement.

hypaphrodisia (hip"af-ro-diz'ĭ-ă) [G. *hypo,* + aphrodisia]. Decreased or deficient sexual desire.

hypaxial (hi-paks'ĭ-al) [" + *axōn,* axis]. Situated beneath the body axis.

hyper- [G.]. Prefix: Above, excessive, or beyond.

hyperacidaminuria (hi"per-as"id-am-in-u'rĭ-ă) [G. *yper,* above, + L. *acidus,* sour, + *amine* + G. *ouron,* urine]. Presence of an excess of amino acids in the urine. SYN: *acidaminuria.*

hyperacid'ity [" + L. *acidus,* sour]. 1. An excess of acid. 2. An excess of acid in the stomach. SEE: *hyperchlorhydria.*

DIET: Three meals and several between-meal feedings per day. Provide protein to combine with the acid. Moderate amt. of fat to inhibit secretion of acid. Avoid bulky foods, condiments, and extremes of temperature in foods.

hyperacuity (hi-per-a-ku'ĭ-tĭ) [" + L. *acuitās,* sharpness]. Abnormal acuteness, as of vision.

hyperacusis (hi-per-ă-ku'sis) [" + *akousis,* hearing]. Abnormal sensitivity to sound. Sometimes found in hysteria.

hyperadenosis (hi"per-ad-ĕ-no'sis) [" + *adēn,* gland, + *ōsis*]. Lymph gland enlargement. SEE: *Hodgkin's disease.*

hyperadiposis, hyperadiposity (hi-per-ad-ĭ-po'sis, -pos'ĭ-tĭ) [" + L. *adeps, adip-,* fat, + *ōsis*]. Excessive fatness.

hyperadrenalemia (hi"per-ad-re"nal-e'mĭ-ă) [" + L. *ad,* toward, + *rēnalis,* pert. to a kidney, + G. *aima,* blood]. Excess of adrenal secretion in the blood.

hyperadre'nalism [" + " + " + G. *ismos,* state of]. Excess of adrenal secretion.

hyperadre'nia [" + " + *rēn,* kidney]. Condition caused by abnormal activity of adrenal glands.

hyperalbuminosis (hi"per-al-bu-min-o'sis) [" + L. *albumen,* white of egg, + G. *ōsis*]. Increased albumin in the blood.

hyperalgesia (hi-per-al-je'zĭ-ă) [" + *algēsis,* pain]. Excessive sensibility to pain; opp. of hypalgesia.

hyperalgia (hi-per-al'jĭ-ă) [" + *algos,* pain]. Excessive sensitivity to pain.

hyperaminoacidemia (hi"per-am"ĭ-no-as"ĭ-de'mĭ-ă). An undue amount of amino acids in the blood.

hyperanacinesia, hyperanacinesis (hi"per-an"ă-sin-e'zĭ-ă, -sis) [" + *anakinēsis,* exercise]. Hyperanakinesis, *q.v.*

hyperanakine'sis [" + *anakinēsis,* exercise]. Excessive function or movement activity of an organ or part such as of the stomach or intestines.

hyperaphia (hi-per-a'fĭ-ă) [G. *yper,* above, + *aphē,* touch]. Excessive sensitiveness to touch.

hyperaphic (hi-per-af'ĭk) [" + *aphē,* touch]. Marked by extreme sensitiveness to touch.

hyperazoturia (hi-per-az-o-tu'rĭ-ă) [" + *a-,* priv. + *zōē,* life, + *ouron,* urine]. Excessive amt. of nitrogenous matter in the urine.

hyperbilirubinemia (hi"per-bil-ĭ-ru-bin-e'mĭ-ă) [" + L. *bilis,* bile, + *ruber,* red, + G. *aima,* blood]. Excessive amt. of bilirubin in the blood.

hyperbrachycephaly (hi"per-brak-ĭ-sef'ă-lĭ) [" + *brachys,* short, + *kephalē,* head]. Excessive degree of brachycephaly; having a cephalic index over 85.

hyperbu'lia [" + *boulē,* will]. Morbid willfulness.

hypercalcemia (hi-per-kal-se'mĭ-ă) [" + L. *calx,* lime, + G. *aima,* blood]. An excessive amt. of calcium in the blood.

hypercalciuria (hi"per-kal-sĭ-u'rĭ-ă) [" + " + G. *ouron,* urine]. An excessive quantity of calcium in the urine.

hypercap'nia [" + *kapnos,* smoke]. Undue amt. of carbon dioxide in the blood.

hypercatharsis (hi-per-kă-thar'sis) [" + *katharsis,* purge]. Excessive bowel movement.

hypercementosis (hi"per-se-men-to'sis) [" + L. *cementum,* cement, + G. *ōsis*]. Overgrowth of tooth cement (*cementum*).

hypercenesthesia (hi-per-sen-es-the'zĭ-ă) [" + *koinos,* common, + *aisthēsis,* sensation]. SYN: *euphoria.* Exaggerated feeling of well-being.

hyperchloremia (hi-per-klor-e'mĭ-ă) [" + *chlōros,* green, + *aima,* blood]. Increase in chloride content of the blood.

hyperchlorhydria (hi-per-klor-hi'drĭ-ă) [" + " + *ydōr,* water]. An excess of hydrochloric acid in the gastric secretion.

The amount secreted above what is needed to combine with albumoid and basic substances is known as free HCl.

The normal amount of free hydrochloric acid averages 0.4 to 0.5%. Total acidity is expressed in terms of clinical units or the number of cc. of 0.1 N sodium hydroxide solution required to bring the stomach contents to end point of titration (neutrality). If stomach contents give values above 60 and after the second hour instead of declining remain high or continue to rise, *hyperchlorhydria exists.* It is common, occurring in about 5% of population. If values are below 20 after test meals, *hypochlorhydria exists.* Excess of HCl causes a burning sensation in the stomach in the absence of ingested foods. It also gives rise to gas from the acid's decomposition, and this may cause gastric ulcer. It is more frequent in nervous types, ulcers and chronic gastritis. Two pathological conditions commonly accompanying hyperacidity are duodenal ulcer and pyloric obstruction. SEE: *hydrochloric acid.*

DIET: Small, frequent meals to absorb the HCl. Bland foods and those which will not stimulate the secretion of this acid. Proteins, such as gelatin, eggs, and milk, but little meat or meat broths. Fats, such as cream and butter, permissible as they inhibit the secretion of gastric juice. No sweets, bulky foods, cabbage, onions, or condiments. Cereals; toast; custards; soft, strained, cooked fruits allowable. SYN: *gastrosuccorrhea.* SEE: *gastritis; hypochlorhydria.*

hyperchlorida'tion [G. *yper,* above, + *chlōros,* green]. A dosing with large amounts of sodium chloride.

hypercholestere'mia [" + *cholē,* bile, + *stereos,* stiff, + *aima,* blood]. Hypercholesterolemia, *q.v.*

hypercholesterine'mia [" + " + *stereos,* solid, + *aima,* blood]. Hypercholesterolemia, *q.v.*

hypercholesterolemia (hi"per-ko-les"ter-ol-e'mĭ-ă) [" + " + " + *aima,* blood]. Excessive amt. of cholesterol in the blood.

hypercholesterolia (hi"per-ko-les"ter-o'-lĭ-ă) [" + " + *stereos,* stiff]. Excessive cholesterol in the bile.

hypercholia (hi-per-ko'lĭ-ă) [" + *cholē,* bile]. Abnormal secretion of bile.

hyperchromasia (hi"per-kro-ma'zĭ-ă) [" + *chrōma,* color]. Hyperchromatism, *q.v.*

hyperchromatic (hi"per-kro-mat'ĭk) [" + *chrōma,* color]. Overpigmented.

h. cell. A cell or a part of a cell which contains more than the normal number of chromosomes and hence stains more densely.

hyperchro'matism [" + " + *ismos,* state of]. 1. Excessive pigmentation. 2. Increased staining capacity of any structure. SYN: *hyperchromatosis.*

hyperchromatopsia (hi"per-kro-ma-top'-sĭ-ă) [" + " + *opsis,* vision]. Defect of vision in which all objects appear colored.

hyperchromatosis [G. *yper,* above, + *chrōma,* color, + *ōsis*]. Excessive pigmentation, esp. of the skin.

hyperchromemia (hi"per-kro-me'mĭ-ă) [" + " + *aima,* blood]. Condition of a high color index of the blood due to increased amount of hemoglobin in red cells.

hyperchromia (hi-per-kro'mĭ-ă) [" + *chrōma,* color]. Excessive pigmentation. SYN: *hyperchromatism.*

hyperchromic (hi-per-krōm'ĭk) [" + *chrōma,* color]. Pert. to excessive pigmentation.

hyperchylia (hi-per-ki'lĭ-ă) [" + *chylos,* juice]. Abnormal secretion of gastric juice.

hypercinesia (hi-per-sin-e'zĭ-ă) [" + *kinēsis,* motion]. Increased function or motion.

h., professional. Occupational neurosis.

hypercri'nism [" + " + *ismos,* state of]. Condition due to excessive activity of any endocrine gland.

hypercryalgesia (hi-per-kri-al-je'zĭ-ă) [G. *yper,* above, + *kryos,* cold, + *algēsis,* pain]. Excessive sensitivity to cold. SYN: *hypercryesthesia.*

hypercryesthe'sia [" + " + *aisthēsis,* sensation]. Excessive allergy to cold. SYN: *hypercryalgesia.*

hypercyanosis (hi"per-si"ă-no'sis) [" + *kyanos,* dark blue, + *ōsis*]. Extreme cyanosis.

hypercyanotic (hi-per-si-ă-not'ik) [" + *kyanos,* dark blue]. Denoting extreme cyanosis.

hypercyesis (hi-per-si-e'sis) [" + *kyēsis,* gestation]. Presence of more than one fetus in a uterus because of fertilization of a second ovum within a short time. SYN: *superfetation.*

hypercythemia (hi-per-si-the'mĭ-ă) [" + *kytos,* cell, + *aima,* blood]. Condition of having an excessive number of red blood corpuscles.

hypercytosis (hi-per-si-to'sis) [" + " + *ōsis*]. Abnormal increase in leukocytes in the blood. SYN: *hyperleukocytosis.*

hyperdactyl'ia [G. *yper,* above, + *dactylos,* finger]. State of having supernumerary fingers or toes.

hyperdiastole (hi"per-di-as'to-le) [" + *diastellein,* to draw apart]. Extreme cardiac diastole.

hyperdicrot'ic [" + *dikrotos,* beating double]. Abnormally dicrotic. SEE: *dicrotic.*

hyperdistention (hi"per-dis-ten'shun) [" + L. *distendere,* to stretch out]. Excessive inflation or distention.

hyperdiure'sis [" + *dia,* through, + *ourein,* to urinate]. Excessive formation of urine. SYN: *polyuria.*

hyperdyna'mia [" + *dynamis,* force]. Muscular restlessness or extreme violence.

h. uteri. Abnormal uterine contractions in labor.

hypereccrisia, hypereccrisis (hi-per-ek-kris'ĭ-ă, -ek'kris-is) [" + *ek,* out, + *krisis,* separation]. Abnormal amt. of excretion.

hypereccritic, hyperecritic (hi-per-ek-rit'-ik) [" + *ekkritikos,* excreting]. Pert. to an abnormal amt. of excretion or hypereccrisis.

hyperemesis (hi-per-em'ĕ-sis) [G. *yper,* above, + *emesis,* vomiting]. Excessive vomiting.

h. gravidarum. One of the toxemias of early pregnancy characterized by excessive vomiting.

ETIOL: Occurs most frequently in highly sensitive, neurotic individuals, and although it may begin on a neurotic basis the constant vomiting brings on the definite toxic changes. In the severe cases there is definite pathological evidence of the condition, the liver showing changes of a necrotic nature in the center of the lobules.

SYM: The condition may start as a simple vomiting of early pregnancy, but with combined vomiting of first gastric contents, and later of bile, there is developed a chloride depletion, an acidosis, and, finally, with severe and continued vomiting the pathological changes in the liver take place.

The findings are those of a patient who is pregnant and who vomits constantly, loses weight rapidly, dehydrates, develops a rapid pulse, has rise in temperature, and acetone in the urine. Liver function tests may reveal evidences of impaired function if the condition is allowed to progress.

TREATMENT: In early cases, rest in bed; restrictions of fluids taken by mouth, fluids given per rectum or by hypodermoclysis; moderate sedation and antiemetic drugs are usually effective. In the average case where nervous irritability is a factor the patient should be kept in a darkened, quiet room free from all visitors.

With careful management of this type, and no relief from symptoms, and if the pulse and temperature rise and there is definite evidence of liver damage (jaundice), therapeutic abortion should be resorted to.

The necessity for emptying the uterus should occur only rarely if the patient is seen early, and the proper treatment instituted at once. When the patient improves and food is again taken by mouth, it should consist of a light solid diet given in frequent small feedings with fruit juice, milk, etc. between feedings.

h. lactentium. Vomiting in nursing infants.

hyperemia (hi-per-e'mĭ-ă) [" + *aima*, blood]. 1. Congestion. An unusual amount of blood in a part. 2. A form of macula; red areas on skin which disappear on pressure. 3. PT: Increase in the quantity of blood flowing through any part of the body; as undue redness of the skin, caused by the application of heat.

h., active, h., arterial. H. caused by increased blood inflow.

h., Bier's, h., constriction. Passive hyperemia* produced by application of an elastic bandage and by suction.

h., leptomeningeal. Pia-arachnoid congestion.

h., passive, h., venous. H. caused by decreased blood outflow.

hyperemization (hi"per-e-mi-za'shun) [G. *yper*, above, + *aima*, blood]. Hyperemia produced artificially for therapeutic purposes.

hyperemotiv'ity [" + L. *ēmotum, ēmovēre*, to move out]. Excessive emotivity or response to stimuli.

hyperendocrin'ia [" + *endon*, within, + *krinein*, to separate]. Pert. to hyperendocrinism.

hyperendocrinism (hi"per-en-dok'rĭ-nizm) [" + " + " + *ismos*, state of]. Abnormal increase of endocrine gland secretion.

hyperendocrisia (hi"per-en-do-kris'ĭ-ă) [" + " + *krisis*, a separation]. Excessive increase of internal secretions. SYN: *hyperendocrinism.*

hypereosinophilia (hi"per-e"o-sin-o-fil'ĭ-ă) [" + *ēōs*, dawn (rose colored), + *philein*, to love]. Excessive leukocytosis with increase of eosinophils.

hyperephidrosis (hi"per-ef-ĭ-dro'sis) [" + *epi*, upon, + *idrōs*, sweating]. Abnormal sweating.

hyperepinephria (hi"per-ep"ĭ-nef'rĭ-ă) [" + " + *nephros*, kidney]. Excessive adrenal secretion with arterial tension.

hyperepinephrine'mia [" + " + *nephros*, kidney, + *aima*, blood]. Undue proportion of adrenalin in the blood. SYN: *hyperadrenalemia.*

hy"perequilib'rium [" + L. *aequus*, equal, + *libra*, balance]. A tendency to vertigo when making even slight turning movements.

hypererethism (hi-per-er'ĕ-thizm) [" + *erethisma*, stimulation]. Excessive irritability.

hyperergasia (hi-per-er-ga'sĭ-ă) [" + *ergasia*, work]. Unusual functional activity.

hyperergia (hi-per-er'jĭ-ă) [" + *ergon*, work]. 1. Excessive or increased functional activity. SYN: *hyperergasia.* 2. Abnormally sensitive to allergens.

hy"perergy (hĭ'per-er-jĭ) [G. *yper*, above, + *ergon*, energy]. Hypersensitivity or condition in which there is an exaggerated response.

hypererythrocythemia (hi"per-er-ĭ-thro-si-the'mi-ă) [" + *erythros*, red, + *kytos*, cell, + *aima*, blood]. Excess of red corpuscles in the blood.

hyperesophoria (hi"per-es-o-fo'rĭ-ă) [" + *eso*, inward, + *phorein*, to bear]. Tendency of the visual axis to deviate upward and inward due to muscular imbalance. A form of heterophoria, *q.v.*

hyperesthesia (hi"per-es-the'zĭ-ă) [G. *yper*, above, + *aisthēsis*, sensation]. Unusual sensibility to sensory stimuli, such as pain or touch. SYN: *algesia.*

h., acoustic, h., auditory. Abnormal sensitivity to sound.

h., cerebral. H. caused by a cerebral lesion.

h., gustatory. Oversensitivity of taste.

h., muscular. Muscular sensitivity to pain and tiredness.

h., optic. Abnormal sensitivity to light.

h. sexualis. Abnormal increase in the sexual impulse.

h., tactile. Abnormal sensitivity of touch.

hyperesthet'ic [" + *aisthēsis*, sensation]. Pert. to hyperesthesia.

hyperexophoria (hi"per-eks-o-fo'rĭ-ă) [" + *exō*, outward, + *phorein*, to bear]. Tendency of visual axis to deviate upward and outward due to muscular imbalance. A form of heterophoria, *q.v.*

hyperextension (hi"per-eks-ten'shun) [" + L. *extendere*, to stretch out]. Extreme or abnormal extension.

hyperfunction. Excessive activity.

hypergalactia (hi-per-gal-ak'shĭ-ă) [" + *gala*, milk]. Excessive milk secretion.

hypergenesis (hi-per-jen'ĕ-sis) [" + *genesis*, development]. Redundancy of organs or parts; overproduction. SYN: *hyperplasia.*

hy"pergen'italism (hi-per-jen'it-al-izm) [G. *yper*, above, + L. *genitalis*, genital, + G. *ismos*, state of]. Excessive development of the genital organs. SYN: *precocious puberty.*

ETIOL: Disturbances in endocrine secretions of the adrenal gland, or gonads, or hypothalamic disorders.

hypergeusesthesia, hypergeusia (hi"per-gu-ses-the'sĭ-ă, -gu'sĭ-ă) [" + *geusis*, taste]. Excessive acuteness of sense of taste.

hyperglan'dular [" + L. *glandula*, a little acorn]. Having excessive glandular secretions.

hyperglobu'lia [" + L. *globulus*, globule]. Having an excessive number of red blood corpuscles. SYN: *hypercythemia; polycythemia.*

hyperglobulinemia (hi-per-glob-u-lin-e'-mĭ-ă) [" + " + G. *aima*, blood]. Excessive globulin in the blood.

hyperglycemia (hi-per-gli-se'mĭ-ă) [" + *glykus*, sweet, + *aima*, blood]. Increase of blood sugar as in diabetes.

This condition increases susceptibility to infection and it often precedes diabetic coma. SEE: *hypoglycemia.*

hyperglycistia (hi-per-glis-is'tĭ-ă) [G. *yper*, above, + *glykus*, sweet, + *istos*, tissue]. Excess of glucose in the tissues.

hyperglycogenolysis (hi-per-gli-ko-jen-ol′-ĭ-sis) [" + " + *gennan*, to form, + *lysis*, dissolution]. Excessive conversion of glycogen into glucose by hydrolysis.

hyperglycoplasmia (hi″per-gli″ko-plas′-mĭ-ă) [" + " + *plasma*, matter formed]. Excessive sugar in the plasma of the blood.

hyperglycorrhachia (hi″per-gli″ko-ra′kĭ-ă) [" + " + *rachis*, spine]. Excess of sugar in the cerebrospinal fluid.

hyperglycosemia (hi-per-gli-ko-se′mĭ-ă) [" + " + *aima*, blood]. Excessive sugar in the blood. SYN: *hyperglycemia.*

hyperglycosuria (hi-per-gli-ko-su′rĭ-ă) [" + " + *ouron*, urine]. Excessive sugar in the urine. SEE: *glycosuria.*

hypergnosis (hi″per-no′sis) [" + *gnōsis*, knowledge]. All that is involved in projection of conflicts with the environment, evidenced in paranoia, *q.v.*

hypergonadism (hi-per-go′nad-izm) [" + *gonē*, semen, + *ismos*, state of]. Excessive internal secretion of the sexual glands.

hyperguanidinemia (hi″per-gwan-ĭ-dēn-e′-mĭ-ă) [" + *guanidine* + *aima*, blood]. Abnormal amt. of guanidine in blood.

hyperhedonia, hyperhedonism (hi-per-he-do′nĭ-ă, -he′don-izm) [" + *ēdonē*, pleasure, + *ismos*, state of]. 1. Abnormal pleasure in anything. 2. Abnormal sexual excitement.

hyperhepatia (hi″per-he-pa′shĭ-ă) [" + *epar, epat-*, liver]. Overfunctioning of the liver.

hyperhidrosis (hi″per-hi-dro′sis) [G. *yper*, above, + *idrōs*, sweat, + *ōsis*]. Excessive sweating.

ETIOL: Functional disorder of sweat glands, caused by debilitating disease, stimulants, neurasthenia. Increased in rheumatic, malarial, relapsing and septic fever. At night, in pulmonary tuberculosis, and at crisis in pneumonia. In Graves' disease, neuralgia, migraine and following certain drugs and hot drinks. Locally (hands and feet), in hysteria, fright, vagitonia, nervous irritability, and exophthalmic goiter. SEE: *sweat.*

h. oleosa. Increased and altered sebaceous secretion. SYN: *seborrhea.*

hyperhor′monism [" + *ormanein*, to arouse, + *ismos*, state of]. Excessive activity of the endocrine glands.

hyperhypocytosis (hi″per-hi″po-si-to′sis) [" + *ypo*, under, + *kytos*, cell, + *ōsis*]. Decrease of white corpuscles (leukopenia), esp. with relative increase of neutrophils.

hyperinose′mia [" + *is, in-*, fiber, + *aima*, blood]. Abnormal coagulability of the blood; excess of fibrinogen in the blood. SYN: *hyperinosis.*

hyperino′sis [G. *yper*, above, + *is, in-* fiber, + *ōsis*]. Excessive fibrinogen in the blood. SYN: *hyperinosemia.*

hyperinsulinism (hi-per-in′su-lin-izm) [" + L. *insula*, island, + G. *ismos*, state of]. An excessive amount of insulin in the blood.

ETIOL: Tumor or islets of Langerhans, or excessive sensitivity of the islet tissue to an increase in blood-sugar level. May also occur following injection of an excess of insulin.

SYM: The hypoglycemic picture: hunger, weakness, sweating, staggering, diplopia—rarely convulsions—coma, and death. Occasionally spontaneous. Symptoms similar to but more chronic than in insulin shock. SEE: *insulin; insulin shock; shock.*

hyperinvolution (hi-per-in-vo-lu′shun) [" + L. *involvere*, to roll in]. 1. Reduction in size of uterus below normal after childbirth. 2. Reduction in size below normal of any organ following hypertrophy. SYN: *superinvolution.*

h. uteri. Extreme atrophy of the uterus seen following prolonged lactation or severe puerperal sepsis.

hyperisoton′ic [" + " + *tonos*, tension]. Noting one of two solutions having greater osmotic pressure. SYN: *hypertonic.*

hy″perkalem′ia. Excessive amount of potassium in blood plasm.

hyperkeratomycosis (hi″per-ker″ă-to-mi-ko′sis) [" + *keras*, horn, + *mykēs*, fungus, + *ōsis*]. Hypertrophy of horny layer of the epidermis due to a parasitic fungus.

hyperkerato′sis [" + " + *ōsis*]. 1. Overgrowth of cornea. 2. Overgrowth of the horny layer of the epidermis. SYN: *keratodermia; keratosis.*

h. congenitalis. Hyperkeratosis in the harlequin fetus.

hy″perketonur′ia. Excessive quantity of ketones in urine.

hyperkine′sia, hyperkine′sis [" + *kinēsis*, motion]. Excessive amt. of mobility. SYN: *hypercinesia.*

hyperlacta′tion [" + L. *lactare*, to suckle]. Excessive milk secretion. SYN: *superlactation.*

hyperleukocyto′sis [" + *leukos*, white, + *kytos*, cell, + *ōsis*]. Excessive quantity of leukocytes. SYN: *leukocytosis.*

hy″perlipe′mia (hi-per-lip-e′mĭ-ă) [G. *yper*, above, + *lipos*, fat, + *aima*, blood]. Excessive quantity of fat in the blood.

hyperlipo′sis [" + " + *ōsis*]. 1. Abnormal fat; adiposity. 2. Excessive fatty degeneration.

hyperlithuria (hi-per-lith-u′rĭ-ă) [" + *lithos*, stone, + *ouron*, urine]. Excessive excretion of lithic (uric) acid in the urine.

hypermas′tia [" + *mastos*, breast]. 1. Excessively large mammary gland. 2. Presence of abnormal number of mammary glands. SYN: *polymastia; polymazia.*

hypermature (hi-per-mă-tūr′) [G. *yper*, above, + L. *maturus*, ripe]. Overmature; past maturity.

hypermegasoma (hi″per-meg-ă-sō′mă) [" + *megas*, large, + *sōma*, body]. Excessive bodily development. SYN: *gigantism.*

hypermenorrhea (hi-per-men-o-re′ă) [" + *mēn*, month, + *roia*, flow]. 1. Too frequent menstrual periods. 2. Abnormal increase in the duration of menstrual flow.

hypermetaplasia (hi-per-met-ă-pla′sĭ-ă) [" + *metaplasis*, transformation]. Overactivity in tissue replacement or transformation from one type of tissue to another, as cartilage to bone.

hyperme′tria [" + *metron*, measure]. Unusual range of movement.

hypermetrope (hi-per-met′rōp) [" + " + *ōps*, eye]. One who is farsighted. SYN: *hyperope.*

hypermetro′pia [" + " + *ōps*, eye]. Farsightedness. Opp. of *myopia.* SYN: *hyperopia.*

hy″permetrop′ic [" + " + *ōps*, eye]. Pert. to farsightedness.

hypermimia (hi″per-mim′ĭ-ă) [" + G. *mimeomai*, to mimic]. Use of a great number of gestures while speaking.

hypermnesia (hi-perm-ne′zĭ-ă) [" + *mnēsis*, memory]. 1. Great ability to remember names, dates, and details. 2. An exaggeration of memory involving minute details of a past experience. It may occur in mentally unstable individuals after a shock.

hypermorph (hi'per-morf) [" + *morphē,* form]. One whose length of limb and consequent standing height is high in proportion to the sitting height. SEE. *hypomorph; mesomorph.*

hypermotil'ity [" + L. *motiō,* motion]. Unusual motility. SYN: *hyperkinesia.*

hypermyatrophy (hi"per-mi-at'ro-fĭ) [" + *mys, myo-,* muscle, + *atrophia,* atrophy]. Unusual wasting of muscle.

hypermyesthesia (hi"per-mi-es-the'sĭ-ă) [" + " + *aisthēsis,* sensation]. Muscular sensitivity.

hypermyotonia (hi-per-mi-o-to'nĭ-ă) [" + " + *tonos,* tone]. Excessive muscular tonus.

hypermyotrophy (hi-per-mi-ot'ro-fĭ) [" + " + *trophē,* nourishment]. Abnormal muscular development.

hyperneocytosis (hi"per-ne"o-si-to'sis) [" + *neos,* new, + *kytos,* cell, + *ōsis*]. Abnormal increase of leukocytes in the blood (*leukocytosis*) including immature forms. SYN: *hyperleukocytosis.*

hy"pernephro'ma [G. *yper,* above, + *nephros,* kidney, + *ōma,* tumor]. A tumor of the kidney which to the naked eye resembles adrenal tissue.

hyperneurotization (hi-per-nū-rot-i-za'-shun) [" + *neuron,* nerve]. Grafting of a motor nerve into a muscle to increase its energy.

hypernitremia (hi-per-ni-tre'mĭ-ă) [" + *nitron,* niter, + *aima,* blood]. Excess of nitrogen in the blood.

hypernoia (hi-per-noy'ă) [" + *nous,* mind]. Excessive mental activity or imagination. SYN: *hyperpsychosis.*

hypernor'mal [G. *yper,* above, + L. *norma,* rule]. Abnormal.

hypernormocytosis (hi"per-nor"mo-sī-to'-sis) [" + " + G. *kytos,* cell, + *ōsis*]. An increased proportion of neutrophils in the blood.

hypernutri'tion [" + L. *nutrire,* to nourish]. Supernutrition; overfeeding.

hyperontomorph (hi-per-on'to-morf) [G. *yper,* above, + *ōn,* being, + *morphē,* form]. A person with a long thin body and with a tendency to hyperthyroidism.

hyperonychia (hi-per-o-nik'ĭ-ă) [" + *onyx,* nail]. Overgrowth (hypertrophy) of the nails.

hyperope (hi'per-ōp) [" + *ōps,* eye]. One who is farsighted. SYN: *hypermetrope.*

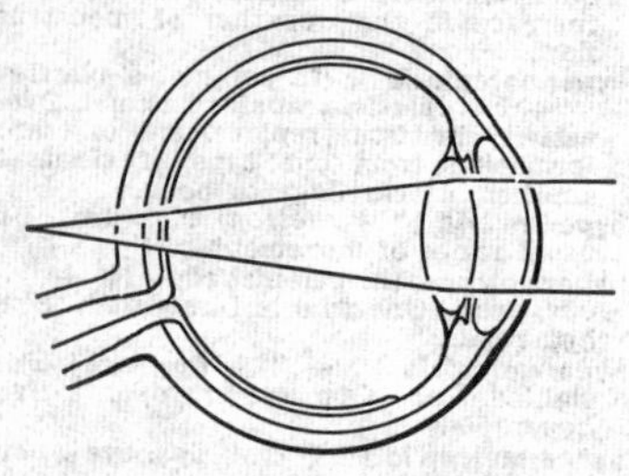

HYPEROPIA

hypero'pia [" + *ōps,* eye]. Farsightedness.

Parallel rays come to a focus behind the retina due to flattening of the globe of the eye, or to error in refraction. SYN: *hypermetropia.*

h., absolute. H. in which the eye cannot accommodate.

h., axial. H. caused by shortness of the eye's anteroposterior axis.

h., facultative. H. which can be corrected by accommodation.

h., latent. H. in which the error of refraction is overcome and disguised by ciliary muscle action.

h., manifest. Total amount of h. which can be measured by a convex lens.

h., relative. H. in which vision is clear only when excessive convergence is made.

h., total. Complete h. combining both latent and manifest types.

hyperorchidism (hi-per-or'kid-izm) [" + *orchis,* testicle, + *ismos,* state of]. Abnormal activity of testicular secretion.

hyperorexia (hi-per-o-reks'ĭ-ă) [" + *orexis,* appetite]. Abnormal hunger.

Usually satisfied by frequent small meals, as in gastric diseases, diabetes, hysteria, psychosis, hyperthyroidism and brain tumors.

It is found in helminthiasis, diabetes, hysteria, convalescence from acute diseases, psychosis, hyperthyroidism, brain tumors, diseases of the stomach in which hypermotility and hypersecretion are present. SYN: *bulimia.*

hyperorthocytosis (hi"per-or"tho-si-to'sis) [" + *orthos,* straight, + *kytos,* cell, + *ōsis*]. Increased white blood cells with normal proportion of various forms and without immature forms.

hyperos'mia [G. *yper,* above, + *osmē,* smell]. Abnormal sensitiveness to odors.

hyperosto'sis [" + *osteon,* bone, + *ōsis*]. Abnormal growth of osseous tissue. SYN: *exostosis.*

h. infantile cortical. Increased growth of subperiosteal bone occurring most frequently in the mandible and clavicles, with fever and other systemic manifestations. SYN: *Caffey's syndrome.*

hyperova'ria [" + L. *ovarium,* ovary]. Precocity of libido in young girls due to excessive ovarian secretion as the result of unusual and premature development of the ovaries.

hyperpancreatism (hi"per-pan'kre-ă-tizm) [" + *pagkreas,* pancreas, + *ismos,* state of]. Abnormal activity of the pancreas with trypsin in excess of other ferments.

hy"perpar'asitism. Condition in which a parasite lives in or upon another parasite.

hyperparathyroidism (hi"per-par-a-thi'-roy-dizm) [" + *para,* beside, + *thyreos,* shield, + *eidos,* form, + *ismos,* state of]. Condition due to increased activity of the parathyroid glands.

hyperpep'sia [" + *pepsis,* digestion]. 1. Unusually rapid digestion. 2. Indigestion with hyperchlorhydria.

hyperpepsinia (hi"per-pep-sin'ĭ-ă) [" + *pepsis,* digestion]. Excess of pepsin in the gastric secretion.

hyperperistalsis (hi"per-per-ĭ-stal'sis) [" + *peri,* around, + *stalsis,* contraction]. Overactive peristalsis.

hyperphalangism (hi-per-fal-an'jizm) [" + *phalagx,* a line, + *ismos,* state of]. Having an extra phalanx on a finger or toe. SYN: *polyphalangism.*

hyperphasia (hi-per-fa'zĭ-ă) [" + *phasis,* speech]. Loss of control of the organs of speech.

hyperphonesis (hi-per-fo-ne'sis) [" + *phonē,* voice]. Increase in voice or percussion sound in auscultation.

hyperphonia (hi-per-fo'nĭ-ă) [" + *phonē,* voice]. Stuttering or stammering due to excessive innervation of vocal muscles.

hyperphoria (hi-per-fo'rĭ-ă) [" + *phorein*, to bear]. Tendency of one eye to turn upward. SEE: *anophoria*.

hyperphosphatemia (hi-per-fos-fă-te'mĭ-ă) [" + L. *phosphās*, phosphate, + G. *aima*, blood]. Abnormal amt. of phosphorus in the blood. SYN: *hyperphospheremia*.

hyperphosphaturia (hi"per-fos-fă-tū'rĭ-ă) [" + " + G. *ouron*, urine]. Increased amt. of phosphates in the urine.

hyperphospheremia (hi"per-fos-fer-e'mĭ-ă) [G. *yper*, above, + L. *phosphās*, phosphate, + G. *aima*, blood]. Abnormal amt. of phosphorous compounds in the blood. SYN: *hyperphosphatemia*.

hyperphrenia (hi-per-fre'nĭ-ă) [" + *phrēn*, mind]. 1. Unusual intellectual activity. 2. Genius.

hyperpiesia, hyperpiesis (hi"per-pi-e'zĭ-ă, -sis) [" + *piesis*, pressure]. Abnormally high blood pressure.

hyperpietic (hi"per-pi-et'ik) [" + *piesis*, pressure]. Rel. to extremely high blood pressure.

hyperpituitarism (hi"per-pi-tu"ĭ-tar'ism) [G. *yper*, above, + L. *pituita*, mucus, + G. *ismos*, state of]. Condition resulting from overactivity of the *hypophysis cerebri* or its ant. lobe. SEE: *acromegaly; gigantism*.

hyperplasia (hī-per-pla'zĭ-ă) [G. *yper*, above, + *plassein*, to form]. An increase in size of a tissue or organ resulting from proliferation of cells or the development of additional tissue of which the organ is composed but excluding tumor formation; excessive formation of tissue.

h., fibrous. Connective tissue cell increase following any inflammation or in chronic visceral fibrosis.

h., lipoid. Increase in cells containing lipoid.

hyperplas'mia [" + *plasma*, matter formed]. 1. Abnormal increase within certain organs of leukocytes which do not appear in the blood. SYN: *aleukemia*. 2. Increase in size of red blood cells through absorption of fluids.

hyperplastic (hi-per-plas'tik) [" + *plassein*, to form]. Rel. to hyperplasia.

hyperpnea (hi-perp-ne'a) [" + *pnoē*, breath]. An increased respiratory rate or breathing which is deeper than that seen in resting subjects. A certain degree of hyperpnea is normal after exercise.

ETIOL: Pain, respiratory disease, febrile or cardiac disease, disease of diaphragm, of blood, of abdominal viscera, or due to certain drugs, hysteria, or atmospheric conditions.

hyperporo'sis [" + *pōros*, callus, + *ōsis*]. Excessive callous formation after a bone fracture.

hyperpragic (hi-per-pra'jik) [" + *praxis*, action]. Denoting excessive activity.

hyperprax'ia [G. *yper*, above, + *praxis*, action]. Excessive activity and restlessness seen in some mental disorders.

hyperprochoresis (hi"per-pro-ko-re'sis) [" + *pro*, forward, + *choreia*, dance]. Unusually rapid passage of food through the alimentary tract due to increased peristalsis. SYN: *hyperperistalsis; hyperanacinesia; tormina nervosa*.

hyperprosexia (hi-per-pro-seks'ĭ-ă) [" + *prosezein*, to heed]. PSY: Fixation of an idea to the exclusion of other ideas, as in compulsion states.

hyperproteinemia (hi"per-pro"te-in-e'mĭ-ă) [" + *prōtos*, first, + *aima*, blood]. Excess of protein in the blood plasma.

hy"perpro"teinu'ria [" + " + *ouron*, urine]. Excess of protein in the urine.

hyperproteosis (hi"per-pro-te-o'sis) [" + " + *ōsis*]. A condition resulting from an excess of protein in the diet.

hyperpselaphesia (hi"perp-sel-ă-fe'zĭ-ă) [" + *psēlaphēsis*, touch]. Morbid sensitivity to touch. SYN: *hyperaphia*.

hyperpsycho'sis [" + *psychē*, mind, + *ōsis*]. Overfunctioning of the mind.

hyperpyre'mia [" + *pyreia*, fuel, + *aima*, blood]. Excess of heat and energy producing substances in the blood.

hyperpyretic (hi"per-pi-ret'ik) [" + *pyrexia*, fever]. Pert. to high body temperature (hyperpyrexia).

hyperpyrexia (hi"per-pi-reks'ĭ-ă) [" + *pyrexia*, fever]. Elevation of systemic temperature, above 106° F.

Produced by following physical agents: Baths, diathermy, radiofrequency current, hot air, radiant heat, electric blankets.

hyperpyrex'ial [" + *pyrexia*, fever]. Denoting high body temperature.

hyperreflex'ia [" + L. *reflexus*, bent back]. Increased action of the reflexes.

hyperres'onance [" + L. *resonāre*, to resound]. Increased resonance caused by percussion.

hy"persaliva'tion. Excessive secretion of saliva.

hypersecretion (hi-per-se-kre'shun) [G. *yper*, above, + L. *secernere*, to secrete]. Abnormal amt. of secretion.

hy"persensibil'ity [" + L. *sensibilitās*, sensibility]. Hypersensitivity of the body to a foreign protein or drug. SYN: *anaphylaxis, q.v.*

hypersensitiveness (hi"per-sen'sĭ-tiv-nes) [" + L. *sensitivus*, sensitive]. Excessive and abnormal susceptibility to the action of a given agent, as pollen or foreign protein. SEE: *allergy; anaphylaxis; hay fever*.

hy"persensitiv'ity. Abnormal sensitivity to a stimulus of any kind.

hypersensitiza'tion [" + L. *sensitivus*, sensitive]. An abnormally increased susceptibility to infection.

hyperskeocytosis (hi"per-ske"o-si-to'sis) [" + *skaios*, left, + *kytos*, cell, + *ōsis*]. Leukocytosis with many immature forms. SYN: *hyperneocytosis*.

hypersom'nia [" + L. *somnus*, sleep]. A toxic condition conducive to sleeping an excessively long time.

hypersphyxia (hi-per-sfiks'ĭ-ă) [" + *sphyxis*, pulse]. High blood pressure with increased activity of the circulation.

hypersthe'nia [" + *sthenos*, strength]. Abnormal strength or excessive tension, as in the insane.

hypersthen'ic [" + *sthenos*, strength]. Denoting excessive strength, or tension.

hypersthenuria (hi"per-sthen-u'rĭ-ă) [" + " + *ouron*, urine]. Dilute condition of the urine with elevation of the freezing point.

hy"persuscep"tibil'ity [" + L. *suscipere*, to take, + *habilis*, apt]. Unusual susceptibility to a disease or to physical, esp. pathological, conditions. SEE: *allergy; anaphylaxis; anatoxic*.

hypersystole (hi-per-sis'to-le) [" + *systolē*, contraction]. Unusual force or duration of the systole.*

hypersystol'ic [" + *systolē*, contraction]. 1. Pert. to hypersystole. 2. Person with undue heart contractions.

hypertarachia (hi-per-tă-rak'ĭ-ă) [" + *tarache*, disorder]. Excessive irritability of the nervous system.

hypertelorism (hi-per-tel'or-izm) [" + *tēlē*, far, + *orizein*, to separate]. Abnormal width between two paired organs.

h., ocular. Abnormal width between the eyes.

hy"pertens'in. Former name for angiotensin, *q.v.*

hy"pertens'inase. An enzyme present in normal kidney tissue which inactivates angiotensin. It is also present in other organs and tissues. SYN: *angiotensinase.*

hy"pertensin'ogen. A globulin present in blood plasma which when acted upon by the enzyme renin forms angiotensin, *q.v.*

hyperten'sion [G. *yper*, above, + L. *tensiō*, tension]. 1. Tension or tonus above normal. 2. A condition in which patient has a higher blood pressure than normal for his age.

ETIOL: The primary factor in hypertension is an increase in peripheral resistance resulting from vasoconstriction or narrowing of peripheral blood vessels.

Systolic pressure of 160 mm. Hg constitutes the beginning of high blood pressure which may run well above 200 or even as high as 280. Persistent high blood pressure may eventuate in apoplexy or heart failure.

h., benign. H. of slow onset which is usually without symptoms.

h., essential. H. which develops without apparent cause. Also called primary or benign hypertension. SYN: *hyperpiesia.*

h., Goldblatt. Hypertension which resembles renal hypertension produced in experimental animals by decreasing the blood flow to the kidney.

h., malignant. Severe form of h. in which occlusion of peripheral vessels occurs resulting from hyperplasia and degenerative changes in intima.

h., renal. H. resulting from kidney disease. H. produced experimentally by constriction of renal arteries. It is due to a humoral substance *renin*, produced in an ischemic kidney.

RS: *blood pressure, diastolic p., hypotension, pulse, pulse pressure, systolic p.*

hyperten'sive [" + L. *tensiō*, tension]. Marked by a rise in blood pressure.

h. diseases. Noninfectious ones with increased blood pressure.

hyperthe'lia [" + *thēlē*, nipple]. The presence of more than two nipples.

hyperthermalgesia (hi"per-therm-al-je'zĭ-ă) [" + *thermē*, heat, + *algesia*, pain]. Unusual sensitiveness to heat.

hyperthermia (hi-per-ther'mĭ-ă) [G. *yper*, above, + *thermē*, heat.] SYN: *hyperpyrexia.* 1. Unusually high fever. 2. Treatment of disease by raising bodily temperature, accomplished by introduction of the malaria organism, injection of foreign proteins, or by physical means.

hyperthermoesthesia (hi-per-therm-o-es-the'sĭ-ă) [" + " + *aisthēsis*, sensation]. Unusual sensitiveness to heat. SYN: *hyperthermalgesia.*

hyperthrombinemia (hi"per-throm-bin-e'mĭ-ă) [" + *thrombos*, clot, + *aima*, blood]. Excess of thrombin in the blood causing coagulation.

hyperthymergastic reaction (hi"per-thi-mer-gas'tik) [" + *thymos*, mind, + *ergasia*, work]. A syndrome of a psychic disorder in which circumscribed attacks exhibit elated excitement, delusions of self-exaltation, euphoria, and other symptoms, including inability to conform to environment, and rebellion against inhibitions.

hyperthymia (hi-per-thi'mĭ-ă) [" + *thymos*, mind]. 1. Morbid sensitiveness. 2. Cruelty or foolhardiness. 3. Moral insanity.

hyperthy'mism, hyperthymiza'tion [" + " + *ismos*, state]. Excess secretion of the thymus gland.

hyperthyrea (hī-per-thi're-ă) [" + *thyreos*, shield]. Excessive activity of the thyroid. SYN: *hyperthyroidism.*

hyperthyreosis (hi"per-thi-re-o'sis) [" + " + *ōsis*]. Overactivity of the thyroid. SYN: *hyperthyrea; hyperthyroidation.*

hyperthyroidation (hi"per-thi-roy-da'-shun) [" + " + *eidos*, form]. Excessive action of thyroid gland. SYN: *hyperthyrea.*

hyperthyroidism (hi-per-thi'royd-izm) [" + " + " + *ismos*, state of]. A condition caused by excessive secretion of the thyroid glands which overstimulates the basal metabolism, causing an increased demand for food to prevent oxidization of body tissues.

It may take two forms: exophthalmic goiter* or Graves' disease and toxic adenoma.

SYM: Autonomic imbalance; exaggeration of all functions, rapid pulse, psychic disturbances, excitement, restlessness, tremors, diarrhea, loss of weight, increased metabolism.

TREATMENT: Surgical, by removal of the thyroid gland following proper medical preparation. Medical, by use of antithyroid drugs (as propylthiouracil, methimazole, or carbimazole), iodide or radioactive iodine (I^{131}).

NP: Mental and physical rest with freedom from worry and excitement imperative. A cool, bracing climate desirable. Exercise during hot weather aggravates symptoms. Winter months often bring improvement.

In severe cases confinement in bed, perhaps for several weeks or months. Light, fresh air, and sunshine are needed and sometimes a change of room desirable. Visitors should not be permitted prior to operation or in severe cases, and the nurse should attempt to allay all nervousness on part of patient. Simple diversions help to allay restlessness. Bedclothes during hot weather reduced to a minimum. Encourage patient to drink plenty of water. Proper elimination should be maintained. Warm baths and frequent rubs are conducive to rest. Patient's position should be changed frequently. Hydrotherapy may be prescribed, and cold applications used to allay palpitation. An accurate record of pulse should be kept and the weight recorded at regular intervals. Regular nursing procedures should be followed for daily care of patient.

DIET: The doctor and the dietition may indicate the needed calories and prescribe the diet. Ordinarily, diet should be light and nourishing, with 2 or 3 pints of milk per day. No coffee or alcohol. Regular nutritive diet.

RS: *Basedow's disease; cretinism; goiter; myxedema; thyroid.*

hyperthyro'sis [" + " + *ōsis*]. Excess of thyroid secretion in the blood. SYN: *hyperthyroidation.*

hyperto'nia [G. *yper*, above, + *tonos*, tension]. Abnormal tension of arteries or muscles.

hyperton'ic [" + *tonos*, tension]. 1. Having a higher osmotic pressure than blood.

Pert. to a solution of higher osmotic pressure than another.

2. Being in a state of greater than normal tension or of incomplete relaxation. Said of muscles. Opp. of *hypotonic.**

hypertonicity (hi″per-ton-ĭ′sĭ-tĭ) [" + *tonos,* tension]. Excess muscular tonus or intraocular pressure. Syn: *hypertonia.*

hypertonus (hi-per-to′nus) [" + *tonos,* tension]. Increased tension, as muscular tension in spasm.

hypertoxic′ity [" + *toxikon,* poison]. The state of being excessively poisonous.

hypertrichiasis (hi″per-trĭk-i′ă-sis) [" + *thrix, trich-,* hair]. Excessive growth of hair.

Etiol: Congenital or obscure causes. May be due to adrenal or gonad disturbances. Syn: *hypertrichosis.*

hypertrichophobia (hi″per-trik-o-fo′bĭ-ă) [" + " + *phobos,* fear]. Fear of hair on the body.

hypertrichophrydia (hi″per-trik-o-frid′ĭ-ă) [" + " + *ophrys,* eyebrow]. Undue length of the eyebrows.

hypertrichosis (hi″per-trĭ-ko′sis) [" + " + *ōsis*]. Excessive growth of hair. Syn: *hypertrichiasis.*

hypertrophia (hi-per-tro′fĭ-ă) [" + *trophē,* nourishment]. Increased size of an organ, or of the body, due to growth. Syn: *hypertrophy.*

hypertrophic (hi-per-trof′ik) [" + *trophē,* nourishment]. Pert. to hypertrophy.

hypertrophy (hi″per′tro-fĭ) [G. *yper,* above, + *trophē,* nourishment]. Syn: *hypertrophia.* Increase in size of an organ or structure which does not involve tumor formation. Term is generally restricted to an increase in size or bulk not resulting from an increase in number of cells or tissue elements, as in the hypertrophy of a muscle. Term sometimes used to apply to any increase in size as a result of functional activity. See: *hyperplasia.*

h., adaptive. H. in which an organ increases in size to meet increased functional demands, as h. of the heart which accompanies valvular disorders.

h., cardiac. H. of the heart; increase in size of the heart resulting from hypertrophy of muscle tissue but without increase in size of cavities.

h., compensatory. H. resulting from increased function of an organ due to a defect, or due to impaired function of the opposite of a paired organ.

h., concentric. H. in which the walls of an organ become thickened, with no enlargement, but with diminished capacity.

h., eccentric. Hypertrophy of an organ with dilatation.

h., false. H. with degeneration of one constituent of an organ and its replacement by another.

h., Marie's. Chronic arthral enlargement subsequent to chronic periostitis.

h., numerical. H. caused by increase in structural elements.

h., physiological. That due to natural rather than pathological factors.

h., pseudomuscular. A disease usually of childhood, characterized by paralysis, depending upon degeneration of the muscles which, however, become enlarged from a deposition of fat and connective tissue. Syn: *pseudohypertrophic muscular dystrophy; Erb's dystrophy.*

Sym: Weakness of muscles, child is awkward, stumbles and seeks support in walking. As paralysis increases, the muscles, particularly those of the calf, thigh, buttocks and back, enlarge. Upper extremities less frequently affected. In erect posture feet are wide apart, abdomen protrudes and spinal column shows a marked curvature with convexity forward. Patient rises from recumbent position by grasping the knees or by resting the hands on the floor in front of him, extending the legs and pushing the body backwards. Gait is waddling. In course of few years paralysis becomes so marked patient is unable to leave his bed; atrophy of muscles follows.

Prog: Unfavorable.

Treatment: Constitutional; graduated exercises, massage.

h., simple. H. due to increase in size of structural parts.

h., true. H. caused by increase in size in all the different tissues composing a part.

h., vicarious. H. of an organ when another organ of allied function is disabled or destroyed.

hypertro′pia [G. *yper,* above, + *tropē,* a turning]. Vertical strabismus upward.

hyperuresis (hi-per-u-re′sis) [" + *ourēsis,* urination]. Excess of urinary secretion. Syn: *enuresis; polyuria.*

hyperuricemia (hi″per-u-ris-e′mĭ-ă) [" + *ouron,* urine, + *aima,* blood]. Abnormal amt. of uric acid in the blood.

hyperuricu′ria [" + " + *ouron,* urine]. Undue amt. of uric acid in the urine.

hypervas′cular [" + L. *vasculus,* vessel]. Excessively vascular.

hypervenosity (hi″per-ve-nos′ĭ-tĭ) [" + L. *venōsus,* pert. to a vein]. Excessive development of the venous system. Syn: *supervenosity.*

hy″perventila′tion [G. *yper,* above, + L. *ventilatio,* ventilation]. Hyperpnea as occurs in forced respiration; increased inspiration and expiration of air as a result of increase in rate or depth of respiration, or both. Results esp. in carbon dioxide depletion (acapnia) with accompanying symptoms (fall in blood pressure, vasoconstriction, and sometimes syncope).

h. syndrome. A condition common during sleep. Faster and deeper breathing causes a loss of carbon dioxide from the lungs producing numbness of the hands, fingers and of other parts of the body, prickling of skin, trembling feeling, racing of heart, light-headedness, fainting, cramps of muscles, esp. of leg, a spastic and painful condition resulting in tetany and possibly death.

hyperviscos′ity [" + L. *viscōsus,* gummy]. Excessive viscosity or exaggeration of adhesive properties. Seen in anemias and inflammatory diseases.

hypervitaminosis (hi″per-vi″ta-min-o′sis) [" + L. *vīta,* life, + *amine* + *ōsis*]. A condition caused by an excessive amount of vitamin. Occurs in cases of administration of massive doses of vitamins A or D.

hypervolemia (hi″per-vol-e′mĭ-ă) [" + L. *volumen,* volume, + G. *aima,* blood]. Plethora of blood.

hypesthesia (hi-pes-the′zĭ-ă) [G. *ypo,* under, + *aisthēsis,* sensation]. Lessened sensibility to touch.

hypha (hi′fă) (pl. *hyphae*) [G. *yphē,* web]. A filament of mold, or part of a mold mycelium.

hyphedonia (hīp-he-do′nĭ-ă) [G. *ypo,* under, + *ēdonē,* pleasure]. Abnormal diminution in gratification of desires.

hyphemia (hi-fe′mĭ-ă) [" + *aima,* blood]. 1. Blood in the ant. chamber of the eye in front of iris. 2. Oligemia, a deficiency of blood.

hyphidrosis (hīp-hid-ro'sis) [" + *idrōs*, sweat]. Diminished secretion of sweat.

Hyphomycetes (hi"fo-mi-se'tēz) [G. *yphē*, web, + *mykes*, fungus]. The *Fungi Imperfecti*. Filamentous fungi with branched or unbranched threads. Do not have sexual spores.

hypinosis (hip-in-o'sis) [G. *ypo*, under, + *is, in-*, fiber, + *ōsis*]. Deficiency of fibrin in the blood.

hypnagogic (hip-nă-goj'ik) [G. *ypnos*, sleep, + *agōgos*, leading]. 1. Inducing sleep or induced by sleep. Syn: *hypnotic*. 2. Psy: Pert. to hallucinations or dreams just before loss of consciousness. See: *hypnogenic zones*.

h. state. A transitional state bet. sleeping and awaking and delusions which may result therefrom.

hypnalgia (hip-nal'jĭ-ă) [" + *algos*, pain]. False sense of pain experienced in a dream.

hypnic (hip'nik) [G. *ypnos*, sleep]. Causing sleep. Syn: *somnifacient; somniferous*.

hyp'nocyst [" + *kystis*, a cyst]. A quiescent cyst or one in which the activity is in abeyance.

hyp"nogenet'ic [" + *gennan*, to produce]. Producing sleep.

h. spots. Areas which, on being stimulated, produce sleep. Syn: *hypnogenic zones*.

hypnogenic zones (hip-no-jen'ik) [" + *gennan*, to produce]. Areas on the body which, when stimulated, produce sleep, esp. a sleep resembling somnambulism.

The area may be the elbow or the popliteal spaces. See: *hypnagogic*.

hypnoidal (hip-noy'dal) [" + *eidos*, resemblance]. Pert. to a condition between sleep and waking, resembling sleep.

hypnoidiza'tion [" + *eidos*, form]. Induction of hypnosis.

hypnolepsy (hip'no-lep-sĭ) [" + *lēpsis*, seizure]. Irresistible sleepiness. Syn: *narcolepsy*.

hypnology (hip-nol'o-jĭ) [" + *logos*, study]. Scientific study of sleep.

hyp"nophob'ia. Morbid fear of falling asleep.

hypnopompic (hip-no-pom'pik) [" + *pompy*, procession]. Dreams persisting after return of consciousness.

hypnosis (hip-no'sis) [" + *ōsis*]. A subconscious condition in which the objective manifestations of mind are more or less inactive, accompanied by abnormal sensibility to impressions, the subject responding to these impressions, unrestrained by the reasoning faculties. See: *autohypnosis; braidism; hypnotism; sleepwalking; somniloquy*.

hypnosophy (hip-nos'o-fĭ) [" + *sophia*, wisdom]. The study of sleep.

hypnother'apy [" + *therapeia*, treatment]. Treatment by hypnotism, or by inducing prolonged sleep.

hypnot'ic [G. *ypnos*, sleep]. 1. Pert. to sleep or hypnosis. 2. An agent that induces sleep or which dulls the senses. Ex: *chloral hydrate, sulfonethylmethane*.

hypnot'ics [G. *ypnos*, sleep]. Drugs which cause insensibility to pain by inhibiting afferent impulses, or the cortical centers of the brain receiving sensory impressions, and thus causing partial or complete unconsciousness.

They include *sedatives, analgesics, anesthetics*, and *intoxicants, q.v.* They should yield not unpleasant aftereffects and result in natural sleep.

They are sometimes called *narcotics, somnifacients*, and *soporifics, q.v.*, when used to induce sleep.

NP: They should not be administered without a physician's order.

Ex: Bromides: sodium bromide, potassium bromide, or ammonium bromide.

Aspirin acts as a mild hypnotic.

Stronger: Trional, Veronal, Sulfonal—this should be given early in the evening, as it takes several hours to act.

Chloral often used in conjunction with bromide to obtain a more powerful hypnotic effect. Chloral is a heart depressant.

Narcotics: Opium, morphine and its derivatives are narcotics. Excessive use of the drugs should be reported to the doctor.

hypnotism (hip'no-tizm) [" + *ismos*, state of]. An induced sleeplike state during which patient is peculiarly susceptible to the suggestions of the hypnotist.

hyp'notist [G. *ypnos*, sleep]. One who practices hypnotism.

hypnotize (hip'no-tīz) [G. *ypnos*, sleep]. To put under hypnotism.

hypo (hī'po) [G. *ypo*, under]. 1. A hypochondriac. 2. Popular name for hypodermic injection.

hypo- [G.]. Prefix: Less than, below.

hy"poacid'ity [G. *ypo*, under, + L. *acidus*, sour]. A condition caused by lowered hydrochloric secretion.

Secondary to other disorders, such as pernicious anemia.

Treatment: Dilute HCl by mouth.

Diet: Fruit juices and meat broths before meals. Nourishing diet.

hypoade'nia [" + *adēn*, gland] Defective activity of the glands.

hypoadre'nalism, hypoadre'nia [" + L. *ad*, to, + *rēnalis*, pert. to kidney, + G. *ismos*, state of]. Adrenal insufficiency.

hypoalimenta'tion [" + L. *alimentum*, nourishment]. Insufficient nourishment. Syn: *subalimentation*.

hypoalonemia (hi"po-al-o-ne'mĭ-ă) [" + *als*, salt, + *aima*, blood]. Lack of salts in the blood.

hypoazoturia (hi"po-az-o-tu'rĭ-ă) [" + *a-*, priv. + *zōe*, life, + *ouron*, urine]. Diminished urea in the urine.

hypobaropathy (hi"po-bar-op'ă-thĭ) [" + *baros*, pressure, + *pathos*, disease]. Symptoms produced by diminished air pressure, mountain sickness, aviator's sickness.

hypoblast (hi'po-blast) [G. *ypo*, under, + *blastos*, germ]. The inner cell layer or *entoderm* which develops during gastrulation. The external layer is called epiblast.

hypoblastic (hi-po-blas'tik) [" + *blastos*, germ]. Pert. to the inner layer of the blastoderm.

hypobulia (hi-po-bu'lĭ-ă) [" + *boulē*, will]. Lack of will power.

hypocalcemia (hi"po-kal-se'mĭ-ă) [" + L. *calx*, lime, + G. *aima*, blood]. Abnormally low blood calcium.

hypocalcia (hi-po-kal'sĭ-ă) [" + L. *calx*, lime]. Lack of calcium in the system.

hypocap'nia [" + *kapnos*, smoke]. Lack of carbon dioxide in the blood.

hypochloremia (hi"po-klo-re'mĭ-ă) [" + *chlōros*, green, + *aima*, blood]. Having deficiency of the chloride contents of the blood.

hypochlorhydria (hi-po-klor-hi'drĭ-ă) [" + " + *ydōr*, water]. Diminished secretion of hydrochloric acid.

Small amount and low acid may be

indicative of carcinoma or anemia. May be found in subacute and chronic gastritis, peptic ulcers, infections, advanced tuberculosis, early carcinoma, and neuroses. SEE: *achlorhydria; hyperchlorhydria.*

hy″pochloriza′tion [" + *chlōros*, green]. Reduction of sodium chloride in the diet in nephritis and epilepsy.

hypochloruria (hi-po-klor-u′rĭ-ă) [G. *ypo*, under, + *chlōros*, green, + *ouron*, urine]. Diminution of chlorides in the urine.

hypocholesteremia (hi″po-ko-les-ter-e′-mĭ-ă) [" + *cholē*, bile, + *stereos*, solid, + *aima*, blood]. Lowered cholesterin in the blood.

hypochon′dria [" + *chondros*, cartilage]. Abnormal concern about health with false belief of suffering from some disease. SYN: *hypochondriasis.*

hypochon′driac [" + *chondros*, cartilage]. 1. Pert. to the region of the hypochondrium,* or upper lateral region on each side of the body and below the thorax; beneath the ribs.

2. One having a morbid fear of disease.

h. region. Part of abdomen beneath lower ribs on both sides of epigastrium. SYN: *hypochondrium.*

hypochondriacal (hi″po-kon-dri′ă-kal) [" + *chondros*, cartilage]. Affected with a morbid interest in health and disease.

hypochondrial reflex (hi-po-kon′drĭ-al). A sudden inspiratory act resulting from sudden pressure below costal border.

hypochondriasis (hi″po-kon-dri′ă-sĭs) [" + *chondros*, cartilage]. Morbid anxiety about one's health; a frequent symptom of depressed states. SYN: *hypochondria.*

hypochon′drium [" + *chondros*, cartilage]. That part of the abdomen beneath the lower ribs on each side of the epigastrium.

hypochromasia (hi″po-kro-ma′sĭ-ă) [" + *chrōma*, color]. Lack of hemoglobin in the red blood cells.

hypochromatosis (hi″po-kro-mă-to′sis) [" + " + *ōsis*]. Disappearance of the chromatin or nucleus in a cell. SYN: *chromatolysis.*

hy″pochrom′ia [G. *ypo*, under, + *chrōma*, color]. Condition of the blood in which the red blood cells have a reduced hemoglobin content.

hypochromic (hi-po-krōm′ik) [" + *chrōma*, color]. Pert. to hypochromia.

hypochro′sis [" + *chrōma*, coloring]. Lack of color in the blood because of low hemoglobin.

hypochylia (hi-po-ki′lĭ-ă) [" + *chylos*, juice]. Lack of normal secretion of gastric juice.

hypocinesia (hi-po-sin-e′zĭ-ă) [" + *kinēsis*, motion]. Diminished power of movement. SYN: *hypokinesia.*

hypocolasia (hi-po-ko-la′zĭ-ă) [" + *kolasis*, hindering]. Functional weakness of the inhibiting mechanism.

hypocondylar (hi-po-kon′dĭ-lar) [" + *kondylos*, condyle]. Below a condyle.

hy′pocone. The distolingual cusp of an upper molar tooth.

hy″pocon′id. The distobuccal cusp of a lower molar tooth.

hypocrinism (hi-po-kri′nizm) [" + *krinein*, to separate, + *ismos*, state of]. Deficient secretion of any gland, esp. an endocrine.

hypocyclosis (hi″po-si-klo′sis) [G. *ypo*, under, + *kyklos*, circle]. Deficient accommodation.

h., ciliary. Weakness of ciliary muscle.

h., lenticular. Lack of elasticity in crystalline lens.

Both forms interfere with accommodation.

hypocystotomy (hi-po-sis-tot′o-mĭ) [" + *kystis*, a bladder, + *tomē*, incision]. Perineal opening of the bladder.

hypocytosis (hi-po-si-to′sis) [" + *kytos*, cell, + *ōsis*]. Lack of normal number of blood corpuscles.

hypodactylia (hi″po-dak-til′ĭ-ă) [" + *daktylos*, finger]. Having a decreased number of fingers or toes.

hypodermatomy (hi-po-der-mat′o-mĭ) [" + *derma*, skin, + *tomē*, incision]. Subcutaneous incision or section, as of a muscle or tendon.

hypoder′mic [" + *derma*, skin]. Under, or inserted under the skin, as a *hypodermic injection.*

It may be given *subcutaneously, intracutaneously* (into the skin), *intramuscularly* (into a muscle), *intraspinally* (into the spinal canal), or *intravenously* (into a vein).

It is given to secure prompt action of a drug when the drug cannot be taken by mouth, when it may not be readily absorbed in the stomach or intestines, when it might be changed by action of the gastric secretions, or to act as an anesthetic about the site of injection.

h., antitoxin, serum, and vaccine. Subcutaneously in infrascapular region, infraclavicular region, or post. portion of axilla. May also be adm. intramuscularly.

h., intracutaneous. Into the skin.

h., intramuscular. Given in gluteal or in lumbar region. Used when a drug is not easily absorbed or when it is irritating and when large quantity of liquid is to be used.

h., intravenous. SITE: Into a vein, the usual site being median basilic, or median cephalic vein.

h., subcutaneous. Given just under the skin, usually in front of thighs, or outer surface of arms and forearm.

hypodermoclysis, hypodermatoclysis (hi″-po-der-mok′lĭ-sis, -mă-tok′lĭ-sis) [" + " + *klysis*, injection]. The injection of fluids into the subcutaneous tissues to supply the body with liquids quickly, as after shock or hemorrhage, diarrhea, or when the blood coagulation time is too long; in fact, it may be given in any condition in which it is impossible to give sufficient water by mouth or by rectum.

When it is necessary to maintain a larger amount of water in the tissues in order to keep up proper metabolism, hypodermoclysis may be ordered. The purpose is about the same as that of intravenous infusions.

SOLUTIONS USUALLY USED: Physiological salt solution. Normal salt solution is generally used because it is one of the principal constituents of the blood.

There are other solutions given by this method as preferred by the attending physician. If the solution is not of the right percentage, hemolysis* may occur. Other solutions adm. intravenously are not generally given by hypodermoclysis.

TEMPERATURE OF SOLUTION: It is very essential that solution be of the proper temperature, which should be from 108°-115° F., in the flask, as it cools rapidly while passing through the tubing. It is very necessary also that it be warm enough during the entire course of the flow.

Site of Injection: The thighs are not used by some authorities as the needles are not supposed to penetrate near the course of large blood vessels. Here the femoral vein is too close to the site of an injection. (a) In the loose tissues at the base of the breasts; (b) in the thighs or buttocks (care being taken to avoid the large blood vessels); (c) in the axillary line (esp. for men); (d) beneath the skin of the abdomen (half way between the navel and the ant. sup. spine); (e) and intraperitoneally in children.

hypodynamia (hi″po-di-na′mĭ-ă) [G. *ypo,* under, + *dynamis,* energy]. Vital debility. Syn: *adynamia.*

hypoeccrisia (hi-po-ek-ris′ĭ-ă) [" + *ek,* out, + *krisis,* separation]. Imperfect excretion.

hypoeccritic (hi″po-ek-krit′ik) [" + *ekkritikos,* secreting]. 1. Retarding normal excretion. 2. Pert. to insufficient or defective excretion.

hypoendocrinism (hi″po-en-dok′rĭ-nizm) [" + *endon,* within, + *krinein,* to separate, + *ismos,* state of]. Insufficiency of internal secretion in one or more glands.

hypoendocrisia (hi″po-en-do-kriz′ĭ-ă) [" + " + *krisis,* separation]. Insufficiency of endocrine secretion. Syn: *hypoendocrinism.*

hypoeosinophilia (hi″po-e″o-sin-o-fil′ĭ-ă) [" + *ēōs,* dawn (rose colored), + *philein,* to love]. Diminished quantity of eosinophil leukocytes of the blood.

hypoepinephria (hi-po-ep-ĭ-nef′rĭ-ă) [" + *epi,* upon, + *nephros,* kidney]. Insufficiency of the adrenal secretion.

hypoergy (hi″po-er′jĭ). Hyposensitiveness to allergens.

hypoesophoria (hi″po-es-o-fo′rĭ-ă) [" + *esō,* inward, + *phorein,* to bear]. Downward and inward deviation of the eye.

hypoesthe′sia [" + *aisthēsis,* sensation]. Dulled sensitivity to touch.

hypoexophoria (hi″po-eks-o-fo′rĭ-ă) [" + *exō,* outward, + *phorein,* to bear]. Downward and outward deviation of the eye.

hypogas′tric [" + *gastēr,* belly]. Pert. to lower middle of the abdomen or hypogastrium.

h. artery. *Arteria iliaca interna.*

h. plexus. Sympathetic nerve plexus in the pelvis.

h. region. The hypogastrium. See: *abdominal region.*

hypogas′trium [" + *gastēr,* belly]. Region below the umbilicus, or navel, between the right and left inguinal regions.

hypogen′esis [" + *genesis,* development]. Cessation of growth or development at an early stage, causing defective structure. Syn: *ateliosis.*

hypogenitalism (hi″po-jen′ĭ-tal-izm) [G. *ypo,* under, + L. *genitalis,* a genital + G. *ismos,* state of]. Condition in which the genital organs are underdeveloped. Characterized by reduced size of genital organs, failure of testes to descend in some cases, and incomplete development of secondary sex characters. See: *hypogonadism.*

Gonadotropic hormones from urine of pregnant mares aid in causing testicular descent and growth of the genitalia.

hypogeusia (hi-po-gū′sĭ-ă) [" + *geusis,* taste]. Blunting of sense of taste.

hypoglobu′lia [" + L. *globulus,* globule]. Lack of cellular elements of the blood. Syn: *cytopenia; hypocytosis.*

hypoglos′sal [" + *glōssa,* tongue]. Situated under the tongue.

h. alternating hemiplegia. Medulla lesion paralyzing the tongue by involving the 12th nerve fibers as they course through the uncrossed pyramid. The pathology may extend across the midline or dorsally, involving the medial fillet, causing contralateral anesthesia.

h. nerve. A mixed nerve, the 12th cranial. It carries afferent proprioceptive impulses as well as efferent motor impulses.

Orig: Medulla oblongata.

Dist: Extrinsic and intrinsic muscles of tongue.

hypoglot′tis [" + *glōssa,* tongue]. 1. Undersurface of tongue. 2. Cystic tumor of floor of mouth. Syn: *ranula.*

hypoglyce′mia [" + *glykos,* sweet, + *aima,* blood]. Deficiency of sugar in the blood.

A condition in which there is less than 80 mg. of sugar per 100 ml. of blood.

Etiol: Hyperfunction of the islets of Langerhans may cause it or injection of excessive quantity of insulin. See: *coma, hyperglycemia, hyperinsulinism.*

Sym: acute fatigue, restlessness, malaise, marked irritability and weakness. In severe cases, mental disturbances, delirium, coma, and possibly death.

hypoglycemic (hi-po-gli-se′mik) [" + " + *aima,* blood]. Pert. to or causing hypoglycemia.

h. shock. Production of shock by artificial production of hypoglycemia by intramuscular adm. of insulin in the treatment of schizophrenia. RS: *insulin, schizophrenia, shock.*

hypoglycogenolysis (hi″po-gli-ko-jen-ol′-ĭ-sis) [" + " + *gennan,* to produce, + *lysis,* solution]. Defective hydrolysis of glycogen (glycogenolysis).

hypognathous (hi-pog′nă-thus) [G. *ypo,* under, + *gnathos,* jaw]. Having a lower jaw longer than the upper one.

hypogonadism (hi-po-go′nad-izm) [" + *gonē,* semen, + *ismos,* state of]. Defective internal secretion of the gonads.

hypohepatia (hi″po-he-pă′tĭ-ă) [" + *ēpar, ēpat-,* liver]. Deficient liver function.

hypohidrosis (hi-po-hi-dro′sis) [" + *idrōs,* sweat, + *ōsis*]. Diminished perspiration. Syn: *hyphidrosis.*

hypohyloma (hi″po-hi-lo′mă) [" + *ylē,* matter, + *ōma,* tumor]. A tumor formed by embryonic tissue. Derived from hypoblast tissue.

hypoinosemia (hi-po-in-o-se′mĭ-ă) [" + *is, in-,* fiber, + *aima,* blood]. Decreased formation of fibrin in the blood.

hypoin′sulinism [" + L. *insula,* island, + G. *ismos,* state of]. Insufficient secretion of insulin. Syn: *diabetes mellitus.*

hypoisotonic (hi″po-i″so-ton′ĭk) [" + *isos,* equal, + *tonos,* tension]. Hypotonic, *q.v.*

hypokalemia (hi″po-kă-le′mĭ-ă). Extreme potassium depletion in the circulating blood, commonly manifested by episodes of muscular weakness or paralysis, tetany, and postural hypotension. Syn: *hypopotassemia.*

hypokinesia (hi-po-kin-e′zĭ-ă) [" + *kinesis,* motion]. Decreased motor reaction to stimulus.

hypokinet′ic [" + *kinēsis,* motion]. Pert. to hypokinesia.

hypokolasia (hi″po-kol-a′sĭ-ă) [" + *kolasis,* hindrance]. Imperfect inhibitory power.

hypolem′nal. Situated below a sheath or membrane.

hypolepidoma (hi-po-lep-ĭ-do′mă) [" + *lepis, lepid-,* rind, + *ōma,* tumor]. A hypoblastic tissue tumor.

hypoleukocytosis (hi″po-lu″ko-si-to′sis) [G. *ypo*, under, + *leukos*, white, + *kytos*, cell, + *ōsis*]. A lessening of leukocytes in blood. SYN: *leukocytopenia*.

hypoliposis (hi″po-li-po′sis) [G. *ypo*, under, + *lipos*, fat, + *ōsis*]. Deficiency of fat in the tissues.

hypologia (hi-po-lo′jĭ-ă) [G. *ypo*, under, + *logos*, word]. A cerebral symptom marked by inadequate speech.

hypolymphemia (hi-po-lim-fe′mĭ-ă) [" + L. *lympha*, lymph, + G. *aima*, blood]. Decreased lymphocytes in the blood with normal number of leukocytes.

hypomania (hi-po-ma′nĭ-ă) [" + *mania*, madness]. Mild mania without much change in behavior, but accompanied by sound associations and distractibility.

hypoma′niac [" + *mania*, madness]. Pert. to maniacal exaltation, or a person so affected.

hypomastia, hypomazia (hi-po-mas′tĭ-ă, -ma′zĭ-ă) [" + *mastos*, *mazos*, breast]. Condition of having abnormally small breasts.

hy″pomelanchol′ia [" + *melas*, black, + *cholē*, bile]. Melancholia without delusions.

hypomenorrhea (hi″po-men-or-re′a) [" + *mēn*, month, + *roia*, flow]. Deficient menstrual flow.

hypomere (hi′po-mēr) [" + *meros*, part]. That portion of the mesoderm that later forms the pleuroperitoneal walls.

hypometabolism (hi″po-mĕ-tab′o-lizm) [" + *metabolē*, change, + *ismos*, state of]. Lowered metabolism.

hypometria (hi-po-me′trĭ-ă) [" + *metron*, measure]. Shortened range or movement.

hypometropia (hi″po-mĕ-trop′ĭ-ă). Myopia or shortsightedness.

hypomicron (hi″po-mi′kron). A submicron; a particle invisible under an ordinary microscope but capable of being recognized under an ultramicroscope.

hypomnesia, hypomnesis (hi-pom-ne′zĭ-ă, -nē′sĭs) [" + *mnēsis*, memory]. Impaired memory.

hypomorph (hi′po-morf) [" + *morphē*, form]. One with short limbs who is short when standing in proportion to when sitting. The opposite of *hypermorph*, *q.v.* SEE: *mesomorph*.

hypomotility (hi-po-mo-til′ĭ-tĭ). Hypokinesia, *q.v.*

hypomyotonia (hi″po-mi-o-to′nĭ-ă) [" + *mys*, *myo-*, muscle, + *tonos*, tension]. Lacking in muscular tonus.

hypomyxia (hi-po-miks′ĭ-ă) [" + *myxa*, mucus]. Diminished secretion of mucus.

hyponanosoma (hi-po-nan-o-so′mă). Extreme dwarfism.

hyponatremia (hi-po-nă-tre′mĭ-ă). Decreased concentration of sodium in the blood.

hyponeocytosis (hi″po-ne″o-si-to′sis) [" + *neos*, new, + *kytos*, cell, + *ōsis*]. Decreased number of leukocytes (leukopenia) with immature cells in the blood.

hyponoia (hi-po-noy′ă) [" + *nous*, mind]. Sluggish mental activity or imagination. SYN: *hypopsychosis*.

hyponychium (hi-po-nik′ĭ-um) [G. *ypo*, under, + *onyx*, *onych-*, nail]. The nail bed. SYN: *matrix unguis*.

hypopallesthesia (hi″po-al″es-the′zĭ-ă) [" + pallesthesia]. Decreased ability to perceive vibratory sense.

hypopancreatism (hi″po-pan′kre-ă-tizm) [" + *pagkreas*, pancreas, + *ismos*, state of]. Diminished activity of the pancreas.

hypoparathyreosis (hi″po-par-ă-thi-re-o′sis) [" + *para*, beside, + *thyreos*, shield, + *ōsis*]. A condition due to lessened or absent secretion of the parathyroids. SYN: *hypoparathyroidism*.

hypoparathyroidism (hi″po-par-ă-thi′royd-izm) [" + " + " + *eidos*, form, + *ismos*, state of]. Insufficient secretion of the parathyroid glands.

hypopep′sia [" + *pepsis*, digestion]. Impaired digestion due to lack of pepsin.

hypopepsinia (hi-po-pep-sin′ĭ-ă) [" + *pepsis*, digestion]. Deficient pepsin in the gastric juice.

hypophar′ynx [G. *ypo*, under, + *pharynx*, pharynx]. The laryngopharynx; the lowermost portion of the pharynx which leads to the larynx and esophagus.

hypophonesis (hi-po-fo-ne′sis) [" + *phōnē*, voice]. A diminished sound in auscultation or in percussion fainter than usual.

hypophonia (hi-po-fo′nĭ-ă) [" + *phōnē*, voice]. Abnormally weak voice due to incoordination of speech muscles.

hypophoria (hi-po-fo′rĭ-ă) [" + *phorein*, to bear]. Tendency of one visual axis to fall below the other one.

hypophosphatemia (hi″po-fos-fă-te′mĭ-ă) [" + L. *phosphas*, phosphate, + G. *aima*, blood]. Phosphates below normal in the blood.

hypophrenia (hi-po-fre′nĭ-ă) [G. *ypo*, under, + *phrēn*, mind]. Subnormal mentality.

hypophren′ic [" + *phrēn*, mind]. 1. Pert. to subnormal mentality. 2. A feebleminded person.

hypophrenosis (hi-po-fre-no′sis) [" + " + *ōsis*]. Feeblemindedness.

hypophyseal (hi-po-fiz′e-al) [" + *physis*, growth]. Pert. to the hypophysis.

hypophysectomy (hi″po-fĭ-sek′to-mĭ) [" + " + *ektomē*, excision]. Excision of the hypophysis cerebri.

hypophysis (hi-pof′ĭ-sis) (pl. *hypophyses*) [" + *physis*, growth]. 1. Any undergrowth. 2. [NA]. The pituitary body.

h. cerebri. A gland of internal secretion lying in the sella turcica of the sphenoid bone. It consists of two portions, the *adenohypophysis* and the *neurohypophysis*. These are differentiated into the anterior and posterior lobes which are attached to the hypothalamus of the brain by the hypophyseal stalk. SYN: *pituitary gland*, *q.v.*

hypophysitis (hi-pof-ĭ-si′tis) [" + " + *-ītis*, inflammation]. Inflammation of the pituitary body.

hypopiesis (hi-po-pi-e′sis) [" + *piesis*, pressure]. Lower than normal blood pressure.

hypopinealism (hi-po-pin′e-al-izm) [" + L. *pineus*, pert. to pine cone, + G. *ismos*, state of]. Diminished secretion of the pineal body.

hypopituitarism (hi-po-pĭ-tu′ĭ-tă-rizm) [G. *ypo*, under, + L. *pituita*, mucus, + G. *ismos*, state of]. A condition resulting from diminished secretion of pituitary hormones, esp. those of the anterior lobe.

hypoplasia (hi-po-pla′zĭ-ă) [" + *plasis*, formation]. Defective development of tissue. RS: *tissue*.

hypoporosis (hi″po-po-ro′sis). Deficient development of a callus at site of a bone fracture.

hypopotassemia (hi″po-po-tas-se′mĭ-ă). Hypokalemia, *q.v.*

hypopraxia (hi″po-prax′ĭ-ă) [" + *praxis*, action]. Decreased and inefficient activity.

hypoproteinemia (hi″po-pro-te-in-e′mĭ-ă) [″ + *prōtos*, first, + *aima*, blood]. Decrease in the normal quantity of protein in the blood.

hypoproteino′sis. Condition resulting from protein deficiency in diet.

hypoprothrombinemia (hi″po-pro-throm″-bin-e′mĭ-ă). Deficiency of prothrombin in the blood.

hypopselaphesia (hi-pop-sel-ă-fe′zĭ-ă) [″ + *psēlaphēsis*, touch]. Blunted tactile sense.

hypopsychosis (hi-po-si-ko′sis) [G. *ypo*, under, + *psychē*, mind, + *ōsis*]. Weakness of the function of thought. Syn: *hyponoia.*

hypoptyalism (hi-po-ti′al-izm) [″ + *ptyalon*, saliva, + *ismos*, state of]. Decreased salivary secretion.

hypopyon (hi-po′pĭ-on) [″ + *pyon*, pus]. Pus in ant. chamber of the eye in front of iris but behind cornea, seen in corneal ulcer.

hyporeflex′ia [″ + L. *reflexus*, bent back]. Diminished function of the reflexes.

hyposalemia (hi-po-sal-e′mĭ-ă) [″ + L. *sal*, salt, + G. *aima*, blood]. Decreased amt. of salts in the blood. Syn: *hypochloremia.*

hypo″saliva′tion. Abnormal decrease in flow of saliva.

hyposar′ca [″ + *sarx*, flesh]. Extreme dropsy (anasarca) of subcutaneous connective tissue.

hyposecre′tion [″ + L. *secrētus; secernere*, to separate]. Lowered amt. of secretion.

hypo″sen′sitive [G. *ypo*, under, + L. *sentīre*, to feel]. Having reduced ability to respond to stimuli.

hy″posensitiza′tion [″ + L. *sentīre*, to feel]. Production of hyposensitiveness.

hyposialadenitis (hi″po-si″al-ad-e-ni′tis) [″ + *sialon*, saliva, + *adēn*, gland, + *-ītis*, inflammation]. Submaxillary salivary gland inflammation.

hyposmia (hi-poz′mĭ-ă) [G. *ypo*, under, + *osmē*, smell]. Defect in sense of smell.

hypospadia, hypospadias (hi-po-spa′dĭ-ă, -as) [″ + *span*, to draw]. Congenital opening of the male urethra upon the undersurface of the penis; also an urethral opening into vagina.

hyposphresia (hi″pos-fre′sĭ-ă). Hyposmia, *q.v.*

hyposphyxia (hi-pos-fik′sĭ-ă) [″ + *sphyxis*, pulse]. Sluggish circulation due to abnormally low blood pressure.

hypostasis (hi-pos′tă-sis) [″ + *stasis*, a halt]. Deposit; sediment. Opposite of *epistasis.**

hypostatic (hi-po-stat′ik) [G. *ypo*, under, + *statikos*, standing). 1. Of or pertaining to hypostasis. 2. In genetics, hidden or suppressed, said of a gene whose effect is suppressed by the presence of another gene.

hyposteatolysis (hi-po-ste-ă-tol′ĭ-sis) [″ + *stear*, fat, + *lysis*, loosening]. Diminished emulsification of fats during digestion.

hyposthenia (hi-pos-the′nĭ-ă) [″ + *sthenos*, strength]. Subnormal strength; an enfeebled state; weakness.

hyposthenia nt (hi-pos-the′nĭ-ant) [″ + *sthenos*, strength]. Reducing vital forces; debilitant.

hyposthenic (hi-pos-then′ĭk) [″ + *sthenos*, strength]. Debilitant.

hyposthenuria (hi-pos-then-u′rĭ-ă) [″ + ″ + *ouron*, urine]. The secretion of urine of low specific gravity, chiefly in chronic nephritis.

h., tubular. H. resulting from disease of renal tubule epithelial cells.

hypostypsis (hi-po-stip′sis) [″ + *stypsis*, a contracting]. State of being slightly astringent.

hypostyptic (hi-po-stip′tik) [″ + *stypsis*, a contracting]. Slightly astringent.

hy″posuprare′nalism [″ + L. *supra*, above, + *rēn*, kidney, + G. *ismos*, state of]. Suprarenal inactivity.

hyposynergia (hi″po-sin-er′jĭ-ă) [″ + *syn*, with, + *ergon*, work]. Poor coordination.

hyposystole (hi-po-sis′to-le) [G. *ypo*, under, + *systolē*, contraction]. A weak or lowered systolic contraction.

hypotaxia (hi-po-taks′ĭ-ă) [G. *ypo*, under, + *taxis*, arrangement]. State of reduced control over voluntary actions such as occurs in early stages of hypnotism.

hypoten′sion [G. *ypo*, under, + L. *tensiō*, tension]. 1. Decrease of systolic and diastolic blood pressure below normal. 2. Deficiency in tonus or tension.

Below 90 systolic and 50 diastolic is usually considered to be below normal. If hypotension follows hypertension the condition is serious. If the diastolic blood pressure drops in proportion to the systolic pressure and the systolic pressure does not go below 80 points, the patient will, in most cases, respond to the administration of stimulants.

A patient with a systolic pressure of 90 points or less should remain in bed for treatment.

It occurs in shock and collapse, in hemorrhages, infections, fevers, cancer, anemia, neurasthenia, Addison's disease and in other debilitating or wasting diseases, and approaching death.

Hypotension causes an accumulation of blood in the veins and slows down the arterial current. Capillary circulation is interfered with as are other functional processes of the body. Thyroid tablets are frequently used for this condition.

h., orthostatic. H. occurring when a person assumes an erect position.

h., postural. H. occurring upon suddenly arising from a recumbent position or from standing still.

hypoten′sive [″ + L. *tensiō*, tension]. Denoting low blood pressure.

hypotensor (hi-po-ten′sor) [″ + L. *tensus, tendere*, to stretch]. Agent that lowers blood pressure.

hypothalamus (hi-po-thal′ă-mus) [G. *ypo*, under, + *thalamos*, chamber]. The portion of the diencephalon comprising the ventral wall of the third ventricle below the hypothalamic sulcus and including structures forming ventricular floor, including the optic chiasma, tuber cinereum, infundibulum, and mammillary bodies. It lies beneath the thalamus and laterally is continuous with the subthalamic regions. It contains neurosecretions which are of importance in the control of visceral activities, such as maintenance of water balance, sugar and fat metabolism, regulation of body temperature and secretion of endocrine glands. It is the chief subcortical region for the integration of sympathetic and parasympathetic activities.

The hypothalamus is the source of the hormones *vasopressin* and *oxytocin* stored and released by the neural lobe of the hypophysis.

hypothenar (hi-poth′ĕ-nar) [″ + *thenar*, palm]. The fleshy prominence on inner side of the palm next to the little finger.

h. eminence. Prominence on palm below little finger.

hypother'mal [" + *thermē*, heat]. 1 Tepid. 2. Subnormal temperature, below 98.6° F.

hypother'mia [G. *ypo*, under, + *thermē*, heat]. 1. Having a body temperature below normal. 2. A technic of lowered body temperature, usually between 78 and 90° F., to reduce oxygen need during surgery (esp. cardiovascular and neurological procedures) and in hypoxia, to reduce blood pressure, and to remedy hyperpyrexia.

hypothesis (hi-poth'ĕ-sis) [G. *ypo*, under, + *thesis*, a placing]. 1. An assumption not proved by experiment or observation. It is assumed for the sake of testing its soundness or to facilitate investigation of a class of phenomena. 2. A conclusion drawn before all the facts are established and tentatively accepted as a basis for further investigation.

hypothrombinemia (hi"po-throm-bin-e'mĭ-ă) [" + *thrombos*, clot, + *aima*, blood]. Deficiency of thrombin in the blood, making hemophilia possible.

hypothymergasia (hi"po-thi"mer-ga'sĭ-ă) [" + *thymos*, mind, + *ergasia*, energy]. A condition of physical and mental depression.

hypothymergastic reaction (hi"po-thi-mer-gas'tik) [" + " + *ergasia*, energy]. Psychic disorder producing a sense of lonesomeness, sadness, and depression. Opp. of *hyperthymergastic reaction, q.v.*

hypothymia (hi-po-thi'mĭ-ă) [" + *thymos*, mind]. Decreased emotional response to stimuli.

hypothymism (hi-po-thi'mizm) [" + " + *ismos*, state of]. Thymus inactivity.

hypothyrea (hi-po-thi're-ă) [" + *thyreos*, shield]. Thyroid insufficiency. Syn: *hypothyreosis*.

hypothyreosis (hi"po-thi-re-o'sis) [" + " + *ōsis*]. 1. Thyroid insufficiency. 2. Condition resulting from lack of thyroid secretion. Syn: *myxedema*.

hypothyroid (hi-po-thi'royd) [" + " + *eidos*, form]. Marked by insufficiency of thyroid secretion.

hypothyroida'tion [" + " + *eidos*, form]. Condition causing insufficient thyroid secretion.

hypothyroidea (hi"po-thi-roy'de-ă) [" + " + *eidos*, form]. Diminished thyroid secretion. Syn: *hypothyreosis*.

hypothyroidism (hi-po-thi'royd-izm) [" + " + " + *ismos*, state of]. A condition due to deficiency of the thyroid secretion, resulting in a lowered basal metabolism. A lesser degree of cretinism.

Sym: May be obesity; dry skin and hair, both of which become lusterless. Low blood pressure, slow pulse, sluggishness of all functions, depressed muscular activity, goiter.

Treatment: Thyroid organotherapy, as adm. of desiccated thyroid* or thyroxin. Increase iodine in diet if iodine is deficient.

NP: Constipation is a marked feature of this disease, as is decreased metabolic rate, with a subnormal temperature. Guard against chilling, as the patient is abnormally sensitive to cold and the pulse is often feeble. Measures for overcoming constipation will be in order. If thyroid extract is ordered, watch for signs of hyperthyroidism. Observe the patient carefully and watch for overexertion during treatment with thyroid extract.

hypothyrosis (hi-po-thi-ro'sis) [G. *ypo*, under, + *thyreos*, shield, + *ōsis*]. Insufficiency of thyroid secretion. Syn: *hypothyreosis*.

hypotonia (hi-po-to'nĭ-ă) [" + *tonos*, tone]. 1. Reduced tension; relaxation of arteries. 2. Loss of tonicity of the muscles or intraocular pressure.

hypotonic (hi-po-ton'ik) [" + *tonos*, tone]. 1. Pert. to defective muscular tone or tension. 2. A solution of lower osmotic pressure than another.

hypotoxicity (hi"po-toks-is'ĭ-tĭ) [" + *toxikon*, poison]. A reduced toxic quality; only slightly poisonous.

hypotrichosis (hi"po-tri-ko'sis) [" + *thrix, trich-*, hair, + *ōsis*]. Abnormal deficiency of hair.

hypotrophy (hi-pot'ro-fĭ) [" + *trophē*, nourishment]. Progressive degeneration and functional loss of cells and tissues. Syn: *abiotrophy*.

hypotropia (hi-po-tro'pĭ-ă) [" + *tropē*, a turning]. Vertical strabismus downward.

hypouresis (hi"po-u-re'sis) [" + *ourēsis*, urination]. Insufficient urination.

hypouricuria (hi"po-u-rĭ-ku'rĭ-ă) [" + *ouron*, urine, + *ouron*, urine]. Deficient uric acid in the urine.

hypourocrin'ia [" + " + *krinein*, to separate]. Deficient urinary secretion.

hypovaria (hi-po-va'rĭ-ă) [" + L. *ovarium*, ovary]. Deficient internal secretion of the ovary and consequent retardation of growth and development in girls.

hypovenosity (hi"po-ven-os'ĭ-tĭ) [" + L. *venōsus*, pert. to a vein]. Incomplete development of the venous system in an area, resulting in atrophy or degeneration.

hy"poventila'tion [" + L. *ventilātiō*, ventilation]. Reduced rate and depth of breathing.

hypovitaminosis (hi"po-vi-tă-min-o'sis) [" + L. *vita*, life, + *amine* + G. *ōsis*]. A condition due to a lack of vitamins in the diet.

hypovolemia (hi"po-vo-le'mĭ-ă) [" + L. *volumen*, volume]. Diminished blood supply. Syn: *oligemia; oligohemia*.

hypoxanthine (hi"po-zan'thin) [" + *xanthos*, yellow]. A leukomaine, $C_5H_4N_4O$, in muscles and tissues in a stage of urea and uric acid formation. It is formed during protein decomposition. In small amts. it is normal in urine.

hypoxemia (hi-poks-e'mĭ-ă) [" + *oxys*, acid, + *aima*, blood]. Insufficient oxygenation of the blood.

hypoxia (hi"pŏks'ĭ-ă). Anoxia; lack of an adequate amount of oxygen in inspired air such as occurs at high altitudes; reduced oxygen content or tension.

hypsibrachycephalic (hip"se-brak-e-sĕ-fal'ĭk) [G. *ypsi*, high, + *brachys*, broad, + *kephalē*, head]. Having a broad and high skull.

hypsicephalic (hip"si-sĕ-fal'ĭk) [" + *kephalē*, head]. Having a skull with a cranial index above 75.1°.

hypsicephaly (hip-si-sef'ă-lĭ) [" + *kephalē*, head]. The condition of having a skull with a cranial index over 75.1°.

hypsiconchous (hip-sĭ-kong'kus) [" + *kogchē*, shell]. Having an orbital index above 85°.

hypsiloid (hip'sĭ-loyd) [G. *ypsilon*, U or Y, + *eidos*, form]. U- or Y-shaped. Syn: *hyoid*.

h. ***cartilage.*** Y-cartilage.

h. ***ligament.*** Ligamentum iliofemorale.

hypsistaphylia (hip-sĭ-staf-il'ĭ-ă) [G. *ypsi*, high, + *staphylē*, uvula]. Having a narrow, high palatal arch.

hypsistenocephalic (hip″sĭ-sten″o-sĕ-fal′-ik) [″ + *stenos*, narrow, + *kephalē*, head]. Having a cranial index over 75.1°. SYN: *hypsicephalic.*

hypsoceph′alous [″ + *kephalē*, head]. Having a cranial index over 75.1°. SYN: *hypsicephalic.*

hypsokine′sis [G. *ypsos*, height, + *kinēsis*, motion]. Tendency to fall backward when standing; seen in paralysis agitans.

hypsonosus (hip-son′o-sus) [″ + *nosos*, disease]. Mountain sickness; balloon sickness.

SYM: Epistaxis, headache, nausea.

hypsophobia (hip-so-fo′bĭ-ă) [″ + *phobos*, fear]. Fear of being at great heights. SYN: *aerophobia.*

hypurgia (hi-pur′jĭ-ă) [G. *ypourgia*, help]. Any minor factors which change the course of a disease, esp. for the better.

hys′tera [G. *ystera*, uterus]. The uterus.

hysteral′gia [″ + *algos*, pain]. Neuralgia of the uterus.

hysterectomy (his-ter-ek′to-mĭ) [G. *ystera*, uterus, + *ektomē*, excision]. Removal of the uterus. The presence of tumors, both benign and malignant, is a common cause. The uterus may be removed through the abdominal wall or through the vagina.

NP: The patient is placed in dorsal position. The table is ready to be tipped into the Trendelenburg position. As soon as incision is made through the peritoneum, table should be put into Trendelenburg position. This procedure is the same for all abdominopelvic surgery.

This position allows the intestines and abdominal organs to fall backwards from pelvis, so that they may be easily packed off with large pads or with a large roll of packing. Watch intake and output of patient closely, prevent bladder distention, turn frequently. SEE: *laparotomy.*

h., abdominal. Removal of the uterus through an abdominal incision.

h., chemical. Destruction of the endometrium by strong caustic substances.

h., Porro. Subtotal hysterectomy following cesarean section.

h., subtotal. Removal of the uterus, leaving the cervix uteri in place.

h., supracervical. Same as subtotal.

h., supravaginal. Same as subtotal.

h., total. Removal of body and cervix.

h., vaginal. Removal of the uterus through the vagina.

hystere′sis [G. *ysterēsis*, a coming too late]. 1. Failure of related phenomena to keep pace with each other. 2. Failure of the manifestation of an effect to keep up with its cause.

hystereurynter (his-ter-u-rin′ter) [G. *ystera*, uterus, + *eurynein*, to stretch]. An instrument for dilating the os uteri.

hysteria (his-te′rĭ-ă) [G. *ystera*, uterus]. A condition presenting somatic symptoms, simulating almost every type of physical disease, and a series of mental manifestations. The condition occurs in the absence of organic disease to account for the symptoms.

The mental attitude is calm; there is a not unfriendly aloofness, but psychotic indifference is quite another matter, and not seen in hysteria. There may be easy laughing and crying—episodes of emotionalism possibly without any apparent explanation, and even occurring in sleep. Episodic states known as fugues (sleepwalking is similar, occurring in sleep). In these, certain dissociated (repressed) ideas, emotions and goals develop a reality sufficient to constitute a secondary personality which now functions apart from the primary personality.

When the primary consciousness reasserts itself, there is a forgetting (amnesia) of the secondary state. The multiplication or alternation of personalities is quite distinct from schizophrenic splitting in which incongruities and confusion result from the co-existence of each phase of the personality more or less continuously.

An accurate definition is difficult because of extreme diversity of symptoms; a psychoneurosis found in a patient of low vitality, characterized by psychic weakness and undue susceptibility to autosuggestion.

ETIOL: Variable, as in most psychic disturbances. It occurs in both sexes before and after adolescence and at periods of emotional and physical stress, as alternating crying and laughing.

SYM: Emotional instability, various sensory disturbances and a marked craving for sympathy which sometimes leads to fraud.

TREATMENT: Hygienic, hydropathic, massage, diet, suggestive therapeutics. Complete isolation from sympathetic individuals. Place patient in a quiet place devoid of spectators. Cold applications to head, face, and neck are helpful. Quiet, firm suggestions are important. Sedatives are to be used under the direction of a physician.

h., anxiety. Hysteria combined with an anxiety neurosis.

h., major. Very severe h. accompanied by epileptiform convulsions.

h., minor. Mild form of h. without loss of consciousness.

hyste′riac [G. *ystera*, uterus]. A hysterical person.

hyster′ic, hyster′ical [G. *ystera*, uterus]. Pert. to hysteria.

h. ataxia. Loss of sensation in leg muscles and skin in hysteria.

h. chorea. A form of h. with choreiform movements.

hystericoneuralgic (his-ter-ik-o-nu-ral′-jik) [″ + *neuron*, nerve, + *algos*, pain]. Pert. to pain of hysterical origin, but resembling neuralgia.

hysteritis (his-ter-i′tis) [″ + *-ītis*, inflammation]. Inflammation of the uterus.

hysterobubonocele (his″ter-o-bu-bon′o-sēl) [″ + *boubōn*, groin, + *kēlē*, hernia]. Inguinal hernia surrounding the uterus.

hysterocat′alepsy [″ + *kata*, down, + *lēpsis*, seizure]. Major hysteria with cataleptic symptoms.

hysterocele (his′ter-o-sēl) [″ + *kēlē*, hernia]. Hernia of the uterus, esp. when gravid.

hysterocervicotomy (his″ter-o-ser-vĭ-kot′-o-mĭ) [″ + L. *cervix*, neck, + G. *tomē*, incision]. Cesarean section through the vagina. SYN: *hysterotrachelotomy.*

hysterocleisis (his-ter-o-kli′sis) [″ + *kleisis*, closure]. Surgical closure of the os uteri.

hysterocystocleisis (his″ter-o-sis″to-kli′-sis) [″ + *kystis*, a bladder, + *kleisis*, a closure]. Operation fastening the cervix uteri in the wall of the bladder.

hysterodynia (his″ter-o-din′ĭ-ă) [G. *ystera*, uterus, + *odynē*, pain]. Uterine pain. SYN: *hysteralgia.*

hysteroepilepsy (his″ter-o-ep′ĭ-lep-sĭ) [″ + *epilēpsia*, seizure]. Major hysteria with violent epileptiform convulsions.

In addition to usual symptoms of epilepsy, anger, disgust, joy, surprise and other emotions are dramatically expressed when final stage (delirium) is reached.

hysterofrenic (his″ter-o-fren′ik) [" + L. *frenāre,* to restrain]. Arresting an attack of hysteria, noting pressure areas on the body having this effect.

hysterogastrorrhaphy (his″ter-o-gas-tror′ă-fī) [" + *gastēr,* belly, + *raphē,* suture]. Fixation of uterus to gastric wall. SYN: *hysteropexy.*

hysterogen′ic [" + *gennan,* to produce]. Causing a hysterical attack.

hysteroid (his′ter-oyd) [" + *eidos,* resemblance]. 1. Resembling hysteria. 2. Pert. to hysteria.

hysterolaparotomy (his″ter-o-lap-ă-rot′-o-mĭ) [" + *lapara,* flank, + *tomē,* incision]. Uterine incision through abdominal wall; abdominal hysterectomy.

hysterolith (his′ter-o-lith) [" + *lithos,* stone]. A calculus in the uterus.

hysterology (his-ter-ol′o-jĭ) [" + *logos,* knowledge]. Sum of what is known about the uterus.

hysterolysis (his-ter-ol′ĭ-sis) [" + *lysis,* loosening]. Operation of loosening the uterus from its adhesions.

hysteromalacia (his-ter-o-mă-la′sĭ-ă) [" + *malakia,* softening]. Uterine softening.

hysteroma′nia [" + *mania,* madness]. 1. Hysterical mania. 2. Nymphomania.*

hysterometer (his-ter-om′ĕ-ter) [" + *metron,* measure]. Device for measuring the uterus.

hysterom′etry [G. *ystera,* uterus, + *metron,* measure]. Measurement of the size of the uterus.

hysteromyoma (his-ter-o-mi-o′mă) [" + *mys, myo-,* muscle, + *ōma,* tumor]. Myoma or fibromyoma of the uterus.

hysteromyomectomy (his″ter-o-mi″o-mek′-to-mĭ) [" + " + *ektomē,* excision]. Excision of a uterine fibroid.

hysteromyotomy (his″ter-o-mi-ot′o-mĭ) [" + " + *tomē,* incision]. Uterine incision for removal of a solid tumor.

hysteroneurosis (his″ter-o-nu-ro′sis) [" + *neuron,* nerve, + *ōsis*]. A reflex neurosis due to uterine irritation.

hystero-oophorectomy (his″ter-o-o″of-o-rek′to-mĭ) [" + *ōon,* ovum, + *phoros,* bearing, + *ektomē,* excision]. Removal of the uterus and one or both ovaries.

hysteropathy (his-ter-op′ă-thĭ) [" + *pathos,* disease]. Any uterine disorder.

hysteropexy (his′ter-o-peks″ĭ) [" + *pēxis,* fixation]. Surgical fixation of uterus.

hystero′pia [" + *ōps,* eye]. A hysterical visual defect.

hysteropsychosis (his″ter-o-si-ko′sis) [" + *psychē,* mind, + *ōsis*]. Mental disorder due to uterine disease.

hysteroptosia, hysteroptosis (his-ter-op-to′sĭ-a, -sis) [" + *ptōsis,* a dropping]. Prolapse of the uterus.

hysterorrhaphy (his-ter-or′ă-fī) [" + *raphē,* sewing]. Suture of womb.

hysterorrhexis (his-ter-o-reks′is) [" + *rēxis,* rupture]. Rupture of the uterus, esp. when pregnant.

hysterosalpingography (his″ter-o-sal-pin-gog′ră-fī) [" + *salpigx,* tube, + *graphein,* to write]. X-ray of the uterus and oviducts after injecting radiopaque material into those organs.

hysterosalpingo-oophorectomy (his″ter-o-sal″pĭn-go-o″o-for-ek′to-mĭ) [" + " + *ōon,* ovum, + *phoros,* bearing, + *ektomē,* excision]. Surgical removal of uterus, oviducts, and ovaries.

hysterosalpingostomy (his″ter-o-sal-ping-os′to-mĭ) [" + " + *stoma,* opening]. Anastomosis of the uterus with the distal end of the fallopian tube after excision of a strictured portion of the tube.

hysteroscope (his′ter-o-skōp) [" + *skopein,* to examine]. Instrument for examining the uterine cavity.

hysteroscopy (his-ter-os′ko-pĭ) [" + *skopein,* to examine]. Inspection of the uterus by use of mirror.

hys′terospasm [G. *ystera,* uterus, + *spasmos,* a spasm]. Uterine spasm.

hysterostomatocleisis (his″ter-o-sto″mă-to-kli′sis) [" + *stoma,* opening, + *kleisis,* closure]. Operation for vesicovaginal fistula.

Closure of the cervix uteri, making the vesical and uterine cavities into a common cavity by means of the opening between them.

hysterostomatomy (his″ter-o-sto-mat′o-mĭ) [" + " + *tomē,* incision]. Surgical enlargement of the os uteri; incision of the os or cervix uteri.

hysterosyph′ilis [" + *syn,* with, + *philein,* to love]. A hysterical manifestation due to syphilis.

hysterosystole (his″ter-o-sis′to-le) [" + *systolē,* contraction]. A delayed contraction of the heart after its normal time; opp. to *extrasystole.*

hysterotabetism (his″ter-o-ta′bet-izm) [" + L. *tabes,* a wasting away, + G. *ismos,* state of]. Condition of hysteria and tabes combined.

hysterotokotomy (his″ter-o-to-kot′o-mĭ) [" + *tokos,* birth, + *tomē,* incision]. Cesarean operation.

hys′terotome [" + *tomē,* incision]. Instrument for incision of the uterus.

hysterotomotokia (his″ter-o-tom″o-to′-kĭ-ă) [" + " + *tokos,* birth]. Cesarean section.

hysterotomy (his-ter-ot′o-mĭ) [" + *tomē,* incision]. 1. Incision of the uterus. 2. Cesarean section, *q.v.*

hysterotrachelorrhaphy (his″ter-o-tra-kel-or′ă-fī) [" + *trachēlos,* neck, + *raphē,* sewing]. A plastic operation for a lacerated cervix by paring the edges and suturing them together.

hysterotrachelotomy (his″ter-o-tra-kel-ot′o-mĭ) [" + " + *tomē,* incision]. Surgical incision of neck of uterus.

hysterotraumatic (his″ter-o-traw-mat′ik) [" + *trauma,* wound]. Pert. to traumatic hysteria.

hysterotraumatism (his″ter-o-traw′mă-tizm) [" + " + *ismos,* state of]. Hysteric symptoms due to or following traumatism.

hysterotris′mus [" + *trismos,* a spasm]. Uterine spasm.

hysterovagino-enterocele (his″ter-o-vaj″-in-o-en′ter-o-sēl) [" + L. *vagina,* sheath, + G. *enteron,* intestine, + *kēlē* hernia]. Hernia surrounding uterus, vagina, and intestines.

hystriciasis, hystricism (his-trĭ-si′ă-sis, his′trĭ-sizm) [G. *ystrix,* hedgehog]. 1. Erection of hairs like the spines of a hedgehog. 2. A skin disease.

SYM: Thickened epidermis, warty growths, elongated and hypertrophied papillae. SYN: *ichthyosis hystrix.*

hyther (hi′ther) [G. *ydōr,* water, + *thermē,* heat]. The combined effect of humidity and temperature of atmosphere upon the body.

Notes

Notes

Notes

I

I. Chem. symb. for *iodine.*

I^{131}. Radioactive iodine. At. wt. 131.

I^{132}. Radioactive iodine. At. wt. 132.

i. Abbr. for *optically inactive.*

iamatology (i″am-ă-tol′o-jĭ) [G. *iama,* remedy, + *logos,* science]. Study of therapeutics and remedies.

ianthinopia (ī-ăn-thĭ-no′pĭ-ă) [G. *ianthinos,* violet colored, + *opsis,* vision]. Violet vision.

-iasis [G.]. Suffix: Same as *-osis,* meaning the state or condition of, as *psoriasis.*

iatraliptics (i-ă-tră-lip′tĭks) [G. *iatreia,* cure, + *aleiphein,* to anoint]. Treatment by inunction.

iatric (i-at′rik) [G. *iatros,* physician]. Medical.

iatrochem′istry [" + *chēmeia,* chemistry]. Seventeenth century opinion that chemistry is the basis of all physiological phenomena.

iatrogenic illness (i″at-ro-jen′ik) [G. *iatros,* physician, + *genein,* to produce]. An undesired mental or physical condition produced in the patient by something the physician has said or due to an undesired effect of the treatment given by the physician.

iatrogeny (i″ă-troj′ĕ-nĭ). Condition induced by a physician.

i. disorder. Condition involving adverse effects induced by a physician in the care of his patients. Term implies that such effects could have been avoided by proper and judicious care on the part of the physician. The development of anxiety neuroses through thoughtless and ill-considered remarks, development of drug habituation, and the injudicious use of therapeutic measures are examples.

iatrology (i-ă-trol′o-jĭ) [" + *logos,* science]. Medical science.

iatrotechnics (i-at-ro-tek′niks) [" + *technē,* art]. The art and technic of medicine and surgery.

ice (īs) [A.S. *īs*]. Water frozen at temperature below 32° F. (0° C.).

i. bag, i. cap, i. collar. Devices for holding ice to be applied to a patient to obtain the effect of continuous cold in a circumscribed area.

The affected part should always be covered with several thicknesses of cloth to prevent freezing.

i. cravat. Ice pack applied around the neck.

i., dry. Carbon dioxide in a solid form. Its temperature is —78.5° C. (—110° F). Used as a commercial refrigerant; also used for therapeutic refrigeration in the treatment of warts.

Iceland moss (īs′land). A lichen. It contains a form of starch; a slightly tonic demulcent. SYN: *Cetraria.*

ichnogram (ik′no-gram) [G. *ichnos,* footstep, + *gramma,* a writing]. A footprint, taken standing.

ichor (ī′kor) [G. *ichōr,* serum]. Thin, fetid discharge from an ulcer or from a wound.

ichoremia (i-kor-e′mĭ-ă) [" + *aima,* blood]. Septic or toxic blood poisoning due to presence of ichorous matter. SYN: *ichorrhemia.*

ichorous (ī′kor-us) [G. *ichōr,* serum]. Resembling ichor or watery pus.

ichorrhea, ichorrhoea (i-ko-re′ă) [" + *roia,* flow]. Profuse discharge of ichorous fluid.

ichorrhemia (i-kor-re′mĭ-ă) [" + *aima,* blood]. Toxic or septic blood poisoning due to presence of ichorous matter. SYN: *ichoremia.*

ichthammol (ik′thă-mol). A reddish brown, viscous fluid obtained by the destructive distillation of certain bituminous shale.

USES: As a mild antiseptic and local stimulant in certain skin diseases.

ichthyism (ik′thĭ-izm), **ichthyismus** (ik″-thĭ-iz′mus) [G. *ichthys,* fish, + *ismos,* state of]. Poisoning from eating stale or unfit fish.

ichthyo- [G.]. Combining form meaning *fish.*

ichthyoid (ik′thĭ-oyd) [G. *ichthys,* fish, + *eidos,* form]. Fishlike.

ichthyol (ik′thĭ-ol) [" + L. *oleum,* oil]. A brand of ichthammol.

ichthyophobia (ik-thĭ-o-fo′bĭ-ă) [" + *phobos,* fear]. Aversion to fish.

ichthyosis (ik-thi-o′sis) [" + *ōsis*]. Fishskin disease. Congenital abnormality of the skin characterized by dryness, harshness, scaliness.

ETIOL: Congenital with hereditary tendency probably as a result of persisting embryonic epidermis. Hypothyroidism may play a part in acquired cases, which are rare.

SYM: As noted, confined to skin, subject to irritation, giving rise to eczema, etc., with formation of spinous, nutmeg-grater-like lesions at pilosebaceous orifices.

PATH: Dermal, affecting horny layer prickle layer, papillae.

PROG: Milder, clear up with adolescence. Severe, may be ameliorated.

TREATMENT: Locally, oils and greases esp. after baths containing bran, borax, or sodium carbonate. SYN: *sauriosis; xeroderma.*

i. follicularis. I. in which sebaceous and epithelial material accumulate about the hair follicles.

i. hystrix. A form with warts.

i. sebacea. Functional disorder of the sebaceous glands. SYN: *seborrhea.*

i. simplex. I. with cutaneous roughening and dryness. SYN: *xeroderma.*

ichthyotic (ik-thĭ-ot′ik) [G. *ichthys,* fish]. Rel. to ichthyosis.

I. C. N. Abbr. for *International Council of Nurses.*

iconolagny (i-kon′o-lag-nĭ) [G. *eikōn,* image, + *lagneia,* lewdness]. Sexual stimulation produced by pictures, statues or objects.

ICSH. Abbr. for *interstitial cell stimulating hormone.* In male, this hormone stimulates the production of testosterone from the interstitial cells of the testes. Same as LH (luteinizing hormone).

ictal (ik′tal) [from L. *ictus,* a blow or stroke]. Pertaining to or caused by a sudden attack or stroke such as acute epilepsy.

icterepatitis (ik-ter-ĕ-pă-tī′tis) [G. *ikteros,* jaundice, + *ēpar,* liver, + *ītis,* inflammation]. Hepatitis associated with jaundice.

icteric (ik-ter'ik) [G. *ikteros*, jaundice] Pert. to jaundice.

i. fever. Jaundice combined with pernicious malaria.

i. index. A number obtained by matching blood serum in a colorimeter against a standard solution of potassium dichromate (1:10,000), which gives a color approximately same as bilirubin.

A test for determining the intensity of the yellow color of blood serum. Since serum color depends upon bile pigment, the index is an indication of the concentration of this pigment in the blood. Valuable in study of jaundice.

The serum is diluted to known strength and then compared; the reading of the standard, divided by the reading of the serum and multiplied by the dilution gives the icteric index. Normal serum gives a value of 5. In patients with visible jaundice values above 15 are obtained.

icteritious (ik-ter-ish'us) [G. *ikteros*, jaundice]. Yellowish; resembling jaundice. Syn: *icteroid.*

icteroane'mia [" + *an-*, priv. + *aima*, blood]. Icterus associated with anemia, hemolysis and splenic enlargement.

icterogenic, icterogenous (ik-ter-o-jen'ik, -oj'en-us) [" + *gennan*, to produce]. Causing jaundice.

icterohepatitis (ik"ter-o-hep-ă-ti'tis) [" + *ēpar*, liver, + *ītis*, inflammation]. Liver inflammation with jaundice.

icteroid (ik'ter-oyd) [" + *eidos*, form]. Resembling jaundice; yellow-hued.

icterus (ik'ter-us) [G. *ikteros*, jaundice]. Jaundice, *q.v.* Pigmentation of the tissues, membranes and secretions with bile pigments.

i. castren'sis gravis. Serious camp jaundice. Syn: *Weil's disease.*

i. castren'sis levis. Mild camp disease of catarrhal form.

i. cythemoly'tic. A form caused by absorption of bile formed in excess quantities due to hemolysis.

i. febri'lis. Weil's disease.

i. gravis. Acute yellow atrophy of liver with cerebral disorders.

i., hemolytic or *nonobstructive.* Rare chronic form, frequently congenital, with periodic attacks of intense hemolysis.

Sym: Much the same as in obstructive icterus,* but staining not so intense. Sometimes found in acute yellow atrophy, the anemias and infectious fevers. Enlarged spleen.

i. me'las. Black jaundice.

i. neonatorum. Jaundice of the newborn. A type of hemolytic jaundice. It may be benign or malignant.

i., obstructive. Jaundice caused by obstruction to the flow of bile in the common or hepatic duct.

Etiol: Duodenal catarrh, cholangitis, carcinoma, gumma, gallstones, cirrhosis of liver, cysts, parasites in ducts, pressure by tumors, hepatic abscess.

Sym: Skin, mucous membrane and secretions stained yellow; first noticed in the conjunctivae. Stool light or clay-colored, urine dark, pulse low, temperature slightly subnormal. In extreme cases, delirium, convulsions, coma.

i. praecox. Jaundice of secondary syphilis.

i., suppression. Etiol: Caused by toxins in body which destroy the liver cells and red blood cells.

Sym: Feces may be darker than normal, not clay-colored; no excessive amount of bile pigment in urine.

Prog: Quick recovery or speedy death.

i. typhoides. Acute yellow atrophy of the liver.

ictom'eter [L. *ictus*, stroke, + G. *metron*, measure]. An instrument for estimating the force of the heart beat at the chest wall.

ic'tus [L. stroke]. 1. A beat or stroke. 2. An attack.

i. cordis. A term applied to heartbeat.

i. epilepticus. Epileptic convulsion.

i. sanguinis. Apoplexy.

i. solis. Sunstroke.

ID. Abbr. for *intradermal, inside diameter.*

id [G. *idios*, own]. 1. Biol: A biological germ structure carrying the heredity qualities; "an ancestral germ plasm."

Psy: The unconscious undominated by its ego, but by its own impulsions, which are of an instinctive nature, such as the pleasure urge. 2. A suffix indicating certain secondary skin eruptions which appear some distance from site of primary infection. If etiologic agent of primary infection is known, the secondary lesion is designated by adding "id" as *tuberculid, trichophytid.*

idant (id'ant) [G. *idios*, own]. A chromosome containing all the ids regarded as hereditary factors.

-ide. Chem: An ending indicating a binary compound, as *sodium chloride.*

ide'a [G. form, from *idein*, to see]. A mental image; a concept.

i., autochthonous (aw-tok'thon-us). An unaccountable one.

i., compulsive. A persistent, obsessional impulse or thought.

i., dom'inant. One controlling all one's actions and thoughts.

i., fixed. One that completely dominates the mind, as a delusion.

i., flight of. Rapid speech, often disconnected and incoherent, in certain mental diseases.

i. of reference. An impression that the conversation or actions of others have reference to oneself.

ideation (i-de-a'shun) [G. *idea*, form, from, *idein*, to see]. The process of thinking; formation of ideas.

It is slow in dementias, depressions, and other organic brain diseases, and in narcotic intoxications, but quickened in early stage of intoxications. It is unduly active in manic-depressive insanity.

idée fixe (ē-dā fēks') [Fr.]. An obsession; a fixed idea. See: *idea.*

iden'tical [L. *identicus*, the same]. Exactly alike.

i. twins. Twins developed from 1 fertilized cell. See: *Hellin's law, twins.*

identifica'tion [" + *facere*, to make]. 1. A kind of daydream, as when one identifies himself with the hero of a book or play. 2. The process of determining the sameness of a thing or person with that described or known to exist.

i., anthropometric. The Bertillon system of i., *q.v.*

i., Bertillon system of. A system based on physical characteristics.

i., Galton system of. A system based on fingerprints.

i., palm and sole system of. A system based on prints of the palmar surface of hand and the plantar surface of the foot.

ideo- (id'e-o, i'de-o). [G.]. Prefix: Pert. to mental images.

ideogenous (i-de-oj'en-us) [G. *idea*, form, + *gennan*, to produce]. Stimulated by an idea.

ideometabolism. Metabolic changes induced by mental or emotional factors.

ideomo'tion [" + L. *motus*, moving]. Muscular automatic movement activated by a dominant idea.

ideomo'tor [" + L. *motus*, moving]. Pert. to ideomotion.

ideophrenic (id-e-o-fren'ĭk) [" + *phrenitikos*, insane]. Marked by abnormal ideas of a perverted nature.

ideoplastia (id-e-o-plas'tĭ-ă). Condition of the mind of a hypnotized person in which he is capable of receiving and responding to suggestions of the hypnotist.

ideovascular (id"e-o-vas'ku-lar). Pertaining to vascular changes induced by ideas, memories, or emotions.

idio- [G.]. Prefix: Individual, distinct, in compound words.

idiocrasy (id"ĭ-ok'ră-sĭ) [G. *idios*, own, *krasis*, temperament]. Peculiarity which renders one susceptible to certain habits or drugs.

idiocratic (id"i-o-krat'ĭk) [" + *krasis*, temperament]. Pert. to idiocrasy.

id'iocy [G. *idiōteia*, uncouthness]. Mental deficiency usually congenital. SEE: *mental deficiency.*

i., amaurotic familial. Term for a group of related familial diseases marked by dementia and impaired vision. SEE: *amaurotic familial idiocy.*

i., Aztec. I. combined with microcephalia.

i., complete or profound. I. in which primitive instincts are lacking, even that of self-preservation.

i., cretinoid. Endemic i. accompanied by goiter.

i., diplegic. I. marked by paralysis of all extremities in infants.

i., epileptic. I. accompanied by epilepsy.

i., genetous. I. of congenital origin.

i., hemiplegic. Hemiplegic manifestations in infants.

i., hydrocephalic. I. accompanied by chronic hydrocephalus.

i., intrasocial. I. in which mentality permits some occupation.

i., microcephalic. SEE: *Aztec i.*

i., mongolian. Congenital form of i. in which person has mongolian features, the nose being broad, the eyes slanting and the skull flat. SYN: *Down's syndrome, q.v.*

i., paralytic. I. combined with paralysis.

i., paraplegic. I. combined with paraplegia.

i., sensorial. Mental deficiency caused by loss of one of the special senses.

i., traumatic. I. caused by an injury received in infancy or in early childhood.

idiog'amist [G. *idios*, individual, + *gamos*, marriage]. One incapable of the sexual act with more than a few persons because of sexual discrimination.

idiogenesis (id-ĭ-o-jen'ĕ-sis). Of self-origin or origin without known cause, esp. with reference to idiopathic disease.

idioglos'sia [" + *glōssa*, tongue]. Inability to articulate properly so that the sounds emitted are like those of an unknown language.

idioisolysin (id"ĭ-o-i-sol'ĭ-sin) [" + *isos*, equal, + *lysis*, solution]. A hemolysin active against the cells of an individual of the same species.

idiolysin (id-ĭ-ol'ĭ-sin) [" + *lysis*, solution]. A lysin in the blood not formed in response to injection of an antigen.

idiometritis (id-ĭ-o-me-tri'tis) [" + *mētra*, uterus, + *itis*, inflammation]. Inflammation of the uterine parenchyma.

idiomus'cular [" + L. *musculus*, a muscle]. Pert. to the muscles independent of nerve control.

i. contraction. Motion produced by degenerated muscles without nerve stimulus.

idioneurosis (id-ĭ-o-nū-ro'sis) [" + *neuron*, nerve, + *ōsis*]. Any functional neurosis arising without stimuli.

idiopathic (id-ĭ-o-path'ik) [" + *pathos*, disease]. Pert. to conditions without clear pathogenesis, or disease without recognizable cause, as of spontaneous origin.

idiopathy (id-ĭ-op'ă-thĭ) [" + *pathos*, disease]. A primary disease without apparent external cause. SYN: *autopathy.*

idiophrenic (id-i-o-fren'ik) [" + *phrēn*, mind]. Pert. to or originating in the mind alone.

i. psychosis. An organic disease of the brain producing a mental disorder.

idioreflex. A reflex resulting from a stimulus which arises within the organ in which the reflex takes place.

idiosome (id'ĭ-o-sōm) [" + *sōma*, body]. Spermatid's attraction sphere.

idiosyncrasy (id-ĭ-o-sin'kră-sĭ) [" + *sygkrasis*, a mixture]. 1. Special characteristics by which persons differ from each other. 2. That which makes one react differently from others. A peculiar or individual reaction to an idea, an action, a drug, a food, or some other substance as unusual susceptibility. SYN: *idiocrasy.*

i. to drug. When no effects are produced from large doses of a drug, or unusual effects from small doses or from certain drugs. EX: *digitalis, hypnotics, mercury, potassium iodide,* and *salicylates.*

i. of effect. When small doses of a drug create a poisonous or opposite effect, an unusual or no effect.

i. to x-ray. Natural or an inherent tendency on the part of the skin to react vigorously to minute doses of x-rays.

idiosyncratic (id"ĭ-o-sin-krat'ĭk) [" + *sygkrasis*, a mixture]. Pert. to an idiosyncrasy. SYN: *idiocratic.*

id'iot [G. *idiōtēs*, an uncouth person]. Former term for severe mental deficiency. SEE: *idiocy; mental deficiency.*

idiot'ic [G. *idiōtēs*, an uncouth person]. Like an idiot; said of an idea or action.

idiotrophic (id"ĭ-o-trof'ĭk) [G. *idios*, own, + *trophē*, nourishment]. Capable of securing its own nourishment.

idiotrop'ic [" + *tropē*, a turning]. Turning inward mentally. Individual.

i. type. An introvert type satisfied by his own emotions, and by inner contemplation and pursuits, who is content to live apart from social contacts.

idiotypic (id-ĭ-o-tip'ĭk) [" + *typos*, type]. Rel. to heredity.

idioventricular (id-ĭ-o-ven-trĭk'ū-lar) [" + L. *ventriculus*, little belly]. Pert. to the cardiac ventricle alone when dissociated from the atrium.

idrosis (id-ro'sis) [G. *idrōs*, sweat]. Excessive sweating. SYN: *hidrosis.*

IDU. Abbr. for 5-iodo-2'deoxyuridine. Used to treat herpes virus infections of the eye.

ig"niextirpa'tion [L. *ignis*, fire, + *exstirpāre*, to root out]. Cautery excision.

ig″niopera′tion [" + *operari,* to work]. An operation by cautery.

ignipuncture (ig″ni-punk′tur) [" + *punctura,* a piercing]. The use of heated needles in cauterization by puncture.

ignis (ig′nis) [L. fire]. Fire; cautery. SYN: *moxa.*

i. infernalis. Ergotism.

i. sa′cer. An inflammatory skin disease. SYN: *herpes zoster.*

i. Sanc′ti Anto′nii. Acute febrile disease with localized inflammation. SYN: *erysipelas; St. Anthony's fire.*

I.H. Abbr. for *infectious hepatitis.*

ileac (il′e-ak) [L. *ileum,* ileum fr. G. *eilein,* to twist]. Pert. to the ileum.

ileectomy (il-e-ek′to-mĭ) [" + G. *ektomē,* excision]. Excision of the ileum.

ileitis (ĭl-ē-i′tis) [L. *ilium,* flank, + G. *-ītis,* inflammation]. Inflammation of the ileum. The membrane becomes inflamed and ulcerates, the affected portion becoming thick, rigid, and edematous and the lumen progressively narrowed. The lymph glands enlarge and the adjacent mesentery becomes thickened. Most often found in the terminal ileum, but it may spread to other parts of the bowel and to the cecum. Adhesions may be formed. Pain is centered around the umbilicus and right lower quadrant with general distention. Diarrhea alternates with constipation. Vomiting may occur. The stools show occult blood, and mucous shreds if bowels are loose.

i., regional. A nonspecific inflammatory, granulomatous lesion involving the terminal ileum. It is nontuberculous. May be acute or chronic. The acute form simulates appendicitis. The chronic form may extend over many years, with diarrhea, abdominal pain, anemia, loss of weight, fistula formation, and eventually obstructive intestinal symptoms. Stools are soft and grayish or brown in color with abundant fecal particles.

ileocecal (il-e-o-se′kăl) [" + *caecus,* blind]. Rel. to the ileum and cecum.

i. valve. Sphincter muscles which guard the aperture of the ileum at the cecum, where the small intestines open into the ascending colon. It prevents food material from reentering the small intestines.

ileocecum (il-e-o-se′kum) [" + *caecus,* blind]. The ileum and cecum combined.

ileocol′ic [" + G. *kōlon,* colon]. Pert. to the ileum and colon. SEE: *ileocecal.*

i. valve. Passage where food is prevented from reëntering small intestines.

ileocolitis (il-e-o-ko-li′tis) [" + " + *-itis,* inflammation]. Inflammation of mucous membrane of the ileum and colon.

ileocolostomy (il-e-o-ko-los′to-mĭ) [" + " + *stoma,* opening]. Anastomosis between ileum and colon.

ileocolotomy (il-e-o-ko-lot′o-mĭ) [" + " + *tomē,* incision]. Incision of ileum and colon.

ileoproctostomy (il″e-o-prok-tos′to-mĭ) [" + G. *prōktos,* rectum, + *stoma,* opening]. Establishment of opening bet. ileum and rectum.

ileorectostomy (il″e-o-rek-tos′to-mĭ) [" + L. *rectum,* rectum, + G. *stoma,* opening]. Formation of passage bet. ileum and rectum. SYN: *ileoproctostomy.*

ileosigmoidostomy (il″e-o-sig-moid-os′to-mĭ) [" + G. *sigma,* letter S, + *eidos,* form, + *stoma,* opening]. Surgical opening between the ileum and sigmoid flexure.

ileostomy (il-e-os′to-mĭ) [" + G. *stoma,* opening]. Creation of a surgical passage through abdominal wall into ileum.

ileotomy (il-e-ot′o-mĭ) [" + G. *tomē,* incision]. Incision into the ileum. SYN: *ileostomy.*

ileotransversostomy (il″e-o-trans-ver-sos′to-mĭ) [" + *transversus,* crosswise, + G. *stoma,* opening]. Connection of the ileum with the transverse colon.

iletin (i′le-tĭn). Insulin, *q.v.*

il′eum (pl. *ilea*) [L. fr. G. *eilein,* to twist]. Lower 3rd portion of small intestines, from the jejunum to the ileocecal valve. It is about 12 ft. long.

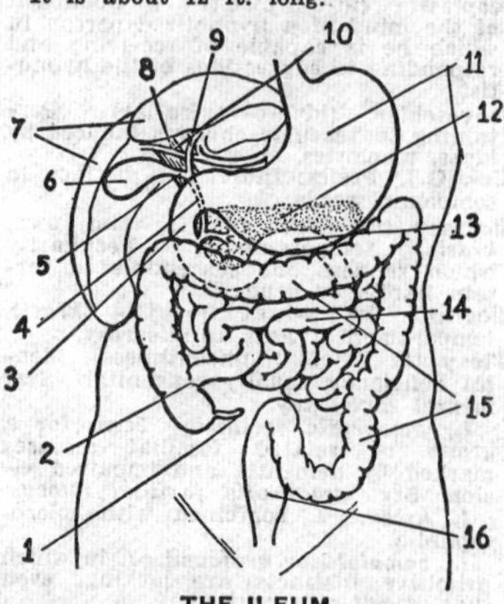

THE ILEUM

1. Appendix. 2. Ileocecal valve. 3. Duodenum. 4. Common bile duct. 5. Cystic duct. 6. Gallbladder. 7. Liver. 8. Portal vein. 9. Hepatic duct. 10. Hepatic artery. 11. Stomach. 12. Pancreas. 13. Jejunum. 14. Ileum. 15. Large intestine. 16. Rectum.

ileus (il′e-us) [G. *eileos,* intestinal colic]. Obstruction of small intestine.

Originally meant colic due to intestinal obstruction.

SYM: Acute obstruction; sudden pain, paroxysmal, then continuous; constipation; persistent fecal vomiting; abdominal distention; collapse.

RS: *intussusception, occlusion, congenital, strangulation, torsion, volvulus.*

i., adynamic. That caused by intestinal muscle paralysis.

i., dynamic, i., hyperdynamic. That caused by intestinal muscle contraction.

i., mechanical. That produced by an obstruction.

i., paralyticus. SEE: *adynamic i.*

il′iac [L. *iliacus,* pert. to ilium]. Rel. to the ilium. SEE: *ilium for illustration.*

i. crest. The hip. Upper free margin of the ilium. SYN: *crista iliaca.*

i. fascia. Transversalis fascia over ant. surface of the iliopsoas muscle.

i. fossa. Fossa iliaca, *q.v.*

i. region. Inguinal region on either side of hypogastrium.

i. roll. Sausage-shaped mass in left i. fossa. Caused by induration of sigmoidal walls.

i. spine. Spina iliaca.

iliocolotomy (il-ĭ-o-kol-ot′o-mĭ) [L. *ilium,* + G. *kōlon,* colon, + *tomē,* incision]. Opening into the colon in the iliac or inguinal region.

iliofemoral (il-i-o-fem′or-al) [" + *femoralis,* pert. to femur]. Pert. to the ilium and femur.

ilioinguinal (il″ĭ-o-in′gwĭ-nal) [“ + *inguinalis,* pert. to groin]. Pert. to the groin and iliac regions.

iliolumbar (il-ĭ-o-lum′bar) [“ + *lumbus,* loin]. Rel. to the iliac and lumbar regions.

iliometer (il-ĭ-om′ĕ-ter) [“ + G. *metron,* measure]. Device for measuring the iliac spines.

iliopectineal (il″ĭ-o-pek-tin′e-al) [“ + *pecten,* a comb]. Rel. to the ilium and the pubes.

iliopsoas (il-ĭ-o-so′as) [“ + G. *psoa,* loin]. The compound iliacus and psoas magnus muscles.

i. abscess. An abscess in the psoas and iliacus muscles.

iliosa′cral [“ + *sacralis,* pert. to sacrum]. Pert. to the sacrum and ilium.

iliotib′ial [“ + *tibialis,* pert. to tibia]. Pert. to the ilium and tibia.

i. band. A thick, wide fascial layer from the iliac crest to the knee joint.

il′ium (pl. *ilia*) [L. flank]. 1. The haunch bone. The wide upper portion of the innominate bone. 2. The flank. SYN: *os ilium.* SEE: *hip bone, Meckel's diverticulum, sacroiliac.*

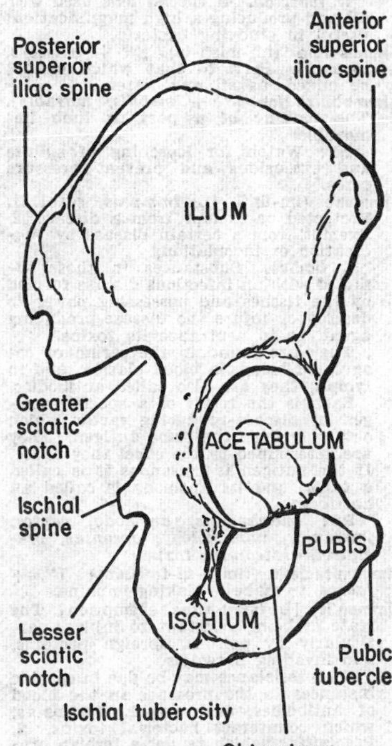

THE ILIUM (Lateral view)

ill (Il) [Ice. *illr,* sick, evil]. Indisposed; not healthy; diseased.

illaqueation (il″ă-kwe-a′shun) [L. *illaqueāre,* to ensnare]. Turning an inverted eyelash by drawing a loop of thread behind it.

illegal (il-le′gal) [L. *in,* not, + *lēgalis,* pert. to law]. Contrary to authorized law.

illegitimate (il″le-jit′ĭ-mit) [“ + *legitimus,* according to law]. 1. Not according to law; not authorized. 2. Born out of wedlock.

illness (il′nes) [Ice. *illr,* sick, + A.S. *-ness,* state of]. 1. State of being sick. 2. Ailment.

illu′minating gas. This is a mixture of various combustible gases, including hydrogen and carbon monoxide.

Its poisonous effects are largely due to carbon monoxide, *q.v.*

TREATMENT: Resuscitation, *q.v.*

illumination (il-lu-min-a′shun) [L. *illumināre,* to light up]. 1. The lighting up of a part for examination or an object under a microscope. 2. Amt. of light thrown upon anything.

i., axial. Light transmitted along the axis of a microscope.

i., central. Axial illumination, *q.v.*

i., darkfield. I. of an object under a microscope in which the central or axial light rays are stopped and the object illuminated by light rays coming from the sides, the object then appearing light against a dark background. Used to observe extremely small objects such as spirochetes, colloid particles, etc.

i., direct. I. of an object under a microscope by directing light rays upon its upper surface.

i., focal. The concentration of light upon an object by means of a mirror or a system of lenses.

i., oblique. Illumination of an object from one side.

i. (by) transmitted light. I. in which the light is directed through the object. Light may come directly from a light source or be reflected by a mirror.

illum′inism. Condition in certain psychotic states in which the patient has delusions of talking or communing with supernatural or exalted beings.

illu′sion [L. *illusiō,* fr. *illudere,* to mock]. PSY: Inaccurate perception; misinterpretation of sensory impressions, whereas a hallucination has no source in fact.

Vague stimuli favor illusions, but essentially it is a disorder of ideation, as in toxic and exhaustive deliria. If an illusion becomes fixed it is said to be a *delusion.*

illu′sional [L. *illusiō,* fr. *illudere,* to mock]. Pert. to, or of the nature of, an illusion.

image (im′ij) [L. *imagō,* likeness]. 1. A mental picture representing a real object. 2. A more or less accurate likeness of a thing or person. 3. The picture of an object such as that produced by a lens or mirror.

i., after. A retinal impression which persists after the stimulus is removed. A *positive* after-image having the same color as the original; a *negative* after-image possesses complimentary colors.

i., direct, i., erect. Picture from rays not yet focused.

i., double. Condition occurring in strabismus when the visual axes of the eyes are not directed toward the same object. The *false* image is formed in the eye that deviates; *true image* in the other eye. SEE: *diplopia.*

i., false. SEE: *i., double.*

i., inverted. I. that is turned upside down.

i., real. I. formed by convergence of rays of light from an object.

i., true. SEE: *i., double.*

i., virtual. SEE: *direct i.*

imagery (im'ij-rĭ) [L. *imagō,* likeness]. Imagination; the calling up of events or mental pictures.

Mental imagery may be of various types, *viz.:*

i., auditory. When sounds can be recalled to mind, as thunder, wind, etc.

i., motor. When movement only is recalled, as the passing of a train. Motor-mindedness is recognized in the mastery of spelling. The constant repetition of movements in writing make for automatic habit formation and fixation of the visual word-image.

i., tactile. When the feel of an object can be readily recalled.

i., taste and ***i., smell.*** Mental conception of taste or odor sensations previously experienced. Often very weak.

i., visual. Mental conception of an object seen previously. This is probably the commonest type of imagery. RS: *afterimage.*

imagination [L. *imagō,* likeness]. The power of forming mental images of things, persons, or situations which are wholly or partially different from those previously known or experienced.

imago (im-a'go) [L. likeness]. 1. An image or shadow. 2. A memory, esp. of a loved one, developed during childhood that has become clouded by idealism and imagination, and which is not always a correct one. 3. The adult, sexually mature form of an insect.

imbal'ance [L. *in,* not, + *bilanx, bilanc-,* two scales]. Out of balance. Without equality in power between opposing forces.

i., autonomic. An i. between sympathetic and parasympathetic divisions of the autonomic nervous system, esp. as pertains to vasomotor reactions.

i., sympathet'ic. Increased excitability of the vagus nerve. SYN: *vagotonia.*

i., vasomotor. Involving impulses to blood vessels resulting in excessive vasoconstriction or vasodilation.

imbecile (im'be-sil) [L. *imbecillus,* weak, silly]. Former term for severe mental deficiency. SEE: *mental deficiency.*

2. Without strength of mind or body; esp. mentally weak. 3. Stupid.

imbecil'ity [L. *imbecillitās*]. A state of severe mental deficiency. SEE: *imbecile.*

imbed' [L. *im,* in, + A.S. *bedd,* bed]. In *histology,* to surround with a firm substance, such as paraffin or collodium, preparatory to cutting sections. SEE: *embed.*

imbibition (im"bĭ-bish'un) [L. *imbibere,* to drink]. The absorption of fluid by a solid body or gel.

imbricate, imbricated (im'brĭ-kāt) [L. *imbricāre,* to tile]. Overlapping, as tiles; overlapping aponeurotic layers.

imbrication (im-brĭ-ka'shun) [L. *imbricāre,* to tile]. 1. Overlapping, as tiles. 2. The overlapping of aponeurotic layers in abdominal surgery.

imida'zole or **imina'zole.** An organic compound characterized structurally by the presence of the heterocyclic ring

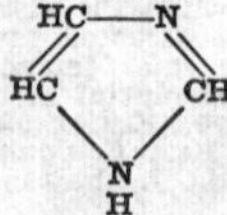

which occurs in histidine and histamine.

imide (im'ĭd). A compound with the bivalent atom group (NH).

immature (im-mă-tūr') [L. *in,* not, + *maturus,* ripe]. Not fully developed or ripened.

imme'diate [" + *mediāre,* to be in middle]. Direct without intervening steps.

i. agglutination. Healing by first intention.

i. auscultation. A. by ear applied to the body. SEE: *auscultation.*

i. cause. A cause directly originating a disease.

i. contagion. Contagion by direct contact.

i. union. Healing by first intention.

immedicable (im-med'ĭ-kă-bl) [" + *medicabilis,* curable]. Incurable.

immersion (im-er'shun) [" + *mergere,* to dip]. Placing a body under water, or another fluid.

In microscopy, the act of immersing the objective (then called an i. lens) in water, oil, etc., preventing total reflection of rays falling obliquely upon peripheral portions of the objective.

i., homogeneous. I. in which the stratum of air between objective and cover glass is replaced by a medium which deflects as little as possible the rays of light passing through the cover glass.

i. lens, oil. A special lens used with oil and producing a high magnification; useful in studying bacteria.

immiscible (im-mis'ĭ-bl) [" + *miscere,* to mix]. Pert. to that which cannot be mixed, as oil and water.

immobiliza'tion [" + *mobilis,* movable]. The making of a part or limb immovable.

NP: Watch for loosening of splints and extensions and prevent pressure sores.

immune (im-ūn') [L. *immunis,* safe]. 1. Protected or exempt from a disease. 2. Exempt from a certain disease by vaccination or inoculation.

i. bodies. Substances in those afflicted with an infectious disease formed by the tissues and possessing power to destroy or injure the disease-producing agent, or to neutralize its toxins.

They are found in the serum of coagulated blood, in blood plasma, and in lymph; they are also called antibodies.

Each is the result of a specific antigen or disease-producing factor which acts only upon the same antigen. They are determined by the effect they cause. If the antigen is poisonous it is called a *toxin,* and its antibody is called an *antitoxin.*

RS: *anaphylaxis, antibody, ceptor, immunity, immunology, opsonins, precipitin, proteolysis, toxin.*

immunifacient (im-u-nĭ-fa'shent) [" + *facere,* to make]. Making immune.

immun'ity [L. *immunitas,* exemption]. The state of being resistant to injury, particularly by poisons, foreign proteins, and invading parasites.

Such resistance may be due in specific instances to the presence in the blood of antibodies, such as: 1. *Antitoxins,* which counteract bacterial toxins. 2. *Precipitins,* which render a foreign protein insoluble. 3. *Opsonins,* which increase the ability of leukocytes to ingest bacteria. 4. *Agglutinins,* which cause clumping of foreign cells. 5. *Lysins,* which dissolve such cells.

i., acquired. I. resulting from the development of active or passive immunity; opp. of natural or innate immunity.

i., active. I. resulting from the development within the body of substances which render a person immune. This may result from having the disease or by the injection of the infectious organism, usually attenuated, or products produced by the organism.

i., congenital. I. present at birth. It may be natural or acquired, the latter being dependent upon antibodies received from the blood of the mother.

i., local. I. which is limited to a given area or tissue of the body.

i., natural. A more or less permanent immunity to disease with which an individual is born, the result of natural inherent factors. It may be the heritage of an individual, a race, or a species. It may be due to the natural presence of immune bodies, but other factors such as diet, differences in metabolism or temperature or adaptive features of infective organisms may be involved.

i., passive. Produced by actual injection of sera containing the antibodies into the subject to be protected.

immunity, *words pert. to:* antianaphylaxis, antivirus, aphylactic, autarcesiology, autarcesis, Ehrlich theory.

immuniza'tion [L. *immunitās,* safety]. Becoming immune or the process of rendering a patient immune. SEE: *autoimmunization; immunity.*

immunizing unit. A unit which expresses an antitoxin's strength. It varies with different antitoxins. SYN: *antitoxic unit.*

immunochemistry (im-mu″no-kem'is-trĭ) [L. *immunis,* safe, + G. *chēmeia,* chemistry]. The chemistry of immunization. The chemistry of antigens, antibodies, and their relation to each other.

immunogenic (im-u-no-jen'ĭk) [" + G. *gennan,* to produce]. Inducing immunity.

immunoglobulins (im″mu-no-glob'u-linz). A group of protein molecules important to the body's immunologic system. In the adult they may be divided into three classes: γM with a molecular weight of one million; γA with a molecular weight of 170,000 to 500,000; γG with a molecular weight of 170,000.

immunologic (im-mu-no-loj'ĭk) [" + G. *logos,* science]. Pert. to immunology.

i. diseases. These are due to the action of antibodies, as in allergic hypersensitiveness to antigens, or to specific reactivity of the tissues.

The phenomenon of anaphylaxis needs to be understood to gain a knowledge of immunology. SEE: *anaphylaxis; serum sickness.*

immunol'ogy [" + *logos,* study]. The study of immunity to diseases, as: 1. I. to microbic diseases. 2. Serology. 3. Immunologic diseases.

SEE: *serology; serum; toxins; vaccination.*

immunopro'tein [L. *immunis,* safe, + G. *protos,* first]. Any protein immune body or substance that confers immunity.

immunotherapy (im-mu-no-ther'ă-pĭ) [" + G. *therapeia,* treatment]. The production of immunity.

immunotox'in [" + G. *toxikon,* poison]. An antitoxin.

immunotransfusion (im-mu-no-trans-fu'-zhun) [" + *trans,* across, + *fusus,* poured]. Transfusion of blood from one who has been immunized by an autogenous vaccine.

immunpro'tein [" + G. *prōtos,* first]. A bacteriolytic substance formed by the injection of attenuated bacterial cultures.

impac'ted [L. *impactus,* pressed on]. Pressed firmly together so as to be immovable. Term may be applied to a fracture in which ends of bones are wedged together; a tooth so placed in jaw bone that eruption is impossible; a fetus wedged in the birth canal; cerumen; calculi, or accumulation of feces in the rectum.

impaction (im-pak'shun) [L. *impactiō,* a pressing together]. 1. Condition of being tightly wedged into a part; overloading of an organ, as the feces in the bowels.

impal'pable [L. *in,* not, + *palpāre,* to touch]. Felt with difficulty; hardly perceptible to the touch.

impal'udism [L. *in,* into, + *palus,* marsh, + G. *ismos,* state of]. Malaria. SYN: *paludism.*

im'par [L. unequal]. Unpaired. SYN: *azygous.*

imparidigitate (im-par-ĭ-dij'ĭ-tāt) [" + *digitus,* finger]. Having uneven number of fingers or toes. SYN: *perissodactylous.*

impatent (im-pa'tent) [" + L. *patere,* to be open]. Closed, not patent.

impe'dance [L. *impedīre,* to hinder]. Resistance met by alternating currents in passing through a conductor; consists of resistance, reactance, inductance, or capacitance.

The resistance due to the inductive and condenser characteristics of a circuit is called *reactance.*

imper'ative [L. *imperatīvus,* commanding]. Obligatory; not controlled by the will; involuntary.

i. concept. An idea which dominates one, as a fear or doubt.

impercep'tion [L. *in,* not, + *percipere,* to perceive]. Inability to form a mental picture; lack of perception.

imper'forate [" + *per,* through, + *forus,* a gangway]. Without an opening.

i. hymen. A hymen without an opening. Seldom discovered before puberty. Menstruation is interfered with and incision of hymen may be necessary. SEE: *hymen.*

imperfora'tion [L. *imperforātus,* not open]. State of being closed or occluded. SYN: *atresia.*

imperious acts. Tics and motions not under control of the will. Urges of compulsion states. SEE: *impulsion.*

imper'meable [L. *in,* not, + *permeāre,* to pass through]. Not allowing passage, as of fluids; impenetrable.

imper'vious [" + *per,* through, + *via,* way]. Unable to be penetrated.

impetiginous (im-pe-tij'in-us) [L. from *impetere,* to attack]. Rel. to impetigo.

impetigo (im-pe-ti'go) [L. from *impetere,* to attack]. Inflammatory skin disease marked by isolated pustules which become crusted and rupture. Occurs principally around mouth and nostrils. SYN: *scrumpox.*

i. contagiosa. A contagious form. Children esp. afflicted.

SYM: Discrete, thin-walled vesicles and bullae which become pustular and thin crusted, appearing in crops. They may be flat and umbilicated with no tendency to rupture, and they are filled with a straw-colored fluid. They dry up as thin yellow crusts. No itching.

ETIOL: Streptococcic or staphylococcic.

PATH: Papillary layer inflammation involving rete and stratum corneum.

TREATMENT: Soaking off crusts with soapy water; warm compresses of potassium permanganate solution; topical antibiotics as neomycin sulfate.

i. ***herpetiformis.*** Rare form occurring usually in puerperal women and accompanied by serious systemic disturbance.

i. ***syphilit'ica.*** A pustular syphilide.

i. ***variolo'sa.*** Pustules in late stage of smallpox. SYN: *melitagra.*

im'plant. 1. To transfer a part, to graft, to insert. 2. That which is implanted, such as a piece of tissue, a pellet of medicine, or a tube or needle of radioactive substance.

implantation (im-plan-ta'shun) [L. *in,* into, + *plantāre,* to plant]. 1. Grafting. 2. Artificial placing of a substance under the skin into the blood, into the uterine canal, etc. 3. Embedding of the developing blastocyst in the uterine mucosa.

i., ***hypodermic.*** Introduction of an implant under the skin.

i., ***parenchymatous.*** Introduction of medicinal substance into a neoplasm.

i., ***teratic.*** Union of an abnormal fetus with a nearly normal fetus.

im'plants [L. *in,* into, + *plantare,* to plant]. Capillary tubes of glass, gold, or platinum, containing radioactive substances for insertion into tissue.

impon'derable [L. *in,* not, + *pondus,* weight]. Having no appreciable weight; incapable of being weighed.

im'potence, im'potency [" + *potentiā,* power]. Weakness, esp. inability of the male to copulate.

i., ***anatomic,*** *i.,* ***organic.*** I. caused by a defect in the genitalia.

i., ***atonic.*** I. resulting from paralysis of nervi erigentes which convey impulses bringing about erection.

i., ***functional.*** I. not due to an organic or anatomical defect; usually of psychogenic origin.

i., ***paretic.*** Failure of impulse.

i., ***psychic.*** Due to mental disturbance.

i., ***symptomatic.*** Due to poor health, drugs, presence of disease, etc.

impotent (ĭm'pō-tĕnt) [" + *potentiā,* power]. 1. Unable to copulate. 2. Sterile; barren.

impoten'tia [" + L. *potentiā,* power]. Impotence.

i. ***coeun'di.*** Inability on part of the male to perform the sexual act.

i. ***erigen'di.*** Loss of power of erection.

impregnate (im-preg'nāt) [L. *impregnāre,* to make pregnant]. 1. To render pregnant. To fertilize an ovum. 2. To saturate.

impreg'nated [L. *impregnāre,* to make pregnant]. 1. Rendered pregnant. 2. Saturated.

i. ***carbon.*** Electrode having a carbon shell with core of various metals or salts of metals for use in a carbon arc lamp.

impregnation (im-preg-na'shun) [L. *impregnāre,* to make pregnant]. Fertilization of an ovum; fecundation.

i., ***artificial.*** Artificial implantation of semen in the female reproductive tract.

impres'sio [L. impression]. A mark, as of one part upon another.

i. ***cardi'aca.*** Depression on surface of liver for the heart. [NA].

i. ***col'ica.*** Depression on under surface of right lobe of liver. [NA].

i. ***digitatae.*** A depression on the inner cranial surface. [NA].

i. ***duodena'lis.*** Depression on under surface of liver beside the gallbladder indicating position of duodenum. [NA].

i. ***gas'trica.*** Hollow under left lobe of liver indicating position of stomach. [NA].

i. ***rena'lis.*** Hollow on under surface of right lobe of liver adjacent to the right kidney. [NA].

impres'sion [L. *impressiō*]. 1. A hollow or depression in a surface. 2. Effect produced upon the mind by external stimuli. 3. Plastic imprint of the jaw and teeth for making a denture.

i., ***digitate.*** I. on inner surface of frontal bone for convolutions of the cerebrum.

impulse (im'puls) [L. *impulsus,* from *impellere,* to drive out]. 1. Act of driving onward with sudden force. 2. An incitement of the mind, prompting an unpremeditated act. 3. PHYS: A change transmitted through certain tissues, esp. nerve fibers and muscles, resulting in physiological activity or inhibition.

i., ***cardiac.*** 1. The heart beat felt at the left side of the chest over the apex of the heart. 2. I. transmitted over the conductile tissue of the heart and responsible for the contraction of the chambers of the heart.

i., ***ectopic.*** A cardiac impulse arising in some part of the heart other than the sinoatrial node.

i., ***enteroceptive.*** Afferent nerve impulses arising from stimuli originating in receptors located in internal organs.

i., ***excitatory.*** One which stimulates activity.

i., ***exteroceptive.*** Afferent nerve impulses arising from stimuli originating in sense organs located on the body surface.

i., ***inhibitory.*** One which lessens activity.

i., ***morbid.*** An uncontrollable desire to perform an abnormal act.

i., ***nervous.*** A self-propagated excitatory state transmitted along a nerve fiber. It is the result of physicochemical changes occurring in the membrane of the nerve fiber. The impulse on reaching the termination of the fiber may (a) induce an impulse in another nerve cell or (b) induce activity in a tissue such as in muscles (contraction) or in glands (secretion), or (c) give rise to a sensation in the higher nervous centers.

i., ***proprioceptive.*** Afferent nerve impulses arising from stimuli originating in joints, muscles, or tendons, or other sensory endings which respond to pressure or stretch.

impul'sion [L. *impulsus,* from *impellere,* to drive out]. Idea to do something or commit some act or crime suddenly imposed upon the subject which tortures him until the act is accomplished.

Clear consciousness of the proposed act followed by an agonizing struggle, defeat, and sense of relief following the act are characteristics of impulsions, obsessions, and of inhibitions. Impulsions may include: (1) *Folie du doute,* or doubting mania; (2) obsessive fears of contact or delirium of touch; (3) agoraphobia; (4) dipsomania; (5) pyromania; (6) kleptomania; (7) homicidal or suicidal impulsion; (8) onomatomania; (9) arithmomania; (10) exhibitionism. SEE: *cerebrifugal, cerebripetal, imperious acts.*

In. Chem symbol for indium.

in- [L.]. Prefix: *Not, in, inside, within;* also *intensive action.*

inac'tivate [L. *in,* not, + *activus,* acting]. To make inactive.

inactiva'tion [" + *activus,* acting]. Rendering anything inert by using heat or other means.

i. of complement. Loss of activity caused by heating serum to about 55° C. (131° F.) for half an hour.

inadequacy (in-ad'e-kwa-sĭ) [" + *adaequare,* to be equal]. Insufficiency; incompetence.

i., renal. Inability of kidney to produce normal amt. of urine with proper proportion of solids and of a sp. gr. more than 1.014.

inalimental (in-al-im-en'tal) [" + *alimentum,* food]. Unfit as food; not nutritious.

inan'imate [" + *animatus,* alive]. 1. Not alive; not animate. 2. Dull, lifeless.

inani'tion [L. *inanis,* empty]. A condition due to lack of any food material essential to the body, such as general underfeeding, undernutrition, or caloric insufficiency.

Etiol: It may be due to causes other than the food supply, such as faulty mastication, stenosis of alimentary canal, etc.

inappetence (in-ap'ĕ-tens) [L. *in,* not, + *appetere,* to long for]. Lack of craving or desire, esp. for food.

inartic'ulate [" + *articulus,* joined]. 1. Not jointed; without joints. 2. Unable to pronounce distinct syllables or express oneself intelligibly. 3. Not given to expressing oneself verbally.

in artic'ulo mor'tis [L.]. At the time of death.

inassim'ilable [L. *in,* not, + *assimilis,* similar]. Not capable of being utilized by the body for nutrition.

inborn. Innate or inherent, said of characteristics both structural and functional which are inherited or developed during intrauterine development.

in'breeding [L. *in,* into, + A.S. *brēdan,* to cherish]. Producing offspring from those closely related.

incandes'cent [L. *incandescere,* to glow]. Glowing with light; white hot.

incar'cerated [L. *in,* into, + *carcer,* prison]. Imprisoned, confined, constricted, as an irreducible hernia.

incarcera'tion [" + *carcer,* prison]. Legal confinement; imprisonment of a part; constriction.

inca'rial bone. Os incae; interparietal bone.

incep'tion [L. *inceptiō,* taking in, beginning]. 1. The beginning of anything. 2. Ingestion. 3. Intussusception.

incest (in'sest) [L. *incestus,* unchastity, incest]. Coitus between those of near relationship.

in'cidence [L. *incidere,* to meet with]. The frequency of occurrence of any event or condition over a period of time and in relation to the population in which it occurs, as i. of a disease; the falling or impinging upon, touching, or affecting in some way.

in'cident [L. *incidere,* to meet with]. 1. A happening, event, or occurrence. 2. Apt to happen, esp. in connection with some other event. 3. Falling or striking, as a ray of light.

incineration (in-sin-er-a'shun) [L. *in,* into, + *cinis, ciner-,* ash]. Destruction by fire. Syn: *cremation.*

incipient (in-sip'ĭ-ent) [L. *incipere,* to begin]. Beginning.

incise' [L. *incisus,* from *incidere,* to cut into]. To cut, as with a sharp instrument.

incised (in-sizd') [L. *incisus,* cut into]. Cut with a knife.

i. wound. One clearly cut.

incision (in-sizh'un) [L. *incisiō,* from *incidere,* to cut into]. A cut made with a knife, esp. for surgical purposes.

incisive (in-si'siv) [L. *incisīvus,* cutting into]. 1. Cutting; having the power of cutting. 2. Rel. to the incisor teeth.

i. bone. Ant. or medial part of the sup. maxilla.

incisor (in-si'zor) [L. *incisor,* a cutter]. 1. That which cuts. 2. That which applies to the incisor teeth. 3. One of the cutting teeth, 4 in each jaw between the cuspids. See: *dentition.*

i., prostatic. Surgical knife for incision of an enlarged prostate.

incisu'ra (pl. *incisurae*) [L. a cutting into]. An incision or notch.

incisure (ĭn-sĭz'ūr) [L. *incisura,* a cutting into]. A notch or slit.

i.'s of Schmidt and Lantermann. Oblique lines on medullated nerve fiber sheaths.

inclina'tion [L. *inclinere,* to slope]. Leaning from the normal, or from the vertical, as a tooth.

inclinometer (in-kli-nom'et-er) [" + G. *metron,* measure]. Device for measuring ocular diameter from vertical and horizontal lines.

inclu'sion [L. *inclusus,* enclosed]. Being enclosed or included.

i., cell. Lifeless, temporary, constituent of the protoplasm of a cell. See: *cell.*

i. blennorrhea. Syn: *ophthalmia neonatorum.* An inflammatory disease of the conjunctiva of newborn infants.

i. bodies. Bodies present in the nucleus or cytoplasm of certain cells in cases of infection by filtrable viruses. See: *Negri bodies.*

i., fetal. Malformed twins in which one, the parasite, is completely enclosed within its host, the *autosite.*

incoercible (in-ko-er'sib-l) [L. *in,* not, + *coercere,* to restrain]. Uncontrollable; not able to be held in check.

i. vomiting. Uncontrollable vomiting

incoherence (in-ko-her'ens) [" + *cohairens,* adhering]. Inability to express oneself coherently, or to present ideas in a related order; sometimes due to interruption of one's thought processes.

incoherent (in-ko-he'rent) [" + *cohairens,* adhering]. Not coherent or understandable.

incombus'tible [" + *combustus,* burned]. Incapable of being burnt.

incompatibil'ity [" + *compatī,* to suffer with]. State which renders admixture of remedies unsuitable through chemical action, insolubility, formation of poisonous or explosive compounds; difference in solubility, or opposite action.

The quality of not being mixed without chemical changes, or without antagonizing the action of ingredients in a compound.

i., physiological. A condition in which 1 or more substances in a mixture have a physiological action different from other substances in the mixture.

incompat'ible [" + *compatī,* to suffer with]. 1. Not capable of uniting in solution. 2. Antagonistic in action, said of some drugs.

i. transfusion. A transfusion in which the isoagglutinins of the recipient react with the red blood cells of the donor resulting in intravascular agglutination and hemolysis.

incom'petence, incom'petency [" + *competere,* to be suitable]. Inadequate ability to perform the function or action normal to an organ or part.

i., aortic. Regurgitation of blood through the aortic valves.

i., ileocecal. Inability of ileocecal valve to stop the return of the material from the colon to the ileum.

i., mental. Mental inability to retain charge of oneself or possessions.

i., muscular. Imperfect closure of the cardiac valve due to weak action of papillary muscles.

i., pyloric. Weakness of pyloric aperture which permits undigested food to leave the stomach and enter the duodenum.

i., relative. Excessive dilatation of a cardiac cavity which makes perfect closure of opposite cardiac valve impossible.

i., valvular. Leaky condition of one or more cardiac valves permitting the return of blood at the time the valves should be completely closed.

incom'petent [" + *competere,* to be suitable]. 1. One legally unable to execute a contract, such as a feebleminded or insane person. 2. Incapable.

incompres'sible [L. *in,* not, + *compressus,* pressed together]. Compact; not compressible.

incon'tinence [" + *continere,* to stop]. 1. Inability to retain urine, semen, or feces, through loss of sphincter control, cerebral or spinal lesions. 2. Lack of sexual restraint.

i., active. Discharge of feces and urine in the normal way at regulated intervals but involuntarily.

i., intermittent. Loss of control of bladder on sudden pressure or movement, because of interruption of voluntary path above the lumbar center.

i. of milk. Excessive milk flow. Syn: *galactorrhea.*

i., overflow. I. caused by pressure of urine retained in the bladder.

i., paralytic. Constant voiding of small amt. of urine and feces due to defective nervous control of sphincters.

i., passive. Urinary i. of a form in which there is a full bladder that doesn't empty normally, but urine drips away upon pressure.

i. of urine. Inability to control urination. Sphincter muscle always relaxed. See: *enuresis, scatacratia.*

incontinen'tia [" + *continere,* to stop]. Incontinence.

i. alvi. Fecal i.

i. urinae. Involuntary continual dripping of urine.

incoor'dinate [" + *coordinãre,* to arrange]. 1. Not able to make coordinate muscular movements. 2. Unable to adjust one's work harmoniously with others.

incoordination (in-co-or-di-na'shun) [" + *coordinãre,* to arrange]. Inability to produce harmonious, rhythmic, muscular action, but not due to weakness.

Etiol: The condition may be sensory, due to failure of afferent impulses to be transmitted from muscles, bones, and joints to coordination centers, or motor, due to disturbance in tone or harmony bet. simultaneously acting muscle groups. Syn: *asynergy.* See: *disdiadokokinesia.*

incorporation. Combining two ingredients to form a homogenous mass.

increment (in'kre-ment) [L. *incrementum*]. 1. Increase or addition. 2. To increase or add to.

incre'tin. A fraction of secretin, a hormone extracted from the duodenal mucosa, which induces hypoglycemia by increasing the output of insulin.

incre'tion [L. *incrētus,* sifted in]. 1. Internal secretion. 2. Functional activity of an endocrine gland.

incretogenous (in-kre-toj'en-us) [" + G. *gennan,* to produce]. Pert. to the internal secretions.

incrusta'tion [L. *in,* on, + *crusta,* crust]. Formation of crusts or scabs.

incubation (in-ku-ba'shun) [L. *incubāre,* to lie on]. 1. The interval between exposure to infection and the appearance of the first symptom. 2. Bact: The period of culture development. 3. The care of a premature infant in an incubator. 4. The development of an impregnated ovum. Syn: *latent period.* See: Table I-11.

in'cubator [L. *incubāre,* to lie on]. 1. Apparatus for rearing premature babies in which the temperature may be regulated. 2. Apparatus for cultivating bacteria. 3. An apparatus for artificially hatching eggs.

incubus (in'ku-bus) [L. *incubāre,* to lie upon]. 1. A burden. 2. A nightmare.

in'cudal [L. *incus,* anvil, from *incudere,* to forge]. Rel. to the incus.

incudectomy (in-ku-dek'to-mī) [" + G. *ektomē,* excision]. Surgical removal of the incus.

incudiform (in-ku'dī-form) [" + *forma,* shape]. Like an anvil in shape.

in"cudomal'leal [" + *malleus,* a hammer]. Rel. to the incus and malleus and articulation of the anvil and hammer in the tympanum.

incudostapedial (in-kū-do-stā-pe'dī-ăl) [" + *stapes,* a stirrup]. Pert. to the incus and stapes and articulation bet. anvil and stirrup in the tympanum.

incu'rable [L. *in,* not, + *curāre,* to care for]. Syn: *immedicable.* 1. Not capable of being cured. 2. A person with an incurable disease.

in'cus (pl. *incī*) [L. *anvil*]. The middle of the 3 ossicles in the tympanum; the anvil.

incyclophoria (in-si-klo-fo-ri'a). Median or negative cyclophoria; the affected eye, when covered, turns inward about its anteroposterior axis.

incyclotrophia (ĭn-sī-klō'trō'fī-ă). Cyclotrophia in which the eye turns inward toward the nose even when both eyes are open.

in d. *In dies;* daily.

indagation (in-da-ga'shun) [L. *indagāre,* to search]. An investigation, esp. examination of the genitalia at termination of puerperium.

indenization (in-den-ī-za'shun) [L. *in,* into, + O. Fr. *deinzein,* from L. *de intus,* from within]. Arrest and development of cells in a part to which they have been carried by metastasis. Syn: *innidiation.*

indenta'tion [" + *dens, dent-,* tooth]. A depression or hollow.

index (in'deks) (pl. *indices*) [L. an indicator]. 1. The forefinger. 2. The ratio between the measurement of a given substance compared with that of a fixed standard.

i., alveolar. Degree of jaw prominence.

i., cephalic. Skull breadth multiplied by 100 and divided by its length.

i., cerebral. Ratio of greatest transverse to the greatest anteroposterior diameter of the cranium.

i., color. The proportion of hemoglobin to each red blood corpuscle, the normal being regarded as 100.

i., gnathic. Degree of jaw prominence expressed by a number.

i., gonoopsonic. Opsonic i. in gonococcal infection.

i., hemorenal. Ratio of blood's electrical resistance to urine's.

i., icteric. The ratio of bilirubin in the blood to a standard.

i., opsonic. The ratio of number of bacteria which are ingested by leukocytes contained in normal serum, compared with the number ingested by leukocytes in the patient's own blood serum.

i., pelvic. Ratio of pelvic conjugate and transverse diameters.

i., phagocytic. Average of bacteria ingested per leukocyte of blood.

i., refractive. Refraction coefficient.

i., thoracic. Ratio of thoracic anteroposterior diameter to transverse diameter.

indican (in'dĭ-kăn). Potassium salt of indoxyl-sulfate, found in sweat and urine, and formed from indole.

When in excess in urine it indicates putrefaction of proteins.

indicanemia (in"dĭ-kan-e'mĭ-ă) [*indican* + G. *aima,* blood]. Indican in the blood.

indicanu'ria [" + G. *ouron,* urine]. Excess of indoxyl-sulfate of potassium, a derivative of indol, in urine.

In normal urine it is found in small quantities.

indica'tion [L. *indicāre,* to point out]. That which indicates the proper treatment.

i., causal. That shown by a knowledge of the cause of a disease.

i., morbid. That shown by diagnosis.

i., symptomatic. That shown by symptoms.

Incubation and Isolation Periods in Common Infections

	Incubation Period	Isolation of Patient
Brucellosis	Usually 5 to 21 days	None
Chickenpox	Two to 3 weeks	One week after onset
Common cold	One to 2 days	None
Conjunctivitis of newborn	Usually 2 days	For 24 hours after administration of antibiotics
Diphtheria	Usually 2 to 5 days	Sixteen days after onset, or until two negative cultures from nose and throat.
Dysentery, amebic	Five days to 4 weeks	None
Dysentery, bacillary	One to 7 days	As long as stools remain positive
Encephalitis, mosquito-borne	Seven to 14 days	None
German measles	Two to 3 weeks	None, except from women in early pregnancy
Gonorrhea	Three to 9 days	No sexual contact until cured
Influenza	One to 3 days	During acute stage
Malaria	Usually 2 weeks	Protected from mosquitoes
Measles	Eight to 10 days	Seven days after appearance of rash
Meningitis	Two to 10 days	Until 24 hours after start of chemotherapy
Mumps	Twelve to 26 days	Until the glands recede
Paratyphoid fevers	One to 10 days	Until 3 stools are negative
Pneumonia, pneumococcal	One to 3 days	Until 24 hours after administration of antibiotics
Poliomyelitis	Three to 21 days	One week from onset
Puerperal infections	One to 3 days	Transfer from maternity wards
Rabies	Usually 2 to 6 weeks	Strict for duration of illness; danger to attendants
Scarlet fever	One to 3 days	Until recovery but not less than 7 days
Septic sore throat	One to 3 days	During disease: no handling of milk!
Smallpox	Seven to 16 days	Strict: in screened hospital wards until all scabs have disappeared
Syphilis	About 3 weeks	Should be enforced until surface lesions are healed in noncooperative patients
Tetanus	Four days to 3 weeks	None
Trachoma	Unknown	Until lesions disappear but usually not practical
Tuberculosis	Variable	In "open" cases until properly educated
Tularemia	One to 10 days	None
Typhoid fever	Usually 1 to 3 weeks	Until 3 cultures of feces and urine are negative
Typhus fever	Six to 14 days	None
Undulant fever	One to 5 weeks	None
Whooping cough	Usually a week	For 3 weeks after spasmodic cough
Vincent's angina	Variable	Preferably during the acute stage

Colors of Indicators

	Color *toward acid*	*toward alkali*	Range of pH
Bromcresol purple	yellow	purple	5.2- 6.8
Bromthymol blue	yellow	blue	6.0- 7.6
Congo red (1)	blue	red	3.0- 5.0
Dimethylaminoazobenzene (2)	red	yellow	2.9- 4.0
Litmus	red	blue	4.5- 8.3
Methyl orange	red	orange	3.1- 4.4
Methyl red	red	yellow	4.2- 6.3
Phenol red	yellow	red	6.8- 8.4
Phenolphthalein (3)	colorless	red	8.3-10.0

in'dicator [L. *indicāre,* to show]. A substance which can be used to distinguish acid from alkali. (In a more general sense, any substance which can be used to determine the completeness of a chemical reaction, as in volumetric analysis.) The colors of indicators in common use are as in the table on p. I-12.

USES: 1. In titration of ammonia and other weak bases. 2. Topfer's reagent, for determining free acid in gastric juice. 3. In titrating weak acids and for determining combined acid in gastric juice.

indif'ferent [L. *in,* not, + *differre,* to differ]. Neutral; tending in no specific direction.

indigenous (in-dij'en-us) [L. *indigenus,* born in]. Native to a country or region.

indigestible (in-dij-es'tĭ-bl) [L. *in,* not, + *digerere,* to separate]. Not digestible.

indiges'tion [L. *in,* not, + *digerere,* to separate]. SYN: *dyspepsia.* Incomplete or imperfect digestion, usually accompanied by one or more of the following symptoms: pain, nausea, and vomiting, heartburn and acid regurgitation, accumulation of gas and belching.

indigitation (in-dĭj-ĭ-ta'shun) [L. *in,* in, + *digitus,* finger]. Displacement of intestines by intussusception.* SYN: *invagination.*

indigouria (ĭn'dĭ-gō-ū'rĭ-ă) [G. *indikon,* Indian dye, + *ouron, urine*]. Indigo in the urine.

indirect' [L. *indirectus,* not kept straight]. Not direct.

i. cell division. Amitosis. Single cell division in which a mitotic figure is not formed.

i. reflexes. 1. Passive flexion of 1 part following flexion of another. 2. Passive flexion of 1 leg causing similar movement of opposite leg.

indisposi'tion [L. *in,* not, + *dispositus,* arranged]. Disorder; any slight or temporary illness.

indium (in'dĭ-um) [from *indigo*]. A rare metallic element. SYMB: In. At. wt. 114.82; at. no. 49.

indole. SYN: *ketol.* A solid, crystalline substance, C_8H_7N, found in feces. It is the product of bacterial decomposition of tryptophan and is largely responsible for the odor of feces. In intestinal obstruction it is absorbed and eliminated in the urine in the form of indican, *q.v.*

indolaceturia (in-dol-as-ē-tu'rĭ-ă) [*indol* + L. *acetum,* vinegar, + G. *ouron,* urine]. Excretion of a considerable amount of indolacetic acid in the urine.

in'dolent [L. *in,* not, + *dolere,* to feel pain]. 1. Indisposed to action. 2. Inactive; not developing; sluggish.

i. ulcer. One that is slow to heal but not painful.

indologenous (in-dol-oj'en-us) [*indol* + G. *gennan,* to produce]. Causing the production of indole.

indolu'ria. The presence of indol in urine.

indoxyl (in-dok'sil) [G. *indikon,* indigo, + *oxys,* sharp]. An oily substance, C_8H_7NO, sometimes found in urine of the apparently healthy, formed from the decomposition of tryptophan.

indoxylemia (in-doks-i-le'mĭ-ă) [" + " + *aima,* blood]. Indoxyl in the blood.

indoxyluria (in-doks-il-u'rĭ-ă) [" + " + *ouron,* urine]. Excretion of indoxyl in urine.

induced (in-dūsd') [L. *inducere,* to lead in]. Produced; caused.

i. abortion. One brought about intentionally.

induc'tance [L. *inducere,* to lead in]. That property of an electric circuit by virtue of which a varying current induces an electromotive force in that circuit or a neighboring circuit.

It is susceptible of measurement. The unit of inductance, or "self-induction," is the *henry.*

induction (in-duk'shun) [L. *inducere,* to lead in]. 1. The process of causing or producing, as labor. 2. The generation of electric current in a body by electricity in another body near it. 3. In embryology the production of a specific morphogenic effect by a chemical substance from one part of the embryo to another. Also called *evocation.*

inductor'ium. An induction coil, *q.v.*

inductotherm (in-duk'to-therm) [" + G. *thermē,* heat]. Device for producing pyrexia by electricity.

inductothermy. Treatment of disease by artificial production of fever by electromagnetic induction.

in'durate [L. *in,* in, + *durus,* hard]. 1. To harden. 2. Hardened.

in'durated [" + *durus,* hard]. Hardened.

indura'tion [" + *durus,* hard]. 1. The act of hardening. 2. An area of hardened tissue.

SEE: *Chaussier's areola, sclerosis, skin.*

i., cyanotic. An i. from long continued venous hyperemia, pressure on vessels causing transudation of blood and serum and formation of a dark, hard mass.

In the liver, spleen, etc., it leads to absorption of more or less of the parenchyma and to formation of new connective tissue.

i., fibrous, of the lung. A form of interstitial pneumonia. Hardened pigment forms red points on the lung.

in'durative [" + *durus,* hard]. Pert. to induration.

indu'sium. 1. A membranous covering. 2. The amnion.

i. griseum. The supracallosal gyrus, a rudimentary gyrus located on the upper surface of the corpus callosum.

inebriant (in-e'brĭ-ant) [L. *inebrius,*

drunken]. 1. Any intoxicant. 2. Making drunk.

ine'briate [L. *inebrius,* drunken]. To make drunk or to become intoxicated.

inebriation (in-e-bri-a'shun). State of intoxication, *q.v.* SYN: *drunkenness, intoxication.*

inelas'tic [L. *in,* not, + G. *elastikos,* elastic]. Not elastic.

inemia (in-e'mĭ-ă) [G. *is, in-,* fiber, + *aima,* blood]. Excess fibrin or presence of inosite (muscle sugar) in the blood. SYN: *inosemia.*

inert' [L. *iners, inert-,* unskilled, idle]. Not active; sluggish.

inertia (in-er'shĭ-ă) [L. inactivity]. 1. Tendency of a body to remain in repose. 2. Sluggishness; lack of activity.

i., uterine. Absence or weakness of uterine contractions in labor.

in extremis (in-eks-tre'mis) [L.]. At the point of death.

in'fant [L. *infans*]. 1. A babe. 2. A child not over 2 years of age. 3. In law, a minor, or one under legal age.

i., artificial feeding of. *Precautions:* 1. An exact time schedule is not considered necessary.

2. Temperature of feeding should be 100° F. Test heat by shaking some of it on the back of the hand. See that bottle is not overheated and that it does not burn infant by coming in contact with it.

3. Nipples should be kept clean and not fitted to bottle until ready to give. They should not be handled more than necessary, and before touching them one should be assured that the hands are clean. See that the hole in nipple permits a free, but not too rapid, flow of milk. The hole should not be too small. It may be enlarged with a heated needle.

4. See that infant is changed before bringing in the feeding.

5. In administering feeding, infant's head and shoulders should be raised higher than its abdomen, but it is better to hold infant while giving the feeding. See that the child is properly protected from drafts or cold. If being fed when in a reclining position the formation of gas may result in belching of the feeding. Change position of bottle as level of the fluid changes.

6. See that nothing disturbs the child while being fed and that the feeding is not interrupted. Close observation is essential, as the baby must receive all the feeding, which will not be the case if it is regurgitated or lost from belching. Interruptions may cause air-swallowing, which results in gas distention and a feeling of fullness that may cause a rejection of necessary nourishment.

7. If an accumulation of gas interferes with the feeding, the usual methods of expelling the gas should be employed, such as holding the child over the shoulder and patting it on the back. This should also be done after each feeding in order to expel any air.

8. Do not rock a baby after it has been fed.

9. Water should be given bet. feedings to maintain elimination and other body needs.

CARE OF NIPPLES AND BOTTLES: Both bottles and nipples should be soaked in cold water. Wash bottles with hot water and soap, using a brush for the purpose, and sterilize them by boiling in hot water. The nipples after being boiled may be kept in a covered, sterile container.

i. development. For 3 days after birth a baby loses weight; in the next 4 days, however, it should regain its loss and weigh as much as it weighed at birth. From 1 year old to 10 years the yearly gain in the child should be 4 or 5 pounds; from 10 to 16 years the yearly growth should be about 8 pounds. Should hold up head by 4th month, sit up before 7th month, walk by 12th to 15th month, talk before 18th month.

Infant Development

Age	Length Inches	Weight Pounds	Girth Inches
At birth	19.5	7	13
1 month	20.5	7.75	..
2 months	21	9.5	..
3 months	22	11	..
4 months	23	12.5	15
5 months	23.5	14	..
6 months	24	15	16
7 months	24.5	16	..
8 months	25	17	..
9 months	25.5	18	..
10 months	26	19	..
11 months	26.5	20	..
12 months	27	21	17

i. feeding. The infant should not go to breast for at least 12 hours after delivery. If this limit is up at night, the next morning will be soon enough for the first nursing. The regular nursing schedule is not necessary until the milk comes in. The 3- or 4-hour nursing interval depends upon the physician, hospital, and the condition of the mother and the baby. The 3-hour interval is advocated by some physicians during the first 2 or 3 weeks. This keeps the breasts emptied, thereby relieving congestion, and increases the amount of the baby's fluid intake in 24 hours. Others prefer the 4-hour interval, especially if the infant is large.

The early cessation of night feedings is an advantage of the 3-hour schedule rarely attained in the 4-hour régime. The individual breast is stimulated by the 15-minute nursing period. Followed by the 6-hour rest period, this combination provides for maximum functioning.

COMPLEMENTARY FEEDING: This is an artificial feeding used to round out a breast feeding that is inadequate. It is better given immediately after the breast feeding rather than before it. It abets the utilization of breast milk without interfering with it, while providing for breast milk deficiency that may exist.

SUPPLEMENTAL FEEDING: An artificial feeding replacing breast feeding, one or several times daily. It is not as generally used as the complementary, since it operates against the stimulation of breast milk production, and so tends to reduce it even further.

COMPOSITION OF ARTIFICIAL FOOD: The basis of artificial infant feedings is cow's milk, which is modified by the addition of water and a carbohydrate. Estimation of the composition of the formula should be based upon the physiologic requirements of the infant. No less than 1½ oz. (45 cc.) of milk per lb. (450 Gm.) of body weight are sufficient for this purpose, and may be increased to 2 oz. (60 cc.) per lb. of body weight within a week or 10 days. Calculation is based upon a 4% fat milk and allows for introducing a weak but sustaining food.

Carbohydrate requirement in 24 hours is 1/10 oz. (3 Gm.) to each lb. (450 Gm.) of body weight, exclusive of the 4% already in the milk. Fluid requirement is 3 oz. (90 cc.) to every lb. of body weight in 24 hours.

Unless an infant is immature or premature, there is no clinical reason for employing concentrated foods, such as evaporated milk, etc.

i., immature. One born near term, but underweight (500-1000 grams) and poorly developed.

i., mature. One born at the end of 270-290 days and weighing 2500 grams or more.

i., postmature. One born two or more weeks after calculated date of confinement. Cannot be judged by size or weight of infant.

i., premature. One born before term, but viable, having a birth weight of 5½ lb. (2500 gm.) or less, with a crown-heel length of 47 cm. or less; the birth weight being the most important factor. Includes larger number of immature infants. The younger the fetus at birth, the greater are its handicaps in carrying out its required body functions, and thus it needs far greater care than a normal or mature infant. SEE: *prematurity.*

ARTIFICIAL FEEDING OF: Oral feedings are usually not given for first 24-48 hours. Then feedings are given by medicine drop dropper or gavage. Glucose in water or plain sterile water, 4-8 cc., usual for first feeding.

Since each infant must be considered individually, the physician will order type of food, which may vary. Breast milk, high-protein low-fat milk, skimmed-milk formula, evaporated milk formula, or formulas from proprietary preparations may be ordered. All feedings should be small, sometimes as little as 5 cc. per feeding according to amount the infant is able to retain, and should be given at 2, 3, or 4 hour intervals.

By end of first week, 40 calories per lb. of body wt. per day are sufficient, and 60 calories per lb. of body wt. per day by the end of second week. After first week, requirements for fluid can be satisfied with 2-2½ oz. per lb. of body weight per day.

Supplemental vitamins and minerals are necessary.

i. pulse. At birth, 120-150 per min.; at the end of 1st year, 120-110; 3rd-4th yr., 100; at puberty, pulse is that of an adult.

i. respiration. At birth, 30-60 per min.; 1st yr., 25-30; 5th yr., 22-25; 14th yr., 20. SEE: *pulse; respiration; temperature.*

i. temperature. Normal (rectal), 98°-99° F. Subnormal more important than in adults.

infanticide (in-fan'tis-īd) [L. *infans*, infant, + *caedere*, to kill]. 1. The killing of an infant. 2. One who takes the life of an infant.

infantile (in'fan-tīl) [L. *infans*, infant]. Pert. to infancy.

i. hernia. Oblique inguinal hernia back of the peritoneal funicular process.

i. paralysis. Acute ant. poliomyelitis.*

i. tet'anus. Tetanus which begins with stiffening of jaw muscles. SYN: *trismus nascentium* or *neonatorum.*

infantilism (in-fan'til-izm) [" + G. *ismos*, condition]. A condition in which the mind and body make slow development. Failure to attain adult characteristics, physical or psychic.

i., angioplastic. I. due to defective development of vascular system.

i., Brissaud's. Infantile myxedema.

i., cachectic. I. caused by chronic infection or poisoning.

i., celiac. I. caused by celiac disease.

i., dysthyroidal. I. caused by defective thyroid.

i., hepatic. I. combined with cirrhosis of liver.

i., hypophyseal. Dwarfism resulting from hyposecretion of growth promoting and gonadotrophic hormones of ant. lobe of the hypophysis. SYN: *pituitary i.; Lorain-Levi dwarfism.*

i., Herter's. I. of the intestines.

i., idiopathic. Variety of arrested physical development, of unknown cause.

i., intestinal. I. associated with chronic intestinal disorder, causing the child to gain no weight nor to grow.

i., Lorain-Levi. Hypophyseal i., *q.v.*

i., lymphatic. A form of i. associated with lymphatism.

i., myxedematous. SYN: *cretinism.* SEE: *Brissaud's i.*

i., pancreatic. I. caused by defect in pancreatic function.

i., partial. Arrest in development of a lone tissue or part.

i., pituitary. Hypophyseal i., *q.v.*

i., renal. I. caused by defect in renal function.

i., reversive. I. commencing subsequent to completion of body growth.

i., sex. Continuation of childish traits, esp. sex characteristics beyond the age of puberty.

i., symptomatic. I. caused by poor tissue development.

i., tardy. SEE: *reversive i.*

i., toxemic. SEE: *intestinal i.*

i., universal. Dwarfed stature, otherwise fairly normal development, except for absence of secondary sexual characteristics.

in'farct [L. *infacire*, to stuff into]. An area of tissue in an organ or part which undergoes necrosis following cessation of blood supply. May result from occlusion or stenosis of supplying artery or more rarely occlusion of vein draining tissue.

i., anemic. I. in which blood pigment is lacking or decoloration had occurred. Also called white or pale infarct.

i., bland. I. in which infection is absent.

i., calcareous. I. in connective tissue in which calcareous salts have been deposited.

i., cicatrized. I. which has been replaced or encapsulated by fibrous tissue.

i., pale. An anemic infarct, *q.v.*

i., red. An i. which is swollen and red as a result of hemorrhage. Also called *hemorrhagic infarct.*

i., uric acid. I. in kidney of a newborn infant due to obstruction of renal tubules by uric acid crystals.

i., white. An anemic infarct, *q.v.*

infarc'tion [L. *infarcire*, to stuff into]. 1. Formation of an infarct. 2. Stoppage of a canal or passage, esp. by engorgement.

i., cardiac. Myocardial infarction, *q.v.*

i., myocardial. I. in cardiac muscle, usually resulting from coronary thrombosis.

i., pulmonary. I. in lung usually resulting from pulmonary embolism.

infect. To cause pathogenic organisms to be present in or upon, as to *infect* a wound.

infection [L. *inficere*, to taint]. The state or condition in which the body or a part of it is invaded by a pathogenic agent (microorganism or virus) which, under favorable conditions, multiplies and produces effects which are injurious.

Localized infection is usually accompanied by inflammation, but inflammation may occur without infection.

The physician is esp. concerned with 3 conditions: (a) Infections arising without known injury; (b) those arising in wounds of accidental origin, and (c) infections of operative wounds.

ETIOL: The principal causes of infections are agents belonging to the following groups of microorganisms: viruses, bacteria, Rickettsias, fungi, and animal parasites.

Known Injury: Many of these are due to wounds. The character of the instrument causing the wound may influence the infection, as in the case of a rusty nail.

Operative Wounds: These infections may occur as the direct result of the operative technic, such as the use of blunt instruments, or too vigorous wiping with sponges, and other surgical causes, and by postoperative exposure to pathogenic microorganisms.

SYM: The symptoms of infection are those of inflammation. The 5 classical symptoms listed by early medical writers are: *Dolor*, pain; *calor*, heat; *rubor*, redness; *tumor*, swelling, and *functio laesa*, disordered function.

Pain: This is esp. prominent when the infection is confined within retaining cavities. The pain is in proportion to the virulence and extent of the infection.

Redness and Swelling: Not evident when infection is within some rigid tissue or deep within some cavity; more apparent when superficial structures are involved. Discoloration would be a better term than "redness," as the color is more bluish or purple in advanced infections, while tuberculosis infections have long been called "white swellings."

Heat: Heat may not be evident on the surface, but there may be considerable elevation of body temperature even with small infections.

Disordered Function: This depends upon the part affected as well as upon the virulence. With almost all acute infections there is an increase of white cells and of polymorphonuclear leukocytes, a percentage of over 85% of the latter being of more import than leukocytosis.*

The degree of prostration is out of proportion to the extent of the injury. There have been many deaths from infection following pricks of needles, small splinters of bone, a trifling cut, or an infection from the bristle of a brush, in which streptococcus was the inciting cause. In this type of infection a red streak may be seen running up the extremity from the site of injury, and following the superficial lymphatics. This red line is absent in staphylococcus infections of the lymphatic vessels.

Infection may be *local* or *general*. Local infections may be at the portal of entry, or remote if transferred by the blood or lymph.

SITE OF: Microorganisms may gain entry to the tissues through the *gastrointestinal tract*, as in typhoid fever, or through the *respiratory tract*, as in tuberculosis and common colds, or through *wounds*, as in rabies, or from *contaminated objects*, as in tetanus, or from *bites of insects*, as in malaria and yellow fever.

Lowered vitality and resistance make possible *subinfection* from bacteria whose normal habitat is in the body. All infections of mucous membranes are mixed infections. Foci of infections may be primary or secondary.

METHODS OF: *Air-borne Infection*: Pathogenic organisms in the respiratory tract, discharged from the mouth or nose, may be borne on the air and settle on food, clothing, walls and floors, and if they are of the type which resists drying for a long period they may remain virulent until transmitted to another person. Coughing, sneezing, and expectorating may be responsible for "droplet infection," as bacteria are expelled into the air.

Animal Carriers: Some microorganisms may be carried from an animal to man by *direct contact, indirect transfer, or by intermediary hosts*.

Contact Infection: This is the result of transmission from person to person, as in kissing, coming in contact with those afflicted with communicable diseases, or with utensils handled by one with an infection.

Food-borne Infection: Bacteria may be communicated through food. Root

The Commoner Protozoal Infections of Man

Disease	Primary Site of Infection	Parasite	Mode of Transmission
Malaria: (1) Benign tertian (2) Benign quartan (3) Malignant tertian	Erythrocytes	(1) *Plasmodium vivax* (2) *Plasmodium malariae* (3) *Plasmodium falciparum*	Mosquito (*Anopheles*)
Sleeping sickness	Blood plasma	*Trypsanosoma gambiense*	Tsetse fly (*Glossina palpalis*)
Rhodesian sleeping sickness	Blood plasma	*T. rhodesiense*	Tsetse fly (*Glossina morsitans*)
Kala-azar	Reticuloendothelial cells and plasma	*Leishmania donovani*	The sand fly (*Phlebotomus argentipes*)
Amebic dysentery	Wall of large intestine	*Entamoeba histolytica*	Fecal (cyst) contamination of food and water

Fungus Infections

Disease	Causative Organisms	Structures Infected	Microscopic Appearances
Ringworm (tinea, otomycosis)	*Microsporum* (*audouini*, etc.)	Horny layer of epidermis and hairs, chiefly of scalp.	Fine septate mycelium inside hairs and scales. Spores in rows and mosaic plaques on hair surface.
	Trichophyton (*tonsurans*, etc.)	Hairs of scalp, beard, and other parts. Also nails.	Mycelium of chained cubical elements and threads in and on hairs. Often pigmented.
Favus (tinea favosa)	*Trichophyton schönleini*	Yellow disks in epidermis round a hair. All parts of body; also nails.	Vertical hyphae and spores in epidermis. Sinuous branching mycelium and chains in hairs.
Epidermophytosis (Dhobie itch, etc.)	*Epidermophyton* (*inguinale*, etc.)	Inflamed patches in inguinal, axillary and interdigital folds. Hairs not affected.	Long, wavy, branched and segmented hyphae and spindle-shaped cells in stratum corneum.
Some systemic infections:			
Thrush and other forms of moniliasis	*Candida albicans*	White patches on tongue, mouth, throat. Also may cause lesions of vagina and skin.	Yeastlike budding cells and oval thick-walled bodies in lesion.
Actinomycosis	*Actinomyces bovis*, *A. israelii*	Chronic, usually in neck.	Branched filaments on radiating rods, forming colonies.
Nocardiosis	*Nocardia asteroides*	Lower extremities or lung.	Closely resemble bacteria. Found in pus.
Blastomycosis	*Blastomyces brasiliensis*, *B. dermatitidis*	Skin and/or lungs.	Yeastlike cells demonstrated in lesion.
Coccidioidomycosis	*Coccidioides immitis*	Respiratory tract.	Nonbudding spheres containing many endospores, in sputum.
Cryptococcosis	*Cryptococcus neoformans*	Meninges, sometimes lungs.	Yeastlike fungus having gelatinous capsule. Demonstrated in spinal fluid.

and salad vegetables may carry bacteria from the soil or from manure. Cooking safeguards by destroying microorganisms on food.

Human Carriers: Some parasites may live in or upon the bodies of those who themselves do not suffer from them, but may be carried by them to others. Carriers may be: (a) *Contact* carriers, or those who never show symptoms; (b) *incubationary* carriers, or those in whom the infection is starting but has not completed the incubation period, and (c) *convalescent* carriers, or those who have recovered but who still harbor the organism causing their disease.

*Insect Vectors**: An insect may act as a physical carrier, as the housefly, which may transmit the typhoid bacillus from one point to another, or one that acts as an active intermediate host, such as the Anopheles mosquito, which transmits malaria by injecting the causative agent into the host while biting that person or animal.

Prenatal Infection: This is the result of the fetus being infected from the mother's blood stream, or from contiguity with the maternal membranes.

Soil-borne Infection: Soil-borne, spore-forming organisms commonly enter the body through wounds, as in tetanus and gas gangrene.

Water-borne Infection: Organisms producing typhoid, dysentery, cholera, and amebic infections may be carried through a water supply, or water in public pools used for bathing. These organisms may pass into the water from the feces of an infected person and be communicated to others.

i., acute. Appears suddenly and runs a short course.

i., a. exacerbation. Recurrence after a period of quiescence.

i., apical. I. located at the tip of root of a tooth.

i., chronic. One having a protracted course.

i., concurrent. Existence of two or more infections at the same time. SEE: *superinfection.*

i., droplet. Acquired by inhalation of a microorganism in the air. Esp. one added to the air by someone's breath or cough.

i., endogenous. I. caused by bacteria, normally nonpathogenic inhabiting the digestive tract.

i., focal. One occurring in a focus or cavity, and acting as a focus for dissemination of infectious material to other parts of the body. Ex: Apical tooth abscess causing infection of heart or joints.

i., food. SEE: *food infections.*

i., local. I. caused by germs lodging and multiplying at one point in a tissue and remaining there, as a *boil.*

i., low grade. Loosely used term for a subacute or chronic infection with only mild inflammation and without pus formation.

i., metastatic. Local i. caused by germs circulated from a focus of infection.

i., mixed. Caused by 2 or more organisms.

i., pyogenic. I. resulting from pus-forming organisms.

i., secondary. Infection by a different organism added to the one already present.

i., simple. Due to a single species of organism.

i., subacute. Intermediate bet. acute and chronic.

i., terminal. One occurring in the late stage of a disease. Generally acute and septic, usually causing death.

infectious (in-fek'shus) [L. *inficere,* to make into]. 1. Capable of being transmitted with or without contact. 2. Pert. to a disease due to a microorganism. 3. Producing infection. SEE: *eruptive.*

i. disease. Any disease caused by growth of pathogenic microorganisms in the body. May or may not be contagious. See table on p. I-11.

NOTE: Period of quarantine varies in different states. SEE: *quarantine;* also, *names of infectious diseases.*

infecundity (in-fe-kun'dĭ-tĭ) [L. *infecunditās,* sterility]. Barrenness; sterility in women.

inferior (in-fe'rĭ-or) [L. *inferus,* below]. Beneath; lower.

inferiority complex. PSY: A repressed state of mind in which one feels himself inferior to others. Such a group of ideas may be manifested by the assumption of superiority, often resulting in over-compensation. OPP: *superiority complex.* RS: *complex.*

infest' [L. *infestāre,* to attack]. The harboring of parasites.

infesta'tion [L. *infestāre,* to attack]. The harboring of animal parasites, esp. macroscopic forms such as ectoparasites and arthropod endoparasites.

infibulation (in-fib-u-la'shun) [L. *in,* in, + *fibula,* clasp]. 1. Fastening the labia of the vagina together, or the prepuce over the glans penis to prevent sexual intercourse. 2. Joining the lips of wounds by clasps.

infiltrate (in-fil'trāt) [L. *in,* into, + *filtrare,* to strain through]. 1. To pass into or through a substance or a space. 2. The material that has infiltrated.

infiltration (in-fil-tra'shun) [L. *in,* into, + *filtrare,* to strain through]. The process of a substance passing into and being deposited within the substance of a cell, tissue, or organ. Ex: I. of a tissue or organ with blood corpuscles, or of a cell by fatty particles.

It must not be confused with degeneration, as in the latter condition the foreign substances are from changes within the cell.

i., amyloid. I. of tissue or viscera with a glycoprotein.

i. anesthesia. Injection of a cocaine or similar solution directly into the tissue. SEE: *anesthesia.*

i., calcareous. Deposits of calcium or magnesium salts within a tissue.

i., cellular. I. of cells, esp. blood cells, into tissues; invasion by cells of malignant tumors into adjacent tissue.

i., fatty. Deposit of fat in the tissues, or oil or fat globules in the cells.

i., glycogenic. Glycogen deposit in cells.

i., pigmentary. Of pigments.

i., purulent. Pus cells in a tissue.

i., serous. With diluted lymph.

i., urinous. With urine.

i., waxy. Amyloid degeneration.

in'finite distance. 1. A distance without limits. 2. In vision, light rays coming from a point of any distance beyond 20 feet are practically parallel and accommodation is unnecessary.

infirm. Weak or feeble, esp. from old age or disease.

infir'mary (L. *infirmarium*). A hospital; a place for the care of sick or infirm persons.

infirmity. 1. Weakness. 2. A sickness or illness.

inflamma'tion [L. *inflammāre,* to flame within]. Tissue reaction to injury, either direct or referred.

It is a defensive reaction to irritation, *chemical, bacterial, mechanical,* or *toxic.* It produces degeneration of the injured area, and repair ensues by aid of the tissue cells.

Inflammation is a conservative process modified by whatever produces the reaction, but it should not be confused with *infection;* the two are relatively different conditions, although one may arise from the other.

ETIOL: The reaction of tissue to injury of any kind may be the result of: (a) Blows and foreign bodies; (b) chemicals; (c) electricity; (d) heat and cold (thermic causes); (e) microorganisms; (f) surgical operations (traumatic causes).

GENERAL SYMPTOMS: *Dolor,* pain; *calor,* heat; *rubor,* redness; *tumor,* swelling, and *functio laesa,* disordered function. In addition to the symptoms mentioned, the absorption of some of the constituents of inflammatory lymph may cause a slight rise of temperature (99°-101° F.), headache, loss of appetite, and a general feeling of discomfort.

PATHOLOGICAL CHANGES: (a) Vascular dilatation and changes in the blood. (b) Exudation of fluid from blood vessels into tissues with comcomitant swelling; migration of leukocytes into the tissues; gelation of fibrinogen in intercellular spaces. If the injury is not too severe, these processes reach their maximum in six to eight hours, after which reparative processes take place. Blood vessels return to normal size, normal blood flow is re-established. Leukocytes degenerate or reenter circulation, cellular disintegration or proliferation occurs in which injured cells are replaced; swelling disappears with resorption of tissue fluid and digestion of fibrin.

Each type of cell has a particular role to play in the inflammatory process. The *monocytes** and *macrophages** are great scavengers for all kinds of dead tissue. The *polymorphs** are active in autolysis* and the destruction of bacteria, and the *lymphocytes** form a barrier against the spread of irritants and probably form the fundamental tissue from which the healing scar develops. These cells appear in inflammatory conditions at stated intervals, and in a definite order or succession; the macrophage, for instance, antedating the polymorph by a week, and the lymphocyte by several days.

NOMENCLATURE: Most words denoting inflammation end with the suffix *itis,* which in itself pertains to inflammatory conditions. This suffix should *not* be pronounced as "etis." The principal inflammations of the various systems are:

Ear: Otitis externa, interna and media, mastoiditis.

The Eye: Conjunctivitis, dacryocystitis, iritis, keratitis, optic neuritis, panophthalmitis, uveitis.

Gastrointestinal Tract: Appendicitis, colitis, cholangitis, cholecystitis, duodenitis, enteritis, gastritis, hepatitis, pancreatitis, peritonitis, periproctitis, peridontitis, parotitis, proctitis.

Miscellaneous Organs: Arthritis, carbuncle, dermatitis, furuncle, myositis, osteitis, osteomyelitis, periostitis, phlegmon, cellulitis, tendovaginitis.

Nervous System: Encephalitis, leptomeningitis, myelitis, neuritis, pachymeningitis, polyneuritis.

Respiratory System: Bronchitis, empyema, laryngitis, pharyngitis, pleurisy, pleuritis, pneumonia, rhinitis.

Urinary System: Balanitis, cystitis, cervicitis, epididymitis, endometritis, myometritis, nephritis, oophoritis, pyelitis, prostatitis, perimetritis, parametritis, pyometra, pyosalpinx, orchitis, seminal vesiculitis, salpingitis, salpingo-oophoritis, urethritis.

Vascular System: Aortitis, endarteritis, endocarditis, epicarditis, lymphangitis, lymphadenitis, myocarditis.

i., acute. I. in which the onset is rapid and the course relatively short.

i., adhesive. One conducive to the healing of wounds.

i., alterative. I. of an organ in which degeneration of parenchymal cells is accompanied by proliferation of other cells. SYN: *parenchymatous.*

i., bacterial. I. induced by the growth of bacteria.

i., catarrhal. I. of a mucous membrane characterized by the excessive secretion of mucus.

i., chronic. I. which progresses slowly, is of long duration, and usually results in the formation of scar tissue.

i., exudative. One in which there is a large accumulation of blood cells and serum.

i., fibrinous. I. in which the exudate is rich in fibrin.

i., hemorrhagic. I. in which red blood cells are conspicous in the exudate.

i., interstitial. I. involving principally the noncellular or supporting elements of an organ.

i., purulent. I. in which pus is formed.

i., reactive. One about a foreign body or a focus of infection.

i., serous. I. in which the exudate is composed principally of serum.

i., suppurative. Purulent i., *q.v.*

i., toxic. This is one due to toxin or poison.

inflam'matory [L. *inflammāre,* to flame within]. Rel. to or marked by inflammation.

inflation (in-fla'shun) [L. *in,* into, + *flāre,* to blow]. Distention of a part by air, gas, or liquid.

inflection (in-flek'shun) [" + *flectere,* to bend]. 1. An inward bending. 2. Change of tone or pitch of the voice; nuance.

influenza (in-flu-en'za) [It. *influence*]. Grippe, an acute, contagious disease characterized by fever, extreme prostration, pain in head and back, and generally by catarrh of respiratory or gastrointestinal tract. SYN: *la grippe.*

ETIOL: The causative agent is a virus, of which several types and subtypes, A, A2, B and C, have been identified. A number of bacteria, esp. Pfeiffer's bacillus (*Hemophilus influenzae*), pneumococci, streptococci, and staphylococci have been found in the lungs in fatal cases, but these are considered to be secondary invaders.

EPIDEMIOLOGY: Usually more prevalent in winter and spring. Young adults, in robust health, appear to be particularly susceptible. The disease is contagious and is spread by discharges from the mouth and nose of infected persons. It may occur sporadically, epidemically, or pandemically.

INCUBATION: One to 3 days.

SYM: Begins abruptly with lassitude, malaise, chilliness, severe pain in head and back, fever from 101°-103° F. Prostration out of proportion to the fever. Eyes injected, sneezing, hoarseness, and hard paroxysmal cough. In most cases, catarrh of respiratory tract is unusually marked. Less frequently, gastrointestinal symptoms predominate. With latter, there may be diarrhea and abdominal pain.

COURSE: Ordinarily runs from 4 to 5 days, and may terminate by crisis or speedy lysis. Pulse rate usually not increased in proportion to fever; may be 90 to 100. Blood pressure low; nosebleed not uncommon. Examination of blood demonstrates a leukopenia. Urinalysis generally demonstrates presence of albumen and casts.

In some epidemics, a striking symptom is a peculiar cyanosis, which is, in all likelihood, of toxic origin. In addition to the respiratory and gastrointestinal forms referred to, nervous and fulminating types are sometimes described. In the latter forms, terms used to designate them are suggestive of predominating symptoms encountered.

Death may occur but mostly in the elderly and those debilitated by chronic diseases.

COMPLICATIONS: Pneumonia, pleurisy, empyema, chronic bronchitis, abscess of lung, sinusitis, otitis media, pericarditis, myocarditis, and very rarely endocarditis; peripheral neuritis, meningitis, and encephalitis are still more rare.

DIFFERENTIAL DIAGNOSIS: Typhoid fever, smallpox in the prodromal stage, cerebrospinal meningitis, and pulmonary tuberculosis.

PROG: As a rule, outcome is favorable in absence of pulmonary complications. In patients with cyanosis, severe nerve disturbances, or bloody expectoration, prognosis must be extremely guarded.

NP: *Prophylactic*: Isolation of patients, disinfection of sputum, and application of aseptic methods in handling sufferers by attendants is of utmost importance; also, sometimes, the wearing of suitable masks. The avoidance of public gatherings and general application of hygienic methods deserve consideration. A vaccine containing influenza viruses types A, B, and the Asian variant strain is available for prophylaxis. In recent years, however, epidemics have been due to serologically new subtypes. This requires a new vaccine which may take so long to prepare that it becomes available only after the epidemic has ended.

Active: Isolation, absolute rest, good ventilation, and a selected diet. No specific treatment; care largely symptomatic. Alcohol and strychnine sometimes recommended as stimulants and codeine may afford relief for cough.

i., *Asian*. Influenza caused by a variant strain of influenza virus type A. SEE: *influenza*.

influenzal (in-flu-en'zal) [It. *influence*]. Relating to influenza.

infolding. Process of enclosing within a fold; an operation employed in the treatment of stomach ulcer in which the walls on either side of the lesion are sutured together.

infra- [L.]. Prefix: *Below*.

infraaxillary (in"fră-aks'il-a-rĭ) [L. *infrā*, beneath, + *axilla*, little axis]. Below the axilla.

in"fraclavic'ular [" + *clavicula*, little key]. Below the clavicle.

infracostal (in-fră-kos'tal) [" + *costa*, rib]. Below a rib.

infraction. An incomplete fracture of a bone in which parts do not become displaced.

infraglenoid (in"fră-glē'noyd) [" + G. *glēnē*, cavity, + *eidos*, form]. Beneath the glenoid fossa. SYN: *subglenoid*.

infrahyoid (in-fră-hi'oid) [" + G. *yoeidēs*, U-shaped]. Below the hyoid bone.

inframam'mary [" + *mamma*, breast]. Below the mammary gland.

inframar'ginal [" + *margō*, a margin]. Below any edge or margin.

***i.* convolution.** The sup. temporal one.

inframax'illary [" + *maxilla*, little jaw]. Below the jaw; submaxillary.

infraocclu'sion [" + *occlusiō*, a shutting up]. Location of a tooth below the line of occlusion.

infraorbital (in-fră-or'bĭ-tal) [" + *orbita*, track]. Beneath the orbit.

infrapatellar (in"fră-pă-tel'ăr) [" + *patella*, a small plate]. Below the patella.

infrapu'bic [" + *pubēs*, hair on genitals]. Below the pubis.

in'frared rays. Invisible heat rays beyond red end of spectrum.

Their wave length ranges from 7,700 to 500,000 Angström units. Long-wave infrared rays (15,000-150,000 A.U.) are emitted by all heated bodies and exclusively by bodies of low temperature such as hot-water bottles and electrical heating pads; short-wave infrared rays (7,200-15,000 A.U.) are those emitted by all incandescent bodies.

SOURCES: The sun, electric arc, incandescent globe, and so-called infrared burners.

USES: Their energy is transformed into heat in a superficial layer of the tissues. They are used therapeutically to stimulate local and general circulation and for relief of pain. They are also used to detect traces of selenium, a deadly poison, in foods, and in alloys and steel. SEE: *radiation, ray*.

The use of a device, *infrared thermograph*, for detecting and photographing infrared rays has been useful in studying the heat of tissues. This device has many applications such as in investigation of the rate of blood flow through a part.

infrascap'ular [L. *infrā*, below, + *scapula*, shoulder blade]. Beneath the shoulder blade.

infraspi'nous [" + *spīna*, a thorn]. Beneath the scapular spine.

infraster'nal [" + G. *sternon*, chest]. Beneath the sternum.

infratrochlear (in"fră-trok'le-ăr) [" + *trochlea*, pulley]. Beneath the trochlea.

infric'tion [L. *in*, on, + *frictiō*, rubbing]. Rubbing of ointments into the skin. SYN: *inunction*.

infundibuliform (in-fun-dib'u-lĭ-form) [L. *infundibulum*, funnel, + *forma*, form]. Funnel-shaped.

***i.* fascia, *i.* process.** The membranous layer investing the spermatic cord.

infundib'ulin [L. *infundibulum*, funnel]. A 20% solution of an extract of the post. lobe of the hypophysis.

infundibulum (in-fun-dib'u-lum) [L. funnel]. 1. Funnel-shaped passage or body. 2. Tube connecting the frontal sinus with the middle nasal meatus. 3. Stalk of the pituitary gland. 4. Any renal pelvis division. 5. Cavity formed by fallopian fimbriae. 6. Terminus of a bronchiole. 7. Terminus at upper end of cochlear canal. 8. Conelike upper ant.

angle of right cardiac ventricle, from which the pulmonary artery arises. SYN: *conus arteriosus.*

infu'sible [L. *infusiō,* an infusion]. 1. Not capable of being fused or melted. 2. Capable of being made into an infusion.

infusion (in-fu'zhun) [L. *infusiō,* from *in,* into, + *fundere,* to pour]. 1. Steeping a substance in cold or hot water below boiling point to obtain its active principles. 2. Product obtained by such a process. SYN: *infusum.* 3. Introduction of a liquid into a vein.

RS: *apothem, autoinfusion, autoreinfusion, infiltration, intravenous.*

i., intravenous. Injection of a solution directly into a vein, usually the cephalic or median basilic vein. Normal saline intravenous solutions are usually temporary in effect due to loss of water in tissues. SEE: *Illustration,* I-20.

infusodecoction (in-fu"zo-de-kok'shun) [" + *dē,* down, + *coquere,* to boil]. 1. Infusion followed by decoction. 2. A medicine made from a crude drug steeped in cold water and then in boiling water.

Infusoria (in-fu-so'rĭ-ă) [L. *infusum,* infusion]. Name formerly applied to a class of *Protozoa,* now called *Ciliata.*

infu'sum [L. infusion]. Liquid preparations made by treating vegetable substances with hot or cold water.

The drug is not subjected to boiling, as in making decoctions. When the strength and method of preparation are not otherwise specified, they are made by treating 5 parts of the coarsely comminuted drug with boiling water to make 100 parts. None is official.

ingesta (in-jes'tă) [L. *ingestum,* from *ingerere,* to carry in]. Food and drink received into the body through the mouth.

inges'tion [L. *ingestum,* from *ingerere,* to carry in]. The process of taking material (particularly food) into the gastrointestinal tract, or by which a cell takes in foreign particles.

Ingrassia's apoph'yses. The lesser wings of the sphenoid.

ingravescent (in-grav-es'ent) [L. *in,* upon, + *gravescī,* to grow heavy]. Becoming more severe.

ingredient [L. *ingrediens,* entering]. Any part of a compound or a mixture; a unit of a more complex substance.

in'growing [L. *in,* into, + A.S. *grōwan,* to grow]. Growing inward.

i. nail. One growing into the flesh. SYN: *onyxia.*

inguen (in'gwen) [L. groin]. The groin.

inguinal (in'gwi-nal) [L. *inguinalis,* pert. to the groin]. Pert. to the region of the groin.

RS: *bubo, bubononcus, groin, hernia, hysterobubonocele.*

i. canal. The one carrying the spermatic cord in the male, and the round ligament in the female. It is 1½ in. long; a potential source of weakness and may be the site of a hernia.

i. glands. Those of the groin.

i. hernia. Hernia in inguinal region.

i. ligament. SYN: *Poupart's ligament.* A fibrous band extending from

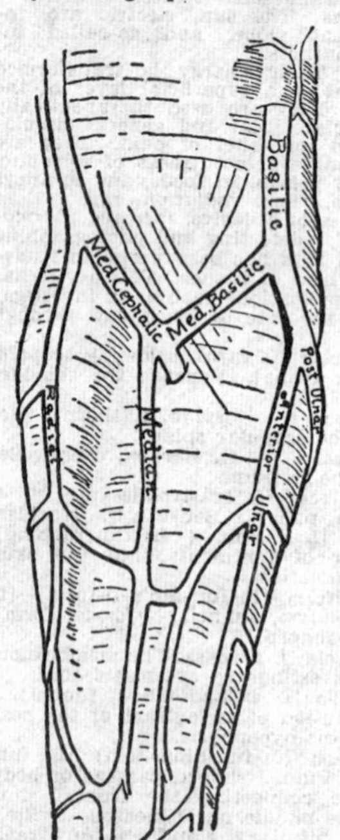

1. The superficial veins of forearm.

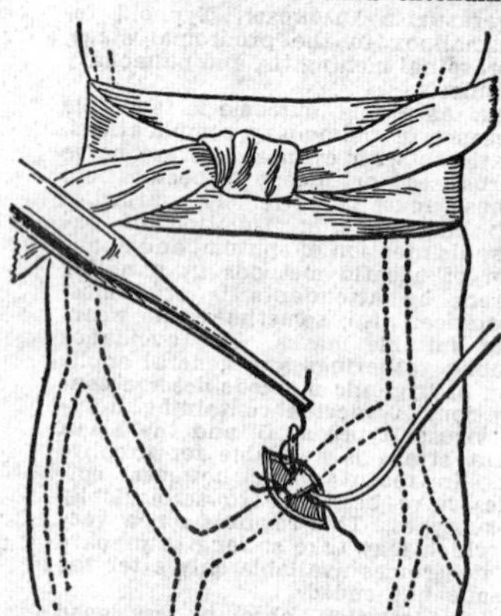

2. Incision method showing the incision made, the distal end of the vein tied, and a second ligature being passed under the proximal end of the vein.

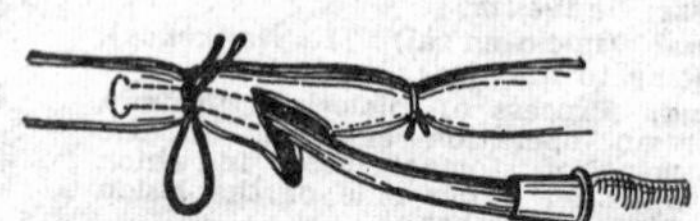

3. Incision method, showing cannula tied in place.

INFUSION, INTRAVENOUS SALINE

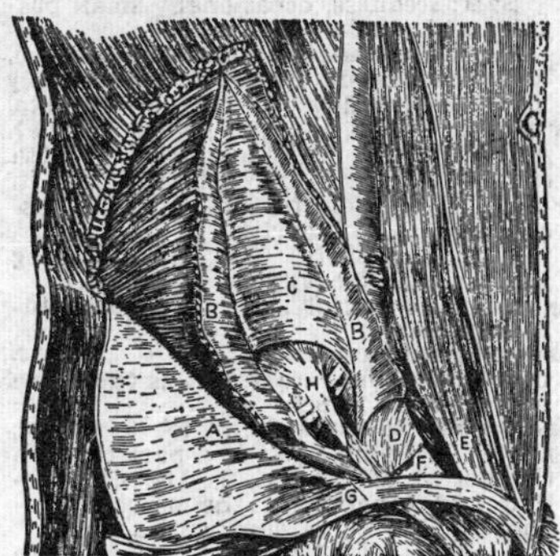

INGUINAL CANAL EXPOSED BY FOLDING BACK COVERING MUSCLES

A, External oblique muscle; B, internal oblique muscle; C, transversalis muscle; D, conjoined tendon; E, rectus abdominis with sheath opened; F, transversalis fascia; G, cremaster; H, infundibular fascia.

ant., sup., iliac spine to the pubic tubercle.

i. reflex. One in females resembling cremasteric* reflex in males.

i. region. The groin. The iliac region on either side of the pubes.

i. ring. Int. opening of the i. canal (abdominal i. ring), and the end of the i. canal (subcutaneous i. ring).

inguinodynia (in″guin-o-din-ĭ-ah). Pain in the groin or inguinal region.

inhal′ant [L. *in,* in + *halāre,* to breathe]. That which may be inhaled.

inhalation (in-ha-la′shun) [" + *halāre,* to breathe]. 1. Act of drawing in of breath, vapor, or gas into the lungs; inspiration. 2. Introduction of dry or moist air or vapor into the lungs for therapeutic purposes, such as *amyl nitrite* to relieve attack of angina pectoris, *aromatic spirits of ammonia* used to overcome fainting.

SUBSTANCES INHALED: *Oxygen* to relieve depressed breathing.

Steam inhalations are given to overcome spastic conditions of the larynx and bronchi, to soften mucus, to aid in absorption of oxygen, to reduce dryness of mucous membranes and to provide heat and moisture to the membranes of the lungs and appendages; also in croup.

Stramonium to relieve spasmodic attacks of asthma.

Stramonium leaves and *belladonna* are used for local effect, the fumes relaxing the involuntary muscles of the bronchial tubes. SEE: *anemopathy, steam tent.*

inhale′ [" + *halāre,* to breathe]. To draw in the breath; to inspire.

inhaler (in-ha′ler) [" + *halāre,* to breathe]. Device for inhaling medicinal vapors or steam.

inhe′rent [" + *haerere,* to stick]. Intrinsic; belonging to anything naturally, originally, not as result of circumstances.

i. cauterization. Deep cauterization.

inheritance. The sum total of all that is inherited; that which is the result of hereditary factors within the egg and sperm.

i., blending. Type of i. in which characteristics of male and female parents appear to be blended in offspring. May result from lack of dominance or equal contributions of several pairs of multiple factors.

i., cytoplas′mic. I. of traits due to self-duplicating mutable units present in the cytoplasm of an egg such as plastids in plants.

inherited. Received from one's ancestors; not acquired.

inhibition (ĭn-hĭb-ĭsh′ŭn) [L. *inhibitus,* from *inhibere,* to restrain]. 1. Act of repressing or state of being repressed; restraint. 2. PHYS: A stopping of an action or function of an organ. 3. PSY: Restraint of 1 mental process almost simultaneously by another opposed mental process; an inner impediment to free activity.

The best example of this important physiological phenomenon is the slowing or stopping of the heart which can be produced by electrical stimulation of the vagus.

i., psychic. Arrest of an impulse, thought, action, or speech. The term is commonly applied to the denial of the sex instinct. SYN: *suppression.*

inhib′itor [L. *inhibere,* to restrain]. That which inhibits. For example: A chemical substance which stops enzyme activity or a nerve which suppresses activity of an organ innervated by it.

inhibitory (in-hĭb′ĭ-to-ri) [L. *inhibere,* to restrain]. Restraining, preventing.

i. nerve. A nerve which carries impulses which act to slow down or inhibit action in the organ or tissue supplied by its fibers.

inhibitrope (in-hib′ĭ-trōp) [" + G. *tropē,* a turning]. One in whom certain stimuli cause partial arrest of function.

iniac, inial (in′ĭ-ak, -ăl) [G. *inion,* nape of neck]. Pert. to the inion.

inion (in′ĭ-on) [G. nape of neck]. 1. Occiput. 2. Back portion of neck. 3. External occipital protuberance.

initial (in-ish′al) [L. *initium,* beginning]. Incipient; rel. to the beginning, or commencing.

initis (in-i′tis) [G. *is, in-,* fiber, + *itis,* inflammation]. 1. Inflammation of fibrous tissue. SYN: *fibrositis.* 2. Inflammation of a tendon. SYN: *tendinitis.* 3. Inflamed condition of a muscle. SYN: *myositis.*

inject′ [L. *injectus,* from *injicere,* to throw in]. To introduce fluid into the body or its parts artificially.

injec′ted [L. *injectus,* thrown in]. Filled by injection of fluid; congested.

injection (in-jeck′shun) [L. *injectus,* from *injicere,* to throw in]. 1. Forcing of a fluid into a vessel or cavity or under the skin. 2. Substance introduced in this manner. 3. State of being injected; congestion.

NP: All equipment to be used must be sterilized and preferably autoclaved if heat sterilization is used. Boiling alone does not destroy the virus of serum hepatitis. The nurse must wash her hands before assembling the syringe and securing the needle. Expel air and measure dosage accurately. Cleanse site of injection with alcohol and sterile cotton before injection and after withdrawal of needle. Rinse syringe and needle, sterilize.

CAUTION: Neither the needle or the syringe should be reused until each of them has been thoroughly cleaned and resterilized. Failure to observe this rule permits transmission by inoculation of the virus of serum hepatitis from person to person.

RS: *aquapuncture, autoplasmotherapy, Casoni's reaction, cirsenchysis, douche, enema.*

i., air. Spinal i. of air to locate a growth, degree of central atrophy in general paresis, and to find cause of epilepsy.

i., epidural. Spinal i. given to relieve pain in limbs in tabes dorsalis or tabes paresis and in gastric crisis.

i., hypodermic. A subcutaneous one, generally in front of thighs, or outer part of arms or forearms.

i., intracardial. Into the heart.

i., intracutaneous. Injections into the skin, a method employed in giving of serums and vaccines when a local reaction is desired.

i., intramuscular. Into intramuscular tissue, usually in front of thigh or in 1 of the buttocks.

i., intra"peritoneal. I. into the peritoneal cavity.

i., intravenous.* Into a vein.

i., lipiodol. Spinal i. to locate spinal cord block or tumor.

i., rectal. Into the rectum; an enema.

i., sclerosing. I. into a vessel or into a tissue of a substance which will bring about obliteration of the vessel or hardening of the tissues.

i. spinal. I. into the spinal canal.

i., subcutaneous. I. beneath the skin. Syn: *hypodermic i.*

i., vaginal. A douche.

inject'ors [L. *injicere,* to throw in]. Various instruments for injecting medicinal fluids, making hypodermic injections and for transfusion of blood and intravenous injection.

in'jury [L. *injuria,* a hurt or wrong]. A hurt or damage.

Sym: There may be progressive fall in blood pressure; subnormal temperature; shallow, rapid breathing; cold, clammy, pale skin constituting shock. Injury may lead to exhaustion of adrenal glands, blood vessel dilatation and bleeding into capillaries, draining arteries and veins, decreasing return flow to the heart and inducing collapse.

NP: Avoid rough handling, the loss of fluids, body heat, and exposure of tissue in burns. Cover all wounded surfaces, apply heat and plenty of fluid if conscious, or, if shock is profound, fluids may be administered intravenously. Solutions of glucose are of great value. Blood transfusion may be necessary if there is hemorrhage. One to 2 pints of hot coffee or tea if patient is conscious. In case of broken bones and laceration, stop hemorrhage, make comfortable, but do not move patient until physician arrives.

See: *transportation of the injured.*

i., egg-white. I. resulting from biotin deficiency. It is produced in experimental animals by feeding raw egg white or its antibiotin component, avidin.

i., steering wheel. I. following automobile accidents in which driver is thrown forward against steering wheel resulting in contusion of heart.

ink poisoning. Many of the poisonings ascribed to ink are in the form of dermatitis. Several types of materials may be responsible. Ordinary ink may cause irritation, either because of irritating nature, or because of susceptibility of particular skins. Sometimes cleaning materials used in removing ink stains have been found to be causative agents.

Sym: Redness, occasionally small pustules and cracking.

F. A. Treatment: Wash with alcohol, soap and water. Rinse carefully, apply a bland dressing, as cold cream, etc.

in'lay [L. *in,* in, + A.S. *lecgan,* to lie]. A solid filling made to the shape of a cavity of a tooth and cemented into it.

in'let [" + A.S. *lǣtan,* to let go]. Passage leading to a cavity.

i. of the pel'vis. The upper opening into the pelvic cavity.

innate' [" + *natus,* born]. Inborn; inherent.

innervate (ĭn-nur'vāt) [" + *nervus.* nerve]. To stimulate a part as the nerve supply of an organ.

innervation (in-er-va'shun) [" + *nervus,* nerve]. 1. Stimulation of a part through the action of nerves. 2. The distribution and function of the nervous system. 3. The nerve supply of a part.

i., collateral. Supply of nervous force through an adjacent nerve tract to a part of which original nerve supply has been injured or destroyed.

i., double. I. of an organ with both sympathetic and parasympathetic fibers.

i., reciprocal. I. of antagonistic muscles of a limb by which impulses of central origin which induce an action such as flexion bring about inhibition of the opposing extensors.

innidiation (in-nid-ĭ-a'shun) [" + *nidus,* nest]. Multiplication of cells in a part to which they have been carried by metastasis.

innocent (in'o-sent) [L. *in,* not, + *nocere,* to injure]. Benign; not malignant. Syn: *innocuous.*

innoc'uous [L. *innocuus*]. Harmless.

innominate (in-nom'ĭ-nāt) [L. *innominatus,* unnamed]. Nameless.

i. artery. Right artery arising from the arch of the aorta, dividing into the right subclavian and right common carotid arteries.

i. bone. *Os innominata.* The hip bone, composed of the *ilium, ischium,* and *pubis;* united to form the pelvis by the sacrum and coccyx.

i. veins. Right and left vein, each formed by union of internal jugular with subclavian veins.

innoxious (in-ok'shus) [L. *in,* not, + *noxius,* harmful]. Not harmful.

inochondritis (in"o-kon-dri'tis) [" + *chondros,* cartilage, + *itis,* inflammation]. Inflammation of a fibrocartilage.

inochondroma (in"o-kon-dro'mă) [" + " + *ōma,* tumor]. A chondroma or tumor with much fibrous tissue; fibrochondroma.

inoculability (in-ok-u-lă-bil'ĭ-tĭ) [L. *inoculāre,* to engraft]. Quality of being susceptible to transmission of infection by inoculation.

inoc'ulable [L. *inoculāre,* to engraft]. 1. Transmissible by inoculation. 2. Susceptible to a transmissible disease. 3. Capable of being inoculated.

inoc'ulate [L. *inoculāre,* to engraft, from *in,* on, + *oculus,* bud]. To inject a pathologic microorganism or virus into the body.

inoculation (in-ok-u-la'shun) [L. *inoculāre,* to engraft]. Intentional introduction of a virus into the system as a preventive against the acquisition of certain diseases; it may be antidiphtheritic, antirabic, antitetanic or antityphoid.

i., animal. The injection of pathogenic organisms into laboratory animals for the purpose of determining their presence, the virulence of the organisms, the action of drugs upon them, or to induce antibody formation.

inoc'ulum [L. *in*, on, + *oculus*, bud]. A substance or virus introduced by inoculation.

inocyst (in'o-sĭst) [G. *is*, *in-*, fiber, + *kystis*, a bladder]. A fibrous capsule.

inocystoma (in"o-sis-to'mă) [" + " + *ōma*, tumor]. Fibrous tumor undergoing cystic degeneration.

inoepithelioma (in"o-ep-ĭ-the-lĭ-o'mă) [" + *epi*, upon, + *thēlē*, nipple, + *ōma*, tumor]. Epithelioma containing fibrous tissue.

ino'genous [" + *gennan*, to produce]. Forming tissue or produced from it.

inohymenitis (in-o-hī-men-i'tis) [" + *ymēn*, membrane, + *ītis*, inflammation]. Inflammation of any fibrous membrane or of an aponeurosis.

inoliomyoma (in"o-li-o-mī-o'mă) [" + *leios*, smooth, + *mys*, *myo-*, muscle, + *ōma*, tumor]. A smooth muscle tissue tumor.

in'olith [" + *lithos*, stone]. A concretion formed from fibrous tissue.

inoma (in-o'mă) [" + *ōma*, tumor]. A fibrous tumor. Syn: *fibroma*.

inomyoma (in-o-mi-o'mă) [" + *mys*, *myo-*, muscle, + *ōma*, tumor]. A fibrous tissue myoma. Syn: *fibromyoma*.

inomyositis (in-o-mi-o-si'tis) [" + " + *ītis*, inflammation]. Chronic muscular inflammation with connective tissue hyperplasia. Syn: *fibromyositis*.

inomyxo'ma [" + *myxa*, mucus, + *ōma*, tumor]. A mixed myxoma and fibroma. Syn: *fibromyxoma*.

inoneuroma (in"o-nu-ro'ma) [" + *neuron*, nerve, + *ōma*, tumor]. A mixed neuroma and inoma. Syn: *fibroneuroma*.

inop'erable [L. *in*, not, + *operārī*, to work]. Unsuitable for being operated upon because of one or more of a variety of reasons. In the case of a tumor, the disease may have spread so extensively as to make surgery useless; or the patient's general condition may be so poor that surgery could cause death.

inopex'ia [G. *is*, *in-*, fiber, + *pēxis*, fixation]. Tendency of the blood to spontaneous coagulation in the vessels.

inorgan'ic [L. *in*, not, + G. *organon*, an organ]. 1. In chemistry, occurring in nature independently of living things, substances not containing carbon. 2. Not pert. to living organisms.

i. acid. An acid composed of inorganic constituents. Syn: *acid, mineral*.

i. chemistry. C. dealing only with inorganic compounds.

i. compound. One without carbon.

inosclerosis (in-o-skle-ro'sis) [G. *is*, *in-*, fiber, + *sklērōsis*, hardening]. Increased fibrous tissue density.

inos'copy [" + *skopein*, to examine]. Diagnosis by examining fibrinous deposits in body fluids.

inos'culating [L. *in*, in, + *osculum*, little mouth]. Directly communicating; anastomosing.

inosculation (in-os-ku-la'shun) [" + *osculum*, little mouth]. Union of two vessels; anastomosis.*

inosemia (ĭn-ō-sē'mĭ-ă) [G. *is*, *in-*, fiber, + *aima*, blood]. 1. An excessive amount of fibrin in the blood. 2. The presence of inositol in the blood.

inosin'ic acid [G. *is*, *in-*, fiber, + L. *acidus*, sour]. A mononucleotide present in muscular tissue which upon hydrolysis yields hypoxanthine and d-ribose-5-phosphoric acid.

inosite (in'o-sīt) [G. *is*, *in-*, muscle]. Inositol, *q.v.*

inositis (in-o-sī'tis) [G. *is*, *in-*, fiber, + *itis*, inflammation]. Inflammation of fibrous tissue.

inositol (in-os'ĭ-tol). Hexahydroxycyclohexane, a sugar-like crystalline substance ($C_6H_6(OH)_6$) found in the liver, kidney, skeletal and heart muscle; and also present in the leaves and seeds of most plants. It is part of the vitamin B complex, deficiency of which in experimental animals results in loss of hair, eye defects, and retardation of growth.

inosituria (in"o-si-tu'rĭ-ă) [" + *ouron*, urine]. Inositol in the urine.

inosteotoma (in-os"te-o-to'mă) [" + *stear*, *steat-*, fat, + *oma*, tumor]. Fatty tumor with fibroma.

inosuria (in-o-su'rĭ-ă) [G. *is*, *in-*, fiber, + *ouron*, urine]. Inositol in the urine. Syn: *inosituria*.

in'quest [L. *in*, into, + *quaerere*, to seek]. 1. In legal medicine, official examination of a corpse to ascertain the cause of death. 2. The act of inquiring.

insaliva'tion [" + *saliva*, spittle]. The process of mixing saliva with food, as in chewing.

insalu'brious [L. *in*, not, + *saluber*, healthful]. Not healthy or contributing to health.

insane (in-sān') [" + *sanus*, sound]. Mentally deranged; pert. to insanity.

insan'itary [" + *sanus*, sound]. Not conducive to health; unhealthful, esp. pert. to filth.

insan'ity [L. *insanitās*]. Legal term for mental derangement; a psychosis. A general term for unsoundness of mind or any mental disorder or psychosis. In legal medicine, the state or mental condition characterized by (1) inability to distinguish between right and wrong; (2) possession of delusions or hallucinations which prevent an individual from looking after his own affairs with ordinary prudence or which render him a menace to others; (3) actions resulting from impulses of such intensity that they cannot be resisted.

The common law recognizes 4 forms: *lunacy, idiocy, accidental loss of understanding,* and *deprivation of understanding*. Only a few states permit divorce for insanity, and then the condition must have continued for a sufficient number of years to indicate incurability.

Lucid Intervals: An insane person during lucid intervals, may enter into a legal contract, a marriage, a business, buying and selling, providing at the time he or she is capable of entering into such matters with an understanding of all that is implied. The mental capacity *at the time* determines the validity of such acts and *not the condition before or after*.

RS: *paresis, phobia, psychosis, restraint.*

i., affective. Affective psychosis, *q.v.*

i., alcoholic. Alcoholic psychosis, *q.v.*

i., alternating. Manic-depressive psychosis, *q.v.*

i., choreic. I. accompanying Huntington's chorea.

i., circular. Alternating i., *q.v.*

i., climacteric. Mental illness occurring during or near the time of the menopause.

i., communicated. Folie a deux in which delusions of one person are transmitted to and accepted by a second person.

i., compulsive. I. in which the actions of a person are the result of obsessions or impulses over which he has no control.

i., cyclic. Circular or alternating insanity, *q.v.*

i., delusional. I. in which delusions or hallucinations are characteristic.

i., emotional. SEE: *psychosis, affective.*

i., imitative. A form of folie a deux in which the insane actions of one are imitated by another.

i., impulsive. I. characterized by the commission of acts, usually of a violent nature, as a result of sudden uncontrollable impulses.

i., induced. Communicated i., *q.v.*

i., manic-depressive. Manic-depressive psychosis, *q.v.*

i., moral. I. characterized by the commission of immoral acts although reasoning and intellectual processes are normal.

i., puerperal. Insanity coming on after childbirth.

i., senile. I. due to degenerative processes of old age.

i., toxic. I. resulting from the effects of a poisonous or toxic substance such as alcohol, opium, or other drugs.

insatiable (in-sā'shĭ-ă-bl) [L. *insatiabilis*]. Incapable of being satisfied or appeased.

inscriptio (in-skrip'shyo) [L. a writing]. Inscription.

i. tendin'ea. Tendinous band traversing a muscle.

inscription (in-skrip'shun) [L. in, *upon,* + *scribere,* to write]. Body of a prescription which gives the names of the drugs prescribed and dosage.

in'sect [L. *insectum*]. Common name for any of the class *Insecta,* of the phylum *Arthropoda.* Insects of medical importance are flies, mosquitoes, lice, fleas, and the true bugs.

i. bites and ***stings.*** In general, insects when they bite inject an acid substance resembling formic acid, consequently they may be relieved by alkalies, such as ammonia water or baking-soda paste rubbed on the wound.

Bees, wasps, and hornets when they sting inject an unknown organic substance for which there is no specific antidote. If a "stinger" is found in the wound it should be removed.

Insecta. A class of the phylum *Arthropoda* characterized by three distinct body divisions (head, thorax, abdomen), three pairs of jointed legs, trachea, and usually two pairs of wings. Insects are of medical significance in that some are parasitic, some serve as carriers or vectors of pathogenic organisms, and some are annoying pests causing injury by their bites or their stings. SYN: *Hexapoda.*

insecticide (in-sek'tĭ-sīd) [L. *insectum,* insect, + *caedere,* to kill]. 1. An agent used to exterminate insects. 2. Destructive to insects.

insemination (in-sem-in-a'shun) [L. *in,* into, + *semen,* seed]. 1. Discharge of semen from the penis into the vagina during coitus. 2. Fertilization of an ovum.

i., artificial. Artificial injection of semen into the uterine canal. Sometimes resorted to in sterility of the husband. Legal complications as to heritage and inheritance may arise and psychological results are not always favorable. SEE: *impregnation.*

insen'sible [L. *in,* not, *sensibilis,* sensible]. 1. Unconscious; without feeling or consciousness. 2. Not perceptible.

inser'tion [L. *in,* into, + *serere,* to plant]. 1. The manner or place of attachment of a muscle to the bone that it moves. 2. A putting into.

i., velamentous. Attachment of the umbilical cord to the edge of the placenta.

insheathed. Enclosed, as by a sheath or capsule; encysted.

insidious (in-sid'ĭ-us) [L. *insidiōsus,* cunning]. Stealthy, treacherous, hidden; not apparent, as a disease that does not exhibit early symptoms of its advent.

in'sight. PSY: Understanding of oneself or of any nervous or mental difficulties one may have.

insipid. Without taste; lacking in spirit or animation.

in si'tu [L.]. In position.

insolation (in-so-la'shun) [L. *insolāre,* to place in the sun]. 1. Any exposure to the rays of the sun. 2. Heat- or sunstroke.

EXPOSURE: Not more than twice a day and not more than five minutes at a time to begin with and never more than 90 minutes. Temperature, pulse, blood and urine should be observed after each treatment in those who are sick.

Dermatitis is always a danger even to the well. The public needs to be warned against undue exposure to the sun's rays which may cause a severe burn of the skin. SEE: *heat, heat exhaustion, heat stroke, heat therapy.*

insoluble (in-sol'u-bl) [L. *in,* not, + *solvere,* to dissolve]. Incapable of solution or of being dissolved.

insomnia (in-som'nĭ-ă) [" + *somnus,* sleep]. Chronic inability to sleep, or sleep prematurely ended or interrupted by periods of wakefulness.

ETIOL: Heavy late meal; with some coffee and other stimulants, including sugar in any form; overtiredness, mental fatigue, worry, excitement and principally the fear of being unable to sleep.

NP & TREATMENT: Remove exciting cause. Train the mind in self-control, remove fear of lack of sleep. Do not try to sleep if too wakeful. Sit up and read until tired. Hot foot bath, drink of hot water or milk before retiring. Small amount of plain food before retiring permitted.

Change of occupation if necessary and possible. Physical exercise during day, and a walk in fresh air at night after dinner. No mental work after dinner. Those complaining about insomnia generally secure more sleep than they realize. Some require much less sleep than others. Inability to sleep continuously through the night is not a pathological condition. SEE: *agrypnotic; anhypnosis; anthypnotic; sleep; somnambulism; vigil.*

inspect' [L. *inspectus;* from *inspicere,* to examine]. To examine visually.

inspec'tion [L. *inspectus;* from *inspicere,* to examine]. Visual examination of the external surface of the body. SEE: *abdomen; chest, and circulatory system.*

inspersion (in-sper'shun) [L. *in,* upon, + *spersus;* fr. *spargere,* to sprinkle]. Sprinkling with powder or a fluid.

inspiration (in-spir-a'shun) [L. *in,* in, + *spirāre,* to breathe]. Inhalation; drawing air into the lungs. Opp. of *expiration, q.v.*

Inspiration may be costal or abdominal, the latter being deeper. The breaking point for breath holding is quite

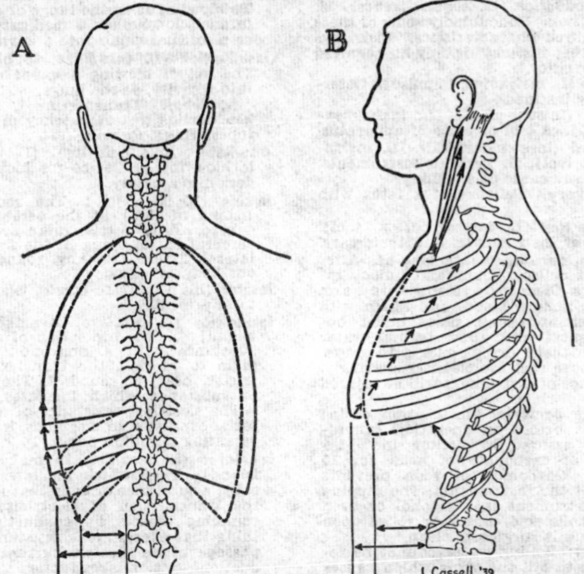

CHANGES IN SIZE OF THORAX DURING INSPIRATION

A. Back view. The contraction of the external intercostal muscles raises the ribs, makes them flare laterally, and so increases the transverse diameter of the thorax.

B. Side view. The contraction of the sternocleidomastoid muscle aids the external intercostals in raising the ribs, and so increases the anteroposterior diameter of the thorax. (Highly schematic.)

variable. Some professional divers are able to prolong this for more than two minutes.

RATE: 16-18 respirations per minute in an adult. SEE: *respiration.*

MUSCLES OF: Ext. intercostals, diaphragm, levatores costarum, pectoralis minor, scaleni, serratus post., sup., sternocleidomastoid.

RS: *air, apnea, asphyxia, breathing, Cheyne-Stokes respiration, dyspnea, hyperpnea, lungs, respiration, ventilation.*

i., crowing. Peculiar noise in laryngismus stridulus* or spasmodic croup.*

i., external. Interchange of gases in the lungs.

i., forcible, difficult, labored. I. in which the muscles of i. are assisted by inspiratory auxiliaries (*i. e.*, muscles attached to chest which by contraction increase the thoracic cavity directly or indirectly by furnishing fixed support whereby other muscles may act more advantageously). If movements become excessively labored, there is brought into coordinate action every muscle in the body which can either directly or indirectly increase the capacity of the thorax.

i., full. I. in which lungs are filled as completely as possible (voluntarily, as in determining the amount of complemental air, or involuntarily, as in cardiac dyspnea).

i., internal. Interchange of gases in the tissues. SEE: *respiration, cell.*

inspirator (in'spĭ-ra-ter). A type of respirator or inhaler.

inspiratory (in-spī'ră-tor-ĭ) [" + *spirāre,* to breathe]. Pert. to inspiration.

inspissate (in-spis'āt) [" + *spissāre,* to thicken]. To thicken by evaporation or absorption of fluid.

inspissated (in'spis-sā-ted) [" + *spissāre,* to thicken]. Thickened by absorption, evaporation or dehydration.

inspissation (in-spis-sa'shun) [" + *spissāre,* to thicken]. 1. Thickening by evaporation or absorption of fluid. 2. Diminished fluidity or increased thickness.

in'step [origin uncertain]. Arch on upper surface of foot in the middle, in front of ankle.

instillation (in-stil-a'shun) [L. *in,* into, + *stillāre,* to drop]. Pouring in a liquid, drop by drop.

in"stillator. An apparatus for introducing, drop by drop, liquids into a cavity.

instinct (in'stinkt) [L. *instinctus,* impulse]. 1. Inherent (racial) patterns of expression normally manifested under suitable conditions, usually heavily loaded with emotional value (libido in its widest sense). Innate urges, principally voluntary, with which one is born and which are necessary for the preservation of life. An innate, complex, coordinated, behavior pattern characteristic of a race or species and usually having an adaptive value. 2. An urge, uncontrolled by reason, to react to stimuli of an emotional nature.

The term is often misapplied to *intuition.* Some only recognize: 1. *Self-preservation.* 2. *Sex.* 3. *Herd instinct.* Others include: 4. ***Flight*** or *fear.* 5. ***Repulsion.*** 6. ***Curiosity.*** 7. ***Pugnacity.*** 8. ***Self-asser-***

tion. 9. *Self-abasement.* 10. *Parental i.* 11. *Reproduction.* 12. *Acquisitiveness.* 13. *Construction.* Undoubtedly some of these are acquired characteristics. Fisk says the "mother instinct" is only an acquired characteristic.

instinct'ive [L. *instinctus,* impulse]. Determined by instinct.

instrument (in'stru-ment) [L. *instrumentum,* tool]. A tool or piece of apparatus.

instrumental (in-stru-men'tal) [L. *instrumentum,* tool]. 1. Pert. to instruments. 2. Being the cause of anything.

i. delivery. Delivery of a fetus with forceps.

instrumenta'tion [L. *instrumentum,* tool]. The use of instruments, and their care.

instruments, care and sharpening of. After operation collect, count and unlock instruments. Cleanse by rinsing with warm water to remove blood, and again with hot water and soap, place under hot water faucet and allow boiling water to run on them, dry at once with gauze.

To remove rust use cleanser sparingly, else surface of instrument will be injured in course of time.

Reliable *bacterial* sterilization of instruments before an operation can always be assured by boiling in a 1% solution of carbonate of soda for 15 minutes. Carbonate of soda prevents rusting of the instruments. The dipping of an instrument into alcohol or even pure carbolic acid cannot be relied upon for making it surgically clean.

CAUTION: Boiling water cannot be relied upon to kill the virus which causes hepatitis. To be certain this virus is destroyed, either autoclaving or the use of some chemical method of sterilization such as ethylene oxide gas is required.

SHARPENING: *Washita stone* is best for dull instruments as it cuts away the metal faster. *Arkansas* stone is better for finishing. Glycerin is best lubricant. Entire edge of knife should be covered in one sweep. Hold knife at angle of 30°. All knives should be honed before used. Blunt instruments should be kept highly polished. Rub with fine emery paper and polish with rouge and chamois skin or gauze. Do not use emery paper on saws. Sharpen with three-cornered files. Silver instruments should not come in contact with rubber, or be exposed to atmosphere. Wrap in dry gauze.

insufficiency (in-suf-fish'en-sĭ) [L. *in,* not, + *sufficiens,* sufficient]. The condition of being inadequate for its purpose.

i., aortic. An imperfect closure of the aortic valves.

i., cardiac. Inability of heart to function normally.

i., gastric. Inability of the stomach to empty itself.

i., hepatic. Inability of the liver to function properly.

i., mitral. In which the mitral valve inefficiently closes with rhythmic action of the heart.

i., muscular. Condition in which a muscle is unable to exert its normal force and bring about normal movement of the part to which it is attached. Term applied esp. to eye muscles.

i. of the ocular muscles. Absence of dynamic equilibrium of ocular muscles.

i., renal. Inability of the kidney to remove waste products from the blood at the normal rate.

i., valvular. Imperfect cardiac valve closure, permitting leakage of blood.

insuf'flate [L. *insufflāre,* to blow into]. 1. To blow in, as in the lungs of a newborn infant. 2. To blow a medicated powder or medicinal vapor into a cavity.

insuffla'tion [L. *insufflāre,* to blow into]. The act of blowing a vapor or powder into a cavity, as the lungs.

i., tubal. Transuterine i. with carbon dioxide to test patency of fallopian tubes. SYN: *Rubin's test.*

insufflator (in'suf-fla-tor) [L. *insufflāre,* to blow into]. Device for blowing powders into a cavity.

in'sula [L. island]. 1. The central lobe (island of Reil) of the cerebral hemisphere. It is a triangular area of the cerebral cortex lying in the floor of the lateral fissure. 2. Any round cutaneous body or patch.

insular (ins'u-lar) [L. *insula,* island]. Rel. to any insula.

insula'tion [L. *insulāre,* to make into an island]. 1. The protection of a body or substance with a nonconducting medium to prevent the transfer of electricity, heat, or sound. 2. The material or substance which insulates.

The electrical resistance of an insulator is expressed in megohms, a unit representing a million ohms.

in'sulator (L. *insulāre,* to make into an island]. That which insulates; specifically, a substance or body that interrupts the transmission of electricity to surrounding objects by conduction; anything that exerts great resistance to the passage of an electric current by conduction. SEE: *nonconductor.*

in'sulin [L. *insula,* island]. 1. A hormone secreted by the beta cells of the islets of Langerhans of the pancreas. Called the *antidiabetic hormone.* It can be readily crystallized as a zinc salt although nickel, calcium, and cobalt also are effective. It is a protein with a molecular weight of approximately 35,000. Insulin is essential for the proper oxidation and utilization of blood sugar (glucose) and for maintenance of the proper blood sugar level. Inadequate secretion of insulin results in improper metabolism of carbohydrates and fats and brings on diabetes characterized by hyperglycemia and glycosuria. Insulin when injected (it is not active orally) into a diabetic produces the following effects: normal storage of glycogen in the liver and muscle tissue; reduction in blood sugar level; disappearance of ketosis and hyperlipemia; prevention of excessive breakdown of protein; increase in respiratory quotient; and increase in resistance to infective diseases. The secretion of insulin is primarily dependent upon the concentration of blood glucose, an increase of blood sugar bringing about an increase in the secretion of insulin.

First discovered and used successfully by Sir F. G. Banting in diabetes. Not a cure, and not necessary in every case. Makes possible a greater metabolism of carbohydrates without evidence of glycosuria. Prepared from animal pancreas.

DOSAGE: Should always be expressed in units rather than in cubic centimeters or minims. There is no average dose of insulin for diabetics; each case must be studied individually. In general, it is advisable to keep the volume per injection at from ½-¾ cc., choosing the strength which will give the required number of units in this volume or less.

ADM: The long-acting (depot) insulins are usually taken in a single dose for the

24 hours before breakfast subcutaneously. The older, short-acting insulins are usually reserved for emergencies (diabetic coma) and for those rare individuals who cannot tolerate the depot type.

i., amorphous. I. to which zinc or other metallic ions have not been added.

i., crystalline. I. which has been precipitated in the presence of zinc or other metallic ions.

i., depot. Insulin that is absorbed slowly from the site of injection.

i., globin. I. combined with globin from blood. It forms a clear solution producing effects longer than those of regular insulin but shorter than those of protamine insulin.

i., hexamine. I. combined with hexamethylene tetramine.

i. histone. Insulin to which has been added the simple protein histone derived from the thymus.

i. histone zinc. Histone insulin to which zinc has been added. The hypoglycemic effect is more prompt, though prolonged, than with protamine zinc insulin. It makes possible a continuously normal blood sugar level and freedom from glycosuria in many.

I., NPH. Abbr. for *neutral-protamine-Hagedorn,* a mixture containing 0.5 mg. of protamine to each 100 units of insulin. Quick-acting, with effects of long duration.

i., protamine. I. combined with protamine, a simple protein derived from the spermatozoa of fishes.

i., protamine zinc. A preparation of insulin, modified by the addition of protamine and a zinc salt.

USES: Same as for unmodified insulin, but has a more prolonged action; its administration is usually but once a day.

i., protamine zinc, clear (soluble). A water-clear preparation with more protamine zinc and glycerin than that present in p. z. insulin.

i. shock. Condition resulting from an overdose of insulin resulting in reduction of blood sugar level below normal (hypoglycemia).

SYM: Excessive hunger, thirst, and nervousness, fear and excitability. Rapid pulse, flushing, pallor and sweating, fainting, convulsions, coma.

TREATMENT: Eating sugar or candy, orange juice, glucose, other carbohydrates and injections of glucose into the blood if patient is unconscious. Adrenalin is of great though transient value.

i. shock therapy. The treatment of schizophrenia and other mental disorders by the injection of insulin. Sufficient insulin is injected to produce unconsciousness, the dosage being carefully regulated during course of treatment. When a deep coma is reached, the patient is brought out of the comatose condition by the administration of glucose followed by a meal rich in carbohydrates.

It is a dangerous procedure with a relatively high mortality and should be employed only by those who are fully equipped, fully qualified, and thoroughly familiar with all aspects of this method. It is essential to have available at all times suitable solutions of dextrose for interrupting the hypoglycemic state which is artificially created.

i. tannate. A combination of insulin with tannic acid.

i. tolerance. The degree to which the body responds to the injection of insulin.

insulinemia (in-su-lin-e'mĭ-ă) [" + G. *aima,* blood]. An undue amt. of insulin in the blood.

insulinogenic (in-su-lin-o-jen'ik) [" + G. *gennan,* to produce]. Caused by hyperinsulinism.

insulinoid (in'su-lin-oid) [" + G. *eidos,* resemblance]. Resembling or having the properties of insulin.

insulogenic (in-su-lo-jen'ik) [" + G. *gennan,* to produce]. Produced by overproduction or overadministration of insulin. SYN: *insulinogenic.*

insulo'ma [" + G. *ōma,* tumor]. A tumor of the island of Reil or of the islands of Langerhans.

insulopath'ic [" + G. *pathos,* disease]. Rel. to or caused by abnormal insulin secretion.

insusceptibility (in"sus-sep"tĭ-bil'ĭ-tĭ) [L. *in,* not, + *susceptus,* undertaken]. Incapability of becoming infected with a germ disease. SYN: *immunity.*

integration (in-tĕ-gra'shun) [L. *integrāre,* to make whole]. 1. Assimilation. 2. A Harmonious relationship of the parts constituting the whole of anything.

i., primary. Early recognition of the body and its psyche as apart from one's environment.

i., secondary. The process involved in developing the adult personality, through sublimation of the sex instinct and its components.

integrator (in'te-gra-tor) [L. *integrāre,* to make whole]. Device for measuring body surfaces.

integument (in-teg'u-ment) [L. *integumentum,* a covering]. 1. A covering. 2. The skin, consisting of the *corium* or ***dermis,*** and *epidermis.*

integumentary (in-teg-ū-men'tă-rĭ) [L. *integumentum,* a covering]. Rel. to the integument. SYN: *cutaneous, dermal.*

in'tellect [L. *intellectus;* from *intelligere,* to understand]. The mind, or understanding; conscious brain function.

intellec'tual [L. *intellectus;* from *intelligere,* to understand]. 1. Pert. to the mind. 2. Possessing intellect.

intel'ligence [L. *intelligere,* to understand]. The capacity to comprehend relationships. The ability to think; the ability to solve problems and to adjust to new situations.

There must be no emotional distortion. If intelligence-testing is to be accurate, a series of graded questions must be asked; the further one can go in answering them correctly, the greater is supposed to be one's intelligence.

i. quotient (IQ). An index of intelligence determined through the subject's answers to arbitrarily chosen questions. IQ is merely a standard score which places an individual in reference to the scores of others within his age group.

i. test. A test designed to determine the intelligence of an individual. A number of tests have been devised including the Binet t., Babcock-Levy t.,

IQ	Classification
Above 140	"Near" genius or genius.
120-140	Very superior intelligence.
110-120	Superior intelligence.
90-110	Normal, or average, intelligence.
80-90	Dullness.
70-80	Border-line deficiency.
Below 70	Definite mental retardation.

Stanford-Binet t., and others. Tests are used as a basis for determining intelligence quotient (IQ), *q.v.*

intem'perance [L. *in,* not, + *temporāre,* to moderate]. Excess in the use of anything; lack of moderation.

inten'sifying [L. *intensus,* intense, + *facere,* to make]. Making intense.

i. screen. A thin sheet of celluloid or other substance coated with a finely divided substance which fluoresces under the influence of roentgen rays and is intended to be used in close contact with the emulsion of a photographic plate or film for the purpose of reinforcing the image. A fluorescent screen.

inten'simeter [" + G. *metron,* measure]. An instrument, often a selenium cell or ionization chamber, designed to measure the intensity of a beam to about 14,000 Angström units.

intensity (in-ten'sĭ-tĭ) [L. *intensus,* tight, intense]. 1. The degree or extent of activity, strength, force, electric current, etc. 2. The state or quality of being intense.

i. of roentgen rays. The attribute of a beam of roentgen rays which determines the rate of ionization of air at a given point, under the conditions stipulated in the definition of roentgen. It is expressed in roentgens per unit of time. SEE: *rays.*

intensive (in-ten'siv) [L. *intensus,* intense]. Rel. to or marked by intensity.

intention (ĭn-tĕn'shŭn) [L. *intensiō,* a stretching]. 1. A natural process of healing. 2. Goal or purpose.

i., first. Healing without granulation or suppuration.

i., second. Healing by adhesion of two granulated surfaces with suppuration.

i., third. Healing of an ulcer, wound, or cavity by filling by granulation and followed by cicatrization. SEE: *first i., granulation, resolution, second i., third i.*

i. tremor. One exhibited or intensified when attempting coordinated movements.

inter- [L.]. Prefix: In the midst, between.

interartic'ular [L. *inter,* between, + *articulus,* joint]. 1. Bet. two joints. 2. Situated bet. two articulating surfaces.

interatrial (ĭn"ter-at'rĭ-ăl) [" + *atrium,* hall]. Located bet. the atria of the heart. SYN: *interauricular.*

interauricular (in"ter-aw-rik'u-lar) [" + *auricula,* auricle]. 1. Situated bet. the auricles or pinnae. 2. Interatrial.

in'terbrain [" + A. S. *braegan,* brain]. The hinder original part of the forebrain including the *thalamus,* pineal body (*epithalamus*) and geniculate bodies (*metathalamus*). SYN: *diencephalon; thalamencephalon.*

intercadence (in-ter-ka'dens) [" + *cadere,* to fall]. A supernumerary pulse wave bet. two regular beats.

intercalary (in-ter'kal-a-rĭ) [" + *calāre,* to call]. 1. Inserted between as something in addition; extraneous. 2. Pert. to an upstroke on a pulse tracing which comes bet. two pulse beats, intercalated.

intercalated (in-ter'kal-at-ed) [L. *inter,* between, + *calāre,* to call]. 1. Inserted between as something in addition; extraneous. 2. Pert. to an upstroke on a pulse tracing which comes between two pulse beats, intercalary.

i. disks. SEE: *disk, intercalated.*

i. ducts. Short, narrow ducts which lie between secretory ducts and the terminal alveoli in the parotid and submaxillary glands and the pancreas.

intercarot'ic [" + G. *karoun,* to stupefy]. Bet. the ext. and int. carotid arteries.

in"tercartilag'inous [" + *cartilāgō,* cartilage]. Connecting or bet. cartilages.

intercellular (in-ter-sel'-u-lar) [" + *cellula,* little cell]. Bet. the cells of a structure.

interchondral (in-ter-kon'dral) [" + G. *chondros,* cartilage]. Bet. cartilages. SYN: *intercartilaginous.*

intercilium (in-ter-sil'ĭ-um) [" + *cilium,* eyelid]. The space bet. the eyebrows. SYN: *glabella.*

interclavic'ular [" + *clavicula,* little key]. Bet. the clavicles.

intercolumnar (in-ter-kŏ-lum'nar) [" + *columna,* column]. Bet. columns.

i. fascia. A membrane bet. pillars of the abdominal ring, enclosing the spermatic cord.

i. fibers. Intercrural fibers.

intercon'dylar, intercon'dyloid, intercon'dylous [" + G. *kondylos,* condyle]. Bet. two condyles (the rounded eminence at the articular end of a bone).

intercos'tal [" + *costa,* rib]. Bet. the ribs.

i. muscles, external. Outer layer of muscles between the ribs, originating on the lower margin of each rib, being inserted on the upper margin of the next rib. They elevate the ribs, enlarging the thorax thus functioning in inspiration. SEE: Fig. p. I-28.

i. muscles, internal. Those bet. the ribs lying beneath the external intercostals; function uncertain.

intercostobrachial (in"ter-kos"tō-brā'kē-al). Pertaining to the intercostal space and the arm, as the posterior lateral branch of the second intercostal nerve supplying the skin of the arm, or a similar branch of the third intercostal nerve. Formerly called intercostohumeralis.

intercos"tohumera'lis. Term formerly used for intercostobrachial, *q.v.*

in'tercourse [" + *cursus,* from *currere,* to run]. Social contacts.

sexual i. The sexual act. SYN: *coitus.*

intercris'tal [" + *crista,* crest]. Bet. two crests of a bone, organ, or process.

intercrural (ĭn"ter-kru'răl) [L. *inter,* between, + *crus, crur-,* limb]. Bet. two crura.

intercur'rent [" + *currere,* to run]. 1. Intervening. 2. Pert. to a disease attacking a patient with another malady.

intercusp'ing. The fitting together of the surfaces of opposing teeth.

interden'tal [" + *dens, dent-,* tooth]. Bet. the teeth.

interdentium (in-ter-den'shĭ-um) [" + *dens, dent-,* tooth]. The space bet. any two contiguous teeth.

interdigita'tion [" + *digitus,* fingers]. 1. Interlocking of toothed or fingerlike processes. 2. Processes so interlocked.

interfascic'ular (in-ter-fas-ik'u-lar) [" + *fasciculus,* bundle]. Bet. fasciculi.

interfem'oral (in-ter-fem'or-ăl) [" + *femoralis,* pert. to the thigh]. Between the thighs.

interference. Clashing or colliding.

i. of impulses. Condition in which two excitation waves, upon approaching each other and meeting in any part of the heart, are mutually extinguished.

interferon (in-ter-fēr'on). A protein or proteins formed when cells are exposed to viruses. Noninfected cells exposed to interferon are protected against viral infection.

interfib'rillar, interfib'rillary [" + *fibrilla,* a small fiber]. Between fibrils.

interfi'lar [" + *filum,* thread]. Between the fibrils of a reticulum.

i. mass. The fluid portion of the protoplasm.

interganglion'ic [" + *gagglion*, a swelling]. Bet. ganglions.

interglob'ular [" + *globulus*, globule]. Bet. globules.

i. spaces. Gaps in dentin due to failure of calcification. SYN: *Czermak's spaces.*

interlo'bar [" + *lobus*, lobe]. Between lobes.

interlobi'tis [" + " + G. *-ītis*, inflammation]. Inflammation of the pleura separating the pulmonary lobes.

interlob'ular [" + *lobulus*, lobule]. Between lobules of an organ.

i. emphysema. Air bet. the lobes of the lung.

intermar'riage [" + *maritāre*, to marry]. 1. Marriage bet. persons of two different races or tribes. SYN: *miscegenation.* 2. Marriage bet. blood relations.

intermax'illary [L. *inter*, between, + *maxilla*, jaw]. Between two maxillae.

intermediary (in-ter-me'dĭ-a-rĭ) [" + *mediāre*, to divide]. 1. Situated between two bodies. 2. Occurring between two periods of time.

i. amputation. One performed during the stage of inflammatory fever.

i. body. An amboceptor; an immune body. SEE: *Ehrlich's side-chain theory.*

i. metabolism. The series of intermediate compounds formed during digestion before the final excretion or oxidation products are formed or eliminated from the body.

intermedin (in-ter-mē'din) [" + *mediāre*, to divide]. Name formerly given to melanocyte-stimulating hormone (MSH).

intermediolat'eral [" + " + *latus, later-*, side]. Intermediate but not central.

i. tract of spinal cord. A lateral tract bet. the dorsal and ventral horns.

intermeningeal (in-ter-men-in'je-al) [" + *mēnigx*, membrane]. Between the meninges.

intermenstrual. Between the menses, or menstrual periods.

intermis'sion [" + *missus;* from *mittere*, to send]. 1. Interval between two paroxysms of a disease. 2. Temporary cessation of symptoms.

intermit'tence [" + *mittere*, to send]. 1. Condition marked by intermissions in the course of a disease or of a process. 2. A loss of one or more pulse beats.

intermittent (in-ter-mit'ent) [" + *mittere*, to send]. Ceasing at intervals.

i. fever. One in which there is complete absence of symptoms bet. paroxysms of the fever. SEE: *malaria; undulant fever; remittent fever for Illus.*

i. pulse. One in which a beat is dropped at intervals.

i. temperature. One that reaches the normal line at intervals during the course of a fever.

intermus'cular [" + *musculus*, muscle]. Between muscles.

intern (in'tern) [L. *internus*, within]. Physician or surgeon on a hospital staff, usually a recent graduate receiving a year of postgraduate training prior to being eligible to be licensed to practice medicine. Cf. *externe.*

inter'nal [L. *internus*, within]. Within the body. Within or on the inside; enclosed, inward. Opp. of external.

i. bleeding. Internal hemorrhage, *q.v.*

i. capsule. SEE: *capsule, brain (internal of).*

i. ear. The vestibule, semicircular canals, and cochlea.

i. injury. Any injury not visible from the outside, as injury to the organs occupying the thoracic, abdominal, or cranial cavities.

SYM: Vary with structures involved. Ordinarily, profound shock, patient is pale, cold, perspiring freely with an anxious expression; may be semicomatose. Pain usually intense at first, and may continue, or gradually diminish as patient grows worse.

In severe injuries, pain may not be manifested. The pulse is very feeble, fast, often irregular. Patient may be very restless, breathless, and usually has shallow respiration.

F. A. TREATMENT: Above all, patient should be kept very quiet and comfortably warm but not hot. Do not give anything by mouth, and do not give stimulants, as they may exaggerate bleeding. Transportation must be done very cautiously. If patient is in shock shoulders should be lowered and extremities elevated at least 45°. This may be done by placing patient on a chair, box, or a folded coat. Most of these patients require operation.

i. medicine. That branch of medicine that deals with diseases not usually treated surgically.

i. secretion. That of the ductless glands which, entering the blood stream, activates other glands and organs. SYN: *hormones, q.v.*

SEE: *secretion, ductless gland, endocrine.*

international unit. One defined and adopted by the International Conference for Unification of Formulae.

international x-ray unit of intensity. SEE: *unit, x-radiation.*

interne (in'tern) [L. *internus*, within]. Intern, *q.v.*

intern'ist [L. *internus*, within]. One who specializes in internal medicine, not a surgeon.

in'ternode [L. *inter*, between, + *nodus*, node]. Space between adjacent nodes.

internun'cial [" + *nuncius*, messenger]. Acting as a connecting medium.

i. neuron. One between two other neurons in a neural pathway.

interocep'tive [L. *inter*, within, + *ceptus:* from *capere*, to take]. In nerve physiology, concerned with sensations arising within the body itself, as distinguished from those (*i.e.*, sight) arising outside the body.

interoceptor (in"tĕr-ō-sĕp'tor) [" + *ceptus;* from *capere*, to take]. A receptor activated by stimuli within the body.

i., general. An end organ carrying sensations of hunger, thirst, visceral pain, nausea, sexual and circulatory sensations.

i., special. One for smell and taste.

interofec'tive [" + *affectus;* from *afficere*, to influence]. 1. Pert. to that which concerns the interior of an organism. 2. Cannon's term concerning the autonomic nervous system.

in"tero-infe'rior. Pert. to an inward and downward position.

interol'ivary [L. *inter*, between, + *oliva*, olive]. Between the olivary bodies.

interor'bital [" + *orbita*, orbit]. Between the orbits.

inteross'eous [" + *os*, bone]. Situated or occurring bet. bones, as some muscles and ligaments.

interosseus (in"ter-os'ē-us) (pl. *interossei*). A muscle lying between bones.

interpalpebral (in-ter-pal'pe-bral) [" + *palpebra*, eyelid]. Between the eyelids.

interpari'etal [" + *paries, pariet-*, wall]. 1. Between walls. 2. Between the parietal bones. 3. Between the parietal lobes of the cerebrum.

i. bone. SYN: *inca bone; incarial bone.*

i. suture. Sagittal suture.

interparoxys'mal [" + G. *paroxysmos,* spasm]. Between paroxysms.

interpeduncular (in"ter-pē-dunk'ū-lar) [" + *pedunculus,* peduncle]. Between peduncles.

interphalangeal (in"ter-fă-lan'jē-ăl) [" + *phalagx,* phalanx]. In a joint between two phalanges.

interpolar (in"ter-po'lar) [" + *polus,* pole]. Between two poles.

i. path. Path of galvanic current through tissues between poles.

interprox'imal [" + *proximus,* next]. Between two adjoining surfaces.

i. space. Triangular space between two adjacent teeth.

interpu'bic [" + *pubes,* pubes]. Between the pubic bones.

interpu'pillary [" + *pupula,* pupil]. Between the pupils.

i. distance. Distance between centers of the two pupils of the eyes.

interre'nal [" + *rēn,* kidney]. Between the kidneys.

interrupt'er [" + *ruptus,* broken]. A device, usually automatic, for making and breaking (closing and opening alternately) an electric circuit. Such a device is ordinarily employed in low voltage, direct current circuits.

interscapil'ium [" + *scapula,* shoulder blade]. Area between the shoulders or scapulae. SYN: *interscapulum.*

interscap'ular [" + *scapula,* shoulder blade]. Between the scapulae.

i. reflex. Scapular muscular contraction following percussion or stimulus between the scapulae.

interscap'ulum [" + *scapula,* shoulder blade]. Section of back between shoulder blades. SYN: *interscapilium.*

intersex. An individual having both male and female characteristics.

in'terspace. The space between two similar parts, as between two ribs.

inter'stice [L. *interstitium,* a thing standing bet.]. A space or gap in a tissue or structure of an organ.

interstitial (in-ter-stish'al) [L. *interstitium,* thing standing bet.]. 1. Placed or lying between; pert. to interstices or spaces. 2. Occupying space between essential parts of an organ which comprises its proper tissue; opp. to *parenchymatous.*

i. cells of testes. Cells of Leydig, located in groups between the seminiferous tubules. They produce the internal secretion (testosterone) of the testes.

intersystole (in-ter-sĭs'tō-lē) [L. *inter,* bet., + G. *systolē,* contraction]. The period between the end of the atrial systole and the commencement of the ventricular systole.

intertrigo (in"ter-trī'gō) [" + *tritum;* from *terere,* to rub]. A superficial dermatitis in the folds of the skin. SEE: *erythema intertrigo.* SYN: *paratrimma.*

intertrochanteric (in"ter-trō-kăn-tĕr'ĭk) [" + G. *trochantēr,* runner]. Between the femur's two trochanters.

i. line. The ridge between the greater and lesser trochanters of femur on posterior aspect of the bone.

intertubular (in-ter-tu'bū-lar) [" + *tubulus,* tubule]. Between or among tubules.

interureteral (in"ter-ū-rē'tĕr-al) [" + G. *ourētēr,* ureter]. Between the two ureters. SYN: *interureteric.*

interureteric (in"ter-u-re-ter'ik) [" + G. *ourētēr,* ureter]. Between the ureters. SYN: *interureteral.*

intervaginal (in-ter-vaj'in-al) [" + *vagina* sheath]. 1. Between sheaths. 2. Within the vagina.

interval (in'ter-val) [" + *vallum,* a breastwork]. 1. The space or time between two objects or periods. 2. Break in the course of a disease or between paroxysms.

i., a-c., atriocarotid i., auriculocarotid i. In a venous pulse-tracing, the interval between onset of the presystolic wave (a) and the systolic (c) wave. It indicates the time required for impulses to travel from S-A node to ventricle, normally about 0.2 sec.

i., A-V. That between beginning of atrial systole and ventricular systole measured in man from an electrocardiogram.

i., c-a., cardio-arterial i. The time between apex beat and radial pulsation.

i., focal. Distance between anterior and posterior focal point of the eyes.

i., isometric. Bet. onset of ventricular systole and opening of the semilunar valves. SYN: *presphygmic, q.v.*

i., lucid. Brief remission of symptoms in a psychosis.

i., passive. The rest period of the heart.

i., postsphygmic. I. bet. closure of semilunar valves and opening of semilunar valves and opening of atrioventricular valves.

i., presphygmic. Brief period bet. the ventricular systole and opening of the semilunar valves.

i., QRST. The ventricular complex of the electrocardiogram.

intervascular (ĭn-tĕr-vas'kū-lar) [" + *vasculum,* a vessel]. Situated between blood vessels.

interventric'ular [" + *ventriculum,* a small cavity]. Between the ventricles.

interver'tebral [" + *vertebra,* joint]. Situated between two adjacent vertebrae.

i. disk. Broad and flattened disk of fibrocartilage between the bodies of vertebrae, as in symphysis, *q.v.*

intes'tinal [L. *intestinum,* intestine]. Pertaining to the intestines.

i. digestion. The mixture of food and secretions described under duodenal* digestion moves on rapidly through the jejunum and is then detained for some hours in the lone remaining part of the small intestine, the ileum.

i. d., chemical. The hydrolysis of starches and sugars to monosaccharides is accomplished by enzymes provided by the pancreatic and intestinal juices. The fats are emulsified by the bile, and then hydrolyzed by the action of the lipase (steapsin) of the pancreatic juice.

The digestion of proteins, begun in the stomach by the pepsin, is carried on by the trypsin of the pancreatic juice, by the erepsin (mixture of enzymes) of the intestinal juice. The result is a rather fluid mixture of food and secretions, stained with bile. The products of the chemical action are monosaccharides, fatty acids, glycerol, and amino acids, and they are actively absorbed.

i. d., mechanical. Both digestion and absorption are accelerated by a continual mixing and moving of the intestinal contents. A column of chyme may be broken into segments by contractions of the circular intestinal musculature; the segments may reunite and then again divide at the same point or elsewhere (rhythmic segmentation). A column may suddenly move several cm., remain stationary for a time, and then either return or advance.

The area of the absorbing surface is increased by the presence of permanent circular folds in the intestine; the entire surface is studded with fine villi which stud the folds as well as the spaces bet. them. At the end of the ileum the advance of the chyme is halted by the ileocolic sphincter. Peristalsis driving chyme towards it thus results in a churning effect. The sphincter opens at intervals to allow chyme to spurt into the first section of the large intestine, the colon. For ensuing phenomena, SEE: *colon, digestion in the;* also *intestines.*

i. flora. Bacteria in intestines of which *Bacillus acidophilus* is the most favorable.

At birth no bacteria are present in the intestines but bacteria are found there very shortly after birth. Favorable bacteria may protect the body from invasion by unfavorable ones, which cannot thrive in an acid condition.

i. gases. Carbon dioxide, hydrogen, methane, methylmercaptan, and sulfurated hydrogen.

i. juice. A secretion of the crypts of Lieberkühn. The secretion is induced by mechanical stimulation of the mucosa which brings about secretion through local reflexes in Meissmer's plexus. A chemical substance, secretin, produced by the intestinal mucosa, also induces secretion of water and bicarbonate.

COMP. I. juice varies in composition and consistency. It is usually cloudy in appearance due to presence of cells and mucus. Its reaction is alkaline (*p*H 7.0-8.5) due to presence of sodium bicarbonate. It contains the following enzymes: an enzyme complex consisting of many peptidases, formerly considered as a single enzyme (*erepsin*), a weak *lipase, maltase, sucrase* (*invertase*), *lactase.* SEE: *intestinal digestion.*

i. obstruction. *Acute*: Small intestine usually involved. Due to intussusception, strangulation, volvulus (twists), foreign bodies, knots, adhesions, tumors, stricture, and gallstones in intestines. It may produce a high-pitched tinkle or no sound at all.

SYM: Pain localized and intense. Temperature subnormal or normal, vomiting, constipation and distention of abdomen.

Chronic: Involves large intestine. Due to stricture, inflammation, abscesses, tumors, fecal matter or chronic peritonitis, and gallstones may obstruct feces. Gradual constipation, pain becoming more severe in few days followed by acute symptoms.

i. putrefaction. The chemical changes by bacteria in the intestine, forming the following: indole, skatole, paracresol, phenol, phenylpropionic acid, phenylacetic acid, paraoxyphenylacetic acid, hydroparacumaric acid, fatty acids, carbon dioxide, hydrogen, methane, methylmercaptan, and sulfurated hydrogen.

i. reflex. Intestinal contraction and relaxation above a portion of bowel which is stimulated.

intestine (ĭn-tĕs′tĭn) [L. *intestinum*]. The alimentary canal extending from the pylorus to the anus.

It is approximately 24 feet long, and is divided into the small intestine and the large intestine or colon.

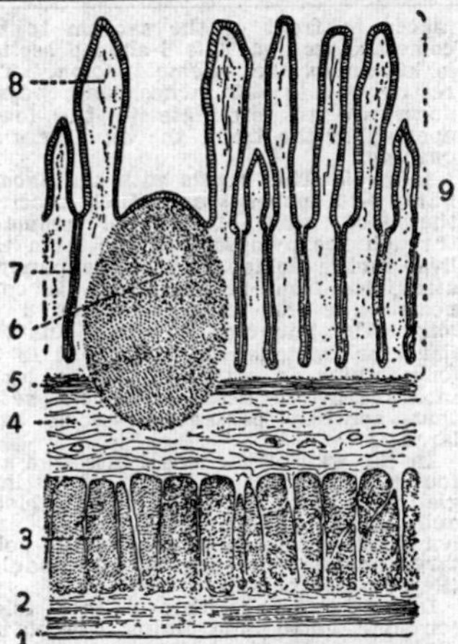

LONGITUDINAL SECTION OF SMALL INTESTINE

1. Serous coat. 2. Longitudinal muscular fibers. 3. Circular muscular fibers. 4. Submucosa. 5. Muscularis mucosae. 6. Solitary nodule. 7. Intestinal gland. 8. Villus. 9. Mucosa.

The total surface of the inside of the intestine is approximately 100 times greater than the surface of the body.

PALPATION OF THE I.: *Fecal accumulations.* Feel like tumor but hard and resistant; but if one finger be pressed steadily upon them for 1 or 2 minutes will at last indent like a large snowball; most frequently collect in descending colon.

PERCUSSION OF I.: In normal condition large intestine furnishes a more amphoric percussion sound than the stomach. When filled with liquid or solid accumulations, the situation of these accumulations can be marked out on the surface by dullness on percussion. As these accumulations most frequently collect in the descending colon the percussion sound over this portion is usually less resonant than over the ascending or transverse colon.

i., large. The large intestine extends from the ileum to the anus, and consists of cecum with vermiform appendix, colon, and rectum.

Mucous coat resembles that of small i., *q.v.*, although glands are smaller.

The beginning of the large intestine is the *cecum,* a pouch situated on right side, about 2x3 inches, adjoining the ascending colon.

Attached to the cecum is the *vermiform appendix,* about 3-4 inches long, function unknown.

The colon avrages 4 to 5 ft. in length. The first portion of *ascending colon* extends from the cecum to the under surface of the liver where it turns to the left as the *transverse colon.* Its bend is the right colic or hepatic flexure. The transverse colon passes horizontally to the left to the region of the spleen where it turns downward as the *descending colon.* This turn is the *splenic flexure.* The descending colon continues downward on the left side of the abdomen until it reaches the pelvic brim and curves like the letter **S** and is placed in front of the sacrum to become the *rectum.* This S-shaped section is known as the *"sigmoid colon."* The rectum, about 4-5 inches long, passes downward to terminate in the lower opening of the tract, the *anus* or *anal opening.*

i., small. This begins with the *duodenum,* 8-10 inches long, which receives the food mass from the stomach through the pylorus, the bile from the liver and gallbladder, and the pancreatic juice from the pancreas. It connects with the *jejunum,* about 8 ft. long. The jejunum, in turn, joins the *ileum* or twisted intestine, about 12 ft. long, which is attached to the large intestine by the *ileocecal* or *colic valve* that controls passage of food into large i.

In the wall of the small intestine are found Brunner's glands, intestinal glands (crypts of Lieberkühn), blood and lymph vessels (lacteals), and lymphatic tissue in the form of solitary nodules or aggregated nodules (Peyer's patches).

Inner surface is thrown into folds (circular folds) and lining the entire surface are minute fingerlike *villi* through which the products of digestion (simple sugars, amino acids, and fatty acids and glycerol) are absorbed. Villi range from 1.48 to ⅛ of an inch in length.

intestinum (ĭn-tĕs-tī'nŭm) [L.]. Intestine.

i. crassum [NA]. The large intestine.

i. rectum. The rectum.

i. tenue [NA]. The small intestine.

in'tima [L. innermost]. Innermost coat of a structure, as a blood vessel. Syn: *tunica intima.*

intimal (in'tim-al) [L. *intima,* innermost]. Pert. to the inner coat of a blood vessel, the intima.

intimi'tis [" + G. *-itis,* inflammation]. Inflammation of an intima.

intol'erance [L. *in,* not, + *tolerāre,* to bear.] Inability to endure or incapacity for bearing, as pain, or the effects of a drug or other substance.

intoxicant. An agent which produces intoxication.

intoxica'tion [" + G. *toxikon,* poison]. 1. State of being intoxicated, esp. of being poisoned by a drug or toxic substance. 2. Intoxicated from overindulgence in alcoholic beverages. 3. Drunk. See: *alcoholism, autointoxication.*

The determination of alcohol content is frequently of value in the diagnosis of intoxication from alcohol, especially in differentiating other disorders. Normally the alcohol content of body tissues and fluids is negligible. Upon ingestion of alcoholic fluids the alcohol rapidly increases in the blood and is excreted in the urine. The urine concentration will generally be slightly less than that of the blood. To be representative the tests must be made immediately. Results are expressed as "milligrams of alcohol per cubic ml. of blood or urine."

i., acid. I. resulting from acidosis.

i., alkaline. I. resulting from alkalosis.

i., intestinal. Autointoxication.

i., water. I. resulting from excessive intake or undue retention of water.

intra- [L.]. Prefix meaning *within.*

in"tra-abdom'inal [L. *intra,* within, + *abdominalis,* pert. to abdomen]. Within the abdomen.

i. pressure. Pressure within the abdomen.

intra-arte'rial [" + G. *artēria,* artery]. Within the artery(ies).

intra-articular (in-tră-ar-tĭk'ū-lar) [" + *articulus,* joint]. Within a joint.

intra-atrial. Within the atrium or atria of the heart.

intracap'sular [" + *capsula,* little box]. Within a capsule.

i. fracture. One occurring within the capsule of a joint.

intracartilaginous (in"tra-kar-tĭ-laj'in-us) [" + *cartilagō,* gristle]. Within a cartilage or cartilaginous tissue.

intracellular (in-tra-sel'ū-lar) [" + *cellula,* cell]. Within cells.

intracra'nial [" + G. *kranion,* skull]. Within the cranium or skull.

intracuta'neous [" + *cutis,* skin]. Within the substance of the skin. Syn: *intradermal.*

i. reaction. One following injection of tuberculin into the skin.

intracys'tic [" + G. *kystis,* bladder]. Inside a bladder or cyst.

intrad (in'trad) [L. *intra,* within]. Inwardly; toward the inner part.

intrader'mal [" + G. *derma,* skin]. Within the substance of the skin. Syn: *intracutaneous.*

intradermoreaction (in"tră-derm"ō-rē-ak'shun) [" + " L. *rē,* back, + *actus;* from *actere,* to do]. One resulting from the injection of a reagent into substance of the skin. Syn: *intracutaneous reaction.*

intraduct (in'tră-dukt) [" + *ductus,* a canal]. Inside a duct

in"traduode'nal [" + *duodeni,* twelve]. Within the duodenum.

intradu'ral [" + *durus,* hard]. Within or enclosed by the dura mater.

intrafeb'rile [" + *febris,* fever] During the febrile stage.

intrafi'lar [" + *filum,* thread]. Within a network.

i. mass. The fluid portion of protoplasm. Syn: *hyaloplasm, paramitome, paraplasm.*

intragas'tric. Within the stomach.

intragem'mal. Within a bud or the expanded ending of a nerve, as a taste bud.

intraglan'dular. Within a gland.

intraintes'tinal. Within the intestine.

intraligamen'tary [" + *ligamentum,* a binding]. Within the leaves of a ligament.

Usually used in referring to fibroid tumors or cysts of the ovary that have grown within the broad ligament.

intraligamentous (in"tra-lig-ă-men'tus) [" + *ligamentum,* a binding]. Within a ligament.

intralo'bar. Within a lobe.

intralob'ular. Within a lobule.

intraloc'ular [" + *loculus,* a cavity]. Within the cavity of any structure.

intralum'bar [" + *lumbus,* a loin]. Within the lumbar region or portion of the spinal cord.

intraluminal (in-tră-lu'mĭ-nal) [" + *lumen, lumin-,* light]. Within interior of any tubular structure. Syn: *intratubal.*

intramastoiditis (in-tra-mas-toid-ī'tis) [" + G. *mastos,* breast, + *eidos,* form, + *-itis,* inflammation]. Inflammation of the antrum and mastoid process. Syn: *endomastoiditis.*

intramu'ral [" + *murus,* a wall]. Within the walls of a hollow organ or cavity.

intramus'cular [" + *musculus,* a muscle]. Within a muscle.

i. injection. Hypodermic injection of drugs into a muscle.

intranas'al. Within the nasal cavity.

intraoc'ular [" + *oculus,* eye]. Within the eyeball.

intraor'al. Within the mouth.

intraor'bital. Within the orbit.

intraosseous (in-tra-os'ē-us). Within the bone substance.

intraparietal (in-tra-pă-ri'ĕ-tal) [" + *pariēs, pariet-,* wall]. 1. Within the parietal lobe of the cerebrum. 2. Intramural.

intraperitone'al [" + G. *peritonaion,* peritoneum]. Within the peritoneal cavity.

intrapleu'ral [" + G. *pleura,* rib]. Within the pleural cavity.

intrapon'tine [" + *pons, pont-,* bridge]. Within the *pons Varolii.*

intrapsychic, intrapsychical (ĭn-tra-sī'kĭk, kĭ-kăl) [L. *intra,* within, + G. *psychē,* mind]. Having a mental origin or basis, such as conflicts and complexes.

intrapul'monary [" + *pulmō, pulmon-,* lung]. Within the lung cavity.

intrapyretic (in-tră-pi-ret'ik) [" + G. *pyretos,* fever]. During the period of fever. SYN: *intrafebrile.*

intraspi'nal [" + *spina,* spine]. 1. Ensheathed, within a sheath. 2. Within the spinal canal. SYN: *intrathecal.*

intrathecal (in-tră-thē'kal) [" + G. *thēkē,* sheath]. Intraspinal; within spinal canal.

intrathoracic (in-tră-thō-ras'ĭk) [" + G. *thōrax, thorak-,* chest]. Within the thorax.

intratracheal (in"tră-trăk'ē-ăl) [" + G. *tracheia,* trachea]. Introduced into, or inside, the trachea.

i. anesthesia. A. administered through a catheter passed down the trachea.

in"tratu'bal [" + *tuba,* hollow tube]. Within a tube, esp. the fallopian tube.

in"tratympan'ic [" + G. *tympanon,* drum]. Within the tympanic cavity.

intrau'terine [" + *uterus,* womb]. Within the uterus.

intravasation (in-trav-ă-sa'shun) [" + *vas,* vessel]. Passage into the blood vessels of matter formed outside of them through traumatic or pathological lesions.

intravas'cular. Within blood vessels.

intravenous (in-tra-ve'nus) [L. *intra,* within, + *vena,* vein]. Within or into a vein. ABBR: I.V.

i. infusion. Injection into a vein of a solution to secure an immediate result as in hemorrhage, shock or collapse.

SOLUTIONS: Normal saline, Ringer's, glucose 5-10%, sodium bicarbonate 4%. Solutions should be at room temperature for infusion.

QUANTITY: 250-500 cc.

SITE: Median basilic or median cephalic vein.

Preparation same as for i. injection but a needle or cannula is used. The vein must be exposed if cannula is used. Introduction of solution should be very slow, usually from 60 drops per minute (using a 19-gauge needle) to 120 drops per minute (using a 26-gauge needle).

i. injection. Surface over skin is sterilized, tourniquet or bandage applied to middle of arm, the median cephalic or median basilic vein at front of elbow being used. Hypodermic needle is inserted in the vein, pointing upward. Pressure should be loosed before injection, which should be given very slowly.

i. medication. The injection of a sterile solution of a drug or an infusion into a vein.

i. treatment. This may consist of (*a*) intravenous injection or (*b*) intravenous infusion. The *injection* is usually known as the introduction of a small amount of solution into a vein with a hypodermic syringe. An *infusion* is usually known as the introduction of a solution in a larger quantity—250 to 500 cc. by means of a bottle connected to the needle by plastic or rubber tubing. The rate of infusion may be regulated by adjusting the number of drops per minute. Flow is usually by gravity but can be given under pressure.

CAUTION: I.V. infusions should be discontinued or infusion fluid replenished when the bottle being administered is depleted.

intraventricular (ĭn-tră-vĕn-trĭk'ū-lar) [" + *ventriculus,* ventricle]. Within a ventricle.

intravi'tal [" + *vita,* life]. During period of living.

i. stain. One which when introduced into a living organism is taken up by living cells.

in'tra vi'tam [L.]. During life.

intravitelline (ĭn-tră-vī-tel'ĭn). Within the vitelline or yolk.

intrin'sic [L. *intrinsicus,* on the inside]. Located entirely within or pertaining exclusively to a part.

i. factor. A substance prepared from animal intestines which, in humans, increases absorption of vitamin B complex.

i. muscles. Those which have their origin and insertion entirely within a structure, as the intrinsic muscles of the tongue, larynx, or eye.

intro- [L.]. Prefix meaning *in* or *into.*

introdu'cer [L. *intrō,* into, + *ducere,* to lead]. Device for controlling, directing and placing an intubation tube within the trachea. SYN: *intubator.*

introflexion (ĭn-trō-flĕx'shŭn). A bending inward.

introitus (in-tro'it-us) [" + *īre,* to go]. An opening or entrance into a canal or cavity, as the abdomen or vagina.

i. canalis sacralis. Terminal opening of spinal canal at end of sacrum.

i. laryngis. Upper opening of larynx.

i. vaginae. Ext. orifice of vagina.

introjec'tion [" + *jectus;* from *jacere,* to throw]. PSY: Identification of the self with another, or with some object, the victim assuming the supposed feelings of the other personality.

intromission (in-tro-mish'un) [" + *missus;* from *mittere,* to send]. An insertion or placing of one part into another.

intromittent (in-tro-mit'ent) [" + *mittere,* to send]. Conveying or injecting into a cavity or body.

introspec'tion. Looking within, esp. examination of one's own mind.

introsusception (in-tro-sus-sep'shun) [" + *suscipere,* to receive]. Intussusception, *q.v.*

introversion (in-tro-ver'shun) [" + *versiō,* a turning]. 1. Turning inside out of a part or organ. 2. PSY: The condition of an introvert, *q.v.* Preoccupation with one's self.

in'trovert [" + *vertare,* to turn]. 1. PSY: A personality reaction type characterized by the withdrawal from reality, fantasy formation, and stress on the subjective side of life adjustments, seen pathologically in extreme form in schizophrenia. OPP: *extrovert, q.v.*

intubate (ĭn'tū-bāt) [L. *in,* into, + *tuba,* a tube]. To insert a tube in a part, esp. the larynx. SYN: *invaginate.*

intubation (in-tū-bā'shun) [" + *tuba,* a tube]. Insertion of a tube into any hollow organ, as into the larynx through the glottis for entrance of air, or to dilate a stricture.

POSITION: Patient held upright in lap of assistant, head upon assistant's left shoulder, arms secured by wrapping sheet about patient's body or being grasped by elbows. Another assistant stands behind patient with hands firmly grasping the head and holding gag in place. Patient so held that body, neck and head are kept naturally in a straight line.

NP: Never leave patient alone, do not feed for two or three hours after intubation; nursing infants may go to breast, soft diet to others; keep on back with head and shoulders elevated to position of greatest comfort in breathing.

in'tubator [" + *tuba*, a tube]. Device used in inserting a tube into the larynx. SYN: *introducer*.

intumesce (in-tū-mes') [L. *intumēscere*, to swell up]. To enlarge or swell.

intumes'cence [L. *intumēscere*, to swell up]. A swelling or the process of enlarging. SYN: *tumefaction*.

intumescent (in-tu-mes'ent) [L. *intumēscere*, to swell up]. Swelling or becoming enlarged.

intussusception (in-tus-sus-sep'shun) [L. *intus*, within, + *suscipere*, to receive]. 1. Growth of cells by deposit of particles bet. those already existing. 2. Invagination.

The slipping of one part of an intestine into another part just below it. Noted chiefly in children—more common in males—usually ileocecal region.

PROG: Good, if surgery is performed immediately. High mortality rate if untreated within 24 hours. SEE: *ileus*.

intussuscep'tum [" + *suscipere*, to receive]. The inner segment of intestine which has been pushed into another segment.

intussuscipiens (in"tus-sus-sip'ĭ-ens) [" + *suscipiens*, receiving]. That portion of intestine which receives the intussusceptum.

inulase (ĭn'ū-lās). An enzyme that converts inulin into levulose.

in'ulin. 1. A polysaccharide found in plants. Yields levulose when hydrolyzed. 2. An agent used to study renal function.

inunction (in-unk'shun) [L. *in*, into, + *unguere*, to anoint]. Ointment or medicated substance rubbed into the skin, to secure a local or a more general or systemic effect.

inustion (in-us'chun) [" + *ustus;* from *urere*, to burn]. 1. To apply cautery. 2. Deep cauterization.

in u'tero [L.]. Within the uterus.

in vac'uo. Within a cavity or a space from which air has been exhausted.

invaginate (in-vaj'ĭn-āt) [L. *in*, into, + *vagina*, sheath]. 1. To ensheath. 2. To insert one part of a structure within a part of the same structure; intussusception. 3. In Emb., to grow in or from an ingrowth or inpocketing, esp. the ingrowth of the wall of the blastula which results in the formation of the gastrula.

invag'inated [" + *vagina*, sheath]. Enclosed in a sheath; ensheathed.

invagina'tion [" + *vagina*, sheath]. 1. The process of becoming ensheathed. SYN: *intussusception*. Opp. to *evagination*.

in'valid [L. *in*, not, + *validus*, strong]. 1. Not well; weak. 2. A sickly person.

invasin. Hyaluronidase, *q.v.*

inva'sion [L. *in*, into, + *vasus;* from *vadere*, to go]. 1. That period of a disease following entrance of infective organisms and preceding the appearance of symptoms. 2. The entrance of bacteria or other infectious organisms into the body and their distribution to the tissues.

invermina'tion [" + *vermināre*, to be wormy]. Infestation by intestinal worms. SYN: *helminthiasis*.

inverse-square law. The intensity of radiation at any distance is inversely proportional to the square of the distance bet. the irradiated surface and a point source.

inversion (in-ver'shun) [L. *in*, into, + *versiō*, a turning].. 1. Turning inside out of an organ, *e. g.*, the uterus. 2. In chemistry, the process of converting sucrose (which rotates the plane of polarized light to the right) into a mixture of dextrose and levulose, which mixture rotates the plane to the left. The resulting mixture is called invert sugar, and the enzyme which catalyzes this conversion is called invertase. SEE: *enzyme*.

i., psychic. Lack of harmony bet. the physical and psychic self or sex.

i., sexual. Deviation from normal sex relationship, diametrically opposite, *i. e.*, sexual interest in one of the same sex. SYN: *homosexuality*.

i., uterine. A condition in which the fundus of the uterus protrudes through the cervix, and in some cases through the vaginal introitus. May be acute or chronic, the acute type usually occurring immediately postpartum as a result of too vigorous placental expression or pulling on the placental cord when the placenta is fixed in the uterus. The chronic type is usually due to tumors of the fundus uteri that pull themselves and the uterus through the cervix.

in'vert [" + *vertere*, to turn]. 1. One who, or that which is opposite the normal. SEE: *homosexual*. 2. (ĭn-vert'). To turn inside out or upside down.

i. sugar. A term usually applied to a mixture of levulose and dextrose, formed by inversion of sucrose by enzyme, invertase. SEE: *carbohydrate, inversion, sugar*.

invertase (in-ver'tās) [" + *vertere*, to turn]. A sugar-splitting ferment or enzyme found in the intestinal juice. It causes the inversion of sugar. SYN: *invertin*.

inver'tebrate. Without a backbone; an animal lacking a spinal column.

invertin (in-ver'tin). An intestinal ferment which converts cane sugar into invert sugar. SYN: *invertase*.

invest'ing [L. *in*, in, + *vestīre*, to clothe]. Ensheathing, encircling with a sheath or coating, as tissue; surrounding.

invest'ment. A covering or sheath.

invet'erate [" + *vetus, veter-*, old]. Chronic; firmly seated, as a disease or a habit.

in vitro (in vī'trō) [L.]. In glass, as in a test tube.

in vivo (in vī'vō) [L.]. In the living body or organism.

in'volucre, involu'crum [L. *in*, in, + *volvere*, to wrap]. 1. A sheath or covering. 2. The covering of newly formed bone enveloping sequestrum in infection of bone.

invol'untary [L. *in*, not, + *voluntās*, will]. Independent of or even contrary to volition.

involution (in-vo-lu'shun) [L. *in*, into, + *volvere*, to roll]. 1. A turning or rolling inward. 2. The reduction in size of the uterus following delivery. 3. The retrogressive change in vital processes or in an organ after fulfilling their functions, such as that which follows the menopause. 4. A backward change. 5. Diminishing of an organ in vital power or in size. 6. In Bact., digression from the usual morphological type such as occurs in certain bacteria esp. when grown under unfavorable conditions; degeneration.

i. forms. Bacteria possessing abnormal and unusual forms.

i. of uterus. Return of uterus by absorption to normal size after childbirth.

i., senile. Shriveling of an organ or part from old age.

i., sexual. Cessation of menstrual function. Syn: *climacteric, menopause.**

involutional (ĭn-vō-lu'shŭn-ăl) [" + *volvere,* to roll]. Concerning involution or a turning inward.

i. melancholia. M. associated with senile and presenile types and manic-depressive group.

Occurs in the climacteric period, somewhat more frequently in women than in men. Stands alone in the classification of the psychoses.

Sym: 1. No evidence of physical disease. 2. Irregular menstruation or cessation. 3. Anemic. 4. Loss of weight. 5. Foul breath. 6. Expression of being miserable. 7. Temperature usually subnormal. 8. Diminished perspiration. 9. Sleeplessness. 10. Movements slow. 11. Dry and sallow skin. 12. Pulse feeble. 13. Flabby muscles. 14. Decreased urine. 15. Shallow respiration. 16. Constipation. 17. Digestion upset. 18. Large joints more or less rigid. 19. Delusions frequent. 20. May refuse food. 21. *May commit suicide.*

Forms of: *Simple*: 19, absent; 21, possible. *Delusional*: Very marked. *Agitated*: Reverse of No. 10, noisy expressions; 18, smaller joints continually in motion; picking at skin.

I. & O. Abbr. for *intake and output.*

Iodamoeba (ī-ŏd-ă-mēb'a). A genus of amebas in the class Sarcodina, found in the intestinal tract. Their cysts are peculiar in that they are irregular in shape, nucleus usually single, and they possess a vacuole filled with glycogen which stains brown in iodine.

I. butschlii. A small, sluggish ameba found in the large intestine of man. Also found in monkeys and pigs. It is usually nonpathogenic. Also called *Endolimax williamsi.*

iodide (ī'ō-dīd). A compound of iodine containing another radical or element, as potassium iodide.

iodine (i'o-dīn, i'o-dēn) [G. *iōdēs,* violet colored]. A nonmetallic element belonging to the halogen group. It is a black, crystalline substance having a density of 4.94. It melts at 113.7 and boils at 183° C., giving off a characteristic violet vapor. Symb: I. At. wt. 126.904; at. no. 53.

Functions: Development and functioning of the thyroid gland, formation of thyroxine and prevention of goiter; regulation of basal metabolic rate. The amount of iodine in the entire body averages 50 mg., of which one-third to one-fifth (10-15 mg.) is found in the thyroid. Butanol-extractable iodine content of the serum varies from 3.6 to 6.5 micrograms per 100 ml. Protein-bound serum iodine varies from 3.5 to 8.0 micrograms per 100 ml. Daily requirement for iodine is about 100 micrograms. A growing child or a pregnant woman needs several times as much as an adult. Those under emotional strain and the adolescents likewise need more iodine.

Sym. of Deficiency: Iodine deficiency in diet may lead to simple goiter characterized by thyroid enlargement and hypothyroidism. This may result in retardation of physical, sexual, and mental development in the young, a condition called *cretinism.*

Sources: In vegetables especially those growing near the seacoast, and in seafoods especially in liver of halibut and cod or the fish liver oils.

Poisoning: Sym: Brown stains on lips and mouth; burning pain in mouth, throat and stomach; vomiting (blue vomitus if stomach contained starches; otherwise yellow vomitus); bloody diarrhea.

F. A. Treatment: Give immediately by mouth a starch solution, barley water or gruel. Lavage with starch solution or 2% sodium thiosulfate solution. Morphine for pain and mild stimulants as indicated.

Incompatibilities: *alkaloids.*

Uses: Tincture of iodine (a 2 or 3% solution in alcohol) is used as a disinfectant and germicide. It is used as a preventative of simple goiter and, in the form of Lugol's solution, is invaluable in the treatment of exophthalmic goiter.

i., radioactive. I^{131}, an isotope of I with an atomic weight of 131. Used in diagnosis of thyroid disorders and in the treatment of toxic goiter and thyroid carcinoma.

i., tincture of. A 2% solution of iodine and sodium iodide in dilute alcohol.

iodinin (ī-ŏd'ĭ-nĭn). $C_{12}H_8O_4N_2$. A purple pigment having antibacterial activity effective against Staphylococcus aureus and Streptococcus hemolyticus.

iodism (ī'ō-dĭzm) [G. *iōdēs,* violet colored]. Condition induced by prolonged and excessive use of iodine or its compounds. See: *iodine poisoning.*

i'odize [G. *iōdēs,* violet colored]. To administer or impregnate with iodine.

i'odized [G. *iōdēs,* violet colored]. Impregnated with iodine.

i. salt. Salt containing 1 part sodium or potassium iodide to 10,000 parts of sodium chloride. See: *salt.*

io'doform [G. *iōdēs,* violet colored, + L. *forma,* form]. CHI_3. USP. Yellow crystals having a disagreeable odor. Produced by the action of iodine on acetone in the presence of an alkali. Syn: *triiodomethane.*

Action and Uses: A local analgesic and antiseptic used as a dressing for wounds or ulcers.

Incompatibilities: Mercuric oxide, calomel, silver nitrate, tannin, balsam of Peru.

io'doformism [" + " + G. *ismos,* state of]. Poisoning caused by iodoform.

iodophilia (ī"ō-dō-fĭl'ĭ-ă). Condition in which certain cells, when stained, esp. polymorphonuclear leukocytes, show a pronounced affinity for iodine, the cells acquiring a brownish-red color. Seen in pathologic conditions such as acute infections and anemia.

i., intracellular. I. in which color changes occur within the cells.

i., extracellular. I. in which substances in the plasma outside the cells are colored.

iodopyracet (i"o-do-pi'ră-set). A radiopaque medium used in intravenous pyelography and urography. Proprietary name: Diodrast.

iodother'apy [" + *therapeia*, treatment]. Use of iodine medication.

io'dum [L.]. Iodine.

i'on [G. *iōn*, going]. Molecular constituent, *i. e.*, one or more atoms, carrying an electric charge.

A particle carrying an electric charge, consisting of an atom or group of atoms into which the molecules of an electrolyte are divided; or one of the electrified particles into which the molecules of a gas are divided by ultraviolet rays, gamma rays, or x-rays, or by other ionizing agents.

Ions occur (1) in gases, esp. at low pressures, under the influence of strong electrical discharges, x-rays, and radium, and (2) in solutions of acids, bases, and salts. Such moving particles render the gas or solution capable of conducting the electric current, and on reaching the electrodes they are discharged.

Ions which carry *positive* charges and which consequently discharge at the negative electrode (cathode) are called cations; examples are the hydrogen in aqueous solutions of acids and the sodium in aqueous solutions of sodium chloride.

Ions which carry *negative* charges will appear at the positive electrode (anode) and are, therefore, called anions; an example is the chlorine in aqueous solutions of hydrochloric acid or of sodium chloride. Thus in the reaction

$$HCl \rightarrow H^+ + Cl^-$$

is represented the ionization of hydrogen chloride (hydrochloric acid) when dissolved in water; it means that when the electric current is passed through the solution hydrogen gas will appear as bubbles at the cathode, while chlorine will appear at the anode.

ion-exchange resins. Synthetic organic substances of high molecular weight. They replace certain negative or positive ions which they encounter in solutions. Have been used to replace sodium ions in cases of edema, or to reduce the acidity of gastric juice.

ion'ic [G. *iōn*, going]. Pert. to ions.

i. medication. The introduction of chemical ions into the superficial tissues for medicinal purposes by means of a direct current.

The basic rules are: Substances of like electric charge repel each other; unlike forms attract each other. Bases, metallic radicals, and alkaloids are electropositive and should be placed at the positive pole. Acids and acid radicals are electronegative and should be placed at the negative pole. Ex: Potassium iodide for the introduction of free iodine should be placed at the negative pole, cocaine hydrochloride for local anesthesia at the positive pole. SYN: *iontophoresis 2, q.v.*

ionization [G. *ion*, going]. The dissociation of compounds (acids, bases salts) into their constituent ions.

ionize [G. *ion*, going]. To separate into ions; ionization, *q.v.*

i"onom'eter [" + *metron*, measure]. An instrument consisting of an ionization chamber, an electroscope and an electric charging current designed to measure the amount of radiation used by roentgen rays or radium and to measure the intensity of the rays themselves.

ionotherapy (i"on-o-ther'ă-pĭ) [" + *therapeia*, treatment]. 1. Introduction of ions into the body. SYN: *iontophoresis.* 2. [G. *ion*, violet]. Treatment of disease with violet rays.

iontophoresis (i-on"to-fo-re'sis) [" + *phorein*, to carry]. 1. Process of electrical current traveling through salt solution causing migration of metal ion to negative pole and radical ion to positive pole. 2. Introduction of various ions into tissues through the skin by means of electricity. SYN: *ionic medication.*

iontoquantimeter (ī"ŏn-tō-kwon-tĭm'ĕ-tĕr) [" + L. *quantus*, how much, + G. *metron*, measure]. Instrument used to measure the amount of radiation used by, and the intensity of, roentgen rays. SYN: *ionometer; iontoradiometer.*

iontoradiometer (ī-on"tō-rā-dĭ-ŏm'ĕ-tĕr). [" + L. *radius*, ray, + G. *metron*, measure]. Instrument for measuring the amount and intensity of roentgen rays. SYN: *ionometer; iontoquantimeter.*

iontotherapy (i-on"to-ther'ă-pĭ) [" + *therapeia*, treatment]. Treatment by forcing ions into the body electrically.

IOP. Abbr. for intraocular pressure.

iophobia (ī-ō-fō'bĭ-ă) [G. *ios*, poison, rust, + *phobos*, fear]. 1. Fear of being poisoned. SYN: *toxicophobia.* 2. Fear of touching any rusty object.

iotacism (ī-ō'tă-sĭzm) [G. *iōta*, letter i]. Defective utterance marked by constant substitution of an ē sound (Greek iota) for other vowels.

iothiouracil sodium (i-o-thi-o-u'ră-sil). Sodium 5-iodo-2-thiouracil. An iodine derivative of thiouracil, it is used as an antithyroid drug.

ipecac (ip'ĕ-kak). USP. A dried root of a plant (*ipecacuanha*), grown in Brazil. It is the source of emetine.

ACTION AND USES: Specific against amebic dysentery. Also an expectorant, emetic, and diaphoretic.

IPPB. Abbr. for *intermittent positive pressure breathing.*

ipral sodium (ip'ral). A proprietary derivative of barbital; a persistent acting hypnotic.

ipsilateral, ipselateral (ip-sĭ-lat'er-al) [L. *ipse*, same, + *latus, later-*, side]. On the same side. Affecting the same side of the body.

Thus, when the right patellar tendon is tapped, a knee-jerk is observed on the same side. Said of findings (paralysis) appearing on same side of body as brain or spinal cord lesion producing them. Opp. of *crossed, contralateral.* SYN: *homolateral.*

IQ. Abbr. for *intelligence quotient, q.v.*

Ir. Chemical symbol for *iridium.*

I.R. Abbr. for *internal resistance* or when written *IR infrared.*

iral'gia [G. *iris*, iris, + *algos*, pain]. Pain felt in the iris. SYN: *iridalgia.*

irascible (ī-ras'ĭ-bl) [L. *irasci*, to be wrathful]. Marked by hot temper or ease of becoming angered.

iridadenosis (ĭr"ĭ-dăd-ĕ-nō'sĭs). A glandular affection of the iris.

iridal (ir'ĭd-al) [G. *iris, irid-*, iris]. Rel. to the iris.

iridalgia (ir-id-al'jĭ-ă) [" + *algos*, pain]. Pain felt in the iris. SYN: *iralgia.*

iridauxesis (ir"ĭ-dawk-se'sis) [" + *auxēsis*, increase]. Increase in thickness of the iris.

iridectome (ir-id-ek'tōm) [" + *tomē*, a cutting]. Instrument for cutting the iris in iridectomy.

iridectomesodialysis (ir-ĭ-dek"tō-mēs"ō-dĭ-al'ĭ-sĭs) [" + *ektomē*, excision, + *mesos*, middle, + *dialysis*, loosening]. Formation of an artificial pupil, by separating adhesions on inner margin of iris.

iridectomize (ir-id-ek'tō-mīz) [" + *ektomē,* excision]. To excise a portion of the iris.

iridec'tomy [" + *ektomē,* excision]. Surgical removal of a portion of iris.

i., optical. I. done for purpose of making an artificial pupil.

iridectropium (ir-ĭ-dek-trō'pĭ-um) [" + *ektropion,* eversion]. Partial eversion of the iris.

iride'mia [" + *aima,* blood]. Bleeding from the iris.

iridencleisis (ir"id-en-klī'sis) [" + *egklein,* to lock in]. Iris inclusion operation; the iris being incarcerated in the wound, thereby forming a fistula lined with iris tissue. Performed in glaucoma.

iridentropium (ir"ĭ-den-trō'pĭ-um) [" + *entropion,* inversion]. Partial inversion of the iris.

irideremia (ir-id-er-ē'mĭ-ă) [" + *erēmia,* lack]. Partial or total congenital absence of the iris. SYN: *aniridia.*

iridesis (i-rid'ĕ-sis [" + *desis,* a binding]. Formation of an iris artificially, by ligation. SYN: *iridodesis.*

iridic (ir-id'ik) [G. *iris, irid-,* iris]. Rel. to the iris. SYN: *iridal.*

iridium (ī-rĭd'ē-ŭm) [L. *iris,* rainbow]. A white, hard metallic element. SYMB: Ir. At. wt. 192.2; at. no. 77.

ir'ido- [G.]. Combining form, pert. to the iris.

iridoavulsion (ir"ĭ-do-av-ul'shun) [G. *iris, irid-,* iris, + L. *avulsiō,* tearing away]. Tearing away (avulsion) of the iris.

iridocapsulitis (ir"id-ō-kap-sŭ-lī'tis) [" + L. *capsula,* little box, + G. *-ītis,* inflammation]. Iritis with inflammation of the capsule of the lens.

iridocele (i-rid'o-sēl) [" + *kēlē,* hernia]. Protrusion of a portion of the iris through a defect in the cornea.

iridochorioiditis, iridochoroiditis (ir"ĭ-do-ko"ri-oy-di'tis) (ir"ĭ-do-ko-roy-di'tis) [" + *chorioeidēs,* skinlike]. Inflamed condition of both iris and choroid.

ir"idocolobo'ma [" + *kolobōma,* mutilation]. Congenital defect or fissure of the iris.

iridocyclectomy (ir"ĭ-dō-sī-klĕk'tō-mĭ) [" + *kyklos,* circle, + *ektomē,* excision]. Surgical removal of iris and ciliary body.

iridocyclitis (ir"id-ō-sī-klī'tis) [" + " + *-ītis,* inflammation]. Inflammation of iris and ciliary body.

iridocystectomy (ir"ĭ-dō-sĭs-tĕk'tō-mĭ) [" + *kystis,* a bag, + *ektomē,* excision]. An operation for removal of a cyst from the iris.

iridodesis (ĭr-ĭ-dod'ĕ-sĭs) [" + *desis,* a binding]. Ligature of part of iris to form an artificial one. SYN: *iridesis.*

ir"idodiagno'sis [" + *dia,* through, + *gnōsis,* knowledge]. Diagnosis of disease by changes in color and form of the iris.

iridodialysis (ir"id-ō-dī-al'ĭ-sĭs) [" + *dialysis,* loosening]. The separation of the outer margin of the iris from its ciliary attachment, usually due to trauma, forming an artificial pupil.

iridodila'tor [" + L. *dilatāre,* to dilate]. Substance causing dilatation of the pupil.

iridodonesis (ir"id-ō-dō-nē'sĭs) [" + *donēsis,* tremor]. Tremulousness of iris, seen in an aphakic eye or one with subluxated lens. SYN: *hippus.*

iridokeratitis (ir"ĭ-do-ker"ă-ti'tis). Inflammation of the iris and the cornea.

iridokinesis (ir"id-ō-kĭn-ē'sis) [" + *kinēsis,* motion]. The contracting and expanding movements of the iris.

iridoleptynsis (ĭr-ĭ-dō-lĕp-tĭn'sĭs). Thinning or atrophy of the iris.

iridology (ir-ĭ-dol'ō-jĭ) [" + *logos,* study]. The study of changes in the iris during course of a disease.

iridomalacia (ir"id-ō-ma-lā'sĭ-ă) [" + *malakia,* softening]. Softening of the iris.

iridomedialysis (ir"id-ō-mēd-ĭ-al'ĭ-sis) [" + L. *medius,* in middle, + G. *dialysis,* loosening]. Separation of inner marginal adhesions of iris. SYN: *iridomesodialysis.*

iridomesodialysis (ir"id-o-mes"o-dī-al'ĭ-sis) [" + *mesos,* middle, + *dialysis,* loosening]. Separation of adhesions around the inner border of iris. SYN: *iridomedialysis.*

iridomo'tor [" + L. *motor,* motion]. Rel. to movements of the iris.

iridon'cus [G. *iris,* iris, + *ogkos,* tumor]. Tumefaction of the iris or development of a tumor.

ir"idoparal'ysis [" + *paralysis,* a loosening]. Paralysis of the iris. SYN: *iridoplegia.*

iridoparelkysis (ir"ĭ-do-par-el'kĭ-sis) [" + *parelkysis,* protraction]. Dislocation of pupil due to prolapse of the iris.

iridoperiphacitis, iridoperiphakitis (ĭr"ĭ-do-per"ĭ-fă-si'tĭs, -per"ĭ-fă-ki'tĭs) [" + *peri,* around, + *phakos,* lens, + *ītis,* inflammation]. Inflammation of the iris and ant. portion of capsule of the lens.

iridoplegia (ir"id-ō-plē'jĭ-ă) [" + *plēgē,* stroke]. Paralysis of sphincter of iris.

i., accommodative. Inability of iris to contract when stimulated by accommodation.

i., complete. I. in which the iris fails to respond to any stimulation.

i., reflex. Absence of light reflex with retention of accommodation reflex (Argyll Robertson pupil, *q.v.*).

iridoptosis (ir-ĭ-dop-to'sis) [" + *ptōsis,* a dropping]. Prolapse of the iris.

iridorrhexis (ir-id-ō-rĕks'ĭs) [" + *rēxis,* rupture]. Rupture of or a tearing of the iris away from its attachment.

iridosclerotomy (ir"id-ō-sklē-rot'ō-mĭ) [" + *sklēros,* hard, + *tomē,* incision]. Piercing of the sclera and of the border of the iris.

iridosteresis (ir"ĭ-dō-stē-rē'sĭs) [" + *sterēsis,* loss]. Removal of the iris or a portion of it.

iridot'asis [" + *tasis,* a stretching]. Stretching the iris for glaucoma.

iridotomy (ir-ĭ-dot'ō-mĭ) [" + *tomē,* incision]. Incision of iris without excising a piece, done for the purpose of making a new aperture in the iris when the pupil is closed. SYN: *iritomy; irotomy; coretomy.*

Indicated in eyes that had been operated on for cataract but which have lost their sight through subsequent iridocyclitis. Also done in seclusio pupillae.

i'ris [G.]. The colored contractile membrane suspended between the lens and the cornea in the aqueous humor of the eye, separating the ant. and post. chambers of the ball and perforated in the center by the pupil. It regulates by contraction and dilatation the entrance of light.

ANAT: The free inner edge rests on the lens when the pupil is contracted or partially dilated. The iris separates the ant. and post. chambers of the eyeball. The iris contains two muscles, the sphincter pupillae (circular fibers) about one millimeter wide, and the dilator pupillae (meridionally arranged fibers) extending from sphincter pupillae to root of iris. The former is supplied through the oculomotor nerve with parasympathetic fibers derived from the ciliary ganglion; the latter by sympathetic fibers from the sup. cervical ganglion.

The color of the iris depends on the pigment in the stroma cells and in the cells of the retinal layers.

SEE: *aniridia, choroidoiritis, heterochromia iridis, "irid-" words.*

i. bombé. Seen in annular post. synechia (seclusio pupillae). The iris is bulged forward by the pressure of the aqueous humor which cannot reach the anterior chamber.

i., chromatic asymmetry of. Difference in color of the two irides (*heterochromia*). One may be blue or gray and the other brown. May occur in early iritis or cyclitis.

i. contraction reflex. Normal contraction on exposure to light.

i., piebald. Dark discoloration in irregularly shaped area. May be in one or both eyes.

I'rish moss. A genus of seaweeds; *Chondrus crispus.* Also called *carrageen,* a demulcent used in pharmacologic preparations.

iritic (i-rit'ik) [G. *iris,* iris]. Rel. to the iris.

iri'tis [" + *itis,* inflammation]. Inflammation of the iris.

SYM: Pain, photophobia, lacrimation, diminution of vision; the iris appears swollen, dull, and muddy; the pupil is contracted, irregular and sluggish in reaction.

TREATMENT: *Constitutional* (sweating, catharsis, etc., internal medication for pain, and directed toward etiological factors). *Local:* atropine and adrenocortical steroids as eye drops or ointment.

i., plastic. I. in which the fibrinous exudate forms new tissue.

i., primary. When the process develops in the iris itself. Seen in general diseases as syphilis, tuberculosis; metastatic in infectious diseases, gonorrhea and focal infections; also occurs in trauma and sympathetic ophthalmia.

i., purulent. One with a purulent exudate.

i., secondary. When the inflammation spreads from neighboring parts as diseases of cornea and sclera.

i., serous. Serum forming the exudate.

iritomy (i-rit'o-mi) [" + *tomē,* incision]. Formation of an artificial pupil. SYN: *iridotomy; irotomy.*

I'ron [A.S. *iren*] (L. *ferrum*). A metallic element widely distributed in nature. SYMB: Fe. At. wt. 55.847; at. no. 26. Its compounds (oxides, hydroxides, salts) exist in two forms: ferrous, in which iron has a valence of two, and ferric in which it has a valence of three. It is widely used in the treatment of certain forms of anemia. Its compounds have an astringent and styptic action.

Iron is essential for the formation of chlorophyll in plants, although it is not a constituent of chlorophyll. It is an essential constituent of hemoglobin.

FUNCTIONS: Iron is necessary for life, being an essential component of hemoglobin and essential for the formation of red blood corpuscles and also a component of certain respiratory enzymes, esp. the cytochrome system. It plays a role in the nutrition of epithelial tissues. There are approximately 4 to 5 gm. of iron in the adult body, distributed as follows: 65% in hemoglobin, 15% in the reticuloendothelial tissues (liver, spleen, bone marrow) and 20% in remaining tissues. Iron is stored in the tissues principally as *ferritin.* Iron is absorbed from the food in the small intestine; it passes, in the blood, to the bone marrow; here it is used in making hemoglobin which is incorporated in the red corpuscles. A corpuscle, after circulating in the blood for approximately 120 days is destroyed, and its iron is used over again. The adult male requires from 0.5 to 1.0 mg. of iron a day. A female of menstrual age will require about double this amount. During pregnancy and lactation she may require treble this amount. Prior to puberty and after menopause the female requires no more iron than the male.

Copper in the food is necessary for the utilization of iron. It is stored in the body and is reused repeatedly. The infant's food is poor in iron so it draws upon its store to such an extent that its reserve supply may be exhausted before the child is six months old. 10-16 mg. of iron per day are necessary in the diet of the average person. 15 mg. is the normal amt. obtained from daily intake of food, this being equal to the daily loss. Two to three times this amount is needed.

Manganese and cobalt, in addition to copper, are necessary for proper utilization of iron.

Iron, as a component of hemoglobin, is essential in the transportation of oxygen. It is needed for tissue respiration and the development of blood cells. Various forms of iron are used in medicine.

DEFICIENCY SYM: Anemia, lowered vitality, pale complexion, retarded development, decreased red blood cells and hemoglobin.

Sometimes a disturbance in iron metabolism occurs in which an iron-containing pigment, *hemosiderin,* and *hemofuscin* are deposited in the tissues. This gives rise to *hemochromatosis.* Excessive deposition of hemosiderin in the tissues such as may occur as a result of excessive breakdown of red cells is called *hemosiderosis.*

SOURCES: *Ex.* Almonds, asparagus, bran, beans, cauliflower, celery, chard, dandelions, Boston brown bread, graham bread, egg yolk, kidney, lettuce, liver, oatmeal, oysters, soy beans, whole wheat. *Good:* Apricots, beans, greens, beets, beef, cabbage, cucumbers, currants, dates, duck, goose, lamb, molasses, oranges, parsnips, peppers, peas, potatoes, prunes, radishes, raisins, rhubarb, pineapples, tomatoes, peanuts, turnips, cornmeal, mushrooms. There is less iron in carrots and milk than in other foods. Only 50% of the iron in spinach and similar vegetables is assimilable by the body.

i.-high diet. Foods rich in iron and blood building substances are emphasized, *i. e.,* liver, beef heart, kidney, red meats, green leafy vegetables, apricots, peaches, raisins, apples, prunes, molasses.

irot'omy [G. *iris,* iris, + *tomē,* incision]. Formation of an artificial pupil. SYN: *iridotomy, iritomy.*

irra'diate [L. *irradiāre,* to illumine]. To administer x-rays or other forms of radiation.

irra'diating [L. *irradiāre,* to illumine]. Diverging or spreading out from a common center.

irradia'tion [L. *irradiāre,* to illumine]. 1. Therapeutic application of roentgen rays, radium rays, ultraviolet rays or other radiation to a patient. 2. Application of form of radiation to an object or substance to give it therapeutic value, or increase that which it already has. 3. Phenomenon in which a bright object on a dark background appears larger than a dark object of the same size on a bright background. 4. The spreading in all directions from a common center, as nerve impulses, the sensation of pain.

RS: *Grenz ray, heliotherapy, radium, roentgen ray and ultraviolet.*

i., interstitial. Therapeutic irradiation by the insertion into the tissues of capillary tubes containing radon.

i. of reflexes. The spread of a reflex to an increasing number of motor units upon increasing the strength of the stimulus.

irreducible (ĭr-rē-dū'sĭ-bl) [L. *in,* not, + *rē,* back, + *ducere,* to lead]. Not capable of being reduced or made smaller.

irrel'evance [" + *relevans,* raising]. Psy: Giving an answer not in harmony with question.

irrespirable (ir"rĕ-spī'ră-bl) [" + *re-,* again, + *spirāre,* to breathe]. Unfit for breathing as a gas, or incapable of being breathed.

ir'rigate [L. *in,* into, + *rigāre,* to carry water]. To wash out with a fluid.

ir"riga'tion [" + *rigāre,* to carry water]. The cleansing of a canal (as the throat, ear, or colon) by the injection of water or other fluids; the washing of a wound.

Solutions should be sterile and have an approximate temperature slightly warmer than body temperature (100 to 115° F.).

i., bladder. Washing out of bladder for treatment of inflammation.

NP: *Articles Needed*: The same as for a catheterization plus: Sterile funnel about 3 in. diameter; solution ordered, in sterile pitcher, covered and warmed to 105° F.; bedpan.

If medication is ordered for instillation following irrigation have it ready in medicine glass covered with fold of sterile gauze.

Procedure: 1. The patient may be placed on the bedpan and catheterized or she may be catheterized first and the pan put in place after that. 2. Catheterize but do not remove catheter. 3. Attach funnel to free end of catheter. Do not put your fingers *inside funnel.* 4. Hold funnel up and pour full of solution, allowing almost all of it to run in, then refilling. Do this 3 times and the 4th time fill funnel and turn it down quickly toward bedpan. This will siphon off contents of bladder. 5. Repeat until amount of solution ordered has been used or until solution returns clear. 6. If irrigating can is used, attach small end of connector to catheter and let 4 oz. of solution flow in gently. Detach catheter and allow fluid to run out into bedpan. Repeat. 7. If return-flow catheter is used just keep solution running gently, as it will return by other side of catheter. 8. Run medication ordered through catheter as soon as irrigation is finished. 9. Care for patient and equipment. 10. Record treatment including the following information:

Bladder Irrigation: *Time. By whom done. Solution used*: Kind. Amount. Temperature. *Appearance of return flow*: Bloody. Mucus shreds, etc. *Medication instilled. Reaction of patient.*

i., colonic. The flushing of the colon with water. See: *colonic i.*

ir"riga'tor [" + *rigāre,* to carry water]. Device with hose attachment used for purpose of flushing or washing a part or cavity with fluids.

ir"ritabil'ity [L. *irritāre,* to tease]. 1. Excitability. 2. The ability to respond in a specific way to a change in environment, a property of all living tissue. 3. Condition in which a person, organ, or a part responds excessively to a stimulus. 4. Quick response to annoyance; impatience.

i., muscular. Normal response of muscle to a stimulus.

i., nervous. Response of a nerve to stimulus.

ir'ritable [L. *irritāre,* to tease]. 1. Capable of reacting to a stimulus. 2. Sensitive to stimuli.

i. heart. A syndrome characterized by forceful uncomfortable heart beats, tachycardia, atrial flutter and fibrillation, faintness, fatigue and other symptoms. Syn: anxiety neurosis; effort syndrome; neurocirculatory asthenia, *q.v.;* soldier's heart.

i. joint. A condition sometimes following a sprain, marked by recurring attacks of acute or subacute inflammation.

ir'ritant [L. *irritāre,* to tease]. An agent which, when used locally, produces more or less local inflammatory reaction. Anything which induces or gives rise to irritation. Ex. *iodine.*

i. poisons. These include a large number of poisons of great variety, not including the corrosive acids or alkalies. They cause pain in the mouth, esophagus, and stomach, nausea, vomiting, and great thirst, abdominal cramping, bloody diarrhea, and diminished urine.

Treatment: Varies. See: *Poisons and Poisoning* in Appendix.

irrita'tion [L. *irritāre,* to tease]. 1. Reaction to that which is irritating. 2. Extreme reaction to pain or pathological conditions. 3. Normal response to stimulus of a nerve or muscle.

i., spinal. A neurasthenic condition characterized by tenderness along the spinal column, numbness and tingling in the limbs, and susceptibility to fatigue.

i., sympathetic. The response of an organ to irritation in another organ.

ir'ritative [L. *irritāre,* to tease]. Pert. to that which causes irritation.

irrumation (ir-ru-ma'shun) [L. *irrumāre,* to give suck]. Intromission of the penis into another individual's mouth. Syn: *fellatio; fellatorism.*

I.S. Abbr. for *intercostal space.*

Isambert's disease (e-zahm-bairz') [Emile Isambert, French physician, 1828-1876]. Tuberculous ulceration of the larynx and pharynx.

ischemia (ĭs-ke'mĭ-ă) [G. *ischein,* to hold back, + *aima,* blood]. Local and temporary anemia due to obstruction of the circulation to a part.

ischesis (is-kē'sis) [G. *ischein,* to hold back]. Suppression of a discharge, esp. a normal one.

ischiac, ischiadic (ĭs'kĭ-ăk, ĭs-kĭ-ăd'ĭk). Ischiatic.

ischial (ĭs'kĭ-al) [G. *ischion,* hip]. Pert. to the ischium.

ischialgia (ĭs-kĭ-al'jĭ-ă) [" + *algos,* pain]. Neuralgic pain in the hip. Syn: *sciatica.*

ischiatic (ĭs-kĭ-at'ĭk) [G. *ischion,* hip]. Pert. to the ischium or hip bone. Syn: *sciatic.*

ischiatitis (ĭs-kĭ-ă-tī'tis) [" + *-ītis,* inflammation]. Sciatic nerve inflammation.

ischidrosis (is-kĭ-dro'sis) [G. *ischein,* to

hold back, + *hidrōsis,* sweat]. Suppression of perspiration.
ischio- [G. *ischion,* hip]. Prefix: pert. to the ischium.
ischiobulbar (is″kĭ-ō-bul′bar) [″ + L. *bulbus,* bulb]. Rel. to the ischium and urethral bulb.
ischiocavernosus (ĭs″kĭ-ō-kav-ĕr-nō′sŭs) [″ + L. *cavernosus,* cavernous]. A muscle extending from the ischium to the penis or clitoris. It assists in the erection of these structures.
ischiocele (ĭs′kĭ-ō-sēl) [″ + *kēlē,* hernia]. Hernia through the sciatic notch.
ischiococcygeus (ĭs″kĭ-ō-kok-sĭj′ē-us) [″ + *kokkyx, coccyx*]. 1. Coccygeus muscle. 2. Post. portion of the levator ani.
ischiofemoral (is″kĭ-ō-fem′or-al) [″ + L. *femur,* thigh]. Rel. to the ischium and femur.
ischiofib′ular [″ + L. *fibula,* buckle]. Rel. to the ischium and fibula.
ischiohebotomy (is″kĭ-ō-hē-bŏt′ō-mĭ) [″ + *hēbē,* pubes, + *tomē,* incision]. Surgical division of the ascending ramus of the pubes and the ischiopubic ramus. SYN: *ischiopubiotomy.*
ischiomenia (ĭs″kĭ-ō-mē′nĭ-ă). Ischomenia, *q.v.*
ischioneuralgia (is-kĭ-o-nu-ral′jĭ-ă) [G. *ischion,* hip, + *neuron,* nerve, + *algos,* pain]. Neuralgic pain in the hip. SYN: *sciatica.*
ischiopubic (is-kĭ-o-pu-bĭk) [″ + L. *pubes,* the pubes]. Rel. to the ischium and pubes.
ischiopubiotomy (ĭs″kĭ-ō-pū-bĭ-ŏt′ō-mĭ). Ischiohebotomy, *q.v.*
is″chiorec′tal [″ + L. *rectus,* straight]. Pert. to the ischium and rectum.
i. abscess. Collection of pus in fatty cavity on either side of rectum.
ischium (is′kĭ-um) (pl. *is′chia*) [G. *ischion,* hip]. Lower portion of the innominate or hip bone.
ischo- (ĭs-kō) [G. *ischein,* to hold back]. Prefix meaning to suppress or restrain.
ischochymia (ĭs″kō-kĭ′mĭ-ă) [″ + *chymos,* chyme]. Retention of food in dilation of the stomach.
ischogalactic (ĭs″kō-gă-lăk′tĭk) [″ + *gala, galakt-,* milk]. 1. Causing suppression of breast milk. 2. Agent which checks milk secretion. SYN: *antigalactic; lactifuge.*
ischomenia (ĭs″kō-mē′nĭ-ă) [″ + *mēn,* month]. Menstrual suppression or retention.
ischuretic (is-ku-ret′ik) [″ + *ouron,* urine]. 1. Relieving or pert. to ischuria. 2. That which relieves urinary retention or suppression.
ischuria (ĭs-kū′rĭ-ă) [″ + *ouron,* urine]. Suppression or retention of the urine.
island (ī′land) [A.S. *igland*]. A structure detached from surrounding tissues, or characterized by difference in structure; an islet.
i′s. of Calleja. Groups of densely packed, small cells in the cortex of the gyrus hippocampi.
i′s. of Langerhans. Clusters of cells in the pancreas. The cells are of three types: alpha, beta, and delta cells. The beta cells are found in greatest abundance and produce insulin. Destruction or impairment of function of the islands may result in diabetes or hypoglycemia.
i., pancreatic. An island of Langerhans, *q.v.*
i. of Reil. The *insula,* a lobe of the cerebral cortex comprising a triangular area lying in the floor of the lateral or sylvian fissure. It is overlapped and hidden by the gyri of the fissure which constitute the operculum of the insula.
islet (ī′lĕt) [Fr. *isle,* island]. A tiny isolated mass of 1 kind of tissue within another type.
i′s. of Calleja. SEE: *islands of Calleja.*
i′s. of Langerhans. SEE: *islands of Langerhans.*
-ism [G. *ismos*]. Suffix: meaning condition, or theory of principle or method.
iso- [G. *isōs,* equal]. Combining form meaning equal.
isoagglutinin (ī″sō-ă-glu′tĭn-ĭn) [G. *isōs,* equal, + L. *agglutināre,* to glue to]. Antibody in a serum which agglutinates the blood cells of those of the same species from which it is derived.
RS: *agglutinin; blood grouping; isohemagglutinin.*
isoagglutinogen (ī″sō-ag″lu-tĭn′ō-jen). One of two substances designated A and B which may be present in red blood cells. Cells containing these substances become agglutinated when mixed with serum containing corresponding isoagglutinins (*a* or *b*).
isobar (i′sō-băr) [″ + *baros,* weight]. In chemistry, one of two or more chemical bodies having same atomic weight, but with different atomic numbers.
isobaric (i″so-bar′ik) [G. *isos,* equal, + *baros,* weight]. Specific gravity equal to that with which it is being compared. Thus an anesthetic solution used in spinal anesthesia if isobaric would be of the same specific gravity as the spinal fluid.
isocel′lular [″ + L. *cellula,* little cell]. Composed of equal and similar cells.
isochromatic (ī-sō-krō-măt′ĭk) [″ + *chrōma,* color]. 1. Having the same color. 2. Of uniform color.
isochromatophil(e (i″so-kro-mat′o-fĭl or fīl) [″ + ″ + *philein,* to love]. Having the same affinity for a dye.
isochronal (ī-sok′rō-nal) [″ + *chronos,* time]. Acting in uniform time, or taking place at regular intervals. SYN: *isochronic; isochronous.*
isochroous (ī-sok′rō-us) [″ + *chroa,* color]. Of uniform color. SYN: *isochromatic, 2.*
isocolloid (ī-so-kol′oyd) [″ + *kollōdēs,* glutinous]. A colloid having the same composition in every transformation.
isocom′plement [″ + L. *complēre,* to complete]. One from the same individual or species which provides the amboceptor.
isocoria (i-so-ko′rĭ-ă) [″ + *korē,* pupil]. Equality of size of both pupils. SEE: *anisocoria.*
i″so-cort′ex. The neopallium or non-olfactory portion of the cerebral cortex. It is composed of six layers of fibrous and cellular tissue having a similar distribution pattern. SYN: *neopallium.*
isocytotoxin (i″so-si″to-tok′sĭn) [″ + *kytos,* cell, + *toxikon,* poison]. A cytotoxin destructive to cells of the same species from which it is derived.
isodactylism (i-so-dak′til-izm) [″ + *daktylos,* finger, + *ismos,* state]. Condition of having fingers and toes of equal length.
isodiametric (i″so-di-a-met′rik) [″ + *aia,* across, + *metron,* measure]. Having equal diameters.
isoelectric (i-so-e-lek′trik) [″ + *elektron,* amber]. Having equal electric potentials.
i″soenerget′ic [″ + *energeia,* energy]. Showing equal force or activity.
isogam′ete [″ + *gametē,* husband or wife]. 1. A cell which, through conjugation

or fusion with a similar cell, reproduces. 2. A gamete of the same size as the one with which it fuses or unites.

isogenesis (i-so-jen'ĕ-sĭs) [" + *genesis*, production]. Similarity in morphological development.

i'sograft [" + L. *graphium*, grafting knife]. A graft taken from another individual or animal of the same species. OPP: *autograft*. SYN: *heterograft; homograft*.

isohemagglutinin (i"so-hem-ag-glu'tin-in) [" + *aima*, blood, + L. *agglutināre*, to glue to]. Substance normally present in most human blood serum and responsible for the clumping of corpuscles observed when incompatible bloods are mixed.

The clumping is ascribed to the interaction of an agglutinogen in the corpuscles with a specific agglutinin in the foreign serum. In transfusions, the corpuscles of the donor are exposed to an overwhelming quantity of the recipient's plasma; therefore the agglutinogen content of the donor's corpuscles and the agglutinin content of the recipient's serum are the factors which determine compatibility.

Assuming that there are but two possible agglutinogens, red corpuscles from a given donor may contain both, either, or neither. If the agglutinin, *alpha*, can react only with agglutinogen A, one can construct a table from which compatibilities can be deduced (Jansky system). SEE ALSO: *agglutinin; blood groups, and table (on B-31)*.

i"sohemol'ysin [" + *aima*, blood, + *lysis*, dissolution]. Substance destroying red blood corpuscles of animals of same species from which it is obtained. SYN: *isolysin*. SEE: *hemolysin*.

i"sohemol'ysis [" + *aima*, blood, + *lysis*, dissolution]. Action of an isohemolysin. SYN: *isolysis*.

isohypercytosis (i"so-hi-per-si-to'sis) [" + *yper*, above, + *kytos*, cell, + *-ōsis*]. Increase of leukocytes, the proportion of varieties being unchanged.

isohypocytosis (i"so-hy-po-si-to'sis) [" + *ypo*, under, + *kytos*, cell, + *-ōsis*]. Decrease in number of leukocytes with proportion of varieties unchanged.

isoikonia (i"so-i-ko'nĭ-ă) [" + *eikōn*, image]. Equality of both retinal images.

isoikonic (i"so-i-kon'ĭk) [" + *eikōn*, image]. Having equal retinal images.

i"soimmuniza'tion. Immunization of an individual against the blood of an individual of the same species, esp. the development of Rh-agglutinins in an Rh-mother in response to agglutinogens present in transfused Rh+ blood or developed in an Rh+ fetus.

i'solate [It. *isolare;* from L. *insulāre*, to detach]. 1. To separate or detach from other persons, as during an infectious disease. 2. To free from a chemical combination.

isola'tion [It. *isolare;* from L. *insulāre*, to detach]. Limitation of movement and social contacts of patient suffering from, or a known carrier of, communicable disease, in contradistinction to *quarantine*, which limits the movements of exposed or contact persons. SYN: *sequestration 2*. SEE: *quarantine*.

NP: When a patient is in isolation, the purpose is to prevent the spread of the disease-causing germs. These general rules should be followed in order to confine the organisms to the isolated area and to protect those caring for the isolated patient:

1. Consider everything contaminated in the room or area with which the patient is in direct or indirect contact.

2. The hands of the nurse or attendant are the commonest means of carrying the infection. Therefore, thorough scrubbing and rinsing and keeping them away from the face are the most important means of control.

3. Burn, boil, or disinfect all contaminated material such as dishes, uneaten food, linens, all body discharges and utensils.

4. The gowns, masks, and caps used in the sickroom should be removed and left at the entrance to the area.

5. Contact the local health authorities, the doctor or hospital in charge of the case for specific information about Isolation Technic.

i. ward. Hospital ward where patients suffering from communicable diseases may be kept apart from the rest of the patients.

isoleucine (ī-sō-lu'sēn). An amino acid formed during hydrolysis of fibrin and other proteins. It is essential in the diet.

isolophobia (ī-sō-lō-fō'bĭ-ă) [L. *insulāre*, to detach, + G. *phobos*, fear]. Fear of being alone.

isolysin (ī-sol'ĭs-ĭn) [G. *isos*, same, + *lysis*, dissolution]. Substance which dissolves red corpuscles of animals of the same species from which it is obtained. SYN: *isohemolysin*.

isol'ysis [" + *lysis*, dissolution]. Destruction of red blood corpuscles produced by an isolysin. SYN: *isohemolysis*. SEE: *hemolysis*.

isolyt'ic [" + *lysis*, dissolution]. Rel. to isolysis.

isomer (i'so-mer) [G. *isos*, same, + *meros*, part]. One of two or more chemical substances which have the same molecular formula but different chemical and physical properties owing to different arrangement of the atoms in the molecule. Dextrose is an isomer of levulose. SEE: *metamer; polymer*.

isomeric (ī-sō-mĕr'ĭk) [G. *isos*, same, + *meros*, part]. Pertaining to isomerism, *q.v.*

isomerism (i-som'er-izm) [" + *meros*, part, + *ismos*, state of]. State of being composed of compounds of the same number of atoms, but having different atomic arrangement in the molecule. SEE: *metamerism, polymerism*.

isomet'ric [G. *isos*, equal, + *metron*, measure]. Having equal dimensions. OPP: *isotonic*.

i. contraction. C. of a muscle in which shortening or lengthening is prevented. Tension is developed, but no mechanical work performed, all energy being liberated as heat.

i. contraction phase. The first phase in contraction of the ventricle in which ventricular pressure increases but there is no decrease in volume of contents because semilunar valves are closed.

i. muscle. PHYS: Contraction in which a muscle increases its tension without shortening.

isometro'pia [" + " + *ōps*, eye]. Same refraction of the two eyes.

isomor'phism [" + *morphē*, form, + *ismos*, state of]. Condition marked by possession of the same form.

isomorphous (ī"sō-mor'fus) [" + *morphē*, form]. Possessing the same shape.

isoniazid (ī"sō-nī'ă-zĭd). USP. $C_6H_7N_3O$. An odorless compound occurring as colorless or white crystals or as a white crystalline powder. An antibacterial, it is effective only against mycobacteria. It is used in the treatment of tuberculosis. Syn: *isonicotinic acid hydrazide; isonicotinylhydrazine.*

isonormocytosis (ī″sō-nor″mō-sī-tō′sĭs) [" + L. *norma*, rule, + G. *kytos*, cell, + *-ōsis*]. State of having leukocytes normal in number and proportion of varieties.

isop′athy [" + *pathos*, disease]. Therapeutic administration of the causative agent of the disease or its products, as the use of variolous matter in smallpox. Syn: *isotherapy.*

isophoria (ī-sō-fō′rĭ-ă) [" + *phorein*, to carry]. Equal tension of vertical muscles of the eyes with visual lines in same horizonal plane, both hyperphoria* and hypophoria* being absent.

iso″plastic. Term applied to a graft taken from one individual and transplanted to another of the same species. See: *isograft.*

i″sose″rother′apy [" + L. *serum*, whey, + G. *therapeia*, therapy]. Treatment with serum from one having had the same disease as the patient.

isose′rum [" + L. *serum*, whey]. A serum from one having the disease for which a patient is to receive treatment.

isosmotic (ī″sŏs-mŏt′ĭk). Isotonic, *q.v.*

Isospora. A genus of Sporozoa belonging to the order Coccidia.

I. hominis. A parasitic protozoon inhabiting the small intestine of man. It is nonpathogenic.

isosthenuria (ī″sŏs-thĕn-ū′rĭ-ă) [" + *sthenos*, strength, + *ouron*, urine]. The decreased variation in specific gravity of urine in renal insufficiency.

isostimula′tion [" + L. *stimulāre*, to excite]. Cell stimulation of an organ by injection of the same cell substance.

isother′apy [" + *therapeia*, treatment]. Treatment by active causal agent of a disease. Syn: *isopathy.*

isother′mal [" + *thermē*, heat]. Of an equal degree of heat.

isothermognosis (ī″sō-thĕrm-og-nō′sĭs) [" + " + *gnosis*, knowledge]. Abnormal perception in which stimulation by pain, heat, and cold are all felt as heat.

isoto′nia [" + *tonos*, tone, tension]. The state of equal osmotic pressure of two or more solutions or substances.

isotonic (ī″sō-ton′ĭk). 1. Having the same tension or tone. Said of muscles in physiology. Opp: *isometric.* 2. Having the same osmotic pressure. Syn: *isosmotic.*

i. solutions. Those having the same osmotic pressure.

isotonicity (ī″sō-tō-nĭs′ĭ-tĭ). The state or condition of being isotonic.

isotope (ī′sō-tōp) [G. *isos*, equal, + *topos*, part]. One of a series of chemical elements which have nearly identical chemical properties but which differ in their atomic weights and electric charge. Many isotopes are radioactive.

isotropic (i-so-tro′pĭk) [" + *tropos*, a turning]. 1. Possessing similar qualities in every direction. 2. Having equal refraction.

isotyp′ical [" + *typos*, type]. Belonging to the same variety or classification.

issue (ĭs′shu) [O. Fr.; from L. *exīre*, to go out]. 1. Offspring. 2. A suppurating sore maintained by a foreign body in the tissue and acting as a counterirritant.

isthmectomy (ĭs-mĕk′tō-mĭ) [G. *isthmos*, narrow passage, + *ektomē*, excision]. Excision of an enlarged isthmus, esp. of the thyroid gland. Syn: *median strumectomy.*

isthmian (ĭs′mĭ-an) [G. *isthmos*, narrow passage]. Rel. to an isthmus.

isthmitis (ĭs-mī′tĭs) [" + *-itis*, inflammation]. Inflammation of the throat or fauces.

is″thmocholo′sis [" + *cholē*, bile, + *-ōsis*]. Catarrh of fauces accompanied by bilious disturbances.

isthmoparalysis (ĭs″mō-pă-ral′ĭ-sĭs) [" + *paralysis*, a loosening]. Paralysis of the muscles of the fauces. Syn: *isthmoplegia.*

isthmoplegia (ĭs″mō-plē′jĭ-ă) [" + *plēgē*, a stroke]. Faucial paralysis.

isth′mospasm [" + *spasmos*, spasm]. Isthmian spasm, as of the fauces or of the fallopian tubes.

isthmus (ĭs′mus) [G. *isthmos*, narrow passage]. 1. A narrow passage connecting two cavities. 2. A narrow structure connecting two larger parts. 3. A constriction bet. two larger parts of an organ, or anatomical structure.

i., aortic. Constriction in fetal aorta between ductus arteriosus and left subclavian artery. Sometimes persists in adults.

i. of eustachian tube. See: *i. tubae auditivae.*

i. faucium [NA]. Isthmus (def. 3) connecting the posterior mouth cavity proper with the pharynx.

i. glandulae thyreoideae [NA]. A narrow portion of the thyroid gland connecting the left and right lobes. Syn: *i. of thyroid.*

i., pharyngeal. See: *i. pharyngonasalis.*

i. pharyngonasalis [NA]. The opening between the naso- and oral pharynx. Syn: *pharyngeal i.*

i. of thyroid. See: *i. glandulae thyreoideae.*

i. tubae auditivae [NA]. Narrowest portion of the eustachian tube. Syn: *i. of eustachian tube.*

i. tubae uterinae [NA]. The constricted portion (the medial third) of the uterine (fallopian) tube nearest the uterus. Syn: *i. of uterine tube.*

i. uteri [NA]. A slight constriction on the surface of the uterus midway between the uterine body and the cervix. Syn: *i. of uterus.*

i. of uterine tube. See: *i. tubae uterinae.*

i. of uterus. See: *i. uteri.*

isuria (ī-sū′rĭ-ă) [G. *isos*, equal, + *ouron*, urine]. Excretion of urine at a uniform rate, hour by hour.

itch [A. S. *giccan*, to itch]. 1. Irritation of skin, inducing desire to scratch. Syn: *pruritus, q.v.* 2. Scabies.

i., army. Chronic i. prevalent during U. S. Civil War (1860-1864).

i., barber's. A fungus infection of the bearded portion of the face and neck. Syn: *tinea barbae.*

i., dhobie. A fungus infection of the groin and perineum. Syn: *jock itch; tinea cruris.*

i., ground. Local irritation produced by penetration of the skin of the foot by hookworm larvae, especially Necator americanus.

i., jock. A fungus infection of the groin and perineum. Syn: *dhobie itch; tinea cruris.*

i. mite. *Sarcoptes scabiei.*

itch′ing. Pruritus; irritation of the skin, causing desire to rub or scratch the part.

-ite [G.]. Suffix denoting *of the nature of.* In chemistry a salt of an acid having the termination *-ous.*

i′ter [L. a way]. Passageway bet. two anatomical parts.

i'teral. Pert. to an iter.

ithycyphosis, ithyokyphosis (ith"ĭ-si-fo'sis, ith"i-o-ki-fō'sis) [G. *ithus*, straight, + *kyphos*, humped]. Kyphosis with backward projection.

ithylordosis (ith"ĭ-lor-do'sis) [" + *lordōsis*, a bending forward]. Lordosis without lateral curvature of the spine.

-itis (ī'tĭs) [G.]. Suffix: *inflammation of.*

I.U. Abbr. for *immunizing unit, International unit.*

I.V. Abbr. for *intravenous(ly).*

i'vy poisoning. Dermatitis caused by contact with poison ivy. SEE: *poison ivy dermatitis.*

Ixo'des. A genus of ticks of the family Ixodidae, *q.v.*, many of which are parasitic on man and animals.

ixodiasis (iks-o-di'a-sis) [G. *ixōdēs*, like birdlime]. 1. Lesions of the skin caused by tick bites. 2. Any disease caused by ticks, as Rocky Mountain fever.

ixodic (iks-od'ik). Pert. to or caused by ticks.

Ixodidae. A family of ticks belonging to the order Acarina, class Arachnida. Comprises the hard-bodied ticks including the genera *Amblyomma, Boophilus, Dermacentor, Haemaphysalis, Hyalomma, Ixodes* and *Rhipicephalus.* All are parasitic and of importance as pests or in the transmission of disease in domestic animals and man. Among diseases transmitted are Rocky Mountain spotted fever, relapsing fever, and tularemia.

ixomyelitis (iks-ō-mī-e-li'tis) [G. *ixōdēs*, like birdlime, + *myelos*, marrow, + *-itis*, inflammation]. Inflammation of the spinal cord in the lumbar region.

Notes

J

J. Symb. for the *joule* and for *Joule's equivalent.*

Jaboulay's button (zhab-oo-lā') [Mathieu Jaboulay, French surgeon, 1860-1913]. Two cylinders which may be screwed together for lateral intestinal anastomosis.

jack'et [Fr. *jaquette;* from Sp. *jaco,* jacket]. A plaster of Paris or leather bandage applied to the trunk to immobilize spine or correct deformities.

j., Sayre's. Plaster of Paris jacket used as a support for deformity of the spinal column.

j., strait. Device for restraining a violently insane person. SYN: *camisole.*

j., Willock's respiratory. A type of jacket for strengthening the respiratory movements in emphysema of the lungs.

jack-knife or reclining position. The patient lies on the back with shoulders elevated, thighs flexed on abdomen, legs on thighs, the thighs being at right angles to the abdomen. Employed when passing a urethral sound.

jack'screw. A threaded screw to expand the arch in regulating teeth.

jackson'ian epi'lepsy. A localized form with spasms confined to one part or one group of muscles. SEE: *epilepsy.*

Ja'cob's mem'brane [Arthur Jacob, Irish ophthalmologist, 1790-1874]. Retinal layer of rods and cones.

J.'s ulcer. Epithelioma, usually of the face, which slowly eats away soft tissue and bones. SYN: *rodent ulcer.**

Ja'cobson's car'tilage. [Ludwig Jacobson, Danish anatomist, 1783-1843]. One of two narrow longitudinal cartilages lying along ant. portion of inferior border of nasal septum. They are rudimentary in man.

J.'s nerve. Nervus tympanicus.

J.'s organ. Rudimentary sac in nasal septum. SYN: *vomeronasal organ.*

J.'s sulcus. Portion of middle ear containing branches of tympanic plexus.

Jacquemier's sign (zhak-me-āz') [Jean Jacquemier, French obstetrician, 1806-1879]. Blue or purplish color of the vaginal mucosa, indicating pregnancy.

jactitation (jak-ti-ta'shun) [L. *jactitāre,* to toss]. Convulsive movements. Restless tossing. Changing from one posture to another, usually characteristic of severe mental and febrile affections.

j., periodic. Chorea.

Jadelot's lines, furrows, or **traits** (zhad-loz') [Francois N. Jadelot, Paris physician, 1791-1830]. Three lines on the face, said to indicate disease in children.

J.'s labial l. Down from corner of mouth; seen in respiratory diseases.

J.'s nasal l. From lower border of ala nasi about outer side of orbicularis oris muscle; seen in abdominal disorders.

J.'s ocular l. From inner canthus toward glenoid fossa; observed in cerebral disease.

Jaeger's test types (ya'gerz) [Edward Jaeger von Jasttha, Viennese ophthalmologist, 1818-1884]. Lines of type of various sizes, printed on a card for testing close visual acuteness.

jail fever. Typhus fever, *q.v.*

Jaksch's anemia or **disease** (yakshs) [Rudolf von Jaksch, Czechoslovakian physician, 1855-1947]. Infantile anemia with lymphatic enlargement and changes in spleen. SYN: *infantile pseudoleukemia.*

jal'ap. The dried tuberous root of the plant of the same name.

ACTION AND USES: Purgative, in the form of compound powder.

James' pow'der. Official antimonial powder.

James'town weed. Antispasmodic and local anodyne. Old name for Jimson weed (stramonium), *q.v.*

POISONING: F. A. TREATMENT: Same as atropine, *q.v.*

Janet's disease (zhă-nez') [Pierre M. Janet, French physician, 1859-1947]. A neurosis characterized by obsessions and phobias. SYN: *psychasthenia.*

jar'gon [O. Fr., a chattering]. Unintelligible speech. SYN: *paraphasia.*

jar"gonapha'sia [" + G. *a-,* priv., + *phasis,* speech]. A form of aphasia* in which words are jumbled so that speech is unintelligible. SYN: *paraphasia.*

Jar'vis' snare [William C. Jarvis, American laryngologist, 1855-1895]. A snare for removing growths.

jaundice (jawn'dis). SYN: *icterus, q.v.* A condition characterized by yellowness of skin, white of eyes, mucous membranes and body fluids, due to deposition of bile pigment resulting from excess bilirubin (hyperbilirubinemia) in the blood. It may result from obstruction of bile passageways, excess destruction of red blood cells, or disturbances in functioning of liver cells.

j., acathectic. Form caused by functional hepatic cell disorder.

j., acholuric. J. without bile pigment in the urine.

j., black. J. to an extreme degree; icterus melas.

j., catarrhal. J. resulting from inflammation of the liver. Now considered identical with infectious hepatitis, *q.v.*

j., congenital. J. occurring at or shortly after birth due to maldevelopment of biliary apparatus.

j., congenital hemolytic. A familial, hereditary disorder characterized by increased fragility of red blood cells, splenomegaly, and hemolytic anemia. SYN: *chronic acholuric j.; spherocytic anemia.*

j., hematogenous. Hemolytic jaundice, *q.v.*

j., hemolytic. An inherited, chronic disease marked by increased fragility of red blood cells. Characterized by anemia, increased destruction of red blood cells, absence of bile pigment in urine, and splenomegaly.

j., hepatocanalicular. J. resulting from changes in the bile canaliculi, the liver cells remaining relatively normal.

j., hepatocellular. J. resulting from changes in liver cells.

j., hepatogenous. ETIOL: Due to catarrh of bile duct and duodenum, pressure from tumors or blood vessels, parasites, stricture of gallduct or obstruction by gallstones.

SYM: Yellow skin and mucous membranes. Light-colored feces, dark urine, nausea, itching, anorexia, and mental depression.

j., homologous serum. A form resembling infectious hepatitis. Follows injection of homologous serum containing inducing agent.

j., infectious. Infectious hepatitis, *q.v.*

j., malignant. Acute yellow atrophied condition of the liver.

j. of newborn. J. affecting newborn infants. SYN: *icterus neonatorum.*

j., obstructive. That due to a mechanical impediment to the bile flow.

SYM: 1. Symptoms of gastroduodenal catarrh usually precede, *i. e.,* coated tongue, anorexia, fetid breath, epigastric distress, vomiting, and perhaps diarrhea; yellow skin and conjunctivae, light stools and dark urine. 2. In acute cases slight fever and swelling of the liver, which is tender to touch.

TREATMENT: Rest, liquid diet, constitutional remedies, surgery.

j., parenchymatous. Hepatocellular j., *q.v.*

j., posthepatic. J. resulting from obstruction of flow of bile ducts. May be incomplete or complete.

j., prehepatic. A rare benign form in which there is no demonstrable liver damage. Also called *familial nonhemolytic jaundice.*

j., regurgitation. J. due to bile entering lymph channels of the liver and thence being conveyed to the blood. May result from biliary obstruction or lesions involving bile capillaries.

j., retention. J. resulting from inability of liver cells to remove bile pigment from circulation.

j., spirochetal. An acute infectious disease due to a spirochete, *Leptospira icterohaemorrhagiae.* SYN: *Weil's disease.*

j., toxic. J. resulting from bacterial toxins or poisons such as phosphorus, arsphenamine, carbon tetrachloride, etc.

j., xanthochromic. J. without bile pigment in the urine, but with yellowish discoloration of soles and palms.

jaw [Mid. Eng. *jawe;* from A. S. *cheowen,* to chew]. Either or both the maxillary and mandibular bones, bearing the teeth and forming mouth framework.

j., dislocation of the. Such dislocations are uncomfortable and extremely embarrassing to the patient. They may occur on either side, in which instance the tip of the jaw is pointed away from the dislocation.

On the normal side, just in front of the ear, may be felt a little hollow or depression which is often tender. If both sides of the jaw are dislocated, the jaw is pushed downward and forward. In either event, there is pain and difficulty in speech and the condition is often accompanied by shock. Backward dislocation of the jaw is rare.

CAUSES: Dislocations of the jaw are most often caused by a blow to the face or a fall on the chin, but occasionally they are caused by chewing large chunks of food, by yawning, or by hearty laughing.

REDUCTION OF: These dislocations are reduced by placing well padded thumbs inside of the mouth on the lower molar (back) teeth with the fingers running along the jawbone as a lever. The thumbs should be pressed downward towards the patient's lips and the fingers upward towards the patient's nose. Give a twisting motion to the jaw and at the same time with the wrist and elbows press backward toward the neck. The jaw gliding over the ridge of bone may be felt and just as this occurs the jaw usually snaps into place. When this motion is noted, it is desirable to move the thumbs outwardly towards the cheeks to avoid the thumbs being crushed bet. the molars.

This snapping into place is due to an involuntary spasm of the muscles pulling the jaw as though an overstretched rubber band were attached to it. Following the reduction, an immobilizing bandage or double cravat should be applied.

j. jerk reflex. Clonic movement resulting from percussing or stroking lower jaw.

j., lock. 1. Tonic spasm of jaw muscles preventing opening of mouth. 2. Tetanus, *q.v.*

j., lumpy. Fungus disease affecting the jaw, brain, lungs and gastrointestinal tract. Common in cattle and sometimes affecting humans. SYN: *actinomycosis, q.v.*

j., swelling of. LOWER: May be due to alveolar abscess, a cyst, gumma, sarcoma, or actinomycosis. UPPER: Occurs in alveolar abscess, parotid tumor, parotitis, carcinoma, sarcoma, and necrosis of bone or disease of antrum.

jaw, words pert. to: admaxillary, alveolar, alveolate, alveolus, anisognathous, biomaxillary, brachygnathia, epulis, gnathic, hypognathous, mandible, maxilla, ramus, submaxillary, tetanus, trismus.

jaw winking. Elevation of the upper eyelid when there is depression of the lower jaw.

jecorize (jĕk'o-rīz). To treat a food substance in such a way that it possesses the therapeutic value of cod liver oil, as the exposure of milk to ultraviolet rays.

jecur (je'kur) [L.]. The liver.

jejunal (je-jū'nal) [L. *jejunum,* empty]. Rel. to the jejunum.

jejunectomy (je"ju-nek'to-mĭ) [" + G. *ektomē,* excision]. Excision of part or all of the jejunum.

jejunitis (je"ju-ni'tis) [L. *jejunum,* empty, + G. *-itis,* inflammation]. Inflammation of the jejunum.

jejuno- [L.]. Combining form referring to the jejunum.

jeju"nocolos'tomy [L. *jejunum,* empty, + G. *kōlon,* colon, + *stoma,* mouth]. Formation of artificial passage bet. jejunum and colon.

jejunoileitis (je-jun"o-il-e-i'tis) [" + " + *-itis,* inflammation]. Inflamed condition of jejunum and ileum.

jejunoileostomy (je-ju"no-il-e-os'to-mĭ) [" + G. *ileum,* ileum, + *stoma,* mouth]. Formation of a passage bet. jejunum and ileum.

jejunojejunostomy (je-ju"no-je-ju-nos'to-mĭ) [" + *jejunum,* empty, + G. *stoma,* mouth]. Formation of a passage bet. two parts of the jejunum.

jejunostomy (je-jū-nos'to-mĭ) [" + G. *stoma,* mouth]. Surgical creation of a permanent opening into the jejunum.

jejunotomy (je-ju-not'o-mĭ) [" + G. *tomē,* incision]. Surgical incision into the jejunum.

jejunum (je-ju"num) [L. empty]. The second portion of the small intestine extending from the duodenum to the ileum. It is about 8 feet in length, comprising about two-fifths of the small intestine.

j., inflammation of. SYM: Absence of diarrhea; colic, distention of abdomen, borborygmus, flocculent or semisolid stools, containing undigested food, unchanged bile, and some mucus. Tenderness over midabdomen relieved by pressure.

jel'ly [L. *gelāre*, to freeze]. A thick semisolid, gelatinous mass.

j., contraceptive. A jelly introduced into the vagina for the prevention of conception. It may act as an occlusive agent or it may serve as a vehicle for spermicidal substances.

j., mineral. Petrolatum, petroleum jelly.

j., petroleum. Petrolatum.

j., vaginal. A jelly introduced into the vagina for therapeutic or contraceptive purposes.

j., Wharton's. Soft gelatinous connective tissue that constitutes the matrix of the umbilical cord.

Jen'ner's stain [Louis Jenner, English physician, 1866-1904]. Eosin methylene blue stain.

jerk (jerk) [Imitative Origin]. 1. A sudden muscular movement. 2. Term applied to certain reflex actions resulting from striking or tapping a muscle or tendon. SEE: *reflex*.

j., elbow. External stimulation of triceps when stretched produces involuntary extension of forearm.

j., jaw. Result of striking lower jaw with mouth open. Indicative of cerebral lesion.

j., knee. Forward jerk of foot upon striking patellar tendon when knee is flexed at right angles. Absent in locomotor ataxia, infantile paralysis, meningitis, diabetes, destructive lesions of lower part of cord and certain forms of paralysis. Increased in affections of pyramidal areas, brain tumors, spinal irritability and sclerosis, lateral or cerebrospinal. SYN: *patellar tendon reflex*.

j., wrist. When hand is held down at arm's length, the hand being in extreme extension, lateral clonic movements of the hand occur; normal phenomenon.

jig'ger (*Dermatophilus penetrans*). Common name for parasitic fleas belonging to the species *Tunga penetrans*, *q.v.* SYN: *chigger; chigoe*.

jim'son weed. Stramonium, *q.v.*

Jocasta complex (jo-kas'tă). A term implying a mother and son complex from part taken by Jocasta, mother in the Oedipus complex, who was the wife and mother of Oedipus.

Joffroy's reflex (zhof-rwah') [Alexis Joffroy, Paris physician, 1844-1908]. Twitching of gluteal muscles when pressure is made against buttocks.

J.'s sign. 1. Absence of facial muscle contraction when eyes turn upward in exophthalmic goiter. 2. Inability to do simple sums in arithmetic. An early sign of general paralysis.

johim'bine. The hydrochloride of yohimbine, it is used as an aphrodisiac.

joint [L. *junctura*, a joining]. An articulation. The point of juncture bet. two bones. SEE: *Table in Appendix*.

A joint is usually formed of fibrous connective tissue and cartilage. It is classified as being immovable (*synarthrosis*), slightly movable (*amphiarthrosis*), and freely movable (*diarthrosis*).

SYNARTHROSIS: Joint in which the two bones are separated only by an intervening membrane, as the cranial sutures.

AMPHIARTHROSIS: 1. Joint having a fibrocartilaginous disk bet. the bony surfaces (*symphysis*), as the symphysis pubis. 2. Joint with a ligament uniting the two bones (*syndesmosis*), as the tibiofibular articulation.

DIARTHROSIS: Joint in which the adjoining bone ends are covered with a thin cartilaginous sheet and joined by ligament lined by a synovial membrane, which secretes a lubricant.

Grouping is according to motion: Ball and socket (*enarthrosis*), hinge (*ginglymus*), condyloid, pivot (*trochoid*), gliding (*arthrodia*), and saddle joint.

Movements of joints are of four kinds: *Gliding*, in which one bony surface glides on another without angular or rotatory movement; *angular*, occurring only bet. long bones, increasing or decreasing the angle bet. the bones; *circumduction*, occurring in joints composed of the head of a bone and an articular cavity, the long bone describing a series of circles, the whole forming a cone, and *rotation*, in which a bone moves about a central axis without moving from this axis. In angular movement, if it occurs forward and backwards, it is called *flexion* and *extension;* away from the body, *abduction*, and toward the median plane of the body, *adduction*.

INJURIES: Contusions, sprains, dislocations and penetrating wounds.

j., amphidiarthrodial. J. both ginglymoid and arthrodial.

j., arthrodial. Diarthrosis permitting a gliding motion. SYN: *gliding joint*.

j., ball and socket. J. in which round end of one bone fits into cavity of another bone. SYN: *enarthrosis; multiaxial joint*.

j., biaxial. J. possessing two chief movement axes at right angles to each other.

j., bilocular. J. separated into two sections by interarticular cartilage.

j., bleeders'. J. hemorrhage in hemophiliacs.

j., Brodie's. Arthrodial neuralgia due to hysteria.

j., Budin's. Congenital cartilaginous band bet. squamous and condylar parts of the occipital bone.

j. capsule. The saclike structure which encloses the ends of bones in a diarthrodial joint. Consists of an outer *fibrous* layer and an inner *synovial* layer and contains synovial fluid.

j. cavity. The articular cavity or space enclosed by the synovial membrane and articular cartilages. It contains synovial fluid.

j., Charcot's. A disease in tabes dorsalis or syringomyelia. Joint enlargement owing to wasting away of muscles below the joint.

j., Chopart's. Union of remainder of tarsal bones with os calcis and astragalus.

j., cochlear. Hinge j. permitting lateral motion.

j., compound. J. made up of several bones.

j., condyloid. J. permitting all forms of angular movements except axial rotation.

j., Cruveilhier's. Atlanto-odontoid j.

j., diarthrodial. A joint characterized by the presence of a cavity within the capsule separating the bony elements, thus permitting considerable freedom of movement.

j., dry. Arthritis of chronic villous type.

j., ellipsoid. J. having two axes of motion through the same bone.

j., enarthrodial. Ball and socket j., *q.v.* SYN: *multiaxial j.*

Joints, Table Comparing Diseases of[1]

	Acute Rheumatism	Rheumatoid Arthritis	Osteoarthritis	Gout
Age	Children and young adults	25 and over	Middle and old age	Middle and old age
Sex	Either	Chiefly women	Either	Chiefly men
Cause	Unknown ? allergic reaction to streptococci	Often focal sepsis (streptococci)	Trauma, old age, degenerative changes	Uric acid in blood, due to disordered purine metabolism
Joints	Usually large joints, subsiding in one and commencing in another	Multiple, including small joints of hands and feet	Usually large weight-bearing joints, *e.g.*, hip, knee, shoulder	Several, *e.g.*, great toe, knee, elbow, hands, ankle
Pyrexia	At onset	In acute stages	Nil	During acute attack
Permanent Deformity	Nil	Spindle-shaped joints. Often gross deformity	Often slight	Deformity mainly from "chalky" deposits
Heart	Often affected	Not affected	Not affected	Often arteriosclerosis

[1]Sears' *Medicine for Nurses.*

j., false. False j. formation subsequent to a fracture.

j., flail. J. which is extremely relaxed, the distal portion of limb being almost beyond the control of the will.

j., ginglymoid. J. having only forward and backward motion as a hinge. SYN: *hinge joint.*

j., gliding. Diarthrosis permitting a gliding motion.

j., hemophiliac. SEE: *bleeders' j.*

j., hinge. J. having only a forward and backward motion, as a hinge. SYN: *ginglymoid joint.*

j., immovable. J. in which a cavity is lacking between the bones. SYN: *synarthrosis.*

j's., intercarpal. Articulations which the carpal bones form in relation to one another.

j., irritable. Inflamed spasmodic condition of joint of unknown cause.

j., Lisfranc's. Tarsometatarsal joints.

j., midcarpal. J. separating the navicular, lunate, and triangular bones from the distal row of carpal bones.

j., mixed. J. with surfaces joined by fibrocartilaginous disks.

j. mouse. Loose cartilage or other body in a joint.

j., movable. Slightly movable or freely movable joint. SYN: *amphiarthrosis* and *diarthrosis,* respectively.

j., multiaxial. Ball and socket j., *q.v.* SYN: *enarthrodial joint; polyaxial joint.*

j., pivot. A joint which permits rotation of a bone, the joint being formed by a pivot-like process which turns within a ring, or by a ringlike structure which turns on a pivot. SYN: *rotary joint; trochoid joint.*

j., polyaxial. Ball and socket j., *q.v.* SYN: *enarthrodial joint; multiaxial joint.*

j., receptive or ***reciprocal.*** Saddle joint, *q.v.*

j., rotary. A pivot joint, *q.v.*

j., saddle. A joint in which the opposing surfaces are reciprocally concavoconvex.

j., simple. J. composed of two bones.

j., spheroid. Multiaxial j. with spheroid surfaces.

j., spiral. SEE: *cochlear j.*

j., synarthrodial. SEE: *immovable j.*

j's., tarsometatarsal. Made up of three arthrodial joints, the bones of which articulate with the bases of the metatarsal bones.

j., trochoid. Pivot joint, *q.v.*

j., uniaxial. J. moving on a single axis.

j., unilocular. J. with a single cavity.

Jolles' test (yol'ĕz) [Adolf Jolles, Austrian chemist]. Test for biliary pigments in urine.

joule (jool). Work done in one second by current of one ampere against a resistance of one ohm.

Joule's equivalent (jools) [James P. Joule, English physicist, 1818-1899]. Amt. of work which, if converted into heat, will raise temperature of one pound of water 1° F.

J.'s law. 1. Rate of heat production in a part of a circuit is equal to the resistance of that part of the circuit multiplied by the square of the current. 2. In gas expansion, with no change in the amount of heat in a given quantity of gas, and no external work performed. there is no change in temperature.

jugal [L. *jugum,* yoke]. 1. Connected or united as by a yoke. 2. Pertaining to the malar or zygomatic bone.

j. bone. Malar or zygomatic bone.

j. process. Temporal bone process forming zygomatic arch. SYN: *zygomatic process.*

juga'le [L. *jugum,* yoke]. The point at the margin of zygomatic process.

jugate [jū'gāt) [L. *jugatus,* joined]. 1. Coupled, yoked. 2. Having ridges.

jugular (jug'u-ler) [L. *jugulum,* throat]. Pert. to the throat.

j. foramen. Opening formed by jugular notches of the occipital and temporal bones

j. fossa. Depression in the petrosal portion of the temporal bone for the jugular vein.

j. ganglion. Nodes of vagus root and glossopharyngeal nerve in j. foramen.

j. process. Projection from occipital bone toward the temporal bone.

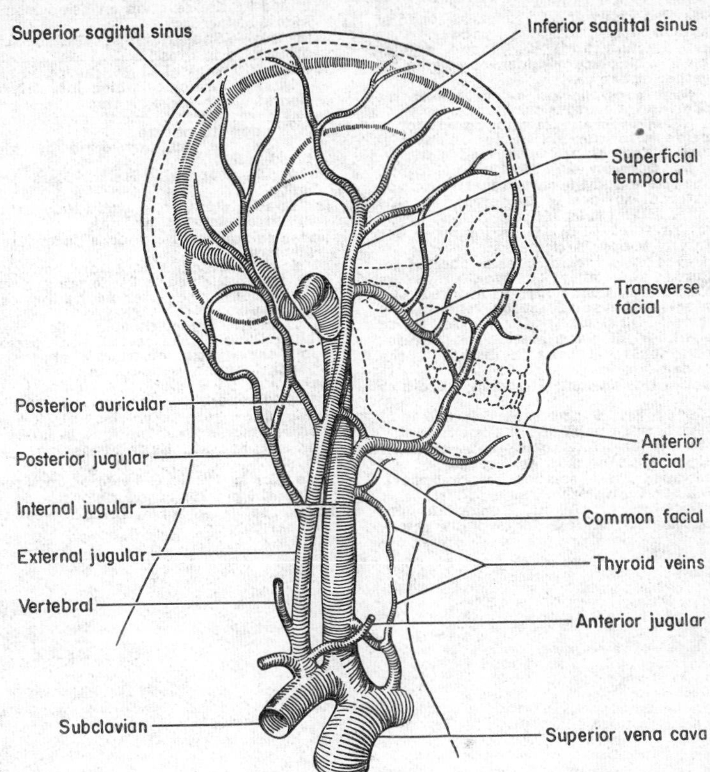

VEINS OF RIGHT SIDE OF NECK

j. veins. *External,* receives the blood from the ext. of the cranium and the deep parts of the face. It lies superficial to the sternocleidomastoid muscle as it passes down the neck to join the subclavian vein. *Internal,* receives blood from the brain and superficial parts of the face and neck. It is directly continuous with the transverse sinus, accompanying the internal carotid as it passes down the neck, and joins with the subclavian vein to form the innominate vein.

They are more prominent during expiration than during inspiration. Also during cardiac decompensation.

jugulate (jug'u-lāt) [L. *jugulāre,* to cut the throat]. To arrest quickly a process or disease by therapeutic measures.

jugula'tion [L. *jugulāre,* to cut the throat]. Sudden arrest of a disease by therapeutic means.

jug'ulum [L. neck]. Neck or throat.

ju'gum [L a yoke]. Ridge or furrow connecting two points.

j. penis. Forceps for temporarily compressing the penis.

j. petrosum. Eminence on petrous section of temporal bone showing the position of sup. semicircular canal. SYN: *arcuate eminence.*

juice [L. *jus,* broth]. Liquid that exudes or is expressed from any part of an organism.

j., alimentary. The digestive juices.

j., gastric. Secretions of the stomach, consisting of water, salts, pepsin, and free hydrochloric acid. See under *gastric.*

j., intestinal. A clear, yellowish, viscid fluid; alkaline in reaction, secreted by Lieberkühn's crypts. SYN: *succus entericus.* See under *intestinal.*

j., pancreatic. A clear, viscid, alkaline digestive juice of the pancreas poured into the duodenum. It contains the enzymes *trypsin, amylase,* and *lipase* or *steapsin.*

jujitsu, jiujitsu (ju-jit'su). A system of physical training for developing the art of self-defense without weapons in which the opponent's weight and strength are used to his disadvantage. Esp. developed in Japan.

jumentous (ju-men'tus) [L. *jumentum,* beast of burden]. Like that of a horse, said of odor of urine.

jum'per. One with nervous disorder who is startled easily or who jumps at sound of a loud noise. SEE ALSO: *palmus.*

junction (junk'shun) [L. *junctiō*, a joining]. The place of union or coming together of two parts.

j., mucocutaneous. A jct. between the skin and a mucous membrane.

j., myoneural. Meeting point of a nerve with the muscle to which it is distributed. SYN: *motor end-plate.*

j., sclerocorneal. Meeting point bet. the sclera and the cornea marked on the external surface of the eyeball by the outer scleral sulcus.

junctura (junk-tu'rā) [L. a joining]. Suture of bones. Articulation.

junk'et [It. *guincata*, cream cheese]. 1. Curds and whey; a type of cream cheese. 2. Commonly, a flavored and sweetened custard set by rennet.

jurymast (ju'rĭ-mast) [L. *jurāre*, to be right, + AS *masc*, a stick]. Apparatus for support of head in disease of the spine.

jusculum (jus'ku-lum) [L. broth]. Broth or soup.

Juster's reflex. Finger extension instead of flexion when palm of hand is irritated.

jus'to ma'jor [L. larger than normal]. Bigger than normal, as a *pelvis.*

justo minor. [L. smaller than normal]. Smaller than normal, as a *pelvis.*

Jus'tus' test [J. Justus, Hungarian dermatologist]. A test for syphilis determined by the reaction on hemoglobin of a dose of mercury.

jute (jūt) [Sanskrit *jūta*, matted hair]. Fiber used in dressings.

juvantia (ju-van'shĭ-ă) [L. *juvāre*, to aid]. Adjuvant medicines which intensify action of other drugs or assist them.

juvenile. 1. Pert. to youth or childhood. 2. Young; immature.

j. cell. A metamyelocyte or white blood cell.

juxta- [L. near to]. Prefix: Close proximity.

jux"ta-artic'ular [" + *articulus*, joint]. Situated close to a joint.

juxtaglomerular. Near or adjacent to a glomerulus.

j. apparatus. A structure consisting of myoepithelioid cells forming a cuff surrounding the arteriole leading to a glomerulus of the kidney.

j. cells. Myoepithelioid cells resembling those of the carotid body present in the juxtaglomerular apparatus. Their function is unknown.

juxtangi'na [" + *angina*, a choking]. Inflamed condition of pharyngeal muscles.

juxtaposition (juks"ta-po-zish'un) [" + *positiō*, place]. Position that is adjacent or side by side. SYN: *apposition; contiguity.*

juxtapylor'ic [" + G. *pylōros*, pylorus]. Near the pylorus or pyloric orifice.

juxtaspi'nal [" + *spina*, thorn]. Near the spinal column.

Notes

Notes

K

K. 1. Chem. symb. for *kalium*, potassium. 2. Symbol for Greek letter *kappa*.

Ka. Also Ca; abbr. for *cathode*.

Ka'der's opera'tion [Bronislaw Kader, Polish surgeon, 1863-1937]. Surgical formation of a gastric fistula with feeding tube inserted through valvelike flap.

Kaes' feltwork [Theodor Kaes, German neurologist, 1852-1913]. Nerve fiber network in cerebral cortex.

kaf'fir pox. Modified smallpox with pustules not umbilicated and without a secondary rise in temperature. SYN: *alastrim.*

Kahn test [Reuben L. Kahn, American bacteriologist, 1887-]. A flocculation test for the diagnosis of syphilis.

Positive reaction based upon appearance of a white precipitate when an alcoholic extract of normal heart muscle is added to the blood serum of one afflicted with syphilis.

kaif (kīf) [Arabic *gaif*, quiescence]. A dreamy, tranquil state induced by drugs.

kainophobia (ki-no-fo'bĭ-ă) [G. *kainos*, new, + *phobos*, fear]. Abnormal aversion to new situations and things. SYN: *neophobia.*

kais'erling, Kais'erling's solution. Liquid used in preserving pathological specimens.

kakidro'sis [" + *idrōsis*, sweat]. Unpleasant odor of the sweat. SYN: *bromidrosis.*

kak'ke [Japanese]. Endemic form of polyneuritis. SYN: *beriberi.*

kakosmia (kak-oz'mĭ-ă) [G. *kakos*, bad, + *osmē*, smell]. Perception of bad odors which do not exist. SYN: *cacosmia, parosmia.*

kakotrophy (kak-ot'rof-i) [" + *trophē*, nourishment]. Malnutrition. SYN: *cacotrophy.*

kala azar (kă"la-a'-zar) [Native, "black fever"]. SYN: *Leishmaniasis.* Visceral leishmaniasis, an infectious disease, common in tropical and subtropical areas of the world. There are several types which differ as to preference for children or adults, incidence in domestic animals, and transmitting agent. The disease is characterized by lesions of the reticuloendothelial system, esp. the liver and spleen. It is often fatal.

ETIOL: *Leishmania donovani*, a flagellated protozoon. The organism is transmitted by sandflies of the genus *Phlebotomus;* however, direct infection through nasal secretions, urine, and feces is possible.

kaliemia (kal-ĭ-e'mĭ-ă) [L. *kali*, potash, + G. *aima*, blood]. Potassium in the blood.

kaligenous (ka-lij'en-us) [" + G. *gennan*, to produce]. Forming potash.

kalimeter (kal-im'e-ter) [" + G. *metron*, measure]. Device for determining degree of alkalinity of a substance. SYN: *alkalimeter.*

ka'lium [L.]. (K) Potassium. A mineral element necessary to the growth of cells, esp. those of the muscles and blood. SEE: *potassium.*

kallikrein (kăl-ĭk'rĕ-ĭn). A vasodilator substance obtained from normal urine. Its origin is unknown, although it is present in the pancreas in considerable amounts.

kaolin (kā'o-lin). A yellowish white powder, occurring as a decomposition product of feldspar. Used internally as an absorbent; externally, as a protective by absorbing moisture.

kaolinosis (kā"o-lin-o'sĭs). Pneumokoniosis caused by inhaling kaolin particles.

kaomagma (kā"ō-mag'ma). A proprietary name of a suspension of kaolin in alumina gel. Used in intestinal inflammation, dysentery, colitis, etc.

kaopectate (kā-ō-pĕk'tāt). A proprietary name of a suspension of kaolin and pectin used for intestinal disturbances.

Kapo'si's disease [Moritz K. Kaposi, Austrian dermatologist, 1837-1902]. Diffuse atrophic skin condition. SYN: *xeroderma pigmentosum, q.v.*

Karell diet (kă'rel) [Philip Karell, Russian physician, 1806-1886]. A saltless diet constituting a fraction of usual normal diet, given in small quantities at definite intervals, gradually increased by adding other foods; intended to relieve the vital organs. For the first 7 days 200 cc. of milk constitutes diet, given every 4 hours between 8 A.M. and 8 P.M., after which soft boiled egg and toast, unsalted butter, cereal, and cream soups are added twice a day, and after 10th day chopped meat, vegetables, and rice boiled in milk, custard, and dextrimaltose are added.

Diet low in calories, vitamins, and iron.

karyo- [G. *karyon*, nucleus]. Prefix: Referring to a cell's nucleus.

kar"yochromat'ophil [" + *chrōma*, color, + *philein*, to love]. Having nucleus which stains.

karyochrome (kar'ĭ-o-krōm) [" + *chrōma*, color]. The cell of a nerve with an easily staining nucleus.

karyoc'lasis [G. *karyon*, nucleus, + *klasis*, a breaking]. The fragmentation of a cell nucleus. SYN: *karyorrhexis.*

karyogamy (kar-ĭ-og'ă-mĭ) [" + *gamos*, marriage]. Union of nuclei in cell conjugation.

karyogen (kar'ĭ-ō-jen) [" + *gennan*, to produce]. A compound of iron in certain cell nuclei.

karyogenesis (kar"ĭ-ō-jĕn'ĕ-sĭs) [G. *karyon*, nucleus, + *genesis*, production]. Formation and development of a cell nucleus.

karyokinesis (kar"ĭ-o-kin-e'sis) [" + *kinēsis*, movement]. 1. Changes taking place in a nucleus during indirect cell division. SYN: *mitosis.* 2. In a narrower sense, nuclear division only.

karyokinetic (ka"rĭ-o-kĭ-net'ĭk) [" + *kinēsis*, movement]. 1. Pert. to karyokinesis. 2. Ameboid.

karyolobism (kar"ĭ-o-lo'bizm) [G. *karyon*, nucleus, + L. *lobus*, lobe, + G. *ismos*, state of]. Condition in which the nucleus of a cell is lobed as in polymorphonuclear leukocytes.

kar'yolymph [" + L. *lympha*, lymph]. Fluid in meshes of the nucleus. SYN: *nuclear sap.*

karyolysis (kar-ĭ-ol'ĭ-sis) [" + *lysis*, dissolution]. The destruction of a nucleus or loss of affinity for basic dyes. SYN: *chromatolysis*.

karyolyt'ic [G. *karyon*, nucleus, + *lysis*, dissolution]. Producing or rel. to karyolysis.

karyomitome (kar-ĭ-om'ĭ-tōm) [" + *mitos*, web]. Network of the cell nucleus.

karyomitosis (kar"ĭ-o-mi-to'sis) [" + " + *-ōsis*]. Nuclear changes in cell division. SYN: *karyokinesis*.

karyomorphism (kar"ĭ-mor'fizm) [" + *morphē*, form, + *ismos*, state of]. The form of a cell nucleus.

karyon (kar'ĭ-on) [G.]. The cell nucleus.

karyophage (kar'ĭ-o-fāj) [G. *karyon*, nucleus, + *phagein*, to eat]. An intracellular protozoan parasite which destroys the nucleus of a cell.

karyorrhexis (kar"ĭ-o-rek'sis) [" + *rēxis*, rupture]. Fragmentation of the chromatin in nuclear disintegration.

karyosome (kar'ĭ-o-sōm) [G. *karyon*, nucleus, + *soma*, body]. SYN: *chromatin nucleolus*. 1. Chromatin mass at nodes of nuclear network. 2. A spherical mass of chromatin designated *false nucleolus* to differentiate it from the true nucleolus.

karyotheca (kar"ĭ-o-the'kă) [" + *thēkē*, sheath]. The enveloping membrane of a cell nucleus.

kata- [G.]. Prefix: Down. Also spelled cata-.

katab'olism [G. *kata*, down, + *ballein*, to throw, + *ismos*, stage of]. Catabolism, *q.v.*

kataphrax'is [" + *phraxis*, a blocking]. Surgical formation of metallic supports for an organ.

kataplasia (kat-ă-pla'sĭ-ă). Cataplasia, *q.v.*

katathermometer (kat"ă-ther-mom'ĕ-ter) [G. *kata*, down, + *thermē*, heat, + *metron*, measure]. A thermometer for measuring the efficiency of ventilation and cooling and drying processes, *i. e.*, the measurement of the cooling power (or, in a very warm atmosphere, of the warming power) of the atmosphere exerted on surface of two thermometers, one a dry bulb and the other wet bulb. Both are heated to 110° F. and the time required for each thermometer to fall from 100° to 90° F. is noted.

The dry kata gives the cooling power by radiation and convection. The wet kata gives the cooling power by radiation, convection, and evaporation.

katatonia (kat-ă-to'nĭ-ă) [" + *tonos*, tension]. Catatonia, *q.v.*

kathisophobia (kath-i-so-fo'bĭ-ă) [G. *kathizein*, to sit down, + *phobos*, fear]. Fear of sitting down, and subsequent inability to sit still.

kation (kat'i-on) [G. *kation*, descending]. Cation, *q.v.*

katotro'pia [" + *tropos*, a turning]. Tendency of the eyeball to drop too far downward. SYN: *katophoria*.

KBr. Potassium bromide.

$KC_2H_3O_2$. Potassium acetate.

KCl. Potassium chloride.

KClO. Potassium hypochlorite.

$KClO_3$. Potassium chlorate.

K_2CO_3. Potassium carbonate.

kefir, kefyr (kef'er) [Caucasian]. A preparation of curdled milk.

kelectome (ke'lek-tōm) [G. *kēle*, tumor, + *tomē*, incision]. Instrument for removing specimen of tumor tissue.

kelis (ke'lis) [G. *kēlis*, stain, spot, blemish]. 1. Skin disease with pigmented pink and purple patches and lesions leaving scars. SYN: *morphea*. 2. Skin tumor of dense tissue. SYN: *keloid*.

Kel'ly's pad [Howard A. Kelly, American surgeon, 1858-1943]. A drainage pad for the operating table or bed made by wrapping one end of a rubber sheet over a rolled small blanket, forming a bolster; the bolster is twisted round like a horseshoe to form the pad, the free part of the sheet forming the apron. Also commercial inflatable rubber pad of horseshoe shape used in same way.

keloid (ke'loyd) [G. *Kēlis*, scar, + *eidos*, form]. 1. Scar tissue. 2. A new growth of the skin consisting of dense tissue occurring esp. in Negroes and members of the yellow race.

k., acne. SYN: *dermatitis papillaris capillitii*. Hypertrophic scars on nape of neck at border of scalp.

ETIOL: Suppurative folliculitis.

k., Addison's. Skin disease with pigmented patches and lesions. SYN: *morphea, q.v.*

k., Alibert's. Growth of fibrous tissue usually at the site of a scar resembling a true keloid.

ETIOL: Predisposition a factor; essential cause unknown.

SYM: Oval, elongated, or irregularly shaped mass, single or lobulated, tender, painful, with burning or pricking sensation. Ranges in size from that of a bean to that of a hand. It sends out clawlike processes as it increases in size.

PROG: Usually good if removed, but sometimes returns.

k. en plaque. Circumscribed hard plate elevated a little over surface and embedded in the skin.

keloidosis (ke-loy-do'sis) [" + *-ōsis*]. The formation of keloids.

kelotomy (ke-lot'o-mĭ) [G. *kēlē*, hernia, + *tomē*, incision]. Operation for strangulated hernia through tissues of the constricting neck.

Kenny treatment. Treatment originated by Sister Kenny, an Australian nurse, for anterior poliomyelitis. Consists of application of hot, moist packs to affected muscles and early re-education of muscles, first through passive exercise and then by active movements as soon as possible. Rigid fixation of paralyzed limbs is disparaged.

kenophobia (ken-o-fo'bĭ-ă) [G. *kenos*, empty, + *phobos*, fear]. Fear of empty spaces.

kephalin (kef'ă-lin) [G. *kephalē*, head]. Cephalin, *q.v.*

ker'asin. A cerebroside isolated from brain tissue.

keratalgia (ker-ă-tal'jĭ-ă) [G. *keras*, *kerat-*, horn, + *algos*, pain]. Neuralgia of the cornea.

keratectasia (ker-ă-tek-tas'sĭ-ă) [" + *ektasis*, extension]. Conical protrusion of the cornea.

keratectomy (ker-ă-tek'to-mĭ) [" + *ektomē*, excision]. Excision of portion of cornea.

keratiasis (ker-ă-ti'a-sis) [G. *keras*, *kerat-*, horn]. Horny wart formation.

kerat'ic [G. *keras*, *kerat-*, horn]. Rel. to horn. SYN: *corneous, horny*.

ker'atin [G. *keras*, *kerat-*, horn]. A scleroprotein substance in hair, nails, and horny tissue, insoluble in gastric juice.

Used for coating pills which should not be dissolved in the stomach.

keratinize (ker'ă-tin-īz) [G. *keras*, horn]. To become hard or horny. Usually said of tissue.

keratinous (ker-at'in-us) [G. *keras*, *kerat-*, horn]. Pert. to or composed of keratin.

keratitis (ker-ă-ti'tis) [" + *-itis*, inflammation]. Inflammation of cornea.

k., aspergillar. K. of cornea due to infection from a mold.

k., band shaped. Whitish or grayish band extending across the cornea.

k. bullosa. The formation of large, quite resistant blebs in the cornea of blind trachomatous eyes with increased tension.

k., deep. SEE: *interstitial k.*

k., dendritic. Superficial branching corneal ulcers.

k. disciformis. Gray disk-shaped opacity in middle of cornea.

k., fascicular. Corneal ulcer resulting from phlyctenules which spread from limbus to center of cornea accompanied by fascicle of blood vessels.

k., herpetic. Vesicular keratitis in herpes zoster.

k., hypopyon. Serpiginous ulcer with pus in ant. chamber.

k., interstitial. Deep form of nonsuppurative k. with vascularization, occurring usually in syphilis and rarely in tuberculosis. Commonly found between 5th and 15th years.

SYM: Pain, photophobia, lacrimation, and loss in vision.

k., lagophthalmic. Desiccation of cornea due to defective closure of lids.

k., mycotic. Produced by mold fungi.

k., neuroparalytic. Dull and slightly cloudy insensitive cornea seen in lesions of fifth nerve.

k., parenchymatous. SEE: *interstitial k.*

k., phlyctenular. Circumscribed inflammation of conjunctiva and cornea accompanied by formation of small projections called phlyctenules which consist of accumulations of lymphoid cells. The phlyctenules soften at the apices, forming ulcers.

k., punctate. Cellular deposits on post. surface of cornea seen in diseases of uveal tract.

k., purulent. K. with formation of pus.

k., sclerosing. Triangular opacity in deeper layers of cornea, associated with scleritis.

k., superficial punctate. Small gray spots in superficial layers of cornea, beneath Bowman's membrane, occurring in young persons.

k., trachomatous. K. with abnormal membrane on cornea. SYN: *pannus.*

k., traumatic. K. caused by wound of the cornea.

k., xerotic. Softening, desiccation and ulceration of cornea. SYN: *keratomalacia.*

kerato-, kerat- [G.]. Combining form: Rel. to horny substances or to the cornea.

keratoacanthoma (ker"ă-to-ak"an-tho'mă) [" + acanthoma]. A papular lesion filled with a keratin plug. It is benign and usually subsides spontaneously. SYN: *molluscum sebaceum.*

keratocele (ker-at'o-sēl) [G. *keras, kerat-,* horn, + *kēlē,* hernia, tumor]. Protrusion or herniation of Descemet's membrane through the floor of corneal ulcer.

keratoconjunctivitis (ker"ă-to-kon-junk-tĭ-vi'tis). Inflammation of the cornea and the conjunctiva.

k., epidemic. An acute, self-limited infection due to a virus.

k., flash. K. resulting from exposure of the eyes to intense ultraviolet irradiation.

k., virus. Epidemic k., *q.v.*

keratoconus (ker-ă-to-ko'nus) [" + *kōnos,* cone]. Conical protrusion of center of cornea without inflammation.

keratoderma (ker-ă-to-der'mă) [G. *keras, kerat-,* horn, + *derma,* skin]. 1. Keratodermia, *q.v.* 2. The cornea.

keratodermatitis (ker"ă-to-der-mă-ti'tis) [" + " + *-itis,* inflammation]. Inflammation of the horny layer of the skin with proliferation.

ker"atoder'mia [G. *keras, kerat-,* horn, + *derma,* skin]. 1. Hypertrophy of the stratum corneum or horny layer of the epidermis, esp. on the palms of hands and soles of feet producing a horny condition of the skin.

keratogenous (ker-ă-toj'en-us) [" + *gennan,* to produce]. Causing horny tissue development.

ker"atoglo'bus [" + L. *globus,* circle]. Globular protrusion and enlargement of cornea seen in congenital glaucoma.

keratohelcosis (ker"ă-to-hel-ko'sis) [" + *elkōsis,* ulceration]. Corneal ulceration.

keratohyalin. A substance present in the form of granules in the cytoplasm of cells in the stratum granulosum and thought to be a precursor of keratin.

ker'atoid [" + *eidos,* form]. Horny or resembling horn or corneal tissue.

keratoiditis (ker"ă-toyd-i'tis) [" + " + *-itis,* inflammation]. Inflammation of the cornea.

keratoiritis (ker"ă-to-i-ri'tis) [" + *iris,* iris, + *-itis,* inflammation]. Inflammation of the cornea and iris.

keratoleptynsis (ker"ă-to-lep-tin'sis) [" + *leptynein,* to make thin]. Removal of the corneal surface, then covering the area with bulbar conjunctiva. A cosmetic operation performed on a sightless eye.

keratoleukoma (ker"ă-to-lu-ko'mă) [" + *leukos,* white, + *ōma,* tumor]. White corneal opacity.

keratolysis (ker-ă-tol'ĭ-sis) [" + *lysis,* loosening]. 1. Loosening of horny layer of the skin. 2. Shedding of the skin at regular intervals.

keratolyt'ic [" + *lysis,* loosening]. Rel. to or causing keratolysis. SYN: *desquamative.*

kerato'ma [G. *keras, kerat-,* horn, + *ōma,* tumor]. 1. A callosity. 2. A horny growth. SYN: *keratosis.*

keratomalacia (ker"ă-to-mă-la'sĭ-ă). Softening of the cornea seen in early childhood due to deficiencies of vitamin A. SYN: *xerotic keratitis.*

keratome (ker'ă-tōm) [" + *tomē,* incision]. Knife for incising the cornea.

keratometer (ker-ă-tom'ĕ-ter) [" + *metron,* a measure]. An instrument for measuring the curves of the cornea.

keratomycosis (ker"ă-to-mī-ko'sis) [" + *mykes,* fungus, + *ōsis*]. Fungus growth on the cornea.

ker"atono'sis [" + *nosos,* disease]. Any noninflammatory disease or deformity of the horny layer of the skin.

keratonyxis (ker"ă-to-niks'is) [" + *nyssein,* to puncture]. Corneal puncture, esp. surgical puncture.

keratoplasty (ker'ă-to-plas"tĭ) [" + *plassein,* to form]. Plastic operation on the cornea.

ker"atopro'tein [" + *prōtos,* first]. The protein of the hair, nails, epidermis, etc.

keratorrhexis (ker"a-to-rek'sis) [" + *rēxis,* rupture]. Corneal rupture.

keratoscleritis (ker"ă-to-skle-ri'tis) [" + *sklēros,* hard, + *-ītis,* inflammation]. Inflammation of both cornea and sclera.

keratoscope (ker'at-o-skōp) [" + *skopein,* to examine]. An instrument for examination of the cornea.

keratos'copy [" + *skopein,* to examine]. Examination of the cornea and its reflection of light.

keratose (ker'ă-tōs) [G. *keras, kerat-,* horn]. Horny.

keratosis (ker-ă-to'sis) (pl. *keratoses*) [G. *keras- kerat-*, horn, + *ōsis*]. 1. Horny growth. 2. Any condition of the skin characterized by the formation of horny growths or excessive development of the horny growth.

k. blennorrhagica. Condition associated with gonorrheal arthritis characterized by development of horny growths, esp. on hands and feet.

k. climatericum. A skin disease occurring in women during the menopause, characterized by a circumscribed hyperkeratosis of the palms and soles.

k. follicular. SYN: *Darier's disease, icthyosis follicularis, psorospermosis.*

k. nigricans. Acanthosis nigricans, *q.v.*

k., palmar and plantar. Chronic disorder showing thickening of horny layer of palms and soles.

ETIOL: Congenital, usually hereditary, occurring in several generations.

PROG: Alleviation but no cure.

k. pilaris. Inflammatory disorder, chronic in course, of area surrounding the hair follicles. SYN: *pityriasis pilaris; ichthyosis follicularis.*

SYM: Accumulation of horny material at follicular orifices, giving to affected surfaces a nutmeg-graterlike appearance, commonly in those with rough, dry skin. Most pronounced in winter, on lateral aspects of thighs and upper arms, with possible extension to legs, forearms and scalp.

TREATMENT: Tonics in anemic and debilitated. Locally, green soap, alkaline baths, rosewater ointment or glycerin lotion. In bearded region soothing cream and "once-over" shaving with very keen razor.

k., seborrheic. Flat, rough, crusted or scaly keratic lesion.

ETIOL: Unknown. SYN: *acanthotic nevus; seborrheic wart; senile wart.*

SYM: Keratoid, nevoid, acanthoid or verrucose types, occurring in elderly and in those with long-standing dry seborrhea, on face, scalp, interscapular or sternal regions and backs of hands, yellowish, grayish, brownish sharply circumscribed lesions covered with a firmly adherent scale, greasy or velvety, on trunk or scalp, but harsh, rough and dry on face or hands. Never disappear spontaneously and are potentially malignant.

TREATMENT: Earlier keratoid lesions removed by bland grease with subsequent occasional lubrication of site. Avoidance of alkaline soaps and water. For verrucose, nevoid, and advanced keratoid forms, carbon dioxide snow. Those showing malignant change are treated as carcinoma of the skin.

k. seni'lis. Dry, harsh skin of the aged.

keratotome (ker-at'o-tōm) [" + *tomē*, incision]. A knife for incising the cornea. SYN: *keratome.*

keratotomy (ker-ă-tot'o-mĭ) [" + *tomē*, incision]. Incision of cornea.

keraunoneurosis (kĕ-raw"no-nu-ro'sis) [G. *keraunos*, lightning, + *neuron*, nerve]. A neurosis from fear of a thunderstorm or from lightning stroke.

keraunophobia (kĕ-raw"no-fo'bĭ-ă) [" + *phobos*, fear]. Dread of thunder and lightning.

Kerck'ring's folds or valves [Theodorus Kerckring, Dutch anatomist, 1640-1693]. Transverse folds of mucous membrane of small intestine. SYN: *plicae circulares; valvulae conniventes.*

kerectomy (ke-rek'to-mĭ) [G. *keras*, cornea, + *ektomē*, excision]. Excision of a portion of the cornea.

kerion (ke'rĭ-on). A form of *tinea tonsurans* with swollen discharging lesions.

k. celsi. Inflammation of the hair follicles of the beard and scalp with formation of pustules. SYN: *tinea kerion.*

kerither'apy [G. *keros*, wax, + *therapeia*, treatment]. Treatment of burns and denuded surfaces with liquid paraffin.

kernic'terus. A form of icterus neonatorum occurring in infants. The basal ganglia and other areas of the brain and spinal cord are infiltrated with a yellow pigment. Develops during the second to eighth day of life. Prognosis is quite poor.

Ker'nig's sign [Vladimir Kernig, Russian physician, 1840-1917]. A symptom of meningitis evidenced by reflex contraction and pain in the hamstring muscles when attempting to extend the leg after flexing the thigh upon the body.

ketogenesis (ke-to-jen'ĕ-sis) [*ketone* + G. *genesis*, production]. Production of ketones or acetone substances.

ketogenic diet (ke-to-jen'ik) [" + G. *gennan*, to produce]. One that produces acetone or ketone bodies, or mild acidosis. Highly beneficial in epilepsy.

This is accomplished by providing a diet wherein the ratio of fatty acid to available carbohydrate is from 3 to 1 to 4 to 1. Thus a 5-year-old child could be given, for a 4 to 1 ratio, 20 gm. protein, 8 gm. carbohydrate, and 120 gm. of fat. To achieve the same ratio a year-old child would require 35 gm. protein, 8 gm. carbohydrate, and 170 gm. of fat.

ketohex'ose. A nonsaccharide consisting of a six-carbon chain and containing a ketone group, in addition to alcohol groups. SYN: *fructose.*

ke'tol. Crystalline substance formed in intestine and pancreas during putrefaction and digestion. SYN: *indole.*

ketol'ysis [" + G. *lysis*, dissolution]. The dissolution of acetone or ketone bodies.

ketolyt'ic [" + *lysis*, dissolution]. Pert. to ketolysis.

ketone (ke'tōn). A substance containing the carbonyl group (CO). Oxidation product of a secondary alcohol. Organic chemical substance of the general formula $\genfrac{}{}{0pt}{}{R}{R}{>}CO$.

Acetone is an example of a simple ketone. The ketone acids in the body are the end products of fat metabolism.

k. bodies. A group of compounds produced during the oxidation of fatty acids, which includes acetoacetic acid, B-hydroxybutyric acid, and acetone. SEE: *ketosis.*

k. threshold. Ketone level in the blood above which ketone bodies appear in the urine.

ketonemia (ke-to-ne'mĭ-ă) [ketone + G. *aima*, blood]. Acetone bodies in the blood. SYN: *acidosis.*

ketonuria (ke-to-nu'rĭ-ă) [" + G. *ouron*, urine]. Acetone bodies in the urine.

ketopla'sia [" + G. *plassein*, to form]. The formation or excretion of ketones.

ketoplas'tic [" + G. *plastikos*, formed]. Pert. to ketoplasia or formation of ketones.

ke'tose. A carbohydrate containing the ketones.

ketosis (ke-to'sis) [*ketone* + G. *-ōsis*, disease]. The accumulation in the body of the ketone bodies: acetone, betahydroxybutyric acid, and acetoacetic acid.

It is frequently associated with acidosis and is often miscalled acidosis. Ketosis results from the incomplete combustion of fatty acids, generally from carbohydrate deficiency or inadequate utilization, and is commonly observed in starvation, high fat diet, pregnancy, following ether anesthesia, and most significantly in diabetes mellitus. Large quantities of these ketone bodies may be eliminated in the urine (ketonuria). The presence of ketosis is easily determined by testing for the presence of acetone or diacetic acid in the urine, a ketonuria being one of the first evidences of beginning acidosis in diabetes.

17-ke'tosteroid. One of a group of neutral steroids having a ketone group in position 17. They are produced by the adrenal cortex and gonads and appear normally in the urine. Among them are androsterone, dehydroisoandrosterone, corticosterone, compound E, and 11-hydroxyisoandrosterone. A greater than normal or less than normal excretion in the urine is abnormal and indicative of certain endocrine disorders.

Key-Ret'zius foram'ina [Ernst A. H. Key, Swedish physician, 1832-1901; Magnus G. Retzius, Swedish histologist, 1842-1919]. Passages in the pia mater carrying the choroid plexus to the fourth ventricle. SYN: *Luschka's foramen.*

kg. Abbr. for *kilogram.*

$KHCO_3$. Potassium bicarbonate.

$KHSO_4$. Potassium bisulfate.

KI. Potassium iodide.

kibe (kīb) [Welsh *cibi*, chilblain]. Inflamed patch on hands or feet caused by exposure to cold. SYN: *chilblain, q.v.*

kid'ney [A. S. *cwith*, womb, + Ice. *nyra*, kidney]. One of two glandular, bean-shaped bodies, purplish-brown in color, situated at the back (retroperitoneal area) of the abdominal cavity, one on each side of the spinal column which excrete end products of metabolism in the form of urine.

The upper level is opp. the 12th thoracic (dorsal) vertebra, the lower level opp. the 3rd lumbar vertebra. The right kidney is slightly lower than the left one.

WEIGHT: 120-180 gm. (4-6 oz). Size, about 11.5 cm. (4½ in.) long, 5-7.5 cm. (2-3 in.) broad, and 2.5 cm. (1 in.) thick.

Each kidney is embedded in fatty tissue known as an adipose *capsule*, and surrounded by the renal fascia, a sheath of fibrous tissue, which helps to hold the kidney in place. The concave border of the kidney faces the median line, the center of the concave border opening into a fissure called the *hilum, q.v.*

The ureter enters the kidney through the hilum into the *pelvis* of the kidney. The outer portion of the kidney is the *cortex*, a mass of cortical substance; the inner portion (medullary substance) is the *medulla.*

Within the cortical substance are found the arteries, veins, convoluted tubules, and glomerular capsules, while the medulla contains the renal pyramids, conical masses with papillae projecting into the cuplike cavities (calyces) of the pelvis.

Each kidney contains from 8 to 18 pyramids made up of collecting tubules, lymphatics, and blood vessels, the pyramids being penetrated by the cortical substance and supporting them; these extensions are known as the renal columns, or columns of Bertini.

The cortical and medullary substance is composed of renal tubules, connective tissue, blood vessels, nerves, and lymphatics. The *renal tubule* or *nephron* constitutes the structural and functional unit of the kidney. Each consists of a *capsule, proximal convoluted portion, loop of Henle* and *distal convoluted portion*, which leads to a collecting duct. The capsule, called the *glomerular* or *Bowman's capsule*, encloses a globular mass of capillaries, the glomerulus. The capsule and the enclosed glomerulus comprise the *malpighian* or *renal corpuscle.* The renal corpuscles are located principally in the cortex.

URINE FORMATION: Urine consists of water (95%) and solids (5%), the latter being in solution. The solids include organic constituents (urea, hippuric acid, uric acid, creatinine) and inorganic constituents, principally salts of sodium and potassium. The kidneys remove these substances from the blood thus acting to maintain homeostasis of the blood and body fluids. Urine is formed by the processes of *filtration* and *reabsorption.* As blood passes through the glomerulus, water and dissolved substances are filtered through the capillary walls and the inner or visceral layer of Bowman's capsule, resulting in formation of the *glomerular filtrate.* Blood cells and colloidal substances such as proteins are retained within the capillaries. The glomerular filtrate passes through the renal tubules to the collecting ducts, during the course of which all of the sugar and some of the salts and other substances are *selectively reabsorbed* into the capillaries surrounding the tubule. There is some evidence that the cells of the tubules may add by the process of secretion some substances such as urea and uric acid to the urine. The final product now known as *urine* passes through straight *collecting ducts* into larger collecting ducts (*papillary ducts*) which open on the tips of the renal papillae. There urine is discharged into the minor calyces of the renal pelvis, and then is conveyed by the ureters to

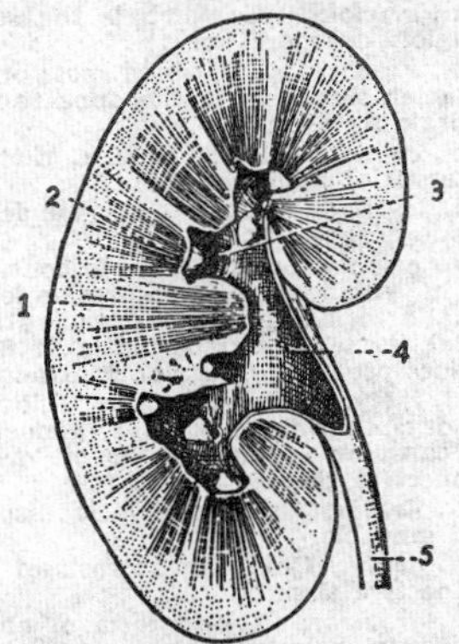

RIGHT KIDNEY, POSTERIOR VIEW OF SECTION

1. Cortex. 2. Renal pyramid. 3. Calyx. 4. Pelvis. 5. Ureter.

the bladder. Periodically the bladder discharges its contents to the outside through the *urethra* (*micturition*).

Substances which are entirely or almost entirely reabsorbed during passage through the tubule are known as *high threshold substances.* These include glucose and chlorides of sodium, potassium, calcium, and magnesium. These are important blood constituents and excreted only when their concentrations in the blood are above normal. *Low* or *nonthreshold substances* are those which are reabsorbed only in limited quantities or not at all. These are usually end products of metabolism such as urea, uric acid, and creatine which appear in considerable quantities in the urine.

The formation of urine is a continuous process, the rate of filtration being dependent primarily upon the blood pressure within the glomeruli and the daily fluid intake. Osmotic pressure exerted by proteins within the blood plasma tends to hold water and dissolved substances within the blood vessels so that the effective filtration pressure (45 mm. Hg) is the difference between capillary blood pressure (70 mm. Hg) and osmotic (25 mm. Hg). General blood pressure and the velocity of blood flow are primary factors in the rate of urine formation.

The volume of urine excreted daily varies from 1000 cc. to 2000 cc. (av. 1500 cc.). The amount varies with water intake, nature of diet, degree of body activity, environmental and body temperature, age, blood pressure, and many other factors. Pathological conditions may affect the volume and nature of the urine excreted.

Nerve Supply: From renal plexuses forming rich networks about renal vessels. Include both sympathetic and parasympathetic (vagal) fibers.

Symptoms of Kidney Disorder: Lumbar pain, renal colic, fever, disturbances in micturition (anuria, oliguria, or pain on micturition), presence of blood, pus, or abdominal substances in the urine, tenderness or swelling in costovertebral region, enlargement or diminution in size of kidney, edema.

Kidney Examination: By palpation, intravenous pyelography, cystoscopy, panendoscopy.

k., amyloid. K. which is the seat of amyloid degeneration.

k., branny. K. in which spots of fatty degeneration give it the appearance of containing bran.

k., contracted. The small k. of chronic interstitial or diffuse nephritis.

k., cystic. One that has undergone cystic degeneration.

k., embolic contracted. A contracted k. in which embolic infarction of the renal arterioles produces degeneration of renal tissue, and hyperplasia of fibrous tissues produces irregular contraction.

k., fatty. One with fatty infiltration or degeneration of tubular, glomerular, or capsular epithelium, or of vascular connective tissue.

k., floating. One which is displaced and movable.

k., gouty. One with necrosis of renal connective tissue.

k., granular. A slow form of chronic nephritis, in which the size is diminished, and color is red with hard, fibrous, and granular texture.

k., hobnail. Granular k.

k., hogback. Pigback k., *q.v.*

k., horseshoe. Congenital malformation with sup. or inf. extremities united by an isthmus of renal or fibrous tissue, in the form of a horseshoe.

k., lardaceous. Chronic nephritis, often secondary to syphilis, with infiltration with lardaceous matter, of the malpighian bodies, arteries, tubes, and epithelium.

k., large mottled. A type of chronic parenchymatous nephritis.

k., large red. One resembling that of acute parenchymatous nephritis.

k., large white. A chronic parenchymatous nephritis, resulting from an acute inflammation, the organ exceeding 12 oz. in weight.

k., movable. Displaced or loosened. Sym: Dragging, heavy pains in abdomen, worse when erect; melancholia, hysteria, gastrointestinal disturbance; sensitive enlarged or abnormally placed k. Treatment: Surgical. Syn: *nephroptosis.*

k., polycystic. K. bearing many cysts.

k., red contracted. Granular kidney, *q.v.*

k., sacculated. A condition in which the organ has been absorbed and only the distended capsule remains.

k., senile. One with atrophy of the glomeruli and tubules seen in old age.

k., small red granular. Granular k.

k. stones. Concretions present in the pelvis of the kidney. They are composed principally of oxalates, phosphates, and carbonates and vary in size from small granular masses to an inch in diameter. Syn: *renal calculus, q.v.; renal lithiasis.* See also: *colloid.*

k., surgical. Suppurative pyelonephritis following operation upon urinary tract.

k., syphilitic. One with fibrous bands running across it, also caseating gummata, due to syphilis.

k., wandering. A floating k.

k., waxy. Lardaceous kidney, *q.v.*

Kienböck unit [Robert Kienböck, Austrian roentgenologist, 1891-1953]. Measurement of x-ray dosage; 1/10 of erythema dose.

Kier'nan's spaces [Francis Kiernan, English physician, 1800-1874]. The spaces between the lobes of the liver.

Kiesselbach's area (ke'sel-bahks) [Wilhelm Kiesselbach, German laryngologist, 1839-1902]. An area on the anterior inferior portion of the nasal septum. The commonest site for septal bleeding.

Kil'ian's pelvis [Hermann F. Kilian, German gynecologist, 1800-1863]. Pelvis affected with osteomalacia. Syn: *pelvis spinosa.*

kilo- [G.]. One thousand.

kil'ogram [G. *chilioi,* a thousand, + gramma, a weight]. One thousand grams or 2.2 lbs. avoirdupois. Abbr: kg.

kiloliter (kil'o-lī-ter) [Fr. *kilolitre*]. One thousand liters.

kil'ometer [Fr. *kilomètre*]. One thousand meters, or 3281 feet (roughly 0.6 of a mile). Abbr: km.

kilonem. A unit of nutrition equivalent to 667 calories, the energy provided by one liter of milk.

kil'ovolt [G. *chilioi,* a thousand, + *volt*]. One thousand volt unit. Abbr: kv.

kil'owatt. A unit of electrical energy equal to one thousand watts. Abbr: kw.

kilurane (kil'u-rān). A unit of radioactivity, equivalent to one thousand uranium units.

kinanesthesia (kin-an-es-the′zĭ-ă) [G. *kinein*, to move, + *an-*, priv., + *aisthēsis*, sensation]. Inability to perceive extent of movement, or direction resulting in ataxia.

kinase (kin′ās) [G. *kinein*, to move]. An organic substance which activates an enzyme.

kinemat′ics [G. *kinein*, to move]. Science of motion.

kineplastic [G. *kinein*, to move, + *plastikos*, formed]. Pert. to kineplasty.

kin′eplasty [" + *plassein*, to form]. A form of amputation so that motion is imparted to an artificial limb.

kinergety (kin′er-jet-ĭ) [" + *ergon*, energy]. The potential capacity for kinetic energy.

kinesalgia (kĭn-ĕ-sal′jĭ-ă) [G. *kinēsis*, movement, + *algos*, pain]. Pain attending muscular movement.

kinesia (kin-e′sĭ-ă) [G. *kinēsis*, motion]. Sickness caused by motion, as seasickness, car sickness. Syn: *kinectosis.*

kinesialgia (kĭ-ne-sĭ-al′jĭ-ă) [" + *algos*, pain]. Pain caused by muscular movements. Syn: *kinesalgia.*

kinesiatrics (kĭ-ne-sĭ-at′riks) [" + *iatrikos*, curative]. Treatment involving active and passive movements. Syn: *kinesitherapy.*

kinesim′eter. An apparatus for determining the extent of movement of a part.

kinesiodic (kĭ-ne-sĭ-od′ik) [" + *odos*, path]. Pert. to paths through which motor impulses pass.

kinesiology (kĭ-nē-sĭ-ol′ō-jĭ) [G. *kinēsis*, motion, + *logos*, study]. The study of muscles and muscular movement.

kinesioneurosis (kĭ-ne-sĭ-o-nu-ro′sis) [" + *neuron*, nerve, + *-ōsis*]. Functional disorder marked by tics and spasms.

k., external. K. affecting external muscles.

k., vascular. K. of the vasomotor system.

k., visceral. K. affecting muscles of internal organs.

kinesiotherapy (kĭ-ne″sĭ-o-ther′ă-pĭ). Therapeutic exercises. Syn: *kinesitherapy.*

kinesis (kin-e′sis) [G.]. Motion.

kinesither′apy [" + *therapeia*, therapy]. Treatment by movements. Syn: *kinetotherapy.*

kinesod′ic [" + *odos*, path]. Rel. to the conveyance of motor impulses.

kinesthesia (kin-es-the′zĭ-ă) [" + *aisthēsis*, sensation]. 1. Ability to perceive extent or direction, or weight of movement. 2. Illusion of gliding through space.

kinesthesiometer (kin″es-thē-zĭ-om′ĕ-ter) [" + " + *metron*, measure]. Instrument for testing the muscular reaction.

kinesthet′ic [" + *aisthēsis*, sensation]. Rel. to kinesthesia.

kinetic (kĭ-net′ĭk) [G. *kinēsis*, motion]. Pert. to or consisting of motion.

kinetosis (kin″ĕ-to′sis) [" + *-ōsis*]. Any disorder caused by motion, such as seasickness, car sickness, etc. Syn: *kinesia.*

kinetotherapy (kĭ-net″o-ther′ă-pĭ) [" + *therapeia*, treatment]. Treatment that employs active and passive movements. Syn: *kinesitherapy.*

king's evil. Constitutional condition characterized by glandular swellings in neck and inflammation of joints and mucosa.

So called, because it was thought curable by touch of a king. Syn: *scrofula.*

kink. Unnatural angle or bend in a duct or tube such as the intestine or ureter.

kinom′eter [G. *kinein*, to move, + *metron*, measure]. Instrument which measures displacements of the uterus.

kinomom′eter [" + *metron*, measure]. Device which measures degree of motion of fingers and toes.

kinone (kĭ′nōn). Quinone.

kiotome (kĭ′o-tōm) [G. *kiōn*, column, + *tomē*, incision]. Instrument for amputating the uvula.

kiotomy (kĭ-ot′o-mĭ) [" + *tomē*, incision]. Use of the kiotome in amputating the uvula.

Kisch's reflex (kĭsh) [Bruno Kisch, German physiologist, born 1890]. Closure of an eye resulting from stimulation of heat or some tactile irritant on the ext. auditory meatus or deeper portions of canal up to tympanum. Syn: *auriculopalpebral reflex.*

Kite apparatus [Joseph H. Kite, American orthopaedic surgeon, born 1891]. Apparatus for re-education of weak muscles and for assistance in overcoming contractures of forearm, wrist and fingers.

KJ. Abbr. for *knee jerk.*

KK. Abbr. for *knee kick* (knee jerk).

kl. Abbr. for *klang* and *kiloliter.*

Klebsiella (klĕb-sĭ-el′ă) [Edwin Klebs, German bacteriologist, 1834-1913]. A genus of bacteria of the family Enterobacteriaceae. They are short, plump, gram-negative bacilli which form capsules. They are nonmotile and do not form spores. Frequently associated with respiratory infections. Commonly called the Friedlander group.

K. ozaenae. Species found in ozena. See: *ozena.*

K. pneumoniae. A cause of pneumonia. Also found as a secondary invader in other respiratory infections such as bronchitis or sinusitis. Syn: *pneumobacillus; Friedländer's bacillus.*

K. rhinoscleromatis. The cause of rhinoscleroma.

Klebs-Loeffler bacil′lus (klebs-lef′ler) [Edwin Klebs; Friedrich Loeffler, German bacteriologist, 1852-1915]. The bacillus of diphtheria. Syn: *Corynebacterium diphtheriae.* See: *diphtheria.*

klepto- (klĕp′tō) [G. *kleptein*, to steal]. Combining form meaning to steal.

kleptolagnia (klep″to-lag′nĭ-ă) [G. *kleptein*, to steal, + *lagneia*, lust]. Sexual gratification derived from stealing.

kleptomania (klep-to-ma′nĭ-ă) [" + *mania*, madness]. Impulsive stealing, the motive not being in the intrinsic value of the article to the patient. There is often deep regret following the act.

kleptoma′niac [" + *mania*, madness]. 1. A psychopathic personality suffering from impulsive stealing. 2. Pert. to kleptomania.

kleptophobia (klep-to-fo′bĭ-ă) [" + *phobos*, fear]. Morbid fear of stealing.

Klieg eye (klēg). Conjunctivitis, lacrimation and photophobia from exposure to the intense lights used in making moving pictures.

Kline test, Kline-Young test [Benjamin Kline, American pathologist, 1886-]. A microscope slide precipitation test for presence of syphilis.

Klon′dike bed. Outdoor sleeping bed that protects patient from draughts.

Klumpke's paralysis (kloomp′kēz) [Madame A. Dejerine Klumpke, Paris neurologist, 1859-1927]. Atrophic paralysis of forearm.

km. Abbr. for *kilometer.*

$KMnO_4$. Potassium permanganate.

Knapp's forceps [Herman J. Knapp, American ophthalmologist, 1832-1911]. A forceps with blades like rollers for expressing trachomatous granulations on the palpebral conjunctiva.

knead'ing [A. S. *cnedan,* to press a man]. A form of massage, consisting of grasping, wringing, lifting, rolling, or pressing part of a muscle or group of muscles. SYN: *pétrissage.*

knee [A. S. *cneōw*]. The ant. aspect of the leg at the articulation of the femur and tibia; also the articulation itself, covered anteriorly with the patella or kneecap. Formed by the femur, tibia, and patella.

RS: *geniculate, geniculum, "genu-" words, "gon-" words, housemaid's k., patella, popliteal.*

k., Brodie's. A chronic, fungoid synovitis of the knee joint in which the affected parts become soft and pulpy.

k. -chest position. Resting upon the knees and chest with forearms supporting the head. SEE: *position.*

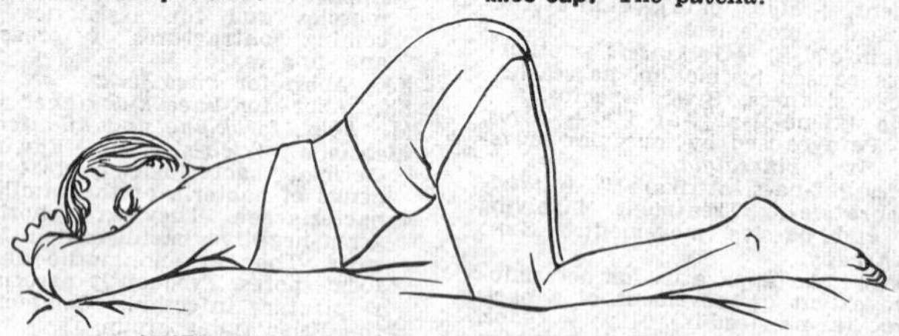

KNEE-CHEST OR GENUPECTORAL POSITION.

k., dislocations of the. Displacement of the knee.

Dislocations of the knee in themselves are unusual. The so-called dislocation of the knee is usually due to various injuries of the joint and of the complicating structures of the knee, such as the tearing of the crushed tendons or ligaments, or slipping of the cartilages, etc., and should be treated either by a straight splint, as in a fracture of the kneecap, or two splints, one on either side of the knee, as in a fracture, and the patient should be transported to a hospital as quickly as possible.

k., game. A lay term for internal derangement of knee joint.

PATH: Usually a torn internal cartilage, a fracture of the tibial spine, or an injury to the collateral or cruciate ligaments.

SYM: Pain or instability, locking, and weakness.

F. A. TREATMENT: Immobilize with a post. splint plus heat and massage. Surgical exploratory arthrotomy may be necessary.

k., housemaid's. Inflamed condition of the bursa in front of the patella, with accumulation of fluid therein, frequently seen in scrubwomen.

k., in-. The condition in which the knees come together while the ankles are far apart, caused by an outward distortion of the leg throwing knee inside the normal line. SYN: *genu valgum; knock-k.*

k. jerk reflex. The reflex contraction or clonic spasm of the quadriceps muscle, produced by sharply striking the ligamentum patellae when the leg hangs loosely flexed at right angles. It is seen normally in health, but is usually absent in locomotor ataxia, multiple neuritis, lesions of the lower portion of the spinal cord, lesions of the ant. gray horns of the cord, meningitis, infantile paralysis, pseudohypertrophic paralysis, atrophic paralysis, etc., and increased in spinal irritability, lesions of the pyramidal tract, cerebral tumors, sclerosis of the brain and cord, etc. SYN: *patellar reflex.* SEE: *jerk.*

k. joint. The articulation of the femur and tibia.

k., knock- In-knee, *q.v.*

k., lawn tennis. A sprain of int. semilunar cartilage of k. joint.

k., locked. Condition in which the leg cannot be extended. Usually due to displacement of semilunar cartilage.

k. of the internal capsule. The curve at the meeting place of the ant. and post. limbs of the internal capsule of the brain.

k., out-. Bowleg. SYN: *genu varum.*

knee'cap. The patella.

Kneipp cure (nīp) [Rev. Father Sebastian Kneipp, 1821-1897]. Application of water in various forms and degrees of temperature in the cure of disease, esp. wading in cold, dewy grass. SYN: *hydrotherapy.*

kneippism (nīp'izm). Walking barefoot in dewy grass, bathing in cold water, etc., as a cure of disease.

knife (nīf) [A. S. *cnīf*]. A cutting instrument.

k., electric. A knife carrying a high frequency cutting current.

knismogenic (nis-mo-jen'ik) [G. *knismos,* tickling of the skin, + *genein,* to produce]. Sensation of tickling.

knit'ting [A. S. *cnittan,* to make knots]. The union of pieces of a fractured bone.

KNO_3. Potassium nitrate, niter, saltpeter.

knock-knee. Condition of having the knees turned inward. SYN: *genu valgum; in-knee, q.v.*

knockout drops. Colloquial name for chloral hydrate given in alcoholic beverages to produce rapid coma.

knot. 1. An intertwining of a cord or cord-like structure to form a lump or knob. 2. In surgery, the intertwining of the ends of a suture, ligature, bandage, or sling so that the ends will not slip or become separated. 3. In anatomy, an enlargement forming a knob-like structure.

k., false. An external bulging of the umbilical cord resulting from the coiling of the umbilical blood vessels.

k., Hensen's. A knoblike structure at the anterior end of the primitive streak. SYN: *Hensen's node.*

k., primitive. Hensen's knot, *q.v.*

k., syncytial. A protuberance formed by many nuclei of the syntrophoblast and found on surface of a chorionic villus.

k., true. A knot formed by the fetus slipping through a loop of the umbilical cord.

knuckle. Prominence of the dorsal aspect of any of the phalangeal joints esp. of the distal heads of the metacarpals when the fist is clenched.

koag'amin. Commercial preparation of blood coagulant.

K. O. C. Abbr. of *cathodal opening contraction.* SYN: *COC.*

Kocher's reflex (ko'kerz) [Theodor Kocher, Swiss surgeon, 1841-1917]. Contraction of abdominal muscles following moderate compression of testicle.

Koch's bacil'lus (kōks) [Robert Koch, German bacteriologist, 1843-1910]. The bacillus of tuberculosis. SYN: *Mycobacterium tuberculosis.*

K.'s law or postulates. To prove an organism the cause of a disease or lesion; 1st, microorganism in question must appear in lesion at all times; 2nd, pure cultures must be obtained from it; 3rd, pure cultures when inoculated into susceptible animals must reproduce the disease or pathological condition; and, 4th, the organism must be obtained again in pure culture from the inoculated animal.

K.'s lymph. Tuberculin.

K.'s phenomenon. Local inflammatory reaction resulting from injection of tuberculin into the skin of a person who has been previously exposed to the tubercle bacillus.

KOH. Potassium hydroxide.

Kohlrausch's fold or **valve** (kōhl'rowshs) [Otto L. B. Kohlrausch, German physician, 1811-1854]. Fold of mucous membrane extending into rectum; rectal valve. SYN: *plica transversales recti; Houston's valves.*

koilonychia (koy-lo-nik'ĭ-ă) [G. *koilos,* hollow, + *onyx, onych-,* nail]. Malformation of the fingernails; outer surface is concave.

koinotropic type (koin'o-trop-ik) [G. *koinos,* common, + *tropos,* a turning]. Term applied to one who can give and take, as the "good mixer."

ko'la. Cardiac and nerve stimulant derived from *Sterculia acuminata.* Its principal ingredients are caffeine, theobromine, and colatin. SYN: *cola.*

Kol'mer test [John Kolmer, Philadelphia pathologist, 1886-]. 1. A modification of the Wassermann test. 2. Complement fixation test for some infectious diseases.

kolp- [G.]. Prefix indicating vagina. Usually spelled *colp-.*

kolpi'tis [G. *kolpos,* vagina, + *-itis,* inflammation]. Inflammation of vaginal mucous membrane. SYN: *colpitis.*

kolpot'omy [" + *tomē,* incision]. A vaginal operation. SYN: *colpotomy; elytrotomy.*

kol'yone [G. *kōlyein,* to hinder]. An organic secretion carried in the blood to other organs. It functions to inhibit growth and function. SYN: *chalone; colyone.*

kolypeptic (ko-lĭ-pep'tĭk) [" + *pepsis,* digestion]. Retarding digestion.

kolyphrenia (kol-ĭ-fre'nĭ-ă) [" + *phrēn,* mind]. Exaggerated mental inhibition.

kolyseptic (ko-lĭ-sep'tĭk) [" + *sēpsis,* putrefaction]. Antiseptic.

kolytic (ko-lit'ĭk) [G. *kōlyein,* to hinder] Hindering or presenting or checking, as a reaction to a stimulus.

Kondoleon's operation (kon-do'le-ŏn). Surgical removal of layers of subcutaneous tissue to relieve elephantiasis.

koniocortex. The cortex of the sensory areas, so named because of its granular appearance.

koniol'ogy [G. *konis,* dust, + *logos,* study]. Science of dust and its effects. SYN: *coniology.*

koniometer (ko-nĭ-om'ĕ-ter) [" + *metron,* measure]. Device for estimating amt. of dust in the air.

koniosis (ko-nĭ-o'sis) [" + *-ōsis,* intensive]. Any morbid condition caused by dust. SYN: *coniosis.*

kopf-tet'anus. Tetanus developing subsequent to head wounds.

kopiopia (ko-pĭ-o'pĭ-ă) [G. *kopos,* fatigue]. Eyestrain. SYN: *copiopia.*

Kop'lik's spots [Henry Koplik, New York pediatrician, 1858-1927]. Small red spots with bluish white centers on the oral mucosa, particularly in the region opposite the molars.

A diagnostic sign in measles before the rash appears. Not infrequently, the spots disappear as the eruption develops.

kopophobia. Abnormal fear of fatigue or exhaustion.

Kopp's asthma. Spasm of the glottis in infants not over two years of age. Thought to be due to an enlarged thymus. SYN: *laryngismus stridulus.*

koronion (ko-rō'nĭ-on) [G. *korōnē,* crest]. Apex of coronoid process of the mandible.

koroscopy (kor-os'ko-pĭ) [G. *korē,* pupil, + *skopein,* to examine]. Shadow test for refraction of the eye.

Korsakoff's psychosis or **syndrome** (kor'să-kofs) [Sergei S. Korsakoff, Russian neurologist, 1854-1900]. One characterized by a psychosis with a polyneuritis, disorientation, muttering delirium, insomnia, illusions and hallucinations, painful extremities, rarely a bilateral wrist drop, more frequently bilateral foot drop with pain or pressure over the long nerves.

Occurs as a sequel to chronic alcoholism but may be due to other intracranial pathology. SYN: *polyneuritic psychosis.*

koumiss (koo'mis) [Tartar]. Fermented milk beverage. Also spelled *kumiss, kumyss.*

Kr. Chemical symbol for krypton.

Kraepelin's classification (kra'pă-linz). A classification of mental disease into two groups: the manic-depressive and the schizophrenic.

kraurosis (kraw-rō'sĭs) [G. *krauros,* dry]. Atrophy and dryness of skin and any mucous membrane, esp. of the vulva.

The subcutaneous fat of the mons pubis and labia disappears, clitoris and prepuce atrophy, and stenosis of the vaginal orifice is common. Fissures may develop. Epithelioma is prone to occur most frequently in postmenopausal women or those who have had ovaries removed.

ETIOL: Probably hypoestrinism.

k. penis. Condition in which the glans penis atrophies and becomes shriveled. SYN: *balanitis xerotica obliterans; Stuhmer's disease.*

k. vul'vae. An atrophy of the skin and mucosa which pathologically consists of a marked atrophy of the vulvar skin, and which is characterized clinically by severe itching. Seen in elderly women.

The skin has a white marblelike appearance, and frequently shows excoriations as a result of the scratching. In a large percentage of these patients, the skin, if allowed to go on without operative interference, may undergo malignant degeneration. SYN: *leukoplakic vulvitis.*

Krause's end bulb [Wilhelm Krause, German anatomist, 1833-1910]. An encapsulated sensory receptor found widely distributed in connective tissue underlying the skin and mucous membranes. It is the end organ for cold sensations.

K.'s glands [Karl Krause, German anatomist, 1797-1868]. Small mucous acinous glands located beneath the fornix conjunctiva. They are accessory lacrimal glands and open into the fornix.

K.'s membrane [Wilhelm Krause]. Thin, dark disk transversely crossing through and bisecting clear zone of a striated muscle and bisecting the clear zone (isotropic disk) of a striated muscle fiber. Also called the Z disk. The portion between two Z disks constitutes a sarcomere.

K.'s valve [Karl Krause]. Mucous membrane fold at juncture where lacrimal sac narrows into nasal duct. SYN: *Béraud's valve.*

kreatinine (kre-at'in-in). Creatinine, *q.v.*

kreotox'in [G. *krĕas,* flesh, + *toxikon,* poison]. Any poisonous substance present in meat due to bacterial action.

kreotox'ism [" + " + *ismos,* state of]. Meat poisoning.

Kromayer lamp (krō'mī-er). Water cooled, mercury quartz lamp for local ultraviolet treatments.

Krompecher's tumor (krōm'pekh-ers). Rodent ulcer. SYN: *Jacob's ulcer.*

Kronecker's center (krōn'ek-ers). The inhibitory center of the heart.

Krönig's area or field (kra'nĭg). Resonant region in the thorax over the apices of the lungs.

Kruk'enberg's tumor [Frederick Krukenberg, German pathologist, 1871-1946]. A malignant tumor of the ovary, usually bilateral, and frequently secondary to malignancy of the gastrointestinal tract.

Histologically these tumors consist of myxomatous connective tissue and cells having a signet ring arrangement of their nuclei. The epithelial tissue resembles malignancy of the original site.

krypton (krip'ton) [G. *kryptos,* hidden]. A gaseous element found in small amts. in the atmosphere. SYMB: Kr. At. wt. 83.80; at. no. 36.

K_2SO_4. Potassium sulfate.

kumiss, kumyss (koo'mis). 1. Cow's milk with sugar and yeast after fermentation. 2. Fermented mare's milk. Also spelled *koumiss.*

Kund'rat's lymphosarco'ma. Lymphosarcoma which affects adjacent glands, but rarely invades neighboring organs.

Kupffer's cells [Karl N. Kupffer, German anatomist, 1829-1902]. SEE: under *cell.*

kuru (koo'roo). A rapidly progressive neurological disease which is invariably fatal. The disease affects mostly adult women and children of both sexes of members of the Fore tribe of New Guinea. Probably due to a slow-acting virus.

kwashiorkor (kwash-ĭ-or'kor) [African word meaning *red hair*]. A disease resulting from a deficiency of protein in infancy or early childhood.

kyestein, kyesthein (ki-es'te-in) [G. *kyēsis,* conception]. A scum or film on stale urine; formerly thought to be a sign of pregnancy. SYN: *cyesthein.*

kyllosis (kil-lō'sĭs) [G. *kyllos,* twisted]. Clubfoot.

ky'matism [G. *kyma,* wave, + *ismos,* state of]. Twitching of isolated segments of muscle. SYN: *myokymia.*

ky'mogram. A tracing or recording made by a kymograph.

kymograph (kī'mō-grăf) [G. *kyma,* wave, + *graphein,* to write]. An apparatus for recording movements of a writing pen. The apparatus is designed so that the pen moves in response to force applied to it. Widely used in physiology to record activities such as blood pressure changes, muscle contractions, respiratory movements, etc. Consists of a drum rotated by a spring or electric motor. Drum is covered by a paper upon which the record is made.

ky'moscope [" + *skopein,* to examine]. Device for measuring variations in blood pressure.

kyogenic (ki-o-jen'ĭk) [G. *kyēsis,* pregnancy, + *gennan,* to produce]. Inducing pregnancy.

kypho- [G.]. Prefix: Humped.

kyphorachitis (ki''fo-ră-ki'tis). Rachitic deformity involving thorax and spinal column. Results in development of anteroposterior hump.

kyphoscoliosis (ki''fo-sko''lĭ-o'sis). Lateral curvature of the spine accompanying anteroposterior hump.

kyphosis (ki-fo'sis) [G. humpback). SYN: *humpback; spinal curvature.* Exaggeration or angulation of normal posterior curve of spine. Gives rise to condition commonly known as humpback, hunchback, or Pott's curvature. Also refers to excessive curvature of the spine with convexity backward. The former may be due to congenital anomaly, disease (tuberculosis, syphilis), malignancy, or compression fracture. The latter may result from faulty posture, osteo- or rheumatoid arthritis, rickets, or other conditions.

kyphotic (ki-fot'ik) [G. *kyphōsis,* humpback]. Affected by or pert. to kyphosis.

ky'rin. A protein resisting tryptic digestion, which yields amino acids when treated with an acid.

kyrtorrhachic (kir-to-rak'ik) [G. *kyrtos,* curved, + *rachis,* spine]. Spinal curvature with concavity backward.

kysthitis (kis-thi'tis) [G. *kysthos,* vagina, + *-itis,* inflammation]. Inflammation of the vagina. SYN: *colpitis; vaginitis.*

kysthoptosis (kis-thop-to'sis) [" + *ptōsis,* a falling]. Prolapse of the vagina.

kyto- [G.]. Prefix; denoting cell. SEE: *cyto-.*

Notes

Notes

L

L. Abbr. for *Latin. Lactobacillus, left, length, lithium, light sense, liter.*
L_+. Symb. for *limes death, q.v.*
L_0. Symb. for *limes zero, q.v.*
l —. In chem., symb. for *levo* (left, or counterclockwise).
La. Symb. for *lanthanum.*
lab, lab ferment. SYN: *zymogen.* One of a number of enzymes produced by bacteria which have the power to coagulate liquid proteins. EXAM: *rennin.*
Labarraque's solution (lăb-ar-ak') [Antoine G. Labarraque, French chemist, 1777-1850]. Chlorinated soda solution; a disinfectant.
Labbe's vein (lă-ba') [Leon Labbé, French surgeon, 1832-1916]. Vein connecting lateral to sup. longitudinal sinus. SYN: *superior anastamotic vein.*
la'bia (pl. of *labium*) [L.]. 1. Lips. 2. The lips of the vulva.
RS: *clitoris, Hottentot's apron, mons veneris, nymphas, nymphoncus, smegma, vagina.*
l. majora. The 2 folds of cellular adipose tissue lying on either side of the vaginal opening and forming the lateral borders of the vulva. Lozenge shaped.
Their medial surfaces unite anteriorly above the clitoris to form the *anterior commissure;* posteriorly they are connected by a poorly defined *posterior commissure.* They are separated by a cleft, the *rima pudendi.* In young girls, their medial surfaces are in contact with each other concealing the labia minora and vestibule; in older women, the labia minora may protrude between them.
l. minora. Two thin folds of integument which lie within the labia majora and enclose the vestibule. Anteriorly each divides into two smaller folds which unite with similar folds from the other side and enclose the clitoris, the more anterior one forming the prepuce (*preputium clitoridis*) of the clitoris, the posterior one forming the *frenulum clitoridis.* In young children they are entirely hidden by the labia majora.
labial (la'bĭ-al) [L. *labium,* lip]. Pert. to the lips.
l. glands. Many racemose glands bet. labial mucosa and orbicularis muscle opening on lip's inner surface.
labialism (la'bĭ-al-izm) [L. *labialis,* pert. to lip, + G. *ismos,* state of]. Defective speech in which labial sounds are stressed.
labile (lab'il) [L. *labī,* to glide]. Not fixed; unsteady; easily disarranged.
l., heat. Easily altered or decomposed by heat. SYN: *thermolabile.*
lability (lab-il'it-ĭ) [G. *labī,* to glide]. State of being unstable or changeable.
labioalveolar (lab"ĭ-ō-ăl-ve'ol-ar) [L. *labium,* lip, + *alveolus,* little hollow]. Pert. to lips and tooth sockets.
labiocervical (lab"ĭ-ō-ser'vĭ-kăl) [" + *cervix, cervic-,* neck]. Pert. to lips, and the neck of a tooth.
labioglossolaryngeal (la"bĭ-o-glos"o-lar-in'je-ăl) [" + G. *glōssa,* tongue, + *larynx,* larynx]. Pert. to lips, tongue, and larynx.
labioglossopharyngeal (la"bĭ-o-glos"o-far-in'je-ăl) [" + " + *pharynx,* throat]. Pert. to the lips, tongue, and pharynx.
labiograph (la'bĭ-o-grăf) [" + G. *graphein,* to write]. Device for registering the lip movements in speaking.
labiology (lā-bĭ-ol'o-jĭ) [" + G. *logos,* study]. Study of the lip movements in speaking or singing.
labiomancy (la'bĭ-o-man"sĭ) [" + G. *manteia,* foretelling]. Interpreting speech by reading lip movements.
labiomental (la-bĭ-ō-men'tal) [" + *mentum,* chin]. Pert. to the lower lip and chin.
labiomycosis (la"bĭ-o-mī-ko'sis) [" + G. *mykēs,* fungus, + *-ōsis*]. Any disease of the lips due to presence of a fungus.
labiopalatine (la"bĭ-ō-pal'ă-tīn) [" + *palatum,* palate]. Relating to the lips and palate.
labioplasty (la'bĭ-o-plas"tĭ) [" + G. *plassein,* to form]. Plastic surgery of the lips. SYN: *cheiloplasty.*
labiotenaculum (la"bĭ-o-ten-ak'u-lum) [L. *labium,* lip, + *tenaculum,* a hook]. Instrument for holding lips during an operation.
la'bium (pl. *labia*) [L. lip]. A lip or a structure like one. SEE: *labia.*
l. cerebri. Margin of the cerebral hemispheres overlapping the corpus callosum.
l. inferius. Lower lip.
l. majus. Labia majora, *q.v.*
l. minus. Labia minora, *q.v.*
l. superius. The upper lip.
l. tympanicum. Outer edge of organ of Corti.
l. urethrae. Lateral margin of meatus urinarius externus.
l. uteri. Thickened margin of the cervix uteri.
l. vestibulare. Vestibular or inner edge of organ of Corti.
la'bor [L. work]. SYN: *parturition, delivery, childbirth.* The physiological process by which the fetus is expelled from the uterus at term.
Normal appearance 280 days after last menstruation.
Labor is divided into three stages:
FIRST STAGE: *Dilatation*: Lasting from the onset of uterine contractions until the cervix uteri is dilated completely.
SECOND STAGE: *Expulsion*: From the time of complete dilatation until the expulsion of the fetus.
THIRD STAGE: *Placental*: From the time of expulsion of the fetus until the expulsion of the placenta.
PREPARATION: Well ventilated, sunny room; temperature 65° during labor, 70° after. Bed with fresh, well-aired linen and a pad previously prepared, of heavy paper covered with cotton wool, the whole covered with cheesecloth, large enough to cover middle third of bed. This receives the discharge and is easily removed and replaced by a similar fresh one, keeping the bed in good condition.
The patient is given enema if bowels have not moved freely within 12 hours; bladder emptied if nature does not attend to it.

The vulva and mons veneris and thighs rendered thoroughly aseptic (patient will have taken a bath as soon as indications appeared that labor was drawing near); shaving or clipping of the hair about the vulvae is optional. Long cotton stockings, made of canton flannel or tennis flannel, reaching to the hips, should be drawn on, protecting limbs from exposure. The gown to be worn turned up and smoothly fastened out of the way above the waist, an old sheet or cloth pinned comfortably about the waist next to body.

After the third stage, by removing soiled pad, stockings and old sheet, gown may be brought down and patient is in good condition for rest without being disturbed.

A large number of old soft white cloths should be at hand aseptically clean, in case of hemorrhage. Also a number of vulval pads prepared for receiving the lochia; vessels of boiled water, cooled and kept tightly covered, should be provided. Many obstetricians carry with them a stout strap with stirruplike ends for the hands, which may be thrown about the foot of bed to aid in expulsive movements.

First Stage: Ascertain amount of dilation and the presentation. In ordinary cases only physician and nurse desired in room; cold water or other cool, refreshing beverage only refreshment required unless protracted.

Ordinarily full dilation is accomplished within 6 hours. Sometimes in a very short time, at others much longer. Patient may walk about or make herself comfortable till second stage. Should then take her position on the pad on left side with breech near edge of bed, thighs flexed at right angles on abdomen and legs on thighs, feet against foot of bed as support during the expulsive efforts. Or the dorsal position (on the back) may be assumed. Pains become stronger and closer together.

Second Stage: During last of first stage or beginning of second, the membranes rupture and a portion of liquor amnii is discharged.

Pains come every 3 minutes or closer; head advances, and fetus is soon expelled; as head appears, attendant should bear the right hand upon the perineum in such a manner as to encircle the labia as much as possible with thumb and fingers, and while drawing down with these upon the labia must press gently forward and upward upon the perineum with the palm of same hand.

Ascertain that cord is not about child's neck. Have at hand a saucer of warm olive oil and as body advances rub it into all the places covered with the vernix which will then easily be removed later. Some form of prophylaxis for ophthalmia neonatorum is required by law in most states. Usually 2 drops of one per cent silver nitrate solution are instilled in the infant's eyes.

If by this time cord has stopped pulsating (usually in about 5 minutes), tie a ligature about 5 inches from the abdomen, another an inch nearer the placenta and cut between them. After thoroughly cleaning the cord and allowing blood to flow from it toward abdomen, take ends of first ligature and tie cord tightly one-half inch from abdomen (after ascertaining that no part of intestine protrudes into cord); this leaves a loop of umbilical cord which prevents hemorrhage or entrance of infection.

As the child is fully expelled the sheet covering the mother should be dropped between her and the child, who should be wrapped in a warm blanket at hand to receive him. The remaining portion of liquor amnii follows the expulsion and uterus contracts upon itself. This ends second stage.

Third Stage: Return of pain (usually a lull after completion of second stage); this marks expulsion of placenta—may occur within 20 minutes or not for hours. Uterus is found low down, hard, globular and size of fetal head.

Expulsion of placenta without retention of shreds of membrane may be accomplished by gentle twisting movement on cord as placenta appears in vulva, contraction of uterus and avoidance of hemorrhage may be aided by gentle massage of uterus through abdominal wall. After expulsion of placenta examine perineum to see if there is any laceration; if deep, repair at once, tie knees together to prevent pulling apart of wound. If tear is slight, leave for nature to heal and avoid infection. Caution used on changing pad at vulva not to tear out stitches by too hasty removal of pad.

Allow few moments' rest, then quickly remove all soiled bedding and apparel, bring down the pinned up gown, draw down shades and leave patient to rest.

From time to time feel if uterus is contracting as desired and that there is no hemorrhage. If labor is complicated by malpositions different tactics must be pursued in the different stages to suit the individual case.

The type of anesthetic used, whether local or general, is determined by the obstetrician. In some cases the mother will have been prepared in advance to have her child by the so-called painless method of childbirth. This method, which can be highly effective, requires no anesthetic.

l., *artificial*. Labor brought on by the use of ecbolics or hydrostatic bags.

l., *complicated*. Any complication occurring during the course of labor.

l., *dry*. Labor after most of the amniotic fluid has been drained away.

l., *false*. Uterine contractions coming on before the onset of actual labor.

l., *induced*. Labor brought on by the use of ecbolic hydrostatic bags, or any other method that may be used.

l., *instrumental*. Labor completed by mechanical means, such as the use of forceps.

l., *missed*. The patient goes through actual labor but the fetus dies and is not expelled.

l., *multiple*. Labor with two or more fetuses.

l., *precipitate*. Rapidly completed labor that occurs without the aid of an accoucheur.

l., *premature*. Labor coming on between the 7th month of gestation and full term.

l., *spontaneous*. Labor that is completed without external aid.

labor, *words pert. to*: abortion; acyesis; "amni-" words; ante partum; aponia; aponic; asynclitism; bag of waters, bag, hydrostatic; ballotment; basilysis; basiotripsy; bipara; biparous; bradytocia; breech presentation; brow presentation; bruit, placental; caput succedaneum; caul; cephalhematoma; cephalic version; cephalotomy; cesarean section; cesarotomy; chorda umbilicalis; cleidotomy; conception; conjugate; Crede's method; cross birth; delivery; disengagement; dystocia; ecbolic; eclampsia; embryectomy; embryo; embryoctony; embryotocia; embryulcia; encyesis; eutocia; fetus; fixity; gestation; Hegar's sign; hourglass contraction; impetigo herpetiformis; maneuver; mimetic; obstetrician; obstetrics; placenta; puerpera; puerperal; puerperium; quintuplets; restitution; Schultze's method; show; synclitism; vagitus; xerotocia.

laboratory (lab'or-a-to-rĭ) [L. *laboratorium,* work place]. A place equipped for analytical or experimental work.

Laborde's method [Jean B. V. Laborde, French physician, 1830-1903] (respiration stimulation). Stimulation of the respiratory center in asphyxiation by a series of rhythmical traction movements upon the tongue.

la'brum (pl. *labra*) [L. lip]. Lip, or liplike structure; the upper lip of an insect.

labyrinth (lab'ĭ-rinth) [G. *labyrinthos,* a maze]. 1. Intricate communicating passages. 2. The internal ear consisting of osseous and membranous labyrinths.

l., bony. Osseous labyrinth, *q.v.*

l. ethmoidal. The lateral mass of the ethmoid bone. Includes the sup. and middle conchae and encloses the ethmoidal air cells.

l., membranous. Structure in osseous labyrinth consisting of utricle and saccule of vestibule, 3 semicircular ducts, and the cochlear duct. All are filled with endolymph.

l., olfactory. The ethmoidal labyrinth, *q.v.*

l., osseous. Consists of vestibule, three semicircular canals, and cochlea. Channeled out of petrous portion of temporal bone.

labyrinthectomy (lab-ĭ-rin-thek'tō-mĭ) [" + *ektomē,* excision]. Excision of the labyrinth.

labyrinthine (lab-ĭ-rĭn'thĭn) [G. *labyrinthos,* a maze]. 1. Pert. to a labyrinth. 2. Intricate or involved, as a labyrinth.

labyrinthitis (lab-ĭ-rĭn-thi'tis) [" + *-itis,* inflammation]. Inflammation (acute or chronic) of labyrinth.

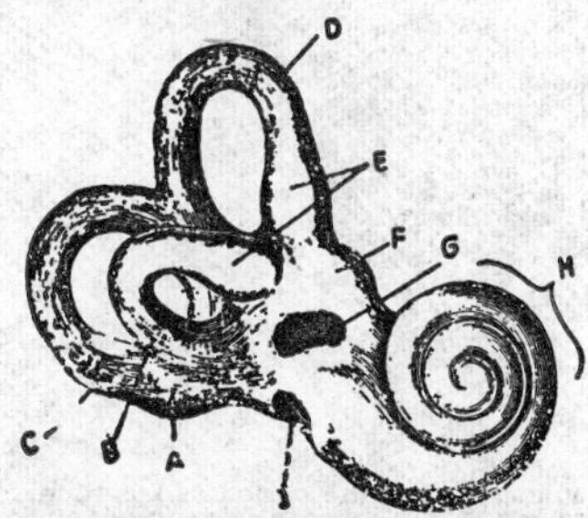

OSSEOUS LABYRINTH, ANTERIOR VIEW

A. Ampulla. B. External semicircular canal. C. Posterior semicircular canal. D. Superior semicircular canal. E. Ampullae. F. Vestibulum. G. Fenestra ovalis. H. Cochlea. I. Fenestra rotunda.

ETIOL: Primary infection, complication of influenza, otitis media, or of meningitis.

SYM: Vertigo, vomiting, nystagmus.

RS: *Meniere's disease.*

labyrinthotomy (lab-ĭ-rin-thot'o-mĭ) [" + *tomē,* incision]. Incision of the labyrinth.

lac (lak) [L.]. 1. Milk. 2. Milky medicinal substance.

lacerate (las'er-āt) [L. *lacerāre,* to tear]. To tear, as into irregular segments.

lacerated (las'er-a-ted) [L. *lacerāre,* to tear]. Torn; broken.

lacera'tion [L. *lacerāre,* to tear]. A wound or irregular tear of the flesh.

l. of cervix. Bilateral, stellate, or unilateral tear of the cervix uteri caused by childbirth.

l. of perineum. Injury to perineum caused by childbirth. If extending through sphincter ani muscle it is *complete.*

lacertus (lă-ser'tus) [L.]. 1. Muscular part of the arm. 2. A muscular or fibrous band.

l. cordis. Muscular tissue bands on inner cardiac surface. SYN: *trabecula carneae.*

l. fibro'sus. Aponeurotic band from the biceps tendon to the bicipital or semilunar fascia of forearm.

lacrimal (lak'rim-ăl) [L. *lacrima,* tear]. Pert. to the tears.

l. apparatus. Structures concerned with secretion and conduction of tears. Includes lacrimal gland and its excretory ducts, lacrimal canaliculi, lacrimal sac, and nasolacrimal duct which empties into nasal cavity.

l. bone. One at inner side of the orbital cavity.

l. duct. SYN: l. *canaliculus.* One of two ducts sup. and inf. which convey tears from lacrimal lake to the lacrimal sac.

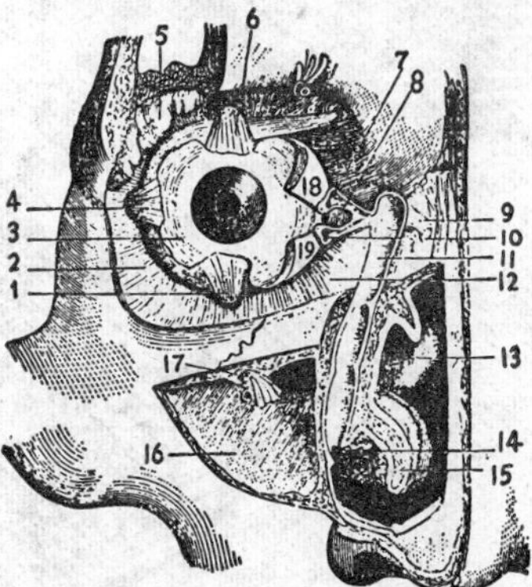

THE LACRIMAL APPARATUS.

1, Inferior rectus muscle; 2, lower eyelid; 3, eyeball; 4, lateral rectus muscle; 5, lacrimal gland; 6, superior rectus muscle; 7, upper lacrimal duct; 8, lacrimal caruncle; 9, medial palpebral ligament; 10, inferior lacrimal duct; 11, lacrimal sac; 12, lower eyelid; 13, middle meatus; 14, opening into inferior meatus; 15, inferior turbinate; 16, maxillary sinus; 17, infraorbital nerve.

l. gland. The gland which secretes the tears. A comp. tubuloalveolar gland located in orbit, superior and lateral to the eyeball. Consists of a large superior portion (pars orbitalis) and a smaller inferior portion (pars palpebralis).

l. reflex. Secretion of fluid resulting from irritation of corneal conjunctiva.

l. sac. Upper dilated portion of nasolacrimal duct situated in groove of lacrimal bone. Upper part is behind internal tarsal ligament. Measures 12 to 15 mm. in length.

lacrima'tion [L. *lacrima,* tear]. Secretion and discharge of tears.

lacrimator. A substance which induces the secretion of tears.

lacrimotomy (lak-rim-ot'o-mĭ) [" + G. *tomē,* incision]. Incision of lacrimal duct.

lactac'idase [L. *lac,* milk]. Enzyme in lactic acid bacteria which causes fermentation of lactic acid.

lactacidemia (lakt-as-id-e'mĭ-ă) [" + *acidus,* sour + G. *aima,* blood]. Lactic acid in the blood. SYN: *lacticemia.*

lactaciduria (lakt-a-sid-ū'rĭ-ă) [" + " + G. *ouron,* urine]. Lactic acid excreted in the urine.

lactagogue (lak'tă-gog) [L. *lac,* milk, + G. *agōgos,* leading]. Agent which induces secretion of milk.

lactalase (lak'tă-lās) [" + *ase,* enzyme]. Ferment converting dextrose into lactic acid.

lactalbu'min [" + *albumen,* coagulated white of egg]. The albumin of milk and cheese; a soluble simple protein.

When milk is heated, the lactalbumin coagulates and appears as a film over the top of the milk.

Lactalbumin is present in higher concentration in human milk than in cow's milk.

COMP: Carbon 52.19, hydrogen 7.18, nitrogen 15.77, oxygen 23.13, and sulfur 1.73.

lac'tase [L. *lac,* milk, + *ase,* enzyme]. An intestinal sugar splitting enzyme converting lactose into dextrose and galactose; found in intestinal juice.

SEE: *enzyme, maltase, sucrase, sugar.*

lactate (lak'tāt). [L. *lac,* milk]. A salt derived from lactic acid.

lactation (lak-ta'shun) [L. *lactatiō,* a suckling]. 1. The period of suckling in mammals. 2. The function of secreting milk.

DIET: The mother during this period needs additional calcium to offset its loss in the milk. One qt. of milk, an egg, and meat are needed once a day. Fruits, vegetables, and whole grain cereal should be added.

lacteal (lak'te-al) [L. *lac,* milk]. 1. Pert. to milk. 2. An intestinal lymphatic that takes up chyle and passes it to the lymph circulation, and by way of the thoracic duct to the blood vascular system.

SEE: *absorption, lymphatic.*

lactescence (lak-tes'ens) [L. *lactescere,* to become milky]. Condition of becoming, or resembling milk.

lac'tic [L. *lac,* milk]. Pert. to milk.

l. acid. A colorless syrupy liquid ($C_3H_6O_3$) formed in milk, sauerkraut, and in certain types of pickles by the fermentation of the sugars by microorganisms. It is also formed in muscles during activity by the breakdown of glycogen (glycolysis). Medicinally, lac-

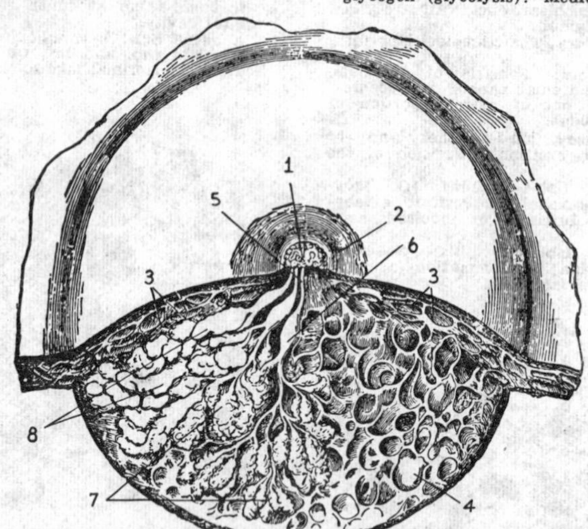

LACTIFEROUS GLANDS.

Dissection of the lower half of the female mamma, during the period of lactation. In the left hand side of the dissected part, the glandular lobes are exposed and partially unravelled; and on the right hand side the glandular substance has been removed to show the reticular loculi of the connective tissue in which the glandular lobules are placed: 1. Upper part of the mammilla or nipple. 2. Areola. 3. Subcutaneous masses of fat. 4. Reticular loculi of the connective tissue which support the glandular substance and contain the fatty masses. 5. One of three lactiferous ducts shown passing toward the mammilla where they open. 6. One of the sinus lactei or reservoirs. 7. Some of the glandular lobules which have been unravelled. 8.Others massed together.

tic acid is used as a spermicidal agent, a caustic antiseptic, and as a dietary constituent. SYN: *hydroxypropionic acid.*

l. acid fermentation. The production of lactic acid from carbohydrates by the action of various bacteria. Occurs commonly in milk and milk products.

lacticemia (lakt-ĭ-se'mĭ-ă) [" + G. *aima,* blood]. Lactic acid in the blood. SYN: *lactacidemia.*

lactiferous (lakt-if'er-us) [" + *ferre,* to bear]. Secreting and conveying milk.

l. ducts. Ducts of the mammary gland.

l. glands. 1. The mammary glands. 2. Montgomery's glands consisting of 20 to 24 glands in the areola of the nipples. SEE: *Ill., p. L-4.*

lactification (lak"tĭ-fĭ-ka'shun) [" + *facere,* to make]. Lactic acid production.

lactifuge (lak'tĭ-fuj) [" + *fugāre,* to expel]. 1. Stopping milk secretion. 2. Agent stopping milk secretion. SYN: *ischogalactic; antigalactic.*

lactigenous (lak-tij'en-us) [" + *gennan,* to produce]. Producing milk.

lactigerous (lak-tij'er-us) [" + *gerere,* to carry]. Secreting or conveying milk.

lac'tin [L. *lac,* milk]. Lactose, sugar of milk.

lactinated (lakt'in-āt-ed) [L. *lac,* milk]. Containing or prepared with milk sugar.

lactivorous (lakt-iv'or-us) [" + *vorāre,* to devour]. Living upon milk.

lactobacillin(e (lakt-o-bas'il-īn) [" + *bacillus,* little rod]. A preparation of lactic acid bacilli (1) to counteract intestinal putrefaction, (2) to cause lactic acid fermentation.

Lactobacillus (lakt-o-bă-sil'us) [" + *bacillus,* little rod]. A genus of bacteria belonging to the family Lactobacteriaceae. They are gram positive, nonmotile rod-shaped organisms which do not produce spores and are acid resisting. They produce lactic acid from carbohydrates. They are responsible for the souring of milk.

L. acidophilus. A lactic acid forming organism found in the intestinal contents of infants. It produces lactic acid fermentation of milk. Nonmotile gram positive rods found in gastric contents especially in cancer of stomach.

L. bulgaricus. The bacillus found in fermented milk. Milk fermented with this organism is known as Bulgarian milk.

L. casei. A type found in milk and cheese.

L. helveticus. Type found in Swiss cheese.

L. panis. Type occurring in sour dough.

lactobutyrometer (lakt"o-bu-tĭ-rom'et-er) [" + G. *boutyron,* butter, + *metron,* measure]. Instrument for estimating the cream content of milk.

lactocele (lakt'o-sēl) [" + G. *kēlē,* hernia]. Cystic tumor of breast due to occlusion of a milk duct. SYN: *galactocele.*

lactocrit (lakt'o-krĭt) [" + *kritēs,* judge]. Instrument for determining the fat content of milk.

lactodensimeter (lakt-o-den-sim'et-er) [" + *densus,* thick, + G. *metron,* measure]. Instrument for determining specific gravity of milk.

lactoflavin. Riboflavin, *q.v.*

lactogenic. Inducing the secretion of milk.

l. hormone. Prolactin, *q.v.*

lactoglobulin (lak"tō-glob'ū-lĭn) [L. *lac,* milk, + *globulus,* globule]. A protein found in milk.

lactolase (lak'to-lās) [L. *lac,* milk, + *ase,* enzyme]. An enzyme forming lactic acid. SYN: *lactacidase.*

lactolin (lakt'o-lĭn) [L. *lac,* milk]. Condensed or evaporated milk.

lactometer (lak-tom'et-er) [" + G. *metron,* measure]. Device for determining the specific gravity of milk.

lactophosphate (lakt'o-fos"fāt) [" + *phosphās,* phosphate]. A salt derived jointly from lactic and phosphoric acid.

lactorrhea (lakt-or-re'ă) [" + G. *roia,* flow]. Discharge of milk between nursings and after weaning of offspring. SYN: *galactorrhea.*

lactoscope (lak'to-skōp) [" + G. *skopein,* to examine]. Device for determining quality of milk.

lac'tose [L. *lac,* milk]. $C_{12}H_{22}O_{11}+H_2O$. A disaccharide which on hydrolysis yields glucose and galactose.

Bacteria can convert it into lactic and butyric acids, as in the souring of milk. 4-7% are found in the milk of all mammals. Its presence in the urine may be indicative of obstruction to flow of milk after cessation of nursing. Commercially, a fine powdered, white substance that will not dissolve in cold water.

USP. Crystalline sugar obtained from evaporation of cow's milk. Used as modified milk for infant feeding, or supplementary food for adults, as a diluent. SYN: *milk sugar.* SEE: *disaccharose.*

lactoserum (lakt-o-sēr'um) [" + *serum,* whey]. 1. Blood serum of an animal inoculated with milk; used to precipitate specific caseins from milk. 2. The whey of milk.

lactosuria (lak-to-su'rĭ-ă) [" + G. *ouron,* urine]. Occurrence of milk sugar (lactose) in the urine.

Frequent during pregnancy and lactation. Identified by osazone crystals.

lactotherapy (lakt-o-ther'ă-pĭ) [" + G. *therapeia,* therapy]. 1. Treatment with milk diet. 2. Medicinal treatment of nursing infant with drugs given to mother to be excreted in milk. SYN: *galactotherapy.*

lac"totox'in [" + G. *toxikon,* poison]. Any toxic substance occurring in milk that has decomposed.

lactovegetarian. 1. Pert. to milk and vegetables. 2. One who lives on a diet of milk and vegetables.

lacuna (la-ku'na) (pl. *lacunae*) [L. a pit]. 1. A small, hollow space, such as that found in bones, in which lie the osteoblasts. 2. A gap or hiatus found in cartilage or bone in which lie cartilage or bone cells.

l., absorption. Howship's l., *q.v.*

l., blood. SEE: *l., trophoblastic.*

l., bone. One of the isolated ovoid spaces bet. osseous lamellae, connected by canaliculi, containing a protoplasmic body or bone cell.

l., Howship's. A pit or groove in bone where resorption or dissolution of bone is occurring. Usually containing osteoclasts.

l., intervil'lous. SYN: *intervillous space.* A space in the placenta occupied by maternal blood and into which fetal placenta villi project.

l. laterales. Irregular diverticula on either side of the sup. sagittal sinus of the brain into which the arachnoidal granulations project.

l. magna. The largest pit-like recess in the fossa navicularis of the distal end of the male urethra.

l. pharyngis. Pit at pharyngeal end of eustachian tube.

l., trophoblastic. Irregular cavities in the syntrophoblast which develop into intervillous spaces or lacunae, *q.v.*

l. of the urethra. One of those in mucous membrane of the urethra, esp. along the floor and in the bulb. They are the openings of urethral glands.

l. vasorum. Internal aperture of femoral canal.

l., venous. Endothelial lined spaces in the dura mater which communicate with the meningeal veins and blood sinuses, esp. the sup. sagittal sinus.

lacunar (la-kū'nar) [L. *lacuna*, pit]. Pert. to lacunae.

lacunula (la-kū'nu-lă) [L. little pit]. Small or minute lacuna.

lacus (la'kus) [L. lake]. Collection of fluid in small hollow or cavity.

l. lacrimalis. Space at inner canthus of eye where tears collect.

Laënnec's cirrhosis (lan-eks') [Rene T. H. Laënnec, French physician, 1781-1826; the inventor of the stethoscope in 1819]. Atrophic cirrhosis of liver. Syn: *hobnail liver.*

L.'s pearls. Round gelatinous masses in asthmatic sputum.

L.'s râle. Modified subcrepitant râle due to mucus in bronchioles.

L.'s thrombus. Globular thrombus in heart.

lag [Welsh *llag*, slow]. 1. Period of time bet. application of stimulus and resulting reaction. Syn: *lag phase.* 2. Early period following bacterial inoculation into culture medium.

lageniform (laj-en'ĭ-form) [" + *forma*, shape]. Flask-shaped.

lagophthalmos, lagophthalmus (lag-of-thal'mos, -mus) [G. *lagōs*, hare, + *ophthalmos*, eye]. Incomplete closure of palpebral fissure when lids are shut, resulting in exposure and injury to bulbar conjunctiva and cornea.

Etiol: Contraction of a scar of eyelid, facial nerve injury, atony of orbicularis palpebrarum, exophthalmos. Incomplete closure of the lids during sleep is seen in hysteria, in exhausted adults, and often in healthy children. Syn: *hare's eye.*

la grippe (la grip') [Fr. the grip]. Acute infectious disease of respiratory or gastrointestinal tract. Syn: *influenza, q.v.*

laity (lā'ĭ-tĭ) [G. *laos*, the people]. The great portion of people as distinguished from those who are a member of a particular profession such as law, medicine, or the clergy.

lake. A small fluid-cavity. See: *lacus.*

laked [A.S. *lacu*, lake]. Said of the blood in hemolysis* or disintegration of the red blood corpuscles, freeing the hemoglobin into the blood plasma.

lak'ing [A.S. *lacy*, lake]. Freeing of hemoglobin from red blood corpuscles.

laliatry (lal-i'a-trĭ) [G. *lallein*, to babble, + *iatria*, therapy]. Study and treatment of speech disorders and defects.

lalla'tion, lal'ling [G. *lallein*, to babble]. A babbling form of stammering. Infantile form of speech. The constant use of "l" instead of "r."

lalognosis (lal-og-no'sis) [" + *gnōsis*, understanding]. Science of understanding speech, particularly lallation.

laloneurosis (lal-o-nū-rō'sis) [" + *neuron*, nerve, + *-ōsis*]. Speech impairment of neurotic origin.

lalop'athy [G. *lallein*, to babble, + *pathos*, disease]. Any disorder affecting the speech.

lalophobia (lal-ō-fō'bĭ-ă) [" + *phobos*, fear]. Morbid reluctance to speak due to fear of stammering or committing errors.

laloplegia (lal-o-ple'jĭ-ă) [" + *plēgē*, a stroke]. A paralysis of speech muscles without affecting action of tongue.

lalorrhea (la-lor-re'ă) [" + *roia*, flow]. Abnormal flow of speech.

lamarckism or **Lamarck's theory** (lam-ark'-ism) [Jean Baptiste P. A. Lamarck, French naturalist, 1744-1829]. Theory that evolutionary changes are the result of environmental changes; that basic inherent needs or changes necessitated by environmental modifications bring about the development of an organ; that use accentuates the development of a structure, disuse brings about its loss or atrophy; that acquired characters are inherited and passed on to descendents. Theory lacks experimental proof and is not generally accepted by Western scientists.

lamb (lăm) [A.S.]. A young sheep.

Cooked, roasted (79% lean, 21% fat): 100 gm. portion contains 319 Calories, protein 24 gm., fat 24 gm., calcium 10 mg., iron 1.6 mg., niacin 5.2 mg.

lambda (lam'dă) [G. *lambda*, letter L]. 1. Letter in Greek alphabet (Λ, λ). Also signified by letter L or l. 2. Point or angle of junction of lambdoid and sagittal sutures.

lambdacism (lam'dă-sizm) [G. *lambda*, letter L]. 1. Stammering of *l* sound. 2. Inability to pronounce *l* sound properly.

lambdoid, lambdoidal (lam'doid, lam-doid'-al) [" + *eidos*, form]. Shaped like Greek letter L.

l. suture. Suture bet. the occipital and 2 parietal bones.

lambert [Johann Lambert, German physicist]. A unit of brightness equal to that seen when a perfectly diffusing surface radiates or reflects one lumen of light per square centimeter.

Lamblia intestinalis (lam'blĭ-ă in-test-ĭ-nal'is) [Wilhelm D. Lambl, Bohemian physician, 1824-1895]. Flagellate protozoan parasite found in intestine. *Giardia lamblia, q.v.*

lambliasis (lăm-blī'ă-sĭs). *Giardiasis, q.v.*

lame. Disabled in limb, esp. in leg or foot; also applied to weak or painful condition as a *lame back.*

lamella (lam-el'a) (pl. *lamellae*) [L. a little plate, leaf]. 1. A medicated disk of gelatin inserted under lower eyelid and against the eyeball used as a local application to eye. 2. A thin plate or scale.

l., bone. Thin layer of ground substance of osseous tissue.

l., circumferential. Syn: *basic lamella, general lamella.* L. found on the external surface or lining the marrow cavity of a bone.

l., concentric. Plate of bone surrounding a haversian canal.

l., intermediate. Bone lamella filling irregular spaces bet. concentric lamellae.

l., interstitial. Syn: *ground lamella.* Bone lamella filling irregular spaces bet. concentric lamellae.

l., medullary. The osseous lamella surrounding and forming wall of medullary cavity of tubular bones.

l., periosteal. Bone lamella next to and parallel with the periosteum, forming ext. portion of bone.

l., triangular. Small fibrous lamina bet. choroid plexuses of 3rd ventricle of the brain.

l., vitreous. Innermost layer of the choroid next to the retina.

SYN: *Bruck's membrane, lamina basalis.*

lamellar (lam-el'lar). Arranged in thin plates or scales.

lameness. Limping, or abnormal gait, hobbling, resulting from partial loss of function in a leg. May be due to maldevelopment, injury, or disease.

lam'ina (pl. *laminae*) [L. a thin plate]. 1. A thin, flat layer or membrane. 2. The flattened part of either side of the arch of a vertebra.

l., alar. Alar plate of spinal cord in human embryo. Later becomes sensory portion.

l., anterior elastic. Thin, tough membrane just below the corneal epithelium. SYN: *Bowman's membrane.*

l., basal. Basal plate of spinal cord in human embryo; later becomes motor portion.

l. basalis of the choroid. The membrane covering the inner surface of the choroid.

l., Bowman's. Basement membrane beneath epithelium of cornea.

l. cartilaginis cricoideae. The posterior portion of the cricoid cartilage.

l. choriocapillaris. Choroid's middle layer containing close mesh of capillaries.

l. cribrosa. Cribriform plate of the ethmoid bone.

l. c. sclerae. Portion of sclera forming a sievelike plate through which pass fibers of the optic nerve to the retina.

l., dental. An epithelial plate which grows gumward from the labial lamina. From it arise the enamel organs of the future teeth.

l. ganglionaris. Ganglionic layer of the isocortex which is the non-olfactory cerebral cortex.

l. granularis externa. External granular layer of the isocortex.

l. granularis interna. The internal granular layer of the isocortex.

l., interpubic fibrocartilaginous. Part of the articulation of the pubic bones; it connects the opposing surfaces of these bones.

l., labial. A thickened band of epithelium which grows from the ectodermal covering of the primitive jaw. It splits into two sheets by development of the labial groove, thus giving rise to the vestibule of the mouth. From it arises the dental lamina, *q.v.*

l., medullary, internal. A layer of white substance which divides the gray substance of the thalamus into three parts—anterior, medial, and lateral.

l. multiformis. Polymorphic layer of the isocortex of the cerebral cortex.

l. papyra'cea. A thin, smooth, plate of bone on lateral surface of lateral mass of ethmoid bone; forms orbital plate.

l., perpendicular. Thin sheet of bone forming perpendicular plate of the ethmoid bone. Supports upper portion of nasal septum.

l. propria. SYN: *tunica propria* (of mucous membranes). A thin layer of fibrous connective tissue which lies immediately beneath the surface epithelium of mucous membranes.

l. pyramidalis. The pyramidal cell layer of the isocortex of the cerebral cortex.

l., rostral. Continuation of the rostrum of the corpus callosum and the lamina terminalis of the third ventricle.

l. spiralis. One which divides the int. of spiral canal of cochlea into 2 scalae and divides into l. spiralis ossea, and l. spiralis membrana.

l. suprachoroidea. Outermost layer of the choroid.

l., terminal. Thin sheet of tissue forming the anterior border of the third ventricle.

l. vitrea. Lamina basalis of the choroid, *q.v.*

l. zonalis. The outer or plexiform layer of the isocortex. Also called plexiform layer.

laminated (lam'in-āt-ed) [L. *lamina*, thin plate]. Arranged in layers or laminae.

lamination (lam-in-ā'shun) [L. *lamina*, thin plate]. 1. Layerlike arrangement. 2. In embryotomy, the slicing of the skull.

laminec'tomy [" + G. *ektomē*, excision]. The excision of a vertebral post. arch.

NP: Keep patient off back in position specified by physician.

laminitis (lă-mĭn-i'tis) [" + G. *-ītis*, inflammation]. Inflammation of a lamina.

lamp [G. *lampein*, to give light]. Device for producing and applying light, heat, radiation, and various forms of radiant energy for the treatment of disease.

l., Gullstrand's. Also called slit lamp. It is constructed so that an intense light is emitted through a slit. It is used for examination of the eye.

l., infrared. Heat lamp; a lamp which develops a high temperature, emitting infrared rays from 7,000 to 16,000 Angström units. Rays penetrate only a short distance (5 to 10 mm.) into the skin. Effect is principally on surface blood vessels and nerve endings.

lamprophonia (lam-pro-fō'nĭ-ă) [G. *lampros*, clear, + *phōnē*, voice]. Marked distinctness or clearness of voice.

lamprophonic (lam-prō-fōn'ik) [" + *phōnē*, voice]. Possessing a clear voice.

lanatoside (lan-at'ō-sīd). Glycoside of Digitalis lanata. An agent used for digitalization.

lance (lans) [L. *lancea*, spear]. 1. Two-edged surgical knife. 2. To incise with a lancet.

Lancefield classification (lans'fēld) [Rebecca Lancefield, American bacteriologist, 1895-]. A classification of hemolytic streptococci into various groups by antigenic structure.

lancet (lan'sĕt) [L. *lancea*, spear]. Pointed surgical knife with 2 edges.

lancinating (lăn'sĭ-nāt-ing) [L. *lancināre*, to tear]. Sharp or cutting, as pain.

Landouzy-Dejerine atrophy (lan-dū-ze'da-zhĕ-rēn'). Atrophy of muscles of face and scapulohumeral group.

Landry's paralysis (lăn-drē'). A form of paralysis in which loss of motor power in lower extremities gradually extends to upper extremities and to circulatory and respiratory centers without sensory manifestations, trophic changes, etc. SYN: *acute ascending paralysis.*

Landsteiner (land'stī-nĕr) [Karl Landsteiner, 1868-1943, Austrian scientist but later a naturalized U. S. citizen]. Discovered the different types of human blood groups. Nobel prize winner in medicine in 1930. SEE: *blood groups.*

Lane's kinks. Bending or twisting of intestine at various points as result of upright position of body.

Langerhans' islands (lahng'er-hahns). SEE: *islets of Langerhans.*

Langer's lines. The structural orientation of the fibrous tissue of the skin. They form the natural cleavage lines which, though present in all body areas, are visible only in certain sites such as the creases of the palm. These lines are of particular importance in surgery. Incisions made parallel to them make a much smaller scar upon healing than will be the case if the incision has been made at right angles to the lines.

Lange's test (lăng'ĕ). Diagnosis of cerebrospinal syphilis by degree of gold precipitation in varying concentrations of colloidal gold solution and spinal fluid.

Lang'hans layer. The cytotrophoblast, a cellular layer present in chorionic villi of the placenta.

languor (lăng'yĕr). Feeling of weariness or exhaustion as from illness; lack of vigor or animation; lassitude.

lanolin, anhydrous (lan'o-lin), USP. The purified, fatlike substance obtained from the wool of sheep.

USES: As an ointment base, having the property of absorbing water, and the advantage of not becoming rancid.

l., hydrous, USP. Wool fat containing about 25% water.

USES: Same as for l., anhydrous.

lanthanum (lan'thă-nŭm). A metallic element. One of a group of elements called lanthanides. At. wt. 138.91; at. no. 57. SYMB: La.

lanuginous (la-nū'jin-ŭs). Covered with lanugo, *q.v.*

lanugo (lan-oo'go) [L. *lana,* wool]. 1. Downy hair covering the body. 2. Fine downy hairs that cover the body of the fetus, esp. when premature.

laparectomy (lap"ă-rĕk'tō-mĭ) [G. *lapara,* loin, + *ektomē,* excision]. Excision of strips or gores in abdominal wall. SYN: *enterectomy.*

laparo- [G.]. Combining form pert. to the *flank* and to operations *through the abdominal wall.*

laparocholecystotomy (lap"ar-o-kol"e-sis-tot'o-mĭ) [" + *cholē,* bile, + *kystis,* bladder, + *tomē,* incision]. Incision into gallbladder through abdominal wall.

laparocolostomy (lap"ar-ō-kō-lŏs'tō-mĭ) [" + *kōlon,* colon, + *stoma,* opening]. Formation of permanent opening into colon through abdominal wall.

laparocolotomy (lap"ar-ō-kō-lot'ō-mĭ) [" + " + *tomē,* incision]. Incision of colon through abdominal wall, forming an artificial opening. SYN: *laparocolostomy.*

laparocolpotomy (lap"ar-ō-kol-pot'ō-mĭ) [" + *kolpos,* vagina, + *tomē,* incision]. Incision over Poupart's ligament dissecting peritoneum to vagina which is incised transversely, enabling dilation of cervix and extraction of child through os uteri. SYN: *celioelytrotomy, laparoelytrotomy.*

laparocystectomy (la"pa-ro-sis-tek'to-mĭ) [" + *kystis,* bladder, + *ektomē,* excision]. Removal of an extrauterine fetus or of contents of a cyst through an abdominal incision.

laparocystidotomy (lap"ar-o-sĭst-ĭ-dŏt'ō-mĭ) [G. *lapara,* loin, + *kystis,* bladder, + *tomē,* incision]. Bladder incision through the abdominal wall.

laparocystotomy (lap"ar-o-sis-tot'o-mĭ) [" +" + *tomē,* incision]. Incision of abdomen to remove contents of a cyst or an extrauterine fetus.

laparoelytrotomy (lap"ar-o-el-ĭ-trot'o-mĭ). Abdominal incision to aid in removal of fetus. SEE: *cesarean operation.*

laparoenterostomy (lăp"ă-rō-ĕn-tĕr-ŏs'tō-mĭ) [" + *enteron,* intestine, + *stoma,* opening]. Formation of aperture into intestine through abdominal wall.

laparoenterotomy (lap"ar-o-en-ter-ot'o-mĭ) [" + " + *tomē,* incision]. Opening into intestinal cavity by incision through the loins.

laparogastrostomy (lăp"ăr-ō-găs-trŏs'tō-mĭ) [G. *lapara,* loin, + *gastēr,* belly, + *stoma,* opening]. Formation of permanent gastric fistula through abdominal wall. SYN: *celiogastrostomy.*

laparogastrotomy (lap"a-ro-gas-trot'o-mĭ) [" + " + *tomē,* incision]. Abdominal incision into stomach.

laparohepatotomy (lăp"ăr-ō-hĕp-ă-tŏt'ō-mĭ) [" + *ēpar, ēpat-,* liver, + *tomē,* incision]. Incision of the liver through abdominal wall from side.

laparohysterectomy (lap"ar-o-his-ter-ek'-to-mĭ) [" + *ystera,* uterus, + *ektomē,* excision]. Abdominal removal of uterus.

laparohystero-oophorectomy (lap"ar-o-his"ter-o-o"o-for-ek'to-mĭ) [" + " + *ōon,* ovum, + *phoros,* bearer, + *ektomē,* excision]. Removal of uterus and ovaries through an abdominal incision.

laparohysteropexy (lap"ar-o-his'ter-o-peks-ĭ) [" + " + *pēxis,* fixation]. Abdominal fixation of the uterus.

laparohysterosalpingo-oophorectomy (lăp"-ăr-ō-hĭs"tĕr-ō-săl-pĭn"gō-ō"ō-fō-rek'tō-mĭ) [G. *lapara,* loin, + *ystera,* uterus, + *salpigx,* tube, + *ōon,* ovum, + *phoros,* bearer, + *ektomē,* excision]. Removal of uterus, fallopian tubes, and ovaries through abdominal incision. SYN: *celiohysterosalpingo-oothecectomy.*

laparohysterotomy (lap"ar-o-his-ter-ot'o-mĭ) [" + " + *tomē,* incision]. Abdominal incision into uterus. SEE: *cesarean section.*

laparoileotomy (lap"ar-o-il-e-ot'o-mĭ) [" + *eilein,* to twist]. Abdominal incision into ileum.

laparokelyphotomy (lăp"ăr-ō-kĕl-ĭ-fŏt'ō-mĭ) [" + *kelyphos,* eggshell, + *tomē,* incision]. 1. Removal of an extrauterine fetus by laparotomy. 2. Suprapubic cystotomy. SYN: *laparocystotomy.*

laparomyitis (lăp"ăr-ō-mī-ī'tĭs) [G. *lapara,* loin, + *mys,* muscle, + *-ītis,* inflammation]. Inflammation of muscular portion of abdominal wall.

laparomyomectomy (lap"ar-o-mi-o-mek'to-mĭ) [" + " + *ōma,* tumor, + *ektomē,* excision]. Abdominal excision of a muscular tumor.

Preparation same as for cesarean operation, minus the obstetrical appliances. POSITION: *Dorsal.*

laparonephrectomy (lap"ar-o-ne-frek'to-mĭ) [" + *nephros,* kidney, + *ektomē,* excision]. Renal excision abdominally.

laparorrhaphy (lăp-ăr-or'ră-fĭ) [" + *raphē,* suture]. Abdominal wall suture SYN: *celiorrhaphy.*

laparosalpingectomy (lap"ar-o-sal-pin-jek'-to-mĭ) [" + *salpigx,* tube, + *ektomē,* excision]. Abdominal excision of a fallopian tube.

laparosalpingo-oophorectomy (lăp"ăr-ō-săl-pĭn"gō-ō"ŏf-ō-rek'tō-mĭ) [" + " + *ōon,* ovum, + *phoros,* bearer, + *ektomē,* excision]. Removal of fallopian tubes and ovaries through abdominal incision. SYN: *celiosalpingo-oothecectomy.*

laparosalpingotomy (lăp"ăr-ō-săl-pĭn-got'-ō-mĭ) [" + " + *tomē,* incision]. Incision of oviduct through abdominal wall. SYN: *celiosalpingotomy.*

laparoscopy (lăp-ăr-os'kō-pĭ) [" + *skopein,* to examine]. Abdominal exploration employing instruments. SYN: *celioscopy*.

laparosplenectomy (lap″ar-o-splen-ek′to-mĭ) [" + *splēn*, spleen, + *ektomē*, excision]. Abdominal excision of the spleen.

laparosplenotomy (lăp″ăr-ō-splēn-ŏt′ō-mĭ) [" + " + *tomē*, incision]. Incision of the spleen through abdominal wall.

laparotomy (lap-ar-ot′o-mĭ) [" + *tomē*, incision]. The surgical opening of the abdomen; an abdominal operation.

PREOPERATIVE PREPARATION: Follow the physician's orders regarding diet, shaving of abdomen and pubic area, enemas, douches and collecting of urine specimens.

POSTOPERATIVE NURSING CARE: Most patients remain in the hospital's recovery room until they are fully conscious. However, when a patient returns to the room, the nurse shall record her observations regarding the patient's general condition, the pulse and respirations, and blood pressure. The attending physician must be notified at once of any unusual symptoms such as shock or bleeding.

Follow the physician's orders as to the patient's position, fluid intake, diet and medications. If catheterization is necessary, use sterile technique.

laparotrachelotomy (lap″ar-o-tra-kĕl-ot′o-mĭ) [G. *lapara*, loin, + *trachēlos*, neck, + *tomē*, incision]. Cesarean section with the incision through the lower segment of the uterus.

laparotyphlotomy (lăp″ăr-ō-tĭ-flŏt′ō-mĭ) [" " + *typhlon*, cecum, + *tomē*, incision]. Incision of cecum through lateral abdominal incision.

laparouterotomy (lăp″ăr-ō-ū-tĕr-ŏt′ō-mĭ) [" + L. *uterus*, womb, + G. *tomē*, incision]. Incision of uterus through abdominal wall. SYN: *laparohysterotomy*.

lapis (la′pis) [L.]. Stone.

laqueus (lak′we-us) [L. noose]. A noose-shaped band, fillet, or cord.

lard [L. fat]. Purified fat from the hog. The sole nutrient is fat. 100 gm. portion contains 902 Calories.

lardaceous (lar-dā′shus) [L. *lardum*, fat]. Resembling lard; waxy, fatty.

larva (lar′vă) [L. ghost, mask]. 1. General term applied to a young animal which differs in form from the parent. 2. An immature stage in insect life after it has emerged from the egg and before it transforms into a pupa from which it emerges as an adult.

l. migrans. SYN: *creeping eruption, sandworm disease*. Caused by larvae of dog-and-cat hookworm, *Ancylostoma braziliense*, but may be caused by the larvae of other nematodes or the larvae of flies.

l. migrans, visceral. Infestation of viscera by larvae of animal nematodes such as *toxocara canis*. These migrate and cause eosinophilia, hepatomegaly, fever and hyperglobulinemia. Occurs mostly in children who play in soil or sand contaminated with dog and cat feces. Disease is self-limiting. No specific treatment is available.

lar′vate. Hidden, concealed.

lar′vicide. An agent which destroys insect larvae.

laryngalgia (lăr-ĭn-găl′jĭ-ă) [G. *larygx*, larynx]. Neuralgia of the larynx.

laryngeal (lar-in′je-al) [G. *larygx*, larynx]. Pert. to the larynx.

l. reflex. Cough as result of irritation of larynx or fauces.

laryngectomy (lar-in-jek′to-mĭ) [" + *ektomē*, excision]. Excision of larynx.

PREPARATION: Similar to tracheotomy, plus additional ligatures, sponge or tampon cannula. Best done in two operations—performing tracheotomy week or two before the main operation.

laryngismal (lar-ĭn-jĭs′măl) [G. *larygx*, larynx]. Concerning or resembling affection with laryngeal spasm.

laryngismus (lar-in-jis′mus) [" + *ismos*, condition of]. Spasm of the larynx.

SYM: Face pale—later cyanosed; eyes rolled up, body arched; thumbs turned into palm, legs extended, soles turned inward. In a few seconds the spasm relaxes.

PROG: Favorable. In very young, death may result from suffocation.

l., infantile. One occurring in children less than one year old, who are poorly nourished.

l. stridulus. A condition characterized by laryngeal stridor of sudden onset, inspiratory dyspnea, temporary apnea, increasing cyanosis, and, in severe cases, unconsciousness, convulsions and possibly death. SYN: *cantus galli*.

ETIOL: Early life (within first 2 years). male sex, and the rachitic diathesis are predisposing causes; often accompanies tetany. The discharge of motor force apparently rises in the medulla and may be excited by reflex irritation as in teething and gastrointestinal troubles.

SYM: Attacks often and sudden; may occur on awakening from sleep — are characterized by a sudden arrest in breathing and tonic muscular swelling; can be detected by finger on throat. Spasm relapses, and air is drawn in through glottis with shrill crowing sound —may occur several times a day or weeks apart.

PROG: Extremely grave.

TREATMENT: Correct diet, cod-liver oil, and calcium lactate to prevent attacks. During attacks, cold cloths over thyroid or hot cloths to nape of neck, a few whiffs of chloroform or ether, ipecac to induce vomiting. When dypsnea persists, tracheotomy may be performed.

laryngitic (lar-ĭn-jĭt′ĭk) [G. *larygx*, larynx]. 1. Resulting from laryngitis. 2. Rel. to laryngitis.

laryngitis (lar-in-ji′tis) [" + *-ītis*, inflammation]. Inflammation of larynx.

l., acute catarrhal. Acute congestive laryngitis; catarrhal inflammation of laryngeal mucosa and the vocal cords.

SYM: Hoarseness and aphonia and occasionally pain on phonation and deglutition.

ETIOL: Improper use or over-use of voice, exposure to cold and wet, extension from infections in nose and throat, inhalation of irritating vapors and dust, associated with systemic diseases as whooping cough, measles, etc.

TREATMENT: Complete rest of voice, promotion of diaphoresis, liquid or soft diet, medicated steam inhalations such as compound tincture of benzoin, codeine for cough and pain. SEE: *croup*.

l., atrophic. L. leading to diminished secretion and glandular atrophy of the mucous membrane.

SYM: Tickling sensation in throat, hoarseness, cough, dyspnea when crusts are thick and accumulate on vocal cords so as to narrow the breathing aperture.

TREATMENT: Iodides internally, inhalants and medicated sprays to loosen the crusts; strict attention to associated nose and throat pathology.

l., chronic. A type due to a recurrent irritation, or following the acute form. Often secondary to sinus or nasal pathology, improper use of voice, excessive smoking or drinking.

SYM: Tickling in throat, amblyphonia and huskiness of voice, dysphonia.

TREATMENT: Correction of preexisting nose and throat pathology, discontinuance of alcohol and tobacco, avoidance of excessive use of voice and proper vocal placement.

l., croupous. Diphtheritic laryngitis, *q.v.*

l., c. hypertrophic. Hypertrophy of tissues accompanying chronic l.

l., diphtheritic. Invasion of larynx by diphtheria bacilli, usually with formation of membrane.

l., membranous. Characterized by inflammation of larynx with the formation of a false membrane of nondiphtheritic origin.

TREATMENT: Free catharsis, inhalation of medicated vapors to loosen the membrane, administration of ipecac for emesis. SEE: *membranous croup.*

l., phlegmonous. Inflamed larynx with purulent infiltration or abscesses.

l., syphilitic. ETIOL: Due to syphilis.

SYM: Hoarseness, cough, simple catarrh, formation of broad condylomata, follicular hyperplasia, syphiloma, syphilitic perichondritis.

Secondary stage in form of mucous patches or tertiary in form of gumma. Secondary syphilis is a diffuse infection and one sees luetic patches spread over large areas of larynx.

In tertiary syphilis the gummatous lesion can occur in any part of larynx. There is marked redness over the infiltrated area as well as in the surrounding mucous membrane. When there is breaking down, the resultant ulceration is deep with sharp edges. Pain is usually absent and fixation of the cord is late. Cicatrization and deformity follow healing of gumma.

TREATMENT: Appropriate antibiotic therapy for syphilis.

l., tuberculous. Secondary to pulmonary tuberculosis.

SYM: Hoarseness, amblyphonia or aphonia, pain in swallowing, cough. Lesion located in: 1. Interarytenoid area. 2. Vocal cords. 3. Epiglottis. 4. False cords. Lesions are relatively pale; ulceration occurs early.

l., ulcerative. Chronic l. with ulceration of the mucous membrane.

laryn'go- [G.]. Prefix: Pert. to the *larynx.*

laryngocele (lar-in'go-sēl) [G. *larygx, larygg-*, larynx, + *kēlē*, hernia]. An air sac connected to the larynx. Is normal in some animals but abnormal in man.

laryngocentesis (lăr-ĭn"gō-sĕn-tē'sĭs) [" + *kentēsis*, puncture]. Incision or puncture of the larynx.

laryngofissure (lar-ing"go-fish'ur) [" + L. *fissura*, a cleft]. The operation of opening the larynx by a median line incision through the thyroid cartilage.

laryngograph (lar-ing'o-grăf) [" + *graphein*, to write]. Device for making a record of laryngeal movements.

laryngography (lăr-ĭn-gŏg'ră-fĭ) [" + *graphein*, to write]. Description of larynx.

laryngologist (lar-ĭn-gol'o-jist) [" + *logos*, study]. Specialist in laryngology.

laryngol'ogy [" + *logos*, study]. The practice of medicine dealing with the treatment of diseases of the larynx.

laryngometry (lăr-ĭn-gŏm'ĕ-trĭ) [G. *larygx, larygg-*, larynx, + *metron*, measure]. Systematic measurement of larynx.

laryngoparalysis (lăr-ĭn"gō-par-ăl'ĭ-sĭs) [" + *para*, beside, + *lyein*, to loosen]. Paralysis of muscles of larynx.

laryngopathy (lăr-ĭn-gop'ă-thĭ) [" + *pathos*, disease]. Any disease of the larynx.

laryngophantom (lăr-ĭn-gō-fan'tŏm) [" + *phantasma*, image]. Plastic model of the larynx.

laryngopharyngeal (lar-ĭn"gō-far-ĭn'jē-ăl) [" + *pharygx*, pharynx]. Rel. jointly to larynx and pharynx.

laryngopharyngectomy (lăr-ĭn"gō-făr-ĭn-jek'tō-mĭ) [" + " + *ektomē*, excision]. Removal of the larynx and pharynx.

laryngopharyngitis (lăr-ĭn"gō-făr-ĭn-jī'tĭs) [" + " + *-itis*, inflammation]. Inflammation of the larynx and pharynx.

laryngopharynx (lăr-ĭn-gō-făr'ĭnks) [" + *pharygx*, pharynx]. Lower portion of the pharynx that extends from the cornua of the hyoid bone or vestibule of the larynx to the lower border of the cricoid cartilage.

laryngophony (lăr-ĭn-gof'ō-nĭ) [G. *larygx, larygg-*, larynx, + *phōnē*, voice]. Voice sounds heard in auscultating the pharynx.

laryngoplasty (lăr-ĭn'gō-plăs-tĭ) [" + *plassein*, to form]. Plastic reparative surgery of larynx.

laryngoplegia (la-ring"go-plē'jĭ-ă) [" + *plēgē*, stroke]. Paralysis of laryngeal muscles.

laryngorhinology (lăr-ĭn"gō-rīn-ŏl'ō-jĭ) [" + *ris, rin-*, nose, + *logos*, study]. Science treating with diseases of the larynx and nose.

laryngorrhagia (lăr-ĭn-gor-ră'jĭ-ă) [" + *rēgnunai*, to flow forth]. Laryngeal hemorrhage.

laryngorrhea (lăr-ĭn-gor-rē'ă) [" + *roia*, flow]. Excessive discharge of laryngeal mucus.

laryngoscleroma (lăr-ĭn-gō-sklē-rō'mă) [" + *sklēros*, hard, + *ōma*, tumor]. Scleroma affecting the larynx.

laryngoscope (lar-in'go-skōp) [" + *skopein*, to examine]. Instrument for examining the larynx.

laryngoscopic (lar-ĭn-gō-skŏp'ĭk) [G. *larygx, larygg-*, + *skopein*, to examine]. Pert. to observation with aid of small long handled mirror for reflecting interior of larynx.

laryngoscopy (lar-in-gos'kō-pĭ) [" + *skopein*, to examine]. Examination of interior of larynx.

NP: Instrument should be warmed.

l., direct. That done with laryngeal speculum or laryngoscope.

NP: Tongue, which is covered with a gauze, is protruded and held in that position by the patient or nurse.

l., indirect. That done with a mirror.

NP: Nurse should stand behind patient with left hand on head, gently holding patient's tongue with right hand to steady it. The tongue is covered with a gauze to prevent its slipping from the fingers.

laryngospasm (lăr-ĭn'gō-spazm) [" + *spasmos*, spasm]. Spasm of laryngeal muscles.

laryngostenosis (lar-ing"go-ste-nō'sis) [" + *stenōsis*, a narrowing]. Stricture of larynx.

l., compression. From causes outside the larynx as result of abscesses, tumors, goiter, etc.

l., occlusion. ETIOL: May be due to congenital bands or membranes, foreign bodies, tumors, cicatricial contraction following ulceration as in diphtheria and tertiary syphilis, penetrating wounds or corrosive fluid.

SYM: Dyspnea, esp. on inspiration and exertion. Loud breathing which becomes a stridulous choking respiration; pulse small and frequent; face anxious and cyanotic.

PROG: Grave.

TREATMENT: Depends on cause. Tracheotomy is often necessary.

laryngostomy (lăr-ĭn-gos'tō-mĭ) [" + *stoma*, opening]. Establishing permanent opening through neck into larynx.

laryngostroboscope (lar-in-go-stro'bo-skōp) [" + *strobos*, whirl, + *skopein*, to view]. Instrument for inspection of vibration of vocal cords.

laryngotomy (lar-in-got'o-mĭ) [" + *tomē*, incision]. Incision of larynx.

laryngotracheitis (lăr-ĭn"gō-tra-kē-ī'tĭs). Inflamed condition of the larynx and trachea.

laryngotracheotomy (lar-in'go-tra-ke-ot'o-mĭ) [" + *tracheia*, windpipe, + *tomē*, incision]. Incision of larynx with section of upper tracheal rings.

laryngoxerosis (lăr-ĭn"gō-zĕr-ō'sĭs) [" + *xērōsis*, dryness]. Abnormal dryness of the larynx.

larynx (lar'inks) (*Pl. larynges*) [G. *larygx*]. The organ of voice, the enlarged upper end of trachea; musculocartilaginous structure lined with mucous membrane.

BLOOD SUPPLY: Inf. thyroid, branch of thyroid axis and sup. thyroid, branch of ext. carotid.

STRUCTURE: Consists of nine *cartilages* bound together by an *elastic membrane* and moved by muscles. *Cartilages* include three single ones (*cricoid, thyroid*, and *epiglottic*) and three paired ones (*arytenoid, corniculate*, and *cuneiform*). The extrinsic muscles include the *omohyoid, sternohyoid, sternothyroid*, and several others; intrinsic muscles include the *cricothyroid, ext.* and *int. thyroarytenoid, trans.* and *obl. arytenoid*, and *ext.* and *int. thyroarytenoid*. The cavity of the larynx contains two pairs of folds, the *ventricular folds* (false vocal cords) and *vocal folds* (true vocal cords), and is divided into three regions (*vestibule, ventricle*, and *inf. entrance to the glottis*. Opening between true vocal folds forms a narrow slit, the *rima glottidis* or *glottis*.

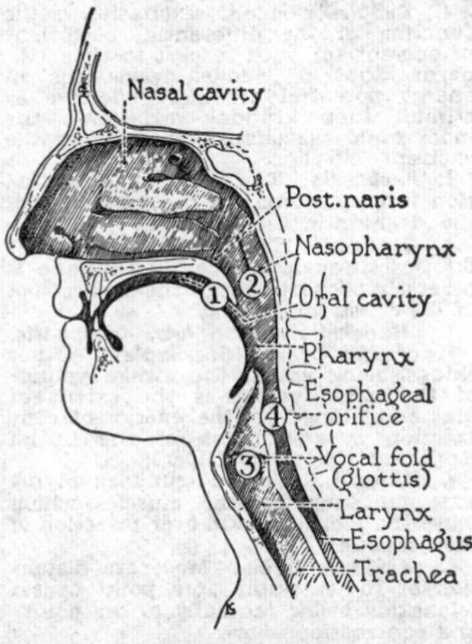

THE LARYNX

Seen in its relation to: 1. The mouth cavity. 2. Nasopharynx. 3. Glottis. 4. Esophagus.

NERVES: From int. and ext. branches of sup. laryngeal.

NP: *Diseases of*: Patient should stay in bed and, in any event, he should avoid changes of atmosphere which may cause an attack of coughing. Room temperature should be maintained at the proper level, and drafts avoided. Movements may set up coughing, so patient should rest quietly. The voice is generally affected in abnormal conditions of the larynx, so voice also should be rested. To keep silence, however, may cause patient to become depressed. The nurse needs to help occupy the patient s time, but she should not ask the patient questions unless they may be answered by a nod of the head. The patient will need encouragement in continuing inhalations ordered.

When possible for the patient to use the voice, instructions should be given to use the diaphragm and abdominal muscles rather than the muscles of the throat. In chronic laryngitis cold water may be applied to the neck morning and night. The nose, throat, and larynx must be kept cleaned by sprays as ordered.

In edema of the larynx sucking ice, or application of ice to the neck may be helpful. Astringent sprays may be ordered by the doctor.

RS: *Bouchut's method, cricoarytenoid, epiglottis, glottis, "laryng-" words, prominentia laryngea, vestibule, vocal cord.*

l., foreign bodies in. SYM: When a foreign body enters it produces violent spasmodic cough and dyspnea; fixed pain at particular spot and loss of voice.

TREATMENT: If on the spot promptly raise patient by the heels and slap him on the back. Search pharynx with finger and extract object. Induce vomiting by inserting finger in throat. Use laryngoscopic mirror and extract substance with forceps. Tracheotomy may be required.

lasciv'ia [L. *lascivire*, to be wanton]. Abnormal sexual desire. SEE: *nymphomania; satyrides.*

Laser (la'zer). Acronym for light amplification by stimulated emission or radiation.

lassitude (las'i-tūd) [L. *lassitūdō*, weariness]. Weariness; exhaustion.

latency (lā'tĕn-sĭ) [L. *latēre*, to be hidden]. State of being concealed or hidden.

la'tent [L. *latēre*, to be concealed]. 1. Lying hidden. 2. Quiet; not active.

l. content. PSY: That part of a dream or unconscious mental content that cannot be brought into the objective consciousness through any effort of will to remember.

l. heat. Caloric or heat energy absorbed by matter changing from solid to liquid or liquid to vapor without a change in temperature.

l. period. 1. Time bet. a stimulus and its response. SYN: *lag phase.* 2. Time during which a disease is supposed to be existent without manifesting itself; period of incubation.

laterad (lat′ĕr-ăd) [L. *latus, later-,* side, + *ad,* toward]. Toward a side or lateral aspect.

lateral (lat′er-al) [L. *latus, later-,* side]. Pert. to the side.

l. sinus. Transverse and sigmoid portion of two cranial venous sinuses. Extends from occipital protuberance to jugular bulb.

latericeous, lateritious (lat-ĕr-ĭ′shŭs) [L. *later,* a brick]. Resembling brick dust.

lateroflexion (lăt″ĕr-ō-flek′shun) [L. *latus, later-,* side, + *flexus;* from *flectere,* to bend]. Bending or curvature toward a side.

lateroprone, laterosemiprone position (lăt″-ĕr-ō-prōn′, -sĕm′ĭ-prōn). Patient on left side leaning on chest, right knee and thigh drawn up, left arm back of patient. SYN: *Sims' position, q.v., for illustration.*

lateropulsion (lat-er-o-pul′shun) [" + *pulsus,* driving]. Involuntary tendency in cerebellar and labyrinthine disease to fall to one side.

lateroversion (lăt-ĕr-ō-vĕr′shun) [" + *versiō,* a turning]. Tendency or a turning toward one side.

lathyrism (lath′ĭr-ĭzm) [G. *lathyros,* vetch]. Chick-pea poisoning. SYN: *lupinosis.*

Nervous disorders and tremors with cramps in arms and legs.

TREATMENT: Provoke vomiting, wash out stomach, stimulants.

latrine (la-trēn′) [L. *latrina*]. A toilet, particularly one in a military camp.

Latrodectus (lăt′rō-dĕkt′us). A genus of small black spiders belonging to the family Theriidae.

L. mactans. The black widow or hourglass spider, a species widely distributed in the United States. The bite of the female produces serious symptoms and may result in death.

la′tus, la′ta, lat′um. [L. broad]. Broad, as the uterine broad ligament.

laud′able [L. *laudabilis,* praiseworthy]. Healthy; normal; said erroneously of *pus.*

laudanum (law′dan-um). Tincture of opium. POISONING: SEE: *morphine.*

laugh (lăf) [M. E. *laughen,* to laugh]. Sound produced by laughing. SYN: *risus.*

l., sardonic. Spasm of facial muscles producing a grinning effect. SYN: *risus sardonicus.*

laughing gas (laf′ing) [M. E. *laughen,* to laugh]. Nitrous oxide gas.

laughter, compulsive. SYN: *obsessive laughter.* L. without cause, occurring in certain psychoses, esp. schizophrenia.

laughter reflex (lăf′tĕr). Uncontrollable laughter resulting from tickling or pretense of tickling.

lavage (la-vazh′) [Fr.; from L. *lavāre,* to wash]. Washing out of a cavity.

l., gastric. Washing out of the stomach. A stomach tube or catheter is used with solution of sterile water, or normal saline, or 1-5% sodium bicarbonate.

QUANTITY OF SOLUTION: Not more than 10 oz. at a time repeated until fluid runs clear.

TEMPERATURE AND TIME: 105° F. Preferably before breakfast. POSITION: Semi-recumbent or low enough to prevent inhalation of returning fluid. In poisoning, save siphoned fluid for examination. If patient is unconscious use a mouth gag.

PURPOSE: To remove irritants or poisons, to relieve nausea or vomiting, to cleanse the stomach preoperatively or postoperatively. In latter case to prevent nausea. SEE: *bladder irrigation, colonic irrigation.*

law [A. S. *laga,* law]. In the scientific sense, a statement which is found to hold true uniformly for a whole class of natural occurrences.

l., all-or-none. The weakest stimulus capable of producing a response produces the maximum response contraction in cardiac and skeletal muscles and nerves.

l., Avoga′dro's. If temperature and ext. pressure are the same, all gases contain same number of molecules in equal volumes.

l., Behring's. Blood and serum of an immunized subject confers immunity when injected into another.

l., Bell's. Ant. spinal nerve roots are motor, and post. roots are sensory.

l's., Berthollet's. 1. When two salts react because of a solvent, if a new salt can be produced less soluble, this salt will be produced. 2. When dry heat is applied to "two salts, if a new salt can be produced more volatile, this salt will be produced."

l. biogenetic. SYN: *recapitulation theory.* Ontogeny recapitulates phylogeny, *i.e.,* an individual in its development recapitulates stages in its racial development.

l., Boyle's. The volume occupied by a fixed quantity of every gas is inversely proportional, and density directly proportional, to pressure applied to the gas.

l., Brew′ster's. For any substance the polarizing angle is equal to that angle of incidence at which the portion of light that is reflected is at right angles to the portion refracted.

l., Charles'. When pressure is constant, volume of a gas varies as the absolute temperature.

l., Courvoisier's. When the common bile duct is obstructed by a calculus, dilatation of gallbladder is rare; when otherwise obstructed, dilatation is common.

l. of definite proportions. Two or more elements when united to form a new substance do so in a constant and fixed proportion by weight.

l., DuBois-Reymond. Excitation is the function of the differential coefficient of current (c) with respect to time (t): dc/dt, that is, sudden variations in energy potential are more effective as stimuli than gradual variations; the more rapid the change, the greater the excitant effect.

l., Fechner's. The intensity of sensation is proportional to the logarithm of the strength of the stimulus.

l., Graham's. The rate at which a gas diffuses through a porous membrane is inversely proportional to the square root of the density of the gas.

l., Haeckel's. SEE: *law, biogenetic.*

l. of the heart (Starling's). Other things being equal, the stroke volume of the heart varies as the extent of diastolic filling; or, the energy of contraction is a function of the initial length of the muscle fibers.

l., Hilton's. A nerve trunk supplying any joint supplies the muscles which move the joint and skin over insertion of such muscles.

l. of the intestine. Moderate distention of the intestine at a point causes relaxation below (aborally to the point) and contraction above.

l., Koch's, Koch's postulate. To prove an organism to be the cause of a given disease or lesion: 1st, the microorganism in question must appear in the lesion at all times; 2nd, pure cultures must be obtained from it; 3rd, cultures must reproduce the disease in animals and pure cultures must be again obtained from these lesions.

l. of Magendie. Same as l. of Bell.

l., Marey's. Heart rate varies inversely to arterial blood pressure; that is, a rise or fall in arterial blood pressure brings about, respectively, a slowing or speeding up of heart rate.

l., Mariotte's. Boyle's law, *q.v.*

l. of mass action. In chemical reactions the amount of change taking place is proportional to action mass of the reacting substance.

l., Mendel's. A number of principles of heredity established by Mendel (1822-1884) which laid the foundation for the modern science of genetics. Includes the principles of unit characters, dominance, segregation, and independent assortment.

l. of molecular weights. The weight of a molecule is the sum of the weights of its atoms and the relative molecular weight of a compound is equal to sum of the atomic weights of its components divided by two.

l., Müller's. SEE: *law of specificity of nervous energy.*

l. of multiple proportions. When two substances unite to form a series of chemical compounds the proportions in which they unite are simple multiples of one another or of one common proportion.

l., Murphy's. If something can go wrong, it will. This law is of the utmost importance in attempting to design and manufacture apparatus or devices which, if they fail, will endanger the patient's safety or life. In other words medical devices and apparatus should be so constructed as to make failure, misapplication, or malfunction virtually impossible.

l., Nysten's. Rigor mortis travels progressively from muscles of mastication, through the face, neck, trunk and arms, reaching the legs and feet last.

l., periodic. The physical and chemical properties of chemical elements are periodic functions of their at. wt.

Natural classification of elements according to their at. wt.; when arranged in order of their at. wt. or atomic numbers, elements show regular variations in most of their physical and chemical properties.

l. of reciprocal proportions. In chemistry, the l. that the proportions in which two elementary bodies unite with a third one are simple multiples or simple fractions of the proportions in which these two bodies unite with each other.

l., Rubner's. 1. *L. of constant energy consumption*: Rapidity of growth is proportional to intensity of the metabolic processes. 2. *L. of constant growth quotient*: The same proportional part, or growth quotient, of total energy is utilized for growth.

l. of specificity of nervous energy. SYN: *Müller's law.* Excitation of a receptor always gives rise to the same sensation regardless of the nature of the stimulus.

l., Waller's, of degeneration. If a spinal nerve is completely divided, the peripheral portion undergoes fatty degeneration, while the proximal part preserves its original character.

l., Weber's. When a stimulus is continually increased the smallest increase of sensation which we can appreciate remains the same, if the proportion of the increase of stimulus to the whole stimulus remains the same.

l., Wolff's. Changes in form and function of bones result in definite changes in their internal structure.

lawrencium (lă-rĕn'si-um). A radioactive chemical element. At. no. 103. SYMB: Lw̄.

lax (lăks) [L. *laxus,* slack]. Without tension.

laxative (lak'să-tĭv) [L. *laxāre,* to loosen]. A mildly purgative medicine; an aperient or mild cathartic.

l. diet. One promoting free intestinal elimination; fresh fruits, lemonade, stewed raisins, prunes, asparagus, cauliflower, spinach, tomatoes, figs, buttermilk, sweet potatoes, sweet corn, pea and bean puree, carrots, greens, nuts, whole grains, yeasts.

layer (lā'ĕr) [M.E. *leyer*]. A stratum; a thin sheetlike structure of more or less uniform thickness.

l., bacillary. Rod and cone layer of retina of the eye.

l., basal. The *basalis,* outermost layer of uterine endometrium lying next to the myometrium.

l., choriocapillary. SEE: *lamina, choriocapillaris.*

l., claustral. Layer of gray matter bet. external capsule and insula.

l., compact. The *compact* surface layer of the uterine endometrium.

l., cuticular, of epithelium. A striated l. secreted by and covering free surface of an epithelial sheet, esp. that on surface of columnar epithelium of the intestine.

l., ependymal. Inner layer of cells of embryonic neural tube.

l., ganglionic. 1. Fifth layer of cerebral cortex. 2. An inner layer of ganglion cells in the retina whose axons form the fibers of the optic nerve.

l., germ. One of the three primary layers of the developing embryo from which the various organ systems develop. SEE: *ectoderm, mesoderm, entoderm.*

l., germinative. SYN: *malpighian layer.* Stratum germinativum, the innermost layer of the epidermis, consisting of basal layer of cells and a layer of prickle cells (stratum spinosum).

l., granular ext. Second layer of cerebellar cortex, lying within molecular layer and separated from it by a single row of Purkinje cells. Consists principally of granule cells.

l., granular int. The fourth layer of the cerebral cortex, consisting principally of closely packed stellate cells.

l., Henle's. A layer of clear cells forming outermost layer of the inner epithelial root sheath of a hair.

l., horny. The stratum corneum, outermost layer of the skin, consisting of clear, dead, scalelike cells, those of the surface layer being constantly desquamated.

l., Huxley's. The middle layer of inner epithelial root sheath of a hair.

l., Langhans'. Cytotrophoblast, *q.v.* SEE: *Langhans' layer.*

l. malpighian. SEE: *l. germinative.*

l., molecular. 1. Outermost layer of cerebral or cerebellar cortex. 2. Inner or outer plexiform layer of the retina.

l., osteogenic. Innermost or bone-forming layer of the periosteum.

l., outer-nuclear. A layer of the retina containing the nuclei of the visual cells (rods and cones).

l., papillary. Superficial layer of the corium lying immediately under the epidermis into which it extends, forming *dermal papillae.*

l., pigment. Outermost layer of the retina. Cells contain a pigment called *fuscin.*

l., Purkinje. A single row of large flash-shaped cells (Purkinje cells) lying between molecular and granular layers of the cerebellar cortex.

l. of pyramidal cells. The ext. pyramidal layer; third layer of cerebral cortex.

l., reticular. The inner layer of the corium lying beneath the papillary layer.

l., somatic. In the embryo, a layer of extra-embryonic mesoderm which forms a part of the somatopleure, the outer wall of the coelom.

l., splanchnic. A layer of extra-embryonic mesoderm, which with the endoderm forms the splanchnopleure.

l., spongy. The stratum spongiosum, the middle layer of the uterine endometrium. Contains dilated portions of uterine glands.

l., subendocardial. Layer of loose connective tissue immediately under the endocardium which binds it to the myocardium. Contains fibers of the conducting system of the heart.

l., subendothelial. Layer of fine fibers and fibroblasts lying immediately under the endothelium of the tunica intima of larger arteries and veins.

lazaret'to [It. *lazzaro,* a leper]. 1. A quarantine station. 2. Hospital for treatment of contagious diseases. SYN: *pesthouse.*

lb. Abbr. for *pound.*

LD. Abbr. for *lethal dose.*

LD_{50}. Abbreviation for lethal dose of a substance which will kill 50% of a group of animals.

L-dopa. L-3,4-dihydroxyphenylalanine. A drug which has been used experimentally in the treatment of parkinsonism. SYN: *levodopa.*

leaching (lēch'ing) [A.S. *leccan,* to wet]. Extraction of a substance from a mixture by washing the mixture with a solvent in which only the desired substance is soluble. SYN: *lixiviation.*

lead (lĕd). SYMB: *Pb.* A metallic element [*plumbum*]. At. no. 82; at. wt. 207.19. Its compounds are poisonous.

l. acetate. USP. Sugar of lead.

ACTION AND USES: An astringent, saturated alcoholic solution; is used as an external lotion in ivy poisoning.

l. colic. That due to lead poisoning.

l. encephalopathy. Disease of brain caused by lead poisoning.

l. line. Bluish line on gums in lead poisoning.

l. pipe contraction. Cataleptic condition during which limbs remain in any position in which placed.

l. poisoning, acute. ETIOL: From large overdosage. SYM: Metallic taste in mouth, burns in throat and gullet. Later abdominal cramps and prostration. F. A.

TREATMENT: Wash out stomach. Adm. of magnesium sulfate (epsom salts) or sodium sulfate which precipitates the lead and helps remove the lead by purging.

l. p., chronic. ETIOL: Exceedingly common. Exposure in the industries; from food when lead vessels are used in its preparation; from cosmetics; or in children from nipple shields, chewing lead toys or objects covered with lead paints.

SYM: Anorexia, nausea, vomiting, salivation, anemia, the lead line on the gums, purging, abdominal pains, muscle cramps and pains in the joints. One of the most typical findings is the abdominal pain known as *lead colic.* There may be impairment of any part of the nervous system, often leading to muscle atrophy and the characteristic foot or wrist drop. Various blood changes may be found, especially the "stippling" of the red cells.

lead (lēd) [A.S. *lǣdan,* to guide]. An electrocardiograph record.

The three common leads are: lead I, right arm to left arm; lead II, right arm to left leg; lead III, left arm to left leg. These are known as *standard leads, bipolar limb leads or indirect leads.*

l., precordial. Record taken when one lead is placed over the precordium, the other over an indifferent region.

l., unipolar. Record made when one lead is placed on chest wall overlying the heart, where potential changes are of considerable magnitude and the other (distant or indifferent electrode) placed where potential changes are of small magnitude.

leaf (lēf) [A.S.]. A plant organ usually shooting out from the side of a stem or branch; somewhat flattened and oval in shape, and green in color. Ex: *Belladonna, hyoscyamus, digitalis.*

lean (lēn) [A.S. *hlǣne,* without flesh]. Without flesh, emaciated.

DIET FOR: Diet as for tuberculosis or neurasthenia. Milk, 2 pints with or bet. meals; 2 eggs; meat, 6-8 oz.; bread, 12 oz.; potatoes, 4 oz.; milk puddings, 4 oz.; thick soup, 5 oz.; butter or other fat, 2 oz.; sugar, 4 oz. in any form; plenty of liquids with meals; tea, coffee, cocoa, water, cod-liver oil. SEE: *macies.*

Leber's disease (lā'bĕr). Congenital atrophy of the optic nerve that is inherited.

L.'s plexus. Plexus of venules in eye bet. Schlemm's canal and Fontana's spaces.

Lecat's gulf (lā-kăts'). Bulbous portion of the urethra.

lechery (letch'er-ĭ) [Fr. *lecher,* to lick]. Lewdness; sensualism.

lechopyra (lek-o-pī'ra) [G. *lechō,* parturient woman, + *pyr,* fever]. Puerperal fever.

lecithin (les'ĭth-ĭn) [G. *lekithos,* egg yolk]. A fatty substance, of the group called phospholipins, found in blood, bile, brain, egg yolk, nerves, and other animal tissues, and yielding stearic acid, glycerol, phosphoric acid, and choline on hydrolysis.

lec"ithin'ase. An enzyme that catalyzes the decomposition of lecithin.

l., cobra. An enzyme present in snake venom which brings about the removal of a molecule of fatty acid from lecithin resulting in production of *lysolecithin, q.v.*

lectual (lekt'ū-ăl) [L. *lectus,* bed]. Pert. to a bed or couch.

l. disease. Bed-confining disease.

leech (lētch) [A.S. *laece*]. A blood-sucking water worm, belonging to the phylum Annelida, class Hirudinea. It is parasitic on man and other animals, producing a condition known as *hirudiniasis, q.v.* Leeches were at one time used as a means of blood-letting, a practice common up to the middle of the 19th century, but which now has been almost completely abandoned. They are a source of *hirudin*, an anticoagulating principle secreted by their buccal glands. SEE: *Hirudo*.

l., artificial. Cup and exhaust pump or syringe for drawing blood.

Lee's ganglion (le). Cervical uterine ganglion formed from 3rd and 4th sacral nerves and hypogastric and ovarian plexuses.

left. SYN: *sinistral*. The opposite of right.

left″-hand′edness. Condition of being more adept in use of left hand. SYN: *sinistrality*.

left lateral recumbent position. The English or obstetrical position. Patient on left side, right knee and thigh drawn up. Used in rectal operations and obstetrics.

leg (lĕg) [M.E.]. One of the 2 lower extremities, including the femur, tibia, fibula, and patella; spec. the part between the knee and ankle.

RS: *acnemia, acragnosis, anxietas tibiarum, Barbadoes, bayonet, bowleg, Buerger's disease, calf, crural, crus, saphena, sura, systremma, tibia.*

l., Anglesey. A form of jointed artificial leg.

l., badger. Inequality in the length of the legs.

l., baker. Genu valgum, or knock-knee.

l., bandy. Same as bowleg.

l., Barbadoes. Elephantiasis of the legs.

l., bayonet. Uncorrected backward displacement of the knee bones, followed by ankylosis at the joint.

l., bird. Reduction in size of the leg from atrophy of the muscles.

l., boomerang. A disease of the leg bones occurring among Australian natives, causing a curvature of the leg resembling a boomerang.

l., bow-. *Genu varum;* an outward curving of the legs at the knees.

l., lawn tennis. Rupture of plantaris muscle accompanied by excruciating disabling pain in the posterior region of the knee.

l., milk. Phlebitis of the femoral vein occasionally following parturition and typhoid fever. It is characterized by swelling of the leg, usually without redness. Called also white leg. SYN: *phlegmasia alba dolens.*

l., scissor. Cross leg deformity; a result of double hip disease, in which the patient walks with the legs crossed.

l., white. SEE: *milk leg.*

leggings (lĕg′ĭngs) [M.E. *leg*, leg]. Sterile leg coverings used on patient while in operating room.

legitimacy (lĕ-jĭt′ĭm-ă-sĭ) [L. *legitimus*, lawful]. 1. Condition of being legal. 2. Condition of being born in wedlock.

legume (lĕ′gūm) [L. *legumen*, pulse]. Fruit or pod of beans, peas, lentils, etc.

COMP: *Nitrogen:* Almost equal to that in meat. It is called *legumin,** forming with water a paste resembling gluten, but easier to digest.

VITAMINS (*Sprouted beans*): A good source of vit. B complex. Vitamin A and ascorbic acid in small amounts.

CARBOHYDRATES: Superior to those in meat. Generally they are in the form of starch in about the same proportion as the cereals, but with more cellulose.

ASH: Twice that of meat or bread. Potash is abundant and soda is present. Alkalinity higher than that of other vegetables. Organic phosphoric acid is high, only exceeded in cheese, oatmeal, and yolk of egg. Iron is found only in the lentils, but lime and magnesium, also nuclein and lecithin, are plentiful in the others as well.

ABSORPTION: They take up large amounts of water. 10.58 oz. of dried peas make 42.38 oz. of puree, while intestinal absorption is lower than that for milk, bread, meat or rice.

EFFECT OF PREPARATION: *Soaking*: The water transforms some of the starch into amylodextrin and modifies the cellulose, assisting in their digestion and absorption.

COOKING: Soft water should be used, as the carbonate of lime in hard water forms an insoluble combination. Add baking soda to hard water. Too much water lowers the nutritive value, wastes the aromatic essences, mineral salts and diminishes digestibility. Cook in small amount of water, over a slow fire.

ACTION: About the same as cereals. Too large quantities may overtax the alimentary canal and cause gaseous and acid fermentation. In the intestines, the albumin and starch react at once on the pancreas and the glandular system, while the cellulose because of its bulk stimulates intestinal activity. They are heavy in nitrogen and nuclein, and should be considered as less expensive substitutes for meat.

IND: *Adolescence and Childhood*: The phosphorus, lime and magnesium in legumes are very valuable in the construction of tissue, as well as in convalescence and tuberculosis. Thick soups may be used when the entire pea or bean might be difficult to digest.

legumelin (leg-u′mel-in) [L. *legumen*, pulse]. An albumin present in many leguminous seeds, as in peas. SEE: *legume, legumin.*

legu′min [L. *legumen*, pulse]. A protein globulin contained in legumes; vegetable casein.

leiodermia (lī-ō-dĕr′mĭ-ă) [G. *leios*, smooth, + *derma*, skin]. Skin disease characterized by abnormal glossiness and atrophy.

leiomyofibroma (lī″ō-mī″ō-fī-brō′mă) [G. *leios*, smooth, + *mys*, my-, muscle, + L. *fibra*, fiber, + G. *oma*, tumor]. A benign tumor composed principally of smooth muscle and fibrous connective tissue.

leiomyoma (lī″ō-mī-ō′mă) [G. *leios*, smooth, + *mys*, my-, muscle, + *oma*, tumor]. Myoma consisting principally of smooth muscle tissue.

leiomyosarcoma (lī″ō-mī″ō-săr-kō′mă) [" + " + *sarx*, flesh, + *ōma*, tumor]. Combined leiomyoma and sarcoma.

leiotrichous (lī″ŏt′rĭ-kŭs). Possessing smooth or straight hair.

Leishmania (lĕsh-măn′-ĭ-ă). A genus of parasitic flagellate protozoans which occur as typical *leishmanian* forms in vertebrate hosts but as *leptomonad* forms in invertebrate hosts or in cultures. They are transmitted by the sandfly, *Phlebotomas.*

L. braziliensis. Causative agent of American leishmaniasis.

L. donovani. Causative agent of kala azar (visceral leishmaniasis).

L. tropica. Causative agent of oriental sore (cutaneous leishmaniasis).

leishmaniasis, leishmaniosis (lĕsh-măn-ī′ă-sĭs, -ĭ-ō′sĭs). Infection with a species of *Leishmania*, affecting the skin, nasal cavities and pharynx, one form causing oriental boil, another kala azar.

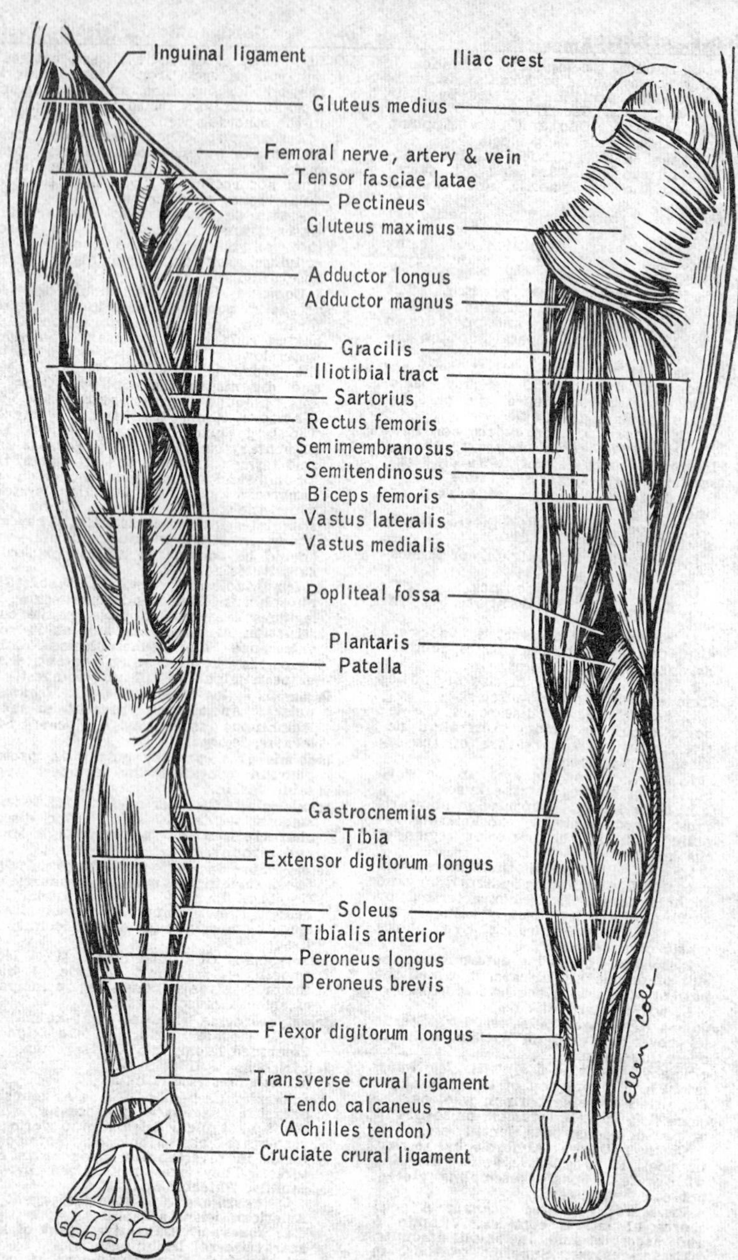

LEG'S ANTERIOR MUSCLES.

LEG'S POSTERIOR MUSCLES.

l., American. L. caused by *L. braziliensis*, involving principally nasopharyngeal and mucocutaneous membranes. Common in Cent. and South America.

l., cutaneous. L. due to infection with Leishmania tropica. SYN: *aleppo boil; oriental sore; Delhi ulcer.*

l., visceral. SYN: *kala azar, dumdum fever.* L. caused by *L. donovani.*

le'ma. SYN: *sebum palpebrale.* The dried secretion of the tarsal glands which collects in the inner canthus of the eye.

-lem'ma. Combining form meaning a membrane, covering, sheath, or envelope.

lemmocyte (lem'mō-sīt) [G. *lemma*, husk, + *kytos*, cell]. A cell which becomes a neurilemma cell.

lemniscus (lem-nis'kŭs) [G. *lēmniskos*, a fillet]. A bundle of sensory fibers (lateral or ext. and median or int.) in the medulla, and pons. SYN: *fillet, laqueus.*

lem'on [Persian *līmūn*, lemon]. Contains citric acid. RAW, PEELED: 100 gm. Calories: 27. Other main values: 1 gm. protein; trace of fat; 8.2 gm. carbohydrates; 7 mg. calcium; 53 mg. ascorbic acid.

l. juice. FRESH: 100 gm. Calories: 25. Other main values: 0.5 gm. protein; 8 gm. carbohydrates; 7 mg. calcium; 46 mg. ascorbic acid.

ACTION: Stimulating and refreshing.

IND: May be used in place of vinegar, spices, and aromatic substances by those who cannot use the latter. Diabetics may use. A fine antiscorbutic.

CONTRA: As they are supposed to increase calcification of arteries and deposit of chalky matter in the tissues, avoid use in pulmonary tuberculosis, and in acute articular rheumatism.

lemoparalysis (le"mo-par-al'ĭs-ĭs) [G. *laimos*, gullet, + *para*, beside, + *lyein*, to loosen]. Paralysis of esophagus.

lemosteno'sis [" + *stenōsis*, a narrowing]. Stricture of esophagus.

lenitive (len'ĭ-tiv) [L. *lenīre*, to soothe]. 1. Demulcent, soothing, slightly laxative. 2. A palliative.

lens (lĕnz) (pl. *lentēs*) [L. *lentil*, lens]. 1. A transparent refracting medium; usually made of glass. 2. The crystalline lens of the eye.

RS: *capsitis, capsulociliary, circle of diffusion, posterior chamber, vitreous chamber.*

l., achromatic. One for correction of chromatic aberration.

l., bifocal. A lens containing in either its upper or lower segment a lens of different power. The main lens is for distant vision; the secondary lens is for near vision.

l., concave spherical. Formed of prisms with their apices together, therefore, thin at the center and thick at the edge. Used in myopia.

l., convex spherical. Formed of prisms with their bases together, therefore, thick at the center and thin at the edge. Used in hyperopia.

l., corneal contact. A type of contact lens which adheres to and covers only the cornea.

l., crystalline. Transparent, colorless structure in eye; biconvex in shape, enclosed in a capsule and held in place just behind the pupil by the suspensory ligament. Consists principally of *lens fibers* which at the periphery are soft, forming the *cortex lentis*, and in the center of harder consistency, forming the *nucleus lentis.* Beneath the *capsule* on ant. surface is a thin layer of cells, the *lens epithelium.* Function is to focus rays so they form a perfect image on the retina.

l., cylindrical. Segment of a cylinder parallel to its axis, used in correcting astigmatism.

lenticonus (len-ti-ko'nus) [" + *conus*, cone]. Conical protrusion of ant. or post. surface of lens.

lentic'ular [L. *lenticulāris*, pert. to a lens]. 1. Lens shaped. SYN: *lentiform.* 2. Pert. to a lens.

l. fossa. Depression in ant. surface of vitreous for reception of the crystalline lens.

l. glands. Small masses of lymphatic tissue in lamina propria of pyloric region of the stomach.

l. nucleus. Mass of gray matter forming part of the corpus striatum. Consists of the putamen and globus pallidus.

lenticulostriate (len-tĭk"ū-lō-strī'āt) [" + *striatus*, streaked]. Rel. to the lenticular nucleus and corpus striatum.

lenticulothalamic. Pert. to lenticular nucleus and the thalamus.

lentiform (lent'ĭ-form) [L. *lens, lent-*, lentil, lens, + *forma*, shape]. Lentil or lens shaped. SYN: *lenticular.*

lentiginous (lĕn-tĭj'ĭn-ŭs) [L. *lentigō*, freckle]. 1. Affected by lentigo. 2. Covered with very small dots.

len'tigo (pl. *lentigines*) [L. freckle]. Small brown macules or yellow-brown pigmented areas on skin sometimes caused by exposure to sun and weather. SYN: *ephelis, freckle.*

lentitis (lĕn-tī'tĭs) [" + G. *-ītis*, inflammation]. SYN: *phakitis.* Inflammation of the crystalline lens.

leontiasis (lē-ŏn-tī'ă-sĭs) [G. *leōn, leont-*, lion]. Lionlike expression about face, accompanying certain diseases.

l. ossea. Enlargement and distortion of facial bones, giving one the appearance of a lion. The condition is rare and not fatal. SYN: *leontiasis.*

leotropic (lē-ō-trop'ĭk) [G. *laios*, left, + *tropos*, a turning]. Running from right to left in a spiral form. OPP: *dexiotropic.*

leper (lĕp'ĕr) [G. *lepros*, scaly]. Person afflicted with leprosy.

lep'ido- [G. *lepis*, scale]. Combining form: Referring to flakes or scales.

Lepidoptera. An order of the class Insecta which includes the butterflies, moths and skippers. Characterized by scaly wings, sucking mouth parts, and complete metamorphosis.

lepidosis (lĕp-ĭd-ō'sis) [" + *-ōsis*, intensive]. Any scaly or desquamating eruption. SYN: *pityriasis.*

lepothrix (lep'o-thriks) [G. *lepos*, scale, + *thrix*, hair]. Condition in which shaft of the hair is encased in hardened, scaly, sebaceous matter.

lepra (lĕp'ră) [G. *lepra*, leprosy]. A term formerly used for leprosy. Now used to indicate a reaction which occurs in leprosy patients. This can occur in any form of leprosy, may be prolonged, and consists of aggravation of lesions accompanied by fever and malaise.

l. alba. Skin is anesthetic and white, and different forms of paralysis follow.

l. anesthetica. Leprosy with anesthetic areas on body.

l. Arabum. True or nodular leprosy.

l. maculosa. Form with pigmented cutaneous areas.

l. mutilans. Final stage of true leprosy, or mutilation stage.

l. nervorum. Maculo-anesthetic leprosy, *q.v.*

leprid(e (lĕp′rēd) [G. *lepra,* leprosy]. Leprous cutaneous lesion.

leprology (lĕp-rol′ō-jĭ) [" + *logos,* study]. The study of leprosy and methods of treating it.

leproma (lĕp-rō′mă) [G. *lepra,* leprosy, + *-ōma,* tumor]. A cutaneous nodule or tubercle characteristic of leprosy.

lep′romin. A substance prepared from lepromatous nodules of leprosy.

l. skin test. One in which lepromin is introduced intradermally. The test was devised to assist in the diagnosis of leprosy but because of false positives and negatives its usefulness is limited. Attempts to refine the test are continuing.

leprosarium. An institution for the care of lepers.

leprosy (lep′ro-sĭ) [G. *lepra,* leprosy]. A chronically communicable disease caused by the acid-fast Mycobacterium leprae. It may occur in various clinical forms. The two principal forms are: 1. *Lepromatous,* characterized by skin lesions and symmetrical involvement of peripheral nerves with anesthesia, muscle weakness and paralysis. In this form, the lesions are limited to the cooler portions of the body such as skin, upper respiratory tract, and testes. 2. *Tuberculoid,* which is usually benign. The nerve lesions are asymmetrical and skin anesthesia is an early occurrence. Visceral involvement is not seen.

Lepromatous leprosy is much more contagious than the *tuberculoid* form. In the latter, Mycobacterium leprae are found only rarely except during reactions.

Between the two major forms are *borderline* and *indeterminate* leprosy. In the borderline group, the clinical and bacteriological features represent a combination of the two principal types. In the indeterminate group, there are fewer skin lesions and bacteria are much less abundant in the lesions.

In many respects, this infection resembles tuberculosis and for many years was regarded as incurable, a conclusion no longer considered true.

Etiol: Caused by Myobacterium leprae. May occur at practically any age.

Incubation: From 1 to 30 years.

Sym: Onset very gradual. The first signs of infection are usually skin changes, but they may be so nonspecific and so slow to progress as to go unrecognized for years.

Complications: Bacterial infections of skin, ulcers, traumatic amputation of fingers due to anesthesia, also fingers may be eaten by rodents while the patient is asleep, tuberculosis is a much more common complication in untreated cases of *lepromatous* leprosy than in the *tuberculoid* form. Amyloidosis may be the cause of death in advanced cases.

Prognosis: With proper therapy the outlook for recovery is good.

Treatment: Diaminodiphenyldisulfone (DDS) is the form of sulfone most commonly used.

Isolation: Segregation of patients in colonies or hospitals until bacterial tests have been negative for six months is *not* the preferred or effective method of isolating patients. Ambulatory treatment of patients at general clinics has been found to be much more effective. Because they are more susceptible to this disease than adults, children should be removed from contact with leprosy patients.

leprotic (lĕp-rot′ĭk) [G. *lepra,* leper]. 1. Rel. to leprosy. 2. Affected with leprosy. Syn: *leprous.*

leprous (lĕp′rŭs) [G. *lepra,* leper]. 1. Pert. to leprosy. 2. Affected by leprosy. Syn: *leprotic.*

leptocephalia. Having an abnormally small head.

leptocephalus. An individual possessing an abnormally small head.

leptodermic (lep-tō-dĕr′mĭk) [G. *leptos,* slender, + *derma,* skin]. Possessing a thin skin.

leptomeninges (lep″to-men-ĭn′jēs) [" + *mēnigx,* membrane]. Pia mater and arachnoid as distinct from dura mater, because of their thinner and more delicate structure.

leptomeningitis (lep″to-men-in-ji′tis) [" + " + *-itis,* inflammation]. Inflammation of the pia and arachnoid membranes. See: *meningitis.*

Etiol: Tubercle bacillus, spirochete of syphilis, and other pathologic organisms.

Sym: Acute headache, pain in back, rigidity of spine, irritability, drowsiness ending in coma.

Clinically, it cannot be distinguished from pachymeningitis, *q.v.*

leptomeninx. Sing. of leptomeninges. The pia and arachnoid mater of the brain.

leptopellic (lep-tō-pel′ĭk) [" + *pellis,* a bowl (pelvis)]. Having an abnormally narrow pelvis.

leptophonia (lĕp-tō-fō′nĭ-ă) [" + *phōnē,* voice]. Weakness or feebleness of voice.

leptoprosopia (lĕp″tō-prō-sō′pĭ-ă). Narrowness of the face.

leptorhine, leptorrhine (lep′tor-rīn) [" + *ris, rin-,* nose]. Having a very thin or slender nose.

leptosome (lĕp′tō-sōm) [" + *soma,* body]. Person of thin, slight stature.

Leptospira (lĕp-tō-spī′ră) [G. *leptos,* thin, + *spaira,* coil]. Genus of spirochetes, thin, spiral, and hook-ended.

L. autumnalis. Species first isolated in Japan. Causes a nonicteric infection in man called *pretibial* or Fort Bragg fever.

L. hebdomadis. Species causing seven-day fever of Japan.

L. icterohaemorrha′giae. Species causing infectious, hemorrhagic spirochetal, jaundice (Weil's disease).

leptospirosis (lĕp″tō-spī-rō′sĭs) [" + " + *-ōsis,* intensive]. Condition resulting from Leptospira infection.

leptothricosis (lep″tō-thri-kō′sĭs) [" + *thrix,* hair]. Disease from Leptothrix infection.

Leptothrix (lĕp′to-thrĭks) [" + *thrix,* hair]. A genus of bacteria often with long filaments. They belong to the family Chlamydobacteriaceae, the so-called iron bacteria.

L. buccalis. A species commonly found in the mouth cavity. Considered non-pathogenic.

L. placoides. Species isolated from a tooth canal.

Leptotrich′ia bucca′lis. An organism inhabiting the buccal cavity normally.

Leptus autumnalis (lep′tŭs) [G. *leptos,* slender]. Parasitic mite larvae causing itch and sometimes wheals. See: *chigger.*

lere′sis. Loquacity in old age; garrulousness.

les'bian [G. *lesbios,* pert. to island of Lesbos]. 1. Pert. to lesbianism, or perverted sexual desire in women for those of their own sex. 2. One who practices lesbianism.

les'bianism. Perversion in which sexual desire of women is for one of their own sex.

Named from the Island of Lesbos wherein the practice of sapphism was reputed to have been general in ancient days. It may be expressed physically or psychically. SEE: *sapphism, tribadism, urningism.*

lesion (le'zhun) [L. *laesio,* a wound]. 1. Morbid change in tissue formation locally. 2. An injury or wound. 3. Single infected patch in a skin disease.

Primary or initial lesions include *macules; vesicles; blebs,* or *bullae; chancres; pustules; papules; tubercles; wheals,* and *tumors, q.v.* Secondary lesions are the result of primary lesions. They may be *crusts, excoriations, fissures, pigmentations, scales, scars,* and *ulcers, q.v.*

RS: *abscess, boil, carbuncle, Cazenave's lupus, cerebropsychosis, chancre, chancroids, Chaussier's areola, felon, gumma, moles, pimples, rash, sebaceous cysts, tumefactions, verruca, wound.*

l., degenerative. L. caused by or showing degeneration.

l., diffuse. L. spreading over a large area.

l., discharging. 1. Brain l. discharging nervous impulses. 2. L. discharging an exudate.

l., focal. L. of small definite area.

l., indiscriminate. L. affecting separate systems of the body.

l., initial, of syphilis. Hard chancre.

l., irritative. L. stimulating or exciting activity in part of body where it is situated.

l., local. L. of nervous origin giving rise to local symptoms.

l., peripheral. One of nerve endings.

l., primary. First l. of a disease, esp. used in referring to chancre of syphilis.

l., structural. One causing change in tissue.

l., systematic. One confined to organs of common function.

l., toxic. One resulting from sepsis.

l., vascular. One of a blood vessel.

le'thal [G. *lēthē,* oblivion]. Pert. to or that which causes death.

lethargic (leth-ar'jĭk) [G. *lēthargos,* drowsiness]. 1. Affected with lethargy. 2. Rel. to lethargy. 3. Sluggish.

lethargy (leth'ar-jĭ) [G. *lēthargos,* drowsiness]. A condition of functional torpor or sluggishness; stupor.

RS: *cataphora, coma vigil, personality, noctambulism, somnambuilism, vigilambulism.*

l., African. Sleeping sickness.

l., hysteric. The sleep of hypnotic lethargy, the state in which many cases of apparent death and resurrection are found.

l. induced. Hypnotic trance.

l., lucid. Retention of intellect but loss of will power with a consequent total lack of muscular response. The subject knows what is going on, resents it, perhaps, but is unable to exercise sufficient will to bring about muscular defense.

ETIOL: Fear, fascination, shock. This unrecognized condition may be responsible for many instances of rape, or of yielding to such an attack.

lethologica (lēth-ō-loj'ĭk-ă) [G. *lēthē,* forgetfulness, + *logos,* word]. Temporary inability to remember a word or name, or an intended action.

Letterer-Siwe's disease. A usually fatal disease of infancy and childhood of unknown cause, with hyperplasia of the reticuloendothelial system without lipoid storage.

let'tuce. The edible leaves of a plant of the genus *Lactuca* esp. *L. sativa.* RAW: 100 gm. of crisp head varieties. Calories: 56. Other main values: 4 gm. protein; 0.4 gm. fat; 12.5 gm. carbohydrates; 86 mg. calcium; 1420 I.U. vitamin A; 28 mg. ascorbic acid.

leuc-. For words beginning thus, see *leuk-* words.

leucine (lū'sēn) [G. *leukos,* white]. Alpha-amino-isobutyl acetic acid, CH_3. $(CH_2)_3$. CH (NH_2). COOH, an amino acid found among the products of the digestion of proteins. It is present in body tissues and is essential for normal growth and metabolism.

leucinosis (lū-sin-ō'sĭs) [" + *-ōsis,* intensive]. Excess of leucine in the body producing leucine in the urine.

leucinuria (lū-sin-ū'rĭ-ă) [" + *ouron,* urine]. Presence of leucine in urine.

leucitis (lū-sī'tis) [" + *-itis,* inflammation]. Inflammation of the sclera. SYN: *scleritis.*

leukanemia (lū-kă-ne'mĭ-ă) [" + *a-,* priv. + *aima,* blood]. Leukemia with marked anemia.

leukasmus (lū-kas'mŭs) [G. *leukasmos,* growing white]. Congenital absence of pigment in bands or patches of the skin. SYN: *leukoderma.*

leukemia (lū-kē'mĭ-ă) [G. *leukasmos,* growing white, + *aima,* blood]. A disease of unknown cause characterized by rapid and abnormal proliferation of leukocytes in the blood-forming organs (bone marrow, spleen, lymph nodes) and the presence of immature leukocytes in peripheral circulation. May be acute or chronic but inevitably fatal.

NP: Watch for local mouth infections, terminal septicemia, and bronchopneumonia as complications. Myelogenous forms are prone to such infections as boils, erysipelas, grippe, influenza and pneumonia. Good nursing care is very important in all forms of this disease. Hemorrhages from nose and mouth often require packing and hemostatics.

l., acute. Leukemia in which onset is sudden and progress rapid. Usually fatal within a period of two or three months.

l., aleukemic. L. in which the total leukocyte count is normal or below normal and in which immature cells are absent.

l., leukemic. L. in which total leukocyte count in peripheral blood is elevated and immature cells of the series involved are present.

l., lymphatic. That in which there is marked increase in the size of the spleen and lymph glands with a great increase in lymphocytes in blood; acute form occurs in children and young adults.

l., monocytic. A rare form of leukemia in which monocytes are the predominant cells involved. Involves the reticulo-endothelial tissues of blood-forming organs.

l., myelogenous. L. involving the hematopoietic bone marrow, esp. that of the ribs, sternum, and vertebrae.

Bone marrow which is normally red in color, becomes gray and assumes a gelatinous consistency. Myeloid elements increase in blood.

SYM: General manifestations of anemia—enlargement of spleen, liver or lymphatic glands. Febrile paroxysms (101°-103° F.), hemorrhage from mucous membranes, digestive disturbances, dimness of vision. There is marked increase in the leukocytes; proportion to red corpuscles may be 1-50 or even 1-10. This leukocytosis results from an increase in all forms of leukocytes, with a concomitant decrease in red blood cells.

PROG: Death usually results in 3 to 4 years.

l., plasma cell. L. in which plasma cells are the predominant cells in the blood.

l., subleukemic. Aleukemic leukemia, *q.v.*

leukemic (lū-kĕm'ĭk) [G. *leukos*, white, + *aima*, blood]. 1. Rel. to leukemia. 2. Affected with leukemia.

leukemoid (lū-kē'moid) [G. *leukos*, white, + *aima*, blood, + *eidos*, form]. Having symptoms of leukemia, but due to other conditions.

leu'ko-, leuk- [G.]. Combining forms signifying *deficiency of color.*

leu'koblast [G. *leukos*, white, + *blastos*, germ]. General term applied to a cell that gives rise to a leukocyte.

leukoblasto'sis. Proliferation of excessive numbers of immature leukocytes.

leukocidin (lū-ko-sid'in) [" + L. *cidus*, from *caedere*, to kill]. A bacterial toxin which destroys leukocytes. SYN: *leukotoxin, q.v.*

leukocytal (lū-kō-sī'tăl) [" + *kytos*, cell]. Rel. to leukocytes.

leukocyte (lū'kō-sīt) [G. *leukos*, white, + *kytos*, cell]. White blood corpuscle. There are two types; (1) *granulocytes* (those possessing granules in their cytoplasm) and (2) *agranulocytes* (those lacking granules). Granulocytes include (a) *juvenile neutrophils* (3-5%), *segmented neutrophils* (54-62%), *basophils* (0-0.75%), and *eosinophils* (1-3%). Agranulocytes include *lymphocytes*, large and small (25-33%) and *monocytes* (3-7%).

The leukocytes act as scavengers and by so doing help to combat infection. They move by ameboid movement and are able to penetrate tissue and then return to the blood stream. The direction of movement is probably due to the stimuli from injured cells. This is called *chemotaxis.* When invading bacteria overcome them, the dead bodies of the white blood corpuscles collect in the form of pus, causing an abscess if a ready outlet is not found. Different types combat various kinds of infection.

One cu. mm. of blood contains 5000-10,000 leukocytes normally.

FUNCTIONS: Leukocytes, esp. the granular forms, are markedly phagocytic, *i.e.*, have the power to ingest particulate substances. Neutrophils ingest bacteria and small particles; other cells such as the monocytes and histiocytes in the tissues ingest larger particles. They are important in both defensive and reparative functions of the body. Basophils most probably function by delivering anticoagulants to facilitate blood clot absorption or to prevent blood coagulation. Eosinophils increase in number in certain conditions such as asthma and infestations of animal parasites. Lymphocytes are not phagocytic. They are thought to be a source of serum globulin and possibly certain immune bodies. Their exact role in immunologic reaction is being extensively studied.

A greatly diminished number of erythrocytes is found in the anemias, and a greatly increased number of leukocytes (leukocytosis) is indicative of the presence of inflammatory products. A leukocyte count is usually a preoperative routine if infection is suspected, such as in appendicitis. A count may also be taken following an operation to be sure that no infection from a wound is present.

HOW TO RECOGNIZE: White blood cells are round, edges occasionally broken, nucleated, granular, having a grayish color, sometimes clumped, and can be stained as polynuclears.

MICROSCOPIC EXAMINATION: They are usually in pieces of mucus and can be stained by ordinary blood stains.

Decrease below normal (5000) is called *leukopenia;* increase above normal (10,000) is called *leukocytosis.*

Two determinations are usually made regarding the leukocytes: their *total number* (total count), and the *percentage of each type* (differential count). Decrease below the normal is called *leukopenia.* Relative increase or decrease of any particular type is denoted by adding the suffix "philia" (denoting increase) or "penia" (denoting decrease), as: neutrophilia, granulocytopenia, neutropenia, eosinophilia, etc.

Sometimes immature white cells are discharged into the blood stream and may be observed in blood smears; myelocytes, myeloblasts, or lymphoblasts. Their presence provides strong suspicion of disease.

In a smear of blood, all of the white cells are not alike; they vary in size, in shape, in appearance, and in color which they assume when stained. Some of the cells contain minute granules, and these cells are called granulocytes, the cytoplasm of others is granular. It is seen that the granules in some cells stain bright red, and the cells are called eosinophils; in others, deep blue, and these are called basophils. In most of the cells, however, the granules take a neutral purplish color, and these are called neutrophils. There are two types of nongranular cells, the lymphocytes and the monocytes.

Not all leukocytes are formed in the same place, nor in the same manner. Granulocytes are formed in the bone marrow, arising from large cells called megakaryocytes. Lymphocytes are formed in the lymph nodes; monocytes from the cells lining the capillaries in various organs, perhaps principally in the spleen and bone marrow.

l., acidophil. An eosinophil l., *q. v.*

l., basophil. L. with cytoplasmic granules which stain with basic dyes. Stain a deep purple with Wright's stain. Comprise 0-0.75% of white cell count.

l., beta. One of those which do not disintegrate during coagulation.

l., eosinophil. L. with cytoplasmic granules which stain with acid dyes. Appear reddish when stained with Wright's stain. Comprise 1-3% of white cell count.

l., granular. SYN: *granulocyte,* L. containing granules in cytoplasm.

l., heterophilic. Neutrophil l. of certain animals whose granules stain with an acid stain.

Tabular Summary of Leukocytes

Cells	Nucleus	Cytoplasmic Granules	Range (in %)
Granulocytes (Polymorphonuclear)			
Juvenile Neutrophils	Unsegmented	Fine, pale stain	3-5
Segmented Neutrophils	Polymorphic	Fine. Neutral stain	54-62
Eosinophils	Polymorphic	Coarse. Stain with acid dye	1-3
Basophils	Polymorphic	Coarse. Stain with basic dye	0-0.75
Agranulocytes			
Lymphocytes, small and large	Spherical (slightly indented)	None	25-33
Monocytes	Kidney shaped	None	3-7

l., neutrophil. L. with fine cytoplasmic granules which do not stain with acid or basic stains but have an affinity for neutral stains.

l., nongranular. An agranulocyte; a lymphocyte or monocyte.

l., polymorphonuclear. L. with a nucleus consisting of several lobes. One of the granulocytes (neutrophil, eosinophil, basophil).

leukocythemia (lū-ko-sī-the'mĭ-ă) [G. *leukos,* white, + *kytos,* cell, + *aima,* blood]. Blood disease characterized by excess of white blood corpuscles and enlargement of spleen, lymphatic glands and bone marrow. SYN: *leukemia, q.v.*

leukocytic (lū-kō-sit'ĭk) [" + *kytos,* cell]. Pert. to leukocytes.

leukocytoblast (lū-kō-sīt'ō-blast) [" + " + *blastos,* germ]. Cell from which leukocytes arise.

leukocytogenesis (lū"kō-sīt"ō-jen'ĕ-sĭs) [G. *leukos,* white, + *kytos,* cell, + *genesis,* formation]. Leukocyte formation. SYN: *leukopoiesis.*

leukocytoid (lū'kō-sī-toid) [" + " + *eidos,* form]. Resembling a leukocyte.

leu"kocytol'ysin. A lysin which destroys leukocytes. SEE: *leukocidin.*

leukocytolysis (lū-kō-sī-tol'ĭ-sĭs) [" + " + *lysis,* dissolution]. Destruction of leukocytes.

leukocytoma (lū-kō-sī-tō'mă) [" + " + *ōma,* tumor]. 1. Tumor composed of cells resembling leukocytes. 2. Tumor-like mass of leukocytes.

leukocytometer (lū"ko-sī-tom'et-er) [" + " + *metron,* measure]. Device for counting white blood corpuscles.

leukocytopenia (lū"kō-sīt"ō-pē'nĭ-ă) [" + " + *penia,* want]. Subnormal number of leukocytes in blood. SYN: *leukopenia.*

leukocytoplania (lū"kō-sīt"ō-plā'nĭ-ă) [" + " + *planē,* wandering]. Wandering of leukocytes through blood vessel walls. SYN: *leukopedesis.*

leukocytopoiesis (lū-kō-sī-poy"ē'sĭs). Formation of white blood cells.

leukocytosis (lū"ko-sī-to'sis) [G. *leukos,* white, + *kytos,* cell, + *-ōsis*]. Increase in the number of leukocytes (above 10,000 per cu. mm.) in the blood, generally caused by presence of infection. It may also accompany or occur after the following conditions: hemorrhage, extensive operations, coronary occlusion, malignant growths, pregnancy, certain intoxications, and toxemias. Eosinophilic leukocytosis occurs in certain allergies, infestation with animal parasites, and Hodgkin's disease.

Leukemias, however, release immature leukocytes due to abnormal condition of blood forming organs. Leukocytosis is present in most infections but not usually in those due to a virus.

Fifteen thousand to thirty thousand is the usual count in leukocytosis, sometimes 50,000 or 75,000; in leukemias 500,000-1,000,000 per cu. mm. Leukocytosis is early and marked in severe infections when the patient's resistance is good; if infection and resistance are less marked it obtains later and in a lesser degree and disappears more quickly. No leukocytosis may occur in unusually virulent infection, such as diphtheria, pneumonia, sepsis, etc.

leukocyturia (lū"ko-sī-tu'rĭ-ă) [" + " + *ouron,* urine]. Leukocytes in the urine.

leukoderma (lū-ko-der'mă) [" + *derma,* skin]. Deficiency of pigmentation of the skin, esp. in patches. SYN: *leukopathia.* Classed as congenital, acquired and syphilitic.

leukodiagnosis (lū-ko-dī-ag-nō'sĭs) [" + *dia,* through, + *gnōsis,* knowledge]. Diagnosis by observance of number, variety, or reaction of leukocytes.

leukoencephalitis (lū-kō-ĕn-sĕf-ă-lī'tĭs). Inflammation of the white matter of the brain.

leukokeratosis (lū"kō-kĕr-ă-tō'sĭs) [" + *keras,* horn, + *-ōsis*]. White patch formation on the surface of mucosa of tongue, cheek and gums. SYN: *leukoplakia.*

leukolysin (lū-kol'ĭ-sĭn) [" + *lysis,* dissolution]. Serum constituent destructive to leukocytes.

leukolysis (lū-kol'ĭ-sis) [" + *lysis,* dissolution]. Destruction of leukocytes. SYN: *leukocytolysis.*

leuko'ma [" + *-ōma,* tumor]. A white, opaque corneal opacity.

l. adherens. Corneal scar with incarcerated iris tissue.

leukomaine (lū-kō'ma-ēn, -ma-ĭn) [G. *leukoma,* whiteness]. Toxic nitrogenous alkaloid developed in living tissue as distinguished from one in dead tissue, or one of vegetable origin.

leukomainemia (lū-kō-mā-ĭn-ē'mĭ-ă) [" + *aima,* blood]. Excess of leukomaines in blood.

leukomatous (lū-kōm'ă-tŭs) [" + *ōma,* tumor]. 1. Pert. to leukoma. 2. Suffering from leukoma.

leukomyelitis (lū"ko-mī-ĕ-li'tis) [G. *leukos,* white, + *myelos,* marrow, + *-itis,* inflammation]. Inflammation of the white matter of the spinal cord.

leukomyelopathy (lū"kō-mī-ĕl-ŏp'ăth-ĭ) [" + " + *pathos,* disease]. Disease involving white matter of spinal cord or myelon.

leukonecrosis (lū"ko-nĕ-krō'sĭs) [" + *nekrōsis*, deadness]. Dry, light colored or white gangrene.*

leukonychia (lū-kō-nik'ĭ-ă) [" + *onyx, onych-*, nail]. "Gift spots," white spots or streaks on the nails.

leukopathia (lū-kō-păth'ĭ-ă) [" + *pathos*, disease]. 1. Absence of pigment in skin. Syn: *leukoderma.* 2. Disease involving leukocytes.

leukopedesis (lū-kō-ped-ĕ'sĭs) [" + *pēdan*, to leap]. Passage of leukocytes through walls of blood vessels. Syn: *leukocytoplania.*

leukopenia (lū-kō-pe'nĭ-ă) [" + *penia*, lack]. Abnormal decrease of white blood corpuscles usually below 5000 per cu. mm.

l., malignant. An acute infection with extreme leukopenia. Syn: *agranulocytosis.*

leukophlegmasia (lū-kō-flĕg-mā'zĭ-ă) [" + *phlegmasia*, inflammation, fever]. Dropsical tendency with general edema and pale, flabby skin.

leukoplakia (lū-kō-plā'kĭ-ă) [G. *leukos*, white, + *plax*, plate]. Formation of white spots or patches on the mucous membrane of the tongue or cheek.

They are smooth, irregular in size and shape, and hard and occasionally fissure. May become malignant. Syn: *leukoma, psoriasis buccalis, smoker's tongue.*

l. buccalis. L. of the mucosa of the cheek.

l. lingualis. L. of the tongue.

l. vulvae. L. of the vulva. See: *kraurosis vulvae.*

leukoplasia (lū-kō-pla'zĭ-ă) [" + *plax*, plate]. White patch formation on buccal mucosa. Syn: *leukoplakia, q.v.*

leukopoiesis (lū"kō-poi-ē'sĭs) [G. *leukos*, white, + *poiēsis*, formation]. Leukocyte production. Syn: *leukocytogenesis.*

leukopoietic (lū"kō-poi-et'ĭk) [" + *poiein*, to make]. Forming leukocytes.

leukoprotease (lū-ko-pro'te-ās) [" + *prōtos*, first, + *ase*, enzyme]. An enzyme in polynuclear leukocytes that digests protein.

leukop'sin. A substance formed in the rods of the retina from rhodopsin under the influence of light.

leukorrhagia (lū-ko-ra'jĭ-ă) [" + *rēgnunai*, to flow forth]. Profuse white vaginal discharge. Syn: *leukorrhea, q.v.*

leukorrhea (lū-kōr-e'ă) [" + *roia*, flow]. White or yellowish mucous discharge from the cervical canal or the vagina.

There is frequently a normal physiological leukorrhea which may be constantly present but somewhat increased preceding and following menstruation. It may be of considerable concern to the young girl at the time of menarche because she has not been told this white fluid would tend to collect on the vulvae. Leukorrhea may be abnormal because of increase in amount, changes in color, variations in consistency, odors, types of bacterial content, and the appearance of blood.

Etiol: Pathological states of the endocervix and vagina. Infection by *Trichomonas vaginalis.*

Sym: Usually indications of acute inflammation, pain, heat, redness of parts involved, which may subside as discharge increases. Pain in groins, hypogastrium, sacral regions and small of back. Urethra often implicated, causing painful micturition. Symptoms which may occur in connection with chronic leukorrhea are innumerable. Reaction of discharge is acid, may be any consistency: thin and watery or viscid and tenacious.

Treatment: Remove the etiological factor. Mild antiseptic douches may be prescribed but their usefulness is questionable.

leukosarcoma (lū-kō-sar-kō'mă) [G. *leukos*, white, + *sarx*, flesh, + *ōma*, tumor]. An unpigmented sarcoma.

leukosis (lū-ko'sis) [" + *-ōsis*, intensive]. 1. Unnatural pallor. 2. Excessive proliferation of leukocyte-producing tissue. On the basis of type of cell involved, leukosis may be *lymphoid, myeloblastic,* or *myelocytic.* See: *leukemia.* 3. Increase in leukocyte forming tissue.

leu"kotac'tic. Possessing the power of attracting leukocytes.

leu"kotax'ine. A nitrogenous substance present in tissues in which inflammatory processes are taking place. It increases capillary permeability and is positively leukotactic.

leu"kotax'is. Possessing the power of attracting (positive l.) or repelling (negative l.) leukocytes.

leukotoxic (lū-kō-toks'ĭk) [" + *toxikon*, poison]. Destroying leukocytes.

leukotrichia (lū-kō-trik'ĭ-ă) [" + *thrix, trich-*, hair]. Whiteness of the hair. Syn: *canities.*

leukous (lū'kŭs) [G. *leukos*, white]. White, esp. rel. to the skin.

levator (le-va'tor) [L. lifter]. 1. A muscle that raises a part; opposed to *depressor.* 2. An instrument which lifts depressed portions.

l. ani. A broad muscle helping to form the floor of the pelvis.

l. palpebrae superioris. A muscle which elevates the upper eyelid.

level of activities. Connector neurons are grouped into "levels" corresponding to different stages of development: (a) spinal cord level; (b) medullary level; (c) midbrain level; (d) basal ganglial level; (e) cortical level. Each level is responsible for certain activities but yet controlled by the one above it.

le'ver. Rigid bar used to modify direction, force and motion. See: *Ill., p. L-24.*

lev"ita'tion. The subjective sensation of rising in the air or moving through the air unsupported. Occurs in dreams and certain mental disorders.

levoduction (lev-ō-dŭk'shun) [" + *ducere*, to lead]. Movement or drawing toward the left, esp. of an eye.

levogyrous (lev-ō-jĭ'rŭs) [" + *gyrāre*, to turn]. Causing to turn toward the left, applied esp. to substances that turn polarized light rays to the left. Syn: *levorotatory.*

levophobia (lev-ō-fō'bĭ-ă) [" + G. *phobos*, fear]. Morbid dread of objects on the left side of the body.

levorotation (lev"ō-rō-tā'shŭn) [" + *rōtāre*, to turn]. Twisting or turning to the left.

levorotatory (lev"ō-rō'tă-tō-rĭ) [" + *rōtāre*, to turn]. Causing to turn toward the left, applied esp. to substances that turn polarized light rays to the left.

levotorsion (lev-ō-tor'shŭn) [L. *laevus*, left, + *torsiō*, a twisting]. A twisting to the left. Syn: *levorotation.*

levoversion (lev-ō-vĕr'shun) [" + *versiō*, a turning]. A turning to the left. Syn: *levotorsion, levorotation.*

lev'ulose [L. *laevus*, left]. Fructose, or fruit sugar, a monosaccharide and a hexose, having the same empirical formula as dextrose, $C_6H_{12}O_6$.

It is an example of the carbohydrates, *q.v.* One of the three simple sugars. It is formed in the body by the digestion of sucrose. It is found in plants and fruits, in honey, corn syrup and syrup resulting from the inversion of sucrose.

levulosemia (lev-ū-lō-sē'mĭ-ă) [" + G. *aima*, blood]. Presence of levulose in the blood.

levulosuria (lev-ū-lō-sū'rĭ-ă) [" + G. *ouron*, urine]. Presence of levulose in the urine, usually in a form of diabetes.

Leyden jar (lī'den) [Ernst V. von Leyden, German physician, 1832-1910]. A glass jar coated partially, inside and out, with metal; it is used as a capacitor or collector of electricity.

Leydig's cells (lī'dig) [Franz von Leydig, German anatomist, 1821-1908]. Interstitial tissue cells in the testicles, believed to be responsible for internal secretion of the testicles, testosterone.

LH. Abbr. for *luteinizing hormone.*

lichen (lī'ken) [G. *leichen*, lichen]. Any form of papular skin disease; usually noting *l. planus.*

l. acuminatus. A form of l. ruber with papulosquamous type of eruption.

l. agrius. Eczema of acute papular type.

l. disseminatus. Form in which the eruption is placed unevenly.

l. pilaris. Form affecting hair follicles. SYN: *lichen spinulosus.*

l. planus. Inflammatory skin disease of many varieties.

SYM: Begins with pinhead size papules, reddish or violaceous, glistening, then coalescing, forming rough, scaly patches; acute, subacute, or chronic itching situated on extremities. According to type of lesion the disease may be *Lichen planus atrophicus, erythematosus, hypertrophicus, linearis, ruber moniliformis,* etc.

ETIOL: Unknown.

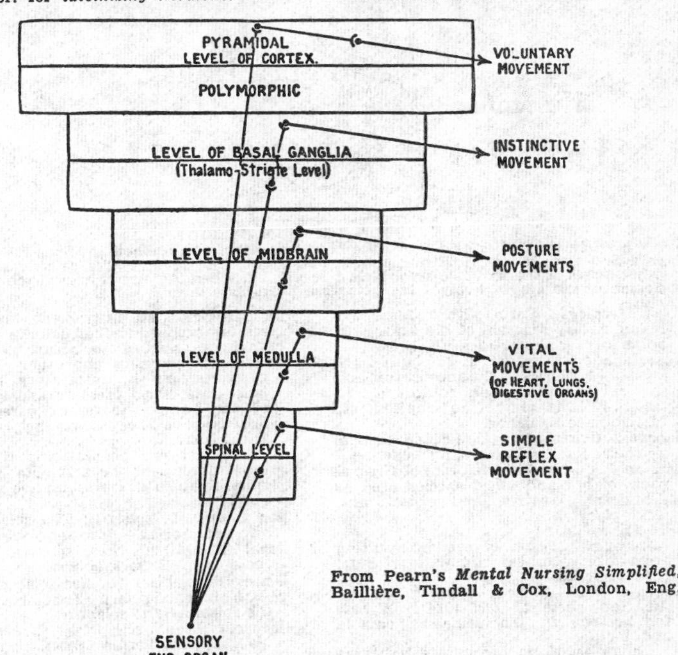

From Pearn's *Mental Nursing Simplified*, Baillière, Tindall & Cox, London, Eng.

LEVEL OF ACTIVITIES

Li. Symbol for *lithium.*

liberomotor (lĭb"ĕr-ō-mō'tōr) [L. *liber*, free, + *motor*, mover]. 1. Pert. to voluntary movement. 2. Free from motor energy.

libidinous (lĭ-bĭd'ĭ-nŭs) [L. *libidinōsus*, pert. to desire]. Characterized by lust or lewdness. SYN: *lascivious, salacious.*

libido (lĭ-bī'dō,-bē-dō) [L. desire]. 1. The sexual drive, conscious or unconscious. 2. In *psychoanalysis*, the energy or force or affect which is the driving force of human behavior. Variously identified as the sex urge, desire to live, desire for pleasure or satisfaction. SEE: *freudian, object choice.*

PROG: Prolonged but favorable.

TREATMENT: Attempt to remove sources of irritation and aggravation in patient's life. Locally, soothing antipruritic ointment.

l. ruber. Form with red, papular lesions and constitutional symptoms. Extremely rare.

SYM: Small, red, glazed, acuminated papules. No tendency to coalesce—associated with itching and failure of general health.

PROG: Chronic course.

l. spinulosus. Form with spine developing in each follicle. SYN: *keratosis pilaris, q.v.*

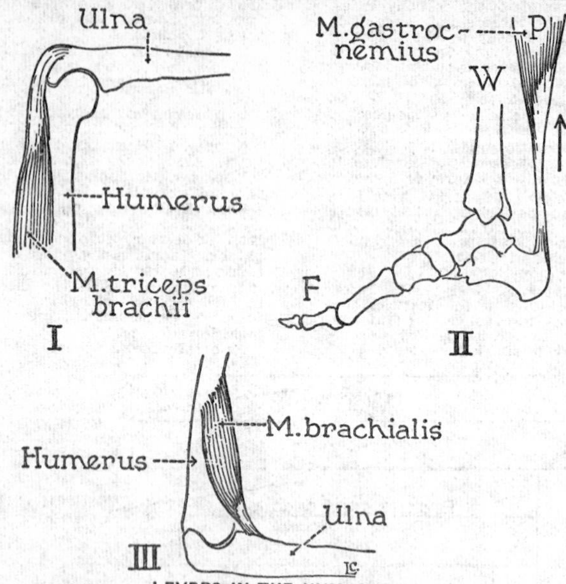

LEVERS IN THE HUMAN BODY

I. When the arm is held above the head, extension of the elbow involves the ulna as a first-class lever. II. Rising on the ball of the foot involves the calcaneus and other bones of the foot as a second-class lever. III. When the arm is held at the side, flexion of the elbow involves the ulna as a third-class lever.

l. tropicus. Form with redness and inflammatory reaction of the skin. SYN: *miliaria rubra, prickly heat.*

lichenification (lī-ken"ĭ-fĭ-kā'shun) [G. *leichēn,* lichen]. 1. Cutaneous thickening and hardening from continued irritation. 2. Changing of an eruption into resemblance to lichen.

lichenoid (li'ken-oid) [G. *leichēn,* lichen, + *eidos,* form]. Resembling lichen.

licorice (lik'ō-ris). A dried root of *Glycyrrhiza glabra* and allied species used as demulcent, laxative, and expectorant. SYN: *glycyrrhiza.*

lid. An eyelid.

l. reflex. Closure of eyelids resulting from direct corneal stimulation. SYN: *corneal reflex.*

Lieben's test (lē'ben) [Adolf Lieben, Austrian chemist, 1836-1914]. A test for acetone in the urine by caustic and iodine.

Yellow iodoform precipitate indicates presence of acetone.

Lieberkuhn crypts (lī'ber-kün) [Johann N. Lieberkuhn, German anatomist, 1711-1756]. SYN: *glands of Lieberkuhn; intestinal glands; Lieberkuhn's follicles.* Simple tubular glands present in the intestinal mucosa. In their epithelium are found *goblet cells, cells of Paneth* and *argentaffine cells.* The glands form minute invaginations opening between the bases of the villi. They lie in the lamina propria, their blind ends extending to the muscularis mucosa. In the large intestine they are longer, contain few if any Paneth cells and more goblet cells. They are arranged vertically with much regularity.

Liebig's extract (lē'big) [Baron Justus von Liebig, German chemist, 1803-1873]. Variety of beef extract.

lie detector. An instrument for determining such minor but definite physical changes assumed to occur under the stress of lying (or any other emotion) as variations in respiratory rhythm, pulse rate, blood pressure and sweating of the hands. Increased perspiration lessens resistance to passage of electrical current.

The test has popular appeal among law-enforcement departments but results obtained are presumptive and not absolute.

lien (li'en) [L. spleen]. The spleen, *q.v.*

l. accessorius. Accessory spleen.

lienal (li'en-ăl) [L. *lien,* spleen]. Rel. to the spleen. SYN: *splenic.*

lienitis (li-en-ī'tis) [L. *lien,* spleen, + G. *-itis,* inflammation]. Inflammation of the spleen. SYN: *splenitis.*

lienocele (li-en'ō-sēl) [" + G. *kēlē,* hernia]. Splenic hernia. SYN: *splenocele.*

lienomalacia (li"en-o-mal-a'sĭ-ă) [" + G. *malakia,* softening]. Softening of the spleen. SYN: *splenomalacia.*

lienomedullary (li"en-ō-med'ū-la-rĭ) [" + *medulla,* marrow]. Rel. to both spleen and bone marrow.

lienomyelogenous (li"en-ō-mī-ĕl-oj'ĕ-nŭs) [" + G. *myelos,* marrow, + *gennan,* to produce]. Derived from both the spleen and bone marrow.

lienomyelomalacia (li"en-ō-mī"el-o-mă-lā'sĭ-ă) [" + " + *malakia,* softening]. Softening of the spleen and bone marrow.

lienopancreatic (li"en-ō-păn-krē-at'ĭk) [" + G. *pagkreas,* pancreas]. Rel. to the spleen and pancreas.

lienopathy (li-en-op'ă-thĭ) [" + G. *pathos,* a disease]. Any disorder of the spleen. SYN: *splenopathy.*

lienorenal (lī″en-ō-rē′nal) [" + *rēnalis,* pert. to a kidney]. Rel. to the spleen and kidney.

lienotoxin (lī″en-ō-toks′ĭn) [" + G. *toxikon,* poison]. Cytotoxin having specific action on splenic cells. SYN: *splenotoxin.*

lienteric (lī-en-ter′ik) [G. *leienteria,* smooth intestine]. 1. Pert. to diarrhea with stools containing undigested food. 2. Affected with lientery.

lientery (lī′en-ter-ĭ) [G. *leienteria,* smooth intestine]. Diarrhea with undigested foods in the stools.

life (līf) [A.S.]. 1. State of being alive; quality manifested by metabolism, growth, reproduction, and adaptation to environment; state in which the organs of an animal or plant are capable of performing all or any of their functions. 2. Time bet. birth and death. 3. The sum total of those properties which distinguish living things (animals or plants) from nonliving inorganic chemical matter or dead organic matter.

RS: *anima, antibiosis, antibiotic, archebiosis, "bio-" words, vital, vitality.*

l., change of. SEE: menopause.

l. expectancy. Expectation of life, the number of years, that a person of a given age may be expected on the average to live as determined by mortality tables.

ligament (lĭg′ă-mĕnt) [L. *ligamentum,* a band]. 1. A band or sheet of strong, fibrous connective tissue connecting the articular ends of bones serving to bind them together and to facilitate or limit motion. 2. A thickened portion or fold of peritoneum or mesentery which supports a visceral organ or connects it to another viscus. 3. A band of fibrous connective tissue connecting bones, cartilages, and other structures and serving for support or for attachment of fascia or muscles. 4. A cordlike structure representing the vestigial remains of a fetal blood vessel.

l., accessory. A l. which supplements another one, esp. one on lateral surface of a joint. One outside of and independent of the capsule of a joint.

l., acromioclavicular. One extending from clavicle to the acromial process of the scapula.

l., alar. SYN: *check l.; odontoid l.* L. connecting odontoid process of atlas to occipital bone.

l., annular. A circular l., esp. (1) l. enclosing head of radius, and (2) l. holding footplate of stapes in fenestra vestibuli.

l., apical. A single median l. extending from odontoid process to occipital bone. Also called apical *odontoid l., suspensory l.*

l., arcuate, lateral and ***medial.*** SYN: *ext. arcuate lig.* L.'s from 12th rib to transverse process of 1st lumbar vertebra to which diaphragm is attached.

l., arcuate popliteal. L. on posterolateral side of knee, extending from head of fibula to joint capsule.

l.'s, auricular. The ant., post., and sup. auricular l.'s uniting external ear to the temporal bone.

l., broad, of the liver. A wide, sickle-shaped fold of peritoneum, attached to lower surface of diaphragm and internal surface of right rectus abdominis muscle, and to the convex surface of liver.

l., broad, of uterus. Folds of peritoneum attached to lateral borders of uterus from insertion of fallopian tube above to the pelvic wall. It consists of 2 leaves between which are found the remnants of the wolffian ducts, cellular tissues, and the major blood vessels of the pelvis.

l.'s, capsular. Heavy fibrous structures, lined with synovial membrane, surrounding articulations.

l.'s, carpal. Those uniting carpal bones.

l., caudal. Bundles of fibrous tissue uniting dorsal surfaces of the 2 lower coccygeal vertebrae and superjacent skin.

l., check. One that restrains motion of a joint, esp. the lateral odontoid l.'s.

l., conoid. Post. portion of coracoclavicular l.

l., coracoacromial. Broad triangular one attached to the outer edge of coracoid process of the scapula, and to tip of acromion.

l., coracoclavicular. One uniting clavicle and the coracoid process of the scapula.

l., coracohumeral. Broad l. connecting coracoid process of scapula to greater tubercle of the humerus.

l., cornicupharyngeal. L. extending from corniculate cartilage of larynx caudally and attaching to mucosa of the pharynx.

l., coronary, of liver. A fold of peritoneum extending from post. edge of liver to diaphragm.

l., costocolic. One attaching splenic flexure of colon to diaphragm.

l., costocoracoid. One joining first rib and coracoid process of the scapula.

l's., costotransverse. One uniting ribs with transverse processes of vertebrae.

l., costotransverse, middle. One consisting of parallel fibers extending bet. a vertebra and its adjacent rib.

l's., costovertebral. Those uniting the ribs and vertebrae.

l., cricopharyngeal. A ligamentous bundle bet. upper and post. border of cricoid cartilage and ant. wall of pharynx.

l's., cricothyroid. Ones uniting cricoid and thyroid cartilages.

l., cricotracheal. The ligamentous structure uniting upper ring of trachea and the cricoid cartilage.

l., cruciate. 1. L. of the ankle passing transversely across dorsum of foot which holds tendons of the anterior muscle group in place. 2. A cross-shaped ligament of the *atlas* consisting of the transverse ligament and sup. and inf. bands, the former passing upwards and attaching to margin of foramen magnum, the latter passing downwards and attaching to the body of the atlas. 3. Two l's. of the *knee* (*ant.* and *post.*), the former passing from tibia to medial aspect of lateral condyle of femur, the latter from tibia to lateral aspect of medial condyle.

l., cruciform. A structure consisting of one l. crossing another.

l., crural. Poupart's l.

l., deltoid. Int. lateral l. of ankle.

l., dentate. Processes of pia mater extending across the subdural space on either side of spinal cord.

l., falciform, of the liver. A wide, sickle-shaped fold of peritoneum, attached to lower surface of diaphragm and internal surface of right rectus abdominis muscle, and to the convex surface of liver.

l., fundiform, of the penis. L. extending from lower portion of the linea alba and Scarpa's fascia to dorsum of penis. Also called *superficial suspensory l.*

l., gastrophrenic. A fold of peritoneum bet. esophageal end of stomach and the diaphragm.

l., Gimbernat's. Triangular flat expansion of aponeurosis of abdominal ext. oblique muscle. Forming medial boundary of femoral ring. Also called *lacunar l.*

l., glenohumeral. Fibers of the coracohumeral l. passing into the joint, and inserted into inner and upper part of bicipital groove.

l., glenoid. One which extends bet. palmar surfaces of phalanges and corresponding metacarpal bone.

l., hepaticoduodenal. A fold of peritoneum from transverse fissure of liver to vicinity of the duodenum and right flexure of colon, forming ant. boundary of foramen of Winslow.

l., ileopectineal. A portion of the pelvic fascia attached to the ileopectineal line and to capsular l. of hip joint.

l., iliofemoral. Bundle of fibers forming the upper and ant. portion of the capsular l. of the hip joint. L. that extends from ilium to intertrochanteric line.

l., iliolumbar. L. extending from 4th and 5th lumbar vertebrae to iliac crest.

l., infundibulopelvic. The upper free edge of the broad l. in which the ovarian artery is found.

l., inguinal. SYN: *Poupart's l.* L. extending from ant. sup. iliac spine to pubic tubercle. Forms lower margin of aponeurosis of ext. oblique muscle.

l., interclavicular. Bundle of fibers bet. sternal ends of the clavicles, attached to interclavicular notch of sternum.

l.'s, interspinal, interspinous. Those extending from sup. margin of a spinous process of one vertebra to lower margin of one above.

l., ischiocapsular. L. extending from ischium to ischial border of acetabulum.

l., lacunar. Gimbernat's l., *q.v.*

l.'s, lateral, of the liver. Folds of peritoneum extending from lower surface of diaphragm to adjacent borders of right and left lobes of the liver. Also called rt. and l. triangular l's.

l., lateral occipitoatlantal. A ligament on each side bet. transverse processes of atlas and jugular process of the occipital bone.

l.'s, lateral odontoid. Strong l.'s extending bet. sides of odontoid process of the axis and inner sides of condyles of the occipital bone.

l., palpebral. Two ligaments, *medial* and *lateral,* extending from tarsal plates of the eyelids to the frontal process of maxilla and the zygomatic bone respectively.

l., Poupart's. Inguinal l., *q.v.*

l., pterygomaxillary. Band of fiber extending bet. apex of internal pterygoid plate of sphenoid bone and the post. extremity of internal oblique line of inferior maxilla.

l., pubic. Those connecting the pubic bones at the symphysis pubis. Include ant. and sup. pubic l's. and the arcuate (inf.) ligament.

l., rhomboid. SYN: *costoclavicular l.,* A strong structure extending from tuberosity of clavicle to outer surface of the cartilage of the first rib.

l., round, of the liver. SYN: *l. teres hepatis.* Fibrous cord extending upward from the umbilicus and enclosed in lower margin of the falciform ligament. Represents obliterated left umbilical vein of the fetus.

l., round, of uterus. SYN: *l. teres uteri.* L. attached to uterus immediately below and in front of the entrance of the fallopian tube. Each extends laterally in the broad ligament to the pelvic wall where it passes through inguinal ring, terminating in the labium majus.

l., sacroiliac. Two ligaments, the ant. and post., which connect sacrum and ilium.

l., sacrospinous. L. extending from spine of ischium to sacrum and coccyx in front of the sacrotuberous ligament.

l., sacrotuberous. L. extending from tuberosity of the ischium to posterior sup. and inf. iliac spines and to lower part of sacrum and coccyx. SYN: *greater sciatic l.; ligamentum sacrotuberale* [NA].

l., sphenomandibular. L. attached superiorly to spine of sphenoid and inferiorly to lingula of mandible.

l., spiral. The thickened periosteum of the peripheral wall of the osseous cochlear canal. The basilar membrane is attached to its inner surface.

l.'s, stomach. The lesser omentum and the phrenicogastric l.

l., stylohyoid. A thin fibroelastic cord bet. lesser cornu of hyoid bone and apex of styloid process of the temporal bone.

l., stylomandibular. A thin fibrous band of tissue extending bet. styloid process of temporal bone and lower part of post. border of ramus of the mandible.

l., stylomaxillary, stylomyloid. A broad fibrous band of tissue extending bet. styloid process of temporal bone and lower part of post. border of ramus of the inferior maxilla.

l., suprascapular. A thin fibrous band of tissue extending from base of coracoid process of scapula to inner margin of suprascapular notch.

l., supraspinal, supraspinous. One uniting apices of spinous processes of vertebrae.

l., suspensory. One suspending an organ.

l., suspensory, of lens. The zonula ciliaris (ciliary zonule); the fibers holding the crystalline lens in position.

l., suspensory, of ovary. SYN: *infundibulopelvic l.* L. extending from tubal end of ovary laterally to pelvic wall. It lies in layers of the broad ligament.

l., suspensory, of the penis. A triangular bundle of fibrous tissue extending from ant. surface of the symphysis pubis and adjacent structures to the dorsum of the root of the penis.

l.'s, suspensory, of the uterus. The broad l.'s, the round ones, and the recto-uterine folds of the uterus.

l.'s, sutural. Thin, fibrous layers interposed bet. articulating surfaces of bones united by suture.

l., transverse, of atlas. A strong l. passing over odontoid process of the axis.

l., transverse crural. L. lying on ant. surface of leg just above the ankle.

l., transverse, of hip joint. A ligamentous band extending across cotyloid notch of the acetabulum.

l., transverse, of knee joint. A fibrous band extending from ant. margin of external semilunar fibrocartilage of knee to extremity of the internal semilunar fibrocartilage.

l., trapezoid. Ant. ext. portion of the coracoclavicular l.

l., triangular, of liver. Two ligaments, right and left, which connect post. aspects of right and left lobes with corresponding portions of the diaphragm.

l., umbilical, lateral. Fibrous cord extending from bladder to umbilicus. Represents obliterated int. iliac artery of fetus.

l., umbilical, median. Fibrous cord extending from apex of bladder to umbilicus. Represents the remains of the urachus of fetus.

l., uterorectosacral. Arises from the sides of the cervix and passes upwards and backwards, passing around the rectum, to the second sacral vertebra. They are enclosed within the recto-uterine folds which demarcate borders of the recto-uterine pouch.

l., ventricular, of larynx. SYN: *vestibular ligament.* The lateral free margin of the quadrangular membrane. It is enclosed within and supports the ventricular fold.

l., vocal, of larynx. The thickened free edges of the elastic cone extending from thyroid angle to vocal processes of arytenoid cartilages. They support the vocal fold, *q.v.*

l., yellow. One of a series of ligaments connecting lamina of adjacent vertebrae. SYN: *ligamenta flavum.*

ligamenta. Plural of ligamentum, *q.v.*

ligamentopexis (lĭg-ă-mĕn"tō-peks'ĭs) [L. *ligamentum,* band, + G. *pēxis,* fixation]. Suspension of uterus on the round ligaments.

ligamentous (lig-ă-men'tŭs) [L. *ligamentum,* band]. 1. Rel. to a ligament. 2. Like a ligament.

ligamentum (lĭg-a-men'tum) (pl. *ligamenta*) [L. a band]. Ligament.

l. arteriosum. A fibrous cord, from pulmonary artery to arch of aorta, the remains of the ductus arteriosus of the fetus.

l. denticulatum. A fibrous band of pia mater extending the length of the spinal cord on each side between the spinal nerves. It has a scalloped appearance as it pierces the arachnoid to attach to the dura mater at regular intervals.

l. flavum. SEE: *ligament, yellow.*

l. nuchae. The upward continuation of the supraspinous ligament, extending from seventh cervical vertebra to occipital bone.

l. palpebrale. Ligamentous band, external and internal, bet. outer margin of the orbit and tissues of eyelids.

l. patellae. A strong, flat band securing the patella to the tibia. It is a continuation of the tendon of the quadriceps femoris muscle.

l. teres femoris. A flat band extending from acetabular fossa to head of femur.

l. teres hepatis. SEE: *l., round, of liver.*

l. teres uteri. SEE: *l., round, of uterus.*

l. venosum. A solid fibrous cord representing obliterated ductus venosus of the fetus. It lies between the caudate and left lobes of the liver and connects the left branch of the portal vein to the interior vena cava.

ligate (lī'gāt) [L. *ligāre,* to bind]. To apply a ligature.

ligation (lī-gā'shun) [L. *ligāre,* to bind]. The application of a ligature. SEE: *cirsodesis.*

ligature (lĭg'a-tūr) [L. *ligatūra,* a binding]. 1. Process of binding or tying. 2. A band or bandage. 3. A ligament. 4. A thread or wire for tying blood vessels.

The cord or material used in tying or binding, as an artery; catgut, kangaroo gut, silk, either the plaited silk or the Chinese twisted silk. In some cases dentists' floss silk as it does not slip easily. SEE: *catgut.*

light (līt) [A. S. *līhtan,* to shine]. The sensation produced by electromagnetic radiation which falls on the retina.

The radiation itself is also called light over the range of wavelengths which produces sensation, and regarding this range it is also called infrared and ultraviolet light. Radiant energy producing a sensation of luminosity on the retina limited to a wavelength of from about 3900 to 7700 angstroms. SEE: *rays.*

l. adaptation. Changes which occur in a dark-adapted eye in order for vision to occur in moderate or bright light. Principle changes are contraction of pupil and bleaching of visual purple in the rods.

l., axial. L. with rays parallel to each other and to optic axis.

l. difference. Abbr. L.D. The difference with respect to sensitiveness to intensity of light between the two eyes.

l., diffused. Rays broken by refraction.

l., Finsen. L. rays given off by a Finsen lamp, consisting principally of violet and ultraviolet rays.

l., polarized. L. in which waves vibrate in one direction only.

l., reflected. Light rays which are thrown back by an illuminated object such as a mirror.

l. reflex. Constriction of the pupil when light is flashed into the eye.

l., refracted. Rays bent from original course.

l. therapy. Phototherapy; the use of light rays in the treatment of disease. Includes use of ultraviolet and infrared radiations. SEE: *heliotherapy, lamp.*

l., transmitted. That which passes through an object.

l. unit. A foot candle. This is the amt. of light measured one foot from a standard candle. The "ideal" amount of light required for work varies with the specific type of work being done. Thus surgery requires a greater intensity of light than would occupations entailing less detailed work. At noon, on a clear day, the sun gives 10,000 candle ft. of light; under a tree we get 1000; on a porch, 500; on a fairly cloudy day, 200. The term *foot candle* took the place of *candle power,* but light intensity is best described by the word *lumen, q.v.*

light, *words pert. to:* aclastic, "actin-" words, anacamptics, catadioptric, circumpolarization, etiolate, Fraunhofer's lines, Grotthus' law, half-value thickness, lambert, lumen, lux, "phot-" words, "radi-" words, ray, reflection, reflector, refraction, spectrum.

light (līt) [A. S. *lēohte,* not heavy]. 1. Not heavy. 2. Pale.

l. diet. All foods allowed in soft diet* plus whole grained cereals, easily digested raw fruits and vegetables. Foods not pureed or ground.

light'ening [A. S. *lēohte,* not heavy]. Uterine descent into pelvis during primary stage of labor.

ligula (lĭg'ū-lă) [L. a strap]. Strip of white substance on the margin of the fourth ventricle.

limb (lĭm) [A.S. *lim*]. 1. An arm or leg. 2. An extremity. 3. A limblike extension of a structure.

RS: *acampsia, acroagnosis, anisomelia, appendicular, artificial, cineplastics, extremity, macrocolia, melagra, melitagra, member.*

l., ant., of internal capsule. The lenticulo-caudate portion which lies between lenticular and caudate nuclei.

l., ascending, of renal tubule. Portion between the bend in Henle's loop, and the distal convoluted portion.

l., descending, of renal tubule. Portion between proximal convoluted portion and the bend in Henle's loop.

l., pelvic. The lower extremity.

l., thoracic. The upper extremity.

limbic (lĭm'bĭk) [L. *limbus,* a border]. Pert. to a limbus or border. SYN: *marginal.*

limbus (lĭm'bŭs) [L. border]. The edge or border of a part.

l. alveolaris. 1. The upper free edge of the alveolar process of the mandible. 2. The lower free edge of the alveolar process of the maxilla. SYN: *arcus alveolaris* [NA].

l., corneoscleral. In the eye, a transitional dome 1 to 2 mm. wide where the cornea joins the sclera and conjunctiva.

l. conjunctivae. The edge of conjunctiva overlapping the cornea.

l. corneae [NA]. The edge of the cornea where it units with the sclera.

l. fossa ovalis. The thickened margin of the fossa ovalis, esp. the rim of the septum secundum bounding the fossa.

l. lamina spiralis. Thickening of the periosteum of the osseus spiral lamina of cochlea to which the tectorial membrane is attached.

l. palpebralis, ant. The ant. margin of the free edge of the eyelid from which the cilia or eyelashes grow.

l. palpebralis, post. The post. margin of the free edge of the eyelid; the region of transition of skin to conjunctival mucous membrane.

l. sphenoidalis. Ridge on ant. portion of upper surface of sphenoid bone.

lime (līm) [A.S. *lim,* glue]. CaO (calcium oxide). A substance obtained from limestone. SEE: *calcium.*

l., chlorinated. Substance resulting from chlorinization of lime, consisting chiefly of calcium chloride and calcium hypochlorite. Used principally as a disinfectant.

l. liniment. Carron oil, *q.v.*

l., slaked. Calcium hydroxide.

l. water. Solution of calcium hydroxide, $Ca(OH)_2$, in water; a weak base and used as an antacid.

lime (fr. *limo*). Fruit of *Citrus aurantifolia.* Its juice is antiscorbutic. JUICE, FRESH: 100 gm. Calories: 26. Other main values: 0.3 gm. protein; trace of fat; 9 gm. carbohydrates; 9 mg. calcium; 32 mg. ascorbic acid.

limen (lī'mĕn) [L. threshold]. Edge, threshold.

limes death. The least amount of toxin which when mixed with one unit of antitoxin and injected into a guinea pig weighing 250 gm. will bring its death within 96 hours. SYMB: L_+.

limes zero. The greatest amount of toxin which when mixed with one unit of antitoxin and injected into a guinea pig weighing 250 gm. will cause no local reaction. SYMB: L_0.

liminal (lĭm'ĭ-năl) [L. *limen, limin-,* threshold]. Hardly perceptible; rel. to a threshold as of consciousness.

limitans (lĭm'ĭ-tăns) [L. *limitāre,* to limit]. 1. Used in conjunction with other words to denote limiting. 2. Used synonymously to indicate membrane limitans.

limo'sis [G. *limos,* hunger]. Abnormal hunger; perverted appetite.

limotherapy (lim-ō-ther'ă-pĭ) [" + *therapeia,* treatment]. Treatment by restriction of diet, or fasting.

lincture (lĭnk'tūr), **linctus** (-tŭs) [L. *linctus,* a licking]. A thick, sweet, syrupy medical preparation given for its effect on the throat. Usually taken in sips or may be licked or sucked as with a throat lozenge. SEE: *electuary.*

line (līn) [L. *linea*]. 1. Any long, relatively narrow mark. 2. A boundary or an outline. 3. A wrinkle.

l., abdominal. Line indicating abdominal muscle boundaries.

l., alveobasilar. One from nasion to alveolar point.

l., alveolonasal. From alveolar point to nasion.

l., auriculobregmatic. From auricular point to bregma.

l., axillary (ant., post. and mid-). Downward from axilla.

l., base. From infraorbital ridge through middle of external auditory meatus to midline of occiput.

l., basiobregmatic. From basion to bregma.

l., Baudelocque's. Ext. conjugate diameter of pelvis.

l.'s, Beau's. Transverse lines on the fingernails.

l., biauricular. From one auditory meatus over vertex to other.

l., blue. One on gums in chronic lead poisoning.

l., costoarticular. From sternoclavicular joint to point on 11th rib.

l., costoclavicular. Line midway bet. nipple and sternum border.

l. of demarcation. Division bet. healthy and diseased tissue.

l. of femur, internal supracondylar. Inner of 2 ridges into which linea aspera of femur divides.

l. of fibula, oblique. Prominent ridge on int. surface of shaft of fibula.

l. of fixation. Imaginary l. drawn from subject viewed to the fovea centralis.

l., gingival. 1. Line of junction of cementum and enamel of a tooth. 2. One on neck of tooth where gum is attached.

l.'s., gluteal. Three lines, *ant., post.,* and *inf.,* on ext. surface of ilium.

l., iliopectineal. Bony ridge marking brim of pelvis.

l. of ilium, intermediate. Ridge upon crest of ilium bet. inner and outer lip.

l. of inferior maxilla, internal oblique. Ridge on int. surface of lower jaw.

l., interauricular. One joining the 2 auricular points.

l., intercondylar, intercondylean. Transverse ridge joining condyles of femur above the intercondyloid fossa.

l., intertrochanteric. Ridge upon post. surface of femur ext. bet. greater and lesser trochanters.

l., intertuberal. One joining inner borders of ischial tuberosities below small sciatic notch.

l., mammary. Horizontal from one nipple to other.

l., mammillary. Vertical line through center of nipple.

l., median. One joining any 2 points in the periphery of the median plane of the body, or one of its parts.

l., milk. The mammary ridge, an ectodermal thickening in embryo ext. between bases of limb buds.

l., nasobasilar. Through basion and nasion.

l., nuchal, sup. and inf. Two curved ridges on occipital bone extending laterally from ext. occipital crest.

l., oblique, of fibula. The medial crest or posteromedial border; a line extending from med. side of head and terminating distally at interosseous crest.

l., oblique, of radius. Faint ridge on ant. surface passing downward and laterally from radial tuberosity.

l., parasternal. Line midway bet. nipple and sternum border.

l., pectineal. L. on post. surface of femur extending downward from lesser trochanter. That portion of iliopectineal l. formed by the os pubis.

l., popliteal. L. of post. surface of tibia, extending obliquely downward from fibular facet on lateral condyle to medial border about middle of bone.

l., scapular. Downward from lower angle of scapula.

l., semilunar. Curved tendinous condensation of aponeurosis of obliquus abdominis externus.

l., sight. From center of pupil to viewed object, imaginary.

l., sternal. Median line of sternum.

l., sternomastoid. From bet. heads of sternomastoid muscle to mastoid process.

l., supracondylar, medial and lateral. Two ridges on post. surface of distal end of femur, formed by diverging lips of the linea aspera.

l., supraorbital. Across forehead above root of ext. angular process of frontal bone.

l., temporal, *sup. and inf.* Two curved l.'s on lateral surface of skull, passing upwards and backwards from zygomatic process of frontal bone and terminating posteriorly at supramastoid crest.

l.'s, test. Those for detecting fracture or shortening of neck of femur.

l., umbilicopubic. That portion of median l. extending from umbilicus to symphysis pubis.

l., visual. One that extends from object to macula lutea passing through the nodal point. SYN: *visual axis.*

linea (lĭn'e-ă) (pl. *lineae*) [L. line]. An anatomical line.

l. alba. The white line of connective tissue in middle of abdomen from sternum to the pubis.

l. aspera. A longitudinal ridge on post. surface of middle third of the femur.

l. costoarticularis. A line bet. the sternoclavicular articulation and point of the 11th rib.

l. ni'gra. Black line or discoloration of the abdomen seen in pregnant women during latter part of term. It runs from above the umbilicus to the pubes.

l. splendens. A thickening of the pia mater extending along ant. median surface of the spinal cord. It ensheaths the ant. spinal artery.

l. sternalis. Median line of the sternum.

l. terminalis. BNA. Bony ridge on inner surface of ilium continued on to pubis which divides true and false pelvis.

l. transversae ossis sacralis. Ridges formed by lines of union of the 5th sacral vertebrae.

lineae albicantes. Lines seen on the abdominal wall. Frequently due to pregnancy but may occur as the result of abdominal distention due to any cause. SEE: *striae.*

linear (lĭn'ē-ar) [L. *linea,* line]. Pert. to, or resembling, a line.

l. measure. Measure of length.

Linear Measure

12 inches (in.)	=1 foot (ft.)
3 feet	=1 yard (yd.)
16.5 feet	=1 rod (rd.)
320 rods	=1 mile (mi.)
1760 yards	=1 mile
5280 feet	=1 mile

lingism (lĭng'ĭzm). Treatment or cure of a condition by use of exercise esp. exercise not involving use of apparatus. SYN: *kinesitherapy.*

Ling's cure, L.'s system (ling) [Peter H. Ling, Swedish poet and gymnast, 1776-1839]. Treatment by movements.

lingua (lĭng'gwă) [L. tongue]. Tongue, or tonguelike structure.

l. fraenata. A tongue with a very short frenum, resulting in tonguetie.

l. nigra. Black tongue, *q.v.*

l. plicata. A fissured tongue.

lingual (lĭn'gwal) [L. *lingua,* tongue]. 1. Pert. to the tongue. 2. Tongue-shaped.

lingula (lĭn'gū-lă) [L. little tongue]. Tongue-shaped process, esp. lingula cerebelli.

l. cerebelli. Tongue of cerebellum prolonged forward on upper surface of sup. medullary velum.

l. of lung. Projection of lung which separates cardia notch from inf. margin of left lung.

l. of mandible. Projection of bone forming medial boundary of mandibular foramen.

l. of sphenoid. Ridge between the body and ala magna of the sphenoid.

l. Wrisbergi. Connecting fibers of motor and sensory roots of the trifacial nerve.

lin'iment [L. *linimentum,* smearing substance]. A liquid containing a medicament and oil, alcohol or water for use externally, applied by friction method or on a bandage.

linimentum (lĭn-ĭm-en'tum) [L. smearing substance]. Liquid preparation for external use and usually applied with rubbing. Four are official.

li'nin [L. *linum,* flax]. An achromatic, threadlike substance which forms the nuclear network of a cell; the nucleoplasm is found in its reticulum, in the form of granules.

linitis (lĭn-ī'tis) [G. *linon,* web, + *-ītis,* inflammation]. Inflamed condition of gastric cellular tissue.

l., plastica. L. with thickening of the wall of the stomach usually due to neoplasmic tissue. Also called leather bottle stomach.

linkage. In genetics, condition in which two or more genes present in the same chromosome tend to remain together and not assort independently in the formation of gametes.

l., sex. Condition in which a character is due to a factor located on the X-chromosomes.

lin'seed [A.S. *linsǣd*]. SYN: *flaxseed.* Seeds of the common flax, *Linum usitatissimum.* It is the source of linseed oil. Linseed is used as a demulcent and emollient, and sometimes as a laxative.

l. poultice. One made from crushed linseed which is heated. Test for heat with hand before applying.

l. tea. A soothing demulcent drink for colds. Add 1 tablespoonful of linseed to 1 pint of water. The juice of a lemon may be added and sugar. Some use ¼ oz. of liquorice and ¼ oz. of candy. It is then simmered in a saucepan for half an hour, strained, and served hot.

lint (lĭnt) [L. *linteum*, made of linen]. 1. Linen scraped until soft and woolly for dressing wounds. 2. Cotton fiber.

lintin (lin'tĭn) [L. *linteum*, made of flax]. Prepared absorbent cotton; fabric used in dressings.

lip [A.S. *lippa*]. 1. Soft structure around the oral cavity, externally. 2. One of the lips of the pudendum (*labium majus* or *minus*). 3. A liplike structure forming border of an opening or groove.

Diagnostic examination incomplete unless lips are everted to expose buccal surfaces. Conditions affecting lip are: *Chancre*: It is not unusual to have the initial lesion of syphilis appear upon the lip as an indurated base, with a thin secretion, accompanied by enlargement of the submaxillary glands. Innocent extragenital syphilitic infection may take place on the lips. *Condyloma latum*: This appears as a mucous patch, flattened, coated with gray exudate, with strictly delimited area, usually at the angle of the mouth. *Eczema*: Dry fissures, often covered with a crust, bleeding easily, and occurring on both lips. *Epithelioma*: May be confused with chancre. Seldom appears before the age of 40, but there are exceptions. It may appear as a common cold sore, a painless fissure or other break of the lower lip. Less than 5% occur on upper lip. A crust or scab covers the lesion, leaving a raw surface if removed. Pain does not appear until well advanced. *Herpes*: Appears on the lips in malaria, pneumonia, typhoid, common cold, other febrile diseases, and idiopathically. *Tuberculous ulcer:* At inner portion of lip close to angle of mouth. Pathological examination necessary for verification.

RS: ***buccal, cheilitis, "chil-" words, labia, labium, labrum.***

l., bluish or purplish. May appear in the aged, in those exposed to great cold, and in carbon monoxide poisoning.

l., cleft. Harelip, *q.v.*

l., dry. May be seen in fevers, or be caused by drugs such as atropine, by thirst, or exhaustion.

l., fissured. May occur after exposure to cold, in avitaminosis, and in children in congenital syphilis. The dribbling of saliva, and a toothless condition may cause fissures in the corners of the mouth.

l., glenoid. Thickened fibrocartilaginous structure surmounting margin of acetabulum.

l., hare. Harelip, *q.v.*

l.'s, oral. Upper and lower lips which surround mouth opening, and form ant. wall of buccal cavity.

l., pale. May be seen in anemia and wasting diseases, in prolonged fever, and after a hemorrhage.

l. rashes. These may be manifestations of typhoid fever, meningitis, or pneumonia. In secondary syphilis, chancre, cancer, and epithelioma, mucous patches may appear.

l. reading. Catching meaning of a speaker by watching movements of his lips without hearing his words.

l. reflex. Reflex movement of li when angle of mouth is suddenly a lightly tapped during sleep.

l., tympanic. Lower border of t sulcus spiralis internus of the cochle

l., vestibule. Upper border of t sulcus spiralis internus of the cochle

lipacidemia (lĭp"ă-sĭ-dē'mĭ-ă) [G. *lipo* fat, + L. *acidus*, acid, + G. *aim* blood]. Fatty acid in the blood.

lipaciduria (lĭp"ă-sĭ-dū'rĭ-ă) [" + " + *ouron*, urine]. Fatty acids in the urin

liparocele (lip'ă-ro-sēl) [" + *kēlē*, he nia]. 1. Scrotal hernia containing fa 2. A fatty tumor.

liparomphalus (lip-ă-rom'fă-lŭs) [" *omphalos*, navel]. Fatty tumor locate at, or involving, the umbilical cord.

liparous (lĭp'ăr-ŭs) [G. *lipos*, fat]. Obes fat.

lipase (lī'pās, lĭ'pās) [G. *lipos*, fat, *ase*, enzyme]. A lipolytic or fat splittin enzyme found in the blood, pancreat secretion and tissues. SEE: *enzyme, di gestive.*

Emulsified fats of cream and egg yol are changed in the stomach to fatt acids and glycerol by gastric lipase.

l., pancreatic. Steapsin, *q.v.*

lipasuria (lĭp-ās-u'rĭ-ă) [" + " + G *ouron*, urine]. Lipase in the urine.

lipectomy (lī-pek'to-mĭ) [" + *ektomē* excision]. Excision of fatty tissues.

lipemia (lī-pē'mĭ-ă) [" + *aima*, blood] Fat in the blood.

l. retinalis. Condition in which retina vessels appear reddish white, or white found in cases of lipemia.

lipfanogens (lĭp-făn'ō-jĕns). Substance producing visible fat or lipoid substances in blood serum, which, when in a free state, are converted by living cell into visible fat.

l., anti-. Substance in blood serum which regulates or reduces or prevents deposition of fat in atherosclerosis. It in part may combine with lipfanogens to form a complex not converted into visible fat.

lipid(e (lip'id) [G. *lipos*, fat]. Any one of a group of fats or fatlike substances characterized by their insolubility in water. Includes (a) *true fats* (esters of fatty acids and glycerol), (b) *lipoids* (phospholipids, cerebrosides, waxes), (c) *sterols* (cholesterol, ergosterol), and (d) *hydrocarbons* (squalene, carotene); also called lipin. SEE: *fat.* SYN: *lipin, lipoid.*

lipidosis. Amaurotic family idiocy (Tay-Sachs disease). Also called *lipoidosis.*

lipin (lĭp'ĭn) [G. *lipos*, *fat*]. SEE: *lipid.*

lipiodol (lĭp-ī'ō-dŏl) [" + " + L. *oleum*, oil]. Proprietary name for an iodized oil obtained by fixation of iodine in poppyseed oil.

It contains 40% of pure iodine by weight. It is opaque to x-rays and used for radiological diagnosis. It is introduced into cavities by a catheter, into the trachea for outlining the bronchial tree by x-ray, and spinally to locate tumors. It is eliminated completely and does not cause iodism.

l. injection. May be cisternal, lumbar, or both, depending upon whether the suspected block is near the cisterna magna or below it. Two cubic centimeters are injected into spinal canal. There are two forms of lipiodol: *ascending* and *descending.* If tumor is near the cisterna, descending lipiodol is given intraspinously; if position is uncertain or halfway bet. cisterna and lumbar region, both forms are given. If there is a block in the canal, the picture shows a dark mass through which the lipiodol has not passed, and a light streak where the lipiodol is present.

lipo-, lip- [G.]. Combining forms pert. to fat.

lipoarthritis (lip-ō-arth-rī'tĭs) [G. *lipos*, fat, + *arthron*, joint, + *-itis*, inflammation]. Inflammation of fatty tissues of joints.

lipoblast (lĭp'ō-blast) [" + *blastos*, germ]. Immature fat cell.

lipoblastoma (lĭp-ō-blast-ō'mă) [" + " + *-ōma*, tumor]. Tumor of fatty tissue. SYN: *adipoma, lipoma.*

lipocardiac (lip"ō-kar'dĭ-ăk) [" + *kardia*, heart]. 1. Pert. to fatty heart degeneration. 2. Sufferer from fatty degeneration of heart.

lipocele (lĭp'ō-sēl) [" + *kēlē*, hernia] Presence of fatty tissue in a hernial sac. SYN: *adipocele, liparocele.*

lipocere (lip'ō-sēr) [" + L. *cera*, wax] Waxy substance resulting from exposure of fleshy tissue to moisture with the exclusion of air. SYN: *adipocere.*

lipochondrodystrophy (lĭp-ō-kŏn-drō-dĭs'-trō-fĭ). Congenital abnormality in the skeletal bones and cartilage, with deranged mucopolysaccharide metabolism, kyphosis and other deformity, possible mental deficiency and cloudy corneae. SYN: *Hurler's syndrome.*

lipochondroma (lĭp"ō-kŏn-drō'mă) [G. *lipos*, fat, + *chondros*, cartilage, + *-ōma*, tumor]. Tumor both fatty and cartilaginous.

lipochrome (lĭp'ō-krōm). Colored substance of fatty nature.

Ex: *Carotene*, the fat-soluble yellow pigment found in carrots, sweet potatoes, egg yolk, butter, body fat and corpus luteum. SEE: *carotene.*

lipoclasis (lĭp-ok'lă-sĭs) [" + *klasis*, breaking]. Splitting up of fat. SYN: *lipolysis, lipodieresis.*

lipoclastic (lĭp-ō-klas'tĭk) [" + *klastikos*, broken]. Fat splitting. SYN: *lipolytic.*

lipocyte (lip'ō-sīt) [" + *kytos*, cell]. Fat cell.

lipodieresis (lip-ō-dī-er'ĕ-sĭs) [" + *dia*, apart, + *airein*, to take]. Splitting or destruction of fat. SYN: *lipoclasis.*

lipodystrophy (lĭp-ō-dĭs'trō-fĭ) [" + *dys*, bad, + *trophē*, nourishment]. Disturbance or defectiveness of fat metabolism.

l., insulin. Atrophy of subcutaneous fat at site of injection of insulin.

l., intestinal. Disease characterized principally by fat deposits in intestinal and mesenteric lymphatic tissue and by fatty diarrhea, loss of weight and strength, and arthritis.

lipoferous (lĭp-ŏf'ĕr-ŭs) [" + *pherein*, to carry]. Causing or carrying fat.

lipofibroma (lip"ō-fī-brō'mă) [G. *lipos*, fat, + L. *fibra*, fiber, + G. *-ōma*, tumor]. Tumor indicating lipoma and fibroma. A fibrolipoma, *q.v.*

lipogenesis (lip-ō-jĕn'ĕ-sĭs) [" + *genesis*, formation]. Fat formation.

lipogenetic (lip-ō-jĕn-ĕt'ĭk) [" + *gennan*, to produce]. Fat producing. SYN: *lipogenic, lipogenous.*

lipogenic (lĭp-ō-jĕn'ik) [" + *gennan*, to produce]. Fat producing. SYN: *lipogenetic, lipogenous.*

lipogenous (lip-ŏj'ĕn-ŭs) [" + *gennan*, to produce]. Producing fat. SYN: *lipogenetic, lipogenic.*

lipogranuloma (lip"ō-gran-ū-lo'mă) [" + L. *granulum*, granule, + G. *-ōma*, tumor]. Inflammation of fatty tissue with granulation and development of oily cysts.

lipoid (lĭp'oid) [" + *eidos*, form]. 1. Substance resembling fats in appearance and solubility, but containing other groups than the glycerol and fatty acids which make up the true fats.

Ex: cholesterol, kephalin and lecithin, *q.v.* SYN: *lipid.*

2. Similar to fat.

lipoidemia (lĭp-oi-dē'mĭ-ă) [" + " + *aima*, blood]. Lipoids in the blood.

lipoidosis (lĭp-oi-dō'sĭs) [G. *lipos*, fat, + *eidos*, form, + *-osis*]. Condition in which lipids accumulate in excessive quantities in body tissues. SEE: *Xanthomatosis.*

l., arterial. Arterosclerosis, *q.v.*

l., cerebral infantile. SEE: *amaurotic familial idiocy, infantile.*

l., cerebroside. SYN: *Gaucher's disease.* A familial disease characterized by deposition of kerasin, a cerebroside, in cells of the reticuloendothelial system.

l., primary. L. of unknown etiology in which (a) serum lipids are abnormal in quantity or in quality, or (b) serum lipids are normal but lipids accumulate intracellularly.

lipoiduria (lĭp-oi-dū'rĭ-ă) [G. *lipos*, fat, + *eidos*, like, + *ouron*, urine]. Lipoids in the urine.

lipolipoidosis (lĭp"ō-lĭp-oi-dō'sĭs) [" + *lipos*, fat, + *eidos*, form, + *-ōsis*]. Infiltration of fats and lipoids into a tissue.

lipolysis (lip-ol'ĭs-ĭs) [" + *lysis*, dissolution]. The decomposition of fat.

lipolytic (lĭp-ō-lĭ'tĭk) [" + *lysis*, dissolution]. Having ability to hydrolyze fats.

l. digestion. The conversion of neutral fats by hydrolysis into fatty acids and glycerol; fat splitting.

l. enzyme. Fat splitting ferment. SYN: *lipase.* SEE: *enzymes.*

lipoma (lĭ-po'mă) [" + *-ōma*, tumor]. A fatty tumor. SEE: *chondrolipoma.*

They are frequently multiple, but not metastatic.

l. arborescens. An abnormal treelike accumulation of fatty tissue in a joint.

l., cystic. One containing cysts.

l., diffuse. One not definitely circumscribed.

l. diffusum renis. Condition in which fat displaces parenchyma of the kidney.

l. durum. One in which there is marked hypertrophy of the fibrous stroma and capsule.

l., hernial. A lipocele.

l., nasal. A fibrous growth of the subcutaneous tissue of the nostrils.

l., osseous. One in which the connective tissue has undergone calcareous degeneration.

l. telangiectodes. A rare form containing a large number of blood vessels.

lipomatosis (lĭp-ō-mă-to'sis) [G. *lipos*, fat, + *-ōma*, tumor, + *-ōsis*, intensive]. Excessive deposit of fat in the tissues. SYN: *liposis, obesity.*

l. renis. Fatty infiltration of renal parenchyma. SYN: *lipoma diffusum renis.*

lipomatous (lĭp-ō'mă-tŭs) [" + *-ōma*, tumor]. 1. Of the nature of lipoma. 2. Affected with lipoma.

lipometabolic (lĭp"ō-met-ă-bol'ĭk) [" + *metabolē*, change]. Rel. to metabolism of fat.

lipometabolism (lĭp-ō-mĕ-tab'ol-ĭzm) [" + " + *ismos*, state of]. Fat metabolism.

lipomyoma. A myoma containing fatty tissue.

lipomyxoma (lĭp″ō-miks-ō′mă) [" + *myxa*, mucus, + *-ōma*, tumor]. Tumor containing both lipoma and myxoma.

lipopectic (lĭp-ō-pek′tĭk) [" + *pēxis*, fixation]. Characterized by lipopexia.

lipopexia (lĭp-ō-pek′sĭ-ă) [" + *pēxis*, fixation]. Accumulation of fat in the body. Syn: *adipopexia*.

lipophage (lip′o-fāj) [" + *phagein*, to eat]. Cell absorbing fat.

lipophagic (lĭp-ō-fā′jik) [" + *phagein*, to eat]. Consuming, destroying, or absorbing fat. Syn: *lipolytic*.

lipophil (ĭp′ō-fĭl) [G. *lipos*, fat, + *philein*, to love]. 1. Having an affinity for fat. 2. Absorbing fat.

lipophrenia (lĭp-ō-frē′nĭ-ă) [" + *phrēn*, mind]. Mental failure or collapse.

lipoprotein. A conjugated protein consisting of a simple protein combined with a lipid.

liposarcoma (lĭp-ō-sar-kō′mă) [" + *sarx*, flesh, + *-ōma*, tumor]. Sarcoma with fatty elements.

lipo′sis [" + *-ōsis*, intensive]. Accumulation of fat in a part.

lipostomy. Congenital absence or extreme smallness of the mouth.

lipothymia (lĭ-po-thĭ′mĭ-ă) [G. *leipein*, to leave, + *thymos*, mind]. Faintness; syncope.*

lipotropic (lĭp-ō-trŏp′ĭk) [G. *lipos*, fat, + *trope*, a turning]. Having an affinity for lipids, said of certain dyes such as Sudan III which stains fat readily.

lipoxeny (lĭp-oks′ĕ-nĭ) [G. *leipein*, to leave, + *xenos*, host]. Desertion of host by parasitic organism after completion of its development.

lipsis (lip′sis) [G. *leipsis*, failing]. Cessation. Fainting. *L. animi.*

lipuria (lĭ-pu′rĭ-ă) [G. *lipos*, fat, + *ouron*, urine]. Fat in the urine.

liquefacient (lik-we-fa′shent) [L. *liquere*, to flow, + *facere*, to make]. 1. Agent which produces a conversion into liquid. 2. Converting into liquid.

liquefaction (lĭk-we-fak′shun) [L. *liquere*, to flow, + *facere*, to make]. 1. The conversion of a solid into a liquid. 2. Conversion of solid tissues to a fluid or semifluid state.

liquescent (lik-wes′sent) [L. *liquescere*, to become liquid]. Becoming liquid. Syn: *deliquescent*.

liqueur (lĭ-ker′) [Fr.]. Alcoholic spirit. Aromatically flavored, often colored, and sweetened. A cordial.

liquid (lĭk′wĭd) [L. *liquidus*, flowing]. 1. Flowing easily. 2. Substance which flows without being melted. See: *emulsion, liquefacient, liquefaction.*

l. air therapy. Therapeutic application of low temperatures. See: *refrigeration.*

l. measure. Measure of liquid capacity.

Liquid Measure

4 gills (gi.)	=1 pint (pt.)
2 pints	=1 quart (qt.)
4 quarts	=1 gallon (gal.)
63 gallons	=1 hogshead
2 hogsheads	=1 pipe
2 pipes	=1 tun

li′quid di′et. Coffee with hot milk, tea, water, milk in all forms, milk and cream mixtures, cocoa, cream soups strained, fruit juices, meat juices, beef tea, clear broths, gruels, meat soups strained, eggnogs. See: *fluid diet.*

l. d., full. Restricted liquid diet plus gruels, strained fruit juice, tomato juice, strained cream soups, milk and cream beverages, plain gelatin, custard, plain ice cream, junket, coffee, tea.

l. d., high caloric. Full liquid diet reinforced with lactose, glucose, dextrimaltose, ice cream, ices, coffee, tea, etc.

l. d., or fluid, without milk. Cereal water, strained fruit and strained vegetable juices, plain gelatin, water ices, ginger ale, clear fat-free broth, beef juice, coffee, tea, etc.

l. d., restricted. Fat-free broth, tea (no cream), ginger ale, bland fruit juice such as pear, white cherry, or peach juice.

l. d., surgical. Strained fruit juices, ginger ale, fat-free broth, strained cream soup, milk and cream beverages, tea, coffee, gelatin beverage if ordered.

liquor (lik′er) [L. a liquid]. 1. Any liquid or fluid. 2. An alcoholic beverage. 3. Pharm: Solution of medicinal substance in water.

l. amnii. The amniotic fluid, a clear, watery fluid which surrounds the fetus in the amniotic sac.

l. folliculi. The fluid contained in the graafian follicle.

l. puris. Liquid portion of pus.

l. sanguinis. Blood serum or plasma.

l. solutions. Aqueous solutions of nonvolatile substances presenting the greatest variety in strength, character, and method of preparation. They are usually very active medicinal preparations.

lisencephalous. Condition in which the brain is smooth owing to failure of development of cerebral gyri.

lisping (lĭsp′ing) [A.S. *wlisp*, stammering or lisping]. Substitution of sounds due to defect in speech, as of *th* sound for *s* and *z*.

lissotrichy (lĭs-sot′rĭ-kĭ) [G. *lissos*, smooth, + *thrix, trich-*, hair]. Condition of having straight hair.

listeriosis (lĭs-tĕr-ē-ō′sĭs). A disease affecting many domestic animals, wild animals, and man. Caused by *Listeria monocytogenes*, a soil saprophyte which becomes pathogenic for animals or man under favorable circumstances. The most common manifestation in the adult is meningitis. It may be transmitted transplacentally to the fetus in which case it may cause abortion. In newborns the disease, known as *granulomatosis infantiseptica*, is much more serious than in the adult. Although man has a high degree of resistance to the bacteria, hygienic precautions should be taken when handling infected animals. Also spelled *listerosis*.

liter (lē′tĕr) [Fr. *litre*, from G. *litra*, a pound]. Metric fluid measure; 1000 milliliters (ml.), 270 fl. drams, 61 cu. in., 33.8 fl. oz., 1.0567 qt. The volume occupied by one kilogram of water at 4° C. and 760 mm. pressure. See: *metric system.*

Note: It is common to define a liter as 1000 cc. This is almost but not quite correct because 1 ml. is equal to 1.000028 cubic centimeters.

lithagogue (lĭth′ă-gŏg) [G. *lithos*, stone, + *agōgos*, leading]. 1. Agent which expels calculi. 2. Expelling calculi.

lithectasy (lith-ek′ta-sĭ) [" + *ektasis*, dilatation]. Removal of a stone from bladder through the dilated urethra.

lithemia (lĭth-e′mĭ-ă) [" + *aima*, blood]. Excess of lithic or uric acid in the blood due to imperfect metabolism of the nitrogenous substances. Syn: *uricemia.* See: *oxypathy.*

lithiasis (lĭth-ī'ă-sĭs) [G. *lithos,* stone]. 1. Formation of calculi and concretions. 2. Uric acid diathesis.

l. biliaris. Gallstones.

l. nephritica. Stone formation in the kidneys. Syn: *nephrolithiasis.*

l. renalis. Kidney stones.

lithicosis. Stone-cutters silicosis; pneumoconiosis.

lithium (lĭth'ē-ŭm) [G. *lithos,* stone]. A metallic element. Symb: Li. At. wt. 6.939; at. no. 3.

litho-, lith- [G.]. Prefixes: Pert. to *stone* or *calculus.*

lithocenosis (lĭth-ō-sĕn-ō'sĭs) [G. *lithos,* stone, + *kenōsis,* evacuation]. Removal of crushed fragments of calculi. Syn: *litholapaxy, lithotrity.*

lithoclast (lĭth'o-klăst) [" + *klan,* to crush]. Forceps for breaking up large calculi. Syn: *lithotrite.*

lithoclasty (lĭth'ō-klăs-tĭ) [" + *klan,* to crush]. The crushing of a stone into fragments that it may pass through natural channels.

lithoclysma (lĭth-ō-klĭs'mă) [" + *klysma,* a clyster]. Injection into urinary bladder substances which have the ability to dissolve calculi.

lithocystotomy (lĭth"ō-sĭs-tot'o-mĭ) [G *lithos,* stone, + *kystis,* bladder, + *tomē,* incision]. Incision of bladder to remove calculus.

lithodialysis (lĭth"ō-dī-al'ĭ-sĭs) [" + *dialysis,* a breaking up]. Fragmentation or solution of calculi. Syn: *litholysis.*

lithogenesis (lĭth-ō-jen'ĕ-sĭs) [" + *genesis,* formation]. Formation of concretions.

lithokonion (lĭth-ō-kō'nĭ-on) [" + *konian,* to pulverize]. Instrument for pulverizing vesical calculi.

litholapaxy (lĭth-ol'a-păks-ĭ) [" + *lapaxis,* removal]. The operation of crushing a stone in the bladder followed by immediate washing out of the crushed fragments through a catheter.

lithology (lĭth-ol'ō-jĭ) [" + *logos,* science]. The science dealing with calculi.

litholysis (lĭth-ol'ĭ-sĭs) [" + *lysis,* dissolution]. Dissolving of calculi. Syn: *lithodialysis.*

lithometer (lĭth-om'ĕ-tĕr) [" + *metron,* measure]. Instrument for estimating size of calculi.

lithometra (lĭth-ō-me'tră) [" + *mētra,* uterus]. Uterine tissue ossification.

lithomyl (lĭth'ō-mĭl) [G. *lithos,* stone, + *mylē,* mill]. Instrument for crushing a vesical stone. Syn: *lithokonion.*

lithonephrotomy (lĭth"o-nĕ-frot'ō-mĭ) [" + *nephros,* kidney, + *tomē,* excision]. Incision of kidney for removal of renal calculus.

lithontriptic (lĭth-ŏn-trip'tĭk) [" + *tribein,* to crush]. An agent that tends to dissolve calculi.

Ex: *Lithium citrate, potassium citrate,* and *ammonium benzoate.*

lithopedion (lĭth"ō-pe'dĭ-ŏn) [" +*paidion,* child]. A fetus which has died and become calcified.

lithophone (lĭth'o-fōn) [" + *phōnē,* sound]. Instrument for determining by sound the presence of calculi in the bladder.

lithoscope (lĭth'o-skōp) [" + *skopein,* to examine]. Instrument for examining stone in bladder.

lithotome (lĭth'o-tōm) [" + *tomē,* incision]. Instrument for performing lithotomy.

lithotomy (lĭth-ot'o-mĭ) [" + *tomē,* incision]. Incision into bladder for removing a stone.

NP: See that retention catheter is kept draining at all times. Record intake and output of urine. Keep dressings clean and dry.

l., bilateral. Incision across perineum.

l., high. Suprapubic incision.

l., lateral. Front of rectum to one side of raphe.

l., median. In median line in front of anus.

l. position. Upon the back with thighs flexed upon abdomen and legs upon thighs, which are abducted. Syn: *dorsosacral.*

l., rectal. Through the rectum.

l., vaginal. Through vaginal wall.

lithotony (lĭth-ot'ō-nĭ) [" + *tonos,* a stretching]. Removal of a calculus through small incision instrumentally dilated.

lithotresis (lĭth-ō-trē'sĭs) [G. *lithos,* stone, + *trēsis,* boring]. Drilling or boring of holes in a calculus to facilitate crushing.

lithotripsy (lĭth'ō-trĭp-sĭ) [" + *tripsis,* a rubbing]. Crushing of a calculus in bladder or urethra.

lithotriptic (lĭth-o-trip'tĭk) [" + *tripsis,* a rubbing]. 1. An agent that dissolves calculi. 2. Pert. to lithotripsy. Syn: *lithontriptic.*

lithotrite (lĭth'o-trīt) [" + L. *tritus,* a rubbing]. Instrument for crushing stone in the bladder. See: *lithotrity.*

lithotrity (lĭth-ot'rĭ-tĭ) [" + L. *tritus,* a rubbing]. Crushing of a stone to small fragments in the bladder. See: *litholapaxy.*

lithous (lĭth'ŭs) [G. *lithos,* stone]. Rel. to a calculus or stone. Syn: *calculous.*

lithoxiduria (lĭth"oks-ĭ-dū'rĭ-ă) [" + *oxide* + G. *ouron,* urine]. Presence of xanthic oxide in the urine.

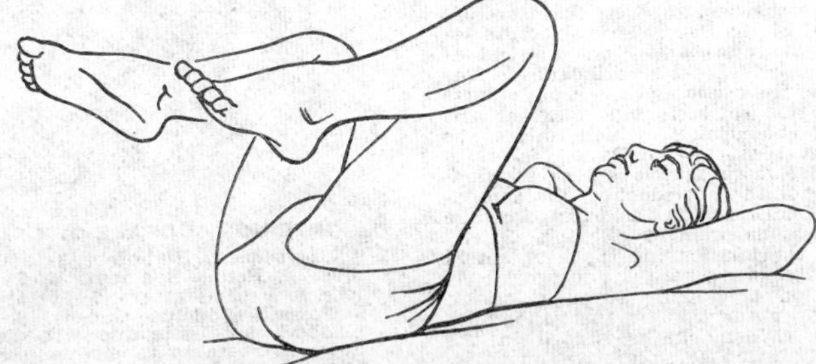

LITHOTOMY OR DORSOSACRAL POSITION.

lithuresis (lith-u-re′sis) [" + *ourēsis,* urination]. Passage of calculus through the urethra during urination.

lithureteria (lĭth″ū-re-tē′rĭ-ă) [" + *ourētēr,* ureter]. Disease of the ureter due to presence of calculi.

lithuria (lĭth-u′rĭ-ă) [" + *ouron,* urine]. Excess of uric acid or of urates in the urine.

litmus (lĭt′mus) [O.N. *litr,* lichen dye, + *mosi,* moss]. A blue dyestuff made by treating coarsely powdered lichens, such as those of the family *Rocella* species, with ammonia.

l. paper. Chemically prepared blue paper which is turned red by acids, and remains blue in alkali solutions; pH range is 4.5 to 8.5. SEE: *indicator.*

litter (lĭt′ter) [Fr. *litiere,* from *lit,* a bed]. A stretcher for carrying the wounded or the sick.

Little's disease (lĭt′tls). Congenital spastic paralysis on both sides (diplegia), although it may be *paraplegic* or *hemiplegic* in form. Cerebral spastic paralysis.

ETIOL: Possible birth injury.

SYM: Child dribbles, is feebleminded, possibly an idiot. Stiff, awkward movements, legs crossed and pressed together, arm adducted, forearm flexed, hand pronated, scissors gait.

livedo (lĭv-ē′dō) [L. a dark spot]. Patchy or general bluish discoloration of the skin. SYN: *lividity.*

l. reticularis. Semipermanent bluish mottling of the skin of the legs and hands. Worse on exposure to cold.

liver (liv′er) [A.S. *lifer*]. Largest gland in the body, approximately 20 to 22.5 cm. in its greatest transverse diameter, 15 to 17.5 cm. in its greatest vertical height, and 10 to 12.5 cm. in its anteroposterior depth, 1200 to 1600 gm., situated on right side beneath the diaphragm; right hypochondriac, epigastric, and part of left hypochondriac regions, level with bottom of sternum, undersurface, concave, covers stomach, duodenum, hepatic flexure of colon, right kidney and suprarenal capsule, secretes bile and aids metabolism.

The liver, the largest organ of the body, is completely covered by a tough fibrous sheath, Glisson's capsule, which is thickest at the transverse fissure. At this point, the capsule carries the blood vessels and hepatic duct which enter the organ at the hilus. Strands of connective tissue originating from the capsule enter the liver parenchyma and form the supporting network of the organ and separate the functional units of the liver, the hepatic lobules.

The many intrahepatic bile passages converge and anastomose, finally leading into the hepatic duct, the excretory channel of the liver. This structure receives the cystic duct on the end of which is situated the gallbladder. The union of the cystic and the hepatic ducts forms the common bile duct or the ductus choledochus, which enters the duodenum at the papilla of Vater. A ring of smooth muscle at the terminal portion of the choledochus, the sphincter of Oddi, permits the passage of bile into the duodenum by relaxing. Briefly stated, the bile leaving the liver enters the gallbladder where it undergoes concentration principally through loss of fluids by absorption by the gallbladder mucosa. When bile is needed in the small intestine for digestive purposes, the gallbladder contracts and the sphincter relaxes, thus permitting escape of the viscid gallbladder bile. Ordinarily, the sphincter of Oddi is contracted, shutting off the duodenal entrance and forcing the bile to enter the gallbladder after leaving the liver.

Within the sinusoids of the liver and attached to their walls are found the cells of Kupffer, which are highly phagocytic. They remove cellular detritus, bacteria, and other foreign particulate substances from the blood stream.

Has four lobes, five ligaments, five fissures, five sets of vessels, and in the fasting state secretes 500 to 700 ml. of bile in 24 hours. The amount of bile secreted is greatly increased during digestion.

BLOOD SUPPLY: From the hepatic artery, a branch of the celiac art. and the hepatic portal vein, which drains the intestine.

FUNCTIONS: The liver receives blood from the portal vein and thus is the first organ to receive blood from the intestines where the blood has absorbed the final products of digestion and decomposition products. From this blood the liver removes glucose from which it synthesizes glycogen which it stores. Glucose not stored as glycogen or used to form amino acids is converted to fatty acids, carbon dioxide, and water. It deaminizes amino acids with the resultant formation of ammonia which is converted into urea. Hippuric acid and uric acid are synthesized in the liver. The liver incorporates amino acids into proteins. The liver probably makes such proteins as albumin, prothrombin component, fibrinogen, transferrin, and glycoprotein. The liver acts to chemically detoxify such substances as indole and skatole which may be absorbed into the blood from the intestine.

The liver excretes bile pigments, *bilirubin* and *biliverdin,* formed in the cells of the reticuloendothelial system in various parts of the body from hemoglobin derived from effete ("exhausted" and no longer functioning) red corpuscles. The liver synthesizes *fibrinogen* and *prothrombin,* blood constituents essential for clotting. It is the source of *heparin,* an anticoagulant. It is the source of red blood cells in the fetus and is the main site for the *production of plasma proteins.* Reticuloendothelial cells (Kupffer cells), present in the linings of the sinusoids, act to

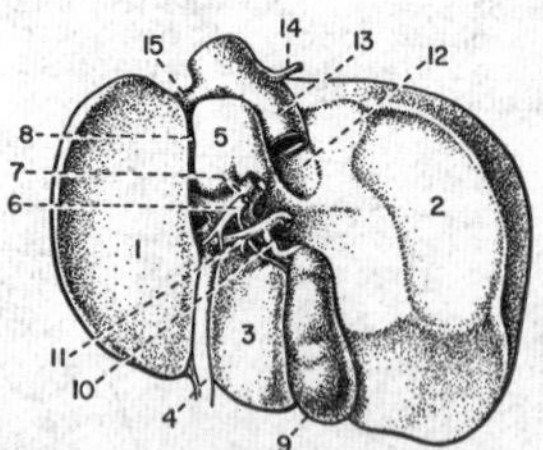

INFERIOR SURFACE OF LIVER

1. Left lobe. 2. Right lobe. 3. Quadrate lobe. 4. Round ligament. 5. Caudate lobe. 6. Hepatic artery. 7. Portal vein. 8. Fossa for ductus venosus. 9. Gallbladder. 10. Cystic duct. 11. Hepatic duct. 12. Fossa for vena cava. 13. Vena cava. 14. Right inferior phrenic vein. 15. Hepatic vein.

filter out and destroy bacteria present in the blood stream.

The liver also performs these additional functions. It is a storage place for the fat-soluble vitamins A, D, E, K, and B_{12}, the anti-pernicious anemia factor. It plays a role in the regulation of blood volume and is one of the main sources of body heat. The liver is important in lipid metabolism. Cholesterol, which is found in most body cells and is a major constituent of bile, is manufactured mainly in the liver.

NERVE SUPPLY: Parasympathetic fibers from the vagi and sympathetic fibers from celiac plexus via hepatic artery.

DISEASES OF:

l., abscess of. Temperature up in evening, low in morning; sweats and chills; liver enlarged, painful, tender, may be bulging and fluctuation. Pus may be detected by aspirating needle.

ETIOL: Pathogenic bacteria, esp. pyogenic organisms such as *Streptococcus, Staphylococcus,* and *Pneumococcus;* traumatism; infection by *Entamoeba histolytica.*

PROG: Embolic (multiple) abscesses generally fatal. Traumatic abscesses, or those due to an amebic dysentery may terminate favorably after spontaneous or induced evacuation.

l., acute yellow atrophy of. A rare and grave disease, characterized anatomically by a rapid destruction of the liver tissues, and manifested by jaundice and hemorrhages, a reduction in size of liver and marked cerebral phenomena. SYM: (1) Malaise, slight fever, coated tongue, nausea, vomiting and jaundice. (2) Nervous symptoms follow, as severe headache, tremor, delirium, convulsions and coma; these sometimes precede the jaundice. (3) Urine is scanty, contains albumin, blood, and casts. (4) Hemorrhages are common, the skin may be covered with ecchymoses and bleeding from the mucous membranes may occur. (5) Hepatic dullness diminished; splenic, increased. PROG: Generally fatal. TREATMENT: Constitutional and palliative.

l., amyloid. An enlargement of liver, due to the deposition of an albuminoid substance. SYM: Failure of general health with anemia. Liver is enlarged, smooth, firm and painless. Spleen and kidneys share in the degeneration so the spleen enlarged and urine albuminous. PROG: Unfavorable. TREATMENT: Remedies must be directed to the causal disease, usually prolonged suppuration, syphilis, tuberculosis or chronic malaria.

l., cancer of. Male sex, heredity and traumatism predisposing factors, Malignancy in the liver as a result of spread from a primary source is many times more frequent than primary tumor of the liver. The liver is the most usual site of metastatic spread of tumors which disseminate through the blood stream. SYM: (1) Severe pain and tenderness; (2) cachexia, *i.e.,* loss of flesh and strength with pallor; (3) pressure symptoms, jaundice common; (4) liver enlarged, surface is nodular and the central depression or umbilications can often be detected; (5) symptoms of the primary growth. Fever generally absent, but secondary perihepatitis or suppuration of cancerous nodules may produce it. PROG: Fatal; duration from few months to year. TREATMENT: Palliative, constitutional in first stage.

l., cirrhosis of, atrophic. A chronic disease characterized anatomically by a hyperplasia of the connective tissue and destruction of the secreting cells shown chiefly by symptoms of portal obstruction. In advanced stage, liver small, firm, gray color and covered with numerous nodular granulations ("hobnails"). SYM: Abdominal swelling due to ascites, jaundice, weakness, weight loss, anorexia, nausea, fetor hepaticus, and mild continuous fever. As obstruction becomes greater, portal blood finds new channels, and the superficial abdominal veins enlarge, notably about the umbilicus, forming the so-called "caput medusae"; hemorrhoids and esophageal varices result from the same cause. In the final stages hepatic encephalopathy develops. This is due in part to substances absorbed from the intestines which have not been metabolized by the liver reaching the brain and producing cerebral intoxication. Clinically the patient is mentally dulled, may have hallucinations and a peculiar type of flapping tremor. PROG: Unfavorable except in first stages.

l., c. of, hypertrophic. In which the connective tissue hyperplasia starts from the periphery of the capillary bile ducts instead of from ramifications of portal vein as in atrophic form. SYM: Jaundice marked, liver large, yellow and surface smooth or finely granular, spleen swollen. Disease may last 1 or 2 years, but abrupt termination may occur at any time in convulsions and coma. TREATMENT: Constitutional.

l., cysts of. May be (a) simple cysts, usually small and single, (b) hydatid cysts (SEE: *hydatid; Echinococcus granulosus*), or (c) cysts associated with cystic disease of the liver, a rare condition usually associated with congenital cystic kidneys.

l., hobnail. That of atrophic cirrhosis, *q.v.*

l., inflammation of (hepatitis). The usual cause of hepatitis is the same as that caused by infectious hepatitis (IH) or serum hepatitis (SH) viruses. The clinical picture may be so mild as to be almost unnoticed or may be so severe that the jaundice is followed rapidly by hepatic encephalopathy and death.

TREATMENT: All patients should be treated as if they were going to progress to the severe form: bed rest, diet as requested by patient but should be high caloric, cortisone should not be given routinely. There is no specific treatment and in general the disease is self-limiting.

liver, words pert. to: anhepatia; anhepatic; anhepatogenic; anticholagogue; arginase; azorubin S; bile; -acids; -calculi; -colic; -pigments; "bili-" words; capsule, Glisson's; cardiohepatic; chloasma; choleresis; cirrhosis; facies hepatica; flexure; "glyco-" words; "hepa-" words; jaundice; perihepatitis.

liver (as food). BEEF (fried): 100 gm. Calories: 229. Other main values: 26 gm. protein 10.6 gm. fat; 11 mg. calcium; about 50,000 I.U. vitamin A but may vary from 100 to 100,000; 27 gm. ascorbic acid.

The liver stores more vitamin A and D than other parts of the animal. Cooked beef liver contains about 9 mg. of iron in each 100 gm. portion.

ACTION: Liver supplies some protective substance necessary for the stroma of red cells but not for the formation of hemoglobin. It does not affect gastric secretion.

IND: In anemias (½ lb. or more per day) and diseases of the bone marrow, neurasthenia, and phthisical persons. Recommended for adolescents and convalescents. Easily digested. One hundred and forty degrees Fahrenheit coagulates the albumin and destroys its useful ferments.

liver extract. SYN: *extractum hepatis.* A dry, brown powder obtained from mammalian livers which contains the hematinic factor (antianemic factor) which stimulates erythropoiesis. Was important in treatment of pernicious anemia until vitamin B_{12} was discovered.

liver "flap." A characteristic flapping type of tremor seen in patients with severe impairment of liver function.

liver fluke, human. *Clonorchis sinensis,* common in Far East. Adults infest biliary and pancreatic ducts. Eggs pass out with feces and continue development in snails of the subfamily Buliminae (Family Hydrobiidae). Cercaria emerge and infest numerous species of freshwater fishes in which they encyst. Infestation results from eating raw fish containing encysted metacercaria.

liver spots. Yellowish-brown spots on skin following some digestive disturbances. SYN: *Chloasma hepaticum.*

livid (lĭv'ĭd) [L. *lividus,* dark in color] 1. Ashen, cyanotic. 2. Discolored.

lividity (lĭv-ĭd'ĭ-tĭ) [L. *lividus,* dark in color]. 1. Skin discoloration, as from a bruise or venous congestion. 2. State of being livid.

Livierato's reflex (lĭv-yār-ā'tō) [Panagino Livierato, Italian physician, 1860-1936]. Reduction of area of cardiac dullness resulting from manual friction of precordial and epigastric areas.

livor (lī'vor) [L. a dark spot]. Lividity, *q.v.*

l. mortis. Cutaneous dark spot on dependent portion of a cadaver.

lixiviation (lĭks"ĭv-ĭ-ā'shŭn) [L. *lixivia* lye]. Separation of soluble from insoluble substances by washing and filtration.

LLQ. Abbr. for *left lower quadrant* (of abdomen).

Loa loa (lō'ă lō'ă). The African eyeworm, a species of filarial worm which infests the subcutaneous tissues and conjunctiva of man. Its migration causes itching and a creeping sensation. Sometimes causes itchy edematous swellings known as "Calabar swellings." It is transmitted by flies of the genus *Chrysops.*

lobar (lō'bar) [G. *lobos,* lobe]. Pert. to a lobe.

l. pneumonia. Inflammation of 1 or more lobes of the lungs. SEE: *pneumonia, lobar.*

lobate (lō'bāt) [L. *lobatus,* lobed]. 1. Pert. to a lobe. 2. Having a deeply undulated border. 3. Producing lobes.

lobe (lōb) [G. *lobos*]. A globular part of an organ separated by boundaries.

l., anterior, of hypophysis. Ant. portion of the hypophysis or pituitary gland, consisting of the pars distalis, and pars tuberalis.

l., caudate. A lobe on post. surface of liver.

l., central. Island of Reil, which forms floor of lateral cerebral fossa.

l.'s of the cerebrum. Frontal, parietal, occipital, and temporal lobes and the insula or island of Reil (central lobe).

l. of the ear. Lower portion of auricle having no cartilage.

l., flocculonodular. A lobe of the cerebellum consisting of the flocculi, nodulus, and their connecting peduncles.

l., frontal. That part of a cerebral hemisphere in front of central and sylvian fissures.

l., insular. SEE: *central l.*

l.'s, lateral, of the prostate. The portions on each side of the urethra.

l.'s, lateral, of thyroid gland. The two main portions, one on each side of trachea, united below by thyroid isthmus.

l., limbic. Marginal section of cerebral hemisphere on medial aspect. SYN: *gyrus fornicatus.*

l. of the lungs. Large divisions of the lungs: *sup.* and *inf. lobes* of the left lung; *sup., mid.,* and *inf. lobes* of the right lung.

l. of the mamma. The 15-20 divisions of the glandular tissue of the breast separated by connective tissue and each possessing a duct (lobar duct) opening on the nipple.

l., occipital. Caudal region of either hemicerebrum.

l., olfactory. A series of convolutions below horizontal portion of the intraparietal fissure of cerebrum, containing olfactory bulb. The rhinencephalon, *q.v.*

l.'s, orbital. The convolutions above the orbit.

l.'s of the pancreas. Roundish aggregations of glandular tissue separated by connective tissue.

l., parietal. Upper and lateral portion of hemisphere of cerebrum.

l. of the parotid, accessory. A small lobe, variable in size, on ant. surface of parotid gland superior to exit of parotid duct.

l., posterior, of hypophysis. The posterior portion of the pituitary gland, consisting of the *pars intermedia* and the *processus infundibuli* (*pars nervosa*).

l.'s of the prostate. The lateral l.'s and the middle l. of the gland.

l., pyramidal, of thyroid. A portion of the thyroid gland extending upward from the isthmus. It is extremely variable in size.

l., quadrate, of liver. An oblong elevation on lower surface of liver.

l., spigelian. SYN: *caudate lobe.* Irregular quadrangular portion of liver behind fissure for portal vein and bet. fissures for vena cava and ductus venosus.

l., temporal. The portion of cerebral hemisphere lying below lateral fissure of Sylvius. It is continuous posteriorly with the occipital lobe.

lobectomy (lō-bĕk'tō-mĭ) [G. *lobos,* lobe, + *ektomē,* excision]. Surgical removal of a lobe of any organ or gland.

lobotomy (lŏb-ŏt'ō-mĭ). A bilateral small trephination in the plane of the coronal suture through which the white matter of the brain is sectioned, disconnecting the diencephalon, esp. the hypothalmic area from the prefrontal cortex by section of the white fiber connecting pathways subcortically in a plane that passes adjacent to ant. tip of lateral ventricle and post. margin of sphenoid wing for relief of mental disturbances.

lob'ular [G. *lobulus,* small lobe]. Composed of small lobes.

lobulate, lobulated (lŏb′ū-lāt, -lāt-ed) [L. *lobulus,* small lobe]. 1. Consisting of lobes or lobules. 2. Pert. to lobes or lobules. 3. Resembling lobes. SYN: *lobular.*

lobule (lŏb′ūl) [L. *lobulus,* small lobe]. A small lobe.

l., central, of the cerebellum. A small lobe at ant. part of sup. vermiform process.

l. of the epididymis. Conelike divisions of the head of the epididymis formed by the much coiled distal ends of the efferent ducts of the testis.

l. of kidney. Subdivision of a renal cortex consisting of a medullary ray and surrounding glandular tissue.

l. of the liver. Structural unit consisting of hepatic cells arranged in irregular, branching and interconnected groups and anastomosing blood channels (sinusoids) surrounding a central vein. Polyhedral in shape with branches of portal vein, hepatic artery, and interlobular bile ducts at its periphery.

l. of the lung. Physiological unit of the lung consisting of a respiratory bronchiole and its branches (alveolar ducts, alveolar sacs, and alveoli).

l., paracentral. Sup. convolution of ascending frontal and parietal convolutions forming a union of both.

l., parietal. One of two subdivisions of the parietal lobe. The *sup. parietal lobule* comprises posterior part of the upper portion; the *inf. parietal lobule* comprises a lateral area continuous with temporal and occipital lobes.

l. of the testis. One of the pyramidal divisions separated from each other by incomplete partitions called septulae. Each consists of one to three much coiled seminiferous tubules.

l. of the thymus. Subdivisions of a lobe each consisting of a cortex and medulla.

lobuli. Plural of lobulus.

lobulus (lŏb′ū-lŭs) (pl. *lobuli*) [L.]. A lobule.

l. centralis vermis superior. A small lobe at ant. part of sup. vermiform process.

l. epididymidis. Segments into which the epididymis is divided by transverse septa from its tunica albuginea.

l., parietalis. One of 2 portions of the parietal lobe.

l. testiculi. Approximately 250 pyramidal compartments which make up glandular structure of the testicle.

lobus (lōb′ŭs) [L., from G. *lobos*]. Lobe.

l. cerebelli anteriores. The lobes forming ant. and sup. portion of hemisphere of the cerebellum.

l. pulmonales. Lobes of the lung.

l. reniculi. Lobes in fetal kidney, later forming malpighian pyramids.

local (lō′kăl) [L. *locus,* place]. Limited to one place or part.

localization (lō-kăl-ĭ-zā′shun) [L. *locus,* place]. 1. Limitation to a definite area. 2. Determination of the seat of an infection. 3. Relation of a sensation to its point of origin.

l., cerebral. Determination of centers of various faculties and functions in particular parts of the brain.

localized (lō′kăl-īzd). Restricted to a limited region.

localizer. Apparatus used for locating solid opaque bodies in the eye by roentgenographic examination.

lochia (lō′kĭ-ă) [G. *lochia,* pert. to childbirth]. The discharge from the uterus of blood, mucus and tissue, during the puerperal period.

SYM: The first 6 days it is distinctly blood-tinged and is known as *lochia rubra* or *cruenta;* the following 3 or 4 days the discharge becomes brownish and is known as *lochia serosa;* after this it becomes yellowish, turning to white and is known as *lochia alba.*

It is diminished or suppressed in high fever. If offensive it is result of contamination with saprophytic organisms. Position should favor drainage.

lochial (lo′kĭ-al). Pert. to the lochia.

lochiocolpos (lō″kĭ-ō-kŏl′pŏs) [G. *lochia,* pert. to childbirth, + *kolpos,* vagina]. Retention of lochia in the vagina.

lochiometra (lō″kĭ-ō-mē′tră) [" + *mētra,* uterus]. Retention of lochia in the uterus.

lochiometritis (lō″kĭ-ō-mē-trī′tis) [" + " + *-ītis,* inflammation]. Puerperal inflammation of the uterus.

lochiopyra (lō-kĭ-op′ĭr-ă) [" + *pyr,* fever]. Puerperal fever.

lochiorrhagia (lo-kĭ-or-ra′jĭ-ă) [" + *rēgnunai,* to break forth]. Excessive flow of lochia.

lochiorrhea (lō″kĭ-or-rē′ă) [" + *roia,* flow]. Abnormal flow of lochia.

lochioschesis (lō-kĭ-os′kē-sĭs) [" + *schesis,* retention]. Retention or suppression of the lochia.

lochometritis (lō″kō-mē-trī′tĭs) [G. *lochos,* childbirth, + *mētra,* uterus, + *-ītis,* inflammation]. Puerperal inflammation of uterus.

lock′jaw. Tonic spasm of muscles of jaw. SEE: *tetanus; trismus.*

locomotion (lō-kō-mō′shun) [L. *locus,* place, + *motus,* moving]. Movement or power of movement from one place to another.

locomotor (lō-kō-mō′tor) [" + *motor,* mover]. Pert. to locomotion.

l. ataxia. A sclerosis affecting the post. columns of the spinal cord. SYN: *tabes dorsalis.* SEE: *ataxia; Charcot's arthropathy.*

locular (lŏk′ū-lăr) [L. *loculus,* a small place]. Divided into small cavities.

loculated (lŏk′ū-lāt-ĕd) [L. *loculus,* a small place]. Containing or divided into loculi. SYN: *locular.*

loc′ulus (pl. *loculi*) [L.]. 1. A cell. 2. A small cavity.

lo′cum ten′ens [L. *locus,* place, + *tenere,* to hold]. A substitute. Physician who substitutes for another temporarily.

lo′cus [L. a place]. 1. A spot or place. 2. In genetics the position of a gene on a chromosome.

l. caeruleus, l. cinereus, l. ferrugineus. A dark-colored depression in floor of 4th ventricle at its upper part.

l. niger. Gray matter separating the crusta and tegmentum of the crura cerebri. SYN: *substantia nigra.*

Loeffler's bacillus (lĕf′lĕr). SYN: *Klebs-Loeffler bacillus.* The bacillus of diphtheria, *Corynebacterium diphtheriae.*

logadectomy. Excision of a portion of the conjunctiva.

logaditis (lō-gă-dī′tĭs) [G. *logades,* conjunctivae, + *-ītis,* inflammation]. Inflammation of the sclerotic coat of the eye. SYN: *scleritis.*

logagnosia (lōg-ăg-nō′sĭ-ă) [G. *logos,* word, + *a-,* priv. + *gnōsis,* knowledge]. Word blindness. SEE: *aphasia.*

logagraphia (lōg-ă-grăf′ĭ-ă) [" + " + *graphein,* to write]. Loss of ability to express ideas in writing. SYN: *agraphia.*

logamnesia (lōg-ăm-nē′zĭ-ă) [" + *amnēsia,* forgetfulness]. Aphasia of a sensory character. Inability to recognize spoken or written words.

logaphasia. Motor aphasia, *q.v.*

logoklony (log'o-klo-nĭ) [" + *klonein*, to agitate]. Intermittent repetition of the last syllable of a word.

logokophosis. Inability to understand spoken language; word deafness.

logomania (lŏg-ō-mā'nĭ-ă) [" + *mania*, madness]. Repetitious, continuous and excessive flow of speech seen in monomania.

logoneurosis (lŏg"ō-nū-rō'sĭs) [G. *logos*, word, + *neuron*, nerve, + *-ōsis*]. Any neurosis marked by speech disorders.

logopathia (lŏg-ō-păth'ĭ-ă) [" + *pathos*, disorder]. Any disorder of speech.

logopedia (lŏg-ō-pē'dĭ-ă) [" + *pais, paid-*, child]. Science dealing with speech defects, and their correction.

logoplegia (lŏg-ō-plē'jĭ-ă) [" + *plēgē*, stroke]. Paralysis of the speech organs.

logorrhea (lŏg-or-ē'ă) [" + *roia*, flow]. Unusual loquacity seen in insanity. Syn: *garrulousness; logomania.*

logospasm (lŏg'ō-spazm) [" + *spasmos*, spasm]. Spasmodic word enunciation.

-logy [G.]. Suffix meaning *discourse, science* or *study of.*

loiasis (lō-ī-ăs'ĭs). Infestation with *Loa loa, q.v.*

loimic (loi'mĭk) [G. *loimos*, plague]. Pert. to pestilence or plague.

loimology (loi-mŏl'ō-jĭ) [" + *logos*, science]. Science concerned with contagious diseases, esp. plague.

loin (loyn) [O.Fr. *loigne*, long part]. Lower part of back and sides bet. the ribs and pelvis.

lol'ism. Poisoning by the seeds of *Lolium temulentum* (darnel ryegrass).

long- [L.]. Prefix meaning *long.*

long flame arc lamp. According to distance bet. electrodes, carbon arc lamps are either short or long flame.

longevity (lŏn-jĕv'ĭ-tĭ) [L. *longaevus*, aged]. 1. Length of life. 2. Unusual length of life. Age was reckoned by the Romans in six stages: *pueritia*, childhood, to 5 years; *adolescentia*, youth, to 18 years; *juventus*, young man, to 25 years; *majores*, man, 25 to 50 years; *senectus*, old man, 50 to 60 years; *crepita aetas*, decrepit, 60 years to death.

longing. An eager desire or craving for something, usually that which is remote or unattainable.

longitudinal. Parallel to the long axis of the body or part.

longsightedness (lawng-sī'tĕd-nĕs) [L. *longus*, long, + A.S. *gesiht*, sight]. Farsightedness. Syn: *hyperopia, q.v.*

Lophotrichea (lō-fō-trĭk'ē-ă) [G. *lophos*, tuft, + *thrix, trich-*, hair]. Microorganisms possessing flagella in tufts.

lophotrichous (lō-fŏt'rĭk-ŭs) [" + *thrix, trich-*, hair]. Having bunches of flagella at one end.

lordoma (lōr-dō'mă) [G. *lordōma*, a bending]. Forward incurvation of the spine. Syn: *lordosis.*

lordoscoliosis (lōr"dō-skō-lĭ-ō'sis) [G. *lordoun*, to bend, + *skoliōsis*, curvation]. Lordosis and scoliosis combined.

lordosis (lor-dō'sĭs) [G. *lordoun*, to bend]. Abnormal ant. convexity of the spine.

lotion (lō'shun) [L. *lotiō*]. Liquid medicinal preparation for local application to or bathing of a part.

loupe (lūp) [Fr.]. A magnifying lens.

louse (lows) [A.S. lūs]. A small wingless insect which lives as an ectoparasite on birds and mammals. Sucking lice belong to the order *Anoplura;* biting or chewing lice belong to the order *Mallophaga.*

Human lice are the primary transmitters of epidemic typhus, trench fever, and relapsing fever. They may also be the mechanical transmitters of other diseases such as plague.

l., body. *Pediculus humanus corporis.* Lives principally in or on clothing.

l., crab. *Phthirus pubis.* Lives principally in hair in pubic region, but also found in beard, eyebrows, and eyelashes.

l., head. *Pediculus humanus capitus.* Lives in hair of the head.

lous'iness [A.S. lus]. Syn: *pediculosis, q.v.* State of being infested with lice.

Loven's reflex (lōv'en). Vasodilation with corresponding increase in size of organ resulting from stimulation of afferent nerve of organ.

low protein diet. Breakfast, 413 calories; lunch, 695; supper, 704. Total daily, 1812. No salt except what is used in cooking, which will equal 3 or 4 gm. per day.

Breakfast: Fruit, cereal with cream and sugar or milk (2 oz.), toast, butter, jelly or jam, cocoa or milk (1 cup), and 1 egg.

Lunch: Cream soup or 1 cup milk, 1 potato, 1 serving of vegetable, large serving salad with mayonnaise, 1 thin slice bread, liberal amt. butter, custard, gelatin, cake, ice cream or blanc mange, 1 serving. One egg may be substituted for cream soup or milk.

Supper: One serving cereal or 1 large serving of potatoes, 3 oz. of cream or milk, sugar and butter as desired, large serving salad, fruit and vegetable, 1 cup cocoa, 1 egg or 1 glass milk.

Foods to be avoided: meat, fish, chicken, meat gravies, soups or broth. Peas and dried beans only 2 or 3 times per week.

Low'man bal'ance board. Tilted board for walking with feet inverted to restore proper muscle balance and to correct static faults.

LOX. Abbreviation for *liquid oxygen.*

loxarthron (lŏks-ar'thron) [G. *loxos*, slanting, + *arthron*, joint]. Oblique deformity of a joint without dislocation.

loxia (loks'ĭ-ă) [G. *loxia*, slanting]. Wry neck. Syn: *torticollis.*

loxotic (lŏks-ot'ĭk) [G. *loxos*, slanting]. Distorted in an awry manner.

loxotomy (lŏks-ot'ō-mĭ) [" + *tomē*, a cutting]. Amputation by oblique section.

lozenge (loz'ĕnj) [Fr. diamond-shaped]. Small, dry, medicinal solid to be held in mouth until it dissolves. Syn: *troche.*

LSD. Abbr. for *lysergic acid diethylamide*, a derivative of an alkaloid in ergot. It is made from a fungus growing on wet grass and grain. LSD is used legally only for experimental purposes. Its illegal use has increased to where it is now a social and legal problem. The use of LSD by persons prior to or during pregnancy has been implicated as a cause of birth defects.

LTH. Abbr. for *luteotrophic hormone.*

lubb (lŭb) [imitative origin]. Word denoting 1st cardiac sound in auscultation. Caused by closure of the atrioventricular valves, the impact of blood rushing into the aorta and pulmonary artery and the contraction of the ventricular muscle. It is pitched low and slightly longer than the 2nd sound. See: *dupp; heart, auscultation of.*

lubb-dupp (lub-dup) [imitative origin]. The two sounds heard in auscultation marking a complete cycle of the heart.

Pause following the cycle is slightly longer than that bet. the two sounds.

lubricant (lūb′rĭ-kănt) [L. *lubricans,* making smooth]. Agent which makes smooth.

lub′ricating en′ema. One given to soften feces and lubricate anal canal after hemorrhoidectomy, or to soften fecal impaction. SEE: *enema.*

Lucas-Championniere disease (lū-ka″-shawn-pē-ōn-yair″). Pseudomembranous bronchitis.

L.-C. method. Early massage and mobilization in treating fractures.

lucid (lū′sĭd) [L. *lucidus,* clear]. Clear, esp. applied to clarity of the mind.

l. interval. Period of normal mentality bet. psychiatric attacks.

lucidity (lū-sĭd′ĭ-tĭ) [L. *lucidus,* clear]. Quality of clearness or brightness, especially with regard to mental conditions. SEE: *lucid.*

lucotherapy (lū-kō-ther′ă-pĭ) [L. *lux, luc-,* light, + G. *therapeia,* treatment]. Therapeutic use of light rays. SYN: *phototherapy.*

Ludwig's angi′na (lūd′wĭg). A suppurative inflammation of subcutaneous connective tissue adjacent to a submaxillary gland. SEE: *angina.*

Luer-Lok syringe. A glass syringe made to permit rapid and firm attachment of the needle.

lues (lū′ēz) [L. pestilence]. Any pestilential disease; the plague, esp. syphilis.

l. venerea. Syphilis.

luetic (lū-et′ĭk) [L. *lues,* pestilence]. 1. Pert. to syphilis. 2. Affected with syphilis. SYN: *syphilitic.*

luetin (lū′et-ĭn) [L. *lues,* pestilence]. A killed culture of Treponema pallidum for the Noguchi skin test for syphilis.

Lugol's caustic (lū′gol) [Jean G. A. Lugol, Paris physician, 1786-1851]. Aqueous solution of 25% each of iodine and potassium iodide.

L.'s solution. Iodine, 5%; potassium iodide, 10%, and water to make 100 cc. Strong iodine solution used in iodine therapy.

INCOMPATIBILITIES: Codeine.

lumbago (lŭm-bā′gō) [L. *lumbus,* loin]. A general nonspecific term for dull, aching pain across the loins.

lumbar (lŭm′băr) [L. *lumbus,* loin]. Pert. to the loins. SEE: *lumbago.*

l. nerves. Five pairs, corresponding with the lumbar vertebrae.

l. puncture. One made by placing an aspiration needle into the subarachnoid space of the spinal cord. Usually done in the lumbar area at the level of the 4th intervertebral space. SYN: *spinal puncture; subarachnoid puncture.*

PURPOSE: For the removal of spinal fluid for diagnostic or other purposes, and for the injection of an anesthetic solution.

NOTE: May be dangerous if done in the presence of increased intracranial pressure. The brain stem may, upon decrease of pressure in the spinal canal, herniate into the foramen magnum of the base of the skull.

Medication (dissolved in fluid previously removed) or anesthetics for cord blocking, etc., may be cautiously introduced.

The part is cleansed and painted with iodine. A sterile puncture needle is then readily passed directly in the midline, to and through the dura. On removing the stylet, spinal fluid will escape and can be collected in 2 or 3 tubes for examination. Explain the procedure and try to reassure patient.

NP: Patient should be turned on side near edge of bed with back to operator. Thighs flexed on trunk and head lowered to chest, back bowed as far as possible. Nurse holds patient in this position. Alternatively the patient may be in a sitting position with head, neck, and thoracic spine flexed. The legs are allowed to dangle over the side of the bed or table. The nurse stands in front of the patient to support him. Articles needed: Sterilized lumbar puncture needles, gloves for physician, alcohol, sterilized gauze and sponge, sterile towel, procaine hydrochloride 0.5% solution, 5 cc. Two sterile test tubes, collodion, cotton. After procedure is completed, patient should remain completely flat, either prone or supine, for 24 hours. SEE: *cerebrospinal fluid; cisternal puncture; spinal puncture; Queckenstedt test.*

The use of a small-gauge needle will lessen the chance that spinal fluid will continue to seep from the spinal canal after the needle is removed, and thus the possibility of development of postspinal tap headache will be diminished.

l. reflex. Irritation of the skin over the erector spinal muscles causing contraction of muscles of the back.

l. region. Each side of umbilical region above the iliac, below the hypochondriac.

l. vertebrae. Five bones of spinal column between sacrum and thoracic vertebrae.

lumbarization (lŭm-băr-ĭ-zā′shŭn) [L. *lumbus,* loin]. Coalescence of the 1st sacral vertebra with the last lumbar vertebra.

lumbo- [L.]. Combining form pert. to the *loins.*

lumbocolostomy (lŭm″bō-kō-los′tō-mĭ) [L. *lumbus,* loin, + G. *kōlon,* colon, + *stoma,* opening]. Colostomy by lumbar incision.

lumbocolotomy (lŭm-bō-kō-lot′ō-mĭ) [" + " + *tomē,* incision]. Incision into the colon through lumbar region.

lumbocostal (lŭm-bō-kos′tăl) [" + *costa,* rib]. Rel. to the loins and ribs.

lumbodynia (lŭm-bō-dĭn′ĭ-ă) [" + G. *odynē,* pain]. Pain and rigidity in the loins. SYN: *lumbago.*

lumbosacral. Pert. to the lumbar vertebrae and the sacrum.

l. plexus. Nerve plexus formed by union of lumbar, sacral, and coccygeal nerves.

lumbrical (lŭm′brĭ-kăl) [L. *lumbricus,* earthworm]. Like a worm. SYN: *vermiform.*

lumbrica′lis [L. *lumbricus,* earthworm]. One of the muscles of the hand or foot which are wormlike in shape.

lumen (lū′mĕn) (pl. *lumina*) [L. light]. 1. The space within an artery, vein, intestine or tube. 2. Unit of light, the amt. of light emitted in a unit solid angle by a uniform point source of 1 international candle.

luminal (lū′mĭ-năl) [L. *lumen, lumin-,* light]. 1. Rel. to lumen of tubular structure, such as a blood vessel. 2. A brand of phenobarbital.*

l. sodium. A brand of soluble phenobarbital.

lunacy (lū′nă-sĭ) [L. *luna,* moon. Insanity was formerly thought to be affected by the moon]. Obsolete term for insanity.

lu′nar [L. *luna,* moon]. Pert. to the moon, a month, or silver.

l. caustic. Silver nitrate.

lu'nate. A bone in the proximal row of the carpus. SYN: *semilunar bone.*

lunatic (lū'nă-tĭk) [L. *luna,* moon]. Obsolete term for an insane person.

lunet, lunette (lū-nĕt') [Fr. *lunette,* from L. *luna,* moon]. A concavo-convex lens for spectacles.

lung (lung) [A.S. *lungen*]. ANAT: One of two cone-shaped, spongy organs of respiration contained within the pleural cavity of the thorax.

Connected with the pharynx through the trachea and larynx. The base rests on diaphragm and apex rises from 2.5 to 5 cm. above the sternal end of the first rib, the collarbone, supported by its attachment to the hilum or root structures.

Right lung has 3 lobes, left one 2. Approximate weight in the adult male: right lung 625 gm., left 570 gm. The lungs contain 300,000,000 alveoli and the respiratory surface is between 70 and 80 square meters. Averages 18 respirations per minute in adult. The total capacity of the lung varies from 3.6 to 9.4 liters in the male and 2.5 to 6.9 in normal females.

The left lung has an indentation for the normal place of the heart, which is called the *cardiac depression.* Behind this is the *hilum* through which the blood vessels, lymphatics and bronchi enter and leave the lung.

Air travels from the mouth and nasal passage to the pharynx and the trachea. Two main bronchi, one on each side, extend from the trachea. The main bronchi divide into smaller bronchi, one for each of five lobes. These further divide into a great number of smaller bronchioles. The pattern distribution of these into the segments of each lobe is important in lung surgery. There are 10 bronchopulmonary segments in the right lung and 8 in the left but the number is variable. There are 50 to 80 terminal bronchioles in each lobe. Each of these divide into two respiratory bronchioles which in turn divide to form 2 to 11 alveolar ducts. The alveolar sacs and alveoli arise from these ducts. The spaces between the alveolar sacs and alveoli are called *atria.*

The alveolus is the point at which the blood and inspired air are separated

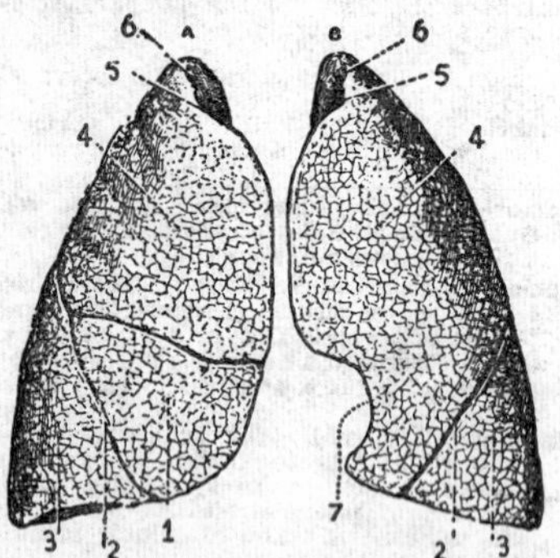

ANTERIOR ASPECT OF LUNGS

A. Right lung. B. Left lung. 1. Middle lobe. 2. Oblique fissure. 3. Lower lobe. 4. Upper lobe. 5. Groove for innominate vein. 6. Groove for subclavian artery. 7. Cardiac notch.

only by a very thin wall or membrane which allows O_2 and nitrogen to diffuse into the blood and CO_2 and other gases to pass from the blood into the alveoli. This wall is so thin (0.07 to 2.0 microns) that it is best seen by using an electron microscope. The alveoli contain small pores, 7 to 10 microns in diameter, which serve to connect adjacent alveoli to each other. Their exact function is unknown.

NERVE SUPPLY: Parasympathetic fibers via vagus nerve and sympathetic fibers from ant. and post. pulmonary plexuses.

BLOOD VESSELS: Bronchial, pulmonary arteries, and pulmonary veins. Blood passing through lungs gives off carbon dioxide and receives oxygen. The lungs include the lobes, lobules, bronchi, bronchioles, infundibula, and alveoli or air cells.

l. abscess. Circumscribed, suppuration of lung. SYM: High and irregular fever, rigors, sweats and pallor. Dyspnea, cough and purulent expectoration. May be bubbling râles and later cavernous breathing and pectoriloquy.

PROG: Fair, except in embolic abscesses.

TREATMENT: Nutritious food. Remedies called for by general condition. Abscess should be opened and drained.

l. cancer. That which may appear in trachea, air sacs and other lung tubes. It may appear as an ulcer in the windpipe, as a nodule or small flattened lump, or on the surface blocking air tubes. It may invade surface of tubes extending to lymphatics into blood vessels.

l., collapse of. Atelectasis. Condition resulting from a lowering of intrapulmonic pressure or an increase in intrathoracic pressure. It may be *focal,* involving only a few lobules, or *massive,* in which an entire lobe or the complete lung is involved. It may result from obstruction of the bronchial tubes (*obstructive atelectasis*) or pressure upon the lung by air or fluid in the pleural cavity, an intrathoracic tumor, or a greatly enlarged heart (*compressive atelectasis*). Air may be introduced artificially into the pleural cavity (artificial pneumothorax) or it may be derived from emphysematous lesions. Collapse may occur in the newborn as a result of blockage of bronchioles by mucus or from failure of the lung to distend because of weak inspiratory movements.

SYM: In a sudden collapse, there are pronounced dyspnea and circulatory collapse. When collapse occurs gradually, symptoms are less pronounced or may not occur at all.

PROG: Depends upon extent of collapse and gravity of preëxisting disease.

TREATMENT: In the newborn, aspirate the excess mucus from the bronchus and gently inflate lung with a catheter. In acquired varieties, direct remedies to the original disease. SEE: *auscultation of lungs, chest; emphysema; tuberculosis.*

l. c., hypostatic. Congestion of dependent portions of the lungs occurring in asthenic diseases which necessitate a protracted recumbent position.

SYM: Dyspnea, cough, scanty expectoration. Slight dullness, subcrepitant râles, and feeble bronchial breathing.

TREATMENT: Development should be prevented by frequent change in position and timely use of cardiac stimulants.

l. c., passive. Results from obstruction to the flow of blood from the lungs to the heart.

SYM: Dyspnea, hard cough, mucous expectoration containing pigmented cells and râles. Slight dullness, feeble breathing.

l., edema of. Effusion of serous fluid into air vesicles and into interstitial tissue of lungs SYN: *pulmonary edema.*

SYM: Extreme dyspnea; rapid, labored breathing; cough with frothy, blood-stained expectoration; cyanosis; cold extremities.

PROG: Grave. Often a final symptom of some pulmonary disease.

TREATMENT: Directed toward altering the condition which caused the difficulty. Usually this includes vigorous treatment of the heart condition, oxygen, and morphine; in extreme cases phlebotomy may be required. But prior to this, tourniquets are applied to the limbs in an attempt to have the excess tissue fluid collect in the extremities rather than the lungs. NOTE: Tourniquets should be applied to only one limb at a time for 15 minutes and with pressure sufficient to block venous return but not enough to interfere with arterial blood flow to the limb.

l. fluke. *Paragonimus westermanii.*

lung-heart disease. Cor pulmonale. A serious respiratory and heart condition caused by pollution of air by soot, gasoline vapor, sulfur dioxide, or unburned droplets of such air. It can cause fatal heart failure. It interferes with flow of blood, especially through the right side of the heart which fails. There are more cases than coronary artery disease and hypertension combined.

l., hemorrhage from. Hemoptysis.*

l. inflammation. Pneumonia.*

l., iron. Device for inducing respiration artificially.

Patient is placed in airtight compartment except for his head and neck, and then atmospheric pressure inside is raised and lowered by a pulmotor. SEE: *Drinker respirator.*

l. motor. An apparatus designed for forcing air or a mixture of air and oxygen into the lungs.

lung, *words pert. to:* aeropleura, air, air vesicle, aluminosis, alveobronchitis, alveolar, alveolus, alveolus pulmoneus, anthracosis, anthrax, anthropotoxin, apicitis, artificial pneumothorax, asbestosis, atelectasis, atmiatrics, atmocausis, atrium, auscultation of, "bronch-" words, byssinosis, byssophthisis, calcicosis, cardiopulmonary, chest, emphysema, hilum, pectoriloquy. "pleur-" words, "pneum-" words, pulmonary, râles, siderosis, silicosis, tuberculosis, vesicular resonance, vomica.

lunula (lu'nu-lă) [L. little moon]. The semilunar white arch or area near the root of the nail.

l. of valves of heart. SYN: *l. valvulae semilunaris.* One of two narrow portions on the free edges of the semilunar valves on each side of the nodulus.

lupiform (lū'pĭ-form) [L. *lupus,* wolf, + *forma,* shape]. Resembling lupus.

lupoma (lū-pō'mă) [" + G. *-ōma,* swelling]. Nodule of lupus, esp. a primary one.

lupous (lū'pŭs) [L. *lupus,* wolf]. 1. Pert. to lupus. 2. Affected with lupus.

lupus (lū'pŭs) [L. wolf]. Originally any chronic, progressive, usually ulcerating, skin disease. In current usage: when the word is used alone it has no precise meaning. SEE: *l. vulgaris.*

l., disseminated follicular. L. of face with small and large papules.

l. erythematosus, disseminated. A chronic and usually fatal disease characterized by pathologic changes in the vascular system, esp. the collagen which serves as a binding substance for capillaries and small blood vessels. A skin rash is usually present, the erythema spreading across bridge of nose and face in a butterfly pattern. Marked constitutional symptoms are manifested. Etiology is unknown. Incidence highest in females between puberty and menopause. Corticosteroid therapy often helpful.

l. hypertrophicus. L. with vegetations.

l. maculo'sus. L. with maculae.

l. nonex'edens. L. without ulcerations.

l., pernio. Sarcoidosis (Boeck's sarcoid).

l. serpigino'sus. L. spreading with creeping ulcerations.

l. tu'midus. L. with edematous infiltrations.

l. verrucosus. Lesion consisting of an elevated plaque with indolent inflammatory base and a warty papillary surface.

l. vulgaris. Tuberculosis of the skin. Characterized by patches which break down and ulcerate, leaving scars on healing. Most common form of lupus.

LUQ. Abbr. for *left upper quadrant* (of abdomen).

Lust's reflex (lŭst). Dorsal flexion and abduction of foot resulting from percussion of ext. branch of sciatic nerve.

lu'teal [L. *luteus,* yellow]. Pert. to the corpus luteum, its cells, or its hormone.

l. hormone. Progesterone, *q.v.* Secreted by the corpus luteum. SEE: *endocrine; hormone; ovary; corpus luteum; estrogen.*

lutein (lū'tē-ĭn) [L. *luteus,* yellow]. 1. Yellow pigment derived from corpus luteum, egg yolk, and fat cells or lipochromes. 2. A proprietary substance prepared from corpora lutea from the ovaries of sows.

l. cells. Ovarian cells which contain a yellow pigment and are involved in the formation of the corpus luteum. They are of two types: *granulosa lutein cells* of follicular origin and *theca lutein cells* from the theca interna.

luteinization (lū-te-in-ĭ-ză'shŭn). Process of development of the corpus within a ruptured graafian follicle.

luteinizing hormone. Hormone secreted by ant. lobe of the hypophysis which stimulates development of the corpus luteum. ABBR: LH. Also called *interstitial-cell stimulating hormone* (ICSH).

luteoma (lū-tē-ō'mă) [L. *luteus,* yellow, + G. *-oma,* tumor]. An ovarian tumor containing lutein cells.

luteotrophin (lu-te-o-tro'fin). SYN: *prolactin, lactogenic hormone.* Hormone of ant. lobe of hypophysis which maintains mature corpora lutea and stimulates secretion of their hormone, progesterone. It also stimulates the secretion of milk by the mammary gland. Also called *luteotropin.*

lutetium (lu-te'shĭ-um). A rare element. SYMB: Lu. At. wt. 174.97; at. no. 71.

luteum (lu'tē-ŭm) [L.]. Yellow.

l., corpus. Yellow cellular mass which forms in position of ruptured graafian follicles in ovary. It persists and enlarges in pregnancy.

lutin (lū'tin). Hormone of corpus luteum which aids in preparation of endometrium for fertilized ovum. SYN: *progestin.*

lux (luks) [L. *light*]. A unit of light intensity equivalent to one lumen per square meter.

luxation (lŭks-ā'shŭn) [L. *luxāre*, to dislocate]. Displacement of organs or articular surfaces; dislocation of a joint.

lux'us [L. excess]. Excess of anything.

Luys' body [Jules B. Luys, French physician, 1828-1898]. Small mass of gray matter lying on dorsal surface of peduncle dorsolateral to substantia nigra. *Luys' nucleus* located in the posterior portion of the thalamus. SYN: *centromedian nucleus.*

lycanthropy (lī-kan'thrō-pĭ) [G. *lykos*, wolf, + *anthrōpos*, man]. Mania in which patient believes himself a wild beast, esp. a wolf. SYN: *lycomania.*

lycomania (lī-kō-mā'nĭ-ă) [" + *mania*, madness]. Delusion of being a wild animal, esp. a wolf. SYN: *lycanthropy.*

lycoperdonosis (li"ko-per"don-o'sis). Respiratory disease caused by inhaling large quantities of spores from the mature mushroom commonly called puffball. *Lycoperdon* is the genus of fungi to which most puffballs belong.

lycopodium (lī-kō-pō'dĭ-ŭm). A yellow powder formed from spores of *Lycopodium clavatum*, a club moss. Used as a dusting powder, and as a dessicant and absorbent.

lye (lī) [A.S. *leáh*]. 1. Liquid from leaching of wood ashes. 2. Any strong alkaline solution, esp. sodium or potassium hydroxide. SEE: *alkalies; NaOH.*

ly'ing-in. 1. The puerperal state. 2. Being in confinement.

lymph (lĭmf) [L. *lympha*]. The lymph is a body alkaline fluid found in the lymphatic vessels and the cisterna chyli.

Lymph is usually a clear, transparent, colorless fluid; however, in vessels draining the intestines it may appear milky owing to presence of absorbed fats. It differs from blood in that red blood corpuscles are absent and its protein content lower. Osmotic pressure and alkaline reserve are slightly higher than in blood plasma; viscosity, slightly less. Sp. gr. 1.016-1.023.

Lymph may vary considerably in composition in different parts of the body. In peripheral vessels it is similar to blood plasma except that the protein content is usually much lower. Lymph contains proteins (serum albumin, serum globulin, serum fibrinogen), salts, organic substances (urea, creatinine, neutral fats, glucose), and water. Cells present are principally lymphocytes, formed in lymph nodes and other lymphatic organs. Lymph from the intestine (called chyle) contains fats and other substances absorbed from the intestine.

The lymph is formed in tissue spaces all over the body and is gathered into small vessels which carry it centrally. All lymph eventually enters into either the *thoracic duct* or *right lymph duct*, each terminating at the junction of the internal jugular and subclavian veins where the lymph reenters the blood stream. The thoracic duct commences in the abdomen as a dilated sac, the *cisterna* (*receptaculum*) *chyli*, which receives lymph vessels from the lower limbs and pelvis and from the intestines and digestive organs. It continues upward through the thorax receiving intercostal vessels and near its termination it receives the *left subclavian trunk*, draining left upper extremity, and the *left jugular trunk*, draining l. side of head and neck. The rt. lymph duct drains the right sides of the thorax, head, and neck.

Lymph in passing from any region of the body to the main lymph ducts must pass through lymph vessels which pass through regional *lymph nodes*. These filter the lymph, freeing it of foreign particulate matter, esp. bacteria.

The absorption of fatty matter chiefly takes place through the *epithelial cells* of the intestines, and those of the villi. These cells carry it to the lacteals when the particles break up into fat and protein matter.

Absorption is most active in the alimentary canal, the digested material passing into the blood stream through the vessels of the portal circulation and into the lacteals.

l., animal. Vaccine l. from an animal.

l. cell or corpuscle. A lymphocyte.

l. channel. A lymph sinus, *q.v.*

l. follicle. Old term for lymph node.

l., inflammatory. Exudate due to inflammation.

l., intercellular. Tissue fluid.

l. node. A lymph node is a rounded body consisting of accumulations of lymphatic tissue found at intervals in the course of lymphatic vessels. L. nodes vary in size from a pinhead to an olive; may occur singly or in groups. One side bears an indentation, the *hilum*, from which blood vessels enter and leave and *efferent vessels* leave. *Afferent vessels* enter on side opposite from hilus.

The node is enclosed in a *capsule*, from which *trabeculae* project inwardly, dividing node into compartments called *ampullae* or *alveoli*. Outer compact region comprises the *cortex;* the inner diffuse portion, the medulla. The cortex is tightly packed with *lymph nodules*, which are separated from capsule by the *cortical sinus*. The lymphatic tissue of the medulla is arranged in the form of *medullary cords*. Irregular tortuous spaces, called *lymph sinuses*, are present throughout the node. The nodes are aggregated in regions, the principal ones of which are in the neck (*cervical*), in the armpit (*axillary*), in the groin (*inguinal*). Lymph nodes as well as vessels are divided into *superficial* and *deep* groups. Among the deep groups are those draining lymph from the visceral organs of the thorax and abdomen.

FUNCTIONS: Lymph nodes produce lymphocytes and monocytes. They act as filters keeping particulate matter, esp. bacteria, from gaining entrance to the blood stream. They may stop cancer cells but in turn may be the seat of cancer.

l. nodule. A small compact, densely staining mass of cells each containing a lighter staining central area in which lymphocytes are formed. They comprise the structural unit of lymphatic tissue. May occur singly, in groups as in Peyer's patches, or in encapsulated organs as lymph nodes.

l. scrotum. Scrotal lymphatic dilatation occurring esp. in elephantiasis.

l. sinuses. Irregular tortuous vessels found in lymphatic organs. Lined with cells belonging to the reticuloendothelial system.

l. spaces. Those esp. in connective tissue filled with lymph.

lymphadenectasis (lĭmf"ă-den-ĕkt'ă-sĭs) [L. *lympha*, lymph, + G. *adēn*, gland, + *ektasis*, dilatation]. Dilatation or distention of a lymph node.

lymphade'nia [" + G. *adēn*, gland]. Hyperplasia affecting lymphatic tissue.

l. ossea. Bone marrow hyperplasia accompanied by Bence-Jones protein in urine.

Sym: Neuralgic pains, followed by painful swellings on ribs and skull, and possible occurrence of spontaneous fractures. Syn: *multiple myeloma.*

lymphadenitis (lĭmf"ad-en-i'tis) [" + " + *-ītis*, inflammation]. Inflammation of a lymphatic gland.

Etiol: Drainage of bacteria or toxic matter into lymph nodes. May be specific, as by the organisms of typhoid, syphilis, or tuberculosis, or nonspecific, in which causative organism is not identified.

Sym: Marked increase of tissue; possible suppuration. Swelling, pain, tenderness. Usually accompanies lymphangitis.*

Treatment: Hot, moist dressings; incision and drainage if abscesses occur. Similar to other severe infections.

l., tuberculous. Etiol: Infection.

Sym: Possible loss of weight and strength; gradual onset and enlargement of lymph nodes; may become adherent, necrotic, and discharge pus through skin.

Treatment: Elimination of foci; exposure of area to sunlight; deep x-ray in some cases. Surgical removal.

NP: If tuberculosis is cause, same as in that condition. Otherwise, same as in lymphangitis, *q.v.*

lymphadenoma (lĭmf"ad-ĕ-no'mă) [" + " + *-ōma*, tumor]. Hyperplasia of the lymph nodes. Syn: *lymphoma.*

lymphadenopathy. Disease of the lymph nodes.

lymphagogue (lĭmf'ă-gŏg) [L. *lympha*, lymph, + G. *agōgos*, leading]. An agent which stimulates the production or flow of lymph.

lymphangiectasis (lĭmf"ăn-jĭ-ek'tă-sĭs) [" + G. *aggeion*, vessel, + *ektasis*, dilatation]. Dilatation of lymphatic vessels. Syn: *lymphectasia.*

lymphangioendothelioma (lĭmf-ăn"jĭ-ō-en"-dō-thĕl-ĭ-ō'mă) [" + " + *endon*, within, + *thēlē*, nipple, + *-ōma*, tumor]. Endothelioma originating from lymph vessels. Syn: *lymphendothelioma.*

lymphangiofibroma (lĭmf-an"jĭ-ō-fĭ-brō'-mă) [" + " + L. *fiber*, fiber, + G. *-ōma*, tumor]. Fibroma and lymphangioma combined.

lymphangioma (lĭmf"ăn-jĭ-ō'mă) [" + " + *-ōma*, tumor]. Tumor composed of lymphatic vessels.

lymphangiophlebitis (lĭmf-ăn"jĭ-ō-flē-bī'-tis) [" + " + *phleps*, vein, + *-ītis*, inflammation]. Inflammation of lymphatic vessels and veins.

lymphangioplasty (lĭmf-an'jĭ-ō-plăs-tĭ) [L. *lympha*, lymph, + G. *aggeion*, vessel, + *plassein*, to form]. Formation of artificial lymphatics.

lymphangiosarcoma (lĭmf-an"jĭ-ō-săr-kō'-mă) [" + " + *sarx*, flesh, + *-ōma*, tumor]. Lymphangioma and sarcoma combined.

lymphangiotomy (lĭmf"an-jĭ-ot'ō-mĭ) [" + " + *tomē*, a cutting]. 1. Dissection of the lymphatics. 2. Anatomy of the lymphatics. Syn: *lymphotomy.*

lymphangitis (limf-an-ji'tis) [" + " + *-ītis*, inflammation]. Inflammation of lymphatic channels or vessels.

Etiol: May be due to a variety of organisms but is frequently due to streptococci.

Sym: Onset chill and high fever, moderate swelling and pain. Deep general flush with raised border on affected area if infection is in deep layers of skin. The red inflamed area is commonly called "blood poisoning" by lay persons.

NP: Applications of heat in the form of baths or fomentations may be ordered. Adm. plenty of fluids. Light diet and rest are important. General care given in febrile and painful conditions.

lymphatic (lim-fat'ĭk) [L. *lymphaticus*, pert. to lymph]. 1. Of or pert. to lymph. 2. A lymph vessel.

A lymph vessel conveys toward the heart; contains valves like the veins. The intestinal parts of the lymphatics which take up some of the products of digestion are called *lacteals.*

After the *chyle* enters the lacteals it is known as *lymph.* The lymphatics, or lacteals, carry the food material in the form of lymph, which has not hitherto been taken directly into the blood vessels of the alimentary canal, into the blood stream.

Fluids exuded from the blood vessels into the tissues are gathered up and carried back again to the blood by the lymphatics, so that they serve two purposes. They appear like small veins with thin walls, and they are provided with valves. They commence as lymph capillaries, microscopic in size, and empty into two trunks which open into the large veins near the heart.

Unlike the blood, the fluid contained in the lymphatics flows only in 1 direction from the small capillaries to the main trunk (the thoracic duct and a smaller duct on the right side) and then to the large veins. When the lymph

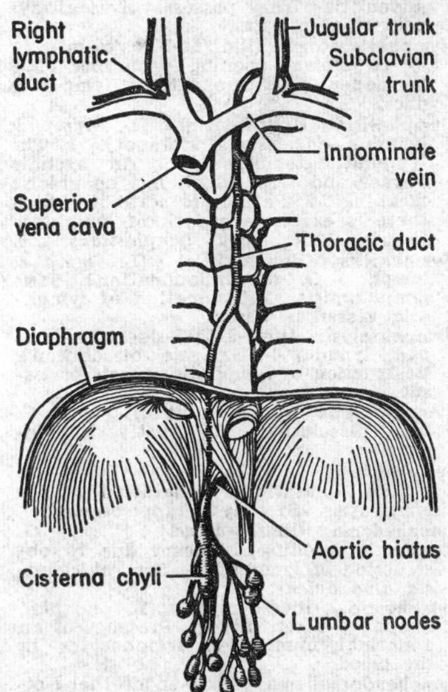

LYMPHATIC DRAINAGE

enters the blood it becomes part of its constituents.

PRINCIPAL GROUPS OF LYMPHATICS: (a) Right internal jugular vein; (b) right subclavian vein; (c) lymphatics of upper extremities; (d) receptaculum chyli; (e) lymphatics of lower extremities; (f) thoracic duct; (g) right subclavian vein; (h) lacteals; (i) lymphatics of lower extremities.

RS: *angioleukasia, angioleukitis, angiolymphitis, angiolymphoma, angiosis, bubo, chylangioma, leukosis, varix, "vas-" words.*

l., afferent. Any of the small vessels carrying lymph to a lymph node.

l. blockade. Local defense mechanism in which minute bits of material, such as fibrinous exudate from injured tissue, enter local lymphatic vessels, tending to obstruct them and thus preventing foreign substances, esp. bacteria, from passing to other parts of the body.

l. capillary. The smallest lymph vessels. Minute tubes consisting of a single layer of endothelium ending blindly in swollen or rounded ends. Tissue fluid enters the lymphatic system through the lymph capillaries. In intestinal villi they are called *lacteals.*

l., efferent. Any of the small vessels carrying lymph from a lymph node.

l. organ. A structure composed principally of lymphatic tissue. Includes lymph nodes, spleen, tonsil, thymus.

l. system. That system including all structures involved in the conveyance of lymph from the tissues to the blood stream. It includes the *lymph capillaries, lacteals, lymph nodes, lymph vessels,* main *lymph ducts* (thoracic and rt. lymphatic duct). For the circulation of lymph, SEE: *lymph.*

l. vessels. Thin-walled vessels conveying lymph from the tissues. They resemble veins in structure, possessing three layers: the intima, media, and adventitia. They possess valves always occurring in pairs.

lymphaticostomy (lĭmf"ăt-ĭ-kos'tō-mĭ) [" + G. *stoma,* opening]. Making of a permanent aperture into a lymphatic duct.

lymphatism (lĭmf'ă-tĭzm) [L. *lympha,* lymph, + G. *ismos,* state of]. 1. The lymphatic temperament. An archaic phrase and term which has no precise meaning. 2. Pathologic state in which there is excessive growth of lymphatic tissues. SYN: *status lymphaticus, q.v.*

lymphatitis (lĭmf-ă-tī'tĭs) [L. *lympha,* lymph, + G. *-itis,* inflammation]. SYN: *lymphangitis.* Inflammation of lymphatic vessel or tissue.

lymphatolysis (lĭmf-ă-tŏl'ĭ-sĭs) [L. *lympha,* lymph, + G. *lysis,* dissolution]. Destruction of lymphatic vessels or tissue.

lymphatolytic (lim-fat-ō-lit'ĭk) [" + G. *lysis,* dissolution]. Destructive to lymphatics.

lymphectasia (lĭmf-ĕk-tā'zĭ-ă) [" + G. *ektasis,* dilatation]. Dilatation of the lymphatics. SYN: *lymphangiectasis.*

lymphedema (lĭmf-ĕ-dē'mă) [" + G. *oidēma,* swelling]. Edema due to obstruction of lymphatics. SEE: *phlegmasia alba dolens.*

lymphemia (limf-e'mi-a) [L. *lympha,* lymph, + *aima,* blood]. Presence of an abnormal number of lymphocytes in the blood.

lymphendothelioma (lĭmf-ĕn"dō-thēl-ĭ-ō'mă) [" + G. *endon,* within, + *thēlē,* nipple, + *-ōma,* tumor]. Tumor from proliferation and dilatation of lymphatics with overgrowth of myxomatous tissue.

lymphenteritis (lĭmf"ĕn-tĕr-i'tĭs) [" + G. *enteron,* intestine, + *-ītis,* inflammation]. Serous infiltration accompanying inflammation of bowels.

lymphnoditis (lĭmf-nōd-ī'tĭs) [" + *nodus,* knot, + G. *-itis,* inflammation]. Inflamed condition of a lymph node.

lymphoadenoma (lĭmf"ō-ad-en-ō'mă) [" + G. *aden,* gland, + *-ōma,* tumor]. 1. A tumor of lymphoid tissue. 2. Hypertrophied condition of the lymphatics. SYN: *lymphadenoma.*

lymphoblast (lĭmf'ō-blăst) [L. *lympha,* lymph, + G. *blastos,* germ]. A cell which gives rise to a lymphocyte.

lymphoblastoma (limf-ō-blast-ō'mă) [" + " + *-ōma,* tumor]. Tumor composed of lymphocytes. SYN: *lymphosarcoma.*

lymphoblasto'sis [" + " + *-ōsis,* intensive]. Excessive number of lymphoblasts in the blood.

lymphocele (lĭmf'ō-sēl) [" + G. *kēlē,* hernia]. Tumor containing lymph. SYN: *lymphocyst.*

lymphocyst (lĭmf'ō-sist) [" + G. *kystis,* cyst]. Tumor containing lymph. SYN: *lymphocele.*

lymphocyte (lĭmf'ō-sīt) [" + G. *kytos,* cell]. Lymph cell or white blood corpuscle without cytoplasmic granules. They normally number from 20 to 50% of total white cells. May increase to 90% in lymphatic leukemia.

Lymphocytes averaging 10 to 12 microns in diameter but may be as large as 20 microns. Characterized by deeply staining, compact nucleus taking a dark blue. The nucleus occupies all or most of the cell, either in center or at one side. The cytoplasm is usually clear but in some cells bright reddish-violet granules are seen.

lymphocythemia (lĭmf"o-sī-the'mĭ-ă) [" + " + *aima,* blood]. Excess of lymph cells in the blood.

lymphocytopenia (lĭmf"ō-sīt"ō-pē'nĭ-ă) [" + " + *penia,* lack]. Less than normal number of lymphocytes in the blood.

lymphocytopoiesis (lĭmf"ō-sīt"ō-poi-ē'sĭs) [" + " + *poiesis,* production]. Lymphocyte production.

lymphocyto'sis [" + " + *-ōsis,* intensive]. Excess of lymph cells. SYN: *lymphocythemia.*

lymphocytotoxin (lĭmf"o-sīt"ō-toks'in) [" + " + *toxikon,* poison]. A toxin destructive to lymphocytes.

lymphodermia (lĭmf-ō-dĕr'mĭ-ă) [L. *lympha,* lymph, + G. *derma,* skin]. Disease of cutaneous lymphatics.

lympho"epithelio'ma. A tumor composed of epithelium and lymphatic tissue which develops usually in the nasal cavity or pharynx.

lymphogenous (lĭmf-oj'en-ŭs) [" + G. *gennan,* to produce] 1. Forming lymph. 2. Derived from lymph.

lymphogonia (lĭmf"ō-go'nĭ-ă) [" + G. *gonos,* offspring]. Large lymphocytes with large nuclei appearing in lymphatic leukemia.

lymphogranuloma venereum. SYN: *l. inguinale, lymphopathia venereum, climatic bubo, fourth venereal disease.* A venereal disease characterized by a small primary lesion, usually on genitalia, inflammation of regional lymph nodes, and constitutional symptoms. It is caused by a virus and readily transmitted by sexual contact.

lymphogranulomatosis (lĭmf″ō-grăn-ū-lō″-mă-tō′sĭs) [" + " + G. *-ōma*, tumor, + *-ōsis*]. 1. Infectious granuloma of the lymphatics. 2. Hodgkin's disease.

lymphoidectomy (lĭmf-oid-ek′tō-mĭ) [L. *lympha*, lymph, + G. *eidos*, form, + *ektomē*, excision]. Surgical removal of lymphoid tissue.

lymphoidocyte (limf-oid′ō-sīt) [" + " + *kytos*, cell]. A hemocytoblast, *q.v.*

lymphology (lĭmf-ol′ō-jĭ) [" + G. *logos*, study]. Science of the lymphatics.

lymphoma (limf-o′ma) [L. *lympha*, lymph, + G. *-oma*, tumor]. A general term for growth of new tissue in the lymphatic system. Included in this general group are Hodgkin's disease, lymphosarcoma, and malignant lymphoma.

l. granulomatosum. Small, white lymphatic nodule in liver in Hodgkin's disease.

lymphomatosis (lĭmf″ō-mă-tō′sis) [" + " + *-ōsis*, intensive]. General lymphatic engorgement; general deposition of lymphomata throughout the body.

lymphomatous (lĭmf-ō′mă-tŭs) [" + G. *-ōma*, tumor]. 1. Pert. to a lymphoma 2. Affected with lymphoma.

lymphopath′ia vene′reum [" + *pathos*, disease]. Venereal disease marked by ulceration and enlargement of lymph nodes in inguinal area. Syn: *lymphogranuloma inguinale.*

lymphopathy (lĭmf-op′ă-thĭ) [" + G. *pathos*, disease]. Any lymphatic disease.

lymphopenia (lĭmf-ō-pē′nĭ-ă) [" + G. *penia*, a lack]. Deficiency of lymphocytes in the blood.

lymphopoiesis (lĭmf-ō-poi-ē′sis) [" + G. *poiēsis*, production]. Formation of lymphocytes.

lymphopoietic (lĭmf-ō-poi-et′ĭk) [" + G. *poiein*, to produce]. Forming lymphocytes.

lymphoprotease. Protein-splitting enzyme secured from a suspension of lymphatic tissue.

lymphorrhagia (limf-or-rā′jĭ-ă) [L. *lympha*, lymph, + G. *rēgnunai*, to burst forth]. Flow of lymph from ruptured lymph vessels. Syn: *lymphorrhea.*

lymphorrhea (lĭmf-or-rē′ă) [" + G. *roia*, flow]. Internal or external discharge of lymph through a wound. Syn: *lymphorrhagia.*

lymphosarcoma (limf-ō-sar-kō′mă) [" + G. *sarx*, flesh, + *-ōma*, tumor]. A malignant disease of lymphatic tissue. Clinically may be quite similar to Hodgkin's disease. Diagnosis is made by biopsy rather than by clinical examination.

lymphosarcomatosis. Condition characterized by the development of lymphosarcoma.

lymphostasis (lĭmf-os′tă-sĭs) [" + G. *stasis*, a stoppage]. Stoppage of flow of lymph.

lymphotome (lĭmf′o-tōm) [" + G. *tomē*, incision]. Instrument for removing glandular growths from tonsils and adenoids.

lymphotrophy (lĭmf-ot′rō-fĭ) [" + G. *trophē*, nourishment]. Lymph nourishment of cells in regions devoid of blood vessels.

lymphuria (lĭmf-ū′rĭ-ă) [" + G. *ouron*, urine]. Lymph in the urine.

lymphvascular (lĭmf-vas′kū-lar) [" + *vasculus*, a little vessel]. Rel. to the lymphatic vessels.

lyo-. Combining form meaning *dissolved, loose.*

lyochrome. Flavin, *q.v.*

lyogel. A gel containing much water.

lyophilization. Process of rapidly freezing a substance at an extremely low temperature and then dehydrating in a high vacuum.

lyophobe, lyophobic. Tending not to go into solution; applied to colloidal systems in which there is a strong affinity between dispersed phase and dispersion medium.

lyotrope. A substance which goes into solution readily.

lyra (lī′ră) [G. *lyra*, lyre]. One of several anatomical structures so called because of their resemblance to the shape of a lyre or lute.

lysimeter (lī-sĭm′ĕ-ter) [" + *metron*, measure]. Apparatus for determining solubilities.

lysin (lī′sĭn) [G. *lysis*, dissolution]. A specific antibody acting destructively upon cells and tissues. See: *immune body.*

lysine (lī′sēn) [G. *lysis*, dissolution]. An amino acid which is a hydrolytic cleavage product of protein through digestion.

It is essential for growth and repair.

lysis (lī′sĭs) [G. dissolution]. 1. The gradual decline of a fever or disease. The opp. of *crisis.** 2. Destruction of blood cells, etc., by a lysin, as when rabbit's red corpuscles are dissolved by dog's serum. 3. Combining form meaning dissolution of, decomposition of (ex. *hydrolysis*), or in medicine, reduction or relief (ex. *paralysis*). See: *crisis, hemolysis.*

lysogenesis (lī-sō-jen′ĕ-sĭs) [G. *lysis*, dissolution, + *genesis*, production]. The production of cell-dissolving substance known as lysin.

lysogenic (lī-sō-jen′ĭk) [" + G. *gennan*, to produce]. Producing lysins.

lysogeny (li-soj′ĕ-nĭ). A special type of virus-bacterial cell interaction maintained by a complex cellular regulatory mechanism. Bacterial strains freshly isolated from their natural environment may contain a low concentration of bacteriophage. This phage will lyse other related bacteria. Cultures which contain these substances are said to be lysogenic.

lysol (lī′sŏl). A proprietary preparation of a mixture of cresols. Used as an antiseptic.

Poisoning: When swallowed it causes corrosion, edema of the lungs, immobility of pupils, and collapse. Vomiting may occur, death sometimes after symptoms have abated.

Treatment: *Prompt emptying of the stomach by aspiration through a stomach tube.*

lysolecithin. A substance obtained from lecithin through the action of an enzyme present in cobra venom. Exerts a powerful hemolytic action.

lysozyme (lī′sō-zīm) [" + *zymē*, leaven]. A substance present in tears, saliva and other body fluids. An enzyme with antibacterial activity.

lyssa (lĭs′să) [G. *lyssa*, frenzy]. An acute infectious disease, transferable by inoculation, which particularly attacks the nervous system. Syn: *hydrophobia; rabies.*

lyssin (lĭs′sĭn) [G. *lyssa*, frenzy]. Virus of lyssa. Syn: *hydrophobin.*

lyssodexis (lĭs-sō-deks′ĭs) [" + *dēxis*, a bite]. The bite of an animal infected with rabies virus.

lyssoid (lĭs′soyd) [" + *eidos*, resemblance]. Resembling lyssa or rabies.

lyssophobia (lĭs-ō-fō′bĭ-ă) [" + *phobos*, fear]. 1. Hysteria resembling rabies. 2. Fear of rabies.

lyterian (lī-tēr′ĭ-an) [G. *lyein*, to dissolve]. Indicative of the lessening of a disease process.

lytic (lĭt′ĭk) [G. *lyein*, to dissolve]. Rel. to lysis or a lysin.

lytta [G. frenzy]. Old term for rabies.

lyze (līz) [G. *lysis*, from *lyein*, to dissolve]. To bring about lysis.

Notes

Notes

Notes

Notes

M

M. Abbr. for *mille,* a thousand; *misce,* mix.

m. Abbr. for *meter* and *minim;* in chemistry, for *meta-,* and for *mol* or *mole, q.v.*

M. A. Abbr. for *Master of Arts.*

MA. Mental age.

Ma. Chem. symbol for *masurium.*

ma. Abbr. for *milliampère.*

M.A.C. Abbr. for *maximum allowable concentration.*

macaro'ni [It.]. Cooked: 1 cup (130 gm.). Calories: 190. Other main values: 6 gm. protein; 39 gm. carbohydrate; 1.4 mg. iron; 0.23 mg. thiamine; 0.14 mg. riboflavin; 1.9 mg. niacin.

mace (mās) [L. *macis*]. A spice from the outer covering of the nutmeg; employed as a condiment.

maceration (măs-ĕr-a'shŭn) [L. *macerāre,* to make soft]. 1. Process of softening a solid by steeping in a fluid.

Mache unit (mä'kĕ). The unit of measurement of concentration of radium emanation. Abbr. *M. u.,* or German, *M. E.* See: *unit.*

machonnement (mash-shōn-mon') [Fr.]. Movement of jaws resembling chewing.

macies (mā'shĭ-ēz) [L. wasting]. Atrophy, wasting, emaciation.

macrencephalia, macrencephaly (mak-ren-sĕ-fa'lĭ-ă, -sef'a-lĭ) [G. *makros,* long, + *egkephalos,* brain]. Abnormal size of brain.

macro-, macr- [G.]. Combining forms meaning *large, long.*

macrobiosis (mak"rō-bī-ō'sĭs) [G. *makros,* large, + *biōsis,* life]. State of surpassing normal span; longevity.

macrobiota (mak"rō-bī-ō'tă). The large living organisms, flora and fauna, of an area, as differentiated from microbiota.

macrobleph"ar'ia. Abnormal largeness of eyelid.

macrobrachia (mak"rō-brā'kĭ-ă). Abnormal largeness of the arm.

macrocephalia (mak-rō-sĕ-fa'lĭ-ă) [G. *makros,* large, + *kephalē,* head]. Abnormal largeness of head.

Etiol: Found in acromegaly, hydrocephalus, rickets, osteitis deformans, leontiasis ossea, myxedema, sporadic cretinism, idiocy, leprosy and hemiatrophy; also in pituitary disturbances.

macrocephalous (mak-ro-sef'ă-lŭs) [" + *kephalē,* head]. Pert. to or having an excessively large head.

macrocephaly (mak-rō-sĕf'al-ĭ) [" + *kephalē,* head]. Abnormal size of head. Syn: *macrocephalia.*

macrocheilia (mak-rō-kī'lĭ-ă) [G. *makros,* large, + *cheilos,* lip]. Abnormal size of lip characterized by swelling of glands of lip. It is a congenital condition. Syn: *hypertrophy of lip.*

macrocheiria (mak-rō-kī'rĭ-ă) [" + *cheir,* hand]. Excessive size of the hands. Syn: *macrochiria.*

macrocornea (mak-rō-kor'nē-ă) [G. *makros,* large, + L. *cornu,* horn]. Abnormal size or projection of the cornea. Syn: *keratoglobus, megalocornea.*

mac'rocyte [G. *makros,* large, + *kytos,* cell]. Erythrocyte larger than normal, exceeding 10 microns in diameter.

macrocythemia (mak-rō-sī-thē'mĭ-ă) [" + " + *aima,* blood]. Abnormal number of macrocytes in the blood.

macrocytosis (mak"rō-sī-tō'sĭs) [" + " + *-ōsis,* intensive]. Development of macrocytes, esp. in greater numbers than normal.

macrodactylia (mak"rō-dak-til'ĭ-ă) [" + *daktylos,* finger]. Excessive size of one or more of the digits.

macrodont (mak'rō-dont) [" + *odous, odont-,* tooth]. Having abnormally large teeth. Syn: *megadont.*

macroesthesia (mak"rō-ĕs-thē'zĭ-ă) [G. *makros,* large, + *aisthēsis,* sensation]. A state in which objects seen or felt appear to be greatly magnified.

macrogam'ete. A large, immobile reproductive cell formed in certain protozoa and simple plants. Corresponds to the ovum in higher forms.

macrogametocyte. A large nonmotile reproductive cell developing from the merozoite of certain protozoans; the female gametocyte. See: *Plasmodium.*

macrogenitosomia (mak"rō-jen"ĭ-tō-sō'-mĭ-ă) [" + L. *genitālis,* genital, + G. *sōma,* body]. Precocious body development in general, with unusually large genitalia.

macroglia (mak-rog'lĭ-ă) [G. *makros,* large, + *glia,* glue]. A type of neuroglia in which cells are called astrocytes, *q.v.* See: *neuroglia, glia cell, spider cell.*

macroglobulinemia (mak-rō-glob"ū-lin-ē'-mĭ-ă). Presence of globulins in blood in concentration greater than 5%. Syn: *Waldenstroem blood disease.*

macroglobulins (mak"rō-glob'ū-lĭnz). A group of proteins of high molecular weight, about 1,000,000, normally present in the blood but increased in disease states such as multiple myeloma, collagen disorders, cirrhosis of the liver, and amyloidosis.

macroglos'sia [" + *glōssa,* tongue]. Hypertrophied condition of the tongue. A congenital disorder.

macrognathia (mak-rō-nā'thĭ-ă) [" + *gnathos,* jaw]. Abnormal size of jaw.

macrogy'ria. Excessively large size of convolutions (gyri) of cerebral hemispheres.

macrolabia (mak-rō-lā'bĭ-ă) [" + L. *labium,* lip]. Abnormal size of lip. Syn: *macrocheilia, q.v.*

macrolymphocyte (mak"rō-limf'ō-sīt) [" + L. *lympha,* lymph, + G. *kytos,* cell]. A large lymphocyte.

macromastia (mak-rō-mas'tĭ-ă) [" + *mastos,* breast]. Abnormal size of the breasts.

macromazia (mak-rō-mā'zĭ-ă) [" + *mazos,* breast]. Abnormal development of breasts. Syn: *macromastia.*

macrome'lia. Excessive size of an organ or a part, esp. an extremity.

macrome'lus. An individual possessing limbs of excessive size.

macromere (mak'rō-mēr) [" + *meros.* a part]. Blastomere of large size.

mac"ronor'moblast (G. *makros,* large, + L. *norma,* rule, + G. *blastos,* germ]. Large, nucleated normoblast.

macrophage, macrophagus (mak'rō-fāj, -rof'ă-gus) [G. *makros,* large, + *phagein,* to eat]. Syn: *clasmatocyte, resting wandering cell, adventitial cell.* A cell of the reticuloendothelial system having the ability to phagocytose particulate substances and to store vital dyes and other colloidal substances. They are found in loose connective tissues and various organs of the body. They include *Kupffer cells* of the liver, *splenocytes* of the spleen, *dust cells* of the lung, *microglia* of spinal cord and brain, and *histiocytes* of loose connective tissue.

m., fixed. A nonmotile macrophage.

m., free. SYN: *wandering m.* A wandering or ameboid macrophage. Found esp. in areas where inflammatory processes are in progress.

macrophallus (mak″rō-făl′ŭs) [″ + *phallos,* penis]. Abnormally large penis.

macrophthalmia (mak″rof-thal′mĭ-ă). Abnormally large eyeballs.

macroplasia (mak″rō-plā′zĭ-ă). Abnormally large size of a part or specific tissue.

macropodia (mak-rō-pō′dĭ-ă) [″ + *pous, pod-,* foot]. Abnormally large feet.

macroprosopia (mak″rō-prō-sō′pĭ-ă) [″ + *prosōpon,* face]. Large facial features.

macropsia (mak-rop′sĭ-ă) [″ + *opsis,* vision]. Condition in which objects look larger than they really are.

macrorhinia (mak-rō-rīn′ĭ-ă) [″ + *rīs, rīn-,* nose]. Excessive size of the nose, either congenital or pathological.

macroscelia (mak-rō-sĕl′ĭ-ă) [″ + *skelos,* leg]. Abnormal size of the legs.

macroscopic (mak-rō-skop′ĭk) [″ + *skopein,* to examine]. Large enough to be seen by the naked eye. OPP: *microscopic.* SYN: *megascopic.*

macroscopy (mak-ros′ko-pĭ) [″ + *skopein,* to examine]. Examination of an object with the naked eye.

macrosomatia (mak″rō-sō-mā′shĭ-ă) [″ + *sōma,* body]. Abnormally large body. SYN: *macrosomia.*

macrosomia (mak-rō-sō′mĭ-ă) [″ + *sōma,* body]. Abnormally large body. SYN: *macrosomatia.*

m. adiposa congenita. An obese type of premature development probably due to hyperfunction of the adrenal cortex.

macrostomia (mak-rō-stō′mĭ-ă) [″ + *stoma,* mouth]. Excessively wide mouth.

macrotia (mak-ro′shĭ-ă) [G. *makros,* large, + *ous, ot-,* ear]. Abnormally large ears.

macrotooth. Abnormally enlarged tooth.

macula (mak′u-lă) (pl. *maculae*) [L. *spot*]. SYN: *macule.* A small spot or colored area. SEE: *roseola.*

m. acusticae. Oval thickened areas in saccule and utricle in which fibers of vestibular branch of acoustic nerve terminate. They are sensory receptors containing hair cells which respond to movement of the endolymph. They include *m. sacculi* and *m. utriculi.*

m. albida. White mark found on liver in some contagious diseases. SYN: *tache blanche.*

m. atrophica. Glistening white spot on skin following a circumscribed hemorrhage.

m. caerulea. Steel gray or blue stain of epidermis, without elevation, which does not disappear on pressure, occurring esp. with pediculosis pubis or bites from fleas.

m., cerebral. Reddened line, becoming deeper and persisting for some time, esp. in tuberculous meningitis, by drawing the fingernail across the skin; tache cérébrale, *q.v.*

m. corneae. Opaque spot in cornea.

m. cribrosa. One of the tiny foramina in wall of vestibule of bony labyrinth of the ear through which pass filaments of the acoustic nerve.

m. flava. A small yellow spot at ventral end of each vocal fold formed by a small mass of elastic tissue or, sometimes, cartilage.

m. gonorrhoeica. Red spot at orifice of Bartholin's gland. Seen in gonorrheal vulvitis.

m. lutea. The yellow spot on the retina, about 1/12 in. (2.08 mm.) to outer side of the optic nerve's exit, the exact center of the retina. Contains a pit, the *fovea centralis,* where retina is reduced to a layer of closely packed cones, which functions as the area of most acute vision (central vision).

m. sacculi. SEE: *m. acusticae.*

m. solaris. A freckle.

m. utriculi. SEE: *m. acusticae.*

macular (mak′ū-lar) [L. *macula,* spot]. 1. Rel. to macules. 2. Having macules.

maculate(d (mak′ū-lāt, -lāt-ĕd) [L. *macula,* spot]. Spotted, as with macules.

maculation (mak-ū-lā′shun) [L. *macula,* spot]. Process of becoming maculate. Development of macules.

macule (mak′ūl) [L. *macula,* spot]. Discolored spot or patch on the skin, neither elevated nor depressed, of various colors, sizes and shapes.

They consist of *hyperemia, roseola, erythema, telangiectasis, nevi vasculosi, areola, achromia, chloasma, purpura, petechiae, ecchymosis, vibices, albinism, vitiligo, lentigines, nevi pigmentosi, nevi spili, discolorations, q.v.*

Macules occur in pellagra, pityriasis rosea, pediculosis corporis, rubella, scurvy, serum sickness, peliosis, anemia, leukemia, cancer, Bright's disease, infectious diseases, poisoning, erysipelas, acne rosacea, nevus pigmentosus, vitiligo, leprosy, morphea, facial hemiatrophy, etc. SYN: *macula, q.v.*

maculopap′ular. Consisting of or pertaining to macules and papules.

mad. SYN: *insane; rabid.* 1. Not rational. 2. Angry. 3. Rash, foolish, frantic. 4. Suffering from infection with rabies.

madarosis (mad-ă-ro′sis) [G. *madaros,* bald]. Loss of eyelashes or eyebrows.

madescent (mad-es′ent) [L. *madescere,* to become moist]. Slightly moist, or becoming so.

madidans (mad′ĭ-dans) [L. *madidus,* wet]. Exuding, moist, as in some skin lesions.

Madu′ra foot. Fungus disease of the foot. SYN: *mycetoma, maduromycosis, q.v.*

maduromycosis (mad-ū-rō-mī-kō′sĭs). Chronic infection of the foot or hand characterized by marked swelling and development of nodules, vesicles, and sinuses.

ETIOL: A variety of fungi, esp. *Monosporium apiospermum* and various species of *Nocardia.* Infections by the latter are usually designated *mycetomas, q.v.*

Magendie's foramen (mă-zhan-de′) [Francois Magendie, French physiologist, 1783-1855]. The median of three openings in the roof of the 4th ventricle which is in front of the cerebellum and behind the *pons varolii,* connecting the ventricle with the subarachnoid space.

magenstrasse (mag″en-stras′ĕ) [Ger. *magen,* stomach, + *strasse,* street]. A groove along lesser curvature of stomach from cardia to pylorus.

mag′got (origin uncertain). Larva of an insect, esp. the soft-bodied, footless larva of flies (order Diptera). Many are parasitic giving rise to *myiasis, q.v.*

m. treatment. An obsolete method of treating septic wounds. Meat maggots, introduced into a sloughing septic wound, ingested the necrotic material, leaving the wound with a clean granulating surface. The maggots were then removed and destroyed. SEE: *osteomyelitis.*

magistery (maj'ĭs-tĕr-ĭ) [L. *magister,* master]. 1. Specially compounded remedy. 2. A precipitate.

magistral (măj'ĭs-trăl) [L. *magister,* master]. Concerning medicines prescribed by a physician for a particular case. SEE: *officinal.*

magma (mag'mă) [G. *magma,* from *massein,* to knead]. 1. Mass left after extraction of principle. 2. Salve. 3. A pulpy mass or paste.

magnesia (măg-nē'zĭ-ă) [G. *magnēs,* a magnet]. Magnesium oxide. MgO.

m., milk of. An aperient composed of magnesium hydroxide and water.

magne'sium [L.]. SYMB: *Mg.* At. wt. 24.312; at. no. 12; sp. gr. 1.738. A white mineral element found in soft tissue, muscles, bones, and to some extent in the body fluids. It is a naturally occurring element on earth, being extracted from wells and sea water.

The entire body contains 0.05% Mg, 70% of which is contained in the bones. The muscles contain less of it than they do calcium. Concentration of Mg in the blood serum averages 2.5 (1.8—3.6) mg. per cent.

Daily minimum requirement, 0.22 gm.

FUNCTIONS: Salts of magnesium and potassium, and other minerals are necessary to maintain osmotic pressure. Magnesium is needed for the ion balance, the activation of enzymes, for muscular activity, nerve stability, and bone structure. It also has a laxative effect.

DEFICIENCY SYM: Convulsions, nervous conditions, retarded growth, digestive disturbances, spasticity of muscles and nerves, accelerated heart beat, arrhythmia, and vasodilation.

SOURCES: It is obtained in sufficient quantities in meat, milk, fruits and vegetables to make special dietary planning to include it unnecessary. From 0.14 to 0.67 gm. have been found in the food for a single day. Indeed, Mg added to a mixed diet, may cause a loss of calcium. Most foods contain almost as much of it as they do of calcium.

m. car'bonate ($MgCO_3.3H_2O$). USP. A bulky, white, odorless powder.

ACTION AND USES: Internally, to neutralize acid in stomach.

m. citrate solution. USP. A solution containing an amount of magnesium citrate corresponding to approximately 1.6% magnesium oxide.

ACTION AND USES: Purgative.

m. hydroxide ($Mg[OH]_2$). A bulky white powder which, in aqueous suspension, is milk of magnesia. Laxative and antacid.

m. oxide (MgO). USP. Calcined magnesia. *Light* magnesia. A white, very bulky, fine powder.

ACTION AND USES: Antacid, laxative.

Heavy. USP. magnesii oxidum ponderosum.

ACTION AND USES: Same as magnesium oxide, light.

m. phosphate tribasic. A white, odorless powder.

USES: As an antacid and laxative.

m. stearate. USP. Compound of magnesium and palmitic and stearic acid. Used in manufacture of pharmaceutical tablets.

m. sul'fate ($MgSO \cdot 7H_2O$). USP. Small, colorless crystals. Saline bitter taste. SYN: *Epsom salt.*

ACTION AND USES: Refrigerant, hydragogue, cathartic, in tetanus and eclamptic conditions.

INCOMPATIBILITIES: Ammonium chloride, soapsuds enema, quinine, ferric chloride, sulfanilamide.

m. trisilicate. USP. Magnesium oxide, slicon dioxide and water. Used as an antacid.

mag'net [G. *magnes*]. Any body which has the property of attracting iron, spec. a mass of iron or steel which has this property given to it artificially. A piece of iron may be magnetized by passage of an electric current through an insulated wire wound about it.

m., horseshoe. One in shape of a horseshoe.

m. operation. Removal of metal particles with a magnet.

magnet'ic [G. *magnēs*]. Pert. to a magnet or having magnetism.

m. field. The space permeated by the magnetic lines of force surrounding a permanent magnet or coil of wire carrying electric current.

m. induction. The production of magnetic properties in magnetic metals such as iron by the influence of a magnetic field or of a magnet.

m. lines of force. The lines indicating the direction of the magnetic force in the space surrounding a magnet or constituting a magnetic field.

magnetism (măg'nĕ-tĭzm) [" + *-ismos,* condition]. The property of repulsion and attraction of certain substances.

magnetotherapy (mag"nĕt-ō-ther'ă-pĭ) [" + *therapeia,* treatment]. Application of magnets or magnetism in treating diseases.

magnification (mag-nĭ-fĭ-kā'shun) [L. *magnus,* great, + *facere,* to make]. Process of increasing apparent size of an object, esp. under microscope.

mag'num [L. large]. 1. Large. (EX: foramen magnum). 2. Old term for capitate bone (os magnum), the largest of the carpals.

maidenhead (mād'en-hĕd). Thin, crescentic fold partly closing vaginal opening and once considered a sign of virginity. SYN: *hymen.*

maieusiomania (mī-ū-sĭ-ō-mā'nĭ-ă) [G. *maieusis,* childbirth, + *mania,* madness]. Insanity following childbirth.

maieusiophobia (mī-ū-sĭ-ō-fō'bĭ-ă) [L. *magnus,* great, + *phobos,* fear]. Extreme fear of childbirth.

maieutics (mī-u'tĭks) [G. *maieusis,* childbirth]. Obstetrics.

maim (mām) [M.E. *maymen,* to cripple]. 1. To injure seriously; to disable. 2. To deprive of the use of a part, such as an arm or leg.

main (măn) [Fr.]. Hand.

m. en griffe (ahn-grēf'). Flexion and atrophy of the hand in a claw shape.

m. succulente (sŭk-kū-lahnt'). Edema of a hand.

Majocchi's disease (mah-yok'ē) [Domenico Majocchi, Italian physician, 1849-1929]. Ringform, purplish eruption of lower limbs; *purpura annularis telangiectodes, q.v.*

make. In elect., to complete an electric circuit. Opp. of *break.*

m. twitch. In physiol., the contraction of a muscle which occurs upon closure of the primary circuit.

makro- [G.]. For words beginning thus, see under *macro-*.

mal-. Combining form meaning ill, bad, poor.

mal (mahl) [Fr. from L. *malum,* an evil]. An evil, a sickness or a disorder.

m. de Cayenne. Elephantiasis.

m. de la rosa. Pellagra.

m. de mer. Seasickness.

m., grand. A major epileptic attack with convulsions.

m. perforant. A perforating ulcer of the foot.

m. p. palatin. A perforating ulcer of the palate.

m., petit. A minor attack of epilepsy without convulsions.

mala (ma'lă) [L.]. 1. The cheek. 2. The cheekbone.

malabsorption syndrome. Disordered or inadequate absorption of nutrients from the intestinal tract. May be due to a disease which affects the intestinal mucosa, as infections, tropical sprue, gluten enteropathy, pancreatic insufficiency, or to antibiotic therapy (neomycin).

malachite green (mal'ă-kīt) [G. *malachē,* a mallow (with green leaves)]. Dye sometimes used in treating trypanosomiasis and as an indicator. Also used as a bacteriological stain.

malacia (mă-la'sĭ-ă) [G. *malakia,* softening]. 1. Abnormal softening of tissues of an organ or of tissues themselves. 2. A morbid appetite for some specific food, esp. condiments.

m. cordis. Softening following infarction of the myocardium.

malacoma (măl-ă-kō'mă) [G. *malakia,* softening]. Softening of an organ or part of the body. Syn: *malacia, malacosis.*

malacoplakia (mal-ă-kō-plā'kĭ-ă) [" + *plax, plak-,* plaque]. Existence of soft patches in mucous membrane of a hollow organ.

m., vesical. Soft, funguslike patches on mucosa of the bladder.

malacosarcosis (măl-ă-kō-sar-kō'sĭs) [" + *sarx,* flesh, + *-ōsis*]. Softness of tissue, especially muscular.

malacosis (măl-ă-kō'sĭs) [" + *-ōsis,* intensive]. Abnormal softening of an organ or part of the body. Syn: *malacia, malacoma.*

malacosteon (mal-ă-kos'tē-ŏn) [G. *malakia,* softening, + *osteon,* bone]. Softening of the bones. Syn: *osteomalacia.*

malacotic (mal-ă-kot'ik) [G. *malakia,* softening]. 1. Soft. 2. Affected with malacia. 3. Rel. to malacia.

m. teeth. Those of soft texture easily affected by caries.

malacotomy (măl-ă-kot'ō-mĭ) [" + *tomē,* incision]. Incision of soft areas of the body, esp. of the abdominal wall.

mal"adjust'ed. Poorly adjusted; unhappy or unsuccessful because of inability or failure to adjust one's desires or needs to one's environment or station in life.

malady (mal'ă-dĭ) [Fr. *maladie,* illness, from L. *malum,* an evil]. A condition of ill health. Syn: *disease.*

malaise (mă-lāz') [Fr.]. Discomfort, uneasiness, indisposition, often indicative of infection.

malar (mā'lar) [L. *mala,* cheek]. Pert. to cheekbones.

m. bone. A 4-pointed bone on each side of the face, uniting the frontal and sup. maxillary bones with the zygomatic process of the maxilla. The zygomatic or cheek bone. See: *zygoma.*

malaria (mă-lā'rĭ-ă) [It. *malaria,* bad air]. An acute and sometimes chronic infectious disease due to the presence of protozoan parasites within red blood cells. The parasites undergo an asexual cycle in man and a sexual cycle in the mosquito. Sporozoites injected by the bite of a mosquito go through an exo-erythrocytic cycle in tissue cells such as liver cells where they undergo schizogony. After an interval of 7-10 days, they invade erythrocytes in which they undergo several divisions (schizogony), forming many merozoites. These break free and invade other corpuscles. The destruction of corpuscles with liberation of pigment and waste products brings on the characteristic paroxysms of chills and fever. This occurs at 48-hr. intervals in tertian and 72-hr. intervals in quartan malaria. After several generations of schizonts, some merozoites develop into micro- and macrogametocytes which when sucked up by a mosquito undergo further development. The microgametocytes produce several "flagellated bodies" which unite with a macrogamete to form a zygote, which elongates forming a vermicule or ookinete, which penetrates the stomach wall of the mosquito forming an oocyst in which sporozoites develop. When mature, the oocyst bursts, liberating sporozoites into body cavity through which the sporozoites make their way to salivary glands. They are discharged through salivary ducts when the mosquito bites a person.

Etiol: Four species of a sporozoan, *Plasmodium* (*P. vivax, P. falciparum, P. malariae, P. ovale*). The causative organism is transmitted through bites of infected mosquitos of the genus *Anopheles;* may be transmitted by blood transfusion.

Incubation Period: *P. falciparum,* 12 d.; *P. vivax* and *P. ovale,* 14 d.; *P. malariae,* 30 d. For some strains of *P. vivax,* may be 8 to 10 months.

Sym: Various derangements of the digestive and nervous systems. Characterized by periodicity, chills, fever and sweats, in the order mentioned, having pathologic manifestations of progressive anemia, splenic enlargement, and deposition in various organs of a melanin, resulting from the biologic activity of the plasmodia.

Treatment: Chloroquine, amodiaquine, quinacrine, pyrimethamine, chloroguanide. Choice of drug depends on type of malaria and stage of the disease.

m., algid. Cold malaria characterized by coldness of skin. See: *m., estivo-autumnal.*

m., cephalgic. Unusually severe headache, nausea, vomiting, etc. Differential Diag: Meningitis and intracranial lesions.

m., cerebral. Falciparum malaria in which brain is affected due to tendency of corpuscles to agglutinate, resulting in clogging of capillaries which in the brain lead to coma or sometimes sudden death.

m., estivoautumnal. Indistinct chill, usually only a chilly sensation. Intense headache, profound weakness, marked muscular aching. Marked mental depression. Coated tongue, feeble and accelerated pulse, rapid respiration. Febrile stages may be 36 hours long. See: *m., falciparum.*

m., falciparum. M. caused by *Plasmodium falciparum.* More prevalent in tropics; also called malignant tertian, subtertian, estivoautumnal malaria. Symptoms more severe than in other types, but runs a shorter course without relapses.

m., latent. Parasites exist within blood stream, but give rise to no recognizable symptoms. Individuals having this form constitute portion of carriers.

m., pernicious. Onset may be sudden, resembling apoplexy; coma usually comes, however, after obvious, severe, and intense symptoms. Hot skin; petechiae; contracted pupils; Cheyne-Stokes respiration; coated tongue; loss of sphincter control; rapid, irregular, weak pulse; elevated temperature. A remission may occur with profuse perspiration, but other paroxysms follow if treatment is inadequate. ETIOL: *Plasmodium vivax.* PROG: In spite of heroic administrations, death sometimes occurs. Often general collapse, with death in cases where no treatment is instituted.

m., quartan. Short and less severe paroxysms. Sporulation occurs each 72 hours, causing seizures with that interval. Caused by *Plasmodium malariae.*

m., quotidian estivoautumnal. Paroxysms occur with daily periodicity due to 24-hour sporulation. Abrupt rise and fall of temperature. Due to multiple infections with the same organism.

m., tertian. Sporulation each 48 hours. Symptoms more common during the day. Paroxysms divided into chill, fever and sweating stages. Cold stage is usually 10-15 minutes, but may last an hour or more. Febrile stage varies from 4-6 hours.

m., t., benign. Caused by *Plasmodium vivax;* malignant tertian by *Plasmodium falciparum.*

m., vivax. SYN: *benign tertian.* Malaria caused by *Plasmodium vivax.*

malarial (mă-lar'ĭ-ăl) [It. *malaria,* bad air]. 1. Affected with malaria. 2. Causing malaria. 3. Resembling malaria. 4. Pert. to malaria. SYN: *malarious.*

malariology (mă-lar-ĭ-ol'ō-jĭ) [" + G. *logos,* study]. The scientific study of malaria.

malariotherapy (mă-lar-ĭ-ō-ther'ă-pĭ) [" + G. *therapeia,* treatment]. Method of treating paresis and parasyphilitic conditions by injecting malarial organisms into the body.

malarious (ma-lar'ĭ-ŭs) [It. *malaria,* bad air]. Of the nature of, or afflicted with malaria. SYN: *malarial.*

Malasse'zia. A genus of fungi.

malassimilation (mal"ă-sim-ĭ-la'shŭn) [L. *malus,* ill, + *assimilāre,* to make like]. Defective, incomplete, or faulty assimilation, esp. of nutritive material.

malaxation (mal-aks-a'shun) [L. *malaxāre,* to soften]. Kneading movement used in massage.

male (māl). 1. Masculine. 2. One of the sex that fertilizes; one potentially capable of producing sperm.

RS: *female, organs, virile, virilescence, virilism.*

m. sex hormone. SYN: *androsterone.** 1. Hormone, found in urine and secreted by the testicles, which regulates development at puberty of male characteristics. 2. An *androgen.* One of a group of steroids which stimulate the development of secondary sex characteristics and accessory sex organs in the male. They are produced principally by the interstitial cells of the testes, although the adrenal cortex and the ovaries also produce androgenic compounds. They are also found in urine. Principal androgenic hormone is testosterone ($C_{19}H_{30}O_2$). Other androgenic substances include adrenosterone, androsterone, and isoandrosterone.

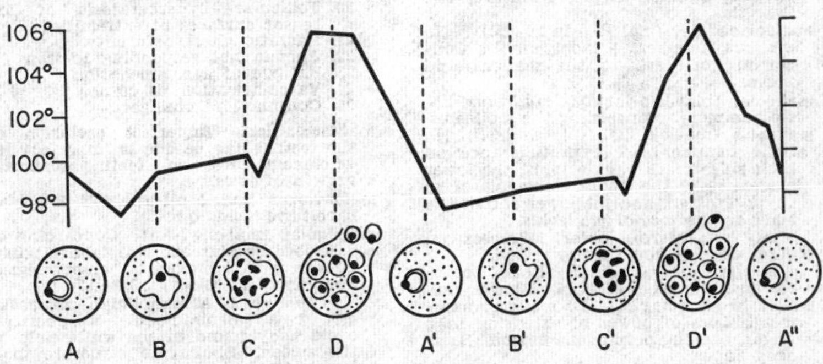

HUMAN CYCLE OF TERTIAN MALARIA.

In the circles A, B, C, D, and A', B', C', and D', which represent red blood corpuscles, malarial parasites are shown growing from the little spore in A and A' to the adult in C and C' and sporulating in D and D'. Above is a temperature curve, the figures on the left indicating the temperature of the patient (given in the centigrade scale) the vertical lines indicating days. The temperature is highest— i. e., there is a paroxysm—each time the parasite reaches the stage of sporulation, D and D'.

malemission (mal-ē-mĭs'shŭn) [L. *malus,* weak, + *ē,* out, + *mittere,* to send]. Failure of semen to be ejaculated from the urethra during coitus.

maleruption (mal-e-rup'shun). Incorrect eruption of teeth.

malformation (măl-for-mā'shŭn) [L. *malus,* bad, + *formatiō,* a shaping]. Deformity; abnormal shape or structure esp. congenital.

malic (ma'lĭk) [L. *malum,* apple]. Pert. to apples.

m. acid. An acid found in some fruits, such as apples. SEE: *acid.*

malign (mă-līn') [L. *malignus,* of bad kind]. Malignant. Tending to injure or harm.

malignancy (mă-lĭg′năn-sĭ) [L. *malignus*, of bad kind]. 1. Opposition to treatment. 2. Severe form of occurrence, tending to grow worse. SYN: *virulence.*

malignant (mă-lig′nănt) [L. *malignus*, of bad kind]. Virulent. Growing worse; resisting treatment, said of cancerous growths. Tending or threatening to produce death; harmful.

malinger (mă-ling′er) [Fr. *malingre*, weak, sickly]. To feign illness, usually to arouse sympathy, escape work, or to continue to receive compensation.

malingerer (mă-lĭng′ger-er) [Fr. *malingrē*, sickly, weak]. 1. One who pretends to be ill or to be suffering from a nonexistent disorder to arouse sympathy. 2. One who pretends slow recuperation from a disease once suffered in order to continue to receive benefits of sick insurance.

malleation (măl-lē-ā′shŭn) [L. *malleāre*, to hammer]. Spasmodic action of the hands in which they seem drawn to strike any near object, as spasmodic rapping against thighs, furniture, etc. SEE: *tic.*

malleoincudal (măl″lē-ō-ĭn′kū-dăl) [L. *malleus*, hammer, + *incus*, anvil]. Concerning or pert. to the malleus and incus.

malleolar (măl-le′o-lar) [L. *malleolus*, little hammer]. Concerning the malleolus.

malleolus (mă-le′o-lus) (pl. *malleolī*) [L. little hammer]. The protuberance on both sides of the ankle joint, the lower extremity of the fibula being known as the *lateral m.*, and the lower end of the tibia as the *medial malleolus.*

m., ext., lateral, outer. Process on outer edge of fibula at lower end.

m., int., inner, medial. Round process on inner edge of tibia at lower end.

mallet finger (mal′let) [L. *malleus*, hammer]. Loss of power of extension in a finger, causing permanent flexion. SYN: *drop-finger.*

m. toe. Abnormal flexion or loss of power of extension of a toe. SYN: *hammer toe.*

malleus (mal′ē-ŭs) (pl. *mallei*) [L. hammer]. [NA]. 1. The largest of the three auditory ossicles in the middle ear, attached to the eardrum, and articulating with the incus. 2. Glanders, an acute febrile disease with suppuration and necrosis of cartilage and bone.

Malloph′aga. An order of insects which includes the biting lice.

malnutrition (mal-nū-trĭ′shun). Lack of necessary food substances in the body or improper absorption and distribution of them.

MALNUTRITION

PHYSICAL SIGNS OF DEFICIENCY STATE*

Infants and Children

1. Lack of subcutaneous fat
2. Wrinkling of skin on light stroking
3. Poor muscle tone
4. Pallor
5. Rough skin (toad skin)
6. Hemorrhage of newborn (K)
7. Bad posture
8. Nasal blackheads and whiteheads
9. Sores at angles of mouth, cheilosis
10. Rapid heart
11. Red tongue
12. Square head, wrists enlarged, rib beading
13. Vincent's angina, thrush
14. Serious dental abnormalities
15. Corneal and conjunctival changes—slit lamp

Adolescents and Adults

1. Nasolabial sebaceous plugs
2. Sores at corners of mouth, cheilosis
3. Vincent's angina
4. Minimal changes in tongue color or texture
5. Red swollen lingual papillae
6. Glossitis
7. Papillary atrophy of tongue
8. Stomatitis
9. Spongy, bleeding gums
10. Muscle tenderness, extremities
11. Poor muscle tone
12. Loss of vibratory sensation
13. Increase or decrease of tendon reflexes
14. Hyperesthesia of skin
15. Bilateral symmetrical dermatitis
16. Purpura
17. Dermatitis; facial butterfly, Casal's necklace, perineal, scrotal, vulval.
18. Thickening and pigmentation of skin over bony prominences
19. Nonspecific vaginitis
20. Follicular hyperkeratosis of extensor surfaces of extremities
21. Rachitic chest deformity
22. Anemia not responding to iron
23. Fatigue of accommodation
24. Vascularization of cornea
25. Conjunctival changes

* Committee on Medical Nutrition, National Research Council.

mal″occlu′sion. Imperfect occlusion of the teeth. May be due to imperfect development, loss of teeth, abnormal growth of jaws.

malonylurea (mal-ō-nil-u′re-ă). Same as barbituric acid, *q.v.*

malpighian (măl-pĭg′ĭ-ăn). Concerning or described by Marcello Malpighi. [Italian microscopist, biologist, embryologist. Founder of histology. 1628-1694.]

m. body. 1. A malpighian corpuscle, *q.v.* 2. A splenic nodule, a spherical, ovoid body found in the white pulp of the spleen. Similar in structure to a lymphatic nodule.

m. corpuscle. SYN: *renal corpuscle.* A spherical body found in cortex of kidney consisting of a glomerulus and Bowman's capsule.

m. layer. SYN: *stratum germinativum, stratum mucosum, stratum Malpighii.* The innermost layer of the epidermis.

m. pyramid. A renal pyramid.

malposition (măl-pō-zĭ′shŭn) [L. *malus*, bad, + *positus*, from *ponere*, to place]. Faulty or abnormal position or placement, esp. of the body or one of its parts.

malpractice (măl-prak′tĭs) [" + G. *praxis*, an action]. Wrong or injurious treatment, esp. applied to performing illegal abortions.

malpresentation (mal-prē-zen-tā′shun) [" + *praesentatiō*, a presenting]. Abnormal position of fetus rendering natural delivery difficult or impossible.

malt (mawlt) [A.S. *mealt*]. Germinated grain, usually barley, used in manufacture of ale and beer. Contains carbohydrates (dextrin, maltose), a diastase, and proteins and is used as a food, esp. in wasting diseases.

m. extract. A viscous, light brown fluid obtained from wort (malt steeped in water).

m. sugar. Maltose, *q.v.*

Malta fever. SYN: *Mediterranean fever, Neapolitan fever, Gibraltar fever, undulant fever.* An infectious disease caused by one of three species of *Brucella* (*Br. melitensis* from goats, *Br. suis* from swine, and *Br. abortus* from cattle).

Transmitted principally from animals to man. May occur in acute or chronic form.

SYM: Swelling of the joints and spleen, excessive perspiration, weakness and anemia, and recurrent febrile attacks. Organisms tend to localize in tissues of the reticuloendothelial system, esp. spleen, liver, bone marrow, and lymph nodes.

maltase (mawl'tās) [A.S. *mealt*, grain]. A salivary and pancreatic enzyme which acts on maltose converting it by hydrolysis to glucose. SEE: *enzyme* and *digestion*.

maltose (mawl'tōs) [A.S. *mealt*, grain]. Malt sugar ($C_{12}H_{22}O_{11}$). A disaccharide present in malt, malt products, and sprouting seeds. It is formed by the hydrolysis of starch and is converted into glucose by the enzyme *maltase, q.v.* SEE: *carbohydrates* and *disaccharose*.

maltosur'ia. Presence of maltose in urine.

mal''turn'ed. Abnormally turned, said of a tooth turned on its long axis.

malum (ma'lŭm) [L. an evil]. A disease.

m. coxae senilis. Hip disease in the aged, exp. osteoarthritis.

m. perforans pedis. Ulcer of the foot of perforating type. It begins with thickening of the epidermis.

m. vene'reum. Syphilis.

malunion (măl-ūn'yŭn) [L. *malus*, bad, + *uniō*, oneness]. Growth of the fragments of a fractured bone in a faulty position, forming an imperfect union.

mamelonation (mam-el-ō-nā'shun) [Fr. *mamelle*, from L. *mamma*, breast]. Nipplelike prominences on a part or organ.

mamma (măm'ă) (pl. *mammae*) [L. breast]. One of two glands and structures in the female secreting milk; situated between the 3rd and 6th ribs when not pendulous. SYN: *breast, mammary gland.*

mammal (mam'al). An animal of the class Mammalis. Characterized by having breast from which milk is available for the nourishment of the newborn.

mammalgia (mam-al'jĭ-ă) [" + G. *algos*, pain]. Pain in the breast. SYN: *mastalgia.*

mammary (mam'ă-rĭ) [L. *mamma*, breast]. Pert. to the breast.

m. glands. Two compound glands of the female breast secreting milk. They are made up of lobes and lobules bound together by areolar tissue.

The main ducts are 15 to 20 in number and are known as *lactiferous* ducts, each one discharging through a separate orifice upon the surface of the nipple. The dilatations of the ducts form reservoirs for the milk during lactation.* The pink, or dark colored, skin around the nipple is called the *areola.** SYN: *mammae.*

RS: *breast; b., caked; galactagogue; gynecomastia; mammectomy; mastectomy; mastopathy; nipple.*

mammectomy (măm-mek'to-mĭ) [" + G. *ektomē*, excision]. Removal of the breast. SYN: *mastectomy.*

mammilla (măm-ĭl'lă) [L. nipple]. 1. Nipple. 2. Any structure resembling a nipple.

mammillary (mam'ĭl-lar-ĭ) [L. *mammilla*, nipple]. Like or concerning a nipple.

mammillated (mam'mĭl-lā-tĕd) [L. *mammilla*, nipple]. Having protuberances like a nipple.

mammillation (măm-ĭl-la'shŭn) [L. *mammilla*, nipple]. 1. Condition of having a granulated appearance or nipplelike projections. 2. A nipplelike protuberance.

mammilliform (mam-mĭl'ĭ-form) [" + *forma*, shape]. Shaped like a nipple.

mammilliplasty (măm-mĭl'ĭ-plăs-tĭ) [" + G. *plassein*, to form]. Plastic operation on a nipple. SYN: *theleplasty.*

mammillitis (măm-mĭl-ī'tĭs) [" + G. *-itis*, inflammation]. Inflammation of a nipple. SYN: *thelitis.*

mammitis (măm-ī'tĭs) [L. *mamma*, breast, + G. *-itis*, inflammation]. Inflamed condition of the breast. SYN: *mastitis.*

mammography (mam-og'ră-fĭ). Study of the breast by use of x-ray.

mammoplasty (mam'o-plas-tĭ). Surgical reconstruction of the breasts sometimes augmented by substances such as fat tissue or silicone to alter the size and shape.

mammose (mam'ōs) [L. *mamma*, breast]. 1. Having unusually large breasts. 2. Shaped like a breast.

mammotomy (măm-ot'ō-mĭ) [" + G. *tomē*, incision]. Surgery of a breast. SYN: *mastotomy.*

mammotropin (măm-ōt'rō-pĭn). Name of lactogenic principle of the ant. pituitary lobe. SYN: *prolactin.*

man (măn) [A.S. *mann*]. 1. Member of the human race; a human being. 2. Male member of the species. 3. The human race, collectively; mankind. SEE: *"anthrop-" words.*

mancinism (man'sĭn-ĭzm) [L. *mancus*, crippled]. State of being left-handed.

mandelic acid (man-del'ik). A crystalline compound derived from benzaldehyde.

USES: In the treatment of urinary infections, esp. pyelitis and cystitis.

It is necessary that the acidity of the urine be controlled; thus an acidifying agent, as ammonium chloride, is usually required when the sodium salt is used.

It is advised, because of renal irritation, that the drug be used not longer than 12-14 days.

Restriction of fluid intake is essential to keep urine volume below 1500 ml. per day in order that an effective concentration of mandelic acid is obtained.

mandible (man'dĭ-bl). The bone forming the lower jaw. SYN: *mandibula.* The inferior maxilla.

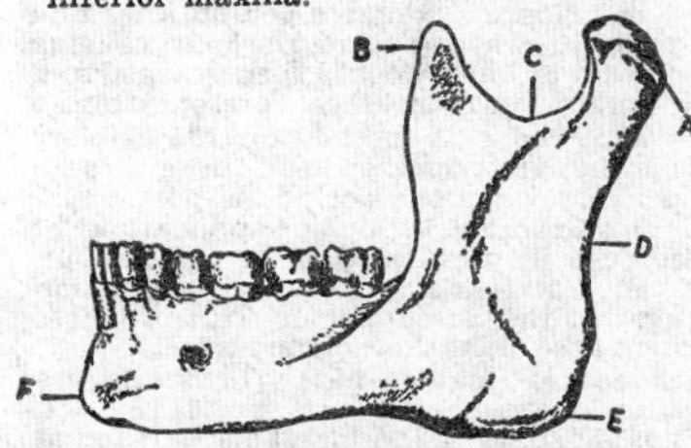

THE MANDIBLE.

A, Condyle; B, Coronoid process; C, Mandibular notch; D, Ramus; E, Angle; F, Mental protuberance.

mandibula (pl. *mandibulae*) (man-dib'-u-lă) [L.] [NA]. The bone of the lower jaw having a somewhat horseshoe shape.

mandibular (măn-dib'ū-lar). Rel. to the lower jaw.

m. reflex. Clonic movement resulting from percussing or stroking lower jaw.

m. and m. enema. One given because its ingredients form gases and distend the bowel, thus causing frequent and copious bowel movements. A mixture of milk and molasses, hence its name. SEE: *enema, m. and m.*

mandrin (man'drĭn) [Fr.]. A guide for a flexible catheter.

manducation (măn-dū-ka'shŭn) [L. *mandu̇cāre,* to chew]. The chewing of food. Syn: *mastication.*

maneuver (măn-ōō'ver) [Fr. *manoeuvre,* from L. *manu operari,* to work by hand]. Obs: Manipulation of the fetus and placenta to aid in delivery. See: *labor.*

m., Crede's. Method of expressing the placenta first described by Crede, in which the hand is placed on the fundus of the uterus with the thumb on the ant. wall and the fingers on the post. wall, the placenta being pushed out by pressure in the direction of the birth canal.

m., Leopold's. Method of abdominal palpation for the diagnosis of presentation and position of the fetus in utero.

m., Mauriceau - Smellie - Veit. Method employed to deliver the aftercoming head in breech presentation. Straddling the baby over the right arm, the index finger of that hand is introduced into the mouth of the child and applied over the maxilla; 2 fingers of the other hand are then hooked over the neck, grasping the shoulders. Downward traction is made until the occiput appears under the symphysis pubis. The body of the child is now raised up toward the mother's abdomen and the mouth, nose, brow and occiput are successively brought over the perineum.

m., Mulier's. Inspiratory effort with a closed glottis at the end of expiration. This produces negative intrathoracic pressure.

m., Munro Kerr. A method for determining the presence of disproportion bet. the fetal head and the maternal pelvis. The fetal head is pushed into the pelvis with the right hand on the abdomen, while with 2 fingers of the left hand in the vagina the possibilities of engagement of the head are noted. At the same time the thumb of the left hand feels over the brim of the pelvis to determine the degrees of overlapping.

m., Pinard's. Fingers behind knee and push it toward and past the body, causing flexion of knee. Foot is then grasped and brought down in breech presentation.

m., Prague. A method for the delivery of the aftercoming head in a breech delivery when the occiput is post.

m., Scanzoni. Double application of forceps in post. position of the occiput.

m., Valsalva's. Forcible expiration against the closed glottis. This produces increased intrathoracic pressure.

manganese (man'gă-nēz) [L. *manganesium*]. Symb: *Mn.* At. wt. 54.938; at. no. 25; sp. gr. 7.2. A metal element found in many foods, and in some plants, and in the tissues of the higher animals.

Functions: Its significance in the diet is not clear. It is believed to supplement copper in aiding in the formation of hemoglobin, although some think it has a nutritional function of its own. It is known to activate certain enzymes, for example, some of the phosphatases, and in experimental animals is essential for normal growth and reproductive activity.

Deficiency Sym: Subnormal growth and deficient tissue respiration.

Sources: *Ex:* Bananas, bran, beans, beets, blueberries, chard, chocolate, peas. *Good:* Leafy vegetables and whole grains.

Poisoning: A rather uncommon industrial poison found usually after prolonged exposure.

Sym: Muscular weakness, peculiar gait, tremors, central nervous system disturbances, salivation.

F. A. Treatment: Removal from source of exposure.

mania (mā'nĭ-ă) [G. *mania,* madness]. 1. Madness, characterized by excessive excitement. 2. A form of psychosis characterized by exalted feelings, delusions of grandeur, elevation of mood, psychomotor overactivity, and overproduction of ideas. See: *psychosis, manic-depressive.*

m. à pótu. Delirium tremens.

m., puerperal. A form of mental derangement occurring occasionally during the puerperium.

m., religious. Mania resulting from excessive religious fervor.

m., transitory. Short attacks of frenzy.

m., unproductive. Behavior characteristic of mania by lack of spontaneity in speech or muteness sometimes seen in manic-depressive psychosis. See: *alcoholism.*

maniac (mā'nĭ-ăk) [G. *mania,* madness]. A person with mental disease, usually one disturbed or excited.

maniacal (mă-nī'ăk-ăl) [G. *mania,* madness]. 1. Like a maniac. 2. Afflicted with mania.

man'ic-depres'sive psychosis. Cyclic or circular affective psychosis in which there are alternating moods of depression and mania. See: *psychosis, manic-depressive.*

man'ikin [D. *manneken,* little man]. 1. A model of the human body or its parts, used especially in teaching nursing procedures.

manipulation (mă-nip"u-la'shun) [L. *manipulāre,* to handle]. Any treatment or procedure involving use of the hands.

RS: *massage, osteopathy, spondylotherapy, Swedish movements.*

manipula'tive surgery. Use of manipulation in surgery, bonesetting, etc.

man'nerism. A peculiar modification of an ordinary movement.

Mann'kopf's sign [Emil W. Mannkopf, German physician, 1836-1918]. Pulse acceleration exhibited on pressing a painful point. Not present in feigned pain.

Mansonia. A genus of mosquito which transmits microfilaria to man.

manometer (măn-om'et-er) [G. *manos,* thin, + *metron,* measure]. Device for determining liquid or gaseous pressure.

mantle (man'tl) [A.S. *mentel,* a garment]. A covering structure or layer. Syn: *pallium.*

Mantoux's reaction, test (man-tooz'). Intracutaneous injection of old tuberculin. Within 24 to 72 hours the area becomes hard (indurated) and red if a tuberculous infection—active or inactive—is present.

manual (man'ū-al) [L. *manus,* hand]. 1. Pert. to the hands. 2. Performed by or with the hands.

manubrium (man-u'brĭ-um) [L. handle]. 1. The upper bone of the sternum articulating with the clavicle and first pair of costal cartilages. 2. That portion of the malleus* resembling a handle. See: *umbo.*

m. sterni. [NA]. Same as *manubrium, 1.*

manus (ma'nus) [L.]. The hand.

manustupration (man"u-stu-pra'shun) [L. *manustupratiō,* defilement by hand]. Masturbation.

marantic (mă-răn′tĭk) [G. *marainein*, to waste]. 1. Pert. to marasmus. 2. Wasting away.

marasmic (mă-raz′mĭk) [G. *marainein*, to waste]. Affected with marasmus; wasting away. Syn: *marantic.*

marasmus (mar-az′mus) [G. *marasmos*, wasting]. Emaciation, wasting. Infantile atrophy which occurs almost wholly as a sequel to acute diseases, esp. diarrheic diseases of infancy.

Most common from 6-18 months of age. Extreme wasting, child becoming a mere living skeleton.

Sym: May be vomiting and diarrhea, sleep restless, child uncomfortable and in pain, constantly hungry, frets, worries, suffers abdominal pain and headache. Feet edematous, urine scanty, anus and nates chafed and sore from urinal acidity and alkalinity or acidity of evacuations. Prostration becomes extreme, heart weak, abdomen distended, and mesenteric glands enlarged.

Prog: Fair, but recovery is slow.

Treatment: Often change of climate or simply from city to country is of great benefit. Keep in fresh air as much as possible. Oil baths.

Diet: Blandest kind of nourishment, as free from starch as possible. Different foods must be tried till one is found to suit the case. Constitutional treatment.

marble bones. Abnormally calcified bones with spotted appearance in a roentgenogram. Syn: *Albers-Schönberg disease, osteopetrosis.*

mareo (mar-ā′ō) [Sp. from L. *mare*, sea]. Seasickness.

m. de la Cordillera. Mountain sickness.

Marfan's syndrome. A hereditary condition of connective tissue, bones, muscles, ligaments and skeletal structures. Sym: Irregular, unsteady gait, lean, tall with stooping shoulders. Lincoln is said by some to have been thus afflicted. Syn: *arachnodactyly; dolichostenomelia.*

margarine. Artificial butter made from refined vegetable oils or a combination of vegetable oils and animal fats. Coloring material and vitamin A are added. Contains about 35 calories per teaspoonful. Syn: *oleomargarine.*

marginal (mar′jĭn-ăl) [L. *margō, margin-*, edge]. Concerning a margin or border.

margination (mar-jĭ-nā′shŭn) [L. *margō, margin-*, edge]. Adhesion of leukocytes to walls of blood vessel in first stages of inflammation.

margin′oplasty [" + G. *plassein*, to form]. Plastic surgery of a border, as of an eyelid.

margo (mar′go) [L.]. A border or edge.

m. acutus. A sharp margin of the heart extending from apex to the right.

m. obtusus. Portion of a line extending from apex to root of pulmonary artery which lies along rounded left side of left ventricle.

Marie's disease (mă-rē′) [Pierre Marie, French physician, 1853-1940]. Chronic condition of enlargement of bones and soft tissues of hands, feet and face. Syn: *acromegaly, hypertrophic pulmonary osteoarthropathy.*

M.'s sign. Hand tremor seen in exophthalmic goiter.

marijuana (mar-ĭ-wă′nă). Also spelled marihuana. An intoxicating excitant drug, used illegally in the U. S. and elsewhere usually in cigarette form. Obtained from top leaves and flowers of the Indian hemp plant (Cannabis sativa). Psychologically habituating but not habit-forming. Withdrawal of marijuana causes no such physical symptoms as opiate withdrawal does. Drug is considered to have no medical value.

Mariotte's law (mar-ē-ot′) [Edme Mariotte, French physician, 1620-1684]. Boyle's* law.

M.'s spot. The blind spot of the eye. Syn: *optic papilla.*

mark [A.S. *mearc*]. A nevus, bruise, cut or spot on the surface of a body.

m., birth-. Blemish on the skin at birth. A nevus.

m., port-wine. A congenital hemangioma or nevus vascularis, *q.v.*

m., strawberry. Same as nevus vascularis, *q.v.*

Marmo's method (mar′mōz) [Serafino Marmo, contemporary Italian obstetrician] (artificial respiration). A manner of performing artificial respiration in asphyxiated infants. The accoucheur places his hands in the infant's axillae and thereby raises the subject up in the air and suddenly releases his hands. A sudden drop of a foot or two will cause inspiration to occur, with expiration being effected by pressure of the accoucheur's hands against the chest wall.

mar′row [A.S. *mearh*]. The soft tissue occupying the medullary cavities of long bones, some haversian canals, and spaces between trabeculae of cancellous or spongy bone. Of two types, *red* and *yellow, q.v.*

In adult bone there are red and fat, or yellow, m. The yellow m. is found esp. in medullary cavity of long bones, and the red in spongy bones.

It consists of both fat and red marrow; from 20-80% fat marrow, to 100% red marrow. The marrow may be as high as 5% of body weight in an adult.

RS: *giant cell; leukomyelitis.*

m., gelatinous. Yellow marrow of old or emaciated persons, almost devoid of fat and having a gelatinous consistency.

m., red. That in cancellous tissue of bone. Concerned with the production of blood cells and hemoglobin.

m., spinal. Spinal cord.

m., yellow. That in the medullary canal of long bones. Consists principally of fat cells.

marsh fever. Malarial fever.

m. gas. Methane, *q.v.*

Marsh's test [James Marsh, English chemist, 1789-1846]. A test to detect the presence of arsenic.

marsupialization (mar-sū″pĭ-al-ĭ-za′shun) [L. *marsupium*, pouch]. Process of raising the borders of an evacuated tumor sac to the edges of the abdominal wound, and stitching them there to form a pouch.

The interior of the sac suppurates and gradually closes by granulation.

maschaladenitis (mas-kal-ad-ĕ-ni′tis) [G. *maschalē*, armpit, + *adēn*, gland, + *-ītis*, inflammation]. Inflammation of axillary glands.

maschaliatry (mas-kal-ĭ-at′rĭ) [" + *iatreia*, healing]. Treatment by axillary inunctions.

masculation (măs-kū-lā′shŭn) [L. *masculus*, a male]. Male sex characteristics formation.

masculine (măs′kū-lin) [L. *masculus*, a male]. Having male characteristics.

masculino″voblasto′ma. A benign ovarian tumor which resembles, microscopically, adrenal cortical tissue. Usually results in virilization.

maser. Initials of word stand for microwave amplification by stimulation emission of radiation. A device which produces a non-diverging radiation beam.

mask [Fr. *masque*]. 1. A covering for the face, as the gauze mask of a surgeon or nurse. 2. The countenance or appearance of the face such as appears in certain pathologic conditions.

m., BLB. A mask for delivering oxygen to aviators or to patients during anesthesia. Invented by Boothby, Lovelace, and Bulbulian.

m., death. A copy of the face molded in plaster of Paris soon after death.

m., ecchymotic. Cyanotic facies accompanying traumatic asphyxia.

m., Hutchinson's. A feeling of compression over face as though one is wearing a mask. A symptom of tabes dorsalis.

m., luetic. Blotchy brown pigmentation of cheeks, forehead and temples, seen in tertiary syphilis.

m., Parkinson's. Immobile facial appearance as a result of paralysis agitans (Parkinson's disease). The face is devoid of expression.

m. of pregnancy. Pigmented spots on the face seen in some pregnant women.

masked (măskd) [Fr. *masque*]. Concealed, esp. as in masked infection. Example: Women exposed to *Rubella* during the first trimester of pregnancy may be given immune globulin. This may prevent the clinical symptoms of *Rubella* in the mother, yet the fetus may still be adversely affected and be born with congenital defects.

masochism (mas'ō-kizm) [Named after Leopold von Sacher-Masoch, 1835-1895, Austrian novelist who described it]. Abnormal sexual passion in which one gains pleasure from the abuse or cruelty of his or her associate; hence any pleasure obtained from being abused or dominated. Opp. to sadism. SEE: *algolagnia; flagellation.*

masochist (mas'ō-kĭst). A person addicted to masochism.*

mass (măs) [L. *massa*, mass]. 1. A quantity of material, such as cells which unite or adhere to each other. 2. Soft, solid preparation for internal use, and of such consistency that it may be molded into pills. It is frequently prescribed alone or with other agents, and may be given in pill form or put into capsules. Two masses are official.

m., cell. An aggregation of cells which serves as the primordium (anlage) of a future organ or part.

m., epithelial. Inner portion of a developing gonad enclosed within the germinal epithelium.

m., inner cell. Mass of cells within the blastocyst from which the embryo, yolk sac, and amnion develop.

m., intermediate cell. A plate of nonsegmented mesoderm lying lateral to the segments (somites) and connecting them to the nonsegmented lateral mesoderm. Also called *nephrotome.*

mas'sa [L.]. Mass, *q.v.*

m. intermedia. The middle commissure, an inconstant mass of gray matter extending across third ventricle and connecting adjacent surfaces of the thalami.

massage (mas-săzh') [G. *massein*, to knead]. Manipulation; methodical pressure, friction and kneading of the body. Must always be applied upon the bare skin.

RS: *anatripsis, effleurage, flagellation, friction, frolement, fustigation, kneading, malaxation, masseur, petrissage, Swedish movements, tapotement, vibration.*

m., auditory. Massage of the eardrum membrane.

m., cardiac. Manual manipulation of the heart to restore heart beat after heart has stopped. Accomplished through an incision in the chest wall.

m., douche. Massage resulting from the application of a douche.

m., electrovibratory. Massage by means of an electric vibrator.

m., external cardiac. Accomplished by manual, rhythmic compression of chest wall and infraxiphoid area. This forces blood out of the heart as if the heart were beating. Also called *external cardiac compression.*

m., general. Consists of centripetal stroking in connection with some muscular kneading from the toes upward. Principally used for nervousness, being an important part of the well known "rest cure." Useful in connection with certain baths, duration 30-40 minutes. As soon as a part is massaged, it should be given a few passive rotary movements and afterwards covered up.

m., hydropneumatic. Massage by means of air forced through a tube at the end of which is a chamber containing water, the water chamber being applied to the part massaged.

m., introductory. Consists of centripetal strokings around the affected part; as in an affection of the knee joint, where introductory massage should be used on lower part of thigh and somewhat below the knee. Very useful in cases where it is impossible for operator to apply treatment directly to diseased parts.

m., local. Consists in treatment confined to particular parts.

m., tremolo. A variety of mechanic massage.

m., vapor. A treatment of a cavity by a medicated and nebulized vapor under interrupted pressure.

m., vibratory. Massage by rapidly repeated light percussion with a vibrating hammer or sound.

masseter (mas-sē'tĕr) [G. *masētēr*, chewer]. The muscle which closes the mouth and is the principal muscle in mastication.

masseur (mă-sur') [Fr.]. 1. A man who gives massages. 2. An instrument for massaging.

masseuse (mă-suz') [Fr.]. A woman who gives massages.

massive (măs'sĭv) [Fr. *massif*]. Bulky; consisting of a large mass; huge.

m. collapse of the lung. Dyspnea and pain in chest, esp. in patients who have suffered severe shock and collapse after abdominal operation or thyroidectomy.

Patient's condition resembles that of postoperative pneumonia, but the collapsed lung expands in 2-3 days. The condition is a dangerous one.

TREATMENT: That used for general collapse, Fowler's position, heat to affected side; inhalations of oxygen and carbon dioxide. SEE: *lung.*

massotherapy (măs-ō-ther'ă-pĭ) [G. *massein*, to knead, + *therapeia*, treatment]. Use of massage in treatment of disease.

mastadenitis (măst-ad-ĕ-ni'tis) [G. *mastos*, breast, + *adēn*, gland, + *-ītis*, inflammation]. A mammary gland inflammation.

mast"adeno'ma. A tumor of the breast.

mastalgia (mast-al'jĭ-ă) [" + *algos*, pain]. Pain in the breast. SYN: *mastodynia.*

mastatrophia (mast-ă-trō′fĭ-ă) [" + *a-*, priv. + *trophē,* nourishment]. Atrophy of breasts. SYN: *mastatrophy.*

mastatrophy (mast-at′rō-fĭ) [" + " + *trophē,* nourishment]. Atrophy of breasts. SYN: *mastatrophia.*

mastauxe (mas-tawk′se) [" + *auxē,* increase]. Excessive size of the breast.

mast cells. Connective tissue cells which contain heparin and histamine in their granules. Important in cellular defense mechanisms needed during injury or infection.

masteechymosis (măs-tĕk″ĭ′mō-sĭs). Ecchymosis of the breast.

mastectomy (mas-tek′to-mĭ) [G. *mastos,* breast, + *ektomē,* excision]. Excision of the breast.

POSTOPERATIVE NP: The doctor will tell the nurse how much information is to be given the patient and her family concerning the physical findings and laboratory reports. One of the nurse's responsibilities will be to recognize the patient's emotional reactions and to reassure her. Fear and anxiety are frequently present after this type of operation. The degree of mobility of the arm and shoulder will be determined by the surgeon and instructions for exercise must be carefully followed. Here again, the nurse is essential to the patient's physical and mental recovery.

masthelcosis (măs-thĕl-kō′sĭs) [G. *mastos,* breast, + *elkōsis,* ulceration]. Ulcerated condition of breast.

mastication (măs-tĭ-kā′shŭn) [L. *masticāre,* to chew]. Chewing. The comminution and insalivation of the food in the mouth is the first stage of digestion.

Certain muscles close the mouth, raise and lower the mandible, tense the cheeks, and accomplish the highly coordinated movements of the tongue.

The smell and taste of food stimulate sensory nerves, which reflexly elicit both motor and secretory activity in various digestive organs. Thus the salivary glands begin to secrete at once, and both the glands and the musculature of the stomach gradually become active. The saliva dissolves some substances, dilutes materials too concentrated for the stomach, hydrolyzes (due to the salivary enzyme, ptyalin) some of the starch to maltose, and lubricates material to be swallowed.

RS: *absorption, amasesis, enzyme, gastric and salivary digestion.*

masticatory (măs′tĭk-ă-tō-rĭ) [L. *masticāre,* to chew]. 1. Pert. to mastication. 2. Any substance chewed to stimulate secretion of saliva.

Mastigophora (măs-tĭ-gŏf′ō-ră). A class of protozoa characterized by the possession of one or more flagella. Includes both free-living and parasitic forms.

mastitis (măs-tī′tĭs) [G. *mastos,* breast, + *-ītis,* inflammation]. Inflammation of the breast.

Most common in women during lactation, but it may occur at any age.

ETIOL: May be due to entry of disease-producing germs through the nipple. In most cases there is a crack or abrasion of the nipple. Infection begins in one lobule but may extend to other areas.

SYM: The earliest sign is a triangular flush generally underneath the breast. There may be a high temperature and pulse rate.

m., cystic. M. resulting in formation of cysts which give the breast a nodular feeling upon palpation.

m., interstitial. Inflammation of connective tissue of the breast.

m., parenchymatous. Inflammation of the glandular substance of the breast.

m., puerperal. M. in later portion of puerperium and often accompanied by suppuration. Breast may become indurated owing to retention of milk.

m., stagnation. Caked breast.

mastocarcinoma (măst″ō-kăr-sĭn-ō′mă) [G. *mastos,* breast, + *karkinos,* crab cancer, + *-ōma,* tumor]. Carcinoma of the breast.

mastochondroma (mast″ō-kon-drō′mă) [" + *chondros,* cartilage, + *-ōma,* tumor]. Cartilaginous breast tumor.

mastodynia (măst-ō-dĭn′ĭ-ă) [" + *odynē,* pain]. Pain in the breast.

mastoid (mas′toid) [" + *eidos,* form]. 1. Pert. to mastoid process of the temporal bone. 2. The mastoid process of temporal bone. 3. Formed like a nipple.

m. antrum. Small chamber by which the mastoid cells communicate with the tympanic cavity.

m. bone. Mastoid process of temporal bone.

m. cells. Mastoid sinuses.

m. disease. Inflammation of mastoid.

m. operation. Outward drainage of mastoid cells.

m. portion of temporal bone. Portion of temporal bone lying behind ext. opening of ear and below temporal line. Contains *mastoid cells* and *antrum* and its inner surface bears a deep curved *sigmoid groove* which transmits a part of the transverse sinus.

m. process. Nipple-shaped process of mastoid portion of temporal bone extending downward and forward behind ext. auditory meatus. Serves for attachment of sternocleidomastoid, splenius capitis, and longissimus capitis muscles.

mastoidal (măs-toi′dăl) [" + *eidos,* form]. Rel. to mastoid process.

mastoida′le [" + *eidos,* form]. The mastoid process' lowest point.

mastoidalgia (mas-toid-al′jĭ-ă) [" + " + *algos,* pain]. Pain in the mastoid.

mastoidec′tomy [" + " + *ektomē,* excision]. Excision of mastoid cells. Rarely indicated since advent of antibiotics. May be *simple,* involving exenteration of the air cells of the mastoid process alone, or *radical,* involving the middle ear.

NP: Patient in dorsal position with small sand bag under shoulders. The area of operation is painted with iodine (3½%). Two sterile towels placed lengthwise under head and shoulders. One is brought up around head and is kept in place with towel clips. The other covers end of table. A laparotomy sheet is placed over patient, with opening over area of operation.

mastoideocentesis (măs-toid-ē-ō-sen-tē′-sĭs) [G. *mastos,* breast, + *eidos,* form, + *kentēsis,* puncture]. Surgical puncture of the mastoid process.

mastoiditis (măs-toid-ī′tis) [G. *mastos,* breast, + *eidos,* form, + *-itis,* inflammation] Inflammation of the air cells of the mastoid process.

COMPLICATIONS: Perisinus abscess, periphlebitis. lateral sinus thrombosis. Involvement is metastatic through blood vessels without erosion of sinus plate or extension of suppuration directly through sinus plate into the sinus.

SYM: Fever, chills, tenderness over emissary vein, leukocytosis, sepsis.

TREATMENT: Surgical.

m., Bezold's. Abscess underneath insertion of sternocleidomastoid muscle due to pus breaking through the tip cell.

m., externa. Inflammation of the periosteum of the mastoid process.

m., sclerosing. M. in which there is thickening and hardening of trabeculae between mastoid cells.

mastoidotomy (mas-toid-ot'ō-mĭ) [" + " + *tomē,* incision]. Incision into mastoid process.

mastology (mast-ol'ō-jĭ) [" + *logos,* study]. Science or study of the breasts.

mastomenia (mas-to-me'nĭ-ă) [" + *mēnēs,* menses]. Vicarious menstruation from the mammary glands.

mastoncus (mas-ton'kŭs) [" + *ogkos,* tumor]. Any tumor of the breast.

mastooccipital (mas"tō-ok-sĭp'ĭ-tăl) [G. *mastos,* breast, + L. *occipitalis,* pert. to occiput]. Rel. to mastoid process and occipital bone.

mastopathy (măs-top'ă-thĭ) [" + *pathos,* disease]. A disease of the mammary glands.

mastopexy (mas'tō-pĕks-ĭ) [" + *pēxis,* fixation]. Surgical correction of a pendulous breast. SYN: *mazopexy.*

mastoplasia (măst-ō-plā'zĭ-ă) [" + *plassein,* to form]. Hyperplasia of mammary gland tissue. SYN: *mazoplasia.*

mastoptosis (mas"to-to'sis). Pendulous breasts.

mastorrhagia (măs-tōr-ā'jĭ-ă) [G. *mastos,* breast, + *rēgnunai,* to burst forth]. Hemorrhage from the breast.

mastoscirrhus (măs-tō-skĭr'ŭs) [" + *skirros,* hardness]. A hard cancer of breast.

mastos'tomy. Incision into the breast.

mastotomy (mas-tot'o-mĭ) [" + *tomē,* incision]. Surgical incision of a breast.

masturbate (mas'ter-bāt) [L. *masturbārī,* to pollute one's self]. To arouse self-excitement through manipulation of the genital organs.

masturbation (măs-ter-bā'shŭn) [L. *masturbārī,* to pollute one's self]. Self-production of an orgasm by manipulating the genitals either by hand or some mechanical means.

RS: *manustupration, onanism, self-abuse.*

masu'rium. Former name of the element *technetium.*

match'es. Lucifer matches are usually made of phosphorus, *q.v.,* and potassium chlorate and may be lit by friction.

"Safety" matches contain antimony, sulfide and potassium chlorate and must be lit by striking on the box which is covered with red phosphorus.

POISONING SYM: Gastrointestinal irritation with blood changes.

F. A. TREATMENT: Wash out stomach with water or very dilute potassium permanganate. Repeated catharsis.

maté (mah'ta) [Sp. *mate,* vessel for preparing leaves]. Paraguay tea made from the leaves of *Ilex paraguayensis.*

Said to contain caffeine and tannin.

USES: Diaphoretic, diuretic, and for headaches.

materia alba. White cheeselike deposit along gum line about the necks of teeth, consisting of mucus, epithelial cells, food particles, leukocytes, and microorganisms.

materia medica (mă-tē'rĭ-ă mĕd'ĭ-kă) [L. medical matter]. That branch of science dealing with all drugs used in treatment of diseases, their source, preparation, dosage and use.

RS: *active principles, drug action, drug administration, medical preparations, pharmacognosy, pharmacology.*

mater'nal [L. *maternus,* pert. to a mother]. 1. Rel. to the mother. 2. From a mother.

maternity (mă-ter'nĭ-tĭ) [L. *mater,* mother]. 1. The condition of motherhood. 2. Lying-in hospital.

maternology (ma-ter-nol'ō-jĭ) [" + G. *logos,* study]. The scientific study of motherhood.

matrix (mā'trĭks) (pl. *matricēs*) [L. mother; womb]. 1. The womb. 2. The formative portion of a tooth or nail. 3. The intercellular substance of a tissue. 4. Mold for casting.

m. unguis. Nail bed.

matrixitis (mā-trĭks-ī'tĭs) [" + G. *-itis,* inflammation]. Inflammation of the bed of a nail. SYN: *onychia.*

matter. 1. Anything that occupies space. May be gaseous, liquid, or solid. 2. Pus, principally.

m., gray. SYN: *substantia grisea.* The gray substance of the spinal cord and brain, consisting principally of nerve-cell bodies, dendrites, and portions of axons. Also found in peripheral ganglia and retina of eye.

m., white. SYN: *substantia alba.* The white substance of spinal cord and brain, consisting principally of nerve fibers (myelinated and unmyelinated).

mattoid (mat'oid) [L. *mattus,* drunken, + G. *eidos,* form]. Person not in full control of mental faculties, but not to extent of insanity.

maturate (mat'u-rāt) [L. *maturus,* ripe]. 1. To ripen; to mature. 2. To suppurate. SYN: *suppurate.*

maturation (măt-ū-rā'shŭn) [L. *maturus,* ripe]. 1. Maturing; ripening, as a *graafian follicle.* 2. Suppuration. 3. The process in the development of germ cells (spermatozoa and ova) occurring in spermatogenesis or oogenesis in which the number of chromosomes is reduced from the diploid number to the haploid number (one half of diploid). Includes two cell divisions, the first qualitative (meiosis), the second quantitative. SEE: *oogenesis, spermatogenesis.*

mature (ma-tūr') [L. *maturus,* ripe]. Fully developed or ripened.

matu'rity [L. *maturus,* ripe]. State of being mature or fully developed; time when a person becomes capable of reproducing.

matutinal (ma-tū'tĭ-năl) [L. *matutinus,* morning]. Occurring early in the day, as *morning sickness;* in the morning.

matzoon (măt-soon') [Armenian]. Milk with a ferment containing lactic acid, bacilli and other organisms.

maxill'a (pl. *maxillae*) [L. jawbone]. [NA]. A jawbone, esp. the upper one; the superior maxilla. SEE: *skeleton.*

m., inferior. The lower jawbone, or mandible.

m., superior. Upper jawbone.

maxillary (măk'sĭ-la-rĭ) [L. *maxillaris,* pert. to the maxilla]. Pert. to the jaw, esp. the upper.

m. bones. Sup. and inf. maxillae; upper and lower jawbones.

m. sinus. The antrum of Highmore, air cavity in sup. maxilla opening into middle meatus of nose.

maxillitis (măks'ĭl-ī'tĭs) [L. *maxilla,* jawbone, + G. *-itis,* inflammation]. 1. Inflammation of maxilla. 2. Inflammation of the submaxillary (submandibular) gland.

maxillofa'cial. Pert. to the lower half of the face.

maximal (maks'ĭ-mal) [L. *maximus,* greatest]. Greatest possible; highest.

maximum (maks'ĭ-mum) [L. greatest]. 1. The greatest quantity. 2. Height of a disease.

Mayo-Robson's point [Arthur Mayo-Robson, London surgeon, 1853-1933]. A point just above and to right of the umbilicus, where pressure causes tenderness in pancreatic disease.

mazopexy (mā'zō-pĕks-ĭ) [G. *mazos,* breast, + *pēxis,* fixation]. Correction of a pendulous breast by surgical fixation. SYN: *mastopexy.*

mazoplasia (mā-zo-plā'zĭ-ă) [" + *plassein,* to form]. Hyperplasia of mammary gland tissue. SYN: *mastoplasia.*

Mc. Abbr. for *megacurie.*

mc. Abbr. for *millicurie.*

McBurney's incision [Charles McBurney, New York surgeon, 1845-1914]. Abdominal incision employed in appendectomy.

An incision is made parallel to the path of external oblique muscle, about 1-2 inches away from ant. sup. spine of right ilium, cutting through the external oblique to the internal oblique and transversalis, separating their fibers.

McB.'s point. Point of tenderness in acute appendicitis, situated on a line bet. the umbilicus and the right ant. sup. iliac spine, about 1 or 2 inches above the latter.

McCarthy's reflex. Contraction of orbicularis palpebrarum with closure of lids resulting from percussion above supraorbital nerve.

McCormac's reflex. Adduction of one leg resulting from percussion of patella tendon of opposite leg.

mcg. Abbr. for *microgram.*

MCH. Abbr. for *mean corpuscular hemoglobin.* The amount of hemoglobin in each red blood cell.

mc.h. Abbr. for *millicurie hour.*

MCHC. Abbr. for *mean corpuscular hemoglobin concentration.* Average hemoglobin concentration in each red blood cell, expressed as a percentage value.

MCV. Abbr. for *mean corpuscular volume.* Expressed as the average volume, in cubic microns, of red blood cells.

M.D. [L. *Medicinae,* doctor]. Abbr. for *Doctor of Medicine.* In spoken and written English shortened to Doctor. This usage, esp. in nonmedical circles, may lead to confusion. *Doctor* may mean dentist, veterinarian or other persons possessing a doctoral degree (*e.g.,* Ph.D., Doctor of Philosophy). Thus, when practical, the word *physician* is preferred over *doctor* when doctor of medicine is intended.

meal (mēl) [A.S. *māēl,* measure, meal]. Portion of food eaten at a particular time to satisfy the appetite. SEE: *test m., von Leube motor test m., von Leube's test m.*

mean (mēn) [L. *medius,* in middle]. In statistics, a number derived from a series of other numbers by a prescribed method of computation. SEE: *median.*

Thus the *arithmetic mean* (commonly called the average) of a series of n numbers is obtained by adding all the numbers and dividing the sum by n.

measles (mē'zls) [Dutch *maselen*]. Rubeola. A highly communicable virus disease characterized by catarrhal symptoms and by a typical eruption on the skin and mucous membranes of the mouth (Koplik's spots). It occurs usually before adolescence. The occurrence of measles before the age of six months is relatively uncommon.

An attack of measles almost invariably confers permanent immunity. Active immunization can be produced by administration of measles vaccine, preferably that containing the live attenuated virus, although measles vaccine containing the inactivated virus is available for individuals in whom the live attenuated type is contraindicated. Passive immunization is afforded by administration of gamma globulin.

INCUBATION: Ten to 14 days.

SYM: Onset gradual; coryza, rhinitis, drowsiness, loss of appetite, gradual elevation of temperature for first 2 days, when fever may rise from 101-103° F. Photophobia and cough soon develop, although some recession in the temperature may occur.

About 4th day, fever usually reaches a higher elevation than previously, at times as high as 104-106° F., and with this recurrence the rash appears.

Eruption first appears on face, being seen early as small maculopapular lesions which rapidly increase in size and coalesce in places, often causing a swol-

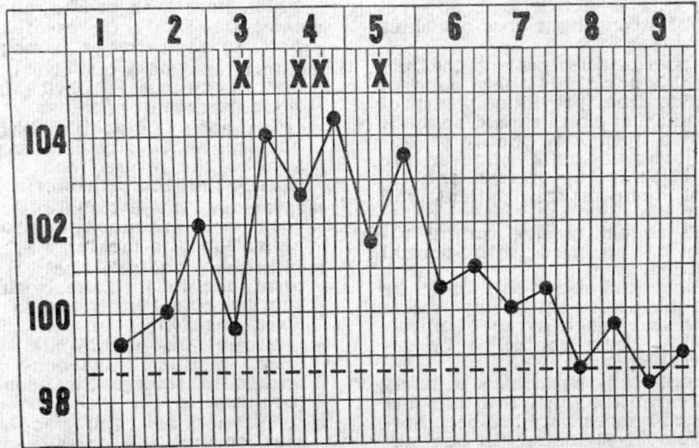

USUAL COURSE OF FEVER IN MEASLES.
(Landon, John F., and Sider, Helen T.: Communicable Diseases, 8th Ed., 1964.)

len, mottled appearance. The rash extends to the body and extremities, and in some areas may assume a deviousness suggestive of scarlet fever.

A cough, present at this time, is due to the bronchitis produced by the inflammatory condition of the mucous membranes that undoubtedly corresponds to the rash seen on the skin. Ordinarily, the rash lasts from 4-5 days and, as it subsides, the temperature declines. Consequently, by the end of 5 days from appearance of rash, temperature should be normal, or approximately normal in uncomplicated cases. Prior to appearance of the eruption, a leukocytosis may be noted. Following presence of rash, a leukopenia may always be expected.

COMPLICATIONS: Encephalitis is the most dreaded complication and has a poor prognosis. Bronchopneumonia is a serious complication of measles. Otitis media, followed by mastoiditis, brain abscess, or even meningitis, is not rare. Cervical adenitis with marked cellulitis sometimes leads to fatal consequences. Tracheitis and laryngeal stenosis, due to edema of glottis, are sometimes seen in the course of measles.

Eye Complications: Not common in measles, although a marked conjunctivitis usually occurs.

DIFFERENTIAL DIAG: Scarlet fever, German measles, the prodromal rash of smallpox, or even cases of confluent smallpox may have to be considered. If the measles patient is observed prior to appearance of rash, or sometimes even after rash has developed, a definite decision may be based on the presence of Koplik's spots, *q.v.*

Hemorrhagic spots are also seen on the hard palate and mucous membranes many times before rash is evident on the skin. These spots probably correspond to the typical maculopapular eruption of the disease.

PROG: While usually favorable in the well-nourished child, the seriousness of the possible complications of measles should not be minimized.

TREATMENT AND NP: Patient isolated in a well-ventilated room, since, when a respiratory infection is being dealt with, good ventilation is of utmost importance. Though a room is frequently darkened, this is not a necessary requirement if strong light does not shine in patient's face.

The average measles patient does not care to eat during first few days of illness. Aside from providing plenty of fluids, no unusual effort should be made to force food upon him. Plenty of water, fruit juices and milk, however, are desirable. With fading of rash and reduction of temperature, patient will soon regain his appetite.

The eyes should receive careful attention, being cleansed with normal saline solution.

The cough and laryngitis may be controlled to some extent by steam inhalations and cough syrup of physician's choice. Fever controlled by aspirin or cool sponges.

QUARANTINE: It is customary in many states to quarantine until rash has disappeared and temperature has been normal for from 24-48 hours. In the uncomplicated cases, this usually means that the duration of the quarantine will be approximately 10 days from the date of onset. Measles is much more contagious before eruption than it is after eruption has appeared. Consequently, it is not at all likely that the quarantine of measles patients exerts any influence on the control of a measles epidemic. On the other hand, quarantine of susceptible contacts is plainly beneficial in limiting exposures and preventing the spread of infection.

Human gamma globulin or immune serum globulin for passive immunization. Measles vaccine• believed to provide safe and effective active immunization.

SEE: *Koplik's spots, rubella, rubeola.*

m., black. A serious form of measles characterized by hemorrhagic areas in the skin and marked constitutional symptoms.

m., German. Rubella, *q.v.*

m., hemorrhagic. Black measles, *q.v.*

measure (mĕ'zhūr) [Fr. *mesure*, from L. *mensura*, a measuring]. 1. A determined extent or quantity. 2. To determine the extent or amount of an area or substance.

meat. 1. The edible portion of anything. 2. The flesh of animals, including poultry, which is used for food.

Meat is an important source of vitamins, esp. those of the B complex (thiamine, riboflavin, niacin). Pork is especially rich in thiamine. Liver has an unusually high vitamin content, esp. of vitamin A. The glandular organs such as liver and kidney contain a considerably higher percentage of certain mineral elements and vitamins than are found in other forms of meat.

Nitrogenous extractives, purines and mineral salts give flavor to meat. Lean meat contains about 1% of mineral ash. Clear fat has almost none. The amount of mineral elements in lean meat is proportional to the amount of protein it contains. It is rich in phosphorus, potassium, iron, and it has a good percentage of other minerals, but is deficient in calcium. The ash constituents differ somewhat in the different groups (beef, pork, etc.), and in the same animals at different ages, but in all meats the acid-forming elements are decidedly in excess of the base-forming.

Meat has been assailed for several reasons: "It forms acids in the body"; "it is hard on the kidneys"; "it is conducive to 'autointoxication,'" all of which have been proved unwarranted.

meatal (mē-ā'tăl) [L. *meatus*, passage]. Pert. to a meatus or passage.

meatometer (mē-ă-tom'ĕt-ĕr) [" + G. *metron*, measure]. Device for measuring a passage or opening.

meatorrhaphy (mē-at-or'af-ĭ) [L. *meatus*, passage, + G. *raphē*, a sewing]. Suture of the severed end of a meatus, usually the *meatus urinarius.*

meatoscopy (mē-ă-tos'kō-pĭ) [" + G. *skopein*, to examine]. Instrumental examination of a meatus.

meatotome (mē-at'ō-tōm) [" + G. *tomē*, incision]. Knife with probe or guarded point for enlarging meatus by direct incision.

meatotomy (mē-at-ot'ō-mĭ) [" + G. *tomē*, incision]. Incision of urinary meatus to enlarge the opening. SYN: *porotomy.*

meatus (mē-ā'tŭs) (pl. *meatūs*) [L. *meatus*, opening]. A passage or opening.

m. acusticus externus. [NA]. External auditory canal from tympanum to pinna.

m. acusticus internus. [NA]. Canal in the petrous portion of temporal bone, containing facial and auditory nerves and vessels.

m. auditorius. SEE: *m. acusticus, ext.* and *int.*

m. nasi communis. Common nasal cavity on either side of septum.

m. nasi inferior. [NA]. Space beneath inf. turbinate.

m. nasi medius. [NA]. Space beneath middle turbinate or concha.

m. nasi superior. [NA]. Space beneath sup. turbinate or concha.

m. nasopharyngeus. [NA]. Posterior portion of nasal cavity which communicates with the nasopharynx.

m. urinarius. External opening of the urethra; usually said of the male.

mechanical rectifier. A device which, by changing contacts at the proper moment in a cycle, changes alternating current into pulsating direct current.

mechanicoreceptor, mechanoreceptor (mĕ-kan″ĭ-co-re-sep′tor, mek″ă-no-re-sep′-tor). A receptor which receives mechanical stimuli such as pressure from sound or touch.

mechanics (mē-kăn′ĭks) [G. *mēchanē,* machine]. Science of force and matter.

mech′anism. PSY: Combination of mental processes by which a result is obtained.

mechanology (mĕk-ăn-ŏl′ō-jĭ) [" + *logos,* study]. Study of force and matter.

mechanoreceptor, mechanicoreceptor. SEE: *mechanicoreceptor.*

mechanotherapy (mĕk″an-ō-thĕr′ă-pĭ) [G. *mēchanē,* machine, + *therapeia,* treatment]. Use of various types of mechanical apparatus to perform passive movements and to exercise various parts of the body. Ex: MacKenzie and Zander apparatus.

meckelectomy (mek-el-ek′tō-mĭ) [G. *ektomē,* excision]. Excision of Meckel's ganglion.

Meckel's cartilage. A cartilaginous bar about which the mandible develops.

M.'s divertic′ulum. A congenital sac or blind pouch sometimes found in lower portion of the ileum. Representing the persistent proximal end of the yolk stalk. Sometimes is continued to the umbilicus as a cord, or as a tube forming a fistulous opening at the umbilicus. Strangulation may cause intestinal obstruction. SEE: *diverticulum, diverticulitis.*

M.'s ganglion. G. located in the sphenomaxillary fossa giving off nerves to eyes, nose and palate. SYN: *sphenopalatine g.*

M.'s space. Area in dura holding the gasserian ganglion.

meclizine hydrochloride (mek′lĭ-zēn). USP. Antiemetic esp. effective for control of nausea and vomiting of motion sickness. Trade name: Bonine.

mecometer (mē-kom′ĕt-ĕr) [G. *mēkos,* length, + *metron,* measure]. Device for measuring an infant's length.

meconism (mek′ō-nizm) [G. *mēkōn,* poppy, + *ismos,* condition of]. 1. Opium poisoning. 2. The opium habit.

meconium (me-kō′nĭ-um) [G. *mēkōnion,* poppy juice]. 1. Opium; poppy juice.

2. First feces of a newborn infant, made up of salts, liquor amnii, mucus, bile and epithelial cells; greenish black to light brown, almost odorless and of a tarry consistency.

Evacuated by 3rd or 4th day after birth. Its disappearance should not be hastened, as it is a preventive of early infection.

mecystasis (mē-sis′tă-sĭs). Process in which a muscle maintains its original degree of tension although its length is increased.

M.E.D. Abbr. for *minimal effective dose.*

medi- [L.]. Prefix: The *middle.*

media (me′dĭ-ă) [L. middle]. 1. Middle or muscular coat of an artery. SYN: *tunica media.* 2. Plural of *medium.*

mediad (me′dĭ-ad). Toward the median line for plane of the body.

me′dial [L. *medius,* middle]. 1. Pert. to middle. 2. Nearer the medial plane.

me′dian [L. *medius,* middle]. 1. Middle; central. 2. In statistics, a number obtained by arranging the given series in order of size and taking the middle number; one then has as many greater as there are less. Thus, in the series 5, 7, 8, 9, 10 the median is 8. SEE: *mean.*

m. artery. A branch of the volar interosseous artery.

m. line. An imaginary line extending longitudinally on the ant. or post. surface of the body marking the edges of the median plane, *q.v.*

m. nerve. One of motion and sensation having its origin in the brachial plexus.

m. plane. The midsagittal plane; a vertical plane through the trunk and head dividing the body into right and left halves.

mediastinal (mē-dĭ-ăs-tī′năl) [L. *mediastinus,* in middle]. Rel. to the mediastinum.

mediastinitis (mē-dĭ-as-tī-nī′tis) [" + G. *-ītis,* inflammation]. Inflammation of tissue of the mediastinum.

mediastinopericarditis (mē-dĭ-ăs″tī-nō-pĕr″ĭ-kăr-dī′tĭs) [" + G. *peri,* around, + *kardia,* heart, + *-ītis,* inflammation]. Inflammatory condition of mediastinum and pericardium.

mediastinum (mē-dĭ-ăs-tī′nŭm) [L. in the middle]. 1. A septum or cavity bet. two principal portions of an organ. 2. [NA]. The folds of the pleura and intervening space bet. right and left lung. The interpleural space. It contains the thoracic viscera. SEE: *chylomediastinum.*

m. testis. [NA]. SYN: *corpus Highmori, or body of Highmore.* The thickened portion of the tunica albuginea on post. surface of testis.

m., thoracic. The space between the pleural cavities which encloses the heart and pericardium; large vessels entering and leaving heart, thoracic duct, vagus and phrenic nerves, trachea, esophagus, and thymus. Extends from sternum to vertebral column. Divided into superior, middle, inferior, anterior, and posterior portions.

mediate (me′dĭ-āt) [L. *mediatus,* in the middle]. 1. Accomplished by indirect means. 2. Between two parts or sides.

medic. A member of the medical team in the U.S. Armed Forces.

medicable (med′ĭ-kă-bl) [L. *medicārī,* to heal]. Amenable to cure.

medical (mĕd′ĭ-kal) [L. *medicārī,* to heal]. Pert. to medicine.

m. jurisprudence. Principles of medicine in their application to questions of law.

m. preparations. SOLID SUBSTANCES: Capsule or *capsula;* cachet, confection or *confectio;* cerate or *ceratum;* extract or *extractum;* lozenge or *trochiscus; lamella**; ointment or *unguentum;* plaster or *emplastrum;* powder or *pulvis;* pill or *pilula;* paper or *charta;* sterule* or *sterula;* suppository or *suppositorium;* tablet or *tabella;* vescette.*

FLUIDS: Fluidextract, or *fluidextractum;* tincture or *tinctura;* infusion or *infusum;* decoction or *decoctum;* wine or *vinum;* oleoresin or *oleoresina.*

SUSPENSIONS: Mixture or *mixtura;* emulsion or *emulsum.*

SOLUTIONS: Water or *aqua;* mucilage or *mucilago;* solution or *liquor;* elixir or *elixir;* syrup or *syrupus;* spirit or *spiritus;* glycerite or *glyceritum;* vinegar or *acetum.*

MISC: Liniment or *linimentum;* oleate or *oleatum.*

RS: *alkaloid, active principle, names of preparations, drugs with two names; antidote; dosage; drug action; drugs and their administration; names of individual drugs in alphabetical order; names of poisons; poison; poisoning; preparations usually given by rectum; prescription writing.*

medical corpsman. An enlisted man in the U.S. Armed Forces who works as a member of the medical team. Also called *corpsman.*

med'icament [L. *medicamentum*]. A medicine or remedy.

RS: *epispastic, errhine, escharotic, evacuant, medical preparations, rubefacient, saponin, sedative, specific, vesicant, vesicatory.*

medicate (mĕd'ĭ-kāt) [L. *medicari,* to heal]. 1. To treat a disease with drugs. 2. To impregnate with medicinal substances.

medication (mĕd-ĭ-kā'shŭn) [L. *medicāri,* to heal]. 1. Treatment with remedies. 2. Impregnation with medicine.

m., hypodermic. Treatment by injection of remedies beneath the skin.

m., ionic. Introduction of ions of drugs into the body by cataphoresis.

m., sublingual. Treatment with an agent, usually in tablet form, placed under the tongue.

m., substitutive. Medical therapy to cause a nonspecific inflammation to counteract a specific one.

ROUTES OF MEDICATION

m. r., inhalation. By use of masks, atomizers, or vaporizers.

m. r., intra-arterial. Introduction of medicaments or blood into an artery.

m. r., intracardiac. Introduction of a drug into heart muscle or one of the heart chambers.

m. r., intracutaneous (intradermal, endermic). Injection of drug between layers of skin.

m. r., intramedullary. Introduction of fluids into bone marrow, esp. that of sternum.

m. r., intramuscular. Introduction of drug into muscles. Usual sites are deltoid or triceps muscles, or gluteus maximus. ABBR: I.M.

m. r., intranasal. Introduction of nosedrops or jellies for antiseptic, antihistaminic, or vasoconstrictive effects.

m. r., intrathecal. Introduction into subdural space of spinal cord. Spinal fluid is withdrawn equal to that introduced.

m. r., intravenous. Injection of fluids into a vein, usually the basilic or median cubital vein. ABBR: I.V.

m. r., iontophoresis (ion transfer). Introduction of drugs into deeper layers of the skin by a galvanic electric current.

m. r., oral. Introduction by mouth. Not available for drugs destroyed by digestion, or those incapable of absorption, or drugs that are irritating to mucous membranes.

m. r., rectal. Drugs may be given in form of liquids or suppositories.

In diseases of the rectum and adjacent parts, medication is often applied by way of the anus, esp. if medication cannot be adm. by mouth, as in persistent nausea or emesis, during unconsciousness or delirium, or on account of the bad taste of the medication.

Almost any drug other than those of a corrosive nature may be adm. through the rectum.

Three points must be kept in mind: (1) The rectum must be free of fecal material. A purgative enema should be given an hour before the rectal medicine in order that peristalsis will subside and there will be no fecal contents to absorb the medicated solution.

(2) The medicinal substance must be readily soluble. The solution must have the consistency of thin starch, and be given at body temperature. A normal salt solution of 4 oz. with 5% glucose is a common medicated enema.

(3) The solution is given slowly through a small catheter attached to a funnel. The patient, who remains on his left side for 10 minutes, is assisted in retaining the fluid by pressure on the anus with cotton or tissues.

m. r., subcutaneous. Injection of drugs or implantation of pellets under the skin.

m. r., sublingual. Absorption of drugs by the sublingual mucosa.

m. r., vaginal. Drugs may be given in liquid form by douche or in the form of suppository, powder, or paint.

medicinal (mĕ-dĭ'sĭn-ăl) [L. *medicina,* medicine]. Pert. to medicine.

m. enema. One to which some drug or medication has been added, for retention or absorption, particularly in cases where medication cannot be adm. by mouth. SEE: *enema.*

medicine (mĕd'ĭ-sĭn) [L. *medicina*]. 1. A drug. 2. The art of preventing, caring for, and assisting in the cure of disease, and the care of the injured. 3. Treatment of disease medically as distinguished from surgery.

m., aerospace. Branch of medicine concerned with pathology and physiology of men and animals who travel in air and space craft, both in the Earth's atmosphere and in outer space, and concerned with the selection of men for duty as pilots or crew members for flight and space missions.

m., clinical. Observation and treatment at the bedside.

m., environmental. Concerned with diseases and conditions peculiar to working conditions. SYN: *occupational medicine, industrial medicine.*

m., experimental. The scientific study of disease or pathologic conditions by experimentation upon laboratory animals, or through clinical research.

m., forensic. Application of medical knowledge to legal affairs.

m., group. (a) The practice of medicine by a group of physicians, usually consisting of specialists in various fields who pool their services and share jointly laboratory and x-ray facilities. Such a group is commonly called a clinic. (b) The securing of medical services by a group of individuals who, upon paying definite sums of money, are entitled to certain medical services or hospitalization in accordance to prearranged rules and regulations.

m., internal. 1. Treatment of diseases involving the internal structures. 2.

Treatment of diseases nonsurgical in nature.

m., legal. Forensic medicine.

m., patent. A medicine for which a patent has been granted. SEE: *patent medicine.*

m., physical. SYN: *physiotherapy, physical therapy.* Treatment of disease by physical agents such as heat, cold, light, electricity, manipulation, or the use of mechanical devices.

m., preventive. The practice of preventing disease.

m., proprietary. Medicine in which proprietary interests have been secured by patent, copyright of labels, or secrecy of composition. SEE: *proprietary medicine.*

m., psychosomatic. Treatment of disease of mental and physical origin, esp. the study of the emotional or psychic conditions as a cause or factor in bodily disorders. SEE: *psychosomatic.*

m., socialized. Practice of medicine under control and direction of the State.

m., state. SYN: *public medicine.* Branch of medical science which is concerned with collection of vital statistics, public health, esp. control of contagious diseases, food and drug control, etc.

m., tropical. Branch of medical science which deals principally with diseases common in tropical or subtropical regions.

m., veterinary. That which deals with the diagnosis and treatment of diseases of animals.

medicine man. Person from a primitive culture whose alleged healing powers are derived from mystical and magical sources. SYN: *shaman.*

medicinerea (měd″ĭ-sĭn-ē′rē-a) [L. *medius,* middle, + *cinerea,* ashen]. Internal gray matter of the claustrum and lenticula of the brain.

medicochirurgical (měd″ĭ-kō-kī-rur′jĭ-kăl) [L. *medicus,* medical, + G. *cheir,* hand, + *ergon,* work]. Concerning both medicine and surgery.

medicolegal (měd″ĭ-kō-lē′găl) [" + *legalis,* legal]. Rel. to medical jurisprudence or forensic medicine.

medicornu (med-ĭ-kor′nu). The inferior horn of the lateral ventricle of the brain.

Medina worm. *Dracunculus medinensis, q.v.*

medio- [L.]. Prefix meaning *the middle.*

mediopontine (mē″dĭ-ō-pon′tĭn) [L. *medius,* middle, + *pons, pont-,* bridge]. Rel. to center of the pons Varolii.

mediotarsal (mē″dĭ-ō-tar′săl) [" + G. *tarsos,* tarsus]. Rel. to the middle of the tarsus.

Mediterranean anemia. Thalassemia, *q.v.* (Cooley's anemia). Also called *M. disease.*

M. fever. Brucellosis, *q.v.;* undulant fever.

medium (mēd′ĭ-ŭm) (pl. *media*) [L. middle]. 1. An agent through which an effect is obtained. 2. Substance used for the cultivation of microorganisms. SYN: *culture medium.* 3. Substance through which impulses are transmitted.

medulla (mĕ-dul′lă) [L. marrow]. 1. The marrow. 2. Inner or central portion of an organ, in contrast to the outer portion or cortex. 3. Medulla oblongata.

m., adrenal. Inner portion of the adrenal gland composed of chromaffin tissue. Secretes epinephrine. SEE: *adrenal.*

m. of hair. Central axis of a hair.

m. of kidneys. Renal pyramids.

m. nephrica. Pyramids of kidneys.

m. oblongata. Enlarged portion of spinal cord in cranium after it enters the foramen magnum of the occipital bone; the lower portion of the brain stem.

m. ossium. Marrow in bone.

m. of ovary. Central portion of the ovary composed of loose connective tissue, blood vessels, lymphatics, and nerves.

m. spinalis. Spinal cord.

medullary (med′ū-lar-ĭ) [L. *medulāris,* pert. to marrow]. Concerning marrow or medulla.

medullated (med′ū-lāt-ĕd) [L. *medulla,* marrow]. Covered by or containing marrow or medulla.

m. nerve fiber. A nerve fiber possessing a myelin or medullary sheath; a myelinated nerve fiber.

medullation. Acquiring of a myelin sheath.

medullitis (mĕd-ū-lī′tĭs) [" + G. *-itis,* inflammation]. Inflammation of marrow. SYN: *myelitis.*

medullization (mĕd-ū-lĭ-zā′shŭn) [L. *medulla,* marrow]. Conversion to marrow abnormally.

medulloarthritis (mĕ-dul″o-ar-thrī′tĭs) [" + G. *arthron,* joint, + *-ītis,* inflammation]. Inflammation of marrow elements of bone ends.

medulloblastoma (mĕ-dul′o-blas-tō′mă) [L. *medulla,* marrow, + G. *blastos,* germ, + *-ōma, tumor*]. A malignant, soft, infiltrating tumor of the roof of the 4th ventricle and cerebellum. Often invades the meninges.

medullocell (mĕ-dul′o-sĕl) [" + *cellula,* little box]. Marrow cell. SYN: *myelocyte.*

medulloepithelioma (mĕ-dul′o-ep″ĭ-thēl-ĭ-ō′mă) [" + G. *epi,* upon, + *thēlē,* nipple, + *-ōma,* tumor]. Tumor composed of retina epithelium and of neuroepithelium. SYN: *neuroepithelioma, glioma.*

mega- [G.]. Combining forms meaning *great, large,* or gravity of one million (10^6).

megabladder (mĕg′ă-blăd-ĕr) [" + A.S. *blaedre*]. Permanent abnormal distention of the urinary bladder. SYN: *megalocystis.*

megacardia. Enlargement of the heart. SYN: *cardiomegaly.*

megacephalic (mĕg-ă-sĕf-al′ĭk) [" + *kephalē,* head]. Having an abnormally large head. SYN: *macrocephalous.*

megacoccus (mĕg-ă-kok′ŭs) [" + *kokkos,* berry]. A large size coccus. SYN: *macrococcus.*

megacolon (meg-ă-ko′lon) [" + *kōlon,* colon]. Extremely dilated colon.

Usually congenital, and occurs also in infancy or childhood. In congenital cases, acetylcholine is used as a diagnostic test. SEE: *Hirschsprung's disease.*

megacoly (meg′ă-kol-ĭ) [" + *kōlon,* colon]. Dilatation of the colon.

megadont (mĕg′ă-dont) [G. *megas,* large, + *odous, odont-,* tooth]. Possessing very large teeth. SYN: *macrodont.*

megadyne (meg′ă-dīn) [" + *dynamis,* power]. A unit equal to one million dynes.*

megakaryoblast (mĕg″ă-kăr′ĭ-ō-blăst). An immature megakaryocyte.

megakaryocyte (mĕg″ă-kar′ĭ-ō-sīt) [" + *karyon,* nucleus, + *kytos,* cell]. Large bone marrow cell with large or multiple nuclei. SYN: *megaloblast, myeloplax.*

megalakria (mĕg-ă-lak'rĭ-ă) [" + *akros*, extremity]. Trophic disorder marked by progressive enlargement of head, hands, feet, and thorax. SYN: *acromegaly*.

megalencephaly (mĕg-ăl-ĕn-sĕf'ă-lĭ). Abnormally large size of the brain, usually accompanied by mental deficiency.

megalgia (mĕg-al'jĭ-ă) [" + *algos*, pain]. Very severe pain.

megalo- [G.]. Combining form meaning *large, great*.

megaloblast (meg'ă-lō-blăst) [G. *megas*, large, + *blastos*, germ]. A large size nucleated red blood corpuscle, from 11-20 microns in diameter, oval and slightly irregular. Found in the blood in cases of pernicious anemia. SYN: *macroblast*.

megalocardia (mĕg-ă-lō-kar'dĭ-ă) [" + *kardia*, heart]. Cardiac hypertrophy. SYN: *cardiomegaly*.

megalocephalic (mĕg-ă-lō-sef-al'ĭk) [" + *kephalē*, head]. Having an abnormally large skull. SYN: *megacephalic, macrocephalic*.

megalocephaly (mĕg"ă-lō-sĕf'ă-lĭ). [G. *megas*, large, + *kephale*, head]. SYN: *macrocephaly*. 1. Abnormal size of the head. 2. *Leontiasis ossea*, a rare disease characterized by hyperostosis of bones of the skull.

megalocornea (mĕg"ă-lō-kor'nē-ă) [G. *megas*, large, + L. *cornū*, horn]. An enlarged cornea.

megalocystis (mĕg"ă-lō-sĭs'tĭs) [" + *kystis*, bladder]. Abnormal, permanent enlargement of the bladder. SYN: *megabladder*.

megalocyte (mĕg'ă-lo-sīt) [" + *kytos*, cell]. Red blood corpuscle larger than average.

megalodactylous (mĕg"ă-lō-dak'tĭl-ŭs) [" + *daktylos*, finger]. Having very large digits.

megalodontia (mĕg"ă-lō-don'shĭ-ă) [G. *megas*, large, + *odous, odont-*, tooth]. Abnormally large teeth.

megalogastria (mĕg"ă-lō-gas'trĭ-ă) [" + *gastēr*, belly]. Excessive size of stomach. SYN: *gastromegaly*.

megaloglossia (mĕg"ă-lō-glos'sĭ-ă) [" + *glōssa*, tongue]. Enlargement of the tongue. SYN: *macroglossia*.

megalohepatia (mĕg"ă-lō-hē-pat'ĭ-ă) [" + *ēpar, ēpat-*, liver]. Abnormal enlargement of the liver. SYN: *hepatomegaly*.

megalokaryocyte (meg-ă-lō-kar'ĭ-ō-sīt) [" + *karyon*, nucleus, + *kytos*, cell]. A large bone marrow cell with multiple nuclei. SYN: *megakaryocyte*.

megalomania (meg"a-lo-mā'nĭ-ă) [G. *megas*, large, + *mania*, madness]. A psychosis characterized by ideas of personal exaltation and delusions of grandeur.

megalomelia (mĕg"ă-lō-mēl'ĭ-ă) [" + *melos*, limb]. Abnormally large size of the limbs. SYN: *macromelia*.

megalonychosis (mĕg"ă-lō-nĭ-kō'sĭs) [" + *onyx, onych-*, nail, + *-ōsis*]. Hypertrophy of the nails.

megalopenis (mĕg"ă-lō-pē'nis) [" + L. *penis*, penis]. Abnormally large penis. SYN: *macrophallus*.

megalophthalmus (mĕg-ă-lŏf-thal'mus) [" + *ophthalmos*, eye]. Abnormally large eyes.

megalopsia (meg-a-lop'sĭ-ă) [" + *opsis*, vision]. An affection of the eyes in which objects appear enlarged. SYN: *macropsia*.

megaloscope (meg'a-lo-skōp) [" + *skopein*, to examine]. A speculum that magnifies.

megalosplenia (mĕg"ă-lō-splēn'ĭ-ă) [" + *splēn*, spleen]. Hypertrophy of the spleen. SYN: *splenomegaly*.

megalosyndactyly (mĕg"ă-lō-sin-dak'til-ĭ) [" + *syn*, with, + *daktylos*, finger]. A condition of large and webbed digits.

megaloureter (meg-ă-lo-u-re'ter, mĕg-ă-lō-ūr'ĕ-tĕr) [G. *megas*, large, + *ourētēr*, ureter]. Increase in diameter of the ureter.

megaprosopus (mĕg"ă-prŏs'ō-pŭs). Possessing a large face.

megarectum (mĕg-ă-rek'tŭm) [" + L. *rectum*, straight]. Excessive dilatation of the rectum.

megaseme (mĕg'ă-sēm) [" + *sēma*, sign]. 1. Having an orbital aperture with an index exceeding 89, said of a skull. 2. A megaseme skull.

megophthalmus (mĕg-of-thal'mŭs) [" + *ophthalmos*, eye]. Abnormally large eyes. SYN: *buphthalmus, megalophthalmus*.

megrim (mē'grĭm) [O.Fr. migraine]. Sick headache. SYN: *migraine, q.v.*

meibomian cyst (mī-bō'mĭ-ăn). Small tumor on eyelid, the result of inflammation of a m. gland. SYN: *chalazion*.*

m. gland. SYN: *tarsal gland*. One of the sebaceous glands between the tarsi and conjunctiva of eyelids.

Meinicke reaction or **test** (mī'nĭk-e). Tests for syphilis. 1. Floccular reaction. 2. Turbidity reaction. 3. Clearing reaction.

meiocardia (mī"ō-kar'dĭ-ă) [G. *meiōn*, less, + *kardia*, heart]. Systole; heart contraction.

Meissner's corpuscles (mīs'nĕr). An encapsulated end organ of touch found in dermal papillae close to epidermis. Each is an ovoid body containing endings of myelinated and unmyelinated nerve fibers. Most numerous in hairless portion of skin, esp. volar surface of hands, fingers, feet, and toes; also present in lips, eyelids, tip of tongue, and nipple.

M.'s plexus. Small aggregations of ganglion cells located in submucosa of intestine.

mel [L.]. Honey.

melaena (mel-e'na) [G. *melaina*, black, black bile]. 1. Black vomit. 2. Tarry evacuations. SEE: *melena*.

melagra (mĕl-a'gră) [G. *melos*, limb, + *agra*, seizure]. Pain in the limbs. SYN: *melalgia*.

melalgia (mĕl-al'jĭ-ă) [" + *algos*, pain]. Neuralgia of the limbs.

melan-, black, + *cholē*, bile]. A mental

melancholia (mĕl-an-ko'lĭ-ă) [G. *melas*, disorder characterized by marked depression, physical and mental apathy, brooding, mournful and doleful notions, and inhibition of activity. Observed in depressed phase of *manic-depressive psychoses*.

m., affective. Involving or due to the emotions.

m. agita'ta. M. with much motor excitement.

m. attonita. Characterized by mental and physical stupor.

m., climacteric. Occurring at the menopause.

m., convulsive. Occurring in connection with jacksonian epilepsy.

m., involutional. Despondency, suicidal tendencies, feelings of unworthiness and mental agitation occurring between 45 and 60 years of age.

m., panphobic. Characterized with dread of everything.

m., paretic. Preceding paresis.

m., sexual. M. associated with fear

of impotence, venereal disease, unsatisfied sexual desires.

m. simplex. Without delusions, a mild form.

m. stuporo'sa. SEE: *m. attonita.*

m., suicidal. Having impulse to commit suicide combined with melancholia.

melanedema (mĕl-an-e-dē'mă) [G. *melas, melan-*, black, + *oidēma*, swelling]. Black deposit in the lungs; melanosis of the lungs. SYN: *anthracosis.*

melanemia (mĕl-an-e'mĭ-ă) [" + *aima*, blood]. Unnaturally dark color of blood, due to presence of melanin or free, dark pigment.

Seen mainly in pernicious anemia.

melanephidrosis (mĕl-ăn-ĕf-ĭ-drō'sĭs) [" + *ephidrōsis*, sweating]. Black sweat. SYN: *melanidrosis.*

mélangeur (mā-lon-jher') [Fr. mixer]. Apparatus for drawing and diluting blood specimens for microscopic examination.

melanidrosis (mĕl-an-ĭd-rō'sĭs) [G. *melas, melan-*, black, + *idrōsis*, sweat]. Black sweat. SYN: *melanephidrosis.*

melaniferous (mĕl-ăn-if'ĕr-ŭs) [" + L. *ferre*, to carry]. Containing melanin or some other black pigment.

mel'anin [G. *melas, melan-*, black]. The pigment which gives color to hair, skin and the choroid of the eye, and is present in some cancers, as in *melanoma.*

Melanin can be prepared chemically.

melanism (mĕl'ăn-ĭzm) [" + *ismos*, state of]. Excessively black pigmentation of the organs and tissues.

melano- [G.]. Prefix meaning *black* or *darkness.*

melanoblast (mĕl"ăn'ō-blăst). A cell found in basal layers of epidermis which elaborates melanin.

melanoblastoma (mĕl"ă-nō-blăs-tō'mă) [" + *blastos*, germ, + *-ōma*, tumor]. A tumor containing melanin.

melanocarcinoma (mĕl"ă-nō-kar-sĭn-ō'mă) [" + *karkinos*, crab cancer]. A cancer which is darkly pigmented.

melanocyte (mĕl"an-ō'sīt) [G. *melas, melan-*, black, *-kytos*, cell]. SYN: *chromatophore.* A phagocyte which has ingested melanin.

melanocyte-stimulating hormone. Hormone from the posterior pituitary which influences melanin formation. ABBR: *MSH.*

melanoderma (mĕl"an-ō-der'mă) [" + *derma*, skin]. A dark skin discoloration.

melanoepithelioma (mĕl-ăn-ō-ĕp-ĭ-the"lĭ-ō'mă). A malignant epithelioma containing melanin.

melanogenesis (mel"an-ō-jĕn'ĕ-sĭs) [" + *genesis*, production]. Formation of melanin.

melanoglossia (mĕl"ăn-ō-glŏs'sĭ-ă) [G. *melas, melan-*, black, + *glōssa*, tongue]. Black tongue. SYN: *glossophytia.*

melanoid (mĕl'ă-noid) [" + *eidos*, form]. 1. Concerning or resembling melanosis. 2. Melanin which is chemically prepared.

melanoleukoderma (mel"an-ō-lū-kō-der'-mă) [" + *leukos*, white, + *derma*, skin]. Mottled skin.

m. col'li. Mottled skin of neck sometimes seen in syphilis. SYN: *collar of Venus, venereal collar.*

melano'ma [" + *-ōma*, tumor]. A pigmented mole or tumor. SYN: *nevus pigmentosus.*

melanomatosis (mĕl-an-ō-mat-ō'sĭs) [" + " + *-ōsis*, intensive]. Formation of melanomas on or beneath the skin.

melanonychia (mĕl-ă-nō-nik'ĭ-ă) [G. *melas, melan-*, black, + *onyx, onych-*, nail]. Black pigmentation of the nails.

melanopathy (mel-an-op'ă-thĭ) [" + *pathos*, disease]. 1. Dark pigmentation of skin. 2. Disease with dark pigmentation of the skin. SYN: *melanoderma, melasma.*

melanophore (mel'an-ō-fōr) [" + *phoros*, a bearer]. Cell carrying dark pigment.

melanoplakia (mĕl"an-ō-plā'kĭ-ă) [" + *plax, plak-*, a flat plate]. Condition marked by pigmented patches on the buccal mucosa.

mel"anorrhag'ia [" + *rēgnunai*, to burst forth]. Black feces. SYN: *melanorrhea.*

melanorrhea (mĕl-an-or-re'ă) [" + *roia*, flow]. Black stools. SYN: *melena, 2.*

melanosarcoma (mĕl"ă-nō-sar-kō'mă) [G. *melas, melan-*, black, + *sarx, sark-*, flesh, + *-ōma*, tumor]. Sarcoma containing melanin. SYN: *malignant melanoma.*

melanoscirrhus (mĕl-ă-nō-skir'rŭs) [" + *skirros*, hard]. Black pigmented cancer. SYN: *melanocarcinoma.*

melanosis (mĕl-an-ō'sĭs) [" + *-ōsis*, intensive]. Unusual deposit of black pigments in different parts of body.

m. lenticularis. Rare skin disease, beginning in early youth, characterized by scattered pigment discolorations, ulcers, atrophy, etc. SYN: *xeroderma pigmentosum.*

melanot'ic [G. *melas, melan-*, black]. 1. Blackish in color. 2. Pert. to melanosis.

melanotrichia linguae (mĕl"ăn-ō-trĭk'ĭ-ă lĭng'gwe). Black, hairy tongue. SEE: *black tongue.*

melanuria (mĕl-an-u'rĭ-ă) [" + G. *ouron*, urine]. Dark pigments in urine.

melasma (mĕl-az'mă) [G. a black spot]. Any discoloration of the skin. SYN: *nigredo cutis.*

m. gravidarum. Discoloration of the skin during pregnancy.

m. suprarenale. Hypofunction of the suprarenals with cutaneous pigmentation and severe anemia. SYN: *Addison's disease, q.v.*

melena (mel'ĕ-nă, mĕl-ē'nă) [G. *melaina*, black, black bile]. 1. Black vomit. 2. Evacuations resembling tar, due to action of intestinal juices on free blood. Common in the newly born.

m. neonatorum. M. in the newborn.

melenemesis (mel-ĕ-nem'ĕ-sĭs) [" + *emesis*, vomit]. Black vomit caused by blood that has been acted upon by the gastric juice. SYN: *melena, 1.*

melicera, meliceris (mĕl-ĭ-sĕr'ă, -ĭs) [G. *meli*, honey, + *kēros*, wax]. Cyst containing matter of honeylike consistency.

melioidosis (mē"lĭ-oi-do'sis) ["a resemblance to distemper in asses"]. An acute or chronic disease due to *Pseudomonas pseudomallei* (formerly called *Malleomyces pseudomallei*). Acute form causes pneumonia, multiple abscesses, septicemia and possibly death. SYN: *Whitmore's disease, pseudoglanders.*

melissopho'bia [G. *melissa*, bee, + *phobos*, fear]. Insane fear of bee or wasp stings.

melitagra (mĕl-ĭ-tag'ră) [G. *meli, melit-*, honey, + *agra*, seizure]. A form of eczema with soft crusts resembling honey.

melitemia (mel-ĭ-te'mĭ-ă) [" + *aima*, blood]. Sugar in the blood. SYN: *glycemia.*

melitensis (mel-ĭ-ten'sis). Brucellosis, *q.v.*

melitis (mĕl-ī'tĭs) [G. *mēlon*, cheek, + *-itis*, inflammation]. Inflammation of cheek.

melitoptyalism (mĕl"it-ō-tī'al-ĭzm) [G. *meli, melit-*, honey, + *ptyalon*, saliva]. Saliva containing glucose. SYN: *glycoptyalism.*

melituria (mel-ĭ-tu′rĭ-ă) [" + *ouron*, urine]. Diabetes mellitus; excretion of sugar in urine.

mellite (mel′īt) [G. *meli, melit-*, honey]. Any medicated preparation of honey.

melodiotherapy (mel-ō″dĭ-ō-ther′a-pĭ) [G. *melōdia*, music, + *therapeia*, treatment]. Treatment by music. Syn: *musicotherapy*.

melomania (mel-ō-mā′nĭ-ă) [G. *melos*, song, + *mania*, madness]. Insane love for music.

melomelus (mē-lŏm′ĕl-ŭs). A monster with rudimentary limb attached to normal limb.

meloncus (mēl-on′kŭs) [G. *mēlon*, cheek, + *ogkos*, tumor]. Tumor of the cheek.

mel′on [G. *mēlon*, apple]. Comp: Principally water and carbohydrates, the latter nearly all in the form of sugar.

Action: A good cleanser. Often used in semi-fasting; esp. watermelon.

Ind: If fully ripened, dyspeptics may use in small quantities. Good in constipation and in clogged conditions of the system.

Contra: The sugar in melons is not sufficient to prohibit for diabetics. In irritable conditions of the digestive system they should be avoided.

meloplasty (mel′ō-plas-tĭ) [G. *mēlon*, cheek, + *melos*, limb, + *plassein*, to form]. Reparative surgery of a cheek or limb.

melt′ing point. Temperature at which conversion of a solid to a liquid begins.

mem′ber [L. *membrum*]. An organ or part of the body, esp. a limb.

membrane (mem′brān) [L. *membrana*]. A thin, soft, pliable layer of tissue which lines a tube or cavity, covers an organ or structure, or separates one part from another.

m., arachnoid. Middle layer of membranes covering brain and spinal cord.

m., atlanto-occipital. One of two fibrous membranes (ant. and post.) extending from the arch of the atlas to borders of the foramen magnum.

m., basement. A delicate, noncellular membrane underlying a layer of epithelial cells and serving for their support and attachment.

m., basilar. M. extending from tympanic lip of osseous spiral lamina to crest of spiral ligament in cochlea of ear. It separates scala tympani from cochlear duct and forms supporting structure for the organ of Corti.

m., Bowman's. Thin homogeneous m. separating corneal epithelium from proper substance of the cornea.

m.'s, brain and spinal cord. The meninges, *pia mater*, inner m.; *dura mater*, outer m.; and *arachnoid*, middle m.

m., cell. Surface layer of the cytoplasm of a cell.

m., chorioid. The chorioid, the portion of the vascular tunic or uvea of the eye which extends posteriorly from the ora serrata.

m., costocoracoid. Dense fascia bet. the pectoralis minor and subclavius muscles.

m., cricothyroid. M. connecting thyroid and cricoid cartilages of the larynx.

m., croupous. False yellowish-white m. in the larynx during croup.

m., decidual. One of the membranes formed in the endometrium of a pregnant uterus. Includes the decidua basalis, decidua capsularis, and decidua parietalis, *q.v.*

m., Descemet's. Elastic m. forming lining surface of the cornea.

m., diphtheritic. Fibrinous false m. on mucous surfaces in diphtheria.

m., drum. The tympanic membrane.

m., egg. One of the protective membranes or envelopes enclosing an ovum. May be *primary* (formed by egg itself, Ex: vitelline membrane); *secondary* (formed by follicle cells, Ex: zona pellucida); or *tertiary* (formed by oviduct or uterus, Ex: albumen and shell of hen's egg).

m., elastic. One formed by elastic tissue fibers.

m., elastic, of the larynx. Consists of upper quadrangular membrane and lower elastic cone.

m., enamel. 1. Cuticula dentis. 2. Thin calcified membrane (primary enamel cuticle) on surface of newly erupted tooth.

m., false. Fibrinous exudate on a mucous surface of a membrane, as in diphtheria.

m., fenestrated. A layer of elastic connective tissue possessing minute round or oval openings. Found in tunica intima and tunica media of medium-sized and large arteries.

m., fetal. In mammals, the chorion, amnion, and allantois and, in addition, accessory structures which include the yolk sac, umbilical cord, and placenta.

m., fibrous. M. composed entirely of connective tissue. Examples are fasciae, aponeuroses, perichondrium, periosteum, dura mater, and capsules of some organs.

m., glassy, of graafian follicle. Transparent capsule which separates membrana granulosa from the theca.

m., glassy, of hair. Internal layer of a hair follicle separating the epithelial and connective tissues.

m., glial. Extremely delicate membrane, formed of foot plates of astrocytes, which surrounds all blood vessels in the brain, spinal cord, and in lining of pia mater separating these vessels from nervous tissue proper. It constitutes the major component of the *blood-brain barrier*.

m., Henle's elastic. See: *m., fenestrated*.

m., homogeneous. A fine m. covering villi of the placenta.

m., Huxley's. See: *layer, Huxley*.

m., hyaline. 1. Basement* m. 2. M. bet. outer root sheath of a hair follicle and inner fibrous layer.

m., hyaloid. One investing the vitreous humor of the eye, seen on longitudinal section. Syn: *membrana vitrea*.

m., hypoglossal. A transverse fibrous lamella uniting tongue to hyoid bone.

m., interosseous. 1. A fibrous m. in the arm connecting ulna to radius. 2. A fibrous m. in the leg connecting tibia to fibula.

m., Krause's. Dark membranous band limiting the sarcomere in striated muscle. Also called *Z* or *intermediate disk*.

m., limiting, external. 1. Outer layer of cells of the developing neural tube. 2. M. in retina of eye separating rods and cones from their cell bodies.

m., limiting, internal. 1. Inner layer of ependymal cells lining neural tube. 2. Glial membrane forming innermost layer of the retina and of the iris.

m., meconic. A m. forming a layer in rectum of the fetus.

m., medullary. Endosteum.*

m., mucous. M. lining cavities and canals communicating with the air and kept moist by secretion of mucus.

m., nictitating. A third eyelid present in lower vertebrates and represented in man by a fold of the conjunctiva, the *plica semilunaris.*

m., nuclear. The *karyotheca* or membrane forming surface layer of a nucleus.

m., obturator. Fibrous m. closing the obturator foramen.

m., oral. Pharyngeal m., *q.v.*

m., oronasal. A double epithelial layer separating the nasal pits from the embryonic oral cavity. Same as *bucconasal membrane.*

m., otolithic. A layer of gelatinous substance containing otoconia or otoliths, found on the surface of maculae in inner ear.

m., peridental. Connective tissue between the root of a tooth and the alveolar bone. SYN: *periodontal m.*

m., permeable. A m. which permits the passage of water and certain substances in solution.

m., pharyngeal. M. closing embryonic gut at oral end.

m., plasma. A cell membrane, *q.v.*

m., pseudoserous. M. resembling a serous membrane in structure. Ex: endothelium.

m., pupillary. Transparent m. closing the fetal pupil. If it persists after birth it is known as persistent p. membrane.

m., pyogenic. Granular lining of an abscess or fistula.

m., pyophylactic. Protective lining of an abscess that prevents reabsorption.

m., quadrangular. Upper portion of the elastic membrane of the larynx, *q.v.*

m., Reissner's. SYN: *membrana vestibularis.* Delicate membrane separating cochlear canal from scala vestibuli.

m., Ruysch's. SYN: *lamina choriocapillaris.* Choroid's middle layer composed of a close capillary network.

m., schneiderian. Mucosa of the nasal fossae. SYN: *membrana pituitosa.*

m., selectively permeable. A membrane which allows a substance like water to pass through more readily than another, like salt or sugar.

m., semipermeable. M. allowing passage of water but not substances in solution.

m., serous. M. consisting of mesothelium lying on thin layer of connective tissue which lines the closed cavities (peritoneal, pleural, and pericardial) of the body. Surface is moistened by a thin fluid similar to lymph.

m., Shrapnell's. That portion of the tympanic m. filling the notch of Rivinus.

m., synovial. M. lining a joint and secreting synovia.

m., tectorial. Thin, jellylike membrane projecting from vestibular lip of osseous spiral lamina and overlying the spiral organ of Corti.

m., theory, of nerve conduction. Theory that the nerve cell membrane and that of its axon is the seat of the electromotive force establishing the resting potential of a cell; that the breakdown of the membrane such as caused by a threshold stimulus abolishes the membrane potential and initiates a wave of depolarization which passes along the nerve fiber and is the nerve impulse.

m., thyrohyoid. One joining the hyoid bone and the thyroid cartilage.

m., tympanic. The drum membrane; membrane separating tympanic cavity from the external auditory canal.

m., virginal. The hymen.

m., vitelline. Membrane that forms surface layer of an ovum.

m., vitreous. Descemet's membrane.

m., yolk. A membrane surrounding the ovum; vitelline membrane or zona pellucida, *q.v.*

membraniform (mem-brăn'ĭ-form) [L. *membrana,* membrane, + *forma,* shape]. Resembling or of the nature of a membrane. SYN: *membranoid, membranous.*

membranocartilaginous (mĕm"brăn-ō-kăr-tĭl-aj'ĭ-nŭs) [" + *cartilāgō, cartilagin-,* cartilage]. 1. Pert. to membrane and cartilage. 2. Derived from both membrane and cartilage.

membranoid (mĕm'bră-noid) [L. *membrana,* membrane + G. *eidos,* resemblance]. Resembling a membrane. SYN: *membraniform, membranous.*

membranous (mem'bran-ŭs) [L. *membrana,* membrane]. 1. Rel. to a membrane. 2. Resembling a membrane. SYN: *membraniform, membranoid.*

membrum muliebre (mĕm'brum mu-lĭ-e'-bre) [L. female member]. The clitoris.

membrum virile (mĕm'brŭm vĭr-il'e) [L. male member]. The penis.

memory [L. *memoria,* memory]. The mental registration of past experience, knowledge, ideas, sensations and thoughts.

Registration of experience is favored by clear comprehension during intense consciousness.

Retention of memory differs greatly with individuals. Memory recall, esp. its intentional recall, means the reproduction of a memory in consciousness. Clear comprehension greatly favors retention. Recall may fail because the memory has been obliterated, or functionally because the stream of ideas is that which one does not wish to remember. Various memory defects occur in many diseases.

Memory is confused or obliterated in *maniacal states,* lively in *paranoia,* abolished in *senile psychosis* and *organic brain disease,* but undisturbed in *depressions.* In dementia from senile causes there is accurate m. for remote events but none for recent occurrences.

RS: *anamnestic, association center, mnemic, mnemonics, retention, r. defect.*

m., anterograde. SYN: *antegrade amnesia.* Ability to remember events occurring in the remote past but lacking ability to remember recent events.

m., retrograde. SYN: *retrograde amnesia.* Ability to recall events of recent occurrence but lacking ability to recall knowledge with which patient had previously been familiar.

menacme (mĕn-ăk'mē) [G. *mēn,* month, + *akmē,* top]. The pinnacle (acme) of the menstrual life of a woman.

menadiol sodium diphosphate. USP. A synthetic water-soluble vitamin, having same activity as natural vitamin K. Used as an antihemorrhagic agent in hypoprothrombinemia or hemorrhagic disorders due to hypoprothrombinemia.

menarche (mĕn-ar'kē) [G. *men,* month, + *archē,* beginning]. Onset of menses. Occurs normally between the 10th and 17th year.

mendelevium (men-dĕ-lē'vē-um). A transuranium element. SYMB: Md. At. wt. 256; at. no. 101.

Mendel's laws. Certain principles of heredity established by Gregor Mendel (1865). He demonstrated that traits were inherited as *unit characters,* each determined by a pair of *determiners* or genes; that when two determiners for contrasting characters were present in a single individual (a hybrid), one character would manifest itself to the exclusion of the other. This character was said to be *dominant* over the other, the recessive character. Mendel established that in the formation of gametes the pairs of determiners separated and only one was present in a gamete (the law of *segregation*); that when determiners for two pairs of characters were present, each pair segregated independently of the other (the law of *independent assortment*).

Although Mendel's principles were subsequently shown not to apply universally, his work laid the foundation for the development of modern genetics and the present chromosome theory of heredity (theory of the gene).

M.'s reflex. Dorsal flexion of 2nd to 5th toes upon percussion of the dorsum of the foot.

menhidrosis (mĕn-hī-drō′sĭs). Vicarious menstruation through the sweat glands. Syn: *menidrosis.*

menidrosis (mēn-ĭ-dro′sĭs) [G. *mēn,* month, + *idrōs,* sweat]. Vicarious menstruation through sweat glands. Syn: *menhidrosis.*

Ménière's disease (mā-nē-ārs′). A recurrent and usually progressive group of symptoms including hearing loss, ringing in the ears, dizziness and a sensation of fullness or pressure in the ears. Syn: *Ménière's syndrome.*

Etiol: Unknown.

Treatment: In acute attacks, bed rest is the most effective treatment, antihistamines, discontinue smoking, rarely surgical treatment may be necessary.

meningeal (men-in′jē-ăl) [G. *mēnigx, mēnigg-,* membrane]. Rel. to the meninges.

meningeorrhaphy (mĕ-nĭn-jē-or′ră-fĭ) [" + *raphē,* a sewing]. Suture of any membranes, esp. those of brain and spinal cord.

meninges (mĕn-ĭn′jēz) (sing. *meninx*) [G. *mēnigx, mēnigg-,* membrane]. 1. Membranes. 2. The three membranes investing the spinal cord and brain: the *dura mater,* external; the *arachnoid,* middle, and *pia mater,* internal.

meningina (men-ĭn-jī′nă) [G. *mēnigx,* membrane]. The pia mater and adjacent layer of the arachnoid combined. Syn: *pia-arachnoid.*

meninginitis (men-ĭn-jĭ-nī′tis) [" + *-ītis,* inflammation]. Inflammation of the pia-arachnoid membrane. Syn: *leptomeningitis, piarachnitis.*

meningioma (men-ĭn-jĭ-ō′mă) [" + *-ōma,* tumor]. Tumor in the meninges.

meningism (men-ĭn′jĭzm) [" + *ismos,* state of]. Irritation of the brain and spinal cord with simulation of meningitis, but without actual inflammation.

meningismus. Meningism.

meningitic (men-in-jit′ĭk) [G. *mēnigx,* membrane]. Pert. to meningitis.

meningitis (men-in-ji′tis) [" + *-ītis,* inflammation]. Inflammation of the membranes of spinal cord or brain.

See: *choriomeningitis, Kernig's sign, leptomeningitis, pachymeningitis.*

m., acute. Sym: Moderate, irregular fever, loss of appetite, constipation, intense headache, intolerance to light and sound, contracted pupils, delirium, retraction of head, convulsions and coma.

Etiol: Caused by bacteria, viruses, or other organisms which reach the meninges from other foci in the body via blood or lymph, through trauma, or from adjacent bony structures (sinuses, mastoid cells).

Prog: Favorable with prompt diagnosis and appropriate therapy.

NP and Treatment: The room should be dark and quiet. Retention of urine must be guarded against, as distention is apt to occur. The eyes and mouth must be kept cleansed, and pressure points upon the back should be guarded against. Headache may be relieved by an icebag or cold compresses. Special nursing technic as may be necessary. Isolation and asepsis are indicated. All discharges should be burned. The eyes should be protected from the light, and all noise and everything that might disturb the patient should be avoided.

A bed cradle may be necessary to relieve pressure and friction. Sudden excitement may cause a convulsion, so quiet is absolutely necessary. Change the patient's position frequently but avoid jarring the bed. Hypostatic pneumonia must be guarded against. A cleansing bath with an alcohol rub should be a daily procedure. All body prominences need special attention to prevent pressure sores. Mouth hygiene is also called for morning and night.

The intake and output of fluids must be recorded. During the acute stage restraints may be necessary.

Diet: A fluid diet is necessary during the acute stage, but later as much nourishment should be given as possible, as the disease is an exhaustive one. Milk, eggs, beef tea, water, fruit juices and sugar may be given freely. A more solid diet may be given during convalescence. With stuporous patients, tube feeding is necessary. Children and some adults may have to be fed with a spoon or a medicine dropper.

Sulfanilamide and its derivatives are used successfully now in pneumococcic, meningococcic and beta hemolytic streptococcus meningitis.

m., acute, aseptic. Lymphocytic choriomeningitis, a nonpurulent form usually running a short benign course with recovery.

m., basilar. Inflammation at base of brain of the meninges.

m., cerebral. Acute or chronic m. of brain membranes.

m., cerebrospinal. M. of brain and cord.

m., listeria. Listeriosis, *q.v.*

m., pneumococcal. M. caused by the pneumococcus. Common in young children.

m. serosa circumscripta. M. accompanied by the formation of cystic accumulations of fluid which simulate tumors.

m., serous. Serous exudation in m. into cerebral ventricles.

m., spinal. M. of spinal cord membranes.

m., sterile. M. in which infectious organisms are absent.

m., traumatic. M. resulting from organisms following injury to the skull or spine.

m., tuberculous. An acute inflammation of the cerebral meninges excited by the tubercle bacillus.

Sym: Loss of flesh, gradual wasting of strength, evening rise of temperature, restlessness, irritability, and sleeplessness may exist for some time before acute symptoms come on. These are severe headache, occasional convulsions, delirium, vomiting, fever, optic neuritis.

meningitophobia (me-nin-jit-ō-fō′bĭ-ă) [G. *mēnigx, mēnigg-,* membrane]. 1. Meningism due to fear of brain disease. 2. Morbid fear of meningitis.

meningoarteritis (me-nĭn-gō-ăr-tĕr-ī'tĭs) [" + *artēria*, artery, + *-ītis*, inflammation]. Inflammatory condition of the meningeal arteries.

meningocele (men-ĭn'gō-sēl) [" + *kēlē*, hernia]. Congenital hernia, the meninges protruding through an opening of the skull or spinal column.

meningocerebritis (me-nĭn-gō-ser-e-brī'tĭs) [" + L. *cerebrum*, brain, + G. *-ītis*, inflammation]. Inflamed condition of brain and meninges. Syn: *meningoencephalitis*.

meningococcemia (me-nĭn-gō-kŏk-sē'mĭ-ă) [" + *kokkos*, berry, + *aima*, blood]. Meningococci in the blood.

meningococcus (men-in-go-kok'us) (pl. *meningococci*) [G. *mēnigx*, *mēnigg-*, membrane, + *kokkos*, berry]. *Neisseria meningitidis*, the causative agent of epidemic cerebral meningitis (cerebrospinal fever, spotted fever). Syn: *Weichselbaum's bacillus*.

meningocortical (me-nin-gō-kor'tĭ-kal) [" + L. *cortex*, *cortic-*, bark]. Pert. to the meninges and the cortex.

meningoencephalitis (men-in"go-en-sef-al-ī'tĭs) [" + *egkephalos*, brain, + *-ītis*, inflammation]. Inflammation of meninges and of the brain.

meningoencephalocele (me-nĭn"gō-en-sĕf'ăl-ō-sēl) [" + *egkephalos*, brain, + *kēlē*, hernia]. Hernia of brain and meninges.

meningoencephalomyelitis (me-nĭn"gō-ĕn-sĕf"ăl-ō-mī-ĕl-ī'tĭs) [" + " + *myelon*, marrow, + *-ītis*, inflammation]. Inflammation of the brain, spinal cord, and their meninges.

meningomalacia (me-nĭn-gō-mă-lā'sĭ-ă) [" + *malakia*, softening]. Softening of any membrane.

meningomyelitis (men-ĭn"gō-mī-ĕl-ī'tĭs) [G. *mēnigx*, *mēnigg-*, membrane, + *myelon*, marrow, + *-ītis*, inflammation]. Inflammation of spinal cord and its membranes; less commonly of the dura mater, also.

meningomyelocele (me-nĭn"gō-mī'ĕl-ō-sēl) [" + " + *kēlē*, hernia]. Hernia of spinal cord and membranes.

meningopathy (me-nĭn-gop'ă-thĭ) [" + *pathos*, disease]. Any pathological condition of the meninges.

meningorrhachidian (me-nĭn"go-ră-kid'ĭ-an) [" + *rachis*, spine]. Concerning the spinal cord and meninges.

meningorrhagia (me-nĭn"go-ră'jĭ-ă) [" + *rēgnunai*, to burst forth]. Meningeal hemorrhage. Syn: *meningorrhea*.

meningorrhea (me-nĭn-go-rē'ă) [" + *roia*, flow]. Meningeal hemorrhage. Syn: *meningorrhagia*.

meningotyphoid (me-nĭn"gō-tī'foid) [G. *mēnigx*, *mēnigg-*, membrane, + *typhos*, stupor, + *eidos*, form]. Typhoid fever with symptoms of meningitis.

meningovascular (me-nin"go-vas'ku-lar). Pert. to blood vessels of the meninges.

meninguria (me-nĭn-gū'rĭ-ă) [" + *ouron*, urine]. Presence of membraniform shreds in urine.

meninx (me'ninks) (pl. *meninges*) [G. *mēnigx*, membrane]. Any membrane, but esp. one of the coverings of the brain or spinal cord.

meniscectomy (men"ĭ-sek'to-mĭ). Removal of meniscus cartilage of the knee.

menisci (men-is'i). Plural of meniscus.

meniscitis (men-ĭ-si'tĭs) [G. *mēniskos*, crescent, + *-ītis*, inflammation]. Inflamed condition of an interarticular cartilage, esp. the semilunar cartilages of the knee joint.

meniscocyte (men-ĭs'kō-sīt) [" + *kytos*, cell]. A crescent-shaped red blood cell.

meniscocytosis (men-is"ko-sīt-ō'sĭs) [" + " + *-ōsis*, intensive]. Crescent cells in the blood; sickle cell anemia.

meniscus (men-is'kus) [G. *mēniskos*, crescent]. 1. Concavo-convex lens. 2. Interarticular fibrocartilage of crescent shape, found in certain joints, esp. the lateral and medial menisci (semilunar cartilages) of the knee joint.

m. articularis. See: *meniscus*, 2.

menolipsis (men-ō-lip'sĭs) [" + *leipsis*, a failing]. Temporary absence or retention of menses.

menometrorrhagia (mĕn"ō-mĕt-ro-rā'jĭ-ă) [G. *mēn*, month, + *mētra*, uterus, + *rēgnunai*, to burst forth]. Irregular and excessive menstrual bleeding. RS: *menorrhagia*, *metrorrhagia*.

menopause (mĕn'ō-pawz) [G. *mēn*, month, + *pausis*, cessation]. That period which marks the permanent cessation of menstrual activity.

Occurs bet. 35 and 58 years of life. The menses may stop suddenly or there may be a decreased flow each month until there is a final cessation, or the interval bet. periods may be lengthened until complete cessation is accomplished.

Natural menopause will occur in 25% of women by age 47, in 50% by age 50, 75% by age 52, and in 95% by age 55. Surgical menopause occurs in almost 30% of U.S. women aged 50 to 64. Source: *Age of Menopause.* U.S. Public Health Service Pub. No. 1000—series 11—No. 19.

Sym: Menopause may be accompanied by hot and cold flashes, feeling of weakness, and in some cases mental depression.

Treatment: Hormone replacement as required, yearly pelvic examination to include Papanicolaou test for cancer of the cervix. Syn: *change of life; climacteric*.

RS: *involution*, *menses*, *menstruation*, *sexual involution*.

m., artificial. M. occurring subsequent to surgical castration, x-ray irradiation, or radium implantation into the uterus.

m., premature. M. either natural or artificial occurring before age 35.

menophania (men-ō-fa'nĭ-ă) [G. *mēn*, month, + *phainein*, to show]. First appearance of the menses at puberty.

menoplania (men-ō-plā'nĭ-ă) [" + *planē*, a wandering]. Vicarious menstruation; menstruation through other than the normal outlet, as through the nose.

menorrhagia (men-ō-ra'jĭ-ă) [" + *rēgnunai*, to burst forth]. Excessive bleeding at the time of a menstrual period, either in number of days or amount of blood or both.

Etiol: *Endocrine Disturbances*: Pituitary gland, thyroid and ovary. *General Systemic Diseases*: Hypertension, diabetes mellitus, blood dyscrasias, chronic nephritis. *Malpositions of the Uterus*: Retroversion and retroflexion. *New Growths of the Uterus*: Particularly fibroids of the intramural and submucous types, adenomyosis of the uterus, fibrosis of the uterus with hyperplastic changes of the endometrium. *Conditions of the Cervix Uteri*: Erosions, polypi. *Inflammations in the Pelvis*: Acute salpingitis, acute metritis, acute endometritis, chronic metritis and endometritis. See: *hemorrhage, uterine*.

menorrhalgia (men-o-ral'jĭ-ă) [G. *mēn*, month, + *roia*, flow, + *algos*, pain]. SYN: *dysmenorrhea*. Painful menstruation or pelvic pain accompanying menstruation, sometimes a symptom of endometriosis.

menorrhea (mĕn-or-ē'ă) [" + *roia*, flow]. 1. Normal menstruation. 2. Free or profuse menstruation. SYN: *menorrhagia*.

menostaxis (men-ō-stak'sĭs) [" + *staxis*, dripping]. Prolonged menstruation.

menotoxin [" + G. *toxicon*, poison]. A substance present in the menstrual flow. Toxic to certain plants but nontoxic to the menstruant or her associates.

menoxenia (men-ok-se'nĭ-ă) [" + *xenos*, strange]. Abnormal menstruation.

menses (men'sēz) [L. pl. of *mensis*, month]. Monthly flow of bloody fluid from the uterus; catamenial flow.

menstrual (men'strū-ăl) [L. *menstruāre*, to discharge the menses]. Pert. to menstruation. SYN: *catamenial*.

m. cycle. The periodically recurrent series of changes occurring in the uterus and associated sex organs (ovaries, vagina) associated with menstruation and the intermenstrual period. The human cycle averages about 28 days in length, measured from the beginning of menstruation. The menstrual cycle is, however, quite variable in length even in the same person from month to month.

The menstrual cycle is divided into four phases characterized by histological changes which take place in the uterine endometrium. They are:

1. MENSTRUATION: Period of uterine bleeding accompanied by shedding of the endometrium. Averages 4 to 5 days in length.

2. PERIOD OF REPAIR AND PROLIFERATION (postmenstrual period): Uterine epithelium is restored to normal; endometrium becomes thicker and more vascular, glands elongate. During this period the ovarian follicle is maturing and secreting estrogens. Period is terminated by rupture of follicle and liberation of ovum at about 14 days before next menstrual period begins. Length of period, 10-13 days. Also called *estrogenic* or *follicular period.*

3. LUTEAL OR SECRETORY PHASE: Endometrium increases in thickness, glands become more tortuous and produce an abundant secretion containing glycogen. Coiled arteries make their appearance, endometrium becomes edematous, stroma becomes compact. During this period the corpus luteum in ovary is developing and secreting progesterone. Also called *luteal phase.* Lasts 10 to 14 days.

4. PREMENSTRUAL OR ISCHEMIC PHASE: A day or two before menstruation, coiled arteries constrict, endometrium becomes anemic and shrinks. Corpus luteum of ovary begins involution. Period lasts about two days and is terminated by opening up of constricted arteries, the breaking off of small patches of necrotic endometrium and the beginning of menstruation with the flow of menstrual fluid.

Variations in the length of the cycle are due principally to variation in the length of the period of repair and proliferation.

m. hygiene. The menstrual cycle should be thoroughly explained to young girls well before menarche. If this is done, they will not be frightened or alarmed when they first menstruate. The availability of and directions for using perineal pads and tampons should also be explained. The m. cycle is a normal event and should be presented to adolescent girls in that manner. There is no medical reason why the m. period should be regarded as being a time of sickness, nor should there be necessity for curtailing the individual's normal activity at work or play.

menstruant (men'strū-ănt) [L. *menstruāre*, to discharge the menses]. 1. In the condition of menstruating. 2. One who menstruates.

menstruate (men'strū-āt) [L. *menstruāre*]. To discharge menses.

menstruation (mĕn-strū-ā'shŭn) [L. *menstruāre*, to discharge the menses]. The periodic discharge of a bloody fluid

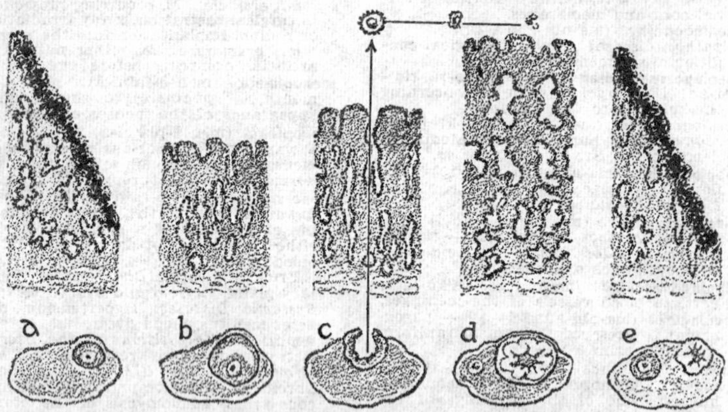

DIAGRAM OF MENSTRUAL CYCLE.

a. Menstruation; graafian follicle beginning to develop. b. Endometrium growing and follicle ripening. c. Endometrium becomes thicker. Follicle ruptures and sets ovum free (ovulation) about 14 days before beginning of next menstrual period. d. Endometrium in premenstrual or luteal phase. Corpus luteum developing. Unfertilized ovum degenerating. e. Corpus luteum degenerating. Menstruation recurs.

from the uterus occurring at more or less regular intervals during the life of a woman from age of puberty to menopause. The discharge contains altered blood, with normal, hemolyzed, and sometimes agglutinated red blood cells, disintegrated endometrial and stroma cells and secretions of glands. In general, menstrual blood does not coagulate, but the passage of occasional clots should not be regarded as being abnormal.

Menstruation is brought on by the reduction in production of ovarian hormones, esp. progesterone, which results from involution of the corpus luteum following failure of the ovum to become fertilized.

Menstruation has its onset at puberty (10-16 years of age). Length of flow varies from 3 to 7 days (ave. 4 to 5 days). It occurs on an average every 27 to 28 days, although time may vary from 18 to 40 days. Menstruation ceases temporarily during pregnancy and may or may not cease during lactation; permanently with onset of menopause. Its failure to occur may result from congenital abnormalities, physical disorders (disease, obesity, malnutrition), emotional or hormonal disturbances, esp. diseases involving the ovaries, hypophysis, thyroid, or adrenal glands.

Menstrual irregularities: absence of flow when normally expected is called *amenorrhea;* scanty flow, *oligomenorrhea;* painful menstruation, *dysmenorrhea.* Excessive loss of blood is termed *menorrhagia. Metrorrhagia* is the loss of blood during intermenstrual periods. Prolongation of menstrual flow is *epimenorrhea.*

m., anovulatory. Menstruation occurring in absence of discharge of ovum from ovary.

m., retrograde. Backflow of menstrual fluid through uterine tubes.

m., suppressed. Failure of menstruation to occur when normally expected.

m., vicarious. Menstruation from other than the uterus.

menstruous (men'strū-ūs) [L. *menstruāre,* to discharge the menses]. Rel. to menstruation.

menstruum (men'strū-um) [L. menstrual fluid; it was believed that this fluid had solvent qualities]. A solvent; a medium. SEE: *vehicle.*

mensuration (men-sū-rā'shŭn) [L. *mensurātiō,* a measuring]. The process of measuring. SEE: *chest, measure.*

mentagra (men-tag'ra) [L. *mentum,* chin, + G. *agra,* seizure]. Inflammation of the hair follicles, esp. of the beard, with pustular eruptions. SYN: *sycosis.*

mentagrophyton (men-tag-rof'i-ton) [" + " + *phyton,* a plant]. The fungus which is the cause of sycosis.

men'tal [L. *mens, ment-,* mind; *mentum,* chin]. 1. Rel. to the mind. 2. Rel. to the chin.

m. age. Age of a person mentally, determined by a group of mental tests.

m. deficiency. The Committee on Nomenclature of the American Psychiatric Association has classified mental deficiency according to intellectual capacity:

m. d., mild. IQ 70-85; functional (vocational) impairment; individual formerly classified as borderline and having lower level of dull normal intelligence; can do laboring jobs.

m. d., moderate. IQ 50-70; intellectual capacity that of 7- to 12-year-old; limited social adjustment; special training and guidance required.

m. d., severe. IQ 0-50; intellectual capacity does not exceed that of 7-year-old; custodial or complete protective care required.

m. disease. A disorder of the mind or intellect. Mild forms are known as *psychoneuroses, q.v.;* more severe forms, *psychoses, q.v.*

m. fog. Clouding of consciousness.

m. hygiene. Science of maintaining healthy mental and emotional responses and preventing development of psychoses.

m. illness. Any disorder which affects the mind or behavior.

m. retardation. Mental deficiency, *q.v.*

mentality. Mental power or activity; keenness of breadth of mind.

men'tha [L.]. Mint.

m. piperita. Peppermint.

m. pulegium. Pennyroyal.

m. viridis. Spearmint.

menthol. An alcohol ($C_{10}H_{19}OH$) obtained from oil of peppermint or other mint oils. May be prepared synthetically. Occurs in crystalline form.

ACTION AND USES: As a counterirritant, antiseptic, and anodyne.

mentula (men'tū-lă) [L.]. The penis.

mentulagra (men-tū-lag'ră) [L. *mentula,* penis, + G. *agra,* seizure]. Painful involuntary erection of the penis, sometimes curved. SYN: *chordee, priapism.*

mentulate (men'tū-lāt) [L. *mentula,* penis]. Possessing a large penis.

mentulomania (mĕn"tū-lō-mā'nĭ-ă) [L. *mens,* mind + G. *mania,* madness]. Mental state characterized by addiction to masturbation.

men'tum [L.]. The chin. SYN: *genion.*

mephenesin (mĕ-fen'ĕ-sin). A centrally acting muscle relaxant. Used only for muscle relaxation.

mephit'ic [L. *mephitis,* foul exhalation]. Noxious, foul, as a poisonous odor.

meprobamate (mep-rō-bam'āt). A tranquilizing agent, used for relief of anxiety and mental tension.

mEq. Abbr. for *milliequivalent.*

meralgia (mer-al'jĭ-ă) [G. *mēros,* thigh, + *algos,* pain]. Neuralgia of the thigh.

m. paresthet'ica. Affection of nerves of the thigh causing itching, tingling, pain, burning, and sometimes numbness.

Mercier's bar or **barrier** (mer-se-ā'). A curved fold at neck of bladder, forming post. margin of trigonum vesicae.

mercupurin (mĕr-kū'pū-rĭn) [L. *mercurius,* mercury, + *purum,* pure, + *uricum.* uric acid]. A proprietary diuretic.

mercurial (mer-kū'rĭ-al) [L. *mercurialis,* pert. to mercury]. 1. Pert. to mercury. 2. A substance containing mercury.

m. diuretics. Organic mercurial compounds that produce diuresis.

m. palsy. Paralysis induced by mercurial poisoning.

m. rash. Rash caused by application of mercurial preparations locally.

mercurialism (mer-kū'rĭ-al-ĭzm) [" + G. *ismos,* state of]. Chronic poisoning by mercury seen as a result of continuous administration of mercury.

Also occurs in workmen who labor on the metal, or inhale its vapors.

SYM: Soreness of gums and loosening of teeth; increased salivation; fetor of breath; griping, and diarrhea.

mercurialization (mer-kū"rĭ-al-ĭ-zā'shŭn) [L. *mercurius,* mercury]. Condition of influencing with mercury.

mercurialized (mĕr-kū'rĭ-ă-līzd) [L. *mercurius,* mercury]. 1. Impregnated with mercury. 2. Influenced by or treated with mercury.

mercuric (mer-ku′rik) [L. *mercurius*, mercury]. Rel. to bivalent mercury.

m. chloride ($HgCl_2$). A common compound of mercury.

One part to 1000 of water is used to free the hands or skin from bacteria. This solution used in strength of 1:2000 or 1:4000 may be used for wound irrigation. It should be remembered that this disinfectant coagulates albumen, that it corrodes metal instruments, and causes local dermatitis. No metallic instrument should ever be placed in contact with mercuric chloride. Since it has been put up in blue coffin-shaped tablets in a notched bottle, poisoning has been less common.

POISONING: SYM: *Acute*: Those of any severe gastrointestinal irritation, with pain, cramping, constriction of the throat, vomiting, and a metallic taste in the mouth. Stronger solution causes a white coating due to coagulation. Abdominal pain may be so severe as to cause fainting, bloody diarrhea, bloody vomitus, scanty urine, prostration, convulsions and unconsciousness. Unless treatment is begun immediately, death is the usual outcome.

SYM: *Chronic*: Bad breath, loosening of teeth, fever, urinary difficulties, nausea, diarrhea, sore tongue, paralyses, weakness and death.

F. A. TREATMENT: Evacuate stomach, wash out with milk or with a baking soda solution made by dissolving a teaspoonful of sodium bicarbonate in six ounces of water. Treatment with BAL (British antilewisite) should begin as soon as possible after poisoning has occurred.

m. oxide (HgO). A powder, usually yellow in color. Used in ointments.

mercurochrome (mer-kū′ro-krōm) [L. *mercurius*, mercury, + G. *chrōma*, color]. A compound containing about 23% mercury, used as an antiseptic in solution.

mercurous (mer-kū′rus, mer′ku-rus) [L. *mercurius*]. Rel. to monovalent mercury.

m. chloride (HgCl) (Calomel). This is a heavy white powder used in small doses in medicine as a laxative.

It is used in powder form as an application in ulcers and skin rashes.

POISONING: SYM: Salivation, abdominal discomfort, and diarrhea.

F. A. TREATMENT: SEE: *mercuric chloride*.

INCOMPATIBILITIES: Iodoform, soluble iodides, soluble hydroxides.

mercury (mer′kū-rĭ) [L. *mercurius*]. SYN: *quicksilver*. A metallic element. SYMB: Hg. At. weight 200.59. At. number 80. Insoluble in ordinary solvents but soluble in hydrochloric acid upon boiling. Forms two series of salts: *mercurous* in which it has a valence of one (univalent) and *mercuric* in which it has a valence of two (bivalent). It is a silvery liquid at ordinary temperatures.

NOTE: Metallic mercury swallowed in small quantities, as from a broken thermometer, is not harmful.

POISONING: SYM: In large doses, increased salivation, abdominal cramps, interference with kidney function, etc. SEE ALSO: *Table of Poisons and Poisoning in Appendix.*

m., ammoniated. SEE: *white precipitate.*

m. bichloride. Corrosive sublimate.

USES: Germicide.

INCOMPATIBILITIES: Albumen, alkalies, borax, etc.

SEE: *mercuric chloride, nephrosis.*

mercuzanthine. A proprietary name for a preparation of mercurophylline sodium, a diuretic.

meridian. A line encircling a globular body at right angles to its equator and passing through the poles, or a half of such a line.

m. of the eye. A circle passing through ant. and post. poles of the eyeball.

meridrosis (mer-id-rō′sĭs) [G. *meros*, part, + *idrōsis*, perspiration]. Local perspiration.

merinthophobia (mĕr-ĭn-thō-fō′bĭ-ă) [G. *mērinthos*, a cord, + *phobos*, fear]. Morbid fear of being tied.

merispore (mer′ĭ-spōr) [G. *meros*, a part, + *sporos*, a seed]. A secondary spore resulting from the division of another spore.

mero- [G.]. Combining form meaning a part, the thigh.

meroblastic (mer-ō-blăst′ĭk) [G. *meros*, a part, the thigh, + *blastos*, germ]. Pertaining to a type of ovum containing considerable yolk or a type of cleavage in which cleavage divisions are restricted to the protoplasmic region of the animal pole. Opp. of *holoblastic.*

merocele (mer′ō-sēl) [G. *mēros*, thigh, + *kēlē*, hernia]. Femoral hernia.

merocoxalgia (mer″ō-koks-al′jĭ-ă) [" + L. *coxa*, hip, + G. *algos*, pain]. Painful condition of the thigh and hip.

merocrine (mer′o-krin, mer′ō-krīn) [G. *meros*, a part, + *krinein*, to secrete]. Pertaining to a type of secretion in which the glandular cell remains intact during the process of elaborating and discharging its product. SEE: *apocrine, holocrine.*

meroergasia (mĕr″ō-ĕr-gā′zĭ-ă) [G. *meros*, a part + *ergasia*, work]. Partial mental disorder with symptoms of emotional instability. SEE: *holergastic.*

merogenesis (mĕr″ō-jen′ĕ-sĭs) [" + *genesis*, production]. Multiplication or reproduction by segmentation.

merology (mer-ol′ō-jĭ) [" + *logos*, study of]. Anatomy of the elementary tissues.

meromicrosomia (mĕr″ō-mī″krō-sō′mĭ-ă) [" + *mikros*, small, + *sōma*, body]. Abnormal smallness of some part or structure of the body.

meronecrosis (mer″ō-nĕk-rō′sĭs) [" + *nekros*, dead]. Necrosis of cells.

meropia (mer-o′pĭ-ă) [G. *meros*, part, + *ōps*, vision]. Partial blindness.

merorrhachischisis (mĕr-or-ră-kis′kĭ-sis) [" + *rachis*, spine, + *schisis*, fissure]. Fissure of a portion of the spinal cord.

meroscope (mer′o-skōp) [G. *meros*, part, + *skopein*, to examine]. Device used in performing meroscopy.

merosmia (mĕr-os′mĭ-ă) [" + *osmē*, odor]. Inability to detect certain odors.

merosystolic (mĕr-ō-sĭs-tol′ĭk) [" + *systolē*, a contraction]. Rel. to a portion of the systole.

merotomy (mer-ot′o-mē) [" + *tomē*, incision]. Division into sections or segments.

merozoite (mer-ō-zō′ĭt) [G. *meros*, part, + *zoon*, animal]. A body formed by segmentation or breaking up of schizont in asexual reproduction of certain sporozoans such as *Plasmodium*. Merozoites when formed are liberated and invade other corpuscles where they repeat the process of schizogony, or develop into gametocytes.

merthiolate (mer-thi'ō-lāt). Proprietary name for thimerosal. An organic combination containing about 50% mercury, and less toxic than bichloride, used as a disinfectant in solutions of 1:5000 to 1:1000, aqueous, or in the form of a tincture, as an ointment, 1:2000. *For ophthalmic use,* 1:5000 ointment, or 1:10,000 aqueous.

Meru'lius lac'rymans. A species of fungi causing dry rot in wood. Spores when inhaled may develop in lungs or respiratory passageways, causing a sometimes fatal disease.

Méry's glands (ma-re') [Jean Mery, Paris anatomist, 1645-1722]. Two bulbourethral glands. SYN: *Cowper's glands.*

mesad (mes'ăd) [G. *mesos,* middle, + L. *ad,* toward]. Toward a median point, line, or plane.

mesal (mes'ăl) [G. *mesos,* middle]. In a middle line or plane.

mesaortitis (mĕs-ā-or-tī'tĭs) [G. *mesos,* middle, + *aortē,* aorta, + *-ītis,* inflammation]. Inflammation of the middle aortic coat.

mesaraic, mesareic (mes-ar-ā'ĭk, -e'ĭk) [" + *araia,* belly]. Rel. to the mesentery. SYN: *mesenteric.*

mesarteritis (mĕs-ar-tĕr-ī'tĭs) [" + *artēria,* artery, + *-ītis,* inflammation]. Inflammation of the tunica media or middle coat of an artery.

mesaticephalic (mĕs-ăt"ĭ-sef-al'ik) [G. *mesatos,* medium, + *kephalē,* brain]. Having a skull with a cephalic index of 75 to 79.9 degrees.

mesatipellic, mesatipelvic (mĕs-ăt"ĭ-pĕl'-lĭk, -pel'vĭk) [" + *pellis,* pelvis]. Having a pelvis with an index bet. 90 and 95 degrees.

mescaline (mĕs'kă-lēn). A poisonous alkaloid, the active ingredient of the mescal cactus which causes hallucinations, esp. those involving color and music. SYN:*Peyote.*

mesectic (mĕs-ek'tĭk) [G. *mesos,* middle, + *echein,* to have]. Using up a normal amount of oxygen. SEE: *mionectic, pleonectic.*

mesectoderm (mĕs-ĕk'tō-derm). The portion of mesenchyme derived from ectoderm, esp. from neural-crest cells ant. to the somites.

mesencephalon (mes-en-sef'al-on) [G. *mesos,* middle, + *egkephalos,* brain]. The midbrain consisting of the corpora quadrigemina, the crura cerebri, and the aqueduct of Sylvius.

mesenchyme (mĕs'ĕn-kīm) [G. *mesos,* middle, + *egchyma,* infusion]. A diffuse network of cells forming the embryonic mesoderm and giving rise to connective tissues, blood and blood vessels, the lymphatic system, and cells of the reticuloendothelial system.

mesenter'ic [" + *enteron,* intestine]. Pert. to the mesentery.

mesenteriolum (mes-en-ter-ĭ-ō'lum) [L. *mesenteriōlum,* little mesentery]. A small mesentery, as that of a diverticulum of the intestine.

mesenteriopexy (mes-en-ter'ĭ-ō-peks-ĭ) [G. *mesos,* middle, + *enteron,* intestine, + *pēxis,* fixation]. Fixation of a torn mesentery.

mesenteriorrhaphy (mes"en-ter-ĭ-or'ra-fĭ) [" + " + *raphē,* a sewing]. Suturing of the mesentery.

mesenteriplication (mĕs"ĕn-tĕr-ĭ-pli-kā'-shun) [" + " + L. *plicāre,* to fold]. Taking tucks in the mesentery surgically.

mesenteritis (mes"ĕn-tĕr-ī'tĭs) [" + " + *-ītis,* inflammation]. Inflamed condition of the mesentery.

mesenteron (mes-en'ter-on) [G. *mesos,* middle, + *enteron,* intestine]. Middle portion of the embryonic digestive tract.

mesentery (mes'en-ter-ĭ) [" + *enteron,* intestine]. A peritoneal fold, connecting the intestine with the post. abdominal wall.

m., proper. That of the small intestine.

Mesocolon is the name given to that of the colon; *mesocecum,* that of the cecum, and *mesorectum,* that of the rectum.

mesiad (mes'ĭ-ad) [" + L. *ad,* toward]. Toward the middle line. SYN: *mesad.*

mesial (mē'sĭ-ăl) [G. *mesos,* middle]. SYN: *median.* Toward the median plane of the body.

mesio-. In dentistry, combining form meaning pertaining to or facing the median plane of the mouth.

mesion (mes'ĭ-on) [G. *mesos,* middle]. The imaginary plane dividing the body into right and left symmetric halves. SYN: *meson.*

mesiris (mes-ī'ris) [" + *īris,* iris]. Middle portion of the iris.

mesmeric (mes-mer'ĭk). Rel. to or induced by hypnotism; fascinating.

mesmerism (mes'mer-izm). Originally the theory of Mesmer, it now means therapeutics employing hypnotism or hypnotic suggestion.

meso-. Combining form meaning (1) middle; (2) in anatomy, pert. to a mesentery; (3) in medicine, secondary or partial.

mesoaortitis (mes"o-ā-or-tī'tis) [G. *mesos,* middle, + *aortē,* artery, + *-ītis,* inflammation]. Inflamed condition of aortic middle coat. SYN: *mesaortitis*

mesoappendicitis (mes-ō-ap-pen-dĭ-sī'tis) [" + L. *appendix,* an appendage, + G. *-ītis,* inflammation]. Inflamed condition of the mesoappendix.

mesoappendix (mes"ō-ap-pen'dĭks) [" + L. *appendix,* an appendage]. Mesentery of the vermiform appendix.

mesobronchitis (mes"ō-bron-kī'tĭs) [G. *mesos,* middle, + *brogchos,* windpipe, + *-ītis,* inflammation]. Inflammation of the middle layer of the bronchi.

mesocardia (mes-ō-kar'dĭ-ă) [" + *kardia,* heart]. Location of the heart in the middle line of the thorax, being a normal position in fetal stage, but a malposition in life.

mesocardium (mes-ō-kar'dĭ-ŭm) [G. *mesos,* middle, + *kardia,* heart]. An embryonic mesentery supporting the heart. The *dorsal m.* connects heart to the foregut; the *ventral m.* connects heart to central body wall.

mesocecum (mes-ō-se'kŭm) [G. *mesos,* middle, + L. *caecum,* blind gut]. Mesentery attaching the cecum.

mesocele (mes'ō-sēl) [" + *koilia,* hollow]. Sylvian aqueduct in the brain.

mesocephalic (mes-ō-sef-al'ik) [" + *kephalē,* head]. 1. Pert. to the midbrain. 2. Having a medium sized head. 3. Having a cranial index of 76.0 to 80.9.

mesocolic (mes-ō-kol'ik) [" + *kōlon,* colon]. Concerning the mesocolon.

mesocolon (mĕs-ō-kō'lon) [" + *kōlon,* colon]. Mesentery connecting colon with post. abdominal wall.

mesocolopexy (mĕs"ō-kō'lō-peks-ĭ) [G. *mesos,* middle, + *kōlon,* colon, + *pēxis,* fixation]. The taking of tucks in the mesocolon and then suturing it to make it shorter. SYN: *mesocoloplication.*

mes'ocord [G. *mesos*, middle, + *chordē*, cord]. A portion of umbilical cord attached to placenta.

mesoderm (mĕs'ō-derm) [G. *mesos*, middle, + *derma*, skin]. A primary germ layer of the embryo lying between ectoderm and entoderm. From it arise all connective tissues, muscular, skeletal, circulatory, lymphatic, and urogenital systems and the linings of the body cavities. SEE: *ectoderm*, *entoderm*.

m., axial. That giving rise to notochord and prechordal plate.

m., extraembryonic. That lying outside the embryo proper. It is involved in formation of amnion, chorion, yolk sac, and body stalk.

m., intermediate. SYN: *mesomere*. M. lying between somite and lateral mesoderm. Gives rise to embryonic and definitive kidneys and their ducts. Also called *nephrotome*.

m., lateral. SYN: *hypomere*. Unsegmented m. lying lateral to the intermediate mesoderm. In it develops a cavity, the *coelom*, separating it into layers, the *somatic* and *splanchnic mesoderm*.

m., paraxial. SYN: *epimere*. M. lying immediately lateral to neural tube and notochord.

m., somatic. Outer layer of lateral mesoderm. Becomes intimately associated with ectoderm, forming *somatopleure* from which ventral and lateral walls of embryo develop.

m., splanchnic. Inner layer of lateral mesoderm. Becomes intimately associated with entoderm forming *splanchnopleure* from which the gut and lungs and their coverings arise.

mesoduodenum (mĕs"ō-dū-ō-dē'nŭm) [" + L. *duodeni*, twelve]. Mesentery connecting duodenum to abdominal wall.

mesogastric (mĕs-ō-gas'trĭk) [" + *gastēr*, belly]. 1. Pert. to umbilical region. 2. Pert. to the mesogastrium.

mesogastrium (mĕs"ō-gas'trĭ-ŭm) [G. *mesos*, middle, + *gastēr*, belly]. 1. The umbilical region. The part of the mesentery of the embryo attached to the primitive stomach.

mesognathic (mĕs-og-nath'ik) [" + *gnathos*, jaw]. Having a gnathic index bet. 98 and 103.

mesognathion (mĕs-og-nath'ĭ-on) [" + *gnathos*, jaw]. The intermaxillary or premaxillary bone.

mesohyloma (mes-ō-hī-lō'mă) [" + *ylē*, matter, + *-ōma*, tumor]. Tumor derived from the mesothelium.

mesoileum (mes-ō-il'ē-ŭm) [" + L. *ileum*, from G. *eilein*, to twist]. Mesentery of the ileum.

mesojejunum (mes-ō-jē-jū'nŭm) [" + L. *jejunum*, empty]. Mesentery of the jejunum.

mesomere. SYN: *nephrotome*, *intermediate mesoderm*. Portion of mesoderm between epimere and hypomere.

mesometritis (mes-o-me-tri'tis) [G. *mesos*, middle, + *mētra*, uterus, + *-itis*, inflammation]. Inflammation of the uterine musculature. SYN: *myometritis*.

mesometrium (mes-o-me'trĭ-um) [" + *mētra*, uterus]. 1. The uterine musculature. 2. [NA]. The broad ligament below the mesovarium.

mesomorph (mes'ō-morf) [" + *morphē*, form]. A well-proportioned person of medium height. SEE: *hypermorph*, *hypomorph*.

meson (mes'on). 1. Particle of mass intermediate between that of the electron and proton. Mesons of more than one variety and of both positive and negative charge occur. SYN: *mesotron*. 2. Mesion, *q.v.*

mesonasal. In the middle of the nose.

mesonephric (mĕs-ō-nef'rĭk) [G. *mesos*, middle, + *nephros*, kidney]. Pert. to the mesonephros.

m. duct. SYN: *wolffian duct*. Embryonic duct which gives rise in the male to reproductive ducts (ductus epididymidis, ductus deferens, seminal vesicle, and ejaculatory duct). In the female, it gives rise to *Gartner's duct of the epoophoron*, a rudimentary structure.

m. tubules. Embryonic tubules consisting of two groups, *cranial* and *caudal*. The cranial group gives rise: (a) in the male to efferent ductules of testes and appendix epididymis; (b) in the female to the epoophoron and vesicular appendices. The caudal group gives rise in the male to the paradidymis and aberrant ductules; in the female to the paroophoron. All structures except the efferent ductules of the testes are vestigial.

mesonephroma (mes"ō-nē-frō'mă). A tumor derived from mesonephric cells developing in reproductive organs, esp. ovary or genital tract.

mesonephros (mĕs"ō-nef'ros). SYN: *wolffian body*, *middle kidney*. A type of kidney which develops in all vertebrate embryos of classes above the Cyclostomes. It is the permanent kidney of fishes and amphibians, but, in reptiles and mammals, is replaced by the metanephros.

mesoneuritis (me-sō-nū-ri'tis) [" + *neuron*, nerve, + *-itis*, inflammation]. Inflammation of the substance of a nerve or of its lymphatics.

mesopexy (mes'ō-peks-ĭ) [" + *pēxis*, fixation]. Operation of shortening the mesentery by taking a tuck in it.

mesophilic (mes-ō-fĭl'ĭk) [G. *mesos*, middle, + *philein*, to love]. Preferring moderate temperature, as some bacteria which develop best at temperatures between 15° and 43° C.

mesophryon (mes-of'rĭ-on) [G. *mesos*, middle, + *ophrys*, eyebrow]. Midpoint in smooth space bet. the eyebrows. SEE: *glabella*.

mesopneumon (mes-ō-nū'mon) [" + *pneumōn*, lung]. Meeting point of two pleural layers at hilus of the lung.

mesoporphyrin. $C_{32}H_{36}N_4$ $(COOH)_2$. An iron-free derivative of hemin.

mesorchium (mes-or'kĭ-um) [" + *orchis*, testicle]. Peritoneal fold which holds fetal testes in place.

mesorectum (mĕs-ō-rĕk'tŭm) [" + L. *rectus*, straight]. Mesentery of the rectum.

mesoropter (mes-ō-rop'ter) [G. *mesos*, middle, + *oros*, boundary, + *optēr*, observer]. Normal eye position with muscles at rest.

mesorrhachischisis (mĕs"o-ră-kĭs'kĭ-sĭs) [" + *rachis*, spine, + *schisis*, cleft]. Fissure of a portion of the spinal cord. SYN: *merorrhachischisis*.

mesorrhaphy (mes-or'ă-fĭ) [" + *raphē*, a sewing]. Suture of the mesentery. SYN: *mesenteriorrhaphy*.

mesorrhine (mes'or-rīn) [" + *ris*, *rin-*, nose]. With a nasal index variously quoted to range anywhere bet. 47 and 53.

mesosalpinx (mĕs"ō-sal'pĭnks) [G. *mesos*, middle, + *salpigx*, tube]. [NA]. The free margin of the upper division of the broad ligament, within which lies the oviduct.

mesoseme (mes'ō-sēm) [" + *sēma*, sign]. Possessing an orbital index bet. 83 and 90.

mesosigmoid (mĕs-ō-sĭg′moid) [" + *sigma*, letter S, + *eidos*, form]. Mesentery of the sigmoid flexure.

mesoskelic (mes-o-skel′ik) [" + *skelos*, leg]. Legs of normal length.

mesosternum (mes″ō-ster′nŭm) [" + *sternon*, chest]. The middle or second section of the sternum. SYN: *gladiolus.*

mesothelium (mĕs-ō-thē′lĭ-ŭm) [" + *thēlē*, nipple]. The layer of cells, derived from the mesoderm lining the primitive body cavity; in the adult it becomes the epithelium covering the serous membranes.

mesothenar (mes-ō-thē′nar) [" + *thenar*, palm]. The adductor pollicis muscle.

mes′otron. A subatomic particle of weight intermediate between light particles (electrons) and heavy particles (protons). SYN: *meson, 1.*

mesovarium (mĕs-ō-va′rĭ-ŭm) [" + L. *ovarium*, ovary]. [NA]. The portion of the peritoneal fold that connects the ant. border of the ovary to the post. layer of the broad ligament.

meta-. Prefix meaning (1) *after, beyond, among,* or *over;* (2) in zool., *later* or *more highly developed;* (3) in chem., the 1-3 position of benzene derivatives.

metabiosis (mĕt-ă-bī-ō′sĭs) [" + *biōsis*, way of life]. Dependence of an organism for its existence upon another and giving no recompense.

metabolic (mĕt-a-bŏl′ĭk) [G. *metabolē*, change]. Pertaining to metabolism.

m. failure. Rapid failure of physical and mental functions ending in death.

m. gradient. A gradient in metabolic activity which exists in certain structures such as the small intestine from duodenum to ileum or in embryos from animal to vegetal poles in which metabolic activity is highest in one region and becomes progressively lower away from this region.

m. rate. SEE: *basal metabolism;* also *metabolism, basal.*

metab′olism [G. *metabolē*, change, + *ismos*, state of]. The sum of all physical and chemical changes which take place within an organism; all energy and material transformations which occur within living cells. It includes *material changes, i. e.,* changes undergone by substances during all periods of life (growth, maturity, senescence) and *energy changes, i. e.,* all transformations of chemical energy of foodstuffs to mechanical energy or heat. It involves two fundamental processes (a) *anabolism* (assimilation or building-up processes), and (b) *catabolism* (disintegration or tearing-down processes). Anabolism is the conversion of ingested substances into the constituents of protoplasm; catabolism is the breakdown of substances into simpler substances, the end-products usually being excreted. *General metabolism* includes all the processes involved in the utilization of substances entering the body; *special metabolism* is the term applied to all the changes involved in the utilization of particular substances, such as carbohydrates, proteins, fats, minerals, or water, and referred to as carbohydrate metabolism, protein metabolism, etc.

m., basal. Lowest level of energy expenditure. This is determined when the body is at complete rest. For an average person, this is, in terms of calories, 1500-1800 per day; in terms of body weight, 1 Cal. per kilogram per hour; in terms of body surface, 40 Cal. per sq. meter per hour.

m., carbohydrate. All carbohydrates are digested to monosaccharides and absorbed as such principally in the form of hexoses of which glucose is the principal one. In the liver and muscles, glucose is converted to *glycogen* or it may be oxidized to carbon dioxide and water, the ultimate fate of all carbohydrates. These reactions require the presence of insulin and other hormones. In the process, many intermediate compounds are formed, among them lactic acid.

The basic reaction is $C_6H_{12}O_6 + 6O_2 \rightarrow 6CO_2 + 6H_2O$ which is the basis for the determination of the *respiratory quotient* (R.Q.), *q.v.*

m., constructive. Anabolism or assimilation. The building-up processes by which complex substances are synthesized.

m., destructive. Catabolism; the breakdown or decomposition of substances into their simple constituents.

m., fat. Fats are digested to fatty acids and glycerol. Following absorption they may be reconverted to neutral fats and stored as adipose tissue or oxidized to CO_2 and H_2O. Fats may be formed from carbohydrates or proteins. In the utilization of fats, the liver plays an important role in the desaturation of fatty acids. Fat metabolism also involves the formation and utilization of substances related to fats, such as sterols and phospholipids.

m., protein. Proteins are digested to amino acids and absorbed as such. In the body these are synthesized into body proteins which form an integral part of protoplasm, hence they are essential for normal growth and the repair of tissues. Those not utilized thus are deaminized, *i. e.,* the amino group is removed. This results in the production of urea which is excreted; the remainder, a fatty acid residue (COOH), may be oxidized or converted to glucose, which may be stored as glycogen or converted to fat.

m., purine. M. involving nucleic acids, present in nuclei of cells in which they are combined with proteins to form nucleoproteins. In the breakdown of nucleic acid, *uric acid,* one of the end products, is formed.

metabolite (mĕ-tab′ō-līt) [G. *metabolē*, change]. Any product of metabolism.

metacar′pal [G. *meta*, beyond, + *karpos*, wrist]. Pert. to the bones of the metacarpus, or bones of the hand. SEE: *skeleton.*

metacarpectomy (met″ă-kar-pek′to-mĭ). Surgical excision of one or more wrist bones.

metacarpus (met-ă-kar′pus) [" + *karpos*, wrist]. The five metacarpal bones of the palm of the hand. SEE: *carpometacarpal.*

metachromasia, metachromatism (mĕt-ă-krō-mă′zĭ-ă, -krōm′ă-tĭzm) [G. *meta*, change, + *chrōma*, color]. Condition in which different substances assume different colors or hues when stained by the same dye.

metachromatic (met″ă-krō-mat′ĭk) [" + *chrōma*, color]. Pert. to metachromatism.

m. bodies* or *granules. Granules in protoplasm which stain deeply and differently from the surrounding ones; seen in various bacteria.

metachromophil (met-a-krōm′ō-fil) [" + " + *philein*, to love]. Not reacting normally to staining.

metachrosis (met-ă-krō′sis) [" + *chrōa*, color]. Change of color in animal life.

DIAGRAM OF NORMAL METABOLIC FOOD CHANGES

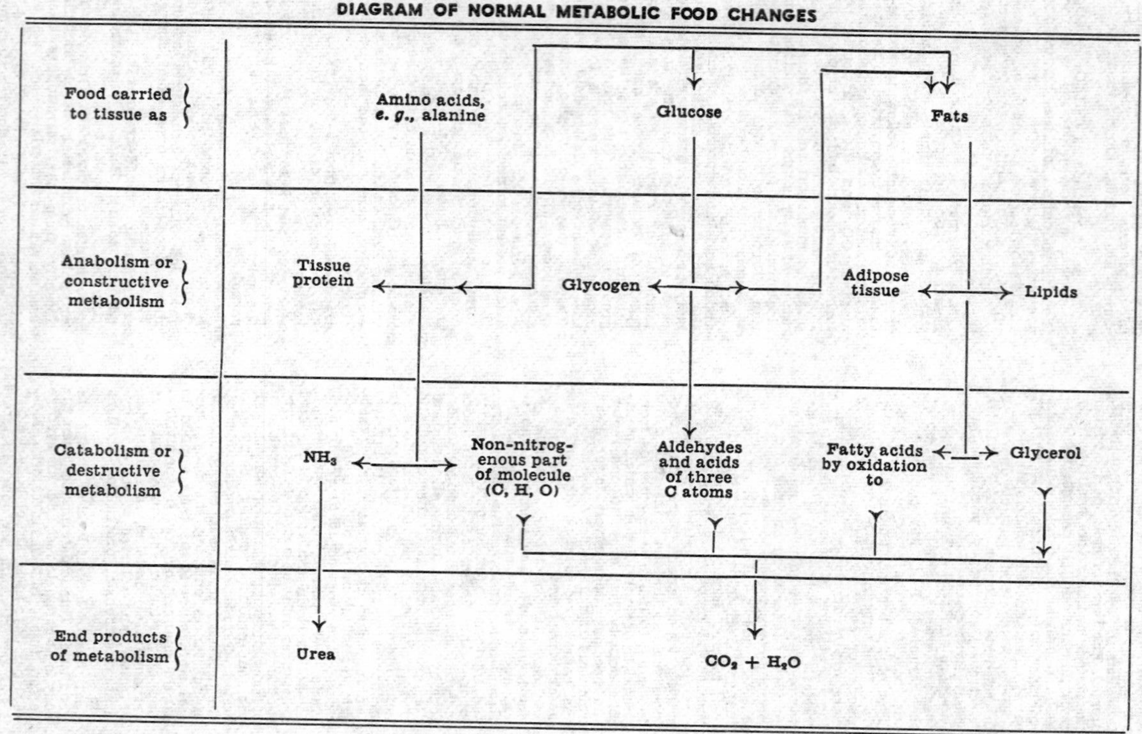

metacone. The distobuccal cusp of an upper molar tooth.

metaconid. The mesiolingual cusp of a lower molar tooth.

metaconule. The distal intermediate cusp of an upper molar tooth.

metacyesis (met-ă-si-ē'sĭs) [" + *kyesis,* pregnancy]. Extrauterine gestation.

metagen'esis [" + *genesis,* formation]. Alternation of generation.

metagglutinin (met-ag-glū'tĭn-ĭn) [G. *meta,* beyond, + L. *agglutināre,* to glue]. A partial agglutinin; an agglutinin present in immune serum which acts on organisms closely related to the one acting as the specific antigen.

Met"agon'imus. A genus of flukes belonging to the family Heterophyidae.

M. yokogawai. A species of intestinal flukes common in the Middle and Far East. Normally infests the intestine of dogs and cats, and other animals, but commonly in man. Intermediate hosts: snails and fishes, esp. a species of trout, *Plecoglossus altivelis.*

metaicteric (met"ă-ik-ter'ik) [" + *ikteros,* jaundice]. Occurring as a consequence of jaundice.

metainfective (mĕt-ă-ĭn-fek'tĭv) [" + L. *infectiō,* an infection]. Occurring as a consequence of an infection.

metakaryocyte (met"ă-kar'ĭ-ō-sīt). A normoblast, *q.v.*

metakinesis (mĕt"ă-kĭn-e'sĭs) [G. *mets,* beyond, -*kinēsis,* motion]. Transition stage in mitosis between prophase and metaphase in which chromosomes move to the equatorial plane. Syn: *metaphase.*

metal fume fever (or braziers' chills). This results from absorbing the fumes in special occupations such as welding, metal founding, torch metal cutting, and galvanizing. Zinc commonest cause of these disturbances.

Sym: Come on late. Chills, weakness, lassitude, profound thirst, followed after some hours by sweating and anorexia; occasionally there is mild inflammation of the eyes and respiratory tract.

F. A. Treatment: Fresh air and symptomatic treatment.

metallesthesia (mĕt"al-ĕs-thē'sĭ-ă) [G. *metallon,* metal, + *aisthēsis,* sensation]. Recognition of metals by touching them.

metallic (mĕ-tal'ik) [G. *metallon,* metal]. 1. Pert. to metal. 2. Composed of or resembling a metal.

m. tinkling. A peculiar ringing or bell-like auscultatory sound in pneumothorax over large pulmonary cavities.

metallophobia (mĕ"tal-ō-fō'bĭ-ă) [" + *phobos,* fear]. Abnormal fear of metals and metallic objects and of touching them.

metalloscopy (mĕ-tăl-os'kō-pĭ) [" + *skopein,* to examine]. Determination of the effects of applying metals to the body, and its sensitivity to them.

metallotherapy (mĕ-tal-ō-ther'ă-pĭ) [" + *therapeia,* treatment]. Treatment by applying metals to the affected part.

metallur'gy [" + *ergon,* work]. Study and methods of using metals.

metamere (met'ă-mēr) [G. *meta,* one after the other + *meros,* part]. One of a series of similar segments arranged in a linear series and making up the body of an animal such as an earthworm.

metameric (met-ă-mer'ik) [G. *meta,* across, + *meros,* part]. Rel. to metamerism. Syn: *isomeric.*

metamerism (mĕ-tam'er-izm). 1. Isomerism, *q.v.* 2. Isomerism consisting of segments or metameres.

metamorphopsia (mĕt"ă-mor-fop'sĭ-ă) [" + *morphē,* form, + *opsis,* vision]. Ophth: Visual distortion of objects; found in refractive errors, esp. astigmatism, retinal disease, choroiditis, detachment of retina, and tumors of retina and choroid.

metamorphosis (met-ă-mor'fō-sĭs) [G. *meta,* across, + *morphē,* form, + *-osis,* intensive]. 1. A change in form or structure, esp. the transition from one form to another as in complete metamorphosis of an insect (egg, larva, pupa, adult). 2. In pathology, a degenerative change.

m., fatty. Fatty degeneration.

metamyelocyte (mĕt"ă-mī-ĭ-lō'sīt). Syn: *juvenile cell.* A cell intermediate in development between a myelocyte and a mature granular leukocyte.

metanephros (met-ă-nĕf'ros) [G. *meta,* across, + *nephros,* kidney]. The permanent kidney of amniotes (reptiles, birds, and mammals). A portion of it develops from caudal portion of intermediate cell mass or nephrotome; the remaining portion is derived from a bud of the mesonephric duct.

metaneutrophil (met-ă-nū'trō-fĭl) [" + L. *neuter,* neither, + G. *philein,* to love]. Not reacting normally with neutral stains.

metaphase (mĕt'ă-fāz) [G. *meta,* beyond, + *phasis,* a shining out]. Stage in mitosis in which the chromosomes are arranged in an equatorial plate. Follows the prophase and precedes the anaphase in which longitudinal halves of chromosomes diverge. Syn: *metakinesis.*

metaphen (mĕt'ă-phĕn). A proprietary name of a preparation of nitromersol.

Uses: In solution, the agent is used as a disinfectant and antiseptic. It is used especially in preoperative preparation of the skin.

metaphysis (mĕ-taf'ĭ-sĭs) [G. *meta,* after, + *physis,* nature]. Portion of a developing long bone between diaphysis or shaft and epiphysis; the growing portion of a bone.

metaplasia (met-ă-plā'zĭ-ă) [" + *plasis,* a molding]. Conversion of one kind of tissue into another.

metaplasm (met'ă-plăzm) [" + *plasma,* a thing formed]. Reserve material present in protoplasm of a cell, esp. stored nutritive substance. Syn: *cell inclusions, paraplasm.*

metaplastic (met-ă-plas'tik) [" + *plastikos,* formed]. Pert. to or formed by metaplasia.

metapneumonic (met-ă-nū-mon'ĭk) [G. *meta,* beyond, + *pneumōnia,* lung infection]. Succeeding or as a consequence of pneumonia.

metapophysis (met-ă-pof'ĭ-sis) [" + *apo,* from, + *physis,* growth]. Mammillary process on the superior articular processes of a vertebra.

metapro'tein [" + *prōtos,* first]. Derived protein resulting from the action of acids or alkalies, in which the molecule is changed to form protein insoluble in neutral solvents but soluble in alkalies and weak acids. See: *protein.*

metapyretic (mĕt"ă-pī-rĕt'ĭk) [G. *meta,* beyond, + *pyretos,* fever]. Performed or occurring after fever; postpyretic.

metarteriole (mĕt"ar-tē'rĭ-ōl). A small vessel connecting an arteriole to a venule from which true capillaries are given off. Syn: *precapillary.*

metastable (met"ă-stā'bl) [G. *meta,* change, + L. *stabilis,* stable]. Changing from one condition to another; unstable. Term used in chemistry and physics.

metastasis (mĕ-tas'tă-sis) [" + *stasis*, a standing]. 1. Movement of bacteria or body cells (esp. cancer cells) from one part of the body to another. 2. Change in location of a disease or of its manifestations or transfer from one organ or part to another.

The usual application is to the manifestation of a malignancy in a secondary growth arising from the primary growth in a new location. Spread is by the lymphatics or blood stream.

metastasize (me-tas'tă-sīz) [" + *stasis*, a standing]. To invade by metastasis.

metastatic (met-ă-stat'ik) [" + *statikos*, standing]. Pert. to metastasis.

metatarsalgia (met-ă-tar-săl'jĭ-ă) [G. *meta*, beyond, *-tarsos*, tarsus]. SYN: *Morton's foot, M's neuralgia.* Severe pain or cramp in ant. portion of metatarsus.

metatarsectomy (met"ă-tar-sĕk'tō-mĭ) [G. *meta*, beyond, + *ektomē*, excision]. Removal of the metatarsus, or a metatarsal bone.

metatarsophalangeal (met"ă-tar"sō-fă-lan'jē-ăl) [" + " + *phalagx, phalagg-*, a phalanx]. Concerning the metatarsus and phalanges.

metatarsus (mĕt-ă-tar'sŭs) [G. *meta*, beyond, + *tarsos*, tarsus]. The region of foot between tarsus and phalanges. Includes the five metatarsal bones.

metathalamus (met-ă-thal'ă-mus) [" + *thalamos*, a chamber]. [NA]. The post. part of the thalamus including the two geniculate bodies.

metathesis (mĕ-tath'ĕ-sis) [G. *meta*, over, + *thesis*, a placing]. 1. A changing of places. 2. Forcible transference of a disease process from one part to another where it will be more accessible for treatment. 3. Double decomposition chemically.

metatro'phic [" + *trophē*, nourishment]. 1. Pert. to metatrophia. 2. Requiring lifeless organic matter for food. SYN: *saprophytic.*

metatrophism (mĕt-ăt'rō-fĭzm) [G. *meta*, change, + *tropē*, a turning, + *ismos*, state of]. Masculine behavior in women and feminine behavior in men.

metatuberculosis (mĕt"ă-tū-ber-kū-lō'sĭs) [" + L. *tuberculum*, a small nodule]. A condition of tuberculous reactions with nontuberculous lesions.

Metazoa. Division of the animal kingdom which includes all multicellular forms, in contrast to unicellular forms or Protozoa.

Metch'nikoff's theory [Elie Metchnikoff, Russian zoologist in France, 1845-1916]. Microorganisms are ingested by living cells, as by leukocytes and other phagocytes. SEE: *phagocytosis.*

metencephalon (met"ĕn-sĕf'ă-lon) [G. *meta*, after, + *egkephalos*, brain]. SYN: *afterbrain, hindbrain.* The ant. portion of the embryonic rhombencephalon from which the cerebellum and pons arise.

meteorism (mē'tē-or-izm) [G. *meteōrizein*, to raise up]. Distention by gas in the abdomen or intestines. SYN: *tympanites.*

me'ter [G. *metron*, a measure]. A linear standard of measurement, 39.37 inches.

met"ergas'is. Change or alteration in function.

met"es'trus. Period following estrus and preceding diestrus.

methadone hydrochloride. A synthetic analgesic drug with potency equal to that of morphine, but the narcotic action is weaker than that of morphine. Methadone is a habit-forming agent and should be administered with care.

methane. CH_4, marsh gas. A colorless, odorless, inflammable gas. It is produced as a result of putrefaction and fermentation of organic matter.

methanol (meth'ă-nol). A poisonous volatile, inflammable alcohol, CH_3OH, which may be mistaken for ethyl alcohol. If ingested, can cause blindness and death. SYN: *wood alcohol; methyl alcohol.*

methemoglobin (met"he-mo-glo'bin) [G. *meta*, across, + *aima*, blood, + L. *globus*, globe]. A compound closely related to oxyhemoglobin found in the blood following poisoning by certain substances.

It gives blood a chocolate-brown color and is useless as a carrier of oxygen.

methemoglobinemia (met"'he-mo-glōb"ĭ-nē'mĭ-ă) [" + " + " + G. *aima*, blood]. Presence of methemoglobin in the blood.

methemoglobinuria (met"he-mo-glōb"ĭ-nū'rĭ-ă) [" + " + " + G. *ouron*, urine]. Presence of methemoglobin in the urine.

methenamine (mĕth"en'ă-mēn). Colorless crystals, with sweetish taste.

USE: Urinary antiseptic.

INCOMPATIBILITIES: Ammonium salts, alkalies, ferric salts.

methionine (meth-ī'ō-nīn). A sulfur-bearing compound; an essential amino acid.

methomania (meth-ō-mā'nĭ-ă) [G. *methē*, drunkenness, + *mania*, mania]. Psychiatric craving for intoxicating drinks. SYN: *dipsomania.*

methyl (meth'ĭl) [G. *methy*, wine, + *ylē*, substance]. In organic chemistry, the radical CH_3, seen, for instance, in the formula for methyl alcohol, CH_3OH.

m. alcohol. A colorless liquid with an alcoholic odor largely used as a solvent for paints, varnishes, etc.

POISONING: SYM: Different from those of ordinary alcoholism. Depression, weakness, nausea, headache, abdominal cramping, difficult breathing, cold sweats, coma, and convulsions. May be confused with cerebrovascular accident. Blindness which often follows may appear in several hours or not for several days. Sometimes the vision remains blurred, or total blindness may take place.

TREATMENT: Intravenous alkali solution (5% sodium bicarbonate) in large amounts, supportive therapy. Washing out stomach is useless.

m. ether. An anesthetic gas without color.

m. salicylate (sal-is'il-āt). USP. Oil of wintergreen, oil of gaultheria. Produced from distillation of leaves of sweet birch; it has a characteristic odor.

ACTION AND USES: Commonly used in preparations in the form of liniment or ointment for topical use as an analgesic balm and counterirritant.

m. violet. Stain employed in histology and bacteriology.

methylcellulose. USP. A tasteless powder which becomes swollen and gummy when wet. Used as a bulk substance in foods and laxatives, also as an adhesive or emulsifier.

methylene blue (meth'ĭ-lēn). USP. Methylthionine chloride. A dark green crystalline powder, producing a distinct blue stain.

USES: As a urinary antiseptic, as a test for kidney function, and as an antidote for carbon monoxide and cyanide poisoning.

It is valuable, also, in the treatment of drug-induced methemoglobinemia (1 mg. of dye per kilogram of body weight).

metopantralgia (met″ō-pan-tral′jĭ-ă) [G. *metōpon*, forehead, + *antron*, cavity, + *algos*, pain]. Pain in frontal sinuses.

metopantritis (met-ō-pan-trī′tis) [" + " + *-ītis*, inflammation]. Inflamed condition of frontal sinuses.

metopic (met-op′ĭk) [G. *metōpon*, forehead]. Rel. to the forehead.

metopion (met-ō′pĭ-on) [G. *metōpon*, forehead]. Craniometric point in forehead midway bet. frontal eminences.

metopism (met′ō-pĭzm) [" + *ismos*, condition of]. Persistence of the metopic suture in an adult.

metopodynia (met-ō-pō-din′ĭ-ă) [" + *odynē*, pain]. Headache in frontal area of head.

metoxenous (mĕ-toks′ĕn-ŭs) [G. *meta*, across, + *xenos*, host]. Denoting a parasite spending each of its two cycles on a different host. Syn: *heterecious*.

metoxeny (me-toks′ĕ-nĭ). Condition of being metoxenous, *q.v.*

metra (mē′tra) [G. *mētra*]. Combining form meaning the uterus. See: *metro-*.

metralgia (me-tral′jĭ-ă) [G. *mētra*, uterus, + *algos*, pain]. Pain in the uterus.

metranoikter (met-ră-nō-ĭk′ter) [" + *anoigein*, to open]. Instrument for dilating cervix uteri by means of two or four spring blades.

metrapectic (met-ră-pek′tĭk) [" + *apechein*, to avoid]. Denoting a disease that is transmitted by the mother, who herself is unaffected by it, for ex., hemophilia.

metratome (met′ră-tōm) [" + *tomē*, incision]. Instrument for incising the uterus.

metratomy (mĕt-răt′ō-mĭ) [" + *tomē*, a cutting]. Surgical incision of the uterus. Syn: *metrotomy*.

metratonia (mē-tra-to′nĭ-ă) [G. *mētra*, uterus, + *a-*, priv. + *tonos*, tone]. Uterine atony occurring after childbirth.

metratrophia (met-ra-tro′fĭ-ă) [" + *atrophia*, atrophy]. Atrophy of the uterus.

metrazol (met′ră-zōl). A proprietary name for a preparation of pentamethylenetetrazol. A white powder, chemically neutral substance.

Uses: As a circulatory and respiratory stimulant. Valuable in treating respiratory and circulatory depression due to overdose of barbiturates.

metre (mē′ter) [G. *metron*, measure]. Meter, *q.v.*

metrechoscopy (mĕt-rĕk-os′kō-pĭ) [" + *ēchō*, sound, + *skopein*, to examine]. Mensuration and auscultation combined with inspection.

metrectasia (mĕt-rĕk-tā′zĭ-ă) [G. *mētra*, uterus, + *ektasis*, dilatation]. Uterine dilatation.

metrectomy (mē-trek′to-mĭ) [" + *ektomē*, excision]. Surgical removal of the uterus. Syn: *hysterectomy*.

metrectopia (met-rek-to′pĭ-ă) [" + *ek*, out, + *topos*, place]. Displacement of the uterus.

metrelcosis (mĕt-rĕl-kō′sĭs) [G. *mētra*, uterus, + *elkōsis*, ulceration]. Uterine ulceration.

metre′mia. Congestion of the uterus.

metreurynter (met-rū-rin′ter) [" + *eurynein*, to stretch]. An inflatable bag which is inserted in the os uteri and distended to dilate the cervix.

metreurysis (me-trū′rĭ-sĭs) [" + *eurynein*, to stretch]. Dilatation of cervix uteri with the metreurynter.

met′ric sys′tem. One based upon the meter (39.37 inches) as the unit of measurement; the gram (15.432 gr.) the unit of weight; the liter (1.057 qt. liquid, or 0.908 qt. dry measure) as the unit of volume.

Conversion Rules: To change grams to grains multiply by 15, or divide by 0.064. To change grains to grams divide by 15, or multiply by 0.064. To change grams to ounces divide by 30. To change ounces to grams or cc. multiply by 30. See: *avoirdupois, household measures, table in Appendix, Troy weight.*

metri′tis [G. *mētra*, uterus, + *-itis*, inflammation]. Inflammation of the uterus. Designated *endometritis* if the endometrium is involved and *myometritis* if the musculature (myometrium) is involved.

m., chronic. Condition in which there is an increase in fibrous tissue and infiltration of lymphocytes.

metro- [G.]. 1. Combining form (*metron*) meaning rel. to measure or measurements. 2. From *metra*, the *uterus*, meaning *rel. to the uterus*.

metrocarcinoma (mĕt″rō-kăr-sĭ-nō′mă) [G. *mētra*, uterus, + *karkinos*, crab cancer, + *-ōma*, tumor]. Uterine carcinoma.

metrocele (met′rō-sēl) [" + *kēlē*, hernia]. Uterine hernia.

metrocolpocele (met″rō-kol′pō-sēl) [" + *kolpos*, vagina, + *kēlē*, hernia]. Protrusion of uterus into the vagina which pushes the vaginal wall downward.

metrocystosis (met″rō-sĭs-tō′sĭs) [" + *kystis*, cyst, + *-ōsis*, intensive]. Formation of uterine cysts.

metrodynia (met-rō-din′ĭ-ă) [G. *mētra*, uterus, + *odynē*, pain]. Uterine pain.

metrofibroma (me-trō-fī-brō′mă) [" + L. *fibra*, fiber, + G. *-ōma*, tumor]. Uterine fibroma.

metromalacia. Softening of the uterus.

metromalacosis (me″trō-mal-ă-kō′sĭs) [" + *malakia*, softening, + *-ōsis*, intensive]. Malacia or softening of uterine tissues.

metronome (met′ro-nōm) [G. *metron*, measure, + *nomos*, law]. Apparatus for recording intervals or periods of time.

metroparalysis (met″rō-pă-ral′ĭ-sĭs) [G. *mētra*, uterus, + *paralysis*, a loosening from the side]. Uterine paralysis.

metropath′ia haemorrhag′ica [" + *pathos*, disease, + *aima*, blood, + *rēgnunai*, to burst forth]. Condition of the uterus characterized by hemorrhage, usually accompanied by hypertrophy of the uterine mucous membranes and ovarian cystic disease. See: *fibrosis uteri*.

metropathic (me-tro-path′ĭk) [" + *pathos*, disease]. Pert. to or caused by uterine disorders.

metropathy (me-trop′ă-thĭ) [G. *mētra*, uterus, + *pathos*, disease]. Any uterine disease.

metroperitonitis (me″trō-per-ĭ-tō-nī′tĭs) [" + *peritonaion*, peritoneum, + *-ītis*, inflammation]. Inflamed condition of uterus and peritoneum.

metrophlebitis (me″trō-flē-bī′tĭs) [G. *metra*, uterus, + *phleps*, *phleb-*, vein, + *-ītis*, inflammation]. Inflamed condition of uterine veins.

metroptosis (met-rop-tō′sĭs) [" + *ptōsis*, a dropping]. Dropping of the uterus.

metrorrhagia (met-ror-ra′jĭ-ă) [" + *rēgnunai*, to burst forth]. Bleeding from the uterus, esp. at any time other than during the menstrual period.

This is most often caused by lesions of the cervix uteri, and its occurrence should always lead one to suspect and search for a malignancy in the genital tract. SEE: *menorrhagia.*

metrorrhea (met-ror-rē'ă) [" + *roia,* flow]. Any morbid discharge from the uterus.

metrorrhexis (met-ror-reks'is) [" + *rēxis,* a rupture]. A uterine rupture.

metrorthosis (me-tror-thō'sĭs) [" + *orthōsis,* a straightening]. Correction of uterine displacement.

metrosalpingitis (met-rō-săl-pĭn-jī'tĭs) [G. *mētra,* uterus, + *salpigx, salpigg-,* tube, + *-ītis,* inflammation]. Inflamed condition of uterus and oviducts.

metroscope (met'ro-skōp) [" + *skopein,* to examine]. Instrument for examining the uterus. SYN: *hysteroscope.*

metrostaxis (me-tro-stak'sĭs) [" + *staxis,* a dripping]. Persistent but slight hemorrhage from the uterus.

metrostenosis (me-trō-stĕn-ō'sĭs) [" + *stēnōsis,* a narrowing]. Contraction or narrowing of the uterine cavity.

metrosteresis (me-trō-ster-ē'sĭs) [" + *sterēsis,* loss]. Removal of the uterus. SYN: *hysterectomy, metrectomy.*

metrother'apy [G. *metron,* measure, + *therapeia,* treatment]. Treatment of a condition by measurement, as in restoration of joint function following injury, measuring the angle of joint motion and recording the progress, has a psychologic effect on patient.

metrotome (mē'trō-tōm) [G. *mētra,* uterus, + *tomē,* a cutting]. Instrument used in incising the uterus.

metrotomy (me-trot'ō-mĭ) [G. *mētra,* uterus, + *tomē,* incision]. Incision of the uterus. SYN: *hysterotomy.*

metrourethrotome (met-ro-u-re'thrō-tōm) [G. *metron,* measure, + *ourēthra,* urethra, + *tomē,* incision]. Device for incising the urethra and measuring depth to be incised.

-metry [G. *metrein,* to measure]. Suffix meaning to measure.

metrypercinesis (met"ri-per-sin-ē'sis) [G. *mētra,* uterus, + *yper,* over, + *kinēsis,* movement]. Excessive contraction of the uterus causing abnormal labor pains.

metycaine (met'ĭ-kān). A white crystalline substance formerly known as neothesin. Proprietary name.

USES: As a local anesthetic, prompt in action as topical application, or subcutaneous injection.

Mev. Abbreviation for *million electron volts.*

Meyer's theory [Adolf Meyer, psychiatrist, born in Switzerland but practiced and taught in the United States, 1866-1950]. That physiologic and psychologic data are considered to be one entity in psychiatry.

Meynert's commis'sure (mi'nerts) [Theodor H. Meynert, professor of neurology and psychiatry at Vienna, 1833-1892]. Fibrous tract extending from subthalamic body to base of 3rd ventricle.

M. F. D. Abbr. for *minimum fatal dose.*

Mg. Symb. for *magnesium.*

mg. Symb. for *milligram.*

mgh. Milligram hour. Dosage obtained by application of 1.0 mg. radium for 1 hr.

miasm, miasma (mī'azm, mī-az'mă) [G. *miasma,* stain]. A foul emanation or odor. Formerly thought to cause disease, esp. fevers such as malaria.

miasmatic (mī-az-mat'ĭk) [G. *miasma,* stain]. Pert. to miasm.

micella, micelle (mī-sĕl'ă) [L. a little crumb]. One of the ultramicroscopic units of protoplasm.

micrencephalon (mĭk-rĕn-sef'ă-lon) [G. *mikros,* small, + *egkephalos,* brain]. 1. Cerebellum. 2. Smallness of brain; cretinism.

micrencephalous (mi-kren-sef'al-ŭs) [G. *mikros,* small, + *egkephalos,* brain]. Possessing a small brain.

micro-, micr- [G.]. Combining forms denoting *small size* or *extent.* Indicates one millionth of a unit; thus microgram is one millionth of a gram.

microaerophilic (mī"krō-a-er-ō-fil'ĭk) [G. *mikros,* small, + *aēr,* air, + *philein,* to love]. Growing at low oxygen tension.

mi"croanal'ysis [" + *analysis,* a loosening apart]. Analytical examination of tiny granules.

microanatomy. Microscopic anatomy.

Micro"bacter'ium. A genus of lactic acid-forming bacteria found in milk. Common species are *M. flavum* and *M. lacticum.*

microbe (mī'krōb) [G. *mikros,* small, + *bios,* life]. 1. A minute one-celled form of life not distinguishable as to its vegetable or animal nature. 2. Bacteria, germs producing fermentation, putrefaction and disease; microorganism.

microbian (mī-krō'bĭ-an) [" + *bios,* life]. Rel. to a microbe. SYN: *microbic.*

microbic (mī-krōb'ĭk) [" + *bios,* life]. Concerning microbes. SYN: *microbian.*

microbicidal (mī-krōb-ĭs-ī'dal) [" + " + L. *cidus,* from *caedere,* to kill]. Destructive to microbes.

microbicide (mī-krōb'is-īd) [" + " + L. *cidus,* from *caedere,* to kill]. An agent which is destructive to microbes.

microbiology (mī"krō-bī-ol'ō-jĭ) [" + " + *logos,* study]. Scientific study of microbes.

microbiophobia (mī"krō-bī-ō-fō'bĭ-ă) [" + " + *phobos,* fear]. An abnormal fear of microbes. SYN: *microphobia.*

microbiota (mi"kro-bi-o'tă). Microscopic organisms of an area. SEE: *macrobiota.*

microbiotic (mī-krō-bī-ot'ĭk) [" + *bios,* life]. Of microbic life, or origin.

microbism (mī'krōb-ĭzm) [" + " + *ismos,* state of]. Infection with microbes.

microblast (mī'krō-blăst) [G. *mikros,* small, + *blastos,* germ]. Minute red blood corpuscle.

microblepharism, microblephary (mī-krō-blef'ar-izm, -ar-ĭ) [" + *blepharon,* eyelid]. Condition of having abnormally small eyelids.

microcalorie (mī"krō-kal'ō-rĭ) [" + L. *calor,* heat]. A unit of heat, the amount required to raise the temperature of 1 cc. of distilled water from 0° to 1° C. NOTE: Caloric value of food is expressed in calories. One thousand microcalories equal one calorie.

microcardia (mī"krō-kar'dĭ-ă) [" + *kardia,* heart]. Unusually small heart.

microcaulia (mī"krō-kaw'lĭ-ă) [" + *kaulos,* penis]. Unusually small size of penis.

microcentrum (mī-krō-sĕn'trum) [" + *kentron,* center]. 1. Centrosome, *q.v.* 2. Motor or dynamic center of a cell.

microcepha'lia [G. *mikros,* small, + *kephalē,* head]. Abnormal smallness of the head.

microcephalic (mī-krō-sef-al'ĭk) [" + *kephalē,* head]. Having or pert. to a small head; one below 1350 cc. capacity.

microcephalous (mĭ-kro-sef'al-us) [" + *kephalē,* head]. Having an abnormally small head.

microcephalus (mik-rō-sef′a-lŭs) [G. *mikros,* small, + *kephalē,* head]. 1. Person with an exceptionally small head, esp. an idiot. 2. Fetus with a very small head.

microcephaly, microcephalism (mī-krō-sef′ă-lĭ, -lĭzm) [" + *kephalē,* head]. Abnormal smallness of head often seen in idiocy; it is congenital.

micro″chei′lia (mī″krō-kī-lĭ-ă). Abnormal smallness of lips.

microchemistry (mī-krō-kĕm′ĭs-trĭ) [G. *mikros,* small + *chēmeia,* chemistry]. Chemical work in which minute quantities are utilized.

microchiria (mī-krō-kī′rĭ-ă). Abnormal smallness of the hand.

Micrococcaceae (mī-krō-kŏk-ā′se-e). A family of bacteria belonging to the order Eubacteriales. Contains the genera *Micrococcus, Gaffkya, Methanococcus, Sarcina,* and *Staphylococcus.*

Micrococcus (mī″krō-kŏk′ŭs) [G. *mikros,* small, + *kokkos,* berry]. A genus of gram-positive bacteria belonging to the family Micrococcaceae. Cells occur singly or in irregular groups.

M. albus. Syn: *Staphylococcus albus, q.v.*

M. aureus. Syn: *Staphylococcus aureus, q.v.*

M. flavus. Syn: *Neisseria flava.*

M. gonorrhoeae. *Neisseria gonorrhoeae.*

M. intracellularis meningitidis. Syn: *Neisseria meningitidis.*

M. lanceolatus. *Diplococcus pneumoniae.*

M. luteus. Nonpathogenic, non-motile and Gram-positive organism. May be found in dairy products.

M. melitensis. Syn: *Brucella melitensis,* cause of undulant fever.

M. meningitidis. Syn: *Neisseria meningitidis.*

M. pneumoniae. Syn: *Diplococcus pneumoniae.*

M. tetragenus. Syn: *Gaffkya tetragena.* An organism of low-grade virulence, occasionally found in blood in septicemia, in pus of abscesses, and in spinal fluid in meningitis.

micro″col′on. Abnormally small colon.

microcor′nea [G. *mikros,* small, + L. *cornū,* horn]. Abnormally small cornea.

microcoulomb (mī-krō-koo′lom) [G. *mikros,* small, + *coulomb*]. One-millionth part of a coulomb.

microcrystalline (mī-krō-kris′tal-īn, -ēn) [" + *krystallos,* ice]. Composed of microscopic crystals.

microcurie. Measure of radiation. One millionth of a curie.

microcyst (mī′krō-sĭst) [" + *kystis,* a cyst]. A very small cyst.

microcytase (mī-krō-sī′tās) [" + *kytos,* cell, + *ase,* enzyme]. Cytase acting on bacteria and formed by leukocytes.

mi′crocyte [G. *mikros,* small, + *kytos,* cell]. 1. A small erythrocyte or red blood corpuscle; one less than 5 microns in diameter. 2. Small, nonnucleated, red blood corpuscle.

micro″cyto′sis. Condition characterized by presence of abnormal numbers of microcytes in the blood.

microdactylia (mī″krō-dak-til′ĭ-ă) [G. *mikros,* small, + *daktylos,* digit]. Abnormal smallness of the digits.

micro″determ′ina′tion. The chemical examination of extremely minute quantities of a substance.

microdissection (mī″krō-dĭ-sĕk′shŭn) [G. *mikros,* small, + L. *dissectio,* a cutting apart]. Dissection with aid of the microscope, esp. by utilization of a micromanipulator.

microdont (mī′krō-dont) [" + *odous, odont-,* tooth]. Possessing very small teeth.

microdontism (mī-krō-don′tĭzm) [" + " + *ismos,* state of]. Unusual smallness of the teeth.

microdose. Minute dose.

micro″electrophore′sis. Electrophoresis of minute quantities of a solution.

microfarad (mī-krō-far′ăd) [G. *mikros,* small, + *farad*]. One-millionth of a farad, *q.v.*

micro″filar′ia. The embryos of filarial worms. They are present in the blood and tissues and are of importance in the diagnosis of filarial infections.

microgamete (mī-krō-gam′ēt) [" + *gametēs,* spouse]. Male element in conjugation of protozoa.

microgametocyte (mī-krō-gam-ē′tō-sīt) [" + " + *kytos,* cell]. Mother cell of the microgamete.

microgamy (mī-krŏg′ă-mĭ). Union of male and female cells in certain lower forms.

microgastria (mī-krō-gas′trĭ-ă) [G. *mikros,* little, + *gastēr,* belly]. Unusual smallness of the stomach.

microgenitalism (mī″krō-jĕn′ĭt-ăl-ĭzm) [" + L. *genitalia,* genitals, + G. *ismos,* state of]. Abnormal smallness of the external genitals.

microglia (mī-krog′lĭ-ă) [" + *glia,* glue]. Neuroglia tissue probably derived from the mesoderm, forming a portion of the adventitial structure of the central nervous system.

microglossia (mī-krō-glos′ĭ-ă) [" + *glossa,* tongue]. Abnormally small tongue.

micrognathia (mī-krog-nā′thĭ-ă) [G. *mikros,* small, + *gnathos,* jaw]. Abnormal smallness of jaws.

microgram (mī′krō-gram) [G. mikros, small, + *gramma,* a small weight]. One-millionth part of a gram. One thousandth of a milligram. Symb: μg. or mcg.

micrograph (mī′krō-graf) [" + *graphein,* to write]. 1. Apparatus for magnifying and recording minute movements. 2. Photograph of an object through a microscope. Syn: *photomicrograph.*

micrography (mī-krog′ră-fĭ) [" + *graphein,* to write]. 1. Study of physical appearance and characteristics of microscopic objects. 2. Very minute writing, engraving, etc. 3. Study of an object by use of a microscope.

microgyria (mī-krō-jir′ĭ-ă) [" + *gyros,* circle]. Smallness of cerebral convolutions.

microhematocrit. Packed red cell volume of blood determined by using very small amount of blood collected in a capillary tube.

microhepatia (mī-krō-hĕ-pat′ĭ-ă) [" + *ēpar, ēpat-,* liver]. Abnormally small size of the liver.

microhm (mī′krōm) [" + *ohm*]. One-millionth of an ohm.

micro″incinera′tion. Determination of presence and distribution of inorganic matter in tissues by subjecting a microscopic section of tissue to a high temperature which destroys organic matter, leaving mineral matter as ash in the form of a spodogram, *q.v.*

micro″injec′tion. Injection of substances into cells or minute vessels by means of a micropipette.

micro″len′tia. Possessing an abnormally small crystalline lens.

mi″croleuk′oblast [G. *mikros,* small, + *leukos,* white, + *blastos,* germ]. Syn: *myeloblast.* A small leukoblast.

microliter (mī'krō-lē-ter) [" + Fr. *litre*, from G. *litra*, a pound]. One-millionth part of a liter.

microlith (mī'krō-lith) [" + *lithos*, stone]. A very tiny calculus.

microlithiasis (mī"krō-lĭ-thī'ă-sĭs) [" + *lithos*, stone]. The development of very minute calculi.

micrology (mī-krol'o-jĭ) [G. *mikros*, small, + *logos*, study]. Science of microscopic investigations.

micromania (mī-krō-mā'nĭ-ă) [" + *mania*, madness]. A delusion that one has become small or infantile or insignificant.

micro"manip'ulator. Apparatus by which extremely minute pipettes or needles can be manipulated under a microscope for microinjection or microsurgery.

micromastia (mĭk-rō-măs'tĭ-ă). Micromazia, *q.v.*

micromazia (mī-krō-mā'zĭ-ă) [" + *mazos*, breast]. Abnormally small size of the breasts.

micrometer (mi'kro-me-ter) [G. *mikros*, small, + *metron*, measure]. SYN: *micron.* A millionth part of a meter. SYMB: μ.

micrometer (mī-krŏm'ĕ-tĕr). Device for making microscopic measurements.

micro"mi'cron. A millionth part of a micron. SYMB: $\mu\mu$.

micromillimeter (mī-krō-mĭl'ĭ-mē-ter) [G. *mikros*, small, + L. *mille*, a thousand, + G. *metron*, measure]. SYN: *millimicron.* One-millionth part of a millimeter. SYMB: μmm.

Micro"monospo'ra. A genus of fungi belonging to the family Streptomycetaceae.

micromyces (mī-krom'ĭ-sēs) (pl. *micromycetes*) [" + *mykēs*, fungus]. Minute fungus.

micromyelia (mī-krō-mī-ē'lĭ-ă) [" + *myelon*, marrow]. Abnormally small size of spinal cord.

micromyeloblast (mī-krō-mī'ĕl-ō-blăst) [G. *mikros*, small, + *myelon*, marrow, + *blastos*, germ]. A very small myeloblast.

micron (mī'kron) [G. *mikros*, small]. SYMB: μ. The millionth part of a meter; the thousandth part of a millimeter; about 1/25,000 part of an inch.

microne (mī'krōn) [G. *mikros*, small]. A colloid particle that is distinguishable with the microscope.

mi"croneed'les. Extremely minute needles used in a micromanipulator for microdissection.

micronize. To pulverize a substance into particles only a few micra in size.

micronucleus (mī-krō-nū'klē-us) (pl. *micronucleī*) [" + L. *nucleus*, kernel]. 1. A small nucleus. 2. The smaller of the two nuclei of infusoria considered as containing the inheritable germ substance.

micronychia (mī-krō"nĭk'ĭ-ă). Possessing abnormally small nails.

microorganism (mi-kro-or'gan-izm) [" + *organon*, organ, + *ismos*, condition]. Minute living body not perceptible to the naked eye, esp. a bacterium or protozoon.

Microorganisms may be carried from 1 host to another as follows:

Animal sources: Some organisms are pathogenic for animals as well as man, and may be communicated to man through direct, indirect or intermediary hosts.

By air: Pathogenic microorganisms in the respiratory tract may be discharged from the mouth or nose and settle on food, dishes, clothing and other places. They may carry infection if they resist drying.

Contact infections: These are the result of direct transmission of bacteria from one to another, as in venereal diseases.

Food-borne: Food and water may contain pathogenic organisms acquired from infected persons handling the food or through fecal or insect contamination.

Human carriers: Persons who have recovered from an infectious disease remain carriers of the organism causing the infection, and may transfer the organism to another host.

Insects: They may be the physical carrier, as the housefly or as vectors *Anopheles* mosquito.

Soil-borne: Spore forming organisms in the soil may enter the body through a cut or wound. Vegetables and fruits, esp. roots, need thorough cleansing before being eaten raw.

m., pathologic. A disease-causing organism. Includes rickettsias, bacteria, spirochetes, yeasts, molds, protozoons, and some helminths.

micropathology (mī"krō-path-ol'ō-jĭ) [G. *mikros*, small, + *pathos*, disease, + *logos*, study]. Study of microorganismal diseases and their cell and tissue changes.

microphage, microphagus (mi'kro-fāj,-krof'ag-us) [G. *mikros*, small, + *phagein*, to eat]. A small phagocyte.

RS: *bacteria, bacteriolysin, leukocyte, opsonin, phagocyte, trephone.*

microphakia (mī"krō-fā'kĭ-ă) [G. *mikros*, small, + *phakos*, lens]. Abnormally small lens.

microphallus (mī-krō-fal'us) [" + *phallos*, penis]. Abnormally small size of penis. SYN: *microcaulia.*

microphobia (mī-krō-fō'bĭ-ă) [" + *phobos*, fear]. Psychopathic fear of microbes. SYN: *microbiophobia.*

microphone (mi'kro-fōn) [" + *phōnē*, sound]. Device for detecting and transmitting sound.

microphonia (mī-krō-fō'nĭ-ă) [G. *mikros*, small, + *phōnē*, voice]. Weakness of voice.

microphonoscope (mī-krō-fō'nō-skōp) [" + " + *skopein*, to examine]. Form of biaural stethoscope for augmenting the sound.

microphotograph (mī"krō-fō'tō-graf) [G. *mikros*, small, + *phos*, phot-, light, + *graphein*, to write]. A photograph of extremely small size. Term sometimes used erroneously for photomicrograph, *q.v.*

microphthalmia (mi-krof-thal'mĭ-ă) [" + *ophthalmos*, eye]. Abnormally small size of eyes.

microphthalmus (mī-krŏf-thal'mus) [" + *ophthalmos*, eye]. 1. Person with unusually small eyes. 2. Condition characterized by abnormally small eyes.

microphysics (mī-krō-fĭz'ĭks) [G. *mikros*, small, + *physis*, nature]. The branch of science dealing with the forces controlling ultimate structure of matter.

microphyte (mī'krō-fīt) [" + *phyton*, plant]. Any microscopic plant, esp. if parasitic.

micropia (mi-kro'pĭ-ă) [" + *opsis*, vision]. A condition in which objects seem diminished in size. SYN: *micropsia.*

micro"pipette. An extremely small pipette used for microinjection.

micropodia (mī-krō-pō'dĭ-ă) [G. *mikros*, small, + *pous*, *pod-*, feet]. Unusually small size of the feet.

micro"polar'iscope. A microscope with a polarizer.

micro″projec′tion. Projection of images of microscopic objects upon a screen.

micro″proso′pia. Abnormal smallness of the face.

micropsia (mi-krop′sĭ-ă) [G. *mikros,* small, + *opsis,* vision]. Condition in which objects seem smaller than they usually are.

Seen in paralysis of accommodation, retinitis and choroiditis. SYN: *micropia.*

micropus (mī-krō′pus) [" + *pous,* feet]. One with unusually small feet.

micropyle (mi′kro-pīl) [" + *pylē,* gate]. The opening in the ovum for entrance of the spermatozoon.

micro″rhin′ia. Abnormal smallness of the nose.

micro″scel′ous. Possessing short legs.

microscope (mī′krō-skōp) [" + *skopein,* to examine]. Instrument which greatly magnifies very minute objects.

m., binocular. M. possessing two eyepieces or oculars.

m., compound. One with 2 or more lenses or lens systems for use in observing the minutest bodies.

m., darkfield. M. using *darkfield illumination, q.v.* An ultramicroscope.

m., electron. A m. which utilizes streams of electrons deflected from their course by an electrostatic or electromagnetic field for the magnification of objects. The final image is viewed on a fluorescent screen or recorded on a photographic plate. Because of greater resolving power, images may be magnified up to 400,000 diameters.

m., fluorescent. SEE: m., ultraviolet.

m., phase, phase-contrast. A compound microscope to which two elements have been added, namely, a diffraction or phase plate and a specialized condenser diaphragm. Such makes visible details of objects characterized by differences in refractive index and thus delineates a change of phase such as brightness or color.

m., polarization. M. for examining specimens which polarize light or have birefringence, or double refraction.

m., simple. One with a simple or single lens.

m., ultraviolet. M. utilizing ultraviolet radiations as a light source and having an optical system for transmitting them. Used in observing a specimen which fluoresces, such as tissues stained with a fluorescent dye.

m., x-ray. M. for utilizing x-rays to reveal structure of objects through which light cannot pass.

microscopic, microscopical (mī-krō-skop′ik, -ĭ-kal) [G. *mikros,* small, + *skopein,* to examine]. 1. Pert. to the microscope. 2. Visible only by using the microscope.

microscopy (mī-krŏs′kōp-ĭ) [" + *skopein,* to examine]. Inspection with the microscope.

m., dark-field. M. in which specimens against a dark background are illuminated by light rays striking from the side. By this means, objects too small to be seen by direct illumination become visible.

microseme (mi′krō-sēm) [" + *sēma,* sign]. Possessing an orbital index less than 83.

microsoma (mi-kro-so′mă) [" + *sōma,* body]. Unusually small stature.

microsome (mī′krō-sōm) [G. *mikros,* small, + *sōma,* body]. A submicroscopic or ultramicroscopic particle present in a cell.

microsomia (mi-kro-so′mĭ-ă) [G. *mikros,* small, + *soma,* body]. Abnormally small size of body.

microspectroscope (mi-kro-spek′trō-skōp) [" + L. *spectrum,* image, + *skopein,* to examine]. A combined spectroscope and microscope.

microspec″trophotom′etry. Method for the histochemical study of substances present in cells such as nucleic acid, based on absorption in the ultraviolet spectrum. Permits quantitative and qualitative studies of certain cellular components with a high degree of sensitivity.

microspherocyte (mi-kro-sfēr′o-sīt). Red blood cells, small and shaped like spheres. Seen in certain kinds of anemia.

microsphygmia, microsphyxia (mi-kro-sfig′mĭ-ă, -sfiks′ĭ-ă) [" + *sphygmos,* pulse, — + *sphyxis,* pulse]. Smallness of the pulse.

microsplenia (mī-krō-splē′nĭ-ă) [G. *mikros,* little, + *splēn,* spleen]. Abnormal smallness of the spleen.

Microsporon (mīk-ros′por-on) [" + *sporos,* seed]. Former name of *Microsporum, q.v.*

Microsporum. A genus of fungi which causes disease of the skin, hair, and nails.

M. audouini. Causative agent of tinea capitis (ringworm of scalp).

M. canis. Cause of ringworm of cats and dogs. May be transmitted to children.

microstomia (mī-krō-stō′mĭ-ă) [" + *stoma,* mouth]. Unusual smallness of the mouth.

micro″sur′gery. Dissection of tissues under the microscope, usually involving the use of a micromanipulator.

microsyringe. A special syringe for injecting very small quantities of solutions.

microtia (mi-kro′shĭ-ă) [" + *ous, ot-,* ear]. Unusually small size of the auricle or external ear.

microtome (mi′kro-tōm) [G. *mikros,* small, + *tomē,* incision]. Instrument for preparing thin sections of tissue for microscopic study.

microtomy (mi-krot′o-mĭ) [" + *tomē,* incision]. The process of cutting thin sections of tissues.

microvolt (mī′krō-volt) [" + *volt*]. One-millionth part of a volt.

micturate (mĭk′tū-rāt) [L. *micturire,* to urinate]. To pass the urine. SYN: *urinate.*

micturition (mĭk-tū-rĭ′shŭn) [L. *micturire,* to urinate]. The voiding of urine. SYN: *urination.*

mid′brain [A.S. *mid,* middle, + *braegen,* brain]. The corpora quadrigemina, the crura cerebri and aqueduct of Sylvius which connect the pons and cerebellum with the hemispheres of the cerebrum. SYN: *mesencephalon, q.v.*

mid′get. A very small person; an adult who has not attained full growth.

midgut (mid′gut) [A.S. *mid,* middle, + *gut,* intestine]. The midportion of the embryonic gut which opens ventrally into the yolk stalk.

midriff (mid′rĭf) [A.S. *mid,* middle, + *hrif,* belly]. The diaphragm.

mid′wife [" + *wif,* wife]. A female who practices the art of aiding in the delivery of children.

midwifery (mid-wīf′er-ĭ) [" + *wif,* wife]. The art of assisting at childbirth. SYN: *obstetrics.*

migraine (mī′grān) [Fr. from G. *ēmikrania,* half skull]. Paroxysmal attacks of headache, frequently unilateral, usually accompanied by disordered vision, and gastrointestinal disturbances.

Thought to be the result of vasodilation of extracerebral cranial arteries.

ETIOL: Unknown. Frequently hereditary. It may be precipitated by allergic hypersensitivity or emotional disturbances.

SYM: As stated. It is also associated with zigzags of light and vomiting, and at times with diplopia, unilateral sweating and focal symptoms. Sharp, stabbing pains frequently in temperofrontal region. Susceptible to light and sound.

PROG: It must be distinguished from other types of headache, but the history, the course of the disorder, and the peculiar combination of symptoms rarely permit of much uncertainty.

TREATMENT: Rest in quiet, darkened room during attack. Ergotamine tartrate proves efficacious in most cases.

migration (mī-grā'shun) [L. *migrāre,* to move from place to place]. Passage of cells, etc., from 1 position to another; *physiological,* as the migration of an ovum from the ovary into the fallopian tube, or *pathological,* as migration of leukocytes through the wall of a blood vessel into surrounding tissues.

m., external, of the ovum. The entrance of an ovum into the oviduct of the opposite ovary.

m., internal, of the ovum. Passage of the ovum through the uterine (fallopian) tube to the uterus.

m. of leukocytes. SYN: *diapedesis.* Passage of white blood corpuscles through walls of capillaries.

m. of the testicle. Descent of testicle into the scrotum. SYN: *descensus testis.*

migratory (mī'grā-tō-rĭ) [L. *migrāre,* to wander from place to place]. 1. Pert. to migrate. 2. Changing or capable of changing positions.

mikro-. For words commencing thus, see *micro-.*

Mikulicz's disease (mik'ū-lits). Chronic hypertrophic enlargement of lacrimal and salivary glands.

M. drain. A method for draining the abdominal cavity after operating.

M.'s mask. Gauze-covered frame worn over nose and mouth during performance of operation.

M.'s pad. Folded gauze pad for packing off the viscera in abdominal operations and used as a sponge in general.

M.'s syndrome. Characteristics of M.'s disease appearing as a complication of another disease.

mil'dew [A.S. *mildeāw*]. A parasitic fungus, and plant disease produced by it.

miliaria (mil-ĭ-a'rĭ-ă) [L *milium,* millet]. Vesicles due to obstruction of the sweat glands. Acute inflammation of the sweat glands. Occurs most commonly in infants, the obese, and in those exposed to excessive heat for prolonged periods. Excessive clothing and hyperhidrosis are contributing factors.

SYN: *heat rash; prickly heat.*

ETIOL: Exposure to excessive heat, infancy, obesity, debility, overclothing and tendency to hyperhidrosis.*

SYM: Sudden appearance of red patches of small papules. Vesicles are discrete and accompanied by red areolae. They usually appear on the trunk and are accompanied by itching and burning; fever of short duration. They occur in hot weather, in tropical countries, in individuals sweating profusely, and the papules may become eczematous if irritated.

TREATMENT: Mild astringent lotions with bland dusting powder.

m. crystallina. SYN: *sudamina.* Form with vesicles opaque and white.

m. rubra. Same as m. crystallina with the addition of inflammation, lesions being on a slightly inflamed base.

miliary (mĭl'ĭ-ā-rĭ) [L. *miliaris,* like a millet seed]. Characterized by presence of small nodules or lesions resembling millet seed.

m. fever. An infectious disease accompanied by fever.

SYM: Fever, profuse sweating, eruption of minute red and white pimples.

m. tubercles. Small gray nodules in first stage of tuberculosis.

m. tuberculosis. Acute, generalized tuberculosis with minute tubercles in the affected part or organ.

milieu (mēl-yew') [Fr.]. Environment.

m. int'erieur. Internal environment of extracellular fluids of the body.

milium (mĭl'ĭ-ŭm) [L. *milium,* millet seed]. Small pink and white nodule below the epidermis, caused by clogged sebaceous glands.

TREATMENT: Mechanical keratolytics (pumice stone, soap), salicylic acid and sulfur ointment, or incision and expression of contents.

m., colloid. Tiny papule formed beneath the epidermis due to colloid degeneration.

milk [A.S. *meolc,* milc]. A secretion of the mammary glands, density about 1.032, for feeding the young.

COMP: Milk consists of water, organic substances, and mineral salts. *Organic substances. Proteins.* The principal proteins are caseinogen, lactoalbumin, and lactoglobulin; in the presence of calcium ions, soluble caseinogen is converted into insoluble casein by the action of acids, rennet, or pepsin. This brings about the curdling of milk. Lactoglobulin is identical with serum globulin of blood and hence contains maternal antibodies. *Carbohydrates:* Lactose or milk sugar is the principal sugar, although small quantities of other sugars are present. *Fats:* The principal fats are glycerides of oleic, palmitic and myristic acid. Smaller quantities of stearic acid and short-chain fatty acids with carbon chains of C_4 to C_{24} are present. Sterols and phosphatides (lecithin and cephalin) are also present. Churning causes the fat globules to unite into a solid mass forming butter. *Mineral salts:* The principal cations are calcium, potassium, and sodium; the principal anions, phosphate, and chloride. Citrates and lactates are present in small quantities. Milk is low in iron and magnesium.

Vitamins: Vitamins A and those of the B complex (thiamine, riboflavin, and pantothenic acid) are present in adequate quantities to meet the needs of a growing child. Milk is low in vitamins C and D.

COW'S, FLUID, WHOLE: 1 cup (244 gm.). Calories: 165. Other main values: 9 gm. protein; 10 gm. fat; 12 gm. carbohydrate; 285 mg. calcium; 390 I.U. vitamin A.

ACTION: Milk makes the smallest demands upon the digestive glands of any food unless it be eggs or meat, and decreases the urinary nitrogen. It is poor in salt and rich in lactose. *Boiled milk* is constipating.

Milk on standing at room temperature sours as a result of the action of lactic bacilli on lactose converting it into lactic acid. When the pH reaches 5.34,

	Mother's Milk (%)	Cow's Milk (%)
Water	87-88	85-88
Minerals	0.2	0.7
Protein	1.0-1.5	3.5-4.0
Fat	3.5-4.0	3.5-4.0
Sugar (lactose, carbohydrate)	6.5-7.0	4.5
Reaction	Alkaline	Acid

coagulation occurs resulting in production of a *curd.* The remaining watery portion is called *whey.*

Milk contains antibodies which are present in the mother's blood. Milk also contains a number of enzymes (catalase, oxidase, reductase, phosphatase).

m., acidophilus. Milk or soy bean oil inoculated with *Lactobacillus acidophilus.*

m. agent. A carcinogenic substance present in the milk of certain strains of mice capable of inducing the development of cancer in offspring.

m., butter-. That left after removal of butter following churning.

m., casein. M. prepared with a large quantity of casein and fat, but little sugar and salts.

m., certified. That certified by a Board of Health as pure.

m., condensed. Partly evaporated and sweetened milk.

m., diabetic. M. with small amt. of lactose.

m., fortified. M. enriched by the addition of cream, albumin, or vitamins.

m., homog'enized. M. with fats combined with the body of the milk; thus the cream does not separate.

m., instant dry non-fat. Dried skim milk. It may be stored at room temperature until needed. Reconstituted by adding water to the granules.

m. leg. Thrombosis of the iliac or femoral vein followed by swelling of the leg. So called because it often is a complication of puerperium. SYN: *phlegmasia alba dolens, q.v.*

m., litmus. M. containing litmus, an indicator. Used in bacteriology.

m. of magnesia. Magnesium hydroxide in permanent suspension. USP.

m., modified. M. altered so that its composition more closely approximates that of human milk.

m., mother's. That from the mammary glands of a woman.

m., non-fat. Same as skimmed milk, *q.v.*

m., pasteurized. M. heated for 30 minutes at 140 to 158° F. (60 to 70°C.) to kill the living pathogenic bacteria. SEE: *pasteurization.*

m., protein. M. with high protein and low carbohydrate and fat content.

m., red. M. contaminated by blood, chromogenic bacteria, or plant pigments.

m., ropy. That which has become viscid due to formation of vegetable gums from carbohydrates or mucinlike substances from proteins as a result of bacterial action.

m., skimmed. M. after removal of cream.

m., sour. M. with lactic acid caused by lactic acid bacteria.

m., sterilized. M. boiled to kill bacteria.

m., sugar of. Lactose.

m. teeth. First or deciduous teeth.

m. tumor. Retention of milk in mammary gland.

m., uterine. Whitish fluid found between villi in placenta of pregnant uterus.

m., uviol. M. sterilized by ultraviolet rays.

m., vegetable. 1. The latex of plants. 2. A synthetic milk prepared from juices expressed from various plants, such as soybean.

m., vitamin D. M. in which vitamin D content had been increased by addition of concentrates, ultraviolet irradiation, or by feeding irradiated yeast to milk-producing animals.

m., witch's. M. secreted by the breasts of the newborn.

milk'pox. Modified form of smallpox prevalent in South Africa. Called *alastrim, q.v.,* in America. SEE ALSO: *amaas.*

Miller-Abbott tube. [Invented by two Philadelphia physicians, T. Grier Miller, 1886- ; W. Osler Abbott, 1902-1943.] A flexible double lumen tube used for diagnosing and treating intestinal disease. Substances may be placed in the intestinal tract by using one lumen; the other lumen may be used for suction.

milli- [L.]. Prefix meaning *a thousandth part.*

milliam'meter [L. *mille,* thousand, + *ampere* + G. *metron,* measure]. Ammeter registering in milliamperes. SEE: *ammeter.*

milliampere (mil"-e-ahm-pair') [" + *ampere*]. P.T. One one-thousandth of an ampere. ABBR: *ma.*

m. minute. An electrical unit of quantity, equivalent to that delivered by 1 milliampere in 1 minute.

millicurie (mil'ĭ-ku'rē) [" + *curie*]. P.T. One-thousandth of a curie.

m. hour. A practical unit of dosage for radon. One millicurie of radon applied for 1 hour. The biologic effect depends on time, filtration, distance.

milliequiv'alent. Weight of a substance contained in 1 milliliter of a normal solution. ABBR: *mEq.*

milligram (mil'ĭ-gram) [L. *mille,* a thousand, + G. *gramma,* a weight]. One-thousandth of a gram. ABBR: *mg.*

mil'lili"ter. One-thousandth of a liter. ABBR: *ml.* For practical purposes it is equivalent to 1 cc.

millimeter (mil'ĭ-mēt-er) [" + G. *metron,* measure]. One-thousandth of a meter.

millimicron (mil-i-mi'kron). One-thousandth of a micron; one-millionth of a millimeter. SYMB: mμ.

millimol (mil'ĭ-mōl). One thousandth of a mol.

milphosis (mĭl-fō'sĭs). Loss of eyebrows or eyelashes.

mime'sis [G. *mimēsis,* imitation]. Imitation, mimicry; term applied to a disease which exhibits symptoms of another disease or to conditions in hysteria which simulate organic disease.

mimetic, mimic (mi-met'ĭk, mĭm'ĭk) [G. *mimētikos,* pert. to imitation]. Imitative.

m. convulsion. Facial convulsion.

m. labor. False labor.

m. spasm. Spasm of facial muscles.

min. Abbr. for *minim; minute.*

mind (mīnd) [A.S. *gemynd*]. Integration of functions of the brain resulting in the ability to perceive surroundings, to have emotions, and to process information in an intelligent manner.

mineral (mĭn'er-ăl) [L.L. *minerale*]. 1. An inorganic element or compound occurring in nature, esp. one that is solid. 2. Inorganic; not of animal or plant origin. 3. Impregnated with minerals, as mineral water. 4. Pertaining to minerals.

m. compounds. Compounds of mineral elements, excepting carbon, constitute the mineral constituents of the body.

Minerals serve the following functions: (a) They are essential constituents of all cells. (b) They form the greater portion of the hard parts of the body (bone, teeth, nails). (c) They are essential components of respiratory pigments, enzymes, and enzyme systems. (d) They regulate the permeability of cell membranes and capillaries. (e) They regulate the excitability of muscular and nervous tissue. (f) They are essential for regulation of osmotic pressure equilibria. (g) They are necessary for maintenance of proper acid-base balance. (h) They are essential constituents of secretions of glands. (i) They play an important role in water metabolism and regulation of blood volume.

Mineral salts and water are excreted daily from the body. These must be replaced through food intake. Daily requirements for principal minerals for a normal adult are as follows: *calcium,* 0.8 gm.; *phosphorus,* 1.4 gm.; *sodium,* 3-6 gm.; *iron,* 12 mg.; *copper,* 1-2 mg. Requirements are greater for growing children and pregnant women and in certain pathologic conditions.

SEE: *acid-base balance; body; names of elements; chemical elements* (in the human body); *buffer.*

m. oil. USP. Liquid petrolatum.

m. spring. A s. whose water contains mineral salts thought to have a therapeutic value in certain diseases, esp. arthritis. SEE: *spa.*

m. water. W. charged with inorganic salts.

mineralocorticoid (min"er-al-o-kor'tĭ-koyd). A biologically active principle of the adrenal cortex, affecting the retention or excretion of sodium or potassium.

minim (min'im) [L. *minimum,* least]. SYN: *drop.* One sixtieth part of a fluidram or 0.06 milliliter. ABBR: *m., min.*

minimal (min'ĭ-mal) [L. *minimum,* least]. Least.

m. dose. Smallest dose producing an effect.

minimum (min'ĭ-mum) [L. least]. Least quantity or lowest limit. SEE: *threshold.*

m. lethal dose. Smallest quantity of a substance producing death.

Minin light (min'in) [A. V. Minin, Russian surgeon]. A lamp for the administration of violet and ultraviolet light.

Minot-Murphy diet (mī'nŏt) [George R. Minot, American physician, 1885-1950; and William P. Murphy, American physician, born 1892]. Diet for pernicious anemia containing large quantities of liver.

mio-. Combining form meaning less, smaller.

miocardia (mī-ō-kar'dĭ-ă) [G. *meiōn,* less, + *kardia,* heart]. Systolic lessening of heart's volume. SYN: *systole.*

mionectic (mī-ō-nek'tik) [G. *mionektikos,* taking less]. Pert. to, having or using a subnormal amount of oxygen, esp. blood. SEE: *mesectic, pleonectic.*

mioplas'mia [G. *meiōn,* less, + *plasma,* a thing formed]. Abnormal lessening of the amount of blood plasma.

miopragia (mī-ō-prā'jĭ-ă) [" + *prassein,* to perform]. Decrease of functional power.

miosis, meiosis (mī-ō'sĭs) [G. *meiosis,* a lessening]. 1. Abnormal contraction of pupils. 2. Period of diminishing symptoms in a disease. 3. Method of cell division which allows each daughter nucleus to receive half the number of chromosomes present in the somatic cells.

miot'ic [G. *meiōn,* less]. 1. An agent that causes the pupil to contract, such as eserine and pilocarpine. 2. Pert. to or causing contraction of the pupil. 3. Diminishing.

miracidium (mī"ră-sĭd'-ĭ-ŭm). A ciliated free-swimming larva of a digenetic fluke. On emerging from an ovum, it penetrates a snail of a particular species and metamorphoses into a sporocyst. SEE: *fluke.*

mire (mīr) [L. *mirāre,* to look at]. OPHTH: An object used as a test, the images of which denote the amount of astigmatism.

mirror drill. Exercise, before a mirror, practicing control of convulsive tics.

Patient sitting in front of mirror tries to control movements. When he does, physician begins to distract his attention from his reflection by having patient do calisthenics.

m. speech. That which reverses the order of words in a sentence or pronounces words backward. SEE: *lalopathy.*

m. writing. Writing in which the words are reversed, as seen in a mirror.

mis- [A.S. *mis,* wrong]. Prefix implying *not, bad, wrong, improper,* etc.

misanthropia (mis"an-thro'pe-ah) [*miso* + *anthrōpos,* man + *ia*]. Hatred of mankind.

miscar'riage [A.S. *mis,* wrong, + L. *carrus,* cart]. A term used synonymously with *abortion,* and referring to the interruption of pregnancy prior to the 7th month.

Usually refers to expulsion of fetus, specifically in period bet. 4th month and viability.

misce (mĭs'e) [L. mix]. ABBR: M. Mix. A direction to the pharmacist placed upon a prescription for mixing the preparation.

miscegenation (mis"ej-en-a'shun) [L. *miscere,* to mix, + *genus,* race]. Sex relations or marriage bet. those of different races.

miscible (mĭs'ĭ-bl) [L. *miscere,* to mix]. Capable of being mixed.

misocainia (mis-o-ki'nĭ-ă) [G. *misein,* to hate, + *kainos,* new]. An aversion to new ideas. SYN: *misoneism.*

misog'amy [" + *gamos,* marriage]. Aversion to marriage.

misogyny (mĭs-oj'ĭn-ĭ) [" + *gynē,* woman]. Abnormal hatred of women.

misologia (mis-o-lo'jĭ-ă) [" + *logos,* word]. Aversion to mental work.

misoneism (mĭ-sō-nē'izm) [" + *neos,* new]. Aversion to new things or new ideas; conservatism.

misopedia (mĭ-sō-pe'dĭ-ă) [" + *pais, paid-,* child]. Abnormal dislike for children or the young.

Mist, mist. Abbr. for *mistura, q.v.*

mistura [L. mixture]. Preparation intended for internal use, and containing suspended insoluble substances which do not unite chemically.

Should always be shaken before using.

mite (mīt) [A.S.]. A minute arachnid, a member of the order Acarina. Some are parasitic and the cause of conditions such as mange and scabies. Some serve as vectors of disease organisms and as intermediate host for certain Cestodes.

m., follicle. *Demodex folliculorum.* M. which lives in hair follicles and sebaceous glands.

m., itch. *Sarcoptes scabei, q.v.*

m., mange. Mites belonging to the families Sarcoptidae and Psoroptidae. The cause of mange and scabies in many species of animals.

m., red. Redbugs or chiggers, members of the family Thrombiculidae. SEE: *chiggers.*

mithridatism (mĭth'rĭ-dāt"ĭzm) [Mithridates, a king of Pontus, B. C., supposed to have acquired immunity in this fashion]. Immunity to a poison acquired by taking it in doses of increasing size.

miticide (mi'tĭ-sīd). A substance which kills mites.

mitigated (mit'ĭ-gāt-ed) [L. *mitigāre,* to soften]. Diminished in severity. SYN: *allayed, moderated.*

mitochondria (mīt"ō-kon'drĭ-ă) (sing. *mitochondrion*) [G. *mitos,* thread, + *chondros,* cartilage]. Granular and filamentous structures in cell cytoplasm.

mito'ma, mi'tome [G. *mitos,* thread]. A fine network support or framework of protoplasm in a cell.

mito'sis (pl. *mitosēs*) [G. *mitos,* thread, + *-ōsis*]. Indirect cell division involving indirect nuclear division (*karyokinesis*) and division of the cell body (*cytokinesis*), the process by which all somatic cells of multicellular organisms multiply.

Mitosis is a continuous process divided into four phases: (1) *Prophase:* the chromatin granules of the nucleus stain more densely and become organized into chromosomes which first appear as long, delicate, spiral structures each consisting of two spiral filaments called *chromatids.* Each chromosome possesses a clear region (*centromere*) usually in the mid-region. As the prophase progresses, the chromosomes become shorter, and more compact and stain densely; the nuclear membrane and the nucleoli disappear. At the same time, the centriole divides and the two daughter centrioles, each surrounded by a centrosphere, move to opposite poles of the cell. They are connected by fine protoplasmic fibrils which form the *achromatic spindle.* (2) *Metaphase:* the chromosomes (paired chromatids) arrange themselves in an equatorial plane midway between the two centrioles forming the *equatorial plate.* (3) *Anaphase:* the chromatids (now called daughter chromosomes) diverge and move toward their respective centrosomes. The end of their migration marks the beginning of the next phase. (4) *Telophase:* the chromosomes at each pole of the spindle undergo changes the reverse of these in the prophase, each becoming a long, loosely spiraled thread. The nuclear membrane reforms and nucleoli reappear. Outlines of chromosomes disappear and chromatin appears as granules scattered throughout nucleus and connected by a lightly staining *linin* net. The cytoplasm becomes separated into two parts, resulting in two complete cells. This is accomplished in animal cells by constriction in the equatorial region; in plant cells a *cell plate* which gives rise to the cell membrane forms in a similar position. The period between two successive divisions is called *interphase.*

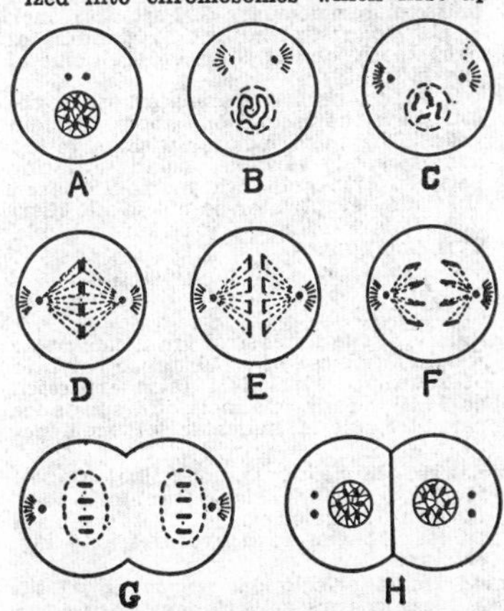

MITOSIS.

Diagram illustrating the four phases of mitotic division in a cell having four chromosomes: A, B, and C illustrate the changes in the centrosome and nucleus during the prophase; D represents the metaphase; E and F, the anaphase; and G and H, the telephase.

Mitosis is of particular significance in that the hereditary determiners (*genes*) are distributed equally to each daughter cell and a constancy in number of chromosomes is maintained in all cells of an organism.

m., heterotypic. The first or reduction division in the maturation of germ cells.

m., homeotypic. The second or equational division in the maturation of germ cells.

mitosome (mī'tō-sōm) [" + *sōma,* body]. 1. A body giving rise to the middle piece of the spermatozoon. 2. Chromatin mass in a cellular nucleus.

mitotic (mī-tot'ĭk) [G. *mitos,* thread]. Pert. to mitosis.

mitral (mi'tral) [L. *mitra,* a miter]. Pert. to the bicuspid or mitral valve. SEE: *facies, mitral.*

m. disease. That of the mitral valve. SEE: *heart.*

m. murmur. One produced at the mitral valve.

m. orifice. Left atrioventricular aperture.

m. regurgitation. Due to failure of valve to close completely, allowing blood to flow back into the auricle.

m. stenosis. Narrowing orifice of the valve obstructing free flow from auricle to ventricle.

m. valve. SYN: *bicuspid valve, valvula bicuspidalis.*

mittelschmerz (mit'el-shmärts) [German]. Pain bet. menstrual periods.

mit'tor [L. *mitere,* to rend]. A neuron terminal which transmits impulses to ceptors of the adjoining neuron.

mixed (mikst) [L. *mixtus,* from *miscere,* to mingle]. Consisting of 2 or more intermingling substances.

m. diet. One consisting of all the food elements in proper proportion. There is no scientific validity to the theory that carbohydrates and proteins should not be eaten together. Over 6000 determinations have been made which proved that the acid response to carbohydrates, to proteins, and to both taken together, is the same and that a mixed diet does not interfere with gastric secretions or with any of the digestive functions. The presence of protein seems to prolong carbohydrate assimilation.

m. marriage. Marriage between persons of different races or different religious beliefs.

m. nerves. The spinal nerves containing sensory or afferent, and motor or efferent fibers.

mix″osco′pia. Sexual perversion in which sexual gratification is obtained through observation of coition.

mixture (mĭks′tūr) [L. *mistura*]. A combination of 2 or more substances without chemical union. SEE: *mistura.*

mks, MKS. Abbr. for *meter-kilogram-second.* Indicates measurements used with meter for length, kilogram for weight, and second for time.

MLD, mld. Abbr. for *minimum lethal dose.*

mm. Abbr. for *millimeter.*

mM. Abbr. for *millimole.*

mmm. Abbr. for *micromillimeter.*

Mn. Symb. for *manganese.*

mne″masthe′nia. Poor memory.

mnemic (ne′mik) [G. *mnēmē,* memory]. Relating to memory.

m. hypothesis or ***theory.*** Stimuli leave engrams (definite traces) on protoplasm, which when frequently repeated set up a habit which persists after the stimuli cease; these engrams possibly may be transmitted to descendants. SYN: *mnemism.*

mnemism (nē′mĭzm) [G. *mnēmē,* memory]. Mnemic hypothesis, *q.v.*

mnemonics (nē-mon′ĭks) [G. *mnēmonikos,* pertaining to memory]. Assisting memory. A device to help recall a series of related data, names, or anatomical terms.

Mo. Chemical symbol for *molybdenum.*

mo. Abbreviation for *month.*

mobile (mo′bil) [L. *mobilis,* movable]. Movable.

m. spasm. Tonic spasm with irregular, slow movements of limbs following hemiplegia. Athetosis.

mobility (mō-bĭl′ĭ-tĭ) [L. *mobilitas*]. State or quality of being mobile; facility of movement.

mobilization (mo″bĭl-ĭ-zā′shŭn) [L. *mobilis,* movable]. 1. The making of a fixed or ankylosed part movable. 2. Restoration of motion to a joint.

In fractures Lucas-Championnière advocated the regular administration of a definite dose of movement followed by a period of rest. This he called mobilization.

3. Freeing an organ or making it movable. 4. The freeing or making available substances held in reserve as glycogen or fat.

m., stapes. Surgical treatment to restore mobility to the stapes. Used in treatment of deafness.

mobilize (mō′bĭl-īz) [L. *mobilis,* movable]. 1. To incite to physiological action. 2. To render movable; to put in movement.

Möbius' sign (me′bĭ-us) [Paul J. Möbius, German neurologist, 1853-1907]. A symptom in Graves' disease in which one eye converges and the other diverges when looking at the tip of one's nose.

modal (mōd′al) [L. *modus,* mode]. Pert. to form without reference to substance.

modal′ity [L. *modus,* mode]. 1. Quality of being modal. 2. A method of application or the employment of any therapeutic agent; limited usually to physical agents. The word is avoided by scholarly writers. 3. Any state that modifies the action of a drug. 4. PSY: Whole character of stimuli or sensations determined by the class to which they belong; that attribute of a sensation by which it is distinguished from all other sensations.

mode (mōd) [L. *modus*]. The value or item of the class occurring most frequently in a series of variables.

modiolus (mō-dī′ō-lŭs) [L. a small measure]. NA. Central pillar or axial part of cochlea extending from the base to the apex.

modulus (mod′ū-lŭs) [L. a small measure]. A unit of physical effects, as a *calorific unit.*

modus (mo′dus) [L. method]. A method or a mode.

m. operandi. Method of performing an act.

mogigraphia (mō-jĭ-grăf′ĭ-ă) [G. *mogis,* with difficulty, + *graphein,* to write]. Writers' cramp.

mogilalia (moj-ĭ-la′lĭ-ă) [" + *lalia,* chatter]. Any speech defect, as *stuttering.*

mogiphonia (moj-ĭ-fō′nĭ-ă) [" + *phōnē,* voice]. Difficulty in emitting vocal sounds.

Mohrenheim's space (mor′en-hīm). Space bet. pectoralis major and deltoid just beneath the clavicle.

moist (moyst) [L. *musteus,* musty]. Damp, wet.

m. chamber. A vessel for keeping microscopic objects moist.

mol(e) (mōl). A quantity of a chemical compound whose weight in grams equals its molecular weight. Thus 18.016 gm. of water would be 1 mol.

mo′lar [L. *molēs,* a mass]. 1. Pert. to a mass; not molecular. 2. Pert. to a mol. 3. [L. *molaris,* grinding]. A grinding or back tooth, one of three on each side of the jaws.

The first permanent one erupts at the 6th year; the second one about the 12th year. The third molars (wisdom teeth) are extremely variable, usually erupting between 17th and 25th years. However, they may erupt later or not at all. SEE: *dentition, teeth.* 4. Gram-molecule. SYN: *mol, q.v.*

m. solution. One in which there is 1 *mol* of the solute dissolved in each liter of the solution.

molarity. The number of gram molecular weights (moles) of a substance per liter of solution. Thus 1/M (also expressed as 1 *M*) means one mole of a substance per liter, 0.1/M indicates 0.1 mole per liter.

molas′ses [L. *mellaceus,* honeylike] (Cane). MOLASSES (*cane, blackstrap*): 1 tbsp. (20 gm.). Calories: 45. Other main values: 11 gm. carbohydrates; 116 mg. calcium.

mold (mōld) [Icelandic *mugga,* mist]. 1. A fuzzy coating of a fungus nature, on the surface of decaying vegetable matter. 2. Any one of a group of parasitic or saprophytic fungi which causes mold. Examples are the *black molds* (Mucorales) and the *blue* and *green molds* (Aspergillales). The latter include *Penicillium,* the source of the antibiotic, *penicillin.* 3. To shape a mass, as a *pill.* 4. To shape the fetal head, adapting it to the pelvic inlet.

mold'ing [L. *modulus,* a small measure]. 1. Shaping of the fetal head, adapting itself to pelvic inlet. 2. Manual shaping of infant's features following delivery. 3. A protective border, used in plastic surgery. 4. Casting of a reproduction.

mole (mōl) [AS. *māl*]. 1. A congenital discolored spot elevated above the surface of the skin. Syn: *nevus.*

Etiol: Not clear. May arise from local or static condition of circulation in a small area. Harmless unless irritated.

Treatment: Protect against irritation. Do not tie a thread about a mole.

See: *acephalocyst, racemose, melanoma.*

2. [L. *mola,* moistened meal]. A uterine mass arising from a poorly developed or degenerating ovum.

m., blood. A mass made up of blood clots, membranes, and placenta, retained following abortion.

m., Breus'. Malformation of the ovum, a decidual tuberous subchorional hematoma.

m., carneous. Blood mole which has assumed a fleshlike appearance, when retained in uterus for some time.

m., false. One formed from a uterine tumor or polypus.

m., fleshy. See: *carneous mole.*

m., hydatid, hydatidiform. A polycystic mass in which the chorionic villi have undergone cystic degeneration.

m., pigmented. *Nevus pigmentosus, q.v.*

m., stone. Calcareous degeneration in the uterus.

m., true. Mole representing the degenerated embryo or fetus.

m., vascular. A hemangioma, *q.v.*

m., vesicular. See: *hydatidiform mole.*

molecular (mō-lek'ū-lar) [L. *molecula,* little mass]. Pert. to a molecule.

m. biology. Branch of biology dealing with the smallest particles of living systems.

m. disease. Disease due to an abnormal molecule. The abnormal hemoglobin molecule found in persons with sickle cell anemia causes the abnormally shaped red cells characteristic of this disease.

m. layer. 1. Cortical l. of cerebellar or cerebral substance. 2. (Inner). Inner retinal plexiform layer. 3. (Outer). Outer retinal plexiform layer.

m. lesion. One not even visible through a microscope.

m. weight. Weight of a molecule attained by totalling the weight of its constituent atoms. See: *atomic weight.*

molecule (mŏl'ĕ-kūl) [L. *molecula,* little mass. 1. The smallest quantity into which a substance may be divided without loss of its characteristics. 2. Any small portions of a substance. 3. A chemical combination of two or more atoms which form a specific chemical compound; the chemical elements are formed by the combination of atoms.

Combinations of dissimilar atoms form chemical compounds. In normal molecules the positive and negative electric charges exactly balance. Excess or deficiency of either positive or negative charge by the loss or acquisition of electrons results in the formation of an ion.

The molecule is designated by the number of atoms it contains, as: *monatomic,* (one atom); *diatomic,* (two); *triatomic,* (three); *tetratomic,* (four); *pentatomic,* (five); *hexatomic,* (six), etc. See: *cleavage.*

moli'men (Pl. *molimina*) [L. effort]. Effort to establish any normal function, esp. the monthly effort to establish the menses and disturbances experienced at the time.

mollities (mol-ĭsh'ĭ-ēz) [L.]. Abnormal softening of a part.

m. ossium. Softening of the bones. Syn: *osteomalacia.*

Moll's glands [Jacob A. Moll, Dutch oculist, 1832-1914]. Modified sweat glands at border of eyelids. Syn: *ciliary glands.*

mol'lusc, mol'lusk. Any member of the phylum Mollusca.

Mollus'ca. A phylum of animals which includes the bivalves (mussels, oysters, clams), slugs, and snails. Snails serve as intermediate hosts of many parasitic flukes. Oysters and clams may transmit the virus of infectious hepatitis, esp. if improperly cooked.

molluscous (mol-lŭs'kŭs) [L. *molluscus,* soft]. Concerning molluscum.

molluscum (mol-us'kum) [L. soft]. A mildly infective skin disease characterized by tumor formations on the skin.

m. contagiosum. The usual mildly contagious form of molluscum.

Sym: Characterized by small waxy globular epithelial tumors containing semifluid caseous matter or solid masses, healing without scarring though they may suppurate and break down, commonly on face, eyelids, breasts, genitalia and inner surface of thigh. On pressure a substance resembling sebum is expressed.

Etiol: A large virus of the pox group.

Treatment: Incision, expression of contents, followed by iodine.

m. fibrosum. A form showing masses of fibrocellular tissue.

m. simplex. See: *m. fibrosum.*

mol. wt. Abbreviation for *molecular weight.*

molybdenum (mō-lĭb'dĕ-nŭm). A hard, heavy, metallic element. Symb: *Mo.* At. wt. 95.94; at. no. 42.

molysmophobia (mō-lĭz"mō-fō'bĭ-ă). Syn: *mysophobia.* Morbid fear of contamination or infection.

momentum (mō-mĕn'tŭm) [L. equilibrium, motion]. 1. Quantity of motion. 2. Force of motion acquired by a moving object as a result of continuance of its motion; impetus.

mon'ad [G. *monas,* a unit]. 1. A univalent element. 2. A unicellular organism. 3. One of the four components of a tetrad.

monarthritis (mŏn-ar-thrī'tĭs) [G. *monas,* single, + *arthron,* joint, + *-itis,* inflammation]. Arthritis affecting a single joint.

monarticular (mŏn-ar-tĭk'ū-lăr) [" + L. *articulus,* joint]. Concerning or affecting one joint.

monaster (mŏn-as'ter) [" + *astēr,* star]. Single starlike figure formed in mitosis.

monathetosis (mŏn"ăth-e-tō'sĭs) [" + *athētos,* not fixed, + *-ōsis*]. Athetosis affecting a single part of the body.

Mondonesi's reflex (mon-dō-na'zĭ) [Filippo Mondonesi, Italian physician]. In coma, contraction of facial muscles following pressure on eyeball. Syn: *bulbomimic reflex, facial reflex.*

monesthetic (mŏn-ĕs-thet'ĭk) [G. *monas,* single, + *aisthēsis,* sensation]. Affecting only one of the senses.

Mongo'lian id'iocy. Congenital form with resemblance to an Asiatic. See: *idiocy.*

Mon'golism. Mongolian idiocy. Now called Down's syndrome or disease, after the English physician Langdon Down, 1828-1896.

monilethrix (mŏn-ĭl'ĕ-thrĭks) [" + G. *thrix*, hair]. Disease in which the hair becomes brittle and nodulated so that it has a beaded appearance.

Monil'ia [L. *monilis*, necklace]. Former name for the genus *Candida*, *q.v.*

moniliasis (mŏ"nĭ-lĭ'ă-sĭs) [G. *monas*, single, + G. *-osis*, intensive]. Infection of the skin or mucous membranes by yeastlike fungi. Usually localized in skin, nails, mouth, vagina, bronchi, or lungs, but may invade blood stream.
ETIOL: Various species of *Candida* but chiefly *C. albicans*.

moniliform (mŏn-ĭl'ĭ-form) [" + *forma*, shape]. Resembling a necklace or string of beads.

moniliosis (mŏn-ĭl-ĭ-ō'sĭs) [" + G. *-ōsis*, intensive]. Moniliasis, *q.v.*

mono, mon- [G.]. Prefixes: *One, single.*

mon"oacid'ic. Having one replaceable hydroxyl (OH) group.

monoanesthesia (mŏn-ō-ăn-ĕs-thē'sĭ-ă) [G. *monos* + *an-*, priv., + *aisthēsis*, sensation]. Anesthesia of a single member or organ.

monobasic (mŏn-ō-bā'sĭk) [G. *monos*, + *basis*, a base]. Having one hydrogen atom replaceable by a metal or positive radical.

mon'oblast. A cell which gives rise to a monocyte.

monoblepsia (mŏn-ō-blĕp'sĭ-ă) [G. *monos*, + *blepsis*, sight]. 1. Condition in which vision is more distinct when only one eye is used, hence tendency to close one eye to see clearly. 2. Color blindness in which only one color can be seen.

monobrachius (mŏn"ō-brā'kĭ-us) [" + *brachiōn*, arm]. 1. State of having only one arm. 2. Fetus with only one arm.

monobromated (mŏn"ō-brō'māt-ĕd) [G. *monos*, single, + *brōmos*, stench]. Pert. to chemical compound with only one atom of bromine in each molecule.

monocalcic (mŏn-ō-kal'sĭk) [" + L. *calx*, *calc-*, lime]. Pert. to a chemical compound containing only one atom of calcium in the molecule.

monocardian (mŏn-ō-kar'dĭ-ăn). Individual possessing a heart with only one atrium and one ventricle.

monocelled (mŏn'ō-sĕld) [" + L. *cella*, a chamber]. Composed of a single cell.

monochord (mŏn'ō-kord) [" + *chordē*, cord]. An instrument for testing upper tone audition by means of friction.

monochorea (mon"ō-kor-ē'ă) [" + *choreia*, dance]. Chorea which affects but a single part.

monochorionic (mŏn-ō-kor-ē"ŏn'ĭk). Possessing a single chorion, as in the case of identical twins.

monochromasy (mŏn"ō-krō-mā'sĭ). Color blindness in which only one color can be perceived.

monochromatic (mŏn"ō-krō-măt'ĭk) [" + *chrōma*, color]. 1. Having but one color. 2. A color-blind person to whom all colors appear to be of one hue.

monochromator (mŏn-ō-krō'mā-tor) [" + *chrōma*, color]. Instrument for selective transmission of homogeneous radiant energy.

monococcus (mŏn-ō-kŏk'ŭs) [" + *kokkos*, berry]. A form of coccus existing singly instead of as part of the usual group or chain.

monocular (mŏn-ŏk'ū-lar) [G. *monos*, single, + L. *oculus*, eye]. 1. Concerning or affecting but one eye. 2. Possessing a single ocular or eyepiece.

monoculus (mŏn-ok'ū-lŭs) [" + L. *oculus*, eye]. 1. A bandage for shielding one eye. 2. A fetus with only one eye.

monocyesis (mŏ-nō-sĭ-ē'sĭs) [" + *kyēsis*, pregnancy]. Pregnancy with a single fetus.

monocyte (mŏn'ō-sīt) [" + *kytos*, cell]. A large mononuclear leukocyte.

monocytic (mŏn-ō-si'tĭk) [" + *kytos*, cell]. Concerning or resembling monocytes.

monocytopenia (mŏn"ō-sīt"ō-pe'nĭ-ă) [" + " + *penia*, lack]. Diminished number of monocytes in the blood.

monocytosis (mŏn"ō-sī-tō'sĭs). Excessive number of monocytes in the blood.

monodactylism (mŏn-ō-dak'tĭl-ĭzm) [" + *daktylos*, digit]. Condition, usually congenital, of having only one digit on a hand or foot.

monodal (mŏ-nod'ăl) [G. *monos*, single, + *odos*, way]. Connected with one terminal of a resonator so that the patient acts as a capacitor for entrance and exit of high frequency currents.

monodiplopia (mŏn"ō-dĭ-plō'pĭ-ă) [" + *diploos*, double, + *ōps*, eye]. Double vision in one eye only.

monodromia. Condition of muscles or nerves in which conduction occurs in one direction only.

monogamy (mo-nog'ă-mĭ [" + G. *gamos*, marriage]. The practice of being married to only one person at a time.

monogony (mŏn-ŏg'ō-nĭ). Asexual reproduction.

monograph (mŏn'ō-grăf) [" + *graphein*, to write]. A treatise dealing with a single subject.

monohy'brid. Offspring of a cross between parents differing in a single pair of characters.

monohydrated (mŏn-ō-hī'drāt-ed) [G. *monos*, single, + *ydor*, water]. United with only one molecule of water.

monoideaism, monoideism (mŏn-ō-ī-dē'ă-ĭzm, -dē'ĭzm) [" + *idea*, idea]. Domination by only one idea.

monolocular (mŏn"ō-lok'ū-lar) [" + L. *loculus*, a small chamber]. Having only 1 cell or cavity. SYN: *unilocular*.

monomania (mŏn-ō-mā'nĭ-ă) [" + *mania*, madness]. Mental illness characterized by distortion of thought processes concerning a single subject or idea.

monoma'niac [" + *mania*, madness]. One afflicted with monomania.

monomastigote (mŏn-ō-măs'tĭ-gōt) [" + *mastix, mastig-*, whip]. Possessing only one flagellum.

monomelic (mŏn-ō-mel'ĭk) [G. *monos*, single, + *melos*, limb]. Affecting a single limb.

monomer (mon'o-mer). A single molecule of a compound formed by uniting several such molecules.

monomeric (mŏn-ō-mĕr'ĭk) [" + *meros*, part]. Consisting of, or affecting a single piece or segment of a body.

monomorphic (mŏn-ō-mor'fĭk) [" + *morphē*, form]. Unchangeable in form.

monomyople'gia [" + *mys, myo-*, muscle, + *plēgē*, stroke]. Paralysis of only one muscle.

monomyositis (mŏn"ō-mĭ-ō-sī'tĭs) [" + " + *-ītis*, inflammation]. Inflamed condition of only one muscle.

mononeural (mŏn-ō-nū'răl) [G. *monos*, single, + *neuron*, nerve]. Supplied by or concerning a single nerve.

mononeuritis (mŏn"ō-nū-rī'tĭs) [" + " + *-ītis*, inflammation]. Inflamed condition of a single nerve.

mononuclear (mŏn-ō-nū'klē-ăr) [" + L.

nucleus, kernel]. SYN: *uninuclear*. Having one nucleus, particularly a blood cell such as a monocyte or lymphocyte.

mononucleosis (mŏn-o-nū-klē-ō'sĭs) [" + L. *nucleus*, kernel]. Presence of more than normal number of mononuclear leukocytes in the blood.

m., infectious. Glandular fever with great increase of atypical or abnormal mononuclear leukocytes in the blood. Cause is unknown, but is most probably infectious. Incubation period may be as long as 4 to 7 weeks.

SYM: Constitutional symptoms, fever, sore throat, and generalized lymphadenopathy; hyperplasia of lymphatic tissue. Blood contains heterophile antibodies.

TREATMENT: There is no specific therapy but for serious complications—hemolytic anemia, pharyngeal swelling interfering with swallowing—cortisone is indicated.

mononucleotide. A product resulting from hydrolysis of nucleic acid consisting of phosphoric acid combined with a glucoside or pentoside.

monoparesis (mŏn-ō-par'es-ĭs) [" + *paresis*, weakness]. Paralysis of a single part of body.

monoparesthesia (mŏn"ō-păr-ĕs-thē'sĭ-ă) [" + *para*, beside, + *aisthēsis*, sensation]. Paresthesia of only one region or limb.

monopathy (mŏn-op'ăth-ĭ) [G. *monos*, single, + *pathos*, disease]. A disease attacking only one part of the body.

monophagia (mŏn-ō-fā'jĭ-ă) (" + *phagein*, to eat]. 1. Appetite for only one kind of food. 2. The habit of eating of just one meal a day.

monophasia (mŏn-ō-fā'zĭ-ă) [" + *phasis*, speech]. Inability to utter anything but one word or phrase repeatedly.

monophobia (mŏn-ō-fō'bĭ-ă) [" + *phobos*, fear]. Abnormal fear of being alone.

monophyletic (mŏn"ō-fīl-ĕt'ĭk) [" + *phylē*, tribe]. Originating from a single source.

monoplegia (mŏn-ō-plē'jĭ-ă) [G. *monos*, single, + *plēgē*, stroke]. Paralysis of a single limb or a single group of muscles.

monopolar (mŏn-ō-pōl'ăr) [" + L. *polus*, pole]. Using 1 terminal only, the ground acting as the 2nd terminal. SEE: *monoterminal*.

monorchid (mŏn-or'kĭd) [" + *orchis*, testicle]. Person having only 1 testicle.

monorchidism, monorchism (mŏn-ōr'kĭd-ĭzm, mŏn'or-kĭzm) [" + *orchis*, testicle]. Condition in which there is only one descended testicle.

monosaccharide (mŏn-ō-sak'ar-id) [G. *monos*, single, + *sakcharon*, sugar]. A sugar which cannot be decomposed by hydrolysis. Ex: *fructose, galactose, glucose, q.v.*

These sugars are absorbed directly. They maintain the glucose content of the blood and provide for the production of glycogen. SYN: *monosaccharose*.

monosaccharoses (mŏn-ō-sak'ă-rōs-ĕs) [" + *sakcharon*, sugar]. A group name for *monosaccharides*. SEE: *disaccharoses, polysaccharoses*.

monosome (mŏn'ō-sōm) [" + *sōma*, body]. An accessory chromosome which, without dividing, goes into only one of the daughter cells. The unpaired sex chromosome.

monospasm (mŏn'ō-spazm) [" + *spasmos*]. Spasm affecting a single part or organ.

Monosporium (mŏn"ō-spōr'ĭ-ŭm). A genus of fungi.

M. apiospermum. Causative agent of maduromycosis, *q.v.*

monosymptomatic (mŏn"ō-sĭmp-tō-mat'ĭk) [" + *symptōma*]. Having only one dominant symptom.

monosyphilide (mŏn-ō-sĭf'il-ĭd) [" + Fr. *syphilide*]. Characterized by only a single syphilitic lesion.

monoter'minal [" + *terma*, a limit]. Using one terminal only in the giving of treatments, the ground acting as the second terminal for the completion of the electrical circuit.

monothermia (mŏn-ō-therm'ĭ-ă) [G. *monos*, single, + *thermē*, heat]. Condition in which body temperature is stable.

Monotricha (mŏn-ot'rĭk-ă) [" + *thrix, trich-*, hair]. Bacteria having a single flagellum at one pole.

monotrichous (mon-ot'rĭ-kus). Pert. to or having a single flagellum.

monovalent (mon-o-va'lent) [" + L. *valēre*, to have power]. Having the combining power of a single hydrogen atom. SYN: *univalent*.

monox'enous. Said of a parasite which has only one species as a host.

monoxide (mŏn-ŏk'sīd) [" + *oxys*, sour]. An oxide having only 1 atom of oxygen.

monozygotic (mŏn"ō-zī-gŏt'ĭk). Originating from a single fertilized ovum, said of identical twins.

Monro's foramen (mŏn-rō') [Alexander Monro, English surgeon, 1737-1817]. Point of communication bet. 3rd and lateral ventricles of the brain.

M.'s sulcus. Sulcus on 3rd ventricle's lateral wall from the foramen interventriculare to the aditus ad aquaeductum cerebri. SYN: *aulix*.

mons (mŏns) (pl. *montēs*) [L. mountain]. An anatomical eminence above the surface of the body.

m. pubis. NA. Pubic eminence. SYN: *m. veneris*.

m. veneris [L. mount of Venus]. A pad of fatty tissue and coarse skin overlying the symphysis pubis in the woman. After puberty covered with short, curly hair called the *escutcheon*. Typically triangular in shape. SEE: *pubes*.

mon'ster [L. *monstrum*]. A grossly deformed individual, usually due to faulty development. The word should never be used when discussing such a patient with those who are emotionally attached to him or her. Terms such as handicapped, congenitally deformed, or abnormal would be more appropriate.

monstripar'ity [" + *parēre*, to give birth to]. To give birth to a monster.

monstros'ity [L. *monstrositās*]. 1. Monster. 2. Congenital malformation.

Montgom'ery's glands [William F. Montgomery, Irish obstetrician, 1797-1859]. Small prominences around the nipple of the breast which enlarge during pregnancy and lactation. SEE: *areola, mamma*.

monthlies (mŭnth'lēs). Slang for the menses.

monticulus (mon-tĭk'u-lus) [L. little mountain]. A protuberance.

m. cerebelli. BNA. Protuberance of the superior vermis whose ant. portion is called the *culmen*, the post. portion the *declive*.

mood (mōōd) [A.S. *mōd*, mind, feeling]. Temporary state of mind in regard to or as result of emotion.

morament (mōr-am'ent) [G. *mōros*, stupid, + *a-*, priv. + L. *mens, ment-*, mind]. A moron of low grade. A person who is mentally defective and without moral sense.

moramentia (mōr-ă-mĕn'shĭ-ă) [" + " + L. *mens, ment-*, mind]. State of being without moral sense.

Morand's disease (mor-an'). Paresis affecting the lower extremities.

Moraxella (mor-ax-ĕl'ă). A genus of Brucellaceae, and are commonly found in diseases of the eye.

M. lacunata. A causative agent of conjunctivitis.

morbid (mor'bĭd) [L. *morbidus,* sick]. 1. Diseased. 2. Pert. to disease.

morbid'ity [L. *morbidus,* sick]. State of being diseased.

m. rate. Number of cases of a specific disease in a specified period of time, usually a year, per unit of population, usually 1,000, 10,000, or 100,000 alive.

morbific (mor-bĭf'ĭk) [" + *facere,* to make]. Causing or producing disease.

morbilli (mor-bil'ī) [L. *morbillus,* little disease]. Measles.

morbilliform. Like measles or its rash.

mor'bus [L. disease]. Disease.

m. addisonii. Addison's disease.

m. caducus. Epilepsy.

m. caeruleus. Cyanosis which is congenital.

m. cardiacus. Cordis, *q.v.*

m. coeliacus. Celiac disease, *q.v.*

m. cordis. Chronic cardiac disease.

m. coxa'rius. Hip joint disease.

m. culliaris. Whooping cough; pertussis.

m. divinua. Epilepsy.

m. dormitivus. Sleeping sickness.

m. elephas. Elephantiasis.

m. gallicus. Syphilis.

m. maculosus neotorum. Hemorrhagic disease of the newborn.

m. miseriae. Condition due to neglect and want.

m. nauticus. Seasickness.

m. regius. Icterus, jaundice.

m. senilis. Arthritis deformans.

m. virgineus. Chlorosis.

m. vulpis. Alopecia.

morcellation, morcellement (mor-sel-ā'-shŭn, -mon') [Fr. *morceller,* to subdivide]. Method of removing a tumor or organ in pieces.

mordant (mor'dănt) [L. *mordere,* to bite]. A substance which fixes a stain or dye, as *alum* and *phenol.*

mores (mo'rāz) [L. plural of *mos,* custom]. Habits and customs of society. Usually those which preserve the social order.

morgagnian (mor-gan'yē-ăn). Pert. to or described by Morgagni.

Morgagni's caruncle (mor-gan'yē) [Giovanni B. Morgagni, Italian anatomist and pathologist, 1682-1771]. The middle prostatic lobe.

M.'s cataract. One that is hypermature with a softened cortex and a hard nucleus. SEE: *cataract.*

M.'s hy'datid. Remains of müllerian duct attached to testicle or oviduct.

M.'s ventricle. Ventriculus laryngis. SEE: *ventricle.*

morgue (morg) [Fr.]. A public mortuary; a place for holding dead bodies before disposing of them. SYN: *mortuary.*

moria (mo'rĭ-ă) [G. *mōria,* folly]. 1. Simple dementia. 2. Foolishness.

moribund (mor'ĭ-bŭnd) [L. *moribundus,* dying]. In a dying condition; dying.

morioplasty (mo'rĭ-ō-plas-tĭ) [G. *morion,* piece, + *plassein,* to form]. Plastic surgery to restore portions of the body which have been lost through accident or disease.

morning or "A. M." care. AIM: Comfort and cleanliness.

ARTICLES NECESSARY: Basin with warm water. Washcloth and face towel. Toothbrush, mouthwash, and water for mouth hygiene. Emesis basin. Comb and brush. Fresh linen as needed. Bath blanket. Rubbing alcohol or suitable back-rubbing lotion and talcum powder.

PROCEDURE: If in ward screen bed or draw curtains. Offer bedpan before beginning procedure, and supply fresh tampon or perineal pad if necessary. Cover patient with bath blanket and fold top bedding to foot of bed. If very disordered, remove to chair. Remove all but one pillow. Assist patient with care of mouth, or care for it if patient is not able to. Wash face and hands. Turn patient on side and rub back with back-rubbing lotion and powder. Patients whose skin is tender should have back washed before the rubbing. If patient is to have bath later the linen need not be changed until that is given. Loosen bottom sheet and draw sheet and pull them tight again, brushing out any crumbs that may be on them. Smooth patient's hair. Fluff and rearrange pillows. Rearrange upper bedding neatly. If patient has a hot water bottle or an ice cap refill it. Leave fresh water within patient's reach. Leave fresh washcloth and towel. Before leaving room, adjust bed position, lighting and ventilation as indicated.

morn'ing sickness. The nausea and vomiting that affect some women during first few months of pregnancy, particularly in the morning. SYN: *hyperemesis gravidarum.*

Headache, dizziness and exhaustion also may be experienced. It may clear up after the 3rd month.

Occurs usually about the 5th or 6th week and symptoms vary from simple morning sickness to pernicious vomiting of pregnancy. Usually clears up without treatment in 1-3 weeks. Occurs in about 50 per cent of pregnancies.

NP & TREATMENT: The anti-nausea drugs and large doses of B complex vitamins usually are the only treatment necessary; however, the following may be helpful where the drugs are not available: Crackers or vanilla wafers on arising. Three to five *small* meals per day. Tea helps, some outdoor activities. Psychic causes aggravate, so mental hygiene is desirable. Good ventilation during sleep; effervescent drinks.

mo'ron [G. *mōros,* stupid]. A feebleminded person, not beyond the Binet age of 12, having the mentality ordinarily attained between 7 and 12. Of greater intelligence than an imbecile. The term implies no moral defect. Possessing an I.Q. of 50 to 70. SEE: *mental deficiency.*

Moro's reaction or **test** [Ernst Moro, German pediatrist, 1874-1951]. Test to determine the presence of tuberculosis, by application of an ointment of 5 cc. of old tuberculin and 5 gm. of anhydrous wool fat to the thorax for 1 minute. An eruption of red papules on the skin appears in 24-48 hours in tuberculosis.

M.'s reflex. A defensive reflex, a response consisting of the drawing of the infant's arms across its chest in an embracing manner, in response to stimuli produced by striking the surface on which the infant rests.

morosis (mo-rō'sĭs) [G. *mōros,* stupid, + *-ōsis*]. The mental state of a moron. Feeblemindedness. SYN: *moronity.*

morphea (mor-fe'ă) [G. *morphē,* form].

Skin disease characterized by discrete, circumscribed, grayish or yellowish patches, firm but not hard, bordered by pinkish or purplish areolae on breasts, head, face, lower extremities, with telangiectases on the lesions.

Plaques disappear spontaneously but may leave cicatrixlike marks. Probably a trophoneurosis. SYN: *Addison's keloid, circumscribed scleroderma.*

mor'phia. Morphine.

morphi'na [L.]. Morphine, *q.v.*

morphine (mor'fēn) [L. *morphina*, from *Morpheus*, god of sleep]. Main alkaloid found in opium, occurring in bitter, colorless crystals. Widely used as analgesic and sedative.

POISONING: *Preliminary Symptoms*: Brief mental exhilaration; languor; followed by weariness, sleepiness, pinpoint pupils; rapid, forcible pulse which becomes slow and feeble. Respiration slow and shallow. Unconsciousness, from which patient may be aroused with difficulty. Muscles become relaxed; reflexes diminished; temperature low; skin pale, cold and moist; pupils dilated; coma and death follow.

F. A. AND EMERGENCY TREATMENT: Gastric lavage with 1:10,000 potassium permanganate solution, high enemas, maintenance of airway. If respiration is depressed, nalorphine hydrochloride, a specific morphine and opiate antagonist, should be administered subcutaneously or I.V. Inhalation of oxygen and artificial respiration may be necessary. SEE: *Table of Poisons and Poisoning in Appendix.*

m. sul'fate. USP. The sulfate of an alkaloid obtained from opium and occurring as white, feathery crystals, incompatible with alkalies, tannic acid and iodides.

ACTION AND USES: Hypnotic and analgesic.

morphinism (mor'fin-ĭzm) [L. *morphina*]. Morbid condition due to habitual or excessive use of morphine. Morphine habit.

morphinomania, morphiomania (mor"fĭn-ō-mā'nĭ-ă, fe-ō-mā'nĭ-ă) [" + G. *mania*, madness]. 1. Morbid desire for morphine. 2. Insanity resulting from use of morphine.

morphogenesis (mor"fō-jĕn'ĕ-sĭs) [G. *morphē*, form, + *genesis*, development]. The various processes occurring during development by which the form of the body and its organs is established.

morphogenetic (mor"fō-jĕn-et'ĭk) [" + *gennan*, to produce]. Stimulating growth and development of form.

m. processes. Those by which morphogenesis is accomplished. Include cell migration; cell aggregation; localized growth; splitting, including delamination and cavitation; folding, including invagination and evagination.

m. substance. Chemical substances present in eggs or early embryos which induce morphologic differentiation. SEE: *induction.*

morphology (mor-fol'ō-jĭ) [" + *logos*, study]. Science of structure and form without regard to function.

morphometry (mor-fom'e-trĭ) [" + *metron*, measure]. The measurement of forms of organisms.

morpio, morpion (mor'pĭ-ō, -pĭ-on) [L.]. The crab louse infesting the pubic area.

mors [L.]. Death.

m. putativa. Apparent death.

m. subita. Sudden death.

m. thymica. Sudden death in children associated with enlarged thymus.

mor'tal [L. *mors, mort-*, death]. 1. Causing death. 2. Subject to death. 3. Human.

mortality (mor-tal'ĭ-tĭ) [L. *mors, mort-*, death]. 1. State of being mortal. 2. The death rate.

mortar (mor'tar) [L. *mortarium*]. Vessel, with a smooth interior, used for powdering or pulverizing drugs with a pestle.

mortician. Undertaker.

mortification (mor"tĭ-fĭ-kā'shŭn) [L. *mors, mort-*, death, + *facere*, to make]. Death or failure of a tissue, organ or part. SYN: *gangrene, necrosis.*

mortinatality (mor"tĭ-nā-tal'ĭ-tĭ) [" + *natus*, birth]. Ratio of stillbirths to normal births.

mort'ise joint. Ankle joint.

Mor'ton's disease. Neuralgia of the metatarsus.

mortuary (mor'tu-a-rĭ) [L. *mortuarium*, a tomb]. 1. Temporary place for keeping dead bodies before burial. SYN: *morgue.* 2. Rel. to the dead or to death.

morula (mor'ū-lă) [L. *morus*, mulberry]. Solid mass of cells, resembling a mulberry, resulting from segmentation of an ovum.

moruloid (mor'u-loid) [" + G. *eidos*, form]. 1. BACT: A colony made up of a mass resembling a mulberry. 2. Resembling a mulberry.

mosa'ic. 1. A picture or design made of many small colored pieces interspersed in some other material. 2. Genetics: an individual whose tissues are of different genetic kinds. 3. BOTANY: Spotted condition in plants as in tobacco mosaic, a disease caused by a virus.

m. bone. B. appearing as small pieces fitted together, characteristic of Paget's disease.

m. development. Type of development exhibited by ova which undergo determinate cleavage in which each blastomere has a characteristic position and unalterable fate.

m. sex. An individual consisting of male tissue in one part and female tissue in another owing to chromosomal abnormalities occurring during development. SEE: *gynandromorph.*

mosquito (mŏs-kē'tō) [Sp. little fly]. 1. A sucking insect belonging to the order Diptera, family Culicidae, *q.v.* Important species are *Anopheles, Culex, Aëdes, Haemagogus, Mansonia,* and *Psorophora.* They serve as transmitting agents of many diseases, including malaria, filariasis, yellow fever, dengue, viral encephalitis, and dermatobiasis.

mosquitocide. Lethal to mosquitoes or their larvae.

mossy cell (maws'ĭ). A protoplasmic astrocyte, a neuroglia cell with many branching processes. SEE: *neuroglia.*

mossy fibers. Afferent fibers to the cerebellar cortex. They give off many collaterals each ending in a glomerulus.

moth'er [A.S. *mōdor*]. 1. Female parent. 2. A structure which gives rise to others.

m. cell. A cell which, by fission or budding, gives rise to similar cells.

m. cyst. An echinococcus cyst enveloping smaller ones.

m., expectant. One who is pregnant.

m. liquor. That left after removal of crystals from a solution.

m.'s mark. A birthmark. SEE: *mark.*

motile (mō'tĭl) [L. *motilis*, moving]. Able to move spontaneously.

motility (mō-tĭl'ĭt-ĭ) [L. *motilis*, moving]. Capability of moving spontaneously.

motion (mō'shun) [L. *motio*, movement]. 1. A change of place or position; movement. 2. Evacuation of the bowels. 3.

(*Pl.*) Matter evacuated. SEE: *"cine-" words, efferent, "kine-" words, circus movements.*

m., active. Movements caused by the patient's own intention.

m., passive. Movements due to an attendant causing the part to be moved.

m. sickness. Nausea, vomiting, and vertigo induced by irregular or rhythmic movements. Ex: seasickness, airsickness, car sickness, swing sickness.

motor (mō'tor) [L. *motus,* moving]. 1. Causing motion. 2. A part or that which induces movements, as *nerves* or *muscles.*

m. aphasia. A condition in which the patient understands but cannot express himself in words, or read aloud.

m. area. Post. part. of frontal lobe ant. to the central sulcus from which impulses for volitional movement arise.

m. end plate. Flat expansion ending a motor nerve fiber where it connects with a muscle fiber.

m. fibers. Axons of motor neurons which innervate skeletal muscles.

m. nerve. A n. composed entirely of motor fibers.

m. neuron. 1. A n. which innervates muscle tissue. 2. A n. which carries impulses initiating muscle contraction.

m. points. Points where the motor nerve enters the muscle, and where visible contraction can be elicited with a minimal amount of stimulation.

m. sense. The kinesthetic sense.

m. unit. A single motor neuron and the muscle fibers its branches innervate.

motorial (mō-tor'ĭ-ăl) [L. *motus,* moving]. Concerning motion or a motor center.

motoricity (mō-tor-ĭs'ĭt-ĭ) [L. *motus,* moving]. Capability of movement.

motorium (mō-tōr'ĭ-ŭm) [L. power of motion]. Motor center of a body or organism.

motorius (mō-tōr'ĭ-ŭs) [L. power of motion]. Any motor nerve.

m. oculi communis. Third cranial nerve. SYN: *motor oculi.*

motorpathy (mō-tōr'păth-ĭ) [L. *motus,* moving, + G. *pathos,* disease]. Treatment of a condition by prescribed movements. SYN: *kinesitherapy, kinetotherapy.*

mottled enamel. Condition in which the enamel of the teeth becomes porous and pigmented owing to excess of fluorine in drinking water. SEE: *fluorosis.*

mottling (mŏt'lĭng) [O.E. *motteley,* many colored]. A condition which is marked by discolored areas.

moulage (moo-lahzh') [Fr.]. 1. A wax model or reproduction, as of a skin condition. 2. Molding of a wax model.

mould (mōld). SEE: *mold.*

moulding (mōld'ĭng). SEE: *molding.*

mounding [origin uncertain]. Lumping, as the mounding of a wasting muscle when struck a quick, firm blow.

mountain fever or ***m. sickness.*** SYN: *hypobaropathy, mareo de la Cordillera, soroche, puna.* Condition occurring in individuals ascending to high altitudes (over 10,000 ft.) or to those subjected to rarefied atmospheres. Due to anoxia resulting from reduced oxygen tension.

SYM: euphoria, tachycardia, headache, nausea, increased respiratory rate, fatigue, and cerebral disorders (loss of memory, errors of judgment).

mounting (mownt'ĭng) [L. *mons, mont-,* mountain]. The arrangement of specimens on slides, frames, chart boards, display boards or any background for study.

mouse unit (mows). Least amount of estrus-producing hormone which induces, in a spayed mouse, a characteristic desquamation of the vaginal epithelium.

mouth (mowth) [A.S. *mūth*]. 1. The opening of any cavity. SYN: *buccal cavity, oral cavity.* 2. The cavity within the cheeks, containing the tongue and teeth, and communicating with the pharynx.

Some conditions involving the mouth cavity are: *abnormalities of tongue:* dry, coated, smooth, strawberry, large, pigmented, geographic, deviated, tremulous, sore; *conditions involving gums and teeth:* gingivitis, sordes, lead line, pyorrhea, atrophy, hypertrophy, dental caries, alveolar abscesses; *conditions involving mucous membrane or other parts of mouth:* eruptions accompanying exanthematous diseases, stomatitis, canker sores, thrush, trench mouth, cysts, tumors, carcinoma, lesions of syphilis such as chancre, mucous patches, gumma, lesions of tuberculosis, abscesses.

Disorders of the mouth cavity may be indications of purely local disease or they may be symptoms of systemic disturbances such as dehydration, pernicious anemia, nutritional deficiencies, esp. avitaminoses.

m. examination. In addition to visual examination, careful digital examination should be made, as such reveals areas of tenderness and alterations of texture characteristic of leukoplakia, cancer, cystic swellings, and lymphadenopathy.

Excessive moisture of the mouth is seen in stomatitis, irritation of pneumogastric nerve, ingestion of irritating drugs or foods, nervous disorders, teething, seeing appetizing foods, smelling pleasant odors.

m., rashes in. Stomatitis, measles, scarlet fever. ON LIPS: Typhoid fever, meningitis, pneumonia. In secondary syphilis, chancre, cancer and epithelioma mucous patches appear. RS: *canker, catarrh.*

m., trench. SYN: *Vincent's angina.* SEE: *trench mouth.*

NP: *Aim*: To keep mouth clean and in good condition. *Articles Necessary*: Small tray with glass of fresh water, glass or cup of mouthwash, applicators, tongue depressors, gauze bandage about 2 in. wide, emesis basin, towel, paper bag, liquid albolene or special ointment, and disposable drinking tube.

Procedure: 1. Have all equipment ready on bedside table. 2. Place towel under patient's chin, across chest. 3. Turn patient's head to side and arrange emesis basin close to corner of mouth. 4. Dip applicators in mouthwash and clean teeth, tongue, gums, and roof of mouth. 5. Discard used applicators into paper bag. Do not dip into mouthwash after using. 6. If teeth are difficult to clean make a larger swab by winding several turns of bandage around tongue depressor. 7. Allow patient to rinse mouth with mouthwash using drinking tube, followed by fresh water. Caution him not to expectorate the fluids forcibly, but to let them run gently out at the corner of his mouth. Keep corner wiped clean. 8. If lips are dry or cracked apply liquid albolene or special ointment. 9. If the patient has a high temperature clean the mouth before each feeding. 10. If he is unconscious hold the mouth open with a tongue depressor padded with gauze. 11. Be gentle and thorough.

RS: *agranulocytosis, Ludwig's; antitrismus; astomatous; bucca; buccal; b. glands; cancrum oris; chalinoplasty; chin jerk; fauces; ora; palate; oral; orifice; os; stoma; stomatitis; tongue; xerostomia.*

movement (mōōv'mĕnt) [L. *movēre,* to move]. 1. Act of passing from place to place or changing position of body or its parts. 2. Evacuation of feces.

m., active. Accomplished without outside assistance.

m., ameboid. Movement resembling that of an ameba in which the protoplasm of a cell flows into a projection of the cell membrane forming a pseudopodium. Characteristic of leukocytes and certain protozoa.

m., associated. Involuntary movement of a part occurring coincident with and subsequent to the movement of another part.

m., autonomic. A spontaneous, involuntary m., independent of ext. stimulation.

m., brownian. The peculiar jiggling or dancing movement of minute particles suspended in liquids or gases when observed under the microscope, due to bombardment of the particles by molecules of their surrounding medium.

m., ciliary. That of the cilia of a ciliated cell or epithelium.

m., circus. A phenomenon in an animal after injury to a corpus striatum, optic thalamus, or crus cerebri, causing it to move about in a circle.

m., disorders of. May be due to injury or disease of (a) muscle, (b) nerve ending, (c) motor nerve, (d) spinal cord, or (e) of the brain.

TYPES OF: Hemiplegia, ataxia, monoplegia, tremors, rigors, choreic, athetosis, convulsions, spasm (clonic or tonic), reflex (hysterical, habit spasm, tics), and spastic paralysis.

m.'s, fetal. Muscular m.'s performed by the fetus in utero.

m., molecular. The movement of molecules of a substance, the basis of the kinetic theory of matter. SEE: *m., brownian.*

m., pendular. Swaying movements of the intestine when exposed, due to rhythmic contractions of the circular layer of muscle.

m., peristaltic. Peristalsis, *q.v.*

m., respiratory. Any m. resulting from the contraction of respiratory muscles or occurring passively as a result of elasticity of the thoracic wall or lungs. SEE: *inspiration, expiration, respiration.*

m. of restitution. A partial rotation of the fetal head, in cases of head presentation.

m., saccadic. Jerky movements of the eyes as in reading.

m., segmenting. M. of the intestine in which annular constrictions occur dividing intestine into ovoid segments.

m., vermicular. Peristalsis.

m., vibratile. Ciliary m.

moxa (mŏk'sa) [Japanese]. Inflammable substance used as a cautery for the skin, or as a counterirritant.

moxibustion (mŏks-ĭ-būst'shŭn) [Japanese *moxa,* + L. *combustus,* burned]. Cauterization by means of a cylinder or cone of cotton wool, called a moxa, placed on the skin and fired at the top. Used to produce counterirritation.

moxosophyra (moks-ō-sof-ĭ'ră) [Japanese *moxa* + G. *sphyra,* hammer]. A hammer heated and used as a cautery.

M.P.H. Abbr. for *Master of Public Health.*

M.P.N. Abbr. for *most probable number* (of bacteria present in a quantity of solution, esp. water).

MSH. Abbr. for *melanocyte-stimulating hormone.*

M.T. Abbr. for *medical technician.*

mu (mū) [Greek letter m]. μ. A micron, 1/1000 of a millimeter or 1/25,000 of an inch.

M. u. Abbr. for Maché unit and mouse unit.

mucedin (mū'se-dĭn) [L. *mucedō,* mucus]. A substance obtained from gluten.

Much-Holzmann reaction (mook-holts'-mahn) [Hans C. R. Much, German physician, 1880-1932; and V. Holzmann, German physician]. Inhibition of hemolysis of erythrocytes by cobra venom in manic-depressive insanity and dementia precox.

muciferous (mū-sĭf'ĕr-ŭs) [L. *mucus,* mucus, + *ferre,* to carry]. Secreting or producing mucus.

muciform (mū'sĭ-form) [" + *forma,* shape]. Appearing similar to mucus.

mucigen (mū'sĭ-jĕn) [L. *mucus,* mucus, + G. *gennan,* to produce]. A substance present in mucous cells which upon being extruded from the cell is converted into mucin.

mucigenous (mū-sĭj'ĕn-ŭs). Producing mucus. SYN: *muciferous.*

mucilage (mū'sĭ-lāj). Vegetable preparation used in pharmaceuticals. SEE: *mucilago.*

mucilaginous (mū-sĭl-aj'ĭn-ŭs) [L. *mucilāgō,* moldy juice]. Resembling mucilage; slimy; sticky.

mucila'go [L. moldy juice]. Thick, viscid, adhesive liquid, containing gum or mucilaginous principles dissolved in water, usually employed to hold insoluble substances in suspension in aqueous liquids or as a demulcent.

mucin (mū'sĭn) [L. *mucus*]. A glycoprotein found in mucus. It is present in saliva and bile and also found in salivary glands, in the skin, connective tissues, tendon, and cartilage. It is formed from mucigen and in water forms a slimy solution.

On decomposition the mucins give dextrose, sulfur and nitrogen among other products.

m., gastric. A commercial preparation made from the gastric mucosa of the hog, used in the treatment of ulcers of the digestive tract.

It forms a protective coating over the ulcer or erosion, which prevents irritation from the passing of bile and acid secretions in the duodenum, and from acid conditions irritating peptic ulcer of the stomach.

mucinemia (mū-sĭn-ē'mĭ-ă) [" + G. *aima,* blood]. Mucin in the blood.

mucinogen (mū-sĭn'ō-jĕn) [" + G. *gennan,* to produce]. A glycoprotein which forms mucin.

mucinoid (mū'sin-oid) [" + G. *eidos,* resemblance]. Appearing similar to mucin.

mucinuria (mū-sĭn-ū'rĭ-ă) [" + G. *ouron,* urine]. Presence of mucin in the urine.

muciparous (mū-sĭp'ăr-ŭs) [L. *mucus,* mucus, + *parēre,* to bring forth]. Producing or secreting mucus. SYN: *muciferous, mucigenous.*

muco- [L.]. Combining form, *having relation to mucus.*

mucocele (mū'kō-sēl) [L. *mucus,* mucus, + G. *kēlē,* swelling]. 1. Enlargement of the lacrimal sac. 2. A mucous cyst. 3. A mucous polypus.

mucocolpos (mū"kō-kŏl-pŏs). Accumulation of mucus in the vagina.

mucocutaneous (mū"kō-kū-tā'nē-ŭs) [" + *cutis*, skin]. Concerning a mucous membrane and the skin.

mucodermal (mū-kō-dĕr'măl) [" + G. *derma*, skin]. Pert. to a mucous membrane and the skin. SYN: *mucocutaneous*.

mucoenteritis (mū"kō-ĕn-tĕr-ī'tĭs) [" + G. *enteron*, intestine, + *-itis*, inflammation]. Inflammation of intestinal mucosa.

mucoglobulin (mū"kō-glŏb'ū-lĭn) [" + *globulus*, globule]. Any protein group to which plastin belongs.

mucoid (mū'koyd) [" + G. *eidos*, resemblance]. 1. Glycoprotein similar to mucin. 2. Muciform similar to mucus.

mucopolysaccharide. Polysaccharides containing hexosamine and sometimes proteins. Thick gelatinous material which is found many places in the body, it glues cells together, lubricates joints, and is found in blood group substances.

mucopurulent (mū-kō-pur'ū-lĕnt) [" + *purulentus*, made up of pus]. Consisting of mucus and pus.

mucopus (mū'kō-pŭs) [" + *pus*, pus]. Mucus combined with or resembling pus.

Mucor (mū'kor) [L. mold]. A genus of mold fungi seen on dead and decaying matter. Sometimes responsible for infections of external ear, skin, and respiratory passageways.

mucoriferous (mū-kor-ĭf'ĕr-ŭs) [" + *ferre*, to carry]. Covered with mold or a moldlike substance.

mucorin (mū'kor-ĭn) [L. *mucor*, mold]. An albuminoid substance derived from molds.

mucormycosis (mū-kor-mī-kō'sĭs) [" + G. *mykēs*, fungus, + *-ōsis*]. A fungus disease due to Mucor.

mucosa (mū-kō'să) (pl. *mucosae*) [L. mucous]. Mucous membrane.

mucosal (mū-kō'săl) [L. *mucōsa*, mucous]. Concerning any mucous membrane.

mucosanguineous (mū"kō-san-gwin'ē-ŭs) [L. *mucus*, mucus, + *sanguineus*, bloody]. Containing mucus and blood.

mucosedative (mū"kō-sĕd'ă-tĭv) [" + *sedativus*, allaying]. Soothing to mucosae of the body. SYN: *demulcent*.

mucoserous (mū"kō-sēr'ŭs) [" + *serum*, whey]. Composed of mucus and serum.

mucosin (mū'kō-sĭn) [L. *mucus*, mucus]. Mucin found in thick, sticky mucus.

mucous (mū'kŭs) [L. *mucus*, mucus]. 1. Having the nature of or resembling mucus. 2. Secreting mucus. 3. Depending on presence of mucus.

RS: *mucitis, mucocele, mucopurulent, mucosa, mucus, "myx-" words.*

m. colitis. Inflammation of the mucosa of the colon. SEE: *colitis*.

m. membrane. That lining passages and cavities communicating with the air. Consists of a surface layer of epithelium, a basement membrane, and an underlying layer of connective tissue, the lamina propria. Mucus-secreting cells or glands are usually present in the epithelium but may be absent.

EXAMINATION OF: Examination should reveal degree of moisture, cyanosis, pallor, hyperemia, pigmentation, lesions, or their absence, and hemorrhage.

PALLOR: Seen in all anemias. If temporary, may indicate shock, vasomotor spasm, or may occur in severe hemorrhages.

BLANCHING AND FLUSHING ALTERNATELY: Accompanies aortic regurgitation.

CYANOSIS: SEE: *skin*.

HYPEREMIA OR EXCESSIVE REDNESS: *Buccal mucous membrane*: Due to decayed teeth, traumatism, stomatitis. SEE: *mouth*.

Nasal mucosa: Ulceration of nose, rhinitis, inflammation. SEE: *nose*.

Eyes (local irritation): Foreign body, ulcer, inflammation. SEE: *jaundice*.

DRYNESS: Seen in fevers, chronic gastritis, some liver disturbances, excitement, shock, prostration, fatigue, thirst and certain drugs.

m. polypus. Small growth from mucous lining of the cervix or uterus.

mucoviscidosis. SEE: *cystic fibrosis*.

mucus (mū'kŭs) [L.]. A viscid fluid secreted by mucous membranes and glands, consisting of mucin, leukocytes, inorganic salts, water and epithelial cells.

A good example is the almost ropy secretion from the sublingual and submaxillary glands. Mucus in feces indicates irritation of mucous lining of the intestines and inflammation. It gives a slimy appearance to the stool. If the inflammation is in the small intestines the mucus will be mixed with the stool; if in the colon it will be on surface.

RS: *amyxorrhea, "blenn-" words, expectorant, expectoration, glairy, goblet cell, "muc-" words.*

mulatto (mū-lăt'tō) [Spanish *mulato*, of mixed breed, from L. *mulus*, mule]. First generation born of pure negro and white parentage; popularly anyone of white and negro blood mixed.

mulieb'ria. The female genitalia.

muliebrity (mū-lī-ĕb'rĭ-tĭ). Femininity; womanliness. The assumption of womanly qualities at puberty. The assumption of female characteristics by a male.

Müller's ducts. Embryonic tubes from which the oviducts, uterus and vagina develop in the female; in the male they become atrophied.

M.'s fibers. SYN: *radial fibers of M.* Fine fibers of neuroglia cells which form supporting elements of the retina.

M.'s muscle. 1. Circular fibers of ciliary muscle. 2. The sup. tarsal muscle of the eyelid. 3. Smooth muscle covering over sphenomaxillary fissure.

M.'s ring. Muscular ring at junction of cervical canal and the gravid uterus.

M.'s trigone. Portion of *tuber cinereum* folding over the optic chiasm.

M.'s tubercle. Projection on dorsal wall of cloaca at which Müller's ducts terminate.

mult-, multi- [L.] Prefixes meaning *many*.

multang'ular. Having many angles.

m. bone, greater. SYN: *trapezium*. The first or outermost of the distal row of carpal bones.

m. bone, lesser. SYN: *trapezoid*. The second in distal row of carpal bones.

multiarticular (mŭl"tĭ-ar-tĭk'ū-lar) [L. *multus*, many, + *articulus*, joint]. Concerning, having, or affecting many joints.

multicapsular (mŭl"tĭ-kap'sū-lar) [" + *capsula*, a little box]. Composed of many capsules.

multicellular (mŭl"tĭ-sĕl'ū-lar) [" + *cellula*, small chamber]. Consisting of many cells.

Mul'ticeps. A genus of tapeworms.

multicuspid, multicuspidate (mul-tĭ-kus'pĭd, -pĭ-dāt) [" + *cuspis*, point]. Having several cusps.

multifactorial. The result of many factors, as in a disease resulting from the combined action of several factors.

multifid (mŭl'tĭf-ĭd) [" + *fidus*, from

findere, to split]. Divided into many sections.

multiform (mŭl'tĭ-form) [" + *forma,* shape]. Having many forms or shapes. SYN: *polymorphous.*

multiglandular (mŭl"tĭ-glănd'ū-lar) [" + *glandula,* a little acorn]. Concerning several glands.

multigrav'ida [L. *multus,* many, + *gravida,* pregnant]. A woman who has been pregnant two or more times. May be written as Gravida II, III, etc. RS: *multipara.*

multi-infection (mŭl"tĭ-ĭn-fek'shŭn) [" + *infectiō,* an infection]. A mixed infection with several organisms developing at the same time.

multilobular (mŭl"tĭ-lōb'ū-lar) [" + *lobulus,* a small lobe]. Formed of, or possessing many lobules.

multilocular (mŭl"tĭ-lok'ū-lar) [" + *loculus,* a cell]. Having many cells or compartments. SYN: *multicellular.*

multimammae (mul"tĭ-mam'mē) [" + *mamma,* a breast]. Condition of possessing more than the normal number of breasts. SYN: *polymastia.*

multinodal (mul-tĭ-nō'dăl) [" + *nodus,* node]. Having many nodes or knots.

multinodular (mŭl-tĭ-nod'ū-lar) [" + *nodulus,* little knot]. Possessing many nodules or small knots.

multinuclear, multinucleate (mul-tĭ-nū'klē-ar, -āt) [L. *multus,* many, + *nucleus,* kernel]. Possessing several nuclei.

multipara (mul-tip'ă-ră) [" + *parēre,* to bear]. A woman who has borne more than one child. May be written Para II, III, etc. RS: *multigravida.*

m., grand. A woman who has given birth seven or more times.

multiparity (mul-tĭ-par'ĭ-tĭ) [" + *parēre,* to bear]. 1. Condition of having borne more than one child. 2. Production of more than one child at birth.

multiparous (mŭl-tĭp'ăr-ŭs) [" + *parēre,* to bear]. 1. Having borne more than one child. 2. Producing more than one child at birth.

multiple (mul'tĭ-pl) [L. *multiplex,* many folded]. 1. Consisting of, or containing more than one; manifold. 2. Occurring simultaneously in various parts of the body.

m. personality. Condition in which the subject may develop two or more personalities. SEE: *dual personality.*

multipolar (mŭl-tĭ-pōl'ar) [L. *multus,* many, + *polus,* a pole]. 1. Possessing more than two poles. 2. Possessing more than two processes, said of neurons.

multiter'minal [" + G. *terma,* a limit]. Providing several sets of terminals, making possible the use of several electrodes.

multivalent (mul-tĭ-vā'lent) [" + *valēre,* to have power]. Having ability to combine with more than two atoms of a univalent element or radical.

mummification (mum"mĭ-fĭ-kā'shun) [Arabian *mūmiyaa,* mummy, + L. *facere,* to make]. 1. Mortification producing a hard, dry mass. SYN: *dry gangrene.* 2. Drying and shriveling of a body, as a dead fetus.

mumps (mŭmps) [Dutch *mompen,* to mumble]. An acute, contagious, febrile disease characterized by inflammation of the parotid glands and other salivary glands.

ETIOL: Mumps virus.

SYM: Onset gradual. There may be chilliness, malaise, headache, pain below ears, moderate fever (101-102° F.), sometimes higher, followed by swelling of one or both parotid glands. Usually swelling in one gland is subsiding as other swells. Swelling is below and in front of the ear.

The lobe of the ear is sometimes pushed forward, surrounding tissues are edematous, the features may be greatly distorted. Movements of the jaw are painful and restricted. Saliva may be increased or diminished. In a third of cases only one parotid is involved. Occasionally, the parotid glands seem to escape, and swelling is confined to the submaxillary gland. Swelling usually lasts from 5 to 7 days.

COMPLICATIONS: When complications set in, they usually develop about the time the swelling in the parotids subsides. The most common complication in the adult male is orchitis; in the female oöphoritis and mastitis. Rarely permanent impairment of hearing follows an attack of mumps.

DIFFERENTIAL DIAGNOSIS: Cases of symptomatic parotitis must be excluded. Instances of trauma, infections about teeth and mouth, or a blocking of Stensen's duct may be suggestive of mumps.

PROG: Favorable, although the possibility of sterility may have to be considered in extremely rare instances of bilateral orchitis.

TREATMENT: Rest in bed, liquid diet; promote elimination; cold, local applications may control swelling of testicles. SYN: *Infectious parotitis.*

mump'simus. Blind and irrational adherence to a custom or practice even though to do so has been proven to be inadvisable or even dangerous to the patient.

mural (mū'ral) [L. *murus,* a wall]. Pert. to a wall of an organ or part.

muriate (mūr'ĭ-āt) [L. *muria,* brine]. An old synonym for any chloride.

muriat'ic acid [L. *muria,* brine]. Commercial hydrochloric acid, *q.v.*

mur'mur [L. *murmur*]. A soft blowing or rasping sound heard on auscultation. An adventitious sound heard on auscultation of the heart. It results from vibrations produced by movement of the blood within the heart and adjacent large blood vessels. May be heard during systole or diastole or both.

Two of the valves give forth a "lubb" sound and the other two a "dupp" sound, known as the first and second heart sounds. A blowing sound is heard if the valve does not close tightly, indicating an incompetent valve. The flow of blood through a narrowed orifice, as in aortic or mitral stenosis, or a great vessel irregularity, such as an aortic aneurysm, may produce a murmur.

A slight sound given off first does not necessarily indicate an organic trouble, and heart disease may not result in any murmur; this may also be true in angina pectoris and coronary disorders. Air in the lungs may simulate sounds similar to heart murmurs.

RS: *auscultation, circulation of blood, heart, hum, venous.*

m., aneurysmal. Whizzing systolic sound heard over an aneurysm.

m., aortic obstructive. Harsh systolic one heard with and after the 1st heart sound. Loudest at the base.

m., a. regurgitant. Blowing, hissing following 2nd heart sound.

m., apex. Inorganic m. over apex of heart.

m., arterial. Soft flowing one, synchronous with pulse.

m., bronchial. M. heard over large bronchi, resembling respiratory laryngeal m.

m., cardiac pulmonary. M. caused by movement of heart against lungs.

m., diastolic. M. during dilation of heart.

m., direct. M. caused by obstruction of blood in normal course.

m., endocardial. M. produced within the heart cavities.

m., exocardial. A cardiac murmur produced outside the cavities of the heart.

m., friction. M. caused by rubbing of two inflamed mucous surfaces.

m., functional. M. occurring in the absence of any pathologic change in structure of heart valves or orifices. They do not indicate organic disease of the heart. They may disappear upon a return to health. They must not be mistaken for true pathological murmurs.

m., hemic. Sound heard on auscultation of anemic persons without a valvular lesion. ETIOL: Abnormal, usually anemic, blood condition.

m., indirect. M. heard when blood flows in abnormal directions.

m., inorganic. M. not due to structural changes.

m., machinery. A continuous rough murmur heard in cases of a patent ductus arteriosus.

m., mitral. M. produced at orifice of mitral or bicuspid valve.

m., organic. M. due to structural changes.

m., pericardial. M. produced within the pericardium.

m., physiologic. A functional murmur, *q.v.*

m., presystolic. M. occurring just before systole.

m., pulmonary. M. produced at the orifice of the pulmonary artery.

m., regurgitant. M. due to backward flow of blood current.

m., systolic. M. heard during contraction of heart, due to obstruction.

m., to-and-fro. M. heard during both systole and diastole.

m., tricuspid. M. produced at orifice of tricuspid valve.

m., vascular. M. occurring within a blood vessel.

m., vesicular. One heard in normal breathing.

Murphy's button. Mechanical device used to connect visceral ends of a divided intestine in anastomosis.

M.'s drip or ***treatment.*** Continuous slow passage of normal saline solution into the rectum; usually used in treating peritonitis.

Mus. A genus of rodents including mice and rats.

M. musculus. The common house mouse.

Musca. A genus of flies belonging to the order Diptera, family Muscidae.

M. domestica. The common house fly, the transmitting agent for causative organisms of typhoid fever, bacillary and amebic dysentery, cholera, trachoma, and many other diseases.

muscae volitantes (mus'sē vol-ĭ-tan'tēz) [L. flitting flies]. Black specks seen floating in the vitreous humor of the eye and visible to the patient; often seen in myopia.

muscle (mus'el) [L. *musculus*]. A type of tissue composed of contractile cells or fibers which effects movement of an organ or part of the body.

The outstanding characteristic of muscular tissue is its ability to shorten or *contract.* It also possesses the properties of *irritability, conductivity,* and *elasticity.* Muscle tissue possesses little intercellular material, hence its cells or fibers lie close together. Three types of muscle differentiated on basis of histologic structure occur in the body, namely, *smooth, striated,* and *cardiac.*

Smooth, Nonstriated, Plain: Cells are fusiform or spindle-shaped, each containing a central nucleus. Cells usually arranged in sheets or layers but may occur as isolated units in connective tissue. Called *involuntary* because they are not under conscious control. Found principally in the internal organs, esp. digestive tract, respiratory passages, urinary and genital ducts, urinary bladder and gallbladder, and walls of blood vessels. Smooth muscle lacks the cross striations characteristic of other types of muscle.

Striated, Striped, Skeletal: The cytoplasm (sarcoplasm) contains numerous *myofibrillae.* The cytoplasmic cell membrane is called the *sarcolemma.* Muscle fibers are grouped into bundles called *fasciculi,* each of which is surrounded by a sheath of connective tissue called *perimysium.* The fibers within a fasciculus are surrounded by and held together by delicate reticular fibrils forming the *endomysium.* Striated muscle is found in all skeletal muscles. It also occurs in the tongue, pharynx, and upper portion of esophagus.

Cardiac: Fibers branch and anastomose, forming a continuous network or syncytium. At intervals, prominent bands or *intercalated disks* cross the fibers. Certain fibers, called *Purkinje fibers,* form the *impulse-conducting system* of the heart.

Tabular Comparison of the Properties of Three Types of Muscle

	Smooth	Cardiac	Striped
Synonyms	Involuntary Visceral Plain	Myocardium	Voluntary Skeletal Striated
Fibers:			
Length in micra	50-200		25,000.
Thickness	4-8		75.
Shape	Spindles		Cylinders
Marking	No striation	Striation	Marked striation
Nuclei	Single	Single	Multiple
Speed of contraction	Very slow	Moderate	Very quick
Effects of cutting related nerve	Slight	Slight	Complete paralysis

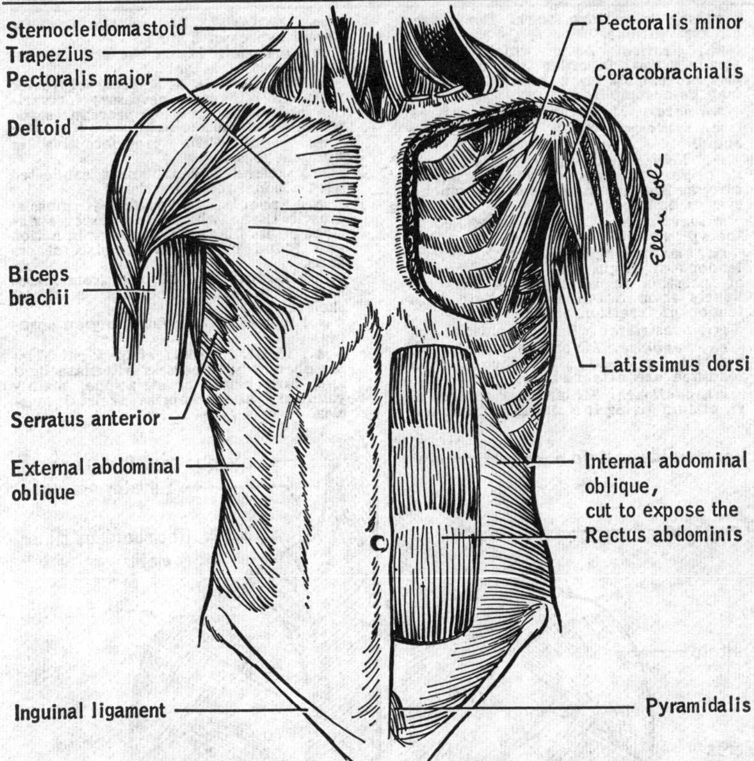

MUSCLES OF THE ANTERIOR CHEST AND ABDOMINAL WALL.

SHAPE: A contractile organ consisting of muscle tissue which effects movements of parts of the body, esp. a structure composed of striated muscle and attached to a part of the skeleton. A typical muscle consists of a central fleshy portion or *belly* and its attachments. One end called the *head* is attached to a fixed structure termed the *origin;* the other end is attached to a movable part called the *insertion.* Some muscles are spindle-shaped, others form flat sheets or bands.

Muscles may be attached directly to the periosteum of bones or they may be attached by means of tough cords of connective tissue (*tendons*) or broad flat sheets (*aponeuroses*). The connective tissue enclosing a muscle is called *epimysium;* it is continuous with the deep *fascia.*

BLOOD SUPPLY: Obtained from small blood vessels which enter the muscular tissue and subdivide into capillaries which permeate throughout.

NERVE SUPPLY: *Voluntary*: From branches of the peripheral cerebrospinal nervous system. It is because of this that the skeletal muscles are under conscious control. *Involuntary*: Smooth and cardiac receive their nerve supply from autonomic nervous system and function involuntarily without conscious control.

FUNCTION: To bring about changes in position.

m., abductor. M. which draws away from the midline.

m., adductor. M. which draws toward the midline.

m., antagonistic. M. which counteracts the action of another muscle. SYN: *Agonistic m.*

m.'s, antigravity. M.'s which pull against the force of gravity to maintain posture.

m., appendicular. One of the skeletal muscles of the limbs.

m., articular. M. attached to capsule of a joint.

m., axial. A skeletal m. of the head or trunk.

m., bipennate. M. in which the fibers converge toward a central tendon on both sides.

m., constrictor, of pharynx. A m. which constricts the pharynx.

m. curve. A tracing of muscular contraction.

m., digastric. M. which lowers the jaw.

m., extensor. M. which straightens a part.

m., extrinsic. M. whose origin lies outside the part moved.

m. fatigue. The reduced capacity of

a muscle to perform work. For causes of, SEE: *fatigue*.

m., fixation. A m. which acts to steady a part in order that more precise movements in a related structure may be accomplished.

m., flexor. M. which bends a part.

m., fusiform. A m. resembling a spindle.

m., intrinsic. A m. which has both its origin and insertion within a structure, as intrinsic muscles of the tongue, eye, or limb.

m., involuntary. M. not controlled by the will; mainly smooth.

m., multipennate. M. with several tendons of origin and several tendons of insertion in which fibers pass obliquely from a tendon of origin to a tendon of insertion on each side.

m., nonstriated. Smooth muscle, *q.v.*

m., papillary. M. on inner surface of ventricle of heart to which chorda tendinae are attached.

m., pectinate. M. on inner surface of rt. atrium giving it a ridged appearance.

m., postaxial. M. on the post. or dorsal aspect of a limb.

m., preaxial. M. on the ant. or ventral aspect of a limb.

m. relaxant. A drug used to provide muscular relaxation necessary for various medical and surgical procedures and for relief of muscle pain.

m. sense. The proprioceptive or kinesthetic sense.

m., skeletal. M. which is connected with a bone; mainly striated.

m., smooth. Nonstriated muscle; muscle tissue which lacks cross striations on its fibers; involuntary in action and found principally in visceral organs.

m., somatic. M. derived from mesodermal somites. Includes most of skeletal m.

m., sphincter. M. controlling an opening.

m., striated. SYN: *striped m.* Muscle fibers which possess alternate light and dark bands or striations; mainly voluntary and comprise skeletal muscles.

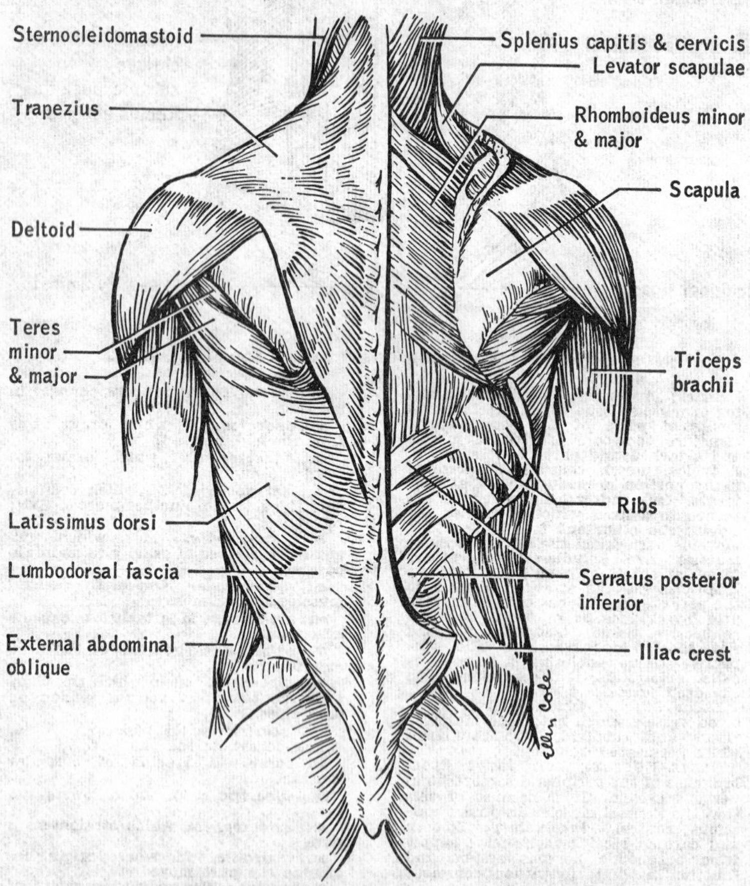

MUSCLES OF THE POSTERIOR NECK, SHOULDER AND BACK.

m.'s, synergistic. M.'s aiding one another in function.

m., unipennate. M. whose fibers converge on only one side of a tendon.

m., unstriated, m., unstriped. SYN: *smooth muscle.* M. without markings; mainly involuntary.

m., voluntary. M. whose action is controlled by will; excepting the cardiac m., all striated m.'s are voluntary.

muscle-bound. Condition in which muscles are less elastic and bulkier than normal. A result of overuse, often from athletics.

mus'cular [L. *musculus,* muscle]. 1. Pert. to muscles. 2. Possessing well developed muscles.

m. contractions, graduated. Accomplished by use of electrical current of varying strength and duration. Used (a) in muscles with an intact nerve supply when muscles are atonic, wasted away, or when voluntary exercise is not feasible, and (b) in denervated muscles as in cases following nerve injury or poliomyelitis.

m. dystrophy. Wasting away and atrophy of muscles. SEE: *dystrophy, progressive muscular.*

m. rheumatism. That affecting white fibrous tissue of the body. SYN: *fibrositis.*

muscularis (mŭs-kū-la'rĭs) [L. muscular]. Muscular layer of an organ or tubule.

m. mucosae. Unstriated muscular tissue layer of mucous membrane.

muscularity. State or quality of being muscular.

mus'culature [L. *musculus,* muscle]. The arrangement of muscles in the body or its parts.

mus'culin [L. *musculus,* muscle]. A globulin in muscle.

musculo- [L.]. Combining form *pert. to a muscle.*

musculoaponeurotic (mŭs-kū-lō-ăp"ō-nū-rŏt'ĭk). Composed of muscle and an aponeurosis of fibrous connective tissue.

musculocutaneous (mŭs"kū-lō-kū-tān'ē-ŭs) [L. *musculus,* muscle, + *cutis,* skin]. 1. Pert. to the muscles and skin. 2. Supplying or affecting the muscles and skin.

musculofascial. Composed of muscle and fascia.

musculomembranous (mŭs"kū-lō-mĕm'-brān-ŭs) [" + *membrana,* membrane]. Pert. to or consisting of muscle and membrane.

mus"culophren'ic. Pertaining to muscles of the diaphragm.

mus"culoten'dinous. Composed of both muscle and tendon.

mus'culus (pl. *musculī*) [L.]. Muscle, *q.v.*

mush'room [Fr. *moucheron,* from L. *muscus,* moss]. Umbrella-shaped fungus belonging to the Basidiomycetes which grows on decaying vegetable matter; common in woods and damp places. The poisonous varieties are commonly called *toadstools, q.v.*

COMP: Low in carbohydrates and fats; high in protein but of little alimentary value. Xanthic bodies and toxic elements are present. Their relationship and similarity to poisonous fungi are so close that only those who are thoroughly capable of distinguishing the poisonous varieties from the edible ones should attempt to gather them.

CANNED (*solids and liquids*): 1 cup 244 gm.). Calories: 30. Other main values: 3 gm. protein; trace of fat; 9 gm. carbohydrate; 17 mg. calcium.

m. and toadstool poisoning. Poisoning resulting from ingestion of mushrooms, such as *Amanita muscaria* which contains muscarine or other species which contain phalloidine, a component of the amanita toxin. SEES *Muscaria mushrooms in Table of Poisons and Poisoning in Appendix.*

musicogenic (mū"zĭ-ko-jen'ik). Caused by music, esp. epileptic convulsions.

mu"sicoma'nia [G. *mousikē,* music, + *mania,* madness]. Insane love of music.

mu"sicother'apy [" + *therapeia,* treatment]. Treatment of mental diseases with music.

musk (mŭsk) [G. *moskos,* from Sanskrit *muska,* testicle]. Substance obtained from musk bag of male musk deer.

musk'melon [" + G. *mēlon,* apple]. Av. SERVING: 200 Gm. Pro. 1.2, Fat 0.2, Carbo. 11.8. VITAMINS: A++, B++, C++ to +++. ASH: Ca 0.017, Mg 0.012, K 0.235, Na 0.061, P 0.015, Cl 0.041, S 0.014, Fe 0.0003. SEE: *cantaloupe, melon.*

mus'sel [L. *musculus,* little mouse]. A fresh-water bivalve mollusc belonging to the class *Pelecypoda.*

m. poisoning. Poisoning common on the Pacific coast resulting from eating mussels or clams which have ingested a poisonous dinoflagellate. Occurs from June to October. The poison is not destroyed by cooking.

mussitation (mŭs-sĭ-tā'shŭn) [L. *mussitāre,* to mutter]. The muttering of delirium or the moving of the lips without sound.

mus'tard [Fr. *moustarde*]. Yellow powder of mustard seed used as a counterirritant, rubefacient, emetic and stimulant. SEE: *plaster.*

As a condiment: Av. SERVING (prepared): 10 Gm. Pro. 0.4, Fat 0.3, Carbo. 0.7. ASH: Ca 0.402, Mg 0.260, K 0.761, Na 0.056, P 0.755, Cl 0.016, S 1.230. No iron. SEE: *condiments.*

m. gas. Dichloro-diethylsulfide, a vesicant war gas.

m. greens. Av. SERVING: 50 Gm. Pro. 1.2, Fat 0.2, Carbo. 2.00. VITAMINS: A+++, B+, riboflavin.

mutant (mū'tănt) [L. *mutāre,* to change]. In heredity, a sport or variation which breeds true.

mutase (mū'tās) [" + *ase,* enzyme]. 1. Enzyme which accelerates oxidation reduction reactions through activation of oxygen and hydrogen. 2. A food preparation made from leguminous plants high in protein content.

mutation (mū-tā'shŭn) [L. *mutāre,* to change]. 1. Change; transformation; instance of such change. 2. Sudden, permanent variation with offspring differing from parents in a marked characteristic as differentiated from gradual variation through many generations. Also person showing such change. 3. A change in a gene potentially capable of being transmitted to offspring.

m., induced. M. resulting from experimental treatment with x-rays, radioactive substances, etc.

m., natural. M. occurring in nature, thought to be a primary factor in evolutionary change.

m., somatic. M. occurring in somatic cells.

mute (mūt) [L. *mutus,* dumb]. 1. One who is unable to speak. 2. Dumb; without ability to speak.

m., deaf. Individual who is unable to hear or to speak.

mu'tilate. To deprive of a limb or a part; to maim or disfigure.

mutism (mū'tizm) [L.]. 1. Condition of being unable to speak. 2. PSY: Persistent inhibition to speech; seen in *dementia praecox.*

mutualism (mu'tu-al-izm) [L. *mutuus,* exchanged]. A form of symbiosis in which organisms of two different species live in close association to the mutual benefit of each.

myalgia (mī-al'jĭ-ă) [G. *mys, my-,* muscle, + *algos,* pain]. Tenderness or pain in the muscles; muscular rheumatism.

myasis (mī-ā'sĭs) [G. *myia,* a fly]. Condition which arises from larvae of flies or maggots in the body or upon mucous membranes. Syn: *myiasis.*

myasthenia (mī-ăs-thē'nĭ-ă) [G. *mys, my-,* muscle, + *astheneia,* weakness]. Muscular weakness.

m., angiosclerotic. Vascular changes producing excessive muscular fatigue.

m. gastrica. Loss of muscular tone in coats of the stomach.

m. gravis. A disease characterized by great muscular weakness (without atrophy) and progressive fatigability. It is due to a functional abnormality, lack of acetylcholine, or excess of cholinesterase at the myoneural junction in which nerve impulses fail to induce normal muscle contractions.

Etiol: Unknown. More common in females. Occurs most frequently between ages of 20 and 50.

Sym: Abnormal fatigability and weakness of muscles. Muscles of the face and neck primarily involved, those of the trunk and extremities secondarily. Onset gradual; symptoms worse in the evening. Patient complains of difficulty in chewing, swallowing, and talking. Expressionless facies and ptosis usually present.

Prog: Some cases mild; other rapidly fatal, death resulting from respiratory failure. Course is variable. Prolonged remissions may occur.

Treatment: Restricted activity; complete rest in severe cases. Soft or liquid diet; tube feedings sometimes essential. Physostigmine and neostigmine given I.M. or orally are effective. Potassium chloride, ephedrine, and guanidine are also used as adjuvants of neostigmine, the drug of choice.

myasthe'nic [" + *astheneia,* weakness]. Marked by muscular weakness.

myatonia (mī-ă-tō'nĭ-ă) [" + *tonos,* tone]. Deficiency or loss of muscular tone.

m. congenita. M. of early childhood; it is not hereditary. Syn: *amyotonia congenita.*

myatrophy (mī-at'rō-fĭ) [" + *atrophia,* atrophy]. Muscular wasting away.

myc-, myco-. Combining form meaning *fungus.*

mycelioid (my-se'lĭ-oid) [G. *mys, my-* muscle, + *atrophia,* atrophy, + *eidos,* form]. Moldlike; resembling mold colonies in which filaments radiate from a center, said of bacterial colonies.

mycelium (mī-se'lĭ-ŭm) [G. *mykēs,* fungus, + *ēlos,* nail]. The mass of filaments (hyphae) which constitutes the vegetative body of fungi such as molds.

myce'tes. The fungi.

mycethemia (mī-se-thē'mĭ-ă) [" + *aima,* blood]. Fungi in the blood. Syn: *mycohemia.*

mycet'in. An antibiotic derived from *Streptomyces violaceus;* effective against gram-positive bacteria.

mycetism, mycetismus (mī'se-tĭzm, -tiz'mŭs) [" + *ismos,* condition]. Poisoning from eating mushrooms.

mycetogenetic, mycetogenic, mycetogenous (mī-sē"tō-jĕn-ĕt'ĭk, -jĕn'ĭk, -toj'ĕn-ŭs) [G. *mykēs,* fungus, + *gennan,* to produce]. Induced by fungi.

mycetoma (mī-se-tō'mă) [" + *ōma,* tumor]. A disease induced by fungi, seen in India, which attacks the foot. Syn: *Madura foot.*

Mycobacte'rium [G. *mykēs,* fungus, + *baktērion,* little rod]. A genus of acid-fast bacteria belonging to the Mycobacteriaceae which includes the causative organisms of tuberculosis and leprosy. They are slender nonmotile rods, gram-positive and do not produce spores or capsules.

M. leprae. Causative agent of leprosy.

M. tuberculosis. Causative agent of tuberculosis in mammals.

my"cocid'in. An antibiotic derived from molds of the family Aspergillaceae.

mycoder'ma [G. *mykēs,* mucus, + *derma,* skin]. Mucous membrane.

mycoid (mī'koyd) [G. *mykēs,* fungus, + *eidos,* form]. Funguslike.

mycology (mī-kol'ō-jĭ) [" + *logos,* study]. Science of fungi.

mycomyringitis (mī"kō-mī-rin-jī'tĭs) [" + *myrigx,* membrane, + *-itis,* inflammation]. Fungus inflammation of membrana tympani.

mycophthalmia (mī-kŏf-thăl'mĭ-ă). Ophthalmia resulting from fungus infection.

Mycoplasma (mī"ko-plaz'mă). Type genus of the family *Mycoplasmataceae.* Usually parasitic in man. Includes the pleuropneumonia-like organisms (PPLO).

mycosis (mī-kō'sĭs) [" + *-ōsis,* intensive]. Any disease induced by a fungus.

m. fungoides. A rare malignant disease that affects the superficial and deep layers of the skin, and occasionally the mucous membrane.

Sym: Urticarial, erythematous or eczematous patches of irregular shape and size, with well-defined margins usually upon scalp and skin of trunk. Itching intense, and frequently the patches become hypertrophic and firm. Hard nodules varying from size of pea to apple, either sessile or pedunculated, develop on them. These eventually break down and form ulcers that contain sensitive, fungating granulation tissue, and discharge thin pus and serum. Death results from progressive cachexia.

Treatment: General supportive measures. X-ray may be used.

m., superficial. A dermatomycosis; a fungus infection of the skin or its appendages. Includes erythrasma; tinea barbae, t. capitis, t. corporis, t. cruris, t. favosa, t. pedis, t. unguium; trichomycosis axillaris.

m., systemic. A deep myocosis; a fungus infection involving various bodily systems or regions. Includes aspergillosis, blastomycosis, chromoblastomycosis, coccidioidomycosis, conidiosporosis, cryptococcosis, geotrichosis, histoplasmosis, maduromycosis, moniliasis, mucormycosis, nocardiosis, para-actinomycosis, penicilliosis, rhinosporidiosis, sporotrichosis.

mycotic (mī-kŏt'ĭk) [G. *mykēs,* fungus]. Caused by or affected with microorganisms.

mycterophonia (mĭk"ter-ō-fō'nĭ-ă). Phonation in which the voice possesses a nasal quality.

mydaleine (mĭd-ā'le-ēn) [G. *mydaleos,* putrid]. A poisonous ptomaine from putrefied visceral organs, acting mainly on the heart.

mydriasis (mid-rī'ăs-ĭs) [G. *mydriasis*]. Abnormal dilation of the pupil.

Etiol: Fright, sudden emotion, anemia, 1st and 3rd stages of anesthesia, drugs, coma, hysteria, botulism, irritation of cervical sympathetic nerve.

m., alternating. M. which affects one eye, then the other. Also called *leaping, springing,* or *bounding m.*

m., paralytic. M. resulting from paralysis of oculomotor nerve.

m., spastic. M. resulting from overactivity of dilator muscle of iris or of sympathetic nerves supplying that muscle. Also called *spasmodic m.*

m., spinal. M. resulting from a lesion of, or irritation of, ciliospinal center of spinal cord.

mydriatic (mid-rī-at'ĭk) [G. *midriasis.* dilatation]. 1. Causing pupillary dilatation. 2. Any drug which dilates the pupil.

Ex: *atropine, cocaine, ephedrine, euphthalmine, homatropine.*

myectomy (mī-ĕk'tō-mĭ). Excision of a portion of a muscle.

myectopia (mī-ĕk-tō'pĭ-ă) [G. *mys, my-,* muscle, + *ek,* out, + *topos,* place]. Muscle dislocation.

myelalgia (mī-el-al'jĭ-ă) [G. *myelos,* marrow, + *algos,* pain]. Pain of the spinal cord or its membranes.

myelanalosis (mī"el-ă-nal-ō'sĭs) [" + *analōsis,* wasting]. Gradual wasting of spinal cord. Syn: *tabes dorsalis.*

myelapoplexy (mī-el-ap'ō-plĕks-ĭ) [" + *apoplēxia,* stroke]. Hemorrhagic effusion into the spinal cord.

myelasthenia (mī-ĕl-ăs-thē'nĭ-ă) [G. *myelos,* marrow, + *astheneia,* weakness]. Spinal exhaustion; neurasthenia arising from spinal causes.

myelatelia (mī-ĕl-ă-tē'lĭ-ă) [" + *ateleia,* imperfection]. Defective development of spinal cord.

myelatrophy (mī-el-at'rof-ĭ) [" + *atrophia,* atrophy]. Wasting of the spinal cord.

myelauxe (mī-ĕl-awks'ē) [" + *auxē,* increase]. Abnormal enlargement of spinal cord.

myelemia (mī-ĕl-ē'mĭ-ă) [" + *aima,* blood]. Abnormal number of marrow cells in the blood. Syn: *myelocytosis.*

myelencephalon (mī"ĕl-ĕn-sĕf'ă-lŏn) [G. *myelos,* marrow, + *egkephalos,* brain]. The most post. portion of the embryonic hindbrain (rhombencephalon) which gives rise to the medulla oblongata.

myel'ic. Pert. to the spinal cord.

my'elin [G. *myelos,* marrow]. 1. A fatlike substance forming the principal component of the myelin sheath of nerve fibers. Composed of cholesterol, certain cerebrosides, phospholipins, and fatty acids. 2. A complex lipoid substance present in the brain in small quantities.

myelination (mī-ĕl-ĭn-ā'shŭn) [G. *myelos,* marrow]. Process of acquiring a myelin sheath. Syn: *myelinization.*

myelinic (mī-ĕl-ĭn'ĭk) [G. *myelos,* marrow]. Concerning or composed of myelin.

myelinization (mī"ĕl-ĭn-ĭ-zā'shŭn) [G. *myelos,* marrow]. Acquirement of myelin sheath for nerve fibers. Syn: *myelination.*

myelinogenetic (mī"ĕl-ĭn-ō-jĕn-et'ĭk) [" + *gennan,* to produce]. Producing myelin or a myelin sheath.

myelinosis (mī"ĕl-ĭn-ō'sĭs) [" + *-ōsis,* intensive]. Fatty degeneration during which myelin is produced.

myelitic (mī-el-it'ĭk) [G. *myelos,* marrow]. Concerning myelitis.

myelitis (mi-el-i'tis) [" + *-itis,* inflammation]. 1. Inflammation of the spinal cord. 2. Inflammation of bone marrow.

Sym: Moderate fever (101°-103° F.), loss of appetite, coated tongue and constipation, followed by pain in back radiating into the limbs. Various forms of paresthesia, as numbness, tingling, burning, etc. Frequently a sense of painful constriction, "girdle pain" at level of the disease. Paralysis soon develops, and may become more or less complete; at first may be retention, later frequently incontinence of feces, anesthesia, more or less complete. Bedsores soon develop. Death may result in few days from extension upward, and involvement of respiratory muscles. In rare cases a spontaneous arrest of inflammation and slow recovery follows, attended with partial paralysis.

See: *axophage, osteomyelitis, poliomyelitis.*

m., acute. Simple acute form which develops following injury.

m., acute ascending. M. which moves progressively upward in the spinal cord.

m., bulbar. M. involving the medulla.

m., central. M. in which the gray matter is esp. involved.

m., c., acute. Resembles acute transverse m., but the trophic disturbances are more marked and duration shorter. Usually fatal in 1 to 2 weeks.

Prog: Always extremely grave.

Treatment: If possible place patient on water bed. Continuous closed drainage of bladder is preferable to intermittent catheterization. In incontinence of urine and feces the discharges should be received on cotton or wool, which should be frequently renewed and parts thoroughly cleansed. In the beginning ice bags or wet cups may be applied to the spine. Frequent baths should be given. Milk, eggs, rice, toast, farina, fruit and blanc mange may be given in early stages of disease. Later, more nutritious diet.

m., chronic. Form progressing slowly but steadily.

Sym: Begin with numbness, tingling or burning in lower extremities, followed by loss of power and sensation. Reflexes generally exaggerated. Sphincters soon become involved. Girdle pain at level of disease. Progress slow, 6 months to 10 years.

Treatment: Patient should be put at rest. Frequent tepid baths; plenty of sleep; good, nourishing food; moderate exercise that stops short of fatigue. Freedom from mental worry. Constitutional treatment, antisyphilitics where indicated.

m., compression. M. caused by pressure on the cord, as by a hemorrhage.

m., cornual. M. affecting the spinal cord's horns of gray matter.

m., descending. M. affecting successively lower areas of the spinal cord.

m., diffuse. M. involving large sections of the cord.

m., disseminated. M. with several separated foci on the cord.

m., hemorrhagic. M. with hemorrhage.

m., parenchymatous. M. of nerve substance.

m., sclerosing. M. with hardening of cord, and interstitial tissue growth.

m., systemic. M. affecting only certain tracts of the cord.

m., transverse. M. involving the whole thickness of the cord.

m., t., acute. Acute form of m. involving entire thickness of cord, developing subsequent injury to spinal cord.

m., traumatic. M. due to cord injury.

myelo- [G.]. Prefix denoting *the spinal cord,* or *bone marrow.*

myeloblast (mī'el-ō-blăst) [G. *myelos,* marrow, + *blastos,* germ]. Bone marrow cell which develops into a myelocyte.

myeloblastemia (mī"ĕl-ō-blăst-ē'mī-ă) [" + " + *aima,* blood]. Occurrence of myeloblasts in the blood.

myeloblastoma (mī"ĕl-ō-blăst-ō'mă) [" + " + *-ōma,* tumor]. 1. Tumor containing myeloblasts. 2. Myelogenic form of leukemia.

myeloblastosis (mī'ĕ-lō-blăs-tō'sĭs). Excess production of myeloblasts and their presence in circulating blood; myeloblastic leukemia.

myelocele (mī'ĕl-ō-sēl) [" + *kēlē,* hernia]. 1. A form of spina bifida with spinal cord protrusion. 2. [" + *koilos,* hollow]. Central canal of spinal cord.

myelocyst (mī'ĕl-ō-sĭst) [G. *myelon,* marrow, + *kystis,* bladder]. Cyst arising from the spinal cord.

myelocystocele (mī"ĕl-ō-sĭst'ō-sēl) [" + " + *kēlē,* hernia]. Cystic tumor of spinal cord.

myelocystomeningocele (mī"ĕl-ō-sĭst"ō-men-ĭn'gō-sēl) [" + " + *mēnigx,* membrane, + *kēlē,* hernia]. Combined myelocystocele and meningocele.

myelocyte (mī'el-ō-sīt) [G. *myelos,* marrow, + *kytos,* cell]. A large cell in red bone marrow, from which leukocytes are derived.

myelocythemia (mī"ĕl-ō-sī-thē'mī-ă) [" + " + *aima,* blood]. Presence of an excess number of myelocytes in the blood. SYN: *myelocytosis.*

myelocytic (mī"ĕl-ō-sĭt'ĭk) [" + *kytos,* cell]. Characterized by presence of, or pert. to, myelocytes.

myelocytoma (mī"ĕl-ō-sīt-ō'mă) [" + " + *-ōma,* tumor]. Leukemia with leukocytes arising from both myeloid and lymphoid substance. SYN: *chronic myelogenous leukemia.*

myelocytosis (mī"ĕl-ō-sī-tō'sĭs) [" + " + *-ōsis,* intensive]. Myelocytes in large quantities in the blood. SYN: *myelocythemia.*

myelodiastasis (mī"ĕl-ō-dī-as'tă-sĭs) [G. *myelos,* marrow, + *diastasis,* separation]. Destruction and disintegration of spinal cord.

myelodysplasia (mī"ĕl-ō-dĭs-plā'zĭ-ă) [" + *dys,* bad, + *plassein,* to form]. Defective formation of the spinal cord.

myeloencephalic (mī"ĕl-ō-ĕn-sĕf-al'ĭk) [" + *egkephalos,* brain]. Concerning the spinal cord and brain.

myeloencephalitis (mī"ĕl-ō-ĕn-sĕf-ă-lī'tĭs) [" + " + *-ītis,* inflammation]. Inflamed condition of spinal cord and brain.

myelofibrosis (mi"ĕ-lo-fi-bro'sĭs). Replacement of bone marrow by fibrous tissue.

myelogenesis (mī"ĕl-ō-jen'ĕ-sĭs) [" + *genesis,* development]. 1. The development of brain and spinal cord. 2. Development of myelin.

myelogenic, myelogenous (mī-ĕ-lō-jen'ĭk, -loj'ĕn-ŭs) [" + *gennan,* to produce]. Producing or originating in marrow.

myelography (mī-ĕl-og'ră-fĭ) [" + *graphein,* to write]. Roentgenographic inspection of the spinal cord by use of a radiopaque medium injected into the intrathecal space.

m., air. M. in which oxygen or air is used instead of radiopaque dye.

myeloid (mī'el-oid) [" + *eidos,* form]. 1. Medullary; like marrow. 2. Resembling a myelocyte, but not necessarily originating from bone marrow.

myeloidosis (mī"ĕl-oid-ō'sĭs) [" + " + *-ōsis,* intensive]. Formation of myeloid tissue, esp. abnormal tissue formation.

myelolymphangioma (mī"ĕ-lō-lĭm-făn"gĭ-ō-mă). Elephantiasis, *q.v.*

myelolymphocyte (mī"ĕl-ō-lĭmf'ō-sīt) [" + L. *lympha,* lymph, + G. *kytos,* cell]. Tiny lymphocyte formed abnormally in bone marrow.

myeloma (mi-el-o'ma) [G. *myelos,* marrow, + *-oma,* tumor]. A tumor originating in cells of the hematopoietic portion of bone marrow.

m., multiple. A neoplastic disease characterized by the infiltration of bone and bone marrow by myeloma cells forming multiple tumor masses. Usually progressive and generally fatal. Accompanied by anemia, renal lesions, and high globulin levels in blood. Common in 6th decade of life. More frequent in males by ratio of 3:1.

myelomalacia (mī"ĕl-ō-mă-lā'sĭ-ă) [" + *malakia,* softening]. Abnormal softening of spinal cord.

myelomatosis (mī"ĕl-ō-mă-tō'sĭs) [" + *-ōma,* tumor, + *-ōsis*]. Disease marked by multiple tumors of the bone marrow, pernicious anemia, and albumosuria. SYN: *multiple myeloma.*

myelomenia (mī-ĕl-ō-mē'nĭ-ă) [" + *mēn,* month]. Vicarious menstrual discharge in the spinal cord.

myelomeningitis (mī"ĕl-ō-men-ĭn-jī'tĭs) [G. *myelos,* marrow, + *mēnigx, mēnigg-,* membrane, + *-ītis,* inflammation]. Inflamed spinal cord and membranes; spinal meningitis.

myelomeningocele (mī"el-ō-men-ĭn'gō-sēl) [" + " + *kēlē,* hernia]. Spina bifida with portion of cord and membranes protruding

myelomyces (mī-el-ō-mī'sēs) [" + *mykēs,* fungus]. Malignant growth resembling brain substance. SYN: *encephaloma.*

myelon (mī'el-on) [G. *myelos,* marrow]. The spinal cord.

myeloneuritis (mī"ĕl-ō-nū-rī'tĭs) [" + *neuron,* nerve, + *-ītis,* inflammation]. Multiple neuritis and myelitis combined.

myelonic (mī-ĕl-on'ĭk) [G. *myelos,* marrow]. Pert. to the spinal cord.

myeloparalysis (mī"ĕl-ō-pă-ral'ĭ-sĭs) [" + *para,* beside, + *lyein,* to loosen]. Paralysis of the spine.

myelopathy (mī-ĕl-op'ă-thĭ) [" + *pathos,* disease]. Any pathological condition of the spinal cord.

myelopetal (mī-ĕl-op'et-ăl) [" + L. *petere,* to seek for]. Proceeding toward the spinal cord.

myelophage (mī'ĕl-ō-fāj) [" + *phagein,* to eat]. A myelin ingesting macrophage.

myelophthisis (mī-ĕl-ŏf'thĭ-sĭs) [G. *myelos,* marrow, + *phthisis,* a wasting]. SYN: *myelanalosis.* 1. Atrophy of the spinal cord. 2. Replacement of the bone marrow by a disease process such as a neoplasm.

my'eloplast [G. *myelos,* marrow, + *plastos,* formed]. A bone marrow cell similar to a leukocyte.

my'eloplax [" + *plax,* plate]. Large, multinuclear, bone marrow cell.

myeloplaxoma (mī"ĕl-ō-plăks-ō'mă) [G. *myelos,* marrow, + *plax,* plate, + *-ōma,* tumor]. Tumor composed of myeloplaxes.

myeloplegia (mī"ĕl-ō-plē'jĭ-ă) [" + *plēgē,* stroke]. Paralysis of spinal origin.

myelopoiesis (mī"ĕl-ō-poy-ē'sĭs) [" + *poiein,* to form]. The development of marrow or myelocytes.

m., ectopic. Extramedullary m., *q.v.*

m., extramedullary. Development of myeloid elements (erythrocytes and granular leukocytes) in regions other than bone marrow.

my′elopore″. An opening in the spinal cord.

myeloradiculitis (mī″ĕ-lō-rā-dĭk″ū-lī′tĭs). Inflammation of spinal cord and dorsal roots of spinal nerves.

myeloradiculodysplasia (mī″ĕ-lō-rā-dĭk″-ū-lō′dĭs-plā′sĭ-ă). Congenital abnormality of spinal cord and spinal nerve roots.

myelorrhagia (mī-ĕl-ŏr-rā′jĭ-ă) [" + *rēgnunai,* to burst forth]. Hemorrhage into myelon.

myelorrhaphy (mī-ĕl-or′ră-fĭ) [" + *raphē,* a sewing]. Suture of a cut or wound of the spinal cord.

myelosarcoma (mī″ĕl-ō-săr-kō′mă) [" + *sarx,* flesh, + *-ōma,* tumor]. Sarcoma of bone marrow cells and tissue. Syn: *osteosarcoma.*

myelos′chisis. Cleft spinal cord resulting from failure of neural tube to close. See: *spina bifida, rachischisis.*

myelosclerosis (mī″ĕl-ō-sklĕr-ō′sĭs) [G. *myelos,* marrow, + *sklērōsis,* hardening]. Sclerosis of the spinal cord.

myelosis (mī-ĕl-ō′sĭs) [" + *-ōsis,* intensive]. Formation of a myeloma or medullary tumor.

myelospongium (mī″ĕl-ō-spon′jĭ-ŭm) [" + *spoggos,* sponge]. Embryonic network from which the neuroglia arises.

myelotome (mī′ĕl-ō-tōm) [" + *tomē,* incision]. Instrument used to dissect the spinal cord.

myelotomy (mī-ĕl-ot′ō-mĭ) [" + *tomē,* incision]. Surgical severance of nerve fibers of spinal cord.

myelotoxic (mī-ĕl-ō-toks′ĭk) [" + *toxikon,* poison]. 1. Destroying bone marrow. 2. Pert. to or arising from diseased bone marrow.

myelotoxin (mī″ĕl-ō-toks′ĭn) [" + *toxikon,* poison]. Toxin which destroys marrow cells.

myenteric (mī-ĕn-ter′ĭk) [" + *enteron,* intestine]. Concerning the myenteron.

m. reflex. Intestinal contraction above and relaxation below the point of stimulation.

myenteron (mī-en′tĕr-ŏn) [" + *enteron,* intestine]. Muscular layer of the intestine.

myesthesia (mī-ĕs-thē′-zĭ-ă) [G. *mys, my-,* muscle, + *aisthēsis,* sensation]. Muscle sense; consciousness of muscle contraction.

myiasis (mī-ĭ′ă-sĭs) [G *myia,* fly]. Condition resulting from infestation by the larvae (maggots) of flies. Infestation may be (a) *cutaneous* (in the skin), (b) *intestinal,* (c) *atrial* (within a cavity such as mouth, nose, eye, sinuses, vagina, urethra), (d) *wound,* or (e) *external.*

myiodesopsia (mī″i-ō-dĕs-op′sĭ-ă) [G. *myiōdēs,* flylike, + *opsis,* vision]. Condition in which spots are seen before the eyes. See: *muscae volitantes.*

myitis (mī-i′tĭs) [G. *mys, my-,* muscle, + *-itis,* inflammation]. Inflamed condition of a muscle. Syn: *myositis.*

mylodus. A molar tooth.

mylohyoid (mī″lō-hī′oid) [G. *mylē,* mill, + *yoeidēs,* U-shaped]. Pert. to the hyoid bone and the molar teeth.

myo- [G.]. Combining form pert. to *muscle.*

myoalbumin (mī″ō-al-bū′mĭn) [G. *mys, myo-,* muscle, + L. *albumen,* white of egg]. Albumin found in muscular tissue.

myoalbumose (mī-ō-al′bū-mōs) [" + L. *albus,* white]. A protein derived from muscle.

myoarchitectonic (mī″ō-ar″kĭ-tĕk-ton′ĭk) [" + *architektōn,* master workman]. Pert. to or resembling structural arrangement of muscle or of fibers.

myoatrophy (mī-ō-ăt′rō-fĭ) [" + *atrophia,* atrophy]. Muscular wasting.

myoblast (mī′ō-blast) [G. *mys, myo-,* muscle, + *blastos,* germ]. An embryonic cell which develops into muscle fiber cell.

myoblasto′ma. A tumor consisting of cells resembling myoblasts.

myobra′dia [" + *bradus,* slow]. Slow muscular reaction to stimulation.

myocardiac, myocardial (mī-ō-kar′dĭ-ăk, -ăl) [" + *kardia,* heart]. Concerning the myocardium.

m. infarction. Development of an infarct in the myocardium, usually the result of myocardial ischemia following occlusion of a coronary artery.

Sym: Pain similar to that of angina pectoris, shock, cardiac dysfunction, and frequently sudden death.

m. insufficiency. Cardiac failure, *q.v.*

myocardiograph (mī″ō-kar′dĭ-ō-grăf) [G. *mys, myo-,* muscle, + *kardia,* heart, + *graphein,* to write]. Instrument for recording heart movements.

myocardiosis (mī-ō-kăr-dĭ-ō′sĭs) [" + " + *-ōsis,* intensive]. Noninflammatory cardiac disorder. Syn: *myocardia.*

myocarditis (mī-ō-kar-dī′tĭs) [" + " + *-itis,* inflammation]. Inflammation of the cardiac muscular tissue.

Etiol: Associated with a number of conditions including many types of infections, nephritis, carbon monoxide poisoning, heat stroke, and burns. Occurs commonly after rheumatic fever and diphtheria or may be idiopathic.

Physical Signs: Apex beat extremely weak and rapid; pulse irregular and weak; tenderness over precordium, percussion negative, auscultation reveals 1st sound of heart resembling 2nd heart sound, high pitched and wanting in muscular quality.

NP: In acute myocarditis absolute rest is essential. Years may be added to the life of the patient with chronic myocarditis if moderation in all things is observed. Plenty of rest and sleep, light diet, and avoidance of all worry, hurry, and physical strains are very important. High altitudes must be avoided and climbing stairs should be reduced to a minimum, and haste avoided. Proper elimination should be maintained. In some instances graduated exercises may be ordered.

m., acute, primary. Acute interstitial inflammation of the myocardium.

m., a., secondary. Acute inflammation of the heart muscle.

Etiol: Secondary to acute inflammation of pericardium or endocardium, or may occur during some infectious disease.

Sym: Marked by primary disease; great weakness; cardiac palpitation with irregularity; small, feeble pulse, and dyspnea; precordial pain and distress.

m., a., septic. Localized, suppurative inflammation of the heart muscle.

Etiol: Distant infection, suppurating pericardium or endocardium.

m., chronic. Characterized by round cell infiltration of interstitial tissue, followed by parenchymatous changes of muscle fibers.

ETIOL: Nephritis, syphilis, grave anemias, diabetes, rheumatic fever, malaria, toxic substance, or excessive use of alcohol and tobacco. Certain wasting diseases, disease of coronary arteries, joint affections, or extension from endocardium and pericardium.

SYM: Cardiac insufficiency. Rapid heart which does not immediately recover from exercise. On first exertion the heart and blood pressure rise quickly but become slower with prolonged exertion.

PHYSICAL SIGNS: Face appears cyanosed, esp. about the lips and ears; also about the fingertips. Apex beat of heart not displaced unless the heart was previously hypertrophied, in which case apex beat will be displaced downward and to the left, or downward if dilatation exists. Pulse weak, blood pressure either low or high. Auscultation reveals a short, feeble 1st sound, lacking in muscular quality with reduplication of that sound. Second sound, esp. the aortic, is accentuated. Systolic murmur at apex over a small area if dilatation exists.

m., Fiedler's. An idiopathic m. of unknown etiology. Also called "isolated myocarditis" as endocardium or pericardium are not affected.

m., fragmentation. F. of the myocardium.

m., indurative. Chronic m. causing hardening of muscular walls of the heart.

myocardosis (mī″ō-kär-dō′sĭs) [G. *mys, myo-*, muscle, + *kardia*, heart, + *-ōsis*, intensive]. 1. A noninflammatory disorder of the myocardium. 2. Any degenerative condition (except myofibrosis) of the heart muscle.

myocele (mī′ō-sēl) [" + *kēlē*, hernia]. 1. Muscular protrusion through a muscle sheath. 2. Cavity within a somite of an embryo.

myocelialgia (mī″ō-sē-lĭ-al′jĭ-ă) [" + *koilia*, belly, + *algos*, pain]. Abdominal muscle pain.

myocelitis (mī-ō-sē-lī′tĭs) [" + " + *-itis*, inflammation]. Inflamed condition of abdominal muscles.

myocellulitis (mī″ō-sĕl-ū-lī′tĭs) [G. *mys, myo-*, muscle, + L. *cellula*, little chamber, + G. *-itis*, inflammation]. Myositis combined with cellulitis.

myocerosis (mī″ō-sē-ro′sĭs) [" + *kēros*, wax]. Waxy degeneration of a muscle.

myochorditis (mī″ō-kor-dī′tĭs) [" + *chordē*, cord, + *-itis*, inflammation]. Inflammation of the muscles of the larynx.

myochrome (mī′ō-krōm) [" + *chrōma*, color]. Reddish pigment derived from hemoglobin and found in muscle. SYN: *myohematin.*

myochronoscope (mī″ō-krō′nō-skōp) [" + *chronos*, time, + *skopein*, to examine] Device for determining time for producing a muscular contraction.

myoclonia (mī-ō-klo′nĭ-ă) [" + *klonos*, tumult]. Condition of intermittent, clonic spasm or twitching of a muscle or muscles.

myoclonus (mī-ok′lō-nŭs) [G. *mys, myo-*, muscle, + *klonos*, tumult]. Twitching or clonic spasm of a muscle or group of muscles. SYN: *paramyoclonus.*

m. multiplex. Condition marked by persistent and continuous muscular spasms.

myocoele (mi′o-sēl) [" + *koilos*, hollow]. SEE: myocele.

myocolpitis (mī″ō-kol-pī′tĭs) [G. *mys, my-*, muscle, + *kolpos*, vagina, + *-itis*, inflammation]. Inflammation of vaginal muscular tissue.

myocomma (mī-ō-kŏm′mă) [" + *komma*, cut]. SYN: *myotome.* Septum dividing the myotomes.

myocrismus (mī-ō-kris′mŭs) [" + *krizein*, to squeak]. A peculiar crackling sound sometimes heard in auscultation resulting from contraction of a muscle.

myocyte (mī′ō-sīt) [" + *kytos*, cell]. A muscular tissue cell.

myocytoma (mī″ō-sī-tō′mă) [G. *mys, myo-*, muscle, + *kytos*, cell, + *-ōma*, tumor]. Tumor containing muscle cells.

myodemia (mī-ō-de′mĭ-ă) [" + *dēmos*, fat]. Fatty degeneration of muscular tissue.

Muscular fiber cells become filled with fat granules and are ultimately destroyed.

myodesopsia (mī″ō-des-op′sĭ-ă) [G. *myiōdēs*, flylike, + *opsis*, vision]. SYN: *myiodesopsia.*

myodiastasis (mī″ō-di-as′tă-sĭs) [G. *mys, myo-*, muscle, + *diastasis*, separation]. Division or rupture of a muscle.

myodynamia (mī″ō-dī-nam′ĭ-ă) [" + *dynamis*, force]. Muscular force or strength.

myodynamometer (mī″ō-dī-nă-mom′ĕt-ĕr) [" + " + *metron*, measure]. Device for measurement of muscular strength.

myodynia (mī-ō-dĭn′ĭ-ă) [" + *odynē*, pain]. Any muscle pain. SYN: *myalgia.**

myoedema (mī″ō-ĕ-dē′mă) [G. *mys, myo-*, muscle, + *oidēma*, swelling]. 1. Lumping in a wasting muscle when struck. SYN: *mounding.* 2. Muscular edema.

my″oelast′ic. Pert. to muscle and elastic tissue. SEE: *tissue, myoelastic.*

myoelectric (mī″ō-ē-lĕk′trĭk) [" + *ēlektron*, amber]. Pert. to muscular electrical properties.

myoendocarditis (mī″ō-ĕn″dō-kar-dī′tĭs) [" + *endon*, within, + *kardia*, heart, + *-itis*, inflammation]. Inflammation of the cardiac muscular wall and membranous lining.

myoepithelial (mī″ō-ĕp-ĭ-thē′lĭ-ăl) [G. *mys, myo-*, muscle, + *epi*, upon, + *thēlē*, nipple]. Pert. to contractile epithelial cells.

m. cells. Spindle-shaped or branched contractile epithelial cells found between glandular cells and basement membrane of sweat, mammary, and salivary glands.

myofascitis (mī″ō-făs-ī′tĭs) [" + L. *fascia*, band, + G. *-itis*, inflammation]. Inflamed condition of a muscle and its fascia.

myofibril, myofibrilla (mī-ō-fī′brĭl, -fī-brĭl′lă) (pl. *myofibrillae*) [G. *mys, myo-*, muscle, + L. *fibrilla*, a small fiber]. A tiny fibril found in muscular tissue, running parallel to the cellular long axis, from one cell to another.

May be the contractile element.

myofibroma (mī″ō-fī-brō′mă) [" + L. *fibra*, fiber, + G. *-ōma*, tumor]. Tumor containing muscular and fibrous tissue.

myofibrosis (mī″ō-fī-brō′sĭs) [" + " + G. *-ōsis*, intensive]. Increase of connective or fibrous tissue with degeneration of muscular tissue.

myogelosis (mī-ō-jel-ō′sĭs) [" + L. *gelāre*, to congeal]. Hardening of a portion of muscle.

myogen (mī′ō-jĕn) [" + *gennan*, to produce]. A protein found in muscle plasma, which is spontaneously coagulable.

myogenesis (mī-ō-jĕn′ĕ-sĭs) [" + *genesis*,

development]. Formation of muscular tissue.

myogenetic (mī″ō-jĕn-et′ĭk) [G. *mys, myo-*, muscle, + *gennan*, to produce]. Having origin in muscle. SYN: *myogenic.*

myogen′ic, myog′enous [" + *gennan*, to form]. Arising from muscle.

myoglia (mī-og′lĭ-ă) [" + *glia*, glue]. A fibrous network in muscular tissue resembling neuroglia in appearance.

myoglobin. Myohemoglobin, *q.v.*

myoglobulin (mī″ō-glob′ū-lĭn) [" + L. *globulus*, globule]. A coagulable globulin seen in muscular tissue.

my′ogram [" + *gramma*, a marking]. A tracing made by the myograph of muscular contractions.

myograph (mī′ō-grăf) [G. *mys, myo-*, muscle, + *graphein*, to write]. Instrument for tracing movements caused by muscular contractions.

myographic (mī-ō-graf′ĭk) [" + *graphein*, to write]. Pert. to a myograph, or the tracings made by it.

m. tracing. A myogram or muscular tracing.

myography (mī-og′ră-fĭ) [" + *graphein*, to write]. 1. Recording of muscular contractions by a myograph. 2. Description of the muscles and their action.

myohematin (mī″ō-hĕm′-ăt-ĭn) [G. *mys, nyo-*, muscle, + *aima*, blood]. Cytochrome, *q.v.*

myo″hemoglob′in. A respiratory pigment in muscle tissue which serves as an oxygen carrier. ABBR. MHb. Also called *myoglobin, myoglobulin.*

myohysterectomy (mī″ō-hĭs-tĕr-ek′tō-mĭ) [" + *ystera*, uterus, + *ektomē*, excision]. Excision of the body of the uterus, leaving the cervix in place. SYN: *subtotal hysterectomy.*

my′oid [" + *eidos*, resemblance]. Resembling muscle.

myoidema (mī-oi-dē′mă) [" + *oidēma*, swelling]. SYN: *myoedema.*

myoischemia (mī″ō-ĭs-kē′mĭ-ă) [" + *ischein*, to hold back, + *aima*, blood]. Local anemia in a muscle.

myokerosis (mī″ō-kĕ-rō′sĭs) [G. *mys, myo-*, muscle, + *kēros*, wax, + *-ōsis*]. Waxy degeneration of muscle or muscular tissue.

my″okinase′. An enzyme present in muscle which catalyzes the synthesis of adenosinetriphosphate.

myokinesis (mī″ō-kĭn-ē′sĭs) [" + *kinēsis*, motion]. 1. Muscular activity. 2. Surgical displacement of muscular fibers.

myokymia (mī-ō-kĭm′ĭ-ă) [" + *kyma*, wave]. Twitching of fibers of a muscle.

It may be functional and is also seen in organic affections and general paresis.

myolipoma (mī″ō-lĭ-pō′mă) [" + *lipos*, fat, + *-ōma*, tumor]. Muscle tissue tumor containing fatty elements.

myology (mī-ol′o-jĭ) [" + *logos*, study]. The science or study of the muscles and their parts.

myolysis (mī-ol′ĭ-sĭs) [G. *mys, myo-*, muscle, + *lysis*, destruction]. Fatty degeneration and infiltration with destruction of muscular tissue accompanied by separation and disappearance of muscle cells.

myoma (mī-ō′mă) [" + *-ōma*, tumor]. A tumor containing muscle tissue. SEE: *chondromyoma.*

m. lymphangiectodes. M. containing dilated lymphatic vessels.

m., nonstriated. A tumor of unmarked muscle tissue. SYN: *leiomyoma.*

m. striocellulare. Fibroma with striated muscular fibers. SYN: *rhabdomyoma.*

m. telangiectodes. Coiled blood vessel tumor in muscular fibers.

myomalacia (mī″ō-mă-lā′sĭ-ă) [" + *malakia*, softening]. Softening of muscular tissue.

m. cordis. Softening of the heart muscle.

myomatosis (mī-ō-mă-tō′sĭs) [" + *-ōma*, tumor, + *-ōsis*]. The development of myomas.

myomatous (mī-ō′mă-tŭs) [" + *-ōma*, tumor]. Pert. to or resembling a myoma.

myomectomy (mī-ō-mek′tō-mĭ) [" + " + *ektomē*, excision]. 1. Removal of a portion of muscle or muscular tissue. 2. Removal of a myomatous tumor, generally uterine, usually by abdominal section, leaving the uterus in place.

NP: Same as for cesarean section. Position, dorsal, possibly followed by Trendelenburg's.

myomelanosis (mī″ō-mĕl-ă-nō′sĭs) [G. *mys, myo-*, muscle, + *melanosis*, blackening]. Darkening of muscle tissue.

myomere (mī′ō-mēr) [" + *meros*, part]. SYN: *myotome.*

myometer (mī-om′ĕt-ĕr) [" + *metron*, measure]. Device for measurement of muscular contractions.

myometritis (mī″ō-me-trī′tĭs) [" + *mētra*, uterus, + *-itis*, inflammation]. Inflamed condition of the muscular part of the uterus.

myometrium (mī″ō-me′trĭ-ŭm) [" + *mētra*, uterus]. Muscular structure of the uterus.

myomohysterectomy (mī-ō″mō-hĭs-tĕr-ĕk′-tō-mĭ) [G. *mys, myo-*, muscle, + *-ōma*, tumor, + *ystera*, uterus, + *ektomē*, excision]. Hysterectomy performed to remove a myomatous uterus.

myomotomy (mī-ō-mot′ō-mĭ) [" + " + *tomē*, excision]. Excision of a myoma, usually uterine. SYN: *myomectomy.*

my′on [G. *mys, myo-*, muscle]. A muscle.

myonarcosis (mī″ō-năr-kō′sĭs) [" + *narkosis*, a numbing]. Muscular numbness.

myonephropexy (mī″ō-nef′rō-pĕk″sĭ) [" + *nephros*, kidney, + *pēxis*, fixation]. Fixation of a movable kidney by attaching it to a portion of muscular tissue with sutures.

my″oneur′al. Pert. to muscle and nerve.

m. junction. Ending of a nerve in a muscle. SEE: *motor end plate.*

myoneurasthenia (mī″ō-nŭr-ăs-thē′nĭ-ă) [" + " + *astheneia*, weakness]. Neurasthenic muscular relaxation.

myoneuroma (mī″ō-nū-rō′mă) [" + " + *-ōma*, tumor]. A neuroma partially composed of muscular elements.

myonosus (mī-on′o-sŭs) [" + *nosos*, disease]. A disease of muscular tissue. SYN: *myopathy.*

myopachynsis (mī″ō-păk-ĭn′sĭs) [" + *pachynsis*, thickening]. Abnormal thickening of muscle tissue.

myopalmus (mī-o-pal′mŭs) [" + *palmos*, a twitching]. Twitching of muscles.

myoparalysis (mī″ō-pă-ral′ĭ-sĭs) [" + *para*, beside, + *lysis*, loosening]. Paralysis in a muscle.

myo″pare′sis. Paralysis of a muscle.

myopathic (mī-ō-path′ĭk) [" + *pathos*, disease]. 1. Pert. to muscular disease. 2. One suffering from a muscular disease.

m. facies. Facial expression caused by relaxation of facial muscles.

myopathy (mī-op′ă-thĭ) [G. *mys, myo-*, muscle, + *pathos*, disease]. Any disease or abnormal condition of striated muscle.

m., cortisone. Myopathy, especially of the limbs, following high dosage of corticosteroid preparations for an extensive period of time. Recovery takes place upon lowering the dose or discontinuing administration of the drug.

m., facial. Atrophy of facial muscles.

SYM: Lips pouted, "twisted" smile. Sometimes ptosis of upper eyelids; inability to whistle or to blow out the cheeks, depending upon the muscles affected.

m., metabolic. Myopathy resulting from enzymatic defects in the muscle walls.

m., thyrotoxic. A chronic disease characterized by progressive muscular weakness and atrophy and hyperthyroidism.

myope (mī'ōp) [G. *myein,* to shut, + *ōps,* eye]. One afflicted with myopia or nearsightedness.

myopericarditis (mī"ō-per-ĭ-kar-dī'tis) [G. *mys, myo-,* muscle, + *peri,* around, + *kardia,* heart, + *-itis,* inflammation]. Inflammation of the pericardium and cardiac muscular wall.

myophone (mī'ō-fōn) [" + *phōnē,* voice]. Device for conveying sound of muscular contractions.

myo'pia [G. *myein,* to shut, + *ōps,* eye]. Defect in vision so that objects can only be seen distinctly when very close to the eyes; nearsightedness.

Light rays come to a focus in front of the retina.

m., axial. M. due to elongation of the axis of the eye.

m., chromic. Color blindness when viewing distant objects.

m. of curvature. M. due to curvature of the eye's refracting surfaces.

m., index. M. resulting from abnormal refractivity of the media.

m., malignant. Pernicious myopia.

m., pernicious. M. with progressive disease of the choroid, terminating in blindness.

m., prodromal. M. in which reading is possible without glasses; seen in incipient cataract.

m., progressive. M. that increases steadily during adult life.

m., stationary. Myopia that comes to a stop after adult growth is attained.

m., transient. M. seen in spasm of accommodation, as in acute iritis or iridocyclitis.

myopic (mī-op'ĭk) [" + *ōps,* eye]. Pert. to or affected with myopia.

m. crescent. Post. crescentic protrusion seen in myopia.

myoplasm (mī'ō-plazm) [G. *mys, myo-,* muscle, + *plasma,* a thing formed]. The contractile part of the muscle cell, as differentiated from the sarcoplasm.

myoplastic (mī-ō-plăst'ĭk) [" + *plassein,* to form]. Pert. to plastic use of muscle tissue or plastic surgery on muscles.

myoplasty (mī'ō-plas-tĭ) [" + *plassein,* to form]. Plastic surgery of muscle tissue.

myoplegia (mī"ō-plē'jĭ-ă) [" + *plēgē,* stroke]. Muscular paralysis.

my"oportho'sis. Correction of myopia or nearsightedness.

myoprotein (mī"ō-prō'tē-ĭn) [" + *prōtos,* first]. A protein found in muscle tissue.

myoproteose (mī"ō-pro'te-ōs) [" + *prōtos,* first]. A protein found in muscle plasma. SYN: *myoalbumose.*

myorrhaphy (mī-or'ă-fĭ) [" + *raphē,* a sewing]. Suture of a muscle wound.

myorrhexis (mī-or-eks'ĭs) [" + *rēxis,* a rupture]. Rupture of a muscle.

myosalgia (mī-ō-sal'jĭ-ă) [" + *algos,* pain]. Pain in a muscle. SYN: *myalgia.*

myosalpingitis (mī"ō-săl-pĭn-jī'tĭs) [" + *salpigx, salpigg-,* tube, + *-itis,* inflammation]. Inflamed condition of muscular tissue of a fallopian tube.

myosarcoma (mī"ō-sar-kō'mă) [" + *sarx, sark-,* flesh, + *-ōma,* tumor]. Tumor containing both muscular tissue and connective tissue cells.

myosclerosis (mī"ō-sklĕr-ō'sĭs) [" + *sklērōsis,* hardening]. Hardening of muscle.

my'osin [G. *mys, myo-,* muscle]. A protein present in muscle fibrils and comprising about 65% of total muscle protein. It consists of long chains of polypeptids joined to each other by side chains. The molecular structure of myosin is thought to be responsible for the properties of muscle tissue, namely, birefringence, double refraction, contractility, and elasticity. Myosin combines with another muscle protein, *actin,* to form *actomyosin.*

m. ferment. A coagulating enzyme in muscle plasma. It converts myosinogen into myosin.

my"osinase'. An enzyme that catalyzes the conversion of myosinogen to myosin.

myosinogen (mī"ō-sĭn'ō-jĕn) [G. *mys, myo-,* muscle, + *gennan,* to produce]. A protein present in muscle tissue, the precursor of myosin. SYN: *myogen.*

myosinose (mī-os'ĭn-ōs) [G. *mys, myo-,* muscle]. A proteose resulting from the hydrolysis of myosin.

myosinuria (mī"ō-sĭn-ū'rĭ-ă). The occurrence of myosin in the urine.

myo'sis [G. *myein,* to close]. Contraction of the pupil. SEE: *miosis, 1.*

ETIOL: Irritation of oculomotor system, paralysis of dilators. Occurs in certain fevers, congestion of iris, in typhus and in early stages of meningitis; also from drug poisoning. Seen in brain lesions, sunstroke and pulmonary congestion.

myositis (mī-ō-sī'tĭs) [G. *mys, myo-,* muscle, + *-itis,* inflammation]. Inflammation of muscle tissue, esp. voluntary muscles.

ETIOL: Infection, trauma, diathetic states, or infestation by parasites. SEE: *fibrositis.*

m., interstitial. M. with hyperplasia of connective tissue.

m. ossificans. M. marked by ossification of muscles.

m., parenchymatous. M. of substance of a muscle.

m. purulenta. Suppurative myositis.

m., traumatic. May be simple, with pain and swelling, or suppurative.

m. trichinosa, m., trichinous. M. due to infestation with trichinae.

myospasm (mī'ō-spăzm) [" + *spasmos,* spasm]. Spasmodic contraction of a muscle.

myosteo'ma [" + *osteon,* bone, + *-ōma,* tumor]. A bony growth found in muscle tissue.

myosuria (mī-ō-sū'rĭ-ă) [" + *ouron,* urine]. Presence of myosin in the urine. SYN: *myosinuria.*

myosuture (mī"ō-sū'chūr) [" + L. *sutura,* a stitch]. Stitching of a muscle.

myosynizesis (mī-ō-sin-ĭ-zē'sis) [G. *mys, myo-,* muscle, + *synizēsis,* sitting together]. Adhesion of muscular layers of tissue.

myotactic (mī"ō-tăk'tĭk) [G. *mys, myo-,* muscle, + L. *tactus,* touch]. Pert. to muscle or kinesthetic sense.

m. reflex. The stretch reflex, *q.v.*

myotasis (mī-ot'ă-sĭs) [" + *tasis,* a stretching]. Stretching of a muscle.

myotat'ic [" + *tasis,* stretching]. Pert. to the stretching of muscles.

myotenontoplasty (mī"ō-ten-on'tō-plast-ĭ) [" + *tenōn, tenont-,* tendon, + *plassein,* to form]. Plastic operation involving muscles and tendons. Syn: *tenontomyoplasty.*

myotenositis (mī"ō-tĕn-ō-sī'tĭs) [" + " + *-itis,* inflammation]. Inflamed condition of a muscle and its tendon.

myotenotomy (mī"ō-tĕn-ot'ō-mĭ) [" + " + *tomē,* incision]. Division of the tendon of a muscle.

myothermic (mī"ō-therm'ĭk) [" + *thermē,* heat]. Pert. to rise in muscle temperature due to its activity.

myot'ic [G. *myein,* to close]. 1. An agent that will contract the pupil of the eye. Ex: *physostigmine, pilocarpine.* 2. Producing contraction of a pupil.

myotility (mī-ō-til'ĭ-tĭ) [G. *mys, myo-,* muscle]. Contractility of a muscle.

myotome (mī'ō-tōm) [G. *mys, myo-,* muscle, + *tome,* incision]. Syn: *muscle plate.* 1. Knife for cutting muscles. 2. That portion of an embryonic somite which gives rise to somatic (striated) muscles.

myotomy (mī-ot'ō-mĭ) [" + *tomē,* incision]. Division or anatomical dissection of muscles.

myotonia (mī-ō-tō'nĭ-ă) [" + *tonos,* tension]. Tonic spasm of a muscle, or temporary rigidity after muscular contraction.

m. atrophica. M. dystrophica, *q.v.*

m. congenita. A disease characterized by tonic spasms of the muscles induced by voluntary movements; usually congenital and transmitted from one generation to another.

Sym: Disease appears in early childhood, is manifested by a tonic spasm of the muscles every time they are put in use, In a few minutes, rigidity wears away and the movements become free from repeated contractions, the muscles becoming firm and extremely well developed; under electrical treatment the muscles contract and relax slowly. Syn: *Thomsen's disease.*

Prog: Incurable.

Treatment: Quinine or procaine amide for relief of myotonia. Avoid obesity, prolonged bed rest and inactivity. Cortisone is contraindicated.

m. dystrophica. An hereditary disease, it is characterized by muscular wasting, myotonia, and cataract. Syn: *myotonia atrophica; Steinert's disease.*

myoton'ic [" + *tonos,* tension]. Pert. to tonic muscular spasm.

myotonometer (mī"ō-tō-nom'ĕt-ĕr) [" + " + *metron,* measure]. Instrument used to measure muscular tonus.

myot'onus [" + *tonos,* tension]. A tonic muscle spasm with temporary rigidity.

myot'rophy [" + *trophē,* nourishment]. Nutrition of the tissues of muscle.

Myriapoda (mĭr-ĭ-ap'ō-dă) [G. *myrios,* numberless, + *pous, pod-,* foot]. Group of arthropods including millepedes and centipedes.

myriapodiasis (mir"i-ăp-ō-dī'ă-sĭs) [" + *pous, pod-,* foot]. Infestation with one of the Myriapoda.

myringa (mĭr-ĭn'gă) [L. drum membrane]. The tympanic membrane.

myringectomy (mĭr-ĭn-jĕk'tō-mĭ) [" + G. *ektomē,* excision]. Syn: *myringodectomy.*

myringitis (mĭr-ĭn-jī'tĭs) [" + G. *-itis,* inflammation]. Inflammation of the tympanum or eardrum.

m. bullosa. M. with blebs or vesicular inflammation of the outer layer.

myringodectomy (mĭr-ĭn-gō-dĕk'tō-mĭ) [L. drum membrane + G. ektomē, excision]. Syn: *myringectomy.* Excision of a part or the entire tympanic membrane.

myringomycosis (mĭr-ĭn"gō-mī-kō'sĭs) [L. *myringa,* drum membrane, + G. *mykes, fungus,* + *-osis*]. Inflammation of the tympanic membrane resulting from infection by parasitic fungi. Syn: *mycomyringitis, otomycosis, mycotic otitis externa.*

myringoplasty (mĭr-ĭn'gō-plăst-ĭ) [" + G. *plassein,* to form]. Plastic operation on membrana tympani.

myringoscope (mĭr-ĭn'gō-skōp) [" + G. *skopein,* to examine]. Instrument used for examination of the eardrum.

myringotome (mĭ-rĭn'gō-tōm) [" + G. *tomē,* incision]. Knife for incising the tympanic membrane.

myringotomy (mĭr-ĭn-got'ō-mĭ) [" + G. *tomē,* incision]. Incision of tympanic membrane.

myrrh (mur) [G. *myrra*]. USP. A gum resinous substance of great antiquity, cherished as a constituent of incense and perfume; most important use today is as an aromatic, astringent mouthwash. Tincture of m. provides symptomatic relief when applied to canker sores.

mysophobia (mī-sō-fō'bĭ-ă) [G. *mysos,* filth, + *phobos,* fear]. Abnormal aversion to dirt or contamination.

mytacism (mī'tă-sĭzm) [G. *mytakismos,* fondness for letter m]. Excessive or incorrect use of the letter *m* or the *m* sound.

mythomania (mĭth-ō-mā'nĭ-ă) [G. *mythos* myth, + *mania,* madness]. Abnormal tendency to lie and exaggerate.

mythophobia (mĭth-ō-fō'bĭ-ă) [" + *phobos,* fear]. Abnormal dread of making a false or incorrect statement.

myxadenitis (mĭks-ad-en-ī'tĭs) [G. *myxa,* mucus, + *adēn,* gland, + *-itis,* inflammation]. Inflammation of mucous gland or glands.

m. labialis. Syn: *Baelz's disease.* M. of the lips.

myxadenoma (miks-ad-en-ō'mă) [" + " + *-ōma,* tumor]. 1. A tumor with the structure of a mucous gland. 2. A tumor of glandular structure containing mucous elements. Syn: *myxoadenoma.*

myxangitis (miks-an-jī'tis) [" + *aggeion,* vessel, + *-itis,* inflammation]. Inflammation of mucous gland ducts.

myxasthenia (mĭks-ăs-thē'nĭ-ă) [" + *asthēneia,* weakness]. Imperfect or insufficient secretion of mucus.

myxedema (mĭks-ĕ-dē'mă) [G. *myxa,* mucus, + *oidēma,* swelling]. Syn: *Gull's disease.* Condition resulting from hypofunction of the thyroid gland. Occurs in older children and adults.

Etiol: Iodine deficiency in diet, surgical excision or atrophy of thyroid gland, excessive use of antithyroid drugs. May occur secondary to hypofunction of ant. pituitary and is complicated by adrenal and gonadal deficiencies.

Sym: Low BMR (—35 to —40), low radioactive iodine uptake by thyroid, decreased protein bound iodine, anemia, myxedematous facies, large tongue, slow speech, puffiness of hands and face, coarse and thickened edematous skin, loss and dryness of hair, mental apathy, drowsiness, and sensitivity to cold.

TREATMENT: Desiccated thyroid.

m., childhood. M. occurring before puberty.

m., operative. SYN: *cachexia strumipriva.* M. following removal of thyroid gland.

m., pituitary. M. occurring secondary to ant. pituitary hypofunction.

myxedematoid (mĭks-ĕ-dĕm′ă-toid) [" + " + *eidos,* resemblance]. Resembling myxedema.

myxedematous (mĭks-ĕ-dĕm′ă-tŭs) [" + *oidēma,* swelling]. Marked by or concerning myxedema.

myxemia (mĭks-ē′mĭ-ă) [G. *myxa,* mucus, + *aima,* blood]. Accumulation of mucin in the blood. SYN: *mucinemia.*

myxidiotic (mĭks-ĭd-ĭ-ot′ĭk) [" + *idiōtēs,* private]. Myxedema with marked mental defects.

myxiosis (mĭks-ĭ-ō′sĭs) [G. *myxa,* mucus]. A mucous discharge or secretion.

myxo-, myx- [G.]. Combining form meaning *of,* or *pert. to mucus.*

myxoadenoma (mĭks″ō-ăd-en-ō′mă) [G. *myxa,* mucus, + *adēn,* gland, + *-ōma,* tumor]. SYN: *myxadenoma.*

Myxobacteriales (mix″o-bak-te-rĭ-a′lēz). An order of bacteria found in soil and dung. Characterized by a slimy spreading colony.

myx″ochon″drofibrosar″co′ma. A malignant tumor composed of myxomatous, chondromatous, fibrous and sarcomatous elements.

my″xochon″dro′ma. A malignant tumor composed of myxomatous and chondromatous elements.

myxocystoma (mĭks″ō-sĭs-tō′mă) [" + *kystis,* cyst, + *-ōma,* tumor]. 1. A cystic tumor containing mucus.

myxoedema (mĭks-ĕ-dē′mă) [G. *myxa,* mucus, + *oidema,* swelling]. Myxadenoma, *q.v.*

myxoenchondroma (mĭks″ō-ĕn-kŏn-drō′mă) [" + *en,* in, + *chondros,* cartilage, + *-ōma,* tumor]. A cartilaginous tissue tumor which has undergone partial mucous degeneration.

myxofibroma (mĭks″ō-fī-brō′mă) [" + L. *fibra,* fiber, + G. *-ōma,* tumor]. Tumor composed of mucous and fibrous elements.

myxoglioma (mĭks″ō-glī-ō′mă) [G. *myxa,* mucus, + *glia,* glue, + *-ōma,* tumor]. Tumor composed of myxomatous and gliomatous elements.

myxoid (mĭks′oid) [" + *eidos,* resemblance]. Similar to or resembling mucus.

myxoinoma (mĭks″ō-ĭn-ō′mă) [" + *is, in-,* fiber, + *ōma,* tumor]. A myxofibroma, *q.v.*

myxolipoma (mĭks″ō-lĭ-pō′mă) [" + *lipos,* fat, + *-ōma,* tumor]. Mucous tumor with fatty tissue elements in it.

myxoma (mĭks-ō′mă) [G. *myxa,* mucus, + *-ōma,* tumor]. A tumor composed of mucous connective tissue similar to that present in the embryo or umbilical cord. Cells are stellate or spindle-shaped and separated by mucoid. The tumors are usually soft, gray, lobulated, and translucent and are not completely encapsulated. May be pure or of mixed types involving other types of tissue.

m., cartilaginous. SYN: *chondromyxoma.*

m., cystic, cystoid. One with parts fluid enough to resemble cysts.

m., enchondromatous. One with nodules of hyaline cartilage.

m., erectile. SEE: *telangiectatic m.*

m., fibrous. SYN: *fibromyxoma.*

m., intracanalicular, of the mamma. One developing in the interstitial connective tissue of the mamma.

m., telangiectatic, vascular. One of highly vascular structure.

myxomatosis (mĭks″ō-mă-tō′sĭs) [G. *myxa,* mucus, + *-ōma,* tumor, + *-ōsis*]. 1. Formation of multiple myxomas. 2. Degeneration of myxomatous type.

Myxomycetes (mĭks″ō-mī-sē′tēz) [G. *myxa,* mucus, + *mykēs,* fungus]. A group of organisms of uncertain classification, but thought to be fungus-like. Includes slime molds.

myxomyoma (mĭks-ō-mī-ō′mă) [" + *mys, myo-,* muscle, + *-ōma,* tumor]. Muscle tissue tumor that has undergone mucous degeneration.

myxoneuroma (mĭks″ō-nū-rō′mă) [" + *neuron,* nerve, + *-ōma,* tumor]. Tumor composed of mucous and nerve tissue elements.

myxopapilloma (mĭks″ō-păp-ĭl-ō′mă) [" + L. *papilla,* nipple, + *ōma,* tumor]. Combination myxomatous and papillomatous tumor or tumors.

myxorrhea (mĭks-or-rē′ă) [" + *roia,* flow]. Free discharge from mucous surfaces. SYN: *blennorrhea.*

m. gastrica. Excessive mucous secretion in the stomach.

m. intestinalis. Secretion of mucus from the bowel in neurotic persons in times of mental stress.

myxosarcoma (mĭks″ō-săr-kō′mă) [" + *sarx, sark-,* flesh, + *-ōma,* tumor]. Mixed tumor, partly myxomatous and partly sarcomatous, having undergone partial degeneration.

myxosarcomatous (mĭks″ō-săr-kō′măt-ŭs) [" + " + *-ōma,* tumor]. Pert. to or of the nature of myxosarcoma.

myxospore (mĭks′ō-spor) [G. *myxa,* mucus, + *sporos,* seed]. Spore embedded in a gelatinous mass, seen in some fungi and protozoa.

Myxosporidia (mĭks-ō-spor-ĭd′ĭ-ă) [" + *sporos,* seed]. Parasitic sporozoans, most commonly found in epithelial cells of lower vertebrates.

myxoviruses. Group name for related viruses which cause influenza, mumps, measles, and parainfluenza.

myzesis (mī-zē′sĭs) [G. *myzein,* to suck]. Sucking.

Notes

Notes

Notes

Notes

Notes

Notes

N

N. 1. Symb. for *nitrogen*. 2. Abbr. for *normal*, esp. with reference to solutions.

n. Symb. for *index of refraction;* abbr. for *nasal*.

NA. Abbr. for *numerical aperature; Nomina Anatomica (Paris)*.

Na. Symb. for *sodium*.

nabothian cysts (na-bō'thĭ-ăn). Retention cysts formed by the n. follicles at neck of uterus. See: *cyst*.

n. follicles, n. glands. Mucous follicles of the external os uteri. They contain a glairy fluid.

Etiol: Due to closing of mouths of glands by new epithelium of a healed erosion. They always denote an erosion has been present.

n. menorrhagia. Accumulated mucus in the pregnant uterus, the result of excessive secretion of the uterine glands.

NaBr. Sodium bromide.

NaCl. Sodium chloride.

NaClO. Sodium hypochlorite.

Na_2CO_3. Sodium carbonate.

nacreous (na'kre-us) [Arabian, *nagir*, hollowed out]. Having an iridescent, pearl-like luster, as bacterial colonies.

N. A. D. Abbr. for *no appreciable disease*.

Naegele's obliquity (na'ge-le). Inclination of fetal head, laterally in a flat pelvis.

N.'s pelvis. An obliquely contracted pelvis, caused by disease in infancy.

N's rule. To estimate the day labor will begin, count back 3 months from the day the last menstrual period began and add 7 days.

NaF. Sodium fluoride.

$NaHCO_3$. Sodium bicarbonate.

$NaHSO_3$. Sodium bisulfite.

nail (năl) [A.S. *naegel*]. Syn: *unguis*. A horny cell structure of the epidermis forming flat plates upon the dorsal surface of the terminal phalanges.

A nail consists of a *body*, the exposed portion, and a *root*, the proximal portion hidden by the *nail fold*, both of which rest on the *nail bed* or *matrix*. The latter consists of epithelium and corium continuous with the epidermis and dermis of the skin of the *nail fold*. The crescent-shaped white area near the root is the *lunula*. The epidermis extending from the margin of the nail fold over the root is called *eponychium;* that underlying the free border of the distal portion is called *hyponychium*.

A nail grows in length and thickness through activity of cells in the stratum germinativum in region of the root. Average rate of growth in fingernails is about 1 mm. per week. It is slower in toenails and slower in summer than in winter. It varies with age and is affected by disease and certain hormone deficiencies.

Changes in the nails, such as ridges, may occur in defective nutrition or after a serious illness. In achlorhydria, hypochromic anemia, excessive spoon-shaped nails with center depression may occur. In chronic pulmonary conditions and congenital heart disease excessive curving of the nails may be associated with clubbed fingers.

Atrophy: May occur as a result of hereditary or congenital tendencies. Permanent atrophy may follow injuries, scars from disease, frostbite, nerve injuries and hyperthyroidism. Nail shedding is due to the same causes.

Nails that are fragile or split often may be congenital or due to prolonged contact with chemicals or to too frequent manicuring.

Discolorations: *Black*: In diabetes and other forms of gangrene. *Blue-black*: Common condition, usually due to hemorrhage, bleeding diseases such as hemophilia, and trauma. May be painful and can be relieved by drilling holes in the nails. *Brown*: May be due to arsenical poisoning. *Brownish-black*: This discoloration often indicates chronic mercurial poisoning, due to formation of sulfide of mercury in the tissues. *Cyanosis*: Usually indicates anemia, poor circulation, or venous stasis. *Slate*: This is an early manifestation of argyria and administration of silver should be stopped at once. *White spots*: Striate lesions may be due to trauma and are more frequent in women. Transverse white bands in all nails may be a sign of acute or chronic arsenical poisoning, or rarely of thallium acetate poisoning. Syn: *leukonychia*.

Dry, Malformed: May result from trophic changes resulting from injury to nerve or finger, neuritis, Raynaud's disease, pulmonary osteoarthropathy, syphilis, onychia, scleroderma, acrodermatitis and granuloma fungoides of the fingers.

Striations, Longitudinal: Often found in those past middle life; frequently associated with onychorrhexis, splitting at the free margins. Note in association with a focus of infection in the bowel or at root of a tooth. Vitamin deficiency may be a cause. Microscopic examination of nail clippings should be made for ringworm. When hard and brittle, gouty conditions are indicated.

Transverse lines (Beau's lines): May result from previous interference of nail matrix growth. May be caused by local or systemic conditions. Approximate date of lesion may be determined, as it takes 4-6 months for the nail to grow.

Ulcers and Ecchymosis: At base of nails noted in chloral addicts, syphilis and scrofula if not due to trauma. Chancre may be suspected if a small, indolent ulcer appears near the nail, esp. if indurated and associated with enlarged lymph glands above the inner condyle.

Quincke's Capillary Pulsation: Rhythmic flushing and blanching most frequent in aortic regurgitation and often in anemia.

n. bed. The end of a finger or toe covered by the nail. Syn: *nail matrix*.

n. biting Syn: onychophagia. A nervous affliction or neurosis in which the free edges of the nails are bitten down to the quick.

n. culture. Test tube culture in which the culture grows in the shape of a nail.

n., eggshell. Nail plate is soft, semitransparent, bends easily, and splits at end. Associated with arthritis, peripheral neuritis, leprosy and hemiplegia. May be the only visible sign of late syphilis.

n. fold. Groove in the cutaneous tissue surrounding the margins and proximal edges of the nail.

n. groove. The space between nail wall and the nail bed.

n., hang. Broken epidermis at edge of the nail. SYN: *agnail, (1)*.

n., ingrowing. Nail with tissue overgrowing its edges.

n. matrix. The nail bed.

n., reedy. One marked by longitudinal fissures.

n. root. Proximal portion of nail covered by nail fold.

n., spoon. A nail with central portion depressed and lateral edges elevated.

n. wall. Epidermis covering edges of the nail. SYN: *vallum unguis*.

naked (nā'kĕd) [A.S. *naced*, nude]. Uncovered, exposed to view, nude, bare.

nalorphine (nal-or'fēn). Generic name for N-allylnormorphine. Used in treatment of narcotic overdose.

nanism (na'nizm) [G. *nanos*, dwarf]. Condition of being dwarflike in build.

n., symptomatic. N. with deficient dentition, sexual development and ossification.

nano- (na'no) [G. *nanos*, dwarf]. Prefix indicating 1 billionth of the unit following. Thus a nanogram is 1 billionth of a gram.

nanocephalism (nan-ō-sef'ăl-ĭzm) [" + *kephalē*, head]. Condition of having an abnormally small head.

nanocephalous (nan-ō-sef'ă-lŭs) [" + *kephalē*, head]. Having an abnormally small head.

nanocormia (na-nō-kor'mĭ-ă) [" + *kormos*, trunk]. Abnormally dwarfed thorax or body.

nanoid (na'noid) [" + *eidos*, like]. Dwarflike.

nanomelus (nā-nōm'ĕ-lĕs). A monster with undersized extremities.

nanosoma. Nanosomia, *q.v.*

nanosomia (na-nō-so'mĭ-ă) [" + *sōma*, body]. State of being a dwarf. SEE: *nanism*.

nanosomus (nā-nō-sō'mŭs). A person of stunted size; a dwarf.

nanous (nan'ŭs) [G. *nanos*, dwarf]. Dwarfed or stunted.

na'nus [G. *nanos*]. 1. A dwarf. 2. Stunted; dwarflike.

NaOH. Sodium hydroxide.

nap (năp) [A.S. *hnappian*, nap]. 1. To slumber. 2. A short sleep; a doze.

napalm (na'palm) [from *na*phthene + *palm*itate]. Gasoline made thick or jelly-like for use in incendiary bombs and flame throwers.

n. burn. Burn due to use of napalm, usually during war.

nape (nāp; năp) [origin uncertain]. Back of neck.

napex (na'peks) [origin uncertain]. Scalp beneath the occipital protuberance.

naphtha (naf'thă) [G. *naphtha*]. 1. A volatile inflammable liquid distilled from carbonaceous substances. 2. Petroleum, esp. more volatile varieties.

naphthalene (naf'thă-lēn) [G. *naphtha*]. A hydrocarbon, one of principal constituents of coal tar. $C_{10}H_8$.

USES: As a disinfectant, in moth balls, and in manufacture of dyes and explosives.

naphthol (năf'thōl). Coal tar substance used as an antiseptic and in certain dyes. Also prepared from naphthalene.

napiform (na'pĭ-form) [L. *napus*, turnip, + *forma*, shape]. BACT: Formed like a turnip, as gelatin liquefaction.

naprapathy (nap-răp'ăth-ĭ) [Czech *naprava*, correction, + G. *pathos*, disease]. Method of manipulation practiced by a certain school in the treatment of disease which is based upon the assumption that disease is due to faulty functioning of ligaments.

narceine (nar'se-ēn). $C_{22}H_{27}O_8N$, an alkaloid obtained from opium. A hypnotic and used as a substitute for morphine.

narcism, narcissism (nar'sĭzm, nar-sĭs'ĭzm) [G. from *Narkissos*, a mythical character who fell in love with his own image]. 1. Self-love or self-admiration. 2. Voluptuous pleasure derived from observing one's own naked body.

narcissistic (nar-sĭs-sĭst'ĭk). Pert. to narcissism.

n. object choice. Selection of another like one's own self as the object of love, friendship or liking.

narco- [G.]. Prefix: *numbness, stupor*.

narcoanesthesia (nar"kō-ăn-ĕs-thē'zĭ-ă) [G. *narkē*, stupor, + *an-*, priv. + *aisthesis*, sensation]. Anesthesia produced by a narcotic, as scopolamine and morphine.

narcohypnia (nar"kō-hĭp'nĭ-ă) [" + *hypnos*, sleep]. Numbness following sleep.

narcohypnosis (när-cō"hĭp-nō'sĭs). SYN: *hypnonarcosis*. Stupor or deep sleep produced by hypnosis.

narcolepsy (nar'ko-lep-sĭ) [" + *lēpsis*, seizure]. Overwhelming attacks of sleep which the victim cannot inhibit, often associated with cataplexy, *q.v.* Electroencephalogram is normal. SYN: *sleep epilepsy; sleep, paroxysmal*.

ETIOL: Unknown.

narcoleptic (nar-kō-lĕp'tĭk) [" + *lēpsis*, seizure]. Pert. to or marked by an overwhelming desire to sleep.

narcoma (nar-kō'mă) [" + *kōma*, coma]. Coma or stupor from use of a narcotic.

narcomania (nar-kō-mā'nĭ-ă) [" + *mania*, madness]. 1. Abnormal craving for alcohol or narcotics. 2. Insanity due to use of alcohol or narcotics.

narcomaniac (nar-kō-mā'nĭ-ăk) [" + *mania*, madness]. 1. Pert. to narcomania. 2. One affected by narcomania.

narcomatous (nar-kō-mă'tus) [" + *kōma*, coma]. Pert. to a state of stupor from use of narcotics.

nar'cose [G. *narkē*, stupor]. In a stuporous state.

narco'sis [G. *narkē*, stupor, + *-ōsis*]. Unconscious state due to narcotics.

n., basal. N. produced prior to administration of a general anesthetic.

n., medullary. General anesthesia induced by a local anesthetic injected in the sheath of the spinal cord in lumbar region. SYN: *spinal anesthesia*.

narcosomania (nar-kō"sō-mā'nĭ-ă) [" + *mania*, madness]. Morbid craving for or insanity produced by narcotics. SYN: *narcomania*.

narcot'ic [G. *narkōtikos*, benumbing]. 1. Producing stupor or sleep. 2. A drug which in moderate doses depresses the central nervous system thus relieving pain and producing sleep but which in excessive doses produces unconsciousness, stupor, coma, and possibly death. Examples are opium, morphine, codeine, papaverine, heroin, and many synthetics. Most are habit forming. 3. Anything that soothes, relieves or lulls. 4. One addicted to the use of narcotics.

Narcotics are more powerful than hypnotics. EX: *chloral hydrate, sulfonal, trional, veronal.*

RS: drug addiction.

narcotism (nar'kŏt-ĭzm) [G. *narkē*, stupor, + *ismos*, condition]. 1. State of stupor induced by a narcotic. SYN: *narcosis.* 2. An addiction to the use of narcotics.

Addiction may be said to exist when discontinuance causes abstinence symptoms relieved speedily by a dose of the drug. It is this addition to the original purpose in taking the drug that so readily aggravates the need.

TREATMENT: Can ordinarily be successful only under sanitarium conditions positively preventing the use of the drug, and then it consists mostly of substituted sedatives to minimize distress of withdrawal. Relapses are frequent and the building up of a new philosophy of life is sometimes of prime importance.

POISONING: Narcotic or sleep producing poisons as opium and its derivatives, chloral combinations, barbital and its myriad subvarieties, etc.

SYM: Depression, slowing of heart and respiration, sleep, followed by coma.

F. A. TREATMENT: Remove poison by vomiting, purging, dilution of blood, diuretics, intravenous hypertonic glucose. Administer stimulants by all routes.

nar'cotize [G. *narkōtikos*, benumbing]. To render unconscious through the use of a narcotic.

naris (na'rĭs) (pl. *nares*) [L. nostril]. The nostril.

n., anterior. BNA. External nostril.

n., posterior. BNA. Either internal opening into pharynx.

RS: *anosmia, epistaxis, hyperosmia, nose, parosmia, septum, smell.*

nasal (nā'zl) [L. *nasus*, nose]. 1. Pert. to the nose. 2. Uttered through the nose. 3. A nasal bone.

n. bones. The 2 small bones forming the arch of the nose.

n. cartilages. C. forming principal portion of framework of external nose.

n. cavity. C. between floor of cranium and roof of mouth.

n. conchae. SEE: *concha, nasal.*

n. douche. Injection of fluid into nostril, with fluid escaping by way of the nasopharynx out of the mouth.

Patient should keep mouth open to prevent fluid from entering the throat. Force must not be great. Atomized spray is safer. Container should not be suspended over 6 inches above patient, who should not blow the nose during treatment.

n. feeding. N. gavage, *q.v.*

n. fossa. One of the two halves of the nasal cavity.

n. gavage. Feeding through a tube in the nasal passage.

This is resorted to when it is the only route available to the stomach, or when the patient refuses to eat. Quite often in the latter case, nasal feeding is necessary to make him realize that it is much easier to eat.

NP: Throughout a course of tube feedings in mental cases, the nurse should frequently experiment to see if the patient will eat. Try him with a fully prepared tray. Also offer the tube feeding in a glass that he may drink it. Again, it should be remembered that suggestion is a very powerful factor in the care of the mental patient, so the nurse may see the reflection of her own attitude in the patient's behavior.

ARTICLES NECESSARY: (a) Tray with feeding (consisting usually of milk, eggs, sugar and malted milk, concentrated broths and purées with milk and cream, and orange juice) heated to 98° F. (b) Pitcher of water (about 100 cc.). (c) Basin with ice and nasal tube and funnel. (d) Medicine glass with glycerine. (e) Gown for doctor. (f) Rubber and draw sheet to protect patient. (g) Face towel. (h) Bowl of water to invert funnel in. (i) Any medication ordered.

PROCEDURE: (a) Have patient in bed or in chair, according to the doctor's wishes, usually in a chair, however. (b) Restrain, if a mental patient, with a blanket sheet or restraining jacket. (c) Protect patient with rubber draw sheet. (d) Attach nasal tube to funnel, pour water into it, and clamp tube so no air will enter. (e) Dip end of nasal tube in glycerine. (f) After tube is inserted, note color of face, invert funnel in water and if air bubbles appear, tube is in the trachea and should be removed immediately. (g) If certain tube is in stomach, fill funnel with feeding and hold slightly above patient's head to allow flow by gravity. (h) Give any medication, also water. (i) Hold towel over patient's mouth and keep head raised slightly as patient is more apt to retain the feeding. (j) Remove tube quickly and keep patient quiet for a few minutes, until desire for regurgitation has passed. (k) Entire amount of fluid given at one feeding should not exceed 1000 cc.

n. height. Distance bet. lower border of nasal aperture and the nasion.

n. index. The greatest width of the nasal aperture in relation to a line from the lower edge of the n. aperture to the nasion.

n. line. L. from lower edge of the ala nasi curving to outer side of the orbicularis oris muscle, seen in abdominal disorders. SYN: *Jadelot's furrow or line.*

n. meatus. SEE: *meatus.*

n. obstruction. Commonest causes: (a) Irregular septum; (b) enlarged turbinates; (c) nasal polypi; (d) in children foreign bodies such as food, buttons, or pins. Many complications result. TREATMENT: Nasal douches, inhalations and operative care: (a) Resection of septum; (b) turbinectomy; (c) removal of polypi; (d) opening and draining sinuses; (e) removal of foreign body.

n. reflex. Sneezing resulting from irritation of nasal mucosa.

n. sinuses, accessory. The paranasal sinuses, *q.v.* SEE: *sinuses, accessory nasal.*

n. width. Maximum width of nasal aperture.

nascent (năs'ĕnt; nā'sĕnt) [L. *nascens*, born]. 1. Just born; incipient or beginning. 2. Pert. to a substance being set free from a compound.

nasion (nā'zĭ-ŏn) [L. *nasus*, nose]. The point where the nasofrontal suture is cut across by the median anteroposterior plane.

nasitis (nā-zī'tĭs) [" + G. *-ītis*, inflammation]. Inflammation of the nose. SEE: *rhinitis.*

Nasmyth's membrane (naz'mĭth) [Alexander Nasmyth, Scotch dental surgeon in London, died 1847]. Epithelial m. enveloping enamel of a tooth for short period after birth.

naso- [L.]. Combining form, *rel. to the nose.*

nasoantritis (nā"zō-ăn-trī'tĭs) [L. *nasus*, nose, + G. *antron*, cavity, + *-ītis*, inflammation]. Inflammation of nose and antrum of Highmore with rhinitis.

nasociliary (nā″sō-sĭl′ĭ-ăr-ĭ). Pert. to nose, eyebrow, and eyes. Applied esp. to nerve supplying these structures.

nas″ofron′tal [“ + *frons, front-*, forehead]. Pert. to nasal and frontal bones.

nas″ola′bial [“ + *labium*, lip]. Connected with or rel. to the nose and lip.

nasolacrimal (nā″zō-lăk′rĭm-ăl) [“ + *lacrima*, tear]. Pert. to nose and lacrimal mechanism.

nasology (nā-zol′ō-jĭ) [“ + G. *logos*, study]. Study of the nose and its diseases.

nasomental (nā″zō-mĕn′tăl) [“ + *mentum*, chin]. Pert. to the nose and chin.

n. reflex. Contraction of mentalis muscle with elevation of lower lip and wrinkling of skin of chin resulting from percussion of side of nose.

nasopalatine (nā″zō-păl′ăt-īn) [L. *nasus*, + *palatum*, palate]. Pert. to both nose and palate.

nasopharyngeal (nā″zō-făr-ĭn′jē-ăl) [“ + G. *pharygx*, pharynx]. Pert. to the pharynx and nose.

nasopharyngitis (nā″zō-făr-ĭn-jī′tĭs) [“ + “ + *-ītis*, inflammation]. Inflamed condition of the nasopharynx. Syn: *rhinopharyngitis.*

nasopharynx (nā″zō-far′ĭnks) [“ + G. *pharygx*, pharynx]. Part of pharynx situated above the soft palate (postnasal space). Syn: *rhinopharynx.*

nasoscope (nā′zō-skōp) [“ + G. *skopein*, to examine]. Electrical device for examination of the nasal cavity.

nasoseptitis (nā″zō-sĕp-tī′tĭs) [“ + *saeptum*, partition]. Inflamed condition of the nasal septum.

nasosinuitis, nasosinusitis (nā″zō-sĭn-ū-ī′tĭs, -sī-nū-sī′tĭs) [“ + *sinus*, cavity]. Inflammation of the nasal accessory sinuses and cavities.

nasospinale (nā″zō-spĭn′-ăl-ē). Point at which med. sagittal plane intersects line joining lowest points on nasal margins.

nasus (nā′sŭs) [L.]. The nose.

natal (nā′tăl) [L. *natus*, birth; *nascī*, to be born]. 1. Pert. to birth or the day of birth. 2. [L. *nates*, buttocks]. Pert. to the nates or buttocks.

natal′ity [L. *natus*, birth; *nascī*, to be born]. The birth rate.

natant (nā′tănt) [L. *natāre*, to swim]. Floating; swimming.

nates (nā′tēz) [L. pl. buttocks]. 1. Gluteal region; fleshy prominences formed by the gluteal muscles and covering of fat and skin. Syn: *buttocks.* 2. The ant., sup. or upper two corpora quadrigemina. See: *testes.*

natimortality (nā″tĭ-mor-tăl′ĭ-tĭ) [L. *natus*, one born, + *mortalitās*]. Rate of stillbirths in proportion to birth rate.

National Formulary. Abbr. N.F. Formulary issued by the Amer. Pharmaceutical Assn.

native (nā′tĭv) [L. *nativus*, born in]. 1. Born with; inherent. 2. Natural, normal. Syn: *indigenous.* 3. Belonging to, as place of one's birth.

n. albumin. A protein group found in tissues. See: *albumin.*

natremia (na-trē′mĭ-ă) [L. *natrium*, sodium, + G. *aima*, blood]. Sodium in the blood.

natrium (na′trĭ-um) [L. sodium]. Symb: Na. Sodium.

This is found abundantly in plants, animal fluids and minerals, as common salt.

natriuresis (na″tre-u-re′sis) [L. “ + G. *ouresis*, make water]. Sodium in the urine.

natriuretic. A drug which causes loss of sodium in the urine. See: *diuretic.*

na′tron. Sodium carbonate.

na′trum. Homeopathic name for soda or sodium.

nat′ural [L. *natura*, nature]. Not abnormal or artificial.

n. selection. A theory of evolution proposed by Chas. Darwin to account for the origin of species. Essential points are that all species tend to overproduce. As food supply is limited, there is a struggle for existence. Variations occur, hence individuals possessing favorable variations would tend to survive; those with unfavorable ones would die out. Through heredity, such variations would be transmitted to successive generations and, in time, new types or species differing from their ancestors would come into existence.

naturetin. An effective oral diuretic and antihypertensive agent, and also used to control edema.

na′turopath [“ + G. *pathos*, suffering]. One who practices naturopathy.

naturopathy (nā-tūr-op′ă-thĭ). A therapeutic system employing natural forces such as light, heat, air, water, massage.

naupathia (naw-path′ĭ-ă) [G. *naus*, ship, + *pathos*, disease]. Seasickness.

nausea (naw′shē-ă; naw′sē-ă) [G. *nausia*, seasickness]. Inclination to vomit; usually preceding emesis.

It is present in seasickness, early pregnancy, diseases of the central nervous system, neurasthenia, hysteria. It may be due to the sight or odor of obnoxious matter or conditions, or to mental images of same. It may be present, without vomiting, in certain gallbladder disturbances and in carsickness.

NP: Report the nature of vomitus, if it occurs, *frequency and time, effect of food and sleep, bilious, fecal, profuse, purulent, watery, mucous* and *hematemesis.* Be prepared to maintain airway if patient is stuporous. See: *vomitus.*

n. gravidarum. Morning sickness of pregnancy.

n. navalis. Seasickness. Syn: *mal de mer, naupathia.*

nauseant (naw′shē-ănt; naw′sē-ănt) [G. *nausia*, seasickness]. 1. Causing nausea. 2. That which causes nausea.

nauseate (naw′shē-āt; naw′sē-āt) [G. *nausia*, seasickness]. To cause or affect with nausea.

nauseous (naw′shus; naw′shē-ŭs) [G. *nausia*, seasickness]. Producing nausea, disgust or loathing. Also to be nauseated.

navel (nā′vĕl) [A.S. *nafela*]. The depression or scar in center of abdomen, where the umbilical cord of fetus was attached. Syn: *umbilicus, q.v.*

RS: *cirsomphalos, umbilical cord, umbilicate.*

n. string. Umbilical cord.

navicula (nă-vĭk′ū-lă) [L. *navicula*, boat]. Fossa naviculàris, *q.v.*

navicular (nă-vĭk′ū-lar) [L. *navicula*, boat]. 1. Shaped like a boat. 2. Scaphoid bones in the carpus and in the tarsus. See: *skeleton.*

n. fossa. See: *fossa navicularis.*

Nb. Chem. symb. for niobium (columbium).

N.C.A. Neurocirculatory asthenia.

Nd. Chem. symb. for neodymium.

Ne. Chem. symb. for neon.

near point. Syn: *punctum proximum.* Abbr: n.p. Closest point of distinct vision, with maximum accommodation.

It recedes with age, varying from 3 in. in 2 yr. to 40 in. at 60 yr.

n. p., absolute. For either eye.

n. p., relative. For both eyes taken together.

nearsight (nēr′sīt). Ability to see clearly only a short distance. SYN: *myopia.*

near′sight″ed. Able to see clearly only a short distance. SYN: *myopia.*

nearsight′edness. Ability to see distinctly only a short distance. SYN: *myopia.*

nearthrosis (nē-ar-thrō′sĭs) [G. *neos,* new, + *arthron,* joint]. A false joint or abnormal articulation.

nebula (nĕb′ū-lă) [L. mist, cloud]. 1. Slight haziness. 2. Cloudiness in urine. 3. Aqueous or oil substance for use in an atomizer.

n. corneae. Grayish opacity of the cornea.

nebuliza′tion [L. *nebula,* vapor]. 1. Treatment with spray method. 2. Conversion into a vapor. SYN: *vaporization.*

nebulizer (nĕb′ū-lī-zĕr) [L. *nebula,* mist]. An atomizer or sprayer.

Ne″ca′tor [L. *murderer*]. A genus of nematode hookworms belonging to the family Ancylostomidae.

N. americanus. A species of hookworm widely distributed in tropical regions, and common in the southern United States. Called the American hookworm. Adults live in small intestine attached to mucosa by their buccal capsules. Adults lay eggs which pass out with feces and under proper conditions of warmth and moisture hatch within 24 hrs. into rhabditiform larvae. After two molts, the larvae becomes strongyliform. After two more molts occurring within five days, they become infective larvae. They enter the body through the skin, pass into the lymph or blood stream and are carried to the lungs. Here they burrow into air spaces from which they pass via bronchial tubes and trachea to the pharynx from which they are expectorated or swallowed. If swallowed, they reach the intestine, bury themselves among the villi, molt again, acquire a mouth capsule and attach themselves to the mucosa. Worms may live 5 years.

necatoriasis (ne-ka″to-ri′ă-sis). Infestation by *Necator americanus, q.v.*

neck (nĕk) [A.S. *hnecca,* nape]. 1. Part of body bet. head and shoulders. 2. The constricted portion of an organ, or that resembling a neck. 3. Region between crown and root of a tooth.

n., anatomical. Constriction just below the head of the humerus. SYN: *collum anatomicum.*

n., back of. Nape. SYN: *nucha, scruff.*

n., Madelung's. Diffuse lipoma of the neck.

n., Nithsdale. Goiter.

n., surgical. Narrow part of humerus below the tuberosity. Fracture here is common.

n. of womb. The cervix uteri.

n., wry. Torsion of the neck caused by contracted muscles. SYN: *torticollis.*

necrectomy (nĕ-krĕk′to-mĭ) [G. *nekros,* dead, + *ektomē,* excision]. Surgical removal of necrosed tissue.

necro- [G.]. Combining form meaning *pertaining to death.*

necrobiosis (nĕk-rō-bī-ō′sĭs) [G. *nekros,* dead, + *biosis,* life]. Gradual degeneration and death of tissue. SEE: *necrosis.*

n. lipoidica diabeticorum. SYN: *Oppenheim-Urbach disease.* A skin disease common in diabetics characterized by necrosis of connective tissue and discoloration of skin.

necrobiotic (nĕ″krō-bī-ŏt′ĭk) [" + *biosis,* life]. Pert. to or affected by necrosis. SYN: *necrotic.*

necrocytosis (nĕ″krō-sī-tō′sĭs) [" + *kytos,* cell, + *-ōsis*]. Cellular death or decomposition.

necrocytotoxin (nek″ro-si″to-toks′in). A toxin which causes death of cells.

necrogenic, necrogenous (nĕ-krō-jĕn′ĭk, -kroj′ĕn-ŭs) [" + *gennan,* to produce]. Caused by, pert. to, or originating in dead matter.

necrologist (nĕk-rol′ō-jĭst) [" + *logos,* study]. A student of mortality statistics.

necrology (nĕk-rol′o-jĭ) [" + *logos,* study]. The study of mortality statistics.

necromania (nĕk-rō-mā′nĭ-ă) [G. *nekros,* dead, + *mania,* madness]. 1. Abnormal interest in dead bodies or in death. 2. Mania with desire for death.

necrometer (nĕk-rom′ĕt-ĕr) [" + *metron,* measure]. Device for measurement of dead organs.

necromimesis (nĕk″rō-mī-mē′sĭs). A delusion in which a person believes himself to be dead or acts as though he were dead.

necronectomy (nĕk-rōn-ĕk′tō-mĭ) [" + *ektomē,* excision]. Excision of a necrotic part, esp. of necrotic ossicles.

necrophagous (nĕ-krŏf′ă-gŭs) [" + *phagein,* to eat]. Feeding or existing on dead bodies or matter.

necrophile (nĕk′rō-fĭl) [" + *philein,* to love]. One who has a morbid interest in or violates dead bodies.

necrophilism (nĕk-rŏf′ĭl-ĭzm) [" + *philein,* to love, + *ismos,* condition]. 1. Sexual perversion in which there is insane love for, or violation of, the dead. 2. Strong desire for death.

necrophilous (nĕk-rŏf′ĭl-ŭs) [" + *philein,* to love]. 1. Having a morbid fondness for, or feeding on, dead tissue. 2. Pert. to or affected with necrophilism.

necrophobia (nĕk-rō-fō′bĭ-ă) [G. *nekros,* dead, + *phobos,* fear]. 1. Abnormal aversion to dead bodies. 2. Insane dread of death. SYN: *thanatophobia.*

necropneumonia (nĕk″rō-nū-mō′nĭ-ă) [" + *pneumon,* lung]. Pulmonary gangrene.

necropsy (nĕk′rŏp-sĭ) [" + *opsis,* view]. The scientific examination of a dead body to determine cause of death or pathological conditions. SYN: *autopsy, necroscopy, postmortem.*

necrosadism (nĕk″rō-sā′dĭzm) [" + *sadism*]. Sexual gratification derived from the mutilation of dead bodies.

necroscopy (nĕ-krŏs′kō-pĭ) [" + *skopein,* to examine]. Scientific inspection of a dead body to find cause of death or pathological condition. SYN: *autopsy, necropsy.*

necrose (nĕk-rōs′) [G. *nekros,* dead]. To cause or to undergo necrosis.

nec″ro′sin. A substance obtained from inflamed tissues which induces inflammatory changes in normal tissue.

necrosis (pl. *necroses*) (nĕk-rō′sĭs) [G. *nekrōsis,* a killing]. Death of areas of tissue or bone surrounded by healthy parts; death in mass as distinguished from *necrobiosis,* a gradual degeneration. SYN: *gangrene, mortification.*

The dead part in bone is called *sequestrum;* in soft tissue, a *slough* or *sphacelus.* Term is usually applied to bone destruction or small areas of tissue, while gangrene is generally applied to destruction of specific parts or larger areas.

ETIOL: Cessation of blood supply; physical agents such as trauma, radiant energy (electricity, infrared, ultraviolet, roentgen and radium rays); chemical agents (exogenous substances acting locally or acting internally following absorption and endogenous substances), or products (toxins) of bacteria.

n., anemic. N. caused by disturbed circulation in a part.

n., Balser's fatty. Pancreatitis with gangrenous areas in the fatty tissues.

n., caseous. SEE: *cheesy n.*

n., central. N. which affects only the center of a part.

n., cheesy. N. with cheeselike formation. Usually due to tuberculosis or syphilis.

n., coagulative. N. occurring esp. in infarcts in which coagulation occurs in necrotic area converting it into a homogenous mass.

n., colliquative. N. caused by liquefaction of tissue due to autolysis or bacterial putrefaction.

n., dry. N. with dryness of the sequestrum.

n., embolic. N. resulting from an embolus which causes anemic n.

n., fat. N. in small scattered areas in the fatty tissue.

n., fibrinous. SEE: *coagulative n.*

n., focal. Coagulative n. in small scattered areas.

n., gummatous. N. resulting from syphilis forming a dry rubbery mass.

n., ischemic. N. resulting from interference in blood supply to a part. Results in development of an infarct, decubitus, or gangrene.

n., liquifactive. SYN: *colliquative necrosis, q.v.*

n., medial. N. of cells in tunica media of arteries.

n., moist. N. with softening and moist condition of the dead bone.

n., putrefactive. N. caused by bacterial decomposition.

n., superficial. N. affecting only the outer layers of bone or any tissue.

n., thrombotic. N. due to thrombus formation.

n., total. N. affecting an entire part.

n. ustilaginea. Dry n. due to ergot poisoning.

nec'ro-sperm'i-a. Condition in which spermatozoa in the ejaculate are immobile or lifeless.

necrot'ic [G. *nekrōsis,* a killing]. Rel. to death of a portion of tissue.

necrotomy (ne-krot'o-mĭ) [G. *nekros,* dead, + *tomē,* a cutting]. 1. Dissection of a cadaver. 2. Excision of a sequestrum or other necrotic tissue.

nectarine (nek"ter-ēn'). AV. SERVING: 125 Gm. Pro. 0.8, Carbo. 19.9. VITAMINS: A+, B_1, C+.

needle (nēd'l) [A.S. *naedl*]. A pointed instrument for stitching, ligaturing or puncturing.

It may be *straight, half curved, full curved, semicircular,* or *double curved,* sometimes called *"S"* or *sigmoid-shaped.* There are two classifications: cutting edge and round point. Cutting edge type is used in skin and dense tissue work, while round point needles are used for more delicate operations. All curved needles are used with a holder, straight usually without a holder.

CARE OF: Wash off, scrub with mild cleanser, benzene and ether, sharpen, oil, and then sterilize.

n., hypodermic. A hollow needle for hypodermic injections.

need'ling [A.S. *naedl*]. Treatment by puncturing with a needle. SYN: *discission.*

n. of aneurysm. Insertion of needles into an aneurysm in an effort to thicken and strengthen walls of the sac. Several fine needles are introduced into sac and left to be played upon by the blood stream, so that the farther wall becomes scratched and irritated, thus setting up an inflammatory thickening.

n., cataract. SYN: *discission.* Puncturing of capsule of lens to allow entrance of aqueous fluid in order to bring about absorption of lens substance.

n. of heart. Cardiocentesis, *q.v.*

n. of kidney. Insertion of a needle into the kidney.

NEFA. Abbr. for *nonesterified fatty acids.*

negative (neg'ă-tiv) [L. *negāre,* to deny]. 1. Without positive statement. 2. Lacking results. 3. PSY: Marked by resistance or retreat, as to a suggestion. 4. Directed away from a source of stimulation. 5. Not affirming presence of an organism, as a negative diagnosis.

n. culture. One not revealing the suspected organism.

n. electricity. Static e. in which elementary unit is the electron, and which is produced by friction.

n. electrode. The pole by which currents leave. SYN: *negative pole.*

n. glow. The luminous glow that is adjacent to the cathode in a vacuum tube through which an electrical discharge is passing.

n. reaction. Absence of a positive indication of disease, as a negative Wassermann reaction for syphilis.

n. sensation. One caused by stimulus not perceived in consciousness.

n. sign. Minus sign (—) used in subtraction and to indicate a lack.

negativism (neg'ă-tiv-izm) [L. *negāre,* to deny, + G. *ismos,* state]. Behavior peculiarity marked by not performing suggested actions (*passive negativism*) or in doing the opposite (*active negativism*), as seen in dementia precox.

A patient may refuse to respond to suggestions because of *sluggish mental reflexes,* or from *fear.* Retardation may be slow, or sudden and intense, as in manic depressive insanity. Opposition from fear must be considered apart from dementia praecox, in which the patient performs acts directly contrary to those suggested.

Negri bodies (na'gre) [Adelchi Negri, Italian physician, 1876-1912]. Very minute bodies formed in nerve cells of the brain of one affected by rabies.

Neisseria (ni-se'rĭ-ă). A genus of bacteria belonging to the family Neisseriaceae. They are gram-negative and usually occur in pairs with flattened sides but may occur singly or in irregular groups. Some are pathogenic.

N. catarrhalis. Species of N. found in catarrhal inflammations of the upper respiratory tract.

N. discoides. Species occurring in alimentary and urinogenital tracts.

N. flava. Species found in nasopharynx; nonpathogenic. Produces a yellow pigment.

N. flavescens. Species found in spinal fluid in meningitis patients.

N. gonorrhoeae. Species causing gonorrhea. SYN: *gonococcus.*

N. intracellularis. SYN: *N. meningitidis, q.v.*

N. meningitidis. SYN: *N. intracellularis, Micrococcus meningitidis, M. intracellularis meningitidis.* Species causing epidemic cerebrospinal meningitis.

N. orbiculata. Species found in alimentary and urinogenital tracts.

N. reniformis. Species found in alimentary and urinogenital tracts.

N. sicca. Species found in mucous membrane of respiratory tract. Thought to be causative agent of kidney infections and endocarditis.

Nelaton's line (na-lă-ton′) [Auguste Nelaton, French surgeon, 1807-1873]. Line from ant. sup. spine of the ileum to tuberosity of the ischium.

nem. A food value unit, the value in calories of 1 gm. of mother's milk, equaling about ⅔ calorie.

nemathelminth (nĕm-ă-thĕl′mĭnth) [G. *nēma,* thread, + *helmins,* worm]. A roundworm belonging to the phylum Nemathelminthes.

Nemathelminthes (nĕm-ă-thĕl-mĭn′thēz). The phylum of the roundworm.

nematocide (nem′ă-tō-sīd) [" + *caedere,* to kill]. An agent that kills nematode worms.

Nematoda (nem″ă-to′dă) [G. *nemat-,* thread, + *eidos,* like]. A class of the phylum Nemathelminthes which includes the true roundworms or threadworms, many species of which are parasitic. They are cylindrical or spindle-shaped worms possessing a resistant cuticle, have a complete alimentary canal, lack a true coelom, sexes usually separate, development usually direct and simple.

nematode (nem′ă-tōd) [G. *nemat-,* thread, + *eidos,* like]. A member of the class Nematoda, *q.v.*

nematodiasis (nem″ă-to-di′ă-sis) [" + " + *iasis,* infection]. Infestation by a parasite belonging to the class Nematoda.

nematoid (nem′ă-toid). Threadlike, like a nematode.

nematology (nem″ă-tol′o-jĭ). The division of parasitology which deals with worms belonging to the class Nematoda.

nembutal (nem′bu-tal). Proprietary name for pentobarbital sodium. Used as a preanesthetic, sedative and hypnotic.

neo- [G.]. Combining form meaning *new* or *recent.*

neoarthrosis (nē″ō-ar-thrō′sĭs) [" + *arthron,* joint, + *-ōsis, increase, invasion*]. A false joint. SYN: *nearthrosis.*

neoblas′tic [" + *blastos,* germ]. Pert. to, or constituting, a new growth of tissue.

neocerebellum (nē″ō-sĕr-ĕ-bĕl′ŭm) [G. *neos,* new, + L. *cerebellum,* little brain]. The portion of the corpus cerebelli of the cerebellum which lies between the primary and prepyramidal fissures. Consists principally of the ansiform lobules. Phylogenetically it develops last in conjunction with cerebral cortex and is concerned with the integration of voluntary movements. The posterior lobe of the cerebellum.

neocinchophen (nē-ō-sĭn′kō-fĕn) [" + *cincophen*]. USP. A tasteless preparation of cinchophen and less likely to cause gastric irritation.

neocortex (nē″ō-kôr′tĕks). The neopallium, *q.v.*

neodiathermy (nē-ō-dī′ă-therm′ĭ). Short wave diathermy.

neodymium (ne″o-dim′e-um). A chemical element. SYMB: Nd. At. wt. 144.24; at. no. 60.

neofetus (nē-ō-fē′tŭs) [" + L. *foetus,* offspring]. Embryo during 8th and 9th week of intrauterine existence.

neoformation (nē″ō-for-mā′shŭn) [" + L. *formātiō,* a shaping]. 1. Regeneration. 2. A neoplasm or new growth.

neogala (ne-og′ă-lă) [" + *gala,* milk]. The first milk following childbirth. SEE: *colostrum.*

neogenesis (nē-ō-jĕn′ĕ-sĭs) [" + *genesis,* formation]. Regeneration or re-formation, as of tissue.

neogenetic (nē″ō-jĕn-ĕt′ĭk) [" + *genesis,* formation]. Newly formed; relating to new formations.

neohydrin (ne-o-hi′drin). Proprietary name for chlormerodrin, a diuretic.

neohymen (nē-ō-hī′mĕn) [" + *ymēn,* membrane]. A false or new membrane. SYN: *pseudomembrane.*

neologism (nē-ol′ō-jĭzm) [" + *logos,* study, + *ismos,* state]. 1. A new word or phrase, or a new meaning attached to an old word or phrase. 2. PSY: A mental condition in which the patient coins new words which are meaningless, or words to which he gives *special* significance without being aware of their normal significance. SEE: *lalopathy.*

neomembrane (nē-ō-mĕm′brān) [" + L. *membrana,* membrane]. A false or a new membrane. SYN: *neohymen.*

neomorph (nē′ō-mŏrf) [" + *morphē,* form]. BIOL: A new formation or development which is not inherited from a similar structure in an ancestor.

neomycin (nē″ō-mī′sĭn) [" + *mykes,* fungus]. An antibiotic from a species of *Streptomyces,* isolated from soil. Active against gram-positive and gram-negative bacteria, as well as streptomycin-resistant strains of *Mycobacterium tuberculosis.* Toxic to kidneys and eighth nerve, and affects hearing.

neon (nē′ŏn) [G. *neos,* new]. SYMB: Ne. An inert, gaseous element in the air derived from liquid argon. At. wt. 20.183; at. no. 10.

neonatal (nē″ō-nā′tăl) [G. *neos,* new, + L. *natāre,* to be born]. Concerning the first 4 weeks after birth.

neonate (ne′o-nāt). A newborn infant.

neopallium (nē″ō-păl′ĭ-ŭm) [G. *neos,* new, + L. *pallium,* cloak]. SYN: *neocortex, isocortex.* That portion of cerebral hemisphere not belonging to the rhinencephalon or corpus striatum, comprising most of the convoluted cortex and its associated white fibers.

Phylogenetically, it is the new part of the pallium.

neopathy (nē-ŏp′ă-thĭ) [" + *pathos,* disease]. 1. A newly found disease. 2. A new complication or new condition of a disease.

neophilism (nē-ŏf′ĭl-ĭzm) [" + *philein,* to love, + *ismos,* state]. Morbid love of novelty and new persons and scenes.

neophobia (nē″ō-fō′bĭ-ă) [" + *phobos,* fear]. Fear of new scenes or novelties; aversion to all that is unknown or not understood. SYN: *cainotophobia.*

neophrenia (nē″ō-frē′nĭ-ă) [" + *phrēn,* mind]. Mental deterioration or primary psychical failure in early youth.

neoplasia (nē″ō-plā′zĭ-ă) [" + *plassein,* to form]. The development of new tissues or neoplasms.

neoplasm (nē′ō-plăzm) [" + *plasma,* a thing formed]. A new and abnormal formation of tissue, as a tumor or growth.

It serves no useful function, but grows at the expense of the healthy organism.

n., benign. A growth not spreading by metastases or infiltration of tissue.

n., histoid. A n. in which structure resembles the tissues and elements which surround it.

n., malignant. A growth, such as cancer, that infiltrates tissue, metastasizes, and often recurs after removal.

n., mixed. A n. composed of tissues from two of the germinal layers.

n., multicentric. A growth arising from a number of distinct groups of cells.

n., organoid. A n. in which the structure is similar to some organ of the body.

n., unicentric. A growth having origin in one group of cells.

neoplastic (nē″ō-plas′tĭk) [G. *neos,* new, + *plastikos,* formed]. Pert. to, or of the nature of, new, abnormal tissue formation.

neoplasty (nē′ō-plăs-tĭ) [" + *plassein,* to form]. Surgical formation or restoration of parts.

neosalvarsan (nē″ō-săl′var-săn). A proprietary name for neoarsphenamine, *q.v.*

neostigmine (ne-o-stig′mēn). USP. A compound similar to physostigmine.

n. bromide. A preparation of neostigmine used for oral administration in the treatment of myasthenia gravis. Ophthalmic solution used for glaucoma.

n. methylsulfate. A preparation of neostigmine used for parenteral administration in treatment of myasthenia gravis.

neostomy (nē-os′tō-mĭ) [G. *neos,* new, + *stoma,* opening]. Formation of opening into an organ or bet. two organs.

neostriatum (nē″ō-strī-ā′tŭm) [G. *neos,* new, + L. *striatum,* grooved]. The caudate nucleus and the putamen considered together.

neo-synephrine hydrochloride (ne″o-sin-ef′rin). Proprietary name for phenylephrine hydrochloride.

nephelometer (nĕf-ĕl-om′ĕ-ter) [G. *nephelē,* mist, + *metron,* measure]. Apparatus for measuring the turbidity of a fluid.

nephelometry (nĕf-ĕl-ŏm′ĕ-trĭ) [" + *metron,* measure]. The employment of the nephelometer.

nephelopia (nĕf-el-ō′pĭ-ă) [" + *ōps,* eye]. Dim or cloudy vision from lessened transparency of the ocular media.

nephradenoma (nĕf-răd-ĕn-ō′mă) [G. *nephros,* kidney, + *adēn,* gland, + *-ōma,* tumor]. Renal adenoma.

nephralgia (nĕf-ral′jĭ-ă) [" + *algos,* pain]. Renal pain.

In absence of other symptoms, may alone be symptomatic of an obstructive renal process, but commonly presents a problem in differential diagnosis.

nephralgic (nĕf-răl′jĭk) [" + *algos,* pain]. Pert. to renal pain.

nephrapostasis (nĕf-ră-pos′tă-sĭs) [" + *apostasis,* suppuration]. Renal abscess or purulent inflammation of the kidney.

nephratony (nĕf-rat′ō-nĭ) [" + *a-,* priv. + *tonos,* tone]. Lack of normal renal tone. Same as *nephrotonia.*

nephrauxe (nĕf-rawks′ē) [" + *auxē,* increase]. Renal hypertrophy.

nephrectasia, nephrectasis, nephrectasy (nĕf-rĕk-ta′zĭ-ă, -rĕk′tă-sĭs, -tă-sĭ) [G. *nephros,* kidney, + *ektasis,* dilatation]. Distention of the kidney.

nephrectomy (nĕf-rek′tō-mĭ) [" + *ektomē,* excision]. Removal of a kidney.

ONP: Patient lies on the good side. Lower thigh is flexed to a right angle at hip and the knee is drawn up to same extent. Other lower limb goes straight down the table. Upper extremity in contact with the table is flexed at the elbow, while the arm lies a little on front at side of body. A kidney bridge or sandbag is placed under the loin. The procedure is routine.

The wound should be redraped after kidney is removed and instruments used in its removal discarded. Plenty of heavy drainage tubing, both of plain and cigarette types, should be ready.

NP: Patient should be kept on back without a pillow. Urine should be measured each day. Bland diet throughout illness. Dressing watched for signs of bleeding and changed often. Drainage tube left in for a few days, removed, and dressings changed. Stitches removed in 10-12 days.

COMPLICATIONS: Suppression of urine and secondary hemorrhage.

nephrelcosis (nĕf-rĕl-kō′sĭs) [" + *elkōsis,* ulceration]. Ulceration of the mucosa of the kidney.

nephrelcus (nĕf-rel′kŭs) [" + *elkos,* ulcer]. Renal ulcer.

nephremia (nĕf-rē′mĭ-ă) [" + *aima,* blood]. Congested state of kidney. SYN: *nephrohemia.*

nephremphraxis (nĕf″rem-fraks′is) [" + *emphraxis,* obstruction]. Obstruction in the renal vessels.

nephric (nĕf′rĭk) [G. *nephros,* kidney]. Pert. to the kidney or kidneys. SYN: *renal.*

nephrine (nef′rin) [G. *nephros,* kidney]. An amino acid derived from protein digestion. SYN: *cystine.*

nephrism (nĕf′rĭzm) [" + *ismos,* condition]. Aggregate of symptoms produced by chronic kidney disease.

nephritic (nĕf-rĭt′ĭk) [G. *nephros,* kidney]. 1. Rel. to the kidney. 2. Pert. to nephritis. 3. An agent used in nephritis.

nephritis (nē-frī′tĭs or nĕf-rī′tĭs) (pl. *nephritides*) [G. *nephros,* kidney, + *-itis,* inflammation]. Inflammation of the kidney.

ETIOL: Bacteria or their toxins, scarlet fever, diphtheria, septicemia, or toxic drugs, such as mercury, arsenic, alcohol. The glomeruli, tubules, or interstitial tissue, or all may be affected. It may be either acute or chronic.

RS: *arteriosclerosis, glomerulonephritis, kidney, nephrosis, nephrotic syndrome, pyelonephritis, nephroscleroses.*

n., acute. An inflammatory form involving the glomeruli, the tubules, or the entire kidney. It is of various types, depending on the portion of the kidney involved, degenerative, diffuse, suppurative, hemorrhagic, interstitial, and parenchymatous.

n., chronic. Progressive form in which entire structure of kidney may be affected, or affection may be confined to the glomerular or tubular processes. One variety of nephritis may merge with another, causing a diffuse nephritis. Symptoms depend upon the tissues involved.

n., diffuse, acute. An inflammatory process involving more or less the entire kidney.

SYM: Acute onset; moderate fever; dull lumbar pain; marked edema and anasarca; hypertension; rapid pulse; vomiting; delirium; scanty, highly colored urine, containing large quantities of albumin and blood; bloody, hyaline and granular casts; uremic symptoms may develop.

PROG: Poor. May become chronic or death through exhaustive uremia or dropsy.

TREATMENT: Absolute rest in bed until albumin has disappeared. Severe cases in pregnancy may require therapeutic abortion or induction of premature labor.

DIET: Milk, buttermilk, citrus fruit juices; later, cereals, fruits, vegetables. Cream and sugar allowed. Limit proteins, salt and fluids.

n., d., chronic. SEE: *interstitial n., chronic.*

n., focal. N. with foci of inflammation distributed throughout the kidney.

n., glomerular. A form involving the renal glomeruli. It may be acute or chronic. SEE: *glomerulonephritis.*

n., g., acute. Acute form in which the pulse is rapid, and hypertension, edema and urine containing albumin, blood and casts are present. There is retention of urea and salt.

n., g., chronic. Form almost always following acute glomerular n. It is marked by hyalinization of the glomeruli, arteriosclerosis, hypertension, albuminuria, edema, and later uremic symptoms. Usually fatal. SEE: *glomerulonephritis, chronic.*

n., g., focal, embolic. N. in which emboli lodge in the capillary loops of the glomeruli, occluding them.

ETIOL: Subacute bacterial endocarditis due to *Streptococcus viridans.*

Glomerulus becomes hyalinized and there is blood in the lumen of tubules. Marked by blood, albumen, and hyaline and granular casts in urine. There is no edema or hypertension. TREATMENT: That of endocarditis.

n., g., f., nonembolic. N. in which not all of the glomeruli are affected and those affected are not equally so.

ETIOL: Streptococcus infections.

Marked by blood, albumin, erythrocytes, leukocytes, and granular and hyaline casts in the urine. Lumbar pain and slightly painful urination. Edema and hypertension absent. TREATMENT: Removal of the etiologic disease.

n., hemorrhagic. Acute n. with tubular hemorrhage and subsequent hematuria.

n., idiopathic. N. of unknown etiology.

n., indurative. Chronic n. marked by atrophy of the renal secreting structure and enlargement of the connective tissue stroma.

n., interstitial, acute. Rare form of acute n. in which there occur areas of cellular infiltration irregularly distributed bet. the tubules and around the glomeruli. SEE: *n., glomerular, focal, nonembolic,* for symptoms and treatment.

n., i., chronic. Glomeruli and interstitial tissue involved.

ETIOL: May follow parenchymatous n., alcoholism, lead poisoning, irritating toxins, bacterial infection, syphilis.

SYM: Headache, weakness, digestive disturbances, retinal hemorrhages and eye disturbances, dry skin. Vasomotor disturbances, such as tingling in fingers, with blanching. Hypertension marked. Low sp. gr. of urine, the quantity of which is considerable; as much by night as by day. Trace of albumin, few narrow hyaline casts, and sometimes granular casts. Retention of urea, uric acid, creatinine and protein waste products in blood.

NP: Rest and general hygienic care. Observe diet strictly, care for skin. Treat symptoms as they arise.

n., lipomatous. Fatty infiltration of the renal parenchyma. SYN: *lipomatosis renis.*

n., parynchmatous, acute. Acute glomerular nephritis with associated changes in tubules.

n., p., chronic. Chronic glomerular nephritis (*q.v.*) with associated changes in renal tubules.

n., saturnine. N. from lead poisoning.

n., suppurative. Purulent form of n.

n., s., acute. Purulent form with abscess formation.

n., s., chronic. Cheesy and tubercular form of n.

n., tubal, n., tubular. N. affecting the renal tubules with little change in glomerular structure.

n., tuberculous. N. due to presence of tubercle bacilli.

nephro- [G.]. Prefix: Pert. to the kidney.

nephroabdominal (něf″rō-ăb-dom′ĭ-năl) [G. *nephros,* kidney, + L. *abdominalis,* pert. to abdomen]. Concerning the kidney and abdomen.

nephrocalcinosis (něf-rō″kăl″sĭn-ō′sĭs). Calcinosis of the kidney characterized by deposits of calcium phosphate in renal tubules.

nephrocapsectomy (něf″rō-kăp-sek′tō-mĭ) [" + L. *capsula,* capsule, + G. *ektomē,* excision]. Renal decapsulation.

nephrocardiac (něf″rō-kar′dĭ-ăk) [" + *kardia,* heart]. Concerning the heart and kidney.

nephrocele (něf′rō-sēl) [" + *kēlē,* hernia]. 1. Renal hernia. 2. Embryonic cavity of a nephrotome.

nephrocolic (něf″rō-kŏl′ĭk) [" + *kōlikos,* pert. to colon]. 1. Severe, colicky pain in ureter due to passage of stone. 2. Concerning the colon and kidney.

nephrocolopexy (něf″rō-kŏl′ō-pěks″ĭ) [" + *kōlon,* colon, + *pēxis,* fixation]. Surgical suspension of kidney and colon using the nephrocolic ligament.

nephrocoloptosis (něf″rō-kō-lŏp-tō′sĭs) [" + " + *ptōsis,* a dropping]. Condition in which the kidney and colon are displaced downward.

nephrocystanastomosis (něf″rō-sĭst-ăn-ăs″-to-mō′sĭs) [" + *kystis,* bladder, + *anastomōsis,* outlet]. Surgical formation of a connection bet. kidney and the bladder, in permanent ureteral obstruction.

nephrocystitis (něf″rō-sĭs-tī′tĭs) [G. *nephros,* kidney, + *kystis,* a bladder, + *-itis,* inflammation]. Inflamed condition of kidneys and bladder.

nephrogenetic, nephrogenic, nephrogenous (něf″rō-jěn-ět′ĭk, -jěn′ĭk, -rŏ′jěn-ŭs) [G. *nephros,* kidney, + *gennan,* to develop]. Arising in or from the renal organs; capable of giving rise to kidney tissue.

n. cord. The intermediate mesoderm, *q.v.*

nephrohydrosis (něf″rō-hī-drō′sĭs) [" + *ydōr,* water, + *-ōsis*]. Accumulation of urine in renal pelvis and calyces due to obstruction.

nephrohypertrophy (něf″rō-hī-pěr′trō-fĭ) [" + *yper,* over, + *trophē,* nourishment]. Overgrowth or dilatation of the kidneys.

nephroid (něf′roid) [" + *eidos,* resembling]. Resembling a kidney; kidney-shaped. SYN: *reniform.*

nephrolith (něf′rō-lĭth) [" + *lithos,* stone]. Stone in the kidney.

nephrolithiasis (něf″rō-lĭth-ī′ă-sĭs) [G. *nephros,* kidney, + *lithos,* stone]. The formation of renal stones. SYN: *lithiasis nephritica, lithiasis renalis.* SEE: *calculus, renal.*

nephrolithotomy (něf″rō-lĭth-ot′ō-mĭ) [" + " + *tomē,* incision]. Renal incision for removal of calculus.

nephrology (nĕf-rŏl′ō-jĭ) [" + *logos*, study]. Science of the structure and function of the kidney.

nephrolysis (nĕf-rol′ĭs-ĭs) [" + *lysis*, loosening]. 1. Surgical detachment of an inflamed kidney from adhesions. 2. Destruction of kidney tissue by action of a nephrotoxin.

nephroma (nĕf-rō′mă) [" + *-ōma*, tumor]. Renal tumor or one of renal tissue.

nephromalacia (nĕf″rō-mă-lā′sĭ-ă) [" + *malakia*, softening]. Abnormal renal softness or softening.

nephromegaly (nĕf″rō-mĕg′ă-lĭ) [" + *megas, megal-*, large]. Extreme enlargement of one or both kidneys.

nephromere (nĕf′rō-mēr) [G. *nephros*, kidney, + *meros*, part]. SYN: *nephrotome.* Segment in embryo from which kidney develops. The intermediate mesoderm in an embryo from which the kidney develops.

nephron (nĕf′ron) [G. *nephros*, kidney]. SYN: *renal tubule, uriniferous tubule.* The structural and functional unit of the kidney, consisting of a *renal (malpighian) corpuscle* (a glomerulus enclosed within Bowman's capsule) and its attached tubule consisting of the *proximal convoluted portion, loop of Henle,* and *distal convoluted portion* which connects by arched collecting tubules with straight collecting tubules. Urine is formed by filtration in renal corpuscle and selective reabsorption and secretion by cells of the renal tubule. There are approximately one million nephrons in each kidney. SEE: *kidney, malpighian corpuscle, urine.*

nephroncus (nĕf-rŏn′kŭs) [" + *ogkos*, tumor]. A renal tumor.

nephroparalysis (nĕf″rō-păr-ăl′ĭ-sis) [" + *paralysis*, a loosening]. Paralyzed renal function.

nephropathy (nĕf-rop′ă-thĭ) [" + *pathos*, disease]. Disease of the kidney.

This term includes inflammatory (nephritis), degenerative (nephrosis), and sclerotic (arteriosclerotic) lesions of the kidney.

nephropexy (nĕf′rō-pĕks-ĭ) [" + *pēxis*, fixation]. Surgical attachment of a floating kidney.

nephrophthisis (nĕf-rŏf′thĭs-ĭs) [" + *phthisis*, a wasting]. 1. Tuberculosis of the kidney, with caseous degeneration. 2. Suppurative nephritis with wasting of the kidney substance.

nephroptosis (nĕf-rŏp-tō′sĭs) [" + *ptōsis*, a dropping]. Prolapse or downward kidney displacement.

ETIOL: Shape of lumbar recess, preg-

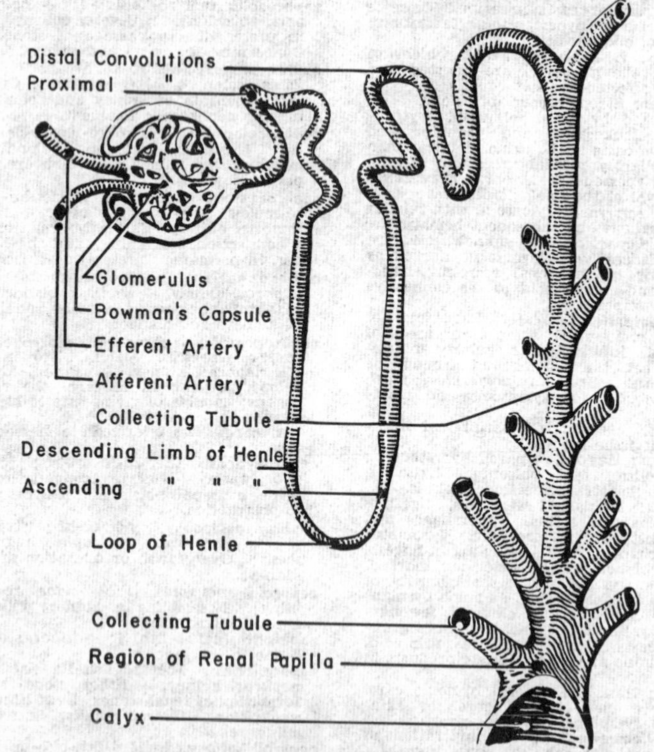

NEPHRON UNIT

(From Rossomando, A. H., and Miles, F. M.: Urological Nursing Manual.)

nancy, emaciation, enteroptosis are predisposing factors.

SYM: (1) None. (2) Symptoms not referable to kidney (nervous and digestive disorders or pain). (3) Painful paroxysms simulating renal colic; albuminuria; painful, scanty and frequent micturition.

TREATMENT: Bed rest, truss, surgery. SEE: *nephrectomy, nephropexy.*

nephropyelitis (něf″rō-pī-ěl-ī′tĭs) [G. *nephros,* kidney, + *pyelos,* pelvis, + *-itis,* inflammation]. SYN: *pyelonephritis.* Inflammation of the renal pelvis and parenchyma of kidney.

nephropyosis (něf″rō-pī-o′sĭs) [" + *piōsis,* suppuration]. Purulence of a kidney.

nephrorrhagia (něf-ror-ā′jĭ-ă) [" + *rēgnunai,* to burst forth]. Renal hemorrhage into pelvis and tubules.

nephrorrhaphy (něf-ror′ă-fĭ) [" + *raphe,* a stitch]. Suture of a floating kidney to the post. wall of the abdomen.

nephros (něf′rŏs). The kidney.

nephrosclerosis (něf″rō-sklě-ro′sĭs) [" + *sklērōsis,* a hardening]. Renal sclerosis or hardening. SEE: *nephritis, chronic interstitial.*

n., arterial. Arteriosclerosis of kidney arteries. Results in ischemia, atrophy of parenchyma, and fibrosis of kidney.

n., arteriolar. Sclerosis of the smaller renal arterioles, esp. the afferent glomerular arterioles with resulting fibrosis, ischemic necrosis and glomerular degeneration and failure. Occurs in most cases of essential hypertension.

n. malignant. N. which develops rapidly in patients with severe hypertension. SEE: *hypertension, malignant.*

nephrosis (nē-frō′sĭs) [G. *nephros,* kidney]. Condition in which there are degenerative changes in the kidneys without the occurrence of inflammation.

n., acute. N. accompanying acute infectious disease or resulting from poisoning or metabolic disturbances such as toxemias of pregnancy or obstructive jaundice.

n., amyloid. N. due to deposition of amyloid within the walls of the renal blood vessels and at the base of the cells of the tubules. Marked degeneration of kidney tissue results.

n., lipoid. A chronic disease of unknown etiology in which large amounts of albumin are lost in urine, resulting in depletion of the plasma protein and development of nephrotic edema.

It is probably due to disordered metabolism. Occurs mainly in children and young adults.

SYM: Gradual development of edema, which reaches a high degree. Oliguria, albumin, casts of hyaline and granular type and lipids in urine. Blood serum proteins markedly reduced, but nitrogenous constituents remain normal. Blood cholesterol and globulin elevated. Hypertension absent. Anemia occurs.

PROG: Guarded.

TREATMENT: Prolonged bed rest is not required. High-protein and low-sodium diet, cortisone may help.

nephrostoma, nephrostome (nē-fros′tō-mă, něf′ros-tōm) [G. *nephros,* kidney, + *stoma,* mouth]. The internal orifice of a Wolffian tubule, connected with the celom in the human embryo.

nephrostomy (něf-ros′to-mĭ) [" + *stoma,* mouth]. Formation of an artificial fistula into the renal pelvis.

nephrotic (něf-rot′ĭk) [G. *nephros,* kidney]. Rel. to, or caused by, nephrosis.

n. syndrome. Term applied to renal disease of whatever cause, characterized by massive edema, proteinuria and usually elevation of serum cholesterol and lipids.

nephrotome (něf′rō-tōm) [G. *nephros,* kidney, + *tome,* a section]. SYN: *intermediate cell mass, mesomere, nephromere.* Embryonic bridge of cells, connecting primitive segments along neural tube to the somatic and splanchnic mesoderm from which arises the urogenital system.

nephrotoxin (něf″rō-tŏks′ĭn) [" + *toxikon,* poison]. A specific toxin which destroys renal cells.

nephrotresis (něf-rō-trē′sis) [" + *trēsis,* piercing]. Formation of a permanent excretory opening in the kidney through the loin.

nephroureterectomy (nef″rō-ū-rē″tĕr-ĕk′tō-mĭ) [" + *ourētēr,* ureter, + *ektomē,* excision]. Surgical excision of kidney with the ureter or part of it.

nephrydrosis (něf-ri-drō′sĭs) [" + *ydōr,* water, + *-ōsis*]. Water collected in the renal pelvis due to obstruction. SYN: *hydronephrosis, nephrohydrosis.*

Nep′tune gir′dle. Compress of linen covered by flannel which encircles the trunk from lower end of sternum to the pubes. Used in applying wet packs, esp. cold.

NP: Linen wrung out of water the temperature of which should be between 42° and 50° F. Linen changed when necessary to maintain this temperature. Cover with blanket. Patient should first be given a foot bath of 104°-110° F. for 5 minutes with cold compress over forehead. Girdle to remain on 1-6 hr. Forehead compress to remain during treatment.

neptun′ium. An element obtained by bombarding uranium with neutrons. At. wt. 237; at. no. 93. SYMB: Np.

nerve (nerv) [L. *nervus,* sinew; probably from G. *neuron,* sinew]. A bundle or a group of bundles of nerve fibers outside the central nervous system which connects the brain and spinal cord with various parts of the body. Nerves conduct *afferent* impulses centrally from receptor organs and *efferent* impulses peripherally to effector organs. The fibers of peripheral nerves are the processes of neurons whose cell bodies are located within the brain, spinal cord, or in ganglia.

A bundle of nerve fibers is called a *fasciculus.* The fibers within a fasciculus are surrounded and held together by delicate connective tissue fibers forming the *endoneurium.* Each fasciculus is surrounded by a sheath of connective tissue, the *perineurium.* The entire nerve is enclosed in a thick sheath of connective tissue, the *epineurium* which may contain numerous fat cells. Small nerves may lack an epineurium.

n., accelerator. N. to the heart carrying sympathetic fibers conveying impulses which accelerate the heart beat.

n., afferent. One which transmits impulses from the periphery to a nerve center.

n., autonomic. A n. of the autonomic nervous system.

n. block. The induction of regional anesthesia by preventing sensory nerve impulses from reaching centers of consciousness. Accomplished by injecting an anesthetic solution (Ex: procaine) about the nerve some distance from the region or by anesthetizing nerve endings in the region itself (*infiltration*).

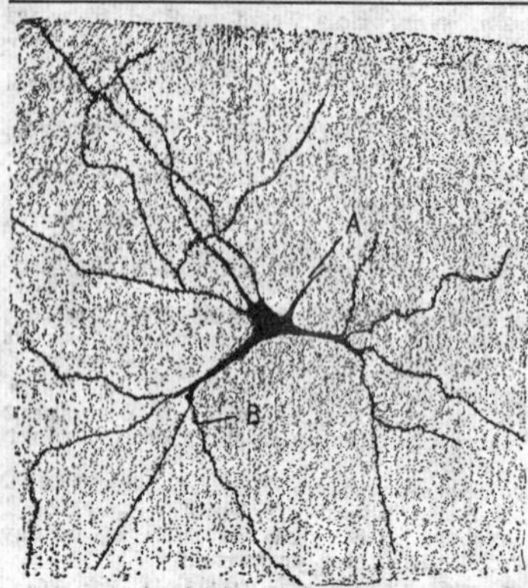

NERVE CELL FROM CEREBRAL CORTEX.

A. Axis cylinder, directed towards periphery. B. Dendrites.

n. cell. A neuron, *q.v.*

n., cerebrospinal. A n. originating from the brain or spinal cord.

n., cranial. One of the 12 pairs of nerves arising from the brain and making its exit through a foramen of the cranium.

n., depressor. Any afferent n. which when stimulated depresses the activity of an organ or nerve center.

n., efferent. One transmitting impulses from a nerve center to the periphery.

n. ending. The termination of a nerve fiber (axon or dendrite) in a peripheral structure. May be *sensory* (receptor) or *motor* (effector). Sensory endings are (a) *nonencapsulated* (Ex: free nerve endings, peritrichal endings, tactile corpuscles of Merkel) or (b) *encapsulated* (Ex: end-bulbs of Krause, Meissner's corpuscles, Vater-Pacini corpuscles, Golgi-Mazzoni corpuscles, neuromuscular and neurotendinous spindles).

n., excitatory. N. transmitting impulses which stimulate function.

n. fiber. SEE: *nerve fiber(s)* (separate entry following *nerve*).

n. fibril. A fine fiber in the cytoplasm and cell processes of a neuron. SYN: *neurofibrilla.*

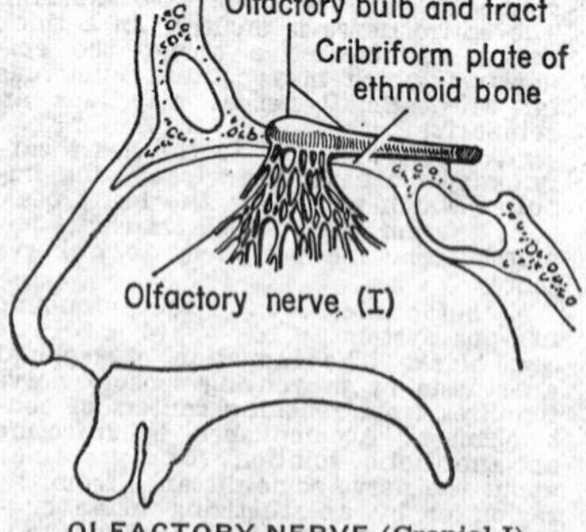

OLFACTORY NERVE (Cranial I)

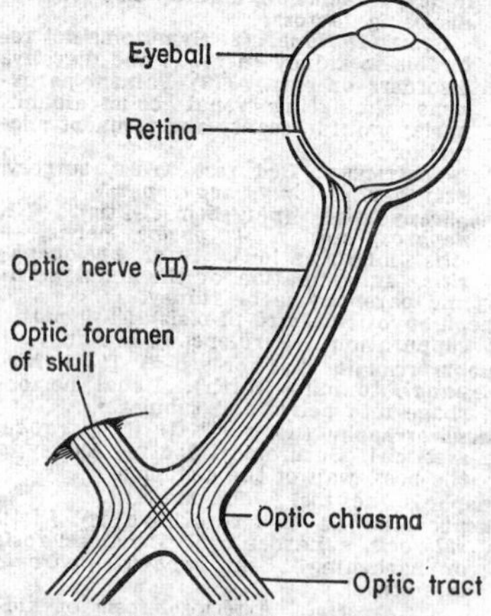

OPTIC NERVE (Cranial II)

n., frigorific. A sympathetic n. causing a lowering in temperature on stimulation.

n. impulse. Name for the excitatory process which travels along a nerve fiber when stimulated.

n., inhibitory. One which, upon stimulation, lessens activity in a part.

n., mixed. One containing both afferent (sensory) and efferent (motor) fibers.

n., motor. One containing motor fibers and conveying motor impulses. SYN. *efferent n.*

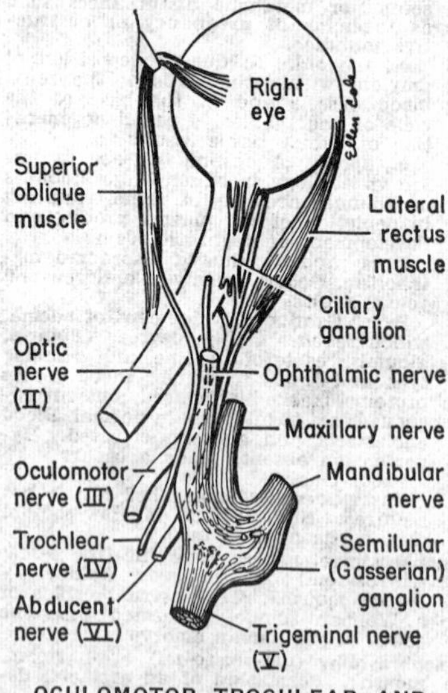

OCULOMOTOR, TROCHLEAR, AND ABDUCENT NERVES (Cranial III, IV and VI)

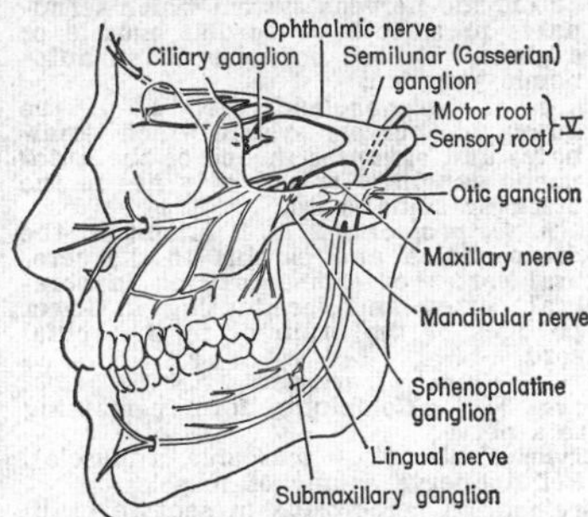

LEFT TRIGEMINAL NERVE (Cranial V)

n., parasympathetic. A n. of the parasympathetic division of the autonomic nervous system.

n., peripheral. Any nerve which connects the brain or spinal cord with peripheral receptors or effectors.

n., pilomotor. A nerve which innervates the arrectores pilorum muscles of hair follicles.

n. plexus. A group of nerves intertwined.

n., pressor. An afferent n. which when stimulated excites the vasoconstrictor center thus increasing blood pressure.

n., secretory. N. whose stimulation excites secretion in a part.

n., sensory. A nerve which conducts afferent impulses from sensory receptors to the brain or spinal cord.

n., somatic. A n. which innervates somatic structures, *i. e.,* those comprising the body wall and extremities.

n., spinal. One of 31 pairs of nerves which connect with the spinal cord. Includes 8 cervical, 12 thoracic, 5 lumbar, 5 sacral, 1 coccygeal.

n., sympathetic. N. of the sympathetic division of the autonomic nervous system. SEE: *autonomic nervous system.*

n. trunk. The main stem of a peripheral nerve.

n., vasoconstrictor. A n. which conducts impulses which bring about constriction of a blood vessel.

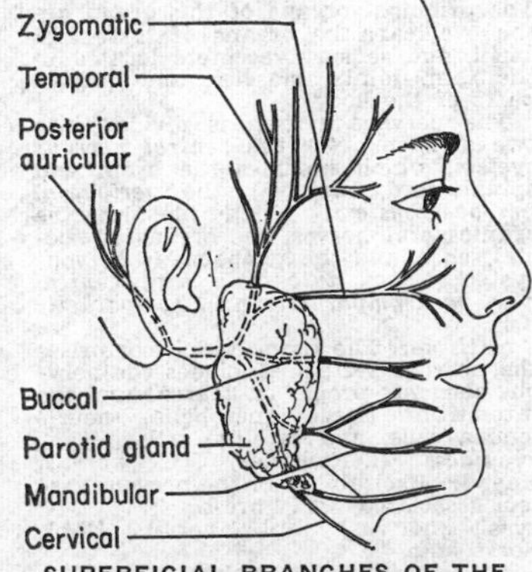

SUPERFICIAL BRANCHES OF THE FACIAL NERVE (Cranial VII)

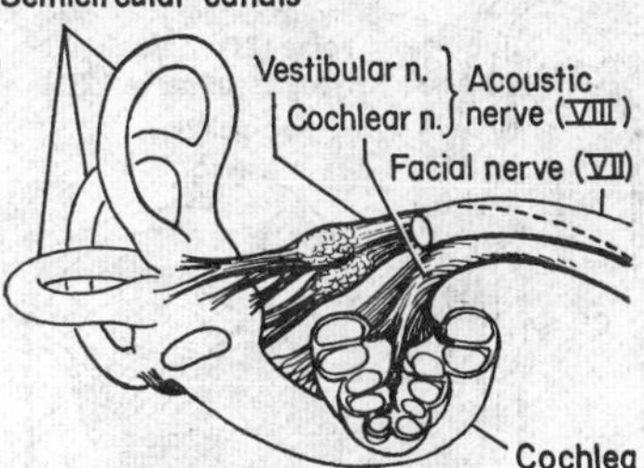

RIGHT ACOUSTIC NERVE (Cranial VIII), front view

n., vasodilator. A n. which conducts impulses which bring about dilation of a blood vessel.

n., vasomotor. N. which controls the caliber of a blood vessel. A vasoconstrictor or vasodilator nerve, *q.v.*

nerve fiber(s). An elongated process of a nerve cell or neuron, usually the axon, concerned primarily with the conduction of impulses. Nerve fibers form the major portion of the white matter of the brain and spinal cord and all nerves. Most fibers in periph-

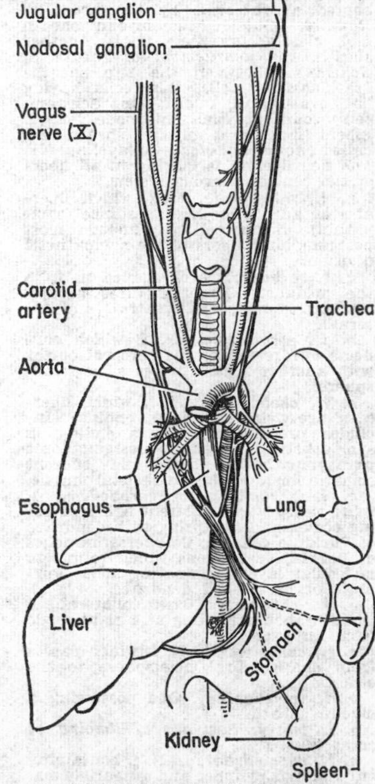

VAGUS NERVE (Cranial X)

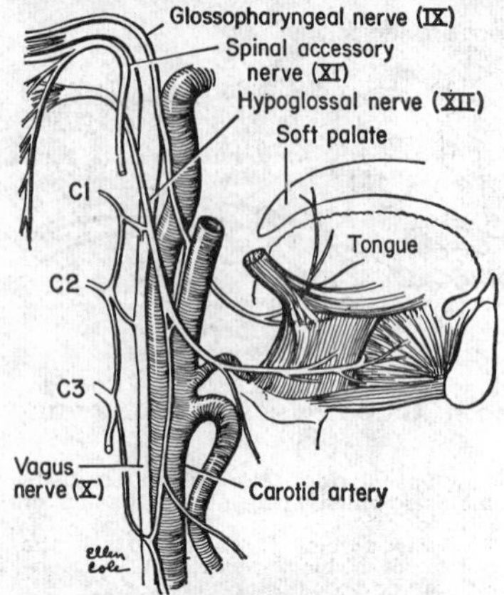

RIGHT GLOSSOPHARYNGEAL, SPINAL ACCESSORY, AND HYPOGLOSSAL NERVES (Cranial IX, XI, XII)

eral nerves are *myelinated* (*medullated, i. e.,* they are covered by an noncellular sheath of myelin, a fatty substance). The myelin sheath is interrupted at intervals by the *nodes of Ranvier*. Outside the myelin sheath and closely investing it is another sheath, the *neurilemma* or *sheath of Schwann*. Between the two sheaths are *Schwann cells,* thin cells having flat, oval-shaped nuclei. One Schwann cell occurs at each internode length. Fibers lacking a myelin sheath are called *nonmedullated* (*unmyelinated*). The neurilemma is lacking in all fibers of the central nervous system.

n. f., adrenergic. N. f. which liberates an adrenaline-like substance (sympathin) at its ending. Include most postganglionic fibers of the sympathetic division.

n. f., arcuate. Arch-shaped n. f. in the medulla. Comprise three groups, the ext. dorsal, ext. ventral, and internal.

n. f., association. N. f. which connects one region of the cerebral cortex with another region in the same hemisphere.

n. f., cholinergic. N. f. which liberates acetylcholine at its ending. Includes preganglionic fibers ending in sympathetic ganglia, postganglionic parasympathetic fibers, and efferent somatic fibers ending in skeletal muscle.

n. f.'s, climbing, of cerebellum. 1. SYN: *mossy fibers.* Afferent n. f.'s entering cortex and synapsing with dendrites of Purkinje cells. 2. Collateral branches of Purkinje cell axons which return to molecular layer terminating about Purkinje or basket-cell dendrites.

n. f., collateral. SYN: collateral. A small branch extending at a right angle from an axon.

n. f., commissural. N. f. which passes from one cerebral hemisphere to the other.

n. f., myelinated. One possessing a myelin sheath.

n. f., mossy. SEE: *n. f.'s, climbing, of cerebellum.*

n. f., nonmedullated. N. f. containing only an axis cylinder and a neurilemma.

n. f., postganglionic. N. f. of the autonomic nervous system which terminates in smooth or cardiac muscle or a gland. Its cell body lies in an autonomic ganglion.

n. f., preganglionic. N. f. of the autonomic nervous system which terminates and synapses in one of the autonomic ganglia. Its cell body lies in the brain or spinal cord.

n. f., projection. N. f. arising in the diencephalon and passing to the cerebral cortex or a fiber arising in cerebral cortex and terminating in lower portions of the brain or in the spinal cord.

nervi. Plural of *nervus.*

nervo- [L.]. Combining form pertaining to a nerve.

nervomus'cular [" + *musculus,* a muscle]. Rel. to nerve supply of muscles.

nerv'one. A cerebroside present in brain tissue; contains nervonic acid.

nervosism (ner'vō-sĭzm) [" + G. *ismos,* state of]. 1. Neurasthenia or nervousness. 2. The idea that morbid conditions depend upon alterations of nerve force.

nervosity. Nervosism (1), *q.v.*

nervous (ner'vus) [L. *nervus,* sinew]. 1. Characterized by instability of nerve action; excitability. 2. Pert. to the nerves.

n. debility. Nervous fatigue with resultant physical exhaustion. SYN: *neurasthenia.*

n. exhaustion. SEE: *nervous debility.*

n. impulse. The excitatory process set up in nerve fibers by stimuli.

It is probably in the nature of a wave of electrochemical disturbance traveling at the comparatively slow rate (even in fastest conducting mammalian nerves) of 50-80 meters per second. The velocity varies in different fibers according to the diameter.

n. prostration. SEE: *nervous debility.*

n. system. A system of extremely delicate nerve cells, elaborately interlaced with each other, collectively consisting of the brain, cranial nerves, spinal cord, spinal nerves, autonomic ganglia, ganglionated trunks and nerves, maintaining the vital function of reception and response to stimuli.

The nervous system regulates and coordinates bodily activities and brings about responses by which the body adjusts to changes of environment, either external or internal. These changes constitute *stimuli* which initiate impulses in receptors or sense organs. The principal organs of this group are the eye, ear, the organs of taste and smell, and sensory receptors located in the skin, joints, muscles, and various parts of the body.

The nervous system is divided into two divisions: (1) the *central nervous system,* which includes the brain and spinal cord, and (2) the *peripheral nervous system,* which includes the craniosacral nerves, the organs of special sense, and the sympathetic nervous system. SEE: *autonomic n.s., central n.s., parasympathetic n.s., sympathetic n.s.*

n. tissue. The tissue which comprises the nervous system. Includes the nervous elements proper or *neurons* and the interstitial tissue (neuroglia, neurilemma cells, and satellite cells).

nervousness (nĕr'vŭs-nĕs) [L. *nervus,* sinew]. Excitability of the nervous system associated with unrest.

nervus (ner'vus) (pl. *nervi*). [NA]. Nerve, *q.v.*

n. erigens. The pelvic nerve. A scattered bundle of craniosacral autonomic fibers originating from the 2nd to 4th sacral nerves and passing to terminal ganglia from which postganglionic fibers pass to the pelvic organs (bladder, colon, rectum, prostate gland, seminal vesicles, ext. genitalia).

n. intermedius. The pars intermedia (intermediate nerve of Wrisberg), a branch of the facial nerve consisting principally of sensory fibers.

n. nervorum. Nerve fibers which innervate sheaths of nerves.

n. terminalis. The terminal nerve, a small nerve accompanying the olfactory nerve to the brain. Consists principally of sensory fibers from mucosa of nasal septum.

n. vasorum. Nerve fibers which innervate the walls of blood vessels.

nest, cell. A small mass of epithelial cells set apart from surrounding cells by connective tissue.

nes'tis [G. *nēstis,* fasting]. Obsolete name for jejunum.

nestither'apy [G. *nēstis,* fasting, + *therapeia,* treatment]. Use of fasting or low calorie diet therapeutically.

n. et m. Abbr. for *nocte et mane,* night and morning.

ne tr. s. num. Abbr. for *ne tradas sine nummo,* do not deliver unless paid.

net'tle rash. Skin rash with intense itching, resembling condition produced by stinging with nettles. Syn: *hives, urticaria.*

net'work [A.S. *net,* net, + *wyrcan,* to work]. Fiber arrangement in a structure resembling a net. Syn: *rete, reticulum.*

Neumann's disease (noi'mănz) [Isidor Neumann, Viennese dermatologist, 1832-1906]. Pemphigus vegetans, *q.v.*

neuragmia (nū-răg'mĭ-ă) [G. *neuron,* sinew, + *agmos,* break]. The tearing or rupturing of a nerve trunk.

neural (nū'răl) [G. *neuron,* sinew]. Pert. to nerves or connected with the nervous system.

n. crest. A band of cells extending longitudinally along the neural tube of an embryo from which cells forming cranial, spinal, and autonomic ganglia arise.

n. fold. One of two longitudinal elevations of the neural plate of an embryo which unite to form the neural tube.

n. plate. A thickened band of ectoderm along the dorsal surface of an embryo, from which the nervous system develops.

n. spine. Spinous vertebral process.

n. tube. Tube formed from fusion of the neural folds from which the brain and spinal cord arise.

neuralgia (nū-ral'jĭ-ă) [" + *algos,* pain]. Severe, lancinating pain along the course of a nerve.

Etiol: Pressure on nerve trunks, faulty nerve nutrition, toxins, neuritis. Usually no morphologic changes can be detected.

Sym: According to the part affected. See: *geniculate, sciatica.*

n., cardiac. Angina pectoris.

n., degenerative. N. caused by degenerative changes in the nerves or nerve cells.

n., epileptiform. Spasmodic facial n. Syn: *tic douloureux.*

n., facial. See: *n., trigeminal.*

n., facialis vera. Geniculate n.

n., Fothergill's. Trigeminal n.

n., geniculate. N. characterized by pain over all or any part supplied by sensory fibers of facial nerve. Pain may be deep in facial muscles, within the ear, or in pharynx. Syn: *herpes zoster auricularis; herpes zoster oticus; Hunt neuralgia or syndrome; Ramsay-Hunt syndrome.*

n., glossopharyngeal. N. along the course of the glossopharyngeal nerve characterized by severe pain in back of throat, tonsils, and middle ear.

n., hallucinatory. Impression of local pain without actual peripheral pain.

n., Hunt's. Geniculate n.

n., idiopathic. N. without structural lesion or pressure from a lesion.

n., intercostal. Pain follows course of intercostal nerves; frequently associated with eruption of herpes zoster; spots of tenderness near vertebral column, in middle of nerve, and near sternum. May be dependent upon spinal caries, or thoracic aneurysm.

n., mammary. N. of the breast. Syn: *mastodynia.*

n., Morton's. N. of joint of 3rd and 4th toes. Syn: *metatarsalgia.*

n., nasociliary. N. of eyes, brows and root of nose.

n., occipital. Involves upper cervical nerves. A spot of tenderness found bet. mastoid process and upper cervical vertebrae. May be due to spinal caries.

n., otic. Geniculate n.

n., reminiscent. Continued mental impression of pain after n. has ceased.

n. (of) sphenopalatine ganglion. Syn: *Sluder's n.* Sym: Pain on one side of face, radiating to eyeballs, ear, occipital and mastoid areas of skull; sometimes to nose, upper teeth and shoulder of same side. Prog: good.

n., stump. Pressure on nerves in stump after amputation, causing pain.

n., symptomatic. N. not primarily involving the nerve structure.

n., trifacial. Old term for trigeminal neuralgia, *q.v.*

n., trigeminal. N. involving the gasserian ganglion or one or more branches of the trigeminal nerve.

Etiol: Unknown. Attacks often precipitated by contact with certain hypersensitive areas called *trigger zones* on face, lips, or tongue.

Sym: Tender points correspond to supraorbital, infraorbital, and mental foramina. Often violent spasm of muscles. In long standing cases hair on affected side sometimes becomes coarse and bleached.

Prog: Good.

Treatment: Alcohol injection or cutting of the nerve. Symptomatic treatment may permit spontaneous remission to occur.

Syn: *tic douloureux; Fothergill disease.*

neuralgic (nū-ral'jĭk) [G. *neuron,* sinew or nerve, + *algos,* pain]. Of, or concerning, neuralgia.

neuramebimeter (nu"răm-ē-bĭm'ĕt-ĕr) [" + *amoibē,* response, + *metron,* a measure]. Device for determining time of response of a nerve to a stimulus.

neurapophysis (nū-ră-pof'ĭ-sĭs) [G. *neuron,* sinew, + *apo,* from, + *physis,* growth]. Either of the two sides of a vertebra which unite to form the neural arch.

neurapraxia (nū-ră-prăks'ĭ-ă). Cessation in function of a peripheral nerve without degenerative changes occurring. Recovery is the usual outcome.

neurasthenia (nū-răs-thē'nĭ-ă) [G. *neuron,* sinew, + *astheneia,* weakness]. An ill-defined disease commonly following depressed states characterized by a sense of weakness or exhaustion, or by the symptoms of various types of organic disease without the existence of organic disease in a degree sufficient to justify the subjective complaints of the patient.

SYM: Fatigue; weakness; headache; sweating; polyuria; tinnitus and vertigo; photophobia; fear; easy exhaustion on the slightest effort; inability to concentrate; irritability and complaint of poor memory; poor sleep; numerous, constantly varying aches and pains; vasomotor disturbances.

The neurasthenic is often physically asthenic with a long, narrow thorax, small muscles and undernourished. The face is thin, alert, and often suggests chronic suffering. Much of this is the result of the neurasthenia, but it suggests also a physical type, inherently predisposed to develop the disease.

Freud believes the disease is probably a frustration (esp. sexual) which possibly complicates the symptoms by an element of renunciation as well.

PROG: Favorable, if cause can be removed.

TREATMENT: Attempt to determine cause. If no specific illness such as anemia or chronic infection can be discovered, then intensive psychotherapy is indicated.

neurastheniac, neurasthenic (nū-răs-thē′nĭ-ăk, -nĭk) [G. *neuron,* sinew, + *astheneia,* weakness]. 1. Suffering from or concerning neurasthenia. 2. Individual suffering from neurasthenia.

neuratrophia, neuratrophy (nū-ră-trō′fĭ-ă, -răt′rō-fĭ) [" + *atrophia,* a wasting]. Atrophy of the nervous tissue or deficient nutrition of the nervous system.

neuraxitis (nū-răks-ī′tĭs) [" + *axon,* axis, + *-itis,* inflammation]. 1. Inflamed condition of a neuraxis. 2. Encephalitis.

n., epidemic. Epidemic encephalitis.

neuraxon(e (nū-răks′ŏn) [" + *axon,* axis]. The axis cylinder process of a nerve cell. SYN: *axon.* SEE: *nerve fiber.*

neurectasy, neurectasia, neurectasis (nū-rĕk′ta-sĭ, -rĕk-tā′zĭ-ă, -rĕk′ta-sĭs) [" + *ektasis,* a stretching]. Surgical nerve stretching.

neurectomy (nū-rĕk′tō-mĭ) [" + *ektomē,* excision]. Partial or total excision or resection of a nerve.

neurectopia, neurectopy (nū-rĕk-tō′pĭ-ă, nūr-ek′tō-pĭ) [" + *ek,* out, + *topos,* place]. Displacement or abnormal position of a nerve.

neurenteric (ū-rĕn-ter′ĭk) [G. *neuron,* sinew, + *enteron,* intestine]. Rel. to the neural canal and intestinal tube of the embryo.

n. canal. Temporary canal of the embryo between the neural and intestinal tubes. In human development, the temporary communication between cavities of the yolk sac and the amnion.

neurepithelium (nur″ep-ĭ-the′lĭ-ŭm) [" + *epi,* upon, + *thēlē,* nipple]. 1. Epithelial structures forming the terminations of nerves of special sense. 2. Embryonic layer from which arises the cerebrospinal axis. SYN: *neuroepithelium.*

neurergic (nū-rer′jĭk) [G. *neuron,* sinew, + *ergon,* work]. Concerning the activity of a nerve.

neurexairesis (nū-rĕks-ī-rē′sĭs) [" + *exairein,* to draw out]. Ripping or tearing out of a nerve to relieve neuralgia.

neuriatry (nū-rī′a-trĭ) [" + *iatreia,* treatment]. Study and treatment of diseases of nervous system. SYN: *neurology.*

neurilemma, neurolemma [G. *neuron,* sinew, + *lemma,* rind]. SYN: sheath of Schwann. A thin membranous sheath enveloping a nerve fiber. SEE: *nerve fiber.*

neurilemmitis (nū″rĭ-lĕm-mī′tĭs) [G. *neuron,* sinew, + *lemma,* sheath, + *-itis,* inflammation]. Inflamed condition of a neurilemma.

neurilemmoma. SYN: *neurinoma, schwannoma, peripheral glioma.* A firm, encapsulated fibrillar tumor of peripheral nerves.

neurilemosarcoma (nū-rĭ-lĕm-ă-sar-kō′mă). A malignant neurilemmoma.

neurimotility (nū-rĭ-mō-tĭl′ĭ-tĭ) [" + L. *motilis,* able to move]. Power of neural motion. SYN: *nervimotility.*

neurimo′tor [" L. *motor,* a mover]. Concerning a motor nerve.

neurinoma (nū-rĭn-ō′mă) [G. *neuron,* sinew, + *-oma,* swelling]. SYN: *neurilemmoma, neurofibroma, schwannoma.* A tumor of a peripheral nerve arising from endoneurium or sheath of Schwann.

neurinomatosis (nū″rĭn-ō-mă-tō′sĭs). Condition of having multiple neurinomas on nerve fibers. SYN: *neurofibromatosis.*

neurite (nu′rīt) [G. *neuron,* sinew]. The axis cylinder process of a neuron. SYN: *axon, neuraxon.*

neuritis (nū-rī′tĭs) [G. *neuron,* sinew or nerve, + *-itis,* inflammation]. Inflammation of a nerve or nerves, usually associated with a degenerative process.

ETIOL: 1. Mechanical factors, compression, contusion, trauma. 2. Infections may be localized involving direct infection of nerves or may accompany diseases such as leprosy, tetanus, or tuberculosis, malaria, measles, etc. 3. Toxins, esp. poisoning by heavy metals (arsenic, lead, mercury), alcohol, carbon tetrachloride, etc. 4. Metabolic factors, as in thiamine deficiency, gastrointestinal dysfunction, diabetes, toxemias of pregnancy, etc. 5. Vascular, as in n. accompanying peripheral vascular disease.

SYM: Neuralgia in part affected; hyperesthesia, paresthesia, dysesthesia, hypesthesia, or anesthesia; muscular atrophy of part supplied by affected nerve; paralysis; lack of reflexes.

NP: Rest in bed, water or air bed. Uniformity of pressure on body. Temperature of water in water bath must be maintained by frequent replacement of cooling water with warm water. Hot water bags or electric heating pads under covers but not next to skin, as lack of sensibility to heat on part of patient may lead to burns. Cradles may be necessary. Padded splints with little bandage compression to affected parts. No sudden change of position. Place limb in suspended towel to move it. No rubbing. Later diathermy under direction of physician, also massage, using mildest of manipulations. Avoid all strain on patient. SEE: *polyneuritis.*

n., adventitial. Inflammation of nerve sheath.

n., ascending. N. along a nerve trunk away from periphery.

n., axial. Parenchymatous n.

n., degenerative. N. with rapid degeneration of nerve.

n., descending. N. along nerve trunk toward the periphery.

n., dietetic. Same as beriberi, *q.v.*

n., diphtheritic. N. following diphtheria.

n., disseminated. Segmental n.

n., endemic. Same as beriberi or multiple n.

n., interstitial. N. involving connective tissue of a nerve.

n., intraocular. N. of retinal fibers of optic nerve.

SYM: Disturbed vision, contracted field, enlarged blind spot, fundus findings such as exudates, hemorrhages and abnormal condition of blood vessels.

TREATMENT: Depends on etiology such as brain tumors, meningitis, syphilis, nephritis, diabetes, etc.

n. migrans. N. which passes along a nerve trunk. May be ascending or descending, *q.v.*

n., multiple. Inflammation of many nerves at the same time.

SYM: *Acute*: Chill; fever, 102-103° F.; headache; pain in back; malaise; coated tongue; loss of appetite; constipation; loss of power, esp. in legs and extensor muscles; abolition of reflexes; atrophy of muscles; more or less anesthesia; tenderness over nerve trunks. *Chronic*: Pains in limbs, hyperesthesia, paresthesia, irregular areas of anesthesia, loss of power, abolition of deep reflexes, tenderness over nerve trunks, wasting of muscles, impaired electrical contractility; edema of hands and feet.

PROG: Guardedly favorable. Acute form may prove fatal from involvement of respiratory muscles.

TREATMENT: Acute cases, absolute rest, limb in splint later, and in chronic cases, massage, electricity, general treatment.

SYN: *polyneuritis.* SEE: *beriberi.*

n. nodosa. N. with formation of nodes on nerves.

n., optic. N. of optic nerve.

n., parenchymatous. N. of nerve fiber substance.

n., peripheral. N. of terminal nerves or of end organs.

n., retrobulbar. N. of optic nerve behind eyeball.

SYM: Loss of vision in affected eye. (a) *Acute*: Seen in sinus disease; orbital cellulitis; poisons, as lead and alcohol; multiple sclerosis. (b) *Chronic, or toxic amblyopia*: Seen in excessive tobacco and alcohol users. SYM: Central scotoma.

n., rheumatic. N. with symptoms of rheumatism.

n., sciatic. Sciatica, *q.v.*

n., segmental. N. affecting segments of a nerve interspersed with healthy segments.

n., senile. N. in feet and legs of the elderly.

n., sympathetic. N. of opposite nerve without attacking nerve center.

n., tabetic. N. in locomotor ataxia.

n., toxic. N. resulting from metallic poisons such as arsenic, mercury, thallium, or nonmetallic poisons (various hydrocarbons and organic solvents).

n., traumatic. N. following an injury.

neuro- [G. *neuron*, sinew, nerve]. Combining form meaning pert. or rel. to a nerve, nervous tissue, or nervous system.

neu″roanat′omy [G. *neuron*, sinew, + *ana*, up, + *tomē*, a cutting]. Study of anatomy of the nervous system.

neuroarthritism (nū″rō-ar′thrĭt-ĭzm) [“ + *arthron*, joint, + *ismos*, condition]. Tendency toward contraction of nervous and gouty disorders.

neuroarthropathy (nū″rō-ar-throp′ăth-ĭ) [“ + *arthron*, joint, + *pathos*, disease]. Disease of a joint combined with disease of the central nervous system.

neurobion (nū-ro-bī′on) [“ + *bios*, life]. A hypothetical particle connected with renewal of nerve tissue.

neurobiotaxis (nu-ro-bi-o-tak′sis) [G. *neuron*, sinew, + *bios*- life, + *taxis*, order]. The phenomenon involving growth of dendrites and migration of nerve-cell bodies during development toward the region from which their dominant impulses are initiated.

neuroblast (nū′rō-blăst) [G. *neuron*, sinew, + *blastos*, germ]. An embryonic cell derived from neural tube or neural crest, which gives rise to a neuron.

neuroblastoma (nū-rō-blăst-tō′mă [G. *neuron*, sinew, + *blastos*, germ, + *oma*, tumor]. A malignant soft and hemorrhagic tumor composed principally of cells resembling neuroblasts which give rise to cells of the sympathetic system, esp. adrenal medulla. Occurs chiefly in young infants and children. SYN: *neuroblastoma sympatheticum; sympathicoblastoma; sympathicogonioma; retinoblastoma.*

neurocanal (nū″rō-kă-năl′) [“ + L. *canalis*, passage]. The central canal of the spinal cord.

neurocardiac (nū″rō-kar′dĭ-ăk) [“ + *kardia*, heart]. 1. Pert. to the nerves supplying the heart or nervous system and the heart. 2. Concerning a cardiac neurosis.

neurocele (nū′rō-sēl) [“ + *koilia*, cavity]. Ventricles and cavities in the cerebrospinal axis.

neurocentral (nū″rō-sĕn′trăl) [“ + *kentron*, center]. Pert. to the centrum of a vertebra and the neural arch.

neurochemistry (nū″rō-kĕm′ĭs-trĭ) [“ + *chēmeia*, chemistry]. Physiological chemistry dealing with nervous tissue.

neurochorioretinitis (nū″rō-kō″rĭ-ō-rĕt-ĭn-ī′tĭs) [“ + *chorion*, skin, + L. *rētē*, a net, + G. *-ītis*, inflammation]. Inflammation of choroid and retina combined with optic neuritis.

neurochoroiditis (nū″rō-kō-roi-dī′tĭs) [“ + *chorion*, skin, + *eidos*, like, + *-ītis*, inflammation]. Inflamed condition of the choroid coat and optic nerve.

neurocirculatory (nū″rō-sur′kū-lă-tō″rĭ) [“ + L. *circulatiō*, circulation]. Pert. to circulation and the nervous system.

n. asthenia. A combination of nervous and circulatory disturbances with fatigue and precordial pain, usually seen in soldiers. SYN: *irritable heart, soldier's heart.* SEE: *asthenia.*

neuroclonic (nū″rō-klon′ĭk) [“ + *klonos*, spasm]. Marked by spasms of nervous origin.

neurocoele (nū′rō-sēl) [“ + *koilia*, cavity]. System of cavities in cerebrospinal axis. SYN: *neurocele.*

neurocranium. (nū″rō-krā′nĭ-ŭm) [“ + *kranion*, skull]. The part of the skull enclosing the brain.

neurocutaneous (nū″rō-kū-tā′nē-ŭs) [“ + L. *cutis*, skin]. Pert. to the nervous system and skin.

neurocyte (nū′rō-sīt) [G. *neuron*, sinew, + *kytos*, cell]. A nerve cell. SYN: *neuron.*

neurocytoma (nū″rō-sī-tō′mă) [“ + “ + *-ōma*, tumor]. A tumor formed of cells, usually ganglionic, of nervous origin. SYN: *neuroma, 2.*

neurodealgia (nū″rō-de-al′jĭ-ă) [G. *neurōdēs*, retina, + *algos*, pain]. Pain in the retina.

neurodendrite, neurodendron (nū″rō-dĕn′-drīt, -dron) [G. *neuron*, sinew, + *den-*

dron, tree]. Protoplasmic branched process of a nerve cell. SYN: *dendrite, dendron.*

neurodermatitis (nū″rō-dĕr-mă-tī′tĭs) [" + *derma,* skin, + *-itis,* inflammation]. Cutaneous inflammation due to nervous disorder, marked by itching.

n., disseminated. Chronic superficial inflammation of skin characterized by thickening, excoriation, and lichenification, beginning usually in infancy. Common in families with high familial incidence in allergic diseases. SYN: *atopic dermatitis; atopic eczema; Brocq disease.*

neurodermatosis (nū″rō-dĕr-mă-tō′sĭs) [" + " + *-ōsis,* condition]. Any skin disease of neural origin. Includes neurofibromatosis (von Recklinghausen's disease), von Hippel-Landau disease, Sturge-Weber syndrome, and tuberous sclerosis.

neurodermatrophia (nū-rō-derm-ă-trŏf′-ĭ-ă). Atrophy of the skin from nervous disease.

neurodiagnosis (nū″rō-dī-ăg-nō′sĭs) [" + *dia,* through, + *gnōsis,* knowledge]. Diagnosis of nervous disorders.

neurodocitis (nū″rō-dō-sī′tĭs) [" + *-itis,* inflammation]. Lesion of nerve roots due to pressure.

neurodynamia (nū″rō-dī-nam′ĭ-ă) [" + *dynamis,* power]. Nervous energy or force.

neurodynamic (nū″rō-dī-nam′ĭk) [" + *dynamis,* power]. Concerning nervous force or energy.

neurodynia (nū″rō-dĭn′ĭ-ă) [G. *neuron,* sinew or nerve, + *odynē,* pain]. Pain in a nerve or nerves. SYN: *neuralgia.*

neuroendocrine (nū′ro-ĕnd′o-krim). Pertaining to the nervous and endocrine system as an integrated functioning mechanism.

neuroepidermal (nū″rō-ĕp-ĭ-dŭr′măl) [" + *epi,* upon, + *derma,* skin]. Pert. to or giving rise to nervous system and epidermis.

neuroepithelioma (nū″rō-ĕp″ĭ-thē-lĭ-ō′mă) [" + " + *thēlē,* nipple, + *-ōma,* tumor]. A tumor of neuroepithelium in a nerve of special sense.

neuroepithelium (nū″rō-ĕp″ĭ-thē′lĭ-ŭm) [" + " + *thēlē,* nipple]. 1. A specialized epithelial structure forming the termination of a nerve of special sense. Includes gustatory cells, olfactory cells, hair-cells of inner ear, and rods and cones of retina. 2. Embryonic layer of the epiblast from which the cerebrospinal axis is developed.

neurofibril, neurofibrilla (nū-rō-fī′brĭl, -fī-brĭl′ă) (pl. *neurofibrils, neurofibrillae*) [" + L. *fibrilla,* a small fiber]. A tiny fiber in the cytoplasm of a neuron which continues on into the nerve processes. SEE: *neuron.*

neurofibroma (nū″rō-fī-brō′mă) (pl. *neurofibromata* or *-mas*) [" + L. *fibra,* fiber, + G. *-ōma,* tumor]. A tumor of connective tissue of a nerve including medullated layer of a nerve fiber. May occur in mouth, pleura or stomach.

SYN: *neuroma, false; pseudoneuroma.*

neurofibromatosis (nū″rō-fī-brō″mă-tō′sĭs) [" + " + " + *-ōsis,* increase]. Condition in which there are tumors of various sizes on peripheral nerves.

They may be neuromas or fibromas.

n., multiple. SYN: *von Recklinghausen's disease, q.v., multiple neurofibroma.*

neurofibrosarcoma (nū-rō-fīb-rō-săr-kō′-mă). SYN: *neurogenic sarcoma.* A malignant neurofibroma.

neurofibrositis (nū″rō-fī″brō-sī′tĭs) [" + " + G. *-itis,* inflammation]. Inflammation of nerve fibers and sensory nerve fibers in muscular tissue.

neurogangliitis (nū″rō-gan-glĭ-ī′tis) [G. *neuron,* sinew, + *gagglion,* knot, + *-itis,* inflammation]. Inflamed condition of a neuroganglion.

neurogenesis (nū″rō-jĕn′ĕ-sĭs) [" + *genesis,* production]. 1. Growth or development of nerves. 2. Development from nervous tissue.

neurogenetic (nūr″ō-jĕn-et′ĭk) [" + *genesis,* production]. 1. Pert. to nerve formation. 2. Pert. to origin in nerves.

neurogenic, neurogenous (nū-rō-jĕn′ĭk, -roj′ĕn-ŭs) [" + *gennan,* to produce]. 1. Originating from nervous tissue. 2. Due to or resulting from nervous impulses.

neurogeny (nū-roj′ĕn-ĭ) [" + *gennan,* to produce]. SEE: *Neurogenesis.*

neuroglia (nū-rŏg′lĭ-ă) [G. *neuron,* sinew, + *glia,* glue]. The tissue which forms the interstitial or supporting elements —cells and fibers—of the nervous system. Neuroglia, also called glia includes: (1) astrocytes, (2) oligodendroglias, (3) microglia (mesoglia), (4) ependyma, (5) neurilemma sheath cells or nerve fibers (cells of Schwann), and (6) satellite (capsule) cells surrounding cranial and spinal ganglia. All except the microglia are of ectodermal origin. Neuroglia functions as connective or supporting tissue and also plays an important role in the reaction of the nervous system to injury or infection.

n. cell. SYN: *Glial cell.* Any of the cells of neuroglia; a neurogliacyte.

n. proper. Astroglia (astrocytes) and oligodendroglia (oligodendrocytes) of the central nervous system.

neurogliacyte (nū-rŏg′lĭ-ă-sīt) [" + " + *kytos,* cell]. Any one of the cells found in neuroglial tissue.

neuroglial (nū-rŏg′lē-al). Pertaining to neuroglia.

neuroglioma (nū″rō-glī-o′mă) [" + " + *-ōma,* tumor]. Tumor of neuroglial tissue. SYN: *glioma.*

n., ganglionar, n., ganglionare. Glioma with ganglion cells.

neurogliosis (nū″rō-glī-ō′sĭs) [" + " + *-ōsis,* increase]. Development of numerous neurogliomas.

neurogram (nū′rō-grăm) [" + *gramma,* a mark]. The impression left upon the physical brain following any cerebral experience which is retained as unconscious memory. SEE: *engram.*

neurography (nū-rog′ră-fĭ) [G. *neuron,* sinew, + *graphein,* to write]. 1. A study or description of the nervous system. 2. Formation of neurograms in the brain.

neurohematology (nū″rō-hem″at-ol′ō-jĭ) [" + *aima,* blood, + *logos,* study]. The study of hemic changes in neural diseases.

neurohistology (nū″rō-hĭs-tol′ō-jĭ) [" + *istos,* tissue, + *logos,* study]. The study of nervous tissue.

neurohumor (nū-rō-hūm′ŏr). A chemical substance liberated at a nerve-ending which excites or activates and adjacent structure (neuron or muscle fiber). Ex: acetylcholine and sympathin (epinephrine). These substances are essential for transmission of impulses across synapses or myoneural junctions.

neurohypophysis (nū″rō-hī-pof′ĭs-ĭs) [" + *ypo,* under, + *physis,* growth]. Post. portion or pars nervosa of the pituitary gland.

neuroinduction (nū″rō-ĭn-dŭk′shŭn) [" + L. *in,* into, + *ductus,* leading]. Suggestion.

neurokeratin (nū″rō-ker′ă-tĭn) [G. *neuron,* sinew or nerve, + *keras, kerat-,* horn]. The variety of keratin found in myelinated nerve fibers.

neurologic, neurological (nū-rō-loj′ĭk, -ĭ-kal) [" + *logos,* study]. Pert. to the study of nervous diseases.

neurologist (nū-rol′ō-jĭst) [" + *logos,* study]. A specialist in diseases of nervous system.

neurology (nū-rol′ō-jĭ) [G. *neuron,* sinew, + *logos,* study]. The branch of medicine that deals with the nervous system and its diseases.

neurolymph (nū′rō-lĭmf) [" + L. *lympha,* fluid]. The cerebrospinal fluid.

neurolysin (nū-rol′ĭs-ĭn) [" + *lysis,* destruction]. A substance which destroys nerve cells.

neurolysis (nū-rol′ĭs-ĭs) [" + *lysis,* a loosening; a degeneration]. 1. Exhaustion of a nerve or nerves from prolonged stimulation. 2. Stretching of a nerve to relieve tension. 3. Loosening of adhesions surrounding a nerve. 4. Disintegration of nerve tissue.

neurolytic (nū-rō-lit′ĭk) [" + *lysis,* destruction]. Concerning neurolysis.

neuroma (nū′rō-mă) [G. *neuron,* sinew, + *-ōma,* tumor]. A tumor along the course of a nerve or at the end of a divided nerve, consisting of coiled masses of axis cylinders, Schwann cells, and fibrous tissue, since classified on a basis of cytology and histology.

n., amputation. N. occurring on a stump after amputation.

n., amyelinic. N. composed principally of unmyelinated nerve fibers.

n., appendiceal. N. found in mucosa and submucosa of the appendix.

n. cutis. N. of the derma.

n., cystic. N. with cystic formations.

n., false. Tumor arising from connective tissue of nerves, including the myelin sheath. SYN: *neurofibroma, pseudoneuroma.*

n., ganglionated. N. composed of nerve cells.

n., myelinic. N. composed of medullated nerve fibers.

n., plexiform. Congenital n. involving all branches of a nerve. Usually found around head and are painless.

n. telangiectodes. N. with an abundance of blood vessels contained within it.

n., traumatic. N. occurring in wounds or on an amputation stump.

neuromalacia (nū″rō-mal-a′sĭ-ă) [" + *malakia,* softening]. Pathological softening of neural tissue.

neuromatosis (nū-rō″mă-tō′sĭs) [" + *-ōma,* tumor, + *ōsis,* increase]. Multiple neuromas occurring in the body.

neuromatous (nū-rō′mă-tŭs) [" + *-ōma,* tumor]. Rel. to a neuroma.

neuromechanism (nū″rō-mĕk′ăn-ĭzm) [" + *mēchanē,* machine]. The neural structure controlling organic and systemic function.

neuromere (nū′rō-mēr) [G. *neuron,* sinew, + *meros,* part]. SYN: *rhombomere.* One of a series of segmental elevations on the ventrolateral surface of the rhombencephalon.

neuromimesis (nū-rō-mĭm-ē′sĭs) [" + *mimēsis,* imitation]. Resemblance of hysteria to organic disease.

neuromuscular (nū″rō-mus′kū-lăr) [" + L. *musculus,* a muscle]. Concerning both nerves and muscles.

neuromyelitis (nū-rō-mī-ĕl-ī′tĭs) [G. *neuron,* sinew, + *myelos,* marrow, + *-itis,* inflammation]. Inflammation of nerves and the spinal cord.

n. optica. A syndrome resulting from demyelinization occurring in the spinal cord, optic nerves, and chiasma; also called *disseminated myelitis with optic neuritis, ophthalmoneuromyelitis, Devic's disease.*

neur″o-my″opath′ic. Pert. to pathologic conditions involving both muscles and nerves.

neuromyositis (nū″rō-mī″ō-sī′tĭs) [" + " + *-itis,* inflammation]. Inflammation of both nerves and muscles of a part.

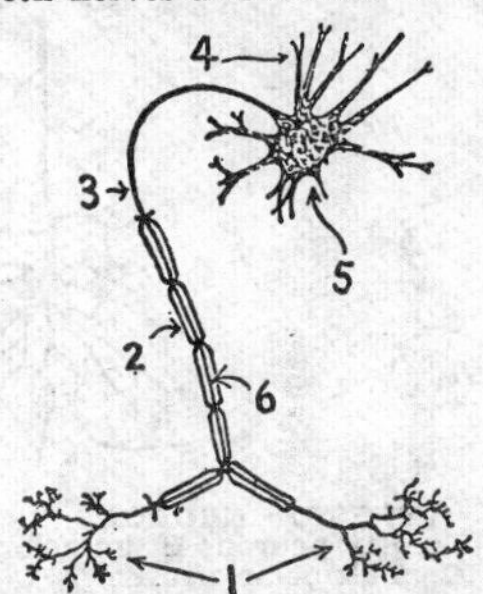

NEURON.
1. Terminal branches. 2. Neurilemma. 3. Axon. 4. Dendrites. 5. Cell body. 6. Myelin sheath.

neuron (nū′rŏn) [G. *neuron,* sinew]. A nerve cell, the structural and functional unit of the nervous system. A n. consists of a *cell body* or *perikaryon* and its processes, an *axon* and one or more *dendrites.* Neurons function in the initiation and conduction of impulses. SEE: *nerve, nerve impulse, nervous system, nervous tissue.*

n., afferent. N. conducting impulses toward brain or spinal cord; a sensory neuron.

n., associative (association). N. which mediates impulses between a sensory and a motor neuron; a central neuron.

n., bipolar. N. bearing two processes, an axon and a dendrite.

n., central. N. confined entirely to central nervous system; an association n.

n., commissural. N. whose axon crosses to opposite side of brain or spinal cord.

n., efferent. N. which conducts impulses away from the brain or spinal cord.

n., motor. N. which conveys impulses initiating muscle contraction.

n., motor, lower. SYN: *ventral horn cells.* N. whose cell body lies in ant. gray column of spinal cord and axon innervates striated muscle fibers.

n., motor, upper. N. whose cell body lies in motor area of cerebral cortex. Its axon passes down spinal cord and synapses with lower motor neurons.

n., multipolar. N. with one axon and many dendrites.

n., peripheral. N. whose process constitutes a part of the peripheral nervous system (cranial, spinal or sympathetic nerves).

n., postganglionic. N. of autonomic nervous system whose cell body lies in central nervous system and axon terminates in peripheral ganglia.

n., preganglionic. N. whose body lies in an autonomic ganglion and axon terminates in an effector organ (smooth or cardiac muscle or glands).

n., pseudounipolar. A unipolar neuron which is derived embryologically from a bipolar neuron. Ex. sensory neurons of spinal nerves.

n., sensory. An afferent n. which conveys impulses which give rise to sensations.

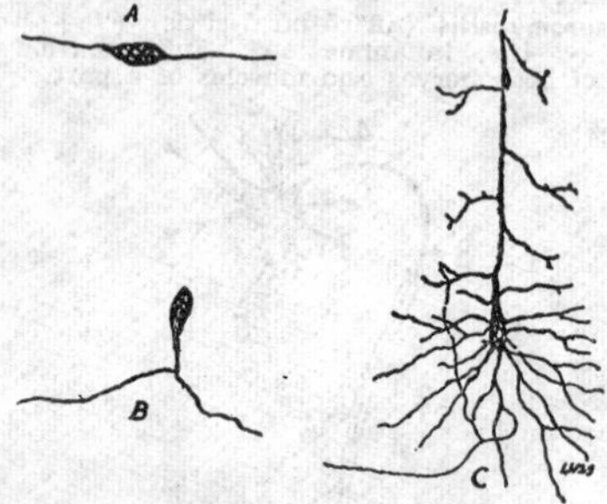

TYPES OF NEURONS
A, Bipolar neuron; B, unipolar neuron; C, multipolar neuron.

n., unipolar. N. whose cell body bears one process.

neuronal (nu'ro-nal). Pertaining to one or more neurons.

neurone. Neuron, *q.v.*

neuronevus (nu"ro-ne'vis). Intradermal nevus.

neuronitis (nū-rōn-ī'tĭs) [" + *-ītis,* inflammation]. Inflammation, or degenerative inflammation of nerve cells.

neuronophage (nū-ron'ō-fāj) [" + *phagein,* to eat]. A phagocyte which destroys neurons.

neuronophagia, neuronophagy (nū-ron-ō-fā'jĭ-ă, -of'ă-jĭ) [+ " + *phagein,* to eat]. Destruction of nerve cells by phagocytes.

neuronyxis (nū-rō-niks'ĭs) [" + *nyxis,* a piercing]. Neural puncture.

neuropath (nū'rō-păth) [G. *neuron,* sinew or nerve, + *pathos,* disease]. One predisposed to neurosis.

neuropathic (nū-rō-păth'ĭk) [" + *pathos,* disease]. Rel. to neuropathy.

neuropathogenesis (nū"rō-păth"ō-jĕn'ĕ-sĭs) [" + " + *genesis,* production]. Development of a neural disease.

neuropathology (nū"rō-pă-thol'ō-jĭ) [" + " + *logos,* study]. The study of the diseases of the nervous system and the structural and functional changes occurring in them.

The diseases are divided into congenital defects in development, those in which an inherent tendency to degeneracy reveals itself only after a period of time, and finally those in which destructive influences act upon a brain initially normal. The last-named are mainly inflammatory, toxic, traumatic, mechanical or neoplastic in type. Circulatory impairment, disuse and overactivity also contribute to the development of nervous diseases.

neuropathy (nū-rop'ă-thĭ) [" + *pathos,* disease]. Any disease of the nerves.

neurophonia (nū"rō-fō'nĭ-ă) [" + *phōnē,* voice]. A tic or spasm of muscles of speech resulting in an involuntary cry or sound.

neurophysiology (nū"rō-fĭz-ĭ-ol'ō-jĭ) [" + *physis,* growth, + *logos,* study]. Physiology of the nervous structure of the body.

neuropil (nū'rō-pil) [G. *neuron,* sinew, + *pilos,* felt]. Network of unmyelinated fibrils into which nerve processes of central nervous system divide.

neuroplasm (nū'rō-plăzm) [G. *neuron,* sinew, + *plasmos,* a thing formed]. SYN: *interfibrillar* or *perifibrillar substance.* The undifferentiated cytoplasmic substance of a neuron which surrounds and separates the neurofibrils.

neuroplasmic (nū"rō-plaz'mĭk) [" + *plasmos,* a thing formed]. Concerning the protoplasm of a neuron.

neuroplasty (nū'rō-plăs-tĭ) [" + *plassein,* to form]. Reparative surgery of the nerves.

neu"ropod'ia (plural of *neuropodium*). SYN: *end feet; terminal buttons.* Small bulblike expansions of axon terminals at a synaptic junction.

neuropore (nū'rō-pōr) [" + *poros,* an opening]. Embryonic opening from neural canal to exterior.

neuropsychiatry (nū"rō-sī-kī'ă-trĭ) [" + *psychē,* mind, + *iatreia,* healing]. Study and treatment of nervous and mental diseases.

neuropsychology (nū"rō-sī-kol'ō-jĭ) [G. *neuron,* sinew, + *psychē,* mind, + *logos,* study]. The science of connection of neurological and psychological facts.

neuropsychopathy (nū"rō-sī-kop'ăth-ĭ) [" + " + *pathos,* disease]. A neurosis in combination with a mental disease.

neurorecidive (nū"rō-rĕs'ĭ-dĭv) [" + L. *recidere,* to fall back]. Neurorelapse, *q.v.*

neurorecurrence (nū"rō-rē-kŭr'ănz) [" + L. *rē,* back, + *currere,* to run]. Nervous manifestation as a sequel to salvarsan injection. SYN: *neurorelapse.*

neurorelapse (nū"rō-rē-lăps') [G. *neuron,* sinew, + L. *relapsus,* fallen back]. Nervous symptoms in syphilis subsequent to an injection of salvarsan. SYN: *neurorecurrence.*

neuroretinitis (nū"rō-rĕt"ĭn-ī'tĭs) [" + L. *rētē,* net, + G. *-ītis,* inflammation]. Inflamed condition of optic nerve and retina.

neurorrhaphy (nū-ror'ă-fĭ) [" + *raphē,* a sewing]. Suturing of ends of a severed nerve.

neurorrhyctes hydrophobiae (nū"rō-rĭk'-tēs hī-drō-fō'bĭ-ē) [" + *oryktēs,* a digger, + *ydōr,* water, + *phobos,* fear]. Supposed microorganisms of rabies. Inclusion bodies usually found in cells of cerebellum and cerebrum in animals infected with rabies. SYN: *Negri bodies.*

neurosarcokleisis (nū"rō-săr"kō-klī'sĭs) [" + *sarx, sark-,* flesh, + *kleisis,* closure]. Operation for relief of neuralgia by resection of a wall of the osseous canal carrying a nerve and transplanting the nerve to soft tissues.

neurosarcoma (nū"rō-săr-kō'mă) [" + " + *-ōma,* tumor]. A sarcoma containing neuromatous components.

neurosclerosis (nū"rō-sklĕ-rō'sĭs) [" + *sklērōsis,* a hardening]. Hardening of nervous tissue.

neurosecretion (nū"rō-sē-krē'shŭn). The elaboration and discharge of a substance by a neuron. Ex: secretion of hormones by cells of the hypothalamus.

neurosensory (nū"rō-sĕn'sō-rĭ) [" + L. *sensōrius,* pert. to a sensation]. Concerning a sensory nerve.

neurosis (nu-ro'sis) [G. *neuron,* sinew, *-osis,* disease]. Also called psychoneurosis. A disorder of the thought processes not due to demonstrable disease of the structure of the central nervous system. Probably due to unresolved internal conflicts which make for an uneasy adjustment to life. Contact with reality is maintained which is not the case in psychosis, *q.v.* The neuroses are usually classified as fatigue (or neurasthenia); simple nervousness (or anxiety); phobic; obsessive compulsive (or psychasthenia); hysteria; hypochondriasis; reactive depression. The disease rarely occurs in one of these pure forms. Thus most neurotic persons would be classed as having *mixed psychoneuroses.*

TREATMENT: Psychotherapy, tranquilizers, and sedatives. It must be remembered that in general a symptom due to a neurotic reaction to a situation is just as real to the patient as if it were due to organic disease. Usually such a symptom is much more difficult to treat than it would be if due to organic disease.

n., accident. A nervous disorder caused by injury or an accident.

n., anxiety. N. in which fear or apprehension is the essential symptom. SEE: *anxiety n.*

n., association. N. in which association of ideas causes mental repetition of an experience.

n., cardiac. Same as neurocirculatory asthenia (see under *asthenia*).

n., compensation. N. developing after an accident in people who think they can obtain compensation by being ill.

n., compulsion. N. marked by overpowering impulse to perform acts against the will.

n., craft. Occupational n., *q.v.*

n., expectation. Condition in which anticipation of an occurrence produces nervous symptoms.

n., fatigue. Neurasthenia, *q.v.*

n., obsessional. Uncontrollable obsessions dominating the victim's behavior.

n., occupational, n., professional. N. due to the occupation or profession of a patient.

n., pension. Compensation n., *q.v.*

n., sexual. N. involving sexual function.

n., traumatic. SEE: *accident n.*

n., war. N. brought on by conditions of war. SYN: *shell shock.*

neurospasm (nū'rō-spăzm) [" + *spasmos,* spasm]. Spasmodic muscular twitching due to a nervous disorder.

Neuros'pora. The pink bread-mold, a fungus belonging to the Ascomycetes. Used experimentally in studies of genetics and in bio-assays.

neurosurgery (nū"rō-sur'jĕ-rĭ) [G. *neuron,* sinew, + L. *chirurgia,* from G. *cheir,* hand, + *ergon,* work]. Surgery of the nervous system.

neurosuture (nū"rō-sū'chūr) [" + L. *sutura,* a stitch]. Stitching of ends of a cut nerve. SYN: *neurorrhaphy.*

neurosyphilis (nū"rō-sĭf'ĭ-lĭs) [" + *syphilis*]. Syphilis affecting the nervous structures. SEE: *dementia paralytica.*

n., asymptomatic. N. preceding symptomatic neurosyphilis but showing no symptoms. Diagnosed by changes in spinal fluid.

n., meningovascular. A form of n. involving the meninges and vascular structures in the brain or spinal cord or both.

neurotension (nū"rō-tĕn'shŭn) [" + L. *tensiō,* a stretching]. Operative stretching of a nerve. SYN: *neurectasis.*

neurothecitis (nū"rō-the-sī'tĭs) [" + *thēkē,* sheath, + *-ītis,* inflammation]. Inflamed condition of a nerve sheath.

neurotherapeutics (nū"rō-thĕr-ă-pū'tĭks) [" + *therapeutikē,* treatment]. Treatment of disorders of the nervous system. SYN: *neurotherapy.*

neurotherapy (nū-rō-ther'ă-pĭ) [" + *therapeia,* treatment]. Treatment of nervous disorders.

neurothlipsis (nū"rō-thlip'sĭs) [" + *thlipsis,* pressure]. Irritation or pressure on a nerve.

neurotic (nū-rot'ĭk) [G. *neuron,* sinew]. 1. One suffering from instability of the nervous system. 2. Nervous or pert. to a neurosis.

neuroticism (nū-rŏt'ĭ-sĭzm) [" + *ismos,* state of]. A condition or trait of neurosis.

neurotization (nū-rot-ĭ-zā'shŭn) [G. *neuron,* sinew]. 1. Acquisition of nervous substance. 2. Regeneration of a nerve after division. 3. Surgical introduction of a nerve into a paralyzed muscle.

neurotology (nū"rō-tŏl'ō-jĭ) [G. *neuron,* sinew, + *ous, ot-,* ear, + *logos,* study]. The division of otology which deals with the inner ear, esp. its nerve supply, nerve connections with the brain, and auditory and labyrinthine pathways and centers within the brain.

neurotome (nū'rō-tōm) [" + *tomē,* a slice]. Fine knife used in the division of a nerve.

neurotmesis (nū"rŏt-mē'sĭs). The severing or division of a nerve.

neurotomy (nū-rot'ō-mĭ) [" + *tomē,* an incision]. Division or dissection of a nerve.

neurotonic (nū"rō-ton'ĭk) [" + *tonos,* tension]. 1. Concerning neural stretching. 2. Having a stimulating effect upon nerves or the nervous system.

neurotony (nū-rot'ō-nĭ) [G. *neuron,* sinew, + *tonos,* a stretching]. Nerve stretching.

neurotoxic (nū"rō-toks'ĭk) [" + *toxikon,* poison]. Poisonous to the nerve cells.

neurotoxin (nū"rō-toks'ĭn) [" + *toxikon,* poison]. A toxin that attacks nerve cells. SYN: *neurolysin.*

neurotrauma (nū-rō-traw'mă) [" + *trauma,* wound]. Wounding of a nerve.

neurotripsy (nū'rō-trip-sĭ) [" + *tripsis,* a rubbing]. Surgical crushing of a nerve.

neurotrophasthenia (nū"rō-trof-ăs-thē'-nĭ-ă) [" + *trophē,* nourishment, + *astheneia,* weakness]. Malnutrition of the nervous system.

neurotrophy (nū-rot'rō-fĭ) [" + *trophē,* nourishment]. Nutrition of the nerves.

neurotroph'ic. Pert. to the influence of nervous impulses upon the well-being of an organ or structure.

neurotropism (nū-rot'rō-pĭzm) [" + " + *ismos,* condition]. Attraction which nutritive elements, basic dyes, and microorganisms have for nervous tissue.

neurotropy (nu-rot'ro-pĭ). Same as neurotropism, *q.v.*

neurotrosis (nū"rō-trō'sĭs) [" + *trōsis,* a wound]. Wounding of a nerve. SYN: *neurotrauma.*

neurovaccine (nū"rō-văk'sēn) [" + L. *vaccinus,* pert. to a cow]. A standardized vaccine virus of specific strength. Usually secured by cultivation in a rabbit's brain.

neurovaricosis (nū"rō-văr-ĭ-kō'sĭs) [" + L. *varicōsus,* pert. to a swollen vein]. Multiple swellings along the pathway of a nerve.

neurovascular (nū″rō-văs′kū-lăr) [" + L. *vasculus,* a small vessel]. Concerning both the nervous and vascular systems.

neurovirus (nu-ro-vi′rus). A neurovaccine.

neurula (nū′rū-lă). Stage in development of an embryo, esp. amphibian embryos, during which the neural plate develops and axial embryonic nervous structures are elaborated.

neutral (nū′trăl) [L. *neuter,* neither]. 1. Neither alkaline nor acid. 2. Indifferent; having no positive properties.

n. fat. One of the fats commonly found in the tissues; an ester of fatty acids with glycerol. Ex: *tristearin, triolein, tripalmitin.*

n. point. *p*H 7, a point on the *p*H scale which represents neutrality, *i. e.,* the solution is neither acid or alkaline in reaction.

n. red. A dye used as an indicator and as a vital stain.

neutralization (nū-tral-ĭ-zā′shŭn) [L. *neuter,* from *ne,* not, + *uter,* either, one of two]. 1. The opposing of one force or condition with an opposite force or condition to such degree as to cause counteraction that permits neither to dominate. 2. In chem. the process of destroying the peculiar properties or effect of a substance, as the neutralization of an acid with a base, or vice versa. 3. In med. the process of checking or counteracting the effects of any agent which produces a morbid effect.

neutralize (nū′tral-īz) [L. *neuter,* from *ne,* not, + *uter,* either, one of two]. 1. To counteract. 2. CHEM: To destroy peculiar properties of or effect of; to make inert.

neutroclusion (nū″trō-klū′zhŭn) [" + *occlusiō,* a closing before]. State in which the anteroposterior occlusal positions of the teeth or the mesiodistal positions are normal, but malocclusion of the other positions exists.

neutron (nū′trŏn) [L. *neuter,* neither]. Subatomic particle equal in mass to a proton but without an electric charge.

It is a constituent of the atomic nucleus.

neutropenia (nū-trō-pē′nĭ-ă) [" + G. *penia,* lack]. Abnormally small number of neutrophil cells in the blood.

neutrophil(e (nū′trō-fĭl, -fīl) [" + G. *philein,* to love]. 1. Staining easily with neutral dyes. 2. A leukocyte which stains easily with neutral dyes. SEE: *polymorphonuclear leukocyte.*

neutrophilia (nū″trō-fĭl′ĭ-ă) [" + G. *philein,* to love]. Increase in the number of neutrophil leukocytes.

neutrophilic, neutrophilous (nū-trō-fĭl′ĭk, -trof′ĭ-lŭs) [" + G. *philein,* to love]. Staining readily with neutral dyes.

nevoid (nē′voyd) [L. *naevus,* birthmark, + G. *eidos,* form]. Resembling a nevus.

nevolipoma (nē-vō-lip-ō′mă) [" + G. *lipos,* fat, + *-ōma,* tumor]. Rare lipoma containing numerous blood vessels, probably a degenerated nevus.

nevose (nē′vōs) [L. *naevus,* birthmark]. Spotted or marked with nevi. SEE: *nevus.*

nevus (nē′vŭs) [L. *naevus,* birthmark]. 1. A congenital discoloration of a circumscribed area of the skin due to pigmentation. SYN: *birthmark, mole.* 2. Circumscribed vascular tumor of the skin, usually congenital, due to hyperplasia of the blood vessels. SEE: *angioma.* PL: *nevi.*

n. angiectodes. SEE: *n. vascularis.*

n. angiomatodes. Extensive diffuse angiomatous condition of the subcutaneous tissues.

n. araneus. Acquired or congenital dilatation of the capillaries, marked by red lines radiating from a central red dot. SYN: *spider n.*

n., capillary. N. of dilated capillary vessels, elevated above the skin. TREATMENT: Ligature, excision.

n., cutaneous. N. formation on the skin.

n. flammeus. Reddish discoloration of the face or neck, usually not elevated above the skin. A serious deformity due to large size and color.

n. lipomatodes. Fatty connective tissue tumor, probably a degenerated nevus, containing numerous blood vessels. SYN: *nevolipoma.*

n. maternus. A birthmark.

n. pigmentosus; pigmented n. Congenital pigment spot varying in color from light yellow to blackish. Intradermal, or common moles, are benign. Other types are, or may become, malignant.

TREATMENT: Malignant or suspicious lesions should be treated by wide surgical excision. Benign lesions do not require treatment, except when located at sites of friction causing bleeding, ulceration, etc.; some are removed for cosmetic reasons.

n. pilosus. A n. covered with hair.

n., spider. SEE: *n. araneus.*

n. spilus. Pigmented n. with smooth surface.

n., strawberry. N. vascularis, *q.v.;* strawberry mark.

n., telangiectatic. N. containing dilated capillaries.

n. vascularis, n. vasculosus. N. in which superficial blood vessels are enlarged.

Nevi are usually congenital and of variable size and shape, slightly elevated, reddish or purplish, on face, head, neck and arms, though no region is exempt. Usually disappear spontaneously, but wrinkling, pigmentation, and scarring are sometimes seen.

SYN: *strawberry n.; strawberry mark.*

n. venosus, n. venous. N. formed of dilated venules.

n. verrucosus. N. with a raised wart-like surface.

new growth. Any morbid new formation, as a tumor. SYN: *neoplasm.*

nexus (neks′us) [L. *nectere,* to bind]. A connection or link; a binding together.

N. F. Abbr. for *National Formulary.*

NH_3. Ammonia.

NH_4Br. Ammonium bromide.

NH_4Cl. Ammonium chloride.

NH_4NO_3. Ammonium nitrate.

NH_4OH. Ammonium hydroxide. Also called aqua ammonia or ammonia water.

Ni. Symb. for *nickel.*

niacin (nī′ă-sĭn). A synonym for *nicotinic acid.*

n. amide. A synonym for *nicotinamide.*

niccolum (nĭk′ō-lŭm) [L.]. Nickel, *q.v.*

niche. A depression or recess.

n., enamel. SYN: *enamel crypt.* One of two depressions which develop between the dental lamina and the enamel organ.

nickel (nĭk′el) [L. *niccolum*]. SYMB: Ni. Metallic element. At. wt. 58.71, at. no. 28.

n. arc. One that emits strongly at 230 and esp. at 350 millimicrons.

Nicolas-Favre disease (nē″kō-lă făvr′). Venereal disease marked by involvement of inguinal lymph glands with an exuding lesion. SYN: *Frei's disease, lymphogranuloma venerea.*

nicotinamide (nĭk″ō-tĭn′ă-mĭd). Member of vitamin-B complex, used in management or prevention of pellagra. The peripheral flush that often accompanies therapy with nicotinic acid, *q.v.*, is avoided with nicotinamide. SYN: *niacinamide.*

nicotine (nĭk′ō-tēn, -tĭn). A poisonous alkaloid found in all parts of the tobacco plant, but esp. in the leaves. When pure, it is a colorless oily fluid with little odor, but a sharp, burning taste. On standing or in crude materials, it becomes deep brown with a characteristic smell.

n. poisoning, acute. SYM: Excitement, restlessness, clonic convulsions, confusion, weakness, increased salivation, nausea and vomiting, abdominal cramps and diarrhea, rapid and irregular pulse, rapid and labored respiration. TREATMENT: If patient is conscious, oral administration of universal antidote (*q.v.*), tannic acid, activated charcoal, or strong tea, followed by gastric lavage or an emetic; in unconsciousness, use gastric lavage. Keep patient warm with external heat. Ephedrine sulfate I.M., for maintenance of circulation; artificial or mechanical respiration and oxygen therapy if necessary.

n. poisoning, mild. Symptoms usually disappear within few hours. In excitement, pentobarbital sodium may be used.

nicotinic acid (nĭk″ō-tĭn′ĭk). The antipellagra principle of vitamin B complex. Occurs as a white crystal or powder. Used orally or parenterally as a preventive and, specifically, as therapy in pellagra. SYN: *niacin.*

nicotinism (nĭk′ō-tēn-ĭzm, -tĭn-izm). Poisoning from excessive use of tobacco or nicotine.

nictation, nictitation [L. *nictitāre,* to wink]. Involuntary winking due to a nervous disorder.

nictitate (nĭk′tĭ-tāt) [L. *nictitāre,* to wink]. To wink.

nictitating (nĭk′tĭ-tāt-ĭng) [L. *nictitāre,* to wink]. Winking or blinking.

n. spasm. Clonic spasm of eyelid with continuous winking.

nidal (nī′dal) [L. *nidus,* nest]. Pert. to a nidus.

nidation (nī-da′shun) [L. *nidus,* nest]. Implantation of the fertilized ovum in the lining of the uterus (endometrium).

nidus (nī′dŭs) [L. nest]. 1. A cluster; nestlike structure. 2. Focus of infection. 3. A nucleus or origin of a nerve.

n. avis cerebelli. A deep sulcus of each side of the inferior vermis separating it from adjacent lobes of hemispheres.

Niemann-Pick disease (nē-man-pĭk). A disturbance of lipoid metabolism characterized by enlargement of liver and spleen (hepatosplenomegaly), anemia, lymphadenopathy, and progressive mental and physical deterioration. A hereditary disease, its onset is in early infancy with death usually before the third year. Typical cell, having a foamy appearance and filled with a lipoid believed to be sphingomyelin, can be found in bone marrow, spleen, or lymph nodes and aids in establishing the diagnosis. SYN: *lipid histiocytosis.*

night blindness (nīt blīnd′nĕs) [A.S. *neaht,* night, + *blind,* without sight]. Absence of or defective vision in the dark. SYN: *nyctalopia, nyctotyphlosis.*

ETIOL: Due to lack of visual purple in the rods or its slowness in regenerating after exposure to light. May result from vitamin A deficiency or hereditary factors.

Nightingale, Florence (nīt′ĭn-gāl). Originator of modern nursing.

N. oath or pledge. "I solemnly pledge myself before God and in the presence of this assembly to pass my life in purity and to practice my profession faithfully. I will abstain from whatever is deleterious and mischievous, and will not take or knowingly administer any harmful drug. I will do all in my power to elevate the standard of my profession, and I will hold in confidence all personal matters committed to my keeping, and all family affairs coming to my knowledge in the practice of my calling. With loyalty will I endeavor to aid the physician in his work and devote myself to the welfare of those committed to my care."

nightmare (nīt′mār) [" + *mara,* incubus]. A bad dream accompanied by great fear and a feeling of suffocation, once believed to be caused by a female monster or spirit that sat upon the dreamer. SYN: *oneirodynia.* SEE: *antephialtic.*

nightshade (nīt′shād) [A.S. *nihtscada*]. Any of the species of *Solanum.*

n., deadly. Belladonna, *q.v.*

night sweat (nīt swĕt) [A.S. *neaht,* night, + *swat,* sweat]. Profuse sweating during sleep at night.

Often an early sign of disease with intermittent temperature. In children, it occurs in rickets, in debilitated states. Patient should be rubbed down, sponged, and changed into dry clothing.

night terrors (nīt tĕr′ĕrs) [" + L. *terror,* state of fear]. Form of nightmare in children causing them to awaken in terror, screaming.

Fear continues for a period after the return to consciousness. SYN: *pavor nocturnus.*

night vision. The ability to see at night or in light of low intensity. Results from dark adaptation in which pupil dilates, visual purple increases and intensity threshold of the retina is lowered. Smoking tobacco decreases ability to see at night. SYN: *scotopic vision.*

nightwalking (nīt″wauk′ĭng) [" + *wealcan,* to revolve]. State in which individual walks about habitually while sleeping. SYN: *somnambulism.*

nigra (nī′gră) [L. black]. Mass of gray matter bet. the dorsal and pedal parts of the crus cerebri. SYN: *substantia nigra.*

nigri-, nigro- [L.]. Combining forms meaning *pert. to blackness.*

nigricans (nī′grĭ-kăns) [L.]. Blackened.

nigrities (nī-grĭsh′ĭ-ēz) [L. blackness]. Blackness; black pigmentation.

n. linguae. A black pigmentation of the tongue. SYN: *glossophytia.*

NIH. ABBR. for *National Institutes of Health.*

nihilism (nī′ĭ-lĭzm) [L. *nihil,* nothing, + G. *ismos,* state of]. 1. Disbelief in beneficial properties of medicine. 2. PSY: A delusion that everything is unreal.

Nikolsky's sign (nĭ-kol′skĭ). Condition of the external layer of the skin in which it can be rubbed off by slight friction or injury. Seen in pemphigus.

ninth cranial nerve. Glossopharyngeal nerve. SEE: *Appendix, cranial nerves.*

niobium (ni-o′be-um). A chemical element. SYMB: Nb. At. wt. 92.906; at. no. 41. Formerly called *columbium.*

niphablepsia (nĭf″ă-blĕp′sĭ-ă) [G. *nipha,* snow, + *ablepsia,* blindness]. Blindness caused by light glare on snow.

niphotyphlosis (nĭf″ō-tĭf-lō′sĭs) [" + *typhlōsis,* blindness]. Snow blindness. SYN: *niphablepsia.*

nipple (nĭp′l) [earlier *neble, nible,* possibly diminutive from A.S. *neb,* a little protuberance]. 1. The protuberance in each breast from which, in the female, the lactiferous ducts discharge. SYN: *mammilla, papilla, teat.* 2. Artificial substitute for female n. to be used on a nursing bottle.

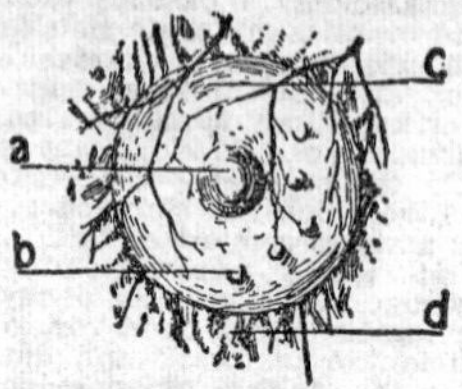

NIPPLE.

a. Nipple; b. areolar glands; c. primary areola; d. secondary areola.

The nipple contains erectile tissue and is surrounded by a pigmented area called the areola. The areola is pink in those who have never borne children and darker in those who have. It is supplied with a row of small sebaceous glands around its base called areolar glands which secrete an oily substance to keep it supple.

NP: During pregnancy, they should be washed well with soap and water and dried with a rough towel. Excessively dry nipples may be massaged with cold cream or lanolin. Cracked and sore nipples result from misuse of the nipple due to the baby's chewing.

Retracted nipples are caused by deficiency of muscle tissue or flattening of the erectile tissue, and are lower than the surrounding area.

RS: *acromastitis, halo, mammary, mammillation, Paget's disease of n., thelalgia, thelitis.*

n., crater. SEE: *n. retracted.*

n. line. SYN: *mammillary line.* A vertical line passing through the nipple.

n., retracted. N. whose tip lies below level of mammary gland.

n. shield. Mechanical device to protect the nipple during lactation period.

Nissl's bodies or granules (nis′el). SYN: *tigroid bodies.* Chromophil substance in the form of granules found in the cell bodies and dendrites of neurons but lacking in the axon and axon hillock. They are stained selectively by toluidin and other basic aniline dyes. They consist principally of the ribose type of nucleic acid and nucleoprotein.

Their physiologic significance is uncertain. They are concerned with active protein and metabolism and their condition varies with physiologic and pathologic conditions. In fatigue and certain pathologic states they may dissolve and disappear, a phenomenon called *chromatolysis.*

nisus (nī′sŭs) (pl. *nisūs*) [L. effort]. 1. An effort or struggle. 2. The desire for coitus on the part of certain animals in the spring. 3. Contraction of the muscles of the abdomen and diaphragm in the expulsion of the feces or urine.

nit (nĭt) [A.S. *hnitu*]. The egg of a louse or any other parasitic insect. SEE: *pediculosis.*

niter (nī′ter) [G. *nitron,* soda]. Sodium nitrate or potassium nitrate (saltpeter). Spelled also *nitre* (British).

niton (nī′tŏn). Radon, *q.v.*

nitrate (nī′trāt) [G. *nitron,* soda]. A salt of nitric acid.

ni′trated [G. *nitron,* soda]. Combined with nitric acid or a nitrate.

nitra′tion [G. *nitron,* soda]. Combination with nitric acid or a nitrate.

nitre (nī′tĕr) [G. *nitron,* soda]. Sodium nitrate or potassium nitrate (saltpeter). Spelled also *niter.*

ni′tric acid. HNO_3. A colorless, corrosive, poisonous liquid in concentrated form, employed as a caustic. It is widely used in industry and in chemical laboratories.

POISONING: SYM: Are essentially same as those produced by sulfuric acid. Pain, burning, vomiting, thirst and shock.

TREATMENT: Dilute with large volumes of water. Neutralize with weak alkalies; give magnesium oxide, milk of magnesia, milk or egg white in large amounts. AVOID: emetics and stomach tubes, because either may cause rupture of the stomach.

n. a., fuming. Combination of nitric acid which emits fumes of a choking nature. SEE: *fumes.*

nitride (nī′trĭd). A binary compound formed by direct combination of nitrogen with another element, as lithium nitride Li_3N.

nitrification (nī″trĭ-fĭ-kā′shŭn) [G. *nitron,* soda, + L. *facere,* to make]. The process by which the nitrogen of ammonia or other compounds is oxidized to nitric or nitrous acid or their salts (nitrates, nitrites). Takes place continually in the soil through the action of nitrifying bacteria.

nitrifying (nī″trĭ-fī′ing [G. *nitron,* soda, + *facere,* to make]. The process of nitrification, *q.v.*

n. bacteria. Bacteria which induce nitrification. Include the nitrite bacteria (*Nitrosomas*) which convert ammonia to nitrites and nitrate bacteria (*Nitrobacter*) which convert nitrites to nitrates.

nitrile (nī′trĭl, nī′trīl). An organic compound in which the nitrogen of ammonia exists with all three of the hydrogen atoms displaced.

nitrite (nī′trīte) [G. *nitron,* salt]. A salt of nitrous acid. In med., nitrites dilate blood vessels, reduce blood pressure, and depress motor centers of the spinal cord. They also act as antispasmodics. Principal nitrites used are amyl, ethyl, potassium, and sodium nitrite, *q.v.*

nitritoid (nī′trĭ-toyd) [" + *eidos,* resemblance]. Resembling a nitrite.

n. crisis. A syndrome resembling symptoms produced by the use of a nitrite, usually occurring after arsphenamine injection.

nitrituria (nī-trĭ-tū′rĭ-ă) [" + *ouron,* urine]. Nitrites or nitrates present in the urine.

nitro-, nitr- [G.]. Combining form denoting (a) combination with nitrogen, (b) presence of the group NO_2.

nitrofurazone (nī-trō-fu′ră-zōn). A synthetic antibiotic for topical application in some skin diseases and in preparation for skin grafting.

nitrogen (nī′trō-jen) [" + *gennan,* to produce]. SYMB: N. A colorless, odorless, tasteless, gaseous element occurring free in the atmosphere, forming 4/5 of its volume. At. wt. 14.0067; at. no. 7.

One of the important elements in all proteins, essential to plant and animal life for tissue building. Nitrogen is generally found in organic nature only in the form of compounds, as ammonia, nitrites, and nitrates which are transformed by plants into proteins, and, being consumed by animals, are converted into animal proteins of the blood and tissues.

RS: *azotation, azote, azotification, azotized.*

n. balance. The difference between intake and outgo of nitrogen. If intake is greater, a *positive balance* exists; if less, there is a *negative balance.* SEE: *n. equilibrium.*

n. cycle. The return of nitrogen from animal life to the soil, from which plants derive their supply, and in turn its return to animal life through plants taken as food.

n. equilibrium. Condition during which nitrogen excreted in the urine, feces, and sweat equals amt. taken in by the body in the food.

n. fixation. Conversion of atmospheric nitrogen into nitrates through the action of bacteria in the soil.

n. lag. Time required after a given protein is ingested until an equal amt. of nitrogen is excreted as that ingested.

n. monoxide. Nitrous oxide. N_2O. Also referred to as *laughing gas.*

n. mustards. A term embracing certain therapeutic mustard compounds. Used in Hodgkin's disease, lymphosarcoma, giant follicular lymphoblastoma, chronic lymphoid and myeloid leukemia, rheumatoid arthritis, and nephritis.

n., nonprotein. A nitrogenous component of the blood that is not a protein.

nitrogenous (nī-troj'ĕn-ŭs) [G. *nitron,* soda, + *gennan,* to produce]. Pert. to or containing nitrogen.

Foods which contain nitrogen are the proteins; those which do not contain nitrogen are the fats and carbohydrates. The retention of nitrogenous products in the blood is marked in kidney diseases.

nitroglycerin (nī″trō-glĭs'ĕr-ĭn) [" + *glycerin*]. Any nitrate of glycerol, specifically the trinitrate, a heavy, oily, explosive, colorless liquid obtained by treating glycerol with nitric and sulfuric acids. SYN: *glyceryl trinitrate.*

USES: Explosive constituent of dynamite and in medicine it has the action of nitrites and is a vasodilator. Used especially in angina pectoris.

nitromuriatic acid (nī″trō-mū-rĭ-at'ĭk) [" + L. *muriaticus,* briny]. A mixture of 1 part nitric and 3 parts hydrochloric acid used in commercial industries because it dissolves all the metals including platinum and gold.

POISONING: SYM: Same as those of nitric acid poisoning. TREATMENT: Same. SYN: *aqua regia.*

nitrous (nī'trŭs) [G. *nitron,* soda]. Containing nitrogen in its lowest valency.

n. oxide. N_2O. Colorless, sweet-tasting gas with pleasing smell causing temporary general anesthesia when inhaled. SYN: *laughing gas.*

In industry, used as a propellent for many aerosol products both food and non-food.

It is not toxic or inflammable. It is given in various amounts with oxygen or other anesthetic agents. If used with ether it may be inflammable. The patient may easily be asphyxiated if it is not administered properly.

SIGNS: Deep signs of nitrous oxide anesthesia are a slight increase in respirations, some dyspnea, cyanosis becomes deeper, eyeballs are fixed, either upward or downward. There is muscular rigidity, cyanosis increases to a grayish pallor, pupils become fixed in a dilated form, and respirations become paralyzed.

ACTION: Little or no effect on body temperature, blood pressure, volume or composition of blood, metabolism, or genitourinary system. Diaphoresis or increased muscle tone or both may occur with induction of anesthesia with nitrous oxide. Prolonged administration of nitrous oxide will cause depression of bone marrow.

Its action as an anesthetic can be potentiated by other classes of drugs: barbiturates, narcotics, tranquilizers, and inhalation agents.

CONTRAINDICATIONS: Not to be given in advanced conditions of anemia, in hypertension of 180 or above, hypotension of 80 or below, decompensated heart lesions, obesity, diabetes, dyspnea, alcoholism, or in advanced pulmonary tuberculosis.

HYPERANESTHESIA FROM: The patient should be given oxygen under pressure, and a respiratory stimulant administered. Carbon dioxide may also be given.

N. L. N. Abbr. for *National League for Nursing.*

NMRI. Abbr. for *Naval Medical Research Institute* (U. S. Navy).

N. N. D. Abbr. for *New and Nonofficial Drugs,* annual publication of the Council of Drugs of the American Medical Association, listing and describing the articles that are proposed for use. Since 1965, has been called *New Drugs.*

No. Abbr. L. *numero,* to the number of.

N_2O. Nitrous oxide.

N_2O_3. Nitrogen trioxide.

N_2O_5. Nitrogen pentoxide.

nobelium [from Nobel Institute, where it was first prepared]. Element obtained from bombardment of curium. SYMB: No. At. wt. 254; at. no. 102.

Nocard'ia. A genus of aerobic fungi belonging to the family Actinomycetaceae.

N. asteroides. Fungus causing actinomycosis.

nocardio'sis. Pathologic condition resulting from infection by *N. asteroides* or other species of *Nocardia.* May occur as a pulmonary infection which may spread, resulting in abscesses in the skin, brain, or other areas. May also give rise to fungus tumors (mycetomas) which occur most frequently in lower extremities especially the foot, in which case it is called maduromycosis or Madura foot. Nocardiosis is distinguishable from actinomycosis by identification of organism.

TREATMENT: Sulfadiazine daily. This may be supplemented by an antibiotic after laboratory determination of the antibiotic agents to which the strain of the causative organism is sensitive.

nociceptive (no″sĭ-sĕpt'ĭv). [L. *nocere, to hurt,* + *ceptus,* receiving]. Pert. to stimuli to the brain.

n. impulses. Impulses giving rise to sensations of pain.

n. reflex. A reflex initiated by painful stimuli.

nociperception (nō″sĭ-pĕr-sĕp'shŭn) [" + *perceptiō,* apprehension]. The perception by the nerve centers of injurious influences or painful stimuli.

Noct. [L.]. Abbr. for *night.*

noctalbuminuria (nok″tal-bū-mĭn-ū'rĭ-ă) [L. *nox, noct-,* night, + *albumen,* white of egg, + G. *ouron,* urine]. Excess of albumin voided in urine at night. SYN: *nyctalbuminuria.*

noctambulism (nŏk-tăm′bū-lĭzm) [" + *ambulāre,* to walk, + G. *ismos,* state of]. Sleep walking. SYN: *somnambulism.*

noctiphobia (nŏk″tĭ-fō′bĭ-ă) [" + G. *phobos,* fear]. Fear of the night and darkness. SYN: *nyctophobia.*

nocturia (nŏk-tū′rĭ-ă) [" + G. *ouron,* urine]. Urination, esp. excessive, during the night. SYN: *nycturia.* SEE: *enuresis.*

noctur′nal [L. *nocturnus,* at night]. Pert. to or occurring in the night. OPP: *diurnal.* SEE: *"nyct-" words.*

*n. enuresis.** Urinary incontinence during sleep at night. SYN: *bedwetting.*

no′cuous. Noxious, injurious, harmful.

nodal (nō′dăl) [L. *nodus,* knot]. Pert. to a protuberance.

n. points. One of 2 points situated on axis of a lens that any incident ray sent through 1 will produce a parallel emergent ray sent through the other.

n. rhythm. Cardiac rhythm with origin at auriculoventricular node.

nodding (nŏd′ĭng) [origin uncertain]. Quick inclination of the head downward. SYN: *nutation.*

n. spasm. Nodding of the head due to spasm of the sternomastoid muscles. SYN: *salaam convulsion.*

node (nōd) [L. *nodus,* knot]. 1. A knot, knob, protuberance or swelling. 2. A constricted region. 3. A small rounded organ or structure.

n., atrioventricular. SYN: *A-V node.* A tangled mass of Purkinje fibers located in lower part of interatrial septum from which the atrioventricular bundle (b. of His) arises.

n., A-V. ABBR. for *atrioventricular node, q.v.*

n's., Bouchard's. N's. on 2nd joints of the fingers in gastric dilatation.

n's., Féréol's. N's that are subcutaneous and seen in acute rheumatism.

n's., Haygarth's. Swelling of joints in arthritis deformans.

n's., Heberden's. N. on fingers seen in osteoarthritis.

n., Hensen's. SYN: *Hensen's knot, primitive knot.* A mass of rapidly proliferating cells at ant. end of primitive streak of embryo.

n., Keith and Flack's. Sinoauricular node.

n., lymph. Mass of lymphoid tissue along the course of lymphatic vessels.

n's., Meynet's. Those in capsules of joints and tendons in rheumatism.

n's., Parrot's. Osteophytes around ant. fontanel seen in hereditary syphilis.

n., piedric. Node on the hair shaft seen in piedra.*

n.'s of Ranvier. Constrictions of the myelin sheath of a myelinated nerve fiber.

n., sentinal. A signal node, *q.v.*

n., signal. SYN: *Virchow's node. Virchow's signal node.* Enlargement of one of the supraclavicular lymph nodes. Usually indicative of primary carcinoma of thoracic or abdominal organs.

n., singer's. Small white node which develops on vocal cords. SEE: *chorditis nodosa.*

n., sinoatrial. SYN: *S-A node.* N. in wall of rt. atrium near entrance of sup. vena cava, consisting of dense network of Purkinje fibers. Source of impulses initiating heart beat. Also called *pacemaker* of the heart.

n., sinoauricular. Sinoatrial node, *q.v.*

n., sinus. Sinoatrial node, *q.v.*

n., syphilitic. Circumscribed swelling at end of long bones due to congenital syphilis. Sensitive and painful during inflammation, esp. at night. SEE: *Parrot's n.*

nodose (nō′dōs) [L. *nodōsus,* knotted]. Swollen or knotlike at intervals; marked by nodes or projections.

nodosity (nō-dŏs′ĭ-tĭ) [L. *nodositās,* a knot]. 1. A protuberance or knot. 2. Condition of having nodes.

nodular (nod′ū-lăr) [L. *nodulus,* a little knot]. Containing or resembling nodules.

nodule (nod′ūl) [L. *nodulus,* a small knot]. 1. A small node. 2. A small aggregation of cells. SEE: *chalarosis, cladosporiosis.*

n.'s, aggregate. A group of solitary lymph nodules. EX: Peyer's patches of small intestine.

n., Albini's. N's. on free edges of auriculoventricular valves in infants.

n's., Arantius'. Central fibrous tubercles in segments of semilunar valves. SYN: *corpora Arantii.*

n., Aschoff's. N. found in myocardium, a characteristic lesion of rheumatic carditis.

n. of cerebellum. SEE: *nodulus.*

n.'s, cortical. Lymph nodules located in cortex of a lymph node.

n's., Gamna. Yellowish-brown ones in the spleen in certain enlargements. SYN: *tabac n's.*

n.'s, juxta-articular. SYN: *Jeanselme's n.'s.* N.'s in subcutaneous tissue around joints seen in syphilis, yaws, and other treponemal diseases.

n., lymph. A mass of densely packed lymphocytes forming the structural unit of lymphatic tissue. Each contains a *germinal center* where new lymphocytes are formed.

n., lymphatic, lymphoid. A lymph nodule, *q.v.*

n's., Morgagni. SEE: *n's. of Arantius.*

n., Schmorl's. N. formed by herniation of nucleus pulposus of intervertebral disc.

n. of semilunar valve. SEE: *n.'s, Arantius.*

n.'s, siderotic. Small brown n.'s, seen in spleen and other organs, consisting of necrotic tissue encrusted by iron salts.

n., solitary. An isolated nodule of lymphatic tissue such as occurs in mucous membranes.

n.'s, typhoid. N.'s characteristic of typhoid fever found in the liver.

nodulus (nod′ū-lŭs) (pl. *noduli*) [L.]. Nodule.

n. of cerebellum. The anterior portion of the vermis.

nodus (nō′dŭs) [L.]. Node.

noematachograph (nō-ē″mă-tak′ō-grăf) [G. *noēma,* understanding, + *tachus,* swift, + *graphein,* to write]. Device for recording time taken in mental activity.

noematachometer (nō-ē″mă-tak-om′ĕt-ĕr) [" + " + *metron,* measure]. Device for measurement of the time taken in a simple perception. SYN: *noematachograph.*

noise (noyz) [O.Fr. *noise,* strife, brawl; possibly derived from G. *nausea,* seasickness]. Sound of any sort, usually a loud, harsh one.

noli-me-tangere (nō′lĭ-mē-tan′jĕ-rē) [L. touch me not]. Cancerous ulcer, generally of the face, which eats away bone and soft tissue.

noma (nō′mă) [G. *nomē,* a spreading]. A gangrenous progressive condition, generally found in children, spreading from the mucous membrane of the cheek or gum to the cutaneous surface. SYN: *cancrum oris, stomatitis, gangrenous.*

n. pudendi, n. vulvae. A similar condition affecting the labia majora.

no'madism [G. *nomas*, roaming about]. PSY: Impulse to wander.

nomenclature (nō'mĕn-klā"chur) [L. *nomenclatura*, a name calling]. System of technical or scientific names. SYN: *terminology.*

nomogram (nŏm'ō-gram) [G. *nomos*, law, + *gramma*, a mark]. Representation by graphs, diagrams or charts of the relationship bet. numerical variables.

nomography (nō-mog'ră-fĭ) [G. *nomographia*, a writing of laws]. A graphic representation of the relation bet. numerical variables.

nomotopic (nŏm-ō-tŏp'ĭk) [G. *nomos*, law, + *topos*, place]. Occurring at the normal site.

non- [L.]. Prefix denoting *not, negation.*

nona-, non-, [L.]. Prefix meaning *ninth.*

nona (nō'nă) [L. *nonus*, ninth]. Acute or chronic infectious disease of central nervous system. SYN: *encephalitis lethargica, sleeping sickness.*

nonan (nō'năn) [L. *nonus*, ninth]. Having increased symptoms or reappearing every 9th day, as the paroxysms of malaria.

non compos mentis (nŏn kŏm'pŏs mĕn'tĭs) [L.]. Not of sound mind.

nonconductor (nŏn"kŏn-dŭk'tŏr) [L. *non*, not, + *con*, with, + *ductor*, a leader]. A substance that does not conduct or conducts with difficulty heat, sound, or electricity.

Strictly speaking, there is no perfect nonconductor. On the application of a sufficiently high voltage, current may be caused to flow through materials usually spoken of as nonconductors. SYN: *insulator.*

non"disjunc'tion. 1. The condition in which one or more pair of homologous chromosomes fail to separate following synapsis. 2. Term also applied to failure of daughter chromosomes to separate during mitosis.

nonelectrolyte (non"e-lek'tro-lĭt) [L. *non*, not, + *ēlectron*, amber, + *lytos*, dissolved]. A nonconducting solution.

nonigravida. SYN: *nonipara, q.v.*

nonipara (nō-nĭp'ăr-ă) [L. *nonus*, ninth, + *parēre*, to bring forth]. A woman who has given birth 9 times.

nonlax'ative diet. Low residue diet* with boiled milk and toasted crackers. No strained oatmeal, vegetable juice, or fruit juice given. Fats and concentrated sweets are restricted.

nonpolar (nŏn-pō'lĕr) [L. *non*, not + *pōlus*, a pole]. Not having separate poles; sharing electrons.

n. compound. One formed by the sharing of electrons.

nonpro'tein [L. *non*, not + G. *prōtos*, first]. Any substance not a protein.

n. nitrogen. 1. A nitrogenous constituent of blood that is not a protein. 2. Sum of all nonprotein nitrogen in the blood. SEE: *nitrogen.*

non repetat [L.]. Do not repeat.

nonrestraint (nŏn"rē-strānt') [L. *non*, not, + *rē*, back, + *stringere*, to bind back]. Treatment of the insane without using mechanical restraint.

nonseptate (nŏn-sĕp'tāt) [" + *saeptum*, a partition]. Having no dividing walls.

nonsexual (nŏn-sĕk'shū-ăl) [" + *sexus*, sex]. Without sex. SYN: *asexual.*

nontoxic (nŏn-tŏks'ĭk) [" + G. *toxikon*, poison]. Not poisonous or productive of poison.

nonunion (nŏn-ūn'yŭn) [L. *non*, not, + *uniō*, oneness]. Failure of bone fragments to knit together.

no'nus [L.]. 1. Ninth. 2. Hypoglossal or ninth cranial nerve.

nonviable (nŏn-vī'ă-bl) [L. *non*, not, + *via*, life]. Incapable of life or of living.

nooklep tia (nō-ō-klep'tĭ-ă) [G. *nous*, mind, + *kleptein*, to steal]. An obsession that one's thoughts are being stolen by others.

noopsyche (no'o-sī-ke) [" + *psychē*, soul]. Reasoning or intellectual processes.

N. O. P. H. N. Abbr. *National Organization for Public Health Nursing.*

norepinephrine (nor-ĕp"ĭ-nĕf'rĭn). A hormone produced by the adrenal medulla similar in chemical and pharmacologic properties to epinephrine but is chiefly a vasoconstrictor and has little effect on cardiac output. SYN: *noradrenalin; levarterenol bitartrate.*

norethindrone. A steroid hormone similar in action to progesterone. Used in progestation agents for birth control.

norm (norm) [L. *norma*, rule]. A type or standard pattern.

nor'ma [L. rule]. A view or aspect, esp. with reference to the skull.

n., anterior. N. facialis or frontalis.

n. basilaris. N. inferior or ventralis. View of underneath surface of skull.

n. facialis. View directed towards the face.

n. frontalis. N. facialis, *q.v.*

n., inferior. View of underneath surface of the skull.

n. lateralis. View as seen from the side; a profile view.

n. occipitalis. View as seen from behind.

n. sagittalis. View as seen in sagittal section.

n., superior. N. verticalis, *q.v.*

n. ventralis. View of inferior surface of skull.

n. verticalis. View of skull as seen from above.

normal (nor'măl) [L. *norma*, rule]. 1. Standard; performing proper functions; natural; regular. 2. BIOL: Not affected by experimental treatment; occurring naturally and not because of a disease or experimentation. 3. PSY: (a) Free from mental disorder; (b) of average development or intelligence. 4. CHEM: A term used to describe a solution so made that 1 liter contains 1 gram equivalent of the solute.

In the case of acids and bases formed by univalent radicals, a normal solution is the same as *molar*, as in the case of HCl. In the case of H_2SO_4, however, the normal solution would be half as strong as the molar, and in the case of H_3PO_4 it would be one-third.

n. body temperature. 98.6° F.

n. pulse. 72-80 beats per minute.

n. respiration. 18-24 per minute.

n. salt. SYN: *neutral salt.* An ionic compound containing no replaceable hydrogen or hydroxyl ions.

n. solution. 1. Solution containing 1 gm., molecular weight, of dissolved substance divided by the hydrogen equivalent of the substance per liter of solution. 2. A sol. which neutralizes an equal volume of a normal solution of any base or acid.

normalization (nŏr-măl-ĭ-zā'shŭn) [L. *norma*, rule]. Modification or reduction to normal.

normergic (norm-ĕr'jĭk). Reacting or pertaining to that which reacts in a normal manner.

normoblast (nor′mō-blăst) [L. *norma,* rule, + G. *blastos,* germ]. A nucleated red blood corpuscle similar in size to an ordinary erythrocyte.

normochromasia (nŏr″mō-krō-mā′zĭ-ă) [" + G. *chrōma,* color]. Average staining capacity in a cell or tissue.

nor″mochro′mia. Blood possessing normal color and hemoglobin content.

normocyte (nor′mō-sīt) [" + G. *kytos,* cell]. An average-sized red blood corpuscle. SYN: *erythrocyte.*

normocytosis (nor″mō-sī-tō′sĭs) [" + " + *-ōsis,* condition]. A normal state of the corpuscular elements of the blood.

normoglycemia (nor″mō-glī-sē′mĭ-ă) [" + G. *glykus,* sweet, + *aima,* blood]. Normal state of sugar content of the blood.

normoglycemic (nor″mō-glī-sē′mik) [" + " + *aima,* blood]. Having a normal amount of sugar in the blood.

normoorthocytosis (nor″mō-or″thō-sī-tō′-sĭs) [L. *norma,* rule, + G. *orthos,* correct, + *kytos,* cell, + *-ōsis,* increase]. Increase in the blood of the number of leukocytes, but with normal proportion of the different varieties.

normoskeocytosis (nor″mō-skē″ō-sī-tō′sĭs) [" + *skaios,* left, + *kytos,* cell, + *-ōsis,* condition]. Normal number of the leukocytes of the blood with deviation to the left, *i. e.,* with immature forms present.

normosthenuria (nor″mō-sthĕn-ū′rĭ-ă) [L. *norma,* rule + G. *sthenos,* strength, + *ouron,* urine]. Urination of normal amount and specific gravity.

normotensive (nor-mo-ten′siv). Normal blood pressure.

normotonic (nor″mō-ton′ik) [" + G. *tonos,* tension]. 1. Having normal muscular tonus. 2. One who has normal muscle tonus.

normotopia (nor″mō-tō′pĭ-ă) [" + G. *topos,* place]. Situation in the regular place.

normotopic (nor″mō-top′ik) [" + *topos,* place]. In the right location; pert. to the normal situation.

normovolemia (nor″mō-vō-lē′mĭ-ă) [" + *volūmen,* volume, + G. *aima,* blood]. Normal state of blood volume.

Norwe′gian itch. Severe form of scabies marked by pustules and crusts.

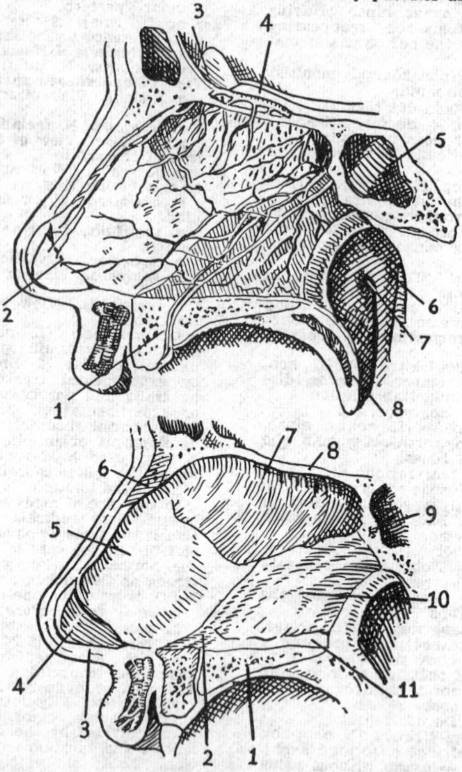

NOSE.

Nasal cavity, showing its structural arrangement, blood, and nerve supply. *Above:* 1. Incisor canal. 2. Little Kisselbach triangle. 3. Crista galli. 4. Olfactory bulb. 5. Sphenoid sinus. 6. Rosenmueller's fossa. 7. Pharyngeal orifice of eustachian tube. 8. Soft palate. *Below:* 1. Hard palate. 2. Septal or medial crest of maxillary bone. 3. Columella. 4. Medial crus of major alar cartilage. 5. Septal cartilage. 6. Nasal bone. 7. Perpendicular plate of ethmoid. 8. Cribriform plate of ethmoid. 9. Rostrum of sphenoid. 10. Vomer. 11. Septal or medial crest of palatine bone.

nose (nōz) [A.S. *nosw*]. Projection in center of face; the organ of olfaction and the entrance which warms, moistens and filters the air for the respiratory tract. SYN: *nasus; organon olfactus.*

ANAT: The external portion of the nose is a triangle of cartilage and bone covered with skin and lined with mucous membrane. Internally, a septum divides nose into 2 chambers. Each chamber contains 3 *meatuses* which are found underneath the corresponding turbinates. Orifices of frontal, ant. ethmoid and maxillary sinuses are in middle meatus. Orifices of posterior ethmoids and sphenoids are in superior meatus.

Sinuses, Communicating: Ethmoidal, frontal, maxillary, sphenoidal.

Nerves: Facial, olfactory, ophthalmic and maxillary.

Blood Supply: External and internal maxillary arteries from the external carotid and ethmoidal artery from the internal carotid.

EXAMINATION OF: Note shape, size, color, state of the alae nasi, discharge, interference with respiration, evidences of injury, deflected or perforated septum, enlarged turbinates, and tenderness over frontal and maxillary sinuses.

DIAG: COLOR: *Chronic red n.*: Dilated capillaries the result of alcoholism, lupus erythematosus, acne rosacea, pustules, boils and digestive disorders. ULCERATION, SUPERFICIAL: Tuberculous ulcer, epithelioma, syphilis. SIZE AND SHAPE: *Broad and Coarse*: Cretinism, myxedema, acromegaly. *Sunken*: Syphilis or injury. *Pinched with Small Nares*: Hypertrophied adenoid tissue or chronic obstructions; also tumors. DISCHARGES: *Inoffensive watery discharge*: Present in nasal catarrh, early stages of measles, hay fever, acute irritation of lining membranes. *Offensive discharges*: Nasopharyngeal diphtheria, lupus, local infection, impacted foreign bodies, caries, rhinitis, glanders, syphilitic infection.

FOREIGN BODY IN THE NOSE: SYM: Irritation of nose resulting in coughing or watery or purulent discharge. Occasionally pain and obstruction of nose. If not recognized immediately it often causes a foul discharge on the affected side of the nose. There may be obstruction to breathing in one nostril. If the foreign body is very small, symptoms may be absent.

TREATMENT: Vigorous blowing of the nose is dangerous as it may spread infection to the various cavities and sinuses about the nose or to the ear. Do not attempt to fish the body out with a hairpin or other object, as attempts to dislodge it may cause it to slip further in the nose or down the throat, from where it occasionally drops into the windpipe. Foreign bodies in the nose rarely need emergency measures. Take the patient to a physician.

n., bridge of. Sup. portion of ext. nose formed by union of the two nasal bones.

n., hammer. Rhinophyma, *q.v.*

n., saddle. Nose with depressed bridge seen in tertiary syphilis due to gummatous destruction of septal supporting structure, and following operations which are complicated by suppuration and destruction of supporting framework.

nose, *words pert. to:* agger nasi; ala nasi; alinasal; anosmia; apostaxis; bulb, olfactory; bulla ethmoidalis; choana; columella nasi; epistaxis; hyperosmia; naris; "nas-" words; nostril; parosmia; rhinalgia; rhinitis; "rhino-" words; septum; sinus, accessory nasal; sinusitis; smell; vestibule of nose; vibrissae; vomer; xeromycteria.

nosebleed (nōz′blēd) [A.S. *nosu,* nose, + *blēdan,* to bleed]. Hemorrhage from nose. SYN: *epistaxis.*

nosema (no-sē′mă) [G. *nosēma,* disease]. 1. Ailment (nosema) or disease. 2. *Nosema,* a genus of Microsporidia.

noso- [G.]. Combining form meaning *pert. to disease.*

nosochthonography (nos″ok-thon-og′ră-fĭ) [G. *nosos,* disease, + *chthōn,* earth, + *graphein,* to write]. Study of geography of diseases; medical geography. SYN: *nosogeography.*

nosocomial (nos″o-ko′mĭ-al) [" + *komein,* to care for]. Pert. to a hospital or infirmary.

n. infection. Infection acquired in a hospital.

nosode (nos′ōd) [" + *eidos,* appearance]. A bacterial vaccine used in treatment of the disease of which it is the causative agent.

nosogenesis, nosogeny (nos″ō-jĕn′ĕ-sĭs, nos-oj′en-ĭ) [" + *gennan,* to produce]. The development and progress of a disease.

nosogeography (nos″ō-jē-og′ră-fĭ) [" + *gē,* earth, + *graphein,* to write]. Study of medical geography. SYN: *nosochthonography.*

nosography (no-sog′ră-fĭ) [" + *graphein,* to write]. The description of a disease.

nosohemia (nŏs-ō-hē′mĭ-ă) [G. *nosos,* disease, + *aima,* blood]. Disease of the blood.

nosology (no-sol′o-jĭ) [" + *logos,* word]. The science of description, or the classification of diseases.

nosomania (nos″ō-mā′nĭ-ă) [" + *mania,* madness]. 1. The delusion that one is diseased. 2. Morbid fear of disease.

nosomycosis (nos″ō-mī-kō′sĭs) [" + *mykēs,* fungus, + *-ōsis*]. Any disease caused by a parasitic fungus or Schizomycete.

nosonomy (nos-on′ō-mĭ) [" + *nomos,* law]. The science of disease classification.

nosophobia (nō″sō-fō′bĭ-ă) [G. *nosos,* disease, + *phobos,* fear]. Abnormal aversion to illness, or to a particular affection.

nosophyte (nōs′ō-fīt). A disease-causing plant microorganism.

nosopoietic (nō″sō-poy-ĕt′ĭk) [" + *poiein,* to form]. Producing or causing disease.

Nosopsyllus (nō″sŏp-sĕl′lŭs). A genus of fleas belonging to the order Siphonaptera.

N. fasciatus. A species of rat fleas responsible for transmission of murine typhus and perhaps of plague.

nosotherapy (nos″ō-ther′ă-pĭ) [" + *therapeia,* treatment]. Treatment of one disease by voluntarily introducing another microorganism into the body.

nosotrophy (nos-ot′rō-fĭ) [G. *nosos,* disease, + *trophē,* nourishment]. Nursing care and feeding of the sick.

nos″otrop′ic. Directed against the symptoms or effects of a disease. SEE: *etiotropic.*

nostalgia (nos-tal′jĭ-ă) [G. *nostos,* a return home, + *algos,* pain]. Homesickness. SEE: *cainotophobia.*

nostomania (nos″tō-ma′nĭ-ă) [" + *mania,* madness]. Nostalgia verging on insanity.

nos′tril [A.S. *nosu,* nose, + *thyrl,* a hole]. One of the external apertures of the nose. SYN: *naris.* SEE: *nose.*

n. reflex. Reduction of opening of naris on affected side in lung disease in proportion to lessened alveolar air capacity on affected side.

nostrum (nŏs′trŭm) [L. our]. A patent or a quack remedy.

notal (nō′tăl) [G. *nōton,* back]. Concerning the back. SYN: *dorsal.*

notalgia (nō-tal′jĭ-ă) [" + *algos,* pain]. Painful condition of the back. SYN: *dorsalgia.*

notch (nŏtsh) [A.S. *nocke*]. A rather deep indentation or narrow gap in the edge of a part. SYN: *incisura.*

n., acetabular. Notch in inferior border of acetabulum.

n., aortic. One in sphygmogram from rebound at aortic valve closure.

n., cardiac. Concavity on ant. border of left lung into which the heart projects.

n., cerebellar, anterior and posterior. A deep notch separating the hemispheres of the cerebellum.

n., clavicular. One at the upper angle of the sternum with which the clavicle articulates.

n., costal. One of seven pairs of indentations on lateral surfaces of the sternum, for articulation with costal cartilages.

n., cotyloid. SEE: *acetabular n.*

n., ethmoidal. N. separating the two orbital portions of frontal bone.

n., frontal. N. on supraorbital arch which transmits frontal artery and nerve.

n., greater sciatic. Large n. on posterior border of hip bone between posterior inferior iliac spine and spine of ischium.

n., interclavicular. A rounded one at top of manubrium of sternum, between surfaces articulating with the clavicles.

n., jugular (of occipital bone). One which forms the posterior and middle portions of jugular foramen.

n., jugular (of sternum). N. on upper surface of manubrium between the two clavicular notches.

n., lesser sciatic. N. immediately below spine of ischium on post. border of hip bone. Converted into a foramen by the sacrotuberous ligament.

n., mandibular. N. on sup. border of ramus of mandible separating coronoid and condyloid processes.

n., nasal. 1. Deep notch on anterior surface of maxilla and forming lateral border of piriform aperture. 2. N. between internal angular processes of frontal bone.

n., pancreatic. N. on lateral surface of head of pancreas for sup. mesenteric artery and vein. It separates uncinate process of head from remaining portion.

n., radial. N. on lat. surface of coronoid process of ulna for receiving circumference of head of radius.

n. of Rivinus. Tympanic notch, *q.v.*

n., scapular. A deep n. on sup. border of scapula. Transmits suprascapular nerve.

n., sciatic. SEE: *greater or lesser sciatic n.*

n., semilunar. N. on ant. aspect of proximal end of ulna for articulation with trochlea of humerus.

n., sphenopalatine. N. between orbital and sphenoidal processes of palatine bone.

n., suprasternal. Jugular n. of the sternum, *q.v.*

n., tentorial. N. in free border of tentorium cerebelli through which brain stem passes.

n., thyroid. Deep n. on sup. border of thyroid cartilage of larynx separating the two laminae.

n., tympanic. SYN: *N. of Rivinus.* N. in sup. portion of the tympanic ring.

n., ulnar. N. on distal end of radius for receiving head of ulna.

n., umbilical. N. on ant. border of liver where it is crossed by falciform ligament.

n., vertebral. Concavity on inf. surface of root of vertebral arch. When two vertebrae are in position, the notches form the *intervertebral foramina.*

note (nōt) [L. *nota,* a mark]. A sound of definite pitch.

n. blindness. Inability to recognize musical notes; due to a central lesion.

notencephalocele (no″tĕn-sef′al-ō-sēl) [G. *nōton,* back, + *egkephalos,* brain, + *kēlē,* hernia]. Protrusion of brain substance at the back of the head.

notifi′able diseases. The laws of the various states require that certain diseases when existing shall be reported to the local health authorities, such as a Board of Health. A fine may be levied for not doing so. Among the diseases generally required to be reported are: All communicable or contagious diseases, such as smallpox, scarlet fever, relapsing fever; diphtheria or membranous croup; enteric fevers, such as typhoid fever; puerperal pyrexia and sepsis; cholera; typhus; meningococcal meningites; acute anterior poliomyelitis; polioencephalitis; encephalitis lethargica; tuberculosis; epidemic of acute diarrheal disease; chickenpox; gonorrhea; syphilis. SEE: *quarantine; reportable diseases.*

notochord (nō′tō-kord) [G. *nōton,* back, + *chordē,* cord]. A rod of cells lying dorsal to intestine and extending from ant. to post. end which forms axial skeleton in embryos of all chordates. In vertebrates it is replaced partially or completely by centra of vertebrae. A remnant persists in man as a portion of nucleus pulposus of intervertebral disk.

no″togen′esis. Development of the notochord.

noumenal (nū′mē-năl) [G. *nooumenon,* a thing perceived]. Pert. to rational intuition opposed to sensual perception.

noumenon (nū′mē-nŏn) [G. *nooumenon,* a thing perceived]. An object of rational apprehension as opposed to perception.

nourishment (nur′ĭsh-mĕnt) [L. *nutrīre,* to nurse]. 1. Act of nourishing or of being nourished. 2. Sustenance; nutriment. SEE: *center, trophic; trophic.*

novocain (no′vo-kan). A proprietary name for procaine hydrochloride, *q.v.*

noxa (noks′ă) (pl. *noxae*) [L. injury]. Anything harmful to health.

noxious (nok′shus) [L. *noxius,* injurious]. Harmful; not wholesome.

NP. Abbreviation for *nucleoplasmin index; nucleoprotein; nursing procedure.*

Np. Chemical symbol for *neptunium.*

NPH insulin. Abbr. for *neutral protamine Hagedorn insulin.* SEE: *insulin, NPH.*

NPN. Abbr. for *nonprotein nitrogen.*

n-rays. Rays discovered by Blondlot in 1903 making certain bodies luminous.

Nt. Symbol for *niton.*

nubecula (nū-bek′ū-la) [L. little cloud]. Cloudiness of the cornea or the urine.

nubile (nū′bĭl) [L. *nubere,* to marry]. Pert. to a girl who has attained puberty and who is thus able to marry.

nubility (nū-bĭl′ĭ-tĭ) [L. *nubere,* to marry]. Marriageableness, said of female at puberty, the final state of sex development.

nucha (nū′kă) [L.]. Nape of neck.

nuchal (nū′kal) [L. *nucha*, back of neck]. Pert. to the neck or *nucha*.

Nuck's canal or diverticulum (nook). An anomalous peritoneal pouch extending for a variable distance into the labium. Homologous to processus vaginalis of the male.

nuclear (nū′klē-ăr) [L. *nucleus*, a kernel]. Resembling or concerning a nucleus.

n. arc. Region of equator of crystalline lens where cells undergo transition into lens fibers. Also called *nuclear zone; lens vortex.*

n. sap. Syn: *karyolymph.* Liquid of a cell nucleus found within the meshwork.

nuclease (nū′klē-ās) [L. *nucleus*, kernel, + *ase*, enzyme]. Any enzyme in animals and plants which facilitates hydrolysis of nuclein and nucleic acids.

nucleate (nū′klē-āt) [L. *nucleatus*, having a kernel]. 1. Having a nucleus. 2. To form a nucleus. 3. A salt or ester of nucleic acid.

nucleic acid. Syn: *nucleinic acid.* One of an important group of substances found in cells, esp. the nuclei. They have a complex chemical structure being formed of sugars (pentoses), phosphoric acid, and nitrogen bases (purines and pyramidines). Most important are *deoxyribonucleic acid* and *ribonucleic acid, q.v.*

nuclein (nu′klē-ĭn) [L. *nucleus*, a kernel]. A normal chemical constituent of a cell nucleus, a colorless, shapeless substance obtained by hydrolysis of nucleoproteins or cells containing nucleic acid and proteins rich in phosphorus.

n. bases. Bases formed from decomposition of nuclein. Ex: adenine, guanine, xanthine, hypoxanthine.

n. therapy. The use of nuclein derived from various glands and blood serum in the treatment of disease. Said to increase white blood cell formation and thus increase resistance to infection.

nucleinase. Syn: *nuclease, q.v.*

nucleo- [L.]. Pertaining to a *nucleus*.

nucleoalbumin (nū″klē-ō-ăl-bū′mĭn) [L. *nucleus*, kernel, + *albus*, white]. A complex of nucleic acid and albumin.

nucleoalbuminuria (nū″klē-ō-al-bu″mĭ-nū′rĭ-ă) [L. *nucleus*, kernel, + *albus*, white, + G. *ouron*, urine]. The presence of nucleoalbumin in urine.

nucleoalbumose (nū″klē-ō-ăl′bū-mōs) [" + *albus*, white]. Partly hydrated nucleoalbumin found in the urine of patients with osteomalacia.

nucleofugal (nū-klē-of′ū-găl) [" + *fugere*, to flee]. Directed or moving away from a nucleus in the cell.

nucleohiston(e (nū″klē-ō-hĭs′ton, -tōn) [" + *istos*, tissue]. A substance in leukocytes, lymph and thymus glands, composed of nuclein and histone.

nucleoid (nū′klē-oyd) [" + G. *eidos*, resemblance]. Resembling a nucleus.

nucleolar (nū-klē′ō-lăr) [L. *nucleolus*, a little kernel]. Pert. to a nucleolus.

n. organizer or ***n. zone.*** One of several constrictions in a nucleolar chromosome which give rise to the nucleoli. Syn: *SAT-zone.*

nucleoliform (nū-klē′ō-lĭ-form) [" + *forma*, shape]. Like a nucleolus.

nucleolin (nū-klē′ō-lĭn) [L. *nucleolus*, little kernel]. The substance composing the nucleolus.

nucleolonucleus (nu″kle-o-lo-nu′kle-us). Nucleololus; a minute point within the nucleolus.

nucleolus (nū-klē′ō-lŭs) (pl. *nucleoli*) [L. little kernel]. A spherical body within the cell nucleus.

n., chromatin. A false nucleolus, *q.v.*

n., false. Dense bodies of chromatin found on chromonemata. Syn: *karyosome, q.v.*

nucleomicrosome (nū″klē-ō-mī′krō-sōm) [L. *nucleus*, kernel, + G. *mikros*, tiny, + *sōma*, body]. Any one of the minute granules making a nucleoplasmic fiber.

nucleons (nu′kle-onz). Collective name of the particles that make up the nucleus of an atom.

nucleopetal (nū-klē-op′ĕt-ăl) [" + *petere*, to seek]. Seeking or moving toward the nucleus.

nu″cleoplas′mic. Pert. to nucleoplasm.

n. index. The ratio of nuclear volume to cytoplasmic volume, expressed thus:

$$NP = \frac{\text{vol. of nucleus}}{\text{vol. of cell} - \text{vol. of nucleus}}$$

nucleoprotein (nū″klē-ō-prō′tē-ĭn) [" + G. *prōtos*, first]. The combination of 1 of the proteins with nucleic acid to form a conjugated protein found in cell nuclei.

nucleoreticulum (nū″klē-ō-rē-tĭk′ū-lŭm) [" + *reticulum*, network]. Any mesh framework in a nucleus.

nucleosidase (nū″klē-ō-sī′dās). An enzyme that catalyzes the hydrolysis of nucleosides.

nu′cleoside. A glycoside formed by the union of a purine or pyrimidine base with a sugar (pentose).

nucleospindle (nū″klē-ō-spĭn′dl) [" + A.S. *spinel*]. Spindle-shaped body occurring in karyokinesis, *q.v.*

nucleotidase (nū″klē-ō-tī′-dās). An enzyme (nucleophosphatase) which splits phosphoric acid from nucleotides leaving a nucleoside.

nucleotide (nū′klē-ō-tīd) [L. *nucleus*, kernel]. Syn: *mononucleotide.* A comp. formed of phosphoric acid, a sugar, and a base (purine or pyrimidine), all of which constitute the structural unit of nucleic acid.

nu″cleotox′in [" + G. *toxikon*, poison]. A toxin acting upon or produced by cell nuclei.

nucleus (nū′klē-ŭs) (pl. *nuclei*) [L. little kernel]. 1. A central point about which matter is gathered, as in a calculus.

2. The vital body in the protoplasm of a cell; the essential agent in growth, metabolism, reproduction and transmission of characteristics of a cell. See: *cell structure.*

3. A group of nerve cells or mass of gray matter in the central nervous system, esp. the brain.

4. Chem: Heavy central atomic particle in which most of the mass and total positive electric charge are concentrated.

n., abducent. A gray n., the origin of abducens nerve, on floor of 4th ventricle, behind trigeminal n. Syn: *abducens nucleus; nucleus of abducens nerve.*

n. ambiguus. [NA]. N. of the glossopharyngeal and vagus nerves in medulla oblongata. Lies in lateral half of reticular formation. Syn: *ambiguous nucleus.*

n., amygdaloid. N. projecting into inf. cornua of lat. ventricle. Constitutes part of basal ganglia.

n., angular. Syn: *Bechterew's n.* The sup. vestibular nucleus.

n., ant., of thalamus. N. located in rostral part of thalamus. Receives fibers of mammillothalamic tract.

n., arcuate. 1. N. located on basal aspect of pyramid of medulla. 2. The posteromedial ventral n. of the thalamus. Also called *semilunar n.*

n., auditory. Nest of nerve cells where auditory nerves arise.

n. of von Bechterew. The sup. vestibular nucleus, *q.v.*

n. of Burdach. The cuneate nucleus, *q.v.*

n., caudate. A comma-shaped mass of gray matter forming part of the corpus striatum. Constitutes part of the basal ganglia.

n., central, of thalamus. SYN: *centromedian n.* A group of nuclei in middle part of thalamus.

n., centromedian. SYN: *n. of Luys.* The central nucleus of the thalamus, *q.v.*

n., cerebellar. One of the nuclei of the cerebellum: *n. fastigii, n. emboliformis, n. globosus,* and *n. dentatus.*

n., cochlear, dorsal. N. in medulla oblongata lying dorsal to restiform body. Receives fibers of cochlear nerve. SEE: *nucleus, cochlear, ventral.*

n., cochlear, ventral. N. in medulla oblongata lying anterior and lateral to restiform body. Receives fibers from cochlear nerve. SEE: *nucleus, cochlear, dorsal.*

n., cornucommissural, posterior. A column of cells extending entire length of spinal cord lying along medial border of post. column near post. gray commissure.

n., cuneate. N. in inf. portion of medulla oblongata in which fibers of the fasciculus cuneatus terminate. SYN: *nucleus cuneatus* [NA]; *nucleus of Burdach.*

n., Deiter's. Lateral vestibular nucleus, *q.v.*

n., dentate. SYN: *n. dentatus.* Large convoluted mass of gray matter in lateral portion of cerebellum. It is folded so as to enclose some of the central white matter. Gives rise to fibers of the sup. cerebellar peduncle.

n., dorsal, of spinal cord. SYN: *Clarke's column.* A column of gray matter lying at base of dorsal horn of gray matter and extending from 7th cervical to 3rd lumbar segments. Cells give rise to fibers of the dorsal spinocerebellar tract.

n., dorsal motor, of vagus. A column of cells in medulla oblongata lying lateral to hypoglossal nucleus. Its cells give rise to most of efferent fibers of vagus nerve.

n., dorsal sensory, of vagus. N. lying lateral to dorsal motor nucleus of vagus. Receives fibers of solitary tract.

n., ectoblastic. One in cells of the epiblast.

n., Edinger-Westfall. N. of midbrain located dorsomedially to oculomotor nucleus. Gives rise to visceral efferent fibers terminating in ciliary ganglion, axons from which innervate ciliary muscle and sphincter iridis.

n., emboliform. N. of cerebellum lying between dentate and globose nuclei. Receives axons of Purkinje cells and sends efferent fibers into brachium conjunctivum.

n., facial motor. N. in medulla oblongata in floor of 4th ventricle giving rise to efferent fibers of facial nerve. SYN: *nucleus nervi facialis* [NA]; *nucleus of facial nerve.*

n., fastigial. N. in medullary portion of cerebellum. Receives afferent fibers from vestibular nerve and sup. vestibular nucleus. Afferent fibers form fasciculus uncinatus and fastigiobulbar tract.

n. funiculi gracilis. BNA. Elongated mass of gray matter in dorsal pyramid of medulla oblongata.

n., germinal. N. resulting from union of male and female pronuclei.

n., globose. N. of the cerebellum located medial to the emboliform nucleus.

n. gracilis. N. in medulla oblongata in which fibers of the fasciculus gracilis terminate.

n., habenular. N. of the diencephalon located in the habenular trigone. Functions as an olfactory correlation center. SYN: *nucleus of habenula; nucleus habenulae* [NA].

n., hypoglossal. An elongated mass of gray matter in the medulla oblongata in floor of 4th ventricle. Gives rise to motor fibers of hypoglossal nerve. SYN: *nucleus of hypoglossal nerve; nucleus nervi hypoglossi* [NA].

n., hypothalamic. One of the nuclei occurring in four groups found in hypothalamus. Includes the following nuclei: dorsomedial, intercalatus, lateral, mamillary (lateral and medial), paraventricular, posterior, supraoptic, tuberal, ventromedial. Cells of these nuclei, esp. the supraoptic and paraventricular, in addition to serving a neural function, are secretory and produce the vasopressor, oxytocic, and antidiuretic principles of the hypophysis. These hormones pass through efferent fibers of the infundibular stalk to the pars nervosa (post. lobe) of the hypophysis where they are stored and liberated. SYN: *nucleus hypothalamicus* [BNA]; *nucleus subthalamicus* [NA].

n., interpeduncular. N. of the midbrain near sup. border of pons. Receives fibers of the habenulopeduncular tract.

n., interstitial, of Cajal. N. in sup. portion of midbrain. Receives fibers from vestibular nuclei, basal ganglia, and occipital regions of cerebral cortex. Efferent fibers pass to ipsi- and contralateral fasciculi and interstitiospinal tracts.

n., intraventricular. SEE: *n., caudate.*

n., lenticular. One of the n. forming part of the basal ganglia of the cerebrum. Consists of *globus pallidus* and *putamen.* With the caudate nucleus, it forms the *corpus striatum.*

n. lentis. N. of crystalline lens.

n., mother. One that divides into two or more parts called *daughter nuclei.*

n., motor. N. giving rise to motor fibers of a nerve.

n., motor, of trigeminal nerve. N. in medulla oblongata near 1st margin of sup. part of 4th ventricle. Gives rise to motor fibers of trigeminal nerve. SYN: *nucleus motorius nervi trigemini* [NA].

n., oculomotor. N. in central gray matter of midbrain lying below rostral end of cerebral aqueduct.

n., olivary, inferior. A large convoluted mass of cells lying in ventral part of medulla oblongata and forming part of the reticular system. Gives rise to fibers of the olivocerebellar tract. SYN: *olivary nucleus; nucleus olivaris inferior; nucleus olivaris* [NA].

n., olivary, superior. A small n. located in mid-lateral tegmental region of pons. Receives fibers from ventral cochlear nucleus. SYN: *nucleus dorsalis corporis trapezoidei* [NA].

n. of origin. N. giving rise to fibers of a nerve or nerve tract.

n., paraventricular. N. of hypothalamus lying in supraoptic portion. Its axons with those of supraoptic n. form supraopticohypophyseal tract. SEE: *nucleus, hypothalamic.*

n., pontine (*pontile*). One of several groups of nerve cells located in the pons. Receives afferent fibers from cerebral cortex; efferent fibers pass through brachium pontis to cerebellum.

n. pulposus. A gelatinous mass in center of an intervertebral disk; remains of the notochord.

n., pyramidal. Band of gray matter near olivary n. in the medulla.

n. quintus. Trigeminal nerve nucleus.

n., red. Large oval pigmented mass in upper portion of midbrain and extending upward into subthalamus. Receives fibers from cerebral cortex and cerebellum; efferent fibers give rise to rubrospinal tracts.

n., reticular. A column of neurons in spinal cord in basal zone of posterior gray column.

n. ruber. BNA. Mass of red colored gray matter in crus cerebri close to optic thalamus.

n., salivatory, inferior. N. located in pons near level of dorsal motor nucleus of the vagus. Gives rise to preganglionic parasympathetic fibers which pass to otic ganglion via hypoglossal nerve. Impulses regulate secretion of parotid gland.

n., salivatory, superior. An ill-defined n. in pons lying dorsomedial to facial nucleus. Gives rise to preganglionic parasympathetic fibers passing through chorda tympani and lingual nerve to submaxillary ganglion. Impulses regulate secretion of submaxillary and sublingual glands.

n., segmentation. N. of zygote formed by fusion of male and female pronuclei.

n., sensory. A nucleus of termination, *q.v.*

n., sensory, of trigeminal nerve. A group of nuclei in pons and medulla oblongata consisting of *spinal nucleus* which extends inferiorly into spinal cord, the *main nucleus* lying dorsal and lateral to motor nucleus, and the *mesencephalic nucleus* lying in lateral wall of 4th ventricle.

n., subthalamic. [NA]. SEE: *n., hypothalamic.*

n., supraoptic. N. of the hypothalamus lying above rostral ends of optic tracts and lateral to optic chiasma. SEE: *nucleus, hypothalamic.*

n. of termination. N. in which fibers of a nerve or nerve tract terminate.

n., thalamic. Any of the nuclei of the thalamus. Include a large number belonging to the following groups: anterior, intralaminar, lateral, and medial thalamic nuclei.

n., vesicular. N. having deeply staining membrane and pale center.

n., vestibular. One of four nuclei in medulla oblongata in which fibers of vestibular nerve terminate. Include *medial* (Schwalbe's), *superior* (Bechterew's), *lateral* (Deiter's) and *inferior.* SYN: *nuclei vestibulares* [NA]; *nuclei nervi vestibularis.*

n., vitelline. One formed by union of male and female pronuclei within the vitellus. SYN: *yolk nucleus.*

n., white. Central white substance of corpus dentatum of olive.

nuclide (nu'klīd). A particular type of atom capable of existing for a measurable length of time.

nude (nūd) [L. *nudāre,* to strip]. 1. Bare; naked; unclothed. 2. An unclothed body.

nud'ism. 1. In psychiatry, morbid desire to remove clothing. 2. The cult or practice of living in a nude condition.

nudo- [L.]. Combining form denoting *uncovered, naked.*

nudomania (nū-dō-ma'nĭ-ă) [L. *nudāre,* to strip, + G. *mania,* madness]. Abnormal desire to be nude.

nudophobia (nū-dō-fō'bĭ-ă) [" + G. *phobos,* fear]. Abnormal fear of being unclothed. SEE: *gymnophobia.*

Nuel's space (nū'ĕl). S. in organ of Corti between outer pillar and outer phalangeal cells (Deiter's cells).

Nuhn's gland (noon). Mucous gland on each side of frenum of the tongue. SYN: *Blandin's gland.*

null hypothesis. The assumption or hypothesis that the observed difference between two groups of patients studied is accidental or due to chance, and is not due to one of the groups having received a specific treatment.

nullipara (nŭl-ĭp'ă-ră) [L. *nullus,* none, + *parēre,* to bear]. A woman who has borne no children.

nulliparity (nŭl-ĭ-par'ĭ-tĭ) [" + *parēre,* to bear]. Condition of not having given birth to a child.

nulliparous (nŭl-lĭp'ăr-ŭs) [" + *parēre,* to bear]. Never having borne a child.

numb (nŭm) [A.S. *numen,* taken]. 1. Insensible; lacking in feeling as from cold. 2. Deadened or lacking in power to move as *numb* with cold.

number (nŭm'bĕr) [L. *numerus,* number]. 1. A total of units. 2. A symbol graphically representing an arithmetical sum.

RS: *mean, median, modality, mode, numeral.*

numbness (nŭm'nĕs) [A.S. *numen,* taken]. Lack of sensation in a part, esp. from cold. SEE: *narcohypnia; obdormition.*

numeral (nū'mĕr-ăl) [L. *numerus,* number]. 1. Denoting or pert. to a number. 2. A word or figure expressing a number.

num'miform, num'mular [L. *nummus,* a coin, + *forma,* shape]. 1. Coin-shaped, said of some mucous sputum. 2. Arranged like a stack of coins.

nummulation (num-u-la'shun) [L. *nummus,* a coin]. The formation of a coin-shaped mass.

nunnation (nŭn-ā'shŭn) [Arabic *nun,* letter N]. Frequent and abnormal use of the n sound.

nupercaine (nu'per-kān). Proprietary name for dibucaine, a white powder or crystals manufactured from cinchoninic acid. Used as a local anesthetic of prolonged action.

nurse (ners) [L. *nutrix,* a nurse]. One who cares for the sick or wounded, esp. a registered nurse.

n., charge. One in charge of a single hospital ward.

n., community, n., district. A visiting nurse.

n., dry. An infant's nurse who does not suckle the child.

n., flight. N. who cares for patients being transported in airplanes.

n., general duty. One not specializing.

n., graduate. One who is a graduate of an accredited school of nursing.

n., head. A supervisor at the head of a hospital nursing staff.

n., health. A community or visiting nurse.

n., practical. One who is licensed to administer care, usually working under direction of a licensed physician or a registered nurse. May be a graduate of an accredited school for practical nursing or one who has practical experience only.

n., private. A nurse in charge of a single patient.

n., private duty. One not a member of a hospital staff who is called in to care for an individual patient in the hospital.

n., probationer. A student nurse during the first part of training.

n., public health. A graduate nurse employed by a Board of Health.

n., registered. A graduate nurse who has been registered and legally licensed to practice by state authority. ABBR: *R.N.*

n., school. A registered nurse whose duties are to supplement the work of the physician in medical inspection of pupils.

n., scrub. N. who is a member of an operating team being surgically clean in order to be able to assist the surgeon.

n., special. A private nurse taking special care of one patient or one who specializes in the care of certain types of patients.

n., student. An individual who is enrolled in a school of nursing.

n., trained. A registered nurse.

n., visiting. A registered nurse, employed by an association to care for the sick poor in their homes.

n., wet. A woman who breast-feeds the infants of others.

nurse (ners) [L. *nutrix,* a nurse]. 1. To feed an infant at the breast. 2. To care for an invalid. 3. To care for a young child.

nursery. Place in hospital where the newborn are cared for.

n., day. A nursery in which children, usually of preschool age, are cared for during the day.

nur'sing [L. *nutrix,* nurse]. 1. Scientific care of the sick by a graduate, registered nurse. 2. Loosely applied to any care of the sick. 3. Breast-feeding. 4. Lactation.

nutation (nū-tā'shŭn) [L. *nutātiō,* a nodding]. Nodding, as of the head.

n. of sacrum. Partial rotation of the sacrum on its transverse axis to give greater space for passage of the fetus.

nutrient (nū'trĭ-ĕnt). 1. Food that supplies the body with its necessary elements. 2. Nourishing.

Those containing carbon are *organic* food nutrients. Organic food nutrients may or may not contain nitrogen. Nutrients used for body fuel are fat, proteins and carbohydrates. Energy is obtained by the oxidation of certain food nutrients.

RS: *calorie, carbohydrate, fat, food, mineral, nitrogen, protein.*

nutriment (nū'trĭ-mĕnt) [L. *nutrimentum,* nourishment]. That which nourishes; nutritious substance.

nutrition (nū-trĭ'shŭn) [L. *nutritiō,* a feeding]. The sum total of the processes involved in the taking in and utilization of food substances by which growth, repair, and maintenance of activities in the body as a whole in any of its parts are accomplished. Includes ingestion, digestion, absorption and metabolism (assimilation).

Nutrients are stored by the body in various forms, and drawn upon when the food intake is not sufficient in the following order: usable gases; water as needed; body carbohydrates, such as sugar or glycogen; lactic acid and then the fats are utilized; large globules of neutral fat, and the fats that bear a relation to other fats, as glycogen does to sugar.

nutritional (nū-trĭsh'ŭn-ăl) [L. *nutritiō,* a feeding]. Rel. to nutrition.

nutritious (nū-trish'ŭs) [L. *nutritius,* feeding]. Affording nutriment. SYN: *nutritive.*

nutritive (nū'trĭ-tĭv) [L. *nutritius*]. Pert. to the process of assimilating food; having the property of nourishing.

n. enema. One of predigested foods to give sustenance to a patient unable to take nourishment in the usual way. SEE: *enema.*

nutriture (nu'trĭ-tūr). The state of body nutrition.

nux vomica (nŭks vom'ī-ka). A poisonous seed from an East Indian tree, containing several alkaloids, the principal ones being brucine and strychnine, *q.v.* USP.

nyctalbuminuria (nĭk"tăl-bū"min-ū'rĭ-ă) [G. *nyx, nykt-,* night, + L. *albus,* white, + G. *ouron,* urine]. A cyclic albuminuria occurring at night. SYN: *noctalbuminuria.*

nyctalgia (nĭk-tal'jĭ-ă) [" + *algos,* pain]. Pain during the night.

nyctalopia (nĭk-tă-lō'pĭ-ă) [" + *alaos,* blind, + *ōps,* eye]. 1. A condition in which person cannot see well in a faint light or at night. Occurs in retinitis pigmentosa and choroidoretinitis. Also may be due to vitamin A deficiency. Smoking tobacco impairs ability to see at night. SYN: *night blindness.* 2. Incorrectly, having better sight at night or in semidarkness than by day; night vision. SEE: *hemeralopia.*

nyctamblyopia (nik"tam-blĭ-ō'pĭ-ă) [" + *amblyōpia,* poor sight]. Poor vision at night without visible eye changes.

nyctaphonia (nĭk-tă-fō'nĭ-ă) [" + *a-,* priv. + *phōnē,* voice]. Hysterical loss of voice during the night.

nycterine (nĭk'tĕr-ĭn) [G. *nyx, nykt-,* night]. 1. Taking place at night. 2. Obscure.

nycthemerus (nĭk-them'ĕ-rŭs) [G. *nychthemeros*]. 1. Space of a day and a night. 2. Pert. to a night and day.

nyctohemeral (nik"to-hē'mer-al) [" + *ēmeraa,* day]. Rel. to both day and night.

nyctophilia (nĭk"to-fil'ĭ-ă) [" + *philein,* to love]. A predilection for darkness or for night. SYN: *scotophilia.*

nyctophobia (nĭk"tō-fō'bĭ-ă) [G. *nyx,* night, + *phobos,* fear]. Abnormal dread of the night, or of darkness. SYN: *scotophobia.*

nyctophonia (nĭk"tō-fō'nĭ-ă) [" + *phōnē,* voice]. Hysterical loss of voice only during the day.

nyctotyphlosis (nĭk"tō-tĭf-lō'sĭs) [" + *typhlōsis,* blindness]. Poor vision at night. SYN: *night blindness; nyctalopia.*

nycturia (nĭk-tū'rĭ-ă) [" + *ouron,* urine]. Urination, esp. excessive, during the night. SYN: *nocturia.* SEE: *enuresis.*

nygma (nĭg'mă) [G. *nygma,* a puncture]. A puncture wound.

nym'pha (pl. *nymphae*) [G. *nymphē,* a maiden]. One of the labia minora,* the small folds of mucous membrane forming the inner lips of the vulva.

So called from the nymphs, or goddesses of the fountain. SYN: *labium minus pudendi.*

n. pendulae. Stretched pendulous nymphae.

nymphectomy (nĭm-fĕk'tō-mĭ) [" + *ektomē,* excision]. Excision of hypertrophied nymphae.

nymphitis (nĭm-fī'tĭs) [" + *-itis,* inflammation]. Inflamed condition of the nymphae.

nymphocaruncular sul'cus (nĭm"fō-kăr-ŭn'-kū-lăr) [" + L. *caruncula*, little mass of flesh]. The depression bet. the caruncula of the hymen and the labium minus.

nymphohymenal sul'cus (nĭm"fō-hī'mĕn-ăl) [" + *ymēn*, membrane]. Trench bet. labium minus and the hymen on either side.

nympholepsy (nĭm'fō-lĕp-sĭ) [" + *lēpsia*, a seizure]. Frenzied ecstasy usually erotic in nature.

nymphomania (nĭm"fō-mā'nĭ-ă) [" + *mania*, madness]. Abnormally excessive sexual desire in the female. Syn: *furor femininus; furor uterinus*. See: *satyriasis*.

nymphomaniac (nĭm"fō-ma'nĭ-ăk) [G. *nymphē*, maiden, + *mania*, madness]. 1. Woman who is afflicted with excessive sexual desire. 2. Marked by excessive sexual desire.

nymphoncus (nĭm-fon'kŭs) [" + *ogkos*, a swelling]. Swelling or tumor of the nymphae.

nymphotomy (nĭm-fot'ō-mĭ) [" + *tomē*, a cutting]. 1. Removal of the nymphae. Syn: *nymphectomy*. 2. Incision into a nympha. 3. Removal of the clitoris.

nystagmic (nĭs-tag'mĭk) [G. *nystazein*, to nod]. Rel. to or suffering from condition of involuntary eyeball movements.

nystagmiform (nĭs-tăg'mĭ-form) [G. *nystazein*, to nod, + L. *forma*, shape]. Like or resembling nystagmus.

nystagmograph (nĭs-tag'mō-grăf) [" + *graphein*, to write]. Apparatus for recording the oscillations of the eyeball in nystagmus.

nystagmoid (nĭs-tag'moyd) [" + *eidos*, resemblance]. Similar to or resembling nystagmus.

nystagmus (nĭs-tag'mŭs) [G. *nystazein*, to nod]. Constant involuntary more or less cyclical movement of the eyeball. Movement may be in any direction.

Etiol: (1) Congenital, seen in bilateral amblyopia. (2) Occupational, as in miners and train dispatchers. (3) Labyrinthine irritability. (4) Neurologic diseases.

n., aural. N. due to disorder in the labyrinth of the ear.

n., convergence. Slow abduction of eyes followed by rapid adduction. Usually accompanies other types of nystagmus.

n., jerk. Rhythmic n., *q.v.*

n., labyrinthine. N. due to disease of the labyrinthine vestibular apparatus.

n., lateral. Horizontal movement of eyes from side to side.

n., miner's. N. occurring in those who work in comparative darkness for long periods.

n., opticokinetic. A rhythmic jerk nystagmus occurring when one is watching from a moving object.

n., oscillating. N. in which irregular, oscillatory movements occur. Also called *pendular n.*

n., pendular. Same as *oscillating nystagmus.*

n. rhythmic. Syn: *jerk nystagmus.* N. in which the eyes move slowly in one direction and then are jerked back.

n., rotatory. Rotation of the eyes about the visual axis.

n., vertical. Up and down ocular movements.

n., vestibular. That due to ear disturbances.

Nysten's law (nĭ'stĕn). Rigor mortis begins with muscles of mastication and progresses down the body affecting legs and feet last. See: *rigor mortis.*

nyxis (niks'ĭs) [G. *nyxis*, a pricking]. Puncture or piercing. Syn: *paracentesis.*

Notes

O

O. Chemical symb. for *oxygen* and abbr. for various terms, as: *oculus*, eye; *octarius*, pint.

o-. Abbr. for *ortho-*, most commonly used in chemical terminology.

O_2. Symb. for the molecular formula of oxygen.

O_3. Symb. for *ozone*.

oakum (ō'kŭm) [A.S. *ācumba*, tow]. Loose fiber obtained from old hemp ropes, formerly used as a surgical dressing.

oarialgia (ō"ăr-ĭ-ăl'jĭ-ă) [G. *ōarion*, little egg, + *algos*, pain]. Ovarian pain. SYN: *oothecalgia; ovarialgia*.

oario-, oari- [G.] Prefix pert. to the ovary. SEE: words beginning with *ovario-* or *oophor-*.

oasis (ō-ā'sĭs) (pl. *oases*) [G. *oasis*, a dry spot]. Area of healthy tissue surrounded by a diseased portion.

oat (ōt) [A.S. *āte*, oat]. Grain or seed of a cereal grass used as an article of diet.

oatmeal (ōt'mēl) [" + *melu*, meal]. COMP: Cellulose heavy. Rich in fats and lecithins.

COOKED: 1 cup (236 gm.). Calories: 150. Other main values: 5 gm. protein; 3 gm. fat; 26 gm. carbohydrate; 21 mg. calcium.

ACTION: Stimulating, laxative, fattening and nutritive.

ob- [L.]. Combining form meaning *towards, against, in the way of*.

O. B., OB. Abbr. for *obstetrics*.

obcecation (ob"se-ka'shun). Partial blindness.

obdormition (ŏb-dor-mĭsh'ŭn) [" + *dormire*, to sleep]. Numbness followed by tingling in a limb produced by pressure of the nerve trunk supplying it.

Limb is commonly referred to as being asleep.

obduction (ŏb-duk'shŭn) [" + *ducere*, to lead]. Scientific inspection of a dead body to learn pathological conditions and cause of death. SYN: *autopsy; necropsy*.

obelion (ō-bē'lĭ-ŏn) [G. *obelos*, a spit]. A craniometric point on the sagittal suture bet. the two parietal foramina.

obese (ō-bēs') [L. *obesus*, fat]. Extremely fat. SYN: *corpulent*.

obesity (ō-bē'sĭ-tĭ) [L. *obesitās*, corpulence]. Abnormal amount of fat on the body. SYN: *adiposity; corpulence; polysarcia*.

Term usually not employed unless individual is from 20-30% over average weight for his age, sex and height. There are two general classifications, *exogenous*, that caused by excessive food intake, and *endogenous*, that caused by some abnormality within the body, endocrine or faulty metabolism.

ENDOCRINE CAUSES: (1) Hypothyroidism, producing a decreased metabolic rate and insufficient energy output to balance the caloric intake; not a very frequent cause; (2) adrenal hyperfunction, apparently causing exaggerated metabolism; (3) testicular and ovarian hypofunction, the most important of the endocrine factors causing obesity.

ETIOL: Sex, obesity being more frequent in the female; race; climate; heredity, and occupation. Common in middle life. The most important factors in obesity not due to a disease process are too much food and too little exercise.

TREATMENT: (1) Prophylaxis, in children of families with a tendency to obesity, in the form of moderate dieting and exercise; (2) dieting; (3) dextroamphetamine in combination with a relatively low calorie diet. Dextroamphetamine stimulates nervous energy, produces a sense of well being, and reduces the desire for food.

Diet should be below maintenance requirements so far as energy units are concerned and must be provided with all other essential nutrients. Maintenance requirements are based on what the average weight should be. 1200-1600 calories per day is a slow reduction regimen; 1000-1200 calories is more rapid.

DIET: The average basic diet is about 9 calories per pound of ideal body weight per day. Thus a 160 pound person whose ideal wt. is 135 should eat a diet of about 1000 calories a day. These calories should be obtained from foods which would provide adequate protein, carbohydrates, fats, minerals, and vitamins and not from a "fad" diet. Adherence to this diet should cause the person to lose the excess weight. After that the diet is adjusted in that caloric intake is just equal to total energy required. Obviously this is different for each individual.

Losing weight by fasting is effective but is not recommended unless done under strict medical and nursing supervision.

RS: *carbohydrate, emaciation, fat, height, protein, starch, sugar, vitamin, weight*.

o., endogenous. O. caused by some abnormality within the body, endocrine, or metabolic.

o., exogenous. O. due to excessive intake of food.

o., hypothalamic. O. resulting from dysfunction of hypothalamus, esp. the appetite-regulating center.

obex (ō'bĕks) [L. a band]. A thin, crescent-shaped band of tissue covering the calamus scriptorius at the point of convergence of nervous tissue at the caudal end of 4th ventricle.

obfuscation (ŏb-fŭs-kā'shŭn) [L. *obfuscāre*, to darken]. 1. The act of making obscure or confusing. 2. Mental confusion.

ob'ject [L. *objectum*, a thing thrown before]. That which is visible or tangible to the senses.

o. blindness. Affection in which brain fails to recognize things seen correctly by eyes. SEE: *apraxia*.

o. choice. Selection of love object decided by a fixation developed in pregenital stage.

o. libido. Love or interest expressed external to oneself upon persons, objects, causes. SEE: *anaclitic choice*.

o. symbolism. A concept formed, or an emotion incited by seeing an object, as in ideas like *heart* of stone, the *brow* of a hill, the *lap* or *bosom* of nature, etc.

objective (ob-jek'tiv) [L. *objectivus*, pert. to something thrown before]. 1. Perceptible to other persons, said of symptoms. 2. Directed toward external things. 3. The lens of a microscope which is closest to the object.

o. symptoms. Those apparent to physical means of diagnosis.

obligate (ob'lĭ-gāt) [L. *obligāre*, to bind to]. 1. To make necessary or to require. 2. Compulsory, bound.

o. aerobe. A microbe that must have oxygen in order to live.

o. anaerobe. A microorganism that lives only without oxygen.

o. parasite. One that can exist only at the expense of another plant or organism.

oblique (o-blēk', o-blīk') [L. *obliquus*, slanting]. Slanting, diagonal.

o. muscles. Two muscles of the eye, two of the abdomen, two of the head, and two of the ears.

obliquimeter (ŏb-lĭk-wim'ĕt-ĕr) [" + G. *metron*, measure]. Apparatus for indicating the angle of the pelvic brim with the upright body.

obliquity (ŏb-lĭk'wĭ-tĭ) [L. *obliquus*, slanting]. The state of being oblique.

o., Litzmann's. Inclining of the fetal head until the post. parietal bone presents to the uterine canal.

o., Nägele's. Presentation of the fetal head with ant. parietal bone toward the uterine canal with oblique biparietal diameter in relation to the pelvic brim.

o. of pelvis. Inclination of pelvis.

o., Roederer's. Presentation of fetal head with occiput at pelvic brim.

obliquus (ŏb-lī'kwŭs) [L. slanting]. A name applied to several muscles. SEE: *Table of Muscles in Appendix.*

o. reflex. Contraction of ext. obliquus muscle in toto on application of stimulus to skin of thigh below Poupart's ligament.

obliteration (ŏb-lit"ĕr-ā'shŭn) [L. *obliterāre*, to deface]. Extinction or complete occlusion of a part by means of surgery, degeneration or disease.

oblongata (ŏb"lon-gā'tă) [L. *ob*, before, + *longus*, long]. The medulla oblongata; the cylindrical extension of the spinal cord as it enters the brain, about an inch long, reaching to the pons, and forming part of base of 4th ventricle.

obmutescence (ŏb-mū-tes'ents) [L. *obmutescere*, to become dumb]. Loss of vocal power. SYN: *aphonia.*

obnubilation (ŏb-nū-bil-ā'shŭn) [L. *obnubilāre*, to befog or darken]. An impaired or confused state of mind.

obscure (ŏb-skūr') [L. *obscurus*, dark]. Hidden, indistinct, as the cause of a condition.

observerscope (ob-zer'ver-skōp). Type of endoscope having two branches, so that two persons can inspect the same place simultaneously.

obses'sion. An uncontrollable desire to dwell on an idea or an emotion, or to perform a specific act.

It is not uncommon among normal persons, but if not banished may become all compelling, developing into a "compulsion neurosis." A dominating condition in certain psychoses.

o.'s, impulsive. Those accompanied by action. They sometimes becomes manias, *q.v.*

o.'s, inhibitory. O.'s accompanied by impediments to action. They represent the phobias, *q.v.*

obses'sional neuro'sis. A psychoneurosis marked by obsessions controlling the behavior of the individual. SYN: *compulsion neurosis.*

obstetric, obstetrical (ŏb-stet'rĭk, -rĭ-kăl) [L. *obstetrix*, a midwife, from *obstāre*, to stand before]. Pert. to obstetrics or midwifery.

o. forceps. Instrument used to facilitate delivery of the fetus.

obstetrician (ŏb-stĕt-rĭsh'ăn) [L. *obstetrix*, *-ic-*, a midwife]. A physician who treats women during pregnancy and parturition. SYN: *accoucheur.*

obstetrics (ob-stet'rĭks) [L. *obstetrix*, a midwife]. Scientific management of women during pregnancy, childbirth and the puerperium. SYN: *maieutics.*

RS: *childbirth, delivery, labor, maneuver, midwife, parturition, pregnancy.*

obstipation (ŏb-stĭp-ā'shŭn) [L. *obstipāre*, to stop up]. 1. The act or condition of obstructing. 2. Obstinate or extreme constipation due to an obstruction. SYN: *absolute constipation.*

obstruction (ŏb-struk'shŭn) [L. *obstructus*, built up before]. 1. Blocking of a structure that prevents it from functioning normally. 2. A thing that impedes; an obstacle.

o., aortic. Blocking of the aorta, thereby preventing flow of blood.

o., intestinal. Blockage of the lumen of the intestine. SEE: *intestinal o.*

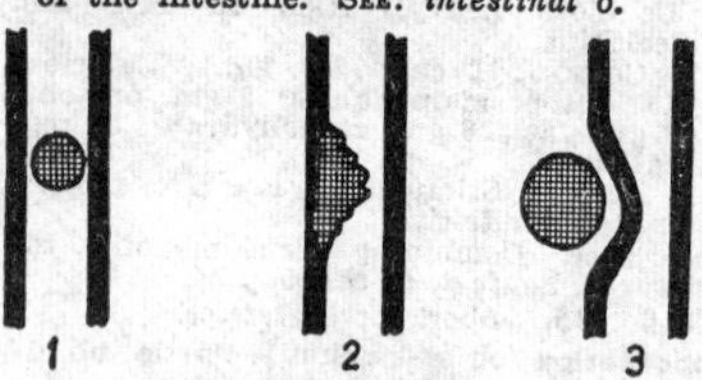

After Sears.

DIAGRAM ILLUSTRATING TYPES OF OBSTRUCTION.

1. Foreign body in the lumen. 2. Disease of the duct wall. 3. Pressure from outside.

obstruent (ŏb'strū-ĕnt) [L. *obstruens*, blocking]. 1. Blocking up. 2. That which closes a normal passage in the body.

obtund (ŏb-tŭnd') [L. *obtundere*, to beat against]. To dull or blunt, as sensitivity or pain.

obtundent (ŏb-tŭn'dĕnt) [L. *obtundere*, to beat against]. 1. Deadening sensibility of a part, or reducing irritability, soothing. 2. A soothing remedy.

obturation (ŏb-tū-rā'shun) [L. *obturāre*, to stop up]. Closure of a passage or opening.

obturator (ob'tū-rā"tor) [L. *obturāre*, to stop up]. 1. Anything that obstructs or closes a cavity or opening. 2. Rel. to the o. membrane. 3. Bridge for spanning the gap in the cleft palate.

o. foramen. O. in the anterior part of the os innominatum bet. pubis and ischium.

o. membrane. Strong o. occluding the o. foramen.

o. muscles. Two muscles on each side in the pelvic region which rotate the thighs outward. SEE: *Table of Muscles in Appendix, psoas for illustration.*

obtuse (ŏb-tūs') [L. *obtusus*, blunted]. 1. Not pointed or acute; dull or blunt. 2. Stupid; dull mentally.

obtusion (ŏb-tū'zhŭn) [L. *obtusiō*, from *obtundere*, to beat against]. Blunting or weakening of normal sensation, as in certain diseases.

occipital (ŏk-sĭp′ĭ-tăl) [L. *occiput,* back of head]. Concerning the back part of the head.

o. bone. Bone in lower back part of skull bet. the parietal and temporal bones.

o. lobe. Post. lobe of the cerebral hemisphere which is shaped like a three-sided pyramid.

occipitalis (ŏk-sĭp″ĭ-tā′lĭs) [L. pert. to back of head]. The posterior portion of the occipitofrontalis muscle at back of the head.

occipito- [L.]. Combining form showing relationship bet. the occiput and another part.

occiput (ok′sĭ-pŭt) [L.]. The back part of the skull.

occlude (ŏ-klūd′) [L. *occludere,* to shut up]. To close up, obstruct or join together, as the masticatory surfaces of the teeth.

occlus′al. Pertaining to the closure of an opening.

o. surface. The masticating surface of a tooth.

occlusion (ŏ-klū′zhŭn) [L. *occlusiō,* a closing up]. 1. The closure, or state of being closed, of a passage. SYN: *imperforation.* May be acquired or congenital. 2. Adsorption of gas by a substance which does not thereby lose its characteristic property. 3. Relation of the teeth when the jaws are closed.

o., coronary. Coronary thrombosis.

oc′cult [L. *occultus,* hidden]. Obscure; hidden, as a hemorrhage.

o. blood. Blood in such minute quantity that it can only be recognized by microscopic or chemical means.

occupa′tion neuro′sis. A functional disorder of a part, caused by certain occupations, as writer's cramp.

occupa′tional ther′apy. Treatment based on utilization of activities calculated to encourage the physically or mentally disabled patient to contribute to his own recovery. On the request of the patient's physician a registered occupational therapist selects and directs the patient's activities.

ochlesis (ŏk-lē′sĭs) [G. *ochlēsis,* a crowding]. Any disease caused by conditions of overcrowding.

ochlophobia (ŏk-lō-fō′bĭ-ă) [G. *ochlos,* crowd, + *phobos,* fear]. Abnormal dread of crowds or populated places.

ochrodermia (ō″krō-der′mĭ-ă) [G. *ōchros,* pale yellow, + *derma,* skin]. A yellow state of the skin.

ochrometer (ō-krom′ĕt-ĕr) [G. *ōchros,* pallor, + *metron,* measure]. Device for estimating the capillary blood pressure by compression of a finger until its skin becomes blanched.

ochronosis, ochronosus (ō-krō-nō′sĭs, -sŭs) [G. *ōchros,* yellow, + *nosos,* disease]. A rare condition marked by dark pigmentation of the ligaments, cartilage, fibrous tissues, skin and urine. May be caused by an inborn error of metabolism, *alkaptonuria.* This allows formation of homogentisic acid, part of which is excreted in the urine and part is stored in the tissues. Can also be due to chronic phenol poisoning.

octa-, octo- [G.]. Combining forms meaning *eight.*

octahedron (ok-tă-he′dron). An eight-sided solid figure.

octan (ŏk′tăn) [G. *oktō,* eight]. Reappearing on every 8th day, as a fever.

octane (ŏk′tān) [G. *oktō,* eight]. A hydrocarbon of the paraffin series. C_8H_{18}.

octarius (ŏk-ta′rĭ-ŭs) [L.]. Pint.

octavalent (ok″tă-vā′lĕnt) [G. *oktō,* eight, + L. *valere,* to have power]. Having a valence of 8.

octipara (ŏk-tĭp′ă-ră) [" + L. *parēre,* to bear]. A woman who has given birth to 8 children.

octogenarian (ok-to-jĕ-na′rĭ-en). A person who is 80 through 89 years old.

octoroon (ŏk-tō-roon′) [G. *oktō,* eight]. One who has one-eighth negro blood and seven-eighths white blood; progeny of a white person and a quadroon.

ocular (ok′ū-lăr) [L. *oculus,* eye]. 1. Concerning the eye or vision. 2. Eyepiece of a microscope.

oculist (ŏk′ū-lĭst) [L. *oculus,* eye]. Old term for ophthalmologist, a physician who is a specialist in diseases of the eye.

oculocephalogyric re′flex (ok″ū-lō-sĕf″-ă-lo-ji′rĭk). Associated movements of eye, head and body in focalizing vision upon an object.

oculogyration (ok″ū-lō-jī-rā′shŭn) [L. *oculus,* eye, + G. *gyros,* circle]. Motions of the eyeball.

oculogyric (ŏk″ū-lō-jī′rik) [" + G. *gyros,* circle]. Producing or concerning movements of the eye. SYN: *ophthalmogyric.*

oculomotor (ŏk″ū-lō-mō′tor) [" + *motor,* mover]. Rel. to eye movements. SYN: *oculogyric.*

o. nerve. The 3rd cranial nerve. FUNCT: Primarily motor but contains proprioceptive fibers. ORIGIN: Medial surface of cerebral peduncle of midbrain. COMPONENTS: General somatic efferent, general visceral efferent, and general somatic afferent fibers. DIST: All extrinsic muscles of eye except ext. rectus and sup. oblique; levator palpebrae superioris of eyelid; ciliary muscle; sphincter muscle of iris.

SEE: *cranial nerves:* Table of Cranial Nerves, Appendix.

oculomotorius (ok″ū-lō-mō-tor′ĭ-ŭs) [L.]. The oculomotor or 3rd cranial nerve. The *motor oculi* of the eye.

FUNCT: Motor. Supplies five of the seven eye muscles.

ORIGIN: Floor, aquaeductus cerebri.

DIST: All eye muscles except ext. rectus and sup. oblique. SEE: *cranial nerves; Table of Cranial Nerves, Appendix.*

oculomycosis (ok″ū-lō-mī-kō′sĭs) [L. *oculus,* eye, + G. *mykēs,* fungus, + *-ōsis*]. Any disease of the eye or its parts caused by a fungus.

oculonasal (ŏk″ū-lō-nā′sal) [" + *nasus,* nose]. Concerning both eye and nose.

oculoreaction (ok″ū-lō-rē-ak′shŭn) [" + *rē,* back, + *actus,* acting]. A reaction in the eye, upon the instillation into the eye of toxins of tuberculosis and typhoid. More severe in persons suffering from the disease. SYN: *ophthalmic reaction; Calmette's reaction.*

oculozygomatic (ok″ū-lō-zī-gō-mat′ĭk) [" + G. *zygon,* yoke]. Pert. to the eye and zygoma.

o. line. Line bet. inner canthus of eye and cheek supposedly indicating neural disorders.

oculus (ok′ū-lŭs) [L.]. Eye.

o. caesius. Glaucoma.

o. dexter. The right eye. Abbr. O.D.

o. lacrimans. Epiphora, *q.v.*

o. sinister. The left eye. Abbr. O.S.

o. uterque. Each eye. Abbr. O.U.

O. D., o. d. Abbr. for *oculus dexter,* right eye.

odaxesmus (o-daks-ēz'mŭs) [G. *odaxēsmos*, a biting]. The biting of the tongue, lip or cheek during an epileptic attack.

odaxetic (o-dăks-ĕt'ĭk) [G. *odaxēsmos*, a biting]. Producing a stinging or itching sensation.

Oddi's sphincter (ŏd'dĭ). A sphincter at the opening of the common bile duct into the duodenum at the papilla of Vater.

odogenesis (ō-dō-jĕn'ĕ-sĭs) [G. *odos*, path, + *genesis*, formation]. The re-establishment of connections bet. the divided ends of a nerve by nerve process attraction. SYN: *neurocladism.*

odontagra (ō-dŏn-tăg'ră) [G. *odous, odont-*, tooth, + *agra*, seizure]. Toothache, esp. when originating from gout.

odontalgia (o-don-tal'jĭ-ă) [" + *algos*, pain]. Toothache. SYN: *odontia; odontodynia.*

o., phantom. Pain felt in the area from which a tooth has been pulled.

odontatrophy (ō"dŏn-tăt'rō-fĭ) [" + *atrophia*, atrophy]. Imperfect development of the teeth.

odontectomy (ō-dŏn-tek'tō-mĭ) [" + *ektomē*, excision]. Surgical removal of a tooth.

odonterism (ō-don'tĕr-ĭzm) [" + *erismos*, quarrel]. Chattering of the teeth.

odontia (ō-dŏn'shĭ-ă) [G. *odous, odont-*, tooth]. 1. Pain in a tooth. SYN: *odontalgia.* 2. Condition or abnormality of the teeth.

odontiasis (ō"dŏn-tī'ăs-ĭs) [" + *iasis*, disease]. 1. Cutting of the teeth. SYN: *dentition, teething.* 2. Disease caused by teething.

odontitis (ō-dŏn-tī'tĭs) [" + *-itis*, inflammation]. Inflammation of a tooth.

odonto-, odont- [G.]. Combining form meaning *tooth.*

odontoblast (ō-dŏn'tō-blăst) [G. *odous, odont-*, tooth, + *blastos*, germ]. One of the cells forming the surface layer of the dental papilla which is responsible for the formation of the dentine of a tooth. After a tooth is formed, the odontoblasts line the pulp cavity and continue to produce dentine for years after the tooth has erupted. From their distal ends Tomes' fibers extend to the periphery of the dentine.

odontoblasto'ma. A blastoma composed principally of odontoblasts.

odontobothrion (ō-don'tō-both'rĭ-ŏn) [" + *bothrion*, pit]. Socket of a tooth.

odon"tobothri'tis. Inflammation of the socket of a tooth.

odon'tocele. An alveolodental cyst.

odontochirurgical (ō-dŏn-tō-kĭ-rur'jĭ-kăl). Pert. to dental surgery.

odontoclasis (ō-dŏn-tŏk'lă-sĭs). The breaking or fracture of a tooth.

odon'toclast. A cell which brings about the absorption of the roots of deciduous teeth.

odontodynia (ō-dŏn"tō-din'ĭ-ă) [" + *odynē*, pain]. Toothache. SYN: *odontalgia; odontia.*

odontogenesis, odontogeny (ō-don"tō-jĕn'ĕ-sĭs, -toj'ĕn-ĭ) [" + *genesis*, production]. The origin and formation of the teeth.

odontoid (ō-don'toyd) [" + *eidos*, resemblance]. Toothlike.

o. process. The toothlike projection from upper surface of the body of the 2nd cervical vertebrae.

odon'tolith. The accretion of a calcareous substance on the teeth; tartar.

odontol'ogist. A dentist or dental surgeon.

odontology (ō-dŏn-tol'ō-jĭ) [" + *logos*, study]. The science of dealing with the teeth and their care. SYN: *dentistry.*

odontoma (ō-dŏn-tō'mă) [G. *odous, odont-*, tooth, + *-ōma*, tumor]. Tumor of a tooth or of the dental tissue.

o., coronary. Bony tumor at crown of a tooth.

o., follicular. Bony shell in gums below tooth margin, usually after 2nd dentition.

ETIOL: Excessive number of dental follicles.

SYM: Crepitating to pressure. They often contain 1 or more teeth. SYN: *cyst, dentigerous.*

o., radicular. Bony tumor at root of a tooth.

odontonecrosis (ō-don"tō-nĕ-krō'sĭs) [" + *nekros*, dead, + *-ōsis*, intensive]. Extensive decay of a tooth.

odontopathy (ō-dŏn-top'ăth-ĭ) [" + *pathos*, disease]. Any disease of the teeth.

odontophobia (ō-don"tō-fō'bĭ-ă) [" + *phobos*, fear]. 1. Abnormal aversion to the sight of teeth. 2. Abnormal fear of dental surgery.

odontoplerosis (ō-don"tō-plē-rō'sĭs) [G. *odous, odont-*, tooth, + *plērōsis*, filling]. The filling of a dental cavity.

odontoprisis (ō-don"tō-pri'sĭs) [" + *prisis*, sawing]. Grinding of the teeth. SYN: *Bruxism.*

odontorrhagia (ō-don"tō-rā'jĭ-ă) [" + *rēgnunai*, to burst forth]. Hemorrhage from a tooth socket following extraction.

odontorthosis (ō-dŏn-tŏr-thō'sĭs) [" + *orthos*, straight]. Operation of straightening irregular teeth.

odontosis (ō-dŏn-tō'sĭs) [" + *-ōsis*, intensive]. 1. Development of teeth. 2. Eruption of teeth.

odontotherapy (ō-don'tō-ther'ă-pĭ) [" + *therapeia*, treatment]. Care of diseased teeth.

odontotripsis (ō-don"tō-trĭp'sĭs) [" + *tripsis*, a rubbing]. Natural abrasion of the teeth.

odontotrypy (ō-dŏn-tot'rĭ-pĭ) [" + *trypan*, to bore]. Drilling of a tooth.

odor (ō'der) [L. smell]. 1. That quality of a substance which renders it perceptible to sense of smell. 2. Any smell, esp. a sweet scent. 3. Any sensation of sense of smell.

Each odoriferous substance causes its own sensation. Odors have been classed as (a) pure odors, (b) those mixed with sensations from the mucous membrane, (c) those mixed with the sensation of taste.

PURE ODORS: These are *aromatic, burning, fragrant, fetid*, or *nauseating*, and *repulsive odors.*

Another classification is *spicy, flowery, fruity, resinous, foul, scorched.*

RS: *antibromic, "brom-" words, deodorant, effluvium, olfactory, osmolagnia, osphresiolagnia, pungent, smell.*

odoriferous (ō"der-ĭf'ĕ-rŭs) [" + *ferre*, to bear]. Bearing scent, having an odor; fragrant; perfumed.

odorime'try. The measurement of the ability of a substance to induce olfactory sensations.

odorous (ō'dŏr-us) [L. *odor*, smell]. Having an odor, scent or fragrance.

odynacusis (ō-dĭn-ă-kū'sĭs) [G. *odynē*, pain, + *akusis*, hearing]. A condition in which noises cause pain in the ear.

odynometer (ō-dĭn-om'ĕt-ĕr) [" + *metron*, measure]. Device for measuring pain.

odynophagia (ō-dĭn-ō-fā'jĭ-ă) [" + *phagein*, to eat]. Pain upon swallowing.

odynophobia (ō″dĭn-ō-fō′bĭ-ă) [" + *phobos*, fear]. Abnormal dread of pain.

Oedipus com′plex (ed′ĭ-pŭs). Abnormally intense love of the child for parent of the opposite sex retained in adulthood.

Usually involves jealous dislike of the other parent. Most commonly love of a son for his mother. SEE: *Electra complex*.

Oertel's terrain cure (er′tel). Graduated exercise, mountain climbing, diet, and reduction of fluids for patients with some types of heart disease, obesity, circulatory diseases, etc.

Oesophagos′tomum. A genus of nematodes belonging to the suborder Strongylata.

O. apiostomum. The nodular worm of monkeys. Occasionally infests man.

offi′cial. Said of medicines authorized as standard in the U. S. Pharmacopeia, and in the National Formulary.

officinal (of-ĭs′in-al) [L. *officina*, shop]. Regularly kept in a druggist's stock. SEE: *magistral*.

Oguchi disease (o-gootch′ē) [Chuta Oguchi, Japanese ophthalmologist, 1875—]. Recessive hereditary night blindness, onset of which is in infancy. Commonly found in Japan; rare in United States.

-OH. Molecular formula for hydroxyl group.

ohm (ōm). Practical unit of resistance, the resistance through which a difference of potential of 1 volt will produce a current of 1 ampere.

The international or legal ohm is the resistance offered by a column of mercury 106.3 cm. long, 14.45 gm. in mass, and of constant cross section at 0° C.

-oid [G.]. Suffix meaning *having the form of, or likeness of*, as *ovoid*.

oidiomycetes (ō-ĭd″ĭ-ō-mī-sē′tēs) [*Oidium* + G. *mykēs*, fungus]. A group of fungi including the Oidium.

oidiomycosis (ō-ĭd″ĭ-ō-mī-kō′sĭs) [*Oidium* + G. *mykēs*, fungus, + *-ōsis*]. Disease due to infection by Oidium.

Oidium (ō-ĭd′ĭ-ŭm) [G. *ōion*, egg]. A genus of fungi, now called *Candida, q.v.*

O. albicans. A microscopic fungus that causes thrush. Now called *Candida albicans, q.v.*

oikofugic (oy-ko-fu′jik) [G. *oikos*, house, + L. *fugere*, to flee]. Having a compulsion to leave home.

oikomania (oy-kō-mā′nĭ-ă) [G. *oikos*, house, + *mania*, madness]. Nervous disorder induced by unhappy home surroundings.

oikophobia (oy″kō-fo′bĭ-ă). Morbid dislike of the home. SYN: *ecomania*.

oil (oyl) [L. *oleum*]. A greasy liquid not miscible with water, usually obtained from a mineral, vegetable or animal source.

According to character, oils are subdivided principally as *fixed* or *fatty*, and *volatile* or *essential*.

Ex: Fixed—*Castor oil, olive oil, cod liver oil.* Volatile—*Oils of mustard, peppermint, rose.*

RS: *oleaginous, oleate, oleic, olein, oleum, unctuous.*

ointment (oynt′mĕnt) [Fr. *oignement*]. A fatty, soft substance having antiseptic or healing properties.

Its base is usually petroleum jelly, lard or lanolin to which the medicament is added. Applied on linen. It should be spread from the center outwards, so that edges are completely covered. SYN: *salve; unguent.*

okra (ō′kra). COOKED: 8 pods (85 gm.). Calories: 30. Other main values: 2 gm. protein; trace of fat; 6 gm. carbohydrate; 70 mg. calcium; 630 I.U. vitamin A.

ol. Abbr. for *oleum*, oil.

O. L. A. Abbr. for L. *occipito laevo anterior*, fetal presentation with the occiput toward the maternal left acetabulum.

old age. Human life after 65 years.

olea (ō′lē-ă) [L. oils, olive]. 1. L. for *olive*. 2. Pl. of *oleum, oils.*

oleaginous (ō-lē-ăj′ĭ-nŭs) [L. *oleaginus*, oily]. Greasy; oily; unctuous.

oleate ((ō′lē-āt) [L. *oleatum*]. 1. Any salt of oleic acid. 2. Salt of oleic acid dissolved in an excess of the acid.

oleatum (ō-lē-at′ŭm) [L.]. Preparation made by dissolving metallic salts or alkaloids in oleic acid. SYN: *oleate, 2.*

olecranal (ō-lĕk′răn-ăl) [G. *ōlekranon*, elbow]. Concerning the olecranon.

olecranarthritis (ō-lek″răn-ar-thrī′tĭs) [G. *ōlekranon*, elbow, + *arthron*, joint, + *-ītis*, inflammation]. Inflamed condition of the elbow joint.

olecranarthrocace (ō-lĕk″răn-ar-throk′ă-sē) [" + " + *kakē*, badness]. Tuberculous ulceration of the elbow joint.

olecranarthropathy (ō-lĕk″răn-ar-throp′-ăth-ĭ) [" + " + *pathos*, disease]. Any disease of the elbow joint.

olecranoid (ō-lĕk′răn-oyd) [" + *eidos*, resemblance]. Similar to the olecranon.

olecranon (ō-lek′răn-ŏn, ō″lē-krā′nŏn) [G. elbow]. [NA]. A large process of the ulna projecting behind the elbow joint and forming the bony prominence of the elbow.

FRACTURE OF: Prevent spasm of triceps muscle to avoid separation of fragments. Latter may have to be wired.

TREATMENT: Similar to that for fracture of patella, *q.v.* SEE: *skeleton.*

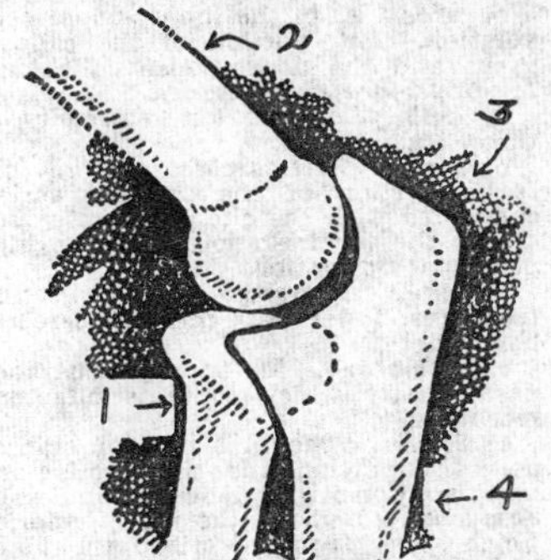

OLECRANON.
1. Radius. 2. Humerus. 3. Olecranon. 4. Ulna.

oleic (ō-lē′ĭk) [L. *oleum*, oil]. Derived from or pert. to oil.

o. acid. A colorless, oily liquid prepared from fats, the salts of which are *oleates*. Formula C_8H_{34} O_2.

olein (ō′lē-ĭn) [L. *oleum*, oil]. An oleate of glyceryl found in nearly all fixed oils and fats; an important part of oils. SYN: *triolein*.

oleo- [L.]. Combining form meaning *oil*.

oleoarthrosis (ō″lē-ō-ar-thrō′sĭs) [L. *oleum*, oil, + G. *arthron*, joint, + *-ōsis*]. Therapeutic introduction of oil into a joint.

oleoinfusion (ō″lē-ō-ĭn-fū′zhŭn) [" + *in*, into, + *fusus*, poured]. Combination of a drug and oil.

oleomargarine (ō″lē-ō-mar′jă-rēn) [" + *margarine*]. Artificial butter made from refined vegetable and animal fats. SYN: *margarine*.

oleoresin (o″le-o-rez′in) [" + *resina*, resin]. Extract of plant containing resinous substance and oil, prepared by dissolving the crude drug in ether, acetone or alcohol.

oleosaccharum (ō-lē-ō-sak′ăr-ŭm) [" + G. *sakcharon*, sugar]. A substance compounded of sugar and volatile oil.

oleotherapy (ō″lē-ō-ther′ă-pĭ) [" + G. *therapeia*, treatment]. Therapeutic injection of oil. SYN: *eleotherapy*.

oleothorax (ō-lē-ō-thō′răks) [" + G. *thōrax*, chest]. Therapeutic injection of oil into the pleural cavity.

oleum (ō′lē-ŭm) [L.]. Oil.

o. *morrhuae*. Cod-liver oil.

o. *olivea*. Olive oil. ABBR: *ol. oliv.*

o. *percomorphum*. Mixture of oils from livers of various members of order Percomorphi. More potent than cod liver oil in vitamins A and D.

o. *ricini*. Castor oil.

olfactie (ŏl-făk′tĭ) [L. *olfacere*, to smell]. Unit of smell; the threshold of stimulation for an odor.

olfaction (ŏl-fak′shŭn) [L. *olfacere*, to smell]. The sense of smell. Smelling.

olfactive (ŏl-fak′tĭv) [L. *olfacere*, to smell]. Pert. to the sense of smell. SYN: *olfactory*.

olfactology (ŏl-făk-tol′ō-jĭ) [" + G. *logos*, study]. Scientific investigation of sense of smell.

olfactometer (ŏl″fak-tom′et-ĕr) [" + G. *metron*, measure]. Apparatus for testing the power of the sense of smell.

olfactory (ŏl-fak′tō-rĭ) [L. *olfacere*, to smell]. Pert. to smell.

o. *area*. A. in the hippocampal convolution. Ant. portion of the callosal gyrus and the uncus. Also called *anterior perforated substance*.

o. *bulb*. Enlarged ant. extremity of the o. tract.

o. *cortex*. SYN: *archicortex* (*allocortex*). Portion of the cerebral cortex concerned with the olfactory sense. Includes the pyriform lobe and the hippocampal formation.

o. *lobe*. A cranial lobe projecting from ant. lower part of each cerebral hemisphere.

o. *membrane*. M. in upper part of nasal cavity which contains olfactory receptors.

o. *nerves*. The first pair of cranial nerves supplying the nasal olfactory mucosa. Consist of delicate bundles of unmyelinated fibers, the *fila olfactoria*, which pass through cribriform plate and terminate in olfactory glomeruli of olfactory bulb. The fila are central processes of bipolar receptor neurons of olfactory mucous membrane.

o. *organ*. The nose.

o. *striae*. Three bands of fibers, lateral, intermediate and medial which form the roots of the olfactory tract.

o. *tract*. Band of fibers extending posteriorly from o. bulb to ant. perforated substance. Here it enlarges and divides into the olfactory striae.

o. *trigone*. Small triangular area between lateral and medial olfactory striae.

o. *tubercle*. An elevation at rostral end of ant. perforated substance. Well developed in lower mammals, rudimentary in man.

oligemia (ol-ig-e′mĭ-ă) [G. *oligos*, little, + *aima*, blood]. Deficient volume of blood in the body. SYN: *oligohemia*.

oligergasia (ol-ĭ-gĕr-ga′sĭ-ă) [" + *ergasia*, work]. Psychic disorder from deficiency due to imperfect development.

olighidria (ŏl-ĭ-gĭd′rĭ-ă). Deficient perspiration. Also spelled *oligidria*.

olighydria (ŏl-ĭ-gĭd′rĭ-ă) [G. *oligos*, little, + *ydōr*, water]. Deficiency of body fluids.

oligo-, olig- [G.]. Combining form meaning *small* or, in the plural sense, *few*.

oligocholia (ol-ĭg-ō-kō′lĭ-ă) [G. *oligos*, little, + *cholē*, bile]. Lack of bile.

oligochromemia (ol″ĭg-ō-krō-mē′mĭ-ă) [" + *chrōma*, color, + *aima*, blood]. Lack of sufficient hemoglobin in the blood.

oligochylia (ol-ĭ-gō-ki′lĭ-ă) [" + *chylos*, juice]. Deficiency of chyle.

oligochymia (ol-ĭg-ō-ki′mĭ-ă) [" + *chymos*, juice]. Deficiency of chyme.

oligocystic (ol-ĭ-gō-sĭst′ĭk) [" + *kystis*, a bladder]. Having just a few cysts, as a tumor.

oligocythemia (ol″ĭ-gō-sī-thē′mĭ-ă) [" + *kytos*, cell, + *aima*, blood]. Deficiency in number of red blood corpuscles.

oligocytosis (ol″ĭ-gō-sī-tō′sĭs) [" + " + *-ōsis*, intensive]. Deficiency of red blood corpuscles. SYN: *oligocythemia*.

oligodactylia (ol-ĭ-gō-dăk-tĭl′ĭ-ă) [" + *daktyllos*, digit]. Subnormal number of fingers or toes.

oligodendrocyte. Neuroglial cells having few and delicate processes.

oligodendroglia (ol″ĭ-gō-den-drog′lĭ-ă) [" + *dendron*, a tree, + *glia*, glue]. Adventitial cells found in central nervous system, with characteristic vinelike processes. SYN: *mesoglia*.

oligodendroglioma ol″ĭ-gō-dĕn-drō-glī-ō′-mă). A malignant tumor occurring principally in the cerebrum, consisting mostly of oligodendrocytes. Calcification frequently occurs. The etiology is unknown.

oligodipsia (ol-ĭ-gō-dĭp′sĭ-ă) [G. *oligos*, few, + *dipsa*, thirst]. Abnormal lack of desire for fluids.

oligodon′tia [" + *odont*, tooth]. A hereditary developmental anomaly characterized by a less-than-normal number of teeth.

oligodynamic (ŏl″ĭ-gō-dī-năm′ĭk) [" + *dynamis*, power]. Effective in a small quantity.

oligoerythrocythemia (ol″ĭ-gō-er″ith-rō-sī-thē′mĭ-ă) [" + *erythros*, red, + *kytos*, cell, + *aima*, blood]. Deficiency of hemoglobin or red blood corpuscles.

oligogalactia (ol″ĭ-gō-gă-lak′tĭ-ă) [" + *gala, galakt-*, milk]. Deficient milk secretion.

oligogenics (ol-ĭ-gō-jĕn′ĭks) [" + *gennan*, to produce]. Limitation of the number of offspring by artificial mediums such as contraceptives. SYN: *birth control*.

oligohemia (ol″ĭ-gō-hē′mĭ-ă) [" + *aima*, blood]. Insufficiency of blood in the body. SYN: *oligemia*.

oligohydramnios (ol″ĭg-ō-hī-dram′nĭ-ōs) [" + *ydor*, water, + *amnion*, amnion]. Abnormally small amount of amniotic fluid.

oligohydruria (ol″ĭ-gō-hī-drū′rĭ-ă) [G. *oligos*, few, + *ydōr*, water, + *ouron*, urine]. Highly concentrated urine.

oligoleukocythemia (ol″ĭ-gō-lū″kō-sī-thē′-mĭ-ă) [" + *leukos*, white, + *kytos*, cell, + *aima*, blood]. Reduction in leukocytic content of blood. SYN: *leukopenia*.

oligomania (ol-ĭ-gō-mā′nĭ-ă) [" + *mania*, madness]. Insanity involving only a few mental faculties.

oligomastigate (ol-ĭ-gō-mas′tĭ-gāt) [" + *mastix, mastig-*, whip]. Characterized by two flagella.

oligomenorrhea (ol″ĭg-ō-mĕn-ō-rē′ă) [" + *mēn*, month, + *roia*, flow]. Scanty or infrequent menstrual flow.

oligopepsia (ol-ĭ-gō-pĕp′sĭ-ă) [" + *pepsis*, digestion]. Insufficient digestive tone.

oligophosphaturia (ol″ĭ-gō-fŏs-făt-ū′rĭ-ă) [" + *phosphas*, phosphate, + *ouron*, urine]. Scanty amount of phosphates in the urine.

oligophrenia (ol″ĭg-ō-frē′nĭ-ă) [G. *oligos*, few, + *phrēn*, mind]. Mental deficiency due to faulty development. SYN: *imbecility*.

oligoplasmia (ŏl″ĭg-ō-plăz′mĭ-ă) [" + *plasmos*, a thing formed]. Insufficient amt. of blood plasma.

oligopnea (ol-ĭg-op′nē-ă) [" + *pnoia*, breath]. Infrequent respiration. SYN: *hypopnea*.

Respiration shallow or abnormally deep; rate as slow as 6-10 per minute. Usually accompanied by slow pulse, although high in some conditions.

ETIOL: Cerebral compression, meningeal or pontine hemorrhage, cerebral or cerebellar tumors, abscess, gumma of meninges, osteoma of cranium, some forms of meningitis, trauma of brain, drug poisoning, shock, constitutional diseases, etc.

oligoposy (ol-ĭ-gop′ō-sĭ) [" + *posis*, drink]. Insufficient use of liquids in the diet. SYN: *oligoposia*.

oligoptyalism (ol-ĭ-gō-tī′ă-lĭzm) [" + *ptyalon*, saliva]. Insufficient secretion of saliva. SYN: *oligosialia*.

oligoria (ol-ĭ-gō′rĭ-ă) [G. *oligoria*, apathy]. A form of melancholia in which there is apathy toward things and people.

oligosialia (ol″ĭ-gō-sĭ-a′lĭ-ă) [G. *oligos*, few, + *sialon*, saliva]. Scanty salivary secretion. SYN: *oligoptyalism*.

oligospermia (ŏl″ĭ-gō-spĕr′mĭ-ă) [" + *sperma*, seed]. Deficient amount of spermatozoa in seminal fluid. It may be temporary or permanent. SYN: *hypospermatogenesis*.

oligotrichia (ol-ĭ-gō-trĭk′ĭ-ă). Scantiness of hair.

oligotrophy (ol-ĭ-got′rō-fĭ) [" + *trophē*, nourishment]. Inadequate nutrition.

oliguresis (ol-ĭg-ū-rē′sĭs) [" + *ourēsis*, urination]. Scantiness of urine; infrequent urination.

oliguria (ol-ĭg-ū′rĭ-ă) [" + *ouron*, urine]. Diminished amt. of urine formation.

ETIOL: Seen after profuse perspiration, bleeding, and diarrhea. Also in retention of urine due to brain disease, drug poisoning, deep coma.

oliva (ō-lī′vă) [L. olive]. NA. An olive-shaped gray body behind the ant. pyramid of the medulla oblongata. SEE: *olivary body*.

ol′ivary [L. *oliva*, olive]. Shaped like an olive; oval.

o. body. SYN: *oliva, inf. olivary nucleus, inf. olive*. A rounded mass located in anterolateral portion of the medulla oblongata. Consists of a convoluted sheet of gray matter enclosing white matter.

olive. PICKLED (*green*): 12 extra large or 7 jumbo (66 gm.). Calories: 70. Other main values: 1 gm. protein; 7 gm. fat; 48 mg. calcium; 170 I.U. vitamin A.

olive (ŏl′ĭv) [L. *oliva*, olive]. Oliva. NA.

o., accessory. SYN: *accessory olivary nuclei, dorsal and medial*. Two masses of gray matter lying adjacent to the inferior olive.

o., inferior. Olivary body.

o., superior. The superior olivary nucleus, *q.v.*

-ology [G.]. Suffix meaning *science of, knowledge, study of*.

olophonia (ol-ō-fōn′ĭ-ă) [G. *oloos*, destroyed, + *phōnē*, voice]. Malformation of vocal organs with resulting unnatural speech.

-oma [G.]. Suffix denoting *a tumor*.

omagra (ō-mag′ră) [G. *ōmos*, shoulder, + *agra*, seizure]. Attack of gout in the shoulder.

omalgia (ō-mal′jĭ-ă) [" + *algos*, pain]. Neuralgia of shoulder.

omarthritis (ō-mar-thrī′tĭs) [" + *arthron*, joint, + *-ītis*, inflammation]. Inflamed condition of the shoulder joint.

ombrophobia (ŏm-brō-fō′bĭ-ă) [G. *ombros*, rain, + *phobos*, fear]. Fear and anxiety induced by storms, threatening clouds, or rain.

ombrophore (om′brō-for) [" + *phoros*, a carrier]. Portable apparatus for administering shower baths.

omental (ō-mĕn′tăl) [L. *omentum*, covering]. Pert. to the omentum, the peritoneal fold supporting the viscera.

o. bursa. SYN: *lesser peritoneal sac*. A cavity within the layers of peritoneum forming the great omentum. Its opening into the main peritoneal cavity is the *epiploic foramen* (*foramen of Winslow*).

omentectomy (ō-mĕn-tĕk′tō-mĭ) [" + G. *ektomē*, excision]. Surgical removal of a portion of the omentum.

omentitis (ō-mĕn-tī′tĭs) [" + G. *-ītis*, inflammation]. Inflamed condition of omentum.

omentopexy (ō-mĕn′tō-pĕks″ĭ) [" + *pēxis*, fixation]. Fixation of the omentum to the abdominal wall or adjacent organ.

omentorrhaphy (ō-mĕn-tor′ră-fĭ) [" + G. *raphē*, a sewing]. Suture of the omentum.

omentosplenopexy (ō-men″tō-splē′nopĕks-ĭ) [" + G. *splēn*, spleen, + *pēxis*, fixation]. Fixation of the spleen and omentum. Omentopexy and splenopexy.

omentotomy (ō-mĕn-tot′ō-mĭ) [" + G. *tomē*, incision]. Surgery of the omentum.

omentum (ō-mĕn′tŭm) (pl. *omenta*) [L. a covering]. A double fold of peritoneum attached to the stomach and connecting it with certain of the abdominal viscera. It contains a cavity, the *omental bursa* (lesser peritoneal cavity).

The omenta are the *great o.*, or *gastrocolic;* and the *lesser, or gastrohepatic o.*

PALPATION OF: Cancerous and tubercular enlargements are distinguished by the fact that they extend across the abdomen; cannot be traced backward; do not ascend behind the ribs; are rough, hard, and uneven.

RS: *abdomen, caul, epiploon, kidney, ovary, spleen*.

o., great. Portion of the o. suspended from greater curvature of the stomach and covering the intestines like an apron. It dips in among the folds of the intestines and is attached to the transverse colon and mesocolon.

It contains fat and aids in keeping the intestines warm, and preventing friction. It also aids in localizing infections. SYN: *epiploon majus*.

o., lesser. It passes from the lesser curvature of stomach to transverse fissure of the liver. SYN: *epiploon minus*.

omitis (ō-mī′tĭs) [G. *ōmos*, shoulder, + *-ītis*, inflammation]. Inflamed condition of the shoulder.

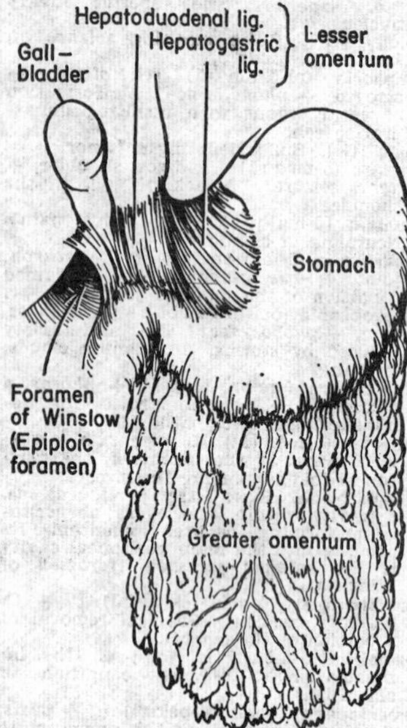

ANATOMIC RELATIONSHIPS OF GREATER AND LESSER OMENTUM

omn. bih. Abbr. for [L.] *omni bihora,* every two hours.

omn. hor. Abbr. for [L.] *omni hora,* every hour.

omn. noct. Abbr. for [L.] *omni nocte,* every night.

omni- (om'nĭ) [L.]. Prefix meaning *all.*

omnip'otence of thought. PSY: Infantile concept of reality whereby one expects his wishes to be instantly accomplished, as a child that gains its objectives through crying, comes to believe in his own omnipotence because of a parent's surrender to his demands.

omnivorous (ŏm-nĭv'ō-rŭs) [L. *omnis,* all, + *vorāre,* to eat greedily]. Living on all kinds of food.

omo- [G.]. Combining form meaning *shoulder* or *pert. to the shoulder.*

omodynia (ō-mō-din'ĭ-ă) [G. *ōmos,* shoulder, + *odynē,* pain]. Pain of the shoulder.

omohyoid (ō-mō-hī'oyd) [" + *yoeidēs,* y-shaped]. 1. Concerning the scapula and the hyoid bone. 2. Muscle attached to the hyoid bone and the scapula. SEE: *Table of Muscles in Appendix.*

omophagia (ō-mō-fā'jĭ-ă) [G. *ōmos,* raw, + *phagein,* to eat]. The custom of eating foods raw, esp. flesh.

OMPA. Abbr. for *octamethyl pyrophosphoramide.*

omphal-, omphalo [G.]. Combining form meaning *relating to the navel.*

omphalectomy (ŏm-făl-ek'tō-mĭ) [G. *omphalos,* navel, + *ektomē,* excision]. Surgical removal of the umbilicus.

omphalic (om-fal'ĭk) [G. *omphalikos,* pert. to the navel]. Concerning the umbilicus.

omphalitis (ŏm-făl-ī'tĭs) [G. *omphalos,* navel, + *ītis,* inflammation]. Inflamed condition of the navel.

omphalocele (ŏm-făl'ō-sēl) [G. *omphalos,* navel, + *kēlē,* hernia]. Hernia of the navel. SEE: *hernia.*

omphalomesenteric (om"fal-ō-mĕs-ĕn-ter'ĭk) [" + *mesenterion,* mesentery]. Concerning the umbilicus and mesentery.

omphaloncus (om-fal-on'kŭs) [" + *ogkos,* tumor]. Umbilical tumor or swelling.

omphalophlebitis (ŏm"făl-ō-flē-bī'tĭs) [" + *phleps,* vein, + *-ītis,* inflammation]. Inflamed condition of umbilical veins.

omphalorrhagia (ŏm"făl-ŏr-rā'jĭ-ă) [" + *rēgnunai,* to burst forth]. Umbilical hemorrhage.

omphalorrhea (om-fal-or-ē'ă) [" + *roia,* flow]. Discharge of lymph at the navel.

omphalorrhexis (om-fal-or-rĕks'ĭs) [" + *rēxis,* rupture]. Rupture of the navel.

omphalos (om'făl-ŏs) [G. navel]. Umbilicus. SYN: *navel.*

omphalosotor (om-fal-ō-sō'tor) [G. *omphalos,* navel, + *sōtēr,* preserver]. Device used in replacing the prolapsed umbilical cord at childbirth.

omphalospinous (om-fal-ō-spī'nŭs) [" + L. *spina,* thorn]. Concerning the navel and the ant. sup. spine of the ilium.

omphalotomy (om-făl-ot'ō-mĭ) [" + *tomē,* incision]. Division of umbilical cord at birth.

DRESSING: Sterile cotton; change on second day of life.

omphalotripsy (om'făl-ō-trĭp'sĭ) [" + *tripsis,* a rubbing]. Severing of the umbilical cord by a crushing method.

o.n. Abbr. for [L.] *omni nocte,* every night.

onanism (ō'năn-ĭzm). Coitus interruptus, so named because it was practiced by the Biblical character Onan, but the term is used also, erroneously, to designate masturbation, *q.v.*

onanist (ō'năn-ĭst). One who practices coitus interruptus or, erroneously, masturbation.

Onanoff's reflex (ŏn-ăh-nŏf'). Contraction of bulbocavernous muscle resulting from compression of glans penis.

Onchocerca (ŏng-kō-ser'kă) [G. *ogkos,* hook, + *kerkos,* tail]. A genus of filarial worms. They live in subcutaneous and connective tissues and are usually enclosed in fibrous cysts or nodules.

O. caecutiens. A species of Onchocerca that causes cutaneous filariasis in man.

O. volvulus. A species of O. which infests man, frequently invading the tissues of the eye. Transmitted by species of the blackfly, *Simulium.*

onchocerciasis (ŏng-kō-ser-kī'ăs-ĭs) [" + " + iasis, infestation]. Condition produced by infestation with one of the species of Onchocerca. SYN: *onchocercosis.*

Oncocerca. Onchocerca, *q.v.*

oncocercosis. Onchocerciasis, *q.v.*

oncogenesis (ong"kō-jĕn'ĕ-sĭs) [G. *ogkos,* mass]. Tumor formation and development.

oncogenous (ŏng-koj'ĕ-nŭs) [" + *gennan,* to produce]. Forming or producing tumors.

oncograph (ŏng'kō-grăf) [" + *graphein,* to write]. Device attached to oncometer for making record of the internal organs' size.

oncology (ŏng-kŏl'ō-jĭ) [" + *logos,* study]. The branch of medicine dealing with tumors.

oncolysis (ŏng-kol'ĭ-sĭs) [" + *lysis,* dissolution]. The absorption or dissolution of tumor cells.

oncolytic (ong-kō-lĭt′ĭk) [" + *lysis*, dissolution]. Destructive to tumor cells.

oncoma (ong-kō′mă) [G. *ogkōma*, a swelling]. A tumor or swelling.

Term is no longer commonly used.

oncometer (ŏng-kom′ĕt-ĕr) [G. *ogkos*, mass, + *metron*, measure]. Apparatus for measurement of variations in size of internal organs. SEE: *plethysmograph.*

oncometric (on-kō-mĕt′rik). Pertaining to oncometry.

oncom′etry. The measurement of variations in size of internal organs.

oncosis (ŏng-kō′sĭs) [" + *-ōsis*, intensive]. 1. A condition characterized by the development of tumors. 2. A swelling or tumor.

oncosphere (ong′kō-sfēr) [G. *ogkos*, hook, + *sphaira*, sphere]. Embryonic stage of a tapeworm in which it has hooks.

oncothlipsis (ŏng-kō-thlĭp′sĭs) [G. *ogkos*, tumor, + *thlipsis*, pressure]. Pressure due to presence of a tumor.

oncotic (ŏng-kŏt-ĭk) [G. *ogkos*, tumor]. Concerning, caused, or marked by swelling.

oncotomy (ŏng-kot′ō-mĭ) [" + *tomē*, incision]. The operation of cutting into a tumor, abscess, or boil.

oncotropic (ong-kō-trop′ĭk) [" + *tropos*, a turning]. Possessing special attraction for tumor cells. SYN: *tumoraffin.*

oneiric (ō-nī′rĭk) [G. *oneiros*, dream]. Resembling, rel. to, or accompanied by dreams.

oneirism (ō-nī′rĭzm) [" + *ismos*, state of]. Dreamlike hallucination in a waking state.

oneirodynia (ō-nī-rō-dĭn′ĭ-ă) [" + *odynē*, pain]. Painful dreaming; nightmare, *q.v.*

oneirology (ō-nī-rol′ō-jĭ) [" + *logos*, study of]. The scientific aspect of dreams.

oneiroscopy (o-nī-ros′kō-pĭ) [" + *skopein*, to examine]. Analysis of dreams in the diagnosis of the individual's mental state.

oniomania (ō-nĭ-ō-mā′nĭ-ă) [G. *ōnios*, for sale, + *mania*, madness]. A psychoneurotic symbolism evidenced by an abnormal urge to spend money.

onion (ŭn′yŭn) [L. *uniō*, onion]. RAW: 1 (110 gm.). Calories: 50. Other main values: 2 gm. protein; trace of fat; 11 gm. carbohydrate; 35 mg. calcium.

onkinocele (ŏng-kĭn′ō-sēl) [G. *ogkos*, mass, + *is*, *in-*, fiber, + *kēlē*, swelling]. Inflammation, with swelling, of a tendon sheath.

onomatology (ŏn-o-mă-tol′ō-jĭ) [G. *onoma*, name, + *logos*, study]. Science of names. SYN: *nomenclature, terminology.*

onomatomania (ŏn-ō-mă-tō-mā′nĭ-ă) [" + *mania*, madness]. An abnormal or morbid impulse to dwell upon and repeat certain words, their imagined hidden meanings and significance, or to try to recall frantically a particular word.

onomatophobia (ŏn-ō-mă-tō-fō′bĭ-ă) [" + *phobos*, fear]. Abnormal fear of hearing a certain name or word because of an imaginary dreadful meaning attached to it.

onomatopoiesis (ŏn-ō-mă-tō-poy-ē′sĭs) [" + *poiein*, to make]. Imitation of natural sounds by the use of created, usually meaningless, imitative words and sounds.

onto- [G.]. Combining form, *being.*

ontogenesis (ŏn″tō-jĕn′ĕ-sĭs). Ontogeny, *q.v.*

ontogeny (ŏn-toj′ĕn-ĭ) [" + *gennan*, to produce]. The history of the development of an individual. SYN: *ontogenesis.*

onychalgia. Pain in the nails.

o. nervosa. SYN: *hyperesthesia unguium.* Extreme sensitivity of nails.

onychatrophia (ŏn″ĭ-kă-trō′fĭ-ă) [G. *onyx*, *onych-*, nail, + *a-*, priv. + *trophē*, nourishment]. Atrophy of the nails.

onychauxis (ŏn″ĭ-kawk′sĭs) [" + *auxein*, to increase]. Hypertrophy of the nails.

onychia (on-ĭk′ĭ-ă) [G. *onyx*, *onych-*, nail]. Inflammation of the nail bed with suppuration and, frequently, loss of the nail. SYN: *matrixitis; onychitis; onyxitis.* SEE: *paronychia.*

o. craquele. Fragility of nails.

o. lateralis. Suppuration of tissues in the area lateral to fingernail.

o. maligna. Type in debilitated persons in which there is fetid ulceration and loss of the nail.

o. parasitica. Any parasitic disease of the nails.

o. punctata. Condition in which a nail possesses small punctiform depressions.

onychitis (on-ĭk-ī′tĭs) [" + *-itis*, inflammation]. Inflammation of the nail bed. SYN: *onychia.*

onychocryptosis (ŏn″ĭ-kō-krĭp-tō′sĭs) [" + *kryptein*, to conceal]. Ingrowing of the toenail.

onychograph (ŏn-ĭk′ō-grăf) [" + *graphein*, to write]. Device for making record of capillary blood pressure under the fingernails.

onychogryposis (on″ĭ-kō-grĭ-pō′sĭs) [" + *grypōsis*, a curving]. Abnormal growth of the nails with inward curvature.

onychoid (on′ĭ-koyd) [" + *eidos*, resemblance]. Similar to a nail, esp. a fingernail.

onycholysis (ŏn-ĭ-kol′ĭ-sĭs) [" + *lysis*, destruction]. Loosening or detachment of the nail from the nail bed.

onychoma (on-ĭ-kō′mă) [G. *onyx*, *onych-*, nail, + *-ōma*, tumor]. Tumor of the nail or the nail bed.

onychomalacia (ŏn″ĭ-kō-mă-lā′sĭ-ă) [" + *malakia*, softening]. Unnatural softening of the nails. SEE: *hapalonychia.*

onychomycosis (on″ĭ-kō-mī-kō′sĭs) [" + *mykēs*, fungus, + *-ōsis*]. Disease of the nails due to a parasitic fungus.

onychonosus (ŏn-ĭ-kon′ō-sŭs) [" + *nosos*, disease]. Any disease of the nails.

onychopathy (ŏn-ĭ-kop′ăth-ĭ) [" + *pathos*, disease]. Any disease of the nails. SYN: *onychonosus.*

onychophagy (ŏn-ĭ-kof′ă-jĭ) [" + *phagein*, to eat]. The practice of nail biting.

onychophosis (ŏn-ĭk-ō-fō′sĭs) [" + *yphē*, web]. Accumulation of horny layers of epidermis under the toenail.

onychophyma (ŏn″ĭ-kō-fī′mă) [G. *onyx*, *onycho*, nail, + *phyma*, a growth]. Painful degeneration of the nail with hypertrophy.

onychoptosis (ŏn-ĭk-ŏp-tō′sĭs) [" + *ptōsis*, a falling]. Dropping off of the nails.

onychorrhexis (ŏn″ĭ-kō-rĕk′sĭs) [" + *rēxis*, a rupture]. Nail splitting. SYN: *brittle nails; fragilitas unguium.*

onychosis (ŏn-ĭ-kō′sĭs) [" + *-ōsis*, disease]. Any diseased condition of the nails. SYN: *onychopathy.*

onychotomy (ŏn-ĭ-kot′ō-mĭ) [" + *tomē*, incision]. Surgical incision of a fingernail or toenail.

onychotrophy (ŏn-ĭ-kŏt′rō-fĭ) [" + *trophē*, nourishment]. Nourishment of the nails.

onyx (on'ĭks) [G. *onyx*, nail]. 1. A fingernail or toenail. SYN: *unguis* [NA]. 2. Pus collection bet. the corneal layers of the eye.

onyxis (ŏn-ĭk'sĭs) [G. *onyx*, nail]. Ingrowing of the nails.

onyxitis (ŏn-ĭk-sī'tĭs) [" + *-itis*, inflammation]. Onychia, *q.v.*

oo- (ō-ō) [G. *ōon*, egg]. Combining form denoting an *egg*, or the *primordial cell* that develops into an ovule. SEE: *ovo-*.

oocyesis (ō"ō-sī-ē'sĭs) [" + *kyēsis*, pregnancy]. Ectopic pregnancy in the ovary.

oocyst (ō'ō-sĭst) [G. *ōon*, egg, + *kystis*, bladder]. The encysted form of a fertilized gamete (zygote) occurring in certain Sporozoa. SEE: *ookinete*.

oocyte (ō'ō-sīt) [" + *kytos*, cell]. The early or primitive ovum before it has developed completely.

o., primary. Cell at end of growth period of oogonium and before 1st maturation division has occurred.

o., secondary. The larger of two cells resulting from first maturation division. SEE: *body, polar*.

oogenesis (ō"ō-jĕn'ĕ-sĭs) [" + *genesis*, formation]. Formation and development of the ovum. SYN: *ovigenesis*.

oogonium (ō"ō-gō'nĭ-ŭm) (pl. *oogonia*) [" + *gonē*, generation]. 1. The primordial cell from which an oocyte originates. 2. Descendant of primordial cell from which the oocyte arises.

ookinesis (ō'ō-kĭn-ē'sĭs) [G. *ōon*, egg, + *kinesis*, movement]. Mitotic phenomena taking place within an ovum during maturation and fertilization.

o"okin'ete. An elongated motile zygote occurring in the life cycle of certain sporozoan parasites, esp. *Plasmodium*. It penetrates stomach wall of a mosquito and gives rise to an *oocyst*.

oophor- [G.]. Form indicating *ovary*.

oophoralgia (ō"ŏf-ō-ral'jĭ-ă) [G. *ōon*, egg, + *phoros*, bearing, + *algos*, pain]. Pain in an ovary.

oophorauxe (ō"ŏf-ō-rawks'ē) [" + " + *auxein*, to increase]. Ovarian enlargement.

oophorectomy (ō"ŏf-ō-rĕk'tō-mĭ) [" + " + *ektomē*, excision]. Excision of an ovary. SYN: *ovariectomy*.

oophoritis (ō"ŏf-o-rī'tis) [" + " + *-ītis*, inflammation]. Inflamed condition of the ovary. SYN: *ovaritis, q.v.*

o., follicular. Inflammation of the graafian follicles.

oophorocystosis (ō-ŏf"ō-rō-sĭs-tō'sĭs) [" + " + *kystis*, cyst, + *-ōsis*]. Development of an ovarian cyst.

oophorohysterectomy (ō-ŏf"ō-rō-hĭs-tĕr-ĕk'tō-mĭ) [" + " + *ystera*, uterus, + *ektomē*, excision]. Surgical removal of the uterus and ovaries. SYN: *ootheco-hysterectomy; ovariohysterectomy*.

oophoroma (ō-ŏf-ō-rō'mă) [" + " + *-ōma*, tumor]. Malignant ovarian tumor.

oophoromania (ō-ŏf"ō-rō-mā'nĭ-ă) [" + " + *mania*, madness]. Insanity arising from an ovarian disease.

oophoron (ō-ŏf'ō-rŏn) [" + *phoros*, bearing]. An ovary. SYN: *ootheca*.

oophoropathy (ō-ŏf-or-ŏp'ă-thĭ). Any pathologic condition of the ovary.

oophoropeliopexy (ō-ŏf"ō-rō-pe'lĭ-ō-pĕk-sĭ) [" + " + *pĕlios*, pelvis, + *pēxis*, fixation]. Suture of a displaced ovary to the pelvic wall.

oophoropexy (ō-ŏf"ō-rō-pĕk'sĭ) [G. *ōon* *phoros*, bearing, + *pēxis*, fixation]. Fixation of a displaced ovary. SYN: *oophoropeliopexy*.

oophorosalpingectomy (ō-ŏf"ō-rō-săl-pĭn-jĕk'tō-mĭ) [" + " + *salpigx*, tube, + *ektomē*, excision]. Excision of an oviduct and ovary. SYN: *ovariosalpingectomy*. POSITION: Dorsal.

oophorosalpingitis (ō-ŏf-or-ō-săl-pĭn-jī'tĭs). Inflammation of the ovary and oviduct.

oophorostomy (ō-ŏf-ō-ros'tō-mĭ) [" + " + *stoma*, opening]. Creation of artificial opening into ovarian cyst for drainage.

oophorrhagia (ō"ŏf-ōr-ra'jĭ-ă) [" + " + *rēgnunai*, to burst forth]. Hemorrhage from an ovulatory site severe enough to cause clinical symptoms or signs.

oophorrhaphy (ō-ŏf-or'ă-fĭ) [" + " + *raphē*, a sewing]. Suture of a displaced ovary to the pelvic wall.

ooplasm (ō'ō-plăsm). The cytoplasm of an ovum.

oosperm (ō'ō-spĕrm) [" + *sperma*, seed]. The cell formed by union of the spermatozoon with the ovum; the fertilized ovum.

Oospora (ō-os'pō-ră). Nocardia, *q.v.*

ootheca (ō-ō-thē'kă) [G. *ōothēkē*, ovary]. An ovary. SYN: *oophoron*.

oothecohysterectomy (ō-ō-thē"kō-hĭs-tĕr-ĕk'tō-mĭ) [" + *ystera*, uterus, + *ektomē*, excision]. Excision of the uterus and ovaries. SYN: *oophorohysterectomy*.

ootherapy (ō"ō-ther'ă-pĭ) [G. *ōon*, egg, + *therapeia*, treatment]. Treatment with ovarian substance.

opacity (ō-păs'ĭ-tĭ) [L. *opacitās*, darkness]. 1. Darkness; shading from light. 2. Lack of transparency.

opaque (ō-pāk') [L. *opacus*, dark]. 1. Dark. 2. Not transparent. 3. Stupid.

OPC. Abbr. for *outpatient clinic*.

OPD. Abbr. for *outpatient department*.

open (ō'pĕn) [A.S.]. 1. Not shut. 2. Uncovered, exposed, as to air. 3. To puncture, as to open a boil. 4. Interrupted, said of an electric circuit, when current cannot pass.

operable (ŏp'ĕr-ă-bl) [L. *operārī*, to work]. 1. Practicable. 2. Admitting of treatment by operation with reasonable expectation of cure.

operate (ŏp'ĕr-āt) [L. *operatus*, worked]. 1. To perform an excision or incision or to make a suture on the body or any of its organs or parts to restore health. 2. To produce an effect, as a drug.

operation (ŏp-ĕr-ā'shŭn) [L. *operatiō*, a working]. 1. The act of operating. 2. A surgical procedure to restore health. 3. Action of a drug.

PREPARATION FOR:

Abdominal: Shave entire abdomen and pubic hair. Cleanse umbilicus.

Anal and perineal: Shave genital area.

Arm: Shave axilla, and from shoulder to below elbow.

Breast: Shave axilla and well around the breast. If radical operation, also chest from sternum to spine, and from costal margin to clavicle.

Cerebellar: In males and children, shave the whole head and back of neck to scapulae; in females, back of head from above ears down to scapulae.

Cerebral: Shave entire head unless otherwise ordered.

Chest: Shave from median line to median line, including back.

Elbow: Shave from middle of upper arm to fingers; also axilla.

Forearm: Shave from hand to shoulder.

Hernia: Shave genital area and lower abdomen to umbilicus; also down front of thighs to middle of thighs.

Kidney: Shave from scapula to sacrum, and spine to ant. median line.

Knee: Shave from thigh to foot.

Leg: Shave from thigh to ankle.

Neck, lateral: Shave 2 inches behind ear on side indicated; cheek in males.

Rectal: SEE: *anal.*

Spine: Shave entire back if necessary.

Thigh: Shave from groin to foot; also genital area.

Thyroid: Shave lower neck in front if necessary.

SEE: *Name of operation, in alphabetical order.*

o., preparation for, in home. If it is impossible for an operation to be performed in a hospital, it may be necessary to set up a room in a home as an operating room. It should be near a water supply and have facilities for boiling surgical instruments, water, and other necessary articles such as pans and basins.

On the day before the operation, remove curtains, rugs, and all unnecessary furniture. Wash the windows, walls, woodwork, tables, and floor by scrubbing with plenty of hot water and soap. Supplies of sterile sheets, towels, handbrushes, masks, caps, and gauze sponges must be prepared also in the following manner.

Make separate packets of each type of supply, and label in pencil on the outside cover. The sheets, towels, gowns, etc., should be washed and ironed, then folded compactly and wrapped in squares of old muslin, pinned with straight pins and labeled in pencil. Then bake these packets in a moderate oven (350° F.) for 30 minutes, or until the outside wrapping shows a light tinge of scorching.

For the operating table, select a kitchen table of the proper height for the surgeon to work comfortably. Cover top with a clean blanket for padding; cover the padding with a sterile sheet. The surgeon will indicate the instruments, which are to be boiled for 10 minutes in a pan with a tight lid.

Everyone in the operating room must wear a sterile gown (nightshirts may be used), a cap to cover the head and hair, and a gauze mask.

Proper ventilation in the room is necessary but there must be no drafts. Keep the temperature of the room between 72°-75° F.

o., ablative. O. in which a part is removed.

o., capital. A grave or serious operation; one in which life is endangered.

o., exploratory. O. performed for diagnostic purposes.

o., major. One involving danger to life.

o., minor. O. not serious or risking life.

o., plastic. O. for reconstruction and repair of surface structures.

o., radical. O. performed to effect complete cure.

o., reconstructive. O. to repair a loss or defect.

o., subtotal. One in which not quite all of the organ is removed, as subtotal removal of thyroid gland.

operative (op'ĕr-ă-tĭv) [L. *operativus*, working]. 1. Effective, active. 2. Pert. to or brought about by an operation. 3. A drug that is acting.

o. procedure. A surgical operation.

opercular (ō-pur'kū-lăr) [L. *operculum*, a cover]. Concerning a covering.

operculum (ō-pur'kū-lŭm) (pl. *opercula*) [L. a covering]. 1. Any covering. 2. Plug of mucus which fills up the opening of the cervix upon impregnation. 3. NA. Convolutions of the cerebrum, the margins of which are separated by the lateral cerebral (Sylvian) fissure. The opercula cover the insula.

ophiasis (ō-fī'ăs-ĭs) [G. *ophis*, snake]. Baldness occurring in winding streaks upon the head.

ophidiophobia (ō-fĭd"ĭ-ō-fō'bĭ-ă) [G. *ophidion*, snake, + *phobos*, fear]. Abnormal fear of snakes.

ophidism (ō'fĭd-ĭzm) [G. *ophis*, snake, + *ismos*, condition]. Poisoning from snake bite.

ophiotoxemia (ō"fī-ō-tŏk-sē'mĭ-ă) [" + *toxikon*, poison, + *aima*, blood]. Poisoning due to venom injected by a snake.

ophritis, ophryitis (ŏf-rī'tĭs, -rē-ī'tĭs) [G *ophrys*, eyebrow, + *-itis*, inflammation]. Inflammation of the eyebrow.

ophryon (o'frē-on) [G. *ophrys*, eyebrow]. Meeting point of the facial median line with a transverse line across the forehead's narrowest portion.

ophthalmagra (ŏf-thăl-măg'ră) [G. *ophthalmos*, eye, + *agra*, seizure]. Gouty or rheumatic inflammation of the eye, with pain.

ophthalmalgia (ŏf-thăl-măl'jĭ-ă) [" + *algos*, pain]. Pain in the eye. SYN: *ophthalmodynia.*

ophthalmatrophy (ŏf-thăl-măt'rō-fĭ) [" + *atrophia*, a wasting]. Atrophy of eyeball.

ophthalmectomy (ŏf-thăl-mĕk'tō-mĭ) [" + *ektomē*, excision]. Surgical excision of an eye.

ophthalmia (ŏf-thăl'mĭ-ă) [G. *ophthalmos*, eye]. Severe inflammation of the eye, usually including the conjunctiva.

o., catarrhal. Conjunctivitis of a severe, frequently purulent, form.

o., Egyptian. Granular conjunctivitis. SYN: *trachoma.*

o., electric. Ophthalmia marked by pain in the eye, intolerance to light, and tearing (lacrimation). Occurs following exposure, usually prolonged, to intense light as that in arc welding.

o., gonorrheal. Severe, purulent form due to infection with gonococcus.

o., granular. Severe purulent conjunctivitis with formation of granules on the eyelids. SYN: *trachoma.*

o., metastatic. Sympathetic inflammation of the choroid due to pyemia or metastasis.

o., migratory. SEE: *sympathetic* o.

o. neonatorum. Severe purulent conjunctivitis in the newborn.

ETIOL: Infection of the birth canal at the time of delivery with gonococcus responsible for great majority of cases. Symptoms present 12-48 hrs. after birth when due to gonorrhea.

PROPHYLAXIS: Introduction of a few drops of a silver nitrate solution or penicillin ophthalmic ointment into each eye of newborn at birth.

o., neuroparalytic. One resulting from injury or disease involving semilunar ganglion or branches of trigeminal nerve supplying eyeball.

o., phlyctenular. Vesicular formations on epithelium of conjunctiva or cornea.

o., purulent. Purulent inflammation of eye, usually due to gonococcus.

o., scrofulous. Phlyctenular o., *q.v.*

o., spring. Conjunctivitis in the spring of the year, usually an allergic reaction to tree pollen. SYN: *vernal conjunctivitis.*

o., sympathetic. Serous uveitis in one eye caused by uveitis in the other eye.

SYM: Photophobia, lacrimation, pain, blurring of vision, eyeball tenderness, deposits on post. surface of cornea. Exudate appears in pupillary area with post. synechia, seclusio pupillae, secondary atrophy with blindness.

TREATMENT: Removal of exciting eye prior to onset of the disease. Mydriatics, analgesics, steroid or other anti-inflammatory therapy.

o., varicose. O. seen in varicose veins of the conjunctiva.

ophthalmiatrics (ŏf-thăl-mĭ-at′rĭks) [G. *ophthalmos,* eye, + *iatreia,* treatment]. The treatment of eye diseases.

ophthalmic (ŏf-thăl′mĭk) [G. *ophthalmos,* eye]. Pert. to the eye.

o. nerve. A branch of the trigeminal or trifacial nerve (5th cranial n.). It is sensory and its branches are the *lacrimal, frontal,* and *nasociliary.*

o. reaction. Reaction of the eye following instillation into the eye of toxins of typhoid or tuberculosis. SYN: *Calmette's reaction; oculoreaction; ophthalmoreaction.*

ophthalmitis (ŏf-thăl-mī′tĭs) [" + *-ītis,* inflammation]. Inflamed condition of the eye.

ophthalmo- [G.]. Combining form *pert. to the eye.*

ophthalmoblennorrhea (ŏf-thăl″mō-blĕn-ŏr-rē′ă) [G. *ophthalmos,* eye, + *blenna.* mucus, + *roia,* flow]. Purulent inflammation of the eye or conjunctiva, usually due to the gonococcus.

ophthalmocele (ŏf-thăl′mō-sēl) [" + *kēlē,* swelling]. Abnormal protrusion of the eyeballs. SYN: *exophthalmos.*

ophthalmocopia (ŏf-thăl-mō-kō′pĭ-ă) [" + *kopos,* fatigue]. Ocular fatigue; eye-strain. SYN: *asthenopia.*

ophthalmodesmitis (ŏf-thăl″mō-dĕs-mī′tĭs) [" + *desmos,* ligament, + *-ītis,* inflammation]. Inflammation of tendons of the eye.

ophthalmodiagnosis (ŏf-thăl″mō-dī-ăg-nō′sĭs) [" + *dia,* through, + *gnōsis,* knowledge]. Diagnosis of eye conditions by means of the ophthalmoreaction, *q.v.*

ophthalmodynia (ŏf-thăl-mō-dĭn′ĭ-ă) [" + *odynē,* pain]. Pain in the eye. SYN: *ophthalmalgia.*

ophthalmofundoscope (ŏf-thăl″mō-fŭnd′ō-skōp) [G. *ophthalmos,* eye, + L. *fundus,* base, + G. *skopein,* to examine]. Apparatus used in examining the fundus of the eye.

ophthalmography (ŏf-thăl-mŏg′răf-ĭ) [" + *graphein,* to write]. Description of the eye.

ophthalmogyric (ŏf-thăl-mō-jī′rĭk) [" + *gyros,* circle]. Causing or concerning ocular movements. SYN: *oculogyric.*

ophthalmolith (ŏf-thăl′mō-lĭth) [" + *lithos,* stone]. A calculus of the lacrimal duct.

ophthalmologist (ŏf-thăl-mŏl′ō-jĭst) [G. *ophthalmos,* eye, + *logos,* study]. A physician who specializes in the treatment of disorders of the eye; an oculist.

ophthalmology (ŏf-thăl-mol′ō-jĭ) [" + *logos,* study]. The science dealing with the eye and its diseases.

ophthalmomalacia (ŏf-thăl″mō-măl-a′sĭ-ă) [" + *malakia,* softening]. Shrinkage or softening of the eye.

ophthalmometer (ŏf-thăl-mŏm′ĕt-ĕr) [G. *ophthalmos,* eye, + *metron,* measure]. Instrument for making measurements of corneal astigmatism.

ophthalmometry (ŏf-thăl-mom′ĕt-rĭ) [" + *metron,* measure]. Measurement of the ocular defects and refractive powers.

ophthalmomycosis (ŏf-thăl″mō-mī-kō′sĭs) [" + *mykēs,* fungus, + *-ōsis*]. Any fungus disease of the eye.

ophthalmomyitis (ŏf-thăl″mō-mī-ī′tĭs) [" + *mys, my-,* muscle, + *-ītis,* inflammation]. Inflammation of the ocular muscles.

ophthalmomyositis (ŏf-thăl″mō-mī-ō-sī′tĭs). Ophthalmomyitis, *q.v.*

ophthalmomyotomy (ŏf-thăl″mō-mī-ot′ō-mĭ) [" + " + *tomē,* incision]. Surgical section of the muscles of the eyes.

ophthalmoneuritis (ŏf-thăl″mō-nū-rī′tĭs) [" + *neuron,* sinew, + *-ītis,* inflammation]. Inflamed condition of the optic nerve.

ophthalmopathy (ŏf-thăl-mop′ă-thĭ) [G. *ophthalmos,* eye, + *pathos,* disease]. Any eye disease.

ophthalmophlebotomy (ŏf-thăl″mō-flē-bŏt′ō-mĭ) [" + *phleps, phleb-,* vein, + *tomē,* incision]. Incision of the eye to overcome congestion of conjunctival veins.

ophthalmophthisis (ŏf-thăl-mŏf′thĭs-ĭs). Ophthalmomalacia, *q.v.*

ophthalmoplasty (ŏf-thăl′mō-plăs″tĭ) [" + *plassein,* to form]. Ocular plastic surgery.

ophthalmoplegia (ŏf-thăl″mō-plē′jĭ-ă) [" *plēgē,* stroke]. Paralysis of ocular muscles.

o. externa. Paralysis of extraocular muscles.

o. interna. Paralysis of iris and ciliary muscle.

o., nuclear. O. due to lesion of nuclei of origin of the ocular motor nerves.

o. partialis. Paralysis of not all of ocular muscles.

o. progressiva. Form in which all muscles become involved slowly.

o. totalis. Paralysis of both internal and external ocular muscles.

ophthalmoptosis (ŏf-thăl-mŏp-tō′sĭs) [" + *ptōsis,* a dropping]. Protrusion of the eyeball. SYN: *exophthalmos.*

ophthalmoreaction (ŏf-thăl″mō-rē-ăk′shŭn) [" + L. *rē,* back, + *actus,* acted]. Reaction of the conjunctiva following instillation of a drop of tuberculin or typhoid fever toxin into the eye of persons suffering from the diseases. SYN: *Calmette's reaction; oculoreaction; ophthalmic reaction.*

ophthalmorrhagia (ŏf-thăl-mō-rā′jĭ-ă) [G. *ophthalmos,* eye, + *rēgnunai,* to break forth]. Ocular hemorrhage.

ophthalmorrhea (ŏf-thăl-mō-rē′ă) [G. *ophthalmos,* eye, + *roia,* flow]. Discharge of watery or purulent matter from the eye.

ophthalmorrhexis (ŏf-thăl-mō-rĕks′ĭs) [" + *rēxis,* rupture]. Rupture of an eyeball.

ophthalmoscope (ŏf-thăl′mō-skōp) [" + *skopein,* to examine]. Instrument for examining interior of the eye.

ophthalmoscopy (ŏf-thăl-mŏs′kō-pĭ) [" + *skopein,* to examine]. The examination of the interior of the eye.

o., direct. Examination in which image in interior of eye is upright.

o., indirect. Examination in which image in interior of eye is inverted.

ophthalmospasm (ŏf-thăl′mō-spăsm). Spasm of ocular muscles.

ophthalmostat (ŏf-thăl′mō-stăt) [" + *statos,* standing]. Instrument used to hold the eye still during an operation.

ophthalmostatometer (ŏf-thăl″mō-stăt-om′ĕt-ĕr) [" + " + *metron,* measure].

Instrument for ascertaining position of eyes.

ophthalmosynchysis (ŏf-thăl″mō-sĭn′kĭ-sĭs). Effusion into one of the cavities of the eye.

ophthalmothermometer (ŏf-thăl″mō-thĕr-mom′ĕt-ĕr). Instrument for determining local temperature in eye diseases.

ophthalmotonometer (ŏf-thăl″mō-tō-nŏm′-ĕt-ĕr) [" + *tonos,* tension, + *metron,* measure]. Instrument for determining tension within globe of eye.

ophthalmotoxin (ŏf-thăl″mō-toks′ĭn) [" + *toxikon,* poison]. Cytotoxin derived on injection of emulsions of the ciliary body.

ophthalmotrope (ŏf-thăl′mō-trōp) [" + *tropē,* a turning]. Instrument or model of the eye used to demonstrate the movements of the extraocular muscles.

ophthalmotropometer (ŏf-thăl″mō-tro-pom′ĕt-ĕr) [" + " + *metron,* measure]. Instrument for measuring the eye movements.

ophthalmovascular (ŏf-thăl-mō-văs′kŭl-ar). Pertaining to blood vessels of eye.

ophthalmoxyster (of-thal-mox-is′ter) [" + *xyster,* scraper]. Instrument used to scrape the conjunctiva.

opiate (ō′pĭ-āt) [G. *opion,* poppy juice]. 1. A drug derived from opium. 2. A drug inducing sleep. 3. To deaden, to put to sleep.

The principal opiates are opium and its derivatives, such as morphine. They are all habit-forming.

o. abstinence syndrome. Symptoms induced by withdrawal of opiate from an addict. In a mild addict, they are restlessness, depression, and mild disturbances in functioning of autonomic nervous system. In a strong addict, an acute illness develops, lasting several days. Emotional reactions may be pronounced.

opiomania (ō″pĭ-ō-mā′nĭ-ă) [" + *mania,* madness]. Morbid addiction to use of opium or its derivatives.

opiophagism (ō-pĭ-ŏf′ă-jizm) [" + *phagein,* to eat, + *ismos,* condition]. Addiction to the use of opium, esp. the eating of it.

opisthenar (ō-pĭs′the-năr) [G. *opisthen,* behind, + *thenar,* palm]. Back of the hand.

opisthion (ō-pĭs′thĭ-ŏn) [G. *opisthion,* rear]. Craniometric point at middle of lower border of foramen magnum.

opistho-, opisth- [G.]. Combining form meaning *backward, behind.*

opisthognathism (ŏp″ĭs-thŏg′nă-thĭzm) [G. *opisthen,* behind, + *gnathos,* jaw, + *ismos,* state of]. Skull abnormality marked by a receding lower jaw.

opisthoporeia (ō-pĭs″thō-pō-rĭ′ă) [G. *opisthen,* behind, + *poreia,* a walking]. Involuntary walking backward due to loss of motor control.

opisthorchiasis (ō-pĭs″thor-kĭ′ă-sĭs). Infestation of the liver by flukes of the genus *Opisthorchis.*

Opisthorchis (ō-pĭs-thor′kĭs) [G. *opisthen,* behind, + *orchis,* testicle]. A genus of parasitic flukes belonging to the family Opisthorchiidae.

O. felineus. A species of liver flukes in dogs, cats, foxes. Occasionally infest man.

O. sinensis. SYN: for *Clonorchis sinensis,* a common liver fluke in man, esp. in the Far East.

opisthotic (ŏp″ĭs-thŏt′ĭk) [" + *ous, ot-,* ear]. Located behind the ear or in the int. ear.

opisthotonos (ŏp″ĭs-thŏt′ō-nŏs) [" + *tonos,* tension]. An arched position of the body with feet and head on the floor caused by a tetanic spasm.

Seen in severe cases of meningitis and tetanus. SEE: *emprosthotonos, pleurothotonos, posture.*

opium (ō′pĭ-ŭm) [G. *opion,* poppy juice]. USP. The dried juice obtained from the unripe capsule of the poppy. *Papaver somniferum.* It has a number of important alkaloids such as morphine, codeine, heroin, and papaverine.

ACTION: Opium is a narcotic, soporific, and astringent. In therapeutic doses, it relieves pain and discomfort and induces a deep sleep.

USES: (1) As a sedative. (2) It diminishes the secretions of bronchial tubes and relieves spasm; given to suppress ineffective coughing. Caution indicated because it is a respiratory depressant. (3) Also a heart depressant, but is administered in some heart cases to produce sleep and so improve condition of heart by relieving anxiety and permitting sleep. It slows the pulse. (4) Sedative to the nervous system; promotes rest and sleep by relieving excitability and fear. It relieves pain. (5) Inhibits all secretions of the body except perspiration, which it increases. It also contracts the pupils, even in small doses.

POISONING: See *morphine* in *Table of Poisons and Poisoning in Appendix.*

opiumism (ō′pĭ-ŭm-ĭzm) [G. *opion,* poppy juice, + *ismos,* state of]. 1. Addiction to use of opium. 2. Physical condition resulting from overuse of opium.

opo- [G.]. Prefix meaning *derived from juice.*

Oppenheim's disease (ŏp′ĕn-hīm). A noninherited but sometimes familial disease characterized by absence of muscular development, with the lower extremities being the first involved. It is first seen at, or shortly after, birth. SYN: *amyotonia congenita; myatonia congenita.* SEE: *Werdnig-Hoffman's disease.*

oppilation (ŏp″pĭ-lā′shŭn) [L. *oppilātiō,* a closure]. 1. An obstruction. 2. Act or state of being obstructed. 3. Constipation.

oppilative (ŏp′pĭ-lā-tĭv) [L. *oppilāre,* to stop up]. 1. Closing the pores. 2. Constipating. 3. Obstructive. 4. A constipating agent.

opponens (op-pō′nĕns) [L. placed against]. Opposing, a term applied to muscles of hand or foot by which one of the lateral

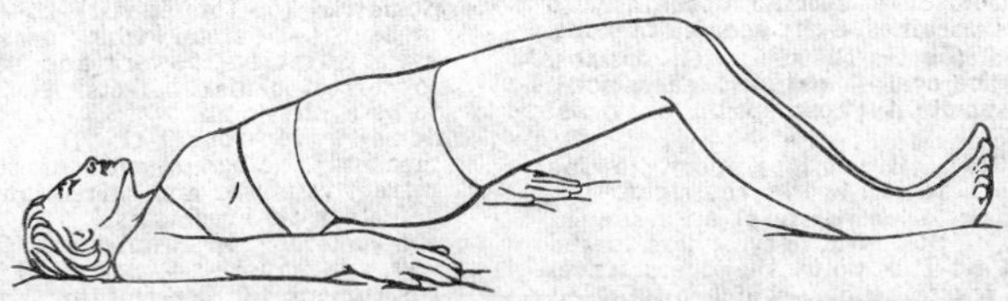

OPISTHOTONOS.

digits may be opposed to one of the other digits. SEE: *Table of Muscles in Appendix.*

opsialgia (ŏp-sĭ-al′jĭ-ă) [G. *ōps*, face, + *algos*, pain]. Neuralgic pain of the face.

opsinogenous (ŏp-sĭn-oj′ĕn-ŭs) [" + *gennan*, to produce]. Capable of forming opsonins.

opsiometer (ŏp-sĭ-ŏm′ĕt-ĕr) [G. *opsis*, vision, + *metron*, measure]. Apparatus for measuring refractive power of the eye. SYN: *optometer.*

opsionosis (ŏp″sĭ-ō-nō′sĭs). A disease or disorder of the eye or vision.

opsiuria (ŏp-sĭ-ū′rĭ-ă) [G. *opson*, food, + *ouron*, urine]. Condition in which excretion of urine is more rapid during fasting than after a meal.

opsomania (ŏp-sō-mā′nĭ-ă) [G. *opson*, food, + *mania*, madness]. Morbid desire for some special article of food.

opsonic (ŏp-son′ik) [G. *opsōnein*, to prepare food for]. Pert. to opsonins or their use in therapy.

o. index. A measure of the resistance of a patient to bacterial invasion.

Determined by the ratio bet. the number of bacteria destroyed and ingested by the leukocytes in normal blood serum, as compared with the number ingested by leukocytes under the influence of the patient's own serum.

A special technic is followed. The white corpuscles are fixed, stained, and examined under the microscope. The number of germs in 100 leukocytes are counted. The total is then divided by 100, showing the patient's phagocytic index. This is divided by average from normal blood serum and result is the opsonic index.

opsonification (ŏp-sŏn″ĭ-fĭ-kā′shŭn) [" + L. *facere*, to make]. Effect of opsonins in rendering cells or bacteria phagocytized more readily.

opsonin (op′sō-nĭn) [G. *opsōnein*, to prepare food for]. Substance in blood serum which acts upon microorganisms and other cells, facilitating phagocytosis.

opsonization (ŏp-sŏn-ĭ-zā′shun) [G. *opsōnein*, to prepare food for]. Action of opsonins to facilitate phagocytosis. SYN: *opsonification.*

opsonize (ŏp′son-īz) [G. *opsōnein*, to prepare food for]. To facilitate phagocytosis.

opsonocytophagic (op″sŏn-o-sĭ-tō-fā′jĭk) [" + *kytos*, cell, + *phagein*, to eat]. Pert. to phagocytic action of blood when serum opsonins are present.

opsonometry (ŏp-sō-nŏm′ĕt-rĭ) [" + G. *metron*, measure]. Estimation of amt. of opsonins in the blood serum. SEE: *opsonic index.*

opsonophilia (ŏp-sŏn-ō-fĭl′ĭ-ă) [" + *philein*, to love]. Attraction for opsonins.

opsonophil′ic [" + *philein*, to love]. Attractive to opsonins.

opsonotherapy (ŏp-sŏn-ō-thĕr′ă-pĭ) [" + *therapeia*, treatment]. Treatment by stimulation of a specific opsonin with bacterial vaccines. SYN: *vaccine therapy.*

optesthesia (ŏp-tĕs-thē′zĭ-ă) [G. *optikos*, pert. to the eye, + *aisthēsis*, sensation]. Visual sensibility; perception of visual stimuli.

optic (op′tik) [G. *optikos*, pert. to the eye]. Pert. to the eye or the sight.

o. chiasm, o. commissure. An x-shaped crossing of the optic nerve fibers in the brain. Past this point the fibers travel in *optic tracts.* Fibers which originated in the outer half of the retina end up on the same side of the brain, those from the inner half cross over.

o. disk. Area in retina for entrance of optic nerve; the blind spot.

o. foramen. Groove for optic nerve and ophthalmic artery at the orbit's apex.

o. nerve. Second cranial n. FUNCT: Special sense of sight. ORIG: Lateral geniculate body of thalamus via optic tract and optic chiasma. DIST: Retina. SEE: *Table of Cranial Nerves, Appendix.*

o. papilla. SEE: *optic disk.*

o. tract. Fibers of optic nerve which continue beyond optic chiasma, most of which terminate in lateral geniculate body of thalamus. Some continue to sup. colliculus of midbrain, others enter hypothalamus and terminate in supraoptic and medial nuclei.

optical (ŏp′tĭ-kăl) [G. *optikos*, pert. to the eye]. Pert. to vision or the eye or optics.

o. activity. CHEM: The property of rotating the plane of polarized light.

Measurement of this property is called polarimetry, and is useful in the determination of optically active substances like dextrose. Particularly the sugars are classified according to this criterion.

Optical activity in a substance can be detected by placing it bet. polarizing and analyzing prisms.

optician (ŏp-tĭsh′ăn) [G. *optikos*, pert. to the eye]. 1. One who makes optical apparatus. 2. One skilled in the grinding of lenses and fitting glasses.

o., dispensing. One who deals in ophthalmic lenses.

optico- [G.]. Combining form meaning *relating to the eye or vision.*

opticociliary (ŏp″tĭ-kō-sĭl′ĭ-ăr-ĭ) [G. *optikos*, pert. to the eye, + L. *ciliaris*, pert. to eyelash]. Concerning the optic and ciliary nerves.

opticonasion (op″tĭ-ko-na′sĭ-on). Length of an imaginary line drawn from the posterior edge of the optic foramen to the nasion.

opticopupillary (ŏp″tĭ-kō-pū′pĭl-ĕr-ĭ) [" + L. *pupilla*, pupil]. Concerning optic nerve and the pupil.

optics (ŏp′tĭks) [L. *optikos*, pert. to vision]. The science dealing with light and its relation to vision.

optimum (ŏp′tĭm-ŭm) (pl. *optima*) [L. *optimus*, best]. The condition which is most conducive to favorable activity. SYN: *optimal.*

o. temperature. That t. which is most suitable for development of bacterial cultures.

opto- [G.]. Combining form meaning *vision or eye.*

optogram (ŏp′tō-grăm) [G. *optos*, seen, + *gramma*, mark]. Image of ext. object fixed on the retina by photochemical bleaching action of light on the visual purple.

optometer (ŏp-tŏm′ĕt-ĕr) [" + *metron*, measure]. Instrument for measurement of the eye's refractive power. SYN: *opsiometer.*

optometrist (ŏp-tŏm′ĕt-rĭst) [" + *metron*, measure]. Person who measures the eye's refractive powers and fits glasses to correct ocular defects. Not required to be a physician.

optometry (ŏp-tom′ĕt-rĭ) [" + *metron*, measure]. Measurement of the visual refractive power and correction of visual defects with eyeglasses.

optomyometer (ŏp″tō-mī-om′ĕt-ĕr) [" + *mys, my-*, muscle, + *metron*, a measure]. Instrument for determining strength of the muscles of the eye.

optophone (ŏp'tō-fōn) [" + *phōnē*, voice]. Instrument converting light energy into sound energy. Used by the blind.

optostriate (ŏp-tō-strī'āt) [" + L. *striatus*, grooved]. Concerning the optic thalamus and the corpus striatum.

ora (ō'ra) [L.] Plural: *oras* or *orae*. 1. Mouth. 2. A border or margin.

o. serrata retinae. Notched ant. edge of sensory portion of retina.

orad (ō'răd) [L. *os, or-*, mouth, + *ad*, toward]. Toward the mouth or oral region.

oral (ō'răl) [L. *os, or-*, mouth]. Concerning the mouth.

orale (ō-rā'lē). Point on hard palate in midsagittal plane where lines drawn tangent to lingual margins of alveoli of medial incisor teeth intersect.

oralogy (ō-răl'ō-jĭ) [" + G. *logos*, study of]. 1. The science of oral hygiene. 2. Study of diseases of the mouth.

orange (ŏr'ĕnj) [Persian *nārang*, orange]. Contains citric acid, sugar and considerable cellulose. RAW: 1 (235 gm.). Calories: 106. Other main values: 2 gm. protein; 0.5 gm. fat; 26 gm. carbohydrate; 78 mg. calcium; 447 I.U. vitamin A; 115 mg. ascorbic acid.

JUICE (fresh): 1 cup (247 gm.). Calories: 100. Other main values: 2 gm. protein; 27 gm. carbohydrate; 47 mg. calcium; 460 I.U. vitamin A; 122 mg. ascorbic acid.

orbicular (ŏr-bĭk'ū-lăr) [L. *orbiculus*, a small circle]. Circular.

o. bone. Ossicle frequently becoming attached to the incus. SYN: *os orbiculare*. SEE: *o. process*.

o. muscle. Muscle about an opening.

o. process. End of long process of the incus. SYN: *lenticular process*.

orbicularis (ŏr"bĭk-ū-la'rĭs) [L. *orbiculus*, little circle]. Muscle surrounding an orifice; a sphincter muscle.

o. ciliaris. SYN: *ciliary ring*. The ciliary muscles of the eye.

o. oculi. Muscle encircling the opening of orbit of the eye.

o. oris. Circular muscle surrounding the mouth.

o. palpebrarum. SEE: *o. oculi*.

orbit (or'bĭt) [L. *orbita*, track]. The bony pyramid-shaped cavity of the skull which holds the eyeball. It is pierced posteriorly by the *optic foramen*, which transmits the optic nerve and ophthalmic artery, the *sup. and inf. orbital fissures*, and several foramina.

It is formed by the frontal, malar, ethmoid, maxillary, lacrimal, sphenoid, and palatine bones.

orbita (or'bĭ-tă) (pl. *orbitae*) [L. wheel track]. NA. Latin term for orbit.

orbital (or'bĭ-tăl) [L. *orbita*, track]. Concerning the orbit.

orbitale (or-bĭ-tā'lē) [L. *orbita*, track]. Lowest point on lower orbital margin.

orbitotomy (or-bĭt-ŏt'ō-mĭ) [" + G. *tomē*, incision]. Surgical incision into the orbit.

orchectomy (ŏr-kĕk'tō-mĭ) [G. *orchis*, testicle, + *ektomē*, excision]. Surgical removal of a testicle.

DRESSINGS, ETC: Small drainage tube, sterilized gauze, borosalicylic acid powder, 4:1.

SYN: *orchidectomy, orchiectomy*.

orcheoplasty (or'kē-ō-plăs-tĭ) [" + *plassein*, to form]. Plastic repair work of the testicle.

orchialgia (or-kĭ-ăl'jĭ-ă) [" + *algos*, pain]. Pain in the testes. SYN: *orchiodynia*.

orchichorea (or"kĭ-kō-rē'ă) [" + *choreia*, a dance]. Involuntary jerking movements of the testicles.

orchidalgia (or-kĭ-dal'jĭ-ă) [G. *orchis, orchid-*, testicle, + *algos*, pain]. Neuralgia in the testicles. SYN: *orchialgia*.

orchidectomy (or"kĭd-ek'tō-mĭ) [" + *ektomē*, excision]. Removal of a testicle surgically. SYN: *orchectomy, orchiectomy*.

orchidic (or-kid'ik). Concerning or rel. to the testes.

orchido- [G.]. Combining form, meaning *testicle*. See also words beg. *orchio-*.

orchidoncus (ŏr-kĭ-dong'kŭs) [" + *ogkos*, mass]. A neoplasm of the testicle. SYN: *orchioncus*.

orchidopexy (or'kĭd-ō-pĕks"ĭ) [" + *pēxis*, fixation]. Surgical transfer of an imperfectly descended testicle into the scrotum and suturing it there. SYN: *orchiopexy*.

orchidoplasty (ŏr'kĭd-ō-plăs"tĭ) [" + *plassein*, to form]. Operative transfer of an undescended testicle to the scrotum.

orchidoptosis (ŏr"kĭd-ŏp-tō'sĭs) [" + *ptōsis*, a falling]. Dropping of the testicle.

orchidotomy (ŏr-kĭd-ŏt'ō-mĭ) [G. *orchis, orchid-*, testicle, + *tomē*, incision]. Incision into the testes.

orchiectomy (ŏr-kĭ-ĕk'tō-mĭ) [" + *ektomē*, excision]. Surgical excision of a testicle. SYN: *orchectomy, orchidectomy*. SEE: *castration*.

orchiencephaloma (or"kĭ-ĕn-sef-ă-lō'mă) [" + *egkephalos*, brain, + *-ōma*, tumor]. Tumor of brainlike substance in the testicle. SEE: *orchiomyeloma*.

orchiepididymitis (or"kĭ-ep"ĭ-dĭd-ĭ-mī'tĭs) [" + *epi*, upon, + *didymos*, testis, + *-ītis*, inflammation]. Inflamed condition of a testicle and epididymis.

orchiocele (or'kĭ-ō-sēl) [" + *kēlē*, mass]. 1. Scrotal hernia. SYN: *orchidocele*. 2. A tumor of the testicle.

orchiodynia (ŏr-kĭ-ō-din'ĭ-ă) [" + *odynē*, pain]. Testicular pain. SYN: *orchialgia, orchidalgia*.

orchiomyeloma (or"kĭ-ō-mī-ĕ-lō'mă) [G. *orchis*, testicle, + *myelos*, marrow, + *-ōma*, tumor]. Tumor of the testicle composed of marrowlike cells.

orchioncus (ŏr-kĭ-ong'kŭs) [" + *ogkos*, tumor]. Neoplasm of the testicle. SYN: *orchidoncus*.

orchioneuralgia (or"kĭ-ō-nū-răl'jĭ-ă) [" + *neuron*, sinew, + *algos*, pain]. Neuralgia of the testicles. SYN: *orchialgia*.

orchiopathy (ŏr-kĭ-op'ăth-ĭ) [" + *pathos*, disease]. Any diseased condition of the testes.

orchiopexy (or'kĭ-ō-peks"ĭ) [" + *pēxis*, fixation]. The suturing of an undescended testicle in the scrotum. SYN: *orchidopexy, orchiorrhaphy*.

orchioplasty (or'kĭ-ō-plas"tĭ) [" + *plassein*, to form]. Plastic repair of the testicle.

orchiorrhaphy (ŏr-kĭ-or'ră-fĭ) [" + *raphē*, a sewing]. The suturing of an undescended testicle to surrounding tissue in the scrotum. SYN: *orchidopexy, orchiopexy*.

orchioscheocele (or-kĭ-os'kē-ō-sēl) [" + *oschē*, scrotum, + *kēlē*, hernia]. Scrotal hernia with enlargement or tumor of testicle.

orchioscirrhus (or-kĭ-ō-skĕr'rŭs) [G. *orchis*, testicle, + *skirros*, hard]. Testicular hardening due to tumor formation.

orchis (ŏr'kĭs) [G.]. A testicle.

orchitic (or-kit'ik) [G. *orchis*, testicle, + *-ītis*, inflammation]. Concerning or caused by orchitis.

orchitis (ŏr-kī'tĭs) [" + *-ītis,* inflammation]. Inflammation of a testis due to trauma, metastasis, mumps, or infection elsewhere in the body.

SYM: Swelling, severe pain, possibly gangrene, chills, fever, vomiting, hiccough, delirium. May end in atrophy of organ.

TREATMENT: In mumps, confine patient to bed first 8 days; locally by immobilization of organ, and ice bag.

o., *gonorrheal.* O. due to gonococcus.

o., *metastatic.* O. due to infection from organisms in blood stream.

o., *syphilitic.* SYM: Begins painlessly in body of gland as a rule, apt to be bilateral; causes dense, irregular, knotty induration, but not much increase in size.

o., *tuberculous.* Form generally arising in the epididymis. It may be accompanied by formation of chronic sinuses, and destruction of tissues.

SYM: Little or no pain. Begins as hard, irregular enlargement at lower and post. aspect of gland, gradually increasing, sometimes extends along vas deferens. Later whole gland undergoes caseous degeneration.

orchitolytic (or"kĭt-ō-lĭt'ĭk) [G. *orchis,* testicle, + *lysis,* destruction]. Destructive to testicular tissue.

orchotomy (ŏr-kŏt'ō-mĭ) [" + *tomē,* incision]. 1. Incision into a testicle. 2. Erroneously, excision of the testes. SYN: *orchectomy.*

orcin, orcinol (or'sĭn, -ol). A substance derived from lichens, used in skin disorders.

order. In biological classification, the main division of a class.

orderly (or'dĕr-lĭ) [L. *ordō,* order]. Male attendant in a hospital, other than doctors or interns, responsible for care or preparation of male patients.

They shave male patients preparatory to operation, catheterize them, and assist nurses in lifting.

ordure (or'dūr). Feces or other excrement.

orexigenic (ō-rĕk-sĭ-jĕn'ĭk) [G. *orexis,* appetite, + *gennan,* to produce]. Stimulating the appetite.

oreximania (ō-rĕk-sĭ-mā'nĭ-ă) [" + *mania,* madness]. Abnormal desire for food.

orf. A disease of sheep which is transmissible to man.

organ (or'găn) [G. *organon,* organ]. A part of the body having a special function.

Most organs are in pairs. Any 1 organ may be extirpated and the remaining 1 will perform all necessary functions peculiar to it. Even half of the brain may be removed without being fatal. From one-third to two-fifths of some organs may be removed without interference with their functions.

o., *accessory.* One having a subordinate function.

o., *acoustic.* SEE: *o. of Corti.*

o. *of Corti.* Terminal acoustic apparatus in the cochlea. SEE: *Claudius' cells, ear.*

o., *enamel.* A knoblike thickening which develops on dental lamina which gives rise to a double-walled, cup-shaped organ that encloses the dental papilla. It functions in the shaping of the tooth and the formation of enamel.

o., *end.* The specialized termination of a sensory nerve fiber which serves as a receptor. May be nonencapsulated or encapsulated.

o., *endocrine.* An organ yielding internal secretions. SEE: *endocrine.*

o., *excretory.* An organ which is concerned with the excretion of waste products from the body.

o.'s *of generation.* The reproductive organs, external and internal. SEE: *genitalia, male and female.*

o. *of Giraldes.* A small body on the spermatic cord, above the epididymis. SYN: *paradidymis.*

o., *Golgi's.* SYN: *neurotendinous spindle, Golgi's corpuscle.* A spindle-shaped structure at junction of a muscle and tendon. Functions as a receptor for proprioceptive sense.

o., *gustatory.* A taste bud. SYN: *organum gustus* [NA].

o. *of Jacobson.* SYN: *vomeronasal organ.* A blind tubular sac which develops in medial wall of nasal cavity; becomes a functional olfactory organ in lower animals but degenerates or remains rudimentary in man.

o., *reproductive.* Any organ concerned with the production of offspring. Includes the *primary organs* (testes and ovaries) and *accessory structures* such as penis and spermatic cord in the male and fallopian tubes, uterus, and vagina in the female.

o. *of Ruffini.* SYN: *corpuscle of Ruffini.* Sensory receptor of warmth located principally at tips of fingers.

o., *sense.* A sensory receptor. A structure consisting of specialized sensory nerve endings which are capable of reacting to a stimulus (an environmental change) by giving rise to nerve impulses which pass through afferent nerves to the central nervous system. These impulses may give rise to sensations or reflexly bring about responses in the body. SYN: *organa sensuum* [NA].

o., *sex.* A reproductive organ.

o., *special sense.* The eye, ear, and organs of smell and taste.

o., *vomeronasal.* SEE: *Jacobson's o.*

o., *Weber's.* Residual prostatic pouch in the male, the remains of the müllerian ducts.

o.'s *of Zuckerkandl.* A pair of o's, appearing in the embryo and persisting until shortly after birth. Located under anterior surface of abdominal aorta.

organelle. A specialized part of a cell which performs a definite function. Ex: mitochondria, Golgi apparatus, endoplasmic reticulum, lysosomes, and cell centriole.

organic (or-găn'ĭk) [G. *organon,* organ]. 1. Pert. to an organ or organs. 2. Structural. 3. Pert. to or derived from animal or vegetable forms of life.

o. *acid.* Any acid containing one or more -COOH or carboxyl groups. Ex: acetic, formic, lactic, and all fatty acids.

o. *chemistry.* Branch dealing with carbon compounds.

o. *disease.* A disease associated with observable or detectable changes in the organs or tissues of the body.

o. *psychoses.* PSY: A general term applied to those psychoses induced by structural brain changes.

In general, a character change is manifested in behavior and disposition. The patient is less stable than before, emotional instability, irritability and anger outbursts being frequent. His attention fluctuates widely; gradually he deteriorates; early or later, memory, comprehension, ideation, and orientation become defective.

Size, Weight, and Capacity of Various Organs and Parts of the Body*

Description	Size (in centimeters)	Weight (in grams)	Capacity (in milliliters)
Adrenal gland	3 to 5 cm. long, 4 to 6 cm. thick	3.5 to 5.0 gm.	
Bladder	12 cm. in diameter		500 ml. (when moderately full)
Blood volume			♂ 4200 ml., ♀ 5000 ml.
Brain		♂ 1430 gm., ♀ 1294 gm.	
Esophagus	23 to 25 cm.		
Fallopian tube	10 cm.		
Gallbladder	7 to 10 cm. long, 2.5 cm. wide		30 to 35 ml.
Heart	12 x 8 to 9 x 6.0 cm.	♂ 280 to 340 gm., ♀ 230 to 280 gm.	
Intestines—small	Quite variable 472 to 970 cm. long		
Intestines—large	150 cm. long		
Intestines—vermiform appendix	2 to 20 cm. long, Average 8.3 cm.		
Intestines—rectum	12 cm. long		
Kidney	11.25 cm. long, 5 to 7.5 cm. broad, 2.5 cm. thick	♂ 125 to 170 gm., ♀ 115 to 155 gm.	
Liver		♂ 1400 to 1600 gm., ♀ 1200 to 1400 gm.	
Lung		Rt. 625 gm.. Lt. 567 gm.	6500 ml.
Ovaries	4 x 2 x 0.8 cm.	2 to 3.5 gm.	
Pancreas	12.5 to 15 cm. long	♂ 74 to 106 gm., ♀ 70 to 100 gm.	
Pharynx	12.5 cm. long		
Prostate	2 x 4 x 3 cm.	20 gm.	
Spinal cord	42 to 45 cm. long	30 gm.	
Spleen	12 x 7 x 3 to 4 cm.	100 to 250 gm. Decreases with age	
Stomach	Quite variable. 25 cm. long, 10 cm. wide		Quite variable. 1000 ml.
Testes	4 to 5 x 2.5 x 3.0 cm.	10.5 to 14 gm.	
Thoracic duct	38 to 45 cm. long		
Thymus		Newborn, 10.9 gm.; 10-15 yrs., 29.5 gm.; 20-25 yrs. 18.6 gm.	
Thyroid	Each lobe 5 x 3 x 2 cm.	30 gm. total	
Trachea	11 cm. long, 2 to 2.5 cm. in diameter		
Ureter	28 to 34 cm. long		
Urethra	♂ 17.5 to 20 cm. long ♀ 4 cm. long		
Uterus	7.5 x 5.0 x 2.5 cm.	30 to 40 gm. (nonpregnant)	
Skeleton		Average adult male, 4957 gm.	
Skull		Average (without teeth), 642 gm.	

*Gray's Anatomy, 27th ed. Lea & Febiger, Philadelphia, 1959; Growth. Federation of American Societies for Experimental Biology, Washington, D. C., 1962.

ETIOL: Alcohol, narcotics, trauma, syphilis, drugs, poisons, chronic infections, encephalitis, brain tumors among many others.

organism (or′găn-ĭzm) [G. *organon*, organ, + *ismos*, condition]. A living thing, plant or animal. May be *unicellular* (bacteria, yeasts, protozoa) or *multicellular* (all complex organisms including man).

organization (or″găn-ĭ-zā′shŭn) [G. *organon*, organ]. 1. Process of becoming organized. 2. Systematic arrangement. 3. That which is organized; an organism.

o. center. 1. A group of cells in an embryo which induces the development of another structure. 2. A region in an ovum which is responsible for the mode of development of the fertilized ovum.

organize (or′găn-īz) [G. *organon*, organ]. To develop from an amorphous state to that having structure and form.

organogenesis, organogeny (or-găn-ō-jen′ĕ-sĭs, -oj′ĕn-ĭ) [" + *gennan*, to produce]. The formation and development of body organs from embryonic tissues.

organography (or-găn-og′ră-fĭ) [" + *graphein*, to write]. The description of the body organs.

organoid. An organelle, *q.v.*

organoleptic (or-găn-ō-lep′tĭk) [" + *lēpsis*, a seizure]. 1. Affecting an organ, esp. the organs of special sense. 2. Susceptible to sensory impressions.

o. test. Subjective test (taste, odor, smell) of drugs, foods, and beverages.

organology (or-găn-ol'ō-jĭ) [" + *logos,* study]. The science dealing with the body organs.

organon (or'găn-ŏn) [G. & L. organ]. Organum, *q.v.*

organopexy (or"găn-ō-pĕk'sĭ) [G. *organon,* organ, + *pēxis,* fixation]. Surgical fixation of an organ that is detached from its proper position.

organoscopy (or-găn-os'kō-pĭ) [" + *skopein,* to examine]. Examination of the internal organs of the body.

organotherapy (or"găn-ō-thĕr'ă-pĭ) [" + *therapeia,* treatment]. The treatment of disease by preparations of the endocrine glands of animals, or by extracts made from the same.

organotrope, organotropic (or-găn'ō-trōp, -trŏp'ĭk) [" + *tropos,* a turning]. Having affinity for tissues, noting substances acting on the organs of the body.

or'ganum (pl. *organa*). NA. An organ.

o. auditus. O. vestibulocochleare, *q.v.*

o. gustus [NA]. Organ of taste.

o. olfactus [NA]. Organ of smell.

o. spirale [NA]. Spiral organ in the cochlea. SYN: *organ of Corti.*

o. vestibulocochleare [NA]. Organ of hearing. SEE: *ear.*

o. visus [NA]. The organ of sight.

o. vomeronasale [NA]. Canal opening into nasal septum. SYN: *Jacobson's organ.*

orgasm (or'găzm) [G. *orgein,* to be passionate]. A state of paroxysmal emotional excitement, esp. that which occurs at the climax of sexual intercourse. In the male it is accompanied by the ejaculation of semen.

orien'tal sore. An ulcerating, chronic, nodular skin lesion prevalent in the Orient and the tropics, due to infection with Leishmania tropica. SYN: *cutaneous leishmaniasis; Aleppo boil; Delhi boil.*

orientation (or"ĭ-ĕn-tā'shŭn) [L. *oriens,* the east]. Ability to comprehend and to adjust one's self in an environment with regard to time, location, and identity of persons.

Partially or completely absent in some psychoses.

orifice (or'ĭ-fĭs) [L. *orificium*]. Mouth, entrance or outlet to any aperture.

o., anal. The anus.

o., atrioventricular. The opening between the atrium and the ventricle on each side of the heart.

o., auriculoventricular. The atrioventricular orifice, *q.v.*

o., cardiac. Opening of esophagus into stomach.

o., mitral. Opening between atrium and ventricle.

o., pyloric. Opening from stomach into the duodenum. SEE: *pylorus.*

o., ureteric. Opening of ureter into bladder.

o., urethral, external. Ext. opening of the urethra. In male, located at tip of glans penis; in female, located anterior and cephalad to vaginal opening.

o., urethral, internal. Opening from which urethra makes its exit from bladder.

orificial (or-ĭ-fĭ'shĭ-ăl) [L. *orificium,* outlet]. Pert. to or forming an orifice.

orificialist (or-ĭ-fĭsh'ăl-ĭst) [L. *orificium,* outlet]. One who practices orificial surgery in the treatment of disease.

origin (or"ĭ-jĭn) [L. *origo,* beginning]. 1. The source of anything; a starting point. 2. The beginning of a nerve. 3. The more fixed attachment of a muscle.

o., deep, ental. The region within the brain where the fibers comprising a cranial nerve terminate.

o., superficial, ectal. Point where a cranial nerve makes its exit from the brain.

orinase (or'ĭ-nās). Proprietary brand of tolbutamide (1- butyl-3, p-tolylsulfonylurea). An antidiabetes agent used in treatment of diabetes mellitus. Administered orally.

Ornithodoros. A genus of ticks belonging to the family Argasidae, which infest mammals including man. Several species serve as transmitters of the causative agents of disease including spotted fever, tick fever, Q fever, tularemia, Russian encephalitis, and relapsing fever.

ornithosis (or-nĭ-tho'sĭs). A virus disease of birds, communicated to man. SYN: *psittacosis, q.v.; parrot fever.*

orodiagnosis (or"ō-dī-ăg-nō'sĭs) [G. *oros,* serum, + *dia,* through, + *gnōsis,* knowledge]. Diagnosis by using serums or serum reactions.

orolingual (ō"rō-lĭn'gwăl) [L. *os, or-,* mouth, + *lingua,* tongue]. Concerning the mouth and tongue.

oronasal (ō"rō-nā'zăl) [" + *nasus,* nose]. Concerning the mouth and nose.

oropharynx (ō"rō-far'ĭnks) [" + G. *pharygx,* pharynx]. Portion of pharynx between the soft palate and upper portion of epiglottis.

orotherapy (ō"rō-thĕr-ă-pĭ) [" + G. *therapeia,* treatment]. 1. Treatment of disease with serums. SYN: *serotherapy.* 2. Use of whey in treatment.

Oro'ya fever [Oroya, a region in Peru]. SYN: *verruga peruana; bartonellosis; Carrion's disease.* An acute infectious disease endemic in Peru and other S.A. countries. The first clinical stage of bartonellosis, *q.v.*

SYM: Intermittent fever; lymphadenopathy; severe anemia; and pains in joints and long bones.

orrhology (or-rol'ō-jĭ) [" + *logos,* study]. The study of serums and their reactions. SYN: *serology.*

orrhomeningitis (or"rō-men-ĭn-jī'tĭs) [" + *mēnigx,* membrane, + *-itis,* inflammation]. Inflammation of a serous membrane.

orrhoreaction (or"rō-rē-ăk'shŭn) [" + L. *rē,* back, + *actus,* acted]. A reaction from injection of serum.

orrhorrhea (or"rō-rē'ă) [" + *roia,* flow]. 1. A flow of serum. 2. A watery discharge.

orrhotherapy (or"rō-thĕr'ă-pĭ) [" + *therapeia,* treatment]. Serum therapy.

ortho- [G.]. Combining form meaning *straight, correct.*

orthocephalic (or"thō-sē-făl'ĭk) [" + *kephalē,* head]. Noting a head with a height-length index bet. 70 and 75.

orthochorea (or"thō-kō-re'ă) [" + *choreia,* dance]. Movements in erect posture of person having chorea.

orthochromatic (or"thō-krō-mat'ĭk) [" + *chrōma,* color]. Having normal color.

orthochromophil (or"thō-krō'mō-fĭl) [" + " + *philein,* to love]. Staining normally with neutral dyes.

orthocrasia (or"thō-krā'sĭ-ă) [" + *krasis,* temperament]. Condition in which the body reacts normally to drugs, proteins, and treatment in general.

orthodiagraph (or"thō-dī'ă-grăf) [" + *dia.* through, + *graphein,* to write]. An instrument for accurately recording the outlines and positions of organs or foreign bodies as seen by radiographic apparatus.

or'thodig'ita. The division of podiatry which deals with the correction of deviated toes; the prevention and correction of deformities of the fingers or toes.

orthodontia (or"thō-don'shĭ-ă) [" + *odous, odont-*, tooth]. Division of dentistry dealing with prevention and correction of irregularities of the teeth such as malocclusion. SYN: *orthodontics.*

orthodontist. A dentist who is an expert in orthodontia, *q.v.*

orthogenesis (or"thō-jĕn'ĕ-sĭs) [G. *orthos*, straight, + *genesis*, development]. A biological principle that variations in an animal species begin to assume a definite direction, resulting in evolution of a new type, irrespective of ext. factors.

orthognathous (or-thog'nă-thŭs) [" + *gnathos*, jaw]. Having straight jaws with a gnathic index of 97.9 or less.

orthograde (or'thō-grād) [" + L. *gradus*, a step]. Walking with the body vertical or upright.

orthometer (or-thom'ĕt-ĕr) [" + *metron*, measure]. Device for determining the degree of protrusion or retraction of the eyes.

orthopedia (orthopaedia) (or"thō-pē'-dĭ-ă) [" + *pais, paid-*, child]. Orthopedics, *q.v.*

orthopedic (orthopaedic) (or"thō-pē'dĭk) [" + *pais, paid-*, child]. Concerning orthopedics; prevention or correction of deformities.

o. surgery. Surgical prevention and correction of deformities.

orthopedics (orthopaedics) (or"thō-pē'-dĭks) [G. *orthos*, straight, + *pais, paid-*, child]. Branch of medical science that deals with treatment of disorders involving locomotor structures of the body, esp. the skeleton, joints, muscles and fascia. Term formerly applied to treatment of deformities in children.

orthopedist (or"thō-pē'dĭst) [G. *orthos*, straight, + *pais, paid-*, child]. A specialist in orthopedics.

orthopercussion (or"thō-pĕr-kŭsh'ŏn) [" + L. *percussiō*, a striking through]. Percussion with the distal phalanx of the percussing finger held perpendicularly to the surface percussed.

orthophoria (or"thō-fō'rĭ-ă) [G. *orthos*, straight, + *pherein*, to bear]. Parallelism of visual axes, the normal muscle balance.

orthophrenia (or"thō-frē'nĭ-ă) [" + *phrēn*, mind]. The normal mental state of one who shares his emotional life with the family or a group.

orthopnea (or-thŏp-nē'ă) [" + *pnein*, to breathe]. Respiratory condition in which breathing is possible only when person sits or stands in erect position.

ETIOL: Seen in grave cardiac diseases, bronchial and cardiac asthma, pulmonary edema, severe emphysema, pneumonia, angina pectoris, spasmodic croup.

SYM: Respiratory rate, slow or rapid; sitting or standing posture necessary, muscles of respiration forcibly used; patient feels necessity of bracing himself in order to breathe. Anxious expression, face cyanosed. Struggle to inhale and exhale.

RS: *dyspnea, hyperpnea, oligopnea, posture, respiration.*

orthopraxy (or'thō-prăk-sĭ) [" + *prassein*, to make]. Correction and prevention of deformities by mechanical means. SYN: *orthopedics.*

orthopsychiatry (or"thō-sī-kī'ă-trĭ) [" + *psychē*, soul, + *iatreia*, treatment]. The study and treatment of emotional and behavioral disorders, esp. in the young.

orthoptic (or-thŏp'tĭk) [G. *orthos*, straight, + *optikos*, pert. to vision]. Pertaining to normal binocular vision.

o. training. Eye muscle exercises for the purpose of correcting squint; orthoptics.

orthop'tics. The science of correcting defects in binocular vision resulting from defects in optic musculature.

orthoroentgenography (or"thō-rĕnt-gĕn-og'ră-fĭ) [" + roentgen, + G. *graphein*, to write]. Measurement of size and position of internal organs accurately, using radiographic apparatus. SEE: *orthodiagraph.*

orthoscope (or'thō-skōp) [G. *orthos*, straight, + *skopein*, to examine]. Instrument for examining the eyes through a layer of water.

orthoscopic (or"thō-skŏp'ĭk) [" + *skopein*, to examine]. 1. Having correct vision. 2. Seen without distortion. 3. Made to correct optical distortion.

orthoscopy (or-thŏs'kō-pĭ) [" + *skopein*, to examine]. Ocular examination with an orthoscope.

ortho'sis. The straightening or correction of a deformity.

orthostatic (or'thō-stăt-ĭk) [" + *statos*, standing]. Concerning an erect position.

orthostatism (or'thō-stăt-ĭzm) [" + " + *ismos*, condition]. An upright standing position of the body.

orthotast (or'thō-tăst) [" + *tassein*, to arrange]. Instrument for straightening bone curvatures.

orthotic. 1. Relating to *orthosis, q.v.* 2. *orthostatic, q.v.*

orthotist. One skilled in *orthosis, q.v.*

orthotonos, orthotonus (or-thŏt'ō-nos, -nŭs) [" + *tonos*, tension]. Tetanic spasm marked by rigidity of the body in a straight line.

orthropsia (or-throp'sĭ-ă) [G. *orthros*, time near dawn, + *opsis*, sight]. Characteristic of human vision by which sight is better at dawn or dusk than in bright sunlight.

orthuria (orth-ū'rĭ-ă) [" + *ouron*, urine]. Average frequency of urination.

oryzanin (ŏ-rĭ'ză-nin) [G. *oryza*, rice]. A glutelin obtained from rice.

O. S., o. s. Abbr. for L. *oculus sinister*, left eye.

Os. Symb. for *osmium.*

os (ŏs) (pl. *ōra*) [L.]. Mouth, opening.

o. uteri. Mouth of the uterus.

o. uteri externum. The opening of cervical canal of uterus into the vagina.

o. uteri internum. The internal opening of the cervical canal into the uterus.

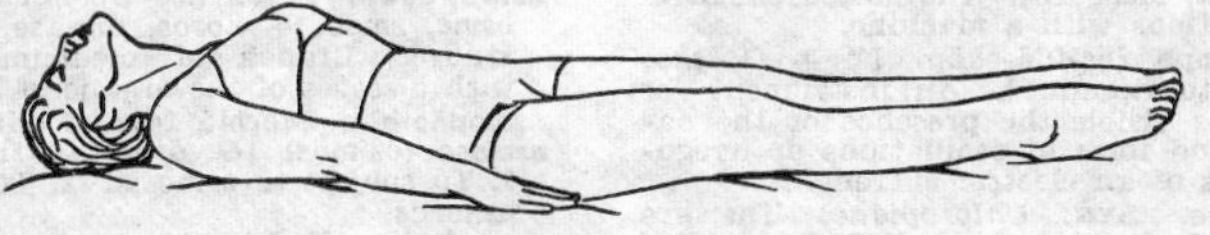

ORTHOTONOS.

o. ventriculi. The cardia of the stomach.

os (ŏs) (pl. *ossa*) [L.]. Bone.

o. calcis. Heel bone. SYN: *calcaneum.*

o. coxae. Hip bone.

o. hamatum. Hooked bone in second row of carpus. SYN: *unciform bone.*

o. hyoideum. U-shaped bone at the base of the tongue. The hyoid bone.

o. ilium. The ilium.

o. innominatum. SEE: *o. coxae.*

o. magnum. SYN: *capitate.* A carpal bone, the third in the second distal row.

o. orbiculare. Tiny bone in the ear which usually becomes attached to the incus, forming the lenticular process.

o. peroneum. Bone occasionally found in tendon of peroneus longus muscle.

o. planum. 1. Flat bone. 2. Orbita plate of ethmoid bone.

o. pubis. The pubic bone.

o. scaphoides. SEE: *scaphoid.*

o. trigonum. Bone which develops from an extra center of ossification along post. surface of talus.

o. unguis. Lacrimal bone.

o. vesalianum. Bone which develops from ossification of the post. tubercle of the fifth metatarsal.

osazone (ō'să-zōn). Any of a series of compounds resulting from heating sugars with acetic acid and phenylhydrazine.

oscedo (os-sē'dō) [L. yawning]. 1. Yawning. 2. White spots on the mucosa of the mouth. SYN: *aphthae.*

oscheal (os'kē-ăl) [G. *oscheon,* scrotum]. Concerning the scrotum.

oscheio-, oscheo- [G.]. Combining forms meaning the *scrotum.*

oscheitis (ŏs-kē-ī'tĭs) [G. *oscheon,* scrotum, + *-ītis,* inflammation]. Inflamed condition of the scrotum. SYN: *oschitis.*

oscheocele (os'kē-ō-sēl) [" + *kēlē,* swelling]. 1. A scrotal swelling or tumor. 2. Scrotal hernia. SYN: *oscheoma.*

oscheohydrocele (os"kē-ō-hī'drō-sēl) [" + *ydōr,* water, + *kēlē,* hernia]. Collection of fluid in the sac of a scrotal hernia.

oscheolith (os'kē-ō-lĭth) [" + *lithos,* stone]. A concretion in the scrotal sebaceous glands.

oscheoma (ŏs-kē-ō'mă) [" + *-ōma,* tumor]. Scrotal tumor. SYN: *oscheoncus.*

oscheoncus (ŏs-kē-on'kŭs) [" + *ogkos,* tumor]. A tumor of the scrotum.

oscheoplasty (os'kē-ō-plăs-tĭ) [" + *plassein,* to form]. Plastic surgical repair of the scrotum.

oschitis (os-kī'tis). Oscheitis, *q.v.*

oscillation (ŏs"sĭl-ā'shŭn) [L. *oscillāre,* to swing]. A swinging, pendulumlike movement; a vibration.

oscillogram (os'il-ō-grăm) [" + G. *gramma,* a mark]. Record made by the oscillograph.

oscillograph (ŏs'il-ŏ-grăf) [" + G. *graphein,* to write]. An instrument either electronic or mechanical or combined for recording electric vibrations, as of the heart or blood pressure.

oscillometer (ŏs-ĭl-om'ĕt-ĕr) [" + G. *metron,* measure]. Machine to measure oscillations.

oscillometry (ŏs-ĭl-om'ĕ-trĭ) [" + G. *metron,* measure]. The measurement of oscillations with a machine.

oscilloscope (ŏs-ĭl'ō-skōp) [" + G. *skopein,* to examine]. An instrument for making visible the presence or the nature and form of oscillations or irregularities of an electric current.

Oscinidae. SYN: *Chloropidae.* The eye flies. A family of small hairless flies which includes the genera Hippelates, Siphunculina, and Oscinis. They are serious pests and transmit a number of infectious diseases.

oscitation (ŏs-ĭ-tā'shŭn) [L. *oscitāre,* to yawn]. Yawning, gaping.

oscula'tion. 1. The union of two vessels or structures by their mouths. 2. Kissing.

osculum (os'kū-lŭm) [L. a little mouth]. Any tiny aperture or pore.

-ose. Chemical suffix indicating (a) carbohydrates, as *glucose;* (b) primary alteration product of a protein, as *proteose.*

-osis [G.]. Suffix denoting *caused by, state of, disease, intensive.*

Osler's disease (ōs'lĕr) [Sir William Osler, professor of medicine, University of Oxford, England, 1849-1919]. Disease of the blood in which the red cells are increased in number, the spleen becomes enlarged, and the face is a deep red rather than truly cyanotic. SYN: *erythremia; polycythemia vera; Vaquez's disease.*

Osler-Weber-Rendu disease. SEE: *telangiectasia, hereditary hemorrhagic.*

os'mate. A salt of osmic acid.

osmatic (ŏz-măt'ĭk) [G. *osmaein,* to smell]. Having a keen sense of smell.

osmesis (ŏz-mē'sĭs) [G. *osmēsis,* smelling] The sense of smell; act of smelling.

osmesthesia (ŏz-mĕs-thē'zĭ-ă) [G. *osmē,* smell, + *aisthēsis,* sensation]. Olfactory sensibility; power of perceiving and distinguishing odors.

osmic acid (ŏz'mĭk) [G. *osmē,* smell]. 1. Volatile, colorless compound formed by heating osmium in air. 2. Compound of osmium trioxide and water (H_2OsO_4).

osmicate (oz'mĭ-kāt) [G. *osmē,* smell]. To impregnate or stain with osmic acid.

osmics (ŏz'mĭks) [G. *osmē,* smell]. The science of odors.

osmidrosis (ŏz-mĭd-rō'sĭs) [" + *idrōsis,* perspiration]. Condition in which perspiration has a very strong odor. SYN: *bromhidrosis.*

osmium (ŏz'mĭ-ŭm) [G. *osmē,* smell]. SYMB. Os. A metallic element; at. wt. 190.2, at. no. 76.

osmo- [G.]. Combining form. 1. (osme) *odor* or *smell,* and 2. (osmos) *thrust* or *push.* 3. Pertaining to osmosis.

osmodysphoria (ŏz-mō-dĭs-fō'rĭ-ă) [" + *dys,* bad, + *pherein,* to bear]. Abnormal dislike of certain odors.

osmolagnia (ŏz-mō-lăg'nĭ-ă) [G. *osmē,* a smell, + *lagneia,* lust]. Erotic satisfaction derived from odors, usually of the body.

osmolality (os-mo-lal'ĭ-tĭ). Osmotic concentration, the characteristic of a solution determined by the ionic concentration of the dissolved substance per unit of solvent.

osmology (ŏz-mŏl'ō-jĭ) [" + *logos,* study]. 1. The study of odors. SYN: *osphresiology.* 2. [G. *ōsmos,* a thrusting]. Study of osmosis.

osmometer (oz-mŏm'ĕt-ĕr) [G. *osmē,* smell, + *metron,* measure]. 1. Device for measuring acuity of sense of smell. 2. [G. *ōsmos,* a pushing]. A device for measuring osmotic pressure.

osmonosology (ŏz"mō-no-sŏl'ō-jĭ) [G. *osmē,* smell, + *nosos,* disease, + *logos,* study]. Branch of medicine dealing with diseases of the organs of smell.

osmopho'bia. Morbid fear of odors.

osmose (ŏz'mōs) [G. *ōsmos,* a thrusting] 1. To subject to osmosis. 2. To undergo osmosis.

osmosis (ŏz-mō'sĭs) [" + *-ōsis,* intensive]. The passage of solvent through a partition separating solutions of different concentrations.

The solvent, usually water, passes through the membrane from the region of lower concentration of solute to that of a higher concentration of solute thus tending to equalize the concentrations of the two solutions.

The rate of osmosis is dependent primarily upon: (1) difference in osmotic pressures of the solutions on the two sides of a membrane, (2) the permeability of the membrane, (3) electric potential across the membrane and charge upon walls of the pores in it.

RS: *absorption, dialysis, diffusion, diosmosis, hypotonic, isotonic.*

osmotic (ŏz-mŏt′ĭk) [G. *ōsmos*, a thrusting]. Pertaining to osmosis.

o. pressure. 1. The pressure which develops when two solutions of different concentrations are separated by a semipermeable membrane. 2. The pressure which would be developed if a solution were enclosed in a membrane impermeable to all solutes present and surrounded by pure solvent.

Osmotic pressure varies with concentration of the solution and with temperature increasing with an increase of each. Animal cells have an osmotic pressure approximately equal to that of the circulating fluid, the blood. Solutions exerting this osmotic pressure are said to be *isotonic* or *isosmotic.* Stronger solutions which cause cells to shrink are *hypertonic,* weaker solutions which cause cells to swell are *hypotonic.*

osphresiolagnia (ŏs-frē″zĭ-ō-lag′nĭ-ă) [G. *osphrēsis*, smell, + *lagneia*, lust]. Excitement of an erotic nature aroused by odors.

osphresiology (ŏs-frē-zĭ-ŏl′ō-jĭ) [" + *logos*, study]. Science of odors and the sense of smell. Syn: *osmology.*

osphresiometer (ŏs-frē-zĭ-ŏm′ĕt-ĕr) [" + *metron*, measure]. Apparatus for measuring the acuteness of the sense of smell. Syn: *osmometer, 1.*

osphresis (ŏs-frē′sĭs) [G. *osphrēsis*, smell]. The sense of smell. Syn: *olfaction.*

osphretic (ŏs-fret′ĭk) [G. *osphrēsis*, smell]. Concerning the sense of smell. Syn: *olfactory.*

osphus (os′fŭs) [G. *osphys*, loin]. Loin.

osphyalgia (ŏs-fĭ-al′jĭ-ă) [" + *algos*, pain]. Pain of the loins or hips. See: *lumbago, sciatica.*

osphyitis (ŏs-fĭ-ī′tĭs) [" + *-itis*, inflammation]. Inflammation in the lumbar region.

osphyomyelitis (ŏs″fĭ-ō-mĭ-ĕl-ī′tĭs) [" + *myelos*, marrow, + *-itis*, inflammation]. Inflamed condition of the lumbar region of the spinal cord.

os pubis (ŏs pū′bĭs) [L. *os*, bone, + *pubis*, pubes]. A bone that in adult life unites the innominate or hip bone with the ilium and ischium to form the pelvis. Irregular shape, divided into a horizontal, ascending, and descending ramus. The outer extremity constitutes approximately one-fifth of the acetabulum. The inner unites in middle line with corresponding part of the bone of opp. side, forming the symphysis pubis.

ossa (ŏs′ă) (sing. *os*). Bones.

ossein (ŏs′ē-ĭn) [L. *ossa*, bones]. The organic substance of bones. Syn: *ostein.*

osseofibrous (os″e-o-fi′brus). Composed of bone and fibrous tissue.

osseous (ŏs′ē-ŭs) [L. *osseus*, bony]. Bone-like; concerning bones. Syn: *bony.*

ossicle (ŏs′ĭ-kl) [L. *ossiculum*, little bone]. Any small bone, as one of the three bones of the ear, the *malleus, incus,* or *stapes.*

ossicula (ŏs-ĭk′ū-lă) [L. pl.]. Little bones.

ossiculectomy (ŏs″ĭk-ū-lĕk′tō-mĭ) [L. *ossiculum*, little bone, + G. *ektomē*, excision]. Excision of an ossicle, especially one of the ear.

ossiculotomy (ŏs″ĭk-ū-lŏt′ō-mĭ) [" + G. *tomē*, incision]. Surgical incision of one or more of the ossicles of the ear.

ossiculum (ŏs-ĭk′ū-lŭm) [L.]. Tiny bone, esp. one of the three in the middle ear.

ossiferous (ŏs-if′ĕr-ŭs) [L. *os*, bone, + *ferre*, to bear]. Composed of, or forming bone or bony tissue.

ossific (ŏs-ĭf′ĭk) [" + *facere*, to make]. Producing or becoming bone.

ossification (ŏs″ĭ-fĭ-kā′shŭn) [" + *facere*, to make]. 1. Formation of bone substance. 2. Conversion into bone. See: *center, epiotic, centrosclerosis.*

o., endochondral. Syn: *intracartilaginous o.* The formation of bone in cartilage as in formation of long bones. It involves (1) the destruction and removal of cartilage and (2) the formation of osseous tissue in space occupied by the cartilage.

o., intramembranous. The formation of bone in or underneath a fibrous membrane, such as occurs in formation of the cranial bones.

o., pathologic. Formation of bone in abnormal sites or abnormal development of bone.

ossiflu′ence. Osteolysis or softening of bone.

ossiform. Resembling bone.

ossify (ŏs′ĭ-fī) [" + *facere*, to make]. To turn into bone.

ostalgia (ŏs-tăl′jĭ-ă) [G. *osteon*, bone, + *algos*, pain]. Pain in a bone. Syn: *osteodynia.*

os′teal. Pert. to bone.

ostealleosis (ŏs″tē-ăl″lē-ō′sĭs). A change in the substance of bone.

osteanabrosis (ŏs″tē-ăn-ă-brō′sĭs) [" + *anabrōsis*, eating up]. Wasting away of bone.

osteanagenesis (ŏs″tē-ăn-ă-jĕn′ĕ-sĭs) [" + *anagenesis*, reproduction]. Regeneration or re-formation of bone.

ostearthrotomy (ŏs″tē-ăr-thrŏt′ō-mĭ) [" + " + *tomē*, incision]. Surgical excision of the articular end of a bone. Syn: *osteoarthrotomy.*

ostectomy, osteectomy (ŏs-tek′tō-mĭ, -tē-ĕk′tō-mĭ) [" + *ektomē*, excision]. Surgical excision of a bone or a portion of one.

osteectopia (ŏs″tē-ĕk-tō′pĭ-ă) [" + *ek*, out, + *topos*, place]. Displacement of a bone.

osteitis (ŏs-tē-ī′tĭs) [" + *-itis*, inflammation]. Inflammation of a bone.

o., condensing. O. in which the marrow cavity becomes filled with osseous tissue. Bone becomes denser and heavier.

o. deformans. Chronic form with thickening and hypertrophy of the long bones and deformity of the flat bones.

Etiol: Unknown.

Sym: Slow and insidious in onset. Pain in lower limbs, esp. the tibia. Frequent fractures. Waddling gait. Skull becomes enlarged, so that the face appears small and triangular in shape with the head pushed forward. Stature shortens.

Treatment: Constitutional and palliative. There is no known specific therapy. Syn: *Paget's disease.*

o. fibrosa cystica. Syn: *von Recklinghausen's disease, hyperparathyroidism.* A condition resulting from overactivity of the parathyroid glands with resulting disturbances in calcium and phosphorus metabolism. Characterized by decalcification and softening of bone, nephrolithiasis, and elevation of blood calcium and lowering of blood phosphorus. Cysts often multiple, and tumors may develop.

o., *gummatous.* Chronic o. associated with syphilis and characterized by the formation of gummas.

o., *rarefying.* SYN: *osteoporosis.* Form in which the bone tissue becomes cancellated.

o., *sclerosing.* SEE: *o., condensing.*

ostembryon (ŏs-tĕm′brĭ-ŏn). A fetus which has become ossified.

ostemia (ŏs-tē′mĭ-ă) [G. *osteon,* bone, + *aima,* blood]. Congestion of blood in a bone.

ostempyesis (ŏs-tĕm-pī-ē′sĭs) [" + *empyēsis,* suppuration]. Purulent inflammation within a bone.

osteo- [G.]. Combining form meaning *bone.*

osteoaneurysm (ŏs″tē-ō-an′ū-rĭzm) [G. *osteon,* bone, + *aneurysma,* a widening]. Aneurysm, or dilatation of a blood vessel filled with clotted blood, occurring within a bone.

osteoarthritis (ŏs″tē-ō-ăr-thrī′tĭs) [G. *osteon,* bone, + *arthron,* joint, + *-itis,* inflammation]. SYN: *degenerative joint disease, hypertrophic arthritis.* A chronic disease involving the joints, esp. those bearing weight. Characterized by destruction of articular cartilage, overgrowth of bone with lipping and spur formation, and impaired function.

osteoarthropathy (ŏs″tē-ō-ar-thrŏp′ă-thĭ) [G. *osteos,* bone, + *arthron,* joint, + *pathos,* disease]. Any disease involving the joints.

o., *hypertrophic pulmonary.* An affection characterized by enlargement of distal phalanges of fingers and toes and a thickening of their distal ends, accompanied by a peculiar longitudinal curving of nails. Wrist and interphalangeal joints may become enlarged as well as distal ends of tibia and fibula and the jaw.

ETIOL: Found in pulmonary tuberculosis, chronic bronchitis, bronchiectasis, congenital heart disease, and chronic cardiac affections.

osteoarthrotomy (ŏs″tē-ō-ar-throt′ō-mĭ) [" + " + *tomē,* incision]. Excision of joint end of a bone. SYN: *ostearthrotomy.*

osteoblast (ŏs-tē-ō-blăst) [G. *osteon,* bone, + *blastos,* germ]. A cell of mesodermal origin which is concerned with the formation of bone.

osteocampsia (ŏs″tē-ō-kămp′sĭ-ă) [" + *kampein,* to bend]. Curvature of a bone, as in osteomalacia.

osteocarcinoma (ŏs″tē-ō-kăr-sĭn-ō′mă) [" + *karkinos,* crab, cancer, + *-ōma,* tumor]. 1. Osteoma and carcinoma combined. 2. Carcinoma of a bone.

osteocephaloma (ŏs″tē-ō-sĕf-ă-lō′mă) [" + *kephalē,* head, + *-ōma,* tumor]. Encephaloma, a malignant neoplasm of brainlike texture in a bone.

osteochondritis (ŏs″tē-ō-kŏn-drī′tĭs) [" + *chondros,* cartilage, + *-ītis,* inflammation]. Inflammation of bone and cartilage.

o. *deformans juvenile.* Chronic inflammation of head of femur in childhood resulting in atrophy and shortening of neck of femur and wide, flat head.

o. *dissecans.* Condition affecting a joint in which a fragment of cartilage and its underlying bone becomes detached from articular surface. Occurs commonly in the knee joint.

osteochondroma (ŏs″tē-ō-kŏn-drō′mă) [" + " + *-ōma,* tumor]. Tumor composed of both cartilaginous and bony substance.

osteoclasia, osteoclasis (ŏs″tē-ō-klā′zĭ-ă, -ŏk′lă-sĭs) [G. *osteon,* bone, + *klasis,* a breaking]. 1. Fracture of a bone, surgically, to remedy a deformity. 2. Bony tissue destruction.

osteoclast (ŏs′tē-ō-klăst) [" + *klan,* to break]. 1. Device for fracturing bones for therapeutic purposes. 2. Giant, multinuclear cell found in depressions on the surface of a bone causing entire resorption of bone substance.

These depressions are called *Howship's lacunae.* The bone appears eroded or as if gnawed.

osteocopic (ŏs″tē-ō-kŏp′ĭk) [" + *kopos,* pain]. Concerning pain in the bone.

osteocranium (ŏs″tē-ō-krā′nĭ-ŭm) [G. *osteon,* bone, + *kranion,* skull]. The portion of the cranium formed of membrane bones in contrast to that formed of cartilage (chondrocranium).

osteocystoma (ŏs″tē-ō-sĭs-tō′mă) [" + *kystis,* a bladder, + *-ōma,* tumor]. Cystic tumor of a bone.

osteodermia (ŏs″tē-ō-dĕr′mĭ-ă) [G. *osteon,* bone, + *derma,* skin]. The formation of bony structure in the skin.

osteodynia (ŏs″tē-ō-din′ĭ-ă) [G. *osteon,* bone, + *odynē,* pain]. Persistent pain in a bone. SYN: *ostealgia.*

osteodystrophia (ŏs″tē-ō-dĭs-trō′fĭ-ă) [" + *dys,* ill, + *trophē,* nourishment]. Defective bone development.

osteoepiphysis (ŏs″tē-ō-ĕp-ĭf′ĭs-ĭs) [" + *epi,* upon, + *physis,* growth]. A small piece of bone which later becomes attached to the larger one.

osteofibroma (ŏs″tē-ō-fī-brō′mă) [" + L. *fibra,* fiber, + G. *-ōma,* tumor]. Tumor of bony and fibrous tissues. SYN: *fibroosteoma.*

osteogen (ŏs′tē-ō-jĕn) [" + *gennan,* to produce]. Substance of the inner periosteal layer from which bone is formed.

osteogenesis, osteogeny (ŏs″tē-ō-jĕn′ē-sĭs, -ŏj′ē-nĭ) [" + *gennan,* to produce]. Formation and development of bone taking place in connective tissue or in cartilage. Ossification.

o. *imperfecta.* A congenital bone disease causing the bones to fracture easily.

osteogen′ic. Pertaining to osteogenesis.

osteography (ŏs-tē-og′raf-ĭ) [G. *osteon,* bone, + *graphein,* to write]. Descriptive treatise on the bones.

osteohalisteresis (ŏs″tē-ō-hăl-ĭs-tĕr-ē′sĭs) [" + *als,* salt, + *sterein,* to deprive]. Deficiency of the mineral constituents in bone causing softening.

osteoid (ŏs′tē-oyd) [" + *eidos,* resemblance]. Resembling bone.

osteology (ŏs-tē-ol′ō′jĭ) [" + *logos,* study]. The science of structure and function of bones.

osteolysis (ŏs-tē-ol′ĭs-ĭs) [" + *lysis,* dissolution]. Softening and destruction of bone, as in caries.

osteoma (ŏs-tē-ō′mă) (pl. *osteomata*) [" + *-ōma,* tumor]. A bony tumor; a hard tumor of bonelike structure developing on a bone, and sometimes on other structures.

o., *cancellous.* One that is soft and spongy. Its thin and delicate trabeculae enclose large medullary spaces similar to cancellous bone.

o., cavalryman's. Bony outgrowth of femur at the insertion of the adductor femoris longus.

o. dentale. A hard, bony outgrowth from the jawbone.

o. medullare. An osteoma containing medullary spaces.

o., osteoid. A benign tumor of bone composed of sheets of osteoid tissue partially calcified and ossified.

o. spongiosum. Soft, spongy tumor in bone.

osteomalacia (ŏs″tē-ō-măl-ā′sĭ-ă) [" + *malakia,* softening]. Softening of the bones. SYN: *malacosteon, mollities ossium.*

A disease marked by increasing softness of the bones, so that they become flexible and brittle and cause deformities. It is attended with rheumatic pains. The limbs, spine, thorax, and pelvis esp. are affected; anemia and signs of deficiency disease present; the patient becomes weak, and finally dies from exhaustion. It occurs chiefly in adults.

ETIOL: Deficiency or loss of calcium salts; vitamin D deficiency.

osteomalacic (ŏs″tē-ō-măl-ā′sĭk) [G. *osteon,* bone, + *malakia,* softening]. Concerning or characterized by softening of the bone.

osteomatoid (ŏs-tē-ō′mă-toyd) [" + *-ōma,* tumor, + *eidos,* resemblance]. Resembling a tumor of bone tissue.

osteomere (os′te-o-mēr) [" + *meros,* part]. One in a series of like bony structures, as vertebrae.

osteometry (ŏs-tē-om′et-rĭ) [" + *metron.* measure]. The study of the measurement of bones.

osteomyelitis (ŏs″tē-ō-mī-ĕl-ī′tĭs) [G. *osteon,* bone, + *myelos,* marrow, + *-ītis,* inflammation]. Inflammation of bone marrow, or of the bone and marrow.

SYM: Pain over affected part, fever, sweats, leukocytosis, overlying muscles usually rigid, skin inflamed, pain on pressure over affected part. Suppuration may occur.

TREATMENT: Prompt and adequate doses of antibiotics. Sedation for pain and anxiety. Aspiration of abscess. Immobilization of affected extremity. Surgery if abscess persists.

osteoncus (ŏs-tē-on′kŭs) [" + *ogkos,* tumor]. A bone tumor. SYN: *exostosis, osteoma.*

osteonecrosis (ŏs″tē-ō-nē-krō′sĭs) [G. *osteon,* bone, + *nekrōsis,* death]. Death of bone tissue in mass.

osteoneuralgia (ŏs″tē-ō-nū-ral′jĭ-ă) [" + *neuron,* nerve, + *algos,* pain]. Pain of a bone.

osteopath (os′tē-ō-păth) [" + *pathos,* disease]. A practitioner of osteopathy, *q.v.*

osteopathic (ŏs″tē-ō-păth′ĭk) [" + *pathos,* disease]. Concerning therapeutic bone manipulation.

osteopathology (os-tē-ō-path-ol′ō-jĭ) [G. *osteon,* bone, + *pathos,* disease, + *logos,* study]. Any bone disease.

osteopathy (ŏs-tē-op′ăth-ĭ) [" + *pathos,* disease]. 1. Any bone disease.

2. "A school of medicine based upon the theory that the body is a vital mechanical organism whose structural and functional integrity are coördinate and that the perversion of either is disease, while its therapeutic procedure is chiefly manipulative correction, its name indicating the fact that the bony framework of the body largely determines the structural relation of its tissues." *Committee on Osteopathic Terminology.*

osteopecilia (ŏs″tē-ō-pē-sĭl′ĭ-ă) [G. *osteon,* bone, + *poikilia,* spottedness]. Osteopetrosis, *q.v.*

osteopedion (ŏs″tē-ō-pe′dĭ-ŏn) [" + *paidion,* child]. A calcified or hardened fetus. SYN: *lithopedion, ostembryon.*

osteoperiosteal (ŏs″tē-ō-per-ĭ-os′tē-ăl) [" + *peri,* around, + *osteon,* bone]. Concerning bone and its periosteum, the protective membrane.

osteoperiostitis (ŏs″tē-ō-per-ĭ-ŏs-tī′tĭs) [" + " + " + *-ītis,* inflammation]. Combined inflammation of a bone and its protective membrane, the periosteum.

osteopetrosis (ŏs″tē-ō-pĕt-rō′sĭs) [G. *osteon,* bone, + L. *petra,* stone, + G. *-osis,* disease]. SYN: *marble bones. Albers-Schönberg disease, osteopoikilosis, osteosclerosis fragilis generalisata.* Excessive calcification of bones causing spontaneous fractures and marblelike appearance.

osteophage (os′tē-ō-fāj) [G. *osteon,* bone, + *phagein,* to eat]. Large multinuclear cell which causes absorption of bone. SYN: *osteoclast, 2.*

osteophagia (os″te-o-fa′jĭ-ă) [" + *phagein,* to eat]. Bone consumption due to a craving for phosphorus.

osteophlebitis (ŏs″tē-ō-flē-bī′tĭs) [" + *phleps, phleb-,* vein, + *-ītis,* inflammation]. Inflammation of veins of a bone.

osteophone (ŏs′tē-ō-fōn) [" + *phōnē,* voice]. Device used by the deaf for conducting sound through facial bones.

osteophyma (ŏs″tē-ō-fī′mă) [" + *phyma,* growth]. A swelling or growth of bone.

osteophyte (ŏs′tē-ō-fīt) [" + *phyton,* plant]. A bony excrescence or outgrowth, usually branched in shape.

osteoplastic (ŏs″tē-ō-plăs′tĭk) [" + *plastikos,* formed]. 1. Pert. to bone repair. 2. Concerning bone formation.

osteoplasty (ŏs″tē-ō-plăs″tĭ) [G. *osteon,* bone, + *plassein,* to form]. Plastic repair of the bones.

osteopoikilosis (ŏs″tē-ō-poy-kĭ-lō′sĭs) [" + *poikilos,* spotted]. Disease of bones marked by excessive calcification in spots, causing spontaneous fractures and spotted marble appearance. SYN: *osteosclerosis fragilis generalisata, q.v.*

osteoporosis (ŏs″tē-ō-por-ō′sĭs) [" + *poros,* a passage]. Increased porosity of bone.

SYM: Softening of bone, widening of haversian canals, absorption of calcareous matter. SEE: *osteomalacia.*

o., parachitic. O. with tendency to develop into rickets. Congenital.

osteoporotic (ŏs″tē-ō-pō-rot′ĭk) [" + *poros,* passage]. Concerning enlarged bone spaces.

osteopsathyrosis (ŏs″tē-op-sath″ĭ-rō′sĭs) [" + *psathyros,* fragile]. Fragility or brittleness of bones. Osteogenesis imperfecta, *q.v.*

Hereditary condition of unknown etiology, in which the long bones seem normal in appearance and chemical composition, but are extremely brittle.

SYM: Breaks may occur upon bathing infant or turning him over, following minor injuries, chewing, bending the knee, etc. Breaks almost painless with slight swelling and only evidence is unwillingness of the child to use his injured limb.

PROG: Condition tends to improve after puberty but may return in later life.

TREATMENT: Good hygiene, nourishing diet, supports to prevent breaks. Bones knit quickly with normal amount of callus. SYN: *fragilitas ossium, osteogenesis imperfecta.*

osteoradionecrosis (ŏs″tē-ō-rā-dĭ-ō-nē-krō′sĭs). Death of bone following irradiation.

osteorrhagia (ŏs″tē-ō-rā′jĭ-ă) [" + *rēgnunai,* to burst forth]. Hemorrhagic flow of blood from a bone.

osteorrhaphy (ŏs-tē-or′ăf-ĭ) [" + *raphē,* a sewing]. Suture of bone or the wiring of bone fragments.

osteosarcoma (ŏs″tē-ō-sar-kō′mă) [G. *osteon,* bone, + *sarx, sark-,* flesh, + *-ōma,* tumor]. A malignant sarcoma of the bone. SYN: *myelosarcoma.*

osteosarcomatous (ŏs″tē-ō-sar-kō′măt-ŭs) [" + " + *-ōma,* tumor]. Concerning or like an osteosarcoma.

osteosclerosis (ŏs″tē-ō-sklē-rō′sĭs) [" + *sklēros,* hard, + *-ōsis,* intensive]. Hardening of bone with increased heaviness.

o. fragilis generalisata. Abnormal calcification of the bones, causing spontaneous fractures and spotted marble-like appearance in a roentgenogram. SYN: *Albers-Schönberg disease; marble bones; osteitis, condensing; osteopetrosis; osteopoikilosis.*

osteoscope (ŏs′tē-ō-skōp) [" + *skopein,* to examine]. Appliance used to test x-ray machines by observing certain bones of the forearm which are considered as a standard.

osteoseptum (ŏs″tē-ō-sĕp′tŭm) [" + L. *saeptum,* a dividing]. The bony area of the nasal septum.

osteosis (ŏs″tē-ō′sĭs) [G. *osteon,* bone, + *-ōsis,* condition]. Formation of bony tissue. SYN: *osteogenesis.*

o. cutis. Diffuse thickening of skin and subcutaneous tissue. Rare.

osteospongioma (ŏs″tē-ō-spon-jĭ-ō′mă) [" + *spoggos,* sponge, + *-ōma,* tumor]. A spongy neoplasm of bone. SYN: *osteoma spongiosum.*

osteosteatoma (ŏs″tē-ō-stē-ăt-ō′mă) [" + *stear, steat-,* fat, + *-ōma,* tumor]. A fatty tumor with bony elements.

osteostixis (ŏs″tē-ō-stiks′ĭs) [" + *stixis,* a puncture]. Therapeutic puncture of a bone.

osteosuture (ŏs″tē-ō-sūt′chūr) [" + L. *sutura,* a stitch]. Suture or wiring of bone fragments. SYN: *osteorrhaphy.*

osteosynovitis (ŏs″tē-ō-sin-ō-vī′tĭs) [" + *syn,* with, + *ōon,* egg, + *-ītis,* inflammation]. Inflammation of a synovial membrane and the surrounding bones.

osteosynthesis (ŏs″tē-ō-sĭn′the-sĭs) [" + *synthēsis,* a joining]. Surgical fastening of the ends of a fractured bone mechanically.

osteotabes (ŏs″tē-ō-tā′bēz) [G. *osteon,* bone, + *tabes,* a wasting]. Atrophy of the bone in infants, beginning with wasting of the marrow and gradually the rest of the bone.

osteotelangiectasia (ŏs″tē-ō-tĕl-ăn″jĭ-ĕk-tā′zĭ-ă) [" + *telos,* end, + *aggeion,* vessel, + *ektasis,* a stretching]. Sarcomatous tumor of the bone containing dilated blood vessels.

osteothrombosis (ŏs″tē-ō-thrŏm-bō′sĭs) [" + *thrombōsis,* a clotting]. Clot formation in the veins of a bone.

osteotome (ŏs′tē-ō-tōm) [" + *tomē,* a cutting]. A chisel bevelled on both sides for cutting through bones.

osteotomy (ŏs-tē-ot′ō-mĭ) [" + *tomē,* incision]. The operation for cutting through a bone.

o., cuneiform. The excision of a wedge of a bone.

o., linear. Lengthwise division of a bone.

o., Macewen's. Supracondylar section of the femur for correction of knock-knee.

o., subtrochanteric. Gant's operation, division of shaft of femur below lesser trochanter to correct ankylosis of hip joint.

o., transtrochanteric. Section of the femur through the lesser trochanter for deformity about the hip joint.

osteotrite (ŏs′tē-ō-trīt) [" + *tribein,* to crush]. Instrument used to scrape away diseased bone.

osteotrophy (ŏs-tē-ot′ro-fĭ). Bone nutrition.

osthexia (ŏs-thĕks′ĭ-ă) [G. *osteon,* bone, + *exis,* condition]. Excessive ossification, esp. in abnormal places.

ostial (os′tĭ-ăl) [L. *ostium,* a little opening]. Concerning an orifice.

ostitis (ŏs-tī′tĭs) [G. *osteon,* bone, + *-ītis,* inflammation]. Inflammation of a bone. SYN: *osteitis, q.v.*

ostium (ŏs′tĭ-ŭm) (pl. *ostia*) [L. a small opening]. [NA]. Any small opening.

o. abdominale tubae uterinae. [NA]. Fimbriated end of fallopian tube. SYN: *o. abdominale.*

o. arteriosum. BNA. Arterial orifice, of ventricle of the heart into the aorta, or pulmonary artery.

o. internum. Uterine end of a fallopian tube. SYN: *o. uterinum tubae uterinae.*

o. pharyngeum. Pharyngeal opening of the auditory (Eustachian) tube.

o. tympanicum. Tympanic opening of the auditory (Eustachian) tube.

o. vaginae. Ext. opening of the vagina.

ostraco, ostrac- [G.]. Combining form meaning *hard shell.*

ostreotoxismus (ŏs″trē-ō-tŏks-ĭz′mŭs) [G. *ostreon,* oyster, + *toxikon,* poison]. Poisoning from eating diseased oysters.

O.T. Abbr. for (1) *old term* in contrast to BNA or NA term, (2) old tuberculin, (3) occupational therapy.

otacoustic (ō″tă-koos′tĭk) [G. *ōtakoustein,* to listen]. 1. Aiding or concerning the hearing. 2. Device to aid hearing; an ear trumpet.

otalgia (ō-tăl′jĭ-ă) [G. *ous, ōt-,* ear, + *algos,* pain]. Pain of the ear. SYN: *earache; otodynia; otoneuralgia.*

TREATMENT: *Local:* Heat in the form of compresses or hot water bottle, warm glycerin dropped in ear. Incision of drum if bulging is present. *General:* Active elimination, sedatives.

otantritis (ō″tăn-trī′tĭs). Inflammation of the mastoid antrum.

otectomy (ō-tĕk′tō-mĭ) [" + *ektomē,* excision]. Surgical excision of the contents of the middle ear.

othelcosis (ō-thĕl-kō′sĭs) [" + *elkōsis,* ulceration]. Ulceration or suppuration of the ear.

othematoma (ō″them-ă-tō′mă) [" + *aima,* blood, + *-ōma,* tumor]. Effusion of blood between perichondrium and cartilage of pinna.

Common in fighters or wrestlers. SEE: *cauliflower ear.* SYN: *hematoma auris.*

othemorrhea (o-them″o-re′ă) [" + *haima,* blood, + *rhoia,* flow]. Bleeding from the ear.

othygroma (ō-thī-grō′mă) [G. *ous, ōt-,* ear, + *ygros,* moist, + *-ōma,* tumor]. Edema of ear lobe.

otic (ō′tĭk) [G. *ous, ōt-,* ear]. Concerning the ear.

oticodinia (ō″tĭk-ō-dĭn′ĭ-ă) [" + *dinē,* a whirl]. Vertigo due to ear disease.

otitic (ō-tĭʹtĭk) [" + *-ītis,* inflammation]. Concerning inflammation of the ear.

otitis (ō-tīʹtĭs) [G. *ous, ōt-,* ear, + *-ītis,* inflammation]. Inflamed condition of the ear.

It is differentiated as *externa, media,* and *interna,* depending upon the portion of the ear which is inflamed.

o., aero-. O. resulting from pressure changes when auditory tubes are obstructed. Occurs commonly in aviators or divers.

o., furuncular. Furuncle formation in ext. meatus.

o. labyrinthica. Inflammation of the labyrinth.

o. mastoidea. Inflamed condition of the middle ear which involves the mastoid spaces.

o. mycotica. Fungus inflammation.

o. parasitica. Inflammation caused by a parasite.

o. sclerotica. Inflammation of inner ear accompanied by hardening of the aural structures.

oto-, ot- [G.]. Combining form meaning *ear.*

otoantritis (ō″tō-ăn-trīʹtĭs) [G. *ous, ōt-,* ear, + *antron,* cavity, + *-ītis,* inflammation]. Inflamed condition of mastoid antrum and the tympanic attic.

otoblennorrhea (ō″to-blĕn-or-rēʹă) [" + *blenna,* mucus, + *roia,* flow]. Mucous discharge from ear.

otocatarrh (ō″tō-kă-tarʹ) [" + *katarrein,* to flow down]. Catarrhal discharge of the ear.

otocleisis (ō-tō-klīʹsĭs) [" + *kleisis,* a closure]. 1. Occlusion of auditory canal. 2. Occlusion of auditory tubes.

otoconium (ō″tō-kōʹnĭ-ŭm) (pl. *otoconia*) [G. *ous, ōt-,* ear, + *konis,* dust]. SYN: *otoliths, ear dust.* Minute particles composed chiefly of calcium carbonate found in otolithic membrane on surface of maculae of inner ear. SYN: *otolith.*

otocyst (ōʹtō-sĭst) [" + *kystis,* bladder]. Primordial chamber from which arises the membranous labyrinth. SYN: *auditory vesicle.*

otodynia (ō″tō-dinʹĭ-ă) [" + *odynē,* pain]. Pain in the ear. SYN: *otalgia; otoneuralgia.*

otogenic, otogenous. Having its origin in the ear.

otolaryngolʹogist. A specialist in otolaryngology.

otolaryngology. The division of medical science which includes otology, rhinology, and laryngology.

otolith (oʹto-lith) [G. *ous, ōt-,* ear, + *lithos,* stone]. SEE: *otoconium.*

otological (ō″tō-lŏjʹĭ-kl) [" + *logos,* study]. Rel. to study of diseases of the ear.

otologist (ō-tŏl-ō-jĭst) [" + *logos,* study]. One versed in diseases of the ear. SYN: *aurist.*

otology (ō-tolʹō-jĭ) [" + *logos,* study]. The science of the ear, its function, and diseases.

otomyasthenia (ō″tō-mī-ăs-thēʹnĭ-ă) [" + *mys, my-,* muscle, + *astheneia,* weakness]. 1. Weakened condition of the ear muscles. 2. Defective hearing caused by paresis of the tensor tympani and stapedius muscles.

otomyces (ō″tō-mīʹsēz) [" + *mykēs,* fungus]. Any fungus infesting the ear.

otomycosis (ō″tō-mī-kōʹsĭs) [" + " + *-ōsis,* condition]. Fungus infection of ext. auditory meatus of the ear. SYN: *otitis mycotica; mycomyringitis; myringomycosis.*

otoncus (ō-tŏngʹkŭs) [" + *ogkos,* tumor]. An aural tumor.

otonecrectomy, otonecronectomy (ō″tō-nĕk-rĕkʹtō-mĭ, -rō-nĕkʹtō-mĭ) [G. *ous, ōt-,* ear, + *nekros,* dead, + *ektomē,* excision]. Excision of necrosed areas from the ear.

otoneuralgia (ō″tō-nū-rălʹjĭ-ă) [" + *neuron,* sinew, + *algos,* pain]. Pain in the ear. SYN: *otalgia; otodynia.*

otoneurasthenia (ō″tō-nū-răs-thēʹnĭ-ă) [" + " + *astheneia,* weakness]. Neurasthenia caused by ear disease.

otoneurology (ō″tō-nū-rŏlʹō-jĭ) [" + " + *logos,* study]. Study of ear conditions in conjunction with neural complications. SYN: *neurotology.*

otopathy (o-topʹăth-ĭ) [" + *pathos,* disease]. Any diseased condition of the ear.

otopharyngeal (ō″tō-far-ĭnʹjē-ăl) [" + *pharygx,* pharynx]. Concerning the ear and pharynx.

o. tube. Passage bet. tympanic cavity and the pharynx. SYN: *eustachian tube.*

otophone (oʹtō-fōn) [G. *ous, ōt-,* ear, + *phōnē,* voice]. Device for assisting deaf to hear.

otopiesis (ō″tō-pī-ēʹsĭs) [" + *piesis,* a pressing]. 1. Sinking in or depression of the membrana tympani. 2. Pressure on the labyrinth causing deafness.

otoplasty (ōʹtō-plăs-tĭ) [" + *plassein,* to form]. Plastic surgery of the ear to correct defects.

otopolypus (ō″tō-polʹĭp-ŭs) [" + *polus,* many, + *pous,* foot]. Smooth growth occurring in the ear.

otopyorrhea (ō″tō-pī-ō-reʹă) [" + *pyon,* pus, + *roia,* a flow]. Purulent ear discharge.

otopyosis (ō″tō-pī-ōʹsĭs) [" + " + *-ōsis,* infection]. Ear disease marked by discharge of pus.

otorhinolaryngology (ō″tō-rī-nō-lăr-ĭn-gŏlʹō-jĭ) [" + *ris, rin-,* nose, + *larygx,* larynx, + *logos,* study]. The science of ear, nose, and larynx and their functions and diseases.

otorhinology (ō″tō-rī-nŏlʹō-jĭ) [" + " + *logos,* study]. Branch of medicine dealing with ear and nose diseases.

otorrhagia (ō-tō-răʹjĭ-ă) [G. *ous, ōt-,* ear, + *rēgnunai,* to flow]. Discharge of blood from ear.

otorrhea (ō-tō-rēʹă) [" + *roia,* flow]. Inflammation of ear with purulent discharge. SEE: *otitis.*

otosalpinx (ō″tō-sălʹpĭnks) [" + *salpigx,* tube]. Passage connecting pharynx and tympanic cavity. SYN: *eustachian tube, otopharyngeal tube.*

otoscleronectomy (ō″tō-sklē-rō-nĕk (ɪɯ-oʇ, [" + *sklēros,* hard, + *ektomē,* excision]. Surgical excision of sclerosed and ankylosed ear ossicles.

otosclerosis (ō″tō-sklē-rōʹsĭs) [G. *ous, ōt-,* ear, + *sklerosis,* a hardening]. Condition characterized by chronic progressive deafness esp. for low tones. Due to the formation of spongy bone, esp. around the oval window with resulting ankylosis of stapes. In late stages atrophy of the organ of Corti may occur. More common in females. May be made worse by pregnancy.

ETIOL: Unknown. In some cases, condition is familial.

otoscope ((ōʹtō-skōp) [" + *skopein,* to examine]. Device for examination of the ear.

otosis (ō-tōʹsĭs) [" + *-ōsis,* intensive]. Mishearing of spoken sounds.

otosteal (ō-tos′tē-ăl) [G. *ous, ōt-*, ear, + *osteon*, bone]. Concerning the bones or ossicles of the ear.

ototomy (ō-tŏt′ō-mĭ) [" + *tomē*, incision]. Incision into or dissection of the ear.

O. U., o. u. Abbr. for L. *oculus uterque*, for each eye.

ouabain (wăh-băh′ĭn). A glucoside prepared from *Strophanthus gratus*. USP. Syn. for *G. strophanthin*.

USES: Same as for digitalis.

Oudin current (oo-dan′) [Paul Oudin, French electrotherapeutist and roentgenologist, 1851-1923]. A high frequency oscillating current of higher voltage than the current used ordinarily, employed in treatment.

O. resonator. A coil of wire with an adjustable number of turns, designed to be connected to a source of high frequency current, such as a spark gap and induction coil, for the purpose of applying a convective discharge of high voltage current to a patient.

oulitis (oo-lī′tĭs) [G. *oulon*, gum, + *ĭtis*, inflammation]. Ulitis, *q.v.*

oulorrhagia (oo-lō-rā′jĭ-ă) [" + *rēgnunai*, to burst forth]. Hemorrhage from the gums. SYN: *ulorrhagia.*

ounce (ouns) [L. *uncia*, a twelfth]. A measure of weight. ABBR: *oz.*

In *apothecaries'* or *troy* weight. 1/12 lb. [480 gr. (31.103 Gm.)]. Symb. ℥.

In *avoirdupois* measure, 1/16 lb. [437.5 gr. (28.349 Gm.)].

o., fluid. Apothecaries' measure for liquid medicines, 8 fluid drams [1/16 pint (29.6 cc.)].

outflow. In neurology, the passage of impulses outwardly from the central nervous system.

o., craniosacral. Impulses passing through parasympathetic nerves.

o., thoracolumbar. Impulses passing through sympathetic nerves.

outlet. The inferior aperture of the true pelvis.

out′patient. One receiving treatment at a hospital, clinic, or dispensary but not occupying a bed.

ova (ō′vă) (pl. of *ovum*) [L., from G. *ōon*, egg]. Reproductive cells of the female. 2. Eggs. SEE: *ovary, ovum.*

oval (ō′văl) [L. *ovum*, egg]. 1. Like or concerning an ovum, the reproductive cell of the female. 2. Shaped like an egg.

o. window. Oval-shaped aperture in the middle ear into which fits the base of the stapes.

ovalbumin (ō-văl-bū′mĭn) [" + *albumen*, white of egg]. Albumin present in egg white.

ovalocyte (o′văl-ō-sīt) [" + G. *kytos*, cell]. Elliptical red blood corpuscle.

ovalocytosis (ō-văl″ō-sī-tō′sĭs) [" + " + *-ōsis*, intensive]. Elliptical red blood corpuscles in the blood.

ovaralgia, ovarialgia (o-var-al′jĭ-ă, -ĭ-al′-jĭ-ă) [L. *ovarium*, ovary, + G. *algos*, pain]. Ovarian pain. SYN: *oothecalgia.*

ovarian (ō-vā′rĭ-ăn) [L. *ovarium*, ovary]. Concerning or resembling the ovary.

o. cyst. A sac containing fluid which develops in the ovary proper.

It consists of 1 or more chambers containing fluid. These *loculi*, or chambers, may contain an enormous amt. of fluid. Not malignant but may prove fatal if not removed, because of twisting of the pedicle which causes gangrene, or because of pressure.

o. follicle. SEE: *follicle.*

ovariectomy (ō-vā-rĭ-ĕk′tō-mĭ) [" + G. *ektomē*, excision]. Excision of an ovary or a portion of it. SYN: *oophorectomy.*

ovario- [G.]. Combining form meaning *ovary.*

ovariocele (ō-va′rĭ-ō-sēl) [L. *ovarium*, ovary, + G. *kēlē*, mass]. Ovarian tumor or hernia.

ovariocentesis (ō-vā-rĭ-ō-sĕn-tē′sĭs) [" + G. *kentēsis*, a piercing]. Puncture and drainage of an ovarian cyst.

ovariocyesis (ō-vā-rĭ-ō-sī-ē′sĭs) [" + G. *kyēsis*, pregnancy]. Pregnancy in the ovary.

ovariodysneuria (ō-va″rĭ-ō-dĭs-nū′rĭ-ă) [" + G. *dys*, ill, + *neuron*, sinew]. Neuralgia in an ovary.

ovariohysterectomy (ō-vā″rĭ-ō-hĭs-tĕr-ĕk′-tō-mĭ) [" + G. *ystera*, uterus, + *ektomē*, excision]. Excision of the ovaries and uterus. SYN: *oophorohysterectomy; oothecohysterectomy.*

ovariorrhexis (ō-vā″rĭ-ō-rĕks′ĭs) [" + G. *rēxis*, a rupture]. Rupture of an ovary.

ovariosalpingectomy (ō-vā″rĭ-ō-săl-pĭn-jĕk′tō-mĭ) [" + G. *salpigx*, tube, + *ektomē*, excision]. Removal of an ovary and oviduct. SYN: *oophorosalpingectomy.*

ovariosteresis (ō-va″rĭ-ō-ster-ē′sĭs) [L. *ovarium*, ovary, + G. *sterēsis*, loss]. Complete eradication of an ovary.

ovariostomy (ō-vā-rĭ-ŏs′tō-mĭ) [" + G. *stoma*, opening]. Creation of an opening in an ovarian cyst for drainage.

ovariotomy (ō-va″rĭ-ŏt′ō-mĭ) [" + G. *tomē*, incision]. Incision into or removal of an ovary, or of an ovarian tumor.

ovariotubal (ō-va″rĭ-ō-tū′băl) [" + *tuba*, a narrow duct]. Concerning the ovary and the oviducts.

ovariprival (ō-vā″rĭ-prī′văl) [" + *privāre*, to remove]. Resulting from loss of the ovaries.

ovaritis (ō-va-rī′tĭs) [L. *ovarium*, ovary, + G. *-ītis*, inflammation]. Inflamed condition of an ovary.

Usually involved secondarily in inflammation of the oviducts or pelvic peritoneum. May involve the substance of the organ (*oophoritis*) or its surface (*perioophoritis*), and may be acute or chronic.

o., acute. Acute, severe inflammation of the ovary.

o., chronic. Inflammation of ovary over a long period of time.

ovarium (ō-va′rĭ-ŭm) (pl. *ovaria*) [L.]. Ovary.

ovary (ō′va-rĭ) [L. *ovarium*, ovary, egg holder]. One of two glands in the female, producing the reproductive cell, the ovum, and two known hormones.

They are almond-shaped bodies lying in the fossa ovarica on either side of the pelvic cavity, attached to the uterus by the uteroovarian ligament and lying close to the fimbria ovarica of the fallopian tube. About 4 cm. long, 2 cm. wide, and 1½ cm. thick. Each ovary is attached to the broad ligament by the *mesovarium*. It is also attached to the side of the uterus by the *ovarian ligament* (*lig. ovarii proprium*) and to the side of the pelvis by the *suspensory ligament* (*lig. suspensorium ovarii* or *infundibulopelvic lig.*).

The ovary is divided into 2 parts, the *cortex* and the *medulla*. In the cortex are the primary oocytes and the developing graafian follicles. The medullary portion consists mainly of the vascular supply of the organ. The outer covering of the ovary is known as the *tunica albuginea ovarii.* The surface of the ovary in early life is smooth and in later life is markedly pitted as an end result of the atrophy of corpora lutea.

STRUCTURE: Each ovary consists of an outer portion or *cortex* which encloses a central *medulla.* The medulla consists of a *stroma* of connective tissue containing nerves, blood and lymphatic vessels, and some smooth muscle tissue at region of hilus. The cortex consists principally of *follicles* in various stages of development (*primary, growing,* and *mature or graafian*). Its surface is covered by a single layer of cells, the *germinal epithelium* beneath which is a layer of dense connective tissue, the *tunica albuginea.* Other structures (*corpus luteum, corpus albicans, q.v.*) may be present.

BLOOD SUPPLY: Mainly derived from the ovarian artery which reaches it through the infundibulopelvic ligament.

FUNCTION: 1. The production of ova. 2. The production of hormones among which are (a) *estrogen* or female sex hormones secreted by the follicles and (b) *progesterone* secreted by the corpus luteum. These hormones are responsible for development and maintenance of secondary sexual characteristics, preparation of uterus for pregnancy and its continuance, and development of the mammary gland.

Functional activity of the ovary is controlled primarily by gonadotrophins of the hypophysis, esp. the follicle-stimulating hormone (FSH) and luteinizing hormone (LH) or interstitial cell hormone (ICH).

ovary, words pert. to: adnexitis; albuginea; castrate; cell, interstitial; conception; corpus albicans; dysovarism; facies ovarica; fimbria ovarica; fimbriation; folliculoma; graafian follicle; hyperovaria; Krukenberg's tumor; menstruation; mesosalpinx; mesovarium; oarialgia; "oophor-" words; "ov-" words; pyoovarium; spay; spermatozoon; stroma; teratoma; tunica albuginea.

overbite. The vertical extension of the upper teeth over the lower anteriorly when the jaws are in centric occlusion.

overcompensation. A compensatory mechanism which goes beyond the extent required to effect compensation.

overcorrection. The use of too powerful a lens to correct the defect in refractive power of the eye.

overdetermination (ō″vĕr-dē-tĕr-mĭ-nā′-shŭn) [A.S. *ofer,* above, + L. *determinare,* to limit]. PSY: The idea that every symptom and dream may have several meanings, being determined by more than a single association.

overexertion. Physical exertion to a state of exhaustion.

overextension. Hyperextension; extension beyond that which usually occurs.

overflow. The continuous escape of fluid from a vessel or viscus, as o. of urine or tears.

overgrowth. Excessive growth; hypertrophy or hyperplasia. In bacteriology, the growth of one type of microorganism on a culture plate so that it covers and obscures the growth of other types.

overlay. Superimposed upon; added to.

o., psychiatric. Mental symptoms added to those present because of the basic disease or defect.

overproduction (ō″vĕr-prō-dŭk′shŭn) [" + L. *producere,* to beget]. Destruction of an organic element is followed by overproduction of the element during the reparative process, as excessive callous development after a bone fracture. SYN: *Weigert's law.*

overri′ding [" + *rīdan,* to ride]. The slipping of one end of a fractured bone past the other part.

ov′ertone [" + G. *tonos,* a stretching]. A harmonic.

o., psychic. A dimly perceived associated impression about a mental image.

overweight. Exceeding normal weight by more than 10-15%. SYN: *obesity.*

overwork (ō′vĕr-wŭrk) [" + *worc,* work]. Excessive work causing exhaustion. SEE: *ergasthenia.*

ovi- [L.]. Combining form meaning *egg.*

ovi albumen (ō″vĭ ăl-bū′mĭn) [L.]. White of egg. SYN: *ovalbumin.*

oviduct (ō′vĭ-dŭkt) [L. *ovum,* egg, + *ductus,* a path]. SYN: *uterine tube, fallopian tube.* One of two tubes extending laterally from sup. angles of the uterus which serve to convey the ovum from the ovary to the uterus. Each consists of (a) *infundibulum,* expanded portion surrounding the *ostium* or opening through which the ovum enters, (b) *ampulla,* and (c) *isthmus,* a straight narrow portion which connects with the uterus.

The border of the infundibulum bears many fingerlike processes called *fimbria.*

Each oviduct is a muscular tube consisting of three layers, *mucosa, muscular layer,* and *serosa.* The mucosa consists of columnar epithelial cells, some ciliated, others glandular. In addition to conveying the ovum, the oviduct serves to transport sperm from the uterus toward the ovary. It is the usual site of fertilization of the ovum.

oviferous (ō-vĭf′ĕr-ŭs) [" + *ferre,* to bear]. Containing or producing ova. SYN: *ovigerous.*

ovification (ō-vĭ-fĭ-kā′shŭn) [" + *facere,* to make]. The production of ova. SYN: *ovulation.*

oviform (ō′vĭ-form) [" + *forma,* shape]. 1. Having the shape of an egg. 2. Resembling an ovum. SYN: *ovoid.*

ovigen′esis. Oogenesis. *q.v.*

ovigen′ous. Giving rise to ova.

ovigerm (ō′vĭ-jĕrm) [" + *germen,* germ]. The cell which produces or develops into an ovum.

ovigerous (ō-vĭj′ĕr-ŭs) [" + *gerere,* to bear]. Producing or carrying ova. SYN: *oviferous.*

oviparous (ō-vĭp′ăr-ŭs) [" + *parēre,* to produce]. Producing eggs hatched outside the body.

oviposition. The laying of eggs as in oviparous reproduction.

ovo- [L.]. Combining form meaning *egg.*

ovo″cent′er. The centrosome of a fertilized ovum.

ovo″flav′in. A flavin derived from eggs; identical to riboflavin.

ovogenesis (ō″vō-jĕn′ĕ-sĭs) [" + G. *genesis,* production]. Production of ova. SYN: *oogenesis.*

ovoglobulin (ō″vō-glŏb′ū-lĭn) [" + *globulus,* globule]. The globulin found in egg white. SEE: *albumen, protein.*

ovoid (ō′voyd) [" + G. *eidos,* form]. Egg shaped. SYN: *oviform.*

ovomucoid (ō″vō-mū′koyd) [" + *mucus,* mucus, + G. *eidos,* form]. A glycoprotein principle from egg white.

ovo″plasm′. Ooplasm, *q.v.*

ovovitellin (ō″vō-vĭ-tĕl′lĭn) [" + *vitellus,* yolk]. Protein found in an egg yolk.

ovoviviparous (ō″vō-vi-vip′ă-rŭs) [" + *vivus*, alive, + *parēre*, to bear]. Reproducing by eggs which have a well-developed shell as in oviparous reproduction, but which hatch inside the maternal organism.

ovula (ō′vū-lă) (sing. *ovulum*) [L.]. Little eggs.

o. nabothi. Distended mucous glands in tissues of the cervix uteri.

ovular (ō′vū-lăr) [L. *ovulum*, little egg]. Concerning an ovule or ovum.

ovulation (ō-vū-lā′shŭn) [L. *ovulum*, little egg]. The periodic ripening and rupture of the mature graafian follicle and the discharge of the ovum from the cortex of the ovary.

Ovulation occurs approximately 14 days before the *next* menstrual period. It is virtually impossible to determine when ovulation will occur by counting from the first day of the preceding menstrual period. Following ovulation, a corpus luteum develops within the collapsed follicle. SEE: *corpus luteum.*

The ovum, being liberated from the follicle, enters the fallopian tube and is slowly transported toward the uterus. If sperm are present, it may become fertilized; if not, the ovum degenerates within the oviduct.

RS: *anovular, conception, menstruation, ovary, ovum, safe period, spermatozoon, fertilization, follicle, corpus luteum.*

ovulatory (ō′vū-lă-tō-rĭ) [L. *ovulum*, a little egg]. Concerning ovulation.

ovulogenous (ō-vū-lŏj′ĕn-ŭs). Giving rise to ovules or ova.

ovum (ō′vum) (pl. *ova*) [L. egg]. The female reproductive or germ cell; a cell which is capable of developing into a new organism of the same species. Fertilization by a spermatozoon is usually necessary although in some lower animals ova develop without fertilization (parthenogenesis).

The various parts of the ovum have been named as follows: The protoplasm is known as the *vitellus* or *yolk;* the outer layer is referred to as the *ectoplasm* or *zona pellucida* or *zona radiata;* the inner layer, the cell membrane, is the *vitelline membrane;* the nucleus is called the *germinal vesicle,* and the nucleolus, the *germinal spot.*

The cellular layers proliferate, becoming cuboid in shape, and in the center a clear albuminous fluid, the *liquor folliculi,* forms. The follicular cells surrounding the fluid-filled cavity are known as the *membrana granulosa.* The layer surrounding the egg cell, or *oocyte,* is known as the *discus proligerus* or *cumulus oophorus.*

As the follicular layer enlarges to form the *graafian follicle,* the term for the developed ovum, containing the above, before it leaves the ovary, there is a slight protrusion of the ovarian surface when the follicle has matured. Its rupture through the ovarian surface frees the ovum, which then proceeds ordinarily into the fallopian tube and into the uterus, which process is known as *ovulation, q.v.* It usually takes the ovum from 5 to 7 days to go from the ovary to the uterus. SEE: *menstruation.*

Normally, only one graafian follicle matures each month, not necessarily in alternate ovaries.

o., alecithal. One in which there is little or no food yolk.

o., centrolecithal. One having a large central food yolk.

o., holoblastic. O. which undergoes complete cleavage.

o., human. The female reproductive cell which develops within the graafian follicle of the ovary. It develops from an *oogonium* which undergoes a process of maturation (*oogenesis*) during which primary and secondary *oocytes* are produced which finally give rise to the mature ovum. During this process the number of chromosomes is reduced from 46 to 23 and the egg is prepared for fertilization.

A mature ovum is approximately 0.130 mm. to 0.140 mm. in diameter. Each in diameter (1/200 of an in.). Each contains a spherical *nucleus,* bounded by a *nuclear membrane* enclosing *chromatin material* and one or more *nucleoli.* The *cytoplasm* is granular and contains yolk granules or *deutoplasm* and the other characteristic organoids of cells. Its surface layer is the *vitelline membrane.* When liberated from the ovary as a primary oocyte (see *ovulation*) it is surrounded by a clear layer, *zona pellucida,* and several layers of adhering follicular cells, the latter constituting the *corona radiata.*

The length of time a human ovum retains its ability to be fertilized and develop is not precisely known but is probably at least 48 hours. If fertilized, it undergoes development. (SEE: *embryo, development of.*) If not fertilized, it degenerates. SEE: *cleavage, follicle, conception, fertilization, menstruation, ovulation, spermatozoa.*

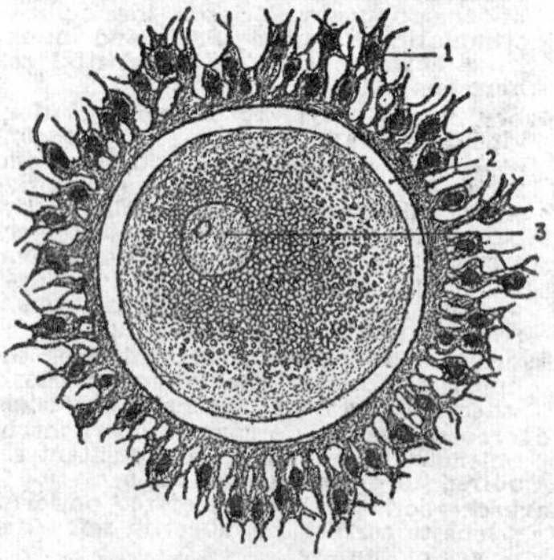

MATURE HUMAN OVUM AFTER DISCHARGE FROM FOLLICLE

1. Cells of corona radiata. 2. Zona pellucida. 3. Nucleus or germinal vesicle.

o., isolecithal. O. in which the yolk is uniformly distributed.

o., meroblastic. O. in which only the protoplasmic region undergoes cleavage; characteristic in ova containing a large amount of yolk.

o., permanent. One ready for fertilization.

o., primordial. Germ cells which arise very early in development of embryo, usually in yolk sac endoderm, and migrate into urogenital ridge and possibly serve as progenitors of functional sex cells.

o., telolecithal. O. in which yolk is fairly abundant and tends to concentrate in one hemisphere.

ox-. 1. Combining form meaning *presence of oxygen.* 2. Abbr. of oxal-.

oxa-. Combining form indicating *presence of oxygen* in place of carbon.

oxacid (ŏk'să-sĭd) [G. *oxys*, sour, + L. *acidum*, acid]. An acid of which oxygen is a constituent.

oxacillin (oks"ă-sil'in). Penicillin derivative used to treat staphylococcal infections resistant to penicillinase.

oxal-, oxalo-. CHEM: Combining forms indicating derivation from *oxalic acid*.

oxalacetic acid (ŏks"ăl-ă-sē'tĭk). SYN: *oxyaloacetic acid*. A product of carbohydrate metabolism resulting from oxidation of malic acid. May be derived from other sources.

oxalate (ŏk'să-lāt) [G. *oxalis*, sorrel]. A salt of oxalic acid.

oxalic acid (ŏk-săl'ĭk) [G. *oxalis*, sorrel]. A white crystalline powder often used about the home as a stain remover or bleach, resembling Epsom salts in appearance.

Investigations have revealed that oxalic acid has the effect of marked and rapid reduction of blood coagulation time, with indication of its value in treating hemorrhage, jaundice, etc.

SOURCES: Cranberries, chard, rhubarb, gooseberries, spinach, beet leaves. When eating these should be accompanied by liberal portions of calcium foods, such as eggs, beans, and milk.

POISONING: SYM: Erosive action on swallowing; sour taste; burning in mouth, throat and stomach; great thirst; bloody vomitus; collapse; sometimes convulsions and coma.

TREATMENT: Soapsuds are of no value against oxalic acid since they form poisonous oxalates which may be absorbed and do further damage. Use powdered chalk, calcium carbonate or magnesium carbonate. Dilute the poison and cause vomiting. Intravenous calcium gluconate or calcium chloride to treat tetany. SEE: *acid, poisoning*.

o. a. diathesis. Chronic state of oxalemia.

oxalism (ok'săl-ĭzm) [" + *ismos*, state of]. Poisoning from oxalic acid or an oxalate.

oxaluria (ok-sa-lū'rĭ-ă) [" + *ouron*, urine]. The abnormal excretion of oxalates in the urine, esp. calcium oxalate.

oxalylurea (ok"sa-lĭl-ū-rē'ă). An oxidation product of uric acid.

oxidase (ŏk'sĭ-dās) [G. *oxys*, sour]. An enzyme which catalyzes an oxidation reaction; a respiratory enzyme.

o., cytochrome. Enzyme present in most cells which oxidizes reduced cytochrome back to cytochrome.

oxidation (ŏk'sĭ-dā'shŭn) [G. *oxys*, sour]. 1. The process of a substance combining with oxygen. 2. The loss of electrons with an accompanying increase in positive valence.

oxide (ŏk'sīd) [G. *oxys*, sharp]. Any chemical compound in which oxygen is the negative radical.

oxidize (ŏk'sĭ-dīz) [G. *oxys*, sour]. 1. To combine with oxygen. 2. To increase the positive valence of, or to decrease the negative valence by bringing about a loss of electrons.

oximeter (ox-im'ĕ-ter). Apparatus for continuously determining the amount of oxygen in the blood. Usually done by measuring the amount of light transmitted through the skin.

o., ear. Oximeter attached to ear.

oxonemia (ŏk"sō-nē'mĭ-ă) [L. *oxone*, acetone, + G. *aima*, blood]. Excess of acetone bodies found in the blood. SYN: *acetonemia*.

oxy- [G.]. 1. Combining form meaning *sharp, keen, acute, acid, pungent*. 2. Presence of oxygen in a compound. 3. Presence of a hydroxyl group.

oxyacusis (ŏk"sĭ-ă-kū'sĭs) [" + *akousis*, hearing]. Abnormally acute hearing. SYN: *hyperacusis*.

oxybenzene (ok"sĭ-ben'zēn). Phenol, *q.v.*

oxyblepsia (ŏk"sĭ-blĕp'sĭ-ă) [" + *bleps*, vision]. Extraordinary acuteness of vision.

oxybutyria (ŏk"sĭ-bū-tĭr'ĭ-ă) [G. *oxys*, sharp, + *boutyron*, butter]. Oxybutyric acid in the blood or in the urine.

oxycalcium (ok"si-kal'sē-um). Of or pertaining to oxygen and calcium.

oxycephalia (ŏk"sĭ-sĕf-ā'lĭ-ă) [" + *kephalē*, head]. State of having a high and pointed skull.

oxycephalous (ŏk-sĭ-sef'ă-lŭs) [" + *kephalē*, head]. Denoting a head that is pointed and conelike.

oxychloride (ŏks"ĭ-klor'īd) [G. *oxys*, sharp, + *chlōros*, green]. A compound consisting of an element or radical combined with (a) oxygen and chlorine or (b) the hydroxyl radical (OH) and chlorine.

oxychromatic (ŏk"sĭ-krō-măt'ĭk) [G. *oxys*, sour, + *chrōma*, color]. Staining readily with acid dyes.

oxychromatin (ŏk"sĭ-krō'mă-tĭn) [" + *chrōma*, color]. That part of chromatin which stains readily with acid dyes.

oxycinesia (oks"ĭ-sĭn-ē'zĭ-ă) [G. *oxys*, keen, + *kinēsis*, movement]. Pain experienced on moving.

oxydase (ŏk'sĭ-dās) [" + *ase*, enzyme]. Old spelling of oxidase, *q.v.*

oxyecoia (ok"sĭ-ĕ-koy'a) [G. *oxys*, sharp, + *akoē*, hearing]. Abnormal sensitivity to noises.

oxyesthesia (ŏk"sĭ-ĕs-thē'zĭ-ă) [" + *aisthēsis*, sensation]. Abnormal acuteness of sensation. SYN: *algesia; hyperesthesia*.

oxygen (ŏk'sĭ-jĕn) [G. *oxys*, sharp, since oxygen was formerly considered an essential element of acids, + *gennan*, to produce]. SYMB: O. A nonmetallic element occurring free in the atmosphere as a colorless, odorless, tasteless gas. At. wt. 15.9994; at. no. 8.

It is a constituent of animal, vegetable and mineral substances comprising by weight 3/4 of the animal, 4/5 of the vegetable, and 1/2 of the mineral world, and by volume, 1/5 of the atmosphere, and by weight 8/9 of water.

It is essential to respiration of most forms of animal and plant life, and is the most important and abundant element, composing about 21% of the atmosphere's total volume. When O combines with another substance, the process is called *oxidation*. When combination takes place rapidly enough to produce light and heat, the process is called burning or *combustion*. O combines readily with other elements to form oxides.

It is the only element that enters the animal organism in a free state. It is absorbed by plants in the form of water and carbon dioxide being converted by them into organic substances utilized for the food of man, and in turn is returned to the atmosphere by man in form of waste products of water and carbon dioxide, thus maintaining the balance of oxygen and carbon dioxide in the atmosphere.

It represents 65% of the elements in the body; 10-16% in venous, and 17-21% in arterial blood at sea level.

USES: In conditions in which there is insufficient oxygen being carried by the blood to the tissues. Thus O would be used in cases of severe anemia, shock or circulatory collapse, pulmonary edema, pneumonia; or by mountain climbers, astronauts, or aviators when at heights where the amount of oxygen present in the atmosphere is insufficient to support life.

Oxygen is administered by mask, nasal tube, tent, or by placing the patient in an airtight chamber in which the pressure may be increased. No matter how much O is given it is important to have it adequately humidified. It is desirable to administer O at whatever rate is necessary to increase the O content of inspired air to 50%.

Oxygen is employed frequently with ether or other agents used for the induction of general anesthesia. Following extensive surgery it reduces reactions to anesthetic. Also employed in septicemia, gas gangrene, peritonitis, and intestinal obstruction.

Oxygen is used under pressure in chambers for cardiac surgery, in treating aerobic infections such as gas gangrene, vascular disorders, carbon monoxide poisoning, and in connection with radiation therapy of tumors. When oxygen is used in this manner it is called *hyperbaric oxygenation.*

o. capacity. The maximum amount of oxygen expressed in volume per cent (cc. per 100 cc.) which a given amount of blood will absorb. For normal blood it is about 20 cc.

o. content. The amount of oxygen in volume per cent which is present in the blood at any one moment.

o. debt. The amount of oxygen required after muscular activity for the removal of lactic acid and other metabolic products which accumulate when the supply of oxygen is below the needs of the organism.

o. dissociation curve. A curve which shows relationship between partial pressure of oxygen and the percentage saturation of hemoglobin with oxygen, *i. e.,* the proportion of oxyhemoglobin to reduced hemoglobin. Factors which favor shift of curve to the right, *i. e.,* which accelerate the decomposition of hemoglobin are a rise in temperature and an increase of H ions which results from liberation of CO_2 and formation of lactic acid.

o. saturation. Oxygen content of blood divided by oxygen capacity and expressed in volume per cent.

o. tent. An air-tight enclosure for a patient's head and shoulders and in which the oxygen content of the air can be raised above normal.

o. therapy. The administration of oxygen for the treatment of conditions resulting from oxygen want. It is used to combat acute arterial anoxia such as results from pneumonia, pulmonary edema, or obstruction to breathing. It is also employed in congestive heart failure, coronary thrombosis, and following surgery.

It may be administered by nasal catheter, mask (nasal or oronasal), funnel or cone, oxygen tent, or special oxygen chamber, and usually in a concentration of 70-100%. Inhalation of high concentrations of oxygen, esp. at pressures of more than one atmosphere may produce deleterious effects such as irritation of respiratory tract, reduced vital capacity, and sometimes neurological symptoms. For premature infants serious eye defects may result. SEE: *retrolental fibroplasia.*

CAUTION: Care must be exercised not to permit a spark or open flame in the vicinity of the apparatus.

o. want. Anoxia, oxygen lack.

oxygenase (ŏk'sĭ-jĕn-ās) [G. *oxys,* sharp, + *gennan,* to produce, + *ase,* enzyme]. An enzyme which enables an organism to use atmospheric oxygen in respiration.

oxygenate (ok'sĭ-jen-āt). To combine or supply with oxygen.

oxygenation (ŏk"sĭ-jĕn-ā'shŭn) [" + *gennan,* to produce]. Impregnation or combination with oxygen, as the aeration of the blood in the lungs.

o., hyperbaric. Administration of oxygen under increased pressure while patient is in an airtight chamber. Used for certain surgical procedures, treatment of aerobic infections such as gas gangrene, and in conjunction with radiation therapy of tumors.

oxygenic (ŏk"sĭ-jĕn'ĭk) [" + *gennan,* to produce]. Concerning, resembling, containing, or consisting of oxygen.

oxygenize [G. *oxys,* sharp, + *gennan,* to produce]. To oxidize, *q.v.*

oxygeusia (ŏk"sĭ-gū'sĭ-ă) [" + *geusis,* taste]. Abnormally keen sense of taste.

oxyhematin. An iron compound which constitutes the coloring matter in oxyhemoglobin. When oxidized it yields hematinic acid; when reduced, hematoporphyrin.

oxyhemoglobin (ŏk"sĭ-hē"mō-glō'bĭn) [" + *aima,* blood, + L. *globus,* a sphere]. The combined form of hemoglobin and oxygen.

Hemoglobin with oxygen is found in arterial blood and is the oxygen carrier to the body tissues.

oxyhemoglobinometer (ŏk"sĭ-hē"mō-glo"-bĭn-ŏm'ĕt-ĕr) [" + " + " + G. *metron,* a measure]. Apparatus for measurement of oxygen in the blood.

oxyhydrocephalus (ŏk"sĭ-hī-drō-sĕf'ăl-ŭs) [G. *oxys,* sharp, + *ydōr,* water, + *kephalē,* brain]. Pointed head shape type of hydrocephalus.

oxyiodide (ŏk"sĭ-ī'ō-dĭd) [" + *iōdēs,* violet colored]. Compound of iodine and oxygen with an element or radical.

oxylalia (ok"sĭ-lā'lĭ-ă) [G. *oxys,* swift, + *lalein,* to speak]. Abnormal rapidity of speech.

oxyntic (ŏk-sĭn'tĭk) [G. *oxynein,* to make acid]. Producing or secreting acid. SEE: *cell.*

oxyopia (ŏk"sĭ-ŏ'pĭ-ă) [G. *oxys,* sharp, + *ōps,* sight]. Unusual acuteness of vision.

oxyopter (ŏk"sĭ-op'tĕr) [" + *opsis,* vision]. A unit of visual acuity, being the reciprocal of the visual angle, in degrees.

oxyosmia (ŏk"sĭ-oz'mĭ-ă) [" + *osmē,* odor]. Unusual acuity of sense of smell.

oxyosphresia (ok"sĭ-ŏs-frē'zĭ-ă) [" + *osphrēsis,* smell]. Abnormal acuity of the sense of smell.

oxypathia, oxypathy (ok"sĭ-păth'ĭ-ă, -sĭp'-ăth-ĭ) [G. *oxys,* sharp, + *pathos,* feeling]. 1. Unusual acuity of sensation. 2. An acute condition. 3. Condition of inability to eliminate unoxidizable acids which combine with fixed alkalies of the tissues and harm the organism.

oxyperitoneum ŏk"sĭ-pĕr-ĭ-tō-nē'ŭm) [" + *peritonaion,* peritoneum]. Introduction of oxygen into the peritoneal cavity.

oxyphil(e (ok'sĭ-fĭl, -fīl) [" + *philein,* to love]. 1. Staining readily with acid dyes. 2. A cell which stains readily with acid dyes.

oxyphilous (ŏk-sĭf'ĭl-ŭs) [" + *philein,* to love]. Having an affinity for acid dyes. SYN: *oxyphil, 1.*

oxyphonia (ok"sĭ-fō'nĭ-ă) [" + *phōnē,* voice]. An abnormally sharp or shrill voice.

oxypurine (ŏk"sĭ-pu'rēn) [G. *oxys,* sharp, + L. *purus,* pure, + *urina,* urine]. An oxidation product of purine.

Group includes hypoxanthine, xanthine, uric acid.

oxyrhine (ŏk'sĭ-rīn) [" + *ris,* nose]. 1. Having a sharp pointed nose. 2. Possessing an acute sense of smell.

oxysparteine (ok"sĭ-spăr'te-ēn) [" + L. *spartium,* broom]. White crystalline oxidation product of sparteine, used as a cardiac stimulant.

oxytetracycline (ox"ĭ-tet"ră-si'klin). One of a group of broad-spectrum antibiotic substances called tetracyclines. Originally obtained from a strain of Streptomyces, it is now prepared synthetically.

oxytocia (ŏk"sĭ-tō'shĭ-ă) [G. *oxys,* swift, + *tokos,* childbirth]. Unusual rapidity of childbirth.

oxytocic (ŏk"sĭ-tō'sĭk) [" + *tokos,* birth]. 1. Agent which stimulates uterine contractions. 2. Accelerating childbirth.

o. principle. A hormone stored in post. lobe of hypophysis which acts specifically on smooth musculature of the uterus increasing tone of and inducing uterine contractions. SYN: *oxytocin, q.v.*

oxytocin (ŏk"sĭ-to'sĭn) [G. *oxys,* swift, + *tokos,* birth]. A pituitary hormone that stimulates the uterus to contract and thus induces parturition. It also acts on the mammary gland to force out the milk.

o. injection. USP. An aqueous solution containing the oxytocic principle of the post. pituitary gland.

oxyuriasis (ŏk"sĭ-ū-rĭ'ăs-ĭs) [G. *oxys,* sharp, + *oura,* tail, + *iasis,* infection]. Infestation with *Enterobius vermicularis* (pinworm), *q.v.*

oxyuricide (ŏk"sĭ-ū'rĭ-sīd) [" + " + L. *caedere,* to kill]. Destructive to, or an agent that destroys pinworms.

oxyurid [G. *oxys,* sharp, + *ours,* tail]. Pinworm or seatworm. SEE: *Enterobius vermicularis.*

Oxyuris [G. *oxys,* sharp, + *ours,* tail]. Old name for genus of nematode worms which includes the pinworms or seatworms. SEE: *Enterobius.*

o. vermicularis. *Enterobius vermicularis, q.v.*

oyster (oi'ster) [G. *ostreon*]. Shellfish eaten raw or cooked. When eaten raw or partially cooked may be source of infectious hepatitis virus.

RAW (*meat only*): 1 cup (240 gm.). Calories: 160. Other main values: 20 gm. protein; 4.3 gm. fat; 8 gm. carbohydrate; 175 mg. sodium; 226 mg. calcium; 740 I.U. vitamin A.

Oz., oz. ABBR. for *ounce.*

oz. ap. ABBR. for the pharmaceutical term *ounce apothecary's.*

oz. av. ABBR. for the term *ounce avoirdupois.*

ozena (ō-zē'nă) [G. *ozein,* to smell]. Disease of the nose characterized by atrophy of the turbinates and mucous membrane accompanied by considerable crusting and discharge and a very offensive odor.

It is present in various forms of rhinitis.

ozochrotia (ō"zō-krō'shĭ-ă) [" + *chrōs,* skin]. Strong odor given off by the skin. SYN: *bromidrosis.*

ozonator (ō'zō-nā-tor) [G. *ozein,* to smell]. Device for generating ozone.

ozone (ō'zōn) [G. *ozein,* to smell]. A form of oxygen in which 3 atoms of the element combine to form the molecule, O_3.

ozonization (ō-zō-nĭ-zā'shŭn) [G. *ozein,* to smell]. The act of converting to, or impregnating with ozone.

ozonize (ō'zō-nīz) [G. *ozein,* to smell]. 1. To convert oxygen to ozone, *i. e.,* 3 atoms to the molecule of free oxygen. 2. To impregnate the air of a substance with ozone.

ozonometer (ō"zō-nom'ĕt-ĕr) [" + *metron,* a measure]. An apparatus for estimating the quantity of ozone in the atmosphere.

ozonoscope (ō-zō'nō-skōp) [" + *skopein,* to examine]. A device for showing the presence or amount of ozone.

ozostomia (ō"zō-stō'mĭ-ă) [G. *ozē,* stench, + *stoma,* mouth]. Fetid breath.

Notes

Notes

Notes

Notes

Notes

P

P. Symb. for *phosphorus.* Abbr. for *position, posterior, postpartum, pressure, pulse, pupil.*

P_2. Abbr. for *pulmonic second sound.*

p. Abbr. for *page, pupil.*

p-. Abbr. for *para-* in chem. formulas.

P-A. Abbr. for *posteroanterior.*

P & A. Abbr. for *percussion and auscultation.*

Pa. Symb. for *protactinium.*

PABA. Abbr. for *para-aminobenzoic acid, q.v.*

pablum (pab′lum). Proprietary or trade name for a cereal food for infants.

pabular (pab′ū-lar) [L. *pabulum,* food]. Pert. to nourishment.

pabulum (păb′ū-lŭm) [L.]. Food; nourishment.

PAC. Abbr. for *phenacetin, aspirin,* and *caffeine.*

pacchionian bodies (păk-ē-ō′nĭ-ăn). Enlarged villi, small pedunculated or rounded growths of fibrous tissue along longitudinal fissure of the cerebrum growing on arachnoid membrane.

p. depressions. Small pits produced on inner surface of skull by protuberance of p. bodies.

p. glands. SEE: *p. bodies.*

pacemaker (pās′māk-ĕr) [L. *passus,* a step, + A.S. *macian,* to make]. 1. The sinoatrial node, so named because cardiac rhythm commences here, taking place near the spot where the large veins empty into the atrium. 2. That which influences the rate of occurrence of an event.

cardiac p., artificial or ***electric.*** An electrical device which can substitute for a defective natural pacemaker and control the beating of the heart by a series of rhythmic electrical discharges. If the electrodes which deliver the discharges to the heart are placed on the outside of the chest, it is called an *external pacemaker.* If the electrodes are placed within the chest wall, it is called an *internal pacemaker.*

pachismus (păk-ĭz′mŭs) [G. *pachys,* thick, + *ismos,* condition]. Condensation or thickening of an organ or part.

pachy-, pach- [G.]. Combining form meaning *thick, large, heavy, massive.*

pachyacria, pachyakria (păk-ĭ-ăk′rĭ-ă) [G. *pachys,* thick, + *akron,* end]. Hypertrophy of soft portions of the extremities.

pachyblepharon (păk″ĭ-blĕf′ăr-ŏn) [G. *pachys,* thick, + *blepharon,* eyelid]. A thickening of border of eyelid.

pachyblepharosis (păk-ĭ-blĕf-ă-rō′sĭs). Chronic thickening of the eyelid.

pachycephalic (păk″ĭ-sĕf-al′ĭk) [" + *kephalē,* brain]. Possessing a thick skull. SYN: *pachycephalous.*

pachycephalous (păk″ĭ-sĕf′ăl-ŭs) [" + *kephalē,* brain]. Thick skulled. SYN: *pachycephalic.*

pachycephaly (păk″ĭ-sĕf′ăl-ĭ) [" + *kephalē,* brain]. Unusual thickness of the walls of the skull.

pachychilia (păk″ĭ-kī′lĭ-ă) [" + *cheilos,* lip]. Unusual thickness of the lips.

pachycholia (păk″ĭ-kō′lĭ-ă) [" + *cholē,* bile]. Thickening or inspissation of the bile.

pachychromatic (păk″ĭ-krō-măt′ĭk) [" + *chrōma,* color]. Possessing a coarse chromatin network.

pachycolpismus (păk-ĭ-kŏl-piz′mŭs) [G. *pachys,* thick, + *kolpos,* vagina, + *ismos,* condition]. Chronic inflammation of vagina with thickened vaginal walls. SYN: *pachyvaginitis.*

pachydactylia, pachydactyly (păk″ĭ-dăk-til′-ĭă, -dak″tĭ-lĭ) [G. *pachys,* thick, + *daktylos,* digit]. Condition marked by unusually large fingers and toes.

pachyderma (păk-ĭ-der′mă) [" + *derma,* skin]. Unusual thickness of the skin.

pachydermatocele (păk″ĭ-dĕr-măt′ō-sēl) [" + " + *kēlē,* swelling]. A pendulous state of the skin with thickening. SYN: *dermatolysis.*

pachydermatosis (păk″ĭ-dĕr-măt-ō′sĭs) [" + " + *-ōsis,* condition]. Chronic hypertrophy of the skin. SYN: *pachydermia.*

pachydermatous (păk-ĭ-der′mă-tŭs) [" + *derma,* skin]. Possessing a thick skin.

pachydermia (păk-ĭ-der-mĭ′ă) [G. *pachys,* thick, + *derma,* skin]. 1. Excessive thickening of the skin. 2. Elephantiasis, *q.v.*

p. laryngis. Irregular thickening and hypertrophy of mucous membrane in the larynx seen in chronic laryngitis.

p. lymphangiectatica. A diffuse form of skin thickening due to blocked or defective lymph drainage.

p., occipital. A disease in which the skin of the scalp, esp. in occipital region, is thrown into thickened folds.

p. vesica. Condition in which there is a thickened mucous membrane in the urinary bladder.

pachyemia (păk-ĭ-ē′mĭ-ă) [G. *pachys,* thick, + *aima,* blood]. Thickness of the blood.

pachyglossia (păk″ĭ-glos′sĭ-ă) [" + *glōssa,* tongue]. Unusual thickness of the tongue.

pachygnathous (păk-ĭg′năth-ŭs) [" + *gnathus,* jaw]. Having a thick or large jaw.

pachygyria (păk-ĭ-jī′rĭ-ă) [" + *gyros,* a circle]. Flat, broad formation of the cerebral convolutions.

pachyhematous (păk-ĭ-hĕm′ăt-ŭs) [" + *aima,* blood]. Having thickened blood.

pachyhemia (păk-ĭ-hē′mĭ-ă) [" + *aima,* blood]. A thickened state of the blood.

pachyleptomeningitis (păk-ĭ-lĕp-tō-mĕn-ĭn-jī′tĭs) [G. *pachys,* thick, + *leptos,* thin, + *mēnigx,* membrane, + *-itis,* inflammation]. Inflammation of pia and dura of the brain and spinal cord.

pachylosis (păk-ĭ-lō′sĭs) [G. *pachylos,* thick]. A rough, dry, thickened, chronic condition of skin. SYN: *xerosis.*

pachymenia [G. *pachys,* thick, + *hymen,* membrane]. Thickening of the skin.

pachymeningitis (păk-ĭ-mĕn-ĭn-jī′tĭs) [G. *pachys,* thick, + *mēnigx, mēnigg-,* membrane, + *-itis,* inflammation]. Inflamed condition of the dura mater.

Inflammation of the pia, dura, or arachnoid membranes is sure to extend to one or both of the others, and the consequence in any form is suppuration, abscess, effusion into the ventricles and softening of cerebral tissue if brain is involved.

p. externa. Inflammation of outer layer of dura mater.

p., hemorrhagic. Circumscribed effusion of blood on inner surface of dura with inflammation. SYN: *chronic subdural hematoma.*

SYM AND SIGNS: Intermittent headache, choked disks, hemiparesis, dilated pupil, unconsciousness in varying degrees.

ETIOL: Usually the result of trauma, such as a blow, which results in a venous tear. Blood oozes into subdural space, a blood clot is formed which becomes encysted, giving rise to a hematoma.

p. interna. Inflammation of inner layer of dura mater.

p., spinal. Inflammation of the dura of the spinal cord.

pachymeningopathy (păk″ĭ-mĕn″ĭn-gŏp′ă-thĭ). Any disease of the dura mater.

pachymeninx (păk-ĭ-mē′nĭnks) [G. *pachys,* thick, + *mēnigx,* membrane]. Membrane known as the dura mater.

pachymeter (păk-ĭm′ĕt-ĕr) [" + *metron,* measure]. Instrument for measuring thickness as of paper.

pachynsis (păk-ĭn′sĭs) [G. *pachynsis,* a thickening]. Thickening of a substance or part, usually abnormal.

pachyntic (păk-ĭn′tĭk) [G. *pachynsis,* a thickening]. Thickening, abnormally thickened.

pachyonychia (păk″ĭ-ō-nĭk′ĭ-ă) [G. *pachys,* thick, + *onyx, onych-,* nail]. Thickening of finger or toe nails.

p. congenita. A congenital condition characterized by thickening of the nails, thickening of the skin on palms of hands and soles of feet, follicular keratosis at knees and elbows, and corneal dyskeratosis.

pachyostosis (păk″ĭ-ŏs-tō′sĭs) [" + *osteon,* bone, + *-ōsis,* disease]. Thickening of the bones.

pachyotia (păk-ĭ-ō′shĭ-ă) [" + *ous, ōt-,* ear]. Abnormal thickness of the ears.

pachypelviperitonitis (păk″ĭ-pĕl″vĭ-pĕr-ĭt-ō-nī′tĭs) [" + L. *pelvis,* basin, + G. *peritonaion,* peritoneum, + *-ītis,* inflammation]. Inflammation of the pelvic and peritoneal membranes with hypertrophy and thickening of their surfaces.

pachyperitonitis (păk-ĭ-pĕr-ĭt-ō-nī′tĭs) [" + *peritonaion,* peritoneum, + *-ītis,* inflammation]. Inflammation of the peritoneum with thickening of the membrane.

pachypleuritis (păk-ĭ-plū-rī′tĭs) [" + *pleura,* a side, + *-ītis,* inflammation]. Inflamed condition of the pleura with thickening of the membrane.

pachypodous (pak-ip′ō-dŭs) [" + *pous, pod-,* foot]. Having massive feet.

pachyrhinic (păk″ĭ-rĭn′ĭk). Having a thick, flat nose.

pachysalpingitis (păk-ĭ-săl-pĭn-jī′tĭs) [G. *pachys,* thick, + *salpigx,* tube, + *-ītis,* inflammation]. Chronic inflammation of an oviduct with thickening of the walls.

pachysalpingoovaritis (păk″ĭ-săl-pĭn″gō-ō-văr-ī′tĭs) [" + " + L. *ovarium,* ovary, + G. *-ītis,* inflammation]. Chronic inflamed condition of an ovary and oviduct with thickening of the membranes.

pachysomia (păk-ĭ-sō′mĭ-ă) [G. *pachys,* thick, + *sōma,* body]. Pathological thickening of the soft parts of the body.

pachyvaginalitis (păk″ĭ-văj-ĭn-ăl-ī′tĭs) [" + L. *vagina,* sheath, + G. *-ītis,* inflammation]. Inflamed condition of the tunica vaginalis of the testes.

pachyvaginitis (păk″ĭ-văj-ĭn-ī′tĭs) [" + " + *-ītis,* inflammation]. Chronic inflammation of the vagina with thickening of the membranes. SYN: *pachycolpismus.*

pacinian corpuscle (pă-sĭn′ĭ-ăn). SYN: *corpuscle of Vater-Pacini.* An encapsulated sensory nerve ending found in subcutaneous tissue and many other parts of the body (pancreas, penis, clitoris, nipple). These corpuscles are stimulated by deep or heavy pressure.

pack (păk) [Gaelic, *pakke*]. 1. A dry or moist, hot or cold blanket or sheet wrapped around a patient. Used for treatment. 2. To fill up a cavity with cotton, gauze or a similar substance.

p., cold wet sheet. This pack is a physiologic sedative and hypnotic employed for relief of restlessness, insomnia, and used extensively in psychiatric conditions.

Patient is wrapped in two or more sheets that have been placed in cold water and wrung out before application. The patient's body is then wrapped in heavy blankets to prevent loss of cooling and evaporation of moisture.

p., dry. Procedure used in combination with hot bath. When patient leaves hot bath he is placed in dry, warm sheet and wrapped in several warm blankets.

p., full. SEE: *pack, wet sheet.*

p., half. Wet sheet pack but in this type the moist fabric and dry blanket extend from the axilla to below the knees.

p., hot bath. SEE: *pack, dry.*

p., hot blanket. The envelopment of a patient in moist blanket wrung from very hot water (150° to 160° F.). Given to relax contracted muscles, relieve convulsions, or induce profuse perspiration.

p., ice. If ice bag is not available, a local cold application may be made by folding a soft towel so it will fit the area and filling it with crushed ice.

p., neutral wet sheet. SEE: *pack, wet sheet.*

p., one sheet. Same as wet sheet pack except only 1 large sheet, 84 x 96 in., is used.

p., partial. SEE: *half* and *three-quarter packs.*

p., three-quarter. Pack using same temperatures as wet sheet pack but the body is enveloped from below upward as far as the armpits.

p., wet sheet. The envelopment of patient in one, two or three linen or soft cotton sheets that have been wrung out of water which is hot, cold or lukewarm, depending on the purpose. These are held against the body by large woolen blankets.

Temperature of the water used for the sheets varies.

packer (păk′ĕr) [Gaelic *pakke,* a pack]. Device for packing a cavity, as the uterus or rectum with gauze, etc.

packing (păk′ĭng) [Gaelic *pakke,* a pack]. 1. The process of filling a cavity or wound with gauze sponges, etc. 2. Material used to fill a cavity or wound.

pad (păd) [origin uncertain]. Soft cushion or bag to relieve or give pressure, support an organ or part, etc.

Usually cotton, oakum, jute or wood wool. Surgical cotton is not suitable for open wounds or broken surfaces. Oakum or marine lint is too irritating to place in direct contact with skin.

p., abdominal. Pad for absorbing fluids from surgical wounds, etc., of abdomen.

p., dinner. Pad placed on stomach prior to application of a plaster cast.

Pad is then removed, leaving space for abdominal distention after meals.

p., kidney. Air or water pad fixed on abdominal belt for compression over a movable kidney.

p.'s, knuckle. Nodules on dorsal sides of the fingers.

p., Malgaigne's. Mass of fat in knee joint on either side of the patella's upper end.

p., Mikulicz's. One of folded gauze used in surgery.

p., perineal. Pad covering the perineum. Used to cover a wound or to absorb the menstrual flow.

p., sucking. A pad of fat seen inside the cheek of infants.

p., surgical. Soft rubber pad with apron and inflatable rim for drainage of escaping fluids, used in operations and obstetrics.

paed-, paedo-. For words beginning in this way, see ped-, pedo-.

Pagenstecher's ointment (pǎhg'ěn-stěk-ěr). Ophthalmic ointment composed of a base of yellow oxide of mercury.

P.'s thread. Suture thread made of linen dipped in celluloid.

Paget's disease (păj'ět). Chronic inflammation of bones with thickening and distortion. SYN: *osteitis deformans.*

of nipple. Carcinoma of the mammary ducts.

pain (pān) [G. *poinē,* penalty]. 1. A sensation in which a person experiences discomfort, distress, or suffering. 2. In the plural, refers to contractions of the uterus in childbirth, or labor pains.

Pain may vary in intensity from that which produces mild discomfort to that of intolerable agony. In most cases, pain stimuli are harmful to the body and tend to bring about reactions by which the body protects itself. Adaptation to pain stimuli does not readily occur. Pain is one of the cardinal symptoms of inflammation.

Later in life, if one had always been well, definite pain may be a danger signal. In a complainer, a new pain may not mean much.

The degree of pain is measured by a dolorimeter in terms of *dol.* Childbirth is registered as 10½ dols; migraine headache, 5 dols; toothache, 2 dols. The average man seldom experiences pain of over 6 dols. A 2-dol pain may cease after taking aspirin. Increasing dosage if pain is over 2 dols will not help.

p., abdominal. Increased with respiration; experienced in appendicitis, broken ribs, intercostal neuralgia, wounds, herpes zoster, pleurisy, pleurodynia, myalgia, periostitis, acute peritonitis, colic; hepatic, gastric, or renal ulcer; gallbladder disorders; carcinoma in late stages, and gummata of this region.

p., aching. Generalized aching may be ushered in with infectious disease such as influenza, smallpox, or rheumatic fever. It is also found in myalgia and various headaches.

p., acute. Same as lancinating pain. Usually associated with acute inflammation, or inflammation of serous membranes as in pleurisy, and pericarditis; also posterior spinal-root pains.

p., after-. That following labor, caused by contraction of uterine muscles during involution.

p., agonizing. May be due to coronary thrombosis, angina pectoris, aortic aneurysm, mediastinitis. May occur in milder form in asthma, tracheobronchitis, or it may be due to referred pain from gallbladder, intestinal obstruction, diaphragmatic hernia, pancreatitis, or a perforated ulcer.

p., angina pectoris. Paroxysmal, severe pain radiating from the heart to shoulder, thence down the arm, or rarely from the heart to the abdomen or ear. Lasts from a few seconds to several minutes.

p., appendicitis. If acute, abdominal pain, usually severe, generally throughout the abdomen, followed by localization of pain in right lower quadrant of abdomen with tenderness over right rectus muscle with rigidity.

p., bearing-down. Straining with uterine contractions. Usually occurs in second stage of labor.

p., Brodie's. That caused near a joint affected with neuralgia when the skin is folded near it.

p., burning. SYN: *causalgia.* Experienced in heat burns, superficial skin lesions, herpes zoster and in circumscribed neuralgias.

p., cardiac. Angina pectoris, *q.v.*

p., causalgic. A spontaneous pain, esp. burning in character, when associated with anesthesia, or hyperesthesia in a given nerve. SEE: *causalgia.*

p., ceiling and threshold of. Ascertained by a low amount of controlled heat to a square centimeter of skin surface for 3 seconds. The *pain threshold* is reached when sensation starts to be painful, or when 220 millicalories or heat units are reached. The ceiling is found by increased heat until 480 millicalories are reached. Beyond this point no increased physical suffering is experienced although burns will result. They occur at 7 or 8 dols, but ordinary pain registers at 2 dols; migraine at 3 to 5 dols; histamine injectors at 6 to 7 dols; passing of a kidney stone or childbirth may register 10½ dols if no pain-relieving drug is given. As this is the pain-ceiling no further physical pain may be felt. Pain greater than 6 dols is rare. A greater pain cancels a lesser one. Heavy doses of a drug, such as aspirin, do not give greater relief than the ordinary dose. The pain threshold is the same for everyone, although emotional reactions simulate increased pain.

p., central. That due to a lesion in the brain or spinal cord.

p., cephalgic. Head pain, *q.v.*

p., chest. Severe pain in chest from exercise may be due to heart trouble. If due to pleurisy it comes with a deep breath, or it may come with a stiff shoulder or neck, due to arthritis or fibrositis. If, after a meal, it comes when bending over, it may be due to diaphragmatic hernia.

p., continuous. May indicate persistent obstruction; also a tendency to suppuration.

p., cramplike. Muscular spasm such as epigastric pain. Significance depends upon location of pain.

p., degree of. SEE: *dol, dolorimeter.*

p., dilating. P. occurring during the first stage of labor accompanying dilatation of the cervix.

p., dull. Continuous mild throbbing.

p., ear. May indicate inflammation of the ext. auditory canal, except in young children. It also may indicate a furuncle in the meatus, or middle ear disease. SYN: *otodynia.*

p., eccentric. P. occurring in peripheral structures due to a lesion involving post. roots of spinal nerves.

p., ecstatic. Unreasonable desire for excitement, pleasurable or painful. A martyrlike pleasure, or a feeling of being unfairly treated may be experienced with satisfaction.

p., epigastric. Severe pain occurring in paroxysms in gastric disorders. In general, may accompany any gastric or intestinal disorder, as well as pleural and some cardiac affections. SEE: *cardialgia.*

p., expulsive. That of the second and third stages of labor.

p., false. One mistaken for a true labor pain; an ineffective pain of labor.

p., fixed. Indicates derangement at some special point.

p., fulgurant. Sudden shooting p., esp. experienced in tabes dorsalis due to syphilis.

p., gallbladder. In upper right abdominal quadrant, dull pain just below the last rib in infection, or sharp pain in same area radiating to the back and up under right shoulder, esp. if calculi are present.

p., gastralgic. Severe pain occurring in paroxysms in gastric disorders. SYN: *epigastric p.*

p., girdle. One resembling sensation of a constricting cord around the waist.

p., growing. That felt in the joints of growing children; may be rheumatic.

p., head. SYN: *headache, cephalalgia.* An ache or pain located in the head, esp. one experienced in region of cranial vault. Headache *may be* a symptom of acute systemic infections; intracranial tumors, infections, or vascular lesions; hypertension; acute and chronic infections of the nose and sinuses, pharynx, eye, and ear; and toxic states (alcoholism, uremia, etc.). Headache may occur after the injection of histamine, following a lumbar puncture, in infections of the meninges, and in subarachnoid hemorrhages. Headache occurs in many febrile diseases, in anemia and oxygen want, and following head injuries (post-traumatic). Migraine, *q.v.*, is a common type, of unknown etiology. Many headaches are psychogenic such as those occurring in conversion hysteria, anxiety states, etc.

p., heterotopic. Referred pain.

p., homotopic. That felt at the point of injury.

p., hunger. Pain due to need for food.

p., hypogastric. Pain in the hypogastrium.

p., ideogenous. Pain of mental origin.

p., imperative. In psychasthenia. A persistent sensation of pain.

p., inflammatory. Pain in presence of inflammation which is increased by pressure.

p., intermenstrual. Pelvic pain occurring during the period between the menses. SYN: *mittelschmerz.*

p., intractable. Pain that cannot be easily relieved, as that occurring from certain neoplastic invasions.

p., joy. Apparent enjoyment of pain during hysterical conditions.

p., labor. That accompanying childbirth.

p., lancinating. A short, sharp, cutting pain.

p., lightning. The cutting, darting pain associated with tabes dorsalis.

p., lingual. Pain in tongue which may be due to local lesions, glossitis, fissures, pernicious anemia.

p., lung. SEE: *pain, pulmonary.*

p., menstrual. Pain, usually cramping, occurring just prior to onset or during (or both) the menstrual period. SYN: *dysmenorrhea.*

p., mental. One of psychic origin; mental distress or grief. May, if persistent, cause true physical pain (psychosomatic pain).

p., middle. Pain bet. menstrual periods. SYN: *mittelschmerz.*

p., migraine. Headache accompanied by nausea and vomiting. It may arise from a number of causes, esp. those of neurological origin.

p., mind. Pain occurring subsequent to a mental operation or of mental origin. SYN: *psychalgia.*

p., mobile. One that moves from one area to another.

p., movement. Kinesalgia.

p., neuralgic. Pain, frequently paroxysmal, occurring along the branches of a nerve. Temporarily relieved by heat or pressure. May be of rheumatic origin, a tic or inflammation of nerves or nerve trauma.

p., niggling. The early ones of puerperal labor.

p., night. Pain in hip or knee during muscular relaxation in sleep.

p., noise. Pain of ear caused by a noise. SEE: *odynacusis.*

p., objective. One excited by some external or internal irritant, by inflammation, or by injury to nerves, organs or other tissues which interfere with the function, nutrition, or circulation of the affected part; usually traceable to a definite pathologic process.

p., organic. Somatalgia.

p., osteocopic. Pain in bones. SEE: *osteocope.*

p., parenchymatous. That felt at the peripheral end of a nerve.

p., paresthesic. Stinging or tingling sensation manifested in central and peripheral nerve lesions. SEE: *paresthesia.*

p., phantom. That felt following an amputation and which seems to be in the missing limb.

p., postprandial. Abdominal pain after eating.

p., premonitory. Ineffective contractions of the uterus prior to the beginning of true labor.

p., pseudomyelic. False sensation of movement in a paralyzed limb or of no movement in a moving limb. Not a true pain.

p., psychic. Mental suffering such as that resulting from a sense of unworthiness or from feelings of guilt.

p., psychogenic. P. of mental origin which occurs in the absence of physical disorders.

p., psychosomatic. Pain due to mental or emotional disorders.

p., pulmonary. Sharp pain in the region of the lungs.

p., rectal, constant. Usually aggravated by defecation. May be due to ischiorectal abscess, anal abscess, inflamed or strangulated hemorrhoids, carcinoma, periproctitis, prostatic abscess, seminal vesiculitis, fecal impaction, acute salpingitis, tabes dorsalis, irritation from diarrhea, foreign bodies, fissures, rectal polyps, or adenoma. ***During defecation:*** Fissure in ano, ulcer, hemorrhoids, anal abscess, stenosis, stricture, dysentery, impaction, foreign body, or any inflammation.

p., referred. Pain seeming to arise in an area or point other than at its origin, as pain from appendicitis which often seems to occur in areas other than that of the appendix. SYN: *synalgia.*

p., reflex. A reflex action resulting from a painful stimulus. Pain reflexes are protective and prepotent, *i.e.,* tend to take precedence over less urgent reflexes.

p., regional. Pain in a specific area and its significance.

p., remittent. P. which subsides temporarily. Characteristic of neuralgia and colic.

p., root. Cutaneous pain caused by disease of sensory nerve roots.

p., shifting. Present in rheumatism, hysteria and locomotor ataxia.

p., shooting. SEE: *p., fulgurant.*

p., sick headache. Migraine, *q.v.*

p.'s, spot. Pains which seem to be located in patches of the integument.

p's., starting. Those accompanied by muscular spasm during early stages of sleep.

***p., subdiaphragmatic* (pleurisy).** A sharp, stitchlike pain occurring during breathing. When the breath is held, the pain ceases. Pressure against the lower costals eases the pain.

p., subjective. One that has no apparent physical basis for its existence. It may be found among the highly imaginative neurotics in whom mild sensations are translated into pain sense.

p., sympathetic. SEE: *p., referred.*

p., tenesmic. P. accompanying urination or defecation. SEE: *tenesmus.*

p., terebrant, p., terebrating. A boring type of pain.

p., thermalgesic. Pain caused by heat.

p., thoracic. A sharp pain over the sternum, often running down the arm to the elbow.

May be indicative of angina pectoris, although it must not be confused with pain from gastric pressure in the region of the heart, caused by an accumulation of gas.

It is increased with respiration, experienced in broken ribs; intercostal neuralgia; wounds, herpes zoster; pleurisy; pleurodynia; myalgia; periostitis; acute peritonitis; colic; hepatic, gastric, or renal ulcer; gallbladder disorders; carcinoma in late stages, and gumma of this region.

p., threshold of. SEE: *p., ceiling and threshold of.*

p., throbbing. Found in dental caries, headache, and associated with phlegmonous inflammation and suppuration.

p., tongue. SEE: *p., lingual.*

p., tracheal. Trachealgia.

p., wandering. One which changes its location repeatedly.

p., worry and anxiety. Worry and anxiety cause muscular tension resulting in pain which if long continued may interfere with nerve and blood circulation.

paint (pānt). A solution of medication for application to skin.

p., Castellani's. A germicide consisting of phenol, resorcinol, boric acid, acetone, and basic fuchsin.

painters' colic (pān'tĕrs). Colic accompanying lead poisoning. SEE: *Lead or its salts* in Table of Poisons and Poisoning in Appendix.

PAL. Abbr. for *posterior axillary line.*

palatable (păl'ăt-ă-bl) [L. *palatum,* palate]. Pleasing to the palate or taste, as food.

palatal (păl'ăt-ăl) [L. *palatum,* palate]. Pert. to the roof of the mouth, the palate.

p. reflex. Swallowing induced by stimulation of soft palate.

palate (păl'ăt) [L. *palatum,* palate]. 1. The horizontal structure separating the mouth and the nasal cavity; the roof of the mouth.

DISORDERS: *Koplik's Spots*: A rash frequently seen upon the palate in measles.

Secondary Syphilis: Indicated by mucous patches on the palate.

Herpes of the Throat: Shown by vesicles in circles upon the pharyngeal walls and soft palate.

Swelling of Uvula: Noted in inflammations of pharynx and tonsil, in nephritis, severe anemia, angioneurotic edema, and general debility. In diphtheria and Vincent's angina, a membranous exudate appears. In purpura hemorrhagica and some hemorrhagic diatheses, bloody extravasation appears.

Paralysis: May result from diphtheria, bulbar paralysis, neuritis, basal meningitis, tumor at base of brain.

Anesthesia: Seen in involvement of 2nd division of the 5th nerve.

RS: *Avellis' syndrome, Bednar's aphthae, cheilognathopalatoschisis, cleft, "palat-" words, "staphyl-" words, "uran-" words, "uvul-" words.*

p., artificial. Hard substance molded to fill a cleft in the palate.

p. bones. Bones forming post. part of hard palate and lateral nasal wall bet. the int. pterygoid plate of sphenoid bone and sup. maxilla.

p., cleft. One with congenital opening bet. 2 parts of palate.

p., falling. Abnormally long uvula.

p., gothic. An excessively high palate arch.

p., hard. Ant. part supported by the maxillary and palatine bones.

p., soft. Post. muscular, membranous fold partly separating the mouth and pharynx. SYN: *velum.*

palatine (păl'ă-tĭn) [L. *palatum,* palate]. 1. Concerning the palate. 2. The palate bones, *q.v.*

p. arches. SYN: *pillars.* Two archlike folds of mucous membrane *(glossopalatine* and *pharyngopalatine arches)* which form the lateral margins of faucial and pharyngeal isthmuses. They are continuous above with the soft palate.

p. artery, greater. A branch of the maxillary artery which supplies the palate, upper pharynx, and pharyngotympanic tube.

p. bone. Palate bones, *q.v.*

palatitis (păl-ăt-ī'tĭs) [" + G. *-itis,* inflammation]. Inflamed condition of the palate.

palatoglossus (păl"ă-tō-glŏs'ŭs) [*palatum,* palate, + G. *glōssa, tongue*]. SYN: *glossopalatinus.* Muscle arising from sides and under surface of tongue. Fibers pass upward through glossopalatine arch and are inserted in palatine aponeurosis. It constricts faucial isthmus by raising root of tongue and drawing sides of soft palate downward.

palatognathous (păl-ăt-og'nă-thŭs) [" + G. *gnathos,* jaw]. Having a congenital cleft in the palate.

palatography (pal"ă-tog'ră-fe). The recording of the movements of the palate in speech.

palatopharyngeus (păl"ăt-ō-far"ĭn-jē'ŭs) [L. *palatum,* palate, + G. *pharygx,*

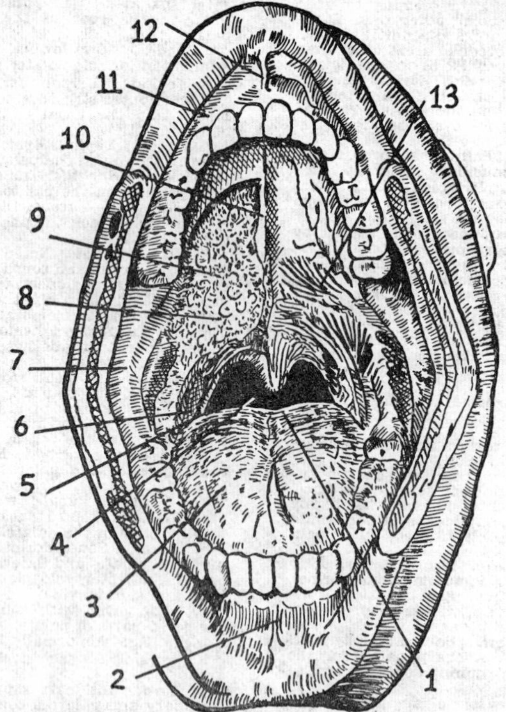

THE MOUTH OR BUCCAL CAVITY SHOWING THE HARD AND SOFT PALATE.

The dissection to the left shows the large mass of glandular tissue extending the full length of the palate; to the right the musculature of the soft palate and faucial pillars. 1. Isthmus of faucies. 2. Inferior lip frenulum. 3. Tongue surface (dorsum linguae). 4. Oropharynx. 5. Uvula. 6. Palatine tonsil. 7. Buccal cavity. 8. Soft palate. 9. Palatine glands. 10. Hard palate. 11. Gum (gingiva). 12. Superior lip frenulum. 13. Levator veli palitini.

pharygg-, pharynx]. Muscle arising from thyroid cartilage and pharyngeal wall and extending upward in post. pillar and inserting into aponeurosis of soft palate. Constricts pharyngeal isthmus, raises larynx, and depresses soft palate.

palatoplasty (păl′ăt-ō-plăs″tĭ) [“ + G *plassein,* to form]. Plastic surgery of the palate, usually to correct a cleft. SYN: *staphylorrhaphy, uranoplasty.*

palatoplegia (păl″ăt-ō-plē′jĭ-ă) [“ + G. *plēgē,* stroke]. Paralysis of muscles of the soft palate. SEE: *palate.*

palatorrhaphy (păl-ă-tor′ă-fĭ) [“ + G. *raphē,* a sewing]. Operation for uniting of a cleft palate. SYN: *staphylorrhaphy.*

palatoschisis (păl-ă-tŏs′kĭs-ĭs) [L. *palatum,* palate, + *schisis,* a fissure]. Palate with cleft in it.

paleencephalon, paleoencephalon (pā″lē-ĕn-sĕf′ă-lŏn, -ō-ĕn-sef′ă-lŏn) [G. *palaios,* old, + *egkephalos,* brain]. Phylogenetically older portion of the brain which includes all of it except the cerebral cortex and its allied structures.

paleo- [G. *palaios,* old, ancient]. Combining form meaning old or ancient.

paleocerebellum (pă″lō-ō-ser″ĕ-bĕl′lŭm). Phylogenetically, the older portion of the cerebellum which includes the flocculi, certain parts of the vermis (lingula, nodulus, uvula) and the lobulus centralis, culmen, pyramis, uvula, and simple lobule. These parts are primarily concerned with equilibrium and movements of locomotion.

paleogenesis (pā″lē-ō-jĕn′ĕ-sĭs) [“ + *genesis,* production]. Reproduction of ancestral characteristics without change, in a later generation, esp. abnormalities.

paleogenetic (pā″lē-ō-jĕn-ĕt′ĭk) [“ + *genesis,* production]. Having origin in a previous generation.

paleokinetic (pā″lē-ō-kĭn-ĕt′ĭk) [“ + G. *kinēsis,* motion]. Noting a peripheral motor nervous system controlling automatic associated movements and phylogenetically older than system controlling voluntary movement.

paleontology (pā″lē-ŏn-tŏl′ō-jĭ) [G. *palaios,* old, + *onta,* existing things, + *logos,* study]. Branch of biology dealing with ancient plant and animal life of the earth. SEE: *phylogeny.*

paleopathology (pā″lē-ō-păth-ŏl′ō-jĭ) [“ + *pathos,* disease, + *logos,* study]. The study of diseases in remains of bodies and fossils of ancient times.

paleostriatal (pā″lē-ō-strī-ā′tăl) [" + L. *striatus,* ridged]. Concerning the primitive portion of the corpus striatum.

paleostriatum (pā″lē-ō-strī-ā′tŭm) [" + L. *striatus,* ridged]. Primitive portion of corpus striatum, the globus pallidus. SEE: *neostriatum.*

paleothalamus (pā″lē-ō-thăl′ă-mŭs) [" + *thalamos,* chamber]. Medial portion of thalamus, the medullary, or noncortical part which is phylogenetically older. SEE: *thalamus.*

palikinesia (păl″ĭ-kĭn-ē′zĭ-ă) [G. *palin,* again, + *kinēsis,* motion]. Continued, involuntary, repetitious movements.

palilalia (păl-ĭ-lā′lĭ-ă) [" + *lalein,* to speak]. Pathologic repetitious use of words and phrases.

palinal (păl′ĭn-ăl) [G. *palin,* backward]. Moved or moving backward.

palindromia (păl-ĭn-drō′mĭ-ă) [" + *dromos,* a running]. The recurrence of a disease or a relapse.

palindromic (păl-ĭn-drŏm′ĭk) [" + *dromos,* a running]. Recurring, as the symptoms of a disease. SYN: *relapsing.*

palinesthesia (păl″ĭn-ĕs-thē′zĭ-ă) [" + *aisthēsis,* sensation]. Return of power of sensation, as after recovery from anesthesia or coma.

palingenesis (păl″ĭn-jĕn′ĕ-sĭs) [" + *genesis,* formation]. 1. Regeneration or restoration of an organism or part of one. 2. Reappearance of ancestral characteristics, esp. abnormal ones. SYN: *atavism, paleogenesis.*

palingraphia (păl″ĭn-grăf′ĭ-ă) [" + *graphein,* to write]. Pathologic repetition of words or phrases in writing.

palinphrasia, paliphrasia (păl-ĭn-frā′zĭ-ă, -ĭ-frā′zĭ-ă) [" + *phrasis,* speech]. Pathological condition in which there is coherent speech but certain words or phrases are frequently repeated. SYN: *palilalia.*

palladium (pă-la′de-ŭm) [the asteroid *Pallas*]. SYMB: Pd. Metallic element. At. wt. 106.4; at. no. 46. Used in dentistry and surgical instruments.

pallanesthesia (păl″ăn-ĕs-thē′zĭ-ă) [G. *pallein,* to shake, + *anaisthēsia,* anesthesia]. Loss of vibration sensation of skin and bones. SYN: *apallesthesia.* SEE: *pallesthesia.*

pallescence (pă-lĕs′ĕns) [L. *pallescere,* to grow pale]. Diminution of body color; a pale appearance. SYN: *pallor.*

pallesthesia (păl-ĕs-thē′zĭ-ă) [G. *pallein,* to shake, + *aisthēsis,* sensation]. The sensation of vibration felt in skin or bones, as that produced by a tuning fork when held against the body.

palliate (păl′ĭ-āt) [L. *pallium,* a cloak]. To ease or reduce in violence, to allay temporarily, as pain, without curing.

palliative (păl′ĭ-a-tĭv) [L. *pallium,* a cloak]. 1. Serving to relieve or alleviate, without curing. 2. An agent which alleviates or eases.

pallid (păl′ĭd) [L. *pallidus,* pale]. Lacking color, pale, wan.

pallidal (păl′ĭ-dăl) [L. *pallidus,* pale]. Concerning the pallidum of the brain.

pallidum (păl′ĭd-ŭm) [L. pale]. The globus pallidus of the lenticular nucleus in the corpus striatum.

pallium (păl′ĭ-ŭm) [L. cloak]. The cerebral cortex with its adjacent white substance, considered as a cover for rest of the brain. SYN: *brain mantle.*

pallor (păl′or) [L. *pallere,* to be pale]. Lack of color; paleness. SEE: *skin.*

palm (pahm) [L. *palma,* hand]. Ant. or flexor surface of the hand from wrist to fingers. SYN: *vola manus.* SEE: *antithenar, thenar.*

palmar (păl′mar) [L. *palma,* hand]. Concerning the palm of the hand.

p. or **darwinian reflex.** A grasping reflex in infants, more highly developed in some than in others. It gradually disappears and is absent after 4 or 5 months.

palmaris (păl-mā′rĭs) [L. *palma,* hand]. One of 2 muscles, *p. brevis* and *p. longus.* SEE: *Table of Muscles in Appendix.*

palm-chin reflex. Scratching the thenar eminence of the hand with a sharp object causes contraction of the chin muscles on the same side.

palmic (pal′mĭk) [G. *palmos,* a beat]. 1. Concerning palpitation or pulse. 2. Concerning palmus, *q.v.*

palmitic acid (pal-mĭt′ĭk). $CH_3(CH_2)_{14}$-COOH. A fatty acid found in solid fats, animal and vegetable, palm oil, some waxes and many fatty oils.

palmitin (pal′mĭt-ĭn). An ester of glycerol and palmitic acid, derived from fat of both animal and vegetable origin.

palmomen′tal reflex. SEE: *palm-chin reflex.*

palmoplantar (păl″mō-plănt′ar). SYN: *volar.* Pert. to the palms of the hands and soles of the feet.

palmus (păl′mŭs) [G. *palmos,* a throb]. 1. Palpitation; a throb. 2. Jerking; a disease with convulsive nervous twitching of the leg muscles, similar to jumping. 3. Heartbeat.

palpable (păl′pă-bl) [L. *palpāre,* to stroke]. Perceptible, esp. by touch.

palpate (păl′pāt) [L. *palpāre,* to touch]. To examine by touch; to feel.

palpation (păl-pā′shŭn) [L. *palpatiō,* a feeling]. Process of examining by application of the hands to the external surface of the body to detect evidence of disease in the various organs.

palpebra (pl. *palpebrae*) (păl′pe-bră, păl-pē′bră) [L. *palpebra,* eyelid]. An eyelid.

p. inferior. The lower eyelid.

p. superior. The upper eyelid.

palpebral (păl′pe-brăl) [L. *palpebra,* eyelid]. Concerning an eyelid.

p. cartilages. Thin plates of condensed tissue forming the framework of the eyelid. SYN: *tarsal cartilages.*

p. commissure. The union of the eyelids at each end of palpebral fissure.

p. fissure. The opening bet. the eyelids.

p. ligament. One of two ligamentous structures (medial and lateral) which fix the two ends of the tarsi to the orbital wall.

p. muscles. 1. Palpebral portion of m. orbicularis oculi. 2. Levator palpebra muscle.

palpebrate (păl′pē-brāt) [L. *palpebra,* eyelid]. 1. To wink. 2. Possessing eyelids.

palpitant (păl′pĭ-tănt) [L. *palpitāre,* to quiver]. Throbbing; trembling.

palpitate (păl′pĭ-tāt) [L. *palpitāre,* to quiver]. 1. To cause to throb. 2. To throb or beat intensely or rapidly, usually said of the heart.

palpitation (păl-pĭ-tā′shŭn) [L. *palpitāre,* to quiver]. Rapid, violent or throbbing pulsation, as an abnormally rapid throbbing, or fluttering of the heart. SEE: *heart.*

p., arterial. That felt in course of an artery.

palsy (pawl′zĭ) [M.E. *palesie,* from G.

paralysis, a disabling at the side]. 1. Temporary or permanent loss of sensation, or of ability to move, or to control movement. 2. A person disabled by palsy. SYN: *paralysis*.

p., Bell's. P. of the facial nerve at its periphery.

p., birth. P. arising from an injury received at birth.

p., cerebral. Bilateral, symmetric, nonprogressive paralysis resulting from developmental defects in brain or trauma at birth. SYN: *cerebral spastic infantile paralysis; Little's disease*.

p., crutch. P. resulting from pressure on nerves in the axilla from use of a crutch.

p., Erb's. A paralysis of the deltoid, biceps, long supinator, and brachialis anticus muscles due to a lesion of the brachial plexus or of the 5th and 6th cervical nerves.

p., lead. Paralysis of extremities in lead poisoning.

p., night. Form of paresthesia in which numbness is a symptom, esp. at night.

p., scrivener's. Writer's cramp.

p., shaking. Progressive muscular weakness and tremor with impaired voluntary motion. SYN: *paralysis agitans, Parkinson's disease*.

p., wasting. Chronic condition in which there is atrophy and paralysis of muscles which grow progressively worse. SYN: *progressive muscular atrophy*.

paludal (păl'ū-dăl) [L. *palus*, a marsh]. Concerning, or originating in, marshes. SYN: *malarial*.

paludism (păl'ū-dĭzm) [" + G. *ismos*, condition]. Swamp fever. SYN: *malaria, q.v.*

pampiniform (păm-pĭn'ĭ-form) [L. *pampinus*, a tendril, + *forma*, shape]. Convoluted like a tendril.

p. plexus. 1. A mesh of spermatic or ovarian veins. 2. Network of nerves supplying the testicles.

pampinocele (păm-pĭn'ō-sēl) [" + G. *kēlē*, swelling]. A swollen, painful condition of the veins of the spermatic cord. SYN: *varicocele*.

pan- [G.]. Combining form meaning *all*.

panacea (păn-ă-sē'ă) [G. *pas, pan-*, all, + *akeisthai*, to heal]. A remedy for all ills.

panagglutinin (păn-ăg-lū'tĭn-ĭn) [" + L. *agglutināre*, to glue to]. Substance capable of agglutinizing corpuscles of every blood group.

panaris (pă-nă'rĭs, pa'nă-rĭs) [L. *panaricium*, whitlow]. Inflammation of the skinfold surrounding the nail. SYN: *paronychia*.

panarthritis (păn-ar-thrī'tĭs) [G. *pas, pan-*, all, + *arthron*, joint, + *-itis*, inflammation]. 1. Inflammation of all parts of a joint. 2. Inflamed condition of all the joints in the body.

panasthenia (păn-ăs-thē'nĭ-ă) [" + *astheneia*, weakness]. Generalized weakness or exhaustion without evidence of organic disease. SYN: *neurasthenia, q.v.*

panatrophy (păn-ăt'rō-fĭ) [" + *a-*, priv. + *trophē*, nourishment]. 1. Wasting away of an entire structure. 2. Generalized wasting away of the body.

pancarditis (păn-kăr-dī'tĭs) [" + *kardia*, heart, + *-itis*, inflammation]. Inflamed condition involving all the structures of the heart.

panchreston (păn-krē'stŏn) [" + *chrestos*, useful]. A remedy for every disease. SYN: *panacea*.

panchromia (păn-krō'mĭ-ă) [" + *chrōma*, color]. Power of staining with numerous dyes.

pancreas (păn'krē-ăs) [G. *pas, pan-*, all, + *kreas*, flesh]. A compound tubulo-acinar or racemose gland situated behind the stomach in front of the 1st and 2nd lumbar vertebrae, in a horizontal position, its head attached to the duodenum and its tail reaching to the spleen. The portion between the head and the tail constitutes the body.

The gland is composed of *lobules* which form lobes connected by strands of tissue, with ducts which lead from

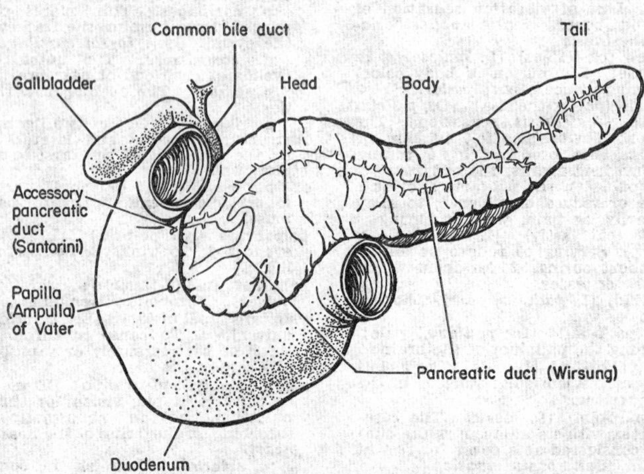

THE PANCREAS, DUCTS, AND DUODENUM.

the lobules into a main one, the *pancreatic duct*, or *duct of Wirsung*, which in turn is connected with the duodenum. Scattered throughout the substance are differentiated masses of cells which are the *islets of Langerhans*. An *accessory pancreatic duct* or *duct of Santorini* is frequently present. It is smaller than the main duct and opens into the duodenum cephalad to the main duct with which it communicates.

FUNCTIONS: The pancreas produces both an external and an internal secretion. The *external secretion*, called *pancreatic juice, q.v.*, is produced by the cells of the acini. It passes through the pancreatic ducts into the duodenum where it plays an important role in the digestion of all classes of foods. The *internal secretion*, which is elaborated by the islets of Langerhans, includes the hormones *insulin* and *glucagon* (hyperglycemic-glycogenolytic factor). These hormones, in conjunction with hormones from other endocrine glands (adrenal cortex and medulla, anterior hypophysis), play a primary role in the regulation of carbohydrate metabolism.

Diminished secretion of insulin by the islets of Langerhans results in a clinical entity called *diabetes mellitus, q.v.* In this disease there are disturbances in the metabolism of carbohydrates and fats resulting in the elevation of blood glucose, cholesterol, and ketones bodies. Urinary output is greatly increased and the urine usually contains glucose and ketone bodies.

Excessive secretion of insulin (*hyperinsulinism)* may sometimes occur. This results in the lowering of blood sugar *(hypoglycemia)*.

RS: *diabetes mellitis, secretin.*

p., accessory. Small mass of tissue close to the pancreas, apparently detached from it.

p., annular. An anomalous condition in which a portion of the pancreas encircles the duodenum.

p., dorsal. a dorsal outpocketing of the embryonic gut which gives rise to the body and tail of the adult pancreas.

p., fibrocystic disease of. SEE: *cystic fibrosis.*

p., little or lesser. Semidetached lobular part of post. surface of head of the p., sometimes having a separate duct opening into the principal one.

p., ventral. An outgrowth at the angle of the hepatic diverticulum and the embryonic gut which migrates and fuses with the dorsal pancreas. It forms the head of the definitive organ.

p., Willis'. SEE: *pancreas, little.*

pancreatalgia (păn″krē-ăt-ăl′jĭ-ă) [G. *pas, pan-*. all, + *kreas*, flesh, + *algos* pain]. Pain in the pancreas.

pancreatectomy (păn″krē-ăt-ĕk′tō-mĭ) [" + " + *ektomē*, excision]. Operation for removal of part or all of the pancreas.

Total pancreatectomy will produce diabetes because of a complete lack of insulin. Following a *subtotal* (or partial) *pancreatectomy*, diabetes will develop some time later because the remaining islets will be unable to take care of the excessive demands placed upon them.

SEE ALSO: *diabetes.*

pancreatemphraxis (păn″krē-ăt-ĕm-frăk′-sĭs) [" + " + *emphraxis*, stoppage]. Congestion of pancreas due to obstruction of pancreatic duct causing swelling of the gland.

pancreathelcosis (păn″krē-ăth-ĕl-kō′sĭs) [" + " + *elkōsis*, ulceration]. Ulcerated condition of the pancreas or its suppurative inflammation.

pancreatic (păn-krē-ăt′ĭk) [G. *pas, pan-*, all, + *kreas*, flesh]. Concerning the pancreas.

p. cystic fibrosis. SEE: *cystic fibrosis.*

p. juice. Its secretion is brought about by two hormones, *secretin* and *pancreozymin*, which are secreted by the duodenal mucosa. P. juice begins to flow when the acid contents of the stomach pass through the pylorus. It is a clear, viscid, alkaline fluid (pH 8.4-8.9) resembling saliva in consistency. It contains water, protein, inorganic salts, and enzymes. Among the enzymes are (a) *trypsinogen* which by the action of intestinal enterokinase is converted into *trypsin*, a proteolytic enzyme, (b) *chymotrypsinogen* which is converted by trypsin into *chymotrypsin*, a milkcurdling enzyme, (c) *amylopsin*, and a maltase which act on carbohydrates, and (d) *steapsin*, a lipase which acts on fats.

From 500 to 800 cc. are secreted every 24 hr. It is discharged into the duodenum through the duct of Wirsung.

Amylopsin hydrolyzes starch to maltose; steapsin hydrolyzes fats to fatty acids and glycerol; trypsinogen, by the action of enterokinase in the duodenum. is converted into the active form trypsin which hydrolyzes proteins to amino acids. The alkali neutralizes the acidity of the chyme entering the duodenum from the stomach.

RS: *duodenal digestion, enzyme, pancreas, secretion.*

pancreatico-enterostomy (păn″krē-ăt″ĭ-kō-en-ter-os′to-mĭ). Surgical creation of a passage between the pancreatic duct and the intestine.

pancreaticojejunostomy (păn″krē-ăt″ĭ-kō-jĕ-jū-nos′to-mĭ). Surgical creation of a passage between the pancreatic duct and the jejunum.

pancreaticocholecystostomy (păn″krē-ăt″-ĭ-kō-kō″le-sĭs-tos′tō-mĭ) [G. *pas, pan-*, all, + *kreas*, flesh, + *cholē*, bile, + *kystis*, bladder, + *stoma*, opening]. Surgical creation of passage bet. the gallbladder and pancreas.

pancreaticoduodenal (păn″krē-ăt″ĭ-kō-dū-ō-dē′năl) [" + " + L. *duodeni*, twelve]. Concerning the duodenum and pancreas.

pancreaticoduodenostomy (păn″krē-ăt″ĭ-kō-dū″ō-dē-nŏs′tō-mĭ) [" + " + " + G. *stoma*, opening]. Surgical creation of a passage bet. pancreas and duodenum.

pancreaticogastrostomy (păn″krē-ăt″ĭ-kō-găs-trŏs′tō-mĭ) [" + " + *gastēr*, belly, + *stoma*, opening]. Surgical creation of a passage bet. pancreas and the stomach.

pancreatin (păn′krē-ăt-ĭn) [" + *kreas*, flesh]. 1. One of the active ferments of the pancreas. 2. N.F. A mixture of enzymes obtained from pancreas of cattle or hog.

ACTION AND USES: Chiefly as a digestant. Inactive in presence of acid, should be adm. in combination with an alkali, as sodium bicarbonate.

pancreatitis (păn″krē-ă-tī′tĭs) [G. *pas, pan-*, all, + *kreas*, flesh, + *-itis*, inflammation]. Inflamed condition of the pancreas.

p., acute. Form characterized by necrosis, suppuration, gangrene, and hemorrhage.

SYM: Sudden and intense pain in epigastric region, vomiting, belching of gas, sometimes hiccough, collapse. Rigidity and tenderness over umbilicus. Constipation, slow pulse, possible jaundice.

p., calcareous. P. with calculi formation.

p., centrilobar. P. about divisions of the pancreatic duct.

p., chronic. Form marked by formation of scar tissue in pancreas associated with malfunction.

Pain mild or severe. Pain has tendency to radiate to the back. Jaundice, weakness, emaciation, diarrhea. SEE: *pancreas.*

p., hemorrhagic. Form with hemorrhage into pancreatic tissue.

SYM: Paroxysms of deep-seated pain in epigastrium, nausea, retching, constipation. Slight rise in temperature, blood and mucus in vomitus, delirium, tympanities, jaundice, hiccough, cyanosis, collapse.

p., interstitial. P. with overgrowth of inter- and intra-acinar connective tissue.

p., perilobar. Fibrosis of the pancreas bet. acinous groups.

p., purulent. P. with suppuration.

p., suppurative. Form marked by development of many small abscesses.

SYM: May be those of acute or chronic form.

pancreatoduodenectomy (păn″krē-ă-tō-dū″ō-dē-nĕk′tō-mĭ) [G. *pas, pan-*, all, + *kreas*, flesh, + L. *duodeni*, twelve, + G. *ektomē*, excision]. Excision of the head of the pancreas and the adjacent portion of the duodenum.

pancreatogenic, pancreatogenous (păn″-krē-ă-tō-jĕn′ĭk, -tŏj′ĕ-nŭs) [" + " + *gennan*, to produce]. Produced in or by the pancreas; having origin in the pancreas.

pancreatolith (păn-krē-ăt′ō-lĭth) [G. *pan*, all, + *kreas*, flesh, + *lithos*, stone]. A calculus of the pancreas.

pancreatolithectomy (păn″krē-ăt-ō-lĭth-ĕk′tō-mĭ) [" + " + " + *ektomē*, excision]. Removal of a concretion from the pancreas. SYN: *pancreatolithotomy.*

pancreatolithotomy (păn″krē-ăt-ō-lĭth-ot′-ō-mĭ) [" + " + " + *tomē*, an incision]. Removal of a concretion from the pancreas. SYN: *pancreatolithectomy.*

pancreatolysis (păn″krē-ăt-ŏl′ĭ-sĭs) [" + " + *lysis*, dissolution]. Destruction of the pancreatic substance.

pancreatolytic (păn″krē-ăt-ō-lĭt′ĭk) [" + " + *lysis*, dissolution]. Destructive to the pancreatic tissues. SYN: *pancreolytic.*

pancreatomy (păn-krē-at′ō-mĭ) [G. *pas, pan-*, all, + *kreas*, flesh, + *tomē*, incision]. Operation into the pancreas. SYN: *pancreatotomy.*

pancreatoncus (păn-krē-ăt-ong′kŭs) [" + " + *ogkos*, tumor]. A pancreatic tumor.

pancreatopathy (păn″krē-ăt-op′ă-thĭ) [" + " + *pathos*, disease]. Any pancreatic disease.

pancreatotomy (păn-krē-ă-tŏt′ō-mĭ) [" + " + *tomē*, incision]. Surgical incision into the pancreas. SYN: *pancreatomy.*

pancreectomy (păn-krē-ek′tō-mĭ) [" + " + *ektomē*, excision]. Partial or total excision of the pancreas.

pancreolithotomy (păn″krē-ō-lĭth-ŏt′ō-mĭ) [" + " + *lithos*, stone, + *tomē*, incision]. Surgical removal of a pancreatic concretion.

pancreolytic (păn-krē-ō-lĭt′ĭk) [" + " + *lysis*, dissolution]. Destructive to the pancreas.

pancreopathy (păn-krē-ŏp′ăth-ĭ) [" + " + *pathos*, disease]. Any diseased condition of the pancreas. SYN: *pancreatopathy.*

pancreozymin (păn″krē-ō-zĭm-ĭn). A hormone extracted from the duodenal mucosa which stimulates the secretion of pancreatic juice, especially increasing its enzymatic concentration.

pancytopenia (pan″si-to-pe′nĭ-ă) [G. *pan*, all, + *-cyte*, cell, + *penia*, poverty]. A reduction in all of the cellular elements of the blood. SEE: *anemia, aplastic.*

pandemia (păn-dē′mĭ-ă) [G. *pas, pan-*, all, + *dēmos*, the people]. Epidemic affecting the major portion of the population of a district.

pandemic (păn-dĕm′ĭk) [" + *dēmos*, the people]. 1. Affecting the majority of the population; said of a disease. 2. A disease affecting the majority of the population of a large region, or which is epidemic at the same time in many different parts of the world.

pandiculation (păn-dĭk-ū-lā′shŭn) [L. *pandiculārī*, to stretch oneself]. Stretching of the limbs and yawning, as on awakening from normal sleep.

Paneth, cells of [Josef Paneth, German physician, 1857-1890]. Large secretory cells containing coarse granules found at the blind end of the crypts of Lieberkuhn (the intestinal glands).

pang (păng) [M.E. *prange*]. 1. A paroxysm of extreme agony. 2. A sudden attack of any emotion.

pangenesis (păn-jĕn′ĕs-ĭs) [G. *pas, pan-*, all, + *genesis*, production]. Darwin's theory of reproduction in which each cell of the parent is represented by a particle in the reproductive cell, and thus each part of the organism reproduces itself in the progeny.

panglossia (păn-glŏs′sĭ-ă). Excessive garrulity, esp. in psychotic persons.

panhidrosis (păn-hĭd-rō′sĭs) [G. *pas, pan-*, all, + *idrōsis*, perspiration]. Perspiration over the entire surface of the body. SYN: *panidrosis.*

panhydrometer (păn″hī-drŏm′ĕt-ĕr) [G. *pan-*, all, + *ydor*, water, + *metron*, measure]. Apparatus for obtaining specific gravity of any fluid.

panhysterectomy (păn-hĭs-tĕr-ĕk′tō-mĭ) [" + *ystera*, uterus, + *ektomē*, excision]. Excision of entire uterus including the cervix uteri.

NP: Preparation same as for ovariohysterectomy. SEE: *hysterectomy.*

panhysterokolpectomy (păn-hĭs″tĕr-ō-kŏl-pĕk′tō-mĭ) [" + " + *kolpos*, vagina, + *ektomē*, excision]. Total excision of the uterus and vagina.

panhystero-oophorectomy. Excision of uterus, cervix uteri, and one or both ovaries.

panhysterosalpingo-oophorectomy. Excision of entire uterus, ovaries, and uterine tubes.

panic. A sudden overwhelming fright, esp. one without a reasonable cause.

panidrosis (păn-ĭd-rō′sĭs) [" + *idrōsis*, perspiration]. Panhidrosis, *q.v.*

panis (păn′ĭs) [L.]. Bread.

p., mica. Bread crumb.

panmyelophthisis (păn″mī-ĕl-of′thĭ-sĭs) [G. *pas, pan-*, all, + *myelos*, marrow, + *phthisis*, a wasting]. General wasting away of the bone marrow.

panmyelosis (păn″mī-ĕl-ō′sĭs) [" + " + *-ōsis*, intensive]. Increase in all the constituents of the bone marrow.

panneuritis (păn″ū-rī′tĭs) [" + *neuron*, sinew, + *-itis*, inflammation]. Generalized neuritis.

p. endemica, p. epidemica. Deficiency disease in which there is lack of vitamin B_1. SYN: *beriberi.*

panniculitis (pan-ĭk-ū-lī'tĭs) [L. *panniculus,* a small piece of cloth, + G. *-itis,* inflammation]. Inflamed condition of a layer of fatty connective tissue in the anterior wall of the abdomen.

SYM: Pain and tenderness and hypertrophy of tissue in parts where fat is the thickest.

panniculus (păn-ik'ū-lŭs) [L. a small piece of cloth]. A layer or sheet of tissue.

p. adiposus. The subcutaneous layer of fat, esp. where fat is abundant; the superficial fascia which is heavily laden with fat cells.

p. carnosus. Thin layer of muscular tissue in superficial fascia. SEE: *platysma myoides.*

pannus (păn'ŭs) [L. cloth]. Newly formed vascular tissue involving the upper half of the front of the cornea.

The area is cloudy, and its surface is uneven as it is covered with a film of new capillary blood vessels. May cover entire cornea. Seen in trachoma, acne rosacea, eczema, and as a result of irritation in granular conjunctivitis.

p. carateus. Pinta, *q.v.*

p. carnosus. SYN: *p. crassus, q.v.*

p. crassus. P. which is highly vascularized, thick, and opaque.

p. degenerativus. *P. siccus, q.v.*

p. siccus. P. accompanying xerophthalmia composed principally of connective tissue and poorly vascularized.

p. tenuis. P. which is thin, poorly vascularized, and with slight opacity.

panophobia (păn-ō-fō'bĭ-ă) [G. *pas, pan-,* all, + *phobos,* fear]. Morbid fear of some unknown evil or of everything in general; general apprehension. SYN: *pantophobia.*

panophthalmia, panophthalmitis (păn-ŏf-thăl'mĭ-ă, -mī'tĭs) [G. *pas, pan-,* all, + *ophthalmos,* eye, + *-itis,* inflammation]. Inflammation of entire eye.

panoptic (păn-ŏp'tĭk) [G. *pas pan.,* all, + *opsis,* sight]. Making every part visible.

p. stain. Stain which causes every part of the tissue to be differentiated.

panoptosis (păn-ŏp-tō'sĭs) [" + *ptōsis,* a dropping]. General prolapse of the abdominal organs.

panosteitis (păn"ŏs-tē-ī'tĭs) [" + *osteon,* bone, + *-itis,* inflammation]. Inflammation of every structure of a bone.

panotitis (păn-ō-tī'tĭs) [" + *ous, ōt-,* ear, + *-itis,* inflammation]. Inflammation involving all the parts of the ear.

panphobia (păn-fō'bĭ-ă) [" + *phobos,* fear]. Groundless fear of everything.

pansinusitis (pan"si-nus-i'tis). Inflammation of all of the paranasal sinuses.

pansphygmograph (păn-sfĭg'mō-grăf) [G. *pas, pan-,* all, + *sphygmos,* pulse, + *graphein,* to write]. Apparatus for registering cardiac movements, the pulse wave, and chest movements at one time.

Panstrongylus (păn-strŏn'jĭ-lŭs). A genus of insects belonging to the order Hemiptera, family Reduviidae.

p. megistus. Species which serves as vector for *Trypanosoma cruzi,* the causative agent of Chagas' disease.

pant (pănt) [O.Fr. *pantaisier,* to be breathless]. 1. To breathe hard; to gasp for breath. 2. A short or labored breath.

ETIOL: Produced by overexertion physically, as in running, or from fear.

pantachromatic (păn"tă-krō-măt'ĭk) [G. *pas, pan-,* all, + *a-,* priv. + *chrōma,* color]. Entirely colorless.

pantalgia (păn-tăl'jĭ-ă) [" + *algos,* pain]. Pain felt over the entire body.

pantatrophia, pantatrophy (păn-tă-trō-fĭ-ă, -tat'rō-fĭ). General wasting and atrophy.

panthodic (păn-thŏd'ĭk) [" + *odos,* way]. Radiating to all parts of the body, esp. applied to nervous impulses.

panting (pănt'ĭng) [O.Fr. *pantaisier,* to be breathless]. 1. Breathing hard; gasping for breath. 2. Labored breathing.

pantophobia (păn-tō-fō'bĭ-ă) [" + *phobos,* fear]. Morbid, groundless fear of everything in general. SYN: *panophobia.*

pantoscopic (păn"tō-skŏp'ĭk) [G. *pas, pan-,* all, + *skopein,* to examine]. Viewing everything; adjusted to both close and far objects.

p. glasses. Glasses with two segments of different focal lengths for near and far objects. SYN: *bifocal lenses.*

pantothenic acid (păn-tō-thĕn'ĭk). A vitamin of the B-complex group widely distributed in nature, occurring naturally in yeast, liver, heart, salmon, eggs, and various grains. It was synthesized in 1940.

pantothermia (păn"tō-thĕr'mĭ-ă). [G. *pan,* all, + *thermē,* heat]. Condition in which there is a variation in bodily temperature without any apparent reason.

pantropic (pan-tro'pik, -trop'ik). Showing affinity to many organs, as pantropic viruses. SYN: *polycytotropic.*

panturbinate (păn-tur'bĭ-nāt) [" + L. *turbinatus,* shaped like a top]. All of the turbinate structure of the nose.

pap (păp) [L. *papa,* infant's cry for food]. Any soft, semiliquid food.

papain (pa-pā'ĭn, pa'pā-ĭn). A digestive ferment containing a proteolytic enzyme. Obtained from the papaw fruit.

USES: A digestant.

Papanicolaou test. A uterine smear to detect cancer cells in the mucus of that organ. Commonly called *Pap test* or *Pap smear.*

papaverine hydrochloride (pă-păv'ĕr-ēn) [L. *papaver,* poppy]. The salt of an alkaloid obtained from opium.

USES: Antispasmodic, especially in gastric and intestinal distress, and recommended in bronchial spasm.

papaya. Fruit of the papaw tree.

paper (pā'pĕr), [G. *papyros,* a paper]. 1. A substance prepared in thin sheets from fibers of wood, rags, and other substances. 2. SYN: *charta.* A piece of paper specially prepared, as by having a medicinal preparation spread out on it.

p., bibulous. P. which absorbs water readily.

p., blistering. A paper saturated with a substance such as cantharides which causes vesiculation.

p., chromatography. Analysis of biological fluids by use of special papers which selectively permit the fluid constituents to migrate up the paper.

p., filter. A porous, unglazed paper used for filtration.

p., indicator. P. saturated with an indicator solution of known strength and then dried. Used for testing the *p*H (acidity or alkalinity) of a solution.

p., litmus. An indicator paper impregnated with litmus, which in alkalies turns blue, in acids red.

p., test. An indicator paper, *q.v.*

papilla (pă-pĭl'ă) (pl. *papillae*) [L. nipple]. A small, nipple-like protuberance or elevation.

p., circumvallate. One of the large

papillae near the base on the dorsal aspect of the tongue, arranged in a V-shape. The taste buds are located in the epithelium of the trench surrounding the papilla.

p., dental. A mass of connective tissue which becomes enclosed by the developing enamel organ. It gives rise to dentine and dental pulp.

p., dermal. Small elevations of the corium which indent the inner surface of the epidermis.

p., duodenal. SEE: *p. of Vater.*

p., filiform. One of the very slender papillae at tip of the tongue.

p., fungiform. One of the broad, flat papillae resembling a fungus, chiefly found on dorsal central area of tongue.

p., gustatory. Taste papilla of tongue; one of those possessing a taste bud.

p. (of) hair. A conical process of the corium which projects into undersurface of a hair bulb. It contains capillaries through which a hair receives its nourishment.

p., lacrimal. An elevation in medial edge of each eyelid for the lacrimal puncta.

p., lenticular. A small rounded elevation underlying lymphatic nodules in mucosa of root of tongue. SYN: *papillae lenticulare.*

p., lingual. Any one of the tiny eminences covering ant. two-thirds of tongue, including circumvallate, filiform, fungiform, and conical papillae.

p. mammae. [NA]. The nipple of the mammary gland. Also called *mammary papilla.*

p. of Vater. The duodenal end of the drainage systems of the pancreatic and common bile ducts. Commonly, but inaccurately, called ampulla of Vater. SYN: *duodenal papilla.*

p., optic. Point at which optic nerve fibers leave the eyeball. SYN: *blind spot; optic disk; papilla nervi optici.*

p., renal. Apex of a malpighian pyramid in the kidney.

p., tactile. A dermal papilla which contains a sensory end-organ for touch.

p., taste. SEE: *gustatory p.*

papillary (păp′ĭ-lar-ĭ) [L. *papilla,* nipple]. 1. Concerning a nipple or papilla. 2. Resembling or composed of papillae.

p. ducts of Bellini. Short ducts which open on tip of renal papilla. They are formed by union of the straight collecting tubules.

p. layer. SYN: *Stratum papillare.* The layer of the corium which adjoins the epidermis.

p. muscles. Muscular eminences in ventricles of the heart.

p. tumor. Neoplasm composed of or resembling enlarged papillae. SEE: *papilloma.*

papillate (păp′ĭl-āt) [L. *papilla,* nipple]. BACT: Having nipplelike growths on the surface, as a culture.

papillectomy (păp-ĭl-ĕk′tō-mĭ) [" + G. *ektomē,* excision]. Excision of any papilla or papillae.

papilledema (păp-ĭl-e-dē′mă) [" + *oidēma,* swelling]. Edema and inflammation of the optic nerve at its point of entrance into the eyeball.

ETIOL: Intracranial pressure, often caused by tumor of the brain pressing on optic nerve.

PROG: Unless relieved, blindness may result very rapidly. SYN: *choked disk.*

papilliferous (păp-ĭl-ĭf′ĕr-ŭs) [" + *ferre,* to carry]. Having or containing papillae.

papilliform (pă-pĭl′ĭ-form) [" + *forma,* shape]. Having the characteristics or appearance of papillae.

papillitis (păp-ĭl-ī′tĭs) [" + G. *-itis,* inflammation]. Inflammation of optic disk with edema. SYN: *choked disk.*

papilloadenocystoma (păp″ĭl-ō-ăd″ē-nō-sĭs-tō′mă) [" + G. *adēn,* gland, + *kystis,* a cyst, + *-ōma,* tumor]. A tumor composed of elements of papilloma, adenoma and cystoma.

papillocarcinoma (păp″ĭl-ō-kăr-sĭn-ō′mă) [" + G. *karkinos,* crab cancer, + *-ōma,* tumor]. 1. A malignant tumor of hypertrophied papillae. 2. Carcinoma with papillary growths.

papilloma (pl. *papillomata*) (păp-ĭ-lō′mă) [" + G. *-ōma,* tumor]. 1. Any benign epithelial tumor. 2. Epithelial tumor of skin or mucous membrane consisting of hypertrophied papillae covered by a layer of epithelium.

Included in this group are *warts, condylomas,* and *polypi.* SEE: *acanthoma.*

p. durum. A hardened p., as a wart.

p., hard. P. which develops from squamous epithelium.

p. molle. A p. with only a thin, horny layer covering it.

p., soft. P. formed from columnar epithelium.

papillomatosis (păp″ĭl-ō-mă-tō′sĭs) [" + " + *-ōsis,* disease]. 1. Widespread formation of papillomata. 2. Condition of being afflicted with many papillomata.

papilloretinitis (păp″ĭl-ō-rĕt-ĭn-ī′tĭs) [" + *rētē,* net, + G. *-itis,* inflammation]. Inflamed condition of the papilla and retina extending to the optic disk.

pappataci fever. SEE: *sandfly fever.*

pap′pose. Covered with fine, downy hair.

pap′pus. The first growth of hair appearing on the cheeks and chin as a fine, downy hair.

paprika (păp′rĭ-ka, păp-rē′kă) [G. *peperi,* pepper]. ASH CONST: Ca 0.229, Mg 0.164, K 2.075, Na 0.178, P 0.341, Cl 0.155. No iron or sulfur. VITAMINS: C+++. Used to add flavor and color to food.

papula (păp′ū-lă) [L.]. A pimple. SYN: *papule.*

papular (păp′ū-ler) [L. *papula,* pimple]. Of the nature of or concerning pimples.

p. fever. Mild fever with maculopapular eruptions and rheumatoid pains.

papulation (păp-ū-lā′shŭn) [L. *papula,* pimple]. 1. The development of papules. 2. The stage of pimple formation in a disease.

papule (păp′ūl) [L. *papula,* pimple]. Red elevated area on the skin, solid and circumscribed.

P.'s often precede vesicular or pustular formation and may appear in erythema multiforme, eczema papulosum, prurigo, syphilis, measles, smallpox, and they may develop after the use of bromides, iodides, coal tar preparations, etc.

In *measles* they are small and run together; in *smallpox* they are hard and feel like shot, terminating in umbilicated vesicles which itch. In *prurigo* they are small, pale, deep seated, and accompanied by intense itching; in *syphilis* they are dark colored and widely distributed, especially on the trunk and surfaces of the extremities. They do not cause itching. In *eczema* they are small, often associated with pustules and vesicles, and are closely aggregated; there is intense itching and the skin is thickened. In *erythema multiforme* they are found with macules and tubercles, and are bright red or purple and flat, appearing especially on the extremities. They do not suppurate or cause itching, but are accompanied by rheumatic pains and prostration.

p., dry. Hard one that is primary lesion of syphilis.

p., moist; p., mucous. A syphilitic eruption of papules with flat tops. Syn: *condyloma lata.*

papuliferous (păp″ū-lĭf′ĕr-ŭs) [L. *papula*, pimple, + *ferre*, to bear]. Having papules or pimples.

papulo- [L.]. Combining form meaning *a pimple, a papule.*

papyraceous (păp-ĭ-rā′shŭs) [L. *papyraceus*, made of papyrus, from G. *papyros*, parchment]. Parchmentlike.

Ob: Denoting a fetus retained in the uterus beyond natural term that has assumed a mummified appearance.

par [L. pair]. A pair, esp. a pair of cranial nerves.

p. vagum. The vagus or 10th pair of cranial nerves.

para (pl. *paras* or *parae*) [L. *parere*, to bring forth, to bear]. Combining form. A woman who has been delivered of living children as in multi*para*. Also used to describe those who have not delivered a living child as in nulli*para*. May also be used as a prefix as in Para-0 or Para-1 to indicate the number of living children a woman has delivered.

para-, par- [G.]. Combining forms meaning *alongside of, by, past, beyond, the opposite, abnormal, irregular.* Abbr: p- when used in chemistry to indicate *para-*.

para-aminobenzoic acid (păr″ă-ăm-ĭ-nō-bĕn-zō′ĭk). Commonly abbrev. *PABA.* A member of the vitamin B complex. Used in arthritis, rheumatic fever, fibrositis, gout, scleroderma, dermatomyositis. Inhibits bacteriostatic action of sulfonamides; hence contraindicated during sulfonamide therapy.

para-aminosalicylic acid (păr″ă-ăm-ĭ-nō-săl-ĭ-sĭl′ĭk). Commonly abbrev. *PAS.* An adjuvant to streptomycin or dihydrostreptomycin in treatment of tuberculosis. Valuable both for inhibitory effect on tubercle bacillus and for ability to delay development of streptomycin-resistant organisms.

para-anesthesia (păr″ă-ăn-ĕs-thē′zhĭ-a) [G. *para*, beside, + *an-*, negative, + *aisthēsis*, sensation]. Anesthesia of two corresponding sides, esp. of lower half of body.

para-appendicitis (păr″ă-ăp-ĕnd-ĭ-sī′tĭs) [" + L. *appendix*, + G. *-ītis*, inflammation]. Inflammation involving the connective tissue adjacent to the appendix. Syn: *perityphlitis.*

parabiosis (păr″ă-bī-ō′sĭs) [" + *biōsis*, living]. 1. Joining together of two individuals. This may occur congenitally as with Siamese twins or by surgical means. 2. Temporary suppression of excitability of a nerve.

parabiotic (păr″ă-bī-ŏt′ĭk) [G. *para*, beside, + *biōsis*, living]. Concerning parabiosis.

parablepsia, parablepsis (păr″ă-blĕp′sĭ-ă, -sĭs) [G. *para*, irregular, + *blepsis*, vision]. Abnormality of the visual sensations.

parabulia (păr-ă-bū′lĭ-ă) [" + *boulē*, will]. Perversion or abnormality of will power.

paracanthoma (păr-ă-kăn-thō′mă). A tumor involving the prickle-cell layer of the epidermis.

paracasein (păr-ă-kā′sē-ĭn). A substance formed when rennin or pepsin acts on the casein of milk. In the presence of calcium ions, an insoluble protein is formed resulting in the curdling of milk.

paracentesis (păr-ă-sĕn-tē′sĭs) [G. *para*, beside, + *kentēsis*, a puncture]. Puncture of a cavity with removal of fluid, as in pleural effusion or ascites.

NP: Watch pulse and respirations for signs of collapse during and following procedure.

p., abdominal. Tapping of the abdomen.

p. capitis. P. of the cranium.

p. cordis. Surgical puncture of the heart.

p. pericardii. P. of the pericardial sac.

p. pulmonis. Removal of fluid from a lung.

p. thoracis. Drainage of fluid from the cavity of the chest. See: *aspiration.*

p. tunicae vaginalis. P. of the tunica vaginalis.

p. tympani. Drainage or irrigation through incision of the tympanic membrane.

p. vesicae. Puncture of the wall of the urinary bladder.

paracentetic (păr″ă-sĕn-tet′ĭk) [G. *para*, beside, + *kentēsis*, a piercing]. Concerning paracentesis.

paracentral (păr″ă-sĕn′trăl) [" + *kentron*, center]. Located near the center.

p. lobule. Cerebral convolution on mesial surface joining the upper terminations of the ascending parietal and frontal convolutions.

paracholia (păr″ă-kō′lĭ-ă) [G. *para*, abnormal, + *cholē*, bile]. Condition of disturbed bile secretion.

parachordal (păr-ă-kord′ăl) [G. *para*, beside, + *chordē*, a cord]. 1. Lying alongside the anterior portion of the notochord. 2. A parachordal cartilage.

p. cartilage. One of a pair of cartilages in head of embryo which in man unite to form a single basal plate which is the forerunner of the occipital bone.

parachroma (păr-ă-krō′mă) [" + *chrōma*, color]. Discoloration, as that of the skin.

parachromatopsia (păr″ă-krō-mă-tŏp′sĭ-ă) [" + " + *opsis*, vision]. Color blindness.

parachromatosis (păr″ă-krō-mă-tō′sĭs) [" + " + *-ōsis*, disease]. Any one of the diseases in which the skin is pigmented.

parachromophoric (păr″ă-krō″mō-for′ĭk) [" + " + *phoros*, a carrier]. Excreting pigment, but retaining it within the organism.

paracinesia, paracinesis (păr″ă-sĭn-ē′zĭ-ă, -sĭs) [G. *para*, abnormal, + *kinēsis*, motion]. Condition in which there is perversion of motor powers; motor abnormality. Syn: *parakinesia.*

paracme [" + *akmē*, point]. Denoting the period of decrease of symptoms.

Paracoccidioides (par″ă-kŏk-sĭd″ē-oy′dēz). A genus of yeastlike fungi.

p. brasiliensis. The causative agent of paracoccidioidomycosis.

paracoccidioidomycosis (par″ă-kŏk-sĭd′ē-oy″dō-mī-kō-sĭs). Syn: *South American blastomycosis.* A chronic granulomatous disease of the skin caused by *Paracoccidiides brasiliensis.*

paracolitis (par-ă-kō-lī′tĭs). Inflammation of the tissue surrounding the colon.

Paracolobactrum. Found in gastroenteritis. Syn: *paracolon bacillus.*

paracolon bacilli. A group of colonlike bacilli which ferment lactose. Their pathogenicity is uncertain.

paracolpitis (păr″ă-kŏl-pī′tĭs) [G. *para*, abnormal, + *kolpos*, vagina, + *-ītis*, inflammation]. Inflammation of tissues adjoining the vagina.

paracolpium (păr"ă-kol'pĭ-ŭm) [G. *para,* abnormal, + *kolpos,* vagina]. The connective tissue adjacent to the vagina.

paracrisis (păr-ak'rĭ-sĭs, păr"ă-krĭ'sĭs) [" + *krisis,* a separation]. Any abnormality of the secretions.

paracusia, paracusis (par"a-kūs'ĭa, -sĭs) [" + *akousis,* a hearing]. Any abnormality or disorder of the sense of hearing.

p. acris. Excessively acute hearing.

p. duplicata. The hearing of one sound as two. SYN: *diplacusis.*

p. loci. Difficulty in estimating the direction of sound.

p. willisiana. An apparent ability to hear better in a noisy place, found in deafness due to stapes fixation and adhesive processes.

paracyesis (păr-ă-sī-ē'sĭs) [G. *para,* beside, + *kyēsis,* pregnancy]. Extrauterine pregnancy.

paracystitis (păr"ă-sĭs-tī'tĭs) [" + *kystis,* bladder, + *-itis,* inflammation]. Inflamed condition of connective tissues and other structures around the urinary bladder.

paracystium (păr-ă-sĭs'tĭ-ŭm) [" + *kystis,* bladder]. The connective tissue surrounding the urinary bladder.

paradenitis (păr"ăd-en-ī'tĭs) [" + *adēn,* gland, + *-itis,* inflammation]. Inflammation of tissues around a gland.

paradidymis (păr-ă-did'ĭ-mĭs) [" + *didymos,* testicle]. BNA. The atrophic remnants of the tubules of the wolffian body, situated on the spermatic cord above the epididymis. SYN: *massa innominata, organ of Giraldès.*

paradione (par-ă-di'ōn). Proprietary name for a preparation of paramethadione, an anticonvulsant drug.

paradoxic, paradoxical (păr"ă-dŏk'sĭk, -sĭkal) [G. *paradoxos,* contrary to opinion]. Seemingly contradictory, but demonstrably true.

paraffin (păr'ă-fĭn) [L. *parum,* too little, + *affinis,* allied]. 1. A waxy, white, tasteless, odorless mixture of solid hydrocarbons obtained from petroleum.

2. One of a series of saturated aliphatic hydrocarbons having the formula C_nH_{2n-2}. Paraffins constitute the *methane* or *paraffin series.*

p., hard. Solid p. with a melting point bet. 45° C. and 60° C.

p., liquid. Liquid hydrocarbon. SYN: *liquid petrolatum.*

p., soft. A semisolid p. SEE: *petrolatum.*

paraffinoma (păr"ă-fĭn-ō'mă) [" + " + G. *-ōma,* tumor]. A tumor which arises at site of injection of paraffin.

paraffinum (păr-ă-fē'nŭm) [L.]. Paraffin, *q.v.*

paraformaldehyde (par"ă-fōr-măl'dĕ-hīd). A white, powdered antiseptic and disinfectant, a polymer of formaldehyde.

paragammacism (păr"ă-găm'mă-sĭzm) [G. *para,* beside, + *gamma,* Greek letter G, + *ismos,* condition]. Inability to pronounce "g," "k," and "ch" sounds, with substitution of other consonants, such as "d" or "t," for them.

paraganglia (păr"ă-găng'lĭ-ă). Plural of paraganglion. Groups of chromaffin cells similar in staining reaction to cells of the adrenal medulla which are associated anatomically and embryologically with the sympathetic system. They are located in various organs and parts of the body.

paraganglioma (păr"ă-găng-lĭ-ō'mă) [G. *para,* beside, + *gagglion,* knot, + *-ōma,* tumor]. A tumor derived from chromaffin cells. Includes tumors of the adrenal medulla and the paraganglia. SYN: *pheochromocytoma.*

paraganglion (pl. *paraganglia*) (păr"ă-găng'lĭ-ŏn) [G. *para,* beside, + *gagglion,* knot]. SEE: *paraganglia.*

parageusia, parageusis (păr-ă-gū'sĭ-ă, -sĭs) [" + *geusis,* taste]. Disorder or abnormality of the sense of taste.

paraglobulin (păr"ă-glŏb'ū-lĭn) [" + L. *globulus,* a small sphere]. A globulin found in blood plasma, lymph, and other body fluids, associated with coagulation.

paraglobulinuria (păr"ă-glŏb-ū-lĭn-ū'rĭ-ă) [" + " + G. *ouron,* urine]. Excretion of paraglobulin in the urine.

paraglossa (păr-ă-glŏs'să) [" + *glōssa,* tongue]. 1. Enlargement of the tongue. 2. Congenital hypertrophy of the tongue.

par"aglos'sia. Inflammation of the tissues underlying the tongue.

paragomphosis. Impaction of the fetal head in the pelvic canal.

Paragonimus (păr"ă-gŏn'ĭm-ŭs). Genus of trematode worms.

P. westermanii. The lung fluke, a common parasite of the mink in the U.S. Human infestation occurs through eating raw crabs or crayfish, the second intermediate host. Infestation endemic in certain parts of Orient.

par"agram'matism. A speech defect characterized by improper use of words and inability to arrange them grammatically.

paragraphia (păr-ă-grăf'ĭ-ă) [G. *para,* besides, + *graphein,* to write]. The writing of letters or words other than those intended.

par"ahem"ophil'ia. A rare congenital, idiopathic disorder due to deficiency of factor V characterized by prolonged prothrombin and coagulation times.

parahepatitis (păr"ă-hĕp-ă-tī'tĭs) [G. *para,* beside, + *ēpar, ēpat-,* liver, + *-itis,* inflammation]. Inflamed condition of parts immediately adjacent to the liver.

par"ahor'mone. A substance which is conveyed through the circulatory system and exerts a stimulating effect like hormones, yet not originating in endocrine tissue.

Ex: *carbon dioxide.*

par"ahypno'sis. Abnormal or disordered sleep.

parainfection (păr"ă-ĭn-fĕk'shŭn) [G. *para,* beside, + L. *in,* into, + *facere,* to make]. The symptomatology of an infectious disease without evidence of the presence of the microorganisms causing the disease.

parakeratosis (păr"ă-kĕr-ă-tō'sĭs) [" + *keras, kerat-,* horn, + *-ōsis,* infection]. Any disorder affecting the horny layer of the epidermis.

p. psoriasiformis. Scab formation resembling that of psoriasis.

p. scutularis. Scalp disease with hairs encircled by epidermic crust formation.

parakinesia. SEE: *paracinesia.*

paralalia (păr-ă-lā'lĭ-ă) [G. *para,* abnormal + *lalein,* to babble]. Any speech defect, characterized by sound distortion.

p., literalis. Stammering, *q.v.*

paralambdacism (păr"ă-lăm'dă-sĭzm) [G. *para,* beside, + *lambda,* Greek letter L, + *ismos,* condition]. Inability to sound the letter "l" correctly, substituting some other letter for it.

paralbumin (păr-ăl-bū'mĭn) [" + L. *albumen,* white of egg]. An albumin found in fluid content in ovarian cysts and in ascites.

paraldehyde (păr-ăl'dĕ-hīd). USP. $C_6H_{12}O_3$. A liquid polymer of acetaldehyde which is colorless, with characteristic unpleasant odor and taste.

Made by action of hydrochloric acid on acetic aldehyde.

ACTION AND USES: Hypnotic, having low toxicity and prompt action as a sedative. Sometimes used as an analgesic in obstetrics, esp. in combination with rectal ether.

POISONING: SYM: Resemble those of chloral hydrate, cardiac and respiratory depression, dizziness, collapse with partial or complete anesthesia. Odor on the breath is a constant distinct sign.

F. A. TREATMENT: Same as for chloral hydrate, *q.v.*

paraldehydism (păr-ăl'dĕ-hīd-ĭzm). Poisoning from an overdose of paraldehyde, *q.v.*

paralepsy (par'ă-lĕp"sĭ) [G. *para*, besides, + *lēpsis*, seizure]. Temporary attack of mental inertia and hopelessness, or sudden alteration in mood or mental tension. SYN: *psycholepsy.*

paralexia (păr-ă-lĕk'sĭ-ă) [G. *para*, abnormal, + *lexis*, speech]. Inability to comprehend printed words or sentences with substitution of meaningless combinations of words.

paralgesia (păr-ăl-jē'zĭ-ă) [" + *algēsis*, pain]. Any unusual sensation which is painful.

paralgia (păr-al'jĭ-ă) [" + *algos*, pain]. Sensation both abnormal and painful.

parallagma (păr-ăl-ăg'mă) [G. *parallagma*, alternation]. Overlapping or displacement of the fragments of a fractured bone.

parallax (păr'ă-lăks) [G. *paraliax*, in turn]. The apparent movement or displacement of objects due to a change in position of the observer or movement of the head or eyes.

paralogia (păr-ă-lō'jĭ-ă) [G. *para*, abnormal, + *logos*, understanding]. A disorder of the reasoning; a psychosis.

paralutein cells. Theca lutein cells. SEE: *Lutein cells.*

paralysis (pă-ral'ĭ-sĭs) [G. *paralyein*, to disable at the side]. Temporary suspension or permanent loss of function, esp. loss of sensation or voluntary motion.

Any voluntary movement depends on the integrity of two motor neurons; one arising in the motor cortex, coursing across the brain stem and ending in the ant. gray horn of the spinal cord, and the lower neurons arising in the ant. horn cell and passing to the muscle. If the latter are destroyed, the muscle loses tone, atrophies (withers away) and shows reaction of degeneration (R. D.).

The flaccidity and absent muscular reflexes reveal the loss of tonus. If the upper neuron is paralyzed, the patient is equally unable to move the affected part, but the intact lower neuron may permit other motor centers to act on the muscle. In addition, tone is increased, there is no R. D. and no atrophy save that of disuse. So-called pathological reflexes may appear in addition to the increase of normal deep reflexes.

Paralyses are divided into 2 groups, *spastic*, when due to lesion of upper motor neuron, and *flaccid*, when due to lesion of lower motor neuron.

Psychic inhibition of motor function occurs most characteristically in hysteria, but the evidence of organic disease is always lacking in these hysterical paralyses.

p. of accommodation. Inability of the eye to adjust itself to various distances due to paralysis of ciliary muscles.

p., acoustic. Deafness, *q.v.*

p., acute ascending. Rapidly progressing form of paralysis which begins in the feet and slowly ascends. Fatal. SYN: *Landry's p.*

p., acute atrophic. SEE: *p., infantile.*

p., acute infectious. SEE: *p. infantile.*

p. agitans. A disease of middle and late life producing a picture of rigid tremulousness progressive in its course, and marked by weakness, delay of voluntary motion, a peculiar festinating gait, and muscular contraction, causing peculiar and characteristic positions of the limbs and head. While movement is slow, there is no true paralysis. The face appears expressionless, there is general flexion attitude, the balance tends to be lost (in a forward direction). Sometimes occurs following encephalitis lethargica; others are due to an unknown cause. SYN: *Parkinson's disease, q.v.*

p., alcoholic. P. due to habitual drunkenness.

p., anesthesia. P. which develops following administration of anesthesia.

p., anterior spinal. SEE: *p., infantile.*

p., arsenical. P. following poisoning from arsenic.

p., ascending. P. beginning with the lower limbs and progressing upward.

p., association. SEE: *p., bulbar.*

p., Bell's. Facial paralysis.

ETIOL: Lesion of the facial nerve or of its nucleus; a neuritis of this nerve. Pressure on nerve as it reaches the face through its bony canal near the ear.

SYM: One side of entire face may be affected, or corner of mouth may drop, eyelid may droop or be unable to close, may be unable to close lips or to speak, or loss of control of eye.

p., Bernhardt's. Pain and hyperesthesia on the outer femoral surface from lesion or disease of the external cutaneous nerve of the thigh.

p., birth. P. caused by injury received at birth.

p., brachial. Paralysis of one or both arms.

p., brachiofacial. P. of the face and an arm.

p., Brown-Sequard's. P. of motion on one side and of sensation on the other.

p., bulbar. P. caused by changes in the motor centers of the brain stem.

p., central. Any paralysis from a lesion of the brain or spinal cord.

p., cerebral spastic infantile. Nonprogressive paralysis resulting from developmental defects in brain or from trauma at birth. SYN: *cerebral palsy; Little's disease.*

p., complete. P. in which there is total loss of function.

p., compression. P. due to pressure on a nerve, as by a crutch or during sleep.

p., crossed. P. of the face on one side of the body and the limbs on the opposite side.

p., crutch. P. due to pressure in the armpit.

p., decubitus. P. due to pressure on a nerve from lying in one position for a long time.

p., diver's. P. due to decrease in

pressure after a diver has been exposed to pressure greater than atmospheric pressure. SYN: *saisson disease* or *bends.*

p., Erb's. 1. SEE: *p., birth.* 2. Partial p. of the brachial plexus.

p., exhaustion. P. due to prolonged voluntary movements involving exhaustion of the nerve centers.

p., facial. SEE: *p., Bell's.*

p., flaccid. P. in which there is loss of muscle tone, loss of or reduction of tendon reflexes, atrophy and degeneration of muscles, and reaction of degeneration is manifest. Due to lesions of lower motor neurons of spinal cord.

p., general. Progressive loss of power and the mental faculties resulting eventually in dementia and death. SYN: *paresis.*

p., ginger. P. of the limbs after drinking Jamaica ginger. SYN: *Jamaica ginger polyneuritis, q.v.*

p., glossolabial. P. of the tongue and lips. Occurs in bulbar paralysis, *q.v.*

p., histrionic. Paralysis of certain facial muscles, producing a facial expression of some emotion.

p., hysteric. One that may simulate any form of paralysis; it appears to have no adequate causative lesion.

p., incomplete. Partial paralysis of the body or a part.

p., infantile. Motor paralysis with atrophy of a group of muscles following an acute infectious disease in children which is transmitted by a filtrable virus. SYN: *acute anterior poliomyelitis.*

p., ischemic. P. resulting from impaired blood supply.

p., jake. SEE: *p., ginger.*

p., Klumpke's. Wasting p. of the arms and hands.

p., Kussmaul's; p., Landry's. SEE: *p., acute ascending.*

p., lead. P. following poisoning by lead.

p., local. P. of a single muscle or one group of muscles.

p., muscular. Loss of the capacity of muscles to contract. May be due to a structural or functional disorder in the muscle, at the myoneural junction, in efferent nerve fibers, in cell bodies of nuclei of origin of brain or gray matter of spinal cord, in conducting pathways of brain or spinal cord, or motor centers of the brain.

p., nuclear. P. caused by lesion of a nerve nucleus in the central nervous system.

p., obstetrical. SEE: *p., birth.*

p., periodic. P. which recurs and abates temporarily.

p., phonetic P. of the vocal cords.

p., progressive bulbar. SEE: *p., bulbar.*

p., pseudobulbar. P. caused by cerebral center lesions, which simulates the bulbar types of paralysis.

p., sensory. Loss of sensation. May be due to a structural or functional disorder of the sensory end-organs, sensory nerves, conducting pathways of spinal cord or brain, or sensory centers in the brain.

p., spastic. P. usually involving groups of muscles and characterized by excessive tone and spasticity of muscles, exaggeration of tendon reflexes but loss of superficial reflexes, positive Babinski response, no atrophy or wasting except from prolonged disuse, and absence of reaction of degeneration. Due to lesions of upper motor neurons or cerebrum.

p., spinal. P. due to injury or disease of the spinal cord.

p., supranuclear. P. resulting from disorders in pathways or centers above nuclei of origin.

p., tick-bite. P. resulting from bites of certain species of ticks, esp. of the genera Ixodes and Dermacentor, presumably due to a toxin present in saliva of tick. Affects domestic animals and humans, esp. children. Causes a progressive ascending, flaccid, motor paralysis. Recovery usually occurs after removal of ticks.

p., Todd's. A transitory paralysis following an epileptic seizure.

p., tourniquet. P., esp. of the arm, resulting from a tourniquet being applied for too long a time.

p., vasomotor. P. of vasomotor centers resulting in lack of tone and vasodilation of blood vessels.

p., Volkmann's. SEE: *p., ischemic.*

p., wasting. Progressive wasting away of the muscles. SEE: *progressive muscular atrophy.*

paralytic (păr-ă-lĭt'ĭk) [G. *para,* beside, + *lyein,* to loosen]. 1. Concerning paralysis. 2. One afflicted with paralysis.

p. dementia. Progressive paralysis with mental deterioration. SYN: *paresis.*

p. ileus. P. of intestinal wall with distention and symptoms of acute obstruction and prostration.

ETIOL: It may occur after any abdominal operation.

paralyzant (păr'ă-līz"ănt) [" + *lyein,* to loosen]. 1. Causing paralysis. 2. A drug or other agent that induces paralysis.

paralyze (păr'ă-līz) [" + *lyein,* to loosen]. 1. To cause temporary or permanent loss of muscular power or sensation. 2. To render ineffective.

paramastitis (păr-ă-măs-tī'tĭs) [" + *mastos,* breast, + *-ītis,* inflammation]. Inflammation around the mamma.

paramedic (par"ă-med'ik). A physician or trained medical assistant who parachutes to areas where medical services are needed.

paramedical. Supplementing the work of medical personnel.

paramenia (păr-ă-mē'nĭ-ă) [" + *mēniaia,* menses]. Irregular, abnormal or difficult menstruation.

parameter (par-am'e-ter) [" + *metron,* measure]. An arbitrary constant characterizing the mathematical expression in which it appears by its values.

paramethadione (par"ă-meth"ă-di'ōn). An anticonvulsant agent. It is used to control petit mal seizures in epilepsy. 3-Dimethyl-5-ethyl + oxozolidine-2,4-dione.

parametric (păr-ă-mĕt'rĭk) [" + *mētra,* uterus]. 1. Concerning the area near the uterus. 2. Rel. to the parametrium, the tissue surrounding the uterus.

parametritis (păr"ă-mē-trī'tĭs) [G. *para,* beside, + " + *-ītis,* inflammation]. Inflamed condition of parametrium, the cellular tissue adjacent to uterus. SYN: *cellulitis, pelvic.*

parametrium (păr-ă-mē'trĭ-ŭm) [" + *mētra,* uterus]. Fat and connective tissue around the uterus.

paramimia (păr-ă-mĭm'ĭ-ă) [G. *para,* beside, + *mimeisthai,* to imitate]. Use of gestures which are inappropriate to the spoken words.

paramnesia (păr-ăm-nē'zĭ-ă) [" + *a-,* priv. + *mnēsis,* memory]. 1. the use of words without meaning. 2. Inability to distinguish imaginary or suggested experiences from those which have actually occurred. 3. Seeming recall of events which never have occurred.

paramorphia (păr-ă-mor′fĭ-ă) [" + *morphē*, form]. Abnormality of shape.

paramusia (păr-ă-mū′zĭ-ă) [G. *para*, beside, + *amousia*, want of harmony]. A form of aphasia in which the ability to render music correctly is lost.

paramyoclonus multiplex [G. *para*, beside, + *mys, my-*, muscle, + *klonos*, tumult]. Sudden and frequent shocklike contractions usually affecting muscles of both legs. The contractions which disappear during sleep and motion, may occur 10 to 50 times each minute.

paramyosinogen (păr″ă-mī″ō-sĭn′ō-jĕn) [" + *mys, my-*, muscle, + *gennan*, to produce]. Protein derived from muscle plasm.

paramyotonia (păr″ă-mī″ō-ō′nĭ-ă) [" + " + *tonos*, tone]. A disorder marked by muscular spasms and abnormal muscular tonicity.

p. ataxia. Tonic muscular spasm when making any movement, with slight ataxia or paresis.

p. congenita. Syn: *Eulenberg's disease.* Congenital condition of tonic muscular spasms when body is exposed to cold.

p., symptomatic. Temporary muscular rigidity when first trying to walk, as in paralysis agitans.

par″anos′al. Situated near or alongside the nasal cavities.

p. sinuses. The frontal, maxillary, ethmoid, and sphenoid sinuses.

paranephritis (păr″ă-ne-frī′tĭs) [G. *para*, beside, + *nephros*, kidney, + *-itis*, inflammation]. 1. Inflamed condition of the suprarenal capsules. 2. Inflammation of connective tissue about kidney. Syn: *perinephritis.*

paranephros (păr-ă-nĕf′rŏs) [" + *nephros*, kidney]. A suprarenal or adrenal capsule.

paranoia (păr-ă-noy′ă) [G. *para*, abnormal, + *nous*, mind]. A chronic, psychotic entity characterized by fixed but ever-expanding systematized delusions of persecution.

General characteristics are sensitive, suspicious, jealous, brooding nature; excessive self-consciousness; fixed ideas, developed into well-systematized, logical delusions, megalomania, rare hallucinations, inability to make concessions.

paranoiac (păr-ă-noy′ăk) [" + *nous*, mind]. 1. One suffering from paranoia. 2. Concerning or afflicted with paranoia.

paranoid (păr′ă-noyd) [G. *para*, not normal, + *nous*, mind, + *eidos*, like]. 1. Resembling paranoia. 2. A person afflicted with paranoia.

p. reaction type. Individual who has fixed, systematized delusions, is suspicious, has a persecution complex and is resentful, bitter, and a megalomaniac.

Many states approach true paranoia and resemble it, but lack one or more of its distinguishing features. Some of these are: (*a*) Transitory p. states due to toxic conditions; (*b*) p. type of schizophrenia; (*c*) p. states due to alcoholism.

NP: In dealing with all types of paranoid patients, do not handle without an assistant.

paranomia (păr-ă-nō′mĭ-ă) [G. *para*, beside, + *onoma*, name]. Form of aphasia in which there is inability to remember correct name of objects shortly after seeing or using them.

paranorm′al. 1. Alongside or aside from the normal. Pertaining to experiences that appear to happen outside of the known. 2. Moderately abnormal.

paranuclein (păr″ă-nū′klē-ĭn) [" + L. *nucleus*, a kernel]. A protein which does not yield nitrogenous bases when decomposed. Syn: *nucleoalbumin.*

paranucleus (păr″ă-nū′klē-ŭs) [" + L. *nucleus*, a kernel]. A small body lying close to a cell nucleus.

paraomphalic (păr″ă-ŏm-făl′ĭk) [" + *omphalos*, navel]. Adjacent to the navel. Syn: *paraumbilical.*

paraoperative (păr″ă-ŏp′ĕr-ă-tĭv) [" + L. *opus, oper-*, work]. Concerning all the details and the accessories of operation and preparation of the patient.

paraosteoarthropathy (păr″ă-ŏs″tē-ō-ăr-thrŏp′ăth-ĭ) [" + *osteon*, bone, + *arthron*, joint, + *pathos*, disease]. Paralysis of lower portion of the body in addition to bone and joint disease.

paraparesis (păr″ă-păr-ē′sĭs, -par′ĕ-sĭs) [" + *paresis*, paralysis]. Partial paralysis affecting the lower limbs.

parapathia (păr-ă-păth′ĭ-ă) [G. *para*, beside, + *pathos*, disease]. Emotional aspects of a disorder.

parapedesis (păr″ă-pĕd-ē′sĭs) [G. *para*, beside, + *pedēsis*, a bending]. Secretion through other than normal channels.

parapeptone (păr″ă-pĕp′tōn) [" + *peptein*, to digest]. Intermediate digestion product of albumin. See: *peptone.*

paraphasia (păr-ă-fā-zĭ-ă) [G. *para*, abnormal, + *a-*, priv., + *phasis*, speech]. The misuse of words or word combinations spoken; a form of aphasia.

paraphemia (păr″ă-fē′mĭ-ă) [" + *phēmē*, speech]. A disorder marked by consistent use of the wrong words, or mispronunciation of words.

paraphia (păr-ă′fĭ-ă) [" + *aphē*, touch]. Abnormality of the sense of touch.

paraphimosis (păr″ă-fĭ-mō′sĭs) [" + *phimoein*, to muzzle]. Strangulation of glans penis due to retraction of foreskin.

p. oculi. Retraction of eyelid in back of eyeball.

paraphobia (păr-ă-fō′bĭ-ă) [G. *para*, abnormal, + *phobos, fear*]. A mild form of phobia.

paraphonia (păr″ă-fō′nĭ-ă) [" + *phōnē*, voice]. Partial loss or weakness or abnormal change of the voice.

p. puberum. A harsh, deep voice that develops in boys at puberty.

paraphora (păr-ăf′ō-ră) [G. a wandering]. A mental disorder of minor degree.

paraphrasia (păr-ă-frā′zĭ-ă) [G. *para*, abnormal, + *phrasis*, speech]. Disorder characterized by incoherent speech. Syn: *paraphasia.*

paraphrenia (păr-ă-fre′nĭ-ă) [" + *phrēn*, mind]. A group of psychoses now called "paranoid conditions."

p. confabulans. P. marked by memory distortions.

p. expansiva. P. with delusions of grandeur, exaltation and moderate excitement.

p., phantastica. P. with unsystematized delusions.

p. systematica. P. with progressive delusions of persecution, followed by delusions of grandeur, but personality shows no deterioration.

paraphrenitis (păr″ă-frē-nī′tĭs) [G. *para*, beside, + *phrēn*, mind, diaphragm, + *-itis*, inflammation]. Inflammation of the tissues around the diaphragm.

paraplasm (păr′ă-plăzm) [" + *plasma*, a thing formed]. 1. Any abnormal new formation or malformation. 2. The fluid portion of protoplasm. Syn: *hyaloplasm.*

paraplastic (păr-ă-plăs′tĭk) [G. *para*, beside, + *plastikos*, formed]. 1. Pert. to fluid portion of protoplasm. 2. Misshapen; deformed.

paraplectic (păr-ă-plĕk′tĭk) [G. *paraplēktikos*, striking at the side]. Afflicted with paralysis of lower extremities. SYN: *paraplegic*.

paraplegia (păr-ă-plē′jĭ-ă) [G. *para*, beside, + *plēgē*, a stroke]. Paralysis of lower portion of the body and of both legs.

ETIOL: A lesion involving the spinal cord which may be due to the following: maldevelopment, epidural abscess, hematomyelia, acute transverse myelitis, spinal neoplasms, multiple sclerosis, or syringomyelia. May also be due to trauma.

p., alcoholic. P. of spinal origin due to excessive use of alcohol.

p., ataxic. Lateral and post. sclerosis of spinal cord, combined, and resulting symptoms.

p., cerebral. P. from bilateral cerebral lesion.

p. dolorosa. P. due to pressure of a neoplasm on post. spinal cord and nerve roots. Very painful.

p., peripheral. P. due to pressure on, injury to, or disease of peripheral nerves.

p., senile. P. resulting from sclerosis of arteries supplying spinal cord.

p., spastic. P. characterized by increased muscular tone, and accentuated tendon reflexes. Seen in multiple sclerosis and other conditions involving the pyramidal tracts.

p., spastic, primary. P. from degeneration in pyramidal tracts.

p., tetanoid. Same as *spastic p.*

paraplegic (păr-ă-plē′jĭk) [G. *para*, beside, + *plēgē*, a stroke]. Concerning, or affected with, paraplegia. SYN: *paraplectic*.

parapleuritis (păr″ă-plū-rī′tĭs) [G. *para*, beside, + *pleura*, a side, + *-ītis*, inflammation]. 1. Inflammation in the thoracic wall. 2. Mild inflammation of the pleura. 3. Pain in the pleura. SYN: *pleurodynia*.

parapoplexy (păr-ăp′ō-plĕk-sĭ) [" + *apoplēxia*, a striking down]. A mild or slight apoplexy with partial stupor; a stupor resembling apoplexy. SYN: *pseudoapoplexy*.

parapraxia, parapraxis (păr-ă-prak′sĭ-ă, -sĭs) [" + *praxis*, a doing]. Disturbed mental processes producing inaccuracy and forgetfulness and tendency to misplace things and make slips of speech or pen.

paraproctitis (păr″ă-prŏk-tī′tĭs) [" + *prōktos*, anus, + *-ītis*, inflammation]. Inflamed condition of tissues near the rectum.

parapsia, parapsis (păr-ăp′sĭ-ă, -sĭs) [G. *para*, beside, + *apsis*, touch]. Any disorder of touch. SYN: *paraphia*.

parapsoriasis (păr″ă-sō-rī′ă-sĭs) [" + *psōriasis*, itching]. A chronic disorder of the skin marked by scaly red lesions.

par″apsychol′ogy. The division of psychology which deals with extrasensory perception, telepathy, psychokinesis, clairvoyance, and associated phenomena.

pararenal (păr-ă-rē′năl) [" + L. *rēn*, kidney]. Near the kidneys.

pararhotacism (păr″ă-rō′tă-sĭzm) [" + *rho*, letter R, + *ismos*, condition]. Constant erroneous use of letter r or the placing of undue emphasis on letter r.

parasalpingitis (păr″ă-săl-pĭn-jī′tĭs) [G. *para*, beside, + *salpigx*, *salpigg-*, tube, + *-ītis*, inflammation]. Inflamed condition of tissues around an oviduct or a eustachian tube.

par″asecre′tion. 1. An abnormality in secretion. 2. A substance abnormally secreted.

parasigmatism (păr″ă-sĭg′mă-tĭzm) [" + *sigma*, letter S, + *ismos*, condition]. Imperfect pronunciation of the letter S. SYN: *lisping*.

parasite (păr′ă-sīt) [" + *sitos*, food]. An organism that lives within, upon, or at expense of another organism known as the host.

p., accidental. One infesting a host which is not its normal host.

p., external. One which lives on the outer surface of its hosts. Ex: fleas, lice, mites, ticks. An ectoparasite.

p., facultative. P. capable of living independently of its host at certain times.

p., incidental. An accidental parasite, *q.v.*

p., intermittent. One which visits its host at intervals.

p., internal. One which lives within the body of the host, occupying the digestive tract or body cavities, or living within body organs, blood, tissues, or even cells. Ex: protozoa, worms.

p., obligate. P. completely dependent on its host.

p., occasional. SYN: *Periodic parasite.* One which seeks its host at intervals to obtain nourishment.

p., periodic. An occasional parasite, *q.v.*

p., permanent. One which lives upon its host until maturity or spends its entire life upon its host. Ex: flukes, itch mites.

p., specific. One which requires a specific host in order to complete its life cycle.

p., temporary. One which is free-living during a part of its life cycle.

parasitic (păr-ă-sĭt′ĭk) [" + *sitos*, food]. Like, caused by, or concerning, a parasite.

parasiticide (păr″ă-sĭt′ĭ-sīd) [" + " + L. *caedere*, to kill]. 1. Killing parasites. 2. An agent that will kill parasites.

parasitism (păr′ă-sīt-ĭzm) [G. *para*, beside, + *sitos*, food, + *ismos*, condition]. The state or condition of being infected or infested with parasites.

parasitize (păr″ă-sĭt′īz). To infest or infect with a parasite.

parasitogenic (păr″ă-sī″tō-jĕn′ĭk) [G. *para*, beside, + *sitos*, food, + *gennan*, to produce]. 1. Caused by parasites. 2. Favoring parasite development.

parasitology (păr″ă-sī-tŏl′ō-jĭ) [G. *para*, beside, + *sitos*, food, + *logos*, study]. The study of parasites and parasitism.

parasitophobia (păr″ă-sī″tō-fō′bĭ-ă) [" + " + *phobos*, fear]. Unusual fear of parasites.

parasitosis (păr″ă-sīt-ō′sĭs). A disease or condition resulting from parasitism.

parasitotropic (păr″ă-sī″tō-trŏp′ĭk) [G. *para*, beside, + *sitos*, food, + *tropos*, turning]. 1. Having attraction for parasites. 2. Having an affinity for parasites such as a drug.

paraspadia (păr-ă-spā′dĭ-ă) [G. *paraspaein*, to draw aside]. Condition in which the urethra has an opening into one side of the penis.

paraspasm (păr′ă-spazm) [G. *para*, beside, + *spasmos*, a spasm]. 1. Muscular spasm of the lower extremities. 2. Spastic paralysis of the lower extremities.

parasteatosis (păr-ă-stē-ă-tō′sĭs) [" + *stear*, *steat-*, tallow, + *-ōsis*, disease].

Any disordered condition of the sebaceous secretions.

parasternal (păr-ă-stern'ăl) [" + *sternon,* chest]. Along the side of the sternum.

p. line. Imaginary vertical line running midway bet. sternal margin and line passing through the nipple.

p. region. Area bet. sternal margin and parasternal line.

parasthenia (păr-ăs-thē'nĭ-ă) [" + *sthenos,* strength]. Condition characterized by abnormal functioning of organic tissue at odd intervals.

parastruma (păr-ă-strū'mă) [" + L. *struma,* goiter]. Goiterlike tumor due to hypertrophy of a parathyroid gland.

parasympathetic (păr"ă-sĭm-pă-thĕt'ĭk) [G. *para,* beside, + *sympathētikos,* suffering with]. Of or pertaining to the craniosacral division of the autonomic nervous system.

p. nervous system. The craniosacral division of the autonomic nervous system. Preganglionic fibers originate from nuclei in the midbrain, medulla, and sacral portion of the spinal cord. They pass through cranial nerves III, VII, IX, and X and the second, third, and fourth sacral nerves and synapse with postganglionic neurons located in autonomic (terminal) ganglia which lie in the walls of or near the organ innervated.

Some effects of parasympathetic stimulation are constriction of pupil, contraction of smooth muscle of alimentary canal, constriction of bronchioles, slowing of heart rate, and increased secretion by glands, except sweat glands. Parasympathetic effects are *specific* rather than general. SEE: *autonomic nervous system, sympathetic nervous system.*

parasympathicotonia (păr-ă-sĭm-pă-thĭk-ō-tōn'ĭ-ă). SYN: *vagotonia.* Condition in which there is an imbalance in functioning of the autonomic nervous system, the parasympathetic division dominating over the sympathetic.

parasympatholytic (păr"ă-sĭm-pă-thō-lĭt'ĭk). Having a destructive effect on or blocking parasympathetic nerve fibers.

parasympathomimetic (păr"ă-sĭm-pă-thō-mĭm-ĕt'ĭk). Producing effects similar to those resulting from stimulation of parasympathetic nervous system.

parasynovitis (păr-ă-sin-ō-vī'tis) [G. *para,* beside, + *syn,* with, + *ōon,* egg, + *-ītis,* inflammation]. Inflamed condition of tissues about a synovial sac.

parasyphilitic (păr"ă-sif-ĭl-it'ĭk) [" + *syn,* with, + *philos,* love]. Being nonsyphilitic but due to syphilis.

parasystole (păr-ă-sĭs'tō-lē) [" + *systolē,* contraction]. Abnormally prolonged interval of rest between the systole and diastole.

paratarsium (păr-ă-tar'sĭ-ŭm) [" + *tarsos,* tarsus]. The covering and connective tissues of the tarsus of the feet.

paratenon (păr-ă-tĕn'ŏn) [" + *tenōn,* tendon]. Fatty and areolar tissue which surrounds the tendon and fills the spaces around the tendon.

paratereseomania (păr"ă-te-rē"sē-ō-mā'-nĭ-ă) [G. *paratērēsis,* observation, + *mania,* madness]. Insane desire to investigate new scenes and subjects.

paratherapeutic (păr"ă-thĕr-ă-pū'tĭk) [G. *para,* beside, + *therapeutikē,* treatment]. Caused by the treatment used for another disease.

parathormone (păr"ă-thor'mōn) [G. *para,* beside, + *thyroid,* + *ormanein,* to excite]. An extract from fresh or frozen parathyroid glands of domestic animals which contains the active principle or principles of these glands.

parathymia (păr"ă-thī'mĭ-ă) [" + *thymos,* mind]. Disordered state of the emotions.

parathyroid (păr-ă-thī'royd) [G. *para,* beside, + *thyreos,* shield, + *eidos,* form]. 1. Located close to the thyroid gland. 2. One of several small endocrine glands about 6 mm. long by 3 to 4 mm. broad on the back of and at lower edge of the thyroid gland or embedded within its substance. These glands secrete a hormone, *parathormone,* which regulates calcium-phosphorus metabolism. *Hyposecretion,* or hypoparathyroidism, results in neuromuscular hyperexcitability as manifested in tetany. Blood calcium falls and blood phosphorus rises. Other symptoms include cataract. teeth defects, bone lesions, maldevelopment of hair and nails, and skin disturbances. *Hypersecretion,* or *hyperparathyroidism,* results in a rise in blood calcium and fall in phosphorus. Calcium is removed from bones, resulting in increased fragility. Muscular weakness, reduced muscular tone and general neuromuscular hypoexcitability occur. Generalized osteitis fibrosa or osteitis fibrosa cystica (von Recklinghausen's disease) is a clinical entity associated with hyperplasia and resulting hypersecretion of the parathyroids. *Parathormone, q.v.,* secreted by these glands contains the active principle or principles.

parathyroidectomy (păr-ă-thī-royd-ĕk'tō-mĭ) [G. *para,* beside, + *thyreos,* shield, + *eidos,* form, + *ektomē,* excision]. Excision of one or more of the parathyroid glands.

parathyroprivia (păr"ă-thī"rō-prĭv'ĭ-ă) [" + " + L. *privus,* deprived of]. Condition which supervenes when the parathyroids are removed or cease functioning.

parathyroprivic, parathyroprivous (păr-ă-thī-rō-prĭv'ĭk, -us) [" + " + L. *privus,* deprived of]. Resulting from loss of function of, or removal of, parathyroid glands.

paratonsilar (păr"ă-tŏns-il'ăr). Near or about the tonsil.

paratrichosis (păr"ă-trĭ-kō'sĭs) [" + *thrix, trich-,* hair, + *-ōsis,* disease]. Abnormality of hair or its location.

paratrimma (păr-ă-trĭm'mă) [" + *tribein,* to rub]. Chafing; irritation of the skin. SYN: *intertrigo.*

paratripsis (păr-ă-trĭps'ĭs). 1. Rubbing, chafing. 2. A slowing of catabolism.

paratrophic (păr-ă-trō'fĭk) [G. *para,* beside, + *trophē,* nourishment]. 1. Requiring living substances for food; parasitic. 2. Pert. to abnormal nutrition.

paratrophy (păr-at'rō-fĭ) [" + *trophē,* nourishment]. 1. Localized fatty swellings and nerve lesions in various regions of the body. SYN: *Dercum's disease, adiposis dolorosa.* 2. Defective nutrition. SYN: *dystrophy.*

paratuberculosis (păr"ă-tū-bĕr"kū-lō'sĭs) [" + L. *tuberculus,* a tubercle, + G. *-ōsis,* disease]. A nontuberculous disease thriving in a tuberculous environment.

paratyphlitis (păr"ă-tĭf-lī'tĭs) [" + *typhlos,* blind, + *-ītis,* inflammation]. Inflammation of the connective tissue close to the cecum.

paratyphoid (păr-ă-ti'foyd) [G. *para,* near, + *typhos,* fever, + *eidos,* like]. Similar to typhoid.

p. fever. An infectious fever resembling typhoid.

ETIOL: Bacteria of the genus *Salmonella*, especially the species *S. paratyphi* (A & B strains) and *S. choleraesuis*.

SYM: Fever rises more quickly than in typhoid, more diarrhea, less cause for hemorrhages and perforation, recovery quicker and disease milder than typhoid. The ulcers are in lower end of small intestine in typhoid but more are in the upper end of the large intestine in paratyphoid. Widal test is negative.

paratypic (păr-ă-tip'ĭk) [G. *para*, beside, + *typos*, type]. Diverging from a type.

paraumbilical (păr"ă-ŭm-bĭl'ĭk-ăl) [" + L. *umbilicus*, navel]. Close to the navel.

paraurethral (păr"ă-ū-rē'thrăl) [" + *ourēthra*, urethra]. Located close to the urethra.

parauterine (păr"ă-ū'tĕr-ĭn) [" + L. *uterus*, womb]. Around the uterus.

paravaginal (păr"ă-văj'ĭn-ăl) [" + L. *vagina*, sheath]. Around the vagina.

paravaginitis (păr"ă-văj-ĭn-ī'tĭs) [" + " + G. *-itis*, inflammation]. Inflammation of the tissue surrounding the vagina.

paravertebral (păr"ă-ver'tĕ-brăl). Alongside or near the vertebral column.

p. anesthesia. Injection of a local anesthetic about roots of spinal nerves.

paravesical (păr"ă-vĕs-ĭk'ăl). Near the urinary bladder.

paravitaminosis (păr"ă-vīt-ăm-ĭn-ō'sĭs). A disease or disorder resulting indirectly from vitamin deficiency.

paraxial (păr-ăk'sĭ-ăl) [" + L. *axis*, axis]. On either side of the axis of the body, or one of its parts.

parazoon (păr-ă-zo'ŏn). An animal which lives as a parasite upon animals.

parched (parchd) [M.E. *parchen*]. Dried to extremity.

parectasia, parectasis (păr"ĕk-tā'sĭ-ă, -sĭs). Excessive dilatation or stretching of a structure.

paregoric (păr-e-gor'ĭk) [G. *parēgoros*, soothing]. 1. Soothing. 2. Camphorated tincture of opium, a narcotic-containing drug which in large doses is poisonous. Used extensively in the symptomatic treatment of diarrhea.

TREATMENT FOR POISONING: Same as for morphine, *q.v.*

parenchyma (păr-ĕn'kĭ-mă) [" + *en*, in, + *chein*, to pour]. The essential parts of an organ which are concerned with its function in contradistinction to its framework.

The uriniferous tubules of the kidneys are a part of that organ's parenchymatous tissue.

p. disease. Disease affecting the principal tissue of an organ.

parenchymatitis (păr-ĕn-kĭ-mă-tī'tĭs) [" + " + " + *-itis*, inflammation]. Inflamed condition of parenchyma, or substance of a gland.

parenchymatous (păr-ĕn-kĭm'ăt-ŭs) [" + " + *chein*, to pour]. Concerning the essential substances of an organ.

parent (pār'ent) [L. *parēre*, to bring forth]. A father or a mother; one who begets offspring.

p. fixation. Continuation of the child-parent affiliation into the adult state, so that the person has an abnormal attachment to a parent.

parenteral (păr-ĕn'tĕr-ăl) [G. *para*, beside, + *enteron*, intestine]. Situated or occurring outside of the intestines.

p. digestion. Digestion of foreign substances by body cells as opposed to *enteral digestion*, which occurs in the alimentary canal.

p. injection. Injection of substances into the body through any route other than via alimentary canal, as subcutaneous, intravenous, intramuscular, or intrathecal injection.

p. therapy. Introduction of a substance, esp. nutritive material, into the body by means other than the intestinal tract.

parepithymia (păr"ĕp-ĭ-thĭ'mĭ-ă). Abnormal desire or craving.

parergastic reactions (păr-ĕr-găst'ĭk) [" + *ergon*, work]. A general term used by A. Meyer for the essentials involved in schizoid types but without relation to prognosis.

paresis (păr'e-sĭs, pă-rē'sĭs) [G. weakness]. 1. Partial or incomplete paralysis. 2. An organic mental disease with somatic, irritative and paralytic focal symptoms and signs running a slow, chronic, progressive course and tending to a fatal termination. SYN: *general paresis of the insane.*

ETIOL: Diffuse and focal involvement of brain and spinal cord due to syphilis, usually occurring from 5 to 15 years after primary infection.

PATH: A diffuse meningoencephalitis with degenerative changes dependent upon vascular and toxic factors.

SYM: May simulate any psychoneuroses or psychoses. Pupillary changes, facial tremors, tremors of the lips and tongue, speech distrubances. Usually Argyll-Robertson pupil, impaired vision, headache, speech slurred with letters and syllables often omitted. Epileptic convulsions. Unequal exaggeration of the reflexes. Always a positive Wassermann reaction of spinal fluid, with increase of protein anl lymphocytes. Colloidal gold curve changes, reading often being 5555543210. Memory defective, expansive delusions, depression, dementia.

TREATMENT: Penicillin.

p., juvenile. General p. due to congenital syphilis, seen in children.

paresthesia (păr-ĕs-thē'zĭ-ă) [G. *para*, beside, + *aisthēsis*, sensation]. Abnormal sensation without objective cause, such as numbness, prickling, and tingling; heightened sensitivity.

Experienced in central and peripheral nerve lesions and in locomotor ataxia.

paretic (pă-rĕt'ĭk, pă-rē'tĭk) [G. *paresis*, weakness]. Affected with or concerning paresis.

pareunia (păr-ū'nĭ-ă) [G. *pareunos*, lying beside]. Sexual intercourse. SYN: *coition; coitus; copulation.*

paridrosis (păr-ĭ-drō'sĭs) [" + *idrōsis*, perspiration]. Any disordered secretion of perspiration.

paries (pā'rĭ-ēs) (pl. *parietes*) [L. a wall]. The enveloping wall of any structure; applied especially to hollow organs.

parietal (pă-rī'ĕ-tăl) [L. *pariēs, pariet-*, wall]. Pert. to, or forming, the wall of a cavity. SEE: *suture, sagittal.*

p. bone. One of two bones which form the roof and sides of the skull.

p. cells. Large cells on margin of the peptic glands of stomach which supposedly secrete hydrochloric acid. SYN: *acid cells; delomorphous cells.*

p. lobe. A central portion of the cerebrum bet. the parieto-occipital and rolandic fissures above the horizontal branch of the fissure of Sylvius.

parietes (pă-rī'ĕ-tēs) [L.]. Plural of paries; walls of an organ or hollow part.

pari passu [L. with equal step]. Occurring at the same time or at the same rate.

Paris green (păr′ĭs grēn). A compound of copper and arsenic, *q.v.*; copper acetoarsenite.

parity (păr′ĭ-tĭ) 1. Equality, similarity. 2. The condition of a woman with respect to the number of children she has borne. SEE: *multiparity, nulliparity, primiparity, secundiparity.*

Parkinson's disease (par′kĭn-sŭn) [James Parkinson, English physician, 1755-1824]. A chronic nervous disease characterized by a fine, slowly spreading tremor, muscular weakness and rigidity and a peculiar gait.

SYM: Onset may be abrupt; generally insidious. First symptom is a fine tremor beginning in hand or foot which may spread till it involves all the members. At first paroxysmal but becomes almost continuous.

Face becomes expressionless. Speech slow and measured, later muscular rigidity. Head bowed, body bent forward, arms flexed, thumbs turned into palms, knees slightly bent. Gait characteristic by this time; steps grow faster and faster, body inclines more and more forward until patient falls, seeks some support; this is termed festination.

Occasionally a tendency to fall backwards, retropulsion replaces festination; numbness, tingling, sensation of heat.

PROG: Recovery rarely if ever occurs. Duration indefinite.

TREATMENT: General supportive measures plus medicines to combat muscle rigidity and lethargy. Destruction of a part of the thalamus on one side by producing extreme cold in a very small area. It is not a cure but alleviates tremors. SYN: *palsy, shaking; paralysis agitans.*

P.'s mask. Expressionless appearance of the face. Eyebrows are raised, wrinkles are smoothed out, and there is immobility of the facial muscles.

A typical symptom seen in P.'s disease and in postencephalitic states.

P.'s syndrome. Symptoms of P.'s disease.

paroccipital (păr-ŏk-sĭp′ĭt-ăl) [G. *para,* near, + L. *occiput,* occiput]. 1. Close to the occipital bone. 2. The paramastoid process.

parodontitis (păr″ō-don-tī′tĭs) [" + *odous, odont-,* tooth, + *-itis,* inflammation]. Inflamed condition of tissues around a tooth.

parodynia (păr-ō-din′ĭ-ă) [L. *parere,* to bring forth, + G. *odynē,* pain]. 1. Labor pains. 2. Difficult or abnormal labor or birth. SYN: *dystocia.*

p. perversa. Presentation with fetus lying transversely across the uterus. SYN: *cross birth.*

parolivary (păr-ŏl′ĭ-va-rĭ) [G. *para,* near, + L. *oliva,* olive]. Situated close to the olivary body.

p. bodies. Nuclei in medulla oblongata, lying close to the olivary bodies.

paromphalocele (păr-om′fă-lō-sēl″) [" + *omphalos,* navel, + *kēlē,* hernia]. Hernia or tumor close to the umbilicus.

paroniria (păr-ō-nī′rĭ-ă) [" + *oneiros,* dream]. Abnormal dreaming of a terrifying nature.

p. ambulans. Sleepwalking.

p. salax. Restlessness in sleep with lascivious dreams and nocturnal emissions.

paronychia (păr-ō-nĭk′ĭ-ă) [" + *onyx, onych-,* nail]. Acute or chronic infection of marginal structures about the nail.

ETIOL: Trauma, infection.

SYM: Redness, swelling and suppuration around nail edge.

TREATMENT: Heat to area unless there is inadequate blood supply; surgery in severe cases.

SYN: *runaround, whitlow.*

p. tendinosa. Inflammation of sheath of a digital tendon. ETIOL: Sepsis.

paronychomycosis (păr″ō-nī-kō-mī-kō′sĭs). Fungus infection about the nails.

paronychosis (păr-ō-nī-kō′sĭs). Growth of a nail in an abnormal position.

paroophoron (păr-ō-ŏf′ō-rŏn) [G. *para,* near, + *ōon,* egg, + *phoros,* bearer]. A group of minute tubules located in mesosalpinx between uterus and ovary. It is a vestigial structure consisting of the remains of the caudal group of mesonephric tubules and is a homolog of the paradidymis of the male.

parophthalmia (păr-ŏf-thăl′mĭ-ă) [" + *ophthalmos,* eye]. Inflamed condition of tissue around the eye.

parophthalmoncus (păr-ŏf-thăl-mōn′kŭs). A tumor located near the eye.

paropsis (păr-op′sĭs) [" + *opsis,* vision]. Any disorder of sense of sight.

parorchidium (păr-ŏr-kĭd′ĭ-ŭm) [" + *orchis, orchid-,* testicle]. Abnormal position or nondescent of a testicle. SYN: *ectopia testis.*

parorexia (păr-ō-rĕk′sĭ-ă) [" + *orexis,* appetite]. An abnormal or perverted craving for special or strange foods. SEE: *appetite, taste.*

parosmia (păr-ŏz′mĭ-ă) [" + *osmē,* odor]. Any disorder or perversion of the sense of smell; a false sense of odors or perception of those which do not exist.

Agreeable ones are considered offensive and disagreeable odors are accepted as pleasant. SEE: *kakosmia.* SYN: *parosphresia.*

parosphresia, parosphresis (păr″ŏs-frē′zĭ-ă, -sĭs) [" + *osphrēsis,* a smelling]. Disordered sense of smell. SYN: *parosmia, q.v.*

parosteitis, parostitis (păr-ŏs-tē-ī′tĭs, -tī′tĭs) [G. *para,* beside, + *osteon,* bone, + *-itis,* inflammation]. Inflammation of tissues next to the bone.

parosteosis, parostosis (păr-ŏs-tē-ō′sĭs, -tō′sĭs) [" + " + *-ōsis,* disease]. 1. Bone formation outside of the periosteum. 2. Bone development in an unusual location.

parotic (pă-rot′ik). Near the ear.

parotid (pă-rŏt′ĭd) [" + *ous, ot-,* ear]. 1. Located near the ear. 2. Parotid gland.

p. duct. Approx. 2 in. long. Extends from ant. border of the parotid gland crossing the masseter and piercing the buccinator, and then runs between the buccinator and the mucous membrane.

It opens in the mouth opposite 2nd upper molar. The transverse facial artery is above the duct and buccal branch of 7th nerve below. SYN: *Stensen's duct.* SEE: *saliva.*

p. gland. A pure albuminous (serous) gland, its secreting tubules and acini being long and branched. It is enclosed in a sheath, the *parotid fascia.*

parotidectomy (pă-rŏt-ĭd-ĕk′tō-mĭ) [" + " + *ektomē,* excision]. Excision of parotid gland.

parotiditis (pă-rŏt-ĭ-dī′tĭs) [" + " + *-itis,* inflammation]. Parotitis, *q.v.*

parotidoscirrhus (pă-rŏt″id-ō-skĭr′ŭs) [" + " + *skirros,* hardness]. 1. Hardening of the parotid gland. 2. A scirrhous cancer of the parotid area.

parotitis (pă-rō-tī′tĭs) [G. *para,* near, +

ous, ot-, ear, + *-itis*, inflammation]. SYN: *mumps*. Inflammation of the parotid gland, either simple or epidemic.

parous (pa'rus) [L. *parēre*, to bring forth]. Parturient; fruitful; having borne at least one child.

parovarian (par-ō-văr'ĭ-ăn) [G. *para*, near, + L. *ovarium*, ovary]. 1. Situated near or beside the ovary. 2. Pert. to the parovarium, a residual structure in the broad ligament.

parovariotomy (păr-ō-vā-rĭ-ŏt'ō-mĭ) [" + " + G. *tomē*, a cutting]. Removal of a parovarian cyst.

parovarium (păr"ō-văr'ĭ-ŭm) [" + L. *ovarium*, ovary]. The epoophoron, *q.v.* Also called *organ of Rosenmuller*.

paroxysm (păr'ŏk-sĭzm) [G. *para*, beside, + *oxynein*, to sharpen]. 1. A sudden, periodic attack or recurrence of symptoms of a disease; an exacerbation of the symptoms of a disease. 2. A fit or convulsion of any kind. 3. Sudden emotional state, as of fear, grief, or joy.

paroxysmal (păr-ŏk-sĭz'măl) [" + *oxynein*, to sharpen]. 1. Occurring in or concerning paroxysms. 2. Of the nature of a paroxysm.

parricide (par'ĭ-sīd). The murdering of one's own parent. SYN: *patricide.*

par'rot fever. SYN: *psittacosis, q.v.*

Parrot's disease (păr-ō') [Jules Marie Parrot, French physician, 1839-1883]. The pseudoparalysis of the extremities in infants caused by syphilis.

P.'s nodes. Bony nodules on skull of infants with syphilis.

P.'s sign. In meningitis, pupils dilate upon pinching the skin of neck.

P.'s ulcer. Lesions of thrush or stomatitis.

Parry's disease (păr-ē) [Caleb H. Parry, English physician, 1755-1822]. SEE: *goiter, exophthalmic.*

pars (parz) (pl. *partes*) [L. *pars, part-*, a part]. A part.

p. anterior hypophyseos. The ant. lobe of the hypophysis.

p. basilaris occipitalis. [NA]. Basilar process of the occipital bone.

p. buccalis hyphyseos. Developmental protrusion in primitive buccal cavity of anterior lobe of hypophysis.

p. caeca oculi. The optic disk.

p. caeca retinae. Parts of the retina not light-sensitive (*pars ciliaris retinae* and *pars iridica retinae, q.v.*).

p. cavernosa urethra. Cavernous portion of urethra of male.

p. cephalica nervi sympathici. Plexuses, ganglia, and nerves derived from sympathetic nerve.

p. ciliaris retinae. [NA]. Portion of retina situated in front of ora serrata and covering the ciliary body.

p. distalis. That part of the hypophysis forming the major portion of the anterior lobe.

p. flaccida. A portion of membrane of the eardrum which fills the notch of Rivinus. SYN: *Shrapnell's membrane.*

p. intermedia. The intermediate lobe of the hypophysis cerebri.

p. iridica retinae. [NA]. Portion of retina on post. surface of iris.

p. membranacea urethrae. The membranous portion of the urethra.

p. nervosa hypophyseos. Post. lobe of the pituitary gland.

p. optica hypothalami. The optic chiasma.

p. optica retinae. The sensory portion of the retina extending from optic disc to ora serrata.

p. tensa. The larger portion of the tympanic membrane, a tightly stretched membrane lying inferior to the maleolar folds.

p. tuberalis. The portion of the ant. lobe of the hypophysis cerebri which invests the infundibular stalk.

pars'ley [M.E. persely, parsley]. A plant, *Petroselinum crispum*, belonging to the carrot family. It is the source of a volatile oil called *apiol.*

PARSLEY (*raw, chopped*): 1 tbsp. (3.5 gm.). Calories: 1. Other main values: trace of protein; trace of fat; trace of carbohydrate; 3 mg. calcium.

pars'nips [M.E. *pasnepe*, parsnip]. PARSNIPS (*cooked*): 1 cup (155 gm.). Calories: 95. Other main values: 2 gm. protein; 1 gm. fat; 22 gm. carbohydrates; 88 mg. calcium. ACTION: Easy to digest.

partes (pär'tēs). Plural of pars, *q.v.*

parthenogenesis (par"then-o-jen'ĕ-sis) [G. *parthenos*, virgin, + *genesis*, origin]. Reproduction arising from a female egg which has not been fertilized by the male.

particulate (par-tĭk'ū-lāt). Made up of particles.

parturient (păr-tū'rĭ-ĕnt) [L. *parturiens*, desiring to bring forth]. 1. Concerning childbirth or parturition. 2. Bringing forth; giving birth.

p. canal. Path from uterine cavity to vulva.

p. woman. One in labor.

parturifacient (păr-tū-rĭ-fā'shĕnt) [" + *facere*, to make]. 1. Inducing or accelerating labor. 2. Drug used to cause delivery of the fetus.

parturition (păr-tū-rĭsh'ŭn) [L. *parturitiō*, childbirth]. Act of giving birth to young. SYN: *childbirth, delivery.*

parturition, *words pert. to:* accouchement, accoucheur, accoucheuse, afterbirth, afterpains, axis traction, bradytocia, childbirth, dystocia, labor, multipara, nullipara, obstetrics, oxytocia, parturient, parturifacient, postpartum.

partus (păr'tŭs) [L. *partus*, from *parēre*, to bring forth]. Labor; parturition.

p. agrippinus. Breech presentation in delivery.

p. caesareus. Delivery by cesarean section.

p. difficilis. Difficult labor. SYN: *dystocia.*

p. immaturus. Premature labor.

p. maturus. Labor at term.

p. precipitat'us. Precipitate labor.

p. serotinus. Prolonged or delayed labor.

p. siccus. Dry labor with little amniotic fluid.

parulis (păr-ū'lĭs) [G. *para*, near, + *oulon*, gum]. Abscess in a gum. SYN: *gumboil.*

parumbilical (păr-ŭm-bĭl'ĭ-kăl) [" + L. *umbilicus*, navel]. Close to the navel.

paruria (păr-ū'rĭ-ă) [" + *ouron*, urine]. Any abnormality in discharge of urine.

parvicellular (păr-vĭ-sĕl'ū-lăr) [L. *parvus*, small, + *cellula*, a little box]. Concerning, or composed of, tiny cells.

parvule (păr'vūl) [L. *parvulus*, very small]. A small pill, pellet, or granule.

PAS. Abbr. for *para-aminosalicylic acid, q.v.*

Paschen bodies (pă'shĕn). Particles thought to be the pathogenic virus of vaccinia and variola found in great numbers in skin exanthemas.

passage (păs'aj) [L. *passus*, a step]. 1. A communication bet. cavities and body structures or with the ext. surface of an organ. 2. Act of passing. 3. An evacuation of the bowels. 4. Introduction of a probe or catheter, etc. 5. Incubation of a pathogenic organism, especially a virus in one or a series of tissue cultures or living organisms.

passion (păsh'ŭn) [L. *passiō*, suffering]. 1. Suffering. 2. Great emotion, esp. sexual excitement.

passional (păsh'ŭn-ăl) [L. *passiō*, suffering]. Exciting or concerning any passion. SEE: *emotional*.

passive (păs'ĭv) [L. *passivus*, enduring]. 1. Submissive. 2. Acted upon. 3. Not active.

p. congestion. Congestion due to obstruction in venous return or, if general, due to myocardial insufficiency.

p. exercise. Muscular exercise without any effort on part of patient.

p. hyperemia. Blood in a part due to decreased outflow.

p. motion. Same as p. exercise.

p. movement. SEE: *p. exercise*.

passivism (păs'ĭ-vĭzm) [" + G. *ismos*, condition]. Sexual perversion with subjugation of the will by that of another, usually of the male by the female.

past pointing. Inability to accurately place finger or some other part of the body on a selected point. Seen in certain neurologic disorders.

paste (pāst) [G. *pastē*, barley broth]. 1. To cause to adhere. 2. Any ointment whose base is a nonfatty material. 3. A mixture of flour and water, used as an adhesive. 4. A moist, doughy, plastic substance.

Pasteur treatment (păs-tĕr') [Louis Pasteur, French chemist and bacteriologist, 1822-1895]. Daily injection of increasingly virulent suspensions prepared from the brain or spinal cord of rabbits which have died of rabies. Suspension is treated so as to kill or inactivate the virus. Used for the prevention of rabies.

CAUTION: In some cases neurologic complications may occur ranging from simple neuritis to serious encephalomyelitis and paralysis which may be fatal. Treatment should be employed only when absolutely necessary. SEE: *rabies*.

Pasteurella (păs-tĕr-ĕl'ă). A genus of bacteria belonging to the tribe Pasteurelleae, family Parvobacteriaceae. The organisms are gram-negative, nonsporulating rods, exhibiting bipolar staining. Many species are pathogenic for animals, a few for man.

P. pestis. Cause of bubonic plague. SYN: *plague bacillus*.

P. tularensis. Organism causing tularemia. Now generally called *Francisella tularensis*.

pasteurellosis (păs-ter-ĕl-ō'sĭs) [G. *-ōsis*, disease]. Disease caused by infection with bacteria of the *Pasteurella* group inducing hemorrhagic septicemia.

pasteurization (păs-tĕr-ī-zā'shŭn). The process of heating a fluid at a moderate temperature for a definite period of time in order to destroy undesirable bacteria without changing to any extent the chemical composition of the fluid except for loss of about 20% of the vitamin C content.

In p. of milk, pathogenic bacteria are destroyed at 140° F. (60° C.) for 20 min. If higher temperatures are used the time of exposure to heat is reduced.

Pasteurization should not be considered as a substitute for cleanliness in milk production. SEE: *milk*.

pastille (pas-tēl', pas-til') [L. *pastillus*, a little roll]. 1. A small cone used to fumigate or scent the air of a room. 2. A medicated disk used for local action on the mucosa of the throat and mouth. SYN: *lozenge, troche*. 3. PT: Small disk of paper coated with barium platinocyanide or other substances, used to estimate the amount of x-rays administered, also for testing the intensity of ultraviolet radiations.

The green color changes to brown when exposed to roentgen rays.

p. radiometer. An instrument consisting of a color index by means of which the color changes in the pastilles, before and after exposure to roentgen rays, may be gauged. At one time it was used frequently to estimate the quantity of roentgen rays but is now practically obsolete.

patagium (pā-tāy'gĭ-ŭm). A weblike membrane extending from one body part to another.

patch (pătsh) [M.E. *pacche*]. A blotch distinct from surrounding surface in character and appearance.

p., herald. Oval patch of efflorescence showing before the general eruption of pityriasis rosea; often several days before.

p., Hutchinson's. Salmon-yellow area seen on cornea in syphilitic keratitis.

p., mucous. A syphilitic eruption having an eroded, moist surface; generally on mucous membrane of mouth or external genitals or on surface subject to moisture and heat. SYN: *condyloma latum*.

p., opaline. Whitish patch in mouth, sometimes observed in syphilis.

p's., Peyer's. Masses of lymphoid follicles found on mucous membrane of small intestine. SYN: *noduli lymphatici aggregati*.

p., salmon. Salmon-colored area of cornea in ocular syphilis.

p., smokers'. Leukoplakia, *q.v.*

p. test. One to detect hypersensitiveness to food, pollen or other substances by applying suspected substance to an area on the skin.

A small square of clean linen cloth should be covered with substance suspected. Cloth is laid on skin of chest or upper arm and another piece of cloth laid over it and fastened with adhesive. Another piece of the cloth containing none of the suspected substance is also applied to the skin. Both pieces are removed at the end of 24 hr. If irritation is present only where the suspected substance was tested, the individual is probably sensitive to it.

Substances with which the patient comes in contact may be used for the test. SEE: *allergy, eczema*.

patella (pă-tĕl'ă) [L. a small pan; kneepan]. The kneecap, or kneepan; a lens-shaped sesamoid bone situated in front of the knee, in the tendon of the quadriceps femoris muscle. [NA].

RS: *housemaid's knee; knee*.

p., floating. A patella which floats up from the condyles due to a large effusion in the knee.

p., fracture of. TREATMENT: Suture of bone fragments. A plaster is then put on, reaching from the toes to the groin, remaining on for 6-8 weeks. Then gradual exercise and weight upon the leg for a few weeks, after which patient may walk.

p., rider's painful. Tenderness and pain in patella from horseback riding.

patellapexy (pă-tĕl'ă-pĕk"sĭ) [L. *patella*, kneepan, + G. *pēxis*, fixation]. Fixation of the patella to the lower end of the femur to stabilize the joint.

patellar (pă-tĕl'ăr) [L. *patella*, kneepan] Concerning the patella.

p. paradoxic reflex. Contraction of ant. muscles when leg is forcibly flexed and immediately released.

p. reflex. Involuntary jerk of leg due to sudden spasm of quadriceps following percussion of patellar ligament. SYN: *knee-jerk reflex.*

patelliform (pă-tĕl'ĭ-form) [" + *forma*, shape]. Of the shape of the patella.

patellofemoral (pă-tĕl"ō-fĕm'or-ăl) [" + *femur, femor-*, thigh]. Concerning the patella and the femur.

patency (pā'tĕn-sē) [L. *patens*, from *patere*, to be open]. The state of being freely open.

patent (păt'ĕnt, pā'tĕnt) [L. *patens*, from *patere*, to be open]. Wide open; evident; accessible.

pat'ent med'icine. Packaged remedy for public use which is protected by letters patent and sold without a physician's prescription.

The law requires that it be labeled with names of active ingredients, the quantity or proportion of the contents, directions for its use, and that it may not have misleading statements as to curative effects on the label. SEE: *prescription.*

paternal (pă-ter'nal). Of, pertaining to, or inherited from the father.

path. SEE: *pathway.*

path-, patho-. Prefix meaning *pertaining to disease.*

pathema (pă-thē'mă) (pl. *pathemas* or *pathemata*) [G. *pathēma*, a suffering]. Disease.

pathergasia (păth-ĕr-gā'zĭ-ă) [G. *pathos*, disease, + *ergon*, work]. Any form of constitutional or structural malfunctioning which inhibits self-adjustment. Part of A. Meyer's theory of psychiatry.

pathergia (path-er'jĭ-ă). Same as pathergy, *q.v.*

pathergy (path'er-jĭ). Condition in which the response to a stimulus is either exaggerated or subnormal. SEE: *hyperergy; hypoergy.*

pathetic (pă-thĕt'ĭk) [G. *pathētikos*, suffering]. Arousing the tender emotions, as sorrow.

pathetism (path'ĕt-ĭzm) [G. *pathein*, to suffer, + *ismos*, condition]. State of overcoming another's will by suggestion. SYN: *hypnotism; mesmerism.*

pathfinder (păth'fīnd-ĕr) [A.S. *paeth*, road, + *findan*, to locate]. Instrument for locating stricture of the urethra.

pathic (păth'ĭk) [G. *pathos*, disease]. A sexual pervert who assumes the passive role in submitting to unnatural desires of another.

pathocrine (păth'ō-krīn, -krēn, -krĭn) [" + *krinein*, to secrete]. Concerning an endocrine disorder.

pathodixia (păth-ō-dik'sĭ-ă) [" + L. *dicere*, to say, from G. *deiknunai*, to show]. Exhibitionism in reference to an injury or to disease.

pathodontia (păth'ō-dŏn'shĭ-ă) [" + *odous, odont-*, tooth]. Branch of dentistry dealing with diseases of the teeth.

pathogen (păth'ō-jĕn) [" + *gennan*, to produce]. A microorganism or substance capable of producing a disease.

pathogenesis (păth-ō-jĕn'ĕ-sĭs) [" + *genesis*, development]. Origination and development of a disease.

p., drug. 1. Morbid symptoms of disease produced by a drug. 2. Observation of all symptoms which may be produced by a drug.

pathogenetic, pathogenic (păth"ō-jĕn-ĕt'ĭk, -jĕn'ĭk) [" + *gennan*, to produce]. Productive of disease. SYN: *morbific.*

p. organism. One that produces disease in the body.

pathogeny (păth-ŏj'ĕn-ĭ) [" + *gennan*, to produce]. The origin or growth of a disease. SYN: *pathogenesis.*

pathognomonic (păth-ŏg-nō-mŏn'ĭk) [" + *gnōmonikos*, showing]. Indicative of a disease, especially of one or more of its characteristic symptoms.

pathologic, pathological (păth-ō-lŏj'ĭk, -ĭ-kăl) [" + *logos*, study]. 1. Concerning pathology. 2. Diseased; due to a disease. SYN: *morbid.*

p. histology. Histology of diseased tissues.

p. reflex. An abnormal reflex indicating an abnormal or diseased state.

pathologist (pă-thŏl'ō-jĭst) [G. *pathos*, disease, + *logos*, study]. A specialist in diagnosing the morbid changes in tissues removed at operations and postmortem examinations.

pathology (pă-thŏl'ō-jĭ) [" + *logos*, study]. 1. Study of the nature and cause of disease which involves changes in structure and function. 2. Condition produced by disease.

p., anatomic. That which deals with structural changes.

p., cellular. That which is based upon microscopic changes in body cells during disease.

p., chemical. The study of chemical changes which occur in disease.

p., comparative. The observation of pathological condition, spontaneous or artificial, in the lower animals or in vegetable organisms as compared to those of human body.

p., experimental. Study of diseases induced intentionally, especially in animals.

p., functional. SYN: *physiologic pathology.* The study of alterations of functions which occur in disease processes.

p., geographical. P. in its relations to geographical conditions.

p., medical. The p. of disorders which are not accessible for surgical procedures.

p., special. The p. of particular diseases or organs.

p., surgical. The p. of surgical diseases.

pathomania (păth-ō-mā'nĭ-ă) [" + *mania*, madness]. Moral insanity; irresistible tendency toward forbidden conduct with retention of reasoning power.

pathometry (păth-ŏm'ĕt-rĭ) [" + *metron*, measure]. The estimate of the incidence of a disease.

pathomimesis (păth"ō-mĭm-e'sĭs) [" + *mimēsis*, imitation]. Intentional or unconscious as well as conscious imitation of a disease.

pathomimicry (path"o-mim'ik-rĭ). Pathomimesis, *q.v.*

pathomorphism (păth-ō-mor'fĭzm) [" + *morphē*, form, + *ismos*, condition]. Study of abnormal form and structure of organisms.

pathonomy (păth-ŏn'ō-mĭ) [" + *nomos*, law]. Science of the laws of diseased conditions.

pathophilia (păth-ō-fĭl'ĭ-ă) [G. *pathos*, disease, + *philein*, to love]. Adjustment of habits to conditions made mandatory by some chronic disease.

pathophobia (păth-ō-fō'bĭ-ă) [" + *phobos*, fear]. Morbid apprehension of disease.

pathophoresis (păth″ō-for-ē′sĭs) [" + *phoros*, carrying]. The transmission of disease-producing organisms.

pathophoric (păth-ō-for′ĭk) [" + *phoros*, carrying]. Carrying or transmitting disease, as certain insects.

pathopoiesis (păth″ō-poy-ē′sĭs) [" + *poiein*, to make]. The method of disease production.

pathopsychology (păth″ō-sī-kŏl′ō-jĭ) [" + *psychē*, soul, + *logos*, study]. The branch of psychology dealing with mental processes during disease.

patho′sis. A diseased state or condition.

pathway. A path or a course; more specifically a pathway formed by neurons (cell bodies and their processes) over which impulses pass from their point of origin to their destination.

p., afferent. One leading from a receptor to the spinal cord and (or) brain.

p., central. One within the brain or spinal cord.

p., conduction. A group of fibers in a nerve, spinal cord, or brain over which impulses are conducted.

p., efferent. One from the central nervous system to an effector.

p., metabolic. The sequence of chemical reactions which occur as a substance is metabolized.

p., motor. P. over which motor impulses are conveyed from a motor center to muscles.

p., sensory. P. over which sensory impulses are conveyed from sense organs or receptors to sensory or reflex centers of the spinal cord or brain.

patient (pā′shĕnt) [L. *patiens, patient-*, suffering]. 1. Enduring pain or injury. 2. A person who is receiving treatment for disease.

patricide (pat′rĭ-sīd). Same as parricide, *q.v.*

patrilineal [L. *pater*, father, + *linea*, line]. Tracing descent through the father.

pattern. 1. A design, figure, model, or example. 2. In psychology, a set or arrangement of ideas or behavior reaction.

patulous (păt′ū-lŭs) [L. *patulus*, open]. SYN: *patent.* Open, distended, spread apart.

paulocardia (pawl″ō-kar′dĭ-ă) [G. *paula*, pause, + *kardia*, heart]. 1. Sensation of momentary stoppage of heartbeat. 2. Undue prolongation of the rest period in the cardiac cycle.

pause. An interruption; a temporary cessation of activity.

p., compensatory. The long interval following an extrasystole, so-called because its duration is such that the next beat occurs at the exact time of the succeeding normal beat.

pavement′ing. Condition occurring during inflammation in which leukocytes adhere to the lining of capillaries.

pavor (pā′vor) [L.]. Anxiety, dread.

p. nocturnus. Night terror during sleep in children and the aged.

Pavy's disease (pā′ve) [Frederick Pavy, English physician, 1829-1911]. Albuminuria which recurs at periodic intervals.

Pb. Chem. symb. for *lead* (*plumbum*).

P.B. Abbr. for *Pharmacopoeia Britannica* (British pharmacopeia).

PBI. Abbr. for *protein-bound iodine.*

P.B.W. Abbr. for *posterior bite wing* (dentistry).

PBZ. Abbr. for *pyribenzamine.*

p.c. Abbr. L. *post cibos*, after meals.

P_{CO_2}. Symb. for *carbon dioxide pressure* or tension.

PCV. Abbr. for *packed cell volume.*

Pd. Chem. symb. for *palladium.*

P.D. Abbr. for *Doctor of Pharmacy.*

pea (pē) [G. *pison*]. COMP: Richer in proteins than other vegetables except lentils, but poorer in carbohydrates. PEAS (*canned, solids and liquid*): 1 cup (249 gm.). Calories: 170. Other main values: 8 gm. protein; 1 gm. fat; 32 gm. carbohydrates; 62 mg. calcium; 1350 I.U. vitamin A.

peach (pētsh) [L. *persicum*, peach]. RAW: 1 peach (114 gm.). Calories: 35. Other main values: 1 gm. protein; trace of fat; 10 gm. carbohydrates; 9 mg. calcium; 1320 I.U. vitamin A.

peanut (pē′nŭt). ROASTED (*shelled, halves*): 1 cup (144 gm.). Calories: 840. Other main values: 39 gm. protein; 71 gm. fat; 28 gm. carbohydrates; 104 mg. calcium.

p. butter. 1 tbsp. (16 gm.). Calories: 90. Other main values: 4 gm. protein; 8 gm. fat; 3 gm. carbohydrate; 80 mg. calcium.

pear (pār) [L. *pirum*]. RAW: 1 pear (182 gm.). Calories: 100. Other main values: 1 gm. protein; 1 gm. fat; 25 gm. carbohydrates; 13 mg. calcium.

ACTION: Heavy in the stomach unless cooked. Dried pears are highly nutritive and contain malic acid.

pearl (pĕrl) [O.Fr. *perle*]. 1. Small, tough mass in sputum in asthma. 2. Small, hollow glass capsule containing a fluid for inhalation, as amyl nitrite.

p., epithelial. Concentric squamous epithelial cells in carcinoma.

p., gouty. Sodium urate concretion on cartilage of the ear seen in people with gout.

peau d'orange [Fr. "orange skin"]. Dimpled skin which resembles an orange.

pecan (pē-kăn′) [Algonquin *paccan*]. PECAN (*halves*): 100 grams. Calories: 687. Other main values: 9.2 gm. protein; 71 gm. fat; 16 gm. carbohydrate; 73 mg. calcium.

peccant (pek′ant) [L. *peccāre*, to sin]. Corrupt; producing disease. SYN: *pathogenic, unhealthy, morbid.*

peccatiphobia (pĕk-ăt-ĭ-fō′bĭ-ă) [" + G. *phobos*, fear]. Abnormal dread of sinning.

pecilo-. For words beginning with pecilo-, see *poikilo-.*

Pecquet's cistern (pē-ka′) [Jean Pecquet, French anatomist, 1622-1674]. A reservoir for chyle at lower end of the thoracic duct. SEE: *receptaculum chyli.*

P.'s duct. Passage from the cisterna chyli to the joining point of the left subclavian and int. jugular veins, acting as a lymph channel.

P.'s reservoir. SEE: *P.'s cistern.*

pectase (pĕk′tās) [G. *pēktos*, congealed, + *ase*, enzyme]. Enzyme facilitating the conversion of pectin to pectic acid and methanol.

pecten (pĕk′tĕn) [L. comb]. 1. The pubic bone. 2. A comblike organ. 3. Middle portion of anal canal.

p. ossis pubis. A sharp ridge on superior ramus of pubis which forms pubic portion of the terminal (iliopectineal) line.

pectic acid (pĕk′tĭk) [G. *pēktos*, congealed]. An acid derived from pectin by hydrolyzing the methyl ester group which is found in many fruits.

pectin (pĕk′tĭn) [G. *pēktos*, congealed]. A white, amorphous plant carbohydrate that forms a gelatinous mass in the cooking of fruits and vegetables, causing them to "jell." SEE: *pectose.*

pectinate (pĕk'tĭn-āt) [L. *pecten*, comb]. Having teeth like a comb.

pectineal (pĕk'tĭn'ē-ăl) [L. *pecten*, comb]. Relating to the os pubis or the pectineus muscle.

p. line. The line or ridge on the os pubis separating the true from the false pelvis. SYN: *iliopectineal line, linea terminalis.*

pectineus (pek-tĭn-ē'-us) [L. *pecten, pectin-*, comb]. A flat, quadrangular muscle at upper and inner part of thigh arising from sup. ramus of pubis and inserted bet. lesser trochanter and linea aspera of the femur, which flexes and adducts the thigh. SEE: *Table of Muscles in Appendix.*

pectiniform (pĕk-tĭn'ĭ-form) [" + *forma*, shape]. Toothed like a comb. SYN: *pectinate.*

pectization (pĕk-tĭ-zā'shŭn) [G. *pēktos*, congealed]. In colloidal chemistry, the conversion of a substance from sol to gel state.

pectoral (pĕk'tō-răl) [L. *pectus, pector-*, breast]. 1. Concerning the chest. 2. Efficacious in relieving chest conditions, as a cough.

pectoralgia (pĕk-tō-ral'jĭ-ă) [" + G. *algos*, pain]. Neuralgic pain in the chest.

pectoralis (pĕk-tō-rā'lĭs) [L.]. One of four muscles of the breast.

p. major. A large triangular muscle extending to the humerus which draws the arm forward and downward and aids in chest expansion.

p. minor. Muscle beneath p. major, extending to scapula, which lowers the scapula and depresses the shoulder point.

pectoriloquy (pĕk-tō-rĭl'ō-kwĭ) [L. *pectus, pector-*, breast, + *loqui*, to speak]. The distinct transmission of vocal sounds to the ear through the chest wall in auscultation, *q.v.*

The words seem to emanate from the spot which is ausculted. Heard over cavities which communicate with a bronchus; areas of consolidation near a large bronchus; over pneumothorax when the opening in the lung is patulous; over some pleural effusions. SEE: *chest.*

p., aphonic. In auscultation, whispered sound heard over a lung with a cavity or pleural effusion.

p., whispering. Sound over a lung with a cavity of limited extent when patient whispers, in auscultation of the chest.

pectorophony (pĕk-tō-rof'ō-nĭ) [" + G. *phōnē*, voice]. Exaggeration of vocal sounds heard on auscultation of the chest. SYN: *pectoriloquy.*

pectose (pĕk'tōs) [G. *pēktos*, congealed]. A substance found in some fruits and vegetables that yields pectin when it is boiled.

pectunculus (pĕk-tun'kū-lŭs) [L. little comb]. One of the tiny longitudinal ridges on the sylvian aqueduct.

pectus (pĕk'tŭs) [L.]. The chest; breast; thorax.

p. carinatum. Abnormal prominence of the sternum. SYN: *chicken* or *pigeon breast.*

p. excavatum. SYN: *funnel breast.* Congenital condition in which sternum is abnormally depressed.

ped- [L. foot]. Combining form denoting foot.

pedal (pĕd'ăl, pē'dăl) [L. *pēs, ped-*, foot]. Concerning the foot.

pedarthrocace (pē"dār-throc'ă-sē). Carious condition of joints of children.

pedatro'phia. SEE: *pedatrophy.*

pedatrophy (pē-dăt'rō-fĭ). 1. Marasmus. 2. Any wasting disease in children. 3. Tabes mesenterica.

pederast (pĕd'ĕr-ăst) [G. *pais, paid-*, youth, + *erastēs*, lover, from *eran*, to love]. A male who indulges in sexual intercourse with men, esp. young boys, through the anus.

pederasty (pĕd'ĕr-ăs-tĭ) [" + *erastēs*, lover, from *eran*, to love]. Illicit coitus by the anus with males, esp. with young boys. SYN: *sodomy.*

pedes (pe'dēz). Plural of pes, *q.v.*

pedesis (pē-dē'sĭs). The incessant dancing or to-and-fro movements of particles in a colloidal system or minute particles of any substance in a liquid or gaseous medium resulting from thermal movement of molecules. Also called brownian movement.

pedi- (ped'ĭ). Combining form denoting foot.

pedialgia (pĕd-ĭ-al'jĭ-ă, pē-dĭ-) [G *pedion*, foot, + *algos*, pain]. Pain of the foot.

pediatric (pē-dĭ-ăt'rĭk) [G. *pais, paid-*, child, + *iatreia*, treatment]. Concerning the treatment of children.

pediatrician (pē-dĭ-ă-trĭsh'an) [G. *pais, paid-*, child, + *iatrikos*, healing]. A specialist in treatment of children's diseases. SYN: *pediatrist.*

pediatrics (pē-dĭ-ăt'rĭks) [" + *iatreia*, treatment]. Medical science relating to hygienic care of children and treatment of diseases peculiar to them. SYN: *pediatry.*

pediatrist (pē"dĭ-ăt'rĭst) [" + *iatrikos*, healing]. Physician who specializes in treatment of children's diseases.

pediatry (pĕd'ĭ-ăt-rĭ, pē-dĭ'ăt-rĭ). The treatment of children's diseases. SYN: *pediatrics.*

pedicellation (pĕd"ĭ-sĕl-ā'shŭn) [L. *pediculus*, a little foot; stalk]. Formation and development of a pedicle.

pedicle (pĕd'ĭ-kl) [L. *pediculus*, a little foot]. 1. The stem which attaches a new growth. 2. The bony process which projects backward from the body of a vertebra connecting with the lamina on each side. Forms the *root* of the vertebral arch.

pedicterus (pē-dĭk'ter-us). Icterus neonatorum or jaundice of the newborn.

pedicular (pē-dĭk'ū-lar) [L. *pediculus*, a louse]. 1. Infested with or concerning lice. 2. [L. *pediculus*, a little foot]. Concerning a stalk or stem.

pediculate (pē-dĭk'ū-lāt) [L. *pediculus*, a little foot]. Having a pedicle or stem. SYN: *pedunculate.*

pediculation (pē-dĭk-ū-lā'shŭn) [L. *pediculus*, a louse; a little foot]. 1. Infestation with lice. 2. Development of a pedicle.

pediculicide (pē-dĭk'ū-lĭ-sīd) [L. *pediculus*, a louse, + *caedere*, to kill]. Destroying or that which destroys lice.

Pedicul'idae. A family of lice belonging to the order Anoplura. Includes the species parasitic on primates including man. SEE: *Pediculus.*

pediculophobia (pē-dĭk"ū-lō-fō'bĭ-ă) [" + G. *phobos*, fear]. Abnormal dread of lice. SYN: *phthiriophobia.*

pediculosis (pē-dĭk-ū-lō'sĭs) [" + G. *-ōsis*, infestation]. Lousiness; infestation with lice. SEE: *Pediculus.*

p. capitis. P. due to infestation with the head louse, Pediculus humanus humanus, *q.v.* Transmission is by personal contact or common use of brushes, combs, or headgear.

SYM: Itching and eczematous dermatitis. In long-standing, neglected cases, scratching may result in marked inflammation and secondary infection by bacteria may occur with formation of pustules, crusts, and suppuration. Hair may become matted and give rise to an unpleasant odor.

TREATMENT: Rub benzyl benzoate emulsion into scalp at night. A day after treatment hair should be shampooed and then combed with a fine-tooth comb to remove nits. In severe infestations or if hair is matted, hair should be cut short. Treatment should be repeated in ten days to kill newly hatched lice. All possible sources of infection should be examined and treated if necessary. Headgear, combs, brushes should be disinfected by heat or use of disinfection solutions.

p. corporis (p. vestimenti). P. due to infestation with the body louse, *Pediculus humanus corporis, q.v.* Transmitted by direct contact or use of infested wearing apparel. Occurs as a result of crowding or unhygienic conditions.

SYM: Intense itching. In heavy infections, generalized red skin eruption, mild fever, tiredness, irritability and, in severe cases, weakness and debility.

TREATMENT: Clothing and bedding should be sterilized by dry heat (140° F. for 5 min.), hot water (150° F. for 5 min.) or by immersion in gasoline or 5% DDT solution, or by dry cleaning. Thorough cleansing of the body and scrubbing with soap followed by a pediculicidal lotion applied to hairy parts of the body.

p. pubis. P. due to infestation with the crab louse, *Phthirus pubis, q.v.* Generally confined to hairs of genital region but hair of the axilla, eyebrows, eyelashes, beard, and, in hairy individuals, body surface may be involved. Lice may be acquired through sexual relations, wearing contaminated clothing, from toilet seats, or from bed clothes.

SYM: Itching, esp. in genital or crural regions. Small pale-blue spots resulting from the action of salivary secretion on hemoglobin are characteristic.

TREATMENT: Cleanse thoroughly with soap and water. Apply DDT powder or lotion. A copper pediculicidal solution (Cuprex) is also effective. All sources of infection should be checked and lice eliminated.

pediculus (pē-dĭk'ū-lŭs) [L. stem, louse]. 1. A pedicle. 2. Louse. SEE: *Pediculus.*

Pedic'ulus. A genus of parasitic insects commonly called *lice* which infest humans and other primates. They are sucking insects belonging to the family Pediculidae, order Anoplura. They are of medical importance in that they are the transmitters of the causative organisms of epidemic typhus, trench fever, and relapsing fever and may also serve as mechanical transmitters of bubonic plague and possibly other diseases.

P. humanus corporis. The body louse which inhabits the seams of clothing worn next to the body and feeds on regions of the body covered by that clothing. Eggs are attached to fibers of the clothing. The cause of *pediculosis corporis* or *vestimenti, q.v.*

P. humanus humanus. SYN: *P. humanus capitis.* The head louse which lives in the fine hair of the head, although beard and eyebrows may be infested. Its eggs, commonly called "nits," are glued to hairs frequently forming "nests" in the vicinity of the ears. Cause of *pediculosis capitis, q.v.*

P. vestimenti. SEE: *P. humanus corporis.*

pedicure (ped-ĭ-kūr) [L. *pēs, ped-*, foot, + *cura,* care]. 1. Care of the feet. 2. A chiropodist or one who cares for the feet. 3. The care, painting, and polishing of the toenails.

pediform (ped'ĭ-form). Having the shape of a foot.

pediluvium (pĕd-ĭ-lū'vĭ-ŭm) [" + *luere,* to wash]. A foot bath.

pedionalgia (pĕd-ĭ-ō'nal'jĭ-ă) [G. *pedion,* foot, + *algos,* pain]. Neuralgic pain in the sole of the foot. SYN: *metatarsalgia.*

pediophobia (pē-dĭ-ō-fō'bĭ-ă) [G. *pais, paid-*, child, + *phobos,* fear]. Unnatural dread of young children or of dolls.

pedobaromacrometer (pē"dō-băr"ō-măk-rŏm'ĕt-ĕr) [" + *baros,* weight, + *makros,* long, + *metron,* measure]. Apparatus for determining measurement and weight of infants.

pedobarometer (pē"dō-băr-om'ĕt-ĕr) [" + " + *metron,* measure]. Apparatus for weighing infants.

pedodontia, pedodontics (pē"dō-don'shĭ-ă, -tĭks) [" + *odous, odont-*, tooth]. Phase of dentistry dealing with care of children's teeth.

pedodontist (pē"dō-dŏn'tĭst) [" + *odous, odont-*, tooth]. Dentist who specializes in care of children's teeth.

pedograph (pĕd'ō-grăf) [L. *pēs, ped-*, foot, + G. *graphein,* to write]. Imprint of the foot on paper.

pedologist (pē-dŏl'ō-jĭst) [G. *pais, paid-*, child, + *logos,* study]. One who has made a study of children and their development.

pedology (pē-dŏl'ō-jĭ) [" + *logos,* study]. The study of children and their development.

pedometer (pē-dom'ĕt-ĕr) [G. *pais, paid-*, child, + *metron,* measure]. 1. Device for measurement of infants. 2. (pĕd-ŏm'-ĕt-ĕr) [L. *pēs, ped-*, foot, + G. *metron,* measurement]. Watch which indicates number of steps taken in walking.

pedomorphism (pē"dō-mor'fizm) [G. *pais, paid-*, child, + *morphē,* form, + *ismos,* condition]. Retention of juvenile characteristics in the adult.

pedonosology (pē"do-nōs-ŏl-ō-jĭ) [" + *nosos,* disease, + *logos,* study]. The study of children's diseases. SYN: *pediatrics.*

pedophilia (pē"dō-fĭl-ĭ-ă) [" + *philein,* to love]. 1. Fondness for children. 2. PSY: Unnatural desire for sexual relations with children.

peduncle (pē-dung'kl) [L. *pedunculus,* a little foot]. 1. A stem or stalk. SYN: *pedicle.* 2. A brachium of the brain; a band connecting parts of the brain. SYN: *pedunculus.* SEE: *cimbia, crus, sessile.*

p., cerebellar, inferior. SYN: *restiform body.* A band of fibers running along lateral border of 4th ventricle which connects spinal cord and medulla with the cerebellum.

p., cerebellar, middle. SYN: *brachium pontis.* A band of fibers connecting cerebellum with basilar portion of the pons.

p., cerebellar, superior. SYN: *brachium conjunctivum.* A band of fibers connecting cerebellum with midbrain.

p., cerebral. SYN: *crus cerebri.* A pair of white bundles from upper part of the pons to the cerebrum. They constitute the ventral portion of the midbrain.

p., mammillary. A band of fibers extending from tegmentum of midbrain to mammillary body.

p. of flocculus. A band of fibers connecting flocculus of cerebellum with vermis.

p. of sup. olive. A slender band of fibers extending from sup. olivary nucleus in medulla to nucleus of abducens nerve.

p., pineal. A band from either side of the pineal gland to the ant. pillars of the fornix.

p., thalamic. One of four groups of fibers known as *thalamic radiations, q.v.*, which connect thalamus with cerebral cortex.

peduncular (pē-dun′kū-lar) [L. *pedunculus,* a little foot]. Concerning a peduncle.

pedunculate, pedunculated (pē-dŭn′kū-lāt, -ed) [L. *pedunculus,* a little foot]. Possessing a stalk or peduncle. Syn: *pediculate.*

peeling. Shedding of surface layer of skin; desquamation.

peer (pēr). The same variety or group; an equal.

peinotherapy (pī-nō-thĕr′ă-pĭ) [G. *peina,* hunger, + *therapeia,* treatment]. Hunger cure for disease. Syn: *pinotherapy.*

pelage (pĕ-lahj′) [Fr.]. The hair of the body collectively.

Pel-Ebstein's fever. Cyclic fever occurring in Hodgkin's disease in which periods of fever lasting from 3 to 10 days are separated by an afebrile period of about the same length.

pelioma (pĕl-ĭ-ō′mă) [G. *peliōma,* a livid spot]. A livid cutaneous patch. Syn: *ecchymosis.*

peliosis (pĕl-ĭ-ō′sĭs) [G. *peliōsis,* a livid spot]. A disease marked by purple patches on the mucous membranes and skin. Syn: *purpura.*

p. rheumatica. An acute affection characterized by inflammation of the joints.

A form of rheumatism. Sym: Sore throat, urticaria, moderate fever, purpuric spots over extremities or trunk. Tenderness, swelling, and pain in joints. Syn: *purpura rheumatica; Schonlein's disease.*

pellagra (pĕl-ă′gră, pĕ-lăg′ră) (L. *pellis,* skin, + G. *agra,* seizure). A deficiency disease or syndrome endemic in certain parts of the world, characterized by cutaneous, gastrointestinal, mucosal, neurologic, and mental symptoms.

Etiol: Due to deficiency in diet or failure of body to absorb niacin (nicotinic acid) or its amide (niacinamide, nicotinamide), and usually associated with a deficiency of proteins containing tryptophane, such as occurs in a high maize or corn diet. It may occur secondary to gastrointestinal diseases and alcoholism.

Sym: In advanced cases, scarlet stomatitis and glossitis, diarrhea, dermatitis, and mental symptoms. Cutaneous lesions include erythema followed by vesiculation, crusting and desquamation. Skin may become dry, scaly, and atrophic. The mucous membranes of mouth, esophagus, and vagina may undergo atrophy, ulcers and cysts may develop. Anemia is common. Nausea, vomiting and diarrhea occur, the latter being characteristic. Involvement of the central nervous system is first manifested by neurasthenia, followed by organic psychosis characterized by disorientation, impairment of memory and confusion. Later delirium and clouding of consciousness may occur.

Treatment: A diet adequate in all vitamins, minerals, and amino acids supplemented by 500 to 1000 mg. of niacinamide given orally three times daily.

p. sine pellagra. Pellagra in which the characteristic erythematous rash is absent.

pellagrazein (pĕl-ă-grā′zē-ĭn). Poisonous substance in cornmeal that has decomposed. Syn: *pellagracein.*

pellagrin (pĕ-lā′grĭn, -lăg′rĭn) [L. *pellis,* skin, + G. *agra,* seizure]. A person afflicted with pellagra.

pellagrous (pĕ-lā′grŭs, -lăg′rŭs) [" + G. *agra,* seizure]. Concerning or affected with pellagra.

pellet (pĕl′ĕt) [L. *pila,* a ball]. A tiny pill or small ball of medicine or food.

pellicle (pĕl′ĭ-kl) [. *pelicula,* a little skin]. Syn: *scum.* 1. A thin piece of cuticle or skin. 2. Film or surface on a liquid. 3. A thin nonliving sheath forming the surface layer of certain one-celled animals.

pellotine (pĕl′ō-tēn). A white, crystalline alkaloid used as a hypnotic.

pellucid (pē-lū′sĭd) [L. *pellucidus,* shining through]. Translucent; transparent.

p. zone. Clear layer covering the oocyte. Syn: *zona pellucida.*

pelvic (pĕl′vĭk) [L. *pelvis,* basin]. Pertaining to a pelvis, usually the bony pelvis.

p. girdle. Arch made by the innominate bones.

p. inlet. Upper pelvic entrance, the brim of the pelvis forming its boundary.

p. outlet. Lower pelvic opening.

pelvilithotomy (pĕl″vĭ-lĭ-thŏt′ō-mĭ) [" + G. *lithos,* stone, + *tomē,* a cutting]. Removal of a stone from the renal pelvis. Syn: *nephrolithotomy, pelviolithotomy, pyelolithotomy.*

pelvimeter (pĕl-vĭm′ĕt-ĕr) [" + G. *metron,* measure]. Device for measuring the pelvis.

pelvimetry (pĕl-vĭm′ĕt-rĭ) [" + G. *metron,* measure]. Measurement of the pelvic dimensions or proportions. Helps determine whether or not it will be possible to deliver the fetus through the normal route. Done by manual or x-ray methods or both. See: *pelvis; Illus., p. P-30.*

p., x-ray. Use of x-ray studies for measurement of the pelvis.

pelviolithotomy (pĕl″vĭ-ō-lĭ-thŏt′ō-mĭ) [" + G. *lithos,* stone, + *tomē,* a cutting]. Incision of the renal pelvis to remove a calculus.

pelvioplasty (pĕl′vĭ-ō-plăs″tĭ) [" + G. *plassein,* to form]. Enlargement of the outlet of the pelvis. Syn: *hebotomy, symphyseotomy.*

pelvioscopy (pĕl″vĭ-ŏs′kō-pĭ) [L. *pelvis,* basin, + G. *skopein,* to examine]. Inspection of the pelvis.

pelviotomy (pĕl-vĭ-ŏt′ō-mĭ) [" + G. *tomē,* a cutting]. 1. Incision of pelvic bones, esp. in case of difficult labor. 2. Incision into the renal pelvis.

pelviperitonitis (pĕl″vĭ-pĕr-ĭ-tō-nī′tĭs) [L. *pelvis,* basin, + G. *peritonaion,* peritoneum, + *-itis,* inflammation]. Inflammation of the peritoneum lining the pelvic cavity.

pelvis (pĕl′vĭs) (pl. *pelves*) [L. basin]. 1. Any basin-shaped structure or cavity. 2. The bony structure formed by the innominate bones, the sacrum, the coccyx, and the ligaments uniting them, which serves as a support for the vertebral column and for articulation with the lower limbs. 3. The cavity included within these bones.

It is separated into a *false,* or superior pelvis, and a *true,* or inferior one, by the iliopectineal line, and the upper margin of the symphysis pubis, the circumference of this area constituting the *inlet* of the true pelvis. Lower border of true pelvis is formed by the coccyx, the protuberances of the ischia, the ascending rami of the ischia, the descending rami of the ossa pubis and the sacrosciatic ligaments, and is termed the *outlet.*

The floor of the pelvis is formed by the perineal fascia, levator ani and the coccygeus.

DIAMETERS: All diameters normally are larger in the female than in the male.

EXTERNAL: *Interspinous*: Distance bet. outer edges of the ant. sup. iliac spines, diameter normally measuring 26 cm. (10 in). *Intercristal*: Distance bet. outer edges of the most prominent portion of the iliac crests, diameter normally being 28 cm. (11 in.). *Intertrochanteric*: Distance bet. most prominent points of the femoral trochanters, 32 cm. (12½ in.). *Oblique* (right and left): Distance from one post. sup. iliac spine to the opposite ant. sup. iliac spine, 22 cm. (8½ in.), right being slightly greater than the left. *External conjugate*: Distance from the undersurface of the spinous process of last lumbar vertebra to the upper margin of ant. surface of the symphysis pubis, 20 cm. (7¾ in.). SYN: *Baudelocque's diameter*.

INTERNAL: *True conjugate*: Anteroposterior diameter of the pelvic inlet, 11 cm. (4¼ in.), the most important single diameter of the pelvis. *Diagonal conjugate*: Distance bet. the promontory of the sacrum to undersurface of symphysis pubis, 13 cm. (5 in.), 2 cm. being deducted for the height and inclination of symphysis to obtain diameter of conjugate. *Transverse*: Distance bet. ischial tuberosities, 11 cm. (4¼ in.). *Anteroposterior* (of outlet): Distance bet. the lower border of symphysis and tip of sacrum, 11 cm. (4¼ in.). *Anterior sagittal*: Distance from undersurface of symphysis to center of line bet. the ischial tuberosities, 7 cm. (2¾ in.). *Posterior sagittal*: Distance from the center of line bet. ischial tuberosities to the tip of the sacrum, 10 cm. (4 in.).

RS: *acanthopelvis, brim, Claudius' fossa, diameter, endopelvic, pelvic cavity, pelvimetry, pelviotomy.*

p. aequabiliter justo major. One symmetrically above standard in all its dimensions.

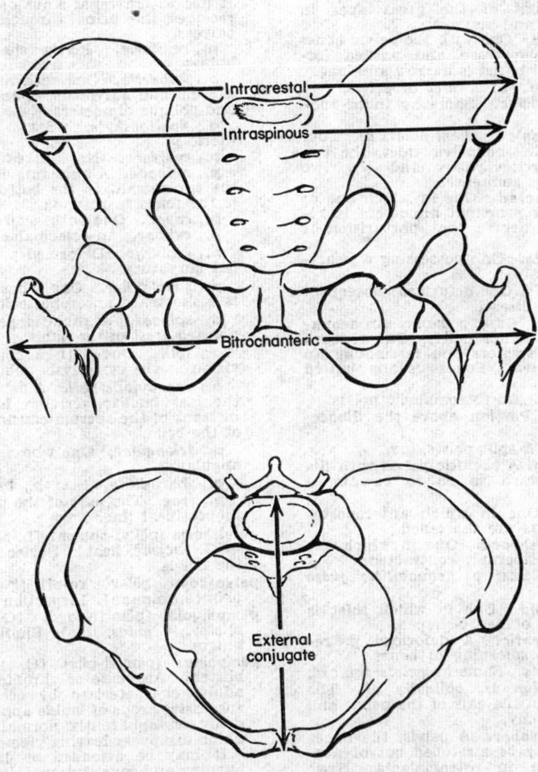

EXTERNAL PELVIMETRY

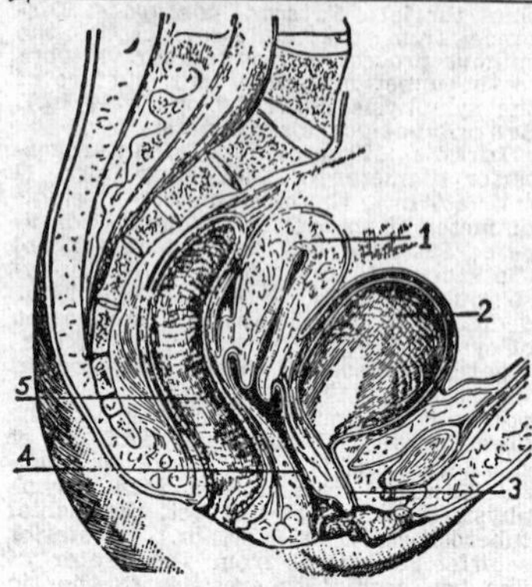

SECTION OF FEMALE PELVIS.

1. Uterus. 2. Bladder. 3. Urethra. 4. Vagina. 5. Rectum.

p. aequabiliter justo minor. One with all equally below standard.

p., android. A female pelvis which resembles that of a male.

p., anthropoid. A female pelvis resembling that of the great apes in being long and narrow.

p., beaked. One with the pelvic bones laterally compressed and pushed forward so that outlet is narrow and long.

p., brim of. SEE: *inlet of pelvis.*

p., caoutchouc. Same as India rubber pelvis.

p., Capuron's cardinal points of. Four points within the pelvic inlet, the two sacroiliac articulations and the two iliopectineal eminences.

p., contracted. One in which one or more of the principal diameters is reduced to a degree that parturition is impeded.

p., cordate. One possessing a heart-shaped inlet.

p., coxalgic. One deformed subsequent to hip joint disease.

p., dwarf. SYN: *p. nana.* An aequabiliter justo minor pelvis. One reduced in all its diameters and resembling an infantile pelvis. Bones usually united by cartilage.

p., elastic. An osteomalacic pelvis.

p., false. Portion above the iliopectineal line.

p. fissa. A split pelvis, *q.v.*

p., fissured. A rachitic pelvis with ilia pushed forward so as to be almost parallel.

p., flat. One in which anteroposterior diameters are shortened.

p., funnel-shaped. One in which the outlet is considerably contracted.

p., giant. SEE: *p. aequabiliter justo major.*

p., gynecoid. One in which inlet is oval instead of heart-shaped.

p., halisteretic. A deformed p. resulting from softening of bones.

p., Hauder's. Same as *pelvis spinosa.*

p., inclination of, obliquity of. The angle between the axis of the pelvis and that of the body.

p., India rubber. A pelvis, the bones of which may be stretched out of normal position in osteomalacia. SYN: *caoutchouc p.*

p., infantile. P. of an adult which retains its infantile characters.

p., Kilian's. SEE: *osteomalacic pelvis.*

p., kyphotic. Deformed p. characterized by increase of the conjugate diameter at the brim with reduction of the transverse diameter at the outlet.

p., lordotic. Deformed p. in which the spinal column has an ant. curvature in the lumbar region.

p., major. The false pelvis, *q.v.*

p., malacosteon. SEE: *rachitic p.*

p., masculine. SYN: *android pelvis.* P. of a female which resembles that of a male, esp. in being narrower, more conical, with heavy bones, and heart-shaped inlet.

p., Naegele. An obliquely contracted pelvis in which conjugate diameter assumes an oblique direction.

p. nana. A dwarf pelvis, *q.v.*

p., osteomalacic. P. distorted as a consequence of osteomalacia.

p., Prague. SEE: *spondylolisthetic p.*

p., pseudoosteomalacic. A rickety pelvis similar to that of a person affected with osteomalacia.

p., rachitic. One deformed from rickets.

p., reduced. SEE: *aequabiliter justo minor.*

p., renal. SYN: *pelvis renalis.* The expanded proximal end of the ureter. It lies within renal sinus of kidney and receives the urine through the major calyces.

p., reniform. Pelvis shaped like a kidney.

p., Robert's. One with an embryonic sacrum and narrowing of the transverse and oblique diameters.

p., Rokitansky's. SEE: *spondylolisthetic p.*

p., rostrate. SEE: *beaked p.*

p., rotunda. A tympanic depression in the inner wall, at the bottom of which is the fenestra rotunda.

p., round. One with a circular inlet.

p., rubber. An osteomalacic p.

p., scoliotic. Deformed p. due to spinal curvature.

p., simple flat. One whose deformity is a shortened anteroposterior diameter.

p. spinosa. A rachitic pelvis with a pointed crest of the pubis.

p., split. One with a congenital division at the symphysis pubis.

p., spondylolisthetic. A pelvis in which the last lumbar vertebra is dislocated in front of the sacrum causing occlusion of the brim.

p., triangular. One whose inlet is triangular.

p., triradiate. SEE: *p., beaked.*

p., true. The part of the p. below the iliopectineal line.

pelvitherm (pĕl'vĭ-thurm) [L. *pelvis*, basin, + G. *thermē*, heat]. Device for heating the pelvis.

pelvoscopy (pĕl-vŏs'kō-pĭ) [" + G. *skopein* to examine]. Inspection of a pelvis.

pemphigoid (pĕm'fĭ-goyd) [G. *pemphix*, blister, + *eidos*, like]. Similar to pemphigus.

pemphigus (pĕm'fĭ-gŭs) [G. *pemphix*, a blister]. An acute or chronic disease of adults characterized by occurrence of successive crops of bullae appearing suddenly on apparently normal skin, and which disappear leaving pigmented spots. It may be attended by itching and burning and constitutional disturbance.

ETIOL: Unknown.

TREATMENT: Care of general health. In severe and extensive cases patient to be kept on air or water mattress; continuous bath therapy, tonics, carron oil bath, ultraviolet irradiation, corticosteroid hormones. In *p. foliaceous* and *p. vegetans*, autogenous serum. Locally, large quantities of powder, soothing lotions.

p. acutus. Constitutional symptoms severe and outcome often fatal. Bullae 1-10 cm. in diameter often containing blood and serum. If coalescing, denuded areas are formed.

p. circinatus. P. with circular eruptions.

p. contagiosa. An infective type of the groin and axilla.

p. disseminatus. P. marked by widely separated bullae.

p. foliaceus. Rare type. Large flaccid bullae developing rapidly, rupture soon, leaving moist, raw surface covered with seropurulent fluid. Bullous contents are purulent from beginning with sickening odor. Chronic course.

p. neonatorum. P. soon after birth, generally due to septic infection but sometimes leutic.

p. pruriginosus. P. with severe, continuous itching.

p. syphiliticus. A form due to syphilis.

p. vegetans. Variant of *p. vulgaris* in beginning, but instead of drying up, the lesions persist, resulting in papillary excrescences with no tendency to heal, secreting foul-smelling seropurulent fluid and sodden decomposing masses of epidermis.

p. vulgaris. Uncomplicated form in which replacement of epidermis follows. Lesions round or oval, thin walled, tense, translucent, contents bilateral in distribution, developing suddenly, without scarring resulting.

penalge'sia. A reduction in number of touch and pain spots in skin in cases of trigeminal neuralgia.

pendular (pĕn'dū-lĕr) [L. *pendulus*, from *pendere*, to hang]. Hanging so as to swing by an attached part; oscillating like a pendulum.

pendulous (pĕn'dū-lŭs) [L. *pendulus*, from *pendere*, to hang]. Swinging freely like a pendulum; hanging.

penetrate (pĕn'e-trāt) [L. *penetrāte*, to go within]. To enter into the interior of.

penetrating (pĕn'e-trāt-ĭng) [L. *penetrāre*, to go within]. Entering beyond the exterior.

p. power. Penetrating capacity of a lens.

p. wound. Wound affecting the interior of an organ or cavity.

penetration (pĕn"e-trā'shŭn) [L. *penetrāre*, to go within]. 1. Process of entering within a part. 2. Capacity to enter within a part. 3. Power of a lens to give a clear focus at varying depths.

penetrometer (pĕn-e-trŏm'ĕt-ĕr) [" + G. *metron*, measure]. FT: An instrument that compares roughly the comparative absorption of roentgen rays in various metals, esp. silver, lead and aluminum; hence, it gives a rough estimation of hardness of roentgen rays. SYN: *penetrameter; qualimeter.*

penicillin (pĕn-ĭs'ĭ-lĭn, pen-ĭ-sĭl'ĭn). One of a group of antibiotics biosynthesized by several species of molds, esp. *Penicillium notatum* and *P. chrysogenum.* They are bacteriostatic inhibiting the growth of most Gram-positive bacteria and certain Gram-negative forms. They are also effective against certain molds, spirochetes, and rickettsias. There are many different penicillins including synthetic ones and their effectiveness varies for different organisms.

penicillinase (pen-ĭ-sil'ĭ-nās). A substance produced by bacteria which inactivates most but not all penicillins. Is used to treat allergic reaction to penicillin.

penicilliosis (pen"is-il-ĭ-o'sis) [L. *penicillum*, pencil]. Infection with the fungi of the genus *Penicillium.*

Penicillium (pen"ĭs-ĭl'ĭŭm) [L. *penicillum*, pencil, brush]. A genus of molds belonging to the Ascomycetes (Sac fungi). They form the blue molds which grow on fruits, bread, cheese, etc. A number of species (*P. chrysogenum, P. notatum* and others) are the source of penicillin. Occasionally in man they produce infections of the external ear, skin, or respiratory passageways. They are common allergens.

penicillus. A group of the branches of arteries in the spleen which are arranged like the bristles of a brush. Each consists of successive portions, the *pulp arteries, sheathed arteries,* and *terminal arteries.*

penile (pē'nīl, -nĭl) [L. *penis*, penis]. Pert. to the penis.

p. reflex. 1. Sudden downward movement of penis when the prepuce or gland of a completely relaxed penis is pulled upward. 2. Contraction of bulbocavernous muscle on percussing dorsum of penis. 3. Contraction of bulbocavernous muscle resulting from compression of glans penis.

penis (pē'nĭs) (pl. *penes*) [L.]. The male organ of copulation. (See illus., p. G-15.)

It is a cylindrical, pendulous organ suspended from the front and sides of the pubic arch. It is composed of three columns of cavernous tissue, the whole being covered with skin, the two lateral columns being known as the *corpora cavernosa penis.* The third or median column contains the urethra, known as the *corpus cavernosum urethrae.*

The head of the penis is known as the *glans penis* in which the urethral orifice is situated, and it is covered with a movable hood known as the *foreskin* or *prepuce,** under which is secreted a lubricating substance called *smegma.** Hyperemia of the genitals fills the corpora cavernosa with blood as the result of sexual excitement or stimulation, thus causing an *erection.** The hyperemia is lowered following ejaculation of the seminal fluid and the organ returns to its normal condition.

p. captivus. One which is held within the vagina during copulation as a result of vaginismus and contraction of the perineal muscles.

p., clubbed. A condition when the penis is curved during erection.

p. lunatus. Painful curved erection in gonorrhea. SYN: *chordee, q.v.*

p. muliebris. Clitoris,* the erectile organ of the female.

p. palmatus. One enclosed by the scrotum.

p. webbed. Same as *p. palmatus.*

penis, words pert. to: balanitis; "balano-" words; cavernitis; cavernosum; chordee; circumcision; condyloma; cord, spermatic; corpus cavernosum; Cowper's glands; ductus deferens; epispadias; erection; foreskin; frenulum preputii; genitalia, male; hypospadias; mentula;

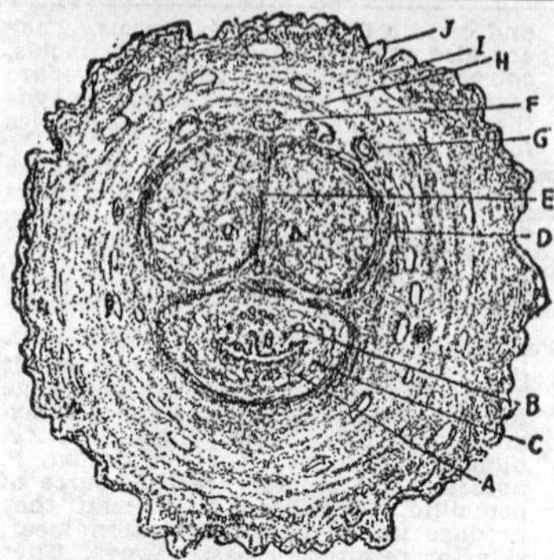

TRANSVERSE SECTION OF PENIS.
A. Lumen of urethra. B. Mucosa urethrae. C. Corpus cavernosum urethrae. D. Corpus cavernosum penis. E. Arteria profunda penis. F. Arteria dorsalis penis. G. Vena dorsalis penis. H. Nervus dorsalis penis with pacinian corpuscles. I. Musculus ischiocavernosus. J. Musculus bulbocavernosus.

nervus erigentes; peotomy; "phall-" words; prepuce; prostate; scrotum; seminal vesicle; testes; Tyson's glands; urethra; vas deferens.

penischisis (pen-ĭs'kĭs'-ĭs). Epispadias, hypospadias, paraspadias, or any fissured condition of the penis.

penitis (pē-nī'tĭs) [L. *penis*, penis, + G. *itis*, inflammation]. Inflammation of the penis.

penniform (pĕn'ĭ-form) [L. *penna*, feather, + *forma*, shape]. Feather-shaped.

pennyroyal (pĕn"ĭ-roi'ăl). Name for various plants, esp. Hedeoma and Mentha, which yield commercial oil used as carminative, and stimulant.

pennyweight (pĕn'ĭ-wāt). Troy weight containing 24 gr. or 1/20 of an ounce.

pension neurosis (pĕn'shan nū-rō-sis). A condition which develops subsequent to an injury in the belief that compensation can be obtained or will be continued by being ill. SEE: *neurosis, compensation.*

penta-, pent- [G.] Combining form meaning *five.*

pentad (pĕn'tăd) [G. *pente*, five]. 1. A radical or element with a valence of 5. 2. Group of 5.

pentamethylenediamine (pĕn"tă-mĕth"ĭl-ēn-dī'ăm-ēn) [G. *pente*, five]. A nontoxic ptomaine occurring in tissue decomposition. SYN: *cadaverine.*

pentane (pĕn'tān) [G. *pente*, five]. C_5H_{12}. One of the hydrocarbons of the methane series. A product of petroleum distillation.

pentavalent (pĕn"tă-vā'lĕnt, -tăv'ă-lent) [G. *pente*, five, + L. *valens*, having power]. Having a valence of 5. SYN: *quinquivalent.*

pentene (pĕn'tēn) [G. *pente*, five]. A liquid hydrocarbon formerly used as an anesthetic. SYN: *amylene.*

pentobarbital sodium (pĕn"tō-bar'bĭ-tăl sō'dĭ-ŭm). A barbituric acid derivative used as an oral or intravenous hypnotic agent in preanesthetic medication.

Used in labor with or without scopolamine. SYN: *nembutal.*

pentosazon (pĕn"tō-sa'zōn). Abnormal substance in urine which is incapable of fermentation.

pentose (pĕn'tōs) [G. *pente*, five]. $C_5H_{10}O_5$. A simple sugar with 5 atoms of carbon in the molecule.

pentosemia (pĕn"to-sē'mĭ-ă) [*pentose* + G. *aima*, blood]. Pentose in the blood.

pentoside (pĕn'tō-sīd). Pentose combined with some other substance.

pentosuria (pĕn"tō-sū'rĭ-ă) [*pentose* + G. *ouron*, urine]. A condition in which pentose is found in the urine.

pentothal sodium (pĕn'tō-thăl so'dĭ-ŭm). Proprietary name for thiopental sodium (USP: *sodium thiopental*), an ultra-short-acting anesthetic.

peonin (pē'ō-nĭn). A dye used as a hydrogen ion concentration test.

peotillomania (pe"ō-til-ō-mā'nĭ-ă) [G. *peos*, penis, + *tillein*, to pull, + *mania*, madness]. A tic resulting in constant pulling at the penis. SYN: *pseudomasturbation.*

peotomy (pē-ŏt'ō-mĭ) [" + *tomē*, incision]. Amputation of the penis.

pepo (pē'pō) [G. *pepōn*, ripe]. USP. Pumpkin seed which is used as an agent to remove tapeworms.

pepper (pĕp'ĕr) [G. *peperi*, pepper]. A spice which is used as a condiment, stimulant, carminative and counterirritant.

PEPPER (*sweet, green*): 1 pod (62 gm.). Calories: 15. Other main values: 1 gm. protein; trace of fat; 3 gm. carbohydrate; 6 mg. calcium; 260 I.U. vitamin A; 79 mg. ascorbic acid.

peppermint (pĕp'ĕr-mĭnt). USP. The top and leaves of the plant Mentha piperita from which oil of peppermint is derived.

USES: Aromatic stimulant, carminative, and flavoring agent.

pepsic (pĕp'sĭk) [G. *peptein*, to digest]. Peptic, *q.v.*

pepsin (pĕp'sĭn) [G. *pepsis*, digestion]. The chief enzyme of gastric juice which converts proteins into proteoses and peptones. It is formed by the chief cells of gastric glands and produces its maximum activity at a *pH* of 1.5 to 2. It is obtainable in granular form and in the presence of HCl, will digest proteins *in vitro.*

USP: An enzyme obtained from the glandular layer of the fresh stomach of the hog. Assayed to digest 3000 times its weight of freshly coagulated egg albumen.

ACTION AND USES: Acts only in acid medium. Useful to aid digestion of protein food in the stomach, sometimes combined with hydrochloric acid in cases of acute dyspepsia.

pepsinogen (pĕp-sin'o-jen) [G. *pepsis*, digestion, + *gennan*, to produce]. The zymogen or antecedent of pepsin existing in the form of granules in the chief cells of gastric glands.

peptic (pĕp'tĭk) [G. *peptein*, to digest]. 1. Concerning digestion. 2. Concerning pepsin.

p. ulcer. An ulcer occurring in lower end of esophagus, in stomach usually along lesser curvature, in duodenum, or on jejunal side of a gastrojejunostomy.

SYM: Pain is the most characteristic symptom, tending to be of uniform quality and usually described as "gnawing." It is localized in the epigastrium and exhibits a rhythmicity and periodicity usually appearing one to three hours after a meal. It is absent before breakfast but may occur during the night. It is relieved by foods and alkalis; it is aggravated by alcohol and condiments. Often periods of remission occur in which pain is absent.

Other symptoms include dyspepsia, heartburn, acid eructations, nausea, vomiting, and anorexia. Diarrhea may occur with loss of weight. In some cases, physical signs may be absent, the first indication of the condition being hemorrhage or perforation. Gastric juice always exhibits hyperacidity.

Prog: Guardedly favorable. Hemorrhage or perforation may occur without warning and relapses from new ulcers not uncommon.

NP: Medicine to reduce acid secretion of stomach. Bed rest, at first, in calm, quiet atmosphere. Daily bath and oral hygiene. Watch for complications of hemorrhage and perforation. Examine vomitus and stools for blood. In hemorrhage, ice cap over epigastric area, no food or fluid by mouth, no movement. Report pain immediately as it is first sign of perforation.

Treatment: Absolute rest in bed, alkaline Sippy treatment. Iron therapy in presence of hemorrhage. Lavage contraindicated. Hemorrhage requires absolute rest, ice bag to stomach; pellets of ice by mouth. Remedies as indicated.

Diet: Frequent feedings; bland, smooth, liquid or semi-liquid foods; high protein feedings to keep the acid in combination; high fat to inhibit acid secretion and increase energy value of food; medicines to combine with HCl to keep stomach neutral. In acute ulcer, Sippy diet recommended, *q.v.* With normal progress, after 1 week at the most, soft, bland foods; purée of vegetable and fruit; custards, and toast may be added. Number of feedings is decreased if increased amount is given at each feeding and intervals of feeding extended to 6 small meals a day, each to consist of from 10 to 12 oz. Syn: *gastric ulcer.*

peptidase. An enzyme which converts peptides to aminoacids.

peptide (pĕp'tīd) [G. *peptein,* to digest]. Compound formed by hydrolytic cleavage of peptones and which contains two or more amino acids.

A class of substances prepared by synthesis from amino acids and intermediate in molecular weight and chemical properties bet. the amino acids, which may be made artificially, and the proteins, which may not.

RS: *dipeptide, polypeptide. tripeptide.*

peptidolytic (pĕp"tĭd-ō-lĭt'ĭk) [" + *lysis,* dissolution]. Causing the splitting up or digestion of peptides.

peptinotoxin (pĕp-tĭn-ō-tŏk'sĭn) [" + *toxikon,* poison]. Poisonous ptomaine found in the body as a result of disordered or defective digestion.

peptization (pĕp-tĭ-zā'shŭn) [G. *peptein,* to digest]. In the chemistry of colloids, the process of making a colloidal solution more stable; conversion of a gel to a sol.

peptogenic, peptogenous (pĕp-tō-jĕn'ĭk, -tŏj'ĕn-ŭs) [" + *gennan,* to produce]. 1. Producing peptones and pepsin. 2. Promoting digestion.

peptoid (pĕp'toyd) [" + *eidos,* resemblance]. A product of protein digestion which does not give the biuret reaction.

peptolysis (pĕp-tŏl'ĭ-sĭs) [G. *peptein,* to digest, + *lysis,* dissolution]. The splitting up or hydrolysis of peptones.

peptolytic (pĕp-tō-lĭt'ĭk) [" + *lysis,* dissolution]. Pert. to the splitting up of peptone.

peptone (pĕp'tōn) [G. *pepton,* digesting]. A secondary protein formed by the action of proteolytic enzymes, acids, or alkalis on certain proteins.

They are nitrogenous compounds soluble in water and are not coagulated by boiling.

peptonemia (pĕp-tō-nē'mĭ-ă) [" + *aima,* blood]. Peptones in the blood.

peptonization (pĕp"tō-nĭ-zā'shŭn) [G. *peptōn,* digesting]. Process of changing protein substance into peptones by action of proteolytic enzymes.

peptonize'. To convert into peptones; to predigest with pepsin.

pep"tonol'ysis. Syn: *peptolysis.* The breakdown of peptones into simpler products, (peptides, or amino acids).

peptonuria (pĕp-tō-nū'rĭ-ă) [" + *ouron,* urine]. Excretion of peptones in the urine.

per- [L.]. A word used as a prefix or by itself meaning *through, by, by means of.* In chemistry the highest valence of an element.

peracidity (pŭr-ăs-ĭd'ĭt-ĭ) [L. *per,* throughout, + *acidus,* sour]. Abnormal acidity.

peracute (pŭr-ăk-ūt') [" + *acutus,* keen]. Very acute or violent.

per anum (pŭr ā'nŭm) [L.]. Through or by way of the anus.

peratodyn'ia. Heartburn; pain in region of cardia of stomach.

percaine (per'kān). Dibucaine hydrochloride (USP). Used for surface and spinal anesthesia.

per cent, percent. By the hundred.

p. c. of a solution. Term which designates the number of grams of solute per 100 cc. of solvent or the number of cc. of a liquid dissolved in 100 cc. of another.

perception (pŭr-sĕp'shŭn) [L. *perceptiō,* a seeing through]. 1. Process of being aware of objects; consciousness. 2. The process of receiving sensory impressions. 3. The elaboration of a sensory impression; the ideational association modifying, defining, and usually completing the primary impression or stimulus.

Vague or inadequate association occurs in confused and depressed states.

p., depth. The ability to recognize that an object has depth, as well as height and width.

p., extrasensory. Perception not through the recognized senses. Also called *paranormal perception.*

p., stereognostic. Recognition of objects by touch.

perceptivity (pŭr-sĕp-tĭv'ĭ-tĭ) [L. *perceptus,* from *percipere,* to see through]. Power to receive sense impressions.

perclu'sion. Inability to perform a movement.

percolate (pŭr'kō-lāt) [L. *percolāre,* to strain through]. 1. To seep through a powdered substance. 2. Any fluid that has been filtered or percolated. 3. To strain a fluid through powdered substances in order to impregnate it with soluble principles of such substances.

percolation (pŭr"kō-lā'shŭn) [L. *percolāre,* to strain through]. 1. Filtration. 2. Process of extracting soluble portions of a drug of powdered composition by filtering a liquid solvent through it.

percolator (pŭr'kō-lā"tŭr) [L. *percolāre,* to strain through]. Apparatus used for extraction of a drug with a liquid solvent.

per contiguum (pŭr kŏn-tĭg'ū-ŭm) [L.]. Touching, as in the spread of an inflammation from 1 part to a contiguous structure.

per continuum (pŭr kŏn-tĭn′ū-ŭm) [L.]. Continuous, as the spread of an inflammation from part to part.

percuss (pŭr-kŭs′) [L. *percussus*, from *percutere*, to strike through]. To tap parts of the body to aid diagnosis by sound emitted.

percussion (pŭr-kŭsh′ŭn) [L. *percussiō*, a striking through]. Tapping the body lightly but sharply to determine position, size and consistency of an underlying structure, the presence of fluid or pus in a cavity and resonance, pitch of the sound emitted, by vibration elicited, or by resistance encountered.

Immediate percussion is performed by striking the surface directly with the fingers.

Mediate p. is performed by using fingers of one hand as a plexor, and those of the opposite hand as a pleximeter.

RS: *abdomen, bladder, boxnote, chest, heart, intestines, kidney, liver, ovary, palpation, spleen, uterus.*

p., auscultatory. Percussion combined with auscultation.

p., direct. Immediate percussion.

p., finger. Striking of the finger resting upon the body with a finger of the other hand.

p., hammer. Syn: *plexor.* A hammer with a rubber head used for percussion.

p., indirect. Mediate percussion.

percussor (pŭr-kŭs′or) [L. striker]. Device used for diagnosis by percussion, consisting of hammer with rubber or metal head. See: *emballometer.*

percutaneous (pŭr″kū-tā′nē-ŭs) [L. *per*, through, + *cutis*, skin]. Effected through the skin, as in inunction. Or to inject through the skin.

pereirine (pĕ-rā′rēn). An alkaloid obtained from pereira bark which is used as a quinine substitute in treatment of fevers.

perflation (pŭr-flā′shŭn) [L. *perflāre*, to blow through]. The process of blowing air into a cavity to expand its walls or to force out secretions or other matter.

perforans (pŭr′fō-răns) [L. boring through]. Perforating or penetrating, as a nerve or muscle.

perforate (pŭr′fō-rāt) [L. *perforāre*, to pierce through]. 1. To puncture or to make holes. 2. Pierced with holes.

perforation (pŭr″fō-rā′shŭn) [L. *perforāre*, to pierce through]. 1. The act or process of making a hole, such as that caused by ulceration. 2. Hole made through substance or part.

p. of stomach or intestine. Sym: Abdominal crisis due to escape of contents of the perforated viscus into the peritoneal cavity. Peritonitis certain unless operated upon in time. Onset is accompanied by acute pain over perforated area spreading all over the abdomen which is rigid. Face is anxious with beads of perspiration on it. Nausea and vomiting will occur. Pulse rapid and feeble, respiration rapid and shallow. Temperature drops, but rises as peritonitis sets in, when pulse becomes fuller.

Treatment: Surgical. Pending operation give no fluids. Complete rest. No talking. Apply warmth. See: *peritonitis.*

perforator (pŭr′fō-rā-tor) [L. a piercing device]. Instrument for piercing the skull and other bones.

p., tympanum. Instrument for perforating the tympanum.

perfrication (pŭr-frĭ-kā′shŭn) [L. *perfricāre*, to rub]. Thorough rubbing with an ointment or embrocation. Syn: *inunction.*

perfusion (pŭr-fū′zhŭn) [L. *perfundere*, to pour through]. 1. Passing of a fluid through spaces. 2. The pouring of a fluid. 3. Supplying an organ or tissue with a field by injection into an artery.

perhydrocyclopentanophenanthrene (per-hi″dro - si″klo - pen - tan″o - phen-an′-thrēn). Name of the ring structure of the chemical nucleus of the steroids.

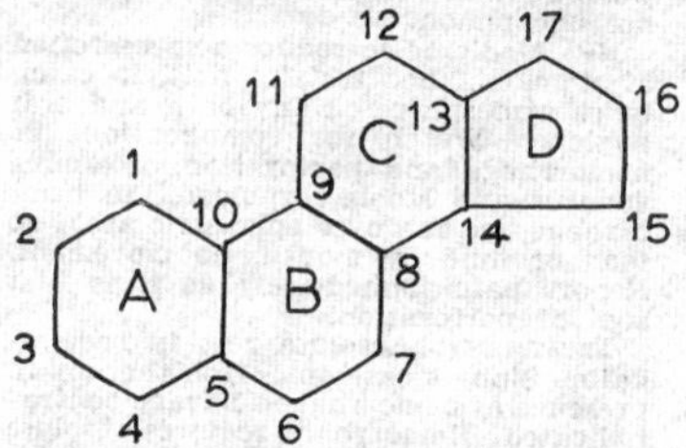

PERHYDROCYCLOPENTANOPHENANTHRENE

peri- [G.]. Prefix meaning *around, about.*

periacinal, periacinous (pĕr″ĭ-ăs′ĭ-năl, -ŭs) [G. *peri*, around, + L. *acinus*, grape]. Placed around an acinus.

periadenitis (pĕr-ĭ-ă-dē-nī′tĭs) [" + *adēn*, gland, + *-ītis*, inflammation]. Inflamed condition of tissues surrounding a gland.

perialienitis (pĕr″ĭ-ā″lĭ-ĕn-ī′tĭs) [" + L. *alienus*, foreign, + G. *-ītis*, inflammation]. Noninfectious inflammation around a foreign body. Syn: *perixenitis.*

periamygdalitis (pĕr″ĭ-ăm-ĭg″dăl-ī′tĭs) [" + *amygdalē*, tonsil, + *-ītis*, inflammation]. Inflammation of connective tissue around the tonsil. Syn: *peritonsillitis.*

periangiitis (per″ĭ-an″jĭ-i′tis) [" + *aggeion*, vessel, + *-ītis*, inflammation]. Inflamed condition of tissue around a blood or lymphatic vessel.

periangiocholitis (pĕr″ĭ-ăn″jĭ-ō-kō-lī′tĭs) [" + *aggeion*, vessel, + *cholē*, bile, + *-itis*, inflammation]. Inflamed condition of tissues around the bile ducts.

periaortitis (pĕr″ĭ-ā-or-tī′tĭs) [" + *aorte*, aorta, + *-ītis*, inflammation]. Inflamed condition of adventitia and tissues around the aorta.

periapical (pĕr″ĭ-ăp′ĭ-kăl) [G. *peri*, around, + L. *apex*, tip]. Around the apex of the root of a tooth.

periappendicitis (pĕr″ĭ-ă-pĕn-dĭ-sī′tĭs) [" + L. *appendix*, that which hangs, + G. *-ītis*, inflammation]. Inflamed condition of appendix with its surrounding tissues.

p. decidualis. Decidual cells in the peritoneum of the appendix vermiformis in cases of tubal pregnancy due to adhesions bet. fallopian tubes and the appendix.

periarterial (pĕr″ĭ-ar-tē′rĭ-ăl) [" + *artēria*, artery]. Placed around an artery.

periarteritis (pĕr″ĭ-ar-tĕr-ī′tĭs) [" + " + *-ītis*, inflammation]. Inflammation of ext. coat of an artery.

p. gummosa. Gummas in the blood vessels in syphilis.

p. nodosa. Widespread focal areas of damage due to inflammation of arteries, especially small and medium-sized ones. Function of organs involved is impaired. When the disease begins, its manifestations are extremely variable. Symptoms of a moderate febrile disease are quite common. Also called *polyarteritis nodosa.*

periarthric (per″ĭ-ar′thrĭk) [″ + *arthron,* joint]. Surrounding a joint. SYN: *circumarticular.*

periarthritis (pĕr″ĭ-ar-thrī′tĭs) [″ + *arthron,* joint, + *-itis,* inflammation]. Inflammation of area around a joint.

periarticular (pĕr″ĭ-ar-tĭk′ū-lăr) [″ + L. *articulus,* a joint]. Surrounding a joint. SYN: *circumarticular.*

periaxial (pĕr-ĭ-ăks′ĭ-ăl) [″ + *axōn,* axis]. Located around an axis.

periaxillary (pĕr″ĭ-ăk′sĭl-ĕ-rĭ) [G. *peri,* around, + L. *axilla,* armpit]. About the axilla.

peribronchiolitis (pĕr″ĭ-brŏng″kĭ-ō-lī′tĭs) [″ + L. *bronchiolus,* bronchiole, + *-itis,* inflammation]. Inflammation of area around the bronchioles.

peribronchitis (pĕr″ĭ-brŏng-kī′tĭs) [″ + *brogchos,* windpipe, + *-itis,* inflammation]. Inflammation of all tissues surrounding the bronchi or bronchial tubes.

pericardiac, pericardial (pĕr-ĭ-kar′dĭ-ăk, -ăl) [″ + *kardia,* heart]. Concerning the pericardium.

pericardicentesis (pĕr″ĭ-kar″dĭ-sĕn-tē′sĭs) [″ + *kardia,* heart, + *kentēsis,* puncture]. Surgical piercing of the pericardium.

pericardiectomy (pĕr″ĭ-kar-dĭ-ĕk′tō-mĭ) [″ + ″ + *ektomē,* excision]. Excision of part or all of the pericardium.

pericardiocentesis (pĕr″ĭ-kar″dĭ-ō-sĕn-tē′-sĭs) [G. *peri,* around, + *kardia,* heart, + *kentēsis,* puncture]. Surgical perforation of the pericardium. SYN: *pericardicentesis.*

pericardiolysis (pĕr″ĭ-kar″dĭ-ŏl′ĭ-sĭs) [″ + ″ + *lysis,* dissolution]. Separation of adhesions bet. the visceral and parietal pericardium.

pericardiomediastinitis (pĕr″ĭ-kar″dĭ-ō-mē-dĭ-ăs″tĭ-nī′tĭs) [″ + ″ + L. *mediastinum* + G. *-itis,* inflammation]. Inflamed condition of the pericardium and mediastinum.

pericardiophrenic (pĕr-ĭ-kar″dĭ-ō-fren′ĭk) [″ + ″ + *phrēn,* diaphragm]. Concerning the pericardium and diaphragm.

pericardiopleural (pĕr″ĭ-kar″dĭ-ō-plū′răl) [″ + ″ + *pleura,* rib]. Concerning the pericardium and pleura.

pericardiorrhaphy (pĕr″ĭ-kar″dĭ-or′ă-fĭ) [″ + ″ + *raphē,* a sewing]. Suture of a wound in the pericardium.

pericardiostomy (pĕr″ĭ-kar″dĭ-ŏs′tō-mĭ) [G. *peri,* around, + *kardia,* heart, + *stoma,* opening]. Formation of an opening into the pericardium for drainage.

pericardiosymphysis (pĕr″ĭ-kar″dĭ-ō-sĭm′-fĭ-sĭs) [″ + ″ + *symphysis,* a joining]. Adhesion bet. the layers of the pericardium.

pericardiotomy (pĕr″ĭ-kar-dĭ-ŏt′ō-mĭ) [″ + ″ + *tomē,* a cutting]. Incision of pericardial sac around heart.

pericarditic (pĕr-ĭ-kar-dĭt′ĭk) [″ + *kardia,* heart]. Concerning the pericardium.

pericarditis (pĕr-ĭ-kar-dī′tĭs) [G. *peri,* around, + *kardia,* heart, + *-itis,* inflammation]. Inflammation of pericardium.

ETIOL: Tuberculosis, mycoses, infection by pyogenic organisms, collagen disease, uremia, myocardial infarction, neoplasms, trauma.

SYM: Moderate fever, precordial pain and tenderness, dry cough, dyspnea and palpitation. Pulse, first rapid, forcible, then weak and irregular.

First stage: Auscultation reveals to and fro friction sound heart over 4th left intercostal space near sternum. Inspection and palpation sometimes reveal a diffuse apex beat. Friction rub may sometimes be palpated.

Second stage: Serofibrinous effusion. Bulging of precordium. Increased area of dullness, triangular in shape, base down. Heart sounds muffled, distant, feeble. Purulent effusion yields similar signs, but in addition high, irregular fever; sweats; chills, and progressive pallor; sometimes edema over the precordium. In doubtful cases the aspirating needle reveals pus.

PROG: Fair in early stages. In purulent and fibrinous, extremely grave.

TREATMENT: *General*: Absolute bed rest, light diet. For the relief of pain apply ice bag over precordium or administer pain-relieving drugs, depending on its intensity. *Specific*: Appropriate antibiotic for specific organisms involved. If purulent effusion occurs, aspiration or surgical drainage. If gallop rhythm or signs of heart failure occur, restrict fluids and salt. For chronic constrictive pericarditis, resection of pericardium.

p., acute fibrinous. P. characterized by fibrinous exudation.

p., acute nonspecific. A disease of unknown etiology usually following respiratory infections.

p. adhesiva. Form in which the layers of pericardium adhere.

p., constrictive. P. in which adhesions form between visceral and parietal layers of the peritoneum.

p. externa. Inflammation of exterior surface of the pericardium.

p., fibrinous. Membrane is covered with butterlike exudate which organizes and unites the pericardial surfaces.

SYM: Precordial bulging, a weak apex beat with loud sounds, a systolic retraction at apex and over large part of precordium, peculiar diastolic collapse of jugular veins, feeble apex beat with a forcible impulse over body of heart. Signs of heart failure, as dyspnea, dropsy, cyanosis.

p., hemorrhagic. P. in which the exudate contains blood.

p., idiopathic. SEE: *p., acute nonspecific.*

p., ischemic. P. resulting from myocardial infarction.

p., neoplastic. P. due to invasion of pericardium by malignant tumors of adjoining structures.

p. obliterans. Pericardial inflammation causing adhesions and obliteration of the pericardial cavity.

p., serofibrinous. P. in which there is a considerable quantity of serous exudate but little fibrin.

p., uremic. P. resulting from uremia.

p., viral. SEE: *p., acute nonspecific.*

pericardium (pĕr″ĭ-kar′dĭ-ŭm) [G. *peri,* around, + *kardia,* heart]. The double, membranous, fibroserous sac enclosing the heart and the origins of the great blood vessels.

It is composed of an inner serous layer, (*visceral pericardium* or *epicardium*) and an outer fibrous layer, (*parietal pericardium*). The space between the two constitutes the *pericardial cavity* which is normally filled with a small amount of serous fluid.

Its base is attached to the diaphragm, its apex extending upward as far as the first subdivision of the great blood vessels. It is attached in front to the sternum, laterally to the mediastinal pleura and posteriorly to the esophagus, trachea, and principal bronchi.

Normally, p. contains a thin serous fluid.

p., adherent. Condition in which fibrous bands form between the two layers obliterating pericardial cavity. SEE: *pericarditis, constrictive.*

p., bread and butter. Condition seen in fibrinous pericarditis in which pericardium has a peculiar appearance due to fibrinous deposits on the two opposing surfaces.

p. externum. The outer fibrous layer of the pericardium.

p. internum. Serous inner layer of the pericardium.

p., parietal. The outer fibrous layer of the pericardium.

p., shaggy. Condition occurring in fibrinous pericarditis in which loose shaggy deposits of fibrin are seen on surfaces of pericardium.

p., visceral. Serous inner layer of the pericardium.

pericecal (pĕr-ĭ-sē′kăl) [" + L. *caecum,* blind]. Situated around the cecum.

pericecitis (pĕr-ĭ-sē-sī′tĭs) [" + " + G. *-ītis,* inflammation]. Inflamed condition of area around the cecum. SYN: *perityphlitis.*

pericementitis (pĕr″ĭ-sĕm-ĕn-tī′tĭs) [" + L. *caementum,* cement, + G. *-ītis,* inflammation]. Progressive necrosis of the alveoli of the teeth. SYN: *periodontitis.*

pericementoclasia (pĕr″ĭ-sĕm-ĕn-tō-klā′-zĭ-ă) [" + " + G. *klasis,* a breaking]. Dissolution of the pericementum with alveolar absorption. SYN: *pyorrhea alveolaris.*

pericementum (pĕr″ĭ-sĕm-ĕn′tŭm) [" + L. *caementum,* cement]. Fibrous tissue covering the root of a tooth.

perichareia (per″ĭ-kă-rĭ′ă). Excessive or abnormal rejoicing, seen in certain psychoses.

pericholangitis (pĕr″ĭ-kō-lăn-jī′tĭs) [G. *peri,* around, + *cholē,* bile, + *aggeion,* vessel, + *-ītis,* inflammation]. Inflammation of tissues surrounding a bile duct. SYN: *periangiocholitis.*

pericholecystitis (pĕr″ĭ-kō-lĕ-sĭs-tī′tĭs) [" + " + *kystis,* a sac, + *-ītis,* inflammation]. Inflammation of tissues situated around the gallbladder.

perichondral, perichondrial (pĕr-ĭ-kon′drăl, -drĭ-ăl) [" + *chondros,* cartilage]. Concerning the membrane covering cartilage.

perichondritis (pĕr-ĭ-kŏn-drī′tĭs) [" + " + *-ītis,* inflammation]. Inflamed condition of perichondrium.

perichondrium (pĕr-ĭ-kŏn′drĭ-ŭm) [" + *chondros,* cartilage]. Membrane of fibrous connective tissue around surface of cartilage.

perichondroma (pĕr″ĭ-kŏn-drō′mă) [" + " + *-ōma,* tumor]. A tumor arising from fibrous tissue which covers cartilage.

perichordal (pĕr-ĭ-kor′dăl) [" + *chordē,* cord]. Placed around the notochord.

perichorioidal, perichoroidal (pĕr″ĭ-kō-rĭ-oy′dăl, -roy′dăl) [G. *peri,* around, + *chorioeidēs,* skinlike]. Situated around the choroid coat.

perichrome (pĕr′ĭ-krōm) [" + *chrōma,* color]. A nerve cell in which the tigroid mass is arranged in rows through the protoplasm.

pericolic (pĕr-ĭ-ko′lĭk) [" + *kōlon,* colon]. Around or encircling the colon.

pericolitis (pĕr″ĭ-kō-lī′tĭs) [" + " + *-ītis,* inflammation]. Inflammation of area around the colon.

pericolonitis (pĕr″ĭ-kō-lŏn-ī′tĭs) [" + " + *-ītis,* inflammation]. Inflamed condition of region around the colon.

pericolpitis (pĕr″ĭ-kŏl-pī′tĭs) [" + *kolpos,* vagina, + *-ītis,* inflammation]. Inflammation of connective tissues surrounding the vagina.

periconchal (pĕr-ĭ-kŏng′kăl) [" + *cogchē,* concha]. Around the concha of the ear.

p. sulcus. Groove on post. surface of the auricle.

periconchitis (pĕr″ĭ-kŏng-kī′tĭs) [" + " + *-ītis,* inflammation]. Inflamed condition of the lining of the orbit.

pericorneal (pĕr″ĭ-kor′nē-ăl) [G. *peri,* around, + L. *cornu,* horn]. Placed around the cornea.

pericranitis (pĕr″ĭ-krā-nī′tĭs) [" + *kranion,* skull, + *-ītis,* inflammation]. Inflamed condition of pericranium.

pericranium (pĕr″ĭ-krā′nĭ-ŭm) [" + *kranion,* skull]. Fibrous membrane surrounding the cranium; periosteum of the skull.

p. internum. Lining surface of the cranium. SYN: *endocranium.*

pericystitis (pĕr″ĭ-sĭs-tī′tĭs) [" + *kystis,* a bladder, + *-ītis,* inflammation]. Inflamed condition of tissues about the bladder.

pericytial (pĕr-ĭ-sĭsh′ăl) [" + *kytos,* cell]. Placed around a cell.

peridectomy (pĕr-ĭ-dĕk′tō-mĭ) [" + *ektomē,* excision]. 1. Operation for relief of pannus. 2. Circumcision. SYN: *peritomy.*

peridendric (pĕr-ĭ-dĕn′drĭk) [" + *dendron,* a tree]. Surrounding a dendrite of a nerve cell.

peridental (pĕr-ĭ-dĕn′tăl) [G. *peri,* around, + L. *dens, dent-,* tooth]. Surrounding a tooth or part of one. SYN: *periodontal.*

peridentitis. Inflammation of tissues surrounding a tooth; periodontoclasia.

periderm. SYN: *epitrichal layer* or *epitrichium.* Thin layer of flattened cells forming a transient layer of embryonic epidermis.

peridesmitis (pĕr″ĭ-dĕz-mī′tĭs) [" + *desmos,* band, + *-ītis,* inflammation]. Inflammation of the areolar tissue around a ligament.

peridesmium (pĕr″ĭ-dĕz′mĭ-ŭm) [" + *desmos,* band]. The connective tissue membrane sheathing a ligament.

peridiverticulitis (pĕr″ĭ-dī-vĕr-tĭk″ū-lī′tĭs) [G. *peri,* around, + L. *diverticulāre,* to turn aside, + G. *-ītis,* inflammation]. Inflammation of tissues situated around an intestinal diverticulum.

periductal (pĕr-ĭ-duk′tăl) [" + L. *ductus,* a passage]. Situated about a duct.

periduodenitis (pĕr″ĭ-dū″o-dē-nī′tĭs) [" + L. *duodeni,* twelve, + *-ītis,* inflammation]. Inflammation around the duodenum often causing adhesions attaching it to the peritoneum.

periencephalitis (pĕr″ĭ-ĕn-sĕf-ă-lī′tĭs) [" + *egkephalos,* brain, + *-ītis,* inflammation]. Inflamed condition of the surface of the brain.

periencephalomeningitis (pĕr″ĭ-ĕn-sĕf-ă-lō-mĕn-ĭn-jī′tĭs) [" + " + *mēnigx,* membrane, + *-ītis,* inflammation]. Inflamed condition of cerebral cortex and the meninges.

periendothelioma (pĕr″ĭ-ĕn″dō-thē-lĭ-ō′-mă) [" + *endon,* within, + *thēlē,* nipple, + *-ōma,* tumor]. A tumor arising from the endothelium of the lymphatics and the perithelium of blood vessels.

perienteritis (pĕr″ĭ-ĕn-tĕr-ī′tĭs) [G. *peri,* around, + *enteron,* intestines, + *-ītis,* inflammation]. Inflamed condition of peritoneal lining of intestines.

periesophagitis (pĕr″ĭ-ē-sŏf-ā-jī′tĭs) [" + *oisophagos*, esophagus, + *-ītis*, inflammation]. Inflamed condition of tissues around the esophagus.

perifistular (pĕr-ĭ-fis′tū-ler) [" + L. *fistula*, pipe]. Located around a fistula.

perifolliculitis (pĕr″ĭ-fō-lĭk″ū-lī′tĭs) [" + L. *folliculus*, a little sac, + *-ītis*, inflammation]. Inflamed condition of area around the hair follicles.

perigangliitis (pĕr″ĭ-găng-lĭ-ī′tĭs) [" + *gagglion*, knot, + *-ītis*, inflammation]. Inflamed condition of region around a ganglion.

perigastritis (pĕr″ĭ-găs-trī′tĭs) [" + *gastēr*, belly, + *-ītis*, inflammation]. Inflammation of peritoneal covering of stomach.

perihepatitis (pĕr″ĭ-hĕp-ă-tī′tĭs) [" + *ēpar, ēpat-*, liver, + *-ītis*, inflammation]. Inflammation of peritoneal covering of the liver, usually occurring in circumscribed areas.

perijejunitis (pĕr″ĭ-jĕj-ū-nī′tĭs) [" + L. *jejunum*, empty, + G. *-ītis*, inflammation]. Inflamed condition of tissues around the jejunum.

perikaryon (pĕr-ĭ-kăr′ĭ-ŏn) [G. *peri*, around, +*karyon*, nucleus]. The cell body of a neuron.

per″ikerat′ic. About the cornea.

perilabyrinthitis (pĕr″ĭ-lab-ĭr-ĭn-thī′tĭs) [" + *labyrinthos*, a maze, + *-ītis*, inflammation]. Inflammation of tissues and parts about the labyrinth.

perilaryngitis (pĕr″ĭ-lăr-ĭn-jī′tĭs) [" + *larygx*, larynx, + *-ītis*, inflammation]. Inflamed condition of tissues around the larynx.

perilymph (pĕr-ĭ-lĭmf) [" + L. *lympha*, serum]. The pale, limpid fluid contained in the space bet. the membranous and bony labyrinth of the internal ear.

perilymphangitis (pĕr″ĭ-lĭmf-ăn-jī′tĭs) [G. *peri*, around, + L. *lympha*, serum, + *aggeion*, vessel, + *-ītis*, inflammation]. Inflammation of tissues around a lymphatic vessel.

perimeningitis (pĕr″ĭ-mĕn-ĭn-jī′tĭs) [" + *mēnigx*, membrane, + *-ītis*, inflammation]. Inflamed condition of the dura mater. Syn: *pachymeningitis*.

perimeter (pĕr-ĭm′ĕt-ĕr) [" + *metron*, measure]. 1. The outer edge or periphery of a body or measure of the same. 2. Device for determining the extent of the field of vision.

perimetritis (pĕr″ĭ-mē-trī′tĭs) [" + *mētra*, uterus, + *-ītis*, inflammation]. Inflammation of the peritoneal covering of the uterus.

May be associated with parametritis.

perimetrium (pĕr-ĭ-mē′trĭ-ŭm) [" + *mētra*, uterus]. Peritoneum covering uterus.

perimetry (pĕr-ĭm′ĕ-trĭ) [" + *metron*, measure]. 1. Circumference, edge, border of a body. 2. Measurement of the scope of the field of vision with a perimeter.

perimyelitis (pĕr″ĭ-mī-ē-lī′tĭs) [" + *myelos*, marrow, + *-ītis*, inflammation]. 1. Inflammation of the pia mater and arachnoid of the brain or spinal cord. Syn: *leptomeningitis*. 2. Inflammation of the endosteum, or membrane around medullary cavity of a bone.

perimyelography (pĕr″ĭ-mī-ĕ-lŏg′ră-fĭ) [" + " + *graphein*, to write]. X-ray examination around the spinal cord.

perimyoendocarditis (pĕr″ĭ-mī″ō-ĕn″dō-kar-dī′tĭs) [" + *mys, my-*, muscle, + *endon*, within, + *kardia*, heart, + *-ītis*, inflammation]. Inflammation of the muscular wall of the heart, its endothelial lining and the pericardium.

perimysial (pĕr-ĭ-mĭs′ĭ-ăl) [G. *peri*, around, + *mys*, muscle]. Concerning, or of the nature of, perimysium; sheathing a muscle.

perimysiitis (pĕr-ĭ-mĭs-ĭ-ī′tĭs) [" + " + *-ītis*, inflammation]. Inflamed condition of the perimysium, the sheath surrounding a muscle.

perimysium (pĕr-ĭ-mĭs′ĭ-ŭm) [G. *peri*, around, + *mys*, muscle]. The connective tissue sheath that envelops each primary bundle of muscle fibers. Sometimes called *p. internum*.

perinatal (per-ĭ-na′tal) [" + *natal*, birth]. Occurring just before or after birth.

p. externum. The epimysium, *q.v.*

perineal (pĕr-ĭ-nē′ăl) [G. *perinaion*, perineum]. Concerning or situated on the perineum.

p. body. Mass of tissue composed of skin, muscle, and fascia bet. vagina and rectum in the female, and the urethra and rectum in the male.

p. fascia. Three layers bet. muscles of perineum.

p. hernia. Hernia perforating the perineum. Syn: *perineocele*.

p. section. Surgical incision through perineum. Syn: *perineotomy*.

perineo- [G.]. Combining form pertaining to the perineum.

perineocele (pĕr-ĭ-nē′ō-sēl) [G. *perinaion*, perineum, + *kēlē*, hernia]. Hernia in the region of the perineum.

perineocolporectomyomectomy (pĕr-ĭ-nē″-ō-kŏl″pō-rĕk″tō-mī-ō-mĕk′tō-mĭ) [" + *kolpos*, vagina, + L. *rectus*, straight, + G. *mys, myo-*, muscle, + *-ōma*, tumor, + *ektomē*, excision]. Excision of a myoma by incising the perineum, vagina, and rectum.

perineometer (per″ĭ-ne-om′ĕ-ter). Apparatus for measuring pressure or force which is produced in the vagina when pubococcygeus and levator ani muscles are voluntarily contracted.

perineoplasty (pĕr-ĭ-nē′ō-plăs″tĭ) [" + *plassein*, to form]. Reparative surgery on the perineum.

perineorrhaphy (pĕr″ĭ-nē-ŏr′ă-fĭ) [" + *raphē*, a sewing]. Suture of the perineum usually following labor.

NP: Give external irrigation to perineum following each use of bedpan as sepsis must be avoided. Keep stitches dry, sterile dressing secured with a T-bandage which is changed frequently, at least twice daily. Swab with antiseptic, dry and put on fresh dressing. Warm glycerin packs are sometimes ordered to relieve pain and reduce edema. Light treatments are ordered by some doctors.

It is difficult for patient to assume a comfortable position in which to lie. Prop up first on one and then the other side. The patient is encouraged to move about. Diet as desired. Prevent hard bowel movements by giving substances to soften feces. Be certain patient is voiding freely.

p., anterior. Rectifying cystocele.*

p., colpo-. Removal of part of post. vaginal wall and suturing torn perineal body.

p., posterior. Removal of rectocele.

perineosynthesis (pĕr-ĭ-nē″ō-sĭn′the-sĭs) [" + *synthesis*, a placing together]. Plastic operation for repair of a lacerated perineum; performed by grafting vaginal mucosa over area.

perineotomy (pĕr″ĭ-nē-ŏt′ō-mĭ) [" + *tomē*, a cutting]. Operation of incising the perineum.

perineovaginal (pĕr-ĭ-nē″ō-văj′ĭn-ăl) [" + L. *vagina*, sheath]. Concerning the perineum and vagina.

perinephric (pĕr-ĭ-nĕf′rĭk) [G. *peri*, around, + *nephros*, kidney]. Located or occurring around the kidney.

p. abscess. Abscess formation in peritoneal membrane surrounding the kidney.

perinephritis (pĕr″ĭ-ne-frī′tĭs) [" + " + *-ītis*, inflammation]. Inflammation of peritoneal tissues around the kidney. Syn: *paranephritis.*

perinephrium (pĕr-ĭ-nĕf′rĭ-ŭm) [" + *nephros*, kidney]. The connective and fatty tissue surrounding the kidney.

perineum (pĕr-ĭ-nē′ŭm) [G. *perinaion*, perineum]. 1. The structures occupying the pelvic outlet and comprising the pelvic floor. 2. The region between the vulva and anus in a female or between scrotum and anus in a male.

It is made up of skin, muscle and fasciae. The muscles of the perineum are the ant. portion of the intact levator ani muscle, the transverse perineal muscle and the sphincter muscles of the vagina. RS: *bodies, perineal, "perine-" words.*

p., tears of the. There are 3 degrees of severity, being caused by overstretching of vagina and perineum in delivery, fetal malposition increasing the tears.

Complications: Hemorrhage, infection, cystocele, rectocele, descent of uterus, perhaps loss of bowel control.

Treatment: Surgery.

p., watering-pot. One riddled with fistulas from urethral stricture.

perineurial (pĕr″ĭ-nu′rĭ-ăl) [G. *peri*, around, + *neuron*, sinew]. Concerning the perineurium, the sheath around a bundle of nerve fibers.

perineuritis (pĕr″ĭ-nū-rī′tĭs) [" + " + *-ītis*, inflammation]. Inflammation of the sheath enveloping nerve fibers.

perineurium (pĕr″ĭ-nū′rĭ-ŭm) [G. *peri*, around, + *neuron*, sinew, + *-itis*, inflammation]. A connective tissue sheath investing a fasciculus or bundle of nerve fibers. Also called *perifascicular sheath.*

periocular (pĕr-ĭ-ŏk′ū-ler) [" + L. *oculus*, eye]. Located around the eye. Syn: *circumocular.*

period (pēr′ĭ-ŏd) [" + *odos*, a way]. 1. The time during which anything or at which anything takes place, which is limited by a recurring event. 2. The menses. 3. Time occupied by a disease in running its course, or by a division of the total, as an incubation period.

p., childbearing. The p. in the female during which she is capable of procreation; puberty to the menopause.

p. (of) development. See: *embryo, development of.*

p., gestation. Period of pregnancy or time from conception to parturition. Average length is 10 lunar months or 280 days measured from onset of last menstrual period. Length varies from 250 to 310 days. See: *gestation; pregnancy table.*

p., incubation. Time from moment of infection until appearance of first symptom.

p's (of an) infectious disease. 1. P. of incubation. 2. P. of prodromal symptoms. 3. P. of invasion. 4. Fastigium or acme. 5. P. of decline or defervescence. See: *infection.*

p., latent. The time bet. stimulation and the resulting response.

p., menstrual. Menstruation.

p., neonatal. The first 30 days of infant life.

p., patent. The time in a parasitic disease during which organisms are demonstrable in the body.

p., puerperal. 1. The period of a woman in labor or one who has just been delivered. 2. Period between labor and involution of pelvic organs.

periodic (pēr-ĭ-od′ĭk) [G. *peri*, around, + *odos*, way]. Recurring after definite intervals.

p. law. That which states that the chemical and physical properties of the chemical elements are periodic functions of their atomic weights.

periodicity (pēr″ĭ-ō-dĭs′ĭ-tĭ) [" + *odos*, way]. 1. State of being regularly recurrent. 2. PT: The rate of rise and fall or interruption of a unidirectional current. 3. Recurrence of the menses.

periodontal (pĕr″ĭ-ō-don′tăl) [" + *odous, odont-*, tooth]. Located about a tooth.

periodontitis (pĕr″ĭ-ō-dŏn-tī′tis) [G. *peri*, around, + *odous, odont-*, tooth, + *-itis*, inflammation]. Syn: *pyorrhea alveolaris, Rigg's disease.* Inflammation or degeneration, or both, of the dental periosteum, alveolar bone, cementum, and adjacent gingiva. Suppuration usually occurs, supporting bone is resorbed, teeth become loose and recession of gingivae occurs. Usually follows chronic gingivitis, Vincent's infection, or poor dental hygiene. Systemic factors may predispose.

p., apical. P. of periapical region usually leading to formation of periapical abscess.

periodontium (pĕr-ĭ-ō-dŏn′shĭ-ŭm). The tissues surrounding and supporting a tooth. They include periodontal membrane, alveolar bone, and gingiva.

periodontoclasia (pĕr-ĭ-ō-don′tō-klā′zĭ-ă) [G. *peri*, around, + *odous, odont-*, tooth, + *klasis*, a breaking]. Condition characterized by inflammation accompanied by degenerative and retrogressive changes in the periodontium.

periodontology (pĕr″ĭ-ō-dŏn-tŏl′ō-jĭ) [" + " + *logos*, disease]. Phase of dentistry dealing with treatment of diseases of the tissues around the teeth.

periodoscope (pĕr″ĭ-od′ō-skōp) [G. *peri*, around, + *odos*, way, + *skopein*, to examine]. Table or dial for calculation of expected date of confinement.

periomphalic (pĕr″ĭ-ŏm-făl′ĭk) [" + *omphalos*, eye]. Located around umbilicus.

perionychia (pĕr″ĭ-ō-nĭk′ĭ-ă). Inflammation about a nail.

perionychium (pĕr″ĭ-ō-nĭk′ĭ-ŭm) [" + *onyx, onych-*, nail]. The epidermis surrounding a nail.

perionyxis (pĕr″ĭ-ō-nĭk′sĭs) [" + *onyx*, nail]. Inflammation of epidermis surrounding a nail.

perioophoritis (pĕr″ĭ-ō-of″ō-rī′tĭs) [" + *oophoron*, ovary, + *-itis*, inflammation]. Inflammation of the surface membrane of the ovary. Syn: *perioothecitis.*

perioophorosalpingitis (pĕr″ĭ-ō-ŏf″ō-rō-sal″pĭn-jī′tĭs) [" + " + *salpigx*, tube, + *-ītis*, inflammation]. Inflamed condition of tissues around an ovary and oviduct.

perioothecitis (pĕr″ĭ-ō″o-the-sī′tĭs) [" + *ōon*, egg, + *thēcē*, box, + *-ītis*, inflammation]. Inflammation of the tissues around the ovary. Syn: *perioophoritis.*

perioothecosalpingitis (pĕr″ĭ-ō″o-the″kō-săl-pĭn-jī′tĭs) [G. *peri*, around, + *thēcē*, box, + *salpigx*, tube, + *-ītis*, inflammation]. Inflammation of peritoneal membrane around the ovary and oviduct. SYN: *perioophorosalpingitis, perisalpingoovaritis.*

perioptometry (pĕr″ĭ-op-tŏm′ĕt-rĭ) [" + *optos,* visible, + *metron,* a measure]. Measurement of the visual field.

perior′al. SYN: *circumoral.* About or surrounding the mouth.

periorbita (pĕr″ĭ-or′bĭ-tă) [" + L. *orbita,* orbit]. Periosteum of the socket of the eye.

periorbital (pĕr″ĭ-or′bĭ-tăl) [" + L. *orbita,* orbit]. Surrounding the socket of the eye. SYN: *circumorbital.*

periorbititis (pĕr″ĭ-or-bĭ-tī′tĭs) [" + " + G. *-ītis,* inflammation]. Inflamed condition of the periorbita.

periorchitis (pĕr″ĭ-or-kī′tĭs) [" + *orchis,* testicle, + *-ītis,* inflammation]. Inflamed condition of the tissues investing a testicle.

p. hemorrhagica. Chronic hematocele of the tunica vaginalis coat of the testis.

periosteal (pĕr-ĭ-os′tē-ăl) [" + *osteon,* bone]. Concerning the periosteum.

periosteitis (pĕr″ĭ-ŏs-tē-ī′tĭs) [G. *peri,* around, + *osteon,* bone, + *-itis,* inflammation]. Inflammation of membrane investing a bone, the periosteum. SYN: *periostitis.*

periosteoedema (pĕr″ĭ-os″tē-ō-ĕ-dē′mă) [" + " + *oidema,* swelling]. Edema of the periosteum, the membrane surrounding a bone.

periosteoma (pĕr″ĭ-ŏs-tē-ō′mă) [" + " + *-ōma,* tumor]. 1. An abnormal growth surrounding a bone. 2. Tumor of the periosteum, the tissue surrounding a bone.

periosteomyelitis (pĕr″ĭ-ŏs″tē-ō-mī′ĕ-lī-tĭs) [G. *peri,* around, + *osteon,* bone, + *myelos,* marrow, + *-itis,* inflammation]. Inflammation of bone including the periosteum and marrow.

periosteophyte (pĕr″ĭ-ŏs′tē-ō-fīt) [" + " + *phyton,* growth]. Abnormal bony growth on periosteum, or arising from it.

periosteorrhaphy (pĕr″ĭ-ŏs-tē-or′ă-fĭ) [" + " + *raphē,* a sewing]. Joining by suture the margins of a severed periosteum.

periosteotome (pĕr″ĭ-ŏs′tē-ō-tōm) [G. *peri,* around, + *osteon,* bone, + *tomē,* a cutting]. Instrument for cutting the periosteum or removing it from the bone.

periosteotomy (pĕr″ĭ-ŏs-tē-ŏt′ō-mĭ) [" + " + *tomē,* an incision]. Incision into the periosteum.

periosteous (pĕr″ĭ-os′tē-ŭs) [" + *osteon,* bone]. Concerning, or of the nature of, periosteum. SYN: *periosteal.*

periosteum (pĕr-ĭ-ŏs′tē-ŭm) [G. *peri,* around, + *osteon,* bone]. The fibrous membrane which forms the investing covering of bones except at their articular surfaces. Consists of a dense *external* layer containing numerous blood vessels and an *inner* layer (cambium layer), less vascular and more cellular. It serves as a supporting structure for blood vessels nourishing bone and for attachment of muscles, tendons, and ligaments.

It extends over the whole surface except at the cartilaginous articulations.

p. externum. P. covering ext. surfaces of bones.

p. internum. Int. p. lining the medullary canal of a bone.

periostitis (pĕr-ĭ-ŏs-tī′tĭs) [" + " + *-ītis,* inflammation]. Inflamed condition of membrane investing a bone, the periosteum.

ETIOL: Infection following infectious diseases, esp. syphilis; also trauma.

SYM: Pain over part, esp. under pressure, fever, sweats, leukocytosis, skin inflamed, rigidity of overlying muscles.

p., albuminous. P. with albuminous serous fluid exudate beneath the membrane affected.

p., alveolar. Inflammation of the peridental membrane. SYN: *periodontitis.*

p., dental. P. of a tooth sheath.

p., diffuse. P. of the long bones.

p., hemorrhagic. P. with extravasation of blood under the periosteum.

periostoma (pĕr″ĭ-ŏs-tō′mă) [G. *peri,* around, + *osteon,* bone, + *-ōma,* tumor]. A bony neoplasm around a bone or arising from its membranous sheath.

periostomedullitis (pĕr″ĭ-ŏs″tō-mĕd-ū-lī′-tĭs) [" + " + L. *medulla,* marrow, + G. *-ītis,* inflammation]. Inflammation of the marrow or sheath of a bone. SYN: *periosteomedullitis, periosteomyelitis.*

periostosis (pĕr″ĭ-ŏs-tō′sĭs) [" + " + *-ōsis,* disease]. A bony neoplasm around a bone or arising from it.

periostotomy (pĕr″ĭ-ŏs-tŏt′ō-mĭ) [" + " + *tomē,* incision]. Incision of the periosteum, the sheath covering a bone. SYN: *periosteotomy.*

periotic (pĕr-ĭ-ŏt′ĭk) [G. *peri,* around, + *ous, ot-,* ear]. Situated around the ear, esp. the internal ear.

p. bone. The mastoid and petrous portions of the temporal bone.

peripachymeningitis (pĕr″ĭ-pak″ĭ-mĕn-ĭn-jī′tĭs) [" + *pachys,* thick, + *mēnigx,* membrane, + *-ītis,* inflammation]. Inflamed condition of connective tissue bet. the dura mater and the bone.

peripancreatitis (pĕr″ĭ-păn-krē-ă-tī′tĭs) [G. *peri,* around, + *pagkreas,* pancreas, + *-ītis,* inflammation]. Inflammation of tissues about or around the pancreas.

peripatetic (pĕr-ĭ-pă-tĕt′ĭk) [" + *patein,* to walk]. Moving from place to place.

periphacitis (pĕr-ĭ-fă-sī′tĭs) [" + *phakos,* lens, + *-ītis,* inflammation]. Inflamed condition of the capsule of the crystalline lens of the eye.

periphakus (pĕr″ĭ-fā′kus). The elastic capsule surrounding the crystalline lens.

peripherad (pĕr-ĭf′ĕr-ăd) [" + *pherein,* to bear, + L. *ad,* to]. In the direction of the periphery.

peripheral (pĕr-ĭf′ĕr-ăl) [" + *pherein,* to bear]. Located at or pert. to the periphery.

peripheraphose (pĕr″ĭf′er-ă-fōs). Subjective sensation of darkness or shadow which originates in peripheral optic structures (optic nerve or eyeball).

peripherophose (per-ĭf′er-ō-fōs). A subjective sensation of light or color which originates in peripheral optic structure (optic nerve or eyeball).

periphery (pĕr-ĭf′ĕ-rĭ) [" + *pherein,* to bear]. Outer part or a surface of a body; part away from the center.

periphlebitis (pĕr″ĭ-flē-bī′tĭs) [G. *peri,* around, + *phleps,* vein, + *-ītis,* inflammation]. Inflamed condition of external coat of a vein or tissues around it.

periphoria (pĕr-ĭ-fō′rĭ-ă) [" + *phoros,* a bearer]. Tendency of the axis of the eye to deviate from the normal. SYN: *cyclophoria.*

periphrastic (pĕr-ĭ-frăs′tĭk) [" + *phrazein,* to speak]. Relating to the use of superfluous words in expressing a thought.

periphrenitis (pĕr″ĭ-frĕn-ī′tĭs) [" + *phrēn,* diaphragm, + *-ītis,* inflammation]. Inflamed condition of the structures around the diaphragm.

Periplaneta (per″ĭ-plă-nē′tă). A genus of cockroaches belonging to the order

Orthoptera. Roaches contaminate food and transmit mechanically infectious bacteria, helminth ova, and cysts of protozoa. They also serve as intermediate host of the tapeworm, *Hymenolepis diminuta.*

P. americana. The American cockroach.

P. australasiae. The Australian cockroach.

periplast (pĕr'ĭ-plăst) [" + *plassein,* to form]. 1. Peripheral protoplasm of a cell exclusive of the nucleus. 2. Matrix of a part or organ. 3. A cell wall.

peripleural (pĕr"ĭ-plū'răl) [" + *pleura,* rib]. Encircling the pleura.

peripleuritis (pĕr-ĭ-plū-rī'tĭs) [" + " + *-ītis,* inflammation]. Inflamed condition of the connective tissues bet. the pleura and wall of the chest.

periproctitis (pĕr"ĭ-prŏk-tī'tĭs) [" + *prōktos,* anus, + *-ītis,* inflammation]. Inflammation of areolar tissues in region of the rectum and anus. Syn: *perirectitis.*

periprostatic (pĕr"ĭ-prŏs-tăt'ĭk) [" + *prostatēs,* prostate]. Surrounding or occurring about the prostate.

periprostatitis (pĕr"ĭ-prŏs-tă-tī'tĭs) [" + " + *-ītis,* inflammation]. Inflamed condition of tissues surrounding the prostate.

peripylephlebitis (pĕr"ĭ-pī"le-flē-bī'tĭs) [" + *pylē,* gate, + *phleps, phleb-,* vein, + *-ītis,* inflammation]. Inflamed condition of tissues about the portal vein.

peripyloric (pĕr"ĭ-pī-lor'ĭk) [G. *peri,* around, + *pylōros,* pylorus]. Extending around the pylorus.

perirectal (pĕr"ĭ-rĕk'tăl) [" + L. *rectus,* straight]. Extending around the rectum.

perirectitis (pĕr"ĭ-rĕk-tī'tĭs) [" + " + G. *-ītis,* inflammation]. Inflamed condition of tissues about rectum and anus. Syn: *periproctitis.*

perirenal (pĕr"ĭ-rē'năl) [" + L. *rēn,* kidney]. Extending around the kidney. Syn: *circumrenal, perinephric.*

perirhinal (pĕr"ĭ-rī'năl) [" + *ris, rin-,* nose]. Located about the nose or nasal fossae.

perirhizoclasia (pĕr"ĭ-rī"zō-klā'zĭ-ă) [" + *riza,* root, + *klasis,* a breaking]. Inflammation and destruction of tissues extending around the roots of a tooth.

perisalpingitis (pĕr"ĭ-săl-pĭn-jī'tĭs) [" + *salpigx, salpigg-,* tube, + *-ītis,* inflammation]. Inflamed condition of peritoneal coat about the oviduct.

perisalpingoovaritis (pĕr"ĭ-săl-pĭn"gō-ō-văr-ī'tĭs) [" + " + L. *ovarium,* ovary, + G. *-ītis,* inflammation]. Inflammation of peritoneal tissues surrounding the fallopian tubes and ovaries. Syn: *perioophorosalpingitis, perioothecosalpingitis.*

periscle'rium [G. *peri,* around, + *sklēros,* hard]. Fibrous tissue encircling ossifying cartilage.

periscopic (pĕr"ĭ-skop'ĭk) [" + *skopein,* to examine]. Viewing on all sides.

perish (pĕr'ĭsh) [L. *perire,* to come to nothing]. To disintegrate or die, esp. by other than natural causes.

perisigmoiditis (pĕr"ĭ-sĭg-moi-dī'tĭs) [G. *peri,* around, + *sigma,* Greek letter S, + *eidos,* like, + *-ītis,* inflammation]. Inflamed condition of peritoneal tissues around sigmoid flexure of the colon.

perisinusitis (pĕr"ĭ-sī-nū-sī'tĭs) [G. *peri,* around, + L. *sinus,* cavity, + G. *-ītis,* inflammation). Syn: *perisinuitis.* Inflammation of membranes about a sinus, esp. a venous sinus of the dura mater.

perispermatitis (pĕr"ĭ-spĕr-mă-tī'tĭs) [" + *sperma,* seed, + *-ītis,* inflammation]. Inflamed condition of tissues about spermatic cord.

p. serosa. Hydrocele of spermatic cord.

perisplanchnic (pĕr"ĭ-splănk'nĭk) [" + *splagchnon,* viscus]. Extending around a viscus or the viscera.

perisplanchnitis (pĕr"ĭ-splănk-nī'tĭs) [" + " + *-ītis,* inflammation]. Inflamed condition of the tissues around the viscera. Syn: *perivisceritis.*

perisplenitis (pĕr"ĭ-splē-nī'tĭs) [" + *splēn,* spleen, + *-ītis,* inflammation]. Inflammation of peritoneal coat of the spleen, the splenic capsule.

p. cartilaginea. Syn: *hyalin capsulitis.* Inflammation of capsule of the spleen resulting in thickening and hardening.

perispondylitis (pĕr"ĭ-spŏn-dĭl-ī'tĭs) [" + *spondylos,* vertebra, + *-ītis,* inflammation]. Inflamed condition of the parts around a vertebra.

perissad (pĕr-ĭs'ăd, per'ĭs-ad) [G. *perissos,* odd]. 1. Radical or element of odd valence. 2. Having odd valence.

perissodactylous (pĕr-ĭs"ō-dăk'tĭ-lŭs) [" + *daktylos,* digit]. Having an odd number of toes.

peristalsis (pĕr-ĭs-tăl'sĭs) [G. *perissos,* odd, + *stalsis,* contraction]. A progressive, wavelike movement which occurs involuntarily in hollow tubes of the body, esp. the alimentary canal. It is characteristic of tubes possessing longitudinal and circular layers of smooth muscle fibers.

P. is induced reflexly by distention of the walls of the tube. The wave consists of contraction of the circular muscle above the distention with relaxation of the region immediately distal to the distended portion. The simultaneous contraction and relaxation progresses slowly for a short distance as a wave which causes the contents of the tube to be forced onward in a spiral fashion.

p., mass. Forced peristaltic movements of short duration moving contents from one section of the colon to another, occurring 3 or 4 times daily.

p., reverse. Syn: *antiperistalsis.* Peristalsis in a direction opposite to the normal direction.

peristaltic (pĕr"ĭ-stăl'tĭk) [G. *peri,* around, + *stalsis,* contraction]. Concerning, or of the nature of, peristalsis.

p. rush. A rapidly moving peristaltic wave which occurs from time to time in the small intestine moving all of the contents before it.

p. unrest. Increased peristalsis or abnormal motility of the intestinal tract.

p. wave. The wavelike movement occurring during peristalsis.

peristaphyline (pĕr"ĭ-stăf'ĭ-lĭn) [" + *staphylē,* uvula]. About the uvula.

peristome (pĕr'ĭs-tōm) [" + *stoma,* mouth]. Channel leading to the cytosome or mouth in certain types of protozoa.

peristrumitis (pĕr"ĭ-strū-mī'tĭs) [" + L. *struma,* goiter]. Inflamed condition of tissues around a goiter. Syn: *perithyroiditis.*

perisynovial (pĕr"ĭ-sĭn-ō'vĭ-ăl) [" + *syn,* with, + *ōon,* egg]. Extending around a synovial structure.

perisystole (pĕr"ĭ-sĭs'tō-lē) [" + *systolē,* contraction]. The period preceding the systole in the cardiac rhythm. Syn: *presystole.*

peritectomy (pĕr″ĭ-tĕk′tō-mĭ) [G. *peri*, around, + *ektomē*, excision]. Surgical removal of a ring of conjunctiva around the cornea.

peritendineum (pĕr-ĭ-tĕn-dĭn′ē-ŭm) [G. *peri*, around, + L. *tendō*, tendon]. A sheath of fibrous connective tissue investing a fiber bundle of a tendon.

peritendinitis (pĕr″ĭ-tĕn-dĭn-ī′tĭs) [" + " + G. *-ītis*, inflammation]. Inflamed condition of the sheath of a tendon. SYN: *peritenonitis.*

p. calcarea. The deposition of calcareous material in tendons and associated regions, characterized by pain, tenderness, and limitation of motion.

peritenonitis (pĕr″ĭ-tĕn-on-ī′tĭs) [" + *tenōn*, tendon, + *-ītis*, inflammation]. Inflammation of sheath investing a tendon. SYN: *peritendinitis.*

perithelioma (pĕr″ĭ-thē-lĭ-ō′mă) [" + *thēlē*, nipple, + *-ōma*, tumor]. A tumor derived from the perithelial layer of the blood vessels.

perithelium (pĕr-ĭ-thē′lĭ-ŭm) [" + *thēlē*, nipple]. Fibrous outer layer of the smaller blood vessels and capillaries.

perithyroiditis (pĕr″ĭ-thī-roy-dī′tĭs) [" + *thyreos*, shield, + *eidos*, form, + *-ītis*, inflammation]. Inflammation of capsule or tissues sheathing the thyroid gland. SYN: *peristrumitis.*

peritomy (pĕr-ĭt′ō-mĭ) [G. *peri*, around, + *tomē*, incision]. 1. Excision of narrow strip of conjunctiva around the cornea in treatment of pannus. 2. Circumcision.

peritoneal (pĕr″ĭ-tō-nē′ăl) [G. *peritonaion*, peritoneum]. Concerning the peritoneum.

p. cavity. Region bordered by parietal layer of the peritoneum containing all the abdominal organs exclusive of the kidney. SEE: *cholascos.*

p. sac, lesser. The omental bursa or cavity of the great omentum.

peritonealgia (pĕr″ĭ-tō-nē-al′jĭ-ă) [" + *algos*, pain]. Pain of the peritoneum.

peritoneocentesis (pĕr″ĭ-tō-nē″ō-sĕn-tē′sĭs) [" + *kentēsis*, a puncture]. Piercing of the peritoneal cavity to obtain fluid. SEE: *paracentesis.*

peritoneoclysis (pĕr″ĭ-tō-nē″ō-klī′sĭs) [" + *klysis*, a washing out]. Introduction of fluid into the peritoneal cavity.

peritonealize. During abdominal surgery, to cover a tissue with peritoneum.

peritoneopathy (pĕr″ĭ-tō-nē-op′ăth-ĭ) [" + *pathos*, disease]. Any disordered condition of the peritoneum.

peritoneopexy (pĕr″ĭ-tō-nē′ō-pĕks″ĭ) [" + *pēxis*, fixation]. Fixation of the uterus by way of the vagina.

peritoneoplasty (pĕr″ĭ-tō-nē′ō-plăs″tĭ) [" + *plassein*, to form]. Reparative surgery to prevent re-formation of loosened adhesions.

peritoneoscope (pĕr″ĭ-tō-nē′ō-skōp) [G. *peritonaion*, peritoneum, + *skopein*, to examine]. Long, slender periscope or telescope device with a light at one end and an eye piece at the other. Used to inspect the peritoneal and abdominal cavities through a small incision in the abdominal wall.

peritoneoscopy (pĕr″ĭ-tō-nē-ŏs′kō-pĭ) [" + *skopein*, to examine]. Examination of peritoneal cavity with the peritoneoscope.

peritoneotomy (pĕr″ĭ-tō-nē-ŏt′ō-mĭ) [" + *tomē*, a cutting]. Process of incising the peritoneum

peritoneum (pĕr-ĭ-tō-nē′ŭm) [G. *peritonaion*]. The serous membrane reflected over the viscera, and lining the abdominal cavity.

PALPATION: If palmar surface of hand be applied to side of abdomen at level of the liquid in ascites, and light percussion be performed on the opposite side, a sense of fluctuation will be communicated to the hand.

p., parietal. P. lining abdominal and pelvic walls and undersurface of diaphragm.

p., visceral. The p. that invests the abdominal organs.

peritonitic (pĕr-ĭ-tō-nĭt′ĭk) [" + *-ītis*, inflammation]. Affected with or concerning peritonitis.

peritonitis (pĕr″ĭ-tō-nī′tĭs) [G. *peritonaion*, peritoneum, + *-ītis*, inflammation]. Inflammation of the peritoneum, the membranous coat lining the abdominal cavity and investing the viscera.

ETIOL: Infectious organisms which gain access by way of: (1) rupture or perforation of viscus or associated structures, (2) female genital tract, (3) piercing of abdominal wall, (4) blood stream or lymphatic vessels, (5) operative incisions and failure to practice aseptic technics.

TREATMENT: Antibiotic therapy. More important than treatment are prophylactic measures to prevent the development of peritonitis.

p., acute diffuse. Generalized p. of a large area.

ETIOL: Rupture of an intraabdominal viscus, as the appendix or stomach. Infection may take place directly from an adjacent organ which is inflamed, or from the blood stream in patients with septicemia.

SYM: Chill; fever, 102°-103° F.; rapid pulse rate; abdominal pain and tenderness so intense abdominal respiration and bodily movement inhibited; patient on back, thighs flexed; features pinched, and anxious; vomiting persistent; bowels usually constipated; hiccough; abdominal distention.

PROG: Guarded.

TREATMENT: Surgical intervention. Absolute bed rest; sips of water by mouth; saline or glucose solution, blood, or plasma parenterally; analgesics for pain; suction to gastrointestinal tract; antibiotic therapy.

p., adhesive. P. in which the visceral and parietal layers stick together by means of adhesions.

p., aseptic. P. due to causes other than bacterial infection, such as trauma, presence of chemicals produced naturally or introduced from without, irradiation.

p., chronic. Usually tuberculous, cancerous or syphilitic; occurs in chronic alcoholism.

SYM: Fever slight or absent. Pain not severe; paroxysms; usually diffuse tenderness; anemia and emaciation may be marked.

PROG: Guarded.

TREATMENT: Rest; light diet; paracentesis. Laparotomy.

p. deformans. Chronic p. with thickened membrane and adhesions contracting and causing retraction of the intestines.

p., diffuse. SYN: *generalized peritonitis.* P. which is widespread involving most of the peritoneum.

p., localized. P. in which only a small area is involved.

p., pelvic. That involving p. of the pelvic region, usually the sequela of uterine tube infection in female.

p., primary. P. resulting from infectious organisms transmitted through blood or lymph.

p., puerperal. P. which develops following childbirth.

p., secondary. P. resulting from extension of infection from adjoining structures, rupture of a viscus, abscess, or trauma.

p., septic. P. caused by a pyogenic bacterium.

p., serous. P. in which there is liquid exudation.

p., traumatic. P. due to injury or wound infection.

p., tuberculous. P. caused by numerous tubercle bacilli on the peritoneum.

peritonsillar (pĕr″ĭ-ton′sĭl-ăr) [G. *peri,* around, + L. *tonsilla,* tonsil]. Extending around a tonsil.

peritonsillitis (pĕr-ĭ-tŏn-sĭl-ī′tĭs) [" + " + G. *-itis,* inflammation]. Inflamed condition of tissues around the tonsils. SYN: *periamygdalitis.*

peritrichous (pĕr-it′rĭk-ŭs) [" + *thrix, trich-,* hair]. BACT: Having cilia or flagella covering the entire surface.

perityphlitis (pĕr″ĭ-tĭf-lī′tĭs) [" + *typhlos,* blind, + *-itis,* inflammation]. Inflamed condition of tissues around the cecum and appendix. SYN: *appendicitis.*

periureteritis (pĕr″ĭ-ū-rē″tĕr-ī′tĭs) [" + *ourētēr,* ureter, + *-itis,* inflammation]. Inflamed condition of parts about the ureter.

periurethral (pĕr″ĭ-ū-rē′thrăl) [" + *ourēthra,* urethra]. Located about the urethra.

periuterine (pĕr″ĭ-ū′tĕr-ĭn) [" + L. *uterus,* womb]. Located about the uterus. SYN: *perimetric.*

perivaginitis (per″ĭ-vaj″ĭ-nī′tis) [G. *peri,* around, + L. *vagina,* sheath, + G. *-itis,* inflammation]. Inflammation of region around the vagina. SYN: *pericolpitis.*

perivascular (pĕr″ĭ-văs′kū-ler) [" + L. *vasculus,* a little vessel]. Located around a vessel, esp. a blood vessel.

perivasculitis (pĕr″ĭ-văs-kū-lī′tĭs) [" + " + G. *-itis,* inflammation]. Inflamed condition of tissues surrounding a blood vessel. SYN: *periangitis.*

perivisceritis (pĕr″ĭ-vĭs″ĕr-ī′tĭs) [" + L. *viscus, viscer-,* internal organ, + G. *-itis,* inflammation]. Inflamed condition of the tissues surrounding the viscera.

perixenitis (pĕr″ĭ-zĕn-ī′tĭs) [" + *xenos.* strange, + *-itis,* inflammation]. Inflammation of the region around a foreign body.

perle (perl). A soft capsule containing a medicine.

perlèche (per-lesh′) [Fr.]. Disorder marked by fissures and epithelial desquamation at corners of the mouth, esp. seen in children. May be due to oral moniliasis or a symptom of dietary deficiency, esp. riboflavin deficiency.

permanent (perm′ă-nent) [L. *per,* through, + *manere,* to remain]. Enduring; without change.

p. teeth. Teeth developing at the second dentition. SEE: *dens permanens.*

permanganate (pĕr-man′găn-āt). Any one of the salts of permanganic acid.

permeability (per″me-ă-bil′ĭ-tĭ). The quality of being permeable.

p., capillary. The condition of capillary wall which enables substances in the blood to diffuse into tissue spaces or into cells or vice versa.

permeable (per′me-ă-bl) [L. *per,* through, + *meare,* to pass]. Capable of or allowing the passage of fluids or substances in solution.

permeation (pĕr″mē-ā′shŭn). Penetration and spread throughout an organ or tissue, or space.

pernicious (pĕr-nĭsh′ŭs) [L. *perniciōsus,* destructive]. Destructive; fatal; harmful.

p. anemia. Severe form of blood disease, marked by progressive decrease in red blood corpuscles, muscular weakness, and gastrointestinal and neural disturbances. May be fatal if not treated with vitamin B_{12}, iron, and diet. SEE: *anemia, pernicious.*

p. trend. PSY: An abnormal departure from conventional ideas and social interests. Pregenital interests are manifested.

pernio (per′nĭ-o) [L. chilblain]. Congestion and swelling of the skin, due to cold.

SYM: Attended with severe burning or itching; ulceration may result from vesicles and bullae which sometimes form. SYN: *chilblain.*

perniosis (per-nĭ-o′sis) [L. *perniō,* chilblain, + G. *-ōsis,* disease]. A skin disorder due to cold. SEE: *chilblain; pernio.*

pero-. Comb. form meaning *deformed.*

perobrachius (pe″rō-brā′kē-ŭs). Condition in which forearms and hands are deformed.

perocephalus. Term applied to an individual with a defective head.

per″om′elus. An individual with stunted, deformed limbs.

peroneal (pĕr-ō-nē′ăl) [G. *peronē,* pin]. Concerning the fibula.

peroneo- [G.]. Combining form, *pert. to the fibula.*

peroneum (pĕr-ō-nē′ŭm) [G. *peronē,* pin]. The fibula. SYN: *os peroneum.*

peroneus (pĕr-ō-nē′ŭs) [L., from G. *peronē,* pin]. One of several muscles of the leg causing motion in the foot.

peronia (pe-rō′nĭ-ă). Malformation.

peroral (pĕr-or′ăl) [L. *per,* through, + *os, or-,* mouth]. Via the mouth.

per os [L.]. By mouth.

pero′sis. Condition due to abnormal or defective development.

peroxidase (per-ŏks′ĭ-dās) [L. *per,* through, + *oxys,* acid, + *ase,* enzyme]. An enzyme which hastens the transfer of oxygen from peroxide to a tissue that requires the oxygen. This process is essential to intracellular respiration.

peroxide (per-oks′īd) [" G. *oxys,* acid]. In chemistry, a compound containing more oxygen than the other oxides of the element in question.

Examples are the peroxides of hydrogen, H_2O_2; sodium, Na_2O_2; magnesium, MgO_2; and nitrogen, NO_2.

perplication (per-plĭ-kā′shŭn) [" + *plicāre,* to fold]. Inserting the cut end of an artery through an incision in its own wall to arrest bleeding.

per primam, per primam intentionem (per prē′măm ĭn-tĕn-tĭ-ō′nĕm) [L.]. By first intention. SEE: *healing, first intention.*

per rectum (per rĕk′tŭm) [L.]. By the rectum; through the rectum.

persalt (per′sawlt). CHEM: A salt containing largest possible amount of an acid radical.

per secundam (per se-kun′dăm) [L.]. By second intention. SEE: *healing, second intention.*

perseveration (per-sĕv-ĕr-ā′shŭn) [L. *perseverāre,* to persist]. Continued repetition of a meaningless word or phrase, or repetition of answers which are not related to successive questions asked.

persimmon (per-sim′en) [Algonquin]. RAW (*seedless*): 1 (125 gm.). Calories:

75. Other main values: 1 gm. protein; trace of fat; 20 gm. carbohydrate; 6 mg. calcium; 2740 I.U. vitamin A.

persona (per-so'nă) [L. mask]. The outer attitude or appearance a person presents to others.

personal [L. *persona,* a person]. Characteristic of an individual.

p. equation. In scientific observation, factors depending on personal qualities of individual observers.

personality (per"son-al'ĭ-tĭ) [L. *persona,* person). The unique organization of traits, characteristics and modes of behavior of an individual which sets him apart from other individuals and at the same time determines how others react to him.

Personality refers to the mental aspects of an individual in contrast to physique.

p., double. SEE: *p., dual.*

p., dual. Mental dissociation in which one individual shows in alternation two very different personalities. SEE ALSO: *dual personality.*

p., extroverted. That in which activities or libido are directed to other individuals or the environment.

p., introverted. One in which activities or libido are directed to the individual himself.

p., multiple. State in which three or more personalities alternate in the same individual. SEE ALSO: *multiple personality.*

p., neurotic. One characterized by behavior intermediate between normal and that of a neurotic individual.

p., psychopathic. One who, while possessing normal intelligence, by reason of heredity or congenital conditions, becomes constitutionally lacking in moral sensibilities, emotional control and inhibitions of the will.

Constitutional imbalance in the pattern of the mind, but not a disorder of function such as is observed in actual neuroses and psychoses. In other words, such a personality represents a borderline state. The inferiority of the psychopath is *emotional and not intellectual.* SYN: *character disorder.*

p., schizoid. One characterized by withdrawal, introspection, odd and unsocial behavior.

p., split. Dissociation of ideas not amenable to conscious control, as in schizophrenia.

RS: *consciousness, dissociation, dual p., multiple p., somnambulism, vigilambulism.*

perspiration (per"sper-a'shun) [L. *per,* through, + *spirāre,* to breathe]. 1. Sweat. 2. Secretion and exudation of fluid by sweat glands of the skin, about 700 cc. per day.

Perspiration is increased by (a) temperature and humidity of the atmosphere; (b) diluted blood; (c) exercises; (d) pain; (e) nausea; (f) nervousness; (g) mental excitement; (h) dyspnea; (i) diaphoretics.

It is decreased by (a) colds; (b) diarrhea; (c) voiding large quantities of urine; (d) using certain drugs.

p., insensible. Evaporation of water vapor through the skin without wetting it.

p., sensible. P. which occurs so as to form drops.

perspiration, *words pert. to:* adiaphoresis, adiapneustia, anhidrosis, anidros, bromohyperhidrosis, bromidrosis, chlorephidrosis, chromidrosis, diaphoresis, meridrosis, panidrosis, polyidrosis, secretion, sudor, sweat, -center, sweating, transpiration, uridrosis.

perspire (per-spīr') [L. *per,* through, + *spirāre,* to breathe]. To excrete fluid through the skin. SYN: *sweat.*

perstriction (pĕr-strĭk'shŭn) [L. *per,* through, + *strictus,* from *stringere,* to tighten]. Ligation of a bleeding vessel for the arrest of hemorrhage.

persulfate (per-sul'fāt). One of a series of sulfates containing more sulfuric acid than the others in same series.

per tertiam intentionem (per tĕr'tĭ-ăm ĭn-tĕn-tĭ-ō'nĕm) [L.]. By third intention. SEE: *healing, third intention.*

Perthes' disease (pār'tās) [Georg C. Perthes, German surgeon, 1869-1927]. One in which changes take place in bone at head of femur with deformity resulting.

SYM: Similar to tuberculous hip joint disease. SYN: *osteochondritis deformans juvenilis.*

per tubam (pĕr tū'băm) [L.]. Through a tube.

perturbation. State of being greatly disturbed or agitated; uneasiness of mind.

pertussis (pĕr-tŭs'ĭs) [" + *tussis,* cough]. An acute, infectious disease characterized by a catarrhal stage, followed by a peculiar paroxysmal cough, ending in a whooping inspiration. SYN: *whooping cough.*

ETIOL: Due to a coccobacillus, *Bordetella pertussis* (Bordet-Gengou bacillus).

INCUBATION: Seven to 10 days.

SYM: A blood count shows a marked lymphocytosis which may vary from 20,000 to 10,000. Often divided into three stages; first, *catarrhal.* At this time the symptoms chiefly suggestive of the common cold—slight elevation of fever, sneezing, rhinitis, and dry cough. Irritability and loss of appetite.

After 7 to 10 days, the second or *paroxysmal stage* sets in. The cough is more violent, and consists of a series of several short coughs, followed by long drawn inspiration, during which the typical whoop is heard, this being occasioned by the spasmodic contraction of the glottis.

With the beginning of each paroxysm, patient often assumes a worried expression, sometimes even one of terror. The face becomes cyanosed, eyes injected, veins distended. With conclusion of the paroxysm, vomiting is common. At this time also, there may be epistaxis, subconjunctival hemorrhages, or hemorrhages in other portions of body.

Number of paroxysms in 24 hours may vary from 3 to 4 up to 40 or 50. Following an indefinite period of several weeks, the stage of *decline* begins, the paroxysms growing less frequent and less violent. Nutrition of child improves, and after a period which may be prolonged for several months, the cough finally ceases.

This disease may be prevented by immunizing infants beginning at 3 months of age.

pertussoid (pĕr-tŭs'oyd) [L. *per,* through, + *tussis,* cough, + G. *eidos,* resemblance]. 1. Of the nature of whooping cough. 2. A cough generally similar to that of whooping cough.

perversion (per-ver'zhun) [L. *per,* through, + *versiō,* a turning]. Deviation from the normal path, whether it be in the area of one's emotions, actions, or reactions.

p., sexual. Maladjustment of sexual life in which satisfaction is sought in ways deviating from the accepted normal. In judging the sexual actions of individuals it is important to remember that what is normal behavior in one society may be regarded as grossly abnormal or perverted in another.

Nevertheless, most social groups regard homosexuality, sexual molesting of children, and sexual exhibitionism as abnormal.

pervert (per-vert') [L. *per*, through, + *vertere*, to turn]. 1. v. To turn from the normal. 2. (per'vert). n. One who has turned from the normal or socially acceptable path, esp. sexually.

p., sexual. One whose sex conduct is not normal.

Many of these individuals suffer from mental diseases, such as dementia, senility, and from general paralysis.

Most of them are mental degenerates suffering from psychic or physical defects. Heredity plays a part in some instances. Diseases of the nervous system, alcoholism, and infections also may be responsible in part.

pervigilium (pĕr-vĭ-jĭl'ĭ-ŭm) [L. *per*, through, + *vigil*, awake]. Inability to sleep. Syn: *insomnia; wakefulness.*

pervious (per'vĭ-us) [L. *per*. through, + *via*, way]. 1. Capable of being penetrated. 2. Penetrating. Syn: *permeable.*

pes (pēz) (pl. *pedes*) [L. *pēs, ped*, foot]. The foot or a footlike structure.

p. anserinus. Three primary branches of the facial nerve after leaving the stylomastoid foramen.

p. cavus. Abnormal hollowness of the sole of the foot.

p. contortus. Clubfoot. Syn: *talipes, q.v.*

p. corvinus. Wrinkles radiating from the outer canthi of the eyes. Syn: *crow's foot.*

p. equinus. Deformity marked by walking without touching heel to the ground. Syn: *talipes equinus, q.v.*

p. gigas. Syn: *macropodia.* An abnormally large foot.

p. hippocampi. Lower portion of the hippocampus major.

p., infraorbital. Terminal radiating branches of the infraorbital nerve after exit from the infraorbital canal.

p. planus. Flatfoot.

p. valgoplanus. P. planus, *q.v.*

p. valgus. Clubfoot in which sole turns outward. Syn: *talipes valgus.*

p. varus. Clubfoot in which sole turns inward. Syn: *talipes varus.*

pessary (pes'ă-rĭ) [G. *pessos*, oval pebble]. A device which is inserted into the vagina. It may function as a supportive structure for the uterus or as a contraceptive device.

p., cup. One which has a cup-shaped hollow that fits over the os uteri.

p., diaphragm. Cup-shaped rubber p. used as a contraceptive device.

p., Gariel's. Inflatable hollow rubber p.

p., Hodge's. P. used to correct retrodeviations of the uterus.

p., lever. P. designed according to the principles of a lever.

p., ring. Round pessary.

p., stem. P. with stem which fits into the uterine canal.

pes'simism. Morbid state of mind in which outlook toward life is gloomy or the worst interpretation is applied to events occurring; lacking in hope. Opp. of *optimism.*

pest (pĕst) [L. *pestis*, plague]. 1. Fatal epidemic disease, esp. the plague. 2. A noxious, destructive insect.

p.-house. Hospital for those infected with a pestilential or communicable disease.

pestiferous (pĕst-ĭf'ĕr-ŭs) [" + *ferre*, to carry]. Producing a pestilence; carrying infection. Syn: *pestilential.*

pestilence (pĕst'ĭl-ĕns) [L. *pestilentia*, a widespread epidemic]. 1. An epidemic contagious disease, specifically bubonic plague. 2. An epidemic caused by such a disease.

pestilential (pĕst-ĭ-lĕn'shăl) [L. *pestilentia*, a widespread disease]. Concerning or causing a pestilence. Syn: *pestiferous.*

pestis (pĕs'tĭs) [L. plague]. The plague.

pestle (pĕs'l) [L. *pistillum*, pestle]. Device for macerating drugs in a mortar.

petechiae (pe-tē'kĭ-ē) (plural of *petechia*) [Italian *peteche*, a flea bite]. 1. Small, purplish, hemorrhagic spots on the skin which appear in certain severe fevers and are indicative of great prostration, as in typhus. May be due to abnormality of blood clotting mechanism. Also applied to similar spots occurring on mucous membranes or serous surfaces. 2. Red spots from bite of a flea.

petechial (pe-tē'kĭ-ăl) [Italian *peteche*, a flea bite]. Marked by presence of petechiae.

pet'iole. A slender stalk or stem, as petiole of the epiglottic cartilage.

petit mal (pĕt'ē măhl) [F. little illness]. Mild form of epileptic attack. Consciousness may be lost, but there is an absence of convulsions. See: *epilepsy, pyknolepsy.*

Petit's canal. Syn: *zonular spaces.* A space or cleft encircling lens between points of attachment of fibers of suspensory ligament.

P.'s sinuses. Hollows in aortic and pulmonary arteries behind semilunar valves.

P.'s triangle. Syn: *trigonum lumbale.* Area on lateral abdominal wall bounded by crest of ilium, post. margin of ext. oblique, and lateral margin of latissimus dorsi.

Petri dish (pe'tre). A shallow dish with cover. Used to hold solid media for culturing bacteria. Made of plastic or glass.

petrifaction (pĕt-rĭ-făk'shŭn) [L. *petra*, stone, + *facere*, to make]. Process of changing into stone or hard substance.

petrified (pĕt'rĭ-fīd) [L. *petra*, stone]. Changed into stone; rigid.

petrify (pĕt'rĭ-fī) [L. *petra*, stone]. Convert into stone; make rigid.

pétrissage (pā-trē-sazh') [Fr.]. A kneading movement in massage.

Performed generally (a) by the tips of the thumbs; (b) with index finger and thumb; (c) with palm of hand.

It is used principally on the extremities. The operator picks up a special muscle or tendon and, placing one finger on each side of the part, proceeds in centripetal motion with a firm pressure. Syn: *kneading.*

petro- [L.]. Combining form meaning *stone.* Pert. to petrous portion of temporal bone.

petrolatoma (pĕt"rō-lā-tō'mă) [L. *petra*, stone, + *oleum*, oil, + G. *-ōma*, tumor]. Tumor or swelling caused by introduction of liquid petrolatum under the skin.

petrolatum (pĕt-rō-lā'tŭm) [" + *oleum,* oil]. USP. A purified semi-solid mixture of hydrocarbons obtained from petroleum. Syn: *petroleum jelly; soft paraffin.*

Action and Uses: As a base for ointments and as a lubricant.

p. liquid. USP. A mixture of liquid hydrocarbons obtained from petroleum.

Action and Uses: A vehicle for medicinal substances for local applications. Light p. employed as a spray. Heavy p. given internally in treatment of constipation.

petroleum (pĕt-rō'lē-ŭm) [L. *petra,* stone, + *oleum,* oil]. An oily inflammable liquid found in the upper strata of the earth, a hydrocarbon mixture.

pet"romas'toid. Pert. to petrous portion of temporal bone and occipital bone.

petrosa (pĕt-rō'să) [L. stony]. The petrous part of the temporal bone.

petrosal (pĕt-rō'săl) [L. *petrōsus,* stony]. Of, pert. to, or situated near the petrous portion of the temporal bone.

petrositis (pĕt"rō-sī'tĭs) [" + *-ītis,* inflammation]. Inflamed condition of the petrous region of the temporal bone.

petro"sphe'noid. Pert. to petrous portion of temporal bone and sphenoid bone.

petro"squa'mous. Pert. to petrous and squamous portions of temporal bone.

petrous (pĕt'rŭs) [G. *petra,* stone]. 1. Resembling stone. 2. Relating to the petrous portion of the temporal bone. Syn: *petrosal.*

p. ganglion. Inf. ganglion of the glossopharyngeal nerve.

Peyer's patch (pī'ĕr). An aggregation of solitary nodules or groups of lymph nodules found chiefly in the ileum near its junction with the colon. They are circular or oval, about 1 cm. wide and 2 to 3 cm. long. They lie in the mucosa and submucosa and always occur on side of intestine opposite to attachment of mesentery. In typhoid fever, they undergo hyperplasia and often become ulcerated. Also called *aggregated* or *agminated nodules* or *follicles.*

Peyronie's disease (pa-ro'ne) [Francois de la Peyronie, French surgeon, 1678-1747]. Hardening of the corpora cavernosa of the penis. This causes distortion or deflection of the penis especially when erect.

Pfeiffer's bacillus (fifer) [Richard F. Pfeiffer, bacteriologist, born in Breslau, 1858-?]. *Hemophilus influenzae, q.v.*

P.'s phenomenon. A discovery announced in 1894 that serum of guinea pigs immunized with cholera vibrios destroyed cholera organisms in peritoneal cavity of immune and nonimmune guinea pigs and that same reaction occurred in vitro. Also that same lytic reaction occurred with typhoid and colon bacteria.

PH. Abbr. for *Pharmacopoeia.*

pH. In chemistry the logarithm of $\frac{1}{cH}$ or hydrogen ion (H+) concentration, a symbol used to express degree of acidity or alkalinity. The pH of a neutral solution is 7 at 25° C. Alkaline or basic solutions range from pH 7 to pH 14; acid solutions range from pH 7 to pH 0. The pH of 14 and 0 exist for solutions of 1 N strength alkali and acid, respectively.

The pH of a solution may be determined electrically by a pH meter or colorometrically by the use of indicators. A list of indicators and the pH range registered by each is given under *indicator, q.v.*

The following table is for orientation:

Material	pH
Decinormal HCl	1.0
Gastric juice	1.0 to 5.0
Thousandth-normal HCl	3.0
Pure water (neutral) at 25° C.	7.0
Blood plasma	7.35 to 7.45
Pancreatic juice	8.4 to 8.9
Thousandth-normal NaOH	11.0
Decinormal NaOH	13.0

phacitis (fă-sī'tĭs) [G. *phakos,* lens, + *-ītis,* inflammation]. Inflamed condition of the crystalline lens. Syn: *phakitis.*

phaco- [G.]. Prefix, *pert. to lens of the eye.*

phacoanaphylaxis (făk"ō-ăn-ă-fĭl-ăk'sĭs) [G. *phakos,* lens, + *ana,* up, + *phylaxis,* a guard]. Hypersensitivity to protein of the crystalline lens.

phacocele (făk'ō-sēl) [" + *kēlē,* swelling]. Displacement of the crystalline lens into the int. chamber of the eye.

phacocyst (făk'ō-sĭst) [" + *kystis,* a sac]. Capsule of the crystalline lens.

phacocystectomy (făk"ō-sĭs-tĕk'tō-mĭ) [" + " + *ektomē,* excision]. Surgical excision of part of crystalline lens capsule for cataract.

phacocystitis (făk"ō-sĭs-tī'tĭs) [" + " + *-ītis,* inflammation]. Inflamed condition of capsule of crystalline lens.

phacoeresis (făk"ō-ĕr-ē'sĭs) [" + *erēsis,* removal]. Removal of crystalline lens by suction method.

phacoglaucoma (făk"ō-glaw-kō'mă) [" + *glaukos,* green, + *-ōma,* tumor]. Glaucoma and the changes it induces in the crystalline lens. See: *glaucoma.*

phacohymenitis (făk"ō-hī-mĕn-ī'tĭs). Inflamed condition of capsule of crystalline lens.

phacoid (făk'oyd) [G. *phakos,* lens, + *eidos,* form]. Lentil or lens-shaped.

phacoidoscope (făk-oyd'ō-skōp) " + " + *skopein,* to examine]. Instrument for observing accommodative changes of the lens. Syn: *phacoscope.*

phacolysis (făk-ol'ĭ-sĭs) [" + *lysis,* dissolution]. 1. Dissection and removal of the lens of the eye in treatment of cataract. 2. Any dissolution or disintegration of the crystalline lens.

phacomalacia (făk"ō-mal-ā'sĭ-ă) [" + *malakia,* softening]. A softening of the lens usually due to a soft cataract.

phacomatosis. Syn: *neurodermatoses.* One of a group of diseases, congenital and probably hereditary in origin, manifested by cutaneous and neurologic syndromes. They include the following: *neurofibromatosis* (von Recklinghausen's disease), *von Hippel-Lindau disease, Sturge-Weber syndrome,* and *tuberous sclerosis.*

phacometachoresis (făk"ō-mĕt-ă-kō-rē'sĭs) [" + *metachōrēsis,* displacement]. Dislocation of the crystalline lens. Syn: *phacocele.*

phacometer (făk-ŏm'ĕt-ĕr) [" + *metron,* measure]. Device for ascertaining refractive power of a lens.

phacoplanesis (făk"ō-plăn-ē'sĭs) [" + *planēsis,* a wandering]. Abnormal mobility of the crystalline lens.

phacosclerosis (făk"ō-sklĕr-ō'sĭs) [G. *phakos,* lens, + *sklērōsis,* a hardening]. Hardening of the crystalline lens of eye.

phacoscope (făk'ō-skōp) [" + *skopein,* to examine]. Instrument for observing change of curvature of crystalline lens during accommodation.

phacoscotasmus (făk″ō-scō-tăs′mŭs). Clouding of crystalline lens of the eye.

phag-, phago-. Combining form meaning an *eater,* or pertaining to ingestion or engulfing.

phage (fāj) [G. *phagein,* to eat]. A particulate, transmissible, ultramicroscopic substance that dissolves or exerts a lytic effect upon bacteria. SEE: *bacteriophage.*

phagedena (făj-ĕd-ē′nă) [G. *phagedaina,* a cancerous sore]. A sloughing ulcer that spreads.

p., sloughing. Hospital gangrene.

phagedenic (făj-e-dĕn′ĭk) [G. *phagedaina,* a cancerous sore.]. Concerning, or of the nature of, phagedena.

phagocyte (făg′ō-sīt) [G. *phagein,* to eat, + *kytos,* cell]. A cell which has the ability to ingest and destroy particulate substances such as bacteria, protozoa, cells and cell debris, dust particles, and colloids. Ex: Cells of the reticuloendothelial system (macrophages or histiocytes, reticular cells of lymph nodes, Kupffer's cells of liver, dust cells of lung) and leukocytes.

There are two classes: *macrophages,* large mononucleated cells which ingest dead tissues and cells, and *microphages,* which ingest bacteria.

RS: *histiocyte; macrophage; reticuloendothelial system.*

phagocytic (făg″ō-sĭt′ĭk) [" + *kytos,* cell]. Concerning phagocytes or phagocytosis.

p. index. The average number of bacteria ingested by each leukocyte after incubation of the bacteria in a mixture of serum and bacterial culture. SEE: *opsonic index.*

phagocytolysis (făg″ō-sī-tŏl′ĭ-sĭs) [" + " + *lysis,* dissolution]. Destruction or disintegration of phagocytes. SYN: *phagolysis.*

phagocytolytic (făg″ō-sī″tō-lĭt′ĭk) [" + " + *lysis,* dissolution]. Destroying phagocytes.

phagocytosis (făg″ō-sī-tō′sĭs) [G. *phagein,* to eat, + *kytos,* cell, + *-ōsis,* intensive]. Ingestion and digestion of bacteria and particles by phagocytes. SYN: *Metchnikoff's theory.*

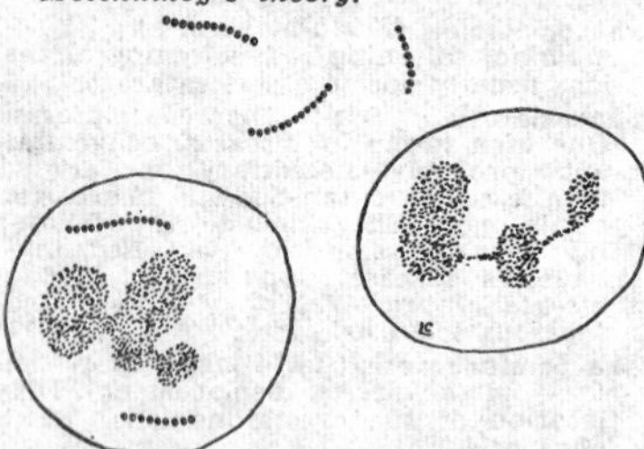

PHAGOCYTOSIS.
A small drop of blood was mixed with a drop of a suspension of dead streptococci; the mixture was kept at 37° C. for 20 minutes. A smear examined under the microscope was found to show (1) polys containing streptococci in their cytoplasm, (2) polys which did not contain streptococci, and (3) a few chains of streptococci which lay free in the medium and must have escaped phagocytosis.

phagodynamometer (fag″o-di″nă-mom′ĕ-ter) [" + *dynamis,* power, + *metron,* measure]. Device that measures energy expended in chewing.

phagokaryosis (făg″ō-kar-ĭ-ō′sĭs) [" + *karyon,* nucleus, + *-ōsis,* intensive]. Phagocytic action which is performed by a cell nucleus.

phagolysis (făg-ol′ĭ-sĭs) [" + *lysis,* dissolution]. Disintegration of phagocytes. SYN: *phagocytolysis.*

phagomania (făg-ō-mā′nĭ-ă) [" + *mania,* madness]. Abnormal craving for food.

phagopyrism (făg″ō-pī′rĭzm) [" + *pyr,* fever, + *ismos,* condition]. Hypersensitiveness to certain foods which induce symptoms of poisoning upon ingestion.

phagotherapy (făg″ō-thĕr′ă-pī) [" + *therapeia,* treatment]. Treatment by feeding or overfeeding.

phakitis (făk-ī′tĭs) [G. *phakos,* lens, + *-itis,* inflammation]. Inflamed condition of the crystalline lens. SYN: *phacitis.*

phakolysis (făk-ol′ĭs-ĭs) [" + *lysis,* dissolution]. Disintegration or removal of the crystalline lens. SYN: *phacolysis.*

phalacrosis (făl-ă-krō′sĭs) [G. *phalakrōsis,* baldness]. Baldness. SYN: *alopecia.*

phalacrotic (făl-ăk-rŏt′ĭk) [G. *phalakrōsis,* baldness]. Bald; baldheaded.

phalacrous (făl-ăk′rŭs) [G. *phalakrōsis,* baldness]. Bald. SYN: *phalacrotic.*

phalangeal (fă-lăn′jē-ăl) [G. *phalagx,* row]. Concerning a phalanx.

p. cells, inner. A row of cells along surface of inner pillar cells in the organ of Corti.

p. cells, outer. SYN: *cells of Deiters.* Cells arranged in rows which support the outer hair cells in the organ of Corti.

phalangectomy (fă-lăn-jĕk′tō-mĭ) [" + *ektomē,* excision]. Excision of one or more phalanges.

phalanges (fă-lăn′jēz) (sing. *phalanx*) [G. *phalagx,* row]. Bones of a finger or toe. SEE: *skeleton.*

phalangitis (fă-lăn-jī′tĭs) [" + *-itis,* inflammation]. Inflamed condition of one or more phalanges.

phalanx (fă′lănks) (pl. *phalanges*) [G. row]. 1. Any one of the bones of fingers or toes. 2. One of a set of plates formed of phalangeal cells (inner and outer) forming the reticular membrane of the organ of Corti.

p., distal. The one most remote from the metacarpus or metatarsus.

p., metacarpal, p., metatarsal. SEE: *p., proximal.*

p., middle. The p. (where there are three) intermediate between distal and proximal phalanges.

p., proximal. The p. articulating with a metacarpal or metatarsal bone.

p., terminal, p., ungual, p., unguicular. SEE: *p., distal.*

phallalgia (făl-ăl′jĭ-ă) [G. *phallos,* penis, + *algos,* pain]. Pain in the penis.

phallic (făl′ĭk) [G. *phallos,* penis]. Concerning the penis.

phallitis (făl-ī′tĭs) [" + *-itis,* inflammation]. Inflamed condition of the penis.

phallocampsis (făl-ō-kămp′sĭs) [" + *kampsis,* a bending]. Painful downward curvature of penis when erect; seen in gonorrhea. SYN: *chordee.*

phallodynia (făl-ō-dĭn′ĭ-ă) [" + *odynē,* pain]. Pain in the penis. SYN: *phallalgia.*

phalloid (făl′oyd) [" + *eidos,* form]. Similar to a penis.

phalloncus (făl-on′kŭs) [" + *ogkos,* a mass]. Tumor or swelling on the penis.

phalloplasty (făl'ō-plăs"tĭ) [" + *plassein*, to form]. Reparative or plastic surgery on the penis.

phallorhagia (făl-ō-rā'jĭ-ă) [G. *phallos*, penis, + *rēgnunai*, to flow forth]. Flow of blood from the penis.

phallus (făl'ŭs) [G. *phallos*, penis]. 1. The penis. 2. An artificial penis, used as a symbol. 3. Embryonic structure developing at tip of genital tubercle which in the male develops into the penis, and in the female, the clitoris.

phanero-, phaner- [G.]. Combining forms meaning *evident, visible.*

phaneromania (făn-ĕr-ō-mā'nĭ-ă) [G. *phaneros*, visible, + *mania*, madness]. Abnormal tendency to bite the nails, pick or scratch, or pull a pimple, wart, or the mustache.

phaneroscope (făn-ĕr'ō-skōp) [" + *skopein*, to examine]. Instrument for securing transparency of skin by illumination.

phaneroscopy (făn-ĕr-ŏs'kō-pĭ) [" + *skopein*, to examine]. Observation of skin by phaneroscope. Use of a lens to concentrate light in examination of skin lesions.

phanerosis (făn-ĕr-ō'sĭs) [" + *-ōsis*, intensive]. The process of becoming visible.

phanic (făn'ĭk) [G. *phanein*, to show]. Manifest; apparent.

phantasia (făn-tā'zĭ-ă) [G. *phantasia*, a showing]. An appearance that is imaginary.

phantasm (făn'tăzm) [G. *phantasma*, appearance]. An optical illusion; an apparition, or illusion of something that does not exist.

phantasmatomoria (făn-taz"măt-ō-mo'rĭ-ă) [" + *moria*, folly]. Dementia with silly fancies; childishness in the demented.

phantasy (făn'tă-sĭ) [G. *phantasia*, appearance]. A daydream.

Phantasy-thinking is a form of wish-fulfillment, a disregard for reality which one would escape through revelling in imaginative possibilities.

RS: *delirium; delusion; hallucination; hysteria; illusion; phobia.*

phantom (făn'tŭm) [G. *phantasma*, an appearance]. 1. An apparition. 2. A model of the body or of one of its parts.

p. corpuscle. A colorless erythrocyte.

p. limb. An illusion following amputation of a limb that the limb still exists. The sensation that pain exists in the removed part is known as *phantom limb pain.*

p. pregnancy. Pseudopregnancy, *q.v.*

p. tumor. An apparent tumor due to muscular contractions or flatus seen in hysteria.

pharmacal (făr'măk-ăl) [G. *pharmakon*, drug]. Concerning pharmacy.

pharmaceutical (făr-mă-sū'tĭk-ăl) [G. *pharmakeutikos*, pert. to a drug]. Concerning drugs or pharmacy.

pharmaceutics (făr-mă-sū'tĭks) [G. *pharmakon*, drug]. Science of dispensing medicines. Syn: *pharmacy.*

pharmacist (făr'mă-sĭst) [G. *pharmakon*, drug]. A druggist; one licensed to prepare and dispense drugs. Syn: *apothecary.*

pharmaco- [G.]. Combining form meaning *drug, medicine, poison.*

pharmacodiagnosis (făr"mă-kō-dī-ăg-nō'sĭs) [G. *pharmakon*, drug, + *dia*, through, + *gnosis*, knowledge]. Use of drugs in making a diagnosis.

pharmacodynamics (făr"mă-kō-dī-năm'ĭks) [" + *dynamis*, power]. Study of drugs and their reactions.

pharmacogenetics (far"mă-ko-jen-et'iks). Study of the influence of hereditary factors on response to drugs.

pharmacognosy (făr"mă-kog'nō-sĭ) [" + *gnōsis*, knowledge]. The science of crude drugs, their physical, botanical and chemical properties.

pharmacography (făr"mă-kog'ră-fĭ) [" + *graphein*, to write]. Treatise on the properties of drugs.

pharmacology (făr-mă-kŏl'ō-jĭ) [G. *pharmakon*, drug, + *logos*, a study]. The study of drugs, their origin, nature, properties and their effects upon living organisms.

pharmacomania (făr"mă-kō-mā'nĭ-ă) [" + *mania*, madness]. Abnormal desire for giving or taking medicines.

pharmacopedia (făr"mă-kō-pē'dĭ-ă) [" + *paideia*, education]. Information concerning drugs and their preparation.

pharmacopeia (făr"mă-kō-pē'ă) [G. *pharmakon*, drug, + *poiein*, to make]. Authorized treatise on drugs and their preparation, esp. a book containing formulas and information concerning drugs which is a standard for their preparation and dispensation.

Pharmacopeia, United States. Abbr: U.S.P.; U. S. Phar. A pharmacopeia issued every five years prepared under supervision of a national committee of pharmacists, pharmacologists, physicians, chemists, biologists, and other scientific and allied personnel.

The United States Pharmacopeia was adopted as standard in 1906.

pharmacophobia (făr"mă-kō-fō'bĭ-ă) [" + *phobos*, fear]. Abnormal fear of taking medicines.

pharmacopsychosis (făr"mă-kō-sī-kō'sĭs) [" + *psychē*, soul, + *-ōsis*, disease]. Addiction to drugs.

pharmacotherapy (făr"mă-kō-thĕr'ă-pĭ) [" + *therapeia*, treatment]. Use of medicine in treatment of disease.

pharmacy (făr'mă-sĭ) [G. *pharmakon*, drug]. 1. The practice of compounding and dispensing medicinal preparations. 2. A drugstore.

pharyngalgia (făr-ĭn-găl'jĭ-ă) [G. *pharygx*, pharynx, + *algos*, pain]. Pain in the pharynx. Syn: *pharyngodynia.*

pharyngeal (far-ĭn'jē-ăl) [G. *pharygx*, pharynx]. Concerning the pharynx.

p. bursa. A small, inconstant, blind sac often present in lower portion of pharyngeal tonsil.

p. hypophysis. A small structure anterior to pharyngeal bursa. It is derived from lower portion of Rathke's pouch and occasionally gives rise to a cyst or tumor.

p. reflex. Attempt to swallow following any application of stimulus to pharynx.

p. tonsil. Lymphoid tissue on post. sup. wall of the pharynx. When hypertrophied called "adenoids."

pharyngectomy (făr-ĭn-jĕk'tō-mĭ) [" + *ektomē*, excision]. Partial excision of the pharynx to remove growths, abscesses, etc.

pharyngemphraxis (făr-ĭn-jĕm-frăks'ĭs) [" + *emphraxis*, stoppage]. Pharyngeal obstruction.

pharyngismus (făr-ĭn-jĭz'mŭs) [" + *ismos*, condition]. Spasm of the muscles in the pharynx. Syn: *pharyngospasm.*

pharyngitis (făr-ĭn-jī'tĭs) [" + *-itis*, inflammation]. Inflammation of pharynx, usually associated with rhinitis.

p., acute. Sym: Malaise, fever, dysphagia, pain in throat, postnasal secretion.

Treatment: *Local:* Gargles, lozenges, topical application to oral pharynx. *General:* Bed rest, adequate fluids, analgesics, appropriate antibiotic after material has been taken for bacterial study, especially beta hemolytic streptococci.

p., atrophic. Chronic form with some atrophy of mucous glands and abnormal secretion. Syn: *p. sicca.*

p., chronic. Associated with pathology in nose and sinuses, mouth breathing, excessive smoking and chronic tonsillitis.

Sym: Dryness and irritation of throat, cough.

Treatment: Intranasal medication and removal of sinus pathology, tonsillectomy.

p., croupous. P. with the false membrane of croup.

p., diphtheritic. Sore throat with general symptoms of diphtheria.

p., follicular. See: *p., granular.*

p., gangrenous. G. inflammation of mucous membrane of pharynx. Syn: *angina maligna; cynanche maligna.*

p., granular. P. with granulations seen on the pharynx.

p. hypertrophica. A chronic form with thickened, red mucous membrane on each side with a glazed central portion.

p. sicca. See: *p., atrophic.*

p. ulcerosa. P. with fever, pain and the formation of ulcerations.

pharyngo- [G.]. Combining form pertaining to the pharynx.

pharyngoamygdalitis (făr-in″gō-ăm-ĭg-dăl-ī′tĭs) [G. *pharygx,* pharynx, + *amygdalon,* tonsil, + *-ītis,* inflammation]. Inflamed condition of the pharynx and tonsil.

pharyngocele (făr-ĭn′gō-sēl) [″ + *kēlē,* hernia]. Hernia through pharyngeal wall.

pharyngodynia (făr-in″gō-dĭn′ĭ-ă) [″ + *odynē,* pain]. Pain in the pharynx. Syn: *pharyngalgia.*

pharyngokeratosis (făr-ĭn-gō-kĕr″ă-tō′sĭs). Thickening and hardening of mucous lining of pharynx.

pharyngolaryngitis (făr-ĭn″gō-lăr-ĭn-jī′tĭs) [″ + *larygx,* larynx, + *-ītis,* inflammation]. Inflamed condition of pharynx and larynx.

pharyngolith (făr-ĭn′gō-lĭth) [″ + *lithos,* stone]. Concretion in pharyngeal walls.

pharyngology (făr-ĭn-gŏl′ō-jĭ) [″ + *logos,* a study]. Branch of medicine dealing with the pharynx.

pharyngolysis (făr-ĭn-gŏl′ĭ-sĭs). Paralysis of the pharynx.

pharyngomycosis (făr-ĭn″gō-mī-kō′sĭs) [″ + *mykē,* fungus, + *-ōsis,* disease]. Disease of pharynx due to fungi.

pharyngoparalysis (făr-ĭn″gō-păr-ăl′ĭ-sĭs) [G. *pharygx,* pharynx, + *paralysis,* a loosening at the side]. Paralysis of the muscles of the pharynx. Syn: *pharyngoplegia.*

pharyngopathy (făr-ĭn-gŏp′ă-thĭ) [″ + *pathos,* disease]. Any disorder of the pharynx.

pharyngoperistole (făr-ĭn″gō-pĕr-ĭs′tō-lē) [″ + *peristolē,* a drawing out]. Narrowing or stricture of the lumen of the pharynx.

pharyngoplasty (făr-in′gō-plăs″tĭ) [″ + *plassein,* to form]. Reparative surgery of the pharynx.

pharyngoplegia (făr-ĭn″gō-plē′jĭ-ă) [″ + *plēgē,* a stroke]. Paralysis of muscles of pharynx. Syn: *pharyngoparalysis.*

pharyngorhinitis (făr-ĭn″gō-rī-nī′tĭs) [″ + *ris, rin,* nose, + *-ītis,* inflammation]. Inflamed condition of the nasopharynx.

pharyngorhinoscopy (făr-ĭn″gō-rī-nŏs′kō-pĭ) [″ + ″ + *skopein,* to examine]. Inspection of the nasopharynx and posterior nares.

pharyngorrhea (făr-ĭn-go-rē′ă). Discharge of mucus from the pharynx.

pharyngoscope (făr-ĭn′gō-skōp) [G. *pharygx,* pharynx, + *skopein,* to examine]. Instrument for examination of the pharynx.

pharyngoscopy (făr-ĭn-gos′kō-pĭ) [″ + *skopein,* to examine]. Examination of the pharynx.

NP: Watch for difficult breathing and cyanosis from edema. Steam inhalations are sometimes ordered.

pharyngospasm (făr-ĭn′gō-spăzm) [″ + *spasmos,* a spasm]. Spasmodic contraction of muscles of the pharynx. Syn: *pharyngismus.*

pharyngotherapy (făr-ĭn″gō-thĕr′ă-pĭ) [″ + *therapeia,* treatment]. Treatment of pharyngeal disturbances or diseases.

pharyngotome (făr-ĭn′gō-tōm) [″ + *tomē,* an incision]. Instrument for incision of the pharynx.

pharyngotomy (făr-ĭn-gŏt′ō-mĭ) [″ + *tomē,* a cutting]. Incision of the pharynx.

pharynx (pl. *pharynges*) (făr′inks) [G. *pharygx, pharynx*]. A musculomembranous tube extending from base of skull above to level of the 6th vertebra below where it becomes continuous with the esophagus. Upper portion is lined with pseudostratified ciliated epithelium, middle portion with stratified columnar epithelium, and lower portion with stratified squamous epithelium.

Communicates with post. nares, eustachian tube, mouth, esophagus and larynx. *Nasopharynx* part above the palate, *oropharynx* bet. palate and hyoid bone, and *laryngopharynx* part below *the hyoid bone.*

Nerves: Autonomic, vagus, glossopharyngeal.

Blood Vessels: Branches from the ext. carotid artery. Veins form an extensive pharyngeal plexus and drain into int. jugular vein.

Function: Serves as passageway for air from nasal cavity to larynx and food from mouth to esophagus. Also acts as a resonating cavity.

phase (fāz) [G. *phasis,* a showing]. 1. A stage of development. 2. A transitory appearance. 3. The state of a component of a heterogeneous system, as when oil is mixed with water, which is homogeneous throughout itself and bounded by an interface with other phases of the system.

p., continuous. State of substance in a heterogeneous system in which particles are continuous. Ex: The water particles in which oil has been dispersed.

p., contrast microscope. See: *microscope, phase.*

p., disperse. State of a substance in a heterogeneous system in which particles are separated from each other. Also called *discontinuous phase.* Ex: Oil particles in water.

phasic (fā′sĭk). Of or pertaining to a phase.

p. irregularity. Periodic slowing of heart beat such as occurs during convalescence from certain diseases. Cause unknown.

phatne (făt′nē) [G. *phatnē*, socket]. Socket of a tooth.

phatnoma (făt-nō′mă) [" + *-ōma*, tumor]. Tumor of a tooth socket.

phatnorrhagia (făt″nō-rā′jĭ-ă) [" + *rēgnunai*, to burst forth]. Hemorrhage from the socket of a tooth.

Ph.D. Abbr. for *Doctor of Philosophy.*

phenate (fē′nāt). A salt of phenic acid.

phenazone (fĕn′ă-zōn). SEE: *antipyrine.*

phengophobia (fĕn-gō-fō′bĭ-ă) [G. *pheggos*, light, + *phobos*, fear]. Abnormal dread of light. SYN: *photophobia.*

phenic acid (fē′nĭk). Carbolic acid, *q.v.*

phenobarbital (fē″nō-bar′bĭ-tăl). Phenylethylbarbituric acid, a white crystalline substance soluble in alcohol. SYN: *phenylethylmalonylurea.*

ACTION AND USES: A hypnotic, sedative and antispasmodic. Used, often in combination with diphenylhydantoin sodium, in treatment of epilepsy because it has depressive effect on motor areas of the cerebral cortex.

p. sodium. Soluble phenobarbital. More rapidly absorbed than phenobarbital but has the same uses.

phenol (fē′nōl). C_6H_5OH, USP. 1. A crystalline, colorless or light pink solid, melting at 43° C., obtained from the distillation of coal tar, having a characteristic odor, and dangerous because of its rapid corrosive action on tissues. When used carefully, it is effective as a bacteriostatic agent. SYN: *carbolic acid.* 2. Any of the aromatic hydroxyl derivatives of benzene of which phenol is the type.

POISONING: SYM: Strong solutions cause burning, pain and later anesthesia. The skin and mucous membrane first become pale, then grayish white, opalescent and finally brown to black. Even a 5% solution may cause local gangrene. It is absorbed from intact skin wounds and mucous membrane to cause general effects, including collapse and coma. When taken by mouth, it causes whitish discoloration of mucous membranes, intense burning, nausea and rarely vomiting, followed shortly by faintness, weakness, and collapse. Pulse slow and weak. Perspiration is increased, and it causes renal damage.

F. A. TREATMENT: Remove poison from stomach as soon as possible. Emetics such as ipecac or mustard may fail to function because of anesthetic effect of phenol or their action may be dangerous if corrosion has occurred. A well-lubricated stomach pump should be used with caution. Give olive oil at once in large quantities. Olive oil dissolves phenol without hastening absorption. Give extensive lavage with olive oil leaving some in stomach. If olive oil is not available, use cottonseed oil or water. Do not use ethyl alcohol as lavage fluid because it speeds absorption of phenol. Following this, demulcents such as olive oil or cream should be given. Lime water is frequently used as a chemical antidote, also the sulfates, sodium sulfate being the salt of choice. About an ounce of the latter preparation may be introduced through the tube after the stomach has been emptied. Large amounts of liquid petrolatum have been recommended as an antidote. Give large amounts of isotonic saline solution I.V., stimulants, artificial respiration, and oxygen if needed. Shock should be combatted. A guarded prognosis should always be given, for should the patient improve at first, damage to the mucous membrane and absorption of phenol may lead to serious complications later. When phenol has been applied to the skin or mucous membrane, it can be effectively neutralized with 50% alcohol or castor oil.

p. red. An indicator used in determining hydrogen ion concentration.

phenolphthalein (fē″nol-thăl′ē-ĭn, fē″nōl-thăl′ēn). USP. A white, yellowish, crystallized powder, produced by the interaction of phenol and phthalic anhydride.

ACTION AND USES: As a laxative.

phenolsulfonphthalein (fē″nol-sul″fōn-thăl′ē-in). Phenol compound used to test renal function and as an indicator of hydrogen ion concentration. SYN: *phenol red.*

phenoltetrachlorphthalein (fē″nol-tĕt″ră-klōr-thăl′ē-in). A phenol compound used to test function of the liver and as a purgative.

phenoluria (fē″nōl-ū′rĭ-ă) [*phenol* + G. *ouron*, urine]. Elimination of phenols in the urine.

phenomenon (fē-nŏm′ĕ-nŏn) [G. *phainomenon*, appearing]. A change perceivable by the senses that occurs in an organ or vital function; a symptom.

p., Bell's. Rolling of the eyeballs upward and outward when an attempt is made to close the eye affected in peripheral facial paralysis.

phenotype (fē′nō-tīp). The physical appearance or makeup of an individual. Some phenotypes, such as the blood groups, are completely determined by heredity, while others, such as hair color, are readily altered by environmental agents. In genetics, a group of individuals who resemble each other in appearance but may differ in genetic makeup. SEE: *genotype.*

phenozygous (fē-nŏz′ĭ-gŭs). Possessing a cranium much narrower than the face.

phenyl (fĕn′ĭl). In chemistry, the univalent radical of phenol C_6H_5.

phenylhydrazine (fĕn″ĭl-hī′dră-zēn). Oily nitrogenous base used as a test for presence of sugar.

phenylketonuria (fĕn-ĭl-kē″tō-nū′rĭ-ă). 1. Phenylpyruvic acid in the urine. 2. A disease caused by the body's failure to oxidize an amino acid (phenylalanine) to tyrosine, perhaps because of a defective enzyme. About 0.5% of mental defectives suffer from this disease.

phenylpyruvic acid (fĕn-ĭl-pī-rū′vĭk). A metabolic derivative of phenylalanine.

p. a. amentia. SEE: *p. a. oligophrenia.*

p. a. oligophrenia. A form of inherited mental deficiency resulting from an inborn error of metabolism. Characterized by inability to oxidize phenylpyruvic acid which is excreted in urine. Defect is congenital and familial.

phenylthiocarbamide (fen″il-thi″o-car′bă-mid). Phenylthiourea. Usually abbreviated PTC. About 70% of the population inherit the ability to note the taste of PTC to be extremely bitter. To the remainder of the population, it is tasteless. The inheritance of this trait is due to a single dominant gene pair. Used as a diagnostic aid in determining sense of taste.

pheochromocytoma (fe′o-kro′mo-si-to′-mah) [G. *phaios*, dusty + *chrōma*, color + *cyto*, cell + *-ōma*, tumor]. A chromaffin cell tumor producing hypertension by excreting epinephrine and norepinephrine. It usually occurs in the adrenal medulla but may arise in other chromaffin tissues. Is usually benign. SYN: *medullary chromaffinoma; medullary paraganglioma.*

Ph.G. Abbr. for *Graduate in Pharmacy; German Pharmacopeia.*

phial (fī′ăl) [G. *phialē*, a bowl]. A small vessel for medicine; a vial.

-philia. Combining form meaning *love for, tendency towards, craving for.*

philoneism (fĭl″ō-nē′ism). Excessive love or fondness for newness or change. Opp. of *misoneism.*

philt′er, philt′re. A potion or drug which is supposed to induce love or promote sexual activity.

philt′rum. A median groove on external surface of upper lip.

phimosis (fī-mō′sĭs) [G. a muzzling]. Stenosis or narrowness of preputial orifice so that the foreskin cannot be pushed back over the glans penis.

TREATMENT: Circumcision. SEE: *capistration.*

p. vaginalis. Narrowness or closure of the vaginal orifice.

pHisoHex (fī′so-heks). Proprietary name for an antibacterial skin cleanser containing hexachlorophene as a main ingredient.

phlebangioma (flĕb-ăn-jĭ-ō′mă) [" + *aggeion*, vessel, + *-ōma*, tumor]. An aneurysm occurring in a vein.

phlebarteriectasia (flĕb″ăr-tē″rĭ-ĕk-tā′-zĭ-ă) [" + *artēria*, artery, + *ektasis*, dilatation]. Varicose aneurysms; dilatation of blood vessels.

phlebarteriodialysis (flĕb″ăr-tē″rĭ-ō-dī-ăl′-ĭs-ĭs) [" + " + *dialysis*, separation]. Arteriovenous aneurysm.

phlebectasia, phlebectasis (flĕb-ĕk-tā′zĭ-ă, -ĕk′tă-sĭs) [" + *ektasis*, dilatation]. Venous dilatation. SYN: *varicosity.*

phlebectomy (flĕb-ĕk′tō-mĭ) [" + *ektomē*, excision]. Surgical removal of a vein.

phlebectopia (flĕb-ĕk-tō′pĭ-ă) [" + *ek*, out, + *topos*, place]. Abnormal position of a vein.

phlebemphraxis (flĕb-ĕm-frăk′sĭs) [G. *phleps, phleb-*, vein, + *emphraxis*, a stopping]. Artificial obstruction of a vein.

phlebismus (flĕb-ĭz′mŭs) [G. *phleps, phleb-*, vein, + *ismos*, condition]. Venous congestion and dilatation.

phlebitis (flĕ-bī′tĭs) [G. *phleps, phleb-*, vein, + *-itis*, inflammation]. Inflammation of a vein. SYN: *phlegmasia alba dolens, milk leg, thrombophlebitis.*

ETIOL: Unknown. May occur in acute or chronic infections or following operations or childbirth.

SYM: Pain and tenderness along course of vein; discoloration of skin; inflammatory swelling, and acute edema below obstruction; rapid pulse; mild elevation of temperature; pain in joints.

p., adhesive. P. in which vein tends to become obliterated.

p., migrating. A transitory p. which appears in a portion of a vein, then clears up only to reappear later in another location.

p. nodularis necrotisans. Circumscribed inflammation of cutaneous veins resulting in nodules which ulcerate.

p., obliterative. P. in which the lumen of a vein becomes closed. Also called *obstructive* or *adhesive phlebitis.*

p., plastic. Adhesive phlebitis, *q.v.*

p., proliferative. Adhesive phlebitis.

p., puerperal. Venous inflammation following childbirth.

p., sclerosing. P. in which the veins become obstructed and hardened.

p., sinus. Inflammation of a sinus of the cerebrum.

p., suppurative. P. characterized by the formation of pus.

phlebo-. Combining form meaning vein.

phlebocholosis (flĕb″ō-kō-lō′sĭs) [G. *phleps, phleb-*, vein, + *chōlos*, maimed]. Diseased condition of a vein.

phleboclysis (flĕb-ŏk′lĭ-sĭs) [" + *klysis*, injection]. The introduction of an isotonic solution of dextrose or other substances into a vein.

p., drip. Injection, intravenously, drop by drop. SEE: *Murphy's drip.*

phlebogram (flĕb′ō-grăm) [G. *phleps, phleb-*, vein, + *gramma*, a mark]. A tracing of the venous pulse.

phlebography (flĕ-bog′ră-fĭ). A study of the structure and function of the veins.

phleboid (fleb′oid). Pert. to, resembling, or of the nature of a vein; venous.

phlebolite, phlebolith (flĕb′ō-līt, -lĭth) [G. *phleps, phleb-*, vein, + *lithos*, a stone]. A calcareous concretion in a vein resulting from calcification of a thrombus.

phle″bolithi′asis. The formation of phleboliths in veins.

phlebology (flĕb-ŏl′ō-jĭ) [" + *logos*, study]. The science of veins and their diseases.

phlebometritis (flĕb″ō-mē-trī′tĭs) [" + *mētra*, uterus, + *-itis*, inflammation]. Inflammation of uterine veins.

phlebomyomatosis (flĕb″ō-mī″ō-mă-tō′sĭs) [" + *mys, my-*, muscle, + *-ōma*, tumor, + *-ōsis*, disease]. Thickening of the tissue of a vein from overgrowth of muscular fibers.

phlebopexy (flĕb′ō-pĕks″ĭ) [G. *phleps, phleb-*, vein, + *pēksis*, fixation]. Extraserous transplantation of the testes for varicocele, with preservation of venous network.

phleboplasty (flĕb′ō-plăs″tĭ) [" + *plassein*, to form]. Plastic repair of a wounded vein.

phle″boplero′sis. Condition in which veins are distended.

phleborrhaphy (flĕb-or′ăf-ĭ) [" + *raphē*, a sewing]. Suture of a vein.

phleborrhexis (flĕb-or-rĕks′ĭs) [" + *rēxis*, a rupture]. Rupture of a vein.

phlebosclerosis (flĕb″o-sklē-rō′sĭs) [" + *sklērōsis*, a hardening]. Fibrous hardening of a vein's walls.

phlebostasia, phlebostasis (flĕb-ō-stā′zĭ-ă, -ŏs′tă-sĭs) [" + *stasis*, a standing]. Compression of veins temporarily removing an amount of blood from the general circulation. SYN: *phlebotomy, bloodless.*

phlebothrombosis (flĕb″ō-thrŏm-bō′sĭs) [" + *thrombos*, a clot]. Clotting in a vein; phlebitis with secondary thrombosis.

phlebotome (flĕb′ō-tōm) [G. *phleps, phleb-*, vein, + *tomē*, a cutting]. Lancet used in cutting a vein.

phlebotomize (flĕ-bot′o-mīz). To take blood from a person.

Phlebot′omus. A genus of insects, the sandflies, belonging to the family Psychodidae, order Diptera. They are annoying bloodsucking insects and transmit various forms of leishmaniasis, sandfly (pappataci) fever, and Oroyo fever.

P. argentipes. In India, the transmitter of *Leishmania donovani*, causative agent of kala-azar.

P. chinensis. Transmitter of kala-azar in China.

P. papatasii. Transmitter of the causative agent of sandfly fever. The virus is capable of being transmitted through the offspring of flies.

P. sergenti. Transmitter of kala-azar in Middle East and India.

P. verrucarum. In So. America, the transmitter of *Bartonella bacilliformis*, causative agent of Oroyo fever (Carrion's disease).

phlebotomy (flĕb-ŏt'ō-mĭ) [" + *tomē*, an incision]. Opening a vein. SYN: *venesection, q.v.*

p., bloodless. Compression of veins of the extremities, cutting off some of the blood from the general circulation. SYN: *phlebostasia.*

phlegm (flĕm) [G. *phlegma*, inflammation]. 1. Thick mucus, esp. that from the respiratory passages. 2. One of the four "humors" of early physiology.

phlegmasia (flĕg-mā'zĭ-ă) [G. *phlegmasia*, inflammation]. Inflammation.

p. alba dolens. Acute edema, esp. of leg from venous obstruction, usually thrombosis. SYN: *milk leg.*

SYM: Usually begins, esp. in women who have recently given birth, with slight fever; pain in lower part of abdomen follows, extends to hips and back, passes under Poupart's ligament and thence down the thigh into calf of leg. Sometimes proceeds from calf upwards. Whole extremity becomes excessively swollen, hot and painful, but not red, hence the name. The lochia and milk may or may not be suppressed. Constitutional disturbance and fever become greatly increased.

Tenderness on pressure most marked along course of femoral vein and veins of the affected region together with associated lymphatics may be felt to be hard and cordlike. Sometimes marked by faint red line. Progress rapid, which frequently doubles size of limb in 24 hours or less; parts within pelvis become irritable; often difficulty in evacuating bladder and rectum; glands in groin sometimes swell and suppurate, and abscesses may form in different parts of limb.

TREATMENT: Elevate limb, protect with a cradle, and apply warm fomentations. Anticoagulants to prevent clot formation. Vasodilator drugs and paracervical block may be used to combat vasospasm. Ligation of main venous channel proximal to thrombus may be done to prevent embolus.

NP: Complete rest, immobilization of the limb. An elastic bandage, usually cotton, may be ordered by the physician. There is danger of a piece of thrombus becoming detached to form an embolus. No excitement. SYN: *milk leg; white leg.*

p., cellulitic. Septic inflammation of connective tissue of the leg following childbirth.

p. malabarica. Inflammation with hypertrophy and induration of the skin. SYN: *elephantiasis.*

p., thrombotic. SEE: *p. alba dolens.*

phlegmatic (flĕg-măt'ĭk) [G. *phlegmatikos*, inflamed]. Of sluggish or calm temperament. SYN: *apathetic.*

phlegmon (flĕg'mŏn) [G. *phlegmonē*, inflammation]. Acute suppurative inflammation of subcutaneous connective tissue, esp. a pyogenic inflammation that spreads along fascial planes or other natural barriers.

p., bronze. Gaseous p. causing bronze spots near incision.

p., diffuse. D. inflammation of subcutaneous tissues with sepsis.

p., gas. P. with extensive emphysema.

p., Holz. A chronic cellulitis of the deep tissues of the floor of the mouth.

phlegmonous (flĕg'mŏn-ŭs) [G. *phlegmonē*, inflammation]. Pert. to inflammation of subcutaneous tissues.

phlogistic (flō-jĭs'tĭk) [G. *phlogistos*, burnt]. Pert. to or inducing inflammation.

phlogogenic, phlogogenous (flō-gō-jĕn'ĭk, -goj'ĕn-ŭs) [" + *gennan*, to produce]. Producing or exciting inflammation.

phlogosin (flō-go'sĭn) [G. *phlogōsis*, inflammation]. Substance, isolated from cultures of *Staphylococcus aureus*, producing suppuration.

phlogosis (flō-gō'sĭs) [G. inflammation]. 1. Inflammation. 2. Erysipelas.

phlyctena (flĭk-tē'nă) (pl. *phlyctenae*) [G. *phlyktaina*, a blister]. A thin ichor- or lymph-containing vesicle, esp. one of many after a first degree burn.

phlyctenoid (flik'tē-noyd) [" + *eidos*, resemblance]. Resembling a blister or pustule.

phlyctenosis (flik"tē-nō'sĭs) [" + *-ōsis*, disease]. Appearance of blisters or pustules.

phlyctenula (flĭk-tĕn'ū-lă) [G. *phlyktaina*, a blister]. A tiny vesicle or pustule, esp. that seen on the cornea.

phlyctenular (flĭk-tĕn'ū-lăr) [G. *phlyktaina*, a blister]. Resembling or pert. to vesicles or pustules.

phlyctenule (flik'ten-ūl) [G. *phlyktaina*, a blister]. A small vesicle or blister, as on cornea or conjunctiva.

phlyctenulosis (flĭk-tĕn-ū-lō'sĭs) [" + *-ōsis*, intensive]. The formation of many phlyctenules.

-phobia [G.]. Suffix meaning *dread, horror, fear.*

phobia (fō'bĭ-ă) [G. *phobos*, fear]. Any abnormal fear, as acarophobia.

RS: *Words beginning with the following forms: acaro-, acro-, aero-, agora-, aichmo-, ailuro-, algo-, amaxo-, amycho-, andro-, anemo-, anthropo-, aphe-, api-, astra-, astro-, ataxo-, auto-, automyso-, bacillo-, ballisto-, basi-, batho-, bato-, belone-, bromidrosi-, cainoto-, carcinomato-, cardio-, carno-, catoptro-, ceno-, chero-, cholero-, claustro-, copro-, dora-, eremo-, ereuto-, ergasio-, ergo-, erythro-, gato-, gephyro-, gymno-, gyne-, haphe-, hemo-, klepto-, lysso-, maieusio-, mono-, myso-, mytho-, necro-, neo-, noso-, nudo-, nycto-, ochlo-, odonto-, ombro-, onomato-, ophidio-, osmo-, pan-, pharmaco-, photo-, poly-, pono-, psychro-, pyro-, rhabdo-, rhypo-, scoto-, sito-, symbolo-, syphilo-, thanato-, topo-, toxico-, tricho-, trichopatho-, xeno-, zoo-.*

phobic (fō'bĭk) [G. *phobos*, fear]. Concerning a phobia.

phobophobia (fō"bō-fō'bĭ-ă) [" + *phobos*, fear]. Morbid fear of acquiring a phobia.

phonacoscope (fō-năk'ō-skōp) [G. *phōnē*, voice, + *skopein*, to examine]. A device for increasing the percussion note or voice sounds.

phonacoscopy (fō-năk-ŏs'kō-pĭ) [" + *skopein*, to examine]. Inspection of the chest with the phonacoscope.

phonal (fō'năl) [G. *phōnē*, voice]. Concerning the voice.

phonasthenia (fō-năs-thē'nĭ-ă) [" + *astheneia*, weakness]. Vocal weakness or hoarseness due to straining the voice.

phonation (fō-nā'shŭn) [G. *phōnē*, voice]. Process of uttering vocal sounds.

phonatory (fō'nă-tō-rĭ) [G. *phōnē*, voice]. Concerning utterance of vocal sounds.

phonautograph (fōn-aw'tō-grăf) [" + *autos*, self, + *graphein*, to write]. Device for registering the voice's vibrations.

-phone. Combining form meaning *sound* or *voice.*

phone. An element of speech; a single speech sound.

phoneme (fō'nēm) [G. *phōnēma,* sound]. Auditory hallucination of voices and spoken words.

May include neologisms. They may repeat a thought or the part of a sentence just read.

phonendoscope (fō-nĕn'dō-skōp) [G. *phōnē,* voice, + *endon,* within, + *skopein,* to examine]. A stethoscope magnifying sounds.

phonendoskiascope (fō-nen"dō-skī'ăs-kōp) [" + " + *skia,* shadow, + *skopein,* to examine]. Device for observing the cardiac movements and for hearing heart sounds.

phonetics (fō-nĕt'ĭks) [G. *phōnētikos,* spoken]. Science of speech and pronunciation. SYN: *phonology.*

pho"niat'rics. The study of the voice and treatment of its disorders.

phonic (fō'nĭk) [G. *phōnē,* voice]. Concerning the voice or sound.

phonism (fō'nĭzm) [" + *-ismos,* condition]. An auditory sensation occurring when another sense is stimulated. SEE: *synesthesia.*

phono- [G.]. Combining form meaning *sound, voice.*

phonocardiography (fō"nō-kar-dĭ-ŏg-ră-fĭ) [" + *kardia,* heart, + *graphein,* to write]. Mechanical or electronic registration of heart sounds.

phonogram (fō'nō-grăm) [" + *gramma,* a mark]. A graphic curve indicating intensity and duration of a sound.

phonograph (fō'nō-grăf) [" + *graphein,* to write]. Instrument used for reproduction of sounds.

phonology (fō-nŏl'ō-jĭ) [" + *logos,* a study]. Science of vocal sounds. SYN: *phonetics.*

phon"oma'nia. Insanity characterized by homicidal tendencies.

-phonomassage (fō"nō-măs-săzh') [G. Combining form meaning *sound, voice,* + *massein,* to knead]. Exciting movements of the ossicles of the ear by means of noise or alternating suction and pressure directed through the ext. auditory meatus.

phonometer (fō-nŏm'ĕt-ĕr) [" + *metron,* measure]. Device for determining intensity of vocal sounds.

phonomyoclonus (fō"nō-mī-ok'lō-nŭs) [G. *phōnē,* voice, + *mys, myo-,* muscle, + *klonos,* a contraction]. Invisible fibrillary muscular contractions revealed by auscultation.

phonomyogram (fō"nō-mī'ō-grăm) [" + " + *gramma,* a writing]. A recording of sound produced by action of a muscle.

phonomyography (fō"nō-mī-og'ră-fĭ) [" + " + *graphein,* to write]. The recording of sounds made by contracting muscular tissue.

phonopathy (fō-nŏp'ăth-ĭ) [" + *pathos,* disease]. Any disease of organs affecting speech.

phon"opho'bia. 1. Morbid fear of sound or noise. 2. Fear of speaking or hearing one's own voice.

phonopsia (fō-nŏp'sĭ-ă) [G. *phōne,* voice, + *opsis,* vision]. The subjective perception of sensations upon hearing certain sounds.

phonoscope (fō'nō-skōp) [G. *phōnē,* voice, + *skopein,* to examine]. Device for recording photographs of heart sounds.

phoresis (fō-rē'sĭs) [G. *phorēsis,* from *phorein,* to bear]. PT: The migration of ions through a membrane by the action of an electric current.

The direction of migration is sometimes distinguished by the use of the terms "cataphoresis" and "anaphoresis" for migrations toward cathode and anode, respectively.

-phoria. In ophth. a combining form meaning a *turning with reference to the visual axis.* Ex: *cyclophoria.*

Phormia. A genus of blowflies belonging to the family Calliphoridae. Their larvae normally live in decaying flesh of dead animals, but they may infest neglected wounds or sores giving rise to myiasis.

phorology (fō-rol'ō-jĭ) [G. *phorein,* to carry, + *logos,* study]. Science dealing with disease carriers.

phorotone (fō'rō-tōn) [" + *tonos,* tension]. Device for exercising eye muscles.

phose (fōz) [G. *phōs,* light]. A subjective sensation of light or color. SEE: *centraphose; centrophose; chromophose.*

phosgene (fos'jēn) [G. *phos,* light, + *genes,* born]. Carbonyl chloride ($COCl_2$), a poisonous gas causing nausea and suffocation when inhaled. Used in chemical warfare, esp. during World War I; now used in industry in preparation of pharmaceutical and chemical products.

phosphatase (fŏs'fă-tās). One of a group of enzymes which catalyzes the hydrolysis of phosphoric acid esters. They are of importance in absorption and metabolism of carbohydrates, nucleotides, and phospholipids and are essential in the calcification of bone.

p., acid. P. whose optimum pH is between 4.0 and 5.4. Present in kidney, semen, serum, and prostate gland.

p., alkaline. P. whose optimum pH is about 9.0. Present in teeth, developing bone, plasma, kidney, and intestine. It is excreted by the liver, hence increases in blood in obstructive jaundice.

phosphate (fŏs'fāt) [G. *phōs,* light, + *pherein,* to carry]. A salt of phosphoric acid.

Phosphates are important in maintenance of acid-base balance of the blood, the principal ones being monosodium and disodium phosphate. The former is acid, the latter alkaline. In the blood, because of their low concentration, they exert a minor buffering action. In the formation of urine, by altering the proportions of acid and alkaline phosphates, an acid urine is formed and the body's fixed base, chiefly Na but also K, Mg, and Ca, is conserved.

Decreased p. excretion in urine occurs: when alkaline reserve is high, in nephritis, tetany (hypoparathyroidism), adrenal cortical deficiency, and certain bone diseases.

Increased p. excretion in urine occurs: when alkali reserve is low, in starvation, hyperparathyroidism, high protein diet and extreme muscular exercise.

p., acid. P. in which only one or two of hydrogen atoms of phosphoric acid have been replaced by a metal.

p.-bond-energy. Energy derived from phosphorylated compounds such as adenosine triphosphate (ATP) and creatine phosphate.

p., normal. P. in which all three hydrogen atoms of phosphoric acid have been replaced by metals.

phosphatemia (fŏs-fă-tē'mĭ-ă) [" + " + *aima,* blood]. Phosphates in the blood.

phosphatide (fŏs′fă-tīd) [G. *phōs*, light, + *pherein*, to carry]. A phospholipid *q.v.*

phosphatoptosis (fŏs-fă-tŏp-tō′sis) [" + " + *ptōsis*, a dropping]. Spontaneous precipitation of phosphates in urine.

phosphaturia (fŏs-fă-tū-rĭ-ă) [G. *phōs*, light, + *pherein*, to carry, + *ouron*, urine]. Phosphates in the urine.

They often cause renal calculi. SYN: *phosphoruria; phosphuria.*

SYM: Cloudy urine, opaque and pale. Reaction alkaline. Pearly or pinkish white deposits of phosphates in standing urine.

phosphene (fŏs′fēn) [" + *phainein*, to show]. A subjective sensation of light caused by pressure upon the eyeball.

p., accommodation. P. resulting from contraction of ciliary muscles in accommodation. Seen esp. in the dark.

phosphide (fŏs′fīd) [G. *phōs*, light, + *pherein*, to carry]. Binary compound of phosphorus with an element or radical.

phosphite (fŏs′fīt) [" + *pherein*, to carry]. A salt of phosphoric acid.

phosphocreatine (fŏs″fō-krē′ă-tēn). A compound, found in muscle, of equal parts of phosphoric acid and creatine.

phospholipid (fŏs″fō-lĭp′ĭd) [G. *phōs*, light, + *pherein*, to carry, + *lipos*, fat]. A lipoid substance containing phosphorus, fatty acids and nitrogenous base, as lecithin. SYN: *phosphatide; phospholipin.*

phospholipin (fŏs-fō-lĭp′ĭn) [" + " + *lipos*, fat]. A lipoid compound containing phosphorus. SYN: *phosphatide; phospholipid.*

phosphonecrosis (fŏs″fō-nē-krō′sĭs) [G. *phōs*, light, + *pherein*, to carry, + *nekros*, dead, + *-ōsis*, disease]. Necrosis of the alveolar process in persons working with phosphorus.

phosphonuclease (fŏs″fō-nū′klē-ās). An enzyme that catalyzes the hydrolysis of nucleotides to nucleosides and phosphoric acid.

phosphopenia (fŏs″fō-pē′nĭ-ă) [" + " + *penia*, lack]. Deficiency of phosphorus in the body.

phosphoprotein (fŏs″fō-prō′tē-ĭn) [G. *phōs*, light, + *pherein*, to carry, + *prōtos*, first]. One of a group of proteins in which the protein is combined with phosphorus-containing compound. Ex: *caseinogen; vitellin.*

Formerly called nucleoalbumin.

phosphorated (fŏs′fō-rā-tĕd) [" + *phorein*, to carry]. Impregnated with phosphorus.

phosphorescence (fŏs-fō-rĕs′ĕns) [" + *phorein*, to carry]. PT: The induced luminescence that persists after cessation of the irradiation that caused it. The emission of light without appreciable heat.

phosphorhidrosis (fŏs″for-hĭd-rō′sĭs) [G. *phōs*, light, + *phorein*, to carry, + *idrōsis*, sweating]. Secretion of phosphorescent perspiration. SYN: *phosphoridrosis.*

phosphoric acid (fŏs-for′ĭk) [G. *phōs*, light, + *phorein*, to carry]. Orthophosphoric acid, H_3PO_4, a tribasic acid.

phosphoridrosis (fŏs″for-ĭd-rō′sĭs) [" + " + *idrōsis*, perspiration]. Secretion of perspiration that is luminous. SYN: *phosphorhidrosis.*

phosphorism (fŏs′for-ĭzm) [G. *phōs*, light, + *phoros*, carrying, + *ismos*, condition]. Chronic poisoning from phosphorus.

phosphorous acid (fŏs-fō′rŭs) [" + *phoros*, carrying]. Crystalline acid formed when phosphorus is oxidized in moist air. H_3PO_3.

phosphoruria (fŏs″for-ū′rĭ-ă) [" + " + *ouron*, urine]. Phosphorus in the urine in excess of normal. SYN: *phosphaturia; phosphuria.*

phosphorus (fŏs′fĕr-ŭs) [G. *phōs*, light, + *phoros*, carrying]. SYMB: P. At. wt. 30.9738; at. no. 15. A nonmetallic element not found in a free state but in combination with alkalies.

The adult body contains from 500 to 700 gm. of phosphorus in various forms, 70 to 80 per cent in bones and teeth principally combined with calcium, 10 per cent in muscle and 1 per cent in nerve tissue. Minimum daily requirement is approx. 0.9 gm., although daily intake should be about 1.5 gm. for safety. Amount should be doubled during pregnancy. Vitamin D is important in the absorption and metabolism of phosphorus. Excesses of phosphorus are excreted by kidney and intestine, about 60 per cent being excreted in urine principally as phosphates.

Phosphorus compounds (adenosine triphosphate and phosphocreatine) are the principal sources of energy in muscle contraction, and phosphorus is essential in the conversion of glycogen to glucose.

DEFICIENCY SYM: Perverted appetite, retarded growth, loss of weight, weakness, rickets, imperfect bone and teeth development.

It is found in the protein of food. Ex: Almonds, beans, barley, bran, cheese, cocoa, chocolate, eggs, lentils, liver, milk, oatmeal, peanuts, peas, walnuts, whole wheat, and rye. *Good*: Asparagus, beef, cabbage, carrots, celery, cauliflower, chards, chicken, clams, corn, cream, cucumbers, egg plant, fish, figs, prunes, pineapples, pumpkin, raisins, string beans; also in meats.

POISONING: SYM: Acute irritation of gastrointestinal tract, followed by symptoms resembling acute yellow atrophy of liver, and marked blood changes. Bloody vomitus, garlic odor of breath, cramps, headache, liver and kidney damage. Profound weakness, hemorrhage, heart failure. Occasionally nervous symptoms predominate. Metabolism changes.

F. A. TREATMENT: Prolonged gastric lavage, part of which should contain a small amount of copper sulfate or potassium permanganate which may aid in oxidizing the phosphorus. This should, of course, be washed out. Oils, creams and fats should be avoided because these promote absorption of phosphorus. Sodium bicarbonate tends to reduce acidosis. Otherwise treat symptomatically. Blood transfusion is helpful. SEE: *Table of Poisons and Poisoning in Appendix.*

phosphorylase (fos-for′ĭ-lās). An enzyme that catalyzes the formation of glucose-1-phosphate from glycogen.

phosphotal (fŏs′fō-tăl). Commercial phosphorus and creosote compound.

phosphuria (fŏs-fū′rĭ-ă) [G. *phōs*, light, + *phoros*, a bearer, + *ouron*, urine]. Excess of phosphorus in the urine. SYN: *phosphaturia; phosphoruria.*

phot (fōt) [G. *phōs*, *phot-*, light]. The unit of photochemical energy equal to 1 lumen per square centimeter or about 929 foot candles. ABBR: *ph.*

photalgia (fō-tăl′jĭ-ă) [G. *phōs*, *phot-*, light, + *algos*, pain]. Pain produced by light. SYN: *photodynia; photophobia.*

photaugiophobia (fō-tăw-jĭ-ō-fō′bĭ-ă) [" + *augē*, glare, + *phobos*, fear]. Intolerance of bright light.

photesthesis (fō-tĕs-thē′sĭs) [" + *aisthesis*, sensation]. Sensitivity to light.

photic (fō′tĭk) [G. *phōs*, *phot-*, light]. Concerning light.

photism (fō′tĭzm) [" + *ismos*, condition]. A subjective sensation of color or light produced by a stimulus of another sense, such as smell, hearing, taste, or touch. SEE: *synesthesia*.

photo- [G.]. Combining form meaning *light*.

photobiotic (fō″to-bī-ŏt′ĭk) [G. *phōs*, *phot-*, light, + *bios*, life]. Capable of living only in the light.

photocauterization (fō″tō-kaw-tĕr-ĭz-ā′-shŭn) [" + *kautērion*, a branding iron]. Cauterization using radioactive means, as x-rays.

photoceptor (fō″tō-sĕp′tor) [" + L. *ceptor*, a receiver]. A nerve ceptor receiving light ray sensations.

photochemistry (fō″tō-kĕm′ĭs-trĭ) [" + *chemeia*, chemistry]. Phase of science dealing with chemical changes produced by light rays.

photodermatitis (fo″to - der - mă - ti′tis). Sensitivity of the epithelium to light.

photodynamic (fō″tō-dī-năm′ĭk) [" + *dynamis*, force]. Pert. to the effect of light on organisms.

p. action. Action exerted by certain dyes such as methylene blue and eosin on certain biological systems when subjected to light.

photodynia (fō″tō-dĭn′ĭ-ă) [" + *odynē*, pain]. Pain produced by rays of light. SYN: *photalgia*.

photodysphoria (fō″tō-dĭs-fō′rĭ-ă) [" + *dys*, bad, + *phorein*, to carry]. Extreme intolerance of light. SYN: *photophobia; phengophobia*.

photoelectricity (fō″tō-ē-lĕk-trĭ′sĭ-tĭ) [G. *phōs*, *phot-*, light, + *ēlektron*, amber]. Electricty formed by action of light.

photofluorography (fo″to-flōō″er-og′ră-fĭ). Photographing the images seen during fluoroscopic examination.

photogene (fō′tō-jēn) [" + *gennan*, to produce]. Prolonged retinal image. SYN: *after-image*.

photogenic, photogenous (fō″tō-jĕn′ĭk, -tŏj′ĕn-ŭs) [" + *gennan*, to produce]. Induced by or inducing light.

photograph′ic radiom′eter. PT: An instrument containing a half-tone color index for strips of photographic paper after exposure to roentgen rays and, after development, used to estimate the quantity of roentgen rays.

photohemotachometer (fō″tō-hem″ō-tăk-ŏm′ĕt-ĕr) [G. *phōs*, *phot-*, light, + *aima*, blood, + *tachus*, swift, + *metron*, measure]. Device for photographing rate of blood flow.

photokinetic (fō″tō-kĭn-ĕt′ĭk) [" + *kinēsis*, motion]. Reacting with motion to stimulus of light.

photoluminescence (fō″tō-lū-mĭn-ĕs′ents) [" + L. *lumen*, light]. PT: The power of an object to become luminescent when acted on by light.

photolysis (fō-tŏl′ĭs-ĭs) [" + *lysis*, dissolution]. Dissolution or disintegration under stimulus of light rays.

photolytic (fō″tō-lĭt′ĭk). Dissolved by stimulus of light rays.

photomania (fō″tō-mā′nĭ-ă) [" + *mania*, madness]. 1. A psychosis produced by prolonged exposure to intense light. 2. A psychotic desire for light.

photometer (fō-tŏm′ĕt-ĕr) [G. *phōs*, *phot-*, light, + *metron*, measure]. PT: A device for measuring the intensity of light.

photometry (fō-tom′ĕt-rĭ) [" + *metron*, measure]. Measurement of light rays.

photomicrograph (fō″tō-mī′krō-grăf) [" + *mikros*, small, + *graphein*, to write]. Photograph of an object under the microscope.

photom′otor. Pert. to muscular contraction induced by light.

photon (fō′tŏn) [G. *phōs*, *phot-*, light]. A light quantum or unit of energy of a light ray or other form of radiant energy.

photonosus (fō-ton′ō-sŭs) [" + *nosos*, disease]. Disease due to prolonged exposure to intense light.

photoperceptive (fō″tō-pĕr-cĕp′tĭv) [" + *percipere*, to receive]. Capable of perceiving light.

photophilic (fō-tō-fĭl′ĭk) [" + *philein*, to love]. Seeking or fond of light.

photophobia (fō″tō-fō′bĭ-ă) [" + *phobos*, fear]. Unusual intolerance of light.

Occurs in measles and rubella, meningitis, and inflammations of the eyes. SYN: *phengophobia; photodysphoria*.

photophone (fō′tō-fōn) [" + *phōnē*, voice]. Device for production of sound by action of light.

pho′topic. Pert. to bright light.

p. vision. Vision in bright light which involves the formation of images and discrimination of color. SEE ALSO: *scotopic vision*.

photopsia, photopsy (fō-tŏp′sĭ-ă, fō′tŏp-sĭ) [" + *opsis*, vision]. Subjective sensation of sparks or flashes of light in retinal, optic, or brain diseases.

photoptarmosis (fō″tō-tar-mō′sĭs) [" + *ptarmōsis*, sneezing]. Sneezing caused by the action of light.

photoptometer (fō-tŏp-tŏm′ĕt-ĕr) [" + *opsis*, vision, + *metron*, measure]. Device for determining the smallest amount of light that will make an object visible.

photoreceptive (fō″tō-rē-sĕp′tĭv) [" + *receptor*, a receiver]. Capable of perceiving light rays.

photoreceptor (fō″tō-rē-sĕp′tor) [G. *phōs*, *phot-*, light, + *receptor*, a receiver]. Sensory nerve endings or cells which are capable of being stimulated by light. In man, rods and cones of the retina.

photoscope (fō′tō-skōp) [G. *phōs*, *phot-*, light, + *skopein*, to examine]. A variety of fluoroscope used to observe light.

photoscopy (fō-tŏs′kō-pĭ) [" + *skopein*, to examine]. Examination with a fluorescent screen. SYN: *fluoroscopy; skiascopy*.

photosensitization (fō″tō-sĕn-sĭ-tĭ-ză′-shŭn) [G. *phōs*, *phot-*, light, + *sensitivus*, feeling]. Condition in which the skin reacts abnormally to light, esp. ultraviolet rays or sunlight; due to the presence of drugs, hormones, or heavy metals in the system.

photosensitizer (fō″tō-sĕn-sĭ-tī′zĕr) [" + *sensitivus*, feeling]. Sensitizing substance used in light therapy to produce photosensitization, such as fluorescein dyes.

photosynthesis (fō″tō-sĭn′thĕ-sĭs) [G. *phōs*, *phot-*, light, + *synthesis*, a placing together]. The process by which plants are able to manufacture carbohydrates by combining carbon dioxide from the air and water from the soil, utilizing light energy in the presence of chlorophyll.

The basic chemical reaction is as follows:

$6CO_2 + 6H_2O +$ energy (4.1 Cal. per gm. of glucose) $C_6H_{12}O_6 + 6H_2O$.

Only plants containing chlorophyll are capable of thus producing sugars. The red and blue waves of the spectrum are absorbed by the chlorophyll, but all other rays are rejected. CO_2 and H_2O are also necessary factors.

When simple sugar is formed, the plant splits up CO_2, uses the carbon by photosynthesis, and liberates the oxygen. The sources of energy for this disruption are the blue and red rays which are absorbed by the plant. To make 1 gm. of natural sugar the plant uses 750 cu. ft. of CO_2.

phototaxis (fō″tō-tăks′ĭs) [″ + *taxis*, arrangement]. PT: The reaction and movement of cells and microorganisms under the stimulus of light.

phototherapy (fō″tō-thĕr′ă-pĭ) [″ + *therapeia*, treatment]. Light therapy, the use of light in treating disease.

By custom the term denotes also the application of the invisible, infrared or heat, and ultraviolet or actinic rays. SEE: *actinotherapy*.

photothermal (fō″tō-thĕr′măl) [G. *phōs, phot-*, light, + *thermē*, heat]. Concerning heat produced by light.

p. radiation. Radiation of heat by a source of light, as that from an electric bulb.

pho″totop′ia. A subjective sensation of light.

phototoxis (fō″tō-toks′ĭs) [″ + *toxikon*, poison]. Disorder produced by effects of overexposure to light or radiation.

pho″totrop′ism. A tendency exhibited by green plants and some microorganisms to turn toward or grow toward light.

photuria (fō-tū′rĭ-ă) [″ + *ouron*, urine]. Excretion of phosphorescent urine.

phren (frēn) [G. *phrēn*, mind, diaphragm]. 1. The mind. 2. The diaphragm.

phrenalgia (frē-năl′jĭ-ă) [″ + *algos*, pain]. 1. Pain of mental origin or caused by a mental process. SYN: *psychalgia*. 2. Pain in the diaphragm.

phrenasthenia (fren-ăs-thē′nĭ-ă) [″ + *astheneia*, weakness]. Mental deficiency.

phrenemphraxis (frĕn-ĕm-frăk′sĭs). Crushing of the phrenic nerve in order to induce temporary paralysis of the diaphragm, a therapeutic measure employed in treatment of pulmonary tuberculosis.

phrenetic (fren-ĕt′ĭk) [G. *phrēn*, mind]. 1. Maniacal; frenzied. 2. A maniac.

-phrenia. Combining form meaning *mental disorder*.

phrenic (fren′ĭk) [G. *phrēn*, mind, diaphragm]. 1. Concerning the diaphragm, as the p. nerve. 2. Concerning the mind.

p. avulsion. Elevation of a side of the diaphragm and semi-collapse of corresponding lung by means of excision of part of the phrenic nerve.

p. nerve. One arising in the cervical plexus entering the thorax and passing to the diaphragm.

A motor nerve to the diaphragm with sensory fibers to the pericardium. SYN: *nervus phrenicus*.

phrenicectomy (fren-ĭs-ĕk′tō-mĭ) [″ + *ektomē*, excision]. Resection of a part of the phrenic nerve.

Used to collapse the lung on one side by paralyzing the diaphragm.

phrenicoexairesis. Same as *phrenicoexeresis*.

phrenicoexeresis (fren″ĭ-ko-eks″er-e′sis) [″ + *ek*, out, + *airein*, to take]. Excision of part of the phrenic nerve.

phrenicotomy (fren-ĭk-ŏt′ō-mĭ) [″ + *tomē*, a cutting]. Cutting of the phrenic nerve to produce immobilization of a lung by inducing paralysis of one side.

This causes the diaphragm to rise, it compresses the lung and diminishes respiratory movement, thus resting the lung on that side.

phrenitis (frē-nī′tĭs) [″ + *-itis*, inflammation]. 1. Acute delirium or frenzy. 2. Inflammation of the brain. SYN: *encephalitis*. 3. Inflammation of the diaphragm.

phreno- [G.]. Combining form meaning *mind, diaphragm*.

phrenocardia (frē″nō-kar′dĭ-ă) [″ + *kardia*, heart]. Cardiovascular neurasthenia.

SYM: Cardiac arrhythmia, dyspnea with psychic disturbances, and submammary pain.

phrenocolopexy (frē″nō-kō′lō-pĕks″ĭ) [″ + *kōlon*, colon, + *pēxis*, fixation]. Suture of the transverse colon to the diaphragm.

phrenodynia (frē″nō-dĭn′ĭ-ă [″ + *odynē*, pain]. Pain in the diaphragm.

phrenograph (fren′ō-grăf) [G. *phrēn*, diaphragm, mind, + *graphein*, to write]. Device for registering movements of diaphragm.

phrenopathy (frē-nŏp′ăth-ĭ) [″ + *pathos*, disease]. Any mental disorder.

phrenopericarditis (frē″nō-pĕr-ĭ-kar-dī′-tĭs) [″ + *peri*, around, + *kardia*, heart, *-itis*, inflammation]. Attachment of the heart by adhesions to the diaphragm.

phrenoplegia (frē-nō-plē′jĭ-ă) [″ + *plēgē*, a stroke]. 1. A sudden psychopathic attack. 2. Paralysis of the diaphragm.

phrenosin (fren′ō-sĭn) [G. *phrēn*, mind, diaphragm]. SYN: *cerebron*. A cerebroside isolated from brain tissue.

phrictopathic (frĭk-tō-păth′ĭk) [G. *phriktos*, shuddering, + *pathos*, disease]. Pert. to or having a shuddering sensation; applied to a shuddering sensation due to irritating a hysterical anesthetic area.

phro″ne′sis. Soundness of mind.

phrynoderma (frĕn-ō-der′mă). Skin disorder characterized by dryness and follicular hyperkeratosis. Due to deficiency of vitamin A. SYN:*toadskin*.

phthiriasis (thĭr-ī′ăs-ĭs) [G. *phtheir*, louse]. Condition of being infested with lice. SYN: *pediculosis*.

phthiriophobia (thĭr″ĭ-ō-fō′bĭ-ă) [″ + *phobos*, fear]. Abnormal dread of lice.

Phthirus (thĭr′ŭs) [G. *phtheir*, louse]. A genus of sucking lice belonging to the order Anoplura.

P. pubis. The crab louse. Infests primarily pubic region but also found in armpits, beard, eyebrows, and eyelashes. SEE: *pediculosis pubis*.

phthisic (tĭz′ĭk) [G. *phthisis*, a wasting]. 1. Affected with pulmonary consumption. 2. Asthma. 3. One afflicted with phthisis or asthma.

phthisical (tĭz′ĭk-ăl) [G. *phthisis*, a wasting]. Concerning, or afflicted with, phthisis.

phthisicky (tĭz′ĭ-kĭ) [G. *phthisis*, a wasting]. Suffering from asthma or phthisis.

phthisis (tī′sĭs) [G. a wasting]. 1. Pulmonary consumption. SEE: *tuberculosis*. 2. Any wasting or atrophic disease.

p., abdominal. Intestinal tuberculosis.

p., black. Lung disease from inhaled coal dust. SYN: *anthracosis*.

p. bulbi. Atrophy of eyeball following intraocular inflammation.

p., fibroid. 1. Interstitial pneumonia. 2. Pulmonary tuberculosis with dense layers of fibrous tissues surrounding a cavity.

p., miner's. SEE: *p., black.*

p., pulmonary. Tuberculosis of the lungs.

p., stonecutter's. A wasting form of bronchopneumonia due to inhalation of stone dust with consequent irritation.

phycology (fi-kol'o-jĭ) [G. *phykos,* seaweed, + *logos,* study]. Study of algae.

phygogalactic (fī"gō-găl-ăk'tĭk) [G. *pheugein,* to avoid, + *gala,* milk]. Checking or that which checks or arrests milk secretion. SYN: *galactophygous; ischogalactic; lactifuge.*

phylacogogic (fī-lăk-ō-gŏj'ĭk) [" + *agōgos,* leading]. Stimulating the formation of protective antibodies.

phylactic (fī-lăk'tĭk) [G. *phylaxis,* protection]. Concerning or producing phylaxis.

p. agent. One with protective power.

p. power. That of an organism to ward off infection.

phylaxin (fī-lăks'ĭn) [G. *phylaxis,* protection]. Antibody. Protecting and defensive substances produced by the body after exposure to bacterial infection.

phylaxis (fī-lăks'ĭs) [G. protection]. The active defense of the body against infection.

phyletic (fī-lĕt'ĭk). SYN: *phylogenetic.* Pert. to a phylum or race.

phyllo- [G.]. Combining form meaning *leaf.*

phylogenesis (fī-lō-jĕn'ĕ-sĭs) [G. *phylon,* tribe, + *genesis,* generation]. The evolutionary development of a group, race or species. SEE: *phylogeny.*

phylogenetic (fī"lō-jĕn-ĕt'ĭk) [" + *genesis,* generation]. Concerning the development of a race or group.

phylogeny (fī-lŏj'ĕ-nĭ) [" + *gennan,* to produce]. Development and growth of a group or race. SEE: *ontogeny.*

phylum (fī'lŭm) [G. *phylon,* tribe]. One of the primary divisions of the animal or plant kingdom.

phyma (fī'mă) (pl. *phymata*) [G. *phyma,* growth]. A small, rounded skin tumor.

phymatoid (fī'măt-oyd) [" + *eidos,* resemblance]. Like a tumor.

phymatorrhysin (fī"mă-tor-hī'sĭn). A pigment present in hair and melanotic tumors.

phymatosis (fī-mă-tō'sĭs) [" + *-ōsis,* disease]. A disease marked by the presence of phymata or small nodules in the skin.

physaliform, physalliform (fĭs-al'ĭ-form) [G. *physallis,* bubble, + L. *forma,* shape]. Resembling a bleb or bubble.

Phy"salop'tera. A genus of nematode worms belonging to the suborder Spiruata.

P. caucasica. Species normally infesting monkeys but common in natives of tropical Africa.

physiatrics (fĭz"ĭ-ăt'rĭks). The curing of disease by natural methods, especially physical therapy.

physic (fĭz'ĭk) [G. *physikos,* natural]. 1. The art of medicine and healing. 2. A medicine, esp. a cathartic. 3. Drugs in general. 4. To treat with a physic, esp. to purge.

physical (fĭz'ĭk-ăl). [G. *physikos,* natural]. 1. Of or pertaining to nature or material things. 2. Concerning or pert. to the body; bodily.

p. examination. Examination of the body by auscultation, palpation, percussion and inspection.

p. signs. Disease symptoms revealed by physical examination.

p. therapist. PT: One skilled in physical therapy.

p. therapy. The therapeutic use of physical agents other than drugs.

It comprises the use of physical, chemical and other properties of heat, light, water, electricity, massage, exercise, and radiation.

p. t. technician or aide. A lay assistant or a nurse trained to apply the physical measures of treatment which have been prescribed by a physician.

p. unit. Coulomb, erg, dyne, etc. SEE: *unit.*

physician (fĭ-zĭsh'ăn) [O. Fr. *physicien,* from G. *physikos,* natural]. A person authorized by law to treat diseases with medicines.

p., house. P. who lives in a hospital and is available at all times.

p., resident. A physician who lives in a hospital to continue his training after internship. Commonly called *resident.*

physicist (fĭz'ĭs-ĭst) [G. *physikos,* natural]. One who is versed in the science of physics.

physico- [G.]. Combining form meaning *physical, natural.*

physics (fĭz'ĭks) [G. *physis,* nature]. The study of forces and properties of matter, and of natural phenomena.

physinosis (fĭz-ĭn-ō'sĭs) [" + *nosos,* disease]. A disease caused by physical agents.

physio- [G.]. Combining form meaning *nature.*

physiocogenic (fĭz"ĭ-ō-kō-jĕn'ĭk). Originating from physical causes.

physiocopyrexia (fĭz-ĭ-ō-kō-pī-rĕks'ĭ-ă). Fever produced artificially by physical means.

physiognomy (fĭz-ĭ-ŏg'nō-mĭ) [G. *physis,* nature, + *gnōmōn,* a judge]. 1. The countenance. 2. Assumed ability to see the mental or moral character and qualities by the face.

physiognosis (fĭz-ĭ-ŏg-nō'sĭs) [" + *gnosis,* knowledge]. Diagnosis determined from one's facial expression and appearance of the eyes.

physiological (fĭz"ĭ-ō-lŏj'ĭk-ăl) [G. *physis,* nature, + *logos,* study]. 1. Normal; not diseased. 2. Concerning body function.

p. chemistry. Chemistry of living organisms. SEE: *biochemistry.*

p. salt solution. An isotonic sterile solution consisting of 0.85% sodium chloride in distilled water. Also called *normal salt solution* or *normal saline.* Abbr: P.S.S. A teaspoonful of table salt in a pint of water approximates a physiological salt solution.

Used (a) in irrigating mucous membranes and raw surfaces, (b) replenishing of body water in dehydration, and (c) in shock or hemorrhage to restore circulating blood volume.

p. s. s. enema. The distention made by this enema excites peristalsis and evacuation. Often ordered when there is dehydration. SEE: *enema.*

physiology (fĭz-ĭ-ŏl'ō-jĭ) [G. *physis,* nature, + *logos,* study]. The science of the functions of cells, tissues, and organs of the living organism.

physiolysis (fiz"ē-ol'ĭ-sis). Natural decay and dissolution of tissue.

physiotherapy (fĭz-ĭ-ō-thĕr'ă-pĭ) [" + *therapeia,* treatment]. Treatment with physical and mechanical means, as massage, electricity, etc. Syn: *physical therapy.*

physique (fĭ-zēk). Body build; the structure and organization of the body.

physo- [G.]. Combining form meaning *bladder, bellows, bubble.*

physocele (fī'sō-sēl) [G. *physa*, air, + *kēlē*, tumor]. 1. A tumor filled with gas or circumscribed swelling due to gas. 2. A gas-distended hernial sac.

physohematometra (fī"sō-hem-ăt-ō-mē'-tră) [" + *aima*, blood, + *mētra*, uterus]. Gas and blood distending the uterus.

physohydrometra (fī"sō-hī-drō-mē'tră) [" + *ydōr*, water, + *mētra*, uterus]. Air or gas and serum in the uterus.

physometra (fī-sō-mē'tră) [" + *mētra*, uterus]. Air or gas in the uterine cavity.

physopyosalpinx (fī"sō-pī"ō-săl'pĭnks) [" + *pyon*, pus, + *salpigx*, tube]. Pus and gas in the fallopian tube.

physostigmine salicylate (fī-sō-stĭg'mēn săl-ĭs'ĭl-āt). USP. The salicylate of an alkaloid obtained from the dried Calabar bean. Syn: *eserine salicylate.*

Action and Uses: It inactivates cholinesterase thus prolonging and intensifying the action of acetylcholine. It improves the tone and action of skeletal muscle, and through its effects on parasympathetic nervous system, it increases intestinal peristalsis and, in the eye, acts as a miotic. It is used in tetanus and strychnine poisoning and in the treatment of myasthenia gravis.

phytalbumose (fī-tăl'bū-mōs) [" + L. *albumen*, white of egg]. An albumose found in plants and vegetables.

phytase (fī'tās) [" + *ase*, enzyme]. A liver and blood ferment that splits phytin.

phytin (fī'tĭn) [G. *phyton*, plant]. A calcium or magnesium salt of inositol, and hexaphosphoric acid, present in cereals. See: *inositol.*

phyto-, phyt- [G.]. Combining forms meaning a *plant*, or *that which grows.*

phytobezoar (fī"tō-bē'zōr) [G. *phyton*, plant, + Persian *bād-zahr*, antidote]. A mass composed of vegetable matter found in the stomach. Syn: *food ball.*

phytogenesis (fī"tō-jĕn'ĕ-sĭs). Syn: *phytogeny.* The origin and development of plants.

phytoid (fī-toyd'). Plantlike.

1. Any disease of vegetable parasitic origin. 2. The production of a disease by plant parasites. 3. The presence of plant parasites in an organism.

phytosterol (fī"tō-ster'ŏl). Any sterol present in vegetable oil or fat.

phytotoxin (fī"tō-tŏks'ĭn). A toxin produced by one of the higher plants. Ex: *ricin*, from castor bean.

pia (pī'ă). [L. tender]. See: *pia mater.*

pia-arachnitis. Piarachnitis, *q.v.*

pia-arachnoid. Piarachnoid, *q.v.*

pial (pi'al). Concerning the pia mater.

pia mater. A thin, vascular membrane closely investing the brain and spinal cord and proximal portions of the nerves. Innermost of the three meninges.

pian (pī-ăn') [Fr.]. Contagious skin disease of the tropics. Syn: *frambesia; yaws.*

pianists' cramp (pē'ăn-ĭsts, pe-an'ists). Spasm or professional neurosis of muscles of fingers and forearms from piano playing.

piarachnitis (pi-ăr-ăk-nī'tĭs) [L. *pia*, tender, + G. *arachnē*, spider, + *-itis*, inflammation]. Inflammation of the arachnoid and pia mater. Syn: *leptomeningitis.*

piarachnoid (pī-ăr-ăk'noyd) [" + " + *eidos*, like]. The pia mater and arachnoid membranes when regarded as one structure. Syn: *leptomeninges; leptomeninx.*

pica (pī'kă) [L. magpie]. A perversion of appetite, with craving for substance not fit for food, as the practice by some women in pregnancy of ingesting starch, clay, ashes, or plaster.

Condition seen in pregnancy, chlorosis, hysteria, helminthiasis and in certain psychoses. See: *appetite, taste.*

piceous (pĭ'sē-ŭs). Like pitch.

Pick's disease. 1. [Arnold Pick, Czechoslovakian physician, 1851-1924]. A brain disorder involving atrophy of cerebral cortex. Sym: asthenia, loss of speech, progressive dementia. 2. Polyserositis. Condition in which fibrous adhesions of peritoneum, pleura, or pericardium form, sometimes undergoing hyalinization. 3. [Ludwig Pick, German physician, 1868-?]. Niemann-Pick's disease, *q.v.*

Pick's syndrome [Friedel Pick, Prague physician, 1867-1926]. A liver disorder accompanied by ascites but not producing cardiac symptoms or icterus.

picrate (pĭk'rāt). A salt of picric acid.

picro-, picr- [G.]. Combining forms meaning *bitter.*

picrocarmine (pĭk-rō-kar'mĭn). A stain used in microscopy.

picroformal (pĭk-rō-for'mal). Solution of picric acid, formaldehyde and water used as a fixing agent.

picrol (pĭk'rōl). Antiseptic powder used as a dressing for wounds.

picrotoxin (pik-ro-tox'in) [G. *pikros*, bitter, + *toxikon*, poison]. A powerful stimulant to the central nervous system, obtained from the seed of *Anamirta cocculus*, a shrub. It is used as a respiratory stimulant.

piebald skin (pī'bawld). Skin with spots or pigmentation or patches with loss of pigment. See: *leukoderma; vitiligo.*

piedra (pī-ā'dră) [Spanish, stone]. Disease in which hard nodules form on the hair shafts.

Composed of fungus masses of *Trichosporon giganteum.*

p., black. P. caused by fungus, *Piedraia hortai.* Occurs in tropical regions and affects hair of scalp.

p. nostras. P. affecting the beard.

p., white. P. caused by fungus, *Trichosporon bigelii.* Occurs in temperate regions and affects hair of face. Syn: *Tinea nodosa.*

piesesthesia (pī-es-ĕs-thē'zĭ-ă) [G. *piesis*, pressure, + *aisthēsis*, sensation]. Sensibility to pressure. Syn: *pressure sense.*

piesimeter, piesometer (pī-ĕ-sĭm'ĕt-ĕr, -sŏm'ĕt-ĕr). Device for measurement of skin's sensitiveness to pressure.

pigeon breast. Projection of sternum anteriorly.

p. toe. Pes varus; walking with feet turned in.

pigment (pĭg'mĕnt) [L. *pigmentum*, paint]. Any coloring matter. See: *albino; "chrom-" words.*

p., bile. P. in bile: bilirubin and biliverdin and their derivatives (*e.g.*, urobilinogen, urobilin, bilicyanin, bilifuscin). See also: *bile pigments.*

p., biliary. Bilirubin, biliverdin, *q.v.*

p., blood. P. in blood (hemoglobin) or a derivative of it (hematin, hemin, methemoglobin, hemosiderin).

p., endogenous. A pigment produced within the body, as melanin.

p., exogenous. A pigment produced outside the human body.

p., hematogenous. P. from hemoglobin of the erythrocytes.

p., hepatogenous. P. from hemoglobin destruction in the liver. SYN: *bile pigment.*

p., skin. Melanin, melanoid, and carotene, *q.v.*

p., urinary. Urochrome, and sometimes urobilin, *q.v.*

p., uveal. That in cells on inner or post. surface of the iris, choroid, and ciliary processes.

pigmentary (pĭg'mĕn-tĕr-ĭ) [L. *pigmentum,* paint]. Concerning, or like, a pigment.

pigmentation (pĭg-mĕn-tā'shŭn) [L. *pigmentum,* paint]. Coloration due to deposition of pigments.

RS: *albinism, carotenemia, "chrom-" words.*

pigmentophage (pĭg-mĕn'tō-fāj) [" + G. *phagein,* to eat]. Cell that absorbs pigment.

pig"ment'um nig'rum. The pigment of the lamina vitrea of the choroid of the eye.

piitis (pī-ī'tĭs) [L. *pia,* tender, + G. *-itis,* inflammation]. Inflamed condition of the pia mater.

Pil. Abbr. of L. *pilula,* pill, or pl. *pilulae,* pills.

pilar, pilary (pī'lar, pĭl'ă-rĭ) [L. *pilaris,* pert. to the hair]. Concerning, or covered with, hair.

pilaster (pĭ-lăs-ter) [L. *pila,* pillar]. A prominent ridge sometimes seen on the femur.

pile [L. *pila,* a ball, a pillar]. 1. A single hemorrhoid. SEE: *piles.* 2. The hair. 3. A battery for production of electricity. 4. An apparatus for producing and regulating a nuclear chain-reaction fission process.

pileous (pī'lē-ŭs) [L. *pilus,* hair]. Hairy; hirsute.

piles (pīls) [L. *pila,* a mass]. Dilated blood vessels in the rectal mucosa forming a vascular tumor. SYN: *hemorrhoids, q.v.*

pileus (pī'lē-ŭs) [L. a cap]. 1. A hemisphere of the cerebellum. 2. Membrane which sometimes covers the head of an infant at birth. 3. A nipple shield. 4. Top of the head of a bird; also *pileum.*

pili (pī'lē). Plural of *pilus.* Hairs.

p. annulata. Condition in which hairs have a ringed appearance; monilethrix.

p. tactiles. Sensitive or tactile hairs.

p. torti. Condition in which hairs are broken and twisted.

piliation (pĭl-ĭ-ā'shŭn) [L. *pilus,* hair]. Formation and development of hair.

piliform (pĭl'ĭ-form) [" + *forma,* shape]. Hairlike.

pilimiction (pī"lĭ-mĭk'shŭn). Passing of urine containing hairlike or filamentous substances.

pill (pĭl) [L. *pilula,* from *pila,* a ball]. Medicine in the form of a tiny mass to be swallowed.

pillar (pĭl'ĕr) [L. *pila,* a column]. An upright support; column, or structure resembling a column.

p. of the abdominal ring. One of the columns on either side of abdominal ring.

p.'s, anterior, of fornix. Two diverging columns extending downward from ant. extremity of body of the fornix.

p. cells. Two groups of cells (inner and outer) resting on basement membrane of organ of Corti in which elongated bodies (pillars) develop. These enclose the inner tunnel (Corti's tunnel).

p.'s of Corti. Two layers resting on membrana basilaris in the ear. SYN: *rods of Corti.*

p.'s of diaphragm. Crura of diaphragm, two bundles of muscle fibers extending from lumbar vertebrae to central tendon and forming sides of hiatus aorticus.

p.'s of the fauces. SYN: *the glossopalatine and pharyngopalatine arches.* Folds of mucous membrane, one on each side of the fauces, *q.v.* and bet. which is situated the tonsil.

p.'s, posterior, of fornix. Two bands forming prolongation of fornix posteriorly.

pilleus, pilleum (pĭl'ē-ŭs, -ŭm) [L. a cap; caul]. A membrane sometimes covering a baby's head at birth. SYN: *caul.*

p. ventriculi. The 1st portion of the duodenum. SYN: *pyloric cap.*

pillion (pĭl'yŭn) [L. *pellis,* skin]. Artificial leg, esp. in form of a stump.

pilo- [L.]. Combining form meaning *hair.*

pilocarpine hydrochlor'ide (pī"lō-kar'pēn). USP. $C_{11}H_{16}N_2O_2 \cdot HCl$. Hydrochloride of an alkaloid obtained from leaves of the plant of the genus *Pilocarpus.*

ACTION AND USES: Causes contraction of the pupil. Used topically as a miotic, esp. in glaucoma.

p. ni'trate. USP. Nitrate of the alkaloid obtained from *Pilocarpus.*

ACTION AND USES: Same as pilocarpine hydrochloride.

pilocystic (pī-lō-sĭs'tĭk) [L. *pilus,* hair, + G. *kystis,* a bladder]. Encysted and containing hair, said of a dermoid cyst.

pilomotor (pī-lō-mō'tor) [" + *motor,* a mover]. Causing the movements of hairs, as the *arrectores pilarum.*

p. reflex. Gooseflesh formation when skin is cooled or as a result of emotional reaction.

pilonidal (pī-lō-nī'dăl) [" + *nidus,* nest]. Containing hairs in a cyst in nest formation.

p. fistula. F. near the rectum resulting from a growth of subcutaneous hair.

p. sinus. A p. fistula.

pilose (pī'lōs) [L. *pilus,* hair]. Hairy, downy.

pilosebaceous (pī"lō-sē-bā'shŭs) [" + *sebaceus,* fatty]. Concerning the hair and sebaceous glands.

pilosis (pī-lō'sĭs) [L. *pilus,* hair, + G. *-ōsis,* intensive]. Excessive formation of hair.

pilosity (pī-lŏs'ĭ-tĭ) [L. *pilus,* hair]. Hairiness.

pilous (pī'lŭs) [L. *pilus,* hair]. Covered with hair; hirsute.

Piltz's reflex (pĭltz) [Jan Piltz, Polish neurologist, 1830-1931]. Change in size of pupil on sudden fixation of attention.

pilula (pĭl'ū-lă) (pl. *pilulae*) [L. pill]. A small, solid body of medicine of a variety of shapes, intended to be swallowed whole and produce medicinal action.

May be ordered to be made extemporaneously by the druggist, or ready-prepared pills may be used. The latter often are coated with sugar, gelatin, chocolate, etc.

pilular (pĭl'ū-lar) [L. *pilula,* pill]. Pert. to, or of the nature of, pills.

pilus (pī'lŭs) (pl. *pili*) [L. hair). A hair.

pimel- [G.]. Combining form or prefix meaning *fat* or *associated with fat.*

pimelitis (pĭm-ĕl-ī'tĭs) [G. *pimelē,* fat, + *-itis,* inflammation]. Inflammation of adipose and of connective tissue in general.

pimeloma (pĭm-ĕl-ō'mă) [" + *-ōma,* tumor]. A fatty tumor. SYN: *lipoma.*

pimelopterygium (pĭm"ĕ-lō-tĕ-rĭj'ē-ŭm). A fatty outgrowth of the conjunctiva.

pimelorrhea (pĭm-ĕl-or-ē'ă) [" + *roia,* flow]. Discharge of fat in loose stools.

pimelorthopnea (pĭm"ĕl-or"thŏp'nē-ă). Difficulty in breathing when lying down, resulting from obesity.

pimelosis (pĭm-ĕl-ō'sĭs) [" + *-ōsis,* intensive]. 1. A conversion into fat. 2. Fatty degeneration of any tissue. 3. Corpulence; obesity.

pimeluria (pĭm-ĕl-ū'rĭ-ă) [" + *ouron,* urine]. Excretion of fat or oil in urine. SYN: *lipuria.*

pimple (pĭm'pl) [A.S. *pimpel*]. Protuberance of the skin, sometimes going on to suppuration. SYN: *papule; pustule.*

Often seen on the skin of the adolescent. They have little diagnostic value. Patients should be warned, when necessary, not to pick at pimples, as infection may take place.

pincement (pans-mong') [Fr. pinching]. Pinching or nipping of the flesh in massage.

pineal (pĭn'ē-ăl) [L. *pineus,* pine cone]. 1. Shaped like a pine cone. 2. The small red gland attached to post. part of 3rd ventricle of brain. 3. Pertaining to the pineal body, *q.v.*

FUNCTION: Unknown. Such knowledge as we have is derived from observation of cases of teratoma. These are sometimes associated with marked sexual and somatic overgrowth leading to the condition known as pubertas praecox or macrogenitosomia praecox. Whether this is due to a lack of pineal secretion or to hyperfunction of the gland is not known. SYN: *epiphysis.*

p. body. SYN: *epiphysis cerebri.* A small ovoid body which extends from the roof of post. extremity of third ventricle of brain. Consists of ependymal cells and neuroglia embedded in connective tissue stroma. Often contains calcareous granules (brain sand).

pinealectomy (pĭn-ē-ăl-ĕk'tō-mĭ) [L. *pineus,* pine cone, + G. *ektomē,* excision]. Removal of the pineal body.

pinealism (pĭn'ē-ăl-ĭzm) [" + G. *ismos,* condition]. Disorder caused by abnormality of the secretion of the pineal body.

pinealoma (pĭn-ē-ă-lōm'ă). A tumor of the pineal body, usually encapsulated. Often associated with precocious puberty.

pinealopathy (pĭn-ē-ăl-op'ăth-ĭ) [" + G. *pathos,* disease]. Any disorder of the pineal gland.

pineapple (pīn'ăp-l) [A.S. *pīn,* pine, + *aeppel,* apple]. A large fruit of the species *Ananas comosus.* It often ranges from 3 to 5 pounds in weight. COMP: Very rich in cane sugar. Contains bromelin, a proteolytic enzyme.

RAW (*diced*): 1 cup (140 gm.). Calories: 75. Other main values: 0.7 gm. protein; trace of fat; 19 gm. carbohydrate; 22 mg. calcium; 100 I.U. vitamin A; 24 mg. ascorbic acid.

ACTION: Easy to digest.

pineoblastoma (pĭn-ē-ō-blăst-ō'mă). A blastoma of the pineal body.

pine tar (pīn). A product obtained from the distillation of pine wood.

ACTION AND USES: Externally, a stimulant in dermatitis; internally, a stimulant to bronchial mucous membrane. SYN: *pix liquida.*

pinguecula (pĭn-gwĕk'ū-lă) [L. *pinguis,* fat]. Yellowish thickening of bulbar conjunctiva, triangular in shape, on inner and outer margins of the cornea.

Base of triangle ti toward the limbus. Yellowish color is due to increase in the elastic fibers.

pinhole (pĭn'hōl) [A.S. *pinn,* a pin, + *hol,* hole]. Small perforation made by, or size of that made by, a pin.

p. os. A very small os uteri in young women.

p. pupil. Extreme contraction of the iris.

It is seen in locomotor ataxia, after use of miotics, in some brain diseases, and in opium poisoning.

piniform (pĭn'ĭ-form) [L. *pineus,* pine cone, + *forma,* shape]. Shaped like a pine cone.

pink disease (pĭnk). Rare disease of children marked by swelling and redness of feet and hands, sweating, itching and polyarthritis. SYN: *acrodynia; erythredema; polyneuritis; Swift's disease, q.v.*

pink eye. Epidemic form of acute conjunctivitis caused by various organisms. Sporadic, noninfectious cases may result from irritation by various agents, such as intense light, or they may accompany exanthematous disease such as measles.

pinna (pĭn'ă) (pl. *pinnae*) [L. wing]. The auricle or projection part of the ext. ear. It collects and directs sound waves into the external acoustic meatus and thence to the tympanic membrane.

p. nasi. Protruding cartilaginous extension on each nostril. SYN: *ala nasi.*

pinocytosis (pī"nō-sī-tō'sĭs) [G. *pinein,* to drink, + *kytos,* cell]. Term for the absorption of liquids by phagocytic cells.

Pins' sign [Emil Pins, Austrian physician, 1845-1913]. In pericarditis, the disappearance of symptoms of pleurisy when patient assumes knee-chest position.

pint (pīnt) [O.Fr. *pinte*]. Measure of capacity equal to one-half a quart; 16 fluid ounces; 473.17 ml. (cc.). SEE: *Table of Weights and Measures in Appendix.*

pinta (pin'tă). A disease caused by the spirochete *Treponema carateum.* Manifested by depigmented spots or patches. SYN: *azul; carate; mal del pinto; spotted sickness.*

pinworm (pĭn'wurm). A parasitic nematode *Enterobius vermicularis,* causing enterobiasis. Formerly called oxyuris.

pionemia (pī-ō-nē'mĭ-ă) [" + *aima,* blood]. Fat in the blood. SYN: *lipemia.*

pioscope (pī'ō-skōp) [" + *skopein,* to examine]. Device for estimating the fat content of milk.

piper (pī'pĕr) [L.]. Pepper.

piperazine (pi-per'ă-zēn). A white crystalline powder. Used in the treatment of ascariasis and enterobiasis.

pipet, pipette (pī-pĕt) [Fr. *pipette,* a tiny pipe]. Narrow glass tube with both ends open for transferring and measuring liquids, using suction principle.

piptonychia (pĭp-tō-nĭk'ĭ-ă). The shedding of nails.

Pirogoff's amputation (pĭr'ō-gŏf) [Nicolai I. Pirogoff, Russian surgeon, 1810-1881]. Foot amputation, removing part of the os calcis.

Piroplasma (pī"rō-plăz'mă) [L. *pirum,* pear, + G. *plasma,* a thing formed]. Former name of *Babesia, q.v.,* a genus of Sporozoa parasitic in domestic animals.

piroplasmosis (pī″rō-plăz-mō′sĭs) [L. *pirum,* near, + G. *plasma,* a thing formed, + -*ōsis,* condition]. Infection by species of the genus *Babesia* or *Theileria,* sporozoan blood parasites.

Pirquet's test (pēr-kā) [Clemens P. Pirquet, Austrian pediatrician, 1874-1929]. Test for tuberculosis by means of a skin reaction.

pisiform (pī′sĭ-form) [L. *pisum,* pea, + *forma,* shape]. 1. Name of small, pealike sesamoid bone of the wrist. 2. Pea-shaped. 3. The smallest carpal bone, located in proximal row on ulnar side.

pit (pĭt) [A.S. *pytt,* hole]. 1. A tiny hollow or pocket. SYN: *depression, fossa.* 2. To be or become marked with a shallow depression; to cause a depression on pressure in edema.

p., auditory. A pit which develops in auditory placode, *q.v.*

p., gastric. One of many minute depressions (foveolae) in gastric mucosa into which the gastric glands open.

p., nasal. One of two horseshoe-shaped depressions on ventrolateral surface of head bounded by lateral and median nasal processes. It gives rise to nostrils and portion of nasal fossa.

p., olfactory. Nasal pit, *q.v.*

p., primitive. Minute depression at ant. end of primitive groove or streak and immediately posterior to primitive knot.

p. of the stomach. 1. Depression at end of the ensiform process. 2. The center of the abdominal region above the navel. SYN: *scrobiculus cordis.*

pitch. That quality of the sensation of sound that enables one to classify it in a scale from high to low. It is dependent principally on frequency of vibrations.

pithecoid (pĭth′ĕ-koyd) [G. *pithēkos,* ape. + *eidos,* like]. Apelike; resembling an ape.

pithiatic (pĭth-ĭ-at′ik) [" + *iatrikos,* healing]. Capable of being soothed or relieved by persuasion or by suggestion.

pithiatism (pĭth-ī′ăt-ĭzm) [G. *peithein,* to persuade, + *iatos,* curable]. 1. Hysteria induced by suggestion. 2. Mental disorder cured by suggestion.

pithing (pĭth′ing). Destruction of the central nervous system by the piercing of brain or spinal cord, as in vivisection. Done on experimental animals to render them insensible to pain and to inhibit controlling effects of the central nervous system. SYN: *decerebration.*

pitocin (pĭ-to′sin). Proprietary name for an aqueous solution containing the oxytocic fraction of the post. pituitary gland. SEE: *oxytocin injection.*

Pitres' sections (pē-trēs′) [Jean A. Pitres, French physician, 1848-1927]. Series of six coronal vertical brain sections for study of this organ.

pitressin (pĭt-rĕs′ĭn). Proprietary name for vasopressin, a product obtained from the post. lobe of the pituitary gland containing pressor and antidiuretic principles. SEE: *principle, antidiuretic; vasopressin.*

USES: For increasing blood pressure, the muscular contraction of the intestinal tract, and diminishing urinary output in diabetes insipidus.

pitting (pĭt′ĭng) [A.S. *pytt,* hole]. The formation of pits or depressions or scars, as in smallpox.

pituicyte (pĭ-tū′ĭ-sīt). A branched, modified, neuroglia cell characteristic of pars nervosa post. lobe of pituitary gland. Also present in infundibular stalk.

pituitarism (pĭt-ū′ĭ-tă-rĭzm) [" + G. *ismos,* condition]. Any disorder of the pituitary gland.

pituitarium (pĭ-tu″ĭ-tăr′ĭ-um) [L.]. Pituitary, *q.v.*

pituitary (pĭt-ū′ĭ-tăr-ĭ) [L. *pituita,* phlegm]. 1. Concerning phlegm. 2. The pituitary body or gland, *q.v.;* the hypophysis cerebri.

p., anterior. Dried, defatted, powdered anterior lobe of pituitary gland of domestic animals.

p. body. SEE: p. gland.

p. disorders. *Hypersecretion of ant. lobe*—gigantism, acromegaly, pituitary basophilism (Cushing's disease). *Hyposecretion of ant. lobe*—dwarfism, pituitary cachexia (Simmond's disease), Sheehan's syndrome, acromicria, eunuchoidism or hypogonadism. *Post. lobe deficiency or hypothalamic lesion*—diabetes insipidus. *Ant. and post. lobe deficiency and hypothalamic lesion*—Frohlich's syndrome (adiposogenital dystrophy), pituitary obesity.

p. gland. SYN: *hypophysis cerebri.* A small, gray, rounded body attached to the base of the brain by the infundibular stalk, a downward extension of the floor of the third ventricle. It averages 1.3 x 1.0 x 0.5 cm. in size and 0.55 to 0.6 gm. in weight.

FUNCTIONS: The pituitary is an endocrine gland secreting a number of hormones which regulate many bodily processes including growth, reproduction, and various metabolic activities. It is often referred to as the "master gland" of the body.

HORMONES OF INTERMEDIATE LOBE: In cold-blooded animals, *intermedin* is secreted which influences the activity of pigment cells (chromatophores) of fishes, amphibians, and reptiles. In warm-blooded animals no effects are known.

HORMONES SECRETED BY ANT. LOBE: *Somatotrophic, or growth, hormone* (STH), which regulates growth; *adrenocorticotrophic hormone* (ACTH), which regulates functional activity of the adrenal cortex; *thyrotrophic hormone* (TTH), which regulates functional activity of thyroid gland; *gonadotrophic hormones* which include: *follicle-stimulating hormone* (FSH), which stimulates development of ovarian follicles and spermatogenesis in the testis; *luteinizing hormone* (LH), also called *interstitial cell stimulating hormone* (ICSH), in conjunction with FSH induces secretion of estrogens, ovulation, and development of corpus luteum; *luteotrophic hormone* (LTH), which maintains mature corpora lutea and induces secretion of progesterone. It also induces secretion of milk in fully developed mammary gland. Because of this action, it is sometimes called the *lactogenic hormone.*

HORMONES OF THE POST. LOBE: These include oxytocin, which acts specifically on smooth muscle of uterus increasing tone and contractility; *vasopressin,* which induces contraction of smooth muscles of the blood vessels, and associated with it an *antidiuretic principle* which prevents excessive loss of water through the kidneys.

Evidence indicates that these hormones are secreted by neurosecretory cells of the hypothalamus and pass through fibers of the supraopticohypophyseal tracts in the infundibular stalk to the neurohypophysis where they are stored.

p., posterior. Dried, powdered posterior lobe of pituitary gland of animals used as food by man.

p., p., injection. SYN: *injectio pituitarii posterioris.* A sterile, aqueous solution of the principles of post. lobe of pituitary from healthy domesticated animals used as food for man.

ACTION: Constricts blood vessels raising blood pressure; stimulates smooth muscles thus increasing intestinal peristalsis and uterine contractions; reduces volume of urine excreted.

p., whole. Dried, defatted, powdered entire pituitary gland of domestic animals.

pituitotrope (pĭt-ū′ĭt-ō-trōp) [L. *pituita,* phlegm, + G. *tropos,* a turning]. A person exhibiting tendencies to being overinfluenced by the pituitary gland.

pituitotropic (pĭt-ū″ĭt-ō-trŏp′ĭk) [" + G. *tropos,* a turning]. Concerning or marked by pituitotropism.

pituitotropism (pĭt-ū″ĭt-ō-trō′pĭzm) [" + " + *ismos,* condition]. Bodily constitution in which the pituitary influence dominates.

pituitrin (pĭt-ū′ĭt-rĭn). Proprietary name for posterior pituitary extract.

ACTION AND USES: Used to stimulate contraction of blood vessels, peristalsis in intestines, and uterine contractions in labor.

pityriasis (pĭt-ĭr-ī′ăs-ĭs) [G. *pityron,* bran, + *iasis,* disease]. A skin disease characterized by branny scales.

p. alba atrophicans. Cutaneous disorder with scaling and atrophy. SYN: *atrophoderma albidum.*

p. capitis. Dandruff. SYN: *dermatitis seborrheica.*

p. lichenoides et varioliformis acuta. A skin disorder characterized by development of pustules and vesicles and formation of crusts and scarring. Noncommunicable.

p. linguae. Transitory benign plaques of the tongue.

p. maculata et circinata. SEE: *p. rosea.*

p. nigra. The dark brown or black patches in p. versicolor in warm climates.

p. pilaris. SEE: *p. rubra.*

p. rosea. A skin disease characterized by development of distributed patches which are circinate in outline. slightly scaly, a faint red color. SYN: *p. maculata et circinata.*

Acute inflammatory disease marked by a macular eruption on the trunk, obliquely to the ribs. Rose red and somewhat scaly with a clearing in the center, or reddish ring-shaped patches symmetrically distributed over the limbs.

ETIOL: Unknown.

SYM: Macular or circinate lesions; yellowish, salmon or red; rounded, oval or irregular; thinly covered with fine branny scales, increasing in size; when centers clear up, giving rise to slightly elevated reddish rings with fawn-colored centers, coalescence of rings resulting in segmental or gyrate lesions of various sizes. Spontaneous disappearance within three to four weeks but may last several months.

TREATMENT: Locally: antipruritics.

p. rubra. Persistent general exfoliative dermatitis.

p. rubra pilaris. A chronic disease with formation of subacute inflammatory papules around the hair follicles. These coalesce and form infiltrated plaques of scaling dermatitis.

p. versicolor. Contagious skin disease marked by yellow patches, scales and itching. Due to a fungus *Malassezia furfur.*

pityroid (pĭt′ĭr-oyd) [G. *pityron,* bran, + *eidos,* like]. Branny; resembling bran.

pix (pĭks) [L.]. Pitch.

PK. Abbr. for *psychokinesis.*

PKU. Abbr. for *phenylketonuria.*

placebo (plă-sē′bō) [L. I shall please]. Inactive substance given to satisfy patient's demand for medicine.

Also used in controlled studies of drugs. The placebo is given to a group of patients, and the drug being tested is given to a similar group; then the results obtained in the two groups are compared.

placenta (plă-sĕn′ta) (pl. *placentae*) [L. a flat cake, from G. *plakous*]. The oval or discoid spongy structure in the uterus through which the fetus derives its nourishment.

ANAT: The placenta consists of a fetal portion, the chorion frondosum, bearing many chorionic villi which interlock with the decidua basalis of the uterus which constitutes the maternal portion. The chorionic villi lie in spaces in the uterine endometrium where they are bathed in maternal blood and lymph. Groups of villi are separated by placental septa forming about twenty distinct lobules called cotyledons.

Attached to the margin of the placenta is a membrane which encloses the embryo. It is a composite of several structures (decidua parietalis, decidua capsularis, chorion laeve, and amnion). At the center of the concave side is attached the umbilical cord through which the umbilical vessels (two arteries and one vein) pass to the fetus. The cord is approx. 50 cm. long at full term.

The mature placenta is 15 to 18 cm. (6 to 7 in.) in diameter and weighs about 450 gm. (1 lb.). When expelled following parturition it is known as the afterbirth.

PHYS: Maternal blood enters the intervillous spaces of the placenta through spiral arteries, branches of the uterine arteries. It bathes the chorionic villi and flows peripherally to the marginal sinus which leads to uterine veins. Food substances, oxygen, and antibodies pass into fetal blood of the villi; metabolic waste products pass from fetal blood into the mother's blood. In general, there is no admixture of fetal and maternal blood. The placenta also serves as an endocrine organ. It produces chorionic gonadotrophins, the presence of which in urine is the basis of pregnancy tests. Estrogen and progesterone are also secreted by the placenta.

p. accreta. A placenta in which the cotyledons have invaded the uterine musculature and, as a result of this, separation of the placenta is very difficult or even impossible.

p., abruption of. Premature separation of placenta.

p., adherent. One that remains adherent to the uterine wall after normal period following childbirth.

p., annular. A p. that extends like a belt around the interior of the uterus.

p., battledore. A form of insertion of the umbilical cord into margin of the p. in which it spreads out to resemble a battledore.

p., bipartite. One that is divided into two separate parts. SYN: *p. bipartita.*

p., circinate. One that is cup-shaped.

p. cirsoides. P. with appearance of varicose veins.

p., cordiform. A p. having a marginal indentation giving it a heart shape.

p., deciduate. A p. of which the maternal part escapes with delivery.

p., discoid. P. which constitutes practically one mass, circumscribed and circular in form.

p., double. A placental mass of the two placentae of a twin gestation.

p. duplex. Same as *p. bipartite.*

p., fetal. That part of the p. formed by aggregation of chorionic villi in which the umbilical vein and arteries ramify.

p., fundal. One attached to the uterine wall within the fundal zone.

p., horseshoe. A formation in which the two placentae of a twin gestation are united.

p., incarcerated. One retained in the uterus by irregular uterine contractions after delivery.

p., lateral. One attached to lateral wall of uterus.

p., maternal. Portion of placenta that develops from decidua basalis of uterus.

p., membranous. A thinning of the p. from atrophy.

p., nondeciduate. One that does not shed the maternal portion.

p. previa. Placenta which is implanted in the lower uterine segment. There are three types: *centralis, lateralis,* and *marginalis. Placenta previa centralis* is the condition where the placenta has been implanted in the lower uterine segment and has grown to completely cover the internal cervical os. *Placenta previa lateralis* is the condition when the placenta lies just within the lower uterine segment. *Placenta previa marginalis* is the condition where the placenta partially covers the internal cervical os.

SYM: Slight hemorrhage, recurrent with greater severity; appears 7th or 8th month; gradual anemia, pallor, rapid weak pulse, air hunger, low blood pressure.

DIAG: Painless bleeding during last 3 months; placenta in lower portion of uterus.

PROG: Depends upon control of hemorrhage and asepsis.

TREATMENT: Conserve blood supply during delivery and before; prevent and control postpartum hemorrhage; combat anemia before and after labor; prevention of sepsis.

p. reniformis. A kidney-shaped placenta.

p., retained. One not expelled for 2 hours after 2nd stage of labor.

p. spuria. An outlying portion of p. which has not maintained its vascular connection with the decidua vera.

p. succenturiata. An accessory p.

p. tripartita. A three-lobed p.

p., triple. A placental mass of three placentae of a triple gestation.

p., velamentous. A placenta with the umbilical cord attached to the membrane a short distance from the placenta, the vessels entering the placenta at its margin.

p., zonary. Same as *annular p.*

placental (plă-sĕn'tăl) [L. *placenta,* a flat cake]. Relating to the placenta.

p. bruit, p. souffle. Sound heard in auscultation over the placenta in pregnancy; due to circulation of the blood.

placentation (plă-sĕn-tā'shŭn) [L. *placenta,* a flat cake]. The process of formation and attachment of the placenta.

placentitis (plă-sĕn-tī'tĭs) [" + G. *-ītis,* inflammation]. Inflamed condition of placenta.

placentography (plă-sĕn-tŏg'ră-fĭ) [" + G. *graphein,* to write]. Examination of the placenta by x-ray.

placentoid (plă-sĕn'toyd) [" + G. *eidos,* like]. Like the placenta.

placentolysin (plă-sĕn-tŏl'ĭs-ĭn) [" + G. *lysis,* dissolution]. A lysin obtained by injecting placental tissue into an animal, the serum thus obtained being destructive to placental cells of the species of animal from which the placenta was taken.

placentoma (plă-sĕn-tō'mă) [" + G. *-ōma,* tumor]. A new growth derived from retained placental tissue.

placentotherapy (plă-sĕn"tō-thĕr'ă-pĭ) [" + G. *therapeia,* treatment]. Therapeutic use of placental extract.

Placido's disk (pla-sē'dō). A disk marked with black and white circles used in determining amt. and character of corneal astigmatism.

placode (plak'ōd). In embryology, a platelike thickening of epithelium, usually ectoderm, which serves as the anlage of an organ or structure.

p., auditory. A dorsolateral placode located alongside hindbrain which gives rise to *otocyst* which in turn develops into *internal* ear.

p., lens. P. developing in ectoderm directly overlying optic vesicle. Forms *lens vesicle* which becomes enclosed in optic cup and eventually becomes lens of eye.

p., olfactory. P. which gives rise to *olfactory pit* and finally major portion of nasal cavity.

pladaroma (plad-ar-ō'mă) [G. *pladaros,* soft, + *-ōsis,* disease]. A soft growth like a wart on the eyelid.

pladarosis (plad-ar-ō'sĭs) [G. *pladaros,* soft, + *-ōsis,* disease]. Pladaroma.

plagiocephalic (plā-jĭ-ō-sĕf-ăl'ĭk) [G. *plagios,* oblique, + *kephalē,* head]. Marked by or relating to plagiocephaly.

plagiocephalism (pla"jĭ-o-sef'ă-lizm). Plagiocephaly, *q.v.*

plagiocephaly (pla"jĭ-o-sef'ă-lĭ). Malformation of the skull producing the appearance of a twisted and lop-sided head. Due to irregular closure of the cranial sutures.

plague (plāg) [G. *plēgē,* a stroke]. 1. A word once used to describe any widespread contagious disease associated with a high death rate. Now applied specifically to disease caused by *Pasteurella pestis* infection. 2. A highly fatal disease with high fever, shock, restlessness, staggering gait, mental confusion, prostration, delirium, and coma. Exists in several forms: *bubonic* with acutely inflamed lymph nodes *(buboes); septicemic* with absence of buboes; *primary pneumonic* characterized by pulmonary symptoms. The pneumonic form may be spread from man to man by droplets. Streptomycin, tetracyclines, and chloramphenicol are effective in treating plague.

p., ambulatory. Syn: *pestis minor.* Mild but often fatal. Patient does not take to his bed.

p., black. Syn: *bubonic plague, black death.* An epidemic disease with high mortality that swept Europe during the 14th century. So called because of appearance of petechiae or black spots about 3rd day of disease.

p., bubonic. The more common form of plague marked by formation of buboes.

p., hunger. Relapsing fever, *q.v.*

p., murine. Plague infecting rats.

p., pneumonic. A highly virulent form of plague occurring as sequela of bubonic plague, or as a primary infection.

p., septicemic. Bubonic plague accompanied by septicemia.

p., sylvatic. Plague infecting various species of rodents. In the U. S., thirty-eight species harbor the plague organism.

plane (plān) [L. *planus,* flat]. 1. A flat or relatively smooth surface. See: *planum.* 2. A flat surface formed by making a cut, imaginary or real, through the body or a part of it. Planes are used as points of reference by which positions of parts of the body are indicated. In the human subject, all planes are based on body being in an upright, anatomic position, *q.v.*

p.'s, Addison's. Planes used as landmarks in thoracoabdominal topography.

p., Aeby's. One perpendicular to the median plane of the cranium through the *basion* and *nasion.*

p., alveolocondylar. One tangent to the alveolar point and most prominent points on lower aspects of condyles of the occipital bone.

p., Baer's. One through upper border of the zygomatic arches.

p., coccygeal. The fourth parallel plane of the pelvis.

p., coronal. Vertical p. at right angles to a sagittal p. dividing the body into anterior and posterior portions.

p., datum. An assumed horizontal plane from which craniometric measurements are taken.

p., Daubenton's. One passing through the opisthion and inferior borders of the orbits.

p.'s, focal. Two planes through anterior and posterior principal foci of a dioptric system and perpendicular to the line connecting the two.

p., frontal. A coronal plane, *q.v.*

p., Hodge's. One parallel to the plane of the pelvic inlet and passing through the 2nd sacral vertebra and upper border of the os pubis.

p., horizontal. A transverse plane at right angles to the vertical axis of body.

p.'s, inclined, of the pelvis. According to Lusk, "The sciatic spines divide the pelvic cavity into two unequal sections. In the larger, anterior section, the lateral walls slope toward the symphysis and arch of the pubes, while posteriorly the walls slope in the direction of the sacrum and coccyx. The declivities in front of the spines are termed the anterior inclined planes of the pelvis, over which rotation of the occiput takes place in the mechanism of normal labor. Behind the spines the lateral slopes are known as the posterior inclined planes."

p., intertubercular. A horizontal plane passing through tubercles of crests of ilia. Lies approximately at level of 5th lumbar vertebra.

p., Listing's. A transverse vertical plane perpendicular to anteroposterior axis of eye, containing center of motion of the eyes; in it also lie the transverse and vertical axes of voluntary ocular rotation.

p., Meckel's. One through the auricular and alveolar points.

p., medial; p., median; p., mesial. One usually anteroposterior dividing a body or organ into two equal and symmetrical parts. The median p. of the body is known as the *meson.*

p., midsagittal. Vertical plane dividing body into symmetrical right and left halves.

p., Morton's. One passing through the most projecting points of the parietal and occipital protuberances.

p.'s, parallel, of the pelvis. Those intersecting at right angles the axis of the pelvic canal. The first plane is that of the superior strait. The second plane is that extending from middle of the sacral vertebra to the level of the subpubic ligament. The third plane is at the level of spines of the ischia, and the fourth plane is at the outlet.

p.'s of the pelvis. Imaginary ones touching the same parts of the pelvic canal on both sides.

p. of refraction. One passing through a refracted ray of light and drawn perpendicular to the surface at which refraction takes place.

p. of regard. One through the fovea of the eye and fixation point.

p., sagittal. Vertical plane parallel to the midsagittal plane; one which divides body into right and left portions.

p., subcostal. Horizontal plane passing through lowest points of 10th costal cartilages. Lies approximately at level of 3rd lumbar vertebra.

p., transverse. A horizontal plane.

p., visual. One passing the visual axis of the eye.

planigram. An x-ray photograph of a layer or section of the body.

planimeter. Apparatus used to measure the area of a plane figure by passing a tracer around the boundaries.

planoconcave (plā″nō-kon′kāv) [L. *planus,* flat, + *concavus,* hollow]. Flat on one side and concave on the other.

planoconvex (plā″nō-kŏn′vĕks) [" + L. *convexus,* arched]. Flat on one side and convex on the other.

planomania (plan″o-mā′nē-ă). Morbid desire to wander and to be free of social restraints.

Planorbis (plan-or′bis). A genus of freshwater snails which serve as intermediate hosts for certain species of blood flukes (*Schistosoma*).

plant (plănt) [L. *planta,* a sprout]. An organism which contains chlorophyll and manufactures carbohydrates from carbon dioxide and water or, if lacking these characteristics, is similar in structure and life history to those organisms which do possess chlorophyll and manufacture food.

planta (plan′tă) (pl. *plantae*) [L. sole].. NA. The sole of the foot.

plantar (plăn′tăr) [L. *planta,* sole]. Concerning the sole of foot.

p. arch. Vascular arch in sole of foot. The union of the plantar and dorsalis pedis arteries in the sole. Syn: *arcus plantaris.*

p. reflex. Contraction of toes upon irritation of the sole.

p. wart. SYN: *verruca plantaris.* Wart occurring on sole of the foot, and usually quite painful.

plantaris (plăn-tăr'ĭs) [L.]. An extensor muscle found in the calf of the leg.

plant'igrade. Type of foot posture in which entire sole of foot is placed on ground in walking. Ex: bear, rabbit, man.

planum (pla'num). A flat or relatively smooth surface. A plane, *q.v*

p. nuchale. Outer surface of occipital bone between foramen magnum and superior nuchal line.

p. occipitale. Outer surface of occipital bone lying above superior nuchal line.

p. orbitale. Portion of maxilla which forms greater part of floor of orbit.

p. popliteum. Smooth triangular area on posterior surface of distal end of femur. Bordered by medial and lat. supracondylar lines and forms floor of popliteal fossa.

p. sternale. Anterior or ventral surface of sternum.

p. temporale. Depressed area on side of skull below inferior temporal line. Underlies the temporal fossa.

planuria (plăn-ū'rĭ-ă) [G. *planē,* a wandering, + *ouron,* urine]. The voiding of urine from an abnormal passage of the body.

plaque (plăk) [Fr. a spot]. 1. A patch on the skin or on a mucous surface. 2. A blood platelet.

plasma (plăz'mă) [G. *plasma,* a thing formed]. 1. The liquid part of the lymph and of the blood. 2. Protoplasm, cell substance outside the nucleus. 3. An ointment base of glycerol and starch.

In the blood, the corpuscles and platelets float in it. It consists of serum and protein substances in solution.

The blood plasma consists of water in which numerous chemical compounds, both solids and gases, are dissolved. Among the important constituents may be mentioned the following: water, electrolytes, sugar, proteins, nonprotein ntrogenous compounds, fats and lipids, bile pigment or bilirubin, gases.

In general, plasma is a medium for circulation of blood cells, carries nutritive substances to various structures, and removes from them waste products of metabolism. It makes possible chemical communication between different portions of the body carrying minerals, hormones, vitamins and antibodies.

Different constituents of the plasma have specific functions within the blood. The proteins, bicarbonates, carbon dioxide, chlorides, phosphates, and ammonia serve to keep the acid-base equilibrium of the blood constant, when acid or base substances are added to it. The proteins, especially albumin, by virtue of their osmotic pressure, tend to prevent undue leakage of fluids out of the capillaries, and to maintain a proper exchange of fluid between capillaries and tissues.

Plasma, if normal, is thin and colorless when free from corpuscles, or it has a faint yellow tinge when seen in thick layers.

After clotting of the blood, the liquid squeezed out by the clot is called blood serum. If whole blood is prevented from clotting either by chilling it or by adding anticoagulants, such as sodium citrate, it can be centrifuged. The clear fluid which then occupies the upper half of the centrifuge tube is called plasma. SEE: *blood; coagulation; serum.*

p., blood. Fluid in which float the corpuscles.

p. cell. Cell found in bone marrow and loose connective tissue, probably derived from lymphocytes. SEE: *plasmocyte.*

p., lymph. Lymph without its corpuscles.

p., normal human. Sterile pooled plasma obtained from citrated whole blood of eight or more healthy human subjects. It is stored as fluid plasma at 4° C. or as dried plasma prepared by lyophilization technique, i.e., drying in a vacuum at low temperatures.

p. pinch. The stuff that fills space. Made up of widely scattered particles. Many of them are ions which carry a positive charge. The parallel threads become pinched. This stuff is neither solid, liquid, nor gas.

p. skimming. Phenomenon observed in capillaries in which plasma lacking corpuscles flows into neighboring capillaries.

plasmacule (plăz'mă-kūl) [L. *plasmacula,* little plasm]. One of the minute particles said to be found in the blood plasma giving it its vital power. SYN: *hemokonia.*

plasmacyte (plăz'mă-sīt) [G. *plasma,* a thing formed, + *kytos,* cell]. A plasma cell, one of those found in connective tissue with an eccentrically placed round nucleus and filled with a chromatin mass that stains deeply.

plasmacytoma (plaz"mă-si-to'mă). A plasma cell myeloma occurring in bone marrow. SEE: *myeloma, multiple.*

plasmagel (plaz'mă-jel). The peripheral portion of the endoplasm of a cell such as in an ameba. It is immobile and of the nature of a gel.

plasmagene (plaz'mă-jēn). A cytoplasmic hereditary determiner.

plasmapheresis (plăz-mă-fĕr'ē-sĭs) [G. *plasma,* a thing formed, + *aphairesis,* a taking away]. The removal of fluid portion of blood from the body by venesection, centrifugalization, and replacement of the corpuscles into the blood stream.

plasmasol. The internal more fluid portion of the endoplasm of a cell.

plasmasome (plăz'mă-sōm) [" + *sōma,* body]. A leukocyte granule; nucleolar substance (nonchromatin-staining) in the cytoplasm.

plasmatherapy (plăs"mă-thĕr'ă-pĭ). The use of blood plasma for therapeutic purposes, as injection in treatment of shock.

plasmatic (plăz-măt'ĭk) [G. *plasma,* a thing formed]. 1. Relating to plasma. 2. Formative or plastic.

p. layer. Blood plasma adjacent to the capillary walls. SYN: *plasmic.*

plasmatorrhexis (plăz"măt-ō-rĕks'ĭs) [" + *rēxis,* a rupture]. Rupture of a cell with loss of its plasma from internal pressure due to swelling.

plasmocyte (plăz'mō-sīt) [G. *plasma,* a thing formed, + *kytos,* cell]. SYN: *plasma cell.* Cells found in bone marrow, connective tissue, and sometimes in blood plasma. Considered by some to be abnormal leukocytes. They are numerous in plasma cell myeloma.

plasmocytoma (plăs-mō-sī-tō'mă). A plasma cell myeloma.

plasmodium (plăz-mō'dĭ-ŭm) (pl. *plasmodia*) [G. *plasma,* a thing formed, + *eidos,* form]. A multinucleate mass of naked protoplasm, occurring commonly among slime molds.

Plasmodium (plăz-mō'dĭ-ŭm) (pl. *plasmodia*) [G. *plasma*, a thing formed, + *eidos*, form]. A genus of protozoa belonging to subphylum Sporozoa, class Telosporidea. Includes causative agents of malaria in man and lower animals. SEE: *malaria; mosquito.*

P. falciparum. Causative agent for malignant tertian (estivo-autumnal) malaria.

P. malariae. Causative agent for quartan malaria.

P. ovale. Causative agent for benign tertian or ovale malaria.

P. vivax. Causative agent for benign tertian or vivax malaria.

plas"mog'amy. The fusion of cells.

plasmogen (plăz'mō-jĕn) [" + *gennan*, to produce]. Essential part of protoplasm.

plasmology (plăz-mŏl'ō-jĭ) [" + *logos*, a study]. The study of the cells and plasma. SYN: *histology.*

plasmolysis (plăz-mŏl'ĭs-ĭs) [" + *lysis*, dissolution]. Shrinking of cytoplasm in a living cell due to loss of water by osmosis.

plasmolyze (plaz'mo-līz). To bring about loss of water by osmosis.

plasmorrhexis (plăz-mor-ĕks'ĭs) [" + *rēxis*, rupture]. Rupture of a cell with loss of plasma. SYN: *erythrocytorrhexis; erythrorrhexis; plasmatorrhexis.*

plasmoschisis (plăz-mos'kĭs-ĭs) [G. *plasma*, a thing formed, + *schisis*, a splitting]. The splitting of a cell.

plasmotomy (plăz-mŏt'ō-mĭ) [" + *tomē*, incision]. Mitosis in which the cytoplasm divides into two or more masses.

plasmotropism (plăz-mŏt'rō-pĭzm) [" + *tropein*, to turn, + *ismos*, condition]. The action of spleen, liver and bone marrow, causing the destruction of red blood cells.

plasson (plăs'ŏn) [G. *plassōn*, forming]. Primitive protoplasm in the cytode or non-nucleated stage.

plaster (plăs'tŭr) [G. emplastron]. Medicinal preparation, to be used externally, in which the constituents are formed into a tenacious mass of substance harder than an ointment and spread upon muslin, linen, skin or paper.

It may be *mustard, belladonna*, to check secretions, to allay pain, or to act as a counterirritant.

p., adhesive. Plaster made of a strong cloth coated on one side with an adhesive substance. Used to immobilize a part, to relieve pressure upon sutures, to protect wounds, to secure traction in fractures, to exert pressure, to hold dressings in place, etc.

Hair on the area should first be removed before applying any plaster. It should never be applied to abraded or raw surfaces. In re-applying, dead skin should be removed. Surface should be dry and clean. Removal should be made by stripping from both ends up to the wound, first moistening with benzine or ether.

p. bandage. Bandage stiffened with plaster of Paris.

p., blistering. P. made of cantharides.

p., court-. P. made of isinglass on silk; used for superficial wounds.

p. jacket. P. for the trunk made of plaster of Paris.

p., mustard. P. made of powdered mustard paste spread on cloth; used as a rubefacient.

p. of Paris. Calcined gypsum mixed with water to form a paste which sets rapidly; used to make casts and stiff bandages.

p., porous. Perforated p.

p., resin; p., rosin. P. containing resin, wax and lead plaster; used as a soothing agent, especially for children.

p., rubber. SEE: *adhesive p.*

p., warming. P. of cantharides and pitch employed as a counterirritant.

plas'ter cast. Rigid dressing made of gauze impregnated with plaster of Paris, used to immobilize an injured part, esp. in bone fractures.

NP: Patient's position is indicated by fracture. A fracture table should be used when possible and various parts should be in readiness. Place a plaster bandage, end up, in tepid water. When about saturated, water is gently squeezed by pressing both ends (otherwise the plaster will be forced out through the ends of bandage). As one bandage is passed to the physician, another is placed in water. There should be extra plaster of Paris in perforated cans so it can be shaken on in smoothing the cast.

plastic (plăs'tĭk) [G. *plastikos*, formed]. 1. Capable of being molded. 2. Contributing to building tissues.

p. bronchitis. Bronchitis with fibrin exudate adhering in the form of a cast to the bronchial tubes.

p. force. The impetus that builds tissues; generative force.

p. linitis. Cirrhosis of the stomach.

p. lymph. The exudate covering inflamed serous surfaces, as in wounds.

p. surgery. The restoration and repair of external physical defects by use of grafts of bone or tissues. SEE: *chalinoplasty.*

plasticity (plăs-tĭs'ĭ-tĭ) [G. *plastikos*, formed]. The ability to be molded.

plastid (plăs'tĭd) [G. *plastidēs*, molded]. A cytoplasmic organoid found in plant cells. Includes *chloroplasts* (which contain chlorophyll), *leukoplasts* (colorless), *chromoplasts* (contain pigment) and *amyloplasts* (store starch). Plastids are centers of chemical activity involved in cell metabolism.

plastron. The sternum and attached cartilages.

plate (plāt) [G. *platys*, flat]. SYN: *lamina; lamella.* 1. A thin flattened part or portion. 2. A flattened process of bone. 3. An artificial denture or structure for holding false teeth. 4. A shallow covered dish for culturing microorganisms. 5. To inoculate and culture microorganisms in a culture plate.

p., approximation. A disk of decalcified bone used in intestinal surgery.

p., auditory. Bony roof of the external auditory meatus.

p., axial. The primitive streak of the embryo.

p., blood. Platelet.

p., bone. Flat, round or oval decalcified bone or metal disk, employed in pairs, used in approximation.

p., culture. A small, covered plastic or glass dish containing a bacterial culture medium such as agar.

p., dorsal. One of two prominences of the notochord in the embryo.

p., end. The terminal mass of a nerve fiber ending on a muscle cell.

p., foot. Flat portion of stapes. SYN: *basis stapedis* [NA].

p., medullary or ***neural.*** Central portion of the ectoderm developing into neural canal.

p., palate. Part of the palate bone

forming the lateral half of roof of mouth.

p., tympanic. Bony plate between anterior wall of the external auditory meatus and the tympanum.

platelet (plāt'lĕt) [G. *platys*, flat]. SYN: *thromboplastid; thrombocyte*. A round or oval disk, ⅓ to ½ the size of an erythrocyte found in the blood.

Platelets number from 150,000 to 450,000 per cc. They contain no hemoglobin. SEE: *blood*.

FUNCTIONS: Platelets play an important role in blood coagulation, hemostasis and blood thrombus formation. When a small vessel is injured, platelets adhere to each other and the edges of the injury and form a plug which covers the area. The plug or blood clot formed soon retracts and stops the loss of blood.

Thrombocytopenia (reduced platelet count) occurs in acute infections, anaphylactic shock, certain hemorrhagic diseases and anemias. *Thrombocytosis* (increased platelet count) occurs after operations, esp. splenectomy, and following violent exercise and also following tissue injury.

plat'ing. In Bact., inoculation of liquefiable, solid media (gelatin or agar) with microorganisms and pouring of medium into a shallow flat dish. Also called *plating out*.

platinum (plăt'ĭn-ŭm) [Spanish *plata*, silver]. Heavy silver-white metal. SYMB: Pt. At. wt. 195.09; at. no. 78. Sp. gr. 21.4.

platy- [G.]. Combining form meaning *broad*.

platycelous (plăt-ĭ-sē'lŭs) [G. *platys*, broad, + *koilos*, hollow]. Concave ventrally and convex dorsally, said of vertebrae.

platycephalic (plăt"ĭ-sē-făl'ĭk) [" + *kephalē*, head]. Having a wide skull with vertical index less than 70.

platycephalous (plat"ĭ-sef'ă-lus). Same as *platycephalic*.

platycnemia (plat-ĭk'nē-mĭ-ă) [" + *knēmē*, knee, + *ia*, condition]. 1. Having an unusually broad tibia. 2. Broadlegged.

platycnemic (plăt-ĭk-nē'mĭk) [" + *knēmē*, knee]. Having unusually broad tibia.

platycnemism (plat"ik'ne-mizm). Same as *platycnemia*.

platycoria (plăt-ĭ-kor'ĭ-ă). Mydriasis; dilatation of the pupil.

platycoriasis (plăt-ĭ-kor-ĭ-ās'ĭs). Platycoria, *q.v.*

Platyhelminthes (plăt"ĭ-hĕl-mĭn'thēz) [G. *platys*, broad, *elmins*, *elminth-*, worm). A phylum of flatworms which includes the classes *Turbellaria*. *Trematoda* (flukes), and *Cestoidea* (tapeworms). The last two are parasitic and include many species of medical importance. SEE: *Cestoda; Cestoidea; fluke; tapeworm; trematode*.

platyhieric (plat-e-hi-er'ĭk). Having a broad sacrum with a sacral index over 100.

platymeric (plăt-ĭ-mē'rĭk) [G. *platys*, broad, + *mēros*, thigh]. Having an unusually broad femur.

platymorphia (plăt-ĭ-morf'ĭ-ă). Having an eye with shortened anteroposterior diameter. Results in hyperopia.

platyopia (plăt-ĭ-ō'pĭ-ă) [" + *ōps*, visage]. Having a very broad face, the nasomalar index being less than 107.5.

platypellic, platypelvic (plăt"ĭ-pĕl'ĭk, -vĭk) [" + *pella*, a basin]. Having a broad pelvis.

platypodia (plăt-ĭ-pō'dĭ-ă) [" + *pous*, *pod-*, foot]. Condition of being flat-footed.

platyrrhine (plăt'ĭr-īn) [" + *ris*, *rin*, nose]. 1. Having a very wide nose in proportion to length. 2. Pertaining to a skull with a nasal index between 51.1 and 58.

platysma myoides (plăt-ĭz'mă mī-oy'dēz) [G. *platysma*, plate, + *mys*, *my-*, muscle, + *eidos*, form]. Broad, thin plate-like layer of muscle which extends from the fascia of both sides of the neck to jaw and muscles around the mouth. Acts to wrinkle the skin of the neck and to depress the jaw.

platysmal reflex. Dilation of pupil resulting from sharp pinching of platysma myoides.

platyspondylisis (plăt"ĭ-spŏn-dĭl'ĭs-ĭs) [G. *platys*, flat, + *spondylos*, vertebra]. Flatness of the vertebral bodies.

platystencephaly (plăt"ĭs-tĕn-sĕf'ă-lĭ). Having a skull wide at occiput.

Plaut's angina (plawt's ăn-jī'nă) [Hugo C. Plaut, Leipzig (Germany) physician, 1858-1928]. Ulceromembranous form of contagious disease of the oral mucosa, with inflammation of the tonsil. SYN: *trench mouth; Vincent's angina*.

pleas'ure prin'ciple. PSY: The avoidance of pain and the seeking of pleasure, indicative of the early stages of man's development. SYN: *hedonism*.

pledget (plĕj'ĕt) [origin uncertain]. Small, flat compress, usually of gauze or absorbent cotton, used to apply or absorb fluid, as a protector, to exclude air, etc.

plegaphonia (pleg-af-ō'nĭ-ă) [G. *plēgē*, stroke, + *a-*, neg. + *phōnē*, voice]. A sound produced in percussion of the larynx when the glottis is open during auscultation of the chest.

-plegia (ple'jĭ-ă). Suffix meaning paralysis or stroke.

pleio-, pleo-, plio- [G.]. Combining forms meaning *more*.

pleochroic (ple-o-kro'ik). Same as *pleochromatic*.

pleochromatic (plē-ō-kro-măt'ĭk) [G. *pleōn*, more, + *chroma*, color]. Pertaining to property of crystals and some other bodies of showing various colors when seen from different axes.

pleocytosis (plē"ō-sī-tō'sĭs) [" + *kytos*, cell, + *-ōsis*, intensive]. Increased number of lymphocytes in the cerebrospinal fluid.

pleomastia, pleomazia (plē"ō-măs'tĭ-ă. -mā'zĭ-ă) [" + *mastos*, *mazos*, breast]. The state of having more than two mammae. SYN: *polymastia*.

pleomorphic (plē-ō-mor'fĭk) [" + *morphē*, form]. Having many shapes.

pleomorphism (plē-ō-mor'fĭzm) [" + " + *ismos*, condition]. 1. Property of crystallizing into two or more different forms. 2. Occurrence of more than one form in a life cycle.

pleomorphous (plē-ō-mor'fŭs) [" + *morphē*, form]. Having many shapes or crystallizing into several forms.

pleonasm (plē'ō-năzm) [G. *pleonasmos*, exaggeration]. State of having more than normal number of organs or parts.

pleonectic (plē-ō-nĕk'tĭk) [G. *pleonexia*, greediness]. 1. Being saturated with more than the normal amount of oxygen, said of blood. 2. Relating to excessive urge to possess; greedy. SEE: *mesectic; mionectic*.

pleonexia (plē"ō-nĕk'sĭ-ă) [G. greediness]. Having morbid desire for possession.

ple"ro'sis. Restoration of lost tissue.

plesiomorphous (plē-sĭ-ō-mor'fŭs) [G. *ple-*

sios, close, + *morfē*, form]. Of, like or nearly the same in form.

plesiopia (plē″sĭ-ō′pĭ-ă). Increase in convexity of lens of eye.

plessesthesia (plĕs-ĕs-thē′zĭ-ă) [G. *plēssein*, to strike, + *aisthēsis*, sensation]. Palpatory percussion with left middle finger pressed against body and the index finger of right hand percussing in contact with left finger.

plessimeter (plĕs-im′et-er) [" + *metron*, a measure]. A disk held over the body which is struck in mediate percussion. SYN: *pleximeter*.

plessor (plĕ′sor) [G. *plēssein*, to strike]. A hammer for performing percussion. SYN: *plexor*.

plethora (plĕth′ō-ră) [G. *plēthōrē*, fullness]. 1. Overfullness of blood vessels or of the total quantity of blood or other fluid in the body. 2. Congestion causing distention of blood vessels. SEE: *sanguine*.

plethoric (plĕth-or′ĭk) [G. *plēthōrē*, fullness]. Pert. to or characterized by plethora; overfull.

plethysmograph (plē-thĭz′mō-grăf) [G. *plēthysmos*, increase, + *graphein*, to write]. Device for finding variations in size of a part due to variations in amount of blood passing through or contained in the part.

pleura (pl. *pleurae*) (plū′ră) [G. *pleura*, a side]. Serous membrane that enfolds lungs and is reflected upon the walls of the thorax and diaphragm. SEE: *mediastinum; thorax*.

p., costal. Same as *p., parietal*.

p. diaphragmatica. That covering upper surface of diaphragm.

p., parietal. Extends from roots of the lungs covering the sides of the pericardium to chest wall and backward to the spine. The visceral and costal pleural layers are separated only by a lubricating secretion. These layers may become adherent or separated by fluid or air in diseased conditions. SYN: *parietal layer of pleura*.

p. pericardiaca. That covering the pericardium.

p. phrenica. Same as *p. diaphragmatica*.

p. pulmonalis. NA. The pleura investing the lungs and fissures bet. the lobes.

p., visceral. Invests the lungs and enters into and lines the interlobar fissures. It is loose at the base and at sternal and vertebral borders to allow for lung expansion.

pleural (plū′răl) [G. *pleura*, a side]. Concerning the pleura.

p. cavity. Space bet. the parietal and visceral layers of the pleura. SEE: *chylothorax*.

p. fibrosis. Condition occurring in pulmonary tuberculosis in which pleura becomes thickened and pleural cavity is often obliterated.

pleuralgia (plū-răl′jĭ-ă) [" + *algos*, pain]. Pain in the pleura, or in the side. SYN: *neuralgia, intercostal*.

pleurapophysis (plū-ră-pof′ĭs-ĭs) [" + *apo*, from, + *physis*, a growth]. A rib or a vertebral lateral process.

pleurectomy (plū-rĕk′tō-mĭ) [" + *ektomē*, excision]. Excision of part of the pleura.

pleurisy (plū′rĭs-ĭ) [G. *pleura*, a side]. Inflammation of pleura—may be primary or secondary; unilateral, bilateral or local; acute or chronic; fibrinous, serofibrinous or purulent. SEE: *Andral's decubitus*.

NP: In simple pleurisy, absolute rest is essential with plenty of sunlight and fresh air. Routine nursing is in order, but the patient should not be permitted to exert himself and he should be kept cheerful. Assistance should be given in moving the patient. Increase fluid intake. The doctor may strap the affected side to help immobilize the chest.

p., acute. Chilliness, stabbing pain or stitch in affected side, intensified by coughing or deep breathing. Fever, 101°-103° F.; cough short, dry, partially suppressed, face pale, anxious; patient usually lies on affected side. An effusion of fluid in the pleural space which remains unabsorbed is characteristic of chronic pleurisy.

p., diaphragmatic. Inflammation of diaphragmatic pleura.

SYM: Intense pain under margin of ribs, sometimes referred into abdomen, with tenderness on pressure; thoracic breathing; tenderness over phrenic nerve referred to supraclavicular region in neck or same side; hiccough; extreme dyspnea.

p., dry. Condition in which the pleural membrane is covered with a fibrinous exudate.

It clings together, causing pain during respiration. There is slight pain when apical pleura is inflamed, but there is acute stabbing pain in costal or diaphragmatic pleural inflammation.

p., encysted. P. with effusion limited by adhesions.

p., fibrinous. Pain severe and continuous. Aspiration gives negative results, later much retraction of affected side.

p., hemorrhagic. P. with hemorrhage.

p., interlobar. P. in interlobar spaces.

p., purulent. High, irregular fever; sweats; chills; anemia; sometimes pitting from edema of surface; purulent effusion found on aspiration.

p., secondary. Infectious pleurisy resulting from some specific inflammation.

p., serofibrinous. P. with fibrinous exudate and serous effusion.

p., suppurative. SEE: *p., purulent*.

p., tuberculous. A common cause of pleurisy that is apparently primary in tuberculosis. May be secondary to pulmonary phthisis. Effusion apt to be bloody, but presents same symptoms as ordinary serofibrinous pleurisy.

pleuritic (plū-rĭt′ĭk) [G. *pleura*, a side]. Relating to, or like, pleurisy.

pleuritis (plū-rī′tĭs) [" + *-itis*, inflammation]. Inflammation of the pleura. SYN: *pleurisy*.

pleurocele (plū′rō-sēl) [" + *kēlē*, a swelling]. 1. Hernia of lungs or of pleura. 2. A serous pleural effusion.

pleurocentesis (plū″rō-sĕn-tē′sĭs) [" + *kentēsis*, a piercing]. Surgical puncture of the pleural cavity. SYN: *thoracentesis*.

pleurocentrum (pl. *pleurocentra*) (plū-rō-sĕn′trŭm) [G. *pleura*, a side, + *kentron*, center]. The lateral half of the centrum of a vertebra.

pleurocholecystitis (plū″rō-kō-lē-sĭst-ī′tĭs) [" + *cholē*, bile, + *kystis*, bladder, + *-itis*, inflammation]. Inflamed condition of the pleura and gallbladder.

pleuroclysis (plū-rŏk′lĭs-ĭs) [" + *klysis*, an injection]. Injection of fluid into the pleural cavity.

pleurodynia (plū″rō-dĭn′ĭ-ă) [" + *odynē*, pain]. Pain in intercostal muscles of sharp intensity, due to chronic inflammatory changes in chest fasciae; pain of the pleural nerves.

p., epidemic diaphragmatic. Epidemic disease with sudden attack of pain in the chest, fever, and a tendency to recrudescence on the 3rd day. SYN: *devil's grip.*

pleurogenic (plū-rō-jĕn'ĭk) [G. *pleura,* a side, + *gennan,* to produce]. Arising in the pleura. SYN: *pleurogenous.*

pleurogenous (plū-roj'ĕn-ŭs) [" + *gennan,* to produce]. Having origin in the pleura. SYN: *pleurogenic.*

pleurography (plū-rog'ră-fĭ) [" + *graphein,* to write]. X-ray examination of the lungs and pleura.

pleurohepatitis (plū"rō-hĕp-ă-tī'tĭs) [" + *ēpar, ēpat-,* liver, + *-ītis,* inflammation]. Inflammation of pleura and the liver.

pleurolith (plū'rō-lĭth) [" + *lithos,* stone]. A calculus in the pleura.

pleurolysis (plū-rŏl'ĭ-sĭs) [G. *pleura,* a side, + *lysis,* a loosening]. Loosening of parietal pleura from intrathoracic fascia to facilitate contraction of the lung or artificial pneumothorax. Also called *Jacobaeus operation.*

pleuroparietopexy (plū"rō-păr-ī'ĕt-ō-pĕk"-sĭ) [" + L. *pariēs, pariet-,* wall, + G. *pēxis,* fixation]. Fastening the lung to the wall of the chest by binding the visceral pleura to the wall of its cavity.

pleuropericarditis (plū"rō-pĕr"ĭ-kar-dī'tĭs) [G. *pleura,* side, + *peri,* around, + *kardia,* heart, + *-ītis,* inflammation]. Pleuritis accompanied by pericarditis.

pleuroperitoneal (plū"rō-pĕr-ĭ-tō-nē'ăl) [" + *peritonaion,* peritoneum]. Relating to the pleura and peritoneum.

p. cavity. The body cavity. SYN: *celom.*

pleuropneumonia (plū"rō-nū-mō'nĭ-ă) [" + *pneumōn,* lung]. Pleurisy accompanied by pneumonia.

pleuropneumonolysis (plū"rō-nū-mōn-ŏl'ĭ-sĭs) [" + " + *lysis,* a loosening]. Resection of one or more ribs from one side to collapse the lung in unilateral pulmonary tuberculosis.

pleurorrhea (plū"rō-rē'ă) [" + *roia,* a flow]. Effusion of fluid into the pleura.

pleuroscopy (plū-rŏs'kō-pĭ) [" + *skopein,* to examine]. Inspection of the pleural cavity through an incision into the thorax.

pleurothotonos (plū-rō-thŏt'ō-nos) [G. *pleurothen,* from the side, + *tonos,* tension]. Tetanic spasm in which the body position is arched to one side.

RS: *emprosthotonos; opisthotonos; orthotonos; position; posture.*

pleurotomy (plū-rŏt'ō-mĭ) [G. *pleura,* a side, + *tomē,* incision]. Incision of the pleura.

pleurotyphoid (plū-rō-tī'foyd) [" + *typhos,* fever, + *eidos,* form]. Typhoid fever with pleural involvement.

pleurovisceral (plū"rō-vĭs'ĕr-ăl) [" + L. *viscus, viscer-,* viscera]. Concerning the pleura and the viscera.

plexal (plĕks'ăl) [L. *plexus,* a braid]. Pertaining to, or of the nature of, a plexus.

plexiform (plĕk'sĭ-form) [" + *forma,* shape]. Resembling a network or plexus.

pleximeter (plĕks-ĭm'ĕt-ĕr) [" + G. *metron,* measure]. Device for receiving the blow of the percussion hammer.

plexor (plĕks'or) [G. *plēxis,* a stroke]. Hammer or other device for striking upon the pleximeter in percussion.

plexus (plĕk'sŭs) (pl. *plexus* or *plexuses*) [L., a braid]. A network of nerves or vessels—blood or lymphatic. SEE: *rete; table of plexuses in Appendix.*

p., cavernous. 1. *Of the nose,* a venous p. in mucosa covering sup. and mid. conchae. 2. *Of the penis,* nerve plexus at root of penis. Gives rise to large and small cavernous nerves. 3. *Of the clitoris,* nerve plexus at base of clitoris formed of fibers from uterovaginal plexus. 4. *Of the cavernous sinus,* a sympathetic plexus supplying fibers to internal carotid artery and its branches within cranium.

p., enteric. One of two plexuses of nerve fibers and ganglion cells which lie in wall of alimentary canal. Include myenteric (Auerbach's) and submucosal (Meissner's) plexus.

p., nerve. SEE: *table of plexuses in Appendix.*

p., pampiniform. In male, a complicated network of veins lying in spermatic cord and draining the testis; in female, a network of veins lying in mesovarium and draining the ovary.

p., prevertebral. One of three plexuses of autonomic division which lie in body cavities. Includes cardiac, celiac, and hypogastric (pelvic) plexuses, *q.v.*

pliability (plī-ă-bĭl'ĭ-tĭ) [Fr. *plier,* to bend]. Capacity of being bent or twisted easily.

plica (plī'kă) (pl. *plicae*) [*L.* a fold]. A fold.

p. circularis. One of the transverse folds in the intestinal mucosa.

p. epiglottica. One of three folds of mucosa bet. the tongue and the epiglottis.

p. lacrimalis. Mucosal fold at the lower orifice of the nasolacrimal duct.

p. neuropathica. Curly hair due to a nervous disorder.

p. palmatae. Radiating fold in the uterine mucosa on ant. and post. walls of cervical canal.

p. polonica. Tangled matted hair in which crusts and vermin are embedded.

p. semilunaris. 1. Mucosal fold at the inner canthus of the eye. 2. Transverse fold of mucosa of large intestine lying between sacculations.

p. synovialis. A fold of synovial membrane which projects into a joint cavity.

p. transversalis recti. One of the mucosal folds in the rectum.

plicate (plī'kāt) [L. *plica,* fold]. Braided or folded.

plication (plī-kā'shŭn) [L. *plicāre,* to fold]. Stitching folds in an organ's walls to reduce its size.

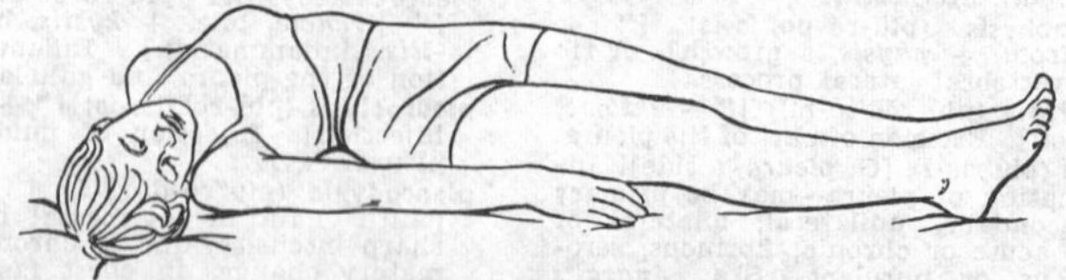

PLEUROTHOTONOS.

plicotomy (plĭ-kŏt′ō-mĭ) [" + G. *tomē*, a cutting]. Section of the post. fold of the tympanic membrane.

plombage (plŭm-bazh′) [Fr. *plomber*, to plug]. A method of collapsing the apex of lung by stripping the parietal pleura from the chest wall at the site of desired collapse and packing the space between the lung and chest wall with an inert substance such as small balls made of certain plastic materials.

plug (plŭg) [M.D. *plugge*, plug]. A mass obstructing or for closing a hole.

p., cervical. One forming in cervix after conception.

p., vaginal. Closed tube for maintaining patency of vagina following operation for fistula.

plumbago (plŭm-bā′gō) [L. lead ore]. Graphite; a native carbon.

plumbic (plŭm′bĭk) [L. *plumbicus*, leaden]. Pertaining to, or containing, lead.

plumbism (plŭm′bĭzm) [L. *plumbum*, lead, + G. *ismos*, condition]. Poisoning from lead, *q.v.*

plumbum (plŭm′bŭm) [L. lead]. Lead; a bluish-white metal.

plumose (plū′mōs) [L. *pluma*, feather]. Having a delicate, feathery growth.

plumper (plŭm′pĕr). Pad for filling out sunken cheeks, sometimes in form of extended artificial dentures.

pluri- [L.] Prefix meaning *several.*

pluriceptor (plū-rĭ-sĕp′tor) [L. *plus*, *plur-*, more, + *ceptor*, a receiver]. A receptor which has more than two groups uniting with the complement.

pluridyscrinia (plū″rĭ-dĭs-krĭn′ĭ-ă) [" + G. *dys*, bad, + *krinein*, to secrete]. Disorder of several endocrine organs at the same time.

pluriglandular (plu″rĭ-gland′u-ler). Pertaining to several glands.

plurigravida (plū-rĭ-grăv′ĭd-ă) [" + *gravida*, pregnant]. A gravid woman who has had two or more pregnancies.

plurilocular (plū-rĭl-ŏk′ū-lar) [" + *loculus*, a cell]. Composed of several compartments or cavities. Syn: *multilocular.*

pluripara (plū-rĭp′ă-ră) [" + *parēre*, to bring forth]. A woman who has given birth to three or more children in at least three pregnancies.

pluripar′ity [L. *plus*, *plur-*, more, + *parēre*, to bring forth]. Condition of having borne three or more children.

plutomania (plū″tō-mā′nĭ-ă) [G. *ploutos*, wealth, + *mania*, madness]. Delusion that one is very rich.

plutonium (plōō-to′nĭ-um) [Named after the planet *Pluto*]. A chemical element. Symb: Pu. At. number, 94. At. wt. 242. Obtained from neptunium which in turn is obtained from uranium.

Pm. Symb. for *promethium.*

PMSG. Abbr. for *pregnant mare's serum gonadotrophin.* See: *gonadotrophin, chorionic.*

pneo- (ne′o). Combining form meaning *pertaining to breath or breathing.*

pneocardiac reflex (nē-ō-kar′dĭ-ăk) [G. *pnein*, to breathe, + *kardia*, heart]. Change in rate and rhythm of heart when an irritant vapor enters air passages.

pneodynamics (nē″ō-dī-năm′ĭks) [" + *dynamis*, force]. The mechanism of breathing. Syn: *pneumodynamics.*

pneograph (nē′ō-grăf) [" + *graphein*, to write]. Apparatus for registering respiratory movements.

pneometer (nē-ŏm′ĕt-ĕr) [" + *metron*, a measure]. Instrument for measuring lung respiration. Syn: *spirometer, q.v.*

pneophore (nē′ō-for) [" + *phoros*, bearing]. Device to aid artificial respiration.

pneopneic reflex (nē-ŏp-nē′ĭk) [" + *pnein*, to breathe]. Change in respiratory depth and rate, coughing, suffocation and pulmonary edema, when an irritant vapor enters air passages.

pneoscope (nē′ō-skōp) [" + *skopein*, to examine]. Device for measuring movements of respiration.

pneum-, pneuma-, pneumato-. Combining form meaning *pert. to air*, or *gas*, or *respiration.*

pneumarthrosis (nū-mar-thrō′sĭs) [G. *pneuma*, air, + *arthron*, joint, + *-ōsis*, intensive]. Accumulation of gas or air in a joint.

pneumascope (nū′mă-skōp) [" + *skopein*, to examine]. 1. Device for estimating gas in expired air. 2. Instrument for internal auscultation of the thorax. 3. Device for discovering foreign bodies in mastoid sinuses. 4. Apparatus for measurement of the movements of respiration. Syn: *pneumatoscope.*

pneumatic (nū-măt′ĭk) [G. *pneumatikos*, pert. to air]. 1. Concerning gas or air. 2. Relating to respiration. 3. Relating to rarefied or compressed air.

p. cabinet. Cabinet for treatment of a part with rarefied or compressed air.

pneumatinuria (nū″măt-ĭn-ū′rĭ-ă) [G. *pneuma*, air, + *ouron*, urine]. Excretion of urine containing free gas. Syn: *pneumaturia.*

pneumatocardia (nū″-măt-ō-kar′dĭ-ă) [" + *kardia*, heart]. Air or gas in the heart chambers.

pneumatocele (nū-măt′ō-sēl) (" + *kēlē*, hernia]. 1. Hernial protuberance of lung tissue. 2. A swelling containing a gas or air, especially a swelling of the scrotum. Syn: *pneumonocele.*

pneumatodyspnea (nū″măt-ō-dĭsp-nē′ă) [" + *dys*, bad, + *pneia*, breath]. Dyspnea caused by pulmonary emphysema.

pneumatogram (nū-măt′ō-grăm) [" + *gramma*, a mark]. A tracing or record made by a pneumatograph.

pneumatograph (nū-măt′ō-grăf) [" + *graphein*, to write]. Device for registering respiratory movements. Syn: *pneograph.*

pneumatology (nū-mă-tŏl′ō-jĭ) [" + *logos*, a study]. Science of gases and air, their chemical properties and use in treatment.

pneumatometer (nū-măt-ŏm′ĕt-ĕr) [G. *pneuma*, air, + *metron*, a measure]. Device for measuring quantity of air involved in inspiration and expiration. Syn: *spirometer.*

pneumatometry (nū-măt-ŏm′ĕt-rĭ) [" + *metron*, measure]. Measurement of respiratory force as a means of diagnosis.

pneumatorachis (nū-măt-or′ă-kĭs) [" + *rachis*, spine]. Air in the spinal canal.

pneumatoscope (nū-măt′ō-skōp) [" + *skopein*, to inspect]. 1. Device for ascertaining presence of foreign bodies in mastoid sinuses. 2. Apparatus used to measure the gas in expired air. 3. Apparatus for internal thoracic auscultation. 4. Instrument used to measure the respiratory movements. Syn: *pneumascope.*

pneumatosis (nu-mă-to′sis). Presence of air or gas in an abnormal location in the body.

p. abdominis. Air in the peritoneal cavity. SYN: *pneumoperitoneum.*

p. cystoides intestinalis. Presence of thin-walled gas-filled cysts in the intestines.

pneumatotherapy (nū"măt-ō-thĕr'ă-pĭ) [" + *therapeia,* treatment]. Treatment by means of rarefied or compressed air.

pneumatothorax (nū"măt-ō-thō'răks) [" + *thōrax,* chest]. Air or gas accumulation in the pleural cavities. SYN: *pneumothorax, q.v.*

pneumaturia (nū-măt-u'rĭ-ă) [G. *pneuma,* air, + *ouron,* urine]. Excretion of urine containing free gas.

pneumatype (nū'mă-tīp) [" + *typos,* type]. Deposit of moisture on glass from the breath exhaled through the nostrils with the mouth closed for purpose of comparing the airflow through the nostrils.

pneumectomy (nū-mĕk'tō-mĭ) [G. *pneumōn,* lung, + *ektomē,* excision]. Excision of all or part of a lung.

pneumo-, pneumono- [G.]. Combining forms meaning *air; lung.*

pneumobacillus (nū"mō-bă-sĭl'ŭs) [" + L. *bacillus,* a little rod]. The bacillus causing pneumonia.

p., Friedlander's. Klebsiella pneumoniae.

pneumocele (nū'mō-sēl) [" + *kēlē,* hernia]. 1. A swelling containing air or gas, esp. of the scrotum. 2. Hernia of lung tissue through chest wall. SYN: *pneumatocele.*

pneumocentesis (nū"mō-sĕn-tē'sĭs) [" + *kentēsis,* a piercing]. Paracentesis, *q.v.*, or surgical puncture of a lung to evacuate a cavity.

pneumocephalus (nū"mō-sĕf'ă-lŭs) [" + *kephalē,* head]. Gas or air in the cavity of the cranium.

pneumochysis (nū-mŏk'ĭs-ĭs) [" + *chysis,* a pouring]. Edema of the lung.

pneumococcal (nū-mō-kŏk'ăl) [G. *pneumōn,* lung, + *kokkos,* berry]. Concerning or caused by pneumococci.

pneumococcemia (nū"mō-kŏk-sē'mĭ-ă). Presence of pneumococci circulating in the blood.

pneumococci (nū-mō-kok'sĭ). Plural of pneumococcus, *q.v.*

pneumococcolysis (nū"mō-kŏk-ŏl'ĭ-sĭs) [" + " + *lysis,* destruction]. Destruction or lysis of pneumococci.

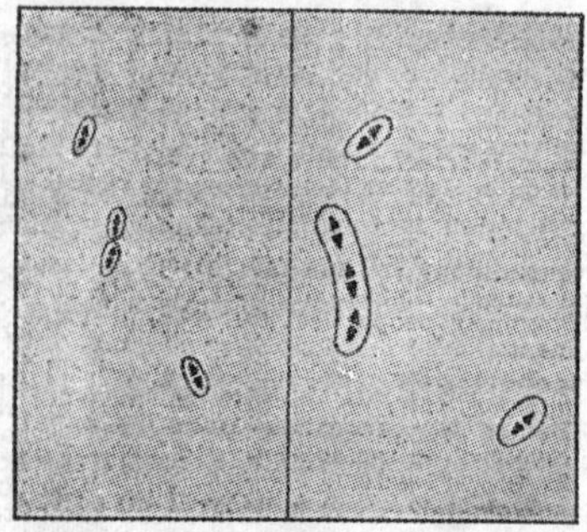

PNEUMOCOCCUS TYPING
(Schematized.)

The sputum is mixed with typing sera. Left, negative reaction; the capsule is thin, the flame-shaped cocci are close together; right, positive reaction; the capsules are much swollen, pushing the cocci apart.

pneumococcus (nū-mō-kŏk'ŭs) (pl. *pneumococci*) [G. *pneumon,* lung, + *kokkos,* berry]. An oval-shaped, encapsulated, nonspore-forming organism occurring usually in pairs (diplococcus) having lancet-shaped ends. There are more than 75 types of pneumococcus. The Neufeld test is used to determine the type. Types 1, 2, 3, 5, 7 and 8 are the types most frequently encountered. Pneumococci are also found to be the cause of infections such as otitis media, mastoiditis, meningitis, bronchitis, bloodstream infections, keratitis and conjunctivitis.

Pneumococcal infections are effectively treated with antibiotics, especially penicillin. SYN: *Diplococcus pneumoniae, q.v.; Diplococcus lanceolatus; Micrococcus lanceolatus; Fränkel's pneumococcus; Fränkel-Weichselbaum pneumococcus.*

pneumoconiosis (nū"mō-kō-nĭ-ō'sĭs) [G. *pneumōn,* lung, + *konis,* dust, + *-ōsis,* disease]. A condition of the respiratory tract due to inhalation of dust particles.

An occupational disorder such as that caused by mining or stonecutting.

RS: *anthracosis, chalicosis, siderosis, silicosis.*

pneumoderma (nū-mō-dĕr'mă) [" + *derma,* skin]. Emphysema under the skin.

pneumodynamics (nū"mō-dī-năm'ĭks) [" + *dynamis,* force]. Branch of science treating with force employed in respiration.

pneumoempyema (nū"mō-ĕm-pī-ē'mă) [" + *en,* in, + *pyon,* pus]. Empyema accompanied by an accumulation of gas.

pneumo"encephalog'raphy. Roentgenographic examination of ventricles and subarachnoid spaces of brain following withdrawal of cerebrospinal fluid and injection of air or a gas via lumbar puncture.

pneumoenteritis (nū"mō-ĕn-tĕr-ī'tĭs) [" + *enteron,* intestine, + *-ītis,* inflammation]. Pneumonia and enteritis combined.

pneumoerysipelas (nū-mō-ĕr-ĭ-sip'e-las). Erysipelas with pneumonia.

pneumogalactocele (nū"mō-găl-ăk'tō-sēl) [" + *gala, galakt,* milk, + *kēlē,* hernia]. A breast tumor containing milk and gas.

pneumogastric (nū"mō-găs'trĭk) [G. *pneumōn,* lung, + *gastēr,* stomach]. Concerning the lungs and stomach.

p. nerve. Term formerly used for the vagus nerve.

pneumogram (nū'mō-grăm) [G. *pneumōn,* lung, + *gramma,* a mark]. 1. A record of respiratory movements. 2. A roentgenogram following injection of air. SYN: *pneumatogram.*

pneumography (nū-mŏg'ră-fĭ) [" + *graphein,* to write]. 1. A descriptive treatise on the lungs. 2. A tracing of the respiratory movements.

pneumohemopericardium (nū"mō-hem"ō-pĕr-ĭ-kar'dĭ-ŭm) [" + *aima,* blood, + *peri,* around, + *kardia,* heart]. The accumulation of air and blood in the pericardium.

pneumohemorrhagia (nū"mō-hem-or-hā'jĭ-ă) [" + " + *rēgnunai,* to burst forth]. Hemorrhage into pulmonary air cells; apoplexy of the lungs.

pneumohemothorax (nū"mō-hem"ō-thō'răks) [" + " + *thōrax,* chest]. Gas or air and blood collected in the pleural cavity.

pneumohydrometra (nū-mō-hī-drō-mē'-

trā) [" + *hydor*, water, + *metra*, uterus]. The accumulation of gas and fluid in the uterus.

pneumohydropericardium (nū"mō-hī"drō-pĕr-ĭ-kar'dĭ-ŭm) [G. *pneumōn*, lung, + *ydōr*, water, + *peri*, around, + *kardia*, heart]. Air and fluid accumulated in the pericardium.

pneumohydrothorax (nū"mō-hī-drō-thō'-rāks) [" + " + *thōrax*, chest]. Gas or air and fluid in the pleural cavity.

pneumohypoderma (nū"mō-hī-pō-dĕr-mă) [" + *ypo*, under, + *derma*, skin]. Air in the tissues under the skin.

pneumokidney (nū"mō-kĭd'nĭ) [" + M.E. *kydney*, kidney]. Air in the pelvis of the kidney.

pneumolith (nū'mō-lĭth) [" + *lithos*, stone]. A pulmonary calculus.

pneumolithiasis (nū"mō-lĭth-ī'ăs-ĭs) [" + *lithos*, stone]. Formation of concretions in the lungs.

pneumology (nū-mŏl'ō-jĭ) [" + *logos*, a study]. The scientific study of diseases of the lungs and air passages.

pneumolysis (nū-mŏl'ĭs-ĭs) [G. *pneumōn*, lung, + *lysis*, a loosening]. Separation of an adherent lung from costal pleura.

pneumomalacia (nū"mō-mă-lā'sĭ-ă) [" + *malakia*, a softening]. Abnormal softening of the lung.

pneumomassage (nū"mō-măs-sazh') [" + *massein*, to knead]. Massage of the tympanum with air to cause movement of the ossicles.

pneumomelanosis (nū"mō-mĕl-ăn-ō'sĭs) [" + *melas*, *melan-*, black, + *-ōsis*, disease]. Pigmentation of lung seen in pneumoconiosis.

pneumometer (nū-mŏm'ĕt-ĕr) [" + *metron*, measure]. Instrument for measuring amount of air inspired and expired in respiration. Syn: *spirometer*, *q.v.*

pneumomycosis (nū"mō-mī-kō'sĭs) [" + *mykēs*, fungus, + *-ōsis*, disease]. A fungus pulmonary disease. Syn: *pneumonomycosis*.

pneumomyelography (nū"mō-mī-ĕl-ŏg'ră-fĭ) [" + *myelos*, marrow, + *graphein*, to write]. X-ray inspection of the spinal canal.

pneumonectasia, pneumonectasis (nū-mōn-ĕk-tā'zĭ-ă, ĕk'tă-sĭs) [G. *pneumōn*, lung, + *ektasis*, dilatation]. Distention of lungs with air.

pneumonectomy (nū-mōn-ĕk'tō-mĭ) [" + *ektomē*, excision]. Removal of a lung. Syn: *pulmonectomy; pneumectomy*.

pneumonemia (nū-mō-nē'mĭ-ă) [" + *aima*, blood]. Congestion of the lungs.

pneumonia (nū-mō'nĭ-ă). Inflammation of the lungs caused primarily by bacteria, viruses, chemical irritants, vegetable dusts and allergy. There are more than 50 different causes; commoner ones are listed in the table on page P-72.

Pneumonias caused by pneumococci, staphylococci, streptococci and bacilli often begin suddenly.

Sym: Chills, high fever, pain in chest, cough, sputum purulent and often bloody. Mortality 30% unless treated with antibiotics.

NP: Bed rest necessary. For restlessness or pain, drugs or other therapeutic agents should be used as prescribed by the physician. All measures to promote comfort should be taken.

A careful watch over the patient's general condition: his color, his general appearance, and his pulse, temperature and respiration. Cyanosis or a rising respiratory rate calls for administration of oxygen, or for increase in the amount of oxygen if it is already being given. The nurse must understand how to regulate the flow of oxygen and to adjust the intranasal tube or the temperature in the oxygen tent. High fever demands tepid sponges, rarely the use of antipyretics. Any marked change in the patient's general condition should be reported to the doctor at once.

Measures to prevent and combat abdominal distention. The bowels should act daily; to accomplish this an enema may be given, or the physician may prescribe a laxative. If distention appears, a rectal tube is inserted.

Unless patient is sensitive, penicillin is drug of choice for pneumococcal and streptococcal pneumonia; otherwise sulfadiazine, erythromycin or tetracycline. Special penicillins for penicillin-resistant staphylococci. Tetracycline for pneumonia caused by Mycoplasma pneumoniae; streptomycin for gram-negative bacillary pneumonias. Anticipate untoward reactions to antibiotics.

p., acute lobar. Pneumonia caused by *Diplococcus pneumoniae*.

p., aspiration. P. after inhaling foreign matter into the lungs.

p., atypical. See: *p., primary atypical*.

p., chronic interstitial. Chronic disease of lung with overgrowth of fibrous tissue.

Sym: Moderate dyspnea and chronic cough, expectoration, slight or profuse, fetid, from being retained in bronchiectatic cavities. No fever. May live years.

p., croupous. See: ***p. acute lobar.***

p., hypostatic. Pneumonia caused by constantly remaining in same position. Gravity causes blood to become congested in one part of the lung. Infection aids development of true pneumonia.

NP: Change position of patient frequently and whenever patient is uncomfortable. Have patient breathe deeply several times each hour for full aeration of lungs. Short, shallow breaths predispose to pulmonary complications. Deep respirations after an upper abdominal incision cause pain.

p., lipid. P. after aspiration of oily substances such as oily nose drops or mineral or other bland oil.

p., migratory. P. in which infected area shifts from one part of the lung to another part.

p., primary atypical. A relatively mild pneumonia characterized by cough, fever, pharyngitis and x-ray evidence of lung infiltration out of proportion to the minimal findings upon examining the lungs. Caused by ***Mycoplasma pneumoniae.***

Treatment: Broad spectrum antibiotics; penicillin, sulfonamides and streptomycin are ineffective.

p., terminal. P. occurring secondary to another disease and resulting in death.

p., tuberculous. Condition which simulates pneumonia caused by tubercle bacilli. May result in rapid and widespread inflammatory exudation. If untreated may run a malignant course ending fatally or it may subside and become chronic.

p., tularemic. P. caused by Pasteurella tularensis. May be primary or associated with tularemia, ***q.v.***

p., viral. Same as ***p., primary atypical, q.v.***

Pneumonias

Specific Microbial Causes	Diseases Accompanied by Pneumonia	Pneumonias Not Caused by Infections
Viruses	Tularemia	Oil aspiration
influenza	Brucellosis	Radiation
adeno-	Rheumatic fever	Chemicals
respiro-	Syphilis	Allergy
syncytial	Typhus	Vegetable dusts
etc.	Rocky Mountain fever	Silo-filler's disease
Mycoplasma pneumoniae	Infectious mononucleosis	
(Mycoplasma mycoides; Eaton agent)	Trichiniasis	
Cocci		
Pneumococcus		
Staphylococcus		
Hemolytic streptococcus		
Bacilli		
Hemophilus influenzae		
Mycobacterium tuberculosis		
Klebsiella		
Gram-negative bacilli		
Fungi		
Histoplasma capsulatum		
Coccidioides immitis		

pneumonic (nū-mon'ĭk) [G. *pneumōn*, lung]. Concerning the lungs or pneumonia.

p. phthisis. Tuberculosis of an entire pulmonary lobe.

pneumonitis (nū-mō-nī'tĭs) [" + *-ītis*, inflammation]. Inflammation of the lung. SYN: *pneumonia.*

pneumono- (nū-mon-ō) [G.]. Combining form pertaining to the lung.

pneumonocele (nū-mō'nō-sēl) [G. *pneumōn*, lung, + *kēlē*, hernia]. A pulmonary hernia. SYN: *pneumocele.*

pneumonocirrhosis (nū"mō-nō-sĭr-ō'sĭs) [" + *kirros*, orange]. Interstitial pneumonia; cirrhosis of the lung.

pneumonoconiosis (nū"mō-nō-kō-nĭ-ō'sĭs) [" + *konis*, dust, + *-ōsis*, disease]. Fibrous inflammation or chronic induration of the lungs resulting from inhalation of dust. SYN: *pneumoconiosis, q.v.*

pneumonograph (nū-mō'nō-grăf) [" + *graphein*, to write]. X-ray photograph of the lungs.

pneumonography (nū-mō-nŏg'ră-fī) [" + *graphein*, to write]. The taking and developing of x-ray pictures of the lungs.

pneumonolysis (nū-mō-nŏl'ĭs-ĭs) [G. *pneumon*, lung, + *lysis*, loosening]. Loosening of an adherent lung from the chest wall to induce collapse of lung. SYN: *pneumolysis.*

p., extrapleural. Separation of parietal pleura from chest wall. SEE: *apicolysis.*

p., intrapleural. Separation of adhering visceral and parietal layers of pleura.

pneumonomelanosis (nū"mō-nō-mĕl-ăn-ō'sĭs) [" + *melas, melan-*, black, + *-ōsis*, disease]. Darkening of the lung tissue as a result of inhalation of black dust particles such as coal dust.

pneumonomycosis (nū-mō-nō-mī-kō'sĭs) [G. *pneumon*, lung, + *mykēs*, fungus, + *-ōsis*, disease]. Disease of the lungs caused by fungi. SYN: *pneumomycosis.*

pneumonopathy (nū-mō-nŏp'ăth-ĭ) [" + *pathos*, disease]. Any diseased condition of the lung.

pneumonoperitonitis (nū"mō-nō-pĕr"ĭ-tō-nī'tĭs) [" + *peritonaion*, peritoneum, + *-ītis*, inflammation]. Peritonitis with gas in the peritoneal cavity.

pneumonopexy (nū-mō"nō-pĕk'sĭ) [" + *pēxis*, fixation]. Surgical attachment of the lung to the chest wall. SYN: *pneumopexy.*

pneumonorrhaphy (nū-mō-nor'ă-fī) [" + *raphē*, a sewing]. Suture of a lung.

pneumonosis (nū-mō-nō'sĭs) [G. *pneumon*, lung, + *-ōsis*, disease]. Any noninfective disease or disorder of the lungs, esp. those resulting from degenerative processes.

p., traumatic. In aviation medicine, a condition resulting from quick deceleration which may result in hemorrhage, emphysema, and other pulmonary changes.

pneumonotomy (nū-mō-nŏt'ō-mĭ) [" + *tomē*, incision]. Incision into the lung. SYN: *pneumotomy.*

pneumono ultramicroscopicsilico volcanoconiosis (nu"mo-no-ul"tră-mi-kro-skop'ik-sil"ĭ-ko-vol-kăn'o-ko"nī-o'sis). Noninfectious form of silicosis, miner's lung disease.

pneumopericardium (nū"mō-pĕr-ĭ-kar'dĭ-ŭm) [" + *peri*, around, + *kardia* heart]. Air or gas in the pericardial sac.

ETIOL: Traumatism or communication bet. the esophagus, stomach, or lungs and the pericardium.

SYM: Unusual metallic heart sounds, tympany over precordial area.

pneumoperitoneum (nū"mō-pĕr-ĭ-tō-nē'ŭm) [G. *pneumōn*, lung, + *peritonaion*, peritoneum]. Condition in which air or gas is collected in the peritoneal cavity.

May be artificially injected to treat tuberculous peritonitis or where pneumothorax is impossible.

pneumoperitonitis (nū"mō-pĕr-ĭ-tō-nī'tĭs) [G. *pneumōn*, lung, + *peritonaion*, peritoneum, + *-itis*, inflammation]. Peritonitis with gas accumulation.

pneumopexy (nū'mō-pĕks"ĭ) [" + *pēxis*, fixation]. Surgical attachment of a lung to the thoracic wall.

pneumopleuritis (nū"mō-plū-rī'tĭs) [" + *pleura*, a side, + *-itis*, inflammation]. Inflamed condition of lungs and pleura.

pneumopleuroparietopexy (nū"mō-plū"rō-pă-rī'ĕt-ō-pĕk"sĭ) [" + " + L. *pariēs*, wall, + G. *pēxis*, fixation]. The operation of attaching the lung with its parietal pleura to the border of a thoracic wound.

pneumopyelography (nū"mō-pī-ĕ-lŏg'ră-fĭ) [" + *pyelos*, pelvis, + *graphein*, to write]. Making of a skiagram of the renal pelvis and ureters after they are injected with oxygen.

pneumopyopericardium (nū"mō-pī"ō-pĕr-ĭ-kar'dĭ-ŭm) [" + *pyon*, pus, + *peri*, around, + *kardia*, heart]. Air, gas and pus collected in the pericardial sac.

pneumopyothorax (nū"mō-pī"ō-thō'răks) [" + " + *thōrax*, chest]. Air and pus collected in the pleural cavity.

pneumoradiography (nū"mō-rā-dĭ-ŏg'ră-fĭ) [" + L. *radius*, a ray, + G. *graphein*, to write]. Injection of air into a part for taking an x-ray picture.

pneumorrachis (nū-mor-rā'kĭs) [G. *pneumōn*, lung, + *rachis*, spine]. Gas accumulation in the spinal canal.

pneumorrhagia (nū-mor-ā'jĭ-ă) [" + *rēgnunai*, to burst forth]. Pulmonary hemorrhage. SYN: *hemoptysis.*

pneumoserothorax (nū"mō-sē-rō-thō'răks) [" + " + G. *thōrax*, chest]. Air or gas and serum collected in the pleural cavity.

pneumotachograph (nū"mō-tăk'ō-grăf) [G. *pneuma*, air, + *tachus*, swift, + *graphein*, to write]. Device for registering velocity of inspiration and expiration of air.

pneumotherapy (nū-mō-ther'ă-pĭ) [G. *pneumōn*, lung, + *therapeia*, treatment]. Treatment of diseases of the lungs. SYN: *pneumatotherapy.*

pneumothermomassage (nū"mō-ther"mō-măs-azh') [G. *pneuma*, air, + *thermē*, heat, + *massein*, to knead]. Application to the body of air of varying temperature and pressure.

pneumothorax (nū-mō-thō'răks) [" + *thōrax*, chest]. A collection of air or gas in the pleural cavity.

The gas enters as the result of a perforation through the chest wall or the pleura covering the lung (visceral pleura). This perforation may be the result of an injury or the rupture of an emphysematous bleb or superficial lung abscess; the most common latter condition is a tuberculous abscess in the presence of pulmonary tuberculosis.

SYM: The onset is sudden, usually with a severe sticking pain in the side and marked dyspnea. Fluid very frequently is found, developing within 48 hours (hydropneumothorax). The physical signs are those of a distended unilateral chest, tympanitic resonance, absence of breath sounds, and with fluid, a splash or succussion on shaking patient.

p., artificial. Pneumothorax induced intentionally by artificial means employed in the treatment of pulmonary tuberculosis or pneumonia.

Pneumothorax gives the diseased lung temporary rest. The lung collapses when the air enters the pleural space which is not possible if there are adhesions. Scattered adhesions may afford only a partial collapse. Effusion may occur in about one third of the cases. Hazards are small.

NP: Explain to patient. Instruct not to cough but to warn physician when so impelled. Patient lies on affected side, arm overhead, and held by nurse. Observe color of face, respiration, and pulse. Record intrapleural pressure. Watch for pleural shock and effusion. Pain in side, weak pulse, dyspnea, sweating are instances. Physician gives or orders hypodermics or inhalation of oxygen. Complications may be: (a) Air embolism from puncture of a vein; (b) puncture of lung; (c) surgical emphysema.

Postoperative care: Rest for an hour after. Record temperature every 4 hours for 48 hours. Report dyspnea because it is serious.

p., spontaneous. Spontaneous entrance of air into the pleural cavity.

The pressure may collapse the lung and displace the heart.

SYM: Sudden sharp pain, dyspnea, and cough. Pain may be referred to the shoulder. Majority of cases are mild and require only rest. Rarely shock and collapse occur.

p., valvular. That which is characterized by an opening through the pleura which has a slit with a valvelike action allowing the air to pass in but not out. SYN: *tension pneumothorax.*

pneumotomy (nū-mŏt'ō-mĭ) [G. *pneumōn*, lung, + *tomē*, a cutting]. Incision of the lung.

pneumotoxin (nū"mō-tŏks'ĭn) [" + *toxikon*, poison]. A toxin produced by the pneumococcus.

pneumotyphus (nū"mō-tī'fŭs) [" + *typhos*, fever]. 1. Typhoid fever with pneumonia at onset. 2. Development of pneumonia during typhoid fever.

pneumouria (nū"mō-ū'rĭ-ă) [G. *pneuma*, air, + *ouron*, urine]. Excretion of urine with free gas. SYN: *pneumaturia.*

pneumoventricle (nū"mō-vĕn'trĭ-kl) [" + L. *ventriculus*, little belly]. Air accumulation in the cerebral ventricles.

pneumoventriculography (nū"mō-vĕn-trĭk"-ū-lŏg'ră-fĭ) [" + " + G. *graphein*, to write]. Radiography of the lateral ventricles of the brain, after removal of fluid content and injection with air. SYN: *ventriculography.*

pneusis (nu'sis) [G. *pneein*, to breathe]. 1. Respiration. 2. Panting. SYN: *anhelation.*

pnigophobia (ni-gō-fō'bĭ-ă) [G. *pnigos*, choking, + *phobos*, fear]. Morbid fear of choking; sometimes experienced in angina pectoris.

pock (pŏk) [A.S. *poc*, pustule, pouch]. A pustule of an eruptive fever, esp. of smallpox.

p.-marked. Pitted or marked with cicatrices of smallpox pustules.

pocket (pŏk'ĕt) [Fr. *pochet*, little pouch]. A saclike cavity.

pocketing (pŏk'ĕt-ĭng) [Fr. *pochet*, little pouch]. Method of treating the pedicle in ovariotomy by enclosing it within the edges of the wound.

podagra (pŏd-ăg'ră) [G. *pous, pod-*, foot, + *agra*, seizure]. Gout, esp. of the joints of the foot or of the great toe.

podalgia (pod-ăl'jĭ-ă) [" + *algos*, pain]. Pain in the feet.

podalic (pŏd-ăl'ĭk) [G. *pous, pod-*, foot]. Pert. to the feet.

p. version. Shifting position of a

fetus to bring the feet to the outlet in labor.

podarthritis (pŏd-ar-thrī'tĭs) [" + *arthron,* joint, + *-ītis,* inflammation]. Inflammation of joints of the feet. Syn: *podagra.*

podiatrist (po-di'ăt-rĭst) [G. *pous, pod-,* foot, + *iatreia,* treatment]. Specialist in foot diseases. Syn: *chiropodist.*

podiatry (po-di'ăt-rĭ) [" + *iatreia,* healing]. Treatment of foot disorders. Syn: *chiropody.*

podo-, pod- [G.]. Combining forms meaning *foot.*

podobromidrosis (pŏd"ō-brō-mĭ-drō'sĭs) [" + *bromos,* stench, + *idrōsis,* perspiration]. Offensive perspiration of the feet.

pododynamometer (pŏd"ō-dī-nă-mŏm'ĕt-ĕr) [" + *dynamis,* force, + *metron,* measure]. A device for testing strength of the leg and foot muscles.

pododynia (pŏd-ō-dĭn'ĭ-ă) [" + *odynē,* pain]. Pain in the feet, esp. a neuralgic pain in the heel with swelling and redness.

podogram (pŏd'ō-grăm) [" + *gramma,* a mark]. An imprint of the sole of the foot.

podology (pŏd-ŏl'ō-jĭ) [" + *logos,* a study]. The study of the anatomy and physiology of the foot.

podophyllum (pŏd-ō-fĭl'ŭm) [G. *pous, pod-,* foot, + *phyllon,* leaf]. USP. Mandrake; May apple. An herb grown extensively in eastern U. S. and parts of the South.

p., resin of. A cathartic.

pogoniasis (pō-gō-nī'ăs-ĭs) [G. *pōgōn,* beard, + *-iasis,* disorder]. 1. Excessive growth of the beard. 2. Growth of a beard in a woman.

pogonion (pō-go'nĭ-ŏn) [G. *pōgōn,* beard]. The most anterior projecting midpoint of the chin.

-poietic (poy-ĕt'ĭk) [G.]. Suffix meaning making or producing.

poikilocyte (poy'kĭl-ō-sīt) [G. *poikilos,* various, + *kytos,* cell]. A large, irregular, malformed blood corpuscle.

poikilocytosis (poy"kĭl-ō-sī-tō'sĭs) [" + " + *-ōsis,* intensive]. Variation in shape of red blood corpuscles; a condition characterized by poikilocytes in the blood.

poikiloderma (poy-kĭl-ō-dĕr'mă). A skin disorder characterized by pigmentation, telangiectasis, purpura, pruritus, and atrophy.

poikilothermal (poy"kĭl-ō-thĕr'măl) [" + *thermē,* heat]. Varying in temperature according to environment.

point (poynt) [O.Fr. *point,* a prick, a dot]. 1. The sharp end of any object. 2. Point at which an abscess is about to rupture on a surface. See: *fixation.* 3. A minute spot. 4. Position in space, time, or degree.

p., anterior focal. Same as focal p.

p., anterior nodal. See: *p.'s, nodal.*

p., auricular. Center of external orifice of auditory canal.

p., Boas'. Tender spot in gastric ulcer left of 12th thoracic vertebra.

p., boiling. The temperature at which a liquid will boil.

p., Broca's. Center of the ext. auditory meatus; the *auricular point.*

p.'s, Capuron's. Four fixed points in pelvic inlet, the two iliopectineal eminences and the two sacroiliac joints.

p.'s, cardinal. 1. Six p.'s determining direction of light rays emerging from and entering the eye. 2. Capuron's points, above. See: *p.'s, principal; p.'s, nodal.*

p.'s, corresponding. Point in the retina of the two eyes which, when stimulated simultaneously, result in a single visual sensation.

p., craniometric. One of the fixed points of the skull used in craniometry.

p., critical, of gases. Temperature at or above which a gas can no longer be liquefied by pressure.

p., critical, of liquids. Temperature above which no pressure may retain a body in a liquid form.

p.'s, deaf, of the ear. Point at lower end of tragus and one where helix intersects line of motion when vibrating tuning fork held in front of ear cannot be heard when started from the lower edge of the zygoma and moved backward toward the occiput.

p., dew. The temperature at which moisture begins to be deposited as dew.

p., disparate. Points on the retinae unequally paired.

p., external orbital. The prominent p. at outer edge of orbit above the frontomalar suture.

p., far. The point (20 ft. or more) at which distinct vision is possible without aid of the muscles of accommodation. It is nearer than 20 ft. according to degree of myopia. There is no far point in the hypermetropic eye.

p., fixation. That at which the two visual axes converge.

p., freezing. Temperature at which liquids become solid.

p.'s, hysterogenic. Circumscribed areas of the body which produce symptoms of a hysterical aura, and eventually a hysterical attack when rubbed or pressed.

p.'s, identical retinal. P.'s in the two retinae upon which the images are seen as one.

p., jugal. Posterior border of frontal process of the malar bone where cut by a line tangent to upper border of zygoma.

p., lacrimal. Outlet of lacrimal canaliculus. Syn: *puncta lacrimalia.*

p., Lanz's. Point on line between two anterior superior iliac spines, one third of the distance from right spine, indicating origin of the vermiform appendix.

p., Lian's. One at junction of outer and middle thirds of a line from the umbilicus to anterior superior spine of ilium where trocar may be introduced safely for paracentesis.

p., malar. The most prominent point on external tubercle of the malar bone.

p., McBurney's. One between 1½ and 2 in. above anterior superior spine of ilium, on line between the ilium and umbilicus, where pressure shows tenderness in acute appendicitis.

p., motor. A point usually about the middle of a muscle where a motor nerve enters the muscle at which a minimal electrical stimulus to the overlying skin will elicit a visible contraction.

p., Munro's. One halfway between left anterior iliac spine and the umbilicus.

p.'s, nasal genital. Point at anterior end of lower turbinated bone, and one at the tuberculum septi, irritation of which, when in a hyperesthetic state, produces pain in the hypogastrium and in sacral region.

p., near. Nearest one at which the eye can accommodate for distinct vision.

p.'s, nodal. An anterior and posterior cardinal point on the surface of lens of the eye so related that every ray directed toward the anterior point is represented after refraction by a ray emanating from the posterior point.

p.'s, painful. Points over which a neuralgic nerve is tender on pressure.

p.'s, pressure. 1. Points on the skin which, when stimulated, give rise to sensation of pressure. 2. Points where arteries come near to the surface and at which pressure may be applied to stop arterial bleeding.

p.'s, principal. Two p.'s so situated that the optical axis is cut by the two principal planes.

p.'s, Valleix's. Tender spots upon pressure over the course of a nerve in neuralgia. SYN: *points douloureux.*

pointillage (pwăhn-tĭ-yahzh') [Fr.]. Massage with the finger tips.

pointing. Reaching a point.

p. of an abscess. An abscess which is about to rupture spontaneously.

p., past. Inability to accurately place finger or some other part of the body on a selected point. Seen in certain neurologic disorders.

Poiseuille's law (pwă-sū-ēz'). The rapidity of the capillary current is in direct proportion to the square of the diameter of the capillary tube, the pressure on the fluid, and indirectly to the viscosity of the liquid and length of the tube.

P.'s layer or ***space.*** The inert capillary current in which leukocytes move slowly, the erythrocytes moving more rapidly in the middle current.

poison (poy'zn) [L. *potiō,* a poisonous draft]. Any substance which, taken into the body whether by ingestion, inhalation, injection, absorption, etc., interferes with normal physiologic functions. Virtually any substance can be poisonous if consumed in sufficient quantity so that the term poison more often implies an excessive degree of dosage rather than any list of substances. Aspirin is not usually thought of as a poison, but overdoses of this drug kill more children accidentally each year than any of the traditional poisons. Since the list of poisonous substances is virtually infinite, it defies classification in any simple way. One of the most widely employed classifications is found in *Standard Nomenclature of Diseases and Operations,* 5th ed., McGraw-Hill Book Co., Inc., New York, 1961. For a list of commonly encountered hazardous substances in the home, SEE: *Poisons and Poisoning Table in Appendix, App. 97.*

p., economic. Pesticides. Chemicals whose toxic properties are commercially exploited in agriculture, industry or commerce to increase quantity, improve quality or generally to promote the consumer acceptability of a variety of products. Common types of economic poisons include insecticides, rodenticides, herbicides, fungicides, insect repellants, molluscicides and some kinds of food additives. The wide variety of economic poisons that are commonly found in and around the home constitutes an important group in accidental poisonings. SEE: *Poisons and Poisoning Table in Appendix, App. 97.*

poison control center. A facility meeting the staffing and equipment standards of the American Association of Poison Control Centers and recognized to be able to give information on, or treatment to patients suffering from, poisoning. A poison information center consists only of a reference library, and does not have treatment facilities. Over 400 poison centers of these two types are scattered throughout the U. S. Staffed largely by volunteer personnel, they offer service at any time of the day or night. By virtue of their function, they are commonly associated with or are part of large hospitals or medical schools. A government agency—the Poison Control Branch of the Division of Accident Prevention, Public Health Service, Department of Health, Education and Welfare—is also active in poison control programs and in coordinating the efforts of individual centers.

poison ivy. A climbing vine, *Rhus toxicodendron,* which on contact produces a severe form of dermatitis. *Rhus* species contain urushiol, an extremely irritating oily resin. Urushiol may also be a potent sensitizer since in many cases subsequent contacts produce increasingly severe reactions.

p. i. dermatitis. Dermatitis resulting from irritation or sensitization of the skin by the resin of the poison ivy plant.

IMMUNITY: There is no absolute immunity though susceptibility varies greatly even in the same individual.

SYM: Always an interval between time of contact of poison with skin and first appearance of symptoms, varying from a few hours to several days, and depending on sensitivity of the patient and possibly condition of skin. Moderate itching or burning sensation soon followed by small blisters; later manifestations vary. Blisters usually rupture and are followed by oozing of serum and subsequent crusting.

FA: Thorough washing of the skin with soap and water and complete change of clothing are advised if there has been known exposure.

TREATMENT: In mild dermatitis, a lotion to relieve itching is usually sufficient. In severe dermatitis, cool wet dressings or compresses, potassium permanganate baths, and perhaps a course of intramuscular or oral corticosteroid therapy are advised. Sedation is also necessary in some cases.

poison oak. A climbing vine, *Rhus radicans* or *R. diversiloba,* closely related to poison ivy and containing the same active principle. The symptoms and treatment are identical with those for poison ivy dermatitis, *q.v.*

poison sumac. A shrub-like plant, *Rhus vernix,* widely distributed in the U. S. as are all *Rhus* species. Since it contains the same active principle as poison ivy, the symptoms and treatment are the same as in poison ivy dermatitis, *q.v.*

poisoning (poy'zn-ing) [L. *potiō,* a poisonous draft]. 1. The state produced by introduction of a poison into the body. 2. Administration of a poison. The symptoms of poisoning vary widely with the agent. SEE: *Poisons and Poisoning Table in Appendix.*

FIRST AID: Avoid becoming excited. Contact a physician or a poison control center immediately and explain the nature of the emergency. Attempt to identify the nature of the poison by looking for the container, questioning the patient, noting burns, stains, odors or symptoms. Do not discard the poison; keep a sample and the original container, but clean up any spilled material which might be a hazard to another member of the family. If the patient vomits, preserve a sample of the vomitus. Take all specimens and containers to the hospital with the patient.

Dilute the poison at once with large quantities of milk, water or a slurry of activated charcoal in water. Diluting delays absorption, and it is easier to induce emesis when the stomach is full. Do not attempt to induce emesis in an unconscious or stuporous patient or if strong alkali, mineral acid or kerosene was ingested.

The following suggestions are to be employed only if they will not delay professional treatment appreciably. The primary emphasis should be directed toward getting the patient to a medical facility in the shortest possible time.

Emesis may be induced by stroking or gently tickling the back of the patient's throat with a finger or the handle of a teaspoon. Sometimes a glass or two of warm water containing either 3 teaspoonsful of table salt or 1 teaspoonful of dry mustard will produce vomiting.

If attempts to induce vomiting are successful, readminister large amounts of milk, condensed milk, egg whites, flour and water or a slurry of activated charcoal in water.

If material was spilled on the patient's skin, clothing, or splashed in the eyes, discard the garments and flush with running tap water. It may be necessary to hold the victim's eyelids open under water to effect good rinsing. If the material is a gas or a vapor, remove the patient and other persons from the area.

Make notes of all that is said by the patient, but do not repeat any of this to anyone except the physician or a court official.

If the patient is unconscious and shows signs of impending vomiting, lay him on his side with his head a few inches below the rest of his body. Watch for difficulty in breathing and be prepared to give artificial respiration if the patient stops spontaneous breathing.

If the patient convulses, do nothing except prevent him from falling or otherwise injuring himself. Blankets, wet compresses and gentle massage can do no harm and may serve some purpose. Strong black coffee or tea should be given if the patient becomes drowsy.

NOTE: Do not be hasty in concluding that a patient has been poisoned. Many disease states can mimic the symptoms of poisoning by a variety of substances. Cerebral hemorrhage, epilepsy, overdose of insulin, diabetic coma, meningitis, thrombosis and uremia may all simulate poisoning. Acute indigestion, appendicitis, gastritis, renal colic, or peptic ulcer may mimic poisoning by corrosive substances.

p., acute. A state of intoxication produced by a single rapidly administered dose. Acute poisoning does not refer to the rapidity with which symptoms develop after exposure to a toxic agent although it follows that a large dose of a poison given rapidly usually produces symptoms within a relatively short time.

p., blood. SEE: *bacteremia; pyemia; septicemia; toxemia.*

p., chronic. A state of intoxication produced by multiple small doses given over a period of time not one dose of which would have produced the full toxic syndrome if given alone.

p., convulsive. SEE: *convulsant poisons.*

p., corrosive. SEE: *corrosive poisons.*

p., cumulative. Chronic poisoning.

p., fish. SEE: *fish poisoning.*

p., food. SEE: *food poisoning.*

p. [by] unknown substances. In cases where no information is available about the nature of the poison taken, and the signs and symptoms are not recognized as being due to any particular substance, it is obvious that specific antidotes cannot be given. There are, however, certain agents which act in a general manner and may be efficacious. One of these is activated charcoal which is available from many sources. Although a slurry of this in water is messy and offensive to the patient, it is a highly effective adsorbent for certain kinds of poisons.

Another material is referred to as the "universal antidote." It consists of a mixture of 2 parts activated charcoal, 1 part magnesium oxide and 1 part tannic acid. The universal antidote has been used empirically for a number of years and pre-packaged units are now commercially available. It is doubtful if this mixture offers any real advantage over activated charcoal alone which has a proven effectiveness against many substances.

Both these materials may be given as a slurry made from several heaping teaspoonsful in a glass of water. Since the ingredients are essentially harmless and since the efficiency is increased by increasing the amount of adsorbent relative to the amount of poison, the dose may be repeated several times.

poi'sonous. Having the properties or qualities of a poison; venomous.

p. plants. *Do not eat:* castor bean, chinaberry, European bittersweet, wild or black cherry, horse chestnuts, poisonous hemlock, laurel, mushroom or death cup, black nightshade or deadly nightshade, Jimson weed. *Do not touch:* poison ivy, poison oak, poison sumac.

poker back. Stiffness of the spine. May result from spondylitis, *q.v.*, or rheumatoid arthritis.

pokeroot (pōk'rōōt). The dried root of Veratrum viride used internally as an antihypertensive agent.

p. poisoning. Poisoning resulting from ingestion of pokeroot.

SYM: Nausea, vomiting, drowsiness, vertigo, and possibly convulsions and respiratory paralysis.

TREATMENT: Emetic or lavage.

polar [L. *polus*, pole, from G. *polos*, axis]. Concerning a pole.

polarimeter (pō-lar-ĭm'ĕt-ĕr) [" + G. *metron*, a measure]. Instrument for measuring amount of polarization of light, or rotation of polarized light.

polarimetry (pō-lar-ĭm'ĕt-rĭ) [" + G. *metron*, a measure]. Measurement of the amount and rotation of polarized light.

polariscope (pō-lar'ĭ-skōp) [" + G. *skopein*, to examine]. Apparatus used in measurement of polarized light.

polarity (pō-lar'ĭt-ĭ) [L. *polus*, pole]. P.T. 1. The quality of having poles. 2. The exhibition of opposite effects at the two extremities.

polarization (pō-lăr-ĭ-zā'shŭn) [L. *polus*, pole]. 1. Condition in a ray of light in which vibrations occur in only one plane or in curves. 2. In a galvanic battery, collection of hydrogen bubbles on negative plate and oxygen on the positive plate, whereby generation of current is impeded. 3. Condition in which ions of opposite charges are separated by a semipermeable membrane such as a cell membrane.

pole (pōl) [L. *polus*, a pole, from G. *polos*, axis]. 1. The extremity of any axis about which forces acting on it are symmetrically disposed. 2. One of two points in a magnet, cell, or battery having opposite physical qualities.

p., animal. One opposite the yolk in an ovum. At this point, polar bodies are formed and pinched off and protoplasm is concentrated and has greatest activity.

p.'s of the eye. The anterior and posterior extremities of the optic axis.

p., frontal. Most projecting part of the anterior extremity of both cerebral hemispheres.

p., germinal. The p. of an ovum at which the development begins.

p.'s of the kidney. The kidney's upper and lower extremities.

p., occipital. The posterior emtremity of the occipital lobe.

p., pelvic. Breech of a fetus.

p., placental, of the chorion. Spot at which the domelike placenta is situated.

p., temporal. The anterior extremity of the temporal lobe.

p.'s of the testicle. The upper and lower extremities of a testicle.

p., vegetal. Part of the egg containing the food yolk. Also called *vegetative* or *antigerminal pole.*

policlinic (pŏl-ĭ-klĭn'ĭk) [G. *polis*, city, + *klinē*, bed]. A city hospital or clinic for outpatients. SEE ALSO: *polyclinic.*

pol'io. Acute anterior poliomyelitis, *q.v.*

polioclastic (pŏl″ĭ-ō-klăs'tĭk) [G. *polios*, gray, + *klastos*, breaking]. Destructive of the gray matter of the nervous system.

polioencephalitis (pŏl″ĭ-ō-ĕn-sĕf-ăl-ī'tĭs) [G. *polios*, gray, + *egkephalos*, brain, + *-itis*, inflammation). Condition characterized by lesions sometimes inflammatory of the gray matter of the brain. SYM: *Fever, vomiting, convulsions.*

p. acuta. Acute inflammation of the cerebral cortex giving rise to infantile cerebral palsy in children.

p., anterior superior. SYN: *Wernicke's encephalopathy.* A disease involving necrotic changes in gray matter about 3rd ventricle, ant. portion of 4th ventricle and aqueduct of Sylvius. Characterized by ocular abnormalities, mental disturbances, and ataxia. Of nutritional origin, probably thiamine (vitamin B_1) deficiency.

p. hemorrhagica. P. accompanied by hemorrhagic lesions.

p., posterior. P. involving gray matter about 4th ventricle.

polioencephalomeningomyelitis (pŏl″ĭ-ō-ĕn-sĕf″ăl-ō-men-ĭng-ō-mī-ĕl-ī'tĭs) [" + *egkephalos*, brain, + *mēnigx*, membrane, + *myelos*, marrow, + *-ītis*, inflammation]. Inflammation of the gray matter of the brain and spinal cord and their meninges.

polioencephalomyelitis (pŏl″ĭ-ō-ĕn-sĕf″ăl-ō-mī-ĕl-ī'tĭs) [" + " + *myelos*, marrow, + *-ītis*, inflammation]. Inflamed condition of the gray matter of the brain and spinal cord. SYN: *Heine-Medin disease.*

polioencephalopathy (pŏl″ĭ-ō-ĕn-sĕf-ăl-ŏp'ăth-ĭ) [" + " + *pathos*, disease]. Diseased condition of the gray matter of the brain.

poliomyelencephalitis (pŏl″ĭ-ō-mī-ĕl-ĕn″-sĕf-ăl-ī'tĭs) [" + *myelos*, marrow, + *egkephalos*, brain, + *-ītis*, inflammation]. Poliomyelitis with polioencephalitis.

poliomyelitis (pŏl″ĭ-ō-mī-ĕl-ī'tĭs) [G. *polios*, gray, + *myelos*, marrow, + *-ītis*, inflammation]. Inflammation of the gray matter of the spinal cord.

p., abortive. P. in which illness is mild with no involvement of central nervous system.

p., acute anterior. An acute infectious inflammation of the anterior horns of the gray matter of the spinal cord. SYN: *spinal paralytic paralysis; acute lateral paralysis; infantile paralysis; epidemic paralysis; polio; Heine-Medin's disease; acute wasting paralysis.*

This is an acute, systemic, infectious disease in which paralysis may or may not occur. In the majority of patients, the disease is mild, being limited to respiratory and gastrointestinal symptoms such constituting the *minor illness* or the *abortive type*, which lasts only a few days. In the *major illness*, paralysis or weakness of muscles occurs with loss of superficial and deep reflexes. In such cases, characteristic lesions are found in the gray matter of the spinal cord, medulla, motor area of cerebral cortex, and cerebellum.

ETIOL: Causative agent is a virus, consisting of particles 8 to 30 millimicrons in diameter. The virus is resistant and stable, remaining viable for months outside the body. Three immunologic types exist, I (Brunhilde), II (Lansing), and III (Leon).

SYM: Onset is often abrupt, though the ordinary manifestations of a severe cold or some gastrointestinal disturbances may come on gradually, accompanied by slight elevation of temperature, frequently enduring for not more than 3 days. At the end of this period, paralysis may or may not develop. The extent of any paralysis necessarily depends upon degree of nerve involvement. Consequently, paralysis may be confined to one small group of muscles or affect one or all extremities. In some instances, the respiratory muscles are also involved, and it is in these cases that death is so likely to ensue. In the average paralytic case it is the extensor muscles in particular that are affected.

COMPLICATIONS: Any paralysis occurring in this disease may be regarded as a complication. Atrophy of muscles and ultimate deformities may likewise be classed in a similar way. Aside from bronchopneumonia, which may develop in very severe cases, other complications are surprisingly few.

DIFFERENTIAL DIAG: Among the diseases confused with this infection are the various types of meningitis, rheumatism, traumatic conditions, tuberculosis involving bones or joints, and occasionally scurvy or rickets in infants.

INCIDENCE: Poliomyelitis is endemic throughout the world but occurs in epidemics in certain countries, including the U.S. Epidemics are seasonal, occurring in summer and fall. Children are more susceptible than adults. Infection is spread by direct contact, the virus probably entering the body via mouth. How it reaches the central nervous system is not known.

INCUBATION PERIOD: From 3 to 21 days, but usually 7 to 12 days.

PROG: Ordinarily, the outcome as to life is good. It is only the bulbar and respiratory types in which death is likely to occur. In fact, these two types constitute nearly all of the fatal cases. Even in those cases in which paralysis is present, complete restoration of the parts may finally be brought about. In the more severe types, however, some paralysis may remain.

PROPHYLAXIS: Passive immunization with gamma globulin gives a limited amount of protection. Active immunization with Salk vaccine has greatly reduced the incidence of paralytic poliomyelitis. 1.0 cc. is administered I.M. twice, 4 to 6 weeks apart, followed by a third injection after an interval of 7 months. Annual booster doses should be given for maintenance of immunity.

The Sabin oral poliomyelitis vaccine is also used for active immunization. Three types of Sabin vaccine (types 1, 2, and 3) are administered at 4-week intervals in the following order: types 1, 3, and 2. Two drops of the vaccine are placed on a sugar cube which is then permitted to melt in the mouth and swallowed. It is believed that permanent immunity is obtained without booster doses; nevertheless children who are immunized as infants should receive a booster dose of vaccine at 15 months of age. This dose should contain all three types of the virus.

PREDISPOSING FACTORS: Tonsillectomy and other nose and throat operations, routine immunizations, excessive physical strain and fatigue. Pregnant women are especially susceptible during epidemics.

NP: No known specific drug treatment. Treatment is systematic, aimed at relieving symptoms, preventing deformities, and saving life. In abortive cases, bed rest for 7 to 10 days and light diet are adequate. In severe cases, muscle tenderness and pain are alleviated by proper positioning, gentle passive movement, and by application of hot, moist packs at 20-min. intervals or by hot baths for children. Mild analgesics and sedatives may be used. Fluid and salt balance should be maintained.

Retention of urine and constipation are troublesome complications. The former may be treated by a parasympathetic stimulating drug, the latter by mild laxatives and warm saline enemas.

Respiratory failure may occur in bulbar poliomyelitis. It may result from paralysis of respiratory muscles, failure of respiratory centers in the medulla, obstruction of air passageways resulting from weakness of pharyngeal or laryngeal muscles, or pulmonary edema. Oxygen administration, tracheotomy, or use of respirator may be indicated.

Convalescence of the paralyzed patient necessitates careful attention, often involving physical and occupational therapy and orthopedic treatment as well as an understanding and amelioration of psychological difficulties. Mechanical supports for weakened structures may be necessary.

p., anterior. Inflamed state of the anterior horns of the spinal cord.

p., ascending. P. in which paralysis begins in lower extremities and progresses up legs, thighs, trunk, and finally involves respiratory muscles.

p., bulbar. P. in which gray matter of the medulla oblongata is involved, resulting in paralysis and usually respiratory failure. Also called *bulbar paralytic poliomyelitis.* See discussion under *p., acute anterior*

p., chronic anterior. Progressive wasting of the muscles. Myelopathic progressive muscular atrophy.

p., epidemic. SEE: *poliomyelitis, acute anterior.*

p., nonparalytic. Pain and stiffness in the muscles of the axial skeleton, especially of the neck and back, mild fever, and increased proteins and leukocytes in the cerebrospinal fluid. Diagnosis depends on the isolation of the virus and serological reactions. SYN: *preparalytic p.*

p., paralytic. Poliomyelitis with a variable combination of signs of damage of the central nervous system. These include weakness, incoordination, muscle tenderness and spasms, flaccid paralysis, and disturbance of consciousness.

p., p., bulbar. See discussion under *p., acute anterior.*

p., p., spinal. Same as *p., acute anterior, q.v.*

poliomyelopathy (pŏl″ĭ-ō-mī-ĕl-ŏp′ăth-ĭ) [G. *polios,* gray, + *myelos,* marrow, + *pathos,* disease]. Any diseased condition of the gray matter of the spinal cord.

polioplasm (pŏl′ĭ-ō-plăzm) [“ + *plasma,* a thing formed]. Granular protoplasm.

poliosis (pŏl-ĭ-ō′sĭs) [“ + *-ōsis,* condition]. Absence of pigment in the hair. SYN: *canities; grayness.*

politzerization (pŏl″ĭ-tsĕr-ĭ-zā′shun). The inflation of the middle ear using a Politzer bag.

Politzer's bag (pŏl′ĭ-tzer) [Adam Politzer, Hungarian otologist, 1835-1920]. Soft rubber bag with rubber tip for inflating the middle ear by increasing the pressure in the nasopharynx.

pollakiuria (pŏl-ăk-ĭ-ū′rĭ-ă) [G. *pollakis,* often, + *ouron,* urine]. Abnormally frequent passage of urine.

pollen (pŏl′ĕn) [L. powder]. The microspores of a seed plant which develop in the anther at tip of stamen. Each pollen grain develops a *pollen tube* and constitutes the *male gametophyte.* Within it develops a *tube nucleus* and two *sperm nuclei,* the latter constituting the male reproductive elements.

pollenogenic (pŏl″ĕn-ō-jen′ĭk) [“ + G. *gennan,* to produce]. Due to the pollen of plants or producing plant pollen.

pollenosis (pŏl-ĕn-ō′sĭs) [“ + G. *-ōsis,* disease]. Pollinosis, *q.v.*

pollex (pŏl′ĕks) [L. thumb]. The thumb.

p. pedis. The great toe. SYN: *hallux.*

p. valgus. Abnormal deviation of thumb toward ulnar side.

p. varus. Abnormal deviation of thumb toward radial side.

pollinosis (pŏl-ĭn-ō′sĭs) [L. *pollen,* powder, + G. *-ōsis,* disease]. Nasal congestion of mucous membranes due to contact with pollen. SYN: *hay fever.*

pollution (pō-loo′shun). 1. State of making impure or defiling. 2. Voluntary or involuntary emission of semen at times other than in coition.

polonium (pō-lo′nĭ-ŭm). Radioactive element isolated from pitchblende. SYMB: Po. At. wt. 210; at. no. 84. SYN: *radium F.*

polus (pō′lŭs) [L.]. Pole.

poly- [G.]. Prefix meaning *many* or *much.*

poly. (pŏl′ĭ). Abbr. for *polymorphonuclear leukocyte.*

polyadenitis (pŏl-ĭ-ad-ĕ-nī′tĭs). Condition of inflamed lymph nodes especially the cervical lymph nodes.

polyadenomatosis (pŏl″ĭ-ăd-ĕ-nō-mă-tō′-sĭs) [" + *aden*, gland, + *-ōma*, tumor, + *-ōsis*, disease]. Adenomas in many glands.

polyadenous (pŏl-ĭ-ad′ē-nŭs) [" + *adēn*, gland]. Involving or relating to many glands.

polyalgesia (pol″ĭ-ăl-je′zĭ-ă) [" + *algēsis*, sensation]. A single stimulus of a part, producing sensation in many parts.

polyandry (pol″ĭ-an′drĭ) [" + *aner, andr-*, man]. The practice of having more than one husband at the same time. SEE: *polygamy*.

polyarteritis (pol″ĭ-ar-ter-ī′tĭs) [" + *artēria*, artery, + *-ītis*, inflammation]. Inflammation of several arteries at the same time.

p. nodosa. Widespread focal areas of damage due to inflammation of arteries, especially small and medium-sized ones. Function of organs involved is impaired. When the disease begins, its manifestations are extremely variable. Symptoms of a moderate febrile disease are quite common. SYN: *periarteritis nodosa*.

polyarthric (pŏl″ĭ-ar′thrĭk) [" + *arthron*, joint]. Affecting or pert. to several joints.

polyarthritis (pol-ĭ-ar-thrī′tis) [G. *polys*, many, + *arthron*, joint, + *-itis*, inflammation]. Inflammation of a number of joints.

polyarticular (pŏl″ĭ-ar-tĭk′ū-lar) [" + L. *articulus*, a joint]. Affecting many joints. SYN: *multiarticular*.

polyatomic (pol″ĭ-ă-tom′ĭk) [" + *atomon*, atom]. Having several atoms or more than two replaceable hydrogen atoms.

polyblast (pŏl′ĭ-blăst) [" + *blastos*, a germ]. Large mononuclear phagocyte present in inflammation derived from an embryonic wandering cell.

polyblennia (pŏl-ĭ-blĕn′nĭ-ă) [" + *blennos*, mucus]. Secretion of more mucus than normal.

polycholia (pŏl-ĭ-kō′lĭ-ă) [" + *cholē*, bile]. Abnormal secretion of bile.

polychrest (pol′ĭ-krĕst) [" + *chrēstos*, useful]. A medicine useful in many diseases.

polychromasia (pŏl″ĭ-krō-mā′zĭ-ă) [" + *chrōma*, color]. Quality of having many colors.

polychromatic (pŏl″ĭ-krō-măt′ĭk) [" + *chrōma*, color]. Multicolored.

polychromatophil (pŏl″ĭ - krō - măt′ō - fĭl) [G. *polys*, many, + *chrōma*, color, + *philein*, to love]. A cell, esp. an erythrocyte, which is stainable with more than one kind of stain.

polychromatophile. Alternate spelling for *polychromatophil, q.v.*

polychromatophilia (pol″ĭ-krō-măt-ō-fĭl′-ĭ-ă) [" + " + *philein*, to love]. 1. The quality of being stainable with more than one stain. 2. Polychromatophil cells in the blood to excess.

polychromemia (pŏl-ĭ-krō-mē′mĭ-ă) [G. *polys*, many, + *chrōma*, color, + *aima*, blood]. Increase in the hemoglobin of the blood.

polychylia (pŏl″ĭ-kī′lĭ-ă) [" + *chylos* juice]. Excessive secretion of chyle.

polyclinic (pŏl-ĭ-klĭn′ĭk) [" + *klinē*, bed] Hospital or clinic treating many diseases; a general hospital.

polyclonia (pŏl″ĭ-klō′nĭ-ă) [" + *klonos*, tumult]. A disease characterized by many clonic spasms but distinct from chorea or tic.

polycoria (pŏl-ĭ-kō′rĭ-ă) [" + *korē*, pupil]. The state of having more than one pupil in one eye.

polycrotic (pŏl-ĭ-krŏt′ĭk) [" + *krotos*, a beat]. Having several pulse waves for each heart beat.

polycrotism (pŏl-ĭk′rōt-ĭzm) [" + " + *ismos*, a beat]. Condition of having several pulse waves for each heart beat.

polycystic (pŏl-ĭ-sĭs′tĭk) [" + *kystis*, a bladder]. Composed of many cysts.

polycythemia (pŏl″ĭ-sī-thē′mĭ-ă) [" + *kytos*, cell, + *aima*, blood]. An excess of red blood cells. SEE: *erythrocytosis*.

p. megalosplenica, p., myelopathic, p. rubra, p., splenomegalic, p. vera. Polycythemia vera, *q.v.*

p., primary. P. in which there is hyperplasia of blood-forming cells in bone marrow. SYN: *p. vera, q.v.*

p., relative. Relative increase in number of erythrocytes which occurs in hemoconcentration.

p., secondary. P. resulting from some physiological condition such as lowered oxygen tension in the blood which stimulates erythropoiesis. SYN: *erythrocytosis; symptomatic p.*

p., splenomegalic. P. in which enlargement of the spleen occurs. SEE: *p. vera.*

p. vera. A slowly progressive disease characterized by an increased number of red blood cells and increase in total blood volume. SYN: *erythremia; p., primary; p. rubra; splenomegalic p.; Osler's disease; Vaquez's disease.*

SYM AND SIGNS: Weakness, fatigue, vertigo, tinnitus, irritability, enlarged spleen, flushing of face, redness and pain of extremities, black and blue spots. Basal metabolism increased and bone marrow shows increased cellularity.

ETIOL: Unknown.

TREATMENT: Permanent cure cannot be achieved today, but remissions of many months can be produced. Venesection and radioactive phosphorus (^{32}P) have proved to be effective.

polydactylism (pŏl″ĭ-dăk′tĭ-lĭzm) [" + *daktylos*, digit, + *-ismos*, condition]. State of having supernumerary fingers or toes.

polydipsia (pŏl-ĭ-dĭp′sĭ-ă) [" + *dipsa*, thirst]. Excessive thirst.

polyemia (pol-ĭ-ē′mĭ-ă) [" + *aima*, blood]. Abnormal amount of blood in the system. SYN: *polycythemia*.

polyesthesia (pŏl″ĭ-ĕs-thē′zĭ-ă) [G. *polys*, many, + *aisthēsis*, sensation]. Abnormal sensation of touch in which a single stimulus is felt at two or more places.

polyesthetic (pŏl″ĭ-ĕs-thĕt′ĭk) [G. *polys*, many, + *aisthēsis*, sensation]. 1. Pert. to polyesthesia, *q.v.* 2. Pert. to several senses or sensations.

polygalactia (pŏl″ĭ-găl-ăk′shĭ-ă) [" + *gala, galakt-*, milk]. Excessive secretion or flow of milk.

polygamy (pō-lĭg′ă-mĭ) [G. *polys*, many, + *gamos*, marriage]. Practice of having several wives or husbands at the same time, esp. wives.

polygastria (pŏl″ĭ-găs′trĭ-ă). Excessive secretion or flow of gastric juice.

polyglandular (pŏl″ĭ-glăn′dū-lar) [" + L. *glandula*, a little kernel]. Pert. to or affecting many glands. SYN: *pluriglandular*.

polyglobulia, polyglobulism (pŏl″ĭ-glō-bū′-lĭ-ă, -glŏb′ū-lĭzm) [" + L. *globulus*, globule, + G. *-ismos*, condition]. Increase in number of red corpuscles in the blood. SYN: *polycythemia*.

polygram (pŏl′ĭ-grăm) [" + *gramma*, a mark]. Sphygmographic record made by polygraph of pulse beats simultaneously.

polygraph (pŏl′ĭ-grăf) [" + *graphein*, to write]. A device which records simultaneously tracings of several different pulsations, as arterial and venous pulse waves, apex beat of heart, and other pulsations. SYN: *sphygmograph.*

polygyria (pŏl-ĭ-jī'rĭ-ă) [" + *gyros,* circle]. Excess of the number of convolutions in the brain.

polyhedral (pŏl-ĭ-hē'drăl) [" + *edra,* base]. Having many surfaces.

polyhemia (pŏl"ĭ-hē'mĭ-ă) [" + *aima,* blood]. Abnormal increase in amount of the blood. SYN: *polyemia.*

polyhidrosis (pŏl-ĭ-hĭ-drō'sĭs) [" + *idrōsis,* perspiration]. Excessive perspiration.

polyhydramnios (pŏl-ĭ-hī-drăm'nĭ-ŏs) [" + *ydōr,* water, + *amnion,* amnion]. An excess of amniotic fluid in the bag-of-waters in pregnancy. SEE: *amnion.*

polyhydruria (pŏl"ĭ-hī-drū'rĭ-ă) [" + " + *ouron,* urine]. Excessive amt. of water in urine.

polyhypermenorrhea (pŏl"ĭ-hī-pĕr-mĕn-ō-rē'ă) [G. *polys,* many, + *yper,* over, + *mēn,* month, + *roia,* flow]. Frequent menstruation with excessive discharge.

polyhypomenorrhea (pŏl-ĭ-hī-pō-mĕn-ō-rē'ă) [" + *ypo,* under, + *mēn,* month, + *roia,* flow]. Frequent menstruation with scanty discharge.

polyinfection (pŏl"ĭ-ĭn-fĕk'shŭn) [" + L. *infectiō,* a making in]. Infection with two or more microorganisms. SYN: *multi-infection.*

polykaryocyte (pŏl-ĭ-kar'ĭ-ō-sīt) [" + *karyon,* nucleus, + *kytos,* cell]. A cell possessing several nuclei.

polyleptic (pŏl"ĭ-lĕp'tĭk) [" + *lēpsis,* a seizure, from *lambanein,* to seize]. Characterized by numerous remissions and exacerbations, as malaria.

polymastia (pŏl-ĭ-măs'tĭ-ă) [" + *mastos, mazos,* breast]. Condition of having more than two breasts.

polymastigote (pŏl-ĭ-măs'tĭ-gōt) [" + *mastix, mastig-,* whip]. Possessing several flagella.

polymazia (pol"ĭ-ma'zĭ-ă). Condition of having more than two breasts.

polymenia (pŏl-ĭ-mē'nĭ-ă) [G. *polys,* many. + *mēn,* month]. Same as polymenorrhea, *q.v.*

polymenorrhea (pŏl"ĭ-mĕn-or-rē'ă) [" + " + *roia,* a flow]. Menstrual flow occurring too frequently. SYN: *polymenia.*

polymer (pŏl'ĭ-mer) [G. *polys,* many, + *meros,* a part]. A substance formed by a combination of two or more molecules of the same substance. Ex: paraformaldehyde $(HCHO)_3$ formed from three molecules of formaldehyde, HCHO.

polymeria (pŏl-ĭ-mē'rĭ-ă) [" + *meros,* a part]. Condition of having supernumerary parts of the body.

polymeric (pŏl-ĭ-mĕr'ĭk) [" + *meros,* a part]. 1. Consisting of the same elements in same proportions by weight, but differing in molecular weight. 2. Said of muscles derived from more than one myotome.

polymerism (pŏl'ĭ-mĕr-ĭzm, pō-lĭm'ĕr-ĭzm) [" + *meros,* part, + *ismos,* condition]. 1. Condition of having more than normal number of parts. SYN: *polymeria.* 2. Isomerism in which the molecular weights of the polymers are multiples of each other.

polymerization (pŏl"ĭ-mĕr-ĭ-zā'shŭn) [" + *meros,* part]. Process of changing into another compound having same elements in same proportions, but a higher molecular weight.

polymitus (po-lim'ĭ-tŭs) [G. *polys,* many, + *mitos,* thread]. Stage in reproduction of microorganisms with threads of protoplasm which, being detached, constitute the microgamete.

polymorph (pol'ĭ-morf). A polymorphonuclear leukocyte.

polymorphic (pŏl-ĭ-mor'fĭk) [" + *morphē,* form]. Occurring in more than one form.

polymorphism (pŏl-ĭ-mor'fĭzm) [" + " + *-ismos,* condition]. 1. Capacity for appearing in many forms. 2. Existence of several types in the same group or species. SYN: *pleomorphism.*

polymorphocellular (pŏl"ĭ-mor-fō-sĕl'ū-lar) [" + " + L. *cellula,* a small chamber]. Composed of cells of many forms.

polymorphonuclear (pŏl"ĭ-mor-fō-nū'klē-ar) [G. *polys,* many, + *morphē,* form, + L. *nucleus,* a kernel]. Possessing a nucleus consisting of several parts or lobes connected by fine strands.

p. leukocyte. A white blood cell which possesses a nucleus composed of two or more lobes or parts; a granulocyte (neutrophil, eosinophil, basophil).

polymorphous (pŏl-ĭ-mor'fŭs) [" + *morphē,* form]. Appearing in many forms. SYN: *polymorphic.*

polymyoclonus (pŏl-ĭ-mī-ŏk'lō-nŭs) [G. *polys,* many, + *mys, myo-,* muscle, + *klonos,* tumult]. A shocklike muscular contraction, occurring in various parts at the same time. SYN: *myoclonus multiplex; paramyoclonus.*

polymyositis (pŏl-ĭ-mī-ō-sī'tĭs) [" + " + *-itis,* inflammation]. Simultaneous inflammation of many muscles.

polymyxin (pŏl-ĭ-mĭks'ĭn). One of several closely related antibiotics isolated from *Bacillus polymyxa* and designated polymyxins A, B, C, D, and E.

p. B. Least toxic of the antibiotic fractions of polymyxin, and the only one used therapeutically.

polynesic (pŏl-ĭ-nē'sĭk) [" + *nēsos,* an island]. Appearing in many separate locations or foci.

polyneural (pŏl-ĭ-nū'răl) [" + *neuron,* sinew]. Pert. to, innervated, or supplied by many nerves.

polyneuralgia (pŏl"ĭ-nū-ral'jĭ-ă) [" + " + *algos,* pain]. Neuralgia in several nerves.

polyneuritic (pŏl"ĭ-nū-rĭt'ĭk) [" + " + *-itis,* inflammation]. Suffering from inflammation of several nerves at once.

p. psychosis. P. seen in chronic alcoholism with disturbed orientation, polyneuritis, hallucinations, falsification of memory, etc.

polyneuritis (pŏl-ĭ-nū-rī'tĭs) [" + " + *-itis,* inflammation]. A neuritis involving two or more nerves, usually a large number.

p., acute idiopathic. SYN: *infectious polyneuritis, Landry's paralysis, Guillain-Barré syndrome.* A disorder of peripheral nerves characterized by ascending muscular weakness, impairment of reflexes, and sensory disorders. Often follows a febrile illness. Cause unknown.

p., Jamaica ginger. P. esp. of nerves of extremities following ingestion of Jamaica ginger. SYN: *ginger paralysis.*

p., metabolic. P. resulting from metabolic disorders such as nutritional deficiency, esp. lack of thiamine, gastrointestinal disorders, or pathologic conditions such as diabetes, pernicious anemia, toxemias of pregnancy, etc.

p., toxic. P. resulting from poisons such as heavy metals, alcohol, carbon monoxide, various organic compounds, etc.

polyneuropathy (pol"ĭ-nu-rop'ă-thĭ). Term applied to any disorder or affection of peripheral nerves but preferably restricted to those of a noninflammatory nature. SYN: *polyneuritis; multiple neuritis.*

p., amyloid. P. characterized by deposition of amyloid in nerves.

p., erythredema. A condition of unknown etiology occurring in children, and characterized by degenerative changes in peripheral nerves, skin disorders, motor and sensory disturbances. SYN: *pink disease; acrodynia; Swift's disease, q.v.; Feer's disease.*

p., porphyric. P. resulting from acute porphyria characterized by pains and paresthesias in the extremities and flaccid paralysis.

p., progressive hypertrophic. A rare familial disease beginning in childhood and characterized by increased size of peripheral nerves due to multiplication and hypertrophy of cells of sheath of Schwann. SYN: *Dejerine-Sottas disease.*

polynuclear (pŏl″ĭ-nū′klē-ar) [G. *polys,* many, + L. *nucleus,* a kernel]. Possessing more than one nucleus. Multinuclear.

polynucleotidase (pol″ĭ-nū″kle-o-tĭd′ās) An enzyme present in intestinal mucosa and intestinal juice that catalyzes the breakdown of nucleic acids to nucleotides.

polynucleotide (pŏl-ĭ-nū′klē-ō-tĭd). Nucleic acid composed of four nucleotides; a tetranucleotide.

polyodontia (pŏl″ĭ-ō-dŏn′shĭ-ă) [" + *odous, odont-,* tooth]. State of having supernumerary teeth.

polyopia, polyopsia (pŏl-ĭ-ō′pĭ-ă, -ŏp′sĭ-ă) [" + *opsis,* vision]. Multiple vision; perception of more than one image of the same object.

polyorchidism (pŏl″ĭ-or′kĭd-ĭzm) [" + *orchis,* testicle, + *-ismos,* condition]. Condition of having more than two testicles.

polyorchis (pŏl-ĭ-or′kĭs) [" + *orchis,* testicle]. One with more than two testicles.

polyorrhomenitis (pŏl-ĭ-or″ro-mĕn-ī′tĭs) [" + *orros,* serum, + *ymēn,* membrane, + *-itis,* inflammation]. Malignant inflammation and wasting of serous membranes. SYN: *Concato's disease.*

polyotia (pŏl-ĭ-ō′shĭ-ă) [G. *polys,* many, + *ous, ot-,* ear]. State of having more than two ears.

polyp (pŏl′ĭp) [G. *polys,* many, + *pous,* foot]. SYN: *polypus.* A tumor with a pedicle. Commonly found in vascular organs such as the nose, uterus, and rectum. Polyps bleed easily and should be removed surgically.

p., bleeding. Angioma of nasal mucous membrane.

p., fibrinous. Polyp containing fibrin and blood, and located in the uterine cavity.

p., mucous. A polyp of soft or jelly-like consistency and exhibiting mucoid degeneration.

p., vascular. A pedunculated angioma.

polyparesis (pŏl″ĭ-par′ĕs-ĭs) [" + *paresis,* relaxation]. General progressive paralysis of paralytic dementia.

polypathia (pŏl-ĭ-păth′ĭ-ă) [" + *pathos,* disease]. The presence of several diseases at one time, or their frequent recurrence.

polypeptide (pŏl-ĭ-pĕp′tĭd) [" + *peptein,* to digest]. A union of three or more amino acids. SEE: *peptide.*

polypeptidemia (pŏl″ĭ-pĕp-tĭd-ē′mĭ-ă) [" + " + *aima,* blood]. Polypeptides present in the blood.

polypeptidorrhachia (pŏl″ĭ-pĕp-tĭd-ō-rā′-kĭ-ă) [" + " + *rachis,* spine]. Polypeptides in the cerebrospinal fluid.

polyphagia (pŏl-ĭ-fā′jĭ-ă) [G. *polys,* many, + *phagein,* to eat]. Eating abnormally large amounts of food at a meal.

RS: *acoria; anorexia; bulimia; parorexia; taste.*

polyphalangism (pŏl″ĭ-făl-ăn′jĭzm) [" + *phalagx,* phalanx, + *ismos,* condition]. An extra number of phalanges on a finger or toe.

polypharmacy (pŏl-ĭ-far′mă-sĭ) [" + *pharmakon,* drug]. 1. Excessive use of drugs or overdose of a drug. 2. Prescription of many drugs given at one time.

polyphobia (pŏl-ĭ-fō′bĭ-ă) [" + *phobos,* fear]. Excessive or abnormal fear of a number of things.

polyphony (pŏl′ĭ-fōn-ĭ). SYN: *pleitropism.* Condition in which a single gene produces several effects in the body.

polyphrasia (pŏl-ĭ-frā′zĭ-ă) [" + *phrasis,* speech]. Excessive talkativeness, a manifestation of insanity. SYN: *verbigeration.*

polyphyletic (pŏl″ĭ-fī-lĕt′ĭk). Having more than one origin. Opp. of *monophyletic, q.v.*

polyplastic (pŏl-ĭ-plăs′tĭk) [G. *polys,* many, + *plastos,* formed]. 1. Having had many evolutionary modifications. 2. Having many substances in cellular composition.

polyplastocytosis (pŏl″ĭ-plăs-tō-sī-tō′sĭs) [" + " + *kytos,* cell, + *-ōsis,* intensive]. Increase of formation of blood platelets.

polyplegia (pŏl-ĭ-plē′jĭ-ă) [" + *plēgē,* a stroke]. Paralysis affecting several muscles.

polyploid (pol′ĭ-ployd). 1. Characterized by polyploidy. 2. An individual in which the chromosome number is a multiple of the haploid number.

polyploidy (pol′ĭ-ployd-ĭ). Condition in which the chromosome number is a multiple of the haploid number found in gametes.

polypnea (pŏl-ĭp-nĭ′ă) [" + *pnoia,* breath]. Very rapid breathing. SYN: *panting.*

polypodia (pŏl″ĭ-pō′dĭ-ă) [" + *pous, pod-,* foot]. Possession of more than the normal number of feet.

polypoid (pŏl′ĭ-poyd) [" + *pous,* foot, + *eidos,* like]. Like a polyp.

polyporous (pŏl-ĭp′o-rus). Possessing many small openings or pores.

polyposis (pŏl-ĭ-pō′sĭs) [" + " + *-ōsis,* intensive]. The presence of numerous polypi.

p. coli. P. of the large intestine.

p. ventriculi. Presence of numerous polyps, sometimes involving entire mucosa, accompanied by chronic atrophic gastritis.

polypotome (pol-ĭp′o-tōm) [G. *polys,* many, + *pous,* foot, + *tomē,* a cutting]. Instrument for excision of polyps.

polypus (pŏl′ĭ-pŭs) (pl. *polypi*) [" + *pous,* foot]. A polyp, *q.v.*

p., bleeding. Angioma of nasal mucous membrane.

p., cellular. Mucous polypus.

p., cervical. A polyp, either fibrous or mucous, on the cervical mucosa.

p., fibrous. A pedunculated fibroid tumor within the uterine or cervical cavities.

p., fleshy. A submucous myoma in the uterus.

p., placental. A polyp composed of retained placental tissue.

polyradiculitis (pol″ĭ-ră-dik″u-li′tis). Inflammation of nerve roots especially those of spinal nerves.

polyrexia (pŏl-ĭ-rĕks′ĭ-ă). Syn: *bulimia.* Insatiable appetite, excessive hunger.

polyrrhea, polyrrhoea (pol-ĭ-rē′ă) [G. *polys,* many, + *roia,* flow]. Excessive secretion of fluid.

polysaccharide (pol″ĭ-sak′ă-rīd) [G. *polys,* many, + *sakcharon,* sugar]. One of a group of carbohydrates which upon hydrolysis yield more than two molecules of simple sugars. They are complex carbohydrates of high molecular weight, usually insoluble in water but, when soluble, form colloidal solutions. Their basic formula is $(C_6H_{12}O_6)x$.

They include two groups: 1. *Starch group* (Ex: starch, inulin, glycogen, dextrin). 2. *Cellulose group* (Ex: cellulose and hemicelluloses). The hemicelluloses include the pentosans (Ex: gum arabic), hexosans (Ex: agar-agar) and hexopentosans (Ex: pectin).

See: *carbohydrates; monosaccharides; disaccharides.*

polysaccharose (pŏl″ĭ-săk′ă-rōs) [G. *polys,* many, + *sakcharon,* sugar]. A polysaccharide, *q.v.*

polysarcia (pŏl″ĭ-sar′shĭ-ă) [" + *sarx, sark-,* flesh]. Fleshiness; obesity.

polysarcous (pŏl″ĭ-sar′kŭs) [" + *sarx, sark-,* flesh]. Very fleshy; fat.

polyscelia (pŏl″ĭ-sē′lĭ-ă) [" + *skelos,* leg]. Condition of having more than the normal number of legs.

polyscope (pŏl′ĭ-skōp) [" + *skopein,* to examine]. Instrument for illumination and examination of cavities.

polyserositis (pŏl″ĭ-sē-rō-sī′tĭs) [G. *polys,* many, + L. *serum,* whey, + *-itis,* inflammation]. Syn: *multiple serositis.* General progressive inflammation, esp. in upper abdominal cavity.

p., chronic. Syn: *Pick's disease.* P. involving fibrous adhesions in pleural and pericardial cavities.

polysinuitis (pol″ĭ-sin″u-i′tis). Same as *polysinusitis, q.v.*

polysinusitis (pŏl″ĭ-sī″nus-i′tis) [" + L. *sinus,* a hollow, + G. *-itis,* inflammation]. Inflammation of several sinuses simultaneously. Syn: *polysinuitis.*

polyspermia (pŏl″ĭ-sper′mĭ-ă) [" + *sperma,* seed]. 1. Excessive secretion of seminal fluid. 2. Entrance of several spermatozoa into one ovum. Syn: *polyspermism.*

polyspermism (pol″ĭ-sperm′izm). Same as *polyspermia, q.v.*

polystichia (pŏl-ĭ-stĭk′ĭ-ă) [" + *stichos,* a row]. Condition in which there are more than two rows of eyelashes.

polystomatous (pŏl-ĭ-stō′mă-tŭs). Possessing many mouths or openings.

polythelia (pŏl-ĭ-thē′lĭ-ă) [" + *thēlē,* nipple, + *-ismos,* condition]. Presence of more than one nipple on a mamma. Syn: *polythelism.*

polythelism (pol″ĭ-thē′lizm). Same as *polythelia, q.v.*

polytocous (pŏl-ĭt′ō-kŭs) [" + *tokos,* birth]. Producing several offspring at one time.

polytrichosis (pŏl-ĭ-trĭ-kō′sĭs) [G. *polys,* many, + *thrix, trich-,* hair, + *-ōsis,* intensive]. Excessive growth of hair. Syn: *hypertrichosis.*

polytrophia (pŏl-ĭ-trō′fĭ-ă) [" + *trophē,* nourishment]. Excessive or abundant nutrition. Syn: *polytrophy.*

polytrophy (pol-it′ro-fe). Same as *polytrophia, q.v.*

pol″ytrop′ic. Affecting more than one type of cell, said of viruses, or affecting more than one type of tissue, said of certain poisons.

polyuria (pŏl-ĭ-ū′rĭ-ă) [" + *ouron,* urine]. Excessive secretion and discharge of urine.

The urine does not, as a rule, contain abnormal constituents. Several hundred ounces a day may be voided. It is pale in color. Sp. gr. 1.000 to 1.002, and higher in diabetes.

Etiol: Occurs in diabetes insipidus, diabetes mellitus, chronic nephritis, nephrosclerosis, following edematous states, esp. those induced by heart failure treated with diuretics, in hyperthyroidism, and following excessive intake of liquids.

polyvalent (pŏl-ĭ-vā′lĕnt, pō-lĭv′ă-lent) [" + L. *valēre,* to be strong]. 1. Multivalent; having a combining power of more than 2 atoms of hydrogen.

p. serum. One with antibodies produced by injecting several strains of microorganisms of the same species or by injecting different species.

p. vaccine. One produced from cultures of a number of strains of the same species.

polyvinylpyrrolidone (pol″ĭ-vi″nil-per-rol′ĭ-dōn). A polymeric substance used to treat conditions associated with decreased blood volume. It is given intravenously. Abbr: *PVP.*

pomade (po-măd′) [Fr. from L. *pomum,* apple]. A perfumed ointment, esp. one for the hair. Syn: *pomatum.*

pomatum (pō-mā′tŭm) [L. *pomum,* apple]. A perfumed unguent, esp. one used on the hair. Syn: *pomade.*

pompholyx (pŏm′fō-lĭks) [G. *pompholyx,* bubble]. Acute inflammatory affection characterized by bullae limited to hands and feet.

Etiol: Not known. Occurs in 2nd to 4th decade, in coffee and tobacco users, and in those with lowered vitality.

Sym: Symmetrical eruptions of crops of deeply seated vesicles and bullae with itching, hyperemia, lasting 4 to 6 weeks. Secondary infection may occur.

Treatment: Hygienic regimen. Locally, soothing lotions, potassium permanganate compresses, salicylic acid in alcohol. X-irradiation in resistant cases.

pomphus (pŏm′fŭs) (pl. *pomphi*) [G. *pomphos,* a blister]. A blister or a circumscribed elevation on the skin; a wheal.

pomum (pō′mŭm) [L.]. An apple.

p. Adami. Syn: *Adam's apple.* Prominence in middle line of throat, caused by junction of two lateral wings of the thyroid cartilage.

ponderal (pon′der-al) [L. *pondus,* weight]. Relating to weight.

p. index. The ratio of an individual's height to the cube root of his weight. Expressed as: $\frac{\text{ht.}}{\sqrt[3]{\text{wt.}}}$.

ponograph (pŏn′ō-grăf) [G. *ponos,* pain, + *graphein,* to write]. Device for measuring and registering sensitiveness to pain or fatigue.

ponopalmosis (pŏn″ō-păl-mō′sĭs) [" + *palmos,* palpitation, + *-ōsis,* intensive]. Palpitation of the heart produced by slight exertion. Syn: *neurocirculatory asthenia.*

ponophobia (pŏn-ō-fō′bĭ-ă) [G. *ponos,* pain, + *phobos,* fear]. 1. Abnormal distaste for exerting one's self. 2. Dread of pain.

pons (ponz) (pl. *pontes*) [L. bridge]. 1. A process of tissue connecting two or more parts. 2. Pons varolii, *q.v.*

p. cerebelli. Pons varolii, *q.v.*

p. hepatis. Part of liver extending

sometimes from quadrate lobe to left lobe across the umbilical fissure.

p. varolii. A rounded eminence on ventral surface of the brain stem. It lies between the medulla and cerebral peduncles, and appears externally as a broad band of transverse fibers. It is connected to the cerebellum by the mid. cerebellar peduncle or brachium pontis. It contains fiber tracts connecting medulla oblongata and cerebellum with upper portions of the brain; the origins of the abducens, facial, trigeminal and cochlear division of the eighth (vestibulocochlear) nerves are at the borders of the pons.

Named for Costanzo Varolio, anatomist of Bologna, 1544-75.

RS: *cerebropontile.*

pontic (pŏn'tĭk) [L. *pons, pont-*, bridge]. An artificial tooth set in a bridge.

pontile (pon'tĭl) [L. *pons, pont-*, bridge]. Pert. to the pons varolii.

p. hemiplegia. One due to lesion of the pons. The arm and leg on one side and face on the other are affected.

p. nuclei. The gray matter in the pons.

pontine (pon'tin, -tēn). Pertaining to the pons varolii.

pont"obulb'ar. Pert. to the pons and the medulla oblongata.

pontocaine hydrochlo'ride (pŏn'tō-kān). A proprietary name for tetracaine hydrochloride. Is available in several forms for use as a topical or spinal anesthetic.

popliteal (pŏp-lĭt-ē'ăl, pop-lĭt'ē-al) [L. *poples, poplit-*, the ham]. Concerning the post. surface of the knee.

popliteus (pŏp-lĭt'ē-ŭs, -lĭt-ē'ŭs). Muscle located in hind part of the knee joint which flexes the leg and aids it in rotating. SEE: *Table of Muscles in Appendix.*

poppy. A plant. *Papaver somniferum*, the source of opium.

poradenitis (pōr-ăd-ĕ-nī'tĭs) [G. *poros*, pore, + *adēn*, gland, + *-itis*, inflammation]. SYN: *lymphogranuloma venereum, q.v.* Formation of small abscesses in the iliac glands.

porcellaneous, porcellanous (pōr-sĕ-lā'nē-ŭs, -sel'ăn-ŭs) [Italian *porcellana*, the porcelain shell]. Translucent or white like porcelain, as the skin.

porcupine disease (por'kū-pīn) [L. *porcus*, swine]. A chronic skin disease with scaly epidermal plates. SYN: *ichthyosis, q.v.*

pore (pōr) [G. *pōros*, a pore]. 1. A minute opening, esp. one on an epithelial surface. 2. Opening of excretory duct of a sweat gland.

RS: *skin; stoma; sweat glands.*

p., alveolar. A minute opening which is thought to exist between adjacent alveoli of the lung.

p., gustatory. A taste pore, *q.v.*

p., taste. The external opening of a taste bud. SYN: *gustatory pore.*

porencephalia, porencephaly (pōr-ĕn-sĕf-a'lĭ-ă, pōr-ĕn-sĕf'ă-lĭ) [G. *pōros*, a pore, + *egkephalos*, brain]. An anomalous condition in which the ventricles of the brain are connected with the subarachnoid space.

porencephalitis (pōr-ĕn-sĕf-ăl-ī'tĭs) [G. *pōros*, a pore, + *egkephalos*, brain, + *-itis*, inflammation]. Inflammation of the brain with development of cavities communicating with the subarachnoid space.

porencephalous (pōr-ĕn-sĕf'ăl-ŭs) [G. *pōros*, a pore, + *egkephalos*, brain]. Pertaining to *porencephalia, q.v.*

pori. Plural of porus, *q.v.*

poriomania. Morbid desire to wander from home.

pork (pōrk) [L. *porcus*, swine]. The meat of hogs. COMP: Roasted, medium-fat pork loin contains, in each 100 gram portion, 362 calories, 24.5 grams protein, 28.5 grams fat, 11 mg. calcium, 3.2 mg. iron. High in amounts of vitamin B_1.

pornography (pōr-nŏg'ră-fĭ) [G. *pornē*, prostitute, + *graphein*, to write]. Obscene writing, painting, or photographs.

porocephaliasis, porocephalosis (pō"rō-sĕf-ăl-ī'ă-sĭs, -ō'sĭs) [G. *pōros*, pore, + *kephalē*, head]. Infection with a species of Porocephalus.

Porocephalus (pō"rō-sĕf'ă-lŭs) [G. *pōros*, pore, + *kephalē*, head]. A genus of wormlike arthropods found commonly in snakes. The young sometimes infest mammals, including man.

porokeratosis (pō"rō-kĕr-ăt-ō'sĭs) [G. *pōros*, callus, + *keras*, a horn, + *-ōsis*, disease]. Skin disease marked by thickening of stratum corneum in linear arrangement, followed by its atrophy.

It appears on smooth areas. It is irregular in form and size, with circumscribed outline and affects hands and feet, forearms and legs, the face, neck and scalp.

poroma (pō-rō'mă) [" + *-ōma*, tumor]. Inflammatory hardening or callosity.

porosis (pō-rō'sĭs) [G. *pōros*, callus, + *-osis*, disease]. Condition marked by formation of pores or cavities and increased translucency to roentgen rays.

porosity (pō-rŏs'ĭ-tĭ) [G. *pōros*, pore]. The state of being porous.

porous (pō'rŭs) [G. *pōros*, a pore]. Full of pores; able to admit passage of a liquid.

por'phin. $C_{20}H_{14}N_4$, the structure forming the framework of all porphyrins. Consisting of four pyrrole rings united by methene couplings.

porphobilin (pōr-fō-bī'lĭn). A derivative of hemoglobin sometimes present in urine.

porphobilinogen (por-fō-bī-lĭn'ō-jĕn). A substance sometimes found in the urine of patients with acute porphyria. The urine may appear to be normal when fresh, but will change to a Burgundy wine color or even to black when heated with dilute hydrochloric acid to 100° C.

porphyria (por-fī'rĭ-ă) [G. *porphyra*, purple]. Porphyrin in the blood.

p., acute intermittent. A rare metabolic disorder characterized by excessive excretion of porphyrins, acute abdominal pain, and neurologic disturbances, inherited as a mendelian dominant trait. Sometimes precipitated by excessive use of sulfonamides, barbiturates, or other drugs. Sensitivity to light is characteristic.

p., congenital. A rare condition due to an inborn error of metabolism. Inherited as a mendelian recessive trait.

p. cutanea tarda hereditaria. Porphyria inherited as a non-sex-linked mendelian dominant characteristic. Onset of symptoms usually occurs between the ages of 10 and 30 years.

p. erythropoietica. P. due to a defect in the synthesis of hemoglobin.

p. hepatica. P. due to disturbance in liver metabolism such as occurs following hepatitis, poisoning by heavy metals, certain anemias, and other conditions.

porphyrin (por'fī-rĭn) [G. *porphyra*, purple]. One of a group forming basis of animal and plant respiratory pigments, obtained from hemoglobin and chlorophyll.

porphyrinuria (por"fĭ-rĭn-ū'rĭ-ă) [" +

ouron, urine]. The excretion of porphyrin in the urine.

porphyrization (por″fĭr-ĭ-zā′shŭn) [G. *porphyra,* purple]. Process of pulverizing.

porphyruria (por-fĭr-ū′rĭ-ă) [″ + *ouron,* urine]. Excretion of porphyrin in urine.

porrigo (pō-rī′gō) [L. dandruff]. Any disease of scalp involving scaling or loss of hair.

p. decalvans. Baldness in patches. Syn: *alopecia areata.*

p. favosa. Tiny, contiguous ulcer and crust formation. Syn: *favus, q.v.*

p. furfurans. Ringworm of the scalp. Syn: *tinea tonsurans, q.v.*

p. larvalis. Eczema of the scalp with impetigo.

Porro's operation (por′ōz) [Edwardo Porro, obstetrician in Milan, 1842-1902]. Removal of a pregnant uterus, the ovaries, and tubes through an incision in the abdominal wall.

porta (por′tăh) [L. gate]. The point of entry of nerves and vessels into an organ or part.

p. hepatis. The fissure of the liver where the portal vein and hepatic artery enter and the hepatic duct leaves.

p. lienis. Hilus of the spleen where vessels enter.

p. pulmonis. Pulmonary hilus for entry and exit of the bronchi, nerves, and vessels.

p. renis. Hilus of the kidney for entry of the vessels.

portal (por′tăl) [L. *porta,* a gate]. 1. Concerning a porta or entrance to an organ, especially that through which the blood is carried to liver. 2. An entryway.

p. circulation. That of blood brought into the liver by the portal vein and out by the hepatic vein.

p. of entry. The avenue by which infectious organisms gain access to the body.

p., intestinal. The opening of the midgut or yolk sac into the foregut or hindgut of an embryo.

p. system. The portal vein and its branches by which blood is collected from abdominal viscera and conveyed to the sinusoids of the liver from which it passes through the hepatic veins to the inf. vena cava.

p. vein. One formed by the veins of the splanchnic area conveying its blood into the liver.

It is made of the combined sup. and inf. mesenteric, splenic, gastric, and cystic veins.

porte-, port- (pōrt) [Fr. *porter,* to carry, from L. *portāre,* to carry]. To carry.

portio (pōr′shĭ-ō) [L. a part]. A part.

p. dura. The 7th cranial nerve; the facial nerve.

p. vaginalis. The part of the cervix within the vagina.

port-wine mark or **stain.** A purplish-red, superficial birthmark. Syn: *nevus, q.v.*

porus (pō′rŭs) [L., from G. *poros,* a passage]. A meatus or foramen; a tiny aperture in a structure; a pore.

p. acusticus externus. The external opening of the external acoustic meatus.

p. acusticus internus. The opening of the internal acoustic meatus into the cranial cavity.

p. lactiferous. Opening of a lactiferous duct on tip of nipple of mammary gland.

p. opticus. Opening in center of optic disk through which retinal vessels (central artery and vein) reach retina through lamina cribrosa of sclera.

p. sudoriferus. Opening of a sweat gland.

posiomania (pos″ĭ-ō-mā′nĭ-ă) [G. *posis,* a drink, + *mania,* madness]. Addiction to alcoholic drinks. Syn: *dipsomania.*

position (pō-zĭsh′ŭn) [L. *positiō,* a placing, from *ponere,* to place]. 1. Place in which a thing is put. 2. Manner in which a body is arranged, as by the nurse or physician for examination. 3. Ob: The relation of some arbitrarily chosen portion of the child in the pelvis to the right or left side of the mother, the occiput, chin, sacrum and scapula being the points that are most common.

Positions of Fetus in Utero

Vertex Presentation (point of designation—occiput):

Left occiput anterior	LOA
Right occiput posterior	ROP
Right occiput anterior	ROA
Left occiput posterior	LOP
Right occiput transverse	ROT
Occiput anterior	OA
Occiput posterior	OP

Breech Presentation (point of designation—sacrum):

Left sacroanterior	LSA
Right sacroposterior	RSP
Right sacroanterior	RSA
Left sacroposterior	LSP
Sacroanterior	SA
Sacroposterior	SP
Left sacrotransverse	LST
Right sacrotransverse	RST

Face Presentation (point of designation—chin [mentum]):

Left mentoanterior	LMA
Right mentoposterior	RMP
Right mentoanterior	RMA
Left mentoposterior	LMP
Mentoposterior	MP
Mentoanterior	MA
Left mentotransverse	LMT
Right mentotransverse	RMT

Transverse Presentation (point of designation—scapula of presenting shoulder):

Left scapuloanterior	LScA
Right scapuloposterior	RScP
Right scapuloanterior	RScA
Left scapuloposterior	LScP

p., anatomic. Position assumed when a person is standing erect with arms at the sides, palms forward.

p., dorsal. P. in which patient is on his back.

p., d. elevated. On back, with head and shoulders elevated at angle of 30° or more. Employed in digital examination of genitalia and in bimanual examination.

p., d. recumbent. On back, extremities moderately flexed and rotated outward. Employed in application of obstetrical forceps, repair of lesions following parturition, vaginal examination, bimanual palpation. See: *dorsal recumbent p. for illustration.*

p., dorsosacral. Same as *p., lithotomy.*

p., Edebohl's. Same as *Simon's p.*

p., Elliott's. P. in which supports are placed under small of back so that patient resembles a double inclined plane.

p., English. See: *p., left lateral recumbent.*

p., erect. Occiput and heels on line, also nose, groins, and great toes in same vertical plane. Employed in practice of ballottement, differentiation of tumors, cystic and solid hernia.

p., Fowler's. Position when the head of the patient's bed is raised above the level about 1½ ft. and knees are elevated. SEE: *Fowler's p. for illustration.*

p., genucubital. Patient on knees, thighs upright, body resting on elbows, head down on hands. Employed when not possible to use the classic knee-chest position.

p., genupectoral. Patient on knees, thighs upright, head and upper part of chest resting on table, arms crossed above head. Employed in displacement of prolapsed fundus, dislodgment of impacted head of fetus, management of transverse presentation, replacement of retroverted uterus or displaced ovary, flushing of intestinal canal.

p., horizontal. Lying supine, feet extended. Employed in palpation, in auscultation of fetal heart and in operative procedures. SEE: *horizontal p. for illustration.*

p., h. abdominal. Patient flat on abdomen, feet extended. Employed in examination of back and spinal column.

p., jackknife. Patient on back, shoulders elevated, legs flexed on thighs, thighs at right angles to abdomen. Employed when passing urethral sound.

p., knee-chest. Same as *p., genupectoral.* SYN: *genupectoral p.* SEE: *knee-chest p. for illustration.*

p., knee-elbow. SEE: *p., genucubital.*

p., kneeling-squatting. Patient stooping, knees pressed on abdomen, trunk erect. Employed in childbirth in difficult cases and in uncivilized nations.

p., lateroprone. Same as *Sims' p.*

p., laterosemiprone. Same as *Sims' p.*

p., left lateral recumbent. Patient on left side, right knee and thigh drawn up. Employed in childbirth.

p., lithotomy. Patient on back, thighs flexed on abdomen, legs on thighs, thighs abducted. Employed in operation on genital tract, in vaginal hysterectomy, diagnosis and treatment of diseases of urethra and bladder.

p., obstetrical. Same as *p., left lateral recumbent.*

p., orthograde. Same as *p., anatomic.*

p., prone. P. in which patient is lying face downward.

p., reclining. Same as *p., jackknife.*

p., side, semiprone. Same as *Sims' p.*

p., Simon's. Exaggerated lithotomy position. Patient flat on back, legs flexed on thighs, thighs on abdomen, hips somewhat elevated, thighs strongly abducted. Employed in operations on vagina.

p., Sims'. Patient on left side, right knee and thigh drawn well up above left, left arm back of patient and hanging over edge of table, chest inclined forward so that patient rests upon it. Employed in curettement of uterus, intrauterine irrigation after labor, tamponade of vagina, rectal exploration, operations on cervix. SEE: *Sims' position for illustration.*

p., Trendelenburg. Dorsal position, body elevated at angle of about 45°, feet and legs hanging over end of table, head down. Employed in abdominal surgery to favor gravitation upward of abdominal viscera.

p., Walcher. The patient with hips on the edge of the table and the lower extremities hanging down.

positioner (po-zish'un-er). Apparatus for holding or placing the body or part, especially the head, in a certain position.

positive (pŏz'ĭt-ĭv) [L. *positivus,* ruling]. 1. Definite; affirmative; opposed to negative. 2. Indicating the reaction in laboratory work. 3. Indicating an abnormal condition in examination and diagnosis. 4. Indicates pathological change in postmortem examination. 5. Noting a quantity greater than zero.

Indicated by the plus (+) sign.

positron (pŏz'ĭ-tron). A particle having the same mass as a negative electron but possessing a positive charge.

posological (pŏs"ō-loj'ĭ-kăl) [G. *posos,* how much, + *logos,* a study]. Concerning dosage.

posology (pō-sŏl'ō-jĭ) [" + *logos,* a study]. Branch of scientific study dealing with dosage.

possession (pō-zĕsh'ŭn) [L. *possessiō,* a sitting before]. State of being dominated by an idea, a passion or a mental obsession.

p., demoniacal. Belief of being under the influence of an evil spirit or demon.

Possum [derived from *p*atient operated *s*elector *m*echanism]. A device that permits a disabled individual to control and operate various machines, such as switches, telephones and typewriters, by breathing into the master control of the apparatus.

post- [L.]. A prefix meaning *behind* or *after.*

postabortal (pōst"ă-bor'tăl) [L. *post,* after, + *abortus,* abortion]. Happening subsequent to abortion.

postaxial (pōst-ăks'ĭ-ăl) [" + G. *axōn,* axis]. Situated or happening behind an axis.

postcapillary (pōst-kăp'ĭl-lā-rĭ). SYN: *venous capillary.* A terminal vessel of a capillary network which leads to a venule.

postcava (pōst-kā'vă) [" + *cavus,* a hollow]. The ascending or inferior vena cava.

postcaval (pōst-kā'văl) [" + *cavus,* hollow]. Concerning the postcava.

postcentral (pōst-sĕn'trăl) [" + G. *kentron,* center]. 1. Situated or happening behind a center. 2. Located behind the fissure of Rolando.

postcibal (pōst-sī'băl) [" + *cibum,* food]. Occurring after meals.

postclavicular (pōst"klă-vĭk'ū-lăr) [" + *clavicula,* a little key]. Located or occurring behind the clavicle.

postclimacteric (pōst-klī-măk-tĕr'ĭk, -mak'tĕr-ĭk) [L. *post,* after, + G. *klimaktēr,* round of a ladder]. Occurring after the menopause.

postcoital (pōst-kō'ĭt-ăl) [" + *coitiō,* a coming together]. Subsequent to sexual intercourse.

postconnubial (pōst-kŏn-ū'bĭ-ăl) [" + *connubium,* marriage]. Occurring after marriage.

postconvulsive (pōst-kŏn-vŭl'sĭv) [" + *convulsiō,* a pulling together]. Occurring after a convulsion.

postdiastolic (pōst-dī-ăs-tŏl'ĭk) [" + *diastolē,* a sending apart]. Occurring after the cardiac diastole.

postdicrotic (pōst-dī-krŏt'ĭk) [L. *post,* after, + G. *dikrotos,* beating double]. Occurring after the dicrotic pulse wave.

p. wave. A recoil or second wave (not always present) in a sphygmographic tracing.

postdiphtheritic (pōst-dĭph-thĕr-ĭt'ĭk). Following diphtheria.

postencephalitis (pōst"ĕn-sĕf-ăl-ī'tĭs) [" + *egkephalos,* brain, + *-itis,* inflammation]. The condition sometimes remaining after convalescence from epidemic encephalitis.

postepileptic (pōst″ĕp-ĭ-lĕp′tĭk) [" + G. *epi,* upon, + *lēpsis,* a seizure]. Following an epileptic seizure.

posterior (pŏs-tē′rĭ-or) [L. after]. 1. Toward the rear or caudal end; opp. of *anterior.* 2. In man, toward the back; dorsal. 3. Situated behind; coming after.

postero- (pos′ter-o) [L.]. Prefix meaning *posterior, situated behind* or *towards the back.*

posteroexternal (pos″ter-o-eks-ter′nal) [L. *posterus,* behind, + *externus,* outer]. Towards the back and outer side.

posterointernal (pos″ter-o-in-ter′nal) [L. *posterus,* behind, + *internus,* inner]. Towards the back and inner side.

posterolateral (pos″ter-o-lat′er-al) [" + *latus, later-,* a side]. Located behind and at the side of a part.

posteromedial (pos″ter-o-me′dĭ-al). Toward the back and toward the median plane.

posteromedian (pos″ter-o-mē′dĭ-en) [L. *posterus,* behind, + *medius,* middle]. Situated posteriorly and in the median plane.

posterosuperior (pos″ter-o-sū-pe′rĭ-or) [" + *superior,* upper]. Located behind and above a part.

postesophageal (pōst″ē-sō-făj′ē-ăl) [L. *post,* after, + G. *oisophagos,* gullet]. Located behind the esophagus.

postethmoid (pōst-ĕth′moyd) [" + G. *ēthmos,* sieve, + *eidos,* form]. Located behind the ethmoid bone.

postfebrile (pōst-fē′brĭl) [" + *febris,* fever]. Occurring after a fever.

postganglionic (pōst″găn-glĭ-ŏn′ĭk). Situated behind or after a ganglion.

p. fiber. The axon of a postganglionic neuron which passes from an autonomic ganglion to a visceral effector.

p. neuron. The second of a series of efferent neurons which transmit impulses from the central nervous system to a visceral effector. Its cell body lies in one of the autonomic ganglia.

posthetomy (pŏs-thĕt′ō-mĭ) [G. *posthē,* prepuce, + *tomē,* a cutting]. Surgical removal of all or part of the foreskin. Syn: *circumcision.*

posthioplasty (pŏs′thĭ-ō-plas″tĭ) [" + *plastos,* formed]. Plastic surgery of the prepuce or foreskin.

posthitis (pŏs-thĭ′tĭs) [" + *-itis,* inflammation]. Inflamed condition of the foreskin.

posthumous (pŏs′tū-mŭs) [L. *postumus,* last]. 1. Occurring after death. 2. Born after death of father. 3. Said of a child taken by cesarean section after death of mother.

posthypnotic (pōst″hĭp-nŏt′ĭk) [L. *post,* after, + G. *ypnos,* sleep]. Occurring or performed subsequent to the hypnotic state.

p. suggestion. One offered during the hypnotic state influencing a later action when individual returns to normal state.

postictal (pōst-ik′tal) [post- + L. *ictus,* a blow or stroke]. Following a sudden attack or stroke, as an epileptic seizure or apoplexy.

posticteric (pōst-ĭc-tĕr′ĭc) [post + G. *ikteros,* jaundice]. Following jaundice.

post-mortem (pōst-mor′tĕm) [L.]. After death.

p. examination. Dissection of a dead body to ascertain cause of death and the changes wrought by disease. Syn: *autopsy.*

postnatal (pōst-nā′tăl) [L. *post,* after, + *natus,* birth]. Happening after birth.

post″necrot′ic. After death of a tissue or a part.

postocular (pōst-ŏk′ū-lar) [" + *oculus,* eye]. Behind the eye.

p. neuritis. Inflammation of the optic nerve behind the eyeball.

postolivary (pōst-ŏl′ĭv-a-rĭ) [" + *oliva,* olive]. Behind the olivary body; back of the anterior pyramid of the medulla.

postoperative (pōst-ŏp′ĕr-ā-tĭv) [" + *operatus,* from *operārī,* to work]. After or following a surgical operation.

Postoperative Care: 1. When you are called to the operating room to get a patient, take a towel and emesis basin with you. 2. See that ether bed is ready and furniture moved so stretcher can be gotten close to it. 3. Be careful when handling unconscious patient. Remember that it will be a difficult task because he is a dead weight and not able to help himself. Get assistance. 4. See that there are no drafts, but plenty of fresh air. Do not let direct light shine on patient's face. 5. When he vomits keep his head turned to one side so vomitus will not be swallowed or inhaled. 6. Change gown when wet or soiled, rubbing patient dry with bath towel under the bedclothes. 7. Watch him carefully when consciousness begins to return, for it is at this time he becomes restless. 8. Note pulse, respiration, blood pressure and other signs as required by the routine of your hospital. It varies with the operation.

postoperculum (pōst-ō-per′kū-lŭm) [" + *operculum,* a cover]. The fold covering the insula that is formed of part of the supertemporal gyrus. Syn: *operculum temporal.*

postoral (pōst-or′al) [" + *os, or-,* mouth]. Behind or in the posterior part of the mouth.

postpallium (pōst-păl′ĭ-ŭm) [L. *post,* after, + *pallium,* cloak]. That part of the cerebral cortex behind the fissure of Rolando.

postpaludal (post-pal′ū-dăl) [" + *palus, palud-,* swamp]. After a malarial attack.

postparalytic (pōst-par-ă-lĭt′ĭk) [" + *para,* beside, + *lyein,* to loosen]. Subsequent to an attack of paralysis.

postpartum (pōst-par′tŭm) [L. *post,* after. + *partus,* birth]. After parturition.

p. hemorrhage. Hemorrhage which occurs after childbirth.

NP: If hemorrhage occurs, regardless of the use of safe and preventive measures, drastic ones for its control must be employed.

Extra hypodermics of oxytocic drugs may be used as ordered. An icebag placed on the fundus is used as early routine postpartum measure by some physicians. Massage of uterus with a piece of ice on the abdomen is frequently used when bleeding persists. Packing the lower segment of uterus and vagina is an excellent method of controlling hemorrhage. The large tubular packer is preferred here to a dressing forceps to avoid contamination of the packing by contact with the vulva and vaginal tract. Packing the vagina may be done by the nurse, if absolutely necessary, when a physician is not available.

If the above procedures fail to halt the hemorrhage, the physician may insert one hand into the fundus and at the same time massage the uterus with the other hand on the abdomen. A sterile pair of long gloves should be ready in this case. Keep the patient warm during this time. Elevate the lower extremities as soon as possible. Oxytocic drugs may be ordered intravenously by some physicians. Note the pulse and general condition frequently. Stimulants are given as necessary.

Blood transfusions are generally given to maintain and increase the patient's resistance. Massage the uterus. The fingertips may be kept lightly on the fundus to discover any relaxation. Give massage only when relaxation occurs. Hypodermoclysis and intravenous injections are used if patient is unable to take and retain fluids. Force fluids as soon as patient's condition warrants, but do not take a chance on making the patient vomit, as retching may start another hemorrhage.

When tolerated, the patient may be given a limited number of oral preparations of ergot, perferably the ones that are not nauseating. These keep the uterus contracted and lessen the chance of infection to which the patient has been predisposed by the loss of blood, lowered resistance, and much manipulation. Perfect asepsis must be maintained at all times. Remember that since this patient is predisposed to sepsis, her general resistance must be built up and maintained by plenty of fluids, nourishing foods and, above all, rest.

postpontile (pōst-pŏn'tĭl) [L. *post,* after, + *pons, pont-,* bridge]. Situated behind the pons varolii.

post"prand'ial. Following a meal.

post"pubes'cent. Following puberty.

postpyramidal post-pĭ-răm'ĭd-ăl). Behind a pyramidal tract.

p. nucleus. Mass of gray matter in post. column of the medulla. SYN: *nucleus funiculi gracilis.*

postulate (pŏst'ū-lāt). A supposition or view, usually self-evident, which is assumed without proof. SEE: *Koch's law* or *postulates.*

postural (pos'tū-răl) [L. *postura,* position]. Pert. to or effected by posture.

p. drainage. Drainage of secretions from the bronchi or a cavity in the lung by placing the patient's head lower than the area to be drained.

Used in bronchiectasis and before operation for lobectomy, *q.v.* The position aggravates coughing, resulting in expectoration of much sputum, 5 to 10 oz. in severe cases. Five to 10 minutes morning and evening is recommended. High protein diet to replace protein lost.

posture (pŏs'tūr) [L. *postura,* position]. Attitude or position of the body.

p., coiled. Body on one side with legs drawn up to meet the trunk. Noted in cerebral diseases and in hepatic, intestinal or renal colic.

p., dorsal inertia. Patient on back, with tendency to slip down in bed or to either side. Seen in great weakness, in acute infectious diseases such as typhoid, in mental apathy or muscular weakness.

p., dorsal rigid. P. on back with both legs drawn up. Seen in peritonitis, meningitis, ascites, tympanites. In appendicitis the right leg is drawn up. Also occurs in pelvic inflammation or peritonitis of right side, renal calculus in right ureter, and in psoas abscess.

p., emprosthotonos. The body is incurved and rests upon the forehead and feet with face downward. It is rarely seen in tetanus and strychnine poisoning.

p., opisthotonos. An uncommon dorsal position in which the body rests upon the head and heels, with the trunk arched upward. It is seen in strychnine poisoning, tetanus, hysteria, epilepsy, the convulsions of rabies, and to a slight extent in meningitis. In the latter case, the neck is rigid and the head retracted, seeming to press into the pillow. SEE: *opisthotonos.*

p., orthopnea. Patient sitting upright, hands or elbows resting upon some support. Seen in spasmodic asthma, emphysema, dyspnea, ascites, effusions into the pleural and pericardial cavities, and in late stages of diseases of the heart.

p., orthotonos. Neck and trunk extended rigidly in straight line; seen in tetanus, strychnine poisoning, rabies or meningitis.

p., pleurothotonos. Lateral position with body arched in acute pleural involvement or spinal affection.

p., prone. Posture assumed after abdominal colic or because of tuberculosis of spine, eroded vertebrae, abdominal pain or gastric ulcer.

p., semireclining. Used in diseases of heart and interference with respiration in asthma and pleural effusions.

p., unilateral. Patient on right side in acute pleurisy, lobar pneumonia of right side and in a greatly enlarged liver, or left side in lobar pneumonia, or pleurisy on that side, and in large pericardial effusions.

postuterine (pōst-ū'tĕr-ĭn) [L. *post,* after, + *uterus,* womb]. Situated behind the uterus.

pot. Slang term for marijuana.

potable (pō'tă-bl) [L. *potabilis,* from *potāre,* to drink]. Suitable for drinking.

Potain's apparatus (po-tān'). A form of aspirator.

P.'s disease. Pulmonary edema.

P.'s sign. Dullness on percussion of the aorta in dilatation, extending from the *manubrium sterni* toward the third costal cartilage on the right, the base of the sternum in segment of a circle to the right marking the upper limit.

potamophobia (pŏt"ăm-ō-fō'bĭ-ă) [G. *potamos,* river, + *phobos,* fear]. A morbid fear of large bodies of water.

potash (pŏt'ăsh). Potassium carbonate, *q.v.*

p., caustic. Potassium hydroxide, *q.v.*

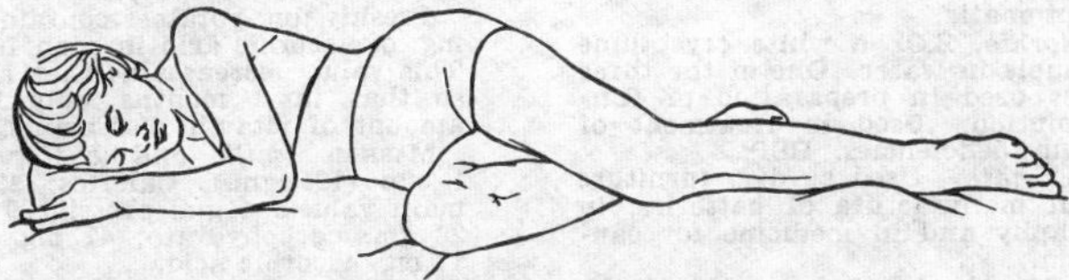

UNILATERAL POSTURE FOR COMFORT.

p., sulfurated. USP. Liver-colored or greenish yellow substance made up of potassium thiosulfate and potassium polysulfides, and containing 12.8% sulfur as a sulfide. A principal ingredient of white lotion (USP).

potassa sulfurata (pō-tas'ă sul-fū-ră'tă). Sulfurated potash. SEE UNDER: *potash*.

potassemia (pō-tăs-sē'mĭ-ă) [L. *potassa*, + G. *aima*, blood]. Presence of excessive quantity of potassium in the blood.

potassic (pō-tas'ĭk) [L. *potassa*, potash]. Composed of or containing potash.

potassium (pō-tas'ĭ-ŭm) [L. *potassa*, potash]. SYMB: K. At. wt. 39.102. Sp. gr. 0.86. Mineral element found in combination with other elements in the body and constituting 0.35% of body weight. SYN: *kalium*.

FUNCTIONS: Potassium is the principal cation in intracellular fluid and is of primary importance in its maintenance. In conjunction with sodium and chloride, it aids in regulation of osmotic pressure and acid-base balance. A proper balance of potassium, calcium, and magnesium ions is essential for normal excitability of muscle tissue, esp. cardiac muscle, and it plays a role in the conduction of nerve impulses.

DEFICIENCY: SYM: Disorders of the nervous system, loss of weight, poor digestion, irregular heart action, and poor muscular control.

SOURCES: Found in most foods. Excellent sources are: cereals, dried peas and beans, fresh vegetables, fresh or dried fruits, nuts, molasses, cocoa, fresh fish, and fresh poultry.

p. acetate. USP. A white powder or crystalline flakes. CH_3COOK.

ACTION AND USES: Alkaline diuretic.

p. bicarbonate. USP. White crystals or powder. $KHCO_3$.

ACTION AND USES: To neutralize acid of stomach and lessen acidity of urine

p. bitartrate. Cream of tartar. White powder or crystalline salt. $KHC_4H_4O_6$.

ACTION AND USES: Diuretic; cathartic; and as a dusting powder, in place of starch, for surgical gloves.

p. bromide. USP. White cubical crystals of powder.

ACTION AND USES: Nerve sedative.

p. carbonate. SYN: *potash*. K_2CO_3, a white crystalline powder used in pharmaceutical and chemical preparations.

p. chlorate. $KClO_3$, an explosive white crystalline salt soluble in water. Formerly used internally in treatment of pharyngitis and stomatitis but its use has been discontinued because of destructive effect on red blood cells. Its use now is limited to mouthwashes and gargles.

POISONING: SYM: Large doses cause abdominal discomfort, vomiting, diarrhea, hematuria with nephritis and disturbances of the blood.

F. A. TREATMENT: Stomach should be washed out. Otherwise treatment must be symptomatic.

p. chloride. KCl, a white crystalline salt, soluble in water. One of the three chlorides used in preparation of Ringer's solution. Used in treatment of potassium deficiencies. USP.

p. chromate. Used as dye, furniture stain, in manufacture of batteries, in photography and in medicine for cauterization.

SYM: May be inhaled or contact the nose from fingers, causing deep, indolent ulcers. When taken by mouth has a disagreeable taste, causes cramping, pain, vomiting, diarrhea, slow respiration; may affect liver and kidneys.

F. A. TREATMENT: Treat as an acid, dilute and give weak alkalies as chalk, baking soda, magnesia, etc., followed by soothing mucilaginous drinks. Treat symptomatically.

p. citrate. Transparent prismatic crystals.

ACTION AND USES: Similar to potassium acetate.

INCOMPATIBILITIES: Caffeine sodium benzoate.

p. cyanide. SEE: *cyanide*.

p. hydroxide. SYN: *caustic potash*. KOH. Grayish-white compound used in preparation of soap. It is used also as a chemical reagent. USP.

POISONING: SYM: Nausea; soapy taste; burning pain in mouth which causes bloody, slimy vomitus; abdominal cramping; bloody purging and prostration.

TREATMENT: Dilute with weak, acidulated water such as vinegar, lemon juice, orange juice, grape juice. Household oils likewise reduce the free alkali, but more slowly. Follow with olive oil, sweet melted butter or lard.

p. iodide. USP. Colorless or white crystals having a faint odor of iodine.

ACTION AND USES: To increase bronchial secretions; to treat certain metallic poisons; to make strong iodine solution.

p. permanganate. USP. Dark purple prisms, odorless, with sweet taste. $KMnO_4$.

ACTION AND USES: Deodorant, germicide and astringent. Internally, an antidote in phosphorus poisoning and snake bite. Used for disinfectant and deodorant action as an application in gangrenous ulcers, cancerous sores, diphtheria and gonorrhea. In diluted solutions it may be used as a gargle or mouthwash (¼%), to disinfect the hands (1%), and for other purposes.

Concentrated solutions irritate and even corrode the skin, and when swallowed induce gastroenteritis. The solutions have considerable power as disinfectants, owing to their oxidizing power which destroys bacteria. They fail to penetrate deeply in an active form and this renders them of less value than many other disinfectants, except for use in very superficial infections.

p. sulfate. USP. A laxative and a purgative, but because of its irritant qualities not to be recommended.

potato (pō-tā'tō). COMP: Deficient in protein and fat; also in salt (sodium chloride) and water is in excess. This lowers the nutritive value. Young potatoes contain more juice and protein and less starch. They should be supplemented with milk, butter and eggs, and always used with salt. Potash and soda make them higher in alkalinity than fresh vegetables.

Freshly dug potatoes contain about 20 mg. of ascorbic acid in each 100 grams. This value decreases as they are stored so that in 3 months only half this amount of vitamin C remains.

MASHED (*milk and butter added*): 1 cup (195 gm.). Calories: 230. Other main values: 4 gm. protein; 9 gm. fat; 28 gm. carbohydrate; 47 mg. calcium; 17 mg. ascorbic acid.

ACTION: The intestinal absorption is imperfect which lessens the food value.

The method of cooking changes the nutritive value and ease of digestion.

COOKING: *Boiled:* The weight is not appreciably diminished by boiling, but part of the essential salts is lost. By adding common salt, or by boiling with the jackets on, much of this loss is compensated. Steaming also helps. *Baked:* Baked, they lose ¼ of their weight of water. The addition of milk and butter and salt adds to their nutritive value. Esp. good for dyspepsia. *Fried:* The addition of fat and the elimination of water doubles their food value, but this process adds to their difficulty of digestion. This also applies to potato salad.

potency (pō′tĕn-sĭ) [L. *potentia,* power]. 1. Strength of a medicine. 2. Ability of male to perform coitus. 3. Strength; force; power.

potent (pō′tĕnt) [L. *potens, potent-,* powerful]. 1. Powerful. 2. Highly effective medicinally. 3. Having power of procreation.

potentia coeundi (pō-tĕn′shĭ-ă kō-ĕ-ŭn′dē). [L.]. Complete ability to perform sexual intercourse in a normal manner.

potential (pō-tĕn′shăl) [L. *potentia,* power]. 1. Latent; existing in possibility. 2. *Elect.,* voltage or electrical pressure; a condition in which a state of tension or pressure exists capable of doing work. When two electrically charged bodies of different potentials are brought together, an electric current passes from the body of high potential to that of low.

p., action. ABBR. *A.P* The electrical changes that are associated with conduction of a nerve impulse or contraction of a muscle. They may be visualized by use of a cathode-ray oscillograph.

p., after. On an oscillograph, smaller waves following a sharp rising curve of action potential. SEE ALSO: *p., spike.*

p., demarcation. SYN: *injury potential.* The difference in potential between an intact longitudinal surface and the injured end of a muscle or nerve.

p., injury. SEE: *p., demarcation.*

p., spike. A change in potential indicated by a sharp spikelike curve indicating a negative deflection.

potentiate (pō-tĕn′shĭ-āt). To augment or increase the potency or action.

po″tentia′tion. SYN: *augmentation.* The synergistic action of two substances, e.g., hormones, in which the total effects are greater than the sum of the independent effects of the two substances.

potion (pō′shŭn) [L. *potiō,* draft]. A drink or draught; a dose of poison or liquid medicine.

potocytosis (pō″tō-sī-tō′sĭs). The submicroscopic imbibing or taking up of water by cells in contrast to *pinocytosis, q.v.*

potomania (pō-tō-mā′nĭ-ă) [G. *potos,* a drinking, + *mania,* madness]. Delirium tremens, *q.v.*

Pott's disease (pŏts) [Percivall Pott, British surgeon, 1713-1788]. Caries or osteitis of the vertebrae, usually of tuberculous origin; tubercular inflammation of bodies of the vertebrae.

The disease is primarily a disease of children and of adults up to age 40. Destruction and compression of affected vertebrae often results in kyphosis with resulting compression of spinal cord and nerves. Often infection spreads to paravertebral tissues giving rise to paravertebral abscesses.

SYM: Child will complain of pain in region supplied by the nerves arising from affected segment of the cord. If disease is lumbar, pains are abdominal and apt to be associated with vesical irritability; if dorsal, pains are epigastric or intercostal, and respiration sometimes irregular and hurried from failure of respiratory muscles to take the full share in the work; if cervical, neuralgic pain or numbness in hands, a tickling cough and difficult swallowing. Pains apt to be symmetrical.

Increase of pain on jumping or flexing or rotating spine is extremely significant. If child can jump painlessly from chair to floor it is almost certain no inflammation of the body of a vertebra exists. If vertebrae be crowded together by pressure on head or shoulders while patient sits or stands, or while he lies face downward across knees of surgeon, pain much increased.

If stretched, so spine is elongated, relief follows. Involuntary immobilization of spine, as a result of pain on movement, is very characteristic military attitude. If child is asked to look at something behind him, he turns whole trunk. If requested to pick up something from floor, he stoops by bending the thighs upon the trunk and knees upon thighs, never by flexing spinal column in usual way.

In *walking,* moves as if on ice, sliding or shuffling along so as to avoid jar of successive steps. In *standing,* he fixes upper portion of column by aid of trapezii and other scapular muscles, action of which at same time raises shoulders and throws arms out from sides. In *standing* or *sitting,* there is an involuntary transfer of the weight of head and shoulders and parts above diseased area to the pelvis, by means of the upper extremities. Hands placed upon the hips and arm muscles are tense. In walking about room, lays hold of furniture for aid. Spinal abscess occurs later, location varying with seat of caries. Paralysis may occur, always motor at first, not affecting sensation at all.

TREATMENT: 1. Endeavor to secure resolution of the tuberculous osteitis. 2. Limit destruction of tissue and resulting deformity. 3. Promote ankylosis. 4. Evacuate pus. 5. Remove a sequestrum or the focus of carious bone. 6. Relieve cord from pressure by pus, bone, or most commonly, by products of an ext. pachymeningitis. Rest in bed in recumbent position. Gentle massage, friction, alcohol baths. Cod-liver oil inunctions. Food nutritious and abundant. Extension — plaster or other jackets — jury masts, etc. Tuberculosis in any part must be dealt with accordingly. Good nourishing food, fresh air, sunshine, and constitutional remedies plus surgical aid, when feasible. Chemotherapy as for pulmonary tuberculosis. *q.v.*

SEE: *gibbosity; kyphosis.*

P.'s fracture. Fracture of lower end of fibula and medial malleolus of the tibia with dislocation of foot outwards and backwards.

After reduction, foot and leg are put in plaster in which a walking iron is incorporated. The patient is able to walk, and plaster is removed in about 6 weeks.

pouch (powch) [Fr. *poche,* pocket]. Any pocket or sac. SYN: *sacculation.*

p., branchial. SEE: *p., pharyngeal.*

p., Broca's. A sac in tissues of the labia majora.

p. of Douglas. SEE: *p., rectouterine.*

p., laryngeal. Blind pouch of mucosa entering the ventral portion of the ventricle of the larynx.

p., Pavlov. A stomach pouch formed surgically for the experimental study of gastric secretion. A section of the stomach is separated from the main stomach left or attached by only a small pedicle, and fistulized so as to drain to exterior of body.

p., pharyngeal. One of a series of five pairs of entodermal outpocketings which develop in lateral walls of pharynx of embryo.

p., Rathke's. An outpocketing of the roof of embryonic stomodeum. Gives rise to ant. lobe of hypophysis cerebri.

p., rectouterine. Pouch between anterior rectal wall and posterior uterine wall. SYN: *cul-de-sac; excavatio rectouterina* [NA]; *p. of Douglas.*

p., rectovesical. A fold of peritoneum that in the male extends downward between bladder and rectum.

poultice (pōl'tĭs) [L. *puls, pult-*, porridge]. A hot, moist mass of linseed, bread, mustard, or soap and oil between two pieces of muslin applied to the skin to relieve congestion or pain and to stimulate absorption of inflammatory products. SYN: *cataplasm.* SEE: *plaster; sinapism.*

p., bread. The crumb of bread is moistened by pouring boiling water over it; the water is then pressed out, and the bread mash spread between old linen and applied.

p., charcoal. Used for foul septic wounds. It can either be made in the same way as a mustard poultice in the proportion of 1 part mustard to 3 parts charcoal, or an ordinary linseed poultice can be made and the charcoal powdered over the top; the former method is the more usual.

p., flaxseed. AIM: To apply moist heat for the relief of congestion.

ARTICLES NECESSARY: Tray. Old muslin twice the size the finished plaster is to be. Flaxseed meal. Tablespoon, teaspoon. Saucepan, 1 to 2 qt. size. Boiling water. Sodium bicarbonate. Petroleum jelly, or mineral oil in medicine glass. Applicators. Oiled muslin a little larger than the finished plaster. Bandage or binder if needed. Towel. Emesis basin or paper bag.

PROCEDURE: 1. Assemble equipment. 2. Put water in saucepan and bring to rapid boil. 3. Spread muslin on tray. 4. Sprinkle flaxseed meal into boiling water, stirring constantly until it is about the consistency of "breakfast cereal," or until it will drop off the spoon in lumps. 5. Take from fire and beat well. 6. Add ½ to 1 teaspoonful of sodium bicarbonate, stir in well but do not beat hard. 7. Spread on one-half the muslin, leaving a 2-in. margin around plaster. 8. Turn edges of muslin up and fold other half over. 9. Lay on tray, cover with towel, add oiled muslin, oil and swabs, and carry to bedside. 10. Cover area to be poulticed (unless poultice is to be put over dressings) with oil or petroleum jelly. Apply poultice, raising it frequently to accustom the patient's skin to the heat. 11. When patient can bear heat without discomfort, cover poultice with oiled muslin and then with towel. Fasten with bandage or binder if needed. 12. Change poultices each ½ hour or as ordered. Do not let them get cold. 13. Make fresh poultice each time. The old one cannot be reheated. 14. Renew oil as necessary. 15. When treatment is completed wipe excess oil from skin and cover area with old flannel or a towel.

p., jacket. One made both for the chest and back; used in acute lobar pneumonia.

p., linseed. Have everything heated before commencing. Pour 1 teacupful of boiling water into hot bowl and add heated linseed (about 3 cupfuls) handful by handful, stirring all the time. Should be a stiff paste which does not stick to the sides of the bowl.

On the flannel spread the paste ¼ to ½ in. thick with the hot moist spatula, fold over the edges of the flannel. The poultice is then rolled on itself, carried bet. 2 hot plates to the bedside. Apply to the part, cover with wool and bandage. The fresh poultice is rolled on as the old one is removed. The skin must not be exposed.

p., mustard. Dry mustard is added to the dry linseed in proportions of 1 part dry mustard to 8 parts dry linseed for adults, but 1 to 12 to 1 to 16 for children; the poultice is then made as for an ordinary linseed poultice.

Mustard acts as a counterirritant and produces erythema. Skin should be examined every 5 min. and plaster removed when a definite pinkness appears, usually within 10 to 20 minutes. Blistering will result if left on too long.

pound (pownd) [L. *pondus,* a weight; pound]. SYMB: lb. A measure of weight, 16 ounces.

p., avoirdupois. Sixteen ounces, 7000 grains and equal to 453.59 grams.

p., foot-. Power necessary to raise 1 pound 1 foot high.

p., troy. Twelve ounces, 5760 grains.

Poupart's ligament (pōō-parz'). The ligament forming the lower border of aponeurosis of external oblique muscle between anterior superior spine of the ilium and spine of the pubis. SYN: *inguinal ligament.*

powder (pow'dĕr) [Fr. *poudre,* powder]. 1. Aggregation of particles. 2. Fine particles of 1 or more substances that may be passed through fine meshes. 3. A dose of such a powder, contained in a paper.

power (pow'er) [M.E. *pouer,* from L. *posse,* to be able]. 1. Rate at which work is done. 2. Capacity for action. 3. In *optics,* the degree to which a lens or optical instrument magnifies. 4. In *microscopy,* the number of times the diameter of an object is magnified, indicated by placing an X after the number. Ex: 10X.

pox (pŏks) [M.E. *pokkes,* pits]. 1. An eruptive, contagious disease. 2. A papular eruption that becomes pustular.

SEE: *chickenpox, smallpox, etc.*

P.P. Abbreviation for *punctum proximum,* near point of accommodation (in vision).

P. P. D. Abbreviation for *purified protein derivative,* substance used in intradermal test for tuberculosis.

P. P. F. Abbreviation for the *pellagra preventive factor* in vitamin B.

PPLO. Pleuropneumonia-like organisms found in the throat, saliva, sputum, bladder, and urine. They may be an underlying cause of some infectious diseases.

Ppt. Abbreviation for *precipitate.*

Pr. Abbreviation for *presbyopia;* chem. symb. for *praseodymium.*

P.R. Abbreviation for *punctum remotum,* far point of visual accommodation.

practice (prăk′tĭs) [G. *praktikē,* business]. The use, by a physician, of medical knowledge and skill in diagnosing and treating disease and sickness.

practitioner (prăk-tĭsh′ŭn-ĕr) [G. *praktikē,* business]. One who practices the profession of medicine.

prae-. For words beginning thus, see *pre-.*

praecox (pre′kox) [L.]. Early.

praevia, praevius (pre′vĭ-ă, pre′vĭ-us) [L.]. Going before in time or place.

pragmatagnosia (prăg″măt-ăg-nō′zĭ-ă) [G. *pragma,* object, + *agnōsia,* lack of recognition]. Inability to recognize objects once familiar.

pragmatamnesia (prăg″măt-ăm-nē′zĭ-ă) [" + *amnēsia,* forgetfulness]. Inability to recall the appearance of an object.

p., visual. Name for the mental condition making possible pragmatamnesia.

pragmatic (prăg-măt′ĭk) [G. *pragma,* a thing done]. Pert. to, or concerned with, the practical side of anything.

pragmatism (prăg′mă-tĭzm) [" + *ismos,* condition]. A belief that the practical application of a principle should be the determining factor.

pragmatist (prăg′mă-tĭst) [G. *pragma,* a thing done]. One who believes that practical application should be the determining factor of a principle.

prandial (pran′dĭ-al) [L. *prandium,* late breakfast]. Relating to a meal.

praseodymium (prā-sē-ō-dĭm′ĭ-ŭm). A metallic element obtained from rare earth. SYMB: Pr. At. wt. 140.907; at. no. 59.

praxinoscope (prăk-sĭn′ō-skōp) [G. *praxis,* action, + *skopein,* to examine]. Contrivance for studying the larynx.

praxiology (prak-sĭ-ol′o-jĭ). Study of behavior.

pre- [L.]. Prefix meaning *before,* or in *front of.*

preagonal (prē-ăg′ō-năl) [L. *prae,* before, + G. *agōnia,* agony]. Pert. to condition immediately before death agony.

prealbuminuric (prē″ăl-bū″mĭn-ū′rĭk) [" + *albumen,* white of egg]. Before the appearance of albuminuria.

preanal (prē-ā′năl) [" + *anus,* anus]. In front of the anus.

preanesthetic (prē″ăn-ĕs-thĕt′ĭk) [" + G. *anaisthēsia,* lack of sensation]. Preliminary drug given to facilitate induction of general anesthesia.

preantiseptic (prē″ăn″tĭ-sĕp′tĭk) [" + G. *anti,* against, + *sēpsis,* decay]. Before the adoption of antisepsis in surgery.

preaortic (prē-ā-or′tĭk) [" + G. *aortē,* aorta]. Located in front of the aorta.

preataxic (prē-ă-tak′sik) [" + G. *ataxia,* disorder]. Before the onset of ataxia.

preaxial (prē-ăk′sĭ-ăl) [" + G. *axōn,* axis]. In front of the axis of a limb or of the body.

precancerous (prē-kan′sĕr-ŭs) [" + *cancer,* crab]. Said of a growth which is not yet but will probably become cancerous.

precapillary. An arterial capillary; one which branches from an arteriole or metarteriole.

precava (pre′ka-vă) [" + *cavus,* hollow]. The descending or superior vena cava.

precentral (prē-sĕn′trăl) [" + G. *kentron,* center]. In front of a center, as the central fissure of the brain.

p. convolution. The ascending frontal convolution.

prechordal (prē-kor′dăl) [" + G. *chordē,* cord]. In front of the notochord.

precipitant (prē-sĭp′ĭt-ănt) [L. *praecipitāre,* to cast down]. A substance bringing about precipitation.

precipitate (prē-sĭp′ĭt-āt). 1. A deposit separated from a suspension or solution by precipitation, the reaction of a reagent, which causes the deposit to fall to the bottom or float near the top. 2. To separate as a precipitate. 3. Hasty.

precipitation (prē-sĭp″ĭ-tā′shŭn). Process of a substance being separated from a solution by action of a reagent.

p. test. One in which positive reaction is indicated by formation of a precipitate in the solution being tested.

precipitin (prē-sĭp′ĭt-ĭn). An antibody formed in the blood serum of an animal due to presence of a soluble antigen usually a protein. When added to a solution of the antigen, it brings about precipitation.

The injected protein is called the *antigen* and the antibody produced is the *precipitin.* SEE ALSO: *autoprecipitin; precipitinogen.*

p. reaction. The formation of a precipitate in a solution containing a soluble antigen upon addition of serum containing the specific precipitin. The reaction is very specific, the test being used for identification of unknown proteins, determining types of pneumococci, meningococci, determination of types of blood stains, whether human or animal, and for diagnosis of plague, anthrax, and echinococcus disease; also called *precipitin test.*

precipitinogen (prē-sĭp″ĭt-ĭn′ō-jĕn) [" + G. *gennan,* to produce]. Any protein which, acting as an antigen, stimulates the production of a specific precipitin.

precipitinoid (prē-sĭp-ĭt-ĭn-oyd) [L. *praecipitāre,* to cast down, + G. *eidos,* form]. Precipitin which can no longer cause precipitation when mixed with its antigen but retains its affinity to the antigen.

precipitophore (prē-sĭp′ĭt-ō-fōr) [" + G. *phoros,* a bearer]. Group in a precipitin which produces precipitation. OPP: *haptophore precipitum.*

precipitum (prē-sĭp′ĭ-tum). The precipitate produced by action of a precipitin.

preclinical (prē-klĭn′ĭ-kăl) [L. *prae,* before, + G. *klinikos,* pert. to a bed]. Before the development or onset of disease.

p. medicine. 1. Medical procedures designed for preventing the development of or postponing the onset of disease or pathologic conditions. 2. Medical training engaged in before the study of patients, usually constituting the first two years of medical study.

preclival (prē-klī′văl) [" + *clivus,* slope]. In front of the cerebellar clivus.

precocity (prē-kos′ĭ-tĭ). Premature development.

p., sexual. Premature genital maturation; precocious sexual maturity.

precoital (prē-kō′ĭt-ăl) [" + *coitiō,* a going together]. Prior to sexual intercourse.

preconscious (prē-kŏn′shŭs) [" + *conscius,* aware]. Not present in consciousness but able to be recalled as desired.

preconvulsive (prē-kŏn-vŭl′sĭv) [" + *convulsiō,* a pulling together]. Before a convulsion.

precordia (prē-kor′dĭ-ă) [L. *praē,* before, + *cor, cord-,* heart]. The precordium, *q.v.*

precordial (prē-kor′dĭ-ăl) [L. *prae*, before, + *cor, cord-*, heart]. Pert. to the precordium or epigastrium.

precordialgia (prē″kor-dĭ-ăl′jĭ-ă) [" + " + G. *algos*, pain]. Pain in the chest or precordial area.

precordium (prē-kor′dĭ-ŭm) [" + *cor, cord-*, heart]. The area on the anterior surface of the body overlying the heart, its great vessels, the pericardium, and whatever pulmonary tissue lies anterior to these structures and the anterior chest wall. SYN: *precordia.*

precornu (prē-kor′nū) [" + *cornu*, horn]. Anterior horn of lateral ventricle of the brain.

precuneus (prē-kū′nē-ŭs) [" + *cuneus*, wedge]. The division of the mesial surface of a cerebral hemisphere between the cuneus and the paracentral lobule.

prediastolic (prē-dī-ăs-tŏl′ĭk) [" + G. *diastolē*, a sending apart]. Before the diastole, or interval in the cardiac cycle that precedes it.

predicrotic (prē-dī-krŏt′ĭk) [" + G. *dikrotos*, beating double]. Preceding the dicrotic wave of the sphygmographic tracing.

predigestion (prē-dĭ-jĕs′chŭn) [L. *prae*, before, + *digestiō*, a carrying apart]. Artificial proteolysis or digestion of proteins and amylolysis of starches before ingestion for use in illness.

predisposing (prē-dĭs-pōz′ĭng) [" + *disponere*, to dispose]. Conferring a tendency to or susceptibility to disease.

predisposition (prē″dĭs-pō-zĭ′shŭn) [" + *disponere*, to dispose]. A tendency to develop a certain disease, either acquired or hereditary.

p., acquired. P. to disease not due to innate or inherited factors, such as that resulting from malnutrition, excessive fatigue, etc.

predormition (prē-dŏrm-ĭ′shŭn). State of unconsciousness immediately preceding actual sleep.

preeclampsia (prē″ĕk-lămp′sĭ-ă) [" + G. *ek*, out, + *lampein*, to flash]. A toxemia of pregnancy characterized by increasing hypertension, headaches, albuminuria, and edema of the lower extremities.

If this condition is neglected or not treated properly, the patient may develop true eclampsia. SEE: *eclampsia.*

prefrontal (prē-fron′tăl) [" + *frons, front-*, front]. 1. The middle portion of the ethmoid bone. 2. In ant. part of the frontal lobe of the brain.

p. leukotomy. P. lobotomy, *q.v.*

p. lobotomy. SEE: *lobotomy.*

preganglionic (prē″găng-lĭ-ŏn′ĭk). Situated in front of or anterior to a ganglion.

p. fiber. The axon of a preganglionic neuron.

p. neuron. The first of a series of two efferent neurons which transmit impulses to visceral effectors. Its cell body lies in the central nervous system. Its axon terminates in an autonomic ganglion.

pregenital (prē-jĕn′ĭt-ăl) [L. *prae*, before, + *genitalia*, genitals]. PSY: Relating to that period when erotic interest is not yet organized about the reproductive organs and functions.

preglobulin (prē-glŏb′ū-lĭn) [" + *globulus*, a small sphere]. A proteid in cell protoplasm derived from cytoglobulin.

pregnancy (prĕg′năn-sĭ) [L. *praegnans*, with child]. The condition of being with child.

SYM AND SIGNS: Amenorrhea, nausea, and vomiting, inordinate appetite, pigmentation of the areola of the breasts, the development of Montgomery's tubercles around the nipple, changes in the uterus (softening and progressive enlargement), vaginal discoloration and frequent urination.

The positive sounds are: hearing and counting the fetal heart beat, finding x-ray evidence of the fetal skeleton, and detection by the physician of movements of the fetus. There are various biological tests for pregnancy, and these are between 90 and 95 per cent accurate.

The duration of pregnancy is approximately 280 days. SEE *Table, page P-94.* To estimate the day of delivery, count back 3 months from the day of onset of the last menstrual period and then add 7 days. For example, if the last menstrual period began June (6/10), subtracting 3 months leaves 3/10 and adding 7 days results in 3/17 (that is, the expected day of delivery would be March 17 of the next year. This method assumes all months have the same number of days; thus the date determined will not agree exactly with that found by using the table on page P-94.

PHYSICAL CHANGES DURING: *The Uterus*: (a) Changes shape, size and consistency. (b) Lining undergoes changes. (c) Peritoneal covering enlarges. (d) Muscles increase enormously. (e) Blood vessels penetrate through uterine muscle. (f) Cervix, vagina, and vulva become softer.

The Vaginal Canal: (a) Elongation caused by rising of uterus in pelvis. (b) Mucosa thickens. (c) Secretion increased. (d) Increased vascularity and elasticity.

Abdominal Changes: (a) Growing distention and flattened navel. (b) Striae gravidarum.

The Breasts: (a) Enlarged and painful. (b) Skin thin and sensitive. (c) Nipples erectile and enlarged, and darker. (d) Escape of colostrum. (e) Primary and secondary areola. (f) Tingling sensation.

Endocrine Glands: (a) Thyroid increases in size and activity. (b) Parathyroids enlarge, secretion increases. (c) Pituitary increases its activity. (d) Placenta gives forth hormones, affecting ovaries and corpus luteum.

Circulatory System: (a) Increased activity. (b) Increased blood volume. (c) Blood pressure should be normal. (d) Varicose veins common.

Skeletal Changes: (a) Pelvic joints soften. (b) Pelvic joints more movable. (c) Bones and teeth affected.

Respiratory Changes: (a) Lungs impeded in late pregnancy. (b) Breathing deeper and more frequent.

Digestive Tract: (a) Nausea and vomiting in early pregnancy. (b) Appetite affected. (c) Loss of weight in early pregnancy with slight anemia. (d) Basal metabolism raised in later pregnancy. (e) Constipation frequent.

The Liver: Enlarged and displaced in late pregnancy.

Skin: (a) Sudoriparous and sebaceous glands very active. (b) Deposit of brown pigment (mask of pregnancy). (c) Linea nigra.

The Weight: (a) Loss during first months. (b) Increased later.

Posture: (a) Changes, as enlargement of abdomen advances. (b) Sacroiliac joints and symphysis pubis more movable. (c) Painful locomotion and backache; waddling gait.

The Urinary Tract: (a) Increased kidney activity. (b) Failure of kidneys produces nephritic toxemia. (c) Ureters, especially right one, dilated. (d) Pressure on bladder with increased circulation. (e) Frequent urination. (f) Bladder lifted into abdomen and pressure diminished. (g) Bladder later pressed upon by presenting part. (h) Urinary output varies. (i) Presence of albumin abnormal. (j) Sugar found in later part of pregnancy. May be diabetes or glycosuria. (k) No blood sugar change.

DISORDERS OF: *Nausea and Vomiting*: (a) May be marked when stomach is empty. (b) May occur at any time. (c) Food may help on arising. (d) Four or five small meals per day. (e) Psychic causes may be responsible.

Constipation and Flatulence: (a) Pressure of uterus on intestines may be a cause. (b) Laxative diet and exercise may aid. (c) Intestinal stasis may cause flatulence. (d) Gas-forming foods should be avoided.

Muscular Cramps: (a) Retention of waste products a cause. (b) Poor circulation may cause (a). (c) Pressure on foot, extension of leg helps. (d) Rest between periods of standing needed. (e) Tetany may ensue because of deficient calcium supply. (f) Calcium and vitamin D indicated.

Pressure Edema: (a) May occur during last weeks. (b) Better in morning; worse at night. (c) Frequent rest and elevation of limbs indicated. (d) May be due to calcium deficiency. (e) Toxemia must be ruled out by frequent blood pressure and urinalysis.

Headache: (a) Intestinal intoxication and constipation causes. (b) Eyestrain may be suspected. (c) Temporary hypertrophy of pituitary common. (d) Sinusitis most common cause. (e) May be due to toxemia. (f) Blood pressure and urinalysis checked.

Neuralgic Pains: (a) Pressure of fetal head upon sciatic nerve suspected. (b) Rest periods and abdominal support indicated. (c) Knee-chest position after retiring.

Toothache: (a) May be due to caries induced by deficient calcium. (b) Acid condition of gums may be a cause. (c) Magnesia as a mouthwash indicated in (b). (d) Frequent dental examinations desirable.

Backache: (a) Abnormal balance caused by protruding abdomen. (b) Proper shoes indicated for (a). (c) Intra-abdominal pressure may be a cause. (d) Flatulence aggravates (c); enemas may help it. (e) Knee-chest position at night may help. (f) Gastric hyperacidity may induce high backaches. (g) Alkalies may temporarily help (f).

Dyspnea: (a) Pressure of uterus upward on transverse colon and stomach. (b) Aggravated by flatulence, especially when lying down. (c) Alkalies may help. (d) Pillows under head and shoulder indicated. (e) Reexamination of heart indicated.

Vaginal Discharge: (a) Increased blood supply to glands of cervix. (b) Cleanliness but no douches indicated. (c) Foul or blood-tinged or profuse discharge should be reported.

Pruritus or Itching: (a) Breasts, abdomen, and vulva may be affected. (b) Stretching of skin of abdomen a cause in that area. (c) If general, a toxic or nervous origin may be cause. (d) Acid-forming organism may cause vulvar itching. (e) Alkaline solutions, bland ointment, talcum for (d). (f) Sugar in urine may cause pruritus of vulva.

Heartburn: (a) Hyperacidity may be responsible, due to oversecretion of hydrochloric acid; also nervous tension. (b) Sedation, frequent small meals, no highly seasoned foods. (c) Organic acids from fermentative changes may be responsible. (d) Alkalies must not be taken too close to a meal. (e) Discomfort may be felt in the back. (f) Hydrochloric acid administered by the doctor.

Salivation: (a) May be associated with extreme nausea and vomiting. (b) Usually an expression of neurosis. (c) Mild astringents may be employed. (d) If due to a toxemia, refer to the physician.

Varicose Veins: (a) Congenitally acquired; aggravated by pregnancy. (b) May occur in pelvis, vulva, and legs; marked on right side. (c) Round garters, tight clothing, standing to be avoided. (d) Rest and supporting stockings indicated. (e) Elevation of lower limbs while sleeping. (f) Sims' position, pillow under hips to shift uterus.

Hemorrhoids: (a) Avoid constipation. (b) Ointments, wet compresses, suppositories on doctor's orders. (c) Carbolized or mentholated petrolatum in absence of (b). (d) Incision by surgeon.

p., abdominal. Implantation of the ovum in the abdominal cavity.

p., ampullar. P. in ampulla of uterine tube.

p., bigeminal. Pregnancy with twins *in utero*.

p., cervical. Implantation of the ovum in the cervical canal.

p., cornual. Pregnancy in one of the horns of a bicornuate uterus.

p., ectopic. SEE: *p., extrauterine.*

p., extrauterine. Pregnancy outside the uterine cavity.

p., false. SEE: *p., phantom.*

p., heterotropic. Combined intrauterine and extrauterine pregnancies.

p., hydatid. P. giving rise to a hydatidiform mole. SEE: *hydatid mole.*

p., interstitial. P. occurring in the uterine wall which forms part of the oviduct.

p., intraligamentary. P. occurring within the broad ligament.

p., intramural. Interstitial p., *q.v.*

p., mask of. Area of brown pigmentation sometimes appearing on the face during pregnancy.

p., membranous. P. in which amniotic sac ruptures and fetus comes to lie in direct contact with uterine wall.

p., mesenteric. Tuboligamentary p., *q.v.*

p., multiple. State of having more than one fetus in the uterus at the same time.

p., ovarian. Implantation of the fertilized ovum in the substance of the ovary.

p., phantom. Enlargement of the abdomen simulating pregnancy. SEE: *pseudocyesis.*

p., sarcofetal. P. involving presence of a fetus and a mole.

p. table. See Pregnancy Table on page P-94 for calculation of expected date of delivery from the first day of the last menstrual period.

PREGNANCY TABLE

Find the date of the last menstrual period in the top line (light-face type) of the pair of lines. The dark number (bold-face type) in the line below will be the expected day of delivery.

Jan.	1	2	3	4	5	6	7	8	9	10	11	12	13	14	15	16	17	18	19	20	21	22	23	24	25	26	27	28	29	30	31	
Oct.	8	9	10	11	12	13	14	15	16	17	18	19	20	21	22	23	24	25	26	27	28	29	30	31	(1	2	3	4	5	6	7	Nov.
Feb.	1	2	3	4	5	6	7	8	9	10	11	12	13	14	15	16	17	18	19	20	21	22	23	24	25	26	27	28				
Nov.	8	9	10	11	12	13	14	15	16	17	18	19	20	21	22	23	24	25	26	27	28	29	30	(1	2	3	4	5				Dec.
Mar.	1	2	3	4	5	6	7	8	9	10	11	12	13	14	15	16	17	18	19	20	21	22	23	24	25	26	27	28	29	30	31	
Dec.	6	7	8	9	10	11	12	13	14	15	16	17	18	19	20	21	22	23	24	25	26	27	28	29	30	31	(1	2	3	4	5	Jan.
Apr.	1	2	3	4	5	6	7	8	9	10	11	12	13	14	15	16	17	18	19	20	21	22	23	24	25	26	27	28	29	30		
Jan.	6	7	8	9	10	11	12	13	14	15	16	17	18	19	20	21	22	23	24	25	26	27	28	29	30	31	(1	2	3	4		Feb.
May	1	2	3	4	5	6	7	8	9	10	11	12	13	14	15	16	17	18	19	20	21	22	23	24	25	26	27	28	29	30	31	
Feb.	5	6	7	8	9	10	11	12	13	14	15	16	17	18	19	20	21	22	23	24	25	26	27	28	(1	2	3	4	5	6	7	Mar.
June	1	2	3	4	5	6	7	8	9	10	11	12	13	14	15	16	17	18	19	20	21	22	23	24	25	26	27	28	29	30		
Mar.	8	9	10	11	12	13	14	15	16	17	18	19	20	21	22	23	24	25	26	27	28	29	30	31	(1	2	3	4	5	6		April
July	1	2	3	4	5	6	7	8	9	10	11	12	13	14	15	16	17	18	19	20	21	22	23	24	25	26	27	28	29	30	31	
April	7	8	9	10	11	12	13	14	15	16	17	18	19	20	21	22	23	24	25	26	27	28	29	30	(1	2	3	4	5	6	7	May
Aug.	1	2	3	4	5	6	7	8	9	10	11	12	13	14	15	16	17	18	19	20	21	22	23	24	25	26	27	28	29	30	31	
May	8	9	10	11	12	13	14	15	16	17	18	19	20	21	22	23	24	25	26	27	28	29	30	31	(1	2	3	4	5	6	7	June
Sept.	1	2	3	4	5	6	7	8	9	10	11	12	13	14	15	16	17	18	19	20	21	22	23	24	25	26	27	28	29	30		
June	8	9	10	11	12	13	14	15	16	17	18	19	20	21	22	23	24	25	26	27	28	29	30	(1	2	3	4	5	6	7		July
Oct.	1	2	3	4	5	6	7	8	9	10	11	12	13	14	15	16	17	18	19	20	21	22	23	24	25	26	27	28	29	30	31	
July	8	9	10	11	12	13	14	15	16	17	18	19	20	21	22	23	24	25	26	27	28	29	30	31	(1	2	3	4	5	6	7	Aug.
Nov.	1	2	3	4	5	6	7	8	9	10	11	12	13	14	15	16	17	18	19	20	21	22	23	24	25	26	27	28	29	30		
Aug.	8	9	10	11	12	13	14	15	16	17	18	19	20	21	22	23	24	25	26	27	28	29	30	31	(1	2	3	4	5	6		Sept.
Dec.	1	2	3	4	5	6	7	8	9	10	11	12	13	14	15	16	17	18	19	20	21	22	23	24	25	26	27	28	29	30	31	
Sept.	7	8	9	10	11	12	13	14	15	16	17	18	19	20	21	22	23	24	25	26	27	28	29	30	(1	2	3	4	5	6	7	Oct.

p., tuboabdominal. P. in which part of fetus is in uterine tube and part in abdominal cavity.

p., tuboligamentary. P. occurring in uterine tube and extending into broad ligament.

p., tuboovarian. P. in which development of fetus occurs in both uterine tube and ovary.

pregnanediol (prĕg″năn-dī-ōl). $C_{21}H_{36}O_2$. The inactive end product of metabolism of progesterone present in the urine. Amount in urine increases during premenstrual or luteal phase of menstrual cycle and during pregnancy.

pregnant (prĕg′nănt) [L. *praegnans,* with child.] Having conceived; with child. SYN: *gravid.*

pregnenolone (prĕg-nĕn′ō-lōn). A synthetic hormone. A direct oxidation product of cholesterol with a formula closely related to that of cortisone.

pregravidic (prē-grăv-ĭd′ĭk) [L. *prae,* before, + *gravida,* pregnant]. Before pregnancy.

prehallux (prē-hăl′ŭks) [" + *hallux,* the great toe]. A supernumerary bone or accessory *naviculare pedis* or sometimes a prolongation inward of it on the foot.

prehemiplegic (prē-hĕm-ĭ-plē′jĭk) [" + G. *emi,* half, + *plēgē,* a stroke]. Occurring before an attack of hemiplegia.

prehensile (prē-hĕn′sĭl) [L. *prehendere,* to seize]. Capable of grasping.

prehension (prē-hĕn′shŭn) [L. *prehensiō,* from *prehendere,* to seize]. The act of grasping or seizing.

preimmunization. (prē-ĭm″ū-nĭ-zā′shŭn) [L. *prae,* before, + *immunis,* safe]. Immunization produced artificially in very young infants.

Preiser's disease (prī′zĕr). A porous condition of bone, osteoporosis, caused by trauma and affecting the carpal scaphoid bone of the wrist.

prelum (prē′lŭm) [L.]. A press.

p. abdominale. Squeezing of abdominal viscera in defecation, urination, and parturition, bet. the diaphragm and abdominal wall.

premature (prē-mă-tūr′). Not mature; before term or full development.

p. beat. A cardiac contraction occurring before the normal one. SYN: *extrasystole.*

p. infant. One born before term.

ETIOL: Uterine disease, shock, accident, toxemia of pregnancy, syphilis or any serious organic disease.

p. labor. Onset of labor before full term.

prematurity. The state of low birth weight of infants.

The normal gestation period for the human being is forty weeks; infants born prior to the thirty-eighth week of intrauterine life are considered premature. As difficulties are encountered in obtaining accurate and objective data as to the exact length of gestation, a birth weight of 2500 grams (5½ pounds) or less has been internationally accepted as the clinical criterion of prematurity regardless of the period of gestation. Other measures suggestive of prematurity are crown-heel length (47 cm. or less), crown-rump length (32 cm. or less), occipitofrontal circumference (33 cm. or less), occipitofrontal diameter (11.5 cm. or less), and ratio of the thorax circumference to the head circumference (less than 93%).

The use of a single criterion measure (birth weight) imposes limitations in accurately identifying those infants born before adequate development of body organs and systems has been achieved; it can easily include mature infants who are of low birth weight for reasons other than a shortened gestation period. The Expert Committee on Prematurity of the World Health Organization (1961) has recommended that the concept of prematurity in the international definition be replaced by that of low birth weight. This term, *low birth weight,* more accurately describes the infant population encompassed by a 2500 gram birth weight criterion than does the term *prematurity;* the latter should be reserved for those neonates within the low birth weight group that show signs of immaturity.

During 1962 there were 4,167,362 live births in the United States. Eight per cent of these infants weighed 2500 grams or less at birth. Chances of survival depend upon degree of maturity achieved, general condition, and quality of care received. (See table, P-95.)

Prematurity is the leading cause of death in the neonatal period; mortality among infants weighing less than 2500 grams at birth is twenty times greater than among infants with birth weight above 2500 grams. Chief causes of mortality are poor abnormal pulmonary ventilation, infection, intracranial hemorrhage, abnormal blood conditions, and congenital anomalies.

The incidence of neonates of low birth weight is more frequent among

PERCENTAGE DISTRIBUTION AND SURVIVAL OF THE LOW BIRTH WEIGHT INFANTS

Birth Weight Group	*Total Live Births* (per cent)*	*Low Birth Weight Infants Only* (per cent)*	*Approximate Survival of Low Birth Weight Infants** (per cent)*
Under 1000 grams	0.5	6.25	10
1001 - 1500 grams	0.7	8.75	50
1501 - 2000 grams	1.5	18.75	85
2001 - 2500 grams	5.3	66.25	95
Total 2500 grams or less:	8.0	100.00	85***
Total 2500 grams or over:	92.0		
Total Live Births:	100.0		

* U. S. National Vital Statistics 1962.
** New York City Infant Mortality Rates 1962.
*** Weighted average.

the female sex; the non-white race; the plural born; and the first and fifth (and over) born infants. Delivery of infants of low birth weight is reported to be more frequent among women who are less than nineteen years of age and more than thirty years of age; are poorly nourished; and have had little or no prenatal care; as well as among those women who are unmarried; are cigarette smokers; and have bacteriuria that has not been treated. Low birth weight infants are also reported to be more frequent among women who work during pregnancy; women who live in high altitude areas; families of lower social classes; families in which pregnancies occur within a two-year period or beyond a six-year period of the previous pregnancy; and families living in urban areas.

Factors contributing to prematurity and/or low birth weight have been shown to be premature rupture of the membranes, antepartum hemorrhage, toxemia of pregnancy, chronic diseases, acute infections, pelvic abnormalities, physical and emotional trauma, blood incompatibilities, malformation of the fetus, and multiple births. In more than 50 per cent of these deliveries, the cause for low birth weight cannot be stated.

Premature infants are frequently handicapped by a number of anatomical and physiological limitations. These limitations vary in direct proportion to the degree of immaturity present, and include weakness of the sucking and swallowing reflexes; small capacity of stomach; lowered tolerance of alimentary tract; impairment of renal function; incomplete development of capillaries of medulla and lungs; immature alveoli of the lungs; weakness of the cough and gag reflexes; weakness of the thoracic cage and muscles used in respiration; inadequate regulation of body temperature; incomplete enzyme systems; hepatic immaturity; and deficient placental transfer and antenatal storage of minerals, vitamins, and immune substances.

Care of low birth weight infants should be individualized and reflect the needs of the developing organism in relation to the presence of anatomic and physiologic handicaps. Evaluation for degree of immaturity present and the identification of special problems appearing after birth will dictate care required by these infants. In general, care revolves around the prevention of infection, stabilization of body temperature, maintenance of respiration, provision for adequate nutrition and hydration, and conservation of energy.

Aseptic technique is practiced to prevent infection. An incubator or heated bed provides a suitable environment for maintenance of body temperature. A high humidity environment may be of value in respiratory difficulties. Gentle suctioning will aid to keep airways clear. Use of oxygen should be restricted to those minimal amounts required for survival of infant. Because of the danger of retrolental fibroplasia, the oxygen concentration should not exceed 40 per cent.

Depending upon the ability of the infant to suck and swallow, gavage feedings may be necessary. Some of these infants may not be given anything by mouth for as long as seventy-two hours following birth. Caloric and fluid intakes are gradually increased until 100-120 calories per kilogram and 140-150 cc. per kilogram, per twenty-four hours, are reached. The time required to achieve these intakes depends upon the size and condition of the baby. Small, frequent feedings may be needed to cope with the small capacity of the stomach, to prevent vomiting and distention, and to meet caloric and fluid requirements of the body. Over-feeding should be avoided. During the early days of life, clyses are sometimes administered to maintain adequate hydration.

The infant should not be allowed to become fatigued either from excessive handling, prolonged feeding procedures, or too much crying. His position should be changed every two to four hours. Minimal handling regimen should not be used indiscriminately; gentle handling, rather than minimal handling, should be practiced.

premaxilla (prē"măks-ĭl'ă) [" + *maxilla*, upper jaw]. The intermaxillary bone forming median anterior part of superior maxillary bones.

premaxillary (prē-măk'sĭ-lĕr-ĭ) [" + *maxillaris*, pert. to the upper jaw]. Located before the maxilla.

p. bone. The intermaxillary bone. SYN: *incisive bone.*

premedication (prē-mĕd-ĭ-kā'shŭn) [" + *medicari*, to heal]. Induction of unconsciousness by internal drugs prior to administration of inhalation anesthesia. SYN: *prenarcosis.*

premenstrual (prē-mĕn'strū-ăl) [L. *prae*, before, + *menstruāre*, to menstruate]. Before menstruation.

premenstruum (prē-mĕn'strū-ŭm) [" + *menstruum*, monthly fluid]. The period prior to menstruation.

premolar (prē-mō'ler) [" + *moles*, a mass]. 1. A bicuspid tooth. 2. Before a molar tooth.

premonition (prē-mō-nĭsh'ŭn) [" + *monēre*, to warn]. A feeling of an impending event.

premonitory (prē-mon'ĭ-tō-rĭ) [L. *praemonitorius*, warning before]. Giving a warning; foreboding or forewarning.

premonocyte (prē-mon'ō-sīt) [L. *prae*, before, + G. *monos*, alone, + *kytos*, cell]. An embryonic cell transitional in development prior to a monocyte.

premunition (prē-mū-nĭsh'ŭn.) [L. *prae*, before, + *munitio*, a fortification]. Immunity depending upon existence of a long-continued latent infection.

premyelocyte (prē-mī'ĕl-ō-sīt) [L. *prae*, before, + G. *myelos*, marrow, + *kytos*, cell]. The cell that is the immediate precursor of a myelocyte.

prenarcosis (prē-nar-kō'sĭs) [" + G. *narkōsis*, stuporous condition]. Induction of unconsciousness by drugs before administration of a general inhalation anesthetic. SYN: *premedication.*

prenatal (prē-nā'tl) [" + *natalis*, pert. to birth]. Before birth.

p. care. The care of the pregnant woman during the period of gestation.

This care consists of periodic examinations for the determination of the blood pressure, weight, urinalysis, changes in the size of the uterus, and condition of the fetus as determined by the heart tones and position. By such examinations, changes in the condition of the patient can be noted and toxemias prevented by the institution of treatment as soon as any abnormal signs are present.

preoperative preparation. 1. Prepare area indicated according to technique of your hospital. 2. Be sure the water and liquid soap you use for shaving and cleansing the skin are warmed; cold liquids on the abdomen give the patient a disagreeable shock. 3. See that patient is attended by his clergyman if this has not already been done before he came to the hospital. This is *absolutely essential* in the case of patients who are members of the Roman Catholic Church or the Church of Jesus Christ of Latter Day Saints (Mormon). 4. Try to have the patient get as much sleep as possible. If he is wakeful and you do not wish to give sedative early, try to find some reading matter for him. 5. Give the enemas ordered for the morning as late as you can if he is asleep so as to give him as much rest as possible. 6. Get order for catheterization if you think it will be needed. 7. *Never* send a patient to the operating table with a full bladder. 8. Give preanesthetic medication, or basal anesthetic, at *exactly* the time specified. 9. See that dentures are removed and placed in a glass of water which is marked with the patient's name and room number. 10. See that women do not have make-up on face or nails and that they are not wearing hair pins or "bobbie" pins. 11. Tie the wedding ring in place. 12. Do not use straight pins in patient's gown or operating cap. 13. Wrap blankets well around neck when he is placed on stretcher to keep drafts out. 14. Do not forget chart when taking him to surgery. 15. Do not chatter with other nurses you meet on the way or while waiting with the patient before he is anesthetized. 16. Do not forget to reassure anxious relatives who may not like to disturb you with many questions and who do not understand all that is going on as well as you do.

preoral (prē-ō'răl) [" + *os, or-*, mouth]. In front of the mouth.

preparation (prep-ă-ra'shun). 1. The making ready, especially of a medicine for use. 2. A specimen set up for demonstration in anatomy, pathology, or histology.

preparalytic (prē"păr-ă-lĭt'ĭk) [" + G. *para*, at the side, + *lyein*, to loosen]. Before the appearance of paralysis.

preparations usually given by rectum. These are the following:

Chloral hydrate: 0.5 to 1.0 gm. dissolved in 3 oz. of olive oil, warmed; or 3 oz. of very warm milk, or 3 oz. of thin, boiled cornstarch water. This makes a good preparation or a base in which to hold the medicine in suspension. The patient's pulse should be taken 5 minutes before and 5 minutes after the administration to determine the heart action. If untoward effects are noticed, action may be taken to prevent further absorption.

Glycerin: This is added, 1 oz. to a pint of plain water. It will cause a good evacuation. One ounce of glycerin to 1 oz. of water will cause irritation of the lower bowel and precipitate an evacuation. This may be given with a bulb syringe.

Alum: The alum enema consists of 1 qt. of warm water and 1 oz. of powdered alum. This enema has a tendency to dry up intestinal fermentations.

Paraldehyde: Dosage, 1 to 4 cc. may be mixed with water in the proportion of 1 to 8 and in this ratio it may be mixed with thin starch water for rectal medication. There should be about 3 oz. of starch water.

Sodium bicarbonate: One tablespoonful or 4 gm. to 500 cc. or 1 pint of water aids in the expulsion of the bowel content. The neutralizing action of the acidity of the bowel content brought about by the sodium bicarbonate solution leaves the bowel soothed and with a bland reaction.

RS: *alkaloids, active principles, drugs with 2 names, names of preparations; antidotes; dosage; drug action; drugs and their administration; medical preparations; names of individual drugs in alphabetical order; names of poisons; poison; poisoning; prescription writing.*

prepatellar (prē-pă-tĕl'ar) [L. *prae*, before, + *patella*, pan]. In front of the patella.

p. bursitis. Inflammation of the bursa in front of patella. SYN: *housemaid's knee.* SEE: *bursitis.*

prepat'ent. Before becoming evident or manifest.

p. period. Period between the time of introduction of parasitic organisms into the body and their appearance in the blood or tissues.

prepuce (prē'pūs) [L. *praeputium*, prepuce]. The foreskin or fold of skin over the glans penis in the male.

Excision constitutes *circumcision*, a common religious practice, but also performed in cases of phimosis and for hygienic purposes. A sebaceous secretion under the prepuce is called *smegma.*

RS: *acrobystiolith, acrobystitis, acroposthitis, aposthia, frenulum, penis, phimosis, smegma, urethra* (of male).

p. of the clitoris. Fold of the labia minora which covers the clitoris. SEE: *clitoris.*

preputial (prē-pū'shăl) [L. *praeputium*, prepuce]. Concerning the prepuce.

p. glands. Small sebaceous glands of the corona of the penis which secrete an odoriferous discharge. SYN: *Tyson's glands.*

preputium (prē-pū'shĭ-ŭm) (pl. *preputia*) [L. *praeputium*, prepuce]. The fold of skin that covers the glans penis. SYN: *prepuce, q.v.*

p. clitoridis. Prepuce of the clitoris, a fold overhanging the glans clitoridis formed by the union of the two labia minora.

prepyloric (pre"pi-lor'ik). Anterior to or preceding the pylorus of the stomach.

presbyacusia, presbyacousia (prĕz"bĭ-ă-kū'sĭ-ă) [G. *presbys*, old, + *akousis*, hearing]. Hearing less acutely, due to old age. SYN: *presbycusis.*

presbyatrics, presbyatry (prĕz-bĭ-ăt'rĭks, prĕz'bĭ-ăt-rĭ) [" + *iatrikos*, healing]. That branch of medicine dealing with the diseases of old age. SYN: *geriatrics.*

presbycusis, presbykousis (prĕz-bĭ-kū'sĭs) [" + *akousis*, hearing]. Impairment of hearing in old age. SYN: *presbyacusia.*

presbyophrenia (prĕz-bĭ-ō-frē'nĭ-ă) [" + *phrēn*, mind]. Senile psychotic syndrome involving confabulation and disorientation with preservation of mobility, loquacity, and good spirits. SYN: *Wernicke's syndrome.*

presbyopia (prĕz-bĭ-ō'pĭ-ă) [" + *ōps*, eye]. Defect of vision in advancing age involving loss of accommodation or recession of near point. Due to loss of elasticity of crystalline lens.

The onset usually occurs between 40 and 45 years of age. SEE: *farsightedness.*

presbytiatrics (prĕz-bĭt-ĭ-ăt'rĭks) [" +

iatrikos, healing]. Science of old age and its treatment. SYN: *geriatrics; presbyatrics; presbyatry.*

prescription (prē-skrĭp′shŭn) [L. *praescriptiō,* a writing before, an order]. A written order for dispensing drugs signed by a physician.

A prescription consists of four main parts.

SUPERSCRIPTION: Represented by the symbol ℞ which signifies *Recipe,* from the Latin *recipere,* meaning to take.

INSCRIPTION: Containing the ingredients. This again is generally constructed of four parts: (a) The *basis* or principal drug; (b) the *adjuvant,* which assists the action of the basis; (c) the *corrective,* which diminishes unpleasant taste or pain or griping, etc.; (d) the *vehicle* to hold the drugs either in solution or suspension.

SUBSCRIPTION: Directions to the dispenser as to the manner of preparation of the drugs.

SIGNATURE: Directions to the patient with regard to the manner of taking, dosage, etc.; finally, the physician's signature, address, telephone number, date, and whether or not the prescription may be refilled. When applicable, the physician's narcotics registry number should be included.

p. carbons. PT: Carbons impregnated with various substances for use in treatment of specific conditions.

p. drug. A medicine which can be obtained only when prescribed by a physician.

p., shotgun. Indiscriminate prescription for a large number of drugs in the hope that at least one of them will accomplish the desired effect.

prescription writing. Modern practice is to write prescriptions entirely in the language of the country in which written (as English in the United States) and to use few, if any, abbreviations. All drug quantities should be shown by using the metric system of weights and measures (grams, milligrams, liters, milliliters, etc.).

Note: The following classical presentation of the art of prescription writing is included primarily for its historical interest.

LATIN USAGE IN PRESCRIPTIONS: An official Latin name is in the nominative case. *Drugs:* Written in the genitive case, as the prescription is an order, meaning "take thou." *Word "of":* This is not written in Latin but is indicated by the ending of a word: *Quinina,* of course, means "quinine," but changing the termination to "ae" we have *"quininae,"* meaning *of quinine.*

ALKALOIDS: Written the same as in English, except that the final "e" is changed to "a" to form the nominative case, as *quinina,* for the English quinine. To form the genitive case, the final "e" is changed to "ae," as *quininae.*

ACTIVE PRINCIPLES: These, such as glucosides, resinoids and others, add "um" to the nominative, and "i" to the genitive, as Strophanthin becomes *strophanthinum* to form the Latin nominative, and *strophanthini,* to form the Latin genitive.

ACIDS: The names of these are formed in the same way as those of alkaloids, except that the adjective is formed in the same way and follows the nominative, as *Acidum Hydrochloricum,* or the genitive, *Acidi Hydrochlorici.*

METALS: Latin names of metals, except those of a few known to the ancients, are the same as English forms ending in "um," as in *Sodium,* forming the Latin nominative, but ending in "i" to form the genitive, *Sodii.*

SALTS: Written first with the name of the *base* in its genitive form, next the *acid radical* in the nominative, followed by the *qualitative adjective,* also in the nominative, as *Ferri Sulfas Exsiccatus,* exsiccated sulfate of iron.

NAMES OF PREPARATIONS: Show the *class* to which it belongs first, the name of the *ingredient* next, and the *qualifying* adjective last, as *Syrupus Scillae Compositus* (Compound Syrup of Squills). First and last words are in nominative case and middle one in genitive.

DRUGS WITH TWO NAMES: Both should be in the genitive, as *Liquor Potassi Arsenitis. -ate endings*: The Latin nominative ends in "as," as *sulfas,* for sulfate, and the genitive in "atis," as *sulfatis. -ite endings*: If the English word ends in "ite," as *"sulfite,"* the Latin nominative ends in "is," as *sulfis,* and the genitive in "itis," as *sulfitis. -ide endings*: If an English word has this ending, as "Bromide," the Latin nominative ends in "um," dropping the final "e" in the English form, as *Bromidum;* the genitive dropping the "um" to add "i," as *Bromidi.*

-a, -us, -um endings: English words with these endings are the same in the Latin nominative, but the genitive is formed by changing "a" to "ae," or the "us" or "um" to "i." *-in endings*: An English word having this ending adds "um" (usually) to form the Latin nominative as Benzoin and *Benzoinum,* the genitive being formed by merely adding "i," as *Benzoini. -ol endings*: The Latin nominative is the same as the English, as in "Phenol," but "is" is added to form the genitive, as *Phenolis. -al endings*: To form the Latin nominative, "um" is added, as Chloral and *Chloralum.* To form the genitive, "i" is added to the English form, as *Chlorali.*

There are, of course, exceptions to the foregoing. Many Latin words have the same form as in English. Fortunately, perhaps, most drugs are indicated in prescription by abbreviations which may not discriminate bet. the Latin nominative and genitive.

RS: *alkaloids, active principles, drugs with 2 names, names of preparations; antidotes; dosage; drug action; drugs and their administration; medical preparations; names of individual drugs in alphabetical order; names of poisons; poison; poisoning; preparations usually given by rectum.*

presentation (prē-zĕn-tā′shŭn) [L. *praesentatiō,* a placing before]. OB: Term applied to the manner of the fetus presenting itself to the examining finger in the vagina or rectum.

Thus longitudinal (normal) and transverse (pathological) presentation.

p., breech. When buttocks of fetus present.

Breech presentation is of three types: *Complete breech,* when the thighs are flexed on the abdomen and the legs flexed upon the thighs; *frank breech,* when the legs are extended over the ant. surface of the body, and *footling,* when a foot or feet present; footling can be single, double, or if the leg remains flexed, knee presentation.

Terms Used in Prescription Writing

Abbreviation	*Word or Phrase*	*English Equivalent*
āā or a	ana	of each
abs. feb.	absente febre	fever being absent
ad	ad	to, up to
add.	adde	add
ad. feb.	adstante febre	fever being present
adhib.	adhibendus	to be administered
ad. lib.	ad libitum	at pleasure
admov.	admove	apply
ad part. dolent.	ad partes dolentes	to the painful parts
agit.	agita	shake, stir
alb.	albus	white
alter	alter	the other
alt. hor.	alternis horis	every other hour
ante cib. or A. C.	ante cibum	before food
aq. bull.	aqua bulliens	boiling water
aq. dest.	aqua destillata	distilled water
aq. font.	aqua fontis	spring water
aq. pur.	aqua pura	pure water
aut	aut	or
bene	bene	well
b. i. d.	bis in die	twice daily
bib.	bibe	drink
bis	bis	twice
bol.	bolus	a large pill
bull.	bulliat	let (it) boil
c̄	cum	with
cap.	capsula	a capsule
chart. or cht.	chartula	a small medicated paper
coch. mag.	cochleare magnum	a tablespoonful
coch. med	cochleare medium	a dessertspoonful
coch. parv.	cochleare parvum	a teaspoonful
collyr.	collyrium	an eyewash
commisce	commisce	mix together
comp.	compositus	compounded of
cong.	congius	a gallon
cont. rem.	continuantur remedia	continue the medicine
cotula	cotula	a measure
cras mane sum	cras mane sumendus	take tomorrow morning
cuj. lib.	cujus libet	of any you please
d., det.	da, detur	give, let be given
d. d. in d.	de die in diem	from day to day
dec.	decanta	pour off
dent. tal. dos.	dentur tales doses	give of such doses
dexter	dexter	the right
dieb. alt.	diebus alternis	every other day
dieb. tert.	diebus tertiis	every 3rd day
dil.	dilue, dilutus	dilute, diluted
dim.	dimidius	one-half
div.	divide	divide
div. in p. aeq.	dividatur in partes aequales	let it be divided into equal parts
donec alv. sol. ft.	donec alvus soluta fuerit	until bowels are open
dos.	dosis	dose
dur. dolor.	durante dolore	while pain lasts
e.m.p.	ex modo prescripto	as directed
emp.	emplastrum	plaster
emuls.	emulsio	an emulsion
en.	enema	an enema
epistom.	epistomium	a stopper
ext.	extende	spread
febris	febris	fever
ferv.	fervens	boiling
filt.	filtra	filter
ft.	fiat	let be made
garg.	gargarisma	a gargle
grad.	gradatim	by degrees
gr.	granum	a grain
gtt.	gutta, guttae	a drop, drops
guttat.	guttatim	by drops
h.	hora	an hour
haust.	haustus	a draught
hor. decub.	hora decubitus	bedtime
hor. som. or h. s.	hora somni	bedtime
hor. 1 spat.	horae unius spatio	one hour's time
idem	idem	the same
ind.	indies	daily
inf.	infusum	let it infuse
int.	intime	thoroughly
lin.	linimentum	a liniment
liq.	liquor	a solution
lot.	lotio	a lotion

Abbreviation	*Word or Phrase*	*English Equivalent*
M.	misce	mix
mac.	macera	macerate
man. prim.	mane primo	first thing in the morning
mas.	massa	mass
med.	medicamentum	a medicine
m. et n.	mane et nocte	morning and night
mitt.	mitte	send
mitt. x tal.	mitte decem tales	send 10 like this
mod.	modicus	moderate sized
mod. praesc.	modo praescripto	in the manner written
moll.	mollis	soft
mor. dict.	more dicto	in the manner directed
mor. sol.	more solito	as accustomed
ne tr. s. num.	ne tradas sine nummo	deliver not without the money
no.	numerus	number
noct. maneq.	nocte maneque	night and morning
non. rep., n. r.	non repetatur	let it not be repeated
nunc	nunc	now
o.	octarius	a pint
O.D.	oculus dexter	right eye
O.L.	oculus laevus	left eye
omn. bih.	omni bihoris	every 2nd hour
omn. hor.	omni hora	every hour
om. ¼ h.	omni quadrantae horae	every 15 minutes
om. mane vel. noc.	omni mane vel nocte	every morning or night
part. vic.	partitus vicibus	individual doses
p. c.	post cibum	after meals
pil.	pilula	a pill
p. p. a.	phiala prius agitata	the bottle being first shaken
p. r. n.	pro re nata	as occasion arises
pro. rat. aet.	pro ratione aetatis	according to patient's age
pulv.	pulvis	powder
q. h.	quaque hora	every hour
q. l.	quantum libet	as much as pleases
q. s.	quantum sufficiat	as much as suffices
quotid.	quotidie	daily
red. in pulv.	redactus in pulverem	reduced to powder
repetat., rep.	repetatur	to be repeated
rub.	ruber	red
sec. a., or s. a.	secundem artem	according to art
semih.	semihora	half an hour
sig.	signa	write
sing.	singulorum	of each
sol.	solutio	solution
s. o. s.	si opus sit	if need exists
solv.	solve	dissolve
ss.	semi or semisse	a half
stat.	statim	immediately
st.	stet or stetem	let it (or them) stand
subind.	subinde	frequently
sum.	sume	take
sum. tal.	sumat talem	take 1 such
suppos.	suppositoria	a suppository
s.v.r.	spiritus vini rectificatus	rectified spirit of wine
tab.	tabella	a tablet
tere	tere	rub
tere bene	tere bene	rub well
t. i. d.	ter in die	three times daily
tinct.	tinctura	a tincture
trit.	tritura	triturate or grind
ult. praes.	ultimus praescriptus	the last ordered
ung.	unguentum	an ointment
ut dict.	ut dictum	as directed
vitel.	vitellus	yolk of an egg

Weights and Measures.

♏ Minimum, -i, n., minim, of a fluidram.
Gtt. Gutta, -ae, f., a drop.
gr. Granum, -i, n., a grain.
℈ Scrupulus, -i, m., a scruple, 20 grains.
ʒ Drachma, -ae, f., a dram, 60 grains.
f ʒ Fluidrachma, -ae, f., a fluidram, 60 minims.
℥ Uncia, -ae, f., a troy ounce, 480 grains.
f ℥ Fluiduncia, -ae, f., a fluidounce, 8 fluidrams.
lb. Libra, -ae, f., a pound (troy), 5760 grains.
O. Octarius, -i, m., a pint, 16 fluidounces.
C. Congius, -i, m., a gallon, 8 pints.
ss. Semis, indecl., a half.

Quantities are designated by Roman numerals following the symbol for denomination
SEE: *charting.*

p., brow. When the brow presents.

p., cephalic. Presentation of the head in any position.

p., face. When the head is sharply extended so that the face presents.

p., footling. Presenting feet first.

p., placental. Presentation of the placenta first. SYN: *placenta previa.*

p., sinciput. When the large fontanel presents.

p., transverse. With fetus lying crosswise.

p., vertex. P. of the upper and back part of the head.

preservative (pre-zerv'ă-tiv). A substance added to medicines or foods to prevent them from spoiling. It may act by interfering with certain chemical reactions or with the growth of molds, fungi, bacteria or parasites. Some common preservatives are sugar, salt, vinegar, ethyl alcohol, sulfur dioxide, and benzoic acid.

presphenoid (prē-sfē'noyd) [L. *prae,* before, + G. *sphēn,* wedge, + *eidos,* form]. Ant. region of the body of the sphenoid bone.

presphygmic (prē-sfĭg'mĭk) [" + G. *sphygmos,* pulse]. Pert. to period preceding the pulse wave.

prespinal (prē-spī'năl) [" + *spina,* thorn]. Before the spine, or ventral to it.

prespondylolisthesis (prē-spŏn"dĭl-ō-lĭs-thē'sĭs) [" + G. *spondylos,* vertebra, + *olisthanein,* to slip]. A congenital defect of both pedicles of the fifth lumbar vertebra without displacement. This predisposes to spondylolisthesis.

pressinervoscopy (prĕs"ĭ-nĕr-vŏs'kō-pĭ) [L. *pressus,* from *premere,* to press, + *nervus,* a nerve, + G. *skopein,* to examine]. Diagnosis by pressing upon the parasympathetic and sympathetic nerves.

pressor (prĕs'ōr) [L. *pressor,* from *premere,* to press]. 1. Stimulating, increasing the activity of a function, especially of vasomotor activity, as a nerve. 2. Inducing an elevation in blood pressure.

p. base or ***amine.*** One of several amines or nitrogenous bases of plant or animal origin which, when injected, have the ability to increase blood pressure.

p. nerves. Nerves which when stimulated bring about an increase in blood pressure.

p. reflex. Any reflex in which the response to stimulation is increased by blood pressure.

pressoreceptor (pres"o-re-sep'tor). Sensory nerve ending such as those in the aorta and carotid sinus which are stimulated by changes in blood pressure.

pressure (prĕsh'ūr) [L. *pressura,* a squeezing]. 1. A compression. 2. Stress or force exerted on a body, as by tension, weight, pulling, etc. 3. PSY: Quality of sensation aroused by moderate compression of the skin. 4. In physics, the quotient obtained by dividing a force by the area of the surface on which it acts.

RS: *atmosphere; blood; hypertonic; isotonic.*

p., after-. A feeling of p. which remains for a few seconds after removal of a weight or other pressure.

p., arterial. P. of blood in the arteries.

For a normal young man at physical and mental rest and in sitting position, systolic blood pressure averages about 120 mm. Hg; diastolic pressure about 80 mm. Hg. There is a wide range of normal variation, due to constitutional, physical, and psychic factors. For women the figures are lower; for older people they are higher. There is little difference in the b.p. of the two arms.

p., atmospheric. P. of weight of atmosphere; at sea level it averages about 760 mm. of mercury.

p., back. P. resulting from interference in flow of blood from the ventricles such as occurs in valvular disorders. Results in reduced venous return to the heart and consequent venous engorgement.

p., blood. P. exerted by blood against the walls of blood vessels. SEE: *blood pressure.*

p., diastolic. Arterial pressure during diastole or dilatation of heart chambers.

p., endocardiac. Blood pressure within the heart. SYN: *p., intracardiac.*

p., hydrostatic. The pressure exerted by a fluid within a closed system.

p., intraabdominal. P. within the abdominal cavity such as that caused by descent of the diaphragm.

p., intracranial. P. of the cerebrospinal fluid in the subarachnoid space between the skull and the brain. The pressure is normally the same as that found during lumbar puncture.

p., intraocular. Normal tension within the eyeball, equal to 20 to 25 mm. of mercury.

p., intrathoracic. P. within the thorax but outside of the lungs. In quiet expiration it is about — 4.5 mm., and in forced inspiration, as high as — 30 mm., but in quiet inspiration, — 7.5 mm.

p., intraventricular. P. within the ventricles of the heart during different phases of diastole and systole.

p., oncotic. Osmotic pressure, *q.v.*

p., osmotic. The force with which a solvent, usually water, passes through a semipermeable membrane separating solutions of different concentrations. It is measured by determining the hydrostatic (mechanical) pressure which must be opposed to the osmotic force to bring the passage to a standstill. The osmotic pressure of blood serum and of solutions isotonic with it is 6.7 atmospheres. SYN: *p., oncotic.*

p. palsy. Temporary paralysis due to pressure on a nerve trunk.

p. paralysis. Paralysis due to pressure on the spinal cord.

ETIOL: Injury, tumor, gummata.

p. points. Areas for exerting pressure to control bleeding.

For control of hemorrhage, pressure above bleeding point when an artery passes over a bone may be sufficient. The principal pressure points are:

(a) Two inches above clavicle, over *common carotid artery,* backwards, against spine. (b) At side of face in front of ear, over *temporal artery.* (c) Behind mastoid process, over *occipital artery.* (d) Behind clavicle, pressing *subclavian artery* down on to 1st rib. (e) The *axillary artery* by compression in axilla. (f) The *brachial artery* compressed by pressure at inner edge of biceps muscle halfway down arm, and also above bend of elbow, before artery divides into *radial* and *ulnar arteries.* (g) On thumb side of wrist against radius, to compress the *radial.* (h) On little finger side of wrist against ulna, to compress *ulnar.* (i) In palm, opp. root of abducted thumb, over *deep palmar arch.* (j) *Abdominal artery* may be compressed against lumbar vertebrae, to left of middle line, when patient lies on his back. (k) By abduction and external rotation of thigh, head of femur is brought forward into groin and *femoral artery* may be compressed against it, in this position. (l) In popliteal space over *popliteal artery.* (m) At front of bend of ankle over *ant. tibial artery.* (n) Behind internal malleolus, over *post. tibial artery,* as it passes into foot.

p., pulse. The difference between systolic and diastolic pressures.

p. sore. A sore caused by pressure as from a splint or other appliance or from the body itself when it has remained immobile in bed for extended periods of time. SYN: *bed sore; decubitus ulcer.*

p., systolic. Arterial pressure at time of the contraction of the ventricles, or the ventricular systole.

p., venous. Pressure of the blood within the veins. It is highest near the periphery, diminishing progressively from capillaries to the heart. Near the heart the pressure may be below zero (a "negative pressure") due to negative intrathoracic pressure.

presternum (prē-ster'nŭm) [L. *prae,* before, + G. *sternon,* chest]. The upper part of the sternum. SYN: *manubrium, sterni.*

presuppurative (prē-sŭp'ū-rā-tĭv) [" + *sub,* under, + *puris,* pus]. Relating to period of inflammation before suppuration.

presylvian fissure (pre-sil'vĭ-ăn) [L. *prae,* before]. The anterior division of the sylvian fissure.

presystole (prē-sĭs'tō-lē) [" + G. *systolē,* contraction]. The period in the heart's cycle just before the systole.

presystolic (prē-sĭs-tol'ĭk) [" + *systolē,* contraction]. Before the systole of the heart.

pretarsal (prē-tar'săl) [" + G. *tarsos,* tarsus]. In front of the tarsus.

pretibial (prē-tĭb'ĭ-ăl) [" + *tibia,* shin]. In front of the tibia.

p. fever. SYN: *Fort Bragg fever.* A viral disease characterized by fever, rash on legs, prostration, splenomegaly, and respiratory disturbances.

preurethritis (prē"ū-re-thrī'tĭs) [" + G. *ourēthra,* urethra, + *-itis,* inflammation]. Inflammation around the urethral orifice of the vaginal vestibule.

prev'alence. The number of cases of a disease present in a specified population at a given time.

preventive (prē-vĕn'tĭv) [L. *praevenīre,* to come before]. Warding off. SYN: *prophylactic.*

p. medicine. That branch of medicine concerned with the prevention of disease.

preventorium (prē-vĕn-to'rĭ-ŭm) [L. *praevenīre,* to come before]. An institution for those threatened with tuberculosis.

prevertebral (prē-ver'te-brăl) [L. *prae,* before, + *vertebra,* vertebra]. In front of a vertebra.

prevertiginous (prē-ver-tĭj'ĭn-ŭs) [" + *vertigo,* dizziness]. Having a tendency to fall forward. SYN: *dizzy.*

prevesical (pre-ves'ĭ-kl). Located in front of the bladder.

pre'via, praevia. Appearing before or in front of.

prezon'ular. Pert. to the post. chamber of the eye, the space between iris and ciliary zonule (suspensory ligament).

priapism (prī'ă-pizm) [G. *Priapos,* god of fertility, + *-ismos,* condition]. Abnormal, painful and continued erection of the penis due to disease, usually without sexual desire.

ETIOL: May be due to lesions of the cord above the lumbar region, or turgescence of corpora cavernosa without erection may exist. It may be reflex from peripheral sensory irritants, from organic irritation of nerve tracts or nerve centers when libido may be lacking, Is sometimes seen in patients with acute leukemia.

RS: *erection; gonorrhea; satyriasis.*

priapitis (prī-ă-pī'tĭs) [" + *-itis,* inflammation]. Inflammation of the penis.

priapus (prī'ă-pus). The penis.

prickle cell (prĭk'l). A cell with rod-shaped processes, intercellular bridges connecting with similar adjoining cells.

p. c. layer. SYN: *stratum germinativum, stratum spinosum, malpighian layer.* The innermost layer of the epidermis.

prickly heat (prĭk'lĭ hēt). Noncontagious cutaneous eruption of red pimples, with itching and tingling of the affected parts, seen usually in hot weather.

ETIOL: Inflammation of skin around sweat glands. SYN: *lichen tropicus; miliaria.*

Priessnitz compress (prēs'nĭtz). A wet cold compress. SEE: *Neptune girdle.*

primae viae (prī'mē vī'ē) [L. first passages]. The alimentary canal; the secondary ones consisting of the lacteals.

primary (prī'mă-rĭ) [L. *primus,* first]. First in time or order. SYN: *principal.*

p. amputation. One before inflammation has set in.

p. bubo. An adenitis, of simple character, of an inguinal gland. SYN: *bubon d'emblée.*

p. cell. PT: A device consisting of a container, two solid conducting elements and an electrolyte, for the production of electric current by chemical energy.

p. dementia. A psychosis of youth. SYM: Extreme apathy, listlessness, without perception of environment.

p. hemorrhage. Bleeding at time of an injury.

p. lesion. 1. An original lesion from which a second one originates. 2. Lesion of syphilis, a chancre.*

p. sore. The initial sore or hard chancre of syphilis.

primate (prī'māt) [L. *primus,* first]. A member of the order Primates.

Primates. An order of vertebrates belonging to the class Mammalia, subclass Theria. Includes the lemurs, tarsiers, monkeys, apes, and man. They are most highly developed with respect to the brain and nervous system.

prime (prīm) [L. *primus,* first]. Period of greatest health and strength.

p. mover. SYN: *agonist, protagonist.* The muscle primarily responsible for a specific action.

primigravida (prī-mĭ-grăv'ĭ-dă) [" + *gravida,* pregnant]. A woman during her first pregnancy.

primipara (prī-mĭp'ă-ră) [" + *parēre,* to bear offspring]. A woman who has had or who is giving birth to her first child.

primiparity (prī-mĭ-par'ĭ-te) [" + *parēre,* to bear offspring]. Condition of having given birth to only one child.

primiparous (prī-mĭp'ă-rŭs) [" + *parēre,* to bear offspring]. Pert. to a primipara, woman giving birth to, or having had, her first child.

primitiae (prī-mĭsh'ĭ-ē) [L. *primus,* first]. Liquor amnii appearing before the fetus at birth. SEE: *amnion; bag of waters; liquor amnii; labor.*

primitive (prĭm'ĭ-tĭv) [L. *primitivus*, from *primus*, first]. Original; early in point of time; embryonic.

p. groove. The longitudinal depression in the dorsum of the embryonic area.

p. streak. A dark, thickened longitudinal band which forms at caudal end of the embryonic disk, consisting of a surface layer of ectoderm overlying a thickened mass of mesoderm cells. It marks the future longitudinal axis of the embryo.

primordial (prī-mor'dĭ-ăl) [L. *primordium*, the beginning]. 1. Existing first. 2. Existing in an undeveloped, primitive, or early form.

primordium. In embryology: the first beginnings of a future organ or part. SYN: *anlage*.

princeps (prĭn'sĕps) [L. *princeps*, chief]. 1. Original; first. 2. The name of certain arteries. Ex: *princeps cervicis*.

principal (prĭn'sĭ-păl) [L. *princeps, princip-*, chief]. 1. Chief. 2. Outstanding.

principle (prĭn'sĭ-pl) [L. *principium*, foundation]. 1. A constituent of a compound representing its essential properties. 2. A fundamental truth. 3. An established rule of action.

p., antianemic. Antianemic factor. SEE UNDER: *factor*.

p., antidiuretic. The antidiuretic hormone (ADH) present in extracts of the post. lobe of hypophysis.

p.'s, gastrointestinal. Substances secreted by mucosa of stomach and intestine which are absorbed by the blood and act as hormones. SEE: *cholecystokinin; gastrin; secretin*.

p., oxytocic. A hormone in extracts of post. lobe of hypophysis which stimulates contraction of uterine muscle.

p., proximate. A substance that may be extracted from its complex form without destroying or altering its chemical properties.

prism (prĭzm) [G. *prisma*]. A solid with sides which are parallelograms whose bases are similar plane figures.

p., enamel. A minute rod of calcareous material deposited at the end of an ameloblast in the formation of the enamel of a tooth.

prismoptometer (prĭz-mŏp-tŏm'ĕt-ĕr) [" + *opsis*, vision, + *metron*, measure]. Device for estimating abnormal refraction of the eye by using prisms.

privates (prī'vĕts) [L. *privatus*, peculiar to an individual]. The external genitalia of the male or female.

p. r. n. [L. *pro re nata*]. As circumstance may require.

pro- [L. & G.]. Prefix meaning *for, in front of, before, from, in behalf of, on account of*, etc.

proactinomycin (prō-ăk"tĭ-nō-mī'sĭn). An antibiotic obtained from *Nocardia gardneri*. Effective against gram-positive bacteria.

proagglutinoid (prō"ăg-glū'tĭ-noyd). An agglutinoid having a greater affinity for the agglutinogen than that possessed by the agglutinin.

proamnion (prō-ăm'nĭ-ŏn) [G. *pra*, before, + *amnion*, amnion]. A region anterior to the head in a vertebrate embryo in which mesoderm is lacking.

proantithrombin (prō"ăn-tĭ-thrŏmb'ĭn). A substance present in blood plasma or serum which, through the action of heparin, is converted into antithrombin.

proband (pro'band). An individual who is actually being studied and whose family history or pedigree is being constructed to determine if other members of the family have had the same disease discovered in the *proband*.

probationary (prō-bā'shŭn-ar-ĭ) [L. *prōbatiō*, a trial]. One who is on trial. Waiting, as for admission or for a test.

p. ward. One for the temporary detention of patients suspected of having a communicable disease.

probationer (prō-bā'shŭn-ĕr) [L. *prōbatiō*, a trial]. A person working during a trial or try-out period, as a student nurse just after entering training.

probe (prōb) [L. *probare*, to test]. An instrument, usually flexible, for exploring the depth and direction of a wound or sinus.

procaine hydrochlor'ide (prō'kān). USP. White, colorless, crystalline compound.

ACTION AND USES: A safe, local anesthetic, less toxic than cocaine. Used in infiltration anesthesia, nerve block, and spinal anesthesia. Its effect is prolonged by simultaneous injection of epinephrine.

procatarctic (prō"kăt-ark'tĭk) [G. *prō*, before, + *katarchein*, to begin]. Predisposing or inciting, as the cause of a disease.

procatarxis (prō"kăt-ark'sĭs) [" + *katarchein*, to begin]. Inception of a disease through a predisposing cause.

procedure (pro-sēd'ūre) [L. *procedere*, to proceed]. A particular way of accomplishing a desired result.

procelous (prō-sē'lŭs) [" + *koilos*, hollow]. Concave anteriorly.

procephalic (prō-sē-făl'ĭk) [" + *kephalē*, a head]. Of or relating to the ant. part of the head.

procercoid (prō-sĕr'koyd). The first larval stage in the development of certain cestodes belonging to order Pseudophillidea. It is an elongated structure which develops in crustaceans.

process (prŏs'ĕs) [L. *processus*, a going before]. 1. A method of action. 2. State of progress of a disease. 3. A projection or outgrowth of bone or tissue.

p., acromion. The acromion, *q.v.*

p., alar. A process of cribiform plate of ethmoid bone which articulates with frontal bone.

p., alveolar. 1. The inferior border of the maxilla containing sockets for upper teeth. 2. The superior border of body of mandible containing sockets for lower teeth.

p., articular, of vertebra. One of four processes (two superior and two inferior) by which vertebrae articulate with each other.

p., basilar. Narrow part of the base of occipital bone, in front of foramen magnum, articulating with the sphenoid bone. SYN: *pars basilaris*.

p., caudate. P. of caudate lobe of liver extending under right lobe.

p., ciliary. One of about 70 prominent meridional ridges projecting from corona ciliaris of choroid coat of eye to which suspensory ligament of lens is attached.

p., condyloid. Post. process on sup. border of ramus of mandible which articulates with temporal bone.

p., coracoid. A beak-shaped process extending upward and laterally from neck of scapula.

p., coronoid. 1. P. extending upward from ant. portion of ramus of mandible. 2. Sharp projection forming ant. and lower border of semilunar notch of ulna.

p., ensiform. The xiphoid process of the sternum.

p., ethmoidal. Small process on superior border of inferior concha which articulates with uncinate process of ethmoid.

p., falciform. An extension of post. edge of sacrotuberous ligament to ramus of ischium.

p., frontal. Upward projection of maxilla which articulates with frontal bone. Forms part of orbit and nasal fossa.

p., frontosphenoidal. Upward projecting process of zygomatic bone.

p., head. SYN: *notochordal plate.* An axial strand of cells in vertebrate embryos extending forward from primitive knot. Forms primitive axis about which embryo differentiates.

p., infraorbital. Medially projecting process of zygomatic bone which articulates with maxilla. Forms inferior lateral margin of orbit.

p., jugular. P. of occipital bone lying lateral to occipital condyle.

p., lacrimal. A short process of inferior concha which articulates with lacrimal bone.

p., lenticular. A knob on the malleus in the ear which articulates with the stapes.

p., lyophile. SEE: *lyophilization.*

p., mandibular. Posterior portion of first branchial arch from which lower jaw develops.

p., mastoid. Projection of mastoid portion of the temporal bone.

p., maxillary. 1. Ant. portion of 1st branchial arch which, with medial nasal processes, forms upper jaw. 2. P. of inf. nasal concha extending laterally and covering orifice of antrum. 3. P. on ant. border of perpendicular portion of palatine bone.

p., odontoid. SYN: *dens.* Toothlike process extending upward from axis about which the axis rotates.

p., olecranon. The olecranon, an extension at proximal end of ulna.

p., orbital. 1. P. at tip of perpendicular portion of palatine bone directed upward and backward. 2. P. of zygomatic bone which forms ant. boundary of temporal fossa.

p., palatine. P. extending transversely from medial surface of maxilla. With corresponding process from other side, it forms major portion of hard palate.

p., postglenoid. P. of temporal bone separating mandibular fossa from external acoustic meatus.

p., pterygoid. P. of sphenoid bone extending downward from junction of the body and great wing. Consists of the *lateral* and *medial pterygoid plates.*

p., styloid. SEE: *styloid process.*

p., transverse. P. extending laterally and dorsally from the arch of a vertebra.

p., vermiform. Vermiform appendix, *q.v.*

p., vocal. P. of arytenoid cartilage which serves for attachment of vocal ligament.

p., xiphoid. SYN: *ensiforme p.* Thin, elongated process extending caudally from body of sternum.

processus (prō-sĕs'ŭs) (pl. *processūs*) [L.]. Process or processes.

p. cochleariformis. Curved portion of a thin plate of bone separating eustachian tube from canal for tensor tympani muscle over which tendon of muscle passes before insertion into manubrium of malleus.

p. retromandibularis. Wedge-shaped portion of parotid gland which projects medially toward the pharynx.

p. uncinatus. 1. Curved process of ethmoid labyrinth projecting from lateral wall of middle meatus which forms inf. border of hiatus semilunaris. 2. SYN: *pancreas of Winslow.* A hooklike portion of the head of pancreas which curves around the sup. mesenteric vessels.

procheilon (prō-hīgh'lŏn). Prominence in central portion of the upper lip.

prochondral (pro-kon'dral). Preceding the formation of cartilage.

prochoresis (pro-ko-re'sis). Movement downward of partially digested food through the pyloric canal.

Prochownick's diet (prō-kŏv'nĭk) [Ludwig Prochownick, German obstetrician, 1851-1923]. A restricted one for women who are pregnant for the purpose of limiting the weight and size of the newborn. Carbohydrates and liquids are reduced.

Prochownick's method (artificial respiration) [Ludwig Prochownick]. A manner of administering artificial respiration in asphyxia of the newborn by compression of the infant's chest while the head hangs backward.

pro"chrom'osome. SYN: *chromocenter; false or chromatin nucleolus; karyosome, q.v.*

procidentia (prō-sĭ-dĕn'shĭ-ă) [L. a falling forward]. A complete prolapse, esp. of the uterus which lies outside of the vulva, with everted vaginal walls.

ETIOL: Generally due to injury of pelvic floor. SEE: *descensus uteri.*

procreate (prō'krē-āt) [L. *prō,* forward, + *crēare,* to create]. To beget; to bring forth young.

procreation (prō"krē-ā'shŭn) [" + *crēare,* to create]. The act or state of bringing forth young. SYN: *reproduction.*

proctagra (prŏk-tag'ră) [G. *prōktos,* anus, + *agra,* seizure]. Sudden rectal pain.

proctalgia (prŏk-tăl'jĭ-ă) [" + *algos,* pain]. Pain in or about the anus and rectum.

p. fugax. Rectal pain due to an unknown cause. May occur following sexual excitement and is sometimes relieved by defecation.

proctatresia (prŏk-tăt-rē'zĭ-ă) [" + *a-,* priv. + *trēsis,* perforation]. Imperforate condition of the anus.

proctectasia (prŏk"tĕk'tā-sĭ-ă). Dilatation of the anus or rectum.

proctectomy (prŏk-tĕk'tō-mĭ) [" + *ektomē,* excision]. Excision of the rectum or anus.

proctenclisis (prŏk-tĕn-klĭ'sĭs) [" + *egkleiein,* to shut in]. Stricture of the anus or rectum.

procteurynter (prŏk-tū-rĭn'tĕr) [" + *eurynein,* to widen]. Instrument for dilation of the anus or rectum.

proctitis (prŏk-tī'tĭs) [" + *-itis,* inflammation]. Inflammation of rectum and anus. SEE: *rectitis.*

ETIOL: Infectious organisms, trauma, radiation injury, drugs esp. broad-spectrum antibiotics, allergy.

p., acute or chronic. SYM: Rectal discomfort, repeated urge to evacuate rectum, accompanied by inability to pass feces, presence of mucus, blood or pus in stools, tenesmus.

p., diphtheritic. Diphtheritic membrane forms over surface of mucous membrane, forms sort of albuminous membrane. Headache, roaring in ears. Constipation, gas, neurasthenia, bloating.

p., dysenteric. May result from ordinary diarrhea, affects upper part the most. May have ulcers, afterwards cicatricial scars.

p., gonorrheal. Gonorrheal infection.

p., traumatic. SYM AND SIGNS: Pain, pressure as if bowels were going to move; irritable; mucous membrane red, eroded. Surface tissues sensitive to touch. Chronic constipation.

procto-, proct- [G.]. Combining forms meaning the *anus* and *rectum*.

proctocele (prŏk'tō-sēl) [G. *prōktos*, anus, + *kēlē*, hernia]. A protrusion of the rectal mucosa.

p., vaginal. Hernia of the rectum into the vagina.

proctoclysis (prŏk-tŏk'lĭ-sĭs) [" + *klysis*, a washing out]. A continuous infusion into the rectum and colon in which the solution is introduced drop by drop.

THERAPEUTIC PURPOSES: (a) To supply fluid in postoperative cases when fluids cannot be taken otherwise. (b) To supply the body with fluid as in hemorrhage, vomiting, or in diarrhea. (c) To relieve thirst as in persistent vomiting. (d) To lower body temperature by giving ice water enemas.

SOLUTIONS USED: The solution usually consists of a normal saline solution, a sodium bicarbonate solution, or plain tap water at body temperature. Normal salt solution half strength is frequently used. This need not be a sterile solution unless so ordered. Sodium bicarbonate of 2% to 5% strength. A glucose solution of 5% to 15% strength may be ordered for its nutritive value. A combination of these may also be ordered: as a normal saline with glucose and sodium bicarbonate, 5% and 2%, respectively, or other combinations may be given as an order.

METHOD: 15 to 30 drops per minute continuously for 36 hr. SEE: *enteroclysis.*

TEMPERATURE: This should be not less than 105° F. to begin with, although some advocate 118° to 120° F. SYN: *Murphy drip.*

proctococcypexia, proctococcypexy (prŏk"tō-kŏk-sĭ-pĕk'sĭ-ă, -kŏk'sĭ-pĕk"sĭ) [" + *kokkyx*, coccyx, + *pēxis*, fixation]. Suture of rectum to the coccyx.

proctocolitis (prŏk"tō-kō-lī'tĭs) [" + *kolon*, colon, + *-ītis*, inflammation]. Inflamed condition of colon and rectum.

proctocolonoscopy (prŏk"tō-kō"lŏn-ŏs'kō-pĭ) [" + *kolon*, colon, + *skopein*, to examine]. Examination of interior of rectum and lower colon.

proctocystotomy (prŏk"tō-sĭs-tŏt'ō-mĭ) [G. *prōktos*, anus, + *kystis*, bladder, + *tomē*, a cutting]. Incision into the bladder through the rectum.

proctodeum (prŏk-tō-dē'ŭm) [G. *prōktos*, anus, + *daiein*, to divide]. An ectodermal depression located caudally which, upon rupture of the cloacal membrane, forms the anal canal.

proctodynia (prŏk-tō-dĭn'ĭ-ă)' [" + *odynē*, pain]. Pain in the rectum or about the anus.

proctologist (prŏk-tŏl'ō-jĭst) [" + *logos*, a study]. One who specializes in diseases of the colon, rectum and anus.

proctology (prŏk-tol'ō-jĭ) [" + *logos*, a study]. Phase of medicine dealing with treatment of diseases of colon, rectum and anus.

proctoparalysis (prŏk-tō-păr-ăl'ĭs-ĭs) [" + *para*, at the side, + *lyein*, to loosen]. Paralysis of the anal sphincter muscle.

proctopexia, proctopexy (prŏk-tō-pĕks'ĭ-ă, prŏk'tō-pĕks"ĭ) [" + *pēxis*, fixation]. Suture of the rectum to some other part.

proctophobia (prŏk"tō-fō'bĭ-ă) [G. *prōktos*, anus, + *phobos*, fear]. Abnormal apprehension in those suffering from rectal disease.

proctoplasty (prŏk'tō-plăs-tĭ) [" + *plastos*, formed]. Plastic surgery of the anus or rectum.

proctoplegia (prŏk"tō-plē'jĭ-ă) [" + *plēgē*, a stroke]. Paralysis of the anal sphincter. SYN: *proctoparalysis.*

proctoptosis (prŏk-tŏp-tō'sĭs) [" + *ptōsis*, a dropping]. Prolapse of the anus and rectum. SEE: *procidentia.*

proctorrhaphy (prŏk-tŏr'ă-fĭ) [" + *raphē*, a sewing]. Suturing of rectum or anus.

proctorrhea (prŏk-tŏr-ē'ă) [" + *roia*, a flow]. Mucous discharge from the anus.

proctoscope (prŏk'tō-skōp) [" + *skopein*, to examine]. Instrument for inspection of the rectum.

proctoscopy (prŏk-tŏs'kō-pĭ) [G. *prōktos*, anus, + *skopein*, to examine]. Instrumental inspection of the rectum.

proctosigmoiditis (prŏk"tō-sĭg-moyd-ī'tĭs) [" + *sigma*, letter S, + *eidos*, form, + *-ītis*, inflammation]. Inflamed condition of the rectum and sigmoid.

proctospasm (prŏk'tō-spăzm) [" + *spasmos*, a contracting]. Rectal spasm.

proctostasis (prŏk"tō-stā'sĭs). Constipation resulting from failure of rectum to respond to defecation stimulus.

proctostenosis (prŏk"tō-stĕn-ō'sĭs) [" + *stēnōsis*, a narrowing]. Stricture of the anus or rectum.

proctostomy (prŏk-tŏs'tō-mĭ) [" + *stoma*, a mouth]. Creation of a permanent opening into the rectum.

proctotome (prŏk'tō-tōm) [" + *tomē*, a cutting]. Knife for incision into rectum.

proctotomy (prŏk-tŏt'ō-mĭ) [" + *tomē*, a cutting]. Incision of the rectum or anus.

POSITION: Simon's.

DRESSING: Iodoform gauze, T-bandage.

proctotoreusis (prŏk-tō-tō-rū'sĭs) [" + *toreusis*, boring]. The making of an opening in an imperforate anus.

proctovalvotomy (prŏk-tō-văl-vŏt'ō-mĭ) [" + L. *valva*, valve, + G. *tomē*, a cutting]. Incision of the rectal valves.

procumbent (prō-kŭm'bĕnt) [L. *procumbere*, to lean forward]. Lying face down. SYN: *prone.*

procursive (prō-kŭr'sĭv) [L. *procursivus*, running forward]. Having an involuntary tendency to run forward, as in procursive epilepsy.

prodromal (prŏd'rō-măl) [G. *prōdromos*, running before]. Pert. to the initial stage of a disease; the interval bet. the earliest symptoms and the appearance of the rash or fever.

p. rash. One that precedes the true rash of an infectious disease.

prodrome (prō'drōm) [G. *prōdromos*, running before]. A symptom indicative of an approaching disease.

product (prŏd'ŭkt) [L. *producere*, to beget]. Anything which is made naturally or artificially. SEE: *catabolite.*

production (prō-dŭk'shŭn) [L. *productiō*, a begetting, a formation]. Development or formation of a substance.

productive (prō-dŭk'tĭv) [L. *producere*, to beget]. Forming, as new tissue.

p. inflammation. Inflammation producing new tissue with or without an exudate.

proenzyme (prō-ĕn'zīm) [G. *prō*, before, + *en*, in, + *zymē*, a leaven]. SYN: *zymogen.* The inactive form of an enzyme found within a cell which, upon leaving the cell, is converted into the active form. Ex: *pepsinogen.*

proerythroblast (prō"ĕ-rĭth'rō-blăst). SYN: *basophilic erythroblast.* The earliest cells which show differentiation in the direction of erythrocyte formation.

proestrus (pro-es-'trus). The period preceding estrus characterized by development of ovarian follicles and concomitant development of uterine endometrium.

proferment (prō-fer'mĕnt) [" + L. *fermentum,* leaven]. 1. Substance which develops into an enzyme. 2. Microorganism causing fermentation.

professional (prō-fĕsh'ŭn-ăl) [L. *professiō,* from *profiteri,* to profess]. 1. Pert. to a profession. 2. Caused by the practice of a profession, as *writer's cramp.*

proflavine powder (prō-flā'vĭn). A powder used for dusting wounds, apparently overcoming infection where sulfanilamide fails.

pro"fluv'ium. An excessive flow or discharge; a flux.

p. lactis. Excessive flow of milk.

p. seminis. Flow of semen from the vagina deposited during coition.

profondometer (prō-fŏn-dŏm'ĕt-ĕr) [L. *profundus,* deep, + G. *metron,* a measure]. Device for locating a foreign body with the fluoroscope.

profunda. Deep seated; term applied to certain deeply located blood vessels.

progenitor (pro-jen'ĭ-tor). An ancestor.

progeny (prŏj'ĕn-ĭ) [L. *progeniēs,* offspring]. Offspring.

progeria (prō-jē'rĭ-ă) [G. *pro,* before, + *gēras,* old age]. Premature senility occurring in childhood.

Etiol: Unknown.

Sym and Signs: Small stature, face looks old and wizened, skin is dry and thin, hair is scanty, and sex organs are infantile.

progesterone (prō-jĕs'tĕr-ōn). $C_{21}H_{30}O_2$, a steroid hormone obtained from the corpus luteum, adrenals, or placenta. It is responsible for: 1. Changes in uterine endometrium in second half of menstrual cycle preparatory for implantation of blastocyst. 2. After implantation, development of maternal placenta. 3. Development of mammary glands.

Uses: In treatment of menstrual disorders (amenorrhea, dysmenorrhea) and threatened abortion. It is ineffective when given orally hence must be administered parenterally.

progestin (prō-jĕs'tĭn). A corpus luteum hormone which prepares the endometrium for the fertilized ovum. This word is now used to cover a large group of synthetic drugs which have a progesterone-like effect on the uterus. Syn: *progesterone.*

proglot'tid or **proglottis.** A segment of a tapeworm. See: *Cestoda; tapeworm.*

prognathism (prŏg'nă-thĭzm) [*pro,* before, + *gnathos,* jaw, + *ismos,* condition]. Projection of jaws beyond upper face.

prognathous (prŏg'năth-ŭs) [" + *gnathos,* jaw]. Having jaws projecting forward beyond rest of the face.

prognosis (prŏg-nō'sĭs) [G. *prognōsis,* foreknowledge]. Prediction of course and end of disease, and outlook based on it.

p. anceps. Doubtful prognosis.

p. fausta. Favorable prognosis.

p. infausta. Unfavorable prognosis.

prognostic (prŏg-nŏs'tĭk) [G. *prognōsis,* foreknowledge]. Affording an indication as to outcome of a disease.

prognosticate (prŏg-nŏs'tĭ-kāt) [G. *prognōstikon,* knowing before]. To make a statement on the probable outcome of an illness.

prog"ono'ma. A tumor such as a hairy mole which develops from displacement of embryonic cells.

pro"gran'ulocyte. A promyelocyte, *q.v.*

pro"grav'id. Before or preceding pregnancy.

p. phase. The secretory phase of the menstrual cycle, *q.v.*

pro"gres'sion. Advancing or moving forward.

p., backward. Syn: *retropulsion.* Walking backward; a symptom seen in certain nervous disorders.

progressive (prō-grĕs'ĭv) [L. *progressus,* stepping forward]. Advancing.

p. muscular atrophy. Gradual advancing atrophy of groups of muscles due to spinal cord degeneration. See: *atrophy.*

p. ossifying myositis. Tendency to bony deposits in the muscles with chronic inflammation.

proiosystole (prō-ĭ-ō-sĭs'tō-lē) [G. *prōi,* early, + *systolē,* contraction]. A cardiac contraction occurring before its normal time.

proiosystolia (prō-ĭ-ō-sĭs-tō'lĭ-ă) [" + *systolē,* contraction]. A condition marked by occurrence of systoles before the normal time.

proiotia (prō-ĭ-ō'shĭ-ă) [G. *prōi,* early]. Genital precocity.

projec'tile vomiting. Vomiting not preceded by nausea in which the stomach contents are forcibly ejected.

projection (prō-jĕk'shŭn) [L. *pro,* forward, + *jacere,* to throw]. 1. The act of throwing forward. 2. A part extending beyond the level of its surroundings. 3. The mental process by which sensations are referred to the sense organs or receptors stimulated or outside the body to the object which is the stimulus. 4. Psy: Distortion of a perception as a result of its repression, resulting in such a phenomenon as hating without cause one who has been dearly loved, or attributing to others one's own undesirable traits. Characteristic of the paranoid reaction.

prolabium (prō-lā'bĭ-ŭm) [L. *pro,* forward, + *labium,* lip]. The entire central portion of the upper lip.

prolactin (prō-lăk'tĭn) [" + *lac,* milk]. Hormone, derived from the ant. pituitary lobe, which stimulates lactation. It also produces luteotrophic effects and is considered identical to luteotrophine. Syn: *galactin; mammotropin.*

prolamin(e (prō-lăm'ĭn, prō'lă-mĭn). Any one of a class of proteins found in seeds, soluble in alcohol, and insoluble in water and absolute alcohol. Syn: *gliadin.*

prolan (prō'lan). A hormone principle formerly believed to be from the anterior pituitary body, but now known to be chorionic gonadotrophins. See: *gonadotrophin, chorionic.*

prolapse (prō-lăps') [L. *pro,* before, + *lapsus,* from *labi,* to fall]. 1. A dropping of an internal part of the body, as of the uterus or rectum. 2. To drop down, noted of an organ. Syn: *ptosis.*

p. (of) anus. See: *prolapsus ani.*

p. of the cord. Expulsion of umbilical cord prematurely. See: *labor.*

p. (of) iris. Protrusion of iris through an injury in the cornea.

p. (of) rectum. Protrusion of rectal mucosa through the anus.

p. (of) uterus. Prolapsus uteri, *q.v.*

prolapsus (prō-lăp'sŭs) [L. a dropping]. A falling or downward displacement of some part of the body, as the uterus.

p. ani. Protrusion of lower portion of digestive tract through external sphincter of anus. SEE: *prolapse (of) rectum.*

p. uteri. Downward displacement of uterus, the cervix sometimes protruding from the vaginal orifice. SYN: *descensus uteri.*

prolepsis (prō-lĕp'sĭs) [G. *pro,* before, + *lēpsis,* a seizure]. Return of paroxysmal attacks at successively shorter intervals.

proleptic (prō-lĕp'tĭk). Recurring before the time expected, said of paroxysms.

proleukocyte (prō-lū'kō-sīt) [" + " + *kytos,* cell]. An undeveloped leukocyte. SYN: *leukoblast.*

proliferate (prō-lĭf'ĕr-āt) [L. *proles,* offspring, + *ferre,* to bear]. To increase by reproduction of similar forms.

proliferation (prō-lĭf"ĕr-ā'shŭn) [" + *ferre,* to bear]. 1. Reproduction rapidly and repeatedly of new parts, as by cell division. 2. Process or result of rapid reproduction. SEE: *auxesis.*

promyelocyte (prō"mī'ĕl-ō-sīt) [G. *pro,* before, + *myelos,* marrow, + *kytos,* cell]. 1. A large mononuclear myeloid cell seen in the blood in leukemia. 2. Cell development bet. myeloblast and a myelocyte, resembling a myeloblast.

pronation (prō-nā'shŭn) [L. *pronāre,* to bend forward]. 1. The act of lying prone or face downward. 2. The act of turning hand so that palm faces downward or backward.

pronator. A muscle which pronates. SEE: *Table of Muscles in Appendix.*

pronaus, pronaeus (prō-nā'us) [G. *pronaios,* the court before a temple]. The vagina or vestibule of the vagina.

prone (prōn) Lying horizontal, with face downward; of the hand, with the palms turned downward. OPP: *supine.*

pronephric (prō-nĕf'rĭk). Pert. to the pronephron, *q.v.*

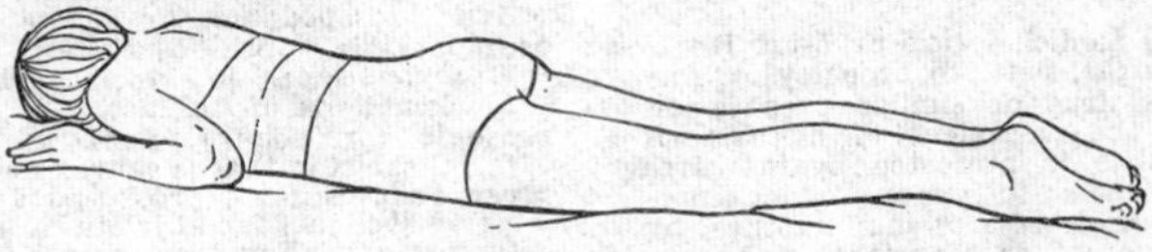

PRONE POSITION.

proliferous (prō-lĭf'ĕr-ŭs) [" + *ferre,* to bear]. 1. Multiplying, as by formation of new tissue cells. 2. Bearing offspring.

p. cyst. One with epithelial lining, proliferating and projecting from inner surface of the cyst.

prolific (prō-lĭf'ĭk) [" + *facere,* to make]. Fruitful; reproductive. SYN: *fertile.*

proligerous (prō-lĭj'ĕr-ŭs) [" + *gerere,* to bear]. Producing offspring. SYN: *germinating.*

pro'linase. An enzyme found in animal tissues and yeast which hydrolyzes proline peptids to simpler peptids and proline.

prolin(e (prō'lēn, -lĭn). An important amino acid, formed by protein decomposition, having the formula: C_4H_8N.-COOH.

prolymphocyte (prō"lĭmf'ō-sīt). A cell intermediate between a lymphoblast and lymphocyte.

promegakar'yocyte. Cell from which a megakaryocyte develops.

promegaloblast (prō"mĕg'ăl-ō-blăst) [G. *pro,* before, + *megas, megal-,* large, + *blastos,* germ]. A cell of the erythrocyte series preceding the megaloblast.

promethium (pro-me'thĭ-um). A chemical element. SYMB: Pm. At. number 61. At. weight 147.

prominentia (prŏm-ĭn-ĕn'shĭ-ă) [L.]. A projection.

p. laryngea. [NA]. The laryngeal prominence; Adam's apple. SYN: *pomum adami.*

p. spiralis. SYN: *spiral prominence.* A small ridge extending entire length of cochlea located on inner surface of spiral ligament. It projects slightly into cochlear canal and contains blood vessels including the vas prominens. [NA].

promontory (prŏm'un-tō-rĭ) [L. *promontorium,* a projection]. A projecting process or part.

p. of sacrum. The ant. projecting portion of the pelvic surface of base of the sacrum. With the 5th lumbar vertebra, it forms the sacrovertebral angle.

p. of tympanic cavity. Projection on medial wall of tympanic cavity produced by first turn of the cochlea.

p. duct. Duct which connects posteriorly to cloaca and to which pronephric tubules are connected.

p. tubules. Several pairs of segmentally arranged tubules which open into cranial portion of pronephric duct. They communicate with coelom through a ciliated funnel-shaped nephrostome. They are vestigial in higher vertebrates.

pronephron, pronephros (prō-nĕf'rŏn, -rŏs) [G. *pro,* before, + *nephros,* kidney]. The earliest and simplest type of excretory organ of vertebrates, functional in simpler forms (cyclostomes) and serving as a provisional kidney in some fishes and amphibians. In reptiles, birds, and mammals, it appears in the embryo as a temporary, functionless structure.

pronograde (prō'nō-grād) [L. *pronāre,* to bend forward, + *gradus,* a step]. Walking on hands and feet or resting with the body in a horizontal position. OPP: *orthograde.*

pronometer (prō-nŏm'ĕt-ĕr) [" + G. *metron,* a measure]. Device for showing amount of pronation or supination of forearm.

pronucleus (prō-nū'klē-ŭs) [L. *pro,* before, + *nucleus,* nut]. Nucleus of the ovum, the female p., or of the spermatozoon, the male p., after the fertilization of the ovum.

prootic (prō-ŏt'ĭk, -ō'tĭk) [G. *pro,* before, + *ous, ot-,* ear]. In front of the ear.

propagation (prŏp-ă-gā'shŭn) [L. *propagāre,* to fasten forward]. Act of reproducing or giving birth. SYN: *generation; reproduction.*

propagative (prŏp'ă-gā-tĭv) [L. *propagāre,* to fasten forward]. Pert. to or taking part in reproduction.

propalinal (prō-păl'ĭn-ăl) [G. *pro,* before, + *palin,* back]. Applied to a backward and forward movement, as of the jaws.

propeptone (prō-pĕp'tōn) [G. *pro,* before, + *peptein,* to digest]. An intermediate product in the digestive conversion of protein into peptone. SYN: *hemialbumose.*

propeptonuria (prō"pĕp-tō-nū'rĭ-ă) [" + " + *ouron,* urine]. Excretion of propeptone in the urine. SYN: *hemialbumosuria.*

properdin (prō-perd′ĭn) [L. *perdere,* to destroy]. A serum protein which, in the presence of magnesium ions and complement, has the ability to help destroy bacteria and neutralize viruses.

prophase (prō′fāz) [G. *pro,* before, + *phasis,* an appearance]. First stage of indirect cell division.

SEE: *centriole; "meta-" words; mitosis; "tele-" words.*

prophylactic (prō-fĭl-ăk′tĭk) [G. *prophylaktikos,* guarding]. 1. Warding off disease. 2. Agent which wards off disease. 3. A chemical substance or physical device used to prevent venereal disease. Usually used during or following sexual intercourse.

prophylaxis (prō-fĭl-ăks′ĭs) [G. *prophylassein,* to guard against]. 1. Observance of rules necessary to prevent disease. 2. In dentistry, cleansing of the teeth's surface.

proprietary medicine (prō-prī′ĕ-tar″ĭ) [L. *proprietarius,* pert. to property]. "Any chemical, drug or similar preparation used in the treatment of diseases, if such article is protected against free competition, as to name, product, composition or process of manufacture, by secrecy, patent or copyright, or by another means." *American Medical Association.* SEE: *patent medicine.*

proprioception (prō″prĭ-ō-sĕp-shŭn). The awareness of posture, movement, changes in equilibrium, and the knowledge of position, weight, and resistance of objects in relation to the body.

proprioceptive (prō″prĭ-ō-sĕp′tĭv) [L. *proprius,* one's own, + *cepius,* from *capere,* to take]. Pert. to proprioception.

p. impulses. Afferent impulses arising in proprioceptors, *q.v.*

p. sense. Muscle sense; kinesthetic sense.

proprioceptor (prō″prĭ-ō-sĕp′tor) [L. *proprius,* one's own, + *ceptor,* a receiver, from *capere,* to take]. A receptor which responds to stimuli originating within the body itself, esp. those responding to pressure, position or stretch. Ex: *muscle spindles, Golgi tendon organs, pacinian corpuscles,* and *labyrinthine receptors.*

proptometer (prŏp-tŏm′ĕt-ĕr) [G. *proptōsis,* protrusion, + *metron,* a measure]. An instrument for measuring extent of exophthalmos.

proptosis (prŏp-tō′sĭs) [G. *proptōsis,* protrusion]. A downward displacement, as of the uterus or of the eyeball in exophthalmic goiter, or in inflammatory conditions of the orbit.

propulsion (prō-pŭl′shŭn) [L. *propulsus,* from *propellere,* to force forward]. 1. A tendency to push or fall forward in walking. 2. A condition seen in paralysis agitans. SEE: *festination.*

propylthiouracil (prō″pĭl-thī-ō-ū′ră-sĭl). Antithyroid drug used in treatment of hyperthyroidism, thyroiditis, and thyrotoxicosis. Also employed for preoperative therapy and in cases where surgery is contraindicated.

pro re nata (prō rā nah′tă) [L.]. According to the circumstances.

prorennin (prō-rĕn′ĭn) [L. *pro,* before, + *rennin*]. The preliminary material which is converted into rennin. SYN: *mother substance; reninogen; zymogen.*

prorrhaphy (pror′ă-fe) [G. *pro* + *raphē,* suture]. Advancement. Surgical movement of a muscle or tendon insertion to a point farther away. Done to change the action of a muscle.

prosecretin (prō″sē-krē′tĭn) [L. *pro,* before, + *secretiō,* a secretion]. Substance present in the duodenal mucosa which, when acted on by hydrochloric acid in chyme, is converted into secretin. SEE: *secretin.*

prosector (prō-sĕk′tor) [" + *sector,* from *secāre,* to cut]. One who prepares cadavers for dissection or dissects for demonstration.

prosencephalon (prŏs-ĕn-sĕf′ăl-ŏn) [G. *pros,* before, + *egkephalos,* brain]. The embryonic forebrain which gives rise to the telencephalon and diencephalon, *q.v.*

prosodemic (prŏs-ō-dĕm′ĭk) [G. *prosō,* forward, + *dēmos,* people]. Spread by individual contact; said of a disease.

prosopalgia (prŏs-ō-păl′jĭ-ă) [G. *prosōpon,* face, + *algos,* pain]. Neuralgic pain in the trigeminal nerve and its branches. SYN: *prosopodynia; tic douloureux.*

prosopectasia (prŏs″ō-pĕk-tā′zĭ-ă) [G. *prosōpon,* face, + *ektasis,* dilatation]. Abnormal size of the face.

prosopic (prō″sŏp′ĭk). Pert. to face or facial skeleton that is convex anteriorly.

prosopoanoschisis (prŏs″ō-pō″ă-nŏ′chĕ-sĭs). Oblique facial cleft, a slanting furrow extending from mouth to eye.

prosopodiplegia (prŏs″ō-pō-dī-plē′jĭ-ă) [G. *prosōpon,* face, + *dis,* double, + *plēgē,* a stroke]. Paralysis on both sides of the face.

prosopodynia (prŏs″ō-pō-dĭn′ĭ-ă) [" + *odynē,* pain]. Pain in the face. SYN: *tic douloureux.*

prosoponeuralgia (prŏs″ō-pō-nū-răl′jĭ-ă) [" + *neuron,* sinew, + *algos,* pain]. Facial neuralgia. SYN: *prosopalgia.*

prosopoplegia (prŏs″ō-pō-plē′jĭ-ă) [" + *plēgē,* stroke]. Paralysis of the face.

prosopoplegic (prŏs″ō-pō-plē′jĭk) [" + *plēgē,* a stroke]. Relating to, or afflicted with, facial paralysis.

prosoposchisis (prŏs-ō-pŏs′kĭ-sĭs) [L" + *schisis,* a cleft]. Congenital cleft of the face.

prosopospasm (prŏs′ō-pō-spazm) [" + *spasmos,* a spasm]. Facial spasm.

prosopotocia (prŏs″ō-pō-tō′shĭ-ă) [" + *tokos,* birth]. Presentation of the face in parturition.

pros′opus va′rus [G. *prosopon,* face, + L. *varus,* crooked]. Congenital obliquity of the face due to atrophy of one side of the head.

prostatalgia (prŏs-tă-tal′jĭ-ă) [G. *prostatēs,* prostate, + *algos,* pain]. Pain of the prostate gland.

prostate (prŏs′tāt) [G. *prostatēs*]. A male body, partly glandular, partly muscular, surrounding proximal portion of the male urethra, the neck of the bladder and the ejaculatory ducts, consisting of a median lobe and two lateral lobes, the glandular matter emptying through ducts into the prostatic urethra.

SIZE: About 2 by 4 by 3 cm., and weighing about 20 grams. It is enclosed in a fibrous capsule containing smooth muscle fibers in its inner layer. Muscle fibers also separate the glandular tissue and encircle the urethra.

FUNCTION: The gland secretes a thin, opalescent, slightly alkaline fluid which forms part of semen.

PATHOLOGY: Inflammation of the prostate may occur, oftentimes the result of gonorrheal urethritis. Enlargement of the prostate is common, esp. after middle age. This results in urethral obstruction, impeding urination and sometimes leading to retention. Tumors, both benign and malignant, calculi, and nodular hyperplasia are common, particularly in men past 60.

prostatectomy (prŏs-tă-tĕk'tō-mĭ) [G. *prostatēs*, prostate, + *ektomē*, excision]. Excision of part or all of the prostate gland. Operation may be performed with an incision in the perineum (perineal p.) or an incision into the bladder (suprapubic p.), or through the urethra (transurethral p.).

After prostatectomy, the patient is unable to ejaculate but his libido is unaffected.

COMPLICATIONS: Retention of urine, hematuria, cystitis, infection of kidney, pyelitis, infective nephritis, renal failure.

prostathelcosis (pros"tat-hel-ko'sis) [prostate gland + G. *helkosis*. ulceration]. Ulceration of prostate gland.

prostatic (prŏs-tăt'ĭk) [G. *prostatēs*, prostate]. Concerning the prostate gland.

p. calculus. A stone in the prostate.

p. plexus. 1. Veins around the base and neck of the bladder and prostate gland. 2. Nerves from the pelvic plexus to the prostate gland, erectile tissue of the penis, and to the seminal vesicles.

p. urethra. Part of the urethra surrounded by the prostate gland.

prostatism (prŏs'tă-tĭzm) [G. *prostatēs*, prostate, + *-ismos*, condition]. Term applied to all conditions which result in obstruction by the prostate gland of flow of urine from the bladder.

ETIOL: Benign hypertrophy, carcinoma, prostatitis, nodular hyperplasia.

SYM: Frequent, uncomfortable urination, nocturia. Retention of urine may occur with development of uremia.

prostatitis (prŏs-tă-tī'tĭs) [" + *-itis*, inflammation]. Inflamed condition of the prostate gland.

May be a complication of gonorrheal infection.

p., acute. Discomfort and pain in perineal area. Frequent urination; later, retention of urine. If severe, marked malaise, rise of temperature, constipation, chills and vomiting.

p., chronic. Dull, aching pain in perineal region. Discharge from the penis.

prostatocystitis (prŏs"tă-tō-sĭs-tī'tĭs) [G. *prostatēs*, prostate, + *kystis*, bladder, + *-itis*, inflammation]. Inflammation of the prostatic urethra involving the bladder.

prostatocystotomy (prŏs"tă-tō-sĭs-tŏt'ō-mĭ) [" + " + *tomē*, a cutting]. Surgical incision of the prostate and the bladder.

prostatodynia (prŏs"tă-tō-dĭn'ĭ-ă) [" + *odynē*, pain]. Pain in the prostate gland. SYN: *prostatalgia*.

pros"tat'olith. A calculus of the prostate gland.

prostatomegaly (prŏs"tă-tō-mĕg'ăl-ĭ) [" + *megas*, *megal-*, large]. Enlargement of the prostate gland.

prostatometer (prŏs-tă-tŏm'ĕt-ĕr) [" + *metron*, a measure]. Device for measuring enlargement of the prostate.

prostatomyomectomy (prŏs"tă-tō-mī-ō-mĕk'tō-mĭ) [" + *mys*, *my-*, muscle, + *ektomē*, excision]. Surgical excision of a prostatic myoma.

prostatomy (prŏs-tăt'ō-mĭ) [" + *tomē*, a cutting]. Incision into the prostate.

prostatorrhea (prŏs-tăt-or-rē'ă) [G. *prostatēs*, prostate, + *roia*, flow]. Abnormal discharge from the prostate gland.

prostatotomy (prŏs-tă-tŏt'ō-mĭ) [" + *tomē*, a cutting]. Incision into prostate gland.

prostatovesiculectomy (prŏs"tă-tō-vĕs-ĭk"-ū-lĕk'tō-mĭ) [" + L. *vesiculus*, a little sac, + G. *ektomē*, excision]. Removal of the prostate gland and seminal vesicles.

prostatovesiculitis (prŏs"tă-tō-vĕs-ĭk-ū-lī'-tĭs) [" + " + G. *-itis*, inflammation]. Inflammation of the seminal vesicles and prostate gland.

prosternation (prō-stĕr-nā'shŭn) [G. *pro*, before, + *sternon*, chest]. Habitual flexion of the trunk forward. SYN: *camptocormia*.

prostheon (prŏs'thē-ŏn) [G. *prosthios*, foremost]. The alveolar point; midpoint of lower border of upper alveolar arch.

prosthesis (prŏs'thē-sĭs) [G. *pros*, to, + *thesis*, a placing]. 1. Replacement of a missing part by an artificial substitute. 2. An artificial organ or part.

p., dental. Mechanical dentistry.

p., maxillofacial. Repair and artificial replacements of face and jaw.

p., paraffin. Subcutaneous injection of paraffin to restore the natural contour of a part or to replace cartilaginous part of the nasal septum.

prosthetics (prŏs-thĕt'ĭks) [" + *thesis*, a placing]. The making and application of an artificial part to remedy a want or defect of the body, as an artificial arm or leg.

prosthetist (prŏs'thē-tĭst) [" + *thesis*, a placing]. 1. Specialist in artificial dentures. 2. Maker of artificial limbs.

prosthodontist (prŏs-thō-dŏn'tĭst) [" + " + *odous*, *odont-*, tooth]. A dentist who specializes in the mechanics of making and fitting artificial teeth.

prostigmin (prō-stĭg'mĭn). Registd. trademark for a brand of neostigmine; a synthetic parasympathetic stimulant for oral and parenteral use. A cholinergic stimulant which inhibits the destruction of acetylcholine by cholinesterase.

USES: To stimulate peristalsis, improve tone and motility of intestine and urinary bladder, and to stimulate skeletal muscle. Used as an antidote to curare, for treatment of myasthenia gravis and glaucoma, for diagnosis of pregnancy and treatment of delayed menstruation.

p. bromide. USES: Orally, for the treatment of myasthenia gravis. USP. Syn: *neostigmine b.*

p. methylsulfate. USES: For prevention and treatment of postoperative distention. USP. Syn: *neostigmine methylsulfate.*

prostitute (prŏs'tĭ-tūt). 1. A woman or, less frequently, a man who gives sexual gratification for a fee. 2. To sell one's self basely, such as to prostitute one's talents.

prostitution (prŏs-tĭ-tū'shŭn) [L. *prostituere*, to prostitute]. Act or practice of prostituting. Said to be the oldest profession, prostitution is a major cause of the spread of venereal disease.

prostrate. 1. Lying with body extended. 2. To deprive of strength or to exhaust.

pros"trat'ed. Depleted of strength, exhausted.

prostration (prŏs-trā'shŭn) [L. *prostratus*, spreading before]. Absolute exhaustion.

p., heat. Exhaustion resulting from exposure to excessive heat.

p., nervous. General physical and nervous exhaustion. SYN: *neurasthenia*.

protactinium (pro-tak-tin'ĭ-um). A radioactive element. SYMB: Pa. At. wt. 231; at. no. 91.

protal (pro'tal) [G. *protos*, first]. Existing from time of birth or before. Hereditary.

protamine (prō'tă-mēn) [" + *amine*]. 1. One of a class of simple proteins which are strongly basic, noncoagulable in heat and yield diamino acids when hydrolyzed. 2. An amine, $C_{16}H_{32}O_2N_9$, isolated from spermatozoa and spawn of fish.

Found in fish sperm and named from the fish from which it is derived. SEE: *salmine; sturine*.

p. insulin, p. zinc insulin. Preparations of insulin which are more slowly dissolved and absorbed by body tissues than ordinary insulin. Act longer and keep the blood sugar normal for 20 to 24 hr. One injection is sufficient for this period.

protanopia (prō-tăn-ō'pĭ-ă) [G. *prōtos*, first, + *an-*, negative, + *opsis*, vision]. Defect in color vision in which there is condition of red blindness.

protean (prō'tē-ăn) [G. *Prōteus*, a god who changed shapes at will]. 1. Having the ability to change form, as the ameba. 2. [G. *prōtos*, first]. One of the primary derivatives of protein resulting from action of water, enzymes or dilute acids.

protease (prō'tē-ās) [G. *prōtos*, first, + *ase*, enzyme]. A protein-splitting enzyme.

protective (prō-tĕk'tĭv) [L. *protectus*, shielding]. 1. Covering or guarding. 2. An agent that will mechanically protect the part to which applied. Ex: *collodion, plaster*. SYN: *dressing*.

proteidogenous (prō"tē-ĭd-ŏj'ĕn-ŭs) [" + *gennan*, to produce]. Producing proteins.

protein (prō'tē-ĭn, prō-tēn) [G. *prōtos*, first]. One of a class of nitrogenous compounds which occur naturally, give amino acids when hydrolyzed, and are essential to all living organisms.

CLASSIFICATION

p., conjugated. Those containing the protein molecule with some other molecule or molecules. *Chromoproteins*: Ex: hemoglobin. *Glycoproteins*: Ex: mucin. *Lecithoproteins*: Compounds of lecithins or similar substances with the protein molecule. *Nucleoproteins. Phosphoproteins*: Ex: casein.

p., derived. Proteins not occurring naturally but derived from them through the action of heat, reagents, enzymes, etc.

p., simple. Those which produce alpha amino acids on hydrolysis. *Albumins*: Soluble in water and coagulated by heat. Ex: egg albumin. *Globulins*: Insoluble in water, soluble in salt solutions, coagulated by heat. Ex: edestin, from hemp seed. *Glutelins, Prolamines* (alcohol-soluble proteins): Ex: gliadin, from wheat. *Albuminoids*: Ex: keratin, from corn. *Histones. Protamines*: Ex: salmon, from the ripe sperm of salmon.

COMPOSITION: Proteins are composed of carbon, hydrogen, oxygen, nitrogen, phosphorus, sulfur, and iron which make up the greater part of plant and animal tissue. Amino acids represent the elements in proteins, 22 of which may be combined to form various proteins. Different protein foods contain a different number and various kinds of amino acids. A complete protein is one that contains all the *essential amino acids* (tryptophane, lysine, methionine, valine, leucine, isoleucine, phenylalanine, threonine, arginine, and histidine). These are necessary for growth and maintenance of body weight.

FUNCTIONS: Proteins are a source of heat and energy to the body; they are essential for growth, the building of new tissue, and the repair of injured or broken-down tissue. They form an integral part of the protoplasm of every cell.

They are oxidized in the body, thus liberating heat. One gm. supplies 4 calories of heat. It is said that 0.65 gm. of protein will care for the wear of 1 kilogram of body tissue or body weight. That amount is the minimum requirement as a basal protein level.

Children require from 2 to 3 gm. per kilogram of body weight. Weight should always be calculated at the normal level. Age also is a factor in determining protein requirements, the amount decreasing with the age. Physical work demands increased protein requirement, as is the case during menstruation, lactation, and convalescence. Excess protein in the diet means an elimination of nitrogen through the urine.

SOURCES: Milk, eggs, cheese, and meat are the best sources. Proteins are found in both vegetable and animal forms. The principal animal proteins are ovalbumin in eggs, lactalbumin in milk, serumalbumin in serum, myogen or myosinogen in striated muscle tissue, crystallins found in the lens of the eye, fibrinogen in blood, ovoglobulin in eggs, lactoglobulin in milk, serum globulin in serum, myosin in striated muscle tissue, thyroglobulin in thyroid, globin in blood, thymus histones in thymus, collagen and gelatin in connective tissue, elastin and keratin. Nucleoprotein is found in the thymus, pancreas, liver, animal cells and glands; chondroprotein is found in tendons and cartilage; mucin and mucoids are found in various secreting glands and animal mucilaginous substances; caseinogen in milk; vitellin in egg yolk; hemoglobin in blood, and lecithoprotein in blood, brain and bile.

p. balance. Equilibrium between protein intake and anabolism and protein catabolism and elimination of nitrogenous products. SEE: *nitrogen equilibrium*.

p., Bence Jones. Protein which occurs in urine; its presence is symptomatic of certain pathologic conditions: multiple myeloma, lymphosarcoma, leukemia, or Hodgkin's disease.

p.'s, blood. Those present in blood. Include *hemoglobin* present in red blood cells and the *plasma proteins*. Normal values are hemoglobin, 14 to 18 grams per 100 ml. in men and 12 to 16 grams per 100 ml. in women; albumin, 4 to 5%; globulin, 1.5 to 3%; fibrinogen, 0.2 to 0.4%. The amount of albumin in relation to the amount of globulin is referred to as the *albumin-globulin (A/G) ratio*, which is normally 1.5 to 2.5 : 1.

p., complete. One containing all the essential amino acids.

p., defensive. Any of the proteins present in blood which render the body immune to infectious disease. SEE: *globulin; alexin*.

p., denatured. P. whose amino acid composition and stereochemical structure has been altered by physical or chemical means.

p. high diet. 1.5 to 2 gm. protein per kg. ideal body weight.

p., incomplete. One lacking one or more of the essential amino acids.

p. low diet. 0.65 gm. protein per kg. ideal body weight. Supplied by means of protein of good biological value.

p., native. A protein in its natural state; one which has not been denatured.

p.'s, plasma. P.'s present in blood plasma, viz., albumins, globulins, fibrinogen.

p. sensitization. Condition in which patient is hypersensitive to foreign proteins, so that severe reaction occurs upon their administration.

p., serum. P.'s present in blood serum, viz., albumins and globulins.

p. sparer. A substance in the diet (carbohydrates or fat) which relieves the body tissues of the necessity of giving up protein for energy.

p., tissue. P. within the solid tissues of the body in contrast to those in circulating blood.

proteinase (prō'tē-ĭn-ās) [G. *prōtos*, first, + *ase*, enzyme]. A proteolytic enzyme; an enzyme that acts on native proteins.

proteinic (prō-tē-ĭn'ĭk) [G. *prōtos*, first]. Relating to protein.

proteinivorus (prō-tē-ĭn-ĭv'ō-rŭs) [" + L. *vorāre*, to devour]. Living on protein.

proteinogenous (prō-tē-ĭn-ŏj'ĕn-ŭs) [" + *gennan*, to produce]. Developing from a protein.

proteinophobia (prō"tē-ĭn-ō-fō'bĭ-ă) [" + *phobos*, fear]. Aversion to foods containing protein.

proteinosis (prō"tē-ĭn-ō'sĭs). Accumulation of proteins in the tissues.

p., lipid. Syn: *lipoidosis cutis et mucosae.* A rare condition resulting from altered fat metabolism. Yellow deposits of a mixture of protein and lipoid occur especially on the mucous surface of the mouth and tongue. Nodules may appear on the face and extremities.

proteinuria (prō-tē-ĭn-ū'rĭ-ă) [" + *ouron*, urine]. Protein, usually albumin, in the urine.

proteogens (prō'tē-ō-jĕns) [G. *prōtos*, first, + *gennan*, to produce]. Preparations of plant proteins for injection hypodermically.

proteolysin (prō-tē-ŏl'ĭs-ĭn) [" + *lysis*, dissolution]. A specific substance causing decomposition of proteins.

proteolysis (prō-tē-ŏl'ĭs-ĭs) [G. *prōtos*, first, + *lysis*, dissolution]. The hydrolysis of proteins usually by enzyme action into simpler substances.

proteolytic (prō-tē-ō-lĭt'ĭk) [" + *lysis*, dissolution]. In the chemistry of enzymes, hastening the hydrolysis of proteins.

proteometabolism (prō"tē-ō-mē-tăb'ō-lĭzm) [" + *metabolē*, change, + *ismos*, condition]. Digestion, absorption, and assimilation of proteins.

proteopeptic (prō"tē-ō-pĕp'tĭk) [" + *peptein*, to digest]. Pert. to the digestion of protein.

proteopexic (prō-tē-ō-pĕks'ĭk) [" + *pēxis*, fixation]. Pert. to fixation of proteins within the organism.

proteopexy (prō"tē-ō-pĕks'ĭ) [G. *prōtos*, first, + *pēxis*, fixation]. The fixation of proteins within the body.

proteose (prō'tē-ōs) [G. *prōtos*, first]. One of the class of intermediate products of proteolysis bet. protein and peptone.

p., primary. First formed products during proteolysis of proteins.

p., secondary. P. resulting from further hydrolysis of primary proteoses.

proteosuria (prō"tē-ōs-ū'rĭ-ă) [" + *ouron*, urine]. Proteose in urine. Syn: *albumosuria.*

proteuria (prō-tē-ū'rĭ-ă) [" + *ouron*, urine]. Proteins in the urine. Syn: *proteinuria.*

Proteus (prō'tē-ŭs) [G. *Prōteus*, a god of many forms]. A genus of family Bacteriaceae found in intestines and decaying material, which cause protein decomposition.

P. morganii. Species isolated from stools of children suffering from summer diarrhea.

P. vulgaris. An essentially saprophytic form but may invade body producing pathologic condition such as pleuritis, peritonitis, cystitis, and suppurative abscesses.

prothesis (prŏth'ĕs-ĭs) [G. *pro*, before, + *thesis*, a placing]. Replacement by an artificial part. Syn: *prosthesis.*

prothrombase (prō-thrŏm'bās) [" + *thrombos*, a clot]. A substance which becomes a fibrin ferment when activated by thrombokinase. Syn: *prothrombin; thrombogen.*

prothrombin (prō-thrŏm'bĭn) [" + *thrombos*, a clot]. A chemical substance existing in circulating blood, and which, through the medium of *thrombokinase*, interacts with calcium salts to produce thrombin. Syn: *thrombogen.*

prothrombinemia (prō-thrŏm"bĭ-nē'mĭ-ă). Presence of prothrombin in the blood.

prothrombinopenia (prō-thrŏm"bĭ-nō-pē'nĭ-ă). Deficiency of prothrombin in the blood. Syn: *hypoprothrombinemia.*

Protis'ta. Term applied to kingdom of organisms including the simpler animals and plants, characterized by being acellular or unicellular; includes bacteria, fungi, spirochetes, protozoa, viruses, and rickettsias.

protistologist (prō-tĭs-tŏl'ō-jĭst) [G. *prōtista*, the very first, + *logos*, study]. One who studies the Protista, the unicellular organisms.

protistology (prō-tĭs-tŏl'ō-jĭ) [" + *logos*, study]. The science of Protista or animal unicellular plant and microorganisms. Syn: *microbiology.*

proto- (pro'to) [G.]. 1. A prefix signifying *first.* 2. The lowest of a series of compounds having the same elements.

protobe (prō'tōb) [G. *prōtos*, first, + *bios*, life]. d'Herelle's term for the bacteriophage. Syn: *protobios.*

protobiology (prō"tō-bĭ-ŏl'ō-jĭ) [" + *bios*, life, + *logos*, study]. The phase of science dealing with the forms more minute than bacteria, as the ultraviruses and bacteriophages.

protobios (prō-tō-bĭ'ŏs) [" + *bios*, life]. A term suggested by d'Herelle for the minute forms parasitic to other organisms. Syn: *bacteriophage.*

protoblast (prō'tō-blăst) [" + *blastos*, a germ]. 1. A naked cell with no cell wall yet formed. 2. Blastomere of segmenting ovum which is parent cell of a part or organ.

protoblastic (prō"tō-blăs'tĭk) [" + *blastos*, germ]. Pert. to a protoblast.

protocol (prō'tō-kŏl) [" + *kolla*, glue (first notes glued)]. 1. A clinical report from first notes taken. 2. Minutes of a meeting. 3. Description of steps taken in an experiment.

protodiastole (prō"tō-dĭ-ăs'tō-lē). The first of four phases of ventricular diastole characterized by drop in intraventricular pressure and closure of semilunar valves.

protogala (prō-tŏg'ăl-ă) [" + *gala*, milk]. A mother's first milk after birth of a child. SYN: *colostrum.*

protogaster (prō"tō-găs'ter) [G. *prōtos*, first, + *gaster*, belly]. The archenteron or gastrocele; the cavity in a gastrula or developing embryo from which the digestive tract develops.

protoleukocyte (prō"tō-lū'kō-sīt) [" + *leukos*, white, + *kytos*, cell]. A minute lymphoid cell in red bone marrow and in the spleen.

Pro"tomastig'ida. An order of flagellate protozoa. It contains several pathogenic forms including *Leishmania* and *Trypanosoma*.

proton (prō'tŏn) [G. *prōtos*, first]. A positively charged particle forming the nucleus of hydrogen and present in the nuclei of all elements, the atomic number of the element indicating the number of protons present. SEE: *atom; atomic theory; electron; element.*

pro"topath'ic. Primitive, undiscriminating. SEE: *sensibility.*

protoplasia (pro"to-pla'zĭ-ă). The primary formation of tissue.

protoplasm (prō'tō-plăzm) [G. *prōtos*, first, + *plasma*, a thing formed]. A thick, viscous colloidal substance which constitutes the physical basis of all living activities, exhibiting the properties of assimilation, growth, motility, secretion, irritability, and reproduction. It is a complex mixture of heterogeneous substances surrounded by an invisible membrane that regulates the interchange of substances with the surrounding medium. It possesses the physical properties of a colloidal mass, the medium of dispersion being water.

It consists of *inorganic substances* (water, mineral compounds) and *organic substances* (proteins, carbohydrates, and lipids). The principal elements present are oxygen, carbon, hydrogen, nitrogen, calcium, and phosphorus which comprise about 99% of protoplasm. Others present in small amounts are potassium, sulfur, chlorine, sodium, magnesium, iron together with trace elements (copper, cobalt, manganese, zinc and others).

RS: *cell; cytoplasm; nucleus.*

protoplasmic (prō"tō-plăz'mĭk) [G. *prōtos*, first, + *plasma*, a thing formed]. Pertaining to protoplasm or composed of it.

protoplast (prō'tō-plăst) [G. *prōtos*, first, + *plassein*, to form]. SYN: *protoplasm.* 1. A cell. 2. A mass of protoplasm.

protoporphyrin (prō"tō-pōr'fĭr-ĭn). $C_{34}H_{34}N_4O_4$, a derivative of hemoglobin containing four pyrrole nuclei. Formed from heme (ferriprotoporphyrin) by deletion of an atom of iron. Occurs naturally.

protoproteose (prō"tō-prō'tē-ōz). A primary proteose which, upon further digestion, is converted to deuteroproteose.

protospasm (prō'tō-spăzm) [" + *spasmos*, a spasm]. One that begins in one area and extends to other parts.

prototoxin (prō"tō-tŏks'ĭn) [" + *toxikon*, poison]. Dissociation product of a toxin, having greatest affinity for the antitoxin.

prototrophic (prō"tō-trō'fĭk) [" + *trophē*, nourishment]. Requiring simple inorganic elements as food.

protovertebra (prō"tō-vĕr'tē-bră) [G. *prōtos*, first, + L. *vertebra*, vertebra]. Primitive vertebra in the notochord. SYN: *metamere; somite.*

protozoa (prō-tō-zō'ă) (sing. *protozoon*) [G. *prōtos*, first, + *zōon*, animal]. The phylum of the animal kingdom which

Table of Pathogenic Protozoa

Subphylum	Genus and Species	Disease Caused
Mastigophora Locomotion by flagella	*Borrelia recurrentis*	Relapsing fever
	Borrelia duttonii	Relapsing fever
	Borrelia bronchialis	Bronchial infection
	Borrelia vincentii	Vincent's disease
	Leptospira icterohaemorrhagiae	Weil's disease
	Leishmania donovani	Kala-azar
	Leishmania braziliensis	American leishmaniasis
	Leishmania tropica	Oriental sore
	Giardia lamblia	Intestinal disturbances
	Trypanosoma gambiense	Sleeping sickness
	Trypanosoma rhodesiense	Sleeping sickness
	Trypanosoma cruzi	Chagas' disease
Sarcodina Locomotion by pseudopodia	*Entamoeba histolytica*	Amebic dysentery
	Dientamoeba fragilis	Diarrhea, fever
Sporozoa No locomotion in adult stage	*Plasmodium malariae*	Quartan malaria
	Plasmodium falciparum	Malignant tertian malaria
	Plasmodium vivax	Benign tertian malaria
	Plasmodium ovale	Ovale malaria
Ciliophora Possess cilia in some stage of life cycle	*Balantidium coli*	Balantidiasis

includes the simplest animals. Most are unicellular, although some are colonial. Reproduction usually asexual by fission, although conjugation and sexual reproduction occur. For subphyla and species of medical importance, SEE: *Table of Pathogenic Protozoa.*

protozoacide (prō-tō-zō'ă-sīd) [" + " + L. *cidus,* from *caedere,* to kill]. Destructive to, or that which kills, protozoa.

protozoal (prō"tō-zō'ăl) [" + *zōon,* animal]. Pert. to protozoa, unicellular organisms.

p. diseases. Those produced by single-celled organisms, such as amebic dysentery, malaria and syphilis.

protozoology (prō"tō-zō-ŏl'ō-jĭ) [" + " + *logos,* study]. Phase of science dealing with study of protozoa.

protozoon (prō"tō-zō'ŏn) (pl. *protozoa*) [" + *zōon,* animal]. Unicellular organism. SEE: *protozoa.*

protozoophage (prō"tō-zō'ō-fāj) [" + " + *phagein,* to eat]. A phagocyte which ingests protozoa.

protractor (prō-trăk'tŏr) [L. *pro,* forward, + *tractōr,* that which draws]. 1. Instrument for removing foreign bodies from wounds. 2. A muscle that draws a part forward. OPP: *retractor.*

protrude. To project; to extend beyond a border or limit.

protrusion. State or condition of being forward or projecting.

protuberance (prō-tū'bĕr-ents) [" + *tuberare,* to bulge]. A part that is prominent beyond a surface, like a knob.

proud flesh (prowd). A mass of excessive granulation, formed when a wound shows no other sign of healing or tendency to cicatrization.

provisional (prō-vĭzh'ŭn-ăl) [L. *provisiō,* a providing before]. Serving a temporary use. Temporary.

provitamin (prō-vī'tăm-ĭn) [L. *pro,* before, + *vita,* life, + *amine*]. A substance that may be inactive, but can be transformed in the body to the corresponding active vitamin. They can function as vitamins.

p. A. Carotene, the precursor of vitamin A.

proximad (prŏk'sĭm-ăd) [L. *proximus,* next, + *ad,* toward]. Toward the proximal or central point.

proximal (prŏks'ĭm-ăl) [L. *proximus,* nearest]. Nearest the point of attachment or center of the body or point of reference. The opposite of *distal.*

proximate (prŏks'ĭm-āt) [L. *proximus,* nearest]. Next to; immediate.

proximoataxia (prŏk-sĭ-mō-ă-tak'sĭ-ă) [L. *proximus,* nearest, + G. *ataxia,* lack of order]. Lack of coordination in muscles of the proximal area of an extremity, as the arm, forearm, thigh, or leg.

pro'zone. That portion of the low dilution range of a homologous serum which fails to agglutinate bacteria that are agglutinated by the same serum in a higher dilution.

prozymogen (prō-zī'mō-jĕn) [G. *pro,* before, + *zymē,* leaven, + *gennan,* to produce]. An intranuclear substance that becomes zymogen. SYN: *prezymogen.*

prune (prōōn) [L. *pruna*]. A dried plum, rich in carbohydrate. Contains a substance which is useful in stimulating the bowel especially for those who suffer from chronic constipation.

COOKED (*unsweetened*): 1 cup (270 gm.). Calories: 305. Other main values: 3 gm. protein; 1 gm. fat; 81 gm. carbohydrate; 60 mg. calcium; 1850 I.U. vitamin A.

pruriginous (prū-rĭj'ĭn-ŭs) [L. *prurigō,* itch, from *prurīre,* to itch]. Pert. to, or of the nature of, prurigo.

prurigo (prū-rī'gō) [L. itch, from *prurīre,* to itch]. A chronic skin disease marked by constantly recurring, discrete, pale, deep-seated, intensely itchy papules on extensor surfaces of limbs.

Superimposed exanthematous manifestations may mask the true nature.

ETIOL: Exciting cause unknown. Hygienic factors are supplementary.

PROG: Guarded. It begins in childhood and may last a lifetime.

TREATMENT: Constitutional and local. Hygienic regimen. Locally, antipruritics.

p. aestivalis. P. recurring every summer and continuing during hot weather.

p. agria. Very severe p. with great itching.

p. infantilis. P. in children during eruption of milk teeth.

p. nodularis. Eruption in skin of hard nodules with great itching.

p. simplex. Simple form of p. with recurring tendency.

pruritus (prū-rī'tŭs) [L. itching, from *prurīre,* to itch]. Severe itching.

May be symptomatic, or occur idiopathically as a neurosis without structural change.

ETIOL: Predisposing factor is cutaneous hyperesthesia. Localized causes are present in pruritus ani, pruritus vulvae, focal infection, intestinal parasites (pinworms), mycotic infection, bath itch, etc.

TREATMENT: Exciting or contributory cause to be located and removed. Hygienic regimen. Pilocarpine, phenacetin, bromide. In anal and vulvar pruritus, examination by competent gynecologist or proctologist before cutaneous therapy is instituted. In bath avoid too sudden changes of temperature. For dry skins, avoid frequent soap and water bathing. Soft, nonirritating underclothing, soothing lotions, oil rubs, antipruritics.

p. aestivalis. P. with prickly heat occurring in hot weather. SYN: *summer itch.*

p. ani. Itching about the anus. May be due to pinworms, fistula in ani, hemorrhoids, contact with soap or detergents which remain in underclothing following improper washing, or irritation.

p., essential. P. without apparent skin lesion.

p. hiemalis. Winter itch, occurring in cold weather.

p. senilis. P. in aged with degenerative skin changes.

p., symptomatic. P. as a symptom of some other disorder.

p. vulvae. Disorder marked by severe itching of external female genitalia. Often an early sign of diabetes mellitus.

Prussak's space (prōōs'ăk) [Alexander Prussak, Russian otologist, 1839-1897]. Tiny space in middle ear between Shrapnell's membrane laterally and neck of malleus medially.

prussic acid (prŭs'ĭk, prōō'sĭk). A violent and rapid poison. SYN: *acid, hydrocyanic, q.v.*

psalterium (săhl-tē'rĭ-ŭm) [G. *psaltērion,* harp]. A transverse band of fibers which connect the crura of the fornix immediately posterior to body of fornix. SYN: *lyre; hippocampal fissure.*

psammoma (săm-ō'mă) [G. *psammos,* sand, + *-ōma,* tumor]. A small tumor of the brain, the choroid plexus and other areas, containing calcareous particles.

p. bodies. Laminated concretions often found in the pineal body. SYN: *corpora arenacea; brain sand.*

psammosarcoma (săm″ō-sar-kō′mă) [G. *psammos,* sand, + *sarx,* flesh, + *-ōma,* tumor]. A sarcoma in which psammoma bodies are present.

psammotherapy (săm″ō-thĕr′ă-pĭ) [″ + *therapeia,* treatment]. The application of sand baths in treatment.

psam′mous. Sandy, gritty.

pselaphesia, pselaphesis (sĕl-ă-fē′zhĭ-ă, -sĭs) [G. *psēlaphēsis,* touch]. 1. Active sense of touch, including muscle sense. 2. Plucking at bedclothes with the fingers, a sign observed in low delirium. SYN: *carphology.*

psellism, psellismus (sĕl′ĭzm, sĕl-ĭz′mŭs) [G. *psellizein,* to stammer]. Defective pronunciation, stuttering or stammering.

p. mercurialis. Jerking, hurried, unintelligible speech in mercurial tremor.

pseudacousma (sū″dă-kūz′mă) [G. *pseudēs,* false, + *akousma,* a thing heard]. Condition in which all sounds are heard falsely, seeming to be altered in quality of pitch, or imaginary sounds are heard.

pseudacusis (sū″dă-kū′sĭs) [″ + *akousis,* hearing]. State in which sounds are heard falsely or imagined. SYN: *pseudacousma.*

pseudagraphia (sū-dă″grăf′ĭ-ă). SYN: *pseudoagraphia.* A form of agraphia in which a person is unable to write independently but is able to copy words or letters.

pseudaphia (sū-dăf′ĭ-ă) [″ + *aphē,* touch]. A false or defective perception of touch. SEE: *paraphia; pseudesthesia.*

pseudarthritis (sū″dar-thrī′tĭs) [″ + *arthron,* joint, + *-itis,* inflammation]. Hysterical disease of the joints.

pseudarthrosis (sū-dar-thrō′sĭs) [″ + ″ + *-ōsis,* disease]. A false joint developing after a fracture that has not united.

pseudesthesia (sū-dĕs-thē′zĭ-ă) [″ + *aisthēsis,* sensation]. 1. An imaginary or false sensation, as that after amputation felt in the lost part. 2. Sense of feeling not caused by external stimulation. SEE: *paraphia; pseudaphia.*

pseudo- (sū′dō) [G. *pseudēs,* false]. A prefix meaning *false.*

pseudoacromia parasitica. Tinea versicolor, *q.v.*

pseudoagglutination (sū-dō-ăg-glū-tĭn-ā′shŭn). The clumping together of red blood cells as in the formation of rouleaux, but differing from true agglutination in that they can be dispersed by shaking.

pseudoagraphia. Pseudagraphia, *q.v.*

pseudoalbinism. Loss of pigment of the skin as occurs in leukopathia or vitiligo.

pseudoanemia (sū″dō-ăn-ē′mĭ-ă) [G. *pseudēs,* false, + *an-,* negative, + *aima,* blood]. Pallor of mucous membranes and skin without other signs of true anemia.

pseudoangina (sū″dō-ăn′jĭ-na, -an-jĭ′nă) [″ + L. *angina,* a choking]. False symptoms resembling angina pectoris of nervous origin.

SYM: Functional attacks in cardiac region but not associated with any disease of the heart or its vessels.

pseudoapoplexy (sū″dō-ăp′ō-plĕk-sĭ). Condition simulating apoplexy but not accompanied by cerebral hemorrhage.

pseudoataxia (sū″dō-ă-tăks′ĭ-ă) [G. *pseudēs,* false, + *ataxia,* lack of order]. Condition resembling **ataxia** not due to *tabes dorsalis.*

pseudobacterium (sū″dō-băk-tē′rĭ-ŭm) [G. *pseudēs,* false, + *baktērion,* a little rod]. Any microscopic cell similar to a bacterium.

pseudoblepsia, pseudoblepsis (sū″dō-blĕp′sĭ-ă, -sĭs) [″ + *blepsis,* sight]. False or imaginary vision. SYN: *parablepsia; pseudopsia.*

pseudobulbar paralysis (sū″dō-bŭl′ber) [″ + *bolbos,* a swollen end]. Paralysis resembling bulbar paralysis, but due to lesion of cortical centers.

pseudocartilaginous (sū″dō-kar-tĭ-lăj′ĭn-ŭs) [G. *pseudēs,* false, + L. *cartilāgō,* gristle]. Pert. to, or formed of, a substance resembling cartilage.

pseudocast (sū′dō-kăst) [″ + M.E. *casten,* a throwing off]. A sediment in urine resembling a true cast.

pseudocele (sū′dō-sēl) [G. *pseudēs,* false, + *koilos,* hollow]. The cavity of the septum pellucidum, the so-called 5th ventricle. SYN: *cavum septi pellucidi* [NA]; *pseudocoele.*

pseudocholinesterase (sū-dō-ko-lin-ĕs′ter-ās). A nonspecific cholinesterase which hydrolyzes noncholine esters as well as acetylcholine. Found in blood serum and pancreatic tissue.

pseudochorea (sū″dō-kō-rē′ă) [″ + *choreia,* a dance]. Hysterical state resembling chorea. SYN: *spurious chorea.*

pseudochromesthesia (sū″dō-krō-mĕs-thē′zĭ-ă) [″ + *chrōma,* color, + *aisthēsis,* sensation]. A condition in which sounds, esp. of the vowels, seem to induce a sensation of a distinct visual color. SEE: *phonism; photism.*

pseudochromidrosis (sū″dō-kro-mid-ro′sĭs). Appearance of colored sweat in which the sweat acquires its color after it is excreted.

pseudocirrhosis (sū″dō-sĭr-ō′sĭs) [″ + *kirros,* orange yellow, + *-ōsis,* disease]. A condition with symptoms of cirrhosis of liver, due usually to pericarditis.

SYM: Cyanosis, ascites, dyspnea.

pseudocoele (sū′dō-sēl) [G. *pseudēs,* false, + *koilos,* hollow]. The 5th ventricle of brain. SYN: *pseudocele.*

pseudocoloboma (sū″dō-kŏl-ō-bō′mă) [″ + *kolōboma,* imperfection]. A scarcely noticeable scar on the iris from an embryonic fissure.

pseudocrisis (sū-dō-krī′sĭs) [″ + *krisis,* a separation]. A temporary fall of body temperature which may be followed by a rise.

pseudocroup (sū′dō-kroop) [″ + A.S. *kropan,* to shout aloud]. False croup. SYN: *laryngismus stridulus.*

pseudocyesis (sū″dō-sī-ē′sĭs) [″ + *kyēsis,* pregnancy]. A condition in which a patient has nearly all of the usual signs and symptoms of pregnancy such as enlargement of abdomen, weight gain, cessation of menses, and morning sickness but is not pregnant. This has also been reported as occurring in men.

Usually seen in women who are either very desirous of having children or wish to avoid pregnancy. When the patient is under anesthesia or hypnosis or is asleep, the abdominal enlargement disappears.

Treatment is usually psychiatric. SYN: *phantom pregnancy.*

pseudocyst (sū′dō-sĭst) [G. *pseudēs,* false, + *kystis,* bladder]. A dilatation resembling a cyst.

pseudodementia (sū″dō-dē-mĕn′shĭ-ă) [″ + L. *de-,* negative, + *mens, ment-,* mind]. Exaggerated indifference to environment without impairment of mind.

pseudodiphtheria (sū″dō-dĭf-thē′rĭ-ă) [" + *diphthera*, membrane]. A condition resembling diphtheria but not due to Klebs-Löffler bacillus.

p. bacillus. A nonpathogenic bacillus resembling the true diphtheria bacillus.

pseudoedema (sū″dō-ē-dē′mă) [G. *pseudēs*, false, + *oidēma*, a swelling]. A puffy condition of the skin simulating edema.

pseudoemphysema (sū″dō-ĕm-fĭz-ē′mă) [" + *emphysēma*, an inflation]. A bronchial condition with blocking simulating emphysema.

pseudoencephalitis (sū″dō-ĕn-sĕf-ă-lī′tĭs) [" + *egkephalos*, brain, + *-itis*, inflammation]. A false encephalitis, due to profuse diarrhea.

pseudoerysipelas (sū″dō-ĕr-ĭ-sĭp′ĕl-ăs) [" + *erythros*, red, + *pella*, skin]. An inflammation of subcutaneous cellular tissue simulating erysipelas.

pseudoesthesia (sū″dō-ĕs-thē′zĭ-ă) [G. *pseudēs*, false, + *aisthēsis*, sensation]. An imaginary sensation or a false one. SYN: *pseudesthesia.*

pseudofracture. A ribbonlike zone of decalcification seen in certain types of osteomalacia, especially milkman's syndrome.

pseudoganglion (sū″dō-găn′glĭ-ŏn) [" + *gagglion*, knot]. A slight thickening of a nerve resembling a ganglion.

pseudogeusesthesia (sū″dō-gū-sĕs-thē′zĭ-ă) [" + *geusis*, taste, + *aisthēsis*, sensation]. A sense of color accompanying sensations of taste.

pseudogeusia (sū″dō-gū′sĭ-ă) [" + *geusis*, taste]. A subjective sensation of taste not produced by external stimulus.

pseudoglioma (sū″dō-glī-ō-mă) [G. *pseudēs*, false, + *glia*, glue, + *-ōma*, tumor]. Inflammatory changes occurring in the vitreous body, due to iridochoroiditis, which simulate glioma of retina.

pseudoglobulin (sū″dō-glŏb′ū-lĭn) [G. *pseudēs*, false, + L. *globulus*, little globe]. One of a class of globulins characterized by being soluble in salt-free water. SEE: *euglobulin.*

pseudoglottis (sū″dō-glŏt′ĭs) [" + *glōttis*, glottis]. Area bet. false vocal cords.

pseudohemophilia (sū-dō-hĕm-ō-fĭl′ĭ-ă). Condition in which coagulation time is normal but bleeding time is prolonged.

pseudohemoptysis (sū″dō-he-mŏp′tĭs-ĭs) [" + *aima*, blood, + *ptyein*, to spit]. Spitting of blood which does not arise from the bronchi or the lungs.

pseudohermaphroditism (sū″dō-hĕr-măf′rō-dīt″ĭzm) [G. *pseudēs*, false, + *Hermaphroditos*, mythical two-sexed god]. A congenital abnormality of the external genitalia and of the body in which one resembles the other sex. SEE: *intersex.*

p. femininus. Condition, in a female, marked by a large clitoris resembling the penis and hypertrophied labia majora resembling the scrotum, thus resembling a male.

p. masculinus. Condition, in a male, marked by a small penis and perineal hypospadias, and scrotum without testes, thereby resembling the vulva.

pseudohydrophobia (sū″dō-hī-drō-fō′bĭ-ă) [" + *ydor, ydr-*, water, + *phobos*, fear]. Disorder simulating hydrophobia in its symptoms. SYN: *lyssophobia.*

pseudohypertrophic (sū″dō-hī-pĕr-trō′fĭk) [" + *yper*, above, + *trophē*, nourishment]. Pert. to a false hypertrophy.

p. paralysis. Paralysis with enlargement and loss of motion of muscles.

pseudohypertrophy (sū″dō-hī-per′trō-fĭ) [G. *pseudēs*, false, + *yper*, above, + *trophē*, nourishment]. Increase in size of an organ or structure due to hypertrophy or hyperplasia of tissue other than parenchyma. Often accompanied by diminution of function.

pseudoisochromatic (sū-dō-ĭ-sō-kro-măt′ĭk). Apparently of the same color, said of certain colors which appear alike to color-blind persons.

pseudoleukemia (sū″dō-lū-kē′mĭ-ă) [G. *pseudēs*, false, + *leukos*, white, + *aima*, blood). Condition in which pathological changes such as enlargement of lymph nodes resemble those in leukemia but in which blood picture remains near normal. Includes Hodgkin's disease, aleukemic myelosis, and others.

p., infantile. SYN: *von Jassch's disease.* A form of anemia in children usually associated with rachitic tendencies and accompanied by mild leukocytosis.

pseudoleukocythemia (sū″dō-lū″kō-sī-thē′mĭ-ă) [" + *leukos*, white, + *kytos*, cell, + *aima*, blood]. Progressive anemia with lymphomata, characteristic of several conditions. SYN: *pseudoleukemia.*

pseudologia (sū-dō-lo′jĭ-ă) [G. *pseudēs*, false, + *logos*, a study]. Falsification in writing or in speech, a form of pathological lying.

p. fantastica. Pathological lying; one of the forms of the psychopathic state.

pseudomania (sū″dō-mā′nĭ-ă) [G. *pseudēs*, false, + *mania*, madness]. 1. A psychosis in which the patient falsely accuses himself of crimes which he thinks he has committed. 2. Pathological lying.

pseudomasturbation (sū″dō-măs-tur-bā′shŭn). A nervous habit of pulling at the penis. SYN: *peotillomania.*

pseudomelanosis (sū″dō-mĕl-ăn-ō′sĭs) [" + *melas, melan-*, black, + *-ōsis*, disease]. Discoloration of tissues after death.

pseudomembrane (sū″dō-mĕm′brān) [" + L. *membrana*, membrane]. A false membrane, as in diphtheria.

pseudomembranous (sū″dō-mĕm′bră-nŭs) [" + L. *membrana*, membrane]. Pert. to or marked by false membranes.

pseudomeningitis (sū″dō-mĕn-ĭn-jī′tĭs) [" + *mēnigx*, membrane, + *-itis*, inflammation]. A condition resembling symptoms of meningitis without lesions of meningeal inflammation.

pseudomenstruation (su″do-men″strōō-ā′shun). Bleeding from the uterus not accompanied by the usual changes in the endometrium.

pseudometamerism (sū - dō - mē - tăm′er - izm). False metamerism such as seen in tapeworms in which the body consists of linear series of proglottids instead of true segments.

pseudomnesia (sū″dŏm-nē′zĭ-ă) [" + *mnēsis*, memory]. A memory perversion in which patient remembers that which never occurred.

Pseudomonas (sū-dō-mō′năs) [G. *pseudēs*, false, + *monas*, single]. A genus of small, motile, gram-negative bacilli belonging to the family Pseudomonadaceae. Most are saprophytic living in soil and decomposing organic matter. Some produce blue and yellow pigments.

Ps. aeruginosa. SYN: *pyocyanea.* A pathogenic species isolated from infections of otitis media, suppurative lesions, and infant diarrhea.

Ps. pyocyanea. Ps. aeruginosa, *q.v.*

pseudomucin (sū-dō-mū′sĭn) [G. *pseudēs*, false, + L. *mucus*, mucus]. A variety of mucin found in proliferative ovarian cysts.

pseudomyelia paresthetica (sū"dō-mī-ē'lĭ-ă păr-ĕs-thĕt'ĭk-ă). False sense of motion in paralyzed limb or of no motion in a moving limb. SEE: *pain.*

pseudomyotonia (sū-dō-mī-ō-tōn'ĭ-ă). Delay in relaxation of the muscle contraction induced by a deep tendon reflex. Characteristic of hypothyroidism.

pseudomyxoma (sū-dō-mĭx'ō-mă). A peritoneal tumor resembling a myxoma and containing a thick viscid fluid.

p. peritonaei. A type of tumor developing in peritoneum from implantation metastases resulting from rupture of ovarian cystadenoma or cells escaping during surgical removal. Numerous papillomas develop attached to abdominal wall and intestine and peritoneal cavity becomes filled with mucuslike fluid.

pseudoneoplasm (sū-dō-nē'ō-plăsm). A false or phantom tumor. A temporary swelling which simulates a tumor, usually of an inflammatory nature.

pseudoneuroma (sū"dō-nū-rō'mă) [G. *pseudēs,* false, + *neuron,* sinew, + *-ōma,* tumor]. SYN: *neurofibroma.* A mass of interlacing, coiled nerve fibers, cells of Schwann and fibrous tissue which forms a mass at end of amputation stump. Also called *amputation* or *traumatic neuroma.* It is not a true neuroma.

pseudonuclein (sū"dō-nū'klē-ĭn) [" + L. *nucleus,* a nut]. A combination of albumin with metaphosphoric acid. SYN: *paranuclein.*

pseudonucleolus (sū"dō-nū-klē-ōl'ŭs). The false nucleolus or karyosome.

pseudoparalysis (sū"dō-pă-răl'ĭ-sĭs) [" + *para,* at the side, + *lyein,* to loosen]. A loss of muscular power not due to lesion of the nervous system.

pseudoparaplegia (sū"dō-păr-ă-plē'jĭ-ă) [" + " + *plēgē,* a stroke]. Seeming paralysis of the lower extremities without impairment of the reflexes.

pseudoparasite (sū"dō-par'ă-sīt) [" + " + *sitos,* food]. 1. Anything resembling a parasite. 2. Organism that can live as a parasite, although it is normally not one. SYN: *commensal.* SEE: *facultative parasite.*

pseudoparesis (sū"dō-par-e'sĭs, -par'e-sĭs) [" + *paresis,* relaxation]. A condition simulating paresis but unlike the ordinary forms and due to hysteria.

pseudopeptone (sū"dō-pĕp'tōn) [G. *pseudēs,* false, + *peptein,* to digest]. Hemialbumose, *q.v.* Also called *propeptone.*

Pseudophyllidea (sū-dō-fĭl-lĭd'ē-ă). An order belonging to the class Cestoidea, subclass Cestoda. Includes tapeworms with scolex bearing two lateral (or one terminal) sucking grooves (bothria). Includes *Diphyllobothrium,* the fish tapeworm of man.

pseudoplegia (sū"dō-plē'jĭ-ă) [G. *pseudēs,* false, + *plēgē,* a stroke]. Paralysis of hysterical origin. SYN: *pseudoparalysis.*

pseudopod (sū'dō-pŏd) [" + *pous, pod-,* foot]. Protruding protoplasmic process of a temporary nature in protozoa for taking up food and aiding in locomotion. SYN: *pseudopodium.*

pseudopodium (sū"dō-pō'dĭ-ŭm) (pl. *pseudopodia*) [G. *pseudēs,* false, + *pous, pod-,* foot]. SYN: *pseudopod.* 1. A temporary protruding process of a protozoan or an ameboid cell such as a leukocyte which aids in locomotion and the engulfing of food particles or foreign substances as in phagocytosis. 2. An irregular projection at the edge of a wheal.

pseudopregnancy (sū-dō-prĕg'năn-sĭ). 1. Condition occurring in lower animals following sterile matings in which anatomical and physiological changes occur similar to those of pregnancy. 2. Phantom pregnancy, *q.v.* SEE: *pseudocyesis.*

pseudopsia (sū-dŏp'sĭ-ă) [" + *opsis,* vision]. Visual hallucinations or false perceptions. SYN: *pseudoblepsis.*

pseudoptosis (sū-dō-tō'sĭs). Apparent ptosis of the eyelid resulting from fold of skin or fat projecting below edge of eyelid.

pseudorabies (sū"dō-rā'bēz, -rā'bĭ-ēz) [G. *pseudēs,* false, + L. *rabere,* to rage]. A condition resembling rabies. SYN: *lyssophobia; pseudohydrophobia.*

pseudoreaction (sū-dō"rē-ăk'shŭn). A false reaction. A response to injection of a test substance into the tissues due to presence of an allergen other than one for which test is made.

pseudorubella (sū-dō-rū-bĕl'lă). SYN: *exanthem subitum, roseola infantum.* An acute disease in infants characterized by high fever which is unaffected by antipyretics and rubelliform eruption which appears just as the fever subsides.

pseudoscarlatina (sū"dō-skar-lă-tē'nă) [" + L. *scarlatina,* scarlet]. A septic febrile condition with rash resembling scarlatina.

pseudosclerosis (sū"dō-sklē-rō'sĭs) [" + *sklērōsis,* a hardening]. A condition with the symptoms, but without the lesions, of multiple sclerosis of the nervous system.

pseudosmia (sū-dŏz'mĭ-ă) [" + *osmē,* smell]. An olfactory hallucination or perversion of the sense of smell.

pseudostoma (sū-dŏs'tō-mă) [" + *stoma,* a mouth]. An apparent aperture between endothelial cells that have been stained.

pseudostratified (sū-dō-străt'ĭ-fīd). Apparently composed of layers.

p. epithelium. E. in which basal ends of all cells rest on basement membrane but distal ends may or may not reach the surface. Their nuclei lie at different levels giving the appearance of being stratified.

pseudosyphilis (sū"dō-sĭf'ĭ-lĭs) [" + *syn,* with love, + *philos,* love]. A nonspecific condition resembling syphilis.

pseudotabes (sū"dō-tā'bēz) [" + L. *tabēs,* a wasting]. A neural disease simulating tabes dorsalis.

pseudotetanus (sū"dō-tĕt'ăn-ŭs) [G. *pseudēs,* false, + *tetanos,* tension]. Persistent muscular contractions resembling tetanus.

pseudotuberculosis (sū"dō-tū-ber"kū-lō'sĭs) [" + L. *tuberculus,* tubercle, + G. *-ōsis,* disease]. Disease like tuberculosis but not caused by the tubercle bacillus.

pseudotympany (sū"dō-tĭm'pă-nĭ). Flattening of arch of diaphragm, swelling of abdomen with increased respiration.

It disappears under anesthesia and is of purely nervous origin. SYN: *accordion abdomen.*

pseudotyphoid (sū"dō-tī'foyd) [" + *typhos,* fever, + *eidos,* resemblance]. Condition resembling typhoid fever, but not caused by the typhoid bacillus.

pseudoxanthoma (sū-dō-zăn-thōm'ă) [G. *pseudēs,* false, + *xanthos,* yellow, + *-ōma,* tumor]. Condition resembling xanthoma.

p. elasticum. Chronic, degenerative cutaneous disease marked by yellow patches and stretching of skin. Associated with hypertension and degeneration of elastic coat of arteries. Angioid streaks in retina common.

psilosis (sī-lō'sĭs) [G. *psilōsis*, a stripping]. 1. Falling out or removal of hair. 2. Tropical diarrhea of severe, often fatal form. SYN: *sprue.*

ETIOL: Disease of pancreas, invasion by bacteria or sensitivity to gluten in diet.

SYM: Diarrhea, large, lightly-colored, acid stools containing fat. No pain or tenesmus. Inflamed, eroded and cracked tongue and mouth.

psittacosis (sĭt-ă-kō'sĭs) [G. *psittakos*, parrot, + *-ōsis*, disease]. An infectious viral disease of parrots and other birds that may be transmitted to man. The tetracyclines or penicillin are effective in treatment. SYN: *ornithosis.*

SYM AND SIGNS (in man): Headache, epistaxis, nausea, chill followed by fever, constipation, sometimes pulmonary disorders.

psoas (sō'ăs) [G. *psoa*. loins]. One of two muscles of the loins. SEE: *Table of Muscles in Appendix; Illus., below.*

p. abscess. A cold abscess in sheath of the psoas major muscle.

It follows the sheath of this muscle until it reaches the surface and points. It generally occurs above Poupart's ligament in the iliac fossa or near the attachment of the psoas muscle to the femur.

ETIOL: Usually tuberculous disease of vertebrae accompanied by pus.

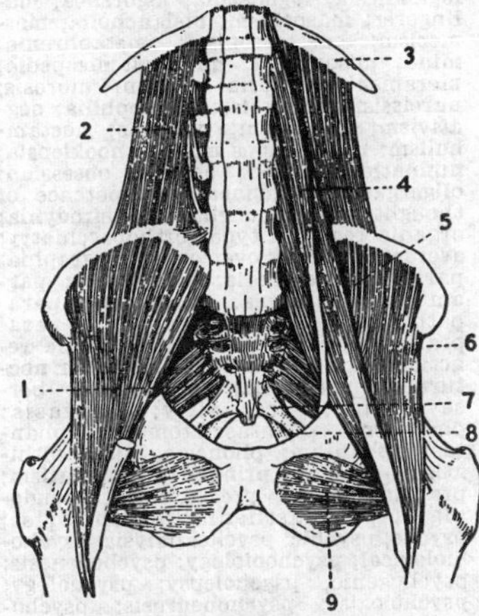

PSOAS, ILIACUS AND QUADRATUS LUMBORUM

1. Pyriformis. 2. Quadratus lumborum. 3. Twelfth rib. 4. Psoas minor. 5. Psoas major. 6. Iliacus. 7. Sarcospinous ligament. 8. Sarcotuberous ligament. 9. Obturator externus.

psoitis (sō-ī'tĭs) [G. *psoa*, loins, + *-itis*, inflammation]. Inflammation of the psoas muscles or of the area of the loins.

psora (sō'ră) [G. *psōra*, itch]. 1. An itching disease of the skin; scabies. 2. Psoriasis, an erythematous, scaling, cutaneous eruption.

psorelcosis (sō-rĕl-kō'sĭs) [" + *elkōsis*, ulceration]. Ulceration occurring as a result of scabies.

psoriasis (sō-rī'ăs-ĭs) [G. *psōriasis*, an itching]. Chronic inflammatory skin disease of many varieties characterized by formation of silvery scaling patches on body.

ETIOL: Unknown.

SYM: Begins in adult life as flat-topped papule covered with thin, grayish-white scale spreading peripherally; lesions coalescing; centers regressing, forming circinate lesions. Under the dry scales are red bleeding points (papillae).

TREATMENT: Hygienic regimen. Daily colloid baths followed by soothing ointment. Locally an ointment such as salicylic acid to promote shedding keratic layer of the skin. SEE: *Bazin's disease.*

p. buccalis. Variety with white patches on tongue and cheek. SYN: *leukoplakia buccalis.*

p. circinata. Form with ring-shaped lesions with healing beginning in the center.

p. diffusa. P. with more or less coalescence of lesions.

p. punctata. P. with papular red eruptions tipped with white scales.

psorophthalmia (sō-rŏf-thăl'mĭ-ă) [G. *psōra*, itch, + *ophthalmos*, eye]. Marginal inflammation of the eyelids with ulceration.

psorous (sō'rŭs) [G. *psōra*, itch]. Related to or affected with itch.

P.S.P. Abbr. for *phenolsulfonphthalein.* A substance used to test kidney function.

psychagogy (sī''kă-gō'jē). A psychotherapeutic, reeducational procedure which stresses proper social adjustment of the individual.

psychalgia (sī-kăl'jĭ-ă) [G. *psychē*, soul, mind, + *algos*, pain]. 1. Mental distress or pain, esp. in melancholia. 2. Pain of hysterical origin. SYN: *mind pain; soul pain; phrenalgia.*

psychanalysis (sī-kăn-ăl'ĭ-sĭs) [" + *analysis*, a loosening apart]. Discovery of the pathogenic links bet. the objective and subjective consciousness by a system of recall. SYN: *psychoanalysis, q.v.*

psychanopsia (sī-kăn-ŏp'sĭ-ă) [" + *an-*, negative, + *opsis*, vision]. Sight with failure to recognize anything seen, due to brain lesion. SYN: *psychic blindness.*

psychasthenia (sī-kăs-thē'nĭ-ă) [" + *astheneia*, weakness]. A neurotic condition marked by sense of inadequacy, unreality, anxiety and doubt.

A neurosis characterized by obsessions, phobias, tics, and compulsions. Obsessions are intrusive ideas which the patient cannot dismiss from consciousness and yet clearly recognizes as pathologic. (Delusions are false ideas not recognized as abnormal.)

There may be associated restlessness, palpitation, fatigue, or irritability. A definite sense of dread or fear is associated with phobias. The anxiety is rationalized, as a fear of syphilis (syphilophobia), or cancer (carcinomatophobia), or insanity (psychopathophobia). or contamination (mysophobia), among many others.

Obsessions and phobias may occur at the onset or during the course of other diseases, notably schizophrenia. Frequently, obsessive impulses dominate behavior. These may be peculiar (touching lampposts, avoiding lines on sidewalk), or distinctly antisocial. In the latter event, it is indicative of a condition more serious than a neurosis. SYN: *anxiety neurosis, q.v.; Janet's disease.*

psychataxia (sī″kă-tăk′sĭ-ă) [G. *psychē*, soul, + *ataxia*, lack of order]. Disordered power of concentration.

psychauditory (sī-kaw″dĭ-tō-rĭ). Pert. to the perception and interpretation of sounds.

psyche (sī′kē) [G. *psychē*, soul, mind]. All that constitutes the mind and its processes.

psychedelic (sī″kĕ-del′ik). Originally used in 1963 to mean mind manifesting. Now used by lay persons to describe some of the subjective respects of intoxication particularly with a drug such as lysergic acid diethylamide (LSD) or other psychotogenic medicines.

psychentonia (sī″kĕn-tō-nĭ-ă). Mental strain or tension.

psychiasis (sī-kē-ī-ăs′ĭs). Spiritual healing.

psychiatric (sī-kĭ-ăt′rĭk) [" + *iatrikos*, healing]. Pertaining to psychiatry, the science dealing with mental ailments.

p. types. *The Confused*: May not realize the incongruity of an act as related to the environment.

The Deluded: May have phobias or specific fears which control some of their habits.

The Depressed: May ignore everything because of their misery, which engages all of their attention.

The Excited: May be unable to concentrate.

The Feeble: May be unable to control themselves because of weakness.

The Hallucinated: Habits may be affected by "voices," etc.

psychiatrist (sī-kī′ă-trĭst) [G. *psychē*, soul, + *iatreia*, healing]. A physician who specializes in study and treatment of mental disorders.

psychiatry (sī-kī′ă-trĭ) [G. *psychē*, soul, + *iatreia*, healing]. The branch of medicine which deals with the diagnosis, treatment and prevention of mental illness.

psychiatry, words pert. to: abalienation; abalienatio mentis; aberration; abnormality; abreaction; abulia; acatalepsia; acatamathesia; acataphasia; acousma; acousmatagnosis; acousmatamnesia; acrasia; Adler's organ inferiority; affect; agnosia; agraphia; agrypnia; ahypnia; akathisia; akinesia; alcoholism; alexia; algesia; algolagnia; algopsychalia; alienation; alienism; alienist; alliteration; allophasis; allopsychic; allotropic; alogia; Alzheimer's disease; ambitendency; ambivalence; amentia; amimia; amnesia; amnestic; amok; amoralia; amusia; anaclitic choice; anacroasia; anal erotic; ananabasia; ananastasia; anandria; anergastic; anhedonia; anoesia; anoia; anomia; anorexia; apandria; apanthropia; apastia; apathy; aphasia; aphemesthesia; aphemia; aphonia; aphrasia; aphrenia; aphronesia; aphthenxia; apodemialgia; apraxia; aprosexia; apsithyria; apsychosis; asemasia; asemia; asitia; association; assonance; asterognosis; asyllabia; asymbolia; asynesia; atactilia; atavism; ataxaphasia; ataxia, intrapsychic; ataxophemia; ateliosis; athymia; atrabiliary; attitude; autism; autistic thinking; autoanalysis; automatism; autoecholalia; autophagy; autophilia; autophobia; autoplastic; autopsychosis; autosuggestion; autosynoia; avulsion; behaviorism; blocking; bradylalia; bradylexis; brain storm; catatonia; catharsis; cenesthesia; censor; chorea; claustrophilia; claustrophobia; complex; compulsion; conation; condensation; confabulation; conflict; constellation; coprolagnia; coprolalia; coprophilia; cretinism; cryptesthesia; cycloid; cyclothymia; deafness; delire de toucher; delirium; delusion; dementia; depersonalization; depression; dereistic; determinism; disassociation; disorientation; displacement; distractibility; divagation; dysbulia; dyschiria; dyscinesia; dysmnesia; dysphremia; dysthymia; echolalia; echomania; echomimia; ego; egocentric; ekphorize; electra complex; emotion; emotivity; empathy; eremophobia; erethism; ergasiomania; ergasiophobia; erotism; erotomania; erythrophobia; eschrolalia; eviration; exhibitionism; extrovert; fabrication; fastidium; fear; feeblemindedness; fixation; folie; free association; fuge; furor amatorius; Ganser's syndrome; geophagia; graphorrhea; hallucination; hallucinosis; haphalgesia; hebephrenia; heterolalia; holergastic; hyperhedonia; hyperognosis; hyperprosexia; hypersthenia; hyperthymia; hypnagogic; hypnoidal; hypnosis; hypnotic; hypnotism; hypochondria; hypochondriac; hypochondriasis; hypophrenia; hysteria; idea; idiocy; idiophrenic psychosis; idiot; idiotropic type; illusion; image; imago; imbecile; imperious act; impulsion; incoherency; incompetent; infantilism; inhibition; insanity; instinct; integration; intelligence; intraphysical; introjection; introversion; introvert; kakergastic reaction; katatonia; kinesthesia; Korsakoff's psychosis; latent content; lethargy; lethologica; logamnesia; logopathia; logorrhea; malingerer; masochism; melancholia; mesmerism; mestatropism; metaphrenia; mind; misocainea; misologiamisopedia; moramentia; moria; moron; morosis; narcissism; narcotism; necrophilia; negativism; neologism; neurosis; noctambulism; non compos mentis; nooklepsia; nunnation; object choice; obsession; oligergasia; oligopnea; omnipotence of thought; oneiric; oneirism; oneirodynia; organic reaction type; orthopsychiatry; overdeterminism; overtone; paragraphia; paralexia; paralogia; paramimia; paramnesia; paranoia; paranomia; parapathia; paraphasia; paraphonia; parapraxis; parent-fixation; parergastic reaction; paresis; pathergasia; pavor nocturnus; pedophilia; periphrastic; perseveration; personality; phantasia; phantasm; phantasmatomoria; phantasy; phantom; phoneme; pica; pithiatism; pleasure principle; pragmatism; pragmatagnosia; preconscious; pseudoalgia; psychasthenia; psychiatrist; psyche; psychic; psychoanalysis; psychobiological; psychobiology; psychogenesis; psychogenic; psycholepsy; psychology; psychologist; psychoneurosis; psychopath; psychopathology; psychosis; psychotherapy; rationalization; reaction; reality principle; recapitulation theory; repression; resistance; restraint; retardation; rut formation; safety symbolism; satyriasis; schizoid; schizophrenia; scotomization; sexual bondage; shell shock; sterotypy; stupor; subconscious; subjective; sublimation; subliminal; suggestion; surrogate; sycophancy; symbiosis; symbol; symbolism; syntonic; threshold of consciousness; transfer; transference; transvestism; trend; twilight state; tyrannism; unconscious; verbigeration; vesania; vigil; vigilambulism; vision; voice; word blindness; word salad; zeloptypia.

psychic (sī′kĭk) [G. *psychē*, soul, mind]. 1. Concerning the mind, or psyche. 2. One said to be endowed with semisupernatural powers, such as the ability to read the mind of others, or to foresee coming events; one apparently sensitive to nonphysical forces.

p. blindness. Sight without recognition of that which is seen.

p. contagion. Communication of another's nervous disorder by imitation, as a tic.

p. deafness. Inability to recognize sounds heard.

p. determinism. The theory that mental processes are determined by conscious or unconscious motives, and are never irrelevant.

p. force. One generated apart from physical energy.

psychical (sī'kĭ-kăl) [G. *psychē,* soul]. Pert. to mind or soul. SYN: *psychic.*

psychinosis (sī-kĭn-ō'sĭs) [G. *psychē,* mind, + *nosos,* disease]. Any functional disease affecting the mind.

psycho-, psych-. Combining form meaning pertaining to the mind, or mental processes.

psychoanalysis (sī"kō-ăn-ăl'ĭ-sĭs) [" + *analysis,* a loosening apart]. Method of obtaining a detailed account of past and present mental and emotional experiences and repressions, in order to determine the source and eliminate the pathologic mental or physical state produced by these mechanisms.

Largely a system that is the creation of Sigmund Freud and was originally the outgrowth of his observations of neurotics. Frequently, the term often is used synonymously with freudianism, but more commonly for a rather more extensive system of psychologic fact and theory applying both to normal and abnormal groups.

In addition to freudian method, other schools of thought or disciplines utilized in analysis of the psyche include *analytical psychology* (Jung), *psychobiology* (Meyer) and *individual psychology* (Adler).

The process is based upon the theory that such abnormal phenomena are due to repression of painful or undesirable past experiences, which, although totally forgotten, later manifest themselves in various abnormal ways. Psychoanalysis, therefore, makes an effort to bring up such forgotten memories into the conscious mind. The patient is thus enabled to view the occurrence in its true perspective, and so loses its harmful effect. There are two main methods: (1) dream analysis; (2) free association.

Includes a study of the ego in relation to reality, and more particularly the herd, and the conflicting goals so created. This conflict is "solved" by repressing one component. This repressed or censored emotion-laden complex of ideas exists in the so-called "subconscious," manifesting itself in the hidden content of dreams, in neuroses and tension states.

Quite unaware of the influence of the subconscious, anger outbursts, rationalization of unfair attitudes, slips of the tongue, etc., occur. Repressed material is largely sexual and the peculiar conditioning of the patient is chiefly determined by the emotional experiences of the earlier years. Reactions of inferiority may result in a compensatory reaction of goodness, ambition, etc. Sublimation is the escape of creative interest on levels not socially taboo. This, however, is not accepted by all psychologists.

psychoanalyst (sī-kō-ăn-ăl'ĭst). One who practices psychoanalysis.

psychobiology (sī"kō-bī-ŏl'ō-jĭ) [G. *psychē,* soul, + *bios,* life, + *logos,* a study). SYN: *biopsychology.* 1. The study of the biology of the psyche, including the anatomy, physiology, and pathology of the mind. 2. A method of psychoanalysis established by Adolf Meyer employing *distributive analysis* which includes a study of all mental and physical factors involved in the growth and development of an individual.

p., objective. P. in which special emphasis is placed on the relationship of the individual to his environment.

psychocardiac reflex (sī"kō-kar'dĭ-ăk). Change in circulatory rate and consciousness of heart thumping resulting from memory of, or subconscious dream state recollection of, an emotional impression or experience.

psychocatharsis (sī"kō-ka-thar'sĭs). The bringing of so-called traumatic experiences and their affective associations into consciousness by interview, hypnosis, or by use of drugs such as sodium amytal.

psychochrome (sī'kō-krōm) [G. *psychē,* soul, + *chrōma,* color]. Color impression resulting from sensory stimulation of a part other than the visual organ. SEE: *psychochromesthesia.*

psychochromesthesia (sī"kō-krōm-ĕs-thē'-zĭ-ă) [" + " + *aisthēsis,* sensation]. Color sensation produced by the stimulus of sense organ other than that of vision.

psychocoma (sī-kō-kō'mă) [" + *kōma,* stupor]. Condition of mental stupor.

psychocortical (sī"kō-kor'tĭ-kăl) [" + L. *cortex,* rind]. Pert. to the cerebral cortex as the seat of sensory, motor, and psychic functions.

psychodiagnostics (sī"kō-dī-ăg-nŏs'tĭks). The Rorschach test used in personality study.

Psychodidae (sī"kŏd'ĭ-dē). A family of the order Diptera which includes the moth flies, owl midges, and sand flies. SEE: *Phlebotomus.*

psychodometry (sī"kō-dŏm'ĕ-trĭ) [" + *odos,* way, + *metron,* measure]. Measurement of rate of mental activity.

psychodrama (si"ko-dram'ă). A form of group psychotherapy. The patients act out assigned rôles and, in so doing, are able to gain insight into their own mental disturbances.

psychodynamics (sī"kō-dī-năm'ĭks) [" + *dynamis,* power]. The scientific study of mental action or force.

psy"choepilepsy. A form of hysterical neurosis accompanied by movements resembling those of epilepsy.

psychogenesis (sī"kō-jĕn'ĕs-ĭs) [G. *psychē,* soul, + *genesis,* formation]. 1. The origin and development of mind; the formation of mental traits. 2. Origination within the mind or psyche.

psychogenetic (sī"kō-jĕn-ĕt'ĭk) [" + *genesis,* to produce]. 1. Originating in the mind, as a disease. 2. Concerning formation of mental traits.

psychogenic (sī-kō-jĕn'ĭk) [" + *gennan,* to produce]. 1. Of mental origin. 2. Concerning the development of the mind. SYN: *psychogenetic.*

psychogeusic (sī"kō-gĕu'sĭk). Pert. to perception of taste.

psychogram (sī'kō-grăm) [" + *gramma,* a writing]. A subjective visualization of a mental concept.

psychograph (sī"kō-grăf'). 1. A chart showing personality traits. 2. A history of the personality of an individual.

psychokinesia (sī″kō-kĭn-ē′zĭ-ă) [″ + *kinēsis,* motion]. Explosive or impulsive maniacal action due to defective inhibition. SYN: *psycheclampsia.*

psychokinesis (sī-kō-kĭn-ē′sĭs). Influence exerted on a system by a subject without any intermediate physical energy or instrumentation.

psycholagny (sī″kō-lăg′nĭ). Sexual excitation brought about by mental imagery; psychic or mental masturbation.

psycholepsy (sī″kō-lĕp′sĭ) [″ + *lēpsis,* a seizure]. Sudden alteration of moods in which mental inertia and hopelessness are manifested.

psycholeptic (sī″kō-lĕp′tĭk) [″ + *lēpsis,* a seizure]. Concerning sudden shifting of moods, particularly to one marked by hopelessness and mental inertia.

psychological (sī″kō-lŏj′ĭ-kal) [G. *psychē,* soul, mind, + *logos,* a study]. Pert. to study of the mind in all of its relationships, normal and abnormal.

psychologist (sī-kŏl′ō-jĭst) [″ + *logos,* study]. One who specializes in the mental phenomena of consciousness and behavior or mental activity.

psychology (sī-kŏl′ō-jĭ) [″ + *logos,* a study]. The science dealing with the mental processes, both normal and abnormal and their effects upon behavior.

There are two main approaches to the study: (1) Introspective, *i. e.,* looking inward, or self-examination of one's own mental processes. (2) Objective, *i. e.,* studying the minds of others. In the latter approach, there are four chief lines of attack: (a) The experimental method; (b) the comparative method; (c) the genetic method; (d) the pathological method. SEE: *esthetic morality; "psych-" words.*

p., abnormal. The study of abnormal behavior and the mental phenomena associated with such.

p., analytic. Psychoanalysis based on the concepts of Carl Jung which deemphasizes sexual factors in motivation and emphasizes the "collective unconscious" and "psychological types" (introvert and extrovert).

p., animal. The study of animal behavior.

p., applied. The application of the principles of psychology to special fields such as clinical, industrial, educational, nursing, or pastoral psychology.

p., depth. P. which pertains to the unconscious.

p., dynamic. The psychology of motivation; that which seeks the causes of mental phenomena.

p., experimental. Study of mental acts by tests and experiments.

p., Gestalt. That which emphasizes the wholeness of psychological processes and behavior and maintaining that such cannot be adequately explained by breaking down into constituent parts.

p., individual. A system of psychological thinking developed by Alfred Adler in which an individual is regarded as having three life goals; physical security, sexual satisfaction, and social integration. Self-evaluations lead to feelings of inferiority and inadequacy which often lead to overcompensation or a striving for superiority.

p., physiologic. That which deals with the structure and function of the nervous system and other bodily organs and their relationship to behavior.

psychometry (sī-kŏm′ĕt-rĭ) [G. *psychē,* soul, mind, + *metron,* a measure]. Capacity to acquire knowledge supernormally by handling objects.

psychomotor (sī-kō-mō′tor) [″ + L. *motor,* a mover]. Concerning, or causing, voluntary movement.

psychoneurosis (sī″kō-nū-rō′sĭs) [G. *psychē,* soul, + *neuron,* sinew, + *-ōsis,* disease]. One of a group of mental disorders of a functional nature in which there is partial disorganization of the psyche, a psychopathological syndrome characterized principally by anxiety states, phobias, compulsions, obsessions, and conversion phenomena. Insight is maintained.

Includes hysteria, psychasthenia and neurasthenia.

SEE: *neurosis; psychoanalysis; psychosis.*

p., defense. Condition due to attempt to dismiss from the mind ideas and sensations that are painful. This results in buried subconscious memories producing psychoneurosis.

psychoneurotic (sī″kō-nū-rŏt′ĭk) [G. *psychē,* soul, mind, + *neuron,* sinew]. Pert. to a functional disorder of mental origin.

psychonomy (sī-kŏn′ō-mĭ) [″ + *nomos,* law]. The science of the laws of the mind and its functions.

psychoparesis (sī″kō-păr-ē′sĭs, -par′ĕ-sĭs) [″ + *paresis,* relaxation]. Weakness or enfeeblement of the mind.

psychopath (sī′kō-păth) [″ + *pathos,* disease]. One with a constitutional lack of moral sensibility, although possessing normal intelligence. SYN: *psychopathic personality; character disorder.*

p., transportation of. 1. Be sure you have necessary legal papers.

2. Learn all you can about patient before starting.

3. Ascertain if destructive or dangerous.

4. If so (No. 3), do not travel with patient without assistance.

5. See that patient has nothing that may be used for violence or self-destruction.

6. If on train or boat, use a compartment.

7. If patient is dangerous, notify the transportation company in advance.

8. Do not hesitate to call upon local police or trainmen if necessary.

9. Be sure you have enough money for the journey and your own return.

10. Ascertain names of physicians who may be called enroute if needed.

11. Secure copy of inventory of patient's effects from hospital, with statement as to any bruises or injuries suffered by patient.

psychopath′ia., Psychopathy, *q.v.*

p. martialis. Shell-shock.

p. sexualis. Sexual perversions.

psychopathic (sī″kō-păth′ĭk) [″ + *pathos,* disease]. 1. Concerning or characterized by a mental disorder. 2. Concerning treatment of mental disorders. 3. Abnormal.

p. personality. "One who, though possessing normal intelligence, is or becomes, by reason of heredity or congenital conditions, constitutionally lacking in moral sensibility, emotional control, and the inhibition of will."—Dr. C. H. Patten.

A constitutional imbalance in the pattern of the mind, but not a disorder of function, such as is observed in the actual neuroses and psychoses. Psychopaths are attractive but cannot be depended upon. Judgment is poor; they are easily pleased or displeased, and are above the average in intelligence. Usually antisocial.

psychopathology (sī″kō-păth-ŏl′ō-jĭ) [G. *psychē*, soul, mind, + *pathos*, disease, + *logos*, a study]. The study of the causes and nature of mental disease or abnormal behavior.

psychopathy (sī-kŏp′ăth-ĭ) [G. *psychē*, soul, + *pathos*, feeling]. Any mental disease, esp. one characterized by defective character or personality.

psychopharmacology (si-ko-farm-ă-kol′-o-jĭ). The science of drugs having an effect on psychomotor behavior and emotional states.

psychophonasthenia (sī″kō-fō″năs-thē′-nĭ-ă). A speech defect of mental origin.

psychophysical (sī″kō-fĭz′ĭ-kăl) [" + *physikos*, natural]. Concerning the relation of the physical and the mental.

p. law. Intensity of sensation increases as the logarithms of the stimuli.

psychophysics (sī″kō-fĭz′ĭks) [" + *physikos*, natural]. 1. The study of mental processes in relation to physical processes. 2. The study of stimuli in relation to the effects they produce.

psychophysiologic (sī″kō-fĭz-ĭ-ō-lŏg′ĭk). Pert. to psychophysiology, *q.v.*

p. autonomic and visceral disorders. Term applied to a large number of disorders of organs and viscera innervated by the autonomic nervous system in which emotional factors are a primary causative factor. Formerly called psychosomatic disease or disorder.

psychophysiology (sī″kō-fĭz-ĭ-ŏl′ō-jĭ) [" + *physis*, nature, + *logos*, study]. Physiology of the mind; science of the correlation of body and mind.

psychoplegic (sī-kō-plē′jĭk) [G. *psychē*, mind, soul, + *plēgē*, a stroke]. An agent reducing excitability of the cerebrum.

psychorhythmia (sī″kō-rĭth′mĭ-ă) [G. *psychē*, soul, mind, + *rythmos*, rhythm]. Mental condition in which involuntary repetition of previous voluntary actions occurs.

psychorrhea (sī-kŏr-ē′ă) [G. *psychē*, soul, mind, + *roia*, a flow]. A mental condition characterized by incoherent stream of thought resulting in vague and often bizarre theories and ideas.

psychosensory (sī″kō-sĕn′sor-ĭ) [" + L. *sensorius*, pert. to sensation]. 1. Understanding and interpreting sensory stimuli. 2. Concerning perceptions not arising in sensory organs, as hallucinations.

psychosexual (sī″kō-sĕks′ū-ăl) [" + L. *sexus*, sex]. Concerning the emotional components of sexual instinct.

p. development. Evolution of personality through infantile and pregenital periods to sexual maturity.

psychosin (sī-kō′sĭn) [G. *psychē*, mind, soul]. A cerebroside occurring in brain tissue.

psychosis (sī-kō′sĭs) (pl. *psychoses*) [G. *psychē*, mind, soul). A term formerly applied to any mental disorder but now generally restricted to those disturbances of such magnitude that there is personality disintegration and loss of contact with reality. They are of psychogenic origin or without clearly defined physical cause or structural change in the brain. They are usually characterized by delusions and hallucinations and hospitalization is generally required.

A condition manifested in the behavior, emotional reaction and ideation of the patient. He fails to mirror reality as it is, reacts erroneously to it, builds up false concepts regarding it, and his behavior responses are peculiar, abnormal, inefficient, or definitely antisocial.

All this does not include amentia, because defective intelligence merely lessens comprehension of reality but does not distort it, or the psychopathic personality, as here the patient reacts badly because of intrinsic emotional differences playing upon an undistorted world of reality.

Delusions or hallucinations strongly suggest a psychosis, as do marked indifference, depression and excitement. Antisocial behavior occurs with psychopathic personalities and mental defectiveness. When epileptic, it suggests the occurrence of an episodic psychosis known as an equivalent.

Classification: Divided into two main groups. 1. Those due to impairment of brain tissue. 2. Those in which any associated brain function disturbance is secondary to the psychiatric disorders.

Treatment: Treatment includes medical, psychological, and sociological procedures. Medical therapy includes shock therapy (insulin, metrazol, electroshock), electronarcosis, psychosurgery (prefrontal lobotomy), physiotherapy (hydrotherapy, electrotherapy massage), biochemotherapy (use of CO_2, hormones, histamine, benzedrine sulfate, ataraxic and tranquilizing agents). Psychotherapy includes psychoanalysis, emotional release, emotional reeducation, hypnotherapy, and occupational and recreational therapy. Sociological therapy involves modification of environment.

p., alcoholic-delusional. A degenerative process marked by delusions.

p., circular. P. with alternating manic and depressive episodes.

p., climacteric. Occurring at the menopause.

p., congenital. From birth.

p., depressive. Syn: *psychotic depressive reaction.* P. characterized by extreme depression, melancholia, and feelings of unworthiness.

p., exhaustion. Syn: *exhaustion or collapsed delirium.* Reaction resulting from extreme physical exertion.

p., famine. P. resulting from starvation.

p., involutional. P. occurring during involutional period of bodily and intellectual decline. In women from ages 40-55; in men from 50-65.

p., manic-depressive. Ordinarily a series of periods of psychotic depression or excessive well-being, appearing in any sequence and alternating with longer periods of relative normalcy.

Though intensity may vary greatly, the manic shows an elated though unstable mood, a flight of ideas, and great physical activity. The case of primary depression finds all exertion exhausting; there is difficulty in thinking or acting and victim is very unhappy.

p., organic. The result of a pathological condition of the central nervous system, such as paresis.

p., postinfectious. P. following an infectious disease such as meningitis, pneumonia, typhoid fever.

p., puerperal. P. occurring during pregnancy or following childbirth.

p., reactive. Syn: *situation psychosis.* P. presumably induced by an environmental condition.

p., senile. Due to old age.

p., situation. Transitory psychosis caused by an unpleasant situation.

p., toxic. One resulting from toxic agents.

p., traumatic. One resulting from head injuries and belonging to the organic group.

psychosomat'ic. Pert. to interrelationship between the mind and body.

p. disorder. A pathological condition due to emotional or psychogenic factors.

p. medicine. The branch of medical science that emphasizes mental factors as the cause of functional and anatomical changes in disease processes.

psychosurgery (sī"kō-sur'jer-ĭ) [G. *psyche,* soul, + G. *cheirourgia,* handwork]. Brain surgery for mental illness. The term includes such procedures as lobotomy, topectomy, and thalamotomy.

psychotechnics (sī"kō-tĕk'nĭks) [G. *psychē,* soul, + *technē,* art]. Application of psychological methods in the study of economic and social problems.

psychotherapy (sī-kō-thĕr'ă-pĭ) [" + *therapeia,* treatment]. Any mental method of treating disease, esp. nervous disorders, by means such as suggestion, hypnotism, psychoanalytic therapy, etc.

psychotogenic (si-kot'o-jen'ik). Producing a psychosis, usually temporary and due to certain powerful drugs.

psychotomimetic (si-ko-to-mim'et-ik). A hallucinogen producing weird illusions and phantasms.

psychroalgia (sī-krō-ăl'jĭ-ă) [G. *psychros,* cold, + *algos,* pain]. Painful sensation of cold.

psychroesthesia (sī"krō-ĕs-thē'zĭ-ă) [" + *aisthēsis,* sensation]. A sensation of cold in a part of the body, although it is warm.

psychrometer (sī-krŏm'ĕ-tĕr) [" + *metron,* a measure]. Device for measuring relative humidity of the atmosphere.

psychrophilic (sī-krō-fĭl'ĭk) [" + *philein,* to love]. Preferring cold, as bacteria which thrive best at low temperatures between 0° and 30° C. (32° and 86° F.).

psychrophobia (sī-krō-fō'bĭ-ă) [" + *phobos,* fear]. Abnormal aversion or sensitiveness to cold.

psychrophore (sī'krō-fōr) [" + *phorein,* to carry]. Apparatus for applying cold to the urethra, or other canal.

psychrotherapy (sī"krō-thĕr'ă-pĭ) [" + *therapeia,* treatment]. Treatment of disease by administration of cold.

psyllium seed (sĭl'ĭ-ŭm). The dried, ripe seed of a plant grown in France, Spain, and India.

Use: As a mild laxative.

ptarmic (tar'mĭk) [G. *ptarmos,* a sneezing]. 1. Causing sneezing. Syn: *sternutatory.* 2. That which causes sneezing.

pterion (tē'rĭ-ŏn) [G. *pteron,* wing]. Point of suture of frontal, parietal, temporal, and sphenoid bones.

pteroylglutamic acid. See: *folic acid.*

pterygium (tĕr-ĭj'ĭ-ŭm) [G. *pterygion,* wing]. Ophth: Triangular thickening of bulbar conjunctiva on the cornea with apex toward pupil.

p., progressive. Stage in which the growth extends toward center of cornea.

p., stationary. Stage in which the head of pterygium remains permanently attached to same point on the cornea.

Treatment: Surgical.

pterygoid (tĕr'ĭ-goyd) [" + *eidos,* appearance]. Wing-shaped. Syn: *alate.*

p. process. One of two large processes of sphenoid bone extending downward from junction of body and great wings, each consisting of lateral and medial pterygoid plates.

pterygomaxillary (tĕr"ĭ-gō-măks'ĭl-ă-rĭ) [" + L. *maxillaris,* pert. to upper jaw]. Concerning the pterygoid process and the upper jaw.

pterygopalatine (tĕr"ĭ-gō-păl'ă-tīn) [" + L. *palatinus,* pert. to the palate]. Relating to the pterygoid process and the palate bone.

PTH. Abbr. for *parathyroid hormone.*

ptilosis (tĭl-ō'sĭs) [G. *ptilon,* feather, + *-ōsis,* disease]. Loss of eyelashes.

P.T.O. Abbr. for *Perlsucht tuberculin original*: Klemperer's tuberculin.

ptomaine (tō'mān) [G. *ptōma,* dead body]. One of a class of nitrogenous organic bases formed in the action of putrefactive bacteria on proteins and amino acids. Ex: *cadaverine,* $NH_2(CH_2)_5NH_2$. See: *aporrhegma.*

ptomainuria (tō"mă-ĭ-nū'rĭ-ă). Presence of ptomaines in urine.

ptosis (tō'sĭs) [G. *ptosis,* a dropping]. Dropping or drooping of an organ or part, as the upper eyelid from paralysis, or the visceral organs from weakness of the abdominal muscles.

RS: *visceroptosis.*

p., abdominal. Sagging of transverse colon, sometimes almost to the pelvic floor.

Etiol: Obesity or lack of abdominal muscle tone.

Treatment: A properly adjusted abdominal belt may help.

Contra: Dependence upon belt rather than on exercising and developing abdominal muscles.

ptyalagogue (tī-ăl'ă-gŏg) [G. *ptyalon,* saliva, + *agōgos,* leading]. Causing or that which causes a flow of saliva. Syn: *sialogogue.*

ptyalin (tī'ă-lĭn) [G. *ptyalon,* saliva]. A salivary amylolytic enzyme converting starch into maltose and dextrin. See: *enzyme; ptyalism; saliva.*

ptyalism (tī'ăl-ĭzm) [" + *-ismos,* condition]. Excessive secretion of saliva.

Etiol: May be due to pregnancy, stomatitis, rabies, exophthalmic goiter, menstruation and other disorders, including epilepsy, hysteria, nervous conditions and gastrointestinal disorders. May be induced by mercury, iodides, pilocarpine and other drugs. Syn: *salivation.* See: *xerostomia.*

ptyalith (tī'ă-lĭth) [" + *lithos,* stone]. A calculus in a salivary gland.

ptyalocele (tī-ăl'ō-sēl) [" + *kēlē,* hernia]. A salivary cystic tumor or cystic dilatation of a salivary duct.

p., sublingual. See: *ranula.*

ptyalogenic (tī"ăl-ō-jĕn'ĭk) [" + *gennan,* to produce]. Of salivary origin.

ptyalogogue (tī"ăl'ō-gŏg) [G. *ptyalon,* saliva, + *agōgos,* leading]. An agent which causes the flow of saliva. Syn: *sialogogue, q.v.*

ptyalogram (tī-ăl'ō-grăm) [G. *ptyalon,* saliva, + *gramma,* a writing]. An x-ray film of the salivary glands.

ptyalography (tī-ăl-ŏg'ră-fĭ) [" + *graphein,* to write]. X-ray inspection of the salivary glands and ducts. Syn: *sialography.*

ptyalolith (tī'ă-lō-lĭth) [" + *lithos,* stone]. A salivary concretion.

ptyalolithiasis (tī"ă-lō-lith-ī'ă-sĭs). Presence of a concretion in a salivary gland or duct.

ptyalolithotomy (tī"ăl-ō-lĭth-ŏt'ō-mĭ) [" + " + *tomē,* a cutting]. Surgical removal of a concretion from a salivary duct or gland.

ptyalorrhea (tī″ă-lō-rē′ă) [" + *roia*, flow]. An excessive flow of saliva.

ptysis (tī′sĭs). Spitting; the ejection of saliva from the mouth.

ptysmagogue (tĭz′mă-gŏg). An agent that induces the flow of saliva.

P.U. Abbr. for *pregnancy urine* which contains chorionic gonadotrophin.

pubarche (pu-bar′ke). 1. Beginning development of pubic hair. 2. The beginning of puberty.

puber (pū′bŭr) [L.]. One at onset of puberty.

puberal (pū′bĕr-ăl) [L. *pubertās*, puberty]. Concerning puberty.

pubertas (pū′ber-tās). Puberty.

p. plena. Complete puberty.

p. praecox. Precocious puberty or puberty at an early age.

puberty (pū′bĕr-tĭ) [L. *pubertās*, puberty]. Period in life at which one of either sex becomes functionally capable of reproduction.

A period of rapid change in boys and girls. It occurs in temperate climates bet. the ages of 13 and 16 in boys, and from 12 to 15 in girls, and ends in the attainment of sexual maturity.

In the boy it is marked by appearance of hair on the face and chest, under the axilla, and on the pubes, change of voice, definite enlargement of the penis, and the appearance of erections and erotic dreams with ejaculation. Other physical and psychic disturbances are normal at this period, and end in the appearance of functional spermatozoa in the semen.

In the girl menstruation begins, the breasts enlarge, and hair appears in axilla and on the pubes.

RS: *hebephrenia; hebetic; interstitial; latency period; menacme; nubility.*

pubes (pū′bēz) (sing. *pubis*) [L. pubic hair]. 1. Anterior part of innominate bone; os pubis. 2. The pubic region. 3. Hair of the pubic region.

pubescence (pū-bĕs′sĕns) [L. *pubescēre*, to become hairy]. 1. Puberty or its approach. 2. Covering of fine, soft hairs on the body. SYN: *lanugo.*

pubescent (pū-bĕs′ĕnt) [L. *pubescēre*, to become hairy]. 1. Reaching puberty. 2. Covered with downy hair.

pubetrotomy (pū″bē-trŏt′ō-mĭ) [L. *pubes*, pubic hair, + G. *ētron*, belly, + *tomē*, a cutting]. Section through the pubes.

pubic (pū′bĭk) [L. *pubes*, pubic hair]. Concerning the pubes.

p. bone. The lower anterior part of the innominate bone. SYN: *os pubis.*

p. hair. Hair over the pubes which appears at onset of sexual maturity. The distribution is somewhat different as compared to women.

pubio-, pubo- [L.]. Combining form meaning the *pubic hair, pubic bone* or *region.*

pubiotomy (pū-bĭ-ŏt′ō-mĭ) [L. *pubes*, pubic hair, + *tomē*, a cutting]. Incision across the pubis in order to enlarge the pelvic passage, facilitating the delivery of the fetus when pelvis is malformed.

pubis (pū′bĭs) [L. pubic hair]. Pubic bone. RS: *os pubis.*

pubofemoral (pū″bō-fĕm′or-ăl) [L. *pubis*, pubic hair, + *femur, femor-*, thigh bone]. Pert. to the os pubis and the femur.

puboprostatic (pū″bō-prŏs-tăt′ĭk) [" + G. *prostatēs*, prostate]. Relating to the os pubis and prostate gland.

pubovesical (pū″bō-vĕs′ĭ-kl) [" + *vesiculus*, a little sac]. Pert. to the os pubis and bladder.

pudenda (pū-dĕn′dă) (sing. *pudendum*) [L. *pudendum*, from *pudere*, to be ashamed]. The external genitalia, especially of the female. SYN: *vulva.*

pudendagra (pū″dĕn-dăg′ră) [" + G. *agra*, seizure]. Pain in the external genitals.

pudendal (pū-dĕn′dăl) [L. *pudendum*, from *pudere*, to be ashamed]. Relating to the external genitals of female.

pudendum (pū-dĕn′dŭm) (pl. *pudenda*) [L.]. The external genitals, especially those of the female; the vulva.

p. muliebre. BNA. External genitals of the female.

pudic (pū′dĭk) [L. *pudicus*, modest]. Concerning ext. female genitalia. SYN: *pudendal.*

Puente's disease. Simple glandular cheilitis.

puericulture (pū-er′ĭ-kŭl″chūr) [L. *puer*, child, + *cultura*, a cultivating]. Science concerned with prenatal care of unborn children and the art of raising and training children.

puerile (pū′ĕ-rĭl) [L. *puer*, boy]. Concerning a child; childlike.

p. respiration. That heard in auscultation of healthy children.

puerilism (pū′ĕr-ĭl-ĭzm) [" + G. *-ismos*, condition]. Childishness.

puerpera (pū-er′pĕr-ă) [L. *puer*, boy, + *parēre*, to bear]. Woman during the period following the 3rd stage of labor, lasting until there is complete involution of the pelvic viscera.

puerperal (pū-er′pur-ăl) [L. *puer*, boy, + *parēre*, to bear]. Concerning puerperium.

p. eclampsia. Convulsions during puerperium.

p. fever. Septicemia following childbirth. SYN: *childbed fever.*

p. insanity. A psychosis resulting during the puerperium.

p. period. Period immediately following childbirth.

p. sepsis. A toxemia of puerperium accompanied by a rise in temperature during the first 21 days after childbirth.

CHARACTERISTICS: (a) Prior to effective antibiotic therapy this was the greatest single cause of death due to childbirth. (b) Lowered resistance a danger. (c) Toxemia, anemia, exhaustion in labor, abrasions and lacerations, loss of blood predisposing factors. (d) May be autogenous or heterogeneous. (e) Other foci aside from genitals may be responsible for invasion. (f) Infection may remain localized or it may spread. (g) Infected thrombi from veins of placental site may enter blood stream. (h) Metastatic areas of infection may be caused by (g). (i) Spreading along mucous membranes the infection may reach the tubes, ovaries and peritoneum. (j) Thrombophlebitis in pelvic veins may lead to thrombophlebitis in veins of the leg. (k) Localized infections indicated by fever, rapid pulse, pain and pelvic tenderness. (l) Fever in (k) about 3rd day, 103° F. to 104° F. (m) In endometritis, tenderness confined to uterus; lochia may be scant without odor. (n) Lochia profuse and foul if any membranes are retained. (o) Parametritis in more severe infections. (p) In (o) swelling due to inflammatory exudate, giving place to suppuration after a few days, accompanied by chill and rise in temperature. (q) Peritonitis possible, especially if gonococcus is present. (r) Every spread of disease indicated by rise in temperature, and perhaps chills. (s)

Drainage may be necessary. (t) Permanent sterility possible.

PREVENTION: 1. Aseptic technique in all obstetric cases. 2. Masking of those who come in contact with patient. 3. Complete bacteriological survey following any infection to determine possible source. 4. Exclusion of all positive carriers from attendance upon maternity cases. 5. Better intrapartum care of patient long in labor, use of least traumatizing type of delivery, avoidance of blood loss and wider use of blood transfusions.

TREATMENT: Active surgical intervention during infection seldom indicated. Good nursing care, high caloric and vitamin diet, restriction of visitors and sources of irritation. All manipulative procedures kept at a minimum. Excellent results have been obtained from use of sulfonamides and antibiotics.

puerperalism (pū-er′pŭr-ăl-ĭzm) [L. *puer,* boy, + *parēre,* to bear, + G. *ismos,* condition]. Pathological conditions of the puerperal state.

p., infantile. Any pathogenic condition of the newborn.

p., infectious. Puerperal disease caused by infection.

puerperant (pū-er′pŭr-ănt) [" + *parēre,* to bear]. A woman in labor or one who recently has been delivered.

puerperium (pū-er-pē′rĭ-ŭm). Period following the 3rd stage of labor, lasting until involution of pelvic organs takes place; usually 3 to 6 weeks.

RS: *childbed; sepsis, puerperal.*

puerperous (pū-ŭr′pŭr-ŭs) [L. *puer,* boy, + *parēre,* to bear]. In the period following childbirth. SYN: *puerperal.*

Pu′lex. A genus of fleas belonging to the order Siphonaptera.

P. irritans. The human flea, which also infests dogs, hogs, and other mammals. May serve as intermediate host of the tape worms *Dipylidium caninum* and *Hymenolepsis diminuta.*

pulicaris (pū″lĭ-kār′ĭs). Marked by spots resembling flea bites.

pulicatio (pū-lĭ-kā′tĭ-ō). Infested with fleas.

Pulicidae (pū-lĭs′ĭ-dē). A family of fleas belonging to the order Siphonaptera which includes the genera *Pulex, Echidnophaga, Ctenocephalides,* and *Xenopsylla.* SEE: *flea.*

pulicide (pū′lĭ-sīd). An agent which kills fleas.

pullulate (pull′u-lāt). To bud or germinate.

pullulation (pull″u-la′shun). The act of budding or germinating, as seen in yeast plant.

pulmo- [L.]. Combining form meaning *lung.*

pulmoaortic (pŭl″mō-ā-or′tĭk) [L. *pulmō,* lung, + G. *aortē,* aorta]. 1. Concerning the lungs and the aorta. 2. Relating to the pulmonary artery and aorta.

pulmometer (pŭl-mŏm′ĕt-ĕr) [" + G. *metron,* a measure]. Device for measuring the lung capacity. SYN: *spirometer.*

pulmometry (pŭl-mŏm′ĕt-rĭ) [" + G. *metron,* a measure]. Determination of capacity of the lungs.

pulmonary (pŭl′mō-na-rĭ) [L. *pulmō, pulmon-,* lung]. Concerning or involving the lungs.

p. circulation. Passage of blood from heart to lungs and back again for purification.

The blood flows from the right cardiac ventricle through the lungs, there to be oxygenated; then back to the left cardiac atrium.

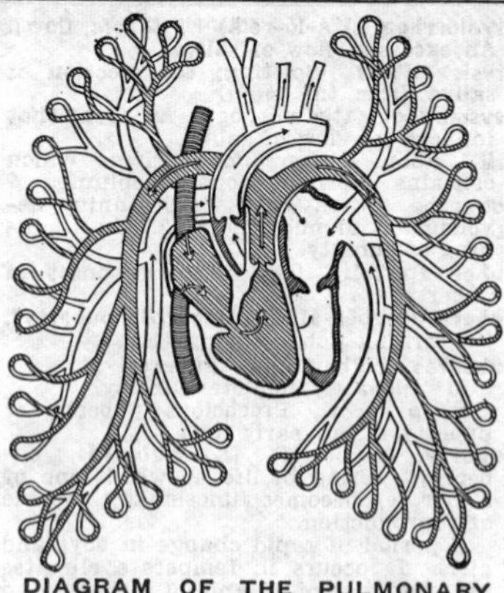

DIAGRAM OF THE PULMONARY CIRCULATION.

The shaded areas represent the course of deoxygenated blood; the unshaded, oxygenated blood.

p. incompetence, p. insufficiency. Failure of the pulmonary valve to close properly.

p. stenosis. Narrowing of opening into the pulmonary artery from right cardiac ventricle.

pulmonectomy (pŭl-mō-nĕk′tō-mĭ) [L. *pulmō, pulmon-,* lung, + G. *ektomē,* excision]. Removal of part or all of a lung's tissue. SYN: *pneumonectomy.*

pulmonitis (pŭl-mō-nī′tĭs) [" + G. *-ītis,* inflammation]. Inflamed condition of the lung. SYN: *pneumonia.*

pulmotor (pŭl-mō′tor) [" + *motor,* a mover]. Apparatus for inducing artificial respiration by forcing oxygen into and out of the lungs.

pulp (pŭlp) [L. *pulpa,* flesh]. 1. The soft part of fruit. 2. The soft part of an organ. 3. Chyme. 4. In dentistry, the soft vascular portion of the center of a tooth.

p. cavity. Hollow space within a tooth containing dental pulp.

p. cells. Those in the pulp cavity of any organ.

p. cords. SYN: *cords of Billroth.* Anastomosing cords of red pulp of the spleen traversed by venous sinuses.

p., digital. Elastic, soft prominence on the palmar or plantar surface of the last phalanx of a finger or toe.

p., enamel. Cells forming a stellate reticulum lying between outer and inner layers of the enamel organ of a tooth.

p., red. The portion of splenic pulp consisting of venous sinuses plus pulp cords.

p., splenic. The soft, spongelike tissue-forming substance of the spleen.

p., white. Portion of splenic pulp consisting of a compact type of lymphatic tissue which forms a sheath about certain arteries.

pulpal (pŭl′păl) [L. *pulpa,* flesh]. Relating to pulp.

pulpefaction (pŭl-pĭ-făk′shŭn) [" + *facere,* to make]. Conversion into pulpy substance.

pulpitis (pul-pi′tis). Inflammation of the pulp of a tooth.

pulpy (pŭl'pĭ) [L. *pulpa*, flesh]. Resembling pulp; flabby. SYN: *pultaceous.*

pulsate (pŭl'sāt) [L. *pulsāre*, to beat]. To throb or beat in rhythm.

pulsatile (pŭl'să-tĭl). Pulsating; characterized by a rhythmic beat. SYN: *throbbing.*

pulsation (pŭl-sā'shŭn) [L. *pulsatiō*, a beating]. The rhythmic beat, as of the heart and blood vessels; a throbbing. SEE: *pulse.*

ABNORMAL CENTERS OF PULSATION: *Epigastric p.*: May result from: 1. Excited action of heart from any cause. 2. Enlargement of right ventricle. 3. A pulsating aorta noted in certain nervous and anemic patients. 4. Aortic aneurysm. 5. Tumors of left lobe of liver resting on the aorta. *P. in left axillary region*: May result from: 1. Enlargement of heart. 2. A tense purulent effusion in left pleural sac (pulsating empyema). 3. Aneurysm. 4. Chronic disease of left lung and pleura, associated with retraction.

Unnatural p. in carotids: May result from: 1. Excitement of heart from any cause. 2. Exophthalmic goiter. 3. Anemia. 4. Valvular disease, especially aortic regurgitation. 5. Aneurysm or dilatation of the vessels. 6. Unnatural elasticity of the vessels, noted in certain nervous and anemic patients. *Jugular p*: The jugular vein often becomes distended in forced expiration and coughing. Sometimes distention noted in adherent pericardium. A true rhythmical venous pulsation usually results from tricuspid regurgitation. A pulsation may be transmitted to the jugular vein from the underlying carotid, but this false pulsation will continue when light pressure is made on root of neck, while the true venous pulse will cease.

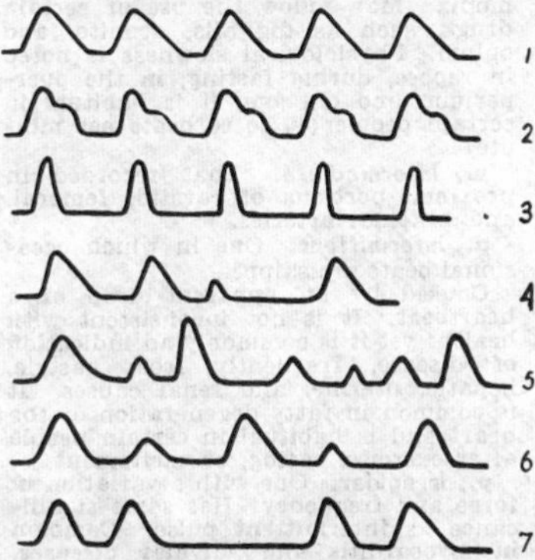

DIAGRAM ILLUSTRATING THE COMMON TYPES OF PULSE.
(After Sears.)

1. Normal pulse. Fairly sharp onset with more gradual falling away of the beat. 2. Dicrotic pulse. Secondary wave as the beat falls away. 3. Waterhammer pulse. Abrupt onset and sharp falling away of the beat. 4. Pulse with extrasystole. A small premature wave followed by a pause before the next normal beat. 5. Pulse in auricular fibrillation, with irregularity in rhythm and volume of all the beats. 6. Pulsus alternans. Large and small beats alternate regularly with each other. 7. Pulsus bigeminus. A coupling of two beats, followed by a pause.

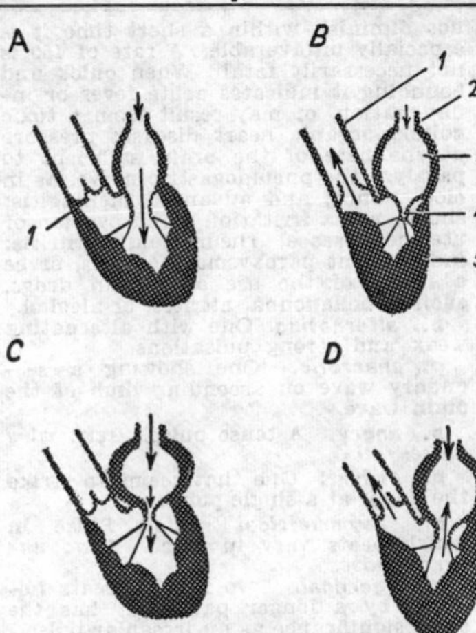

PULSE.
(After Sears.)

A. Normal diastole. Mitral valve open. 1. Aortic valve. B. Normal systole. Mitral valve closed, aortic valve open. 1. Aorta. 2. Pulmonary veins. 3. Atrium. 4, Mitral valve, 5. Ventricle. C. Mitral stenosis. Hypertrophied left atrium forcing blood through narrowed mitral valve. D. Mitral regurgitation. Ventricular systole forcing blood into aorta, with regurgitation into left atrium owing to inadequate closure of mitral valve.

pulse (pŭls) [L. *pulsus*, from *pulsāre*, to beat]. 1. Rate, rhythm, condition of arterial walls, compressibility and tension, and size and shape of the wave. 2. Rhythmical throbbing. 3. Throbbing caused by the regular contraction and alternate expansion of an artery; the periodic thrust felt over arteries in time with the heartbeat.

Normal pulse rate of adult is 70 to 72 in men and 78 to 82 in women, and is usually felt in radial artery of the wrist.

POINTS TO BE OBSERVED: Hour, frequency, pressure, regularity, force. Temperature and respiration are of clinical importance to the physician. Right and left radial arteries are usually tested, and differences, if any or absent, should be noted. Pressure should not be too great on artery. Thumb should not be used because examiner may be counting pulse in own thumb rather than patient's. Count for at least one-half minute.

A tracing of this is called a sphygmogram and consists of a series of waves in which the upstroke is called the *anacrotic* limb, and the downstroke (on which is normally seen the dicrotic notch), the *catacrotic.*

p., accelerated. A common symptom in all fevers. The pulse of the adult rarely exceeds 150 beats per minute even in acute inflammatory infections; when it exceeds 170 it *may* portend a fatal issue.

A pulse of 170 is known as *tachycardia*, and in some diseases it is a common symptom. If such an acceleration does not diminish within a short time it is especially unfavorable. A rate of 150 is not necessarily fatal. When quick and bounding it indicates acute fever or inflammation, or may result from a toxic goiter; organic heart disease; pressure at the base of the brain sufficient to paralyze the pneumogastric nerve, as in clot, tumor, and advanced meningitis; shock; reflex irritation, as in ovarian or uterine disease; rheumatoid arthritis; independent paroxysmal neurosis, or be a result of the use of certain drugs, such as belladonna, nitrites, or alcohol.

p., alternating. One with alternating weak and strong pulsations.

p., anacrotic. One showing a secondary wave on ascending limb of the main wave.

p., angry. A tense pulse. SYN: *wiry pulse.*

p., ardent. One that seems to strike the finger at a single point.

p., asymmetrical radial. Pulse in which beats vary in force. SYN: *unequal pulse.*

p., bigeminal. Two regular beats followed by a longer pause. It has the same significance as an irregular pulse.

p., bounding. SYN: *collapsing pulse.* P. which reaches a higher level than normal, then disappears quickly. Best detected when arm is held aloft. Due to shortened ventricular systole and reduced peripheral pressure.

p., capillary. Alternating redness and pallor of capillary region, as in the matrices beneath the nails, occurring chiefly where an excessive cardiac impulse coincides with general arterial narrowing.

p., catacrotic. One showing 1 or more secondary waves on descending limb of the main wave.

p., central. P. recorded near the origin of the carotid or subclavian arteries.

p., collapsing. One feebly striking the finger, then subsiding abruptly and completely. SEE: *p., bounding, q.v.*

p., Corrigan's. One of aortic insufficiency. SEE: *p., waterhammer.*

p., decurtate. Pulse which gradually decreases in force. SYN: *myurous p.*

p., deficit. The number of pulse beats counted at the wrist is less than those counted in the same period of time at the heart. Seen in *auricular fibrillation.*

p., dicrotic. A double beat, 1 heartbeat for 2 arterial pulsations, or a seeming weak wave bet. the usual heartbeats. This weak wave should not be counted as a regular beat. It is indicative of low arterial tension, and is noted in fevers, in low states of the nervous system, and sometimes in typhoid fever.

p., entopic. Intermittent subjective sensations of light which accompany the heartbeat.

p., febrile. A full, bounding pulse at onset of fever, becoming feeble and weak when fever subsides or on prostration.

p., female. More frequent than male p. by 8 to 10 beats. There is an important correlation bet. the pulse, respiration and temperature which must be considered in most disease states.

p., filiform. SEE: *p., thready.*

p., formicant. A small, feeble pulse.

p. frequency. Depends upon sex, age, exertion, position of body, and health. It is higher in children and increases with very old age. It is slower in tall persons than it is in short ones. It is 10 to 12 beats more frequent in standing than sitting. Physical exertion will raise it from 75 to 125 or higher. Eating and drinking likewise increase heart action. It is less frequent when sleeping or lying down.

p., full. A distended one in an artery giving a tense feeling; observed in sthenic inflammation.

p., gaseous. A soft, full pulse.

p., goat-leap. A weak pulsation following a strong one.

p., hard. One with sensation of hardness due to changes in the arterial wall or to vascular distention.

p., hepatic. One due to expansion of veins of the liver at each ventricular contraction.

p., high-tension. One in which force of beat is relatively increased and which may be roughly estimated by noting the amount of pressure of the fingers that is required to arrest the beat. It is observed in many conditions, notably: cardiac diseases, such as hypertrophy; chronic nephritis; cerebral affections; irritation of the vasomotor center, as in apoplexy, tumors, and beginning meningitis; also after the use of certain drugs, such as digitalis, ergot, and alcoholic stimulants; and in chills, angina pectoris, epileptic and hysterical seizures, gout, and uremia.

p., incident. One with 2nd beat weaker than 1st, the 3rd weaker than the 4th, followed by a stroke as strong as the 1st.

p., infrequent. Observed in organic heart disease, especially fatty degeneration, and fibroid induration; jaundice; pressure at base of brain sufficient to irritate the vagus, as in beginning meningitis; and at the close of febrile diseases, as in typhoid fever, and pneumonia. May follow the use of certain drugs, such as digitalis, aconite, and opium. Physiological slowness is noted in repose, during fasting, in the puerperium, and old age; it is habitual in certain people (40 to 60 beats per minute).

p., intermediate. That recorded in proximal portions of carotid, femoral, and brachial arteries.

p., intermittent. One in which occasional beats are skipped.

Caused by an apparent drop of a heartbeat. It is not inconsistent with health; yet it is commonly an indication of disease, frequently from gastric, hepatic, uterine, and renal causes. It is common in fatty degeneration of the heart and is habitual in certain people after exercise, eating, or excitement.

p., irregular. One with a variation in force and frequency. Has same significance as intermittent pulse. Common in myocarditis and valvular diseases, especially in mitral regurgitation. Heart trouble may be noted by long continued irregular pulse.

p., jerky. That of aortic regurgitation, because from a state of emptiness the artery is suddenly filled with blood.

p., jugular. Venous pulse felt in jugular vein.

p., long. One in which duration of the systolic wave is comparatively long.

p., low-tension. One with sudden onset, short duration and rapid decline; esp. noted in degeneration of the heart, collapse, debility, fevers, and low states of the nervous system.

p., male. From 70 to 72 beats per minute, but not an invariable rule, as some are healthy with a pulse rate of 50 or even 90.

p., monocrotous. One with a sphygmogram showing a simple ascending and descending, uninterrupted line and no dicrotism; indicative of a grave condition of the circulation and of impending death.

p., myurous. Pulse which decreases in force. SYN: *decurtate p.*

p., paradoxical. One which is more or less suppressed at close of each full inspiration. Thought to be due to compression of the great vessels by inflammatory adhesions, the latter being stretched during act of inspiration. Frequently noted in adherent pericardium.

p., peripheral. Pulse recorded in arteries (radial or pedal) in distal portion of limbs.

p., pistol-shot. Pulse resulting from rapid distention and collapse of an artery as occurs in aortic regurgitation.

p., plateau. One slowly rising but which is maintained.

p. pressure. The difference bet. the systolic and the diastolic pressure.

This is really expressive of the tone of the arterial walls. Ex:

120 is systolic pressure.
100 is diastolic pressure.
20 is the pulse pressure.

130 is the systolic pressure.
90 is the diastolic pressure.
40 is the pulse pressure.

Normal pulse pressure: The systolic pressure is normally about 40 points greater than the diastolic. *Abnormal pulse pressure*: A pulse pressure over 50 points or under 30 points is considered abnormal.

p., quick, full, bounding. Indicates inflammation or fever of acute inflammatory character.

p., quick, hard. Characteristic of diphtheria and scarlatina. It also indicates inflammation or fever of acute inflammatory nature.

p., Quincke's. SEE: *p., capillary.*

p., rapid. SEE: *p., accelerated.*

p. rate.

Average Normal Beats/Minute

P. of embryo	150
At birth	140-130
During 1st year	130-115
During 2nd year	115-100
During 3rd year	100- 90
About 7th year	90- 85
About 14th year	85- 80
In middle life	75- 70
Old age	65- 50

p., regular. When the force and frequency are the same, that is, when the length of beat and number of beats per minute and the strength are the same.

p., respiratory. Alternate dilatation and contraction of the large veins of the neck occurring simultaneously with inspiration and expiration following rapid exercise.

p., running. A weak rapid pulse with one wave continuing into the next.

p., senile. That of the aged. The sphygmogram shows a high position of the secondary waves in descent with great size of the 1st secondary wave as compared with the 2nd.

p., short. One with a short, quick systolic wave.

p., shuttle. One that feels as though it is floating something solid as well as fluid.

p., slow. A very slow pulse, fully accentuated, often found among the aged, and it is a habitual rate among those inclined to be slow and easy in their actions. Such a pulse rate ranges bet. 40 and 60 beats per minute.

p., sluggish, full. Common in diseases attended with coma resulting from concussion or compression of brain and chronic softening.

p., small and rapid. Seen in great prostration from wasting diseases or hemorrhage.

p., soft. One which may be stopped by digital compression.

p., thready. A fine, scarcely perceptible pulse.

p., tremulous. One in which a series of oscillations is felt with each beat.

p., trigeminal. Three regular beats followed by a pause. SEE: *p., irregular.*

p., undulating. One that seems to have several successive waves.

p., unequal. Pulse in which beats vary in force.

p., vagus. A slow pulse resulting from vagus inhibition of the heart.

p., venous. Pulse in a vein, esp. one of the large veins near the heart such as the internal and external jugular. Normally is undulating and scarcely palpable. In conditions such as tricuspid regurgitation, it is pronounced.

p., vermicular. A small, frequent one with a wormlike feeling.

p., waterhammer. Characterized by a short, powerful, jerky beat which suddenly collapses. The peculiar pulsation may be distinctly visible, not only in the carotids, but throughout the brachial artery. It is diagnostic of aortic regurgitation during the period of compensation, and its force is due to excessive ventricular hypertrophy and to the large amount of blood expelled with each systole; its sudden recession is due to the incompetent valves failing to support the column of blood. SYN: *Corrigan's p.*

p. wave. A wave in the blood column and the arterial walls which is initiated by the ejection of blood from the left ventricle into the aorta. It travels at a rate of 7 to 9 m. per sec.

p., wiry. A tense one that feels like a wire or firm cord. SYN: *angry p.*

pulse, *words pert. to:* acrotic, acrotism, Adams-Stokes syndrome, anacrotic, anadicrotic, anadicrotism, anatricrotic, arrhythmia, artery, asphyctic, auricular, bisferious, bradycrotic, bradydiastole, bradysphygmia, cacosphyxia, caprizant, cardiopuncture, catacrotism, catadicrotic, catadicrotism, centesis, Corrigan's, diastasis, diastole, diastolic pressure, dicrotic, heart, -block, hemisystole, infant, intercadence, intercalary, phlebogram, pulsate, pulsation, pulsus, respiration, spinal, sphygmoid, sphygmogram, sphygmomanometer, systaltic, systole, systolic pressure, systolic temperature, thermometry, vein.

pulsimeter (pŭl-sĭm'ĕt-ĕr) [L. *pulsus,* a beat, + G. *metron,* measure]. Contrivance for measuring frequency and force of the pulse. SYN: *sphygmometer.*

pul'sion [L. *pulsus*]. Driving or propelling in any direction.

p., lateral. Movement, particularly walking as if pulled to one side.

pulsus (pŭl'sŭs) [L.]. Pulse.

p. alternans. A succession of strong and weak beats alternating.

p. bigeminus. Paired beats.

p. celer. Fast pulse, particularly that associated with high pulse pressure in aortic regurgitation.

p. paradoxus. One in which the pulse becomes weaker during inspiration.

p. tardus. Slow pulse, especially that felt in aortic stenosis.

pultaceous (pŭl-tā'shŭs) [L. *puls, pult-*, pap]. Resembling a poultice. Syn: *pulpy.*

pulv. [L.]. Abbreviation for *pulvis*, powder.

pulverization (pŭl-vĕr-ĭ-zā'shŭn) [L. *pulvis*, powder]. The crushing of any substance to powder or tiny particles.

pulverulent (pŭl-vĕr'ū-lĕnt) [L. *pulvis, pulver-*, powder]. Of the nature of, or resembling, powder. Syn: *powdery.*

pulvinar (pŭl-vī'nĕr) [L. cushioned seat]. Part of the thalamus comprising a portion of the posterior nuclei. Projects posteriorly and medially partially overlying midbrain.

pulvinate (pŭl'vĭn-āt) [L. *pulvinus*, cushion]. Very convex; shaped like a cushion.

pulvis (pŭl'vĭs) [L.]. Powder.

pump (pŭmp) [M.E. *pumpe*]. 1. Apparatus that transfers fluids or gases by pressure or suction. 2. To force air or fluid into a cavity, as heart pumps blood.

p., air. Device for forcing air in or out of a chamber.

p., breast. Apparatus for removing milk from the breasts.

p., dental. Apparatus for removing saliva from the mouth during operation on teeth or jaws.

p., stomach. Apparatus for removing contents of stomach.

pumpkin (pŭmp'kĭn) [G. *pepōn*, ripe]. Canned: 1 cup (228 gm). Calories: 340. Other main values: 10 gm. protein; 3.0 gm. fat; 80 gm. carbohydrate; 160 mg. calcium; 66,188 I.U. vitamin A.

punch drunk. Abnormal condition of brain function due to multiple concussions. Characterized by slow body movement and impairment of intellect. Seen in boxers, particularly those who began boxing before the head was fully developed.

punched out. Appears as if holes have been made; used to describe appearance of bones (as seen on x-ray film) in certain pathological states.

puncta (pŭnk'tă) (sing. *punctum*) [L. *punctum*, point]. Points.

p. dolorosa. Painful points in course of or at exit of nerves affected by neuralgia.

p. lacrimalia. Orifices of lacrimal ducts situated at tip of lacrimal papillae located on inner margins of eyelids about 6 mm. from medial canthus.

p. vasculosa. Minute red areas which mark the cut surface of white central substance of the brain, from blood escaping from divided blood vessels.

punctate (pŭnk'tāt) [L. *punctum*, point]. Having pinpoint punctures or depressions on the surface; marked with dots.

p. rash. One with minute red points.

punctiform (pŭnk'tĭ-form) [" + *forma*, shape]. 1. Formed like a point. 2. Bact: Referring to pinpoint colonies of less than 1 mm. in diameter.

punctograph (pŭnk'tō-grăf) [" + G. *graphein*, to write]. Device employing radiography for localization of foreign bodies in the tissues.

punctum (pŭnk'tŭm) (pl. *puncta*) [L.]. Point.

p. caecum. Spot in fundus of the eyeball where the optic nerve enters. Syn: *blind spot.*

p. lacrimale. Outlet of lacrimal canaliculus.

p. nasale inferius. Lower portion of suture joining the nasal bones. Syn: *rhinion.*

p. proximum. Visual accommodation near point. Abbr: P.P.

p. remotum. Visual accommodation far point. Abbr: P.R.

p. saliens. First trace of the embryonic heart.

puncture (pŭnk'chūr) [L. *punctura*, a point]. 1. A hole or wound made by a sharp pointed instrument. 2. To make a hole with such an instrument.

p., diabetic. Syn: *Bernard's puncture.* Puncture in floor of 4th ventricle which results in glycosuria.

p., exploratory. Removal of fluid or pus from a cavity or cyst for examination by piercing it.

p., lumbar. Puncture of the lumbar spinal membranes to relieve dropsy or for examination of spinal fluid. See: *cisternal puncture; lumbar puncture; cerebrospinal fluid.*

p., ventricular. Puncture of a ventricle of the brain for purpose of withdrawing fluid or introducing air for ventriculography.

p. wound. A wound made by piercing with a sharp instrument. See also under: *wound, puncture.*

pungency (pŭn'jĕn-sĭ) [L. *pungere*, to prick]. Quality of being sharp, strong or bitter, as an odor or taste.

pungent (pŭn'jĕnt) [L. *pungere*, to prick]. Acrid, sharp, as applied to an odor or to taste.

P. U. O. Abbr. for *pyrexia of unknown origin.*

pupa (pū'pă). Stage in complete metamorphosis of an insect which follows the larva and precedes the adult or imago. Insect does not feed in this stage and is usually inactive.

pupil (pū'pĭl) [L. *pupilla*, pupil]. The contractile opening at the center of the iris of the eye.

It contracts when exposed to strong light, and when the focus is on a near object. It dilates in the dark, and when the focus is on a distant object. Average diameter is 4 to 5 mm. Both pupils should be equal.

Constriction of: Occurs in old age, in photophobia. Also induced by morphine, pilocarpine, physostigmine, eserine and other miotic drugs.

Dilatation of: May occur in blindness or deficient sight from any cause, from distress or strong emotion, in fevers and comatose states, oculomotor nerve paralysis, glaucoma.

May be induced by belladonna (atropine), cocaine, eucatropine, homatropine, hyoscine (scopolamine), and other mydriatic drugs.

RS: *accommodation, adaptation, anissocoria, cat's eye pupil, ciliospinal center, corectasis, corencleisis, eye, hippus, iridoplegia, isocorial, miosis, miotic, mydriasis, mydriatic, myosis, myotic, occlusio pupillae, reflex, seclusio pupillae.*

p., Argyll Robertson. P. which reacts to accommodation but not to light. Seen in tabes dorsalis and occasionally in other diseases affecting midbrain.

p., artificial. P. made by iridectomy when normal pupil is occluded.

p., bounding. Rapid dilatation of pupil alternating with contraction.

p., cat's-eye. One narrow and slit-like.

p., occlusion of. One with opaque membrane shutting off the pupillary area.

p., pinhole. A pupil of minute size; one excessively constricted. Seen after use of miotics, in opium poisoning, and in certain brain disorders.

p., tonic. One which reacts slowly in accommodation-convergence reflexes.

pupillary (pū'pĭ-lĕr"ĭ) [L. *pupilla,* a pupil]. Concerning the pupil.

p. reflex. 1. Constriction of pupil upon stimulation of retina by light. 2. Syn: *accommodation reflex.* Constriction of pupil upon accommodation for near vision and dilatation upon accommodation for far vision. 3. Syn: *commensual light reflex.* Constriction of pupil of one eye in response to stimulation of the other by light. 4. Syn: *Westphal's pupillary reflex.* Constriction of pupil upon attempted closure of eyelids which are held apart. Also called *lid or orbicularis reflex.* See: *ciliospinal reflex; hippus.*

pupillometer (pū-pĭl-ŏm'ĕt-ĕr) [L. *pupilla,* a pupil, + G. *metron,* a measure]. Device for measurement of diameter of a pupil.

pupilloscopy (pū-pĭl-os'kō-pĭ) [" + G. *skopein,* to examine]. 1. Measurement of eye refraction by effect of light and shadow on the retina. Syn: *skiascopy.* 2. Examination of the pupil.

pupillostatometer (pū"pĭl-ō-stăt-ŏm'ĕt-ĕr) [" + G. *statos,* placed, + *metron,* a measure]. Device for measuring distance between centers of the pupils.

pure. 1. Free from pollution; uncontaminated. 2. Chaste.

p. line. The progeny of a single homozygous individual obtained by self-fertilization. 2. The progeny of an individual reproducing asexually by simple fission or by buds, runners, stolons, etc. 3. The progeny of two homogyzous individuals reproducing sexually.

purgation (pŭr-gā'shŭn) [L. *purgatiō,* from *purgāre,* to cleanse]. 1. Evacuation of the bowels caused by action of a purgative medicine. Syn: *catharsis.* 2. Cleansing.

purgative (pŭr'gă-tĭv) [L. *purgāre,* to cleanse]. 1. Cleansing. 2. An agent that will cause watery evacuation of the intestinal contents. Ex: *castor oil, magnesium sulfate.* See: *catharsis; cathartic.*

Simple: Produces free discharge from bowels with some griping. *Drastic*: Produces violent action of bowels with cramps and griping. *Saline*: Produces copious watery discharges. *Cholagogue*: Stimulates flow of bile, producing green stools.

p. enema. A strong, high colonic one that produces evacuation when other enemas fail. See: *enema.*

purge (pŭrj) [L. *purgāre,* to cleanse]. 1. To evacuate the bowels by means of a cathartic. 2. A drug that causes evacuation of the bowels.

puriform (pū'rĭ-form) [L. *pus, pur-,* pus, + *forma,* shape]. Resembling pus.

purin(e (pū'rēn, -rĭn) [L. *purum,* pure, + *uricum,* uric acid]. Parent of a group of heterocyclic nitrogen compounds including purine itself, $C_5H_4N_4$, and caffeine, theobromine, theophylline, xanthine, prepared from uric acid.

Purines are the end products of nucleoprotein digestion and may be synthesized in the body. They are divided into the following groups: xanthine, hypoxanthine, and uric acid, belonging to the *oxypurines;* guanine and adenine, belonging to the *aminopurines;* and theophylline, theobromine, and caffeine, belonging to the *methylpurines.* Purines break down to form uric acid. See: *meat.*

p. body. Purine or any base derived from it. Syn: *p. base.* Those mentioned in the foregoing paragraph plus paraxanthine and heteroxanthine.

Purines in Food

Group A: High concentrations (150 to 1000 mg. per 100 grams)

Liver	Sardines (in oil)
Kidney	Meat extracts
Sweetbreads	Consomme
Brains	Gravies
Heart	Fish roes
Anchovies	Herring

Group B: Moderate amounts (50 to 150 mg. per 100 grams)

Meat, game and fish other than those mentioned in Group A

Fowl	Asparagus
Lentils	Cauliflower
Whole grain cereals	Mushrooms
Beans	Spinach
Peas	

Group C: Very small amounts. Need not be restricted in diet of persons with gout.

Vegetables other than those mentioned above

Fruits of all kinds	Coffee
Milk	Tea
Cheese	Chocolate
Eggs	Carbonated beverages

Refined cereals, spaghetti & macaroni
Butter, fats, nuts & peanut butter*

Sugars and sweets	Tapioca
Vegetable soups	Yeast

* Fats interfere with the urinary excretion of urates and thus should be limited when attempting to control the excretion of uric acid.

p., endogenous. P. originating from nucleoproteins within the tissues.

p., exogenous. P. present in or derived from foods.

p. -free diet. Diet which excludes the following: meat, esp. sweetbreads, liver, kidney; poultry; fish; condiments; alcohol; and foods that are difficult to digest as concentrated sweets, rich pastries, and fried foods.

p. -low diet. Excludes foods such as meat, fish, fowl, spinach, lentils, mushrooms, peas, asparagus.

Purkinje cells (per-kin'je) [Johannes E. Purkinje, Bohemian physiologist, 1787-1869]. Large neurons which have dendrites extending to the molecular layer of the cerebellar cortex and into the white matter of the cerebellum.

P. fibers. Atypical muscle fibers lying beneath endocardium of heart which constitute the impulse-conducting system of the heart.

P's. figures. Dark lines produced by the vessels of the retina.

P's. network. Fibrous network of large muscle cells found in cardiac muscle beneath the endocardium.

P. phenomenon, pupillomotor. When the eye adapts from light to dark conditions, the maximum pupillary movement is caused by green instead of yellow light.

P. vesicle. The nuclear portion of an ovum. SYN: *germinal vesicle.*

Purkinje-Sanson's images (poor-kĭn'yĕ-săhn-son'). Three images of one object seen in the pupil of the eye.

purohepatitis (pū"rō-hep-ă-tī'tĭs) [L. *pus, pur-,* pus, + G. *ēpar, ēpat-,* liver, + *-ītis,* inflammation]. Purulent inflammation of the liver.

puromucous (pū"rō-mū'kŭs) [L. *pus, pur-,* pus, + *mucus,* phlegm]. Mucopurulent, containing both mucus and pus.

purpura (pūr'pū-ră) [L. purple]. An affection with various manifestations and obscure etiology, characterized by hemorrhages into the skin, mucous membranes, internal organs, and other tissues.

Hemorrhage into the skin shows red, darkening into purple, then brownish-yellow and finally disappearing in from 2 to 3 weeks. Areas of discoloration do not disappear under pressure.

p. annularis telangiectodes. Eruption of ring-shaped spots on lower limbs with pronounced telangiectasia.

p., fibrinolytic. P. resulting from excess fibrinolytic activity of blood.

p. fulminans. A rapidly progressing form occurring principally in children; of short duration and frequently fatal.

p., hemorrhagic. SEE: *p., idiopathic thrombocytopenic.*

p., idiopathic thrombocytopenic. SYN: *land scurvy; primary splenic thrombocytopenia; Werlhof's disease.* ABBR: ITP. A hemorrhagic disorder in which there is a pronounced reduction in circulating blood platelets, due to presence in blood plasma of a substance which agglutinates platelets. Primary cause unknown.

SYM: Bleeding from mouth and skin upon slight injury. Bleeding may also occur from mucous membranes, in serous membranes and sometimes into brain. Increased bleeding time and poor clot retractility.

p., nonthrombocytopenic. SYN: *p. simplex.* P. of intestine accompanied by bleeding. Associated with abdominal pain, diarrhea, and vomiting.

p., rheumatic. SYN: *Schonlein's p.; peliosis rheumatica.* P. with fever, swelling and severe rheumatic pains.

p., senile. In debilitated and aged persons; ecchymoses and petechiae on legs.

p., symptomatic. SYN: *secondary p.* P. which results from effects of various chemical, vegetable, animal, or physical agents, certain infectious diseases, or is a part of certain blood disorders.

p., thrombocytopenic. SEE: *p., idiopathic thrombocytopenic.*

purpuric (pūr-pū'rĭk) [L. *purpura,* purple]. Pert. to, resembling, or suffering from, purpura.

purpurin (pūr'pū-rĭn) [L. *purpura,* purple]. 1. An acid dye used to stain nuclei. 2. *Uroerythrin,* a red pigment sometimes present in urine.

purpurinuria (pūr"pū-rĭn-ū'rĭ-ă) [" + G *ouron,* urine]. Purpurin in urine. SYN: *porphyrinuria.*

purring thrill (pūr'ĭng). Thrill or vibration, like a cat's purring, due to mitral stenosis, aneurysm, or valvular erosion of the heart felt by palpation over the precordium.

purulence (pūr'ū-lĕns) [L. *purulentia.* a pus condition]. The state of containing pus. SYN: *suppuration.*

purulency (pūr'u-len-sĭ). Same as purulence.

purulent (pūr'ū-lĕnt) [L. *purulentia,* a pus condition]. Suppurative; forming or containing pus. SEE: *sputum.*

puruloid (pūr-ū'loyd) [L. *pus, pur-,* pus, + G. *eidos,* form]. Like pus. SYN: *puriform.*

pus (pus) [L.]. Liquid product of inflammation composed of albuminous substances, a thin fluid, and leukocytes or their remains, generally yellow in color.

If *red* it suggests rupture of small vessels. If *blue* or *green* it indicates presence of *Pseudomonas aeruginosa.*

ETIOL: Streptococci, staphylococci, gonococci, and pneumococci and other species of bacteria.

p. cells. Leukocytes, generally dead and showing degenerative changes. Found in suppurative inflammation.

p., cheesy. Very thick pus.

p., concrete. Fibropurulent coagula seen in infective endocarditis.

p., ichorous. P. that is thin with shreds of sloughing tissue. It may have a fetid odor.

p., sanious. Pus colored by blood.

p., serous. Pus mostly of thin serum containing flakes.

p. in urine. Condition when there are more than the normal number of pus or white blood cells in the urine. It may be due to cystitis, pyelitis, urethritis, tuberculosis of the kidney, or any infection of the genitourinary tract. May also be caused by trauma. SYN: *pyuria.*

Freshly passed urine may be cloudy due to presence of phosphates or pus. If the former, the addition of acid will cause it to clear; if pus is present it will not clear but may become gelatinous.

pus, *words pert. to:* apogenous, apyetous, apyous, archepyon, biocytoculture, burrowing, cell, clap threads, empyema, empyesis, pyemia, "pyo-" words, resorption, saprogenic, suppurate, suppuration.

pustulant (pŭs′tū-lănt) [L. *pustulāre*, to blister]. 1. Causing pustules. 2. Agent which produces the formation of pustules, such as croton oil and antimony; seldom used any more.

pustular (pŭs′tū-lĕr) [L. *pustulāre*, to blister]. Pert. to, or characterized by, pustules.

pustulation (pŭs-tū-lā′shŭn) [L. *pustulāre*, to blister]. The development of pustules.

pustule (pŭs′tūl) [L. *pustulāre*, to blister]. Small elevation of skin filled with lymph or pus.

Pustules may be circumscribed, flat, rounded or umbilicated. They occur in eczema pustulosum, acne vulgaris, dermatitis herpetiformis, impetigo simplex, ecthyma, varicella, syphilis, or in smallpox.

RS: *Chaussier's areola; pus; pustulant.*

p., malignant. Severe infectious disease with formation of hard pustule and symptoms of collapse. SYN: *anthrax, q.v.*

pustulocrustaceous (pŭs″tū-lō-krŭs-tā′-shŭs) [L. *pustulāre*, to blister, + *crusta*, a shell]. Characterized by formation of pustules and crusts.

pustulosis (pŭs-tū-lō′sĭs) [" + G. *-ōsis*, disease]. A generalized eruption of pustules.

putamen (pū-tā′mĕn) [L. shell]. BNA. The darker, outer layer of the lenticular nucleus.

putrefaction (pū″trē-făk′shŭn) [L. *putrefacere*, to putrefy]. Decomposition of animal matter, esp. protein, associated with malodorous and poisonous products, such as the ptomaines, mercaptans, and hydrogen sulfide, caused by certain kinds of bacteria and fungi.

Decomposition occurring spontaneously in sterile tissue after death is called autolysis. SEE: *intestinal putrefaction; sepsis.*

putrefactive (pū-trē-făk′tĭv) [L. *putrefacēre*, to putrefy]. 1. Causing, or pert. to, putrefaction. 2. Agent promoting putrefaction.

p. alkaloid. A ptomaine, a base formed by action of bacteria on an amino acid.

putrefy (pū′trĕ-fī) [L. *putrefacere*, to putrefy]. To undergo putrefaction.

putrescence (pū-trĕs′ĕns) [L. *putrescere*, to grow rotten]. Decay; rottenness.

putrid (pū′trĭd) [L. *putridus*, rotting]. Decayed; rotten; foul.

putrilage (pū′trĭl-āj) [L. *putrilāgō*, putrefaction]. Product of putrefaction.

pyarthrosis (pī-ar-thrō′sĭs) [G. *pyon*, pus, + *arthron*, joint]. Pus in the cavity of a joint.

pycnemia (pĭk-nē′mĭ-ă) [G. *pyknos*, thick, + *aima*, blood]. Thickening of the blood. SYN: *pyknemia.*

pycno- (pĭk′no) [G.]. Combining form meaning *dense, thick.* SEE: words beginning with *pykno-*.

pyecchysis (pī-ĕk′ĭs-ĭs) [G. *pyon*, pus, + *ek*, out, + *chein*, to pour]. An effusion of pus.

pyelectasia, pyelectasis (pī-ĕl-ĕk-tā′zĭ-ă, -ek′tăs-ĭs) [G. *pyelos*, pelvis, + *ektasis*, dilatation]. Dilatation of the renal pelvis.

pyelitic (pī-ĕ-lĭt′ĭk). Relating to or affected with pyelitis.

pyelitis (pī-ĕl-ī′tĭs) [" + *-ītis*, inflammation]. Inflammation of the kidney pelvis and its calices.

p., calculous. P. resulting from a calculus.

pyelo- [G.]. Combining form meaning the *pelvis.*

pyelocystitis (pī″ĕl-ō-sĭs-tī′tĭs) [G. *pyelos*, pelvis, + *kystis*, bladder, + *-ītis*, inflammation]. Inflamed condition of the kidney, pelvis and bladder.

pyelocystostomosis (pī″ĕl-ō-sĭs″tō-sto-mō′-sĭs) [" + " + *stoma*, mouth, + *-ōsis*]. Establishment of surgical communication between the kidney and the bladder.

pyelogram, pyelograph (pī′ĕl-ō-grăm, -grăf) [" + *gramma*, a mark]. A roentgen picture of the ureter and renal pelvis.

pyelography (pī-ĕ-lŏg′ră-fī) [" + *graphein*, to write]. X-ray examination of a renal pelvis and ureter.

pyelolithotomy (pī″ĕl-ō-lĭth-ŏt′ō-mĭ) [" + *lithos*, stone, + *tomē*, incision]. Removal of calculus from the pelvis of a kidney through an incision.

pyelometer (pī-ĕl-ŏm′ĕt-ĕr) [" + *metron*, a measure]. Device to measure the pelvic diameters. SYN: *pelvimeter.*

pyelometry (pī-ĕl-ŏm′ĕ-trĭ) [" + *metron*, a measure]. 1. Measurement of the kidney's pelvis. 2. Measurement of the diameters of the pelvis. SYN: *pelvimetry.*

pyelonephritis (pī″ĕl-ō-nef-rī′tĭs) [G. *pyelos*, pelvis, + *nephros*, kidney, + *-itis*, inflammation]. Inflammation of kidney substance and pelvis.

ETIOL: Bacterial, metastatic or urogenous (ascending from bladder).

SYM: Pain in the loins, vesical irritability, swelling, chills and fever, urine cloudy and decreased in amount with increased frequency in acute p., increased in amount in chronic p. and pyelonephritis; albumin and sediment with pus cells, bacteria, and fatty or hyaline casts, and sometimes red blood corpuscles.

PROG: Depends upon character and virulence of infection, accessory etiological factors, drainage of kidney, presence or absence of complications, and general physical condition.

TREATMENT: Recognition and removal of cause (focal infection, etc.), measures to increase resistance of patient, bed rest, avoidance of drugs irritating to kidney, condiments, and alcohol. Hot water bag, antipyretic drugs, urinary antisepsis. Surgery if necessary (nephrotomy, nephrectomy, pyelotomy). If both kidneys and pelvis are affected, urine generally is acid, and pus in form of slugs or balls passes in the urine.

pyelonephrosis (pī″ĕl-ō-nef-rō′sĭs) [" + " + *-ōsis*, disease]. Disease of the pelvis of the kidney.

pyelopathy (pī-ĕl-ŏp′ăth-ĭ) [" + *pathos*, disease]. Any disease of the pelvis of the kidney. SYN: *pyelonephrosis.*

pyeloplasty (pī′ĕl-ō-plăs″tĭ) [" + *plastos*, formed]. Reparative operation on the kidney pelvis.

pyeloplication (pī″ĕl-ō-plĭ-kā′shŭn) [" + L. *plicāre*, to fold]. Shortening of the wall of a dilated renal pelvis by taking tucks in it.

pyeloscopy (pī-ĕl-ŏs′kō-pĭ) [" + *skopein*, to examine]. Examination of the pelvis of the kidney using an x-ray.

pyelostomy (pī-ĕl-ŏs′tō-mĭ) [" + *stoma*,

mouth]. Creation of an opening into the renal pelvis.

pyelotomy (pī-ĕl-ŏt′ō-mĭ) [G. *pyelos*, pelvis, + *tomē*, incision]. Incision of renal pelvis.

NP: Keep patient dry, watch skin for decubitus. If retention catheter present, keep draining at all times. Accurate record of intake and output of urine.

pyelovenous backflow (pī-ĕl-ō-vē′nŭs) [" + L. *vena*, vein]. Drainage from the renal pelvis into the venous system because of back pressure.

pyemesis (pī-ĕm′ĭs-ĭs) [G. *pyon*, pus, + *emesis*, vomiting]. The vomiting of pus.

pyemia (pī-ē′mĭ-ă) [G. *pyon*, pus, + *aima*, blood]. A form of septicemia due to presence of pus-forming organisms in the blood, manifested by formation of multiple abscesses of a metastatic nature.

Sym: High intermittent temperature with recurrent chills; sweetish odor to breath. Metastatic processes in various parts of the body, especially in lungs. Septic pneumonia, empyema. Results may be fatal.

Treatment: Antibiotics. Prophylactic treatment consists in prevention of suppuration. When possible all metastatic abscesses or suppurating joints should be laid open and thoroughly disinfected. Internal remedies. Easily digested food given unsparingly.

p., arterial. P. resulting from dissemination of emboli from a thrombus in cardiac vessels.

p., cryptogenic. P., the focus of which is hidden in the deeper tissues.

p., metastatic. Multiple abscess resulting from infected pyemic thrombi.

p., portal. Suppurative inflammation of portal vein.

pyemic (pī-ē′mĭk) [G. *pyon*, pus, + *aima*, blood]. Relating to or affected with blood poisoning.

pyencephalus (pī-en-sef′al-us) [" + *egkephalos*, brain]. A brain abscess with suppuration within the cranium. Syn: *pyocephalus.*

pyesis (pī-ē′sĭs) [G. *pyon*, pus]. The formation of pus. Syn: *suppuration.*

pygal (pī′găl) [G. *pygē*, rump]. Concerning the buttocks.

pygalgia (pī-găl′jĭ-ă) [" + *algos*, pain]. Pain in the rump or buttocks.

pygmalionism (pĭg′mā-lĭ-ŏn-ĭzm) [Pygmalion, a sculptor and king, in Greek mythology, who fell in love with a figure he had carved]. Psychopathic condition in which a person is in love with a creation of his own.

pygo- [G.]. Combining form meaning the *rump.*

pyin (pī′ĭn) [G. *pyon*, pus]. A substance of albuminous nature sometimes present in pus.

pyknic type (pĭk′nĭk) [G. *pyknos*, thick]. One with broad head, thick shoulders, large chest, short neck and stocky body.

They are often happy, carefree persons whose emotional reactions are obvious. They are interested in others apart from themselves. They are extroverts. See: *asthenic body type.*

pykno-. Combining form meaning *thick, compact, dense, frequent.* See also words beginning with *pycno.*

pyknocardia (pĭk-nō-kar′dĭ-ă) [" + *kardia*, heart]. Rapid pulse. Syn: *tachycardia.*

pyknohemia (pĭk-nō-hē′mĭ-ă) [" + *aima*, blood]. Thickening of the blood. Syn: *pyknemia.*

pyknolepsy (pĭk-nō-lĕp′sĭ) [" + *lēpsis*, seizure]. Attacks similar to petit mal or minor epileptic seizures, usually occurring in childhood.

pyknometer (pĭk-nŏm′ĕt-ĕr) [" + *metron*, measure]. Device for determining specific gravity of liquids.

pyknomorphous (pĭk″nō-morf′ŭs) [" + *morphē*, form]. Characterized by compact arrangement of the stainable portions, said esp. of certain nerve cells.

pyknophrasia (pĭk″nō-frā′zĭ-ă) [" + *phrasis*, speech]. Thickness of words uttered in speech.

pyknosis (pĭk-nō′sĭs) [" + *-ōsis*, intensive]. Inspissation; thickness, esp. shrinking of cells through degeneration. See: *pycnosis.*

pyle- (pi′le) [G. *pyle*, gate]. Combining form meaning *orifice*, especially that of the portal vein.

pylemphraxis (pī-lĕm-frăk′sĭs) [G. *pylē*, gate, + *emphraxis*, stoppage]. Occlusion of the portal vein.

pylephlebectasia, pylephlebectasis (pī-le-flē-bĕk-tā′zĭ-ă, -bĕk′tă-sĭs) [" + *phleps, phleb-*, vein, + *ektasis*, dilatation]. Distention of the portal vein.

pylephlebitis (pī-le-flē-bī′tĭs) [" + " + *-itis*, inflammation]. Inflamed condition of the portal vein, generally suppurative.

p., adhesive. Thrombosis of the portal vein.

p. obturans. P. with obstructed flow in the portal vein.

pylethrombosis (pī-le-thrŏm-bō′sĭs) [" + *thrombos*, a clot, + *-ōsis*, intensive]. Occlusion of portal vein by a thrombus.

pylometer (pī-lŏm′ĕt-ĕr) [" + *metron*, a measure]. Device for measuring obstructions at vesical opening.

pyloralgia (pī″lō-răl′jĭ-ă) [G. *pylōros*, gatekeeper, + *algos*, pain]. Pain around the pylorus.

pylorectomy (pī-lō-rĕk′tō-mĭ) [" + *ektomē*, excision]. Surgical removal of the pylorus.

pyloric (pī-lor′ĭk) [G. *pylōros*, gatekeeper]. Pert. to the opening bet. the stomach and duodenum.

p. antrum. Syn: *p. vestibule; p. sinus.* The first part of the pyloric portion of the stomach; portion leading to pyloric canal.

p. canal. The narrow constricted region of pyloric portion of stomach which opens through pylorus into duodenum.

p. gland. A gland of the stomach near the pylorus.

p. orifice. Opening or passage bet. the stomach and duodenum.

p. stenosis. Narrowing of the pyloric orifice. Also due to excessive thickening of circular muscle of pylorus (*hypertrophic pyloric stenosis*), or hypertrophy and hyperplasia of mucosa and submucosa.

pyloristenosis (pī″lō-rĭ-stĕn-ō′sĭs) [" + *stenōsis*, a narrowing]. Constriction of the pylorus.

pyloritis (pī-lō-rī′tĭs) [" + *-itis*, inflammation]. Inflamed condition of the pylorus.

pyloro- [G.]. Combining form meaning *gatekeeper;* applied to the *pylorus.*

pyloroduodenitis (pī″lor-ō-dū″ō-dē-nī′tĭs) [G. *pylōros,* gatekeeper, + L. *duodeni,* twelve, + G. *-ītis,* inflammation]. Inflammation of the mucosa of the pylorus and duodenum.

pylorogastrectomy (pī-lō″rō-găs-trĕk′tō-mĭ) [" + *gastēr,* belly, + *ektomē,* excision]. Excision of pyloric portion of the stomach.

pyloromyotomy (pī-lō″rō-mī-ŏt′ō-mĭ) [" + *mys, my-,* muscle, + *tomē,* a cutting]. Incision and suture of the pyloric sphincter.

pyloroplasty (pī-lor′ō-plăs″tĭ) [" + *plassein,* to form]. Operation to repair the pylorus, esp. one to increase the caliber of the pyloric opening by stretching.

pyloroptosia, pyloroptosis (pī-lo″rŏp-tō′-sĭ-ă, -rŏp′tō-sĭs) [" + *ptōsis,* a dropping]. Displacement downward of the pyloric end of the stomach.

pyloroschesis (pī′lor-o-shē′sĭs). Obstruction of pyloric orifice.

pyloroscopy (pī-lō-rŏs′kō-pĭ) [" + *skopein,* to examine]. Fluoroscopic examination of the pylorus.

pylorospasm (pī-lō′rō-spăzm) [" + *spasmos,* a spasm]. Spasmodic contraction of the pyloric orifice. Usually due to a disturbance in motor mechanism of pylorus. May occur secondary to lesions of stomach and duodenum near to pylorus.

pylorostenosis (pī-lō″rō-stĕn-ō′sĭs) [G. *pyloros,* gatekeeper, + *stenosis,* narrowing]. Abnormal narrowing or stricture of the pyloric orifice. SEE: *pyloric stenosis.*

pylorostomy (pī-lor-ŏs′tō-mĭ) [G. *pylōros,* gatekeeper, + *stoma,* opening]. Formation of an opening through the abdominal wall into the pylorus.

pylorotomy (pī-lor-ŏt′ō-mĭ) [" + *tomē,* a cutting]. Incision of the pyloric submucosa to relieve hypertrophic stenosis.

pylorus (pī-lōr′ŭs) [G. *pylōros,* gatekeeper]. The lower orifice of the stomach opening into the duodenum. The pylorus is closed most of the time but opens at intervals permitting acid chyme to enter duodenum. The primary factor in the opening of pylorus is elevation of gastric pressure over duodenal pressure.

p., spasm of. Same as *pylorospasm, q.v.*

pyo-, py- [G.]. Combining forms meaning *pus.*

pyocele (pī′ō-sēl) [G. *pyon,* pus, + *kēlē,* hernia]. A hernia or distended cavity containing pus.

pyocelia (pī-ō-sē′lĭ-ă) [" + *koilia,* cavity]. Pus formation in the abdominal cavity.

pyocephalus (pī″ō-sĕf′ă-lŭs) [" + *kephalē,* head]. Effusion of purulent nature within the cranium.

p., circumscribed. Abscess of the brain.

p., external. Suppuration of the meninges.

p., internal. Pus in the cerebrospinal fluid.

pyochezia (pī″ō-kē′zĭ-ă) [" + *chezein,* to defecate]. Pus in the feces.

pyococcus (pī″ō-kŏk′ŭs) [" + *kokkos,* berry]. A micrococcus which causes suppuration, as the *Streptococcus pyogenes.*

pyocolpocele (pī-ō-kŏl′pō-sēl) [" + *kolpos,* vagina, + *kēlē,* mass]. A vaginal tumor containing pus. SEE: *pyocolpos.*

pyocol′pos [" + *kolpos,* vagina]. Accumulation of pus in the vagina.

pyoculture (pī′ō-kŭl-chūr) [G. *pyon,* pus, + L. *cultura,* growth]. Comparative tests for cultivation of pus from a wound, a portion being left in the collecting tube and a portion being cultivated on bouillon.

If the test is positive, it indicates a struggle bet. the bacteria and the body forces which need therapeutic assistance.

pyocyanase (pī″ō-sī′ă-nāze). An antibiotic obtained from *Pseudomonas aeruginosa.* Active principally against gram-positive organisms on which it has a lytic action.

pyocyanic (pī″ō-sī-ăn′ĭk) [G. *pyon,* pus, + *kyanos,* dark blue]. Pert. to pyocyanin or blue pus.

pyocyanin (pī-ō-sī′ă-nĭn). An antibiotic obtained from *Pseudomonas aeruginosa,* effective principally against gram-positive organisms.

pyocyst (pī′ō-sĭst) [" + *kystis,* sac]. A cyst holding pus.

pyoderma (pī-ō-der′mă) [G. *pyon,* pus, + *derma,* skin]. Any acute inflammatory skin disease caused by pus-forming bacteria.

p. faciale. P. of the face characterized by erythema (red or cyanotic) and deep abscesses.

p. gangrenosum. P. usually associated with ulcerative colitis. Occurs principally on the trunk.

pyodermatitis (pī″ō-dŭr-mă-tī′tĭs) [" + *derma,* skin, + *-ītis,* inflammation]. Pyogenic infection of the skin causing a dermatitis.

pyodermatosis (pī″ō-dĕr-mă-tō′sĭs) [" + " + *-ōsis,* condition]. Any skin condition of pyogenic origin. SYN: *pyodermia.*

pyodermia (pī″ō-der′mĭ-ă) [" + *derma,* skin]. Any suppurative skin disease.

pyofecia (pī″ō-fē′sĭ-ă) [" + L. *faeces,* feces]. Pus in the stools.

pyogenesis (pī″ō-jĕn′ĕs-ĭs) [G. *pyon,* pus, + *genesis,* formation]. The formation of pus.

pyogenic (pī-ō-jĕn′ĭk) [" + *gennan,* to produce]. Producing pus.

p. microorganisms. M. forming pus. The principal ones are *Staphylococcus aureus, S. albus, Streptococcus hemolyticus, Bacillus anthracis, B. subtilis, Clostridium perfringens, Pseudomonas aeruginosa,* and *Neisseria gonorrhoeae.*

pyohemothorax (pī″ō-hĕm-ō-thō′răks) [" + " + *thōrax,* chest]. Pus and blood in the pleural cavity.

pyoid (pī′oyd) [" + *eidos,* like]. Resembling pus.

pyolabyrinthitis (pī″ō-lăb-ĭ-rĭn-thī′tĭs) [" + *labyrinthos,* a maze, + *-ītis,* inflammation]. Inflammation with suppuration of the labyrinth of the ear.

pyometra (pī-ō-mē′tră) [G. *pyon,* pus, + *mētra,* uterus]. Retained pus accumulation in the uterine cavity.

pyometritis (pī″ō-mē-trī′tĭs) [" + " + *-ītis,* inflammation]. Purulent inflammation of the uterus.

pyonephritis (pī″ō-nef-rī′tĭs) [" + *nephros,* kidney, + *-ītis,* inflammation]. Inflammation of the kidney, suppurative in character.

pyonephrolithiasis (pī″ō-nef-rō-lĭth-ī′ăs-ĭs) [" + " + *lithos,* stone]. Pus and calculi formation in the kidney.

pyonephrosis (pī″ō-nef-rō′sĭs) [" + " + *-ōsis,* condition]. Pus accumulation in the pelvis of kidney.

pyo-ovarium (pī″ō-ō-vā′rĭ-ŭm) [G. *pyon*, pus, + L. *ovarium*, ovary]. Abscess formation in an ovary.

pyopericarditis (pī″ō-pĕr-ĭ-kar-dī′tĭs) [" + *peri*, around, + *kardia*, heart, + *-itis*, inflammation]. Pericarditis with suppuration.

pyopericardium (pī″ō-pĕr-ĭ-kar′dĭ-ŭm) [" + " + " *kardia*, heart]. Pus formation in the pericardium.

pyoperitoneum (pī″ō-pĕr-ĭ-tō-nē′ŭm) [" + *peritonaion*, peritoneum]. Pus formation in the peritoneal cavity.

pyoperitonitis (pī″ō-pĕr-ĭ-tō-nī′tĭs) [" + " + *-itis*, inflammation]. Purulent inflammation of the lining of peritoneum.

pyophagia (pī″ō-fā′jĭ-ă) [" + *phagein*, to eat]. Swallowing of purulent substance.

pyophthalmia, pyophthalmitis (pī″ŏf-thăl′mĭ-ă, -thăl-mī′tĭs) [" + *ophthalmos*, eye, + *-itis*, inflammation]. Suppurative inflamed condition of the eye.

pyophylactic (pī″ō-fī-lăk′tĭk) [G. *pyon*, pus, + *phylaxis*, protection]. Guarding against formation of pus.

p. membrane. Lining membrane of an abscess cavity separating it from healthy tissue.

pyophysometra (pī″ō-fī-sō-mē′tră) [" + *physa*, air, + *mētra*, uterus]. Pus and gas accumulation in the uterus.

pyoplania (pī″ō-plā′nĭ-ă) [" + *planos*, wandering]. Spreading of pus by infiltration into tissue.

pyopneumocholecystitis (pī″ō-nū″mō-kō-lē-sĭs-tī′tĭs) [" + *pneuma*, air, + *cholē*, bile, + *kystis*, sac, + *-itis*, inflammation]. Distention of the gallbladder with air and pus.

pyopneumocyst (pī″ō-nū′mō-sĭst) [" + " + *kystis*, a bladder]. A cyst enclosing pus and gas.

pyopneumopericardium (pī″ō-nū″mō-pĕr-ĭ-kar′dĭ-ŭm) [" + " + *peri*, around, + *kardia*, heart]. Pus and air or gas in pericardium.

pyopneumoperitonitis (pī″ō-nū″mō-pĕr-ĭ-tō-nī′tĭs) [" + " + *peritonaion*, peritoneum]. Pus and air in the peritoneal cavity complicating peritonitis.

pyopoiesis (pī″ō-poy-ē′sĭs) [G. *pyon*, pus, + *poiein*, to make]. Formation of pus. SYN: *pyogenesis; suppuration.*

pyopoietic (pī″ō-poy-ĕt′ĭk) [G. *pyon*, pus, + *poiein*, to make]. SYN: *suppurative.* Pert. to formation of pus.

pyoptysis (pī-ŏp′tĭs-ĭs) [" + *ptyein*, to spit]. Spitting of pus.

pyorrhagia (pī-or-ā′jĭ-ă) [" + *rēgnunai*, to burst forth]. Profuse flow of pus, as when an abscess ruptures.

pyorrhea (pī-ō-rē′ă) [" + *roia*, a flow]. A discharge of purulent matter.

p. alveolaris. SYN: *periodontoclasia; periodontosis; Riggs' disease.* A periodontal disease characterized by inflammatory or degenerative changes of the periosteum, alveolar bone, and tooth cementum. Resorption of alveolar bone occurs, resulting in loosening of teeth and recession of gums.

pyosalpingitis (pī″ō-săl-pĭn-jī′tĭs) [G. *pyon*, pus, + *salpigx*, tube, + *-itis*, inflammation]. Retained pus in the oviduct with inflammation.

pyosalpingo-oophoritis (pī″ō-săl-pĭn″gō-ō-ŏf-ō-rī′tĭs) [" + " + *ōon*, ovum, + *phoros*, a bearer, + *-itis*, inflammation]. Inflammation of ovary and oviduct with suppuration.

pyosalpinx (pī″ō-săl′pĭnks) [" + *salpigx*, tube]. Pus in the fallopian tube. SEE: *pyosalpingitis.*

pyosis (pī-ō′sĭs) [" + *-ōsis*, intensive]. Formation of pus. SYN: *suppuration.*

pyospermia (pī″ō-spĕr′mĭ-ă) [" + *sperma*, seed]. Pus in the semen.

pyostatic (pī″ō-stăt′ĭk) [" + *statikos*, standing]. 1. Agent checking the development of pus. 2. Preventing pus formation.

pyotherapy (pī″ō-thĕr′ă-pĭ) [" + *therapeia*, treatment]. Treatment of disease with pus.

pyothorax (pī″ō-thō′răks) [" + *thōrax*, chest]. Pus in the pleural cavity. SYN: *empyema.*

pyotorrhea (pī″ō-tor-ē′ă) [" + *ous*, *ot-*, ear, + *roia*, flow]. Purulent discharge from the ear.

pyotoxinemia (pī″ō-tŏk-sĭ-nē′mĭ-ă) [G. *pyon*, pus, + *toxikon*, poison, + *aima*, blood]. Infection from toxic products of pus organisms in the blood.

pyoturia (pī″ō-tū′rĭ-ă) [" + *ouron*, urine]. Pus cells in the urine. SYN: *pyuria.*

pyourachus (pī″ō-ū′ră-kŭs) [" + *ourachos*, fetal urinary canal]. Accumulation of pus in the urachus.

pyoureter (pī″ō-ūr′ĕt-ĕr, -ū-rē′tĕr) [" + *ourēter*, ureter]. Pus collection in a ureter.

pyovesiculosis (pī″ō-vĕs-ĭk-ū-lō′sĭs) [" + L. *vesiculus*, a small vessel, + G. *-ōsis*, condition]. Pus collection in the seminal vesicles.

pyoxanthin (pī″ō-zăn′thĭn). A yellow pigment resulting from oxidation of pyocyanin. Sometimes present in pus.

pyramid (pĭr′ăm-ĭd) [G. *pyramis*, a pyramid]. 1. A solid on a base with 3 or more sides, the triangular planes of which meet at an apex. 2. Any part of the body resembling a pyramid. 3. A compact bundle of nerve fibers in the medulla oblongata. 4. Petrous portion of temporal bone.

p. of cerebellum. A median ventral projection of vermis of cerebellum lying between tuber and uvula.

p., malpighian. A renal pyramid, *q.v.*

p. of the medulla. A pair of elongated tapering prominences on ant. surface of medulla oblongata, composed of descending corticospinal fibers.

p., renal. SYN: *p. of Malpighi; malpighian p.* One of number 8-18 of cone-shaped structures comprising medulla of the kidney. Their apices (*papillae*) bear openings of papillary ducts through which urine enters renal pelvis.

p. of the thyroid. SYN: *pyramidal or median lobe.* A conical process sometimes present extending cephalad from the isthmus of the thyroid gland.

p. of temporal bone. The pyramis or petrous portion.

p. of the tympanum. SYN: *pyramidal eminence.* A hollow projection on inner wall of the tympanum through which passes the stapedius muscle.

pyramidal (pĭ-răm′ĭd-ăl) [G. *pyramis*, *pyramid-*, pyramid]. In the shape of a pyramid.

p. cell. Pyramid-shaped cell of cerebral cortex.

p. tract. SYN: *cortispinal tract.* One of three descending tracts (lateral, ventral, ventrolateral) of the spinal cord. Consists of fibers arising from giant pyramidal cells of Betz present in motor area of cerebral cortex.

pyramidalis (pĭ-răm-id-al'ĭs) [G. *pyramis,* pyramid). The muscle which arises from the crest of the pubis and is inserted into the linea alba upward about half way to the navel.

p. auriculae. Small muscle inserted into auricle of ear. Often absent.

p. nasi. SYN: *procerus muscle.* Small muscle overlying nasal bone. Inserted into skin at root of nose.

pyramidon (pĭ-răm'ĭd-ŏn). Proprietary preparation of amidopyrine; a yellowish-white powder.

USES: As an antipyretic.

pyram'in. 2-methyl-4-amino-5-hydroxymethylpyrimidine, a product of thiamine metabolism and excreted in urine in cases of excess dosage of thiamine.

pyran (pi'ran). C_5H_6O, a heterocyclic compound to which certain sugars are related.

pyrectic (pī-rĕk'tĭk) [G. *pyrektikos*]. Feverish. SYN: *pyretic.*

pyrenemia (pī-rē-nē'mĭ-ă) [G. *pyrēn,* fruit stone, *aima,* blood]. Condition in which there are nucleated red cells in the blood.

pyrenin (pī-rē'nĭn) [G. *pyrēn,* fruit stone]. The oxyphilic substance found in a nucleolus.

pyrenoid (pī'rē-noyd) [" + *eidos,* like]. A colorless, highly refractive body in certain protozoan chromatophores.

pyretherapy (pī-rē-thĕr'ă-pĭ) [G. *pyr,* fever, + *therapeia,* treatment]. Artificial fever treatment.

pyrethrins (pi-re'thrinz). General name of substances derived from certain flowers. Used as insecticides.

pyretic (pī-rĕt'ĭk) [G. *pyretos,* fever]. Concerning fever.

p. therapy. Treatment of disease by artificial induction of fever, either by heat or the inoculation of malarial organisms.

pyreticosis (pī-rĕt-ĭ-kō'sĭs) [" + *-ōsis,* intensive]. Feverishness.

pyreto- (pi-ret'o) [G.]. Prefix meaning *fever.*

pyretogen (pī-rĕt'ō-jĕn) [G. *pyretos,* fever, + *gennan,* to produce]. A substance producing fever.

pyretogenesia, pyretogenesis (pī"rĕt-ō-jĕn-ē'zĭ-ă, -jĕn'ĕs-ĭs) [" + *genesis,* production]. Origin and production of fever.

pyretogenic, pyretogenous (pī"ret-ō-jĕn'ĭk, -ŏj'ĕn-ŭs) [" + *gennan,* to produce]. Producing or causing fever.

p. bacteria. Pathogenic bacteria causing fever.

p. stage. Period in a fever when it is rising slowly.

pyretography (pī-rĕt-ŏg'ră-fĭ) [" + *graphein,* to write]. A treatise on fever.

pyretology (pī-rĕt-ŏl'ō-jĭ) [" + *logos,* a study]. Science of fevers and their characteristics.

pyretolysis (pī-rĕt-ŏl'ĭs-ĭs) [" + *lysis,* a disintegration]. 1. Reduction of fever. 2. Hastening of lysis by elevation of temperature.

pyretotherapy (pī"rē-tō-thĕr'ă-pĭ) [" + *therapeia,* treatment]. 1. Treatment by artificially raising the patient's temperature. 2. Treatment of fever.

pyretotyphosis (pī-rĕt-ō-tī-fō'sĭs) [" + *typhōsis,* delirium]. The delirious or stuporous symptom of fever.

pyrexia (pī-rĕk'sĭ-ă) [G. *pyressein,* to be feverish]. Condition in which the temperature is above normal. SYN: *fever.*

Some classify it as:

Low	99°—101° F.
Moderate	101°—103° F.
High	103°—105° F.

p., local. Acute inflammation of a part.

pyrexial (pī-rĕks'ĭ-ăl) [G. *pyressein,* to be feverish]. Concerning fever.

pyrexin (pī'rĕks'ĭn). A substance extracted from inflammatory exudates which induces fever.

3-pyridinecarboxylic acid (pĭr"ĭd-ēn-kar"-bŏk-sĭl'ĭk). Organic substance obtained by oxidizing nicotine. SYN: *nicotinic acid.* SEE: *pellagra.*

pyridoxal (pĭr"ĭ-dŏks'ăl). One of the vitamin B_6 group; an analog of pyridoxine.

p. phosphate. A derivative of pyridoxine which serves as a coenzyme of certain amino-acid decarboxylases in bacteria and, in animal tissues, of dioxyphenylalanine (DOPA) decarboxylase.

pyridoxamine (pĭr"ĭ-dŏks'ă-mīn). One of the vitamin B_6 group; a 4-aminoethyl analog of pyridoxine.

pyridoxic acid (pĭr"ĭ-dŏks'ĭk). The principal end product of pyridoxine metabolism which is excreted in urine of humans.

pyridoxine (pĭ-rĭ-dŏks'ēn). SYN: *eluate factor, rat acrodynia factor, adermin.* One of the vitamin B_6 group of the B complex. Term used as a synonym of vitamin B_6. Its role in human nutrition has not been established but in rats and bacteria it is a growth factor. Deficiency in rats causes acrodynia and dermatitis. Called *antidermatitis vitamin.*

pyriform (pĭr'ĭ-form) [L. *pyrum,* pear, + *forma,* shape]. Shaped like a pear.

pyrimidine (pĭ-rĭm'ĭd-ēn). The parent of a group of heterocyclic nitrogen compounds. $C_4H_4N_2$, including uracil, cytosine, and thymine, some of which are components of nucleic acid.

pyrithiamine (pĭr"ĭ-thī'ă-mēn). A synthetic analog of thiamine acts as an antithiamine substance. When administered, it produces many of the symptoms of thiamine deficiency.

pyro- (pi'ro) [G.]. Prefix meaning *heat* or *fire.*

pyrocatechin (pī"rō-kăt'ĕ-kin). Pyrocatechol, *q.v.*

pyrocatechinuria (pī"rō-kăt-ĕ-kĭn-ū'rĭ-ă) [G. *pyr,* fire, + *catechin,* + G. *ouron,* urine]. Pyrocatechin in the urine.

pyrocatechol (pī"rō-kat'ĕ-kōl). A crystalline substance, $C_6H_4(OH)_2$, obtained from catechu. An astringent and antiseptic. Sometimes found in urine. Also called *catechol.*

pyrogallol, pyrogallic acid (pī"rō-găl'ŏl, -ĭk). USP. A poisonous substance obtained by the decomposition of gallic acid. $C_6H_3(OH)_3$.

USES: Topically in skin diseases, as psoriasis, although an active irritant and internally a poison.

pyrogen (pī"rō-jĕn) [G. *pyr,* fire, + *gennan,* to produce]. A substance of unknown nature, but probably protein, found in distilled water used in preparation of blood substitutes and responsible for rise of temperature sometimes following blood transfusions or other fluids given intravenously. It stimulates the hypothalamus into action in the heat-regulation center.

NP: Do not give fluids intravenously which have been previously opened and allowed to stand even though the top may have been closed tightly.

pyrogenic (pī″rō-jĕn′ĭk) [G. *pyr*, fire, + *gennan*, to produce]. Producing fever.

pyrolagnia (pī″rō-lăg′nĭ-ă) [" + *lagneia*, lust]. Insane desire to see or produce fires; accompanied by sexual gratification.

pyrolysis (pī-rŏl′ĭs-ĭs) [" + *lysis*, dissolution]. Disintegration of organic matter when there is a rise in temperature.

pyromania (pī″rō-mā′nĭ-ă) [" + *mania*, madness]. Fire madness; mania for setting fires or seeing them.

pyrometer (pī-rŏm′ĕt-ĕr) [" + *metron*, measure]. Device for measuring extreme degrees of heat.

pyronyxis (pī-rō-nĭks′ĭs) [" + *nyxis*, a piercing]. Treatment or cauterization by puncturing a part with hot needles. SYN: *ignipuncture*.

pyrophobia (pī-rō-fō′bĭ-ă) [" + *phobos*, fear]. Abnormal fear of fire.

pyroptothymia (pī-rŏp-tō-thī′mĭ-ă) [G. *pyr*, fire, + *ptoein*, to scare, + *thymos*, mind]. A psychosis in which one imagines himself surrounded by flames.

pyropuncture (pī″rō-pŭnk′chūr) [" + L. *punctūre*, a piercing]. Treatment by puncture of a part with hot needles. SYN: *pyronyxis*.

pyrosis (pī-rō′sĭs) [G. *pyrōsis*, burning]. A burning sensation in the epigastric and sternal region, with raising of acid liquid from stomach. SYN: *heartburn; waterbrash*.

NP: Note whether it occurs before or after food is taken, the time and duration, and whether different foods give rise to it. SEE: *taste*.

pyrotic (pī-rŏt′ĭk) [G. *pyrōsis*, burning]. 1. Caustic. 2. Pert. to pyrosis.

pyrotoxin (pī-rō-tŏks′ĭn) [G. *pyr*, fire, + *toxikon*, poison]. A toxin generated by a febrile process.

pyroxylin (pī-rŏk′sĭl-ĭn) [" + *xylon*, wood] (soluble gun cotton). A product obtained by the action of a mixture of nitric and sulfuric acids on cellulose.

USES: In the preparation of collodion.

INCOMPATIBILITIES: Sulfides, alkalies.

pyrrol cells. SYN: *histiocytes*. Cells of the reticuloendothelial system so called because of their ability to ingest colloidal dyes (pyrrol blue).

pyrollic amino acids. Proline and oxyproline.

pyruvate (pi-roo′vāt). A salt or ester of pyruvic acid.

pyruvic acid (pi-roo′vik). $CH_3CO.COOH$, an organic acid which plays an important role in Krebs cycle, it being an intermediate product in the metabolism of carbohydrates, fats, and amino acids. It increases in quantity in the blood and tissues in thiamine deficiency, thiamine being essential for its oxidation.

pyuria (pī-ū′rĭ-ă) [G. *pyon*, pus, + *ouron*, urine]. Pus in the urine; evidence of renal disease.

ETIOL: Lesion of urethra, ureters, bladder, kidneys, infection.

RS: *cystitis, kidney, pyelitis, ureteritis, urethritis*.

PZI. Abbr. for *protamine zinc insulin*.

Notes

Notes

Notes

Notes

Notes

Notes

Q

Q. 1. Abbr. for *electric quantity; quart.* 2. Symb. for *coulomb.*

Q_{CO_2}. Number of microliters of CO_2 given off per milligram of dry weight of tissue per hour.

Q_{O_2}. Number of microliters of O_2 taken up per milligram of dry weight of tissue per hour.

q. d. Abbr. for L. *quaque die,* every day.

Q disk. SYN: *Q band, Q stripe, A disk.* A dark, doubly refractile, anisotropic band of a striated muscle myofibril.

Q fever. SYN: *Nine-mile fever, quadrilateral fever.* An acute infectious disease characterized by headache, fever, malaise, myalgia, and anorexia. Caused by *Coxiella burnetii.* Contracted by inhaling infected dusts, drinking unpasteurized milk from infected animals, or by handling infected animals such as goats, cows, or sheep. An effective vaccine is available for prevention of infection.

q. h. Abbr. for L. *quaque hora,* every hour.

q. i. d. Abbr. for *quater in die,* four times a day.

q. l. Abbr. for *quantum libet,* as much as one pleases.

Q law. As temperature decreases, chemical activity decreases. A principle used in treatment of gastric ulcers. 50° F. for 48 hrs. stops bleeding and secretion of acid.

q. m. Abbr. 'for L. *quaque matin,* every morning.

q. n. Abbr. for L. *quaque nox,* every night.

QRS complex. The Q, R, and S waves or deflections of an electrocardiogram produced during the transmission of the excitation wave through the conductile tissue of the heart. Normal duration is 0.06-0.08 sec.

QRST complex. The Q, R, S, and T waves of an electrocardiogram. Duration is approximately same as that of mechanical systole. Also called *ventricular complex.*

q. s. Abbr. for *quantum sufficit,* as much as necessary.

qt. Abbr. for *quart.*

Q wave. A downward or negative wave of an electrocardiogram following the P wave. It is usually not prominent and may be absent without significance.

quack (kwăk) [Dutch *kwaksalven,* to peddle salve]. One who pretends to have knowledge or skill in medicine. SYN: *charlatan.*

quackery (kwăk'ĕr-ĭ) [Dutch *kwaksalven,* to peddle salve]. The practice or pretensions of a quack. SYN: *charlatanry.*

quadrangular (kwŏd-răng'ū-lĕr) [L. *quadri,* four, + *angulus,* angle]. Having four angles and four sides.

q. lobe. A region forming sup. portion of each cerebellar hemisphere.

q. membrane. The upper portion of the elastic membrane of the larynx. Extends from aryepiglottic folds above to level of ventricular folds below.

quadrant (kwŏd'rănt) [L. *quadrans,* a fourth]. 1. The 4th of a circle. 2. One of four corresponding regions, as of the abdomen, divided for descriptive and diagnostic purposes.

quadrantanopsia (kwŏd-rănt-ăn-ŏp'sĭ-ă) [" + G. *an-,* negative, + *opsis,* vision]. Loss of sight in approximately one fourth of the visual field.

quadrate (kwŏd'rāt) [L. *quadratus,* squared]. Square or having four equal sides.

q. lobe. A small lobe of liver located on visceral surface and lying in contact with pylorus and duodenum.

q. lobule. The square lobule of the upper surface of the cerebellum.

quadri-, quadr- [L.]. Combining forms meaning *having four; consisting of four.*

quadriceps (kwŏd'rĭ-sĕps) [L. *quadri,* from *quattuor,* four, + *ceps,* from *caput,* head]. Four-headed as a quadriceps muscle.

q. femoris. A large muscle on anterior surface of thigh composed of four muscles, *rectus femoris, vastus lateralis, vastus medialis, and vastus intermedius,* which are inserted by a common tendon on tuberosity of tibia. It is an extensor of the leg. SEE: *Table of Muscles in Appendix.*

q. reflex. SYN: *knee jerk; patellar reflex.* Extension of the leg following contraction of the quadriceps muscle resulting from a quick tap of the patellar tendon.

quadrigemina (kwŏd-rĭ-jĕm'ĭn-ă) [" + *geminus,* twin]. The corpora quadrigemina.

quadrigeminal (kwŏd-rĭ-jĕm'ĭn-ăl) [" + *geminus,* twin]. Fourfold; having four symmetrical parts.

quadrilateral (kwŏd-rĭ-lăt'ĕr-ăl) [" + *latus, later-,* side]. Having four sides.

quadripara (kwŏd-rĭp'ă-ră) [" + *parēre,* to bear]. A woman in her fourth confinement or who has had four children.

quadripartite (kwŏd-rĭ-par'tīt) [" + *partīre,* to divide]. Divided into four parts.

quadriplegia (kwŏd-rĭ-plē'jĭ-ă) [L. *quadri-,* from *quattuor,* four, + G. *plēgē,* a stroke]. Paralysis affecting all four limbs.

quadrisect (kwŏd'rĭ-sĕkt) [" + *sectiō,* a cutting]. To divide into four parts.

quadritubercular (kwŏd"rĭ-tū-bur'kū-lĕr) [" + *tuberculum,* a tubercle]. Having four tubercles or cusps.

quadrivalent (kwŏd-rĭ-vā'lĕnt, -rĭv'ăl-ĕnt) [" + *valens,* powerful]. Having ability to replace four atoms of hydrogen in a compound.

quadroon (kwŏd-rōōn') [Spanish *cuarterón*]. The offspring of a white person and a mulatto; a person having one-quarter Negro blood.

quadrupedal reflex (kwod-rōōp'ĕd-ăl) [L. *quadri-,* from *quattuor,* four, + *pēs,* foot]. Extension of flexed arm on assuming quadrupedal posture.

quadruplet (kwŏd'rū-plĕt) [L. *quadruplus,* fourfold]. One of four children born of the same mother at same labor. SEE: *Hellin's law.*

quale (kwā'lē) [L. of what kind]. The quality of anything, as of a sensation.

qualimeter (kwŏl-ĭm'ĕt-ĕr) [L. *qualis,* how constituted, + G. *metron,* a measure]. Device to determine hardness of the x-rays. SEE: *penetrometer.*

qualitative (kwŏl'ĭ-tā-tĭv) [L. *qualitativus,* pert. to quality]. Referring to the quality of anything.

q. analysis. CHEM: One that determines the nature of the elements of a compound, or the identity of the components of a mixture. SEE: *quantitative.*

quality (kwŏl'ĭ-tĭ) [L. *qualitās,* quality]. That which constitutes or characterizes a thing; nature.

quanta (kwŏn'tă) [L. as much as]. Plural of quantum, *q.v.*

quantimeter (kwŏn-tĭm'ĕt-ĕr) [L. *quantus,* how great, + G. *metron,* a measure]. Colorimetric standard for measuring quantity of x-rays to which a subject is exposed.

quanti-Pirquet (kwŏn-tĭ-pēr'kā). Quantitative cutaneous test of amt. of sensitiveness to tuberculin by use of graduated dilutions.

quantitative (kwon-tĭ-tā'tĭv) [L. *quantitatīvus,* pert. to quantity]. Concerning quantity.

q. analysis. One that determines the proportionate parts of elements in a compound, or the percentage of components of a mixture. SEE: *qualitative.*

quantity (kwŏn'tĭ-tĭ) [L. *quantitās,* quantity]. Amount; portion.

q., unit of. Coulomb, the measure of amt. of electric current passing a given point in a conductor in a given time.

quantum (kwŏn'tŭm) [L. how much]. 1. A unit of radiant energy. 2. A definite amount.

q. libet. [L.]. As much as desired.

q. limit. Shortest wave length in x-ray spectrum. SYN: *minimum wave length.*

q. sufficit. [L.]. As much as needed. ABBR: *q.s.*

q. theory. Radiation is an intermittent emission of energy in varying multiples of quanta action; not continuous.

quarantine (kwor'ăn-tēn) [Italian *quarantina*]. 1. The period of debarring from entrance to a country, or the isolation of persons exposed to infectious diseases: formerly 40 days. 2. Period of isolation from public communication following onset of a contagious disease. 3. As defined by Amer. Pub. Health Assn.: Limitation of freedom of movement of such well persons or domestic animals as have been exposed to a communicable disease, for a period of time equal to the longest incubation period of the disease, in such a manner as to prevent effective contact with those not so exposed. SEE: *contagious diseases; isolation.*

quart (kwort) [L. *quartus,* a fourth]. Abbr. *qt.* A unit of fluid or dry measure; one fourth part of a gallon or two pints; one eighth part of a peck.

quartan (kwor'tăn) [L. *quartus,* a fourth]. 1. Occurring every 4th day. 2. Malarial fever with a paroxysm every 4th day, figuring from and including the 1st day of paroxysm. SEE: *fever; malaria.*

q., double. Malaria in which there are two concurrent cycles resulting in fever occurring on two successive days.

q., triple. Malaria in which there are three concurrent cycles resulting in fever occurring every day.

quartile (kwor'tĭl) [L. *quartus,* a fourth]. One of the two middle values of each half of a series of variables.

quartipara (kwor-tĭp'ă-ră) [" + *parēre,* to bear]. A woman who has borne her fourth child.

quartiparous (kwor-tĭp'ăr-ŭs) [" + *parēre,* to bear]. Having given birth to four children or having been in labor four times.

quartz (kwortz) [uncertain origin]. Silicon dioxide, the principal ingredient of sandstone (crystallized silica; rock crystal).

When crystal is clear and colorless it permits the passage of ultraviolet radiations in large proportions.

q. applicator. Quartz rod of various shapes and angles to conduct (by total internal reflection) ultraviolet radiation from a water-cooled mercury arc quartz lamp.

q. glass. Crystalline quartz is used for prisms and lenses, fused quartz for windows, etc., through which ultraviolet radiations are freely transmitted.

quassation (kwă-sā'shŭn) [L. *quassāre,* to shake]. A beating, a shaking; breaking up of crude materials into small pieces.

quassia (kwŏsh'ă, kwosh'e-ă). The wood of a tree grown chiefly in Jamaica.

USES: Once considered valuable as a bitter tonic, and as an injection for certain intestinal parasites.

quassin. $C_{22}H_{30}O_6$. A bitter principle extracted from the wood of Quassia.

quater in die (quă'ter in dĭ'ĕ) [L.]. Four times a day. ABBR: *q.i.d.*

quaternary (kwă-tĕr'nă-rĭ) [L. *quaterni,* four each]. 1. The 4th in order. 2. Composed of four elements.

Queckenstedt's sign (qwek'en-stet, qvek'-en-stet) [Hans Queckenstedt, German physician, 1887(?)-1918]. Upon compression of the veins of the neck, unilaterally or bilaterally, cerebrospinal fluid pressure rises rapidly in healthy persons; this disappears when pressure is released. In vertebral canal block, the pressure is scarcely affected by this procedure.

querulent (kwĕr'ū-lĕnt) [L. *querulārī,* to complain]. 1. Complaining; fretful. 2. One who is dissatisfied, complaining, and suspicious.

quick. 1. A part susceptible to keen feeling, esp. part of a finger or toe to which nail is attached. 2. Pregnant.

quickening (kwĭk'ĕn-ĭng) [A.S. *cwic,* living]. First movements of the fetus felt in utero.

Occurs from 18th to 20th week of pregnancy. Movements have been felt as early as the tenth week and rarely are not felt during the entire pregnancy.

quicklime. CaO. Calcium oxide, unslaked lime. Forms calcium hydroxide when water is added to it.

quicksilver (kwĭk'sĭl-vĕr) [" + *silver*]. The metal, mercury.

quillaja (kwĭl-ā'yă) (soap bark). The inner bark of a tree grown in Chile.

USES: As an emulsifying agent. It has been used unwisely in the production of foam on nonalcoholic beverages.

quinacrine hydrochloride. SYN: *Atabrine, q.v.* An agent used in the treatment of malaria. Also used in infestations of *Giardia lamblia,* a parasite.

quince (kwĭns) [M.E. *quyne*]. COMP: Contains 3 times as much cellulose as cherries. Also contains tannin.

AV. SERVING: 240 gm. Pro. 1.0, Fat 0.3, Carbo. 37.0. VITAMIN: C 35 mg.

Quincke's disease (kvĭng'kĕh) [Heinricus I. Quincke, German physician, 1842-1922]. Angioneurotic edema of skin; urticaria; giant hives.

Q's. pulse. Capillary pulse. Seen under fingernails and indicated by alternate reddening and blanching; a sign of aortic insufficiency.

Q's. puncture. Lumbar p. to determine tension of, or to remove some of, the spinal fluid.

quinidine sulfate (kwĭn'ĭd-ēn). USP. The sulfate of an alkaloid obtained from cinchona bark, being a white, crystalline substance with a bitter taste.

ACTION AND USES: To regulate heart rhythm, especially to prevent fibrillation.

quinine (kwī'nīn, kwī'nēn) [Spanish *quina*]. Bitter, crystalline, white alkaloid derived from cinchona bark.

USES: Analgesic, antipyretic, antimalarial. Usually administered in the form of its salts.

q. bisulfate. USP. The acid sulfate of quinine.

ACTION AND USES: Same as quinine sulfate, but having greater solubility.

q. dihydrochloride. The dihydrochloride of quinine, freely soluble in water, 1 gm. dissolving in 0.6 cc. of water. Suitable for intravenous injection.

q. hydrochloride. USP. The hydrochloride of quinine. Used in treatment of malaria.

q. sulfate. USP. The sulfate of an alkaloid obtained from cinchona.

ACTION AND USES: Antipyretic and specific in malaria.

INCOMPATIBILITIES: Tea (tannin), coffee (caffeine), magnesium sulfate, Fowler's solution, ferrous iodide, fluidextract of cascara sagrada.

q. tannate. USP. A nearly tasteless and odorless compound of quinine and tannic acid. A means of administering quinine to young children.

q. and urea hydrochloride. Local anesthetic and used in treatment of malaria, by intramuscular or intravenous injections. In solutions of 5% or higher, used as a sclerosing agent for injection treatment of hemorrhoids and varicose veins.

quininism (kwī'nīn-ĭzm, kwī-nēn'ĭzm) [Spanish *quina*, + G. *-ismos*, condition]. Poisoning by cinchona or its alkaloids. SYN: *cinchonism.*

quinisal (kwĭn'ĭs-ăl). A commercial compound of quinine and salicylic acid.

USES: In rheumatism and other conditions where the effects of its components are desired.

quin'oline. C_9H_7N, a tertiary amine derived from coal tar. It is a solvent and antiseptic and many of its salts are used medicinally as antipyretics, analgesics, and in the treatment of amebic dysentery and other infections.

quinone (kwĭn-ōn'). 1. Yellow, crystalline oxidation product of quinic acid. 2. Class of organic compounds in which two atoms of hydrogen are replaced by oxygen.

quinoxyl (kwĭn-ŏk'sĭl). SEE: *chiniofon.*

quinqu- [L.]. Combining form meaning *five.*

Quinquaud's disease (kăn-kōz') [Charles E. Quinquaud, French physician, 1841-1894]. Purulent inflammation of scalp's hair follicles with bald patches as a result.

quinquina (kwĭn-kwī'nă, kĭn-kē'nă). Cinchona, *q.v.*

quinsy (kwĭn'zē) [G. *kynanche,* sore throat]. Acute inflammation of the tonsil and of the peritonsillar tissue usually forming an abscess. SYN: *peritonsillar abscess; angina tonsillaris.*

SYM: Sore throat, pain on swallowing, sense of suffocation because of swelling of throat, the tonsil area being enlarged, inflamed and red. Usually unilateral. Local lymphatics swollen and tender.

TREATMENT: Horizontal incision at point of greatest fluctuation. Incision need not be deep but blunt forceps are inserted and spread, which produce a large opening with little danger of hemorrhage.

NP: Heat mouthwashes, gargle if possible. Antibiotics and sulfonamide drugs by mouth. Warn against swallowing pus if abscess breaks.

q., lingual. Phlegmonous inflammation of the lingual tonsil.

quintan (kwĭn'tăn) [L. *quintanus,* pert. to a fifth]. 1. Occurring every fifth day. 2. Intermittent fever, the paroxysms occurring every 5th day with intermission of three days.

quinti- [L.]. Combining form meaning *fifth.*

quintipara (kwĭn-tĭp'ă-ră) [L. *quintus,* fifth, + *parēre,* to bear]. A woman in her 5th confinement or who has had five children.

quintuplet (kwĭn'tū-plĕt) [L. *quintuplex,* fivefold]. One of five children born of one mother during the same confinement. SEE: *Hellin's law; twins.*

quotidian (kwō-tĭd'ĭ-ăn) [L. *quotidianus,* daily]. Occurring daily.

q. fever. A malarial fever characterized by daily paroxysms.

quotient (kwō'shĕnt) [L. *quotiens,* how many times]. Number of times one number is contained in another.

q., caloric. Result obtained by dividing heat (in calories) by the oxygen consumed (in milligrams) in metabolism.

q., D. The ratio of glucose to nitrogen in the urine.

q., growth. Percentage of the food energy utilized for growth; estimated to be 5%.

q., intelligence. Division of the patient's mental age by his actual age.

q., protein. The number obtained by dividing the amount of globulin by the albumin in a specimen of blood plasma.

q., respiratory. The result of dividing amt. of carbon dioxide in expired air by the oxygen inhaled, normally 0.9.

q. v. 1. Abbr. for L. *quantum vis,* as much as you like. 2. Abbr. for L. *quod vide,* meaning *which see.*

Notes

R

R. Abbr. for *roentgen, respiration, right.* In chem., a radical. ℞. Symb. for L. *recipe,* to take.

R—. Abbr. used in organic chemistry to indicate part of a molecule.

—R. Rinne negative. SEE: *Rinne's test.*

+R. Rinne positive. SEE: *Rinne's test.*

℞. Symb. for L. *recipe,* to take.

RA. Abbr. for *rheumatoid arthritis.*

Ra. Chemical symb. for *radium.*

rabbetting (răb'ĕt-ĭng) [Fr. *raboter,* to plane]. Interlocking of the jagged edges of a fractured bone.

rabbit fever. Tularemia, *q.v.*

rabiate (rā'bĭ-āt) [L. *rabere,* to rage]. Suffering from rabies. SYN: *rabid.*

rabic (răb'ĭk) [L. *rabere,* to rage]. Concerning rabies.

rabicidal (răb-ĭ-sī'dăl) [" + *cidus,* from *caedere,* to kill]. Destructive to causative virus of rabies.

rabid (răb'ĭd) [L. *rabidus,* raving]. Pert. to or affected with rabies. SYN: *rabiate.*

rabies (rā'bēz) [L. *rabies,* to rave]. SYN: *hydrophobia.* An acute infectious disease of animals, especially carnivores (dog, wolf, bat, fox, cat), characterized by involvement of central nervous system resulting in paralysis and finally death. May be communicated to man through the bite of a rabid animal, usually a dog.

PERIOD OF INCUBATION: Usually 4-6 weeks, but sometimes longer depending on deepness of laceration and site of wound.

ETIOL: A neurotropic filtrable virus present in saliva of rabid animals.

PREVENTION: Thoroughly clean all bites or scratches made by any animal with strong (20%) medicinal soap solution. Deep puncture wounds should be opened to permit access of solution.

TREATMENT: If animal is caught, confine and observe for 10 days. Give vaccine to exposed person at first sign of physical or laboratory evidence of rabies in the observed animal. If animal is not caught and rabies is known to be present in the area, start vaccination immediately. In severe bites, rabies hyperimmune serum may be used in addition to the vaccine.

SEE: *dog bite.*

race (rās) [Italian *razza*]. 1. A class of individuals with common interests, characteristics, appearance, habits, etc., as if derived from a common ancestor. 2. Division of mankind with traits sufficient to mark it as a distinct human type.

racemose (răs'ē-mōs) [L. *racemōsus,* full of clusters]. Resembling a clustered bunch of grapes, as a gland, divided and subdivided, ending in a bunch of follicles.

rachi-, rachio- [G.]. Combining forms meaning *rib of a leaf, ridge, spine.*

rachialbuminimeter (rā"kĭ-ăl-bū-mĭn-ĭm'ĕt-ĕr) [G. *rhachis,* spine, + L. *albumen,* white of egg, + G. *metron,* measure]. Device for determining the amount of albumin in the cerebrospinal fluid.

rachialbuminimetry (rā"kĭ-ăl-bū-mĭn-ĭm'ĕt-rĭ) [" + " + G. *metron,* measure]. Determining the amount of albumin in the cerebrospinal fluid.

rachianalgesia (rā"kĭ-ăn-ăl-jē'zĭ-ă) [" + *analgesia,* lack of pain]. Spinal anesthesia. SYN: *rachianesthesia.*

rachialgia (rā-kĭ-ăl'jĭ-ă) [" + *algos,* pain]. Pain in the spine.

rachianesthesia (rā"kĭ-ăn-ĕs-thē'zĭ-ă) [" + *an-,* negative, + *aisthēsis,* sensation]. Spinal anesthesia.

rachicele (rā'kĭ-sēl). Protrusion of contents of spinal canal in spina bifida.

rachicentesis (rā"kĭ-sĕn-tē'sĭs) [" + *kentēsis,* a piercing]. Puncture into the spinal canal.

rachidian (ra-kĭd'ĭ-ăn) [G. *rhachis, rachid-,* spine]. Relating to the spinal column.

rachigraph (rā'kĭ-grăf) [" + *graphein,* to write]. Device for outlining the curves of the spine.

rachilysis (rā-kĭl'ĭs-ĭs) [" + *lysis,* a loosening]. Mechanical treatment of lateral curvature of the spine.

rachiocampsis (rā-kĭ-ō-kamp'sĭs) [" + *kampsis,* a bending]. Curvature of spine.

rachiochysis (rā-kĭ-ok'ĭs-ĭs) [" + *chysis,* a pouring]. Accumulation of fluid within the spinal canal.

rachiodynia (rā-kĭ-ō-dĭn'ĭ-ă) [" + *odynē,* pain]. Painful condition of spinal column. SYN: *rachialgia.*

rachiometer (rā-kĭ-ŏm'ĕt-ĕr) [" + *metron,* measure]. Instrument for measuring a curvature of the spine.

rachiopagus (ra-ke-op'ă-gus). Twins united back to back but involving only the spinal column.

rachioplegia (rā"kĭ-ō-plē'jĭ-ă) [" + *plēgē,* a stroke]. Paralysis of spine.

rachioscoliosis (rā"kĭ-ō-skō"lĭ-ō-sĭs). Lateral curvature of the spine.

rachiotome (rā'kĭ-ō-tōm) [" + *tomē,* a cutting]. Instrument for dividing the vertebrae.

rachiotomy (rā-kĭ-ŏt'ō-mĭ) [" + *tomē,* a cutting]. Surgical cutting of the vertebral column.

rachis (rā'kĭs) (pl. *rachises*) [G. spine]. The spinal column.

rachischisis (rā-kĭs'kĭs-ĭs) [G. *rhachis,* spine, + *schisis,* cleft]. Spinal column fissure; congenital. SYN: *spina bifida; cleft spine.*

rachitic (rā-kĭt'ĭk) [G. *rhachis,* spine]. Pert. to or affected with rickets.

***r.* beads.** Rachitic rosary, *q.v.*

***r.* flat pelvis.** Pelvic deformity due to having had rickets in childhood.

***r.* rosary.** Beadlike prominences at junction of the ribs with their cartilages.

rachitis (ra-ki'tis [G. *rhachis,* spine, + *-itis,* inflammatory]. 1. Inflammation of the spine, commonly rickets. 2. Rickets, *q.v.* SEE: *rachitic beads.*

***r.* fetalis annularis.** Enlargement of epiphyses of long bones; congenital.

***r.* fetalis micromelica.** Congenital shortness of the bones.

rachitism (rak'ĭ-tism). Tendency towards rickets.

rachitogenic (răk"ĭ-tō-jĕn'ĭk). Causing or inducing development of rickets.

rachitome (rā'kĭ-tōm) [" + *tomē,* a cutting]. Instrument employed for opening spinal canal.

raclage (răk-klăj'). SYN: *raclement.* Destruction and removal of a soft growth by scraping or rubbing.

radectomy (rā-dĕk'tō-mĭ). Surgical removal of a tooth or a part of one.

radiability (rā-dĭ-ă-bĭl'ĭ-tĭ) [L. *radius*, ray]. Capability of being penetrated readily by the x-ray.

radiad (rā'dĭ-ăd) [L. *radius*, spoke, + *ad*, toward]. In direction of the radial side.

radial (ra'dĭ-ăl) [L. *radius*, spoke]. 1. Radiating out from a given center. 2. Pert. to the radius.

r. reflex. Flexion of forearm resulting when lower end of radius is percussed.

radiant (rā'dĭ-ănt) [L. *radiāre*, to emit rays]. 1. Emitting beams of light. 2. Transmitted by radiation. 3. Emanating from a common center.

RS: *energy; flux; heat.*

radiate (rā'dĭ-āt) [L. *radius*, spoke]. To spread from a common center.

radiation (rā-dĭ-ā'shŭn) [L. *radiāre*, to emit rays]. 1. Process by which energy is propagated through space or matter not affected by it. 2. Emission of rays in all directions from a common center. 3. Treatment with a radioactive substance. 4. In neurology, a group of fibers which diverge from a common origin.

A general term for any form of radiant energy emission or divergence, as of energy in all directions from luminous bodies, roentgen ray tubes, radioactive elements and fluorescent substances.

r., acoustic. SEE: *r., auditory.*

r., auditory. SYN: *acoustic r.; thalamotemporal r.* A band of fibers which connects auditory areas of cerebral cortex with medial geniculate body of thalamus.

r. of corpus callosum. Total of fibers radiating from corpus callosum into each cerebral hemisphere.

r., heterogeneous. R. containing waves of various wave lengths.

r., homogeneous. R. containing waves of only one wave length.

r., infrared. Near or short infrared extends from 7200 A. U. to 14,000 A. U. Far or long infrared from 15,000 to 120,000.

r., interstitial. R. accomplished by insertion of radium or radon directly into tissues.

r., ionizing. R. which induces either directly or indirectly ionization of radiation-absorbing material.

r., irritative. Overdosage of ultraviolet irradiation resulting in erythema, and, in exceptional cases, blister formation.

r., mitogenetic. SYN: *Gurvich r.* Hypothetical radiations given off by cells during mitosis which induce mitosis.

r., occipitothalamic. SEE: *r., optic.*

r., optic. SYN: *geniculocalcarine tract.* A system of fibers extending from lateral geniculate body of thalamus through sublenticular portion of internal capsule to the calcarine occipital cortex (striate area).

r., photochemical. From a therapeutic standpoint the electromagnetic spectrum divided into photothermal and photochemical radiations. Photochemical r's. penetrate only to fractions of millimeters, are absorbed by protoplasm, and cause physical and biological changes.

r., photothermal. Photothermal radiations penetrate subcutaneous tissues, heat the blood, accelerate vital reactions and act instantaneously. SEE: *r., photochemical.*

r., solar. Radiations of the sun, 60% in infrared region and 40% visible and ultraviolet, shortest wave length.

r., striomesencephalic. Fibers originating in corpus striatum and terminating principally in substantia nigra of midbrain.

r., striosubthalamic. SYN: *ansa lenticularis.* A system of fibers consisting of three groups emerging from medial aspect of lentiform nucleus and entering subthalamic region, most terminating there but some continuing into the midbrain.

r., striothalamic. Groups of fibers connecting the corpus striatum with thalamus and subthalamus.

r. sickness. SEE: *r. syndrome.*

r. syndrome. SYN: *radiation sickness.* 1. Illness resulting from exposure of body tissue to ionizing radiations from radioactive substances (radium, radon) or roentgen rays. Mild acute illness is manifested by anorexia, headache, nausea, vomiting, and diarrhea. Delayed effects resulting from repeated or prolonged exposure may result in amenorrhea, sterility, disturbances in blood cell formation, cataract formation, carcinogenesis, and leukemia. 2. Illness resulting from effects of explosion of an atomic bomb. Effects include destruction of lymphatic tissue, extensive hemorrhages, aplastic bone marrow, prolonged clotting and bleeding times, loss of hair and teeth, and possible genetic changes. In massive exposure to radiation such as would occur in persons close to the center of the atomic bomb explosion, death may occur within several weeks if the individual is not fortunate enough to die immediately from the physical effects of the explosion.

r., thalamic. SYN: *t. peduncles or stalks.* Groups of fibers which connect thalamus with cerebral hemispheres. Include frontal, centroparietal occipital, and optic radiations.

r., ultraviolet. Radiant energy extending from 3900 to 200 A. U. Divided into "near ultraviolet," extending from 3900 to 2900 A. U., and "far ultraviolet," from 2900 to 200 A. U.

r. unit. SEE: *angstrom unit; maché unit.*

r., visible. Visible spectrum may be broken up into different wave lengths representing different colors:

Violet	4000-4500 A. U.
Blue	4500-4900 " "
Green	4900-5500 " "
Yellow	5500-5900 " "
Orange	5900-6300 " "
Red	6300-7800 " "

SEE: *spectrum.*

RS: *heliotherapy; helium.*

radiator (rā'dĭ-ā-tor) [L. *radiator*]. Device for radiating heat or light.

r., infrared. Device for transmitting infrared rays. SEE: *heater, radiant.*

radical (răd'ĭ-kăl) [L. *radix, radic-*, root]. 1. A group of atoms acting as a single unit, passing without change from one compound to another, but not able to exist in a free state. 2. Anything that reaches the root or origin; original. 3. A foundation or principle.

r. treatment. A treatment that seeks an absolute cure, as r. surgery; not palliative. Opp. of *conservative treatment.*

radicle (răd'ĭ-kl) [L. *radix, radic-*, root]. 1. A structure resembling a rootlet, as a r. of a nerve or vein. 2. Group of elements unaffected by chemical change, unable to exist in the free state. 3. SEE: radical.

radicotomy (răd-ĭ-kŏt'ō-mĭ) [" + G. *tomē*, a cutting]. Section of spinal nerve roots. SYN: *rhizotomy.* SEE: *radiculectomy.*

radiculalgia (răd-ĭ-kū-lăl′jĭ-ă) [" + G. *algos,* pain]. Neuralgia of roots of nerves.

radicular (răd-ĭk′ū-lar) [L. *radix, radic-,* root]. Concerning a root or radicle.

radiculectomy (răd-ĭk-ū-lĕk′tō-mĭ) [" + G. *ektomē,* excision]. 1. Excision of a spinal nerve root. 2. Resection of post. spinal nerve root. SEE: *radicotomy.*

radiculitis (răd-ĭk-ū-lī′tĭs) [" + G. *-ītis,* inflammation]. Inflammation of spinal nerve roots, accompanied by pain and hyperesthesia.

radiculomeningomyelitis (răd-ĭk″ū-lō-mē-nĭn″gō-mī-ĕl-ī′tĭs) [" + G. *mēnigx,* membrane, + *myelos,* marrow, + *-ītis,* inflammation]. Inflamed condition of nerve roots, meninges, and spinal cord. SYN: *rhizomeningomyelitis.*

radiculomyelopathy (rā-dĭk″ū-lō-mī″ă-lŏp′ă-thĭ). Any diseased condition involving spinal cord and roots of spinal nerves.

radiculoneuritis (rā-dĭk″ū-lō″nū-rī′tĭs). Inflammation of roots of spinal nerves.

radiculopathy (rā-dĭk″ū-lŏp′ă-thĭ). Any diseased condition of roots of spinal nerves.

radio-. Combining form meaning *pert. to radiant energy,* or *radioactive substances.*

radioactinium (rā-dĭ-ō-ăk-tĭn′ĭ-ŭm). A radioactive product formed from disintegration of actinium.

radioactive (ră″dĭ-ō-ăk′tĭv) [L. *radius,* ray, + *activus,* acting]. Capable of emitting radiant energy.

r. decay. The shift from high-energy-level unstable nuclei to low-energy-level stable nuclei accompanied by emission of energy or particles.

radioactivity (rā″dĭ-ō-ăk-tĭv′ĭ-tĭ) [L. *radius,* ray, + *activus,* acting]. The ability of a substance to emit rays or particles (alpha, beta, gamma) from its nucleus.

r., artificial. SYN: *induced r.* Radioactivity resulting from bombardment of a substance with high-energy particles in a cyclotron, betatron, or other apparatus.

r., induced. Temporary r. of a substance which has been within the sphere of influence of a radioactive element.

r., natural. That possessed by a number of elements which are continuously disintegrating and emitting alpha particles (helium nuclei) or beta particles (electrons) atom by atom. Ex: radium.

radioautograph (rā″dĭ-ō-aw′tō-grăf). A photograph of a histologic section of a tissue which shows the distribution of radioactive substances in the tissue.

radiobe. A peculiar structure formed in sterilized bouillon as a result of radium radiation. It resembles bacteria in appearance.

radiobiology (rā-dĭ-ō-bĭ-ŏl′ō-jĭ). Branch of biology which deals with the effects of radiations on living organisms.

radiocarpal (rā″dĭ-ō-kar′păl) [L. *radius,* spoke, + G. *karpos,* wrist]. Concerning the radius and carpus.

radiochemistry (rā″dĭ-ō-kĕm′ĭs-trĭ) [" + G. *chemeia,* chemistry]. The phase of chemistry dealing with radioactive phenomena.

radiochroism (rā″dĭ-ō-krō′ĭzm) [" + G. *chroa,* color]. The ability of a substance to absorb radioactive rays.

radiochrometer (rā″dĭ-ō-krŏm′ĕt-ĕr) [" + G. *chrōma,* color, + *metron,* measure]. Device for measuring penetrating powers of x-rays and the character of roentgen tubes. SEE: *penetrometer.*

radiocystitis (rā-dĭ-ō-sĭs-tī′tĭs) Inflammation of the bladder following treatment by radium or roentgen rays.

radiode (rā′dĭ-ōd) [L. *radius,* ray]. Metal container for radium, used in therapeutic application.

radiodermatitis (rā″dĭ-ō-der″mă-tī′tĭs) [" + G. *derma,* skin, + *-ōsis,* condition]. Inflammation of the skin caused by roentgen rays or radiation from radioactive elements.

radiodiagnosis (rā″dĭ-ō-dĭ-ăg-nō′sĭs) [" + G. *dia,* through, + *gnōsis,* knowledge]. Diagnosis by means of x-ray.

radiodontia (rā-dĭ-ō-dŏn′shĭ-ă). Roentgenography of the teeth.

radioelement (rā″dĭ-ō-ĕl′e-mĕnt) [" + *elementum*]. An element possessing power of radioactivity.

radioepidermitis (rā″dĭ-ō-ĕp-ĭ-der-mī′tĭs) [" + G. *epi,* upon, + *derma,* skin, + *-ītis,* inflammation]. Irritation of the skin caused by radioactive rays.

radioepithelitis (rā″dĭ-ō-ĕp-ĭ-thē-lī′tĭs) [" + " + *thēlē,* nipple, + *-ītis,* inflammation]. Disintegration of epithelium due to exposure to irradiation.

radiogram (rā′dĭ-ō-grăm) [" + G. *gramma,* a writing]. X-ray picture, especially of internal organs.

radiograph (rā′dĭ-ō-grăf) [" + G. *graphein,* to write]. 1. A record produced on a photographic plate, film, or paper by the action of roentgen rays or radium; specifically an x-ray photograph. 2. To make a radiograph of. SEE: *skiagraph.*

radiographer (rā″dĭ-ŏg′ră-fer) [" + G. *graphein,* to write]. A person skilled in making roentgenograms, or radiographs.

Usually, but at the present time not necessarily, applied to physicians who practice diagnostic roentgenology.

radiography (rā-dĭ-ŏg′ră-fĭ) [" + G. *graphein,* to write]. The making of x-ray pictures. SYN: *roentgenography; skiagraphy.*

radiohumeral (rā″dĭ-ō-hū′mĕr-ăl) [" + *humerus*]. Concerning the radius and humerus.

radioiodine (rā-dĭ-ō-ī′ō-dīn). A radioactive isotope of iodine. Used in the diagnosis and treatment of thyroid disorders.

radioisotopes (rā-dĭ-ō-ī′sō-tōps). Radioactive forms of chemicals such as radioactive cobalt.

radiologist (rā-dĭ-ŏl′ō-jĭst) [" + G. *logos,* a study]. One who practices diagnosis and treatment by radiant energy.

radiology (rā-dĭ-ol′ō-jĭ) [L. *radius,* ray, spoke, + G. *logos,* study]. The branch of science which deals with roentgen rays, radium rays, and other radiations, and their curative properties.

radiolucency (rā″dĭ-ō-lū′sĕn-sĭ) [" + *lucere,* to shine]. Property of being partly or wholly permeable to radiant energy.

radiolus (rā-dĭ′ō-lŭs) [L. *radiolus,* a little spoke]. A sound; a probe.

radiometer (ra-dĭ-om′ĕ-ter). Instrument for measuring intensity of radiation.

radiomimetic (ra″di-o-mim-et′ik) [" + G. *mimetikos,* imitation]. Imitating the biological effects of radiation.

radion (rā′dĭ-ōn) [" + G. *ōn,* being]. One of the particles of the alpha, beta rays, or cathode rays, given off by radioactive matter.

radionecrosis (rā″dĭ-ō-nĕ-krō′sĭs) [" + G. *nekrōsis,* death]. Disintegration of tissue by exposure to radiant energy.

radioneuritis (rā″dĭ-ō-nū-rī′tĭs) [" + G. *neuron,* sinew, + *-ītis,* inflammation].

Neuritis caused by exposure to radioactive substance.

radiopaque (rā-dĭ-ō-pāk') [" + *opacus*, dark]. Impenetrable to the x-ray or other forms of radiation.

radioparent (rā"dĭ-ō-par'ĕnt) [" + *parere*, to appear]. Penetrable by the x-ray or other rays.

radiopathology (rā-dĭ-ō-pă-thŏl'ō-gĭ). Study of pathologic changes induced by radiation.

radiopelvimetry (rā"dĭ-ō-pĕl-vĭm'ĕt-rĭ) [L. *radius*, ray, spoke, + *pelvis*, basin, + G. *metron*, measure]. Measurement of the pelvis by the x-ray.

radiopraxis (rā"dĭ-ō-prăks'ĭs) [" + G *praxis*, practice]. Diagnosis or use in treatment of some radioactive substance, as x-ray or ultraviolet ray.

radioresistant. Resistant to the action of radiation, especially of a tumor which cannot be destroyed by treatment with radiation.

radioscopy (rā-dĭ-ŏs'kō-pĭ) [" + G. *skopein*, to examine]. Inspection and examination of the inner structures of the body by means of roentgen rays.

radiosensibility (rā"dĭ-ō-sĕn"sĭ-bĭl'ĭ-tĭ) [" + *sensibilitās*]. Quality of sensitivity to radioactive substances.

radiosensitive (rā"dĭ-ō-sĕn'sĭ-tĭv) [" + *sensitīvus*, feeling]. Capable of being destroyed by radiation, as a tumor by x-rays.

radiosurgery (rā"dĭ-ō-sur'jer-ĭ) [L. *radius*, ray, + G. *cheirurgia*, handwork]. The use of radium in surgery.

radiotelemetry (ra"dĭ-o-tel-em'ĕ-trĭ). Transmission of data, including biological data, via radio. Developed in order to be able to monitor heart rate, ECG, and body temperature data from astronauts. Now used also in hospitals.

radiotherapist (rā"dĭ-ō-ther'ă-pĭst) [" + G. *therapeia*, treatment]. One trained in use of radiant energy for therapeutic purposes.

radiotherapy (rā"dĭ-ō-ther'ă-pĭ) [" + G. *therapeia*, treatment]. The treatment of disease by application of roentgen rays, radium, ultraviolet and other radiations.

radiothermy (rā"dĭ-ō-ther'mĭ) [L. *radius*, ray, + G. *thermē*, heat]. 1. Use of radiant heat or heat from radioactive substances for therapeutic purposes. 2. Short-wave diathermy.

radiotoxemia (rā"dĭ-ō-tŏks-ē'mĭ-ă) [" + G. *toxikon*, poison, + *aima*. blood]. Toxemia produced by exposure to radioactive substance. SYN: *actinotoxemia.*

radiotransparent (rā"dĭ-ō-trăns-par'ĕnt) [" + *trans*, across, + *parere*, to appear]. Penetrable by x-ray or other forms of radiation.

radiotropic (rā"dĭ-ō-trŏp'ĭk) [L. *radius*, ray, spoke, + G. *tropos*, a turning]. Affected by radiation.

radioulnar (rā"dĭ-ō-ŭl'nar) [" + *ulna*, arm]. Concerning the radius and ulna.

radish (răd'ĭsh) [L. *radix*, an edible root]. COMP: High in oxalic acid; little food value, but desirable for its minerals.

RAW: 4 radishes (40 gm.). Calories: 7. Other main values: trace of protein; trace of fat; 1.5 gm. carbohydrate; 15 mg. calcium.

radium (rā'dĭ-ŭm) [L. *radius*, rays]. SYMB: Ra. A metallic element found in very small quantities in pitchblende. At. wt. 226; at. no. 88. SEE: *"actin-" words.*

It does not seem to exist in a free state. It is radioactive and fluorescent. becoming darker on exposure to light.

Radiation is of 3 kinds: (1) The *alpha rays;* (2) *beta rays;* (3) *gamma rays* which are analogous to the x-rays.

r. intratumoral application. Implanting radium into tumors for therapeutic purposes.

r. needles. Slender containers for radium. These are inserted into tissue in order to kill the malignant cells.

radiumization (rā"dĭ-ŭm-ĭ-za'shŭn) [L. *radius*, ray]. Exposure to action of radium rays.

radiumologist (rā"dĭ-ŭm-ŏl'ō-jĭst) [" + G. *logos*, a study]. One who specializes in radium therapy.

radiumology (rā"dĭ-ŭm-ŏl'ō-jĭ) [" + G. *logos*, a study]. The science of radium therapy.

radium therapy (rā'dĭ-ŭm ther'ă-pĭ) [" + G. *therapeia*, treatment]. The treatment of disease by means of radium, radon, its emanation, or its active deposit.

radius (rā'dĭ-ŭs) [L. *radius*, a spoke, ray]. 1. The outer and shorter bone of the arm which revolves partially about the ulna.

Its head articulates with the *capitulum* of the humerus. Its lower extremity articulates by the ulnar notch with the ulna, and by another articulation with the navicular and lunate bones of the wrist. 2. A line extending from a circle's center point to its circumference.

r., fracture of. Colles' fracture. A fracture and dislocation of lower end of radius, generally caused by falling on the outstretched hand.

radix (ra'dĭks) (pl. *radices*) [L. root]. 1. The root portion of a cranial or spinal nerve. 2. The root of a plant.

radon (ra'don) [L. *radius*, ray]. SYMB: Rn. At. wt. 222; at. no. 86. A radioactive gaseous element resulting from disintegration of radium. Also called *niton.*

rage. Violent anger.

ragsorters' disease (răg'sort'ers). A febrile pulmonary disease arising in persons who sort paper and rags, due to inhalation of bacillus causing anthrax, *q.v.*

ragweed. One of several species of the genus *Ambrosia* whose pollen is an important allergen. Pollen-producing period of grasses is, in temperate zones, from middle of August to the first hard or "killing" frost, usually the middle of October.

Raillietina (rī"lē-ē-tī'nă). A genus of cyclophyllidean tapeworms belonging to family Davaineidae.

R. demerariensis. SYN: *R. quitensis.* A species which infests humans, reported from several S. American countries, esp. Ecuador.

railway sickness. Motion sickness resulting from movement of a train.

raised (rāzd) [M.E. *reisen*, to rise]. BACT: Having a thick, elevated growth with terraced edges.

raisin. DRIED: 1 cup (160 gm.). Calories: 460. Other main values: 4 gm. protein; trace of fat; 124 gm. carbohydrate; 99 mg. calcium.

rale (rahl) [Fr. rattle]. An abnormal sound heard on auscultation of the chest produced by passage of air through bronchi which contain secretion or exudate or which are constricted by spasm or a thickening of their walls. May be heard on either inspiration or expiration.

CLASS: There is no general agreement as to classification of the sounds. They are designated *moist* and *dry.* Moist rales are also called *crackling* and these in turn, *coarse, medium,* or *dry.* If loud and sharp, they are *consonating.* Dry rales are sometimes designated *musical* and may be *tinkling, sonorous, snoring,* or *low pitched* or they may be *whistling, piping,* and *high pitched.*

r., atelectatic. Crepitant r., *q.v.*

r., bronchiectatic. Heard over bronchiectatic cavities filled with accumulated secretion. Disappears with expectoration.

r., bubbling medium. Heard in inspiration and expiration; produced by passage of air through mucus in the larger tubes; *character,* larger than the small bubbling moist r.; heard in capillary bronchitis, esp. in children.

r., cavernous. Heard in inspiration and expiration; produced by passage of air through a small cavity with flaccid walls that collapse with expiration; *character,* hollow and metallic.

r., clicking. Heard in inspiration only; produced by passage of air through softening material in smaller bronchi; *character,* small, sticky; heard in pulmonary tuberculosis, early stage.

r., coarse. Originates in the larger bronchi.

r., consonating. A loud, sharp rale sounding as though close to the ear. Usually associated with consolidation of tissues about bronchial tubes.

r., crackling, medium. Heard chiefly in inspiration; produced by fluid in the finer bronchi; *character,* larger than the small, crackling, dry; heard in softening of the tubercular deposit, or pneumonic exudation.

r., crepitant. Heard at end of inspiration; produced by passage of air into collapsed vesicles containing fibrinous exudation, usually at base of lungs; *character,* small, like rubbing hair between the fingers; heard in pneumonia, in early stage edema of lungs, hypostatic pneumonia. It is localized in pulmonary tuberculosis.

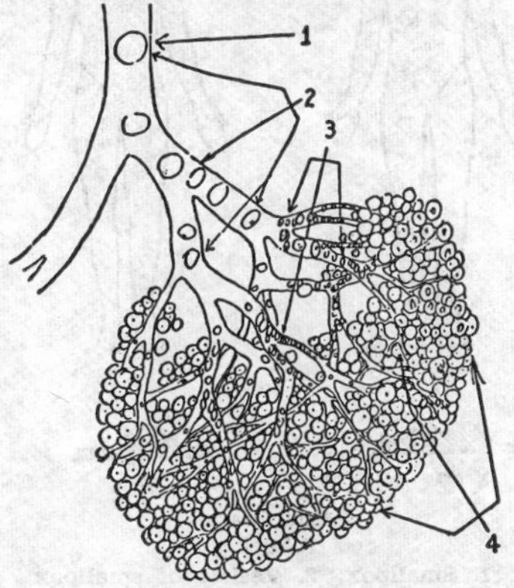

RALES.

1. Death rattle. 2. Large moist rales, 3. Small moist rales. 4. Subcrepitant rales.

r., dry. Heard in inspiration and expiration; produced by narrowing of the bronchial tubes from thickening of their mucous lining, from spasmodic contraction of the muscular coat, viscid mucus within or pressure from without; *character,* large and sonorous, small, hissing or whistling; heard in bronchitis, asthma, and localized in beginning pulmonary tuberculosis.

r., gurgling. Heard in inspiration and expiration; produced by passage of air through fluid in cavities of large bubbles; heard in pulmonary tuberculosis after formation of cavities.

r., moist. Produced by passage of air through bronchi containing fluid.

r. redux, r. de retour. Heard in inspiration and expiration; produced by passage of air through fluid in bronchial tubes; *character,* crackling, unequal; heard in pneumonia, in the stage of resolution.

r., sibilant. High pitched, whistling, and frequent at end of inspiration.

r., sonorous. Low snoring, greater in volume, continuing during inspiration.

r., subcrepitant. Heard in inspiration and expiration; produced by passage of air through mucus in the capillary bronchial tubes; *character,* small, moist; heard in capillary bronchitis.

r., submucous. Higher pitched and more numerous than large mucous rale. Heard in interscapular and supramammary regions and indicating involvement of many tubes of small caliber.

r., vesicular. Crepitant r., *q.v.*

rami (rā'mī) (L. *ramus*]. Plural of *ramus, q.v.*

ramification (răm-ĭ-fĭ-kā'shŭn) [L. *ramus,* branch, + *-ficāre,* to make]. 1. Process of branching. 2. A branch. 3. Arrangement in branches.

ramify (răm'ĭ-fī) [L. *ramificāre,* to make in branches]. To branch; to spread out in different directions.

ramisection (răm'ĭ-sĕk"shŭn) [L. *ramus,* branch, + *sectio,* a cutting]. Surgical division of a ramus communicans between a spinal nerve and a ganglion of the sympathetic trunk.

ramisectomy (răm-ĭs-ĕk'tō-mĭ) [" + G. *ektomē,* excision]. Excision of a ramus, specifically ramus communicans. SEE: *ramisection.*

ramollissement (rah"mo-lēs-mon') [Fr. *ramollir,* to soften]. Morbid softening of some organ or tissue, especially of brain.

ramose. Branching. Having many branches.

ram'ulus (pl. *ramuli*). A small branch or ramus.

ramus (rā'mŭs) (pl. *rami*) [L. *ramus,* a branch]. 1. A branch of one of the divisions of a forked structure. 2. Posterior portion of lower jawbone. 3. Primary division of a blood vessel or nerve.

r., anterior. A primary division of a spinal nerve which supplies the lateral and ventral portions of body wall, the limbs, and perineum. Also called *ventral ramus.*

r., bronchial. Collateral branches of each primary bronchus.

r. communicans. One of the primary branches of a spinal nerve which connects with a sympathetic ganglion. Each consists of a *gray* portion (*gray ramus communicans*) of myelinated preganglionic sympathetic fibers and a *white* portion (*white ramus communicans*) composed of unmyelinated postganglionic fibers [NA].

r., meningeal. SYN: *recurrent branch.* One of the primary branches of a spinal nerve which reenters vertebral foramen and supplies meninges and vertebral column.

r., posterior. One of the primary branches of a spinal nerve which supplies muscles and skin of the back. Also called *dorsal ramus.*

rancid (răn'sĭd) [L. *rancere,* to be rancid]. Offensive; having a sour smell or taste from partial decomposition, as a *fat.*

range. The difference between the highest and lowest values in a set of variables or in a series of values or observations.

r. of accommodation. Difference between least and greatest distance of distinct vision. SEE: *accommodation.*

ranine (rā'nīn) [L. *rana,* a frog]. 1. Pert. to a ranula or to the region beneath the tip of the tongue. 2. Branch of the lingual artery supplying that area. 3. Pertaining to frogs.

ranula (răn'ū-lă) [L. *ranula,* little frog]. A large cystic tumor seen on underside of tongue on either side of the frenum; a retention cyst of the submaxillary or sublingual ducts.

The swelling may be small or as large as an egg.

SYM: Semitranslucent; soft, large, dilated veins coursing over it. Fullness and discomfort. Usually no pain. Contains clear, glairy fluid, due to dilatation of ducts of salivary glands and to obstruction of those of sublingual mucous glands.

TREATMENT: Periodic emptying of sac by careful needle aspiration will provide temporary relief. Surgical intervention is required to completely remove.

r., pancreatic. Cystic disease of pancreas due to obstruction of its ducts.

Ranvier's nodes (ron-vē-āz') [Louis A. Ranvier, French pathologist, 1835-1922]. Constrictions in the medullary substance of a nerve fiber at more or less regular intervals. SEE: *nerve fiber.*

rape (rāp) [L. *rapere,* to snatch]. 1. Coitus with a female without her consent or when she is too young or without sufficient intelligence to give legal consent.

It is a crime punishable by death in some states. It is very difficult legally to prove rape. Rape of a vigorous girl by an unassisted male is considered almost impossible if the victim is conscious and free to defend herself.

RS: *age of consent; coitus; sexual intercourse; virginity.*

raphania (răf-ā'nĭ-ă) [G. *rhaphanos,* radish]. A spasmodic disease caused by eating seeds of the wild radish; allied to ergotism, *q.v.* SYN: *rhaphania.*

raphe (rā'fē) [G. *rhaphē,* a seam]. A crease, ridge or seam noting union of the halves of a part.

r., buccal. R. on cheek indicating line of fusion of maxillary and mandibular processes.

r., palatine. A line or ridge in median line of palate.

r. of penis. A median ridge on post. surface of penis, a continuation of raphe of scrotum.

r., perineal. A line or ridge in midline of perineum.

r. of scrotum. A ridge in midline of scrotum.

r. of tongue. A median groove on dorsum of tongue.

rapport (ră-por') [Fr. *rapporter,* to bring back]. A relationship of mutual sympathy and understanding, especially between patient and physician.

raptus (rap'tus). A sudden seizure or attack; rape.

r. hemorrhagicus. A sudden hemorrhage.

r. maniacus. A sudden maniacal attack.

r. melancholicus. A sudden attack of agitation occurring during melancholia.

r. nervorum. A sudden attack of extreme nervousness; a cramp or spasm.

rarefaction (rar"ĕ-făk'shŭn) [L. *rarefacere,* to make thin]. Process of decreasing density and weight, as of *air.*

The farther from the surface of the earth, the less dense the atmosphere becomes.

r. of bone. The process of making bone more porous because of absorption of mineral substances.

ETIOL: Disturbed calcium-phosphorus metabolism possibly resulting from excess parathyroid hormone. SEE: *osteoporosis; parathyroid.*

rarefy (rār'ĕ-fī). To make less dense or to increase porosity of.

rar'efy"ing os"tei'tis. Chronic bone inflammation marked by development of granulation tissue in marrow spaces with absorption of surrounding hard bone. SEE: *osteitis.*

rash (rash) [O. Fr. *rasche,* eruption]. SYN: *exanthema.* General term applied to any eruption of the skin, esp. those associated with communicable diseases. Usually temporary. SEE: *eruption; lesion; roseola.*

NP: *Color,* usually a shade of red which varies with disease. *Extent,* whether localized, discrete, diffuse, or confluent. *Character,* whether consisting of macules, papules, wheals, vesicles, pustules, bullae, or petechia.

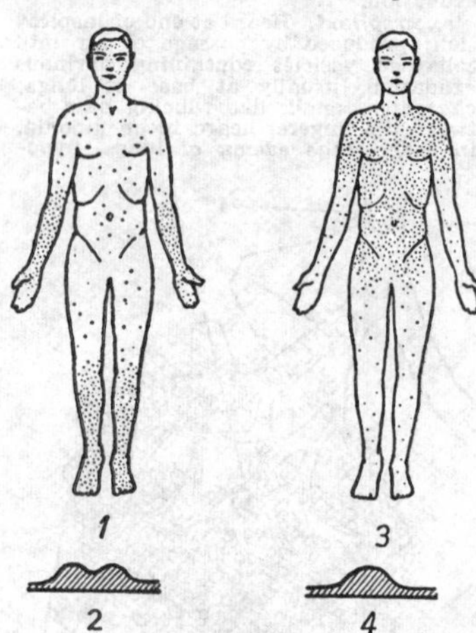

After Sears.

RASH.

1. Smallpox. 2. Vesicle of smallpox with umbilication. 3. Chickenpox. 4. Vesicle of chickenpox, no umbilication.

Course, whether onset is gradual or sudden. Note changes in character.

r., cable. An acneiform eruption caused by contact with chlorinated waxes.

r., canker. Scarlet fever, *q.v.*

r., diaper. SYN: *erythema gluteale.* Inflammation of skin of infants in the diaper area due to one or more diverse primary irritants. Improperly processed diapers and metabolic by-products of wastes are probable irritant sources.

r., drug. SYN: *dermatitis medicamentosa, q.v.* One caused by use of certain drugs, such as bromide or iodine. SEE: *idiosyncrasy; drug rashes.*

r., ecchymotic. A hemorrhagic rash, *q.v.*

r., enema. One caused by soap in an enema.

r., gum. A red, papular eruption of the chin and anterior chest area of children seen during teething. A form of miliaria due to excess saliva coming in contact with the skin. SYN: *strophulus.*

r., heat. Miliaria, *q.v.*

r., hemorrhagic. A rash consisting chiefly of hemorrhages or ecchymoses.

r., mulberry. R. seen in typhus fever; dusky in color.

r., nettle. Smooth, elevated, itchy, white patches. SYN: *hives; urticaria.*

r., red. SEE: *gum rash.*

r., rose. Any rose-colored rash. SYN: *roseola.*

r., serum. Rash accompanying serum sickness resulting from injection of a foreign serum. SEE: *serum sickness.*

r., tooth. SEE: *gum rash.*

r., vaccination. One that sometimes follows vaccination.

r., wandering. SEE: *geographic tongue.*

raspatory (răs′pă-tō″rĭ) [L. *raspatorium*]. File used in surgery, esp. for trimming surfaces of bone. SYN: *xyster.*

raspberry (răz′bĕr-ĭ) (red). COMP: Contains 3 times as much cellulose and less ash than strawberry.

RED: 100 gram portion. Calories: 57. Protein: 1.2 gm. Fat: 0.5 gm. Carbohydrate: 13.6 gm. Calcium: 22 mg. Iron: 0.9 mg. Vitamin A: 130 I.U. Ascorbic acid: 25 mg.

rasura, rasure (rā-sū′ră, rā′zhur) [L. *rasura*, a scraping]. 1. Process of scraping or shaving. 2. Scrapings or filings.

rat (răt) [A.S. *raet*]. A rodent (*rattus rattus*) found in and around human habitations. In addition to causing enormous economic loss, rats are of primary importance in the spread of human and animal diseases in that they serve as (1) hosts of various protozoans, flukes, tapeworms, and threadworms and (2) reservoirs of amebiasis, murine and scrub typhus, plague (bubonic, septicemic, pneumonic). The latter are transmitted to man principally through arthropods (rat flea). Rats also transmit *ratbite fever, q.v.* SEE: *flea.*

ratbite fever. Two diseases. One is caused by *Streptobacillus moniliformis* and the other *Spirillum minus.* Both are acute infectious diseases which occur following rat bite. *Spirillum minus* disease is rare in the U.S.A.

rate (rāt) [L. *rata*, a fixed amount]. The speed or frequency of occurrence of an event. Usually expressed with respect to time or some other known standard.

r., case fatality. The number of deaths per 100 cases of a specific disease.

r., morbidity. The number of cases per year of a certain disease in relation to the population in which they occur.

r., mortality. The frequency of deaths over a period of time in relation to the population (sick and well) in which the deaths occur. SYN: *death rate; mortality.*

ratio (rā′shĭ-ō) [L.]. Proportion.

r., A-G. Albumin-globulin ratio, *q.v.*

r., albumin-globulin. Ratio of albumin to globulin in blood plasma or serum. Normally 1.3:1 to 3.0:1. Values less than one (1) are indicative of pathologic conditions.

r., body-weight. Body weight in grams divided by body height in centimeters.

r., cell-color. Percentage of erythrocytes divided by percentage of hemoglobin.

r., concentration. Concentration of a solid in urine divided by its concentration in blood.

r., curative. Therapeutic ratio, *q.v.*

r., D-N. Dextrose-nitrogen ratio, *q.v.*

r., dextrose-nitrogen. Ratio of dextrose to nitrogen in urine.

r., G-N. Glucose-nitrogen ratio. SEE: *ratio, dextrose-nitrogen.*

r., mendelian. A ratio obtained between groups of offspring of parents which differ in certain unit characters. Ratios will vary depending on degree of dominance of one character over the other, whether parents are homozygous, etc.

r., sex. Ratio of males to females in a given population. Usually expressed as number of males per 100 females.

r., therapeutic. Ratio obtained by dividing effective therapeutic dose by minimum lethal dose.

ration (rā′shŭn) [L. *ratiō*, proportion]. Fixed allowance of food and drink for a certain period.

rational (răsh′ŭn-ăl) [L. *rationalis*, reasoning]. 1. Of sound mind. SYN: *sane.* 2. Reasonable or logical. 3. Employing treatments based on reasoning or general principles, opposed to empiric.

rationalization (răsh-ŭn-ăl-ĭ-zā′shŭn) [L. *rationalitās*, reasoning]. PSY: Rational or plausible explanation to justify behavior or belief actually determined by some process other than reason.

rattle (răt′l) [M.E. *ratelen*, probably of imitative origin]. A sound or rale heard on auscultation.

r., death. A gurgling sound or subcrepitant rale heard in the trachea of the dying.

raucous (raw′kŭs) [L. *racus*, hoarse]. Hoarse, strident, as the sound of a voice.

Rauwolfia (ro-wolf′ĭ-ă) [Named for Leonhard Rauwolf, a German botanist, 16th century]. The dried roots of *Rauwolfia serpentina.* Extracts are potent hypotensive agents and sedatives with low toxicity. Derivatives are *serpentine, serpentinine,* and *reserpine, q.v.*

rave (rāv) [O.Fr. *faver*, to rave]. To talk irrationally, as in delirium.

raving (rāv′ĭng) [O.Fr. *raver*, to rave]. 1. Irrational utterance. 2. Talking irrationally.

ray (rā) [L. *radius*, a rod, spoke]. 1. One of a number of lines diverging from a common center. 2. Line of propagation of any form of radiant energy, esp. light or heat; loosely, any narrow beam of light.

RS: *energy; e., radiant; fluorescence; heat; radiation; "roentgen-" words; spectrum; x-ray.*

r., actinic. A solar ray of the spectrum capable of producing chemical changes.

r., alpha. Ray composed of positively charged particles of helium derived from atomic disintegration of radioactive elements.

Velocity one-tenth that of light. They are completely absorbed by a thin sheet of paper, and possess powerful fluorescent, photographic and ionizing properties. They are less penetrative than the beta rays.

r., antirachitic. Ultraviolet ray from 2700 to 3020 A. U.

r., bactericidal. Ray between 1850 and 2600 A. U. which is strongly bactericidal.

r.'s, Becquerel's. Those from radium, uranium, and other radioactive substances.

r.'s, beta. Negatively charged electrons expelled from atoms of disintegrating radioactive elements.

r.'s, border, r.'s, borderline, r.'s, Bucky. SEE: *grenz rays.*

r.'s, canal. Positive rays in a vacuum tube going from anode toward cathode. Old name for positive ray.

r.'s, cathode. Negatively charged electrons discharged by the cathode through a vacuum, moving in a straight line and, upon hitting solid matter, producing roentgen rays.

r., characteristic. Secondary roentgen rays, the wavelengths of which are determined by the chemical constitution of the object that emits, transmits, or scatters them.

r., chemical. Actinic ray, *q.v.*

r., cosmic. Electromagnetic waves (radiation) coming from unknown sources in outer space. Cosmic rays have a short wavelength and exceptionally high velocity and penetrative power. SYN: *Millikan rays.*

r.'s, delta. Highly penetrative ether waves given off by radioactive substances.

r.'s, dynamic. Rays which are physically or therapeutically active.

r., erythema-producing. Ray bet. 1800 and 4000 A. U., which produces erythema, with those around 2540 and between 2050 and 3100 A. U. being most effective.

r., Finsen (or light). Ultraviolet radiation from the Finsen lamp.

r.'s, fluorescent roentgen. Secondary rays whose wavelengths are characteristic of the substance which emits them.

r. fungus. Genus of parasitic fungi with radiating formation.

r., gamma. Heterogeneous vibrations caused by electronic disturbance in atoms of radioactive elements during their disintegration; they appear identical with roentgen rays except that the wavelengths range from about 1.4 to 0.01 angstroms. They have high velocity and penetrative power. They lie bet. ultraviolet and roentgen rays.

r., grenz. Soft roentgen ray with an average wavelength of 2 angstroms (range from 1 to 3 angstroms); obtained with peak voltage of less than 10 kilovolts.

r.'s, hard. X-rays of short wavelength and great penetration.

r.'s, heat. Visible rays from 4000 to 7000 A. U. and infrared rays from 6000 to 14,000 A. U. The heating effect of visible rays on deeper tissue is proportionately stronger than that of infrared rays, because the visible rays have greater penetrating power. SEE: *heat.*

r.'s, Hertzian. Electromagnetic waves of great wavelength. Used in radio communication.

r.'s, infrared. Radiations just beyond the red end of the spectrum. Their wavelengths range between 7700 and 500,000 angstroms. The therapeutic range extends from about 7700 to about 14,000 angstroms.

r.'s, Lenard's. Cathode rays that have passed outside the discharge tube. SEE: *cathode ray.*

r., luminous. Visible ray.

r., medullary. SYN: *pars radiata, processes or rays of Ferrein.* One of many slender processes composed of straight tubules which project into the cortex from the bases of renal pyramids.

r.'s, Millikan. Cosmic rays, *q.v.*

r.'s, monochromatic. Rays characterized by a definite wavelength, as secondary rays.

r.'s, pigment-producing. Rays at 2500 and 3000 A. U. are most effective in causing pigmentation, a local response to irritation of cutaneous prickle-cells.

r., positive. Ray of positively charged ions which, in a discharge tube, go from the anode toward the cathode.

r., primary. Ray discharged directly from a radioactive substance, as the alpha, beta, and gamma rays.

r., roentgen. X-rays discovered by Wilhelm Konrad Roentgen. They have a penetrative power through opaque substances; used for photographing internal organs and parts, and for diagnostic and therapeutic purposes.

r.'s, scattered. Roentgen rays or gamma rays which, in their passage through a substance, have deviated in direction and also may have been changed by an increase in wavelength.

r.'s, Schumann. Rays in the region bounded bet. 1220 and 1850 angstroms.

r.'s, secondary. Roentgen rays emitted in all directions by any matter irradiated with roentgen rays.

r.'s, ultraviolet. Invisible rays of the spectrum which are beyond the violet rays, and of varying wavelengths. Of luminous ether which may be refracted, reflected, and polarized, but which will not traverse many substances impervious to the rays of the visible spectrum. They do not affect the retina, but rapidly destroy the vitality of bacteria. They produce photochemical and photographic effects.

r.'s, x. SEE: *roentgen rays.*

Raynaud's disease or syndrome (ra-nōz') [Maurice Raynaud, Paris physician, 1834-1881]. A condition caused by an abnormal degree of spasm of the blood vessels of the extremities, especially in response to cold temperature which would not affect a normal person.

Venous stasis follows in three stages: Local syncope, asphyxia, and gangrene. A vasomotor neurosis, characterized by local anemia, congestion or gangrene.

SYM: In one form, a part, usually a finger or toe, becomes pale, cold, anesthetic. After a time these phenomena disappear and are followed by redness, heat and tingling. Attacks may be excited by cold and come and go without damaging the part. In another form, affected part becomes swollen, dark, red, painful; if attack persists, bullae may appear and gangrene develop. Gangrenous areas often symmetrical, involving a finger on each hand, toe on each foot, or both ears. Hemoglobinuria may occur in, or replace, an attack.

PROG: Attacks persist, but life not endangered. In rare instances extensive gangrene develops and death follows. Gangrene may be absent in mild forms.

TREATMENT: Patients liable to attacks should be well protected from cold, frequent bathing and friction.

Rb. Symb. for *rubidium.*

RBC, rbc. Abbr. for *red blood count.*

R.C.D. Abbr. for *relative cardiac dullness.*

R. C. P. Royal College of Physicians.
R. C. S. Royal College of Surgeons.
R. D. A. Right dorsoanterior presentation position of the fetus.
R. D. P. Right dorsoposterior presentation position of the fetus.
R. E. Abbr. for *radium emanation* and for *right eye.*
Re. Symb. for *rhenium.*
re- [L.]. Prefix meaning *back* or *again.*
reaction (rē-ăk'shŭn) [L. *re,* back, + *actus,* acting]. 1. Response of an organism or part of it to a stimulus. 2. In Chem., a chemical process or change; the result of a test to determine the pH (hydrogen-ion concentration) of a solution and designated acid, neutral, or alkaline. 3. An opposing or counteraction. For reactions not listed here or given under their name, see *method, reflex, response, test.* 4. Emotional and mental state created by a situation.

FORMS OF REACTIONS: *Anesthesia Dolorosa*: Pain associated with anesthesia of a part, as in thalamic lesions.

Subjective Sensations: These may include causalgia, paresthesia, pseudomyelia paresthetica, a false sensation, as of movement in a paralyzed limb or part, or sensation of lack of movement in a moving limb.

r., affective. SEE: *affective psychosis; manic-depressive psychosis.*

r., alarm. The first stage in the *general adaptation syndrome* (G-A-S) which includes changes occurring in the body when subjected to stressful stimuli. Physiologic changes which occur are direct results of damage and/or shock or reactions of the body to defend itself against shock.

r., allergic. A reaction resulting from hypersensitivity to an antigen.

r., anamnestic. The reappearance of antibodies which may occur when an antigen is injected a considerable time after the first injection.

r., anaphylactic. That which follows injection or administration of a foreign substance to an animal which has been sensitized to it. The principal manifestation of the antigen-antibody reaction, *q.v.* Also called *anaphylaxis.*

r., anaphylactoid. R. similar to an anaphylactic reaction but not as severe. Induced by introducing into subject a substance to which he has not become hypersensitive.

r., antigen-antibody. The combination of molecules of an antigen with one or more molecules of its specific antibody.

r., atopic. SEE: *sensitivity, atopic.*

r., complement fixation. A test based on the principle that the complement enters into combinations formed between soluble or particulate antigens and antibody. Used for diagnosis of certain diseases, esp. syphilis.

RS: *complement.*

r., consensual. 1. An involuntary action. 2. A crossed reflex.

r., cross. A reaction between an antibody and an antigen which is not specific for the antibody but closely allied to the one which is.

r. of degeneration. The change in muscle reactivity to electricity, seen in lower motor neuron paralysis.

r., delayed. One occurring a considerable time after a stimulus, esp. a reaction such as inflammation of the skin occurring hours or days after exposure to the allergen.

r., false-positive. A positive reaction in a test, esp. test for syphilis, which is due to faulty technique or to presence of another disease.

r. formation. The checking of infantile impulses and tendencies, which might become those of an antisocial nature later or which might hold the individual upon an infantile level, and the attributes developed from such partial repressions as modesty, shame, or disgust.

r., immune. A reaction which demonstrates the presence of antibodies in the blood. Indicative of a high degree of immunity.

r., inflammatory. SEE: *inflammation.*

r., local. R. occurring at point of stimulation or injection of exciting substances.

r., myasthenic. Gradual decrease and eventually cessation of muscle contractions when a muscle is stimulated repeatedly by direct current.

r., neutral. In chemistry a reaction indicating absence of acid or alkaline properties. Expressed as pH 7.0.

r., ophthalmic. Local reaction of conjunctiva to introduction of toxins of tuberculosis and typhoid fever; more severe in those having the diseases.

r., quellung. SYN: *Neufeld's reaction.* The swelling of capsules of bacteria when mixed with their specific immune serum.

r., time. Time elapsing between application of a stimulus and the response to it.

r., transfusion. Reaction following transfusion of incompatible blood resulting from agglutination and hemolysis of red blood cells.

reactivate. To make active again, esp. the process of reactivating immune serum which has lost its potency by the addition of fresh normal serum, thus restoring the complement which had become inactive through age, heat, or other factors.

reactive depression (rē-ăk'tĭv dē-prĕsh'ŭn). PSY: A psychosis resulting from bereavement, sadness or a situation causing such emotions, lasting longer and more marked than the normal reaction.

reagent (rē-ā'jĕnt) [L. *rē,* again, + *agere,* to act]. 1. A substance involved in a chemical reaction. 2. A substance used to detect the presence of another substance. 3. PSY: Subject of a psychological experiment, esp. one reacting to a stimulus.

reagin (re-a'jin). 1. An antibody associated with atopic hypersensitivity; one associated with manifestations of hay fever, asthma, urticaria, angioedema, and infantile eczema. SEE: *sensitivity, atopic.* 2. A substance present in serum and cerebrospinal fluid which induces flocculation in complement fixation and similar tests.

r., atopic. Antibodies, present in naturally hypersensitive persons, which will produce passive hypersensitivity when injected into a normal subject.

reality principle (rē-ăl'ĭ-tĭ) [Fr. *réalité*]. The effect of necessity or external consideration, acting to control self-gratification, or of the ego's self-protective influences.

re"amina'tion. The restoration of an amino group to a compound from which one had previously been removed.

reanimate. To reactivate, restore to life, revive, resuscitate.

reapers' keratitis (rēp'ĕrs kĕr-ă-tī'tĭs). Keratitis caused by dust from grain.

Réaumur's thermometer (rā'o-mur). A thermometric scale having 0° for the freezing point, and 80° for the boiling point of water.

Readings changed to Centigrade by multiplying by 5/4, to Fahrenheit by multiplying by 9/4 and adding 32. SEE: *Thermometric Scale, Comparative.*

rebound. Response seen in reflexes in which sudden withdrawal of stimulus is followed by fresh activity such as a strong contraction following a moderate one, marked relaxation following moderate relaxation, or contraction replacing inhibition.

r. phenomenon. When a limb or a part is acting against a resistance and the resistance is suddenly removed, the limb will move forcibly in direction toward which effort was being directed.

recalcification (rē″kăl-sĭ-fĭ-kā′shŭn). The restoration of mineral salts to tissues from which they have been withdrawn.

recall (rē-kawl′) [" + A.S. *ceallian,* to call]. PSY: Act of bringing back to mind that which has been previously learned or experienced; reproduction.

recapitulation theory (rē″kă-pĭt-ū-lā′-shŭn) [L. *rē,* again, + *capitulum,* a section]. The theory that an individual in its development from the ovum to maturity passes through successive stages which approximate the series of adult ancestors from which that organism has descended. Summarized in the statement *ontogeny recapitulates phylogeny.*

receiver (rē-sēv′er) [L. *rē,* back, + *capere,* to take]. 1. Container for holding a gas or a distillate. 2. Apparatus for receiving electrical waves or current, for example, a radio receiver.

receptaculum (rē-sĕp-tăk′ū-lŭm) [L. a container]. A vessel or cavity in which a fluid is contained.

r. chyli. SYN: *cisterna chyli.* Inferior, pear-shaped, expanded portion of the lower end of the thoracic duct, near 1st and 2nd lumbar vertebrae, into which the right and left lumbar trunks, an intestinal trunk, and some thoracic vessels empty.

receptor (rē-sĕp′tor) [L. a receiver]. 1. Molecular group in cells which have a special affinity for toxins, amboceptors, etc. SEE: *Ehrlich's side chain theory.* 2. Group of cells functioning in reception of stimuli; a sense organ; endings of afferent (sensory) nerves.

r., auditory. The hair cells in the organ of Corti in cochlea of ear.

r., contact. A receptor which gives rise to a sensation such as touch, temperature, pain which can be localized in or on surface of body.

r., cutaneous. One which is located in the skin.

r., distance. SYN: *telereceptor.* A receptor which responds to stimuli originating at a distance from the body. Includes visual, auditory, and olfactory sense organs.

r., gravity. The hair cells of macula of utricle and saccule which respond to changes in position of the head and linear acceleration.

r., olfactory. The olfactory cells, bipolar nerve cells, found in olfactory epithelium, whose axons form fibers of olfactory nerve.

r., optic. The rods and cones of the retina.

r., proprioceptive. Muscle and tendon spindles, the receptors of the muscle or kinesthetic sense.

r., rotary. The hair cells in the cristae of the ampulla of semicircular ducts, which are stimulated by angular acceleration or rotation.

r., sensory. A sensory nerve-ending, a cell or group of cells, or a sense organ which, when stimulated, gives rise to an afferent or sensory impulse.

CLASSIFICATION: (a) *Exteroceptors,* those located on or near surface which respond to stimuli of outside world. Include eye and ear (*distance receptors*) and touch, temperature, and pain receptors (*contact receptors*). (b) *Interoceptors,* those in mucous linings of alimentary and digestive tracts which respond to internal stimuli. Also called *visceroceptors.* (c) *Proprioceptors,* those responding to stimuli arising within body tissues.

Receptors are also classified on the basis of nature of stimuli to which they respond: (a) *chemoreceptors,* those that respond to chemical substances (taste buds, olfactory cells, receptors in aortic and carotid bodies); (b) *pressoreceptors,* those that respond to pressure (receptors in aortic arch and carotid sinus); (c) *photoreceptors,* those that respond to light (rods and cones); (d) *tangoreceptors,* those that respond to touch (Meissner's corpuscle).

r., stretch. Neuromuscular and neurotendinar spindles and organs of Golgi which are stimulated by stretch. SEE: *receptor; proprioceptor.*

r., taste. The gustatory cells of the taste buds.

r., temperature. Krause's end-bulbs (receptors of cold) and Ruffini's corpuscles (receptors for warmth).

r., touch. Merkel's disks, Meissner's corpuscles, and nerve plexus about the roots of hairs.

re′cess. A small indentation, depression, or cavity. SEE: *recessus.*

r., cochlear. A small concavity lying between the two limbs of the vestibular crest in vestibule of ear which lodges the beginning of the cochlear duct.

r., elliptical. A small concavity lying superiorly and posteriorly on medial wall of vestibule which lodges the utricle.

r., epitympanic. SYN: *attic.* That portion of the tympanic cavity which lies above the level of tympanic membrane. It contains the head of the malleus and short limb of incus.

r., infundibular. A small projection of third ventricle which extends into infundibular stalk of hypophysis.

r., lateral, of fourth ventricle. One of two lateral extensions of the 4th ventricle, forming narrow pockets on each side and around upper portions of the restiform bodies.

r., lineal. SEE: *recess, omental.*

r., nasopalatine. A small depression on floor of nasal cavity near nasal septum. Lies immediately over incisive foramen.

r., omental. One of three pocket-like extensions of the omental bursa. The *superior recess* extends upward behind caudate lobe of liver, the *inferior recess* extends downward into great omentum, the *lienal recess* extends laterally to hilus of spleen.

r., optic. A pocket of the 3rd ventricle lying anterior to infundibular recess. It is bound inferiorly by optic chiasma.

r., pharyngeal. SYN: *fossa of Rosenmüller.* Recess in lateral wall of nasal pharynx lying above and behind opening to auditory tube.

r., pineal. A recess of roof of 3rd ventricle extending into stalk of pineal body.

r., pyriform. A deep depression in wall of laryngeal pharynx lying lateral to orifice of larynx. It is bounded laterally by thyroid cartilage and medially by cricoid and arytenoid cartilages. It is a common site for lodgement of foreign objects.

r., sphenoethmoidal. Small space in nasal fossa lying above sup. concha. Lies between ethmoid bone and ant. surface of body of sphenoid bone and posteriorly receives opening of sphenoidal sinus.

r., spherical. Recess on medial wall of vestibule of inner ear which accommodates the saccule.

r., suprapineal. A posterior extension of roof of 3rd ventricle forming a small cavity above pineal body.

r., tympanic membrane. One of two pouches of tympanic mucous membrane (anterior and posterior) lying between tympanic membrane and anterior and posterior malleolar folds.

r., umbilical. A dilatation on left main branch of portal vein which marks position where umbilical vein was originally attached.

reces'sion. The withdrawal of a part from its normal position.

r. of gums. SYN: *ulatrophia.* Shrinkage of gums away from necks of teeth.

recess'ive. Tending to recede or go back; lacking control.

r. character. In genetics a character which is a cross between two pure races or species does not express itself in the hybrid offspring being suppressed or "dominated" by its allelomorph. SEE: *gene; factor; heredity.*

r. gene. A gene which in the presence of its dominant allelomorph does not express itself.

recessus (rē-sĕs'ŭs) [L. cavity]. A small hollow or recess.

recidivation (re-cid"ĭ-va'shun). 1. The relapse of a disease. 2. The relapsing into crime.

recid'ivism. Habitual criminality; repetition of antisocial acts.

recid'ivist. A confirmed criminal. Also a patient, especially one with mental illness, who has repeated relapses, especially a mentally ill patient who relapses into behavior marked by antisocial acts.

recidiv'ity. Tendency to relapse or to return to a former condition.

recipe (rĕs'ĭ-pē) [L. *recipere,* to receive]. 1. [L.]. Take, indicated by the sign ℞. 2. A prescription or formula for a medicine

recipient (rē-sĭp'ĭ-ĕnt) [L. *recipiens,* receiving]. One who receives anything, especially the blood in transfusion. SEE: *donor.*

reciprocal (rē-sĭp'rō-kăl) [L. *reciprocus* turning backward and forward]. Interchangeable in character.

r. reception. Articulation with convex surface in one direction and concave surface in another.

Recklinghausen's canals [Friedrich D. von Recklinghausen, German pathologist, 1833-1910]. Rootlets of the lymphatics, minute spaces in connective tissue.

R.'s disease, and syndrome. Pigmentation of skin, multiple small fibrous tumors on same with tenderness along nerves, pain in joints, sluggishness, multiple neurofibromatosis.

R.'s tumor. An adenoleiomyofibroma on wall of the fallopian tube, or posterior uterine wall.

reclination (rĕk-lĭ-nā'shŭn) [L. *reclināre,* to lean back]. The turning of the eye lens covered with a cataract over into the vitreous to remove it from line of vision. SYN: *couching.*

recline (rē-klīn') [L. *reclināre,* to lean back]. To be in recumbent position; to lie down.

Reclus' disease (rĕ-klū'). Multiple, benign, cystic growths in the mammary gland.

recomposi'tion. The recombining of constituents or parts.

recompres'sion. Resubjecting a person to increased atmospheric pressure, a procedure used in the treatment of caisson disease (bends).

reconstituent (rē"kŏn-stĭt'ū-ĕnt) [L. *rē,* again, + *constituens,* constituting]. An agent that improves or strengthens one or more parts or functions of the body by replacing lost material. Ex: *calcium; iron; phosphorus.* SYN: *tonic.*

recover. To regain health after illness; to regain a former state of health. To regain a normal state as to *recover* from fright.

recovery. The process or act of recovering.

recrement (rĕk'rē-mĕnt) [L. *recrementum,* that which is separated back]. Secretion which, after having performed its function as the saliva or part of the bile, is reabsorbed into the blood.

recrementitious (rĕk"rē-mĕn-tĭsh'ŭs) [L. *recrementum,* that which is separated back]. Of the nature of a secretion which, having performed its function, is reabsorbed into the blood.

recrudescence (rē-krū-dĕs'ĕns) [L. *recrudescere,* to become raw again]. Return of symptoms. SYN: *relapse.*

recrudescent (rē-krū-dĕs'ĕnt) [L. *recrudescere,* to become raw again]. Assuming renewed activity.

recruitment (rē-kroot'mĕnt). Condition in which response in a reflex action increases to a maximum when a stimulus is prolonged even though strength of stimulus is unchanged; due to activation of increasingly greater numbers of motor neurons. Ex: If, while testing the patellar reflex, the normal patient clasps his hands together and attempts to pull them apart, the intensity of the reflex response will be increased.

r. of end organs. Increase in discharge from sensory end organs resulting from increase of stimulus accounted for by increase in number of end organs discharging and increase in frequency in discharge from each.

rectal (rĕkt'ăl) [L. *rectus,* straight]. Pert. to the rectum.

r. alimentation. Rectal feeding, *q.v.*

r. anesthesia. Introduction of anesthetic into rectum for local desensitization, used esp. in labor. SEE: *anesthesia, labor.*

r. crisis. Tenesmus and rectal pain in locomotor ataxia.

r. feeding. The introduction of nutrients in fluid form into the colon through the rectum. SYN: *nutrient enema, q.v.*

r. reflex. The normal desire to evacuate feces present in rectum.

rectalgia (rĕk-tăl'jĭ-ă) [L. *rectus,* straight, + G. *algos,* pain]. Pain in rectum.

rectectomy (rĕk-tĕk'tō-mĭ) [" + G. *ektomē,* excision]. Excision of the rectum or anus. SYN: *proctectomy.*

rectification (rĕk"tĭ-fĭ-kā'shŭn) [" + *-ficāre,* to make]. 1. The process of refining or purifying a substance. 2. Act of straightening or correcting.

rectified (rĕk'tĭ-fīd) [" + *-ficāre,* to make]. Made pure or straight. Set right.

r. spirit. One resulting from fractional or repeated distillation of alcohol, as whisky.

rectifier (rĕk'tĭ-fī"ĕr) [" + *-ficāre*, to make]. Transformation of an alternating current into a direct one.

rectitis (rĕk-tī'tĭs) [" + G. *-itis*, inflammation]. Inflamed condition of the rectum. SYN: *proctitis*.

recto- [L.]. Combining form meaning *straight, the rectum*.

rectocele (rĕk'tō-sēl) [L. *rectus*, straight, + G. *kēlē*, hernia]. Protrusion or herniation of posterior vaginal wall with anterior wall of rectum through the vagina. SEE: *cystocele*.

rectoclysis (rĕk-tŏk'lĭs-ĭs) [" + G. *klysis*, a washing out]. Slow introduction of fluid into rectum. SYN: *Murphy drip; proctoclysis*.

rectococcypexia (rĕk"tō-kŏk-sĭ-pĕks'sĭ-ă) [" + G. *kokkyx*, coccyx, + *pēxis*, fixation]. Fixation of rectum by suturing it to coccyx.

rectocolitis (rĕk"tō-kō-lī'tĭs) [" + G. *kōlon*, colon, + *-ītis*, inflammation]. Inflamed condition of rectum and colon. SYN: *proctocolitis*.

rectocystotomy (rĕk"tō-sĭs-tŏt'ō-mĭ) [" + G. *kystis*, bladder, + *tomē*, a cutting]. Incision of the bladder through rectum, usually to remove a calculus.

rectopexy (rĕk'tō-pĕks-ĭ) [" + G. *pēxis*, fixation]. Fixation of rectum by suturing to another part. SYN: *proctopexy*.

rectophobia (rĕk"tō-fō'bĭ-ă) [" + G. *phobos*, fear]. Morbid fear in those patients with rectal disease.

rectoplasty (rĕk'tō-plăs"tĭ) [L. *rectus*, straight, + G. *plassein*, to form]. Plastic operation on the anus and rectum. SYN: *proctoplasty*.

rectorrhaphy (rĕk-tor'ră-fĭ) [" + G. *raphē*, a sewing]. Suture of rectum and anus. SYN: *proctorrhaphy*.

rectoscope (rĕk'tō-skōp) [" + G. *skopein*, to examine]. A speculum to examine the rectum.

rectosigmoid (rĕk"tō-sĭg'moyd) [" + G. *sigma*, letter S, + *eidos*, form]. Upper part of rectum and adjoining portion of the sigmoid colon.

rectostenosis (rĕk"tō-stĕn-ō'sĭs) [" + G. *stenōsis*, a narrowing]. Stricture of the rectum.

rectostomy (rĕk-tŏs'tō-mĭ) [" + G. *stoma*, a mouth]. Creation of an artificial opening into the rectum to relieve stricture. SYN: *proctostomy, q.v.*

rectotomy (rĕk-tŏt'ō-mĭ) [" + G. *tomē*, an incision]. Incision for stricture of the rectum or other purposes. SYN: *proctotomy, q.v.*

rectourethral (rĕk"tō-ū-rē'thrăl) [L. *rectus*, straight, + G. *ourēthra*, urethra]. Concerning the rectum and urethra.

rectouterine (rĕk"tō-ū'ter-ĭn) [" + *uterus*, womb]. Concerning the rectum and uterus.

rectovaginal (rĕk"tō-văj'ĭn-ăl) [" + *vagina*, sheath]. Concerning the rectum and vagina.

rectovesical (rĕk"tō-vĕs'ĭk-ăl) [" + *vesica*, a small vessel]. Concerning the rectum and bladder.

rectum (rĕk'tŭm) [L. straight]. Lower part of large intestine, about 5 in. (12 cm.) long, bet. sigmoid flexure and the anal canal.

The centers for the defecation reflex are located in the medulla and 2nd, 3rd and 4th sacral segments.

PREPARATIONS SOMETIMES GIVEN BY RECTUM:

(1) *Chloral Hydrate:* Prescribed dose dissolved in 3 oz. of warm olive oil, 3 oz. of very warm milk, or 3 oz. of thin, boiled cornstarch water. This makes a good preparation or base in which to hold the medicine in suspension. The patient's pulse should be taken 5 minutes before and at 5-minute intervals for one-half hour after the administration, to observe the heart action. If untoward effects are noticed, action should be taken to prevent further absorption.

(2) *Paraldehyde:* Prescribed dose may be mixed with water in the proportion of 1 to 8, and in this ratio it may be mixed with thin starch water for rectal medication. There should be about 3 oz. of starch water.

(3) *Sodium Bicarbonate:* One teaspoonful, or 4 gm. to 500 cc., or 1 pint, of water aids in the expulsion of the bowel content. The neutralizing action on the acidity of the bowel content brought about by the sodium bicarbonate solution leaves the bowel soothed and with a bland reaction.

(4) *Glycerin:* One oz. is added to a pint of plain water. It will cause a good evacuation. One oz. of glycerin to 1 oz. of water will cause irritation of the lower bowel and precipitate an evacuation. This may be given with a bulb syringe.

(5) *Alum:* The alum enema consists of 1 quart of warm water and 1 oz. of powdered alum. This enema has a tendency to dry up intestinal flora and check fermentation.

RS: *anorectal; anus; archocele; archoptosis; archoptima; archorrhagia; archostenosis; caribi; cloaca; colon; feeding; hemorrhoid; "proct-" words; "rect-" words; sigmoid.*

rectus (rĕk'tŭs) [L. straight]. 1. Straight; not crooked. 2. Any straight muscle.

r. muscles. 1. Two external abdominal muscles, one on each side, from pubic bone to the ensiform cartilage and 5th, 6th, and 7th ribs. 2. Four short muscles of the eye, *exterior, interior, superior*, and *inferior*.

recumb'ency. State of leaning or reclining.

recumbent (rē-kŭm'bĕnt) [L. *recumbere*, to lean back]. 1. Lying down. SEE: *left lateral recumbent position, prone.* 2. Inactive, idle.

recuperation (rē-kū"per-ā'shŭn) [L. *recuperāre*, to recover]. Restoration to normal health.

recurrence (rē-kŭr'ĕns) [L. *rē*, again, + *currere*, to run]. Return of symptoms after a period of quiescence, as in recurrent fever and in yellow fever. SYN: *relapse*.

recurrent (rē-kur'ĕnt) [" + *currere*, to run]. Returning at intervals, as a fever.

r. fever. Relapsing fever, *q.v.*

re"curva'tion. The act of bending backwards.

recurve (rē-kurv') [" + *curvus*, curved]. Bend backward.

red (rĕd) [A.S. *rēad*]. A primary color of the spectrum.

r. blindness. Inability to see red hues. The most frequent color blindness.

r. blood cell. Blood corpuscle containing hemoglobin. SYN: *erythrocyte, q.v.*

r. lead. Lead tetroxide, Pb_3O_4; minium.

r. nucleus. Gray matter in the tegmentum of midbrain. SYN: *nucleus ruber*.

r. precipitate. Red mercuric oxide.

POISONING: SYM: Similar to mercuric chloride.

r. softening. Hemorrhagic softening of the brain and cord.

red. in pulv. Abbr. for *reductus in pulverum,* reduced to powder.

redia. Stage in life cycle of a trematode which follows the sporocyst. The organisms are sac-like structures, possessing an oral sucker and a blind gut. They arise parthenogenetically from germ masses within the sporocyst and in turn give rise to 2nd or 3rd generation rediae or to cercaria.

redintegration (rĕd-ĭn-tē-grā'shŭn) [L. *rē,* again, + *integrāre,* to make whole]. 1. Restitution of a part. 2. Restoration to health. 3. Recall by mental association.

red-out (red'out). A term used in aerospace medicine to describe what happens to the vision and central nervous system, i.e., seeing red and perhaps experiencing unconsciousness when the aircraft is doing part or all of an outside loop at high speed. The condition is due to engorgement of the vessels of the head including those of the retina.

redox. Abbr. for *oxidation-reduction.*

redressment (rē-drĕs'mĕnt) [Fr. *redressement*]. 1. Correction of a deformity. 2. Dressing of a wound more than once.

reduce (rē-dūs') [L. *rē,* back, + *ducere,* to lead]. 1. To restore to usual relationship, as the ends of a fractured bone. 2. To weaken, as a solution. 3. To diminish, as in bulk or weight.

reducible (rē-dūs'ĭ-bl) [" + *ducere,* to lead]. Capable of being replaced in a normal position, as a dislocated bone, a hernia, etc.

reducing agent. A substance which loses electrons easily, hence causes other substances to be reduced. Ex: *hydrogen sulfide, sulfur dioxide.*

reductase (rē-dŭk'tās) [" + " + *ase,* enzyme]. An enzyme accelerating process of reduction of chemical compounds.

reduction (rē-dŭk'shŭn) [L. *reductiō,* a leading back]. 1. Restoration to normal position, as a fractured bone or a hernia. 2. CHEM: A type of reaction in which hydrogen is taken up by the given compound, or oxygen is removed, or the valence of the metallic element is lowered. *Cf. oxidation.*

r. diet. One which reduces the caloric content sufficiently to cause loss of weight.

Normal metabolism must be preserved. Bulk, mineral, protein, vitamin, and water requirements must be maintained. Energy value should be 600 to 1500 calories below maintenance requirements. For a person of average size, this could be accomplished by a diet containing the following amounts of nutrients: Protein 60 gm.; carbohydrate 50 gm.; fat 45 gm.

r. division. SYN: *meiosis; miosis.* Division occurring in gametogenesis following synapsis in which diploid number of chromosomes is reduced to the haploid number (one half the diploid number).

redundant (re-dun'dent). More than necessary.

reduplicated (rē-dū'plĭ-kā"tĕd) [L. *rē,* back, + *duplicāre,* to double]. 1. Doubled. 2. Bent backward upon itself, as a fold.

reduplication (rē-dū"plĭ-kā'shŭn) [" + *duplicāre,* to double]. 1. A doubling, as of the heart sounds in some morbid conditions. 2. A fold.

Reduviidae (rĕd"ū-vē'ĭ-dē). A family of the order Hemiptera which includes the assassin bugs.

Reduvius (rē-dū'vĭ-ŭs). A genus of true bugs belonging to the family Reduviidae.

R. personatus. SYN: *masked hunter; kissing bug.* A species which normally feeds on other insects but sometimes attacks man inflicting painful bites about the face. In some individuals, these bugs may cause severe allergic symptoms.

re-education (rē"ĕd-ū-kā'shŭn) [L. *rē,* again, + *educāre,* to educate]. 1. Training of a disabled or mentally disordered individual to restore to him at least partial competence. 2. Physical means for restoring muscular tone and activity.

refec'tion. 1. Act of restoring after fatigue or exhaustion. 2. Recovery from symptoms of vitamin B-complex deficiency on a diet deficient in vitamin B. Thought to be due to bacterial synthesis of vitamins by intestinal bacteria.

referred pain (rē-ferd' pān). Pain felt in a part removed from its point of origin. SYN: *synalgia.*

refine (rē-fīn') [L. *rē,* back, + M.E. *fine,* finished]. To purify or render free from foreign material.

reflection (rē-flĕk'shŭn) [" + *flectere,* to bend]. 1. Condition of being turned back upon itself, as when the peritoneum passes from wall of a body cavity to and around an organ and back to the body wall. 2. The throwing back of a ray of radiant energy from a surface not penetrated. 3. Mental consideration of some subject matter.

reflector (rē-flĕk'tor) [" + *flectere,* to bend]. Device or surface which reflects waves of radiant energy or sound.

reflex (rē'flĕks) [L. *reflexus,* bent back]. An involuntary response to a stimulus; a reflex action. Reflexes are *specific* and *predictable* and are usually *purposeful* and *adaptive.* Reflexes depend upon an intact neural pathway between point of stimulation and responding organ (muscle or gland). This pathway is called *reflex arc.* In a simple reflex this includes: (a) a sensory receptor, (b) afferent or sensory neuron, (c) reflex center in brain or spinal cord, (d) one or more efferent neurons, and (e) an effector organ (muscle or gland). Most reflexes, however, are more complicated and include *internuncial* or *associative neurons* intercalated between afferent and efferent neurons.

RS: *Achilles jerk; areflexia; chemoreflex; chin jerk; conditioned; consensual; individual name; intestinal; jerk; reaction; reinforcement; Setschenow's center.*

r., abdominocardiac. A change in heart rate, usually a slowing, resulting from mechanical stimulation of abdominal viscera.

r., acquired. A conditioned reflex, *q.v.*

r. action. An involuntary response to a stimulus, a reflex, *q.v.*

r., after-discharge of. Reflex activity which persists for a time after cessation of the stimulus.

r's, allied. Reflexes initiated by several stimuli originating in widely separated receptors whose impulses follow the final common path to effector organ and reinforce one another.

r's, antagonistic. Two or more reflexes initiated simultaneously in different receptors which involve the same motor center but produce opposite effects. The most important or adaptive response takes place.

r. arc. The neural pathway or circuit between point of stimulation and responding organ in a reflex action. SEE: *reflex.*

r., autonomic. Any reflex involving the response of a visceral effector (cardiac muscle, smooth muscle, glands). Such reflexes always involve two efferent neurons (a preganglionic and postganglionic).

r., autonomic, true. A visceral response in which afferent impulses do not pass through central nervous system, but instead enter prevertebral ganglia where connections are made with efferent neurons.

r., axon. A reflex which does not involve a complete reflex arc, hence is not a true reflex. The afferent and efferent limbs of the reflex are branches of a single nerve fiber, the axon (axon-like dendrite) of a sensory neuron. Ex: vasodilation resulting from stimulation of skin.

r., biceps. Flexion of forearm upon percussion of tendon of biceps brachii.

r. center. A region usually in brain or spinal cord where impulses from an afferent limb of a reflex arc initiate impulses in the efferent limb.

r., conditioned. SYN: *conditioned response.* A reflex acquired as a result of training in which the cerebral cortex is an essential part of the neural mechanism. Any reflex not inborn or inherited.

r., consensual. SEE: *r., crossed.*

r., convulsive. Condition in which a weak stimulus will induce a convulsion resulting in widespread uncoordinated and purposeless actions. Seen in strychnine poisoning.

r., cranial. Any reflex whose center lies in the brain.

r., crossed. Reflex in which stimulation of one side of body results in response on opposite side.

r., deep. One caused by stimulation of parts beneath skin, like tendons or bones, as the jaw, elbow, wrist, triceps, knee and ankle jerk reflexes.

r., delayed. One not taking place until some seconds after application of stimulus.

r., elbow. Triceps reflex, *q.v.*

r., elementary. A typical reflex common to all vertebrates. Includes postural, flexion, stretch and extensor thrust reflexes.

r., extensor thrust. A quick and brief extension of a limb upon application of pressure to plantar surface.

r., inborn. An unconditioned reflex; an innate or inherited reflex.

r., indirect. A crossed reflex, *q.v.*

r's, inhibition of. The stoppage or prevention of a reflex action, as inhibiting a sneeze by pressure on facial nerve just under upper lip or through action of higher cerebral centers.

r., intersegmental. One in which several segments of spinal cord are involved.

r., intestinal. Myenteric reflex, *q.v.*

r., intrasegmental. One which involves only a single segment of the spinal cord.

r's, irradiation of. The spreading of reflexes through the central nervous system whereby impulses entering the cord in one segment activate motor neurons located in many segments.

r., kinetic. A labyrinthine reflex, *q.v.*

r., knee jerk. Extension of the leg resulting from percussion of patellar tendon. This is an example of a myotactic or stretch reflex of importance in the maintenance of posture.

The reflex is diminished or abolished in (a) lesions of the nerve supplying the muscle and tendon, (b) lesions of post. roots involving sensory pathway as in tabes dorsalis, (c) lesions of ant. root involving motor pathways, or (d) lesions of lower motor neurons in ant. horns of gray matter of spinal cord, as in poliomyelitis. If, however, the upper motor neuron is destroyed, muscle tone and the motor response are greatly increased. So-called pathologic reflexes under these conditions may appear (see Babinski's sign). Reflexes are also modified by higher centers—e.g., emotional tension increases the knee jerk (and muscle tension generally).

r., labyrinthine. A reflex, esp. a postural reflex, resulting from stimulation of receptors in semicircular ducts, utricle, and saccule of inner ear. Also called *kinetic* or *accelerator* reflex.

r., local. One which does not involve the central nervous system. Ex: the myenteric reflex which occurs even though extrinsic nerves to intestine have been cut.

r., long. One involving many segments of the spinal cord.

r., mass. Condition following a section of spinal cord in which a weak stimulus through irradiation brings about widespread responses due to release from inhibition of higher cortical centers.

r., monosynaptic. One involving only two neurons, an afferent and efferent.

r., myenteric. SYN: *intestinal reflex.* One caused by distention of intestine resulting in contraction above point of stimulation and relaxation below it.

r., myotatic. A stretch reflex, *q.v.*

r., near. Accommodation reflex, *q.v.*

r., nociceptive. A reflex initiated by a painful stimulus.

r., palm-chin. Vigorous stroking or scratching of the thenar eminence, producing contraction of the skin and lower lip muscles on the same side.

r., patellar. SEE: *knee jerk r.*

r., pathologic. Abnormal reflex due to disease and seen as one of its symptoms.

r., postural. Any reflex which is concerned with maintenance of posture.

r., pressor. A reflex which results in elevation of blood pressure brought about by constriction of arterioles.

r., pupillary. A beam of light striking the retina normally causes the pupil to contract (protective against excessive stimulation). The same effect results with accommodation to near objects.

r., righting. Any of the many reflexes which enable an animal to maintain the body in a definite relationship to the head and thus maintain its body right side up.

r., sexual. Reflexes concerned with sexual activities, esp. erection and ejaculation.

r., short. One involving one or a few segments of spinal cord.

r., somatic. One induced by stimulation of somatic sensory nerve endings.

r., spinal. A reflex whose center is in the spinal cord.

r., static. Those concerned with establishment and maintenance of posture when body is at rest.

r., statokinetic. Those occurring when body is moving, i.e., walking or running.

r., stretch. SYN: *myotatic reflex.* Contraction of a muscle as a result of stretching the same muscle.

r., superficial (cutaneous). R. caused by irritation of the skin or areas depending upon the spinal cord as a motor center, such as the *scapular, epigastric, abdominal, cremasteric, gluteal,* and *plantar reflexes,* or upon *centers in the medulla,* as *conjunctival, pupillary* and *palatal reflexes.*

r., tendon. Deep r. obtained by tapping skin over tendon of a muscle sharply.

It is exaggerated in disease of an upper neuron, and diminished or lost in disease of lower neuron.

r., triceps. Sharp extension of forearm resulting from tapping of triceps tendon while arm is held loosely in bent position.

r., unconditioned. A natural or inherited reflex action; one not acquired.

r., vascular. A vasomotor reflex, *q.v.*

r., vasomotor. Constriction or dilatation of a blood vessel in response to a stimulus.

r., visceral. Any reflex induced by stimulation of visceral nerves.

r., visceromotor. Contraction or tenseness of skeletal muscles resulting from painful stimuli originating in visceral organs.

reflexogenic (rē-flĕks"ō-jĕn'ĭk) [L. *reflexus,* bent back, + G. *gennan,* to produce]. Causing a reflex action.

reflexograph (rē-flĕks'ō-grăf) [" + G. *graphein,* to write]. Device for charting a reflex.

reflexometer (rē-flĕks-ŏm'ĕt-ĕr) [" + G. *metron,* a measure]. Instrument for measuring force of the tap required to excite a reflex.

reflexophil (rē-flĕks'ō-fĭl) [" + G. *philein,* to love]. Characterized by activity of, or exaggerated, reflexes.

reflexotherapy (rē-flĕks-ō-ther'ă-pĭ) [" + G. *therapeia,* treatment]. Treatment by manipulation, anesthetizing, or cauterizing an area distant from seat of the disorder. SEE: *spondylotherapy; zone therapy.*

reflux (rē'flŭks) [L. *rē,* back, + *fluxus,* flow]. A return or backward flow. SYN: *regurgitation, 2.*

refract (rē-frăkt') [L. *refractus,* from *refringere,* to break back]. 1. To turn back. 2. To deflect a light ray. 3. To detect errors of refraction in the eyes and to correct them.

refracta dosi (rē-frak'tă dō'sī) [L.]. In divided doses, denoting a definite amt. of a drug taken within a given time in a number of fractional equal parts.

refraction (rē-frăk'shŭn) [L. *refractiō,* from *refringere,* to break back]. 1. Deflection from a straight path, as of light rays as they pass through media of different densities; the change of direction of a ray when it passes from one medium to another of a different density. 2. Determination of amount of ocular refractive errors and their correction.

RS: *ametropia; anisometropia; astigmatism; emmetropia; hypermetropia; myopia; presbyopia.*

r., angle (of). The angle formed by a refracted ray of light with a line perpendicular to surface at point of refraction.

r., coefficient of. The quotient or sine of angle of incidence divided by sine of angle of refraction.

r., double. Birefringence or possessing more than one refractive index.

r., dynamic. Static refraction of the eye plus that accomplished by accommodation; the reciprocal of the near-point distance.

r., errors of. SYN: *ametropia.* Condition in which parallel rays of light are not brought to a focus upon the retina because of a defect in shape of eyeball or in refracting media of the eye.

r., index of. 1. Ratio of angle made by incident ray with the perpendicular (angle of incidence) to that made by emergent ray (angle of refraction). 2. The ratio of speed of light in air to its speed in another substance. The refractive index of water is 1.33 of crystalline lens, 1.413.

r., ocular. Refraction of the eye, *q.v.*

r. of the eye. Ocular refraction. Refraction brought about by refractive media of the eye (cornea, aqueous humor, crystalline lens, vitreous body).

r., static. Refraction of the eye when accommodation is at rest or paralyzed.

refractionist (rē-frăk'shŭn-ĭst) [L. *refractiō,* from *refringere,* to break back]. One skilled in determining and correcting ocular refractive errors by means of glasses.

refractive (rē-frăkt'ĭv) [L. *refractus,* from *refringere,* to break back]. Concerning refraction.

r. index. SEE: *refraction, index of.*

r. power. The degree to which a transparent body deflects a ray of light from a straight path. SEE: *diopter.*

refractometer (rē-frăk-tŏm'ĕt-ĕr) [" + G. *metron,* a measure]. Device for measuring the refractive power, as of the eye.

refractory (rē-frăk'tō-rĭ) [L. *refractus,* from *refringere,* to break back]. 1. Obstinate, stubborn. 2. Resistant to ordinary treatment. 3. Resistant to stimulation, said of muscle or nerve.

r. period, relative. Period of relaxation of a muscle during which excitability is depressed. If stimulated, it will respond but a stronger stimulus is required and response is less.

refracture (rē-frăk'chūr) [L. *rē,* again, + *frangere,* to break]. 1. To break again, as a bone set wrongly. 2. Rebreaking of a fracture united in the wrong position.

refrangible (rē-frăn'jĭ-bl) [" + *frangere,* to break]. Capable of refraction.

refresh (rē-frĕsh') [O.Fr. *refreschir,* to renew, from L. *rē,* again, + *friscus,* new]. 1. To restore strength; to relieve from fatigue; to renew; to revive. 2. To scrape epithelial covering from two opposing surfaces of a wound to cause them to unite.

refrigerant (rē-frĭj'ĕr-ănt) [L. *rē,* again, + *frigerāre,* to make cold]. 1. Allaying heat or fever; cooling. 2. Medicine or agent which relieves thirst and is cooling or reduces a fever. SEE: *algefacient.*

r. gases. A number of these gases are used in ordinary household refrigerators; poisoning due to leaks, faulty connections or breakage, and gas dissipated into atmosphere may occur.

refrigeration (rē-frĭj"ĕr-ā'shŭn) [L. *rē,* back, + *frigerāre,* to make cool]. Cooling; reduction of heat.

r. anesthesia. Anesthesia resulting from cold such as that produced in a limb by immersion in cold water.

r. therapy. SYN: *cryotherapy.* Use of low temperatures as a therapeutic procedure. SEE: *hypothermia.*

refringent. Refractive, *q.v.*

refusion (rē-fū'zhŭn) [L. *rē,* back, + *fusiō,* a pouring]. The return of blood into the circulatory system after having been removed from the same patient.

regeneration (rē-jĕn″ĕr-ā′shŭn) [" + *generāre,* to beget]. Repair, regrowth, or restoration of a part, as tissues. Opp. of *degeneration, q.v.*

regimen (rĕj′ĭ-mĕn) [L. guidance, from *regere,* to rule]. 1. Regulation of diet, sleep, exercise, and manner of living to improve or maintain health. 2. Hygiene.

region (rē′jŭn) [L. *regiō,* a boundary line]. A portion of the body with natural or arbitrary boundaries. SEE: *abdomen.*

RS: *epigastrium; inguinal; Kiesselbach's area; temple.*

regional (rē′jŭn-ăl) [L. *regiō,* a boundary line]. Concerning a region.

register. 1. The compass or range of a voice. 2. A series of tones of like quality or character, as low or high register, chest or head register, etc.

registrant (rĕj′ĭs-trănt) [L. *registrans* registering]. A nurse who is named on the books of a registry as being "on call" or available to be called for duty.

registrar (rĕj′ĭs-trar) [L. *registrans,* registering]. The official manager of a registry.

registra′tion. The act of recording, such as births, deaths, etc.

registry (rĕj′ĭs-trĭ) [Fr. *registrer,* from L. *registrum*]. An office or book where a list of nurses ready for duty is kept; a placement bureau for nurses.

regression (rē-grĕsh′ŭn) [L. *regressiō,* a going back]. 1. A turning back or return to a former state. 2. A return of symptoms. 3. Retrogression. 4. IN PSY. an abnormal return to earlier reaction, characterized by mental state and behavior inappropriate to the situation. Regression may occur as a result of frustration or in states of fatigue, dreams, hypnosis, intoxication, illness, and in certain psychoses (schizophrenia).

r., filial. In biology, tendency of offspring to deviate less from the average of a population than their parents.

regressive (rē-grĕs′sĭv) [L. *regressiō,* a going back]. Concerning or marked by regression.

regular (rĕg′ū-lar) [L. *regula,* a rule]. 1. Conforming to rule or custom. 2. Methodical, steady in course, as pulse. SYN: *normal; typical.*

regula′tion. 1. State of being controlled or directed. 2. The ability of an individual such as a developing embryo to develop normally in spite of experimental modifications.

r. development. IN EMBRY., condition in which a single blastomere or a portion of an embryo can give rise to an entire whole embryo. Opp. of *mosaic development, q.v.*

regula′tive. Pert. to regulation.

regulator. A device for adjusting or controlling the rate of flow or administration of fluids, oxygen, blood, etc.

regurgitant (rē-gŭr′jĭt-ănt) [L. *rē,* back, + *gurgitāre,* to flood]. Throwing or flowing back in a direction opposite to the normal.

regurgitation (rē-gŭr-jĭ-tā′shŭn) [L. *rē,* back, + *gurgitāre,* to flood]. 1. Return of solids or fluids to the mouth from the stomach. It may be a complication of diphtheria and it occurs in paralysis of the soft palate, and in some digestive disorders. SEE: *taste.* 2. Return of blood backward through a defective heart valve.

r., aortic. Backflow of blood into left ventricle as a result of incompetent aortic valves.

r., cardiac. Backward flow of blood through the aortic, mitral, or tricuspid valves due to incomplete closure.

r., duodenal. Return flow of chyme from duodenum to stomach.

r., functional. R. not due to valvular disorder but to dilatation of ventricles, the great vessels, or valve rings.

r., mitral. Backflow of blood from left ventricle into left atrium resulting from imperfect closure of mitral or bicuspid valve.

r., pulmonic. Backflow of blood from pulmonary artery into the right ventricle.

r., tricuspid. Backflow of blood from the right ventricle into the right atrium.

rehabilitation (rē″hă-bĭl″ĭ-tā′shŭn) [L. *rehabilitāre*]. Process of restoring, or of undergoing restoration, to health or efficiency, as a person physically handicapped.

rehalation (rē-ha-lā′shŭn) [L. *rē,* again, + *halāre,* to breathe]. Rebreathing process occasionally employed in anesthesia.

Reichert's cartilage (rī′kerts) [Karl Bogislaus Reichert, German anatomist, 1811-1884]. The second branchial arch of the embryo which gives rise to stapes, styloid process, stylohyoid ligament, and lesser cornua of hyoid bone.

Reichmann's disease (rīk′mahnz). Excessive gastric secretion without intermission. SYN: *gastrochronorrhea; gastrorrhea; gastrosuccorrhea.*

Reid's base line (rēds) [Robert W. Reid, Scottish anatomist, 1851-1938]. One extending from lower edge of the orbit to center of aperture of external auditory canal backward to center of occipital bone.

Reil's island (rīlz) [Johann C. Reil, German anatomist, 1759-1813]. Three or more small convolutions at bottom of fissure of Sylvius. SYN: *insula* [NA]; *island of Reil, q.v.*

reimplantation (rē″ĭm-plăn-tā′shŭn) [L. *rē,* again, + *in,* into, + *plantāre,* to set]. Replacement of a part from where it has been taken out, as a tooth.

reinfection (rē″ĭn-fĕk′shŭn) [" + *inficere,* to make into]. A second infection with the same organism.

reinforcement (rē″ĭn-fors′mĕnt) [L. *rē,* again, + O. Fr. *enforcier,* to strengthen]. Strengthening; augmentation of force.

r. of reflex. Strengthening of the response to one stimulus by concurrent action of another; the exaggeration of a reflex by nervous activity elsewhere.

Thus, during the raising of a heavy weight the knee jerk is stronger.

re″infu′sion. The reinjection of blood serum or cerebrospinal fluid.

reinnervation (rē″ĭn-ner-vā′shŭn) [L. *rē,* again, + *in,* into, + *nervus,* nerve]. 1. Anastomosis of a paralyzed part with a living nerve. 2. Grafting of a fresh nerve for restoration of function in a paralyzed muscle.

reinoculation (rē″ĭn-nŏk-ū-lā′shŭn) [L. *rē,* again, + *in,* into, + *oculus,* bud]. A second inoculation with the same virus or organism following a previous one. SEE: *reinfection.*

Reinsch's test (rīnsh'ez). [Adolf Reinsch, German physician, 1862-1916]. A test for presence of arsenic, antimony, or mercury.

re"integra'tion. In Psy., the resumption of normal behavior and mental functioning following disintegration of personality in mental illness.

reinversion (rē"ĭn-ver'shŭn) [L. *rē*, again, + *in*, into, + *versiō*, a turning]. Correction of an inverted organ, as of an inverted uterus, by pressure on the fundus.

Reissner's membrane. Syn: *membrana vestibularis.* Delicate membrane separating the cochlear canal from scala vestibuli.

rejuvenation (rē-jū-ve-nā'shŭn) [L. *rē*, again, + *juvenis*, young]. A return to youthful conditions or to the normal.

rejuvenescence (rē-jū-ve-nĕs'ĕns) [" + *juvenis*, young]. The renewal of youth or return to earlier stage of existence.

relapse (re-lăps') [L. *relapsus*, slipping back]. Recurrence of a disease or symptoms after apparent recovery.

relapsing (rē-lăps'ĭng) [L. *relapsus*, slipping back]. Recurring after apparent recovery.

r. fever. An infectious disease marked by intermittent attacks of high fever.

Etiol: Several species of spirochetes belonging to genus *Borrelia* and transmitted by head lice, body lice, and ticks of the genus *Ornithodorus.*

Treatment: Symptomatic treatment with bed rest. Penicillin and broad-spectrum antibiotics have replaced the use of arsenicals except in cases where spirochetes are resistant. The use of antipyretics and antinauseants may be indicated and dehydration and electrolyte imbalance should be combated by parenteral injections.

relax [L. *relaxare*, to ease]. To decrease tension or intensity, or to be rid of strain, anxiety and nervousness.

relaxant (rē-lăks'ănt) [L. *rē*, back, + *laxāre*, to loosen]. 1. Related to or producing relaxation. 2. A drug which reduces tension. 3. A laxative.

relaxation (rē-lăks-ā'shŭn) [" + *laxāre*, to loosen]. 1. A lessening of tension or activity in a part. 2. Phase or period in a single muscle-twitch following contraction in which tension decreases, fibers lengthen, and muscle returns to resting position.

r., general. R. which includes practically the entire body lying down.

r., heat of. That portion of initial heat about 35% in muscle activity produced during relaxation.

r., local. R. limited to a particular muscle group or to a part.

relaxed move'ment (rē-lăksd'). Form of bodily movement which the operator carries through without the assistance or resistance of the patient. Syn: *passive exercise.*

relaxin (rē-lăks'ĭn). A hormone present in the serum of pregnant animals and corpus luteum of sows. In those animals it facilitates delivery of the young by relaxing the pelvic ligaments and dilating the cervix.

relief (rē-lēf') [O.Fr. *relief*]. Alleviation or removal of a distressing or painful symptom.

relieve [L. *relevare*, to lighten]. To provide relief.

R.E.M. Abbreviation for *rapid eye movement.* Movement of the closed eyes observed or recorded during sleep. Movements occur while the subject is dreaming.

rem. Abbreviation for roentgen equivalent (in) man.

Remak's axis cylinder (ra'mahk). The conducting part of a nerve.

R's. band. The axis cylinder of a neuron.

R's. fibers. The nonmedullated nerve fibers.

R's. ganglion. A group of nerve cells in coronary sinus near its entry into right atrium.

R's. sign or symptom. 1. Polyesthesia. A single stimulus is perceived as if it were several stimuli applied in separate locations. 2. Delay in perception of stimuli. Both are seen in *tabes dorsalis.*

remedial (rē-mē'dĭ-ăl) [L. *remedialis*, pert. to a remedy]. Curative; intended for a remedy.

remedy (rĕm'ĕd-ĭ) [L. *remedium*]. 1. Anything that relieves or cures a disease. 2. To cure or relieve a disease.

r., local. Agent to relieve a local condition, as a sore.

r., systemic. Agent to relieve or cure a disease affecting the entire organism.

remission (rē-mĭsh'ŭn) [L. *remissiō*, a sending back]. Lessening of severity, or abatement of symptoms.

remittent (rē-mĭt'ĕnt) [L. *rē*, back, + *mittere*, to send]. Alternately abating and returning at certain intervals.

r. fever. A fever alternately abating and returning, without intervals of afebrility. See: *malaria.*

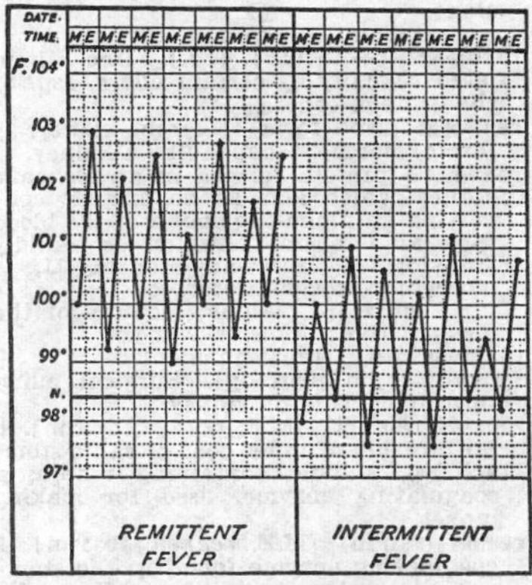

ren (pl. *renes*) [L.]. The kidney.

r. amyloidens. Amyloid degeneration of the kidneys.

r. mobilis. Movable kidney.

r. unguiformis. Horseshoe kidney.

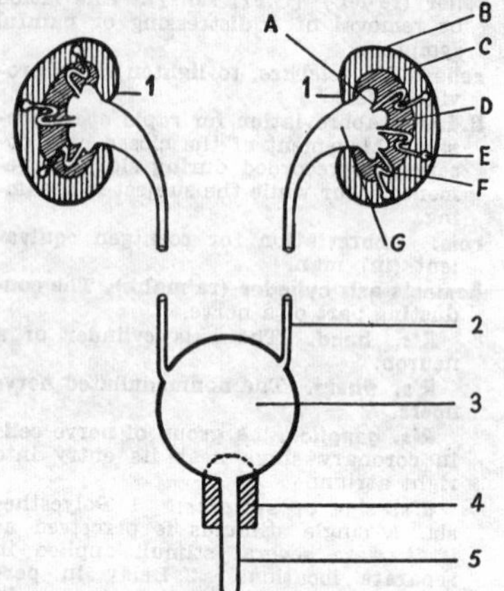

After Sears.

RENAL TRACT. DIAGRAM OF THE
1. Kidney. 2. Ureter. 3. Bladder. 4. Prostate. 5. Urethra. A. Pyramid. B. Capsule. C. Cortex. D. Medulla. E. Glomerulus. F. Tubule. G. Pelvis.

renal (rē'năl) [L. *rēnalis*, pert. to kidney]. 1. Pert. to the kidney. 2. Shaped like a kidney.

r. clearance test. A kidney function test based on the ability of the kidney to eliminate a given substance in a standard time. Urea, phenolsulfonphthalein (PSP), Diodrast and other substances are employed. Normal urea clearance is 75, i.e., the quantity of urea removed from circulation in one minute equals that contained in 75 cc. of blood. Diodrast clearance is 500 to 700 cc./min. in females and 560 to 830 in men.

r. insufficiency. The reduced capacity of the kidney to perform its functions.

r. tubule. A nephron, *q.v.*

renifleur (rā-nĭ-flur') [Fr.]. One stimulated sexually by certain odors, esp. by the urine of others.

reniform (ren'ĭ-form) [L. *rēn*, kidney, + *forma*, shape]. Shaped like a kidney.

ren'in. A protein formed in an ischemic kidney which acts as an enzyme converting an alpha-2-globulin of the blood into angiotensin I which is rapidly transformed into angiotensin II, a powerful vasoconstrictor.

r. substrate. $Alpha_2$ globulin of the plasma. SYN: *hypertensinogen.*

renipuncture (rĕn"ĭ-pŭnk'chŭr) [" + *punctūra*, a piercing]. Surgical puncture of capsule of kidney.

rennet (rĕn'nĕt) [M.E. *rennen*, to run]. 1. An infusion of inner coat of calf's stomach. 2. A fluid containing rennin, a coagulating enzyme, used for making junket.

rennin (rĕn'ĭn) [M.E. *rennen*, to run]. A coagulating enzyme found in the stomach of ruminants, which curdles milk. It is the active principle of rennet. It acts on caseinogen in the presence of calcium ions converting it to insoluble casein.

renninogen, rennogen (rĕn-ĭn'ō-jĕn, rĕn'ō-jĕn) [A.S. *rennen*, to run, + G. *gennan*, to produce]. Antecedent or zymogen from which rennin is formed. The inactive form of rennin.

renogastric (rĕn-ō-găs'trĭk) [L. *rēn*, kidney, + G. *gastēr*, belly]. Concerning the kidney and stomach.

renogram (re'no-gram). 1. List of the results of a group of kidney function tests. 2. Record of rate of removal from the blood by the kidneys of an intravenously injected dose of radioactive iodine (I^{131}).

renography (rē-nŏg'ră-fĭ) [" + G. *graphein*, to write]. Study of the kidney by means of an x-ray picture.

renointestinal (rĕn"ō-ĭn-tĕs'tĭn-ăl) [" + *intestinum*, intestine]. Concerning the kidney and the intestine.

renopathy (rĕn-ŏp'ăth-ĭ) [" + G. *pathos*, disease]. Any pathological condition of the kidneys.

renotrophic (rĕn-ō-trŏf'ĭk). Having the ability to induce hypertrophy of the kidney.

reovirus (re'o-vi-rus). Viruses found in the respiratory and digestive tracts of apparently healthy persons. Their exact importance in producing disease is not known. This group of viruses was formerly classed as *Echo virus, type 10.*

repair (rē-pār') [L. *reparāre*, to prepare again]. To remedy, replace or heal, as a wound or a lost part.

repell'ance. Condition in which certain individuals are relatively immune to bites of arthropods.

repellent (rē-pĕl'ĕnt) [L. *repellere*, to drive back]. 1. An agent which repels noxious organisms such as insects, ticks, and mites. Repellents may be applied to surface of body as a liquid, or dust, or they may be used to impregnate clothing. 2. Reducing a swelling. 3. That which lessens a swelling.

repercolation (rē"per-kō-lā'shŭn) [L. *re*, again, + *percolāre*, to filter]. Repeated percolation using same materials.

repercussion (rē-per-kŭsh'ŭn) [" + *percussiō*, a striking]. 1. Reciprocal action. 2. Action involved in causing subsidence of a swelling, tumor or eruption. 3. OB: Diagnosis of pregnancy by insertion of a finger into the vagina to push the uterus, causing embryo to rise and fall. SYN: *ballottement.*

re"percuss'ive. Causing repercussion; an agent which repels; a repellent.

replacement. The act of replacing.

r. bone. SYN: *substitution bone, cartilage bone, endochondral bone.* Bone which is formed in cartilage which precedes the definitive bone.

replanta'tion. Planting again.

r. of a tooth. Replacement of a tooth which has been removed accidentally or otherwise from its socket.

repletion (rē-plē'shŭn) [L. *repletiō*, a filling up]. 1. Condition of being full or satisfied. 2. Fullness of blood. SYN: *plethora.*

re"polariza'tion. Reestablishment of a polarized state in a muscle or nerve fiber following contraction or conduction of a nerve impulse.

report'able diseases. Diseases which must be reported by the physician to the health authorities. There are six diseases which, by international sanitary regulations, are universally required to be reported. They are *cholera, plague, louse-borne relapsing fever, smallpox, louse-borne typhus fever,* and *yellow fever.*

List of Reportable Diseases

1. Actinomycosis.
2. Acute infectious conjunctivitis (ophthalmia neonatorum).
3. Ankylostomiasis (hookworm).
4. Anthrax.
5. Botulism and other forms of food poisoning.
6. Chancroid.
7. Chickenpox.
8. Cholera (Asiatic).
9. Dengue.
10. Diphtheria.
11. Dog bites.
12. Dysentery (amebic).
13. Dysentery (bacillary and other infectious types).
14. Epidemic (lethargic) encephalitis.
15. Erysipelas.
16. Favus.
17. German measles.
18. Glanders.
19. Gonorrhea.
20. Granuloma inguinale.
21. Impetigo contagiosa (in institutions).
22. Influenza, epidemic.
23. Leprosy.
24. Malaria.
25. Measles.
26. Meningitis, epidemic (cerebrospinal fever, meningococcus meningitis).
27. Mumps.
28. Pellagra.
29. Paratyphoid fever.
30. Plague.
31. Pneumonias, the primary and the pneumonias complicating influenza, measles and whooping cough.
32. Poisonings, heavy metals, drugs, occupational and other poisonings.
33. Poliomyelitis, acute anterior (infantile paralysis).
34. Psittacosis.
35. Puerperal septicemia.
36. Rabies.
37. Rocky Mountain spotted or tick fever.
38. Scarlet fever.
39. Septic sore throat.
40. Smallpox.
41. Syphilis.
42. Tetanus.
43. Trachoma.
44. Trichinosis.
45. Tuberculosis (pulmonary).
46. Tuberculosis (other than pulmonary).
47. Tularemia.
48. Typhoid fever.
49. Typhus.
50. Undulant fever and Malta fever (brucellosis).
51. Vincent's angina and other anginas.
52. Whooping cough.
53. Yellow fever.

reposition (rē-pō-zish'ŭn) [L. *repositio*, a replacing]. Restoration of an organ or tissue to its correct or original position.

repositor (rē-pŏz'ĭt-or) [L. *repositio*, a replacing]. Instrument for restoring a tissue or an organ to its normal position.

***r.*, *inversion*.** Instrument for replacement of an inverted uterus.

***r.*, *uterine*.** A lever to replace the uterus when out of normal position.

repression (rē-prĕsh'ŭn) [L. *repressus*, from *reprimere*, to check]. Psy: Refusal to entertain distressing or painful ideas, thus submerging them in the unconscious where they continue to exert their influence upon the individual. Psychoanalysis seeks to discover and to release these repressions.

reproduction (rē-prō-dŭk'shŭn) [L. *rē*, again, + *productio*, production]. 1. Process by which plants and animals give rise to offspring. 2. The creation of a similar structure or situation; the act of duplicating.

***r.*, *asexual*.** R. in which sex cells are not involved, as by fission or budding.

***r.*, *sexual*.** Syn: *syngamy*. R. by means of sexual or germ cells. Usually a male cell (spermatozoon) fuses with a female cell egg or ovum. Sometimes ova may develop without fertilization. See: *parthenogenesis*.

reproductive (rē-prō-dŭk'tĭv) [L. *rē*, again, + *producere*, to produce]. Concerning, or employed in, reproduction.

repulsion (rē-pŭl'shŭn) [L. *repulsio*, a thrusting back]. 1. Act of driving back. 2. The force exerted by one body on another to cause separation.

RES. Abbr. for *reticuloendothelial system*.

research [Fr. *rechercher*, to research]. Scientific and diligent study, investigation or experimentation in order to establish facts and analyze their significance.

***r.*, *clinical*.** Research done more or less at the bedside rather than just in the laboratory.

***r.*, *laboratory*.** Research done principally in the laboratory.

***r.*, *medical*.** Research concerned with any phase of medical science.

resect. To cut off or to cut out a portion of a structure or organ, as to cut off the end of a bone or to remove a segment of the intestine.

resectable (re-sek'tă-bl). Able to be removed, especially by surgical means. Usually used in reference to malignant growths which can be completely removed by use of surgery.

resection (rē-sĕk'shŭn) [L. *resectio*, a cutting off]. Partial excision of a bone or other structure.

***r.*, *window*.** Resection of a portion of the nasal septum after reflection of a flap of mucous membrane; also called *submucous resection*.

resectoscope (rē-sĕk'tō-skōp) [L. *resectus*, cutting back, + G. *skopein*, to examine]. An instrument for resection of prostate gland through the urethra.

resectoscopy (rē-sĕk-tŏs'kō-pĭ) [" + G. *skopein*, to examine]. Resection of the prostate through the urethra.

reserpine (rē-serp'ĭn). A chemically pure derivative of *Rauwolfia serpentina*. An old snake root remedy used in India for centuries for snake bite, mental illness, anxiety states. It lowers blood pressure and acts to cause the person to become tranquil.

reserve (rē-zerv') [L. *reservāre*, to keep back]. 1. That which is held back for future use. 2. Self control of one's feelings and thoughts.

***r. air*.** Additional amount of air that can be expelled from the lungs over the normal quantity, 1200-1600 cc.

***r.*, *alkali*.** Alkali content of body available for neutralization of acid. See: *alkaline reserve*.

***r.*, *cardiac*.** The ability of the heart to increase cardiac output to meet the needs of the body.

reservoir of infection. A source of supply of an infectious agent or disease. These may be man, animals, plants or organic matter which will allow an infectious agent to live. For example, the reservoir for *tuberculosis* is usually man but may be in other animals such as the milk from tubercular cows.

res′ident. A physician who continues to further his training after his internship.

r. physician. A resident receiving further training, past his internship, in a hospital.

residual (rē-zĭd′ū-ăl) [L. *residuum*, that is left behind]. 1. Relating to that which is left as a residue. 2. Psy: Any internal aftereffect of experience influencing later behavior.

r. air. That remaining in the lungs after the strongest possible (forced) expiration.

r. urine. That left in bladder after urination; occurring in cases of enlarged prostate.

residue (rĕz′ĭd-ū) [L. *residuum*, that which remains]. That which remains after a part is removed.

r. free diet. One without cellulose or roughage.

Purées and semisolids and bland foods are included.

r., high, diet. A diet with increased amounts of cellulose (fiber), water, mineral salts, and vitamins (esp. vitamin B).

r., low, diet (solid). An inadequate diet including solid food in which residue is reduced to a minimum. See: *nonlaxative diet.*

residuum (rē-zĭd′ū-ŭm) [L.]. Residue; the remainder.

resilience (rē-zil′ĭ-ĕns) [L. *resiliens*, leaping back]. The quality of coming back to normal after straining, as a stretched rubber band when released. Syn: *elasticity.*

resilient (rē-zĭl′ĭ-ĕnt) [L. *resiliens*, leaping back]. Elastic.

resin (rĕz′ĭn) [L. *resina*]. 1. An amorphous, nonvolatile solid or soft solid substance, a natural exudation from plants; it is practically insoluble in water, but soluble in alcohol. Ex: *Guaiac, rosin.* 2. Amorphous synthetic substance of high molecular weight.

r., ion-exchange. Ionizable synthetic substances which may be acid or basic, and used accordingly to remove either acid or basic ions from solutions. Thus *anionic-exchange resins* may be used to absorb acid in the stomach. *Cationic-exchange resins* have the ability to remove basic, or alkaline, ions from solutions.

resinous (rĕz′ĭn-ŭs) [L. *resina*]. Of the nature of or pert. to resin.

resistance (rē-zĭs′tăns) [L. *resistens*, standing back]. 1. Opposition to or the ability to oppose anything, as the power of a fluid to retard that which is passing through it, as the resistance of the air, or opposition of the body to passage of an electric current. Incorrectly used in reference to immunity; or ability of the body to resist infection or disease. 2. The sum total of body mechanisms which interpose barriers to the progress of invasion or multiplication of infectious agents or to damage by their toxic products. *Immunity* is resistance associated with the presence of antibodies having a specific action on infectious microorganisms. *Inherent resistance* is the ability to resist disease independently of antibodies. 3. The force exerted to penetrate the Unconscious or to submerge memories in the Unconscious. 4. In Psy., condition in which patient avoids bringing into consciousness conflicts and unpleasant events responsible for his neurosis, or reluctance of subject to give up old patterns of thought and behavior.

resolution (rĕz-ō-lū′shŭn) [L. *resolūtio*]. 1. Decomposition; absorption or breaking down of the products of inflammation. 2. Cessation of inflammation without suppuration. The return to normal. 3. The ability of the eye or series of lenses to distinguish fine detail.

resolve. To return to normal as after a pathologic process; to separate into component parts.

resolvent (rē-zŏl′vĕnt) [L. *resolvens*, dissolving]. 1. Promoting disappearance of inflammation. 2. That which causes dispersion of inflammation.

resonance (rĕz′ō-năns) [L. *resonantia*, an echo]. 1. Quality or act of resounding. 2. *In physical diagnosis*, the quality of the sound heard on percussion of a hollow structure such as chest or abdomen. Absence of resonance is termed *flatness*, diminished resonance, *dullness.* 3. *In physics*, modification of sound due to vibrations of a body which are set up by waves of another vibrating body. 4. *In elect.*, state in which two electrical circuits are in tune with each other.

r., amphoric. Sound, as that when blowing across the mouth of an empty bottle.

r., bandbox. See: *r., tympanitic.*

r., bell-metal. Sound heard in pneumothorax in auscultation when coin is held against chest wall and it is struck by another coin.

r., cracked-pot. A sound having a peculiar "clinking" quality sometimes heard on percussion of chest in cases of advanced tuberculosis when cavities are present.

r., skodaic. Increased percussion sound over upper lung when there is pleural effusion in lower part.

r., normal. See: *r., vesicular.*

r., tympanitic. That obtained by percussion of a hollow structure such as the stomach or colon when moderately distended with air.

r., vesicular. Normal pulmonary resonance.

r., vocal. The vibrations of the voice transmitted to the ear, normally more marked over the right apex.

Abnormally increased in: (1) Pneumonic consolidation; (2) lungs infiltrated with tuberculosis; (3) cavities which freely communicate with a bronchus.

Vocal r. is diminished or absent in: (1) Pleural effusion — air, pus, serum, lymph or blood; (2) emphysema; (3) pulmonary collapse; (4) pulmonary edema; (5) egophony, a modified bronchophony, characterized by a trembling, bleating sound usually heard above the upper border of dullness of pleural effusions; occasionally heard in beginning pneumonia; (6) bronchophony; extreme exaggeration of vocal resonance, the sounds, but not words, are transmitted. Esp. noted over marked consolidations and over certain cavities.

r., whispering. Auscultation sound heard when patient whispers.

resonat′ing. Vibrating sympathetically with a source of sound or electrical oscillations.

r. cavities. The resonator of the human voice. Includes upper portion of larynx, pharynx, nasal cavity, paranasal sinuses, and mouth cavity.

resonator (rĕz″ō-nā′tôr) [L. *resonare*, to resound]. 1. A structure which is capable of being set into sympathetic vibration when sound waves of the same frequency from another vibrating body strike it. 2. *In elect.*, an apparatus consisting of an electrical circuit in which oscillations of a certain frequency are set up by oscillations of the same frequency in another circuit. When this occurs, the circuits are said to be in syntony.

resorbent (rē-sor'bĕnt) [L. *resorbens*, sucking in]. An agent that promotes the absorption of abnormal matter, as exudates or blood clots. Ex: *Potassium iodide, ammonium chloride.*

resorption (rē-sorp'shŭn) [L. *resorbere*, to drink in]. 1. Act of removal by absorption, as resorption of an exudate or pus. 2. Removal of hard parts of a tooth as a result of lysis and phagocytic action.

respirable (rē-spīr'ā-bl, rĕs'pĭr-ā-bl) [L. *respirāre*, to respire]. Fit or adapted for respiration.

respiration (rĕs-pĭr-ā'shŭn) [L. *respiratio*, breathing]. 1. The interchange of gases between an organism and the medium in which it lives. More specifically the taking in of oxygen and its utilization in the tissues and the giving off of carbon dioxide. 2. The act of breathing.

Adventitious Sounds: Friction sounds produced by the rubbing together of roughened pleural surfaces, may be heard both in inspiration and expiration and often resemble subcrepitant râles,

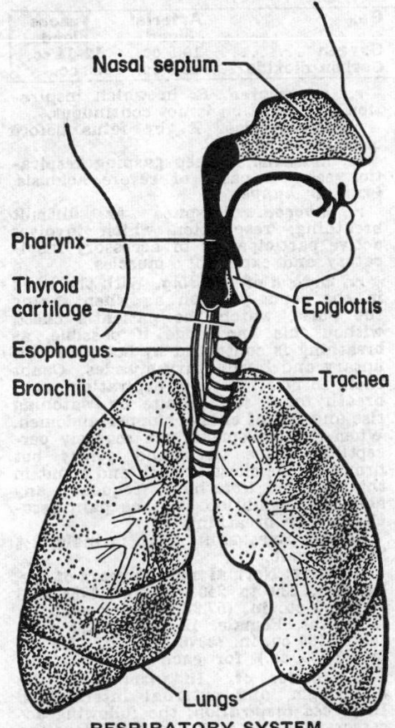

RESPIRATORY SYSTEM

but are more superficial and localized than the latter, and are not modified by cough or deep inspiration.

Metallic tinkling: Silvery bell-like sounds heard at intervals over a pneumohydrothorax or large cavity. Speaking, coughing and deep breathing usually induce them. Must not be confounded with similar sound produced by liquids in the stomach.

Râles: Abnormal bubbling sounds heard in air cells or bronchial tubes, *q.v.*

Succussion-splash or hippocratic succussion: A splashing sound produced by the presence of air and liquid in the chest, may be elicited by gently shaking the patient while auscultating. Nearly always indicates either a hydro- or a pyopneumothorax, although it has been detected over very large cavities. Air and liquid in stomach produce similar sounds. See: *respiration, also heart, for auscultation.*

Auscultation of Respiratory Organs: Normal respiration. Vesicular breathing is heard over the body of the lungs and is characterized by a soft, breezy inspiration, and a short, low pitched expiration. Normally, expiration is not more than ½ as long as inspiration. Auscultation over trachea or main bronchi in the interscapula space yields bronchial breathing.

Modification of the Respiratory Murmur: Amphoric and cavernous breathing. These two are almost identical. Sounds loud, expiration prolonged and hollow. Pitch of amphoric breathing a little higher than cavernous. May be imitated by blowing over the mouth of an empty jar. Heard in: (a) Phthisical or bronchiectatic cavities; (b) pneumothorax, when the opening to the lung is patulous; (c) area of consolidation near a large bronchus; (d) sometimes over lung compressed by a moderate effusion.

r., abdominal. R. where the diaphragm chiefly exerts itself, while walls of chest are nearly at rest. Utilized in normal quiet breathing, esp. by males, and in pathological conditions as in pleurisy, pericarditis, and fracture of ribs. Also called ***diaphragmatic breathing.***

r., absent. R. in which respiratory sounds are suppressed.

r., accelerated. Considered accelerated when more than 25 per minute, after 15 years of age.

Frequently occurs in disease. In disease it may be preternaturally frequent, or slow, rising to 60 or 80, or falling to 8 or 10 per minute. Increased frequency may, in health, result from exercise or physical exertion or from mental disturbances. It is present in many disorders of the *lungs*, as in pneumonias, bronchiectasis, advanced pulmonary tuberculosis, consolidation or compression of a lobe or of entire lung, congestion, asthma, emphysema, abscess, tumors, aneurysms, diseases of the chest wall, hernia of the diaphragm, and partial obstruction to the entrance of air into the lungs. It may be seen in diseases of the *blood*, such as the anemias; in *kidney* troubles; *febrile disease;* diseases of the *heart*, and as a result of drugs or nervous conditions.

r., aerobic. R. in which air or free oxygen is utilized.

r., amphoric. R. having amphoric resonance, *q.v.*

r., anaerobic. R. in which oxygen is obtained from chemical reactions not involving the liberation of free oxygen.

r., apneustic. Breathing characterized by prolonged inspiration unrelieved by attempts to expire. Seen in patients who have had the upper part of the *pons* of the brain removed or damaged.

r., artificial. Artificial methods to restore respiration in cases of suspended breathing. SEE: *artificial respiration.*

r., Biot's. Breathing with irregularly alternating periods of apnea and hyperpnea. Occurs in meningitis and disorders of the brain which cause increased intracranial pressure.

r., cell. SYN: *biological* or *intracellular oxidation.* The combination of oxygen with various substances within cells resulting in formation of CO_2 and H_2O and release of energy. There are many intermediary reactions in which substances other than oxygen act as oxidizing agents, *i.e.,* hydrogen or electron acceptors. Reactions are catalyzed by respiratory enzymes which include the flavoproteins, cytochromes, and other enzymes. Certain vitamins (nicotinamide, riboflavin, thiamine, pyridoxine, and pantothenic acid) are essential in the formation of components of various enzyme systems.

r., Cheyne-Stokes. Respirations gradually increase in rapidity, and volume, until they reach climax, then gradually subside and cease entirely for from 5 to 50 seconds, when they begin again.

Due to some disturbance of respiratory center, exact nature of which is as yet undetermined. Usually forerunner of death but may last several months, or few days, and disappear.

r., cogwheel. SEE: *r., interrupted.*

r., costal. Costal breathing. R. in which chest cavity is enlarged by raising the ribs.

r., decreased. It obtains in uremia, diabetic coma, affections of the brain, in shock, hysteria, stenosis of the larynx, in chronic fibroid phthisis, on approaching death, and in poisoning with opium or its derivatives.

r., diaphragmatic. Abdominal respiration, *q.v.*

r., difficult. Dyspnea, *q.v.*

r., direct. R. in which an organism such as a one-celled ameba secures its oxygen and gives up carbon dioxide directly to the surrounding medium.

r., external. SYN: *pulmonary respiration.* The processes involved in ventilating the lungs (breathing) and the exchange of gases (O_2 and CO_2) between the air in lungs and the blood within capillaries in the walls of alveoli.

Inspiration or drawing in of air is accomplished by enlargement of the thoracic cavity. This is brought about by contraction of the diaphragm and by raising the ribs and sternum. *Expiration* or the expulsion of air may be active or passive. In ordinary breathing, it is passive, no muscular effort being needed to bring chest wall back to normal position. In forced or labored respiration, muscular effort is involved.

The chemical changes in the air thus taken into the lungs are given under *air*: the volumes of air involved in respiratory movements are given under *spirometry.* If the aspiration of air is accomplished chiefly by contraction of the diaphragm, the abdomen will bulge with each inspiration, for the diaphragm, forming at once the floor of the thorax and the roof of the abdominal cavity, is dome-shaped, with its concavity downward; in contracting, it pushes the abdominal viscera down. This type of respiration is called diaphragmatic or abdominal. Its opposite is the thoracic type, in which the ribs and sternum must be raised and which is seen when the abdomen is confined by tight clothing.

RS. *breathing, diaphragm, expiration, inspiration, air, spirometry.*

r., fetal. Exchange of gases in the placenta between blood of fetus and maternal blood.

r., forced. Voluntary hyperpnea (increase in rate and depth of breathing).

r., forms of. Jerking, spasmodic, stertorous, stridulous, whistling, wavy, lack of evenness, abdominal, or thoracic.

r., frequent. Common in all febrile and inflammatory diseases, esp. in children. As a rule, rapid breathing is a sign of thoracic disease. In hysteria patient often breathes 60 to 70 times per minute. It may occur in acute respiratory affections, lesions of medulla, or it may be induced by atropine, carbon dioxide, cocaine.

r., internal. The passage of oxygen from the blood into the cells, its utilization by the cells and the passage of carbon dioxide from cells into the blood.

Oxygen is carried in combination with hemoglobin; oxyhemoglobin gives arterial blood its red color, reduced hemoglobin gives venous blood its blue color. Carbon dioxide is carried in combination with metallic elements in the blood as bicarbonates and also as carbonic acid.

The following table gives the number of cc. of each gas contained in 100 cc. of blood. The higher of the two figures for carbon dioxide represents conditions during exercise:

Gas	Arterial Blood	Venous Blood
Oxygen	19.5 cc.	12-14 cc.
Carbon dioxide	48.0 cc.	58 cc.

r., interrupted. R. in which inspiration or expiration is not continuous.

r., intrauterine. R. by fetus before birth. SEE: *r., fetal.*

r., Kussmaul's. Deep gasping respiration seen in cases of severe acidosis. SEE: *air hunger.*

r., labored. Dyspnea or difficult breathing; respiration which involves active participation of accessory inspiratory and expiratory muscles.

r., method of counting. With the hand in the same position as when taking the pulse, watch the patient's chest, without his knowledge if possible, as breathing is controlled by both the voluntary and involuntary muscles. Count each inspiration and expiration as 1 breath for 1 full minute by watching rise and fall of chest or upper abdomen. When the movements are scarcely perceptible, place the hand gently but firmly on the chest or back and count in this manner. *Note* hour, frequency, any abnormal condition such as pain associated with breathing.

NORMAL EXPANSION: 2 in. in male, 2½ in. in female.

CAPACITY: Normal male 22 years of age, 5.8 feet, 230 to 240 cu. in. (3769-3933 cc.), 3.5 cu. in. (57.36 cc.) for each in. in height. Female, 19 years, 5.25 feet, 145 to 150 cu. in. (2376-2458 cc.), 2.3 cu. in. (37.69 cc.) for each in. in height.

r., muscles of. In *inspiration,* the diaphragm, and external intercostals. In *forced inspiration,* the following accessory muscles may assist in elevating ribs and sternum: the scaleni, levatores costorum, sternocleidomastoideus, pectoralis major, platysma myoides, and serratus posterior superior. In *expiration* (voluntary deep breathing or forced expiration), rectus abdominis, external and internal oblique, transverse abdominis. The following accessory muscles may assist in depressing the ribs: internal intercostals, serratus posterior inferior, quadratus lumborum. SEE: *diaphragm, expiration, inspiration.*

r., paradoxical. 1. R. occurring in open pneumothorax in which lung fills on expiration and is deflated on inspiration. 2. Condition seen in paralysis of diaphragm in which diaphragm ascends during inspiration.

r., periodic. Breathing of uneven rhythm as in Cheyne-Stokes respiration, *q.v.*

r. pigment. A pigment that carries oxygen. Ex: hemoglobin and hemocyanin.

r., placental. Fetal respiration, *q.v.*

r. quotient. SEE: *quotient, respiratory.*

r., rate of. It may be preternaturally frequent, or slow, rising to 60 or 80, or falling to 8 or 10 per minute.

In newly born	30-60 per m.
1st year, about	25-30 " "
2nd year, about	20-26 " "
15th year, about	20 " "
21st year:	
Men	16-18 per m
Women	18-20 " "
50th year	16 " "
70th year	14-16 " "
Usual ratio to pulse.......	1- 4 " "

Respiration, Pulse and Temperature Ratio

Respiration	Pulse	Temperature
18	80	99° F.
19 (plus)	88	100
21	96	101
23	104	102
25 (minus)	112	103
27	120	104
28	128	105
30	136	106

r., slow. Generally result of some structural or functional derangement of the nervous system.

Observed in apoplexy, in effusion of serum within cranium, softening of the brain and in most of the circumstances that occasion coma. It may occur in brain compressions and hemorrhage, and in uremia or be induced by carbon monoxide and opium or its derivatives.

r., stertorous. Rattling or bubbling sounds which obscure normal respiratory sounds. Usually caused by breathing with mouth open with resultant vibration of soft palate.

r., stridulous. A high-pitched, crowing or barking sound heard during inspiration caused by an obstruction in vicinity of glottis or in respiratory passageway.

r. system. The *lungs* and the *respiratory passages.* The latter include *nasal cavities, pharynx, mouth* (if open), *larynx, trachea, bronchi,* and *bronchioles.*

r., thoracic. R. when abdomen does not move, being performed entirely by expansion of the chest. Observed when peritoneum or diaphragm is inflamed or when abdominal cavity is physically restricted by tight bandages, clothes or the weight of the surgical team during procedures involving the abdominal cavity.

respiration, words pert. to: air, complementary (complemental); a., minimal; a., reserve; a., residual; a., supplemental; a., tidal; anapnea; apnea; asphyxia; Biot's breathing; blowing; Bouchut's respiration; chest; Cheyne-Stokes; diaphragmatic; dyspnea; eupnea; hyperpnea; hypopnea; infant; inspiration; oligopnea; orthopnea; polypnea; respirator; respiratory; stridor; stridulus; tachypnea; thermometry.

respirator (rĕs′pĭ-rā″tor) [L. *respirāre,* to breathe]. 1. A device by which inspired air is purified, warmed, or medicated when passing through it. 2. A machine for prolonged artificial respiration. SEE: *Drinker respirator.*

respiratory (rē-spīr′ă-tō-rĭ, rĕs′pĭ-ră-tō-rĭ) [L. *respirāre,* to breathe]. Pertaining to respiration.

r. center. A region in the medulla oblongata which regulates movements of respiration. Consists of an *inspiratory center* located in rostral half of reticular formation overlying olivary nuclei and an *expiratory center* located dorsal to inspiratory center. A *pneumotaxic center,* located in the pons; also is concerned with respiratory movements.

r. minute volume. ABBR: *RMV.* The amount of air breathed in one minute.

r. system. The lungs, pleura, bronchi, pharynx, larynx, tonsils, and the nose.

respirometer (rĕs″pĭr-ŏm′ĕt-ĕr) [" + G. *metron,* a measure]. Instrument to ascertain character of respirations.

response. 1. A reaction such as contraction of a muscle or secretion of a gland resulting from a stimulus. SEE: *reaction.* 2. The sum-total of reactions of an individual to specific conditions as the *response* (favorable or unfavorable) of a patient to a certain treatment.

r., inverse. The acquisition of a refractoriness to repeated injections of parathyroid hormone. Results in osteopetrosis or marble bones.

r., triple. Three phases of vasomotor reactions occurring when a pointed instrument is drawn across the skin. Includes (1) red reaction, (2) flare or spreading flush, (3) wheal.

rest (rĕst) [A.S. *raestan,* to rest]. 1. Repose of body due to sleep. 2. Freedom from activity, as of mind or body. 3. To lie down; to cease from motion. 4. A remnant of embryonic tissue that persists in the adult. Also called *epithelial* or *fetal rest.*

restiform (rĕs′tĭ-form) [" + *forma,* shape]. Ropelike; rope-shaped.

r. body. SYN: *corpus restiforme.* Inferior cerebellar peduncle.

resting. Inactive, motionless, at rest.

r. cell. 1. A cell not in the process of dividing. 2. A cell when *not* performing its normal function, as a nerve cell which is not conducting an impulse, or a muscle cell which is not contracting.

r. potential. The potential difference which exists across a cell membrane between the outside and the inside of a resting cell.

restitutio integrum. Complete restoration to health.

restitution (rĕs-tĭ-tū′shun) [L. *restitutio*]. 1. A return to a former status. 2. The act of making amends. 3. The turning of the fetal head to the right or left after it has completely emerged through the vagina.

restorative (rē-stor′ă-tĭv) [L. *restaurāre,* to fix]. 1. Pert. to restoration. 2. An agent that is effective in the regaining of health and strength.

restraint (rē-strānt′) [O.Fr. *restraindre*]. 1. Process of hindering from any action, mental or physical. 2. State of being hindered. 3. That which hinders or restricts; device or method used to keep a patient from injuring himself. SEE:

knot. Various states have laws concerning the restraint of patients.

r. in bed. Move bed against wall, place straight backed chairs along open side of bed. Tie them into place by interlacing with rope and then tying to foot and head of bed, or place a wide board the length of bed on either side and fasten through 3 or 4 holes bored near ends of the boards. Fold sheet lengthwise to width of 1 foot. Place under patient's chest and cross in front below armpits. At sides secure hem ends to side bar or springs of bed. This allows some freedom for turning from side to side. The hands and feet may be restrained by a clove hitch of wide bandage around wrists and ankles and tied to side or foot of bed.

r. (of the) lower extremities. Tie a sheet across knees and tie feet together with a figure-of-eight bandage. (Start loop under ankles, cross between feet and bring ends around feet and tie on top.)

r., mechanical. Restraint by physical devices, esp. restraint of insane.

r., medicinal. Restraint of mentally ill who are violent by use of narcotics, or sedatives.

resuscitation (rē-sŭs-ĭ-tā'shŭn) [L. *resuscitātio*]. Act of bringing one back to full consciousness.

r., heart-lung. The American Heart Association recommends the following:

IF UNCONSCIOUS: Be certain there is an adequate airway. Elevate head, and push jaw up. Then clear vomitus, false teeth or other matter from mouth and pharynx.

IF NOT BREATHING: Use *oral* (mouth-to-mouth) *resuscitation* described below.

IF PULSE IS ABSENT: And the pupils are dilated and there is a deathlike appearance, massage the heart by using the following *closed chest* (i.e., not surgical method) *compression method:* Press on the sternum with sufficient force to depress it 1½ to 2 inches. Do this once per second. At the same time continue *mouth-to-mouth resuscitation.* Continue both *mouth-to-mouth* resuscitation and intermittent chest compression until spontaneous pulse and respiration return. If one person is doing the resuscitation, alternate two quick inflations with 15 chest compressions. If there are two operators, do these maneuvers at the rate of one inflation for every fifth chest compression.

r., oral (mouth-to-mouth). SEE: Illustration, *A-91.* Adopted by Red Cross. (a) Wipe from mouth and pharynx any foreign matter. (b) Bend head back, chin pointing up. (c) Pull or push jaw outward moving tongue from back of throat. (d) Open mouth wide and place your mouth tightly over victim's mouth. Close patient's nostrils by pinching them together with the fingers. Blow into victim's mouth. If mouth has been damaged hold mouth and lips shut and blow into patient's nose. In small children place mouth over child's nostrils and mouth, and blow into both. (e) Remove your mouth, turn head to side and listen for return rush of air. Repeat blowing. (f) Blow vigorously at rate of 12 breaths a minute. For a child about 20 shallow breaths a minute. (g) If initial failure to get air exchange, recheck head and jaw position. A child can be up-ended holding ankles and slapping 2 or 3 times between shoulder blades.

RS: *anabiosis, anastasis, artificial respiration, revivification.*

resuscitator (rē-sŭs'ĭ-tā"tor). An automatic breathing machine that forces oxygen into the lungs under pressure of 4 ounces per square inch when back pressure of 3 ounces trips the machine for exhalation. May be used for several patients at the same time.

retardation (rē-tar-dā'shŭn) [L. *retardare,* to delay]. 1. A holding back or slowing down; delay. 2. Delayed mental or physical response due to pathological conditions.

retard'ed depres'sion. The depressed state of manic-depressive psychosis.

retch (rĕtch) [A.S. *hrǣcan,* to clear the throat]. To make an involuntary attempt to vomit, *q.v.*

retching (rĕtch'ĭng) [A.S. *hrǣcan,* to clear the throat]. An involuntary attempt to vomit.

rete (rē'tē) (pl. *retia*). A network. A plexus of nerves or blood vessels.

r., articular. R. about a joint, esp. a deep anastomosis at knee joint.

r., cutaneum. A network of blood vessels at junction of the corium and superficial fascia.

r. mirabile. NA. A plexus formed by sudden division of a vessel into small twigs which unite again to form one vessel, as in the glomeruli of the kidneys.

r. olecrani. A network of vessels at back of elbow formed by divisions of the recurrent ulnar arteries.

r. ovarii. A group of rudimentary cell-cords lying in broad ligament and mesovarium of ovary. They are homologous to rete testes in male.

r., patella. A superficial network of vessels lying about the patella. Formed by branches of genicular arteries.

r. subpapillare. A network of vessels between papillary and reticular layers of the dermis.

r. testis. A network of tubules in mediastinum testis which receive sperm through the *tubuli recti* from the seminiferous tubules. From the rete testis, *efferent ducts* convey sperm to the epididymis.

r., vertebral. SEE: *retia, venous, of the vertebra.*

retention (rē-tĕn'shŭn) [L. *retentio,* a holding back]. Retaining in the body that which does not belong there, or which should be excreted, as urine, feces, or perspiration. SEE: *chloruremia.*

r. cyst. One caused by retention of a secretion in a gland.

ETIOL: Closure of the gland's duct.

r. defect. Inability to recall a name, number, or fact shortly after the subject was requested to remember it.

r. enema. Enema to be retained to provide nourishment, medicate the mucosa or for anesthesia. SEE: *enema, retention.*

r. of urine. This is failure of ability to empty bladder.

This may be due to a number of causes, such as (a) loss of muscle tone of the bladder from anemia, old age, exposure to cold, prolonged operation, or a greatly distended bladder without voiding for a considerable length of time; (b) lesions involving nervous pathways to and from the bladder; (c) lesions involving reflex centers in brain and spinal cord; (d) obstruction of the urethra which may result from inflammation, stricture, stones, diverticula, cysts, tumors, or pressure from the outside as in cases of hypertrophy of the prostate; (e) psychogenic factors.

INDICATIONS: Disease of spinal cord if not induced by obstruction such as that from calculi, enlarged prostate, or from nervousness.

r. with overflow. Spasm of sphincter, causing failure to empty the bladder at one voiding, only overflow dribbling away, due to above causes.

retia. Plural of rete.

r., venous, of the vertebrae. Two plexuses within vertebral canal extending from foramen magnum to coccyx. They lie posteriorly and laterally to dura and between latter and arches of vertebrae.

reticula. Plural of reticulum.

reticular rĕ-tĭk'ū-lăr) [L. *reticula*, net]. Meshed or in the form of a network.

r. apparatus of Golgi. SEE: *Golgi apparatus.*

r. cells. 1. Phagocytic cells present in lymphatic and myeloid tissues. 2. The cells of reticular connective tissue. SEE: *reticular tissue.*

r. fibers. SYN: *lattice fibers, argyrophil fibers.* Extremely fine argyrophilic (i.e., silver-staining) fibers found in reticular tissue, *q.v.*

r. formation. SEE: *formation, reticular.*

r. layer. Layer of connective tissue forming deeper portion of dermis. Lies beneath papillary layer.

r. membrane. Membrane formed by cuticular plates of distal ends of supporting cells in the organ of Corti.

r. tissue. A form of connective tissue consisting of a network of reticular fibers and cells. Cells are stellate with protoplasmic processes anastomosing with adjacent cells. Protoplasm also encloses and extends along the fibers. Found principally in bone marrow and lymphatic organs (lymph nodes), spleen and also in various organs (liver, kidney), in tissue underlying mucous membranes, and in walls of blood vessels.

retic'ulate. Of the nature of a network

r. substance. Reticular formation, *q.v.*

reticulated (rē-tĭk'ū-lā-tĕd) [L. *reticula*, network]. Netlike; pert. to a reticulum. SYN: *reticular.*

reticulation (rē-tĭk-ū-lā'shŭn) [L. *reticula*, a net]. The formation of a network mass.

reticulin (rē-tĭk'ū-lĭn) [L. *reticula*, net]. An albuminoid or scleroprotein substance in the connective tissue framework of lymphatic tissues.

reticulocyte (rĕ-tĭk'ū-lō-sīt) [L. *reticula*, net, + G. *kytos*, cell]. A red blood cell containing a network of granules or filaments representing an immature stage in development. Normally comprise about 1% of circulating red blood cells.

reticulocytopenia (re-tĭk"ū-lō-sī"tō-pē'-nĭ-ă) [" + " + *penia*, lack]. Lowering of the number of the reticulocytes of the blood.

reticulocytosis (re-tĭk"ū-lō-sī-tō'sĭs). [L. *reticula*, net, + G. *kytos*, cell, + *-ōsis*, intensive]. SYN: *reticulosis.* Increase in number of reticulocytes in circulating blood. Indicative of active erythropoiesis in red bone marrow. Occurs after hemorrhage, in high altitudes, and following treatment for pernicious anemia.

reticuloendothelial. Pert. to the reticuloendothelial system, *q.v.*

r. cell. SYN: *histiocyte, macrophage.* A phagocytic cell of the reticuloendothelial system, *q.v.*

r. system. ABBR: RES. Term applied to those cells scattered throughout the body which have the power to ingest (phagocytose) particulate matter (bacteria, colloidal particles). Includes *macrophages* (*histiocytes, clasmatocytes*, or *resting wandering cells*) of loose connective tissue, *reticular cells* of lymphatic organs and myeloid tissues, *Kupffer cells* of the liver, *cells* lining blood sinuses of spleen, bone marrow, adrenal cortex and hypophysis, *microglia* of central nervous system, *adventitial cells* about blood vessels and *dust cells* of the lungs. The above types are called *fixed R.E. cells.* Under certain conditions, esp. inflammatory stimuli, fixed cells may become *wandering R.E. cells*, i.e., they become actively motile. Monocytes of the blood also are included in this group. R.E. cells function in elimination of worn out cells, esp. red blood cells, in repair of injured tissue, and in defense mechanisms, both local and general, of the body.

Diseases of the RES. include lymphosarcoma, reticulum cell sarcoma, Hodgkin's disease, follicular lymphoma, mycosis, fungoides, Gaucher's disease, and Niemann-Pick's disease.

reticuloendotheliosis (re-tĭk"ū-lō-ĕn"dō-thē-lĭ-ō'sĭs) [" + " + " + *-ōsis*, intensive]. Hyperplasia of reticuloendothelium.

reticuloendothelium (re-tĭk"ū-lō-ĕn"dō-thē'lĭ-ŭm) [" + " + *thēlē*, nipple]. Tissue of the reticuloendothelial system.

reticulosis (re-tĭk-ū-lō'-sĭs) [L. *reticula*, network, + G. *-ōsis*, intensive]. Reticulocytosis, *q.v.*

reticulum (re-tĭk'ū-lŭm) (pl. *reticula*) [L. *reticulum*, a little net]. A network.

r. of nucleus. A fine network of linin threads on which are arranged masses of chromatin.

r., stellate. The enamel pulp consisting of stellate cells lying between inner and outer epithelial layers of enamel organ of developing tooth.

retiform (rĕt'ĭ-form) [L. *rētē*, net, + *forma*, shape]. Resembling a network. SYN: *reticular.*

retina (rĕt'ĭ-nă) (pl. *retinae*) [L. *rētē*, a net]. Innermost or 3rd tunic of the eye which receives image formed by the lens and is immediate instrument of vision.

It is a light-sensitive structure upon which light rays come to a focus. It extends from the point of entrance of the optic nerve anteriorly to the margin of the pupil, completely lining the interior of the eye. It consists of three parts: (1) *pars optica*, the nervous or sensory portion extending from optic disc forward to *ora serata*, a wavy line immediately behind ciliary process; (2) *pars ciliaris*, part lining inner surface of ciliary process; and (3) *pars iridica*, part forming post. surface of iris. Slightly lateral to post. pole of the eye is a small, oval, yellowish spot, the *macula lutea*, in center of which is a depression, the *fovea centralis.* This region contains only cones and is the region of most acute vision. About 3.5 mm. nasally from the fovea is the *optic papilla* (optic disk), point at which nerve fibers from retina make their exit and form *optic nerve.* This region is devoid of rods and cones and is insensitive to light, hence named the *blind spot.*

The layers of the retina from without inward are:

(1) Layer of pigment epithelium; (2) layer of rods and cones; (3) external

limiting membrane; (4) external nuclear layer; (5) external plexiform layer; (6) internal nuclear layer; (7) internal plexiform layer; (8) layer of ganglion cells; (9) layer of nerve fibers; (10) internal limiting membrane.

COLOR: Normally a purplish red tint, varying with complexion. It is colorless in severe anemia or in ischemia. It is reddened in hyperemia.

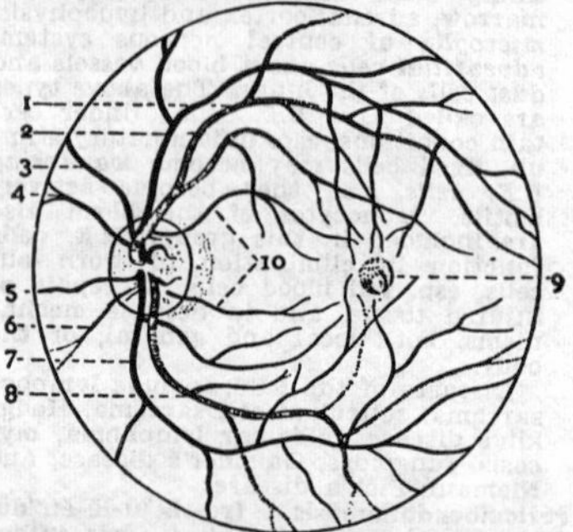

RETINAL VESSELS, DIAGRAM OF

1. Superior temporal artery. 2. Superior temporal vein. 3. Superior nasal vein. 4. Superior nasal artery. 5. Inferior nasal vein. 6. Inferior nasal artery. 7. Inferior temporal vein. 8. Inferior temporal artery. 9. Macula lutea. 10. Macular veins.

VESSELS: The arteries shown are branches of a single *central artery*, a branch of the *ophthalmic artery*. The central artery enters at the center of the optic papilla and it supplies the inner layers of retina. The outer layers, including rods and cones, are nourished by capillaries of the choroid layer. The veins lack muscular coats. They parallel the arteries, blood leaving by a *central vein* which leads to the *superior ophthalmic vein*.

r., coarctate. Condition in which there is an effusion of fluid between retina and choroid giving retina a funnel shape.

r., detachment of. Complete or partial separation of retina from the choroid. May follow trauma, or choroidal hemorrhages, or tumors.

r., shot silk. R. having an opalescent appearance sometimes seen in young persons. SYN: *watered silk r.*

r., tigroid. R. having a spotted or striped appearance seen in retinitis pigmentosa.

retinaculum (rĕt-ĭn-ăk′ū-lŭm) (pl. *retinacula*) [L. halter]. A band or membrane holding any organ or part in its place. Thickenings of the deep fascia in distal portions of limbs which hold tendons in position when muscles contract. Called *retinaculum tendinum.*

r. cutis. A fibrous band connecting the corium with underlying fascia.

r., extensor, of ankle. 1. The *sup. extensor retinaculum,* a band which crosses the extensor tendons of foot and is attached to lower portion of tibia and fibula. 2. The inf. *extensor retinaculum,* a band located on dorsum of foot. Consists of two "limbs" having common origin or lat. surface of calcaneum. The *upper limb* is attached to medial malleolus; *lower limb* curves around instep and is attached to fascia of abductor hallucis on medial side of foot.

r., extensor, of wrist. An oblique band attached medially to styloid process of ulna, hammate bone, and medial ligament of wrist joint. Laterally it is attached to ant. border of radius. Contains 6 separate compartments for passage of extensor tendons to hand.

r., flexor, of ankle. R. extending from medial malleolus to medial tubercle of calcaneum.

r., flexor, of wrist. R. extending from trapezium and scaphoid bones laterally to hammate and pisiform bones medially.

r. of hip joint. Any one of three flat bands lying along neck of femur and continuous with capsule of hip joint. Also called *cervical ligaments.*

r. mammae. Strands of connective tissue in mammary gland extending from glandular tissue through fat towards the skin where they are attached to deep fascia. Over cephalic portion of mammae they are well developed and called *suspensory ligaments of Cooper.*

r., patellar. Two fibrous bands (*medial* and *lateral r.*) lying on either side of knee joint and forming part of joint capsule. They are extensions of the insertions of the medial and lateral vastus muscles.

r., peroneal. Two fibrous bands on lateral side of foot which contain tendons of peroneus longus and brevis muscles. The *sup. peroneal r.* extends from lat. malleolus to lat. surface of calcaneum; the *inf. peroneal r.* is attached below to calcaneum, above to lower border of inf. extensor retinaculum.

r. tendinum. SEE: *retinaculum.*

retinal (rĕt′ĭn-ăl) [L. *rētē,* net]. Concerning the retina.

r. correspondence. Condition in which simultaneous stimulation of points in the retinas of two eyes results in formation of a single visual sensation. Such points are called *corresponding points.* These lie in the foveas of the two retinas or in the nasal half of one retina and the temporal half of the other.

Abnormal correspondence results in double vision (*diplopia*) and is usually the result of inequality of ocular muscles. SEE: *strabismus.*

r. purple. Rhodopsin or visual purple, *q.v.*

retinene. SYN: *xanthopsin, visual yellow.* An orange-yellow carotenoid pigment formed in retina as a result of the action of light on rhodopsin; an aldehyde of vitamin A. In dark adaptation, rhodopsin is regenerated from retinene.

retinitis (rĕt-ĭn-ī′tĭs) [" + G. *-itis,* inflammation]. Inflamed condition of the retina.

SYM: Diminished vision, contractions of fields or scotomata, alteration in size of objects, photophobia.

TREATMENT: Absolute rest of eyes, protection from light, treat underlying cause.

r., actinic. R. due to exposure to intense light or other forms of radiant energy.

r. albuminurica. R. associated with chronic kidney disease and malignant hypertension.

Shows not only general signs of retinitis but is distinguished by white patches in the fundus, esp. surrounding the papilla and in the macular region.

r., apoplectic. R. associated with hemorrhaging of retinal vessels.

r. circinata. R. in which there is a circle of white spots about the macula.

r. circumpapillaris. R. in which there is a proliferation of outer layers of retina about optic disk.

r., diabetic. R. occurring in diabetics, esp. that of long duration. Characterized by aneurysmal dilatation of blood vessels, hemorrhages, and waxy and cotton-wool exudates.

r. disciformis. R. accompanied by degeneration of retina in region of macula.

r., exogenous purulent. R. following introduction of infectious organisms into eye as a result of perforating wound or ulcer.

r., external exudative. Syn: *ext. hemorrhagic r., Coats' disease.* Condition in which large masses of white and yellow crystals occur beneath retina as a result of organization of hemorrhages.

r., metastatic. Acute purulent retinitis resulting from lodgement of infective emboli in retinal vessels.

r. pigmentosa. Syn: *primary pigmentary degeneration of retina.* A chronic progressive disease characterized by degeneration of retinal neuroepithelium, esp. rods, atrophy of optic nerve, and widespread pigmentary changes in retina. A degenerative condition without inflammation. Etiology unknown but a hereditary tendency is manifested. Usually appears in childhood.

r. proliferans. Vascularized masses of connective tissue which project from retina into the vitreous. End result of recurrent hemorrhage from retina into the vitreous.

r. punctata albescens. Syn: *degeneratio punctata albescens.* A nonprogressive degenerative, familial disease characterized by presence of innumerable, minute, white spots scattered over entire retina and without pigmentary changes. Usually starts early in life.

r., punctate, central. R. characterized by numerous white or yellow spots in fundus of eye.

r. septica. Syn: *r. of Roth.* A mild benign condition occurring in patients with systemic infections. Characterized by white spots usually surrounded by hemorrhagic areas and seen near the optic disk. These are called *Roth's spots.*

r., solar. R. resulting from exposure of retina to rays of sun.

r., stellate. Syn: *toxic exudative r., pseudonephritic r.* R. characterized by presence of exudates and hemorrhages, blurring of optic disk, and formation of a star-shaped figure about macula.

r., syphilitic. R. resulting from or associated with syphilis. May involve not only retina but also optic nerve (syphilitic neuroretinitis).

retinoblastoma. A malignant glioma of the retina. Occurs in young children and shows a hereditary pattern. Usually unilateral.

retinochoroiditis (rĕt″ĭn-ō-kō-royd-ī′tĭs) [L. *rētē,* net, + G. *chorioeidēs,* skinlike, + *-itis,* inflammation]. Inflamed condition of retina and choroid.

retinocystoma (rĕt″ĭn-ō-sĭs-tō-mă) [" + G. *kystis,* sac, + *-ōma,* tumor]. Glioma of the retina.

retinoid (rĕt′ĭn-oyd) [" + *eidos,* resemblance]. Like the retina.

retinopapillitis (rĕt″ĭ-nō-pă-pĭl-ī′tĭs) [" + *papilla,* nipple, + G. *-itis,* inflammation]. Inflamed condition of retina and optic papilla. Syn: *papilloretinitis.*

retinopathy. Any disorder of the retina.

r., arteriosclerotic. R. accompanying generalized arteriosclerosis and moderate hypertension.

r., diabetic. R. occurring in diabetics.

r., hypertensive. That associated with hypertension, toxemia of pregnancy, glomerulonephritis.

r., syphilitic. R. occurring in later stages of syphilis.

retinoscope (rĕt″ĭn-ō-skōp) [" + G. *skopein,* to see]. An instrument used in performing retinoscopy.

retinoscopy (rĕt-ĭn-ŏs′kō-pĭ) [" + G. *skopein,* to examine]. Shadow test or refraction of eyes by effect of lights and shadows. Syn: *skiascopy.*

retisolution (rĕt-ĭ-sō-lū′shŭn) [L. *rētē,* net, + *solutio,* dissolution]. Dissolution of the Golgi structures.

retispersion (rĕt″ĭ-sper′zhŭn) [" + *spersio.* a scattering]. Transference of Golgi structures to periphery of the cell.

retort (rē-tort′) [L. *retortus,* bent back]. A flasklike, long-necked vessel used for distilling.

retothelium (rē″tō-thē′lĭ-ŭm) [" + G. *thēlē,* nipple]. Cellular layers covering reticular tissue. Syn: *reticuloendothelium, reticulothelium.*

re″tract′. To draw back.

retractile (rē-trăkt′ĭl) [L. *retractilis,* able to be drawn back]. Capable of being drawn back or in.

retraction (rē-trăk′shŭn) [L. *retractio,* from *retrahere,* to draw back]. A shortening. The act of drawing backward or state of being drawn back.

r. ring. A ridge sometimes felt on uterus above the pubes, marking line of separation bet. upper contractile and lower dilatable segments of the uterus. Seen in prolonged or obstructed labor. Syn: *Bandl's ring.*

r., uterine. The process by which muscular fibers of the uterus remain permanently shortened to a small degree following each contraction or labor pain.

retractor (rē-trăk′tor) [L. from *retrahere,* to draw back]. 1. Instrument for holding back the margins of a wound. 2. Muscle which draws in any organ or part.

re″treat′. Act of retiring or withdrawing from difficult life situations. May be *direct* as in physical flight or *indirect* as in malingering, illness, abnormal preoccupation, and self-deception.

retrenchment [Fr. *retrancher,* to cut back]. Procedure used in plastic surgery to remove excess tissue.

retro- [L.]. Prefix meaning *backward.*

retroaction (ret-ro-ak′shun). Action in a reverse direction.

retroauricular (rē″trō-aw-rĭk′ū-lar) [L. *rētrō,* backward, + *auricula,* ear]. Behind the auricle or ear.

retrobuccal (rē″trō-bŭk′ăl) [L. *rētrō,* backward, + *bucca,* cheek]. Concerning the back part of the mouth or area behind the mouth.

retrobulbar (rē″trō-bŭl′bar) [" + G. *bolbos,* a bulb]. 1. Behind the eyeball. 2. Post. to the medulla oblongata.

retrocedent (rē″trō-sē′dĕnt) [" + *cedere,* to go]. Going backward; returning.

retrocervical (rē″trō-sĕr′vĭ-kăl) [" + *cervix,* neck]. Back of the cervix uteri.

retrocession (rē″trō-sĕsh′ŭn) [" + *cessio,* from *cedere,* to go]. 1. A going back; a relapse. 2. Metastasis of a condition from the surface to an internal organ. 3. Indication of an abnormal (further back) position of the uterus.

retrocolic (rē″trō-kol′ĭk) [" + G. *kōlon*, colon]. Back of the colon.

retrocollic (rē″trō-kŏl′ĭk) [" + *collum*, neck]. Concerning the back of the neck.

r. spasm. Wryneck with spasms affecting post. muscles of neck.

retrocollis (rē″trō-kŏl′ĭs) [L. *rētrō*, backward, + *collum*, neck]. Spasm of post. muscles of the neck with torsion. SYN: *torticollis.*

retrocursive (rē″trō-kŭr′sĭv) [" + *cursio*, from *currere*, to run]. Stepping or turning backward.

retrodeviation (rē″trō-dē″vĭ-ā′shŭn) [" + *deviāre*, to turn aside]. Backward displacement, as of an organ.

retrodisplacement (rē″trō-dĭs-plās′mĕnt) [" + Fr. *déplacer*, to displace]. Displacement backwards of a part.

retroesophageal (rē″trō-ē-sŏf-ă′jē-ăl) [" + G. *oisophagos*, gullet]. Located behind the esophagus.

retroflexed (rē′trō-flĕkst) [" + *flexus*, bent, from *flectere*, to turn]. Bent backward.

retroflexion (rē″trō-flĕk′shŭn) [L. *rētrō*, backward, + *flexio*, a bending]. A bending or flexing backward.

r. of uterus. A condition of the womb in which its body is bent backward at an angle with the cervix whose position usually remains unchanged.

retrogasserian (rē″trō-găs-sē′rĭ-ăn) [L. *rētrō*, backward, + *gasserian*]. Referring to the post. root of the gasserian ganglion.

retrograde (rĕt′rō-grād, rē′trō-grād) [" + *gradi*, to step]. Moving backward; degenerating from better to worse state.

r. amnesia. Loss of memory for events and situations just preceding time of patient's illness.

r. flow. The flow of fluid in a direction opposite to that which is considered normal.

retrography (rē-trŏg′ră-fĭ) [" + G. *graphein*, to write]. Mirror writing, a symptom of certain brain diseases.

retrogression (rĕt″rō-grĕsh′ŭn) [L. *rētrō*, backward, + *gressus*, stepping]. 1. A going backward as in the involution, degeneration, or atrophy of a tissue or structure. 2. Passing from a more complex to a simpler type of structure in the development of an organ, an individual, or a race. 3. The return of symptoms in recovery from a disease.

retrogressive changes (rē″trō-grĕs′ĭv) [" + *gressus*, stepping]. Changes to lower type of organization, such as in atrophy, degeneration, necrosis, hypertrophy, etc.

retroinfection (rē″trō-ĭn-fĕk′shŭn) [" + *infectiō*, infection]. Infection communicated by the fetus *in utero* to the mother.

retroinsular (rē″trō-ĭn′sū-lar) [" + *insula*, island]. Situated behind the island of Reil.

retrojection (rĕt-rō-jĕk′shŭn). Washing out a cavity from within by injection of a fluid.

retrolabyrinthine (rē″trō-lăb-ĭ-rĭn′thĭn) [L. *rētrō*, backward, + G. *labyrinthos*, a maze]. Situated behind the labyrinth of the ear.

retrolent′al. Behind the crystalline lens.

r. fibroplasia. ABBR: RLF. Condition in which an opaque fibrous membrane develops on post. surface of the lens. Occurs chiefly in premature infants weighing less than 2000 gm., especially those subjected to high oxygen concentrations while in an incubator for a considerable period of time.

retrolingual (rē″trō-lĭng′gwal) [" + *lingua*, tongue]. Behind the tongue.

retromammary (rē″trō-măm′mă-rĭ) [" + *mamma*, breast]. Located behind the mammary gland.

retromandibular (rē″trō-măn-dĭb′ū-lar) [" + *mandibulum*, jaw]. Located behind the lower jaw.

retromastoid (rē″trō-măs′toyd) [L. *rētrō*, backward, + G. *mastos*, breast, + *eidos*, like]. Situated behind the mastoid process.

retromorphosis (rē″trō-mor′fō-sĭs) [" + G. *morphē*, form, + *-ōsis*, intensive]. 1. Change in shape accompanying a transition from a higher to a lower type of structure. 2. Retrogressive changes within cells or tissues; catabolism, *q.v.*

retronasal (rē″trō-nā′zăl) [" + *nasus*, nose]. Relating to or situated at the back part of the nose.

retroocular (rē″trō-ŏk′ū-lar) [L. *rētrō*, backward, + *oculus*, eye]. Located behind the eye.

retroperitoneal (rē″trō-pĕr-ĭ-tō-nē′ăl) [" + G. *peritonaion*, peritoneum]. Located behind the peritoneum.

retroperitoneum (rē″trō-pĕr-ĭ-tō-nē′ŭm) [" + G. *peritonaion*, peritoneum]. The space behind the peritoneum.

retroperitonitis (rē″trō-pĕr-ĭ-tō-nī′tĭs) [" + " + *-ītis*, inflammation]. Inflammation behind the peritoneum.

retropharyngeal (rē″trō-făr-ĭn′jē-ăl) [" + G. *pharygx*, pharynx]. Behind the pharynx.

retropharyngitis (rē″trō-făr-ĭn-jī′tĭs) [L. *rētrō*, backward, + G. *pharygx*, pharynx, + *-ītis*, inflammation]. Inflammation of the retropharyngeal tissue.

retroplacental (rē″trō-plă-sĕn′tăl) [" + *placenta*, a flat cake]. Behind the placenta, or behind both the placenta and the uterine wall.

retroplasia (rē″trō-plā′zĭ-ă) [" + G. *plassein*, to form]. Degenerative change of a cell or tissue into a more primary form.

retroposed (rē-trō-pōsd′) [" + *posus*, from *ponere*, to place]. Displaced backward.

retropulsion (rē″trō-pŭl′shŭn) [L. *rētrō*, backward, + *pulsiō*, a thrusting]. 1. Pushing back of any part, as of the fetal head in labor. 2. A walking or running backward, involuntarily, seen in some nervous disorders.

retrosternal (rē″trō-ster′năl) [" + G. *sternon*, chest]. Behind the sternum.

r. pulse. Venous pulse felt over suprasternal notch.

retrotarsal (rē-trō-tar′săl) [" + G. *tarsos*, edge of eyelid]. Located behind the tarsus of the eye.

retrouterine (rē″trō-ū′tĕr-ĭn) [" + *uterus*, womb]. Located behind the uterus.

retrovaccination. Vaccination with virus obtained from a calf inoculated with smallpox virus obtained from a human.

retroversion (rĕt″rō-ver′shŭn, rē″trō-ver′-shŭn) [" + *versio*, a turning]. A turning or state of being turned back.

r. of uterus. Displacement of the uterus backward with cervix pointing forward toward symphysis pubis.

Normally, the cervix points toward the lower end of the sacrum with the fundus toward the suprapubic region.

re″trude′. To force inward or backward.

re″tru′sion. 1. Process of forcing backward, esp. with reference to teeth. 2. Condition in which teeth are retroposed.

Retzius, lines of (ret′zē-ŭs). Brownish, concentric lines in the enamel of a tooth.

R., space of. SYN: *prevesical space, retropubic space, cavum Retzii.* Space in lower portion of abdomen between bladder and pubic bones and bounded superiorly by peritoneum. Contains areolar tissue, fat, and a plexus of veins.

R., veins of. SYN: *retroperitoneal veins.* Veins forming communications bet. the mesenteric veins and inf. vena cava.

Reuss' test (rois'ez). Test for atropine employing sulfuric acid and an oxidizing agent.

revellent (rē-vel'ent) [L. *rē*, back, + *vellere*, to draw]. 1. Producing revulsion, the diversion of disease or blood from one part of the body to another. 2. Agent producing revulsion.

re"verbera'tion. Process by which closed chains of neurons when excited by a single impulse will continue to discharge impulses from collaterals of its cells.

re"vers'al. 1. A change or turning in the opposite direction. 2. *In Psych.* a change in an instinct to its opposite, as from love to hate.

re"versi'on. 1. Return to a previously existing condition. 2. In genetics, the appearance of traits possessed by a remote ancestor. SEE: *atavism.*

revivification (rē-vĭv"ĭ-fĭ-kā'shŭn) [" + *vivere*, to live, + *-ficāre*, to do]. 1. Attempt to restore life to those apparently dead; restoration to life or consciousness. Also restoring life in local parts, as a limb after freezing. 2. Paring of surfaces to facilitate healing, as in a wound.

revulsant (rē-vŭl'sănt) [" + *vulsio*, a pulling]. 1. Causing transfer of disease or blood from one part of the body to another. 2. Drug which draws blood to an inflamed part.

revulsion (rē-vŭl'shŭn) [L. *revulsio*, a pulling back]. 1. Act of driving backward, as diverting disease from one part to another by a quick withdrawal of the blood from that part. 2. PT: Circulatory changes obtained by sudden and intense reactions to heat and cold.

The Scotch douche is a powerful revulsive measure. SEE: *counterirritation.*

revulsive (rē-vŭl'sĭv) [L. *revulsio*, a pulling back]. 1. Causing revulsion. 2. A counterirritant.

RF. Abbr. for rheumatoid factor, *q.v.*

Rh. 1. Chemical symbol for *rhodium.* 2. Abbr. for *rhesus*, a monkey (*Macaca rhesus*) in which the Rh factor was first identified.

Rh antiserum. SYN: *anti-Rh-serum.* Human serum which contains Rh antibodies.

Rh-Hr agglutinogens (antigens). Substances present on red blood cells which stimulate antibody formation.

Rh blood factor. A factor discovered in erythrocytes of the rhesus monkey and present in about 85% of human population, such individuals being designated Rh+ (Rh positive). In the remaining 15% (Rh—, or Rh negative) it causes, when injected, the formation of anti-Rh agglutinin. Subsequent transfusions of Rh+ blood may result in serious transfusion reactions (agglutination and hemolysis of red blood cells). A pregnant woman may become sensitized by blood of a Rh positive fetus. In subsequent pregnancies, if the fetus is Rh positive, Rh antibodies produced in maternal blood may cross the placenta and destroy fetal cells giving rise to *erythroblastosis fetalis.*

Rh genes. A series of eight allelic genes which are responsible for the various Rh blood types and designated by Wiener as R^1, R^2, R^o, R^z, *r*, *r'*, *r"*, and r_y. Genes represented by small r's are responsible for Rh negative persons; those by large R's for Rh positive persons.

Rhabditis (răb-dī'tĭs) [G. *rhabdos*, rod]. A genus of small nematode worms, some of which are parasitic.

rhabdo- [G. *rhabdos*, rod]. Combining form meaning *rod.*

rhabdomyoma (răb"dō-mī-ō'mă) [" + *mys, my-*, muscle, + *-ōma*, tumor]. A striated muscular tissue tumor.

rhabdophobia (răb-dō-fō'bĭ-ă) [" + *phobos*, fear]. Abnormal fear of being chastised, or of anything that might be used for such a purpose, as a *rod.*

rhachialgia (rā"kĭ-ăl'jĭ-ă) [G. *rhachis*, spine, + *algos*, pain]. Pain in the spine.

rhachiocampsis (rā"kĭ-ō-kămp'sĭs) [" + *kampsis*, a bending]. Curvature of spine.

rhachioplegia (rā"kĭ-ō-plē'jĭ-ă) [" + *plēgē*, a stroke]. Spinal paralysis.

rhachioscoliosis (rā"kĭ-ō-skō-lĭ-ō'sĭs) [" + *skoliōsis*, a bending]. Curvature of the spine laterally.

rhachis (rā'kĭs) [G.]. Spinal column.

rhachischisis (rā-kĭs'kĭs-ĭs) [G. *rhachis*, spine, + *schisis*, fissure]. A congenital cleft in the spinal column.

rhachitis (rā-kī'tĭs) [" + *-itis*, inflammation]. Constitutional disease of infancy marked by faulty nutrition and bone deformity. SYN: *rachitis, rickets, q.v.*

rhacoma (rā-kō'mă) [G. *rhakoein*, to rend]. 1. Ragged, irregular abrasion, usually of the skin. 2. Relaxation of integument of scrotum.

rhagades (răg'ăd-ēz) [G. *rhagadēs*, tears]. Linear fissures appearing in skin, esp. at the corner of the mouth or anus, causing pain.

If due to syphilis, they form a radiating scar on healing.

rhagadiform (răg-ăd'ĭ-form) [" + L. *forma*, shape]. Fissured; having cracks.

-rhage, -rhagia [G.]. Suffix meaning *bleeding.*

rhaphania (răf-ā'nĭ-ă) [G. *rhaphanos*, radish]. Spasmodic disease caused by eating the wild radish. SYN: *raphania.*

rhaphe (rā'fē) [G. *rhaphē*, a seam]. A seam or ridge. SYN: *raphe.*

-rhea. [G. *rhoia*, flow]. Suffix meaning *to flow.*

rhegma (rĕg'mă) [G. *rhēgma*, a tear]. Rupture, fracture or rent, as of vessel walls, a bone, or of an abscess.

rhembasmus (rĕm-băs'mŭs). Wandering of mind; indecision.

rhenium (re'nĭ-um). A metallic element similar to manganese. SYMB: Re. At. wt. 186.2; at. no. 75.

rheo- [G.]. Combining form meaning *current, stream,* or *to flow.*

rheobase (rē'ō-bās) [G. *rheos*, current, + *basis*, step]. In unipolar testing with the galvanic current using negative as active pole, the minimal voltage required to produce a stimulated response.

This is the rheobase, or threshold of excitation. SEE: *chronaxie.*

rheochord (rē'ō-kord) [" + *chordē*, cord]. Type of rheostat used for measuring resistance of an electric current. SEE: *rheostat.*

rheometer (rē-ŏm'ĕt-ĕr) [" + *metron*, a measure]. 1. Instrument for qualitative determination of presence of an electric current. SYN: *galvanometer.* 2. Device for measuring rapidity of the blood current.

rheonome (rē'ō-nōm) [" + *nemein*, to distribute]. Device for ascertaining the effect of irritation on a nerve.

rheophore (rē'ō-fōr) [" + *phoros*, a carrier]. A cord conducting an electrical current, as one bet. patient and electrical apparatus. SYN: *electrode.*

rheoscope (rē′ō-skōp) [" + *skopein,* to examine]. Device indicating the existence of an electric current. SYN: *galvanoscope.*

rheostat (rē′ō-stăt) [" + *statos,* standing]. A device maintaining fixed or variable resistance for controlling the amount of current entering a circuit.

rheostosis (rē-ŏs-tō′sĭs) [G. *rheos,* current, + *osteon,* bone]. A hypertrophying and condensing osteitis in streaks, involving long bones.

rheotachygraphy (rē-ō-tă-kig′ră-fī) [" + *tachys,* swift, + *graphein,* to write]. Graphic recording of variation of electromotive force in a muscle.

rheotaxis (rē″ō-tăks′ĭs) [" + *taxis,* arrangement]. Reaction to a current of fluid causing the part acted upon to move against the current.

rheotome (rē′ō-tōm) [" + *tomē,* a cutting]. A device for interrupting electrical current at required intervals.

rheotrope (rē′ō-trōp) [" + *tropos,* a turning]. An instrument for automatically reversing a current of electricity.

rhestocythemia (rĕs″tō-sī-thē′mĭ-ă) [G. *rhaistos,* destroyed, + *kytos,* cell, + *aima,* blood]. Condition of degenerated red blood cells in the peripheral circulation.

rheum, rheuma (rūm, rūm′ă) [G. *rheuma,* a flowing]. Any catarrhal or watery discharge.

r., salt. Moist tetter and similar skin eruptions; chronic eczema.

rheumatic (rū-măt′ĭk) [G. *rheuma,* a flowing]. Pert. to rheumatism.

r. chorea. SEE: *chorea, Sydenham's.*

r. fever. A systemic, febrile disease, inflammatory and nonsuppurative in nature, variable in severity, duration, and sequelae. It is frequently followed by serious heart disease.

ETIOL: Unknown, but its onset usually follows a preceding infection with a strain of group A beta hemolytic streptococci. Attacks usually occur in childhood; an individual is especially susceptible to subsequent attacks. Onset gradual or acute.

SYM: Preceding streptococcal respiratory infection, fever, migratory polyarthritis, pain upon motion, abdominal pain, Sydenham's chorea (St. Vitus' dance), cardiac involvement (pericarditis, myocarditis, and endocarditis). Later gives rise to precordial discomfort and development of heart murmurs. Skin manifestations include *erythema marginatum* and development of subcutaneous nodules. Epistaxis is common.

TREATMENT: Enforced bed rest until signs of active rheumatic fever have disappeared. Salicylates for symptomatic relief. Penicillin administered to eradicate streptococci. Complications, especially those involving heart, require special treatment.

PROPHYLAXIS: Prompt and adequate treatment of streptococcal infections with penicillin preferably, or erythromycin in appropriate dose *for a minimum of 10 days.* Following an attack of rheumatic fever, individuals should receive continuous prophylaxis with penicillin or sulfadiazine for an indefinite period.

rheumatism (rū′măt-ĭzm) [G. *rheuma,* a flowing, + *-ismos,* condition]. A general term commonly applied to conditions acute and chronic, characterized by soreness and stiffness of muscles and pain in joints and associated structures. It includes arthritis (infectious, rheumatoid, gouty), arthritis due to rheumatic fever or trauma, degenerative joint disease, neurogenic arthropathy and degenerative joint disease, hydroarthrosis, myositis, bursitis, fibromyositis, and many other conditions. SEE: *arthritis, rheumatic fever.*

r., acute articular. SEE: *rheumatic fever.*

r., chronic. R. associated with a joint disorder such as rheumatoid arthritis, gout, or degenerative joint disease which usually results in deformity of the joint.

r., gonorrheal. Arthritis resulting from gonorrheal infection. SEE: *gonorrhea.*

r., muscular. Term applied to a number of muscular conditions characterized by tenderness, soreness, pain, and local spasm. Includes such conditions as fibromyositis, myositis, myalgia, and torticollis, *q.v.*

r., palindromic. Recurring attacks of acute arthritis and periarthritis at irregularly spaced intervals.

r., psychogenic. R. of psychic origin, esp. that occurring under emotional stress; common among soldiers.

rheumatoid (rū′mă-toyd) [" + *eidos,* like]. Of the nature of rheumatism.

r. arthritis. Form with inflammation of the joints, stiffness, swelling, cartilaginous hypertrophy, and pain. SEE: *arthritis.*

r. factor. About 85% of adults with rheumatoid arthritis have an immunoglobulin (I, M) termed *rheumatoid factor* present in their serum. This factor, though not specific for rheumatoid arthritis, is quite helpful in diagnosing and investigating this disease.

rhexis (rĕks′ĭs) [G. *rhēxis,* a rupture]. The rupture of any organ, blood vessel, or tissue.

rhic″no′sis. Wrinkling of the skin due principally to atrophy of subcutaneous tissue, esp. elastic fibers.

rhinal (rī′năl) [G. *rhis, rhin-,* nose]. Concerning the nose. SYN: *nasal.*

rhinalgia (rī-năl′jĭ-ă) [" + *algos,* pain]. Pain in nose; nasal neuralgia.

rhinencephalon (rī-nĕn-sĕf′ăl-ŏn) [G. *rhis, rhin-,* nose, + *egkephalos,* brain]. Portion of brain concerned with reception and integration of olfactory impulses. Includes *olfactory bulb, olfactory tract* and *striae, intermediate olfactory area, pyriform area, paraterminal area, hippocampal formation,* and *fornix.* It constitutes the *paleopallium* and *archipallium.*

rhinesthesia (rī-nĕs-thē′zĭ-ă) [" + *aisthēsis,* sensation]. The sense of smell.

rhineurynter (rī-nū-rĭn′tĕr) [" + *eurynein,* to dilate]. Elastic bag used for dilating the nostrils.

rhinion (rin′ĭ-on) [G. *rhinion,* nostril]. Lower end of the suture bet. nasal bones. A craniometric point. SYN: *punctum nasale inferius.*

rhinitis (rī-nī′tĭs) [G. *rhis, rhin-,* nose, + *-itis,* inflammation]. Inflammation of the nasal mucosa. SEE: *endorrhinitis, ozena.*

r., acute. SYN: *common head cold, coryza.* Acute congested condition of nose with increased secretion of mucus.

TREATMENT: No specific treatment is known. General measures include rest, adequate fluids, well-balanced diet. Analgesics and antipyretics may be used to make patient comfortable. Sulfonamides and antibiotics are of no value and should not be administered.

Antihistamines may relieve early symptoms but do not "abort" or alter course. Vasoconstrictors in form of inhalants or nasal sprays or drops may give temporary relief. Their use helps prevent the development of middle ear infections by helping to maintain the patency of the *eustachian tubes.*

r., allergic. SYN: *atopic rhinitis, vasomotor rhinitis, hay fever.* Rhinitis due to sensitivity of nasal mucosa to an allergen.

r., atrophic. Chronic inflammation with marked atrophy of mucous membrane with considerable dry crusting and disturbance in the sense of smell.

Usually accompanied by ozena. The throat is dry and, as a rule, contains crusts. A husky voice or hoarseness is often a common accompaniment.

SYM: Fetid odor from nose and throat, with considerable crusting.

TREATMENT: Irrigation of nose with warm alkalinized saline solution twice daily. General hygienic measures. Correction of any associated disorders. Surgical treatment seldom helpful.

r. caseosa. Unilateral rhinitis characterized by accumulation in nose and sinuses of offensive cheeselike masses and accompanied by a seropurulent discharge.

r., chronic hyperplastic. Chronic inflammation of mucous membrane accompanied by polypoid formation and underlying sinus pathology. SEE: *sinus.*

r., chronic hypertrophic. Inflammation of the mucous membrane of the nose characterized by hypertrophy of the mucous membrane of the turbinates and the septum.

SYM: Those of nasal obstruction, postnasal discharge and recurrent head colds.

TREATMENT: Consists in surgical removal of hypertrophic or mulberry ends of inf. turbinates and cauterization of mucosa of inf. turbinates and septum.

r., fibrinous. R. characterized by formation of a false membrane in nasal cavities.

r., perennial. SYN: *vasomotor r.; hyperesthetic r.* Rhinitis which is nonseasonal but continues indefinitely with variations in severity.

r., periodic. Allergic rhinitis, *q.v.*

r., pseudomembranous. Fibrinous r., *q.v.*

r., vasomotor. Rhinitis with rhinorrhea due to increased secretion of mucus from the nasal mucosa. May be caused by allergy or neurovascular imbalance.

rhino- [G.]. Combining form meaning *the nose.*

rhinoantritis (rī"nō-ăn-trī'tĭs) [G. *rhis, rhin-*, nose, + *antron*, cavity, + *-itis*, inflammation]. Inflamed condition of the nasal cavities and one or both maxillary antra.

rhinobyon (rī-nō-bī'ŏn) [" + *byein*, to plug]. A tampon or plug for the nose.

rhinocanthectomy (rī"nō-kăn-thĕk'tō-mĭ) [" + *kanthos*, corner of the eye, + *ektomē*, excision]. Excision of inner canthus of the eye. SYN: *rhinommectomy.*

rhinocele (rī'nō-sēl) [" + *koilos*, hollow]. The ventricle or hollow of the olfactory lobe or *rhinoencephalon.*

rhinochiloplasty (rī"nō-kī'lō-plăs-tĭ) [" + *cheilos*, lip, + *plastos*, formed]. Plastic surgery of the nose and upper lip.

rhinocleisis (rī-nō-klī'sĭs) [" + *kleisis*, closure]. Nasal obstruction.

rhinodacryolith (rī-nō-dăk'rĭ-ō-lĭth) [" + *dakryon*, tear, + *lithos*, stone]. A nasal calculus.

rhinodynia (rī-nō-dĭn'ĭ-ă) [G. *rhis, rhin-*, nose, + *odynē*, pain]. Nasal pain. SYN: *rhinalgia.*

Rhinoestrus (rī-nĕs'trŭs). A genus of flies belonging to family Oestridae. Larvae may be deposited in eye or nasal and buccal cavities of mammals.

R. purpureus. Russian gad-fly, whose larvae sometimes cause naso- and ophthalmomyiasis in man.

rhinogenous (rī-nŏj'ĕn-ŭs) [" + *gennan*, to produce]. Originating in the nose.

rhinokyphosis (rī"nō-kī-fō'sĭs). A nose with an excessively prominent bridge.

rhinolalia (rī-nō-lā'lĭ-ă) [" + *lalia*, speech]. Nasal quality of voice.

r. aperta. R. caused by undue patency of posterior nares.

r. clausa. R. caused by closure of nasal passages.

rhinolaryngitis (rī"nō-lăr-ĭn-jī'tĭs) [" + *larygx*, tube, + *-itis*, inflammation]. Inflammation of mucosa of nose and larynx at the same time.

rhinolite (rī'nō-līt) [" + *lithos*, a stone]. A nasal calculus; stone in the nose.

rhinolith (rī'nō-lĭth) [" + *lithos*, stone]. Nasal concretion.

rhinolithiasis (rī"nō-lĭth-ī'ă-sĭs) [" + " + *-iasis*, condition]. The formation of nasal calculi.

rhinologist (rī-nŏl'ō-jĭst) [G. *rhis, rhin-*, nose, + *logos*, study]. A specialist in diseases of the nose.

rhinology (rī-nŏl'ō-jĭ) [" + *logos*, study]. Science of the nose and its diseases.

rhinomanometer (rī"nō-măn-ŏm'ĕt-ĕr) [" + *manos*, thin, + *metron*, a measure]. A device for measuring the amount of nasal obstruction.

rhinometer (rī-nŏm'ĕt-ĕr) [" + *metron*, a measure]. Device for measurement of the nose or its cavities.

rhinomiosis (rī-nō-mī-ō'sĭs) [" + *meiōsis*, a lessening]. Surgical reduction in size of the nose. Also spelled *rhinomeiosis.*

rhinommectomy (rī-nŏm-mĕk'tō-mĭ) [" + *omma*, eye, + *ektomē*, excision]. Surgical excision of the inner canthus.

rhinomycosis (rī"nō-mī-kō'sĭs) [" + *mykēs*, fungus, + *-ōsis*, condition]. Fungi in mucous membranes and secretions of the nose.

rhinonecrosis (rī"nō-nē-krō'sĭs) [G. *rhis, rhin-*, nose, + *nekrōsis*, death]. Necrosis of the nasal bones.

rhinopathy (rī-nŏp'ă-thĭ) [" + *pathos*, disease]. Any nasal diseases.

rhinopharyngitis (rī"nō-făr-ĭn-jī'tĭs) [" + *pharygx, pharygg-*, pharynx, + *-itis*, inflammation]. Inflamed condition of the nasopharynx.

rhinopharyngocele (rī"nō-făr-ĭn'gō-sēl) [" + " + *kēlē*, a mass]. A nasopharyngeal tumor.

rhinopharyngolith (rī"nō-făr-ĭn'gō-lĭth) [" + " + *lithos*, stone]. Concretion in the nasal pharynx.

rhinopharynx (rī"nō-făr'ĭnks) [" + *pharygx*, pharynx]. Upper portion of pharynx continuous with the nasal passages.

rhinophonia (rī"nō-fō'nĭ-ă) [" + *phōnē*, voice]. A nasal tone in speaking.

rhinophyma (rī-nō-fī'mă) [G. *rhis, rhin-*, nose, + *phyma*, growth]. Lobular hypertrophy of nose, with red coloration, congestion and retention of sebum. SYN: *acne rosacea.*

rhinoplasty (rī'nō-plăs-tĭ) [" + *plastos*, formed]. Plastic surgery of the nose.

rhinopolypus (rī-nō-pŏl′ĭp-ŭs) [" + *polys,* many, + *pous,* foot]. Polypus of the nose.

rhinoreaction (rī″nō-rē-ăk′shŭn) [" + L. *rē,* back, + *actio,* an acting]. Moeller's test for tuberculosis, a nasal tuberculin reaction.

rhinorrhagia (rī-nō-rā′jĭ-ă) [" + *rhēgnūnai,* to burst forth]. Profuse hemorrhage from nose. SYN: *epistaxis, nosebleed.*

rhinorrhea (rī-nō-rē′ă) [" + *rhoia,* a flow]. Thin, watery discharge from nose.

r., cerebrospinal. Discharge of spinal fluid from nose due to defect in cribriform plate.

rhinosalpingitis (rī″nō-săl″pĭn-jī′tĭs) [" + *salpigx, salpigg-,* tube, + *-itis,* inflammation]. Inflammation of the mucosa of the nose and eustachian tube.

rhinoscleroma (rī-nō-skle-rō′mă) [G. *rhis, rhin-,* nose, + *sklēros,* hard, + *-ōma,* tumor]. A chronic, infectious disease involving nose and upper portions of respiratory tract in which growths of almost stony hardness develop, sometimes leading to marked deformity.

ETIOL: *Klebsiella rhinoscleromatis.* A gram-negative encapsulated bacillus.

SYM: The disease presents a hard, nodular growth, which usually begins at ant. end of nose and spreads to the lower respiratory tract. There is usually no pain and no tendency to ulceration.

TREATMENT: Surgical, in combination with streptomycin.

rhinoscope (rī′nō-skōp) [" + *skopein,* to examine]. Instrument for examination of the nose.

rhinoscopy (rī-nŏs′kō-pĭ) [" + *skopein,* to examine]. Examination of nasal passages.

r., anterior. E. through anterior nares.

r., posterior. E. through posterior nares usually with small mirror in nasopharynx.

rhinosporidiosis (rī″nō-spō-rĭd″ĭ-ō′sĭs). Condition caused by a fungus, *Rhinosporidium seeberi,* which causes development of pedunculated polyps on mucous membranes of nose, larynx, eyes, penis, vagina and sometimes skin of various parts of body. Disease is contracted from cattle. Found in India, Ceylon, and other parts of the world.

Rhinosporidium (rī″nō-spō-rĭd′ĭ-ŭm). A genus of fungi which is pathogenic to man.

R. seeberi. Causative agent of *rhinosporidiosis, q.v.*

rhinostenosis (rī″nō-sten-ō′sĭs) [" + *stenōsis,* a narrowing]. Obstruction of the nasal passages. SYN: *rhinocleisis.*

rhinotomy (rī-nŏt′ō-mĭ) [" + *tomē,* incision]. Incision of the nose.

rhinovaccination (rī″nō-văk-sĭn-ā′shŭn) [" + L. *vaccinus,* pert. to a cow]. Vaccine applied to the mucosa of the nose.

Rhipicephalus (rī″pĭ-sĕf′ă-lŭs). A genus of ticks belonging to the family Ixodidae. Several species, esp. *R. sanguineus,* serve as vectors for the organisms of spotted fever, boutonneuse fever, and other rickettsial diseases.

rhitidectomy (rĭ-tĭ-dĕk′tō-mĭ) [G. *rhytis,* wrinkle, + *ektomē,* excision]. Removal of wrinkles by operation. SYN: *rhytidectomy.*

rhitidosis (rĭ-tĭ-dō′sĭs) [" + *-ōsis,* condition]. 1. Wrinkling of face without corresponding signs of age. 2. Wrinkling of the cornea, indicating its disintegration. SYN: *rhytidosis.*

rhizo- [G.]. Combining form meaning *root.*

rhizodontropy (rī-zō-dŏn′trō-pĭ) [G. *rhiza,* root, + *odous, odont-,* tooth, + *tropē,* a turning]. Process of pivoting an artificial crown upon the root of a tooth.

rhizodontrypy (rī-zō-dŏn′trĭ-pĭ) [" + " + *trypē,* a hole]. Puncture of root of a tooth.

rhizoid (rī′zoyd) [G. *rhiza,* root, + *eidos,* form]. 1. Rootlike. 2. A rootlike structure, usually one-celled, occurring in lower forms of plant life. 3. In bacteriology, term applied to a colony showing an irregular rootlike system of branching.

rhizome (rī′zōm) [G. *rhizōma,* a mass of roots]. SYN: *root, stock.* An underground stem.

rhizomelic (rī-zō-mĕl′ĭk) [G. *rhiza,* root, + *melos,* limb]. Concerning the hips and shoulders, in man the roots of the extremities.

Rhizopoda (rī-zop′ō-dā) [G. *rhiza,* root, + *pous,* pod-foot]. A subclass of the class Sarcodina, phylum Protozoa, characterized by possession of lobose pseudopodia and lacking a central filament. Includes the amebae and foraminifera.

rhizotomy (rī-zŏt′ō-mĭ). [G. *rhiza,* root, + *tomē,* a cutting]. SYN: *Dana's operation.* Section of a root, as of a nerve or tooth.

r., anterior. Section of ventral root of spinal nerve.

r., posterior. SYN: *Dana's operation.* Section of dorsal root of spinal nerve for the relief of pain.

rhodium (ro′dĭ-um). A rare metallic element. SYMB: Rh. At. wt. 102.905; at. no. 45.

rhodogenesis (rō″dō-jĕn′ĕs-ĭs) [" + *genesis,* formation]. Regeneration of visual purple bleached by light.

rhodophane (rō′dō-fān) [" + *phainein,* to show]. A red pigment found in retinal cones of birds and fishes.

rhodophylaxis (rō-dō-fī-lăks′ĭs) [" + *phylaxis,* protection]. Ability of the retinal epithelium to regenerate visual purple which has been bleached by light.

rhodopsin (rō-dŏp′sĭn) [" + *opsis,* vision]. Visual purple, a pigment in outer segment of retinal rods.

rhombencephalon (rŏm-bĕn-sĕf′ă-lŏn) [G. *rhombos,* rhomb, + *egkephalos,* brain]. SYN: *hindbrain.* A primary division of the embryonic brain which gives rise to metencephalon and myelencephalon. Includes the pons, cerebellum, and medulla oblongata.

rhombocele (rŏm′bō-sēl) [G. *rhombos,* rhomb, + *koilos,* a hollow]. The cavity of the rhombencephalon.

rhomboid (rŏm′boyd) [" + *eidos,* shape]. An oblique parallelogram.

r. fossa, r. sinus. The 4th ventricle of the brain.

rhomboideus (rŏm-boi′dē-ŭs) [L.]. One of 2 muscles beneath the trapezius muscle. SEE: *Table of Muscles in Appendix; muscles, back, for illustration.*

rhoncal, rhonchial (rong′kal, rŏng′kĭ-ăl) [G. *rhogchos,* a snore]. Pert. to or produced by a rhonchus, or rattle in the throat.

rhonchus (rŏn′kŭs) [G. *rhogchos,* a snore]. A râle or rattling in the throat, esp. when it resembles snoring.

rhotacism (rō′tăs′ĭzm) [G. *rhōtakizein,* to overuse letter r]. Overuse or improper utterance of *r* sounds, with too much emphasis upon this letter.

rhubarb (rū′barb) [L. *rhabarbarum,* wild rhubarb]. USP. Extract made from roots and rhizome of *Rheum officinale, R. palmatum,* and other species.

ACTION AND USES: Cathartic and astringent.

COMP: High in oxalic acid. Of little food value but desirable for its mineral content.

COOKED *(sugar added):* 100 grams. Calories: 141. Protein: 0.5 gm; trace of fat; carbohydrate: 63 gm.; calcium: 78 mg.

Rhus (rus). A genus of trees and shrubs, some of which are poisonous as poison ivy (*Rhus toxicodendron*) or poison sumac (*R. venenala*).

rhyostomaturia (rī″ō-sto-mă-tū′rĭ-ă) [G. *rhyas*, fluid, + *stoma*, mouth, + *ouron*, urine]. The elimination of urinary elements by the salivary glands.

rhyparia (rī-pa′rĭ-ă) [G. *rhyparia*, filth]. 1. Foul substance in mouth in low fevers. SYN: *sordes*. 2. Filth.

rhypophagy (rī-pŏf′ă-jĭ) [G. *rhypos*, filth, + *phagein*, to eat]. The eating of filth. SYN: *scatophagy*.

rhypophobia (rī-pō-fō′bĭ-ă) [" + *phobos*, fear]. Abnormal disgust at the act of defecation, feces, or filth.

rhythm (rĭth′ŭm) [G. *rhythmos*, measured motion]. 1. A measured time or movement; regularity of occurrence of action or function. 2. Marking the intermenstrual periods of fertility and sterility in the female. SEE: *cacorhythmic*.

r., alpha. SYN: *Berger rhythm or wave, alpha wave*. In electroencephalography, rhythmical oscillations in electric potential occurring at a rate of 8 to 12 per sec. Characteristic of inattentive brain or in drowsiness or narcosis.

r., atrioventricular nodal. SYN: *A-V nodal rhythm*. Rhythmic discharge of impulses from atrioventricular (A-V) node which occurs when activity of S-A node is depressed or abolished. If impulses arise in upper or atrial portion of node, the atria are activated slightly before ventricles (*upper nodal rhythm*); if in middle portion, atria and ventricles contract simultaneously (*middle nodal rhythm*); if in lower or ventricular portion, atria are activated slightly before ventricles (*lower nodal rhythm*).

r., Berger. Alpha rhythm, *q.v.*

r., beta. SYN: *beta waves*. In electroencephalography, waves ranging in frequency from 15 to 30 per sec. and of lower voltage than alpha waves. More pronounced in frontomotor leads.

r., bigeminus. The coupling of extrasystoles with previously normal beats.

r., cantering. Gallop rhythm, *q.v.*

r., coupled. One in which every other heartbeat produces no pulse at the wrist.

r., delta. SYN: *delta waves*. In electroencephalography, slow waves with a frequency of ½ to 3 per sec. and of relatively high voltage (20 to 200 microvolts). Occur in sleep.

r., ectopic. A cardiac rhythm originating outside S-A node. May be *homotropic* or *heterotropic, q.v.*

r., gallop. Abnormal heart rhythm with three sounds in each cycle resembling gallop of a horse.

r., idioventricular. Rhythm of ventricles occurring in heart block resulting from establishment of a new center of rhythmicity in ventricular myocardium usually in bundle of His.

r., nodal. SEE: *r., atrioventricular*.

r., pendulum. R. with the 2 heart sounds alike, with the sound of a ticking clock.

r., sinus. The normal cardiac rhythm proceeding from the sinoatrial node.

r., tic-tac. A state of cardiac distress in which the first and second heart sounds are the same quality. SYN: *embryocardia*.

r., ventricular. Very slow ventricular contractions in heart block.

rhyth′mic. Rhythmical; pertaining to or marked by rhythm.

rythmicity (rĭth-mĭs′ĭ-tĭ). Characterized by rhythmic activity.

rhytidectomy (rĭt-ĭd-ĕk′tō-mĭ) [G. *rhytis*, wrinkle, + *ektomē*, excision]. Excision of wrinkles by plastic surgery.

rhytidosis (rĭt-ĭd-ō′sĭs) [" + *-ōsis*, condition]. 1. Wrinkling of the skin. 2. Wrinkling of cornea.

Occurs in cases of great diminution in tension of eyeball, particularly after the escape of aqueous or vitreous, usually near death. SYN: *rhitidosis*.

rib (rib) [A.S. *ribb*]. One of a series of 12 pairs of narrow, curved bones extending laterally and anteriorly from sides of thoracic vertebrae and forming a part of the skeletal thorax. With the exception of the floating ribs, they are connected to the sternum by means of costal cartilages.

r., asternal. A false rib, *q.v.*

r., bicipital. Condition usually involving the first rib. Results from fusion of two ribs.

r., cervical. A supernumerary rib sometimes developing in connection with a cervical vertebra, usually the lowest.

r.'s, false. Five ribs on each side not directly attached to the sternum.

r.'s, floating. Two lower ribs not attached to the sternum.

r., lumbar. A rudimentary rib which develops in relation to a lumbar vertebra.

r., sternal. A true rib.

r.'s, true. The upper 7 ribs on each side which join the sternum by separate cartilages.

riboflavin (rĭb″ō-flāv-ĭn). SYN: *vitamin* B_2, *vitamin G, lactoflavin, ovoflavin, hepatoflavin*. A water-soluble vitamin of the B complex group. It is an orange-yellow crystalline powder ($C_{17}H_{20}N_4O_6$), comparatively stable to heat and air but unstable in light.

SOURCES: Milk and milk products, leafy green vegetables, liver, beef, fish, dry yeast. Also synthesized by bacteria in body.

DAILY REQUIREMENT: 1.0 to 2.0 mg. depending on activity. For pregnant and lactating women, should be increased.

EFFECTS OF DEFICIENCY: Eye disorders, cheilosis, glossitis, seborrheic dermatitis, esp. of face and scalp.

FUNCTIONS: It is a constituent of certain flavoproteins which function as coenzymes in cellular oxidations. Essential for tissue repair.

ribonuclease (rĭb-ō-nū′klē-ās). An enzyme which catalyzes the depolymerization of ribonucleic acid (RNA) with formation of mononucleotides. ABBR: *RNA-ase*.

rib″onu″cle″ic′ acid. ABBR: *RNA*. A nucleic acid found principally in the nucleolus, microsomes, and mitochondria of cells. It appears to play an important role in synthetic reactions within cells.

ribose. $C_5H_{10}O_5$, a pentose sugar present in ribonucleic acids, riboflavin, and some nucleotides.

rice (rīs) [G. *oryza*]. 1. A cereal grass (*Oryza sativa*) raised extensively in warm climates for its seed or grain. 2. The seeds of rice plant widely used as a food.

COMP: Poor in nitrogen and fats, high in carbohydrates. Lowest of all cereals in albumin. Polished rice contains half as much phosphorus and lime as white bread, while magnesium is lower and iron a little higher. Potassium much higher than in other cereals. Cellulose is higher than in bread and residue greater.

RICE *(cooked, parboiled):* 100 gm. Calories: 106; protein: 2.1 gm; fat: 0.1 gm.; carbohydrate: 23 gm.; calcium: 19 mg.

POTENTIAL ACIDITY: 9 cc. per 100 gm., 2.6 cc. per 100 cal.

ACTION: Easier to digest than bread, but large quantities tax the digestive system. In cooking, the starch is partly converted into dextrin. It is highly nutritive and strengthening.

r., polished. Rice which has been milled to produce the white product commercially available in Western countries. This treatment removes the hull which contains the majority of the vitamin B_1.

r. water stools. Those of cholera which resemble water in which rice has been boiled.

ricin (ris′in). A white, amorphous, highly toxic protein (albumin) present in the seed of the castor bean, *Ricinus communis.*

ricinine (rĭs′ĭn-ēn, -in). A poisonous alkaloid present in the leaves and seeds of castor bean plant, *Ricinus communis.*

ricinoleic acid. 12-hydroxy-9-octadecenoic acid. An unsaturated hydroxy acid comprising about 80% of fatty acids in the glycerides of castor oil. Has a strong laxative action.

rickets (rĭk′ĕts). SYN: *rachitis, avitaminosis D.* A form of osteomalacia in children resulting from deficient deposition of lime salts in developing cartilage and newly formed bone, resulting in abnormalities in shape and structure of bones.

ETIOL: Due primarily to vitamin D deficiency which affects the absorption of calcium and phosphorus from the intestine and the reabsorption of phosphorus by the renal tubules. May also result from inadequate intake or excessive loss of calcium.

SYM: Restlessness and slight fever at night (101-102° F.), free perspiration about head, diffuse soreness and tenderness of body, pallor, slight diarrhea, enlargement of liver and spleen, delayed dentition and eruption of badly formed teeth, head large and more or less square in outline, craniotabes or skull bones often so thin they crackle like parchment.

Sides of thorax flattened; sternum prominent; nodules can be felt at sternal ends of ribs, forming rachitic rosary. Deformity may be kyphosis, lordosis or scoliosis. Liver and spleen may be considerably enlarged, long bones are curved and prominent at their extremities.

PROG: Serum phosphatase studies are helpful in making diagnosis and prognosis. Usually favorable. Deformity disappears in 90% of cases.

PROPHYLAXIS AND TREATMENT: Exposure to ultraviolet light (sunlight or artificial light) and administration of vitamin D in quantities to provide 400 International Units of vitamin D activity per day are effective in prevention of rickets.

For active rickets, careful regulation of diet to meet nutritive requirements of the child plus administration of 1600 I.U. of vitamin D per day is usually effective. Some bone deformities may require surgery.

CAUTION: Excessive use of vitamin D (in infants, over 20,000 I.U. daily; in adults over 100,000 I.U. daily) is to be avoided because of danger of hypervitaminosis D.

r., renal. SYN: *renal osteitis fibrosa generalisata.* A disturbance in epiphyseal growth during childhood due to severe chronic renal insufficiency resulting in persistent acidosis.

Dwarfism and failure of gonadal development result.

PROG: Poor.

TREATMENT: Diet low in meat, milk, cheese and egg yolk and adm. of calcium lactate or calcium gluconate in large doses.

rickettsia (rĭk-ĕt′sĭ-ă). Term applied to any of the microorganisms belonging to the genus Rickettsia, *q.v.*

Rickettsia. Generic name applied to a group of microorganisms, family Rickettsiaceae, order Rickettsiales, which occupy a position intermediate between viruses and bacteria. They differ from bacteria in that they are obligate parasites requiring living cells for growth and differ from viruses in that they are retained by the Berkefeld filter. They are the causative agents of many diseases and are usually transmitted by arthropods (lice, fleas, ticks, mites) which serve as vectors. SEE: *rickettsial diseases, rickettsiosis.*

rickettsial disease. A disease caused by an organism of the genus Rickettsia. The most common types are: spotted-fever group (Rocky Mt. spotted fever, African tick fever, rickettsialpox); typhus group (endemic typhus, epidemic typhus, Brill's disease, and scrub typhus).

rickettsialpox (rĭk-ĕt″sĭ-ăl-pŏks). An acute, febrile, self-limited disease caused by *Rickettsia akari.* It is transmitted from mouse to man by a small colorless mite, *Alloderma-anyssus sanguineus.*

rickettsiosis. Infection with Rickettsia.

riders' bone (rī′derz). Bony formation in adductor muscle of leg. Seen in those who ride horses extensively. SYN: *cavalry bone.*

r. leg, r. sprain. Sprain of adductor muscles of the thigh.

ridge (rĭj) [M.E. *rigge,* from A.S. *hrycg,* back of an animal]. An elongated projecting structure or crest.

r., carotid. A sharp ridge between carotid canal and jugular fossa.

r., epicondylic. One of 2 ridges for muscular attachments on the humerus.

r., gastrocnemial. A ridge on post. femoral surface for attachment of gastrocnemius muscles.

r., genital. R. which develops on ventromedian surface of urogenital ridge and gives rise to gonads.

r., gluteal. A ridge extending obliquely downward from great trochanter of femur for the attachment of the gluteus maximus muscle.

r., interosseous. A ridge on the fibula for attachment of the interosseous membrane.

r., mesonephric. Ridge which develops on lat. surface of urogenital ridge and gives rise to mesonephros.

r., pronator. Oblique ridge on the ant. surface of ulna, giving attachment to the pronator quadratus.

r., pterygoid. One at angle of junction of temporal and infratemporal surface of great wing of the sphenoid bone.

r., superciliary, r., supraorbital. Curved ridge of the frontal bone over supraorbital arch.

r., supracondylar. One of two ridges (lateral and medial) on distal end of humerus extending upward from lat. and med. epicondyles.

r., tentorial. One on upper inner surface of the cranium to which is attached the tentorium.

r., trapezoid. An oblique ridge on the upper surface of the clavicle giving attachment to the trapezoid ligament.

r., urinogenital. SYN: *urogenital fold, wolffian ridge.* Ridge on dorsal wall of coelom which gives rise to genital and mesonephric ridges, *q.v.*

r., wolffian. *Mesonephric ridge, q.v.*

ridgel, ridgil, ridgeling, ridgling (rĭj'ĕl, -ĭl, -lĭng) [origin uncertain]. A male human being or animal with only one testicle.

Riedel's lobe (rē'dĕl). A tongue-shaped process of liver, frequently found protruding over gallbladder in cases of chronic cholecystitis.

Riga's disease (rē'gă). Ulceration of frenum of the tongue with membrane formation.

right. Dexter. Pertaining to the side of the body opposite to the left. ABBR: *R.*

right-handed. Voluntary preference for use of the right hand.

rigid. Stiff, hard, unyielding.

rigidity (rĭj-ĭd'ĭ-tĭ) [L. *rigidus,* stiff]. 1. Tenseness; immovability; stiffness; inability to bend or be bent. 2. In psychiatry, refers to one who is excessively resistant to change.

r., cadaveric. Rigor mortis.

r., cerebellar. Stiffness of body and extremities resulting from lesion of middle lobe of cerebellum.

r., cogwheel. Condition noted upon passively stretching a hypertonic muscle in which resistance is jerky.

r., decerebrate. Sustained contraction of extensor muscles of limbs resulting from a lesion in the brain stem between sup. colliculi and vestibular nuclei.

rigor (rĭ'gōr, rĭg'or) [L. *rigor,* stiffness]. 1. A sudden, paroxysmal chill with high temperature, called the *cold stage,* followed by a sense of heat and profuse perspiration, called the *hot stage.* 2. A state of hardness and stiffness, as in a muscle. Rigor chills may be coarse, fine, diffuse, trembling.

r. mortis. The stiffness seen in corpses. SEE: *dead, care of the; Nysten's law.*

rima (rī'ma) (pl. *rimae*) [L. *rima,* a slit]. A slit, fissure, or crack.

r. cornea'lis. Groove in the sclera holding edge of the cornea. SYN: *corneal cleft.*

r. glottidis. An elongated slit between the vocal folds.

r. oris. Aperture of the mouth.

r. palpebrarum. Slit bet. the eyelids.

r. pudendi. Space bet. the labia majora. SYN: *pudendal slit, vulvar slit, urogenital cleft.*

r. respiratoria. Space behind the arytenoid cartilages.

r. vestibuli. BNA. Space bet. the false vocal cords. SYN: *glottis spuria.*

r. vocalis. SEE: *r. glottidis.*

rimose (rī'mōs) [L. *rimōsus,* full of cracks]. Fissured or marked by cracks.

rimous (rī'mŭs) [L. *rimōsus,* full of cracks]. Filled with cracks or fissures. SYN: *rimose.*

rimula (rĭm'ū-lă) [L. *rimula,* a little crack]. A minute fissure or slit, esp. of the spinal cord or brain.

rind (rīnd) [A.S. bark]. The skin or cortex of an organ or person.

r. tumor. Neoplasm arising from lining membrane tissue of the embryo. SYN: *lepidoma.*

ring (rĭng) [A.S. *hring*]. 1. Any round organ or band around a circular opening. 2. BACT: A growth like a ring around upper margin of a liquid culture, adhering to the glass more or less closely. SEE: *annulus.*

r., ciliary. SYN: *orbicularis ciliaris.* Portion of ciliary body consisting of a bandlike zone lying directly anterior to ora serrata.

r., femoral. The sup. aperture of femoral canal.

r., inguinal, abdominal. SYN: *internal abdominal ring.* The abdominal opening of the inguinal canal.

r., inguinal, subcutaneous. SYN: *ext. abdominal ring.* The external opening of inguinal canal.

r., tympanic. SYN: *tympanic annulus.* A ring of bone formed by three elements, squamous, petro-mastoid and tympanic which develops into tympanic plate.

Ringer's solution (rĭng'er). An aqueous solution containing sodium, calcium, and potassium chlorides.

USES: In forms of dehydration, and for improving circulation.

ringworm (rĭng'wŭrm). A dermatomycosis due to various species of fungi belonging to the genera *Microsporum, Epidermophyton* and *Trichophyton.*

Ringworm of the scalp is called *Tinea capitis;* of the body, *Tinea corporis;* of the beard, *Tinea barbae;* of the nails, *Tinea unguium.* SEE: *tinea.*

SYM: Red ringed patch of vesicles, itching, pain, scaling.

TREATMENT: Griseofulvin may be helpful in certain types. Preparations containing undecylenic acid, zinc undecylenate, and triethanolamine.

r., crusted. SYN: *favus; Tinea favosa, q.v.*

r., honeycomb. SEE: *Tinea favosa.*

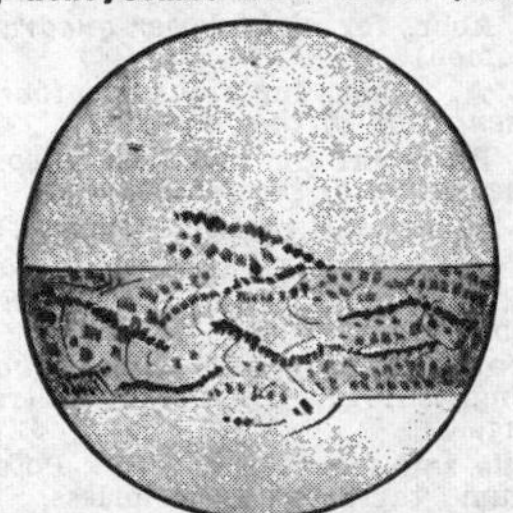

RINGWORM OF HAIR.

Granular threads of the parasite invade and destroy the hair shaft.

Rinne's test (rĭn'nĕh). Use of tuning fork to compare bone conduction hearing with air conduction. The vibrating fork is held by its stem on the mastoid process of the ear until it is no longer heard by the patient. Then it is held close to the external auditory meatus. If the subject still hears the vibrations this is called a *positive Rinne test.*

If the fork is not heard by air conduction, the test is repeated but first air conduction is tested until the sound is no longer heard, then the stem of the fork is placed on the mastoid process of the ear. If the sound is still heard, this is called a *negative Rinne test.*

Riolan's arch (rē-ō-lahn'). Arch of transverse mesocolon.

R.'s bouquet. Two ligaments and 3 muscles attached to styloid process of temporal bone.

R.'s muscle. Ciliary portion of orbicularis oculi. Syn: *musculus ciliaris.*

ripa (rī'pă) [L. *ripa,* bank]. Any line of reflection of the ependyma of the brain from the ventricular wall to the choroid plexus.

Ripault's sign (rē-pōz'). Change in shape of pupil produced by unilateral pressure upon eyeball, transitory phase during life, but permanent after death.

risorius (rĭ-sō'rĭ-ŭs) [L.]. Muscular fibrous band arising over masseter muscle and inserted into tissues at the corner of the mouth. See: *Table of Muscles in Appendix.*

risus (rī'sŭs) [L.]. Laughter; a laugh.

r. sardonicus. A peculiar grin, as seen in tetanus, caused by acute spasm of facial muscles.

Ritter's disease (rĭt'ĕr). Severe inflammation of skin with scaling, seen in infants. Syn: *dermatitis exfoliativa infantum.*

Ritter-Valli law (rĭt"ĕr-văl'ĭ). Increased irritability from center outward if a nerve is cut off from its center or if the latter is destroyed.

Irritability is soon lost.

ri'valry strife. Alternate sensations of color and shape when the fields of vision of the two eyes cannot combine in one visual image.

Rivinus' canals or ducts (re-ve'nŭs). Ducts of sublingual gland.

R.'s glands. Sublingual glands.

R.'s ligament. Small portion of the drum membrane in notch of Rivinus. Syn: *Shrapnell's membrane.*

riziform (rĭz'ĭ-form) [Fr. *riz,* rice, + *forma,* form]. Resembling rice grains.

RLF. Abbr. for *retrolental fibroplasia, q.v.*

RLQ. Abbr. for *right lower quadrant* (of abdomen).

R. M. A. Abbr. for *right mentoanterior presentation of the fetal face.*

R. M. P. Abbr. for *right mentoposterior presentation of the fetal face.*

R. N. Abbr. for *registered nurse.*

RNA. Abbr. for *ribonucleic acid, q.v.*

Robertson's pupil. Same as *Argyll Robertson pupil.*

roborant (rŏb'ō-rănt) [L. *roborans,* strengthening]. 1. A tonic. 2. Strengthening.

Rochelle salt (rō-shĕll'). USP. Potassium sodium tartrate, a colorless, transparent powder, having a cooling and saline taste.

Action and Uses: Saline cathartic.

Rocky Mountain spotted fever. An infectious disease caused by a parasite, *Rickettsia rickettsii,* and transmitted by a wood tick; marked by fever, pains in bones and muscles, and profuse reddish eruption.

In the Rocky Mountains and on the Pacific Coast the mortality is no longer high. See: *spotted fever, tick fever.*

rod (rŏd) [A.S. *rodd,* club]. 1. Slender, straight bar. 2. One of the slender, long sensory bodies in retina responding to faint light. 3. Bacterium shaped like a rod.

r.'s and cones. The light-sensitive portions of rod and cone visual cells of the retina. They form the 2nd layer lying between ext. limiting membrane and pigment epithelium. The rods contain visual purple (rhodopsin), essential for vision in dim light.

r.'s, enamel. Minute calcareous rods or prisms laid down by ameloblasts and forming enamel of a tooth.

rodent ulcer (rō'dĕnt) [L. *rodere,* to gnaw]. A slow growing, gnawing cancer which steadily eats into tissues, causing great destruction.

The most usual sites are on outer angle of the eye, near side and on tip of nose, and edges of the scalp. See: *ulcer, rodent.*

rodenticide. An agent which kills rodents.

rodonalgia (rō-dŏn-ăl'jĭ-ă) [G. *rhodon,* rose, + *algos,* pain]. Vasomotor condition marked by redness and neuralgic pain of the extremities and swelling, and fever. Syn: *erythromelalgia.*

roentgen (rĕnt'gĕn). The international unit of roentgen radiation. The unit of dose of x- and gamma rays.

r. equivalent man. The dose of ionizing radiation which produces the same biological effect in man as one unit of x- and gamma rays. Abbr: *rem.*

roentgenography (rent-gen-og'ră-fĭ). The process of obtaining pictures by use of roentgen rays.

roentgenologist (rĕnt-gĕn-ŏl'ō-jĭst) [*roentgen* + G. *logos,* study]. A physician skilled in roentgen diagnosis, roentgen therapy, or both.

roentgenology (rĕnt-gĕn-ŏl'ō-jĭ) [*roentgen* + G. *logos,* study]. The science of applying roentgen rays for diagnostic and therapeutic purposes.

roentgenotherapy, roentgentherapy (rĕnt-gĕn-ō-ther'ăp-ĭ, rĕnt-gĕn-ther'ă-pĭ) [*roentgen* + G. *therapeia,* treatment]. The treatment of disease by exposure of the patient to roentgen rays.

roentography (rĕn-tŏg'ră-fĭ) [*roentgen* + G. *graphein,* to write]. The making of x-ray pictures. Syn: *roentgenography, skiagraphy.*

roetein, roetheln (ret'ĕln). German measles, *q.v.* Syn: *rubella.*

Rokitansky's disease (rō-kĭt-ăn'skĭ). Acute yellow atrophy of the liver.

Rolan'do's area. Motor area in the cerebral cortex.

R. fissure. Fissure bet. parietal and frontal lobes. Syn: *sulcus centralis.*

roller (rōl'er) [L. *rotula,* a little wheel]. 1. Strip of muslin or other cloth rolled up in cylinder form for surgeon's use. 2. A roller bandage. See: *bandage.*

Rollier technic (rōl'ē-ā). Method of using heliotherapy in which the body is gradually exposed to the sun's rays.

romaine (rō-mān') [Fr. *romaine,* Roman]. A leafy vegetable in the lettuce family. Also called *cos* or *cos lettuce.* Average serving: 50 gm. Protein: 0.7 gm.; carbohydrate: 1.8 gm.

Roman numerals. Those used by the Romans in contradistinction to the Arabic numerals which we now use.

In Roman notations values are increased either by adding 1 or more symbols to the initial symbol, as III for 3, or by subtracting a symbol from 1 or more to the right of it, as IV for 4, IX for 9, etc., as shown in the following table:

Arabic	Roman	Arabic	Roman
1	I	18	XVIII
2	II	19	XIX
3	III	20	XX
4	IV	30	XXX
5	V	40	XL
6	VI	50	L
7	VII	60	LX
8	VIII	70	LXX
9	IX	80	LXXX
10	X	90	XC
11	XI	100	C
12	XII	500	D
13	XIII	900	CM
14	XIV	1,000	M
15	XV	1,900	MCM
16	XVI		
17	XVII	1,000,000	$\overline{M}$

A line placed over a letter increases its value 1000 times, as $\overline{M}$ is equal to 1000 times 1000 for which the M stands.

romanopexy (rō-man'ō-pĕks"ĭ) [L. *romanum*, the sigmoid, + G. *pēxis*, fixation]. Fixation of the sigmoid flexure for prolapse of the rectum. Syn: *sigmoidopexy.*

romanoscope (rō-măn'ō-skōp) [" + G. *skopein*, to examine]. Instrument for examining the sigmoid flexure.

Romberg's sign (rŏm'bĕrg). Inability to maintain the body balance when the eyes are shut and the feet close together; seen in tabes dorsalis, severe alcoholic neuritis, etc.

rongeur (ron-zhŭr') [Fr. *ronger*, to gnaw]. A gouge forceps, an instrument for removing tiny fragments of bone.

roof nucleus (rūf nū'klē-ŭs). Small mass of gray matter in white substance of vermis of the cerebellum. Syn: *nucleus fastigii.*

rooming-in. The housing of mothers in the same hospital room as their infants, beginning immediately following birth.

root (rūt) [A.S. *rōt*]. 1. The underground part of a plant. Ex: *Stillingia, Glycyrrhiza, Belladonna.* 2. Proximal end of a nerve. 3. Portion of an organ implanted in tissues.

r., anterior. Syn: *ventral root.* One of two roots by which a spinal nerve is attached to spinal cord. Contains efferent nerve fibers. Also called motor root.

r. arteries. A. accompanying nerve roots into the spinal cord. Syn: *radicular vessels.*

r. canal. Pulp cavity of root of tooth.

r., posterior. Syn: *dorsal root.* One of two roots by which a spinal nerve is attached to spinal cord. Contains afferent nerve fibers. Also called *sensory root.*

r. sheath. Epithelium covering the hair follicle.

r. zone. Burdach's column of the spinal cord. Outer tract of post. funiculus or white column of the cord. Syn: *fasciculus cuneatus.*

R. O. P. Abbr. for *right occipitoposterior presentation, i. e.*, the occiput of fetus being in relation to the right sacroiliac joint of the mother.

rosa (rō'ză) [L.]. Rose.

r. asturica. Deficiency disease due to lack of vitamin B_2. Syn: *pellagra.*

rosacea (rō-zā'sē-ă) [L. *rosaceus*, rosy]. Chronic hyperemic disease of the skin, esp. of the nose. Syn: *acne rosacea.*

rose cold or rose fever. Summer or June cold; hay fever of early summer attributed to inhaling rose pollen. See: *hay fever.*

Rosenbach's sign (rō'zĕn-băhk). Absence of abdominal skin reflex in intestinal inflammation.

Rosenmüller's body (rō'zĕn-mū-ler). Rudimentary tubule in the mesosalpinx bet. the fallopian tube and ovary. Syn: *epoophoron, parovarium.*

R.'s cavity, R.'s fossa. Slitlike depression in the pharyngeal wall behind opening of the eustachian tube.

roseo- [L.]. 1. Combining form meaning *rose-colored.* 2. A prefix in chemical terms.

roseola (rō-zē'ō-lă) [L. *roseus*, rosy]. 1. Skin condition marked by maculae or red spots of varying sizes on the skin; a rose-colored rash. 2. Measles or German measles. Syn: *rose rash.*

r. idiopathica. Macular eruptions not associated with any well-defined symptoms.

r. infantum. Syn: *exanthem subitum.* A noninfectious roseola occurring in infants; characterized by high fever, splenomegaly, and a rash which appears just as the fever subsides.

r. symptomatica. Macular eruption occurring in well-defined diseases.

roseolous (rō-zē'ō-lŭs) [L. *roseus*, rosy]. Resembling or pert. to roseola.

rose rash (rōz răsh). Any red colored eruption. Syn: *roseola.*

rosette. 1. Something that resembles a rose. 2. A spherical group of fine red vacuoles surrounding cytocentrum of a monocyte.

rose water (rōz wau'ter). Saturated aqueous solution of the oil of rose.

Action and Uses: To impart agreeable odor to lotions, etc.

rosin (rŏz'ĭn) [L. *resina*]. Substance distilled from oil of turpentine and used as adhesive and stimulant on plasters.

Rossbach's disease (rŏs'băhks). Excessive secretion of gastric acid. Syn: *gastroxynsis; hyperchlorhydria.*

Rossolimo's reflex (rŏs-ō-lē'mō). Plantar flexion of 2nd to 5th toes in response to percussion of plantar surface of the toes.

Ross' bodies (rŏs). Bodies sometimes found in tissue fluids in syphilis.

They are copper-colored, round and dark granules sometimes exhibiting ameboid movements.

rostellum (rŏs-tĕl'lŭm) [L. *rostellum*, little beak]. A fleshy protrusion on anterior end of scolex of tapeworms bearing one or more rows of spines or hooks.

rostral (rŏs'trăl) [L. *rostrum*, beak]. 1. Resembling a beak. 2. Toward the front or cephalic end of the body.

rostrate (rŏs'trāt) [L. *rostrum*, beak]. Having a beak or hook formation.

rostrum (rŏs'trŭm) [L. beak]. Any hooked or beaked structure.

rosulate (rŏs'ū-lāt) [L. *rosulatus*, like a rose]. Shaped like a rosette.

rot. To decay or decompose.

r., jungle. Common term for certain fungus diseases of the skin occurring in the tropics.

rotate (rō'tāt) [L. *rotāre*, to turn]. To twist or revolve.

rotation (rō-tā'shŭn) [L. *rotatio*, a turning]. Process of turning on an axis.

r., fetal. Twisting of the fetal head as it follows the curves of the birth canal, downward.

rotator (rō-tā'tor) (pl. *rotatores*) [L. that which turns]. A muscle revolving a part on its axis.

r., uterine. An elevator or replacer used to push or rotate the uterus when it is out of its natural position.

röteln, rötheln (re'teln) [Ger. *rot,* red]. German measles. SYN: *rubella.*

Rothera's test (rŏth'ĕ-ră). Method for finding acetone bodies in urine. SEE: *acetone.*

Rouget cells. Contractile cells which surround the capillaries, observed in frogs and salamanders.

roughage (rŭf'ij) [M.E. *rough,* from A.S. *rūh*]. Indigestible fiber of fruits, vegetables, and cereals which acts as a stimulant to aid intestinal peristalsis.

Plenty of water should be added to consumption of roughage. Should not be used in colitis or in intestinal irritation. SEE: *cellulose.*

r. diet. Diet with large amounts of cellulose, water, mineral salts and vitamins. SYN: *high residue diet.*

rouleau (roo-lō') (pl. *rouleaux*) [Fr. roll]. A group of red blood corpuscles arranged like a roll of coins.

round (rownd) [L. *rotundus,* round]. Circular in shape.

r. ligament. 1. Curved fibrous cord attached to center of articular surface of head of femur. 2. Two round cordlike structures passing from front of the body of the uterus in ant. wall of broad ligament, below the fallopian tubes, outward through the inguinal canals to soft tissues of the labia majora. 3. Fibrous cord which is the remnant of umbilical vein.

roundworm. SYN: *threadworm.* Any member of the phylum Nemathelminthes (Aschelminthes), esp. one belonging to the class Nematoda, *q.v.*

RPF. Abbr. for *renal plasma flow.*

RPS. Abbr. for *renal pressor substance.* SEE: *renin.*

R. Q. Abbr. for *respiratory quotient.*

-rrhagia (rā'jĭ-ă) [G. *-rrhagia,* from *rhēgnunai,* to burst forth]. Combining form indicating *abnormal discharge, hemorrhage.*

R.S.A. Abbr. for *right sacroanterior* position of fetus.

R.T. Abbr. for *reading test, registered technician.*

R.U. Abbr. for *rat unit.*

Ru. Chem. symbol for *ruthenium.*

rubber dam. Thin rubber tissue used by dentists to seal off the tooth being treated from the saliva in the mouth.

rubedo (rū-bē'dō) [L.]. Temporary redness of the skin. SYN: *blushing.*

rubefacient (rū"be-fā'shĕnt) [L. *rubefaciens,* making red]. 1. Causing redness, as of the skin. 2. Agent which reddens the skin, producing a local congestion, the vessels becoming dilated and the supply of blood increased.

The rubefacients include: (a) *mustard;* (b) *turpentine;* (c) *capsicum;* (d) *flaxseed;* (e) *arnica,* and (f) *liniments.*

rubella (rū-bĕl'lă) [L. *rubellus,* reddish]. Acute infectious disease, resembling both scarlet fever and measles, but differing from these in its short course, slight fever and freedom from sequelae. SYN: *German measles; röteln; three-day measles.*

INCUBATION: 14-21 days. It produces a maculopapular rash which vanishes by slight desquamation in from 2 to 3 days.

SYM: Prodromes, slight or altogether absent. Drowsiness, slight fever, sore throat. Eruption 1st or 2nd day. In some cases, rash composed of pale red, scarcely elevated papules, more or less discrete rubella morbilliforme; in others, rash is bright red and diffuse like that of scarlet fever, rubella scarlatiniforme. Begins on face, spreads rapidly over whole body, but fades so rapidly that face may be clear before extremities are affected. Slight desquamation frequently present, though not always. Superficial cervical and posterior auricular glands more swollen than in measles. Duration, 3 to 5 days.

COMPLICATIONS: Rubella in pregnant women, esp. in first two or three months of gestation, is serious in that it may give rise to fetal anomalies, esp. congenital cataract.

PROG: Good.

TREATMENT: Nonspecific. Local antipruritics for itching. Rest. Liquid diet. Sponging with tepid water.

rubeola (rū-bē'ō-lă) [L. *rubeus,* reddish]. 1. Acute, contagious disease, marked by fever, catarrhal symptoms and a typical cutaneous eruption. SYN: *measles.* 2. Term occasionally applied to acute infectious disease with mild symptoms and rose-colored macular eruption. SYN: *rubella, q.v.*

rubescent (rū-bĕs'ĕnt) [L. *rubescere,* to grow red]. Growing red; flushing.

rubidium (rū-bĭd'ĭ-ŭm) [L. *rubidus,* red]. A soft, silvery metal which decomposes water with violence and bursts into flame spontaneously in air. Its salts are used medicinally. SYMB: Rb. At. wt. 85.47; at. no. 37.

rubiginous (rū-bĭj'ĭn-ŭs). Rusty or rust-colored.

rubigo (rū-bī'gō) [L. rust, mildew]. Rust; mildew.

Rubin's test (rū'bĭn). Transuterine insufflation with carbon dioxide of the fallopian tubes to test their patency. SEE: *sterility.*

rubor (rōō'bor) [L. redness]. Discoloration or redness due to inflammation.

One of the classical symptoms of inflammation. RS: *calor, dolor, tumor.*

rubrospinal (rū"brō-spī'năl) [L. *ruber,* red, + *spina,* thorn]. A descending tract consisting of a small bundle of nerve fibers in lateral funiculus of spinal cord. Fibers arise in cells of the red nucleus of midbrain and terminate in ventral horn of gray matter.

rubrum (ru'brum) [L. red]. Reddish nucleus of gray matter in crus cerebri near optic thalamus.

r. scarlatinum. Scarlet red, a substance used as a healing agent and stain.

ructus (rŭk'tŭs) [L.]. Belching of air from stomach.

rudiment (rū'dĭm-ĕnt) [L. *rudimentum,* a wild thing]. 1. That which is undeveloped. 2. BIOL: A part just beginning to develop. 3. An organ arrested in an early stage of development. 4. Remains of a part functional only at an earlier stage of an individual or in his ancestors.

rudimentary (rū-dĭm-ĕn'tă-rĭ) [L. *rudimentum,* a wild thing]. 1. Elementary. 2. Undeveloped; not fully formed; remaining from an earlier stage. SYN: *vestigial.*

Ruffini's corpuscles. Encapsulated sensory nerve endings found in subcutaneous tissue, thought to mediate sense of warmth.

rufous (rū'fŭs) [L. *rufus,* red]. Ruddy; having a ruddy complexion and reddish hair.

ruga (rū'gă) (pl. *rugae*) [L.]. A fold or crease, esp. one of the folds of mucous membrane seen on internal surface of stomach.

r. of the vagina. SYN: *rugae vaginales.* Small ridges on inner surface of vagina extending laterally and upward from the *columna rugarum* (long ridges on ant. and post. walls).

Ruggeri's reflex. Increase in pulse rate when eyes are strongly converged on a near object.

rugose, rugous (rū'gōs, -gŭs) [L. *rugōsus,* wrinkled]. Wrinkled and rough in short, irregular folds. SYN: *corrugated.*

rugosity (rū-gos'ĭ-tĭ) [L. *rugōsitas,* wrinkled condition]. 1. Condition of being folded or wrinkled. 2. A ridge or wrinkle.

R.U.L. Abbr. for *right upper lobe* (of lung).

rule. A guide or principle based on experience or observation.

rumination (rū-mĭn-ā'shŭn) [L. *rumināre,* to chew the cud]. 1. Regurgitation, esp. with rechewing, of previously swallowed food. 2. In PSYCH., obsessional preoccupation of mind by a single idea, or a set of thoughts and inability to dismiss or dislodge them.

rump (rŭmp) [M.E. *rumpe*]. Post. end of the back; the gluteal region or buttocks.

Rumpf's symptom (rŭmpf). 1. In neurasthenia, the pulse is quickened when pressure is exerted over a painful spot. 2. Twitching, after strong faradization, in traumatic neuroses.

run (rŭn) [A.S. *rinnan,* to flow]. To exude pus or mucus.

run-around, runround (rŭn'ă-rownd. -rownd). Superficial infection encircling the fingernail. SYN: *felon, paronychia, whitlow.*

rupia (rū'pĭ-ă) [G. *rhypos,* filth]. A cutaneous eruption, usually of tertiary syphilis, which manifests itself at first by large elevations of the epidermis, filled with a clear or bloodstained serum, soon becoming turbid and purulent.

The bulla bursts, allows some fluid to escape and as it desiccates is covered with a crust, which dries, accumulates new layers and becomes covered with greenish-brown scales, sometimes to depth of ½ in. Thickest of all syphilides and presents most extensive ulcerations.

TREATMENT: Constitutional, antisyphilitics.

rupophobia (rū"pō-fō'bĭ-ă) [" + *phobos,* fear]. Abnormal dislike for dirt or filth. SYN: *rhypophobia.*

rupture (rŭp'tūr) [L. *ruptūra,* a breaking]. A breaking apart, as of an organ. SYN: *hernia, q.v.*

r. of membranes. R. of amniotic sac as normal result of dilatation of the cervix uteri in labor.

r. of perineum. Rupture of p. in labor, a condition the obstetrician seeks to avoid; more frequent in *primiparae.*

r. of tubes. Rupture of a fallopian tube; a serious event in extrauterine pregnancy which may occur without the woman's knowledge of her pregnancy.

r. of uterus. Rare and due to unrelieved obstructed labor.

RUQ. Abbr. for *right upper quadrant* (of abdomen).

Russell's bodies (rŭs'ĕl). Hyaline, small, spherical bodies in cancerous and simple inflammatory growths.

Russian bath. Hot vapor bath followed by friction and plunge in cold water.

rusts. Members of an order of parasitic fungi (Uredinales) all of which are parasitic on plants; many are allergens.

Rust's disease (rŭst). Tuberculosis of 2 upper cervical vertebrae and their articulations.

rusty (rŭst'ĭ) [A.S. *rustig*]. Reddish in color. Resembling or containing rust. SYN: *rubiginous.*

r. sputum. Reddish sputum expectorated in pneumonia.

rut. SYN: *estrus, heat.* Period of sexual excitement in lower animals during which ovulation and mating usually take place.

rutabaga (rū"tă-bā'gă) [Swedish *rotabagge*]. A large variety of turnip. AVERAGE SERVING: 120 gm. Calories: 55. Protein: 1.3 gm.; fat: 0.1 gm.; carbohydrate: 13.0 gm. Vitamins: A, B, C.

rut-formation. Loss of interest in environment, fixation upon a single object, and concentration of emotional or other interests in a groove or rut.

ruthenium (rū-thē'nĭ-ŭm). A hard, brittle, metallic element of platinum group. SYMB: Ru. At. wt. 101.07; at. no. 44.

ruth'erford. ABBR: *rd.* A unit of radioactivity representing 10^6 disintegrations per sec.

rutidosus (rŭt-ĭ-dō'sŭs) [G. *rhytis,* wrinkle]. Contraction or puckering of cornea just before death.

rutilizm (rū'tĭl-ĭzm) [L. *rutilis,* red, + G. *-ismos,* condition]. Having red or auburn-colored hair.

rutin. A crystalline glucoside of quercetin, closely related to hesperidin. Derived from buckwheat; said to be a constituent of thirty-eight specific plants.

USES: To restore increased capillary fragility to normal, preventing vascular accidents in patients with hypertension; in various hemorrhagic conditions in which permeability, or capillary fragility is involved.

Rx. Symbol for "take," "recipe." SEE: *prescription.*

rye (rī) [A.S. *ryge*]. COMP: Contains cellulose and sometimes ergot.

WAFERS: 2 wafers (13 gm.). Calories: 45. Other main values: 2 gm. protein; trace of fat; 10 gm. carbohydrate; 6 mg. calcium.

ACTION: Hard to digest. Cellulose may be desirable in constipation.

rytidosis (rĭt-ĭ-dō'sĭs) [G. *rhytis,* a wrinkle, + *-ōsis,* condition]. Wrinkling or contraction of cornea preceding death. SYN: *rutidosis.*

Notes

Notes

Notes

Notes

Notes

S

S. Abbr. for *signa,* mark, term used in prescription writing; *sinister,* left; *semis,* half; *spherical* or *spherical lens.*

S. Symb. for *sulfur;* also L. *sine,* without.

saber shin. Ant. border of the tibia marked with sharp convexity found in hereditary syphilis.

sabulous (săb′ū-lŭs) [L. *sabulum,* sand]. Gritty; sandy.

saburra (să-bŭr′ră) [L. *saburra,* sand]. Foulness of stomach or mouth due to decayed food. SYN: *sordes.*

saburral (să-bŭr′ăl) [L. *saburra,* sand]. 1. Pert. to foulness of mouth or stomach due to accumulation of decayed food. 2. Pertaining to sand, as in application of a hot sand bath for relief from pain, as in muscular rheumatism.

sac (săk) [G. *sakkos,* a bag]. A baglike part of an organ; a cavity or pouch, sometimes containing fluid. SEE: *cyst.*

s., air. An alveolar cell in the lung.

s., allantoic. SYN: *vesicle, allantoic.* The expanded end of the allantois, well developed in birds and reptiles.

s., alveolar. SYN: *air sac.* The terminal portion of an air passageway within the lung. Its wall contains pocketlike structures (*alveoli*) and each alveolar sac is connected to a respiratory bronchiole by an *alveolar duct.*

s., amniotic. A thin membrane, containing a serous fluid, enclosing the embryo. SYN: *amnion.*

s., chorionic. SYN: *chorionic vesicle.* Saclike structure consisting of chorion which encloses the developing embryo.

s., conjunctival. The cavity lined with conjunctiva which lies between the eyelids and ant. surface of the eye.

s., dental. The mesenchymal tissue surrounding a developing tooth.

s., endolymphatic. The expanded distal end of the endolymph duct.

s., hernial. A saclike protrusion of the peritoneum containing a herniated organ. SEE: *hernia, hernial sac.*

s., lacrimal. Upper dilated portion of the nasolacrimal duct.

s., lesser peritoneal. SYN: *omental bursa.* A large sacculation developing from an invagination of the dorsal mesogastrium which gives rise to the great omentum. It communicates with greater peritoneal cavity through the epiploic foramen.

s., vitelline. The yolk sac, *q.v.*

s., yolk. SYN: *umbilical vesicle.* An extra-embryonic membrane which encloses the yolk in reptiles, birds, and monotremes. It is formed of an inner layer of entoderm invested by splanchnic mesoderm. In marsupials and placental mammals which lack a yolk mass, the yolk sac is a rudimentary vesicle lying within the chorionic sac.

saccate (săk′āt) [L. *saccatus,* baglike]. 1. Pert. to, like, or enclosed in a sac. SYN: *encysted.* 2. BACT: Marking a sac-shaped form, as in a type of liquefaction.

sac′charase. An enzyme which catalyzes the breakdown of disaccharides to monosaccharides, esp. the hydrolysis of sucrose to dextrose. EX: *sucrase, invertase.*

saccharide (săk′ă-rīd) [G. *sakcharon,* sugar]. One of the carbohydrate group containing sugar, made up of monosaccharoses, disaccharoses, and polysaccharoses, *q.v.*

sacchariferous (săk-ă-rĭf′ĕr-ŭs) [" + L. *ferre,* to carry]. Producing or containing sugar.

saccharin (săk′ă-rĭn) [G. *sakcharon,* sugar]. USP. ($C_6H_4SO_2$-NHCO.) A sweet, white, powdered, synthetic product derived from coal tar, 300 to 500 times as sweet as sugar.

USES: In diabetes as sugar substitute.

saccharine (săk′ă-rĭn, -rīn) [G. *sakcharon,* sugar]. Of the nature of, or having the quality of, sugar. SYN: *sweet.*

saccharo- [G.]. Combining form meaning *sugar.*

saccharogalactorrhea (săk″ă-rō-găl-ăk-tō-rē′ă) [G. *sakcharon,* sugar, + *gala, galakt-,* milk, + *rhoia,* flow]. Excessive lactose secreted in milk.

saccharolytic (săk″ă-rō-lĭt′ĭk) [" + *lysis,* dissolution]. Able to split up sugar.

Saccharomyces (săk″ă-rō-mī′sēz) (pl. *saccharomycetes*) [" + *mykēs,* fungus]. A genus of fungi, reproducing by budding. SYN: *yeasts.*

saccharomycosis (săk″ă-rō-mī-kō′sĭs) [G. *sakcharon,* sugar, + *mykēs,* a fungus, + *-ōsis,* condition]. SYN: *blastomycosis.* Any disease or pathologic condition due to yeasts or *Saccharomycetes.*

saccharorrhea (săk-ă-rō-rē′ă) [G. *sakcharon,* sugar, + *rhoia,* flow]. Secretion of sugar in the body fluids, as in urine or perspiration. SEE: *diabetes mellitus, glycosuria.*

saccharose (săk′ăr-ōs) [G. *sakcharon,* sugar]. 1. Sucrose; cane, beet, or maple sugar. 2. One of the group of carbohydrates having the same chemical formula, $C_{12}H_{22}O_{11}$.

saccharosuria (săk″ă-rō-sū′rĭ-ă) [" + *ouron,* urine]. Saccharose in the urine.

saccharum (săk′ăr-ŭm) [L. sugar]. Sugar, the term being used in the pharmacopeia.

s. album. Pure or white crystallized sugar.

s. canadense. Maple sugar.

s. candidum. Rock candy.

s. lactis. Sugar of milk. SYN: *lactose.*

s. purificatum. Pure white sugar.

s. ustum. Burnt sugar; caramel.

saccharuria (săk-ă-rū′rĭ-ă) [G. *sakcharon,* sugar, + *ouron,* urine]. Sugar in the urine.

sacciform (săk′sĭ-form) [G. *sakkos,* bag, + L. *forma,* shape]. Bag-shaped or like a sac. SYN: *saccate.*

sacculated (săk′ū-lāt-ĕd) [L. *sacculātus,* baglike]. Consisting of small sacs or saccules.

sacculation (săk″ū-lā′shŭn) [L. *sacculus,* a little bag]. 1. Formation into a sac or sacs. 2. Group of sacs, collectively.

saccule (săk′ūl) [L. *sacculus,* a little bag]. 1. A small sac. 2. The smaller of two sacs comprising the portion of the membranous labyrinth occupying the vestibule of inner ear. It communicates with the utricle, cochlear duct and endolymphatic duct all of which are filled with endolymph. In its wall is the *macula sacculi*, a sensory area.

s. of the larynx. SYN: *ventricular appendix*. A small diverticulum extending ventrally from the laryngeal ventricle lying between ventricular fold and thyroarytenoid muscle.

s., vestibular. SEE: *saccule, 2.*

sacculus (săk'ū-lŭs) (pl. *sacculi*) [L. a small bag]. A saccule or little sac.

saccus (săk'ŭs) [L. a bag). A sac or pouch.

s. endolymphaticus. NA. Dilated, blind end of the *ductus endolymphaticus.*

s. lacrimalis. NA. The lacrimal sac, into which empty the 2 lacrimal ducts.

sacrad (sā'krăd) [L. *sacrum*, sacred, + *ad*, toward]. In the direction of the sacrum.

sacral (sā'krăl) [L. *sacrum*, sacred]. Relating to the sacrum.

s. bone. A triangular bone made up of 5 fused vertebrae just above the coccyx.

s. canal. Continuation of the vertebral canal in the sacrum.

s. flexure. Rectal curve in front of the sacrum.

s. index. Sacral breadth multiplied by 100 and divided by sacral length.

s. nerves. Five pairs of spinal nerves, the upper four of which emerge through the post. sacral foramina, the 5th pair through the sacral hiatus (termination of sacral canal). All are mixed nerves (motor and sensory).

s. plexus. Plexus of sacral nerves from which sciatic nerve originates. It is a part of the lumbosacral plexus.

s. vertebra. Fused segments forming the sacrum.

sacralgia (sā-krăl'jĭ-ă) [" + G. *algos*, pain]. Pain in the sacrum. SYN: *hieralgia.*

sacralization (sā-krăl-ĭ-zā'shŭn) [L. *sacrum*, sacred]. Union of the sacrum and the 5th lumbar vertebra.

sacra media (sā'kră mē'dĭ-ă) [L.]. Middle sacral artery.

sacrectomy (sā-krĕk'tō-mĭ) [" + G. *ektomē*, excision]. Excision of part of sacrum.

sacrificial operation. One in which some organ is removed for the patient's good.

sacro- (sā'krō) [L.]. Prefix denoting the *sacrum.*

sacroanterior (sā"krō-ăn-tē'rĭ-or) [L. *sacrum*, sacred, + *anterior*, comparative of *ante*, before]. Denoting a fetus having the sacrum directed forward.

sacrococainization (sā"krō-kō-kān-ĭ-zā'-shŭn) [" + *cocaine*]. Injection of cocaine through the sacrolumbar space into the spinal cord.

sacrococcygeal (sā"krō-kŏk-sĭj'ē-ăl) [" + G. *kokkyx*, coccyx]. Concerning the sacrum and coccyx.

sacrococcygeus (săk"rō-kŏk-sĭj'ē-ŭs). One of two small muscles (ant. and post.) extending from sacrum to coccyx.

sacrocoxalgia (sā"krō-kŏks-ăl'jĭ-ă) [" + *coxa*, hip, + G. *algos*, pain]. Pain in sacroiliac joint, usually due to inflammation. SEE: *sacrocoxitis.*

sacrocoxitis (sā"krō-kŏks-ī'tĭs) [" + " + G. *-itis*, inflammation]. Inflammation of the sacroiliac joint, frequently tuberculous.

sacrodynia (sā-krō-dĭn'ĭ-ă) [" + *odynē*, pain]. Pain in the region of the sacrum.

sacroiliac (sā"krō-ĭl'ĭ-ăk) [L. *sacrum*, sacred, + *iliacus*, pert. to the hipbone]. Of, or pert. to the sacrum and ilium.

s. disease. Tuberculous disease of the sacroiliac joint.

s. joint. The articulation bet. the hipbone and sacrum.

It is a diarthrodial joint, a narrow joint cavity being present; however, joint movement is limited because of interlocking of articular surfaces.

sacrolumbar (sā"krō-lŭm'bar) [L. *sacrum*, sacred, + *lumbus*, loin]. Of, or concerning the sacrum and loins.

s. angle. Angle formed by articulation of the last lumbar vertebra and the sacrum.

sacroposterior (sā"krō-pŏs-tē'rĭ-or) [" + *posterior*, comparative of *posterus*, coming after]. Having the fetal sacrum directed backward.

sacrosciatic (sā"krō-sĭ-ăt'ĭk) [" + *sciaticus*, pert. to hip joint]. Concerning the sacrum and ischium.

sacrospinalis. A large muscle lying on either side of vertebral column extending from sacrum to head. Its two chief components are the iliocostalis and longissimus muscles. SEE: *Table of Muscles in App.*

sacrotomy (sā-krŏt'ō-mĭ) [" + G. *tomē*, a cutting]. Surgical excision of the lower part of the sacrum.

sacrouterine (sā"krō-ū'tĕr-ĭn) [" + *uterus*. womb]. Concerning the sacrum and uterus.

sacrovertebral (sā"krō-ver'tē-brăl) [" + *vertebra*, vertebra]. Concerning the sacrum and the vertebrae.

s. angle. Angle formed by base of sacrum and 5th lumbar vertebra.

sacrum (sā'krŭm) [L. *sacrum*, sacred]. The triangular bone situated dorsal and caudal from the 2 ilia bet. the 5th lumbar vertebra and the coccyx.

It is formed of five united vertebrae and is wedged between the two innominate bones, its articulations forming the sacroiliac joints. It forms the base of the vertebral column and, with the coccyx, forms the post. boundary of the true pelvis. The sacrum in a male is narrower and more curved than in a female.

sactosalpinx (săk"tō-săl'pĭnks) [G. *saktos*, stuffed, + *salpigx*, tube]. Dilated fallopian tube due to retention of secretions, as in pyosalpinx or hydrosalpinx.

saddle joint (săd'l). Joint with articulating surfaces convex in 1 direction and concave in the other. Ex: *carpometacarpal joint of the thumb.*

s. nose. A nose with a depressed bridge.

sadism (sā'dĭzm, săd'ĭzm) [Fr. *sadisme*]. A morbid phenomenon named after the Marquis de Sade, a French pervert of the 18th century, in which gratification is obtained by hurting others. SEE: *masochism; algolagnia.*

sadist (sa'dist, sad'ist). One who practices sadism.

sadomasochism (sa"do-mas'ĕ-kizm, sad"o-mas'ĕ-kizm). Sexual pleasure related to both sadism and masochism.

Saemisch's ulcer (sā'mĭsh). Serpiginous, infectious ulcer of the cornea.

Saenger's operation (seng'er). A form of cesarean section by which the uterus is taken out before the fetus.

safety symbolism. Engagements to marry, the engagement ring, the wedding, the wedding ring, marriage itself, the public announcement of wedding anniversaries, the advent of children, are all symbols which announce to the world that a man or a woman is the possession of one or the other; a warning, as it were, to protect the other partner from the attentions of one of the opposite sex.

sagittal (săj′ĭ-tăl) [L. *sagitta,* arrow]. Arrowlike; in an anteroposterior direction.

s. *plane.* A vertical plane through the longitudinal axis of the trunk dividing the body into right and left portions. If it is through the midaxis dividing body into right and left halves, it is called a *median* or *midsagittal plane.*

s. *sinus.* The sup. longitudinal sinus.

s. *sulcus.* Groove on inner surface of parietal bones which forms a channel for the sup. sagittal sinus.

s. *suture.* Suture bet. the 2 parietal bones.

sago (sā′gō) [Malay *sagu*]. A substance prepared from various palms, consisting principally of starches. Used as a demulcent and as a food with little residue

ACTION: Easy to digest. Fattening. Leaves little residue.

IND: Convalescence, emaciated conditions and when little residue is desired. SEE: *starch, carbohydrate.*

Saint Anthony's fire. Any of certain inflammations or gangrenous skin conditions, esp. erysipelas, hospital gangrene, and ergotism, *q.v.*

Saint Gotthard's disease. Condition due to presence of hookworms in intestinal tract. SYN: *ankylostomiasis.*

Saint Vitus' dance. Nervous disease with involuntary, jerking motions. SYN: *chorea.*

sal (săl) [L. salt]. Salt; or a substance resembling salt.

s. *ammoniac.* Chloride of ammonia.

salaam convulsion (sa-lahm′) [Arabic *salām,* peace]. Clonic muscular spasm of the trunk resulting in a bowing movement. SYN: *nodding spasm.*

salacious (sa-lā′shŭs) [L. *salax, salac-,* lustful]. Lustful or inciting to lust.

salicylate (săl′ĭ-sĭl″ăt, săl-ĭs′ĭl-āt). Any salt of salicylic acid.

s., *methyl.* The principal constituent of oil of wintergreen. It is applied externally for acute rheumatism.

s., *sodium.* White crystalline substance with disagreeable taste, in some cases even nauseating.

USES: To reduce pain and temperature.

salicylated (săl-ĭs′ĭl-āt-ĕd). Impregnated with salicylic acid.

salicylism (săl′ĭs-ĭl-ĭzm) [*salicylic acid* + G. *-ismos,* condition]. Toxic condition caused by an overdose of salicylic acid or its derivatives.

salicyl-sulfonic acid test. Test for albumin in urine. SEE: *albumin.*

salicyluric acid (săl-ĭs-ĭl-ū′rĭk). Acid in urine after taking salicylic acid or its derivatives.

salifiable (săl-ĭf-ĭ′ă-bl) [L. *sal,* salt, + *fieri,* to be made]. Capable of forming a salt by combining with an acid.

salimiter (săl-ĭm′ĭt-er) [L. *sal,* salt, + G. *metron,* a measure]. Device for testing strength of saline solutions.

saline (sā′lĭn) [L. *salinus,* of salt]. 1. Containing or pert. to salt; salty. 2. A mineral salt that produces evacuation of the intestinal contents. Ex: *magnesium sulfate, sodium sulfate,* and *potassium citrate.*

s. *enema.* E. used to excite peristalsis and evacuation.

Magnesium sulfate, 1 oz. in 2 oz. of very warm water (115° F.), given with a small bore tube. SEE: *enema, physiological salt solution.*

s. *purgative.* Any salt producing evacuation, as Epsom salts.

s. *solution.* A solution of sodium chloride and distilled water; in biological laboratory parlance, a 0.9% solution of sodium chloride. An isotonic solution.

A normal saline s. consists of 0.85% salt solution, which is necessary to maintain osmotic pressure and the stimulation and regulation of muscular motion. SYN: *physiological salt solution, q.v.*

saliva (să-lī′vă) [L. saliva]. The 1st digestive secretion emitted from the salivary glands into the mouth. SYN: *spittle.*

CHARACTER: It is tasteless, clear, odorless, viscid, and weakly alkaline, being neutralized after being acted upon by the gastric juice in the stomach. Sp. gr. 1.002-1.006. Amount secreted in 24 hr., 1000-1500 cc.

CONSTITUENTS: Saliva consists of *inorganic substances* including water, 99.5% salts (chlorides, carbonates, phosphates, and sulfates), gasses in solution, and sometimes abnormal substances being excreted from body, *e.g.,* acetone. *Organic substances* include enzymes (ptyalin, maltase, lysozyme), proteins (serum albumin and globulin, mucin) and small amounts of urea, uric acid, creatine and amino acids. *Cellular elements* include epithelial cells and leukocytes.

FUNCTION: (a) To moisten food facilitating mastication and deglutition, (b) to moisten and lubricate mouth parts, (c) to act as a solvent, (d) for excretion of waste products, (e) to initiate digestion of starches, (f) to assist in regulation of water balance.

RS: *angiosialitis, aptyalia, aptyalism, asialia, glycosialia, insalivation, parotid, ptyalin, ptyalinogen, ptyalism, salivary digestion, s. glands, sialagogue.*

salivary (săl′ĭv-ĕr-ĭ) [L. *saliva,* saliva]. Pert. to, producing, or formed from saliva.

s. *amylase.* Ptyalin, *q.v.* SEE ALSO: *salivary digestion.*

s. *calculus.* Concretion in a salivary duct.

s. *corpuscles.* Nucleated, spherical bodies in saliva thought to be modified leukocytes from lymphatic tissue.

s. *digestion.* That occurring in the mouth resulting from action of salivary enzymes. *Ptyalin,* a salivary amylase, acts on boiled starch converting it successively by hydrolysis to *erythrodextrin, achrodextrin, maltose,* and *isomaltose.* Small quantities of maltose may be converted to glucose by action of *maltase* in saliva. Digestion is limited because of the short time food remains in the mouth but is continued in the stomach until food becomes acidified by gastric juice. Ptyalin is active at a *p*H of 6.7 to 6.8 but inactivated by a *p*H below 6.

s. *glands.* Three pairs of glands including the: (1) *Parotid* glands, 1 on each side of the face below the ear; (2) *submaxillary* glands, principally in the floor of mouth; (3) *sublingual* glands, principally in floor of mouth; (4) *buccal* glands, scattered beneath the mucous membrane of lips and cheeks. They form a secretion that is mixed with the saliva.

Salivary secretion is under nervous control being reflexly initiated by mechanical, chemical, or radiant stimuli acting on taste buds (gustatory receptors) in the mouth, olfactory receptors, visual receptors (eyes) or other sense organs. Secretion may also occur as a result of conditioned reflexes as when one thinks about food or hears a dinner bell.

NERVES: Facial and glossopharyngeal, also the autonomic system.

BLOOD SUPPLY: Branches from the ext. carotid artery. SEE: *saliva, salivary digestion.*

salivation (săl-ĭ-vā'shŭn) [L. *salivātio*, a secreting of saliva]. Excessive secretion of saliva. SYN: *ptyalism.*

salivatory (săl"ĭ-vă'tō-rĭ) [L. *salivātio*, a secreting of saliva]. Producing secretion of saliva.

sallow (săl'ō) [A.S. *salu*]. Of a pale, yellowish gray color, usually said of complexion or skin.

sallowness (săl'ō-nĕs) [A.S. *salu*]. Brownish-yellow tint combined with pallor of skin; normal to brunettes. SEE: *skin, face, facies.*

salmin(e (săl'mēn, -mĭn). $C_{30}H_{57}N_{14}O_6$. A protamine obtained from spermatozoa of salmon. SEE: *protamine, protein.*

salmon (săm'ŭn) (pl. *salmon*) [M.E. *salmon* from L. *salmo, salmon-*, salmon]. CANNED (liquid and solids; pink): 100 grams. Calories: 141. Protein: 20.5 gm.; fat: 5.9 gm.; calcium: 196 gm.

salmon patch (săm'ŭn). Salmon-colored area of the cornea in syphilitic keratitis. SYN: *Hutchinson's patch.*

Salmonella (săl-mō-nĕl'ă) [L.]. A genus of bacteria belonging to the family *Enterobacteriaceae.* They are gram negative, usually motile rods. Several species are pathogenic, some producing mild gastroenteritis, others producing a severe and often fatal food poisoning. Also called *paratyphoid bacilli.*

S. aertrycke (ā-ĕr'trĭk-ĕ). A medium-sized, motile, gram negative rod present in meat poisoning and in paratyphoid fevers.

S. entiritidis. Salmonella gastroenteritis and Salmonella food poisoning in man. SYN: *Gartner's bacillus.*

S. paratyphi A. Causative agent of paratyphoid fever in man.

S. paratyphi B. Causative agent of paratyphoid fever and certain acute food poisonings in man.

S. paratyphi C. Causative agent for certain enteric fevers in Europe, Asia, and Africa.

S. schottmülleri. Species causing paratyphoid fever, Type B.

S. typhosa. The causative agent of typhoid fever. SYN: *Eberth's bacillus.*

salmonellosis (săl-mō-nĕ-lō'sĭs) [L. *salmonella* + G. *-ōsis*, condition]. Infestation with bacteria of genus *Salmonella.*

salpingectomy (săl-pĭn-jĕk'tō-mĭ) [G. *salpigx, salpigg-*, tube, + *ektomē*, excision]. Excision of an oviduct.

salpingemphraxis (săl"pĭn-jĕm-frăks'ĭs) [" + *emphraxis*, a stoppage]. Obstruction of the eustachian tube causing deafness, or of a fallopian tube.

salpingian (săl-pĭn'jĭ-ăn) [G. *salpigx, salpigg-*, tube]. Concerning an oviduct, or the eustachian tube.

salpingion (săl-pĭn'jĭ-ŏn) [G. *salpigx, salpigg-*, tube]. A point at inf. surface of the apex of the petrous portion of temporal bone.

salpingitis (săl-pĭn-jī'tĭs) [G. *salpigx, salpigg-*, tube, + *-itis*, inflammation]. Inflammation of the fallopian tube or, less commonly, of the eustachian tube.

ETIOL: The condition may be acute, subacute, or chronic. The organisms most often associated with salpingitis are the gonococcus, staphylococcus, streptococcus, colon bacillus, and tubercle bacillus.

s., eustachian. SYN: *eustachitis.* Inflammation of the eustachian tube.

salpingo- [G.]. Combining form meaning *trumpet* or *tube.*

salpingocatheterism (săl-pĭng"gō-kăth'ĕt-ĕr-ĭzm) [G. *salpigx, salpigg-*, tube, + *katheter*, catheter, + *-ismos*, process]. Catheterization of the eustachian tube.

salpingocele (săl-pĭn'gō-sēl) [" + *kēlē*, hernia]. Hernial protrusion of an oviduct.

salpingocyesis (săl-pĭng"ō-sī-ē'sĭs) [" + *kyēsis*, pregnancy]. Pregnancy where fetus begins to develop in an oviduct; tubal pregnancy.

salpingo-oophorectomy (săl-pĭng"gō-ō"o-for-ĕk'tō-mĭ) [" + *ōōn*, ovum, + *phoros*, a bearer, + *ektomē*, excision]. Excision of an oviduct and ovary.

OPER. NP: The needle layout, sutures and operating procedure identical with those for hysterectomy. In the operation for a ruptured ectopic pregnancy it is well to have 3 times the usual number of laparotomy pads and packs ready, as well as an extra amount of very warm saline solution for flushing out the abdominal cavity. This is because there may be a great quantity of both fresh and clotted blood to be removed. POSITION: Horizontal.

salpingo-oophoritis (săl-pĭng"ō-ō"o-for-ī'tĭs) [G. *salpigg*, tube, + *ōōn*, ovum, + *phoros*, a bearer, + *-ītis*, inflammation]. Inflammation of the tube and ovary. SYN: *salpingo-oothecitis.*

salpingo-oophorocele (săl-pĭng"gō-ō-of'or-ō-sēl) [" + " + " + *kēlē*, hernia]. Hernia enclosing the ovary and fallopian tube.

salpingo-oothecitis (săl-pĭng"gō-ō"ō-thē-sī'tĭs) [G. *salpigx, salpigg-*, tube, + *ōon*, ovum, + *thēkē*, box, + *-ītis*, inflammation]. Inflammation of a fallopian tube and ovary. SYN: *salpingo-oophoritis.*

salpingo-oothecocele (săl-pĭng"gō-ō"o-thē'kō-sēl) [" + " + " + *kēlē*, hernia]. Hernia of both ovary and fallopian tube.

salpingo-ovariectomy (săl-pĭng"gō-o"var-ĭ-ĕk'tō-mĭ) [" + L. *ovarium*, ovary, + G. *ektomē*, excision]. Surgical removal of an oviduct and ovary. SYN: *salpingo-oophorectomy.*

salpingopexy (săl-pĭng'ō-pĕks"ĭ) [" + *pēxis*, fixation]. Fixation of a fallopian tube.

salpingopharyngeus (săl-pĭng"ō-făr-ĭn'jē-ŭs) [" + *pharygx, pharygg-*, pharynx]. The muscle arising near opening of the eustachian tube. Raises nasopharynx.

salpingorrhaphy (săl-pĭng-or'ă-fĭ) [" + *rhaphē*, a seam]. Suture of an oviduct.

salpingosalpingostomy (săl-pĭng"gō-săl-pĭng-gŏs'tō-mĭ) [" + *salpigx*, tube, + *stoma*, a mouth]. The operation of attaching 1 fallopian tube to the other.

salpingoscope (săl-pĭng'gō-skōp) [G. *salpigx, salpigg-*, tube, + *skopein*, to see]. Device for examining the nasopharynx and eustachian tube.

salpingostenochoria (săl-pĭn-gō-stĕn-ō-kor'ĭ-ă). Stenosis or stricture of auditory tube.

salpingostomatomy (săl-pĭng"gō-stō-măt'ō-mĭ) [" + *stoma*, a mouth, + *tomē*, a cutting]. Creation of an artificial opening in a fallopian tube after it has been occluded as a result of inflammation and scarring.

salpingostomy (săl-pĭng-ŏs'tō-mĭ) [" + *stoma*, a mouth]. Surgical opening of a fallopian tube which has been occluded, or for drainage.

salpingotomy (săl-pĭng-ŏt'ō-mĭ) [" + *tomē*, a cutting]. Incision of a fallopian tube.

salpingo-ureterostomy (săl-pĭng"ō-ūr-ēt"-ĕr-ŏs'tō-mĭ) [" + *ourēter*, ureter, + *stoma*, opening]. Surgical connection of the ureter and the fallopian tube.

salpingysterocyesis (săl-pĭn-jĭs"ter-ō-sī-ē'-sĭs) [" + *hystera*, uterus, + *kyēsis*, pregnancy]. Pregnancy partly in a fallopian tube and partly in the uterus.

salpinx (săl'pĭnks) (pl. *salpinges*) [G. *salpigx*]. The fallopian or eustachian tube.

salsify (săl'sĭ-fĭ) [Italian *sassefrica*, goat's beard]. COMP: Large portion of carbohydrate in the fresh product is in the form of insulin and thus may not be available for metabolism. During storage, insulin is converted to sugars. It is a fibrous food, heavier in carbohydrates, protein and fat than carrots, turnips, beets or celery, but it contains less ash than any of them.

AV. SERVING (cooked): 100 gm. Protein: 2.6 gm.; fat: 0.6 gm.; carbohydrate: 15.1 gm.

salt (sawlt) [A.S. *sealt*]. SYMB: NaCl. 1. White crystalline compound occurring in nature, known chemically as sodium chloride. 2. Containing, tasting of, or treated with salt. 3. To treat with salt. 4. *plural*. Any mineral salt or saline mixture used as an aperient or cathartic, esp. Epsom salts or Glauber's salt. 5. CHEM: A compound consisting of a positive ion other than hydrogen, and a negative ion other than hydroxyl. 6. A chemical compound, usually crystalline, resulting from the interaction of an acid and a base.

Salts and water are the inorganic or mineral constituents of the body. They play specific roles in the functions of cells and are indispensable for life. The principal salts are chlorides, carbonates, bicarbonates, sulfates, and phosphates which are compounds of sodium, potassium, calcium, magnesium, and iron with chlorine, CO_2, sulfur, and phosphorus. In general, salts serve the following roles in the body: 1. Maintenance of proper osmotic conditions. 2. Maintenance of water balance and regulation of blood volume. 3. Maintenance of proper acid-base balance. 4. Provide essential constituents of tissue, esp. bones and teeth. They are essential for normal irritability of muscle and nerve cells and essential for coagulation of the blood. 5. They are essential components of certain enzyme systems, respiratory pigments, and hormones. 6. They regulate cell membrane and capillary permeability.

RS: *chlorite, normal, rheum, sal, saline, salt-free diet, salt glow, secretion, "sial-" words.*

s., buffer. A salt found in the blood which fixes excess amounts of acid or alkali, without a change in hydrogen-ion concentration.

s., Epsom. Magnesium sulfate.

s., Glauber's. Sodium sulfate.

s., iodized. Salt containing 1 part sodium or potassium iodide to 5000 parts of sodium chloride. An important source of iodine in the diet. The use of this form of salt will prevent goiter. Salt which has not been iodized should not be used in the diet.

s., Rochelle. Sodium and potassium tartrate.

s., rock. Native sodium chloride.

s. solution, normal. SEE: *physiological salt solution.*

s. s., physiological. A sterile solution containing 0.85% of sodium chloride in chemically pure distilled water (8.5 gm. sodium chloride in 1000 ml. or one liter of distilled water).

NP: When salt solution is given intravenously or hypodermically, rigid aseptic precautions must be observed. Usually injected in front of thighs or under breasts, as loose tissue is found in these areas. The temperature of the solution is about 100° F., so that when the blood is reached solution will be at body temperature. If the disadvantage of slowness is not very important, administration via the rectum is the least risky, as it is not painful and there is no risk of infection. The patient placed on left side, hips are elevated by a pillow, and the solution, by means of a rectal tube, is instilled into the rectum. The solution is allowed to run in at the rate of about 1 quart per hour.

saltation (săl-tā'shŭn) [L. *saltātio*, a leaping]. 1. Act of leaping or dancing, as in chorea. 2. Abrupt variation in character of a species. SYN: *mutation.* 3. A spurting forth of arterial blood.

saltatory (sal'tă-tō-rĭ) [L. *saltātio*, a leaping]. Marked by dancing or leaping.

s. conduction. Skipping from node to node, said of movement of the potential along myelinated neurons.

s. spasm. Tic of muscles of lower extremity, causing convulsive leaping upon attempt to stand. SEE: *palmus.*

salt-free diet. It is impractical to attempt to maintain a diet absolutely free of sodium chloride. Thus "Salt free" means a *low sodium* diet. A diet which allows 500 mg. (0.5 gm.) of salt per day. On this diet, table salt should not be added to the food. Also, it is important to know the amount of salt in the drinking water, because some areas have water containing a large amount of sodium. Some medicines (for example, sodium salicylate) are quite high in sodium content. Exclusion of sodium-containing medicines is important in attempting to regulate the amount of sodium consumed.

RS: *salt, sodium chloride.*

salt glow. Name given to a rub of the entire body with moist salt for stimulation.

salting out. A method of separating a specific protein from a mixture of proteins by the addition of a salt (*e.g.*, ammonium sulfate).

salt, low-, diet. No salt allowed on patient's tray. No salty food served.

saltpeter. Also spelled *saltpetre* (sawlt' pē'ter) [O.Fr. *salpetre*, from L. *sal*, salt, + *petra*, rock]. A common name for potassium nitrate.

s., Chile. A common name for sodium nitrate. $NaNO_3$. Crystalline powder, saline in taste and soluble in water.

salt-poor diet. All food prepared and served without the addition of salt, including salt-free bread and butter. Milk intake is limited.

salt rheum (sawlt room). Any one of a variety of skin affections of the eczematous type. SEE: *eczema.*

salts. Plural of salt. SEE: *salt, 4.*

salubrious (săl-ū'brĭ-ŭs) [L. *salubris*, healthy]. Promoting or favorable to health. SYN: *wholesome.*

salutary (săl'ū-ta-rĭ) [L. *salutaris*, healthy]. Healthful; promoting health; curative.

salvarsan (săl′var-săn) [L. *salvus,* saved, + G. *arsen,* arsenic]. An arsenical, yellowish powder preparation (606) given intramuscularly or intravenously for syphilis.

RS: *arsphenamine, autoserosalvarsan.*

salve (săv) [A.S. *sealf*]. 1. An ointment applied to wounds. 2. PHARM: Any ointment or cerate made with a base of a fat, oil, petrolatum, resin, etc.

samarium. A rare metallic element. SYMB: Sm. or Sa. At. wt. 150.35; at. no. 62. Sp. gr. 7.54.

sanative (săn′ă-tĭv) [L. *sanāre,* to heal]. Of a healing nature. SYN: *curative.*

sanatorium (săn-ă-tō′rĭ-ŭm) (pl. *sanatoriums* or *-ria*) [L. *sanatōrius,* healing]. An establishment for preservation of health or the treatment of the chronically sick. SYN: *sanitarium.*

sanatory (săn′ă-tō-rĭ) [L. *sanatōrius,* healing]. Curative; conducive to health.

sand (sănd) [A.S.]. Fine grains of disintegrated rock.

s., auditory. Calcareous concretion in labyrinth of the ear. SYN: *otolith.*

s. bath. Therapeutic covering of the body with hot sand.

s., brain. Concretion of matter near base of the pineal gland. SYN: *acervulus cerebri.*

s. tumor. One in membrane of the brain, choroid plexus, and other areas made up of calcareous particles. SYN: *psammoma.*

sandflies. Flies of the order *Diptera* belonging to the genus *Phlebotomus.* They transmit sandfly fever, Oroya fever and various types of leishmaniasis.

sandfly fever. SYN: *three-day fever, pappataci fever.* A mild virus disease which clinically resembles influenza except for absence of respiratory symptoms. The causative virus is transmitted by the common sand fly *phlebotomus papatasii,* a small hairy blood sucking midge which bites at night and has a limited flight range. The disease occurs in tropical and subtropical areas which experience long periods of hot, dry weather.

Sandwith's bald tongue. Abnormally clean tongue seen in late stages of pellagra.

sane (sān) [L. *sanus,* sane, healthy]. Sound of mind; mentally normal.

sanguicolous (săng-gwĭk′ō-lŭs) [L. *sanguis,* blood, + *colere,* to dwell]. Inhabiting the blood, as a parasite.

sanguifacient (săng-gwĭf-ā′shĕnt) [" + *facere,* to make]. Making blood.

sanguiferous (săng-gwĭf′ĕr-ŭs) [" + *ferre,* to carry]. Conducting blood, as the circulatory organs.

sanguification (săng-gwĭf-ĭk-ā′shŭn) [" + *facere,* to make]. Conversion into, or formation of, blood. SYN: *hematopoiesis.*

sanguimotor, sanguimotory (săng″gwĭ-mō′tor, -tō-rĭ) [" + *motor,* a mover]. Pert. to the blood circulation.

sanguine (săng′gwĭn) [L. *sanguineus,* bloody]. 1. Hopeful. 2. Plethoric, bloody; marked by abundance and active blood circulation. 3. Pert. to or consisting of blood.

sanguineous (săng-gwĭn′ē-ŭs) [L. *sanguineus,* bloody]. 1. Bloody; relating to blood. 2. Having an abundance of blood. SYN: *plethoric.*

sanguinolent (săng-gwĭn′ō-lĕnt) [L. *sanguinolentus,* from *sanguis,* blood]. Containing, or tinged with, blood.

sanguinopoietic (săng″gwĭn-ō-poy-ĕt′ĭk) [L. *sanguis,* blood, + *poiein,* to form]. Generating blood. SYN: *hematopoietic, sanguifacient.*

sanguirenal (săng″gwĭ-rē′năl) [" + *rēn,* kidney]. Pert. to the blood supply of the kidneys.

sanguis (săng′gwĭs) [L.]. Blood.

sanguisuga (săng-gwĭs-ū′gă). [L. *sanguis,* blood, + *sugere,* to suck]. A leech or bloodsucker. SEE: *Hirudo.*

sanies (sā′nĭ-ēz) [L. diseased blood]. A thin, fetid, greenish discharge from a wound or ulcer, presenting appearance of pus tinged with blood.

saniopurulent (sā″nĭ-ō-pū′rū-lĕnt) [L. *sanies,* diseased blood, + *purulentus,* full of pus]. Having characteristics of sanies and pus; pert. to a fetid, serous, blood-tinged discharge containing pus.

sanioserous (sā″nĭ-ō-sē′rŭs) [" + *serum,* whey]. Composed of sanies* and serum.

sanious (sā′nĭ-ŭs) [L. *sanies,* diseased blood]. Of the nature of fetid, purulent fluid from an ulcer; sanies.

sanitarium (săn-ĭ-tā′rĭ-ŭm) (pl. *sanitariums* or *-ria*) [L. *sanatōrius,* giving health]. Institution for treatment and recuperation of persons having physical or mental disorders; occasionally limited to place where conditions are prophylactic rather than therapeutic. SYN: *sanatorium.*

sanitary (săn′ĭ-tar-ĭ) [L. *sanitas,* health]. Promoting, or pert. to, conditions improving health.

sanitation (săn″ĭ-tā′shŭn) [L. *sanitas,* health]. The use of measure to promote and establish conditions favorable to health, esp. public health. SEE: *assanation, hygiene.*

sanity (săn′ĭt-ĭ) [L. *sanitas,* health, from *sanus,* sound]. Soundness of health or mind; normal mentality. SEE: *sane.*

santal oil (săn′tăl) [L. *santalum,* sandalwood]. USP. Sandalwood oil. A volatile oil distilled from the wood of the plant.

ACTION AND USES: Expectorant, local and genitourinary irritant with possible antiseptic properties.

INCOMPATIBILITIES: Alkalies.

santonin (săn′tō-nĭn) [L. *santoninum*]. USP. A colorless crystalline substance obtained from the unexpanded flower heads of species of the plant *Artemisia cina.*

ACTION AND USES: A vermifuge against the roundworm.

sap (săp) [A.S. *saep*]. 1. Any fluid essential to life and vitality of a living structure. 2. To cause gradual exhaustion of, as the strength.

s., cell. Hyaloplasm, *q.v.*

s., nuclear. Liquid portion of a cell nucleus. SYN: *karyolymph.*

saphena (să-fē′nă) (pl. *saphenae*) [G. *saphēnēs,* manifest]. Name given to two large veins of the leg.

saphenous (saf′ē-nŭs) [G. *saphēnēs,* visible]. Pert. to or associated with a saphenous vein or nerve in the leg. Superficial, manifest.

s. nerve. A deep branch of the femoral nerve. In lower leg, it follows the long saphenous vein supplying medial side of leg, ankle, and foot.

s. opening. An aperture in the fascia, oval in shape, in inner and upper part of thigh transmitting the saphenous vein below Poupart's ligament. SYN: *fossa ovalis.*

s. veins. Two veins, long and short, passing up the leg, the long from the foot to the saphenous opening, the short one behind outer malleolus up back of leg joining the popliteal. SEE: *vein.*

sapid (săp′ĭd) [L. *sapidus,* tasty]. Savory; tasty; opp. of insipid.

sapo (sā'pō) [L.]. USP. Soap prepared from pure olive oil and sodium hydroxide.

saponaceous (săp-ō-nā'shŭs) [L. *saponaceus,* soapy]. Soapy; resembling soap in feel or quality.

saponatus (să-pō-nā'tŭs). Mixed with soap.

saponification (sa-pŏn"ĭ-fĭ-kā'shŭn) [Fr. *saponifier,* from L. *sāpo, sāpōn-,* soap, + *-ficāre,* to make]. 1. Conversion into soap; chemically, the hydrolysis or the splitting of fat by an alkali yielding glycerol and 3 molecules of alkali salt of the fatty acid, the soap. 2. CHEM: Hydrolysis of an ester into corresponding alcohol and acid (free or in form of a salt).

s. number. In analysis of fats, the number of milligrams of potassium hydroxide needed to neutralize the fatty acids in 1 Gm. of oil or fat. Also called *saponification value.*

saponify (sa-pŏn'ĭ-fī) [L. *sāpo, sāpōn-,* soap, + *-ficāre,* to make]. To convert into a soap, as when fats are treated with an alkali to produce a free alcohol plus the salt of the fatty acid.

Thus, stearin, saponified with sodium hydroxide, yields the alcohol glycerol plus the soap sodium stearate.

saponin (săp'ō-nĭn) [L. *sāpo, sāpōn-,* soap]. Unabsorbable glucoside contained in the roots of some plants forming a lather in an aqueous solution.

Saponins cause hemolysis of red blood cells even in high dilutions. When taken orally, can produce diarrhea and vomiting.

saporific (săp"ō-rĭf'ĭk) [L. *saporificus,* producing taste]. Imparting a taste or flavor.

sapphism (săf'ĭzm) [G. *Sapphō,* Greek poetess]. Sexual desire of women for their own sex.

From Sappho, the reputed instigator of lesbianism.

RS: *amor lesbicus, homosexual, tribadism, urningism.**

sapremia (săp-rē'mĭ-ă) [G. *sapros,* rotten, + *aima,* blood]. A toxic condition caused by the absorption into the blood of toxins or poisons produced by saprophytes or putrefactive bacteria. SEE: *septicemia.*

sapro- [G.]. Combining form meaning *putrid.*

saprodontia (săp-rō-dŏn'shĭ-ă) [G. *sapros,* rotten, + *odous, odont-,* tooth]. Caries of the teeth; tooth decay.

saprogen (săp'rō-jĕn) [" + *gennan,* to produce]. Any microorganism causing or produced by putrefaction.

saprogenic (săp"rō-jĕn'ĭk) [" + *gennan,* to produce]. Causing putrefaction or resulting from it.

saprophilous (săp-rof'ĭl-ŭs) [" + *philein,* to love]. Living on decaying or dead substances, as a microorganism. SYN: *saprophytic.*

saprophyte (săp'rō-fīt) [G. *sapros,* rotten, + *phyton,* plant]. Any organism living on decaying or dead organic matter.

Most of the higher fungi are saprophytes. SEE: *parasite.*

saprophytic (săp-rō-fĭt'ĭk) [" + *phyton,* growth]. Living or growing in decaying or dead matter; characteristic of a saprophyte.

saprozoic (săp-rō-zō'ĭk) [" + *zōon,* animal]. Living on decaying or dead organic matter.

sarapus (sar'ă-pus) [G. *sarapous,* splayfooted]. A person having flat feet.

sarcitis (sar-sī'tĭs) [G. *sarx,* flesh, + *-ītis.* inflammation]. Inflammation of muscle tissue. SYN: *myositis.*

sarco- [G.]. Combining form meaning *flesh.*

sarcoadenoma (sar"kō-ăd"en-ō'mă) [G. *sarx, sark-,* flesh, + *adēn,* gland, + *-ōma,* tumor]. A fleshy tumor of a gland. SYN: *adenosarcoma.*

sarcobiont (sar"ko-bi'ont) [G. " + *bious,* life, + *on,* being]. A microorganism which lives on flesh.

sarcoblast (sar'kō-blăst) [" + *blastos,* a germ]. SYN: *myoblast.* Embryonic cell which develops into a muscle cell.

sarcocarcinoma (sar"kō-kar-sĭn-ō'mă) [" + *karkinos,* crab cancer, + *-ōma,* tumor]. A tumor of malignant growth of sarcomatous and carcinomatous types.

sarcocele (sar'kō-sēl) [" + *kēlē,* a mass]. A fleshy tumor of the testicle.

Sarcocystis (sar"kō-sĭs'tĭs) [" + *kystis,* bladder]. A genus of sporozoons found in the muscles of higher vertebrates (reptiles, birds, and mammals).

S. lindemanni. A species infesting muscles of man.

Sarcodina (sar-kō-dī'nă) [" + *eidos,* form]. A class of Protozoa characterized by absence of a thick pellicle and movement by pseudopodia. They are typically holozoic and reproduce principally by asexual methods. Includes the families Amoebidae and Endamoebidae, the latter including many forms parasitic and pathogenic in man.

sarcogenic (sar"kō-jĕn'ĭk) [" + *gennan,* to produce]. Producing flesh or muscle.

sarcoid (sar'koyd) [" + *eidos,* form]. 1. Resembling flesh. 2. A small epithelioid tubercle-like lesion characteristic of sarcoidosis. *q.v.*

sarcoidosis (sār"koid-ō'sĭs). A chronic granulomatous disease of unknown etiology characterized by the formation of tubercle-like lesions in the organs most generally affected, which are the skin, lymph nodes, lungs, and bone marrow. The term now includes a number of diseases previously considered as separate entities (*Boeck's sarcoid; Schaumann's disease.*

sarcolemma (sar"kō-lĕm'ă) [" + *lemma,* a rind]. A delicate membrane surrounding each striated muscle fiber.

sarcology (sar-kŏl'ō-jĭ) [G. *sarx, sark-,* flesh, + *logos,* a study]. Branch of medicine dealing with study of the soft tissues of the body.

sarcolysis (sar-kŏl'ĭ-sĭs) [" + *lysis,* a dissolution]. Decomposition of the soft tissues or flesh.

sarcolytic (sar"kō-lĭt'ĭk) [" + *lyein,* to dissolve]. Decomposing flesh.

sarcoma (sar-kō'mă) (pl. *sarcomas, -mata*) [G. *sarx, sark-,* flesh, + *-ōma,* tumor]. Cancer arising from underlying tissue; muscle, bone and other connective tissue.

May affect the bones, bladder, kidneys, liver, lungs, parotids, and spleen.

s., botryoid. S. of uterus composed of polypoid mass of soft edematous tissues.

s., chondro-. One composed of masses of cartilage.

s., Ewing's. A diffuse endothelioma or endothelial myeloma forming a fusiform swelling on a long bone.

s., fibro-. A malignant tumor with fibrous tissue and many spindle cells and dilated vessels.

s., giant cell. S. from cancellous bone tissue with large cells with many nuclei. A special type called an epulis is seen in the jaw. SYN: *osteoclastoma.*

s., lipo-. A rare tumor of bone containing cells of various types containing small vacuoles of fat.

s., lymphangio-. S. arising from endothelium of lymph vessels in a lymph gland.

s., myeloid. Same as giant cell sarcoma.

s., myxo-. SYN: *myxoma.* A benign tumor of mucoid tissue such as that of the umbilical cord.

s., osteogenic. One composed of osseous tissue containing variously shaped cells.

s., reticulum cell. SYN: *Hodgkin's sarcoma.* A variety of malignant lymphoma involving the lymph nodes and other lymphatic tissue.

s., rhabdomyo-. An embryonal tumor of striated muscle containing multinucleated cells with a striated cytoplasm.

s., spindle cell. One consisting of small and large spindle-shaped cells.

sarcomatoid (sar-kō'mă-toyd) [G. *sarx, sark-,* flesh, + *-ōma,* tumor, + *eidos,* form]. Resembling a sarcoma.

sarcomatosis (sar-kō-mă-tō'sĭs) [" + " + *-ōsis,* condition]. Condition marked by presence and spread of a sarcoma; sarcomatous degeneration.

sarcomatous (sar-kō'măt-ŭs) [" + *-ōma,* tumor]. Of the nature of, or like, a sarcoma.

sarcomere (sar'kō-mēr) [G. *sarx, sark-,* flesh, + *meros,* a part]. The portion of a striated muscle fibril lying between two adjacent dark lines (*Krause's membranes*) considered to be the structural and functional muscular unit.

sarcomphalocele (sar-kŏm-făl'ō-sēl) [" + *omphalon,* umbilicus, + *kēlē,* mass]. Fleshy tumor at the umbilicus.

sarcomyces (sar"kō-mī'sēz). A fleshy growth having the appearance of a fungus.

Sarcophagidae (sar"kō-fădj'ĭ-dē). The family of the order *Diptera* which includes the flesh flies. Females deposit their eggs or larvae on decaying flesh of dead animals. Larvae of two genera *Sarcophaga* and *Wohlfahrtia* frequently infest open sores and wounds of man giving rise to cutaneous myiasis.

sarcophagy (sar-kŏf'ă-jĭ) [" + *phagein,* to eat]. Practice of eating flesh.

sarcoplasm (sar'kō-plăzm) [" + *plasma,* a thing formed]. Hyaline, semifluid, interfibrillary substance of striated muscle fibers.

sarcopoietic (sar"kō-poy-ĕt'ĭk) [" + *poiein,* to form]. Forming muscle or flesh.

Sarcoptidae (sar"kŏp'tĭ-dē). A family of mites of the order *Acarina,* class *Arachnida,* which includes *Sarcoptes scabiei,* the causative agent of scabies or itch in man and mange and scab in other animals.

sarcosis (sar-kō'sĭs) [" + *-ōsis,* condition]. 1. The development of multiple fleshy tumors. 2. Abnormal formation of flesh.

sarcosome (sar'kō-sōm) [G. *sarx, sark-,* flesh, + *sōma,* body]. A minute granular element found in sarcoplasm of skeletal and cardiac muscle.

Sarcosporidia (sar"kō-spō-rĭd'ĭ-ă) [G. *sarx, sark-,* flesh, + *sporos,* a seed]. An order of protozoa belonging to the class *Sporozoa* which are parasitic in the muscles of higher vertebrates. Includes the genus *Sarcocystis.*

sarcosporidiosis (sar"kō-spō-rĭd-ĭ-ō'sĭs) [" + " + *-ōsis,* condition]. Infestation with *Sarcosporidia* or condition produced by them.

sarcostosis (sar-kŏs-tō'sĭs) [" + *osteon,* bone, + *ōsis,* condition]. Ossification of fleshy or muscular tissue.

sarcostyle (sar'kō-stīl) [G. *sarx, sark-,* flesh, + *stylos,* a column]. Any one of the fine longitudinal fibrillae of a striated muscle fiber.

sarcotic (sar-kŏt'ĭk) [G. *sarx, sark-,* flesh]. 1. Producing or pert. to flesh formation. 2. Agent producing growth of flesh.

sarcous (sar'kŭs) [G. *sarx, sark-,* flesh]. Concerning flesh or muscle.

s. substance. Substance of a sarcous element.

sardine (sar-dēn') [L. *sardina*]. SARDINES (CANNED IN OIL; SOLIDS AND LIQUIDS): 100 gm. Calories: 311. Protein: 20.6 gm.; fat: 24.4 gm.; calcium: 35+ mg.; vitamin A: 180 I.U.

sardon'ic laugh. Old term for a spasmodic affection of facial muscles, giving an appearance of laughter. SYN: *risus sardonicus.*

sartorius (sar-tō'rĭ-ŭs) [L. *sartor,* tailor]. A long, ribbon-shaped muscle of the thigh.

It aids in flexing the knee; longest muscle in the body. So-called from its use in crossing the legs, as tailors do. SEE: *Table of Muscles in Appendix.*

SAT. 1. Abbr. for *satellite.* 2. Abbr. for L. *sine acido thymonucleinico,* without thymonucleic acid.

sat. Abbr. for *saturated.*

SAT-chromosome. One possessing a satellite.

SAT-zone. SYN: *nucleolar zone; nucleolar organizer.* One of several constrictions in a nucleolar chromosome which give rise to the nucleoli.

satellite (săt'ĕl-īt) [L. *satelles,* companion]. A small structure attached to a larger one, esp. a minute body attached to a chromosome by a slender chromatic filament. Also called *trabant.*

s., bacterial. A bacterial colony that grows best when close to a colony of another microorganism.

s. cells. SYN: *capsular cells.* 1. Certain astrocytes which lie close to bodies of neurons in central nervous system. 2. Neuroglial cells enclosing the cell bodies of neurons in spinal ganglia. Also called *amphicytes.*

satellitosis (săt-ĕl-ī-tō'sĭs) [L. *satelles,* companion, + *-ōsis,* condition]. The accumulation of satellite cells about neurons of the central nervous system, seen in certain degenerative and inflammatory conditions.

satiety (sa-tī'ĕt-ĭ) [Fr. *satiété,* from L. *satis,* enough]. Fullness or gratification beyond desire.

saturated (săt'ū-rā-tĕd) [L. *saturāre,* to saturate]. 1. Holding all that can be absorbed, received, combined, etc. 2. Term applied to a solution in which no more of a substance can be dissolved. 3. Term applied to carbon compounds in which all the atoms are linked by single bonds.

s. compounds. Those incapable of additional products, as any in the methane series. SEE: *unsaturated compounds.*

s. solution. One containing as much of the solid drug as it can dissolve.

s. time. Time required for peripheral blood of a person inhaling pure oxygen to become saturated. Normal time is 10-15 sec.

saturation (săt"ū-rā'shŭn) [L. *saturatio*]. The holding in solution of all of a solid that can be dissolved therein.

saturnine (săt'ŭr-nīn) [L. *saturnus*, lead]. Concerning or produced by lead.

*s. **breath***. Sweet breath produced by lead* poisoning.

saturnism (săt'ŭrn-ĭzm) [" + G. *ismos*, condition]. Lead poisoning, *q.v.* SYN: *plumbism*.

satyriasis (sat-ĭ-rī'ă-sĭs) [G. *satyriasis*]. Excessive sex drive and desire in men.

Sauerbruch's cabinet (sow'ĕr-brook). An airtight cabinet for operation on the chest under negative pressure.

The patient's head is outside the cabinet and his body and the surgeon's are within it.

sauerkraut (sow'ĕr-krowt) [Ger. *sauer*, sour, + *kraut*, cabbage]. SERVING: 100 gm. (solid and liquids). Calories: 17. Protein: 1.0 gm.; fat: 0.2 gm.; carbohydrate: 4.0 gm.; vitamin A: 50 I.U.; vitamin C: 14 mg.

sausage (saw'saj) (pork) [M.E. *sausige*]. SERVING: 100 gm. (cooked). Calories: 476. Protein: 18.1 gm.; fat: 44.2; carbohydrate: trace.

savory (sā'vō-rĭ) [O.Fr. *savouré*, tasty]. Having a pleasant or appetizing taste or odor.

saw (saw) [A.S. *sagu*]. Instrument for cutting, esp. bone, its cutting edge being toothed.

saxifragant (săks-ĭf'ră-gănt) [L. *saxum*, rock, + *frangere*, to break]. Dissolving or breaking calculi, esp. in the bladder.

Sayre's jacket (sārz). A jacket of plaster-of-Paris worn to support the spine in vertebral diseases.

Sb. Symb. for *antimony*.

$SbCl_3$. Antimony trichloride.

Sb_2O_5. Antimonic oxide; antimony pentoxide.

Sb_4O_6. Antimonious oxide.

Sc. Chemical symbol for *scandium*.

s.c. Abbr. for *subcutaneously*. Also sometimes S.C.

scab (skăb) [M.E. *scabbe*]. 1. Crust of a cutaneous sore, wound, ulcer or pustule formed by drying up of the discharge. 2 To become covered with a crust.

scabicide (skā'bĭ-sīd). An agent which kills mites, esp. the causative agent of scabies, *q.v.*

scabies (skā'bĭ-ēz, -bēz) [L. *scabere*, to scratch]. SYN: *itch; seven-year itch.* A highly communicable skin disease caused by an arachnid, *Sarcoptes scabiei*, the itch mite.

SYM: Papules, vesicles, pustules, burrows and intense itching resulting in eczema.

The impregnated females live in burrows which appear as slightly discolored lines several millimeters to several centimeters in length. Eggs deposited within the tunnel hatch within 4-8 days.

Parts most commonly affected are hands, bet. the fingers, the wrists, axillae, genitalia, beneath the mammae and inner aspect of the thighs.

PROG: Favorable.

TREATMENT: Benzyl benzoate 25% solution applied to the entire body, except the eyes, nose and mouth, after the patient has taken a prolonged hot bath or shower. The affected areas are thoroughly scrubbed, and then the medicine is applied. A second application is made the following morning.

scabiphobia (skă'bĭ-fō-bĭ'ă). SYN: *acarophobia.* Morbid fear of acquiring scabies.

scabrities (skă-brĭsh'ĭ-ēz) [L.]. 1. Scaly, roughened condition of the skin. 2. A morbid roughness of inner surface of eyelids, causing sensation as if sand were in eyes.

*s. **unguium***. Morbid degeneration of the nails, making them rough, thick, distorted and separated from the flesh at the root. Symptomatic of syphilis and leprosy.

scala (skā'lă) [L. ladder]. Any one of the 3 spiral passages of the cochlea. SEE: *cochlea.*

*s. **media***. The cochlear duct, which lies between the s. tympani and s. vestibuli. Its floor contains the spiral organ of Corti. It extends from saccule to tip of cochlea and is filled with endolymph.

*s. **tympani***. Canal filled with perilymph lying below spiral lamina of cochlea. Extends from tip of cochlea to round cochlear window.

*s. **vestibuli***. A canal forming the upper portion of the osseous canal of the cochlea. It lies above the spiral lamina and extends from floor of vestibule to tip of cochlea where it communicates with *scala tympani* through an aperture, the *helicotrema*.

scald (skawld) [M.E. *scalden*, from L. *ex*, out, + *calidus*, hot]. 1. Burn to skin or flesh caused by moist heat and hot vapors, as steam. 2. To cause a burn with hot liquid or steam. 3. Cutaneous disease marked by scab formation on the head.

It is deeper than dry heat, and should be treated as a burn, *q.v.* Healing is slower and scar formation greater.

Emergency treatment of a scalded area should be the immediate application of cold in the most readily available form, *i.e.*, ice packs or very cold water. This should be continued for at least an hour.

scale (skāl) [A.S. *sceale*, scale]. 1. A small, thin, dry exfoliation shed from upper layers of skin. 2. Film of tartar encrusting the teeth. 3. To form a scale on. 4. To shed scales.

5. [M.E. *scole*, balance]. An instrument for weighing.

6. [L. *scala*, ladder]. A graduated or proportioned measure, series of tests, or instrument for measuring quantities or for rating, as individual intelligence. SEE: *Binet.*

Shedding of scales from skin in small amounts is normal. It is also seen in cutaneous disorders such as squamous eczema, seborrhea sicca, psoriasis, ichthyosis, syphilis, lupus erythematosus, pityriasis rosea, and tinea tonsurans. SEE: *macule; rash.*

*s., **absolute***. A scale used for indicating low temperatures based on absolute zero. SEE: *absolute temperature; absolute zero.*

*s., **centigrade***. Thermometric scale running from 0°, the melting point of ice, to 100°, the boiling point of water. SYN: *Celsius scale.* SEE: *centigrade; thermometer, comparative scale.*

*s., **Fahrenheit***. One in which the freezing point of water is 32° and the boiling point is 212°. SEE: *Fahrenheit; thermometer, comparative scale.*

*s., **Réaumur***. Scale which runs bet. freezing point of water at 0° and the boiling point at 80°. SEE: *Réaumur; thermometer, comparative scale.*

scalene (skā-lēn') [G. *skalēnos*, uneven]. 1. Having unequal sides and angles, said of a triangle. 2. Designating a scalenus muscle.

s. tubercle. One on upper surface of 1st rib, the insertion of the scalenus anticus muscle. SYN: *tubercle, Lisfranc's.*

scaleniotomy (skā-lĕn″ĭ-ŏt′ō-mĭ) [" + *tomē,* a cutting]. Incision of scalenus muscles near their insertion to check expansive movements in tuberculosis of the apex of the lung.

scalenus (skā-lē′nŭs) [L. from G. *skalēnos,* uneven]. One of 3 deeply situated muscles on each side of the neck, extending from the transverse processes of 2 or more cervical vertebrae to the 1st or 2nd rib; known as scalenus anterior, medius, posterior. SEE; *Table of Muscles in Appendix.*

s. anticus syndrome, s. syndrome. A symptom complex characterized by brachial neuritis with or without vascular or vasomotor disturbance in the upper extremities.

SYM: Not clearly defined, but pain, tingling and numbness may occur anywhere from shoulder to fingers. Atrophy of small muscles of the hand or even the deltoid or other muscles of arm.

TREATMENT: Correction of posture, avoidance of fatigue and sometimes immobilization of arm and shoulder. When relief is not obtained, operative interference may be considered.

scall (skawl) [Norse, *skalli,* bald head]. Dermatitis of the scalp producing a crusted, scabby eruption.

scalp (skălp) [M.E.]. The hairy integument of the head.

In anat. includes skin, dense subcutaneous tissue, occipitofrontalis muscle with the galea aponeurotica, loose subaponeurotic tissue and the cranial periosteum.

scalpel (skăl′pĕl) [L. *scalpellum,* little knife]. A straight, small surgical knife with a convex edge and thin, keen blade.

scalpriform (skăl′prĭ-form) [L. *scalprum,* chisel, + *forma,* shape]. In the shape of a chisel.

scalprum (skăl′prŭm) (pl. *scalpra*) [L. *scalprum,* knife]. 1. A toothed instrument for removal of carious bone or for trephining. 2. A large scalpel. 3. Cutting edge of an incisor tooth.

scaly (skā′lĭ) [A.S. *sceale,* scale]. Resembling or characterized by scales.

scand′ium. SYMB: Sc. At. wt. 44.956; at. no. 21. A rare metal belonging to the aluminum group.

scanning. Recording, on a photographic plate, the emission of radioactive waves from a specific substance injected into the body. The radioactive agent selected is one that is concentrated in a specific tissue such as thyroid, brain, or liver.

scan′ning speech. Pronunciation of words in syllables, or slowly and hesitatingly; a symptom of disseminated sclerosis.* SEE: *speech.*

scanty (skăn′tĭ) [M.E. *skant,* short]. Not abundant; insufficient, as a secretion.

scapha (skā′fă) [L. from G. *skaphē,* boat]. NA. Elongated depression of the ear bet. the helix and anthelix.

scapho- [G.]. Combining form meaning *boat.*

scaphocephalic, scaphocephalous (skăf″ō-sĕf-ăl′ĭk, -sĕf′ăl-ŭs) [G. *skaphē,* boat, + *kephalē,* head]. Having a deformed head, projecting like a boat's keel.

scaphocephalism (skăf″ō-sĕf′ăl-ĭzm) [" + " + *-ismos,* condition]. Condition of having a deformed head, projecting like the keel of a boat.

scaphoid (skăf′oyd) [G. *skaphē,* boat, + *eidos,* resemblance]. SYN: *os scaphoides, navicular bone.* A proximal, boat-shaped bone of the carpus on radial side. 2. SYN: *navicular bone.* A boat-shaped bone on inner side of the tarsus between the talus and three cuneiform bones. 3. Boat-shaped, navicular, hollowed.

s. abdomen. One with hollowed anterior wall.

s. bone. SEE: *scaphoid, 1 and 2.*

scaphoiditis (skăf-oyd-ī′tĭs) [G. *skaphē,* boat, + *eidos,* form, + *-itis,* inflammation]. Inflamed condition of the scaphoid bone.

scapula (skăp′ū-lă) (pl. *scapulae, -as*) [L. shoulder blade]. The large, flat, triangular bone of the shoulder.

It articulates with the clavicle and the humerus. SYN: *shoulder blade.* SEE ALSO: *triceps.*

s., winged. SYN: *scapula alata.* Condition in which medial border of scapula is prominent, usually the result of paralysis of serratus anterior or trapezius muscles.

RS: *acromial, a. angle, acromioclavicular, acromiocoracoid, acromion, angel's wing, glenoid cavity.*

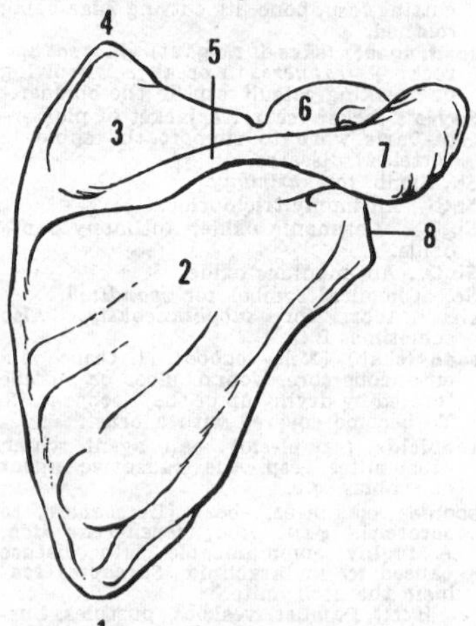

SCAPULA.

1. Inferior angle. 2. Infraspinatous fossa. 3. Supraspinatous fossa. 4. Superior angle. 5. Spine. 6. Coracoid process. 7. Acromion process. 8. Anterior angle.

scapulalgia (skăp-ū-lăl′jĭ-ă) [L. *scapula,* + G. *algos,* pain]. Pain in the region of the shoulder blade.

scapular (skăp′ū-lar) [L. *scapula,* shoulder blade]. Of or pert. to the shoulder blade.

s. reflex. Scapular muscular contraction following percussion or stimulus bet. the scapulas.

scapulary (skăp′ū-la-rĭ) [L. *scapula,* shoulder blade]. A shoulder bandage bifurcated with the 2 ends over the shoulders, the single end passing down the back, the 3 fastened to a body bandage.

scapulectomy (skăp-ū-lĕk′tō-mĭ) [" + G. *ektomē,* excision]. Surgical excision of the scapula.

scapulo- [L.]. Combining form meaning *shoulder.*

scapuloclavicular (skăp″ū-lō-klă-vĭk′ū-lar) [L. *scapula,* shoulder blade, + *clavicula,* a little key]. Concerning the scapula and the clavicle.

scapulodynia (skăp″ū-lō-dĭn′ĭ-ă) [" + *odynē,* pain]. Inflammation and pain in the shoulder muscles.

scapulohumeral (skăp″ū-lō-hū′mer-ăl) [" + *humerus,* shoulder]. Concerning the scapula and the humerus.

s. reflex. When vertebral border of scapula is percussed upper arm is adducted and rotated outwards.

scapulopexy (skăp″ū-lō-pĕks′ĭ) [" + G. *pēxis,* fixation]. Fixation of the scapula to the ribs.

scapulothoracic (skăp″ū-lō-thō-răs′ĭk) [" + G. *thōrax, thōrak-,* chest]. Concerning the scapula and the thorax.

scapus (skā′pŭs) [L. *scapus,* stalk]. The shaft or body of a hair (*s. pili*) or the penis (*s. penis*).

scar (skar) [G. *eschara,* scab]. Mark left in skin or internal organ by healing of a wound, sore or injury because of replacement by connective tissue of the injured tissue.

Scars may result from wounds that have healed, lesions of diseases, or surgical operations.

When first developed it is red or purple, later whitish and glistening. When on the head they may be the result of wounds which have healed or of skin disease. On the skin they may be the result of trauma or of surgical operation. SYN: *cicatrix.* SEE: *cicatricotomy, keloid.*

s., cicatricial. A scar or cicatrix with considerable contraction.

It may be necessary to divide the scar and graft on new skin, as in burns.

s., keloid. A red, raised, smooth scar containing blood vessels, often irritable.

s., painful. One due to involvement of a nerve during healing.

The end of the nerve may become bulbous. TREATMENT: Dissection of scar or excision of nerve.

scarabiasis. SYN: *Beetle disease.* Condition in which intestine is invaded by the dung beetle. Occurs principally in children.

scarfskin (skarf′skĭn) [Fr. *écharpe,* scarf, + O. Norse *skinn*]. Epidermis* or outermost layer of the skin.

scarification (skăr-ĭ-fĭ-kā′shŭn) [L. *scarificatio,* from G. *skariphasthai,* to scratch]. Making of numerous slight incisions in the skin, over a part.

scarificator (skăr′ĭf-ĭk-ā-tor) [L. from G. *skariphasthai,* to scratch]. Instrument for making small incisions in the skin.

scarlatina (skar-lă-tē′nă) (L. *scarlatina,* from *scarlatum,* red]. Scarlet fever, *q.v.*

s. simplex. Mild type of scarlet fever.

scarlatinal (skar-lă-tē′năl) [L. *scarlatum,* red]. Concerning or due to scarlatina.

scarlatinella (skar-lă-tĭn-el′lă) [L.]. A mild disease resembling measles and scarlet fever. SYN: *fourth disease, rubella scarlatinosa.*

scarlatiniform, scarlatinoid (skar-lă-tĭn′ĭ-form, -lăt′ĭ-noyd) [L. *scarlatina* + *forma,* shape, + G. *eidos,* form]. Resembling scarlatina or its rash.

scarlet fever (skar′lĕt) [L. *scarlatum,* red]. An acute contagious disease characterized by sore throat, strawberry tongue, fever, punctiform scarlet rash, and rapid pulse. SYN: *scarlatina.*

ETIOL: Many strains (over 40) of Type A hemolytic, toxin-producing streptococci have been recovered from scarlet fever patients.

The erythema-producing toxin was discovered by Dick and Dick (1924-25).

INCUBATION: Probably never less than 24 hr. May be from 1 to 3 days, rarely longer.

SYM: Onset sudden, rarely with a chill, but sometimes with a convulsion in very young children. As a rule, begins with sore throat, temperature from 101° to 105° F., frequent vomiting, followed within 12 to 36 hr. by a rash, first on neck and chest, rapidly extends over body, lastly involving the extremities. Face flushed and may be characterized by the well-known circumoral pallor, the punctiform rash on the remainder of the body, seldom seen on face.

With first eruption, throat is markedly injected, tonsils are swollen, tongue heavily coated, and the papillae are enlarged, projecting through it; the tongue properly described as a "strawberry" tongue. In mild or average case duration of rash is from 2 to 3 days. By the end of 3rd day, the coating has disappeared from tongue, though the papillae are still enlarged, the remainder of tongue presenting a deep red appearance. In this stage, the tongue may be referred to as the "raspberry" tongue.

With disappearance of rash in an uncomplicated case, the temperature closely approaches normal and recovery is uneventful. Extremely mild cases occur in which the rash is very faint and of very short duration, possibly not exceeding 24 hr. Scarlet fever may actually occur without any rash whatsoever. In any form, a leukocytosis is to be expected in the average case. Number of leukocytes may range from 10,000 to 20,000 with 75% to 90% neutrophils.

SPECIFIC TREATMENT: Penicillin is the agent of choice although other antibiotics may be used to combat the septic factor in the disease; however these have little effect on toxic manifestations. *Penicillin should be given for a minimum of 10 days no matter how mild the infection* in order to prevent the subsequent development of complications such as rheumatic fever and acute glomerulonephritis. Immune serum and antitoxin are effective against toxic manifestations but exert little effect against the streptococcal organisms. Serum therapy has largely been abandoned because of dangers of serum sickness. It is reserved for rare cases in which toxic manifestations suggest a possible fatal outcome.

GENERAL TREATMENT: Isolation, rest, and diet are of utmost importance. Patient with uncomplicated scarlet fever should be kept in bed during acute phase of the illness.

s. f., afebrile. S. f. without fever.

s. f., anginal. S. f. with severe throat symptoms.

s. f., hemorrhagic. S. f. with blood extravasated into mucous membranes and the skin.

s. f., latent. S. f. without rash but complicated by nephritis.

s. f., malignant. S. f. with great prostration and severe symptoms.

s. f., rheumatic. S. f. with joint pain.

s. f. without angina. S. f. without sore throat.

RS: *Amato bodies; Dick method.*

scarlet rash. A rose-colored rash, specifically that of German* measles.

scar'let red. An azo dye, of the color its name suggests.

USES: To stimulate healing of indolent ulcers, burns, wounds, etc.

SYN: *rubrum scarlatinum.*

Scarpa's fascia (skar'pa). Deep layer of superficial abdominal fascia around edge of the subcutaneous inguinal ring.

S's. fluid. Fluid in membranous labyrinth of the ear. SYN: *endolymph.*

S's. foramina. Bony passages opening into the incisor canal for passage of the nasopalatine nerves.

S's. ganglion. The vestibular ganglion, *q.v.*

S's. liquor. SEE: *S's. fluid.*

S's. membrane. Membrane that closes the fenestra rotunda of the tympanic cavity.

S's. triangle. Triangular space bounded laterally by inner edge of sartorius, above by Poupart's ligament, and medially by the adductor longus.

scatacratia (skăt-ă-krā'shĭ-ă) [G. *skōr, skat-*, dung, + *akratia*, lack of control]. Fecal incontinence.

scatemia (skăt-ē'mĭ-ă) [" + *aima*, blood]. Intestinal toxemia from retained fecal matter.

scatology (skăt-ŏl'ō-jĭ) [" + *logos*, a study]. 1. Scientific study and analysis of the feces. SYN: *coprology.* 2. Interest in obscene things, esp. literature.

scatoma (skă-tō'mă) [" + *-ōma*, tumor]. Mass of inspissated feces in colon or rectum resembling an abdominal tumor. SYN: *coproma; fecaloma; stercoroma.*

scatophagy (skă-tŏf'ăj-ĭ) [" + *phagein*, to eat]. The eating of excrement. SYN: *coprophagy.*

scatoscopy (skă-tŏs'kō-pĭ) [" + *skopein*, to examine]. Examination of excreta for diagnostic purposes.

scavenger cell (skăv'ĕn-jer) [O.Fr. *escauwage*, inspection]. A phagocytic cell such as a macrophage or a neutrophil leukocyte which functions in the removal of disintegrating tissues.

Schafer's method of artificial respiration (shā'fer). A method of artificial respiration in which the subject lies prone with both arms extended forward with one flexed so that hand rests under cheek and mouth. Operator kneels astride one or both thighs and places palms of hands on back over lower ribs. Operator rhythmically applies pressure on the hands by raising body at a rate of 12 times per minute.

This method was formerly widely used but has been replaced by more effective methods such as back pressure-arm lift (Nielsen) method, and mouth-to-mouth breathing. SEE: *artificial respiration; resuscitation.*

Schäffer's reflex (shā'fer). Dorsal flexion of toes and flexion of foot resulting when middle portion of tendo achillis is pinched.

schematic (skē-măt'ĭk) [L. *schematicus*, planned]. Pert. to a diagram or model; showing part for part in a diagram.

scheroma (shē-rō'mă). A condition caused by lack of lacrimal fluid. SYN: *xerophthalmia.*

Schick test (shĭk). Injection intradermally of 0.1 ml. of dilute diphtheria toxin (1/50 MLD). MLD—*minimum lethal dose* or the amount of diphtheria toxin which would kill a small guinea pig in four days.

Results 3 to 4 days later. Susceptibility (*positive test*) is indicated by the development of a red, inflamed area at point of injection, which slowly disappears after a few days. A *negative test*, (little or no reaction) indicates the presence of antibodies sufficient to neutralize the toxin, hence the person is immune. SEE: *diphtheria.*

Schilder's disease. Encephalitis periaxilaris diffusa, a progressive familial paraplegia. Also called *progressive subcortical encephalopathy.*

Schiller's test (shĭl'er). One for superficial cancer, esp. of the cervix uteri.

Paint tissue with solution of iodine. Cancer cells not containing glycogen fail to stain, thus revealing their presence.

Schilling test. A test, utilizing radioactive vitamin B_{12}, for gastrointestinal absorption of vitamin B_{12}.

Schilling's method. SYN: *Schilling's hemogram, S's count.* Method of taking a differential blood count by separating the polymorphonuclear neutrophils into four categories according to number and arrangement of the nuclei in the cells.

schindylesis (skĭn-dĭ-lē'sĭs) [G. *schindylēsis*, a splintering]. A form of synarthrosis (wedge and groove suture) in which a crest of one bone fits into a groove of another.

schistocelia (skĭs-tō-sē'lĭ-ă) [" + *koilia*, belly]. Congenital abdominal fissure.

schistocyte (skĭs'tō-sīt) [" + *kytos*, a cell]. A fragmented segment of a red blood cell. Seen in patients with hemolytic anemia.

schistocytosis (skĭs"tō-sī-tō'sĭs) [" + " + *-ōsis*, condition]. Schistocytes in the blood.

schistoglossia (skĭs"tō-glos'ĭ-ă) [" + *glōssa*, tongue]. A cleft tongue.

schistoprosopia (skĭs"tō-prō-sō'pĭ-ă) [" + *prosōpon*, face]. Congenital fissure of the face.

schistorrhachis (skĭs"tor'ă-kĭs) [" + *rhachis*, spine]. Protrusion of membranes through a congenital cleft in lower vertebral column. SYN: *spina bifida.*

Schistosoma (skĭs"tō-sō'mă) [G. *schistos*, a cleft, + *soma*, body]. A genus of blood flukes belonging to the family Schistosomatidae, class Trematoda. Adults live in blood vessels of visceral organs. Eggs make their way into bladder or intestine and are discharged in urine or feces. Eggs hatch into miracidia which enter snails and transform into sporocysts. These develop daughter sporocysts which give rise to fork-tailed cercaria. These leave snail and enter final host directly through skin or through mucous membrane.

S. haematobium. A species common in Africa and southwestern Asia. Adults infest pelvic veins of vesicle plexus. Eggs work their way through bladder wall and are discharged through urine. Cause of urinary bilharziasis.

S. japonicum. A species common in many parts of Orient. Adults live principally in branches of sup. mesenteric vein. Eggs work their way through intestinal wall into lumen and are discharged with feces. Cause of Oriental schistosomiasis.

S. mansoni. A species occurring in many parts of Africa and tropical America (W. Indies, northern part of S.A.). Adults live in branches of inf. mesenteric veins. Eggs discharged through either intestine or bladder.

Cause of bilharzial dysentery or Manson's intestinal schistosomiasis.

schistosome dermatitis (skĭs'tō-sōm). SYN: *swimmer's itch.* Dermatitis resulting from penetration of skin of humans by cercariae of non-human blood flukes. Common in lake region of northern U.S.

schistosomiasis (skĭs"tō-sō-mī'ăs-ĭs) [G. *schistos,* a cleft, + *sōma,* body, + *-iasis,* infection]. SYN: *bilharziasis.* A parasitic disease due to infestation with blood flukes belonging to the genus *Schistosoma, q.v.* The disease is widespread throughout Asia, Africa, and tropical America. Man becomes infested by wading or bathing in water containing cercaria which have issued from snails.

schistothorax (skĭs"tō-thō'răks) [" + *thōrax,* chest]. Fissure of the thorax.

schizamnion (skĭz-ăm'nĭ-ŏn). An amnion formed by development of a cavity in the inner cell mass.

schizaxon (skĭs-ăks'ŏn). An axon that divides in 2 equal or nearly equal branches.

schizo- [G.]. Combining form meaning *to split.*

schizoblepharia (skĭz-ō-blĕf'ă-rĭ-ă). Fissure of an eyelid.

schizocytosis (skĭs"ō-sī-tō'sĭs) [" + " + *-ōsis,* condition]. SYN: *schistocytosis.*

schizogenesis (skĭz"ō-jĕn'ĕs-ĭs) [" + *genesis,* production]. BIOL: Reproduction by fission.*

schizogyria (skĭz-ō-jī'rĭ-ă) [" + *gyros,* a circle]. A break or cleft in the cerebral convolutions.

schizoid (skĭz'oyd) [G. *schizein,* to split, + *eidos,* resemblance]. Resembling schizophrenia.

s. personality. The type of person characterized by seclusiveness, inability to develop close emotional attachments to others, reduced initiative, morbid introspection, and oftentimes queer behavior. The so-called "shut-in" type.

Schizomycetes (skĭz"ō-mī-sē'tēz) [" + *mykēs,* fungus]. Class of plant microorganisms or fungi which multiply by fission. Includes the bacteria.

schizont (skĭz'ont) [G. *schizein,* to split]. 1. Form appearing in the life cycle of a sporozoan protozoon resulting from multiple division or schizogony. 2. Stage in asexual phase of life cycle of *Plasmodium* found in red blood cells. By schizogeny, each gives rise to 12-24 or more merozoites. (See Fig. of Human cycle of tertian malaria, p. M-5). An early schizont is called a *presegmenter,* a mature schizont is called a *rosette* or *segmenter.*

schizonychia (skĭz"ō-nĭk'ĭ-ă) [G. *schizein,* to split, + *onyx, onych-,* nail]. Split condition of the nails.

schizophasia (skĭz-ō-fā'zĭ-ă) [" + *phasis,* speech]. Muttered and incomprehensible speech of the schizophrenic.

schizophrenia (skĭz-ō-frē'nĭ-ă) [G. *schizein,* to split, + *phrēn,* mind]. The most important of the psychoses, characterized by loss of contact with the environment and by disintegration of personality.

This term includes all cases of dementia precox of the older writers. Possibly, it may also apply to numerous borderline cases which would not have been included in dementia precox.

Four types of schizophrenic reactions are usually differentiated although the dominant reaction in any patient may vary from time to time. The types are: *simple, paranoid, catatonic,* and *hebephrenic.* In the simple type, the patient becomes dull emotionally, loses ambition, and tends to withdraw; however, there is no serious intellectual impairment. The paranoid type develops extensive delusions of persecution; the catatonic may show stereotyped excitement or simulate a stupor, though lucid and clearly recalling the episode if recovery occurs. A vague sense of being 2 personalities and "changed" occurs in all types. The hebephrenic shows mannerisms, speech anomalies, hysteroid symptoms, delusions, hallucinations, and often childish behavior and mannerisms.

ETIOL: Unknown.

PROG: Always guarded.

NP: Expert and careful nursing care is required during the hospital stay.

TREATMENT: Hospitalization is essential in most cases. Psychotherapy and shock treatment (insulin, metrazol, and electric) are utilized. Drug therapy involving use of tranquilizing agents such as chlorpromazine or reserpine is effective in certain cases. SEE: *hypoglycemic shock, insulin shock therapy, shock therapy.*

schizophrenic (skĭz"ō-frĕn'ĭk) [G. *schizein,* to split, + *phrēn,* mind]. Afflicted with or person afflicted with schizophrenia.

schizoprosopia (schĭz-ō-prō-sō'pĭ-ă). Fissure of the face as harelip, or cleft palate.

Schizophrenia (Symptoms)

1. Occurs in young men and women.
2. Memory better than it seems.
3. Hallucinations common, especially of hearing.
4. Loss of emotion or, if shown, it is out of place.
5. Affect absent or inappropriate.
6. May revert to stereotype.
7. Impulsive destructive acts.
8. Negativism.
9. May be catatonic.
10. May be hebephrenic.
11. May recover sufficiently to be discharged.
12. Cold, blue, and edematous extremities.
13. Conscious, but takes little cognizance of what is going on about them.
14. Delusions frequent but absurd, often of grandeur and persecution.
15. May have attacks of tears or laughter.
16. May have excited activity.
17. May remain in stupor.
18. Grimaces and mannerisms frequent.
19. May pay no attention to calls of nature if disease is advanced.
20. May be paranoid.
21. Disease sometimes changes its form.
22. Complete recovery rare.

Principal Signs: Moodiness, solitary habits, stupor and excitement, delusions and hallucinations.

schizotrichia (skĭz″ō-trĭk′ĭ-ă) [" + *thrix, trich-*, hair]. Splitting of the tips of the hair.

Schlemm's canal (shlĕm). SYN: *sinus venosus sclera.* Irregular space or spaces in the sclerocorneal region of the eye. It receives the aqueous humor from the ant. chamber of the eye.

Schmidt's intestinal test (shmĭt). Test diet given for indigestion.

For breakfast the following may be served: Milk, ½ liter, or an equal quantity of cocoa made with milk; 1 cooked or raw egg; zwieback or roll, 50 Gm.; butter, 10 Gm.

The midmorning meal consists of ½ liter of oatmeal gruel, made from oatmeal, 40 Gm.; water, 200 cc., and milk, 300 cc.

Dinner consists of chopped beef, 125 Gm., lightly broiled in butter and raw inside; strained potato purée made from mashed potato, 190 Gm.; milk, 100 cc., and butter, 10 Gm.

The midafternoon meal is the same as the breakfast, and supper is the same as the midmorning meal.

This diet is usually maintained for about 3 days. All the food used must be weighed or measured *accurately*. Should the patient not eat the entire amount the portion not eaten must be weighed or measured. All the urine and feces passed are measured and sent to the laboratory for examination. It is also sometimes required that the foods used must first be analyzed.

Schmorl's disease. Herniation of the nucleus pulposus.

schneiderian membrane (shnī-dē′rĭ-ăn). The nasal mucosa. SYN: *pituitary membrane.*

Schönlein's disease (shen′lĭn). SYN: *Schonlein-Henock purpura, purpura hemorrhagica.* An allergic or anaphylactic purpura occurring in individuals, esp. children, with drug sensitivities, serum sickness, and other allergic disorders. It is usually accompanied by pains in joints and abdomen.

Schott method (shŏt). Resisting exercises and special baths in the treatment of heart disease.

Schroeder's method (shrōd′er) (resuscitation). A manner of resuscitating asphyxiated infants by placing the patient in a bath and then bending the body over the abdomen. This movement compresses the thorax and produces a forceful expiration. SEE: *artificial respiration; resuscitation.*

Schueller's method (shil′er) [Karl Heinrich Anton Max Schueller, Berlin surgeon, 1843-1907]. (artificial respiration). A manner of performing artificial respiration by a series of rhythmic raisings of the thorax by the operator hooking his fingers under the lower ribs. SEE: *artificial respiration; resuscitation.*

Schultze's bundle. Longitudinal mass of descending fibers shaped like a comma, in the fasciculus cuneatus of spinal cord.

S's. cells. Olfactory cells.

S's. granule masses. Fine, granular masses formed by breaking up of plaques in the blood.

Schwabach test (shvah′bahkh). A test for hearing by use of 5 tuning forks, each of a different tone. SEE: *test.*

Schwann's cells. Cells of ectodermal origin which comprise the neurilemma.

S.'s sheath. The neurilemma of a nerve fiber. SYN: *neurilemma.*

S.'s white substance. Myelin of a medullated nerve fiber.

sciage (se-ahzh′) [Fr. a sawing]. A movement in massage resembling that in sawing.

sciatic (sī-ăt′ĭk) [G. *ischiadikos*, pert. to the ischium]. 1. Pert. to the hip or ischium. 2. Pert. to, due to, or afflicted with, sciatica.

s. nerve. Largest nerve in the body arising from sacral plexus on either side, passing from pelvis through greater sciatic foramen, down back of thigh, where it divides into tibial and peroneal nerves. Lesions cause paralysis of flexion and of adduction of toes, abduction and adduction of toes, rotation inward and adduction of foot; of plantar flexion and lowering of ball of foot; anesthesia in cutaneous distribution (ext. popliteal nerve); paralysis of dorsal flexion and adduction of foot; of rotation of ball of foot outward and of raising external border of foot and of extension of toes; also anesthesia in cutaneous distribution.

SYN: *great sciatic nerve; nervus ischiadicus* [BNA]. SEE ALSO: *Table of Nerves in Appendix.*

s. n., small. The posterior femoral cutaneous nerve, a cutaneous nerve supplying skin of buttocks, perineum, popliteal region, and back of thigh and leg.

sciatica (sī-ăt′ĭ-kă) [L. from G. *ischiadikos*, pert. to the ischium]. Severe pain in the leg along the course of the sciatic nerve felt at back of thigh running down the inside of the leg. SEE: *meralgia, sciatic nerve, lesions of.*

ETIOL: 1. Compression or trauma of the sciatic nerve or its roots, esp. that resulting from ruptured intervertebral disk or osteoarthrosis of lumbosacral vertebrae. 2. Inflammation of sciatic nerve resulting from metabolic, toxic, or infectious disorders. 3. Pain referred to sciatic nerve from other parts of body.

SYM: May begin abruptly or gradually and is characterized by a sharp, shooting pain running down back of thigh. Movement of limb generally intensifies the suffering. Pain may be uniformly distributed along the limb, but not infrequently there are certain spots where it is more intense; numbness, tingling; nerve may be extremely sensitive to touch. Symptoms grow worse at night and on approach of stormy weather. Duration of attack varies from few days to several months. In long standing cases, muscles grow atrophied and rigid.

PROG: Recovery follows in majority of cases when treatment is instituted early, and is persistently carried out.

TREATMENT: Surgical intervention if due to ruptured intervertebral disk. In acute stage, rest is essential. Hot fomentations. Morphine or Demerol may be required to control pain, but the danger of habituation must be kept in mind. In rheumatic patients, full doses of salicylate or sodium are useful. In chronically ill patients, prolonged rest. Improve general health; good, nourishing diet; bags of hot salt; covering part with flannel and running hot iron over it often provides relief. Some patients are relieved by the spraying of ethyl chloride over course of nerve. Nerve stretching by pulling affected leg. Lift in shoe of affected limb.

scieropia (sī-ĕr-ō′pĭ-ă) [G. *skieros*, shadow, + *opsis*, vision]. Abnormal vision in which things appear to be in shadow.

scintillascope (sĭn-tĭl′ă-skōp) [L. *scintilla*, spark, + G. *skopein*, to examine]. Device for viewing the effect of ionizing radiation, alpha particles, on a fluorescent screen.

scintillation (sĭn-tĭl-lā'shŭn) [L. *scintilla*, spark]. 1. Sparkling; a subjective sensation, as of seeing sparks. 2. The emissions which come from radioactive substances.

scirrho- [G.]. Combining form meaning *hard*, as *scirrhus*, a hard tumor.

scirrhoid (skĭr'oyd) [G. *skirrhos*, hard, + *eidos*, form]. Pert. to or like a hard carcinoma or scirrhus.

scirrhoma (skĭr-ō'mă) [" + *-ōma*, tumor]. A hard carcinoma or scirrhus.

scirrhosarca (skĭr-ō-sar'kă) [" + *sarx*, *sark-*, flesh]. Hardening of the flesh, esp. of the newly born. SYN: *sclerema neonatorum*, *scleroderma*.

scirrhous (skĭr'rŭs) [G. *skirrhos*, hard]. Hard, like a scirrhus.

scirrhus (skĭr'ŭs) [G. *skirrhos*, hard]. A hard, cancerous tumor due to overgrowth of fibrous tissue. A hard form of cancer.

scissor leg (sĭz'or lĕg). Abnormal crossing of both legs, the result of adduction at both hips. SYN: *x-leg*.

s. l. gait. Crossing the legs in walking. SEE: *gait*.

scissors (sĭz'ors) [L. *cisorium* from *caedere*, to cut]. A cutting instrument composed of 2 opposed cutting blades with handles, held together by a central pin.

scissura. A fissure or cleft; a splitting.

sclera (sklē'ră) (pl. *sclerae*) [G. *sklēros*, hard]. NA. The white or sclerotic outer coat of the eye.

It extends from optic nerve to cornea. SYN: *sclerotica*.

scleradenitis (sklē-rad-ĕn-ī'tĭs) [" + *adēn*, gland, + *-ītis*, inflammation]. Inflammation and induration of a gland.

scleral (sklē'răl) [G. *sklēros*, hard]. Concerning the sclera.

sclerectasia (sklĕr-ĕk-tā'zĭ-ă) [" + *ektasis*, dilatation]. Protrusion of the sclera.

sclerectoiridectomy (sklĕr-ĕk"tō-ĭr-ĭ-dĕk'tō-mĭ) [" + *iris*, *irid-*, iris, + *ektomē*, excision]. Formation of a filtering cicatrix in glaucoma by combined sclerectomy and iridectomy.

sclerectoiridodialysis (sklĕr-ĕk"tō-ĭr-ĭd-ō-dī-ăl'ĭ-sĭs) [" + " + *dialysis*, a loosening]. Sclerectomy and iridodialysis for relief of glaucoma.

sclerectomy (sklē-rĕk'tō-mĭ) [" + *ektomē*, excision]. 1. Excision of a portion of the sclera. 2. Removal of adhesions in chronic otitis media.

scleredema (skle"rē-dē'mă). SYN: *scleredema adultorum of Buschke*, *scleriasis*. A condition usually following an acute infection characterized by edema and induration of the skin. It is a benign, self-limited disease occurring more frequently in females than males. It is often confused with scleroderma, *q.v.*

sclerema (sklē-rē'mă) [G. *sklēros*, hard]. Hardening of the skin. SYN: *scleroderma*.

s. adiposum. S. neonatorum, *q.v.*

s. adultorum. Scleroderma, *q.v.*

s. neonatorum. Progressive hardening of the skin in the newly born; usually fatal.

sclerencephalia (skler"ĕn-sĕf-ăl'ĭ-ă). Sclerosis of the brain.

scleriasis (sklē-rī'ăs-ĭs) [" + *-iasis*, disease]. 1. Progressive hardening of the skin. SYN: *scleroderma*. 2. Hardening of the eyelid.

scleriritomy (sklĕr-ĭ-rĭt'ō-mĭ) [" + *iris*, iris, + *tomē*, a cutting]. Incision of iris and sclera.

scleritis (sklē-rī'tĭs) [" + *-ītis*, inflammation]. Inflammation of the sclera; superficial and deep. SEE: *episcleritis*.

s., annular. Inflammation limited to the area surrounding the limbus of the cornea. A complete ring is formed.

scleroblastema (sklē"rō-blăs-tē'mă) [" + *blastēma*, a sprout]. The embryonic tissue from which formation of bone takes place.

scleroblastemic (sklē"rō-blăs-tĕm'ĭk) [" + *blastēma*, a sprout]. Relating to or derived from scleroblastema.

sclerocataracta (sklē"rō-kăt-ă-rak'tă) [" + *katarraktēs*, a pouring down]. A hard cataract.

sclerochoroiditis (sklē"rō-kō-roy-dī'tĭs) [G. *sklēros*, hard, + *chorioeidēs*, skinlike, + *-ītis*, inflammation]. Inflammation of the sclera and choroid coat of the eye.

s., posterior. Myopic choroiditis, posterior staphyloma.

scleroconjunc'tival. Pertaining to the sclera and conjunctiva.

sclerocornea (sklē"rō-kor'nē-ă) [" + L. *cornu*, a horn]. The sclera and cornea together considered as one coat.

sclerodactylia (sklē"rō-dăk-tĭl'ĭ-ă) [" + *daktylos*, digit]. Induration of the skin of the fingers and toes.

scleroderma (sklē-rō-der'mă) [G. *sklēros*, hard, + *derma*, skin]. SYN: *dermatosclerosis*, *sclerema adultorum*, *hidebound skin*, *progressive systemic sclerosis*. A progressive disease of the skin involving collagen tissue resulting in diffuse leathery induration of the skin frequently followed by atrophy and pigmentation. The localized form is known as *morphea*. Involvement of internal organs is to be expected.

ETIOL: Unknown.

SYM: Diffuse symmetrical form, more common in adult women (30 to 50 years old) than in men, following exposure to cold or wet. Smooth, waxy, edematous skin; later becomes hard, yellowish, and adherent to underlying tissue, causing masklike expression (face) or clawlike appearance of hands (sclerodactylia). When chest is involved respiration may be interfered with. Renal and cardiac involvement produce the usual signs of impaired function of these organs.

PROG: Better in circumscribed form than in extensive scleroderma, but the disease is usually slow to progress.

TREATMENT: Physiotherapy for comfort and prevention of fixation where applicable; frequent small feedings for dysphagia. Adrenal steroids do not cure this disease but are of considerable help in controlling the swelling and inflammation. This therapy may be required for months or years. Be alert for systemic bacterial infections; if these occur they are treated with appropriate antibiotic drugs.

s., circumscribed. Skin disease with pink, firm patches which atrophy, leaving scars. SYN: *morphea*.

s. neonatorum. Hardness and tightness of the skin in early infancy. SYN: *sclerema*.

sclerodermatitis (sklē"rō-der-mă-tī'tĭs). Inflammation of the skin accompanied by thickening and hardening.

sclerogenous (sklē-rŏj'ĕn-ŭs) [" + *gennan*, to produce]. Causing sclerosis or hardening of tissue.

scleroid. Having a hard or firm texture.

scleroiritis (sklē"rō-ī-rī'tĭs) [" + *iris*, iris, + *-ītis*, inflammation]. Inflammation of both sclera and iris.

sclerokeratitis (sklē"rō-ker-ă-tī'tĭs) [" + *keras*, *kerat-*, horn, + *-ītis*, inflammamation]. Cellular infiltration with inflammation of the sclera and cornea.

sclerokeratoiritis (sklē"rō-ker"ă-tō-ī-rī'tĭs) [" + " + *iris*, iris, + *-ītis*, inflammation]. Inflamed condition of the sclera, cornea, and iris.

scleroma (sklē-rō'mă) [" + *-ōma*, tumor]. Indurated, circumscribed area of granulation tissue in mucous membrane or skin. SEE: *sclerosis*.

scleromalacia (sklē"rō-mă-lā'sĭ-ă). Softening of the sclera.

s. perforans. Scleromalacia accompanied by perforation.

scleromere (sklē'rō-mēr) [G. *sklēros*, hard, + *meros*, a part]. The caudal half of a sclerotome, *q.v.*

scleronychia (sklē-rō-nĭk'ĭ-ă). Thickening and hardening of the nails.

scleronyxis (sklē-rō-nĭks'ĭs) [G. *sklēros*, hard, + *nyxis*, a piercing]. Puncture of the sclera.

sclero-oophoritis (sklē"rō-ō"ŏf-or-ī'tĭs) [" + *ōon*, egg, + *phoros*, a bearer, + *-ītis*, inflammation]. Induration and inflammation of the ovary.

sclerophthalmia (sklēr-ŏf-thăl'mĭ-ă) [" + *ophthalmos*, eye]. Congenital condition in which opacity of the sclera advances over the cornea.

scleroplasty (sklē-rō-plăst'ĭ). Plastic surgery of the sclera.

scleroprotein (sklē"rō-prō'tē-ĭn) [" + *prōtos*, first]. One of group of simple proteins* forming the skeletal structure of animals marked by their insolubility.

They are not suitable for food. Elastin and keratin are examples. SYN: *albuminoid*.

sclerosed (sklē-rōsd', sklē'rōsd) [G. *sklēros*, hard]. Having sclerosis; hardened. SYN: *indurated*.

sclerosing (sklē-rō'sĭng) [G. *sklēros*, hard]. Causing or developing sclerosis.

sclerosis (sklē-rō'sĭs) [G. *sklērosis*, a hardening]. 1. A hardening or induration of an organ or tissue, esp. that due to excessive growth of fibrous tissue. 2. Hardening within nervous system, esp. brain and spinal cord resulting from degeneration of nervous elements, as the myelin sheath. 3. Thickening and hardening of the layers in wall of an artery. SEE: *atherosclerosis* and *arteriosclerosis*.

RS: *cerebrosclerosis, Charcot's disease, scleritis*.

s., Alzheimer's. Hyaline degeneration affecting the small blood vessels of brain.

s., amyotropic lateral. Progressive muscular atrophy resulting from disease conditions, degenerative in nature, involving anterior horn cells and the pyramidal tracts. It is rapidly progressive, usually ending in bulbar paralysis.

s., annular. S. in which sclerosed substance forms a band about spinal cord.

s., arterial. Hardening of the coats of the arteries. SYN: *arteriosclerosis*.

s., arteriolar. S. of arterioles.

s., diffuse. S. affecting large areas of the brain and spinal cord.

s., disseminated. Multiple s., *q.v.*

s., hyperplastic. Medial s., *q.v.*

s., insular. Multiple sclerosis, *q.v.*

s., intimal. Atherosclerosis, *q.v.*

s., lateral. S. of a lateral column of the spinal cord. SEE: *sclerosis, amyotropic lateral*.

s., lobar. Sclerosis of cerebrum resulting in mental disturbances.

s., medial. SYN: *Mönckeberg's sclerosis*. S. involving the tunica media of arteries, usually the result of involutional changes accompanying aging.

s., multiple. A chronic, slowly progressive disease of the central nervous system characterized by development of disseminated demyelinated glial patches called *plaques*. Symptoms and signs are numerous, but common in later stages are those of Charcot's triad (nystagmus, scanning speech, and intention tremor). Occurs in the form of many clinical syndromes, the most common being the *cerebral, brainstem-cerebellar*, and *spinal*. A history of remissions and exacerbations is diagnostic. Etiology is unknown and there is no specific therapy.

s., neural. S. with chronic inflammation of a nerve trunk with branches.

s., posterior spinal. SEE: *tabes dorsalis*.

s., renal. Nephrosclerosis, *q.v.*

s., vascular. Sclerosis of the walls of blood vessels; arterial and venous sclerosis.

s., venous. Phlebosclerosis, *q.v.*

scleroskeleton (sklē"rō-skĕl'ĕ-tŏn) [G. *sklēros*, hard, + *skeleton*, skeleton]. Skeletal parts resulting from ossification of fibrous structures, such as ligaments, fasciae, and tendons.

sclerostenosis (sklē"rō-stĕn-ō'sĭs) [G. *sklēros*, hard, + *stenōsis*, a narrowing]. Contraction and induration of tissues, esp. those about an orifice.

s. cutanea. Induration of the skin. SYN: *scleroderma*.

sclerostomy (sklē-rŏs'tō-mĭ) [" + *stoma*, an opening]. Formation of an opening in the sclera.

sclerothrix (sklē'rō-thrĭks) [" + *thrix*, hair]. Brittleness of the hair.

sclerotic (sklē-rŏt'ĭk) [L. *scleroticus*, from G. *sklēros*, hard]. 1. Pert. to or affected with sclerosis. 2. Hard.

s. acid. An amorphous, brown powder from ergot. A hemostatic and oxytocic.

s. coat. The membrane forming the ext. coat of the eye. SYN: *sclera, sclerotica*.

s. teeth. Hard, yellowish ones almost immune to caries.

sclerotica (sklē-rŏt'ĭ-kă) [L. from G. *sklēros*, hard]. The ext. white coat of the eye. SYN: *sclera, sclerotic coat*.

scleroticectomy (sklē-rŏt-ĭ-sĕk'tō-mĭ) [L. *sclerotikus*, sclerotic, + G. *ektomē*, excision]. Excision of a part of the sclera. SYN: *sclerectomy*.

scleroticochoroiditis (sklē-rŏt"ĭ-kō-kō"-roy-dī'tĭs) [" + G. *chorioeidēs*, skin-like, + *-ītis*, inflammation]. Inflammation of sclerotic and choroid coats of the eye. SYN: *sclerochoroiditis*.

scleroticonyxis (sklē-rŏt-ĭk-ō-nĭks'ĭs) [" + G. *nyxis*, a piercing]. Puncture of the sclera. SYN: *scleronyxis*.

scleroticopuncture (sklē-rŏt"ĭk-ō-pŭnk'-tūr) [" + *punctūra*, a piercing]. Surgical puncture of the sclera. SYN: *scleronyxis, scleroticonyxis*.

scleroticotomy (sklē-rŏt-ĭk-ŏt'ō-mĭ) [" + G. *tomē*, a cutting]. Incision of the sclerotic coat of the eye. SYN: *sclerotomy*.

sclerotitis (sklē-rō-tī'tĭs) [G. *sklēros*, hard + *-ītis*, inflammation]. Inflammation of the sclera. SYN: *scleritis*.

sclerotium (sklē-rō'shĭ-ŭm) [L. from G. *sklēros*, hard]. Hardened mass formed of mycelium and food débris, the resting stage of certain fungi.

sclerotome (sklē'rō-tōm) [G. *sklēros*, hard + *tomē*, a cutting]. 1. Knife used in incision of the sclera. 2. One of a series of segmentally arranged masses of mesenchymal tissue lying on either side of the notochord. They give rise to the vertebrae and ribs.

sclerotomy (sklē-rŏt'ō-mĭ) [" + *tomē*, a cutting]. Simple division of sclera.

s., anterior. Incision at angle of anterior chamber in glaucoma.

s., posterior. Opening through sclera into the vitreous for detached retina, removal of foreign body, etc.

sclerotrichia (sklē-rō-trĭk'ĭ-ă). Hardness and brittleness of the hair.

sclerous (sklē'rŏs). Hard; indurated.

scobinate (skō'bĭn-āt) [L. *skobina*, rasp] Having a rough, uneven, nodular surface.

scolex (skō'lĕks). The portion of a tapeworm, the so-called "head," by which it attaches itself to the wall of the intestine. They usually possess holdfast organs such as hooks, suckers or grooves (bothria).

scoliometer (skō-lĭ-ŏm'ĕt-ĕr) [G. *skolios*, crooked, + *metron*, measure]. Device for measuring curves, esp. lateral ones of the spine.

scoliorachitic (sko"lĭ-ō-ră-kit'ik) [" + *rachis*, spine]. Pert. to or afflicted with spinal curvature from rickets.

scoliosiometry (skō"lĭ-ō-sĭ-ŏm'ĕ-trĭ) [" + *metron*, a measure]. Measurement of degree of spinal curvature.

scoliosis (skō-lĭ-ō'sĭs) [G. *skoliōsis*, curvature]. Lateral curvature of the spine.

Usually consists of two curves, the original one and a compensatory curve in the opp. direction.

s., cicatricial. S. due to cicatricial contraction resulting from necrosis.

s., congenital. That present at birth, usually the result of defective development of the spine.

s., coxitic. S. in the lumbar spine due to tilting of the pelvis in hip disease.

s., empyematic. S. following empyema and retraction of one side of the chest.

s., habit. S. due to habitually assumed improper position.

s., inflammatory. S. due to disease of the vertebrae.

s., ischiatic. S. due to hip disease.

s., myopathic. Weakening of spinal muscles causing a lateral curvature.

s., ocular, s., ophthalmic. S. from tilting of the head due to visual defects or extraocular muscle imbalance.

s., osteopathic. Same as s., myopathic, *q.v.*

s., paralytic. Lateral curvature of the spine due to paralysis of the muscles.

s., rachitic. S. due to rickets.

s., rheumatic. S. due to rheumatism of dorsal muscles.

s., sciatic. Lateral curvature in sciatica.

s., static. That due to difference in length of legs.

scoliosometry (skō"lĭ-ō-sŏm'ĕt-rĭ) [G. *skoliōsis*, curvature]. Determination of degree of spinal curvature. SYN: *scoliosiometry*.

scoliotic (skō-lĭ-ŏt'ĭk) [G. *skoliōsis*, curvature]. Suffering from or related to scoliosis.

scoliotone (skō'lĭ-ō-tōn) [G. *skolios*, curved, + *tonos*, a stretching]. An apparatus for correcting the curve in scoliosis by stretching the spine.

-scope. Combining form meaning *an instrument or device for viewing or examining*.

scoop (skōōp) [M.E. *scope*, a ladle]. Surgical spoon-shaped instrument.

s., bone. Instrument for scraping or removing necrosed bone or contents of suppurative tracts. Volkmann's, Schede's, Von Brun's, Hebra's, Treve's.

s., bullet. Instrument for dislodging bullets.

s., cataract. Instrument for removing fluids, foreign growths, for exerting pressure or center pressure.

s., ear. Instrument for removing middle ear granulations.

s., lithotomy. Instrument for dislodging encysted calculi, removing stones, débris, etc.

s., mastoid. Instrument used in mastoid operations.

s., renal. Instrument to dislodge or remove small stones from pelvis of kidney.

scopolamine hydrobromide (sko-pol'ă-mēn hī"drō-brō'mīd) [G. *skopolamin*]. USP. The hydrobromide of alkaloids obtained from plants of the nightshade family.

ACTION AND USES: As a cerebral sedative and locally as a mydriatic, and with morphine and pentobarbital in labor to produce twilight sleep. SYN: *hyoscine hydrobromide*.

scopophobia (skō"pō-fō'bĭ-ă) [G. *skopos*, a watcher, + *phobos*, fear]. Abnormal fear of being seen.

scopophobiac (skō"pō-fō'bĭ-ăk) [" + *phobos*, fear]. One who is afraid of being seen.

scoptophilia (skŏp-tō-fĭl'ĭ-ă) [" + *philein*, to love]. Sexual pleasure derived from visual sources, such as nudity, obscene pictures, etc. SYN: *scopophilia*.

scoptophobia (skŏp-tō-fō'bĭ-ă) [" + *phobos*, fear]. Aversion to being seen.

scoptophobiac (skŏp"tō-fō'bĭ-ăk) [" + *phobos*, fear]. One who dreads being seen.

-scopy [G.]. Combining form meaning *examination*.

scoracratia (skōr-ăk-rā'shĭ-ă) [G. *skōr*, dung, + *akratia*, lack of control]. Inability to retain the feces. SYN: *scatacratia*.

scorbutic (skor-bū'tĭk) [L. *scorbutus*, scurvy]. Concerning or affected with scurvy.

scorbutus (skor-bū'tŭs) [L. scurvy]. A deficiency disease due to lack of vitamin C in fresh vegetables and fruits. SYN: *scurvy, q.v.* SEE: *deficiency disease, vitamin*.

scordinema (skor-dĭn-ē'mă) [G. yawning]. Yawning and stretching with heaviness of the head, a prodrome of an infectious disease.

scoretemia (skōr-ē-tē'mĭ-ă) [G. *skōr*, dung, + *aima*, blood]. Autointoxication resulting from absorption of feces in the intestine or absorption of substances from feces retained in the intestine.

scorp'ion. An arachnid belonging to the order *Scorpionida* confined principally to warm countries. They are capable of inflicting a dangerous and sometimes fatal sting by means of a caudal fang, the venom containing neurotoxins, hemolysins, cardiac toxins and agglutinins.

s. sting. Symptoms resemble those of black widow spider bite or strychnine poisoning. Severity of symptoms depends on age of victim. Stings often are fatal to children under 3 years of age; adults usually recover.

TREATMENT: Same as for black widow spider* bite. Apply tourniquet with caution. Apply ice or freeze with ethyl chloride to slow dissemination of venom. Specific antivenin should be administered if available. In S. W. United States, it can be secured from Poisonous Animals Research Laboratory, Arizona State College, Tempe, Arizona.

scotodinia (skō-tō-dĭn'ĭ-ă) [G. *skotos,* darkness, + *dinos,* a whirl]. Vertigo with black spots before the eyes and faintness.

scotoma (skō-tō'mă) (pl. *scotomata*) [G. *skotōma,* darkness]. Islandlike blind gap in the visual field.

s., absolute. An area in the visual field in which there is absolute blindness.

s., annular. A scotomatous zone which encircles the point of fixation like a ring, not always completely closed, but leaves the fixation point intact.

s., central. One which involves the point of fixation, seen in lesions of the macula.

s., color. Color blindness in a limited portion of visual field.

s., eclipse. An area of blindness in the visual field due to having looked directly at the sun during an eclipse.

s., flittering. Same as scintillating scotoma.

s., negative. One not perceptible by the patient.

s., physiological. Blind spot due to absence of rods and cones where optic nerve enters retina.

s., positive. One which patient perceives in his visual field as a dark spot.

s., relative. One in which perception of the object is impaired but not completely lost.

s., scintillating. An irregular outline around a luminous patch in the visual field following mental or physical labor or eyestrain or in migraine. SYN: *teichopsia.*

scotomata (skō-tō'mă-tă) [G.]. Plural of *scotoma.*

scotomatous (skō-tom'ă-tŭs) [G. *skotōma,* darkness]. Relating to, of the nature of, or afflicted with, scotoma.

scotometer (skō-tŏm'ĕt-ĕr) [" + *metron,* a measure]. Device for detecting and measuring a dark spot in visual field.

scotometry (skō-tom'ĕ-trĭ) [" + *metron,* a measure]. The locating and measurement of scotomata.

scotomization (skō-tō-mĭz-ā'shŭn) [G. *skotōma,* darkness]. PSY: A sadistic expression seen in compulsion neuroses and schizophrenia by which the victim indulges in self-punishment as an expression of hatred for another.

scotophilia (skō-tō-fĭl'ĭ-ă) [G. *skotos,* darkness, + *philein,* to love]. Preference for darkness or for the night. SYN: *nyctophilia.*

scotophobia (skō-tō-fō'bĭ-ă) [" + *phobos,* fear]. Abnormal dread of darkness.

scotopia (skō-tō'pĭ-ă) [" + *ōps,* eye]. The adjustment of vision for darkness.

scotopic (skō-tŏp'ĭk). Pert. to scotopia.

s. vision. Dark adaptation; the adjustment of the eyes for vision in dark or dim light.

scotoscopy (skō-tŏs'kō-pĭ) [" + *skopein,* to examine]. Examination of internal organs by use of the fluoroscope. SYN: *skiascopy.*

scratch (skrătsh) [M.E. *cracchen*]. A mark or superficial injury produced by scraping with the nails or a rough surface.

screatus (skre-ā'tŭs) [L. *screātus,* a hawking]. A neurosis characterized by paroxysmal fits of hawking or snorting.

screen. A flat area suitable for projecting pictures upon or for visualizing x-ray pictures.

s., intensifying. An apparatus for intensifying the image produced by x-rays.

screening. Testing or examining an individual or large groups of people by utilizing only a portion of the usual examining procedures. For example, chest x-rays are used in screening for presence of pulmonary or cardiac diseases, urinalysis is used for detection of diabetes, and determination of intraocular pressure is used for diagnosing glaucoma.

scriveners' palsy (skrĭv'ner). Occupational neurosis caused by excessive use of the hand in writing. SYN: *writers' cramp.*

scrobiculate (skrō-bĭk'ū-lāt) [L. *scrobiculus,* a little pit]. Having shallow depressions; pitted.

scrobiculus (skrō-bĭk'ū-lŭs) [L. a little pit]. A small groove or pit.

s. cordis. Pit of the stomach; precordial or epigastric depression.

scrofula (skrŏf'ū-lă) [L. *scrofula,* a breeding sow]. A variety of tuberculous adenitis that is most frequently encountered. It is thought to be a secondary involvement of cervical lymph nodes as a result of a localized hematogenous spread from a pulmonary lesion. Most common in childhood.

TREATMENT: Responds to specific antituberculosis chemotherapy.

scrofulid(e). Scrofuloderma.

scrofuloderma (skrŏf'ū-lō-der'mă) [L. *scrofula,* a breeding sow, + G. *derma,* skin]. A skin manifestation of tuberculous origin, usually secondary to scrofula. Marked by ulcers usually resulting from a tuberculous sinus. Occurs most commonly on chest, neck, and in the axillae and groins, especially in children and adolescents. Now very rare. TREATMENT: Responds to ultraviolet light treatments and specific chemotherapy for tuberculosis. SYN: *tuberculosis cutis colliquativa.*

scrofulosis. Scrofula.

scrofulous (skrŏf'ū-lŭs) [L. *scrofula,* a breeding sow]. Of the nature of, or afflicted with, scrofula.

scrotal (skrō'tăl) [L. *scrotum,* a bag]. Concerning the scrotum.

s. reflex. Slow vermicular contraction of scrotal muscle when perineum is stroked or cold applied.

s. tongue. A furrowed tongue.

scrotectomy (skrō-tĕk'tō-mĭ) [" + G. *ektomē,* excision]. Excision of part of the scrotum.

scrotitis (skrō-tī'tĭs) [" + G. *-ītis,* inflammation]. Inflamed condition of the scrotum.

scrotocele (skrō'tō-sēl) [" + G. *kēlē,* hernia]. Hernia in the scrotum.

scrotum (skrō'tŭm) (pl. *scrota*) [L. *scrotum,* bag]. The double pouch containing the testicles and part of the spermatic cord.

RS: *chimney-sweeps' cancer, chyloderma, dartos, oscheal, oscheitis, oscheoncus, rhacoma, urocele.*

scrub'bing. Term applied to washing the hands, fingernails, and lower arms in preparing to perform surgery. The precise procedure to follow is usually posted in the special area where the washing is done.

METHOD: Scrubbing with soap and water and a nail brush, immersion in a mild germicidal solution and the wearing of sterilized rubber gloves, cap, gown, and mask. SEE: *sterilization.*

scrub nurse. Term applied to operating room nurse who hands instruments to the surgeon, and who has previously sterilized her hands and wears sterile rubber gloves.

scrub typhus. SYN: *tsutsugamushi disease, mite-borne typhus.* An acute febrile illness caused by *Rickettsia tsu-*

tsugamushi transmitted by several species of mites, including *Trombicula akamushi* and *T. deliensis.* Common in the Asiatic-Pacific area. If untreated, fever lasts for about 14 days. Fatality rate varies in untreated cases from 1% to 40%.

TREATMENT: Tetracycline or chloramphenicol.

scruple (skrū'pl) [L. *scrupulus,* a small stone]. Twenty grains in apothecaries' weight; 1.296 gm. ABBR: scr. SYMB: ℈.

scultetus bandage (skŭl-tē'tŭs). A many-tailed bandage used in compound fractures.

Scultetus' position. One with head low and the body on an inclined plane.

scum (skum) [M.E. *scume*]. BACT: Slimy floating islands of bacteria or impurities on the surface of a culture; an interrupted pellicle of bacterial growth.

scurf (skurf) [A.S. *scurf,* a gnawing]. A branny desquamation of the epidermis, esp. on the scalp. SEE: *dandruff.*

scurvy (skur'vĭ) [origin uncertain]. A deficiency disease characterized by hemorrhagic manifestations and abnormal formation of bones and teeth.

ETIOL: Deficiency of vitamin C usually resulting from lack of fresh fruits and vegetables in diet.

SYM: Preceded by period of ill health; sallow; loss of energy; pains in legs, limbs and joints. Anemic; great weakness; spongy, bleeding gums; fetor of breath, and loosening of teeth; subcutaneous hemorrhages and hemorrhages from mucous membranes; painful, brawny indurations of muscles.

PROG: Favorable in early stages.

TREATMENT: For infants, 300 mg. of vitamin C (ascorbic acid) daily for one week, then 150 mg. daily for one month, or 4-8 oz. of orange juice or 12-24 oz. of tomato juice daily. For adults, 300 to 500 mg. of ascorbic acid daily until symptoms have disappeared.

s., infantile. A form of scurvy which sometimes follows the prolonged use of condensed milk, sterilized milk or proprietary foods. SYN: *Barlow's disease.*

SYM: Anemia, immobility of legs, pseudoparalysis, extreme tenderness, swelling without pitting, thickening of bones from subperiosteal hemorrhage, ecchymoses and tendency to epiphyseal fractures at epiphyses of bones.

scute (skūt) [L. *scutum,* shield]. 1. A thin plate or scale, esp. the horny plates found on the carapace of turtles. 2. Term formerly applied to the tegmen tympani, *q.v.*

scutiform (skū'tĭ-form) [" + *forma,* a shield]. Shield-shaped.

scutulum (skū'tū-lŭm) (pl. *scutula*) [L. a little shield]. 1. Any of the thin crusts of favus. 2. The shoulder blade. SYN: *scapula.*

scutum (skū'tŭm) [L. shield]. Plate of bone resembling a shield.

scybalous (sĭb'ăl-ŭs) [G. *skybalon,* dung]. Of the nature of hard fecal matter.

scybalum (sĭb'ăl-ŭm) (pl. *scybala*). [G. *skybalŏn,* dung]. A hard, rounded mass of fecal matter.

scypho- [G.]. Combining form meaning *cup.*

scyphoid (sĭ'foyd) [G. *skyphos,* cup, + *eidos,* like]. Cup-shaped.

Se. Chemical symbol for *selenium.*

searcher (serch'er) [M.E. *serchen,* from L. *circāre,* to go about]. Instrument for locating opening of ureter previous to inserting catheter, exploring sinuses, and esp. for detecting stones in the bladder. SYN: *sound.*

seasickness (sē'sĭk-nĕs) [A.S. *sae,* sea, + *sēocness,* illness]. Disorder due to motion of a vessel at sea, or riding in cars, trains, and elevators. A similar condition affects some air travelers. SYN: *motion sickness.*

ETIOL: Motion affects the middle ear and the vomiting center in the brain stem is stimulated. There is wide individual variation in susceptibility.

SYM: Giddiness, vomiting, headache, nausea, and often extreme drowsiness, retching, prostration.

PREVENTION: Select position in craft where up and down motion is least; avoid dietary and alcoholic excesses; avoid reading or unusual visual stimuli; assume a supine or recumbent position.

TREATMENT: Specific anti-nausea and anti-motion sickness medicine. These include several forms of antihistamines. Sedatives and supportive therapy such as intravenous fluids may be required in severe and prolonged cases.

Generally, anti-nausea pills should not be given to pregnant women during early pregnancy.

RS: *nausea; motion sickness.*

seatworm (sēt'worm). SYN: *pinworm.* A species of nematode worms, *Enterobius vermicularis,* which occurs commonly in man. Adult worms inhabit large intestine in region of cecum and appendix. Gravid females migrate nightly to anus where they deposit eggs in perianal region. Movement of the worms about anus causes intense itching.

sebaceous (sē-bā'shŭs) [L. *sebaceus,* fatty]. Containing or pert. to sebum, an oily, fatty matter secreted by the sebaceous glands.

s. cyst. A cyst filled with sebaceous material from a distended sebaceous gland.

These are sometimes known as *wens.* They frequently form on the scalp, and consist of a small sac containing sebaceous matter, which may grow to a

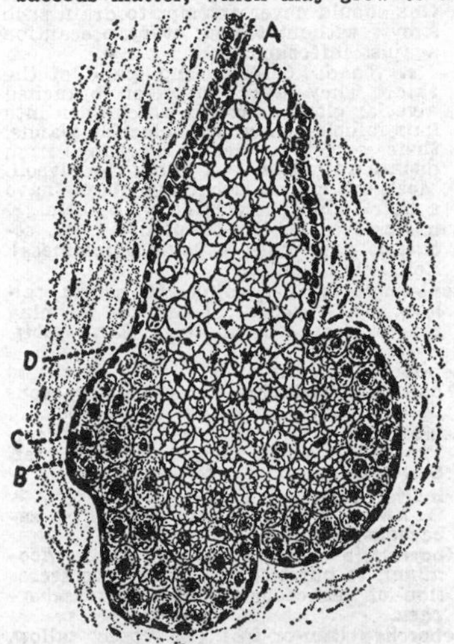

SEBACEOUS GLAND.

A. Epidermis of hair follicle. B. Germinating layer. C. Sebaceous cells in stage of beginning fatty metamorphosis. D. Particles of sebaceous material.

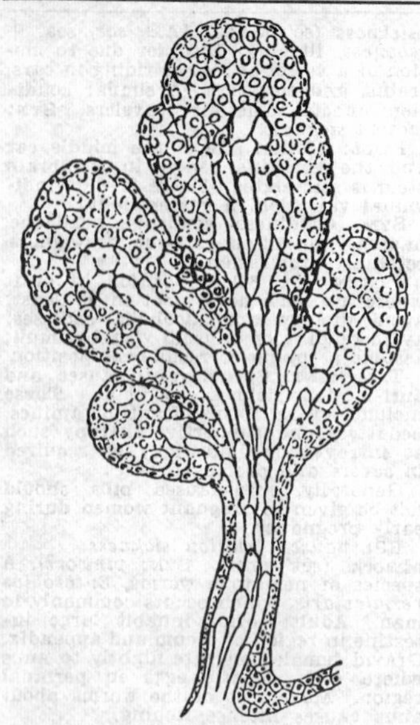

SEBACEOUS GLAND FROM HUMAN SKIN.

large size. They may result from impairment of localized circulation and closure of sebaceous glands or ducts. Drainage does not remove them permanently, as they will recur unless entirely extirpated,* which should be done with an electric current or cutting knife. One should never attempt to drain such a cyst without taking every precaution against infection.

s. gland. Oil-secreting gland of the skin. They are simple or branched alveolar glands most of which open into hair follicles. They are holocrine glands, their secretion, sebum, arising from disintegration of cells filling the alveoli. Most, but not all, sebaceous glands have a hair follicle associated with them.

sebastomania (sē-băs-tō-mā′nĭ-ă) [G. *sebastos,* reverend, + *mania,* madness]. Religious insanity.

sebiagogic (seb-ĭ-ă-goj′ĭk) [L. *sebum,* tallow, + G. *agōgos,* leading]. Forming fat or sebaceous matter. SYN: *sebiferous, sebiparous.*

sebiferous (sē-bĭf′ĕr-ŭs) [" + *ferre,* to carry]. Producing fatty or sebaceous matter. SYN: *sebiagogic, sebiparous.*

sebip′arous [" + *parēre,* to produce]. Producing sebum or sebaceous matter. SYN: *sebiagogic, sebiferous.*

sebolite, sebolith (sĕb′ō-līt, -lĭth) [" + G. *lithos,* a stone]. Concretion in a sebaceous gland.

seborrhagia (sĕb-ō-rā′jĭ-ă) [" + G. *rhēgnūnai,* to burst forth]. Excessive secretion of sebaceous glands. SYN: *seborrhea.*

seborrhea (sĕb-or-ē′ă) [L. *sebum,* tallow, + G. *rhoia,* a flow]. Functional disease of the sebaceous glands marked by increase in the amount and often alteration of the quality of the sebaceous secretion.

RS: *dermatitis seborrhoeica, sebaceous, sebum.*

s. capiti. Scalp seborrhea.

s. congestiva. Facial form with elevated patches with red borders and covered with crusts and scars. SYN: *lupus erythematosus.*

s. corporis. S. of the trunk.

s. faciei. S. of the face.

s. furfuracea. Seborrheic dermatitis, *q.v.*

s. nigra, s. nigricans. Dark-colored crusts in seborrhea.

s. oleosa. S. in which fat elements predominate. Shows shiny skin with widely dilated follicular orifices, many of which contain comedones.

s. sicca. S. with grayish-brown or yellow scale and crust formation in addition to abnormal oiliness.

Differentiation from seborrheic dermatitis is difficult. This form most frequently observed on scalp and constitutes what is popularly called dandruff.

Examination reveals an encrustation composed of thin, yellowish-gray scales. In uncomplicated cases the skin is pale, but often from irritation may become hyperemic or inflamed. When allowed to continue, nutrition of hair is interfered with, and baldness results. On the body s. sicca appears as yellowish-gray, slightly elevated patches covered with greasy scales. Outlets of follicles are often dilated. There is generally more or less redness of the skin from hyperemia (seborrheal eczema).

seborrheic (sĕb-or-rē′ĭk) [L. *sebum,* tallow, + G. *rhoia,* flow]. Afflicted with or like seborrhea.

s. dermatitis. SYN: *dermatitis seborrhoeica, seborrhea furfuracea, seborrhea sicca.*

seborrhoic (sĕb-or-ō′ĭk) [" + G. *rhoia,* a flow]. Suffering from or like seborrhea.* SYN: *seborrheic.*

sebum (sē′bŭm) [L. *sebum,* tallow]. A fatty secretion of the sebaceous glands of the skin.

It varies in different parts of the body; that from the ears is called *cerumen,** that from the foreskin is called *smegma* praeputii.*

RS: *sebaceous, seborrhea, smegma.*

secernent (sē-ser′nĕnt) [L. *secerneus,* secreting]. 1. Secreting. 2. A secreting organ.

seclusio pupillae [L.]. Shutting off of the pupil due to adherence of iris to the lenticular capsule. SYN: *synechia, annular posterior.*

s. p. siderosis bulbi. Deposit of iron pigment within the eyeball.

Seen in cases of retained iron foreign body in the eye.

seconal (sĕ′kōn-ăl). A proprietary barbituric acid derivative.

USES: Same as for the barbiturates.

second cranial nerve (sĕk-ŭnd) [L. *secunda*]. A sensory nerve which conveys visual impulses from eye to thalamus. The two optic nerves undergo partial decussation at the optic chiasma. SEE: *Table of Nerves in Appendix.*

s. intention. Healing by granulation or indirect union. SEE: *healing.*

Granulation tissue is formed to fill the gap bet. the edges of the wound with a thin layer of fibrinous exudate. It bars out bacteria and aids in checking bleeding by the coagulation of the blood. Connective tissue cells support the new capillaries. This form of healing is slower than that by first intention and its grayish-red surface may become pale and flabby if the healing is too long delayed. If the granulations show above the surface they may have to be removed with caustics. If the granulations first form at the top instead of the bottom of the wound, it may have to be kept open with drainage.

RS: *healing, intention, resolution.*

s. sight. Alteration in refractive powers of the lens so that reading again is possible without glasses in incipient cataract. Syn: *gerontopia.**

s. stage of labor. Period bet. complete dilatation of cervix and delivery of the child. See: *labor.*

During this stage pains become severe. It lasts normally 2-4 hr. in primiparae and up to 1 hr. in multiparae.

s. wind. Condition occurring following strenuous exercise in which breathlessness and a feeling of distress subside and the heart beats more regularly. Thought to be the result of the adjustment of the various organs of the body to the increased oxygen demands of the muscles.

secondary (sek'ŭn-dar-ĭ) [L. *secondarius,* second]. 1. Next to or following; second in order. 2. Produced by a primary cause. Syn: *subordinate.*

s. areola. Pigmentation around the nipples during pregnancy. See: *areola.*

s. disease. One following a previous disease.

s. hemorrhage. 1. One after an injury or operation coming on more than 24 hr. afterward and which is due to sepsis and septic ulceration into a blood vessel. 2. Uterine bleeding due to septic infection or from infant's umbilicus due to same cause. See: *hemorrhage.*

secreta (sē-krē'tă) [L.]. The products of secretion.

secretagogue (sē-krē'tă-gog) [L. *secretum,* secretion, + G. *agogos,* leading]. 1. Causing secretion. 2. That which stimulates secreting organs, as "substances present in food or produced by the digestion or decomposition of food which excite the secretion of digestive juice either by acting locally or by being absorbed into the blood or lymph or by causing a hormone to be formed." (A. C. Ivy.)

secrete (sē-krēt') [L. *secretus,* separated]. To separate from the blood, living organism, or gland; more specifically to form a secretion, *q.v.*

secretin (sē-krē'tĭn) [L. *secretiō,* a separation]. 1. A hormone formed in the mucous membrane of the duodenum through the influence of acid contents from the stomach whose function is to stimulate the flow of pancreatic juice. 2. A substance of unknown chemical composition, prepared by extraction from the mucous membrane of the duodenum and causing, when injected intravenously, an increased secretion of pancreatic juice. The first hormone to be isolated.

Probably formed from a precursor, prosecretin.*

See: *digestion, duodenal and intestinal; gastrin.*

secretion (sē-krē'shŭn) [L. *secretiō,* a separation]. A process in physiology whereby certain materials are separated, by the activity of a gland, from the blood and (a) made into something useful to the body or (b) eliminated. 2. Substance secreted.

If the useful material flows out through a duct (*e. g.,* saliva) it is called an *external secretion;* if it is returned to the blood or lymph (*e. g.,* insulin) it is called an *internal secretion* or autacoid.*

Fluids of Body

Blood: Is composed of 14 elements, 79% water, 21% solids, 500 to 600 red blood cells to 1 white blood cell.

Bile: Emulsifies fats and precipitates soluble peptones, 20 to 24 oz. Sp. gr. 1.026-1.032. Reaction alkaline.

Chyle: Absorbed by lacteals, resembles lymph. Begins to be formed in duodenum.

Chyme: Food that has undergone gastric digestion only.

Gastric Juice: An antiseptic juice in the stomach that converts proteids into peptones. 1000 to 1500 ml. per day. Specific gravity 1.010. Reaction acid.

Intestinal Juice: Has combined action of saliva, gastric and pancreatic juices. Converts cane into grape sugar and maltose into glucose. Also contains a milk curdling ferment, 10 oz. Sp. gr. 1.011. Reaction alkaline.

Lymph: Clear, transparent, yellowish fluid devoid of smell with saline taste. Specific gravity 1.012 to 1.022, alkaline.

Menstrual: Menstrual blood. Average 60 ml. during each period.

Pancreatic Juice. Contains enzymes which act on fats, proteins or products of protein digestion, and carbohydrates. 500-800 ml. per day. Sp. gr. 1.010 to 1.015. Alkaline.

Perspiration: The secretion of sweat glands of skin. About 500-1000 ml., under normal conditions. May be as high as 10 to 15 liters each 24 hours in extremely hot and dry conditions.

Saliva: Converts starch into sugar. Secreted by salivary glands. Specific gravity 1.002 to 1.006. Alkaline.

Urine: 1200 to 1500 ml. each 24 hours, but highly variable. Specific gravity 1.003 to 1.025. Acid. Contains 50 to 70 grams of solids, 20 to 30 grams of urea, and 10 to 15 grams of chlorides. See: *urine.*

s., antilytic. Watery saliva excreted continuously by submaxillary gland with intact nerves after division of the chorda tympani of the other side.

s. antiparalytic. Secretion, antilytic, *q.v.*

s., apocrine. That in which the apical end of a secreting cell is broken off and its contents extruded, as in the mammary gland.

s., external. A secretion which passes through duct and is discharged upon an epithelial surface, either internal or external.

s., holocrine. That in which the entire cell and its contents are extruded as a part of the secretory product, as in sebaceous glands.

s., internal. S. imparted to the blood instead of being eliminated by a duct.

s., merocrine. That in which the product is elaborated within cells and discharged through the cell membrane, the cell itself remaining intact.

s., paralytic. Abundant watery secretion continuously from a gland after section of its secretory nerves.

secretion, words pert. to: acrinia, amyxia, anorrhorrhea, apolepsis, asteatosis, athyrea, athyria, athyroidism, cerumen, ceruminal, ceruminosis, ceruminous, choleresis, chromocrinia, crinogenic, diacrisis, errhine, exsiccant, hormone, interstitial, saliva, sebum, secretagogue, secrete, secretin, semen, smegma, succorrhea.

secretogogue (sē-krē′tō-gŏg) [" + G. *agogos,* leading]. 1. Causing secretion. 2. That which stimulates secretion.

secret′or. An individual in which certain blood-group substances (A & B factors) can be extracted with aqueous solutions from tissues and organs, esp. salivary glands and gastric mucosa.

secretory (sē-krē′tō-rĭ, sē′kre-tō-rĭ) [L. *secretiō,* a separation]. Pert. to or promoting secretion; secreting.

s. capillaries. Very small canaliculi receiving secretion discharged from gland cells.

s. fibers. Centrifugal nerve fibers which excite secretion.

s. granules. SEE: *granules, zymogen.*

sectarian (sĕk-tār′ĭ-ăn) [L. *sectum,* from *secāre,* to cut]. A medical man who "follows a dogma, tenet, or principle based on the authority of its promulgator to the exclusion of demonstration and practice" (Judicial Council A. M. A.).

sectile (sĕk′tĭl) [L. *sectilis,* able to be cut]. Capable of being cut.

section (sĕk′shŭn) [L. *sectio,* from *secāre,* to cut]. 1. Process of cutting. 2. A division or segment of a part. 3. A surface made by cutting.

s., abdominal. Any abdominal operation. SYN: *laparotomy, q.v.*

s., cesarean. Incision of uterus for delivery of a fetus through abdominal wall or through the vagina. SEE: *cesarean section.*

s., coronal. A frontal section, *q.v.*

s., frontal. One dividing the body into 2 parts, *dorsal* and *ventral.*

s., frozen. A thin section of the body, an organ, or a piece of tissue which has been frozen before being sectioned and then studied microscopically.

s., midsagittal. One which divides the body into right and left halves.

s., paraffin. A section of a tissue which has been infiltrated with paraffin.

s., perineal. External incision into urethra to relieve stricture.

s., Pitres'. One of a series of sections made through the brain for postmortem examination.

s., sagittal. A section cut parallel to the median plane of the body.

s., serial. Microscopic sections made and arranged in consecutive order.

s., vaginal. Incision into the abdominal cavity through the vagina.

sectioning (sĕk-shŭn′ĭng) [L. *sectio,* a cutting]. The slicing of thin sections of tissue for examination under the microscope.

RS: *microtome.*

s., ultrathin. The cutting of sections extraordinarily thin (less than 1 micron in thickness) especially for use in electron microscopy.

sector (sĕk′tor) [L. *sector,* a cutter]. The area of a circle included bet. 2 radii and an arc.

sectorial (sĕk-tō′rĭ-ăl) [L. *sector,* a cutter]. Having cutting edges, as teeth.

secundigravida (sē-kŭn″dĭ-grăv′ĭd-ă) [L. *secundus,* second, + *gravida,* a pregnant woman]. A woman in her 2nd pregnancy.

secundines (sĕk′ŭn-dēnz, se-kun′-) [L. *secundinae,* things following]. The placenta and fetal membranes expelled during the 3rd stage of labor. SYN: *afterbirth.*

secundipara (sĕk″ŭn-dĭp′ă-ră) [L. *secundus,* second, + *parēre,* to give birth]. A woman who has borne 2 children at separate labors.

secundum artem (sē-kun′dŭm ar′tĕm) [L.]. In an approved manner; according to rule or science.

S. E. D. Abbr. for *skin erythema dose.*

Sed. [L.]. Abbr. of *sedes,* stool.

sedation (sē-dā′shŭn) [L. *sedatio,* from *sedāre,* to calm]. 1. Process of allaying nervous excitement. 2. State of being calmed.

Usually effected by means of a drug.

sedative (sĕd′a-tĭv) [L. *sedativus,* calming]. 1. An agent allaying irritability or nerve action. 2. Quieting.

They may be *general, local, nervous,* or *vascular.*

TYPES AND EX: *Cardiac*: Bromides, chloral, pilocarpine. *Respiratory*: Chloral, opium. *Gastric*: Bismuth, belladonna. *Nervous*: Antipyrine. *Cerebral*: Bromides and all hypnotics. *Intestinal*: Bismuth, opium. *General*: Opium and all hypnotics.

s., cardiac. One that decreases the heart's force.

s. enema. Retention enema given for its soothing action and to allay irritability. SEE: *enema, sedative.*

s., nervous. S. affecting nervous system.

sedentary (sĕd′ĕn-ta-rĭ) [L. *sedentarius,* from *sedere,* to sit]. 1. Sitting. 2. Pert. to an occupation or mode of living requiring minimal physical exercise.

sediment (sĕd′ĭ-mĕnt) [L. *sedimentum,* a settling]. The substance settling at bottom of a liquid. SYN: *hypostasis.* SEE: *precipitate.*

sedimentation (sĕd″ĭ-mĕn-tā′shŭn) [L. *sedimentum,* a settling]. Formation or depositing of sediment.

s. rate. Laboratory test of speed at which erythrocytes settle when an anticoagulant is added to blood.

In this test, blood to which an anticoagulant has been added is placed in a long, narrow tube, and the speed at which the red cells settle is observed. Various methods of determining the rate have been devised. Some pathologists determine the time required for the cells to settle a certain distance (sedimentation time), while others determine the distance the cells settle in a given time (sedimentation rate), both normally about 5 min. per millimeter. The speed at which the cells settle depends upon the size of the clumps into which the red cells aggregate, and the size of the clumps appears to depend upon the amount of fibrinogen in the blood. The speed of settling is increased in a variety of infections, in cancer, and in pregnancy, and may be decreased in liver disease.

sedimentator (sĕd-ĭ-mĕn-tā′tor) [L. *sedimentum,* a settling]. A centrifuge for separating urinary sediment.

seed (sēd) [A.S. *saed,* seed]. 1. The ripened ovule of a spermatophyte plant usually consisting of the embryo (germ), and a supply of nutrient material enclosed within the seed coats. It is a resting sporophyte. 2. Sperm; semen. 3. Capsule containing radon, radium, etc., for use in treatment of cancer. 4. Offspring. 5. To introduce microorganisms into a culture medium.

segment (sĕg′mĕnt) [L. *segmentum,* a portion]. 1. A part or section, esp. a natural one, of an organ or body. 2. One of the serial divisions of an animal.

s., body. SYN: *metamere, somite.* In the embryo, a somite; in the adult, a portion derived from a somite.

s., interannular. Portion of a neuron between two nodes of Ranvier.

s., mesodermal. A somite.

segmental (sĕg-mĕn′tăl) [L. *segmentum,* a portion]. Pertaining to, resembling, or composed of segments.

s. reflex. A reflex action in which afferent impulses enter the cord in the same segment or segments from which the efferent impulses emerge.

s. static reactions. Postural reflexes in which movements of one extremity result in a movement in an opposite extremity.

segmentation (sĕg″mĕn-tā′shŭn) [L. *segmentum,* a portion]. 1. Division into similar parts. 2. Syn: *cleavage.* The division of a fertilized egg into many smaller cells or blastomeres. See: *embryo, cleavage, blastomere.*

s. cavity. Central space in blastula stage of segmentation of an ovum.

s., rhythmic. Division of the intestine and the chyme within it into segments by contraction of circular muscle fibers; also called *segmenting contractions.*

segmenter. Syn: *rosette, mature schizont.* Stage in development of the malarial organism (*Plasmodium*) in which the organism is undergoing schizogony.

segregation. 1. Setting apart, separating. 2. In genetics, the process which takes place in the formation of germ cells (gametogenesis) in which each gamete (egg or sperm) receives only one of each pair of genes.

segregator (sĕg′rē-gā-tor) [L. *segregāre,* to separate]. Instrument composed of 2 catheters for securing urine from each kidney separately.

Séguin's signal symptom (sa-ganz′). Involuntary contractions of muscles just before an epileptic attack.

Seidlitz powder (sĕd′lĭts, sĭd′lĭtz). Effervescent cathartic composed of tartaric acid, sodium bicarbonate, and sodium and potassium tartrate.

seisesthesia (sī-zĕs-thē′zĭ-ă) [G. *seisis,* concussion, + *aisthēsis,* sensation]. The perception of a concussion.

seismesthesia (sīz-mĕs-thē′zĭ-ă) [G. *seismos,* earthquake, + *aisthēsis,* sensation] Perception of vibrations.

seismotherapy (sīz-mō-thĕr′ă-pĭ) [" + *therapeia,* treatment]. Treatment of disease by vibratory massage. Syn: *sismotherapy.*

seizure (sē′zhŭr) [M.E. *seizen,* to take possession of]. A sudden attack of pain or of a disease, or of certain symptoms.

s., convulsive. 1. A convulsion, *q.v.* 2. An attack of epilepsy.

s., larval. A seizure indicated by abnormal brain waves in an electroencephalogram but not evidenced by clinical symptoms.

selec′tion. 1. Choice; the process of choosing or selecting. 2. In biology, any process by which a group of individuals such as a species is enabled to survive or to avoid extermination.

s., artificial. Process by which man selects individuals possessing desirable characteristics and endeavors to produce through selective breeding a race or strain homozygous for these characteristics.

s., natural. 1. Process by which individuals possessing characteristics which adapt them to their environment survive, whereas those lacking these characteristics die or fail to leave progeny. 2. Darwin's theory of evolution or origin of species. See: *natural selection.*

s., sexual. A theory originated to account for differences in secondary sex characteristics between males and females. It assumes that individuals preferentially select for mating individuals of the opposite sex who possess these characteristics.

selen′ium. A chemical element resembling sulfur. Symb: Se. At. wt. 78.96, at no. 34. Selenium is poisonous to certain animals which feed on plants grown on seleniferous soil.

self-diges′tion. Destruction or disintegration of a cell or tissue by its own juice, as that of the walls of the stomach by the gastric juice occurring in certain diseases of that organ. Syn: *autodigestion.*

self-lim′ited disease. Disease that, without treatment, runs a definite course within a limited time.

sella turcica (sĕl′ă tur′sĭ-kă) [L. Turkish saddle]. Syn: *hypophyseal or pituitary fossa.* A concavity on superior surface of body of sphenoid bone which houses the hypophysis cerebri (pituitary gland) [NA].

Selter's disease. Feer's disease, erythredema polyneuropathy.

semeiology (sē″mī-ŏl′ō-jĭ) [G. *sēmeion,* sign, + *logos,* study]. The branch of medicine dealing with the study of symptoms. Syn: *symptomatology.*

semeiosis (sē-mī-ō′sĭs) [" + *-ōsis,* intensive]. Study of disease by symptoms.

semeiotic (sē″mī-ot′ĭk) [G. *sēmeiōtikos,* pert. to a sign]. Of or pert. to symptoms. Syn: *symptomatic.*

semeiotics (sē″mī-ŏt′ĭks) [G. *sēmeiōtikos,* pert. to a sign]. 1. Phase of medical science treating of symptoms. 2. Symptoms of a disease in a particular case considered as a whole. Syn: *semiotics, symptomatology.*

semelincident (sĕm-ĕl-ĭn′sĭd-ĕnt) [L. *semel,* once, + *incidens,* falling upon]. Occurring only once in the same person.

semen (sē′mĕn) (pl. *semina*) [L. *sēmen,* seed]. A thick, opalescent, viscid secretion discharged from the urethra of the male at the climax of sexual excitement (orgasm). Contains the spermatozoa.

It is the mixed product of various glands (prostate and bulbourethral) plus the spermatozoa which, having been produced in the testicles, are stored in the seminal vesicles.

RS: *aspermatic; aspermatism; aspermous; azoospermia; bradyspermatism; coition; coitus; coitus interruptus; copulation; ejaculation; emissio seminis; emission; erection; excitation; fertilization; insemination; libido; orgasm; penis; prostate; sexual intercourse; sperm; sperma; spermatemphraxis; spermatic; spermatorrhea; spermatozoon; vesicle, seminal.*

semenuria (sē″mĕn-ū′rĭ-ă) [L. *sēmen,* seed, + G. *ouron,* urine]. Excretion of semen in the urine. Syn: *seminuria, spermaturia.*

semi- [L.]. Prefix meaning *half.*

semicanal (sĕm″ĭ-kăn-ăl′) [L. *semis,* half, + *canalis,* passage]. A duct open on one side.

semicircular (sĕm″ĭ-sĭr′kū-lar) [" + *circulus,* a ring]. In the form of a half circle.

s. canals. Superior, posterior, and inferior passages forming part of inner ear.

semicoma (sĕm″ĭ-kō′mă) [" + G. *kōma,* lethargy]. Mild degree of coma from which it is possible to arouse the patient.

semicomatose (sĕm″ĭ-kō′măt-ōs) [" + G. *kōma,* lethargy]. In a condition of unconsciousness from which patient may be aroused.

semilunar (sĕm″ĭ-lū′nar) [" + *luna*, moon]. Crescentic in shape.

s. bone. Halfmoon-shaped bone of carpus.

s. cartilages. Two crescentic cartilages (medial and lateral) in the knee joint between the femur and tibia.

s. ganglions. Two small nervous ganglions of the abdominal cavity, supplying solar plexus. The gasserian g.

s. lobe. One on upper surface of the cerebellum.

s. notch. A notch at proximal end of ulna for articulation with trochlea of humerus.

s. valves. Valves of aorta and pulmonary artery. SEE: *Arantius' body.*

semimembranosus (sĕm″ĭ-mĕm-brăn-ō′sŭs) [L.]. Large muscle of inner and back part of thigh. SEE: *Table of Muscles in Appendix.*

seminal (sĕm′ĭn-ăl) [L. *sēmen, semin-*, seed]. Concerning the semen.

s. duct. SYN: *spermatic duct.* Any duct which conveys sperm, especially the ductus deferens and the ejaculatory duct.

s. emission. Involuntary loss of seminal fluid, usually during sleep, esp. in the adolescent male.

s. filament. Male seed. SYN: *spermatozoon.*

s. fluid. Semen, male fertilizing fluid.

s. vesicle. One of two sac-like structures in the male lying behind the bladder and connected to the ductus deferens on each side. They secrete a thick viscous fluid which forms a part of the semen.

semination (sĕm-ĭn-ā′shŭn) [L. *seminatio*, a begetting]. Introduction of semen into the female genital tract during sexual intercourse or artificially. SYN: *insemination.*

s., artificial. Introduction of prepared semen into the uterus. SYN: *artificial insemination.*

seminiferous (sĕm-ĭn-ĭf′ĕr-ŭs) [L. *sēmen, semin-*, seed, + *ferre*, to produce]. Producing or conducting semen, as the tubules of the testes.

seminoma (sĕm-ĭ-nō′mă) [" + G. *-ōma*, tumor]. A tumor of the testis.

seminormal (sĕm″ĭ-nor′măl) [L. *semis*, half, + *norma*, rule]. One-half the normal standard.

s. solution. One having half the quantity of the substance in the normal solution. "Indicated thus: 0.5 N or N/2."

seminuria (sē″mĭn-ū′rĭ-ă) [L. *sēmen*, seed, + G. *ouron*, urine]. Seminal discharge present in the urine. SYN: *semenuria, spermaturia.*

semiology (sē″mĭ-ŏl′ō-jĭ) [G. *sēmeion*, sign, + *logos*, a study]. Phase of medicine dealing with study of symptoms. SYN: *semeiology, symptomatology.*

semiotic (sē-mĭ-ŏt′ĭk) [G. *sēmeiōtikos*, pert. to a sign]. Like or pert. to symptoms of disease. SYN: *semeiotic, symptomatic.*

semiotics (sē″mĭ-ŏt′ĭks) [G. *sēmeiōtikos* pert. to a sign]. Scientific study of symptoms as a whole or in one particular case. SYN: *semiology, symptomatology.*

semipermeable (sĕm″ĭ-per′mē-ă-bl) [" + *per*, through, + *meāre*, to pass]. Half permeable; said of a membrane which will allow fluids but not the dissolved substance to pass through it. SEE: *membrane, osmosis.*

semiprone (sĕm-ĭ-prōn′) [" + *pronus*, prone]. In a position on left side and chest, with both thighs flexed on abdomen, the right higher than the left, and left arm back. SYN: *Sims' position, q.v., for illustration.*

semirecumbent (sĕm″ĭ-rē-kŭm′bĕnt) [" + *recumbere*, to lie down]. Reclining, but not fully recumbent.

semis (sē′mĭs) [L. *semis*, half]. Half.

Abbreviated to *ss* after sign indicating the measure in prescriptions.

semisideratio, semisideration (sĕm″ĭ-sĭd-ĕr-ā′shĭ-ō, -ā′shŭn) [" + *sideratio*, a blight]. Paralysis on one side of the body. SYN: *hemiplegia.*

semisopor (sĕm-ĭ-sō′por) [" + *sopor*, deep sleep]. Light coma from which patient can be roused. SYN: *semicoma.*

semispinalis (sĕm″ĭ-spī-na′lĭs) [L.]. Deep layer of muscle of back on either side of spinal column, divided into 3 parts. SEE: *Table of Muscles in Appendix.*

semisupination (sĕm″ĭ-sū-pĭn-ā′shŭn) [" + *supinus*, bent back]. A position halfway bet. supination and pronation.

semitendinosus (sĕm″ĭ-tĕn-dĭn-ō′sŭs) [L.]. Fusiform muscle of post. and inner part of thigh. SEE: *Table of Muscles in Appendix.*

semper- [L.]. Combining form meaning *always.*

senescence (sĕn-es′ĕns) [L. *senescere*, to grow old]. The process of growing old, or the period of old age.

senile (sē′nĭl, -nīl) [L. *senilis*, old]. Pert. to growing old or to the aged.

senilism (sē′nĭl-ĭzm, -nīl-ĭzm) [" + G. *-ismos*, condition]. Old age, particularly when premature. SEE: *progeria.*

senility (sē-nĭl′ĭ-tĭ) [L. *senilis*, old]. 1. The state of being old. 2. Weakness of old age, mental or physical.

s., premature. Onset of characteristics before the normal time, as early as 40 years.

May be due to dissipation, privation, or congenital structural defects.

s., psychosis of. Mental disorder in old age.

senium (sē′nĭ-ŭm) [L.]. Old age, esp. its debility.

s. precox. PSY: Mental disorder resembling senile dementia occurring before 60, usually marked by incoherent delusions.

senna (sĕn′a) [Arabic *sana*]. USP. The dried leaves of the plant *Cassia acutifolia* and *C. angustifolia.*

ACTION AND USES: As a purgative acting on the large intestine.

senopia (sĕn-ō′pĭ-ă) [L. *senilis*, old, + G. *ōps*, eye]. Improvement in visual power of old people. SYN: *gerontopia.*

sensation (sĕn-sā′shŭn) [L. *sensatio*, a feeling]. A feeling or awareness of conditions within or without the body resulting from the stimulation of sensory receptors.

s., common. The sum total of all bodily sensations.

s., cutaneous. S. through medium of the skin.

s., delayed. S. not experienced immediately following a stimulus.

s., epigastric. A sinking feeling in the stomach.

s., external. Effect upon the mind of any stimuli from peripheral nerves.

s., girdle. A painful s., as a bandage tightened about a limb or the trunk as in spinal disease. SYN: *zonesthesia.*

s., internal. A subjective one.

s., palmesthetic. S. felt in the skin from vibration.

s., referred. Same as reflex sensation.

s., subjective. S. not resulting from

any external stimulus and perceptible only by the subject.

s., tactile. S. produced through the sense of touch.

sense (sĕns) [L. *sensus,* a feeling]. 1. To perceive through a sense organ. 2. The general faculty by which conditions outside or inside the body are perceived. 3 Any special faculty of sensation connected with a particular organ. 4. Normal power of understanding.

The most important of the senses are (1) Sight; (2) hearing; (3) smell; (4) taste; (5) touch and pressure; (6) temperature; (7) weight, resistance, and tension (muscle sense); (8) pain; (9) visceral and sexual sensations; (10) equilibrium; (11) hunger and thirst.

s., color. The perception of various colors.

s., cutaneous. Sensation felt through the skin.

s., genesic. The sexual instinct.

s., kinesthetic. SEE: *s., muscular.*

s., light. Perception of degree of light.

s., muscle, muscular. Consciousness of muscular movement required in a given act.

s. organ. The organ which gives rise to a nerve impulse which reaching the brain registers in consciousness as a particular sensation.

s., posture. Ability through muscle sense to differentiate positions of the body or its structures.

s., pressure. Faculty of feeling various degrees of pressure on the body surface.

s., seventh. Subjective sensations of internal organs.

s., sixth. General feeling of normal functioning of the bodily organs. SYN: *cenesthesia.*

s., space. That sense by which we recognize objects in space, their relationship and dimensions.

s's., special. Sight, hearing, smell, touch, and taste.

s., stereognostic. Ability to judge consistency and shape of objects held in the fingers.

s., temperature. Ability to detect differences of temperature.

s., time. Ability to detect differences in time intervals, as in sound.

s., tone. Ability to distinguish bet. different tones.

s., visceral. Perception of the sensations of the internal organs. SYN: *seventh sense.*

sensibilin (sĕn'sĭ-bĭl-ĭn) [L. *sensibilis,* feeling]. A specific antibody formed at first injection of a foreign protein. SYN: *anaphylactic reaction body.*

sensibility (sĕn-sĭ-bĭl'ĭ-tĭ) [L. *sensibilitās*]. Capacity to receive and respond to stimuli.

s., deep. 1. The sensibility existing after an area of the skin is made anesthetic. 2. Sensation by which the position of a limb and estimation of difference in weight and tension are apparent.

s., mesoblastic. SEE: *s., deep.*

s., palmesthetic. The sensibility existing in the skin to vibration.

s., protopathic. The sensibility to strong stimulations of pain and temperature, which exists in the skin and in the viscera. Now obsolete.

sensibilization (sĕn-sĭ-bĭl-ĭz-ā'shŭn) [L. *sensibilitās,* feeling]. 1. The process of making sensitive; sensitization. 2. Production of hypersusceptibility to a foreign substance by injecting it into the body. SYN: *anaphylaxis; sensitization.*

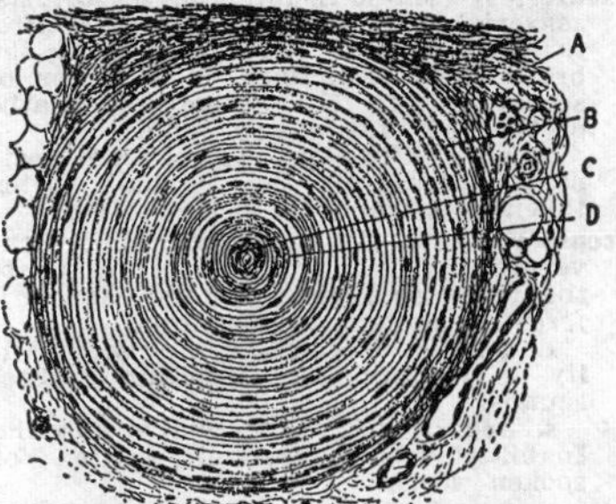

SENSE ORGAN, CUTANEOUS

Transverse section of pacinian corpuscle. Sole of foot of man. A. Connective tissue. B. Outer lamellose sheath. C. Central core. D. Axis cylinder.

sensibilizer (sĕn'sĭ-bĭl-ī-zer) [L. *sensibilitās,* feeling]. Substance in blood serum normally or after inoculation which is active in cytolysis. SYN: *amboceptor.*

sensible (sĕn'sĭ-bl) [L. *sensibilis,* feeling]. 1. Capable of being perceived by the senses; perceptible. 2. Capable of receiving sensations. SYN: *sensitive.* 3. Having reason. SYN: *intelligent.* 4. Conscious, as opposed to insensible.

sensiferous (sĕn-sĭf'ĕr-ŭs) [L. *sensus,* a feeling, + *ferre,* to bear]. Causing, conducting, or transmitting sensations.

sensigenous (sĕn-sĭj'ĕn-ŭs) [" + G. *gennan,* to produce]. Causing or starting a sensory impulse.

sensimeter (sĕn-sĭm'ĕ-ter) [" + G. *metron,* a measure]. Machine for recording the degree of sensitiveness of various areas of the body.

sensitinogen (sĕn-sĭ-tĭn'ō-jen) [L. *sensus,* feeling, + G. *gennan,* to produce]. The antigens collectively which sensitize the body.

sensitive (sĕn'sĭ-tĭv) [L. *sensitivus,* feeling]. 1. Capable of transmitting a sensation. 2. Able to feel a sensation. 3. Subject to destructive action of a complement. 4. Susceptible to suggestions, as a hypnotic. 5. Abnormally susceptible to a substance, as a drug or foreign protein. SEE: *allergic.*

sensitization (sĕn"sĭ-tĭ-zā'shŭn) [L. *sentīre,* to feel]. 1. A condition of being made sensitive to specific stimulus. 2. Rendering of a cell sensitive to the action of a complement by uniting it with a specific amboceptor. 3. Process of making a person susceptible to a substance by repeated injections of it, as a serum. SYN: *anaphylaxis.*

sensitized (sĕn'sĭ-tīzd). Made susceptible to a specific substance.

s. vaccine. A live culture which has been mixed with its antiserum before introduction.

sensitizer (sĕn'sĭ-tī"zer) [L. *sensitivus,* feeling]. An antibody producing susceptibility to cytolysis. SYN: *amboceptor.*

sensitometer (sĕn-sĭ-tŏm'ĕt-ĕr) [L. *sensitivus,* perceiving, + G. *metron,* a measure]. Device for determining the penetrating power of light.

sensorial (sĕn-sō'rĭ-ăl) [L. *sensus,* a sensation]. Pert. to the sensorium, the seat of sensation.

sensorimotor (sĕn-sō-rĭ-mō'tor) [" + *motor,* motion]. Both sensory and motor. SYN: *sensomotor.*

sensorium (sĕn-sō′rĭ-ŭm) (pl. *sensoriums, sensoria*) [L. *sensōrium,* from *sentire,* to perceive]. 1. That portion of the brain which functions as a center of sensations. 2. The sensory apparatus of the body taken as a whole.

s. area. The precentral and postcentral areas of the cerebral cortex taken as a whole.

sensory (sĕn′sō-rĭ) [L. *sensorius*]. 1. Conveying impulses from sense organs to the reflex or higher centers. SYN: *afferent.** 2. Pert. to sensation.

s. amusia. Musical deafness; inability to comprehend music or musical sounds.

s. aphasia. SYN: *perceptive aphasia.* Inability to understand written or spoken words.

s. area. Any area of the cerebral cortex in which sensations are perceived.

s. area, somesthetic. Area occupying postcentral gyrus of cerebral cortex and extending into adjacent areas in which sensations of general somatic sensibility are perceived.

s. decussation. The sup. pyramidal decussation.

s. ending. SYN: *sensory end-organ, receptor.* A termination of an afferent nerve fiber which upon stimulation gives rise to a sensation.

s. epilepsy. Disturbances of sensation that replace epileptic convulsions.

s. nerve. An afferent nerve conveying sensory impulses to the sensorium, or one composed of sensory fibers.

s. unit. A single sensory nerve fiber with all its branches and their terminal nerve endings.

sensual (sĕn′shū-ăl) [L. *sensus,* sense]. Concerning or consisting in the gratification of the senses; indulgence of the appetites; not spiritual or intellectual; carnal, worldly.

sensualism (sĕns′ū-ăl-ĭzm). State or condition of being sensual; condition in which one's actions are dominated by primitive instincts.

sensuous (sĕn′shū-ŭs) [L. *sensus,* sense]. Pert. to or affecting the senses; susceptible to influence through the senses.

sentient (sĕn′shĭ-ĕnt) [L. *sentīre,* to perceive]. Capable of perceiving sensation. SYN: *sensitive.*

sentiment (sĕn′tĭ-mĕnt). Feeling, sensibility, esp. susceptibility to tender feelings; an emotional attitude toward an object or a group of objects.

separation. The process of disconnecting, disuniting, or severing.

s., epiphyseal. S. of the epiphysis from the diaphysis or shaft of a bone.

separator (sĕp′ar-ā-tor) [L. *separator,* a separator]. 1. Anything which prevents 2 substances from mingling. 2. Any device or instrument used for bringing about a separation of two objects.

separatorium (sĕp-ar-ā-tō′rĭ-ŭm) [L. *separatorium,* from *separāre,* to separate]. Instrument for separating pericranium from skull.

sepsis (sĕp′sĭs) [G. *sēpsis,* putrefaction]. SYN: *septicemia, bacteremia.* Pathologic state usually febrile, resulting from the presence of microorganisms or their poisonous products in the blood stream. May be manifested as *cellulitis* (local dissemination of infection), *lymphangitis* or *lymphadenitis* (dispersion along lymphatic channels) or *bacteremia* (widespread dissemination by way of blood stream). The latter is commonly called *"blood poisoning."*

s., gas. That resulting from infection by gas gangrene bacilli (*Clostridium perfringens*) and others.

s., puerperal. SYN: *puerperal infection, childbed fever.* Infection of the genital tract following childbirth.

The infection may be brought about by exogenous or endogenous means. The organisms most commonly associated with this type of infection are *streptococcus, staphylococcus, bacillus coli,* and a putrefactive group of *saprophytic organisms.* The infection may be localized in the uterine cavity, lymphatics, veins and mucous membrane of the vaginal tract.

PATH: In the minor cases of ulceration in the vaginal tract covered by a dirty membrane. In streptococci infection the endometrium is smooth, and the lymphatics are congested with the invading organism. As a rule, the uterine cavity is filled with very little lochia. The saprophytic type shows an endometrial cavity filled with greenish, purulent, foul-smelling shreds. Microscopically, there is a thick layer of leukocytes under the necrotic layer. The uterus shows poor involution. In the event that the infection extends further than the uterus, the parametrium or cellular tissues show edema, serum and in the saprophytic cases, purulent infiltration. Extension of the process to the veins produces infectious thrombi which in turn produce localized abscesses in other parts of the body.

SYM: Onset may be gradual or sudden. Patient begins to have general malaise, headache, chilly sensations or true rigors and rise in temperature. The uterus is tender, there is some abdominal distention, and the lochia in the saprophytic type is profuse and foul-smelling, while in the streptococcic type it is decreased in amount and of a serous character. Occasionally there is swelling of the lower limb accompanied by high fever, rapid pulse rate and chills. Upon palpation the femoral vein is found to be tender and cordlike. This is an infectious thrombosis of the femoral vein, and the condition is known as phlegmasia alba dolens.

COURSE: Early diagnosis and appropriate therapy will effectively control the course of the disease in most cases.

TREATMENT: General measures include absolute bed rest, light or liquid diet, maintenance of fluid balance by parenteral injections if necessary, blood transfusion may be required, analgesics for pain. Check for nutritional deficiencies, esp. of vitamins or minerals.

septal (sĕp′tăl) [L. *saeptum,* a dividing wall]. Concerning a septum.

septan (sĕp′tăn) [L. *septem,* seven]. Recurring every 7th day, as the paroxysms of malarial fever.

septate (sĕp′tāt) [L. *saeptum,* a partition]. Having a dividing wall.

septectomy (sĕp-tĕk′tō-mĭ) [" + G. *ektomē,* excision]. Excision of a septum, esp. the nasal septum or a part of it.

septemia (sĕp-tē′mĭ-ă) [G. *sēptos,* putrid, + *aima,* blood]. Invasion of the blood by pathogenic bacteria or their toxins. SYN: *septicemia.*

septic (sĕp′tĭk) [G. *sēptos,* putrid]. 1. Pert. to sepsis. 2. Pert. to pathogenic organisms or their toxins.

s. fever, s. infection. Fever or infection due to presence of pathogenic organisms or their products in the blood. SYN: *septicemia.*

s. sore throat. Streptococcic inflammation of throat with fever and marked prostration.

septicemia (sĕp-tĭ-sē'mĭ-ă) [G. *sēptikos,* putrid, + *aima,* blood]. Morbid condition from absorption of septic products into blood and tissues or of pathogenic bacteria which may rapidly multiply there. SYN: *blood poisoning.*

Symptoms and signs usually include chills and fever, petechia, purpuric pustules, and abscesses.

s., bronchopulmonary. S. following operation on the larynx resulting in infected secretions from the wound entering the bronchial tubes.

s., cryptogenic. S. in which cannot be found any primary focus of infection.

s., puerperal. S. occurring following prolonged and difficult labor or incomplete abortion. SYN: *septic abortion; postabortal sepsis; puerperal infection.*

septicemic (sĕp-tĭ-sē'mĭk) [G. *sēptikos,* putrid, + *aima,* blood]. Relating to, resulting from, or of the nature of, septicemia.

septicophlebitis (sĕp"tĭ-kō-flē-bī'tĭs) [" + *phleps,* vein, + *-itis,* inflammation]. Septic inflammation of a vein.

septicopyemia (sĕp"tĭ-kō-pī-ē'mĭ-ă) [" + *pyon,* pus, + *aima,* blood]. Septicemia and pyemia together.

septigravida. A woman pregnant for the seventh time.

septimetritis (sĕp"tĭ-mē-trī'tĭs) [G. *sēptos,* putrid, + *mētra,* uterus, + *-itis,* inflammation]. Inflammation of uterus due to sepsis.

septipara (sĕp-tĭp'ă-ră) [L. *septem,* seven, + *parēre,* to bring forth]. A woman who has borne 7 children separately.

septivalent (sĕp-tĭ-vā'lĕnt, -tĭv'ă-lĕnt) [" + *valēre,* to be strong]. Having a valency of 7 or combining with or replacing 7 hydrogen atoms.

septomarginal. Pert. to the margin or the border of a septum.

septometer (sĕp-tŏm'ĕt-ĕr) 1. [L. *saeptum,* a partition]. Calipers for measuring width of nasal septum. 2. [G. *sēptos,* putrid, + *metron,* a measure]. Device for determining atmospheric impurity.

septotome (sĕp'tō-tōm) [L. *saeptum,* a partition, + G. *tomē,* a cutting]. An instrument for cutting or removing a section of the nasal septum.

septotomy (sĕp-tŏt'ō-mĭ) [" + G. *tomē,* a cutting]. Incision of a septum, esp. the nasal septum.

septu'la. Plural of *septulum, q.v.*

s. testis. Thin partition extending inward from mediastinum testis and separating testis into the *lobuli testis.*

septulum. A small partition or septum.

septum (sĕp'tŭm) (pl. *septa*) [L. *saeptum,* a partition]. A membranous wall dividing two cavities.

s., atrial. A wall bet. the atria of the heart.

s. atriorum cordis, s. auricularum. A wall bet. the atria of the heart.

s., crural. A mass of fat obstructing the femoral ring.

s., femoral. Mass of fatty connective tissue closing femoral ring.

s., interatrial. The atrial septum, *q.v.*

s., intermuscular. 1. A connective tissue septum which separates two muscles, esp. one from which muscles may take their origin. 2. One of two connective tissue septa which separate the muscles of the leg into ant., post. and lat. groups.

s., interventricular. The ventricular septum, *q.v.*

s., lingual. A sheet of connective tissue separating the halves of the tongue.

s. lucidum. 1. A translucent s., the int. boundary of lateral ventricles of the brain. SYN: *septum pellucidum.* 2. The stratum corneum layer of the epidermis.

s., mediastinal. SEE: *mediastinum.*

s., nasal. The partition which divides the nasal cavity into two nasal fossae.

Bony portion formed by the perpendicular plate of ethmoid and the vomer bone; cartilaginous portion formed by septal and vomeronasal cartilages and medial crura of greater alar cartilages.

s., orbital. A fibrous sheet extending partially across the anterior opening of the orbit partially closing it.

s. pectiniforme. Comblike partition that separates the corpora cavernosa.

s. pellucidum. A thin triangular sheet of nervous tissue consisting of two lamina attached to corpus callosum above and the fornix below. It forms the medial wall of the lateral ventricles. [NA].

s., rectovaginal. Partition bet. the rectum and the vagina.

s. scroti. Partition dividing the chambers of the scrotum. SYN: *s. of scrotum.*

s., ventricular. Partition between the ventricles of the heart.

septuplet (sĕp'tŭp-lĕt) [L. *septuplum,* a group of seven]. One of 7 children born from the same gestation.

sequela (sē-kwē'lă) (pl. *sequelae*) [L. a following]. A condition following and resulting from a disease.

sequence. The order or occurrence of a series of phenomena as symptoms.

sequester (sē-kwĕs'tĕr) [L. *sequestrāre,* to separate]. 1. To isolate. 2. A piece of necrosed bone separated from surrounding tissue. SYN: *sequestrum.*

sequestration (sē-kwĕs-tra'shŭn) [L. *sequestrātio,* a separation]. 1. The formation of sequestrum. 2. Isolation of a patient for treatment or quarantine. 3. Reduction of hemorrhage of head or trunk by temporarily stopping the return of blood from the extremities by applying tourniquets to the thighs and arms.

sequestrectomy (sē-kwĕs-trĕk'tō-mĭ) [" + G. *ektomē,* excision]. Excision of a necrosed piece of bone.

sequestrotomy (sē-kwĕs-trŏt'ō-mĭ) [" + G. *tomē,* a cutting]. Operation for removal of a sequestrum, a fragment of necrosed bone. SYN: *sequestrectomy.*

sequestrum (sē-kwĕs'trŭm) [L. *sequestrum,* from *sequestrāre,* to separate]. Fragment of a necrosed bone that has become separated from surrounding tissue. Designated *primary* if piece is entirely detached, *secondary* if still loosely attached, and *tertiary* if it is partially detached but still remaining in place.

sera (sē'ră) [L.]. Plural of *serum.*

seralbumin (sēr-ăl-bū'mĭn) [L. *serum,* whey, + *albumen,* white of egg]. Albumin of the blood.

serial (sē'rĭ-ăl) [L. *series,* a succession]. In numerical order, in continuity or sequence, as in a series.

sericeps (sĕr'ĭ-sĕps) [L. *sericus,* silken, + *caput,* head]. Silk sac used in making traction on fetal head.

series (sēr'ēz) [L. *series,* a succession]. 1. Arrangement of objects in succession or in order. 2. ELECT: A mode of arranging the parts of a circuit by connecting them successively end to end to form a single path for the current. The parts so arranged are said to be "in series."

serine. a-amino-B-hydroxypropionic acid, an amino acid present in many proteins including casein, vitellin, and others. Found in the urine of normal human beings.

seriscission (sĕr-ĭ-sĭsh'ŭn) [L. *sericum,* silk, + *scindere,* to cut]. Division of soft tissues, as a pedicle, by tying a silk ligature around it.

sero- [L.]. Combining form *pertaining to serum.*

seroalbuminuria (sē"rō-ăl-bū-mĭn-ū'rĭ-ă) [L. *serum,* whey, + *albumen,* white of egg, + G. *ouron,* urine]. Serum albumin in the urine.

serobacterin (sē"rō-băk'ter-ĭn) [" + G. *bakterion,* a small rod]. Bacterial vaccine sensitized with serum from an animal partially immunized against the same microorganism. SEE: *vaccine.*

serochrome (sē'rō-krōm) [" + G. *chrōma,* color]. The pigment of normal serum.

serocolitis (sē"rō-kō-lī'tĭs) [" + G. *kōlon,* colon, + *-itis,* inflammation]. Inflammation of serous coat of the colon. SYN: *pericolitis.*

seroculture (sē'rō-kŭl-chūr) [" + *cultura,* cultivation]. A bacterial culture on blood serum.

serocystic (sē"rō-sĭs'tĭk) [" + G. *kystis,* a cyst]. Composed of cysts containing serous fluid.

serodermatosis (sē"rō-der-mă-tō'sĭs) [" + G. *derma,* skin, + *-ōsis,* condition]. Skin disease with serous effusion into tissues of the epidermis.

serodiagnosis (sē"rō-dī-ăg-nō'sĭs) [L. *serum,* whey, + G. *dia,* through, + *gnōsis,* knowledge]. Diagnosis by observing the reactions of blood serum.

seroenteritis (sē"rō-ĕn-ter-ī'tĭs) [" + G. *enteron,* intestine, + *-itis,* inflammation]. Inflammation of serous covering of the intestine.

serofibrinous (sē"rō-fīb'rĭn-ŭs) [" + *fibra,* fiber]. 1. Composed of both serum and fibrin. 2. Denoting a serofibrinous exudate.

serohepatitis (sē"rō - hĕp - ă - tī'tĭs) [L. *serum,* whey, + G. *hēpar, hepat-,* liver, + *-itis,* inflammation]. Inflammation of the peritoneal covering of the liver.

serolipase (sē"rō-lĭp'ās) [L. *serum,* whey, + G. *lipos,* fat, + *ase,* enzyme]. Lipase found in blood serum.

serologic, serological (sē-rō-lŏj'ĭk, -ăl) [" + G. *logos,* a study]. Pert. to or the study of sera.

serologist (sē-rŏl'ō-jĭst) [" + G. *logos,* a study]. One versed in serology.

serology (sē-rŏl'ō-jĭ) [L. *serum,* whey, + G. *logos,* a study]. The science of serum reactions, diagnosis and treatment.

It treats of the relation of antibodies and antigens, an antigen being a substance which, inoculated into the body, is capable of causing the creation of antibodies.

serolysin (sē-rŏl'ĭs-ĭn) [" + G. *lysis,* dissolution]. A bactericidal substance or lysin found in the blood serum.

seromembranous (sē"rō-mĕm'brăn-ŭs) [" + *membrana,* membrane]. Both serous and membranous; relating to a serous membrane.

seromucous (sē"rō-mū'kŭs) [L. *serum,* whey, + *mucus,* mucus]. Pert. to or composed of both serum and mucus.

seronegative. Producing a negative reaction to serological tests.

seroperitoneum (sē"rō-pĕr-ĭ-tō-nē'ŭm) [" + G. *peritonaion,* peritoneum]. Fluid in the peritoneum. SYN: *ascites, hydroperitoneum.*

seropositive. Producing a positive reaction to serological tests.

seroprognosis (sē"rō-prŏg-nō'sĭs). [L. *serum,* whey, + G. *prō,* before, + *gnōsis,* knowledge]. Prognosis of disease determined by seroreactions.

seroprophylaxis (sē"rō-prō-fī-lăks'ĭs) [" + G. *prō,* before, + *phylaxis,* protection]. Prevention of a disease by injection of serum. SYN: *seroprevention.*

seropurulent (sē"rō-pū-rū-lĕnt) [L. *serum,* whey, + *purulentus,* full of pus]. Composed of serum and pus, as an exudate.

seroreaction (sē"rō-rē-ăk'shŭn) [L. *serum,* whey, + *re,* back, + *actio,* action]. SYN: *serum sickness.* 1. Any reaction taking place in or involving serum. SEE: *deviation of complement, fixation of complement.* 2. Reaction to an injection of serum marked by rash, fever, pain, etc.

seroresistance. Failure of a serum reaction to become negative or be reduced in titer following treatment.

serosa (sē-rō'să) [L. from *serum,* whey]. SYN: *tunica serosa.* A serous membrane, *q.v.* Examples are peritoneum, pleura, and pericardium.

serosamucin (sē-rō"să-mū'sĭn) [L. *serosus,* serous, + *mucus,* mucus]. Mucoid in serous fluids.

serosanguineous (sē"rō-săn-gwĭn'ē-ŭs) [L. *serum,* whey, + *sanguineus,* bloody]. Containing or of the nature of serum and blood.

seroscopy (sē-rŏs'kō-pĭ) [" + G. *skopein,* to examine]. Examination of serum for diagnostic purposes.

seroserous (sē"rō-sē'rŭs) [L. *serosus,* serous, + *serum,* whey]. Pert. to 2 serous surfaces.

serositis (sē"rō-sī'tĭs) [" + G. *-itis,* inflammation]. Inflamed condition of a serous membrane.

serosity (sē-rŏs'ĭ-tĭ) [Fr. *sérosité,* from L. *serum,* whey]. The quality of being serous.

serosynovitis (sē"rō-sĭn-ō-vī'tĭs) [L. *serum,* whey, + G. *syn,* with, + *ōon,* egg, + *-itis,* inflammation]. Synovitis with increase of synovial fluid.

serotherapy (sē"rō-thĕr'ă-pĭ) [L. *serum,* whey, + G. *therapeia,* treatment]. The injection of blood serum, either human or animal, containing antibodies as a therapeutic measure in the treatment of disease.

Concerned with producing artificial immunity in a person by injecting the blood serum of an animal which has acquired active immunity* to the disease in question. The degree of protection is not great, usually being limited to days or weeks.

serotonin (sĕr"ō-tōn'ĭn). 5-Hydroxytryptamine, a vasoconstrictor. Substance that can be extracted from blood.

serotype. Serological type.

serous (sē'rŭs) [L. *serum,* whey]. 1. Having the nature of serum. 2. Producing a serous secretion, or containing serum or a serumlike substance.

s. cavity. A cavity lined by a serous membrane, specifically the pleural, peritoneal, and pericardial cavities.

s. cell. A cell which secretes a thin, watery, albuminous secretion.

s. effusion. One of serum.

s. exudate. One consisting mostly of serum.

s. fluids. Liquids of the body, similar to blood serum, which are in part secreted by serous membranes.

s. gland. A gland secreting a watery, albuminous fluid. Ex: parotid gland.

s. inflammation. One with a serous exudate or inflammation of a serous membrane.

s. membrane. A membrane lining a serous cavity.

RS: *membrane, serous.*

serovaccination. Combined serum for immediate passive immunization and for vaccination to produce active immunity.

serozymogenic (sē″rō-zī-mō-jĕn′ik) Pert. to a serous fluid and enzymes.

s. cell. A cell which produces a serous secretion containing an enzyme.

serpiginous (ser-pĭj′ĭn-ŭs) [L. *serpere,* to creep]. Creeping from one part to another.

s. ulcer. One extending in one direction, while healing in another direction.

serpigo (ser-pī′gō) [L. *serpere,* to creep]. A creeping eruption, esp. ringworm. Syn: *herpes, ringworm.*

serrate (sĕr′rāt) [L. *serratus,* toothed]. Notched; toothed. Syn: *dentate.*

serration (ser-ā′shŭn) [L. *serratio,* a notching]. 1. Formation with sharp projections like the teeth of a saw. 2. Notch resembling one bet. teeth of a saw.

serratus muscle (sĕr-ā′tŭs) [L. *serratus,* toothed]. Any of several muscles arising from the ribs or vertebrae by separate slips. See: *Table of Muscles in Appendix.*

serrefine (sār-fēn′) [Fr.]. A small, spring wire forceps for compressing bleeding vessels.

serrenoeud (sār-nōōd) [Fr. *serrer,* to squeeze, + *noeud,* knot]. Device for tightening ligatures especially those placed in deep cavities.

Sertoli's cells (sĕr-tō′lē). Supporting, elongated cells of seminiferous tubules which nourish spermatids.

serum (sē′rum) (pl. *serums, sera*) [L. *serum,* whey]. 1. Any serous fluid, esp. the fluid which moistens the surfaces of serous membranes. 2. The watery portion of the blood after coagulation; a fluid found when clotted blood is left standing long enough for the clot to shrink. 3. Serum from an animal rendered immune against a pathogenic organism, to be injected into a patient with the disease resulting from the same organism. It consists of plasma minus fibrogen.

s. albumin. A protein found in blood serum. For properties, see *proteins;* for amount, see *blood.*

s., anticrotalus. S. to overcome the effect of rattlesnake poison.

s., antidiphtheritic. One used to overcome the effects of diphtheria.

s., antimeningococcus. S. antagonistic to meningococcus infection.

s., antipneumococcus. S. for pneumococcus infection.

s., antitetanic. S. given to overcome tetanus toxin.

s., antitoxic. One containing the antitoxin of the microorganism against which it is supposed to be protective.

s., antityphoid. S. containing antibodies of the typhoid bacillus.

s., bactericidal. One having no effect on toxins but which destroys bacteria.

s., bacteriolytic. A serum containing a lysin that destroys certain bacteria.

s., blood. The liquid clear portion of blood without its fibrin and corpuscles.

s., convalescent. Blood serum from one convalescent from an infection to be used on others having the same disease.

s., foreign. Serum from one animal injected into another animal of another species, or into man.

s. globulin. A protein found in blood serum. See: *globulin, serum.*

s., immune. A serum containing antibodies for specific antigens.

s., polyvalent. Serum containing antibodies to several types of the same bacterial species.

s., pooled. Blood s. from several persons, which has been mixed.

s., pregnancy. Blood serum from pregnant women given to premature infants in food.

s., pregnant mare's. Abbr. PMS. A source of hormones, esp. chorionic gonadotrophin.

s. protein. Any protein in blood serum.

Serum p. forms weak acids mixed with alkali salts and this increases the buffer effects of the blood but to a lesser extent than cell protein.

s. rash. One first seen at site of an injection of serum.

It remains thickest there but it may invade other parts of the body. It resembles a combination of *urticarial, morbilliform* and *scarlatiniform rashes.*

Sym: Severe irritation; marked swelling of skin, esp. of the face; malaise, and constitutional symptoms.

s. sickness. An eruption of purpuric spots, with pain in limbs and joints, following administration of serum, esp. horse serum.

Sym: Symptoms appear 5 to 12 days after the injection. Slight fever, skin eruptions, swelling and pain in joints may develop. Hay fever and asthma victims are hypersensitive to serum injections. Adrenalin is used to combat such reactions. Antihistamines are of benefit. In severe cases, adrenal cortical steroids are quite effective. Syn: *serum reaction.*

s. test. Uhlenhuth's test, *q.v.*

serum, words pert. to: agglutinin, agglutinogen, aggressin, antigen, antitropin, antivenin, autoserodiagnosis, autoserotherapy, autoserous, autoserum, chromodiagnosis, complement, icteric index, isohemagglutinin, "lymph-" words, opsonic index, opsonin, orrhorrhea, serology, serous.

serum-fast. Resistant to the action of serum.

serumal (sē-rū′măl) [L. *serum,* whey]. Relating to serum.

s. calculus. One formed about the teeth from serous exudate.

sesamoid (ses′am-oyd) [G. *sēsamon,* sesame, + *eidos,* form]. Resembling in size or shape a grain of sesame.

s. bone. An oval nodule of bone or fibrocartilage in a tendon playing over a bony surface.

The patella is the largest one.

s. cartilage. Syn: *accessory nasal cartilages.* One or more small cartilage plates present in fibrous tissue between lateral nasal and greater alar cartilages of the nose.

sesqui- [L.]. Prefix meaning *one and a half.*

sesquihora (sĕs-kwĭ-hō′ră). Every hour and a half.

sessile (sĕs′ĭl) [L. *sessilis,* low]. Having no peduncle but attached directly by a broad base.

set. 1. To fix firmly in place, as to set a bone in reduction of a fracture. 2. To allow an amalgam or plaster to harden.

setaceous (sē-tā'shŭs) [L. *setaceus,* bristly]. Resembling a bristle; bristly, hairy.

seton (sē'tŏn) [L. *seto, seton-,* a thread]. A thread or threads drawn through a fold of skin to act as a counterirritant, or a fistulous tract so produced.

setose (sē'tōs) [L. *seta,* bristle]. Having bristlelike appendages.

Setschenow's inhibitory centers (sĕtsh'ĕn-ŏf). Centers in the spinal cord and oblongata for inhibiting reflex movement.

seven basic foods. 1. Leafy green and yellow vegetables. 2. Citrus fruit, tomatoes, raw cabbage. 3. Potatoes and other vegetables and fruits. 4. Milk, or milk products. 5. Meat, poultry, fish, eggs. 6. Bread, flour, cereals, wholegrain, enriched or restored. 7. Butter and fortified margarine.

seven year itch. Scabies, *q.v.*

sev'enth cra'nial nerve. Facial nerve; *nervus facialis.*

sevum (sē'vŭm) [L. suet]. Tallow or suet.

sewer gas. Foul air of a sewer. SEE: *carbon monoxide gas.*

sex (sĕks) [L. *sexus,* sex]. 1. The distinctive quality which differentiates bet. male and female. 2. Males or females, collectively.

s. chromosomes. Chromosomes in a cell determining sex.

s., nuclear. The genetic sex of an individual determined by the absence or presence of sex chromatin in the body cells, particularly blood cells.

sexdigital (sĕks-dĭj'ĭ-tăl) [L. *sex,* six, + *digitus,* digit]. Having 6 fingers or toes.

sexivalent (sĕks-ĭ-vā'lĕnt, -ĭv'ăl-ĕnt) [" + *valēre,* to be strong]. Capable of combining with 6 atoms of hydrogen.

sex-limited. Expression of a genetic character or trait in one sex only.

sex-linked. A character which is controlled by genes in the sex chromosomes.

sexology. Scientific study of sexuality.

sextan (sĕks'tăn) [L. *sextanus,* of the sixth]. Occurring every 6th day.

sextigravida (sĕks-tĭ-grăv'ĭd-ă) [L. *sextus,* six, + *gravida,* a pregnant woman]. A woman pregnant for the 6th time.

sextipara (sĕks-tĭp'ă-ră) [" + *parēre,* to bear a child]. A woman who has borne 6 children at different pregnancies.

sextuplet (sĕks'tū-plĕt) [L. *sextus,* six]. One of 6 children born of a single gestation.

sexual (sĕks'ū-ăl) [L. *sexualis,* pert. to sex]. 1. Pert. to sex. 2. Having sex.

s. bondage. An abnormal phenomenon (not perverse) of dependence of one person upon another of the opposite sex, one dominating the other.

s. intercourse. Sexual congress bet. a male and a female. SYN: *coition, coitus, concubitus, copulation.*

RS: *clitoris, coitus interruptus, dyspareunia, ejaculation, emission, excitation, penis, semen, telegony, vagina.*

s. inversion. A perversion in which an abnormal affection for one of the same sex is experienced.

s. involution. The menopause.

s. metamorphosis. A perversion in which one adopts the habits and dress of the opposite sex.

s. psychopathy. A term for the group in which exist perversions of sex, such as *bestiality,* coprolagnism,* exhibitionism,* fetishism,* frottage,* homosexualism,* lesbianism,* masochism,* masturbation,* onanism,* pedophilia,* renifleurs,* sadism,* sodomy,* transvestism,* voyeur.**

s. reflex. Erection and ejaculation resulting from genital stimulation or indirectly from emotion whether asleep or awake.

sexuality (sĕks-ū-ăl'ĭ-tĭ) [L. *sexus,* sex]. 1. State of having sex; the collective characteristics which mark the differences between the male and the female. 2. Constitution and life of individual as related to sex; all the dispositions related to the love life whether associated with the sex organs or not.

shad (shăd) [A.S. *sceadd*]. A herringlike fish having a comparatively deep body. It is valuable as a food fish. COMP: E. P. Pro. 18.8%, Fat 9.5%. FUEL VALUE: 100 gm. equal 164 Cal.

shad'ow. SYN: *phantom cell, ghost cell.* A hemolyzed erythrocyte.

shadowgram, shadowgraph (shăd'ō-grăm, -grăf) [M.E. *shadowe,* darkness, + G. *graphein,* to write]. A print on a photographic plate exposed to x-rays. SYN: *skiagraph.*

shaft. 1. The principal portion of any cylindrical body. 2. The diaphysis of a long bone.

s. hair. The keratinized portion of a hair which extends from a hair follicle beyond the surface of the epidermis.

shakes (shāks) [A.S. *scacan,* to shake]. 1. Shivering caused by a chill, esp. in an intermittent fever. 2. SYN: *jitters.* State of tremulousness and extreme irritability often seen in chronic alcoholics.

shaking (shāk'ĭng) [A.S. *scacan,* to shake]. A passive movement in Swedish massage.

s. palsy. A basal ganglion disease with progressive rigid tremulousness, peculiar gait, muscular contraction and weakness. SYN: *paralysis agitans; Parkinson's disease.*

shaman (sham'in) [Persian, idolator]. One who heals or attempts to heal by the use of magic.

shank (shăngk) [A.S. *sceanca*]. The tibia or leg from knee to ankle. SYN: *shin.*

shape (shāp) [A.S. *sceapan,* to shape]. 1. To mold to a particular form. 2. Outward form; contour.

RS: *aliform, arcate, arciform, arcuation, arenoid, asbestiform, asteroid, bacciform, belemnoid, bilateralism, bosselated, bosselation, bulbiform, calculus, capreolary, capreolate, carinate, caudate, circle, circumvallate.*

sharkskin. Condition seen in pellagra (nicotinic acid deficiency) in which openings of sebaceous glands become plugged with a dry yellowish material.

Sharpey's intercrossing fibers (shar'pē). Fibers forming the lamellae constituting the walls of the haversian canals in bone.

S. perforating fibers. 1. Fibers extending from the periosteum into the lamellae of bone. 2. F. extending from peridontal membrane into cementum of a tooth.

sheath (shēth) [A.S. *scēath*]. A covering structure of connective tissue, usually of an elongated part, such as the membrane covering a muscle, etc.

s., arachnoid or ***arachnoidean.*** Delicate partition bet. pial sheath and dural one of the optic nerve.

s., axon. The myelin sheath and (or) neurilemma.

s., carotid. Portion of cervical or pretracheal fascia enclosing carotid artery, int. jugular vein, and vagus nerve.

s., crural. The femoral sheath.

s., dentinal. One lining the dental canals.

s., dural. A fibrous membrane or ext. investment of the optic nerve.

s., femoral. The fascial covering of femoral vessels.

s. of Henle. The endoneurium, a delicate sheath enveloping nerve fibers within a fasciculus.

s. of Key and Retzius. The endoneurium, *q.v.*

s., lamellar. Connective tissue sheath covering bundle of nerve fibers. SYN: *perineurium.*

s., medullary. Myelin s. surrounding the axis cylinder.

s., myelin. A fatty, semifluid covering of a nerve fiber which serves to insulate the fiber and to speed the rate of impulses. It is interrupted at intervals by constrictions, the nodes of Ranvier. SEE: *neuron, nerve fiber.*

s., nerve. SEE: *s., lamellar.*

s. of Neumann. A layer of dentine which lies adjacent to a dentinal tubule.

s., pial. Extension of the pia, closely investing surface of the optic nerve.

s., root. The layers of a hair follicle derived from the epidermis, includes the *outer root sheath* which is a continuation of the stratum germinativum and the *inner root sheath* which consists of three layers of cells closely investing the root of the hair. SEE: *hair.*

s. of Schwann. Membranous covering of myelin sheath of a nerve fiber. SYN: *neurilemma.*

s. of Schweigger-Seidel. The thickened wall of a sheathed artery of the spleen.

s., synovial. A double-walled tubelike bursa which encloses a tendon. Consists of an inner *visceral* layer lying to and adhering to a tendon and an outer *parietal* layer the two being separated by a space filled with synovial fluid. Found especially in the hands and feet where tendons are confined to osteofibrous canals or pass over bony surfaces.

s., tendon. A dense fibrous sheath which confines a tendon to an osseous groove converting it into an osteofibrous canal.

Found principally in the wrist and ankle. SEE: *synovial sheath.*

shedd'ing. 1. The loss of deciduous teeth. 2. Casting off of surface layer of the epidermis.

sheet (shēt) [A.S. *sciete,* piece of cloth]. Linen or cotton bedcovering next to the sleeper.

s., draw. One folded under patient so it may be withdrawn without lifting the patient.

shell shock. PSY: A form of psychoneurosis which was formerly believed to result from the explosion of shells during war; however, it is now believed to be caused by the physical and emotional stress experienced during war or general military duty. SYN: *war neurosis.*

shield (shēld) [A.S. *scild,* shield]. 1. Any protecting device. 2. BIOL: A protective plate.

s. bone. The scapula.

s., Buller's. A watch glass to be worn over the eye to protect it from gonorrheal or ophthalmic infection.

s., embryonic. SYN: *embryonic disk, q.v.* The two-layered blastoderm or blastodisk from which a mammalian embryo develops.

s., nipple. A protective covering to protect sore nipples.

s., phallic. An antiseptic covering for the male genitals during operations.

shift. A change in position or direction.

s., chloride. The shift of chloride ions (Cl^-) from the plasma into red blood cells upon the addition of carbon dioxide from the tissues and the reverse movement when carbon dioxide is released in the lungs. It is a mechanism for maintaining constant *p*H of the blood.

s. to the left. An increase in the number of young polymorphonuclear leukocytes in the blood.

s. to the right. An increase in the number of older polymorphonuclear leukocytes in the blood.

Shiga's bacillus (shē'gă). SYN: *Shigella dysenteriae.* The bacillus causing a form of dysentery.

Shigella (shĭ-gel'lă). A genus of nonlactose fermenting, nonmotile, gram-negative rods belonging to the family *Enterobacteriaceae.* It contains a number of species which cause digestive disturbance ranging from mild diarrhea to a severe and often fatal dysentery.

S. dysenteriae. The Shiga bacillus, a virulent form isolated during a severe epidemic of dysentery in Japan in 1896.

shin (shĭn) [A.S. *scinu,* shin]. Anterior edge of tibia. Also, leg bet. the ankle and knee. SYN: *shank.*

s., saber. Condition seen in congenital syphilis in which anterior edge of tibia is extremely sharp.

shingles (shĭng'lz) [L. *cingulus,* a girdle]. Eruption of acute, inflammatory, herpetic vesicles on the trunk of the body along a peripheral nerve; occasionally elsewhere. SYN: *herpes zoster, q.v.*

ship fever. A fever due to unhygienic conditions aboard ship, usually typhus fever or yellow fever occasionally.

shiver (shĭv'ĕr) [M.E. *chiveren*]. 1. A slight tremor of the skin, as from cold, or from fear. 2. To tremble or shake, as from fear or cold.

shock (shŏk) [M.E. *schokke*]. A state of collapse resulting from acute peripheral circulatory failure. It may occur following hemorrhage, severe trauma, surgery, burns, dehydration, infections, or drug toxicity.

It may be immediate or delayed, slight or severe, even fatal. May also result from an injury, bleeding, pain, fear, fright, anesthesia, or many other causes.

Every injury is accompanied by some degree of shock and so should be treated promptly. Syncope is caused by insufficient blood supply to the brain in certain persons and resembles shock in symptoms and treatment.

RS: *anaphylactic, catalepsy, cataleptic, insulin.*

SYM: The most outstanding symptoms are: (a) Marked paleness of the skin; (b) a bluish or grayish discoloration (cyanosis of the lips, nails, tips of the fingers and lobes of the ears; (c) the face is pinched and without expression; (d) there may be a staring of the eyes which often lose their characteristic luster; and (e) the pupils may be dilated; (f) the pulse is weak and rapid; (g) the breathing is increased in rate and it is shallow; and (h) the blood pressure is decreased and may be unobtainable; (i) there may be urinary retention and incontinence of feces; (j) occasionally there is an unusual restlessness or excitement, and (k) very often the patient expresses an extreme thirst. If conscious the patient seems quite disinterested in the surroundings and complains little of pain even though he may be groaning.

TREATMENT: Keep patient lying down with head lower than body. The lower extremities can be slightly elevated by placing the lower half of the body on pillows, or by elevating the foot of the bed.

Patient should be kept comfortably warm, but application of external heat is not advisable. Avoid disturbing by any noise, questions, or transportation. Do not move patient unnecessarily.

Even though thirst is present, give fluids by mouth sparingly in order to reduce the possibility of vomiting and aspirating vomitus. If bleeding is present it should be controlled. If internal hemorrhage is suspected, or presence of head injuries, no stimulants are permissible.

A physician should be called promptly. The use of hypodermics and intramuscular and intravenous injections, such as epinephrine, ephedrine, caffeine, strychnine, etc., or hot enemata, may be recommended by the doctor.

Oxygen may be necessary. Blood transfusion or even artificial respiration may be required, depending on the seriousness of the condition.

Relieve pain by splints, posture, supporting bandages and drugs. Morphine is valuable. Maintain circulation by posture, have patient flat. Lower head and shoulders, elevate all extremities. Blood transfusions may be lifesaving. If blood is not available, plasma or blood substitutes may be used.

Respiration may be aided by administration of oxygen preferably mixed with 4 to 10% carbon dioxide as a respiratory stimulant. Constant, kindly, tactful encouragement and extreme gentleness in all procedures are of importance.

F. A. TREATMENT: Depends on accuracy of diagnosis. In general, treat specific etiologic factor, maintain body heat by hot blankets, water bottles, etc. If permissible, a hot bath, hot enemas and hot drinks, and massage (do not expose patient unduly). Stimulants used generously except in presence of suspected bleeding or head injury. Strong and moderately hot black coffee or tea by mouth and/or by rectum are esp. recommended.

s., anaphylactic. Reaction from injection of protein substance to which patient is sensitized.

s., anesthesia. This is not surgical shock, but is due to an overdosage of anesthetic and calls for the immediate cessation of anesthesia.

Artificial respiration and appropriate stimulants should be given at once. The condition is manifested by a weak, rapid pulse; a fall or drop in blood pressure; by cold, clammy skin, and by shallow respirations.

s. (from) burns. SEE: *Burn, treatment.*

s., colloid. One causing symptoms of anaphylaxis when colloids are injected.

s., deferred or delayed. Late manifestation following injury or burns.

May appear in 3 to 30 hours and may be due to transportation, emotional stress, hemorrhage, dehydration, acidosis, or toxemia.

s., electric. The result of passage of electric current. SEE: *electric shock.*

s., epigastric. Result of a blow or other trauma (surgery) in upper abdomen.

s., hypoglycemic. SEE: *insulin shock.*

s., insulin. Condition resulting from overdosages of insulin.

F. A. TREATMENT: Give orange juice, glucose, candy, lump of sugar, etc. If unconscious, inject glucose intravenously. SEE: *insulin.*

s., mental. SEE: *s., psychic.* Due to emotional stress or seeing injury, accidents, etc.

s., peptone or ***protein.*** Reaction resulting from parenteral administration of a protein.

s., psychic. S. due to excessive fear, joy, anger, grief.

s., secondary. Same as *deferred shock.*

s., sense. A mild nightmare.

s., serum. One occurring as part of reaction to injection of serum.

s., shell. SEE: *shell shock.*

s., surgical. Following operations and including traumatic shock, *q.v.*

s. therapy. Form of treatment in mental illness. Three types are widely used: 1. *Electric shock therapy,* in which convulsions are induced by passage of electricity through the brain; used chiefly in manic depressive psychoses, anxiety states, depression, involutional melancholia, and certain types of schizophrenia. 2. *Insulin shock therapy,* in which hypoglycemia and coma are induced by injection of insulin; used chiefly in schizophrenia. 3. *Metrazol shock therapy,* in which convulsions are induced by injection of metrazol; used chiefly in schizophrenia.

s., traumatic (broad interpretation). Shock due to injury or surgery.

May occur as result of *abdominal injury* from any cause. Shock is proportional to extent of injury. Esp. severe in upper abdomen and more marked when viscera are damaged.

If prolonged, indicates hemorrhage or peritonitis or both.

Cerebral injury: Concussion of brain or skull fracture. May come on immediately or later from edema or intracranial hemorrhage.

Chemical injury: Esp. corrosives, due to pain and effect of chemical and absorption of altered tissue.

Crushing injuries: The nearer the visceral area, the greater the shock.

Fracture: Esp. in compound fracture. Often extensive blood loss into tissues and hence body is not able to maintain circulation.

Heart damage: As in angina pectoris, coronary occlusion, or acute dilatation.

Inflammation: As acute general peritonitis or fulminating sepsis anywhere in the body.

Intestinal obstruction: Shock is present when obstruction is acute.

Nerve injury: Contusion of highly sensitive parts, as testicle, solar plexus, eye, urethra, etc.

Operations: May occur even after minor operations, as paracentesis, catheterization, etc.

Perforation or rupture of viscera, as: Acute pneumothorax, ruptured aneurysm, perforated peptic ulcer, perforation in appendicitis, ectopic pregnancy.

Strangulation: As in hernia, intussusception, volvulus.

Thermal injury: As burns, frostbite, heat exhaustion.

Torsion of viscera: As of an ovary, testicle.

s., wound. Same as *traumatic shock.*

shoe'makers' cramp or **spasm.** Spasm of muscles of hand and arm occurring in shoemakers.

shortsightedness (short-sĭt'ĕd-nĕs). A condition of not being able to see very far. Due to light rays coming to a focus in front of the retina. SYN: *myopia, nearsightedness.*

shot'gun prescrip'tion. One containing many drugs given with hope that one of them may prove effective. Not a recommended approach to the treatment of disease.

shoulder (shōl'dĕr) [A.S. *sculdor*]. The junction of the clavicle and scapula where the arm meets the trunk.

RS: *omalgia, omarthritis, omitis, scapula.*

s. blade. The scapula.

s., dislocation of. Displacement of shoulder joint.

Very frequently accompanied by a fracture. It is believed by all surgeons that it is wiser to have an x-ray examination of the affected bones because fractures are so often present and attempts to reduce fractured dislocations without knowing of fractures present are very dangerous, sometimes resulting in serious paralysis of the entire upper extremity, or of grave damage to the large blood vessels in the armpit.

CAUSES: The causes of a dislocation of a shoulder are usually those of falling on an outstretched arm, or a blow to the arm in some unusual position. It is very common among athletes, esp. among football and basketball players. A patient with a dislocated shoulder usually has a deformity with a hollow in place of the normal bulge of the shoulder. There seems to be a slight depression at the outer end of the clavicle, and the patient cannot place his hand at his opposite shoulder and still place his elbow onto his chest. Always compare both sides.

TREATMENT: Send for a doctor as soon as possible. Lay the patient on the back, with a pillow bet. the shoulders (or folded pad). Place a large, soft pad under the elbow on the affected side and then bind the forearm horizontally across the chest, using an open sling which is reinforced by a broad cravat; bandage, and then apply cold applications to the affected shoulder. Treat for shock.

s. girdle. The 2 scapulae and 2 clavicles attaching the bones of the upper extremities to the axial skeleton.

s. joint. Formed by humerus and glenoid cavity of scapula.

show (shō) [A.S. *scēawian*, to look]. The sanguinoserous discharge from the vagina during the first stage of labor or just preceding menstruation.

Shrapnell's membrane (shrăp'nĕl). SYN: *pars flaccida.* A small triangular portion of the tympanic membrane lying above the malleolar folds. It is thin and lax and attached directly to the petrous bone at the tympanic notch (notch of Rivinus).

shred'ded wheat. Av. SERVING: 100 gm. Calories: 354. Protein: 9.9 gm.; carbohydrate: 79.9 gm.; fat: 2.0 gm.; iron: 3.5 mg.; sodium: 3.0 mg.; calcium: 43 mg.

shreds. Slender strands of mucus seen in urine indicative of inflammation of urinary tract or associated organs.

shrimp (shrĭmp) [M.E. *shrimppe*]. Any of numerous, small, long-tailed crustaceans, many varieties of which are used for food. SERVING: 100 gm. (raw). Calories: 91. Protein: 18.1 gm.; carbohydrate: 1.5 gm; fat: 0.8 gm.; calcium: 63 mg.; sodium: 140 mg.

shud'der. A temporary convulsive tremor resulting from fright, horror, or aversion.

shunt (shŭnt) [M.E. *shunten*, to avoid]. 1. To turn away from; to divert. 2. Anomalous passage or one artificially constructed to divert flow from one main route to another. 3. Electric conductor connecting two points in a circuit to form a parallel circuit through which a portion of the current may pass.

Si. Symb. for *silicon.*

siagonantritis (sī"ăg-ō̆n-ăn-trī'tĭs) [G. *siagōn*, jawbone, + *antron*, cavity, + *-itis*, inflammation]. Inflammation within the antrum of Highmore.

sialaden (sī-ăl'ăd-ĕn) [G. *sialon*, saliva, + *adēn*, gland]. A salivary gland.

sialadenitis (sī-ăl-ăd-ĕn-ī'tĭs) [" + " + *-itis*, inflammation]. Inflamed condition of a salivary gland.

sialadenoncus (sī-ăl-ăd-ĕn-ŏng'kŭs) [" + " + *ogkos*, tumor]. Tumor of salivary gland.

sialagogue (sī-ăl'ă-gŏg) [" + *agōgos*, leading]. Agent increasing flow of saliva. Also spelled sialogogue.

sialaporia (sī"al-ap-ō'rĭ-ă) [" + *aporia*, lack]. Deficiency in secretion of saliva.

sialemesis (sī"ăl-ĕm'ĕs-ĭs) [" + *emesis*, vomiting]. Vomiting of saliva or vomiting caused by an excessive secretion of it.

sialine (sī'ăl-ĭn) [G. *sialon*, saliva]. Concerning the saliva.

sialism, sialismus (sī'ăl-ĭzm, sī-ăl-ĭz'mŭs) [" + *-ismos*, condition]. An excessive secretion of saliva. SYN: *ptyalism, salivation.*

sialoadenitis (sī"ăl-ō-ăd-ĕn-ī'tĭs) [" + *adēn*, gland, + *-itis*, inflammation]. Inflammation of a salivary gland. SYN: *sialadenitis.*

sialoaerophagy (sī"ăl-ō-ā-ĕr-ŏf'ă-jĭ) [" + *aēr*, air, + *phagein*, to eat]. Constant swallowing, thus taking saliva and air into the stomach.

sialoangitis (sī"ăl-ō-ăn-jī'tĭs) [" + *aggeion*, vessel, + *-itis*, inflammation]. Inflamed condition of the salivary ducts.

sialocele (sī'ă-lo-sēl). Cyst or tumor of a salivary gland.

sialodochitis (sī"ăl-ō-dō-kī'tĭs) [" + *dochē*, receptacle, + *-itis*, inflammation]. Inflamed condition of salivary ducts.

s. fibrinosa. S. with duct obstructed by a fibrinous exudate.

sialoductitis (sī"ăl-ō-dŭk-tī'tĭs) [" + L. *ductus*, duct, + G. *-itis*, inflammation]. Inflamed condition of Stensen's duct.

sialogenous (si-al-oj'en-us) [G. *sialon*, saliva, + *gennan*, to produce]. Forming saliva.

sialogogic (sī-ăl-ō-gŏj'ĭk). Producing or promoting a secretion of saliva.

sialogogue (si-al'o-gog) [G. *sialon*, saliva, + *agōgos*, leading]. 1. An agent that stimulates the secretion of saliva. 2. Producing or promoting the secretion of saliva.

sialography (sī-ăl-ŏg'ră-fĭ) [" + *graphein*, to write]. Examination of salivary ducts and glands with x-rays. SYN: *ptyalography.*

sialolith (sī-ăl'ō-lĭth) [" + *lithos*, a stone]. A salivary concretion or calculus.

sialolithiasis (sī-ăl-ō-lĭth-ī'ăs-ĭs) [" + " + *-iasis*, condition]. Presence of salivary calculi.

sialolithotomy (sĭ″ăl-ō-lĭth-ŏt′ō-mĭ) [" + " + *tomē*, a cutting]. Removal of a calculus from a salivary gland or duct.

sialoncus (sī-ăl-ŏng′kŭs) [" + *ogkos*, tumor]. A tumor under the tongue caused by obstruction of a salivary gland or duct.

sialoporia (sī″ăl-ō-pō′rĭ-ă) [G. *sialon*, saliva, + *aporia*, lack]. Deficient secretion of saliva.

sialorrhea (sī-ăl-or-ē′ă) [" + *rhoia*, a flow.] Excessive flow of saliva. Syn: *sialism*.

sialoschesis (sī-ăl-ŏs′kĕs-ĭs) [" + *schesis*, suppression]. Suppression or retention of saliva.

sialosemeiology (sī″ăl-ō-sē-mī-ŏl′ō-jĭ) [" + *semeion*, sign, + *logos*, a study]. Diagnosis based upon examination of the saliva.

sialosis (sī-ăl-ō′sĭs) [" + *-ōsis*, condition]. The flow of saliva.

sialostenosis (sī″ăl-ō-stĕn-ō′sĭs) [" + *stenōsis*, a narrowing]. Closure of a salivary duct.

sialosyrinx (sī″ăl-ō-sī′rĭnks) [" + *syrigx*, a pipe]. 1. Fistula into the salivary gland. 2. A syringe for washing out salivary ducts. 3. Drainage tube for a salivary duct.

sialotic (sī-ăl-ŏt′ĭk) [G. *sialon*, saliva]. Concerning the flow of saliva.

sialozemia (sī″ăl-ō-zē′mĭ-ă) [" + *zēmia*, loss]. Involuntary loss of saliva. Syn: *salivation*.

Siamese twins (sī-ă-mēz′). Congenitally united twins, usually at the hips or buttocks, the members being capable of activity.

sib. Syn: *sibling*. A brother or sister.

sibilant (sĭb′ĭl-ănt) [L. *sibilans*, hissing]. Hissing or whistling, as a sound heard in a certain râle, *q.v.*

sibila′tion. Pronunciation in which the sound of "s" is predominant.

sibilis′mus. A hissing sound.

s. aurium. Tinnitus, *q.v.*

sibilus (sĭb′ĭl-ŭs) [L. a hissing]. A hissing râle.

sibling (sĭb′lĭng) [A.S. *sibb*, kin, + *-ling*, having the quality of]. One of 2 or more children of same parents.

sibship. Brothers and sisters of a single family considered as a single group.

siccant (sĭk′ănt) [L. *siccus*, dry]. Drying.

siccative (sĭk′ă-tĭv) [L. *siccativus*, drying]. Drying or that which dries. Syn: *siccant*.

sicchasia (sĭ-kā′shĭ-ă). Nausea.

siccus (sĭk′ŭs) [L. dry]. Not moist; dry.

sick (sĭk) [A.S. *seōc*, ill]. 1. Not well. Syn: *ill*. 2. Nauseated or "sick at the stomach." 3. Menstruating.

s. headache. One with nausea, vomiting, anorexia, etc. Syn: *migraine, q.v.*

s. at the stomach. Inclined to vomit. Syn: *nauseated*.

sick′le cell. Abnormal red blood corpuscle of crescent shape.

s. c. anemia. A form of anemia in which are present abnormal sickle or crescent-shaped erythrocytes. Due to the presence of abnormal type of hemoglobin in the red blood cells. See: *anemia*.

sicklemia (sĭk-lē′mĭ-ă) [A.S. *sicol*, sickle, + G. *aima*, blood]. Sickle cells in the blood.

sickling. Tendency of red blood cells to be sickle shaped. See: *sickle cell anemia*.

sick′ness [A.S. *seōc*, ill]. State of being unwell. Syn: *illness*.

s., bleeding. Abnormal tendency to bleed. Syn: *hemophilia*.

s., car. Nausea and malaise from riding in vehicles such as trains or automobiles. Syn: *motion sickness*.

s., falling. Epilepsy.

s., green. Form of anemia with greenish pallor. Syn: *chlorosis*.

s., monthly. Menstruation.

s., morning. Nausea of early pregnancy.

s., mountain. Nausea and dyspnea caused by being on great elevations.

s., sea. S. caused by motion of a vessel while at sea.

s., serum. S. following injection of serum.

s., sleeping. 1. Infection with genus of Trypanosomes with involvement of central nervous system and ultimately continuous sleeping. Syn: *trypanosomiasis*. 2. Acute infectious disease with increasing lethargy. Syn: *lethargic encephalitis*.

side (sīd) [A.S. *sīde*]. 1. Left or right part of wall of trunk of body. 2. An outer portion considered as facing in a particular direction.

s.-chain theory. Theory concerning cell dissolution and immunity; complex molecules react with one another through their side chains when they have definite correspondence in structure. See: *Ehrlich's side-chain theory*.

s. effect. The action or effect, usually of a drug, other than that desired. Commonly this is an undesirable effect such as an allergic reaction to penicillin.

s. position. Lying on one side, thighs flexed, with underarm behind back. Syn: *Sims' position, q.v.*

sideration (sĭd-ĕr-ā′shŭn) [L. *siderārī*, to be struck by a planet]. 1. Therapeutic application of electric sparks. 2. A sudden stroke of disease, as in apoplexy. 3. Lightning stroke.

siderism, siderismus (sĭd′ĕr-ĭzm, -ĭz′mŭs) [G. *sidēros*, iron, + *-ismos*, condition]. Therapeutic application of metals to the skin. Syn: *metallotherapy*.

sidero- (sid′er-o) [G.]. Combining form meaning *iron* or *steel*, as *siderosis*.

siderocyte (sid′er-ō-sīt). A red blood cell containing iron in a form other than hematin.

sideroderma (sĭd″ĕr-ō-der′mă) [G. *sidēros*, iron, + *derma*, skin]. Bronzed coloration of the skin from disordered hemoglobin disintegration.

siderodromophobia (sĭd″ĕr-ō-drō″mō-fō′bĭ-ă) [" + *dromos*, a way, + *phobos*, fear]. Morbid fear of railway travel.

siderofibrosis (sĭd″ĕr-ō-fī-brō′sĭs) [" + L. *fibra*, fiber, + G. *-ōsis*, condition]. Fibrosis associated with deposits of iron.

siderogenous (sĭd-ĕr-ŏj′ĕn-ŭs) [" + *gennan*, to produce]. Producing or forming iron.

sideropenic (sid″er-o-pe′nik). Being deficient of iron in the blood.

siderophilous (sĭd-ĕr-of′ĭl-ŭs) [" + *philein*, to love]. Having a tendency to absorb iron, as the red blood corpuscles.

sideroscope (sĭd′ĕr-ō-skōp) [" + *skopein*, to examine]. Instrument for finding metal particles in the eye.

siderosis (sid″er-ō′sĭs) [G. *sidēros*, iron, + *-ōsis*, condition]. A form of pneumoconiosis resulting from inhalation of dust or fumes containing iron particles. It is benign and constitutes no serious health hazard. Also called *arc-welders disease*.

Sigault's operation (sē-go′). Division of the symphysis pubis to aid delivery. Syn: *symphyseotomy*.

sigh. Syn: *suspirium.* A deep inspiration followed by a slow audible expiration.

sight (sīt) [A.S. *sihth*]. 1. Power or faculty of seeing. Syn: *vision.* 2. Range of sight. 3. A thing or view seen.

s., day. Night blindness. Syn: *nyctalopia.*

s., far-. Rays of light focusing behind the retina. Syn: *hypermetropia.*

s. meter. Device for measuring intensity of light in foot candles.

s., near-. Rays of light focusing before the retina. Syn: *myopia.*

s., night. Day blindness. Syn: *hemeralopia.*

s., old. Loss of accommodation of near point. Syn: *presbyopia.*

s., second. Alteration in refractive powers of the lens of the eye so that reading again is possible without glasses in incipient cataract.

sight, words pert. to: achromatopsia. afterimage, alexia, amaurosis, amblyopia, ametropia, aniseikonia, anisocoria, anisoiconia, anisometropia, anorthopia, aprosexia, asthenopia, astigmatism, blindness, brachymetropia, Burns' amaurosis, hemeralopia, hypermetropia, hyperopia, myopia, nyctalopia, photophobia, presbyopia, squint.

sigmatism (sĭg'mă-tĭzm) [G. *sigma*, letter S, + *-ismos*, condition]. Excessive or defective use of *s* sounds in speech.

sigmoid (sĭg'moyd) [G. *sigma*, letter S, + *eidos*, form]. 1. Shaped like the Greek letter *sigma*, *s*. 2. Pert. to the sigmoid flexure of the colon.

s. flexure. The lower part of descending colon, bet. iliac crest and the rectum, shaped like the letter S.

RS: *cecosigmoidostomy, colon, "sigmoido-" words.*

sigmoidectomy (sĭg-moy-dĕk'tō-mĭ) [" + " + *ektomē*, excision]. Removal of all or part of the sigmoid flexure.

sigmoiditis (sĭg-moy-dī'tĭs) [" + " + *-ītis*, inflammation]. Inflammation of the sigmoid flexure of the colon.

sigmoidopexy (sĭg-moyd'ō-pĕks"ĭ) [" + " + *pēxis*, fixation]. Fixation of the sigmoid to an abdominal incision for prolapse of the rectum.

sigmoidoproctostomy (sĭg-moyd"ō-prŏk-tos'tō-mĭ) [" + " + *prōktos*, rectum, + *stoma*, passage]. Establishment of artificial passage by anastomosis of the sigmoid flexure with the rectum.

sigmoidorectostomy (sĭg-moyd"ō-rĕk-tŏs'-tō-mĭ) [" + " + L. *rectus*, straight, + G. *stoma*, passage]. Anastomosis of sigmoid flexure with the rectum to establish an artificial passage. Syn: *sigmoidoproctostomy.*

sigmoidoscope (sĭg-moy'dō-skōp) [" + " + *skopein*, to examine]. Tubular speculum for examination of sigmoid flexure.

sigmoidostomy (sĭg-moyd-ŏs'tō-mĭ) [G. *sigma*, letter S, + *eidos*, form, + *stoma*, passage]. Creation of an artificial anus in the sigmoid flexure.

sign (sīn) [L. *signum*, mark]. 1. Symbol or abbreviation, esp. one used in pharmacy. 2. Any objective evidence of an abnormal nature in the body or its organs.

They are more or less definitive and obvious, and apart from the patient's impressions. Symptoms* are subjective.

s., objective. One recognized by an observer. Syn: *physical s.*

s., physical. One revealed by auscultation, percussion, inspection, etc.

signa (sĭg'nă) [L. *signa*, mark]. A term used in writing prescriptions,* meaning mark. Usually designated S or sig.

signature (sĭg'nă-tūr) [L. *signatura*]. The part of a prescription giving instructions to the patient.

silent. Free from noise; mute; still.

s. disease. A disease which produces no clinically obvious symptoms or signs.

s. period. Period in a tendon reflex which immediately follows the contraction of the responding muscles during which the motor neurons do not respond to afferent impulses entering the reflex center.

silica (sĭl'ĭ-kă) [L. *silex*, flint]. Silicon dioxide, SiO_2.

silicate (sĭl'ĭ-kāt) [L. *silicus*, flintlike]. A salt of silicic acid.

silicic (sĭl-ĭs'ĭk) [L. *silex*, flint]. Pert. to silica or silicon.

s. acid. One of a number of colloid acids.

silicon (sĭl'ĭ-kon) [L. *silex*, flint]. Symb: Si. A nonmetallic element found in the soil. At. wt. 28.086; at. no. 14. Sp. gr. 2.33.

Silicon comprises approximately 25% of the earth's crust being exceeded only by oxygen. It occurs in traces in skeletal structures (bones and teeth). Its physiological significance is unknown. Silicon is commonly combined with oxygen to form silicon dioxide, SiO_2, which occurs in many forms, both crystalline and amorphous. In a pure state it forms *quartz* or *rock crystal.* It is present in many abrasive materials and is the principal constituent of glass.

silicosis (sĭl-ĭ-kō'sĭs) [L. *silex, silic-*, flint, + G. *-ōsis*, condition]. A form of pneumoconiosis resulting from inhalation of silica (quartz) dust, characterized by formation of small discrete nodules. In advanced cases, a dense fibrosis and emphysema with impairment of respiratory function may develop.

silicotic (sĭl-ĭ-kŏt'ĭk) [L. *silex, silic-*, flint]. 1. Relating to silicosis. 2. One affected with silicosis.

silicotuberculosis (sĭl"ĭ-kō-tū-bĕr-kū-lō'sĭs) [" + *tuberculus*, a tubercle, + G. *-ōsis*, condition]. Silicosis associated with pulmonary tuberculosis.

siliquose (sĭl'ĭ-kwōs) [L. *siliqua*, pod]. Resembling a 2-valve capsule.

s. cataract. Cataract with a dry, wrinkled capsule.

s. desquamation. Shedding of dried vesicles from the skin.

silver (sĭl'ver) [A.S.*siolfor*]. Symb: Ag. At. wt. 107.870; at. no. 47. A white soft ductile malleable metal, its salts being widely used in medicine for their caustic, astringent, and antiseptic effects.

s. arsphenamine. A brownish black arsphenamine derivative, containing 19% arsenic and 14% silver.

Uses: Same as those of arsphenamine.

s. nitrate. USP. A toxic preparation made from silver. Most of its former uses have passed out of vogue, but it remains important as a germicide and local astringent.

Incompatibilities: Aspirin, sodium chloride.

Poisoning: When taken by mouth, causes a grayish discoloration of mucous membranes.

Sym: Burning in throat and stomach; rather prompt vomiting. When small amounts of silver are taken over a long period, as in nose or eye drops, patient develops argyria, a peculiar bluish discoloration of all the exposed tissues of body.

F. A. Treatment: Large volumes of ordinary table salt in water precipitate the silver as a slightly soluble chloride; follow with egg whites, oils, and other demulcents.

s. picrate. A compound of silver and picric acid, containing 30% silver. Useful as an antiseptic, similar to other preparations of silver.

s. protein. USP. A combination of silver and protein, containing from 7 to 19% silver. Two strengths are official, the strong and mild.

sil'ver-fork deformity or **fracture.** Deformity in Colles' fracture of wrist and hand resembling curve on back of a fork.

Silves'ter's method. A method of artificial respiration in which patient lies on back, and arms are raised to sides of head, held there temporarily, then brought down and pressed against chest. Movement repeated 16 times per minute. This method is no longer the preferred or effective method of producing artificial respiration. See: *artificial respiration; resuscitation.*

simesthesia (sĭm-ĕs-thē'zĭ-ă) [G. *aisthēsis*, sensation]. Sensibility felt in a bone.

similia similibus curantur (sĭm-ĭl'ĭ-ă sĭm-ĭl'-ĭ-bŭs kū-rahn'tŭr) [L. likes are cured by likes]. The homeopathic doctrine that a drug producing pathological symptoms in those who are well will cure such symptoms in disease states.

Simmonds' disease or **syndrome** (sĭm'-mond). Condition in which complete atrophy of the pituitary body causes premature senility and psychic symptoms. Syn: *cachexia, pituitary, q.v.*

Simon's position (zē'mōn). An exaggerated lithotomy position in which the hips are somewhat elevated with thighs strongly abducted. Employed in operations on the vagina.

simple (sĭm'pl) [L. *simplex*, simple]. 1. Not complex; not compound. 2. Deficient in intellect. 3. A medicinal plant.

s. fracture. Fracture without rupture of ligaments and skin.

s. inflammation. Inflammation without pus or other inflammatory exudates.

s. reflex. A reflex in which only two or possibly three neurons are interposed between receptor and effector organ.

Sims' position (sĭmz). A semiprone position. For detailed description see: *position, Sims'.*

simul. (sī'mŭl) [L.]. At once or at the same time.

simulation (sĭm-ū-lā'shŭn) [L. *simulātio*, imitation]. Pretense of having a disease; feigning of illness. Imitation of symptoms of one disease by another. See: *malingerer.*

Simulium. A genus of insects of the order *Diptera* which includes the black flies (buffalo gnats) which are important annoyers of domestic animals and man. The females are vicious blood suckers.

S. damnosum. Species which serves as intermediate host of a filarial worm *Onchocerca volvulus.*

S. venustum. A very annoying species common in eastern portions of the U. S.

Sinapis (sĭ-na'pĭs) [G. *sinapi*, mustard]. A genus of plants, the mustard plant.

sinapiscopy (sĭn-ăp-ĭs'kō-pĭ) [" + *skopein*, to examine]. Use of mustard in testing for sensory disturbance.

sinapism (sĭn'ăp-ĭzm) [" + *-ismos*, process]. A mustard plaster.

Used to relieve congestion or pain, headache, neuralgia, flatulence, nausea, etc.

Proportions: *Adult*: 3-4 parts wheat flour to 1 of mustard flour. *Child*: 8-10 parts wheat flour to 1 of mustard flour. *Infant*: 10-12 parts wheat flour to 1 of mustard flour.

sinapized (sĭn'ăp-īzd) [G. *sinapi*, mustard]. Containing mustard.

sincipital (sĭn-sĭp'ĭ-tăl) [L. *sinciput*, half a head]. Concerning the sinciput.

sinciput (sĭn'sĭp-ŭt) [L. *sinciput*, half a head]. 1. Fore and upper part of the cranium. 2. Upper half of the skull. Syn: *calvaria.*

sinew (sĭn'ū) [A.S. *sinu*]. A tendon.

sing. [L.]. Abbr. of *singulorum*, meaning *of each.*

singer's node or **nodule** (sĭn'gerz nōd, nŏd'-ūl). A swelling bet. the arytenoid cartilages of singers. Syn: *chorditis nodosa.*

singultus (sĭng-gŭl'tŭs) [L. *singultus*, hiccup]. Hiccup, *q.v.*

sinistrad (sĭn'ĭs-trăd) [L. *sinister, sinistr-*, left, + *ad*, toward]. Toward the left.

sinistral (sĭn'ĭs-trăl) [L. *sinister, sinistr-*, left]. 1. Pert. to or showing preference for the left hand, eye, or foot in certain actions. 2. On the left side.

sinistrality (sĭn"ĭs-trăl'ĭ-tĭ) [L. *sinister, sinistr-*, left]. Left-handedness.

sinistraural (sĭn-ĭs-traw'răl) [" + *auris*, ear]. Having better hearing with the left ear.

sinistro- (sĭn'ĭs-trō) [L.]. Prefix meaning *left.*

sinistrocardia (sĭn-ĭs-trō-kar'dĭ-ă) [L. *sinister, sinistr-*, left, + G. *kardia*, heart]. Displacement of the heart to left of the medial line; opp. of *dextrocardia.*

sinistrocerebral (sĭn-ĭs-trō-sĕr'ĕ-brăl) [" + *cerebrum*, brain]. Located in the left cerebral hemisphere.

sinistrocular (sĭn-ĭs-trok'ū-lar) [" + *oculus*, eye]. Having stronger vision in the left eye.

sinistrocularity (sĭn-ĭs-trŏk-ū-lăr'ĭ-tĭ) [" + *oculus*, eye]. Condition of having better vision in the left eye.

sinistrogyration (sĭn-ĭs-trō-jī-rā'shŭn) [" + G. *gyros*, a circle]. Inclination to the left.

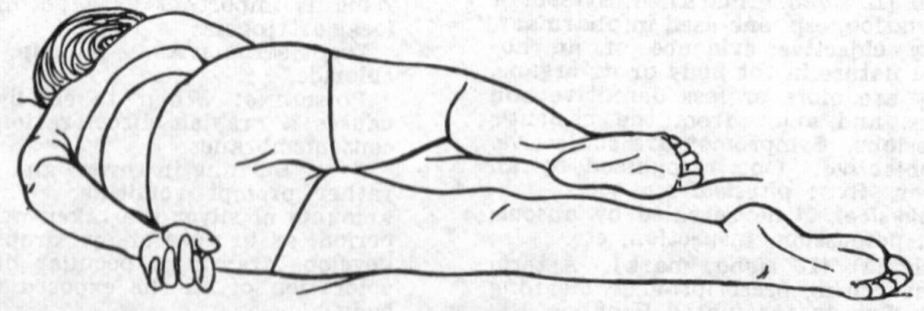

SIMS' POSITION.

sinistromanual (sĭn-ĭs-trō-măn'ū-ăl) [" + *manus*, hand]. Left-handed.

sinistropedal (sĭn-ĭs-trŏp'ĕd-ăl) [" + *pes, ped-*, foot]. Left-footed.

sinistrosis (sĭn-ĭs-trō'sĭs) [L. *sinister, sinistr-*, left, unlucky, + G. *-ōsis*, condition]. Shell shock, *q.v.*

sinistrotorsion (sĭn-ĭs-trō-tor'shŭn) [" + *torsio*, a turning]. A twisting or turning toward the left.

sin'istrous. Awkward, clumsy, unskilled the opposite of dextrous.

sinoatrial (sĭn"ō-ā'trĭ-ăl). Syn: *sinoauricular.* Pertaining to the sinus venosus and the atrium.

s. node. Node at junction of sup. vena cava with right cardiac atrium, regarded as starting point of the heartbeat. Syn: *S-A node.*

sinoauricular. Sinoatrial, *q.v.*

sinuitis (sĭ-nū-ī'tĭs) [L. *sinus*, a curve, + G. *-itis*, inflammation]. Inflammation of a sinus. Syn: *sinusitis.*

sinuotomy (sĭn-ū-ŏt'ō-mĭ) [" + G. *tomē*, a cutting]. Surgical incision into a sinus.

sinuous (sĭn'ū-ŭs) [L. *sinōsus*, winding]. Winding; wavy; tortuous.

sinus (sī'nŭs) (pl. *sinuses, sinūs*) [L. *sinus*, a curve]. 1. A canal or passage leading to an abscess. 2. A cavity within a bone. 3. Dilated channel for venous blood. 4. Any cavity having a relatively narrow opening.

RS: *antritis, antronasal, antrotympanic, antrum, cephalhematocele, lateral sinus, sinusitis, transillumination.*

s's., accessory nasal. The paranasal sinuses; frontal, maxillary, ethmoidal, and sphenoidal. *Anterior group*: Frontal, maxillary and anterior ethmoids. *Posterior group*: Posterior ethmoids and sphenoid.

Sinuses develop embryologically from nasal cavities, are lined with same type of epithelium, are filled with air, and communicate with nasal cavities through their various ostia.

Function of sinuses not definitely known. Various theories give them the same function as nasal cavities, *viz.* (warming, moistening and filtering the air).

s., aortic. Saclike dilatation of the aorta.

s. arrhythmia. Irregularity of heartbeat due to interference with impulses from the sinoatrial node.

s., basilar. See: *transverse s.*

s., cavernous. A large s. from sphenoidal fissure to apex of petrous portion of temporal bone.

s., circular. A venous s. around the pituitary body, communicating on each side with the cavernous s.

s., coronary, of the heart. A vein in transverse groove bet. left cardiac auricle and ventricle.

s's., cranial. Venous canals bet. folds of the dura.

s's., ethmoidal. Air cavities in the ethmoid bone.

s., frontal. An irregular cavity in frontal bone on each side of midline above the nasal bridge. One may be larger than the other. A duct carries secretions to upper part of nostrils.

s., genitourinary. See: *s., urogenital.*

s., inferior longitudinal. A venous s. along post. half of lower border of the falx cerebri.

s., inferior petrosal. A large venous s. from cavernous s., running along lower margin of the petrous portion of the temporal bone.

s's., intercavernous. The ant. and post. halves of the circular s.

s., lateral. One of 2 large venous s's. in inner side of skull passing near the mastoid antrum, emptying into the jugular vein.

s's., lymph. Small spaces throughout the parenchyma of a lymphatic gland.

s., maxillary. A cavity in the maxillary bone opening at upper part of antrum into the nose. Syn: *antrum of Highmore.*

s., occipital. A small venous s. in attached margin of the falx cerebelli extending to margin of the foramen magnum.

s's., paranasal. Accessory nasal sinuses.

s's., pleural. Spaces in pleural sac along the lower and inf. portions of lung which the lung does not occupy.

s. pocularis. Lacuna in prostatic part of the urethra.

s. prostaticus. See: *s. pocularis.*

s., rhomboid. The 4th cranial ventricle.

s. rhythm. Normal cardiac rhythm commencing at the sinoatrial node.

s's., sphenoidal. Air s's. which occupy the body of sphenoid bone and connect with nasal cavity.

s., sphenoparietal. 1. A venous sinus uniting the cavernous sinus and a meningeal vein. 2. The portion of the cavernous sinus below the ensiform process.

s., straight. One which is continuous with the inf. longitudinal s. and running along junction of the falx cerebri and tentorium.

s., superior longitudinal. A triangular one along upper edge of the falx cerebri.

s., superior petrosal. A venous canal running in a groove in the petrous portion of the temporal bone.

s., terminal. A vein encircling the vascular area of the blastoderm.

s., transverse. 1. S. that unites the 2 inf. petrosal sinuses. 2. Venous network in the dura over basilar process of occipital bone.

s., urinogenital or ***urogenital.*** 1. Duct into which, in the embryo, the wolffian ducts and bladder empty and which opens into the cloaca. 2. The common receptacle of genital and urinary ducts.

s's., uteroplacental. Slanting venous channels from the placenta serving to convey the maternal blood from the intervillous lacunae back into the uterine veins.

s. of Valsalva. A dilatation of the aorta or pulmonary artery opp. segment of the semilunar valve. Syn: *aortic s.*

s., venous. One conveying venous blood.

s's., vertebral. Veins within the vertebrae.

sinusitis (sī-nus-ī'tĭs) [L. *sinus*, a curve, a hollow, + G. *-itis, inflammation*]. Inflammation of a sinus, esp. a paranasal sinus.

Etiol: A number of causative agents including viruses, bacteria, or allergy.

Predisposing factors: Inadequate drainage which may result from presence of polyps, enlarged turbinates, deviated septum, etc.; chronic rhinitis, general debility, or dental abscess in maxillary bone.

s., acute catarrhal. Inflammation accompanying a similar process in the nose.

s., acute suppurative. Purulent inflammation with symptoms of pain over the sinus, fever, chills, headache, etc.

TREATMENT: Conservative, shrinkage in the nose for ventilation, and drainage of the sinus, aeration, constitutional treatment, capillary suction. Rest in bed, catharsis, force fluids, anodynes for pain.

s., chronic hyperplastic. Polyps present in sinuses and nose and underlying osteitis of sinus walls.

TREATMENT: *Surgical*: Conservative: removal of polyps and intranasal opening into sinuses for adequate ventilation and drainage. *Radical*: Complete removal of sinus mucosa either through external or intranasal route.

s., chronic hypertrophic. Inflammation found in conjunction with chronic hypertrophic rhinitis.

Living in a climate where the temperature fluctuations are not extreme may be beneficial.

sinusoid (sī'nŭs-oyd) [L. *sinus,* a hollow, a curve, + G. *eidos,* like]. 1. Resembling a sinus. 2. A minute blood vessel found in such organs as the liver, spleen, adrenal glands, and bone marrow. They are slightly larger than capillaries and they lack a continuous lining endothelium.

sinusoidal (sī-nŭs-oyd'ăl) [" + G. *eidos* like]. Pert. to a sinusoid.

s. current. Alternating induced electric current, the 2 strokes of which are equal.

sinusoidalization (sī-nŭs-oyd-al-ĭ-zā'shŭn) [" + G. *eidos,* like]. Use of a sinusoidal current.

sinusotomy (sī-nŭ-sŏt'ō-mĭ) [" + G. *tomē,* a cutting]. The operation of incising a sinus.

SiO_2. Silicon dioxide.

siphon (sī'fŏn) [G. *siphōn,* tube]. A tube bent at an angle to form 2 unequal lengths for removing liquids by atmospheric pressure.

Siphonaptera (sī"fō-năp'ter-ă). An order of insects which includes the fleas. They are wingless, undergo complete metamorphosis, and have piercing and sucking mouth parts, their food being the blood of birds and mammals. The body is compressed laterally and their legs are adapted for leaping. In addition to being annoying pests, they transmit the causative organisms of several diseases (bubonic plague, endemic or murine typhus, and among rodents, tularemia). They also serve as intermediate hosts of certain tapeworms. SEE: *flea.*

siphonoma (sī-fon-ō'mă) [" + *-ōma,* tumor]. A tumor made up of fine tubes.

Sippy diet (sĭp'ē). Treatment of gastric ulcer by diet checking acidity of gastric juice.

Small amounts of milk and cream every hour and alkaline powders every ½ hr.

Average mixture: 1½ oz. each of cream and milk given once each hour for a total of 13 feedings during the day. Then for the next 3 to 4 days continue these feedings but substitute an egg and fine cereal for one feeding in the morning and one at night. Next day, 3 oz. soft cereal added to afternoon feeding; another egg the next day, and finally 3 servings of cereal and 3 eggs per day added to the milk and cream. Purée, custards, toast added the next week. Decreased feedings as amount of each feeding is increased until 6 feedings are given per day. Each feeding replaces the scheduled milk and cream.

This schedule is monotonous, deficient in vitamins, and provides no feeding at night. It is usually modified to compensate for these deficiencies.

siriasis (sĭ-rī'ă-sĭs) [G. *seirian,* to be hot]. Sunstroke, *q.v.*

sismotherapy (sĭs-mō-ther'ă-pĭ) [G. *seismos,* a shake, + *therapeia,* treatment]. Therapeutic employment of vibration. SYN: *seismotherapy, vibrotherapeutics.*

sister. A term used by the British for nurses.

site. Position or location.

sitieirgia (sĭt-ĭ-īr'jĭ-ă) [G. *sition,* food, + *eirgein,* to bar out]. Hysterical refusal to take food.

sitio-, sito- [G.]. Combining forms meaning *bread,* or *made from grain; food,* as *sitomania.*

sitiology (sĭt-ĭ-ŏl'ō-jĭ) [G. *sition,* food, + *logos,* a study]. Science of nutrition. SYN: *sitology.*

sitiomania (sĭt-ĭ-ō-mā'nĭ-ă) [" + *mania,* madness]. Periodic abnormal appetite or craving for food. SYN: *sitomania.*

sitology (sī-tŏl'ō-jĭ) [G. *sitos,* food, + *logos,* a study]. Science of nutrition and food. SYN: *sitiology.*

sitomania (sī"tō-mā'nĭ-ă) [" + *mania,* madness]. 1. Periodic abnormal craving for food. SYN: *sitiomania.* 2. Periodic abnormality of appetite.

sitophobia (sī"tō-fō'bĭ-ă) [" + *phobos,* fear]. Psychoneurotic abhorrence of food, or morbid dread of, or repugnance to food, whether generally or only to specific dishes.

sitotherapy (sī"tō-ther'ă-pĭ) [" + *therapeia,* treatment]. The therapeutic use of food.

sitotoxism (sī"tō-tŏks'ĭzm) [" + *toxikon,* poison, + *ismos,* condition]. Poisoning by vegetable foods infested with molds or bacteria.

sitotropism (sī-tŏt'rō-pĭzm) [" + *tropos,* a turning, + *-ismos,* condition]. Response of cells to the attraction or repulsion of food elements.

situs (sī'tŭs) [L. position]. A position.

s. inversus viscerum. Displacement of viscera abnormally to opposite side of the body.

s. perversus. Malposition of any visceral structure.

sitz bath (sĭtz bath). Bath to sit in with water above and covering the hips. The tub or fixture is usually shaped to allow the legs to be out of the water. SYN: *hip bath.* SEE: *bath.*

sixth cranial nerve. Abducens nerve which supplies the external rectus of the eye. SEE: *cranial nerves.*

skatol(e (skăt'ŏl) [G. *skōr, skat-,* dung]. Beta-methyl indole, C_9H_9N, a malodorous, solid, heterocyclic nitrogen compound found in feces, formed by protein decomposition in the intestines and giving them their odor.

skelalgia (skē-lăl'jĭ-ă) [G. *skelis,* leg, + *algos,* pain]. Pain in the leg.

skeletal (skĕl'ĕ-tăl) [G. *skeleton,* skeleton]. Pert. to the skeleton.

s. muscle. SYN: *striated muscle, voluntary muscle.* Muscle fibers which with few exceptions are attached to parts of the skeleton, and involved primarily in movements of the parts of body.

s. traction. Traction exerted directly on long bones.

skeletization (skĕl-ĕt-ĭ-zā'shŭn) [G. *skeleton,* skeleton]. 1. Excessive emaciation.

2. Removal of soft parts of the body leaving only the skeleton.

skeleto- [G.]. Prefix meaning *skeleton.*

skeletogenous (skĕl-ĕt-ŏj′ĕn-ŭs) [G. *skeleton,* skeleton, + *gennan,* to produce]. Forming skeletal structures or tissues.

skeleton (skĕl′ĕt-ŏn) [G. *skeletos,* dried up]. The bony framework of the body, consisting of 206 bones, 80 axial and 126 appendicular. This number does not include the teeth.

The various bones are as follows:

AXIAL GROUP (80 Bones)

8 cerebral cranials.
14 visceral cranials.
1 os hyoideum (hyoid).
6 ossicula auditus (ossicles, ear bones)
26 columna vertebralis (vertebrae).
24 costae (ribs).
1 sternum (chest).
80 Total

APPENDICULAR GROUP (126 Bones)

64 extremitas sup. (32 in each upper extremity).
62 extremitas inf. (31 in each lower extremity).
126 Total

TRUNK (51 Bones)

Columna vertebralis (vertebrae), 26 Bones
7 cervicales (cervicals).
12 thoraces (dorsals).
5 lumbales (lumbar).
1 os sacrum.
1 os coccygis.
26 Total

Ribs (24 Bones)

14 costae verae (true ribs).
6 costae spuriae (false ribs).
4 costae vertebrales (floating ribs).
24 Total
1 sternum (chest bone).

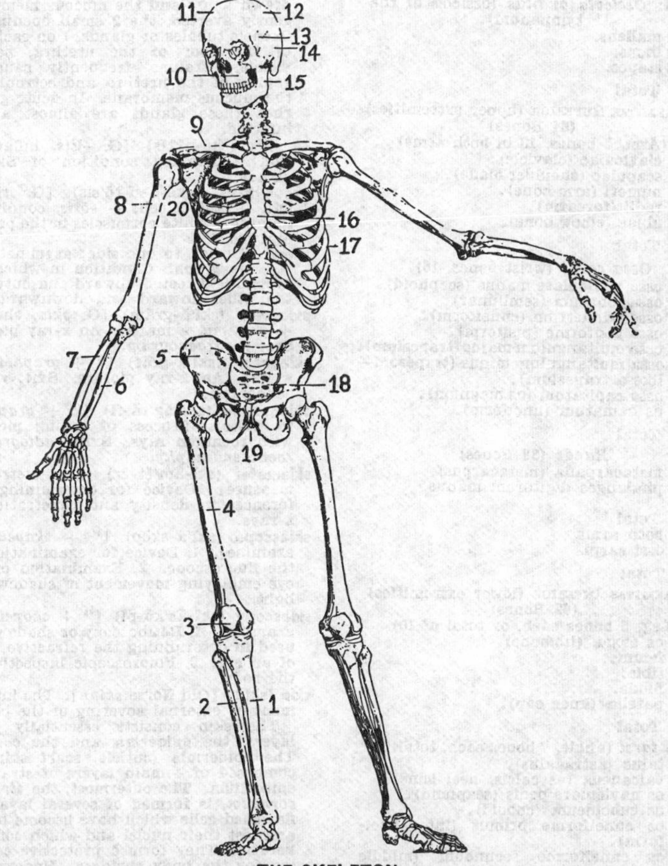

THE SKELETON.
1. Tibia. 2. Fibula. 3. Patella. 4. Femur. 5. Innominate. 6. Ulna. 7. Radius. 8. Humerus. 9. Clavicle. 10. Maxilla. 11. Frontal. 12. Parietal bone. 13. Great wing of sphenoid. 14. Temporal. 15. Mandible. 16. Sternum. 17. Rib. 18. Sacrum. 19. Coccyx. 20. Scapula.

HEAD (29 Bones)

Cerebral cranials (8 Bones)

1 os frontale (frontal).
2 ossa parietalia (parietals).
1 ossa occipitale (occipital).
2 ossa temporales (temporal).
1 os sphenoidale (sphenoid).
1 os ethmoidale (ethmoid).

8 Total

Visceral cranials (facial) (14 Bones)

2 ossa maxillae (sup. maxillary).
1 os mandibula (inf. maxillary).
2 ossa zygomatica (malar).
2 ossa lacrimales (lacrimal).
2 ossa nasalia (nasal).
2 conchae nasales inferiores (turbinates).
1 os vomer.
2 ossa palatina (palate).

14 Total

1 os hyoideum (hyoid).

EAR: *Ossicula auditus* (ossicles of the tympanum).

2 malleus.
2 incus.
2 stapes.

6 Total

EXTREMITAS SUPERIOR (upper extremities) (64 Bones)

(Arm, 5 bones, 10 in both arms)
2 claviculae (clavicle).
2 scapulae (shoulder blade).
2 humeri (arm bone).
2 radii (forearm).
2 ulnae (elbow bone).

10 Total

Ossa carpi (wrist bones, 16)

2 ossa naviculare manus (scaphoid).
2 ossa lunatum (semilunar).
2 ossa triquetrum (cuneiform).
2 ossa pisiforme (pisiform).
2 ossa multangulum majus (trapezium).
2 ossa multangulum minus (trapezoid—like a trapezium).
2 ossa capitatum (os magnum).
2 os hamatum (unciform).

16 Total

Hands (38 Bones)

10 metacarpalia (metacarpus).
28 phalanges digitorum manus.

38 Total
10 both arms.
16 ossi carpi.

64 Total

EXTREMITAS INFERIOR (lower extremities) (62 Bones)

(Leg, 5 bones each, or total of 10)
2 os coxae (hipbone).
2 femur.
2 tibia.
2 fibula.
2 patella (knee cap).

10 Total

Ossa tarsi (ankle, 7 bones each, total 14)

2 talus (astragalus).
2 calcaneus (os calcis, heel bone).
2 os naviculare pedis (scaphoid).
2 os cuboideum (cuboid).
2 os cuneiforme primus (int. cuneiform).
2 os cuneiforme secundum (middle cuneiform).
2 os cuneiforme tertium (ext. cuneiform).

14 Total

14 ossa tarsi (as above).
10 ossa metatarsalia (metatarsal).
28 phalanges digitorum pedis.
10 leg and hip.

62 Total

SUMMARY

28 Head.
1 Hyoid.
51 Trunk.
64 Extremitas superior.
62 Extremitas inferior.

206 Total bones in skeleton.

s., axial. Bones of the head and trunk.

s., cartilaginous. Structure from which the bones have been formed through ossification.

Skene's glands (skēn). SYN: *paraurethral glands.* Glands lying just inside of and on the post. floor of the urethra, in the female.

If the margins of the urethra are drawn apart and the mucous membrane gently averted, the 2 small openings of Skene's tubules or glands, 1 on each side of the floor of the urethra, become visible. Trauma frequently causes a gaping of the urethra and ectropion of the mucous membrane. In acute gonorrhea these glands are almost always infected.

skenitis (skē-nī'tĭs) [G. *-itis,* inflammation]. Inflamed condition of Skene's glands.

skeocytosis (skē-ō-sī-tō'sĭs) [G. *skaios,* left, + *kytos,* cell, + *-ōsis,* condition]. Immature white corpuscles in the peripheral blood.

skew. Turned to one side; asymmetrical.

s. deviation. Condition in which one eyeball is directed upward and outward; the other inward and downward.

skiagram (skī'ă-grăm) [G. *skia,* shadow, + *gramma,* a mark]. An x-ray picture. SEE: *roentgenogram.*

skiagraph (skī'ă-grăf) [" + *graphein,* to write]. An x-ray picture. SYN: *roentgenograph.*

skiagraphy (skī-ăg'ră-fĭ) [" + *graphein,* to write]. Process of taking pictures with roentgen rays. SYN: *radiography, roentgenography.*

skiameter (skī-ăm'ĕt-ĕr) [" + *metron,* a measure]. Device for determining differences in density and penetration of x-rays.

skiascope (skī'ă-skōp) [" + *skopein,* to examine]. 1. Device for examination by the fluoroscope. 2. Examination of the eye employing movement of shadow and light.

skiascopy (skī-ăs'kō-pĭ) [" + *skopein,* to examine]. 1. Retinoscopy or shadow test used in determining the refractive error of an eye. 2. Fluoroscopic inspection of the body.

skin (skĭn) [Old Norse *skinn*]. The integument or external covering of the body.

The skin consists essentially of 2 layers, the *epidermis* and the *corium.* The epidermis (cuticle, scarf skin) is composed of 4 main layers of stratified epithelium. The outermost, the *stratum corneum,* is formed of several layers of flattened cells which have become horny and lost their nuclei and which contain keratin. They form a protective covering for the body surfaces. Underneath this layer is the *stratum lucidum,* which is formed of translucent flattened cells. The 3rd layer, the *stratum granulosum,* consists of two or three layers of flat-

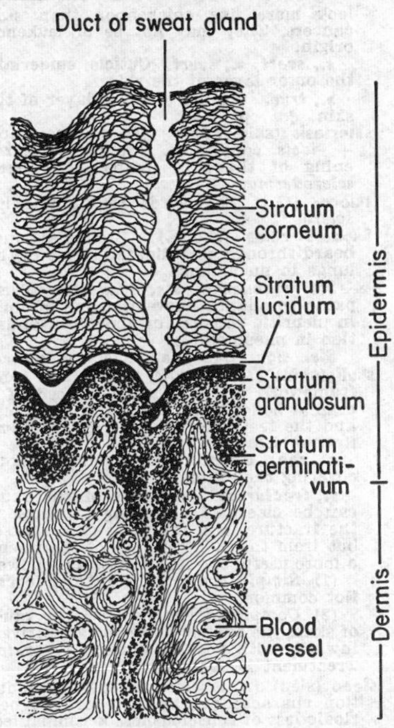

LAYERS OF SKIN.

tened cells containing granules of *eleidin,* the precursor of *keratin.* The 4th and last layer is the *stratum germinativum* (*stratum mucosum, stratum Malpighi*). The cells in upper portion of this layer are cuboidal, those nearest the corium are columnar. Cells of this layer possess well-defined intercellular bridges which appear as "spines" projecting from the surface; hence these cells are often called *prickle cells* and the entire layer, *stratum spinosum.* These cells contain peculiar fibrils, *tonofibrils,* which pass through the intercellular bridges. The color of the skin is due principally to the presence of a pigment, *melanin,* present as granules in stratum germinatum.

The corium (cutis, dermis, derma, true skin) is formed of connective tissue containing lymphatics, nerves and nerve endings, blood vessels, sebaceous and sweat glands, and elastic fibers. It is divided into 2 layers, a *superficial papillary layer* and a *deep reticular layer.* The papillary layer contains conical protuberances, the papillae, which fit into corresponding depressions in the epidermis. Within each papilla is a capillary loop which furnishes the epidermis with a blood supply. The reticular layer is made up in the main of white fibrous tissue supporting the blood vessels and other structures in it. It rests on the subcutaneous connective tissue.

Appendages of the skin are the hair* and nails.*

FUNCTION: 1. Protection against injuries and parasitic invasion. 2. Regulation of body temperature. 3. Aids in elimination. 4. Prevention of dehydration. 5. Reservoir for food and water. 6. Sense organ for the cutaneous senses. 7. Source of antirachitic vitamin (vitamin D).

SYM: *Abnormal dryness*: May indicate abnormal deficiency of thyroid function, diabetes and other causes. *Ashy*: Malignant diseases, severe anemia, cancer, scrofula, chronic interstitial nephritis.

DIAGNOSIS: *Ashy*: Malignant diseases, cancer, scrofula, chronic interstitial nephritis, anemia.

Bronzing: Addison's disease, dyes or metals, early stages of pellagra.

Brownish-yellow Spots (liver spots): Noted in pregnancy (chloasma uterinum), in exophthalmic goiter, and uterine and liver malignancies; also freckles, sunburn, cosmetics, mustard, turpentine, and other irritants.

Cherry Red: Carbon monoxide poisoning.

Cold Sweats: Indicate great prostration, fear or depression of spirits.

Cyanosis: May be congenital; if acquired may be due to asthma, pulmonary tuberculosis, whooping cough, advanced emphysema, croup, tracheal obstruction, aneurysm, goiter, flushing (hyperemia), emotion, febrile disorders, pulmonary tuberculosis, during convulsions, large ovarian tumor, plethora, polycythemia.

Cyanosis Alternating with Pallor: Cerebrospinal diseases, typhoid, vasomotor disturbances, menopause, Gray's argyria, silver salts. May be noted in lips, mucous membranes, fingertips and external ear. If extreme, entire body shows dusky, leaden tint. Indicates lack of oxygen and excess of carbon dioxide in blood. May be due to inflammation of pharynx and larynx, abscess of same, angina Ludovici, croup and disorders affecting respiration. Also to overdose of drugs and asphyxiation by gas.

Discolorations: Seen in icterus, chlorosis, leprosy, resulting from administration of silver nitrate, malignant diseases, and asphyxia from gas.

Edema: Seen in anemia, hydremia, obstruction, inflammation, cardiac, circulatory and renal decompensation. If local, may be due to obstruction of return circulation, heart failure, in which case it will be evident in ankles and often legs, esp. at night. May also be due to renal diseases.

Emphysema: Due to air or gas in cellular tissue.

Hot and Dry: Indicates fever, mental excitement, or excessive use of salted provisions.

Moisture: Lack of noted in ichthyosis. Increased perspiration (hyperhidrosis) may be due to malarial fever; rheumatic, relapsing and septic fever; pneumonic crisis; pulmonary tuberculosis; Graves' disease; neuralgia; migraine; drugs; hot drinks; exercise.

Paleness: Nervous prostration, dropsy, paralysis, malnutrition.

Pallor: Obtains in those living an indoor life, esp. in prisoners and night workers. May be due to lowered circulation, decrease of red blood corpuscles, nonfilling capillaries. Obtains in all anemias. Temporary pallor occurs in syncope, chills, shock, rigors and some vasomotor spasms. If sudden and persistent may be sign of internal hemorrhage. Also seen in lead poisoning, toxic febrile affections. If it gradually becomes permanent may indicate chronic febrile disease, chronic gastrointestinal disease, cancer, arsenical poisoning, chronic suppuration, chronic mercurial poisoning, hemorrhages, leukemia, cachexia, nephrosis, nephritis, syphilis, parasitic diseases, tuberculosis, malaria.

Purplish: Interference of circulation common in asthma and typhus.

Rashes: SEE: *rash.*

Temperature: Usually corresponds with internal temperature, unless raised by local applications of heat. If generally cold may be due to poor circulation or obstruction of same, vasomotor spasms, venous or arterial thrombosis, exposure to cold. General abnormal heat seen in febrile disorders, although some of them present a cold and clammy skin.

Redness: Red spots upon pale cheeks, tubercular involvement, worms. Local redness seen in inflammation, skin diseases, chronic alcoholism, vasomotor disturbances, pyrexia and chlorosis. One side of face, lobar pneumonia. Local redness with pain indicates inflammation. Sunburn (*actinic dermatitis*).

Sallowness: Cachexia, syphilis, chronic gallbladder disease, arthritis deformans, constipation, some anemias, gastric, pancreatic, enteric, or hepatic disorders.

Wrinkling: If permanent may be due to aging; temporary due to prolonged immersion in water, or dehydration.

Yellow: Jaundice, liver derangements. If jaundiced, plethoric, hyperemic, or pigmented, it should be noted in any examination. Rashes, scars, and their cause are also diagnostic. Texture and temperature of skin are important signs. Undue moisture, cold or hot spots on body, dryness of skin are other points to look for in diagnosis. SEE: *face; bacterial endocarditis; pernicious anemia; biliousness; liver condition.*

s., alligator. Severe scaling of the skin with formation of thick plates resembling hide of an alligator.

s. cancer. That of the skin. It may arise on surface of body as a small ulcer, pimple or mole. May be red, brown, black, or white, according to type. May be single or in a group, open or ulcerated. May be localized or invade blood vessels, lymph glands and connecting ducts.

s., deciduous. Shedding of the epidermis. SYN: *keratolysis.*

s., elastic. Skin which has property of great elasticity.

s., fish. SEE: *ichthyosis.*

s., glossy. Shining atrophy of the skin.

s. grafting. Grafting of skin from another part of body to repair a defect or trauma. SEE: *Thiersch's graft.*

ONP: Position of patient indicated by location of graft. The appropriate areas of both donor and recipient are prepared in the usual manner for surgical procedure. Patient is draped with sterile sheets and towels so that both areas are exposed. A dressing is applied to area from which the skin is removed. The area receiving skin is covered with a paraffin-coated mesh.

s., hidebound. Scleroderma, *q.v.*

s., loose. Hypertrophy of the skin.

s., parchment. Atrophy of the skin with stretching.

s., piebald. SEE: *vitiligo.*

s. rashes. They may cover one small area or most of the body surface if they represent blood cell tumors. Sometimes the patches tend to bleed. They look more like chickenpox than skin cancers. They may not be of leukemic origin.

s., scarf, s., scurf. Cuticle, epidermis, the outer layer of the skin.

s., true. Corium or inner layer of the skin, *q.v., p. S-41.*

skleriasis (sklē-rī'ăs-ĭs) [G. *sklēros,* hard, + *-iasis,* condition]. Progressive hardening of the skin in patches. SYN: *scleroderma.*

sklero- [G.]. See words beginning with *sclero-*.

Skoda's râles (skō'dă). Bronchial ones heard through consolidated tissue of the lungs in pneumonia.

S's. resonance, S's. tympany. Tympanic resonance above the line of fluid in pleuritic effusion, or above consolidation in pneumonia.

S's. sign. Same as *Skoda's resonance.*

skull (skŭl) [M.E. *skulle,* bowl]. The bony framework of the head, composed of 8 cranial bones, the 14 bones of the face, and the teeth. SYN: *calvaria, cranium.* SEE: *skeleton.*

s. cap. Upper round portion of skull covering the brain.

s., fractured. Fractures of the skull can be classified according to whether the fracture is in the vault or the base, but from the point of view of treatment a more useful classification is as follows:

(1) *Simple Uncomplicated Fractures*: Not common.

(2) *Compound Fractures*: If in vault of skull, the bone is depressed and driven inwards with possible damage to brain. Treatment is operative.

sleep (slēp) [A. S. *slǣp,* sleep]. A condition characterized by more or less periodic loss of consciousness accompanied by reduced cortical and physical activities.

It is easily differentiated from the lessened consciousness of stupor, in that normal awareness can completely reassert itself when danger threatens and ordinarily continue until sleep can again be resumed.

Emotionalism and anxiety (*e.g.* fear) are the great enemies of sleep, and the most common cause of insomnia. Hypersomnia may be a symptom of hypopituitarism.

s., crescendo. Normal sleep with increased movement during the night.

s. drunkenness. The stupor of sleep in drunkenness. SYN: *somnolentia.*

s. epilepsy. Uncontrollable desire to sleep at periodic intervals. SYN: *narcolepsy.*

s., hypnotic. S. induced by hypnotic suggestion.

s. paralysis. Temporary p. of a part due to pressure during sleep.

s., paroxysmal. SEE: *sleep epilepsy.*

s., pathologic. A term used in encephalitis lethargica (sleeping sickness); here sleep reasserts itself excessively and under conditions not to the best interests of the patient.

s., physiologic standards. Metabolic rate reduced 10-15% below basal level. Systolic pressure falls 10 to 30 mm. of mercury. Pulse rate slows from 10 to 30 beats. Respiration slowed and typically irregular. Temperature drops sharply; lowest about the middle hours of sleep. Muscles relax. Pupils constricted, eyeballs turned upward and outward. Increased sweating. Lacrimal, salivary secretions and volume of urine reduced. Spec. gr. raised. Newborn

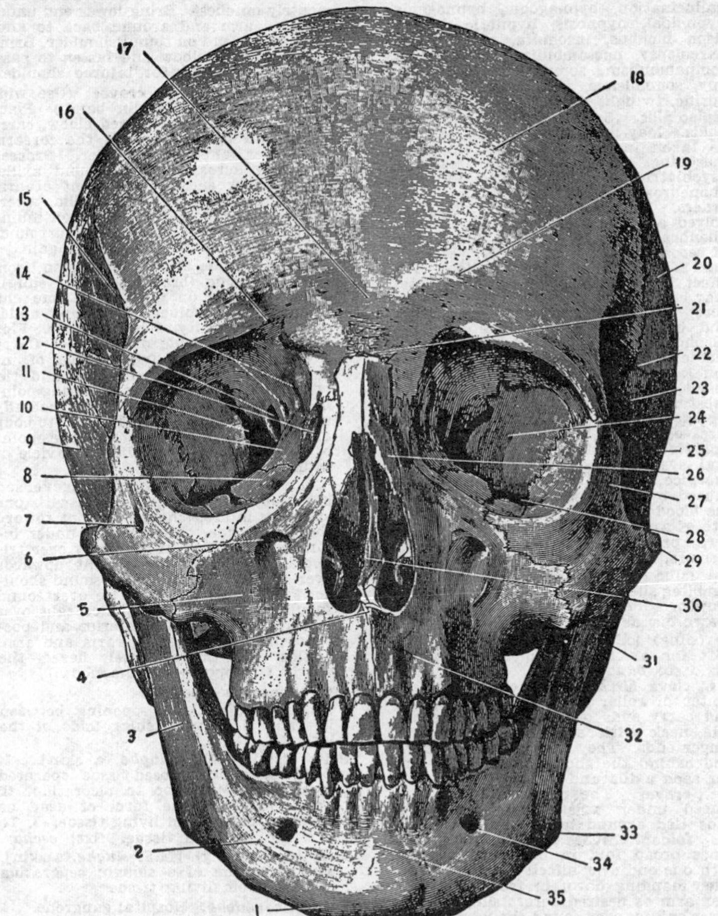

SKULL, FRONT VIEW.

1, Mental tubercle; 2, body of mandible; 3, ramus of mandible; 4, anterior nasal spine; 5, canine fossa; 6, infraorbital foramen; 7, zygomaticofacial foramen; 8, orbital surface of maxilla; 9, squamous temporal; 10, lateral surface of ethmoid; 11, superior orbital fissure; 12, lacrimal bone and groove; 13, optic foramen; 14, ethmoidal foramina; 15, temporal line; 16, supraorbital notch; 17, glabella; 18, frontal eminence; 19, superciliary arch; 20, parietal bone; 21, nasofrontal suture; 22, pterion; 23, great wing of sphenoid; 24, orbital surface of great wing; 25, squamous part of temporal; 26, left nasal bone; 27, zygomatic bone; 28, inferior orbital fissure; 29, zygomatic arch; 30, apertura piriformis; 31, mastoid process; 32, incisive fossa; 33, angle of mandible; 34, mental foramen; 35, symphysis menti. (Robinson, Editor: *Cunningham's Textbook of Anatomy,* 6th Ed., Oxford University Press, New York City.)

sleeps 18-20 hrs. a day; growing child 12-14 hrs., adult 7-9 hrs. Older persons 5-7 hrs. but it is not necessarily true that older persons require much less sleep than they did when they were young. Women require more sleep than men. Depth of sleep varies from hour to hour. Lessens from the second hour.

s., *R.E.M.* Sleep during which Rapid Eye Movements are noted. These eye movements are related to dreams.

s., *twilight.* A procedure of injection of scopolamine and morphine to abolish the subsequent memory of pain felt during childbirth, but it does not completely abolish pain at the time. The patient is delivered in delirium-like state.

s. *walking.* Walking in one's sleep. SYN: *somnambulism.*

sleep, *words pert. to:* agrypnia, ahypnia, antilethargic, anypnia, carotic, carus.

hallucination, hypnagogic, hypnogenic, hypnoidal, hypnosis, hypnotic, hypnotism, incubus, insomnia, narcohypnia, narcolepsy, noctambulism, oneirodynia, somnambulism, somnifacient, somniloquy, somnolence, somnolent, sopor, soporific, twilight sleep.

sleeping pills. Several forms of barbituric acids. May be habit-forming or may be taken in excess resulting in acute poisoning. Habitual use may result in psychiatric disorders, especially psychoneuroses, liver and kidney disorders. The drugs most commonly involved are Nembutal, Seconal, Amytal, phenobarbital, and barbital. The action of *seconal* is quick but brief. *Nembutal* has a slower but longer action. The effect is cumulative, so repeated doses may be fatal. In nonfatal cases of overdose, respiratory disorders (atelectasis and bronchopneumonia) are common. Alcohol should not be taken with them. Sudden withdrawal of drug from a person taking 0.8 gm. or more daily may result in marked withdrawal symptoms (abstinence syndrome).

sleep'ing sick'ness. 1. Acute, infectious disease marked by increasing lethargy, drowsiness, muscular weakness and cerebral symptoms. Syn: *encephalitis lethargica, q.v.* 2. African trypanosomiasis caused by a protozoon introduced into the blood and cerebrospinal fluid by the bite of a tsetse fly; characterized by fever, protracted lethargy, weakness, tremors, and wasting.

slimy (slīm'ĭ) [A.S. *slīm,* smooth]. Resembling slime or a viscid substance; of a growth, adhering to needle so it can be drawn out as a long thread.

sling (slĭng) [A.S. *slingan,* sling]. A support for an injured upper extremity. See also: *bandage.*

s., clove hitch. Make clove hitch in center of roller bandage. Fit to hand and carry ends over shoulder. Tie beside neck with square knot, making longer ends. They may be carried over and behind the shoulders, brought under each axilla and tied over chest.

s., cravat. The center of cravat is placed under wrist or forearm and ends tied around neck.

s., folded cravat (lesser arm sling). Place broad fold in position on chest with one end over affected shoulder and other hanging down in front of chest. Flex arm as desired across sling. Bring lower end up over sound shoulder. Knot with other end on affected shoulder.

s., open. The point of the triangle is placed at tip of elbow. The ends are brought around at back of neck and tied. The point should be brought forward and pinned or tied in a single knot, forming a cup to prevent elbow from slipping out.

s., simple figure-of-eight roller arm. Flex arm on chest in desired position, then fix bandage with single turn toward uninjured side around arm and chest, crossing elbow just above external epicondyle of humerus. Make 2nd turn overlapping 2/3 of 1st and bring bandage forward under tip of elbow, then upwards, along flexed forearm to root of neck of sound side. Then bring downward over scapula and cross chest and arm horizontally, overlapping, turn above and continue as in progressive figure-of-eight.

s., St. John's. Apply triangle with point downwards under elbow, upper end over sound shoulder. Flex arm acutely on chest. Bring lower end under affected arm and around back to knot with upper end on sound shoulder. Bring point up over elbow and fasten to base. Support is wholly for injured shoulder.

s., swathe arm or cravat. (Use wide cravat or folded muslin band.) Place center under acutely flexed elbow, carry front and upwards across the forearm and over affected shoulder. Proceed obliquely across back to sound axilla. Bring other end around front of arm and across body to sound axilla, where it is pinned to other end, continuing around back to part of sling surrounding affected elbow and pinned again.

s., triangular. With suspension from uninjured side (brachioscapular sling). Place triangle on chest with one end over sound shoulder, the point under affected extremity, fold the base. Flex injured arm outside of triangle. Carry lower end upward under axilla of injured side, back of shoulder and tie with upper end behind back. Bring point of triangle anteriorly and medially around back of elbow and fasten to body of bandage. (This bandage changes point of carrying and also relieves clavicle of injured side of a load.)

s., triangular, reversed (reversed brachiocervical sling). Apply with one end over injured shoulder, point toward the sound side, base vertical under injured elbow. Flex arm acutely over triangle. Lower end is brought upwards over front of arm and over sound shoulder. Pull ends taut and tie over sound shoulder. The point is pulled taut over forearm and fixed to anterior and posterior layers between forearm and arm. (Holds elbow more acutely flexed—the weight is supported by the elbow.)

slit. A narrow opening.

s., vestibular. The opening between left and right ventricular folds of the larynx.

slough (slŭf) [M.E. *slughe,* a skin]. 1. Dead matter or necrosed tissue separated from living tissue or an ulceration. 2. To separate in the form of dead or necrosed parts from living tissue. 3. To cast off, as dead tissue. See: *eschar.*

sloughing (slŭf'ĭng) [M.E. *slughe,* a skin]. The formation of a slough; separation of dead from living tissue.

s. phagedena. Hospital gangrene.

slow (slō) [A.S. *slāw,* dull]. 1. Mentally dull. 2. Exhibiting retarded speed, as the pulse. 3. Of a morbid condition or fever, not acute. See: *"brady-" words.*

slows (slōz). An infectious disease of cattle transmitted to man through milk or butter, marked by severe neural symptoms, constipation, vomiting; frequently fatal. Syn: *milk sickness, trembles.*

sludge (slujh). The semisolid matter deposited in sewage.

s., activated. Sludge from well-aerated sewage, exposed to oxidizing bacteria, supplying oxidizing organisms sufficient to activate another supply of sewage.

s., dewatered. Sludge that has been dried.

sludged blood. Condition of the blood in certain abnormal states such as tissue injury or shock in which volume of plasma is reduced and the cells show a pronounced tendency to agglutinate and form large clumps or masses which move slowly through the vessels and sometimes clog the smaller vessels.

slurry (slur'ĭ). A thin watery mixture.

Sm. Chemical symbol for *samarium.*

smallpox (smawl'pŏks) [A.S. *smael,* tiny, + *poc,* pustule]. An acute, contagious, febrile disease, the constitutional symptoms of which are followed by the appearance of an eruption. SYN: *variola, q.v.*

smear, smear culture (smēr) [A.S. *smerian,* to anoint]. 1. BACT: Material spread on a surface, as a microscopic slide or a culture medium. 2. One obtained from infected matter spread over solid culture media.

smegma (smĕg'mă) [G. *smēgma,* soap]. Secretion of sebaceous glands, specifically, the thick, cheesy, ill-smelling secretion found under the labia minora about the glans clitoridis and under the male prepuce from Tyson's glands. SYN: *sebum.*

s. clitoridis. Odoriferous secretion of the glands of the clitoris.

s. embryonum. Vernix caseosa.

s. praeputii. Cheesy odoriferous substance collecting under prepuce in the male, secreted by Tyson's glands.

smegmatic (smĕg-măt'ĭk) [G. *smēgma,* soap]. Pert. to or made up of smegma.

smegmolith (smĕg'mō-lĭth) [" + *lithos,* a stone]. Calcareous mass in the smegma.

smell (smĕl) [M.E. *smellen,* to reek]. 1. To perceive by stimulation of the olfactory nerves. 2. To emit an odor, pleasant or offensive. 3. A chemical sense dependent upon end organs on the surface of the upper part of the nasal septum and the superior nasal conch. 4. Property of a thing affecting the olfactory organs, pleasant or unpleasant. SYN: *odor, scent, stench.*

The sense of smell may be affected by many conditions, some of which are the following:

*Anosmia**: A loss of the sense of smell. It may be a local and a temporary condition resulting from acute and chronic rhinitis, mouth breathing, nasal polyps, dryness of the nasal mucous membrane, pollens, or very offensive odors. It may also result from the following causes. Disease or injury of the olfactory tract, bone disease near the olfactory nerve. disease of the nasal accessory sinuses, basal meningitis, or tumors or gumma affecting the olfactory nerve. It is sometimes found in locomotor ataxia, and frequently in hysteria and neurasthenia. Disease of 1 cranial hemisphere or of 1 nasal chamber may account for anosmia.

Hyperosmia: An increased sensitivity to odors.

*Kakosmia**: The perception of bad odors where none exist and it may be due to head injuries or occur in hallucinations in certain psychoses.

*Parosmia**: A perverted sense of smell. Odors that are considered agreeable are assumed to be offensive and disagreeable odors may be found pleasant to those suffering from certain functional derangements and in some catarrhs.

smell, *words pert. to:* anodmia, anosmatic, anosmia, anosphrasia, aroma, aromatic, cacosmia, dysosmia, hyperosmia, jumentous, kakosmia, odor, odoriferous, olfaction, olfactory, osmesthesia, osphresis, oxyosphresia.

smog. Dense fog combined with smoke and other forms of air pollution.

smok'er's can'cer. Cancer of the lip or throat due to irritation from a pipe stem or excessive smoking.

smudging. A speech defect in which difficult consonants are omitted.

Sn. [L. *stannum*]. Symb. for *tin.*

snail. A small mollusk having a spiral shell and belonging to the class *Gastropoda.* They are important as intermediate hosts of many species of parasitic flukes.

snake. SYN: *serpent.* A creeping reptile possessing scales and lacking limbs, external ears, and functional eyelids.

s. bite. All snakes should be considered poisonous, although there are only a few that secrete an amount of venom sufficient to inoculate poison deeply into the tissues.

F. A. TREATMENT: Apply tourniquet, just tight enough to stop venous return of blood; it should not be tight enough to prevent arterial circulation. Then incise, and induce bleeding. Immobilize patient immediately in order to delay spread of venom. If swelling persists, incise again. This may be necessary repeatedly. Inject antivenin. If the type of snake cannot be determined, use mixed antivenin. Release tourniquet cautiously at 15- to 20-minute intervals and observe effect.

A tourniquet should not be applied too tightly or remain on too long. Alcoholic stimulants must not be taken and nothing should be done to increase circulation. Do not cauterize with strong acids or depend upon home remedies. Antibiotics and tetanus prophylaxis are essential.

s., poisonous. A venom-producing snake. Venom is produced in a poison

Differential Diagnosis Between Smallpox and Chickenpox

	Smallpox	Chickenpox
General symptoms	May be severe, with pyrexia, backache, prostration, etc., for 3 to 4 days before appearance of eruption.	Mild. Appear at same time as rash.
Eruption	About 4th day of illness.	Maculopapular for few hours, then vesicular. First day.
Type	Papules before vesicles. Deep, often "shotty."	
Appearance	All spots at same stage of development. Pustules appear on the 8th day.	Successive crops; therefore, all stages present at the same time. Pustules on 3rd or 4th day.
Distribution	Maximum on distal parts, not in axillae or groins.	Maximum on trunk, present in axillae.

gland which is connected by a tube or groove to a poison fang, one of two sharp, elongated teeth present in upper jaw. The following are poisonous snakes of the U. S.: *coral snake, copperhead, water moccasin* (cottonmouth), and *rattle-snake,* of which there are 15 species. All except the coral snake belong to a group known as *pit vipers* because of presence of a distinct pit between eye and nostril. SEE: *venom, snake.*

A polyvalent antivenin serum for bites by pit vipers is prepared by Wyeth. Inc., Philadelphia, Penna. Antivenin for coral snake bite is available from the Florida State Dept. of Health, Jacksonville, Florida.

Information concerning the nearest source of antivenin may be obtained from the National Institutes of Health, Bethesda, Md.; the Reptile Institute, Silver Springs, Florida; or from large zoos.

RS: *antivenene, antivenom, antivenomous, ophidiophobia, ophidism ophiotoxemia, venenation, venene, veneniferous, venom.*

snap'ping hip. Slipping of the hip joint with a snap due to displacement over the great trochanter of a tendinous band.

snare (snār) [A.S. *sneare,* noose]. Device for excision of polyps, tumors, etc., by tightening wire loops around them.

sneeze (snēz) [M.E. *snesen,* from A.S *fneōsan,* to pant]. 1. To expel air forcibly through the nose and mouth by spasmodic contraction of muscles of expiration due to irritation of nasal mucosa. 2. The act of sneezing.

RS: *sternutation, sternutator, sternutatory.*

Snellen's chart (snĕl'ĕn). One used for testing visual acuity.

S's. reflex. Congestion of ear on same side resulting when distal end of the divided auriculotemporal nerve is stimulated.

snore (snōr) [A.S. *snora,* snoring]. 1. To breathe noisily during sleep, due to vibration of the uvula and soft palate. 2. Noisy breathing in sleep or coma. SYN: *rhonchus, stertor.*

snoring râle (snōr'ing rahl). A sonorous râle, low in pitch, resembling a snore.

snow blind'ness. Irritation of the conjunctiva caused by reflection of the sun on the snow.

SYM: Photophobia, blepharospasm, burning pain in the eyes, hyperemia or temporary blindness. SYN: *chionablepsia, niphablepsia, niphotyphlosis.*

snuffles (snŭf'ls) [Middle Dutch *snuffen,* to snuff]. Obstructed nasal breathing with discharge from the nasal mucosa, esp. in infants, chiefly in congenital syphilis.

soap (sōp) [A.S. *sāpe,* soap]. A cleansing chemical compound formed by an alkali acting on a fatty acid; example: sodium stearate, $NaC_{18}H_{35}O_2$. SEE: *saponification.*

Castile soap is made by saponifying olive oil with sodium hydroxide, and contains mainly sodium oleate, $NaC_{18}H_{33}O_2$.

s., green. SEE: *soap, soft medicinal.*

s. liniment. USP. Liquid opodeldoc. A solution of soap and camphor in alcohol and water.

ACTION AND USES: Stimulant and rubefacient.

s., soft medicinal. SYN: *green soap.* A liquid soap made by saponification of vegetable oils excluding coconut oil and palm kernel oil and without removal of glycerine. Used in the treatment of skin diseases.

s. suds enema. One given so that the irritating action of the soap will stimulate bowel motion. SEE: *enema.*

sob. 1. To weep with convulsive movements of the chest. 2. A cry or wail resulting from a sudden convulsive inspiration accompanied by spasmodic closure of glottis.

sociology (sō-sĭ-ŏl'ō-jĭ) [L. *socius,* companion, + G. *logos,* a study]. Science of the forms, institutions and functions of human groups.

sociomedical. Pertaining to sociology and medicine, esp. the interrelationships between the two.

socket (sŏk'ĕt) [M.E. *soket,* a spearhead]. A hollow in a joint or part for another corresponding organ, as a bone socket or an eye socket.

s., dry. Alveolitis following tooth extraction characterized by extreme pain but without suppuration.

s., tooth. A dental alveolus of the maxilla or mandible; a cavity which contains the root of a tooth.

soda (sō'dă) [Middle Latin *soda,* headache]. 1. Term loosely applied to various salts of sodium, esp. to caustic soda (sodium hydroxide) and baking soda (sodium bicarbonate). SEE: *sodium.* 2. Short for soda water, which is water charged with carbon dioxide.

s. ash. Commercial sodium carbonate.

s., baking. Sodium bicarbonate.

s., caustic. Sodium hydroxide.

s. lime. A white granular substance consisting of a mixture of calcium hydroxide and sodium hydroxide or potassium hydroxide or both. Used to absorb carbon dioxide.

s., lye. Sodium hydroxide.

s., niter. Nitrate of soda.

s., washing. SYN: sal soda, sodium carbonate.

s. water. A solution of carbon dioxide under pressure; carbonic acid.

sodic (sō'dĭk) [Middle Latin *soda,* headache]. Relating to or containing soda or sodium.

sodio-. Prefix denoting a *compound containing sodium.*

sodium (sō'dĭ-ŭm) [Middle Latin *soda,* headache]. SYMB: Na. At. wt. 22.9898, at. no. 11. Sodium constitutes approximately 0.15% of elements of the body. Sodium (Na^+), K^+, Ca^{++}, and Mg^{++} constitute the principal cations of the body, their relative concentration determining the integrity of cell membranes and the bioelectric potentials of tissues. Na^+ is the principal cation found in extracellular fluids.

FUNCTIONS: Sodium salts are found in the fluids of the body, serum, blood, and lymph, and in the tissues, the concentration being lower in the tissues. They are necessary to preserve a balance bet. calcium and potassium to maintain normal heart action and the equilibrium of the body. They regulate osmotic pressure in the cells and fluids, act as an ion balance in tissues, produce a buffer action in the blood, and guard against an excessive loss of water from the tissues.

DEFICIENCY SYM: Weakness, nerve disorders, loss of weight, "salt hunger," miner's cramps, disturbed digestion.

SOURCES: SEE: *names of foods.*

s. acetate. USP. Colorless, odorless, translucent crystals, saline in taste and soluble in water. $NaC_2H_3O_2$.

ACTION AND USES: Diuretic and laxative.

s. aleurate. The monosodium salt of allyl isopropyl barbituric acid.

ACTION AND USES: Oral or rectal adm. as preanesthesia medication.

s. amytal. The monosodium salt of isoamylethylbarbituric acid.

ACTION AND USES: Sedative and hypnotic in control of insomnia; preliminary to surgical anesthesia and in labor.

s. barbital. SEE: *barbital.*

s. benzoate. USP. A white, odorless powder with sweet taste.

ACTION AND USES: Internally in treatment of rheumatism and as a food preservative.

s. bicarbonate. USP. White, odorless powder with saline taste. $NaHCO_3$.

ACTION AND USES: Parenterally for acidosis. Externally, mild alkaline wash.

INCOMPATIBILITIES: Acids, acid salts, ammonium chloride, lime water, ephedrine, hydrochloride, iron chloride.

s. biphosphate. USP. Sodium acid phosphate.

ACTION AND USES: To render urine acid thereby assisting the action of urotropin.

s. bisulfite. Granular or crystalline powder, sulfurous taste and odor, soluble in water.

ACTION AND USES: Gastric and intestinal fermentation.

s. borate. USP. Borax.

ACTION AND USES: Antiseptic and astringent.

s. bromide. USP. NaBr. White crystalline powder with saline taste.

ACTION AND USES: Nerve sedative and cerebral depressant.

INCOMPATIBILITIES: Tincture ferric chloride.

s. cacodylate. USP. The sodium salt of cacodylic acid.

ACTION AND USES: Similar to arsenic.

s. carbonate. USP. Na_2CO_3. White crystalline powder (washing soda).

ACTION AND USES: An alkali employed chiefly in alkaline baths.

s. chloride. USP. NaCl. Common salt.

ACTION AND USES: In preparation of normal saline solution, emetic and to add flavor to foods.

INCOMPATIBILITIES: Silver nitrate.

s. citrate. White granular powder, saline in taste and soluble in water.

ACTION AND USES: Diuretic and antilithic.

s. fluoride. White crystalline powder, saline in taste, soluble in 25 parts of water. USP. NaF.

ACTION AND USES: In drinking water and in solution for local application to teeth for prevention of dental caries. Commercially, in etching glassware, for eradication of rats, insects, ants, and other pests.

POISONING: SYM: Optical: conjunctivitis; oral: retching, vomiting, nausea, later cardiac weakness, kidney disturbances, and interference with coagulation of blood.

F. A. TREATMENT: In addition to washing affected areas, precipitate by addition of soluble calcium salts, as lime water, calcium gluconate, calcium lactate. Give emetics and soothing drinks, as milk, cream, egg whites, etc.

s. hexametaphosphate. A salt of metaphosphoric acid.

ACTION AND USES: Water softener, antiperspirant, and in dermatoses due to oil or soap irritation.

s. hydroxide. A whitish solid; soluble in water, making a clear solution. USP. NaOH.

USES: Antacid and caustic. In the laundry and in commercial compounds, in cleaning sink traps, toilets, etc., and in the preparation of soap.

ACTION: Use great care in handling it as it rapidly destroys organic tissues.

POISONING: SEE: *potassium hydroxide.*

s. hyposulfite. Same as s. thiosulfate.

s. iodide. USP. NaI. A salt resembling in appearance and action potassium iodide.

s. morrhuate. The sodium salt of the fatty acids, found in cod-liver oil. USP.

USES: For the obliteration of varicose veins.

s. nitrate. SEE: *saltpeter, Chile.*

s. nitrite. USP. $NaNO_2$. White crystalline powder, characteristic properties of nitroglycerine; effects more lasting.

s. oleate. A white, soft mass; sodium salt of oleic acid.

s. pentothal. SEE: *pentothal s.*

s. phosphate. USP. $Na_2HPO_4.12H_2O$. White crystalline powder.

ACTION AND USES: Similar to magnesium sulfate, but with less disagreeable taste.

s. phosphate effervescent. USP. A mixture of sodium phosphate, sodium bicarbonate, and tartaric acid.

s. salicylate. USP. White powder or scales with sweet saline taste. $C_7H_5NaO_3$.

ACTION AND USES: As an analgesic and antipyretic.

INCOMPATIBILITIES: Caffeine citrate, caffeine sodium benzoate.

s. sulfate (Glauber's salt). USP. Resembles magnesium sulfate in appearance and action.

s. tartrate. $Na_2C_4H_4O_6 . 2 H_2O$. White soluble crystals.

USES: Diuretic and laxative.

s. taurocholate. Extract of bile from carnivora; a yellowish gray powder soluble in water.

USES: Cholagogue.

s. thiocyanate. NaSCN. A sodium salt.

USES: Reducing high blood pressure, relieving insomnia due to hypertension, in narcotic addiction, and in crises of tabes dorsalis.

s. thiosulfate. USP. White crystalline substance, having a cooling taste.

ACTION AND USES: Externally, for ringworm, in dermatitis, to remove stains of iodine. Intravenously, as an antidote for metallic poisons.

s. valerianate. White crystalline powder with faint odor and taste of valerian. Soluble in water and of unctuous feel.

USES: Nerve tonic.

sodokosis (sŏd-ō-kō'sĭs) [Japanese, rat poison]. Infectious febrile disease caused by infection from bite of a rat. SYN: *ratbite fever, sodoku.*

sodoku (sō-do'koo) [Japanese, rat poison]. Infectious febrile disease due to rat bite. SYN: *ratbite fever, sodokosis.*

sodomy (sŏd'ō-mĭ) [O.Fr. *Sodome*, Sodom]. Anal coitus, usually bet. males; bestiality (*concubitus cum bestia*), and pederasty* (*concubitus cum persona ejusdem sexus*).

Soemmering's bone. Marginal process of malar (zygomatic) bone.

S's. foramen. The fovea centralis, *q.v.*

S's. spot. The macula lutea of the retina.

soft or **convalescent diet.** Fish, egg and cheese dishes, chicken, cereals, bread, toast, butter, nothing not soft, semisolid or liquid. No red meats, vegetables or fruits having seeds or thick skins. No cellulose, raw fruits, or salads.

s. diet, cold. Suitable for tonsillectomies. All forms of milk and cream, iced cocoa, coffee and tea iced, gelatin, junket, custard, strained cereals and fruits if not seeded, such as berries. No fruit juices unless ordered.

s. d., light. Medical liquids; cream soups, strained; toast; cream; poached or coddled eggs; mashed potatoes; carrots, peas, and spinach purées; gelatins; junkets; custards; stewed fruits; soufles; jellies; gruels; cereals if strained; ice cream; sherbets.

s. d., l., surgical. Fluids plus thick water gruels, toast, stewed fruits if strained but no seeded fruits.

s. d., modified. Small meals, frequent feedings, gradual additions to full liquid diet—crackers, baked potato, soft cooked egg, cream of wheat, farina, strained oatmeal, applesauce, puréed pears, jelly, simple desserts; later, cottage cheese, puréed vegetables, minced tender meat.

soft (sŏft) [A.S. *sōfte*]. Not hard, firm or solid.

s. palate. The soft post. part of the palate. Syn: *palatum molle, velum pendulum palati.*

s. sore. A venereal sore, not due to syphilis, caused by Ducrey's bacillus. Syn: *chancroid.*

softening (sŏf'ĕn-ĭng) [A.S. *sōfte,* soft]. Process of becoming soft. Syn: *malacia, mollities.* RS: *words ending in malacia.*

s., anemic. White softening of the brain from lack of blood.

s. of bones. Osteomalacia.

s. of brain. Paresis with progressive dementia. Syn: *encephalomalacia.*

s. colliquative. The liquefying of tissues.

s., gray. S. of the brain with absorption of fat following yellow s.

s. of heart. Myomalacia cordis.

s., hemorrhagic. Red softening, *q.v.*

s., mucoid. Myxomatous degeneration.

s., red. S. of the brain with bleeding into necrosed portions.

s. of stomach. Gastromalacia.

s., white. Same as anemic s.

s., yellow. S. of brain in a late stage with deposit of changing pigment and fatty degeneration of cells.

sol (sŏl, sōl) [G. *sole,* salt water]. 1. Abbr. for *solution.* 2. State of a colloid system in which the dispersion medium or solvent forms a continuous phase in which the particles of the solute are dispersed forming a fluid mass. It is called a *hydrosol* if dispersion medium is a liquid, *aerosol* if a gas.

solanine (sō'lăn-ĭn). A poisonous narcotic alkaloid obtained from potatoes.

solar (sō'lar) [L. *sol,* sun]. Pert. to the sun or its rays.

s. plexus. The celiac plexus behind the stomach and bet. the suprarenal glands, and consisting of 2 large ganglia, the *celiac* and *sup. mesenteric ganglia,* from which sympathetic fibers pass to visceral organs.

s. therapy. Treatment with the sun's rays. Syn: *heliotherapy.*

solargentum (sol-ar-jĕn'tŭm). A brand of mild silver protein, containing 19-23% colloidal silver.

solarium (sō-lā'rĭ-ŭm) [L. from *sol,* sun]. A room designed for heliotherapy or for the application of artificial light.

solation (sō-lā'shŭn) [L. *sol,* sun]. In colloidal chemistry, the transformation of a gel into a sol.

solbisminol (sŏl-bĭz'mĭn-ōl). An antisyphilitic drug which can be taken by mouth.

soldier's heart. See: *asthenia, neurocirculatory.*

sole (sōl) [A.S. *sole,* from L. *solum,* ground]. Syn: *planta.* 1. Underpart of the foot. 2. The portion of a motor end plate at termination of a motor nerve fiber which is directly adjacent to the contractile substance of a muscle fiber. Here are usually aggregated a large number of muscle nuclei. See: *antithenar, thenar.*

s. reflex. Syn: *plantar reflex.* Contraction of muscles when tickling the sole.

soleus (sō'lē-ŭs) [L. *solea,* sole of foot]. A flat, broad muscle of calf of leg. See: *Table of Muscles in Appendix.*

solid (sŏl'ĭd) [L. *solidus,* a solid]. 1. Not gaseous, hollow, or liquid. 2. A substance not gaseous, liquid, or hollow.

s. carbon dioxide therapy. Therapeutic application of solid carbon dioxide. See: *refrigeration.*

solipsism (so'lip-sizm) [L. *solus,* alone, + *ipse,* one's self]. The theory that the self may know only its own feelings and changes and there then is only subjective reality.

solitary (sŏl'ĭ-tăr-ĭ). Alone; single or existing separately.

s. lymph nodules or follicles. Small spherical lymphatic nodules found in lamina propria of small and large intestine.

solubility (sŏl"ū-bĭl'ĭ-tĭ) [L. *solubilis,* from *solvere,* to dissolve]. Capability of being dissolved.

soluble (sŏl'ū-bl) [L. *solubilis,* from *solvere,* to dissolve]. Able to be dissolved.

solum tympani. The floor of the tympanic cavity.

solute (sŏl'ūt) [L. *solutus,* dissolved]. The substance that is dissolved in a solution.

solution (sō-lū'shŭn) [L. *solutio,* a dissolving]. 1. Liquid containing dissolved substance. 2. Process by which a solid is homogeneously mixed with a fluid, or a solid or gas, so that the dissolved substances cannot be distinguished from the resultant fluid. 3. Mixture so formed. 4. Termination of a disease.

The liquid in which the substances are dissolved is called the *solvent** and the substance dissolved, the *solute.** The strength represents the amt. of substance dissolved, represented by ratio, percentage, or grains to the ounce.

s., buffer. A solution of a weak acid and its salt (for ex., carbonic acid sodium bicarbonate) of importance in maintaining a constant *p*H, esp. of the blood.

s., colloidal. That in which the solute is suspended and not dissolved, such as gelatin, albumin.

s., hypertonic. One which has a greater osmotic pressure than that of cells or body fluids; a solution which draws water out of cells thus inducing plasmolysis.

Ex: A concentrated solution of sodium chloride.

s., hypotonic. A solution having an osmotic pressure *less* than that of cells or body fluids; a solution which will cause water to enter cells thus inducing turgor, and possibly hemolysis.

Ex: A sodium chloride solution containing less than 0.9 Gm. of NaCl in each 100 ml. of water.

s., isohydric. A solution having the same hydrogen-ion concentration or *p*H as another.

s., isosmotic. An isotonic solution, *q.v.*

s., isotonic. One which has the same osmotic pressure as that of body cells or fluids.

Ex: A sodium chloride solution containing 0.9 Gm. of NaCl in each 100 ml. of water.

s., Locke-Ringer's. A buffered isotonic solution containing sodium chloride, 9.0 Gm.; potassium chloride, 0.42 Gm.; calcium chloride, 0.24 Gm.; sodium bicarbonate, 0.5 Gm.; magnesium chloride, 0.2 Gm.; dextrose, 0.5 Gm.; distilled water, to make 1000 ml.

s., molar. One containing a gram molecular weight or mole of the reagent dissolved in one liter (1000 ml.) of solution. Designated 1M.

s., normal. One containing one gram equivalent weight of reagent in one liter (1000 ml.) of solution. Designated 1N.

s., normal saline. An isotonic saline solution. SEE: *solution, isotonic.*

s., physiological saline. An isotonic solution of sodium chloride. SEE: *solution, isotonic.*

s., Ringer's. A solution containing chlorides of sodium, calcium, and potassium in most favorable concentration. For mammals it contains sodium chloride, 8.6 Gm.; calcium chloride, 0.33 Gm.; potassium chloride, 0.3 Gm.; distilled water to make one liter (1000 ml.).

s., saline. A solution of a salt; usually sodium chloride. SEE: *s., isotonic; s., physiological saline; s., normal saline.*

s., saturated. A solution that contains all the solute it can dissolve. This limit is called the *saturation* point.

s., seminormal. Abbr. 0.5N or N/2. A solution containing one-half of a gram equivalent weight of reagent in one liter (1000 ml.) of solution.

s., standard. A solution containing a definite amount of a substance as a normal solution.

s., supersaturation. S. in which the saturation point is reached, but when heated it is possible to dissolve more of the solute.

s., test. Abbr. T.S. A reagent solution; one used in performing a particular test.

s., Tyrode's. A modified Ringer's solution containing, in addition, a small amount of *magnesium-chloride* and *acid* and *sodium phosphates.*

s., volumetric. Abbr. V.S. A standard solution containing a definite amount (1/2, 1/10, etc.) gram-equivalent of a substance in one liter (1000 ml.) of solution. Used in volumetric analysis.

solv. [L.]. Abbr. of *solve,* meaning *dissolve.*

solvate (sŏl′vāt). A compound formed by reaction between solvent and solute.

solvation (sŏl-vā′shŭn). The formation of a solvate.

solvent (sŏl′vĕnt) [L. *solvens,* from *solvere,* to dissolve]. 1. Producing a solution; dissolving. 2. A liquid holding another substance in solution. 3. A liquid which reacts with a solvent bringing it into solution.

soma (sō′mă) [G. *sōma,* body]. 1. Body tissues distinguished from germinal or reproductive ones. 2. The body without its appendages. 3. PSY: The body as differentiated from the psyche.

somasthenia (sō-măs-thē′nĭ-ă) [G. *sōma,* body, + *astheneia,* weakness]. A condition of chronic bodily weakness. SYN: *somatasthenia.*

somatasthenia (sō-măt-ăs-thē′nĭ-ă) [" + *astheneia,* weakness]. Chronic bodily weakness usually with low blood pressure, but *not* neurasthenia. SYN: *somasthenia.*

somatesthesia (sō-măt-ĕs-thē′zĭ-ă) [" + *aisthēsis,* sensation]. The consciousness of the body; bodily sensation.

somatic (sō-măt′ĭk) [G. *sōma,* body]. 1. Pertaining to nonreproductive cells or tissues. 2. Pert. to the body. 3. Pert. to structures of the body wall, *e.g.* skeletal muscles (*somatic musculature*) in contrast to structures associated with the viscera, *e.g.* visceral muscles (*splanchnic musculature*).

somatoceptors (sō-măt-ō-sĕpt′ors). Term applied to proprioceptors and exteroceptors collectively.

somatochrome (sō-măt′ō-krōm) [G. *sōma,* body, + *chrōma,* color]. Term applied to neurons which possess abundant cytoplasm containing Nissl bodies. SEE: *gyrochrome* and *stichochrome.*

somatology (sō-mă-tol′ō-jĭ) [G. *sōma,* body, + *logos,* a study]. Comparative study of structure, functions and development of the human body.

somatopathic (sō-măt-ō-păth′ĭk) [" + *pathos,* disease]. Organically ill, as distinguished from neuropathic or psychopathic diseases.

somatoplasm (sō-măt′ō-plăzm) [G. *sōma,* body, + *plasma,* a thing formed]. The protoplasm of all the body cells as distinguished from that of the germ plasm; the soma.

somatopleure (sō-măt′ō-plūr) [G. *sōma,* body, + *pleura,* a side]. The lateral and ventral body wall of an embryo consisting of the outer ectoderm and a layer of somatic mesoderm underlying it. It continues beyond the embryo as the amnion and chorion.

somatopsychic (sō-măt-ō-sī′kĭk) [G. *soma,* body, + *psyche,* mind]. Pert. to both body and mind.

somatopsychosis (sō″mă-tō-sī-kō′sĭs) [" + " + *-ōsis,* condition]. Any mental disorder which is a symptom of a bodily disease.

somatoscopy (sō-măt-ŏs′kō-pĭ) [G. *sōma,* body, + *skopein,* to examine]. Physical examination of the body.

somatotrophic (sō″măt-ō-trŏf′ĭk) [" + *tropos,* a turning]. 1. Having selective attraction for, or influencing body cells. 2. Stimulating growth.

s. hormone. Abbr. STH. Hormone produced by ant. lobe of hypophysis which regulates growth of body.

somatotype (sō′mă-tō-tīp). A particular build or type of body.

s. theory. A theory that certain body types (endomorphy, mesomorphy, ectomorphy) are associated with certain personality types.

somatropin (sō-măt′rō-pĭn) [G. *sōma,* body, + *tropos,* a turning]. The anterior pituitary lobe's growth-stimulating principle.

somesthesia (som-es-the′sĭ-ă) [G. *sōma,* body, + *aisthēsis,* sensation]. Awareness of bodily sensations. SYN: *somatesthesia.*

somesthetic (sō-mĕs-thĕt′ĭk) [" + *aisthēsis,* sensation]. Pert. to sensations and sensory structures of the body.

s. area. The region in the cortex in which lie the terminations of the axons of general sensory conduction paths.

s. path. General sensory conduction path leading to the cortex.

somite (sō′mīt) [G. *sōma,* body]. 1. Embryonic blocklike segment formed on either side of the neural tube and its underlying notochord. 2. Any one of the embryonic segments.

Each somite gives rise to a *muscle mass* supplied by a spinal nerve and each pair gives rise to a *vertebra.*

somnambulism (sŏm-năm′bū-lĭzm) [L. *somnus,* sleep, + *ambulāre,* to walk]. 1. A form of hysteria in which behavior and purposeful actions are not subsequently remembered. 2. Sleepwalking, an affection that prompts the sleeping person to perform, unconsciously, acts that naturally belong to the waking state. SYN: *noctambulism, q.v.*

The term has a more comprehensive meaning in psychiatry than that of noctambulism.

somnambulist (sŏm-năm′bū-lĭst). One who is subject to sleepwalking.

somnarium (sŏm-nā′rĭ-ŭm) [L. *somnus,* sleep]. A sanitarium in which sleep therapy is employed in the treatment of neuroses.

somnifacient (sŏm-nĭ-fā′shĕnt) [" + *facere,* to make]. 1. Producing sleep. SYN: *hypnotic.* 2. A medicine producing sleep. SYN: *soporific, q.v.*

somniferous (sŏm-nĭf′ĕr-ŭs) [" + *ferre,* to bear]. Sleep-producing; pert. to that which promotes sleep.

somnific (sŏm-nĭf′ĭk) [" + *facere,* to make]. Producing sleep.

somniloquist (sŏm-nĭl′ō-kwĭst). One who talks in his sleep.

somniloquy (sŏm-nĭl′ō-kwĭ) [" + *loqui,* to speak]. Act of talking during sleep or in a hypnotic condition.

somnipathy (sŏm-nĭp′ă-thĭ) [" + G. *pathos,* disease]. 1. Any disorder of sleep. 2. Hypnotism.

somnocinematograph (sŏm-nō-sĭn-ĕ-măt′ō-grăf) [" + G. *kinema,* motion, + *graphein,* to write]. Device for recording motions of those who are asleep.

somnolence (sŏm′nō-lĕns) [L. *somnolentia,* sleepiness]. Prolonged drowsiness or a condition resembling trance which may continue for a number of days; sleepiness.

somnolent (sŏm′nō-lĕnt) [L. *somnolentus,* sleepy]. Sleepy; drowsy.

somnolentia (sŏm-nō-lĕn′shĭ-ă) [L. *somnolentia,* sleepiness]. 1. Drowsiness. 2. The sleep of drunkenness in which the faculties are only partially in repose.

sone. A unit of loudness.

sonic boom (sŏn′ĭk) [L. *sonus,* sound]. Noise caused by shock waves from the nose of an airborne object traveling at a speed in excess of the speed of sound. When the waves hit the ground they may break windows and affect the hearing.

sonitus (sŏn′ĭ-tŭs) [L. *sonitus,* sound]. Subjective noises in the ear. SYN: *tinnitus aurium, q.v.*

sonometer (sō-nŏm′ĕtĕr) [L. *sonus,* sound, + G *metron,* a measure]. 1. Device for testing the hearing. 2. Device to cause sound for production of anesthesia; used by dentists.

sonorous (sō-nō′rŭs) [L. *sonor,* sound]. Giving forth a loud and rounded sound.

s. rale. A dry or low pitched rale often caused by vibration of mucous secretion in a bronchus.

sophistication (sō-fĭs-tĭ-kā′shŭn) [G. *sophistikos,* deceitful]. Adulteration of any substances.

sopor (sō′por) [L. *sopor,* deep sleep]. Deep, lethargic sleep. SYN: *stupor.*

soporific (sō-por-ĭf′ĭk) [" + *facere,* to make]. 1. Inducing sleep. 2. Narcotic; a drug producing sleep.

soporose, soporous (sō′por-ōs, -ŭs) [L. *sopor,* deep sleep]. Marked by or resembling sound sleep or coma.

sorbefacient (sor″bē-fā′shĕnt) [L. *sorbere,* to suck, + *facere,* to make]. Causing or that which causes or promotes absorption.

sordes (sor′dēz) [L. *sordere,* to be dirty]. 1. Foul, brown crusts or accumulations on the teeth and about the lips from foul stomach or secretions of the mouth in low forms of fever. 2. Filth.

NP: A solution of half glycerin or mineral oil and half lemon juice carefully applied with applicators will remove the condition and prevent further accumulation.

sore (sōr) [A.S. *sār,* sore]. 1. Tender; painful. 2. A tender or painful ulcer or lesion of the skin.

s., bed. Gangrene of skin due to pressure. SYN: *decubitus, q.v., pressure sore.*

s., canker. SYN: *aphthous ulcer, aphthous stomatitis.* A small lesion of the mucous membrane of the mouth. They often accompany a number of systemic conditions. Cause unknown.

s., cold. Blister on the lips. SYN: *herpes* facialis.*

s., hard. Syphilitic chancre,* primary lesion of syphilis.

s., Oriental. SYN: *tropical sore, Delhi boil.* Cutaneous leishmaniasis.

s., pressure. A bedsore, *q.v.*

s., soft venereal. Soft, nonsyphilitic, venereal sore occurring on the genitalia. SYN: *chancroid.**

s. throat. Any inflammation of the tonsils, pharynx or larynx.

s. t., diphtheritic. Croupous tonsillitis.

s. t., quinsy. Peritonsillar abscess. SEE: *quinsy.*

s. t., septic. Severe, epidemic, pseudomembranous inflammation of fauces and tonsils caused by the hemolytic streptococcus.

s. t., spotted. Follicular tonsillitis.

s. t., ulcerated. Pharyngitis with formation of gangrenous patches.

s., tropical. SEE: *Oriental sore.*

s., venereal. SEE: *soft venereal sore.*

soroche (sō-rō′kā, or skā). Mountain sickness, esp. that occurring in the Andes.

sororiation (so-ror-ĭ-ā′shŭn) [L. *sororiāre,* to increase together]. Growth of the breasts at puberty.

s.o.s. Abbr. for *si opus sit,* if necessary or required.

souffle (soof′fl) [Fr. *souffle,* a puff]. A soft blowing sound heard in auscultation; a bruit; an auscultatory murmur.

s., cardiac. Heart murmur.

s., fetal. The soft blowing sound heard over the location of the umbilical cord of the fetus *in utero* and synchronous with the fetal heartbeat during late pregnancy.

s., funic, s., funicular, s., umbilical. Same as fetal souffle.

s., splenic. Sound heard over spleen in malaria.

s., uterine. Sound caused by blood entering dilated arteries of uterus in last months of pregnancy; synchronous with maternal pulse. It is more frequent than the fetal souffle and is heard as a loud blowing murmur along left side of uterus, and frequently all over it. An enlarged uterus may cause it. That of pregnancy is variable, whereas other forms are constant.

sound (sownd) [L. *sonus,* sound]. 1. Auditory sensations produced by vibrations; noise. It is measured in decibels.

which is the logarithm of the intensity of sound; thus 20 d. represents not twice 10 d., but ten times as much. Conversation represents 90 d's. Exposure to 130 d. for ten minutes in any 24 hrs. should call for a weekly hearing test. A 90 d. noise over an extended period may permanently injure one's hearing. SEE: *decibel, noise, sonic boom.* 2. A form of vibrational energy that gives rise to auditory sensations. SEE: *sonic boom, cochlea, ear, organ of Corti.* 3. Healthy, not diseased. 4. Heart sounds. 5. [Fr. *sonder,* to probe]. Instrument for introduction into a cavity or canal for diagnosis or treatment. SEE: *diastole, systole, sonic boom.*

s., anasarcous. Moist sound heard on auscultation when skin is edematous.

s., blowing. Organic murmur as of air from an aperture expelled with moderate force.

s., bottle. Noise as of fluid in a bottle. SYN: *amphoric* murmur.*

s's., breath. Respiratory sounds heard on auscultation of the chest. In a normal chest they are classified as *vesicular, tracheal,* and *bronchovesicular.*

s., bronchial. Sound not heard in normal lung but occurring in pulmonary disease indicating infiltration and solidification of lung.

s's., bronchovesicular. A mixture of bronchial and vesicular sounds.

s., cracked-pot. A tympanic resonance heard over pulmonary cavities.

s., fetal heart. One made by the fetal heart.

s., friction. One produced by rubbing together of 2 inflamed mucous surfaces.

s's., heart. The two sounds "lubb" and "dupp" resulting from closure of atrioventricular and semilunar valves. SEE: *heart, auscultation of.*

s., to and fro. Rasping friction sounds of pericarditis.

s., tracheal. That normally heard over the trachea of larynx.

s., tubular. Sound heard over the trachea, or large bronchi.

s., vesicular. Sound heard over entire lung during inspiration resulting from distention of alveoli with air.

sound, words pert. to: amphoric, anacamptics, aphthongia, aspirate, auscultation, bell-metal resonance, bourdonnement, capotement, caverniloquy, clang, clapotage, clapotement, heart, hyperacusis, murmur, râle, resonance, souffle, stridulous, succussion, uterus.

soybean (soi'bēn) [Japanese, *shōyū*]. The seed of several varieties of glycine. Contains proteins and a fixed oil (soya oil) and very little starch.

COOKED: 100 gm. Calories: 118. Other values: 9.8 gm. protein; 5.1 gm. fat; 60 mg. calcium; 690 I.U. vitamin A; 10.1 gm. carbohydrate.

sp. Abbr. for 1. L. *spiritus,* spirit. 2. *Species.*

spa. A mineral spring, esp. one having healing properties.

space (spās) [L. *spatium,* space]. An area, region, or segment.

RS: *chondroporosis, circumscribed.*

s., axillary. The axilla or space beneath the arm.

s., circumlental. Space between equator of lens and ciliary body.

s., epidural. S. bet. the dura mater and vertebral periosteum, or bet. the bones of the cranium and the dura mater, assumed to be lymph spaces.

s's. (of) Fontana. Spaces in scleral meshwork in angle of iris through which aqueous humor passes from anterior chamber to canal of Schlemm.

s., interfascial. Space of Tenon, *q.v.*

s., intervillous. Space in placenta which develops from early chorionic trophoblast. It forms a blood sinus in which chorionic villi of fetus are bathed in maternal blood received from uterine vessels.

s., Nuel's. Space bet. outer hair cells and rods in the organ of Corti.

s., perforated. S. pierced by blood vessels at base of brain. SYN: *substantia perforata.*

s's., perivascular. SYN: *Spaces of Virchow-Robin.* Spaces within adventitia of larger blood vessels of the brain. They communicate with subarachnoid space.

s., plantar. S. (1 of 4) bet. fascial layers of the foot. When the foot is infected, pus may be found here.

s., popliteal. S. back of knee joint containing the popliteal artery and vein, and small sciatic and popliteal nerves.

s., prezonular. The ant. portion of the posterior chamber of the eye.

s., Prussak's. S. in tympanum behind Shrapnell's membrane.

s., retropharyngeal. SYN: *retropharyngeal fascial cleft.* Space behind pharynx separating prevertebral from visceral fascia.

s's. subarachnoid. SYN: *intraleptomeningeal spaces.* S. bet. the pia mater and arachnoid containing the cerebrospinal fluid. The spaces, esp. in the cranium, are transversed by numerous trabeculae.

s., subdural. Narrow space between dura and the arachnoid.

s., suprasternal. SYN: *space of Burns.* Triangular space immediately above sternum between layers of deep cervical fascia.

s., Tenon's. Lymph s. bet. the sclera and Tenon's capsule.

s., thenar. SYN: *lateral palmar space.* A deep fascial space in the hand lying anterior to adductor pollicis muscle.

s., tissue. Any space within tissues not lined with epithelium and containing tissue fluid.

s's., zonular. Spaces within zonule (suspensory ligament of lens).

spaghetti (spă-gĕt'ĭ) [Italian *spaghetto,* little cord]. COOKED: 100 gm. Calories: 148. Other values: 0.5 gm. protein; 0.1 gm. fat; 65 mg. calcium; 30.1 gm. carbohydrate.

Spanish fly (spăn'ĭsh flī). A strong rubefacient and blistering agent. SYN: *cantharides.*

spanogyny (spăn-ŏj'ĭ-nĭ) [G. *spanos,* scarce, + *gynē,* a woman]. More males than females; decrease in female births.

sparer (spār'er) [A.S. *sparian,* to refrain]. A substance destroyed by catabolism, but which, nevertheless, lessens catabolic action upon other substances.

s., protein. Carbohydrates and fats, so designated because their presence in diet prevents tissue proteins from being utilized as a source of energy.

sparganosis (spar-gă-nō'sĭs). Infestation with a variety of *Sparganum.*

Sparganum. The plerocercoid larva of tapeworms, esp. those of the genus *Dibothriocephalus.*

S. mansoni. An elongated plerocercoid, 3-14 in. in length found in muscles and connective tissue, esp. that around eye. Common in Far East.

S. mansonoides. Species occasionally occurring in U.S. The adult form is unknown.

S. proliferum. Minute form infesting man and producing acne-like nodules. It is thought to proliferate by means of budlike outgrowths. Adult form unknown.

spargosis (spar-gō′sĭs) [G. *spargōsis,* swelling]. 1. Distention of the female breasts with milk. 2. Swelling or thickening of the skin. SYN: *elephantiasis.*

spark coil. Coil consisting of primary and secondary coils with an interrupted current passing through them. SYN: *induction coil.*

s. gaps. Arrangement of opposed points or surfaces, between which an electric spark may jump.

An adjustable gap between needle points or between spheres is used to measure high potentials.

s. g., quenched. A multiple spark gap with numerous electrodes about 0.3 mm. apart and equipped with a copper air-cooling device.

sparteine sulfate (spar′tēn) [L. *spartium,* broom]. The salt of an alkaloid obtained from Scoparius.

USES: Once regarded as of value in cardiac diseases, and as a diuretic. Also has limited usefulness in obstetrics to stimulate the uterus to contract.

spasm (spăzm) [G. *spasmos,* a convulsion]. An involuntary, sudden movement or convulsive muscular contraction.

Spasms may be *clonic* (characterized by alternate contraction and relaxation) or *tonic* (sustained). They may involve either visceral (smooth) muscle or skeletal (striated) muscle. When contractions are strong and painful, they are called *cramps.*

The effect depends upon the part affected. *Asthma* is assumed to be due to spasm of muscular coats of smaller bronchi; *renal colic* to spasm of muscular coat of the ureter.

TREATMENT: General measures to reduce tension, induce muscle relaxation and improve circulation. Specific measures include analgesics for relief of pain, physiotherapy (heat, diathermy, electrical therapy). Special orthopedic supports or braces are sometimes effective. For vascular spasm, chemical sympathectomy may give relief. Dietary and hygienic factors should be checked.

s., Bell's. Convulsive tic of the face.

s. center. Point in the oblongata where it meets the pons.

s., choreiform. Spasmodic movements resembling chorea.

s., clonic. Intermittent contractions and relaxation of muscles.

s. of esophagus. Paroxysmal dysphagia (inability to swallow), often associated with a sense of constriction in the chest. Little or no loss of flesh.

PROG: For life, good, but indefinite as regards duration.

TREATMENT: Search for exciting cause and remove. Treatment largely dietetic, hygienic and psychologic. Systematic passage of a bougie may be of great value. A mild electrical current may be applied through the bougie.

Characterized by intense dyspnea and occurs in spasmodic croup, true croup, ulceration of larynx, laryngismus stridulus, whooping cough, tetany, hysteria, hydrophobia, laryngeal crises of locomotor ataxia, when foreign bodies have lodged in larynx, when aneurysms or mediastinal tumors press on recurrent laryngeal nerve and irritate it.

s., habit. Spasms due to habit.

s., nodding. A psychogenic condition in adults, causing nodding of the head from clonic spasms of the sternomastoid muscles. A similar nodding in babies with head turning from side to side.

s., saltatory. Term employed to designate a condition allied to hysteria, in which a violent spasm seizes the muscles of the leg as soon as the feet touch the ground and as a result patient is thrown violently in the air.

s., tetanic. S. in which contractions continue for a time without interruption.

s., tonic. Continued involuntary contractions.

s., torsion. Spasm characterized by a turning of a part, esp. the turning of the body at the pelvis.

s., toxic. S. due to poison.

s., winking. *Spasmus nictitans, q.v.*

spasm, *words pert. to:* campospasm, cardiospasm, carpopedal, child crowing, chirospasm, Chvostek's sign, clonic, clonospasm, clonus, facial, habit, hypertonus, mobile, Raynaud's disease, spasticity, tetanus, tetany, tic douloureux, tonic spasm, trismus.

spasmatic, spasmodic (spăz-măt′ĭk, -mŏd′-ĭk) [G. *spasmos,* a convulsion]. Pert. to, like, or marked by, spasm. SEE: *cholepathia spastica.*

s. asthma. A. caused by spasm of the bronchioles.

s. croup. Laryngismus stridulus.

s. stricture. Temporary narrowing of any canal, as the urethra, due to localized spasmodic muscular contraction of its coat.

spasmology (spăz-mŏl′ō-jĭ) [" + *logos,* a study]. The study of spasms, their nature and cause.

spasmolygmus (spăz-mō-lĭg′mŭs) [" + *lygmos,* a sob]. 1. Spasmodic hiccup. 2. Spasmodic sobbing.

spasmolytic (spăz-mō-lĭt′ĭk) [" + *lysis,* dissolution]. Checking or that which checks spasms.

spasmomyxorrhea (spăz″mō-mĭks-or-re′ă) [" + *myxa,* mucus, + *rhoia,* flow]. Excessive secretion of intestinal mucus. SYN: *myxorrhea intestinalis.*

spasmophemia (spăz-mō-fē′mĭ-ă) [G. *spasmos,* convulsion, + *phēmē,* speech]. A spasmodic disorder of speech. SYN: *stuttering.*

spasmophilia (spăz-mō-fĭl′ĭ-ă) [" + *philein,* to love]. A tendency to tetany and convulsions; almost always associated with rickets.

spasmous (spăz′mŭs) [G. *spasmos,* convulsion]. Of the nature of a spasm.

spasmus (spăz′mŭs) [L. from G. *spasmos,* convulsion]. A spasm.

s. agitans. Paralysis agitans, *q.v.*

s. bronchialis. Bronchial asthma.

s. caninus. Spasm of face causing a constant grin. SYN: *risus sardonicus.*

s. coordinatus. Imitative or compulsive movements, as mimic tics or festination.

s. cynicus. Spasmodic contraction of muscles on both sides of the mouth.

s. Dubini. Rhythmic contractions, in rapid succession, of a group or groups of muscles, starting at an extremity or half of the face, and covering a large part or all of the body. PROG: Usually fatal. SYN: *electric chorea.*

s. glottidis. Spasm of larynx. SYN: *laryngismus stridulus.*

s. intestinorum. Pain in intestines. SYN: *enteralgia.*

s. nictitans. A winking movement of the eyelid.

s. nutans. Nodding spasm.

spastic (spăs'tĭk) [G. *spastikos,* convulsive]. Resembling or of the nature of spasms or convulsions.

s. gait. A stiff movement with toes seeming to catch together and to drag.

s. hemiplegia. Partial hemiplegia with spasmodic muscular contractions.

s. paralysis. Muscular rigidity accompanying partial paralysis. Usually due to a lesion involving upper motor neurons.

s. paraplegia. P. due to transverse lesions of the cord or sclerosis.

spasticity (spăs-tĭs'ĭ-tĭ) [G. *spastikos,* convulsive]. Hypertension of muscles causing stiff and awkward movements; the result of upper motor neuron lesion.

spatial (spā'shăl). Pertaining to space.

s. discrimination. Syn: *two-point discrimination.* Ability to perceive as separate points of contact the two blunt points of a compass when applied to the skin.

spatula (spăt'ū-lă) [L. *spatula,* a little sword]. Instrument for spreading or mixing semisolids.

It is usually flat, thin, somewhat flexible and shaped like a knife.

s., eye. Blades for separating lips of corneal wounds, arresting hemorrhage or for making pressure; sheet metal or rubber.

s., nasal. Device for holding mucous flaps in place or to guard against burning from cautery.

spay (spā) [Gael. *spoth,* castrate]. Surgical removal of ovaries, usually said of animals. See: *castration.*

specialist (spĕsh'ăl-ĭst) [L. *specialis,* special]. A physician who has had postgraduate training in and practices a particular branch of medicine such as surgery, internal medicine, pediatrics, obstetrics, etc.

species (spē'shēz) [L. *species,* a kind]. Biol: Category of classification, a subdivision between a genus and a variety in which all the individuals are almost identical.

specific (spē-sĭf'ĭk) [L. *specificus,* pert. to a kind]. 1. A remedy having a curative effect on a particular disease or symptom. 2. Pert. to a species. 3. A disease always caused by the same organism. 4. Restricted, explicit; not generalized.

s. dynamic action. Abbr. SDA. The increase in metabolic rate resulting from absorption of food. For protein it amounts to about 30%, for carbohydrates, 7%, and for fats, 4%.

s. gravity. Weight of a substance compared with an equal volume of water. Water is represented by 1.000.

specificity (spĕ-sĭ-fĭs'ĭ-tĭ) [L. *specificus,* pert. to a kind]. State of being specific; having a relation to a definite result, or to a particular cause.

specillum (spē-sĭl'lŭm) [L. *specillum*]. 1. Lens. 2. Button-shaped silver probe.

specimen (spĕs'ĭ-mĕn) [L. from *specere,* to look]. A part of a thing intended to show kind and quality of the whole, as a specimen of urine.

spectacles (spĕk'tăk-lz) [L. *spectāre,* to see]. Two lenses supported by a nose bridge and side pieces passing over the ears, to aid vision or protect the eyes.

spectro- [L.]. Combining form meaning *appearance, image, form, spectrum.*

spectrocolorimeter (spĕk-trō-kŭl-or-ĭm'ĕt-ĕr) [L. *spectrum,* image, + *color,* color, + G. *metron,* measure]. Device for detecting color blindness by isolating a single spectral color.

spectrograph (spĕk'trō-grăf) [" + G. *graphein,* to write]. An instrument designed to photograph spectra on a sensitive photographic plate.

spectrometer (spĕk-trŏm'ĕt-ĕr) [" + G. *metron,* a measure]. A spectroscope so constructed that angular deviation of a ray of light produced by a prism or by a diffraction grating thus indicates the wave length.

spectrophotometer (spĕk"trō-fō-tŏm'ĕt-ĕr) [" + G. *photos,* light, + *metron,* a measure]. Device for measuring amt. of color in a solution by comparison with the spectrum.

spectrophotometry (spĕk"trō-fō-tŏm'ĕt-rĭ) [" + " + *metron,* a measure]. Estimation of coloring matter in a solution by use of the spectroscope, or spectrophotometer.

spectropyrheliometer (spĕk"trō-pīr-hē-lĭ-ŏm'ĕ-tĕr) [" + G. *pyr,* fire, + *hēlios,* sun, + *metron,* a measure]. Instrument to measure solar radiation.

spectroscope (spĕk'tro-skōp) [" + *skopein,* to examine]. An instrument for separating radiant energy into its component frequencies or wave lengths by means of a prism or grating to form a correct spectrum for inspection.

spectroscopy (spĕk-trŏs'kō-pĭ) [" + G. *skopein,* to examine]. The branch of physical science that treats of the phenomena observed with the spectroscope, or those principles on which its action is based; also, the art of using the spectroscope.

spectrum (spĕk'trŭm) [L. image]. Charted band of wave lengths of electromagnetic vibrations obtained by refraction and diffraction of ray of white light.

The visible spectrum consists of the colors from red to violet with wave lengths of 3900 A° to 7700 A°. When white light is passed through a prism, the various colors, because of different wave lengths, are refracted to various degrees giving rise to the diverse colors of the rainbow. These are violet, indigo, blue, green, yellow, orange, and red.

The invisible spectrum includes rays less than 3900 A° in length (ultraviolet, roentgen or X, gamma, and cosmic rays) and those exceeding 7700 A° in length. The latter include: infrared rays, high frequency oscillations used in short and long wave diathermy, radio, hertzian and very long waves. These range in length from 7700 A° to 5,000,000 meters.

s., invisible. Spectral portion either below the red (infrared) or above the violet (ultraviolet), which is invisible to the eye, the waves being too long or too short to affect the retina.

s., visible. Portion of spectrum which is visible; consists of wavelengths between 3900 A° and 7000 A°.

speculum (spĕk'ū-lŭm) (pl. *specula*) [L. *speculum,* a mirror]. 1. Instrument for examination of canals. 2. Membrane separating ant. cornua of lateral ventricles of brain. Syn: *septum pellucidum.*

s., ear. Short, funnel-shaped tubes, tubular or bivalve; former preferable.

s., eye. Device for separating eyelids. Plated steel wire, plain, Von Graefe's, Steven's or Luer's most common.

speech. 1. Verbal expression of one's thought. 2. The act of uttering articulate words or sounds. 3. Words that are spoken. Primitively, certain crude sounds served as warnings or threats in much the same way as did facial and bodily expressions. As sounds became highly differentiated, each became associated, and gradually identified with a certain idea.

These word-symbols are a most valuable tool in ideation and thinking is very largely dependent on this internal speech. Further identifications have made possible visual symbols (written language); though primitive written language was entirely unrelated—a series of pictures and crude representations.

External speech requires the coordination of larynx, mouth, lips, chest, and abdominal muscles. These have no special enervation for speech but the upper neurons respond to complex motor pattern fields which convert the idea into suitable motor stimuli.

s. abnormalities. Speech failure results in *motor aphasia* in which the patient is speechless but there is no paralysis of muscles of articulation. Although unable to express his thoughts in words, the patient can still understand what he hears and reads.

Labialism is the excessive use of labial sounds.

Absent speech or hoarseness may be part of a hysteria; in epilepsy one finds a monotonous "woody" sound. Aphasias are also described as sensory.

When a word is heard, but the patient has no idea of its meaning, we speak of word-deafness. Similarly, word-blindness means that the written symbol might as well be a foreign word. This is sometimes called *alexia.** *Aphasia** in right-handed patients is classically referable to left-handed brain lesions, but the concept of centers for internal speech esp. is rather misleading. It is probably a diffuse cortical activity and countless minor distortions occur in addition to those mentioned. Chief of those not enumerated is the slurring speech of *paresis**; here letters and syllables are omitted without recognition of defect, and this further identifies the abnormality. *Dysarthria** describes any defect of articulation; muscular tone disturbances as seen in cerebellar disease, chorea, paralysis agitans, lenticular degeneration, multiple sclerosis producing jerky, monotonous or scanning speech.

Paralysis due to bilateral medullary pathology results in indistinct enunciation (mouthful speech) often entirely unintelligible. *Pseudobulbar palsy* (as in cases of double hemiplegia) adds a slow spastic characteristic. Peripheral nerve lesions, cleft palate, adenoids, myasthenia gravis, merely suggest the many possible modifications.

Stammering and stuttering are probably psychogenic.

Emotional values may be added to speech qualities; tremulousness and tension may render the voice high-pitched, irritating, or unsustained and broken. Emotional flattening may occur in the neuroses and psychoses. In the latter, diagnostic changes may occur in the stream of talk.

Slowing is common in all depressed states. When complete (mutism) it suggests the negativism esp. likely to occur in schizophrenia. Aphonic-like aphasia patients will find some means of communication.

Excessive talk flow is seen in mania and excited states generally. When merely voluble but relevant, it constitutes circumstantiality. If the goal ideal is lost, irrelevancy is associated with a "flight of ideas"—in extreme form a "word salad." The manner of speech often mirrors the mood.

Neologisms are words created by the patient, often of no apparent significance.

Stereotyped speech is constant repetition of a word or phrase. It should be distinguished from *perseveration* in which the repetition is against the intention or wishes of the patient.

*Amentia** invariably delays speech appearance and its faulty development is of diagnostic value. Its delayed or nonappearance may be referable to deafness (deaf-mutism). Childish indistinctness (*e. g.*, r's replaced by w's) may persist in feebleminded adults (*lalling-smudging*).

s., aphonic. Whispering.

s., ataxic. Defective speech resulting from muscular incoordination usually the result of cerebellar disorder.

s., clipped. Same as scamping speech.

s., echo. Parrotlike repetition of words spoken by others. SYN: *echolalia.*

s., interjectional. Speech characterized by inarticulate sounds.

s., mirror. Reversing the order of syllables of a word.

s., scamping. Omission of consonants or syllables when unable to pronounce them.

s., scanning. A staccato-like speech with pauses bet. syllables.

s., slurring. Slovenly articulation of letters difficult to pronounce.

s., staccato. Slow and laborious speech with each syllable pronounced separately, as in multiple sclerosis.

speech, words pert. to: acataphasia, alliteration, allolalia, alogia, anarthria literalis, anchone, angophrasia, aphasia, aphemia, aphonia, aphrasia, aphthenxia, aphthongia, articulation, asaphia, ataxophemia, baryglossia, barylalia, baryphonia, betacism, bradyarthria, bradylalia, bradyphrasia, bradyphrenia, bredouillement, cataphasia, deaf mute, divagation, dyslalia, dyslexia, dysphasia, dysphemia, dysphonia, egophony, hyperplasia, labialism, lallation, lalopathy, laloplegia, monophasia, mute, mutism, nyctophonia, onomatomania, onomatopoiesis, oxylalia, palilalia, palinphrasia, perseveration, scanning speech, speech center, stammering, stutter, tachyphasia, Wernicke's syndrome.

sperm (sperm) [G. *sperma*, seed]. 1. The ejaculate from the male; contains spermatozoa. SYN: *semen, q.v.* 2. Spermatozoa, *q.v.*

s. cell. A spermatozoon or spermatid.

s. center. The spermatozoon's centrosome during fertilization.

s. nucleus. That of a spermatozoon.

sperma (sper'mă) [G. *sperma*, seed]. 1. Testicular secretion containing the male reproductive cells, spermatozoa. SYN: *semen.* 2. Individual male germ cell.

spermacrasia (spĕr"măk-rā'zĭ-ă) [" + *akrasia*, bad mixture]. Lack of spermatozoa in the semen.

spermatemphraxis (sper-măt-ĕm-frăks'ĭs) [" + *emphraxis*, stoppage]. An obstruction to emission of semen.

spermatic (sper-măt'ĭk) [G. *sperma*, semen]. Pert. to semen or sperm.

s. arteries. Two long, slender vessels, branches of the abdominal aorta, following each spermatic cord to the testes.

s. cord. The cord suspending the testis composed of *veins, arteries, lymphatics, nerves,* and the *ductus deferens.* SEE: *cord, infundibuliform, varicocele.*

s. duct. Canal for passage of semen, esp. the *ductus deferens* and the *ejaculatory duct.*

s. vein. One of two veins draining the testes. The right one empties into the inferior vena cava, the left one into the left renal vein. In the spermatic cord, each forms a dilated *pampiniform plexus.*

spermaticidal (sperm"ăt-ĭ-sīd'ăl). Destructive to or causing the death of spermatozoa.

spermatid (sper'mă-tĭd) [G. *sperma,* seed]. A cell arising by division of the secondary spermatocyte to become a spermatozoon.

spermatin (sperm'ă-tĭn) [G. *sperma,* seed]. A mucilaginous substance in the semen.

spermatism (sper'mă-tĭzm) [G. *sperma,* seed, + *-ismos,* condition]. Ejaculation of semen, voluntarily or otherwise.

spermatitis (sper"mă-tī'tĭs) [" + *-itis,* inflammation]. Inflammation of the spermatic cord or of the ductus deferens. SYN: *deferentitis, funiculitis.*

spermato- [G.]. Combining form meaning *sperm, to sow seed.*

spermatoblast (sper-măt'ō-blăst) [G. *sperma, spermato-,* seed, + *blastos,* germ]. The rudimentary spermatozoon SYN: *spermatid.*

spermatocele (sper-măt'ō-sēl) [" + *kēlē,* mass]. A cystic tumor of the epididymis containing spermatozoa.

spermatocidal (sper"mă-tō-sī'dăl) [" + L. *cidus,* from *caedere,* to kill]. Destroying spermatozoa.

spermatocyst (sper-măt'ō-sĭst) [" + *kystis,* a sac]. 1. A seminal vesicle. 2. Tumor of epididymis containing semen. SYN: *spermatocele.*

spermatocystectomy (sper"măt-ō-sĭs-tĕk'tō-mĭ) [" + " + *ektomē,* excision]. Removal of the seminal vesicles.

spermatocystitis (sper"măt-ō-sĭs-tī'tĭs) [" + " + *-itis,* inflammation]. Inflammation of a seminal vesicle. SYN: *seminal vesiculitis.*

spermatocystotomy (sper"măt-ō-sĭs-tŏt'ō-mĭ) [" + " + *tomē,* a cutting]. Incision into a seminal vesicle for drainage.

spermatocyte (sper-măt'ō-sīt) [" + *kytos,* cell]. A cell originating from a spermatogonium, and which forms by division the spermatids which give rise to spermatozoa.

s., primary. Cell arising by growth and development from a spermatogonium.

s., secondary. Cell arising from primary spermatocyte by a miotic division. It undergoes a second miotic division, giving rise to two *spermatids* with haploid number of chromosomes.

spermatogenesis (sper-măt-ō-jĕn'ĕ-sĭs) [" + *genesis,* produce]. The formation of mature functional spermatozoa. In the process, undifferentiated *spermatogonia* become *primary spermatocytes* each of which divides to form two *secondary spermatocytes.* Each of these divide to form two *spermatids* which transform into functional motile *spermatozoa.* In the process the chromosome number is reduced from the diploid to the *haploid* number. SEE: *gametogenesis, maturation, miosis.*

spermatogonium (sper-măt-ō-gō'nĭ-ŭm) (pl. *spermatogonia*) [" + *gonē,* generation]. A large unspecialized germ cell which in spermatogenesis gives rise to a primary spermatocyte. SEE: *spermatogenesis.*

spermatoid (sper'măt-oyd) [" + *eidos,* form]. Resembling a spermatozoon.

spermatology (sper-mă-tŏl'ō-jĭ) [" + *logos,* a study]. The study of the seminal fluid.

spermatolysin (sper-măt-ŏl'ĭ-sĭn) [" + *lysis,* dissolution]. A lysin destroying spermatozoa.

spermatolysis (sper-măt-ŏl'ĭ-sĭs) [" + *lysis,* dissolution]. Dissolution or destruction of spermatozoa.

spermatolytic (sper-măt-ō-lĭt'ĭk) [" + *lysis,* dissolution]. Destroying spermatozoa.

spermatopathia, spermatopathy (sper"mă-tō-păth'ĭ-ă, sper-măt-ŏp'ă-thĭ) [" + *pathos,* disease]. Disease of sperm cells or their secreting glands or ducts.

spermatophobia (sper-măt-ō-fō'bĭ-ă) [" + *phobos,* fear]. Abnormal fear of being afflicted with spermatorrhea, involuntary loss of semen.

spermatopoietic (sper-măt-ō-poy-ĕt'ĭk) [" + *poiein,* to make]. Promoting the formation and secretion of semen.

spermatorrhea (sper-măt-or-ē'ă) [" + *rhoia,* a flow]. Abnormally frequent, involuntary loss of semen without orgasm.

spermatoschesis (sper-măt-ŏs'kĕ-sĭs) [" + *schesis,* a checking]. Suppression of the semen.

spermatospore (sper-mat'ō-spōr) [" + *sporos,* a seed]. A primitive cell from which spermatozoa arise. SYN: *spermatogonium.*

spermatotoxin (sper-măt-ō-tŏks'ĭn) [" + *toxikon,* poison]. A toxin which destroys spermatozoa. SYN: *spermatoxin.*

spermatovum (sper-măt-ō'vŭm) [" + L. *ovum,* egg]. A fecundated or impregnated ovum.

spermatoxin (sper-mă-tŏks'ĭn) [" + *toxikon,* poison]. A toxin which causes destruction of spermatozoa.

It is formed by injecting spermatozoa from animal of another species.

spermatozoa (sper"măt-o-zō'ă) [" + *zōon,* life]. Plural of *spermatozoon.*

spermatozoon (sper"măt-ō-zō-ŏn) (pl. *spermatozoa*) [" + *zōon,* life]. The mature male sex or germ cell formed within the seminiferous tubules of the testes.

The spermatozoon has a broad, oval, flattened head with a nucleus and a protoplasmic neck or middle piece and tail. It is about 1/500 in. in length and resembles a tadpole.

It has the power of self-propulsion by means of a flagellum. Developed after puberty from the *spermatids* in the testes in enormous quantities. The head pierces the envelope of the ovum and loses its tail when fusion of the 2 cells takes place. This process is called *fertilization.*

RS: *acrosome; fertilization; gamete; ovum; semen; sperm; zygote.*

spermaturia (sper-măt-ū'rĭ-ă) [G. *sperma,* seed, + *ouron,* urine]. Semen discharged with the urine.

spermectomy (sper-mĕk'tō-mĭ) [" + *ektomē,* excision]. Resection of a portion of the spermatic cord and duct.

spermic (sper'mik) [G. *sperma,* seed]. Concerning sperm, male reproductive cells.

spermicidal (sper"mĭ-sī'dăl) [" + L. *cidus,* from *caedere,* to kill]. Killing spermatozoa.

spermicide (sper'mĭ-sīd) [" + L. *cidus,* from *caedere,* to kill]. An agent which kills spermatozoa.

spermidine. A protein isolated from spermatozoa.

spermiduct (sper'mĭ-dŭkt) [" + L. *ductus*, a duct]. The ejaculatory duct and ductus deferens considered as one.

spermine. A protein isolated from spermatozoa.

spermiogenesis. The processes involved in the transformation of a spermatid to a functional spermatozoon.

spermium. A spermatozoon, *q.v.*

spermoblast (sper'mō-blăst) [" + *blastos*, a germ]. A cell developing into a spermatozoon. SYN: *spermatoblast* or *spermatid.*

spermolith (sper'mō-lĭth) [" + *lithos*, stone]. A calculus in the seminal vesicle or spermatic duct.

spermolysin (sper-mō"lĭs'ĭn). A cytolysin formed following the inoculation of spermatozoa.

spermolytic (sper-mō-lĭt'ĭk) [" + *lysis*, dissolution]. Causing the destruction of spermatozoa.

spermoneuralgia (sper"mō-nū-răl'jĭ-ă) [" + *neuron*, nerve, + *algos*, pain]. Neuralgic pain in the testicles and spermatic cord.

spermophlebectasia (sper"mō-flē-bĕk-tā'zĭ-ă) [" + *phleps, phleb-*, vein, + *ektasis*, dilatation]. Varicosity of the spermatic veins.

spermoplasm (sper'mō-plăzm) [" + *plasma*, a thing formed]. The protoplasm of a male germ cell.

spermosphere (sper'mō-sfēr) [" + *sphaira*, a circle]. Mass of spermatoblasts derived from spermatogonia.

spermospore (sper'mō-spōr) [" + *sporos*, seed]. A primitive cell from which spermatozoa originate. SYN: *spermatogonium, spermatospore.*

sp. gr. Abbr. for *specific gravity.*

spes phthisica (spēz' tĭz'ĭk-ă) [L. *spēs*, hope, + *phthisis*, consumption]. A sense of well-being, happiness, and hopefulness in patients ill with tuberculosis.

The cause may be an underlying fear from which the patient tries to escape, and accomplishes it by repression, which manifests itself by characteristic behavior of the opposite extreme.

sphacelate (sfăs'ĕl-āt) [G. *sphakelos*, gangrene]. 1. To affect with gangrene. 2. Gangrenous. SYN: *mortified, necrosed.*

sphacelation (sfăs-ĕl-ā'shŭn) [G. *sphakelos*, gangrene]. Mortification; formation of a mass of gangrenous tissue. SYN: *gangrene, necrosis.*

sphacelism (sfăs'ĕl-ĭzm) [" + *-ismos*, condition]. Condition of being affected with sphacelus, or gangrene. SYN: *necrosis.*

sphaceloderma (sfăs"ĕl-ō-der'mă) [" + *derma*, skin]. Gangrene of the skin, esp. when symmetrical. SEE: *Raynaud's disease.*

sphacelotoxin (sfăs"ĕl-ō-tŏks'ĭn) [" + *toxikon*, poison]. Poisonous principle obtained from ergot used to produce abortion. SYN: *spasmotin.*

sphacelous (sfăs'ĕl-ŭs) [G. *sphakelos*, gangrene]. Pert. to a slough or patch of gangrene. SYN: *gangrenous, necrosed, necrotic.*

sphacelus (sfăs'ĕl-ŭs) [G. *sphakelos*, gangrene]. 1. A necrosed mass of tissue. SYN: *slough.* 2. Process of becoming gangrenous. SYN: *gangrene, mortification, necrosis.*

sphagiasmus (sfā-jē-ăz'mŭs) [G. *sphagiasmos*, a slaying]. Spasm of neck muscles occurring in an epileptic seizure.

sphagitis (sfă-jī'tĭs) [G. *sphagē*, throat, + -itis]. Inflammation of the throat.

sphenion (sfē'nĭ-ŏn) [G. *sphēn*, wedge]. Point at apex of the sphenoidal angle of the parietal bone.

spheno- [G.]. Combining form meaning a *wedge*, the *sphenoid bone.*

sphenoethmoid (sfē"nō-ĕth'moyd) [" + *ēthmos*, sieve, + *eidos*, form]. Pert. to the sphenoid and the ethmoid bones.

s. recess. Groove back and above the sup. concha, or turbinate bone.

sphenoid (sfē'noyd) [G. *sphēn*, wedge, + *eidos*, form]. Cuneiform, or wedge-shaped.

s. bone. Large bone at base of skull bet. *occipital* and *ethmoid* in front, and the *parietals* and *temporal* bones at the side.

s. fissure. Fissure in sphenoid and frontal bones for nerves and blood vessels.

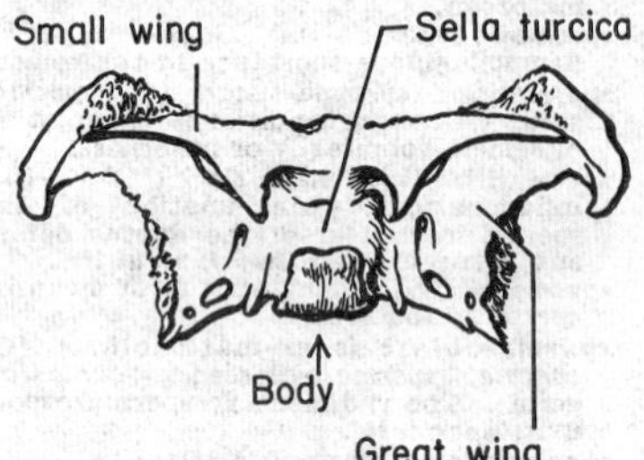

SPHENOID BONE, SUPERIOR SIDE

sphenoiditis (sfē-noy-dī'tĭs) [G. *sphēn*, wedge, + *eidos*, form, + *-itis*, inflammation]. 1. Inflammation of the sphenoidal sinus. 2. Necrosis of the sphenoid bone.

sphenoidotomy. Incision into sphenoid bone.

sphenomaxillary (sfē"no-măks'ĭl-lā-rĭ) [" + L. *maxilla*, jaw]. Concerning the sphenoid and the maxilla.

sphenopalatine (sfē"nō-păl'ăt-ēn) [" + L. *palatum*, palate]. Concerning the sphenoid and palatine bones.

sphenosis. Condition in which fetus becomes wedged in pelvis.

sphenotresia (sfē-nō-trē'zĭ-ă) [" + *trēsis*, a boring]. Perforating of the basal part of the fetal skull in craniotomy.

sphenotribe (sfē'nō-trīb) [" + *tribein*, to crush]. Instrument for breaking up basal part of fetal cranium.

sphere (sfēr) [G. *sphaira*, a globe]. 1. A ball or globelike structure. 2. The limited space of one's action, esp. that in which one is most capable.

s., attraction. SYN: *cell center.* A clear region in cytoplasm close to nucleus and usually containing a *centriole* or *diplosome* (a divided centricle).

spheresthesia (sfēr-ĕs-thē'zĭ-ă) [" + *aisthēsis*, sensation]. A morbid sensation, as of being in contact with a ball.

spherical (sfĕr'ĭ-kăl) [G. *sphaira*, a globe]. Having the form of, or pert. to, a sphere. SYN: *globular.*

spher'ocyte. An erythrocyte which assumes a spheroid shape.

spherocytosis (sfēr-ō-sī-tō'sĭs). Condition in which erythrocytes assume a spheroid shape. Occurs in certain hemolytic anemias.

spheroid (sfē'royd) [" + *eidos*, form]. 1. A body shaped like a sphere. 2. Sphere-shaped.

spherolith (sfē'rō-lĭth) [" + *lithos*, a stone]. A minute concretion in the kidney of the newborn.

spheroma (sfē-ro'mă) [" + *-ōma*, tumor]. A tumor of spherical form.

spherometer (sfē-rŏm'ĕt-ĕr) [" + *metron*, a measure]. Device to ascertain curvature of a surface.

spherospermia (sfē"rō-sper'mĭ-ă) [" + *sperma*, seed]. Round spermatozoa without tails.

spherule (sfĕr'ūl) [L. *sphaerula*, a little globe]. 1. A very small sphere. 2. A minute granule found in center of a centromere of a chromosome.

sphincter (sfĭngk'tĕr) [G. *sphigktēr*, a binder]. Circular muscle constricting an orifice.

s. ampullae. Delicate network of fibers about papilla of Vater, occasionally present in adults, a part of *s. of Oddi.*

s. ani. S. that closes the anus, the *external* one being of striated muscle, the *internal* one, of plain muscle.

s., bladder. Plain muscle about opening of bladder into the urethra.

s., cardiac. Plain muscle about the esophagus at cardiac opening into the stomach.

s. choledochus. Smooth muscle investing common bile duct just before its junction with pancreatic duct; a part of *s. of Oddi.*

s., ileocecal. Plain muscle about the ileum at its opening into the cecum.

s. of Oddi. Contracted region in common bile duct at papilla of Vater.

s. pancreaticus. Smooth muscle encircling pancreatic duct just before it joins ampulla.

s., pyloric. A thickening of the muscular wall around the pyloric orifice.

sphincteralgia (sfĭngk-tĕr-ăl'jĭ-ă) [G. *sphigktēr*, a binder, + *algos*, pain]. Pain in the sphincter ani muscles.

sphincterectomy (sfĭngk-tĕr-ĕk'tō-mĭ) [" + *ektomē*, excision]. 1. Excision of any sphincter muscle. 2. Excision of part of the iris' pupillary border; oblique blepharotomy.

sphincterismus (sfĭngk-tĕr-ĭz'mŭs) [" + *ismos*, condition]. Spasm of sphincter ani muscles.

sphincteritis (sfĭngk-tĕr-ī'tĭs) [" + *-ītis*, inflammation]. Inflammation of any sphincter muscle.

sphincterolysis (sfĭngk-tĕr-ŏl'ĭ-sĭs) [" + *lysis*, dissolution]. Freeing of the iris from the cornea in anterior synechia affecting only the pupillary border.

sphincteroplasty (sfĭngk'tĕr-ō-plăs"tĭ) [" + *plassein*, to form]. Plastic operation upon any sphincter muscle.

sphincteroscope (sfĭngk'tĕr-o-skōp) [" + *skopein*, to examine]. Instrument for inspection of a sphincter.

sphincteroscopy (sfĭngk-tĕr-ŏs'kō-pĭ) [G. *sphigktēr*, a binder, + *skopein*, to examine]. Inspection of the internal anal sphincter.

sphincterotomy (sfĭngk-tĕr-ŏt'ōmĭ) [" + *tomē*, a cutting]. Cutting of a sphincter muscle.

sphygmic (sfĭg'mĭk) [G. *sphygmos*, pulse]. Relating to the pulse.

sphygmo- [G. *sphygmos*, pulse]. Combining form meaning the *pulse.*

sphygmobolometer (sfĭg"mō-bō-lŏm'ĕ-tĕr) [G. *sphygmos*, pulse, + *bōlos*, mass, + *metron*, a measure]. Device to measure force of the pulse rather than the blood pressure.

sphygmocardiogram (sfĭg"mō-kar'dĭ-ō-grăm) [" + *kardia*, heart, + *gramma*, a mark]. A tracing made by a sphygmocardiograph of the heartbeat and radial pulse.

sphygmocardiograph (sfĭg"mō-kar'dĭ-ō-grăf) [" + " + *graphein*, to write]. Device for recording the radial pulse and the heartbeat.

sphygmocardioscope (sfĭg"mō-kar'dĭ-ō-skōp) [" + " + *skopein*, to examine]. Device for recording the action of the pulse and heart. SYN: *sphygmocardiograph.*

sphygmochronograph (sfĭg"mō-krō'nō-grăf) [" + *chronos*, time, + *graphein*, to write]. A sphygmograph recording graphically time bet. the heartbeat and the pulse.

sphygmogram (sfĭg'mō-grăm) [" + *gramma*, a mark]. A tracing of the pulse made by using the sphygmograph.

sphygmograph (sfĭg'mō-grăf) [" + *graphein*, to write]. Instrument for recording the shape and force of the pulse wave.

sphygmoid (sfĭg'moyd) [" + *eidos*, form]. Resembling the pulse.

sphygmology (sfĭg-mŏl'ō-jĭ) [" + *logos*, a study]. The study of the pulse.

sphygmomanometer (sfĭg"mō-măn-ŏm'ĕt-ĕr) [" + *manos*, thin, + *metron*, a measure]. Instrument for determining arterial pressure.

sphygmometer (sfĭg-mŏm'ĕt-ĕr) [" + *metron*, a measure]. Instrument for measuring the pulse. SYN: *sphygmograph.*

sphygmophone (sfĭg'mō-fōn) [" + *phōnē*, a voice]. Instrument for hearing the pulse beat.

sphygmoplethysmograph (sfĭg"mō-plĕth-ĭz'mō-grăf) [" + *plēthysmos*, increase, + *graphein*, to write]. Device which traces the pulse with its curve of fluctuation in volume.

sphygmoscope (sfĭg'mō-skop) [" + *skopein*, to examine]. Instrument for showing the heart's movements or pulsations of arteries and veins.

sphygmosystole (sfĭg"mō-sĭs'tō-lē) [" + *systolē*, contraction]. The segment of the pulse wave that corresponds to the heart's systole.

sphygmotonograph (sfĭg"mō-tō'nō-grăf) [" + *tonos*, tone, + *graphein*, to write]. An instrument for simultaneous recording and timing the arterial blood pressure, jugular or carotid pulse and the brachial pulse.

sphygmotonometer (sfĭg"mō-tō-nŏm'ĕt-ĕr) [" + " + *metron*, a measure]. Instrument for ascertaining elasticity of walls of an artery.

sphygmus (sfĭg'mŭs). A pulse or pulsation.

sphyrectomy (sfī-rĕk'tō-mĭ) [G. *sphyra*, malleus, + *ektomē*, excision]. Surgical excision of the malleus.

sphyrotomy (sfī-rŏt'ō-mĭ) [" + *tomē*, a cutting]. Partial excision of the malleus.

spica (spī'kă) [L. *spica*, ear of grain]. A reverse spiral bandage, the turn of which crosses like letter V. SEE: *bandage.*

spicular (spĭk'ū-lar) [L. *spiculum*, a dart]. Pert. to, or resembling, a spicule; dartlike.

spicule (spĭk'ūl) [L. *spiculum*, a dart]. A small, needle-shaped body.

s., bony. A needle-shaped fragment of bone.

spiculum (spĭk'ū-lŭm) (pl. *spicula*) [L. *spiculum*, a dart]. A sharp, small spike. SYN: *spicule.*

spider (spī'der). An insect, belonging to the order *Araneae*, sub-class *Arachnida*, class *Arachnoidea*, phylum *Arthropoda.* Body is divided into cephalothorax and abdomen joined by narrow waist, usually possess four pairs of legs, poison fangs, breathes by both lungs and trachea, and often possesses spinerettes.

s. bites or poisoning. All spider bites are not dangerous.

SYM: In general, the victim is often bitten about the genitalia. Local symptoms are slight burning followed in about half an hour by severe radiating pains, often extending long distances from puncture. Sloughing at site and along lymphatics may occur. Collapse, unconsciousness, convulsions, and death sometimes follow.

s., black widow. The female of *Latrodectus mactans.* It is glossy black in color with a brilliant red or yellow spot, usually shaped like an hour-glass or two triangles, on under surface of the abdomen. Its bite causes excruciating pain and may prove fatal.

SYM: Initially, the sensation resembles the prick of a pin. This pain usually lasts for a short period of time, subsides and later the abdominal muscles become rigid. Within a half hour severe abdominal cramps begin. The venom which is neurotoxic causes an ascending motor paralysis. Because of the extreme abdominal pain the patient may be suspected of having an acute condition requiring abdominal surgery.

Avoid all stimulants. Suction is of little value as the toxin is rapidly absorbed. Calcium gluconate intravenously often gives relief from pain. Large doses of morphine, repeated when necessary, given slowly by vein, also control pain. Heat, a hot tub, and forcing fluids also recommended. Specific antivenin is available from Merck Sharp and Dohme, West Point, Pa. This horse serum containing preparation should be given intramuscularly as soon as the diagnosis is made. SEE: *bites.*

s. cells. Branching cells in neuroglia. SEE: *Deiter's cell, neuroglia cell.*

s. fingers. Abnormally long phalanges of the fingers. SYN: *arachnodactyly.*

s. nevus. A branched growth on the skin of dilated capillaries, resembling a spider. SYN: *nevus araneus, vascular s.*

Spies' diet. One for pellagra.

Brewer's yeast, milk, eggs, lean meat and perhaps calves' liver, all in greater abundance than in Goldberger's* diet.

spigelian line (spī-jē'lĭ-ăn). SYN: *linea semilunaris* or *semilunar line.* Line on abdomen lying parallel to median line and marking edge of rectus abdominis muscle.

s. lobe. A small lobe behind right lobe of liver. SYN: *lobus caudatus of liver.*

spill (spĭl) [A.S. *spillan*, to squander]. An overflow.

s., cellular. Dissemination of cells through lymph or the blood resulting in metastasis.

spiloma, spilus (spī-lō'mă, spī'lŭs) [G. *spilōma*, spot]. A mole or discoloration of skin. SYN: *nevus.*

spiloplania [G. " + *plane*, a wandering about]. Transient and wandering erythema of the skin.

spiloplaxia (spī"lō-plăks'ĭ-ă) [G. *spilos*, spot, + *plax*, plate]. A red spot appearing in leprosy.

spina (spī'nă) (pl. *spinae*) [L. *spina*, thorn]. 1. Any spinelike protuberance. 2. The spine.

s. bifida. Congenital defect in walls of spinal canal caused by lack of union bet. the laminae of the vertebrae.

Lumbar portion is part chiefly affected.

SYM: As result of this deficiency the membranes of the cord are pushed through the opening, forming a tumor known as spina bifida, on account of condition of spine which gives rise to the deformity, and hydrorrhachis due to the fluid contained in the tumor.

s. bifida occulta. Failure of vertebrae to close but lacking hernial protrusion.

spinach (spĭn'ach) [Spanish *espinaca*]. COMP: Oxalates prevail. COOKED: 1 cup (180 gm.). Calories: 45. Other main values: 6 gm. protein; 1 gm. fat; 6 gm. carbohydrate; 223 mg. calcium; 21,200 I.U. vitamin A; 54 mg. ascorbic acid.

ACTION: Laxative, antitoxic and valuable for its mineral content. SEE. *atriplicism.*

spinal (spī'năl) [L. *spina*, a thorn]. Pert. to the spine or spinal cord.

s. anesthesia. An anesthetic injected into the spinal canal.

RS: *anesthesia, cisternal puncture, lumbar puncture, spinal puncture.*

s. canal. Canal of the vertebral column. RS: *intrathecal, spina bifida, spinal puncture.*

s. column. The vertebral column enclosing spinal cord. Thirty-three bones in all, 7 cervical, 12 dorsal or thoracic, 5 lumbar, 5 sacral vertebrae forming 1 bone and 4 coccygeal vertebrae which, like the sacrum, are fused into 1 bone.

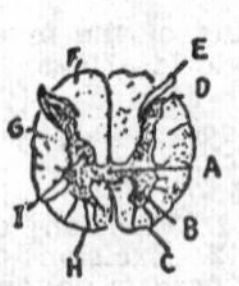

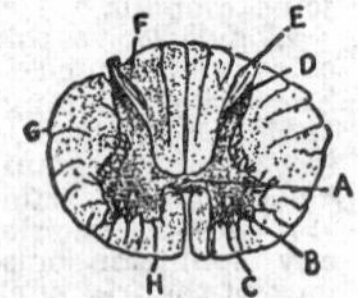

1 2

SPINAL CORD, CROSS SECTION OF

1. Thoracic Portion.

A. Central canal. B. Anterior horns. C. Anterior roots. D. Posterior horns. E. Posterior roots. F. Posterior columns. G. Lateral columns. H. Anterior columns. I. Clarke's columns.

2. Cervical Enlargement.

A. Central canal. B. Anterior horns. C. Anterior roots. D. Posterior horns. E. Posterior roots. F. Posterior columns. G. Lateral columns. H. Anterior columns.

s. cord. An ovoid column of nervous tissue about 44 cm. long, flattened anteroposteriorly, extending from the medulla to the 2nd lumbar vertebra in the spinal canal. From the spinal cord issue all nerves to the trunk and limbs. It serves as a center for spinal reflexes and as a conducting pathway to and from the brain.

In cross section, it does not fill the vertebral space, being surrounded by the pia mater, the cerebrospinal fluid, the arachnoid, and the dura mater, which fuses with the periosteum of the inner surfaces of the vertebrae.

The gray substance forms an "H," there being a post. and ant. horn in either half. The ant. horn is composed of motor cells from which the fibers, making up the motor portions of the peripheral nerves arise. Sensory neurons enter posteriorly.

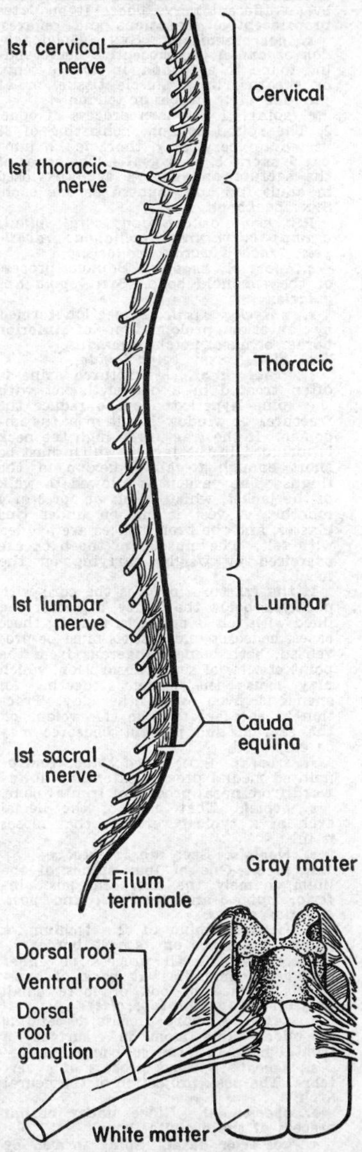

SPINAL CORD, LATERAL VIEW

The "H" also divides the surrounding white matter into post., lateral and ant. bundles. These serve to connect brain and cord in both directions (*i.e.* with efferent and afferent nerves) as well as various portions of the cord itself.

From the spinal cord issue all nerves to the trunk and limbs, and it is the center of reflex action containing the conducting paths to and from the brain.

s. *curvature*. Abnormal curvature of the spine, frequently constitutional in children.

It may be *angular* (caries), or *lateral* (scoliosis), or *anteroposterior* (kyphosis,* lordosis*).

s. *c., angular*. Caries of the spine SYN: *Pott's disease, q.v.*

s. *c., lateral*. Deviation of spine to one or other side causing a twist of the spine.

s. *fluid*. Cerebrospinal fluid, *q.v.*

It contains 55 to 75 mg. of sugar per 100 cc. when normal. The sugar content is lower than that in the blood.

DIAG: *Cell count*: If normal, 0-10 cells per cu. mm. in adults and 0-20 in children. Increased in all diseased states, several hundred or thousands in meningitis, when fluid becomes opaque.

Lymphocytes found in encephalitis and tuberculous meningitis; polymorphonuclears predominate in septic meningitis and epidemic meningitis.

Bloody fluid: Brain hemorrhages due to arteriosclerosis, high blood pressure, tumors and other causes. Spinal fluid may contain blood due to the needle having punctured a small blood vessel.

Encephalitis: Sugar content is increased, fluid clear, cell count 100 plus. SEE: *meningitis.*

Globulin: Absent during health, positive in disease.

Microorganisms: Meningococci, streptococci, pneumococci, tubercle bacilli, and influenza bacilli may be present, any of which may be indicative of meningitis. Epidemic meningitis indicated by gram-negative, intracellular diplococcus, biscuit-shaped microorganisms. Typhoid bacilli may produce meningeal symptoms in typhoid fever. Long chains of hemolytic, green-producing streptococci enter the meninges through the ear, the lungs being the invading point of pneumococci, influenza bacilli, and pneumobacilli. All these may be found in smears, though sometimes missed and found in cultures.

*Meningitis**: Lower spinal fluid sugar than sugar content of blood; 25 to 15 mg. If suppurative m., spinal fluid is puslike and turbid, but it is clear in tuberculous m., encephalitis and poliomyelitis.

*Poliomyelitis**: Same as in encephalitis, *q.v.*

RS: *anhydromyelia, calcinorrhachia, cerebrospinal fluid.*

s. *fusion*. After removal of herniated disks, the adjacent vertebrae are immobilized by surgical procedure. SEE: *spondylosyndesis.*

s. *ganglion*. Enlargement on dorsal or posterior root of a spinal nerve composed principally of cell bodies of somatic and visceral afferent neurons.

s. *nerves*. Those arising from the spinal cord; 31 pairs, consisting of 8 *cervical*, 12 *thoracic*, 5 *lumbar*, 5 *sacral*, and 1 *coccygeal*, corresponding with the spinal vertebrae. SEE: *skeleton.*

Each spinal nerve is attached to the spinal cord by two roots: a *dorsal* or *posterior sensory root* and a *ventral* or *anterior root.* The former consists of afferent fibers conveying impulses to the cord; the latter of efferent fibers conveying impulses from the cord. A typical spinal nerve, on passing through the intervertebral foramen, divides into four branches, a *recurrent branch,* a *dorsal ramus* or post. primary division, a *ventral ramus,* or ant. primary division, and two *rami communicantes* (white and gray) which pass to ganglia of the sympathetic trunk.

s. puncture. Puncture of the spinal cavity with a needle to extract the spinal fluid for diagnostic purposes, or to relieve tension aroused by pressure of the fluid, or to induce anesthesia, or to prevent an excess of fluid when a liquid is to be injected. SYN: *spinal tap.*

SITE OF PUNCTURE: To prevent injury of the nerve fibers, the puncture usually made at the juncture bet. the 3rd and 4th lumbar vertebrae. A line drawn posteriorly from the crest of one ilium over the crest of the other will usually pass over the tip of the spinous process of the 4th lumbar vertebra. The point for the needle injection is directly above this line (*i.e.* toward the head).

NP: Drape a small table with a sterile sheet. Doctor's gown and gloves, flat gauze and iodine sponges are placed on the table. Sterile sponges and adhesive plaster should be in readiness. Patient may be placed sitting with feet over side of table, arms crossed with elbows on knees and head well forward; or in a lateral recumbent "curled-up" position with head and legs flexed. This allows maximum separation of the vertebrae.

If spinal puncture is done in order to administer spinal anesthesia, position of the patient is quite important. Anesthetic materials which are heavier than the spinal fluid will flow "down-hill" and those which are of less specific gravity than the spinal fluid will flow "up-hill." Failure to be aware of this could lead to inadvertent paralysis of the vital centers of the brain. Thus the position of the patient must be specified by the anesthetist and changed only under his or her direction.

Caution: If the cerebrospinal fluid pressure is elevated it may be dangerous to perform spinal puncture.

s. reflex. Any reflex centering in the spinal cord.

s. shock. Effects resulting from transverse section of spinal cord and which occur in segments below level of section. Principal effects are (a) anesthesia, (b) paralysis, (c) loss of muscle tone, and (d) suppression of reflexes, both visceral and somatic.

spinalgia (spī-năl'jĭ-ă) [L. *spina,* thorn, + G. *algos,* pain]. Pain in a vertebra under pressure.

spinalis (spī-nā'lĭs). A muscle attached to the spinal process of a vertebra. SEE: *Table of Muscles in Appendix.*

spinant (spī'nănt) [L. *spina,* thorn]. Any agent which increases spinal cord excitability.

spinate (spī'nāt) [L. *spina,* thorn]. Having spines or shaped like a thorn.

spindle (spĭn'dl) [A.S. *spinel*]. 1 A fusiform-shaped body. 2. The portion of the achromatic apparatus seen in mitosis consisting of a bundle of delicate fibrils which connect the two centrosomes or asters. The chromosomes arrange themselves on the spindle in an equatorial plate.

s., aortic. A dilatation of the aorta following the aortic isthmus.

s. cells. Fusiform cells.

s. legged. Having long, thin legs.

s., neuromuscular. A complex sensory nerve ending consisting of muscle fibers enclosed within a capsule and supplied by an afferent nerve fiber. It mediates proprioceptive sensations and reflexes.

s., neurotendinous. SYN: *Golgi tendon organ.* A proprioceptive nerve ending found in a tendon, in muscle septa or sheaths, in a muscle tissue, or at junction of a muscle or tendon.

spine (spīn). 1. A sharp process of bone. 2. The spinal column, consisting of 33 vertebrae: cervical 7, thoracic 12, lumbar 5, sacral 5, coccygeal 4. The bones of the sacrum and coccyx are ankylosed in adult life and counted as one each. SYN: *backbone.*

RS: *cephalorhachidian; cord, spinal; cramp; curvature; rachialgia; rachilysis, "rach-" words, scoliosis.*

s., alar, s., angular. Spinous process of the sphenoid bone. SYN: *spina angularis.*

s., anterior nasal. Projection formed by anterior prolongation of inferior border of nasal notch of maxilla.

s., bifid. SEE: *spina bifida.*

s., fracture of. A fractured spine is often treated in a plaster jacket with the spine hyperextended to reduce the fracture. A window is cut over the abdomen. If the fracture is high the neck is included in the jacket, which must be short enough to allow flexion of the thighs. The patient is allowed to walk in the jacket, which is left on for 3 or 4 months. A vest is put on under this plaster, and the prominences are padded with felt. The muscles of the back are exercised by weight carrying on the head.

If the fracture involves the cord with paralysis below the injury, a plaster bed lined with felt is made. In nursing these cases, bedsores and cystitis must be prevented, both being dangerous from the point of view of septic absorption, which may cause the patient's death. An enema is given every other day. Traction to the legs to take the weight off the sacrum and prevent bedsores may be employed.

s., frontal. SYN: *nasal spine.* Sharp-pointed medial process extending downward from nasal process of frontal bone.

s., hemal. That part of the hemal arch of a typical vertebra that closes it in.

s., Henle's. SEE: *suprameatal s.*

s., iliac. One of four spines of the ilium, namely the *ant.* and *post. inferior spines* and the *ant.* and *post. superior spines.*

s., ischial. Spine of the ischium, a pointed eminence on its post. border.

s., mental. Small process on inner surface of mandible at back of symphysis formed of one or more small projections (*genial tubercles*).

s., nasal. A sharp process descending in middle line from inf. surface of frontal bone bet. the sup. maxillae.

s., neural. Spinous process of a vertebra. The post. projection of the neural arch.

s., pharyngeal. Ridge under basilar process of the occipital bone.

s., posterior nasal. Spine formed by medial ends of horizontal processes of palatine bones.

s. of the pubes. A prominent tubercle on upper border of the pubis.

s. of the scapula. An osseous plate projecting from the post. surface of the scapula.

s., sciatic. Same as ischial spine.

s. of the sphenoid. Spinous process of greater sphenoid wing.

s., suprameatal. A small spine at junction of sup. and post. walls of the ext. auditory meatus. SYN: *Henle's spine.*

s., typhoid. Acute arthritis due to infection causing spinal ankylosis during or following typhoid fever.

spinifugal (spī-nĭf'ū-găl) [L. *spina,* thorn, + *fugāre,* to flee]. Moving away from the spinal cord.

spinobulbar (spī"no-bŭl'bar) [" + G. *bulbos,* a bulb]. Concerning the spinal cord and medulla oblongata.

spinocellular (spī"nō-sĕl'ū-lar) [" + *cellula,* a little chamber]. Pert. to or like prickle cells.

spinocerebellar (spī"nō-sĕr-ĕ-bĕl'ar) [" + *cerebellum,* little brain]. Concerning spinal cord and cerebellum.

spinocortical (spī"nō-kor'tĭ-kăl) [" + *cortex, cortic-,* rind]. Pert. to the spinal cord and cerebral cortex. SYN: *corticospinal.*

spinoglenoid (spī"nō-glen'oyd) [L. *spina,* thorn, + G. *glēnē,* cavity, + *eidos,* form]. Relating to the spine of scapula and glenoid cavity.

s. ligament. Ligament joining spine of the scapula to the border of the glenoid cavity.

spinous (spī'nŭs) [L. *spina,* thorn]. Pert. to or resembling a spine.

s. point. Spot over a spinous process very sensitive to pressure.

s. process. Prominence at post. part of each vertebra.

spinotectal (spīn-ō-tĕkt'ăl). Pertaining to the spinal cord and the tectum, the dorsal portion (corpora quadrigemina) of the midbrain.

spintherism (spĭn'ther-ĭzm) [G. *spintherizein,* to emit sparks]. Sensation of sparks before the eyes.

spintheropia (spĭn-thĕr-ō'pĭ-ă) [" + *ōps,* eye]. Subjective sensation of sparks before the eyes.

spiradenitis (spī-răd-ĕn-ī'tĭs). A funiculus beginning in coil of a sweat gland. SYN: *hidrosadenitis phlegmonous.*

spiradenoma (spī-răd-en-ō'mă) [G. *speira,* coil, + *adēn,* gland, + *-ōma,* tumor]. Tumor of the sweat glands.

spiral (spī'răl) [G. *speira,* coil]. Coiling like the thread of a screw.

s. bandage. Roller bandage to be applied spirally.

s. canal of the cochlea. The osseous (bony) cochlea enclosing the scala tympani, scala vestibuli, and cochlear duct.

s. canal of modiolus. One that runs spirally around the modiolus and containing spiral ganglion.

s. lamina. SYN: *lamina spiralis.* A thin bony plate projecting from the modiolus into the cochlear canal dividing it into two portions, the upper scala vestibuli and lower scala tympani.

s. organ of Corti. SEE: *organ of Corti.* Structure in floor of cochlear duct resting on basilar membrane. It contains *hair cells* which serve as receptors for the sense of hearing.

spirilla (spī-rĭl'ă) [L.]. Plural of *spirillum.*

spirillicidal (spī-rĭl"ĭ-sīd'ăl) [L. *spirillum,* coil, + *cidus,* from *caedere,* to kill]. Destroying spirochetes or spirilla.

spirillicide (spī-rĭl'ĭ-sīd) [" + *cidus,* from *caedere,* to kill]. Destructive to spirilla.

spirillolysis (spī-rĭl-lŏl'ĭ-sĭs) [" + G. *lysis,* dissolution]. The destruction of spirilla.

spirillosis (spī-rĭl-ō'sĭs) [" + G. *-ōsis,* condition]. A disease caused by presence of spirilla in the blood.

spirillotropic (spī-rĭl-lō-trŏp'ĭk) [" + G. *tropē,* a turning]. Having an attraction to spirilla.

spirillotropism (spī-rĭl-lŏt'rō-pĭzm) [" + " + *ismos,* condition]. The ability to attract spirilla.

Spirillum (spī-rĭl'ŭm) (pl. *Spirilla*) [L. coil]. A genus of spiral shaped motile microorganisms belonging to the family Pseudomonadacea, tribe Spirilleae. Found in fresh and salt water.

S. minus. Found in the blood of rats and mice. The causative agent of one form of ratbite fever.

spirit (spĭr'ĭt) [L. *spiritus,* breathing]. 1. Any distilled or volatile liquor or a solution of volatile liquid in alcohol. 2. Alcohol.

s. (of) ammonia. A mixture of ammonia, alcohol, various flavoring oils, and distilled water, employed as a stimulant for persons who feel faint. A pledget of cotton moistened with the spirit is held to the nose. SYN: *aromatic spirit of ammonia.*

s. (of) bitter almond. A mixture of oil of bitter almond, almond, and distilled water, employed as flavoring agent.

s. (of) camphor. A mixture of camphor and alcohol, employed locally as a counterirritant.

s. (of) chloroform. A mixture of chloroform and alcohol, employed in relief of pain due to colic and similar affections.

s. (of) ether. A mixture of ether and alcohol, employed as a stimulant and carminative.

s. (of) ethyl nitrite. SYN: *sweet s. of niter.* An alcoholic solution of ethyl nitrite, employed as sedative, diuretic, and diaphoretic.

s. (of) glyceryl trinitrate. An alcoholic solution of glyceryl trinitrate, employed in angina pectoris, asthma, and as a relaxant in arterial spasm.

s. (of) juniper. A mixture of oil of juniper and alcohol.

s. (of) lavender. A mixture of oil of lavender flowers and alcohol, employed as a flavoring agent.

s. (of) mustard. A solution of volatile oil of mustard in alcohol, employed as a counterirritant.

s. (of) peppermint. A mixture of oil of peppermint, peppermint and alcohol, employed as a carminative.

spir'itual ther'apy [L. *spiritus,* breathing, + G. *therapeia,* treatment]. The application of spiritual knowledge in the treatment of all mental and physical disorders, based upon the assumption that man is a spiritual being living in a spiritual universe; that in proportion to his acceptance of this idea, and in proportion to his success in demonstrating it, he may control the body and the material elements in harmony with a Divine plan.

spirituous (spĭr'ĭt-ū-ŭs) [L. *spiritus,* breathing]. Alcoholic; pert. to alcohol.

spiritus (spĭr'ĭt-ŭs) [L. breathing]. Alcoholic solution of a volatile substance.

Usually, 5-10% strength. Thirteen are official. SYN: *spirit.*

s. frumenti. Whisky.
s. juniperi. Gin.
s. myrciae. Bay rum.
s. vini gallici. Brandy.

Spirochaeta (spī″rō-kē′tă) [G. *speira*, coil, + *chaitē*, hair]. A genus of slender spiral motile microorganisms belonging to the family Spirochaetaceae, order Spirochaetales.

S. icterohaemorrhagiae. SYN: *Leptospira icterohemorrhagiae.* Species found in Weil's disease or acute febrile jaundice.

S. nodosa. SYN: *Spirillum minus, q.v.* Assumed pathogenic organism of Weil's disease.

S. pallida. *Treponema pallidum*, the microorganism which causes syphilis.

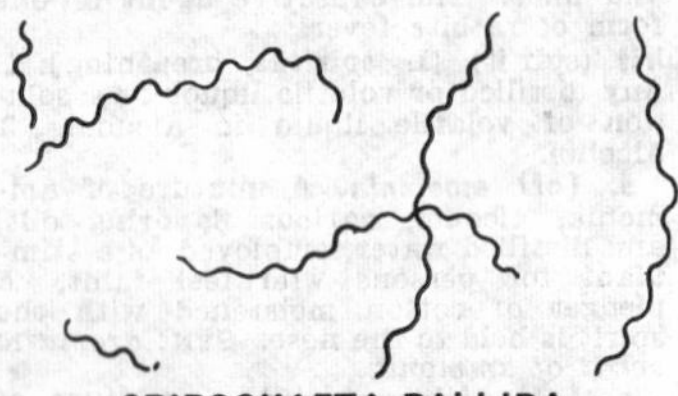

SPIROCHAETA PALLIDA.

Spirochaetales (spī″rō-ke-ta′lēs). An order of slender, flexuous spiral organisms belonging to the class Schizomycetes. It includes the families Spirochaetaceae and Treponemataceae.

spirochetal (spī″rō-kē′tăl) [G. *speira*, coil, + *chaitē*, hair]. Pert. to spirochetes, esp. infections caused by them.

spirochetalytic (spī″rō-kē-tă-lĭt′ĭk) [" + " + *lysis*, dissolution]. Destructive of spirochetes.

spirochete (spī″rō-kēt) [G. *speira*, coil, + *chaitē*, hair]. Any member of the order Spirochaetales.

spirochetemia (spī″rō-kē-tē′mĭ-ă) [" + " + *aima*, blood]. Spirochetes in the blood.

spirocheticidal (spī″rō-kē-tĭ-sī′dăl) [" + " + L. *cidus*, from *caedere*, to kill]. Destructive to spirochetes.

spirocheticide (spī″rō-kē′tĭs-īd) [" + " + L. *cidus*, from *caedere*, to kill]. Anything which destroys spirochetes.

spirochetolysis (spī″rō-kē-tŏl′ĭ-sĭs) [" + " + *lysis*, dissolution]. The destruction of spirochetes by specific antibodies.

spirochetosis (spī″rō-kē-tō′sĭs) [G. *speira*, coil, + *chaitē*, hair, + *-ōsis*, condition]. Any infection caused by spirochetes.

spirochetotic (spī″rō-kē-tŏt′ĭk) [" + " + *-ōsis*, condition]. Pert. to or marked by spirochetosis.

spirocheturia (spī″rō-kē-tū′rĭ-ă) [" + " + *ouron*, urine]. Spirochetes in the urine.

spirogram (spī′rō-grăm) [L. *spirāre*, to breathe, + G. *gramma*, a mark]. A tracing made by a spirograph of respiratory movements.

spirograph (spī′rō-grăf) [" + G. *graphein*, to write]. Device for recording graphically respiratory movements.

spiroid (spī′royd) [G. *speira*, coil, + *eidos*, form]. Resembling a spiral.

spiroma (spī-rō′mă) [G. *speira*, coil, + *-ōma*, tumor]. Multiple, benign, cystic epithelioma of the sweat glands. SYN: *spiradenoma.*

spirometer (spī-rŏm′ĕt-ĕr) [L. *spirāre*, to breathe, + G. *metron*, measure]. An apparatus consisting of a cylindrical bell immersed in water and so equipped with outlets that gases can be exhaled into it or inhaled out of it while measurements of volume are made.

The following are typical measurements made on normal men by using the spirometer:

Complemental air (*Inspiratory reserve volume*): 1600 cc., the amount which a subject can still inhale, by a special effort, after a normal inspiration.

Dead space air: 150 cc., the air which, taken in through the nose, gets only as far as nasopharynx or trachea and does not reach the lungs.

Functional residual air (*Functional residual capacity*): About 2600 cc., the sum of the supplemental and residual air.

Minimal air: Less than 1000 cc., that which remains in the lungs after complete collapse, as in pneumothorax.

Reserve air: Same as *supplemental air.*

Residual air (*Residual volume*): 1000 cc. that are left in the lungs after a complete expiration.

Supplemental air (*Expiratory reserve volume*): 1600 cc. which can still be exhaled after a normal exhalation.

Tidal air: 500 cc., the amount exhaled in a normal inhalation.

spirometry (spī-rŏm′ĕ-trĭ) [L. *spirāre*, to breathe, + G. *metron*, a measure]. Measurement of air capacity of the lungs.

spirophore (spī′rō-fōr) [L. *spirāre*, to breathe, + G. *phoros*, a bearer]. Device for artificial respiration. SYN: *iron lung.*

spiroscope (spī′rō-skōp) [L. *spirāre*, to breathe, + G. *skopein*, to examine]. Device for measuring air capacity of the lungs.

spiroscopy (spī-rŏs′kō-pĭ) [L. *spirāre*, to breathe, + *skopein*, to examine]. The use of the spiroscope to measure respiratory capacity of the lungs.

spissated (spĭs′ā-ted) [L. *spissāre*, to thicken]. Thickened. SYN: *inspissated.*

spissitude (spĭs′ĭ-tūd) [L. *spissitūdo*, a thickening]. Condition of being inspissated, as a fluid thickened by evaporation almost to a solid; thickness.

spit (spĭt) [A.S. *spittan*, to spit]. 1. Saliva. SYN: *expectoration, sputum, spittle.* 2. To expectorate spittle.

spit′tle [A.S. *spāētan*]. The digestive fluid of the mouth. SYN: *saliva.*

splanch′na. The intestines or the viscera.

splanchnapophysis (splăngk-nă-pŏf′ĭ-sĭs) [G. *splagchnon*, viscus, + *apo*, from, + *physis*, shoot]. 1. Any skeletal element connected with the alimentary canal, as the hyoid bone. 2. Outgrowth of a vertebra on opp. side of a vertebral axis, enclosing some viscus.

splanchnectopia (splăngk-nĕk-tō′pĭ-ă) [" + *ektopos*, out of place]. Dislocation of a viscus or of the viscera.

splanchnemphraxis (splăngk-nĕm-frăks′ĭs) [" + *emphraxis*, stoppage]. Obstruction of any internal organ, particularly of the intestine.

splanchnesthesia (splăngk-nĕs-thē′zĭ-ă) [" + *aisthēsis*, sensation]. Visceral sensation.

splanchnesthetic (splăngk-nĕs-thĕt′ĭk) [" + *aisthēsis*, sensation]. Relation to visceral consciousness or sensation.

splanchnic (splăngk'nĭk) [G. *splagchnon,* viscus]. Pert. to the viscera.

s. nerves. Three nerves from the thoracic sympathetic ganglia distributed to the viscera.

splanchnicotomy (splăngk-nĭ-kŏt'ō-mĭ) [" + *tomē,* a cutting]. Section of a splanchnic nerve.

splanchnoblast (splăngk'nō-blăst) [" + *blastos,* germ]. Incipient rudiment of a viscus. SEE: *anlage, proton.*

splanchnocele (splăngk'nō-sēl) [" + *koilos,* a hollow]. 1. That part of the coelom persisting in the adult, giving rise to the visceral cavities. SYN: *splanchnocoele.* 2. [" + *kēlē,* hernia]. Protrusion of any abdominal viscus.

splanchnocoele (splăngk'nō-sēl) [" + *koilos,* a hollow]. Rudimentary embryonic cavity from which the visceral cavities arise.

splanchnocranium (splănk"nō-krā'nĭ-ŭm). The portion of the skull derived from the visceral or branchial skeleton.

splanchnodiastasis (splăngk-nō-dī-ăs'tăs-ĭs) [" + *diastasis,* dilatation]. Displacement or separation of any viscus.

splanchnodynia (splăngk-nō-dĭn'ĭ-ă) [" + *odynē,* pain]. Pain in the abdominal region.

splanchnography (splăngk-nŏg'ră-fĭ) [" + *graphein,* to write]. Descriptive treatise on anatomy of the viscera.

splanchnolith (splăngk'nō-lĭth) [" + *lithos,* stone]. An intestinal calculus.

splanchnology (splăngk-nŏl'ō-jĭ) [G. *splagchnon,* viscus, + *logos,* a study]. The study of the viscera.

splanchnopathia (splăngk-nō-păth'ĭ-ă) [" + *pathos,* disease]. Pathological conditions of the viscera.

splanchnopleure (splăngk'nō-plūr) [" + *pleura,* a side]. The embryonic layer formed by the union of the visceral layer of the mesoderm with the entoderm. SEE: *somatopleure.*

splanchnoptosia, splanchnoptosis (splăngk-nŏp-tō'sĭ-ă, -sĭs) [" + *ptōsis,* a dropping]. Prolapse of the viscera. SYN: *abdominal ptosis, enteroptosia, visceroptosia.*

splanchnosclerosis (splăngk-nē-sklē-rō'sĭs) [" + *sklerōsis,* a hardening]. Hardening of any of the viscera through overgrowth of connective tissue.

splanchnoscopy (splăngk-nŏs'kō-pĭ) [G. *splagchnon,* viscus, + *skopein,* to examine]. Examination of the viscera with aid of roentgen rays or transillumination.

splanchnoskeleton (splănk"nō-skĕl'ĕ-tŏn) [G. *splagchnon,* viscus, + *skeleton,* skeleton]. SYN: *visceral* or *branchial skeleton.* 1. In primitive vertebrates, such as fishes, the cartilaginous or bony arches (branchial) which encircle pharyngeal portion of digestive tract. 2. In higher vertebrates, the bones derived from the branchial arches which include the maxilla, mandible, maleus, incus, stapes, hyoid bone, and cartilages of the larynx.

splanchnotomy (splăngk-nŏt'ō-mĭ) [" + *tomē,* a cutting]. Dissection of the viscera.

splanchnotribe (splăngk'nō-trīb) [" + *tribein,* to crush]. A crushing instrument for temporarily closing the lumen of the intestine prior to resection.

splayfoot (splā'foot) [M.E. (*dis*)*plaien,* to spread out, + A.S. *fōt,* foot]. A flatfoot or the deformity flatfoot. SYN: *pes planus, talipes valgus.*

spleen (splēn) [G. *splēn*]. The largest collection of reticuloendothelial cells in the body, an elongated, dark red, ovoid body lying in upper left quadrant of abdomen posterior and inferior to the stomach. It is composed of spongelike tissue (*splenic pulp*) consisting of lymphatic tissue differentiated into *white pulp* and pulp infiltrated with red blood cells (*red pulp*). It is enclosed by a dense capsule from which *trabeculae* extend into substance of spleen. On one side is the *hilus* through which enter splenic vessels and nerves.

FUNCTIONS: 1. *Blood formation.* In the embryo all types of blood cells are formed but in the adult only lymphocytes and monocytes. 2. *Blood storage.* Smooth muscle and elastic tissue fibers in capsule and trabeculae enable spleen to contract and discharge blood cells into circulation. 3. *Blood filtration* by which bacteria and particulate matter, esp. worn-out red blood cells are removed from circulation.

DISORDERS OF: Acute and chronic infections and certain infection-like states, hypersplenism, primary splenic thrombocytopenia, primary splenic neutropenia, Felty's syndrome, Banti's disease, congestive splenomegaly, tumors, etc. SEE: *thrombosis.*

s., accessory. Splenic tissue nodules near the spleen.

s., floating or wandering. An enlarged movable one not protected by the ribs.

s., lardaceous. Enlargement of spleen from lardaceous matter. SEE: *degeneration, amyloid.*

s. pulp. The spleen's soft parenchyma.

s., sago. One having appearance of sago* grains.

splenadenoma (splē'nad-en-ō'mă) [G. *splēn,* spleen, + *adēn,* gland, + *-ōma,* tumor]. Enlargement of the spleen caused by hyperplasia of its pulp.

splenalgia (splē-năl'jĭ-ă) [" + *algos,* pain]. Pain in the spleen. SYN: *splenodynia.*

splenceratosis (splĕn-sĕr-ă-tō'sĭs) [" + *keras, kerat-,* horn, + *-ōsis,* condition]. Induration of the spleen.

splenectasia (splē-nĕk-tā'zĭ-ă) [G. *splēn,* spleen, + *ektasis,* dilatation]. Enlargement of the spleen.

splenectasis (splē-nĕk'tă-sĭs) [" + *ektasis,* dilatation]. Enlargement of the spleen. SYN: *splenectasia.*

splenectomy (splē-nĕk'tō-mĭ) [" + *ektomē,* excision]. Surgical excision of the spleen.

splenectopia, splenectopy (splē-nĕk-tō'pĭ-ă, -nĕk'tō-pĭ) [" + *ektopos,* out of place]. Displacement or mobility of the spleen. SYN: *spleen, floating.*

splenelcosis (splē-nĕl-kō'sĭs) [" + *elkōsis,* ulceration]. Ulceration or abscess of the spleen.

splenemia (splē-nē'mĭ-ă) [" + *aima,* blood]. 1. Leukemia with splenic hypertrophy. 2. Splenic congestion.

splenemphraxis (splē"nĕm-frăks'ĭs) [" + *emphraxis,* stoppage]. Congested condition of the spleen.

splenepatitis (splĕn-ĕp-ă-tī'tĭs) [G. *splēn,* spleen, + *ēpar, ēpat-,* liver, + *-itis,* inflammation]. Inflammation of both spleen and liver.

splenetic, splenic (splē-nĕt'ĭk, splĕn'ĭk) [G. *splēn,* spleen]. 1. Pert. to the spleen. 2. Suffering with chronic disease of the spleen. 3. Surly, fretful, impatient.

s. cords. SYN: *cords of Billroth.* Poorly defined cords of red pulp of the spleen.

s. flexure. Junction of transverse and descending colon, making a bend on the left side near the spleen.

s. nodule. Syn: *splenic corpuscle; Malpighian corpuscle.* A concentrated mass of white pulp in the spleen.

s. sinus. Syn: *terminal veins; cavernous veins.* One of a series of wide channels with thin walls forming an anastomosing plexus throughout red pulp of spleen.

s. vein. One carrying blood from spleen to the portal vein.

splenicterus (splē-nĭk'tĕr-ŭs) [" + *ikteros,* jaundice]. Inflammation of spleen associated with jaundice.

splenification (splĕn-ĭf-ĭ-kā'shŭn) [" + L. *facere,* to make]. Change in a structure whereby it resembles splenic tissue. Syn: *splenization.*

splenitis (splē-nī'tĭs) [" + *-itis,* inflammation]. Inflamed condition of the spleen.

Comprises acute and chronic hypertrophy, proliferative splenitis and suppurative inflammation, result of acute infectious disease.

Sym: Indefinite or absent, usually little pain or tenderness unless perisplenitis exists. Considerable enlargement may be attended by sense of weight, tension or distress in left hypochondrium, accompanied perhaps by slight dyspnea, sudden pain appearing in gastric region followed by vomiting of pus and blood in course of infectious disease with splenic enlargement which may be due to abscess of spleen.

Prog: Depends upon systemic condition.

splenium (splē'nĭ-ŭm) [G. *splēnion,* bandage]. 1. A compress or bandage. 2. A structure resembling a bandaged part.

s. corporis callosi. The thickened post. end of the corpus callosum.

splenius (splē'nĭ-ŭs) [G. *splēnion,* bandage]. A flat muscle on either side of back of neck and upper thoracic area. See: *muscles, back, for illustration; Table of Muscles in Appendix.*

splenization (splĕn-ĭ-zā'shŭn) [G. *splēn,* spleen]. The change in a tissue, as of the lung, when it resembles splenic tissue.

splenocele (splē'nō-sēl) [" + *kēlē,* mass, hernia]. 1. A hernia of the spleen. 2. A splenic tumor.

splenoceratosis (splē"nō-sĕr-ă-tō'sĭs) [" + *keras, kerat-,* horn, + *-ōsis,* condition]. Induration of the spleen.

splenocleisis (splē"nō-klī'sĭs) [" + *kleisis,* a closure]. Friction on the surface of the spleen or wrapping with gauze to induce the formation of fibrous tissue.

splenocolic (splē"nō-kŏl'ĭk) [" + *kōlon,* colon]. Pert. to the spleen and colon or reference to a fold of peritoneum bet. the two viscera.

splenocyte (splē'nō-sīt) [" + *kytos,* cell]. A unicellular leukocyte or lymphocyte of the spleen, which probably originates elsewhere in the body.

splenodiagnosis (splē"nō-dī-ăg-nō'sĭs) [" + *dia,* through, + *gnōsis,* knowledge]. Injection of typhoid bacilli extract in the spleen to diagnose typhoid fever.

splenodynia (splē"nō-dĭn'ĭ-ă) [" + *odynē,* pain]. Pain in the spleen. Syn: *splenalgia.*

splenogenic, splenogenous (splē"nō-jĕn'ĭk, splē-nŏj'ĕn-ŭs) [" + *gennan,* to produce]. Originating or found in the spleen.

splenography (splē-nog'ră-fĭ) [" + *graphein,* to write]. A treatise on or a description of the spleen.

splenohemia (splē"nō-hē'mĭ-ă) [" + *haima,* blood]. Congestion of the spleen. Syn: *splenemia, 2.*

splenohepatomegaly (splē"nō-hĕp"ă-tō-mĕg'ă-lĭ) [" + *hēpar, hēpat-,* liver, + *megas, megal-,* large]. Enlargement of both spleen and liver.

splenoid (splē"noyd) [" + *eidos,* resemblance]. Resembling the spleen.

splenokeratosis (splē"nō-kĕr-ă-tō'sĭs) [" + *keras,* horn, + *-ōsis,* condition]. Induration of the spleen.

splenology (splē-nŏl'ō-jĭ) [" + *logos,* study]. The study of the spleen, its functions and diseases.

splenolysin (splē-nŏl'ĭ-sĭn) [" + *lysis,* dissolution]. An antibody which destroys splenic tissue.

splenolysis (splē-nŏl'ĭ-sĭs) [" + *lysis,* dissolution]. Destruction of splenic tissue.

splenoma (splē-nō'mă) [" + *-ōma,* tumor]. A tumor of the spleen. Syn: *splenocele.*

splenomalacia (splē"nō-măl-ā'sĭ-ă) [" + *malakia,* softening]. Softening of the spleen.

splenomegalia, splenomegaly (splē"nō-mĕg-ă'lĭ-ă, -mĕg'ă-lĭ) [G. *splēn,* spleen, + *megas, megal-,* large]. Enlargement of the spleen.

splenomyelomalacia (splē"nō-mī"ĕl-ō-mă-lā'sĭ-ă) [" + " + *malakia,* softening]. Abnormal softening of the spleen and the bone marrow.

splenonephric (splē"nō-nĕf'rĭk) [" + *nephros,* kidney]. Relating to the spleen and the kidney. Syn: *lienorenal.*

splenonephroptosis (splē"nō-nĕf-rŏp-tō'sĭs) [" + " + *ptōsis,* a dropping]. Displacement of the spleen and kidney downward.

splenopancreatic (splē"nō-păn-krē-ăt'ĭk) [" + *pagkreas,* pancreas]. Relating to the spleen and pancreas.

splenopathy (splē-nŏp'ă-thĭ) [" + *pathos,* disease]. Any disorder of the spleen.

splenopexy (splē'no-pĕks-ĭ) [" + *pēxis,* fixation]. Artificial fixation of a movable spleen.

splenopneumonia (splē"nō-nū-mō'nĭ-ă) [" + *pneumōnia,* inflammation of lung]. Pneumonia with splenization of the lung.

splenoptosis (splē-nop-tō'sĭs) [" + *ptosis.* a dropping]. Displacement of the spleen downward.

splenorenal (splēn"ō-rē'năl). Pert. to the spleen and kidney.

s. shunt. Anastomosis of splenic vein to renal vein to enable blood from portal system to enter general venous circulation. Performed in cases of portal hypertension resulting from obstruction.

splenorrhagia (splē"nō-rā'jĭ-ă) [" + *-rrhagia,* from *rhēgnynai,* to burst forth]. Hemorrhage from a ruptured spleen.

splenorrhaphy (splē-nor'ăf-ĭ) [G. *splēn,* spleen, + *rhaphē,* a seam]. Suture of wound of the spleen.

splenotomy (splē-nŏt'ō-mĭ) [" + *tomē,* a cutting]. Incision of spleen.

splenulus (splĕn'ū-lŭs) [L. *splenulus,* a little spleen]. A rudimentary or accessory spleen.

splint (splĭnt) [Middle Dutch *splinte,* a wedge]. An appliance made of bone, wood, metal and/or plaster of Paris, used for the fixation, union, or protection of an injured part of the body.

They may be movable or immovable.

s., aeroplane. An appliance usually used on ambulatory patients in the treatment of fractures of the humerus, and it takes its name from the elevated (abducted) position in which it holds the arm suspended in air.

s., Agnew's. A splint for fracture of the patella and metacarpus.

s., anchor. A splint for fracture of the jaw, with metal loops fitting over the teeth and held together by a rod.

s., Ashhurst's. A bracketed splint of wire with a footpiece to cover the thigh and leg after excision of the knee joint.

s., Balkan. One for extension in fracture of the femur.

s., banjo traction. Made out of a steel rod bent to resemble the shape of a banjo, and is used for the treatment of contractures and fractures of the fingers.

s., Bavarian. An immovable dressing in which the plaster is applied bet. 2 layers of flannel.

s., Bond's. A splint for fracture of the lower end of the radius.

s., Bowlby's. One for fracture of shaft of humerus.

s., bracketed. A splint composed of 2 pieces of metal or wood united by brackets.

s., Cabot's. A posterior wire splint.

s., Carter's intranasal. A steel bridge with wings connected by a hinge; used for operation of depressed nasal bridge.

s., coaptation. Small splint adjusted about a fractured limb to produce coaptation of fragments.

s., Dupuytren's. A splint to prevent eversion in Pott's fracture.

s., Fox's. A splint for fractured clavicle.

s., Gibson walking. Modification of Thomas' splint.

s., Gordon's. A side splint for the arm and hand in Colles' fracture.

s., Jones' nasal. A splint for fracture of the nasal bones.

s., Kanavel. One for stiff hands.

s., Levis'. A splint of perforated metal extending from below the elbow to the end of the palm; shaped to fit the arm and hand.

s., McIntire's. A post. splint for the leg and thigh like a double inclined plane.

s., Sayre's. One of 3 varieties of splint, for the ankle, for the knee, and for use in hip joint disease.

s., Stromeyer's. A splint of 2 hinged portions which can be fixed at any angle.

s. technology. The scientific study of splints.

s., Thomas' knee. A splint for removing the pressure of the body weight from the knee joint by transferring it to the ischium and perineum.

s., Thomas' posterior. A splint used in hip joint disease.

s., Volkmann's. One for fracture of lower extremity.

splinter (splĭn′ter) [Middle Dutch *splinte*, a wedge]. 1. A fragment from a fractured bone. 2. A slender, sharp piece of wood piercing the skin.

splinting (splĭnt′ĭng) [Middle Dutch *splinte*, a wedge]. Fixation of a fracture or dislocation with a splint.

split (splĭt) [Middle Dutch *splitten*, to divide]. 1. A longitudinal fissure. 2. Characterized by a deep fissure.

s. foot. Congenital deformity, the division of the toes extending into the metatarsal region.

s. hand. Congenital deformity, the division bet. the fingers extending into the metacarpal region. SYN: *cleft hand.*

s. pelvis. Congenital failure of pubic bones to form a union at the symphysis.

s. tongue. A cleft or bifid tongue resulting from developmental arrest.

splitting (split′ĭng) [Middle Dutch *splitten*, to divide]. In chemistry the breaking up of complex molecules into two or more simpler compounds.

spodogenous (spō-dŏj′ĕn-ŭs) [" + *gennan*, to produce]. Caused by waste material.

s. splenomegaly. Enlargement of the spleen due to degenerated red blood cells.

spodogram (spŏd′ō-grăm) [G. *spodos*, ashes, + *gramma*, mark]. The pattern formed of the ash on microincineration of tissue or other matter.

spodophagous (spō-dŏf′ă-gŭs) [" + *phagein*, to eat]. Destroying the waste matters in the body; said of scavenger cells.

spondylalgia (spŏn″dĭl-ăl′jĭ-ă) [G. *spondylos*, vertebra, + *algos*, pain]. Painful condition of a vertebra.

spondylarthritis (spŏn″dĭl-ar-thrī′tĭs) [" + *arthron*, joint, + *-ītis*, inflammation]. Inflammation of a vertebra.

spondylarthrocace (spŏn″dĭl-ar-thrŏk′ă-sē) [" + " + *kakē*, badness]. Tuberculous condition of the vertebrae.

spondyl(e (spŏn′dĭl) [G. *spondylos*, a vertebra]. A vertebra.

spondylexarthrosis (spŏn″dĭl-ĕks″ar-thrō′-sĭs) [" + *ex*, out, + *arthron*, joint, + *-ōsis*, condition]. Displacement of a vertebra.

spondylitis (spŏn-dĭl-ī′tĭs) [" + *-itis*, inflammation]. Inflammation of one or more vertebrae; esp. tuberculous disease of the vertebrae, Pott's disease.

s. ankylosing. SEE: *spondylitis, rheumatoid.*

s. deformans. Inflammation of the vertebral joints resulting in the outgrowth of bonylike deposits on the vertebrae which may fuse and cause rigid and distorted spine.

s., hypertrophic. Condition occurring in most people over 50 in which bodies of vertebrae hypertrophy and bony changes, such as slipping at their bases, development of bony outgrowths on articular processes, etc., occur.

s., Kummell's. Traumatic spondylitis in which the symptoms do not appear until some time after the injury.

s., Marie-Strumpell. Ankylosing or rheumatoid spondylitis, *q.v.*

s., rheumatoid. A chronic progressive disease involving the joints between articular processes, costovertebral joints, and sacroiliac joints. Bilateral sclerosis of sacroiliac joints is a diagnostic sign. Changes occurring in joints are similar to those seen in rheumatoid arthritis. Ankylosis may occur giving rise to stiff back (poker spine).

s. rhizomelica. Progressive rigidity of the spine caused by ankylosis of the vertebrae from below upward.

s. tuberculosa. Tuberculosis of the vertebral joints. SYN: *vertebral caries, Pott's disease.*

spondylizema (spŏn″dĭl-ĭ-zē′mă) [G. *spondylos*, vertebrae, + *izēma*, depression]. Downward settlement of a vertebra caused by the disintegration of the one below it.

spondylo- [G.]. Combining form meaning a *vertebra.*

spondylocace (spŏn-dĭ-lŏk′ă-sē) [G. *spondylos*, vertebrae, + *kakē*, badness]. Tuberculosis of the vertebrae. SYN: *spondylarthrocace.*

spondylodiagnosis (spŏn″dĭ-lō-dī-ăg-nō′-sĭs) [" + *dia*, through, + *gnōsis*, knowledge]. Diagnosis by means of visceral reflexes obtained by percussion of the vertebrae.

spondylodynia (spŏn″dĭl-ō-dĭn′ĭ-ă) [" + *odynē*, pain]. Pain in a vertebra.

spondylolisthesis (spŏn″dĭl-ō-lĭs-thē′sĭs) [" + *olisthēsis*, a slipping]. Forward subluxation of the lower lumbar vertebrae, usually on the sacrum, with consequent pelvic deformity.

spondylolysis (spŏn-dĭ-lŏl′ĭ-sĭs) [" + *lysis*, a dissolution]. The breaking down of a vertebral structure.

spondylopathy (spŏn″dĭl-ŏp′ă-thĭ) [" + *pathos*, disease]. Any disorder of the vertebrae.

spondylopyosis (spŏn″dĭl-ō-pī-ō′sĭs) [" + *pyōsis*, suppuration]. Suppuration with inflammation of a vertebra.

spondyloschisis (spŏn-dĭl-ŏs′kĭ-sĭs) [G. *spondylos*, vertebra, + *schisis*, a cleft]. Congenital fissure of one or more of the vertebral arches. Syn: *rhachioschisis*.

spondylosis (spŏn-dĭ-lō′sĭs) [" + *-ōsis*, condition]. Vertebral ankylosis.

s., rhizomelic. Ankylosis interfering with movements of hips and shoulders.

spondylosyndesis (spŏn″dĭ-lō-sĭn′dĕ-sĭs) [" + *syndesis*, a binding together]. Surgical formation of an ankylosis bet. vertebrae.

spondylotherapy (spŏn″dĭl-ō-thĕr′ă-pĭ) [" + *therapeia*, treatment]. Spinal therapeutics; spinal manipulation in the treatment of disease.

spondylotomy (spŏn-dĭl-ŏt′ō-mĭ) [" + *tomē*, a cutting]. Removal of part of the vertebral column to correct a deformity or facilitate delivery of a fetus.

sponge (spŭnj) [G. *spongos*, sponge]. 1. Elastic, porous mass forming internal skeleton of certain marine animals, or rubber or synthetic substance having absorbent qualities, used in bathing or in surgery to mop up fluids. 2. An absorbent pad made of gauze and cotton. 3. Short for sponge bath.

s., abdominal. Flat sponges from ½ to 1 in. thick, 3 to 6 in. in diameter, used as packing, to prevent closing or obstruction by intrusion of viscera, as covering to prevent tissue injury, and as absorbents.

s., artificial. Constructed of antiseptic gauze.

s. bath. Bathing of the body with a wet sponge or wash cloth.

s., gelatin. Spongy substance prepared from gelatin. It is a nonantigenic, readily absorbable material and used especially to stop internal bleeding. Sold under trade name of Gelfoam.

s. graft. S. placed in an ulcer to cause granulation.

s. tent. One impregnated with mucilage of acacia, dried in desired shape, to dilate the os uteri or sinuses by absorbing moisture and expanding.

spongiform (spŭn′jĭ-form) [" + L. *forma*, form]. Having the appearance or quality of a sponge.

spongioblast (spŭn′jĭ-ō-blăst) [" + *blastos*, germ]. Cell which develops from embryonic neural tube and serves as forerunner of ependymal cells and astrocytes.

spongioid (spŭn′jĭ-oyd) [" + *eidos*, resemblance]. Resembling a sponge. Syn: *spongiform*.

spongioplasm (spŭn-jĭ-ō-plăzm) [" + *plasma*, a thing formed]. Fibrillar network supporting protoplasm. Syn: *cytoreticulum*.

spongy (spŭn′jĭ) [G. *spongos*, sponge]. Resembling a sponge in texture.

spontaneous (spŏn-tā′nē-ŭs) [L. *spontaneus*, voluntary]. Occurring unaided or without apparent cause; voluntary.

s. fracture. Fracture due to the state of the bone and causing little or no injury.

Etiol: *Fragilitas ossium*, nerve conditions, *i. e., tabes*, secondary malignant growths, *atrophy* in bones of the aged.

s. version. The unaided conversion of a transverse presentation into a vertex or breech presentation.

spoon (spōōn) [A.S. *spōn*, a chip]. Instrument consisting of a small bowl on a handle, used in scooping out tissues, tumors, etc., or in measuring quantities.

s. nail. A nail having a concave outer surface.

sporadic (spō-răd′ĭk) [G. *sporadikos*, scattered]. Occurring occasionally or in scattered instances, as a disease.

RS: *endemic, epidemic, pandemic.*

sporangiophore (spō-răn′jĭ-ō-fōr) [G. *sporos*, seed, + *aggeion*, vessel, + *phoros*, a bearer]. Bact: The supporting stalk for a spore sac of certain fungi.

sporangium (spō-răn′jĭ-ŭm) [" + *aggeion*, vessel]. A sac enclosing spores, seen in certain fungi.

spore (spōr) [G. *sporos*, a seed]. 1. A reproductive cell, usually unicellular, produced by plants and some protozoons. Spores are usually asexual but sexual spores (oospores, zygospores, or ascospores) are formed by certain fungi. Spores usually possess a thick wall enabling the cell to withstand unfavorable environmental conditions.

Sporing is an asexual method of reproduction in many unicellular animals and plants. Certain bacteria also form spores, but more in the nature of a defensive mechanism than for reproduction.

The spores of bacteria are difficult to destroy, as they are very resistant to heat and require prolonged exposure to high temperatures to destroy them.

RS: *apospory, asporogenic, asporous.*

sporicidal (spor-ĭ-sī′dăl) [" + L. *cidus*, from *caedere*, to kill]. Destructive to spores.

sporicide (spor′ĭ-sīd) [" + L. *cidus*, from *caedere*, to kill]. An agent which destroys spores.

sporiferous (spor-ĭf′ĕr-ŭs) [" + L. *ferre*, to bear]. Producing spores.

sporoblast (spōr′ō-blăst) [" + *blastos*, germ]. Structure within the oocyst of certain parasitic protozoons (Eimeria and Isospora) which gives rise to a sporocyst, and eventually a spore.

sporocyst (spor′ō-sĭst) [" + *kystis*, sac]. 1. Sac secreted by certain protozoons prior to spore production. 2. Stage in life cycle of a trematode worm usually found in tissues of 1st intermediate host, a mollusk. It develops from a miracidium and is essentially a germinal sac containing germ cells. It gives rise to daughter sporocysts or redia.

sporogenesis (spôr″ō-jĕn′ĕ-sĭs) [" + *genesis*, production]. The production or formation of spores.

sporogenic (spor″ō-jĕn′ĭk) [" + *gennan*, to produce]. Having the ability of developing into spores.

sporogony (spor-ŏg′ō-nĭ) [" + *gonē*, generation]. Reproducing by development of spores. Syn: *sporogenesis*.

sporophyte (spor′ō-fīt) [" + *phyton*, plant]. The spore-bearing stage of a plant exhibiting alternation of generation.

sporotrichin (spôr-ă-trĭk′ĭn). Antigenic substance derived from *Sporotrichum* and used for diagnostic purposes.

sporotrichosis (spôr-ō-trĭk-ō′sĭs). A chronic granulomatous infection usually involving the skin and superficial lymph nodes characterized by formation of abscesses, nodules and ulcers. It is caused by a fungus *Sporotrichum schenckii, q.v.*

Sporotrichum (spō-rŏt′rĭ-kŭm) (pl. *Sporotricha*) [" + *thrix, trich-*, hair]. A yeastlike genus of microorganisms.

Of the pathogenic species, one is the causative agent of sporotrichosis.*

S. schenkii. The causative agent of sporotrichosis.

Sporozoa (spor″ō-zō′ă) [G. *sporos,* seed, + *zōon,* animal]. A subphylum of the phylum Protozoa which includes a miscellaneous assortment of organisms which are parasitic, usually with complicated life-cycles including sexual and asexual forms and lacking locomotor organs in the adult forms. It includes the classes Telosporidea, Cnidosporidea, and Acnidosporidea.

sporozo′an. Pert. to the sporozoa; a sporozoon.

sporozo′on. A protozoon belonging to the subphylum Sporozoa.

sporozoite (spor″ō-zō′ĭt) [" + *zōon,* animal]. 1. An animal spore. 2. An elongated sickle-shaped cell which develops from a sporoblast within the oocyst in the life cycle of the malaria organism (*Plasmodium*). Upon bursting of oocyst, sporozoites are released into body cavity and make their way to salivary gland. They are introduced into human blood by a mosquito and almost immediately enter tissue cells. Here they go through two schizogonic divisions and then reenter blood stream and infect erythrocytes.

sport (spōrt) [O.Fr. (*de*) *sporter,* to carry away]. An individual organism which spontaneously differs from the accepted limits of normal variation. Syn: *mutation.*

sporulation (spor-ū-lā′shŭn) [L. *sporula,* little spore]. Production of spores or method of reproduction of unicellular organisms.

spot (spŏt) [M.E. a small bit]. A small area of surface differing from surrounding parts in appearance. Syn: *loculus, macula, papule, pustule.*

s., blind. The optic disk where optic nerve enters the retina.

s., blue. Mongolian s., *q.v.*

s., cherry-red. Red spot occurring on retina in cases of amaurotic familial idiocy.

s., cold. An area on surface of skin which, when stimulated, gives rise to sensation of coldness.

s., corneal. Syn: *leukoma.* An opaque area on the cornea.

s's., Filatow's; s's., Flindt's. See: *Koplik's s.'s.*

s., genital. Area on nasal mucosa which tends to bleed during menstruation. See: *menstruation, vicarious, q.v.*

s., germinal. Old term for nucleolus of ovum.

s., hot. See: *warm s.*

s., hypnogenic. A point which, when pressed, will throw a susceptible person into hypnosis or sleep.

s., hysterogenic. A point which, upon pressure, will induce in a susceptible subject an attack of hysteroepilepsy.

s's., Koplik's. Minute white spots or bluish-white ones on mucous membrane of mouth before appearance of the rash of measles.

s., liver. Chloasma, *q.v.*

s., milk. 1. A thickened and opaque area seen on epicardium in postmortems. 2. A dense area of macrophages in the omentum.

s., Mongolian. Bluish or mulberry colored spots usually located in sacral region.

s's., rose. Rose-colored maculae of eruption in typhoid fever.

s., ruby. A senile angioma. See: *angioma.*

s., temperature. A cutaneous area which responds to temperature changes. See: *warm s.*

s., warm. Areas on surface of skin which when stimulated give rise to sensation of warmth.

s., white. Light-colored, elevated areas of various sizes occurring on ventricular surface of ant. leaflet of mitral valve.

s., yellow. Area surrounding and including the *fovea centralis* in the retina. Syn: *macula lutea.*

spot′ted fe′ver. Popular name for various eruptive fevers: 1. Typhus. 2. Tick fever. 3. Cerebrospinal meningitis.

s. f., Rocky Mountain. Syn: *tick fever.* A febrile disease occurring in eastern and northwestern United States caused by *Rickettsia rickettsii,* transmitted by dog and wood ticks.

s. f., South American. Syn: *San Paulo* or *Colombian fever.* A febrile disease occurring in South America, esp. Brazil. It is caused by *Rickettsia pijperi* transmitted by the dog tick.

spotting. Appearance of blood-tinged discharge from the vagina usually between menstrual periods.

sprain (sprān) [O.Fr. *espreindre,* to wring]. Trauma to a joint which causes pain and disability depending upon degree of injury to ligaments. In severe sprain ligaments may be completely torn. The ankle joint is most often sprained. See: *fracture, strain.*

Sym: The signs of a sprain are rapid swelling, heat, and disability; often discoloration and limitation of function.

Treatment: Hot or cold compresses and bandaging; elevate the joint. If recovery proves slow, immobilization of the joint is indicated followed by careful massage. Very cold water helps to alleviate the pain and acts to prevent further swelling.

s. of back. Overstretching of muscles, ligaments or other structures of spinal mechanism, often associated with small fractures.

Sym: Pain, esp. on extreme movements; tenderness; muscle spasm.

F. A. Treatment: Have patient lie down on rigid support, do not allow to sit up or walk until fracture is ruled out; intermittent heat, rest, with adhesive strapping, brace, etc.

s. of foot. Tearing of the ligaments of the foot or ankle.

Sym: Pain, tenderness, swelling, discoloration.

Treatment: Sprain is best treated as a fracture, by complete immobilization until proven otherwise by x-ray examination.

s. fracture. The separation of a tendon or ligament from its insertion, taking with it a piece of the bone.

s., riders'. Sprain of the adductor longus muscles of the thigh, resulting from strain in riding horseback.

spray (sprā) [Middle Dutch *sprayen,* to sprinkle]. 1. A jet of fine medicated vapor applied to a diseased part or discharged into the air. 2. An instrument for applying such a spray. SYN: *atomizer*. 3. To discharge fluid in a fine stream.

s. tube. Device for converting liquid into a spray.

spreading (sprĕd'ĭng) [A.S. *sprǣdan*, to strew]. BACT: Noting a growth extending much (several mm. or more) beyond the site of inoculation.

s. factor. SYN: *hyaluronidase, Duran-Reynal's factor*. A substance produced by staphylococci which increases the permeability of connective tissue.

spring (sprĭng) [A.S. *spring*, a rising]. 1. The 1st of the 4 annular seasons. SYN: *vernal season*. 2. A flying back of a body to its original position through its elasticity.

s. conjunctivitis. A form recurring each year in the spring but disappearing with the first frost. SYN: *vernal catarrh*.

s.-finger. Arrested movement of a finger in flexion or extension followed by a jerk. SYN: *trigger finger*.

s. ligament. Int. calcaneoscaphoid ligament of the sole of the foot.

It joins the os calcis to the scaphoid bone.

sprue (sprū) [Dutch *sprouw*]. SYN: *psilosis*. A disease, endemic in many tropical regions and occurring sporadically in temperate countries, characterized by weakness, loss of weight, steatorrhea, and various digestive disorders, esp. impaired absorption of glucose, fats, and vitamins. It occurs in two forms, *tropical* and *idiopathic* or *non-tropical* sprue. Its cause is unknown.

spud (spŭd) [M.E. a knife]. Short, flattened, spadelike blade to dislodge a foreign substance.

spur (spŭr) [A.S. *spora*, a pointed instrument]. SYN: *calcar*. A sharp or pointed projection. 2. A sharp horny outgrowth of the skin.

s., calcaneal. An exostosis of the heel, often painful and resulting in disability.

s., femoral. Spur sometimes present on medial and underside of neck of femur.

s., scleral. A pointed portion of sclera which projects into the deeper part of cornea immediately behind canal of Schlemm at angle of iris.

spurious (spū'rĭ-ŭs) [L. *spurius*, false]. Not true or genuine; adulterated; false.

sputum (spū'tŭm) (pl. *sputa*) [L. *sputum*, from *spuere*, to spit]. Substance expelled by coughing or clearing the throat. It contains a variety of material from the respiratory tract including cellular debris, mucus, blood, pus, caseous material and microorganisms.

Its appearance depends upon the underlying condition as follows:

AMOUNT: *Copious*: This is seen in chronic inflammations of bronchial and pulmonary systems.

Scanty: This obtains in all pulmonary bronchial acute inflammations, and in the early stages of lobar pneumonia, and beginning bronchopneumonia.

COLOR: This depends upon its origin, cause, and amount of decomposition.

CONDITIONS: *Anthracosis* (coal dust): The sputum is black.

Bronchiectasis: The sputum is mucopurulent, and foul if expectoration is infrequent.

Bronchial asthma: Scanty sputum and frothy, later becoming purulent and grayish, containing eosinophils.

Bronchitis: The sputum is mucous, later purulent, and in chronic cases, greenish-yellow and thick.

Bronchopneumonia: It is frothy, mucoid, thin, mucopurulent, copious, often with blood, or prune juice in color.

Calcinosis: Shows a sputum containing particles of lime, or chalky deposits such as plaster of Paris.

Sputum: Varieties of[1]
The Character and Diseases in Which They Occur

Variety of Sputum	Character of Sputum	Diseases in Which the Various Types Occur
Mucoid.	Clear, thin, may be somewhat viscid.	Early stages of bronchitis.
Mucopurulent.	Thick, viscid, greenish color, inoffensive, frothy, may have sweetish odor.	Later stages of bronchitis, phthisis, pneumonia.
Purulent.	Thick, viscid yellow; often offensive.	Abscess of lung, empyema, advanced phthisis, bronchiectasis.
Nummular.	Mucopurulent, with small, round, semisolid masses which sink in water.	Advanced tuberculosis.
Rusty.	Mucopurulent, very viscid and gelatinous; rusty tinge.	Pneumonia.
Prune juice.	Dark brown, offensive, often semisolid.	Later stages of pneumonia, gangrene of lung, new growth of lung.
Red currant jelly.	Blood clots resembling currant jelly.	New growth in lung.
Blood (hemoptysis).	Bright red, frothy, with air bubbles; blood may be in streaks or mixed with sputum, fluid or clotted, or sputum may consist of pure blood.	Tuberculosis (ulceration of a vessel in a cavity; other diseases of the lung (pneumonia, new growth, gangrene, abscess, bronchiectasis); mitral stenosis; aneurysm rupturing into the bronchial tubes.

[1] Faber's *Nurses' Pocket Encyclopedia*.

Empyema: If accompanied by perforations, the sputum resembles that of pulmonary abscess.

Gangrene of lung and putrid bronchitis: The sputum has an obnoxious odor and is purulent, separates on standing into 3 layers containing pus cells, hematoidin crystals and leukocytes.

Lobar pneumonia: It is scanty and viscid, yellowish, and somewhat mucopurulent during early stages, and in later stages, rusty, bloody, tenacious and viscid, esp. near or soon after crisis.

Pulmonary abscess: Usually purulent and fetid with many pus cells, and pieces of lung tissue.

Pulmonary tuberculosis: In early stages, scanty, whitish, or grayish-yellow, frothy and expectorated in small quantities during coughing. Later, when consolidation takes place, it becomes more copious, tenacious and yellowish-gray, and in the late stages, it becomes mucopurulent, musty and fetid, containing fibers and tubercle bacilli, sometimes blood-tinged or mixed with blood.

Pneumonoconiosis: Depends upon the character of dust inhaled which produced the disease.

Siderosis: It contains particles of iron or other metals, and it resembles that of chronic bronchitis. It also contains alveolar cells.

Silicosis: Produces a sputum containing particles of silica, or other stone dusts.

NP: Instruct patients always to cover mouth and nose while coughing and to avoid exposing other persons to their cough. Sputum should be collected in covered disposable containers which may be easily burned. Boil cotton and linen handkerchiefs in soapy water for 20 minutes. Sputum may be disinfected with 5% phenol or 5% formalin by 1 hour's exposure.

Paper sputum cups should be disposed of if there is any evidence of dried sputum on them. Handkerchiefs and gauze should not be used unless disposed of immediately after using. A paper bag should be attached to the bed or the bedside table. Paper wipes or squares of cloth, or soft tissues may be used for wiping away the discharge and disposing of it in the bag. The bag may be made of newspaper in a conical shape and pinned on; then, as the deposit accumulates, it is removed and another bag replaced. The patient should be instructed to fold the paper well over the material deposited. When removing, the paper should be well folded over and placed in the waste can or burned at once.

RS: *albuminoptysis, albuminoreaction, Charcot-Robin crystals.*

s., bloody. This is seen, of course, in hemorrhages. If the blood is mixed with the sputum the hemorrhage is in the finer bronchioles. Large quantities of blood indicate rupture of larger vessel.

s., currant jelly or ***raspberry.*** Indicates tumor of a lung. If of a fetid odor, bronchitis.

s., fruity. This precedes rupture of an echinococcus cyst. The sputum may be bloody, mucous, mucopurulent, purulent, serous, frothy and in plugs, or it may contain elastic fibers and fibrinous bronchial casts; also bacteria, tubercles, pneumococci, influenza bacteria, diphtheria bacteria, staphylococci, streptococci, and pneumococci.

s., nummular. Round, coin-shaped, flat forms which sink in water; seen in bronchiectasis and advanced pulmonary tuberculosis.

s., prune juice. Thin, reddish, bloody s. in gangrene, cancer of the lung and certain pneumonias.

s., rusty. This is seen in lobar pneumonia.

s., septicemia. S. acquired from inoculation with organisms in saliva or sputum.

squama (sqwā'mă) (pl. *squamae*) [L. *squama*, a scale]. 1. A thin plate of bone. 2. A scale from the epidermis.

squamoparietal (skwā"mō-pă-rī'ĕ-tăl) [" + *paries, pariet-*, wall]. Relating to the squamous and parietal bones.

squamosa (skwā-mō'să) [L. *squamōsa*, scaly]. The squamous part of temporal bone.

squamous (skwā'mŭs) [L. *squama*, scale]. Scalelike.

s. bone. Upper anterior portion of temporal bone.

s. cell. Flat, scaly, epithelial cell.

s. epithelium. Flat form of epithelial cells.

s. suture. Line uniting squamosa and parietal bone.

square knot (skwār). Double knot in which ends and standing parts are together and parallel to each other.

This is used universally because it holds well. The knot is quite easy to tie but may be very difficult to untie.

Hold one end in each hand, carry right end over left end and make a loop or simple knot. Now reverse, carry left end over right end and again tie, thus forming a simple symmetrical knot. If this is not done, a false or "granny" knot results which usually slips. To untie, steady the knot, take one end and draw it over knot and then continue pulling this direction until knot slips or jumps, forming two half hitches, when it may be slipped off.

s. lobe. 1. The quadrate lobe of the liver. SYN: *lobus quadratus.* 2. A lobe on upper surface of the cerebellum.

squarrose, squarrous (skwăr'ōs, -ŭs) [L. *squarrōsus*, scurfy]. Scurfy or scaly; full of scabs or scales.

squash (skwŏsh) [Algonquin *asquash*, raw]. Several kinds of squash are available and they vary considerably in nutrient value. Frozen yellow squash which has been cooked and drained contains in 100 gm.: Calories: 21; 1.4 gm. protein; 0.1 gm. fat; 14 mg. calcium; 4.7 gm. carbohydrate; 140 I.U. vitamin A; 8 mg. vitamin C.

squat'ting position. One in which patient stoops with knees pressed on abdomen. SYN: ***kneeling-squatting position.***

squill (skwĭl) [G. *skilla*]. USP. A drug once popular as an expectorant and diuretic.

squint (skwĭnt) [origin uncertain]. 1. Abnormality in which both the visual axes do not bear toward an objective point simultaneously. SYN: *strabismus.* 2. To close the eyes partly, as in excess light. 3. To be unable to direct both eyes simultaneously toward a point.

s., convergent. Condition existing when eyes are turned toward the medial line. SYN: *esotropia.*

s., divergent. Condition existing when eyes are turned outwards. SYN: *exotropia.*

s., external. Same as *divergent.*

s., internal. Same as *convergent.*

Sr. Symb. of *strontium.*

SR. Abbr. for *sedimentation rate.*

ss. [L.]. Abbr. for *semis,* half.

s. s. & p. enema. A mixture of 1 dram of peppermint added to a soapsuds solution given to relieve flatulence. SEE: *enema.*

s. s. & t. enema. Compound cleaning enema using a mixture of thick liquid soap and turpentine. SEE: *enema.*

ST. 37. Proprietary germicide and disinfectant. SYN: *caprokol, hexylresorcinol, q.v.*

stab (stăb) [Gaelic *stob,* to pierce]. 1. To pierce with a knife. 2. Inoculum plunged deeply into a solid culture medium with a wire or needle; also, the culture so produced.

s. culture. Bacterial culture in which organism is introduced into a solid gelatin medium with a wire or needle.

stabile (stā'bĭl) [L. *stabilis,* standing]. Not moving; fixed.

s. current. An electric current generated by holding stationary electrodes in a fixed position.

stable (stā'bl) [L. *stabilis,* standing]. Firm; steady.

staccato speech or **utterance** (stă-kă'tō) [Italian *staccato,* separated]. Jerky pronunciation with words and syllables separated by pauses. SYN: *scanning speech.* SEE: *speech.*

stactometer (stăk-tŏm'ĕt-ĕr) [G. *staktos,* dropping, + *metron,* a measure]. Instrument for measuring fluid in drops.

stadium (stā'dĭ-ŭm) [G. *stadion,* a measure]. A stage or period, as of a disease.

s. acmes. The height of a disease.

s. augmenti. Period of rising temperature or other symptoms.

s. decrementi. Period of defervescence or decrease of symptoms.

s. florescentiae. Stage of eruption in an exanthematous disease.

s. frigoris. Cold stage in intermittent fevers, as malaria.

s. incrementi. Period of increase of fever or symptoms.

s. invasionis. Incubation period of an infectious disease.

s. sudoris. Sweating stage of a paroxysm of malaria.

staff (stăf) [A.S. *staef,* a stick]. 1. An instrument to be introduced into the urethra and bladder as a guide to a surgical knife. 2. The medical personnel attached to a hospital.

s., attending. Attending physicians and surgeons of a hospital.

s., consulting. Physicians and surgeons attached to a hospital who may be consulted by members of the attending staff.

s. of Wrisberg. Prominence of the cuneiform cartilage seen in the normal larynx during examination.

stage (stāj) [O.Fr. *estage* from L. *stāre,* to stand]. 1. A period in the course of a disease. SYN: *stadium.* 2. The platform of a microscope.

s., algid. Period of chilliness at the beginning of a fever.

s., amphibolic. Stage which intervenes bet. acme of a disease and its outcome.

s., asphyxial. Preliminary stage of Asiatic cholera.

s., cold. Chill or rigor of a malarial paroxysm.

s., defervescent. Period in which temperature is declining.

s., eruptive. Period in which an exanthem appears.

s., expulsive. Stage of dilatation of the cervix uteri during which the child is expelled from uterus.

s., first. Period when the fetal head is molded and the cervix dilated.

s., hot. Febrile s. in a malarial paroxysm.

s. of invasion. Period in which a morbific influence precedes the onset of a disease.

s. of latency. The incubation period of an infectious disease.

s., placental. Period of labor during which placenta and fetal membranes are discharged. Also called *third stage.*

s., preeruptive. Stage following infection and before appearance of eruption.

s., pyrogenetic. Stage of onset in a febrile disease.

s. resting. A stage of relative inactivity between periods of activity as in a cell between mitotic divisions; a dormant stage.

s., second. Expulsive s., *q.v.*

s., sweating. The 3rd or terminal s. of malaria during which sweating occurs.

s., third. Stage, placental, *q.v.*

stagnation (stăg-nā'shŭn) [L. *stagnāre,* from *stagnum,* pool]. 1. Cessation of motion. 2. PATH: A stoppage of motion of any fluid in the body, as blood. SYN: *stasis.*

stain (stān) [M.E. *(di) steinen,* from L. *dis,* apart, + *tingere,* to color]. 1. Any discoloration. 2. A pigment or dye used in coloring microscopic objects and tissues. 3. To apply pigment to a tissue or microscopic object.

s., acid. One in which the color-bearing ion (*chromatophore*) is the anion.

Ex: *eosin.* Commonly used for staining the cytoplasmic or basic elements of cells.

s., acid-fast. SYN: *Ziehl-Neelsen stain.* A stain used in bacteriology especially for staining tuberculosis bacteria. A special solution of carbolfuchsin is used which the organism retains in spite of washing with acid alcohol; a decolorizing agent.

s., basic. One in which the color-bearing ion is the cation.

Ex: *methylene blue.* Commonly used to stain the nucleic or acidic elements of cells.

s., Commission Certified. Abbr. C.C. A stain that has been certified by the Biological Stain Commission.

s., contrast. One used to color one part of a tissue or cell unaffected when another part is stained by another color.

s., counter. A stain, usually a contrast stain, which is used following the staining of specific elements of a tissue.

s., differential. In bact., a stain such as Gram's stain which enables one to differentiate between different types of bacteria.

s., double. A mixture of two contrasting dyes, usually an acid and a basic stain.

s., Gram's. Gram's method, *q.v.*

s., intravital. SYN: *vital stain.* A nontoxic dye which when introduced into an organism selectively stains certain cells, or tissues.

s., inversion. A basic stain which, under the influence of a mordant, acts as an acid stain.

s., metachromatic. A stain which stains the constituents of cells or tissues a color different from the stain itself.

s., neutral. A combination of an acid and a basic stain.

s., nuclear. A basic stain affecting nuclei.

s.'s., *removal from linen.* SEE: *anti-stain formulary.*

s., *substantive.* A stain which is directly absorbed by the tissues when they are immersed in the staining solution.

s., *supravital.* A stain which will color living cells or tissues which have been removed from the body.

s., *vital.* An intravital stain, *q.v.*

s., *Wright's.* A polychrome stain used for staining blood smears. SEE: *staining, Wright's technic.*

staining (stān'ĭng) [M.E. (*di*) *steinen*, from L. *dis*, apart, + *tingere*, to color]. Process of impregnating a substance, esp. a tissue, with pigments so that its component parts may be visible under a microscope.

Wright's technic for blood smears. 1. Cover the dried blood smear with 5 to 10 drops of Wright's stain. Let stand one minute. 2. Add to the stain an equal amount of neutral distilled water. Let diluted stain stand for 3 to 10 minutes. A metallic sheen should appear. 3. Remove stain by gently washing with distilled water. 4. Stand slide on end and allow to dry. 5. Mount in balsam or methacrylate. If staining results are good, red cells will have a pinkish or copper color; white cells will have densely stained blue nuclei, and the cytoplasmic granules will stain variously in the different types of leukocytes. SEE: *leukocytes.*

staircase phenomenon. SYN: *treppe, staircase effect.* That exhibited by skeletal and heart muscle when subjected to rapidly repeated maximal stimuli following a period of rest. In the resulting series of contractions each is greater than the preceding one until a state of maximum contraction is reached.

stalagmometer (stă-lăg-mŏm'ĕ-tĕr) [G. *stalagmos*, dropping, + *metron*, a measure]. Instrument for measuring number of drops in a given amount of fluid.

stalk. An elongated structure usually serving to attach or support an organ or structure.

s., *belly.* Structure in embryo which develops into umbilical cord.

s., *body.* A bridge of mesoderm which connects the caudal end of embryo with chorion. Into it grow the allantois and embryonic blood vessels, the latter forming the umbilical arteries and vein which connect the embryo with placenta.

s., *cerebellar.* One of the cerebellar peduncles which connect the cerebellum with brain stem.

s., *infundibular.* SYN: *infundibulum.* Stalk which connects diencephalon with neural lobe of hypophysis.

s., *optic.* Structure which connects optic vesicle or cup to the forebrain.

s., *yolk.* SYN: *vitelline duct.* The narrow constricted portion by which the yolk sac is connected to midgut of embryo.

stamina (stăm'ĭn-ă) [L. *stamina*, fibers]. Inherent force; constitutional energy; strength; endurance.

stammering (stăm'er-ĭng) [A.S. *stamerian*]. Hesitant or faltering speech disorder.

May be due to hesitation, mispronunciation, transposing the letters l, r, or s, and repetition. SEE: *speech.*

RS: *lalling, mytacism.*

s. *of bladder.* Interrupted and irregular flow of urine, the muscles acting spasmodically.

standard (stăn'dard) [O.Fr. *estandart*]. That which is established by custom or authority as a model, criterion or rule for comparison of measurement.

s. *deviation.* ABBR: S.D.; SYM: σ (*small sigma*). A commonly used measure of scatter or variability from the mean.

s. *error.* ABBR: S.E. A measure of variability which could be expected of a statistical constant following the taking of random samples of a given size in a particular set of observations. An important S.E. is that of the difference between the means of two samples.

standardization. The process of standardizing, esp. that of determining the strength or scale value of a substance or device by comparing with some standard, as standardization of solutions or thermometers.

s., *biological.* The standardization of drugs or biological products (vitamins, hormones, antibiotics) by testing their effects upon animals. Utilized when chemical analysis is impossible or impracticable.

standstill. A cessation of activity.

s., *atrial.* SYN: *auricular standstill.* Cessation of atrial contractions.

s., *cardiac.* Cessation of contractions of heart.

s., *inspiratory.* Temporary cessation of inspiration normally following each inspiration resulting from stimulation of proprioceptors in alveoli of lungs. SEE: *Hering-Breuer reflex.*

s., *respiratory.* Cessation of respiratory movements.

s., *ventricular.* Cessation of ventricular contractions.

stannum (stăn'ŭm) [L.]. Tin; a metallic element. SYMB: Sn. At. wt. 118.69; at. no. 50.

stapedectomy (stā-pē-dĕk'tō-mĭ) [L. *stapes*, stirrup, + G. *ektomē*, excision]. Excision of the stapes in the ear.

stapedial (stā-pē'dĭ-ăl) [L. *stapes*, stirrup]. Relating to the stapes.

stapediotenotomy (stā-pē"dĭ-ō-tĕn-ŏt'ō-mĭ) [" + G. *tenōn*, tendon, + *tomē*, a cutting]. Division of the tendon of the stapedius muscle.

stapediovestibular (stā-pē"dĭ-ō-vĕs-tĭb'ū-lar) [" + *vestibulum*, an antechamber]. Relating to the stapes and vestibule of the ear.

stapedius (stā-pē'dĭ-ŭs) [L. *stapes*, stirrup]. A small muscle of the middle ear inserted in the stapes. SEE: *Table of Muscles in Appendix.*

stapes (stā'pēz) [L. *stapes*, stirrup]. Ossicle in middle ear which articulates with the incus. Commonly called *stirrup.*

The footplate of the stapes fits into oval window. SEE: *ear.*

staphyle (stăf'ĭ-lē) [G. *staphylē*, bunch of grapes]. Pendulous, fleshy mass hanging from the soft palate. SYN: *uvula, q.v.*

staphylectomy (stăf-ĭl-ĕk'tō-mĭ) [" + *ektomē*, excision]. Amputation of the uvula. SYN: *staphylotomy, uvulotomy.*

staphyledema (stăf-ĭl-ē-dē'mă) [" + *oidēma*, swelling]. Swelling of the uvula.

staphyline (stăf'ĭ-lĭn) [G. *staphylē*, a bunch of grapes]. 1. Relating to the uvula. SYN: *uvular.* 2. Resembling a bunch of grapes. SYN: *botryoid.*

staphylinopharyngeus (stăf-ĭ-lĭ"nō-făr-ĭn'-jē-ŭs) [" + *pharygx*, pharynx]. Muscle in undersurface of soft palate which contracts the fauces and elevates back of the tongue. SEE: *Table of Muscles in Appendix.*

staphylinus (stăf-ĭ-lĭ'nŭs) [G. *staphylē*, a bunch of grapes]. One of 2 muscles which elevate the soft palate and make it tense. SEE: *Table of Muscles in Appendix.*

staphylion (stăf-ĭl′ĭ-ŏn) [G. *staphylion*, little grape]. 1. Craniometric point at median line of posterior border of hard palate. 2. Uvula. 3. A nipple or teat.

staphylitis (stăf-ĭl-ĭ′tĭs) [G. *staphylē*, a bunch of grapes, + *-itis*, inflammation]. Inflammation of uvula.

staphylo- [G.]. Combining form meaning: 1. Pert. to the uvula. 2. Pert. or resembling a bunch of grapes. 3. Pert. to *Staphylococcus.*

staphyloangina (stăf″ĭl-ō-ăn-jĭ′nă) [G. *staphylē*, bunch of grapes, + L. *angina*, sore throat]. Sore throat due to staphylococcus.

staphylococcal (stăf-ĭl-ō-kŏk′ăl). Pert. to or caused by staphylococci.

s. actinophytosis. Botryomycosis; a condition characterized by granulomatous lesions, resembling those of actinomycoses; however, organisms, recovered from the lesions and cultured, grow as staphylococci.

s. food poisoning. Poisoning by food containing a heat-stable enterotoxin produced by certain strains of staphylococci. When ingested the toxin causes nausea, vomiting, diarrhea, intestinal cramps, and in severe cases prostration and shock. Attack usually lasts 3 to 6 hours. Fatalities are rare.

staphylococcemia (stăf″ĭl-ō-kŏk-sē′mĭ-ă) [" + *kokkos*, berry, + *aima*, blood]. The presence of staphylococcus in the blood. SEE: *staphylomycosis.*

staphylococci (stăf-ĭl-ō-kŏk′sĭ). Plural of staphylococcus.

Staphylococcus (stăf-ĭl-ō-kŏk′ŭs) [G. *staphyle*, bunch of grapes, + *kokkos*, berry]. SYN: *Micrococcus.* A genus of micrococci belonging to the family Micrococcaceae, order Eubacteriales. They are gram-positive and on agar produce white, yellow, or orange colored colonies. Some species are pathogenic causing suppurative conditions and elaborating endotoxins destructive to tissue cells. Some produce *enterotoxins* and are the cause of a common type of food poisoning.

S. albus. SYN: *Micrococcus pyogenes* var. *albus.* A form of low pathogenicity characterized by formation of white colonies.

S. aureus. SYN: *Micrococcus pyogenes* var. *aurens.* A species commonly present on skin and mucous membranes, esp. those of nose and mouth, characterized by production of a golden-yellow pigment. A cause of suppurative conditions such as boils, carbuncles, and internal abscesses in man.

S. cereus aureus. Species found in nasal mucus in córyza.

S. cereus flavus. Species found in pus causing yellow color.

S. citreus. SYN: *Micrococcus citreus.* A form producing pale yellow colonies. Mildly pathogenic.

S. pyogenes albus. Form causing suppuration.

S. pyogenes aureus. A pus-producing form.

S. viridis flavescens. Species found in lesions of varicella, causing greenish-yellow color.

staphylococcus (stăf-ĭl-ō-kŏk′ŭs). Term applied loosely to any pathogenic micrococci, esp. *Micrococci pyogenes* var. *albus* and *aureus.* SEE: *Staphylococcus.*

staphylodermatitis (stăf-ĭl-ō-dĕrm″ă-tĭ′tĭs). A dermatitis caused by staphylococci.

staphylodialysis (stăf-ĭ-lō-dĭ-ăl′ĭ-sĭs) [G. *staphylē*, a bunch of grapes, + *dialysis*, a loosening]. Relaxation of the uvula.

staphylohemia (stăf-ĭ-lō-hē′mĭ-ă) [" + *haima*, blood]. Staphylococci in the blood. SYN: *staphylococcemia.*

staphylolysin (stăf-ĭ-lol′ĭ-sĭn) [" + *lysis*, dissolution]. The hemolysin thrown off by a staphylococcus.

staphyloma (stăf-ĭl-ō′mă) [G. *staphylōma*, grape tumor]. A protrusion of the cornea or sclera of the eye.

s., anterior. Globular enlargement of ant. part of the eye. SYN: *keratoglobus.*

s., ciliary. S. in region of ciliary body.

s. corneae. Thinning and bulging of the cornea.

s., equatorial. S. in equatorial region of the eye.

s., intercalary. S. in the region of union of sclera with periphery of iris.

s., partial. Extends in one direction displacing the pupil; the remainder of the cornea is clear.

s., posterior, s. posticum. Bulging of sclera backward.

s., total. Opaque, protuberant cicatrix found in place of cornea.

ETIOL: Perforation of cornea. Result: Poor vision, increased tension, rupture of thin scar.

TREATMENT: Prophylaxis, incision, excision, ablation.

s. uveale. Protrusion of any portion of the uvea through the sclera.

staphyloncus (stăf-ĭ-long′cŭs) [G. *staphylē*, a bunch of grapes, + *ogkos*, tumor]. A tumor or enlargement of the uvula.

staphylopharyngeus (stăf-ĭ-lō-făr-ĭn′jē-ŭs). [" + *pharygx*, pharynx]. SYN: *pharyngopalitinus, palatopharyngeus, q.v.* Muscle of soft palate narrowing fauces and occluding nasopharynx.

staphyloplasty (stăf′ĭ-lō-plăs-tĭ) [" + *plassein*, to form]. Plastic surgery of the uvula or soft palate.

staphyloptosia, staphyloptosis (stăf″ĭ-lŏp-tō′sĭ-ă, -sĭs) [" + *ptōsis*, a dropping]. Relaxation or elongation of the uvula SYN: *staphylodialysis.*

staphylorrhaphy (stăf-ĭl-or′ă-fĭ) [" + *rhaphē*, a seam]. Suture of a cleft palate.

staphyloschisis (stăf-ĭ-los′kĭ-sĭs) [" + *schisis*, a fissure]. Fissure of the uvula. SYN: *cleft palate.*

staphylotomy (stăf-ĭ-lŏt′ō-mĭ) [" + *tomē*, a cutting]. Amputation of the uvula.

staphylotoxin (stăf-ĭl-ō-tŏks′ĭn). A toxin elaborated by one of the staphylococci. Among some of the toxins produced are an *enterotoxin*, a cause of food poisoning, and *exotoxins* including a hematoxin which lyses red blood cells, a lethal toxin, a dermonecrotic toxin, and leukocidins.

star. Any structure resembling a star. SYN: *aster.*

s., lens. A starlike structure developing in lens of eye as a result of unequal growth of lens fibers.

s's. of Verheyen. Star-shaped masses of veins in renal cortex. SYN: *venae stellatae.*

starch [M.E. *starche*, from A.S. *stearc*, stiff]. Noncrystalline carbohydrate of the polysaccharose* group found in plants.

The polysaccharoses include *vegetable starches, animal starch* (glycogen), *celluloses, pectins, dextrins,* and *gums,* among which it is difficult to make distinctions. All of them are rather easily decomposed, have high molecular weights

Classification of Starches

Groups

Group	(a)	(b)	(c)
I. Potato Group	Canna	Potato	Arrowroot
II. Leguminous Group	Beans	Peas	Lentils
III. Wheat Group	Wheat	Barley	Rye
IV. Sago Group	Sago	Cassava	Arum
V. Rice Group	Rice	Maize	Oats

Starches

Name	From
1. Cornflour	Maize or corn.
2. Arrowroot	Maranta.
3. Cassava	Brazilian arrowroot.
4. Curcuma	East Indian arrowroot.
5. Arum	Portland arrowroot.
6. Tous-les-mois	Canna (West India).
7. Sago	Palm (East India).
8. Inulin	Dahlia tubers.
9. Lichen	Iceland moss.
10. Glycogen	Animal livers.

NOTE: Starch is soluble at 150° F. Only slightly so in cold water.
IODINE acting on starch paste gives a deep blue.
BROMINE acting on starch paste gives an orange-yellow.

The Percentage of Starch in Various Foods

Article	Per cent	Article	Per cent
Arrowroot	23	Oatmeal	68
Bananas	22	Peanuts	18
Barley	79	Peas, dried	60
Beans	61	Peas, green	14
Beans, green	26	Potatoes	17
Bread fruit	7.1	Potatoes, sweet	26
Buckwheat flour	73	Rice, uncooked	80
Chestnuts, dried	78	Rye flour	73
Lentils	60	Wheat flour	74

and yield monosaccharoses on complete hydrolysis.

Those which the body is able to hydrolyze into hexoses are useful as concentrated energy-giving foods. They all must be reduced to simple sugars, except cellulose, before they may be absorbed. What is not needed is stored in the liver as glycogen. They are heat- and energy-producing foods. In some fruits the starch is changed to sugar when they ripen, while some vegetables (peas and corn) change sugar into starch as their seeds develop.

The amylases of saliva and pancreatic juice hydrolyze starches to dextrins and maltose. These in turn are hydrolyzed to glucose, which is absorbed into the blood stream. Glucose not immediately needed for energy is converted into glycogen, a form of starch which is stored in the liver or in muscle tissue.

Pure starches, having the formula $(C_6H_{10}O_5)n$, if normally metabolized, leave no residue and give rise only to carbon dioxide and water. Starches yield an acid ash.

s., animal. Glycogen.

s., corn. Starch obtained from ordinary corn or maize (*Zea mays*). It is used as a dusting powder and an absorbent and is a constituent in many pastes and ointments. It is widely used in industry and as a food.

stare (stăr) [A.S. *starian*, to stiffen]. To gaze fixedly at anyone or anything.

Starling's law of intestine. A stimulus within the intestine, as the presence of food, initiates a band of constriction on proximal side and relaxation on distal side. This results in a peristaltic wave.

S's. law of heart. The force of the heart beat is determined primarily by the length of the fibers comprising its muscular wall, *i.e.*, an increase in diastolic filling increases force of heartbeat.

start'er. A pure culture of bacteria or other microorganism used to initiate a particular fermentation as in the making of cheese.

starvation (star-vā'shŭn) [A.S. *steorfan*, to die]. 1. The condition of being without food for a long period of time.

When everything but air and water is withheld, the sequence of events is as follows: (a) *Hunger*, beginning about 4 hours after the last meal, accompanied by special activity of the stomach and general restlessness, becoming more acute periodically, esp. at times when meals were customarily taken; (b) *loss of weight;* (c) *utilization of glycogen* stored in liver and muscles; (d) *utilization of stored fat;* (e) *spells of nausea*, and *diminishing acuteness of the sensation of hunger;* (f) *destruction of body protein. The greatest loss of weight* is in: (a) The fatty tissues; (b) the spleen, and (c) the liver. The nervous system loses little and the heart least of all. 2. Condition in which the supply of a specific food or food accessory is below minimum bodily requirements (Ex: *protein starvation*). 3. Condition resulting from failure of the body to digest and absorb essential foodstuffs. SEE: *diet, dietetics, deficiency disease.*

stasibasiphobia (stā"sĭ-bā"sĭ-fō'bĭ-ă) [G. *stasis*, a standing, + *basis*, step, + *phobos*, fear]. Delusion of one's inability to stand or walk or fear to make the attempt.

stasiphobia (stā-sĭ-fō′bĭ-ă) [" + *phobos,* fear]. Delusion of one's inability to stand erect or to make the attempt.

stasis (stā′sĭs) [G. *stasis,* halt]. Stagnation of normal flow of fluids, as of the blood, urine, or of the intestinal mechanism.

s., diffusion. S. with diffusion of lymph or serum.

s., intestinal. Condition in which peristaltic movements fail to move food along the intestine.

s., venous. S. of blood caused by venous congestion.

stat [L.]. Abbr. of *statim,* immediately.

state. 1. A condition. 2. A mode or condition of being.

s., anxiety. A condition characterized by more or less continuous anxiety and apprehension. SEE: *anxiety neurosis.*

s., central excitatory. ABBR: c.e.s. A condition of increased excitability in the central nervous system, esp. in the spinal cord, following an excitatory stimulus.

s., central inhibitory. ABBR: c.i.s. A condition of decreased excitability in the central nervous system, esp. in the spinal cord, resulting from an inhibitory stimulus.

s., fatigue. Neurasthenia, *q.v.*

static (stăt′ĭk) [G. *statikos,* standing]. At rest; in equilibrium; not in motion.

s. electricity. Electricity produced by friction.

s. equilibrium. Equilibrium concerned with recognition of position of head in relation to gravity. Opp. of *dynamic equilibrium.*

s. reflex. A reflex action having to do with maintenance of posture or maintenance of muscle tone.

statics (stăt′ĭks) [G. *statikos,* standing]. Study of matter at rest and forces bringing about equilibrium. SEE: *dynamics.*

statim (stăt′ĭm) [L.]. Immediately; at once.

station (stā′shŭn) [L. *statio,* a standing]. 1. The manner of standing. 2. A stopping place.

s., aid. One in the army for collecting the wounded in battle.

s., dressing. A temporary one for wounded soldiers in the field.

s., rest. A temporary relief station for the sick on a military road or railway.

stationary (stā′shŭn-ar-ĭ) [L. *stationarius,* belonging to a station]. Not moving.

statistical. Pert. to statistics.

s. constant. A value such as the mean, standard deviation, coefficient of variation, or standard error which characterizes a particular series of numerical data.

statistics. The systematic collection of numerical data pertaining to any subject.

s., medical. S. pertaining to medical sciences, esp. data pert. to human disease.

s., morbidity. S. pertaining to sickness.

s., vital. That which deals with births, deaths, marriages, etc.

statokinetic (stăt-ō-kĭn-ĕt′ĭk) Pertaining to reactions of the body produced by movement.

s. reflexes. SYN: *kinetic* or *accelerator reflexes.* Reactions which are the result of movement of the body (positive or negative acceleration) or movements of the head.

statometer (stăt-ŏm′ĕt-ĕr) [G. *statos,* standing, + *metron,* a measure]. Instrument for measuring amount of abnormal protrusion of eyeball.

stature (stăt′ūr) [L. *statura,* size of body]. Height of the body in a standing position.

status (sta′tŭs) (pl. *statuses*) [L. *status,* from *stare,* to stand]. 1. A state or condition. 2. A long sustained abnormal or pathological condition.

s. anginosus. A sustained attack of angina pectoris.

s. arthriticus. Predisposition toward having attacks of gout.

s. asthmaticus. Persistent and intractable asthma.

s. dysraphicus. Condition resulting from imperfect closure of neural tube of embryo.

s. dysmyelinisatus (of Vogt). Condition marked by demyelination of the globus pallidus, and various nuclei of the brain, esp. the hypothalamic nuclei and dentate nucleus of cerebellum.

s. epilepticus. Rapid succession of epileptic attacks without regaining consciousness during the intervals.

s. lymphaticus. A hyperplastic condition of all lymphatic tissue, the spleen, bone marrow, and thymus. Previously thought to be related to sudden unexpected death of infants.

The thymus enlarges together with lymph glands and lymphoid tissue elsewhere in the body. It is often unsuspected and may cause sudden death.

Such individuals have a delicate framework, slight musculature, delicate cardiovascular system, low blood pressure, low blood sugar, and lymphocytosis. They are particularly susceptible to shock and infection.

PROG: Sudden death possible, esp. in surgical anesthesia. SYN: *lymphatism.*

s. parathyreoprivus. Condition resulting from loss of parathyroid tissue.

s. praesens. The state of a patient at time observed.

s. raptus. A state of ecstasy.

s. thymicolymphaticus. Condition resembling *s. lymphaticus,* but with enlarged thymus as primary factor.

s. thymicus. Same as *s. thymicolymphaticus.*

s. typhosus. Condition in wasting fevers in which symptoms are stupor; great prostration; coma; vigil or muttering delirium; feeble, frequent pulse; involuntary discharge of urine and feces; sordes, and dry, brownish tongue. SYN: *typhoid s.*

s. vertiginosus. Persistent condition of vertigo.*

staunch. To stop the flow of blood from a wound.

staurion (staw′rĭ-ŏn) [G. *stauros,* across]. Craniometric point where transverse palatine suture crosses the median one.

stauroplegia (staw-rō-plē′jĭ-ă) [" + *plēgē,* a stroke]. Hemiplegia of a part on one side of the body and another part on the other side. SYN: *hemiplegia, crossed.*

S.T.D. Abbr. for *skin test dose.* SEE: *Dick test.*

steam (stēm) [A.S. *stēam,* vapor]. 1. Invisible vapor into which water is converted at boiling point by heat. 2. Mist formed by condensation of water vapor. 3. Any vaporous exhalation.

s. tent. A device for inhalation of vapors.

Various methods may be improvised but care should be taken not to burn the patient. 1. Tie an old umbrella to the head of the bed, place a pitcher of boiling water in a box alongside of the patient. Vapors tend to fill the umbrella. Solution may be kept hot by placing in a double boiler or wrapping pitcher in an old woolen cloth or newspapers.

2. Window screens may be used by fastening them about head of bed and then covering with a blanket or sheet lined with newspapers. Solution may be used as above or a steaming teakettle placed alongside of bed with the spout directed under tent.

3. A rod or rope fastened across head of bed and down to foot of bed. Place a blanket across rod to cover patient and use inhalation as above.

4. Fasten ropes to all 4 corners of bed, covering with blankets, etc., forming enclosure for patient. Numerous variations will quickly suggest themselves.

Solutions to be used are about a quart of boiling water to which is added a teaspoonful of compound tincture of benzoin or a teaspoonful of tincture benzoin (this does not contain aloe), a few crystals of menthol or camphor, or a few drops of methyl salicylate. These ingredients are pleasant but have relatively little therapeutic effect. Most of the value is in the water vapor. SEE: *croup.*

steapsin (stē-ăp'sĭn) [G. *stear,* fat, + *pepsis,* digestion]. SYN: *pancreatic lipase.* A lipolytic enzyme present in pancreatic juice that hydrolyzes fats to fatty acid and glycerine.

The bile salts prepare the fats for the action of steapsin by emulsifying them. SEE: *enzyme, pancreas.*

ste'arate. An ester or salt of stearic acid.

stearic acid (stē-ăr'ĭk) [G. *stear,* fat]. A white, fatty acid found in solid animal fats and a few vegetable fats.

steariform (stē-ăr'ĭ-form) [" + L. *forma,* shape]. Resembling fat.

stearin (stē'ăr-ĭn) [G. *stear, steat-,* fat]. $C_3H_5(C_{18}H_{35}O_2)_3$. A white, crystalline solid in animal and vegetable fats; any of the esters of glycerol and stearic acid, specifically glyceryl tristearate.

One of the commonest fats in the body, esp. the solid ones. It breaks down into stearic acid and glycerol.

stearodermia (stē"ăr-ō-der'mĭ-ă) [" + *derma,* skin]. Disease of the sebaceous glands of the skin.

stearopten(e (stē-ăr-ŏp'tĕn) [G. *stear, steat-,* fat, + *ptēnos,* volatile]. The more solid portion of a volatile oil as distinguished from the more fluid portion or eleoptene. Ex: *menthol, thymol.*

stearrhea (stē-ăr-ē'ă) [" + *rhoia,* flow]. Excessive secretion of sebum or fat. SYN: *seborrhea oleosa.*

s. flavescens. S. with yellow sebaceous matter deposited on the skin.

s. nigricans. S. with black sweat due to presence of indican. SEE: *chromidrosis, chromodermatosis.*

s. simplex. Excessive discharge of sebum.

steatadenoma (stē-ăt-ăd-ĕ-nō'mă) [" + *adēn,* gland, + *-ōma,* tumor]. Tumor of the sebaceous glands.

steatitis (stē-ă-tī'tĭs) [" + *-itis,* inflammation]. Inflammation of adipose tissue.

steato- (stē-ăt-ō) [G.]. Prefix meaning *fatty.*

steatocele (stē-ăt'ō-sēl, stē'ăt-ō-sēl) [G. *stear, steat-,* fat, + *kēlē,* tumor]. Fatty tumor within the scrotum.

steatocryptosis (stē"ăt-ō-krĭp-tō'sĭs) [" + *kryptē,* a sac, + *-ōsis,* disorder]. Any disease of sebaceous glands. SEE: *stearodermia.*

steatocystoma multiplex (stē-ă-tō-sĭs'-tō-mă). SYN: *steatomatosis.* A skin disorder characterized by development of many sebaceous cysts.

steatogenous (stē-ă-toj'ĕn-ŭs) [" + *gennan,* to produce]. Causing fatty degeneration or any sebaceous gland disease.

steatolysis (stē-ăt-ŏl'ĭs-ĭs) [G. *stear, steat-,* fat, + *lysis,* dissolution]. SYN: *lipolysis.* 1. The process by which fats are first emulsified and then hydrolyzed to fatty acids and glycerine preparatory to absorption. 2. The decomposition of fat.

steatolytic (stē"ăt-ō-lĭt'ĭk) [" + *lysis,* dissolution]. Concerning steatolysis.

steatoma (stē-ăt-ō'mă) [G. *stear, steat-,* fat, + *-ōma,* tumor]. 1. Sebaceous cyst. SYN: *wen.* 2. Benign tumor composed of fat cells. SYN: *lipoma.*

Called a chalazion when on eyelid and meibomian gland.

Smooth, shiny, globular, cutaneous or subcutaneous tumor from pea to orange size arising from sebaceous glands. single or multiple, usually on neck, scalp, back, or scrotum.

ETIOL: Duct occlusion is causative in some.

PROG: Prolonged irritation may cause suppuration.

TREATMENT: Surgical excision by dissection without perforating sac. Packing in suppurative cases.

steatonecrosis (stē"ăt-ō-nē-krō'sĭs) [" + *nekros,* corpse, + *-ōsis,* condition]. Necrosis of fatty tissue in small patches.

steatopathy (stē-ă-tŏp'ă-thĭ) [" + *pathos,* disease]. Disease of the sebaceous glands of the skin.

steatopygia (stē-ăt-ō-pī'jĭ-a, -pĭj'ĭ-ă) [" + *pygē,* buttock]. Abnormal fatness of the buttocks. Seen to an extreme degree in certain parts of Africa. Location of this excess fat accumulation in the buttocks represents adaptation to a very hot climate. If this fat were generally spread throughout the subcutaneous tissue, normal cooling of the skin would be severely limited.

steatorrhea (stē-ăt-or-rē'ă) [" + *rhoia,* flow]. 1. Increased secretion of sebaceous glands. SYN: *seborrhea.** 2. Fatty stools, as seen in pancreatic diseases.

s., idiopathic. SYN: *secondary sprue.* Term applied to gastrointestinal disorders characterized by impaired absorption.

s. simplex. Excessive secretion of sebaceous glands of the face.

steatosis (stē-ăt-ō'sĭs) [" + *-ōsis,* condition]. 1. Fatty degeneration. 2. Disease of the sebaceous glands.

steclin. A proprietary name for tetracycline.

stegnosis (stĕg-nō'sĭs) [G. *stegnōsis,* a closing]. 1. Checking of a secretion or discharge. 2. Closing of a passage. SYN: *stenosis.* 3. Constipation. SYN: *costiveness.*

stegnotic (stĕg-nŏt'ĭk) [G. *stegnōsis,* a closing]. Bringing about stegnosis. SYN: *astringent, constipating.*

Stegomyia (steg"ō-mī'ĭ-ă). A subgenus of mosquito of the genus *Aedes,* family Culicidae, suspected of transmitting the causative organism of yellow fever.

stel'la [L.]. Star.

s. lentis hyaloidea. Post. pole of crystalline lens of eye.

s. lentis iridica. Ant. pole of crystalline lens of eye.

stellate (stĕl′āt) [L. *stella*, star]. Star-shaped; arranged with parts radiating from a center.

s. bandage. One wound on the back, crossways.

s. cell. Any cell that appears star-shaped.

Ex: neurons of molecular layer of cerebellum, Kupffer's cells of the liver sinusoids, astrocytes.

s. fracture. One with numerous fissures radiating from central point of injury.

s. ganglion. Syn: *cervicothoracic ganglion.* A sympathetic ganglion formed by the fusion of inferior cervical and first thoracic ganglions.

s. ligament. Syn: *radiate ligament.* One of the ant. costovertebral ligaments.

s. veins. Venous plexuses beneath the kidney's capsule. Syn: *stars of Verheyen.*

Stellwag's sign (stĕl′vahg). Widening of palpebral aperture with absence or lessened frequency of winking, seen in Graves' disease.

stem (stĕm) [A.S. *stemm*, trunk]. 1. Any stalklike structure. 2. Offspring. 3. To derive from. 4. To check.

s., brain. The lower portion of the brain excluding the cerebrum and cerebellum. Includes the medulla oblongata, pons, midbrain and diencephalon.

s. cell. A cell which gives rise to a specific type of cell as in hematopoiesis

stenion (stĕn′ĭ-ŏn) [G. *stenos*, narrow]. Craniometric point at extremities of the smallest transverse diameter in the temporal region.

steno- [G.]. Combining form meaning *narrow, short*, as *stenosis, stenography.*

stenocardia (stĕn-ō-kar′dĭ-ă) [G. *stenos*, narrow, + *kardia*, heart]. Angina* pectoris.

stenocephaly (stĕn-ō-sĕf′ăl-ĭ) [" + *kephalē*, head]. Narrowness of the cranium in one or more diameters.

stenochoria (stĕn-ō-kō′rĭ-ă) [" + *chōros*, space]. Partial constriction, esp. of the lacrimal duct. Syn: *stenosis.*

stenocompressor (stĕn-ō-kŏm-prĕs′or) [" + L. *compressor*, that which presses together]. An instrument for compressing Stensen's ducts to stop the flow of saliva.

stenocoriasis (stĕn-ō-kō-rī′ăs-ĭs) [" + *korē*, pupil]. Narrowing of pupil of the eye.

stenopaic, stenopeic (sten-o-pā′ĭk, -pē′ĭk) [G. *stenos*, narrow, + *opē*, opening]. Having a narrow opening.

stenosed (stē-nōst′, stĕn′ōzd). Characterized by stenosis; constricted.

stenosis (stĕn-ō′sĭs, stē-nō′sĭs) [G. *stenōsis*, a narrowing]. Constriction or narrowing of a passage or orifice. Syn: *stricture.*

Etiol: May result from embryonic maldevelopment, hypertrophy and thickening of a sphincter muscle, inflammatory disorders, or excessive development of fibrous tissue. It may involve almost any tube or duct.

s., aortic. Constriction of the aortic orifice at cardiac base or narrowing of the aorta.

s., cardiac. A narrowing or constriction of any of the orifices leading into or from the heart or between chambers of the heart.

s., cicatricial. S. resulting from any contracted cicatrix.

s., mitral. S. of mitral valve or orifice of heart, or of both. Usually the result of rheumatic heart disease.

s., pyloric. Obstruction caused by hypertrophy of walls of the pyloric orifice.

s., subaortic. Congenital constriction of aortic tract below aortic valves.

stenostomia (stĕn″ō-stō′mĭ-ă) [G. *stenos*, narrow, + *stoma*, mouth]. Narrowing of the mouth.

stenothermal (stĕn″ō-ther′măl) [" + *thermē*, heat]. Resisting only a small change of temperature.

stenothorax (stĕn″ō-thō′răks) [" + *thōrax*, chest]. An unusually narrow thorax.

stenotic (stĕn-ŏt′ĭk) [G. *stenōsis*, a narrowing]. Produced by or characterized by stenosis.

Stensen's duct (stĕn′sĕn). The excretory duct of parotid gland.

S's. foramina. Incisive foramina of sup. maxillary bone transmitting ant. branches of descending palatine vessels.

stentorophonous (stĕn-tō-rŏf′ō-nŭs). Having a loud voice.

stephanion (stē-fā′nĭ-ŏn) [G. *stephanos*, crown]. Point at intersection of sup. temporal ridge and coronal suture.

step′page gait. The high-stepping gait seen in diabetic neuritis of the peroneal nerve and in tabes dorsalis.

Patient lifts the foot very high in walking to raise the drooping toes from the ground or floor.

sterco- [L.]. Combining form indicating a relationship to feces.

stercobilin (stĕr″kō-bī′lĭn) [L. *stercus*, dung, + *bilis*, bile]. A brown pigment derived from the bile giving the characteristic color to feces. See: *urobilin.*

stercobilinogen (stĕr″kō-bī-lĭn′ō-jĕn). A colorless substance derived from stercobilin. It is present in the feces and turns brown on oxidation. Syn: *urobilinogen.*

stercoraceous (stĕr-kō-rā′shŭs) [L. *stercoraceus*, like dung]. Having the nature of, pert. to or containing, feces.

stercoral (ster′kō-ral) [L. *stercus*, dung]. Pert. to feces. Syn: *stercoraceous.*

stercorolith (ster′kō-rō-lĭth) [" + G. *lithos*, stone]. A fecal concretion. Syn: *coprolith, fecalith.*

stercoroma (ster-kō-rō′mă) [" + G. *-ōma*, tumor]. A fecal tumorlike mass in the rectum. Syn: *coproma, fecaloma, scotoma.*

stercorous (ster′kōr-ŭs) [L. *stercus, stercor-*, dung]. Resembling excrement. Syn: *stercoral, stercoraceous.*

stercus (ster′kŭs) [L.]. Feces. Syn: *excreta, excrement.*

stere (stēr, stār) [Fr. *stère*, from G. *stereos*, solid]. A measure of capacity. Syn: *cubic meter, kiloliter.*

stereo- [G.]. Combining form meaning *solid.*

stereoanesthesia (stĕr″ē-ō-ăn-ĕs-thē′zĭ-ă) [G. *stereos*, solid, + *an-*, negative, + *aisthesis*, sensation]. Inability to recognize objects by feeling their form.

stereoarthrolysis (stĕr″ē-ō-ar-thrŏl′ĭ-sĭs) [" + *arthron*, joint, + *lysis*, a loosening]. Surgical formation of a movable new joint in bony ankylosis.

stereochemical (stĕr″ē-ō-kĕm′ĭ-kăl) [" + *chēmeia*, chemistry]. Concerning stereochemistry.

stereochemistry (ster″ē-ō-kĕm′is-trĭ) [" + *chēmeia*, chemistry]. That branch of chemistry dealing with atoms in their space relation.

stereocilia (stĕr-ē-ō-sĭl′ĭ-ă). Nonmotile protoplasmic projections from free surfaces of cells of ductus epididymis and ductus deferens.

stereognosis (stĕr-ē-ŏg-nō′sĭs) [" + *gnōsis*, knowledge]. Ability to recognize form of solid objects by touch.

stereoisomerism (stĕr″ē-ō-ī-sŏm′ĕr-ĭsm). Condition in which two or more substances may have the same *empirical* formula but a different *structural* formula; structural formulas being mirror images of each other.

Ex: *dextrose* and *levulose*. Such differ in optical activity with regard to their effect on a plane of polarized light.

stereometry (stĕr-ē-ŏm′ĕt-rĭ) [" + *metron*, a measure]. The measurement of a solid body or the cubic contents of a hollow body.

stereoorthopter (stĕr″ē-ō-ŏr-thŏp′ter) [" + *orthos*, straight, + *opsis*, vision]. A mirror-reflecting device for treatment of strabismus.

stereophantoscope (stĕr″ē-ō-făn′tō-skōp) [G. *stereos*, solid, + *phantos*, visible, + *skopein*, to examine]. A stereoscopic device with rotating disks for testing vision.

stereophorometer (stĕr″ē-ō-for-ŏm′ĕ-ter) [" + *phoros*, a bearer, + *metron*, a measure]. A prism-refracting device for use in correcting defective vision.

stereophotography (stĕr″ē-ō-fō-tŏg′ră-fĭ) [" + *phōs*, *phot-*, light, + *graphein*, to write]. Photography which produces effect of solidity or depth of pictures.

stereophotomicrograph (stĕr″ē-ō-fō″tō-mī′-krō-grăf) [" + " + *mikros*, tiny, + *graphein*, to write]. A photograph showing solidity or depth of a microscopical subject.

stereoscope (ster′ē-ō-skōp). [G. *stereos*, solid, + *skopein*, to see]. Instrument which creates an impression of solidity or depth of objects seen by combining images of 2 pictures.

stereoscopic, stereoscopical (ster-ē-ō-skŏp′ĭk, -ĭ-kăl) [" + *skopein*, to see]. Pert. to the stereoscope or its use.

s. vision. Vision in which things have the appearance of solidity and relief as though seen in 3 dimensions. Such is the result of binocular vision.

stereotaxis [G. " + *taxis*, arrangement]. A method of precisely locating areas in the brain; use of this technique is essential in certain neurosurgical procedures.

stereotropism (stĕr″ē-ŏt′rō-pĭzm). Syn: *thigmotropism*. A response toward (*positive s.*) or away from (*negative s.*) a solid object.

stereotypy (stĕr-ē-ō-tī′pĭ) [" + *typos*, type]. Repetition of words, posture, or movement without meaning; seen in catatonic partial stupors.

sterile (stĕr′ĭl) [L. *sterilis*, barren]. 1. Free from living microorganisms. Syn: *aseptic*. 2. Not fertile; unable to reproduce young. Syn: *barren*.

sterility (stĕr-ĭl′ĭ-tĭ) [L. *sterilitās*, barrenness]. Syn: *barrenness*, *infertility*. Inability to produce offspring.

Investigation into the cause of sterility includes investigation of both husband and wife. A routine examination for sterility includes a study of the vaginal secretions, a bimanual examination, visualization of the cervix, and in some cases a test for patency of the tubes.

A history of pelvic disorder in the past is of great importance and any information as to the use of strong chemical douches for the purpose of contraception may be vital.

Treatment: The treatment of sterility depends upon the finding and correction of any or all causes of the condition. A high percentage of couples who have an infertility problem in the first year of marriage will have produced an offspring if they are followed for two to three years, even without treatment.

s., absolute. Complete inability to produce offspring as a result of anatomical or physiological factors which prevent production of functional germ cells, conception or normal development of a zygote.

s., acquired (secondary s.). The failure of further conception after once having given birth to a child.

s., facultative. Voluntary sterility; that resulting from contraceptive practices.

s., female. Inability to give birth to living young.

Etiol. Factors: Congenital Abnormalities: Absence or maldevelopment of the uterus tubes, or ovaries; infantile uterus.

Acquired Local Conditions: (a) *Vagina*: Inflammation. (b) *Cervix*: Narrowing of the internal os; acute and chronic endocervicitis; polyps occluding the cervical canal; cervical mucus which due to either its chemical or physical qualities is "hostile" to sperm. (c) *Body of the uterus*: Fibroids of the uterus which block the canal; diseased endometrium, particularly endometritis. (d) *Fallopian tube*: Chronic salpingo-oophoritis with closure of the tubal ostium and where the ovary is embedded in adhesions. (e) Ovarian dysfunction which may result from congenital conditions or be secondary to endocrine disorders, infections, trauma, neoplasms, x-ray or surgical castration, or effects of toxic agents. (f) Psychological and emotional disturbances. (g) Coital difficulties. (h) Dietary deficiencies and starvation.

s., male. Inability of a male to bring about conception. May result from (a) congenital factors such as cryptorchidism, maldevelopment of testis ducts or testis, etc.; (b) acquired factors (See: *sterility*, female); or (c) lack of libido or impotence.

s., one-child. Sterility in a woman following the birth of one child.

s., primary. S. resulting from failure of testis or ovary to produce functional germ cells.

s., relative. S. due to causes other than defect of sex organs.

sterilization (ster″ĭl-ĭ-zā′shŭn) [L. *sterilis*, barren]. 1. Process of destruction of all microorganisms on a substance by exposure to chemical or physical agents, exposure to ionizing radiation, or by filtering gas or liquids through porous materials which remove microorganisms. 2. Process of rendering barren. Can be accomplished by (a) surgical removal of testis or ovary (castration) or inactivation by irradiation, (b) tying off or removal of a portion of reproductive ducts (ductus deferens or uterine tubes). See: *vasectomy*, *salpingectomy*.

s., dryheat. S. accomplished in ovens by subjection to high heat (165° to 170° C.) for two to three hours. (Def. 1.)

s., fractional. S. in which heating is done at separated intervals, so that spores can develop into bacteria and be destroyed. Usually accomplished by subjecting organisms to free-flowing steam for 15 min. or three or four successive days. Also called *tyndallization* or *intermittent sterilization*. (Def. 1.)

s., gas. Exposure to gases which destroy microorganisms. For example, formaldehyde, ethylene oxide.

s., intermittent. SYN: *fractional sterilization, q.v.*

s., steam, by flowing. Exposure at 212° F. (100° C.) to steam in an unsealed receptacle. (Def. 1.)

s., steam under pressure. Exposure to steam in an autoclave. (Def. 1.)

sterilize (ster'ĭl-īz) [L. *sterilis,* barren]. 1. To free from microorganisms. 2. To make barren.

sterilizer (ster'ĭl-ī-zer) [L. *sterilis,* barren]. Oven or appliance for sterilizing.

s., Arnold steam. A sterilizer using live or streaming steam at atmospheric pressure.

s., steam. An autoclave or steam-pressure cooker which sterilizes by steam under pressure at temperatures above 100 degrees C.

sternal (ster'năl) [G. *sternon,* chest]. Relating to the sternum or breastbone.

sternalgia (stĕr-năl'jĭ-ă) [" + *algos,* pain]. Pain in the sternum. SYN: *sternodynia.*

sternebra. Parts of the sternum prior to fusion.

sterno- [G.]. Combining form meaning *sternum.*

sternoclavicular (ster"nō-klă-vĭk'ū-lar) [G. *sternon,* breast, + L. *clavicula,* a little key]. Concerning the sternum and clavicle.

sternocleidomastoid (ster"nō-klī-dō-măs'toyd) [" + *kleis,* clavicle, + *mastos,* breast, + *eidos,* like]. One of 2 muscles arising from sternum and inner part of clavicle. SEE: *Table of Muscles in Appendix.*

sternocostal (ster"nō-kŏs'tăl) [" + L. *costa,* rib]. Relating to sternum and ribs.

sternodynia (ster"nō-dĭn'ĭ-ă) [" + *odynē,* pain]. Pain in the sternum. SYN: *sternalgia.*

sternohyoid (ster"nō-hī'oyd) [" + *hyoeidēs,* U-shaped]. Muscle from medial end of clavicle and sternum to hyoid bone. SEE: *Table of Muscles in Appendix.*

sternoid (ster'noyd) [" + *eidos,* resemblance]. Resembling the breastbone.

sternomastoid (ster-nō"măst'oid). Pert. to the sternum and mastoid process of temporal bone.

s. region. SYN: *carotid region.* Wide area on lateral region of neck covered by sternocleidomastoid muscle.

sternopericardial (ster"nō-per"ĭ-kar'dĭ-al) [" + *peri,* around, + *kardia,* heart]. Concerning the sternum and pericardium.

sternoschisis (ster-nŏs'kĭ-sĭs). A cleft or fissured sternum.

sternothyroid (ster"nō-thī'royd) [G. *sternon,* breast, + *thyreos,* shield, + *eidos,* like]. Muscle extending beneath the sternohyoid which depresses thyroid cartilage. SEE: *Table of Muscles in Appendix.*

sternotomy (ster-nŏt'ō-mĭ) [" + *tomē,* a cutting]. The operation of cutting the sternum.

sternotrypesis (ster"nō-trī-pē'sĭs) [" + *trypēsis,* a boring]. Surgical perforation of the sternum.

sternum (ster'nŭm) [G. *sternon,* breast]. The narrow, flat bone in the median line of the thorax in front. SYN: *breastbone.*

It consists of 3 portions, distinguished as the *manubrium,* the *gladiolus,* and the *ensiform* or *xiphoid process.*

RS: *chicken breast, chondrosternal, chondroxiphoid, cleft, gladiolus, ensiform, manubrium, xiphoid process.*

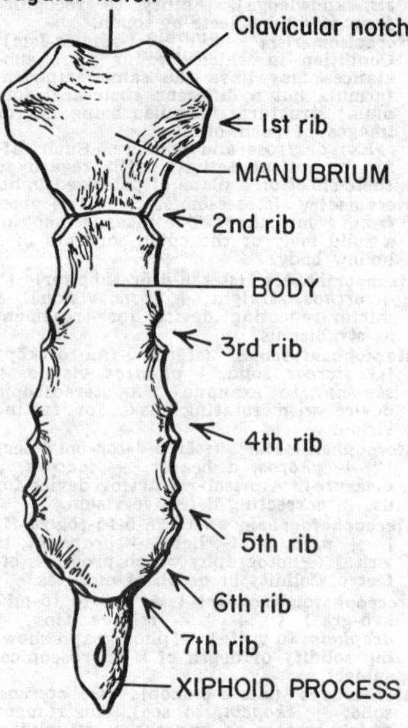

STERNUM, POSTERIOR VIEW
A. Clavicular notch. B. Manubrium. C. Body of gladiolus. D. Xiphoid process.

s., cleft. Congenital fissure of the sternum.

sternutament (ster-nū'tăm-ĕnt) [L. *sternutāre,* to sneeze]. A substance causing sneezing.

sternutatio (stĕr-nū-tā'shē-ō) [L. sneezing]. Sneezing.

s. convulsiva. Paroxysmal sneezing, as in hay fever.

sternutation (ster-nū-tā'shŭn) [L. *sternutāre,* to sneeze]. Act of sneezing.

s., convulsive. Spasmodic or paroxysmal sneezing with profusion of watery secretion from the nose.

sternutator (ster'nū-tāt"or). An agent, such as a war gas, which induces sneezing.

sternutatory (ster-nū'tă-tō"rĭ) [L. *sternutāre,* to sneeze]. Causing sneezing.

steroid (ster'oid). 1. An organic compound containing in its chemical nucleus the perhydrocyclopentanophenanthrene ring. See illus., page P-34. 2. Term applied to any one of a large group of substances chemically related to sterols. Includes sterols, D vitamins, bile acids, certain hormones, saponins, glucosides of digitalis, and certain carcinogenic substances.

s. hormones. The sex hormones and hormones of the adrenal cortex.

sterol (stĕr'ōl) [G. *stereos,* solid, + L. *oleum,* oil]. One of a group of substances related to fats and belonging to the lipoids. They are alcohols with a cyclic nucleus (cyclopentanoperhydrophenanthrene) and are found free or esterified with fatty acids (cholesterides). They are found in animals (*zoosterols*) or in plants (*phytosterols*).

Generally colorless, crystalline compounds, nonsaponifiable and soluble in certain organic solvents. Ex: *cholesterol.*

stertor (stĕr'tōr) [L. *stertor,* a snore]. Snoring or laborious breathing due to obstruction of air passages in the head, seen in certain diseases, as apoplexy.

stertorous (stĕr'tō-rŭs) [L. *stertor,* a snore]. Pert. to laborious breathing provoking a snoring sound.

stetho- [G.]. Combining form meaning the *chest.*

stethogoniometer (steth"ō-gō-nĭ-ŏm'ĕt-ĕr) [G. *stēthos,* chest, + *gōnia,* angle, + *metron,* measure]. Device for measuring the curvature of the chest.

stethograph (stĕth'ō-grăf) [" + *graphein,* to write]. Device to record chest movements in respiration.

stethokyrtograph (stĕth"o-kir'tō-grăf) [" + *kyrtos,* bent, + *graphein,* to write]. Device for measuring and recording the dimensions and amount of curves of the chest.

stethometer (stĕth-ŏm'ĕt-ĕr) [" + *metron,* measure]. Device for measuring the chest's expansion during respiration.

stethophonometer (stĕth"ō-fō-nŏm'ĕt-ĕr) [" + *phōnē,* voice, + *metron,* a measure]. Instrument for determining intensity of sound emitted in auscultation.

stethoscope (stĕth'ō-skōp) [G. *stēthos,* chest, + *skopein,* to see]. Instrument used in auscultation to convey to the ear the sounds produced in the body.

Ordinarily consists of rubber tubing in a Y shape.

s., binaural. S. designed for use with both ears.

s., compound. More than 1 set attached to the same fork and chest piece.

s., double. S. with 2 earpieces and tubes.

s., percussion. Solid cylinder of wood, 1 end wedge-shaped, other enlarged into an earpiece adapted for intercostal use.

s., single or ***monaural.*** For 1 ear only; rigid or flexible.

stethoscopy (stĕth-ŏs'kō-pĭ) [G. *stēthos,* chest, + *skopein,* to see]. Examination by means of the stethoscope.

stethospasm (stĕth'ō-spăzm) [" + *spasmos,* spasm]. Spasm of the pectoral or chest muscles.

STH. Abbr. for *somatotrophin,* the growth hormone.

sthenia (sthē'nĭ-ă) [G. *sthenos,* strength]. Normal or unusual strength, the opp. of *asthenia.*

sthenic (sthĕn'ĭk) [G. *sthenos,* strength]. Active; strong.

sthenometer (sthĕn-ŏm'ĕ-tĕr) [" + *metron,* a measure]. Device for measuring muscular strength.

sthenometry (sthĕn-ŏm'ĕ-trĭ) [" + *metron,* a measure]. Determination of bodily strength.

stibialism (stĭb'ĭ-ăl-ĭzm) [L. *stibium,* antimony, + G. *-ismos,* condition]. Antimonial poisoning.

stibium (stĭb'ĭ-ŭm) [L.]. Antimony.

stichochrome (stĭk'ō-krōm) [G. *stichos,* row, + *chrōma,* color]. A nerve cell in which the stainable bodies (tigroid mass) are arranged in parallel rows.

stictacne (stĭk-tăk'nē) [G. *stiktos,* pointed, + *akmē,* point]. Acne with red base and black pointed comedo at apex. Syn: *acne punctata.*

stiff (stĭf). Rigid, firm, inflexible.

s. joint. One with reduced mobility.

s. neck. *Torticollis, wryneck.* Rigidity of neck resulting from spasm of neck muscles. It is a symptom of many disorders.

s.-n. fever. 1. Dengue. 2. Cerebrospinal meningitis.

stigma (stĭg'mă) (pl. *stigmata*) [G. *stigma,* a mark]. 1. A mark or spot on the skin. 2. Spot on ovarian surface where rupture of a graafian follicle will occur. 3. Red spot due to extravasation of blood produced by nervous influence. 4. Mark characterizing a specific disease.

s. of degeneration. Any of the bodily variations from the normal. Formerly thought to be associated with mental degeneracy.

Degenerative Changes: *Face*: May be unusually hairy in the female and abnormally smooth in the male. *Fingers and toes*: May be an extra one, or adherent or webbed. *Forehead*: May be sloping and very low. *Eyes*: May be different in color or set at different levels. *Ears*: Unusual in many ways. *Jaws*: Either may project unusually. *Head*: May be unusually large or small. *Teeth*: May be irregular or project. *Roof of mouth*: May be high and pointed or unusually narrow. Only several of these irregularities may be considered as indicative of defective mentality.

s., hysterical. Any of the peculiar marks or symptoms of hysteria such as spots on the skin, areas of hyper- or anesthesia, impairment of sensory functions, etc.

s., psychic. Mental state characterized by susceptibility to suggestion.

stigmatic (stĭg-măt'ĭk) [G. *stigma,* mark]. Pert. to or marked with a stigma.

stigmatism. 1. Condition characterized by possession of stigmata. 2. Condition in which the rays of light are accurately focused on retina. See: *astigmatism.*

stigmatization (stĭg"măt-ĭ-zā'shŭn) [G. *stigma,* mark]. The formation of stigmata, esp. hysterical s. on the skin.

stigmatometer (stĭg-mă-tŏm'ĕ-tĕr) [G. *stigma,* mark, + *metron,* a measure]. Device for testing eye refraction. Syn: *astigmatometer.*

stilbestrol. Diethylstilbestrol, *q.v.*

stilet, stilette (stĭl-ĕt') [Fr. *stilette*]. 1. Small, sharp-pointed instrument for probing. 2. Wire used to pass through or stiffen a flexible catheter.

stillbirth (stĭl'birth) [A.S. *stille,* quiet, + M.E. *burth,* birth]. Birth of a dead fetus.

stillborn (stĭl'born) [" + *beran,* to bring forth]. Dead at birth.

stillicidium (stĭl-ĭ-sĭd'ĭ-ŭm) [L. *stilla,* drop, + *cadere,* to fall]. A dribbling or flowing, drop by drop.

s. lacrimarum. Watering of the eye. Syn: *epiphora.*

s. narium. Watery mucus discharged at onset of coryza.

s. urinae. Urinary incontinence from a distended bladder. Syn: *strangury.*

stimulant (stĭm'ū-lănt) [L. *stimulus,* a goad]. Any agent temporarily increasing functional activity.

Stimulants may be classified according to the organ upon which they act as follows: Cardiac, bronchial, gastric, cerebral, intestinal, nervous, motor, vasomotor, respiratory, and secretory.

stimulate (stĭm'ū-lāt) [L. *stimulāre,* to goad on]. To increase functional activity of an organ or structure.

stim'ulating en'ema. One given to excite activity in shock or unconscious state. SEE: *enema.*

stimulation (stĭm″ū-lā′shŭn) [L. *stimulāre,* to goad on]. 1. Process of being stimulated. 2. Irritating action of agents on muscles, nerves or sensory end organs by which activity in a part is evoked.

stimulus (stĭm′ū-lŭs) (pl. *stimuli*) [L. *stimulus,* a goad]. 1. Any agent or factor able to influence directly living protoplasm, as one capable of causing muscular contraction or secretion in a gland, or of initiating an impulse in a nerve. 2. A change of environment of sufficient intensity to evoke a response in an organism. 3. An excitant or irritant.

s., adequate. 1. Any stimulus capable of evoking a response, *i.e.,* an environmental change possessing a certain intensity, acting for a certain length of time and occurring at a certain rate. 2. A stimulus capable of initiating a nerve impulse in a specific type of receptor.

s., chemical. A chemical substance, liquid, gaseous, or solid, which is capable of evoking a response.

s., conditioned. A stimulus which gives rise to a conditioned response. SEE: *reflex, conditioned.*

s., electric. A stimulus resulting from the initiation of, or cessation of, a flow of electrons as from a battery, induction coil, or generator.

s., homologous. A stimulus which acts only on specific sensory end organs.

s., liminal. A threshold stimulus, *q.v.*

s., mechanical. SYN: *physical stimulus.* A stimulus produced by a physical change such as contact with objects, changes in pressure, etc.

s., minimal. A threshold stimulus, *q.v.*

s., nociceptive. A painful and usually injurious stimulus.

s., subliminal. Less than a threshold stimulus.

s., thermal. One produced by a change in temperature of the skin, a rise giving sensations of warmth; a fall giving rise to sensations of coldness.

s., threshold. SYN: *s., liminal; s., minimal.* The least or weakest stimulus that is capable of initiating a response or giving rise to a sensation.

sting (stĭng) [A.S. *stingan,* to stick]. 1. Sharp, smarting sensation, as of a wound or astringent. 2. A sharp offensive weapon of an insect such as a bee or wasp. 3. A wound made by a sting.

S-T interval. The interval in an electrocardiogram which represents the initial and final ventricular complexes.

stippling (stĭp′lĭng) [Dutch *stippelen,* to spot]. A spotted condition, as in retina in certain ocular diseases or in basophilic red corpuscles.

stirrup, stirrup bone (stir′ŭp) [A.S. *stigrāp,* a stirrup]. Stapes of the ears.

stitch (stĭch) [M.E. *stiche,* from A.S. *stice,* a pricking]. 1. A local, sharp, lancinating, or spasmodic pain 2. A single loop of suture material passed through skin or flesh by a needle, to facilitate healing of a wound. 3. To unite skin or flesh with a needle and suture material.

Some are removed after a few days and other types are absorbed by the body. SYN: *suture.*

s. abscess. One developing in a suture; due to infection.

stochastic model [G. *stochastikos,* skillful in guessing]. A statistical model which attempts to reproduce that sequence of events which would be expected to occur in a real-life situation. This technique has some usefulness in predicting the importance and extent of disease in a specified population.

stock (stŏk) [A.S. *stocc,* a trunk]. The original individual, race, or tribe from which others have descended.

s. culture. Permanent culture of a microorganism reinforced from time to time by fresh media.

Stokes-Adams syndrome (stōks-ăd′ăms). A series of symptoms in those suffering from heart block. Onset is sudden, resembling epilepsy, for which it is sometimes mistaken. SYN: *Adams-Stokes syndrome.*

ETIOL: Due to complete heart block with consequent decrease in blood flow to the brain.

TREATMENT: Intracardiac epinephrine, a sharp blow to the precordium or use of an external electric pacemaker.

Stokes' law (stōks). A muscle is frequently a seat of paralysis if lying above an inflamed serous or mucous membrane.

S's. lens. Device used to diagnose astigmatism.

stoma (stō′mă) (pl. *stomata*) [G. *stoma,* a mouth]. 1. A mouth or small opening or a pore. 2. Artificially created opening bet. 2 passages or body cavities or bet. a cavity or passage and the body's surface. 3. A minute opening between cells of certain epithelial membranes, esp. peritoneum and pleura.

stomach (stŭm′ăk) [G. *stomachos,* stomach]. A dilated, saclike, distensible portion of the alimentary canal below the esophagus, 12x4 in., below the diaphragm to right of spleen, partly under the liver.

It is composed of a *fundus,* or round part; a *body,* or middle portion, and pyloric portion which is small end.

It has 2 openings: the upper *cardiac orifice* opens into the esophagus and the lower *pyloric orifice* opens into the duodenum. The stomach is composed of 4 layers: Outer *serous coat* covers almost all of the organ; the *muscular layer* just beneath is formed of 3 layers of smooth muscle fibers; an outer longitudinal layer; a medial circular layer,

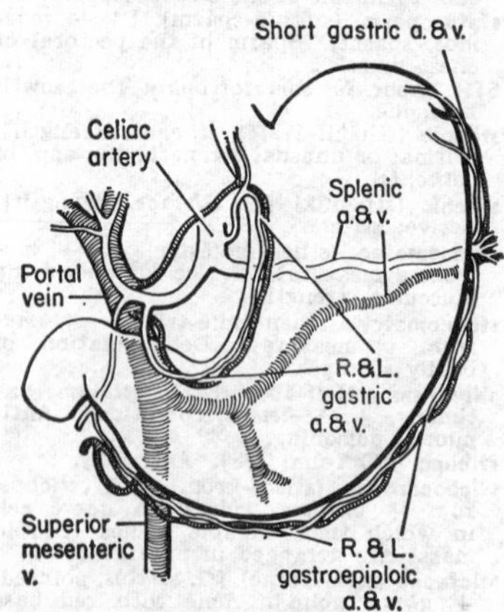

STOMACH.
(Anterior View)

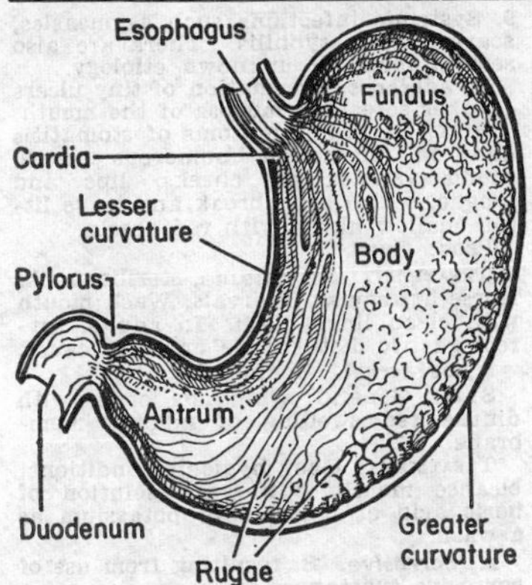

THE STOMACH.

and an inner oblique layer. *Submucous layer* is a connecting medium between the muscular and the *mucous layer*, which is the inner lining of the stomach.

The cardiac, fundic (parietal or oxyntic) and pyloric glands of the stomach are composed of columnar and tubular cells which secrete gastric juice containing hydrochloric acid, pepsin, etc.

FUNCTIONS: It secretes the gastric juice and converts proteins into peptones. In addition to serving strictly as an organ of digestion (SEE: *gastric digestion*), the stomach has the following functions: (1) Acting as a reservoir, it regulates the admission of food to the remainder of the gut; (2) its acid kills a large proportion of the microbes present in most food; (3) it has some power to absorb, SEE: *absorption;* (4) secreting acid, it is important in the acid-base equilibrium of the body; (5) it can excrete some drugs, administered parenterally, into the gastric juice; (6) it acts as a kind of receptor in chemical and nervous mechanisms by which secretion and movement are stimulated in lower parts of the gastrointestinal tract (SEE: *secretagogue* and *reflex, gastrocolic*), and (7) by the action of an *intrinsic factor* (present in gastric juice) on an *extrinsic factor* (vitamin B_{12}) present in foods, a *hematinic principle* (*antianemic factor*) is formed. This is effective in prevention of pernicious anemia.

S. CANCER: May be due to carcinoma, lymphoma, sarcoma, etc.

SYM: General symptoms of dyspepsia with following characteristic symptoms: Continued pain, often tenderness; vomiting of partially digested food; absence of free hydrochloric acid in gastric juice; hematemesis or blood in stools, slight in amount and blood altered so it presents a coffee grounds appearance; presence of tumor; loss of flesh and strength; extreme anemia; involvement of superficial lymph glands. When the pylorus is involved symptoms of gastric dilatation will be added.

PROG: Very poor.

TREATMENT: Early treatment, surgical. Liquid or semiliquid diet. Rest. Constitutional treatment as indicated.

PYLORIC OBSTRUCTION AND DILATATION: Pyloric obstruction increases the resistance offered to the expulsion of food and in its efforts to overcome this the stomach first becomes hypertrophied, then dilated. *Causes of dilatation*: (1) Pyloric obstruction; (2) laxness of walls from simple atony; (3) excessive ingestion of food or drink.

SYM: The general symptoms of dyspepsia, together with the following relating to the vomit: Vomiting occurs long after eating, sometimes several hours or days. Amount often excessive, sometimes several quarts; is sour and fermented, and on standing separates into a sediment of undigested food and a turbid, frothy liquid. Ejected fluid rich in torulae and sarcinae, forms of bacteria. Obstinate constipation.

PHYSICAL SIGNS: Bulging over epigastrium; in thin subjects the outline of stomach may be visible. Palpation gives a splashing fremitus.

PERCUSSION: Increased area of gastric tympany.

AUSCULTATION: Splashing sounds often audible at some distance.

MENSURATION: Ordinarily an esophageal sound may be inserted a distance of 60 cm. from the teeth. In dilatation may be inserted 65 to 70 cm.

PROG: Guarded. More favorable in dilatation without obstruction.

TREATMENT: Diet light, nutritious, not bulky, and should be given in small amounts at frequent intervals. Lavage 2 or 3 times weekly. An abdominal support often relieves some of distressing symptoms.

FOREIGN BODIES: These ordinarily should give no concern. Symptoms are usually absent. The patient may be alarmed. Give nothing by mouth. Salts, cathartics, and enemas should under no circumstances be used, inasmuch as they can only make the condition worse. Such foreign bodies usually pass through the alimentary tract without disturbance. These patients should always be under the care of a doctor.

DIET IN OTHER DISEASES OF STOMACH: *Atony and Hypomobility*: Food is retained longer than normal and if hydrochloric acid is deficient, decomposition may occur. Liquids are retained longer than solids. Diet should consist of quickly and easily digested foods, cream, butter, soft cooked vegetables, chicken, fish, strained beef and moderate amount of milk. Avoid liquids, pastries and rich gravies.

Hypermotility: The stomach empties too rapidly; therefore, diet should be soft and liquid in small amounts and in frequent feedings. Fats delay the emptying of the stomach.

Hyperacidity: Protein to combine with acid, inhibiting its secretion by moderate amt. of fat, and to avoid stimulating secretion of acid. Five small meals, or 3 meals and 2 lunches.

s. ache. Pain in the stomach. SYN: *gastralgia, gastrodynia, stomachalgia, stomachodynia.*

s., bilocular. SEE: *hourglass stomach.*

s., cardiac. Fundus of the stomach.

s., cascade. A form of hourglass stomach in which there is a constriction between cardiac and pyloric portions. Cardiac portion fills first and then contents cascade into pyloric portion. Also called *cup and spill stomach.*

s., cow horn. A high transversely placed stomach. Also called *steer horn s.*

s., dumping. A condition sometimes following gastroenterostomy in which food is rapidly discharged through new opening into intestine with resulting intestinal distention and accompanying discomfort. SYN: *dumping.*

s., hourglass. One resembling an hourglass, caused by constriction from a band of fibrous exudate.

s. *intubation.* Passage of a tube into the stomach: 1. To obtain gastric contents for examination. 2. For prophylaxis and treatment of ileus. 3. To remove ingested poisons.

s., leather bottle. One caused by hypertrophy of the s. walls or their infiltration with malignant tissue.

s. *pump.* Device for removing contents of the stomach through a tube inserted through the mouth.

s., thoracic. Condition in which stomach lies above diaphragm. May result from embryonic anomaly in which stomach fails to descend, or from hernia of diaphragm. Latter results in so-called *upside-down stomach.*

s. *tooth.* A lower canine one during first dentition.

s. *tube.* One for washing out or feeding the stomach.

s., water-trap. One with the pylorus unusually high, causing slow emptying.

stomach, *words pert. to:* abdominal cavity; achylia gastrica; acidity; anachlorhydria; anadenia; anticardium; atony; atretogastria; bead test; Bouchard's nodules; capotement; cardialgia; cardiodiosis; cardiopyloric; cardiospasm; catastalsis; chlorhydria; cholangiogastrostomy; clapotement; clapotage; digestion; ectasia; endogastritis; feeding, artificial; fractional test meal; gastric juice; gastric lavage; gastric motor meals; "gastr-" words; gavage; hourglass stomach; hunger; lavage; linitis; myxorrhea gastrica; oxyntic glands; pneumatosis; pneumogastric; pylorus; saburra; ulcer; ventriculus.

stomachal (stŭm'ăk-ăl) [G. *stomachos,* stomach]. 1. Relating to the stomach. 2. A gastric tonic.

stomachalgia (stŭm-ăk-ăl'jĭ-ă) [" + *algos,* pain] Pain in the stomach.

stomachic (stō-măk'ĭk) [G. *stomachos,* stomach]. 1. Concerning the stomach. 2. Medicine exciting action of the stomach. SYN: *stomachal.*

stomachoscopy (stŭm-ăk-os'kō-pĭ) [" + *skopein,* to inspect]. Examination of the stomach. SYN: *gastroscopy.*

sto'mata. Plural of *stoma, q.v.*

stomatalgia (stō-măt-ăl'jĭ-ă) [G. *stoma, stomat-,* mouth, + *algos,* pain]. Pain in the mouth. SYN: *stomatodynia.*

stomatic (stō-măt'ĭk). Pert. to or relating to the mouth.

stomatitis (stō-mă-tī'tĭs) [G. *stoma, stomat-,* mouth, + *-itis,* inflammation]. Inflammation of the mouth.

SYM: Heat, pain, increased flow of saliva, fetor of breath, restlessness, languor, disinclination to nurse in infants, sometimes fever. RS: *gangrene, noma, thrush.*

ETIOL: S. may be caused by many factors or conditions. Among them are: 1. Pathogenic organisms, including bacteria and viruses. 2. Mechanical trauma. 3. Irritants, such as alcohol, tobacco, hot foods, spices. 4. Sensitization to chemical substances in tooth pastes, mouthwashes, etc. 5. Nutritional deficiencies, esp. avitaminoses. 6. Blood disorders. 7. Poisoning by drugs, esp. heavy metals. 8. Certain skin disorders. 9. Systemic infections such as measles, scarlet fever, syphilis. There are also several forms of unknown etiology.

s., aphthous. Formation of tiny ulcers (canker sores) on mucosa of the mouth.

SYM: General symptoms of stomatitis and on inspection numerous small, round vesicles on cheeks, lips and tongue, which soon break and leave little, shallow ulcers with red areola.

PROG: Good.

TREATMENT: For infants, sterilize milk. Nurse at regular intervals. Wash mouth with clean linen cloth. In adults, correct gastric disturbance or other cause.

s., catarrhal. Simple stomatitis.

SYM: General symptoms of s. with diffuse red swelling of mucous membrane.

TREATMENT: Good hygienic conditions; cleanse mouth with weak solution of boric acid or chlorate of potassium as a wash.

s., corrosive. S. resulting from use of corrosive substances.

s., diphtheritic. Diphtheria of mucous membranes of the gums or cheeks. SYN: *buccal diphtheria.*

s., follicular. SEE: *s., aphthous.*

s., gangrenous. This form seen in debilitated children from 2 to 6 years; usually follows one of the specific fevers, esp. measles and whooping cough.

SYM: General; an inspection shows cheek is affected. Externally, swollen, hard, red and glazed; internally, irregular, sloughing ulcer.

COMPLICATIONS: Perforation, septicemia, lobular pneumonia from aspirated sloughs, and diarrhea from swallowing fetid material.

PROG: Grave. Death common from exhaustion or complications. Recovery often attended with deformity.

TREATMENT: Excision with electrocautery knife early. Nutritious food, good hygiene. SYN: *cancrum oris, noma.*

s., herpetic. S. characterized by cold sores (fever blisters).

s., membranous. S. accompanied by the formation of a false or adventitious membrane.

s., mercurial. This form is seen in artisans who work in mercury; after the administration of very large doses of mercurials, and after small doses where there has been unnatural susceptibility.

PREMONITORY SYMPTOMS: Tenderness of gums, redness near insertion of teeth, metallic taste, increase of saliva.

LATER SYM: Profuse salivation, fetor of breath, redness, swelling and tenderness of gums. Tongue may be similarly affected and protrude from mouth. In severe cases ulceration of mucous membrane, loss of teeth and necrosis of jaw result.

TREATMENT: If due to acute poisoning, early administration of British antilewisite will be helpful. If chronic, remove patient from source of poison and treat symptomatically. SEE: *ptyalism.*

s., myotic. SYN: *thrush, q.v.*

s. *parasitica.* SYN: *thrush.* S. caused by a yeastlike fungus, *Candida albicans.*

SYM: Of general s. with milk-white elevations on tongue and mouth which on removal leave a raw surface. Disease may extend to pharynx, esophagus and larynx. Microscopic examination reveals fungus.

PROG: Good.

TREATMENT: Correct hygiene. Treat any gastric disturbance; locally, mild alkaline mouthwash. Dilute gentian violet mouthwash is also effective. Topical application of dilute nystatin solution may be necessary.

s., simple. Erythematous inflammation of the mouth occurring in patches on the mucous membranes.

s., traumatic. S. resulting from mechanical injury as from ill-fitting dentures, sharp jagged teeth, biting cheek, etc.

s., ulcerative. Thought by some to be an infectious disease, as it often occurs in epidemics and attacks both children and adults when congregated and subjected to bad hygienic conditions.

SYM: Of the general form; gums of lower jaw chiefly affected, are swollen, red and spongy. Linear ulcers soon form and may extend to cheek; gland under jaw swollen. In severe cases loosening of teeth and necrosis of jaw may follow.

PROG: Guardedly favorable.

TREATMENT: Correct hygiene; antiseptic mouthwashes such as hydrogen peroxide; no smoking. SYN: *trench mouth.*

s., vesicular. SEE: *aphthous* s.

s., Vincent's. Ulcerative stomatitis.

stomato- [G.]. Combining form meaning *mouth.*

stomatodynia (stō″mă-tō-dĭn′ĭ-ă) [G. *stoma, stomat-*, mouth, + *odynē*, pain]. Pain in the mouth. SYN: *stomatalgia.*

stomatodysodia (stō″mă-tō-dĭs-ō′dĭ-ă) [" + *dysōdia*, stench]. Foul odor from the mouth.

stomatogastric (stō″mă-tō-găs′trĭk) [" + *gastēr*, belly]. Concerning the stomach and mouth.

stomatography (stō″mă-tŏg′ră-fĭ) [" + *graphein*, to write]. A treatise on the mouth.

stomatologist (stō″mă-tŏl′ō-jĭst) [" + *logos*, a study]. Specialist in treatment of diseases of the mouth.

stomatology (stō″mă-tol′ō-jĭ) [" + *logos*, a study]. Science of the mouth and teeth and their diseases.

stomatomalacia (stō″mă-tō-mă-lā′sĭ-ă) [" + *malakia*, softening]. Pathological softening of any structures of the mouth.

stomatomy (stō-măt′ō-mĭ) [" + *tomē*, a cutting]. Surgical nicking of the edges of the os uteri to facilitate delivery.

stomatomycosis (stō″mă-tō-mī-kō′sĭs) [G. *stoma, stomat-*, mouth, + *mykēs*, fungus, + *-ōsis*, condition]. Any mouth disease resulting from fungi.

stomatonecrosis, stomatonoma (stō″mă-tō-nē-krō′sĭs, -nō′mă) [" + *nekrosis*, death, — + *nomē*, a spreading]. Gangrenous, ulcerative inflammation of the mouth. SYN: *cancrum oris, noma.*

stomatopathy (stō-mă-tŏp′ă-thĭ) [" + *pathos*, disease]. Any mouth disease.

stomatoplasty (stō-măt′ō-plăs″tĭ) [" + *plassein*, to form]. Plastic operation upon the mouth.

stomatorrhagia (stō″mă-tor-rā′jĭ-ă) [" + *-rrhagia*, from *rhēgnynai*, to burst forth]. Hemorrhage from the mouth or gums.

stomatoscope (stō′măt-ō-skōp) [" + *skopein*, to examine]. Instrument for examining the mouth.

stomato′sis. Any disease of the mouth.

stomodaeum, stomodeum (stō″mō-dē′ŭm) [G. *stoma, stomat-*, mouth, + *daiein*, to divide]. An external depression lined with ectoderm and bounded by frontonasal, mandibular, and maxillary processes of the embryo. It forms ant. portion of oral cavity. Its floor, the *pharyngeal membrane*, separates stomodeum from the foregut.

stone (stōn) [A.S. *stān*]. Hardened mineral matter, as *gallstones.** SYN: *calculus, q.v.*

stool (stōōl) [A.S. *stōl*, a seat]. 1. Evacuation of the bowels. 2. Waste matter discharged from the bowels. SYN: *feces, q.v.*

COLOR: Iron and bismuth turn the stool black and certain vegetables and berries darken it or produce a distinct color. Pathological stools are usually grayish or a whitish glistening color, and tarry in hemorrhage or show fresh blood.

CHARACTER OR NATURE OF STOOLS: *Fatty stools*: These are observed in obstructive jaundice, cancer of the pancreas, pancreatic calculi, and in indigestion or overfeeding in infants.

Frothy, poorly formed stools: They may indicate a spastic colon, the presence of gas, or intestinal inflammation.

Lienteric stools: These contain much undigested food and are noted in inflammatory conditions of the stomach and upper bowel.

Tarry stools: They are indicative of gastric hemorrhage, or may result from swallowing blood from the nose or lungs. They also may denote duodenal ulcer, or ulcer of the intestines, hepatic cirrhosis, or cancer.

Membranous shreds: They may exist in cancer of the colon, dysentery, relapsing fever, acute proctitis, and in sloughing of intestinal mucosa.

Mucous stools: Exist in catarrhal or inflamed conditions of the intestines or rectum, in dysentery, enterocolitis, proctitis, impaction, and ulcerative colitis.

SHAPE OF: *Cylindrical*: If of small caliber, they may be indicative of prolapsus ani, annular rectal stricture, or intestinal spasms.

Ribbon-shaped: Indicative of stricture or cancer of the rectum; possibly enlargement of the prostate in males, hemorrhoids, spasm of the lower bowel and anus, prostatic abscess, and prolapse of the uterus.

Scybala: Rounded masses or balls of fecal matter or hardened feces, the result of habitual constipation, atony or sacculation (diverticulum) of the colon, gastric ulcer, or dilation, and rectal cancer, or dysentery.

s., bilious. Yellowish or yellowish-brown discharges in diarrhea becoming darker on exposure.

s., fatty. Fat in the feces, as in pancreatic disease.

s., pea soup. Liquid stools of typhoid.

s., rice water. Watery serum stools with detached epithelium, as in cholera.

stop needle. One with eye at tip and a disk to prevent penetration deeper than desired.

stoppage (stŏp′ăj) [A.S. *stoppian*]. Obstruction of an organ. SEE: *cholestasia.*

storm. A sudden outburst or exacerbation of symptoms of a disease.

s., renal. A sudden attack of renal symptoms accompanying a neurosis sometimes occurring in patients suffering from aortic regurgitation.

stout (stowt) [M.E. stout; bold]. Having a bulky body. SYN: *corpulent.*

stovarsol (stō′var-sol). A commercial brand of acetarsone* used in spirochetal infections.

STP. Abbr. for *standard temperature and pressure.*

strabismic (stră-bĭz′mĭk) [G. *strabismos,* a squint]. Pert. to or afflicted with strabismus.

strabismometer (stră-bĭz-mŏm′ĕt-ĕr) [" + *metron,* a measure]. Instrument for determining amount of strabismus.

strabismus (stră-bĭz′mŭs) [G. *strabismos,* a squinting]. Disorder of eye in which optic axes cannot be directed to same object, due to lack of muscular coordination. SYN: *squint.*

The squinting eye always deviates to the same extent when the eyes are carried in different directions. *Unilateral,* when same eye always deviates. *Alternating,* when either deviates, the other being fixed. *Constant,* when the squint remains permanent. *Periodic,* when eyes are occasionally free from it. Muscles may lead to squint, but prime factor is found in errors of refraction, in hypermetropia or in myopia with or without astigmatism. SYN: *squint, heterotropia.*

s., accommodative. S. due to disorder of ocular accommodation.

s., alternating. S. affecting either eye alternately.

s., bilateral. Same as accommodative s.

s., concomitant. Form in which both eyes move freely, but retain false relation to each other.

s., convergent (internal squint). The deviating eye turns inward.

s. deorsum vergens. Vertical strabismus, the deviating eye turning downward. SYN: *hypotropia.*

s., divergent. Deviating eye turns outward.

s., intermittent. One recurring at intervals.

s., monolateral. When the squinting eye is always the same.

s., monocular. When the same eye habitually deviates.

s., paralytic. That which is due to paralysis of a muscle. The deviation is present only in the sphere of action of the paralyzed muscle. In paralytic squint the secondary deviation is greater than the primary.

This condition is due to paralysis of one or more ocular muscles and may point to grave cerebral disease or to presence of some constitutional disease.

This form is recognized by the fact that if a candle or the finger of the surgeon is carried from right to left before the face of the patient the deviating eye fails to follow to its proper limit, and leads us to look for lesions of the 6th nerve in failure of external rectus, of 3rd nerve in failure of internal rectus of either side, of 4th nerve in impairment of superior oblique muscles. In adults this is usually due to syphilitic disease involving the nerve centers or trunks, or to rheumatism.

PROG: In general, guarded.

TREATMENT: Directed to the cause. Use of glasses.

s., spastic. S. due to contraction of an ocular muscle.

s. sursum vergens. Vertical squint upward. SYN: *hypertropia.*

ETIOL: Defects of fusion faculty, errors of refraction, poor vision in 1 eye, anisometropia.

TREATMENT: Refraction with prescribing of glasses, orthoptic training (training of fusion), operative.

s., vertical. Eye turns upward. The vision is double (diplopia), unless there is unconscious suppression of the image in squinting eye, and expression of face is bizarre and sometimes malign. It is usually the result in childhood of ametropia, or in adult life of central nervous disease.

strabometer (stră-bŏm′ĕt-ĕr) [G. *strabos,* squinting, + *metron,* a measure]. Instrument to ascertain the degree of strabismus.

strabotomy (stră-bŏt′ō-mĭ) [" + *tomē,* a cutting]. Operation for strabismus.

strain (strān) [A.S. *strēon,* begetting]. 1. A stock, said of bacteria or protozoa from a specific source and maintained in successive cultures or animal inoculation. 2. Hereditary streak or tendency. 3. [M.E. *stranen,* from L. *stringere,* to draw tight]. To pass through, as a filter. 4. To injure by making too strong an effort or by excessive use. 5. Excessive use of a part of the body so that it is injured. 6. Trauma to the muscle or the musculotendinous unit from violent contraction or excessive forcible stretch. May be associated with failure of synergistic action of muscles. SEE: *sprain.*

F. A. TREATMENT: Apply cold applications and a firm dressing. Immobilize for some time. Adhesive strapping helpful. Operative repair sometimes necessary.

strainer (strān′er) [M.E. *stranen,* from L. *stringere,* to draw tight]. Device used for retaining solid pieces while liquid passes through. SYN: *filter.*

strait (strāt) [M.E. straight, narrow, from L. *strictus,* tight]. A constricted or narrow passage.

s., inferior. The lower outlet of the pelvic canal.

s.-jacket. Shirt with long sleeves laced on patient and fastened to restrain the arms. SYN: *camisole.*

s's. of the pelvis. The inferior and superior openings of the true pelvis.

s., superior. The upper opening or inlet of the pelvic canal.

stramonium (stră-mō′nĭ-ŭm) [L.]. USP. Jamestown weed, Jimson weed. The dried leaves of *Datura stramonium.*

USES: An ingredient in asthma powder for its antispasmodic effect. Local anodyne.

POISONING: Related to atropine, *q.v.*

strangalesthesia (strang″ăl-ĕs-thē′zĭ-ă) [G. *strangalizein,* to choke, + *aisthēsis,* sensation]. A girdlelike sensation of constriction. SYN: *zonesthesia.*

strangle (strang′gl) [G. *strangalē,* a halter]. To choke or suffocate or be choked from compression of the trachea.

strangulated (străng′ū-lā″tĕd) [L. *strangulāre,* from G. *strangalē,* a halter]. Constricted so that air or blood supply is cut off, as a s. hernia.

strangulation (străng-ū-lā′shŭn) [L. *strangulāre,* from G. *strangalē,* a halter]. Compression or constriction of a part, as the bowel or throat, such as causes suspension of breathing or of passage of contents; congestion accompanies condition.

s., internal. Slipping of a coil of the intestine through the diaphragm or an abnormal opening.

strangury (străng′ū-rĭ) [G. *stragx, stragg-,* a drop, + *ouron,* urine]. Painful and interrupted urination in drops, produced by spasmodic muscular contraction of urethra and bladder.

strap (străp) [A.S. *stropp,* from G. *strophos,* a cord]. 1. A band, as one of adhesive plaster, used to hold dressings in place or to approximate surfaces of a wound. 2. To bind with strips of adhesive plaster.

strapping (străp'ĭng) [A.S. *stropp*, from G. *strophos*, a band]. 1. Adhesive plaster or other substance used to bind surfaces together or hold dressings in place. 2. Application of adhesive plaster strips on a part so as to give it support or compress it.

stratified (străt'ĭ-fīd) [L. *stratificāre*, to arrange in layers]. In strata or in the form of layers.

s. epithelium. E. in superimposed layers with differently shaped cells in the various layers.

stratiform (străt'ĭ-form) [L. *stratum*, layer, + *forma*, shape]. Arranged in layers, as manner of liquefaction of gelatin stab culture, in which there is liquefaction to the walls of the tube at the top and then downward horizontally.

stratum (strā'tŭm, străt'ŭm) (pl. *strata*) [L. *stratum*, layer]. A layer.

s. basale. The innermost or deepest layer of the endometrium of uterus.

s. compactum. The superficial or outermost layer of the endometrium.

s. corneum. Outermost horny layer of the epidermis.

s. disjunction. The outermost layer of the stratum corneum which is being constantly shed.

s. germinativum. Innermost layer of epidermis, a row of columnar cells, which divide to replace rest of the epidermis as it wears away. SEE: *prickle cell.*

s. granulosum. A layer of cells containing deeply staining granules of *keratohyalin* found in epidermis of skin and lying between stratum germinativum and stratum lucidum.

s. lucidum. A translucent layer of the epidermis lying between stratum corneum and stratum granulosum. It is frequently absent.

s. Malpighii. Inner layer of the epidermis. SYN: *rete mucosum, s. germinativum.*

s. mucosum. Same as *s. malpighii.*

s. papillare. The papillary of the corium lying adjacent to the epidermis.

s. reticulare. The reticular layer of the corium lying just beneath the papillary layer.

s. spinosum. Same as *s. malpighii.*

s. spongiosum. Middle layer of decidua.

s. submucosum. Layer of smooth muscle fibers of the myometrium lying contiguous with endometrium.

s. subserosum. Layer of smooth muscle fibers of myometrium which lies immediately under serous coat.

s. supravasculare. A layer of circular and longitudinal muscle fibers lying between s. subserosum and s. vasculare.

s. vasculare. A layer of smooth muscles in myometrium lying between s. submucosum and s. supravasculare.

strawberry (straw'bĕr"ĭ) [A.S. *strēawberige*, hay berry]. COMP: Contain little cellulose. Sugar is low. They contain much lime and a salicylic element.

FROZEN, SLICED, SWEETENED: 100 gm. Calories: 109. Other values: 0.5 gm. protein; 0.2 gm. fat; 14 mg. calcium; 27.8 gm, carbohydrate; 53 mg. vitamin C.

ACTION: The salicylic element is irritating to many and may result in a skin rash.

strawberry mark. SYN: *cavernous angioma.* A soft, nodular, vascular nevus usually present on face or neck, occurring at birth or shortly afterwards. They usually disappear without treatment. SYN: *simplex hemangioma.*

straw'berry tongue. The peculiar, red, papillated tongue of scarlatina, *q.v.* SEE: *tongue.*

straw itch. A skin condition accompanied by itching due to working in straw or sleeping on a straw mattress.

streak (strēk) [A.S. *strica*, a line]. A line or stripe. SYN: *stria.*

s., angioid. A dark streak seen in retina in individuals with pseudoxanthoma elasticum.

s. culture. A bacterial culture in streaks.

s., medullary. Deep longitudinal groove on dorsal surface of the embryo which becomes the medullary tube. SYN: *dorsal groove.*

s., meningitic. A red line across the skin formed by drawing a pointed article across it; seen in meningitis and nerve center affections. SYN: *tache cérébrale.*

s. reflex. A white, shining streak along center of retinal vessels.

strephosymbolia (strĕf-ō-sĭm-bō'lĭ-ă). Difficulty in distinguishing between letters which are similar but in opposite directions, for ex. p-q, b-d, or perception of objects reversed as in a mirror.

strephotome (strĕf'ō-tōm) [G. *strephein*, to twist, + *tomē*, a cutting]. Instrument for invagination of a hernial sac.

strepitus (strĕp'ĭt-ŭs) [L. *strepitus*, noise]. A sound or noise, as that heard on auscultation.

strepticemia (strĕp-tĭ-sē'mĭ-ă) [G. *streptos*, twisted, + *aima*, blood]. Streptococci present in the blood stream causing infection. SYN: *streptococcemia.*

strepto- [G.]. Combining form meaning *twisted.*

streptoangina (strĕp"tō-ăn-jī'nă) [G. *streptos*, twisted, + L. *angina*, a choking]. Sore throat with membranous formation due to streptococci.

streptobacillus (strĕp-tō-bă-sĭl'ŭs). A bacillus in which individual bacilli form a chainlike colony.

streptococcal (strĕp"tō-kŏk'ăl) [" + *kokkos*, berry]. Caused by or pert. to streptococci.

streptococcemia (strĕp"tō-kŏk-sē'mĭ-ă) [" + " + *aima*, blood]. Presence of streptococci in the blood causing infection.

streptococcic (strĕp"tō-kŏk'sĭk) [" + *kokkos*, berry]. Resembling, produced by, or pert. to streptococci.

s. sore throat. Severe epidemic form with membranous formation caused by *Streptococcus haemolyticus.*

streptococcicosis (strĕp"tō-kŏk-sĭ-kō'sĭs) [G. *streptos*, twisted, + *kokkos*, berry, + *-ōsis*, condition]. Any streptococcal infection.

streptococcolysin (strĕp"tō-kŏk-ŏl'ĭ-sĭn) [" + " + *lysis*, dissolution]. A lysin produced by streptococci.

Streptococcus (strĕp"tō-kŏk'ŭs) (pl. *Streptococci*) [G. *streptos*, twisted, + *kokkos*, berry]. A genus of bacteria belonging to the family Lactobacillaceae, tribe Streptococcaceae. They are gram-positive cocci occurring in chains.

Most species are harmless saprophytes but some are among the most common and dangerous pathogens of man. They are differentiated on the basis of their reactions on blood-agar plates into three types: ***alpha*** (α), ***beta*** (β), and ***gamma*** (γ). Those of the *alpha* type

(*Streptococcus viridans*) form a greenish coloration about colonies and partially hemolyze blood; those of the *beta* or hemolytic type form clear zones about colonies and completely hemolyze blood (Ex: *Str. pyogenes*); those of the *gamma* type are nonhemolytic and produce a grayish coloration about colonies (Ex: *Str. anhemolyticus*).

Str. anhemolyticus. A species of low pathogenicity, often found as secondary invaders.

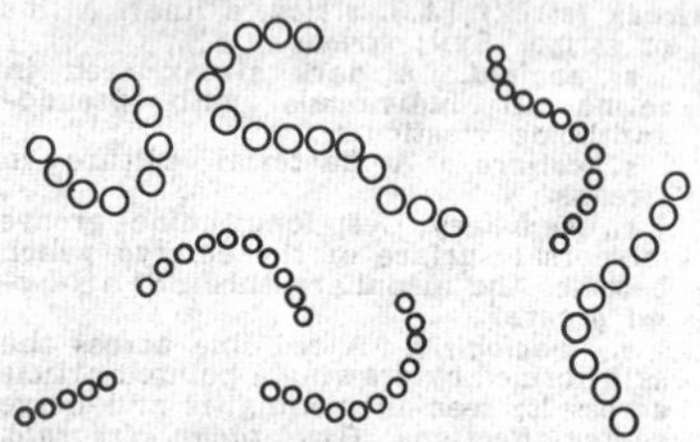

STREPTOCOCCUS.
Cocci of varying size in chains.

Str. cardioarthritidis. Variety found in blood and throat secretion cultures in cases of rheumatic fever.

Str. epidemicus. Hemolytic variety seen in throat cultures in cases of epidemic sore throat. SYN: *Str. pyogenes.*

Str. equinus. Variety found in intestines of horses, and in bovine and in human feces.

Str. haemolyticus, Str., hemolytic. Any of the streptococci causing complete hemolysis of erythrocytes; majority of pathogenic varieties are in this group.

Str. mitis. SYN: *Str. viridans, q.v.*

Str. parvulus. An organism which is found in the respiratory tract.

Str. pyogenes. Any of the hemolytic streptococci causing suppurative processes. The causative agent of scarlet fever, erysipelas, septic sore throat, puerperal sepsis, and various pyogenic infections.

Str. salivarius. Hemolytic variety which normally occurs in the nose, mouth and throat of human beings.

Str. scarlatinae. Probable causative agent of scarlet fever.

Str. thermophilus. An organism found in dairy products.

Str. viridans. Nonhemolytic form producing green colonies on blood agar which frequently is the cause of focal infection, which in turn leads to symptoms of arthritis, neuritis, endocarditis, etc. A form normal in the mouth. Found in the blood of 40 per cent of people after tooth extraction, and in 11 per cent of those with dirty mouths. In 75 per cent of cases, penicillin will kill the germ.

streptocolysin (strĕp″tō-kŏl′ĭ-sĭn) [G. *streptos*, twisted, + *lysis*, dissolution]. A hemolysin produced by streptococci.

streptodermatitis (strĕp″tō-der-mă-tī′tĭs) [" + *derma*, skin, + *-ītis*, inflammation]. Inflammation of the skin caused by streptococci.

streptodornase (strĕp″tō-dor′nās). One of the enzymes (*streptokinase* is another) elaborated by certain strains of hemolytic streptococci, and capable of liquefying fibrinous and purulent exudates. Useful in pneumococcic and tuberculous empyema.

streptokinase (strĕp″tō-kī′nās). SEE: *streptodornase.*

streptoleukocidin (strĕp″tō-lū-kō-sī′dĭn) [" + *leukos*, white, + L. *cidus*, from *caedere*, to kill]. A toxin produced by streptococci destructive to leukocytes.

streptolysin (strĕp-tŏl′ĭ-sĭn) [" + *lysis*, dissolution]. A hemolysin excreted by a streptococcus. SYN: *streptococcolysin, streptocolysin.*

s. O. A streptolysin resistant to heat and acid but sensitive to oxygen.

s. S. A streptolysin insensitive to oxygen but rapidly destroyed by heat and acid.

streptomycin (strep″tō-mī-sĭn). An antibiotic derived from a soil microbe (*Streptomyces griseus*).

streptomycosis (strĕp″tō-mī-kō′sĭs) [" + *mykēs*, fungus, + *-ōsis*, condition]. Infection caused by microorganisms of the genus *Streptomyces.*

streptosepticemia (strĕp″tō-sĕp-tĭ-sē′mĭ-ă) [" + *sēptikos*, putrid, + *aima*, blood]. Septicemia resulting from streptococcus infection. SYN: *streptococcemia, streptomycosis.*

streptothricin (strĕp-tō-thrī′sĭn). An antibiotic biosynthesized by *Streptomyces lavendulae*. It is effective against both Gram-negative and Gram-positive bacteria and some fungi. It is more toxic than streptomycin.

streptothricosis (strĕp-tō-thrĭ-kō′sĭs) [" + *thrix*, hair, + *-ōsis*, condition]. Infection caused by a species of Streptothrix.

SYM: Chronic suppurative inflammation.

Streptothrix (strĕp′tō-thrĭks) [" + *thrix*, hair]. A genus of Chlamydobacteriaceae, of which one form is the cause of actinomycosis and another is assumed to be cause of ratbite fever.

stress. 1. Strain or intense force. 2. An intense force, strain, agent or mental condition which produces a defense reaction. This reaction may be physiological or within normal limits and harmless, but if continued or intensified may lead to pathological lesions.

stress′or. An agent or condition capable of producing stress.

s., systemic. One which produces generalized systemic responses.

s., topical. One which causes mild inflammation or local damage.

stretch. To draw out or extend to full length.

s. receptor. A proprioceptor located in a muscle or tendon which is stimulated by a stretch or pull.

s. reflex. SYN: *myotactic reflex.* The contraction of a muscle as a result of a pull exerted upon the tendon of the responding muscle. Stretch reflexes are of primary importance in maintenance of posture.

stretcher (strĕch′er) [A.S. *streccan*, to reach]. A litter for carrying the sick, injured or dead.

stretch′ing of contrac′tures. Process performed to loosen contracted ligaments, muscles and adhesions in stiff joints.

There should be a slow, steady and gradually increasing pull by the operator or with gradually increasing weights.

stria (strī′a) (pl. *striae*) [L. *stria*, a channel or groove]. A line or band elevated above or depressed below surrounding tissue, or differing in color and texture.

s. acusticae. SYN: *striae medullares.* One of the horizontal white stripes on floor of the 4th ventricle of the brain.

s. atrophica. Fine pinkish-white or

gray lines usually 14 cm. in length seen in parts of body where skin has been stretched. Commonly seen on thighs, abdomen, and breasts of women who are or have been pregnant; in persons whose skin has been stretched by obesity, tumor, or dropsy; or in persons who have taken adrenocortical hormones for a prolonged period.

s. cerebellares. *Striae medullares, s., acusticae, q.v.*

s. gravidarum. Same as *s. atrophica.*

s. longitudinalis lateralis. One of the longitudinal bands of gray matter, slightly elevated on upper part of the corpus callosum.

s. medullares. Same as *s. acusticae.*

s. terminalis. A band of fibers in roof of inf. horn running to floor of body of the lateral ventricle.

striate, striated (strī'āt, strī'āt-ĕd) [L. *stria,* channel]. Striped; marked by streaks or striae.

s. arteries. Branches of the middle cerebral artery which supply basal nuclei of brain.

s. body. Mass of gray and white bands in each cerebral hemisphere. SYN: *corpus striatum.*

s. muscle. Skeletal muscle, consisting of fibers marked by cross striations. SEE: *muscle.*

s. veins, inferior. Branches of basal vein which drain corpus striatum.

striation (strī-ā'shŭn) [L. *stria,* channel]. 1. State of being striped or streaked. 2. One of a series of streaks. SYN: *stria.*

striatum (strī-ā'tŭm) [L. *striatum,* grooved]. The caudate and lentiform nuclei of the brain considered as one. SYN: *corpus striatum.*

stricture (strĭk'chŭr) [L. *strictura,* a tightening]. A narrowing or constricture of the lumen of a tube, duct, or hollow organ such as the esophagus, ureter, or urethra. Strictures may be congenital or acquired. Acquired strictures may result from infection, trauma, fibrosis resulting from mechanical or chemical irritation, muscular spasm, or pressure from outside from adjacent structures or tumors. They may be *temporary* or *permanent,* depending on cause.

s., annular. Ringlike obstruction involving entire circumference of structure.

s., anorectal. Fibrotic narrowing of the anorectal canal.

s., bridle. One caused by a band across a tube, partially occluding it.

s., cicatricial. One resulting from a scar or wound.

s., functional. One due to muscular spasm.

s., impermeable. One closing the lumen of a tube or canal.

s., irritable. One causing pain when an instrument is passed.

s., spasmodic. Same as *functional s.*

s. of urethra. Most common in men. May be partial or complete.

SYM: Straining to pass urine, esp. at commencement of urination.

ETIOL: Spasm of urethral muscle, congestion of urethra and fibrous formation.

stricturotome (strĭk'chŭr-ō-tōm) [L. *strictūra,* a contraction, + G. *tomē,* a cutting]. Instrument for cutting strictures.

stricturotomy (strĭk-chŭr-ŏt'ō-mĭ) [" + G. *tomē,* a cutting]. Operation of cutting strictures.

stridor (strī'dor) [L. a harsh sound]. Harsh sound during respiration; high-pitched and like the blowing of the wind due to obstruction of air passages.

s., congenital or **laryngeal.** Inspiration at birth or during first 3 weeks giving forth a crowing sound.

s. dentium. Noise from grinding of the teeth.

s. serraticus. Sound of respiration like that of sawing, when heard through a tracheotomy tube.

stridulous (strĭd'ū-lŭs) [L. *stridulus,* harsh, creaking]. Making a shrill grating sound.

string-of-pearls deformity. Fusiform enlargement of proximal and middle phalanges seen in rickets.

string sign. A greatly narrowed terminal ileum seen in roentgenologic examination of abdomen in regional enteritis.

strip (strĭp) [A.S. *strȳpan,* to strip off]. To remove all contents from, esp. by gentle pressure, as to strip the seminal vesicles.

strobila (strō-bī'lă) [G. *strobilē,* a twisted plug]. Consecutive segments of body of a tapeworm.

stroke (strōk) [A.S. *strāk,* a going]. 1. A sudden, severe attack of affliction, as apoplexy; a sharp blow. 2. [A.S. *strākian,* a going]. To rub gently in one direction, as in massage. 3. Gentle movement of the hand across a surface.

s., apoplectic. Sudden loss of consciousness resulting from intracranial hemorrhage, thrombosis, or embolism. SEE: *apoplexy.*

s., back. Ventricular recoil of the heart during systole. SYN: *basculation, 2.*

s., heat. SEE: *heatstroke.*

s., paralytic. Sudden onset of paralysis resulting from injury to brain or spinal cord.

s. volume. SYN: *systolic discharge.* The amount of blood ejected by the left ventricle at each beat. Normally about 60 ml.

stroma (strō'mă) (pl. *stromata*) [G. *strōma,* a bed]. 1. Foundation supporting tissues of an organ. 2. Spongy, colorless framework of an erythrocyte.

stromal, stromatic (strō'măl, strō-măt'ĭk) [G. *strōma,* a bed]. Concerning or resembling the stroma of an organ.

Stromeyer's splint (strō-mī-ĕr). A hinged splint for a joint, which can be fixed at an angle.

stromuhr (strō'moor) [Ger.]. Device for measuring velocity of blood flow. SYN: *rheometer.*

Strongylata. A suborder of nematode worms which includes the hookworms, strongyles, gapeworms and lungworms.

strongyle. A nematode belonging to the suborder Strongylata.

Strongyloides (strŏn-jĭ-loy'dēz) [G. *stroggylos,* round, + *eidos,* form]. A genus of roundworms frequently found in the intestines.

S. intestinalis. An intestinal roundworm.

S. stercoralis. SYN: *S. intestinalis.* An intestinal parasite of man similar to the hookworm both in distribution and life cycle.

strongyloidosis (strŏn"jĭ-loy-dō'sĭs) [" + " + *-ōsis,* condition]. Infestation with Strongyloides.

strongylosis (strŏn-jĭ-lō'sĭs) [G. *stroggylos,* round, + *-ōsis,* condition]. Infestation with Strongylus.

strontium (strŏn'shĭ-ŭm). SYMB: Sr. At. wt. 87.62; at. no. 38. sp. gr. 2.6. A metallic element sometimes used in medicine as a carrier of therapeutically active acids. Its salts are also used medicinally.

Strophanthus (strō-făn'thŭs) [G. *strophos*, cord, + *anthos*, flower]. USP. Plant yielding a poisonous, white, crystalline glucoside; used chiefly in the form of alkaloid; strophanthin.

ACTION AND USES: Similar to digitalis.

strophulus (strŏf'ū-lŭs) (L. *strophulus*, from G. *strophos*, a twisted cord]. An infantile red eruption. SYN: *gum rash, red rash, tooth rash*.

s. albidus. Small, white nodule below the epidermis. SYN: *milium*.

s. infantum. Urticaria in infants.

s. pruriginosus. A form with itching papules.

structural (strŭk'tū-răl) [L. *structūra*, a building]. Pert. to organic structure.

s. disease. A disease effecting changes in any structure.

struma (strū'mă) [L. a mass]. Enlargement of the thyroid gland. SYN: *goiter*.

s. aberranta. S. of the accessory thyroid glands.

s., cast iron. Chronic thyroiditis accompanied by extreme development of fibrous tissue.

s. congenita. Goiter present at birth.

s. lingualis. Presence of thyroid tissue in tongue in region of foramen cecum.

s. lymphomatosa. SYN: *Hashimoto's struma*. Rare form involving a diffuse and extensive infiltration of the entire gland.

s. maligna. Carcinoma of the thyroid gland.

s., ovarii. A form of ovarian teratoma in which mass is composed of typical thyroid follicles filled with colloid.

s., Riedel's. A form of chronic thyroiditis in which gland becomes enlarged, hard, and adherent to adjacent tissues. Follicles become atrophic and fibrosis occurs.

strumiprivous (strū"mĭ-prī'vŭs) [L. *struma*, a mass, + *privāre*, to deprive]. Referring to or caused by removal of the thyroid gland. SEE: *cachexia*.

strumitis (strū-mī'tĭs) [" + G. *-ītis*, inflammation]. Inflammation of a thyroid gland with goiter. SYN: *thyroiditis*.

strumous (strū'mŭs) [L. *strumo*, a mass]. 1. Affected with scrofula. SYN: *scrofulous*. 2. Affected with goiter.

Strümpell-Marie disease (strĭm'pĕl). Ankylosing or rheumatoid spondylitis, *q.v.*

Strümpell's sign. Dorsiflexion of foot when thigh is flexed on abdomen.

strychnine (strĭk'nīn, -nēn, -nĭn) [G. *strychnos*, nightshade]. A poisonous alkaloid obtained from plants, as nux vomica.

It is a marked stimulant, causing the heart to beat more strongly. When taken in small doses for some time the mental powers become sharpened and sensibility intensified. Bowel movements become less sluggish and gastric secretion augmented. The spinal cord is affected in a marked degree, reflex action being increased and the muscle tone improved.

USES: As a tonic in convalescence from weakening diseases, in some nervous conditions, and for the debility caused by excessive overstrain. Contraindicated in diseases connected with overactivity of spinal cord. When heart failure threatens the drug is often used hypodermically. Its stimulating action causes it to be a useful adjunct to purgative medicines.

When the nervous system is depressed owing to poisons or toxins, such as alcohol, lead, tobacco, and diphtheria, it is a much-ordered remedy.

POISONING: The fatal dose of strychnine by mouth is probably between 1 and 2 gr., although patients have recovered following much larger doses.

SYM: When swallowed, symptoms usually develop within 15 to 20 minutes. This time element depends largely upon the drug being in solution and the stomach being empty. Given by needle in toxic amounts, the development of symptoms is remarkably prompt. The usual course is, first, a hyperesthesia followed by a modification of the reflexes, especially shown as a tendency for a single stimulus to produce exaggerated reactions and to involve apparently unrelated muscle groups.

If a sufficient amount has been taken, there rapidly develop nervous twitchings followed by convulsions. The seizures are tonic in character, further characterized by cyanosis and opisthotonos, followed by relaxation and exhaustion. The duration of a seizure may be from a few seconds to about a minute. Consciousness may not be lost, so that the tonic contractions may be very painful. They tend to recur in 5 to 15 minutes and may be precipitated by almost any stimulus such as physical contact or unusual noise. In favorable cases, convulsions gradually lessen in severity. Should death occur, it is usually by asphyxiation during one of the early attacks or later by exhaustion following repeated paroxysms.

TREATMENT: Consists in thoroughly emptying the stomach; best done with a small stomach tube. An ideal chemical antidote is *potassium permanganate*, used in a solution of about 1:10,000; about a pint of this left in the stomach. Other measures are keeping patient quiet, free from any disturbing factors, such as noise and confusion. Medication depends upon the administration of antispasmodics. *Barbituric acid salts* are used intravenously, or *chloral hydrate* and *bromides* given by mouth or rectum. Inhalation anesthesia may be given during convulsions. Inhalations of *oxygen* have been used in this condition with apparent benefit. Artificial respiration, either by machine or mouth-to-mouth, may be required. Elimination favored particularly by diuretics.

s. nitrate. USP. The nitrate of the alkaloid strychnine.

ACTION AND USES: Same as strychnine sulfate.

s. sulfate. USP. The sulfate of an alkaloid obtained from nux vomica.

POISONING: An extremely bitter alkaloid used as an animal poisoning to destroy pests.

SYM: Begin shortly after administration. Tightness of chest, a feeling of impending calamity, and shortly violent convulsions with weak, irregular pulse; dilated pupils.

F. A. TREATMENT: Wash out stomach; anesthesia is given cautiously to diminish convulsions. Tannic acid to precipitate the alkaloid. Sedatives, as barbital, desirable, esp. those varieties that may be given intravenously, as sodium amytal and sodium pentobarbital. SEE: *strychnine*.

strychninism (strĭk'nĭn-ĭzm) [G. *strychnos*, nightshade, + *-ismos*, condition]. Chronic strychnine poisoning. SYN: *strychnism*.

strychnism (strĭk'nĭzm). Poisoning from use of strychnine. SYN: *strychninism.*

STS. Abbreviation for *serological test for syphilis; standard test for syphilis.*

STU. Abbreviation for *skin test unit.*

stump (stŭmp) [M.E. *stumpe*]. Basal part of limb left after amputation.

s. hallucination. Consciousness of still being possessed of a limb or arm after its amputation. SYN: *phantom limb.*

stun (stŭn) [M.E. *stunein,* to stun]. To render unconscious or stupified by a blow.

stupe (stūp) [L. *stupa,* tow, from G. *stypē*]. Cloth of flannel wrung out of hot water for a fomentation, often saturated with a counterirritant such as turpentine. SEE: *fomentation.*

s., opium. 30-60 minims of opium sprinkled over stupe after it has been wrung out.

s., turpentine. 1-2 drams of turpentine sprinkled evenly over dry flannel before water is poured on.

stupefacient (stū-pē-fā'shĕnt) [L. *stupefaciens,* stupefying]. Causing or that which causes stupor. SYN: *narcotic; soporific.*

stupemania (stū-pē-mā'nĭ-ă) [L. *stupor,* numbness, + G. *mania,* madness]. Insanity with symptoms of numbness.

stupor (stū'por) [L. *stupor*]. 1. Condition of unconsciousness, torpor, or lethargy with suppression of sense or feeling. 2. PSY: A state of lessened responsiveness.

Stupor occurs in visceral and infectious diseases, melancholia, catatonia, epilepsy, paresis, poisonings, and hysteria. A benign form is seen in manic-depressive psychosis.

s., anergic. Stupor accompanied with immobility seen in certain psychoses.

s., delusional. S. accompanied by delusions.

s., epileptic. S. sometimes following an attack of epilepsy.

s., lethargic. S. accompanied by lethargy. SEE: *trance.*

s. melancholicus. S. associated with mental depression.

s. vigilans. Catalepsy, *q.v.*

RS: *carotic, catatonia, collapse, coma, lethargy, narcoma, narcose, syncope, unconsciousness.*

stuporous (stū'pôr-ŭs). Affected with stupor.

s. depression. An extremely depressed phase of manic-depressive psychosis characterized by extreme psychomotor retardation and unresponsiveness to surrounding conditions.

stupration, stuprum (stū-prā'shŭn, stū'-prŭm) [L. *stuprum,* defilement]. Sexual intercourse with a woman without her consent and by overpowering force, or intimidation. SYN: *rape.*

sturine (stū'rĭn) [L. *sturio,* sturgeon]. Protamine obtained from sperm of sturgeon. Has bactericidal action.

stutter (stŭt'er) [M.E. *stutten,* to strike]. To hesitate and repeat or stumble spasmodically in speaking, due to difficulty in pronouncing initial consonants caused by spasm of lingual and palatal muscles.

stuttering (stŭt'er-ĭng) [M.E. *stutten.* to strike]. Defect in speech in which there is stumbling and spasmodic repetition of same syllable. RS: *battarism, mogilalia.*

s., urinary. Irregular, spasmodic urination. SYN: *stammering* of the bladder.*

sty(e (stī) (pl. *styes* or *sties*) [A.S. *stīgan.* a rising]. Acute localized bacterial infection of one of several sebaceous glands of the eyelid. In external hordeolum the glands of *Zeiss* or *Moll* at the edge of the lid are inflamed. Internal hordeolum affects the *meibomian* or *tarsal* glands under the eyelid.

SYM: General edema of lid, pain, localized conjunctivitis.

TREATMENT: Hot fomentations. When suppuration has taken place, free incision and pressure to evacuate sac Local and systemic antibiotics will hasten resolution and healing in severe cases. When a succession of styes occurs Staphylococcus toxoid or vaccine or an autogenous vaccine may be helpful.

s., meibomian. Inflammation of a meibomian gland.

s., Zeissian. Inflammation of one of Zeiss' glands.

styles, stylet (stīles, stī'lĕt) [L. *stylus,* a pointed instrument]. 1. A slender, solid or hollow plug of metal for making permanent a canal after operation or for stiffening or clearing a cannula or catheter. 2. A thin probe.

styliscus (stī-lĭs'kŭs) [G. *styliskos,* pillar]. A slender, cylindrical plug for dilating a channel or for keeping a wound open.

styloglossus (stī-lō-glŏs'ŭs) [G. *stylos,* pillar, + *glōssa,* tongue]. A muscle connecting the tongue and styloid process which raises and retracts the tongue. SEE: *Table of Muscles in Appendix.*

stylohyoid (stī-lō-hī'oid). Pert. to the styloid process of temporal and the hyoid bone.

stylohyoideus (stī-lō-hī-oyd'ē-ŭs). A muscle having its origin on styloid process and insertion on hyoid bone. It draws the hyoid bone upward and backward. SEE: *Table of Muscles in Appendix.*

styloid (stī'loyd) [G. *stylos,* pillar, + *eidos,* form]. Resembling a stylus or pointed instrument.

s. process. 1. A pointed process of the temporal bone, projecting downward, and to which some of the muscles of the tongue are attached. 2. A pointed projection behind the head of the fibula. 3. A protuberance on distal end of radius' outer portion. 4. An ulnar projection on inner side of the distal end.

styloiditis (stī-loyd-ī'tĭs) [G. *stylos,* pillar, + *eidos,* form, + *-ītis,* inflammation]. Inflammation of a styloid process.

stylomandibular (stī"lō-măn-dĭ'bū-lăr). Concerning the styloid process of the temporal bone and the mandible.

stylomastoid (stī"lō-măs'toyd) [" + *mastos,* breast, + *eidos,* form]. Concerning the styloid and mastoid processes of the temporal bone.

stylomaxillary (stī"lō-măks'ĭ-lă-rĭ) [" + L. *maxilla,* jaw]. Concerning the styloid process of the temporal bone and the mandible.

stylopharyngeus (stī"lō-far-ĭn'jē-ŭs) [" + *pharygx.* pharynx]. Muscle connecting the styloid process and pharynx which elevates and dilates the pharynx. SEE: *Table of Muscles in Appendix.*

stylus (stī'lŭs) [L. *stylus,* a pen, from G. *stylos,* a pillar]. 1. A probe or slender wire for stiffening or clearing a canal or catheter. 2. Pointed medicinal preparation in stick form for external application.

stype (stīp) [G. *stypē,* tow]. A pledget or tampon of cotton or other material.

stypsis (stĭp′sĭs) [G. *stypsis*, a steeping in an astringent]. Astringency or the use of an astringent.

styptic (stĭp′tĭk) [G. *styptikos*, contracting]. 1. Contracting a blood vessel; stopping a hemorrhage by astringent action. 2. Anything that checks a hemorrhage. SYN: *astringent, hemostat.*

Ex: *ferrous sulfate, alum, tannic acid*

sub- [L.]. Combining form meaning *under, beneath, in small quantity, less than normal.*

subabdominal (sŭb-ăb-dŏm′ĭ-năl) [L. *sub*, beneath, + *abdōmen*, abdomen]. Below the abdomen.

subacetate (sŭb-ăs′ĕt-āt) [" + *acetum*, vinegar]. A basic acetate.

subacromial (sŭb-ă-krō′mĭ-ăl) [" + G. *akron*, point, + *omos*, shoulder]. Under the acromion process.

subacute (sŭb-ă-kūt′) [" + *acutus*, sharp] Bet. acute and chronic, but with some acute features, said of the course of a disease.

subalimentation (sŭb-ăl-ĭ-mĕn-tā′shŭn) [" + *alimentum*, food]. A state of insufficient nourishment.

subanconeus (sŭb-ăn kō′nē-ŭs) [" + G. *agkōn*, elbow]. 1. Below the elbow. 2. Muscle beneath the elbow which contracts its post. ligament. SEE: *Table of Muscles in Appendix.*

subaponeurotic (sŭb″ap-ō-nū-rŏt′ĭk) [" + G. *apo*, from + *neuron*, tendon]. Below an aponeurosis.

subarachnoid (sŭb-ă-răk′noyd) [L. *sub*, under, + G. *arachnē*, spider, + *eidos*, form]. Below the arachnoid membrane.

s. cisternae. Spaces at the base of the brain where the arachnoid becomes widely separated from the pia giving rise to large cavities.

s. space. Space between the pia proper and arachnoid containing the cerebrospinal fluid.

subarcuate (sŭb-ar′kū-āt) [" + *arcuatus*, bow-shaped]. Slightly arched.

s. fossa. Depression beneath the arcuate eminence.

subastragalar (sŭb-ăs-trăg′ă-lar) [" + G. *astragalos*, one of a set of dice]. Beneath the astragalus.

subastringent (sŭb-ăs-trĭn′jĕnt) [" + *astringere*, to contract]. Mildly astringent.

subaural (sŭb-aw′răl) [" + *auris*, ear]. Below the ear.

subcapsular (sŭb-kăp′sū-lar) [" + *capsula*, a little box]. Below any capsule, especially the capsule of the brain, or a capsular ligament.

subcarbonate (sŭb-kar′bŏn-āt) [" + *carbo, carbon*, coal]. A basic carbonate; one having proportion of carbonic acid radical less than the normal carbonate.

subcartilaginous (sŭb-kar-tĭl-ăj′ĭn-ŭs) [L. *sub*, beneath, + *cartilāgo*, cartilage]. 1. Beneath a cartilage. 2. Cartilaginous in part.

subchronic (sŭb-krŏn′ĭk) [" + G. *chronos*, time]. Noting a condition bet. subacute and chronic; almost chronic.

subclavian (sŭb-klā′vĭ-ăn) [" + *clavis*, a key]. Under the clavicle or collarbone. SYN: *subclavicular.*

s. artery. Large artery at base of neck which supplies blood to arm. The right subclavian a. branches from the innominate artery; the l. subclavian a. branches from aortic arch.

s. triangle. One of the neck formed by the clavicle, and the omohyoid and sternomastoid muscles.

s. vein. Large vein draining arm. It unites with int. jugular to form the innominate vein.

subclavicular (sŭb-klăv-ĭk′ū-lar) [" + *clavicula*, a little key]. Beneath the clavicle. SYN: *subclavian.*

subclavius (sŭb-klā′vĭ-ŭs) [" + *clavis*, a key]. A tiny muscle from the 1st rib to the undersurface of the clavicle. SEE: *Table of Muscles in Appendix.*

subclinical (sŭb-klĭn′ĭ-kal) [" + G. *klinikos*, pert. to a bed]. Pert. to a period before appearance of typical symptoms of a disease.

subcollateral (sŭb-kō-lăt′ĕr-ăl) [L. *sub*, under, + *con*, with, + *latus, later-*, side]. Below the collateral fissure, indicating a cerebral convolution.

subconjunctival (sŭb-kŏn-jŭnk-tī′văl) [" + *conjunctiva*, a joining]. Beneath the conjunctiva.

subconscious (sŭb-kŏn′shŭs) [" + *conscius*, aware]. Not clearly conscious; pert. to activities of which the mind is not aware or to that which is not cognized through the physical senses; below the threshold of objective consciousness; that which is activated by involuntary processes; intuitional. Now almost obsolete.

s. mind. A hypothetical mind acting below the threshold of objective consciousness.

subconsciousness (sŭb-kŏn′shŭs-nĕs) [" + *conscius*, aware]. 1. The state of being partially unconscious. 2. Noting of impressions and ideas without conscious knowledge of them.

subcontinuous (sŭb-kŏn-tĭn′ū-ŭs) [" + *continuus*, holding together]. Almost continuous; with periods of abatement, but no interruptions to continuity.

s. fever. Fever with periods of remission and exacerbation. SYN: *remittent fever.*

subcoracoid (sŭb-kor′ă-koyd) [" + G. *korakoeidēs*, crowlike]. Beneath the coracoid process.

subcortex (sŭb-kor′tĕks) [" + *cortex*, rind]. White substance of the brain underlying the cortex.

subcortical (sŭb-kor′tĭ-kal) [L. *sub*, under, + *cortex, cortic-*, rind]. Pert. to the region beneath the cerebral cortex.

subcostal (sŭb-kŏs′tăl) [" + *costa*, rib] Beneath the ribs.

subcostalgia (sŭb-kŏs-tăl′jĭ-ă) [" + " + G. *algos*, pain]. Pain in region over the subcostal nerve.

subcranial (sŭb-krā′nĭ-ăl) [" + G. *kranion*, skull]. Beneath or below the cranium.

subcrepitant (sŭb-krep′ĭ-tănt) [" + *crepitāre*, to rattle]. Partially crepitant or crackling in character; noting a rale.

subcrureus (sŭb-krū-rē′ŭs) [" + *crus, crur-*, leg]. Small muscle bet. ant. surface of femoral shaft and synovial membrane of knee joint. SEE: *Table of Muscles in Appendix.*

subculture (sŭb-kŭl′chūr) [" + *cultūra*, cultivation]. To make a culture of bacteria with material derived from another culture.

subcutaneous (sŭb-kū-tā′nē-ŭs) [L. *sub*, under, + *cutis*, skin]. Beneath or to be introduced beneath the skin. SYN: *hypodermic.*

s. surgery. Operation performed through a small opening in the skin.

s. wound. A wound with only a small opening through the skin.

subcuticular (sŭb-kū-tĭk′ū-lar) [" + *cuticula*, little skin]. Beneath the cuticle or epidermis. SYN: *subepidermal.*

subcutis. The layer of connective tissue beneath the skin.

subdelirium (sŭb-dē-lir'ĭ-ŭm) [" + *dē*, away from, + *lira*, track]. A mild or not continuous delirium.

subdermal. Below the skin.

subdiaphragmatic (sŭb-dī-ă-frăg-măt'ĭk) [" + G. *dia*, across, + *phragma*, wall]. Beneath the diaphragm.

subdural (sŭb-dū'răl) [" + *durus*, hard]. Beneath the dura mater.

s. space. Space bet. the arachnoid and dura mater.

subendocardial (sŭb"ĕn-dō-kar'dĭ-ăl) [" + G. *endon*, within, + *kardia*, heart]. Below the endocardium.

subendothelial (sŭb"ĕn-dō-thē'lĭ-ăl) [L. *sub*, under, + G. *endon*, within, + *thēlē*, nipple]. Beneath endothelium.

subepidermal (sŭb"ĕp-ĭ-der'măl) [" + G *epi*, upon, + *derma*, skin]. Beneath the epidermis. SYN: *subcuticular*.

subepithelial (sŭb"ĕp-ĭ-thē'lĭ-ăl) [" + " + *thēlē*, nipple]. Beneath the epithelium.

subfascial (sŭb-făsh'ĭ-ăl) [" + *fascia*, band]. Beneath a fascia.

subfebrile (sŭb-fē'brĭl) [" + *febris*, fever]. Somewhat feverish.

subflavous (sŭb-flā'vŭs) [" + *flavus*, yellow]. Yellowish.

s. ligament. Yellowish ligament connecting the laminae of the vertebrae. SYN: *ligamentum subflavum*.

subfrontal (sŭb-frŭn'tăl) [L. *sub*, beneath, + *frons, front-*, forehead]. Below a frontal convolution or lobe of the brain.

subglenoid (sŭb-glē'noyd) [" + G. *glēnē*, cavity, + *eidos*, form]. Below the glenoid fossa or glenoid cavity.

subglossal (sŭb-glos'ăl) [" + G. *glōssa*, tongue]. Under the tongue. SYN: *hypoglossal, sublingual*.

subglossitis (sŭb-glos-sī'tĭs) [" + " + *-itis*, inflammation]. Inflammation of the undersurface or tissues of the tongue.

subgrondation, subgrundation (sŭb-gron-dā'shŭn, -grŭn-dā'shŭn) [Fr.]. Depression of one fragment of a broken bone beneath the other, as of the cranium.

subhyoid (sŭb-hī'oyd) [L. *sub*, beneath, + G. *hyoeidēs*, U-shaped]. Beneath the hyoid bone.

subiculum (sū-bĭk'ū-lŭm) [L. *subiculum*, a small support]. A division of hippocampal convolution, composed of a thick layer of myelinated fibers on its surface, and containing the olfactory association centers. SYN: *convolution, uncinate; uncus gyri hippocampi*.

subiliac (sŭb-ĭl'ĭ-ăk) [L. *sub*, under, + *iliacus*, pert. to the hip]. 1. Below the ilium. 2. Pert. to the subilium.

subilium (sŭb-ĭl'ĭ-ŭm) [" + *ilium*, haunch bone]. The lowest part of the ilium.

subinfection (sŭb-ĭn-fĕk'shŭn) [" + *infectio*, a putting into]. Mild infection with minimal clinical signs or symptoms.

subinflammation (sŭb"ĭn-flăm-ā'shun) [" + *inflammatio*, a setting on fire]. Very mild inflammation. SYN: *irritation*.

subinflammatory (sŭb"ĭn-flăm'ă-tō-rĭ) [" + *inflammatio*, a setting on fire]. Very mildly inflammatory.

subintimal. Beneath the intima.

subintrant (sŭb-ĭn'trănt) [L. *subintrans*, stealing into]. Having cycles or paroxysms in such rapid succession that they intermingle.

s. fever. Intermittent fever in which the paroxysms occur so rapidly that one comes on before the previous one has disappeared.

subinvolution (sŭb"ĭn-vō-lū'shŭn) [L. *sub*, beneath, + *involutio*, a turning into]. Imperfect involution; incomplete return of a part to normal dimensions after physiological hypertrophy, as when the uterus following childbirth fails to reduce to normal size. SEE: *uterus*.

subia'cent. Lying underneath.

subject (sŭb'jĕkt) [L. *subjectus*, thrown or lying under]. 1. A patient undergoing treatment, observation, or experiment. 2. A body used for dissection.

subjective (sŭb-jĕk'tĭv) [L. *subjectivus*]. Arising from or concerned with the individual; not perceptible to an observer. OPP: *objective*.

s. sensation. A sensation occurring when stimuli due to internal causes excite the nervous system; one not of objective origin.

s. symptoms. Those which are of internal origin and evident only to the patient.

subjugal (sŭb-jū'găl) [L. *sub*, beneath, + *jugum*, yoke]. Below the malar bone or *os zygomaticum*.

sublatio (sŭb-lā'shĭ-ō) [L. *sublatio*, a taking away]. Removal, elevation, or detachment of a part.

s. retinae. Detachment of the retina.

sublethal (sŭb-lē'thăl) [L. *sub*, under, + G. *lēthē*, oblivion]. A little less than lethal; almost fatal.

s. dose. Dose containing not quite enough toxin to cause death.

sublimate (sŭb'lĭ-māt) [L. *sublimāre*, to elevate]. 1. A substance obtained or prepared by sublimation. 2. To vaporize a solid substance by heat and condense it again without liquefying, for purification. 3. PSY: To overcome the libido by diverting it into nonsexual or higher activities.

sublimation (sŭb-lĭ-mā'shŭn) [L. *sublimatio*, an elevation]. 1. CHEM: To convert a solid into a vapor and condense it again without liquefying to purify it. 2. PSY: Conversion of the libido into nonsexual channels.

Adequate expression for organic needs, removed from the primitive satisfaction in such a way that the "herd" regards the outlet as "superior," *i. e.*, best suited to the social interests (demands).

A freudian term pert. to unconscious mental processes whereby the sex instinct finds an outlet through creative mental work.

sublime (sŭb-lĭm') [L. *sublimāre*, to elevate]. CHEM: To evaporate a substance directly from the solid into the vapor state and condense it again.

Thus, metallic iodine on heating does not liquefy, but forms directly a violet gas.

subliminal (sŭb-lĭm'ĭn-ăl) [L. *sub*, under, + *limen*, threshold]. 1. Below the threshold of sensation; too weak to arouse sensation or muscular contraction. 2. Below the normal consciousness.

s. self. PSY: Part of a normal individual's personality in which his mental processes function without consciousness under normal waking conditions.

sublingual (sŭb-lĭng'gwăl) [" + *lingua*, tongue]. Beneath or concerning the area beneath the tongue.

s. gland. The smallest of the salivary glands, located bet. side of tongue and the mandible, one on each side.

It has about 20 ducts opening for the most part directly above the gland.

sublinguitis (sŭb"lĭng-gwī'tĭs) [" + " + G. *-itis*, inflammation]. Inflammation of the sublingual gland.

sublobular (sŭb-lŏb'ū-lar) [" + *lobulus*, a lobule]. Beneath a lobule.

sublumbar (sŭb-lŭm′bar) [" + *lumbus,* loin]. Below the lumbar region.

subluxation (sŭb″lŭks-ā′shŭn) [" + *luxatio,* dislocation]. A partial or incomplete dislocation.

submammary (sŭb-mam′ă-rĭ) [L. *sub,* under, + *mamma,* breast]. Below the mammary gland.

submandibular (sŭb-măn-dĭb′ū-lăr). Beneath the mandible or lower jaw.

s. gland. The submaxillary gland, *q.v.*

submarginal. Close to or next to a margin or border of a part.

submaxilla (sŭb-măks-ĭl′ă) [" + *maxilla,* jaw]. The lower jaw or mandible. SYN: *maxilla, inferior.*

submaxillaritis (sŭb-măks-ĭl-ar-ī′tĭs) [" + " + G. *-ītis,* inflammation]. Inflammation of the submaxillary gland.

submaxillary (sŭb-măks′ĭl-a-rĭ) [" + *maxillaris,* pert. to the jaw]. Beneath the lower jaw or inferior maxilla.

s. gland. SYN: *submandibular gland.* One of the salivary glands, a mixed tubuloalveolar gland about the size of a walnut which lies in digastric triangle beneath the mandible. Its main duct (*Wharton's duct*) opens at side of the frenulum linguae.

submaxillitis (sŭb-măks-ĭl-lī′tĭs) [" + " + G. *-ītis,* inflammation]. Inflammation of or mumps affecting the submaxillary gland.

submental (sŭb-mĕn′tăl) [" + *mentum,* chin]. Under the chin.

submerge. To be or to be placed under water.

submicron (sŭb-mī′krŏn) [" + G. *mikros,* tiny]. A tiny particle invisible except with the ultramicroscope. SYN: *ultramicron.*

submicroscopical (sŭb″mī-krō-skŏp′ĭ-kal) [L. *sub,* under, + G. *mikros,* tiny, + *skopein,* to examine]. Too minute to be visible under the microscope.

submorphous (sŭb-mor′fŭs) [" + G. *morphē,* form]. Neither completely amorphous nor crystalline, as some calculi.

submucosa (sŭb-mū-kō′să) [" + *mucosus,* mucous]. The layer of areolar connective tissue under a mucous membrane.

submucous (sŭb-mū′kŭs) [" + *mucus,* mucus]. Beneath a mucous membrane.

subnarcotic (sŭb-nar-kŏt′ĭk) [" + G. *narkōtikos,* numb]. Mildly narcotic.

subnasal (sŭb-nā′zăl) [" + *nasus,* nose]. Under the nose.

s. point. Craniometric point at base of nasal spine.

subneural (sŭb-nū′răl) [" + G. *neuron,* nerve]. Beneath the neural axis or the central nervous system.

subnormal (sŭb-nor′măl) [L. *sub,* under, + *norma,* rule]. Below normal.

subnucleus (sŭb-nū′klē-ŭs) [L. *sub,* under, + *nucleus,* a nut]. One of the secondary nuclei into which a nucleus of the central nervous system is sometimes divided.

suboccipital (sŭb-ŏk-sĭp′ĭ-tăl) [" + *occiput,* back of head]. Situated below the occiput or occipital bone.

suboperculum (sŭb-ō-per′kū-lŭm) [" + *operculum,* covering]. Portion of occipital convolution overlapping the insula. SEE: *operculum.*

suborbital (sŭb-or′bĭ-tăl) [" + *orbita,* track]. Beneath the orbit.

subpapular (sŭb-păp′ū-lar) [" + *papula,* pimple]. Very slightly papular, as papules elevated being scarcely more than macules.

subpatellar (sŭb-pă-tĕl′ar) [" + *patella,* a pan]. Beneath the patella.

subpeduncular (sŭb″pē-dŭn′kū-lar) [L. *sub,* under, + *pedunculus,* a stem]. Below a peduncle.

s. lobe. Tiny lobe on undersurface of either cerebellar hemisphere. SYN: *flocculus.*

subpericardial (sŭb″pĕr-ĭ-kar′dĭ-ăl) [" + G. *peri,* around, + *kardia,* heart]. Beneath the pericardium.

subperiosteal (sŭb″pĕr-ĭ-ŏs′tē-ăl) [" + " + *osteon,* bone]. Beneath the periosteum.

s. operation. Bone surgery without removal of the periosteum.

subperitoneal (sŭb″pĕr-ĭ-tō-nē′ăl) [" + G. *peritonaion,* peritoneum]. Beneath the peritoneum.

subpharyngeal (sŭb-făr-ĭn′jē-ăl) [" + G. *pharygx,* pharynx]. Beneath the pharynx.

subphrenic (sŭb-frĕn′ĭk) [" + G. *phrēn,* diaphragm]. Beneath the diaphragm. SYN: *subdiaphragmatic.*

s. abscess. Collection of pus beneath the diaphragm.

subplacenta (sŭb-plă-sĕn′tă) [" + *placenta,* a flat cake]. Part of the decidua directly lining the uterus. SYN: *decidua vera.*

subpleural (sŭb-plū′răl) [L. *sub,* under, + G. *pleura,* a side]. Beneath the pleura.

subpontine (sŭb-pŏn′tĭn, -tīn) [" + *pons, pont-,* bridge]. Below the pons Varolii.

subpreputial (sŭb″prē-pū′shăl) [" + *praeputium,* prepuce]. Under the prepuce.

subpubic (sŭb-pū′bĭk) [" + *pubes,* pubis]. Beneath the pubic arch, as a ligament.

subpulmonary (sŭb-pŭl′mō-na-rĭ) [" + *pulmōn,* lung]. Below the lung.

subretinal (sŭb-rĕt′ĭ-năl) [" + *rētē,* a net]. Beneath the retina.

subscapular (sŭb-skăp′ū-lar) [" + *scapula,* shoulder]. Below the scapula.

subscription (sŭb-skrĭp′shŭn) [L. *subscriptio,* a writing under]. Part of a prescription containing direction to a pharmacist.

subserous (sŭb-sē′rŭs) [L. *sub,* under, + *serum,* whey]. Beneath a serous membrane.

subsibilant (sŭb-sĭb′ĭl-ănt). Having the sound of a muffled whistle.

subsidence (sŭb-sīd′ĕnts). The gradual disappearance of symptoms or manifestations of a disease.

subspinous (sŭb-spī′nŭs) [" + *spina,* thorn]. 1. Beneath any spine. 2. Anterior to or beneath the spinal column.

s. dislocation. Dislocation with head of the humerus resting below spine of the scapula.

substage (sŭb′stāj) [" + O.Fr. *estage,* a landing]. Attachment to the microscope beneath the stage by which attachments are held in place.

substance (sŭb′stăns) [L. *substantia,* material]. That of which any material thing is composed; matter.

s., accelerator. One of two substances called Factors V and VII which are essential for rapid conversion of prothrombin to thrombin.

s., agglutinable. S. in red blood corpuscles and bacteria which unites with agglutinin producing specific agglutination.

s., anterior perforated. Portion of rhinencephalon lying immediately anterior to optic chiasma. It is perforated by numerous small arteries.

s., anterior pituitary-like. SYN: *APL substance.* Chorionic gonadotrophin (SEE UNDER: *gonadotrophin*).

s., basophilic. SEE: *chromophilic s.*

s., chromidial. SEE: *chromophilic s.*

s., chromophilic. SYN: *basophilic, chromophil,* or *chromidial substance.* Substance found in the cytoplasm of certain cells which stains similar to chromatin with basic dyes. Includes Nissl bodies of neurons and granules in serozymogenic cells.

s., colloid. Jellylike s. in colloid degeneration.

s., depressor. Any substance whose action is that of reducing arterial blood pressure. SEE: *vasopressin.*

s., gray. Gray matter of the brain and spinal cord.

s., ground. The matrix or intercellular substance in which the cells of an organ or tissue are embedded.

s., intercellular. The substance occupying the spaces between cells.

s., ketogenic. A substance which, in its metabolism, gives rise to ketone bodies.

s., Nissl. Chromatophilic substance of nerve cells. SEE: *Nissl bodies.*

s., posterior perforated. A triangular area forming floor of the interpeduncular fossa. It lies immediately behind the corpora mammillaria and contains numerous openings for blood vessels.

s., pressor. A substance which elevates arterial blood pressure.

s., reticular. SEE: *formation, reticular.*

s., specific soluble. ABBR: SSS. A polysaccharide hapten obtained from the capsules of pneumococci.

s., threshold, high. A substance such as glucose or sodium chloride present in the blood which is excreted by the kidney only when its concentration exceeds a certain optimum value. SEE: *renal threshold.*

s., threshold, low. A substance such as urea or uric acid which is excreted from the blood almost in its entirety. They occur in the urine in high concentrations.

s., white. White matter of brain and spinal cord.

s., w., of Schwann. A nerve fiber's medullary sheath.

substantia (sŭb-stăn′shĭ-ă) [L. *substantia,* material]. Substance.

s. alba. White substance of the brain.

s. cinerea. Gray substance of brain and spinal cord.

s. ferruginea. Elongated mass of pigmented cells in the locus ceruleus.

s. gelatinosa. Gray matter of the cord surrounding central canal and capping head of post. horns of spinal cord.

s. grisea. NA. Gray matter of the spinal cord.

s. nigra. NA. Black substance in a section of the crus cerebri. SYN: *locus niger.*

s. propria membranae tympani. Fibrous middle layer of drum membrane.

substernal (sŭb-ster′năl) [L. *sub,* beneath, + G. *sternon,* chest]. Situated beneath the sternum.

substitution (sŭb-stĭ-tū′shŭn) [L. *substitutio,* a placing under]. 1. CHEM: Displacing an atom (or more than one) of an element in a compound by atoms of another element, equivalently. 2. PSY: The turning from an obstructed desire to one whose gratification is socially acceptable. 3. The turning from an obstructed form of behavior to a more primitive one, as a substitution neurosis. 4. The replacement of a substance by another. 5. In pharmacy, the replacement of one drug by another drug in dispensing.

s. bone. Endochondral of cartilage bone.

s. products. Compounds formed by an element or a radical replacing another element or radical in a compound.

s. therapy. The use in treatment of a substance such as a product of glandular secretion (hormone or enzyme) to replace natural substance in body. This method is employed when glands fail to secrete properly or substance secreted is unavailable to tissues.

substitutive (sŭb′stĭ-tū-tĭv) [L. *substitutivus,* conditional]. Causing a change or substitution of characteristics.

s. therapy. Treatment to overcome an inflammation of a specific character by exciting an acute nonspecific inflammation.

substrate, substratum (sŭb′strāt, sŭb-strā′tŭm) [L. *substratum,* a strewing under]. 1. An underlying layer or foundation. 2. A base, as of a pigment. 3. The substance acted upon, as by an enzyme. SYN: *zymolyte.* SEE: *enzyme.*

subsultus (sŭb-sŭl′tŭs) [L. *subsultus,* from *sub,* under, + *salīre,* to leap]. Any morbid tremor or twitching, as of the tendons; a grave symptom in certain fevers.

s. clonus, s. tendinum. Involuntary twitchings of muscles, esp. of arms and feet, causing movement of tendons, observed in certain febrile conditions.

subsylvian (sŭb-sĭl′vĭ-ăn) [L. *sub,* beneath]. Below the fissure of Sylvius.

subtarsal (sŭb-tar′săl) [" + G. *tarsos,* tarsus]. Below the tarsus.

subthalamic (sŭb-thă-lăm′ĭk) [" + G. *thalamos,* chamber]. Located below the thalamus.

s. nucleus. SYN: *Body of Luys.* An elliptical mass of gray matter lying in ventral thalamus above cerebral peduncle and rostral to substantia nigra. It receives fibers from the globus pallidus.

subthalamus (sŭb-thăl′ă-mŭs) [L. *sub.* beneath, + G. *thalamos,* chamber]. SYN: *ventral thalamus.* Portion of the diencephalon lying below the thalamus and above the hypothalamus.

subtile, subtle (sŭb′tĭl, sŭt′l) [M.E. *sotill,* from L. *subtilis,* woven fine]. 1. Very fine or delicate. 2. Very acute. 3. Mentally acute or crafty or piercing, as sharp. 4. Operating without attracting attention, as subtle poisons.

subtilin (sŭb′tĭl-ĭn). An antibiotic biosynthesized by *Bacillus subtilis.* It is of low toxicity and effective against gram-positive organisms.

subtotal (sŭb-tō′tăl) [L. *sub,* beneath, + *totus,* whole]. Just less than total, as subtotal removal of a gland.

subtrochanteric (sŭb-trō-kăn-ter′ĭk) [" + G. *trochantēr,* a runner]. Below a trochanter.

subtuberal (sŭb-tū′bĕr-ăl) [" + *tuber,* a knot]. Located under a tuber.

subtympanic (sŭb-tĭm-păn′ĭk) [" + G. *tympanon,* drum]. Below the tympanum.

sububeres (sŭb-ū′ber-ēz) [" + *ubera,* breast]. Suckling children.

subumbilical (sŭb-ŭm-bĭl′ĭ-kăl) [L. *sub,* beneath, + *umbilicus,* navel]. Below the umbilicus.

s. space. Space within the body cavity below the navel resembling a triangle in shape.

subungual, subunguial (sŭb-ŭng′gwăl, -gwĭ-ăl) [" + *unguis,* nail]. Situated beneath nail of a finger or toe. SEE: *hyponychium.*

suburethral (sŭb-ū-rē′thrăl) [" + G. *ourēthra*, urethra]. Below the urethra.

subvaginal (sŭb-văj′ĭn-ăl) [" + *vagina*, sheath]. 1. Below the vagina. 2. On inner side of any tubular sheathing membrane.

subvertebral (sŭb-ver′tĕ-brăl) [" + *vertebra*, vertebra]. Beneath or on ventral side of the vertebral column or of a vertebra. SYN: *subspinal.*

subvirile (sŭb-vĭr′ĭl, -vī′rĭl) [" + *virilis*, male]. Of lowered or inferior virility.

subvitrinal (sŭb-vĭt′rĭn-ăl) [" + *vitrina*, vitreous body]. Located beneath the vitreous body.

subvolution (sŭb-vō-lū′shŭn) [" + *volutus*. from *volvere*, to turn]. Method of surgically turning over a flap to prevent adhesions.

succagogue [L. *succus*, juice, + G. *agogus*, a leading]. 1. To stimulate glandular secretion. 2. A substance which stimulates glandular secretion.

succedaneous (sŭk-sē-da′nē-ŭs) [L. *succedaneus*, substituting]. Acting as a substitute or relating to one.

succharase. Sucrase, *q.v.*

succi. Plural of *succus.*

succinylsulfathiazole. 2-N$_4$-succinylsulfanilamido)-thiazole. Member of the sulfonamide family valuable as an antibacterial agent for use in the intestinal tract. Less than 5% is absorbed from the gastrointestinal tract. White crystalline powder sparingly soluble in alcohol, acetone, and water; readily soluble in aqueous bases, as sodium bicarbonate solution.

succorrhea (sŭk-kor-rē′ă) [L. *succus*, juice, + G. *rhoia*, a flow]. Unnatural increase in secretion of any juice, esp. of a digestive fluid.

succus (sŭk′kŭs) [L. *succus*, juice]. A juice or fluid secretion.

s. entericus. The intestinal juice of the body. It is alkaline. Sp. gr. 1.010. The secretion of the minute glands lining the small intestine.

s. gastricus. The gastric juice.

s. pyloricus. An alkaline secretion by the pyloric end of the stomach.

succussion (sŭk-ŭs′shŭn) [L. *succussio*, a shaking]. Shaking of a person to detect the presence of fluid in the bodily cavities by listening for a splashing sound, esp. in the thorax.

suck (sŭk) [A.S. *sūcan*, to suck]. 1. To draw fluid into the mouth, as from the breast. 2. To exhaust air from a tube and thus siphon fluid from a container. 3. That which is drawn into the mouth by sucking.

suckle. To nurse at the breast.

suck′ing pad. Mass of fat in cheeks, esp. well developed in an infant, aiding it to suck. SEE: *myzesis.*

sucrase (sū′krās) [Fr. *sucre*, sugar]. SYN: *invertase, succharase.* An enzyme in the intestinal juice which splits cane sugar into glucose and fructose, which are absorbed into the portal circulation.

sucroclastic (sū-krō-klăs′tĭk) [" + G. *klastos*, destroyed]. Splitting up or hydrolyzing a sugar.

sucrose (sū′krōs) [Fr. *sucre*, sugar]. SYN: *saccharum, sugar.* A saccharose $C_{12}H_{22}O_{11}$ obtained from sugar cane, sugar beet and other sources. It is hydrolyzed in the intestine to glucose and fructose by sucrase present in intestinal juice.

ACTION: Only a little is retained by the stomach and it is all absorbed in the intestines. The lack of residue tends to cause constipation. The mucous membrane of the stomach is apt to be irritated by too much sugar. It and glucose may also set up fermentation. It is stored by the hepatic cells of the liver in the form of glycogen for future use. No chemical changes take place with the simple sugars, as they are directly absorbed. Any hydrolyzation in the stomach is supposed to be due to regurgitation of intestinal juice. Sugar is superior to starch, which requires more digestion. Sugar stimulates. As a rule, alcoholic drinkers do not care for much sugar, and one of the drink cures is the frequent use of candy. Excessive use causes fermentation.

USES: Reduction of intracranial pressure, as in brain tumor, brain abscess.

RS: *carbohydrates, disaccharose, fructose, galactose, glucose, lactose, levulose, maltose.*

suction (sŭk′shŭn) [L. *suctus*, from *sugere*, to suck]. The act of or capacity for sucking up by reduction of air pressure over part of the surface of a substance.

s., post-tussive. Suction sound over a lung cavity heard on auscultation after a cough.

sudamen (sū-dā′mĕn) (pl. *sudamina*) [L. *sudamen*, sweat]. Noninflammatory eruption from sweat glands characterized by whitish vesicles caused by the retention of sweat in corneous layer of the skin, appearing after profuse sweating or in certain febrile diseases, disappearing by absorption.

sudamina (sū-dăm′ĭn-ă). Plural of su damen.*

Sudan (sū-dăn′). One of a number of related biological stains which have a special affinity for fats. Includes Sudan II, Sudan III (G), Sudan IV, and Sudan R.

sudanophil (sū-dăn′ō-fĭl) [*sudan*, + G. *philein*, to love]. A leukocyte which stains readily with Sudan III, indicative of fatty degeneration.

sudanophilia (sū-dăn-ō-fĭl′ĭ-ă) [" + G. *philein*, to love]. A condition in which minute fat droplets contained in the leukocytes take a brilliant red stain, probably indicative of suppuration.

sudation (sū-dā′shŭn) [L. *sudatio*, a sweating]. 1. The act of sweating. 2. Excessive perspiration.

sudatoria (sū-dă-to′rĭ-ă) [L. *sudatorius*, sweating]. Excessive sweating. SYN: *ephidrosis, hyperidrosis.*

sudatorium (sū-dă-tō′rĭ-ŭm) [L. *sudatōrium*, a sweating room]. 1. A hot air bath or any bath to induce perspiration. 2. A room used to induce sweat baths.

sudokeratosis (sū″dō-ker-ă-tō′sĭs) [L. *sudor*, sweat, + G. *keras, kerat-*, horn, + *-ōsis*, condition]. Circumscribed, horny overgrowths obstructing the sweat ducts.

sudomotor (sū″dō-mō′tōr) [" + *motor*, a mover]. Pert. to stimulating the secretion of sweat; noting certain nerves.

sudor (sū′dor) [L. *sudor*, sweat]. Secretion from the sweat glands. SYN: *perspiration, sweat.*

RS: *anhidrosis, bromidrosis, chromidrosis, hydrosis, hematidrosis, perspiration, pore, skin, sweat, sudorific, uridrosis.*

s. cruen′tus. Blood-tinged sweat. SYN: *hematidrosis.*

sudoral (sū′dōr-ăl) [L. *sudor* sweat]. Pert. to, caused by, or marked by perspiration.

sudoresis (sū-dō-rē′sĭs) [L. *sudorēsis*, excessive sweating]. Profuse sweating. SYN: *diaphoresis*.

sudoriferous (sū-dor-if'ĕr-ŭs) [L. *sudor*, sweat, + *ferre*, to bear]. Conveying or producing sweat.

s. glands. Sweat-secreting glands of the skin.

sudorific (sū-dōr-ĭf'ĭk) [L. *sudorificus*, producing sweat]. 1. Secreting or promoting the secretion of sweat. 2. Agent which produces sweating. SYN: *diaphoretic*.

sudoriparous (sū-dor-ĭp'ă-rŭs) [L. *sudor*, sweat, + *parēre*, to produce]. Secreting sweat. SYN: *sudoriferous*.

suet (sū'ĕt) [M.E. from L. *sebum*, suet]. Hard fat from the ox or sheep's kidneys and loins, used as the base of certain ointments and as an emollient.

suffocate (sŭf-ō'kāt). To asphyxiate.

suffocation (sŭf"ō-kā'shŭn) [L. *suffocāre*, to choke]. 1. State of being choked by obstruction of air passages by drowning, smothering, throttling, or inhalation of noxious gases. SYN: *asphyxia*.* Generally from gases. 2. Act of obstructing the air passages.

SYM: Insensibility, breathing slight, face purple and swollen, livid lips. Symptoms not always present.

TREATMENT: Dash cold water in face. Slap chest. Apply ammonia to nostrils. Artificial respiration. Tracheotomy may be required. RS: *resuscitation, unconsciousness*.

suffusion (sŭf-ū'zhŭn) [L. *suffusio*, a pouring over]. 1. Spreading of a bodily fluid into surrounding tissues. SYN: *extravasation*. 2. Pouring of a fluid over the body as treatment.

sugar (shu'gar) [M.E. *suger*, from L. *saccharum*, from G. *sakcharon*, sugar]. A sweet-tasting carbohydrate belonging to the monosaccharose and disaccharose groups. Crystalline carbohydrates of comparatively low molecular weight and generally having a sweet taste.

CLASSIFICATION: First, as to the number of atoms of simple sugars yielded on hydrolysis by a molecule of the given sugar and, secondly, as to the number of carbon atoms in the molecules of the simple sugars so obtained. Thus, *dextrose* (which see) is a monosaccharide because it cannot be hydrolyzed to a simpler sugar; it is a hexose because it contains 6 carbon atoms per molecule. *Sucrose* is a disaccharide because on hydrolysis it yields 2 molecules, 1 of dextrose and 1 of levulose.

s., beet. Sucrose obtained from sugar beets.

s., blood. The carbohydrate present in the blood; principally glucose.

s., brain. Cerebrose (galactose).

s., cane. Sucrose obtained from sugar cane.

s., diabetic. Glucose in the urine of diabetics.

s., fruit. Levulose, or fructose.

s., grape. Glucose.

s., invert. One consisting of one molecule of glucose and one of fructose resulting from the hydrolysis of sucrose.

s., liver. Glycogen.

s., malt. Maltose.

s., milk. Lactose.

s., muscle. Inositol. It is not a true sugar.

sugar, words pert. to: aglycosuric, biose, blood, carbohydrate, dextrose, diabetin, disaccharide, disaccharose, Fehling's tests, fructose, fruit s., galactose, glucide, "gluco-" words. "glyco-" words, hypoglycemia, invert, invertase, lactose, levulose, mannite, melitemia, monosaccharide, monosaccharose, pentose, pentosuria, polysaccharide, polysaccharose, "sacchar-" words, sucrose, xylose.

suggestibility (sŭg-jĕs"tĭ-bĭl'ĭ-tĭ) [L. *suggestus*, suggested]. A condition in which a person responds readily to suggestions or opinions of another.

suggestible (sŭg-jĕs'tĭ-bl) [L. *suggestus*, suggested]. Very susceptible to the opinions or suggestions of others.

suggestion (sŭg-jĕs'chŭn) [L. *suggestio*, from *suggerere*, to supply]. 1. Imparting of an idea in any indirect way. 2. The idea so conveyed. 3. The acceptance or the effect of the statements or actions of one person upon another, depending on the emotional set-up of the recipient and his psychic relationship to the other person.

s., auto-. Self-suggestion as distinguished from that coming from another person, esp. in hypnotic state.

suggestive (sŭg-jĕs'tĭv) [L. *suggestus*, suggested]. Stimulating or pert. to suggestion.

s. medicine. Therapy by suggestion either during consciousness or hypnosis.

s. therapeutics. The practice of treating disease by suggestion or hypnotism.

suggillation (sŭg-jĭl-ā'shŭn) [L. *sugillāre*, to beat black and blue]. A bruise or black and blue mark. SYN: *ecchymosis*.

suicide (sū'ĭ-sīd) [L. *sui*, of oneself, + *cidus*, from *caedere*, to kill]. 1. Act or instance of taking one's own life voluntarily. 2. One who attempts or commits self-murder.

These individuals often have attacks of temporary insanity or mental depression which may lead to suicide. In addition to the usual F. A. Treatment for injuries, kindly interrogation and soothing, tranquil conversation are invaluable. In their after-care, such patients should be watched and kept free from needless questioning or emotional display. Sedatives are useful. Persons who have attempted suicide should be carefully observed because of the danger of their attempting to commit suicide later. SEE: *hysteria*.

MENTAL STATES CONDUCIVE TO: Those with sudden impulses. The depressed. Those with delusions: (a) of persecution; (b) of being ruined; (c) voices suggesting; (d) incurable disease. In melancholia. Schizophrenia. Epilepsy. Confusional states. Alcoholics. Through accidents: (a) Acute delirium; (b) mania; (c) general paralysis.

METHODS RESORTED TO: 1. Hanging. 2. Drowning (in tub or otherwise). 3. Poisoning. 4. Cutting an artery. 5. Burning. 6. Jumping from window. 7. Overdose of various medications. 8. Bombs. 9. Deliberately crashing vehicles or airplane. INSTRUMENTS USED: (a) Matches; (b) knives and spoons; (c) glass; (d) cord, rope, suspenders, bedclothing, etc.; (e) harmless articles converted into dangerous tools; (f) nail files. All must be removed if patient is inclined to harm self or others.

sulcal (sŭl'kăl) [L. *sulcus*, groove]. Pert. to a sulcus.

s. artery. A tiny branch of ant. spinal artery.

sulcate, sulcated (sŭl'kāt, -ed) [L. *sulcatus*, grooved]. Furrowed or grooved.

sulcus (sŭl'kŭs) (pl. *sulci*) [L. *sulcus*, groove]. A furrow or groove, or slight depression or fissure, esp. of the brain.

s. centralis. NA. Fissure dividing the frontal and parietal lobes of each cerebral hemisphere. SYN: *fissure of Rolando.*

s., *intraparietal.* One that separates the inf. from the sup. parietal bones and lobes.

s. *precentra'lis.* NA. An interrupted one generally parallel with the fissure of Rolando and ant. to it.

s. *pulmona'lis.* Depression on either side of the vertebral column.

s. *spira'lis cochleae.* Groove bet. the labium tympanicum and labium vestibulare.

sulf-, sulfo-. Prefix showing that a compound with this prefix contains sulfurous anhydride or the group SO.

sulfa drugs. Drugs of the sulfonamide group possessing bacteriostatic properties. SEE: *sulfonamides.*

sulfabenzamine (sŭl″fă-bĕn′ză-mēn). A sulfonamide drug effective against anaerobic bacteria which cause gas gangrene. It has some antibacterial action against streptococci, staphylococci, and pneumococci.

sulfacetimide (sŭl-fă-sĕt′ĭ-mīd). A sulfonamide used in treatment of *B. coli,* gonorrhea, and infections of the urinary tract, esp. when resistant to sulfanilamide and sulfathiazole.

sulfadiazine (sŭl″fă-dī′ă-zēn). One of a group of diazine derivatives of sulfanilamide.

sulfamerazine (sul″fa-mer′ă-zēn). A sulfur derivative which may be given orally for pneumococci, streptococci, meningococci, and gonococci.

sulfamethazine (sŭl-fă-mĕth′ă-zēn). A near relative of sulfadiazine. Nausea and vomiting less than with sulfapyridine; solubility good, and damage to kidneys slight.

sulfamethylthiazol (sŭl″fă-mĕth″ĭl-thī′ă-zōl). A sulfanilamide derivative which is less toxic than sulfapyridine; effective against staphylococcic organisms.

sulfanilamide (sŭl″făn-ĭl′ă-mīd) (para-amino-benzene-sulfonamide). A white, slightly bitter, crystalline substance from coal tar, the parent of the azo dyes. It was formerly widely used in the treatment of a number of infections but, because of its toxic reactions and its tendency to produce acidosis, it has been superseded by more effective and less toxic sulfonamides.

sulfapyridine (sŭl″fă-pĭr′ĭ-dēn). A sulfonamide, one of the first drugs to have a curative effect upon pneumonia; formerly used extensively in the treatment of streptococcal, gonococcal, and staphylococcal infections, but its use has been supplanted by other sulfonamides which are less toxic and more effective.

sulfapyr'idine so'dium monohy'drate. A soluble salt of sulfapyridine for intravenous use only.

sulfarsphenamine (sŭlf″ars-fĕn′ă-mēn). An arsenic compound; 19% arsenic.

USES: Same as for neoarsphenamine, but said to have more reaction.

sulfasuxidine (sŭl-fă-sŭx′ĭ-dēn). Proprietary name for succinylsulfathiazole, a bacteriostatic for infections of the gastrointestinal tract; very poorly absorbed from the gastrointestinal tract.

sulfate (sŭl′fāt) [L. *sulphas,* sulfur salt]. A salt or ester of sulfuric acid.

s., *iron.* Green vitriol; copperas. Fatal in large dosage.

POISONING: Magnesia and diluents.

s., *magnesium.* Magnesium sulfate, *q.v.*

sulfathiazole (sŭl-fa-thī′ă-zōl). A sulfanilamide compound; largely replaced by less toxic sulfonamides.

sulfhemoglobin (sŭlf″hēm-ō-glō′bĭn). Substance formed by action of hydrogen sulfide on blood.

sulfhemoglobinemia (sŭlf″hēm-ō-glō″bĭn-ē′mĭ-ă). Persistent cyanotic condition due to sulfhemoglobin in blood.

sulfhydryl (sŭlf-hī′drĭl). The univalent radical, SH, of sulfur and hydrogen. Also called *SH group.*

sulfo-. A combining form usually indicating the presence of divalent sulfur or of the sulfo group, $-SO_2OH$.

sulfonal (sŭl′fō-năl). A proprietary hypnotic and sedative.

sulfonalism (sŭl′fō-năl-ĭzm). 1. Sulfonal poisoning and its symptoms. 2. Addiction to sulfonal.

sulfonamides. A group of compounds consisting of amides of sulfanilic acid derived from their parent compound sulfanilamide. They are bacteriostatic, their action on bacteria resulting from interference with functioning of enzyme systems necessary for normal metabolism growth, and multiplication.

sulfonethylmethane (sŭl″fōn-ĕth″ĭl-mĕth′-ān). USP. Trional. White powder or crystalline substance with a bitter taste.

ACTION AND USES: As a hypnotic.

sulfonmethane (sŭl″fōn-mĕth′ān). USP. Crystalline compound with hypnotic and sedative properties. SYN: *sulfonal.*

sulfourea (sŭl″fō-ū-rē′ă) [L. *sulfur,* sulfur, + *urea*]. Urea with oxygen replaced with sulfur. SYN: *thiourea.*

sulfur (sŭl′fŭr) [L.]. SYMB: S. At. wt. 32.064, at. no. 16. Sp. gr. 2.07. It is a pale yellow, crystalline element which burns with a blue flame, producing sulfur dioxide.

The amount of sulfur excreted in the urine varies with amount of protein in diet but more or less parallels the amount of nitrogen excreted as both are derived from protein catabolism. The S:N ratio is approx. 1:14, *i.e.,* for each gram of sulfur excreted, 14 grams of nitrogen are excreted. The amount of sulfur excreted daily in the form of sulfates averages about 2.5 grams. It aids in the ion balance of tissues when oxidized to sulfate and is required for the synthesis of body proteins as cystine or cysteine or their combination.

DEFICIENCY SYM: Dermatitis, imperfect development of hair and nails. Deficiency of cystine or cysteine proteins in diet restricts growth and may be fatal. Tissue oxidation of cystine forms inorganic sulfate if the protein intake is sufficient.

s. *dioxide.* An irritating gas used in industries to manufacture acids, also used in electrical refrigerators. A bactericide and important disinfectant.

POISONING: SYM: Suffocation from a highly irritating gas which forms sulfuric acid when in contact with moisture of the mouth, eyes, and respiratory passages, with resultant pain, swelling, burning, etc.

TREATMENT: Remove patient from the vitiated atmosphere. Oxygen by intermittent positive pressure breathing apparatus or artificial respiration may be necessary. Give heart and respiratory stimulants as needed. Wash affected areas with large amounts of water and weak alkalies, as chalk magnesia, lime water, soapsuds. Follow by bland diet.

sulfurated, sulfureted (sŭl′fŭ-rā-ted, -rĕt-ĕd) [L. *sulfur,* sulfur]. Combined or impregnated with sulfur.

s. hydrogen. A colorless, inflammable gas of disagreeable odor resulting from decomposition of organic matter containing sulfur; used as a chemical reagent. SYN: *hydrogen sulfide.* H_2S.

sulfuric acid (sŭl-fū′rĭk) [L. *sulfur,* sulfur]. SYN: *oil of vitriol.* A colorless, odorless, liquid of heavy, oily consistency. It is extremely caustic and corrosive. It is widely used in manufacturing.

POISONING: Sometimes accidentally taken by mouth, as it resembles syrup or glycerin.

SYM: Local effects—burning, with destruction of skin. If it strikes eye it may result in blindness. If taken by mouth, intense pain extending from mouth to esophagus and down to stomach, causing marked, excruciating pain; swelling of affected tissues; salivation; painful swallowing; often gasping for breath, and hoarse voice. Mucous membrane has a grayish-white coating. There is persistent, painful vomiting. Patient quickly develops shock.

TREATMENT: Dilute acid with large volumes of water. Neutralize acid with milk of magnesia, baking soda or other well-diluted alkalies. Follow by soothing substances, as raw eggs.

s. a., dilute. An aqueous 10% solution of H_2SO_4. Used as an astringent and for gastric hypoacidity.

summation (sŭm-ā′shŭn) [L. *summatio,* an adding]. Cumulative action or effect, as of stimuli.

Thus, an organ reacts to 2 or more weak stimuli as if they were a single strong one.

summer (sŭm′ĕr) [A.S. *sumer*]. The hot season of the year.

sunburn (sŭn′burn) [A.S. *sunne,* sun, + *bernan,* to burn]. Dermatitis due to excess exposure to the actinic rays of the sun. SEE: *burn.*

Sunday morning paralysis. SYN: *Saturday night paralysis.* Radial nerve palsy sometimes the indirect result of acute alcoholism resulting from stuporous patient lying immobile with arm pressed over a projecting surface.

sunstroke (sŭn′strōk) [A.S. *sunne,* sun, + M.E. *strok,* a blow]. An affection from undue exposure to rays of the sun or excessive heat.

SYM: Extreme prostration, high fever, other symptoms of heatstroke, delirium, collapse, loss of mind, or death. SYN: *thermic fever.* SEE: *heatstroke.*

super- [L.]. Combining form meaning *above, beyond, superior.*

superalimentation (sūp″er-ăl-ĭ-mĕn-tā′shŭn) [L. *super,* above, + *alimentum,* food]. Therapeutic forcing of food in excess of body needs or appetite.

superalkalinity (sūp″er-ăl-kă-lĭn′ĭ-tĭ) [″ + *alkalinus,* alkaline]. Excessive alkalinity.

superciliary (sūp-er-sĭl′ĭ-ă-rĭ) [L. *supercilium,* eyebrow]. Pert. to or in the region of an eyebrow.

supercilium (sū-pĕr-sĭl′ĭ-ŭm) [L. *supercilium,* eyebrow]. 1. Eyebrow. 2. A hair of the eyebrow.

superego (sūp″er-ē′gō) [L. *super,* above, + *egō,* I]. An inner, subconscious censor. SEE: *ego.*

superfecundation (sū″pĕr-fē-kŭn-dā′shŭn) [″ + *fecundāre,* to fertilize]. Successive fertilization, by more than one coitus, of two or more ova formed during the same menstrual cycle. Fertilization may be by the same or two different males.

super female. A female having 3 X chromosomes.

superfetation (sū″pĕr-fē-tā′shŭn) [″ + *foetus,* fetus]. Fertilization of two ova in the same uterus at different menstrual periods within a short interval.

superficial (sū-pĕr-fĭsh′ăl) [″ + *facies,* shape]. 1. Confined to the surface. 2. Not thorough; cursory.

s. reflex. One induced by very light stimulus such as stroking skin lightly with soft cotton wad.

superficialis (sū″pĕr-fĭsh-ĭ-ā′lĭs) [L. *superficialis,* superficial]. Superficial; noting a superficial artery, vein, or nerve, or structure near the surface.

superimpregnation (sū″pĕr-ĭm″prĕg-nā′shŭn) [L. *super,* over, + *impregnatio,* impregnation]. Conception during pregnancy; fertilization from 2 different ovulations. SYN: *superfecundation, superfetation.*

superinduce (sū″pĕr-ĭn-dūs′) [″ + *in,* into, + *ducere,* to lead]. To bring in over or above that already existing condition or situation.

superinfection (sū″pĕr-ĭn-fĕk′shun) [″ + *infectio,* a putting into]. A new infection by the same organism, in addition to a similar one already existing.

superinvolution (sū″pĕr-ĭn-vō-lū′shŭn) [″ + *in,* into, + *volutus,* from *volvere,* to roll]. Excessive reduction of the uterus following childbirth to less than its normal size. SYN: *hyperinvolution.*

superior (sū-pē′rĭ-or) [L. comparative of *super,* beyond]. 1. Higher than; situated above something else. 2. Better than. 3. One in charge of others.

superior′ity com′plex. An exaggerated conviction of one's own superiority; a pretense of superiority in order to compensate for supposed inferiority.

superlactation (sū-pĕr-lăk-tā′shŭn) [L. *super,* above, + *lactāre,* to suckle]. Oversecretion of milk, or continuance of lactation beyond normal time.

superlethal (sū″pĕr-lē′thăl) [″ + L. *lethum,* death]. A dose of a drug or exposure to trauma greater than that required to produce death.

supermoron (sū″pĕr-mō′rŏn) [″ + G. *mōros,* stupid]. One slightly subnormal but above a moron mentally.

supermotility (sū″pĕr-mō-tĭl′ĭ-tĭ) [″ + *motilis,* able to move]. Excessive motility in any part. SYN: *hypercinesia.*

supernatant (sū″pĕr-nā′tănt) [″ + *natāre,* to float]. 1. Floating on surface, as oil on water. 2. The clear liquid remaining at the top after a precipitate settles.

supernate (sū-pĕr-nāt′) [″ + *natāre,* to float]. A supernatant fluid.

supernumerary (sū″pĕr-nū′mĕr-a-rĭ) [L. *supernumerarius,* above the number]. Exceeding the regular number.

supernutrition (sū″pĕr-nū-trĭ′shŭn) [L. *super,* above, + *nutritio,* nourishment]. More than normal nutrition.

supersaturated solution (sū″pĕr-săt′ū-rāt″-ĕd) [″ + *saturāre,* to sate]. One containing more salt or other substance than it can dissolve at normal temperature.

superscription (sū″pĕr-skrĭp′shŭn) [″ + *scriptio,* a writing]. The beginning of a prescription noted by the sign ℞, signifying L. *recipe,* take.

supersecretion (sū″pĕr-sē-krē′shŭn) [″ + *secretio,* a separating]. An excess of any secretion.

supersensitiveness (sū″per-sĕn′sĭ-tĭv″nĕs) [″ + *sensitivus,* sensitive]. Excessive susceptibility to a foreign protein or pollen. SYN: *hypersensitiveness.*

supersoft (sū″pĕr-sŏft′) [" + A.S. *sōfte,* soft]. Exceptionally soft; noting roentgen rays of extremely long wave length and low penetrating power.

supersonic. SYN: *ultrasonic.* 1. Pertaining to vibrations of sound space waves of frequencies above 20,000 cycles which are inaudible to the human ear. 2. Used to describe speeds greater than that of sound.

supertension (sū′pĕr-tĕn′shŭn) [" + *tensio,* a stretching]. Extremely high tension. SYN: *hypertension.*

supervenosity (sū″pĕr-vē-nŏs′ĭ-tĭ) [" + *venosus,* pert. to a vein]. Incomplete oxidation of the blood; a condition of excessive venosity.

supervention (sū″pĕr-vĕn′shŭn) [L. *superventio,* a coming over]. Additional condition developing besides something already existing, as a complication to an existing disease.

supervirulent (sū″pĕr-vĭr′ū-lĕnt) [L. *super,* above, + *virulentus,* poisonous] More virulent than usual.

supervisor. A person, usually a nurse, who is responsible for a certain department, ward or activity in a hospital or nursing school.

supervitaminosis. Excess accumulation of vitamins in the body due to an acute or chronic overdose. SYN: *hypervitaminosis.*

supinate (sū′pĭ-nāt) [L. *supināre,* to lay on the back]. 1. To turn the forearm or hand so that the palm faces upward. 2. To rotate the foot and leg outward. 3 To cause to assume, or to assume, a position of supination.

supination (sū-pĭn-ā′shŭn) [L. *supināre,* to lay on the back]. 1. Turning of the palm or foot upward. 2. Act of lying flat upon the back. 3. Condition of being on the back or having the foot or palm facing upward.

supinator (sū″pĭn-ā′tor) [L.]. A muscle producing the motion of supination of the forearm. SEE: *Table of Muscles in Appendix.*

s. longus reflex. Flexion of the forearm caused by tapping of the tendon of the supinator longus.

supine (sū-pīn′) [L. *supinus,* bent back; lying on the back]. 1. Of position, lying on the back or with the face upward. 2. Of the hand or foot noting position with the palm or foot facing upward. OPP: *prone.* SEE: *position.*

supplemental (sŭp-lē-mĕn′tăl) [L. *supplementum,* an addition]. Referring to something added to supply a need or to reinforce.

s. air. SYN: *Reserve air.* The air which by the most forcible effort can be expelled after an ordinary expiration which has followed a normal inspiration. In adult males it averages about 1500 cc.

suppository (sŭp-pŏz′ĭ-tō-rĭ) (pl. *suppositories*) [L. *suppositorium,* that which is placed underneath]. A semisolid, fusible substance for introduction into the rectum, vagina, or urethra, where it dissolves. It often serves as a vehicle for medicines to be absorbed.

Commonly shaped like cylinder or cone and made of soap, glycerinated gelatin or cocoa butter (oil of theobroma).

s., rectal, anodyne. For local or general effects to reduce pain.

s., r., astringent. To contract blood vessels and tissues.

s., r., evacuant. To cause evacuation

suppression (sū-prĕsh′ŭn) [L. *suppressio,* a pressing under]. 1. Repression of the ext. manifestation of a morbid condition. 2. Complete failure of a natural secretion or excretion. OPP: *retention.* 3. PSY: Conscious inhibition of an idea or desire, as distinguished from repression which is considered an unconscious process.

s. of menses. 1. Amenorrhea in which menstruation ceases after once being established and from some cause other than pregnancy or the climacteric. 2. Any suppression of the menses.

s. of urine. Suppression of urine resulting from renal conditions.

suppurant (sŭp′ū-rănt) [L. *suppurans,* from *suppurāre,* to cause to suppurate]. 1. Producing, tending to produce, or characterized by pus formation. 2 Agent causing pus formation. SYN: *suppurative.*

suppurate (sŭp′pū-rāt) [L. *suppurāre,* to cause to suppurate]. To form or generate pus.

suppuration (sŭp-ū-rā′shŭn) [L. *suppurātio,* from *sub,* under, + *pus, pur-,* matter, pus]. 1. The process of pus formation. 2. The discharge produced by suppuration. SYN: *pus.*

One of the terminations of inflammation due to the presence of certain microorganisms called pyogenic* (pus-forming) bacteria. Suppuration does not always obtain even though microorganisms are present in the affected part, as may be the case in erysipelas and acute joint affections where exudate is serous.

The liquefaction of tissues and formation of pus will continue so long as the microorganisms are alive. They cause the death of the leukocytes (white cells) and the cells of the part, liquefying the tissue so that the area becomes filled with a liquid (liquor puris) holding the dead and dying cells. Combination of liquor puris and the dead cells is called "pus."

An abscess may form by the accumulation of this liquid which is indicated by redness, swelling, heat and pain. It will show fluctuation which may be felt by touching it. When the abscess reaches the surface it will burst and discharge its contents.

RS: *abscess, gangrene, inflammation, infection, purulent, pus. pustulant, pustule.*

suppurative (sŭp′ū-rā″tĭv, -ră-tĭv) [L. *suppuratus,* from *suppurāre,* to cause to suppurate]. 1. Producing or associated with generation of pus. 2. Agent producing pus formation.

s. fever. Pus in the blood causing fever; a form of septicemia. SYN: *pyemia.*

supra- [L.]. Combining form meaning *above.*

supra-acromial (sū-pră-ă-krō′mĭ-ăl) [L. *supra,* above, + G. *akron,* point, + *ōmos,* shoulder]. Located above the acromion.

supra-auricular (sū″pră-aw-rĭk′ū-lar) [" + *auricula,* ear]. Located above an auricle.

supracerebellar (sū″pră-sĕr-ē-bĕl′ar) [L. *supra,* above, + *cerebellum,* little brain]. On or above the upper surface of the cerebellum.

suprachoroid (sū″pră-kō′royd) [L. *supra,* above, + G. *chorioeidēs,* skinlike]. SYN: *lamina suprachoroidea, epichoroid.* 1. Situated upon or above the choroid layer of the eyeball. 2. The suprachoroid lamina, *q.v.*

s. lamina. SYN: *epichoroid, lamina suprachoroidea.* The superficial layer of the choroid consisting of thin transparent layers, the outermost adhering to the sclera.

suprachoroidea (sū″pră-ko-roy′dē-ă) [" + G. *chorioeidēs,* skinlike]. Outermost layer of the choroid. SYN: *suprachoroid lamina.*

supraclavicular (sū″pră-klă-vĭk′ū-lar) [" + *clavicula,* a little key]. Located above the clavicle.

s. fossa. Depression on either side of neck reaching down behind the clavicle.

s. point. A stimulation point over the clavicle at which contraction of arm muscles may be produced.

supracondylar (sū″pră-kŏn′dĭl-ar) [" + G. *kondylos,* knuckle]. Above a condyle.

supracotyloid (sū″pră-kŏt′ĭ-loyd) [L. *supra,* above, + G. *kotyloeidēs,* cup-shaped]. Above the acetabulum.

supradiaphragmatic (sū″pră-dī″ă-frăg-mat′ĭk) [" + G. *dia,* across, + *phragma,* wall]. Above the diaphragm.

supraglenoid (sū″pră-glē′noyd) [" + G. *glēnē,* cavity, + *eidos,* form]. Above the glenoid cavity or fossa.

s. tuberosity. A rough surface of the scapula above glenoid cavity to which is attached the long head of biceps muscle.

suprahyoid (sū″pră-hī′oyd) [" + *hyoeidēs,* U-shaped]. Located above the hyoid bone; denoting accessory thyroid glands within the geniohyoid muscle.

s. muscles. The digastric, geniohyoid, mylohyoid, and stylohyoid muscles.

suprainguinal (sū″pră-ĭn′gwĭn-ăl) [" + *inguinalis,* pert. to the groin]. Above the groin.

supraliminal (sū″pră-lĭm′ĭ-năl) [L. *supra,* above, + *limen, limin-,* threshold]. PSY: 1. Above the threshold of consciousness; conscious. 2. Exceeding the stimulus threshold. SEE: *subliminal.*

supralumbar (sū″pră-lŭm′bar) [" + *lumbus,* loin]. Above the lumbar region.

supramalleolar (sū″pră-mal-lē′ō-lar) [" + *malleōlus,* little hammer]. Located above either malleolus.

supramarginal (sū″pră-mar′jĭn-ăl) [" + *margo, margin-,* margin]. Above any border.

s. convolution, s. gyrus. A cerebral convolution on lateral surface of the parietal lobe above post. part of sylvian fissure.

supramastoid (sū″pră-măs′toyd) [" + *mastos,* breast, + *eidos,* like]. Above the mastoid process of the temporal bone.

s. crest. A ridge on the temporal bone. Also called *temporal line.*

supramaxilla (sū″pră-măks-ĭl′lă) [" + *maxilla,* jaw]. The upper jawbone. SYN: *maxilla.*

supramaxillary (sū″pră-măks′ĭl-lā-rĭ) [" + *maxillaris,* pert. to the jaw]. 1. Relating to the upper jaw. 2. Located above the upper jaw.

suprameatal (sū″pră-mē-ā′tăl) [L. *supra,* above, + *meatus,* passage]. Above a meatus, esp. the ext. auditory meatus, noting the spine of Henle, a small, bony projection at post. sup. margin of ext. auditory meatus.

s. spine. SYN: *spine of Henle.* Small bony projection at post. sup. margin of ext. auditory meatus marking the ant. superior apex of the suprameatal triangle, *q.v.*

s. triangle. Triangular space bordered by upper half of post. wall of ext. auditory meatus, and the supramastoid crest used to locate the mastoid antrum.

supraoccipital (sū″pră-ŏk-sĭp′ĭ-tăl) [L. *supra,* above, + *occiput,* back of head]. Lying above or in upper portion of the occiput.

s. portion (of occipital bone). Portion lying immediately above the foramen magnum and forming lower part of squamous portion of occipital bone.

supraorbital (sū″pră-or′bĭ-tăl) [" + *orbita,* track, circuit]. Located above the orbit.

s. neuralgia. N. of the supraorbital nerve. SYN: *hemicrania.*

s. notch. A notch in sup. margin arch of orbit for transmitting supraorbital vessels and nerve.

s. reflex. Contraction of orbicularis oculi muscle with closure of lids resulting from percussion above supraorbital nerve.

suprapelvic (sū″pră-pĕl′vĭk) [L. *supra,* above, + *pelvis,* basis]. Located above the pelvis.

suprapontine (sū″pră-pŏn′tĭn) [" + *pons, pont-,* bridge]. Located above the pons Varolii.

suprapubic (sū″pră-pū′bĭk) [" + *pubis,* pubis]. Above the pubic arch.

s. cystotomy. Surgical opening of the bladder from just above the symphysis pubis.

s. reflex. Deflection of linea alba toward stroked side when abdomen is stroked above Poupart's ligament.

suprarenal (sū″pră-rē′năl) [" + *rēn,* kidney]. 1. Above the kidney. 2. Tiny gland above each kidney. SYN: *adrenal, suprarenal body, s. capsule, s. gland.* 3. Pert. to the suprarenal gland.

s. gland. SYN: *adrenal gland; glandula suprarenalis.* An endocrine gland lying cephalad and mediad to each kidney. SEE: *adrenal, ACTH, adrenalin, endocrine gland, epinephrine, corticosterone, cortisone.*

suprarenalopathy (sū″pră-rē-năl-ŏp′ă-thĭ) [" + " + G. *pathos,* disease]. A disorder due to abnormal functioning of the suprarenal glands.

suprarenopathy (sū″pră-rē-nŏp′ă-thĭ) [" + " + G. *pathos,* disease]. Any disorder of the suprarenal glands.

suprascapular (sū″pră-skăp′ū-lar) [L. *supra,* above, + *scapula,* shoulder]. Located above the scapula.

suprasegmen′tal. Above the segmented portion.

s. brain. The cerebrum, midbrain, and cerebellum as distinguished from the *segmental portion* (pons and medulla oblongata).

suprasellar (sū″pră-sĕl′ar) [" + *sella,* saddle]. Above or over the sella turcica.

suprasonic (sū″pră-sŏn′ĭk) [" + *sonus,* sound]. Noting sound with frequencies of vibration above 20,000 per second.

supraspinal (sū″pră-spī′năl) [" + *spina,* a thorn]. Above a spine.

supraspinous (sū″pră-spī′nŭs) [" + *spina,* thorn]. Above any spine.

s. fossa. A groove above the spine of the scapula.

suprasternal (sū″pră-ster′năl) [" + G. *sternon,* chest]. Above the sternum. SYN: *episternal.*

supra″ster′ol. An end product sometimes resulting from over-irradiation of ergosterol.

supratrochlear (sū″pră-trok′lē-ar) [" + *trochlea,* pulley]. Above a trochlea, esp. that of the humerus.

supravaginal (sū″pră-văj′ĭ-năl) [" + *vagina,* sheath]. Above the vagina or any sheathing membrane.

supravergence (sū-prā-verg'ĕns). Condition in which one eye moves upward in the vertical plane while the other does not.

sura (sū'ră) [L. *sura*, calf of the leg]. The calf of the leg.

sural (sū'răl) [L. *sura*, calf of the leg]. Relating to the calf of the leg.

suralimentation (sŭr-ăl-ĭm-ĕn-tā'shŭn) [Fr. *sur*, from L. *super*, above, + *alimentum*, nourishment]. Treatment by overfeeding. Syn: *gavage, superalimentation.*

surdity (sŭr'dĭ-tĭ) [L. *surditās*, deafness]. Inability to hear. Syn: *deafness.*

surdomute (sŭr'dō-mūt") [L. *surdus*, deaf, + *mutus*, dumb]. 1. A deaf-mute. 2. Deaf and dumb.

surface (sur'făs) [Fr. *sur* from L. *super*, over, + *faciēs*, face]. 1. The exterior of a body having length and breadth. 2. The external or internal exposed portions of a hollow structure as the outer or inner surfaces of the cranium or stomach. 3. The face or faces of a body such as a bone.

s. tension. Abbr: *S.T.* Condition at the surface of a liquid in contact with a gas or another liquid which causes its surface to act as a stretched rubber membrane. It is the result of mutual attraction of the molecules to each other thus producing a cohesive state which causes liquids to assume a shape presenting the smallest surface area to the surrounding medium. This accounts for the spherical shape assumed by fluids, such as drops of oil or water.

surfer's knots. Nodular swelling of area of lower leg and foot exposed to pressure and trauma while on a surfboard. Nodules may be painful.

surgeon (sŭr'jŭn) [Fr. *chirurgien*, from L. *chirurgus*, from G. *cheir*, hand, + *ergon*, work]. A medical practitioner who specializes in surgery.

s., dental. A dentist authorized to operate on the mouth and teeth. Syn: *stomatologist.*

s., house. A surgeon in training who works under the supervision of the attending surgeon.

surgery (sur'jur-ĭ) [M.E. *surgerie*, from G. *cheirourgia*, handwork]. 1. Branch of medicine dealing with manual and operative procedures for correction of deformities and defects, repair of injuries, diagnosis and cure of diseases, relief of suffering and prolongation of life. Syn: *chirurgery, chirurgia.* 2. Surgeon's operating room.

s., aseptic. Operative procedures carried on under aseptic conditions or in the absence of pathogenic organisms.

s., aural. That pertaining to the ear.

s., conservative. That in which as much as possible of a part or structure is retained.

s., major. Important and serious operations involving risk to life.

s., minor. Simple, less serious operations.

s., oral. That pertaining to the mouth and associated structures, esp. the teeth and jaws.

s., orificial. Surgery of the orifices of the body such as the mouth, anus, vagina, etc.

s., orthopedic. S. for correction of deformities.

s., plastic. S. concerned with the repair or restoration of defective or missing structures, frequently involving the transference of tissue from a part or person to another.

surgical (sŭr'jĭk-ăl) [G. *cheirourgia*, handwork]. Of the nature of or pert. to surgery.

s. diathermy. The use of high-frequency electrical oscillations in such a way that animal tissues are destroyed.

s. dressing. Sterile protective covering of gauze or other substance applied to an operative wound. See: *chemise.*

s. fever. Fever following an operation or injury.

s. kidney. Suppuration or tuberculosis of the kidney.

s. neck. Constricted part of shaft of humerus below the tuberosities; commonly the seat of fracture.

surrogate (sŭr'rō-găt) [L. *surrogāre*, to substitute]. Something that replaces another; a substitute.

Psy: The representation of one whose identity is concealed from conscious recognition, as in a dream; a figure of importance may represent one's loved one.

sursumduction (sŭr"sŭm-dŭk'shŭn) [L. *sursum*, upward, + *ducere*, to lead]. Elevation, as the power or act of turning an eye upward independently of the other one.

sursumvergence (sŭr"sŭm-vĕr'jĕns) [" + *vergere*, to turn]. An upward turning, as of the eyeballs.

sursumversion (sŭr"sŭm-vĕr'shŭn) [" + *versio*, from *vertere*, to turn]. Process of turning upward; simultaneous movement of both eyes upward.

susceptible (sŭs-sĕp'tĭ-bl) [L. *susceptibilis*, from *suscipere*, to take up]. 1. Having little resistance to a disease or foreign protein. 2. An individual with little resistance to an infectious disease or who is not known to have become immune to one. 3. Easily impressed or influenced.

suscitate (sŭs'sĭ-tāt) [L. *suscitāre*, to rouse]. To arouse to increased activity; to stimulate.

suscitation (sŭs"sĭ-tā'shŭn) [L. *suscitatio*, from *suscitāre*, to rouse]. Act of stimulating to greater activity. Syn: *excitation.*

suspended (sŭs-pĕnd'ĕd) [L. *suspendere*, to hang]. 1. Hanging. 2. Temporarily inactive.

s. animation. A cessation of the vital functions temporarily.

suspension (sŭs-pĕn'shŭn) [L. *suspensio*, a hanging]. 1. A condition of temporary cessation, as of any vital process. 2. Treatment by immobilization of a part or whole of a patient by hanging in desired position. 3. State of a solid when its particles are mixed with, but not dissolved in, a fluid or another solid; also a substance in this state.

s., cephalic. Supported suspension of a patient by the head to extend the vertebral column.

s., colloidal. A colloidal solution in which particles of the dispersed phase are relatively large.

s. stability. Degree of speed with which erythrocytes sink to bottom in a mass of citrated blood. Syn: *sedimentation rate.*

s., tendon. Tenodesis; fixation of a tendon.

s. of the uterus. The operation of attaching the uterus to the abdominal wall.

suspensoid (sŭs-pĕn'soyd) [L. *suspens*, hanging, + G. *eidos*, form]. A colloid solution in which the dispersed particles are solid, as distinguished from *emulsoid.* Syn: *suspension, colloidal.*

suspensory (sŭs-pĕn′sōr-ĭ) [L. *suspensorius*, hanging]. 1. Supporting a part, as a muscle, ligament, or bone. 2. A structure of the body which supports a part. 3. Bandage or sac for supporting or compressing a part, esp. the scrotum.

s. bandage. A sling for support of the testicles.

s. ligament. Any one of a number of ligaments which support a specific organ or structure. SEE: *ligament, suspensory.*

suspiration (sŭs″pĭr-ā′shŭn). A sigh or the act of sighing.

suspirious (sŭs-pī′rĭ-ŭs) [L. *suspirāre*, to sigh]. Breathing with apparent effort; sighing.

sustentacular (sŭs-tĕn-tăk′ū-lar) [L. *sustentaculum*, support]. Supporting; upholding.

s. cell. A supporting cell such as those found in the acoustic macula, organ of Corti, olfactory epithelium, taste buds, or testes. SEE: *Sertoli cells.*

s. fibers (of Muller). Fibers forming the supporting framework of the retina.

sustentaculum (sŭs-tĕn-tăk′ū-lŭm) [L. a support]. A supporting structure.

s. hepatis. A fold of peritoneum upon which rests the right margin of the liver.

s. lieni. Phrenocolic ligament which apparently supports the spleen.

s. tali. A process of the calcaneum which supports part of the astragalus.

susurrus (sū-sŭr′ŭs) [L. a whisper]. A murmur.

sutura (sū-tū′rā) (pl. *suturae*) [L. *sutura*, a stitch]. Suture.

s. denta′ta. One with interlocking of bony processes resembling the teeth of a saw.

s. harmo′nia. Simple apposition of 2 contiguous bones.

s. limbosa. Beveled suture in which opposing margins fit in parallel ridges as between parietal and frontal bones.

s. no′tha. A false suture with ill-defined projections.

s. serra′ta. One with deeper and more irregular indentations than a dental s.

s. squamosa. That formed by overlapping of contiguous bones by broad beveled edges as in suture between squamous portion of temporal and parietal bones.

s. vera. A true suture.

sutural (sū′tū-răl) [L. *sutura*, a stitch]. Relating to a suture.

s. joint. Articulation bet. 2 bones.

s. ligament. Fibers uniting opposed bones forming a cranial suture.

suturation (sū″tū-rā′shŭn) [L. *sutura*, a stitch]. Application of sutures; stitching.

suture (sū′tūr) [L. *sutura*, a stitch]. 1. Line of union in an immovable articulation, as those bet. the skull bones; also such an articulation itself. SYN: *synarthrosis.* 2. Operation of uniting parts by stitching them together. 3. The thread or wire or other material used in the operation of stitching parts of the body together. 4. The seam or line of union formed by surgical stitches. 5. To unite by stitching, as *to suture a wound.* SEE: *raphe.*

s., absorbable. S. which is gradually removed by body tissues and cells. Suture material made of gut tissue is the best example.

s., basilar. The one bet. the occipital bone and sphenoid bone.

s., bifrontal. SEE: *coronal s.*

s., biparietal. SEE: *sagittal s.*

s′s., buried. Those completely covered by skin and not involving that structure at all.

s., button. One in which the threads are passed through buttons on the surface and tied to prevent the thread from cutting into the skin.

s., catgut. Material used in suturing, made from a portion of the small intestine of sheep. It may be sterilized. Once inserted it is eventually absorbed.

s., coaptation. One uniting as distinguished from one intended to relieve tension.

s., cobbler's. A s. in which the thread has a needle at each end.

s., continuous. The closure of a wound by means of 1 continuous thread, usually by transfixing first 1 lip and then the other, alternately, from within outward.

s., coronal. The junction of the frontal and parietal bones.

s′s., cranial. Those s′s. bet. the bones of the skull.

s., dentate. An articulation of long and toothlike processes.

s., ethmoidofrontal. The one bet. the ethmoid and frontal bones.

s., ethmoidolacrimal. The one bet. the ethmoid and lacrimal bones.

s., ethmosphenoid. The one bet. the ethmoid and sphenoid bones.

s., false. Any form of suture in which one surface is smooth.

s., figure-of-eight. S. which has configuration of the figure 8.

s., frontal. An occasional one in the frontal bone from the sagittal s. to root of nose.

s., frontolacrimal. The one bet. the frontal and lacrimal bones.

s., frontomalar. The one bet. the frontal and malar bones

s., frontomaxillary. The one bet. the frontal bone and sup. maxilla.

s., frontonasal. The one bet. the frontal bone and the alae of the sphenoid bone.

s., frontoparietal. The coronal suture.

s., frontotemporal. The one bet. the frontal and temporal bones.

s., Glover's. A continuous s. in which the needle is, after each stitch, passed through the loop of the preceding stitch.

s., harmonic. One in which there is simple apposition of bone.

s., horsehair. S. adapted for light, superficial sutures, alternated with heavier ones and for exposed places like the face, where scar tissue is to be avoided.

s., implanted. A s. formed by placing pins opposite each other on the 2 sides of a wound, and approximating the lips by winding thread or other similar material about the pins.

s., intermaxillary. The s. bet. the sup maxillae.

s., internasal. The one bet. the nasal bones.

s., interparietal. SEE: *sagittal s.*

s., interrupted. A s. formed by single stitches inserted separately, the needle being usually passed through 1 lip from without inward, and through the other from within outward.

s., jugal. SEE: *sagittal s.*

s., lambdoid. The one bet. the parietal bones and the 2 sup. borders of the occipital bone.

s., longitudinal. SEE: *sagittal s.*

s., mattress. A continuous s. in which a stitch is taken with a needle, the thread tied, and then needle inserted upon the same side as that from which it emerged and passed in opposite direction through both lips of the wound, the direction of the needle being reversed at each stitch.

s., *maxillolacrimal.* The one bet. the maxilla and lacrimal bone.

s., *mediofrontal.* SEE: *frontal s.*

s., *metopic.* SEE: *frontal s.*

s., *nasomaxillary.* The one bet. the nasal bone and sup. maxilla.

s., *nonabsorbable.* Silk, silkworm gut, horsehair and wire.

s., *occipital.* SEE: *lambdoid s.*

s., *occipitomastoid.* The one bet. the occipital bone and mastoid portion of temporal bone.

s., *occipitoparietal.* SEE: *lambdoid s.*

s., *palatine.* One bet. the palate bones.

s., *palatine transverse.* One bet. the palate processes and sup. maxilla.

s., *parietal.* SEE: *sagittal s.*

s., *parietomastoid.* The one bet. parietal bone and mastoid portion of the temporal bone.

s., *petrooccipital.* The one bet. the petrous portion of the temporal bone and occipital bone.

s., *petrosphenoidal.* The one bet. petrous portion of the temporal bone and ala magna of sphenoid bone.

s., *purse-string.* One going in and out around a circular opening, closing when the 2 are drawn taut.

s., *quilled, s., quill.* An interrupted s. in which a double thread is passed deep into the tissues, even quite below the bottom of the wound, needle being so withdrawn as to leave a loop hanging from 1 lip and the 2 free ends of the thread from the other. A quill, or, more commonly, a piece of bougie, is passed through the loops, which are tightened upon it, and the free ends of each separate thread are tied together over a second quill to bring the deep parts into firm coaptation and to relieve tension.

s., *relaxation.* A s. that may be loosened to relieve excessive tension.

s., *relief.* A row of supplementary s's. including the tissues to the extent of 1 or 1½ in. on each side of a fistula or a deep wound, for the purpose of lessening the strain on the coaptation s's.

s., *right-angled.* A s. used in sewing intestine. The needle is passed in the same direction as the long axis of the incision and the process repeated on the opposite side of the incision, the suture being continuous.

s., *sagittal.* Suture between the two parietal bones.

s., *serrated.* An articulation by s. in which there is an interlocking of bones by small, fine and delicate projections and indentations.

s., *shotted.* A s. in which both ends of a wire or silkworm gut are passed through a perforated shot that is then compressed tightly over them.

s., *silk.* Does not produce suppuration if sterilized. Twisted, braided and floss.

s., *silkworm gut.* Causes little friction, pliable, does not curl or twist, less liable to produce irritation.

s., *sphenoparietal.* The one bet. the parietal bone and ala magna of the sphenoid bone.

s., *sphenosquamous.* Articulation of the great wing of the sphenoid with squamous portion of the temporal bone.

s., *sphenotemporal.* The one bet. the sphenoid and temporal bones.

s., *squamoparietal, s., squamosal.* The one bet. the parietal and squamous portion of the temporal bone.

s., *squamosphenoidal.* One bet. the squamous portion of the temporal bone and great wing of sphenoid.

s., *subcuticular.* A buried continuous s. in which the needle is passed horizontally under the epidermis into the cutis vera, emerging at the edge of the wound but beneath the skin, then in a similar manner passed through cutis vera of opposite side of the wound, and so on until the other angle of the wound is reached.

s., *temporooccipital.* SEE: *occipitomastoid s.*

s., *temporoparietal.* One bet. the temporal and parietal bones.

s., *twisted.* A s. in which pins are passed through the opposite lips of a wound, at right angles to direction of wound, and material is wound about the pins, crossing them first at one end and then at the other in a figure-of-eight fashion, thus holding the lips of the wound firmly together.

s., *uninterrupted.* SEE: *continuous s.*

s., *wire.* Usually silver. Adapted for cases where there is much tension, ends of bones, resection, etc.

swab (swŏb) [Dutch *zwabber,* to wipe]. 1. Cotton or gauze on end of slender stick used for cleansing cavities, applying remedies or for obtaining a piece of tissue or secretion for bacteriological examination. 2. To wipe with a swab, as to *swab a wound.*

s., *test tube.* For cleansing tubes, etc.

s., *urethral.* Slender rod for holding cotton, used in examinations with speculum, in treating ulcers, removing secretions, etc.

s., *u., male.* About 7 in. long.

s., *uterine.* For absorbing or wiping away discharges. Slender, flattened wire, plain rod or one with coarse thread on distal end.

swallow (swŏl'ō) [A.S. *swelgan,* to swallow]. To pass into the stomach through the mouth and throat.

swallowing (swŏl'ō-ĭng) [A.S. *swelgan,* to swallow]. SYN: *deglutition.* A complicated act usually initiated voluntarily but always completely reflexly whereby food is moved from the mouth through the pharynx and esophagus to the stomach. It occurs in three stages as follows. In the *first stage,* food is placed on surface of tongue. Tip of tongue is placed against hard palate, then elevation of larynx and backward movement of tongue forces food through isthmus of fauces into pharynx. In the *second stage,* the food passes through the pharynx. This involves constriction of the walls of the pharynx, backward bending of the epiglottis, and an upward and forward movement of the larynx and trachea. This may be observed from the outside by watching the bobbing of the Adam's apple. Food is kept from entering nasal cavity by elevation of soft palate and from entering larynx by closure of the glottis and backward inclination of epiglottis. During this stage, respiratory movements are reflexly inhibited. In the *third stage,* food moves down the esophagus and into the stomach. This movement is accomplished by the momentum given the food during the second stage, and peristaltic contractions aided by gravity. These forces are sufficient to allow liquids to be drunk even when the head is lower than the stomach. Liquids pass rapidly and do not require assistance from the esophagus.

Difficulty in swallowing is called *dysphagia, q.v.* It may be caused by congenital defects such as cleft palate or esophageal obstruction, neuro- and psychogenic disturbances, muscular dysfunction or local conditions such as presence of tumors, abscesses, inflammation, etc.

RS: *acataposis, acnalasia, aglutition, air s., aphagia, choking, deglutition, dysphagia.*

s., air. Syn: *aerophagia.*

s. reflex. Swallowing induced by stimulation of soft palate.

s., tongue. Condition in which the tongue has a tendency to fall backward obstructing openings to larynx and esophagus. The tongue is not actually swallowed, thus the term is inaccurate. Nevertheless it is commonly used. It is due to excessive flaccidity of tongue during unconsciousness. This requires forceful elevation of the chin and extension of the head during artificial respiration in order to help provide an airway.

swallow's nest (swŏl'ōz). Cerebral depression bet. the uvula and the post. velum. Syn: *nidus hirundinis.*

sweat (swĕt) [A.S. *swāt*, sweat]. 1. The secretion of the sudoriparous glands of the skin. Syn: *perspiration, sudor.* See: *glands, Moll's.* 2. Condition of perspiring or of being made to perspire freely, as to order a sweat for a patient. 3. To emit moisture through the skin's pores. Syn: *perspire.* 4. To cause to emit moisture through the pores.

The perspiration is a colorless, slightly turbid, salty, aqueous fluid, although that from the sweat glands in the axillae, and around the anus, and that of the ceruminous glands have an oily consistency. It contains urea, fatty substances and sodium chloride. This salty, watery fluid is difficult to collect without contamination with sebum.*

Function: To cool the body by evaporation, and to rid it of what waste may be expressed through the pores of the skin. The amount per day is about a liter; this figure is subject to extreme variation according to muscular activity and atmospheric conditions and in extreme conditions may be as much as 10 to 15 liters per 24 hours.

Phys: Perspiration is controlled by the sympathetic nervous system through true secretory fibers supplying the sweat glands.

s., bloody. S. tinged with blood. Syn: *hematidrosis.*

s. centers. Principal centers are located in the hypothalamus; secondary centers are present in the spinal cord.

s., colliquative. Profuse sweat of a clammy nature.

s., colored. S. tinged with a pigment. Syn: *chromidrosis.*

s., fetid. S. with foul odor. Syn: *bromidrosis.*

s. glands. Simple, coiled, tubular glands found on all body surfaces except margin of lips, glans penis and inner surface of prepuce. The coiled secreting portion lies in the corium or subcutaneous portion of skin; the excretory duct follows a straight or oblique course through the dermis but becomes spiral in passing through epidermis to its opening, a *sweat pore.* Most sweat glands are merocrine; those of the axilla, areola or mammary gland, labia majora and circumanal region are *apocrine.*

They are most numerous on the palms of the hands and soles of the feet, averaging about 2800 to the sq. in. or over 2,000,000 to the body.

s., night. Sweating during the night; may be a symptom of pulmonary tuberculosis.

s., profuse. Excessive perspiration. Syn: *hyperhidrosis.*

s., scanty. Abnormally small amount or lack of sweat. Syn: *anhidrosis.*

sweat, words pert. to: anaphoresis, antisudoral, antisudorin, bromidrosis, chromidrosis, chylidrosis, diaphoresis, diaphoretic, dyshidria, dysidrosis, ephidrosis, hematidrosis, hidradenitis, hidrorrhea, hidrosis, hydradenitis, hydradenoma, hyphidrosis, hyperidrosis, hypoidrosis, ischidrosis, melanidrosis, perspiration, phosphorhidrosis, sudor, sudorific, sudoriparous, uridrosis.

sweating (swĕt'ĭng) [A.S. *swāt*, sweat]. 1. Act of exuding sweat. 2. Emitting sweat. 3. Causing profuse sweating.

To induce, paint 2 in. square of skin under each axilla with mixture of equal parts of olive oil and guaiacol solution. Cover with several layers of gauze, then flannel, and hold with adhesive tape. Wrap patient in warm blankets.

s., deficiency of. Syn: *anhidrosis.* Seen in profuse diarrhea, polyuria, vomiting, hemorrhage, diabetes insipidus, myxedema, general anasarca, ichthyosis and in high temperature.

s., excessive. Syn: *hyperhidrosis.* Seen in rheumatic, malarial and relapsing fever, septic fevers, pneumonia at crisis, pulmonary tuberculosis, Graves' disease, migraine, neuralgia. Local of hands and feet in hysteria, neurasthenia, vagotonia, nervous irritability, exophthalmic goiter, fright and other emotions.

s. sickness. Miliary fever, *q.v.*

s., urinous. Syn: *uridrosis.* Often found in uremia.

RS: *anhidrosis, bromidrosis, chromidrosis, hidrosis, perspiration, pores, skin, sudor, sudorific, sweat, uridrosis.*

Swedish gymnastics, movements. System of active and passive exercise of the various muscles and joints of the body without using apparatus.

Types: *Active*: Taken by the patient with the assistance or resistance of the operator. *Duplicated active*: Performed by the patient with the operator's assistance. *General active*: Performed by the patient exclusively. *Passive*: All given to the patient by the operator. *General passive*: May be performed while the patient is dressed.

The Principal Movements: 1. *Bending.* 2. *Depression* and *elevation.* 3. *Flexion* and *extension.* 4. *Pressing* and *shaking.* In pressing, the operator uses the tips of his fingers in vertical motion over the principal nerves. In shaking the arm, the operator grasps the hand and shoulder, keeping the arm in an extended position, and shakes as quickly as possible. In shaking the leg, he grasps the foot with one hand and the thigh as high as possible with the other and shakes quickly. These movements are always passive and are principally used in nervous affections. 5. *Pulling.* 6. *Raising.* 7. *Rotation.* This is a rotary movement by which the different joints are brought into motion within their natural limits. Rotation is to lengthen and shorten the veins so as to produce a sucking of their contents, thus stimulating the circulation and assisting the heart in its action. 8. *Separating* and *closing*. 9. *Turning*.

POSITIONS: The movements may be performed in 5 different positions. Kneeling, lying, sitting, standing, or suspending. These are called ground positions and have many subdivisions. There are 47 derivative positions—about 800 movements in all.

S. massage. Massage combined with S. gymnastics.

sweet (swēt) [A.S. *swēte*, sweet]. 1. Pleasing to the taste or smell. SEE: *taste*. 2. Free from excess of acid, sulfur, or corrosive salts.

sweetbread (swēt'brĕd) [origin uncertain]. The thymus and pancreas glands, esp. of the calf, used as food.

COMP: Nuclein and purines are high.

AV. SERVING OF COOKED BRAISED CALF SWEETBREADS: 100 gm. Calories: 168. Other values: 3.2 gm. protein; 3.2 gm. fat.

swelling (swĕl'ĭng) [A.S. *swellan*, to grow larger]. A morbid enlargement, esp. one appearing on the surface of the body.

TREATMENT: *Local*: Ice water with salt in it applied to area reduces swelling rapidly.

RS: *anthorism, detumescence, node, nodule, turgescence, turgid.*

s., albuminous. Same as cloudy s.

s., Calabar. Swellings occurring in infestations by the nematode, *Loa loa*. They are temporary and painless and thought to be the result of temporary sensitization.

s., cloudy. Degeneration of tissues marked by cloudy appearance, swelling, and appearance of tiny albuminoid granules in the cells as observed with the microscope.

s., fugitive. Temporary swellings such as those occurring in infestations of *Loa loa* which appear at one place, persist for two or three days, then disappear possibly to recur at another position.

s., glassy. SYN: *amyloid degeneration, pink disease, erythredema, polyneuropathy*. That occurring in amyloid degeneration of tissues.

s., white. Swelling seen in tuberculous arthritis, esp. of the knee.

Swift's disease (swĭft). Condition occurring in very young children characterized by irritability and restlessness; redness and swelling of the hands and feet, esp. on the palms and soles; desquamation; a sensation of tingling or burning; loss of appetite, and the appearance of a rash, mainly on the trunk, and loss of muscle tone. SYN: *acrodynia*.

Swiss chard. AV. SERVING COOKED: Calories: 18. Other values: 5.9 gm. protein; 0.2 gm. fat; 3.3 mg. carbohydrate; 5400 I.U. vitamin A; 16 mg. vitamin C.

switch, foot. In the application of surgical, high-frequency currents where both hands of the operator are needed, the current is started and cut off by a foot switch.

s., pole-changing. P.T. A switch by which the polarity of a circuit may be reversed.

swoon (swōōn) [M.E. *swounen*, from A.S. *geswōgen*, in a swoon]. 1. A syncope* or fainting fit. 2. To sink into a fainting fit.

sycoma (sī-kō'mă) [G. *sykon*, fig, + *-ōma*, tumor]. A large, soft wart. SYN: *condyloma*.

sycophancy (sĭk'ō-făn-sĭ) [G. *sykophantēs*, a false adviser]. PSY: Characteristics of one maturely intelligent who has not developed a sense of responsibility and who is more or less dependent upon others.

sycophant (sĭk'ō-fănt) [G. *sykophantēs*, a false adviser]. One who seeks to incur favor by flattery and praise.

sycosiform (sī-kō'sĭ-form) [G. *sykōsis*, figlike disease, + L. *forma*, shape]. Resembling sycosis.

sycosis (sī-kō'sĭs) [G. *sykōsis*, figlike disease]. Chronic inflammation of hair follicles.

ETIOL: *Staphylococcus aureus* and *albus* entering through hair follicles, trauma, debility, etc., as predisposing factors.

SYM: As stated, on hairy regions, and, if severe, may result in alopecia and scarring, characterized by an aggregation of papules and pustules, each of which is pierced by a hair. Pustules show no disposition to rupture but dry to yellow brown crusts; more or less itching and burning. If disease persists may lead to extreme destruction of hair follicles and permanent alopecia.

PROG: Disease is curable under prolonged treatment; relapses prone to occur.

TREATMENT: Local treatment includes topical use of antibiotics. Organism should be cultured and tested to determine agent of choice. Generally systemic treatment is also called for with special attention given to diet, possible foci of infection, allergens, etc. X-ray treatment is sometimes effective. Systemic antibiotics and adrenal cortical hormones may be required.

s. barbae. Sycosis of the beard, marked by papules and pustules perforated by hairs, and surrounded by infiltrated skin. SYN: *folliculitis barbae*.

s., hypogenic. *Tinea barbae, q.v.*; barber's itch, usually due to species of *Trichophyton*.

s. tinea. A form due to infection with ringworm commonly affecting the beard.

s. vulgaris. SYN: *folliculitis barbae, barber's itch*. SEE: *sycosis*.

Sydenham's chorea (sĭd'ĕn-hăm). Simple chorea with irregular involuntary movements of the face and extremities.

S's. cough. C. produced in hysteria by spasm of the respiratory muscles.

syllabic utterance (sĭl-ab'ĭk) [G. *syllabē*, a syllable]. A staccato accentuation of syllables, slowly but separately, observed in multiple sclerosis. SYN: *scanning speech*.

syllable stumbling (sĭl'ă-bl) [G. *syllabē*, a syllable]. Hesitating utterance (dysphasia) with difficulty in pronouncing certain syllables.

syllabus (sĭl'ă-bŭs) [G. *syllabos*, a collection]. Abstract of a lecture or outline of a course of study or of a book.

syllepsiology (sĭl-lĕp-sĭ-ol'ō-jĭ) [G. *syllēpsis*, conception, + *logos*, study]. The study of conception and pregnancy.

syllepsis (sĭl-ĕp'sĭs) [G. *syllēpsis*, conception]. Conception; impregnation, or pregnancy.

sylvat'ic plague. Bubonic plague which is enzootic among wild rodents, esp. in western U. S. The causative organism is transmitted by fleas.

Sylvester's method. Method of artificial respiration by drawing arms of a supine patient out above head, and then bringing them down folded onto the chest.

with pressure on the abdomen and ribs to cause expiration.

This and other methods of artificial respiration should *not* be used for the resuscitation of babies born with asphyxia neonatorum. SEE: *artificial* respiration.*

sylvian aqueduct (sĭl′vĭ-ăn). A narrow canal from 3rd to 4th ventricle. SYN: *aqueduct of Sylvius.*

s. artery. Middle cerebral artery in the fissure of Sylvius.

s. fissure. The fissure separating the temporal lobe from the frontal and parietal lobes.

s. line. One on ext. of cranium marking direction of the sylvian fissure.

sym-, syn- [G.]. Combining form meaning *with, along, together with, beside.*

symbion, symbiont (sĭm′bĭ-ŏn, -ŏnt) [G. *syn,* together, + *bios,* life]. SYN: *commensal.* An organism which lives with another in a state of symbiosis.

symbiosis (sĭm-bĭ-ō′sĭs) [G. *symbiōsis,* a living together]. The living together in close association of two organisms of different species. If neither organism is harmed, such is referred to as *commensalism;* if the association is beneficial to both, it is *mutualism;* if one is harmed and the other benefited, it constitutes *parasitism.*

symblepharon (sĭm-blĕf′ă-rŏn) [G. *syn,* together, + *blepharon,* eyelid]. Adhesion bet. conjunctivae of lid and eyeball due to injuries, esp. burns from lime, acids, etc.

Also seen in trachoma, pemphigus, and following operations.

SYM: Interference with movement of eyeball, conjunctival irritation.

TREATMENT: Division of cicatricial bands and keeping raw surfaces separated. Mucous membrane grafts.

symbol (sĭm′bŏl) [G. *symbolon,* a sign]. 1. A representation of an idea or quality in the form of an object or that which stands for something beside itself.

2. PSY: An object used as an unconscious substitute and which is not connected consciously with the libido, but into which the libido is concentrated.

3. CHEM: A mark or letter representing an atom of an element.

s., phallic. An object which bears some resemblance to the penis.

SEE: *Table of Symbols in App.* Also see symbols of weights and measures used in prescription writing.

SEE: *Table of Physical Constants of Elements in App.* and for the symbols of chemical elements.

symbo′lia. Ability to identify or recognize an object by the sense of touch.

symbolism (sĭm′bŏl-ĭzm) [" + *-ismos,* condition]. PSY: 1. Unconscious substitutive expression of subconscious thoughts of sexual significance in terms recognized by the objective consciousness.

2. An abnormal condition in which everything that occurs is interpreted as a symbol of the patient's own thoughts.

symboliza′tion. An unconscious process by which, on the basis of similarity or association, an object or idea comes to represent or stand for, *i.e.,* symbolize, another object or idea.

symbolophobia (sĭm-bō-lō-fō′bĭ-ă) [" + *phobos,* fear]. Fear of expressing one's self in words or action that may be interpreted as possessing a symbolic meaning.

Syme's operation (sĭm). 1. Amputation of the foot at the ankle joint with removal of the malleoli. 2. Excision of the tongue. 3. External urethrotomy.

symmel′ia. Fusion of limbs.

symmetric, symmetrical (sĭm-ĕt′rĭk, -rĭ-kl) [G. *symmetrikos,* measuring with]. 1. Exhibiting correspondence in size and shape of parts. 2. CHEM: Denoting an atomic arrangement in a molecule at equal relative intervals.

s. gangrene. Gangrene affecting corresponding parts simultaneously and similarly. SYN: *Raynaud's disease, q.v.*

symmetromania (sĭm″ĕ-trō-mā′nĭ-ă) [G. *symmetria,* from *syn,* with, + *metron,* a measure]. An abnormal impulse to make symmetrical motions with the arms.

symmetry (sĭm′ĕt-rĭ) [G. *symmetria,* from *syn,* with, + *metron,* a measure]. Correspondence in shape, size, and relative position of parts on opposite sides of a body.

s., bilateral. That symmetry of an organism (a) whose right and left halves are mirror images of each other, or (b) in which a median longitudinal section divides the organism into equivalent right and left halves.

s., radial. That of an organism whose parts radiate from a central axis.

sympathectomy (sĭm-pă-thĕk′tō-mĭ) [G. *sympathētikos,* suffering with, + *ektomē,* excision]. Excision of a portion of the sympathetic division of the autonomic nervous system. It may include a nerve, plexus, ganglion, or a series of ganglia of the sympathetic trunk.

s., chemical. The use of chemicals to destroy or temporarily inactivate part of the sympathetic nerve.

s., periarterial. Removal of sheath of an artery in which are the sympathetic nerve fibers, used in trophic disturbances.

sympatheoneuritis (sĭm-păth″ē-ō-nū-rī′tĭs) [" + *neuron,* nerve, + *-itis,* inflammation]. Inflammation of the sympathetic nerve.

sympathetic (sĭm-pă-thĕt′ĭk) [G. *syn,* with, + *pathos,* suffering]. 1. Pert. to sympathetic nervous system, *q.v.* 2. Caused by or pert. to sympathy.

s. irritation. I. of a structure caused by irritation of another related structure.

s. nervous system. A division of the autonomic nervous system.

RS: *nervous system, parasympathetic nervous system, systema.*

s. ophthalmia. Inflammation of the uveal tract in one eye due to similar inflammation in the other eye.

s. plexuses. Plexuses formed at intervals by the sympathetic nerves and ganglia.

sympatheticalgia (sĭm-pă-thĕt-ĭ-kal′jĭ-ă) [G. *sympathētikos,* suffering with, + *algos,* pain]. Pain in the cervical sympathetic ganglion.

sympatheticless (sĭm-pă-thĕt′ĭk-lĕs) [" + A.S. *lēas,* without]. Noting absence of the abdominal sympathetic chain.

sympatheticoparalytic (sĭm-pă-thĕt″ĭk-ō-par-ăl-ĭt′ĭk) [" + *paralysis,* a loosening at the sides]. Resulting from paralysis of the sympathetic nervous system.

sympatheticopathy (sĭm-pă-thĕt-ĭ-kŏp′ă-thĭ) [" + *pathos,* disease]. Any condition resulting from disorder of the sympathetic nervous system.

sympatheticotonia (sĭm-pă-thĕt″ĭk-ō-tō′nĭ-ă) [" + *tonos,* tone]. Condition characterized by excessive tone of the sympathetic nervous system with unusually high blood pressure and tendency to vascular spasm. SYN: *sympathicotonia.*

sympatheticotonic (sĭm-păth-ĕt″ĭk-ō-ton′-ĭk) [" + *tonos,* tension]. Marked by increased arterial tone or vasoconstriction due to overaction of the sympathetic nervous system.

sympatheticotripsy (sĭm-pă-thĕt″ĭk-ō-trĭp′sĭ) [" + *tripsis,* a crushing]. Surgical crushing of the sup. cervical ganglion in treatment of mental diseases.

sympathicectomy (sĭm-păth-ĭs-ĕk′tō-mĭ) [G. *sympathētikos,* suffering with, + *ektomē,* excision]. Excision of part of the sympathetic nerve. SYN: *sympathectomy.*

sympathicoblast (sĭm-păth′ĭ-kō-blăst) [" + *blastos,* a germ]. A primitive sympathetic nerve cell. SEE: *sympathoblast.*

sympathicoblastoma (sĭm-păth″ĭk-ō-blăs-tō′mă) [" + " + *-ōma,* tumor]. A tumor made up of sympathicoblasts.

sympathicolytic. Interfering with, opposing, inhibiting or destroying impulses from the sympathetic nervous system. SYN: *sympathelytic.*

sympathicomimetic (sĭm-păth″ĭk-ō-mĭm-ĕt′ĭk) [G. *sympathētikos,* suffering with, + *mimētikos,* imitating]. Producing effects resembling those resulting from stimulation of the sympathetic nervous system, such as effects following the injection of epinephrine.

sympathiconeuritis (sĭm-păth″ĭk-ō-nū-rī′-tĭs) [" + *neuron,* nerve, + *-itis,* inflammation]. Inflammation of the sympathetic nerves.

sympathicotonia (sĭm-păth″ĭ-kō-tō′nĭ-ă) [" + *tonos,* tone]. Increased tonus of the sympathetic system with marked tendency to vascular spasm and heightened blood pressure. OPP: *vagotonia.**

sympathicotripsy (sĭm-păth″ĭk-ō-trĭp′sĭ) [" + *tripsis,* a crushing]. Crushing of the sup. cervical ganglion in treatment of mental diseases. SYN: *sympatheticotripsy.*

sympathicotropic (sĭm-păth″ĭ-kō-trop′ĭk) [" + *tropos,* a turning]. Having a special affinity for the sympathetic nerve.

sympathicus (sĭm-păth′ĭ-kŭs) [G. *sympathētikos,* suffering with]. The sympathetic nervous system. SYN: *systema nervorum sympathicum.*

sympathin (sĭm′păth-ĭn) [G. *syn,* with, + *pathos,* suffering]. A term formerly used to denote a postganglionic sympathetic excitor substance, *Sympathin E* and an inhibitor substance at the same site, *Sympathin I.* These supposedly pure substances have never been discovered. SEE: *epinephrine, norepinephrine.*

sympathism (sĭm′păth-ĭzm) [" + " + *-ismos,* condition]. Condition of susceptibility to suggestion. SYN: *suggestibility.*

sympathoblast (sĭm-păth′ō-blăst) [" + " + *blastos,* germ]. A primitive cell from which arises a sympathetic ganglion cell.

sympathoblastoma (sĭm″păth-ō-blăs-tō′-mă) [" + " + " + *-ōma,* tumor]. A malignant tumor made up of sympathetic nerve cells.

sympathoglioblastoma (sĭm″păth-ō-glī″ō-blăs-tō′mă) [" + " + *glia,* glue, + *blastos,* germ, + *-ōma,* tumor]. A tumor made up primarily of sympathoblasts, with scattered neuroblasts and spongioblasts.

sympathogonia (sĭm″păth-ō-gō′nĭ-ă) [" + " + *gonē,* seed]. Primitive cells from which sympathetic cells are derived.

sympathogonioma (sĭm″păth-ō-gō-nĭ-ō′-mă) [" + " + " + *-ōma,* tumor]. A tumor containing sympathogonia.

sympathoma (sĭm-păth-ō′mă) [G. *syn,* with, + *pathos,* suffering, + *-ōma,* tumor]. A tumor composed of tissue similar to that of the sympathetic nervous system.

sympathomimetic (sĭm″păth-ō-mĭm-ĕt′ĭk) [" + " + *mimētikos,* imitating]. SYN: *sympathicomimetic, q.v.*

sympathy (sĭm′pă-thĭ) [G. *sympatheia,* from *syn,* with, + *pathos,* suffering]. 1. Relationship bet. 2 organs or parts through which 1 unaffected part is affected or becomes disordered from disease in the other part without actual transmission of morbific cause. 2. In Psychol., an affective reaction to, and like that of, another person. It may be *imitative sympathy* in which the reaction is like that of another person as perceived or thought (for example, weeping because another person is weeping), or *reflective sympathy* in which the reaction is like that of another person as his situation is understood. 3. Feeling as another feels. SEE: *empathy.*

sympexion (sĭm-pĕks′ĭ-on) [G. *sympēxis,* concretion]. A concretion in certain sites such as the prostate or seminal vesicles.

sympexis (sĭm-pĕks′ĭs) [G. *sympēxis,* concretion]. Term for arrangement of red blood cells due to the effect of surface tension.

symphalangism (sĭm-făl′ăn-jĭzm) [G. *syn,* together, + *phalagx, phalagg-,* phalanx]. 1. Ankylosis of joints of the fingers or toes. 2. Web-fingered or web-toed condition.

symphyseal (sĭm-fĭz′ē-ăl) [G. *symphysis,* a growth together]. Pert. to symphysis.

symphyseotomy (sĭm-fĭz-ē-ŏt′ō-mĭ) [" + *tomē,* incision]. Section of symphysis pubis to enlarge the pelvic diameters during delivery.

symphysiectomy (sĭm-fĭz-ĭ-ĕk′tō-mĭ) [" + *ektomē,* excision]. Section of the symphysis pubis to facilitate delivery.

symphysion (sĭm-fĭz′ĭ-ŏn) [G. *symphysis,* a growth together]. Most ant. point of the alveolar process of the lower jaw.

symphysiotomy (sĭm″fĭz-ĭ-ŏt′ō-mĭ) [" + *tomē,* a cutting]. Section of the symphysis pubis to facilitate delivery by enlarging the pelvic diameters.

symphysis (sĭm′fĭs-ĭs) (pl. *symphyses*) [G. *symphysis,* a growth together]. 1. A line of fusion between two bones which are separate in early development, as *s. of mandible.* 2. A form of synchondrosis in which the bones are separated by a disk of fibrocartilage, as in joints between bodies of vertebrae or between pubic bones. SEE: *intervertebral disk.*

s. *cartilaginosum.* A synchondrosis.

s. *of jaw.* An ant., median, vertical ridge upon outer surface of lower jaw representing line of union of its 2 halves.

s. *ligamentosa.* A syndesmosis.

s. *mandibulae.* S. menti, *q.v.*

s. *menti.* SYN: *symphysis mandibulae.* The symphysis of the chin or the ridge marking line of union of the two halves of the mandible.

s. *pubis.* The junction of the pubic bones on midline in front; bony eminence under the pubic hair. SEE: *disk, interpubic.*

sympodia (sĭm-pō′dĭ-ă) [G. *syn,* together, + *pous, pod-,* foot]. Condition in which lower extremities are united.

symptom (sĭmp′tŭm) [G. *symptōma,* anything that has befallen one]. Any perceptible change in the body or its functions which indicates disease or the kind or phases of disease.

They may be classified as *objective, subjective, cardinal,* and sometimes as *constitutional*. Another classification considers all symptoms as being subjective, the objective indications being called signs.*

Some of the symptoms affecting different parts are the following:

Abdomen*: May be distended, rigid, flat, flabby, adipose, tympanitic, shiny, enlarged, or bulging in certain areas, and certain discolorations, stripings, or markings. Muscles may be tensed and little affected by pressure. May be cold areas, and various sounds may be heard, such as splashings, roarings, and rumblings (*borborygmus,* also known as *intestinal flatus*). Closely associated with abdominal symptoms is pain. Locate exact area affected, and note nature, time of duration, time when it arises, and any causes that might be responsible.

Emesis is another condition associated with symptoms pert. to the abdominal region. This may be watery, clear, or containing mucus or undigested food; may be stertorous, bilious, frothy, profuse, purulent, colored from food or medication, and showing blood in small amounts (hematemesis). If blood is present in large quantity and has been acted on by gastric juices it may resemble coffee grounds. It may be sour, or have odor of feces, or garlic, or may be ammoniacal or have odor characteristic of some food or drug. The genital crease may show edema, lesions, discolorations, discharge, malformations, inflammations, infection, or growths.

The patient may complain of abdominal distention, gas, and pain caused by gas, crowding in the region of the heart, and interference with respiration. Heartburn may be present, or gastritis, and regurgitation. Pain may be felt when food enters the stomach, or relieved by eating or shortly after eating or by changing body position. Distention after eating should be noted, or desire to eructate or to expel flatus from the stomach. Colicky pains in the abdomen may be accompanied by pain in the shoulder. Pain at pit of stomach and in lower right quadrant may be indicative of appendicitis. When over lower right ribs or little below, the gallbladder may be suspected.

Back*: The dorsal side of the body may reveal edema, deformities, irregularities of the spine, discolorations eruptions, impaired motion, decubitus or any condition affecting the skin.

Breath*: May have a fecal odor, a sweet (acetone) odor, or one of wet hay, an odor of fish, or ammonia, urine, blood, or pus. Respiration may be abdominal or thoracic, and show *dyspnea, orthopnea, apnea,* or it may be normal (*eupnea*).

Chest*: The chest may show abnormalities and deformities. Coughing may be *whooping, hacking, crowing, hoarse, dry, rasping* or *hysterical.* There may or may not be expectoration. A cough may be spasmodic or occur on awakening; during deep sleep it may awaken patient, or it may occur when swallowing food, when in a horizontal position, or when subjected to change of temperatures. If singultus* is present note when it occurs. Sputum may be *mucoid, yellowish, thick, tenacious, ropy, gelatinous, dark green, offensive in odor, copious, streaked with bright ("brick red") or dark blood* (hemoptysis), or it may resemble *cheesy lumps.* It may be clear and watery, scanty, or profuse.

Frequency of coughing and clearing throat should be noted. Patient's respirations may be low pitched, *dyspnea* may be present, inability to expand the lungs or complaints of irritation, sticking pains, or catchy pains on inspiration. There may be an accumulation of phlegm in the air passages, or a tickling in throat. Patient may not be able to take deep inspirations, or may be constantly yawning. There may be migrating, knifelike pains in region of heart or throughout chest. "Heart-consciousness" may be present, or a fluttering feeling about the heart, or cardiac pain. Queer sensations, the loud beating of the heart, and heaviness in cardiac region are other symptoms.

Defecation*: Symptoms to observe are the frequency of defecation; the presence of constipation; hemorrhoids; the nature of the feces, such as formation, as ribbon-shaped, soft, semiformed, hard or scybala, cylindrical, and whether watery, liquid, or semiliquid; the color, whether dark brown, light brown, clay-colored, green, yellowish, black, bloody; and whether lienteric, serous, mucous, purulent, tarry, or containing membranous shreds, calculi, or foreign substances. The amount should be noted, as *small, medium, large,* or *copious.* The odor may be characteristic of various conditions: *sour, putrid, offensive,* or *fetid.* The nature of the evacuation should be noted, as *natural, difficult, involuntary,* or *painful.*

Dentition: Teeth may be irregular, missing, or showing a Hutchinson condition, or affected by caries. There may be a partial or complete denture. Dental hygiene may be good or poor. There may be a loosening of teeth, a film over them, or they may show the presence of sordes.*

Ears*: *Tinnitus aurium,* or ringing in the ears, occurs in certain diseases. Pain in ear, about ears, or swelling under either or both should be noted. Impacted cerumen, or foreign bodies or insects may be present in auditory canals.

Nose*: May appear *deformed, discolored, edematous,* or *enlarged.* Nostrils may discharge or show obstruction; may be inability to breathe through one or both. Patient may complain of odors not usually manifested as objective symptoms, or for which there is no known cause.

Eyes*: May be staring, or show an excited look, or they may be expressionless. Nystagmus, strabismus, and coma vigil may be indicated. Pupils may be contracted or dilated, or 1 pupil affected. Patient may keep eyes closed constantly, or keep 1 open and the other closed. Eyes may be sunken or protruding. Lacrimation may be present. Eyelids may be edematous, and eyeball soft to the touch. Accommodation may be faulty. Nictating or squinting, or tremor of the eyelids should always be recorded. Blurring of vision is usually associated with other symptoms. Patient may complain of specks dancing before the eyes (*muscme volitantes*). These may be colorless or colored.

GAIT*: May be faltering, "scissors," festinating, unsteady, staggering, weakened, swaying, or movements may be stiff, awkward, or unusual; may be total disability or immobility.

GENERAL APPEARANCE: The face may show an expression of anxiety, a pinched look, or a "drawn" expression. Patient may have air of apathy, a distorted or a blank look, an emotional expression, a *risus sardonicus*, or sudden lack of all expression (masklike).

GENERAL SYMPTOMS: Burning sensations may be complained of in various parts of the body, as in the head, throat, arms, chest, or abdomen. They may or may not be accompanied by tenderness. The complaint may be of feeling too hot or too cold without apparent cause, or of having a general feeling of distress.

Anorexia, nausea upon taking food or at the thought of food, or with no reference to food are significant and should be noted; also when nausea obtains, on awakening, when taking fluids, after eating, when changing a position, when taking medication, or in the presence of odors. There always should be an explanation for nausea either somatic or psychiatric.

Fear of death (angor animi), anxiety, agitation, or panic may be present.

LIMBS*: The symptoms pert. to the skin, of course, apply to skin of the limbs. Note if there are deformities, abnormalities, impaired motion, discolorations, sensitivity, varicosities.

LIPS*: May be *pale, dry, cyanotic, edematous, drawn, deformed*, out of proportion, motionless and expressionless, *flushed, fissured*, or show other lesions or growths.

MOUTH AND GUMS*: May be pale or ulcerated, highly inflamed and red, infected, discolored, edematous, or abnormal. Pyorrhea or edema may be present. Patient may complain of certain tastes, such as bitter, sweet, salty, sour, fishy, or flat tastes, or an absence of taste. Medication may have much to do with temporary disorders of taste.

PAIN*: The exact area affected must be ascertained, and the wording of the patient's complaint of pain must be charted or reported. Note if pain is in nature of a cramp or spasm, if *dull, superficial*, or *deep, remittent, shifting, shooting, lancinating, gnawing, fixed, sharp, inflammatory*, or if there is an absence of pain, especially in conditions in which pain usually occurs. Note whether pain is relieved or increased by pressure, by heat, or by cold, change of body position or environment, or by other causes. When is pain experienced, how often does the same type of pain recur, and does it awaken the patient from sleep, especially at night? Observe the facial expression during an attack of pain and listen carefully to the patient's description.

Headache: The patient may locate the pain around the eyes and nose, in the center of the forehead above the nose, in 1 or both temples accompanied by throbbing, at the top of the head, or at the base of the brain. It may be felt as a tight, bandlike sensation around the head above the eyes, it may be in the center of the forehead above the eyebrow line or in the upper region of the center forehead, or all over the top of the head, or over 1 or both ears, or back of both ears. Pain may be sharp or dull, or shifting and accompanying head noises, or a roaring in the head may be experienced without pain. Vertigo may be present or a sensation of fainting. Pulsations may perhaps be felt in the occiput or in the temporal region. A patient may be very sensitive to light and sound, and headaches may be accompanied by nausea and vomiting and the sensation of flashing lights, also by chills. Tenderness or soreness may be associated with rigidity.

POSITIONS AND POSTURES*: An inability to lie down, to arise, or to lie on one side or on the back, or in any special position reveals much to the doctor. Whether lying on the affected or unaffected side is also important to observe. The left leg may be flexed or the right one, or both, or there may be an inclination to lie with the arms above the head.

SKIN*: May appear pale, flushed all over or in spots; may be *cyanotic, jaundiced, shiny, erupted, burned, blistered, sunburned, wrinkled, lacerated, nodular, bruised*, or exhibit dermographia, lesions, growth, or deformities, or be *puffy* and *edematous, ashy, gray*, wet with perspiration, or *discolored*.

THROAT*: May show abnormalities, discoloration, inflammation, diseased tonsils, and presence of adenoids. Dysphagia and hoarseness, or aphonia and other conditions affecting the voice may be present. A lump in the throat (*globus hystericus*), or a dry, scratchy irritation or fullness or pulsations may be present.

TONGUE*: May be coated, clean, smooth, atrophic, shiny, dry on top and moist on the sides, or dry all over; may look like raw beef or appear *furry, glossy, tremulous*, or sharp pointed. It may be *edematous* or abnormal in size, there may be fissures, the papillae may have disappeared, there may be a "*strawoerry-tongue*," or it may have various colors.

URINE*: It may be blue, milky, pale, lemon, smoky, brick-colored, clear, amber, straw-colored, orange, or almost any other color. *Hematuria* may be present. *Polyuria* or *oliguria* may be indicated, or there may be frequent urination of small amounts. The odors may be ammoniacal, aromatic, stercorous, or like that of new-mown hay, ripe apples, or violets. There may be retention or suppression, or dribbling, and urination may be painful.

SEE: *Each part or organ in text.*

s., accessory. A minor symptom, or one not pathognomonic.

s., accidental. One incidentally occurring during course of a disease but having no relationship to the disease.

s., assident. An accessory symptom, *q.v.*

s's., cardinal. Those pert. to pulse, respiration, and temperature.

s. complex. The entire group of symptoms presenting a clear picture of a disease. SYN: *syndrome.**

s., concomitant. One occurring along with the essential symptoms of a disease.

s., constitutional, s., general. One caused by or indicating disease of the whole body.

s., delayed. S. appearing sometime after precipitating cause.

s., direct. S. resulting from direct effects of disease.

s., dissociation. Anesthesia to heat, cold, and pain without loss of tactile sensibility. Seen in syringomyelia.

s., equivocal. 1. One that may occur in several diseases, hence of doubtful significance. 2. One of such degree as to be doubtful of its presence.

s., focal. One at a specific location.

s., general. A constitutional symptom, *q.v.*

s., indirect. One occurring secondarily as a result of a disease.

s., labyrinthine. One such as tinnitus, vertigo, or nausea indicating a disease or lesion of the inner ear.

s., local. One indicating specifically the seat of the disease or morbid process.

s., negative pathognomonic. One which never occurs in a certain disease or condition; hence its occurrence rules out the existence of that disease.

s., objective. One apparent to the observer. Also called *sign.*

s., passive. A static symptom, *q.v.*

s., pathognomonic. One which unmistakably points out presence of a particular disease.

s's., prodromal. Those which indicate an approaching disease. Syn: *prodrome.**

s., rational. A subjective symptom, *q.v.*

s., signal. A symptom which is premonitory of an impending condition such as the aura which precedes an attack of epilepsy or migraine.

s., static. One pertaining to the condition of a single organ or structure without reference to remainder of body.

s., subjective. One apparent only to the patient.

s., sympathetic. A symptom for which there is no specific inciting cause and usually occurring at a point more or less remote from the point of disturbance.

s's., withdrawal. Those following sudden withdrawal of a stimulant from an addict, generally excitement and collapse.

symptomatic (sĭmp-tō-măt'ĭk) [G. *symptōmatikos,* pert. to a symptom]. Of the nature of or concerning a symptom.

symptomatology (sĭmp-tō-mă-tŏl'ō-jĭ) [G. *symptōma,* symptom, + *logos,* a study]. 1. Science of symptoms and indications. Syn: *semeiology.* 2. All of the symptoms of a given disease as a whole.

symptomatolytic (sĭmp"tō-măt"ō-lĭt'ĭk) [" + *lysis,* destruction]. Causing the removal of symptoms.

symp'tom com'plex. A group of symptoms which occur together and thus characterize a specific disease. Syn: *syndrome.*

symptomolytic (sĭmp-tō-mō-lĭt'ĭk) [G. *symptōma,* symptom, + *lysis,* destruction]. Pert. to the removal of symptoms. Syn: *symptomatolytic.*

symptosis (sĭmp-tō'sĭs). Emaciation; wasting away.

syn- [G.]. Prefix meaning *joined, together.* See: *prefix con-.*

syn"acto'sis. Malformation resulting from the abnormal fusion of parts.

synalgia (sĭn-ăl'jĭ-ă) [G. *syn,* with, + *algos,* pain]. Referred or reflex pain felt in a part distant from the site of its origin.

synalgic (sĭn-ăl'jĭk) [" + *algos,* pain]. Pert. to or characterized by referred pain.

synanche (si-nang'ke). Syn: *diphtheria.* Severe throat infection.

synanastomosis (sĭn"an-as"tō-mō'sĭs) [" + *anastomōsis,* a connecting mouth]. The connection of several vessels.

synanthema (sĭn-ăn-thē'mă) [" + *anthein.* to bloom]. Exanthem made up of several different forms of eruption.

synapse (sĭn'ăps) [G. *synapsis,* from *syn,* with, + *aptein,* to touch]. The point of junction in a neural pathway between two neurons where the end arborizations of the axon of one neuron come into close proximity with the cell body or dendrites of another. At this point, where the relationship of the two neurons is one of contact only, the impulse travelling in the first neuron initiates an impulse in the second neuron. Synapses are *polarized, i.e.,* the impulses pass in one direction only. They are susceptible to fatigue, offer a resistance to the passage of impulses and are markedly susceptible to the effects of oxygen deficiency, anesthetics and other drugs.

synapsis (sĭn-ăp'sĭs) [G. *synapsis,* from *syn,* with, + *aptein,* to touch]. The process in first maturation division in gametogenesis in which there is conjugation of pairs of homologous chromosomes forming double or *bivalent* chromosomes. In the resulting miotic division, the chromosome number is reduced from the diploid to the haploid number. It is at this stage that crossing over occurs.

RS: *crossing over, miosis, oogenesis, spermatogenesis.*

synap'tic. Pertaining to a synapse or synapsis.

s. field. A field in cerebral cortex, cerebellar cortex and retina where large numbers of contacts between neurons can take place.

synaptolemma (sĭn-ăp-tō-lĕm'mă). The membrane at a synapse separating two neurons.

synarthrodia (sĭn-ăr-thrō'dĭ-ă) [G. *syn,* with, + *arthron,* joint, + *eidos,* form]. Type of immovable cartilaginous joint without a joint cavity in which bones are separated by only a connective tissue membrane; a fixed articulation. Syn: *synarthrosis.* See: *joint.*

synarthrodial (sĭn-ar-thrō'dĭ-ăl) [" + " + *eidos,* form]. Pert. to an immovable articulation bet. bones.

synarthrophysis (sĭn-ăr-thrō-fĭ'sĭs) [" + *arthrōsis,* joint, + *physis,* growth]. Progressive ankylosis of joints.

synarthrosis (sĭn"ar-thrō'sĭs) (pl. *synarthroses*) [" + *arthrōsis,* joint]. A type of joint in which the skeletal elements are united by a continuous intervening substance (cartilage, fibrous tissue, or bone). Movement is absent or limited and a joint cavity is lacking. It includes the *synchondrosis, suture,* and *syndesmosis* types of joints.

syncanthus (sĭn-kăn'thŭs) [G. *syn,* with, + *kanthos,* angle]. Adhesion of eyeball to the structures of the orbit.

synchilia (sĭn-kĭ'lĭ-ă) [" + *cheilos,* lip]. Adhesion or imperforation (*atresia*) of the lips.

synchiria (sĭn-kĭ'rĭ-ă) [" + *cheir,* hand]. Disorder of sensibility in which stimulus applied to one side of the body is referred to both. Syn: *allochiria.* RS: *achiria, dyschiria.*

synchondroseotomy (sĭn-kŏn-drō-sē-ŏt'ō-mĭ) [" + *chondros,* cartilage, + *tomē,* a cutting]. An operation of cutting through the sacroiliac ligaments and closing the arch of the pubes in congenital absence of the ant. wall of the bladder (*exstrophy*).

synchondrosis (sĭn-kŏn-drō'sĭs) [" + *chondros,* cartilage, + *-ōsis,* condition]. An immovable joint having the surfaces bet. the bones connected by cartilages. This may be temporary, in which case the cartilage eventually becomes ossified, or permanent.

synchondrotomy (sĭn-kŏn-drŏt'ō-mĭ) [" + " + *tomē,* a cutting]. 1. Division of articulating cartilage. 2. Section of the symphysis pubis to facilitate childbirth. SEE: *symphyseotomy.*

synchronism (sĭn'krō-nĭzm) [" + *chronos,* time, + *-ismos,* condition]. Occurrence of acts or events simultaneously.

synchronous (sĭn'krŏn-ŭs) [G. *syn,* with, + *chronos,* time]. Occurring simultaneously.

synchysis (sĭn'kĭs-ĭs) [G. *synchysis,* from *syncheein,* to confound]. Fluid state of vitreous of the eye.

s. *scintillans.* Bright flashes of light resulting from presence of crystals of cholesterol or fat substances in vitreous body.

syncinesis (sĭn-sĭn-ē'sĭs) [G. *syn,* with, + *kinēsis,* motion]. An involuntary movement produced in association with a voluntary one. Synkinesis, *q.v.*

s., *imitative.* Occurs on sound side when movement is attempted on paralyzed side.

s., *spasmodic.* Occurs on hemiplegic side when muscles of opp. side are voluntarily moved.

sinciput (sĭn'sĭp-ŭt) [L.]. Ant. upper half of the cranium. SYN: *sinciput.*

synclitism (sĭn'klĭt-ĭzm) [G. *sygklinein,* to lean together]. Parallelism bet. the planes of the fetal head and those of the maternal pelvis.

synclonus (sĭn'klō-nŭs) [G. *syn,* with, + *klonos,* tumult]. 1. Clonic contraction of several muscles together. 2. A disease marked by muscular spasms.

s. *ballismus.* Paralysis agitans.

s. *tremens.* Generalized tremor.

syncopal (sĭn'kō-păl) [G. *sygkopē,* fainting]. Relating to or marked by syncope.

syncope (sĭn'kō-pē) [G. *sygkopē,* fainting]. SYN: *fainting, swoon.* A transient loss of consciousness due to inadequate blood flow to the brain.

ETIOL: Syncope or fainting may be due to deficient blood flow resulting from (1) peripheral circulatory failure, (2) cardiac failure or disturbances or (3) altered quality of the blood as in hyperventilation of hypoglycemia. Predisposing factors include fatigue, prolonged standing, nausea, pain, emotional disturbances, anemia, dehydration, poor ventilation, and many others.

TREATMENT: Stimulate the heart action, fresh air, treat underlying cause. If seated, depress head bet. knees, compressing abdominal viscera. Remove tight clothing. Apply sudden dash of cold water or cold towel which should be removed immediately. Aromatic spirits of ammonia inhalations for a moment or two, only. Test to see it is not too strong. External heat. When recovered, give hot drinks, strong coffee or tea. Keep lying down. Ten to 20 drops of ammonia by mouth in half a glass of water. Call a physician if recovery is not prompt. SEE: *unconsciousness.*

s. *angio'sa.* Syncope occurring with anginal pain.

s., *cardiac.* Syncope of cardiac origin as in Adams-Stokes syndrome, aortic stenosis, tachycardia, bradycardia, myocardial infarction, etc.

s., *carotid sinus.* S. resulting from pressure on, or hypersensitivity of, carotid sinus. May result from turning head to one side or from too tight a collar.

s. *cough.* S. which occurs during a coughing spell. SYN: *tussive syncope.*

s., *hysterical.* That resulting from purely psychologic mechanisms.

s., *laryngeal.* Brief unconsciousness following coughing and tickling in the throat. SYN: *vertigo, laryngeal.*

s., *local.* Numbness of a part with sudden blanching, as of the fingers; a symptom of Raynaud's disease or of local asphyxia.

s., *vasovagal.* SYN: *vasodepressor syncope, carotid sinus syncope.* S. resulting from fall in blood pressure due to failure of peripheral resistance with concomitant, reduced, venous return, or due to slowing of the heart. May be caused by psychogenic faint, pain, acute loss of blood, fear or by assuming an upright position after having been in bed for a prolonged period.

syncytial (sĭn-sĭ'shĭ-ăl). Of the nature of a syncytium.

s. *trophoblast.* Syntrophoblast, *q.v.*

syncytiolysin (sĭn-sĭt-ĭ-ol'ĭ-sĭn) [G. *syn,* with, + *kytos,* cell, + *lysis,* destruction]. A cytolysin that is formed from injections of emulsions of placental tissue.

syncytioma (sĭn-sĭt-ĭ-ō'mă) [" + " + *-ōma,* tumor]. A tumor of the chorion. SYN: *chorioma, deciduoma.*

s. *benig'num.* A mole.

s. *malig'num.* A tumor formed of cells from the syncytium and chorion, occurring frequently after abortion or in the puerperium at site of placenta.

syncytium (sĭn-sĭt'ĭ-ŭm) [G. *syn,* with, + *kytos,* cell]. SYN: *coenocyte.* 1. A multinucleated mass of protoplasm, for example, a striated muscle fiber. 2. A group of cells in which the protoplasm of one cell is continuous with that of adjoining cells. EX: mesenchyme cells of the embryo.

syndactylism (sĭn-dăk'tĭl-ĭzm) [" + *daktylos,* digit, + *ismos,* condition]. A fusion of 2 or more toes or fingers.

syndectomy (sĭn-dĕk'tō-mĭ) [" + *dēin,* to bind, + *ektomē,* excision]. Excision of a circular strip of the conjunctiva around cornea to relieve *pannus.* SYN: *peritomy.*

syndesis (sĭn-dē'sĭs) [G. *syn,* with, + *desis,* a binding together]. 1. Condition of being bound together. 2. Surgical fixation or ankylosis of a joint.

syndesmectomy (sĭn-dĕs-mĕk'tō-mĭ) [" + *desmos,* band, + *ektomē,* excision]. Excision of a section of a ligament.

syndesmectopia (sĭn"dĕs-mĕk-tō'pĭ-ă) [G. *syndesmos,* ligament, + *ektopos,* out of place]. Abnormal position of a ligament.

syndesmitis (sĭn-dĕs-mī'tĭs) [" + *-itis,* inflammation]. 1. Inflammation of a ligament or ligaments. 2. Inflammation of the conjunctiva.

syndesmochorial (sĭn-dĕs"mō-kor'ĭ-ăl). Pertaining to a type of placenta found in ungulates in which there is destruction of surface layer of uterine mucosa thus allowing chorionic villi to come into direct contact with maternal blood vessels.

syndesmography (sĭn-dĕs-mŏg'ră-fĭ) [G. *syn,* with, + *graphein,* to write]. Treatise on the ligaments.

syndesmology (sĭn-dĕs-mŏl'ō-jĭ) [" + *logos,* a study]. Study of the ligaments and their disorders.

syndesmoma (sĭn-dĕs-mō′mă) [G. *syn*, with, + *-ōma*, tumor]. A connective tissue tumor.

syndesmopexy (sĭn-dĕs′mō-pĕks-ĭ) [" + *pēxis*, fixation]. Joining of 2 ligaments or fixation of a ligament in a new place, used in correction of a dislocation.

syndesmoplasty (sĭn-dĕs′mō-plăs-tĭ) [" + *plassein*, to form]. Plastic surgery on a ligament.

syndesmorrhaphy (sĭn-dĕs-mor′ăf-ĭ) [G. *syndesmos*, ligament, + *rhaphē*, a seam]. Repair or suture of a ligament.

syndesmosis (sĭn-dĕs-mō′sĭs) (pl. *syndesmoses*) [" + *-ōsis*, condition]. Articulation in which the bones are united by ligaments. Ex: the distal tibiofibular articulation.

syndesmotomy (sĭn-dĕs-mŏt′ō-mĭ) [" + *tomē*, a cutting]. Surgical section of ligaments.

syndrome (sĭn′drōm, -drō-mē) [G. *syndromē*, a running together]. A complexus of symptoms. For syndromes not listed, look under noun.

s., Adair-Dighton. A familial condition characterized by fragility of bones and blue scleras.

s., Adams - Stokes. Bradycardia and intermittent convulsive seizures with loss of consciousness due to complete heart block.

s., adiposogenital. SEE: *Fröhlich's s.*

s., adrenogenital. S. characterized by pubertas praecox in children, overmasculinization in adults, virilism, and hirsutism, due to oversecretion of adrenal cortical hormones. SEE: *Cushing's syndrome.*

s., Angelucci's. Palpitation, excitable temperament and vasomotor disturbance in some of those who experience spring conjunctivitis.

s., dumping. Symptom complex which may follow partial or complete gastrectomy. Appears to be related to rapid emptying of gastric pouch. Occurs immediately after eating. Consists of weakness, varying degrees of syncope, nausea, sweating, and palpitation, and, sometimes, diarrhea and sensation of warmth. Lying down usually affords some relief.

s., Fröhlich's. Increase in fat, atrophy of the genitals, transition to feminine type due to lesions of the hypophysis.

s., Gradenigo's. External rectus paralysis, temporoparietal pain and suppurative otitis media on same side.

s. of Horner. Contracted pupil, ptosis, enophthalmos and dry, cool face on affected side produced by paralysis of sympathetics.

ETIOL: Tumors in neck, trauma, apical tuberculosis, tabes, syringomyelia, and neuritis of cervical plexus.

s., Korsakoff's. A psychosis, ordinarily due to chronic alcoholism, with polyneuritis, disorientation, insomnia, muttering delirium, hallucinations, and a bilateral wrist or foot drop.

s., Marfan's. A hereditary condition of connective tissue, bones, eyes, muscles, ligaments and skeletal structures. SYM: Irregular, unsteady gait, lean, tall with stooping shoulders.

s., skin-eye. Deposits on the anterior surface of the lens and posterior cornea, and skin pigmentation. Due to extensive medication with some of the phenothiazine type tranquilizers.

s., Weber's. Paralysis of hypoglossal nerve on one side and of oculomotor nerve on other with paralysis of limbs due to lesion of a cerebral peduncle.

syndromic (sĭn-drom′ĭk) [G. *syn*, with, + *dromos*, a running]. Pert. to or occurring as a syndrome.

synechia (sĭn-ē′kĭ-ă) [G. *synecheia*, continuity]. Adhesion of parts, esp. adhesion of iris to lens and cornea.

s., annular. Adhesion of the iris to the lens throughout its entire pupillary margin.

s., anterior. Adhesion of iris to cornea.

s., posterior. Adhesion of iris to capsule of lens.

s., total. Adhesion of entire surface of the iris to the lens.

synechotomy (sĭn-ĕk-ŏt′ō-mĭ) [" + *tomē*, a cutting]. Division of a synechia or adhesion.

synecology (sĭn-ē-kŏl′ō-jĭ) [G. *syn*, with, + *oikos*, house, + *logos*, a study]. The study of organisms in relation to their environment in group form.

syneresis (sĭn-ĕr′ĕs-ĭs) [" + *airesis*, a taking]. Contraction of a gel resulting in its separation from the liquid, as a shrinkage of fibrin when blood clots.

synergetic (sĭn-ĕr-jĕt′ĭk) [G. *syn*, with, + *ergon*, work]. Exhibiting cooperative action, said of certain muscles; working together. SYN: *synergic.*

synergia. The association and correlation of the activity of synergetic muscle groups.

synergic (sĭn-ĕr′jĭk) [" + *ergon*, work]. Relating to or exhibiting cooperation, as certain muscles.

synergism (sĭn′er-jĭz-ĭm). The harmonious action of two agents such as drugs, or organs such as muscles producing an effect which neither alone could produce, or an effect may result which is greater than the total effects of each agent operating by itself.

synergist (sĭn′ĕr-jĭst) [" + *ergon*, work]. 1. A remedy that stimulates the action of another. SYN: *adjuvant.* 2. A muscle or organ functioning in cooperation with another, as the flexor muscles.

synergy (sĭn′ĕr-jĭ) [" + *ergon*, work]. Action of 2 or more agents or organs cooperating with each other; cooperation. Combined action; coordinated action.

synesthesia (sĭn-ĕs-thē′zĭ-ă) [" + *aisthēsis*, sensation]. 1. A sensation in an area from a stimulus applied to another part. 2. A subjective sensation of another sense than the one being stimulated. Hearing a sound may also produce the sensation of smell. SEE: *chromatism, phonism.*

s. al′gica. Painful synesthesia.

synesthesialgia (sĭn″ĕs-thē-zĭ-ăl′jĭ-ă) [" + " + *algos*, pain]. A painful sensation giving rise to a subjective one of different character. SEE: *synesthesia.*

synezesis (sĭn-ĕ-zē′sĭs) [G. *synizēsis*, a sitting together]. Closure of the pupil.

Syngamus (sĭn′gă-mŭs). A genus of nematode worms parasitic in respiratory tract of birds and mammals.

S. laryngeus. Species normally parasitic in ruminants but sometimes accidentally infesting man.

syngamy (sĭn′gă-mĭ) [G. *syn*, with, + *gamos*, marriage]. Sexual reproduction; cell union, as of gametes in fertilization.

syngenesious (sĭn-jĕ-nē′shus). Derived from an individual of the same species, said of tissue transplants.

syngignocism (sĭn-jĭg′nō-sizm) [" + *gignōskein*, to know]. Hypnotism and its results.

synhidrosis (sĭn″hĭ-drō′sĭs). [" + *hidros*, sweat]. Sweating, esp. excessive sweating associated with another condition.

synizesis (sĭn-ĭz-ē'sĭs) [" + *izein*, to sit]. A closure of shutting.

s. pupillae. Closure of the pupil of the eye with loss of vision.

synkaryon (sĭn-kar'ĭ-ŏn) [" + *karyon*, kernel]. A nucleus resulting from fusion of 2 pronuclei.

synkinesis (sĭn-kĭ-nē'sĭs) [G. *syn*, with, + *kinēsis*, motion]. 1. An involuntary movement of a part occurring simultaneously with a movement, either reflex or voluntary, of another part. 2. An involuntary movement in a healthy or normal muscle accompanying an attempted movement of a paralyzed muscle on the opposite side. Called *imitative synkinesis.*

synonym (sĭn'ō-nĭm) [G. *syn*, with, + *onoma*, name]. (In this volume, abbreviated SYN.) A word which has the same or very similar meaning as another word. An additional or substitute name for the same disease, sign, symptom, anatomical structure.

synophrys (sĭn-ŏf'rĭs). Condition in which the eyebrows are continuous.

synopsia (sĭn'ŏp-sĭ-ă). Condition in which there is congenital fusion of the eyes.

synopsis (sĭn-ŏp'sĭs). A summary; a general review of the whole.

synoptophore (sĭn-ŏp'tō-for) [G. *syn*, with, + *ōps, opt-*, sight, + *phoros*, a bearer]. Apparatus for diagnosing and treating strabismus.

synoptoscope (sĭn-ŏp'tō-skōp) [" + " + *skopein*, to examine]. An instrument for diagnosis and treatment of strabismus. SYN: *synoptophore.*

synorchidism, synorchism (sĭn-or'kĭd-ĭzm, -kĭzm) [" + *orchis, orchid-*, testicle, + *-ismos*, condition]. Union or partial fusion of the testicles.

synosteosis, synostosis (sĭn"ŏs-tē-ō'sĭs, -tō'-sĭs) [G. *syn*, with, + *osteon*, bone, + *-ōsis*, condition]. 1. Articulation by osseous tissue of adjacent bones. 2. Union of separate bones by osseous tissue.

synosteotomy (sĭn-ŏs-tē-ŏt'ō-mĭ) [G. *syn*, with, + *osteon*, bone, + *tomē*, a cutting]. Dissection of joints.

synotia (sĭn-ō'shĭ-ă). The union of or approximation of the ears occurring in embryonic development, usually associated with absence of, or incomplete development of, the lower jaw.

synovectomy (sĭn-ō-vĕk'tō-mĭ) [" + L. *ovum*, from G. *ōon*, egg, + G. *ektomē*, excision]. Excision of synovial membrane.

synovia (sĭn-ō'vĭ-ă) [" + L. *ovum*, from G. *ōon*, egg]. A colorless, viscid, lubricating fluid of joints, bursae, and tendon sheaths secreted within synovial membranes. SYN: *synovial fluid.*

It contains mucin, albumin, fat, and mineral salts. SEE: *asynovia.*

synovial (sĭn-ō'vĭ-ăl) [G. *syn*, with, + L. *ovum*, from G. *ōon*, egg]. Pert. to synovia, the joint lubricating fluid.

s. bursa. SYN: *bursa mucosa.* A cleft in connective tissue between muscles, tendons, ligaments, and bones lined by a synovial membrane and containing synovia. SEE: *bursa.*

s. crypt. Diverticulum of a synovial membrane of a joint.

s. cyst. Accumulation of synovia in a bursa, s. crypt, or sac of a synovial hernia, causing a tumor.

s. fluid. Lubricating, clear fluid secreted by the synovial membrane of a joint. SYN: *synovia.*

s. folds. SYN: *plicae synoviales.* Smooth folds of synovial membrane on inner surface of joint capsule.

s. hernia. Protrusion of a portion of synovial membrane through a tear in the stratum fibrosum of a joint capsule.

s. membrane. One lining the capsule of a joint.

s. tendon sheaths. SYN: *vaginae mucosae.* Sheaths which develop in osteofibrous canals through which tendons pass. Each is a double layered tube, the space between the two layers being occupied by synovial fluid.

s. villi. SYN: *haversian fringes.* Slender avascular processes on the free surface of a synovial membrane projecting into the joint cavity.

synovioma (sĭn"ō-vĭ-ō'mă) [G. *syn*, with, + L. *ovum*, + G. *-ōma*, tumor]. A tumor arising from a synovial membrane.

synovitis (sĭn-ō-vĭ'tĭs) [G. *syn*, with, + L. *ovum*, egg, + G. *-ītis*, inflammation]. Inflammation of a synovial membrane.

ETIOL: As a result of an aseptic wound, of a subcutaneous injury (contusion or sprain), of the irritation produced by floating cartilage, or of exposure to cold and dampness, simple inflammation may attack the synovial membrane.

SYM: Joint painful, severely so on motion, esp. at night. Swollen, tense; may be fluctuating. At the knee, patella is floated up from condyles, can be readily depressed, to rise again when pressure is taken off. The part is never in full extension, as this increases the pain. Skin, which is very sensitive to pressure only at certain points, is neither thickened nor reddened. After a few days, pain lessens, swelling diminishes as the effusion and extravasated blood are absorbed, the limb takes its natural position and recovery follows.

s., chronic. The active congestion largely disappears, but there is an undue amount of fluid in the cavity and the membrane itself is edematous. Later, if disease does not subside, membrane and articular structures become irregularly thickened by plastic exudation and formation of fibrous tissue. Joint is weak, but not esp. painful except on pressure; may not be even then; movements, esp. in extension, are restricted, and generally attended by some grating or creaking. When there is great accumulation of liquid, symptoms are well marked. Fluid, which is straw-colored, somewhat viscid, sometimes flocculent and more or less blood stained, may be drawn off with the hypodermic needle.

s., dendritic. S. with villous growths developing in the sac.

s., dry. S. with little or no effusion.

s., fungus. Tuberculosis of a joint. SYN: *arthritis fungosa.*

s., purulent. S. with purulent effusion within the sac.

s., serous. S. with nonpurulent, copious effusion.

s. sicca. Same as *dry* synovitis.*

s., simple. S. with effusion only slightly turbid if not clear.

s., tendinous. Inflammation of a tendon sheath.

s., vaginal. Same as *tendinous* synovitis.*

s., vibration. S. resulting from a wound near a joint.

synovium. A synovial membrane.

synpneumonic (sĭn-nū-mŏn'ĭk) [G. *syn*, with, + *pneumōnia*, pneumonia]. Concurrent with pneumonia; complicating pneumonia.

syntasis [G. " + *teinein*, to stretch]. Stretching.

syntaxis (sĭn-tăks′ĭs) [" + *taxis,* arrangement]. A junction bet. 2 bones. SYN: *articulation.*

syntexis [G. melting together]. Wasting or cachexia.

synthermal (sĭn-thĕr′măl) [" + *thermē,* heat]. Having the same temperature.

synthesis (sĭn′thĕs-ĭs) [" + *tithenai,* to place]. CHEM: The union of elements to produce compounds; the process of building up; the opposite of analysis or decomposition. In general, the process or processes involved in the formation of a complex substance from simpler elements or compounds as the *synthesis* of proteins from amino acids.

synthetic (sĭn-thĕt′ĭk) [G. *synthetikos,* placed together]. Relating to or made by synthesis; artificially prepared.

syntone (sĭn′tōn) [G. *syn,* with, + *tonos,* tone]. An individual temperamentally responsive to his environment and its social demands. SEE: *syntonic.*

syntonic (sĭn-tŏn′ĭk) [" + *tonos,* tone]. Pert. to a reaction type in which the subject responds strongly to emotional stimuli in harmony with the situation.

The type is exaggerated in maniclike states and in depressions.

syntonin (sĭn′tō-nĭn) [" + *tonos,* tense]. An acid albumin; esp. one formed by the action of dilute hydrochloric acid on muscle during gastric digestion.

syntoxoid (sĭn-tŏks′oyd) [" + *toxikon,* poison, + *eidos,* form]. A toxoid having the same degree of affinity for an antitoxin as the toxin has.

syntripsis (sĭn-trĭp′sĭs) [" + *tripsis,* a crushing]. A comminuted fracture or act causing it.

syntropan (sĭn′trō-păn). Registered trademark for a brand of amprotropine phosphate.

USES: In spastic disorders of gastrointestinal and genitourinary tracts, also in parkinsonism.

syntrophoblast (sĭn-trŏf′ō-blăst). The outer syncytial layer of the trophoblast. SEE: *trophoblast, syncytial.*

synulotic (sĭn-ū-lot′ĭk) [" + *oulē,* scar]. 1. An agent stimulating cicatrization. 2. Promoting cicatrization.

syphilelcosis (sĭf-ĭl-ĕl-kō′sĭs) [*syphilis* + G. *elkōsis,* ulceration]. Syphilitic ulceration.

syphilelcus (sĭf-ĭl-ĕl′kŭs) [*syphilis* + G. *elkos,* ulcer]. A syphilitic ulcer or chancre.

syphilide (sĭf′ĭl-ĭd) [Fr.]. Skin eruption caused by syphilis.

syphilionthus (sĭf-ĭl-ĭ-ŏn′thŭs) [" + G. *ionthos,* eruption]. A copper-colored, branny-scaled syphilide.

syphiliphobia (sĭf-ĭl-ĭ-fō′bĭ-ă) [" + G. *phobos,* fear]. Morbid fear of syphilis. SYN: *syphilophobia.*

syphilis (sĭf′ĭ-lĭs) [origin uncertain; possibly from G. *syn,* with, + *philos,* love, or from *Syphilus,* a shepherd, in a poem, who had the disease]. SYN: *lues venera, morbus gallicus, pox.* An infectious, chronic, venereal disease characterized by lesions which may involve any organ or tissue. It usually exhibits cutaneous manifestations, relapses are frequent, and it may exist without symptoms for years.

ETIOL: *Treponema pallidum,* a spirochete, which is transmitted by direct contact between humans, contact with freshly contaminated material, by transfusion of infected blood or plasma, or in utero by passage of organism from mother to fetus. The organism may enter through any broken place in skin or mucous membrane.

PRIMARY STAGE SYM: Initial lesion appears 2 to 4 weeks after inoculation, changing from a small red papule to a small ulcer, to a hard chancre. Usually upon prepuce or vulva. Lymph nodes enlarge about 2 weeks after appearance of lesion.

Almost positive signs of syphilis are inflammation at mouth of Stensen's duct and enlargement of epitrochlear lymph nodes.

SECONDARY STAGE SYM: Symptoms appear about 6 weeks after appearance of primary lesion, principally in the form of lesions of the skin and mucous membranes. The character of the skin lesions is protean, syphilis often being called the "Great Imitator." Systemic symptoms such as headache, fever, and malaise are common but may be absent. Enlargement and induration of regional lymph nodes occurs. Eruptions of skin, maculae (roseola), syphilide, reddish brown "coppery" spots, continuing for a week or two, recurring possibly later.

TERTIARY STAGE SYM: The heart and blood vessels (cardiovascular syphilis) and the central nervous system (neurosyphilis) are frequently involved. Tabes dorsalis, paresis (general paralysis of the insane), and various types of psychoses may result.

DIAG: Laboratory tests for syphilis are based on three procedures: 1. Microscopic: Darkfield demonstration of spirochetes, in material taken from a chancre or other early lesion. 2. Biopsy: Examination of cerebrospinal fluid. 3. Serologic tests for syphilis (S.T.S.) done on blood and spinal fluid. These include flocculation tests (Kahn, Eagle, Mazzini, Kline, Hinton), complement-fixation technics (Wassermann test and its modifications). The VDRL (Venereal Disease Research Laboratory), treponema pallidum immobilization (TPI), and fluorescent treponemal antibody (FTA) tests are also useful in diagnosing syphilis and distinguishing it from biologic false positive serologic reactions.

CAUTION: A person who contracts gonorrhea may have also been exposed to syphilis at the same time. Because the clinical signs and symptoms of gonorrhea develop several weeks prior to those of syphilis, the patient will be treated for that disease. The treatment for gonorrhea may be sufficient to mask or delay the signs of syphilis, but insufficient to rid the patient of the spirochetes. When this occurs syphilis will develop and may be unnoticed by the patient. It is therefore of vital importance either to treat each case of gonorrhea as if syphilis had also been contracted or to test the patient for serologic evidence of syphilis each month for at least four months following the treatment for gonorrhea.

TREATMENT: Penicillin is the treatment of choice for all types and stages. Should allergic reactions occur, other antibiotics (oxytetracycline, chlortetracycline, or erythromycin) may be substituted. The use of arsenicals, bismuth, and mercurials has been almost completely supplanted by antibiotics.

s., cardiovascular. Syphilis involving the heart and great blood vessels, especially the aorta. Saccular aneurysms of the aorta and aortic insufficiency frequently result.

s., congenital. S. present at birth.

s., extragenital. Syphilis in which

the primary chancre is located elsewhere than on genital organs.

s. innocen'tium, s. inson'tium. S. not contracted through coition.

s., latent. Phase in which symptoms are absent and the disease can be diagnosed only by serological tests.

s., marital. Syphilis acquired in wedlock.

s., meningovascular. A form of neurosyphilis in which the meninges and vascular structures of the brain and spinal cord are involved. May be localized or general.

s., neuro-. Involvement of the nervous system by syphilis.

s., prenatal. Syphilis transmitted from mother to child; congenital syphilis.

s., venereal. Syphilis acquired through illicit sexual relations.

s., visceral. Syphilis in which visceral organs are involved.

syphilitic (sĭf-ĭl-lĭt'ĭk) [*syphilis*]. Related to, caused by, or affected with syphilis.

s. fever. Rise in temperature in early stage of secondary syphilis.

s. macules. Small red eruptions manifested in secondary syphilis which often cover the entire body.

Sym: Associated with chancre or scar, alopecia, pain in bones, swollen glands, and sore throat.

syphiloderm, syphiloderma (sĭf-ĭl-ō-derm, sĭf"ĭl-ō-der'mă) [*syphilis* + G. *derma*, skin]. A syphilitic cutaneous disorder.

syphilogenesis, syphilogeny (sĭf"ĭl-ō-jĕn'ĕ-sĭs, sĭf-ĭl-ŏj'ĕn-ĭ) [*syphilis* + G. *gennan*, to produce, — + *genesis*, production]. The development or origin of syphilis.

syphilographer (sĭf-ĭl-ŏg'ră-fer) [*syphilis* + G. *graphein*, to write]. One who writes about syphilis.

syphilography (sĭf-ĭl-ŏg'ră-fĭ) [*syphilis* + G. *graphein*, to write]. A treatise on syphilis.

syphiloid (sĭf'ĭl-oyd) [*syphilis* + G. *eidos*, form]. 1. Resembling syphilis. 2. A disease akin to syphilis.

syphilologist (sĭf-ĭl-ŏl'ō-jĭst) [*syphilis* + G. *logos*, a study]. A specialist in syphilis.

syphilology (sĭf-ĭl-ŏl'ō-jĭ) [*syphilis* + G. *logos*, a study]. The study of syphilis and its treatment.

syphiloma (sĭf-ĭl-ō'mă) [*syphilis* + G. *ōma*, tumor]. A syphilitic tumor. A gumma.

syphilomania (sĭf-ĭl-ō-mā'nĭ-ă) [*syphilis* + G. *mania*, madness]. Morbid fear of syphilis or inference that one is suffering with it. Syn: *syphilophobia*.

syphilopathy (sĭf-ĭl-ŏp'ă-thĭ) [*syphilis* + G. *pathos*, disease]. Any syphilitic disorder.

syphilophobia (sĭf-ĭl-ō-fō'bĭ-ă) [*syphilis* + G. *phobos*, fear]. Morbid fear of syphilis or delusion of having the disease.

syphilophobic (sĭf"ĭl-ō-fō'bĭk) [*syphilis* + G. *phobos*, fear]. Pert. to or affected with syphilophobia.

syphilophyma (sĭf"ĭl-ō-fī'mă) [*syphilis* + G. *phyma*, a growth]. 1. Any growth or excrescence due to syphilis. 2. Syphiloma of the epidermis.

syphilopsychosis (sĭf"ĭl-ō-sī-kō'sĭs) [*syphilis* + G. *psychē*, soul, + *-ōsis*, condition]. Any mental disease caused by syphilis.

syphilosis (sĭf-ĭ-lō'sĭs) [*syphilis* + G. *-ōsis*, disease]. Generalized syphilitic disease.

syphilotherapy. Treatment of syphilis.

syphilotropic (sĭf-ĭl-ō-trŏp'ĭk) [*syphilis* + G. *tropos*, a turning]. Especially susceptible to syphilis.

syphilous (sĭf'ĭl-ŭs) [*syphilis*]. Of the nature of or pert. to syphilis. Syn: *syphilitic*.

syphionthus (sĭf-ĭ-ŏn'thŭs) [*syphilis* + G. *ionthos*, eruption]. The copper-colored patches seen in syphilis.

syrigmophonia (sĭr"ĭg-mō-fō'nĭ-ă) [G. *syrigmos*, a whistle, + *phōnē*, voice]. 1. A sibilant râle. 2. A whistling sound in pronunciation of *s* due to a denture peculiarity.

syrig'mus. A subjective sound such as a hissing or ringing heard in the ears.

syringadenoma (sĭr-ĭng-ăd-en-ō'mă) [G. *syrigx*, pipe, + *adēn*, gland, + *-ōma*. tumor]. Tumor of a sweat gland.

syringe (sĭr-ĭnj', sĭr'ĭnj) [G. *syrigx*, pipe]. 1. Instrument for injecting fluids into cavities or vessel. 2. To wash out or introduce fluid with a syringe.

syringectomy (sĭr-ĭn-jĕk'tō-mĭ) [G. *syrigx*, pipe, + *ektomē*, excision]. Removal of the walls of a fistula.

syringitis (sĭr-ĭn-jī'tĭs) [" + *-itis*, inflammation]. Inflammation of eustachian tube.

syringobulbia (sĭr-ĭn-gō-bul'bĭ-ă) [G. *syrigx*, pipe, + *bulbos*, a bulb]. A chronic progressive disease characterized by development of cavities in the medulla oblongata. See: *syringomyelia*.

syringocele (sĭr-ĭn'gō-sēl) [" + *koilia*, a hollow]. 1. The central canal of the myelon or spinal cord. 2. A form of meningomyelocele which contains a cavity in the ectopic spinal cord.

syringocystadenoma (sĭr-ĭn"gō-sĭs-tad-ĕn-ō'mă) [" + *kystis*, a bladder, + *adēn*, gland, + *-ōma*, tumor]. Adenoma of sweat glands characterized by tiny, hard, papular formations.

syringocystoma (sĭr-ĭn"gō-sĭs-tō'mă) [" + " + *-ōma*, tumor]. Cystic tumor having its origin in ducts of the sweat gland.

syringoid (sĭr-ĭng'oyd) [" + *eidos*, form]. Fistulous. Resembling a tube.

syringoma (sĭr-ĭn-gō'mă) [" + *ōma*, tumor]. Tumor of the sweat glands.

syringomeningocele (sĭr-ĭn"gō-men-ĭn'gō-sēl) [" + *menigx*, membrane, + *kēlē*, hernia]. Meningocele which is similar to a syringomyelocele.

syringomyelia (sĭr-ĭn-gō-mĭ-ē'lĭ-ă) [G. *syrigx*, tube, + *myelos*, marrow]. A chronic progressive disease of the spinal cord characterized by the development of cavities and gliosis of surrounding tissue. Usually begins before age of 30, and is more common among males. Its cause is unknown.

Sym: Cavitation occurs in cervical and lumbar regions and soon involves pathways of the cord carrying impulses of pain and temperature sensations, resulting in dissociated sensory loss. Destruction of lateral and anterior gray matter causes muscular atrophy, weakness, and autonomic anomalies.

Treatment: There is no satisfactory treatment. Sudden enlargement of cavity may warrant surgical intervention with decompression of cavity. Persistent pain may necessitate chordotomy or medullary tractotomy for relief.

syringomyelitis (sĭr-ĭn"gō-mī-ĕ-lī'tĭs) [" + " + *-itis*, inflammation]. Inflammation coincident with abnormal dilation of the central canal of spinal cord.

syringomyelocele (sĭr-ĭn"gō-mī'ĕl-ō-sēl) [" + " + *kēlē*, tumor]. A form of spina bifida in which the cavity of the projecting portion communicates with the central canal of the spinal cord.

syringomyelus (sĭr-ĭn″gō-mī′ĕl-ŭs) [" + *myelos,* marrow]. Abnormal dilatation of central canal of spinal cord.

syringopontia (sĭr-ĭn″gō-pŏn′shĭ-ă) [" + L. *pons, pont-,* bridge]. Cavities in the pons Varolii similar to *syringomyelia.*

syringosystrophy (sĭr-ĭn″gō-sĭs′trō-fĭ) [" + *systrophē,* a twist]. Twisting of the oviduct.

syringotome (sĭr-ĭng′ō-tōm) [" + *tomē,* a cutting]. Instrument for incision of a fistula.

syringotomy (sĭr-ĭn-gŏt′ō-mĭ) [G. *syrigx,* tube, + *tomē,* a cutting]. Operation for cure of fistula by cutting.

syrinx (sĭr′ĭnks) [G. *syrigx,* pipe]. 1. The eustachian tube. 2. Pathological cavity in the spinal cord or brain. 3. A fistula.

syrup (sĭr′ŭp) [L. *syrupus*]. Concentrated solution of sugar in water. Usually specific medicinal substances are added.

They usually do not represent a very high percentage of the active drug. Some are used principally to give a pleasant odor and taste to solutions.

syssarcosis (sĭs-ar-kō′sĭs) [G. *syn,* with, + *sarkōsis,* flesh condition]. The union of bones by means of muscles; muscular articulation, as of the *hyoid* and *patella.*

systaltic (sĭs-tăl′tĭk) [G. *systaltikos,* contracting]. Contracting and dilating alternately; having a systole. Syn: *pulsating.*

system (sĭs′tĕm) [G. *systēma,* an arrangement]. 1. An organized grouping of related structures. 2. A group of structures or organs related to each other and functioning together in the performance of certain functions, as the digestive system. 3. A group of cells or aggregations of cells which perform a particular function, as the reticuloendothelial system.

s., autonomic nervous. That portion of the peripheral nervous system which innervates all smooth muscle, cardiac muscle, and glands, the activities of which are involuntary. It includes the *craniosacral (parasympathetic)* and *thoracolumbar* (*sympathetic*) divisions, each of which provides fibers for most of the visceral structures or organs.

s's., of body. Skeletal, muscular, digestive, circulatory, hematopoietic, lymphatic, respiratory, urinary, integumentary, endocrine, nervous, reproductive.

s., cardiovascular. The heart and blood vessels (aorta, arteries, arterioles, capillaries, venules, veins, vena cavae).

s., centimeter-gram-second. Abbr: *cgs.* A system of units of length, mass, and time. Syn: *metric system.*

s., central nervous. The brain and spinal cord. See under: *central.*

s., chromaffin. See: *chromaffin system.*

s., circulatory. Syn: *vascular system.* System concerned with circulation of body fluids. It includes the cardiovascular and lymphatic systems.

s., cytochrome. Cytochrome oxidase and three hemochromogen-like pigments (cytochromes a, b, and c), which make molecular oxygen available for the oxidation of hydrogen liberated from cellular metabolites.

s., digestive. The alimentary canal (mouth, teeth, tongue, pharynx, esophagus, stomach, small and large intestines) and accessory glands (salivary glands, liver, pancreas).

s., endocrine. The ductless glands or the glands of internal secretion.

s., enzyme. A group of enzymes essential for the completion of a series of metabolic and other reactions.

s., extrapyramidal motor. That which includes all descending fibers arising in cortical and subcortical motor centers which reach the medulla and spinal cord by pathways other than recognized pyramidal tracts. They are of importance in maintenance of equilibrium and muscle tone.

s., genital. The reproductive system.

s., genitourinary. That of the genitals and urinary organs.

s., haversian. The structural unit of bone. See: *haversian system.*

s., hematopoietic. The blood-forming tissues and organs of the body. Includes the bone marrow, spleen, and lymphatic tissue.

s., impulse-conducting. A system of atypical muscle fibers (Purkinje fibers) within the heart which conducts impulses regulating contractions of the atria and ventricles. Includes S-A and A-V nodes and bundle of His.

s., integumentary. The skin and its derivatives (hair, nails, etc.).

s., lymphatic. That concerned with the circulation of lymph. Includes lymph vessels and ducts and lymphatic organs (lymph nodes, tonsils, thymus, spleen).

s., muscular. That which includes all the muscles (smooth, cardiac, striated or skeletal). As generally used, the term refers to the skeletal muscles.

s., nervous. That which includes the brain, spinal cord, ganglia, and nerves. See: *nervous system.*

s., osseous. The bony structures of the body; the skeleton.

s., portal. The hepatic portal vein and all of its branches.

s., reproductive. Syn: *genital system.* The gonads and their associated structures and ducts.

s., reproductive, female. The ovaries, uterine tubes (oviducts), uterus, vagina, and vulva.

s., reproductive, male. The testes, efferent ducts, epididymus, ductus deferens, ejaculatory duct and urethra with the *accessory glands* (bulbourethral, prostate, seminal vesicles) and penis.

s., respiratory. The air passageways (nasal cavities, oral cavity, pharynx, larynx, trachea, and lungs, including bronchi, bronchioles, alveolar ducts, and alveoli).

s., reticuloendothelial. Collectively, all the phagocytic cells of the body excepting the leukocytes. Includes macrophages, histiocytes, Kupffer's cells of the liver, reticular cells of lymphatic organs, microglia of the brain, and many others.

s., sympathetic nervous. The thoracolumbar or sympathetic division of the autonomic nervous system.

s., urinary. The kidneys, ureters, bladder, and urethra.

s., urogenital. The urinary and reproductive systems combined.

s., vascular. That of the heart, blood vessels, and lymphatics.

s., vegetative nervous. The autonomic nervous system, *q.v.*

s., visceral efferent. That which includes all efferent nerve fibers conveying impulses to the visceral organs; the autonomic nervous system, *q.v.*

systema (sĭs-tē′mă) [G. *systēma,* an arrangement]. System.

systemic (sĭs-tĕm'ĭk) [G. *systēma*, arrangement]. Pert. to a whole body rather than to one of its parts; somatic.

s. *circulation*. The blood flow from the left ventricle through the aorta and all its branches (arteries) to the capillaries of the tissues and its return to the heart through veins and the vena cavae which empty into the right atrium.

s. *death*. Death of the body as a whole. SYN: *somatic death*.

s. *remedies*. Remedies which will act on the body as a whole.

systemoid (sĭs'tĕ-moyd) [G. *systēma*, an arrangement, + *eidos*, form]. 1. Resembling a system. 2. Pert. to tumors made up of several types of tissues.

systole (sĭs'tō-lē) [G. *systolē*, contraction]. That part of the heart cycle in which the heart is in contraction, *i. e.*, the myocardial fibers are tightening and shortening.

RS: *murmur, presystole, diastole.*

s., *aborted*. A premature cardiac systole. Arterial pressure is increased little if at all because of inadequate filling of ventricles due to shortening of preceding diastole.

s., *anticipated*. One that is aborted because it occurs before the ventricle is filled.

s., *arterial*. The rebound or recoil of the stretched elastic walls of the arteries following ventricular systole.

s., *atrial*. The contraction of the atria.

s., *electrical*. The total duration of the QRS-T complex in an electrocardiogram. Approximately the same as that of the mechanical systole.

s., *extra-*. A premature one occurring in addition to the fundamental rhythm.

s., *premature*. SYN: *extrasystole*. One slightly preceding a normal systole.

s., *ventricular*. Ventricular contraction.

systolic (sĭs-tŏl'ĭk) [G. *systolē*, contraction]. Pert. to the systole.

s. *discharge*. The amount of blood ejected by the heart at each systole.

s. *murmur*. A cardiac one during systole.

s. *pressure*. Blood pressure is expressed in terms of the systolic pressure; the greatest force exerted by the heart and the highest degree of resistance put forth by the arterial walls.

RS: *blood pressure, diastolic p., pulse p., pulse, systole.*

systolometer (sĭs-tō-lŏm'ĕt-ĕr) [" + *metron*, a measure]. Device for determining quality and character of cardiac murmurs.

systremma (sĭs-trĕm'ă) [G. *systremma*, a twist]. Cramp in calf of the leg, the muscles assuming form of a hard ball.

syzygial (sĭ-zĭj'ĭ-ăl) [G. *syzygia*, conjunction]. Pert. to a syzygium.

syzygiology (sĭ-zĭj"ĭ-ŏl'ō-jĭ) [" + *logos*, a study]. Interdependence or interrelationships of the whole as opposed to isolated functions or separate parts.

syzygium (sĭ-zĭj'ĭ-ŭm) [G. *syzygia*, conjunction]. Fusion of two parts or structures without loss of identity of the parts.

syzygy (sĭz'ĭ-jĭ) [G. *syzygia*, yokel] Fusion of organs, each remaining distinct.

Szabo's test (sah'bō). A test for hydrochloric acid.

Notes

Notes

Notes

Notes

Notes

Notes

T

t. Abbr. for *temporal*, and for Latin, *ter, three times.*
T. Abbr. for *temperature, time, tension* (intraocular). T+ indicates increased tension; T—, diminished tension.
T₁, T₂, etc. First thoracic vertebra, second thoracic vertebra, etc.
T-bandage. Bandage resembling the letter T. SEE: *bandage.*
T-wave. One of the waves or elevations in an electrocardiogram due to ventricular activity.
TA. Abbr. for alkaline tuberculin.*
T. A. Abbr. for *toxin-antitoxin.*
Ta. Chemical symbol for *tantalum.*
tabacism (tăb'ă-sĭzm) [L. *tabacum*, tobacco, + G. *-ismos*, condition]. Chronic tobacco poisoning. SYN: *tabacosis.*
tabacosis (tăb-ă-kō'sĭs) [" + G. *-ōsis*, condition]. Chronic tobacco poisoning, esp. from inhaling tobacco dust.
tabacum (tăb-ăk'ŭm) [L.]. Tobacco.
tabagism (tăb'ăj-ĭzm) [L. *tabacum*, tobacco, + G. *-ismos*, condition]. Tobacco poisoning. SYN: *tabacosis.*
Tabanidae (tă-băn'ĭ-dē). A family of insects belonging to the order *Diptera.* It includes the horse flies, gadflies, deer flies, and mango flies, which are blood-sucking insects attacking man and other warm-blooded animals. They are of medical importance in that they serve in the transmission of the filaria worm, *Loa loa*, tularemia, anthrax and other diseases; their bites are extremely painful and heal with difficulty.
tabardillo (tab'ar-dēl'yo). Mexican typhus. SEE: under *typhus.*
tabatière anatomique (tah-bah-tē-air' ahn-ah-tō-mēk') [Fr. anatomic snuffbox]. Depression at back of hand at base of thumb.
tabella (tă-bĕl'ă) (pl. *tabellae*) [L. *tabella*, tablet]. A medicated mass of material formed into a small disk.

RS: *disk, lozenge, tablet, troche.*

tabes (tā'bēz) [L. *tabes*, a wasting]. 1. A gradual, progressive wasting in any chronic disease. 2. *Tabes dorsalis, q.v.*

SYM: Postural instability, esp. when eyes are closed, and a staggering, wide-base gait are characteristic, hence the name: *locomotor ataxia.* Pains and paresthesias are common, esp. "lightning" pains, described as sharp, stabbing, and paroxysmal. Ankle and knee reflexes are diminished or lost. Many symptoms characteristic of syphilis such as pupillary changes, optic atrophy, bladder disturbances, development of trophic ulcers esp. on feet, make diagnosis certain.

TREATMENT: Antiluetic treatment for which SEE: *syphilis.* Special measures should be taken to relieve pains which are most troublesome. Rehabilitation measures are often essential for those with disturbed gait.

t., cerebral. Chronic degenerative brain disease with physical and mental deterioration. SYN: *paresis, general.*

t., cervical. T. first affecting the upper extremities.

t., diabetic. Peripheral neuritis, affecting diabetics. May affect spinal cord and simulate tabes dorsalis.

t. dorsalis. SYN: *locomotor ataxia, tabetic neurosyphilis.* A form of neurosyphilis characterized by chronic and usually progressive degeneration of ascending fibers of sensory neurons in posterior columns of spinal cord and usually also involving dorsal roots and ganglia of spinal nerves.

t. ergotica. T. resulting from the use of ergot.

t., marantic. T. with great emaciation.

t. mesenterica. Emaciation and general disorder of the functions of nutrition due to engorgement and tubercular degeneration of the mesenteric glands.

tabetic (tă-bĕt'ĭk) [L. *tabes*, a wasting]. Pert. to or afflicted with tabes or tabes dorsalis.

t. ataxia. Occurs when there are lesions of first order of sensory neurons.

t. crises. Paroxysms of pain or other acute manifestations of episodic character in tabes dorsalis.

t. foot. Twisted foot in locomoto ataxia.

tabetiform (tăb-ĕt'ĭ-form) [L. *tabes*, a wasting, + *forma*, shape]. Resembling or characteristic of tabes.
table (tā'bl) [L. *tabula*, a board]. 1. A flat-topped structure, as an operating table. 2. A thin, flat plate, as of bone.

t's. of skull. Inner and outer condensed layers of the cranial bone separated by diploe (cancellous bony tissue).

t., vitreous. The inner cranial table.

t's. of weights and measures. SEE: *weights and measures in Appendix.*

tablespoon (tā'bl-spoon). ABBR: *tbsp.* A rough measure utilizing a household spoon. When instructed to administer a tablespoon of medicine give 15 ml. of the substance.
tablet (tăb'lĕt) [O.Fr. *tablete*, from L. *tabula*, a table]. A small, disklike mass of medicinal powder.

t., coated. Usually made by coating compressed tablets with sugar, chocolate, etc.

t., compressed. Made by forcibly compressing the powdered substances into the desired shape; usually made to contain from 1 to 10 gr. of the active drug.

They are frequently very hard and sometimes not readily soluble.

t., dispensing. Those that contain a comparatively large amount of the active drug, as 1 gr. of strychnine sulfate.

Used by pharmacists and dispensing physicians to avoid the necessity of weighing small amounts of a potent drug in filling prescriptions.

t., hypodermic. Usually made as are tablet triturates, frequently containing, in addition, some agents that produce chemical action when water is added, thus causing a rapid disintegration of the mass.

t. triturates. Made by moistening the powder with a volatile liquid, as alcohol, and then molding into shape and allowing the liquid to evaporate.

They seldom contain more than 1 gr. of the active agent. They will usually disintegrate readily and are a very desirable form for administering certain drugs.

tablier [Fr. apron]. Pudendal apron. Enlarged vulvae.

taboo [Polynesian *tabu*]. An act, object, or social custom separated or set aside as being sacred or profane, thus forbidden for general use.

taboparalysis (ta"bō-păr-ăl'ĭs-ĭs) [L. *tabes*, a wasting, + *paralysis*, a loosening at the sides]. Tabes associated concurrently with general paralysis.

taboparesis (ta"bō-păr-ē'sĭs, -par'ĕ-sĭs) [" + G. *paresis*, relaxation]. SYN: *taboparalysis*. General paralysis in combination with tabes.

tabophobia (tā"bō-fō'bĭ-ă) [" + G. *phobos*, fear]. A morbid fear of being afflicted with tabes, a common symptom of neurasthenia.

tabular (tăb'ū-lar) [L. *tabula*, a table]. 1. Resembling a table. 2. Set up in columns, as a *tabulation*.

t. bone. A flat one, or one with two compact bonelike parts with cancellous tissue bet. them.

tache (tahsh) [Fr. spot]. A colored spot or macule on the skin, as a freckle.

t. blanche. A white spot seen on liver in some infectious diseases.

t. bleuâtre (blu-ăhtr'). A blue spot on skin usually due to bite of cutaneous parasites. SYN: *macula caerulea*.

t. cérébrale. The red line which occurs in meningitis and other nervous disorders, when the fingernail is drawn across the skin, *q.v.*

t. motrice. The motor end plate of a striated muscle fiber.

t. noire. A small round or oval ulcer covered by a black scab; the primary lesion of fievre boutonneuse and rickettsialpox.

tachetic (tăk-ĕt'ĭk) [Fr. *tache*, spot]. Marked by purple or reddish blue patches (*taches*).

tachogram (tăk'ō-grăm) [G. *tachos*, swiftness, + *gramma*, a mark]. A graphic tracing of rate of flow of blood.

tachography (tăk-ŏg'ră-fĭ) [" + *graphein*, to write]. The recording of the speed of the blood circulation.

tachy- [G.]. Combining form meaning *swift*.

tachyauxesis (tăk"ĭ-awks-ē'sĭs). Condition in which a part of an organism grows more rapidly than the whole.

tachycardia (tăk"ĭ-kar'dĭ-ă) [G. *tachys*, swift, + *kardia*, heart]. Abnormal rapidity of heart action.

t., atrial. SEE: *auricular fibrillation*.

t., atrioventricular. T. arising from stimuli in the A-V node characterized by sudden onset and cessation.

t., ectopic. T. resulting from causes other than disorders in conducting tissue of heart.

t., essential. Rapid, persistent heart action due to functional disturbance.

t., extrinsic. T. caused by factors outside the heart, as increased metabolism or instability of the nervous system.

t., intrinsic. T. caused by infection, as from rheumatism.

t., nodal. T. resulting from an increase in rhythmicity of A-V node over the S-A node, often the result of digitalis therapy.

t., paroxysmal. Sudden and abrupt acceleration of cardiac rate, ceasing abruptly.

Due to stimulus of cardiac contraction having its origin at an abnormal point. May go as high as 250 beats per minute. SEE: *arrhythmia, bradycardia.*

t., p. atrial. Paroxysmal tachycardia originating in an ectopic or abnormal focus in the atria. Occurs commonly in early childhood or early adulthood and usually in the absence of heart disease. Its cause is unknown.

t., p. ventricular. Paroxysmal tachycardia originating in an ectopic or abnormal focus in the ventricles. Occurs most commonly after age 50.

t., reflex. Tachycardia resulting from stimuli outside the heart reflexly accelerating heart rate or depressing vagal tone.

t., sinus. Uncomplicated tachycardia when sinus rhythm is faster than 100 beats per minute, as that due to exercise. Causes other than exercise include hyperthermia, thyrotoxicosis, hemorrhage, anoxia, infections, cardiac failure, and certain drugs such as atropine, epinephrine, and nicotine.

TREATMENT: Tachycardia sometimes ceases following procedures which cause vagal stimulation. Among these are pressure on one or both carotid sinuses, pressure on eyeballs, induction of gagging or vomiting, attempted expiration with glottis closed, lying down with feet in air, and bending over. If above procedures when employed singly are unsuccessful, two or more combined may produce desirable results.

t. strumosa exophthalmica. Tachycardia occurring as a symptom of exophthalmic goiter.

t., ventricular. Rapid contractions of the ventricle, the atrial rhythm remaining unchanged.

tachycardiac (tăk-ĭ-kar'dĭ-ăk) [" + *kardia*, heart]. Pert. to or afflicted with tachycardia.

tachylalia (tăk"ĭ-lā'lĭ-ă) [" + *lalein*, to babble]. Rapid speech.

tachymeter (tăk-ĭm'ĕ-ter) [" + *metron*, a measure]. Instrument for estimating the rapidity of any body in motion.

tachyphagia (tăk-ĭ-fā'jĭ-ă) [" + *phagein*, to eat]. Rapid eating.

tachyphasia (tăk"ĭ-fā'zĭ-ă) [" + *phasis*, speech]. Very rapid or voluble speech. SYN: *tachyphrasia*.

tachyphrasia (tăk"ĭ-frā'zĭ-ă) [" + *phrasis*, speech]. Excessive volubility or rapidity of speech, as seen in mental disorders. SYN: *tachyphasia*.

tachyphrenia (tăk"ĭ-frē'nĭ-ă) [G. *tachys*, swift, + *phrēn*, mind]. Abnormally rapid mental activity.

tachyphylaxis (tăk"ĭ-fĭl-ăk'sĭs) [" + *phylaxis*, protection]. Rapid immunization to a toxic dose of a substance by previously injecting tiny doses of the same substance.

tachypnea (tăk-ĭp-nē'ă) [" + *pnoia*, breath]. Abnormal rapidity of respiration.

t., nervous. Forty or more respirations per minute.

It occurs in hysteria, neurasthenia, etc. If prolonged, this will cause excess loss of CO_2 and the hyperventilation syndrome will develop. SEE: *hyperventilation syndrome* and *alkalosis, respiratory*.

tachypsychia (tăk-ĭ-sī'kĭ-ă) [" + *psychē*, soul]. Rapid action of psychic processes.

tachyrhythmia (tăk-ĭ-rĭth'mĭ-ă) [" + *rhythmos*, rhythm]. 1. SYN: *tachycardia*. Rapid heart action. 2. Increase in frequency of brain waves in electroencephalography up to 12 to 50 per sec.

tachysterol(e (tă-kĭs'tĕ-rōl). One of the isomers of ergosterol* obtained by irradiation.

tachysystole (tăk″ĭ-sĭs′tō-lē) [G. *tachys*, swift, + *systolē*, contraction]. Abnormally rapid systole. SEE: *extrasystole.*

tachytrophism (tăk″ĭ-trō′fĭzm) [″ + *trophē*, nourishment, + *-ismos*, condition]. Accelerated metabolism.

tactile (tăk′tĭl) [L. *tactilis*, tangible, from *tangere*, to touch]. Perceptible to the touch.

t. corpuscles. SYN: *Meissner's corpuscle.* Minute elongated bodies enclosing the endings of several afferent nerve fibers and serving as the receptor for slight pressure or touch. They are located in dermal papillae just beneath the epidermis and are most numerous on finger tips, toes, soles, palms, lips, nipples, and tip of tongue.

t. disk. SYN: *Merkel's disk.* Tiny expanded end of a sensory nerve fiber found in epidermis and in epithelial root-sheath of a hair.

t. system. That portion of the nervous system concerned with the sensation of touch. Includes sensory nerve endings (Meissner's corpuscles, Merkel's tactile disks, hair-root endings), afferent nerve fibers, conducting pathways in the cord and brain, and sensory (somesthetic) area of cerebral cortex.

tactometer (tăk-tŏm′ĕt-ĕr) [L. *tactus*, touch, + G. *metron*, a measure]. Instrument for determining acuity of tactile sensitiveness.

tactual (tăk′tū-al) [L. *tactus*, touch]. Relating to the sense of touch. SYN: *tactile.*

tactus (tăk′tus) [L. touch]. Touch.

t. eruditus, t. expertus. Sensitiveness of touch acquired by long practice, as by a diagnostician or surgeon.

taedium vitae [L. irksomeness, disgust with life]. Weariness of life. Suicidal inclination.

taenia (tē′nĭ-ă) [L. *taenia*, a flat band]. 1. Any bandlike structure. 2. A tapeworm.

t. coli. NA. One of 3 bands of the large intestines into which muscular fibers are collected, *i. e., t. mesocolica* (mesenteric insertion), *t. libera* (opp. mesocolic band), and *t. omentalis* (at place of adhesion of omentum to transverse colon).

t. of the fimbriae. The folded or recurved lateral edge of the fimbria to which the epithelium covering the choroid plexus of the inferior horn of the lateral ventricle is attached.

t. pontis. SYN: *fila lateralia.* One or two small transverse bands of fiber at rostral border of the pons.

t. semicircularis. SYN: *stria terminalis* (*terminal striae*).

t. thalami. Structure separating superior surface from lateral surface of thalamus, its lateral portion containing the stria medullaris.

t. ventriculi quarti. SYN: *ligula.* The thickened line of attachment of the arachnoid to lateral surface of the medulla.

t. ventriculi tertii. SYN: *stria medullaris thalami.* The taenia of the third ventricle.

Taenia (te′nĭ-ă). A genus of parasitic flatworms belonging to the class *Cestoda*, phylum *Platyhelminthes.* They are elongated, ribbonlike worms consisting of a scolex, usually armed, and a chain of segments (proglottids). Adults live as intestinal parasites of vertebrates; larvae parasitize both vertebrates and invertebrates which serve as intermediate hosts. SEE: *taeniasis, tapeworm.*

T. rata. *Diphyllobothrium latum.* SYN: *fish tapeworm.* Causes vitamin B_{12} deficiency in the host.

T. saginata. SYN: *beef tapeworm.* Tapeworm whose larval stages live in cattle, the adult living in the intestine of man. Humans acquire it by eating insufficiently cooked beef infested with the encysted larval form (*cysticercus* or *bladder worm*). Adult worms may reach a length of 15 to 20 ft. or longer.

T. solium. SYN: *pork tapeworm.* Tapeworm whose larval stages live in hogs, the adult living in the intestine of man. Humans acquire it by eating insufficiently cooked pork infested with larval form. Infected pork containing the bladder worm (*Cysticercus cellulosae*) is called *measly* pork. The cysticerci may also develop in humans, infection occurring from self-infection with eggs from contaminated hands or by hatching of eggs liberated in the intestine.

taeniacide (tē′nĭ-ă-sīd). An agent which kills tapeworms.

taeniasis (tē″nī′ă-sĭs). Condition of being infested with tapeworms of the genus *Taenia, q.v.* SEE: *tapeworm.*

taeniform (tē′nĭ-form). Having the structure of, or resembling a tapeworm.

taenifuge (tē″nĭ′fūj). An agent which expels tapeworms.

taeniophobia (tē″nĭ-ō-fō′bĭ-ă). Morbid fear of becoming infested with tapeworms.

tagging. Making a chemical or organic material easily measured or detected by using isotopes of the substance or by introducing radioactive elements into the formula. This technic is used to follow the metabolic path of substances as they travel through the body.

tagliacotian operation (tăl-yă-kō′shăn). Plastic operation on the nose in which skin is used from another part of the body. SYN: *rhinoplasty.*

tagma (tăg′mă) (pl. *tagmas, tagmatas*) [G. *tagma*, a thing arranged]. An aggregate of molecules; protoplasm.

tail (tāl) [A.S. *taegel*]. Posterior, long, flexible terminus, as the extremity of the spinal column. SEE: *cauda.*

t. bone. Bone at caudal end of spine. SYN: *coccyx.*

tailor's cramp or spasm (tā′lor) An occupational neurosis characterized by spasm of the muscles of the arms and hands.

Tait's law (tāt). Exploratory laparotomy should be made in every case of obscure abdominal or pelvic disease which is a threat to health or life.

T's. operation. Repair of a torn perineum. SYN: *perineorrhaphy.*

take. A non-medical term used to indicate satisfactory response to smallpox vaccination or skin graft.

talalgia (tăl-ăl′jĭ-ă) [L. *talus*, heel, + G. *algos*, pain]. SYN: *pternalgia.* Pain in the heel or ankle.

talc, talcum (tălk, tălk′ŭm) [L. *talcum*, powder]. Powdered soapstone; a soft, soapy powder; native hydrous magnesium silicate used as a dusting powder.

talipes (tăl′ĭ-pēz) [L. *talus*, heel, + *pēs*, foot]. Any of a number of deformities of the foot, esp. those occurring congenitally; a nontraumatic deviation of the foot in the direction of one or the other of the four lines of movement, or of two of these combined.

t. arcua′tus. Exaggerated normal arch of the foot. SYN: *t. cavus.*

t. calcaneus (flexion). Heel alone touching the ground, the patient walking on inner side of heel. Often follows infantile paralysis of muscle of tendo Achillis.

t. cavus. Same as *t. arcuatus.*

t. equinus (extension). Form with walking on the toes.

t. percavus. Excessive plantar curvature.

t. valgus (abduction). Form with everted foot.

t. varus (adduction). With inverted foot.

talipomanus (tăl-ĭp-ŏm'ăn-ŭs) [L. *talus*, ankle, + *pēs*, foot, + *manus*, hand] Deformity of the hand in which it is twisted out of shape. SYN: *clubhand.*

talocalcaneal (tā''lō-kăl-kā'nē-ăl) [" + *calcaneum*, heel bone]. Pertaining to the talus and calcaneus, bones of the tarsus.

talocrural (tā-lō-krū'răl) [" + *crus, crur-*, leg]. Pertaining to the talus and leg bones.

t. articulation. The ankle joint, a ginglymus or hinge joint.

talonid (tal'ō-nĭd) [M.E. *talon*, from L. *talus*, heel]. The crushing region, the post. part of a lower molar tooth.

talus (tā'lŭs) [L. *talus*, ankle]. [NA]. The ankle bone articulating with the tibia, fibula, calcaneus, and navicular bone. SYN: *astragalus.*

tambour (tam'boor) [Fr. *tambour*, drum]. A shallow, drum-shaped appliance used in transmitting and registering arterial pulsations, blood pressure, respiratory movements, peristaltic contractions and other slight movements.

tampol. A medicated tampon.

tampon (tam'pon) [Fr. *tampon*, plug]. A roll or pack made of various absorbent substances, cotton, rayon, wool, gauze, used to arrest or absorb secretions or hemorrhage from a wound or body cavity.

Mikulicz drain or tampon is a capillary drain on a large scale and consists of a square piece of iodoform gauze of requisite size, placed in a cavity and filled with narrow strips of plain gauze until the necessary degree of compression is secured. Used where there is parenchymatous oozing. Serves as a tampon to arrest bleeding and also acts as a capillary drain.

Rectal tampon made of piece of rubber tubing, size of thumb, 12 in. in length, covered with iodoform gauze. Into this tube is inserted a glass cylinder 3 in. in length, over which the rubber tubing should extend 2 in. An umbrella of iodoform gauze, 12x12 in., is fastened to the tube by tying a silk ligature over it at a point corresponding with the glass cylinder. Strips of sterilized gauze are used in packing the space bet. the tube and umbrella or mantle of gauze after the tube has been inserted into rectum.

t., menstrual. An absorbent material suitably shaped and prepared to provide a hygienic means of absorbing menstrual fluid in the vagina. A cord is attached and this remains outside the vagina to facilitate removal. Most of these tampons are provided with hygienic disposable paper applicators.

t., nasal. Soft rubber bulb, dilated with compressed air, for plugging nostrils to stop hemorrhage from the nose.

tamponade, tamponage (tăm-pŏn-ād', tăm'pŏn-āj) [Fr. *tampon*, plug]. To use or make use of a tampon.

t., cardiac. Condition resulting from accumulation of excess fluid in the pericardium. May result from pericarditis or injuries to the heart or great blood vessels, with accumulation of blood.

tannin (tăn'ĭn). 1. Acid substance found in bark of certain plants and trees or their products, usually from nutgall. Found in coffee and to a greater extent in tea. 2. Any of several substances containing tannin.

ACTION AND USES: Astringent, antidote for various poisons, for burns, and as a hemostatic. It is constipating. It is partly eliminated in the urine as gallic acid.

tantalum (tan'tă-lŭm). A metallic element derived from tantalite. SYMB: Ta. At. wt. 180.948; at. no. 73. Because it is non-corrosive and malleable, it has been used to repair cranial defects and as a wire suture.

tap (tăp) 1. [A.S. *taeppa*, tap]. To puncture or to empty of fluid by paracentesis. 2. [O. Fr. *taper*, of imitative origin]. A slight blow.

tape. To wrap a part with a long bandage made of adhesive tape or other types of material such as linen.

tapetum (tă-pē'tŭm) [L. *tapete*, a carpet]. A layer of fibers from the corpus callosum forming roof and lateral walls of inf. and post. horns of lateral ventricles of the brain. Fibers pass to temporal and occipital lobes.

tapeworm (tāp'worm) [A.S. *taeppe*, a narrow band, + *wurm*, worm]. Any of the species of parasitic worms belonging to the class *Cestoda*, phylum *Platyhelminthes.* A typical tapeworm consists of a *scolex*, with hooks and suckers for attachment, and a series of segments or *proglottids*, which vary in number from a few to several thousand. New proglottids are budded off of the scolex, so that a worm is actually a linear colony consisting of *immature, mature* and *ripe* or *gravid proglottids.*

Adults live as endoparasites in the intestine. The terminal ripe proglottids containing the ova break off and pass out with the feces. Upon disintegration eggs develop into minute six-hooked *oncospheres* which when ingested by proper intermediate host, usually another vertebrate, develop in muscle tissues into an encysted larva known as a *cysticercus* or *bladder worm.* Infestation occurs when uncooked meat containing bladder worms is eaten. These develop into the mature adult in the primary host.

Species of medical importance are: *Diphyllobothrium latum, Echinococcus granulosus, Hymenolepis nana, H. diminuta, Taenia saginata,* and *T. solium, q.v.*

Also see *cysticercus, cysticercosis hydatid, parganum, taeniasis.*

SYM: Often absent. If numerous, may cause intestinal obstruction. Occasionally mild systemic symptoms may occur from absorption of metabolic wastes. Sometimes there are dyspeptic symptoms.

t., armed. *Taenia solium*, the pork tapeworm, whose scolex possesses a row of hooks about the rostellum.

t., beef. *Taenia saginata, q.v.*

t., dog. *Dipylidium caninum, q.v.*

t., dwarf. *Hymenolepis nana, q.v.*

t., fish. *Diphyllobothrium latum, q.v.*

t., mouse. *Hymenolepis diminuta.*

t., pork. *Taenia solium, q.v.*

t., rat. *Hymenolepis diminuta.*

taphephobia, taphophobia (tăf″ĕ-fō′bĭ-ă, -ō-fō′bĭ-ă) [G. *taphos,* grave, + *phobos,* fear]. Abnormal fear of being buried alive.

tapinocephalic (tăp″ĭn-ō-sĕf-al′ĭk) [G. *tapeinos,* lying low, + *kephalē,* head]. Pert. to flatness of top of cranium.

tapinocephaly (tăp″ĭn-ō-sĕf′ă-lĭ) [" + *kephalē,* head]. Flatness of top of the skull.

tapioca (tăp″ĭ-ō′kă) [Portuguese]. COMP: The starchy substance of the cassava plant; a strictly carbohydrate food.

COOKED AS CREAM PUDDING: 100 gm. Calories: 134. Other values: 5.0 gm. protein; 5.1 gm. fat; 17.1 gm. carbohydrate; 105 mg. calcium.

tapiroid (tā′pĭr-oyd) [Spanish *tapir,* tapir, + G. *eidos,* form]. Resembling a tapir's snout; said of an elongated cervix uteri.

tapotement (tă-pōt-mon′) [Fr.]. Percussion in massage.

It is divided into: (a) *Beating* with the clenched hand; used for sciatica and muscular atrophy. (b) *Clapping,* performed with the palm of the hand; used to reach superficial nerves. (c) *Hacking,* with the ulnar border of the hand; used principally around a nerve center and upon the muscles. (d) *Punctuation,* with the tips of the fingers; used principally around the heart and upon the head.

The strength of the manipulations is a principal point in the massage treatment, and care must be taken not to bruise the patient. As a rule, begin with moderate pressure, ascertaining from the patient his sensation. White petrolatum or some other oleaginous substance should be used to avoid abrading the skin. SEE: *massage.*

tapping (tăp′ĭng) [O.Fr. *taper,* of imitative origin]. Percussion in massage. SYN: *tapotement.* 2. [A.S. *taeppa,* tap]. Removal of fluid from a cavity. SYN: *paracentesis.* SEE: *thoracentesis.*

tarantism (tăr′ăn-tĭzm) [Italian *Taranto,* tarantula, + G. *-ismos,* condition]. A nervous affection marked by stupor, melancholy and uncontrollable dancing mania.

Popularly attributed to bite of tarantula.

tarantula (tă-răn′tū-lă). A large venomous spider much feared by many people; however, its bite is relatively harmless. SEE: *spider bite.*

tarassis (tă-ras′is) [G. *tarakis,* disturbance]. Hysteria in the male.

Tardieu's ecchymoses or **spots** (tar-dyu′). Subpleural spots of ecchymosis following death by strangulation.

tardive. Descriptive of a disease wherein the characteristic sign or symptom appears late in the course of the disease.

target (tar′gĕt) [O.Fr. *targette*]. 1. PT: The electrode on which cathode rays within an x-ray tube are focused and from which roentgen rays are emitted; usually of a heavy metal such as tungsten. 2. A tiny figure on an ophthalmometer's arm whose image is used to determine the amount of corneal astigmatism. SYN: *mire, q.v.*

t. cell. An abnormal erythrocyte with rounded central area which stains deeply, surrounded by a lightly staining area which in turn is surrounded by denser cytoplasm at the periphery of the cell, the whole somewhat resembling a target with a bull's eye; found in certain types of anemia and after splenectomy.

t. cell anemia. Thalassemia, *q.v.*

t. organ. The organ or structure toward which the effects of a drug, hormone, or therapeutic agent are primarily directed.

Tarnier's sign (tahr-ne-ā′). A sign of coming abortion; the disappearance of angle bet. upper and lower uterine segments in pregnancy.

tarsadenitis (tar-săd″ĕ-nī′tĭs). Inflammation of the tarsal or meibomian glands of eyelid.

tarsal (tar′săl) [G. *tarsos,* flat of foot, edge of eyelid]. 1. Pertaining to the tarsus or supporting plate of the eyelid. 2. Pertaining to the ankle or tarsus.

t. arches. Two branches, sup. and inf. of the median palpebral artery supplying the eyelid.

t. bones. The seven bones of the ankle.

t. cartilage. SYN: *palpebral cartilage.* The dense connective tissue of the tarsus of eyelid. It is not cartilage.

t. glands. SYN: *meibomian glands.* Branched alveolar, sebaceous glands embedded in tarsus and opening on margin of eyelid.

t. lacrimal glands. Accessory lacrimal glands located on inner surface of eyelids, esp. upper lid.

tarsalgia (tar-săl′jĭ-ă) [G. *tarsos,* flat of the foot, + *algos,* pain]. Pain in tarsus or ankle. May be due to flatfoot, shortening of Achilles tendon, or other causes.

tarsalia (tar-sā′lĭ-ă) (sing. *tarsale*) [L.]. The tarsal bones.

tarsalis (tar-sā′lĭs) [L.]. One of the tarsal muscles. SEE: *Table of Muscles in Appendix.*

tarsectomy (tar-sĕk′tō-mĭ) [G. *tarsos,* flat of the foot, edge of eyelid, + *ektomē,* excision]. 1. Excision of tarsus or a tarsal bone. 2. Removal of tarsal plate of an eyelid.

tarsitis (tar-sī′tĭs) [" + *-itis,* inflammation]. 1. Inflammation of tarsus of the foot. 2. Inflammation of eyelid's border. SYN: *blepharitis.*

tarso- [G.]. Combining form meaning the *flat of the foot, edge of the eyelid.*

tarsocheiloplasty (tar″sō-kī′lō-plăs-tĭ) [G. *tarsos,* edge of eyelid, flat of the foot, + *cheilos,* lip, + *plassein,* to form]. Plastic surgery of borders of the eyelid.

tarsoclasia, tarsoclasis (tar″sō-klā′sĭ-ă, tar-sŏk′lăs-ĭs) [" + *klasis,* a breaking]. Surgical fracture of the tarsus for correction of clubfoot.

tarsomalacia (tar″sō-mă-lā′sĭ-ă) [" + *malakia,* a softening]. Softening of the tarsal cartilages of the eyes.

tarsometatarsal (tar″sō-mĕt-ă-tar′săl) [" + *meta,* between, + *tarsos,* flat of the foot]. Pert. to the tarsus and the metatarsus.

tarsophyma (tar″sō-fī′mă) [" + *phyma,* a growth]. Any tarsal tumor of the eyelid. SYN: *hordoleum, sty.*

tarsoplasia, tarsoplasty (tar″sō-plā′zĭ-ă, tar′sō-plăs″tĭ) [" + *plassein,* to form]. Plastic surgery of margin of the eyelid. SYN: *blepharoplasty.*

tarsoptosis (tars-ŏp-tō′sĭs) [" + *ptōsis,* a dropping]. Falling of the tarsus. SYN: *flatfoot.*

tarsorrhaphy (tar-sor′ă-fĭ) [G. *tarsos* edge of eyelid, flat of the foot, + *rhaphē,* a seam]. The operation of uniting the edges of the lids at the outer commissure for the purpose of reducing the width of the palpebral fissure.

tarsotomy (tar-sŏt′ō-mĭ) [" + *tomē,* a cutting]. 1. Incision of tarsal cartilage of an eyelid. 2. Any surgical incision of the tarsus of the foot.

tarsus (tar'sus) (pl. *tarsi*) [G. *tarsos*, a flat structure]. 1. The ankle, with its seven bones located between bones of lower leg and metatarsus. It forms the proximal portion of the foot. It consists of the following bones: *calcaneus* (os calcis), *talus* (astragalus), *cuboid* (os cuboideum), *navicular* (scaphoid), and *first, second*, and *third cuneiform* bones. The talus articulates with the tibia and fibula; the cuboid and cuneiform bones with the metatarsals.

SEE: *foot, skeleton, names of individual bones.* 2. SYN: *tarsal plates.* A curved plate of dense white fibrous tissue forming supporting structure of eyelid.

tartar (tar'ter) [G. *tartaron*, dregs]. Calcareous matter deposited upon the teeth

t., cream of. Potassium bitartrate.

tartaric acid (tar-tar'ĭk). An acid derived from lees of wine and certain plants, occurring in 4 forms. Sometimes used in artificial lemonades or in effervescent drinks and is rarely toxic unless taken in large doses.

tart cells. Certain cells containing altered nuclear material appearing along with L.E. cells in suspensions of leukocytes or bone marrow cells from patients with disseminated lupus erythematosus.

tartrate. A salt of tartaric acid.

taste (tāst) [O.Fr. *taster*, to feel, to taste]. 1. To try or perceive by touch of the tongue. 2. A chemical sense dependent upon sense organs on the surface of the tongue when they are in contact with a substance to ascertain its attributes, the nervous impulses being carried to the brain by the lingual (from the anterior two-thirds of the surface) and the glossopharyngeal (from the posterior third) nerves.

Taste sensation is experienced through stimulation of gustatory nerve endings in the tongue. There are 4 fundamental taste sensations: *sweet, bitter, sour*, and *salt*.

Loss of taste may be due to bilateral disease of chorda tympani nerve and of gustatory fibers of the glossopharyngeal nerve.

RS: *ageusia, agnosia, alliaceous, allotriogeustia, amblygeustia, appetite, cacogeusia, calyculus gustatorii, degustation, dysgeusia, gustation, gustatory, hypergeusia, hypogeusia, oxygeusia, parageusia, pseudogeusia.*

t., after. The persistence of a taste sensation after removal of original stimulus.

t. area. Area in cerebral cortex at lower end of somesthetic area.

t. blindness. Inability to taste certain substances such as phenylthiocarbamide (PTC). May be due to a hereditary factor which is transmitted as a mendelian recessive trait.

t. buds. Sensory end organs which mediate the sensation of taste. They are oval structures located on surface of tongue, esp. sides of circumvallate papillae, on soft palate, epiglottis, and portions of pharynx. Each contains sensory, gustatory (taste) cells and supporting (sustentacular) cells. When stimulated by chemical stimuli, they give rise to sense of taste. SEE: *taste cells.*

t. cells. SYN: *gustatory cells.* Neuroepithelial cells within a taste bud which serve as receptors for the sense of taste. Each possesses a terminal *taste hair* which projects through the inner *taste pore.*

T. A. T. Abbr. for *toxin-antitoxin* or *tetanus antitoxin.*

tattooing. Indelible marking of the skin produced by introducing minute amounts of pigments into the skin, usually done to form decorative patterns. Technic may also be used to conceal a corneal leucoma or to mask pigmented areas of skin.

taurocholemia (taw"rō-kō-lē'mĭ-ă) [G. *tauros*, a bull, + *cholē*, bile, + *aima*, blood]. Taurocholic acid in the blood.

tauto- [G.] A form meaning *the same.*

tautomeral, tautomeric (taw-tŏm'ĕr-ăl -to-mĕr'ĭk) [G. *tauto*, the same, + *meros*, a part]. Noting certain neurons which send processes to the white matter on the same side of the spinal cord.

tautomerism (taw-tŏm'ĕr-ĭzm) [" + " + *-ismos*, condition]. Phenomenon in which two formulae are possible and exist in dynamic equilibrium so that as the amount of one substance is altered the second is changed into the other form in order to maintain the equilibrium.

tautorotation (taw"tō-rō-tā'shŭn) [" + L. *rotāre*, to turn round]. A change in specific rotation which occurs when a solution of certain sugars stands a while.

taxis (tăk'sĭs) [G. *taxis*, arrangement]. 1. Manual replacement of displaced structures. 2. The response of an organism to its environment; a turning toward (*positive taxis*) or away from (*negative taxis*) a particular stimulus, e.g. *chemotaxis, q.v.*

t., bipolar. Replacing of a retroverted uterus by drawing down the cervix in the vagina and pressing upward through the rectum.

taxonomy (tăks-ŏn'ō-mĭ) [" + *nomos*, law]. Laws and principles of classification of animals and plants.

Tay-Sachs disease [Warren Tay, English physician, 1843-1927; Bernard Sachs, American neurologist, 1858-1944]. The infantile form of amaurotic family idiocy characterized by a cherry-red macula lutea. It is a disorder of lipid metabolism. SEE: *amaurotic familial idiocy, infantile.*

T. b. Abbr. for ***tubercle bacillus*** and for ***tuberculosis.***

Tb. Abbr. for *terbium.*

tbsp. Abbr. for *tablespoon.*

Tc. SYMB. for *technetium.*

t. d. s. Abbr. meaning *take 3 times a day.*

Te. 1. SYMB. for *tellurium.* 2. Abbr. for *tetanus.*

tea (tē). 1. An infusion of a medicinal plant. 2. Leaves of plant *Thea chinensis*, from which a beverage is made.

COMP: It contains dextrin, gum, nitrogenous extracts, oxalates, phosphate of potassium, and its active principle, *theine*, a trimethyl xanthine resembling caffeine. Tea also contains tannin, an astringent, the amount in tea being two to three times that in coffee.

t., black. Tea made from leaves which have been fermented before they are dried.

t., green. Tea prepared by heating leaves in open trays.

t., Paraguay copper. A tea made from the leaves and stems of the *Ilex paraguaiensis.* It is a stimulating drink and contains volatile oil, tannin, and caffeine.

TEAB. Abbr. for *tetraethylammonium bromide.*

TEAC. Abbr. for *tetraethylammonium chloride, q.v.*

tear (tār). To separate or pull apart by force.

tears (tērz) [A.S. *tēar*]. 1. The watery saline solution secreted by the lacrimal glands, *q.v.* 2. Hardened lumps or tearlike drops of any gummy or resinous material.

tease (tēz) [A.S. *taesan*, to pluck]. To separate a tissue into minute parts with a needle to prepare it for the microscope.

teaspoon. Abbr. *tsp.* A spoon holding approximately 5 ml. (cc.). Teaspoons used in the home vary from 3 to 6 ml. When a teaspoon dose is prescribed or ordered, give 5 ml. of the substance.

teat (tēt) [M.E. *tete*, from A.S. *tit, teat*]. 1. The nipple of the mammary gland. SYN: *papilla mammilla.* 2. Any protuberance resembling a nipple.

teatulation (tēt"ū-lā'shŭn) [A.S. *tit*, teat]. The development of a nipplelike elevation.

technic (tĕk-nēk') [Fr. from G. *technē*, art]. Expertness in performing or carrying out the details of a procedure or of an operation.

technical (tĕk'nĭ-kal) [G. *technikos*, skilled]. Requiring technic or special skill.

technician (tĕk-nĭsh'ăn) [G. *technē*, art]. One skilled in a special art.

t., medical laboratory. A person who has received special training in medical laboratory procedures.

technique (tek-nēk'). Same as *technic*, *q.v.*

techno- [G.]. Combining form meaning *art, skill.*

technologist (tĕk"nŏl'ō-jĭst). A technician, esp. one who is highly trained.

t., medical. A medical technician who is certified by the Registry of Medical Technologists of the American Society of Clinical Pathologists.

tecno- [G.]. Combining form meaning *child.*

tectocephaly (tĕk-tō-sĕf'ăl-ĭ) [L. *tectum*, roof, + G. *kephalē*, head]. Possession of a boat-shaped cranium. SYN: *scaphocephalism.*

tectonic (tĕk-tŏn'ĭk) [G. *tektōn*, a builder]. Relating to plastic surgery.

tectorial (tĕk-tō'rĭ-ăl) [L. *tectum*, roof]. Pert. to a roof or covering. SYN: *tegmental.*

tectorium (tĕk-tō'rĭ-ŭm) [L. *tectōrium*, a covering]. 1. Any rooflike structure. 2. Corti's membrane. SYN: *membrana tectoria.*

tectospinal (tĕk"tō-spī'năl) [L. *tectum*, roof, + *spina*, thorn]. From the tectum mesencephali to the spinal cord.

t. tract. A tract of white fibers of the spinal cord passing from the tectum of midbrain and going down through the medulla to the spinal cord. It begins on one side and crosses to the other.

tectum (tĕk'tŭm) [L. *tectum*, roof]. 1. Any structure serving as, or resembling, a roof. 2. The dorsal portion of the midbrain consisting of the sup. and inf. colliculi (corpora quadrigemina).

t. mesencephali. Roof of the midbrain including the corpora quadrigemina.

teeth (tēth) (sing. *tooth*) [A.S. *tōth*, tooth]. Hard, bony projections in jaws serving as organs of mastication, there being 32 permanent teeth, 16 in each jaw. They include the following types: incisors, canines, (cuspids), premolars (bicuspids), and molars. (See table below.) An *average* child should have 6 teeth at 1 year, 12 at 18 months, 16 at 2 years, and 20 at 2½ years. A child may be born with teeth, and in other cases the teeth may not appear until 16 months.

t., anterior. Two canine and four incisors in each jaw.

t., auditory. SYN: *Husch'ke's a. teeth.* Minute toothlike projections along the free margin of the labium vestibulare of the cochlea.

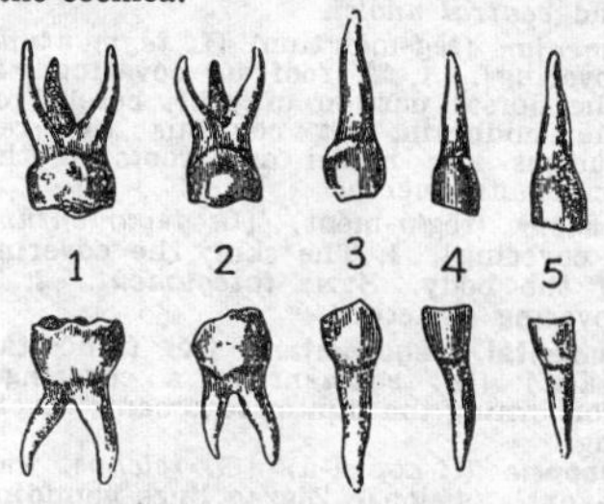

TEETH, DECIDUOUS.
1. Second molar. 2. First molar. 3. Canine. 4. Second incisor. 5. First incisor.

t., back. All posterior teeth (to the canines) of the molar series.

t., deciduous. Temporary or milk teeth; those comprising the first set which are shed.

t., Hutchinson's. Lateral incisors of upper jaw when pegged and central incisors of same jaw having convex sides and crescentic notches on their cutting edges; noted only on permanent teeth, indicating hereditary syphilis.

t., malacot'ic. Those which are apt to decay, soft in structure and white in color.

t., milk. SYN: *deciduous teeth.* The first set of teeth.

t., permanent. Those of the second dentition, replacing the deciduous teeth.

t., sclerotic. Yellowish teeth that are naturally hard and not subject to ready decay.

t., secondary. The permanent teeth erupting about the 6th year and being complete about the 15th year.

DECIDUOUS TEETH

Name	*Erupt (months)*
Lower central incisors	5-9
Upper central incisors	8-12
Upper lateral incisors	10-12
Lower lateral incisors	12-15
Anterior (first) molars	12-15
Canines	18-24
Posterior (second) molars	24-30

PERMANENT TEETH

Name	*Erupt (years)*
First molars	6-7
Central incisors	7-8
Lateral incisors	7-8
First premolars	9-10
Second premolars	9-10
Canines	12-14
Second molars	12-15
Third molars	17-25

t., temporary. Those of the first dentition; the milk or deciduous teeth.

teething (tēth′ĭng) [A.S. *tōth,* tooth]. Eruption of the teeth. Syn: *dentition.*

tegmen (tĕg′mĕn) (pl. *tegmina*) [L. *tegmen,* covering]. A structure that covers a part.

t. mastoideum. Bony roof of mastoid cells.

t. tympani. NA. Roof of tympanum separating middle ear from cranial cavity.

t. ventriculi quarti. The roof of the fourth ventricle.

tegmental (tĕg-mĕn′tăl) [L. *tegmentum,* covering]. Relating to a tegument or tegmentum; covering.

t. field of Forel. Three masses of fibers (fields H, H_1, H_2) located in the ventral thalamus.

t. nuclei. Several masses of gray matter lying in tegmentum of midbrain and upper portion of the pons. Include the *dorsal, pedunculopontile, reticular,* and *ventral nuclei.*

tegmentum (tĕg-mĕn′tŭm) [L. *tegmentum,* covering]. 1. A roof or covering. 2. The dorsal portion of cruri cerebri of the midbrain. It contains the red nucleus and nuclei and roots of the oculomotor nerve.

tegument (tĕg′ū-mĕnt) [L. *tegumentum,* a covering]. 1. The skin; the covering of the body. Syn: *integument.* 2. A covering structure.

tegumental, tegumentary (tĕg″ū-mĕn′tăl, -tă-rĭ) [L. *tegumentum,* a covering]. Concerning the skin or tegument; covering.

teichopsia (tī-kŏp′sĭ-ă) [G. *teichos,* wall + *opsis,* vision]. Zigzag lines bounding a luminous area appearing in the visual field causing a temporary blindness in that portion of the eye, sometimes accompanying migraine headaches and mental or physical strain. Syn: *scotoma, scintillating; scotoma, fortification spectra.*

teinodynia (tī″nō-dĭn′ĭ-ă) [G. *tenōn,* tendon, + *odynē,* pain]. Pain in the tendons. Syn: *tenodynia.*

tela (tē′lă) [L. *tēla,* web]. Any weblike structure.

t. choroi′dea. Part of the pia mater covering roof of the 3rd and 4th cerebral ventricles.

t. subcutanea. Subcutaneous connective tissue; superficial fascia.

t. submucosa. The submucosa of the intestine.

telalgia (tĕl-ăl′jĭ-ă) [G. *tēle,* far away, + *algos,* pain]. Pain felt at a distance from its stimulus. Syn: *pain, referred.*

telangiectasia, telangiectasis (tel-ăn″jĭ-ĕk-tā′zhĭ-ă, -ĕk′tă-sĭs) [G. *telos,* end, + *aggeion,* vessel, + *ektasis,* dilatation]. Dilatation of capillaries and sometimes of terminal arteries producing an angioma of macular appearance, or hyperemic spot.

It may be as a birthmark, or become apparent in young children. May occur anywhere in the skin but is seen most frequently on the face and thighs.

t. faciei. Acne rosacea, *q.v.*

t., hereditary hemorrhagic. Syn: *Osler-Weber-Rendu disease.* A hereditary disease characterized by thinness of walls of blood vessels of nose, skin, and digestive tract and tendency to hemorrhage.

t. lymphat′ica. Tumor composed of dilated lymph vessels.

t., spider. A stellate angioma (nevus araneus).

telangiectoma (tĕl-ăn-jĭ-ĕk-tō′mă) [" + " + " + *-ōma,* tumor]. Angioma from dilatation of capillaries or arterioles. Syn: *telangioma.*

telangiitis (tĕl-ăn-jĭ-ī′tĭs) [" + " + *-itis,* inflammation]. Inflammation of the capillaries.

telangioma (tĕl″ăn-jĭ-ō′mă) [" + " + *-ōma,* tumor]. A tumor made up of dilated capillaries or arterioles.

telangiosis (tĕl-ăn-jĭ-ō′sĭs) [" + " + *-ōsis,* condition]. Disease of capillary vessels.

tele-, tel- [G.] Combining forms meaning *at a distance, far off.*

telecardiogram (tel″ē-kar′dĭ-ō-grăm) [G. *tēle,* distant, + *kardia,* heart, + *gramma,* a writing]. A cardiogram which records at a distance from the patient. Syn: *telelectrocardiogram.*

telecardiography (tĕl″ĕ-kar″dĭ-og′ră-fĭ) [" + " + *graphein,* to write]. Process of taking telecardiograms.

telecardiophone (tĕl″ĕ-kar′dĭ-ō-fōn) [" + " + *phōnē,* voice]. A stethoscope will magnify heart sounds so that they may be heard at a distance from patient.

teleceptive (tĕl-ĕ-sĕp′tĭv) [" + L. *-ceptivus,* receiving, from *capere,* to take]. Relating to a teleceptor.

teleceptor (tĕl′ĕ-sĕp-tor) [G. *tēle,* distant, + L. *ceptor,* a receiver]. Syn: *teloceptor.* A distance receptor; a sense organ that responds to stimuli arising some distance from the body. Ex: eye, ear, nose.

telecinesia (tĕl″ĕ-sĭn-ē′zĭ-ă) [" + *kinēsis,* movement]. Apparent automatic movement of an object produced without contact with any stimulus or power. Syn: *telekinesia.*

telecurietherapy (tĕl-ĕ-kū-rĭ-thĕr′ă-pĭ) [G. *tēle,* distant, + *curie* + G. *therapeia,* treatment]. Application of radium rays from a distance from a patient.

teledendrite, teledendron (tĕl-ĕ-dĕn′drīt, -dĕn′drŏn) [G. *tēle,* distant, + *dendron,* a tree]. Syn: *telodendron.* The terminal processes of an axon.

telediastolic (te″lē-dĭ-as-tol′ĭk) [G. *telos,* end, + *diastolē,* a dilatation]. Concerning the last phase of the diastole.

telegony (tĕl-ĕg′ō-nĭ) [G. *tēle,* distant, + *gonē,* offspring]. An alleged theory that the male sperm from a dam's first sexual contact modifies the blood of the female, thus influencing the offspring resulting from mating with another sire.

This is supposed to be due to the absorption of the male sperm by the mucous tissue of the female's genitals, then entering the lymphatics and blood stream.

telelectrocardiogram (tĕl″ē-lĕk″trō-kar′dĭ-ō-grăm) [" + *ēlektron,* amber (electricity), + *kardia,* heart, + *gramma,* a writing]. One taken with a galvanometer attached to the patient by a wire some distance from the instrument. Syn: *telecardiogram.*

telemeter [" + *metron,* measure]. To transmit information to a distant point by using electronic devices.

telencephalic (tĕl-ĕn-sĕf-al′ĭk) [" + *egkephalos,* brain]. Pert. to the endbrain (telencephalon).

telencephalon (tĕl-ĕ-sĕf′ă-lŏn) [G. *telos,* end, + *egkephalos,* brain]. The embryonic endbrain or ant. division of the prosencephalon from which the cerebral hemispheres, corpora striata, and rhinencephalon develop.

teleo- [G.]. Combining form meaning *perfect, complete.*

teleology (tĕl-ē-ŏl′ō-jĭ) [G. *telos,* end, + *logos,* a study]. The belief that everything is directed toward some final purpose. The doctrine of final causes.

teleopsia (tĕl-ē-ŏp′sĭ-ă). A visual disorder in which objects perceived in space have excessive depth or close objects appear far away.

teleorganic (tĕl″ē-or-găn′ĭk) [" + *organon*, organ]. Necessary to organic life. SYN: *vital*.

teleotherapeutics (tĕl″ē-ō-ther-ă-pū′tĭks) [" + *therapeutikē*, treatment]. The use of hypnotic suggestion in the treatment of disease. SYN: *suggestive therapeutics*.

telepathist (tĕl-ĕp′ă-thĭst) [G. *tēle*, distant, + *pathos*, feeling]. One who claims the ability to read the mind of others.

telepathy (tĕl-ĕp′ă-thĭ) [" + *pathos*, feeling]. Supposed communication of one mind with another at a distance without any means known to physical or psychological science.

teleradiography (tĕl″ĕ-rā-dĭ-og′ră-fĭ) [G. *tēle*, distant, + L. *radius*, ray, + G. *graphein*, to write]. Radiography with the tube about 2 meters (6½ ft.) from the body. Done to minimize distortion by having rays virtually parallel at that distance. SYN: *teleroentgenography*.

telergy (tĕl′er-jĭ) [" + *ergon*, work]. 1. Action without conscious exercise of the will. SYN: *automatism*. 2. Hypothetical action of one individual's thoughts upon brain of another by transmission of some unknown form of energy.

teleroentgenography (tĕl″ĕ-rĕnt″gĕn-ŏg′răf-ĭ) [" + *roentgen* + G. *graphein*, to write]. Radiography in which the tube is about 2 meters (6½ ft.) from the body. SYN: *teleradiography*.

telesthesia (tĕl-ĕs-thē′zĭ-ă) [" + *aisthēsis*, sensation]. 1. An impression received at a distance without normal operation of organs of sense. 2. Distance perception. SYN: *telepathy*.

telesystolic (tĕl″ĕ-sis-tol′ĭk) [G. *telos*, end, + *systolē*, contraction]. Pert. to the termination of the cardiac systole.

teletactor [" + *tactus*, touch]. A device used by the deaf to transmit vibrations to the skin.

teletherapy (tĕl-ĕ-thĕr′ă-pĭ) [G. *tēle*, distant, + *therapeia*, treatment]. Absent treatment; treatment of disease by telepathy*; method of mental healers.

tellurium (tĕl-ū′rĭ-ŭm) [L. *tellus*, *tellur-*, earth]. SYMB: Te. At. wt. 127.60. At. no. 52. A nonmetallic element used as an electric rectifier and in coloring glass.

POISONING: SYM: Garlic odor of all secretions and excretions. A disagreeable odor to the breath with suppression of perspiration and saliva, resulting in dry skin and mouth. Anorexia, nausea, drowsiness, and weakness often found.

F. A. TREATMENT: Saline cathartics, increase fluid intake, induce perspiration, otherwise treatment is symptomatic.

teloceptor. Teleceptor, *q.v.*

telodendron (tĕl-ō-dĕn′drŏn) [G. *telos*, end, + *dendron*, a tree]. The more or less diffuse arborizations at the end of an axon or its collaterals.

telolecithal (tĕl-ō-lĕs′ĭ-thăl). Term applied to an ovum in which the yolk is concentrated at one end.

telolemma (tĕl″ō-lĕm′mă). The membrane covering motor end plate in a striated muscle fiber.

telophase (tĕl′ō-fāz) [G. *telos*, end, + *phasis*, a phase]. The final phase or stage of mitosis (karyokinesis) during which reconstruction of the daughter nuclei takes place and the cytoplasm of the cell divides giving rise to two daughter cells.

telosynapsis (tĕl″ō-sĭn-ăp′sĭs). End-to-end union of pairs of homologous chromosomes during gametogenesis.

telotism (tĕl′ō-tĭzm) [" + *-ismos*, process]. The entire performance of a function, as that of one of the senses.

TEM. Abbr. for *triethylene melamine*. SEE: *nitrogen mustard*.

temperament (tĕm′per-ă-mĕnt) [L. *temperamentum*, mixture]. Individual peculiarity of physical and mental organization.

t., bilious. Temperament characterized by olive or dark skin, brunet hair, well-developed physique, a hot or quick temper.

t., choleric. Same as *bilious t.*

t., melancholic. Temperament characterized by a state of depression; melancholia.

t., sanguine. Temperament marked by a ruddy complexion, fair hair, light-colored eyes, active blood circulation, and a generally optimistic mental outlook.

temperate (tĕm′per-ĭt) Moderate; not excessive.

temperature (tĕm′per-ă-tūr) [L. *temperatura*, proportion]. 1. Degree of heat of a living body; loosely, body heat above normal. 2. Degree of hotness or coldness of a substance.

(a) Body temperature varies with different organs' areas, and with the time of day. The temperature in the *liver* may be 105.1° F., while that under the *tongue* is 98.6° F.; the temperature under the *arm* at 2 P. M. may be 99.0° F. and at 2 A. M. 96.7° F.; the *rectal* temperature is likely to be 0.5 to 1.0° F. above the oral.

One of the mechanisms for raising temperature is muscular work (as in shivering); one for lowering it is sweating. The interplay of such processes keeps the body temperature constant.

(b) Body temperature may be measured by a clinical thermometer placed in the mouth, rectum, or under the arm. Rectal temperature is usually from 0.5 to 1.0° F. higher than by mouth; axillary temperature about 0.5° F. lower than by mouth. Oral temperature may be inaccurate if taken just after the patient has eaten or drunk cold substances.

Body temperature is the result of the balance between *heat production* and *heat loss*. 85% of body heat is lost through the skin, the remainder via lungs and through digestive and urinary excretions. Regulation of body temperature is accomplished principally through thermoregulatory centers located in the hypothalamus. Elevation of temperature above normal is designated fever (pyrexia), subnormal temperature is *hypothermia*.

Temperature Indications

107° F. Generally fatal except in intermittent fever.
106° F. Intense fever.
105° F. High fever, dangerous.
104° F. Severe fever.
102° F. Moderate fever.
101° F. Slight fever.
98.6° F. Normal.
98° F. Subnormal.
96° F. Subnormal.
94° F. Algid collapse.
93° F. Fatal collapse except in cholera.
80-84° F. Fatal.

t., absolute. T. measured from absolute zero, which is minus 273° C.

t., axillary. Thermometer is placed in apex of axilla with arm pressed closely to side of body. Temperature obtained by this method is usually 0.5 to 1.0° F. lower than oral.

t., body. The t. of the body.

t., critical. The t. below which a gas may be converted to liquid form by pressure.

t. curve. Line indicating the fluctuations of t. for a given period.

t. equivalents. SEE: *Fahrenheit scale.* To convert Fahrenheit t. to Centigrade use this formula: $°C = \frac{(F. - 32)}{9} \times 5.$ To convert Centigrade t. to Fahrenheit use this formula: $°F = \frac{9}{5}\ C. + 32.$

t., inverse. Condition in which body temperature is higher in the morning than in the evening.

t., maximum. BACTERIAL: T. above which growth will not take place.

t., mean. The average t. for a stated period in a given locality.

t., minimum. BACTERIAL: T. below which growth will not take place.

t., normal. T. of the body in health, 98.6° F. (37° C.) in man.

t., optimum. T. at which an operation is best carried out, as the culture of a given organism or the action of a new enzyme.

t., oral. Thermometer is held for three minutes under patient's tongue with the lips closed. It should not be taken for at least 10 min. after ingestion of hot or cold liquids. It is *not* advisable for infants, mouth-breathers, comatose patients, or those extremely ill.

t., rectal. The thermometer should be inserted at least 1½ in. and allowed to remain 3-5 minutes. Do not take following a rectal operation or if rectum is diseased. Rectal temperature is more accurate than either oral or axillary temperatures. It averages about 1° F. higher than by mouth.

t., room. T. bet. 65-80° F.

t. scale. Graduated device marked at regular intervals on a thermometer to register temperature.
RS: *thermometer scale.*

t. scale, absolute. One in which absolute zero (minus 273° C. or minus 459.4° F.) is taken as zero. This is the point at which gases theoretically are without volume, molecular motion has ceased, and there is complete absence of heat.

t. senses. The sensations of *warmth* resulting from raising the temperature of the skin and that of *cold* aroused by lowering it. The sensation of warmth is mediated by *Ruffini's corpuscles,* that of cold by *end-bulbs of Krause.* These receptors are distributed so as to form *cold* and *warm spots* on the skin. There are an estimated 250,000 cold spots, 30,000 warm spots. Afferent impulses from receptors, on reaching the thalamus, may give rise to crude uncritical temperature sensations; on being relayed to the somesthetic area of the cortex they result in discrete and fairly well localized sensations of heat and cold. Adaptation is rapid.

t., subnormal. T. below the normal of 98.6° F.

t., zero. T. at which heat and cold are not felt by a sensory end organ.

temperature, *words pert. to:* algid, a. stage, algogenic, Baruch's sign, chauffage, cold, enthermic, frigid, frigidity, frigorific, hardening, heat, infant, myothermic, pseudocrisis, respiration, temperature scale, "therm-" words.

template. A pattern, mold, or form used as a guide in duplicating a shape, structure, or device.

temple (tĕm'pl) [O.Fr. from L. *tempora,* pl. of *tempus,* temple]. The region of head in front of ear and over the zygomatic arch.

tempolabile (tĕm"pō-lā'bl) [L. *tempus,* time, + *labilis,* unstable]. Becoming altered spontaneously within a definite time.

temporal (tĕm'por-ăl) [L. *temporalis,* pert. to time; pert. to temples]. 1. Pert. to or limited in time. 2. Relating to the temples.

t. bone. A bone on both sides of the skull at its base. SYN: *os temporale.* SEE: *Arnold's canal, mastoid, petrosa, petrosal, squamous, styloid process.*

Composed of squamous, mastoid, and petrous portions, the latter enclosing the organ of hearing.

t. line. One of two lines on lateral surface of frontal and parietal bones which mark upper limit of temporal fossa.

t. lobe. Lobe of cerebrum located laterally and below frontal and occipital lobes. Contains auditory receptive areas.

temporalis (tĕm"pō-rā'lĭs) [L.]. Muscle in temporal fossa which elevates the mandible. SEE: *Muscles, Table of, in Appendix.*

temporo- [L.]. Combining form meaning *temples of the head.*

temporomaxillary (tĕm"por-ō-măks'ĭl-lā-rĭ) [L. *tempus, tempor-,* temple]. Pert. to the temporal and maxillary bones.

temporooccipital (tĕm"por-ō-ŏk-sĭp'ĭ-tăl) [" + *occipitalis,* pert. to the occiput]. Pert. to the temporal and occipital bones or their regions.

temporosphenoid (tĕm"por-ō-sfē'noyd) [" + G. *sphēn,* wedge, + *eidos,* form]. Pert. to the temporal and sphenoid bones.

temulence (tĕm'ū-lĕns) [L. *temulentia,* intoxication]. Drunkenness; intoxication.

tenacious (tē-nā'shŭs) [L. *tenax, tenac-,* holding]. Adhering to; adhesive; retentive.

tenaculum (tĕn-ăk'ū-lŭm) [L. *tenaculum,* a holder]. Sharp, hooklike, pointed instrument with slender shank for grasping and holding a part, as an artery.

t., abdominal. Longer than others with smaller hook. *Sim's, Emmet's, Kelly's,* etc.

t., uterine. Heavier and shorter hook used for manipulating uterus.

tenalgia (tĕn-ăl'jĭ-ă) [G. *tenōn,* tendon, + *algos,* pain]. Pain in a tendon. SYN: *tenodynia.*

t. crepitans. Inflammation of a tendon sheath which on movement results in a crackling sound. SYN: *tendosynovitis crepitans.*

tenderness (tĕn'dĕr-nĕs) [M.E. *tendre,* from L. *tener,* tender]. Sensitiveness to pain upon pressure, usually cutaneous.

t., rebound. Production of or intensification of pain when pressure is released.

tendinitis (tĕn-dĭn-ī'tĭs) [L. *tendo,* tendon, + G. *-itis,* inflammation]. Inflammation of a tendon. SYN: *tenonitis, 1, tenontitis.*

tendinoplasty (tĕn'dĭ-nō-plăs"tĭ) [" + G. *plassein,* to form]. Plastic surgery of tendons. SYN: *tenontoplasty, tenoplasty.*

tendinosuture (tĕn″dĭn-ō-sū′tūr) [" + *sutura*, a seam]. The suturing of a divided tendon. Syn: *tenorrhaphy.*

tendinous (tĕn′dĭn-ŭs) [L. *tendinōsus*, like a tendon]. Pert. to, composed of, or resembling tendons.

t. synovitis. Inflammation of a tendon's synovial sheath.

tendo (tĕn′dō) (pl. *tendines*) [L. *tendo*, tendon]. A tendon.

t. Achil′lis. The tendon of the soleus and gastrocnemius muscles inserted into tuberosity of the os calcis. See: *leg for Illustration.*

t. calca′neus. NA. Same as *t. Achillis.*

tendolysis (tĕn-dŏl′ĭ-sĭs) [" + G. *lysis*, a loosening]. The process of freeing a tendon from adhesions.

tendon (tĕn′dŭn) [L. *tendo*, tendon] Fibrous connective tissue serving for the attachment of muscles to bones and other parts. Syn: *sinew.*

RS: *Achilles' jerk, achillobursitis achillotomy, aponeurotomy, chorda sinew, "teno-" words.*

t., Achilles. The large tendon at lower end of gastrocnemius muscle, inserted into the *os calcis.*

It is the strongest and thickest one in the body.

t., calcaneous. Achilles* tendon.

t. cells. Fibroblasts of white fibrous connective tissue of tendons arranged in parallel rows.

t., central. The central portion of the diaphragm consisting of a flat aponeurosis in which fibers of the diaphragm are inserted.

t. reflex. Reflex act in which a muscle contracts when its tendon is percussed.

t. r., patellar. Syn: *patellar reflex, knee jerk.* Slight extension of the leg when tendon of quadriceps muscle is tapped immediately below the patella. Tested with the leg slightly bent at the knee if patient is in bed. May be tested while leg hangs free when patient is sitting on edge of bed.

t. spindle. Fusiform nerve ending in a tendon.

t., superior (of Lockwood). Portion of fibrous ring from which sup. oblique muscle of eye originates.

t. of Zinn. Portion of the fibrous ring (*annulus tendineus communis*) from which inf. rectus muscle of eye originates.

tendoplasty (tĕn′dō-plăs″tĭ) [L. *tendo*, tendon]. Reparative surgery of an injured tendon. Syn: *tenoplasty, tenontoplasty.*

tendosynovitis (tĕn″dō-sĭn″ō-vī′tĭs) [" + *syn*, with, + L. *ovum*, egg, + G. *-itis*, inflammation]. Inflammation of a sheath of a tendon or the tendon. Syn: *tendovaginitis, tenontothecitis.*

t. crepitans. T. accompanied on movement by a crackling sound.

tendotome (tĕn′dō-tōm) [" + G. *tomos*, a cutting]. Instrument for severing a tendon. Syn: *tenotome.*

tendotomy (tĕn-dŏt′ō-mĭ) [" + G. *tomē*, a cutting]. Division of a tendon. Syn: *tenotomy.*

tendovaginal (tĕn″dō-văj′ĭ-năl) [" + *vagina*, sheath]. Relating to a tendon and its sheath.

tendovaginitis (tĕn″dō-văj″ĭn-ī′tĭs) [" + " + G. *-ītis*, inflammation]. Inflamed condition of a tendon and its sheath. Syn: *tenontothecitis.*

Tenebrio (tĕ-nĕb′rĭ-ō). A genus of beetles including the species of *T. molitor* which serves as intermediate host of the tapeworm *Hymenolepis diminuta.*

tenec′tomy. Excision of a lesion of a tendon or tendon sheath; removal of a ganglion or xanthoma.

tenesmic (tĕn-ĕz′mĭk) [G. *teinesmos*, a stretching]. Pert. to or like tenesmus.

tenesmus (tē-nĕz′mŭs) [G. *teinesmos*, a stretching]. Spasmodic contraction of anal or vesical sphincter with pain and persistent desire to empty the bowel or bladder, with involuntary, ineffectual straining efforts.

teni-. For words beginning with *teni* not listed here, see *taeni.*

teniasis (tē-nī′ăs-ĭs) [" + G. *-iasis*, a condition]. Presence of tapeworms in the body.

tenifuge (tĕn′ĭf-ūj) [" + *fugāre*, to put to flight]. Causing or that which causes expulsion of tapeworms. Syn: *teniafuge.*

ten′nis el′bow. An obscure, insidious, distressing complaint after playing tennis following a period of muscular inactivity of the arm or following a long duration of play.

Syn: *radiohumeral bursitis, epicondylitis.*

Etiol: It may involve inflammation of the radiohumeral bursa or partial avulsion of the common extensor tendon with consequent periostitis.

Sym: Pain over lat. epicondyle of humerus radiating to outer side of arm and forearm and aggravated by dorsiflexion and supination of wrist. Weakness of wrist and difficulty in grasping objects.

Treatment: In mild cases, immobilization by a splint or adhesive strapping, supplemented by heat or diathermy. In long continued cases, surgical intervention is indicated.

teno- [G.]. Combining form meaning *tendon.*

tenodesis (tĕn-od′ĕ-sĭs) [G. *tenōn*, tendon, + *desis*, a binding]. Suturing of the end of a tendon to a point of attachment.

tenodynia (tĕn-ō-dĭn′ĭ-ă) [" + *odynē*, pain]. Pain in a tendon. Syn: *tenalgia.*

tenomyoplasty (tĕn′ō-mī′ō-plăs″tĭ) [" + *mys, my-*, muscle, + *plassein*, to form]. Reparative operation upon a tendon and muscle. Syn: *tenontomyoplasty.*

tenomyotomy (tĕn″ō-mī-ŏt′ō-mĭ) [" + " + *tomē*, a cutting]. Excision of lateral portion of a tendon or muscle.

tenonec′tomy. Excision of a portion of a tendon.

tenonitis (tĕn-ŏn-ī′tĭs) 1. [G. *tenōn*, tendon, + *-ītis*, inflammation]. Inflammation of a tendon. Syn: *tenontitis.* 2. [*Tenon* + G. *-ītis*, inflammation]. Inflammation of Tenon's capsule.

tenonometer (tē″nō-nŏm′ĕ-ter) [G. *teinein*, to stretch, + *metron*, a measure]. Device for measuring amount of intraocular tension.

Tenon's capsule (tē-non′). A thin connective tissue envelope of the eyeball behind the conjunctiva.

T's. space. One bet. the post. surface of the eyeball and Tenon's capsule.

tenontitis (tĕn-ŏn-tī′tĭs) [G. *teinein*, to stretch, + *-itis*, inflammation]. Inflammation of a tendon. Syn: *tendinitis, tenositis.*

tenontodynia (tĕn-ŏn-tō-dĭn′ĭ-ă) [" + *odynē*, pain]. Pain in a tendon. Syn: *tenalgia, tenodynia.*

tenontography (tĕn-ŏn-tog′ră-fĭ) [" + *graphein*, to write]. A treatise on the tendons.

tenontology (tĕn-ŏn-tŏl′ō-jĭ) [" + *logos*, a study]. The study of the tendons.

tenontomyoplasty (tĕn-ŏn″tō-mī′ō-plăs″tĭ) [" + *mys, my-*, muscle, + *plassein*, to form]. Plastic surgery, including muscle and tendon repair, in treatment of hernia. SYN: *tenomyoplasty*.

tenontomyotomy (tĕn-ŏn″tō-mī-ŏt′ō-mĭ) [" + " + *tomē*, a cutting]. Cutting of the principal tendon of a muscle, with excision of the muscle in part or in whole. SYN: *myotenotomy*.

tenontoplasty (tĕn-ŏn′tō-plăs″tĭ) [G. *tenōn, tenont-*, tendon, + *plassein*, to form]. Plastic surgery of defective or injured tendons. SYN: *tenoplasty*.

tenontothecitis (tĕn-ŏn-tō-thē-sī′tĭs) [" + *thēkē*, sheath, + *-ītis*, inflammation]. Inflammation of a tendon and its sheath. SYN: *tendosynovitis, tendovaginitis, tenosynovitis*.

t. steno′sans. A chronic form of t. with narrowing of the sheath.

tenophyte (tĕn′ō-fīt) [" + *phyton*, a growth]. A cartilaginous or osseous growth on a tendon.

tenoplasty (tĕn′ō-plăs″tĭ) [" + *plassein*, to form]. Reparative surgery of tendons. SYN: *tenontoplasty*.

tenorrhaphy (tĕn-or′ă-fĭ) [" + *rhaphē*, a seam]. Suturing of a tendon.

tenositis (tĕn-ō-sī′tĭs) [" + *-ītis*, inflammation]. Inflammation of a tendon. SYN: *tenontitis*.

tenostosis (tĕn-ŏs-tō′sĭs) [" + *osteon*, bone, + *-ōsis*, condition]. Conversion of a tendon into bony tissue.

tenosuspension (ten-o-sus-pen′shun) [G. *tenōn*, tendon, + L. *suspensiō*, a hanging under]. Suspension of the humerus by a layer of a tendon to the acromion process.

tenosuture (tĕn″ō-sū′tūr) [" + L. *sutura*, a stitch]. Reunion of a divided tendon. SYN: *tenorrhaphy*.

tenosynovectomy (tĕn-ō-sĭn-ō-vĕk′tō-mĭ). Excision of a tendon sheath.

tenosynovitis (tĕn″ō-sĭn-ō-vī′tĭs) [" + *syn*, with, + L. *ovum*, egg, + G. *-ītis*, inflammation]. Inflammation of a tendon and its sheath.

t. crepitans. Inflammation of a tendon sheath in which a cracking sound is heard on motion.

ETIOL: May follow puncture wounds, contusions, and lacerations, or from lymphatic extension from an abrasion.

SYM: Pain, finger rigid, excessive tenderness.

Most commonly affects flexor tendons.

TREATMENT: Early drainage, rest.

t. hyperplastica. Painless swelling of extensor tendons over the wrist joint.

tenotome (tĕn′ō-tōm) [" + *tomos*, a cutting]. Instrument for section of a tendon.

tenotomist (tĕn-ŏt′ō-mĭst) [" + *tomos*, a cutting]. Specialist in tenotomy.

tenotomy (tĕn-ŏt′ō-mĭ) [" + *tomē*, a cutting]. Section of a tendon.

tenovaginitis (tĕn″ō-văj-ĭn-ī′tĭs.) [G. *tenōn*, tendon, + L. *vagina*, sheath, + G. *-itis*, inflammation]. SYN: *tenontothecitis*. Inflammation of a tendon sheath.

tension (tĕn′shŭn) [L. *tensio*, a stretching]. 1. Process or act of stretching; state of being strained or stretched. 2. Pressure, as arterial tension. 3. Expansive force of a gas or vapor.

Thus, to say that the tension of oxygen in arterial blood is 100 mm. of mercury means that the blood contains as much oxygen as it would absorb if exposed to pure oxygen at a pressure of 100 mm. of mercury long enough to reach equilibrium, or if exposed to a gaseous mixture in which the partial pressure of oxygen was 100 mm. of mercury. This method of expression is very convenient in explaining the direction in which the respiratory gases diffuse within the body.

t., arterial. SYN: *arterial blood pressure*. Tension resulting from the force exerted by the blood on the walls of arteries.

t. of gases. Gas pressure measured in millimeters of mercury (mm. Hg).

When in solution, gases are measured by gas pressure in surrounding medium sufficient to prevent gas from escaping from the solution.

t. headache. Headache caused by sustained tension of muscles of the face, neck, and scalp.

t., intraocular. Internal pressure of liquid within eyeball.

t., intravenous. Force exerted by the blood on the walls of a vein.

t., muscular. That condition of a muscle in which fibers tend to shorten and thus perform work, or liberate heat.

t., premenstrual. Condition occurring periodically usually a week or ten days before menstruation characterized by extreme nervousness and irritability, emotional instability, headaches, and sometimes depression. Usually disappears a few hours after onset of menstrual flow.

t., surface. Molecular property of film on surface of a liquid to resist rupture, the particles tending to pull inward.

t. suture. One used to reduce pull of the edges of a wound.

tensiophone (tĕn′sĭ-ō-fōn) [L. *tensio*, tension, + G. *phōnē*, sound]. Device for obtaining blood pressure readings by auscultation and palpation.

tensor (tĕn′sor) [L. *tensor*, a stretcher]. A muscle making a part tense. SEE: *Muscles, Table of, in Appendix*.

tent (tĕnt) [O.Fr. *tente*, from L. *tenta*, stretched out]. 1. To keep open with a tent. 2. A portable covering or shelter composed of fabric.

t., oxygen. A tent which can be placed over a bed for the administration of oxygen usually to the very sick, restless, and uncooperative patients.

tentative (tĕn′tă-tĭv) [L. *tentativus*, from *tentāre*, to try]. Noting a diagnosis subject to change because of insufficient data; experimental.

tenth cranial nerve. Nerve supplying most of the abdominal viscera, the heart, lungs, and esophagus. SYN: *vagus nerve, q.v.* SEE: *cranial nerves in Appendix*.

tentigo (tĕn-tī′gō) [L.]. Abnormal sexual desire. SYN: *lasciviousness, lust, nymphomania, satyriasis*.

tentorial. Pertaining to a tentorium.

t. notch. SYN: *foramen ovale of Pacchioni*. An arched cavity formed by the anterior and inner border of the tentorium cerebelli.

t. pressure cone. Projection of a portion of temporal lobe of cerebrum through the incisure of the tentorium due to increased intracranial pressure.

tentorium (tĕn-tō′rĭ-ŭm) [L. *tentōrium*, tent]. A tentlike structure or part.

t. cerebelli. NA. The process of the dura mater bet. the cerebrum and cerebellum supporting the occipital lobes.

tentum (tĕn′tŭm) [L. *tentum*, from *tendere*, to stretch]. The penis.

tenuate (tĕn′ū-āt). To make thin.

tenuity (tĕn'ū-ĭ-tĭ). The state or condition of being thin.

tenuous (tĕn'ū-ŭs). Thin, slender, minute.

tephromalacia (tĕf"rō-măl-ā'sĭ-ă) [G. *tephros*, gray, + *malakia*, softening]. Softening of the gray substance of brain or spinal cord.

tephromyelitis (tĕf"rō-mī-ĕl-ī'tĭs) [" + *myelos*, marrow, + *-itis*, inflammation]. Inflammation of the gray matter of the spinal cord. SYN: *poliomyelitis*.

tephrosis (tĕf'rō'sĭs) [" + *-ōsis*, condition]. Incineration; cremation.

tephrylometer (tĕf-rĭ-lom'ĕ-ter) [" + *ylē*, matter, + *metron*, a measure]. Device for measuring the thickness of the cerebral cortex, the gray matter of brain.

tepid (tĕp'ĭd) [L. *tepidus*, lukewarm]. Slightly warm; lukewarm.

t. bath. One about 86° F. (30° C.).

tepidarium (tĕp-ĭd-ā'rĭ-ŭm) [L. pert. to a warm bath]. A place for a warm bath.

TEPP. Abbr. for *tetraethylpyrophosphate*.

ter- [L.]. Combining form meaning *thrice*.

teramorphous (tĕr-ă-morf'ŭs) [G. *teras*, monster, + *morphē*, form]. Similar to, or of the nature of a monster.

ter'as. A severely deformed monster or fetus. Pl. *terata*.

teratic (tĕr-ăt'ĭk) [G. *teratikos*, monstrous]. Pertaining to a severely malformed fetus.

teratism (tĕr'ă-tĭzm). An anomaly or structural abnormality either inherited or acquired.

t., acquired. One resulting from a prenatal environmental influence.

t., atresic. One in which natural openings such as the mouth or anus fail to form.

t., casemic. One in which a normal union of parts fails to occur.

t., ectogenic. One in which parts are absent or defective.

t., ectopic. One in which a part becomes displaced.

t., hypergenetic. One in which a part is exceptionally large.

t., symphysic. One in which parts which are normally separate are fused.

terato- [G.]. Combining form meaning a *severely malformed fetus*.

teratoblastoma (tĕr"ă-tō-blăs-tō'mă) [G. *teras, terat-*, monster, + *blastos*, germ, + *-ōma*, tumor]. A tumor containing embryonic material but which is not representative of all 3 germinal layers. SEE: *teratoma*.

teratogenesis (tĕr-ă-tō-gĕn'ĕs-ĭs). The development of abnormal structures in an embryo; the development of a severely deformed fetus.

teratoid (tĕr'ă-toyd) [G. *teras, terat-*, monster, + *eidos*, form]. Resembling a severely malformed fetus.

t. tumor. Tumor of embryonic remains from all of the germinal layers. SYN: *teratoma*.

teratology (tĕr-ăt-ŏl'ō-jĭ) [" + *logos*, a study]. Branch of science dealing with the study of congenitally deformed fetuses.

teratoma (tĕr-ă-tō'mă) [" + *-ōma*, tumor]. Congenital tumor containing embryonic elements of all 3 primary germ layers, as hair, teeth, etc. SYN: *dermoid*.

teratomatous (ter-ă-tō'mă-tus) [" + *-ōma*, tumor]. Pert. to or resembling a teratoma.

teratophobia (ter"ă-tō-fō'bĭ-ă) [" + *phobos*, fear]. Abnormal fear of giving birth to a malformed fetus or of being in contact with one.

teratosis (tĕr-ă-tō'sĭs) [" + *-ōsis*, condition]. A deformed fetus.

ter'bium. SYMB: Tb. At. wt. 158.924; at. no. 65. A metal of the rare earths.

tere (te're) [L. rub]. Rub.

terebinthinate (ter"ĕ-bĭn'thĭ-nāt) [L. *terebinthus*, turpentine]. Containing or agent containing turpentine.

terebrant, terebrating (ter'ē-brant, -brāt-ing) [L. *terebrāre*, to bore]. Boring or piercing, said of pain.

terebration (tĕr-ē-brā'shŭn) [L. *terebrāre*, to bore]. 1. The act of boring. SYN: *trephining*. 2. A boring pain.

teres (tē'rēz) [L. *teres*, rounded, polished]. 1. Round and smooth; cylindrical. 2. A cylindrical muscle.

t. major. A muscle that draws the arm down and back.

t. minor. A muscle inserted in the great tuberosity of the humerus, which rotates the humerus outward and abducts it.

tereti- [L.]. Combining form meaning *round*.

tergo- [L.]. Combining form, *the back*.

tergum (ter'gŭm) [L.]. The back.

ter in die [L.]. Three times a day. ABBR: t.i.d.

term (term) [L. *terminus*, a boundary]. 1. A limit or boundary. 2. A definite period. 3. The normal period of pregnancy, approximately nine calendar months.

t. birth. One occurring at expected time of delivery; one not premature.

terminal (ter'mĭn-ăl) [L. *terminus*, a boundary]. Pert. to or placed at the end.

t. arteriole. One with no branches, but which splits into capillaries.

t. bars. Minute bars of dense intercellular cement which occupy and close spaces between epithelial cells and bind them together.

t. ganglia. Those of the parasympathetic division of the autonomic nervous system that are located in or close to walls or visceral structures such as heart, intestines, etc.; also called *peripheral ganglia*.

t. infection. One appearing in the late stage of another disease; often fatal.

t. veins. One of two veins (ant. and post.) draining portions of the brain and emptying into int. cerebral veins.

termination. 1. The distal end of a part. 2. The cessation of anything.

terminology (ter-mĭn-ŏl'ō-jĭ) [L. *terminus*, term, + G. *logos*, word]. The special terms used in any field, as an art or science. SYN: *nomenclature*.

ternary (ter'na-rĭ) [L. *ternarius*, triple]. 1. Threefold; triple; third. 2. Composed of 3 elements.

t. acid. An inorganic acid containing hydrogen and 2 other elements.

teropterin (ter-ŏp'ter-ĭn). Trade name for sodium pteroyl triglutamate solution. Used for palliation of certain symptoms of malignancy in treatment adjunctive to x-ray, radium, and surgery.

ter'pin hy'drate. USP. White crystalline substance with a turpentine taste made by the interaction of rectified spirits of turpentine, alcohol, and nitric acid.

ACTION AND USES: As an expectorant.

terra (tĕr'ă) [L.]. Earth; soil.

t. al'ba. White clay.

t. fullon'ica. Fuller's earth.

terracing (ter'ăs-ĭng) [O.Fr. *terrace*]. Suturing in several rows through thick tissues in closing a wound.

terramycin (ter"ră-mī'cĭn). A proprietary name for the oxy derivative of tetracycline. An antibiotic biosynthesized by *Streptomyces rimosus*. It is a broad spectrum antibiotic effective against both gram negative and gram positive bacteria, rickettsias, and some viruses. SEE: *oxytetracycline; tetracycline.*

terror (ter'or) [L. *terror,* fear]. Very great fear.

t., night. Nightmare or night terror, esp. of children.

tertian (ter'shŭn) [L. *tertianus,* pert. to the third]. Occurring every 3rd day.

t. fever. A malarial fever with paroxysms every other day.

t. malaria. Caused by *Plasmodium vivax, q.v.* SEE: *malaria.*

tertiary (ter'shĭ-a-rĭ) [L. *tertius,* third]. Third in order or stage.

t. alcohol. One containing the trivalent group COH.

t. syphilis. Third and most advanced stage of syphilis.

tertipara (tĕr-tĭp'ă-ră) [L. *tertius,* third, + *parēre,* to bring forth]. A woman who has given birth to 3 children.

tessellated (tĕs'ĕl-ā-tĕd) [L. *tessella,* a square]. Composed of little squares.

test (test) [L. *testum,* an earthen vessel]. 1. An examination. 2. Method to determine the presence or nature of a substance, or the presence of a disease. 3. A chemical reaction. 4. A reagent or substance used in making a test.

t., acetone. Test for presence of acetone in the urine; made by adding a few drops of sodium nitroprusside to the urine along with strong ammonia water. Presence of acetone causes formation of a magenta ring at outline of contacts.

t., Allen-Doisy. Test to determine amount of estrogen content in female blood serum by its reaction on secretions of mice.

t., Aschheim-Zondek. Test for pregnancy by injecting the patient's urine subcutaneously in immature female mice.

t., Binet-Simon. Method of ascertaining the mental capacity of children by asking a series of suitable questions. SEE: *Binet age.*

t., biuret. Test for the presence of proteins or urea.

t., Friedman. Test for pregnancy by injecting urine of the patient into unmated mature female rabbits, a positive reaction being indicated by formation of corpora lutea and corpora haemorrhagica.

t., Gelle's. Test for ear lesions by employing rubber tubing and a tuning fork.

t., Huhner. Aspiration of vagina within an hour after coitus, to investigate sperm activity.

t., Kahn's. Precipitation test for syphilis.

t. paper. Paper used in making tests, as litmus paper.

t., pregnancy. Test to determine pregnancy.

t., Rubin. Test for patency of the fallopian tubes by insufflation with carbon dioxide; used to determine cause of sterility.

t., Schiller's. Test for cancer of the cervix by painting with iodine solution; since cancer cells do not stain with iodine, they turn white or yellow.

t., Schneider's. A pregnancy test using female rabbits.

t., Schwabach's. Test for hearing using tuning forks.

t. solution. A standard solution used in making a test.

t. tube. A plain tube of thin glass, closed at 1 end, used for simple tests.

t., urea balance. Test of the kidney function by measuring intake and output of urea.

t., Wassermann. Diagnostic test for syphilis based on principle of fixation of complement.

testectomy (tĕs-tĕk'tō-mĭ) [L. *testis,* testicle, + G. *ektomē,* excision]. 1. Removal of a testicle. SYN: *castration.* 2. Removal of a corpus quadrigeminum.

testes (tĕs'tēs) (sing. *testis*) [L.]. The plural of *testis, q.v.*

testicle (tĕs'tĭ-kl) [L. *testiculus,* a little *testis*]. A *testis, q.v.*

testicular (tĕs-tĭk'ū-lar) [L. *testiculus,* a little testis]. Relating to a testicle.

testis (tes'tĭs) (pl. *testes*) [L. *testis,* testicle]. SYN: *testicle.* The male gonad. One of two reproductive glands located in the scrotum which produce the male reproductive cells or *spermatozoa* and the male hormone, *testosterone.*

Each is an ovoid body about 4.0 cm. long and 2 to 2.5 cm. in width and thickness, enclosed within a dense inelastic fibrous *tunica albuginea.* The testis is divided into numerous *lobules* separated by *septa,* each lobule containing one to three *seminiferous tubules* within which the spermatozoa arise. The lobules lead to *straight ducts* which join a plexus, the *rete testis,* from which 15-20 *efferent ducts* lead to the *epididymis.* The epididymis leads to the *ductus deferens* through which sperm are conveyed to the urethra.

Between the seminiferous tubules are located the *interstitial cells* (cells of Leydig) which are considered to be the source of the male hormone(s).

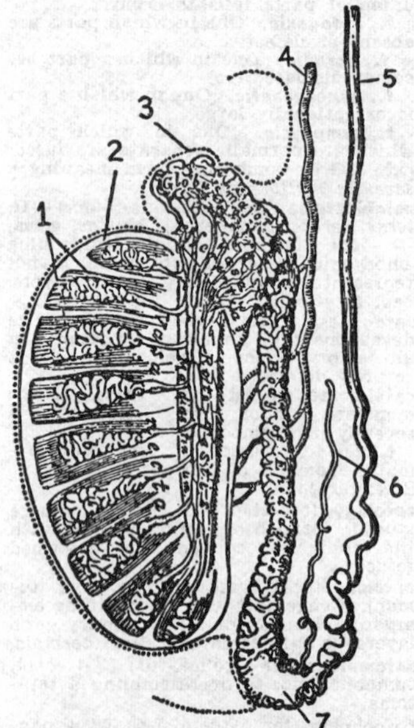

TESTIS AND EPIDIDYMIS

1. Septa. 2. Tunica albuginea. 3. Tunica vaginalis. 4. Spermatic artery. 5. Ductus deferens. 6. Caudal aberrant ductule. 7. Tail of epididymis.

The testes are suspended from the body by the *spermatic cord,* a structure extending from inguinal ring to testis. It contains the ductus deferens, testicular vessels (spermatic artery, vein, lymph vessels) and nerves.

Hyperfunction (hypergonadism) may cause early maturity, such as dentition, large sexual organs with early functional activity, and growth of hair.

Hypofunction (hypogonadism) is indicated by undeveloped testes, absence of body hair, high-pitched voice, sterility, smooth skin, loss of sex desire, low metabolism, and eunuchoid or eunuch type.

t., abdominal. An undescended testis which remains within body cavity.

t. compression reflex. Contraction of abdominal muscles following moderate compression of testis.

t., descent of. Change in position of the testis from abdominal cavity to scrotum during fetal life.

t., displaced. A testis within (abnormally) the inguinal canal, or pelvis.

t., femoral. An inguinal testis which is near or over the femoral ring.

t., inverted. One reversed in the scrotum so that the epididymis attaches to the ant. instead of post. part of gland.

t., perineal. One which is located in the perineal region outside the scrotum.

t., puboscrotal. One located over pubic tubercle.

t., undescended. One or both remain in the inguinal canal or abdominal cavity at birth.

testitis (tĕs-tī'tĭs) [L. *testis,* testicle, + G. *-ītis,* inflammation]. Inflammation of a testis. Syn: *orchitis.*

testitoxicosis (tĕs"tĭ-tŏks-ĭ-kō'sĭs) [" + G. *toxikon,* poison, + *-ōsis,* condition]. A toxic state sometimes following ligation of the ductus deferens.

test meal. A meal usually small and of definite quality and composition, given to aid in chemical analysis of the stomach contents or x-ray diagnosis of the stomach.

testosterone (tĕs-tŏs'ter-ōn) [L. *testis,* testicle]. An androgen isolated from the testes of a number of animals including man and considered to be the principal testicular hormone produced in man. It is a steroid produced by the interstitial cells of Leydig. It has been prepared synthetically by conversion of other sterols, esp. cholesterol.

Action: It accelerates growth in tissues upon which it acts and stimulates blood flow. It stimulates and promotes the growth of secondary sexual characters and is essential for normal sexual behavior and the occurrence of erections. It is essential for normal growth and development of the male accessory sexual organs. It is responsible for deepening of the male voice at puberty, greater muscular development in men, development of beard and pubic hair, and distribution of fat in adult men. It also affects many metabolic activities.

tetanic (tē-tăn'ĭk) [G. *tetanikos,* pert. to a stretching]. 1. Pert. to or producing tetanus. 2. Any agent producing tetanic spasms.

t. convulsion. A tonic one with constant muscular contraction.

tetaniform (tē-tan'ĭ-form) [G. *tetanos,* tetanus, + L. *forma,* shape]. Resembling tetanus.

tetanigenous (tĕt"ă-nĭdj'ĕ-nŭs). Causing tetanus or tetanic spasms.

tetanilla (tĕt-ăn-ĭl'lă) [L.]. 1. Mild form of tetany* without rigidity. 2. Twitchings of a limited group of muscular fibers with clonic paroxysmal contractions.

tetanism (tĕt'ăn-ĭzm) [G. *tetanos,* tetanus, + *-ismos,* condition]. Persistent muscular hypertonicity resembling tetanus, esp. in infants.

tetanization (tĕt-ăn-ĭ-zā'shŭn) [G. *tetanos,* tetanus]. 1. Production of tetanus or tetanic spasms by induction of the disease. 2. Induction of tetanic contractions in a muscle by electrical stimuli.

tetanize (tĕt'ăn-īz) [G. *tetanos,* tetanus]. To induce tonic muscular spasms.

tetanode (tĕt'ă-nōd) [" + *eidos,* form]. 1. Resembling tetanus. Syn: *tetanoid.* 2. Noting interval bet. recurrent tonic spasms in tetany.

tetanoid (tĕt'ă-noyd) [" + *eidos,* form]. Resembling tetanus. Syn: *tetaniform.*

t. paraplegia. Paralysis of lower extremities due to lateral sclerosis of spinal cord. Syn: *spastic paraplegia.*

tetanolysin (tĕt"ă-nol'ĭ-sĭn). A hemolytic component of the toxin produced by *Clostridium tetani,* causative organism of tetanus.

tetanomotor (tĕt"ăn-o-mō'tor) [" + L. *motor,* a mover]. Appliance for the production of tetanic motor spasms mechanically by shocking a nerve.

tetanophil, tetanophilic (tĕt'ăn-ō-fĭl, tĕt"ăn-ō-fĭl'ĭk) [" + *philein,* to love]. Possessing an affinity for tetanus toxin.

tetanospasmin (tĕt"ă-nō-spăs'mĭn). A component of the toxin produced by tetanus bacillus which is responsible for tetanic convulsions.

tetanus (tĕt'ă-nŭs) [G. *tetanos,* tetanus]. 1. An infectious, acute disease due to the toxin of tetanus bacillus, *Clostridium tetani,* growing anaerobically at the site of injury. There is a state of more or less persistent, painful tonic spasm of some of the voluntary muscles. 2. A state of sustained contraction of a muscle, especially that induced experimentally.

Usually begins gradually, but may begin suddenly; may be of brief duration or last some weeks. The first sign is stiffness of the jaw and esophageal muscles and some of the muscles of neck. Soon the jaws become rigidly fixed (trismus, or lockjaw), the voice is altered, muscles of the face contract, producing a wild, excited expression, a compound of bitter laughter and crying (risus sardonicus). The muscles of back, extremities, and penis become tetanic.

If the patient be bent back in a bow, the condition is termed *opisthotonos;* if he be bent to the side, *pleurothotonos;* if he be bent forward, *emprosthotonos.*

The paroxysms are reflex, and are excited by noises, currents of air, and even irritation of bedclothes. The temperature usually rises and may attain remarkable height. The pain is great, patient also suffering from hunger, thirst, and want of sleep. The mind is clear. This disease is usually, but not always, fatal, the patient expiring from asphyxia or exhaustion.

RS: *emprosthotonos, lockjaw, opisthotonos, pleurothotonos, posture, risus sardonicus.*

t., anticus. Form in which the body is bowed forward.

t. antitoxin. An antibody which develops in the blood of man or other animals (horse) as a result of infection by the tetanus organism (*Clostridium tetani*) or inoculation with tetanus toxin or toxoid. 2. A sterile solution of antibody globulins derived from the blood of horses or cattle immunized against tetanus toxin. It is used to produce passive immunity to prevent the development of tetanus and in the treatment of active tetanus. Prophylactic dose is 1500 units injected subcutaneously; for active tetanus, 5000 to 20,000 units injected intravenously or subcutaneously.

t., artificial. Form produced by a drug like strychnine or by mechanical appliance.

t., ascending. Tetanus in which muscle spasms occur first in lower part of body, then spread upward finally involving muscles of head and neck.

t., cephalic. Form due to a wound of the head, esp. one near the eyebrow. It is marked by trismus, facial paralysis on one side, and pronounced dysphagia; resembles rabies; often fatal.

t., cerebral. A form produced by inoculating the brain of animals with tetanus antitoxin, marked by epileptiform convulsions and excitement.

t., chronic. SYN: *delayed tetanus.* 1. A latent infection in a healed wound which is reactivated upon opening the wound. 2. A form of tetanus in which onset and progress of the disease is slower and more prolonged and symptoms less severe.

t., descending. Tetanus in which muscle spasms occur first in head and neck and later are manifested in other muscles of body.

t. dorsalis. Tetanus in which the body is bent backward.

t., extensor. That which affects the extensors especially.

t., head. Cephalic t., *q.v.*

t., hydrophobic. Cephalic t., *q.v.*

t., idiopathic. That which occurs without any visible lesion.

t., imitative. Hysteria which simulates tetanus.

t. infantum. Tetanus of young infants, due to infection of umbilicus.

t., intermittent. SYN: *tetany.*

t., kopf. Cephalic t., *q.v.*

t. lateralis. Form in which the body is bent sideways.

t., local. Tetanus characterized by spasticity of a group of muscles near the wound. Trismus (contraction of jaw muscles) is usually absent.

t. neonatorum. Tetanus of very young infants, usually due to infection of navel.

t. paradoxus. Cephalic tetanus in which condition is combined with paralysis of the facial or other cranial nerve.

t. posticus. Same as *t. dorsalis.*

t., postoperative. T. which follows an operation.

t., puerperal. T. which occurs following childbirth.

t., rheumatic. Form due to exposure to cold and wet.

t., Ritter's. Tetanic contractions at opening of a constant current which has been passing along a nerve for some time; seen in tetany.

t., toxic. Produced by overdose of nux vomica or strychnine.

t. toxoid. Tetanus toxin modified by treatment with formaldehyde so that its toxicity is greatly reduced but its capacity to promote active immunity has been retained.

t., traumatic. T. which follows wound poisoning.

tetany (tĕt'ă-nĭ) [G. *tetanos,* tetanus]. A nervous affection, characterized by intermittent tonic spasms, which are usually paroxysmal and involve the extremities; most frequent in the young; frequently associated with pregnancy or lactation.

ETIOL: Tetany is induced by changes in *p*H and extracellular calcium which increase nervous and muscular excitability. Causative factors are parathyroid deficiency or operative removal of parathyroids in thyroidectomy, alkalosis or vitamin-D deficiency.

SYM: Characterized by nervousness, irritability and apprehension, numbness and tingling of the extremities, cramps of the various muscles, particularly those of the hands, producing a typical accoucheur type of hand and extreme extension of the feet. Bilateral tonic spasms in arms and legs, jaws rarely involved. Contractions usually paroxysmal and are attended with pain. Electrocontractility of muscles greatly exaggerated. May be slight edema. Sensation not disturbed; mind clear, fever slight or absent.

SIGNS: Characteristic diagnostic signs are (a) Trousseau's sign, (b) Chvostek's sign, and (c) the peroneal sign, *q.v.* Prolongation of the isoelectric phase of the ST segment of the ECG is usually indicative of low calcium.

PROG: Usually favorable. Attacks following thyroidectomy sometimes fatal.

t., alkalotic. That resulting from respiratory alkalosis as in hyperventilation, or from metabolic alkalosis induced by excessive intake of sodium bicarbonate or excessive loss of chlorides by vomiting, gastric lavage, or suction.

t., duration. Continuous contraction, esp. in degenerated muscles, in response to a continuous electric current.

t., epidemic. SYN: *rheumatic tetany.* A form of tetany occurring in Europe, esp. in the winter season. It is of short duration and seldom fatal.

t., gastric. Severe t. from stomach disorders accompanied by tonic, painful spasms of extremities.

t., gutturotetany. Stammering resulting from tetanoid laryngeal spasm.

t., hyperventilation. T. caused by continued forced respiration.

t., hypocalcemic. Tetany due to low serum calcium and high serum phosphate levels. May be due to (a) lack of vitamin D, (b) factors which interfere with calcium absorption, such as steatorrhea or infantile diarrhea, or (c) defective renal excretion of phosphorus.

t., latent. That which requires mechanical or electrical stimulation of nerves to show characteristic signs of excitability.

t., manifest. When characteristic symptoms such as carpopedal spasm, laryngospasm, and convulsions are present.

t., parathyroid. SYN: *hypoparathyroidism.* T. resulting from excision of the parathyroid gland or from hyposecretion of the parathyroid gland as a result of disease or disorders of the gland.

t., rachitic. That due to hypocalcemia accompanying vitamin D deficiency.

t., thyreoprival. That resulting from removal of thyroid gland accompanied by removal of parathyroid glands.

tetarcone (tĕt'ar-kōn) [G. *tetartos,* fourth, + *kōnos,* cone]. Fourth or distolingual cusp of an upper molar tooth. SYN: *tetartocone.*

tetartanopia, tetartanopsia (tĕt"ar-tăn-ō'pĭ-ă, -ŏp'sĭ-ă) [" + *ōps,* eye, — + *opsis,* vision]. Symmetrical blindness in the same quadrant of each visual field. Syn: *quadrantanopia.*

tetartocone (tĕt-ar'tō-kōn) [" + *kōnos,* cone]. The distolingual cusp of an upper molar tooth. Syn: *tetarcone.*

tethelin (tĕth'ĕ-lĭn) [G. *tethēlos,* flourishing]. A substance derived from the ant. lobe of the pituitary having an accelerating effect on growth.

tetmil (tĕt'mĭl). Ten millimeters; a unit of measurement.

tetra-, tetr- [G.]. Combining forms meaning *four.*

tetrabasic (tĕt"ră-bā'sĭk) [G. *tetra,* four, + *basis,* base]. Having 4 replaceable hydrogen atoms, said of an acid or acid salt.

tetrablastic (tĕt"ră-blăs'tĭk) [" + *blastos,* germ]. Having 4 germinal layers, the *ectoderm, endoderm,* and 2 *mesodermic* layers.

tetrabromofluorescein (tĕt"ră-brōm"ō-flū-or-ĕs'ĭn, -ē-ĭn). A dye, $C_{20}H_8Br_4O_5$, obtained from action of bromine on fluorescein, used as a stain in microscopy. Syn: *eosin.*

tetracaine hydrochloride. A surface, infiltration, and intraspinal anesthetic.

tetrachlorethylene (tĕt"ră-klor-ĕth'ĭl-ēn). A clear, colorless liquid with a characteristic odor. An anthelmintic.

tetracid (tĕ-trăs'ĭd) [G. *tetra,* four, + L. *acidus,* sour]. 1. Able to react with 4 molecules of a monoacid or 2 of a diacid to form a salt or ester, said of a base or alcohol; term disapproved by some authorities. 2. Having 4 hydrogen atoms replaceable by basic atoms or radicals, said of acids.

Tetracoccus (tĕt"ră-kŏk'ŭs) [" + *kokkos,* berry]. Genus of micrococcus arranged in groups of 4 by division into 2 planes.

tetracrotic (tĕt"ră-krŏt'ĭk) [" + *krotos,* a beat]. Noting a pulse or pulse tracing with 4 upward strokes in the descending limb of the wave. Syn: *catatricrotic.*

tetracycline (tĕt-ră-sī'klēn). A member of the tetracycline group of broad-spectrum antibiotics having similar pharmacologic activity (*i.e.,* tetracycline, chlortetracycline, oxytetracycline). Especially effective in treatment of Q fever, typhus fever, psittacosis, acute brucellosis, granuloma inguinale.

tetrad (tĕt'răd) [G. *tetras, tetrad-,* number four]. 1. A group of 4 things with something in common. 2. An element having a valence or combining power of 4. 3. A group of 4 similar bodies. 4. A group of 4 parts, said of cells produced by division in 2 planes, or of a chromosome in 4 parts in preparation for 2 mitotic divisions in maturation.

tetraethylammonium chloride (tĕt-ră-ĕth-ĭl-am-ō'nĭ-ŭm klō'rīd). A quaternary ammonium compound used as a ganglionic blocking agent in diagnosis and treatment of circulatory diseases. Abbr: TEAC.

tetraethylpyrophosphate (tĕt-ră-ĕth'ĭl-pi-rō-fōs'fāt). Abbr: TEPP. A powerful cholinesterase inhibitor used as an insecticide; poisonous to man. Has had some use in treatment of myasthenia gravis.

tetragenous (tĕt-răj'ĕn-ŭs) [G. *tetra,* four, + *gennan,* to produce]. Pertaining to organisms, esp. bacteria, which divide into groups of four.

tetralogy of Fallot. An anomaly of the heart consisting of pulmonary stenosis, interventricular septal defect, dextroposed aorta which receives blood from both ventricles, and hypertrophy of the right ventricle.

tetramastia (tĕt"ră-măs'tĭ-ă) [G. *tetra,* four, + *mastos,* breast]. Condition characterized by presence of 4 breasts. Syn: *tetramazia.*

tetramazia (tĕt"ră-mā'zĭ-ă) [" + *mazos,* breast]. Condition of having 4 breasts. Syn: *tetramastia.*

tetrameric, tetramerous (tĕt"ră-mĕr'ĭk, tĕt-răm'ĕr-ŭs) [" + *meros,* a part]. Having four parts.

tetranopsia (tĕt-ră-nŏp'sĭ-ă) [" + *an-,* priv. + *opsis,* vision]. Obliteration of visual field by one-quarter.

tetraplegia (tĕt-ră-plē'jĭ-ă) [" + *plēgē,* a stroke]. Paralysis of both arms and legs.

tetrasomic (tĕt-ră-sō'mĭk). Possessing four instead of the usual two of a pair of chromosomes, that is, having a chromosome number of 2n + 2.

tetraster (tĕt-răs'ter) [" + *astēr,* star]. A figure in which there are 4 asters, instead of more commonly 2; occurring abnormally in mitosis.

tetravalent (tĕt-ră-vā'lĕnt). Syn: *quadrivalent.* Having a valence or combining power of four.

tetter (tĕt'ĕr) [A.S. *teter*]. 1. Obsolete term for various vesicular cutaneous diseases, as herpes, ringworm, or eczema. 2. A pimple or blister.

textiform (tĕks'tĭ-form) [L. *textum,* web, + *forma,* shape]. Resembling a network, web or mesh.

textoblastic (tĕks"tō-blăs'tĭk) [L. *textus,* tissue, + G. *blastos,* germ]. Forming adult tissue; regenerative; noting cells.

textural (tĕks'tū-răl) [L. *textura,* a weaving]. Concerning the texture or constitution of a tissue.

T fracture. One in which bone splits both longitudinally and transversely.

Th. Chemical symbol for *thorium.*

thalamic (thăl-ăm'ĭk) [G. *thalamos,* chamber]. Pert. to the thalamus.

t. syndrome. Sensory disturbances and pain in conjunction with mild hemiplegia. Syn: *Dejerine-Roussy syndrome.*

Etiol: Optic thalamus lesion.

thalamo- [G.]. 1. Combining form meaning *chamber, part of brain at which a nerve originates.* 2. Pert. to the *thalamus.*

thalamocele, thalamocoele (thăl'ăm-ō-sēl) [G. *thalamos,* chamber, + *koilia,* a hollow]. The 3rd ventricle of the brain.

thalamocortical (thăl"ăm-ō-kor'tĭ-kăl) [" + L. *cortex, cortic-,* rind]. Pert. to the optic thalamus and the cerebral cortex.

thalamolenticular (thăl"ăm-ō-lĕn-tĭk'ū-lar) [" + L. *lenticula,* a small lentil]. Concerning the optic thalamus and the lenticular nucleus.

thalamotomy (thăl-ă-mŏt'ō-mĭ) [G. *thalamos,* chamber, + *tome,* incision]. A psychosurgical procedure for mental illness. A wire electrode is passed down into the thalamus, and a portion about the size of an almond is coagulated. Said to produce fewer unpleasant personality changes than *lobotomy, q.v.*

thalamus (thăl'ă-mŭs) (pl. *thalami*) [G. *thalamos,* chamber]. [NA]. The largest subdivision of the diencephalon on either side, consisting chiefly of an ovoid, gray nuclear mass in the lateral wall of the 3rd ventricle.

Each consists of a number of *nuclei* (anterior, medial, lateral, and ventral), the *medial* and *lateral geniculate bodies* and the *pulvinar.*

Functions: All sensory impulses with the exception of olfactory impulses, are received by the thalamus. These are associated and synthesized and then relayed, through thalamocortical radiations, to specific cortical areas. Impulses are also received from the cortex, hypothalamus, and corpus striatum and relayed to visceral and somatic effectors. The thalamus is also the center for appreciation of primitive, uncritical sensations of pain, crude touch, and temperature.

t. opticus. Same as *thalamus.*

thalassemia (thal-ă-se'mĭ-ă). Anemia due to a genetic abnormality. *T. major* is characterized by mongoloid facies, splenomegaly, severe anemia, and slight jaundice. Prognosis varies. *T. minor* is a mild disease which may be difficult to detect. Prognosis is excellent. The genetics of this disease are poorly understood. There is no specific therapy available.

SYN for *T. major*: *Cooley's anemia, erythroblastic anemia, Mediterranean disease, hereditary leptocytosis.*

thalassophobia (thăl-ăs"sō-fō'bĭ-ă) [G. *thalassa,* sea, + *phobos,* fear]. Abnormal fear of the sea.

thalassotherapy (thăl-ăs"sō-ther'ă-pĭ) [" + *therapeia,* treatment]. Treatment of disease by living at the seaside, by sea bathing, sea voyages, or sea air.

thalidomide (thă-lid'ō-mīd). A chemical substance, *alpha* (N-phthalimido) glutarimide, used extensively as a sedative and sleeping pill in Europe in the early 1960's. Its use was discontinued when its ability to cause phocomelia (failure of limbs to develop) in fetuses exposed to the drug at a certain time in their very early intrauterine life was discovered.

thallinization (thăl-ĭn-ĭ-zā'shŭn) [G. *thallos,* a young shoot]. Treatment with doses of thalline or its salts.

thallium (thăl'lĭ-ŭm) [L. from G. *thallos,* a young shoot]. A metallic element. SYMB: Tl. At. wt. 204.37; at. no. 81.

thamuria (thă-mū'rĭ-ă) [G. *thamus,* often, + *ouron,* urine]. Abnormally frequent urination. SYN: *pollakiuria.*

thanato- [G.]. Combining form meaning *death.*

thanatobiological (thăn"ă-tō-bī-ō-lŏj'ĭk-ăl) [G. *thanatos,* death, + *bios,* life, + *logos,* study]. Relating to the processes of life and death.

thanatognomonic (thăn"ăt-ŏg-nō-mŏn'ĭk) [" + *gnōmonikos,* knowing]. Indicative of the approach of death.

thanatoid (thăn'ă-toyd) [" + *eidos,* form]. Resembling death.

thanatology (thăn"ă-tol'ō-jĭ) [" + *logos,* science]. The science of death.

thanatomania (thăn"ă-tō-mā'nĭ-ă) [" + *mania,* madness]. Condition of homicidal or suicidal mania.

thanatometer (thăn-ă-tŏm'ĕt-ĕr) [" + *metron,* a measure]. Instrument for determining occurrence of death by internal temperature.

thanatophobia (thăn"ă-tō-fō'bĭ-ă) [" + *phobos,* fear]. Morbid fear of death.

thanatopsia, thanatopsy (thăn"ă-top'sĭ-ă, thăn'ăt-ŏp"sĭ) [" + *opsis,* view]. Examination of a dead body to determine cause of death. SYN: *autopsy, necropsy.*

thanatos (thăn'ă-tōs). The death instinct. In psychoanalysis. All the instinctive tendencies leading to senescence and death.

thaumato- [G.]. Combining form meaning *wonder, marvel.*

theaism (thē'ă-ĭzm) [L. *thea, tea,* + G. *-ismos,* condition]. Chronic poisoning from excess of tea drinking. SYN: *themism, theism.*

thebaism (thē'bă-ĭzm) [G. *Thebai,* Thebes (opium of)]. Condition produced by opium.

Thebesius' foramina (thē-bē'zĭ-ŭs). Orifices of the Thebesius veins, opening into the right auricle of the heart.

T's. valve. An endocardial fold at entrance of the coronary sinus into right auricle.

T's. veins. Venules conveying blood from the myocardium to the auricles or ventricles.

theca (thē'kă) [G. *thēkē,* a box]. A sheath of investing membrane,

t. cell tumor. Thecoma, *q.v.*

t. cor'dis. Pericardium, which sheathes the heart.

t. follic'uli. Outer wall of a graafian follicle. It consists of an inner vascular layer, the *theca interna,* and outer fibrous layer, the *theca externa.*

thecal (thē'kăl) [G. *thēkē,* a box]. Pert. to a sheath.

thecitis (thē-sī'tĭs) [" + *-itis,* inflammation]. Inflammation of the sheath of a tendon.

theco- [G.]. Combining form meaning *sheath, case, receptacle.*

thecodont (thē'kō-dont) [G. *thēkē,* box, + *odous, odont-,* tooth]. Having teeth which are inserted in sockets.

theco'ma. A tumor of the ovary usually occurring during or following the menopause. Only rarely is it malignant. Also called *theca-cell tumor* or *theca-lutein-cell tumor.*

thecostegnosia, thecostegnosis (thē"kō-stĕg-nō'sĭ-ă, -nō'sĭs) [" + *stegnōsis,* a narrowing]. Constriction of a tendon sheath.

theelin (thē'lĭn) [G. *thēlys,* female]. Proprietary name for estrone, an estrogenic substance obtained from pregnancy urine and also synthesized from cholesterol. SEE: *estrone.*

SYN: *estrin, estrone, female sex hormone, folliculin, progynon.*

USES: Chiefly in menopausal disturbances, functional amenorrhea, and delayed puberty.

theelol (thē'lōl) [G. *thēlys,* female]. SYN: *estriol.* An estrus-exciting hormone similar to but more active than theelin, found in urine of pregnant women.

theine (thē'ēn). Caffeine, *q.v.*

thelalgia (thē-lăl'jĭ-ă) [G. *thēlē,* nipple, + *algos,* pain]. Pain in the nipples.

thelarche (thēl-ar'kē) [G.*thēlys,* female, + *archē,* beginning]. The beginning of breast development at puberty.

thelasis (thē-lăs'ĭs). The act of sucking.

Thelazia (thē"lā'zĭ'ă). A genus of nematodes which inhabits the conjunctival sac and lacrimal ducts of various species of vertebrates. They occasionally are found in man.

thelaziasis (thē"lā'zĭ'ă-sĭs). Condition of being infested by worms of the genus *Thelazia.*

theleplasty (thēl'ĕ-plăs"tĭ) [" + *plassein,* to form]. Plastic surgery of the nipple.

thelerethism (thēl-ĕr'ĕ-thĭzm) [" + *erethisma,* stimulation]. Erection of the nipple.

thelitis (thē-lī'tĭs) [" + *-itis,* inflammation]. Inflammation of the nipples.

thelium (thē'lĭ-ŭm) [L. from G. *thēlē,* nipple]. 1. A papilla. 2. A nipple. 3. A cellular layer.

thelon'cus. A tumor of a nipple.

thelophlebostemma (thē-lō-flĕb"ō-stĕm'-mă). A dark or venous circle of veins about the nipple.

thelorrhagia (thē"lor-rā'gĭ-ă). Hemorrhage from a nipple.

thelothism (thē′lō-thĭzm). Erection of a nipple brought about by contraction of smooth muscle fibers. SEE: *thelerethism.*

thenad (thē′năd) [G. *thenar,* palm, + L. *ad,* toward]. Toward the palm or thenar eminence.

thenal (thē′năl) [G. *thenar,* palm]. Pert. to the palm or thenar prominence.

t. aspect. Outer side of the palm.

t. eminence. Ball of the thumb. SYN: *thenar.*

thenar (thē′nar) [G. *thenar,* palm]. 1. Palm of hand or sole of foot. 2. Fleshy eminence at base of thumb. 3. Concerning the palm.

t. cleft. SYN: *thenar space.* A fascial cleft of the palm overlying volar surface of adductor pollicis muscle.

t. eminence. One at the base of the thumb.

t. fascia. A thin membrane covering the short muscles of the thumb.

t. muscles. Abductor and flexor muscles of the thumb.

theobromine (thē-ō-brō′mēn) [" + *brōma,* food]. A white powder obtained from Theobroma cacao.

ACTION AND USES: Dilates blood vessels in the heart and peripherally. Used as a mild stimulant and as a diuretic.

t. with sodium salicylate. USP. Diuretin. Combination of sodium salicylate and theobromine.

ACTION AND USES: Same as theobromine but more soluble.

theocalcin (thē″ō-kăl′sĭn) [" + L. *calx,* lime]. A double salt or mixture of calcium theobromine and calcium salicylate.

ACTION AND USES: Same as theobromine.

theomania (thē-ō-mā′nĭ-ă) [G. *theos,* god, + *mania,* madness]. Religious insanity; esp. that in which patient thinks he is the Deity or is inspired.

theophobia (thē″ō-fō′bĭ-ă) [" + *phobos,* fear]. Abnormal fear of the wrath of God.

theophylline (thē″ō-fĭl′ēn, -ĭn) [L. *thea,* tea, + G. *phyllon,* plant]. USP. A white crystalline powder with action resembling caffeine and theobromine.

theory. A supposition or an assumption based on certain evidence or observations but lacking scientific proof. When a theory becomes generally accepted and firmly established, it then becomes a *doctrine* or *principle.*

theotherapy (thē″ō-thĕr′a-pĭ) [G. *theos,* god, + *therapeia,* treatment]. Treatment of disease by spiritual and religious methods.

therapeutic (thĕr-ă-pū′tĭk) [G. *therapeutikos,* treating]. 1. Pert. to results obtained from treatment. 2. Having medicinal or healing properties. 3. A healing agent.

t. exercise. Scientific supervision of bodily movements for the purpose of preventing muscular atrophy, to restore joint and muscle motility, and to increase muscular strength. SEE: *exercise.*

therapeutics (thĕr″ă-pū′tĭks) [G. *therapeutikē,* treatment]. That branch of medicine concerned with the application of remedies and the treatment of disease. SYN: *therapy, q.v.*

t., suggestive. Treatment of a condition by using hypnotic suggestion.

therapeutist (thĕr-ă-pū′tĭst) [G. *therapeuein,* to treat medically]. One who practices therapeutics.

therapia sterilisans magna (thĕr″ă-pĭ′ă stē-rĭl′ĭ-săns măg′nă) [L.]. Ehrlich's method of administering chemical agent which will destroy in 1 large dose all the parasites in the body of a patient without causing serious injury to the patient.

therapy (thĕr′ă-pĭ) [G. *therapein,* treatment]. Treatment of a disease or pathological condition.

t., light. Treatment with radiation from the visible spectrum.

t., maggot. Use of maggots in suppurating wounds of bones and soft tissues to remove necrotic areas.

t., mental. The use of suggestion in the treatment of disease.

t., nonspecific. Use of injections of foreign proteins, bacterial vaccines, etc., in treatment of infection to stimulate general cellular activity. SEE: *therapy, specific.*

t., opsonic. Use of bacterial vaccines to elevate the opsonic index of the blood.

t., physical. Use of physical agents in the treatment of disease, as massage, heat, hydrotherapy, radiation, electricity, and exercise.

t., serum. Use of injections of blood serum from immunized animals or persons in the treatment of disease. SYN: *serotherapy.*

t., specific. Administration of a remedy acting directly against the cause of a disease, as arsphenamine or mercury for syphilis, or quinine for malaria

t., spiritual. The application of spiritual knowledge in the treatment of disease. SEE: *spiritual therapy.*

t., substitution. Use of glandular extracts to balance the deficiency of secretion of a gland.

t., vaccine. Injection of bacteria or their products to produce active immunization against a disease. SYN: *therapy, opsonic.*

t., zone. Mechanical manipulation or stimulation of an area in the same longitudinal zone as disorder causing distress.

therm (therm) [G. *thermē,* heat]. Term used to indicate a variety of quantities of heat.

thermacogenesis (thĕr″mă-kō-jĕn′ĕs-ĭs) [" + *genesis,* production]. Production of an increase of body temperature by drug therapy.

thermaerotherapy (thĕr-mā″er-ō-ther′ă-pĭ) [" + *aēr,* air, + *therapeia,* treatment]. Therapeutic application of hot air.

thermal (ther′măl) [G. *thermē,* heat]. Pert. to heat.

t. capacity. Heat necessary to raise any body from 0° to 1° C.

t. death point. Degree of heat that will kill a fluid culture in 10 minutes.

t. radiation. Heat radiation.

t. sense. Capacity for recognition of heat. SYN: *thermesthesia.*

thermalgia (thĕr-măl′jĭ-ă) [" + *algos,* pain]. Neuralgia accompanied by intense burning sensation, pain, redness, and sweating of the area involved. SYN: *causalgia.*

thermanalgesia (thĕr″măn-ăl-jē′zĭ-ă) [" + *an-,* priv. + *algēsis,* pain]. Inability to experience reaction to heat because of cerebral lesion.

thermanesthesia (thĕr″măn-ĕs-thē′zĭ-ă) [" + *an-,* priv. + *aisthēsis,* sensation]. Inability to recognize sensations of heat and cold; insensibility to heat changes.

It sometimes occurs in syringomyelia. SYN: *thermoanesthesia.*

thermatology (thĕr-mă-tŏl′ō-jĭ) [" + *logos*, science]. The study of heat in treatment of disease.

thermelometer (thĕr-mĕl-ŏm′ĕt-ĕr) [" + *electric* + G. *metron*, a measure]. An electric thermometer used to indicate temperature changes too slight to be measured on an ordinary thermometer.

thermesthesia (thĕr-mĕs-thē′zĭ-ă) [" + *aisthēsis*, sensation]. Sensitiveness to heat; temperature sense. SYN: *thermoesthesia*.

thermesthesiometer (thĕr″mĕs-thē-zĭ-ŏm′-ĕt-ĕr) [G. *thermē*, heat, + *aisthēsis*, sensation, + *metron*, a measure]. Device for determining sensibility to heat.

thermhypesthesia (thĕrm-hī-pĕs-thē′zĭ-ă) [" + *hypo*, under, + *aisthēsis*, sensation]. Lessened sensibility of the temperature sense. SYN: *thermohypesthesia*.

thermic (thĕr′mĭk) [G. *thermē*, heat]. Pert. to heat.

t. fever. Sunstroke, collapse and high cutaneous temperature after long exposure to the sun. SYN: *insolation, siriasis*.

t. sense. The temperature sense; ability to react to heat stimuli.

thermo- [G.]. Combining form meaning *hot, heat*.

thermoalgesia (thĕr″mō-ăl-jē′zĭ-ă) [G. *thermē*, heat, + *algēsis*, pain]. Condition in which pain is caused by application of moderate heat. SYN: *thermalgesia*.

thermoanalgesia (thĕr″mō-ăn-ăl-jē′zĭ-ă) [" + *an-*, priv. + *algēsis*, pain]. Loss of heat sensation. SYN: *thermanalgesia*.

thermoanesthesia (thĕr″mō-ăn-ĕs-thē′zĭ-ă) [" + *an-*, priv. + *aisthēsis*, sensation]. 1. Inability to distinguish bet. heat and cold. 2. Insensibility to heat or temperature changes.

thermobiosis (thĕr-mō-bī-ō′sĭs) [" + *biōsis*, a living]. Ability to withstand high temperature.

thermobiotic (thĕr″mō-bī-ot′ĭk) [" + *bios*, life]. Able to exist at high temperature.

thermocauterectomy (thĕr″mō-kaw-tĕr-ĕk′tō-mĭ) [" + *kautērion*, branding iron, + *ektomē*, excision]. Excision by thermocautery.

thermocautery (thĕr″mō-kaw′tĕr-ĭ) [" + *kautērion*, branding iron]. 1. Cautery by application of heat. 2. Cauterizing iron. SEE: *actual cautery*.

thermocoagulation (thĕr″mō-kō-ăg-ū-lā′-shŭn) [G. *thermē*, heat, + L. *coagulāre*, to clot]. The use of high frequency currents to produce coagulation to destroy growths.

thermocouple (thĕr′mō-kŭp-ĕl) [" + L. *copula*, a bond]. Device for measuring slight temperature changes. SYN: *thermopile*.

thermoduric (thĕr″mō-dū′rĭk) [" + L. *durus*, resistant, hard]. Able to live in high temperatures. SEE: *thermophylic*.

thermoesthesia (thĕr″mō-ĕs-thē′zĭ-ă) [" + *aisthēsis*, sensation]. Ability to recognize temperature differences. SYN: *thermesthesia*.

thermoexcitory (thĕr″mō-ĕk-sĭ′tō-rĭ) [G. *thermē*, heat, + L. *excitāre*, to irritate]. Exciting the production of heat in the body.

thermogenesis (thĕr″mō-jĕn′ĕ-sĭs) [" + *genesis*, production]. The production of heat, esp. in the body.

thermograph (thĕr′mō-grăf) [" + *graphein*, to write]. Device for registering variations of heat.

thermohyperalgesia (thĕr″mō-hī″pĕr-ăl-gē′zĭ-ă) [" + *hyper*, above, + *algesis*, pain]. Unbearable pain upon the application of heat.

thermohyperesthesia (thĕr″mō-hī″pĕr-ĕs-thē′zĭ-ă) [G. *thermē*, heat, + *hyper*, above, + *aisthēsis*, sensation]. Exceptional sensitiveness to heat.

thermohypesthesia (thĕr″mō-hī″pĕs-thē′-zĭ-ă) [" + *hypo*, under, + *aisthēsis*, sensation]. Diminished perception of heat.

thermoinhibitory (thĕr″mō-ĭn-hĭb′ĭ-tō″rĭ) [" + L. *inhibere*, to restrain]. Arresting or impeding the generation of body heat.

thermolabile (thĕr″mō-lā′bĭl) [" + *labilis*, unstable]. Destroyed or changed easily by heat; unstable. SEE: *heat; heat, latent*.

thermolysis (thĕr-mŏl′ĭs-ĭs) [" + *lysis*, destruction] 1. Loss of heat from the body, as by evaporation. 2. Chemical decomposition by heat.

thermometer (thĕr-mŏm′ĕ-tĕr) [G. *thermē*, heat, + *metron*, a measure]. An instrument for indicating the degree of heat or cold.

t., air or gas. One filled with air or gas, the expansion of which registers high temperatures.

t., alcohol. One containing alcohol.

t., Celsius. Centigrade t.

t., centigrade. Temperature of boiling water at sea level 100° and freezing point 0°, with 100° bet. Generally used in Latin America and in Europe, and in scientific work.

t., clinical. One for measuring temperature of body and in which the mercury remains stationary at registration point until shaken down.

t., differential. One recording slight variations.

t., Fahrenheit. Boiling point 212°, freezing point 32°. Used in English-speaking countries and in Holland.

t., mercury. One containing mercury.

t., Réaumur. Used in some parts of Germany and in Russia. Zero is same as 0° C. or same as 32° F., having 80° instead of 100 like the Centigrade t. SEE: *Comparative Thermometric Scale, below*.

t. scale. Graduated device on a thermometer to indicate a temperature.

Comparative Thermometric Scale

	Centigrade	Fahrenheit	Réaumur
Boiling point of water ...	100°	212°	80°
	90°	194°	72°
	80°	176°	64°
	70°	158°	56°
	60°	140°	48°
	50°	122°	40°
	40°	104°	32°
	30°	86°	24°
	20°	68°	16°
	10°	50°	8°
Freezing point of water	0°	32°	0°
	—10°	14°	—8°
	—20°	—4°	—16°

CONVERSION: *F. to Centigrade*: Subtract 32 and multiply by 5/9. *C. to Fahrenheit*: Multiply by 9/5 and add 32.

To convert R. into F. *multiply* by 9, *divide* by 4, and *add* 32.

t., self-registering. One recording variations of temperature.

t., spirit. One filled with alcohol instead of mercury for registering low temperatures.

Thermometric Equivalents

C	F	C	F	C	F	C	F
0	32	27	80.6	54	129.2	81	177.8
1	33.8	28	82.4	55	131	82	179.6
2	35.6	29	84.2	56	132.8	83	181.4
3	37.4	30	86.0	57	134.6	84	183.2
4	39.2	31	87.8	58	136.4	85	185
5	41	32	89.6	59	138.2	86	186.8
6	42.8	33	91.4	60	140	87	188.6
7	44.6	34	93.2	61	141.8	88	190.4
8	46.4	35	95	62	143.6	89	192.2
9	48.2	36	96.8	63	145.4	90	194
10	50	37	98.6	64	147.2	91	195.8
11	51.8	38	100.4	65	149	92	197.6
12	53.6	39	102.2	66	150.8	93	199.4
13	55.4	40	104	67	152.6	94	201.2
14	57.2	41	105.8	68	154.4	95	203
15	59	42	107.6	69	156.2	96	204.8
16	60.8	43	109.4	70	158	97	206.6
17	62.6	44	111.2	71	159.8	98	208.4
18	64.4	45	113	72	161.6	99	210.2
19	66.2	46	114.8	73	163.4	100	212
20	68	47	116.6	74	165.2		
21	69.8	48	118.4	75	167		
22	71.6	49	120.2	76	168.8		
23	73.4	50	122	77	170.6		
24	75.2	51	123.8	78	172.4		
25	77	52	125.6	79	174.2		
26	78.8	53	127.4	80	176		

t., surface. One for showing temperature of the body's surface.

t., wet and dry bulb. A device for determining relative humidity consisting of two thermometers, the bulb of one being kept saturated with water vapor. The difference in temperatures between the two is dependent upon relative humidity.

thermometric (thĕr″mō-mĕt′rĭk) [G. *thermē*, heat, + *metron*, a measure]. Pert. to heat measurement or a thermometer.

thermometry (thĕr-mŏm′ĕt-rĭ) [G. *thermē*, heat, + *metron*, a measure]. Measurement of temperature.

t., clinical. Temperature of body, taken orally, in a state of health ranges between 96.6° and 100° F. During a 24 hr. period, a person's body temperature may vary 0.5° to 2.0° F. It is highest in late afternoon, lowest during sleep in early hours of the morning.

Slightly increased by eating, exercising and external heat; reduced about 1½° during sleep. In disease the temperature of body deviates several degrees above and below the average of health. When it moves upwards it is far less dangerous than when it moves downward, particularly in children. Even in adults 1° below the standard of health represents more danger than 2½° above, and 2° below more than 4° above, and so on.

In facial erysipelas, acute meningitis, pneumonia, scarlatina, typhus, smallpox, and intermittent fever it sometimes rises as high as 106° or 107° F. In other febrile diseases rarely reaches 104° F. Temperature may reach height of 110° F., as seen in sunstroke, and patient recovers.

The lowest extreme of temperature is sometimes found in cold stage of cholera, when temperature may be very low (90°-85° F.) for several days. Subnormal temperatures below 98° F. are observed in the following conditions:

During convalescence from certain febrile conditions, after pneumonia and typhoid fever, temperature may remain subnormal for several days. In collapse: This may result from shock, from hemorrhage, or from rupture of a viscus, as the bowel in typhoid, the lung in phthisis or stomach in perforating ulcer.

In general, for every degree of fever the pulse rises 10 beats per minute, but rise of temperature to 99.5° F. gives more evidence of disease than rising of pulse from 70 to 90 beats per minute. If temperature remains above normal after general symptoms denote convalescence. patient is in danger of a relapse or the supervention of some other disease. The range of the increase of heat in different febrile diseases extends to 110° F. and as a rule the amount of increase is a criterion of the intensity of the disease.

Artificial fever induced through diathermy, continuous hot bath, or malarial injections utilized in some diseases.

thermoneurosis (thĕr″mō-nū-rō′sĭs) [G. *thermē*, heat, + *neuron*, nerve, + *-ōsis*, condition]. Elevation of body temperature in hysteria and other nervous conditions.

thermopenetration (thĕr″mō-pĕn-ĕ-trā′-shŭn) [" + L. *penetrāre*, to penetrate]. Application of heat to the deeper tissues of the body by diathermy.

thermoperiodicity (thĕrm-ō-pĕr-ĭ-ō-dĭs′-ĭ-tĭ). Condition in which an organism grows better when exposed to alternating high and low temperatures.

thermophagy (thĕrm′ō-fā-gĭ). Swallowing extremely hot foods.

thermophilic (thĕr″mō-fĭl′ĭk) [" + *philein*, to love]. Preferring or thriving best at high temperatures, said of bacteria which thrive best at temperatures between 40° and 70° C. (104° and 158° F.).

thermophobia (thĕr″mō-fō′bĭ-ă) [" + *phobos*, fear]. Abnormal dread of heat.

thermophore (thĕr′mō-fōr) [" + *phoros*, a bearer]. Apparatus for applying heat to a part, consisting of water heater and tubes conveying water to a coil and returning to heater, or salts which produce heat when moistened.

thermophylic (thĕr″mō-fĭ′lĭk) [" + *phylakē,* guard]. Resistant to destruction by heat, noting certain bacteria.

thermopile (thĕr′mō-pīl) [G. *thermē,* heat, + L. *pila,* pile]. PT: A thermoelectric battery used in measuring small variations in the degree of heat.

It consists of a number of dissimilar metallic plates connected together in which, under the influence of heat, an electric current is produced.

thermoplegia (thĕr″mō-plē′jĭ-ă) [" + *plēgē,* a stroke]. Heatstroke; sunstroke. SYN: *insolation, siriasis.*

thermopolypnea (thĕr″mō-pŏl-ĭp-nē′ă) [" + *polys,* many, + *pnoia,* breath]. Quickened breathing caused by high fever or great heat.

thermoradiotherapy (thĕr″mō-rā″dĭ-ō-thĕr′ă-pĭ) [" + L. *radius,* ray, + G. *therapeia,* treatment] Application of heat to deep tissues by diathermy. SYN: *thermopenetration.*

thermoreceptor (thĕrm-ō-rē-sĕpt′or). A sensory receptor which is stimulated by a rise of body temperature.

thermoregulatory (thĕrm″ō-rĕg′ū-lă-tōr-ĭ). Pertaining to the regulation of temperature, especially body temperature.

t. centers. Centers in the hypothalamus which regulate heat production and heat loss, especially the latter, so that a normal body temperature is maintained. They are influenced by nervous impulses from cutaneous receptors and by the temperature of the blood flowing through them.

thermoresistant (thĕr″mō-rē-zĭs′tănt) [" + L. *resistentia,* resistance]. Able to resist high temperature, but not develop in it, noting bacteria.

thermostabile (thĕr″mō-stā′bl) [" + L. *stabilis,* stationary]. Not changed or destroyed by heat.

thermostat (thĕr′mō-stăt) [G. *thermē,* heat, + *statos,* standing]. An automatic device for regulating the temperature.

thermosteresis (thĕr″mō-stē-rē′sĭs) [" + *sterēsis,* deprivation]. The deprivation or loss of heat.

thermosystaltic (thĕr″mō-sĭs-tăl′tĭk) [" + *systellein,* to contract]. Pert. to contraction of the muscles under stimulus of heat.

thermotactic, thermotaxic (thĕr″mō-tăk′-tĭk, -tăks′ĭk) [" + *taktikos,* regulating, — + *taxis,* order]. Relating to regulation of the body temperature.

thermotaxis (thĕr″mō-tăks′ĭs) [" + *taxis,* arrangement]. 1. Regulation of bodily temperature. 2. Reaction of organisms or of protoplasm in the living body to heat. 3. SYN: *thermometropism.* The movement of certain organisms or cells toward (positive thermotaxis) or away from (negative thermotaxis) heat.

thermotherapeutics (thĕr″mō-thĕr-ă-pū′-tĭks) [" + *therapeutikē,* treatment]. Use of heat in treatment of disease. SYN: *thermotherapy.*

thermotherapy (thĕr″mō-thĕr′ă-pĭ) [G. *thermē,* heat, + *therapeia,* treatment]. PT: The therapeutic application of heat. Heat may be applied locally by radiant heating devices which give off infrared rays and by conductive heating which utilizes hot water bottles, paraffin baths, hot packs, etc. or the temperature of the body may be increased (hyperthermia, *q.v.*) by artificial fever induced by raising environmental temperature or preventing heat loss from the body. SEE: *heat.*

thermotolerant (thĕr″mō-tŏl′ĕr-ănt) [G. *thermē,* heat, + L. *tolerāre,* to tolerate]. Able to live normally in high temperature.

thermotoxin (thĕr″mō-toks′ĭn) [" + *toxikon,* poison]. A poison formed in the tissues by excessive heat.

thermotropism (thĕrm-ō-trō′pĭsm). Thermotaxis, *q.v.*

thesaurismosis [G. *thesaurosis,* treasure, + *-osis,* condition]. Abnormal or excessive storage of substances in certain cells. Usually due to a metabolic disease such as lipoidosis.

thesis (thē′sĭs) [G. *thesis,* proposition]. An essay on a given subject offered by a candidate for a collegiate degree.

thi′amin(e). SYN: *vitamin* B_1. A white crystalline compound ($O_{12}H_{17}N_4OS$), occurring naturally and also produced synthetically. It is widely distributed in various animal and plant foods, dry yeast and wheat germ being the richest natural resources. It occurs in the outer layers of seeds and in nuts, legumes, and most vegetables, and in some meats (pork, muscle, livers, hearts, and kidneys).

FUNCTION: It is essential for the normal metabolism of carbohydrates and fats. It acts as a coenzyme of carboxylases in the carboxylation of pyruvic acid, hence is essential for the liberation of energy and disposal of pyruvic acid.

EFFECTS OF DEFICIENCY: Moderate deficiency results in impaired functioning of nervous, circulatory, digestive, and endocrine systems. Neurasthenia, neurologic disorders, cardiac, and gastrointestinal symptoms may result. Loss of appetite, fatigue, muscle tenderness, and increased irritability are symptoms. Severe and prolonged deficiency results in *beriberi.*

DAILY REQUIREMENTS: 1.5 to 3 mg. depending on activity and carbohydrate intake.

Thiersch's graft or **method** (tērsh). A method of skin grafting using epidermis and a portion of the dermis.

thigh (thī) [A.S. *thioh,* thigh], The proximal portion of the lower extremity; the portion lying between the hip joint and the knee. SEE: *hip, pectineus, sartorius.*

t. bone. The femur.

t. joint. The hip joint. SYN: *articulatio coxae.*

thigmesthesia (thĭg-mĕs-thē′zĭ-ă) [G. *thigma,* touch, + *aisthēsis,* sensation]. The sense of touch.

thigmotaxis (thĭg″mō-tăks′ĭs) ["+ *taxis,* arrangement]. Arrangement in which some cells are attracted by contact with solids. SYN: *thigmotropism.*

thigmotropism (thĭg-mŏt′rō-pĭzm) [" + *tropos,* a turning, + *-ismos,* condition]. The attraction exerted by contact with solids over certain cells. SYN: *thigmotaxis.*

thio- [G.]. Prefix denoting *presence of sulfur replacing oxygen.*

thiogenic (thī-ō-jĕn′ĭk) [G. *theion,* sulfur, + *gennan,* to produce]. Able to convert hydrogen sulfide into higher sulfur compounds, said of bacteria in the water of some mineral springs.

thioneine (thī′ō-nēn) [G. *theion,* sulfur, + *neos,* new]. Crystalline sulfur-containing compound found in ergot and red blood cells.

Structurally identified as thiolhistidine.

thiopectic, thiopexic (thī-ō-pĕk′tĭk, -pĕks′-ĭk) [" + *pēxis,* fixation]. Pert. to the fixation of sulfur.

thiopexy (thī′ō-pĕks-ĭ) [" + *pēxis,* fixation]. The fixation of sulfur.

thiophil, thiophilic (thī′ō-fĭl, thī-ō-fĭl′ĭk) [" + *philein,* to love]. Thriving in the presence of sulfur or its compounds, as some bacteria.

thiouracil (thī-ō-ū′ră-sĭl). An antithyroid drug used in treatment of hyperthyroidism, thyrotoxicosis, and thyroiditis.

thiourea (thī″ō-ū-rē′ă) [" + urea]. Colorless crystalline compound of urea in which sulfur replaces the oxygen.

third cranial nerve. Oculomotor nerve. SEE: *Appendix.*

t. intention. Healing of a wound by filling with granulations. SEE: *resolution.*

t. ventricle. Third ventricle of the brain, a narrow cavity bet. the 2 optic thalami. SYN: *ventriculus tertius.*

thirst. 1. Desire for fluid, esp. for water.

This may obtain in fevers and certain other maladies, or it may be entirely lacking in some conditions. The nurse should note whether the intake of fluids allays the patient's thirst. 2. The sensation resulting from the lack of or the need of water. Thirst may result from drying of mucous membranes especially those of the pharynx or from reduced salivary secretion. It also results from general dehydration as may occur following hemorrhage, profuse sweating, vomiting, or excessive loss of urine as in diabetes.

RS: *adipsia, adipsous, adipsy, anadipsia, aposia, taste.*

t., absence of. Adipsia, aposia.

t., excessive. Polydipsia.

t., false. Pseudodipsia; not sated by drinking water.

t., morbid. Dipsosis.

Thiry's fistula (tē′rē). An artificial fistula in a dog's intestines for obtaining intestinal juice for experimental purposes.

Thomsen's disease (tŏm′sĕn). SYN: *myotonia congenita, q.v.*

thoracalgia (thō-răk-ăl′jĭ-ă) [G. *thōrax, thōrak-,* chest, + *algos,* pain]. Pain in the chest wall. SYN: *pleurodynia.*

thoracectomy (thō-ră-sĕk′tō-mĭ) [" + *ektomē,* excision]. Incision of the chest wall with resection of a portion of rib.

thoracentesis (thō″răs-ĕn-tē′sĭs) [" + *kentēsis,* a puncture]. Surgical puncture of the chest wall for removal of fluids. Usually done by using a large-bore needle. SYN: *pleurocentesis, q.v.*

NP: Have patient well supported. Watch for signs of collapse during and following treatment.

thoracic (thŏr-ăs′ĭk) [G. *thōrax, thōrak-,* chest]. Pert. to the chest or thorax.

t. cavity. The space lying above the diaphragm and enclosed within the walls of the thorax; the space occupied by the thoracic viscera. It includes the *pleural cavities* occupied by the lungs and the *mediastinum,* the space between the lungs occupied by the heart lying within the pericardium, the thoracic aorta, pulmonary artery and veins, vena cavae, thymus gland, lymph nodes, trachea, bronchi, and thoracic duct. It is separated from the abdominal cavity by the diaphragm.

t. duct. The main lymph duct of the body having its origin at the *cisterna chyli* on the abdomen. It passes upward through the diaphragm into the thorax, continuing upward alongside aorta and esophagus to the neck where it turns to the left and enters the left subclavian vein near its junction with the left internal jugular vein. It receives lymph from all parts of the body except right side of head, neck, and thorax and right upper extremity.

t. limbs. Upper extremities.

RS: *lacteals, lymphatic, lymphatic system, chyle, cisterna chyli.*

thoraco- [G.]. Combining form meaning *chest, chest wall.*

thoracobronchotomy (thō″răk-ō-brŏn-kŏt′-ō-mĭ) [G. *thōrax, thorak-,* chest, + *brogchos,* windpipe, + *tomē,* a cutting]. Incision through the thoracic wall into the bronchus.

thoracocautery (thō″răk-ō-kaw′tĕr-ĭ) [" + *kautērion,* branding iron]. The use of cautery in breaking up pulmonary adhesions to collapse the lung.

thoracoceloschisis (thō″răk-ō-sē-lŏs′kĭ-sĭs) [" + *koilia,* belly, + *schisis,* a fissure]. Congenital fissure of the thoracic and abdominal cavities.

thoracocentesis (thō″răk-ō-sĕn-tē′sĭs) [" + *kentēsis,* a puncture]. Tapping of the thorax. SYN: *thoracentesis.*

thoracocyllosis (thō″răk-ō-sĭl-ō′sĭs) [" + *kyllōsis,* crippling]. Deformity of the chest.

thoracocyrtosis (thō″răk-ō-sĭr-tō′sĭs) [" + *kyrtōsis,* curvature]. Excessive curvature of the chest.

thoracodynia (thō″răk-ō-dĭn′ĭ-ă) [" + *odynē,* pain]. Pain in the thorax.

thoracogastroschisis (thō″răk-ō-găs-trŏs′-kĭs-ĭs) [G. *thōrax, thorak-,* chest, + *gastēr,* belly, + *schisis,* a cleft]. Congenital fissure of abdomen and thorax.

thoracolumbar (thō″răk-ō-lŭm′bar) [" + L. *lumbus,* loin]. Pert. to the thoracic and lumbar parts of the spine; noting their ganglia and the fibers of the sympathetic nervous system.

thoracolysis (thō″răk-ŏl′ĭs-ĭs) [G. *thōrax, thorak-,* chest, + *lysis,* loosening]. SYN: *pneumonolysis.* The freeing of a lung which is attached to the chest wall.

thoracometry (thō″ră-kŏm′ĕt-rĭ). The measurement of the thorax.

thoracomyodynia (thō″ră-kō-mī″ō-dĭn′ĭ-ă) [" + *mys, my-,* muscle, + *odynē,* pain]. Pain in chest muscles.

thoracopagus [" + G. *pagos,* fixed]. Two malformed fetuses joined at the thorax.

thoracopathy (thō″răk-ŏp′ăth-ĭ) [" + *pathos,* disease]. Any disease of the thorax, thoracic organs, or tissues.

thoracoplasty (thō′ră-kō-plăs″tĭ, thō-ră′-kō-plăs″tĭ) [G. *thōrax, thorak-,* chest, + *plassein,* to form]. A plastic operation upon the thorax; removal of portions of the ribs in stages to collapse diseased areas of the lung. SEE: *empyema.*

thoracopneumoplasty (thō″ră-kō-nū′mō-plăs-tĭ) [" + *pneumon,* lung, + *plassein,* to form]. Plastic surgery involving the chest and lung.

thoracoschisis (thō-ră-kŏs′kĭ-sĭs) [" + *schisis,* a cleft]. Congenital fissure of the chest wall.

thoracoscope (thō-ră′kō-skōp, -răk′ō-skōp) [" + *skopein,* to examine]. 1. An instrument used in auscultation to convey the sounds of the chest to the ear. SYN: *stethoscope.* 2. Instrument, for inspecting the thoracic cavity, which has an electric light and is inserted through an intercostal space.

thoracoscopy (thō″ră-kŏs′kō-pĭ) [" + *skopein,* to examine]. Diagnostic examination of the pleural cavity with an endoscope.

thoracostenosis (thō″ră-kō-stĕn-ō′sĭs) [" + *stenōsis*, a contraction]. Narrowness of the thorax. SYN: *waspwaist.*

thoracostomy (thō-răk-ŏs′tō-mĭ) [" + *stoma*, mouth]. Resection of chest wall to allow room for enlarged heart or for drainage.

thoracotomy (thō″răk-ŏt′ō-mĭ) [G. *thōrax, thorak-*, chest, + *tomē*, a cutting]. Surgical incision of the chest wall.

thorax (thō′răks) (pl. *thoraces* or *thoraxes*) [G. *thōrax*]. That part of the body bet. the base of the neck superiorly and the diaphragm inferiorly. SYN: *chest.*

The surface of the thorax is divided into regions as follows:

ANTERIOR SURFACE: *Supraclavicular*, above the clavicles; *suprasternal*, above the sternum; *clavicular*, over the clavicles; *sternal*, over the sternum; *mammary*, the space bet. the 3rd and 6th ribs on either side; *inframammary*, below the mamma and above the lower border of the 12th rib on either side.

POSTERIOR SURFACE: *Scapular*, over the scapulae; *interscapular*, bet. the scapulae; *infrascapular*, below the scapulae.

ON SIDES: *Axillary*, above the 6th rib.

RS: *acromiothoracis, cholohemothorax, "thorac-" words.*

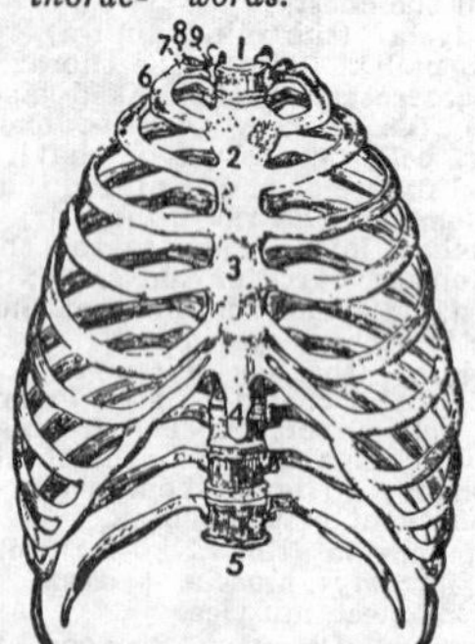

THE SKELETAL THORAX

1. First thoracic vertebra. 2. Manubrium. 3. Gladiolus. 4. Xiphoid processus. 5. Last thoracic vertebra. 6. First rib.

t., Amazon. A chest with only 1 breast.

t., barrel-shaped. A malformed chest rounded like a barrel seen in pulmonary emphysema.

t., fusiform. A chest deformed by long continued tight lacing.

t. paralyticus. The long, flat chest of patients with constitutional visceroptosis.

t., Peyrot's. A chest that has an obliquely oval, deformed shape, seen in large pleural effusions

thorazine (thōr-ă′zēn). A proprietary name for chlorpromazine hydrochloride. It is a central nervous system depressant and employed as a sedative and antiemetic. It potentiates the effects of sedatives and general anesthetics and is of value in quieting severely excited psychiatric patients.

thorium (thō′rĭ-ŭm). SYMB: Th. A metallic element occurring in combination. At. wt. 232.038; at. no. 90.

It is radioactive. Once used to outline blood vessels.

thoron (thō′rŏn). A gaseous, radioactive element; an emanation or transformation product of thorium. SYMB: Tn. At. wt. 220; at. no. 86.

threadworm. 1. Common name applied to the pinworm, *Enterobius vermicularis.*

three-day fever. SYN: *pappataci fever, sandfly fever.* A viral disease transmitted by the sandfly, *Phlebotomus papatasii.* It resembles dengue but is less severe.

thremmatology (thrĕm-ă-tŏl′ō-jĭ) [G. *thremma*, nursling, + *logos*, science]. Science of breeding according to the laws of heredity and variation.

threonine (thrē′ō-nĭn). Alpha-amino-beta-hydroxybutyric acid. One of the essential amino acids.

threpsology (thrĕp-sŏl′ō-jĭ) [G. *threpsis*, nutrition, + *logos*, study]. Science of nutrition.

threshold (thrĕsh′ōld) [A.S. *therscwold*]. 1. Point at which a psychological or physiological effect begins to be produced. 2. A measure of the sensitivity of an organ or function which is obtained by finding the lowest value of the appropriate stimulus that will give the response.

t., absolute. The stimulus of least intensity that will give rise to a sensation or a response.

t., auditory. Minimum audible sound.

t. of consciousness. PSY: Point at which a stimulus is just barely perceived.

t., differential. The lowest limit at which two stimuli can be differentiated from each other.

t., erythe′ma. Stage in which e. of the skin due to radiation just begins.

t., ketosis. The lower limit at which ketone bodies (acetoacetic acid, hydroxybutyric acid, and acetone), upon their accumulation in the blood, are excreted by the kidney. Such indicates that ketone bodies are being produced faster by the liver than the body can oxidize them.

t., renal. The concentration at which a substance in the blood normally not excreted by the kidney begins to appear in the urine. The renal threshold for *glucose* is 160-180 mg. per 100 ml. SEE: *threshold.*

t., sensory. The minimal stimulus for any sensory receptor which will give rise to a sensation.

t., stimulus. SYN: *liminal stimulus, rheobase.* The least or minimal stimulus that will give rise to a sensation or bring about a response such as a muscle contraction.

t. substance. A substance present in the blood which serves a useful function which on being filtered through glomeruli of the kidney is reabsorbed by the tubules up to a certain limit, that being the upper limit of the concentration of the substance in "normal" plasma. *High-threshold* substances are those which are entirely or almost entirely reabsorbed; Ex: *glucose, chlorides; low-threshold* substances are those which are reabsorbed in limited quantities; Ex. *urea, phosphates; no-threshold substances* are those excreted in their entirety. Ex: *creatinine sulfate.*

thrill (thrĭl) [M.E. *thrillen*, to pierce]. 1. Abnormal tremor accompanying a vascular or cardiac murmur felt on palpation. SYN: *fremitus.* 2. A tingling or shivering sensation of tremulous excitement, as from pain, pleasure, or horror.

t., aneurysmal. One felt on palpation of an aneurysm.

t., aortic. One heard over aortic aperture in lesions of valves.

t., arterial. One heard over an artery.

t., diastolic. One felt over the heart during diastole of the ventricle.

t., hydatid. Peculiar tremor felt on palpation of a hydatid cyst.

t., presystolic. One sometimes felt over apex of the heart preceding ventricular contraction.

throat (thrōt) [A.S. *throte*]. 1. The pharynx and the fauces. 2. Cavity from arch of palate to glottis and sup. opening of the esophagus. 3. The front of the neck. 4. Any narrow orifice.

t., sore. SYN: *odynophagia, pharyngitis, tonsillitis.* Inflammation of tonsils, larynx, or pharynx.

FOREIGN BODIES IN: The symptoms depend somewhat on the location and size of the foreign body, and vary from simple discomfort to distressing coughing, difficulty in breathing, retching and cyanosis, and, if not relieved, suffocation resulting in unconsciousness.

TREATMENT: If not causing serious distress, the patient should lie down with the head lower than the body. The common practice of a sudden slap on the back often helps to dislodge bodies in the trachea or throat, and in youngsters is esp. efficacious when the child is inverted. If this does not succeed, it is possible to introduce a finger through the mouth into the throat, possibly to the larynx, and so dislodge the foreign body. It has been possible in this way to dislodge a bean from the larynx of an unconscious child.

Summon a physician immediately. Make sure to tell him the nature of the case so that he may bring the proper instruments, as it may be necessary for him to open the trachea. Cathartics and enemas are of no value whatever, and may be dangerous. SEE: *symptoms, throat.*

throb (thrŏb) [M.E. *throbben*, of imitative origin]. 1. A beat or pulsation, as of the heart. 2. To pulsate.

throbbing (thrŏb'ĭng) [M.E. *throbben*, of imitative origin]. Pulsation; a beating; rhythmic movement.

Throckmorton's reflex (thrŏk'mor"tŭn). Extension of great toe and flexion of others when dorsum of foot is percussed in metatarsophalangeal region.

throe (thrō) [A.S. *thrauu*, suffering]. A severe pain or pang, esp. one in childbirth.

thrombasthenia (thrŏm-băs-thē'nĭ-ă) [" + *astheneia*, weakness]. Deficiency of the blood platelets.

thrombectomy (thrŏm-bĕk'tō-mĭ) [" + *ektomē*, excision]. Excision of a thrombus.

thrombi. Plural of thrombus.

thrombin (thrŏm'bĭn) [G. *thrombus*, a clot]. 1. An enzyme formed in shed-blood from prothrombin which reacts with soluble *fibrinogen* converting it to *fibrin* which forms the basis of a blood clot. SEE: *coagulation.*

thrombin'ogen. SYN: *prothrombin, serozyme, thrombogen, proserozyme.* A factor in the blood essential for clotting; the precursor of thrombin, *q.v.*

thrombo- [G.]. Combining form meaning *clot of blood;* a *thrombus.*

thromboangiitis (thrŏm-bō-ăn-jĭ-ī'tĭs) [G. *thrombos*, clot, + *aggeion*, vessel, + *-itis*, inflammation]. Inflammation of inner coat of a blood vessel with clot formation. SEE: *thrombosis.*

t. obliterans. Chronic recurring inflammatory occlusive disease, chiefly of the peripheral arteries and veins, with an extraordinary affinity for young men. SYN: *Buerger's disease.*

SYM: Occlusion; thrombosis; excruciating pain in leg or foot, worse at night; cyanotic, clammy cold extremity; diminished sense of heat and cold; gangrene of toes or foot may set in.

thromboarteritis (thrŏm"bō-ar-tē-rī'tĭs) [" + *artēria*, artery, + *-itis*, inflammation]. Inflammation of an artery in connection with thrombosis.

thromboblast (thrŏm'bō-blăst) [" + *blastos*, a germ]. A small basophilic cell, said to be the mother cell of the blood platelet.

thromboclasis (thrŏm-bŏk'lă-sĭs) [" + *klasis*, a breaking]. The breaking up of a thrombus. SYN: *thrombolysis.*

thromboclastic (thrŏm-bō-klăs'tĭk) [" + *klasis*, a breaking]. Pert. to or producing the dissolution of a thrombus. SYN: *thrombolytic.*

thrombocyst, thrombocystis (thrŏm'bō-sĭst, -sĭs'tĭs) [" + *kystis*, a sac]. A membranous sac enveloping a thrombus.

thrombocyte (thrŏm'bō-sīt) [G. *thrombos*, a clot, + *kytos*, cell]. One of the pale disks found in normal blood, 200,000 to 400,000 per cu. mm. which aid in coagulation. SYN: *blood platelet.*

They are much smaller than the corpuscles. SEE: *blood, erythrocyte, leukocyte.*

thrombocytocrit (thrŏm"bō-sī'tō-krĭt) [" + *kytos*, cell, + *krinein*, to separate]. Device for estimating the platelet content of the blood.

thrombocytolysis (thrŏm"bō-sī-tŏl'ĭ-sĭs) [" + " + *lysis*, dissolution]. Dissolution of thrombocytes.

thrombocytopenia (thrŏm"bō-sī"tō-pē'nĭ-ă) [" + " + *penia*, lack]. Abnormal decrease in number of the blood platelets. SYN: *thrombopenia.*

thrombocytopoiesis (thrŏm"bō-sī"tō-poy-ē'sĭs) [" + " + *poiēsis*, production]. The development of blood platelets.

thrombocytosis (thrŏm"bō-sī-tō'sĭs). Increase in number of thrombocytes.

thromboembolism (thrŏm"bō-ĕm'bō-lĭsm). An embolism; the blocking of a blood vessel by a thrombus which has become detached from its site of formation.

thromboendocarditis. Formation of a clot on inflamed surface of a heart valve.

thrombogen (thrŏm'bō-jĕn) [" + *gennan*, to produce]. A substance believed to be present in blood plasma which is the precursor of thrombin. SYN: *prothrombin.*

thrombogenesis (thrŏm"bō-jĕn'ĕs-ĭs) [G. *thrombos*, a clot, + *genesis*, production]. The formation of a blood clot.

thrombogenic (thrŏm"bō-jĕn'ĭk) [" + *gennan*, to produce]. Producing or tending to produce a clot.

thromboid (thrŏm'boyd) [" + *eidos*, form]. Resembling a thrombus or clot.

thrombokinase (thrŏm"bō-kĭn'ās) [G. *thrombos*, a clot, + *kinēsis*, motion]. SYN: *thromboplastin, q.v.*

thrombokinesis (thrŏm"bō-kĭn-ē'sĭs) [" + *kinēsis*, motion]. The coagulation of the blood.

thrombolymphangitis (thrŏm"bō-lĭm-făn-jī'tĭs) [" + L. *lympha*, lymph, + G. *aggeion*, vessel, + *-itis*, inflammation]. Inflammation of a lymphatic vessel due to obstruction by thrombus formation.

thrombolysis (thrŏm-bŏl'ĭ-sĭs) [" + *lysis*, destruction]. The breaking up of a thrombus. SYN: *thromboclasis.*

thrombolytic (thrŏm″bō-lĭt′ĭk) [G. *thrombos,* clot, + *lysis,* dissolution]. Pert. to or causing the breaking up of a thrombus.

thrombopathy (thrŏm-bŏp′ăth-ĭ) [" + *pathos,* disease]. A defect in the coagulation apparatus of the blood. SYN: *hemophilia, q.v.*

thrombopenia (thrŏm-bō-pē′nĭ-ă) [" + *penia,* lack]. Lessening of the number of blood platelets.

thrombophilia (thrŏm-bō-fĭl′ĭ-ă) [" + *philein,* to love]. A tendency to the occurrence of clot formation.

thrombophlebitis (thrŏm″bō-flē-bī′tĭs) [G. *thrombos,* a clot, + *phleps, phleb-,* vein, + *-itis,* inflammation]. Inflammation of a vein developing before the formation of a thrombus. SYN: *phlebitis, thrombophlebitis, milk leg, phlegmasia, alba dolens, venous thrombosis.*

NP: Immobilize the affected limb, elevate it and support with a pillow. The weight of bedclothes should be removed by supporting them on a cradle. Fomentations may be ordered. All applications should be kept in place by a many-tailed bandage made so movement of the limb is prevented in changing dressings. Limb should be kept from pressure and well wrapped to keep it warm. It should be inspected daily to see that skin is in good condition.

TREATMENT: Absolute rest to avoid the greatest danger, which is an embolus. Leg elevated so hip and knee are in flexion and heat is applied. Patient must not get up until the temperature has been normal for at least a week; if there have been infarcts, for about 2 weeks. Anticoagulants and ligation of large vein proximal to the thrombus are often used.

thromboplastic (thrŏm″bō-plăs′tĭk) [G. *thrombos,* clot, + *plassein,* to form]. Pert. to or causing acceleration of clot formation in the blood.

thromboplastin (thrŏm″bō-plăs′tĭn) [" + *plassein,* to form]. A substance found in the tissues which accelerates clotting of the blood.

thrombopoiesis (thrŏm″bō-poy-ē′sĭs) [" + *poiēsis,* production]. The formation of blood platelets.

thrombosed (thrŏm′bōzd) [G. *thrombos,* a clot]. 1. Coagulated; clotted. 2. Denoting a vessel containing a thrombus.

thrombosin (thrŏm-bō′sĭn) [G. *thrombos,* clot]. A substance derived from the cleavage of fibrinogen which can be converted into fibrin.

thrombosinusitis (thrŏm″bō-sī-nŭs-ī′tĭs) [" + L. *sinus,* cavity, + G. *-itis,* inflammation]. Thrombus formation of a dural sinus.

thrombosis (thrŏm-bō′sĭs) [G. *thrombos,* clot, + *-ōsis,* condition]. The formation of a blood clot or *thrombus.*

RS: *embolus, "thromb-" words, angina pectoris.*

It is a solid aggregation formed in circulating blood and such changes constitute *thrombosis.* When a thrombus is detached from its original site and found in another part, it is called a *thrombotic embolus.** The simpler forms of *thrombi* do not contain clotted blood.

ETIOL: Trauma, esp. following an operation and parturition; cardiac and vascular disorders, obesity, heredity, increasing age, an excess of erythrocytes and of platelets, an overproduction of fibrinogen, and sepsis are predisposing causes.

SYM: *Lungs*: Obstruction of smaller vessels in the lungs causes an infarct manifested by sudden pain in the side of the chest, similar to pleurisy; also the spitting of blood, a pleural friction rub, and signs of consolidation. *Kidneys*: Blood appears in the urine, and small hemorrhagic spots in the skin. *Spleen*: Pain is felt in the left upper abdomen. *Extremities*: If a large artery in one of the extremities, such as the brachial, is suddenly obstructed, the part becomes cold, pale, bluish, and the pulse disappears below the obstructed site. Gangrene of the digits or of the whole limb may ensue. Same symptoms may apply to embolisms, *q.v.*

NP: In thrombosis of a limb rest in bed is essential. Patient must not be permitted to move himself; not even the upper portion of his body. Elevate the affected limb on a pillow and steady it with sandbags. Cotton or wool may be wrapped about the limb and held in place by a many-tailed bandage, extending from groin to foot. Any application to the limb must be kept in place by a similar bandage.

If limb is badly swollen watch for pressure sores. Guard against burning with hot water bottle or electric pad. From 6 days to several weeks bedrest may be necessary depending on condition of patient.

Anticoagulant therapy necessary. When a thrombus or embolus is large, surgical removal may be necessary.

t., atrophic. T. resulting from malnutrition.

t., cardiac. Thrombosis of the heart.

t., coagulation. T. due to coagulation of fibrin in a blood vessel.

t., compression. T. due to compression bet. a thrombus and the heart.

t., coronary. T. of the coronary arteries. A common cause of myocardial infarction.

SYM: Sudden onset of severe and prolonged substernal oppression and pain, the pain arising over the precordium and being referred to the upper and middle sternum and often radiating to the left and sometimes right arm and into the neck. Blood pressure usually falls, pulse becomes rapid, fever and leukocytosis usually observed within 24 hrs. Erythrocyte sedimentation rate becomes elevated and electrocardiographic changes occur.

TREATMENT: Complete physical and mental rest for first week. Special nursing care is desirable. Prompt and complete relief from pain by use of morphine sulfate; oxygen administration sometimes necessary. Vasopressor drugs to elevate blood pressure; digitalis when there is evidence of congestive heart failure; treatment of cardiac arrhythmias, esp. tachycardia; anticoagulants. Treatment in coronary care unit is highly desirable.

DIET: Low protein and carbohydrate intake of approx. 1000 cal. Fluids to produce urinary output of 1500 cc. daily. Restrict salt intake.

POSSIBLE COMPLICATIONS: Shock; acute pulmonary edema; paroxysmal ventricular tachycardia; congestive heart failure.

t., dilatation. T. due to dilatation of a vein.

t., embolic. T. due to an embolus obstructing a vessel.

t., infective. T. due to bacterial infection.

t., marasmic. T. due to wasting diseases of infancy and old age.

t., placental. Thrombi in the placenta and veins of the uterus.

t., plate. Thrombus formed from an accumulation of blood platelets.

t., puerperal. Coagulation in veins following labor.

t., sinus. T. of a venous sinus.

LATERAL: ETIOL: Associated with middle ear disease. SYM: Sudden rise of temperature with remission, chills, prostration, sweats, headache, mental symptoms, dullness or delirium, high leukocyte count.

CAVERNOUS: Sinus structures involved, edema and venous stasis in and about the eye.

t., traumatic. T. due to a wound or injury of a part.

t., venous. T. of a vein.

thrombostasis (thrŏm-bŏs′tă-sĭs) [G. *thrombos,* clot, + *stasis,* a checking]. Stasis of blood in a part causing or due to formation of thrombus.

thrombotic (thrŏm-bŏt′ĭk) [G. *thrombos,* clot]. Related to, caused by, or of the nature of, a thrombus.

thrombus (thrŏm′bŭs) [G. *thrombos*]. A blood clot obstructing a blood vessel or a cavity of the heart.

Anticoagulants are being used in prevention and treatment of this condition.

t., annular. One whose circumference is attached to the walls of a vessel, an opening still remaining in the center.

t., antemortem. A clot formed before death in heart or large vessels.

t., ball. A round clot in the heart, esp. in the auricles.

t., hyaline. One having a glassy appearance usually occurring in smaller blood vessels.

t., Laennec's. A globular thrombus which forms in the heart, usually in cases of fatty degeneration.

t., lateral. A mural one, *q.v.*

t., milk. A curdled milk tumor in the female breast due to obstruction in a lactiferous duct.

t., mural. SYN: *lateral t., parietal t.* One attached to the wall of a vessel or the heart.

t., obstructing. One completely occluding the lumen of a vessel.

t., progressive. One which increases in size.

t., stratified. SYN: *fibrolaminar.* One composed of layers.

t., white. SYN: *antemortem thrombus, q.v.*

through drainage. (thrū). Drainage by passing a perforated tube into cavity to be drained and flushing cavity by injection of fluids.

t. illumina′tion. Passage of light through the walls of an organ or cavity, for medical examination. SYN: *transillumination.*

thrush (thrŭsh) [Dutch *tröske,* rotten wood]. Fungus infection of mouth or throat, esp. in infants and young children, characterized by formation of white patches, ulcer formation, and frequently fever and gastrointestinal inflammation. SYN: *aphtha, sprue, stomatitis, q.v.*

ETIOL: *Candida (Monilia) albicans.*

thrypsis (thrĭp′sĭs) [G. *thrypsis,* a breaking in pieces]. A comminuted fracture.

thulium (thū′lĭ-ŭm). A rare metallic element found in combination with minerals. SYMB: Tm. At. wt. 168.934; at. no. 69.

thumb (thŭm) [A.S. *thūma,* thumb]. The short, thick, first finger on radial side of the hand, having but 2 phalanges and greater freedom of movement than other fingers. SYN: *pollex.*

thus (thŭs). Frankincense.

thylacitis (thī″lă-sī′tĭs) [G. *thylax,* pouch, + *-itis,* inflammation]. Inflammation of the sebaceous glands of the skin.

thymectomy (thī-mĕk′tō-mĭ) [G. *thymos,* thymus, + *-ektomē,* excision]. Surgical removal of the thymus gland.

thymelcosis (thī-mĕl-kō′sĭs) [" + *elkōsis,* ulceration]. Ulceration of the thymus gland.

thymergastic reaction (thī-mĕr-găs′tĭk) [G. *thymos,* mind, + *ergasia,* work]. Name for psychic disorders most equivalent to manic-depressive or affect psychosis.*

thymic (thī′mĭk) [G. *thymos,* thymus]. Relating to the thymus gland.

thymicolymphatic. Relating to the thymus and lymph glands.

thymion (thĭm′ĭ-ŏn) [G. *thymion,* wart]. A wart.

thymitis (thī-mī′tĭs) [G. *thymos,* thymus, + *-itis,* inflammation]. Inflammation of the thymus gland.

thymo- [G.]. Combining form meaning *thymus.*

thymocyte (thī′mō-sīt) [G. *thymos,* thymus, + *kytos,* cell]. A lymphocyte having origin in the thymus gland.

thymokesis (thī″mō-kē′sĭs) [G. *thymos,* thymus]. Abnormal enlargement and persistence of the thymus in the adult.

thymol (thī′mōl) [G. *thymos,* thyme, + L. *oleum,* oil]. USP. White crystals obtained from oil of thyme.

ACTION AND USES: Antiseptic and deodorizer. It is used also as an anthelmintic specifically in ancylostomiasis.

t. iodide. USP. A reddish-brown powder.

USES: As a substitute for iodoform, as a dusting powder in various skin diseases.

thymolysis (thī-mŏl′ĭ-sĭs) [G. *thymos,* thymus, + *lysis,* dissolution]. Dissolution of thymus tissue.

thymolytic (thī″mō-lĭt′ĭk) [" + *lysis,* dissolution]. Destructive to thymus tissue.

thymoma (thī-mō′mă) [" + *-ōma,* tumor]. A tumor originating in epithelial tissues of the thymus gland.

thymopexy (thī″mō-pĕks′ĭ). Fixation of an enlarged thymus in a new position.

thymotoxic (thī″mō-tŏks′ĭk) [" + *toxikon,* poison]. Poisonous to thymus tissue.

thymus (thī′mŭs) [G. *thymos*]. An unpaired organ located in the mediastinal cavity anterior to and above the heart. It consists of two flattened symmetrical lobes each enclosed in a capsule, from which trabeculae extend into the gland dividing each lobe into many lobules, each consisting of a *cortex* and *medulla.* The cortex is composed of dense lymphoid tissue containing many cells (thymocytes) closely packed together. The *medulla* also contains thymocytes but they are less numerous. It also contains characteristic *thymic* (Hassall's) *corpuscles.*

At birth the thymus weighs 12 to 15 gm. Growth is rapid during the first two years, then slow, attaining a weight of about 40 gm. at puberty, after which it begins to undergo involution and the thymic tissue is replaced with adipose and connective tissue.

FUNCTIONS: Important in development of immune response in newborn. Its removal has been associated with an increased susceptibility to acute infectious diseases at a later time.

PATH: Sometimes it is much larger than it should be and is then known as enlarged or persistent thymus. Children having these enlarged structures should be carefully followed. The practice of routinely treating the enlarged thymus with x-irradiation is not advisable. Children who have been so treated frequently develop thyroid cancer.

SEE: *status thymicolymphaticus, thymic asthma.*

t., accessory. A lobule isolated from the mass of the thymus gland.

t. persistens hyperplastica. A thymus persisting into adulthood, sometimes hypertrophying.

thymusectomy (thī″mŭs-ĕk′tō-mĭ) [G. *thymos,* thymus, + *-ektomē,* excision]. Surgical excision of the thymus.

thyreoplasia congenita. Defective functioning of the thyroid gland due to abnormal development.

thyro-, thyreo- [G.]. Combining forms meaning *oblong, shield, thyroid.*

thyroadenitis (thī″rō-ăd-en-ī′tĭs) [G. *thyreos,* shield, + *adēn,* gland, + *-ītis,* inflammation]. Inflammation of thyroid gland.

thyroaplasia (thī″rō-ă-plā′zĭ-ă) [" + *a-,* priv. + *plasis,* a molding]. Imperfect development of the thyroid gland.

thyroarytenoid (thī″rō-ă-rĭt′en-oyd) [" + *arytaina,* pitcher, + *eidos,* form]. Relating to the thyroid and arytenoid cartilages.

thyrocardiac (thī″rō-kar′dĭ-ăk) [" + *kardia,* heart]. 1. Pert. to the heart and thyroid gland. 2. A person suffering from thyroid disease complicated by heart disorder.

thyrocele (thī′rō-sēl) [" + *kēlē,* mass]. Enlarged condition of the thyroid gland. SYN: *goiter.*

thyrochondrotomy (thī″rō-kŏn-drŏt′ō-mĭ) [" + *chondros,* cartilage, + *tomē,* a cutting]. Surgical incision of thyroid cartilage. SYN: *laryngotomy.*

thyrocricotomy (thī-rō-krī-kot′ō-mĭ) [G. *thyreos,* shield, + *krikos,* ring, + *tomē,* a cutting]. Tracheotomy; division of the cricothyroid membrane.

thyroepiglottic (thī″rō-ĕp-ĭ-glŏt′ĭk) [" + *epi,* upon, + *glōttis,* glottis]. Relating to the thyroid and epiglottis.

t. muscle. Muscle arising on inner surface of thyroid cartilage. It extends upward and backward and is inserted on epiglottis. It depresses the epiglottis.

thyroepiglottideus (thī″rō-ĕp″ĭ-glŏt-ĭd′ē-ŭs) [" + " + *glōttis,* glottis]. Muscle in the thyroid cartilage that depresses the epiglottis.

thyroglobulin (thī″rō-glŏb′ū-lĭn) [G. *thyreos,* shield, + L. *globulus,* a tiny sphere]. SYN: *iodothyroglobulin.* An iodine-containing protein secreted by the thyroid gland and stored within its colloid substance.

thyroglos′sal. Pertaining to the thyroid gland and the tongue.

t. duct. A duct which in the embryo connects the thyroid diverticulum with the tongue. It eventually disappears, its point of origin being indicated as a pit, the *foramen cecum.* It sometimes persists as an anomaly.

thyrohyoid (thī″rō-hī′oyd) [" + *hyoeidēs* U-shaped]. Rel. to thyroid cartilage and hyoid bone. SYN: *hyothyroid.*

thyroid (thī′royd) [G. *thyreos,* shield, + *eidos,* form]. 1. Thyroid extract, *q.v.* 2. A gland of internal secretion in the neck, ant. to and partially surrounding the thyroid cartilage and upper rings of the trachea. SEE: *t. gland.* 3. Muscle which depresses hyoid bone or elevates thyroid cartilage if hyoid bone is fixed. SEE: *Table of Muscles in Appendix.*

t. axis. SYN: *thyrocervical trunk.* A short thick branch of the subclavian artery. Its branches are the *inf. thyroid, suprascapular* and *transverse cervical* which supply the thyroid gland and neck region.

t. cachexia. Exophthalmic goiter.

t. cartilage. The principal cartilage of the larynx consisting of two broad lamina united anteriorly to form a V-shaped structure. It forms a subcutaneous projection, the *laryngeal prominence* or *Adam's apple.*

t. crisis. SEE: *thyroid storm.*

t. extract. USP. The dried thyroid glands of the ox or sheep.

ACTION AND USES: Used in cases of deficient action of the gland, *i.e. hypothyroidism.*

ADMINISTRATION: Tablet form by mouth. The maximum effect of a dose level will not be obtained for at least 7 to 10 days. It is advisable to start with a small dose and increase it gradually until the proper dose is established. Because the patient may take thyroid extract for all of his life, the least expensive form of therapy, which is Thyroid, USP, should be used.

t. gland. A gland of internal secretion located in the base of the neck on both sides of the lower part of the larynx and upper part of trachea.

It consists of two *lateral lobes* connected by an *isthmus.* Sometimes a third *medial* or *pyramidal lobe* extends upward from the isthmus. Histologically it consists of a large number of closed vesicles called *follicles* which contain a homogeneous substance called *colloid* which contains the active principles secreted by the gland. Enlarged in goiter. It may pulsate.

RS: *endocrine gland, hormone hyperthyroidism, hypothyroidism, iodine, struma, thyroxine, thyrotrophic hormone.*

t. storm. SYN: *thyroid crisis.* Fulminating increase in all the signs and symptoms of thyrotoxicosis.

t. therapy. Thyroid ext. treatment.

thyroidectomized (thī-roy-dĕk′tō-mīzd) [G. *thyreos,* shield, +*eidos,* form, + *-ektomē,* excision]. With the thyroid gland removed.

thyroidectomy (thī-royd-ĕk′tō-mĭ) [" + " + *-ektomē,* excision]. Excision of the thyroid gland.

POST. NP: Patient in sitting position as soon as recovered from anesthesia, head and arms well supported. Watch for edema. Steam inhalations sometimes ordered. Give absolute mental and physical rest as much as possible.

thyroiditis (thī″roy-dī′tĭs) [G. *thyreos,* shield, + *eidos,* form, + *-itis,* inflammation]. Inflammation of the thyroid gland. SEE: *Riedel's struma.*

t., giant cell. Thyroiditis characterized by presence of giant cells, round-cell infiltration, fibrosis, and destruction of follicles.

thyroidization (thī″roy-dī-zā′shŭn) [G. *thyreos,* shield, + *eidos,* form]. Thyroid extract therapy.

thyroidotomy (thī-royd-ŏt′ō-mĭ) [" + " + *tomē,* a cutting]. Incision of thyroid gland.

thyroidotoxin. A substance which is toxic for cells of the thyroid gland.

thyrolytic (thī″rō-lĭt′ĭk) [" + *lysis,* dissolution]. Causing destruction of thyroid tissue.

thyroparathyroidectomy (thī″rō-par-ă-thī-roy-dĕk′tō-mĭ) [" + " + *para*, beside, + *thyreos*, shield, + *eidos*, form, + *ektomē*, excision]. Surgical removal of the thyroid and parathyroid glands.

thyropenia (thī″rō-pē′nĭ-ă) [" + " + *venia*, lack]. Defective thyroid secretion with no clinical symptoms.

thyroprival (thī-rō-prī′văl) [" + L. *privus*, lacking]. Pert. to a condition resulting from loss of function or removal of the thyroid gland.

thyroptosis (thī-rŏp-tō′sĭs) [" + *ptōsis*, a dropping]. Downward displacement of a goitrous thyroid into the thorax.

thyrosis (thī-rō′sĭs) [" + *-ōsis*, condition]. Any condition due to abnormal thyroid action.

thyrotherapy (thī″rō-ther′ă-pĭ) [" + *therapeia*, treatment]. Treatment with thyroid gland extracts.

thyrotome (thī′rō-tōm) [" + *tomos*, a piece]. Knife for cutting the thyroid cartilage.

thyrotomy (thī-rŏt′ō-mĭ) [" + *tomē*, a cutting]. 1. The splitting of the thyroid cartilage anteriorly in midline in order to expose laryngeal structures. SYN: *laryngofissure*. 2. Surgery on the thyroid gland.

thyrotoxic (thī″rō-tŏks′ĭk) [G. *thyreos*, shield, + *toxikon*, poison]. Pert. to, affected by, or marked by toxic activity of the thyroid gland.

thyrotoxicosis (thī″rō-tŏks-ĭ-kō′sĭs) [" + " + *-ōsis*, condition]. The condition of intoxication due to excessive thyroid secretion. SYN: *exophthalmic goiter, q.v.*

SYM: Rapid heart action, tremors, elevated basal metabolism, enlarged gland, exophthalmos, nervous symptoms, and loss of weight.

thyrotropic (thī-rō-trŏp′ĭk) [G. *thyreos*, shield, + *tropē*, a turning]. That which has an affinity for or stimulates the thyroid gland.

t. hormone. ABBR: TTH. The thyroid-stimulating hormone secreted by the ant. lobe of hypophysis. Also called *thyroid-stimulating hormone*. ABBR: TSH.

thyrotropin (thī-rot′rō-pĭn). The thyrotropic hormone, *q.v.*

thyroxin (thī-rŏks′ĭn) [G. *thyreos*, shield]. Proprietary name for the active principle of the thyroid gland; one of the constituent amino acids of thyroglobulin. Has also been made synthetically. Used in the treatment of thyroid deficiency.

thyroxine (thī-rŏks′ĕn) [G. *thyreos*, shield]. 3:5:3:5-Tetraiodothyronine, an amino acid obtained from the thyroid gland considered to be the principal thyroid hormone. Used in the treatment of hypothyroidism.

t.-binding protein. ABBR: TBP. The globin protein responsible for binding the greater part of thyroxine in the plasma.

Ti. Chemical symbol for *titanium*.

tibia (tĭb′ĭ-ă) [L. *tibia*, shinbone]. The inner and larger bone of the leg bet. the knee and ankle articulating with the femur above and with the talus below. Also called shin bone

t., Lannelongue's. A syphilitic tibia.

t., saber-shaped. A deformity of the tibia due to gummatous periostitis (syphilitic) in which it curves outward.

tibialis (tĭb-ĭ-ā′lĭs) [L.]. One of 2 muscles of the calf of the leg.

tibioadductor reflex (tĭb″ĭ-ō-ăd-dŭk′tor) [L. *tibia*, shinbone, + *adducere*, to lead to]. Adduction of either the stimulated leg or the opposite one when the tibia is percussed on the inner side.

tibiofemoral (tĭb″ĭ-ō-fem′ō-răl) [" + *femur, femor-*, thigh]. Relating to the tibia and femur.

tibiofibular (tĭb″ĭ-ō-fĭb′ū-lar) [" + *fibula*, buckle]. Relating to the tibia and fibula.

tibiotarsal (tĭb″ĭ-ō-tar′săl) [" + G. *tarsos*, flat of the foot]. Relating to the tibia and tarsus.

tic (tĭk) [Fr.]. A spasmodic muscular contraction, most commonly involving the face, head, neck, or shoulder muscles. SYN: *habit spasm*.

The spasms may be tonic* or clonic.* The movement appears purposeful, is often repeated, involuntary, can be inhibited for a short time, only to burst forth with increased severity.

ETIOL: Certain of these cases are due to structure changes, many psychogenic, the expression of frustration, and its correlated muscular tension. The former group most commonly encountered in patients who have suffered from lethargic encephalitis. SEE: *tiqueur*.

t., convulsive. Facial muscle spasm.

t. douloureux (doo-loo-ru′). Degeneration of or pressure on the trigeminal nerve, resulting in neuralgia of that nerve. *RS: neuralgia*. The pain is excruciating. Usually occurs after forty. Pain is paroxysmal, radiating from angle of the jaw along one of the involved branches. If the first branch, a shocklike pain is felt along the eye and back over the forehead. If it is the middle fiber, the upper lip, nose, and cheek under the eye are affected. If it is the third branch, pain is in the lower lip and outer border of tongue on affected side. Pain is momentary but returns again and again.

TREAT: Injection of the nerve with alcohol. Other measures as anticonvulsants or chlorpromazine may be helpful to shorten attacks or cause remission.

t., facial. Same as *convulsive tic*.

t., habit. Habitual repetition of a grimace or muscular action.

t. rotatoire. Spasmodic torticollis in which head and neck are forcibly rotated or turned from one side to the other.

t., spasmodic. Tonic contractions and paralysis of muscles of one or both sides of the face.

tick (tĭk) [M.E. *tike*]. Any of the numerous bloodsucking arachnids of the order Acarida. Ixodidae is the hard tick family and Argas the soft. They transmit specific diseases to man and lower animals.

t. fever. 1. Any infectious disease transmitted by the bite of a tick. 2. African relapsing fever. 3. Specifically, an acute infectious disease transmitted by the bite of a wood tick in the Rocky Mountain region. SYN: *Rocky Mountain spotted fever, spotted fever*.

ETIOL: A microorganism (*Rickettsia rickettsii*) transmitted by a tick.

SYM: *Incubation period*: From the bite to the first symptom, 5-7 days. Onset may be gradual or sudden, but generally for a period of 1 or more days; if so, it is preceded by weakness, chilly sensations and then a definite chill.

Other symptoms are nausea and vomiting; headache in front and back of head, or both; more or less bloodshot eyes with sensitivity to light; eyeballs sore to touch; deep, dusky flush on face; pain in muscles, bones, and joints; backache, esp. in lower portion;

bronchial cough; nosebleed; constipation, and marked weakness. The skin becomes spotted bet. the 3rd and 5th day after onset. The spots resemble those of measles but differ in distribution. In Rocky Mountain spotted fever spots are apt to be concentrated on the wrist, ankles, and feet, instep, soles, and then spread to the trunk. The spots appear to disappear on pressure but later become hemorrhagic, changing to a rust color due to disintegration. Relative bradycardia may be present during fever. Development of hypotension is a grave prognostic sign.

tickle (tĭk'l) [origin uncertain]. 1. Peculiar sensation caused by titillation or touching, esp. in certain regions, resulting in reflex muscular movements, laughter, or hysteria. 2. To arouse such a sensation by touching a surface lightly.

tickling (tĭk'ling) [origin uncertain]. Gentle stimulation of a sensitive surface and its reflex effect, such as involuntary laughter, etc. SYN: *titillation.*

tictology [G. *tiktein,* to give birth, + *logos,* science]. Obstetrics.

t. i. d. [L. *ter in die*]. Three times a day.

tidal (tī'dăl). Periodically rising and falling, increasing and decreasing.

t. air. That which is inhaled and exhaled during normal quiet breathing. SEE: *air, respiration.*

t. drainage. The drainage of a paralyzed bladder by use of an automatic irrigation apparatus.

tide [A.S. *tīd,* time]. Alternate rise and fall; a space of time.

t., acid. A temporary increase in acidity of urine due to increased secretion of alkaline substances into the duodenum.

t., alkaline. Temporary decrease in acidity of urine following awakening and after meals. The former results from hyperpnea in which excess CO_2 is eliminated; the latter results from increase of base in the blood following the secretion of HCl into gastric juice.

Tietze's disease or **syndrome.** Inflammation of the costochondral cartilage. A self-limiting disease of unknown etiology. Pain may be confused with that of myocardial infarction. There is no specific therapy.

tigering [G. *tigris,* tiger]. Tiger-like striped appearance of heart muscle due to irregular areas of fatty degeneration. Seen in conditions which cause severe anoxemia such as anemia. SYN: *tiger-heart, tiger-lily heart.*

tigretier (tē-grĕt-ē-ā') [Fr.]. A dancing mania or form of tarantism due to bite of a poisonous spider occurring in Tigré, Abyssinia.

tigroid (tī'groyd) [G. *tigroeidēs,* spotted]. Striped, spotted, or marked like a tiger

t. bodies. SYN: *Nissl bodies.* Masses of chromophil substance present in the cell bodies of neurons.

tigrolysis (tĭg"rol'ĭ-sĭs). SYN: *chromatolysis.* Dissolution and disappearance of chromophil substance of a nerve cell. May occur following injury to an axon (retrograde degeneration) or subsequent to direct injury to a nerve cell.

tilmus (tĭl'mŭs) [G. *tilmos,* a plucking]. Delirious picking at the bedclothes by the patient. SYN: *carphology, floccillation.*

tiltometer (til-tom'ĕ-ter). A device for measuring the degree of tilt of a bed or operating table. Used when spinal anesthesia has been given.

timbre (tĭm'ber, tahn'br) [Fr. a bell to be struck with a hammer]. Resonance quality of a sound by which it is distinguished, other than pitch or intensity, depending upon the number and character of vibrating body's overtones.

time (tīm) [A.S. *tīma,* time]. Interval bet. beginning and ending; measured duration. Age.

t., bleeding. Time required for bleeding from a small wound to cease. Usually tested by puncturing lobe of ear. Normal time, 1-3 min.

t., clot retraction. Time required following withdrawal of blood for a clot to completely contract and express the serum entrapped within the fibrin net. Normal time, about 1 hour. Clot retraction is dependent upon number of platelets.

t., coagulation. Time required for clotting to occur after removal of blood from the body. Average time, 5-8 min.

t., prothrombin. That needed for oxalated plasma to clot, measured in seconds, after adding thromboplastin and recalcifying.

t., reaction. Period bet. application of a stimulus and the response.

t., thermal death. Time required to kill all microorganisms at a certain temperature.

timer. A device for measuring, signaling, recording, or regulating time. Various forms of timers are used in x-ray, surgical, and laboratory work.

tin (tĭn) [A.S.]. SYMB: Sn. At. wt. 118.69; at. no. 50. A metallic element, used in medicine.

POISONING: Tin in tinned or soldered containers in the past has occasionally been responsible for poisoning. This is exceedingly rare and for practical purposes need not be considered.

SYM: Metallic taste, gastrointestinal irritation, nausea, vomiting, cramping, and diarrhea.

F. A. TREATMENT: Wash out stomach and administer bland or soothing drinks.

tinctorial (tĭnk-tō'rĭ-al) [L. *tinctorius,* dyeing]. Relating to staining or color.

tincture (tĭngk'tūr) [L. *tinctura,* a dyeing]. Diluted alcoholic solutions of nonvolatile substances (tincture of iodine being an exception), 10% being standard strength for powerful drugs and 20% for weaker ones.

The name of any fluid contained in the tincture other than alcohol is added to the name of the tincture.

This class of preparations contains tannic acid, so, in most instances, cannot be employed with agents that are incompatible with that drug. Those tinctures that contain much resinous matter or oils will precipitate with water. Some examples are tinctures of *ginger, benzoin, guaiac,* etc. Tinctures of the most potent drugs usually represent 10% of the crude drug, as tinctures of *opium, digitalis, aconite,* etc. Where more than a teaspoon of a 10% tincture would have to be taken to get a dose of the drug, the tincture is usually made to represent 20%, or more, of the agent.

t. iodine. POISONING: This commonly used antiseptic is sometimes taken by mouth.

SYM: Very strong irritation of mouth, esophagus, and stomach. Stains membranes dark brown or black. Pain intense, and leads to early vomiting and purging; extreme thirst, often collapse.

TREATMENT: Give large amounts of water, milk and starchy paste; gruels, as boiled rice or cream of wheat.

tinea (tĭn′ē-ă) [L. *tinea,* worm]. Any fungus skin disease, esp. ringworm, occurring in various parts of the body, name indicating the part affected, as *t. barbae, t. corporis,* etc. A dermatomycosis, *q.v.*

SYM: Superficial or deep types. Superficial is marked by scaling; slight itching; reddish or grayish patches; dry, brittle hair which is easily extracted with hair shaft. Deep type is characterized by flat, reddish, kerionlike tumors, the surface studded with dead or broken hairs or by gaping follicular orifices. Nodules may be broken down in center, discharging pus, etc., through dilated follicular openings.

TREATMENT: Griseofulvin, *q.v.,* for all types of true trichophyton infections. Vaccines. Parasiticides for general body surface. That attacking palms and soles is resistant. Fuchsin paint, salicylic and sulfur mixture; avoid soap and water. In tinea cruris, iodine in carbon tetrachloride, salicylic and benzoic acids, iodine. In ringworm of crotch, soothing remedies, antipruritic powders, followed by antiseptics (sod. hyposulfite, carbolized resorcin, iodine, mercuric chloride, formalin), then soothing lotions. Ringworm of the scalp, *T. capitis,* is particularly resistant if due to *M. audouini.* Do not treat topically. Griseofulvin is quite effective.

t. barbae. A fungus skin disease of the bearded portions of neck and face. SYN: *barber's itch.*

t. capitis. A fungus skin disease of the scalp; ringworm of the scalp. May be due to one of several types of *Microsporum.*

t. circinata. On the body—red, slight, elevated, scaly patches, which on examination reveal minute vesicles or papules. New patches spring from the periphery while central portion clears up. Often considerable itching.

t. corporis. A fungus skin disease of the body.

t. cruris. A fungus skin disease of surfaces of contact in the scrotal, crural, anal, and genital areas. SYN: *dhobie itch; jock itch.*

t. favosa. A fungus disease of skin, typically on scalp, due to a specific fungus; characterized by peculiar saucer-shaped, sulfur yellow crusts. Rare in the U.S.A.

t. nodosa. Sheathlike, nodular masses in hair of beard and mustache from growth of an unknown fungus. They surround the hairs, which become brittle, and hair may be penetrated by fungus and thus split.

t. pedis. A fungus skin disease of the foot; ringworm of the foot. SYN: *dermatophytosis; athlete's foot.*

t. trichophytina. Local infectious disease of skin, produced by the trichophyton fungus. The organism grows in the horny epithelium. The lesions vary according to part of body attacked, and whether the hairs are involved. SYN: *ringworm.*

t. versicolor. Fungus infection of skin which produces branny patches which are yellow or fawn-colored. SYN: *pityriasis versicolor.*

tine test. A skin test for tuberculosis. The tuberculin is on metal tines which are pressed into the skin. The unit is sterile and disposable and is therefore very useful in mass surveys.

tingle. A prickling or stinging sensation. May be caused by cold or nerve injury.

tinnitus (tĭn-ī′tŭs) [L. *tinnitus,* a jingling]. A ringing or tinkling sound that is purely subjective.

t. aurium. Ringing, tinkling, buzzing, or other sounds in the ear.

Found in conditions of ext., middle, or inner ear.

ETIOL: Impacted cerumen, myringitis, otitis media, labyrinthitis, Ménière's symptom complex, otosclerosis, hysteria, etc. Also follows overdosage of drugs such as quinine.

t. cere′bri. Noises in the head.

t., telephone. Tinnitus resulting from excessive use of the telephone.

tintometer (tĭn-tŏm′ĕ-ter) [L. *tinctus,* a dyeing, + G. *metron,* a measure]. A scale of different shades of color to determine by comparison the intensity of color of the blood or other fluid.

tintometric (tĭn″tō-mĕt′rĭk) [" + G. *metron,* a measure]. Relating to tintometry.

tintometry (tĭn-tŏm′ĕ-trĭ) [" + G. *metron,* a measure]. Estimation of a color by comparison with a scale of colors.

-tion. O.E. and L. suffix forming abstract names.

-tious. O.E. suffix forming adjective.

tip. A point or apex of a part.

tiqueur (tē-kur′) [Fr.]. One afflicted with a tic.

tire (tīr) [A.S. *tyrian,* to tire]. 1. Exhaustion; fatigue. 2. To exhaust or fatigue. 3. To become fatigued.

tirefond (tēr-fon′) [Fr.]. Appliance like a corkscrew for raising depressed portions of bone or for removing foreign bodies.

tires (tīrz). Condition marked by constipation, vomiting, muscular tremors, and pain. SYN: *milk sickness, trembles.*

tissue (tĭsh′ū) [O. Fr. *tissu,* from L. *texere,* to weave]. A group or collection of similar cells and their intercellular substance which act together in the performance of a particular function. The primary tissues are (a) epithelial, (b) connective, (c) muscular, and (d) nervous.

t., adipose. SYN: *fat.* Areolar tissue containing aggregations of densely packed fat cells.

t., areolar. A form of loose connective tissue consisting of interlacing *collagenous* and *elastic fibers* embedded in a semifluid *matrix* together with fibroblasts, histiocytes, mast cells, plasma cells, and other cellular elements. It is widely distributed forming the interstitial tissue of most organs, the membranes surrounding blood vessels and nerves, and constituting the principal portion of fascia.

t., cartilage. SEE: *cartilage.*

t., chondroid. Embryonic cartilage.

t., chromaffin. Tissues containing cells which give the chromaffin reaction. Found in the adrenal medulla. SEE: *chromaffin system.*

t., chromophil. Those tissues which give a chromophil reaction; found in the medulla and sympathetic ganglia.

t., connective. T. which supports and connects other tissues and parts.

The cells of connective tissue are comparatively few in number, the bulk of the tissue consisting of intercellular substance or *matrix,* the nature of which gives each type of connective tissue its particular properties. Connective tissues are highly vascular with the exception of cartilage. *Connective tissue proper* includes the following types: (a) mucous, (b) fibrous (areolar, white fibrous, yellow fibrous or elastic), (c) reticular, and (d) adipose. *Dense con-*

nective tissue includes cartilage and bone (osseous tissue).

t., elastic. A form of connective tissue in which yellow elastic fibers predominate. Found in certain ligaments, and the walls of blood vessels, esp. the larger arteries.

t., embryonic. SEE: *tissue, mucous.*

t., epithelial. SYN: *epithelium.* A form of tissue composed of cells arranged in a continuous sheet consisting of one or several layers. It forms epidermis of skin, covers surfaces of organs, lines cavities and canals, forms tubes and ducts and secreting portions of glands.

t., erectile. Spongy tissue, the spaces of which fill with blood, causing it to harden and expand. Found in the penis, clitoris, and nipples.

t., fibrous. Connective tissue consisting principally of fibers. Includes three types: (1) areolar or loose connective, (2) white fibrous, and (3) yellow fibrous or elastic. SEE: *specific types listed.*

t., interstitial. Connective t. forming a network with the cellular elements of an organ.

t., mucous. Jelly-like tissue from which connective tissue is derived.

t., muscular. *Voluntary:* Striped or striated tissue principally connected with the bony framework. In animals it is known as "lean meat" or "flesh." It is a cross-striped, muscular tissue, the fibers like a long cylinder with flattened sides and conical ends, enveloped in a delicate sheath, the *sarcolemma. Involuntary:* Smooth or unstriped, or nonstriated, not under control of the will. Principally found in walls of hollow organs, tubes, arteries, and veins.

t., osseous or bone. Connective tissue with intercellular substance impregnated with phosphate and carbonate of calcium, the mineral substances being 2/3 of the bone's dry weight.

t., reticular or retiform. A type of connective tissue consisting of delicate fibers forming interlacing networks. Fibers stain selectively with silver stains and are called argyrophil fibers.

It supports lymph nodes and is found in muscular tissue and in bone marrow, the spleen, liver, lungs, kidneys, and mucous membranes of the gastrointestinal tract.

t., subcutaneous. Areolar tissue under and becoming part of the corium.

t., s. adipose. Adipose tissue within subcutaneous tissue.

t., white fibrous. Connective t. with white, inelastic fibers, forming tendons, ligaments, and resistant membranes.

t., w. nervous. Nervous tissue of medullated nerve fibers.

t., yellow elastic. Same as *elastic tissue.*

titanium (tī-tā'nĭ-ŭm) [L.]. A metallic element found in combination in minerals. SYMB: Ti. At. wt. 47.90; at. no. 22.

titer (tī'ter) [Fr. *titre*]. Standard of strength per volume of volumetric test solution.

t., agglutination. The highest dilution of a serum which will cause clumping or agglutination of the bacteria being tested.

t. of a serum. Amount of specific antibody in an antiserum, or strength of a serum.

titillation (tĭt-ĭl-ā'shŭn) [L. *titillatio*, a tickling]. 1. Act of tickling, as in the throat. 2. State of being tickled. 3. Sensation produced by tickling.

titration (tī-trā'shŭn) [Fr. *titre*, a standard]. 1. Determining strength of a solution by use of solutions of known strength. 2. Determination of quantity of antibody in an antiserum.

titre. SEE: *titer.*

titrimetric (tī"trĭ-mĕt'rĭk) [" + G. *metron*, a measure]. Employing the process of titration.

titubation (tĭt-ū-bā'shŭn) [L. *titubatio*, a staggering]. A staggering gait, seen in diseases of the cerebellum.

t., lingual. Stuttering, stammering.

Tl. Symb. of *thallium.*

Tm. 1. Chem. symbol for *thulium.* 2. Symbol for *maximal tubular excretory capacity.*

Tn. 1. Symb. of *normal intraocular tension.* 2. Chem. symbol for *thoron.*

T.O. Abbr. for *original* or *old tuberculin.* Also abbr. *O.T.*

toadskin. Condition characterized by excessive dryness, wrinkling, and scaling of skin sometimes seen in vitamin deficiencies. SEE: *phrynoderma.*

toadstool (tōd'stool). Any of various fungi with an umbrella-shaped cap; popularly a poisonous mushroom.

POISONING: SYM: Usually come on from a few minutes to 15 hours after ingestion, characterized by marked abdominal pain, vomiting and intense diarrhea associated with blood and mucus. Profound weakness comes early and remains. Sometimes perspiration and lacrimation present and occasionally nervous symptoms.

F. A. TREATMENT: Absolute bed rest. Empty stomach and bowels promptly and completely with gastric lavage and quick acting cathartic and enemata. Atropine is especially helpful and may be given by any route. Fluid and sodium chloride intake should be maintained intravenously if required. Coffee, tea, and milk are helpful. Charcoal may be given early if available. Treat for shock.

tobacco (tō-băk'ō) [Spanish *tabaco*]. Dried leaves of *Nicotiana tabacum* and other species.

It is a narcotic containing *nicotine, pyridine, picoline,* and *collidin.* SEE: *nicotine.*

Widely used in forms of cigars, cigarettes, pipe tobacco, snuff, and chewing. During its combustion, various products are given off, the most important being *nicotine, q.v.* The use of tobacco products may be injurious to health.

t., Indian. Lobelia.

tocodynamometer (tō"kō-dī-năm-ŏm'ĕ-ter) [G. *tokos*, birth, + *dynamis*, power, + *metron*, a measure]. Device for estimating expulsive force of uterine contractions in childbirth.

tocogony (tō-kŏg'ō-nĭ) [" + *gonē*, seed]. Parental generation as opposed to abiogenesis.

tocograph (tŏk'ō-graf) [" + *graphein*, to write]. A device for estimating and recording the force of uterine contractions.

tocology (tō-kŏl'ō-jĭ) [" + *logos*, science]. Science of parturition and obstetrics.

tocomania (tō"kō-mā'nĭ-ă) [" + *mania*, madness]. Puerperal insanity.

tocometer (tō-kŏm'ĕt-ĕr) [" + *metron*, a measure]. Device for estimating expulsive force of the uterus in labor. SYN: *tocodynamometer.*

tocopherol (tō-kŏph'ĕr-ŏl). One of three substances collectively referred to as vitamin E, *q.v.*

tocophobia (tō″kō-fō′bĭ-ă) [" + *phobos*, fear]. Abnormal fear of childbirth.

tocus (tō′kŭs) [L. from G. *tokos*, birth]. Parturition; childbirth.

toe (tō) [A.S. *tā*]. A digit of the foot. RS: *acroataxia, acrodynia, bunion, camptodactylia, clavus, dactyl, dactylus, digit, gout, hallux, metatarsus.*

t., claw. Hammer toe, *q.v.*

t. clonus. Contraction of the big toe in sudden extension of the first phalanx.

t., dislocations of. These are treated essentially same as dislocations of the fingers, *q.v.*

t. drop. Inability to lift the toes. DISEASES: Thromboangiitis obliterans, gangrene, deformities, rashes, bromidrosis.

t.'s, fanning of. Spreading of toes, esp. when sole is stroked.

t., hammer. SEE: *hammer toe.*

t., Morton's. Metatarsalgia, *q.v.*

t., pigeon. Walking with the toes turned inward.

t. reflex. When great toe is strongly flexed all muscles below knee become tense.

toilet (toy′lĕt) [Fr. *toilette*, a little cloth]. Cleansing of a wound after operation or of an obstetrical patient.

toko- [G.]. Combining form meaning *birth.* See words beginning *toco-*.

tolerance (tol′ĕr-ăns) [L. *tolerantia*, tolerance]. Capacity for enduring a poison, or a food or drug which may be harmful if taken in excess; power of resistance to such, or point at which such resistance ends; amount of a drug or food which may be so tolerated.

t., glucose. The ability of the body to absorb and utilize glucose. SEE: *glucose tolerance test.*

t. test. Master's exercise tolerance test for circulatory efficiency consists in ascending and descending 2 steps a variable number of times and in a given period. Blood pressure and pulse readings are recorded before and after the test. Electrocardiogram may be taken continuously during the test or just before and after the exercise.

tol′erant. Capable of enduring or withstanding drugs without experiencing ill-effects.

tomato. A plant the fruit of which may be eaten raw or cooked. COMP: Raw 100 gm. Calories: 22. Other values: 1.1 gm. protein; 0.2 gm. fat; 4.7 gm. carbohydrate.

-tome [G.]. Combining form meaning *a cutting, a cutting instrument.*

tomomania (tō″mō-mā′nĭ-ă) [G. *tomē*, a cutting, + *mania*, madness]. 1. Tendency of a surgeon to resort to unnecessary surgical operations. 2. Abnormal desire to be operated upon.

tomotocia (tō″mō-tō′sĭ-ă) [" + *tokos*, birth]. Cesarean section delivery by incising the uterus.

tonaphasia (tō-nă-fā′zhĭ-ă) [L. *tonus*, from G. *tonos*, a stretching, + *a-*, priv, + *phasis*, speech]. Inability to remember a tune due to cerebral lesion. SYN: *amusia, vocal.*

tone (tōn) [L. *tonus*, from G. *tonos*, a stretching]. 1. PHYS: That state of a body or any of its organs or parts in which the functions are healthy and performed with due vigor. 2. Normal tension or responsiveness to stimuli, as of arteries or muscles, seen particularly in involuntary muscle (such as the sphincter of the urinary bladder). 3. A musical or vocal sound.

t. deafness. Inability to detect differences in musical sounds. SYN: *amusia.*

t., muscular. Condition in which a muscle is in a steady state of contraction; the ability of a muscle to resist a force for a considerable period of time without change in length.

tongue (tŭng) [A.S. *tunge*]. A freely-movable muscular organ lying in the floor of the mouth. Its surface is covered with mucous membrane.

ANAT: It consists of a *body* and *root* and is attached by muscles to the hyoid bone below, the mandible in front, the styloid process behind, and the palate above, and by mucous membrane, to the floor of the mouth, the lateral walls of the pharynx, and the epiglottis. A median fold, the *frenulum linguae*, connects the tongue to the floor of the mouth. The surface of the tongue bears numerous papillae of three types, *filiform, fungiform*, and *vallate. Taste buds* are present on the surfaces of many of the papillae, esp. the vallate papillae. *Mucous* and *serous glands* (lingual glands) are present, their ducts opening on the surface. Lymphoid tissue comprising the *lingual tonsils* is present in the post. third of the tongue. A median fibrous *septum* extends the entire length of the tongue.

RS: Words beginning with *glosso-; macroglossia, microglossio lingual.*

FUNCTIONS: Manipulation of food in mastication and deglutition, speech production, taste.

ARTERIES: Lingual, ext. maxillary, and ascending pharyngeal.

MUSCLES: *Extrinsic muscles* include *genioglossus, hypoglossus, and styloglossus. Intrinsic muscles* consist of four groups: superior, inferior, transverse, and vertical *lingualis muscles.*

NERVES: Lingual nerve (containing fibers from trigeminal and facial nerves), glossopharyngeal, vagus, and hypoglossal.

PAIN: Occurs in local lesions, fissures, glossitis, malignancies, and pernicious anemia.

PROTRUSION: This occurs with very sick patients, as in advanced typhoid fever and toxemia. The tongue is tremulous in early typhoid and in meningitis. In chorea it is thrust out suddenly and at once withdrawn. If it is protruded very slowly or if left exposed after being shown, it is a sign of great exhaustion, congestion, or other pressure on the brain.

SCARS: These may be the result of injury or bulbar palsy causing ulceration and resulting in scars.

SHARP-POINTED T: Observed in irritation and inflammation of the brain, smoker's tongue, leukoplakia.

SPASM: Occurs in multiple sclerosis, general paresis, melancholia, and in stuttering.

TREMORS: Noted in asthenia, alcoholism, bulbar palsy, Graves' disorder, and in hemiplegia it is turned toward the paralyzed side if face is affected. If turned toward the unaffected side, it denotes lesion of the medulla.

TREMULOUS: In all acute diseases but no particular significance in chronic nervous disorders.

COLOR OF TONGUE: *Black coating*: Glossophytia; may be due to stain or presence of microphytes. In dysentery, indicates exhaustion, mortification, death. In jaundice, denotes organic disease of liver. In smallpox, is unfavorable sign.

Bluish: Denotes impeded circulation. Interference with respiration. Heart disease, asthma, cyanosis.

Dark brown: Malignant fever, Addison's disease.

Gray-coated and flabby t: With an oval bare spot in center, which is red and glossy, sometimes seen in children; indicative of gastrointestinal catarrh.

Lead-colored: Found in cholera and mortification of lungs and stomach; with thrush, it denotes death.

Pale: Indicates severe anemia; the tongue appears smaller than normal.

Red: Redness along center indicates intestinal irritation. An early sign in typhoid fever. If glassy, very unfavorable.

Red, cracked t: Points to kidney trouble.

Bright red t: Indicates inflammation of gastric or intestinal mucous membrane, glossitis, stomatitis.

Clean, red t: With papillae prominent, or a white-coated tongue with papillae projecting through the fur, indicates scarlatina.

Red tip and edges, or having red, dry streak in center typical of typhoid and gastric fever.

Scarlet t: Acute in inflammation usually of the stomach, if red along edges and tip.

Strawberry t: White fur through which project bright red and prominent papillae. Seen in early stage of scarlet fever.

White coating: This denotes gastric derangement.

Yellow, with thick fur covering the tongue indicates biliary derangement.

SIZE: *Macroglossia,* or large tongue, is generally congenital, or may result from inflammation of lymphatics, Ludwig's angina, glossitis, actinomycosis, acromegaly, myxedema. If localized, may be due to gumma, carcinoma, foot and mouth disease, and local trauma.

Microglossia, small tongue, atrophy due to hemorrhage, in anemia, emaciation, convalescence from typhoid. These conditions are temporary.

POSITION AND CONDITIONS: If thick and flabby, showing imprints of the teeth, indicates gastric and nervous irritation. *Thrust to one side:* Indicates hemiplegia if continually held in this position.

t., beefy. Occurs in chronic inflammation of the bowels, liver, or mucous surfaces.

t., bifid. One with a cleft at its anterior end; a forked tongue.

t., black, hairy. SYN: *hyperkeratosis linguae, lingua nigra, lingua villosa nigra.* Condition in which tongue possesses a brown, furlike area on its dorsum. The area is composed of hypertrophied filiform papillae pigment, and possibly microorganisms. Sometimes results from excessive use of oxygen-liberating mouthwashes or antibiotic therapy.

t., burning. *Glossopyrosis.*

t., clearing of. If it clears slowly, commencing at tip and edges, leaving natural appearance, permanent recovery may be expected. If fur comes off in patches, leaving smooth, red surface, recovery will be slow. If fur disappears rapidly, leaving glassy, cracked surface, it is unfavorable.

t., cleft. A bifid or trifid tongue, *q.v.*

t., coated. One covered with layer of whitish or yellowish material consisting of desquamated epithelium, bacteria, food debris, etc. Significance is difficult to interpret. May mean only that patient slept with mouth open or has not eaten because of loss of appetite. If *darkly* coated, it may indicate a fungus infection.

t., deviation of. Marked turning of tongue from the midline when protruded. Indicative of lesions of the hypoglossal nerve.

t., dry. One that is dry and shriveled, usually indicative of a dehydration. May also be the result of mouth breathing.

t., fern-leaf. One possessing a prominent central furrow and lateral branches.

t., filmy. One possessing symmetrical whitish patches.

t., fissured. SYN: *furrowed tongue, lingua plicata.* One bearing deep furrows in its epithelium. May be normal. Causes obscure. If deep and inflamed, may be due to syphilitic infection, or dissecting glossitis, a broken tooth, chronic dysentery, hepatic disease, or diabetes mellitus.

t., forked. SEE: *t., bifid.*

t., furred. Coated tongue on which surface epithelium appears as a coat of white fur. Seen in nearly all fevers.

Brown fur: Nervous prostration, putrefaction; a bad indication; deeper the color the worse the omen. If dry with fissures, condition is grave. Circumscribed furring often indicates local disturbance, as from a jagged tooth, or from tonsillitis.

Unilateral furring: May result from disturbed innervation, as in condition affecting the 2nd and 3rd branches of the 5th nerve. Has been noted in neuralgia of those branches and in fractures of the skull involving the foramen rotundum.

Yellow fur: Jaundice.

t., geographic. One possessing white, raised areas resembling mountain ranges on a relief map. Areas consist of heaped-up epithelium surrounding areas of atrophy.

t., hairy. One possessing fine elongated papillae.

t., magenta. One magenta-colored seen in cases of riboflavin deficiency.

t., parrot. A dry shriveled tongue, seen in typhus.

t., scrotal. Furrowed and fissured. Resembling skin of scrotum.

t., smoker's. SYN: *leukoplakia.* Condition characterized by white, opaque patches of thickened epithelium later thickening and becoming fissured.

t., smooth. One resulting from atrophy of papillae. Characteristic of many conditions such as anemia, gastrointestinal disorders, etc.

t., strawberry. Tongue which first has a white coat except at tip and along edges, with enlarged papillae standing out distinctly against white surface. Later white coat disappears leaving a bright red surface. Characteristic of scarlet fever.

t., tremulous. Due to hyperthyroidism.

t., trifid. One in which anterior end is divided into three parts. SEE: *symptoms, throat.*

tongue, words pert. to: circumvallate papillae, cleft, frenulum, "gloss-" words, hypoglossal, lingua, macroglossia, microglossia, ranula, strawberry, sublingual, s. gland.

tongue-swallowing. The tendency, in an unconscious person lying on the back, for the relaxed tongue to slip back into the pharynx. This blocks the airway and seriously interferes with respiration. To correct, elevate the shoulders and extend the head; this maneuver will open the airway. Also a mechanical airway device may be used to hold or push the tongue forward. Unless this is done, attempts to apply artificial respiration to an unconscious person may be in vain.

tongue-tie (tŭng'tī). This is a congenital shortening of the frenum.

SYM: Interference in sucking and in articulation.

TREATMENT: Surgical.

tonic (tŏn'ĭk) [G. *tonikos*, pert. to tone]. 1. Pert. to or characterized by tension or contraction, esp. muscular tension. 2. Restoring tone. 3. A medicine that increases strength and tone.

They are subdivided according to action, as *cardiac, general*, etc. Ex: *iron, digitalis.*

t. spasm. A persistent, involuntary, firm or violent muscular contraction. SEE: *clonic.*

tonicity (tō-nĭs'ĭ-tĭ) [G. *tonos*, tone]. 1. Property of possessing tone, esp. muscular tone. 2. State of normal tension or partial contraction of muscle fibers while at rest. SYN: *tone.*

tonoclonic (tŏn"o-klŏn'ĭk) [G. *tonos*, tone, + *klonos*, tumult]. Both tonic and clonic, said of muscular spasms.

tonograph (tŏn'ō-grăf) [" + *graphein*, to write]. Device for recording blood pressure.

tonometer (tŏn-ŏm'ĕ-ter) [" + *metron*, a measure]. Instrument for measuring the intraocular tension or blood pressure.

tonometry (tŏn-ŏm'ĕ-trĭ) [" + *metron*, a measure]. The measurement of tension of a part, as intraocular tension. This test is extremely useful in detecting glaucoma, *q.v.*

tonophant (tŏn'ō-fănt) [" + *phainein*, to show]. Device for visualizing sound waves.

tonoplast (tŏn'ō-plăst) [" + *plastos*, a thing formed]. An intracellular body. SYN: *vacuole.*

tonsil (tŏn'sĭl) [L. *tonsilla*, almond]. 1. A mass of lymphatic tissue located in depressions of the mucous membrane of fauces and pharynx. SEE: *lingual, palatine*, and *pharyngeal tonsil.* 2. A rounded mass on inferior surface of cerebellum lying lateral to the uvula.

FUNCTION: Acts as filter to protect body from invasion of bacteria, and aids in the formation of white cells.

t., cerebellar. One of a pair of cerebellar lobules on either side of the uvula* projecting from inf. surface of cerebellum.

t., faucial. Same as *tonsil*, (def. 1).

t., lingual. A mass of lymphoid tissue located in root of tongue.

t., Luschka's. Same as *pharyngeal t.*

t., pharyngeal. Lymphoid tissue on post. sup. wall of pharynx. SEE: *adenoid.*

t., nasal. Lymphoid tissue on the nasal septum.

t., palatine. A mass of lymphoid tissue which lies in *tonsillar fossa* on each side of oral pharynx between glossopalatine and pharyngopalatine arches. The free surface of each tonsil is covered with stratified squamous epithelium which forms deep indentations or *crypts* extending into substance of tonsil. The lateral surface of each tonsil is invested by a firm fibrous *capsule.* Efferent lymph vessels convey lymph from the tonsil. No afferent vessels are present.

t., tubal. Lymphatic tissue present in mucous membrane of auditory tube near its opening into pharynx.

tonsillar (tŏn'sĭ-lar) [L. *tonsilla*, almond]. Pert. to a tonsil, esp. the faucial or palatine t.

t. crypt. A deep indentation into pharyngeal surface of a tonsil. It is lined with stratified epithelium.

t. fossa. A depression between the glossopalatine and pharyngopalatine arches in which the palatine tonsil is situated.

t. ring. SYN: *Waldeyer's ring.* The almost complete ring of tonsilar tissue encircling the pharynx. Includes the palatine, lingual and pharyngeal tonsils.

t. sinus. Space lying between plica triangularis and anterior surface of palatine tonsil.

tonsillectomy (tŏn-sĭl-ĕk'tō-mĭ) [" + G. *ektomē*, excision]. Surgical removal of the tonsils.

OPER. NP: Patient is placed in dorsal position with head extended and covered with a sterile sheet up to neck in usual manner; over sterile sheet, at neck, place a sterile towel.

Immediately following operation patient is turned on side or face down, so that vomitus or blood is not inhaled, and ice compress is placed around throat. Pulse rate should be taken frequently and any marked increase that might indicate a possible hemorrhage should be reported to the doctor immediately. It is important for nurse to test suction apparatus before operation. Cold water should be flushed through the suction tip into bottle after operation to prevent stoppage through clotting of blood.

tonsillitis (tŏn-sĭl-ī'tĭs) [L. *tonsilla*, almond, + G. *-itis*, inflammation]. Inflammation of a tonsil, esp. the faucial tonsil.

t., acute. SYN: *scarlet fever, scarlatina, epidemic sore throat, septic sore throat.* Inflammation of the lymphatic tissue of the pharynx, esp. the palatine or faucial tonsils. May occur sporadically or in epidemic form.

ETIOL: May be caused by a variety of organisms. If due to group A hemolytic streptococci, its clinical importance because of possible sequelae must be considered. SEE: *treatment*, below.

SYM: Onset is sudden usually accompanied by chills. Temperature may reach 105° F. Malaise, headache, pains and aches in back and extremities. Pain in tonsils, esp. when swallowing. Tonsils appear enlarged, red, and yellowish exudate projects from crypts.

PROG: Usually self-limited but serious complications may occur such as sinusitis, otitis media, mastoiditis, or peritonsillar abscess.

TREATMENT: (General) Bedrest, liquid diet, antipyretics, hot saline or 30% glucose gargles or throat irrigations. (Specific) Procaine penicillin or tetracycline drugs.

If the disease is thought to be due to group A hemolytic streptococci, the throat should be cultured and then penicillin therapy instituted for a full ten-day course. If in the meantime the report of the culture is negative for these organisms, the penicillin therapy may be discontinued when clinical signs of infection have subsided.

If throat culture technic is not available and infection with group A hemolytic streptococci is suspected, then a full ten-day course of penicillin should be given. This regimen will prevent the streptococci from elaborating the toxic substances which cause rheumatic fever, rheumatic heart disease, and certain kidney diseases. Administration of penicillin for *less than* ten days when tonsillitis is due to group A hemolytic streptococci is *not* advisable, even though clinical signs of infection may disappear within the first several days of treatment.

tonsillolith (tŏn′sĭl-ō-lĭth) [L. *tonsilla,* almond, + G. *lithos,* stone]. A concretion within a tonsil. SYN: *amygdalolith.*

tonsilloscopy (tŏn″sĭl-los′kō-pĭ) [" + G. *skopein,* to examine]. Inspection of the tonsils.

tonsillotomy (tŏn-sĭl-ŏt′ō-mĭ) [" + G. *tomē,* a cutting]. Excision of the tonsils. SEE: *amygdalotomy.*

tonus (tō′nŭs) [L. from G. *tonos,* tone]. That partial, steady contraction of muscle which determines tonicity or firmness. SYN: *tone, tonicity.*

tooth (tooth), (pl. *teeth*) [A.S. *tōth*]. One of the conical hard structures in the upper and lower jaws used for mastication.

A tooth consists of a *crown* or portion above gum, a *root,* portion embedded in socket (alveolus) of jaw bones, and *neck* or *cervix,* constricted region between crown and root which is covered by the *gum* or *gingiva.* The major portion of a tooth consists of *dentin,* an ivorylike substance harder than bone, which surrounds the *pulp cavity.* A layer of *enamel* covers the crown and *cementum* covers the dentin of the root. A *periodontal membrane* surrounds the root and holds the tooth firmly in its socket. The pulp cavity contains *dental pulp* which consists of connective tissue, capillaries, lymph vessels and nerve endings. SEE: *dentition, teeth,* words beginning with *odonto-.*

toothache. SYN: *odontalgia, odontodynia.* Pain in a tooth or the region about a tooth.

topagnosis. Loss of ability to localize tactile sensations.

topectomy (tō-pĕkt′ō-mĭ). A modified form of frontal lobotomy in which small incisions are made through the thalamofrontal tracts. A psychosurgical procedure used in the treatment of certain mental diseases.

topesthesia (to-pes-the′zĭ-ă) [G. *topos,* place, + *aisthēsis,* sensation]. Ability through tactile sense to determine any part that is touched.

tophaceous (tō-fā′shŭs) [L. *tophaceus,* sandy]. 1. Relating to a tophus. 2. Sandy, gritty.

tophus (tō′fŭs) (pl. *tophi*) [L. *tophus,* porous stone]. 1. Deposit of sodium biurate in tissues near a joint in gout. 2. A salivary calculus. 3. Tartar on the teeth.

tophyperidrosis (tŏf″ĭ-pĕr″ĭ-drō′sĭs) [G. *topos,* place, + *hyper,* above, + *idrōsis,* perspiration]. Excessive sweating in local areas.

top′ical [G. *topos,* place]. Pert. to a definite area; local.

topoalgia (tō-pō-ăl′jĭ-ă) [" + *algos,* pain]. Localized pain; common in neurasthenia following emotional upsets.

topoanesthesia (tō″pō-ăn-ĕs-thē′zĭ-ă) [" + *an-,* priv. + *aisthesis,* sensation]. Loss of ability to recognize the location of a tactile sensation.

topognosia, topognosis (tō-pŏg-nō′sĭ-ă, -sĭs) [" + *gnosis,* knowledge]. Recognition of the location of a tactile sensation. SYN: *topesthesia.*

topographic (top-ō-grăf′ĭk) [" + *graphein,* to write]. Pert. to description of special regions.

t. anatomy. SYN: *regional anatomy.* A study of all the structures and their relationships in a given region, for example, the axilla.

topography (tō-pŏg′ră-fĭ) [" + *graphein,* to write]. Description of a part of the body.

toponarcosis (tō″pō-nar-kō′sĭs) [" + *narkōsis,* stupor]. Local anesthesia.

toponeurosis (tō″pō-nū-rō′sĭs) [G. *topos,* place, + *neuron,* nerve, + *-ōsis,* condition]. Neurosis of a limited area.

topophobia (tō-pō-fō′bĭ-ă) [" + *phobos,* fear]. A fear of psychoneurotic origin in relation to a particular locality.

topothermesthesiometer (top″ō-ther-mĕs-thē-zhĭ-ŏm′ĕ-ter) [" + *thermē,* heat, + *aisthēsis,* sensation]. Device for measuring local temperature sense.

torantil (tō-răn′tĭl). A biologically standardized histamine-destroying enzyme, obtained from the mucosa of the small intestines and kidneys of hogs.

USES: In hay fever, some forms of dermatitis, serum sickness, and allergic conditions.

tormen (tor′mĕn) (pl. *tormina*) [L. *tormen,* a twisting]. Griping pain in the bowels.

tormina (tor′mĭn-ă) (sing. *tormen*) [L. twistings]. Intestinal colic with griping pains.

Tornwaldt's disease (torn′vahlt) [Ludwig Tornwaldt, German physician, 1843-1910]. Inflammation of crypt of the pharyngeal tonsil with formation of a pus-containing cyst and nasopharyngeal stenosis.

torose, torous (tō′rōs, -rŭs) [L. *torosus,* full of muscle]. Knobby or bulging; tubercular.

torpent (tor′pĕnt) [L. *torpens,* numbing]. 1. Medicine which modifies irritation. 2. Not capable of active functioning; dormant.

torpid (tor′pĭd) [L. *torpidus,* numb]. Not acting vigorously; sluggish.

torpidity (tor-pĭd′ĭ-tĭ) [L. *torpidus,* numb]. Sluggishness; inactivity.

torpor (tor′por) [L. *torpor,* numbness]. Abnormal inactivity; dormancy; numbness; apathy.

t. intestino′rum. Constipation.

t. peristal′ticus. Atonic constipation.

t. retinae. Reduced sensitivity of retina to light stimuli.

torsion (tor′shŭn) [L. *torsio,* a twisting]. 1. Act of twisting or condition of being twisted. 2. Rotation of the vertical meridians of the eye.

torsive (tor′sĭv) [L. *torsio,* a twisting]. Twisted, as in a spiral.

torso (tor′sō) [Italian]. The trunk of the body.

torsoclusion (tor-sŏk-lū′zhun) [" + L. *occlusio,* a shutting out]. 1. Acupressure in combination with torsion to stop a bleeding vessel. 2. Malocclusion characterized by rotation of a tooth on its long axis.

torticollis (tor-tĭk-ŏl′ĭs) [L. *tortus,* twisted, + *collum,* neck]. Stiff neck caused by spasmodic contraction of neck muscles drawing the head to one side with chin pointing to the other side. Congenital or acquired. SYN: *wryneck.*

ETIOL: Result of scars, disease of cervical vertebrae, adenitis, tonsillitis, rheumatism, enlarged cervical glands, retropharyngeal abscess, cerebellar tumors. It may be spasmodic (clonic) or permanent (tonic). The latter type may be due to Pott's disease.

The muscles affected are principally those supplied by the spinal accessory nerve.

t., fixed. Abnormal position of head due to organic shortening of the muscles.

t., intermittent. Same as *spasmodic t.*

t., ocular. T. from inequality in sight of the two eyes.

t., rheumatic. Same as *symptomatic t.*

t., spasmodic. T. with recurrent but transient contractions of muscles of neck and esp. of the sternocleidomastoid.

t., spurious. T. from caries of the cervical vertebrae.

t., symptomatic. Rheumatic stiff neck.

tortipelvis (tor″tĭ-pĕl′vĭs) [L. *tortus*, twisted, + *pelvis*, basin]. Muscular contractions distorting the spine and hip. SYN: *dystonia musculorum deformans.*

Torula (tor′ū-lă). Former name of a genus of yeastlike organism, now called *Cryptococcus.*

toruloid (tor′ū-loyd) [L. *torulus*, a little bulge, + G. *eidos*, form]. BACT: Beaded; noting an aggregate of colonies like those seen in the budding of yeast.

torulosis (tor-ū-lō′sĭs) [Torula + G. *-ōsis*, condition]. Infestation with Torula or yeast cells. SYN: *cryptococcosis.*

torulus (tor′ū-lŭs) [L. *torulus*, a little elevation]. A very small elevation. SYN: *papilla.*

t. tac′tilis. A tactile cutaneous elevation on palms and soles.

torus [L. swelling]. A linear elevation, a ridge.

totipotent [L. *totus*, all, + *potentin*, power]. A cell capable of differentiating into a large variety of cells. The fertilized ovum has this ability.

touch (tŭtsh) [O.Fr. *touchier*]. 1. To perceive by the tactile sense; to feel with the hands, to palpate. 2. The sense by which pressure on the skin or mucosa is perceived; the tactile sense. 3. Examination with the hand. SYN: *palpation.*

Various disorders may disturb or impair the tactile sense or the ability to feel normally. There are a number of words pert. to sensation and its modifications, a few of the more important ones being listed as follows: *algesia, -algia, anesthesia, dysesthesia, -dynia, esthesia, esthesioneurosis, hyperesthesia, paresthesia.*

t., abdominal. Palpation of the abdomen.

t., after. Persistence of the sensation of touch after contact with stimulus has ceased.

t., double. Vaginal and rectal examination made at same time.

t., rectal. Digital exploration of the rectum.

t., vaginal. Digital exploration of the vagina.

t., vesical. Digital exploration of the bladder.

touch, *words pert. to:* amblyaphia, anaphia, anaptic, astereognosis, atopognosis, delire de toucher, dysaphia, hallucinations, haphephobia, haptic, polyesthesia, stereognosis, tactile.

tour de maître (toor″deh mā′tr) [Fr. the master's turn]. A method of introducing a catheter or sound into the male bladder or into the uterus.

Tourette's disease (too-rĕt′). Convulsive tic, with echolalia and coprolalia, associated with motor incoordination. Also called *Gilles de la Tourette's disease.*

Tournay's sign (toor-nā′). Dilatation of the pupil of the eye on unusually strong lateral fixation.

tourniquet (tŭr′nĭ-kĕt) [Fr. a turning]. Any constrictor used on an extremity to make pressure over an artery and to control bleeding; also used to distend veins to facilitate venipuncture or intravenous injections.

Tourniquets are made more effective by placing a firm object such as a padded stone or a padded piece of wood over an artery to concentrate pressure at that point. A figure-of-eight knot pulled tight is also an excellent method for making firm such an object.

Tourniquet should never be left in place too long. Ordinarily, it should be released from 12 to 18 minutes to determine whether bleeding has ceased. If it has, leave tourniquet loosely in place so that it may be retightened if necessary. If not retighten at once.

In general, a tourniquet should not be used if steady, firm pressure over the bleeding site will stop the flow.

Arterial hemorrhage: Apply bet. the wound and the heart, close to the wound, placing a hard pad over point of pressure. Should be discontinued not later than 1 hour and a tight bandage substituted under the loosened tourniquet.

Venous hemorrhage: Place below bleeding point, but close to the wound. The tourniquet should remain in place with periodic momentary loosening until released by a physician.

t. paralysis. Injury to a nerve due to a tourniquet's having been applied for too long a period or too tightly.

t. test. Test for determining the ability of capillaries to withstand increased pressure.

Touton cells (toot′ŏn). Giant multinucleated cells found in lesions of xanthomatosis.

tow (tō) [A.S. *tow*, a weaving]. Coarse fibers of flax, used for surgical dressings.

towelette (tow-ĕl-ĕt′) [M.E. *towele*, towel]. A small towel for surgical or obstetrical use.

toweling, towelling (tow′ĕl-ĭng) [M.E *towele*, a towel]. Friction with a coarse towel.

toxalbumin (tŏks″ăl-bū′mĭn) [G. *toxikon*, poison, + L. *albumen*, white of egg]. A poisonous albumin or protein.

toxalbumose (tŏks-ăl′bū-mōs) [″ + L. *albumen*, white of egg]. A poisonous albumose.

toxamin (tŏks′ăm-ĭn) [″ + *amine*]. One of a class of injurious substances said to be present in grain food, which are harmful unless counteracted by vitamins.

toxanemia (tŏks″ă-nē′mĭ-ă) [G. *toxikon*, poison, + *an-*, priv. + *aima*, blood]. Toxemia, *q.v.*

toxemia (tŏks-ē′mĭ-ă) [G. *toxikon*, poison, + *aima*, blood]. Distribution throughout body of poisonous products of bacteria growing in a focal or local site, thus producing generalized symptoms.

SYM: Constitutional disturbances, rigors, increased temperature, diarrhea, vomiting, pulse and respiration quickened or depressed, prostration.

In *tetanus*, the nervous system is esp. affected; in *diphtheria*, nerves and muscles.

t., eclamptogenic. Toxemia of pregnancy, *q.v.* Also see *eclampsia.*

t. of pregnancy. Various conditions affecting women in pregnancy.

ETIOL: Unknown.

FORMS: Simple vomiting, pernicious vomiting (hyperemesis gravidarum), acute yellow atrophy of the liver, nephritic toxemia, renal failure, pre-eclampsia, and eclampsia.

toxenzyme (tŏks-ĕn′zīm) [G. *toxikon*, poison, + *en*, in, + *zymē*, leaven]. A poisonous enzyme.

toxic (tŏks′ĭk) [G. *toxikon*, poison]. Pert. to, resembling or caused by poison. SYN: *poisonous*.

t. erythema. Redness of skin or a rash resulting from toxic agents such as drugs.

toxicant (tŏks′ĭ-kănt) [G. *toxikon*, poison]. 1. Poisonous; toxic. 2. Any poison.

toxicide (tŏks′ĭ-sīd) [" + L. *cidus*, from *caedere*, to kill]. 1. Destructive to toxins. 2. A chemical antidote for poisons.

toxicity (tŏks-ĭs′ĭ-tĭ) [G. *toxikon*, poison]. 1. Poisonous. 2. The extent, quality, or degree of being poisonous.

toxico- [G.]. Combining form meaning *poison*.

toxicoderma (tŏks″ĭ-kō-der′mă) [G. *toxikon*, poison, + *derma*, skin]. Any skin disease resulting from a poison.

toxicodermatitis (tŏks″ĭ-kō-derm-ă-tī′-tĭs). Inflammation of the skin due to a poison.

toxicodermatosis (tŏks″ĭ-kō-derm-ă-tō′-sĭs). Toxicoderma, *q.v.*

toxicogenic (tŏks-ĭk-ō-jĕn′ĭk) [" + *gennan*, to produce]. Caused by, or producing, a poison.

toxicoid (tŏks′ĭ-koyd) [" + *eidos*, resemblance]. Of the nature of a poison.

toxicologist (tŏks-ĭ-kŏl′ō-jĭst). A specialist in the field of poisons or toxins.

toxicology (tŏks-ĭ-kŏl′ō-jĭ) [" + *logos*, science]. The science of poisons, their nature, effects, and antidotes.

toxicomania (tŏks″ĭ-kō-mā′nĭ-ă) [" + *mania*, madness]. Abnormal craving for narcotics, intoxicants, or poisons.

toxicopathic (tŏks″ĭ-kō-păth′ĭk) [" + *pathos*, disease]. Pert. to any condition caused by a poison.

toxicopathy (tŏks″ĭ-kop′ă-thĭ) [G. *toxikon*, poison, + *pathos*, disease]. Any disease caused by a poison.

toxicophobia (tŏks″ĭk-ō-fō′bĭ-ă) [" + *phobos*, fear]. Abnormal fear of being poisoned by any medium: food, gas, water, drugs, etc.

toxicosis (tŏks″ĭ-kō′sĭs) [" + *-ōsis*, condition]. A diseased condition resulting from poisoning. SYN: *toxicopathy*.

t., endogen′ic. Disease due to poisons generated within the body. SYN: *autointoxication*.

t., exogen′ic. Any disease resulting from a poison not generated in the body.

t., retention. T. from retained products which normally are excreted as formed.

toxidermitis (tŏks″ĭ-der-mī′tĭs) [G. *toxikon*, poison, + *derma*, skin, + *-itis*, inflammation]. Any inflammatory skin disease due to poisoning. SYN: *toxicodermatitis*.

toxiferous (tŏks-ĭf′ĕr-ŭs) [" + L. *ferre*, to carry]. Containing a poison. SYN: *poisonous*.

toxigenic (tŏks″ĭ-jĕn′ĭk) [" + *gennan*, to produce]. Producing toxins or poisons.

toxigenicity (tŏks″ĭ-jĕn-ĭs′ĭ-tĭ). The virulence of a toxin-producing pathogenic organism.

toxignomic (tŏks-ĭg-nŏm′ĭk) [" + *gnomikos*, knowing]. Having the toxic action peculiar to a poison.

toxin (tŏks′ĭn) [G. *toxikon*, poison]. A poisonous substance of animal or plant origin.

RS: *antibody, antitoxin, bacteria, phytotoxin, toxoid*.

t., bacterial. T. produced by bacteria. Includes exotoxins which diffuse from bacterial cells into surrounding medium, and *endotoxins* which are liberated only when bacterial cell is destroyed. SEE: *bacteria, toxin production*.

t., extracellular. Same as *exotoxin*.

t., intracellular. Same as *endotoxin*.

toxin-antitoxin (tŏks′ĭn-ăn″tĭ-tŏks′ĭn) [G. *toxikon*, poison, + *anti*, against, + *toxikon*]. Diphtheria toxin with its antitoxin in a nearly neutral mixture, the diphtheria toxin being about 85% neutralized.

Used for immunization against diphtheria. Also known as *T. A. T. mixture*.

toxinemia (tŏks″ĭn-ē′mĭ-ă) [" + *aima*, blood]. Blood poisoning. SYN: *toxemia*.

toxinfection (tŏks-ĭn-fĕk′shŭn) [" + L. *infectio*, a putting into]. Infection caused by toxins or other poisons.

toxinicide (tŏks-ĭn′ĭs-īd) [" + L. *cidus*, from *caedere*, to kill]. That which is destructive to toxins.

toxinosis (tŏks-ĭn-ō′sĭs) [" + *-ōsis*, condition]. Disease due to a toxin.

toxipathy (tŏks-ĭp′ă-thĭ) [" + *pathos*, disease]. Any disease due to poison.

toxiphobia (tŏks″ĭ-fō′bĭ-ă) [" + *phobos*, fear]. Abnormal fear of being poisoned.

toxitabellae (tŏks-ĭ-tăb-ĕl′ē) [G. *toxikon*, poison, + L. *tabella*, tablet]. Poisonous tablets. Usually designated by having an angular shape or by having the word "poison" or the "skull and crossbones design" stamped upon them.

toxitherapy (tŏks″ĭ-ther′ă-pĭ) [" + *therapeia*, treatment]. Use of toxins in treatment of disease.

toxituberculid (tŏks-ĭ-tū-bĕr′kū-lĭd). A skin lesion resulting from action of toxin of tuberculosis organism.

toxoalexin (tŏks″ō-ăl-ĕks′ĭn) [" + *alexein*, to ward off]. An alexin which counteracts bacterial toxins.

toxogenin (tŏks″ŏj′ĕn-ĭn) [" + *gennan*, to produce]. Hypothetical substance in the blood caused by injection of antigens, innocuous in itself, but causing anaphylaxis upon addition of fresh antigen.

toxoid (tŏks′oyd) [" + *eidos*, form]. A toxin treated so as to destroy its toxicity, but still capable of inducing formation of antibodies on injection. SEE: *Ehrlich's side-chain theory*.

t., alum-precipitated. T. of diphtheria or tetanus precipitated with potash-alum.

t., diphtheria. Diphtheria toxin detoxified by formaldehyde treatment.

toxolecithin (tŏks-ō-lĕs′ĭ-thĭn). A compound of lecithin with a toxin such as snake venom.

toxolysin (tŏks-ŏl′ĭ-sĭn) [" + *lysis*, dissolution]. Substance destroying toxins. SYN: *antitoxin, toxicide*.

toxomucin (tŏks″ō-mū′sĭn) [" + L. *mucus*, mucus]. Specific toxic albuminoid from cultures of tubercle bacilli.

toxon, toxone (tŏks′ŏn, -ōn) [G. *toxikon*, poison]. A bacterial toxin with lessened activity, producing paralysis and delayed death.

toxonoid (tŏks′ō-noyd) [" + *eidos*, form]. A nontoxic substance with a weak affinity for antitoxin.

toxonosis (tŏks-ō-nō′sĭs) [" + *-ōsis*, condition]. A disease caused by poisoning. SYN: *toxicosis, toxinosis*.

toxopeptone (tŏks-ō-pĕp′tōn) [" + *peptōn*, digesting]. A protein derivative produced by action of a toxin on peptones.

toxopexic (tŏks″ō-pĕks′ĭk) [" + *pĕxis,* fixation]. Pert. to the neutralization of a toxin.

toxophil(e (tŏks′ō-fĭl, -fīl) [" + *philein,* to love]. Having a special affinity for toxins, said of certain haptophore groups.

toxophore (tŏks′ō-fōr) [G. *toxikon,* poison, + *phoros,* a bearer]. That portion of a toxin which gives to a toxin its poisonous qualities. SEE: *Ehrlich's side-chain theory.*

toxophore group (toks′ō-for) [" + *phoros,* a bearer]. Poison-bearing group of a toxin. SEE: *Ehrlich's side-chain theory.*

toxophylaxin (tŏks-ō-fī-lăks′ĭn) [" + *phylaxis,* protection]. A defensive protein that neutralizes bacterial poisons. SYN: *toxicophylaxin.*

Toxoplasma (tŏks-ō-plăs′mă). A genus of protozoa of undetermined relationship.

T. gondii. The causative agent of toxoplasmosis, *q.v.*

toxoplasmosis (tŏks-ō-plăs-mō′sĭs). A disease due to infection with *Toxoplasma gondii.*

toxosozin (tŏks″ō-sō′zĭn) [" + *sōzein,* to save]. A normal defensive protein that neutralizes bacterial poisons. SEE: *sozin.*

TPI test. Abbr. for *Treponema pallidum immobilizing* test (for syphilis).

TPN. Abbr. for *triphosphopyridine nucleotide.*

t.p.r. Abbr. for *temperature, pulse,* and *respiration.*

tr. Abbr. for L. *tinctura,* tincture.

trabecula (tră-bĕk′ū-lă) (pl. *trabeculae*) [L. *trabecula,* a little beam]. Fibrous cord of connective tissue, serving as supporting fiber by forming septum extending into an organ from its wall or capsule.

t. carneae. NA. Thick muscular tissue bands attached to inner walls of the ventricles of the heart.

trabs, trabs cerebri (trăbz ser′ē-brī) [L. *trabs,* a beam]. Arched band of white fibers connecting the cerebral hemispheres. SYN: *corpus callosum.*

trace (trās) [Fr. *tracer,* from L. *tractus,* a drawing]. 1. A very small quantity. 2. A mark.

t. elements. Organic elements normally found in minute traces in foods and tissues, such as fluorine, copper, manganese, zinc, cobalt, nickel, aluminum, silicon, bromine, and other physiologically rare minerals.

t., primitive. Pale white streak in germinal area indicating beginning of development of the blastoderm. SYN: *primitive streak.*

tracer. A radioactive isotope, capable of being incorporated into compounds, which when introduced into the body "tags" a specific portion of the molecule so that its course may be traced. Used in absorption and excretion studies, for determination of intermediary products of metabolism, and determination of distribution of various substances in the body. Radioactive carbon (C^{14}), calcium (Ca^{42}) and iodine (I^{131}) are some of tracers used.

trachea (trā′kē-ă) (pl. *tracheae*) [G. *tracheia,* rough]. A cylindrical cartilaginous tube, 4½ inches long, from the larynx to the bronchial tubes. SYN: *windpipe.*

It extends from the sixth cervical to the fifth dorsal vertebra. Here it divides into 2 bronchi, 1 for each lung. It is lined with mucous membrane. Its inner surface is lined with ciliated epithelium.

tracheaectasy (trā″kē-ă-ĕk′tă-sĭ) [G. *tracheia,* rough + *ektasis,* dilatation]. Dilatation of the trachea.

tracheal (trā′kē-ăl) [G. *tracheia,* rough]. Pertaining to the trachea.

t. tugging. Pulsation of the larynx or downward pull of the trachea, symptomatic of thoracic aneurysm.

trachealgia (trā″kē-ăl′jĭ-ă) [" + *algos,* pain]. Pain in the trachea.

trachealis (trā-kē-ā′lĭs) [L.]. A muscle composed of smooth muscle fibers which extends between the ends of the tracheal rings. Its contraction reduces the size of the lumen.

tracheitis (trā-kē-ī′tĭs) [G. *tracheia,* rough + *-itis,* inflammation]. An inflammation of the trachea.

It may be acute or chronic and may be associated with bronchitis and laryngitis.

NP: It is necessary to keep patient in bed, as the condition may spread and give rise to bronchial complications. As the middle aged are more apt to be afflicted, cardiac strain from constant coughing and loss of sleep must be avoided. Inflammation of the chest must be guarded against. Pulse and temperature must be carefully checked and recorded. Camphorated oil may be rubbed on the chest, which is then covered with warm wool. Lemonade should be within reach of the patient as constant small sips will help relieve irritation from coughing. Diet should be light.

trachelagra (trā-kĕl-ăg′ră) [G. *trachēlos,* neck + *agra,* seizure]. Rheumatism or gout of neck muscles resulting in torticollis.

trachelectomopexy (trā″kĕl-ĕk-tom″o-peks′ĭ) [" + *ektome,* a cutting out + *pexis,* fixation]. Fixation of uterine neck with partial excision.

trachelectomy (trā-kĕl-ĕk′tō-mĭ) [" + *ektomē,* excision]. Amputation of the cervix uteri.

trachelematoma (trā″kĕl-ĕ-mă-tō′mă) [" + *haima,* blood + *-ōma,* tumor]. A hematoma situated on the neck.

trachelism, trachelismus (trā′ke-lĭzm, trā-ke-lĭz′mŭs) [" + *-ismos,* condition]. Backward spasm of the neck, sometimes preceding an epileptic attack.

trachelitis (trā-kē-lī′tĭs) [" + *-itis,* inflammation]. Inflammation of mucous membrane of the cervix uteri. SYN: *cervicitis.*

trachelo- [G.]. Combining form, meaning *neck.*

trachelobregmatic (trā″kē-lō-brĕg-măt′ĭk) [G. *trachēlos,* neck, + *bregma,* front of the head]. Pert. to the neck and the bregma.

trachelocystitis (trā″kĕl-ō-sĭs-tī′tĭs) [" + *kystis,* bladder, + *-itis,* inflammation]. Inflammation of neck of bladder.

trachelodynia (trā″kē-lō-dĭn′ĭ-ă) [" + *odynē,* pain]. Pain in the neck.

trachelokyphosis (trā-kĕl-ō-kī-fō′sĭs). Excessive anterior curvature of cervical portion of spine. Pott's disease.

trachelology (trā″ke-lŏl′ō-jĭ) [" + *logos,* study]. Scientific study of the neck, its diseases and injuries.

trachelomastoid (trā″ke-lō-măs′toyd) [G. *trachēlos,* neck, + *mastos,* breast, + *eidos,* form]. SYN: *longissimus capitus.* A muscle of the neck. SEE: *Muscles, Table of, in Appendix.*

trachelomyitis (trā″ke-lō-mī-ī′tĭs) [" + *mys, my-,* muscle, + *-itis,* inflammation]. Inflammation of muscles of neck.

trachelopexy (trā-kel-ō-pĕks′ĭ) [" + *pexis,* fixation]. Surgical fixation of the cervix uteri to an adjacent part.

tracheloplasty (trā'kel-ō-plas"tĭ) [G. *trachēlos*, neck, + *plassein*, to form]. Plastic surgery of the cervix uteri.

trachelorrhaphy (trā-kel-or'ă-fĭ) [" + *rhaphē*, seam]. Suturing of a torn cervix uteri.

trachelotomy (trā-kel-ŏt'ō-mĭ) [" + *tomē*, a cutting]. Incision of the cervix of the uterus.

tracheo- [G.]. Combining form meaning *trachea, windpipe.*

tracheoaerocele (trā"kē-ō-ā'er-ō-sēl) [G. *tracheia*, rough, + *aēr*, air, + *kēlē*, hernia.] Hernia or cyst of trachea containing air.

tracheobronchoscopy (trā"kē-ō-brŏng-kŏs'kō-pĭ) [" + *brogchos*, tube, + *skopein*, to examine]. Inspection of the trachea and bronchi through a bronchoscope.

tracheocele (trā'kē-ō-sēl) [" + *kēlē*, hernia]. Protrusion of mucous membrane through the wall of the trachea.

tracheoesophageal (trā"-kē-ō-ē-so-faj'ē-ăl, -ē-sŏf'ă-jē-ăl) [" + *oisophagos*, esophagus]. Pert. to the trachea and esophagus.

tracheolaryngotomy (trā"kē-ō-lăr-ĭn-gŏt'ō-mĭ) [" + *larygx*, larynx, + *tomē*, a cutting]. Incision into larynx and trachea.

tracheopathia, tracheopathy (trā"kē-ō-păth'ĭ-a, -op'ă-thĭ) [" + *pathos*, disease]. Diseased condition of the trachea.

tracheopharyngeal (trā"kē-ō-far-in'jē-ăl) [" + *pharygx*, pharynx]. Pert. to both the trachea and pharynx.

tracheophonesia (trā"kē-ō-fōn-ē'zhĭ-ă) [G. *tracheia*, rough, + *phōnēsis*, a sounding]. Cardiac auscultation at the sternal notch.

tracheophony (trā-kē-ŏf'ō-nĭ) [" + *phōnē*, a sound]. Sound heard over the trachea in auscultation.

tracheoplasty (trā'kē-ō-plăs-tĭ) [" + *plassein*, to form]. Plastic operation on the trachea.

tracheopyosis (trā"kē-ō-pī-ō'sĭs) [" + *pyon*, pus, + *-ōsis*, condition]. Tracheitis with suppuration.

tracheorrhagia (trā-kē-or-ā'jĭ-ă) [" + *rhēgnūnai*, to burst forth]. Tracheal hemorrhage.

tracheoschisis (trā-kē-ŏs'kĭs-ĭs) [" + *schisis*, a cleft]. Fissure of the trachea.

tracheoscopy (trā-kē-ŏs'kō-pĭ) [" + *skopein*, to examine]. Inspection of interior of trachea, by means of reflected light.

tracheostenosis (trā"kē-ō-sten-ō'sĭs) [" + *stenōsis*, a narrowing]. Contraction or narrowing of lumen of the trachea.

tracheostomy (tra"kē-os'to-mĭ). Same as tracheotomy, *q.v.*

tracheotome (trā'kē-ō-tōm) [G. *tracheia*, rough, + *tomē*, a cutting]. Instrument used in opening of trachea.

tracheotomy (trā-kē-ŏt'ō-mĭ) [" + *tomē*, a cutting]. Operation of cutting into the trachea usually for insertion of tube to overcome tracheal obstruction. Syn: *tracheostomy.*

NP: Temperature of tracheotomy room must be not less than 80° F. and atmosphere should be saturated with steam. The outer tube should not be removed by nurse, but inner one should be removed every hour or oftener if so directed by physician. It is held in place by a tape connected to each side and joined at the back of the patient's neck. This prevents the tube's being coughed out. The movable or inner tube should be washed, rinsed, and dried thoroughly. Usually there are two or more inner tubes available. Thus each can be sterilized and ready for replacement when a soiled one is removed. Before replacing inner tube, the tube remaining in trachea should also be cleaned to remove mucus that collects in and around tube. The patient will require almost continual observation during the acute phase of the condition which necessitated the tracheotomy. The nurse must check the suctioning apparatus and be familiar with its operation. See: *diphtheria.*

t. tube. T. to insert into opening made in tracheotomy.

trachitis (trā-kī'tĭs) [G. *tracheia*, rough, + *-itis*, inflammation]. Inflammation of the trachea. Syn: *tracheitis.*

trachoma (tră-kō'mă) [G. *trachōma*, roughness]. A chronic contagious form of conjunctivitis, noted by hypertrophy of conjunctiva, formation of follicles with subsequent cicatricial changes. Syn: *conjunctivitis, granular; ophthalmia, Egyptian.*

Etiol: A virus which is readily transmitted especially in early stages of disease. Transmission is by direct contact with trachomatous material or indirectly through contaminated articles such as towels, handkerchiefs, etc.

Complications: Pannus, ptosis, corneal ulcers.

Sequelae: Trichiasis, entropion, ectropion, symblepharon, corneal opacities, staphyloma, blindness.

Treatment: Topical application of tetracycline antibiotics in oil or ointment form. Oral sulfonamides may be required in resistant cases. Surgery may be necessary when lid deformities occur.

t., brawny. T. with general lymphoid infiltration without granulation of the conjunctiva.

t. deformans. Vulvitis with cicatricial contractions.

t., diffuse. T. with large granulations.

trachychromatic (trā"kĭ-krō-mat'ĭk) [G. *trachys*, rough, + *chrōma*, color]. Pert. to a nucleus with very deeply staining chromatin.

trachyphonia (trā-kĭ-fō'nĭ-ă) [" + *phōnē*, voice]. Roughness of the voice.

tract (trăkt) [L. *tractus*, a track]. 1. A course or pathway. 2. A group or bundle of nerve fibers within the spinal cord or brain which constitutes an anatomical and functional unit. See: *fasciculus.* 3. A group of organs or parts forming a continuous pathway.

t., afferent. An ascending tract, *q.v.*

t., alimentary. The canal or passage from the mouth to the anus.

t., ascending. Afferent white fibers in spinal cord.

t., descending. Efferent fibers in the spinal cord.

t., digestive. See: *alimentary tract.*

t., genitourinary. The genital and urinary pathways.

t., motor. Descending pathway conveying motor impulses from brain to lower portions of spinal cord.

t., olfactory. A narrow white band extending from olfactory bulb to anterior perforated substance of brain.

t., optic. A band of fibers extending from optic chiasma to lateral geniculate body of thalamus. Some fibers of the tract continue on to midbrain and hypothalamus.

t., pyramidal. Any of columns of motor fibers in the spinal cord which are continuations of pyramids in the medulla.

t., respiratory. The respiratory organs in continuity.

t., rubrospinal. A descending tract of fibers arising from cell bodies located in red nucleus of midbrain. Fibers terminate in gray matter of spinal cord.

t., sensory. Any tract of fibers conducting sensation to the brain.

t., supraopticohypophyseal. A tract consisting of fibers arising from cell bodies located in supraoptic and paraventricular nuclei of hypothalamus and terminating in post. lobe of hypophysis.

t., urinary. The urinary passageway from kidney to the outside. Includes the pelvis of kidney, ureter, bladder, and urethra.

traction (trăk'shŭn) [L. *tractio,* a drawing]. Process of drawing or pulling.

t., axis. Traction in line with the long axis of a course through which a body (fetus) is to be drawn.

t., elastic. Traction exerted by elastic devices such as rubber bands.

t., head. Traction applied to the head as in the treatment of injuries to cervical vertebrae.

t., weight. Traction exerted by means of weights.

tractotomy (trăk-tŏt'ō-mĭ). Surgical section of a fiber tract of the central nervous system. Sometimes resorted to for relief of intractable pain.

tractus (trăk'tŭs) (pl. *tractūs*) [L., a tract.] A tract or path.

tragacanth (trag'ă-kănth) [G. *tragakantha,* a goat thorn]. The dried gummy exudation from a plant grown in Asia, used in the form of mucilage as a greaseless lubricant, and as an application for chapped skin.

tragal (trā'găl) [G. *tragos,* goat]. Relating to the tragus.

tragi. Plural of tragus, *q.v.*

t., lamina. The cartilage of the tragus.

tragicus (trăj'ĭk-ŭs) [L.]. Muscle on the outer surface of the tragus. SEE: *Muscles, Table of, in Appendix.*

tragomaschalia (trag"ō-măs-kāl'ĭ-ă) [G. *tragos,* goat, + *maschale,* axilla]. Odorous perspiration (bromidrosis) of the axilla.

tragophonia, tragophony (trăg"ō-fō'nĭ-ă, -of'ō-nĭ) [" + *phōnē,* voice]. A bleating sound heard in auscultation at level of fluid in hydrothorax. SYN: *egophony.*

tragopodia (trăg-ō-pō'dĭ-ă) [" + *pous, pod-,* foot]. Knock-knee.

tragus (trā'gŭs) [G. *tragos,* goat]. 1. Cartilaginous tonguelike projection in front of the ext. meatus of the ear. 2. One of the hairs at the entrance of the ext. auditory meatus.

train. To participate in a special program of instruction in order to attain competence in a certain occupation or profession.

trait. A distinguishing feature; a characteristic or property of an individual.

t., acquired. One that is not inherited; one resulting from effects of environment.

t., inherited. One due to hereditary determiners or genes transmitted through germ cells.

trajector (tra-jĕk'tor) [L. *trajectus,* thrown across]. Device for determining approximate location of a bullet in a wound.

trance (trăns) [L. *transitus,* a passing over]. A sleeplike state, as in deep hypnosis, appearing also in hysteria and in some spiritualistic mediums, with limited sensory and motor contact with the ordinary surroundings, and with subsequent amnesia of what has occurred during the state.

t., coma. Hypnotic lethargy.

t., death. Trance simulating death.

t., induced. Hypnotic or somnambulistic t.

t., somnambulistic. T. with anesthesia, or catalepsy, or paralysis induced by hypnotism.

tranquilizer. A drug which acts to reduce mental tension and anxiety without interfering with normal mental activity. This ideal state of tranquilization is difficult to attain. Thus patients, taking these medicines may find that their reactions are slowed. The use of tranquilizers has facilitated the treatment of severely disturbed psychiatric patients. Among the drugs in use are chlorpromazine (Thorazine), reserpine (Serpasil), meprobamate (Miltown, Equanil), promazine (Sparine), hydroxyzine (Atarax). azacyclonal (Frenquel).

Side effects, particularly from chlorpromazine and reserpine, have included jaundice, Parkinson's disease, nausea, rashes, and in some surprising instances severe mental depression. The U. S. Public Health Service has warned of "a significant incidence of severe depression, with suicidal tendencies in some instances," in persons under heavy reserpine dosage.

trans- [L.]. Prefix meaning *across, over, beyond, through.*

transamidation. The transfer of an amidine group from one amino acid to another.

transaminase. An enzyme that catalyzes transamination.

t., glutamic-oxalacetic. ABBR: GOT or SGOT for serum GOT and ***t., glutamic-pyruvic.*** ABBR: GPT or SGPT for serum GPT. Enzymes present in many tissues; the highest concentrations are found in the liver and cardiac muscle. Injury of either of those tissues liberates the enzymes into the bloodstream. Thus measurement of their levels in the serum (SGOT or SGPT) provides a valuable test for hepatic cell or myocardial injury.

transamination (trăns"ăm-ĭ-nā'shŭn). The transfer of an amino group from one compound to another or the transposition of an amino group within a single compound.

transanimation (trans"ăn-ĭ-mā'shŭn) [L. *trans,* across, + *anima,* breath]. Resuscitation of a stillborn infant.

transaudient (trăns"aw'dĭ-ent) [" + *audire,* to hear]. Permeable to sound waves.

transcalent (trăns-kā'lĕnt) [" + *calere,* to be hot]. Permeable to heat rays. SYN: *diathermanous.*

transcapillary (trăns"kăp'ĭl-lă-rĭ). Across the endothelial wall of a capillary.

t. exchange. The passage of substances between blood and tissue (interstitial) fluid.

transducer [L. *trans,* across + *ducere,* to lead]. A device which converts one form of energy to another. Used in medical electronics to receive the energy produced by sound or pressure and relay it as an electrical impulse to another transducer which can reverse the process. The telephone is an example of this.

transduction (trăns-dŭk'shŭn). A phenomenon causing genetic change in bacteria in which DNA is carried from one bacterium to another by bacteriophage. SEE: *transformation.*

transection (trăn-sĕk'shŭn) [" + *sectio,* a cutting]. A cutting made across a long axis; a cross section.

transfer, transference (trans'fer, trans-fer'ĕns) [L. *trans*, across, + *ferre*, to bear]. 1. PSY: Transmission of any affect from one idea to another, or from one object or person to another, unconscious identifications being the activating motive. 2. State in which the symptoms of one area are transmitted to a similar area on the other side, as in hysteria.

t. neuroses. Compulsion neuroses and hysteria.

t. situation. The emotional state of a patient existing bet. him and his physician during psychoanalysis.

Either affection or distrust is transferred by the patient to the physician, although such feelings are not related to reality.

t., thought. Transference of one's thoughts to another. SYN: *telepathy.*

transfix (trăns-fĭks') [L. *trans*, across, + *figere*, to fix]. To pierce through or impale with a sharp instrument.

transfixion (trăns-fĭk'shŭn) [L. *trans*, across, + *figere*, to fix]. Maneuver in performing an amputation in which a knife is passed into the soft parts and cutting is from within outward.

transforation (trăns"for-ā'shŭn) [" + *forāre*, to pierce]. The perforation of the fetal skull at the base in craniotomy.

transforator (trăns'fo-rā-tor) [" + *forāre*, to pierce]. Instrument for perforating fetal skull.

transformation (trăns"for-mā'shŭn) [" + *formatio*, a forming]. 1. Change of shape or form. SYN: *metamorphosis*. 2. Change of one tissue into another. 3. Degeneration. 4. A type of mutation occurring in bacteria. It results from DNA of a bacterial cell penetrating the host cell and becoming incorporated into the genotype of host.

transformer (trăns-form'er) [L. *trans*, across, + *formāre*, to form]. PT: A stationary induction apparatus to change electrical energy at one voltage and current to electrical energy at another voltage and current through the medium of magnetic energy, without mechanical motion.

transfusion (trăns-fū-zhŭn) [L. *trans*, across, + *fusio*, a pouring]. 1. Injection of the blood of one person into the blood vessels of another. SEE: *blood transfusion.*

2. Injection of saline or other solutions into a vein for a therapeutic purpose. SEE: *donor.*

t., direct. Transfer of blood directly from one person to another.

t., indirect. T. of blood from a donor to a suitable storage container and then to the patient.

t., replacement. Procedure in treatment of erythroblastosis fetalis of the newborn in which major portion of total blood volume is withdrawn in small amounts at a time and replaced with Rh-negative blood.

t., subcutaneous. Infusion of saline solution or other fluid beneath the skin.

transiliac (trăns-ĭl'ĭ-ăk) [L. *trans*, across, + *iliacus*, pert. to a haunch bone]. Extending bet. the 2 ilia.

transillumination (trăns"ĭl-lū"mĭ-nā'shŭn) [L. *trans*, across, + *illumināre*, to enlighten]. Inspection of a cavity or organ by passing a light through its walls.

When pus or lesion or degeneration is present, the reflection of light is diminished or absent.

transition (trănz-ĭ'shŭn) [L. *transitio*, a going across]. Passage from one state or position to another, or from one part to another part. SEE: *transitional.*

transitional (trănz-ĭsh'ŭn-ăl) [L. *transitio*, a going across]. Marked by or relating to a transition.

transitionals (trănz-ĭsh'ŭn-ăls) [L. *transitio*, a going across]. Mononuclear leukocytes, characterized by their large size, often 3 times as large as a red cell.

Commonly slightly irregular and found in from 2 to 4% of a normal differential white blood cell count. The nucleus is oval, lobulated or a horseshoe, and stains an even dirty blue color. Protoplasm likewise stained a dirty blue tint. It has neutrophilic granules which take a lilac shade.

translucent (trăns-lū'sĕnt) [L. *trans*, across, + *lucens*, shining]. Not transparent but permitting passage of light.

transmethylation. Process in the metabolism of amino acids in which a methyl group is transferred from one compound to another; for example, the conversion in the body of homocysteine to methionine. In this case the methyl group is furnished by choline or betaine.

transmigration (trăns"mī-grā'shŭn) [L. *trans*, across, + *migratio*, migration]. Wandering across or through, especially the passage of white blood cells through capillary membranes into the tissues.

t., external. Transfer of an ovum from an ovary to an opp. tube through the pelvic cavity.

t., internal. Transfer of an ovum through the uterus to the opposite oviduct.

transmissible (trăns-mĭs'ĭ-bl) [L. *transmissio*, a sending across]. Capable of being carried from one person to another, as an infectious disease.

transmission (trăns-mĭsh'ŭn) [L. *transmissio*, a sending across]. Transfer of anything, as a disease or hereditary characteristics.

t., biological. Condition in which organism transmitting causative agent of disease plays an essential role in the life history of a parasite or germ.

t., duplex. Passage of impulses through a nerve trunk in both directions.

t., mechanical. The passive transfer of causative agents of disease, esp. by arthropods. May be *indirect*, as when flies pick up organisms from excreta of a man or animals and deposit them on food, or *direct*, as when they pick up organisms from body of a diseased individual and directly inoculate them into body of another individual by bites or through open sores.

t., neuromyal. The transmission of excitation from a motor neuron to a muscle fiber at a neuromyal (myoneural) junction.

t., placental. The transmission of substances in the mother's blood to the blood of the fetus by way of the placenta.

t., synaptic. The mechanism by which an impulse in one neuron gives rise to an impulse in another neuron.

t., transovarial. The transmission of causative agents of disease to offspring following invasion of ovary and infection of eggs. Occurs in ticks and mites.

transmutation (trăns-mū-tā'shŭn) [L. *transmutātio*, a changing across]. A transformation or change, as of one species into another.

transonance (trăns-ō'năns). Transmission of sounds through an organ, as heart sounds through the lungs and chest wall.

transparent (trăns-păr'ĕnt) [L. *trans*, across, + *parere*, to appear]. 1. Transmitting light rays so that objects are visible through the substance. 2. Pervious to radiant energy. SEE: *clearing agent.*

transpirable (trăns-pī'ră-bl) [" + *spirāre,* to exhale]. Permitting excretion through the skin or membranes, as perspiration.

transpiration (trăns-pī-rā'shŭn) [" + *spiratio,* exhalation]. 1. Act of exhaling water, gas, or vapor through the skin or a membrane. SEE: *perspiration.* 2. Substance exhaled.

t., cutaneous. Giving off sweat from pores of the skin. SYN: *perspiration.*

t., pulmonary. Escape of watery vapor from the blood to the air in the lungs.

transplantation (trăns-plăn-tā-shŭn) [" + *plantāre,* to plant]. The taking of a portion of living tissue from its normal position in the body or from the body of another person and uniting it with like tissue in another place, to lessen defect or remedy deformity or injury. SEE: *autotransplantation, graft.*

t., autoplastic. Transplantation of tissue from one part to another part of the same body.

t., hetero. The transplantation of an organ or tissue from one individual to another of a different species.

t., heteroplastic. The transplantation of a part from one individual to another individual of the same or a closely related species.

t., heterotopic. One in which transplant is placed in a different location in host than it had in donor.

t., homo-. Transplantation of tissue from one individual of the same species to another.

t., homoplastic. An autoplastic transplant, *q.v.*

t., homotopic. One in which transplant occupies same location in host that it had in donor.

t. of cornea. Keratoplasty, *q.v.*

t., tenoplastic. Transplantation of tissue between individuals belonging to different genera.

transportation of the injured. *Carrying in arms*: Patient is picked up in both arms as a child.

One-arm assist: Patient's arm is placed about neck of bearer and bearer's arms are placed about waist, thus assisting patient to walk.

Chair carry: SEE: *chair stretcher.*

Chair stretcher: Any ordinary firm chair should be tested. Patient is placed seated upon it tilted back. One bearer grasps back of the chair and the other the legs of the chair (either the front or rear, depending on the construction of the chair). Both bearers face in the same direction. Patient's head rests either on chest or back of the head bearer. Turn two chairs to the ground; overlap the backs and tie or wire them together, using the legs as handles.

Double loop: A sheet is rolled on its long axis, tied and placed over the shoulder of both bearers. Patient sits on the long loop and rests his back against a short upper loop with the bearers supporting him. The weight is thus distributed on shoulders of both bearers.

Fireman's drag: Patient's wrists are crossed and tied with tie, belt, etc. Bearer kneels astride patient, places his head under patient's wrists and walks on all fours dragging patient beneath him.

Fireman's lift: Bearer grasps patient's left wrist with right arm; places patient's head under left armpit drawing patient's body over his left shoulder. Left arm should encircle both thighs, then lift patient. Patient's wrist is transferred to bearer's left hand, thus leaving 1 hand free to remove obstacles or to open doors, etc.

Four-handed basket seat: Each bearer grasps his own wrist and then grasps partner's free wrist. Patient sits upon this support.

Pack-strap carry: Patient lies on bearer's back. Patient's right arm is brought over bearer's right shoulder and held by his left hand. Left arm is brought over left shoulder and held by his right hand. Patient is thus carried on the back with arms resembling pack straps.

Pickaback carry: This is the pack strap carry only bearer supports patient's knees in flexed position. This leaves patient practically in a sitting position astride bearer's back with his arms around the bearer's neck or trunk.

Saddle-back carry: Bearer places arm under patient's armpit around his back and grasps it around armpit. Patient's body is across bearer's back. Rescuer's free arm grasps both thighs, allowing patient to rest across the bearer's back.

Shirt-tail carry: Bearer grasps patient's coat, blouse, or shirt tail, twists it to make a handle and brings it over his shoulder thus carrying patient back to back.

Six- or eight-man carry: This is done as the 3-man carry except 3 or 4 bearers are on each side of patient, thus dividing weight more uniformly.

Three-handed basket seat: Bearer grasps his own wrist, partner grasps the other wrist and leaves 1 arm free for supporting patient.

Three- or four-man carry: The little carry used by emergency squads. Three men kneel on one side of patient, place their hands under him and lift him up. The head bearer supports head and shoulders, center bearer lifts waist and hips, and third bearer lifts both lower extremities. If a fourth man is available, he should help steady patient while he is being lifted.

Triangular or greater arm sling, or branchiocervical sling: Place triangle on chest with 1 end over the sound shoulder, the point at elbow of affected side. Fold the base. Flex injured arm outside of triangle above the horizontal. Carry other end upward outside of arm back over shoulder of affected side. Tie to side of neck with square knot. Bring point anteriorly around back of elbow and fasten to ascending base or tie forming a cup at elbow. (In this bandage the weight is taken from entire length of forearm.)

Two-handed seat: Bearers kneel on either side of patient. Each passes one arm around back (under armpits) and other arm under knees and lifts him carefully. Patient is in a sitting position.

Wheel chair, improvised: Fastening casters to ordinary chair: Tie on a broom handle or similar stick for footrest by placing chair legs on parallel boards and fastening roller skates, wheels, etc.

Fastening as rocker to roller skates: Remove legs from an old chair and fasten to frame of a baby carriage, or play wagon.

t. by vehicle. Ambulances are desirable if available and usually contain appropriate stretchers. When not obtainable, stretchers may be made with poles, chairs or ladders. SEE: *stretchers.* When entering or leaving an airplane one must remember that patient must be tied to the stretcher.

t. by automobile. This is difficult except in a station wagon or similar vehicle. One bearer should be in the car and one or two outside to assist patient. A small chair stretcher can sometimes be used with advantage. A door or ladder slung across the open windows or from front to rear seats may be used. The large rear seat can be used, a stretcher being placed diagonally and supported at one end by the seat and the other end on a box or folded blankets.

transposition (trăns-pō-zĭ'shŭn) [L. *trans,* across, + *positio,* a placing]. 1. A transfer of position from one spot to another. SEE: *metathesis.* 2. Displacement of an organ, esp. a viscus, to the opposite side. 3. Transplantation of a flap of tissue without severing it entirely from its original position until it has united in the new position.

transsegmental (trăns"sĕg-mĕn-tăl) [" + *segmentum,* a cutting]. Extending across or beyond a segment as of a limb.

transseptal (trăns-sĕp'tăl) [" + *saeptum,* septum]. Across a septum.

transtemporal (trăns-tĕm'pōral) [" + *temporalis,* pert. to a temple]. Crossing the temporal or the cerebrum.

transthalamic (trăns"thăl-ăm'ĭk) [" + *thalamos,* chamber]. Passing across the optic thalamus.

transthermia (trăns-thĕr'mĭ-ă) [" + *thermē,* heat]. Production of heat in the deep tissues by electric currents. SYN: *diathermy, thermopenetration.*

transthoracic (trăns-thō-răs'ĭk) [" + *thorax,* chest]. Across the thorax.

transthoracotomy (trăns"thō-răk-ŏt'ō-mĭ) [L. *trans,* across, + *thorax,* chest, + *tomē,* a cutting]. The operation of incising across the thorax.

transubstantiation (trăns-sŭb-stăn'shĭ-ā'-shŭn). The process of replacing one tissue by another.

transudate (trăns'ū-dāt). [L. *trans,* across, + *sudare,* to sweat]. The fluid which passes through the pores of a membrane, especially that which passes through capillary walls. Compared to an *exudate, q.v.,* a transudate has fewer cellular elements and would be of a lower specific gravity.

transudation (trăns-ū-dā'shŭn) [" + *sudātio,* a sweating]. Oozing of a fluid through pores or interstices, as of a membrane.

transurethral (trăns"ū-rē'thrăl) [" + *ourēthra,* urethra]. Pert. to an operation performed through the urethra.

transvaginal (trăns-văj'ĭn-ăl) [" + *vagina,* sheath]. Through the vagina.

transversalis. Transverse to or at right angles to the long axis of the body.

t. fascia. A thin membrane forming the peritoneal surface of the transversus muscle and its aponeurosis.

transverse (trăns-vĕrs') [L. *transversus,* turned across]. Lying across; crosswise.

t. fora'men. Canal in each transverse process of a cervical vertebra for the arteries and veins.

transversectomy (trăns-vĕr-sĕk'tō-mĭ) [" + G. *ektomē,* excision]. Excision of a transverse vertebral process.

transversospinalis (trăns-vĕr"sō-spĭ-nā'lĭs) [L. *transversus,* turned across, + *spina,* thorn]. Semispinalis capitus, s. cervicis. SEE: *Muscles, Table of, in Appendix.*

transversus (trăns-vĕr'sŭs) [L. turned across]. 1. Any of several small muscles. SEE: *Muscles, Table of, in Appendix.* 2. Lying across the long axis of a part or organ.

transvestism, transvestitism (trăns-vĕst'ĭzm, -ĭ-tĭzm) [L. *trans,* across, + *vestitus,* clothed, + G. *-ismos,* condition]. A sexual perversion in which a person chooses to dress in clothes of the opposite sex. SYN: *eonism, q.v.*

trapezium (tră-pē'zĭ-ŭm) [G. *trapezion,* a little table]. SYN: *greater multangular bone; os trapezium.* The first bone in the distal row of carpal bones. It lies between navicular and first metacarpal bones.

trapezius (tră-pē'zĭ-ŭs) [G. *trapezion,* a little table]. A flat, triangular muscle covering posterior surface of neck and shoulder. SEE: *Muscles, Table of, in Appendix.*

trapezoid (trăp'ĕ-zoyd) [G. trapezoeidēs, table-shaped]. A plane four-sided figure having two sides parallel.

t. body. SYN: *corpus trapezoideum.* A bundle of transverse fibers in the ventral portion of tegmentum of pons.

t. bone. SYN: *lesser multangular bone.* The second bone in the distal row of carpal bones. It lies between the greater multangular and capitate.

t. ligament. The lateral portion of the coraco-clavicular ligament.

Trapp-Hässer formula (trăp-hă'sĕr). To estimate the grains of solids in urine, multiply last 2 figures of the sp. gr. by 2.33, which gives the solids in 1000 cc.

trauma (traw'mă) (pl. *traumata* or *traumas*) [G. *trauma,* wound]. An injury or a wound.

t., psychic. A painful, emotional experience, which may cause a neurosis.

traumatic (traw-măt'ĭk) [G. *trauma,* wound]. Caused by or relating to an injury.

t. fever. One following an injury.

t. psychosis. One resulting from physical injuries or emotional shock.

traumatism (traw'mă-tĭzm) [" + *-ismos,* condition]. 1. Morbid condition of system due to an injury or wound. 2. Incorrectly, a trauma.

traumatology (traw-mă-tŏl'ō-jĭ) [" + *logos,* science]. The science of wounds and their care.

traumatopnea (traw"mă-tŏp-nē'ă) [" + *noie,* breath]. Passage of air in and out of a wound in the chest wall.

treatment (trēt'ment) [M.S. *treten,* to handle]. 1. Medical, surgical or psychiatric management of a patient. 2. Any specific procedure used for the cure or the amelioration of a disease or pathological condition. SEE: *therapy.*

t., active. Treatment directed specifically toward cure of a disease.

t., after. That employed during convalescence following an operation or an illness.

t., causal. Treatment directed toward removal of the cause of the disease.

t., conservative. 1. The withholding of administration of medicine or utilization of operative procedures until such procedures are clearly indicated. 2. In surgical cases, the preservation of the organ or part if at all possible with the least possible mutilation.

t., dietetic. Treatment based on regulation of diet.

t., electric shock. Electroshock therapy, shock therapy, *q.v.*

t., empiric. One based on observation and experience rather than having a scientific basis.

t., expectant. Relief of symptoms as they arise, *i.e.*, not directed at the specific cause.

t., hypoglycemic shock. Insulin shock therapy, shock therapy, *q.v.*

t., palliative. One designed for the relief of symptoms of the disease rather than curing the disease.

t. paralysis. A serious and sometimes fatal complication following the administration of antirabic vaccine.

t., preventive, prophylactic. T. directed to prevention of disease.

t., rational. One based on scientific principles.

t., shock. Shock therapy, *q.v.*

t., specific. T. directed to the cause of a disease.

t., starvation. Treatment employed in which food is withheld as in cases of bacillary dysentery, following hemorrhage, etc. 2. The treatment of diabetes in which there are days of fasting followed by a restricted and carefully controlled diet.

t., supportive. Special measures employed to supplement specific therapy.

t., surgical. T. by means of operation.

t., symptomatic. Treatment directed toward constitutional symptoms such as pyrexia, shock, and pain.

tree. In anatomy, a treelike structure.

t., bronchial. The right or left bronchus with its branches and their terminal arborizations.

Tre'mato'da. A class of flatworms commonly called *flukes* belonging to the phylum Platyhelminthes. It includes two orders, (1) the *Monogenea*, which are external or semi-external parasites having direct development with no asexual multiplication, and (2) the *Digenea*, internal parasites with asexual generation in its life cycle. The Digenea usually require two or more hosts, the hosts alternating. SEE: *fluke.*

trematode (trĕm'ă-tōd) [G. *trēmatōdēs*, full of holes]. A fluke, a parasitic flatworm belonging to the class *Trematoda.* SEE: *fluke, cercaria.*

trematodiasis (trĕm"ă-tō-dī'ă-sĭs). Infestation with a trematode.

tremble. 1. An involuntary quivering or shaking. 2. To shiver, quiver, or shake.

trembles. SYN: *milk sickness.* A condition resulting from ingestion of plants such as snakeroot (*Eupatorium urticaefolium*) or jimmey weed (*Aploppus heterophyllus*). Common in domestic animals and may occur in humans as a result of ingesting the plants or more commonly from drinking milk or eating the meat of poisoned animals. Symptoms are weakness, anorexia, nausea and vomiting, prostration, and possibly death.

tremetol (trĕm'ĕ-tŏl). A poisonous substance occurring in snakeroot, rayless goldenrod, and other plants which causes trembles in animals or man. SEE: *trembles.*

tremogram (trĕm'ō-grăm) [L. *tremere*, to shake, + G. *gramma*, a mark]. Graphic representation made by a tremograph.

tremograph (trĕm'ō-grăf) [" + *graphein*, to write]. Device for recording tremors.

tremolabile (trē"mō-lā'bl) [" + *labilis*, unsteady]. Easily destroyed or inactivated by shaking; said of a ferment.

tremophobia (trĕm"ō-fō'bĭ-ă) [" + G. *phobos*, fear]. Abnormal fear of trembling.

tremor (trĕm'or, trē'mor) [L. *tremor*, a shaking]. 1. A quivering, esp. continuous quivering of a convulsive nature. 2. An involuntary movement of a part or parts of the body resulting from alternate contractions of opposing muscles.

Tremors may be classified as *involuntary, static, dynamic, kinetic, hereditary,* and *hysteric.* Pathologic tremors are independent of the will. The trembling may be fine or coarse, rapid or slow, may appear on movement (intention tremor) or improve when the part is employed. Often due to organic disease; trembling may express an emotion (*e.g.*, fear).

TREATMENT: Varies with underlying cause. SEE: *subsultus.*

t., alcoholic. The visible t. exhibited by alcoholics.

t., coarse. One in which oscillations are relatively slow.

t., continuous. One that resembles tremors of paralysis agitans.

t., fibrillary. One caused by consecutive contractions of separate muscular fibrillae, rather than of a muscle or muscles.

t., fine. A rapid tremor.

t., flapping. Coarse tremor of a muscle group. The supported part momentarily loses its support and there is an attempt to regain the support. When seen in the outstretched arm and hand the part flaps like a wing. Seen in hepatic coma and other diseases which cause encephalopathy. SYN: *asterixis.*

t., forced. T. continuing after voluntary motion has ceased.

t., hysterical. A fine rapid tremor occurring in hysteria. May be limited to one extremity or generalized.

t., intention. T. when voluntary motion is attempted.

t., intermittent. One common to paralyzed muscles in hemiplegia when attempting voluntary movement.

t., muscular. Slight oscillating muscular contractions in rhythmical order.

t., physiologic. A transient tremor occurring in normal individuals, resulting from excessive physical exertion, excitement, hunger, fatigue, or other causes.

t., rest. One present when the involved part is at rest but absent or diminished when active movements are attempted.

t., senile. A tremor occurring in old age.

t., static. SYN: *rest tremor.* One present when muscles involved are at rest.

t., volitional. Trembling of limbs or of body when making a voluntary effort. Seen in multiple sclerosis and other nervous diseases. SEE: *intention tremor.*

tremulous (trĕm'ū-lŭs) [L. *tremulāre*, to tremble]. Trembling or shaking.

trench fever. SYN: *Wolhynian fever.* A rickettsial disease occurring in central Europe caused by *Rickettsia pediculi* transmitted by the body louse.

trench foot. A condition resembling frostbite affecting feet of soldiers who are obliged to stand in cold water for long periods of time.

trench mouth. Infection of tonsils and floor of the mouth with Vincent's bacillus, characterized by inflammation, ulceration, and painful swelling. SYN: *ulceromembranous angina, Vincent's angina, q.v.*

trend. The inclination to proceed in a certain direction or at a certain rate. Used to describe the prognosis of a symptom or disease.

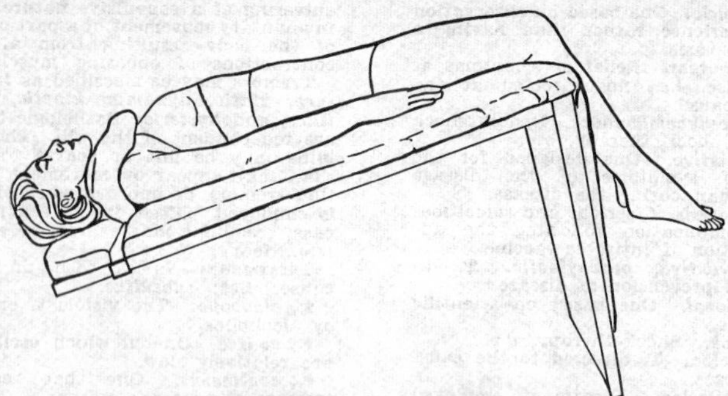

TRENDELENBURG POSITION.
Shoulder braces on table prevent patient from slipping

Trendelenburg position (trĕn-dĕl′ĕn-burg). The bed or table is raised from the foot, greatly elevating the knees, the legs projecting on an extended leg rest.

In this position the abdominal organs are pushed up toward the chest by gravity. The legs are elevated at an angle of 45°. The head is lower than the hips and legs. The foot of the bed may be elevated by resting upon blocks or pins.

This position is assumed in some abdominal surgery, in case of shock, or low blood pressure. In surgical cases, the legs and feet hang over the end of the table. (*Illus., page T-46.*)

trepan (trē-păn′) [G. *trypanon*, a borer]. 1. To perforate the skull with a trepan to relieve brain from pressure. 2. An instrument resembling a carpenter's bit for incision of the skull. SYN: *trephine.*

trephination (trĕf-ĭn-ā′shŭn) [Fr. *tréphine*, a bore]. Process of cutting out a piece of bone with the trephine.

trephine (trē-fīn′) [Fr. *tréphine*, a bore]. 1. To perforate with a trephine. 2. A cylindrical saw for cutting circular piece of bone out of skull. SYN: *trepan.*

trephin′ing. The process of cutting bone with a trephine. 2. The removal of a piece of cornea for the relief of glaucoma.

trephone (trĕf′ōn) [G. *trephein*, to nourish]. Hypothetical growth-promoting substance in the blood serum, used by cells as food material.

trepidant (trĕp′ĭ-dănt) [L. *trepidans*, trembling]. Marked by tremor.

trepidation (trĕp-ĭ-dā′shŭn) [L. *trepidatio*, a trembling]. 1. Fear, anxiety. 2. Trembling movement, esp. when involuntary.

Treponema (trĕp-ō-nē′mă) [G. *trepein*, to turn, + *nēma*, thread]. A genus of spirochetes, parasitic in man, with undulating or rigid bodies. They belong to the family Treponemataceae.

T. carateum. The causative agent of pinta, an infectious disease of the skin.

T. pallidum. Causative organism of syphilis. SYN: *Spirochaeta pallida.*

T. pertenue. Causative organisms of yaws (frambesia).

Treponemataceae. A family of spiral organisms belonging to the order Spirochaetales. Includes the genera *Borrelia, Leptospira*, and *Treponema.*

treponemiasis (trĕp″ō-nē-mī′ă-sĭs) [G. *trepein*, to turn, + *nēma*, thread, + *iasis*, infection]. Infestation with Treponema.

treponemicidal (trĕp″ō-nē-mĭ-sī′dăl) [" + " + L. *cidus*, from *caedere*, to kill]. Destructive to Treponema.

trepopnea (trĕp-ŏp′nē-ă). Difficult breathing when one is in a certain recumbent position.

treppe (trĕp′eh) [Ger. *treppe*, staircase]. Increase in height of contractions when the heart or a muscle is stimulated rapidly at regular intervals. SYN: *staircase phenomenon, q.v.*

tresis (trē′sĭs) [G. *trēsis*, perforation]. Perforation.

tri- [G.]. Combining form meaning *three.*

triad (trī′ăd) [G. *trias*, three]. 1. Any three things having something in common. 2. A trivalent element. 3. Trivalent.

t., Hutchinson's. Notched teeth, interstitial keratitis, and eighth-nerve deafness due to meningeal involvement; a syndrome characteristic of prenatal syphilis.

triage [Fr. *trier*, sort out]. The classification of wounded or injured persons in order to insure the efficient use of medical and nursing manpower, equipment, and facilities. Classification is concerned with the casualties who would live without therapy of any kind, those who would die no matter what treatment is provided, and those who would survive if given adequate care.

triakaidekaphobia (trī″ăk-ī-dĕk-ă-fō′bĭ-ă) [" + *kai*, and, + *deka*, ten, + *phobos*, fear]. Superstition regarding the number 13.

triangle (trī′ăng-l) [L. *três*, three, + *angulus*, angle; *triangulum*]. A figure or area formed by 3 angles and 3 sides.

t., anal. SYN: *rectal triangle.* Triangle with base between the two ischial tuberosities and apex at coccyx.

t., anterior, of the neck. The space bounded by the middle line of the neck, the ant. border of the sternocleidomastoid, and a line running along the lower border of the mandible and continued to the mastoid process of the occipital bone.

t., carotid, inferior. The space bounded by the middle line of the neck, the sternomastoid and the ant. belly of the omohyoid muscle.

t., carotid, superior. The space bounded by the ant. belly of the omohyoid muscle, the post. belly of the digastricus and the sternomastoid.

t., cephalic. A t. on the anteroposterior plane of the skull formed by lines joining the occiput and forehead and chin, and 1 uniting the 2 latter.

t., facial. A t. bounded by lines uniting the basion and the alveolar and nasal points, and 1 uniting the 2 latter.

t., femoral. T. on the inner part of the thigh, bounded by the sartorius and adductor longus muscle, and above by inguinal ligament.

t., frontal. A t. bounded by the maximum frontal diameter and lines joining its extremities and the glabella.

t., Hesselbach's. The interval in the groin bounded by Poupart's ligament, edge of rectus muscle, and deep epigastric artery.

t., inferior occipital. Area having the bimastoid diameter for its base and the inion for its apex.

t., inguinal. SEE: *femoral t.*

t., Lesser's. Space bounded below by ant. and posterior bellies of the digastric muscle and above by the hypogastric nerve.

t., lumbocostoabdominal. The space bounded in front by the obliquus abdominis externus, above by the lower border of the serratus posticus inferior and the point of the 12th rib, behind by the outer edge of the erector spinae, and below by the obliquus abdominis internus.

t., muscular. SEE: *inferior carotid t.*

t., mylohyoid. The triangular space formed by the mylohyoid muscle and the 2 bellies of the digastric muscle.

t., occipital, of the neck. The space bounded by the sternocleidomastoid, the trapezius, and the omohyoid.

t., omoclavicular. SEE: *subclavian t.*

t., omohyoid. SEE: *superior carotid t.*

t. of Petit. The space above the hipbone, bet. the ext. oblique muscle, the latissimus dorsi, and int. oblique muscle.

t., posterior cervical; t., posterior, of the neck. The space bounded by the upper border of the clavicle, the posterior border of the sternocleidomastoid muscle, and the anterior border of the trapezius muscle.

t., pubourethral. A triangular space in the perineum, bounded externally by the ischiocavernous muscle, internally by the bulbocavernous muscle, and posteriorly by the transversus perinei muscle.

t., Scarpa's. Femoral triangle, *q.v.*

t., subclavian. A space bounded by the post. belly of the omohyoid, the upper border of the clavicle, and the post. margin of the sternocleidomastoid.

t., submaxillary. The space between the lower border of the inf. maxilla, the parotid gland, and the mastoid process of the temporal bone above, the post. belly of the digastric and the stylohyoid below, and the middle line of the neck in front.

t., supraclavicular. SEE: *subclavian t.*

t., suprameatal. Triangle slightly above and behind ext. auditory meatus. It is bounded above by root of zygoma and anteriorly by post. wall of ext. auditory meatus.

t., urogenital. Triangle with base formed by line between the two ischial tuberosities and its apex just below symphysis pubis.

t., vesical. The trigone, *q.v.*

triang'ular. Having three sides; shaped like a triangle.

t. ligament. One of two ligaments, right and left, connecting posterior portions of right and left lobes of liver with corresponding portions of diaphragm.

t. nucleus (of Schwalbe). SYN: *medial nucleus.* The chief or dorsal nucleus of the vestibular division of the eighth cranial nerve. Located in pons occupying most of area acoustica of rhomboid fossa.

triangular bandage. One folded diagonally. When folded, the several thicknesses afford support. (*Illus.*, T-48.)

triangularis (trī-ăng-ū-lā'rĭs) [L.]. A muscle of the chin. SEE: *Muscles, Table of, in Appendix.*

Triatoma (trī-ăt'ō-mă). A genus of blood-sucking bugs belonging to the order Hemiptera, family Reduviidae. Commonly called cone-nosed bugs or assassin bugs. It includes the species *T. braziliensis, T. dimidiata, T. infestans, T. protracta, T. recurva, T. rubida* and others. They are house-infesting pests and some species especially *T. infestans* serve to transmit *Trypanosoma cruzi,* causative agent of Chagas' disease.

tribade (trĭb'ăd). A woman, usually one with an enlarged clitoris, who plays the part of a male in homosexual practices.

tribadism (trĭb'ăd-ĭzm) [G. *tribein,* to rub, + *-ismos,* condition]. A form of perversion in which women attempt to imitate heterosexual intercourse with each other.

tribasilar (trī-băs'ĭl-ar). Having three bases.

t. synostosis. Condition resulting from premature fusion of three skull bones, the occipital, sphenoid, and temporal. Results in arrested cerebral development and mental deficiency.

tribe (trīb). In biology, an occasional subdivision of a family; often equal to or below subfamily.

tribromide (trī-brō'mīd). A compound having three atoms of bromine in the molecule.

tribromoethanol (trī-brō-mō-eth'an-ōl). USP. Generic name for avertin.

tricephalus (trī-sĕph'ă-lŭs) [*tri-* + G. *kephalē*]. A fetal monster having three heads.

triceps (trī'sĕps) [L. *trēs,* three, + *caput,* head]. A muscle arising by 3 heads with a single insertion. SEE: *Muscles, Table of, in Appendix.*

t. reflex. Sharp extension of forearm resulting from tapping of triceps tendon while arm is held loosely in bent position.

Tricercomonas (trī"sĕr-cŏm'ō-năs). SEE: *Enteromonas.*

trichangiectasia, trichangiectasis (trik"ăn-jī-ĕk-ta'zī-ă, -ĕk'tă-sĭs) [G. *thrix, trich-,* hair, + *aggeion,* vessel, + *ektasis,* dilatation]. Dilatation of capillaries. SYN: *telangiectasia.*

trichatrophia (trĭk-ă-trō'fī-ă). Brittleness of hair resulting from atrophy of root of hair.

trichauxe, trichauxis (trĭk-awk'sē, -sĭs) [" + *auxē,* increase]. Excessive growth of hair. SYN: *hypertrichosis.*

trichi-, tricho- [G.]. Combining forms meaning *hair.*

trichiasis (trĭk-ī'ăs-ĭs) [G. *trichiasis,* hair condition]. Inversion of eyelashes so that they rub against the cornea, causing a continual irritation of the eyeball.

SYM: Photophobia, lacrimation, and feeling of foreign body in eye.

TREATMENT: Epilation, electrolysis and operation, such as correcting the underlying entropion with which this condition is usually associated.

Trichina (trĭk-ī'nă) [G. *trichinos,* of hair]. A nematoid, parasitic worm usually found in the intestinal tract of certain lower animals and man.

Trichinella (trĭk-ĭ-nĕl'lă) [G. *trichinos,* of hair]. A genus of nematode worms belonging to the suborder Trichurata.

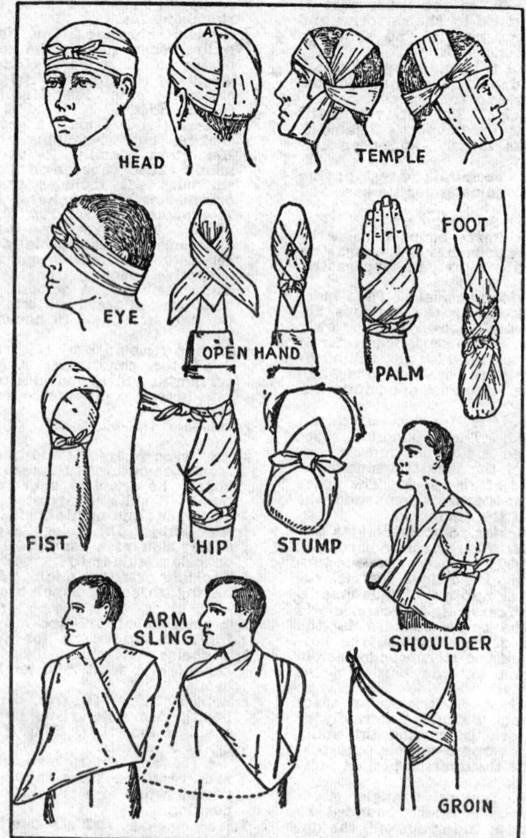

TRIANGULAR BANDAGES.

They are parasitic in humans, hogs, rats, and many other mammals.

T. spiralis. The species of *Trichinella* which commonly infests man causing trichinosis. Infection occurs when raw or improperly cooked meat, particularly pork, containing cysts is eaten. Larvae encyst in the duodenum and invade mucosa of small intestine becoming adults in 5 to 7 days. After fertilization, each female deposits 1000 to 2000 living larvae which enter blood or lymph vessels and are circulated to various parts of the body where they encyst in striated muscle. SEE: *trichinosis.*

trichinelliasis (trĭk-ĭ-nĕl-lī'ă-sĭs). Same as trichinosis, *q.v.*

trichinellosis (trĭ-kĭ-nĕl-lō'sĭs) [" + *-ōsis,* condition]. Disease caused by *Trichinella spiralis.* SYN: *trichinosis, q.v.*

trichinization (trĭk"ĭn-ĭ-zā'shŭn) [G. *trichinos,* of hair]. Infestation with trichinae.

trichinophobia (trĭk"ĭn-ō-fō'bĭ-ă) [" + *phobos,* fear]. Abnormal fear of developing trichiniasis.

trichinosis (trĭk-ĭn-ō'sĭs) [G. *trichinos,* of hair, + *-ōsis,* condition]. Disease caused by the ingestion of *Trichina spiralis* into the system through eating raw or insufficiently cooked pork.

SYM: Sometimes lacking. When large numbers have been ingested, gastrointestinal symptoms develop in a few days. These are pain, nausea, vomiting and serous diarrhea.

In from 1 to 2 weeks muscular symptoms develop, muscles become swollen, firm, extremely painful; movement is inhibited, and dyspnea results from involvement of respiratory muscles. Edema, esp. of face, is a prominent symptom. Profuse sweating sometimes observed and high fever commonly present. Blood shows an eosinophilia.

PROG: Depends on number of worms ingested. Majority recover.

TREATMENT: There is no specific therapy. In later stages after worms have involved muscles, muscle pains should be relieved by analgesics. Treatment is in general symptomatic and supportive to enable patient to survive the acute toxemia following invasion of muscles. After encystment the only symptom is vague muscular pains which may persist for weeks.

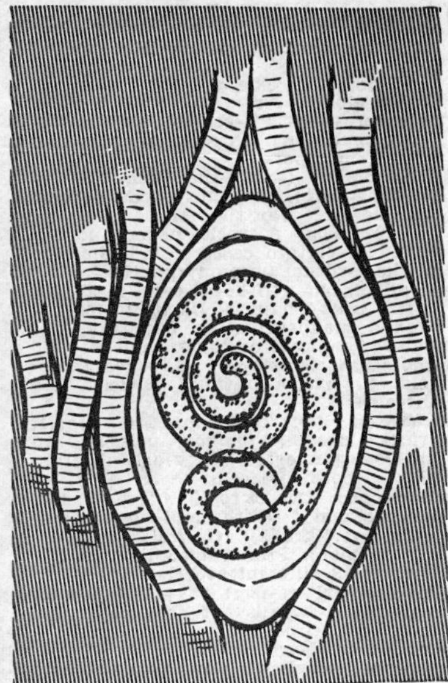

TRICHINELLA SPIRALIS LARVA ENCYSTED IN MUSCLE OF MAN

trichinous (trĭk′ĭn-ŭs) [G. *trichinos,* of hair]. Infested with trichinae.

trichitis (trĭk-ī′tĭs) [G. *thrix, trich-,* hair, + *-itis,* inflammation]. Inflammation of hair bulbs.

trichloroethylene (trī″klor-ō-ĕth′ĭl-ēn). A colorless, clear, volatile liquid with a specific gravity of 1.47 at 59° F. (15° C.). Used as an analgesic and anesthetic agent. It is a halogenated hydrocarbon having the chemical formula CCl_2:CHCl. Marketed under the trade names Trilene and Trimar, this agent has been widely used for the production of analgesia in labor. Its chief advantages are its nonflammability, its production of good analgesia, its portability, and the ease with which it may be combined with other agents. It should not be used with epinephrine.

trichobacteria (trĭk″ō-băk-tē′rĭ-ă) [G. *thrix, trich-,* hair, + *baktērion* rod]. 1. Filamentous bacteria. 2. Bacteria possessing flagella.

trichobezoar (trĭk″ō-bē′zō-ar) [" + Persian *bezoar*]. A hair ball or concretion in the intestine or stomach.

trichocardia (trĭk-ō-kar′dĭ-ă) [" + *kardia,* heart]. Pericardial inflammation with elevations resembling hair. SYN: *cor hirsutum, hairy heart, shaggy pericardium.*

trichocephaliasis (trĭk″ō-sĕf-ăl-ī′ă-sĭs) [" + *kephalē,* head]. Infestation with *Trichuris.*

Trichocephalus (trĭk-ō-sĕf′ăl-ŭs) [" + *kephalē,* head]. A genus of parasitic worms infesting the colon. Now called *Trichuris.*

trichoclasia, trichoclasis (trĭk″ō-klā′zĭ-ă, -ok′lăs-ĭs) [" + *klasis,* a breaking]. Brittleness of the hair. SYN: *trichorrhexis.*

trichocryptosis (trĭk″ō-krĭp-tō′sĭs) [" + *kryptos,* concealed]. Any disease of the hair follicles.

trichoepithelioma (trĭk″ō-ĕp″ĭ-thē-lĭ-ō′mă) [G. *thrix, trich-,* hair, + *epi,* upon, + *thēlē,* nipple, + *-ōma,* tumor]. A benign skin tumor originating in the hair follicles.

trichoesthesia (trĭk″ō-ĕs-thē′zĭ-ă) [" + *aisthēsis,* sensation]. 1. Sensation felt when a hair is touched. 2. A paresthesia causing a sensation of the presence of a hair on a mucous membrane or on the skin.

trichoesthesiometer (trĭk″ō-ĕs-thē-zĭ-ŏm′ĕ-ter) [" + " + *metron,* a measure]. Device for testing sensibility of the scalp by means of the hair.

trichogen (trĭk′ō-jĕn) [" + *gennan,* to produce]. An agent stimulating growth of hair.

trichogenous (trĭk-ŏj′ĕn-ŭs) [" + *gennan,* to produce]. Promoting hair growth.

trichoglossia (trĭk-ō-glŏs′sĭ-ă) [" + *glōssa,* tongue]. Hairy condition of the tongue.

trichoid (trĭk′oyd) [" + *eidos,* resemblance]. Hairlike.

trichokryptomania (trĭk″ō-krĭp″tō-mā′nĭ-ă) [G. *thrix, trich-,* hair, + *kryptos,* hidden, + *mania,* madness]. Abnormal desire to break off the hair or beard with the fingernail. SYN: *trichorrhexomania.*

trichology (trĭk-ŏl′ō-jĭ) [" + *logos,* a study]. Study of the hair and its care and treatment.

trichoma (trĭk-ō′mă) [G. *trichōma,* hairiness]. 1. Inversion of 1 or more eyelashes. SYN: *entropion.* 2. Matted, verminous, encrusted state of the hair. SYN: *plica polonica.*

trichomatosis (trĭk-ō-mă-tō′sĭs) [" + *-ōsis,* condition]. Entangled, matted hair due to fungus disease of scalp and want of cleanliness. SYN: *plica polonica.*

trichomatous (trĭk-o′mă-tŭs) [G. *trichōma,* hairiness]. Of the nature of, or affected with trichoma.

Trichomonas (trĭk-ŏm′ō-năs) [G. *thrix, trich-,* hair, + *monas,* unit]. Genus of flagellate parasitic protozoa.

T. hom′inis. Species in human intestines sometimes causing diarrhea and bacillary dysentery.

T. vaginalis. Vaginitis caused by a species of T. in secretions of the vagina. A fairly common condition in women especially during pregnancy or following vaginal surgery. It is sometimes found in the male urethra and is communicated through intercourse.

SYM: Persistent burning and itching of the vulvar tissue, associated with a profuse white frothy discharge. Occasionally T. vaginalis is present but asymptomatic.

TREATMENT: Metromidazole taken orally by the female and her sex partner.

trichomoniasis (trĭk″ō-mō-nī′ăs-ĭs) [" + " + *-iasis,* infection]. Infestation with a parasite of genus Trichomonas.

trichomycosis (trĭk-ō-mī-kō′sĭs) [" + *mykēs,* fungus, + *-ōsis,* condition]. Any disease of the hair due to a fungus.

t. axillaris. SYN: *trichomycosis nodosa, q.v.* An affection of the axillary region and sometimes pubic hairs caused by *Nocardia tenuis.*

t. nodosa. Disease marked by nodule formations on the hair shafts. SYN: *piedra.*

trichonosis, trichonosus (trĭk-ō-nō′sĭs, -ŏn′ō-sŭs) [" + *nosos,* disease]. Any diseased condition of the hair.

trichopathophobia (trĭk″ō-păth-ō-fō′bĭ-ă) [" + *pathos,* disease, + *phobos,* fear]. Morbid fear of hair on the face experienced by women, or any abnormal anxiety regarding hair.

trichopathy (trĭk-ŏp'ăth-ĭ) [" + *pathos,* disease]. Any disease of the hair.

trichophagia, trichophagy (trĭk-ō-fā'jĭ-ă, -of'ă-jĭ) [" + *phagein,* to eat]. The habit of swallowing hair.

trichophobia (trĭk-ō-fō'bĭ-ă) [G. *thrix, trich-,* hair, + *phobos,* fear]. Abnormal dread of hair or of touching it.

trichophytic (trĭk"ō-fĭt'ĭk) [" + *phyton,* growth]. 1. Relating to Trichophyton. 2. Promoting hair growth.

trichophytid (trĭk-ō-fĭt'ĭd). A skin disorder considered to be an allergic reaction to fungi of the genus *Trichophyton.*

trichophytin (trĭk-ō-fĭt'ĭn). An extract prepared from fungi of the genus *Trichophyton.* Used as an antigen for skin tests and for the treatment of certain trichophytid infections.

trichophytobezoar (trĭk-ō-fī"tō-bē'zŏr). A hair ball found in stomach or intestine composed of hair, vegetable fibers, and miscellaneous debris.

Trichophyton (trĭk-ŏf'ĭt-ŏn). [G. *thrix, trich-* hair, + *phyton,* growth]. A genus of parasitic fungi which lives in or on the skin or its appendages (hair and nails) and is the cause of various dermatomycoses and ringworm infections. Species which produce spores arranged in rows on the outside of the hair are designated *ectothrix;* if spores are within the hair, *endothrix.*

T. gypseum. Causative agent of tinea favosa, *q.v.*

T. schoenleinii. Causative agent of favus of the scalp.

T. tonsurans. Causative agent of ringworm of the scalp. SEE: *tinea capitis.*

T. violaceum. Causative agent of barber's itch (tinea barbae, *q.v.*).

trichophytosis (trĭk"ō-fī-tō'sĭs) [" + " + *-ōsis,* condition]. Infestation with trichophyton fungi; mostly in children.

t. barbae. Tinea barbae, *q.v.*

t. capitis. Tinea capitis, *q.v.*

t. corporis. Tinea corporis, *q.v.*

t. cruris. Tinea cruris, *q.v.*

t. pedis. Tinea pedis, *q.v.*

trichoptilosis (trĭk"ŏp-tĭl-ō'sĭs) [" + *ptilon,* feather, + *-ōsis,* condition]. 1. The splitting of hairs at their ends, giving them a featherlike appearance. 2. Disease of hair marked by development of nodules along the hair shaft at which point it splits off. SYN: *trichorrhexis nodosa.*

trichorrhea (trĭk-or-ē'ă) [" + *rhoia,* a flow]. Rapid falling of the hair.

trichorrhexis (trĭk"ō-rĕks'ĭs) [" + *rhēxis,* a breaking]. Condition in which the hair splits. SYN: *fragilitas crinium, trichoschisis.*

t. nodo'sa. Longitudinal splitting of hair at nodules formed on the shaft. SYN: *clastothrix, trichoclasia.*

trichorrhexomania (trĭk"ō-rĕks"ō-mā'nĭ-ă) [" + " + *mania,* madness]. The abnormal habit of breaking off the hair with the fingernails.

trichoschisis (tri-kos'kis-is) [G. *thrix, trich-,* hair, + *schisis,* a fissure]. Splitting of the hairs.

trichoscopy (trĭk-ŏs'kō-pĭ) [" + *skopein,* to examine]. Inspection of the hair.

trichosis (trĭ-kō'sĭs) [" + *-ōsis,* condition]. Any disease of the hair or its abnormal growth or development in an abnormal place.

t. dec'olor. Any abnormal coloring or lack of coloring of the hair. SYN: *canities.*

t. seto'sa. Coarse hair.

Trichosporon (trĭ-kŏs'pō-rŏn) [G. *thrix, trich-,* hair, + *sporos,* a seed]. A genus of fungi which grows on hair causing piedra.

T. beigelii. The causative agent of white piedra, *q.v.*

trichosporosis (trĭk"ō-spō-rō'sĭs) [" + " + *-ōsis,* condition]. Infestation of the hair with Trichosporon.

Trichothecium (trĭk"ō-thē'sĭ-ŭm) [" + *thēkē,* a box]. A genus of mold fungi causing disease of the hair.

T. ro'seum. A species of mold fungus found in certain cases of inflammation of the eardrum (mycomyringitis).

trichotillomania (trĭ-kō-tĭl-ō-mā'nĭ-ă) [G. *thrix, trich-,* hair, + *tillein,* to pull, + *mania,* madness]. The unnatural impulse to pull out one's own hair.

trichotomy (trī-kŏt'ō-mĭ) [G. *tricha,* threefold, + *tomē,* a cutting]. Division into three parts.

trichotoxin (trĭk"ō-tŏks'ĭn) [G. *thrix, trich-,* hair, + *toxikon,* poison]. An antibody or cytotoxin which destroys ciliated epithelial cells.

trichotrophy (trĭ-kŏt'rō-fĭ) [" + *trophē,* nourishment]. Nutrition of the hair.

trichroic (trī-krō'ĭk) [G. *treis,* three, + *chroa,* color]. Presenting 3 different colors from 3 different aspects.

trichroism (trī'krō-ĭzm) [" + " + *-ismos,* condition]. Quality of showing a different color from each of 3 positions.

trichromatic (trī"krō-măt'ĭk) [" + *chroma,* color]. Relating to or able to see the 3 primary colors; noting normal color vision.

trichromic (trī-krō'mĭk) [" + *chrōma,* color]. Pert. to normal color vision or ability to see the 3 primary colors. SYN: *trichromatic.*

trichuriasis (trĭk"ū-rī'ă-sĭs) [G. *thrix, trich-,* hair, + *oura,* tail]. Presence of worms of genus Trichuris in the colon, or in the ileum. SYN: *trichocephaliasis.*

Trichuris (trĭ-kū'rĭs) [" + *oura,* tail]. A genus of Trematoda.

T. trichiur'ia. The whipworm. SYN: *Trichocephalus dispar.*

tricipital (trī-sĭp'ĭ-tăl) [L. *trēs, tria,* three, + *caput,* head]. Three-headed, as the triceps muscle.

tricornic, tricornute (trī-kor'nĭk, -nūt) [" + *cornu,* horn]. Having 3 horns or cornua.

tricrotic (trī-krŏt'ĭk) [G. *treis,* three, + *krotos,* a beat]. Condition in which three accentuated waves or notches occur on a sphygmograph tracing from one beat of the pulse.

tricrotism (trī'krŏt-ĭzm) [" + " + *-ismos,* condition]. Condition of being tricrotic.

tricuspid (trī-kŭs'pĭd) [L. *tres, tria,* three, + *cuspis,* a point]. 1. Pert. to the tricuspid valve. 2. Having 3 points or cusps. 3. A tooth having 3 cusps.

t. area. Lower portion of body of sternum where sounds of right atrioventricular orifice are best heard.

t. atresia. Stenosis of the tricuspid valve. A fairly uncommon congenital malformation which causes cyanosis and clubbing.

SYM: Paroxysmal dyspnea. Difficulty in feeding.

t. murmur. One caused by stenosis of the tricuspid valve or by its incompetency.

t. orifice. Right atrioventricular cardiac aperture.

t. tooth. One with a crown having three cusps.

t. valve. Right atrioventricular valve. SYN: *valvula tricuspidalis.*

trident, tridentate (trī'dĕnt, trī-dĕn'tāt) [L. *trēs, tria,* three, + *dens, dent-,* tooth]. Having three prongs.

tridermic (trī-der'mĭk) [G. *treis,* three, + *derma,* skin]. Developed from the ectoderm, endoderm, and mesoderm.

tridermoma (trī"dĕr-mō'mă) [" + " + *-ōma,* tumor]. A teratoid growth containing all three germ layers.

trielcon (trī-ĕl'kŏn) [" + *elkein,* to draw] Instrument with 3 branches for removing foreign substances from wounds.

triethylene melamine. Commonly abbr. *TEM.* One of the nitrogen mustard compounds. SEE: *nitrogen mustard.*

trifacial (trī-fā'shăl) [L. *trēs, tria,* three, + *facialis,* facial]. Pert. to the 5th pair of cranial nerves. SYN: *trigeminal.*

t. neuralgia. N. of 1 of the branches of the 5th cranial nerve; often severe. SYN: *tic douloureux.*

trifid (trī'fĭd) [L. *trifidus,* split thrice] Split into 3; having 3 clefts.

trigastric (trī-găst'rĭk). Having three bellies, as certain muscles.

trigeminal (trī-jĕm'ĭn-ăl) [L. *trēs, tria,* three, + *geminus,* twin]. Pert. to the trigeminus or 5th cranial nerve.

t. cough. A reflex cough from irritation of the trigeminal nerve terminations in respiratory upper passages.

t. nerve. SYN: *nervus trigeminus.* The fifth cranial nerve, a large mixed nerve arising superficially from the side of the pons near its superior border. It is attached to the brain stem by two roots: a large *sensory root* and a small *motor root.* The sensory root bears an enlargement, the *semilunar Gasserian ganglion,* from which three large branches arise. These are (1) *ophthalmic,* purely sensory, from skin of upper part of head, mucous membranes of nasal cavity and sinuses, cornea and conjunctiva; (2) *maxillary,* purely sensory, from dura mater, gums and teeth of upper jaw, upper lip, and orbit; (3) *mandibular,* the largest division containing sensory fibers from tongue, gums and teeth of lower jaw, skin of cheek, lower jaw, and lip, and motor fibers supplying principally muscles of mastication.

t. neuralgia. Facial neuralgia. SYN: *tic* douloureux.*

t. pulse. One with longer or shorter interval after each 3 beats because the 3rd beat is an extrasystole. SYN: *pulsus trigeminus.*

trigeminus (trī-jĕm'ĭ-nŭs) [L. *trēs, tria,* three, + *geminus,* twin). SYN: *trigeminal nerve, q.v.* The fifth cranial nerve. SEE: *Table of Cranial Nerves in Appendix.*

trigeminy (trī-jĕm'ĭ-nĭ). Occurring in threes, especially three pulse beats in rapid succession.

trigenic (trī-jĕn'ĭk). In genetics, condition in which three instead of two alleles are present such as occurs in trisomic or triploid individuals.

trigger. To initiate or start with suddenness.

t. action. A physiologic process or a pathologic change initiated by a sudden stimulus.

t. finger. State in which flexion or extension is arrested temporarily, but finally completed with a jerk.

t. material. SEE: *trigger substance.*

t. substance. A chemical substance which initiates a functional activity.

t. zone. 1. An area which when stimulated will initiate an attack of neuralgia. 2. An area of cerebral cortex which when stimulated produces abnormal reactions similar to those in acquired epilepsy. Also called *epileptogenous zone.*

trigylceride. Combination of glycerol with the three fatty acids stearic, oleic, palmitic. Most animal and vegetable fats are triglycerides.

trigonal (trĭg'ō-năl) [G. *trigōnon,* a three-cornered figure]. Triangular; pert. to a trigone.

trigone (trī'gŏn) [G. *trigōnon,* a three-cornered figure]. A triangular space, esp. one at the base of the bladder. SYN: *trigonum.*

trigonid (trī-gō'nĭd). The first three cusps of a lower molar tooth.

trigonitis (trī-gō-nī'tĭs) [" + *-ītis,* inflammation]. Inflammation of trigone of bladder confined to its mucous membrane.

trigonocephalic (trī"gō-nō-sef-ăl'ĭk) [" + *kephalē,* head]. Having a head shaped like a triangle.

trigonum (trī-gō'nŭm) [L. from G. *trigōnon,* a three-cornered figure]. Any triangular area. SYN: *trigone.*

trihybrid (trī-hī'brĭd). In genetics, the offspring of a cross between two individuals differing in three unit characters.

trilabe (trī'lāb) [G. *treis,* three, + *labē,* a handle]. Three-pronged forceps for removing foreign substances from the bladder. SEE: *lithotrite.*

trill (trĭl) [Italian *trillare,* probably imitative]. A tremulous sound, esp. in vocal music.

trilocular. Having three compartments.

trimanual (trī-măn'ū-ăl) [L. *trēs, tria,* three, + *manualis,* by hand]. Performed with three hands, as an obstetrical maneuver.

trimensual (trī-mĕn'shū-ăl) [" + *mensualis,* monthly]. Occurring quarterly or every 3 months.

trimorphous (trī-mor'fŭs) [G. *treis,* three, + *morphē,* form]. 1. Having three different forms as the larva, pupa, and adult of certain insects. 2. Having three different forms of crystals.

trinitrophenol (trī-nī-trō-fē'nōl). USP. Picric acid, a yellow crystalline powder, explosive when heated.

ACTION AND USES: An astringent and antiseptic. Used chiefly in the treatment of burns as a saturated solution.

triorchid, triorchis (trī-or'kĭd, -kĭs) [G. *treis,* three, + *orchis,* testicle]. One having 3 testicles.

triorchidism (trī-or'kĭd-ĭzm) [" + " + *-ismos,* condition]. The condition of having 3 testicles.

triose. A monosaccharide having three carbon atoms in its molecule.

tripara (trip'ă-ră) [L. *trēs, tria,* three, + *parēre,* to bear]. A woman who has had 3 children in separate pregnancies. SYN: *tertipara.* Designated *Para III.*

tripeptid(e (trī-pĕp'tĭd) [G. *treis,* three, + *peptōn,* digested]. Product of combination of 3 amino acids formed during proteolytic digestion.

triphalangia (trī-fă-lan'jĭ-ă) [" + *phalagx, phalagg-,* phalanx]. Deformity marked by presence of 3 phalanges in a thumb or great toe.

triphasic (trī-fā'sĭk) [" + *phasis,* phase]. Consisting of 3 phases or stages, said of electric currents.

Tripier's amputation (trĭp-ē-ā'). Amputation of a foot with part of the calcaneus removed.

triple. Consisting of three; threefold; treble.

t. response. The three reactions of the skin to injury consisting of: (1) A red reaction along line of injury; (2) A red area (flare or erythema) about injury; (3) An elevated area (welt or wheal) resulting from localized edema.

triplegia (trī-plē′jĭ-ă) [G. *treis,* three, + *plēgē,* stroke]. Hemiplegia with paralysis of 1 limb on the other side of the body.

triplet (trĭp′lĕt) [L. *triplus,* threefold]. 1. One of 3 persons born of the same mother from 1 pregnancy. SEE: *Hellin's law.* 2. A combination of 3 of a kind.

triplex (trī′plĕks, trĭp′lĕks) [L. *trēs, tria,* three, + *plexus,* folded]. Triple; threefold.

triploblastic (trĭp-lō-blăst′ĭk). Consisting of three germ layers: ectoderm, entoderm, and mesoderm.

triplokoria (trĭp-lō-kor′ĭ-ă). Possessing three pupillary openings in one eye.

triplopia (trĭp-lō′pĭ-ă) [G. *triploos,* triple, + *opsis,* vision]. Condition in which 3 images of the same object are seen.

triquetral (trī-kwē′trăl). Triangular; the triquetral bone, *q.v.*

t. bone. SYN: *os triquetrum, cuneiform bone.* 1. The third carpal bone in the proximal row, enumerated from radial side. 2. Any wormian bone.

triquetrous (trī-kwē′trŭs) [L. *triquetrus,* triangular]. Triangular.

t. bone. 1. A wormian bone. 2. The Cuneiform bone of the carpus.

trisaccharide (trī-săk′kă-rīd). A carbohydrate which upon hydrolysis yields three molecules of simple sugars (monosaccharides).

trismoid (trĭz′moyd) [G. *trismos,* trismus, + *eidos,* form]. 1. Of the nature of trismus. 2. A form of trismus nascentium; once thought to be due to pressure on occiput during delivery.

trismus (trĭz′mŭs) [G. *trismos,* grating]. 1. Tonic contraction of the muscles of mastication. May occur in mouth infections, encephalitis, inflammation of salivary glands, and tetanus. 2. Old term for tetanus (lockjaw).

trisomic (trī-sōm′ĭk). In genetics, an individual possessing 2n plus 1 chromosomes, that is, one with three chromosomes of a given kind with two only of each of the remaining chromosomes of the haploid set.

trisplanchnic (trī-splănk′nĭk) [G. *treis,* three, + *splagchna,* viscera]. Pert. to the 3 visceral cavities, the *skull, thorax,* and *abdomen.*

t. nervous system. Sympathetic nervous system.

tristichia (trī-stĭk′ĭ-ă) [" + *stichos,* row]. The presence of 3 rows of eyelashes.

tristimania (trĭs-tĭm-ā′nĭ-ă) [L. *tristis,* sad, + *mania,* madness]. Melancholia.

trisulcate (trī-sŭl′kāt) [L. *trēs, tria,* three, + *sulcus,* groove]. Having 3 grooves or furrows.

tritanopia (trī-tăn-ō′pĭ-ă) [G. *tritos,* third, + *an-,* priv. + *opsis,* vision]. Color blindness in which blue and yellow appear gray.

tritiate. To treat with tritium.

triticeous (trĭt-ĭsh′ŭs) [L. *triticeus,* of wheat]. Shaped like a grain of wheat.

t. cartilage, t. nodule. A cartilaginous nodule in the thyrohyoid ligament.

tritium (trit′ĭ-um) [L.]. The mass 3 isotope of hydrogen; triple-weight hydrogen.

tritotoxin (trī″tō-tŏks′ĭn) [G. *tritos,* third, + *toxikon,* poison]. A toxin, according to Ehrlich, which is the 3rd or lowest in order of toxicity.

triturable (trĭt′ū-ră-bl) [L. *triturāre,* to pulverize]. Susceptible of being powdered.

triturate (trĭt′ū-rāt) [L. *triturāre,* to pulverize]. 1. To reduce to a fine powder by rubbing. 2. A finely divided substance made by rubbing.

trituration (trĭt-ū-rā′shŭn) [L. *triturātio,* a rubbing to powder]. Powdered preparation containing 10% of the active drug and 90% of sugar of milk. None is official. The act of reducing to a powder.

trivalent (trī-vā′lĕnt, trĭv′ăl-ĕnt) [L. *trēs, tria,* three, + *valens,* powerful]. Combining with or replacing 3 hydrogen atoms.

trocar (trō′kar) [Fr. *troisquarts,* three-quarters]. Instrument with a triangular tip used for aspiration or removal of fluids from cavities.

troch. Abbr. for *trochiscus.* SEE: *troche.*

trochanter (trō-kăn′ter) [G. *trochantēr,* a runner]. Either of the 2 bony processes below the neck of the femur.

t., greater. SYN: *trochanter major, q.v.*

t., lesser. SYN: *trochanter minor, q.v.*

t. major. NA. A thick process at upper end of the femur projecting upward externally to union of neck and shaft.

t. minor. NA. A conical tuberosity upon inner and post. surface of upper end of femur, at junction of shaft and neck.

t. tertius. The gluteal ridge of the femur when it is unusually prominent. [NA].

t., third. SYN: *trochanter tertius, q.v.*

trochanterian, trochanteric (trō″kăn-tē′rĭ-ăn, trō-kăn-ter′ĭk) [G. *trochantēr,* a runner]. Relating to a trochanter.

troche (trō′kē) [G. *trochē,* a round object]. Solid, discoid, or cylindrical mass consisting chiefly of medicinal powder, sugar, and mucilage.

They are intended to be used by placing them in the mouth and allowing them to remain until, through slow solution or disintegration, their purpose of mild medication is effected. SYN: *lozenge, trochiscus.*

trochlea (trok′lē-ă) (pl. *trochleae*) [L. *trochlea,* pulley]. 1. A structure having the function of a pulley; a ring or hook through which a tendon or muscle projects. 2. The articular smooth surface of a bone upon which glides another bone.

trochlear. Pertaining to, or of the nature of a pulley.

t. fovea. A depression on orbital plate of frontal bone for attachment of cartilaginous pulley of sup. oblique muscle.

t. nerve. SYN: *nerve trochlearis, 4th. cranial nerve.* A small mixed nerve making its exit from dorsal surface of midbrain. It contains efferent motor fibers to sup. oblique muscle of eye and afferent sensory fibers conveying proprioceptive impulses from the same muscle. SEE: *Table of Cranial Nerves in Appendix.*

trochlearis (trō-klē-ā′rĭs) [L.]. Sup. oblique muscle of the eye. SEE: *Muscles, Table of, in Appendix.*

trochocardia (trō″kō-kar′dĭ-ă) [G. *trochos,* a wheel, + *kardia,* heart]. Rotary displacement of the heart on its axis.

trochocephalia, trochocephaly (trō″kō-se-fā′lĭ-ă, -sĕf′ă-lĭ) [" + *kephalē,* head]. Roundheadedness, a deformity due to premature union of frontal and parietal bones.

trochoid (trō'koyd) [G. *trochos*, a wheel, + *eidos*, resemblance]. Rotating or revolving, noting an articulation resembling a pivot or pulley.

t. joint. A pivot joint, *q.v.*

trochoides (trō-koy'dēz) [G. *trochoeidēs*, wheellike]. A pivot or rotary joint.

Troglotrematidae (trŏg"lō-trē-măt'ĭ-dē). A family of flukes which includes *Paragonimus* (human lung fluke) and *Troglotrema* (SYN: *Nanophyetus*), the fluke associated with salmon poisoning in dogs.

Trombicula (trŏm-bĭk'ū-lă). A genus of mites belonging to the Trombiculidae. The larvae called redbugs or chiggers are annoying pests causing an irritating dermatitis. They may serve as vectors of various diseases.

T. akamushi. Species of mite transmitting causative agent of scrub typhus.

trombidiiasis, trombidiosis (trŏm-bĭ-dĭ-ī'ă-sĭs, -bĭd-ĭ-ō'sĭs). Infestation with the *Trombidium irritans*.

Trommer's test (trŏm'er). Test for sugar in the urine.

tromomania (trŏm"ō-mā'nĭ-ă) [G. *tromos*, a trembling, + *mania*, madness]. Delirium tremens.

troph-, tropho- [G.]. Combining forms meaning *nourishment*.

trophedema, trophoedema (trŏ-fĕ-dē'mă) [G. *trophē*, nourishment, + *oidēma*, a swelling]. Localized edema due to congenital hypoplasia of lymphatic vessels or resulting secondarily from obstruction to lymph flow by external pressure or to repeated low grade infection. Also called *Milroy's disease* or *hereditary trophedema*.

trophic (trŏf'ĭk) [G. *trophē*, nourishment]. Concerned with nourishment.

Applied particularly to a type of efferent nerves believed to control the growth and nourishment of the parts they innervate. SEE: *autotrophic*.

trophoblast (trŏf'ō-blăst) [G. *trophē*, nourishment, + *blastos*, germ]. SYN: *trophectoderm*. The outermost layer of the developing blastocyst (blastodermic vesicle) of a mammal. It differentiates into two layers, the *cytotrophoblast* and *syntrophoplast*, the latter coming into intimate relationship with the uterine endometrium with which it establishes nutrient relationships.

trophoblastoma (trof"ō-blăs-tō'mă) [" + " + *-ōma*, tumor]. A neoplasm due to excessive proliferation of chorionic epithelium. SYN: *chorioepithelioma*.

trophoderm (trŏf'ō-derm) [G. *trophē*, nourishment, + *derma*, skin]. Term applied to the trophoblast and its underlying layer of mesoderm. It is homologous to the serosa of birds, reptiles, and lower mammals.

trophology (tro-fŏl'ō-jĭ) [" + *logos*, a science]. The science of nutrition.

trophoneurosis (trŏf"ō-nū-rō'sĭs) [" + *neuron*, nerve, + *-ōsis*, condition]. Any trophic disorder due to defective function of the nerves concerned with nutrition of the part.

t., disseminated. Thickening and hardening of the skin. SYN: *sclerema scleroderma*.

t., facial. Progressive facial atrophy.

t., muscular. Muscular changes in connection with nervous disorders.

trophoneurotic (trŏf"ō-nū-rŏt'ĭk) [" + *neuron*, nerve]. Relating to a trophoneurosis.

trophonosis (trŏf"ō-nō'sĭs) [" + *nosos*, disease]. Any disease due to a nutritional defect.

trophonucleus (trŏf"ō-nū'klē-ŭs) [G. *trophē*, nourishment, + L. *nucleus*, kernel]. Protozoan nucleus concerned with vegetative functions in metabolism and not reproduction. SYN: *macronucleus*.

trophopathia, trophopathy (trŏf"ō-path'-ĭ-ă, trof-op'ă-thĭ) [" + *pathos*, disease]. 1. Any disorder of the nutrition. 2. A trophic disease.

trophotaxis (trŏf"ō-tăks'ĭs) [" + *taxis*, arrangement]. The movement of cells away from or toward nutrients. SYN: *trophotropism*.

trophotherapy (trŏf"o-ther'ă-pĭ) [" + *therapeia*, treatment]. The therapeutic use of foods. SYN: *dietotherapy*.

trophotonos (trŏf-ŏt'ŏn-ŏs) [" + *tonos*, tension]. A rigid state of contractile tissue resulting from trophic disorder.

trophotropism (trŏf-ot'rō-pĭzm) [G. *trophē*, nourishment, + *tropē*, a turning, + *-ismos*, condition]. Attraction and repulsion of cells to nutritive substances. SYN: *trophotaxis*.

trophozoite (trŏf"ō-zō'ĭt) [" + *zōon*, animal]. A sporozoan nourished by its host during its growth stage.

tropia [G. *trope*, turn]. Deviation of the eye or eyes away from the visual axis. Observed with the eyes open and uncovered. *Esotropia* indicates inward or nasal deviation; *exotropia*, outward; *hypertropia*, upward; *hypotropia*, downward. SYN: *manifest squint, strabismus*.

tropical (trŏp'ĭ-kăl) [G. *tropikos*, turning]. Pert. to the tropics.

t. lichen. Prickly heat, acute inflammation of the sweat glands.

tropin. A substance present in blood serum which stimulates the engulfment of foreign organisms by phagocytic cells. SEE: *bacteriotropin*.

tropism (trŏ'pism) [G. *tropē*, a turn, + *-ismos*, condition]. SYN: *taxis*. 1. Reaction of living organisms involuntarily toward or away from light, darkness, heat, cold, or other stimuli. 2. The involuntary response of an organism as a bending, turning, or movement toward (*positive tropism*) or away from (*negative tropism*) an external stimulus. SEE: *chemotropism, phototropism, galvanotropism*.

-tropism. Combining form meaning a *response to* or *a turning towards* an external stimulus.

tropometer (trŏp-om'ĕ-ter) [G. *tropē*, a turn, + *metron*, a measure]. 1. Device for measuring the rotation of the eyeballs. 2. Instrument for measuring torsion in long bones.

Trousseau's sign (trū-so'). Muscular spasm resulting from pressure applied to nerves and vessels of the upper arm. It is indicative of latent tetany. Also occurs in osteomalacia.

T's. spots. Streaking of the skin with the fingernail, seen in meningitis and other cerebral diseases. SYN: *meningitic streak*.

T's. symptom. Spasmodic muscular contractions indicative of tetany, on pressing the principal vessel and nerve of the limb.

troy weight (troi). A system of weighing gold, silver, precious metals, and jewels, and in making philosophical experiments. 5,760 gr. equal 1 lb.

24 grains (gr.) equal.....1 pennyweight
20 pennyweights equal.....1 ounce (oz.)
12 oz. equal................1 pound (lb.)

SEE: *Appendix for apothecaries, avoirdupois and household measures, and metric system.*

TRU. Abbr. for *turbidity reducing unit.*

true (trū) [A.S. *trēowe,* faithful]. Not false; real; genuine.

t. pelvis. Portion below the iliopectineal line.

t. ribs. The 7 upper ones on each side with cartilages articulating directly with the sternum. SYN: *costa vera.* SEE: *ribs.*

truncal (trŭng'kăl) [L. *truncus,* trunk]. Relating to the trunk.

truncate (trŭng'kāt) [L. *truncāre,* to cut off]. 1. Having a square end as if it were cut off; lacking an apex. 2. To cut off; to amputate.

truncus. Trunk.

trunk (trŭnk) [L. *truncus,* trunk]. 1. The body exclusive of the head and limbs. SYN: *torso.* 2. Main stem of a lymphatic, nerve, or blood vessel.

truss (trŭs) [O.Fr. *trousser,* to bundle]. Device for holding a hernia in its place.

truth serum. One of several hypnotic drugs supposedly having the effect of causing a person upon questioning to talk freely and without inhibition.

trypanocide, trypanocidal (trĭp-ăn'ō-sīd, trĭp"ăn-ō-sī'dăl) [G. *trypanon,* a borer, + L. *cidus,* from *caedere,* to kill]. 1. Destructive to trypanosomes. 2. An agent which kills trypanosomes. SYN: *trypanosomicide.*

trypanolysis (trĭp-an-ŏl'ĭ-sĭs) [" + *lysis,* dissolution]. The dissolution of trypanosomes.

Trypanoplasmia (trī"păn-ō-plăz'mă) [" + *plasma,* a thing formed]. A genus of protozoan parasites resembling trypanosomes.

Trypanosoma trī"păn-ō-sō-mă) [G. *trypanon,* a borer, + *sōma,* a body]. A genus of parasitic, flagellate protozoa found in the blood of many vertebrates including man. They are transmitted by insect vectors.

T. brucei. The causative agent of trypanosomiasis in horses and other domestic animals. Nonpathogenic in man.

T. cruzi. The causative agent of American trypanosomiasis in many animals and specifically Chagas' disease in humans. It is transmitted by blood-sucking insects (triatomids) belonging to the family Reduviidae.

T. gambiense. The causative agent of African sleeping sickness. It is transmitted by the tsetse fly.

T. rhodesiense. An organism parasitic in wild game and domestic animals of portions of Africa. May cause East African sleeping sickness in humans.

trypanosomal (trī-păn-ō-sō'măl) [" + *sōma,* body]. Pert. to trypanosomata.

trypanosome (trī'păn-ō-sōm). Any protozoan belonging to the genus *Trypanosoma.*

t. fever. Sleeping sickness.

trypanosomiasis (trī-păn-ō-sō-mī'ă-sĭs) [G. *trypanon,* a borer, + *sōma,* body, + *-iasis,* infection]. Any of the several diseases occurring in man and domestic animals caused by a species of *Trypanosoma.* SEE: *sleeping sickness.*

t., African. African sleeping sickness, caused by *Trypanosoma gambiense, q.v.*

t., American. Trypanosomiasis in the western hemisphere. In man, Chagas' disease is caused by *Trypanosoma cruzi* transmitted by blood-sucking triatomids.

trypanosomid(e (trī-pan'ō-sō-mĭd) [" + *sōma,* body]. A skin eruption in any disease caused by a trypanosome.

tryparsamide (trĭp-ars'ă-mĭd, -mīd). An arsenic compound containing about 25% arsenic.

USES: Chiefly in neurosyphilis and sleeping sickness.

trypesis (trĭp-ē'sĭs) [G. *trypēsis,* a boring]. An incision of the skull to reduce pressure by removing a disk of bone. SYN: *trephining.*

trypsin (trĭp'sĭn) [G. *tripsis,* a rubbing]. A proteolytic enzyme formed in the intestine from the action of enterokinase of the intestinal juice (succus entericus) on *trypsinogen* secreted by the pancreas and present in pancreatic juice. It catalyzes the hydrolysis of peptide bonds in partly digested proteins and some native proteins, the final products being amino acids and various polypeptides. SEE: *chymotrypsin, digestion, enzyme, pancreas.*

trypsinized (trĭp'sĭ-nīzd) [G. *tripsis,* a rubbing]. Subjected to action of trypsin, thus having antitryptic power abolished.

trypsinogen (trĭp-sĭn'ō-jĕn) [" + *gennan,* to produce]. The proenzyme, or inactive form of trypsin found in pancreatic juice. Activated when mixed in the intestine with the enterokinase of the *succus entericus.*

tryptic (trĭp'tĭk) [G. *tripsis,* a rubbing]. Relating to trypsin.

tryptolysis (trĭp-tŏl'ĭ-sĭs) [G. *tripsis,* a rubbing]. The hydrolysis of proteins or their derivatives by trypsin.

tryptonemia (trĭp"tō-nē'mĭ-ă) [" + *aima,* blood]. Tryptones in the blood.

tryptophan(e (trĭp'tō-făn). An amino acid in proteins needed for tissue repair and growth; a product of tryptic digestion.

tryptophanuria (trĭp-tō-fă-nū'rĭ-ă) [*tryptophan* + G. *ouron,* urine]. Tryptophan in the urine.

T.S. Abbr. for *test solution; triple strength.*

TSD. Abbr. for *target skin distance.*

tsetse fly (tsĕt'sē) [South African]. One of several species of blood-sucking flies belonging to the genus *Glossina,* order Diptera, confined to Africa south of the Sahara Desert. They are important transmitters of trypanosomes, the causative agents of African sleeping sickness in man, and nagana and other diseases of cattle and game animals. SEE: *Trypanosoma, trypanosomiasis.*

TSH. Abbr. for *thyroid-stimulating hormone.*

tsp. Abbr. for *teaspoon.*

tsutsugamushi disease (soot"soo-gă-moosh'ĭ). Scrub typhus, *q.v.*

TT. Abbr. for *transit time* of blood through heart and lungs.

T. U. Abbr. for *toxic unit; transmission unit.*

tub (tŭb) [Middle Dutch *tubbe*]. 1. A receptacle for bathing. 2. The use of the cold bath. 3. To treat by using a cold bath.

tubal (tū'băl) [L. *tuba,* tube]. Pert. to a tube, esp. the fallopian tube.

t. nephritis. Inflammation of kidney tubules.

t. pregnancy. Pregnancy in one of the oviducts.

tubatorsion (tū"bă-tor'shŭn) [" + *torsio,* a twisting]. The twisting of an oviduct.

tube (tūb) [L. *tuba,* a tube]. A long, hollow, cylindrical structure.

t., cathode-ray. A vacuum tube with a thin window at the end opposite the cathode to allow the cathode rays to pass outside. More generally, any discharge tube in which the vacuum is fairly high.

t., Coolidge. A kind of hot cathode tube, which is so highly exhausted that the residual gas plays no part in the production of the cathode stream, and which is regulated by variable heating of the cathode filament.

t., Crookes'. One with an exhausted vacuum, used in producing roentgen rays.

t., drainage. A glass or rubber tube which, when inserted into a cavity, drains away its fluid contents.

t., esophageal. Same as *stomach t.*

t., eustachian. The tube passing from the throat to the middle ear.

t., fallopian. One of 2 oviducts.

t., hot-cathode. A vacuum tube in which the cathode is electrically heated to incandescence and in which the supply of electrons depends on the temperature of the cathode.

t., h.-c. roentgen - ray. A vacuum roentgen-ray tube in which the electron stream is supplied by a heated cathode. The cathode stream may be regulated by varying the current through the cathode filament.

t., intubation. A tube for passing into the larynx to facilitate breathing.

t., Leónard. SEE: *cathode-ray tube.*

t., oscillator vacuum. Method of producing alternating current. Current produced by this is a continuous sine wave current in contradistinction to the damped harmonic wave of spark gap diathermy machine.

t., Southey's. Very small tube pushed into tissue to help drain edema fluid. Used in severe congestive heart failure to relieve edema of the legs.

t., stomach. A rubber tube for introducing food into the stomach or for washing out the stomach.

t., tracheotomy. A tube for inserting into the trachea.

tuber (tū'ber) (pl. *tubers, tubera*) [L. *tuber,* a swelling]. A swelling or enlargement.

tubercle (tū'ber-kl) [L. *tuberculum,* a little swelling]. 1. A small rounded elevation or eminence on a bone. 2. A small nodule, esp. a circumscribed solid elevation of the skin or mucous membrane. 3. The characteristic lesion resulting from infection by tubercle bacilli. It consists typically of three parts: a central giant cell, a midzone of epithelioid cells, and a peripheral zone of nonspecific structure. SEE: *tuberculosis.*

t., adductor. That part of femur to which is attached the tendon of the adductor magnus.

t. bacillus. Organism causing tuberculosis.

t., deltoid. One in clavicle for attachment of deltoid muscle.

t., genial. One on either side of lower jawbone.

t., genital. The embryonic structure that becomes the clitoris, or the penis.

t., lacrimal. One on upper jawbone.

t., laminated. The cerebellar nodule.

t., Lisfranc's. T. for scalenus anticus muscle on the 1st rib.

t., miliary. A small tubercle resembling a millet seed; the lesion of tuberculosis.

t., zygomatic. One on the zygoma at junction of ant. root.

tubercular (tū-ber'kū-lar) [L. *tuberculum,* a little swelling]. 1. Relating to or marked by nodules. 2. Incorrectly pert. to tuberculosis. 3. Person with tuberculosis. SEE: *torose.*

tuberculate, tuberculated (tū-ber'kū-lāt, -lāt"ed) [L. *tuberculum,* a small swelling]. Covered with nodules. SYN: *tubercular.*

tuberculation (tū-ber"kū-lā'shŭn) [L. *tuberculum,* a little swelling]. The formation of tubercles.

tuberculid(e (tū-ber'kū-lĭd, -līd) [L. *tuberculum,* a small nodule]. A tuberculous cutaneous eruption due to toxins of tuberculosis.

t., follicular. That characterized by presence of groups of follicular lesions, esp. on trunk.

t., papulonecrotic. Form characterized by symmetrically distributed bluish papules, esp. on extremities. These undergo central necrosis and, on healing, leave deep scars.

tuberculigenous (tū-ber-kū-lĭj'ĕn-ŭs) [" + G. *gennan,* to produce]. Causing or predisposing to tuberculosis.

tuberculin (tū-bĕr'kū-lĭn) [L. *tuberculum,* a little swelling]. A soluble cell substance prepared from the tubercle bacillus, usually the human type, which is used to determine the presence of a tuberculosis infection. SEE: *tuberculin test.* It has also been used as a therapeutic agent but results are questionable. Among the types of tuberculin used are: (1) Koch's original or old tuberculin (ABBR: OT or TO); (2) tuberculin purified protein derivative (ABBR: PPD).

t. test. A test to determine the presence of a tuberculous infection based on positive reaction of subject to tuberculin. Tests commonly used are: *Mantoux test,* injection intradermally of tuberculin; *von Pirquet test,* rubbing tuberculin on scarified skin; and *Vollmer "patch" test,* the application to skin of a piece of gauze impregnated with dried tuberculin. In all three tests a local inflammatory reaction is observed in infected persons after 48-96 hours. Tests do not reveal whether infection is active or inactive. SEE: *tine test.*

tuberculoderma (tū-ber"kū-lō-der'mă) [" + G. *derma,* skin]. A tuberculous lesion of the skin. SYN: *tuberculide.*

tuberculofibroid (tū-ber"kū-lō-fī'broyd) [" + *fibra,* fiber, + G. *eidos,* form]. Denoting fibroid degeneration of tubercles.

tuberculofibrosis (tū-ber"kū-lō-fī-brō'sĭs) [" + " + G. *-ōsis,* condition]. 1. Chronic pulmonary inflammation with formation of fibrous tissue. 2. Interstitial pneumonia.

tuberculoid (tū-ber'kū-loyd) [" + G. *eidos,* resemblance]. Resembling tuberculosis or a tubercle.

tuberculoidin (tū-ber-kū-loy'dĭn) [" + G. *eidos,* form]. A form of tuberculin treated with alcohol.

tuberculol (tū-ber'kū-lol) [L. *tuberculum,* a little swelling]. Tuberculin which is free from secondary products.

tuberculoma (tū-ber-kū-lō'mă) [" + G. *-ōma,* tumor]. 1. A tuberculous abscess. 2. Any tuberculous neoplasm.

tuberculomucin (tū-ber"kū-lō-mū'sĭn) [" + *mucus,* mucus]. A mucinlike substance prepared from old cultures of tubercle bacilli.

tuberculophobia (tū-ber"kū-lō-fō'bĭ-ă) [" + G. *phobos,* fear]. An abnormal fear of becoming affected with tuberculosis.

tuberculopro'tein. A protein derived from tubercle bacilli.

tuberculosis (tū-bĕr″kū-lō′sĭs) [L. *tuberculum,* a little swelling, + G. *-osis,* disease]. An infectious disease caused by the tubercle bacillus, *Mycobacterium tuberculosis,* and characterized pathologically by inflammatory infiltrations, formation of tubercles, caseation, necrosis, abscesses, fibrosis, and calcification.

It most commonly affects the respiratory system but other parts of the body such as gastrointestinal and genitourinary tracts, bones, joints, nervous system, lymph nodes, and skin may become infected. Fish, amphibians, birds, and mammals (cattle) are subject to the disease, three types of the tubercle bacillus existing, namely *human, bovine* and *avian.* Man may become infected by any of the three types but in the U. S. the human type predominates. Infection is usually acquired from contact with an infected person or an infected cow or through drinking contaminated milk.

Tuberculosis may occur in an acute generalized form (*miliary tuberculosis*) or in a chronic localized form. In man, the primary infection usually consists of a localized lesion and regional adenitis, these constituting the *primary complex.* From this state, lesions may heal by fibrosis and calcification and the disease exist in an arrested or inactive stage. Reactivation or exacerbation of the disease or reinfection gives rise to the chronic progressive form.

Note: Many varieties of *Mycobacteria* which were previously thought to be non-pathogenic for man have been found to cause chronic progressive pulmonary disease closely resembling pulmonary tuberculosis. These organisms have been termed "anonymous" or "atypical" Mycobacteria. They have been classified into four groups: I. *photochromogens;* II. *scotochromogens;* III. *non-photochromogens;* IV. *rapid growers.*

Treatment: Sanitorium care is recommended for active cases; however, recent developments in chemotherapy have greatly altered time-honored views. In advanced cases, bed rest, adequate well-balanced diet, relief from emotional tension, collapse therapy (pneumoperitoneum, pneumothorax, phrenemphraxis) and, in some cases, surgery (thoracoplasty) may be required. Among chemotherapeutic drugs, three are widely used: streptomycin, para-aminosalicylic acid (PAS), and isoniazid. Pyrazinamide (PZA), viomycin, cycloserine, and ethionamide have also been used. Symptomatic treatment is necessary for cough, hemoptysis, chest pain, and other symptoms. RS: *tuberculin, tuberculin test, tubercle* (def. 3), *tubercle bacillus, Mycobacterium.*

tuberculostatic. Arresting the growth of tubercle bacillus.

tuberculous (tū-ber′kū-lŭs) [L. *tuberculum,* a little swelling]. Relating to or affected with tuberculosis, or conditions marked by infiltration of a specific tubercle, as opposed to the term tubercular, referring to nonspecific tubercle.

tuberculum (tū-ber′kū-lŭm) (pl. *tubercula*) [L. a little swelling]. A small knot or nodule; a tubercle.

t. acus′ticum. Dorsal nucleus of the cochlear nerve.

t. majus humeri. NA. Larger tuberosity of the humerus at upper end of its lateral surface giving attachment to infraspinatus, supraspinatus, and teres minor muscles.

t. minus humeri. NA. The projection at proximal end of humerus' ant. surface giving attachment to subscapularis muscle.

tuberin (tu′ber-ĭn) [L. *tuber,* a swelling]. A simple protein; a globulin in potatoes.

tuberositas (tū-ber-ŏs′ĭt-ăs) (pl. *tuberositates*) [L. a nodule]. A projection, nodule, or prominence.

tuberosity (tū-ber-ŏs′ĭ-tĭ) [L. *tuberositas,* tuberosity]. 1. An elevated round process of a bone. 2. A tubercle or nodule.

tuberous. Pertaining to or having tubers.

tubo- [L.]. Combining form meaning *tube.*

tuboabdominal (tū″bō-ăb-dŏm′ĭn-ăl) [L. *tuba,* tube, + *abdominalis,* pert. to the abdomen]. Pert. to the fallopian tubes and the abdomen.

t. pregnancy. Ectopic gestation with embryo partly in tube and partly in the abdominal cavity.

tuboligamentus (tū″bō-lĭg-ă-mĕn′tŭs) [" + *ligamentum,* a band]. Pert. to the fallopian tube and broad ligament of the uterus.

tuboovarian (tū″bō-ō-vā′rĭ-ăn) [" + *ovarium,* egg holder]. Pert. to the fallopian tube and the ovary.

tuboovariotomy (tū″bō-ō-vā-rĭ-ŏt′ō-mĭ) [" + " + G. *tomē,* a cutting]. Excision of ovaries and oviducts. Syn: *salpingo-oothecotomy.*

tuboperitoneal (tū″bō-pĕr-ĭ-tō-nē′ăl) [" + G. *peritonaion,* peritoneum]. Relating to the oviduct and peritoneum.

tuborrhea (tū-bor-rē′ă) [" + G. *rhoia,* a flow]. Discharge from the eustachian tube.

tubotympanal (tū″bō-tĭm′pă-năl) [" + G. *tympanon,* a drum]. Relating to the tympanum of the ear and the eustachian tube.

tubouterine (tū″bō-ū′tĕr-ĭn) [" + *uterīnus,* pert. to the uterus]. Relating to the oviduct and the uterus.

tubular (tū′bū-lar) [L. *tubularis,* like a tube]. Relating to or having the form of a tube or tubule.

t. excretory capacity, maximum. Abbr. Tm. The difference between the amount of a substance that is filtered and that appearing in urine per minute. Tm. gives valuable information concerning glomerular and tubular activity.

tubule (tū′būl) [L. *tubulus,* a tubule]. A small tube or canal.

t., collecting. T. in renal medulla which is part of the discharging tubule.

t., excretory. The uriniferous tubules in medullary portion of kidneys.

t., junctional. Short part of a uriniferous t. connecting with a collecting t.

t's., seminiferous. Very small channels of the testes in which spermatozoa develop and through which they leave the testes.

t., uriniferous. Minute canals forming the glandular substance of the kidney, originating in Bowman's capsules and emptying into pelvis of kidney.

tubuloalveolar. Consisting of tubes and alveoli.

t. gland. Syn: *tubuloacinar gland.* Branched, compound glands in which some of the terminal secreting portions are tubular, others alveolar (acinar); for example, salivary glands.

tubulodermoid (tū″bū-lō-der′moyd) [L. *tubulus,* tubule, + G. *derma,* skin, + *eidos,* form]. A dermoid tumor due to the persistent embryonic tubular structure.

tubulus (tū′bū-lŭs) (pl. *tubuli*) [L. a tubule]. A tubule; a small tube.

tuft. A small clump, cluster, or coiled mass.

t., enamel. Abnormal structure formed in development of enamel consisting of poorly calcified twisted rods.

tug'ging. A dragging or pulling.

t., tracheal. An indication of thoracic aneurysm.

SYM: A sense of downward pulling of larynx with cardiac systole when thyroid cartilage is gently raised bet. the finger and thumb.

tularemia (too-lăr-ē'mĭ-ă) [*Tulare*, part of California where disease was first discovered, + G. *aima*, blood]. Deer fly fever transmitted to man from rodents and rabbits bitten by a blood-sucking insect infected with *Pasteurella tularensis*, or by direct contact.

SYM: Three days after infection headache, chilliness, vomiting, aching pains, and fever. Site of infection develops into an ulcer. Glands at elbow or in armpit become enlarged, tender, and painful; later may develop into an abscess. Sweating, loss of weight, and debility.

tumbu fly. Species of African fly belonging to the genus Cordylobia. Their larvae develop in the skin of wild and domesticated animals, and man is frequently attacked.

tumefacient (tū-mĕ-fā'shĕnt) [L. *tumefaciens*, producing swelling]. Producing or tending to produce swelling; swollen.

tumefaction (tū"mĕ-făk'shŭn) [L. *tumefactio*, a swelling]. 1. A swelling. 2. Act of swelling or the state of being swollen.

tumentia (tū-mĕn'shĭ-ă). Swelling.

t., vasomotor. Irregular swellings in lower extremities associated with vasomotor disturbances.

tumescence (tū-mĕs'ĕns). 1. Condition of being swollen or tumid. 2. A swelling. 3. Deposit of semen in the testicles.

tu'mid. Swollen.

tumor (tū'mor) [L. *tumor*, a swelling]. SYN: *neoplasm*. 1. A swelling or enlargement. 2. An autonomous, new growth of tissue forming an abnormal mass which performs no physiologic function. It is with few exceptions of unknown cause, noninflammatory, and develops independent of, and unrestrained by normal laws of growth and morphogenesis. SEE: *cancer*.

TYPES OF TUMORS: *Myeloid Sarcomata, Giant Celled S*: Consist of elements formed chiefly of protoplasm containing 2 or more nuclei, up to 20 or even 50; with a varying number of round, spindle, or mixed cells. Vary in consistency from that of jelly to that of muscle. More frequently occurs on lower jaw, femur, and tibia.

Round Celled Sarcomata: Usually soft, vascular, rapidly growing, become large, and early give rise to metastatic deposits in distant parts and in viscera. Occur in periosteum, bone, lymphatic glands, subcutaneous tissue, testicle, eye, ovary, uterus, lung, kidneys; though may occur wherever fibrous tissue exists.

Glioma: Grows from the connective tissue of nerve centers and its basic substance resembles that structure. Occurs in retina and brain.

Melanotic Sarcoma: In which cells may be either of round or spindle variety. Is the most malignant form.

Spindle-cell Sarcoma: Cells vary much in size, from small oat-shaped cells to greatly elongated bodies with long, fine, tapering extremities. Chiefly in bones.

Endotheliomata: Attack, in different forms, the testicle, pia mater, pleura, and peritoneum.

Acinous or Spheroidal-celled Carcinoma: (1) Hard, spheroidal-celled (scirrhus or chronic c.). SEE: *scirrhus*. (2) Soft, spheroidal celled (encephaloid, or acute c.); resembles brain tissue in appearance and consistency. Occurs in testicle, liver, bladder, kidney, ovary, fundus oculi, more rarely in the breast.

Colloid Carcinoma: Really one of preceding varieties which has undergone mucoid degeneration, and so distended the alveoli they may be seen by naked eye. Occurs in stomach, intestine, omentum, ovary.

Epithelial Carcinoma: (1) The squamous-celled epitheliomata which always spring from skin or mucous membranes, or their glands, esp. at junctions of mucous and cutaneous surfaces. Are not encapsulated. Commence as wart-like growth, flattened tubercle, or fissure, ulceration in all these forms setting in early. (2) Cylindrical or columnar-celled. Less common form of carcinoma. Originates from either the cylindrical surface epithelium of a mucous membrane, or of its glands, closely imitating these structures in microscopic appearance. These growths form indurated, infiltrating masses in the walls of organs attacked, producing considerable stenosis of lumen, of hollow viscera; as rectum and small intestinal obstruction. Occur in uterus and intestinal tract. (3) Tumors composed of epiblastic, hypoblastic, and mesoblastic elements.

Warty or Villous Growth (Papillomata): Resemble in their structure hypertrophied papillae of skin—or mucous membrane. These include condylomata and mucous tubercles. Occur about anus and genitals, or in mouth and throat. Warts and warty growths on skin of hands and genitalia, and mucous surface of larynx. Villous growths, bladder, rectum, and larynx.

Teratoma: Tumors containing bone, hair, teeth, etc., usually situated in ovaries or testicles but may also be present in other tissues.

tumoraffin (tū'mor-ăf-ĭn) [L. *tumor*, a swelling, + *affinis*, related]. Having an affinity for tumor cells. SYN: *oncotropic*.

tumultus (tū-mŭl'tŭs) [L.]. Excessive or agitated activity.

t. cordis. Irregular heart action with palpitation.

t. sermo'nis. Extreme stuttering due to pathologic cause.

tuna fish (tū'nă). CANNED IN OIL, solids and liquids: 100 gm. Calories: 288. Other values: 24 gm. protein; 20 gm. fat; 6 mg. calcium.

Tunga. A genus of fleas commonly called chiggers. It belongs to the family Tungidae, order Siphonaptera.

T. penetrans. SYN: *chigger, chigoe, jigger, sand flea*. A small flea common in tropical regions which infests man, cats, dogs, rats, pigs, and other animals. They produce a severe local inflammation frequently liable to secondary infection.

tungsten. A metallic element. SYMB: W (for wolfram). At. wt. 183.85; at. no. 74.

tunic (tū'nĭk) [L. *tunica*, a sheath]. An investing membrane.

tunica (tū'nĭ-kă) (pl. *tunicae*) [L. *tunica*, a sheath]. An enveloping or covering membrane.

t. adventitia. NA. Outer coat of an artery or any tubular structure.

t. albuginea. The white fibrous coat of the eye, testicle, ovary, or spleen.

t. externa. Outer coat of an artery.

t. interna. SEE: *t. intima.*

t. intima. Lining coat of an artery.

t. media. Middle muscular coat of an artery.

t. propria. NA. Deep portion of the corium containing blood vessels, nerves, glands, and hair follicles.

t. vaginalis. Serous lining of the testicles.

tun'nel. A narrow channel or passageway.

t. anemia. A disease due to ankylostoma, and resembling idiopathic anemia.

t. disease. 1. Caisson disease, *q.v.* 2. Ancylostomiasis, *q.v.*

t., inner. SYN: *tunnel of Corti.* Triangular canal lying between the inner and outer pillars of Corti in the organ of Corti of inner ear.

tunnel vision. 1. A condition seen in hysteria wherein the field of vision is the same regardless of distance from the visual screen. SYN: *tubular vision.* 2. Severe constriction of the visual field due to advanced chronic glaucoma. 3. An expression used to indicate a lack of ability to visualize the broad or long-range aspects of a problem or situation. When used this way the term has no reference to actual visual difficulty.

turbid. Cloudy; not clear. SEE: *turbidity.*

turbidimeter (tür-bĭ-dĭm'ĕ-ter) [L. *turbidus,* disturbed, + G. *metron,* a measure]. Device for estimating degree of turbidity of a fluid.

turbidimetry (tür-bĭ-dĭm'ĕ-trĭ) [" + G. *metron,* a measure]. Estimation of the turbidity of a liquid.

turbidity (tür-bĭd'ĭ-tĭ) [L. *turbiditas,* turbidity]. 1. BACT: Quality of not having translucent appearance of liquid due to growth of microorganisms. 2. Having flaky or granular particles suspended in a clear liquid giving it a cloudy appearance. SEE: *clarificant.*

turbinate(d (tur'bĭ-nā"tĕd) [L. *turbo, turbin-,* a whirl]. Top- or cone-shaped.

t. bones. SYN: *conchae.* SEE: *conchae, nasal.*

turbinectomy (tür-bĭn-ĕk'tō-mĭ) [" + G. *ektomē,* excision]. Excision of a turbinated bone.

turbinotome (tür-bĭn'ō-tōm) [" + G. *tomē,* a cutting]. Instrument for excision of a turbinated bone.

turbinotomy (tür-bĭn-ŏt'ō-mĭ) [" + G. *tomē,* incision]. Surgical incision of a turbinated bone.

Turck's bundle. A pathway of descending projection fibers from cerebral cortex.

turgescence (tur-jĕs'ĕns) [L. *turgescens,* swelling]. Swelling or enlargement of a part.

turgescent (tur-jĕs'ĕnt) [L. *turgescens,* swelling]. Swelling; inflated.

turgid (tur'jĭd) [L. *turgidus,* swollen]. Swollen; bloated.

turgor (tur'gor) [L. *turgor,* a swelling]. 1. Normal tension in a cell. 2. Distention, swelling.

t. vita'lis. Normal fullness of the capillaries and blood vessels.

tur'key. COOKED (roasted light meat): 100 gm. Calories: 126. Other values: 33 gm. protein; 4 gm. fat. Dark meat has about 15% more calories than white meat.

turning (turn'ĭng) [A.S. *turnian,* to turn]. Process of manually changing position of fetus in utero to permit normal delivery. SYN: *version.*

turnip. COOKED: 100 gm. Calories: 23. Other values: 0.8 gm. protein; 0.2 gm. fat; 5.0 gm. carbohydrate; 35 mg. calcium; 22 mg. vitamin C.

turnip greens. COOKED (boiled and drained): 100 gm. Calories: 20. Other values: 2.2 gm. protein; 0.2 gm. fat; 3.3 gm. carbohydrate; 174 mg. calcium; 5700 I.U. vitamin A; 47 mg. vitamin C.

turpentine (tur'pĕn-tīn) [G. *terebinthos,* turpentine tree]. Oleoresin obtained from various species of pine trees.

A mixture of terpenes and other hydrocarbons obtained from pine trees used externally in liniments and counter irritants. The source of oil of turpentine or "spirits of turpentine."

POISONING: May occur from inhalation.

SYM: Warm or burning sensation in the gullet and stomach, followed by cramping, vomiting, and diarrhea. Pulse and respiration become weak, slow, and irregular; irritation of urinary tract and central nervous system resembling alcoholic intoxication.

F. A. TREATMENT: Gastric lavage, soothing drinks, and stimulants. Increase fluid intake.

turunda (tu-run'dă) [L.]. 1. A surgical tent, drain, or tampon. 2. A suppository.

tussal (tŭs'ăl) [L. *tussis,* cough]. Relating to a cough. SYN: *tussive.*

tussis (tŭs'ĭs) [L. *tussis,* a cough]. A cough, as bronchial tussis, senile tussis, etc.

t. convulsi'va. Pertussis* or whooping cough.

t. stomacha'lis. Reflex cough from irritation of the mucosa of the stomach.

tussive (tŭs'ĭv) [L. *tussis,* cough]. Relating to a cough. SYN: *tussal.*

twelfth cranial nerve. One of a pair of cranial nerves distributing to the base of the tongue. SEE: *hypoglossal nerve,* and *Table of Nerves in Appendix.*

twilight sleep (twī'līt slēp). A state of partial anesthesia and hypoconsciousness in which pain sense has been greatly reduced by the injection of morphine and scopolamine.

Patient responds to pain, but afterward memory of pain is dulled or effaced, as following childbirth. SEE: *labor.*

t. state. PSY: One in which consciousness is disordered, making possible actions subsequently forgotten.

Evidenced in hysteria, epilepsy, and dementia precox.

twin (twĭn) [A.S. *twinn*]. One of 2 children developed within the uterus at the same time from the same impregnation. SEE: *Hellin's law.*

RS: *enzygotic, fetus papyraceous.*

t's., biovular. Dizygotic twins, *q.v.*

t's., conjoined. Twins which are united. SEE: *Siamese twins.*

t's., dizygotic. Those from 2 separate ova fertilized at the same time.

t's., fraternal. *Dizygotic twins, q.v.*

t's., identical. Twins which develop from a single fertilized ovum. Twins of this type have the same genetic makeup, consequently are of the same sex and resemble each other strikingly in physical, physiological, and mental traits. They develop within a common chorionic sac and have a common placenta. Each usually develops its own amnion and umbilical cord. They may result from (a) development of two inner cell masses within a blastocyst, (b) development of two embryonic axes on a single blastoderm, or (c) the division of a single embryonic axis into two centers.

t's., interlocked. Twins in which the neck of one becomes interlocked with the head of the other making vaginal delivery impossible.

t's., monozygotic. Those developing from a single fertilized ovum. These give rise to *identical twins, q.v.* Also called *monochorionic, uniovular,* or *similar twins.*

t., parasitic. The smaller of a pair of conjoined twins when there is a marked disparity in size.

t's., Siamese. Symmetrical conjoined twins. SEE: *Siamese twins.*

t's., true. Monozygotic twins.

t's., uniovular. Those developing from a single ovum.

twinge (twĭnj) [A.S. *twengan,* to pinch]. A sudden, keen pain.

twitch (twĭch) [M.E. *twicchen*]. 1. A simple, quick, spasmodic contraction of a muscle. 2. To jerk convulsively. SEE: *myokymia, myopalmus.*

tylion (tĭl'ĭ-ŏn) [G. *tyleion,* knot]. Point at middle of ant. edge of the optic groove.

tyloma (tī-lō'mă) [G. *tylos,* knot, + *-ōma,* tumor]. A callosity.

tylosis (tī-lō'sĭs) [" + *-ōsis,* condition]. 1. A callosity. SYN: *tyloma.* 2. Formation of a callus.

tympanal (tĭm'păn-ăl) [G. *typanon,* drum]. Relating to the tympanum. SYN: *tympanic.*

tympanectomy (tĭm-păn-ĕk'tō-mĭ) [" + *ektomē,* excision]. Excision of the tympanic membrane.

tympanic (tĭm-păn'ĭk) [G. *tympanon,* drum]. 1. Pert. to the tympanum. 2. Resonant.

t. membrane. SYN: *drum membrane.* Membrane serving as the lateral wall of the tympanic cavity and separating it from the ext. acoustic meatus. SEE: *tympanum.*

tympanism (tĭm'păn-ĭzm) [G. *tympanon,* drum, + *-ismos,* condition]. Abdominal inflation from gas. SYN: *tympanites.*

tympanites (tĭm-păn-ī'tēz) [G. *tympanitēs,* distention]. Abdominal distention due to intestinal gas.

tympanitic (tĭm-păn-ĭt'ĭk) [G. *tympanitēs,* distention]. 1. Pert. to or characterized by tympanites. 2. Resonant. SYN: *tympanic.*

t. resonance. A sound produced by percussion over an air- or gas-filled cavity.

tympanitis (tĭm-păn-ī'tĭs) [G. *tympanon,* drum, + *-ītis,* inflammation]. Inflammation of the middle ear. SYN: *otitis media.*

tympano- [G.]. Combining form meaning *eardrum, tympanum of the ear.*

tympanomastoiditis (tĭm"păn-ō-măs-toy-dī'tĭs) [" + *mastos,* breast, + *eidos,* form, + *-ītis,* inflammation]. Inflammation of the tympanum and mastoid cells.

tympanosis (tĭm-pă-nō'sĭs). Tympanites, *q.v.*

tympanotomy (tĭm"păn-ŏt'ō-mĭ) [" + *tomē,* a cutting]. Incision of the membrana tympani. SYN: *myringotomy.*

tympanous (tĭm'păn-ŭs) [G. *tympanon,* a drum]. Marked by abdominal distention with gas.

tympanum (tĭm'păn-ŭm) [G. *tympanon*]. SYN: *cavum tympani, ear drum.* The middle ear or tympanic cavity. SEE: *ear, middle.*

t. antrum. The space by which the epitympanic recess of the tympanic cavity proper communicates with the mastoid cells.

t. cavity. The cavity of the middle ear. SEE: *tympanum.*

tympany (tĭm'pă-nĭ) [G. *tympanon,* drum]. 1. Abdominal distention with gas. 2. Tympanic resonance on percussion.

It is a clear hollow note like that of a drum having no vesicular quality. It indicates a pathologic condition of the lung or of a cavity.

type (tīp) [G. *typos,* type]. The general character of a person, a disease, or substance.

RS: *Aztec, koinotropic, sexual psychopathy, syntonic.*

t., asthenic. One who is slender with a long chest that is flat and who has poor muscular development.

t., pyknic. One with a rounded body, thick shoulders, large chest, short neck, and broad head.

t., vagotonic. One with deficient adrenal stimulus, slow pulse, low blood pressure, and high sugar tolerance.

typhlatonia, typhlatony (tĭf-lă-tō'nĭ-ă, -lăt'ō-nĭ) [G. *typlon,* cecum, + *tonos,* tone]. Deficient motor activity of the cecum.

typhlectasis (tĭf-lĕk'tă-sĭs) [" + *ektasis,* dilatation]. Cecal distention.

typhlectomy (tĭf-lĕk'tō-mĭ) [" + *ektomē,* excision]. Excision of the cecum. SYN: *cecectomy.*

typhlenteritis (tĭf-lĕn-ter-ī'tĭs) [" + *enteron,* intestine, + *-ītis,* inflammation]. Inflammation of the cecum. SYN: *typhlitis.*

typhlitis (tĭf-lī'tĭs) [" + *-ītis,* inflammation]. Inflammation of the cecum.

typhlodicliditis (tĭf"lō-dĭk-lĭ-dī'tĭs) [" + *diklis,* door, + *-ītis,* inflammation]. Inflammation of the ileocecal valve.

typhloempyema (tĭf"lō-ĕm-pī-ē'mă) [" + *en,* in, + *pyon,* pus, + *aima,* blood]. An abdominal abscess following typhlitis.

typhloenteritis (tĭf"lō-ĕn-ter-ī'tĭs) [G. *typhlon,* cecum, + *enteron,* intestine, + *-ītis,* inflammation]. Inflammation of the cecum. SYN: *typhlenteritis, typhlitis.*

typhlolexia (tĭf"lō-lĕks'ĭ-ă) [G. *typlos,* blind, + *lexis,* speech]. Inability to recognize written or spoken words. SYN: *word blindness.*

typhlolithiasis (tĭf"lō-lĭ-thī'ă-sĭs). Formation of a concretion in the cecum.

typhlology (tĭf-lŏl'ō-jĭ) [" + *logos,* study]. Study of blindness, its causes and effects.

typhlopexy (tĭf'lo-pĕks"ĭ) [G. *typhlon,* cecum, + *pēxis,* fixation]. Suturing of a movable cecum to the abdominal wall.

typhlosis (tĭf-lō'sĭs) [G. *typhlos,* blind, + *-ōsis,* condition]. Blindness.

typhlospasm (tĭf'lō-spăsm). Spasm of the cecum.

typhlostenosis (tĭf-lō-stĕn-ō'sĭs) [G. *typhlon,* cecum, + *stenōsis,* a narrowing]. Stenosis or stricture of the cecum.

typhlostomy (tĭf-lŏs'tō-mĭ) [" + *stoma,* opening]. Establishment of a permanent cecal fistula.

typhlotomy (tĭf-lŏt'ō-mĭ) [" + *tomē,* a cutting]. Incision of the cecum.

typhloureterostomy (tĭf"lō-ū-rē"ter-ŏs'tō-mĭ) [" + *ourētēr,* ureter, + *stoma,* opening]. Implantation of a ureter in the cecum.

typho- [G.]. Combining form *pert. to fever, typhoid.*

typhobacillosis (tī"fō-băs-ĭl-ō'sĭs) [G. *typhos,* stupor, + L. *bacillus,* little stick, + G. *-ōsis,* condition]. Poisoning due to toxins produced by the typhoid bacillus.

typhohemia (tī"fō-hē'mĭ-ă) [" + *haima,* blood]. Degeneration of the blood due to presence of bacilli.

typhoid (tī'foyd) [G. *typhos*, stupor, + *eidos*, form]. Resembling typhus.

t. fever. An acute, infectious disease characterized by definite lesions in Peyer's patches, mesenteric glands, and spleen accompanied by fever, headache, and abdominal symptoms.

Etiol: Causative organism *Salmonella typhosa* (*Eberthella typhi*), a gram-negative, motile bacillus. Common in early adult life and esp. prevalent during fall and early winter. It may be transmitted by infected water or milk supplies. Well water in country districts sometimes contaminated through the soil from outhouses. Human carriers, particularly when food handlers, may be responsible for spread of infection. Body discharges from active or convalescent cases may be the means of infecting others.

Incubation: Average, two weeks; varies from one to three weeks.

Sym: *Early*: Headache, general weakness, indefinite pains, nosebleed; constipation may occur.

Within a few days to a week the temperature may reach a maximum of 104° to 105° F. and during this time, or up to the 10th day, rose spots can usually be seen, particularly on the abdomen, though they may be observed on the chest and back. They disappear on pressure and usually come out in crops during a period of several days. Abdominal tenderness develops and with it, generally, distention. Splenomegaly will be found in more than half of the cases by the end of the first week.

During following weeks fever is characterized by marked daily remissions, evening temperature being from 1° to 3° F. higher than the morning. In the young, the temperature often rises very abruptly. When the diurnal remissions are slight, a protracted case is forecast. As defervescence advances, the temperature becomes more irregular. Remissions are more decided and not infrequently a higher temperature is recorded in the morning. Hurried respiration, slight cough, and bronchial râles are common. Pulse is usually slow in comparison with the temperature, and is dicrotic. Heart sounds often feeble, expression dull and heavy, cheeks somewhat flushed, conjunctivae clear, pupils dilated. Tongue tremulous; at first red at tip and edges, and covered posteriorly with a whitish fur.

In severe cases, tongue becomes dry, brown and fissured, and sordes collect on teeth. Gastric symptoms not common, but obstinate. Vomiting sometimes develops and becomes a serious complication. Abdomen tympanitic, tenderness on palpation, esp. in iliac fossa. Diarrhea generally present, though not a constant symptom. Discharges vary from 3 to 6 or more a day; thin, offensive, yellowish. Stupor, muttering, delirium, twitching of the tendons, carphologia, and coma vigil may be present. Urine usually shows albumin. Retention common.

White blood count demonstrates a leukopenia. Convalescence marked by anemia, falling of hair, often desquamation. The patient gives evidence of having suffered from a protracted illness that has produced general enfeeblement of mind and body.

Varieties: *Abortive*: Abrupt onset with severe symptoms, but convalescence follows within a few days. Often seen in children.

Mild form: Moderate fever with marked remissions, diarrhea slight, nervous symptoms often absent, rash usually present and often abundant.

Ambulatory type ("walking" typhoid): Symptoms mild and often disregarded by patient, who refuses to go to bed. However, grave symptoms may suddenly develop and even death from intestinal perforation may follow.

Typhoid of children: Rash often absent, fever rises abruptly, cerebral symptoms may be sufficiently marked to suggest meningitis.

Relapses: These are common in typhoid. There may be a complete repetition of all symptoms experienced during primary attack, but they are usually of shorter duration.

Recrudescence: This is a sudden, temporary elevation of temperature occurring during convalescence, and is not associated with a return of other symptoms. It may be due to constipation, excitement, or irritating food.

Complications: These occur in approximately 25% of cases and account for the majority of the deaths. The most frequent and dangerous complications are intestinal hemorrhage and intestinal perforation. An abrupt fall of several degrees in temperature is suggestive of intestinal hemorrhage or perforation. Usually occurs during 3rd or 4th week.

Differential Diag: Paratyphoid, pneumonia, dysentery, meningitis, smallpox, appendicitis. Diagnostic points of value will be the presence of rose spots, splenomegaly, leukopenia, the Widal test, blood culture and examination of feces for presence of causative organism.

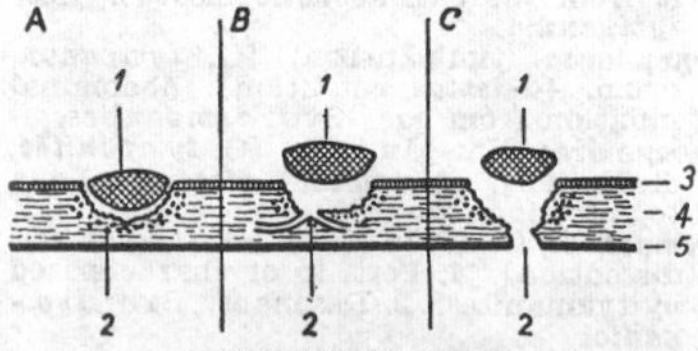

TYPHOID ULCERS.

A. In Peyer's patch. 1. Slough in ulcer. 2. Lymphoid tissue. B. Erosion of blood vessel, with separation of slough, causing hemorrhage. 1. Slough separated. 2. Eroded artery. C. Perforation of ulcer through peritoneum. 1. Slough separated. 2. Peritoneal perforation. 3. Mucous membrane. 4. Muscle layer. 5. Peritoneum.

Prog: Should always be guarded, no matter how mild the case appears to be. Fatality rate varies in different epidemics. Hemorrhages in any form, together with excessive diarrhea, are unfavorable omens.

Prophylaxis: Safeguards adopted for the supply of drinking water in large cities and the more or less general pasteurization of milk are probably chief factors in the great reduction of typhoid fever in well-governed communities. Active immunization is a factor in reduction of mortality. Individual immunity can ordinarily be established by administering two injections of high-antigenicity vaccine spaced by several weeks. See: *typhoid vaccine*.

Treatment of the Active Case: General care, isolation of patient, and disinfection of all discharges are of primary importance. Those caring for the typhoid patient should be immunized against the disease. All precautions applicable to such infections must be adopted. Articles in contact with the patient must be sterilized or disinfected before being handled by other persons than the immediate attendant. It is necessary to guard against development of bedsores. Since delirium is not infrequent, patient may require constant watching to prevent his leaving the bed, which might result in fatal consequences. The mouth should be kept as clean as possible to prevent development of sordes.

Specific Treatment: Chloramphenicol (Chloromycetin) is the drug of choice. It greatly shortens the febrile period and toxicity is markedly reduced, especially if adrenalcortical therapy is used in conjunction with it. Tetracycline drugs are also effective.

Diet: A bland or liquid diet of 3000 calories should be given until the patient improves, then frequent relatively high-caloric feedings. If intestinal symptoms prevent oral feedings intravenous fluids and feedings will be required.

The starvation diet, which was once so common in the treatment of typhoid fever, is seldom followed in the present day.

Ice bags and cold sponging are little used at the present time. On the other hand, sponging with tepid water, or with alcohol, is sometimes used when the temperature has reached unusual heights. In case of severe hemorrhage or intestinal perforation, if antibiotics and bowel decompression fail to control the symptoms surgical intervention will be necessary.

NP: The objectives are: (a) *To support the patient's strength,* (b) *to lessen toxemia,* and (c) *to prevent complications and the spread of the disease. Strict isolation technic should be followed.*

Quiet is essential; visitors, excitement, and noise are not conducive to quiet or peace of mind. Bright lights, heavy bedclothing, and everything that might irritate the patient should be avoided. An airy, well-ventilated room is essential. The bed must be comfortable and protection provided in case of incontinence. If the patient becomes emaciated an air bed may be necessary.

Position of patient: Usually he lies on one side with knees drawn up, so if sores are apt to develop the knees should be wrapped in wool to prevent chafing when together. Extra pillows are permissible if desired by the patient. The patient should make no muscular effort while the bed is being made.

Care of the mouth: Frequent soft swabs and bland lotions should be used, as sordes gather on the teeth and the mouth is dry, brown, and fissured. Keeping the mouth moist cannot be overemphasized.

Care of the skin: A morning and night cleansing bath should be given. In the meantime, tepid sponging will remove perspiration, and help maintain the function of the skin and also assist in elimination. As the secretion of the skin carries infection, water used for bathing should be disposed of and the basin disinfected. The patient's hands should be kept scrupulously clean to prevent them from being contaminated with excreta. Ointment should be used to protect the skin in cases of incontinence.

Headache and backache: A severe frontal headache may last from 10 to 14 days from inception of the fever. The light should be shaded and cold compresses applied. The legs and back should be supported with pillows.

Restlessness: This may induce sleeplessness. A change of position; a sponge bath; taking off a cover if the patient is hot, or adding one if cold; washing the face, and brushing the hair will do much to rest the patient.

Urine: This should be measured and tested daily for albumin. Watch for sign of retention due to atony of the bladder's muscular wall in the latter weeks of illness.

Stools: Inspection for presence of undigested food, for blood, and flatus is very important. Frequency should be noted. Four or 5 movements per day is normal in diarrhea, but 8 to 12 indicate complications. Constipation is not unusual with these patients; nevertheless, laxatives and enemas should not be used. Stool softeners may be used. When complicated by hemorrhages, and frequent stools, the patient may be too exhausted to use a bedpan, in which case the excreta should be received on pads.

Abdominal distention: This may become a dangerous complication; in any event it is distressing. Decompression by gastric or intestinal drainage may be used, but this is hazardous because of the danger of causing perforation or hemorrhage.

Bathing: Baths, their nature, and frequency should be left to the discretion of the physician; otherwise routine care, such as cleansing and sponge baths, may be used unless contraindicated.

Delirium: This is usually of the low muttering type, and the patient stares with a fixed gaze upon the ceiling and plucks on the bedclothing. Utensils and other articles should not be left within his reach and *he must not be left alone.*

Charting: A 4-hour chart should be kept of temperature, pulse, and respiration, although the pulse should be taken much more frequently than this. In the 3rd week, the temperature should be taken every 2 hours. A sudden drop in temperature indicates hemorrhage.

Disinfection: The usual methods of disinfection should be observed in handling all excreta and secretions, linens, and utensils. Disinfection for the nurse is also very important.

t. state. Condition in many diseases marked by profound prostration and other symptoms like those of typhus or typhoid fever.

t. vaccine. A vaccine containing killed typhoid bacilli. Even though its effectiveness in preventing typhoid fever is debatable, its use is advisable in persons who will be exposed to typhoid bacilli.

t., walking. T. fever with mild general constitutional symptoms, the patient being able to be up and to walk. Syn: *ambulatory typhoid.*

typhoidal (tī-foy'dăl) [G. *typhos*, stupor, + *eidos*, resemblance]. Resembling typhoid.

typholysin (tī-fŏl′ĭ-sĭn) [" + *lysis*, dissolution]. A lysin destructive to typhoid bacilli.

typhomalarial (tī″fō-mă-lā′rĭ-ăl) [" + Italian *malaria*, bad air]. Having symptoms of both typhoid and malarial fever.

typhomania (tī-fō-mā′nĭ-ă) [" + *mania*, madness]. Muttering delirium characteristic of typhoid fever and typhus.

typhopneumonia (tī″fō-nū-mō′nĭ-ă) [" + *pneumŏnia*, inflammation of lungs]. 1. Pneumonia occurring in typhoid fever. 2. Pneumonia with typhoid symptoms.

typhous (tī′fŭs) [G. *typhos*, stupor]. Pert. to typhus fever.

typhus, typhus fever (tī′fŭs) [G. *typhos*, stupor]. One of a group of acute, infectious diseases characterized by great prostration, severe headache, generalized maculopapular rash, sustained high fever, and usually progressive neurologic involvement, ending in a crisis in 10 to 14 days.

Three diseases are included in the group: *epidemic (louse-borne) typhus, Brill-Zinsser disease (recrudescent typhus)*, and *murine (flea-borne) typhus*. Although clinically and pathologically similar, they differ in intensity of symptoms, severity, and mortality rate.

Epidemic typhus is particularly prevalent amid unsanitary conditions. It often develops on shipboard, in army camps, and where living conditions are unfavorable and congestion is marked. The disease is rare in the United States, infection being found principally at the seaboard as a result of imported cases.

Incubation: Six to 14 days.

Sym: Onset sudden. Severe headache, pain in back and limbs, extreme prostration. Fever rises rapidly, often reaching 104° to 105° F. in from 2 to 3 days. Remains high for about 10 days, when it falls by crisis. Pulse rapid, weak, often dicrotic. Tongue tremulous, may be covered with whitish fur; in severe cases becomes black and rolled up like a ball in back of mouth. Face dusky, conjunctivae injected, pupil contracted, headache, stupor, delirium, subsultus tendinum, carphologia.

From 4th to 5th day, bluish spots appear over body, esp. on abdomen. These are petechial in character and do not disappear on pressure. The extent of eruption is indicative of severity of attack. Sometimes there is a diffuse, dark red, subcuticular mottling. Bowels are constipated, urine is scanty, high-colored, and often albuminous.

Complications: Bronchopneumonia more frequent than lobar, hypostatic congestion of lungs, nephritis, and parotid abscess.

Differential Diag: Typhoid fever, hemorrhagic smallpox, Henoch's purpura, epidemic meningitis of fulminating type, and ulcerative endocarditis may have to be considered.

Prog: Variable. Mortality may be quite high in epidemic typhus and almost nonexistent in murine typhus. Broad-spectrum antibiotics will be life saving if given early enough.

Treatment: *Preventive*: Absolute cleanliness, sterilization of clothing, and the use of apparel to prevent infestation of the body louse. The delousing camps, so common during the late war, were examples of the precautions necessary to prevent its spread. Patient must be isolated. Absolute rest necessary, and a liquid diet. *Specific:* Broad-spectrum antibiotics, such as the tetracyclines and chloramphenicol, give excellent results. PABA (para-aminobenzoic acid) is also useful.

t., endemic. Murine typhus, *q.v.*

t., epidemic (louse-borne). Syn: *jail fever, war fever, camp fever, Fleck typhus, European typhus, classic typhus, historic typhus.* An infectious disease caused by *Rickettsia prowazekii* and transmitted by the human body louse *(Pediculus humanus corporis).*

t., flea-borne. Murine typhus, *q.v.*

t., Mexican. Syn: *tabardillo.* A louse-borne epidemic typhus present in certain portions of Mexico.

t., mite-borne. Tsutsugamushi disease or scrub typhus.

t., murine. Syn: *endemic, rat, flea-borne, urban,* or *shop typhus.* A disease caused by *Rickettsia mooseri* and occurring in nature as a mild infection of rats and transmitted from rat to rat by the rat-louse or flea. Humans may acquire it by being bitten by infected rat-fleas or ingesting food contaminated by rat-urine or flea-feces.

t., rat. Murine typhus.

t., recrudescent. Syn: *Brill's disease, Brill-Zinsser disease.* A recurrence or recrudescence of a preceding attack of epidemic typhus after initial attack.

t., rural. Scrub typhus, *q.v.*

t., scrub. Syn: *mite-borne* or *rural typhus; Japanese river fever; Tsutsugamushi disease.* A self-limited febrile disease of two weeks duration caused by *Rickettsia tsutsugamushi* and transmitted by two species of mites (chiggers) of the genus *Thrombicula.* Occurs principally in Pacific-Asiatic area.

t., shop. Murine typhus.

t., urban. Epidemic typhus, *q.v.*

typical (tĭp′ĭ-kăl) [G. *typikos*, pert. to type]. Having the characteristics of, pert. to, or conforming to, a type or condition or group.

typing. The determination of the specific blood group to which an individual belongs. Also the determination of the specific type or subdivision of a species to which certain bacteria (*e.g., Salmonella* or *Diplococcus pneumoniae*) belong. See: *blood transfusion.*

typo- [G.]. Combining form meaning *a type.*

typoscope (tī′pō-skōp) [" + *skopein*, to examine]. Device to aid patients with amblyopia and cataract in reading.

tyramine (tī-răm′ĭn). Intermediate product in the conversion of tyrosine to epinephrine.

tyrannism (tĭr′ăn-ĭzm) [G. *tyrannos*, tyrant, + *-ismos*, condition]. Abnormal tendency to exercise cruelty. Syn: *sadism, q.v.*

ty reflex (tī). Sudden reflex grasping of mother's body by infant when startled. Syn: *Moro reflex.*

tyremesis (tī-rĕm′ĕ-sĭs) [G. *tyros*, cheese, + *emesis*, vomiting]. Infant vomiting of curdy or cheesy substances.

tyrogenous (tī-rŏj′ĕn-ŭs) [" + *gennan*, to produce]. Having origin in cheese or produced by it.

Tyroglyphus (tī-rŏg′lĭ-fŭs). A genus of sarcoptoid mites commonly known as *cheese mites.* They infest cheese and dried vegetable food products and occasionally infest man causing a pruritus. Contains species causing *grocer's itch, vanillism,* and *copra itch.*

tyroid (tī′royd) [" + *eidos*, form]. Caseous; cheesy.

tyromatosis (tī-rō-mă-tō′sĭs) [" + " + *-ōsis*, condition]. Cheesy degeneration. Syn: *caseation.*

tyrosinase (tī-rō′sĭn-ās) [G. *tyros*, cheese]. A ferment that acts on tyrosine.

tyrosine (tī′rō-sĭn). An amino acid present in many proteins, esp. casein. It serves as a precursor of epinephrine, thyroxine, and melanin. Two vitamins, ascorbic acid and folic acid, are essential for its metabolism.

tyrosinosis (tī-rō-sĭn-ō′sĭs. Condition resulting from faulty metabolism of tyrosine, whereby its oxidation products appear in the urine.

tyrosinuria (tī-rō-sĭn-ū′rĭ-ă) [" + *ouron*, urine]. Tyrosine in the urine.

tyrosis (tī-rō′sĭs) [" + *-ōsis*, condition]. 1. Curdling of milk. 2. Vomiting of cheesy substance by infants. SYN: *tyremesis.** 3. Cheesy degeneration. SYN: *tyromatosis.*

tyrothricin (tī-rō-thrī′sĭn). An antibiotic isolated from a soil bacteria, *Bacillus brevis.* It contains *gramicidin* and *tyrocidin,* both of which are effective against gram-positive bacteria. Applied topically as an ointment or cream.

tyrotoxism (tī-rō-tŏks′ĭzm) [" + " + *-ismos,* condition]. Poisoning produced by a milk product or by cheese.

Tyrrell's fascia (tĭr′ĕl). An ill-defined fibromuscular layer from the middle aponeurosis of the perineum, behind the prostate gland. SYN: *rectovesical fascia.*

Tyson's glands (tī′sŭn). SYN: *preputial glands.* Modified sebaceous glands located on neck of penis and inner surface of prepuce. Their secretion is one of the components of *smegma.*

Tzank test. Test of cells obtained from floor of pemphigus bulla to substantiate the diagnosis.

Notes

Notes

Notes

Notes

Notes

U

U. 1. Chem. symbol of *uranium.* 2. Abbr. for *unit.*

uarthritis (ū″ar-thrī′tĭs) [G. *arthron,* joint, + *-itis,* inflammation]. Gout supposed to result from excess of uric acid. SYN: *arthritis urica.*

uaterium (wā-tē′rĭ-ŭm). A medical preparation to be used in the ear.

uberous (ū′bĕr-ŭs) [L. *uber,* udder]. Prolific; fruitful; fertile.

uberty (ū′bĕr-tĭ) [L. *uber,* udder]. Fruitfulness; fertility.

UBI. Abbr. for *ultraviolet blood irradiation.*

Uffelmann's test (oof′ĕl-mahn). Test for determination of lactic acid in gastric juice.

Uhlenhuth's test (oo′len-hoot). SYN: *biologic test, Bordet's test, serum test, precipitin reaction, precipitin test.* A test for blood, meat, etc. Substance tested for is used as an antigen and injected into a rabbit. Serum of rabbit is then added to saline solution of suspected material. Solution becomes cloudy if suspected substance is of the same nature as antigen.

Uhthoff's sign (oot′hof). The nystagmus which occurs in multiple disseminated sclerosis.

ulaganactesis (ū-lăg″ă-năk′tē-sĭs) [G. *oulon,* gum, + *aganektesis,* irritation]. Disagreeable sensations or irritation in or about the gums.

ulalgia (ū-lăl′jĭ-ă) [G. *oulon,* gum, + *algos,* pain]. Pain in the gums.

ulatrophia (ū″lăt-rō′fĭ-ă). Shrinking of gums; recession of the gums.

ulcer (ŭl′ser) [L. *ulcus, ulcer-,* ulcer]. An open sore or lesion of the skin or mucous membrane of the body, with loss of substance, sometimes accompanied by formation of pus.

Simple ulcers may result from trauma, caustics, or intense heat or cold. They may accompany varicose veins in the aged.

In syphilis, they are deep seated, having an offensive secretion; in epithelioma, they appear late in life with a single center and a thickened, infiltrated edge with a scanty, bloody secretion; in lupus vulgaris, they appear early in life, but they are superficial.

RS: *abscission, anabrosis, anthracosis, aphtha, argema, carcinelcosis, carcinomelcosis, chalarosis, dieresis, duodenal u., helicoid, peptic, phagedena, rodent u., slough, stomach, vomicose.*

u., amputating. One which destroys tissue to the bone by encircling the part.

u., atonic. A chronic ulcer.

u., callous. A chronic u. with indurated, elevated edges and no granulations, which does not heal.

u., Curling's. A peptic ulcer due to the stress associated with severe and widespread body burn or injury. SYN: *stress ulcer.*

u., decubitus. A bedsore; a pressure sore.

u., duodenal. An ulcer on the mucosa of the duodenum, due to the action of the gastric juice.

u., erethistic. One with an inflamed, red, painful surface.

u., follicular. A tiny ulcer having its origin in a lymph follicle and affecting a mucous membrane.

u., fungus. One in which the granulations protrude above edges of wound and bleed easily.

u., gastric. SEE: *peptic u.*

u., healthy. An u. which tends toward healing, its surface being soft and smooth with tiny red granulations.

u., indolent. Nearly painless u. usually found on leg, characterized by indurated and elevated edge, and nongranulating base.

u., peptic. An ulcer of the mucosa of the duodenum or stomach.

u., perforating. An ulcer which permeates the entire thickness of the part, as the foot or intestine.

u., phagedenic. An ulcer which sloughs particles, spreading rapidly and disintegrating the tissues.

u., rodent. A deeply infiltrating ulcer which slowly eats away the bones and soft tissues; commonly affects the upper part of the face.

u., round. SEE: *peptic ulcer.*

u., serpiginous. A creeping ulcer which heals in one part and extends to another.

u., simple. A local ulcer with no severe inflammation or pain.

u., specific. An ulcer caused by a specific disease, as syphilis or lupus.

u., stercoral. 1. Ulcer caused by pressure from impacted feces. 2. Ulcer through which feces escape.

ulcerate (ŭl′sĕr-āt) [L. *ulcerāre,* to ulcerate]. To produce or become affected with an ulcer.

ulcerated (ŭl′sĕr-ā″tĕd) [L. *ulcerāre,* to ulcerate]. Of the nature of an ulcer or affected with one.

u. sore throat. Putrid sore throat, a gangrenous inflammation.

u. tooth. Suppuration of the alveolar periosteum with ulceration of gum surrounding the decaying root of a tooth.

ulceration (ŭl″sĕr-ā′shŭn) [L. *ulcerāre,* to ulcerate]. Suppuration taking place on a free surface, as on the skin or on a mucous membrane.

A termination of inflammation.

ulcerative (ŭl′sĕr-ā-tĭv) [L. *ulcerāre,* to form ulcers]. Pert. to or causing ulceration.

u. scrofuloderma. Tubercular scrofuloderma.

ulceromembranous (ŭl″sĕr-ō-mĕm′brăn-ŭs) [" + *membrana,* membrane]. Pert. to ulceration and formation of a fibrous pseudomembrane.

u. tonsillitis. Tonsillitis that ulcerates and develops a membranous film.

ulcerous (ŭl′sĕr-ŭs) [L. *ulcerāre,* to ulcerate]. Pert. to or affected with an ulcer.

ulcus (ŭl′kŭs) (pl. *ulcera*) [L.]. Ulcer.

u. cancro'sum. Cancerous ulcer which eats away the tissues. SYN: *rodent ulcer.*

u. cruris. Indolent ulcer of the leg.

u. durum. Lesion of syphilis. A hard ulcer. SYN: *chancre.*

u. induratum. A chancre, *q.v.*

u. molle. Chancroid or soft chancre, *q.v.*

u. tuberculo'sum. Tuberculosis of the skin. SYN: *lupus.*

ulectomy (ū-lĕk'tō-mĭ) 1. [G. *oulē*, scar, + *ektomē*, excision]. Excision of scar tissue, esp. in secondary iridectomy. 2. [G. *oulon*, gum]. Removal of gum tissue, as in pyorrhea alveolaris. SYN: *gingivectomy.*

ulegyria (ū''lē-gī'rĭ-ă). Condition in which gyri of the cerebral cortex are abnormal due to scar tissue from injuries usually occurring in early development.

ulemorrhagia (ū-lē-mor-ā'jĭ-ă). [G. *oulon;* gum, + *haimorrhagia*, bleeding]. Bleeding from the gums.

ulerythema (ū-lĕr-ĭ-thē'mă) [G. *oulē*, scar, + *erythēma*, redness]. An erythematous disorder with atrophic scar formation. SEE: *lupus erythematosus.*

u. centrifugum. Lupus erythematosus.

u. ophryog'enes. Folliculitis of eyebrows.

SYM: Falling out of hair and scarring

u. sycosiforme. Keloid sycosis.

uletic (ū-lĕt'ĭk) [G. *oulon*, gum]. Pert. to the gums.

uletomy (ū-lĕt'ō-mĭ) [G. *oulē*, scar, + *tomē*, a cutting]. Incision of a scar to relieve tension. SYN: *cicatricotomy.*

uliginous (ū-lĭj'ĭn-ŭs) [L. *uliginosus*, wet]. Muddy; slimy.

ulitis (ū-lī'tĭs) [G. *oulon*, gum, + *-itis*, inflammation]. Inflammation of the gums.

u., interstitial. Inflammation of connective tissue of gums about the necks of the teeth.

ulna (ŭl'nă) [L. *ulna*, elbow]. The inner and larger bone of the forearm, bet. the wrist and the elbow, on the side opposite that of the thumb.

It articulates with the head of the radius and humerus above and with the radius below.

RS: *coronoid process, cubital, cubitus, olecranon process, skeleton.*

ulnad (ŭl'năd) [" + *ad*, toward]. In the direction of the ulna.

ulnar (ŭl'nar) [L. *ulna*, elbow]. 1. Relating to the ulna, or to nerve or artery named from it. 2. Cuneiform carpal bone. SYN: *ulnare.*

ulnocarpal (ŭl''nō-kar'păl) [L. *ulna*, elbow, + G. *karpos*, wrist]. Relating to the carpus and ulna, or to the ulnar side of the wrist.

ulnoradial (ŭl''nō-rā'dĭ-ăl) [" + *radius*, spoke of a wheel]. Relating to the ulna and radius, as their ligaments and articulations.

ulocace (ū-lŏk'ă-sē) [G. *oulon*, gum, + *kakē*, badness]. Ulcerative inflammation of the gums.

ulocarcinoma (ū''lō-kar-sĭn-ō'mă) [" + *karkinos*, cancer, + *-ōma*, tumor]. Carcinoma of the gums.

ulodermatitis (u''lo-derm-ă-ti'tis). Skin inflammation with scar formation.

uloglossitis (ū''lō-glos-ī'tĭs) [" + *glossa*, tongue, + *-itis*, inflammation]. Inflammation of the gums and tongue.

uloid (ū'loyd) [G. *oulē*, scar, + *eidos*, resemblance]. 1. Scarlike. 2. A scarlike lesion caused by subcutaneous degeneration.

u. cicatrix. Same as *uloid, 2.*

uloncus (ū-lŏn'kŭs) [G. *oulon*, gum, + *ogkos*, mass]. Swelling or tumor of the gums. SEE: *epulis.*

ulorrhagia (ū-lor-ā'jĭ-ă) [" + *-rrhagia*, bleeding]. Bleeding from the gums.

ulorrhea (ū-lor-rē'ă) [" + *rhoia*, a flow]. Slow bleeding from the gums.

ulosis (ū-lō'sĭs) [G. *oulē*, scar, + *-ōsis*, condition]. Formation of scar tissue. SYN: *cicatrization.*

ulotic (ū-lŏt'ĭk) [G. *oulē*, scar]. Causing cicatrization. SYN: *cicatricial.*

ulotomy (ū-lŏt'ō-mĭ) 1. [" + *tomē*, a cutting]. The cutting of scar tissue to relieve deformity or tension. 2. [G. *oulon*, gum]. Incision of the gums.

ulotrichous (ū-lŏt'rĭk-ŭs) [G. *oulos*, woolly, + *thrix, trich-*, hair]. Having short, woolly hair, as a negro.

ulotripsis (u''lo-trip'sĭs) [G. *oulum*, gum. + *tripsis*, massage]. Stimulation of the gums by massage.

ultex (ŭl'tĕks). A bifocal glass in which the near section is ground with the spherical curve.

ultimate (ŭl'tĭm-ăt) [L. *ultimus*, last]. Final or last.

ultimobranchial bodies (ŭl-tĭ-mō-brăng'kē-ăl). Two embryonic pharyngeal pouches usually considered as rudimentary fifth pouches. They become separated from the pharynx and incorporated into substance of the thyroid gland where they lose their identity. Also called *postbranchial bodies, lateral thyroids.*

ultra- [L.]. Prefix meaning *beyond, excess.*

ultrabrachycephalic (ŭl''tră-brăk''ĭ-sē-făl'ĭk) [L. *ultra*, beyond, + G. *brachys*, short, + *kephalē*, head]. Having a cephalic index of 90 or over.

ultracentrifuge (ŭl-tră-sĕn'trĭ-fūzh). A high speed centrifuge capable of producing centrifugal forces more than 100,000 times gravity. Used in the study of proteins, viruses, etc.

ultrafilter (ŭl-tră-fĭlt'ĕr). A filter by which colloidal particles may be separated from their dispersion medium or from crystalloids.

ultrafiltration (ŭl''tră-fĭl-trā'shŭn) [" + *filtrum*, a filter]. Filtration of a colloidal substance in which the dispersed particles, but not the liquid, are held back.

ultraligation (ŭl''tră-lī-gā'shŭn) [" + *ligāre*, to bind]. Ligation of a blood vessel beyond the origin of a branch.

ultramicrobe (ŭl''tră-mī'krōb) [" + G. *mikros*, tiny, + *bios*, life]. A microorganism too small to be visible by the ordinary microscope.

ultramicroscope (ŭl''tră-mī'krō-skōp) [" + " + *skopein*, to examine]. Microscope by which objects invisible through an ordinary microscope may be seen by means of powerful side illumination. A darkfield microscope, *q.v.*

ultramicroscopy (ŭl''tră-mī-krŏs'kō-pĭ) [" + " + *skopein*, to examine]. The use of the ultramicroscope for scientific purposes.

ultrasonic (ŭl-tră-sŏn'ĭk) SYN: *supersonic.* Pertaining to sounds of frequencies above 20,000 cycles per second which are inaudible to the human ear.

ultrasonics (ŭl-tră-sŏn'ĭks). SYN: *supersonics.* Sounds with frequencies greater than 20,000 cycles per sec. Biological effects may result depending on intensity of beams. *Heating effects* are produced by beams of low intensity, *paralytic effects* by those of moderate intensity, and *lethal effects* by those of high intensity. The lethal action of ultrasonics is primarily the result, either directly or indirectly, of cavitation. Ultrasonics are utilized clinically for therapeutic and diagnostic purposes.

ultraviolet (ŭl″tră-vī′ō-lĕt) [" + *violet*]. Beyond the visible spectrum at its violet end, said of rays. SEE: *infrared rays.*

u. rays. Invisible rays emitted by very hot bodies and ionized gases with wave lengths between 3900 A° and 1800 A°. From a therapeutic standpoint, physiological effects include (a) erythema production, (b) pigmentation of skin, (c) antirachitic effect through production of vitamin D, (d) bactericidal effects, and (e) various effects on metabolism. In clinical practice, dosage is measured in terms of *minimum erythemal dose* (ABBR: M.E.D.).

u. therapy. Treatment with ultraviolet radiation. SEE: *heliotherapy, light therapy.*

ultravirus (ŭl″tră-vī′rŭs) [" + *virus*, poison]. A virus which is filtrable but which can be demonstrated by inoculation test. SEE: *virus, filtrable.*

umbilical (ŭm-bĭl′ĭ-kăl) [L. *umbilicus*, navel]. Pert. to the umbilicus.

u. cord. The attachment connecting the fetus with the placenta, artificially severed at birth of the child.

It leaves a depression on the abdomen of the child called the navel or *umbilicus,** where the cord was attached to the fetus. It contains two arteries and one vein protected by Wharton's jelly. The embryo receives nourishment from the blood. This is supplied by the arteries of the umbilical cord which go from the placenta to the fetus.

Cord should not be cut or tied until umbilical vessels have ceased pulsating. This gives the infant a better blood supply. SEE: *Wharton's jelly.*

u. fissure. Portion of hepatic longitudinal fissure in which the umbilical vein is lodged.

u. hernia. A hernia in the region of the umbilicus.

u. souffle. A hissing sound said to arise from the u. cord.

u. vesicle. That part of the embryonic yolk sac leading from the umbilicus.

umbilicate (ŭm-bĭl′ĭ-kāt) [L. *umbilicātus*, dimpled]. Pert. to or shaped like the navel, noting a bacterial colony with a central depression resembling an umbilicus.

umbilication (ŭm-bĭl-ĭ-kā′shŭn) [L. *umbilicātus*, dimpled]. 1. A depression resembling a navel. 2. Formation at apex of a pustule or vesicle of a pit or depression.

umbilicus (ŭm-bĭ-lī′kŭs, -bĭl′ĭ-kŭs) (pl. *umbilici*) [L. a pit]. A depressed point in the middle of the abdomen; the scar which marks the former attachment of the umbilical cord to the fetus.

RS: *angiolysis; funic; f. souffle; funiculus; funis; hydromphalus; mesogastrium; navel; "omphal-" words; umbilical cord; varicocomphalus; Wharton's jelly.*

umbo (ŭm′bō) [L. boss]. Projecting center of a round surface.

u. of tympanic membrane. The central depressed portion of concavity on lateral surface of tympanic membrane. It marks the point where the handle (manubrium of malleolus) is attached to inner surface.

umbrascopy (ŭm-brăs′kō-pĭ) [L. *umbra*, shadow, + G. *skopein*, to view]. Use of shadows in refraction of the eye or use of roentgen rays. SYN: *skiascopy.*

un- [A.S.]. Prefix meaning *back, reversal, annulment of, not.*

uncia (ŭn′sĭ-ă) [L. *uncia*, the twelfth part of a whole]. An ounce, or an inch.

unciform (ŭn′sĭ-form) [L. *uncus*, hook, + *forma*, shape]. Hook-shaped.

u. bone. Hook-shaped bone on ulnar side of distal row of the carpus. SYN: *os hamatum.*

u. fasciculus. Bundle of fibers connecting frontal cerebral lobes with the temporosphenoid ones.

u. process. 1. Long, thin lamina of bone from orbital plate of the ethmoid articulating with the inf. turbinate. 2. Hook at ant. end of hippocampal gyrus. 3. Hooked end of unciform bone.

Uncinaria (ŭn-sĭn-ā′rĭ-ă) [L. *uncus*, a hook]. Former term applied to a genus of hookworms which included species now in the genera Necator and Ancylostoma.

uncinariasis (ŭn-sĭ-nă-rī′ă-sĭs) [L. *uncus*, hook]. Hookworm disease. SYN: *ancylostomiasis, q.v.*

u. of skin. Vesicular dermatitis generally of the feet from invasion by the *Uncinaria duodenale.*

uncinate (ŭn′sĭn-āt) [L. *uncinātus*, hooked]. Hook-shaped; hooked.

u. bundle of Russell. SYN: *fastigiobulbar tract.* Fibers arising in fastigial sup. cerebellar peduncle and pass inferiorly to vestibular nuclei and reticular formation by which impulses are carried to muscles, esp. those of neck and body.

u. convolution. SEE: *u. gyrus.*

u. epilepsy. Form of e. occurring in disease of uncinate area of the temporal lobe.

u. fasciculus. Bundle of fibers connecting orbital gyri of frontal lobe with rostral portion of temporal lobe. They curve sharply as they pass over lateral fissure of cerebrum.

u. fits. Episodic attacks characterized by olfactory and gustatory hallucinations, usually disagreeable, a sense of unreality, and sometimes convulsions and temporary loss of senses of taste and smell. Associated with lesions of uncinate gyrus.

u. gyrus. SYN: *uncinate convolution, uncus.* A gyrus of the temporal lobe consisting of recurved rostral portion of hippocampal gyrus.

unconditioned reflex. An inborn or natural reflex; one not dependent upon previous experience or training.

unconscious (ŭn-kŏn′shŭs) [A.S. *un*, not, + L. *conscius*, conscious], 1. Insensible; lacking in awareness of the environment. 2. State in which a person experiences no sensory impressions and has no subjective experiences. SEE: *unconsciousness.* 3. PSY: That part of our personality consisting of a complex of feelings and drives of which we are unaware and which are not available to our consciousness.

unconsciousness (ŭn-kŏn′shŭs-nĕs) [A.S. *un*, not, + L. *conscius*, aware]. State of being insensible or without conscious experiences.

Unconsciousness physiologically occurs in *sleep;* pathologically it may occur temporarily as in *syncope* (fainting) or be prolonged and vary in depth from *stupor* (semiconsciousness) to *coma* (profound unconsciousness).

CAUSES: Anoxia; alcohol, barbiturate and bromide intoxication; brain tumor, cerebral accident (hemorrhage, thrombosis, embolism), concussion, cardiac decompensation, carbon monoxide poisoning, diabetes, epilepsy, eclampsia, fear, fracture of skull, fright, heat stroke, hemorrhage (especially subarachnoid), hypertensive encephalopathy, meningitis, neurosyphilis, opium poisoning, pneumonia, subdural hematoma, severe infections, uremia.

SYM: Patient unable to swallow; eyes do not react, insensible to surroundings.

If face is flushed, or if hemorrhage is present or suspected, do not lower head and do not give stimulants. In all other instances, it is desirable to lower head and shoulders, loosen clothing and keep patient comfortably warm but not hot. Turn head to one side to prevent vomit, if any, from being drawn into lungs. Loosen clothing. Fresh air and, if necessary, artificial respiration. Look for fractures, paralysis. Test pulse, respiration, odor of breath, condition of skin and pupils of eyes. Make a diagnosis prior to further treatment.

TO MOVE AN UNCONSCIOUS PATIENT FROM STRETCHER TO BED: *Method I*: 1. Fold draw sheet in half lengthwise and place it across center of stretcher, pleating the excess and tucking the ends under for about 6 in. before patient is put on stretcher. 2. When patient is on stretcher this sheet should be under the buttocks. 3. Place stretcher parallel with bed and as close as you can get it. Get 3 other people to help you. 4. Have one person at patient's head, one at feet, one at side, and one at far side of bed. The ones at the sides take firm hold of the ends of the draw sheet and all 4 lift together, the person at the far side pulling the draw sheet toward her.

Method II: 1. This takes 3 people. 2. Place stretcher at right angles to the foot of the bed. Patient's head at end nearest bed. 3. Standing side by side the 3 people put their arms under patient, lift him, and swing him around onto the bed.

unconsciousness, words pert. to: aochlesia, aphrenia, aphronia, apoplexy, apopsychia, asphyctic, asphyxial, asphyxiation, catalepsy, collapse, coma, fainting, gas, shock, sleep, stupor, syncope, trance, twilight sleep.

unction (ŭnk'shŭn) [L. *unctio*, ointment]. 1. The application of an ointment. 2. Substance used for anointing. SYN: *unguent*.

unctuous (ŭnk'chū-ŭs) [L. *unctus*, an ointment]. Oily; greasy.

uncus (ŭn'kŭs) [L. *uncus*, hook]. 1. Any structure that is hook-shaped. 2. Hooked ant. end of hippocampal gyrus.

undernutri'tion. 1. A deficiency in one or more of the essential dietary constituents. 2. As generally used, a state of nutritional deficiency principally in calories and protein.

SYM: Loss of body weight, representing at first mostly loss of body fat, then loss of protein manifested by atrophy of muscles, weakness, hypothermia, bradycardia, lowered BMR, edema, psychoneuroses.

undertoe (ŭn'dĕr-tō) [A.S. *under*, beneath, + *tā*, toe]. Condition of displacement of the great toe underneath the others.

underweight. Condition in which body weight is at least 10% less than average weight for persons of the same age, sex, height, and body build.

undifferentiation (ŭn-dĭf-ĕr-ĕn-shĭ-ā'shŭn) [A.S. *un*, not, + L. *differens*, bearing apart]. Alteration in cell character to a more embryonic type or toward a malignant state. SYN: *anaplasia*.

undine (ŭn'dĭn). A small glass flask used for irrigating the conjunctiva and in removal of a cataract.

undinism (ŭn'dĭn-ĭzm). Awakening of the libido by running water, as by urination or at sight of urine.

undulant (ŭn'dū-lănt) [L. *undulatus*, wavy]. Rising and falling like waves, or moving like them.

u. fever. SYN: *brucellosis, Malta fever*. An infectious disease characterized by fever which rises to 104° or 105° F. in the evening and drops gradually to normal in the morning. Other symptoms are weakness, sweats, chills, anorexia, general malaise, and nervous symptoms. Caused by one of three species of *Brucella* affecting animals: *Br. abortus*, cattle, hogs), *Br. suis*, (hogs), and *Br. melitensis* (goats).

undulate (ŭn'dū-lāt) [L. *undulatus*, wavy]. Wavy; having a wavy border with shallow sinuses, said of bacterial colonies.

undulation (ŭn-dū-lā'shŭn) [L. *undulatus*, wavy]. A continuous wavelike motion or pulsation.

u., jugular. A venous pulse.

u., respiratory. Fluctuations in blood pressure due to respiratory movements.

ung. [L.]. Abbr. of *unguentum*, ointment.

ungual (ŭng'gwăl) [L. *unguis*, nail]. Pert. to or resembling the nails. SYN: *unguinal*.

u. phalanx. Terminal phalanx of each finger and toe.

u. tuberosity. Spatula - shaped extremity of the terminal phalanx which supports the nails of fingers and toes.

unguent (ŭng'gwĕnt) [L. *unguentum*, ointment]. A lubricant or salve for sores, burns, etc. SYN: *ointment*.

unguentum (ŭn-gwĕn'tŭm) [L. *unguentum*, ointment]. 1. Fatty, soft, solid preparation intended to be applied to the skin by inunction.

2. Simple ointment. SYN: *ointment, q.v.*

unguis (ŭng'gwĭs) (pl. *ungues*) [L. *unguis*, nail]. 1. A finger- or toenail. SYN: *onyx*. 2. The lacrimal bone. 3. Pus mass in cornea. 4. A white prominence on floor of the lateral ventricle's post. horn. SYN: *hippocampus minor*.

u. incarnatus. An ingrowing nail, esp. a toenail.

ungula (ŭn'gū-lă) [L. *ungula*, claw]. Instrument for removal of dead fetus.

uni- [L.]. Combining form meaning *one*.

uniarticular (u"nĭ-ar-tik'u-lar). Pertaining to a single joint. SYN: *monoarticular*.

unicellular (ū"nĭ-sĕl'ū-lar) [L. *unus*, one, + *cellula*, a little box]. Having only one cell.

uniceps (u'nĭ-seps). Having a single head or origin, as in muscles.

unicorn (ū'nĭ-korn) [" + *cornū*, horn]. Having a single cornu or horn.

u. uterus. A uterus with but 1 horn perfectly formed.

unicornous (ū-nĭ-kor'nŭs) [" + *cornū*, horn]. Having but 1 horn or cornu.

unigravida (ū"nĭ-grăv'ĭ-dă) [" + *gravida*, pregnant]. Woman who is pregnant for the first time.

unilateral (ū"nĭ-lăt'ĕr-al) [L. *unus*, one, + *latus, later-*, side]. Affecting or occurring on only one side. SEE: *ipsilateral; homolateral; contralateral*.

unilocular (ū"nĭ-lŏk'ū-lar) [" + *loculus*, a little place]. Having but one cavity.

uninuclear, uninucleate(d (ū"nĭ-nū'klē-ar, -āt, -ā-tĕd) [" + *nucleus*, a kernel]. Having only one nucleus.

uniocular (ū"nĭ-ok'ū-lar) [" + *oculus*, eye]. Pert. to or having only one eye.

union (ūn'yŭn) [L. *unio*, oneness, union]. 1. Act of joining 2 or more things into 1 part, or state of being so united. 2. Growing together of severed or broken parts, as of bones or lips of a wound. SEE: *healing*.

u. of granulations. A healing by third* intention with wound filling up with granulations.

u., non-. Failure to unite, as a fractured bone.

u., secondary. A healing by second* intention with adhesion of granulating surfaces.

u., vicious. Union of ends of a broken bone in such a way as to cause deformity.

unioval (ū"nĭ-ō'văl) [L. *unus*, one, + *ovum*, egg]. Developed from 1 ovum, as identical twins.

unipara (ū-nĭp'ă-ră) [" + *parere*, to bring forth]. A woman who has had only 1 child.

uniparous (ū-nĭp'ă-rŭs) [" + *parere*, to bring forth]. 1. Having produced but 1 child. 2. Giving birth to 1 offspring at a time.

unipolar (ū"nĭ-pō'lar) [L. *unus*, one, + *polus*, pole]. 1. Having or pertaining to one pole. 2. Having a single process as a *unipolar neuron*.

unit (ū'nĭt) [L. *unus*, one]. 1. One of anything. 2. A determined amount adopted as a standard of measurement.

u., Allen-Doisy. SEE: *unit, mouse; unit, rat.*

u., amboceptor. The smallest amount of amboceptor required in the presence of which a given quantity of red blood corpuscles will be dissolved by an excess of complement.

u., Angström. An internationally adopted unit of measurement of wave length, 1/10,000,000 of a millimeter, or 1/254,000,000 of an inch. ABBR: A° or A. u.

u., antigen. Smallest quantity of antigen required to fix 1 unit of complement, preventing hemolysis.

u., antitoxic. A unit for expressing the strength of an antitoxin. Originally the various units were defined biologically but now are compared to a weighed standard specified by the U. S. Public Health Service and the World Health Organization.

u., British thermal. The amt. of heat necessary to raise 1 pound of water at 39° F. one degree.

u. of capacity. Capacity of a condenser which gives a difference of potential of 1 volt when charged with 1 coulomb. SYN: *curie; farad.*

u., cat. The amount of a drug per kg. of weight of animal just sufficient to kill a cat when injected intravenously slowly and continuously.

u., complement. Smallest quantity of complement required for hemolysis of a given amount of red blood corpuscles with 1 amboceptor unit present.

u., electrical. SEE: *ampere, ohm, volt, watt, etc.*

u., Hampson. An x-ray unit of measurement, ¼ the erythema dose.

u., hemolytic. The amount of inactivated immune serum which causes complete hemolysis of 1 cc. of a 5% emulsion of washed red blood corpuscles, in the presence of complement.

u., Holzknecht. An x-ray unit of measurement, 1/5 the erythema dose. ABBR: *H.*

u., immunizing. SEE: *antitoxic unit.*

u., international. One defined and adopted by the International Conference for Unification of Formulae.

u., i., of vitamin A. The vitamin activity of 0.0006 mg. of the international standard carotene.

u., i., of vitamin B. The vitamin activity of 10 mg. of the international standard absorption product.

u., i., of vitamin C. The vitamin activity of 0.05 mg. of the international standard levo-ascorbic acid.

u., i., of vitamin D. The vitamin activity of 1 mg. of the international standard solution of irradiated ergosterol.

u., Kienböck. Measurement of x-ray dosage, 1/10 the erythema dose.

u., light. A foot-candle, or the amount of light 1 ft. from a standard candle.

u., Mache. Unit of measurement of radium emanation. ABBR: *M. u.*

u., mouse. Least amount of estrus-producing hormone which induces, in a spayed mouse, a characteristic desquamation of the vaginal epithelium.

u., physical. SEE: *coulomb, erg, dyne, household measures, metric system, apothecaries' s., avoirdupois s., troy weight.*

u., radiation. SEE: *unit, Mache.*

u., rat. Greatest dilution of an estrus-producing hormone which will cause desquamation and cornification of vaginal epithelium during 1st day, if given to a mature spayed rat in 3 injections, 1 every 4 hours.

u., toxic. A vague term used to define the minimum lethal dose of a toxin.

u., x-ray. SEE: *Kienböck u.*

unitarian (ū-nĭ-tā'rĭ-an) [L. *unitarius*]. Composed of a single unit.

u. theory. That of Bordet that assumes only 1 alexin or complement in the serum of an animal, despite the fact that the alexins in different species differ.

unitary (ū'nĭ-tā-rĭ) [L. *unitarius*]. Relating to a unit. SYN: *unitarian.*

uniterminal (ū"nĭ-ter'mĭn-ăl) [L. *unus*, one, + *terminus*, end]. Having only 1 terminal. SEE: *monoterminal.*

univalent (ū"nĭ-vā'lĕnt, ū-nĭv'ă-lĕnt) [" + *valens*, to be powerful]. 1. Possessing the power of combining or replacing 1 atom of hydrogen. 2. Single, noting a chromosome which lacks or fails to unite with a synaptic mate.

universal (ū"nĭ-ver'săl) [L. *universalis*, combined into one whole]. General.

u. antidote. 2 parts activated charcoal; 1 part tannic acid; 1 part magnesium oxide. Give orally a paste of 5 heaping teaspoonsful of the mixture dissolved in a glass of water. After the patient has swallowed the antidote, the stomach contents should then be removed by gastric lavage. Use in cases of poisoning where specific antidote is unknown or not available.

u. donor. A person belonging to blood group O whose blood as a rule may be transfused without danger of untoward reactions into persons belonging to any of the other blood groups.

NOTE: Because there are multiple blood type factors in addition to those of ABO, it would be dangerous to assume that group O blood could, without further tests of compatibility, be given to persons of different blood type.

u. recipient. A person belonging to blood group AB, whose serum will not agglutinate the cells of any blood group.

unofficial (ŭn-of-ĭsh'ăl) [A.S. *un,* not, + L. *officialis,* doing work]. Not listed by the pharmacopeia or National Formulary, with reference to drugs.

unorganized (ŭn-or'găn-īzd) [" + L. *organizāre,* to form a structure]. 1. Not organized into an organic structure. 2. Without the characteristics of a living organism; inorganic.

unphysiological. Contrary to physiological principles.

unrest. Turbulence, instability, or irregularity.

unsaturated (ŭn-săt'ū-rāt"ĕd) [" + L. *saturāre,* to sate]. 1. Capable of dissolving or absorbing to a greater degree. 2. Not combined to the greatest possible extent.

u. compound. An organic compound having double or triple bonds between the carbon atoms.

unsex (ŭn-sĕks') [A.S. *un,* not, + L. *sexus,* sex]. To castrate; to spay or excise the ovaries.

unstriated (ŭn-strī'āt-ĕd) [" + *striātus,* striped]. Unstriped, as smooth muscle fiber.

unwell (ŭn-wĕl') [" + *wel*]. 1. Sick; ill; indisposed. 2. Menstruating.

upsiloid (ŭp'sĭ-loyd) [G. *upsilon,* letter U, + *eidos,* form]. Shaped like the letter U or V.

urachal (ū'ră-kăl) [G. *ourachos,* fetal urinary canal]. Relating to the urachus.

urachus (ū'ră-kus) [G. *ourachos,* fetal urinary canal]. An epithelioid cord surrounded by fibrous tissue extending from apex of bladder to umbilicus. In the embryo it is continuous with the allantoic stalk; postnatally it forms the *middle umbilical ligament* (of the bladder).

u., patent. Condition in which urachus remains as a hollow tube connecting vertex of bladder with umbilicus resulting in an umbilical urinary fistula.

uracil (u'ră-sil). A base found combined with D-ribose and phosphoric acid in yeast nucleic acid.

uracrasia (ū-ră-kră'sĭ-ă) [G. *ouron,* urine, + *akrasia,* incontinence]. 1. A disordered condition of urine. 2. Inability to retain the urine. SYN: *urinary incontinence.*

uracratia (ū-ră-kră'shĭ-ă) [G. *ouron,* urine, + *akratia,* incontinence]. Incontinence of the urine.

uragogue (ū'ră-gog) [" + *agogos,* leading]. Increasing the secretion of urine. SYN: *diuretic.*

uranalysis (ū"răn-ăl'ĭs-ĭs) [G. *ouron,* urine, + *ana,* apart, + *lysis,* a loosening]. Urinalysis, *q.v.*

uraniscomitis (ū-răn-ĭs"kon-ī'tĭs) [G. *ouraniskos,* palate, + *-itis,* inflammation] Inflammation of the palate.

uraniscoplasty (ū-răn-ĭs'kō-plăs"tĭ) [" + *plassein,* to form]. Operation for repair of cleft palate. SYN: *uranoplasty, uranorrhaphy.*

uraniscorrhaphy (ū-răn-ĭs-kor'ră-fĭ) [" + *rhaphē,* a seam]. Operation for suturing of a cleft palate. SYN: *uraniscoplasty.*

uraniscus (ū-răn-ĭs'kŭs) [G. *ouraniskos,* palate]. Palate, or roof of mouth.

uranism (ū'răn-ĭzm) [G. *ouranos,* heaven, + *-ismos,* condition]. Homosexuality.

uranist (ū'răn-ĭst) [G. *ouranos,* heaven]. A homosexual.

uranium (ū-rā'nĭ-ŭm) [G. *ouranos,* sky]. SYMB: U. Primary radioactive element, the parent of radium and other radioelements. At. wt. 238.04, at. no. 92.

uranoplasty (ū'răn-ō-plăs"tĭ) [G. *ouranos,* palate, + *plassein,* to form]. Operation for cleft palate. SYN: *uraniscoplasty.*

uranoplegia (ū"ră-nō-plē'gĭ-ă) [G. *ouranous,* vault, + *plēgē,* stroke]. Paralysis of muscles of the soft palate.

uranorrhaphy (ū-răn-or'ră-fĭ) [" + *rhaphē,* a seam]. Operation for suture of a cleft palate. SYN: *uraniscorrhaphy.*

uranoschisis (ū-răn-ŏs'kĭs-ĭs) [" + *schisis,* a fissure]. Cleft palate.

uranostaphyloplasty (ū"răn-ō-stăf'ĭl-ō-plăs"tĭ) [" + *staphylē,* uvula, + *plassein,* to form]. Operation for correction of a defect of the soft and hard palates.

uranostaphylorrhaphy (ū"răn-ō-stăf-ĭl-or'-ă-fĭ) [" + " + *rhaphē,* a seam]. Operation for repair of cleft of hard and soft palates.

urapostema (u-ră-pos-te'mă) [G. *ouron,* urine, + *apostema,* abscess]. An abscess containing urine.

uraroma (ū-ră-rō'mă) [G. *ouron,* urine, + *aroma,* spice]. Aromatic, spicy odor of the urine.

urase. Urease, *q.v.*

urate (ū'rāt) [G. *ouron,* urine]. Combination of uric acid with a base; a salt of uric acid.

Urates in urine insignificant unless excessive. Urates can be dispersed by boiling the urine. SEE: *antiuratic.*

uratemia (ū"ră-tē'mĭ-ă) [" + *aima,* blood]. Urates, esp. sodium urate, in the blood.

uraturia (ū"ră-tū-rĭ'ă) [G. *ouron,* urine]. Excess of urates in the urine. SYN: *lithuria.*

urceiform (ŭr-se'ĭ-form) [L. *urceus,* pitcher, + *forma,* shape]. Pitcher shaped.

urea (ū-rē'ă) [G. *ouron,* urine]. The diamide of carbonic acid, a crystalline solid having the formula $CO(NH_2)_2$; found in blood, lymph, and urine.

It is formed in the liver from ammonia derived from amino acids by deamination. It may also be formed directly from arginine.

It is the chief nitrogenous constituent of urine and final product of protein metabolism in the body, and carrying off 85% of the nitrogen excreted.

It is without odor and is colorless, appearing as white prismatic crystals, and forming salts with acids. Its excess is one of the causes of *uremia, q.v.* The amount excreted per day varies from 20-70 Gm., or about an ounce (30 Gm.) on the average. The amount of excreted urea is less on a low protein diet. From 8 to 10 Gm. per day may be excreted on a low protein diet of 50 Gm. per day.

USES: As a diuretic.

INCOMPATIBILITIES: Chloral hydrate, lead acetate.

INCREASED UREA: Observed in (a) fevers and loss of weight; (b) in increased protein intake; (c) following a large intake of water or beer; (d) during and after parturition.

DECREASED UREA: Observed in (a) reduced elimination; (b) low protein intake; (c) pregnancy; (d) gain in weight.

U. CONCENTRATION TEST: Performed for estimating renal efficiency.

It depends upon fact that when healthy kidneys are presented with an extra amount of urea in blood, they will excrete an equal amount of urea into urine.

Method: The patient urinates, and is then given a solution of 15 Gm. of urea in 2 or 3 oz. of water to drink. After 1 hr. patient urinates again, and also after the 2nd hr. The 2 specimens are then tested for the amount of urea, which should rise above 2%.

u. frost. White flaky deposits of urea seen on skin in patients with advanced uremia.

u. nitrogen. Abbr. *BUN*. The nitrogen of urea as distinguished from nitrogen in blood proteins.

ureagenetic (ū-rē"ă-jĕn-ĕt'ĭk) [urea + G. *genesis*, production]. Pert. to or producing urea.

ureal (ū-rē'ăl) [urea from G. *ouron*, urine]. Relating to or containing urea.

ureameter (ū-rē-ăm'et-er) [urea + G. *metron*, a measure]. Device for determining amount of urea in urine. SYN: *ureometer*.

ureametry (ū-rē-ăm'ĕt-rĭ) [urea + G. *metron*, a measure]. Determination of amt. of urea in urine.

ureapoiesis (ū-rē"ă-poy-ē'sĭs) [urea + G. *poiēsis*, formation]. Formation of urea. SYN: *ureopoiesis*.

urease (ū'rē-ās) [urea, from G. *ouron*, urine]. An enzyme which accelerates hydrolysis of urea into ammonium carbonate and hippuric acid into glycocoll and benzoic acid.

It is found in alkaline fermentation of urine, produced by many microorganisms, and is also found in seeds, as the soybean.

It is used in determining the amount of urea in blood or in urine.

urecchysis (ū-rĕk'ĭs-ĭs) [G. *ouron*, urine, + *ekchysis*, a pouring out]. Effusion of urine into areolar tissue.

uredema (ū-re-dē'mă) [" + *oidēma*, a swelling]. Urine in the subcutaneous tissues distending them.

uredo (ū-rē'dō) [L. *uredo*, a blight]. 1. Burning sensation in the skin. 2. Skin disorder marked by smooth, white elevations which itch severely. SYN: *hives*, *urticaria*, *q.v.*

ureide (ū'rē-īd) [urea from G. *ouron*, urine]. Any compound of urea in which acid radicals have taken the place of 1 or more of its hydrogen atoms.

urelcosis (ū-rĕl-kō'sĭs) [" + *elkōsis*, ulceration]. Ulceration of the urinary tract.

uremia (ū-rē'mĭ-ă) [G. *ouron*, urine, + *aima*, blood]. Toxic condition associated with renal insufficiency and the retention in the blood of nitrogenous substances normally excreted by the kidney. SEE: *azotemia*.

ETIOL: Result of disturbed kidney metabolism seen in nephritis and due to suppression or deficient secretion of urine from any cause.

SYM: Nausea, vomiting, headache, dizziness, dimness of vision, coma or convulsions, urinous odor of breath, and perspiration. Stupor, stertorous respiration. No change in pupillary reaction; dry skin; hard, rapid pulse; elevated blood pressure; scanty urine containing casts and albumin. There is a reduction of urea, and presence of tube casts in uremic coma. Urea retention 150 to 500 mg. or more per 100 ml. SEE: *coma, uremic*.

u., extrarenal. Uremia, prerenal, *q.v.*

u., prerenal. Uremia occurring not as a result of primary renal disease but due to other conditions such as disturbances in circulation, fluid balance, or metabolism arising in other parts of the body. Also called *prerenal azotemia*.

uremic (ū-rē'mĭk) [G. *ouron*, urine, + *aima*, blood]. Pert. to or caused by uremia.

uremide (ū're-mīd) [" + *aima*, blood]. The skin lesions of uric acid poisoning.

uremigenic (ū-rē-mĭ-jĕn'ĭk) [" + " + *gennan*, to produce]. Caused by uremia or producing it.

ureometer (ū"rē-ŏm'ĕt-ĕr) [G. *ouron*, urine, + *metron*, a measure]. Appliance used to determine the amt. of urea in urine. SYN: *ureameter*.

ureometry (ū-rē-ŏm'ĕt-rĭ) [" + *metron*, a measure]. Estimation of amt. of urea in urine.

ureopoiesis (ū-rē"ō-poy-ē'sĭs) [" + *poiēsis*, formation]. Formation of urea. SYN: *ureapoiesis*.

urerythrin (ūr-er'ĭ-thrĭn) [" + *erythros*, red]. A red pigment in the urine in rheumatic and certain other fevers. SYN: *uroerythrin*.

uresiesthesia, uresiesthesis (ū-rē"sĭ-ĕs-thē'-zĭ-ă, -sĭs) [G. *ourēsis*, urination, + *aisthēsis*, sensation]. The normal inclination to void urine.

uresis (ū-rē'sĭs) [G. *ourēsis*, urination]. The excretion of urine. SYN: *urination*.

ureter (ū'rē-ter, ū-rē'tĕr) [G. *ourētēr*, ureter]. One of 2 tubes carrying urine from the kidneys to the bladder, beginning with the pelvis of the kidney, and emptying into the base of the bladder.

Each ureter averages about 11 inches in length and about ¼ in. in diameter. Its wall consists of three layers: the mucous, muscular, and fibrous coats.

RS: *autonephrectomy, kidney, urelcosis, "uret-" words*.

ureteralgia (ū-rē-ter-ăl'jĭ-ă) [G. *ourētēr*, ureter, + *algos*, pain]. Pain in the ureter.

uretercystoscope (ū-rē"tĕr-sĭs'tō-skōp) [" + *kystis*, bladder, + *skopein*, to examine]. A cystoscope combined with a ureteral catheter.

ureterectasis (ū-rē"tĕr-ĕk'tă'sĭs) [" + *ektasis*, dilatation]. Dilatation of the ureter.

ureterectomy (ū-rē"tĕr-ĕk'tō-mĭ) [" + *ektomē*, excision]. Excision of a ureter.

ureteritis (ū-rē"tĕr-ī'tĭs) [" + *-itis*, inflammation]. Inflammation of the ureters.

ureterocele (ū-rē'tĕr-ō-sēl) [G. *ourētēr*, ureter, + *kēlē*, hernia]. Cystlike dilatation of ureter near its opening into the bladder usually due to congenital stenosis of ureteral orifice.

ureterocolostomy (ū-rē"tĕr-ō-kō-lŏs'tō-mĭ) [" + *kōlon*, colon, + *stoma*, passage]. The implantation of the ureter into the colon.

ureterocystoneostomy (ū-rē"tĕr-ō-sĭst"ō-nē-ŏs'tō-mĭ) [G. *ourētēr*, ureter, + *kystis*, bladder, + *neos*, new, + *stoma*, passage]. Ureteroneocystostomy.

ureterocystostomy (ū-rē"tĕr-ō-sĭs-tŏs'tō-mĭ) [" + *kystis*, bladder, + *stoma*, passage]. Ureteroneocystostomy, *q.v.*

ureterodialysis (ū-rē"tĕr-ō-dī-ăl'ĭ-sĭs) [" + *dialysis*, a separation]. Rupture of a ureter. SYN: *ureterolysis*.

ureteroenterostomy (ū-rē"tĕr-ō-ĕn-ter-ŏs'-tō-mĭ) [" + *enteron*, intestine, + *stoma*, passage]. Formation of a passage bet. a ureter and the intestine.

ureterography (ū-rē"tĕr-ŏg'ră-fĭ) [" + *graphein*, to write]. X-ray photography of the ureter after injection of some opaque substance into the ureter.

ureterohydronephrosis (ū-rē"tĕr-ō-hī"drō-nē-frō'sĭs) [" + *ydōr*, water, + *nephros*, kidney, + *osis*]. Dilatation of ureter and pelvis of kidney resulting from an obstruction, either mechanical or of an inflammatory nature, in the urinary tract.

ureterolith (ū-rē'ter-ō-lĭth) [" + *lithos,* stone]. A stone or calculus in the ureter.

ureterolithiasis (ū-rē"ter-ō-lĭth-ī'ăs-ĭs) [" + " + *-iasis,* condition]. Development of a calculus in the ureter.

ureterolithotomy (ū-rē"ter-ō-lĭth-ŏt'ō-mĭ) [" + " + *tomē,* a cutting]. Surgical incision for removal of a calculus from ureter.

ureterolysis (ū-rē"ter-ŏl'ĭ-sĭs) [G. *ourētēr,* ureter, + *lysis,* loosening]. 1. Rupture of the ureter. SYN: *ureterodialysis.* 2. Paralysis of the ureter. 3. The process of loosening adhesions around the ureter.

ureteroneocystostomy (ū-rē"ter-ō-nē"ō-sĭs-tŏs'tō-mĭ) [" + *neos,* new, + *kystis,* bladder, + *stoma,* passage]. Surgical formation of a new passage bet. a ureter and the bladder. SYN: *ureterocystoneostomy, ureterocystostomy.*

ureteroneopyelostomy (ū-rē"ter-ō-nē"ō-pī-ĕ-lŏs'tō-mĭ) [" + " + *pyelos,* pelvis, + *stoma,* passage]. Excision of a portion of the ureter with attachment of the severed end of the lower portion to a new aperture in the renal pelvis. SYN: *ureteropycloneostomy.*

ureteronephrectomy (ū-rē"ter-o-nef-rĕk'-tō-mĭ) [" + *nephros,* kidney, + *ektomē,* excision]. Removal of a kidney and its ureter.

ureteropathy (ū-rē-ter-ŏp'ă-thĭ) [" + *pathos,* disease]. Any diseased condition of the ureter.

ureterophlegma (ū-rē"ter-ō-flĕg'mă) [" + *phlegma,* phlegm]. Mucous accumulation in the ureter.

ureteroplasty (ū-rē'ter-ō-plăs"tĭ) [" + *plassein,* to form]. Plastic surgery of the ureter.

ureteroproctostomy (ū-rē"ter-ō-prŏk-tŏs'-tō-mĭ) [G. *ourētēr,* ureter, + *prōktos,* anus, + *stoma,* passage]. Formation of a passage from the ureter to the anus.

ureteropyelitis (ū-rē"ter-ō-pī-ĕl-ī'tĭs) [" + *pyelos,* pelvis, + *-itis,* inflammation]. Inflammation of the pelvis of the kidney and a ureter.

ureteropyeloneostomy (ū-rē"ter-ō-pī"ĕl-ō-nē-ŏs'tō-mĭ) [" + " + *neos,* new, + *stoma,* passage]. Ureteroneopyelostomy, *q.v.*

ureteropyelonephritis (ū-rē"ter-ō-pī"ĕl-ō-nef-rī'tĭs) [" + " + *nephros,* kidney, + *-itis,* inflammation]. Inflammation of the renal pelvis and the ureter.

ureteropyeloplasty (ū-rē"ter-ō-pī'ĕl-o-plăs"tĭ) [" + " + *plassein,* to mold]. Plastic surgery of the ureter and renal pelvis.

ureteropyosis (ū-rē"tĕr-ō-pī-ō'sĭs) [" + *pyon,* pus, + *-ōsis,* condition]. Suppurative inflammation within a ureter.

ureterorrhagia (ū-rē"ter-or-rā'jĭ-ă) [" + *-rrhagia,* from *rhēgnunai,* to burst forth]. Hemorrhage from the ureter.

ureterorrhaphy (ū-rē"ter-or'ră-fĭ) [G. *ourētēr,* ureter, + *rhaphē,* a seam]. Suture of the ureter, as for fistula.

ureterosigmoidostomy (ū-rē"ter-ō-sĭg-moyd-ŏs'tō-mĭ) [" + *sigma,* letter S, + *eidos,* shape, + *stoma,* passage]. Surgical implantation of the ureter into the sigmoid flexure.

ureterostenosis (ū-rē"ter-ō-stĕn-ō'sĭs) [" + *stenōsis,* a narrowing]. Stricture of a ureter.

ureterostomy (ū-rē"ter-ŏs'tō-mĭ) [" + *stoma,* passage]. Formation of a permanent fistula for drainage of a ureter.

ureterotomy (ū-rē"ter-ŏt'ō-mĭ) [" + *tomē,* a cutting]. Incision or surgery of the ureter.

ureteroureterostomy (ū-rē"ter-ō-ū-rē"ter-ŏs'tō-mĭ) [G. *ourētēr,* ureter, + *ourētēr,* ureter, + *stoma,* passage]. 1. Formation of a connection from 1 ureter to the other. 2. Reestablishment of a passage bet. the ends of a divided ureter.

ureterovaginal (ū-rē"ter-ō-văj'ĭ-năl) [" + L. *vagina,* sheath]. Relating to a ureter and the vagina, noting a fistula connecting them.

ureterovesical (ū-rē"ter-ō-vĕs'ĭ-kăl) [" + L. *vesica,* bladder]. Pert. to a connection bet. the ureter and the bladder.

ureterovesicostomy (ū-rē"ter-ō-vĕs"ĭ-kŏs'-tō-mĭ) [" + " + G. *stoma,* passage]. Reimplantation of a ureter into the bladder.

urethra (ū-rē'thră) [G. *ourēthra,* urethra]. A canal for the discharge of urine extending from the bladder to the outside. In the female its orifice lies in the vestibule between vagina and clitoris; in the male, the urethra transverses the penis opening at the tip of the glans penis. In the male it carries semen as well as urine. (*Illus.,* p. U-9)

Its inner lining, the *mucosa,* is thrown into folds and contains openings of *lacunae* into which *glands of Littre* open. Surrounding the mucosa is a *lamina propria* containing many elastic fibers and blood vessels, outside of which is an indefinite muscular layer.

u. mulie'bris. The female urethra. SYN: *u. femina* [NA].

u. viri'lis. The male urethra. SYN: *u. masculina* [NA].

urethra, words pert. to: aerourethroscopy; anaspadias; ankylurethria; atreturethria; blennurethria; bulb; bulbourethral glands; Carcasonne's ligament; corpus spongiosum; gleet; habenula urethralis; hypospadias; meatus urinarius; Skene's glands; urelcosis; "urethr-" words.

urethral (ū-rē'thrăl) [G. *ourēthra,* urethra]. Relating to the urethra.

urethralgia (ū-rē-thrăl'jĭ-ă) [G. *ourēthra,* urethra, + *algos,* pain]. Urethral pain; pain in the urethra.

urethratresia (ū-rē-thră-trē'zĭ-ă) [" + *atrēsis,* imperforation]. Occlusion, or imperforation of the urethra.

urethrectomy (ū-rē-thrĕk'tō-mĭ) [" + *ektomē,* excision]. Surgical excision of the urethra or part of it.

urethremphraxis (ū-rē-thrĕm-frăk'sĭs) [" + *emphraxis,* obstruction]. Urethral obstruction. SYN: *urethrophraxis.*

urethreurynter (ū-rē-thrū-rĭn'ter) [" + *eurynein,* to dilate]. Appliance for dilating the urethra.

urethrism, urethrismus (ū'rē-thrĭzm, ū"rē-thrĭz'mŭs) [" + *-ismos,* condition]. Irritability or spasm of the urethra.

urethritis (ū-rē-thrī'tĭs) [G. *ourēthra,* urethra, + *-itis,* inflammation]. Inflammation of the urethra.

u., anterior. Inflammation of that portion of the urethra ant. to the ant. layer of the triangular ligament.

u., gonococcal. U. caused by gonococcus.

u., posterior. Inflammation of membranous and prostatic portions of the urethra.

u., simple. Catarrhal inflammation of the urethra. SYN: *blennorrhea.*

u., specific. Urethritis occurring in gonorrhea.

urethro- [G.]. Combining form meaning *urethra.*

urethrocele (ū-rē'thrō-sēl) [G. *ourēthra,* urethra, + *kēlē,* hernia]. 1. Pouchlike protrusion of the urethral wall in the

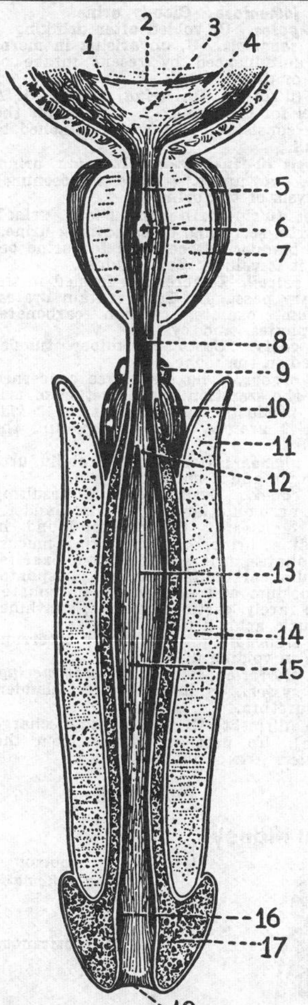

URETHRA, INTERIOR OF MALE, SHOWING THE FLOOR

1. Bell's muscle. 2. Interuretic ridge. 3. Internal trigone. 4. Left ureteric opening. 5. Crest. 6. Opening of utricle. 7. Prostate gland in section (surrounding prostatic portion of urethra). 8. Membranous portion of urethra. 9. Bulbourethral gland of left side. 10. Left half of bulb of urethra. 11. Left crus penis. 12. Openings of ducts of bulbourethral glands. 13. Spongy portion of urethra. 14. Left corpus cavernosum. 15. Urethral glands and lacunae. 16. Fossa navicularis urethrae. 17. Left half of glans penis. 18. Orifice of urethra.

female. 2. Thickening of connective tissue around the urethra in the female.

urethrocystitis (ū-rē″thrō-sĭs-tī′tĭs) [" + *kystis*, bladder, + *-itis*, inflammation]. Inflammation of urethra and bladder.

urethrography (ū-rē-thrŏg′ră-fĭ) [" + *graphein*, to write]. X-ray photography of the urethra, after the injection of an opaque medium.

urethrometer (ū-rē-thrŏm′et-er) [" + *metron*, a measure]. Instrument for measuring diameter of urethra or lumen of a stricture.

urethropenile (ū-rē″thrō-pē′nīl) [" + L. *penis*, penis]. Relating to the urethra and penis.

urethroperineal (ū-rē″thrō-pĕr-ĭ-nē′ăl) [" + *perinaion*, perineum]. Relating to the urethra and perineum.

urethroperineoscrotal (ū-rē″thrō-pĕr-ĭ-nē″-ō-skrō′tăl) [" + " + L. *scrotum*, pouch]. Relating to the urethra, perineum, and scrotum.

urethropexy (u-rēth′ro-pex-ĭ) [" + G. *pexis*, fixation]. Surgical fixation of the ureter.

urethrophraxis (ū-rē-thrō-frăks′ĭs) [G. *ourēthra*, urethra, + *phrassein*, to obstruct]. Urethral obstruction. Syn: *urethremphraxis*.

urethrophyma (ū-rē-thrō-fī′mă) [" + *phyma*, growth]. A neoplasm in the urethra.

urethroplasty (ū-rē′thrō-plăs″tĭ) [" + *plassein*, to mold]. Reparative surgery of the urethra.

urethrorectal (ū-rē″thrō-rĕk′tăl) [" + L. *rectus*, straight]. Relating to the urethra and the rectum.

urethrorrhagia (ū-rē″thror-ā′jĭ-ă) [" + *-rrhagia*, from *rhēgnunai*, to burst forth]. Hemorrhage from urethra.

urethrorrhaphy (ū-rē-thror′ăf-ĭ) [" + *rhaphē*, a seam]. Suture of the urethra, as a urethral fistula.

urethrorrhea (ū-rē″thror-ē′ă) [" + *rhoia*, a flow]. Morbid discharge from the urethra.

u. **ex libidine.** The discharge of normal glandular secretions resulting from sexual stimulation, esp. that preceding sexual intercourse.

urethroscope (ū-rē′thrō-skōp) [G. *ourēthra*, urethra, + *skopein*, to examine]. Device for examining interior of urethra

urethroscopic (ū-rē″thrō-skŏp′ĭk) [" + *skopein*, to examine]. Relating to the urethroscope or urethroscopy.

urethroscopy (ū-rē-thrŏs′kō-pĭ) [" + *skopein*, to examine]. An examination of the mucous membrane of the urethra with a urethroscope.

urethrospasm (ū-rē′thrō-spăzm) [" + *spasmos*, a spasm]. Spasmodic stricture of the urethra.

urethrostaxis (ū-rē″thrō-staks′ĭs) [" + *staxis*, a dropping]. Oozing of blood from the urethral mucous membrane.

urethrostenosis (ū-rē″thrō-sten-ō′sĭs) [" + *stenōsis*, a narrowing]. Stricture of the urethra.

urethrostomy (ū-rē-thrŏs′tō-mĭ) [" + *stoma*, opening]. Formation of a permanent fistula opening into the urethra by perineal section and fixation of membranous urethra in perineum.

urethrotome (ū-rē′thrō-tōm) [G. *ourēthra*, urethra, + *tomē*, a cutting]. An instrument for incision of urethral stricture.

urethrotomy (ū-rē-thrŏt′ō-mĭ) [" + *tomē*, a cutting]. Incision of a urethral stricture.

urethrovaginal (ū-rē″thrō-văj′ĭ-năl) [" + L. *vagina*, sheath]. Pert. to the urethra and vagina.

urhydrosis (ūr-ĭ-drō′sĭs). Condition in which urinary urea, uric acid occurs in excess in sweat.

uric (ū′rĭk) [G. *ouron*, urine]. Of or pert. to urine.

u. acid. $C_5H_4N_4O_3$, a crystalline acid, occurring as an end-product of purine metabolism. It is formed from purine bases derived from nucleoproteins.

It is a common constituent of urinary and renal calculi, and gouty concretions.

OUTPUT: Bet. 0.5 and 1 gm. per day on ordinary mixed diet. Uric acid must be excreted, as it cannot be destroyed within the body.

INCREASED ELIMINATION: Observed in: (1) Ingestion of proteins; (2) gout; (3) leukemia; (4) acute articular rheumatism; (5) after exercise, and (6) the ingestion of nitrogenous foods.

DECREASED ELIMINATION: Observed in: (a) Nephritis; (b) chlorosis; (c) lead poisoning; (d) protein-free diet.

u. a., endogenous. Uric acid derived from purines undergoing metabolism from the nucleoprotein of body tissues.

u. a., exogenous. Uric acid derived from those purines from food made up of free purines and nucleoproteins.

SEE: *urate, uraturia.*

uricacidemia (ū″rĭk-ăs-ĭd-ē′mĭ-ă) [G. *ouron*, urine, + L. *acidus*, sour, + G. *aima*, blood]. Excess uric acid in the blood.

uricaciduria (ū″rĭk-ăs-ĭd-ū′rĭ-ă) [" + " + G. *ouron*, urine]. Excessive amount of uric acid in the urine.

uricase (ū′rĭ-kāz) [G. *ouron*, urine, + *ase*, enzyme]. A hydrolytic enzyme capable of changing uric acid into allantoin.

uricemia (ū-rĭ-sē′mĭ-ă) [G. *ouron*, urine, + *aima*, blood]. SYN: *uricacidemia.* Excess uric acid in the blood.

uricocholia (ū″rĭk-ō-kō′lĭ-ă) [" + *cholē*, bile]. Uric acid in the bile.

uricolysis (ū-rĭk-ŏl′ĭs-ĭs) [" + *lysis*, dissolution]. The decomposition of uric acid.

uricolytic (ū″rĭk-ō-lĭt′ĭk) [" + *lysis*, dissolution]. Decomposing uric acid.

u. index. The amt. of uric acid converted into allantoin.

uricometer (ū-rĭk-ŏm′ĕ-tĕr) [" + *metron*, a measure]. Apparatus for quantitative estimation of uric acid in the urine.

uricopoiesis (ū″rĭk-ō-poy-ē′sĭs) [" + *poiēsis*, formation]. The development of uric acid.

uricosuria (ū-rĭk-ō-sū′rĭ-ă). The excessive excretion of uric acid in the urine.

uricosuric (u″rĭ-kōs-u′rik). Potentiating the excretion of uric acid in the urine.

u. agent. A drug (such as probenecid) that increases the urinary excretion of uric acid, thereby reducing the concentration of uric acid in the blood. Used in treatment of gout.

uricoxydase (ū″rĭk-oks′ĭ-dās) [G. *ouron*, urine, + *oxys*, sharp, + *ase*, enzyme]. An enzyme capable of oxidizing uric acid.

uridrosis (ū-rĭd-rō′sĭs) [G. *ouron*, urine. + *idrōsis*, a sweating]. The presence of urea in the sweat.

Evaporation may show white scales, the crystals of urinary solids.

u. crystalli′na. White powder of uric acid deposited on the skin. SYN: *urea frost.*

uriesthesis (ū-re-ĕs-thē′sĭs) [" + *aisthēsis*, sensation]. Normal desire to void urine.

urina (ū-rī′nă) [L.]. Urine.

u. cibi. Urine voided after a full meal.

u. cruenta. Bloody urine.

u. galactodes. Urine of a milky color.

u. hysterica. Watery, pale urine following hysteria.

u. jumentosa. Cloudy urine.

u. potus. U. voided after drinking.

u. sanguinis. U. on arising in morning uninfluenced by recent intake of food or drink.

urinal (ū′rĭn-ăl) [L. *urina*, urine]. 1. A vessel for the urine. 2. A toilet for the male consisting of a vessel attached to a wall.

urinalysis (ū-rĭn-ăl′ĭs-ĭs) [L. *urina*, urine, + G. *ana*, apart, + *lysis*, a loosening]. Analysis of the urine.

urinary (ū′rĭn-a″rĭ) [L. *urina*, urine]. Pert. to, secreting, or containing urine.

u. bladder. Receptacle for urine before it is voided. SEE: *bladder.*

u. calculi. Concretions formed in the urinary passages. They contain urates, calcium, oxalate, calcium carbonate, phosphates, and cystine.

u. casts. Casts of kidney tubules passed in the urine.

u. organs. The structures concerned with the secretion and excretion of urinary products, consisting of the *2 kidneys, 2 ureters,* the *bladder,* and the *urethra.*

u. pigments. Urochrome, urobilin, uroerythrin, and hematoporphyrin.

u. reflex. Desire to void resulting from accumulation of urine in bladder.

u. sediments. Substances found in standing urine, *i.e.*, bacteria, mucus, phosphates, uric acid, calcium oxalate, calcium carbonate, calcium phosphate. magnesium and ammonium phosphate; more rarely, cystine, tyrosine, xanthine, hippuric acid, hematoidin.

u. stammering. Temporary interruptions in voiding urine.

u. stuttering. Same as *u. stammering.*

u. system. Kidneys, ureters, bladder, and urethra.

urinate (ū′rĭn-āt) [L. *urinãre*, to discharge urine]. To pass the urine from the bladder. SYN: *micturate.*

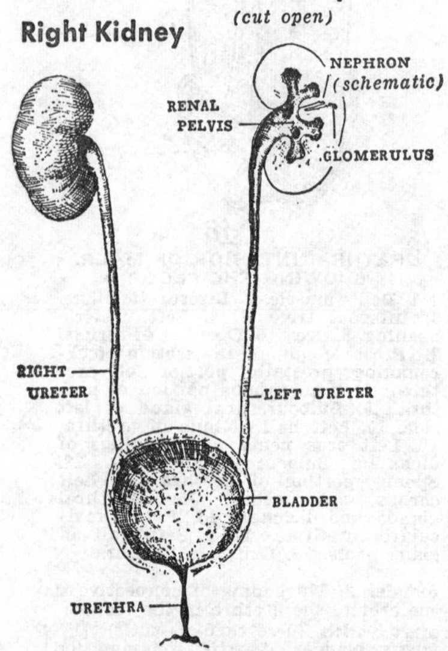

ENTIRE URINARY TRACT

urination (ū-rĭn-ā'shŭn) [L. *urinātio*, a discharging of urine]. The act of voiding urine. Syn: *micturition.*

Although this act is somewhat under voluntary control, it is accomplished chiefly by the action of involuntary muscles. The musculus sphincter vesicae relaxes, while the general musculature of the wall of the urinary bladder contracts to force out its contents.

Increased Frequency: Seen in polyuria; nervous excitement; irritation of bladder, urethra, or urinary meatus; disease of spinal cord; enlarged prostate in male; pregnancy in female; beer drinking; interstitial nephritis; diabetes; phimosis.

Decreased Frequency: After sweating, diarrhea, or bleeding; in anuria, oliguria, uremia, brain disease, drug poisoning, coma, and parenchymatous nephritis. See: *urine.*

urination, words pert. to: aconuresis, acraturesis, anisuria, bacilluria, bladder, bradyuria, catheterization, chaudepisse, diuresis, diuretic, dysuria, enuresis, kidney, melanuria, micturate, micturition, nocturia, nycturia, oliguria, polyuria, strangury, uracratia, urea, "uret-" words, uric acid, "urin-" words, void.

urine (ū'rĭn) [L. *urina*, from G. *ouron*, urine]. The fluid secreted from the blood by the kidneys, stored in the bladder, and discharged, usually voluntarily, through the urethra.

It is conveyed to the bladder by 2 ureters from the kidneys. In health, urine is of amber color, slightly acid reaction, and it has a peculiar odor, with a bitter, saline taste, frequently depositing a precipitate of phosphates when fresh, but especially on standing, and having a specific gravity that varies from 1.005 to 1.030.

The greater the amt. excreted, the lower is the specific gravity. The normal amt. of nonprotein nitrogen is from 25-35 mg. per 100 cc. of blood. The amount of this substance present in the blood is related to how well the kidneys are functioning.

The daily output is equally variable, being adapted to the amt. of water taken in, and to the amt. lost by evaporation from the respiratory and cutaneous surfaces.

Constituents of Urine

Urine consists of water (95%) and solids (5%). Solids amount to 40-50 gm. per liter and include the following (figures are grams per liter):

Organic substances: urea (23), hippuric acid (0.6), uric acid (0.6), creatine (1.5), other solids (2.0). *Inorganic substances:* sodium chloride (9), potassium chloride (2.5), sulfuric acid (1.8), phosphoric acid (1.8), ammonia (0.6) calcium (0.2), magnesium (0.2). In addition to the above, many other substances may be present depending on diet and state of health of the individual. Among substances indicating pathologic states are albumin, glucose, ketone bodies, blood, pus, casts, and bacteria.

Diagnosis

Color of Urine: Normal urine is amber color. Its color is imparted by urobilin,* a pigment mainly derived from bilirubin* in the bile. This pigment is found in more than normal quantities in fever, and it may be indicative of blood destruction. The effect of food and medication must be considered before concluding that the color of the urine reflects a pathological condition.

Black: Melanuria. Malignant pigmented tumor, melanotic cancer or carbolic acid poisoning.

Bile-colored: Seen in jaundice.

Blue: This may result from methylene blue or the presence of indigo.

Colorless urine: This is known as achromaturia.

Milky urine: May be due to chyluria, lipuria, or pus.

Orange-red urine: It may indicate the presence of pyridine dyes.

Pale urine: This indicates an excess of water. It is found in conditions causing polyuria.

Red or reddish color: This may be due to the presence of blood in the urine, hematuria, to senna or rhubarb, which may color the urine either brown or orange.

Condition of Urine: *Acid urine*: It may be found in acidosis and pyelonephritis.

Alkaline urine: This shows a white sediment.

Bacteria in urine: It appears cloudy.

Bloody urine: It shows a smoky sediment, and is reddish-brown.

Pus in urine: This is mucoid and shows a white sediment. It is found in bacterial infections of the urinary tract.

Odor of Urine: *Ammoniacal*: This may result from decomposition products.

Aromatic urine: This is the odor of a normal urine.

Fecal odor: This is due to fistulous communication bet. the intestinal and urinary tracts.

Fishy odor: Cystitis.

New-mown hay odor: Indicative of diabetes.

Overripe apple odor: Indicative of acetonuria, or the presence of acetone bodies in the urine.

Violet odor: This may be caused by turpentine.

Urinary Products in Disease: *Albumin*: Due to nephritis and inflammation of mucous membrane of any portion of the urinary apparatus.

Acetone: Its presence represents the by-products of excessive fat metabolism excreted by the kidneys and known as *ketonuria.*

Animal parasites: Rare, found as result of contamination.

Bacteria: Usually regarded as being of little importance if fewer than 100,000 can be cultured from each ml. of urine.

Bile: Bile in the urine indicates abnormal retention of bile.

Blood: Indicates hemorrhagic nephritis, calculi, congestion of a kidney, renal carcinoma, tuberculosis of kidney, chronic infections.

Casts: These indicate renal disease. A few hyaline casts in the aged denote slight damage to the kidneys. Casts are found in large numbers in nephritis. The less acute the disease, the finer are the granular casts.

Crystals: Acid urine produces crystals, calcium oxalate, and urates; alkaline urine, ammonium biurate and phosphates. Crystals have little significance, excepting leucine and tyrosine crystals which indicate yellow atrophy of the liver, or phosphorus poisoning, or other serious liver damage.

Cylindroids: They have no special significance.

Diacetic acid: Indicates deficient carbohydrate metabolism of an advanced stage. It is preceded by the presence of acetone.

Epithelial cells (squamous): If in large numbers from urinary bladder and ureters they indicate inflammation of these parts; *renal epithelial cells of kidney*: Serious damage to the same.

Fat droplets: Indicate fatty degeneration of kidneys and lipemia.

Froth around standing urine indicates presence of bile.

Indican: It has small significance but is seen in intestinal putrefaction and constipation.

Lipoids, double refractile: Epstein's lipoidal nephrosis.

Mucus: If visible and in quantity, urethritis is indicated. No special significance in women if the quantity is small.

Mucous threads: Mucoid, ribbonlike structures of no great significance.

Pus cells: Their presence may be normal if not many. If accompanied by red cells, they indicate inflammation.

Red blood cells: Stones or inflammation of kidney or urinary tract. No sig-

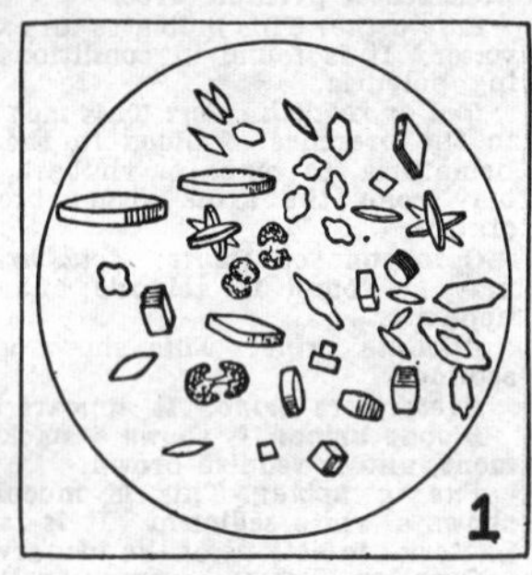

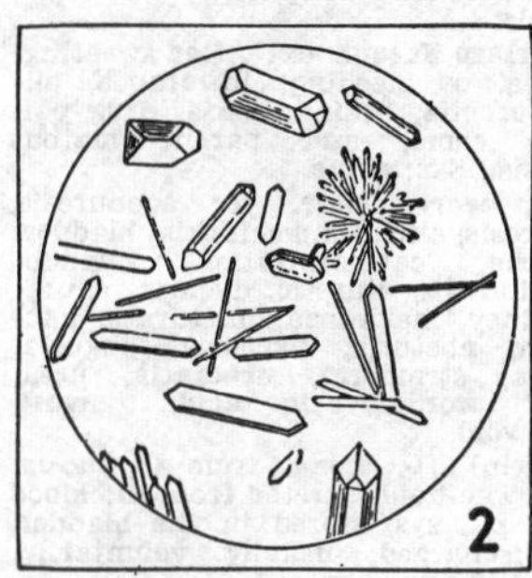

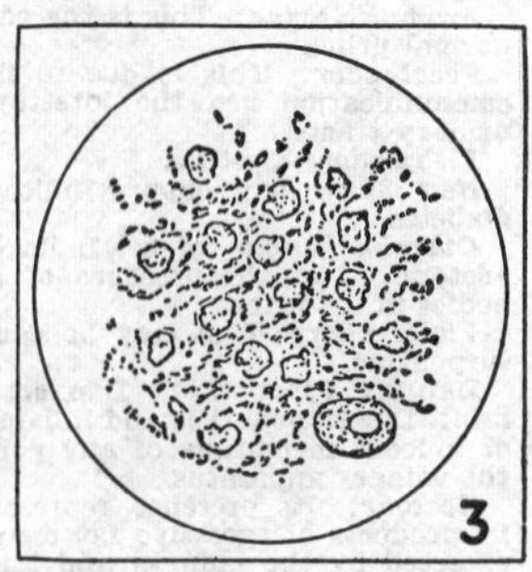

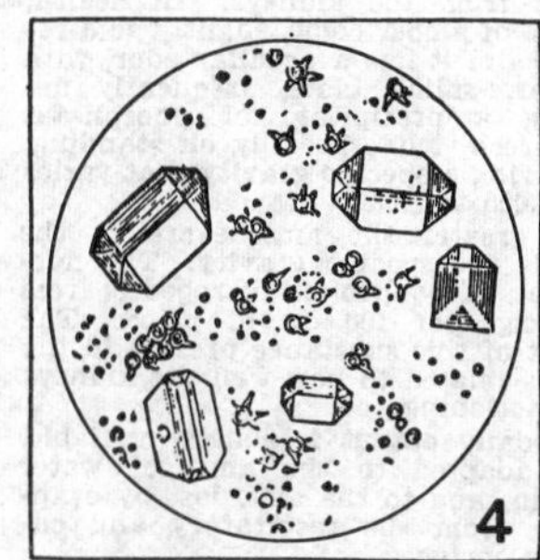

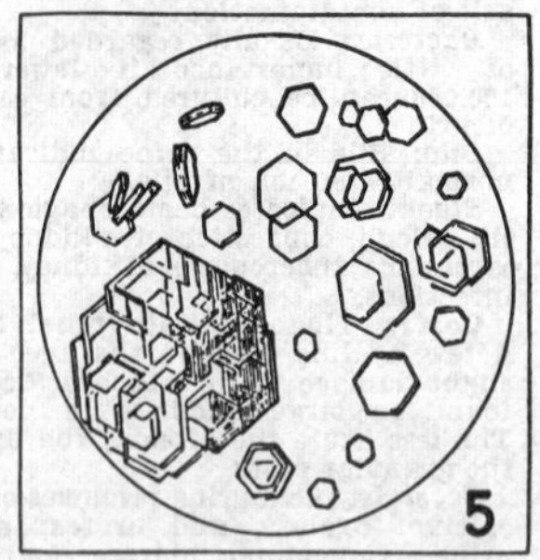

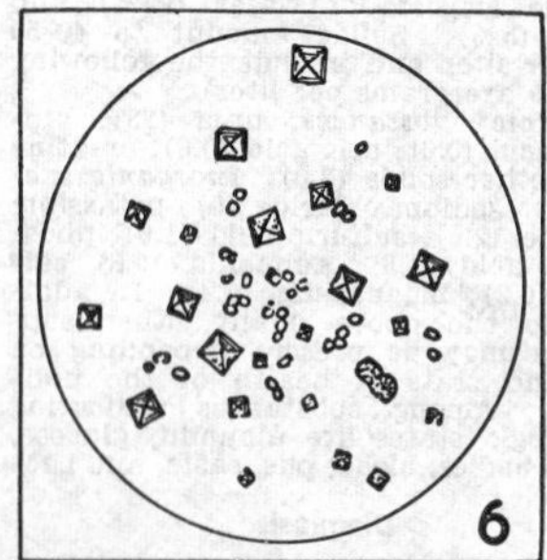

URINARY CONSTITUENTS

1. Various forms of uric acid crystals. 2. Crystals of hippuric acid. 3. Mucus deposited from urine. 4. Urinary sediment of triple phosphates (large, prismatic crystals) and urate of ammonium, from urine which had undergone alkaline fermentation. 5. Crystals of cystine. 6. Crystals of calcium oxalate.

nificance if due to contamination by menstrual fluid.

Sediment: Pinkish due to excess of urates, white, caused by phosphates.

Sugar (glucose): Denotes faulty carbohydrate metabolism as seen in diabetes mellitus.

Urea:* This is the principal end product of protein metabolism.

Yeasts and molds: Result of contamination. SEE: *urinary conditions*.

EXCRETION: *Increased in*: Fevers, esp. if weight is lost, after pregnancy, during parturition, after the intake of large quantities of liquid and after protein intake.

Diminished in: Pregnancy, convalescence with gain in weight, in disease of the liver, and in low protein intake.

URINARY CONDITIONS: *Difficult urine*. Found in urethral stricture, enlarged prostate, atony and impairment of the bladder's muscular power, and in gonorrhea and other inflammatory conditions involving the urethra, bladder, or lower ureter.

Diminished u. (oliguria). Cardiac failure. Scanty in all fevers, accompanies acute and chronic and parenchymatous nephritis, obstruction of return venous circulation of kidney, thrombosis of renal vein or inf. vena cava, loss of fluids through hemorrhages, vomiting or diarrhea, obstruction or pressure upon ureter, lead poisoning, or melancholia.

Frequent u. Excess of urea (azoturia) or of uric acid and urates (lithuria) Reflex of renal calculus in ureter; pyelitis.

Incontinence. SYN: *Enuresis, q.v.* Inability to retain urine. (a) Paralysis or relaxation of sphincters or (b) contraction of longitudinal muscular layer of bladder. Paralysis of both a and b, retention, incontinence and dribbling are

Significance of Changes in Urine

Quantity

Normal	Abnormal	Significance
1000-1500 cc. (96% H_2O)		Depends upon water and fluid foods consumed, exercise, temperature, kidney function, etc.
	High (polyuria)	Diabetes mellitus, diabetes insipidus, nervous diseases, certain types of chronic nephritis (kidney disorder), diuretics (drugs as caffeine, calomel, digitalis, causing increased urinary excretion).
	Low (oliguria)	Acute nephritis, heart disease, fevers, eclampsia, diarrhea, vomiting.
	None (anuria)	Uremia (urinary substances in blood), acute nephritis, metal poisoning, *e. g.*, due to bichloride of mercury.

Color

Normal	Abnormal	Significance
Yellow to amber		Depends upon concentration of pigment (urochrome).
	Pale	Diabetes insipidus, granular kidney, due to a very dilute urine.
	Milky	Fat globules, pus corpuscles in genitourinary infections.
	Reddish	Blood pigments, drugs, or food pigments.
	Greenish	Bile pigment, associated with jaundice.
	Brown-black	Poisoning (mercury, lead, phenol), hemorrhages.

Transparency

Normal	Abnormal	Significance
Clear		No significance.
Cloudy on standing		Precipitation of mucin from urinary tract. Not pathological.
Turbid		Precipitation of calcium phosphate. Not pathological.
	Milky	Presence of fat globules. Pathological.
	Turbid	Presence of pus as result of inflammation of urinary tract. Pathological.

Odor

Normal	Abnormal	Significance
Faintly aromatic		No significance.
	Pleasant (sweet)	Acetone, associated with diabetes mellitus.
	Unpleasant	Decomposition or ingestion of certain drugs or foods.

Specific Gravity

Normal	Abnormal	Significance
1.015 to 1.025 sp. gr.		Ordinarily, sp. gr. inversely proportional to volume.
	Low	Dilution, if volume is large, otherwise nephritis.
	High	Concentrated if volume is small; otherwise if volume is large and light colored, diabetes mellitus. Acute nephritis.

Acidity

Normal	Abnormal	Significance
Acid (slight)		Diet of acid-forming foods (meats, eggs, prunes, wheat, etc.) overbalancing the base-forming foods (vegetables and fruits).
	High acidity	Acidosis, diabetes mellitus, many pathological disorders (fevers, starvation).
	Alkaline	Putrefying bacteria change urea into ammonium carbonate. Infection or ingestion of alkaline compounds.

results. All forms of coma, shock, sunstroke and some forms of insanity, typhoid, typhus. Injuries to spinal cord and tumors of same and lesions; transverse myelitis, spinal meningitis, locomotor ataxia, paralysis. Reflex excitability of nervous system. Local irritation. Cystitis, phimosis, vesical calculus, meatus contracted, ascarides, diabetic or too concentrated urine. Relaxation of vesical sphincters. Hydrocyanic acid poisoning.

Increased u. (polyuria). May be indicative of chronic interstitial nephritis, diabetes (mellitus or insipidus), amyloid disease of kidney; reabsorption of effusions, functional disease of nervous system, as hysteria, neurasthenia, migraine, etc. Persistent in bulbar, cerebellar and spinal tumors, locomotor ataxia and meningitis.

Obstructive u. Result of occlusion of one or both ureters.

Painful urination. Dysuria.* Vesical tenesmus. There is a persistent desire to urinate.

Residual u. That remaining in bladder after urination. Usually indicative of a pathologic condition such as prostatic disease, cystocele, etc.

Retention of u. SYN: *ischuria.* Inability to urinate. Almost same diseases and injuries of cord producing incontinence. All forms of coma, typhoid, in peritonitis, and hysteria, atony, prostatic enlargement; urethral stricture, urethritis, cystitis or tumors of bladder or calculus in urethra.

Strangury. Painful and spasmodic. May be indicative of cystitis, neuralgia, tuberculosis, cancer or ulceration of bladder, urethritis, urethral stricture, hypertrophied, cancerous or inflamed prostate, prolapsus uteri, pelvic peritonitis and abscess, metritis, cancer of cervix, dysmenorrhea, vesical tenesmus. Pain and burning often caused by the concentrated or acid urine. May be a symptom of acute nephritis.

Suppression of u. Failure of kidneys to secrete urine. May be complete (*anuria*) or partial (*oliguria*). Failure of kidneys to secrete the urine or failure to reach the bladder if secreted may be found in acute nephritis or congestion, renal abscess, last stages of chronic nephritis. Renal damage caused by patient's having received the wrong type of blood. Inhalation of ether, lead, phosphorus, cantharides or turpentine poisoning, may occur in connection with Asiatic cholera, cholera infantum or cholera morbus, gastrointestinal perforations, shock or collapse. Typhoid or yellow fever, pernicious malaria, acute yellow atrophy of liver, hysteria.

SEDIMENT, HOW TO OBTAIN: The examination should be made quickly after urine is voided by centrifuging for 3 minutes.

urine, *words pert. to:* acathectic; acetone; a. bodies; a., tests for; acetonuria; achromaturia; acidaminuria; acromaturia; adrenaluria; albiduria; albinuria; albuminaturia; albuminorrhea; albuminuria; albumosuria; alkalinuria; alkaluretic; alkaptone; alkaptonuria; allantoinuria; allotriuria; alloxuria; Almen's test; aminosuria; ammoniuria; amylosuria;

amyluria; anisuria; antidiuresis; antidiuretic; anuresis; anuria; arabinosuria; ardor urinae; azoturia; baruria; Bence-Jones protein; Benedict's test; bilirubinuria; bladder, urinary; bladder stammering; bladder percussion; blennuria; blood, test for; brick dust; calcariuria; carbohydraturia; carboluria; carbonuria; cast; ceramuria; cerebrosuria; chlorides, test for; chloriduria; chloruremia; chloruria; cholerythrin; choleuria; choluria; chondroituria; chromaturia; chyluria; clap threads; diacetic acid test; epithelium; erythruria; Esbach's method; galactosuria; galacturia; glucose; glycosuria; Haines formula; Heller's test; hemoglobinuria; hippuria; hyaline casts; hydruria; incontinence; ischuria; jumentous; ketonuria; ketosis; kidney; lactosuria; lipuria; lithuria; litmus; melanuria; mucus; myosinuria; oliguresis; oxaluria; pentosuria; polydruria; pus; pyuria; residual; residuum; retention; Rothera's test; secretion; tyrosinuria; uraturia; urea; urechysis; uredema; uremia; ureter; uric acid; urinalysis; "uro-" words.

urinemia (ū-rĭn-ē′mĭ-ă) [L. *urina*, urine, + G. *aima*, blood]. Contamination of the blood with urinary constituents. SYN: *uremia, q. v.*

uriniferous (ū-rĭn-ĭf′ĕr-ŭs) [" + *ferre*, to bear]. Carrying urine.

u. tubules. Small tubes of the kidneys for passage of kidney products.

uriniparous (ū-rĭn-ĭp′ăr-ŭs) [" + *parere*, to bear]. Producing or secreting urine.

urinogenital (ū″rĭn-ō-jĕn′ĭt-ăl) [" + *genitalia*, genitals]. Pert. to the genital and urinary organs. SYN: *urogenital.*

urinogenous (ū″rĭn-ŏj′ĕn-ŭs) [" + G. *gennan*, to produce]. 1. Producing urine. 2. Originating in urine. SYN: *urogenous.*

urinoglucosometer (ū″rĭn-ō-glū″kōs-ŏm′ĕ-tĕr) [" + G. *glukus*, sweet, + *metron*, a measure]. Apparatus for estimating amt. of glucose in the urine.

urinology (ū-rĭn-ŏl′ō-jĭ) [" + G. *logos*, study]. Scientific study of the urine. SYN: *urology.*

urinoma (ū″rĭn-ō′mă) [L. *urina*, urine, + G. *-ōmo*, mass]. A cyst containing urine.

urinometer (ū-rĭn-ŏm′ĕt-ĕr) [" + G. *metron*, a measure]. Device for determining urine's specific gravity.

urinometry (ū″rĭn-ŏm′ĕt-rĭ) [" + G. *metron*, a measure]. Determination of specific gravity of the urine.

urinophil (ū′rĭn-ō-fĭl) [" + G. *philein*, to love]. Capable of existing in the urine, as bacteria which grow best in urine.

urinoscopy (ū-rĭn-ŏs′kō-pĭ) [" + G. *skopein*, to examine]. Examination of the urine.

urinose, urinous (ū′rĭn-ōs, ū′rĭn-ŭs) [L. *urina*, urine]. Having the characteristics of, or containing urine.

urisolvent (ū″rĭ-sŏl′vĕnt) [" + *solvens*, dissolving]. Dissolving uric acid or causing it to be dissolved.

urning (oorn′ĭng) [Ger.]. One exhibiting and conscious of sexual inversion. SYN: *homosexual, uranist.* SEE: *urningism.*

urningism, urnism (oorn′ĭng-ĭzm, oorn′ĭzm) [Ger.]. Perversion in which sexual desire is only for one of the same sex. SYN: *lesbianism, sapphism, tribadism, amor lesbicus, homosexualism, q. v.*

uro- [G.]. Combining form meaning *pert. to urine.*

uroacidimeter (ū″rō-ăs-ĭ-dĭm′ĕ-tĕr) [G *ouron*, urine, + L. *acidus*, sour, + G. *metron*, a measure]. An apparatus for measuring the degree of acidity of the urine.

urobilin (ū″rō-bĭl′ĭn) [G. *ouron*, urine, + L. *bilis*, bile]. A brown pigment formed by the oxidation of urobilinogen, a decomposition product of bilirubin. Urobilin may be formed in stools or in urine after exposure to air.

u. jaundice. J. said to be result of urobilin in the blood.

urobilinemia (ū″rō-bĭ″lĭn-ē′mĭ-ă) [" + " + G. *aima*, blood]. Urobilin in blood.

urobilinicterus (ū″rō-bĭ-lĭn-ĭk′tĕr-ŭs) [" + " + G. *ikteros*, jaundice]. Jaundice resulting from urobilinemia. SYN: *urobilin jaundice.*

urobilinogen (ū-rō-bĭ-lĭn′ō-jĕn) [" + " + G. *gennan*, to produce]. A colorless derivative of bilirubin from which it is formed by the action of intestinal bacteria. SYN: *stercobilinogen.*

urobilinogenemia (ū″rō-bĭ″lĭn-ō-jĕn-ē′mĭ-ă) [" + " + " + *aima*, blood]. Urobilinogen in the blood.

urobilinuria (ū″rō-bĭ″lĭn-ū′rĭ-ă) [" + " + G. *ouron*, urine]. Excess of urobilin in the urine.

urocele (ū′rō-sēl) [G. *ouron*, urine, + *kēlē*, hernia]. Effusion of urine into the scrotum.

urocheras (ū-rŏk′ĕr-ăs) [" + *cheras*, gravel]. Gravel or calcareous sediment in the urine. SYN: *uropsammus.*

urochesia (ū-rō-kē′zĭ-ă) [" + *chezein*, to defecate]. A discharge of urine in the feces.

urochrome (ū′rō-krōm) [" + *chrōma*, color]. The substance which gives urine its characteristic color. It is derived from urobilin.

uroclepsia (ū-rō-klĕp′sĭ-ă) [" + *kleptein*, judge]. A diagnosis by inspection of the urine.

urocrisis (ū-rŏk′rĭs-ĭs) [" + *krisis*, crisis]. 1. Change (generally favorable) which supervenes in the crisis of a disease accompanied by copious urination. 2. A crisis marked by excessive urination. 3. Pain in bladder in locomotor ataxia.

urocyanogen (ū″rō-sĭ-ăn′ō-jĕn) [" + *kyanos*, blue, + *gennan*, to produce]. A blue pigment in urine, esp. in cholera patients.

urocyanosis (ū″rō-sĭ-ăn-ō′sĭs) [G. *ouron*, urine, + *kyanos*, blue, + *-ōsis*, condition]. SYN: *indicanuria.* Blue discoloration of the urine. May be due to presence of indigo blue from oxidation of indican, or from ingestion of drugs such as methylene blue.

uroedema (ū″rō-ē-dē′mă) [" + *oidēma*, a swelling]. Extravasation of urine distending the tissues. SYN: *uredema.*

uroerythrin (ū″rō-er′ĭth-rĭn) [G. *ouron*, + *erythros*, red]. A reddish pigment sometimes present in urine. SYN: *urerythrin.*

uroflavin (ū″rō-flăv′ĭn). SYN: *aquaflavin.* A fluorescent substance present in the urine of persons taking riboflavin. It is not thought to be a degradation product of riboflavin.

urofuscin (ū″rō-fŭs′ĭn). A reddish-brown pigment sometimes found in samples of urine, esp. in cases of porphyrinuria.

urofuscohematin (ū″rō-fŭs″kō-hĕm′ăt-ĭn) [" + L. *fuscus*, brown, + G. *haima*, blood]. A red-brown pigment in urine in some diseases.

urogastrone (ū″rō-găs′trōn). A hormone-like substance present in urine which has an inhibitory effect on gastric secretion.

urogenital (ū″rō-jĕn′ĭ-tăl) [G. *ouron*, + L. *genitalia*, genitals]. SYN: *urinogenital.* Pertaining to the urinary and reproductive organs.

urogenous (ū-rŏj′ĕn-ŭs) [" + *gennan*, to produce]. SYN: *urinogenous*. 1. Producing urine. 2. Originating in urine.

uroglaucin (ū″rō-glaw′sĭn) [" + *glaukos*, green]. Indigo blue, a pigment sometimes occurring in the urine, assumed to be result of chromogen oxidation, as in *scarlatina*.

urogram (ū′rō-grăm) [" + *gramma*, a mark]. An x-ray photograph of any part of the urinary tract.

urography (ū-rŏg′ră-fĭ) [G. *ouron*, urine, + *graphein*, to write]. Roentgenography of any part of the urinary tract, after introduction of an opaque medium.

urogravimeter (ū″rō-grăv-ĭm′ĕt-ĕr) [" + L. *gravis*, heavy, + G. *metron*, a measure]. Apparatus for estimating sp. gr. of urine. SYN: *urinometer*.

urohematin (ū″rō-hĕm′ăt-ĭn) [" + *haima*, *haimat-*, blood]. Pigment in urine, considered as identical with hematin,* which alters color of urine in proportion to degree of oxidation.

urohematonephrosis (ū-rō-hĕm″ă-tō-nē-frō′sĭs). Pathological condition of kidney in which pelvis is distended with blood and urine.

urohematoporphyrin (ū″rō-hĕm″ăt-ō-por′-fĭr-ĭn) [" + " + *porphyra*, purple]. Iron-free hematin in urine when hemolysis occurs.

urokinase (u-ro-ki′nās). An enzyme obtained from human urine. Used experimentally for dissolving intravascular clots. It is administered intravenously.

urokinetic (ū-rō-kĭ-nĕt′ĭk). Resulting reflexly from stimulation of the urinary organs.

urolagnia (ū-rō-lăg′nĭ-ă). Sexual excitation associated with urine or urination.

urolith (ū′rō-lĭth) [" + *lithos*, stone]. A concretion in the urine.

urolithiasis (ū″rō-lĭth-ī′ăs-ĭs) [" + " + *iasis*, condition]. Formation of urinary calculi and the illness associated with the presence of calculi in the urinary tract. SEE: *calculus, renal*.

urolithology (ū″rō-lĭth-ŏl′ō-jĭ) [" + " + *logos*, a study]. Science dealing with urinary calculi.

urologic (ū-rō-lŏj′ĭk) [G. *ouron*, urine, + *logos*, study]. Pert. to urology.

urologist (ū-rŏl′ō-jĭst) [" + *logos*, a study]. One who specializes in the practice of urology.

urology (ū-rŏl′ō-jĭ) [" + *logos*, a study]. The branch of medicine concerned with the urinary tract in both sexes and the genital tract in the male.

urolutein (ū″rō-lū′tē-ĭn) [" + L. *luteus*, yellow]. A yellow pigment seen in the urine.

uromelanin (ū-rō-mĕl′ăn-ĭn). A black pigment occurring in urine resulting from the decomposition of urochrome.

urometer (ū-rŏm′ĕt-ĕr) [" + *metron*, a measure]. Instrument for determining specific gravity of urine. SYN: *urinometer*.

uroncus (ū-rŏn′kŭs) [" + *ogkos*, a mass]. A swelling or cyst containing urine.

uronephrosis (ū″rō-nĕf-rō′sĭs) [G. *ouron*, urine, + *nephros*, kidney, + *-ōsis*, condition]. Dilatation of renal structures from obstruction of urinary flow. Distention of renal pelvis and tubules with urine. SYN: *hydronephrosis*.

uronology (ū-rŏn-ŏl′ō-jĭ) [" + *logos*, a study]. The science of urine and genitourinary diseases. SYN: *urology*.

urononcometry (ū″rŏn-ŏn-kŏm′ĕ-trĭ) [" + *ogkos*, mass, + *metron*, a measure]. Measurement of amt. of urine voided in 24 hours.

uronophile (ū-rŏn′ō-fĭl) [" + *philein*, to love]. Developing best in a culture containing urine, noting a microorganism.

uropathy (ū-rŏp′ă-thĭ) [" + *pathos*, disease]. Any disease affecting the urinary tract.

u., obstructive. Any disease resulting from obstruction of the urinary tract.

uropenia (ū-rō-pē′nĭ-ă) [" + *penia*, a lack]. Lack of urinary secretion.

urophan (ū′rō-făn). A substance which when taken into the body appears unchanged in the urine.

urophanic (ū-rō-făn′ĭk) [" + *phainein*, to appear]. Appearing in the urine.

urophein, urophaein (ū″rō-fē′ĭn) [G. *ouron*, urine, + *phaios*, gray]. Gray pigment in urine said to cause its characteristic odor.

urophosphometer (ū″rō-fŏs-fŏm′ĕ-tĕr) [" + L. *phosphas*, phosphorus]. Device for estimating amt. of phosphorus in the urine.

uroplania (ū″rō-plā′nĭ-ă) [" + *planē*, a wandering]. Condition in which urine is present or discharged from parts other than the urinary organs.

uropoiesis ((ū″rō-poy-ē′sĭs) [" + *poiēsis*, production]. Secretion of urine by the kidneys.

uropoietic (ū″rō-poy-ĕt-ĭk) [" + *poiein*, to form]. Concerned in the formation of urine, or uropoiesis.

uroporphyrin (ū-rō-por′fĭ-rin). A reddish pigment present in the urine and feces in cases of porphyria. May also be present in the urine of persons taking certain drugs.

uropsammus (ū″rō-săm′ŭs) [" + *psammos*, sand]. Gravel or calcareous sediment in the urine. SYN: *urocheras*.

uropyonephrosis (ū″rō-pī-ō-nĕf-rō′sĭs) [G. *ouron*, urine, + *pyon*, pus, + *nephros*, kidney, + *-ōsis*, condition]. Urine and pus in the renal pelvis.

uropyoureter (ū″rō-pī″ō-ū-rē′tĕr) [" + " + *ourētēr*, ureter]. Mass of urine and pus in the ureter.

urorosein (ū″rō-rō′zē-ĭn) [" + L. *roseus*, rosy]. A rose-colored pigment in urine, which is increased in certain diseases. SYN: *urorrhodin*.

urorrhagia (ū-ror-ā′jĭ-ă) [" + *-rrhagia*, a flowing]. Excessive secretion of urine. SYN: *polyuria*.

urorrhea (ū-ror-ē′ă) [" + *rhoia*, a flow]. Involuntary flow of urine. SYN: *enuresis*.

urorrhodin (ū-rō-rō′dĭn) [" + *rhodon*, rose]. A rose-colored pigment in the urine. SYN: *urorosein, q.v.*

urorrhodinogen (ū-rō-rō-dĭn′ō-jĕn) [" + " + *gennan*, to produce]. A chromogen of the urine which, when decomposed, forms urorrhodin.

urorubin (ū-rō-rū′bĭn) [G. *ouron*, urine, + L. *ruber*, red]. A red pigment obtained from urine, by treatment with hydrochloric acid.

urorubrohematin (ū″rō-rū″brō-hĕm′ă-tĭn) [" + " + G. *haima*, *haimat-*, blood]. A reddish pigment occasionally found in the urine in some chronic diseases.

urosacin (ū-rō′sa-sĭn) [G. *ouron*, urine]. A red pigment in the urine. SYN: *urorrhodin*.

uroscheocele (ū-rŏs′kē-ō-sēl) [G. *ouron*, urine, + *oscheon*, scrotum, + *kēlē*, mass]. Swelling of scrotum from extravasation of urine into scrotal sac. SYN: *urocele*.

uroschesis (ū-rŏs′kĕs-ĭs) [" + *schesis*, a holding]. 1. Suppression of urine. 2. Retention of the urine.

uroscopy (ū-rŏs′kō-pĭ) [" + *skopein,* to examine]. 1. Examination of the urine. 2. Diagnosis by examination of the urine.

uroselectan (ū″rō-sĕ-lĕk′tăn) [G. *ouron,* urine]. A pyridine derivative for intravenous pyelography.

urosemiology (ū″rō-sē-mĭ-ŏl′ō-jĭ) [" + *sēmeion,* sign, + *logos,* study]. Examination of the urine as an aid to diagnosis.

urosepsin (ū-rō-sĕp′sĭn) [" + *sēpsis,* putrefaction]. A septic poison formed from decomposition of urine in the tissues.

urosepsis (ū-rō-sĕp′sĭs) [" + *sēpsis,* putrefaction]. Septic poisoning due to retention and absorption of urinary products in the tissues.

urospectrin (ū-rō-spĕk′trĭn) [" + L. *spectrum,* image]. A pigment derived from normal urine seen when shaken with acetic ether.

urostealith (ū″rō-stē′ă-lĭth) [" + *stear,* fat, + *lithos,* stone]. A fatty substance in some urinary calculi.

urotoxicity (ū″rō-tŏks-ĭs′ĭ-tĭ) [G. *ouron,* urine, + *toxikon,* poison]. The toxic character of the urine.

uroureter (ū″rō-u′rē-tĕr, -ū-rē′tĕr) [" + *ourētēr,* ureter]. Distention of the ureter with urine, due to stricture or obstruction.

urous (ū′rŭs) [G. *ouron,* urine]. Having the nature of urine.

uroxanthin (ū″rō-zăn′thĭn) [" + *xanthos,* yellow]. Yellow coloring matter of the urine; an indigo-forming substance.

uroxin (ū-rŏk′sĭn) [" + *oxys,* sharp]. A derivative of alloxan.*

urtica (ur′tĭk-ă). A wheal.

urticaria (ŭr-tĭ-kā′rĭ-ă) [L. *urtica,* nettle]. A vascular reaction of the skin characterized by the eruption of pale, evanescent wheals, which are associated with severe itching. SYN: *hives; nettle rash.* SEE: *allergy, angioneurotic edema (giant hives).*

ETIOL: Contact with an ext. irritant, as the nettle rash, physical agents, foods, insect bites, serum sickness, pollens, drugs, neurogenic factors.

SYM: Sudden general eruption of papules or wheals associated with intense itching.

TREATMENT: *General measures.* Because the skin manifestation is an allergic reaction, identify and remove the antigenic offender if possible. Check diet for common offenders such as wheat, milk, eggs, chocolate and other food allergens. Avoid unnecessary medication as drugs are often causative factors. *Specific measures.* Antihistaminic drugs often give quick relief. Injection of epinephrine (subcutaneous). Ephedrine may be used. In severe cases ACTH or cortisone used with caution has proved effective. *Locally,* antipruritic lotions and baths are frequently beneficial.

u. bullo′sa. Eruption of temporary vesicles with infusion of fluid under the epidermis.

u. facti′tia. Wheals following slight irritation of the skin. SYN: *dermatographia.*

u. haemorrhagica. U. with lesions infiltrated with blood.

u. maculo′sa. A chronic form of u. with red-colored lesions.

u. mariti′ma. U. due to salt water bathing.

u. medicamento′sa. U. due to certain drugs.

u. papulosa. In this form the wheal is followed by a lingering papule which is attended by considerable itching. Most commonly observed in debilitated children. SYN: *lichen urticatus, prurigo simplex.*

u. solaris. Urticaria occurring in certain individuals following exposure to sunlight.

u. vesiculo′sa. Same as *u. bullosa.*

urticarial, urticarious (ŭr-tĭk-ā-rĭ-ăl, ŭr-tĭk-ā′rĭ-ŭs) [L. *urtica,* a nettle]. Pert. to urticaria.

urtication (ŭr-tĭk-ā′shŭn) [L. *urtica,* a nettle]. 1. Flogging of a part with nettles to induce counterirritation. 2. Burning or itching sensation. 3. Eruption of itching wheals. SYN: *urticaria.*

urushiol (oo′roo-she-ol″). The principal toxic irritant substance of plants such as poison ivy which produce severe dermatitis upon contact.

U. S. A. N. Abbr. for *United States Adopted Name.* A non-proprietary name for a drug.

U. S. P., U. S. Phar. Abbr. for *United States Pharmacopeia.*

U. S. P. H. S. Abbr. for *United States Public Health Service.*

ustilaginism (ŭs-tĭl-ăj′ĭn-ĭzm) [L. *ustulatus,* scorched]. Poisoning resulting from eating corn infected with smut fungus, *Ustilago maydis.*

Ustilago (us-tĭl-ā′gō). A moldlike fungus, *Ustilago maydis,* commonly called smut.

ustion (ŭs′chŭn) [L. *ustio,* a burning]. 1. Cauterization with actual cautery. 2. Incineration.

ustulation (ŭs-tū-lā′shŭn) [L. *ustulāre,* to scorch]. Roasting, parching, or drying of a moist substance.

ustus (ŭs′tŭs) [L.]. Burned. SEE: *calcination.*

uta (oo′tă). American leishmaniasis, *q.v.*

ut. dict. Abbr. for L. *ut dictum,* as directed.

utend. Abbr. for L. *utendus,* to be used.

uter-, utero. Combining forms, denoting *pertaining to the uterus.*

uteralgia (ū-tĕr-ăl′jĭ-ă) [L. *uterus,* womb, + G. *algos,* pain]. Uterine pain.

uterectomy (ū-tĕr-ĕk′tō-mĭ) [" + G. *ektomē,* excision]. Removal of uterus through the abdomen or vagina. SYN: *hysterectomy, q.v.*

uterine (ū′tĕr-ĭn, -īn) [L. *uterinus,* pert. to the womb]. Pert. to the uterus.

u. bleeding. Bleeding from the uterus. Physiologic bleeding via the vagina occurs in normal menstruation. Abnormal forms include excessive menstrual flow (*hypermenorrhea, menorrhagia*) or too frequent menstruation (*polymenorrhea*). Nonmenstrual bleeding is called *metrorrhagia. Pseudomenstrual or withdrawal bleeding* may occur following estrogenic therapy. "Breakthrough" bleeding is the term used for intermenstrual bleeding which sometimes occurs in women who take progestational agents.

u. cake. The placenta.

u. glands. The tubular glands in the endometrium.

u. milk. A milky, white substance bet. the gravid uterus and the placental villi.

u. souffle (soof′l). Vascular sound in the pregnant uterus heard with stethoscope.

u. subinvolution. Failure of the uterus to return to normal size after childbirth. A uterus which weighs more than 100 gm. is considered to be enlarged.

u. tubes. Small tubes attached to either side of the uterus, and leading from the region of the ovary. SYN: *fallopian tubes.*

uterismus (ū"ter-ĭs-mŭs). Painful contractions of the uterus.

uteritis (ū-tĕr-ī'tĭs) [L. *uterus*, womb, + G. *-itis*, inflammation]. Inflammation of the uterus. SYN: *metritis.*

uteroabdominal (ū"tĕr-ō-ăb-dŏm'ĭn-ăl) [" + *abdominalis*, pert. to abdomen). Pert. to both the uterus and abdomen.

uterocele (ū-tĕr'ō-sēl) [" + G. *kēlē*, hernia]. Hernia containing the uterus.

uterocervical (ū"tĕr-ō-sĕr'vĭ-kăl) [" + *cervix*, neck]. Relating to the uterus and the cervix.

uterocystostomy (ū"tĕr-ō-sĭs-tŏs'tō-mĭ) [" + G. *kystis*, bladder, + *stoma*, mouth]. Formation of a passage bet. the uterine cervix and the bladder.

uterofixation (ū"tĕr-ō-fĭks-ā'shŭn) [" + *fixātio*, a fixing]. Fixation of a displaced uterus. SYN: *hysteropexy.*

uterogestation (ū-tĕr-ō-jĕs-tā'shŭn) [L. *uterus*, womb, + *gestātio*, a carrying]. Pregnancy in the uterus; normal pregnancy.

uterography (ū"tĕr-ŏg'ră-fĭ) [" + G. *graphein*, to write]. Roentgenography of the uterus.

uterolith (ū'tĕr-ō-lĭth) [" + G. *lithos*, stone]. A uterine concretion.

uterologist (ū"tĕr-ŏl'ō-jĭst) [" + G. *logos*, a study]. One who specializes in the practice of gynecology and obstetrics. Obsolete term.

uterology (ū-tĕr-ŏl'ō-jĭ) [" + G. *logos*, a study]. Gynecology combined with obstetrics. Obsolete term.

uterometer (ū"tĕr-ŏm'ĕt-ĕr) [" + G. *metron*, a measure]. Device for measuring the uterus and for determining its position.

uteroovarian (ū"tĕr-ō-ō-vā'rĭ-ăn) [L. *uterus*, womb, + *ovarium*, ovary]. Relating to the uterus and ovary.

uteropexia, uteropexy (ū"tĕr-ō-pĕks'ĭ-ă, ū'tĕr-ō-pĕks-ĭ) [" + G. *pexis*, fixation]. Fixation of the uterus to the abdominal wall. SYN: *hysteropexy.*

uteroplacental (ū"tĕr-ō-plă-sen'tăl) [" + *placenta*, a flat cake]. Relating to the placenta and uterus.

uteroplasty (ū"tĕr-ō-plăs'tĭ) [" + G. *plassein*, to form]. Reparative operation upon the uterus.

uterosacral (ū"tĕr-ō-sā'krăl) [" + *sacralis*, pert. to the sacrum]. Relating to the uterus and sacrum.

uterosalpingography (ū"tĕr-ō-săl-pĭng-ŏg'-ră-fĭ) [" + G. *salpigx*, tube, + *graphein*, to write]. Visualization of the interior of the uterus and fallopian tubes by x-ray.

uteroscope (ū'tĕr-ō-skōp) [L. *uterus*, womb, + G. *skopein*, to examine]. Device for viewing the uterine cavity.

uterotome (ū'tĕr-ō-tōm) [" + G. *tomē*, a cutting]. An instrument used for uterotomy. SYN: *hysterotome.*

uterotomy (ū-tĕr-ŏt'ō-mĭ) [" + G. *tomē*, a cutting]. Incisions of the uterus.

uterotonic (ū"tĕr-ō-tŏn'ĭk) [" + G. *tonos*, tone]. Giving muscular tone to the uterus.

uterotractor (ū"tĕr-ō-trăk'tor) [" + *tractor*, a drawer]. An instrument for making traction on the cervix uteri.

uterotubal (ū"tĕr-ō-tū'băl) [" + *tuba*, tube]. Relating to the uterus and the oviducts.

uterovaginal (ū"tĕr-ō-văj'ĭ-năl) [" + *vagina*, sheath]. Relating to the uterus and vagina.

uterovesical (ū"tĕr-ō-vĕs'ĭ-kăl) [" + *vesica*, bladder]. Relating to the uterus and bladder.

uterus (ū'tĕr-ŭs) [L. *uterus*, womb]. An organ of the female for containing and nourishing the embryo and fetus from the time the fertilized egg is implanted to the time of birth of the fetus. SYN: *womb.*

ANAT: A muscular, hollow, pear-shaped structure of the female. It is partly covered by peritoneum, the cavity lined by mucous membrane which is the *endometrium.*

The uterus consists of three areas: the *body* or expanded upper portion, the *isthmus* or constricted central area, and the *cervix*, the lowermost cylindrical portion at the upper end of the vagina. The rounded portion of the body lying above the openings of the two uterine tubes is the *fundus.*

It is supported in this position by the *pelvic diaphragm*, supplemented by two *broad ligaments*, two *round ligaments*, and two *uterosacral ligaments*, as well as other lesser ligaments.

The upper part of the body is called the *fundus* and the ends of the fundus to which the tubes are attached are called the *cornual ends.* The cavity of the uterus is triangular in shape, with the base of the triangle in the fundal portion. The canal of the cervix is long and narrow, and is constricted at the upper end by the internal os and at the lower end by the external os.

The largest portion of the uterus is made up of musculature which is longitudinal and circular. The outer covering of the uterus is peritoneum with the exception of that part upon which the bladder rests and the vaginal portion of the cervix. The inner lining of the body of the uterus varies in form and histological structure with the period of life in which it is studied, the prepuberty stage, the actively menstruating stage and the menopausal stage each having its own characteristics.

The uterus is situated in the midpelvis approximately halfway bet. the sacrum and the *symphysis pubis.* It is supported in this position by the 2 broad ligaments, the round ligaments, the uterosacral ligaments, and the ligaments attached to bladder. The uterus is normally anteflexed. The blood supply of the uterus is derived from the uterine and ovarian arteries.

POSITIONS: *Anteflexion*: Bending forward. *Anteversion*: Forward displacement of fundus towards pubis, while cervix is tilted up towards sacrum. *Retroflexion*: Bending backward, at junction of body and cervix. *Retroversion:* Inclination backward with retention of normal curve; opposed to anteversion.

AUSCULTATION: After the 4th month of gestation if uterus contains a living fetus 3 distinct sounds may be heard. *Fetal heart sounds*: Consist of a succession of short, rapid, double pulsations varying in frequency from 120 to 140 per minute. First sound is short, feeble, and obscure, while the 2nd, the one usually heard, is loud and distinct; sounds like ticking of a watch wrapped in a napkin. Sound is usually transmitted over space of 3 or 4 inches square. Location is determined by position of fetus.

Generally, when maximum intensity is on level of, or above umbilicus, a breech presentation; when low down in front on left side, 1st position; low in front on right side, in 2nd position. During labor, examinations, if made, should be bet. uterine contractions. In protracted labors is of value in indicating the time for manual or instrumental interference to save life of child.

Sounds: Irregularity and feebleness of sound are the most threatening to the life of the child.

Funic souffle: A sound usually heard at a point quite remote from the uterine bruit. It is short, blowing in character, and corresponds in pregnancy with the fetal pulsation. Supposed to depend upon obstruction to the transmission of blood through the umbilical arteries, as from twirling or knotting of the umbilical cord or from external pressure. Is not a constant or even frequent sound, the conditions of production being rarely met with.

Uterine bruit: This sound is single, intermitting and in character a combination of blowing and hissing sounds. Increases in intensity up to the period of labor. Believed to depend upon rapid passage of blood from the arteries into the distended venous sinuses of the uterus. Synchronous with maternal pulse, subject to same variations, and is always heard before the pulsations of the fetal heart; area over which is audible varies, greatest point of intensity in median line a little above pubes.

PALPATION: During pregnancy: In 3rd month, if walls of abdomen are not too thick, by placing patient upon her back, with head raised and thighs flexed, and pressing points of fingers gently downward and backward above the pubes, a hard, round mass will be found on the median line, rising out of the pelvis. In 2 or 4 weeks later the increase is much more strongly marked. As pregnancy advances, the mass loses more and more of its hardness, and becomes more and more elastic, like a cyst filled with water. In doubtful cases where decided enlargement of abdomen is present, exploration *per vaginum* becomes of great importance.

"Touch," or really internal palpation, signifies the means by which knowledge is obtained of internal conditions by vaginal or anal examination with the finger. By vaginal touch may be able to diagnose the stage of gestation, stage of parturition, or whether the woman is in that state, the progress of labor, the presentation and position of the child and the position of uterus. May be practiced with the woman standing, lying on either side, or back. The sensation of the tip of cervix of unimpregnated uterus to the touch is like that imparted to the finger by touching the tip of the nose, firm and cartilaginous; of the impregnated, like that of touching the lips. Feels soft like velvet, but deeper, beyond the softness, is a hardness, as of board.

PERCUSSION: Unimpregnated uterus is inaccessible to touch externally, or to percussion. In pregnancy at end of 2nd month a dull sound on percussion just above pubes indicates the enlarging uterus; later, as uterus increases in volume and rises into abdomen, able, by oval tumor felt in hypogastrium and by circumscribed area of dullness corresponding to situation of the tumor, to establish strong presumptive evidence of pregnancy. This presumption becomes strengthened if the area of dullness increases with the regularity proper to gestation. Palpation and percussion, however, are not sufficient to determine whether the enlargement is due to pregnancy or to some other form of new growth. After the 5th month both these methods are inferior to auscultation.

U., TUMORS OF: (a) May cause sterility, abortion, or obstruct labor. (b) May become infected or twisted on their attachments. (c) Myomata possible, but not common in young women. (d) Fibroids common beyond 30 and in negro race. (e) Subserous tumors do not affect pregnancy. May bar labor. (f) May disappear following labor. (g) Interstitial and submucous type may interfere with pregnancy and produce abortion

EFFECTS UPON LABOR: (a) Usually have no effects. (b) If low, may cause malpresentation or impossible labor. (c) Labor pains weak and inefficient. (d) Often severe pains and rupture of uterus. (e) Submucous tumors may protrude before or after birth. (f) Placenta may be retained. (g) Tumor may be infected postpartum. (h) Knee-chest position helps patient, if tumor is in pelvis. (i) If in fundus, delivery is through vagina; if not, cesarean section may be needed. (j) Control hemorrhage by packing.

UTERUS, CANCER OF: (a) Extremely rare in pregnancy; growth increases with pregnancy. (b) May produce sterility or abortion, hemorrhage, sepsis. (c) Detected by size, intermittent bleeding, purulent discharge, vaginal or Papanicolaou smear, or cervical or endometrial biopsy.

UTERUS, RUPTURE OF, IN PREGNANCY: (a) Rare but serious. (b) Etiology: weakness of uterine wall, or obstruction. (c) Scars may be cause of weakness of wall. (d) May be spontaneous or traumatic. (e) Child and amniotic sac may be expelled into peritoneal cavity. (f) Spontaneous rupture may occur without warning. (g) Abdominal pains, shock, hemorrhage may occur. (h) Child easily palpated. (i) Active movements of child which cease with death ensuing. (j) Obstruction usually precedes symptoms. (k) Combat shock and hemorrhage.

SUBINVOLUTION: The lack of involution of the uterus following childbirth. It is manifested by a large uterus and a continuation of lochia rubra beyond the usual time. The factors in its causation are usually puerperal infection, multiparity, overdistention of the uterus by multiple pregnancy or polyhydramnios, lack of lactation, malposition of the uterus, and retained secundines. Involution is aided by being certain that the placenta is intact at the time of delivery, and the use of ecbolics to cause contraction of the uterus.

u. acollis. Uterus without a cervix.

u. arcuatus. Uterus with a depressed arched fundus.

u. bicornis. Uterus in which the fundus is divided into 2 parts.

u. biforis. Uterus in which the ext. os is divided into 2 parts by a septum.

u. bilocularis. Uterus in which the cavity is divided into 2 parts by a partition.

u., bipartite. Uterus in which body is partially divided by a median septum.

u., cancer of. Malignant neoplasm of the uterus.

u. cordiformis. A heart-shaped uterus.

u. didelphys. Double uterus.

u. duplex. A double uterus resulting from failure of union of mullerian ducts.

u., fetal. One which is retarded in development and possessing an extremely long cervical canal.

u. gravid. Pregnant uterus.

u. masculinus. The prostatic utricle, *q.v.*

u. parvicollis. Normal uterus with disproportionately small vaginal portion.

u., prolapse of. Downward displacement of uterus, the cervix sometimes protruding from the vaginal orifice.

u., pubescent. An adult uterus which resembles a uterus of a prepuberal female.

u. septus. SEE: *u. bilocularis.*

u. unicornis. Uterus which possesses only one lateral half and usually having only one uterine tube.

utricle (ū′trĭk-l) [L. *utriculus*, a little bag]. One of two sacs of the membranous labyrinth in the bony vestibule of the inner ear.

The utricle communicates with the semicircular ducts by 5 openings on posterior wall and with the sacculus and endolymphatic duct by an opening on ant. wall. On its inner surface is an area of sensory epithelium, the *macula utriculi* containing cells which respond to movement of *otoliths* due to changes in position.

u., prostatic. SYN: *uterus masculinus.* A small blind pouch of the urethra extending into substance of prostate gland. It is a remnant of the embryonic mullerian duct.

u. of the urethra. The prostatic vesicle of the male.

u. of vestibule. Vestibular cavity connecting with the semicircular canals.

utricular (ū-trĭk′ū-lar) [L. *utriculus*, a little bag]. 1. Pert. to the utricle. 2. Like a bladder.

utriculitis (ū-trĭk-ū-lī′tĭs) [L. *utriculus*, a little bag, + G. *-itis*, inflammation]. Inflammation of the utricle, either that of the vestibule or the prostatic utricle.

utriculoplasty (ū-trĭk′ū-lō-plăs″tĭ) [" + G. *plassein*, to form]. Reduction of the uterus by excision of a longitudinal, wedge-shaped section.

utriculosaccular (ū-trĭk″ū-lō-săk′ū-lar) [" + *sacculus*, a small cavity]. Pert. to the utricle and saccule of the labyrinth.

u. duct. A duct uniting the utricle and saccule.

utriculus (ū-trĭk′ū-lŭs) (L. *utriculus*, a little bag]. A utricle, *q.v.*

u. masculin′us. SEE: *utricle, prostatic.*

u. prostaticus. SEE: *utricle, prostatic.*

utriform (ū′trĭ-form) [L. *uter, utri-*, a skin bag, + *forma*, shape]. Having a shape like a bottle.

uvea (ū′vē-ă) [L. *uva*, grape]. The 2nd or vascular coat of the eye lying immediately beneath the sclera.

It consists of iris, ciliary body and choroid, forming pigmented layer.

uveal (ū′vē-ăl) [L. *uva*, grape]. Pert. to the middle coat of the eye, or uvea.

uveitic (ū-vē-ĭt′ĭk) [L. *uva*, grape, + G. *-itis*, inflammation]. Marked by or pert. to uveitis.

uveitis (ū-vē-ī′tĭs) [" + G. *-itis*, inflammation]. Inflammation of the iris, ciliary body, and choroid, or the entire uvea.

uveoparotitis (ū″vē-ō-păr-ō-tī′tĭs) [" + G. *para*, near, + *ous, ot-*, ear, + *-itis*, inflammation]. Parotitis with uveitis.

uveoplasty (ū′vē-ō-plăs″tĭ) [" + G. *plassein*, to form]. Reparative operation or the uvea.

uviofast (ū′vĭ-ō-făst). Unaffected by ultraviolet radiation.

uviol (ū′vĭ-ŏl). Glass which is unusually transparent to ultraviolet rays.

u. lamp. Electric l. with uviol glass globe.

uviolize (ū′vē-ō-līz). To use ultraviolet rays therapeutically.

uvioresistant (ū″vĭ-ō-rē-zĭs′tănt). Resistant to effects of ultraviolet rays. SYN: *uviofast.*

uviosensitive (ū″vĭ-ō-sĕn′sĭ-tĭv). Sensitive to effects of ultraviolet rays.

uvula (ū′vū-lă) [L. *uvula*, a little grape]. Small, soft structure hanging from free edge of soft palate in midline above the root of the tongue. It is composed of muscle, connective tissue and mucous membrane.

RS: *cion, cionitis, cionotomy, staphyle.*

u. of cerebellum. A small lobule of the cerebellum lying on inferior surface of inf. vermis, anterior to the pyramis.

u. fissa. A cleft uvula.

u. palatine. SEE: *uvula.*

u. vesicae. NA. A median projection of mucous membrane of urinary bladder located immediately anterior to orifice of urethra.

uvulaptosis (ū″vū-lăp-tō′sĭs) [" + G. *ptōsis*, a dropping]. A relaxed condition of the uvula. SYN: *uvuloptosis.*

uvular (ū′vū-lar) [L. *uvula*, little grape]. Pert. to the uvula.

uvularis (ū-vū-lā′rĭs) [L.]. The azygos uvulae muscle. SEE: *Muscles, Table of, in Appendix.*

uvulatome (ū′vū-lă-tōm) [L. *uvula*, little grape, + G. *tomē*, a cutting]. Instrument for removal of uvula.

uvulatomy (ū-vū-lăt′ō-mĭ) [" + G. *tomē*, a cutting]. Excision of the uvula.

uvulitis (ū″vū-lī′tĭs) [" + G. *-itis*, inflammation]. Inflammation of the uvula.

uvuloptosis (ū-vū-lŏp-tō′sĭs) [" + G. *ptōsis*, a dropping]. Relaxed condition of the palate.

uvulotome (ū′vū-lō-tōm) [" + G. *tome*, a cutting]. Instrument for performing uvulotomy. SYN: *uvulatome.*

uvulotomy (ū-vū-lŏt′ō-mĭ) [" + G. *tomē*, a cutting]. Amputation of the uvula.

Notes

Notes

V

V. Abbr. for *vision, visual acuity, Vibrio,* and for *volt.* Symb. for *vanadium.*

vaccigenous (văk-sĭj'ĕn-ŭs) [L. *vaccinus,* pert. to a cow, + G. *gennan,* to produce]. Producing vaccine. Syn: *vaccinogenous.*

vaccin (văk'sĭn) [L. *vaccinus,* pert. to a cow]. Vaccine, *q.v.*

vaccina (văk-sī'nă) [L. *vaccinus,* pert. to a cow]. A disease resulting from inoculation with cowpox virus. Syn: *vaccinia, q.v.*

Papules form about 3rd day after vaccination which change to umbilicated vesicles and then to pustules. They dry and form scabs which fall about the 21st day. See: *Paschen bodies.*

vaccinal (văk'sĭn-ăl) [L. *vaccinus,* pert. to a cow]. Relating to vaccine or to vaccination.

v. fever. A mild fever that may follow vaccination.

vaccinate (văk'sĭn-āt) [L. *vaccinus,* pert. to a cow]. 1. To inoculate with cowpox vaccine to prevent or mitigate an attack of smallpox. 2. To inoculate with any vaccine to produce immunity against disease.

vaccination (văk-sĭn-ā'shŭn) [L. *vaccinus,* pert. to a cow]. 1. Inoculation against smallpox. 2. Inoculation with any vaccine as a preventive measure.

Vaccination against smallpox was introduced by Edward Jenner in 1798.

Note: Vaccination should not be done on children with extensive skin lesions or eczema. Also these children should not be allowed near children who have been recently vaccinated.

Time of Performance: In normal infant of good health, about 4th month, unless definite exposure to smallpox is known, when vaccination should be performed regardless of age. It is advisable to revaccinate children about every 5 years.

Method: *Site of selection*: Usually, the left arm, just above point of insertion of deltoid. Not advisable to vaccinate on leg, as secondary infections are much more likely to develop. If vaccination is performed on the leg, the outer muscles at the midthird are the proper point for inoculation. The skin should be cleansed with soap and water, then rendered aseptic by sponging with ether and allowed to dry. The vaccine lymph is expelled from the capillary tube by means of a small rubber bulb, and a sterile needle is selected for the purpose of abrading the epidermis through the drop of vaccine. This may be readily accomplished by the multiple pressure method which consists of holding the needle almost parallel to the skin and gently pressing it down until it touches the skin and just depresses it. This is done 30 times in an area no larger than 2 mm. in diameter. It is not necessary to make the area bleed. Cross scratching or vertical scratching with needle is totally unnecessary and often produces a needlessly large scar. Following inoculation vaccine may be wiped away. Celluloid shields, or any appliance which encircles the arm and causes constriction not only inadvisable, but many times proves to be dangerous, inasmuch as possibilities of secondary infection are promoted by such appliances.

Sym: From the 3rd to the 5th day following inoculation, a papule should develop. This is surrounded by a red areola. By 6th to 7th day, the papule is converted into a pearly vesicle, the center of which becomes depressed. The surrounding tissue may be red and tender with considerable infiltration. From 10th to 12th day the vesicle becomes a pustule, when there may be some swelling and tenderness of the axillary glands, as well as elevation of temperature. From 12th to 25th day, the pustule passes through the stage of desiccation and scab drops off, leaving a pitty scar at its former site. A potent vaccine should always produce a reaction in a susceptible individual. The fact that the vaccination does not take in one who has never been successfully vaccinated, or who has never had smallpox, does not indicate that such an individual is immune.

RS: *arm-to-arm v., autovaccination, autovaccine, vaccina, vaccine, variola.*

v., accelerated. Syn: *vaccinoid, seccondary vaccinia.* That in which the whole course of the reaction is accelerated and shortened. Indicates partial immunity and is designated a "mild take."

v., primary. Vaccinia or "take" with results indicating absence of immunity.

v. rash. One sometimes following vaccination.

vaccine (văk'sēn) [L. *vaccinus,* from *vacca,* a cow]. Killed or modified live virus, bacteria, or rickettsiae prepared in suspension for inoculation. Used to prevent or treat certain infectious diseases.

Vaccines are of four general classes: (1) those containing living attenuated infectious organisms; (2) those containing infectious agents killed by physical or chemical means; (3) those containing soluble toxins of microorganisms, sometimes used as such, but generally forming toxoids; and (4) substances extracted from infectious agents.

Examples of the first class are the BCG vaccine for tuberculosis and vaccines for smallpox and yellow fever.

Examples of the 2nd class are vaccines used to protect human beings against typhoid fever, rabies, and whooping cough. Vaccines of this class have been prepared for use in preventing several other diseases including pneumonia, cholera, dysentery, undulant fever, and plague, but they are less reliable as preventives against these.

In the 3rd class comes toxoid used in the prevention of diphtheria and tetanus.

Examples of the 4th class are capsular polysaccharides extracted from pneumococci.

Function: To stimulate the development in the body of specific defensive mechanism which results in more or less permanent protection against a disease. An attack of smallpox or diphtheria, for example, usually leaves the recovered patient permanently immune to those diseases. As a result of infection, the body succeeds in building up its own defenses, so that a new infection causes no illness. A successful vaccine does same thing without risk of illness.

v., aqueous. V. employing physiological salt solution as the vehicle.

v., autogenous. Bacterial v. taken from the individual to be inoculated.

v., bacterial. Any substance for preventive inoculation, esp. a suspension of bacteria, killed or attenuated, in saline solution used for injection into body to induce development of active immunity to the same organism.

v., BCG (Calmette-Guéron bacillus). Substance used in prophylactic vaccination of infants against tuberculosis with virulence reduced by repeated cultures on glycerinated ox bile.

v., heterologous. One prepared from organisms obtained from a source other than the person to be inoculated.

v., homologous. An autogenous vaccine, *q.v.*

v., humanized. Vaccine obtained from vaccinia vesicles in human beings.

v., influenza. A polyvalent vaccine containing antigenic variants of the influenza virus is available for use in areas which can be expected to have epidemics. Its use is particularly helpful to the aged and chronically ill.

v., killed. One consisting of killed infectious agents.

v., live, attenuated, measles virus. SYN: *Edmonston B vaccine.* V. for immunization against measles. This type of measles vaccine is the preferred form except in patients who have one of the following: lymphoma, leukemia, or other generalized malignancy; pregnancy; active tuberculosis; prolonged treatment with drugs which suppress the immune response; administration of gamma globulin, blood, or plasma.

v., measles virus inactivated. V. for immunization against measles. This preparation should be used only when there are contraindications to the use of the *live, attenuated measles vaccine, q.v.*

v., mixed. One prepared from more than one infectious agent.

v., multivalent. A polyvalent vaccine, *q.v.*

v., mumps. A live, attenuated vaccine used to prevent mumps.

v. point. A needle or quill coated with vaccine lymph at its tip.

v., polyvalent. V. made from several strains of the same species of bacterium or virus.

v., rabies. Vaccine prepared from fixed virus of rabies, used prophylactically following bite by a rabid animal. SEE: *rabies.*

v. rash. One due to vaccination.

v., Sabin. Oral poliomyelitis vaccine. SEE: *poliomyelitis* (*prophylaxis*).

v., Salk. One against poliomyelitis. SEE: *poliomyelitis* (*prophylaxis*).

v., sensitized. V. made more active by treatment of the bacteria with their specific immune serum. SYN: *serobacterin.*

v., smallpox. V. made from lymph of cowpox vesicles obtained from healthy vaccinated bovine animals.

v., stock. Bacterial v. made from same species as that causing the infection, but not autogenous.

v., TAB. A mixture of typhoid, paratyphoid A, and paratyphoid B vaccines.

v. therapy. Treatment of a disease by inoculation with a vaccine specific for that disease.

v., triple (for typhoid). TAB vaccine.

v., virus. An emulsion containing substance from pustules of vaccinia used for inoculation.

vaccinia (văk-sĭn'ĭ-ă) [L. *vaccinus,* pert. to a cow]. A contagious disease resulting from inoculation with cowpox virus.

Papules form about 3rd day after vaccination which change to umbilicated vesicles about the 5th day and then, at end of 1st week, to umbilicated pustules surrounded by a red areola. They dry and form scabs, which fall about the 2nd week, leaving a white, pitted depression.

Inoculation with this virus confers upon man more or less immunity against smallpox. SYN: *cowpox.*

RS: *vaccination, variola, varicella.*

vaccinia immune globulin. Hyperimmune gamma globulin. The therapeutic agent of choice for dermal complications of vaccination for smallpox.

vaccinia necrosum. Spreading necrosis at the site of smallpox vaccination. May be accompanied by similar necrotic areas elsewhere on the body.

vacciniform (văk-sĭn'ĭ-form) [L. *vaccinus,* pert. to a cow, + *forma,* shape]. Of the nature of vaccinia or cowpox.

vacciniola (văk-sĭn-ĭ-ō'lă) [L. diminutive of *vaccinia,* from *vaccinus,* pert. to a cow]. Secondary general eruption after local eruption from vaccine.

vaccinization (văk"sĭn-ĭ-zā'shŭn) [L. *vaccinus,* pert. to a cow]. Vaccination by repeated inoculations until the virus has no effect.

vaccinogenous (văk"sĭn-ŏj'ĕn-ŭs) [" + G. *gennan,* to produce]. Producing vaccine or pert. to its production.

vaccinoid (văk'sĭn-oyd). A mild "take." SEE: *vaccination, accelerated.*

vaccinotherapeutics, vaccinotherapy (văk"-sĭn-ō-thĕr-ă-pū'tĭks, -thĕr'ă-pĭ). Treatment by injection of bacterial vaccines.

vacuolar (vak'ū-ō-lăr). Pertaining to or possessing vacuoles.

v. degeneration. Swelling of cells with increase in number and size of vacuoles. Also called *parenchymous, albuminous,* or *hydropic degeneration;* or *cloudy swelling.*

vacuolated. Possessing or containing vacuoles.

vacuolation (văk-ū-ō-lā'shŭn) [L. *vacuolum,* a tiny empty space]. Formation of vacuoles. SYN: *vacuolization.*

vacuole (văk'ū-ōl) [L. *vacuolum,* a tiny empty space]. A clear space in cell protoplasm filled with fluid or air.

v., plasmocrin. A vacuole present in cytoplasm of secretory cell which is filled with crystalloid material.

v., rhagiocrin. A vacuole present in cytoplasm of secretory cell which is filled with colloid material.

vacuolization (văk"ū-ō-lĭz-ā'shŭn) [L. *vacuolum,* a tiny space]. Vacuolation, *q.v.*

vacuome (văk'ū-ōm). The internal reticular apparatus, *q.v.*

vacuum (văk'ū-ŭm) [L. *vacuum,* empty]. A space exhausted of its air content.

v. extractor. Device, using a suction cup attached to the fetal head, for applying traction to the fetus during delivery. Its use may be hazardous except in the hands of experts.

v. treatment. Insertion of a limb in a partial vacuum.

v. tube. A vessel of insulating material (usually glass) provided with metal electrodes, which has been so highly evacuated that the residual gas does not affect the current passing bet. metal electrodes projecting from the outside.

vag'abond's disease. Discoloration of skin caused by exposure and scratching due to presence of lice. SEE: *pediculosis corporis: melanoderma.*

vagal (vā'găl) [L. *vagus,* wandering]. Pert. to the vagus nerve.

v. attack. A condition of dyspnea, cardiac distress, a fear of impending death, and a sinking sensation assumed to be the result of vasomotor spasm.

v. escape. Condition in which one or more beats of the heart occurs even though the vagus nerve is being continuously stimulated. Stimulation of the vagus normally inhibits heart beat.

v. substance. Substance liberated at termination of vagus nerve fibers in the heart. SEE: *acetylcholine.*

v. tone. Condition in which impulses over the vagus nerve exert a continuous inhibitory effect upon the heart.

vagi. Plural of vagus.

vagina (vă-jī'nă) (pl. *vaginae, vaginas*) [L. *vagina,* sheath]. 1. A sheathlike part. 2. A musculomembranous tube which forms the passageway between the uterus and the external orifice between the vulvae.

ANAT: It is divided into four walls: two lateral, one anterior, and one posterior. In the uppermost part, the cervix divides the vagina into four *fornices,* the two lateral, the anterior and the posterior.

The bladder is situated adjacent to the anterior wall of the vagina and the rectum is behind the posterior wall. The vagina represents a potential space, the walls of which are in contact with each other. Close to the cervix uteri the walls form a horizontal crescent shape, at the midpoint an H shape, and close to the vulva the shape of a vertical slit. The vagina is lined by mucous membrane made up of squamous epithelium. It is surrounded by fascias which allow for easy distensibility. The blood supply of the vagina is furnished from the inferior vesical, inferior hemorrhoidal, and uterine arteries.

FUNCTION: A passage for the intromission of the penis, the reception of the semen, and for the discharge of the menstrual flow; also as the passageway through which the fetus is delivered.

v., bulb of. Small erectile body on each side of the vaginal vestibule. SYN: *bulbi vestibuli, Bartholin's glands.*

v. fibrosa tendinis. A fibrous sheath surrounding a tendon which usually confines it to an osseous groove.

v. masculinus. The prostatic utricle, *q.v.*

v. mucosa tendinis. A synovial sheath which develops about a tendon.

v., septate. Congenital condition in which the vagina is divided longitudinally into two parts. Division may be partial or complete.

vagina, words pert. to: aerocoly, bulbi vestibuli, "colp-" words, Duverney's gland, "elytr-" words, endocolpitis, enterocele, esthiomene, fistula, fornix, fourchette, gynatresia, hematocolpometra, hydrocolpos, hymen, kysthoptosis, leukorrhea, lochiocolpos, pachycolpismus, pachyvaginitis, paravaginal, pronaus, supravaginal, transvaginal, "vagin-" words.

vaginal (văj'ĭn-ăl) [L. *vagina,* sheath]. Pert. to the vagina or to any enveloping sheath.

v. hysterectomy. Surgical removal of uterus through vagina.

vaginalectomy (văj"ĭn-ăl-ĕk'tō-mĭ) [" + G. *ektomē,* excision]. Excision of the tunica vaginalis. SYN: *vaginectomy.*

vaginalitis (văj-ĭn-ăl-ī'tĭs) [L. *vagina,* sheath, + G. *-itis,* inflammation]. Inflammation of *tunica vaginalis testis.*

vaginapexy. Repair of a relaxed and prolapsed vagina. SYN: *colpopexy; vaginofixation.*

vaginate (văj'ĭn-āt) [L. *vagina,* sheath]. Sheathed.

vaginectomy (văj-ĭn-ĕk'tō-mĭ) [L. *vagina,* sheath, + G. *ektomē,* excision]. 1. Resection of tunica vaginalis. 2. Excision of the vagina or a part of it.

vaginicoline (văj-ĭn-ĭk'ō-lĭn) [" + *colere,* to dwell]. Living in the vagina, as microorganisms.

vaginismus (văj-ĭn-ĭz'mŭs) [L.]. Painful spasm of vagina from contraction of the muscles surrounding the vagina. May interfere with coitus.

It may indicate neurotic aversion to the act. Extraordinary hyperesthesia of nerve supply to mucous membrane of vagina at or near site of the hymen, resulting in spasmodic constriction of sphincter vaginae muscle, preventing coitus. May also be due to local trauma, ulceration, lack of physiological lubrication, vaginitis, menopausal involution, or congenital malformation.

SYM: Extreme sensitiveness. Spasmodic closure of vaginal orifice on slightest touch. In severe cases, sterility.

TREATMENT: Psychotherapy; correction of primary causative factors; education correcting misinformation and fear.

v., mental. V. resulting from repugnance to cohabitation.

v., posterior. V. due to contraction of the levator ani muscle.

vaginitis (văj-ĭn-ī'tĭs) [L. *vagina,* sheath, + G. *-itis,* inflammation]. 1. Inflammation of a sheath. 2. Inflammation of vagina.

ETIOL: May be caused by (a) microorganisms, *e.g.,* gonococci, staphylococci, streptococci, spirochetes; (b) chemical irritation, *e.g.,* use of too strong chemicals in douching; (c) fungus infection (moniliasis) caused by *Candida albicans;* (d) protozoan infection (*Trichomonas vaginalis*); (e) irritation from foreign bodies (pessaries, etc.); (f) vitamin deficiency as in pellagra; (g) conditions involving vulva and surrounding areas, as uncleanliness, intestinal worms, masturbation, etc.

SYM: Free, purulent vaginal discharge, sometimes offensive and occasionally stained with blood. There is irritation and itching of the vulvae and perineum, frequency of micturition, and smarting pain on the passage of urine. The vaginal mucous membrane is reddened and there may be superficial ulceration.

TREATMENT: Specific therapy as indicated. Improve perineal hygiene by instructing in: proper method of cleaning anus after a bowel movement; proper use of menstrual protection materials; necessity of drying vulvae following urination. Douching is not essential to the maintenance of vaginal health or cleanliness.

v. adhaesiva. Inflammation with mucous membrane exfoliation causing adhesions and partial obliteration of the vaginal lumen.

v., atrophic. SYN: *postmenopausal* or *senile vaginitis.* That following the menopause, whether natural or artificial.

v., diphtheritic. V. with membranous exudate.

v., emphysematous. V. with gas in connective tissues.

v., glandular. V. when the follicles alone seem affected, when mucous membrane shows no traces of change and when secretion appears more copious and of a yellowish-white or grayish color.

v., granular. V. with infiltrated cells and enlarged papillae. The most common form of v.

v., papulous. Vagina and neck of womb covered with papulae or follicles more or less developed or resembling fleshy granulations.

v., postmenopausal. Atrophic vaginitis, *q.v.* Usually due to insufficient estrogens.

v., pustulous. May result from appearance of pustules in persons affected with pustulous affections of the skin.

v., senile. Atrophic vaginitis, *q.v.*

v. testis. Inflammation of the tunica vaginalis of the testis.

v., Trichomonas vaginalis. That associated with, or caused by infection by *Trichomonas vaginalis,* a flagellate protozoon.

vaginoabdominal (văj"ĭn-ō-ăb-dŏm'ĭn-ăl) [L. *vagina,* sheath, + *abdominalis,* abdominal]. Relating to the vagina and abdomen.

vaginocele (văj'ĭn-ō-sēl) [" + G. *kēlē,* hernia]. Vaginal hernia. SYN: *colpocele.*

vaginodynia (văj"ĭn-ō-dĭn'ĭ-ă) [" + G. *odynē,* pain]. Pain in the vagina.

vaginofixation (văj"ĭn-ō-fĭks-ā'shŭn) [" + *fixātio,* a fixing]. 1. Process of rendering the vagina immovable. 2. Attachment of uterus to vaginal peritoneum.

vaginogenic (văj"ĭn-ō-jĕn'ĭk) [" + G. *gennan,* to produce]. Developed from or originating in the vagina.

vaginography (văj-ĭn-ŏg'ră-fĭ) [" + G. *graphein,* to write]. The taking of x-ray pictures of the vagina.

vaginolabial (văj"ĭn-ō-lā'bĭ-ăl) [" + *labium,* lip]. Relating to the vagina and the labia. SYN: *vaginovulvar, vulvovaginal.*

vaginometer (văj-ĭn-ŏm'ĕ-tĕr) [L. *vagina,* sheath, + G. *metron,* a measure]. Device for measuring the length and expansion of the vagina.

vaginomycosis (văj"ĭn-ō-mī-kō'sĭs) [" + G. *mykēs,* fungus, + *-ōsis,* disease]. A fungus infection (mycosis) of the vagina.

vaginoperineal (văj"ĭn-ō-pĕr-ĭ-nē'ăl) [" + G. *perinaion,* perineum]. Relating to the vagina and perineum.

vaginoperineorrhaphy (văj"ĭn-ō-pĕr-ĭ-nē-or'ăf-ĭ) [" + " + *rhaphē,* a sewing]. Repair of a perineal laceration in the vagina. SYN: *colpoperineorrhaphy.*

vaginoperineotomy (văj"ĭn-ō-pĕr-ĭn-ē-ŏt'-ō-mĭ) [" + " + *tomē,* a cutting]. Separation of the vagina and perineum.

vaginoperitoneal (văj"ĭn-ō-pĕr-ĭ-tō-nē'ăl) [" + G. *peritonaion,* peritoneum]. Relating to the vagina and peritoneum.

vaginopexy (vă-jī'nō-pĕk"sĭ) [" + G. *pēxis,* fixation]. Fixation of the vagina. SYN: *colpopexy.*

vaginoplasty (vă-jī'nō-plăs"tĭ) [L. *vagina,* sheath, + G. *plassein,* to form]. Reparative surgery on the vagina.

vaginoscope (văj'ĭn-ō-skōp) [" + G. *skopein,* to examine]. Instrument for inspection of the vagina.

vaginoscopy (văj-ĭn-ŏs'kō-pĭ) [" + G. *skopein,* to examine]. Visual examination of the vagina.

vaginotome (văj-ī'nō-tōm) [" + G. *tomē,* a cutting]. An instrument for making an incision in the vaginal walls.

vaginotomy (văj-ĭn-ŏt'ō-mĭ) [" + G. *tomē,* a cutting]. Incision of vagina.

vaginovesical (văj"ĭn-ō-vĕs'ĭk-ăl) [" + *vesica,* bladder]. Relating to the vagina and the bladder. SYN: *vesicovaginal.*

vaginovulvar (văj"ĭn-ō-vŭl'var) [" + *vulva,* a covering]. Pert. to the vulva and vagina.

vagitis (vă-jī'tis). Inflammation of the vagal nerve.

vagitus (vă-jī'tŭs) [L. *vagire,* to squall]. First cry of newly born infant.

v. uterinus. Crying of the fetus before birth while still in the uterus.

v. vaginalis. Cry of a child or infant with head still in the vagina.

vagomimetic (vā"gō-mĭm-ĕt'ĭk) [L. *vagus,* wandering + G. *mimetikos,* imitating]. Resembling action of stimulated vagus nerve.

vagosympathetic (vā"gō-sĭm-pă-thĕt'ĭk) [" + G. *sympathētikos,* suffering with]. The cervical sympathetic and the vagus nerves considered together.

vagotomy (vā-gŏt'ō-mĭ) [" + G. *tomē,* a cutting]. Section of the vagus nerve.

vagotonia (vā-gō-tō'nĭ-ă) [L. *vagus,* wandering, + G. *tonos,* tone]. Hyperirritability of the parasympathetic nervous system. SYN: *vasomotor instability, constipation, sweating.* SEE: *sympatheticotonia*

vagotonic (vā"gō-tŏn'ĭk) [" + G. *tonos,* tone]. Pertaining to vagotonia.

vagotropic (vā"gō-trŏp'ĭk) [" + G. *tropos,* a turning]. Acting upon the vagus nerve.

vagotropism (vā-gŏt'rō-pĭzm) [" + " + *-ismos,* condition]. Affinity for the vagus nerve, as a drug.

vagrant (vā'grănt) [L. *vagrans,* from *vagāre,* to wander]. 1. Wandering from place to place. 2. A vagabond.

v's. disease. Cutaneous discoloration and irritation caused by filth and body lice. SYN: *vagabond's disease.*

vagus (vā'gŭs) (pl. *vagi*) [L. *vagus,* wandering]. The pneumogastric or 10th cranial nerve.

It is a mixed nerve having motor and sensory functions and a wider distribution than any of the cranial nerves.

v. pneumonia. P. caused by trauma of the vagus nerve.

v. pulse. A slow pulse caused by the slowing action of the heart due to inhibition of the vagus nerve. SEE: *vagotomy, vagotonia.*

valence, valency (vā'lĕns, -lĕn-sĭ) [L. *valens,* powerful]. 1. Property of an element or radical combining with or replacing other elements or radicals in definite proportion. 2. Degree of the combining power or replacing power of an element or radical, the hydrogen atom being unit of comparison.

The number indicates how many atoms of hydrogen can unite with 1 atom of another element.

SEE: *artiad, atomicity.*

Valentin's ganglion (văl'ĕn-tēn). A small ganglion at junction of mid. and post. branches of the sup. dental plexus.

valetudinarian (văl-e-tū-dĭn-ā'rĭ-ăn) [L. *valetudinarius*, pert. to ill health]. 1. Sickly; ailing. 2. One subject to frequent illness, or feebleness. SYN: *invalid*.

valgus (văl'gŭs) [L. *valgus*, bowlegged]. 1. A term denoting position meaning *bent outward* or *twisted*, applied especially to deformities in which a part is bent outward and away from the midline of the body, as *talipes valgus, q.v., hallux valgus, q.v.*

valine (văl'ēn, vă'lēn). An amino acid derived from digestion of proteins. $C_5H_{11}NO_2$.

vallate (văl'āt) [L. *vallātus*, walled]. Having a rim around a depression.

v. papilla. A circumvallate papilla; one of a group of papillae forming a V-shaped row on post. dorsal surface of tongue.

vallecula (văl-lĕk'ū-lă) [L. *vallecula*, a depression]. A depression or crevice.

v. cerebel'li. NA. A deep fissure on inf. surface of the cerebellum.

v. epiglottica. Depression lying lateral to the median epiglottic fold and separating it from the pharyngo-epiglottic fold. [NA].

v. ova'ta. A depression in the liver in which rests the gallbladder.

v. syl'vii. A depression marking beginning of the fissure of Sylvius.

v. un'guis. Fold of skin in which the proximal and lateral edges of the nails are embedded.

valley of the cerebellum (văl'ē). Hollow on inf. surface of cerebellum. SYN: *vallecula cerebelli.*

vallum unguis (văl'um ŭng'gwĭs). NA. Fold of skin overlapping the nail.

Valsalva's maneuver or **experiment** (văl-săl'vă). Attempt to forcibly exhale with the nose and mouth closed. If the eustachian tubes are not obstructed the pressure on the tympanic membranes will be increased. Maneuver can also be done with the glottis closed. This causes increased intrathoracic pressure, slowing of the pulse, decreased return of blood to the heart, and increased venous pressure.

V's. sinuses. Three dilatations in wall of the aorta behind the flaps of the three aortic semilunar valves.

valvate (văl'văt) [L. *valva*, valve]. Pert. to or provided with valves. SYN: *valvular.*

valve (vălv) [L. *valva*, a fold]. Any one of various structures for temporarily closing an orifice or passage, or for allowing movement of fluid in 1 direction only.

v., aortic. The semilunar valve preventing regurgitation at the entrance of the aorta to the heart, composed of 3 segments.

v., bicuspid. Valve closing orifice bet. left cardiac atrium and left ventricle.

v., ileocecal. Valve bet. ileum and large intestine to prevent regurgitation of intestinal contents; composed of 2 membranous folds.

v., Houston's. Mucosal folds of the rectum. SYN: *plicae transversales recti.*

v., mitral. Bicuspid valve, *q.v.*

v., pulmonary. Valve composed of 3 cusps separating pulmonary artery and right ventricle.

v., pyloric. Prominent circular membranous fold at pyloric orifice of the stomach.

v., semilunar. Valve bet. heart and the aorta and valve bet. the heart and the pulmonary artery.

v., tricuspid. Valve bet. the right cardiac atrium and right ventricle.

v. tube. An electric valve consisting of a vacuum tube having for 1 electrode a hot filament.

v. of Varolius. Ileocecal valve, *q.v.*

valvotomy [L. *valva*, a fold, + G. *tome*, a cutting]. SYN: *diclidotomy*. Incision into a valve, esp. Houston's valves of the rectum.

valvula (văl'vū-lă) [L. *valvula*, a tiny fold]. A valve, specifically a small valve.

v. bicuspidalis. Valve bet. left cardiac atrium and left ventricle.

v. coli. Valve bet. ileum and large intestine. SYN: *ileocecal valve.*

v. pylori. Prominent mucosal fold at pyloric entrance of the stomach.

v. semilunaris. NA. Valve separating heart and aorta and heart and pulmonary artery.

v. tricuspidalis. Valve bet. the right atrium and right ventricle of the heart.

valvulae. Plural of *valvula.*

valvulae conniventes (văl'vū-lē kon-nĭ-vĕn'-tēs) [L.]. Circular membranous folds projecting into lumen of small intestine; they do not disappear on distention of bowel, and act by retarding passage of the food along the bowel; they also provide a greater absorbing area. SYN: *plica circularis.*

valvular (văl'vū-lar) [L. *valvula*, a small fold]. Relating to or having a valve. SYN: *valvate.*

valvulitis (văl-vū-lī'-tĭs) [" + G. *-itis*, inflammation]. Inflammation of a valve, especially a cardiac valve. SYN: *dicliditis.*

valvulotome (văl'vū-lō-tōm) [" + G. *tomē*, a cutting]. An instrument for incising a valve.

valvulotomy (văl-vū-lŏt'ō-mĭ) [" + G. *tomē*, a cutting]. Process of cutting through a valve, as a too rigid rectal fold. SYN: *valvotomy.*

vanadium (văn-ā'dĭ-ŭm). A light gray metallic element. SYMB: V. At. wt. 50.942; at. no. 23.

van Buren's disease (văn bū'rĕn). Induration of the corpora cavernosa.

van den Bergh's test. A direct or indirect test to detect the presence of bilirubin in blood serum in assumed cases of obstructive jaundice or impaired liver functioning.

vanillism (văn-ĭl'lĭzm). Irritation of the skin, mucous membranes and conjunctiva sometimes experienced by workers handling vanilla. It is caused by a mite.

vapor (vā'por) [L. *vapor*, smoke]. 1. Gaseous state of any substance. 2. Medicinal substance for administration in form of inhaled vapor.

v. bath. Exposure of body to hot vapor.

v. cabinet. Cabinet in which to give vapor baths.

v. douche. Treatment with a jet of hot vapor.

SEE: *halitus, nebulization.*

vaporium (vā-pō'rĭ-ŭm) [L. *vaporium*]. Apparatus for applying hot or cold or medicated vapors.

vaporization (vā"por-ĭ-zā'shŭn) [L. *vapor*, smoke]. 1. The conversion of a liquid or solid into vapor. 2. Therapeutic use of a vapor. SYN: *nebulization.*

vaporizer (vā'por-īz-ĕr) [L. *vapor*, smoke]. Device for converting liquids into a vapor spray.

vaporous (vā'por-ŭs) [L. *vapor*, smoke]. Consisting of, pert. to, or producing vapors.

Vaquez's disease (vă-kā'). Continuous excessive erythrocyte formation by the diseased bone marrow with enlargement of the spleen. SYN: *polycythemia vera.*

V's. nodes. Small painful nodules occurring on tips of fingers in cases of bacterial endocarditis.

varicella (var-i-sel'ă) [L. *varicella,* a tiny spot]. An acute, highly contagious disease characterized by an eruption that makes its appearance in crops and passes through successive stages of macules, papules, vesicles, and crusts. SYN: *chickenpox.*

ETIOL: Varicella virus which resembles the virus of herpes zoster in morphology and antigenic properties. May occur at any age, though far less common in adults than in children. Epidemics most frequent in winter and spring. One attack nearly always confers immunity.

INCUBATION: 14 to 21 days.

SYM: *Onset:* There may be but slight elevation of temperature, followed within 24 hours by appearance of the eruption after which time temperature usually rises still further. Eruption first appears on back and chest, crops continuing to make their appearance for a period of from 2 to 3 days on an average.

Each crop requires about 36 hours to pass through the several stages. Because of this, in the same general locality, macules, papules, vesicles and crusts may be found side by side. Lesions are superficial and rupture very easily.

They have a tendency to be ovoid and on the chest their distribution is often particularly marked along the course of the intercostal nerves. Some, though possibly few, scars nearly always remain as evidence of a chickenpox attack. The extremities are relatively free as compared with the trunk.

COMPLICATIONS: Secondary infections, due to scratching, which may result in abscess formation, or at times development of erysipelas or even septicemia. Occasionally lesions in the vicinity of the larynx may cause edema of the glottis and threaten the life of the patient. Encephalitis is a rare complication.

DIFFERENTIAL DIAG: Confusion bet. this disease and smallpox is responsible for the chief importance given chickenpox. Impetigo, dermatitis herpetiformis, herpes zoster, and furunculosis may require consideration.

PROG: Always favorable except in a very severe type which is described as varicella gangrenosa. In this variety, gangrene may develop about the site of the lesions.

TREATMENT: Isolation. Restrain the hands in the case of infants or young children in order that the lesions may not be scratched. Use of calamine lotion locally may alleviate irritation. Keep the skin, bedclothes, and sheets clean to help prevent skin infections. Also keep patient's fingernails well trimmed. Ordinarily, no internal remedies are necessary. The usual duration of the disease is from 2 to 3 weeks. Cases usually classed as contagious until the skin is free of all crusts.

v. gangrenosa. V. in which necrosis occurs around the vesicles resulting in gangrenous ulceration. SEE: *vaccinia necrosum.*

v. inoculata. That resulting from vaccination with fluid from vesicles of varicella lesions. This practice may be dangerous and is therefore not indicated.

varices (var'is-ēz) (Sing. *varix*) [L. *varicēs,* dilated veins]. Plural of varix, *q.v.*

variciform (văr-ĭs'ĭ-form) [L. *varix, varic-,* a twisted vein, + *forma,* shape]. Resembling a varix. SYN: *varicose.*

varicoblepharon (văr-ĭ-kō-blĕf'ă-ron) [" + G. *blepharon,* eyelid]. Varicose tumor of the eyelid.

varicocele (văr'ĭ-kō-sēl) [L. *varix, varic-,* a twisted vein, + G. *kēlē,* hernia]. Enlargement of the veins of the spermatic cord (pampiniform plexus), commonly occurring on the left side in adolescent males; these seldom require treatment.

SYM: Vessels on affected side of scrotum are full, feeling like a bundle of worms, sometimes purplish in color. Dull ache along the cord. Slight dragging sensation in groin.

TREATMENT: Dragging sensation from exceptionally large varicocele may be relieved by a suspensory. Surgery is required for persistent symptomatic varicocele.

v., ovarian. Varicosity of veins of the ovarian or pampiniform plexus of the broad ligament.

v., utero-ovarian. Varicosity of the veins of the ovarian (pampiniform) plexus and uterine plexus of the broad ligament.

varicocelectomy (văr-ĭ-kō-sē-lĕk'tō-mĭ) [L. *varix, varic-,* twisted vein, + G. *kēlē,* hernia, + *ektomē,* excision]. Excision of portion of scrotal sac with ligation of the dilated veins to relieve varicocele.

varicography (văr-ĭ-kŏg'ră-fĭ) [" + G. *graphein,* to write]. X-ray photography of varicose veins.

varicomphalus (văr-ĭk-ŏm'făl-ŭs) [" + G. *omphalos,* navel]. Varicose tumor of the navel.

varicophlebitis (văr"ĭ-kō-flē-bī-tĭs) (" + G. *phleps, phleb-,* vein, + *-itis,* inflammation]. Phlebitis combined with varicose veins.

varicose (văr'ĭ-kōs). Pert. to varices; distended, swollen, knotted veins.

v. veins. Enlarged twisted veins most commonly found on leg and thigh.

ETIOL: Congenitally defective venous valves, pregnancy, occupations requiring standing positions, and obesity.

SYM: Pain in feet and ankles, swelling, ulcers on skin. Severe bleeding, if a vein is injured.

F. A. TREATMENT: Elevation of extremity and gentle pressure over wound will always stop bleeding. The use of a tourniquet is undesirable. Sterile dressing should be held in place with a firm bandage. Patient should not be permitted to walk for some time.

GENERAL: Rest, elevation of extremity, and use of an external support. The use of elastic stockings is much preferred to elastic bandages. Unna's paste boots recommended for elderly or debilitated persons. Injection of sclerosing solutions may be utilized for small varicosities. High ligation and removal of vein by stripping may be necessary for major varicosities.

RS: *cirsenchysis, cirsodesis, cirsomphalos, cirsotomy.*

varicosity (văr-ĭ-kŏs'ĭ-tĭ) [*varix, varic-,* vein]. 1. Condition of being varicose. 2. A swollen, twisted vein. SYN: *varix.*

varicotomy (văr-ĭ-kŏt'ō-mĭ) [" + G. *tomē* a cutting]. Excision of a varicose vein.

varicula (văr-ĭk'ū-lă) [L. *varicula,* a tiny dilated vein]. A small varix, especially of the conjunctiva.

vari'ety. A subdivision of a species.

variola (vă-rī′ō-lă) [*variola*, a small spot]. An acute contagious disease characterized by a prodromal stage during which the constitutional symptoms are usually severe, and followed by an eruption which passes through the successive stages of macules, papules, vesicles, pustules, and crusts. SYN: *smallpox*.

ETIOL: Causative agent is a virus, which closely resembles the vaccinia virus. More common during colder seasons. No age exempt. May occur in utero. No preference as to sex. Acquired chiefly by direct contact with patient. May also be spread through the handling of articles contaminated by the patient. Susceptibility practically universal in those unprotected by proper vaccination, or before a first attack of smallpox, although second attacks have been reported.

INCUBATION: Seven to 16 days. Usually 9 to 12 days to onset of illness and 3 to 4 more days to onset of rash.

SYM: Onset abrupt with chill or chilliness. Headache usually frontal, intense lumbar pains, elevation of temperature, which may rise to 104° or higher, nausea, or more frequently, vomiting. Fever remains high until evening of 3rd or morning of 4th day, when it falls sharply, often to normal.

With drop in temperature, the eruption makes its appearance, coming out first as a rule, about the face, and soon afterward on extremities and to lesser extent on trunk. Eruption is of same character in any one general location, in this respect differing markedly from eruption of chickenpox.

About 2nd day of eruption, the macules become papular, and from 3rd to 5th day these papules become vesicles. The vesicles increase in size and from 7th to 8th day, well developed pustules are present, having appearance of being deep-seated and areola may, or may not, be markedly evident.

The fever of suppuration, so commonly referred to, which is generally anticipated at the time pustules develop, is not always present in the discrete type of smallpox. From 8th to 11th day, desiccation occurs and by end of 21st day in the average discrete case the skin is likely to be free of crusts. The customary observation that smallpox papules when found on the palmar or plantar surfaces feel like shot underneath the skin is a fact to which too much importance is commonly attached.

It may always be expected that the lesions will predominate on the head and extremities, the trunk being relatively free in the discrete type.

The lesions of smallpox, being deep-seated, do not rupture easily, for two reasons. First, the smallpox lesion is not single celled, but multilocular. Second, because of a deeper invasion, there is a thicker protective covering. It is because of the first of these reasons that the smallpox lesion does not collapse when pricked by a needle. If properly treated, the majority of discrete cases will show little evidence of the disease some months after recovery.

Pitting is not an inevitable misfortune in all cases, but depends principally on extent to which the true skin is involved. However, though pitting does not occur, marked pigmentation may exist at the sites of the lesions and continue to attract attention for many weeks following recovery from an acute attack.

Several other types are described and often classified under one heading—the malignant or hemorrhagic.

COMPLICATIONS: Abscesses, iritis, conjunctivitis, cervical adenitis, nephritis, and pneumonia are among the more common ones.

PROG: In modified (*varioloid*) smallpox, the outcome may be considered favorable in practically all instances. In confluent smallpox, recovery is always doubtful and in the hemorrhagic types, death is almost inevitable.

TREATMENT: *Prophylactic*: Successful vaccination against smallpox is an absolute preventive. However, this should always be repeated in the presence of an epidemic or when knowledge of recent exposure is possessed.

General: Absolute isolation of patient in a cool, well-ventilated room. If there are many lesions on mucous membranes a liquid diet may be essential. In the discrete type, patient need not be limited as to diet, unless there is some contraindication. Plenty of water, fruit juices and vegetables should be given. Milk is often soothing as well as nourishing in those cases in which the throat symptoms are severe.

Closest attention should be given to the eyes. They may be irrigated several times each day with 2% sodium bicarbonate solution. It is not advisable to use ointments on the skin before desiccation is complete, as such treatment only blocks the surface and increases likelihood of abscess formation.

The itching commonly associated with smallpox is seldom complained of: when present, calamine lotion may be applied. In the confluent type, weak iodine baths, or weak permanganate tubbings are often necessary not merely for cleansing skin but for purpose of acting as a deodorant.

v., black. Same as *hemorrhagic v.*

v., coherent. V. in which pustules are not confluent,* but coalesce at edges.

v., confluent. V. in which pustules run together. In confluent smallpox, the onset may be no different than in the discrete variety. However, as eruption develops, lesions are so numerous that their presentation may be mistaken for measles. As this eruption progresses, the lesions enlarge until destroyed by breaking down of their walls and so pustular material flows together into small pools.

The temperature does not show the same remission as in the discrete type, the toxemia is much more profound, the throat symptoms are likely to be unusually severe, and swallowing may be practically impossible.

Lesions frequently develop on the conjunctiva, or even on the cornea itself, resulting in the destruction of sight. Death may be due directly to profound toxemia, or to a complicating anemia. Delirium of a violent character is common in these patients who frequently die between the 7th and 12th day of eruption. Death, however, is not inevitable, and if patient recovers, severe pitting is likely to remain.

v., discrete. V. when pustules are distinct.

v., hemorrhagic. V. with hemorrhage into the vesicles.

In the hemorrhagic type, following customary onset, an extensive eruption of skin may develop, suggestive of scarlet fever. Profuse subconjunctival hemorrhages, profuse hemorrhages from nose and mouth may develop and patient die within 24 to 48 hours with no prior loss of consciousness. In some cases of hemorrhagic smallpox, there may be seen only a few, or sometimes many spots, followed by death within 24 hours of their appearance. In still a 3rd type of the hemorrhagic variety lesions progress in the customary manner until pustular stage is reached, when hemorrhages take place in the lesions.

v. major. Ordinary unmodified severe smallpox.

v., malignant. A fatal form of hemorrhagic v., *q.v.*

v. minor. Mild smallpox. SYN: *alastrim.*

v., modified. Type of the disease commonly called varioloid. Case of modified smallpox seen in patients who have been vaccinated some years previously, but have not retained a complete immunity to the disease.

As a result, the infection is usually mild as to number and character of lesions, though at times the onset is somewhat severe.

variolar (văr-ī'ōl-ar). Pertaining to smallpox.

variolate (văr'ĭ-ō-lāt) [L. *variola,* a tiny mark]. 1. To vaccinate with smallpox virus. 2. Having lesions like those of smallpox.

variolation, variolization (văr-ĭ-ō-lā'shŭn, văr-ĭ-ō-lĭ-zā'shŭn) [L. *variola,* a tiny spot]. Inoculation with smallpox.

varioloid (văr'ĭ-ō-loyd) [" + G. *eidos,* form]. 1. Resembling smallpox. 2. Pert. to varioloid. 3. A mild but contagious type of smallpox in those who have had smallpox or have been vaccinated.

variolous (văr-ī'ō-lŭs) [L. *variola,* a tiny mark]. Relating to smallpox.

varix (vă'rĭks) (pl. *varices*) [L. *varix,* a dilated twisted vein]. 1. A tortuous dilatation of a vein. SEE: *varicose veins.* 2. Less commonly, dilatation of an artery or lymph vessel.

v., aneurysmal. A direct communication bet. an artery and a varicose vein without an intervening sac.

v., chyle. A varix of a lymphatic vessel which conveys chyle.

v. lymphaticus. Dilatation of lymphatic vessel.

v., turbinal. Permanent dilatation of veins of turbinate bodies.

varolian (vă-rō'lĭ-ăn). Relating to the pons Varolii.

v. bend. Ant. extension of hindgut on its ventral surface in the fetus.

varus (vā'rŭs) [L. *varus,* bent inward]. 1. Turned inward; bowlegged. 2. A condition in which a clubfooted person walks on outer border of the foot. SYN: *talipes varus.* SEE: *valgus.*

vas (văs) (pl. *vasa*) [L. *vas,* vessel]. A vessel or duct.

v. aberrans. 1. A narrow tube varying in length from 1½ to 14 inches, occasionally found connected with the lower part of the canal of the epididymis or with the commencement of the vas deferens. 2. Vestige of the biliary ducts sometimes found in the liver.

v. afferens. An afferent vessel of a lymph node.

v. afferens glomeruli. The afferent arteriole which conveys blood to the glomerulus of a renal corpuscle.

v. capillare. NA. A capillary blood vessel.

v. deferens. The excretory duct of the testis, the continuation of the epididymis, terminating at *ductus ejaculatorius* at prostatic urethra. SYN: *ductus deferens* [NA].

RS: *ampullitis, cord, spermatic, deferentitis.*

v. lymphaticum. NA. One of the vessels carrying the lymph.

v. prominens. NA. Blood vessel on the cochlea's accessory spiral ligament.

v. spirale. A large blood vessel beneath the tunnel of corti in the basilar membrane.

vasa (vā'să) [L. *vas,* vessel]. Plural of *vas.*

v. afferen'tia. The lymphatic vessels entering a lymph node.

v. bre'via. Branches of the splenic artery going to greater curvature of the stomach.

v. efferen'tia. 1. Lymphatics which leave a lymph node. 2. Excretory ducts of the testis to the head of the epididymis.

v. prae'via. The blood vessels of the umbilical cord presenting before the fetus.

v. rec'ta. 1. Tubules which become straight prior to entering the mediastinum testis. 2. Straight collecting tubules of the kidney.

v. vaso'rum. NA. Tiny blood vessels which are distributed to walls of larger veins and arteries.

v. vortico'sa. Stellate veins of the choroid, carrying blood to the sup. ophthalmic vein. SYN: *venae chroideae oculi* [NA].

vasal (vā'săl) [L. *vas,* vessel]. Relating to a vas or vessel.

vasalgia (vă-sal'jĭ-ă). Pain in a vessel of any kind.

vascular (văs'kū-lăr) [L. *vasculum,* a small vessel]. Pert. to or composed of blood vessels.

v. reflex. Constriction or dilation of vascular trunk or area resulting from mental or physical irritation.

v. system. The heart, blood vessels, lymphatics and their parts considered collectively.

It includes the pulmonary and portal systems.

v. tuft. One of the vascular processes on the chorion in the fetus at an early stage of development. SYN: *villi, chorionic.*

v. tumor. One containing dilated blood vessels. SYN: *angioma, telangioma.*

vascularization (văs"kū-lă-rĭ-zā'shŭn) [L. *vasculum,* a tiny vessel]. Development of new blood vessels in a structure.

vascularize (văs'kū-lă-rīz) [L. *vasculum,* a tiny vessel]. To become vascular by development of new blood vessels.

vasculitis (văs-kū-lī'tĭs) [" + *-itis,* inflammation]. Inflammation of a vessel. SYN: *angiitis.*

vasculum (văs'kū-lŭm) [L. a small vessel]. A tiny vessel.

vasectomy (văs-ĕk'tō-mĭ) [L. *vas,* vessel, + G. *ektomē,* excision]. Removal of all or a segment of the vas deferens.

vasifactive (văs-ĭ-făk'tĭv) [" + *facere,* to make]. Forming new vessels. SYN: *vasofactive, vasoformative.*

vasiform (văs'ĭ-form) [" + *forma,* shape]. Resembling a tubular structure or vas.

vas'o- [L.]. Combining form meaning *a vessel,* as a blood vessel.

vasoactive (vas-o-ak'tiv). Affecting blood vessels.

vasoconstrictive (văs″ō-kŏn-strĭk′tĭv) [L. *vas*, vessel, + *constrictus*, bound]. Causing constriction of the blood vessels.

vasoconstrictor (văs″ō-kŏn-strĭk′tor) [" + *constrictor, a* binder]. 1. Causing constriction of blood vessels. 2. That which constricts or narrows the caliber of blood vessels, as a drug or a nerve.

vasodentin (văs″ō-dĕn′tin) [" + *dentīnus*, pert. to a tooth]. Modified dentine provided with blood capillaries.

vasodepression (văs″ō-dē-prĕsh′ŭn) [" + *depressio*, a pushing down]. Vasomotor depression or collapse

vasodepressor (văs″ō-dē-prĕs′or) [L. *vas*, vessel, + *depressor*, that which pushes down]. 1. Having a depressing influence on the circulation, lowering blood pressure by dilatation of blood vessels. 2. An agent which depresses circulation.

vasodilatation (văs″ō-dĭl-ă-tā′shŭn) [" + *dilatāre*, to widen]. Dilatation of blood vessels, esp. small arteries and arterioles.

v., *antidromic*. Vasodilatation resulting from stimulation of dorsal root of a spinal nerve.

v., *reflex*. Blood vessel dilation due to stimulation of its dilator nerves or inhibition of its constrictor substance or nerves. This can be done by stimulating the sensory reflex arc.

vasodilatin (văs″ō-dī-lā′tĭn) [L. *vas*, vessel, + *dilatāre*, to widen]. A vasodilator substance said to be present in organic extracts, which depresses nerves and blood vessels. It is similar to or possibly identical with histamine.

vasodilator (văs″ō-dī-lā′tor) [" + *dilatāre*, to widen]. 1. Causing relaxation of the blood vessels. 2. A nerve or drug which dilates the blood vessels.

vasoepididymostomy (văs″ō-ĕp″ĭ-dĭd-ĭ-mŏs′tō-mĭ) [" + G. *epi*, upon, + *didymos*, testicle, + *stoma*, passage]. Formation of a passage bet. the vas deferens and the epididymis.

vasoexcitor (văs-ō-ĕks-sĭt′or). Stimulating vasoconstriction.

v. *material*. Abbr. VEM. A pressor principle formed in the kidney which appears in circulation of animals in shock or after prolonged anoxia.

vasofactive (văs″ō-făk′tĭv) [" + *facere*, to make]. Forming new blood vessels. SYN: *vasifactive, vasoformative.*

vasoformative (văs″ō-for′mă-tĭv) [" + *formāre*, to form]. Forming new blood vessels. SYN: *vasofactive, vasifactive.*

vasography (văs-ŏg′ră-fĭ) [L. *vas*, vessel, + G. *graphein*, to write]. X-ray photography of the blood vessels.

vasohypertonic (văs″ō-hī-pĕr-tŏn′ĭk) [" + G. *hyper*, over, + *tonikos*, pert. to tension]. Causing or that which causes constriction of blood vessels. SYN: *vasoconstrictor.*

vasohypotonic (văs″ō-hī-pō-tŏn′ĭk) [" + G. *hypo*, under, + *tonikos*, pert. to tension]. Relaxing or that which relaxes blood vessels. SYN: *vasodilator.*

vasoinhibitor (văs″ō-ĭn-hĭb′ĭ-tor) [" + *inhibere*, to restrain]. An agent that depresses vasomotor nerves.

vasoinhibitory (văs″ō-ĭn-hĭb′ĭ-tor-ĭ) [" + *inhibere*, to restrain]. Restricting vasomotor activity.

vasoligation (văs″ō-lī-gā′shŭn) [" + *ligāre*, to bind]. Ligation of a vessel, specifically the vas deferens.

vasomotion (văs″ō-mō′shŭn) [" + *motio*, a moving]. Change in caliber of a blood vessel.

vasomotor (văs″ō-mō′tor) [L. *vas*, vessel, + *motor*, a mover]. Pert. to the nerves having muscular control of the blood vessel walls.

The circularly arranged fibers of the muscles of arteries and veins can contract or relax; the affected region is accordingly either blanched or flushed. The former effect can commonly be produced by stimulating sympathetic fibers, and is consequently called vasoconstrictor; certain other nerves on stimulation cause vasodilation, examples being the nervus chorda tympani and the nervi erigentes.

A vasomotor reflex is one in which the stimulus, *e. g.*, a horrifying sight, results in a change in vasomotor stage, *e. g.*, pallor. SEE: *vasoconstrictor, vasodilator.*

v. *epilepsy*. E. with vasomotor changes in the skin.

v. *nerves*. Those which cause either contraction or dilation of blood vessels.

v. *spasm*. Spasm of smaller arteries.

vasomotory (văs″ō-mō′tor-ĭ) [L. *vas*, vessel, + *motor*, a mover]. Controlling changes in the size of the blood vessels. SYN: *vasomotor.*

vasoneurosis (văs″ō-nū-rō′sĭs) [" + G. *neuron*, nerve, + *-ōsis*, condition]. A neurosis affecting blood vessels; a disorder of the vasomotor system. SEE: *angioneurosis.*

vasoorchidostomy (văs″ō-or-kĭd-ŏs′tō-mĭ) ["+G. *orchis, orchid-*, testicle, + *stoma*, mouth]. Surgical connection of the epididymis to the severed end of the vas deferens.

vasoparesis (văs″ō-păr-ē′sĭs) [" + G. *paresis*, relaxation]. Partial paralysis or weakness of the vasomotor nerves.

vasopressin (văs″ō-prĕs′ĭn). SYN: *antidiuretic hormone* (Abbr. *ADH.*); *pitressin.* A hormone formed in supraoptic and paraventricular nuclei of hypothalamus and transported to post. lobe of hypophysis through the hypothalamohypophyseal tract. It has an antidiuretic and a pressor effect elevating blood pressure. SEE: *oxytocin.*

vasopuncture (văs′ō-pŭnk-chūr) [L. *vas*, vessel, + *punctura*, a piercing]. Puncture of the vas deferens.

vasorelaxation (văs″ō-rē-lăks-ā′shŭn) [" + *relaxāre*, to loosen]. Lessening of vascular pressure.

vasorrhaphy (văs-or′ă-fĭ) [" + G. *rhaphē*, a seam]. Surgical suture of the vas deferens.

vasosection (văs″ō-sĕk′shŭn) [" + *sectio*, a cutting]. Surgical division of the vasa deferentia.

vasosensory (văs″ō-sĕn′sō-rĭ) [L. *vas*, vessel, + *sensōrius*, pert. to sensation]. Related to sensation in the blood vessels.

vasospasm (văs″ō-spăzm) [" + G. *spasmos*, a spasm]. Spasm of any vessel, esp. of a blood vessel. SYN: *angiospasm, vasoconstriction.*

vasostimulant (văs″ō-stĭm′ū-lănt) [" + *stimulāre*, to goad]. Exciting vasomotor action.

vasostomy (va-zos′to-mĭ) [L. *vas*, vessel, + G. *stoma*, mouth]. Surgical procedure of making an opening into the vas deferens.

vasotomy (văs-ŏt′ō-mĭ) [" + G. *tomē*, a cutting]. Incision of the vas deferens.

vasotonic (văs″ō-tŏn′ĭk) [" + G. *tonikos*, pert. to tone]. Pert. to the tone of a vessel.

vasotribe (văs′ō-trīb) [" + G. *tribein*, to crush]. Pressure forceps used for controlling hemorrhages. SYN: *angiotribe.*

vasotripsy (văs'ō-trĭp-sĭ) [" G. *tripsis*, a crushing]. Arrest of hemorrhages with a strong forceps by crushing an artery. SYN: *angiotripsy*.

vasotrophic (văs"ō-trŏf'ĭk) [L. *vas*, vessel, + G. *trophē*, nourishment]. Concerned with the nutrition of blood vessels.

vasovesiculectomy (văs"ō-vĕs-ĭk-ū-lĕk'tō-mĭ) [" + *vesicula*, tiny sac, + G. *ektomē*, excision]. Excision of the vas deferens and seminal vesicles.

vasovesiculitis (văs"ō-vĕs-ĭk-ū-lī-tĭs) [" + *vesicula*, tiny sac, + G. *-itis*, inflammation]. Inflammation of the vas deferens and seminal vesicles.

vast'us. 1. Great, large, extensive. 2. One of three muscles of the thigh. SEE: *Table of Muscles in Appendix*.

Vater (fah'ter) [Abraham Vater, German anatomist, 1684-1751].

V., ampulla of. Former name for papilla of Vater, *q.v.*

V.'s corpuscles. Ovoid end organs of nerves supplying the skin. SYN: *Vater-Pacini corpuscles*.

V., papilla of. The duodenal end of the drainage systems of the pancreatic and common bile ducts. Also called *vaterian segment*. Formerly called ampulla of Vater.

V.D. Abbr. for *venereal disease*.

V.D.G. Abbr. for *venereal disease—gonorrhea*.

V.D.H. Abbr. for *valvular disease of the heart*.

VDM. Abbr. for *vasodepressor material*.

VDRL. Abbr. for *Venereal Disease Research Laboratories*.

V.D.S. Abbr. for *venereal disease—syphilis*.

veal (vēl) [ME *veel*]. The flesh of a calf. To be distinguished from beef which is the flesh of a full-grown cow or bull.

COOKED: 100 gm. Calories: 235. Other values: 28 gm. protein; 13 gm. fat; 6 mg. niacin.

vection (vĕk'shŭn) [L. *vectio*, a carrying]. Carrying of disease germ from the sick to well persons.

v., circumferen'tial. Transference through an intermediate host.

v., ra'dial. Direct transference of disease germs from one individual to another.

vectis (vĕk'tĭs) [L. *rectis*, pole]. A curved lever for making traction on the presenting part of the fetus.

vector (vĕk'tor) [L. *vector*, a carrier]. An animal, usually an arthropod (insect or tick) which transmits the causative organisms of disease from infected to noninfected individuals, esp. one in which the organism goes through one or more stages in its life cycle.

v., cardiac. SEE: *vectorcardiogram*.

v., circumferen'tial. One carrying infection from the sick to the well.

vectorcardiogram. At any moment the electrical activity of the heart can be represented as an electrical vector with a specific direction and magnitude. This is called the instantaneous *cardiac vector*. These vectors may be established for the entire cardiac cycle. By joining the tips of these vectors with a continuous line, the vectorcardiogram loop is formed. The configuration so obtained may be projected on the frontal plane or viewed as a three-dimensional loop.

Three vectorcardiogram loops are formed during each cardiac cycle: one for the electrical activity of the auricle; one for ventricular depolarization; one for ventricular repolarization. Analysis of the configuration of these loops permits certain statements to be made about the state of health or disease of the myocardium.

vectorial (vĕk-tō'rĭ-ăl) [L. *vector*, a carrier]. Relating to a vector.

vegetable (vĕj'ĕt-ă-bl) [O. Fr. from L. *vegetus*, active]. 1. Pert. to, of the nature of, or derived from plants. 2. A herbaceous plant, esp. one cultivated for food. 3. The edible part or parts of plants which are used as food. Such includes the leaves, stems, seeds and seed pods, flowers, roots, tubers, and fruits.

Vegetables play an important dietary role as they (a) are important sources of minerals and vitamins, (b) provide bulk which stimulates intestinal motility, (c) and are sources of energy. Caloric value is indirectly proportional to water content.

CONTENTS: Vegetables in general are valuable for their mineral content and for their cellulose. *Copper* is estimated at 1.2 milligrams per kg. for leafy vegetables, and 0.7 milligram per kg. for nonleafy ones. They are deficient in fat, which can be corrected by adding milk, cream, butter in their preparation. SEE: *names of minerals*.

CHEMICAL CHANGES: 1. Dry heat changes starch to dextrin. 2. Heat and acid or a ferment change dextrin to dextrose. 3. In germinating grain, starch is changed to dextrin and dextrose. 4. Dextrose in fermentation turns to alcohol and carbon dioxide. 5. Raw starch is not digestible. All starches must be changed to sugars before they can be absorbed in the system. SEE: *sugar, classification of*.

vegetal (vĕj'ĕt-ăl). Trophic or nutritional, esp. with reference to that part of an ovum which contains the yolk. SEE: *pole, vegetal*.

vegetarian (vĕj-ĕ-tā'rĭ-ăn) [L. *vegetabilis*, quickening]. One who eats no animal products, but who lives on vegetables.

vegetarianism (vĕj-ĕ-tā'rĭ-ăn-ĭzm) [" + G. *-ismos*, condition]. The belief and practice of eating vegetables and fruits only.

vegetate (vĕj'ĕ-tāt). 1. To grow luxuriantly with the production of fleshy or warty outgrowths such as a polyp. 2. To lead a passive existence either mentally or physically; to do little more than eat and maintain basic body processes.

vegetation (vĕj-ĕ-tā'shŭn) [L. *vegetātio*, animation]. A morbid luxurious outgrowth on any part, esp. wartlike projections made up of collections of fibrin in which are enmeshed white and red blood cells; sometimes seen on denuded areas of the endocardium covering the valves of the heart.

v., adenoid. Fungus-like masses of lymphoid tissue in nasopharynx.

vegetative (vĕj'ĕ-tā"tĭv) [L. *vegetāre*, to animate). 1. Having the power to grow, as plants. 2. Functioning involuntarily. 3. Quiescent, passive, noting a stage of development.

v. nervous system. The sympathetic* nervous system.

v. pole. Area at end of ovum containing nutritive matter.

vehicle (vē'ĭ-kl) [L. *vehiculum*, that which carries]. A substance, usually inactive therapeutically, used in a medicinal preparation as the agent for carrying the active ingredient, for ex., a syrup in liquid preparations.

veil (vāl) [L. *velum*, a covering]. 1. Any veil-like structure. 2. A piece of the amniotic sac occasionally covering the face of a newborn infant. SYN: *caul*. 3. Slight obscuration of the voice.

v., acquired. Slight imperfection of the voice due to strain or exposure.

v., Hottentot. Elongated labia present in Hottentot women. SYN: *Hottentot apron*.

v., uterine. Device for covering the cervix uteri to prevent impregnation.

vein (vān) [L. *vena*]. Vessel carrying dark red (unaerated) blood to the heart, except for pulmonary vein.

Veins have 3 coats. They differ from arteries in their larger capacity and greater number; also in their thinner walls, larger and more frequent anastomoses and presence of valves which prevent backward circulation. They consist of 2 sets, *superficial* or *subcutaneous* and the *deep* veins with frequent communications. The former do not usually accompany an artery, as do the latter. The systemic veins consist of 3 groups: Those entering the heart through the (a) *superior vena cava*, (b) those through the *inferior vena cava*, and (c) those through the *coronary sinus*. Blood from the capillary plexuses enters the right auricle of the heart. SEE: *circulation, Table of Veins in Appendix*.

vein, words pert. to: basilic, cava, innominate, intravenous, janitrix, jugular, phlebectomy, phlebitis, phlebogram, phlebotomy, phlegmasia alba dolens, portal, thrombophlebitis, thrombus, "varic-" words, varix, vascular, vasoconstrictor, vasodilator, vasomotor, vasoparesis, vena, vena cava, venesection, venosity, veinlet, venostomy, venule, venous.

veinlet. A small vein or venule.

velamen (věl-ā'měn) (pl. *velamina*) [L. *velamen*, veil]. Any covering membrane.

v. nativum. The skin covering the body.

v. vul'vae. Abnormal elongation of the nymphae. SYN: *Hottentot apron* or *veil*.

velamentous (věl-ă-měn'tŭs) [L. *velamen*, veil]. Expanding like a veil, or sheet.

velamentum (věl-ă-měn'tŭm) (pl. *velamenta*) [L. *velamentum*, a cover]. A membranous covering.

velar (vē'lar) [L. *velum*, a veil]. Pert. to a veil or veil-like structure.

vellication (věl-ĭk-ā'shŭn) [L. *vellicāre*, to twitch]. Spasmodic twitching of muscular fibers.

velosynthesis (věl-o-sĭn'thěs-ĭs) [L. *velum*, veil, + G. *synthesis*, a placing together]. Suture of a cleft palate, particularly the soft palate. SYN: *staphylorrhaphy*.

Velpeau's bandage (věl-pō'). A bandage for the shoulder. SEE: *bandage*.

V's deformity. D. seen in Colles'* fracture in which lower fragment is displaced backward.

velum (vē'lŭm) [L. *velum*, veil]. Any veil-like structure.

v. palati'num. NA. The soft palate.

VEM. Abbr. for *vasoexcitor material, q.v.*

vena (vē'nă) (pl. *venae*) [L. *vena*, vein]. A vein. SEE: *Table of Veins in Appendix*.

v. cava, inferior. The principal vein draining lower portion of the body. It is formed by junction of the two common iliac veins and terminates in rt. atrium of the heart. SEE: *heart*.

v. cava, superior. The principal vein draining the upper portion of the body. It is formed by the junction of the rt. and left innominate veins and empties into rt. atrium of the heart. SEE: *heart*.

vena'tion. The distribution of veins to an organ or structure.

venenation (věn-ē-nā'shŭn) [L. *venenum*, poison]. 1. Condition of being poisoned. 2. Act of poisoning.

venene (vē-nēn') [L. *venenum*, poison] A mixture of venoms from poisonous snakes.

veneniferous (věn-ĕ-nĭf'ĕr-ŭs) [" + *ferre*, to carry]. Transmitting or carrying poison.

venenific (věn-ĕ-nĭf'ĭk) [" + *facere*, to make]. Producing poison.

venenous (věn'ĕn-ŭs) [L. *venenum*, poison]. Poisonous.

venepuncture (věn'ĕ-pŭnk"chūr) [L. *vena*, vein, + *punctura*, a piercing]. Venipuncture, *q.v.*

venereal (vē-nē'rē-ăl) [L. *venereus*, from *Venus*, goddess of love]. Pert. to or resulting from sexual intercourse.

v. bubo. Enlarged lymph node in the groin, the result of a venereal disease.

v. collar. Mottled condition of the neck seen occasionally in syphilis.

v. disease. One acquired ordinarily as a result of sexual intercourse with an individual who is afflicted.

The diseases are gonorrhea, syphilis and chancroid. *Trichomonas vaginalis vaginitis* can be, but is not always, contracted through sexual intercourse.

v. sore, v. ulcer. Chancroid.

v. urethritis. Urethritis occurring in gonorrhea.

v. wart. Moist reddish elevation on genitals and anus. SYN: *verruca acuminata, condyloma*.

venereologist (vē-nēr"ē-ŏl'ō-jĭst) [L. *venereus*, venereal, + G. *logos*, a study]. A doctor who specializes in the treatment of venereal diseases.

venereology (vē-nēr"ē-ŏl'ō-jĭ) [" + G. *logos*, a study]. The scientific study and treatment of venereal diseases.

venereophobia (vē-nēr"ē-ō-fō'bĭ-ă) [" + G. *phobos*, *fear*]. Abnormal fear of venereal disease. SYN: *cypridophobia*.

venery (věn'ĕr-ĭ) [L. *Venus, Vener-*, Venus, goddess of love]. Sexual intercourse. SYN: *coitus*.

venesection (věn"-ĕ-sěk'shŭn) [L. *vena*, vein, + *sectio*, a cutting]. Opening of a vein for withdrawal of blood.

venin(e (věn'ĭn) [L. *venenum*, poison]. Toxic substance in snake venom. SYN: *venene*.

venin-antivenin (věn"ĭn-ăn"tĭ-věn'ĭn). Vaccine to counteract snake poison.

veniplex (věn'ĭ-plěks) [L. *vena*, vein, + *plexus*, a braid]. A plexus of veins.

venipuncture (věn"ĭ-pŭnk'chūr) [" + *punctura*, a piercing]. Puncture of a vein for any purpose.

venisection (věn"ĭ-sěk'shŭn) [" + *sectio*, a cutting]. Opening of a vein for removal of blood. SYN: *phlebotomy*.

venisuture (věn-ĭ-sū-chūr) [" + *sutura*, a stitch]. Suture of a vein. SYN: *phleborrhaphy*.

venoatrial (venoauricular) (vē"nō-āt'rĭ-ăl, -aw-rĭk'ū-lăr) [L. *vena*, vein, + *atrium*, corridor]. Relating to the vena cava and the atrium.

venoclysis (vē-nŏk'lĭ-sĭs) [" + G. *klysis*, injection]. The continuous injection of medicinal or nutrient fluid intravenously. SYN: *phleboclysis*.

venogram (vē′nō-grăm) [" + G. *gramma*, a writing]. 1. A roentgenogram of the veins. SYN: *phlebogram*. 2. A tracing of the venous pulse.

venography (vē-nŏg′ră-fĭ) [" + G. *graphein*, to write]. 1. Roentgenography of veins. 2. The making of a tracing of the venous pulse.

venom (vĕn′ŏm) [L. *venenum*, poison]. A poison excreted by some animals, such as insects or snakes, and transmitted by bites or stings.

v., snake. The poisonous secretion of the labial glands of certain snakes. Venoms contain proteins, chiefly toxins and enzymes, which are responsible for their toxicity. They are classified as *neurocytolysins, hemolysins, hemocoagulins, proteolysins*, and *cytolysins* on the basis of the effects produced.

ven″omot′or. Pert. to constriction or dilatation of veins.

venomous. Poisonous.

v. snake. In the USA, the coral snakes and pit vipers (copperhead, cottonmouth moccasin, and rattlesnakes). SEE: *snakes, poisonous.*

venoperitoneostomy (vē″nō-pĕr″ĭ-tō-nē-ŏs′tō-mĭ) [L. *vena*, vein, + G. *peritonaion*, peritoneum, + *stoma*, passage]. Surgically inserting the cut end of the saphenous vein into the cavity of the peritoneum. This is done to allow ascitic fluid from the peritoneal cavity to drain into the vein.

venopressor (vē′nō-prĕs″or) [" + *pressor*, that which squeezes]. Pert. to venous blood pressure.

venosclerosis (vē″nō-sklē-rō′sĭs) [" + G. *sklērōsis*, a hardening]. Sclerosis of veins. SYN: *phlebosclerosis.*

venosity (vē-nŏs′ĭ-tĭ) [L. *vena*, vein]. 1. Condition in which there is an excess of venous blood in a part causing venous congestion. 2. Deficient aeration of venous blood.

venostasis (vē-nŏs-tā′sĭs) [L. *vena*, vein, + G. *stasis*, a standing]. The trapping of blood in an extremity by compression of veins, a method sometimes employed for reducing the amount of blood in circulation.

venostat (vē′nō-stăt) [" + G. *statikos*, standing]. Appliance for performing venous compression.

venothrombotic (vē-nŏ-thrŏm-bŏt′ĭk). Having the property of inducing the formation of thrombi in veins.

venotomy (vē-nŏt′ō-mĭ) [L. *vena*, vein, + G. *tomē*, a cutting]. Incision of a vein.

venous (vē′nŭs) [L. *vena*, vein]. Pert. to the veins or blood passing through them.

v. blood. The dark blood in the veins.

v. hum. Murmur heard upon auscultation over larger veins of the neck.

v. hypere′mia. Excess of venous blood in a part. SYN: *venosity.*

v. return. The amount of blood returning to the atria of the heart.

v. sinus. A channel which carries venous blood. Important venous sinuses are those of the dura mater draining the brain and those of the spleen.

v. sinus of sclera. The canal of Schlemm, *q.v.*

venovenostomy (vē-nō-vē-nŏs′tō-mĭ) [L. *vena*, vein, + *vena*, vein, + G. *stoma*, mouth]. Formation of an anastomosis of a vein into a vein.

vent (vĕnt) [O. Fr. *fente*, slit]. An opening in any cavity, esp. one for excretion.

v., alveolar. An opening between adjacent alveoli of the lung.

venter (vĕn′ter) [L. *venter*, belly]. SYN: *belly.* 1. A belly-shaped part. 2. The cavity of the abdomen. 3. The belly of a muscle.

ventilation (vĕn-tĭl-ā′shŭn) [L. *ventilāre*, to air]. 1. Circulation of air or amt. of fresh air in a room and withdrawal of foul air. 2. Oxygenation of blood. 3. PHYS: The amt. of air inhaled per day.

This can be estimated by spirometry, multiplying the tidal air by the number of respirations per day. An average figure is 10,000 liters. This must not be confused with the total amt. of oxygen consumed, which is on the average only 490 liters.

v. coefficient. The amount of air that must be respired for each liter of oxygen absorbed.

v., pulmonary. The inspiration and expiration of air from the lungs.

v. rate. ABBR: *VR.* The amount of air breathed in one minute. Also called *respiratory minute volume (RMV).*

ven′trad [L. *venter*, belly, + *ad*, toward]. Toward the ventral aspect, opp. to *dorsad.*

ventral (vĕn′trăl) [L. *ventralis*, pert. to the belly]. Pertaining to the belly, hence, in quadrupeds, pertaining to the *lower* or *underneath* side of the body; in man, pertaining to the anterior portion or the front side of the body.

v. hernia. One through the abdominal wall, esp. at points other than the umbilicus and groin.

ventricle (vĕn′trĭk-l) [L. *ventriculus*, a little belly]. 1. A small cavity. 2. One of 2 lower chambers of the heart which propel blood into the arteries. The right v. forces it into the pulmonary artery and the lungs; the left, through the aorta. 3. One of the cavities of the brain.

RS: *Arantius', aula, aulatela, carneous columns, heart.*

v., aortic. Left v. of the heart.

v. of the larynx. The space bet. the true and false vocal cords.

ventricornu (vĕn-trĭ-kor′nū) [L. *venter*, belly, + *cornu*, horn]. The ant. ventral horn of gray matter of the spinal cord.

ventricose (vĕn′trĭ-kōs) [L. *ventricōsus*, big-bellied]. 1. Inflated on 1 side. 2. Corpulent.

ventricular (vĕn-trĭk′ū-lar) [L. *ventriculus*, a little belly]. Pert. to a ventricle.

v. folds. The false vocal cords or folds of mucous membrane parallel or above the true vocal cords.

v. ligament. A narrow band of fibrous tissue lying within each *ventricular fold.*

v. tertius. Third ventricle of the brain.

ventriculography (vĕn-trĭk-ū-lŏg′ră-fĭ) [L. *ventriculus*, a little belly, + G. *graphein*, to write]. An x-ray process used for visualizing the size and shape of the cerebral ventricles by injecting air to displace the cerebrospinal fluid which normally fills these cavities.

ventriculometry (vĕn-trĭk″ū-lŏm′ĕ-trĭ) [" + G. *metron*, a measure]. The measurement of the intraventricular cerebral pressure.

ventriculonector (vĕn-trĭk″ū-lō-nĕk′tor) [" + *nector*, a joiner]. The atrioventricular bundle.

ventriculoscopy (vĕn-trĭk″ū-lŏs′kō-pĭ) [" + G. *skopein*, to examine]. Examination of the ventricles of the brain with an endoscope.

ventriculus (vĕn-trĭk′ū-lŭs) [L. a little belly]. NA. 1. The stomach. 2. A ventricle of the brain or heart.

ventricumbent (vĕn-trĭ-kŭm′bĕnt) [L. *venter*, belly, + *cumbere*, to lie]. Lying on the belly. SYN: *prone*.

ventriduct (vĕn′trĭ-dŭkt) [" + *ductus*, leading]. To draw toward the abdomen.

ventrimeson (vĕn-trĭ-mĕs′ŏn) [" + G. *mesos*, middle]. The median line on the ventral surface of the body.

ventripyramid (vĕn″trĭ-pir′ă-mĭd) [" + G. *pyramis*, pyramid]. An ant. pyramid of the medulla oblongata.

ven′tro-. Combining form denoting the *abdomen* or *ventral (anterior) surface* of the body.

ventrocystorrhaphy (vĕn-trō-sĭs-tor′ă-fĭ) [" + G. *kystis*, sac, + *rhaphē*, a seam]. Suture of a cyst or the bladder to the abdominal wall.

ventrofixation (vĕn″trō-fĭks-ā′shŭn) [" + *fixāre*, to fix]. The suture of a displaced viscus to the abdominal wall.

ventrohysteropexy (vĕn″trō-hĭs′tĕr-ō-pĕks″ĭ) [" + G. *hystera*, uterus, + *pēxis*, fixation]. Attachment of the uterus to the abdominal wall.

ventroscopy (vĕn-trŏs′kō-pĭ) [L. *venter*, belly, + G. *skopein*, to examine]. Examination of the abdominal cavity by illumination. SYN: *celioscopy*.

ventrose (vĕn′trōs) [L. *venter*, belly]. Having a belly or swelling like one.

ventrosity (vĕn-trŏs′ĭ-tĭ). [L. *venter*, belly]. Having an enlarged belly; corpulence.

ventrosuspension (vĕn″trō-sŭs-pĕn′shŭn) [" + *suspensio*, a hanging]. Fixation of displaced uterus to abdominal wall.

ventrotomy (vĕn-trŏt′ō-mĭ) [" + G. *tomē*, a cutting]. Incision into abdominal cavity. SYN: *celiotomy, laparotomy, q.v.*

ventrovesicofixation (vĕn″trō-vĕs-ĭ-kō-fĭks-ā′shŭn) [" + *vesica*, bladder, + *fixāre*, to fix]. Suture of uterus to abdominal wall and bladder. SYN: *hysterocystopexy*.

venturimeter (ven″tūr-im′ĕ-ter) [Giovanni Battista Venturi, 1746-1822, Italian physicist]. Device for measuring flow of fluids through vessels.

venula (vĕn′ū-lă) [L. little vein]. Venule.

venule (vĕn′ūl) [L. *venula*, little vein]. A veinlet, a tiny vein continuous with a capillary.

venus (vē′nŭs). The Roman goddess of love.

v.′s collar. Pigmentation around the neck in eruption due to syphilis.

v., crown of. An eruption around the hairline caused by syphilis.

v., mount of. The mons pubis (mons veneris), *q.v.*

verbigeration (vĕr-bĭj-ĕr-ā′shŭn) [L. *verbigerāre*, to chatter]. Repetition of words which are either meaningless or have no significance.

verbomania (vĕr″bō-mā′nĭ-ă) [L. *verba*, word, + G. *mania*, madness]. The flow of talk in some forms of psychosis.

verdigris (vĕr′dĭg-rĭs) [O.Fr. *vert de Grece*, green of Greece]. 1. Mixture of basic copper acetates. 2. Deposit of copper carbonate upon copper and bronze vessels. These are of a greenish gray color.

POISONING: TREATMENT: Same as for copper sulfate.

verdohemoglobin (vĕr″dō-hēm′ō-glōb-ĭn). A greenish pigment occurring as an intermediate product in the formation of bilirubin from hemoglobin.

Verga's ventricle (vĕr′gă). Cleftlike space bet. the callosum and fornix of the brain.

vergence (vĕrg″ĕns) [L. *vergere*, to bend]. A turning of one eye with reference to the other. May be horizontal (convergence or divergence) or vertical (infravergence or supravergence).

ver′gens. Inclining.

v. deorsum. Inclining downward.

v. sursum. Inclining upward.

Verheyen's stars (fĕr-hī′ĕn). Starlike venous plexuses on surface of the kidney below its capsule.

vermicidal (vĕr″mĭ-sī′dăl) [L. *vermis*, worm, + *cidus*, from *caedere*, to kill]. Destroying worms parasitic in the intestines.

vermicide (vĕr′mĭ-sīd) [" + *cidus*, from *caedere*, to kill]. 1. Destroying worms. 2. An agent that will kill intestinal worms. Ex: *santonin, chenopodium oil.*

vermicular (vĕr-mĭk′ū-lăr) [L. *vermicularis*, like a worm]. Resembling a worm.

v. movements. The wormlike movements of peristalsis.

v. pulse. Small, rapid one resulting in wormlike feeling in the fingers.

vermiculation (vĕr-mĭk″ū-lā′shŭn) [L. *vermiculāre*, to wriggle]. A wormlike motion, as in the intestines. SEE: *peristalsis.*

vermiculose, vermiculous (vĕr-mĭk′ū-lōs, vĕr-mĭk′ū-lŭs) [L. *vermicularis*, wormlike]. 1. Infested with worms or larvae. 2. Wormlike.

vermiform (vĕr′mĭ-form) [L. *vermis*, worm, + *forma*, shape]. Contoured like a worm.

v. appendix. A small tube of variable length, average about 8 cm., connected to the cecum. Its distal end is closed. It is lined with mucosa similar to that of the large intestine.

Its inflammation is called *appendicitis.**

vermifugal (vĕr-mĭf′ū-găl) [" + *fugāre*, to put to flight]. Expelling worms from the intestines.

vermifuge (vĕr′mĭ-fūj) [" + *fugāre*, to put to flight]. Agent for expelling intestinal worms. SEE: *anthelmintic, vermicide.*

vermilion border. The junction of the pinkish red area of the lips with the surrounding skin.

vermin (vĕr′mĭn) [L. *vermis*, worm]. Parasitic insects and animals, such as mice, lice, bedbugs.

vermination (vĕr-mĭn-ā′shŭn) [L. *vermis*, worm]. Vermin or worm infestation.

verminosis (vĕr-mĭn-ō′sĭs) [" + G. *-ōsis*, condition]. Infestation with vermin.

verminous (vĕr′mĭn-ŭs) [L. *vermis*, worm]. Pert. to or infested with worms.

vermiphobia (vĕr-mĭ-fō′bĭ-ă) [" + G. *phobos*, fear]. An abnormal fear of being infested with worms.

vermis (vĕr′mĭs) [L. *vermis*, worm]. 1. A worm. 2. Median connecting lobe of the cerebellum.

v. cerebel′li. NA. Same as vermis, 2.

v., inferior. The anterior inferior portion of the vermis of the cerebellum. Includes the *nodule, uvula, pyramis,* and *tuber*.

v., superior. The posterior, dorsal portion of the vermis. Includes the *folium, declive, culmen,* and *central lobule*.

vernal (vĕr′năl) [L. *vernalis*, pert. to spring]. Occurring in or pert. to the spring.

vernix (vĕr′nĭks) [L.]. Varnish.

v. caseo′sa. A sebaceous deposit covering the fetus due to secretion of skin glands. Most abundant in creases and flexor surfaces. Consists of exfoliations of outer skin layer, lanugo, and secretions of sebaceous glands. It is not necessary to remove this after the fetus is delivered. SEE: *sebum.*

veronal (vĕr′ō-năl). USP. A proprietary brand of barbital, a white crystalline substance. Used as an hypnotic.

v. sodium. A brand of soluble barbital.

veronalism (vĕr′ō-năl-ĭzm). Addiction to the use of veronal and the resultant symptoms.

verruca (vĕr-rū′kă) (pl. *verrucae*) [L. *verruca,* wart]. Elevation of the skin, small, circumscribed, formed by hypertrophy of the papillae and of various forms according to location. SYN: *wart.*

ETIOL: Caused by a filtrable virus, but predisposing factors are not known.

PROG: Essentially benign and may disappear spontaneously, particularly in children and young adults. In elderly with longstanding dry seborrhea, lesions may have potential malignancy.

TREATMENT: Removal with sharp spoon curet under local anesthesia. If elevated, clip off with sharp scissors and touch with iodine. Freezing with carbon dioxide snow, fulguration and, if multiple, x-ray therapy.

v. acuminata. A pointed reddish moist wart about the genitals and the anus. SYN: *venereal wart.*

Develops near mucocutaneous junctures, forming pointed, tufted, or pedunculated, pinkish or purplish projections of varying lengths and consistence.

Venereal warts should be treated with applications of podophyllum resin followed by removal of the resin by washing with soap and water about 6 hours after application.

v. digitata. Form seen on face and scalp, possibly serving as starting point of cutaneous horns, forming several filiform projections with horny caps closely grouped on a comparatively narrow base which in turn may be separated from skin surface by slightly contracted neck.

v. filiformis. Small threadlike growths on neck and eyelids covered with smooth and apparently normal epidermis.

v. gyri hippocampi. One of the small wartlike protuberances on the convex surface of the gyrus hippocampi.

v. plana. Flat oily wart, pigmented, on backs of old people.

v. plantaris. Warts on the soles of the feet. SYN: *plantar wart*

v. senilis. V. plana, *q.v.*

v. simplex. V. vulgaris, *q.v.*

v. vulgaris. Common warts, usually on backs of hands and fingers.

verruciform (vĕr-ū′sĭ-form) [L. *verruca,* wart, + *forma,* shape]. Wartlike.

verrucose, verrucous (vĕr′rū-kōs, vĕr-rū′-kŭs) [L. *verrucōsus,* wartlike]. Wartlike, with raised portions.

verruga peruana (vĕ-roo′gă pĕr-wăn′ă) [Sp. Peruvian wart]. The eruptive second clinical stage of bartonellosis, *q.v.* *Oroya fever* is the first or febrile stage.

versicolor (vĕr′sĭ-kŭl″er) [L. *versicolor,* of changing colors]. 1. Having many shades or colors. 2. Changeable in color SEE: *tinea versicolor.*

version (ver′zhŭn) [L. *versio,* a turning]. 1. Condition of uterus in which its axis is deflected from the normal position without being bent on itself. SEE: *anteversion, lateroversion, retroversion.* 2. Process of turning the fetus in the uterus to facilitate delivery.

v., cephalic. Turning of fetus so that the head presents.

v., pelvic. Manipulation of a cross presentation until it is changed to a pelvic presentation.

v., podalic. Manipulation of fetus by the feet so that the breech presents.

v., spontaneous. V. of fetus by uterine muscular contraction without artificial assistance.

vertebra (ver′tē-bră) (pl. *vertebrae*) [L. *vertebra*]. Any one of the 33 bony segments of the spinal column.

The vertebrae are comprised of 7 cervical, 12 thoracic (dorsal), 5 lumbar, 5 sacral, and 4 coccygeal. In adults, the five sacral vertebrae fuse to form a single bone, the *sacrum,* and the four rudimentary coccygeal vertebrae fuse to form the *coccyx.*

A typical vertebra consists of a ventral *body* and a dorsal or *neural arch.* In the thoracic region the body bears on each side two *costal pits* for reception of the head of a rib. The arch which encloses the *vertebral foramen* is formed of two *roots* or *pedicles* and two *lamina.* The arch bears seven processes: a dorsal

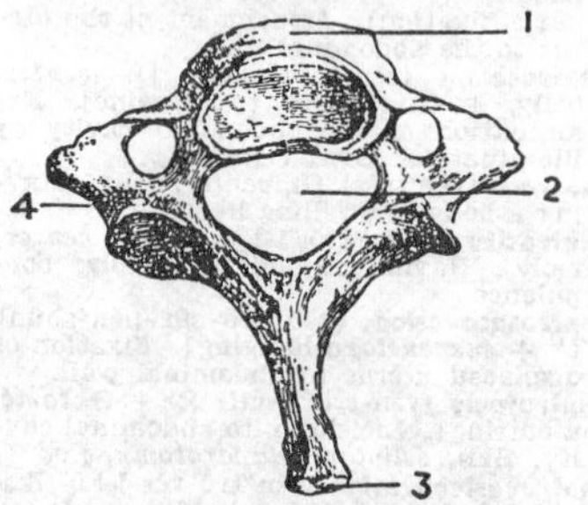

CERVICAL VERTEBRA

1. Body. 2. Vertebral foramen. 3. Spinous process. 4. Transverse process.

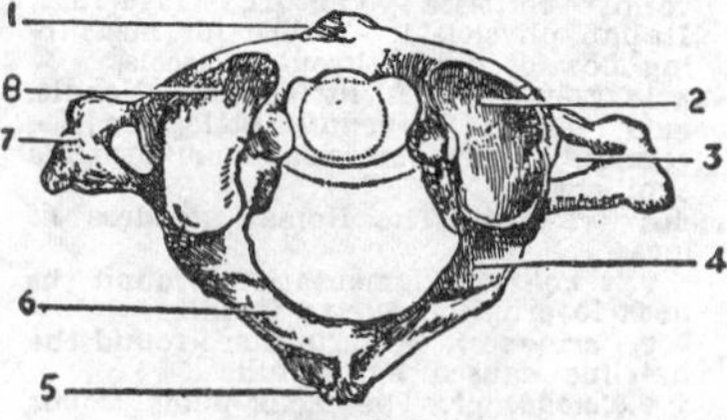

ATLAS

1. Anterior tubercle. 2. Lateral mass. 3. Foramen transversarium. 4. Groove for vertebral artery. 5. Posterior tubercle. 6. Posterior arch. 7. Transverse process. 8. Superior articular surface.

spinous process, two lateral *transverse processes,* and four *articular processes* (two superior and two inferior). A deep concavity, *inf. vertebral notch.* on the inferior border of the arch transmits a spinal nerve. The successive vertebral foramina lodge the spinal cord.

The bodies of successive vertebrae articulate with one another and are separated by *intervertebral disks,* disks of fibrous cartilage enclosing a central mass, the *nucleus pulposus.* The inf. articular processes articulate with the sup. articular processes of the next succeeding vertebra in the caudal direction. Several ligaments (supraspinous, interspinous, ant. and post. longitudinal, and the ligaments flava) hold the vertebrae in position yet permit a limited degree of movement.

RS: *acantha, anapophysis, anticlinal, atlas, axis, cervical v., lamina, spondyle, spondylitis, spondylotherapy.*

v., basilar. The lowest of the lumbar vertebrae.

v., cervical. The 7 vertebrae of the neck.

v., coccygeal. The rudimentary vertebrae of the coccyx.

v., codfish. Abnormal vertebrae seen in cases of osteoporosis in which there are concave deformities of endplates of bodies of vertebrae resulting from pressure from the nucleus pulposus.

v. dentata. The 2nd cervical vertebra. SYN: *axis.*

v., false. One of the segments of the sacrum and the coccyx.

v., fixed. False vertebrae, *q.v.*

v., flexion. All except the atlas and axis.

v., lumbar. The 5 vertebrae bet. the dorsal vertebrae and the sacrum.

v. magnum. The sacrum.

v., odontoid. Same as *v. dentata.*

v. prominens. The 7th cervical vertebra.

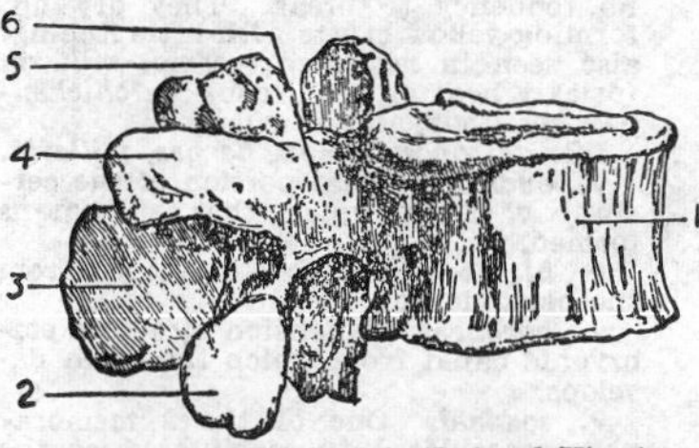

LUMBAR VERTEBRA (Lateral View)
1. Body. 2. Inferior articular process. 3. Spinal process. 4. Transverse process. 5. Inferior articular process. 6. Pedicle.

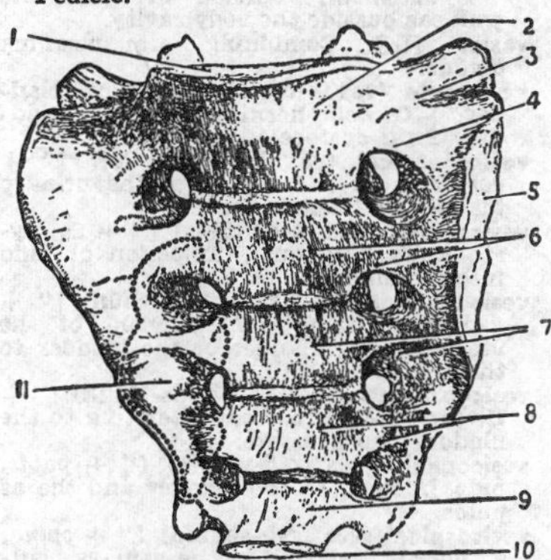

SACRUM (Pelvic Surface)
1. Superior articular process. Articulates with fifth lumbar vertebra. 2. Body of first sacral vertebra. 3. Ala. 4. First anterior sacral foramen. 5. Lateral articular process. 6. Body and foramen of second sacral vertebra. 7. Body and foramen of third sacral vertebra. 8. Body and foramen of fourth sacral vertebra. 9. Body of fifth vertebra. 10. Inferior articular process (area enclosed by dotted line). 11. Attachment of the piriformis muscle. Articulates with coccyx.

v., rotation. The first two cervical vertebrae, the atlas and axis.

v., sacral. The 5 fused segments forming the sacrum.

v., sternal. The segments of the sternum.

v., thoracic. The 12 vertebrae which connect the ribs and form part of the post. wall of the thorax. SYN: *dorsal v.*

v., true. The vertebrae which remain unfused through life.

vertebral (ver'tĕ-brăl) [L. *vertebra,* vertebra]. Pertaining to a vertebra or the vertebral column.

v. arch. The thoracic portion of a vertebra which encloses a vertebral foramen.

v. canal. Cavity of the spinal (vertebral) column which contains the spinal cord.

v. column. Spinal column.

v. foramen. 1. The hollow space enclosed by a vertebral arch. 2. A vertebrarterial foramen.

v. groove. Groove lying on either side of the spinous processes of the vertebrae.

v. notch. Notch on inferior surface of vertebral arch for transmission of a spinal nerve.

v. ribs. The lower 2, or floating ribs.

Vertebrata (vĕr"tĕ-brăt'ă). A subphylum of the phylum Chordata characterized by possession of segmented backbone or spinal column. They possess an axial notochord at some period of their existence. Includes the following classes: *Agnatha* (cyclostomes). *Chondrichthyes* (cartilaginous fishes) *Osteichthyes* (bony fishes), *Amphybia, Reptilia, Aves,* and *Mammalia.*

vertebrate, vertebrated (ver'tē-brāt, ver'-tē-brā-tĕd) [L. *vertebra*]. Having or resembling a vertebral column.

vertebrectomy (ver-tē-brĕk'tō-mĭ) [" + G. *ektomē,* excision]. Excision of a vertebra or part of one.

vertebrochondral (ver"tē-brō-kŏn'drăl) [" + G. *chondros,* cartilage]. Denoting the false ribs (8th, 9th, 10th) connected with a vertebra at 1 end and the costal cartilages at the other.

vertebrocostal (ver"tē-brō-kŏs'tăl) [" + *costa,* rib]. Pert. to a vertebra and a rib. SYN: *costovertebral.*

vertebromammary (ver"tē-brō-măm'mă-rĭ) [" + *mammarius,* pert. to a breast]. Pert. to the vertebral and mammary area.

v. diameter. The anteroposterior diameter of the thorax.

vertebrosternal (ver"tē-brō-ster'năl) [" + G. *sternon,* chest]. Pert. to a vertebra and the sternum.

vertex (ver'tĕks) [L. *vertex,* summit]. The top of the head. SYN: *crown.*

v. cordis. Apex of the heart.

v. presentation. Presentation in labor of vertex of the fetal skull.

vertical (ver'tĭk-ăl) [L. *vertex, vertic-,* summit]. 1. Pert. to or situated at the vertex. 2. Perpendicular to the plane of the horizon of the earth; upright.

verticillate (ver-tĭs'ĭl-āt, -tĭs-ĭl'āt) [L. *verticillus,* a little whirl]. Arranged like the spokes of a wheel or a whorl.

vertiginous (ver-tĭj'ĭn-ŭs) [L. *vertigo, vertigin-,* a turning round]. Pert. to or afflicted with vertigo.

vertigo (ver'tĭg-ō, ver-tī'gō) [L. *vertigo,* a turning round]. True vertigo is the sensation either of moving around in space or of having objects moving about the person. The subject has difficulty maintaining equilibrium. This is due to a disturbance of the sense of balance. Vertigo is not faintness, lightheadedness, or dizziness.

ETIOL: May be caused by a variety of entities including middle ear disease; toxic conditions such as those caused by salicylates; alcohol; streptomycin; sunstroke; postural hypotension; toxemia due to food poisoning or infectious diseases.

v., auditory, v., aural. V. due to disease of the ear.

v., cerebral. V. due to brain disease.

v., epileptic. V. attending an epileptic attack or following it.

v., essential. V. from an unknown cause.

v., gastric. V. from gastric disturbance.

v., hysterical. V. accompanying hysteria.

v., labyrinthine. V. due to disease of labyrinth of the ear. SYN: *Ménière's disease.*

v., laryngeal. V. accompanying laryngeal spasm.

v., objective. V. when objects seen appear to be moving when stationary.

v., ocular. V. caused by disease of the eye.

v., organic. V. from a brain lesion.

v., peripheral. V. from disturbance distant from the brain.

v., subjective. V. in which patient seems to be turning or rotating.

v., toxic. V. from presence of a toxin in the body.

verumontanitis (ver"ū-mŏn-tăn-ī'tĭs) [L. *verumontānum,* mountainous ridge, + G. *-itis,* inflammation]. Inflammation of the verumontanum. SYN: *colliculitis.*

verumontanum (ver"ū-mŏn-tā'nŭm) [L. *verumontānum,* mountainous ridge]. An elevation on the floor of the prostatic portion of the urethra where the seminal ducts enter.

vesalianum (vĕs-a-lĭ-ā'nŭm). One of the sesamoid bones in the tendon of origin of the gastrocnemius muscle, and another on outer border of foot in the angle bet. the cuboid and fifth metatarsal.

Vesalius, foramen of (vĕs-ā'lĭ-ŭs). One in base of the skull transmitting an emissary vein.

v., vein of. Small emissary vein from cavernous sinus passing through foramen of Vesalius and conveying blood to the pterygoid plexus.

vesanic (vĕs-ăn'ĭk) [L. *vesania,* insanity]. Pertaining to insanity.

vesica (vĕs-ī'kă) [L. *vesica,* a bladder]. A bladder.

v. fellea. NA. The gallbladder.

v. prostat'ica. A minute pouch in the prostatic urethra, remnant of müllerian duct. SYN: *utriculus prostaticus.*

v. urinaria. NA. The urinary bladder.

vesical (vĕs'ĭk-ăl) [L. *vesica,* a bladder]. Pert. to or shaped like a bladder.

v. reflex. Inclination to urinate caused by moderate bladder distention.

vesicant (vĕs'ĭk-ănt) [L. *vesicāre,* to blister]. 1. Blistering; causing or forming blisters. 2. Agent used to produce blisters. It is much less severe in its effects than escharotics. 3. A blistering gas used in chemical warfare.

Vesicants draw the deeper fluids to the surface in the form of blisters.

vesication (vĕs-ĭ-kā'shŭn) [L. *vesicāre,* to blister]. 1. Process of blistering. 2. A blister.

vesicatory (vĕs'ĭk-ă-tor"ĭ) [L. *vesicāre,* to blister]. 1. Causing or pert. to blisters. 2. Agent causing blisters. SYN: *vesicant.*

vesicle (vĕs'ĭ-kl) [L. *vesicula,* a little bladder]. 1. A small sac or bladder containing fluid. 2. A blisterlike small elevation on the skin from the size of a pinhead to that of a split pea, containing serous fluid.

Vesicles may be round, transparent, opaque, or dark elevations of the skin, sometimes containing seropurulent or bloody fluid.

They are seen in *sudamina* as the result of sweat which cannot escape from the skin; in *herpes,* mounted on an inflammatory base, having no tendency to rupture but associated with burning pain. In *herpes zoster* they follow the line of the nerve trunks. They are also seen in *dermatitis venenata,* as the result of poison ivy or oak, and accompanied by great itching, in *dermatitis herpetiformis* or *multiformis,* in *impetigo contagiosa,* occurring especially in children in discrete form, flat and umbilicated, filled with straw-color fluid with no tendency to break. They dry up, forming yellow crusts with little itching; also seen in *vesicular eczema, miliaria* (prickly heat or heat rash), in *chickenpox, smallpox,* and in *scabies.*

RS: *chiropompholyx, herpes, miliaria.*

v., auditory. That portion of the cerebral v. from which the ext. ear is formed.

v., blastodermic. Sac developed from the blastoderm.

v., cerebral. Expansion of neural embryonic canal from which the brain develops.

v., seminal. One of the 2 membranous, sacculated tubes situated at the base of the bladder, bet. it and the rectum, serving as a reservoir for the semen and having a secretion of its own.

v., umbilical. Portion of embryonic yolk sac outside the body cavity.

vesico- [L.]. Combining form meaning *bladder.*

vesicocele (ves'ĭk-ō-sēl) [L. *vesica,* bladder, + G. *kēlē,* hernia]. Hernia of bladder. SYN: *cystocele.*

vesicocervical (vĕs"ĭk-ō-ser'vĭ-kăl) [" + *cervix,* neck]. Relating to the urinary bladder and cervix uteri.

vesicoclysis (vĕs-ĭk-ŏk'lĭs-ĭs) [" + G. *klysis,* a washing out]. Injection of fluid into the bladder.

vesicofixation (ves"ĭk-ō-fĭks-ā'shŭn) [" + *fixātio,* a fixing]. Attachment of the uterus to the bladder or the bladder to the abdominal wall.

vesicoprostatic (vĕs"ĭk-ō-prŏs-tăt'ĭk) [" + G. *prostatēs,* prostate]. Relating to the bladder and prostate.

vesicopubic (vĕs"ĭk-ō-pū'bĭk) [" + *pubis,* pubis]. Pert. to the bladder and the os pubis.

vesicospinal (vĕs"ĭk-ō-spī'năl) [" + *spina,* a thorn]. Relating to the urinary bladder and spinal cord.

vesicotomy (vĕs-ĭ-kŏt'ō-mĭ) [L. *vesica,* a bladder, + G. *tomē,* a cutting]. Incision of the bladder.

vesicouterine (ves"ĭk-ō-ū'ter-ĭn) [" + *uterinus,* pert. to the womb]. Pert. to the urinary bladder and the uterus.

v. pouch. SYN: *uterovesical pouch.* Downward extension of the peritoneal cavity located between bladder and uterus.

vesicovaginal (vĕs"ĭk-ō-văj'ĭ-năl) [" + *vagina,* a sheath]. Pert. to the urinary bladder and vagina.

vesicula (vĕs-ĭk'ū-lă) (pl. *vesiculae*) [L. *vesicula,* a tiny bladder]. A small bladder, or vesicle.

v. seminalis. NA. Tiny reservoir of semen at base of the bladder. SYN: *vesicle, seminal, q.v.*

vesicular (vĕs-ĭk'ū-lar) [L. *vesicula,* a tiny bladder]. Pert. to vesicles or small blisters.

v. breathing. Murmur heard in normal breathing.

v. eczema. E. accompanied by formation of vesicles.

v. fellea. The gallbladder.

v. murmur. The normal sound of respiration heard on auscultation. Same as *v. breathing.*

v. prostatica. The prostatic utricle.

v. rale. The crepitant rale, a crackling sound heard at end of inspiration.

v. resonance. Percussion sound heard over the normal lung.

v. seminalis. The seminal vesicle. SEE: *vesicle, seminal.*

vesiculase (vĕs-ĭk'ū-lās) [L. *vesicula,* tiny bladder]. An enzyme in prostatic fluid said to coagulate semen.

vesiculation (vĕs-ĭk-ū-lā'shŭn) [L. *vesicula,* a tiny bladder]. Formation of vesicles or state of having or forming them.

vesiculectomy (vĕs-ĭk"ū-lĕk'tō-mĭ) [" + G. *ektomē,* excision]. Partial or complete excision of a vesicle, particularly a seminal vesicle.

vesiculiform (vĕs-ĭk'ū-lĭ-form) [" + *forma,* shape]. Having the shape of a vesicle.

vesiculitis (vĕs-ĭk"-ū-lī'tis) [" + G. *-itis,* inflammation]. Inflammation of a vesicle, particularly the seminal vesicle.

vesiculocavernous (vĕs-ĭk"ū-lō-kăv'ĕr-nŭs) [" + *cavernōsis,* hollow]. Vesicular and cavernous.

vesiculogram (vĕs-ĭk'ū-lō-grăm [" + G. *gramma,* a mark]. An x-ray picture of the seminal vesicles.

vesiculography (vĕs-ĭk"ū-lŏg'ră-fĭ) [" + G. *graphein,* to write]. X-ray photography of the seminal vesicles.

vesiculopapular (vĕs-ĭk"ū-lō-păp'ū-lăr) [L. *vesicula,* a tiny bladder, + *papula,* a pimple]. Composed of vesicles and papules.

vesiculopustular (vĕs-ĭk"ū-lō-pŭs'tū-lăr) [" + *pustula,* pustule]. Having both vesicles and pustules.

vesiculotomy (vĕs-ĭk"ū-lŏt'ō-mĭ) [" + G. *tomē,* a cutting]. Surgical incision into a vesicle, as a seminal vesicle.

vesiculotympanic (vĕs-ĭk"ū-lō-tĭm-păn'ĭk) [" + G. *tympanon,* drum]. Having both vesicular and tympanic qualities.

vespajus (vĕs-pā'jŭs). Follicular, suppurative inflammation of the hairy part of the scalp.

vessel (vĕs'ĕl) [O. Fr. from L. *vascellum,* a little vessel]. A tube, duct, or canal to convey the fluids of the body. SYN: *vas.*

RS: *anastomose; anastomosis; angiitis; angiodystrophia; arrosion; atresic; endothelial; intima; rhegma; vas; vascular.*

v.'s, absorbent. The lacteals, lymphatics and capillaries of the intestines.

v.'s, blood. Arteries, veins, and capillaries.

v.'s, chyliferous. V.'s arising in the villi of the intestinal walls carrying chyle and terminating in the thoracic duct.

v.'s, lymphatic. Vessels conveying lymph.

v.'s, nutrient. Those supplying interior of the bones.

v., radicular. Branch of a vertebral artery supplying cerebral nerve root.

vestibular (vĕs-tĭb'ū-lăr) [L. *vestibulum,* vestibule]. Pert. to a vestibule.

v. bulbs. Two sacculated collections of veins, lying on either side of the vagina beneath the bulbocavernosus muscle, connected anteriorly by the *pars intermedia,* and through this strip of cavernous tissue communicating with the erectile tissue of the clitoris.

Injury during labor may give rise to troublesome bleeding. The vestibular bulbs are the homologues of the male corpus spongiosum. SEE: *vestibule, Bartholin's glands, vagina.*

v. nerve. A main division of the auditory nerve. Arises in vestibular ganglion. Is concerned with equilibrium.

vestibule (vĕs'tĭb-ūl) [L. *vestibulum,* vestibule]. A small space or cavity at the beginning of a canal, such as the aortic v.

v. of ear. The middle part of the inner ear, behind the cochlea, and in front of the semicircular canals; it contains the utriculus and sacculus.

v. of larynx. The portion of the larynx above the vocal cords.

v. of nose. The anterior part of the nostrils containing the vibrissae.

v. of vagina. An almond-shaped space bet. the lines of attachment of the labia minora. At the ant. angle the *clitoris* is situated; the post. boundary is the *fourchette.* The vestibule appears approximately 4 or 5 cm. long and 2 cm. in greatest width when the labia minora are separated. Four major structures open into vestibule: The *urethra anteriorly,* the *vagina posteriorly,* and the two *excretory ducts of the glands of Bartholin,* laterally. The covering membranes are pink in color and constructed of delicate stratified squamous epithelium. Collections of cavernous tissue are disposed beneath the integument. SEE: *vestibular bulbs, Bartholin's glands, vagina.*

vestibulitis (vĕs-tĭb-ū-lī'tĭs). A dermatitis of the nasal vestibule; common in diabetics.

vestibulotomy (vĕs-tĭb"ū-lŏt'ō-mĭ) [L. *vestibulum,* vestibule, + G. *tomē,* a cutting]. Surgical incision into the vestibule of the inner ear.

vestibulourethral (vĕs-tĭb"ū-lō-ū-rē'thrăl) [" + G. *ourēthra,* urethra]. Relating to the vestibule of vagina and urethra.

vestibulum (vĕs-tĭb'ū-lŭm) (pl. *vestibula*) [L. *vestibulum,* vestibule]. Vestibule.

vestige (vĕs'tĭj) [L. *vestigium,* footstep]. A small degenerate or incompletely developed structure which has been more fully developed in the embryo or in a past generation.

vestigial (vĕs-tĭj'ĭ-ăl) [L. *vestigium,* a footstep]. Of the nature of a vestige. SYN: *rudimentary.*

vestigium (vĕs-tĭj'ĭ-ŭm) [L. a footstep]. Vestige.

veta (vā'ta). Mountain sickness.

veterinarian (vĕt-ĕr-ĭ-nā'rĭ-ăn). One who practices veterinary medicine.

veterinary (vĕt'ĕr-ĭ-nā'ry). Pertaining to the diseases of animals and their treatment. 2. A veterinarian.

v. medicine. That which deals with diseases of animals and their treatment.

via (pl. *viae*) [L. way]. Any passage in the body such as nasal, intestinal, or vaginal.

V.H. Abbr. for *viral hepatitis.*

viability (vī-ă-bĭl′ĭ-tĭ) [L. *vita,* life, + *habilis,* fit]. Ability to live, grow and develop.

viable (vī′ă-bl) [L. *vita,* life, + *habilis,* fit]. Capable of living, as a 7 months' fetus.

vial (vī′ăl) [G. *phialē,* a drinking cup]. A small glass bottle for medicines or chemicals.

vibex (vi′bex) (pl. *vibices*) [L. *vibix,* mark of a blow]. Narrow linear mark, as a line of blood in subcutaneous tissue.

vibratile (vī′bră-tĭl) [L. *vibrāre,* to shake]. Adapted to or used in vibratory motion; moving to and fro. SEE: *vibratory.*

vibration (vī-brā′shŭn) [L. *vibrāre,* to shake]. 1. A to and fro movement. SYN: *oscillation.* 2. Therapeutic shaking of the body, a form of massage.

Consists of a quick motion of the fingers or the hand vertical to the body or use of a mechanical vibrator.

vibrator (vī′brā-tor) [L. *vibrator,* a shaker]. Device for causing artificial vibration of body or its parts.

v., mechanical. Machine driven by hand or motor to give general shake-up of part desired.

v., ossicle. Instrument for breaking up aural adhesions.

vibratory (vī′bră-tō″rĭ) [L. *vibrator,* a shaker]. Having a vibrating or oscillatory movement.

v. sense. The ability to perceive vibrations transmitted through the skin to deep tissues. Usually tested by placing a vibrating tuning fork over bony prominences.

Vibrio (vib′rĭ-ō) [L. from *vibrāre,* to shake]. A genus of short, rigid, motile bacteria, shaped like an "S" or a comma, belonging to the Spirillaceae. They are small, actively motile, curved rods possessing a single polar flagellum. They are gram negative and nonspore forming.

V. chol′erae asiat′icae. The spirillum of Asiatic cholera. SYN: *V. comma.*

V. comma. The causative organism of Asiatic cholera.

vibrion septique (vē-brē-on′sĕp-tēk) [Fr., *septic vibrio*]. Bacillus causing malignant edema. *Clostridium septicum, q.v.*

vibrissae (vī-brĭs′ē) (sing. *vibrissa*) [L. *vibrissa,* that which shakes]. Stiff hairs within the nostrils at the ant. nares.

vibromassage (vi″bro-mă-sazh′). Massage given by a mechanical vibrator.

vibromasseur. Instrument used to produce vibratory massage of the ear.

vibrometer (vī-brŏm′ĕt-ĕr) [L. *vibrāre,* to shake, + G. *metron,* a measure]. Device for the treatment of deafness which produces rapid vibrations of the membrana tympani.

vibrotherapeutics (vī″brō-thĕr-ă-pū′tĭks) [" + G. *therapeutikē,* treatment]. The therapeutic application of vibration.

vicarious (vī-kā′rĭ-ŭs) [L. *vicarius,* substitute]. Acting as a substitute; pert. to assumption of the function of 1 organ by another.

v. menstruation. Menstruation through some channel other than the vagina, as hemorrhage from the nose, from the breast, or eyes, or in form of a leukorrhea at menstrual period.

v. respiration. Increased r. in 1 lung when respiration in the other is lessened or abolished.

Vicq d'Azyr's tract (vĭk da-zēr′). SYN: *mammallothalamic tract.* A large myelinated bundle arising in mammillary nuclei and terminating in ant. thalamic nuclei.

vidian artery (vĭd′ĭ-ăn). Branch of int. maxillary artery passing through the vidian canal.

v. canal. SYN: *pterygoid canal.* A canal in medial pterygoid plate of the sphenoid bone for transmission of pterygoid (vidian) vessels and nerve.

v. nerve. A branch from the sphenopalatine ganglion. SEE: *Nerves, Table of, in Appendix.*

vigil (vĭj′ĭl) [L. *vigil,* awake]. Insomnia; wakefulness.

v., coma. Condition of muttering delirium in which patient is partially conscious and not completely comatose. SEE: *vigilambulism.*

vigilambulism (vĭj-ĭl-ăm′bū-lĭzm) [L. *vigil,* awake, + *ambulāre,* to walk, + G. *-ismos,* condition]. The secondary state of dual or multiple personality, occurring in a state resembling somnambulism, but not during sleep.

According to Charcot, an attack of transformed hysteria producing a primary state in which the subject is normal, and a secondary state, in which vigilambulism takes place, during which all the automatic acts of life continue to take place, but during which the victim assumes a personality entirely unlike the normal personality, each living 2 distinct existences, 1 of them always ignorant of the other, or both ignorant of each other. The secondary state appears to be analogous to hysteric somnambulism.

vigintinormal (vī-jĭn″tĭ-nor′măl) [L. *viginti,* twenty, + *norma,* rule]. Consisting of one-twentieth of what is normal, as a solution.

vigor (vig′or) [L.]. Active force or strength of body or mind.

villi (vĭl′ī) [L. *villus,* tuft of hair]. Plural of *villus.*

v., chorionic. Tiny branching processes of surface of chorion which become vascular and help to form the placenta.

villiferous (vĭl-ĭf′ĕr-ŭs) [" + *ferre,* to bear]. Having villi, or tufts of hair.

villoma (vĭ-lo′mă). A villous tumor.

villose, villous (vĭl′ōs, vĭl′ŭs) [L. *villus,* tuft of hair]. Pert. to or furnished with villi or with fine hairlike extensions.

villositis (vĭl-ōs-ī′tĭs) [L. *villus,* tuft of hair, + G. *-itis,* inflammation]. A bacterial disease causing inflammation of the placental villi.

villus (vĭl′ŭs) (pl. *villi*) [L. *villus,* tuft of hair]. The short filamentous processes found on certain membranous surfaces.

v., chorionic. Tiny vascular projections on the chorionic surface which help to form the placenta. SEE: *chorion.*

Vincent's angina (vĭn′sĕnts ăn-jī′nă). Painful pseudomembranous ulceration of the gums, oral mucous membranes, pharynx and tonsils. SYN: *trench mouth; necrotizing ulcerative gingivostomatitis.* SEE: *Borrelia vincentii.*

ETIOL: *Fusobacterium fusiforme* and *Borrelia vincentii.* Poor oral hygiene, mental and physical stress, nutritional deficiencies. Absorption of heavy metals, such as mercury and bismuth, predisposes to development of the disease. Not considered to be a contagious disease.

SYN: Painful swelling of lymphatic nodes, inf. of tonsils extending to floor of mouth. Pseudomembranous exudate, later ulceration; fever.

vinculum (vĭn′kū-lŭm) [L. *vinculum*, a band]. A uniting band or bundle. SYN: *frenulum, frenum, ligament*.

v. ten′dinum. 1. NA. Tendinous, slender filaments connecting the phalanges with the flexor tendons. 2. The ringlike ligament of the ankle or wrist.

vinegar (vĭn′ĕ-găr) [M.E. *vinegre*, from Fr. *vin*, wine, + *aigre*, sour]. The product of the fermentation of cider, wine, or beer used as a condiment. A weak and impure solution of acetic acid. Usually contains 4 to 6% acetic acid. SYN: *acetum*. SEE: *condiment*.

vinethene (vĭn′ĕth-ēn). Proprietary general anesthetic, acting rapidly, but of short duration.

USES: Chiefly in dentistry and minor surgery.

vinous (vī′nŭs) [L. *vinum*, wine]. Containing or of the nature of wine.

vinum (vī′nŭm) [L. *vinum*, wine]. Wine. The medicated wines are solutions of medicinal substances in wine. They are not often prescribed. None are official.

vioform (vī′ō-form). A proprietary product (iodochlorhydroxyquin, USP) containing 41% iodine and having antibacterial and antifungal action. This is an almost odorless substitute for iodoform.

violate [L. *violatus*, to injure]. To harm or injure a person, especially to rape a female.

violence (vī′ō-lĕnts) [L. *violentia*]. The use of force or physical compulsion.

It may be expected in: *Acute delirious mania*. *Epileptic furor*: Patients have no memory of their violent attacks. *Schizophrenia*: Some patients may become violent.

Many attacks of violence may be averted by recognizing warning signs and by knowing the patient.

violet (vī′ō-lĕt) [ME. *violett*, from L. *viola*, violet]. One of the colors of the spectrum resembling purple.

v. blindness. Inability to see violet tints. SYN: *amianthinopsy*.

viomycin (vī-ō-mī′sĭn). An antibiotic that exerts a suppressive effect against tubercle bacilli. Effective against streptomycin-resistant organisms. Not suitable for routine use, since renal irritation. vestibular impairment, and deafness may result.

viosterol (vī-ŏs′tĕr-ŏl). A solution of irradiated ergosterol in vegetable oil. SYN: *calciferol*.

USES: Same as cod liver oil.

viraginity (vĭr-ăj-ĭn′ĭ-tĭ) [L. *virāgo*, an amazon or manlike woman]. Presence in a woman of masculine qualities and sexual tendencies.

viral. Pertaining to or caused by a virus.

v. disease. One which is caused by a virus. SEE: *virus diseases*.

viremia (vi″rēm′ĭ-ă). Virus in the blood.

virgin (vĭr′jĭn) [L. *virgo*, a maiden]. 1. A woman (or man) who has had no sexual intercourse. 2. Uncontaminated; fresh; new.

virginal (vĭr′jĭn-ăl) [L. *virgo*, a maid]. Relating to a virgin or to virginity.

v. membrane. The membrane around the entrance to the vagina. SYN: *hymen*.

virginity (vĭr-jĭn′ĭt-ĭ) [L. *virginitas*, maidenhood]. The state of being a virgin; not having experienced sexual intercourse.

viricidal (vī-rĭ-sī′dăl) [L. *virus*, poison, + *cidus*, from *caedere*, to kill]. Destructive to or inhibiting a virus. SYN: *virucidal*.

virile (vĭr′ĭl) [L. *virilis*, masculine]. Having characteristics of a mature male. Able to procreate. SYN: *masculine*.

v. reflex. 1. Sudden downward movement of penis when the prepuce or gland of a completely relaxed penis is pulled upward. SYN: *bulbocavernous reflex*. 2. Contraction of bulbocavernous muscle on percussing dorsum of penis. 3. Contraction of bulbocavernous muscle resulting from compression of glans penis.

virilescence (vĭr-ĭl-ĕs′ĕns) [L. *virilis*, masculine]. The acquisition of masculine characteristics in the female.

virilia (vĭr-ĭl′ĭ-ă) [L. *virilia*, male genitalia]. The male generative organs.

virilism (vĭr′ĭl-ĭzm) [L. *virilis*, masculine, + G. *-ismos*, condition]. Presence or development of male secondary characteristics in a woman.

virility (vĭr-ĭl′ĭ-tĭ) (L. *virilitas*, masculinity]. 1. The state of possessing masculine qualities. 2. Normal power of procreation in the male sex.

viripotent (vĭr-ĭp′ō-tĕnt) [L. *vir*, man, + *potens*, able]. 1. Sexually mature, noting male sex. 2. Marriageable, applied only to a female. SYN: *nubile*.

virology (vĭr-ŏl′ō-jĭ) [L. *virus*, poison, + G. *logos*, study]. The phase of biology dealing with viruses and virus diseases.

virose, virous (vī′rōs, vī′rŭs) [L. *virus*, poison]. Having poisonous qualities or effects. SYN: *poisonous*.

virtual (vĭr′tū-ăl) [L. *virtus*, excellence]. Being in effect, but not in fact; potential.

virucidal (vī-rū-sī′dăl) [L. *virus*, poison, + *cidus*, from *caedere*, to kill]. Destructive of a virus.

virulence (vĭr′ū-lĕns) [L. *virulentia*, a stench]. 1. Relative power and degree of pathogenicity possessed by organisms to produce disease. 2. Property of being virulent; venomousness, as of a disease. SEE: *attenuation, avirulent*.

virulent (vĭr′ū-lĕnt) [L. *virulentus*, full of poison]. 1. Very poisonous. 2. Infectious; able to overcome the host's defensive mechanism.

viruliferous (vĭr-ū-lĭf′ĕr-ŭs) [L. *virus*, poison, + *ferre*, to bear]. Conveying or producing a virus.

virus (vī′rŭs) [. *virus*, poison). 1. Originally this word meant any organism capable of causing an infection, but this usage is obsolete. 2. Minute organisms not visible with ordinary light microscopy. They are parasitic and depend on nutrients inside cells for their metabolic and reproductive needs. They cause a variety of infectious diseases and stimulate host antibodies.

A virus was synthesized in the laboratory for the first time in 1967. This was done by using natural virus DNA (deoxyribonucleic acid) as a template for forming the synthetic virus DNA.

v., A_2. One of the several strains of viruses which cause influenza.

v., attenuated. A virus so treated that its pathogenicity is decreased.

v., dehumanized. Vaccine obtained by the inoculation of a heifer with virus from a human being.

v. diseases. Smallpox, chickenpox, measles, mumps, the common cold, poliomyelitis, rabies, epidemic encephalitis, and v. pneumonia are only a few of the virus diseases of man.

v., filtrable. A virus causing infectious disease, the essential elements of which are so tiny that they retain infectivity after passing through a filter of the Berkefeld* type.

v., neurotropic. Those that seek out the nerves.

virusemia (vi-rus-ēm'ĭ-ă). Virus in the blood. SYN: *viremia.*

virustatic. Stopping the growth of viruses.

vis (vĭs) (pl. *vires*) [L. *vis,* force]. Force, strength, energy, power.

v. afron'te. Force that attracts.

v. formati'va. Energy resulting in development of new tissue.

v. medica'trix natu'rae. The healing power of nature.

viscera (vĭs'ĕr-ă) (sing. *viscus*) [L. *viscus, viscer-,* viscus]. Internal organs, esp. the abdominal.

RS: *celosomia, evisceration, splanchnic.*

viscerad (vĭs'ĕr-ăd) [" + *ad,* toward]. Toward the viscera.

visceral (vĭs'sĕr-ăl) [L. *viscus, viscer-,* viscus]. 1. Pert. to viscera. 2. Pertaining to or derived from the gill arches of vertebrates.

v. arches. Branchial arches, *q.v.*

v. cavity. Body cavity containing the viscera.

v. clefts. The fissures separating the visceral arches.

v. skeleton. The pelvis, ribs and sternum enclosing the viscera.

visceralgia (vĭs-ĕr-ăl'jĭ-ă) [L. *viscus, viscer-,* viscera, + G. *algos,* pain]. Neuralgia of any of the viscera.

vis'cero-. Combining form meaning *pertaining to the viscera.*

viscerogenic (vĭs"ĕr-ō-jĕn'ĭk) [" + G. *gennan,* to produce]. Originating in the viscera.

visceroinhibitory (vĭs"ĕr-ō-ĭn-hĭb'ĭ-tō-rĭ) [" + *inhibere,* to restrain]. Checking the action of the viscera.

visceromegaly (vis"er-o-meg'ă-lĭ). Generalized enlargement of the abdominal visceral organs.

visceromotor (vĭs"ĕr-ō-mō'tor) [" + *motor,* a mover]. Conveying motor impulses to the viscera. SYN: *viscerimotor.*

v. reflex. Increase in tonus of abdominal muscles resulting from painful stimuli originating in a viscus.

visceroparietal (vĭs"ĕr-ō-pă-rī'ĕ-tăl) [" + *paries, pariet-,* wall]. Relating to the viscera and the abdominal wall.

visceroperitoneal (vĭs"ĕr-ō-pĕr"ĭ-tō-nē'ăl) [L. *viscus, viscer-,* viscus, + G. *peritonaion,* peritoneum]. Relating to the abdominal viscera and peritoneum.

visceropleural (vĭs"ĕr-ō-plū'răl) [" + G. *pleura,* a side]. Relating to the thoracic viscera and the pleura. SYN: *pleurovisceral.*

visceroptosis (vĭs-ĕr-ŏp-tō'sĭs) [" + G. *ptosis,* a dropping]. Downward displacement of a viscus. SEE: *Glénard's disease.*

visceroreceptors. A group of receptors which includes those located in visceral organs. Their stimulation gives rise to poorly localized and ill-defined sensations. In hollow visceral organs they are stimulated principally by excessive contraction or by distention.

viscerosensory (vĭs"ĕr-ō-sĕn'sō-rĭ) [L. *viscus, viscer-,* viscus, + *sensorius,* sensory]. Pertaining to sensations aroused by stimulation of visceroreceptors.

v. reflex. Pain or tenderness elicited in somatic structures (skin and muscle) due to visceral disorder. SEE: *referred pain.*

visceroskeletal (vĭs"ĕr-ō-skĕl'ĕt-ăl) [" + G. *skeleton,* skeleton]. Relating to the visceral skeleton.

viscerosomatic (vĭs"ĕr-ō-sō-măt'ĭk) [" + G. *sōma,* body]. Relating to the viscera and the body.

v. reaction. A reaction occurring in muscles of the body-wall as a result of stimulation of visceroreceptors.

viscerotonia (vis"er-o-tōn'ĭ-ă). A personality type typical of the endomorphic; characterized by predominance of social over intellectual and physical traits. Individual is sociable, convivial, and exhibits gluttony for food, company, affection, and social support.

viscerotrophic (vĭs"ĕr-ō-trŏf'ĭk). Pertaining to trophic conditions related to or associated with visceral conditions.

viscerovisceral reaction (vĭs-ĕr-ō-vĭs'-ĕr-ăl). A reaction taking place in the viscera as a result of stimulation of visceral receptors. Such reactions are usually below the level of consciousness.

viscid (vĭs'ĭd) [L. *viscidus,* sticky]. Adhering, glutinous, sticky.

BACT: Said of a growth that follows the needle when it is touched to the culture and withdrawn. The sediment rises in a coherent whirl when the liquid culture is shaken.

viscidity (vĭs-ĭd'ĭ-tĭ) [L. *viscidus,* sticky] The property of being viscid or sticky. SYN: *viscosity.*

viscosimeter (vĭs-kŏs-ĭm'ĕt-ĕr) [L. *viscōsus,* sticky, + G. *metron,* a measure] Device for estimating the viscosity of a fluid, esp. of blood.

viscosity (vĭs-kŏs'ĭ-tĭ) [L. *viscōsus,* sticky]. 1. State of being sticky or gummy. 2. Resistance offered by a fluid to change of form or relative position of its particles due to attraction of molecules to each other.

v., specific. The internal friction of a fluid, measured by comparing the rate of flow of the liquid through a tube with that of some standard liquid, or by measuring the resistance to rotating paddles.

viscous (vĭs'kŭs) [L. *viscōsus,* sticky]. Sticky, gummy, gelatinous.

viscus (vĭs'kŭs) (pl. *viscera*) [L. *viscus,* viscus]. Any internal organ enclosed within a cavity, such as the thorax or abdomen. SEE: *viscera.*

visibility. Quality of being visible.

visible. Capable of being seen.

visile (vĭz'ĭl) [L. *visum,* seeing]. 1. Pert. to vision. 2. Readily recalling what is seen, more than that which is audible or motile.

vision (vĭzh'ŭn) [L. *visio,* a seeing]. 1. Act of viewing external objects. SYN: *sight.* 2. Sense by which light and color are apprehended. 3. An imaginary sight.

v., achromatic. Complete color blindness.

v., binocular. Visual sensation which is produced when the images fall on symmetrical points of each retina.

v., central, v., direct. Vision with the fovea centralis.

v., day. Condition in which patient sees better during the day than at night, found in peripheral lesions of the retina, such as retinitis pigmentosa.

v., double. Seeing of one object as two. SYN: *diplopia.*

v., field of. The space within which an object can be seen while the eye remains fixed on some one point.

v., half. Blindness in one or both eyes for half of the visual field. SYN: *hemianopia.*

v., indirect, v., peripheral. Vision with the retina outside of the macular field.

v., monocular. Utilizing only one eye.

v., multiple. Seeing of one object as two or more. Syn: *polyopia.*

v., night. Condition in which patient sees better after dusk, found in lesions of the macula.

vision, *words pert. to:* aberration, chromatic, accommodation, aftercataract, afterimage, ambiopia, amblyopia, ametropia, anopsia, astigmatic, astigmatism, autophony, amphodiplopia, amplitude of accommodation, anianthinopsy, anopsia, anotropia, asthenope, asthenopic, bifocal, caligation, caligo, chloropia, chloropsia, chromatopsia, convergence, cyanopia, chromopsia, cyclophoria, diplopia, emmetropia, erythropsia, farpoint, farsightedness, field, fogging, gerontopia, glare, halation, hypermetropia, hypometropia, ianthinopia, image, macropsia, metamorphosis, micropsia, mire, monoblepsia, muscae volitantes, myometrium, myope, myopia, nyctalopia, nyctamblyopia; nyctotyphlosis, ocular, oculist, orthophrenia, oxyblepsia, polyopia, second sight, scintillation, scotoma, spintherism, strabismus, vergency, visile, visual, words ending in *-phoria,* xanthopsia.

visual (vĭzh'ū-ăl) [L. *visio,* a seeing]. 1. Pert. to vision. 2. One whose learning and memorizing processes are largely of a visual nature.

v. acuity. A measure of the resolving power of the eye. Usually determined by having the subject read letters of various sizes at a standard distance from the test chart. The result is expressed as a fraction. For example, 20/20 is normal vision. This means the subject's eyes have the ability to see from a distance of 20 feet what the normal eye would see at that distance. 20/40 means that a person sees at 20 feet what the normal eye could see at 40 feet, etc.

v. angle. Angle bet. line of sight and the extremities of object seen.

v. axis. The line of vision, from object seen through the pupil's center to macula lutea.

v. cone. The cone whose vertex is at the eye and whose generating lines touch the boundary of a visible object.

v. field. The area within which objects may be seen when the eye is fixed.

v. line. The visual axis.

v. plane. The plane in which both optic axes lie.

v. point. Center of vision.

v. purple. A purple pigment in retinal rods. Syn: *rhodopsin.*

visuoauditory (vĭzh"ū-ō-aw'dĭ-tor-ĭ) [L. *visio,* a seeing, + *auditōrius,* pert. to hearing]. Relating to sight and hearing, as connecting nerve fibers bet. auditory and visual centers.

visuognosis (vĭzh-ū-ŏg-nō'sĭs) [" + G. *gnōsis,* knowledge]. The recognition and appreciation of what is seen.

visuometer (vĭzh-ū-ŏm'ĕ-tĕr) [" + G. *metron,* a measure]. Device for ascertaining the range of vision.

visuopsychic (vĭzh"ū-ō-sī'kĭk) [" + G. *psychē,* soul]. Both visual and psychic noting cerebral area involved in apprehension of visual sensations.

visuosensory (vĭzh"ū-ō-sĕn'sō-rĭ) [" + *sensorius,* sensory]. Relating to the recognition of visual impressions.

visus (vī'sus) [L.]. Vision.

vitaglass (vī'tă-glăs). Window glass containing quartz for transmitting the ultraviolet antirachitic rays of sunlight.

vital (vī'tăl) [L. *vitalis,* pert. to life]. 1. Pert. to or characteristic of life. 2. Contributing to or essential for life.

v. capacity. Volume of air that can be expelled following full inspiration.

v. center. Respiratory center in medulla.

v. signs. Respiration, pulse, and temperature.

v. statistics. A record of births, marriages, disease, and deaths in an area.

vitalism (vī'tăl-ĭzm) [L. *vitalis,* pert. to life, + G. *-ismos,* condition]. The opinion that a vital force neither chemical nor mechanical is responsible for the phenomenon of life.

vitalist (vī'tăl-ĭst) [L. *vitalis,* pert. to life]. One who believes in vitalism.

vitalistic (vī-tăl-ĭs'tĭk) [L. *vitalis,* pert. to life]. Relating to vitalism.

vitality (vī-tăl'ĭ-tĭ) [L. *vitalitas*]. 1. Principle of life. 2. Animation, action. Syn: *strength.* 3. State of being alive.

vitals (vī'tăls) [L. *vita,* life]. Organs of the body, esp. the heart, liver, lungs, and brain, essential to life.

vitamers (vī'tă-mers). Compounds which differ in structure from vitamins but which exert vitaminlike function.

vitamin (vī'tă-mĭn) [L. *vita,* life, + *amine*]. Any of a group of organic substances other than proteins, carbohydrates, fats, minerals, and organic salts which are essential for normal metabolism, growth, and development of the body.

Vitamins are not sources of energy nor do they contribute significantly to the substance of the body, but they are indispensable for normal functions and the maintenance of health. They are effective in minute quantities. They act principally as regulators of metabolic processes and play a role in energy transformations, usually acting as coenzymes in enzymatic systems.

Vitamins are extremely complex chemical substances, but the nature, chemical structure, and composition of most of them are known. Most have been isolated and some have been synthesized. In general, none of the vitamins can be formed in the body but must be obtained preformed from animal or plant sources. Exceptions to the above are the formation of Vitamin A from its precursor, carotene; the formation of vitamin D by the action of ultraviolet light on the skin; and the formation of vitamin K by symbiotic bacteria of the intestines.

Vitamins are unstable, being readily destroyed by oxidation; by heat, esp. in an alkaline medium; strong acids, light, and aging. See: *Vitamin Tables in Appendix.*

RS: *avitaminosis, deficiency disease.*

v., antiberiberi. Thiamine (vitamin B_1). See: *thiamine.*

v., antidermatitis. Vitamin B_6.

v., antihemorrhagic. Vitamin K.

v., anti-infective. Vitamin A.

v., antineuritic. Thiamine (B_1), *q.v.*

v., antipellagra. Nicotinamide (pellagra-preventing factor).

v., antirachitic. The vitamin D group.

v., antiscorbutic. Vitamin C.

v., antixerophthalmic. Vitamin A.

v., coagulation. Vitamin K.

vitamin A. Syn: *vitamin, anti-infective; v., antixerophthalmic.*

A fat-soluble vitamin formed in the body from precursors, yellow pigments of plants (alpha, beta, and gamma carotene). It is essential for normal growth and development, the integrity of epithelial tissues, and for normal teeth and bone development. It is stored in the liver. SEE: *Vitamin Tables in Appendix.*

ACTION: Essential to the normal function of epithelial cells and visual purple.

STABILITY: Resists boiling for some time if not exposed to oxidation. Quite stable to heat but not to continued high temperatures (above 100° C.). Vit. A is present in most canned fruits and vegetables.

VIT. A DEFICIENCY DISORDERS: Interference with growth, reduced resistance to infections, interference with nutrition of cornea, conjunctiva, trachea, hair follicles, renal pelvis. Thus these tissues have an increased susceptibility to infections. Interference with ability of eyes to adapt to darkness (night blindness). Visual acuity will also be impaired. Children will experience impaired growth and development.

VIT. A FOODS: Butter, and butter fat in milk and cod liver oil are rich sources, as are egg yolks. Green leafy and yellow vegetables and some fruits; prunes, pineapples, oranges, limes, cantaloupes, liver.

Recommended Daily Allowances for Vitamin A

	International Units
Man (70 kg.); woman (56 kg.)	5000
Pregnancy, latter half	6000
Lactation	8000
Children:	
Under 1 year	1500
1 to 3 years	2000
4 to 6 years	2500
7 to 9 years	3500
10 to 12 years	4500
12 to 15 years	5000
16 to 20 years	6000

vitamin A_1. Form found in the eye tissues of marine fish.

vitamin A_2. A compound found in the livers of fresh-water fish. Similar in properties to vitamin A but with different absorption spectrum in the ultraviolet.

vitamin B complex. A large number of water-soluble vitamins isolated from liver, yeast, and other sources. Among vitamins included are: thiamine (B_1), riboflavin (B_2), niacin (nicotinic acid), pyridoxine (B_6), biotin, inositol, p-aminobenzoic acid (PABA), cyanocobalamine (B_{12}), and folic acid.

ACTION: Affects growth, appetite, lactation, gastrointestinal, nervous and endocrine systems; aids in marasmus and lymphocytosis, stimulates appetite, reduces sugar content in diabetes, stimulates biliary action, aids in tuberculosis, and is necessary for carbohydrate metabolism.

Only grain-made yeast that is dried at once preserves its potency.

B_1, *thiamine*, for growth and nutrition and carbohydrate metabolism. B_2, *riboflavin*, for growth and cellular metabolism. *Nicotinic acid* prevents pellagra.

Although not destroyed by ordinary cooking, it may be destroyed by excessive heating for 2-4 hours. Soda in cooking aids destruction. Riboflavin and nicotinic acid are more stable than thiamine; are not destroyed by heat or oxidation.

VIT. B DEFICIENCY DISORDERS: Beriberi, pellagra, digestive disturbances, enlargement of liver, reduction of pancreas, affects the thyroid, causes degeneration of sex glands, reduces catalysis of tissues, affects the nervous system, deranges the endocrines; induces edema, affects the heart, liver, spleen and kidneys; enlarges the adrenals and deranges function of the pituitary and salivary glands, and cause of some disorders in diabetes.

Polyneuritis, gastrointestinal disorders, achlorhydria, anorexia, and failure of lactation have been attributed to deficiency of B_1.

SOURCES OF VIT. B FACTORS: *Thiamine:* Whole grains, wheat embryo, brewer's yeast, legumes, nuts, egg yolk, fruits and vegetables.

Riboflavin: Brewer's yeast, liver, meat, especially pork, fish, poultry, eggs, and milk; green vegetables.

Nicotinic Acid: Brewer's yeast, liver, meat, poultry, and green vegetables.

Pyridoxine: Rice, bran, yeast.

Folic Acid: Leafy, green vegetables, organ meats, lean beef and veal, wheat cereals.

STABILITY: Long-continued cooking or high temperature destroys and soda in cooking aids its destruction. Not destroyed by ordinary cooking or heat.

vitamin B_c. Folic acid, *q.v.*

vitamin B_t. SYN: *carnitine*. A vitamin found in muscle and liver.

vitamin B_x. Para-aminobenzoic acid.

vitamin B_1. Thiamine, or thiamine hydrochloride. Also SEE: *Table of Vitamins in Appendix.*

Also called *aneurine, antineuritic factor* or *vitamin, antiberiberi vitamin.*

Recommended Daily Allowances for Vitamin B_1 (Thiamine)

	mg. per 1000 cal.
All ages	0.6
Pregnant women	0.6
Lactating women	0.8

vitamin B_2. Riboflavin, *q.v.* Also called *vitamin G, lactoflavin, ovoflavin, hepatoflavin, antipellagra factor or vitamin.* SEE: *Table of Vitamins in Appendix.*

vitamin B_3. Also called *chick pellagra factor.*

vitamin B_4. Prevents muscular weakness in rats and chicks. Thought to be a mixture of arginine, glycine, and cystine.

vitamin B_5. Necessary for growth in pigeons.

vitamin B_6. Pyridoxine. Found in rice, bran, and yeast. SYN: *antidermatitis v.*

vitamin B_7. A factor in rice polishings that prevents digestive disturbances in pigeons. Called *rice polish factor.*

vitamin B_8. Usually not classified as a vitamin.

vitamin B_{10}, B_{11}. Folic acid compounds affecting chicks.

vitamin B_{12}. SYN: *cyanocobalamin, antipernicious anemia principle.* A red, crystalline substance extracted from liver which is essential for the formation of red blood cells. Its deficiency results in pernicious anemia. It is used for prophylaxis and treatment of these and other diseases in which there is defective red cell formation. Recommended daily requirement: 3-5 micrograms per day.

vitamin B_{14}. A crystalline compound isolated from human urine. It has high cell-proliferating activity in bone-marrow cultures. The effect upon certain suspensions of neoplastic cells is inhibitory.

vitamin B_{15}. Pangamic acid.

vitamin C. SYN: *cevitamic acid, antiscorbutic factor or vitamin.* Ascorbic acid, a factor necessary for formation of intercellular substance of connective tissue and essential in maintenance of integrity of intercellular cement in many tissues, especially capillary walls. Deficiency leads to scurvy. SEE: *Table of Vitamins in Appendix.*

STABILITY: Destroyed easily by heat in the presence of oxygen, as in open-kettle boiling. Less affected by heat in an acid medium; otherwise stable.

VIT. C DEFICIENCY DISORDERS: Scurvy, imperfect prenatal skeletal formation; defective teeth, pyorrhea, anorexia, anemia, undernutrition, injury to bone, cells, and blood vessels.

VIT. C FOODS: Raw cabbage, young carrots, orange juice, lettuce, celery, onions, tomatoes, radishes and green peppers. Citrus fruits are especially rich in this vitamin. Strawberries are about as rich a source as tomatoes, apples, pears, apricots, plums, peaches, and pineapples. Rutabagas are also rich in this vitamin.

Recommended Daily Allowances for Vitamin C

	Mg.
Infants and growing children	30-80
Adults	70

vitamin conversion tables. For vitamins A, B_1, B_2, and C:

Vitamin A:
1 international unit = 2 Sherman units
= 0.6 microgram of carotene

Vitamin B_1:
1 international unit = 3 micrograms
= 0.003 mg.
= 2 Sherman units

Vitamin B_2:
1 mg. = 333 Sherman-Bourquin units
= 1000 micrograms

Vitamin C:
1 mg. = 20 international units
= 2 Sherman units

vitamin D. One of several vitamins having antirachitic activity. The *vitamin D group* includes D_2 (calciferol), D_3 (irradiated 7-dehydrocholesterol), D_4 (irradiated 22-dihydroergosterol) and D_5 (irradiated dehydrositosterol). It is essential in calcium and phosphorus metabolism; consequently it is essential for normal development of bones and teeth.

ACTION: Related to utilization of calcium and phosphorus in blood and bone building. It is called the antirachitic vitamin because deficiency of it interferes with calcium and phosphorus utilization, which in turn causes rickets.* Exposure to the sun or ultraviolet ray synthesizes this vitamin in the body. Necessary for most efficient absorption of calcium and phosphorus. A specific in treatment of infantile rickets, spasmophilia (infantile tetany), and softening of bone; valuable also in prevention. Important in normal growth and mineralization of skeleton and teeth.

VIT. D DEFICIENCY DISORDERS: Imperfect skeletal formation, bone diseases, rickets, caries.

VIT. D FOODS: Milk, cod liver oil, salmon and cod livers, egg yolk, butter fat; ergosterol activated by sunlight or the ultraviolet ray possesses vit. D potency.

STABILITY: Not affected by oxidation or by heat unless over 100° C. or long-continued cooking.

Recommended Daily Allowances for Vitamin D

Infants artificially fed	400 I.U.
Infants breast fed	
Children	
Adults	

vitamin E. Tocopherol, a group of three tocopherols (alpha, beta, and gamma) which prevent sterility and muscular dystrophy in experimental animals. It is essential for the development of spermatozoa and in its absence death and resorption of fetuses occur. *Its role in human nutrition has not been definitely established.*

vitamin K. An antihemorrhagic factor whose activity is associated with compounds derived from naphthoquinone. Vit. K is from alfalfa; vit. K_2 from fishmeal; vit. K_3 is synthesized as menadione sodium bisulfite USP. Vit. K aids blood coagulation, and is necessary for formation of prothrombin. Its deficiency prolongs blood-clotting time and causes hemorrhages.

ACTION: Helps to eliminate prolonged bleeding in operations and in biliary tract of jaundiced patients. Bile salts necessary for its absorption.

VIT. K SOURCES: Found in fats, fishmeal, oats, wheat, rye and afalfa. Synthesized from coal tar, and is 4 times as potent as the natural. SYN: *antihemorrhagic v.*

vitamin loss. Commercial canning destroys from 50 to 85 per cent of vit. C. in peas, lima beans, spinach, and asparagus. The wheat embryo is removed from wheat flour in milling. As the wheat embryo is rich in vitamin B_1, this vitamin is lost in milling. Apple pie and freshly prepared applesauce retain only from 20 to 30 per cent of the vit. C value of the apple. Pickling, salting, curing, or fermenting usually causes complete loss of vit. C. Pasteurization, unless special precautions are observed, causes a loss of from 30 to 60 per cent of vit. C.

vitamin M. Obsolete name for folic acid, *q.v.*

vitamin P. SYN: *citrin, permeability factor* or *vitamin.* A substance associated with vit. C. in citrus fruits which is essential for normal integrity of capillary membranes and normal permeability. Not considered to be a vitamin.

vitamin P-P. Pellagra-preventing factor, or niacinamide, *q.v.*

vitaminoid (vī'tăm-ĭn-oyd) [L. *vita,* life, + *amine,* + G. *eidos,* resemblance]. Of the nature of vitamin.

vitaminology (vī"tăm-ĭn-ŏl'ō-jĭ) [" + " + G. *logos,* a study]. The science dealing with vitamins.

vitellary (vĭt'ĕl-ă-rĭ) [L. *vitellus,* yolk of an egg]. Pert. to the vitellus. SYN: *vitelline.*

vitellin (vī-tĕl'ĭn) [L. *vitellus,* yolk of egg]. A protein which can be extracted from egg yolk and contains lecithin. SEE: *nucleoprotein, ovovitellin.*

vitelline (vī-tĕl'ēn) [L. *vitellus,* yolk of egg]. Pert. to the yolk of an egg or the ovum.

v. circulation. The embryonic circulation of blood to the yolk sac via *vitelline arteries* and its return to general circulation through the *vitelline veins.*

v. duct. The narrow duct connecting the yolk sac with the embryonic gut.

v. membrane. 1. The membrane forming the surface layer of an ovum. 2. In a chicken egg, the membrane forming the surface layer of the *vitellus* or *yolk.*

v. veins. SYN: *omphalomesenteric veins.* Two veins conveying blood from the yolk sac.

vitellorubin (vī-tĕl"lō-rū'bĭn). A red pigment present in yolk of an egg.

vitellus (vĭ-tĕl'ŭs) [L. *vitellus*, yolk of egg]. The yolk of an ovum, especially the yolk of a hen's egg.

vitiation (vĭsh"ĭ-ā'shŭn) [L. *vitiāre*, to corrupt]. Injury, contamination, impairment of use or efficiency.

vitiligo (vĭt-ĭl-ī'gō) [L.]. SYN: *leukoderma, leukasmus, leukopathia, piebald skin.* An acquired cutaneous affection characterized by milk-white patches, surrounded by areas of normal pigmentation. More common in tropics and in the colored race. Cause unknown.

v. capitis. Vitiligo of the scalp with depigmentation of the hairs of the affected area.

v. perinevoid. Vitiligo surrounding a nevus.

vitiligoidea (vĭt-ĭl-ĭg-oyd'ē-ă) [L. *vitiligō*, tetter, + G. *eidos*, appearance]. Disease marked by formation of tiny yellow patches or nodules on the skin, as on the eyelids. SYN: *xanthoma.*

vitium (vĭsh'ĭ-ŭm) (pl. *vitia*) [L. *vitium*, fault]. A fault, defect, or vice.

v. cordis. An organic heart lesion.

vitreocapsulitis (vĭt"rē-ō-kăp-sū-lī'tĭs) [L. *vitreus*, glassy, + *capsula*, capsule, + G. *-itis*, inflammation]. Inflammation of the vitreous humor. SYN: *hyalitis.*

vitreous (vĭt'rē-ŭs) [L. *vitreus*, glassy]. 1. Glassy. 2. Pertaining to the vitreous body of the eye. 3. The vitreous body, *q.v.*

v. body. A transparent jellylike mass that fills the cavity of the eyeball, enclosed by the hyaloid membrane.

v. chamber. The portion of the cavity of the eyeball behind the lens.

v. degeneration. SYN: *hyaline degeneration, q.v.* Retrogressive change of a part into a translucent shining substance, esp. of a blood vessel wall.

v. humor. The clear, watery fluid filling the interstices of the stroma of the vitreous body.

v. membrane. 1. Inner one of the choroid. 2. SYN: *hyaline layer.* The innermost layer of the connective tissue sheath surrounding a hair follicle.

v. table. The inner layer of compact tissue characteristic of most of the bones of the cranium.

vitrescence (vĭ-trĕs'ĕns). Becoming hard and transparent like glass.

vitriol (vĭt'rē-ol) [L. *vitriolum*]. A sulfate of any of various metals.

v., blue. Copper sulfate, *q.v.*

v., green. Ferrous sulfate, *q.v.*

v., oil of. Sulfuric acid, *q.v.*

v., white. Zinc sulfate, *q.v.*

vitro, in. SEE: *in vitro.*

vitropression (vĭt"rō-prĕsh'ŭn) [L. *vitrum*, glass, + *pressio*, a squeezing]. Method of temporarily eliminating redness of the skin caused by hyperemia by pressure with a glass slide on the skin for purpose of studying any lesions or discolorations.

Vitus' dance, St. (vī'tŭs). A functional nervous disorder causing muscular spasms. SYN: *chorea, q.v.*

vivi- [L.]. Combining form meaning *alive.*

vividiffusion (vĭv-ĭ-dĭf-ū'zhŭn) [L. *vivus*, alive, + *diffusio*, a pouring apart]. The process of removing diffusible substances from blood of a living animal by allowing it to flow through dialyzing membranes immersed in saline solution.

vivification (vĭv-ĭ-fĭ-kā'shŭn) [" + *facere*, to make]. 1. Trimming of the surface layer of a wound to aid union of tissues. 2. Transformation of protein food through assimilation into the living matter of cellular organisms.

viviparous (vĭv-ĭp'ăr-ŭs) [" + *parēre*, to bear young]. Developing young within the body, the young being expelled and born alive, the opposite of *oviparous.*

vivisect (vĭv'ĭ-sĕkt) [" + *sectio*, a cutting]. To dissect a living animal for experimental purposes.

vivisection (vĭv"ĭ-sĕk'shŭn) [L. *vivus*, alive, + *sectio*, a cutting]. Cutting of or operation upon a living animal for physiological investigation and the study of disease. The operations are usually performed upon an anesthetized animal under conditions similar to those encountered in an operating room of a hospital.

vivisectionist (vĭv"ĭ-sĕk'shŭn-ĭst) [" + *sectio*, a cutting]. One who practices or believes in vivisection. SEE: *antivivisectionist.*

vivisector (vĭv-ĭs-ĕk'tor) [" + *sector*, a cutting]. One who practices vivisection.

Vleminckx's solution (flĕm'ĭnks). A solution of sulfurated lime.

USES: In various skin diseases.

vivo, in. SEE: *in vivo.*

vo'cal. Pert. to the voice.

v. cords, false. The ventricular folds, *q.v.*

v. cords, true. The vocal cords, *q.v.*

v. folds. The thin edges of the vocal lips, each of which encloses the vocal ligament. They form the edges of the rima glottidis, and are concerned with the production of sound.

v. frem'itus. Chest-wall vibration felt on palpation while patient is speaking.

v. ligament. A strong band of elastic tissue lying within vocal fold.

v. lips. Two shelflike projections of lateral walls of the larynx. Their edges bear the vocal folds, *q.v.*

v. muscle. The inner portion of the thyroarytenoid muscle which lies in vocal lip lateral to and in contact with the vocal ligament.

v. process. That of the arytenoid cartilage to which are attached the vocal cords.

v. res'onance. Sound heard in auscultation of lung while patient is speaking.

v. signs. Indication of disease by changes in the voice.

voice (voys) [L. *vox, voc-*, voice]. Sound uttered by human beings, produced by vibration of the vocal cords

voice, words pert. to: *amphoricity, amphoriloquy, amphorophony, anepia, apsithyria, arytenoid. cacophonia, caverniloquy, heterophonia, hoarseness, mogiphonia, paraphonia, phonation, resonance, rhinolalia, rhinophonia, trachyphonia.*

voices (voys'ĕs). Verbal, auditory hallucinations. SYN: *phoneme.*

void (voyd) [O. Fr. *voider*, to empty]. To evacuate the bowels or bladder.

vol. Abbr. for *volume.*

vol%. Abbr. for *volume per cent.*

vola (vō'lă) [L.]. The sole of foot or palm of the hand.

v. manus. Palm of hand.

v. pedis. Sole of foot.

volar (vō'lăr) [L. *vola*, palm, sole]. Relating to the palm, or sole of foot.

volatile (vol'ă-tĭl) [L. *volatilis*, from *volāre*, to fly]. CHEM: Easily vaporized or evaporated.

Examples of volatile liquids are ether (boiling point, 34.5° C.) and ethyl chloride (b. p. 12.2° C.).

volatilization (vŏl"ă-tĭl-ĭ-zā'shŭn) [L. *volatilis*, from *volāre*, to fly]. Conversion of a solid or liquid into a vapor.

volition (vō-lĭsh'ŭn) [L. *volitio,* will]. The act or power of willing or choosing.

Volkmann's contracture (fōlk'mahn). Degeneration, contracture, fibrosis, and atrophy of a muscle resulting from injury to its blood supply. Usually seen in the hand.

volley (vŏl'ē) [L. *volāre,* to fly]. The simultaneous or nearly simultaneous discharge of a number of nerve impulses from a center within the brain or spinal cord.

volsella (vŏl-sĕl'ă) [L. *volsella,* a tweezer]. Forceps with sharp pointed hooks at end of each blade.

volt (vōlt). An electrical unit of pressure, the electromotive force required to produce 1 ampere of current through a resistance of 1 ohm.

voltage (vōlt-āj). Electromotive force or difference in potential expressed in volts.

Voltolini's disease (vōl-tō-lē'nē). Primary labyrinthitis in children with symptoms of meningitis, and subsequently a staggering gait and deaf-mutism.

volubil'ity [L. *volubilitas,* flow of discourse]. Psy: Excessive speech.

volume. The space occupied by a substance. Usually expressed in cubic units.

v. index. Abbr. *V.I.* The mean volume of an average erythrocyte compared with the mean volume of the normal erythrocyte. Varies from 0.9 to 1.10. Indices below this indicate abnormally small red cells; above, abnormally large ones. The volume index is found by dividing the percentage of red cells into the hematocrit* percentage. See: *color index.*

v., mean corpuscular. The mean volume of an average erythrocyte. Normal values range from 82 to 92 cubic microns. Abbr: *M.C.V.*

v., minute. The amount of blood discharged from one ventricle in one minute.

v., packed cell. Syn: *hematocrit.* The volume of packed erythrocytes in a sample of centrifuged blood. Average volume equals 47% of blood volume in men, 42% in women.

v. per cent. Abbr: *vol.%.* The number of cubic centimeters (milliliters) of a substance (usually O_2 or CO_2) contained in 100 cc. (or ml.) of another substance, *e.g.,* blood.

v., stroke. The amount of blood discharged by a ventricle in one contraction. Determined by dividing the minute volume by the number of heartbeats occurring in one minute.

volumetric (vŏl″ū-mĕt'rĭk) [L. *volūmen,* a volume, + G. *metron,* a measure]. Pert. to measurement of volume.

voluntary (vŏl'ŭn-tā-rĭ) [L. *voluntas,* will]. Pert. to or under control of the will.

v. muscles. Voluntary muscles are generally attached to the skeleton, are innervated by myelinated nerves coming directly from the brain or spinal cord, and under the microscope are seen to consist of long cylindrical fibers bearing crosswise striations.

Voluntary, striped, striated, cross-striated, and skeletal are practically synonymous when applied to muscle.

voluptuous (vō-lŭp'tū-ŭs) [L. *voluptas,* pleasure]. 1. Pert. to, arising from, or provoking consciously or otherwise, sensual desire, usually applied to the female sex. 2. Given to sensualism.

volupty (vŏl'ŭp-tĭ) [O. Fr. *volupté,* pleasure]. Sexual pleasure.

volute (vō-lūt') [L. *volutus,* rolled]. Spiral, rolled up. Syn: *convoluted.*

volvulus (vŏl'vū-lŭs) [L. *volvere,* to roll]. A twisting of the bowel upon itself causing obstruction.

Etiol: Prolapsed mesentery predisposing cause. Usually occurs at sigmoid and ileocecal areas of intestines.

vomer (vō'mer) [L. *vomer,* plowshare]. The plow-shaped bone which forms the lower and post. portion of the nasal septum, articulating with the ethmoid, sphenoid, the 2 palate bones, and 2 sup. maxillary bones.

vomerine (vō'mĕr-ĭn) [L. *vomer,* plowshare]. Pert. to the vomer.

vomeronasal (vō″mĕr-ō-nās'ăl). Pertaining to the vomer and the nasal bones.

v. cartilages. Two narrow strips of cartilage lying along ant. portion of inferior border of septal cartilage of nose.

v. organ (of Jacobson). A small tubular epithelial sac lying on anterior inferior surface of nasal septum. Rudimentary in man.

vomica (vŏm'ĭk-ă) [L. *vomica,* ulcer]. 1. A cavity in the lungs, as from suppuration. 2. Sudden and profuse expectoration of putrid, purulent matter.

vomicose (vŏm'ĭk-ōs) [L. *vomica,* ulcer]. Marked by many ulcers; ulcerous; purulent.

vomit (vŏm'ĭt) [L. *vomere,* to vomit]. 1. Matter ejected from stomach through the mouth. 2. To yield up gastric and intestinal contents through the mouth.

Phys: The act is usually reflex involving coordinated activity of both voluntary and involuntary muscles. A certain position is assumed, the glottis is closed, the diaphragm and abdominal muscles contract, and the cardiac sphincter of the stomach relaxes while antiperistaltic waves course over the duodenum, stomach and esophagus.

RS: *melena, nausea, vomiting.*

v., bilious. Bile forced back into the stomach and ejected with vomited matter.

v., black. Vomit containing blood acted on by the gastric juice. Seen in worst form of yellow fever.

v., coffee-ground. V. having the appearance and consistency of coffee grounds because of blood mixed with gastric contents. Occurs in conditions such as cancer of stomach.

vomiting (vŏm'ĭt-ing) [L. *vomere,* to vomit]. Ejection through the mouth of the gastric contents. Syn: *emesis.*

Emesis may result from:

1. Toxins from ptomaines, drugs, uremia and specific fevers.

2. Cerebral tumors and meningitis. This form often is unaccompanied by nausea and it does not relieve associated headache.

3. Diseases of the stomach, such as ulcer, cancer, dilatation, dyspepsia, etc.

4. Reflex from pregnancy, uterine or ovarian disease, irritation of the fauces, worms, biliary colic.

5. Intestinal obstruction.

6. Motion sickness.

7. Nervous affections, as hysteria and migraine.

8. Periodic vomiting may be in itself a neurosis or associated with the gastric crises of locomotor ataxia.

9. Esophageal vomiting results from obstruction, and the vomitus* is alkaline in reaction.

Treatment: Antinausea medicines by mouth if possible, otherwise intramuscularly or intravenously. Fluids may be given by mouth if patient will accept them. If vomiting continues, fluids and electrolytes intravenously will be required to replace those lost in the vomitus.

In pregnancy: The diet should be dry and high in carbohydrates and water and liquids should be taken only bet. meals and in small quantities. Do not construe this to mean that all pregnant women should be subjected to this regimen, as it is only intended for women subject to emesis.

POSTOPERATIVE: NP. At first sign restrict fluids for ½ hr., then resume in gradually increasing amts. In certain cases (gastric) record *time, color, amt.*, whether *regurgitant* or *projectile*. Save specimen for examination. Wash mouth frequently. Take specimen of urine, if vomiting is persistent. (May be due to acidosis. If so, alkalies and glucose may be given.) Odor, *ammoniacal, fecal, garlic*, etc., should be charted. Fecal v. indicates intestinal obstruction. SEE: *hematemesis*.

POISONS: Emesis may result from taking arsenic, aconite, antimony, barium, colchicum, cantharides, copper, corrosive alkalis, acids, digitalis, iodine, mercury, phenol, phosphorus, veratrum, wood alcohol, food poisons, and zinc.

RS: *anacatharsis; antiemetic; cyclic v.; emesis; emetic; hyperemesis; tyremesis; vomit; vomitus.*

v., cyclic. Recurring paroxysms of vomiting.

v., dry. Nausea without vomitus.

v., incoercible. Uncontrollable vomiting.

v., pernicious. Severe vomiting of pregnancy.

v. of pregnancy. That of morning sickness.

v., projectile. Ejection of vomitus with great force.

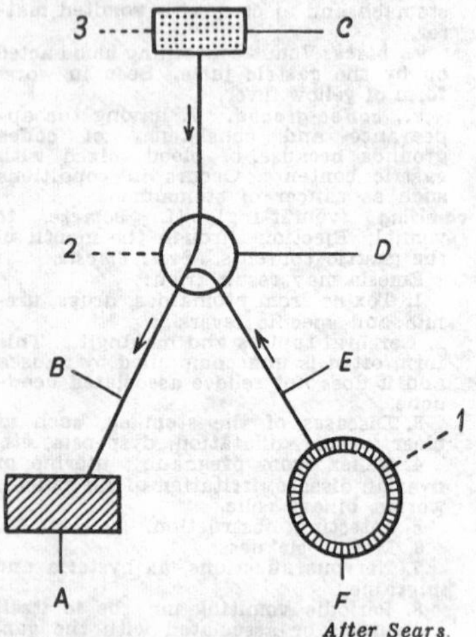

After Sears.

DIAGRAM ILLUSTRATING THE MECHANISM OF VOMITING

1. Focal causes act here. 2. Toxic causes act here. 3. Nervous causes act here. A. Diaphragm and abdominal muscles. B. Efferent nerve. C. Higher centers of brain. D. Vomiting center in medulla. E. Afferent nerve. F. Stomach and other abdominal organs.

v., stercoraceous. Vomiting of fecal matter.

vomitory (vŏm′ĭ-tō-rĭ) [L. *vomitōrius*, pert. to vomit]. 1. Causing vomiting. 2. An agent inducing emesis. 3. A vessel to receive ejecta.

vomiturition (vŏm″ĭ-tū-rĭsh′ŭn) [L. *vomitus*, vomit]. Repeated ineffective efforts to vomit. SYN: *retching.*

vomitus (vŏm′ĭt-ŭs) [L. *vomitus*, vomiting]. 1. Act of ejecting matter from the stomach through the mouth. 2. Material ejected from the stomach by vomiting.

NATURE OF VOMITUS: *Bilious*: Green or greenish-yellow, containing bile, appears after frequent and violent vomiting; if early in the act of vomiting, it may be grass-green; a symptom of peritonitis which also precedes fecal vomiting in intestinal obstruction.

Fecal: This is indicative of intestinal obstruction, general peritonitis, and abnormal communication bet. the intestines and stomach.

Garlic odor: Denotes phosphorus poisoning.

Hematemesis: The vomiting of blood. If bright and fluid it has not been long in the stomach; otherwise, it has the appearance of coffee grounds, reddish-brown, or it forms in clots. This may indicate, also, rupture of aneurysms into the stomach or esophagus, or various esophageal veins; gastric ulcer, cirrhosis of liver, enlarged spleen, carcinoma of the stomach. It is not necessarily fatal.

It may result from swallowed blood. It may occur in vicarious menstruation, gastritis, corrosive poisoning, in the presence of strong alkalies or acids, or it may result from anemia, leukemia, Hodgkin's disease and it is sometimes present in chronic nephritis, scurvy, purpura haemorrhagica, acute yellow atrophy of the liver, and in malarial fevers.

Ammoniacal odor: Indicates uremia.

Profuse: The ejection of large quantities of frothy fermented material is highly significant of gastric dilatation.

Purulent: This may result from the rupture of an abscess into the esophagus or stomach.

Without nausea, distress, or other phenomena: This may occur in certain neuroses of the stomach, in hysteria, uremia, brain disease, as from a tumor, or as a precursor of apoplexy. The vomitus may be colored by certain fruits, by wine, coffee, cocoa, soups and bile. SEE: *blennemesis, cholemesis.*

v., coffee-ground. Vomitus of dark red or black granular material (resembling coffee grounds) which is blood. The blood has been in the stomach or intestinal tract long enough to be changed from red to black by the action of gastric and intestinal juices.

v. cruentus. Bloody vomit.

v. matutinus. The vomiting of morning sickness.

v. mari′nus. Seasickness.

von Gierke's disease (fōn gĕr′kĕ). SYN: *glycogen storage disease, glycogenosis.* Condition in which excessive amounts of glycogen are stored in tissues and body is unable to use it. Results in excessive production of ketones.

von Graefe's sign (fōn gra′fē). Failure of lid to move downward promptly with eyeball, the lid moving tardily and jerkily; seen in exophthalmic goiter.

von Leube motor test meal (fōn loy′be). Soup, 400 cc.; beef, 200 Gm.; water, 200 cc. If at end of 6 hours a gastric lavage fails to show a residue, the motility of the stomach is normal.

v. L.'s test meal. Clear soup, 200 cc.; beefsteak, 200 Gm.; bread, 50 Gm.; water, 200 cc. The stomach contents are expressed in 6 hours. This is a gastric test meal.

Von Pirquet's test (fŏn pēr'kă). A diagnostic test for tuberculosis, in which a little tuberculin is applied to a scarified area of the skin of the arm.

A positive reaction is seen if a red papillar eruption appears at the site of inoculation.

Von Recklinghausen's disease (fŏn rĕk'ling-how"zĕn). 1. Multiple neurofibromata occurring on the skin along the course of the nerves; associated with marked cutaneous pigmentation. 2. Generalized fibrocystic disease of the bones. Syn: *molluscum fibrosum.*

Voorhees' bag (voor'ēz). An inflatable rubber bag for dilating the cervix uteri to induce labor.

voracious (vō-rā'shŭs) [L. *vorāre*, to devour]. Having an insatiable or ravenous appetite.

vortex (vor'tĕks) (pl. *vortices*) [L .*vortex*, a whirlpool]. A structure having a spiral or whorled appearance.

v., coccygeal. Syn: *vortex coccygeus.* The region over coccyx where lanugo hairs of embryo come to a point.

v. lentis. Lens star, *q.v.*

v. of the heart. Region at apex of heart where muscle fibers of the ventricles make a tight spiral and turn inward.

vortices. Pl. of *vortex.*

v. pilorum. Hair whorls as in arrangement of hairs on the scalp.

vorticose (vor'tĭk-ōs) [L. *vortex, vortic-*, a whirlpool]. Whirling or having a whorled arrangement.

v. veins. Four veins (2 sup. and 2 inf.) which receive blood from all parts of the choroid of the eye. They empty into post. ciliary and sup. ophthalmic veins.

vox (vŏks) (pl. *voces*) [L. *vox*]. Voice.

v. abscissa. Loss of voice.

v. capitus. Falsetto voice or a voice in the upper register.

v. choler'ica. The suppressed voice of last stages of cholera.

v. rauca. A hoarse voice.

voyeur (voi-ŭr') [Fr. one who sees]. One whose erotic stimulus is derived from looking at sexual objects or situations, such as watching others during coitus.

V.R. Abbr. for *vocal resonance, right vision, ventilation rate.*

VRI. Abbr. for *virus respiratory infection.*

V.S. Abbr. for *vesicular sound, vital sign, volumetric solution.*

V & T. Abbr. for *volume and tension* (of the pulse).

vril (vrĭl) [L. *virilis*, masculine]. The initial energy with which man is supposed to be endowed from birth and which makes it possible for him to reach full maturity and to reproduce his kind; also applied to all living organisms.

vuerometer (vū"ĕr-ŏm'ĕt-ĕr) [Fr. *vue*, sight, + G. *metron*, a measure]. Apparatus for measuring distance bet. the eyes.

vulgaris (vŭl-gā'rĭs) [L. *vulgaris*, common.] Ordinary.

vulnerable (vŭl'nĕr-ă-bl) [L. *vulnerāre*, to wound]. Easily injured or wounded.

vulnerary (vŭl'nĕr-ăr-ĭ) [L. *vulnerāre*, to wound]. 1. Pert. to wounds. 2. A remedy used to heal wounds.

vulnerate (vŭl'nĕr-at) [L. *vulnerāre*, to wound]. To wound.

vulnus (vul'nus) (pl. *vulnera*) [L. *vulnus*, wound]. A wound or injury.

Vulpian-Sherington phenomenon. Contraction of denervated skeletal muscle by stimulating autonomic cholinergic fibers innervating its blood vessels. Also called *pseudomotor phenomenon.*

vulsella, vulsellum (vŭl-sĕl'ă, vŭl-sĕl'ŭm) [L. *vulsella*, tweezers]. A forceps with a hook on each blade. Syn: *volsella.*

vulva (vŭl'vă) (pl. *vulvae*) [L. *vulva*, a covering]. The ext. female genitalia lying beneath the mons veneris consisting of the labia majora, labia minora, clitoris, vestibule of the vagina, and bulbs of the vestibule.

v. connivens. Vulva in which the labia majora are in apposition.

v. hians. Vulva in which labia majora are gaping.

vulvar (vŭl'var) [L. *vulva*, covering]. Relating to the vulva.

v. leukoplakia. Condition characterized by diffuse or focal, translucent thickening of the vulva. Often gives rise to carcinoma.

vulvectomy (vŭl-vĕk'tō-mĭ) [" + G. *ektomē*, excision]. Excision of the vulva.

vulvismus (vŭl-vĭz'mŭs) [" + G. *-ismos*, condition]. Painful spasm of the vagina. Syn: *vaginismus.*

vulvitis (vŭl-vī'tĭs) [L. *vulva*, covering, + G. *-itis*, inflammation]. Inflammation of the vulva.

v., acute nongonorrheal. V. resulting from chafing of opposed lips of vulva or from accumulated sebaceous material around the clitoris.

v., follicular. Inflammation following infection (usually by Staphylococcus aureus) of hair follicles of vulva.

v., gangrenous. Necrosis and sloughing of areas of vulva, often a complication of infectious diseases such as diphtheria, scarlatina, typhoid fever.

v., leukoplakic. A chronic atrophic vulvitis. See: *kraurosis vulvae.*

v., mycotic. V. caused by various fungi, most commonly by Candida albicans.

vulvo- (L.]. Combining form meaning *a covering, the vulva.*

vulvocrural (vŭl"vō-krū'răl) [L. *vulva*, covering, + *cruralis*, pert. to the leg]. Relating to the vulva and the thigh.

vulvopathy (vŭl-vŏp'ă-thĭ) [" + G. *pathos*, disease]. Any disorder of the vulva.

vulvouterine (vŭl"vō-ū'tĕr-ĭn) [" + *uterinus*, pert. to the uterus]. Relating to the vulva and uterus.

vulvovaginal (vŭl"vō-văj'ĭn-ăl) [" + *vagina*, a sheath]. Pert. to the vulva and vagina.

v. glands. Small glands on either side of the vulvar orifice. See: *Bartholin's glands.*

vulvovaginitis (vŭl"vō-văj"ĭn-ī'tĭs) [" + " + G. *-itis*, inflammation]. Inflammation of both the vulva and vagina at the same time, or of the vulvovaginal glands.

v., diabetic. Mycotic vulvar infection commonly occurring with diabetes.

vv. Abbr. for *veins.*

Notes

W

W. Chemical symbol for *tungsten.*

w. Abbr. for *watt,* a unit of electric energy, *week, wife, with.*

Wachendorf's membrane (vahk'ĕn-dōrf). 1. A thin membrane occluding the pupil of the embryo. Syn: *membrana pupillaris.* 2. The outer membrane ensheathing a cell.

wafer (wā'fer) [ME. *wafre*]. 1. A thin sheet of flour paste used to enclose a medicinal dose of powder. 2. A flat vaginal suppository.

Wagstaffe's fracture (wăg'stăf). One with separation of the internal malleolus.

waist (wāst) [ME. *wast,* growth]. Small part of body bet. thorax and hips. See: *cincture sensation.*

Walcher's position (vahl'ker). The patient assumes the dorsal recumbent position with hips at the end of the bed and the legs hanging down.

Wald cycle. The transformations involved in the breakdown and resynthesis of rhodopsin.

Waldeyer's ring. The ring of tonsillar (lymphatic) tissue which encircles the naso- and oropharynx. Consists of the two palatine tonsils, lingual and pharyngeal tonsils.

walking (wauk'ĭng) [A.S. *wealcan,* to turn]. Act of moving on foot.

RS: *abasia; a. paralytic; akathisia; astasia; a. abasia; atremia; basophobia; claudication; dysbasia; gait.*

w. typhoid. Typhoid fever in which the symptoms are mild so that the patient is ambulatory.

Wallenberg's syndrome. A complex of symptoms resulting from occlusion of posterior inferior cerebellar artery or one of its branches supplying lower portion of brain stem. Dysphagia, muscular weakness or paralysis, impairment of pain and temperature senses, and cerebellar dysfunction are characteristic.

wallerian degeneration (wŏl-ē'rĭ-ăn). Degeneration of a nerve fiber (axon) which has been severed from its cell body. The myelin sheath also degenerates and is transformed into a chain of lipoid droplets which stains by the Marchi method, a method utilized in tracing the course of injured nerve fibers. The neurilemma does not degenerate but forms a tube which directs the growth of the regenerating axon.

walleye (wawl'ī). 1. Eye in which iris is light-colored or white. 2. Leukoma or dense opacity of cornea. 3. Squint in which both visual axes diverge. Syn: *divergent strabismus.*

walnut (wawl'nŭt) [A.S. *wealhhnutu,* a foreign nut]. Black and English. A tree and its nuts of the *Juglans* genus.

English Walnuts: Raw, 100 gm. Calories: 651. Other values: 14.8 gm. protein; 64 gm. fat; 15.8 gm. carbohydrate.

wan'dering. Moving about; not fixed.

w. abscess. One that burrows and comes to the surface at a point distant from its origin.

w. cell. A leukocyte which moves about the substance of an organ.

w. kidney, w. spleen. Dislocated floating kidney or spleen.

w. mind. Daydream or reverie.

Wangensteen's method (wăng'ĕn-stēn). Technic for relieving postoperative distention, nausea and vomiting and certain cases of mechanical bowel obstruction.

It involves use of an intranasal catheter in combination with a suction siphonage apparatus. See: *decompression, distention.*

Warburg apparatus. A capillary manometer used for determining oxygen consumption and CO_2 production. Widely used in metabolism studies.

ward (ward) [A.S. *weard,* a guarding]. A large room or hall in a hospital.

w., accident. One reserved for accident cases.

w., isolation. One for isolation of those suspected of being affected with an infectious disease.

w., psychopathic. One in a general hospital for temporary reception of mentally ill patients.

Wardrop's disease (war'drŏp). Acute inflammation of matrix of the nail in scrofulous children. Syn: *onychia maligna.*

W.'s operation. Ligation of an artery for aneurysm at a distance beyond the sac.

warehousemen's itch (wār'hows-mĕnz ĭtsh). Eczema of hands from touching irritating substances.

war gases. Any chemical substances, whether solid, liquid, or vapor, used to produce poisonous or irritant effects. See: *gases, war.*

wart (wort) [A.S. *wearte*]. A circumscribed cutaneous elevation resulting from hypertrophy of the papillae and epidermis. It is caused by a filtrable virus. Syn: *verruca.*

RS: *condyloma, keratosis seborrheica, sycoma, venereal, verrucose.*

w., fig. Syn: *verruca acuminata, condyloma acuminatum, venereal wart.* A growth of filiform projections usually occurring on genitalia. They are frequently covered with a foul-smelling secretion.

w., plantar. One on pressure-bearing areas, esp. sole of foot.

w., seborrheic. Patch of corneous hypertrophy on face of the aged.

w., senile. See: *seborrheic wart.*

w.'s, venereal. Vegetating growths upon skin, esp. on the mucocutaneous juncture of the genitals, having an offensive discharge. Syn: *verruca acuminata.*

wash. Act of cleaning, especially a part or all of the body.

w., eye. A lotion for the eyes. Syn: *collyrium.*

washerwoman's itch (wash'ĕr-wŭm"ăn). Eczema of the hands of laundry workers.

wash-leath'er skin. A trophic change in the skin in which silver drawn across it leaves a black mark.

wasp. Term sometimes applied to all insects belonging to the suborder Apocrita, order Hymenoptera (except the Formicidae or ants), but more generally restricted to the superfamilies Scolioidea, Vespoidea, and Specoidea. Members have base of abdomen constricted and females have a piercing ovipositor which in many species is modified into a sting. Many are social, living in large colonies. Common representatives are yellow jackets and hornets.

w. sting. The injection of wasp venom into the skin, resulting in a painful wound and sometimes mild systemic reaction. Multiple stings may be dangerous especially to sensitized individuals

TREATMENT: Apply bicarbonate of soda paste or household ammonia solution locally. If pain is severe, infiltrate area with 2% procaine solution. Severe allergic reaction may require injection of epinephrine.

w. waist. Condition seen in some cases of muscular dystrophy in which atrophy of trunk muscles is pronounced.

wasserhelle cell (vŏs'ĕr-hĕl-ĕ). A large vacuolated (water-clear) cell, a variant of chief cells, found in the parathyroid gland.

Wassermann-fast (wahs'ĕr-man). Indicating a positive reaction shown by a Wassermann test which continues after adequate antisyphilitic medication.

W. reaction. Serum complement fixation test as a diagnosis of syphilis. A general term loosely applied to almost any serological test for syphilis.

The results are designated as 1, 2, 3, and 4 plus, the intensity of the reaction usually corresponding to the severity of the infection. The disease may still exist with a negative reaction. Several such reactions would indicate its absence. Several years, after treatment and after last "negative" is obtained, should pass before cure is definitely accepted.

waste (wāst) [L. *vastāre,* to devastate]. 1. To shrink in physical bulk or strength, as from disease. SYN: *cachexia.* 2. Loss by breaking down of bodily tissue. 3. Refuse material no longer useful to an organism.

w. products. Carbon dioxide, organic and inorganic salts, water, dead skin, hair, nails, undigested foods.

w. p.'s, metabolic. Soluble salts in the form of nitrogenous salts (urea) and inorganic salts (sodium chloride); gas in form of carbon dioxide, and liquid in the form of water.

They are excreta, removed by the process of elimination, *q.v.*

wasting (wāst'ĭng) [L. *vastāre,* to devastate]. Enfeebling; causing loss of strength or size; emaciating. SEE: *marasmus.*

w. palsy or ***paralysis.*** Chronic disease marked by gradual atrophy of muscular tissue with paralysis. SYN: *progressive muscular atrophy.*

water (waw'ter) [A.S. *waeter*]. 1. A solution in water of a volatile substance. 2. The urine. 3. H_2O, hydrogen and oxygen, a tasteless, clear odorless fluid, constituting bet. 75% and 90% of all tissues.

It freezes at 32° F. (0° C.) and boils at 212° F. (100° C.).

Water is the principal chemical constituent of the body comprising approx. 75%, and is distributed within the *intracellular fluid* and outside of the cells in the *extracellular fluid.* Water is indispensable for metabolic activities within cells as it is the medium in which chemical reactions can take place. Outside of cells, water is the principal transporting agent of the body. Among the properties of water which are of importance to living organisms are the following:

(a) It is the most *universal solvent.* (b) It is a medium in which acids, bases, and salts *ionize,* and the concentrations of these substances (*electrolytes*) must be and are normally regulated quite precisely by the body. (c) It possesses a *high specific heat* and has a *high latent heat of vaporization,* of importance in regulation and maintenance of a constant body temperature. (d) It possesses a *high surface tension.* (e) It is an important *reacting agent* and essential in all *hydrolytic reactions.*

In the body, water is the principal constituent of all body fluids (blood, lymph, tissue fluid), of all secretions (salivary juice, gastric juice, bile, sweat, etc.), and all excretory fluids (urine). Intake of water is determined principally by the sense of thirst. Excessive intake may lead to *water intoxication;* excessive loss to *dehydration.*

w. balance. Condition in which intake of water equals output.

w.-bed. A rubber mattress, filled 3 parts full with warm water (temp. 100° F.); must not be too full or it will be hard. Fracture boards are placed across the wire mattress to produce a firm foundation and prevent sagging; it should be refilled every fortnight.

w., bound. Water which in protoplasm is attached to organic substances. It is not available for metabolic processes.

w. (on) brain. Disease marked by abnormal increase in cerebral fluid. SYN: *hydrocephalus.*

w. brash. Gastric burning pain with eructations. SYN: *heartburn.*

w.-cure. Use of water in treatment. SYN: *hydrotherapy.*

w., deionized. Water that has been passed through a substance which removes cations and anions present. Final product is equivalent to distilled water.

w.-hammer pulse. Pulse marked by quick powerful beat, collapsing suddenly. SYN: *Corrigan's pulse, q.v.* RS: *pulse.*

w., heavy. SYN: *deuterium oxide.*

w. (for) injection. *Aqua pro injectione.* Water for parenteral use that has been distilled and sterilized within 24 hrs. or water that has been distilled (sometimes redistilled), sterilized, and placed in sealed containers so that it remains free of pyrogens. SEE: *water, pyrogen-free.*

w. intoxication. That resulting from ingestion of large quantities of water or in cases of kidney disorder when urinary secretion is reduced.

SYM: *headache, dizziness, vomiting, convulsions, coma,* and *possibly death.*

w. itch. Schistosome dermatitis, *q.v.*

w., pyrogen-free. Water that has been rendered free of fever-producing proteins (bacteria and their metabolic products). SEE: *water (for) injection.*

water balance diet. Water content of diet is calculated to individual prescription. The water content of foods as well as beverages is calculated as part of the fluid allowance given in the diet prescription.

water cress (waw'tĕr krĕs). A plant with green leaves and white flowers; usually grows in fresh running water. The leaves are much used in salads.

RAW: 100 gm. Calories: 19. Other values: 2.2 gm. protein; 0.3 gm. fat; 3.0 gm. carbohydrate; 4900 I.U. vitamin A; 79 mg. vitamin C.

watermelon (waw'tĕr-mel"ŏn). The large, round or oblong fruit of a vine of the same name. Its red, sweet, juicy center is eaten.

RAW: 100 gm. Calories: 26. Other values: 0.5 gm. protein; 0.2 gm. fat; 6.4 gm. carbohydrate; 13 mg. vitamin

waters (waw'ters). Common term for the amniotic fluid surrounding the fetus.

w., bag of. Sac enclosing liquor amnii surrounding the fetus. SYN: *amniotic sac.*

wave (wāv) [A.S. *wafian*, to wave]. 1. A disturbance of the equilibrium of a body or medium propagated from point to point with a continuous motion through a closed curve. 2. An undulating or vibrating motion. 3. An oscillation seen in the recording of an electrocardiogram, electroencephalogram, or other graphic record of physiological activity.

w., A. Alpha wave; rhythm, alpha, *q.v.*

w., a. Atrial wave of venous pulse.

w., excitation. The excitatory impulse(s) which originate in the sinuatrial node of the heart and sweep through the musculature of the atria stimulating the atrioventricular node and then continuing through the conductile tissue of the ventricles. They bring about the contraction of the chambers of the heart.

w., hertzian. Electromagnetic radiations used in radio and wireless transmission.

w., pulse. 1. The pressure wave originated by the systolic discharge of blood into the aorta. It is not due to the passage of the ejected blood but is the result of the impact being transmitted through the arterial walls. Its speed of transmission varies with nature of the arterial wall increasing with age as the arteries become less resilient. In arteriosclerosis, the velocity is higher.

w's., sound. Vibrations of a vibrating medium which, upon stimulating sensory receptors of the cochlea, are capable of giving rise to sensations of sound. Velocity: In air 1090 ft. per sec. at 0° C.; in water, approx. 4 times faster than in air.

w's., Traube-Hering. Slow rhythmical waves appearing in a blood pressure tracing as a result of interference in blood flow to the medulla. They are probably due to alterations in tone of vasomotor center.

wax (wăks) [A.S. *weax*]. 1. A substance secreted by bees. SYN: *cera.* 2. Anything having the physical properties of, or resembling beeswax. 3. Earwax. SYN: *cerumen.* SEE: *ceroplasty.*

waxy (wăks'ĭ) [A.S. *weax*, wax]. Resembling or pert. to wax.

w. cast. Dense, highly refractile urinary cast.

They have clean-cut contours, sometimes irregular curves and notches. Obtained in severe chronic renal disease.

w. degeneration. Amyloid degeneration seen in wasting diseases.

W.B.C. Abbr. for *white blood count, white blood cells.*

weak (wēk) [ME. *weik*, from Old Norse *veiker*]. Deficient in strength of body; infirm.

RS: *asthenia, atony, cardiasthenia, enervation, ergasthenia, fatigue, lassitude, lipothymia.*

wean (wēn) [A.S. *wenian*, to accustom]. To accustom to loss of breast milk by substitution of other nourishment.

weanling. A young child or infant recently changed from breast to formula feeding.

w. diarrhea. Severe gastroenteritis which sometimes occurs in infants who have been recently weaned.

webbed (wĕbd) [A.S. *webb*, a fabric]. Having a membrane connecting adjacent structures, as the duck's feet.

w. fingers, w. toes. Two or more toes or fingers connected by a membrane.

Weber-Christian disease (wĕb'ĕr krĭs'-chĕn). Relapsing, febrile, nodular, nonsuppurative panniculitis, a generalized disorder of fat metabolism characterized by recurring episodes of fever and development of crops of subcutaneous fatty nodules.

Weber's paralysis (wĕb'ĕr). Paralysis of oculomotor nerve on one side with contralateral spastic hemiplegia.

ETIOL: Lesion of the *crus cerebri.*

weeping (wēp'ĭng) [A.S. *wēpan*, to lament]. 1. Shedding tears. 2. Moist, dripping.

w. eczema. Dermatitis with eruption of vesicles exuding serum.

w. sinew. Circumscribed cystic swelling of a tendon sheath.

Weidel's reaction (vī'dĕl). Test for presence of xanthine bodies or uric acid.

Weigert's law (vī'gĕrt). Loss or destruction of organic elements is usually followed by excessive production during reparative process.

weight (wāt) [A.S. *gewiht*]. 1. The property of matter which causes it to fall to the earth by gravitation. 2. Amt. of such a tendency.

Weight of the body progressively increases in pathological obesity; and progressively decreases in Addison's disease, cancer, chronic diarrhea, chronic suppurations, diabetes, hysteria, anorexia, fevers, lactation when prolonged, marasmus, obstruction of pylorus or thoracic duct, tuberculosis, ulcer of stomach.

Desirable Weights for Men of 25 and Over*

Height (with shoes on) 1-inch heels Ft.	In.	Small Frame	Medium Frame	Large Frame
5	2	112-120	118-129	126-141
5	3	115-123	121-133	129-144
5	4	118-126	124-136	132-148
5	5	121-129	127-139	135-152
5	6	124-133	130-143	138-156
5	7	128-137	134-147	142-161
5	8	132-141	138-152	147-166
5	9	136-145	142-156	151-170
5	10	140-150	146-160	155-174
5	11	144-154	150-165	159-179
6	0	148-158	154-170	164-184
6	1	152-162	158-175	168-189
6	2	156-167	162-180	173-194
6	3	160-171	167-185	178-199
6	4	164-175	172-190	182-204

Desirable Weights for Women of 25 and Over*

Height (with shoes on) 2-inch heels Ft. In.	Small Frame	Medium Frame	Large Frame
4 10	92- 98	96-107	104-119
4 11	94-101	98-110	106-122
5 0	96-104	101-113	109-125
5 1	99-107	104-116	112-128
5 2	102-110	107-119	115-131
5 3	105-113	110-122	118-134
5 4	108-116	113-126	121-138
5 5	111-119	116-130	125-142
5 6	114-123	120-135	129-146
5 7	118-127	124-139	133-150
5 8	122-131	128-143	137-154
5 9	126-135	132-147	141-158
5 10	130-140	136-151	145-163
5 11	134-144	140-155	149-168
6 0	138-148	144-159	153-173

*Weight in pounds, according to frame (in indoor clothing).

(*Courtesy of Metropolitan Life Insurance Company.*)

w., *atomic*. W. of an atom of an element compared with that of oxygen which is taken as 16; the mean value of the isotopic weights of an element.

w., *molecular*. ABBR: *M*. The sum of all the atomic weights of all the elements in one molecule of a compound.

weights and measures. SEE: *Appendix*.

Weil's disease. SYN: *epidemic jaundice; leptospirosis icterohaemorrhagica; spirochetosis icterohaemorrhagica.*

ETIOL: *Leptospira icterohaemorrhagiae*, an organism found in rat urine and feces. Acquired by man through contaminated food or water or by contact of broken skin with rat feces or urine.

It is a specific infection accompanied by muscular pains, fever, jaundice, and enlargement of liver and spleen.

TREATMENT: Rest in bed, liquid diet. otherwise largely symptomatic.

Weil-Felix reaction. The agglutination of certain *Proteus* organisms due to the development of *Proteus* antibodies in certain rickettsial diseases. Also called *Weil-Felix test.*

Weir Mitchell's treatment (wēr mĭt'shĕl). Rest in bed, massage, nourishing diet and isolation for hysteria and neurasthenia.

Welch's bacillus (wĕlsh). *Clostridium welchii, q.v.*, the causative organism of gas gangrene.

wen (wĕn) [A.S. *wenn*]. A cyst resulting from the retention of secretion in a sebaceous gland. SYN: *steatoma.*

SYM: One or more rounded or oval elevations, varying in size from a pea to a large walnut; slowly appears on scalp, face or back; painless, rather soft; contains a yellowish-white caseous mass.

TREATMENT: Sac and contents should be carefully dissected out. SEE: *sebaceous gland.*

Werdnig-Hoffmann's disease. Infantile muscular atrophy, considered by some to be identical with amyotonia congenita.

Werlhof's disease (verl'hof). Form of progressive purpura marked by hemorrhages from the mucous membranes and severe prostration. SYN: *purpura, idiopathic thrombocytopenic.*

SYM: Large reduction of blood platelets, spontaneous hemorrhages into and from tissues, enlargement of spleen, marked prostration.

Wernicke's syndrome (ver'nĭk-ē). Condition of old age frequently seen, marked by loss of memory and disorientation with confabulation. SYN: *presbyophrenia, q.v.*

Westphal-Edinger nucleus. Small group of nerve cells in rostral portion of nucleus of oculomotor nerve. Efferent fibers pass to ciliary ganglion conveying impulses destined for intrinsic muscles of the eye.

Westphal's phenom'enon, W's. sign. Loss of the knee jerk, the patellar reflex.

wet (wĕt) [A.S. *wǣt*]. Soaked with moisture.

w. *brain*. Increased amt. of cerebrospinal fluid with edema of the meninges, due to alcoholism.

w. *cup*. A cupping glass used after scarification.

w. *dream*. Nocturnal seminal emission.

w. *nurse*. A woman who breast-feeds another's child.

w. *pack*. A form of bath, given by wrapping patient in hot or cold wet sheets, covered with a blanket, used esp. to reduce fever.

WEUP. Abbr. for *willful exposure to unwanted pregnancy.*

Wharton's duct (hwar'ton). That of the submandibular salivary gland opening into the mouth at side of the *frenum linguae.*

W's. *jelly*. A gelatinous basic substance in the umbilical cord.

wheal (hwēl) [A.S. *hwele*]. More or less round and evanescent elevation of the skin, white in center with pale red periphery, accompanied by itching.

Seen in urticaria, insect bites, anaphylaxis, angioneurotic edema. SYN: *pomphus.*

wheat (hwēt) [A.S. *hwǣte*]. FLOUR made from hard wheat, 100 gm. Calories: 333. Other values: 13.3 gm. protein; 2.0 gm. fat; 71 gm. carbohydrate; 33 mg. iron; 41 mg. calcium; 372 mg. phosphorus; 4.3 mg. niacin.

STRUCTURE OF A GRAIN OF WHEAT: 1. Husk or outer coat. Removed before grinding. 2. Bran coats removed in making white flour contains the mineral substances. 3. Gluten. Contains the fat and protein. 4. Starch. The center of the kernel.

ACTION: See bread for a comparison of flours made from wheat and other cereals. Boiled whole wheat is a most excellent food.

WHEAT PREPARATIONS AND PASTES: Macaroni, vermicelli, noodles, etc., are made from flour and water, molded, dried, and slightly baked. They are easy to digest and not over 10% of nitrogen content is lost.

wheeze (hwēz) (M. E. *whesen*, to hiss). A whistling or sighing sound resulting from narrowing of the lumen of a respiratory passageway. Often only noted by use of stethoscope. Occurs in asthma, croup, hay fever, mitral stenosis, and pleural effusion. May result from presence of tumors, foreign obstructions, bronchial spasm, tuberculosis, obstructive emphysema or edema.

wheezing (hwē'zĭng) (M. E. *whesen*, to hiss). Production of whistling sounds during difficult breathing such as occurs in asthma, coryza, croup and other respiratory disorders. SEE: *wheeze.*

whelk (hwĕlk) [A.S. *hwylca*, a suppuration]. A wheal; a protuberance on the face, as a nodule or tubercle.

whey (hwā) [A.S. *hwaeg*]. The liquid left after milk has been coagulated by the aid of rennet. It is diuretic, laxative, and mineralizing.

Liquid, 100 gm. Calories: 26. Other values: 0.9 gm. protein; 0.3 gm. fat; 5.1 gm. carbohydrate; 51 mg. calcium.

See: *buttermilk; milk.*

whiff. 1. A slight gust or puff of air, esp. one conveying an odor. 2. A quick inhalation or exhalation, as of tobacco smoke.

Whipple's disease [George Hoyt Whipple, American pathologist, 1878-]. Intestinal lipodystrophy, characterized by fatty stools, loss of weight and strength, chronic arthritis, a distinctive lesion of the mucosa of the jejunum and ileum, and other signs of a malabsorption syndrome. It resembles idiopathic steatorrhea. It is a rare disease.

Treatment: *Tetracycline.*

whipworm (hwĭp'worm) [named from its shape]. A roundworm often parasitic in the human intestines. Syn: *Trichuris trichiuri.*

whirl (hwirl) [M.E. *whirlen*]. To revolve rapidly; to feel giddiness.

whirlbone (hwirl'bōn). 1. The kneecap. Syn: *patella.* 2. The head of the femur.

whisky, whiskey (hwĭs'kē). A distilled alcoholic liquor made from grain. The alcohol present in ethyl alcohol. Syn: *spiritus frumenti.*

whisper (hwĭs'per) [A.S. *hwisprian*]. 1. Speech without voice; a low, sibilant sound. 2. To utter in a low, nonvocal sound.

w., cavernous. Direct transmission of a whisper through a cavity in auscultation.

white (hwīt) [A.S. *hwit*]. 1. The achromatic color of highest brilliance. 2. Of the color of milk.

w. cell, w. corpuscle. The leukocyte. See: *blood, corpuscle.*

w. gangrene. G. due to local anemia.

w. leg. Phlebitis of femoral vein marked by white swelling of the leg. Syn: *phlegmasia alba dolens, q.v.*

w. line. White tendinous attachment of abdominal oblique and transverse muscles. Visible in the midline of the skin covering the anterior wall of the abdomen. Syn: *linea alba.*

w. precipitate. Syn: *mercury, ammoniated.* A white amorphous powder used principally in ointments for external treatment of some skin diseases.

w. matter, w. substance. Any nervous structure composed of white medullated nerve fibers.

w. softening. Stage of softening of any substance in which the affected area has become white and anemic.

whites (hwīts). A medical colloquialism. A thick, whitish vaginal discharge. Syn: *leukorrhea, q.v.*

white'fish. Smoked, 100 gm. Calories: 155. Other values: 20.9 gm. protein; 7.3 gm. fat; no carbohydrate.

White's operation (hwīt). Castration for relief of enlarged prostate.

whitlow (hwĭt'lō) [origin uncertain]. Suppurative inflammation at the end of a finger or toe. Syn: *felon, panaris, paronychia, q.v.*

It may be deep seated, involving the bone and its periosteum, or superficial, affecting parts of the nail.

whoop (hoop) [O.Fr. *houper*, to whoop]. The sonorous and convulsive inspiratory crow following a paroxysm of whooping cough.

whooping cough (hoop'ĭng kawf). An acute infectious disease with recurrent spasms of coughing ending in a whooping inspiration. Syn: *pertussis, q.v.*

whorl (hwurl) [M.E. *wharle*, whirl of a spindle]. 1. Spiral arrangement of cardiac muscular fibers. Syn: *vortex.* 2. A type of fingerprint in which the central papillary ridges turn through at least 1 complete circle.

whortleberry (hwur'tl-bĕr″ĭ) [A.S. *horte*, whortleberry]. A sweet European blueberry. For food value, see *blueberry.*

Widal's reaction or **test** (vē-dal'). An agglutination test for typhoid fever.

wild cherry (*prunus virginiana*). USP. The dried bark of the plant, used principally in the form of the syrup as a vehicle for cough medicine.

will (wĭl) [A.S. *willa*]. Power of controlling one's actions or emotions.

RS: *acrasia, bulesis, volition, voluntary.*

Willis' cords (wĭl'ĭs). Those crossing the sup. longitudinal sinus, transversely.

W., circle of. Syn: *circulus arteriosus.* An intercommunicating set of arteries which encircles optic chiasma and hypophysis from which the principal arteries supplying the brain are derived. It receives blood from the two internal carotid arteries and the basilar artery formed by union of the two vertebrals.

Wilson's disease (wil'sun). A rare disease of degeneration of corpus striatum and cirrhosis of the liver, characterized by tremulous distortion of the muscles (increased by activity), dysarthria, dysphagia, and emotionalism. It is thought to be the result of abnormal copper metabolism.

Winckel's disease (vĭn'kĕl). A fatal disease of the newborn characterized by profuse hemorrhages, hematuria, jaundice, enlarged spleen, and punctiform hemorrhages upon the skin. Results from entry of colon bacilli through stump of umbilical cord (omphalitis).

window. 1. An aperture for the admission of light or air or both. 2. A small aperture into a cavity, especially that of inner ear. See: *fenestra.*

w., cochlear. The *fenestra rotunda, q.v.* Syn: *round window, fenestra cochlea.*

w., oval. The *fenestra ovalis, q.v.* Also called *fenestra vestibuli.*

w., round. The *fenestra rotunda, q.v.* Also called *fenestra cochlea.*

w., vestibular. The *oval window.* Syn: *fenestra ovalis, q.v.*

windpipe (wĭnd'pīp). Air passage from the larynx to the lungs. Syn: *trachea, q.v.*

wine (wīn) [L. *vinum*, wine]. 1. Fermented grape juice or fermented juice of any fruit. 2. Solution of a medicinal substance in wine. Syn: *vinum.*

Table Wine, about 12% alcohol by volume, 100 gm. (slightly more than three fluid ounces). Calories: 85. Other values: 0.1 gm. protein; no fat; 4.2 gm. carbohydrate; 9.0 mg. calcium,

w. glass. A fluid measure of approximately two fluid ounces (60 cc.).

wing. A structure resembling the wing of a bird, especially the great and small wings of the sphenoid bone, *q.v.* See: *ala.*

winged scapula. Scapula, winged, *q.v.*

wink (wĭnk) [A.S. *wincian*]. 1. To close and open the eyelids quickly. 2. Act of closing and opening the eyelids quickly. SEE: *mication, nictitation.*

Winslow, foramen of. The epiploic foramen.

W., ligament of. The oblique popliteal ligament located at back of knee.

W., pancreas of. The processus uncinatus of the pancreas.

win'ter itch. Itching occurring only in cold weather. SYN: *pruritus hiemalis.*

Wirsung, duct of (vēr'soong). Excretory duct of the pancreas. SYN: *pancreatic duct.*

wisdom tooth (wĭz'dŏm). The hindmost or last molar tooth on each side of the jaw, which may appear as late as the 25th year.

witches' milk (wĭtsh'es). Milk secreted by the newly born infant's breast, stimulated by the lactating hormone circulating in the mother.

Wohlfahrtia (vōl-fāhr'tĭ-ă). A genus of flesh flies belonging to the family Sarcophagidae, order Diptera.

W. magnifica. Species found in SE Europe. The larvae may occur in human and animal wounds.

W. opaca. Species occurring in Canada, a common parasite of wild animals. Human babies may become infested.

W. vigil. Species found in Canada and N. United States.

wolffian body (wool'fĭ-ăn). An embryonic organ on each side of the vertebral column. SYN: *mesonephros.* SEE: *archinephron, embryo, paroöphoron, parovarium.*

w. cyst. One of the broad ligaments of the uterus.

w. duct. SYN: *mesonephric duct.* Duct in embryo leading from mesonephros to cloaca. From it develop the ductus epididymis, ductus deferens, seminal vesicle, ejaculatory duct, ureter and pelvis of kidney.

w. tubules. SYN: *mesonephric tubules.* One of 30 to 34 tubules which develop within the mesonephros and empty into mesonephric duct. Most are transitional persisting for only a short time. Some persist in adult males as the *efferent ductules* of the testis, others persist only as vestigial structures. SEE: *paradidymis, epoophoron, paroophoron.*

Wolhynian fever. Trench fever, *q.v.*

womb (woom) [A.S. *wamb*]. Female organ for protection and nourishment of the fetus. SYN: *uterus, q.v.*

wood alcohol (wud al'kō-hōl). (CH_3OH) Alcohol obtained by distillation from wood.

It is a poisonous substance and frequently causes loss of sight. SEE: *methyl alcohol.*

wood tick. *Dermacentor andersoni,* an important N. American species of tick which causes tick paralysis and transmits causative organisms of Rocky Mountain spotted fever and tularemia.

Wood's rays. Ultraviolet rays. Used to detect fluorescent materials in the skin and hair in certain disease states such as *tinea capitis.* The terms *Wood's light* and *Wood's lamp* have become synonymous for *Wood's rays,* even though these are misnomers.

wool fat. Anhydrous lanolin. A fatty substance obtained from sheep's wool. Used as a base for ointments.

woolsorter's disease (wool'sor-ter). A pulmonary form of anthrax which develops in those who handle wool contaminated with *Bacillus anthracis.*

word blindness. Inability to comprehend written words; a form of aphasia, *q.v.* SYN: *alexia.*

w. salad. The use of words with no apparent meaning attached to them or to their relations one with another; usually found in schizophrenia.

work (wurk) [A.S. *worc*]. For definition, SEE: *erg.* For comparison of various energy units, SEE: *calorie, unit.*

worm (werm) [A.S. *wyrm*]. 1. SYN: *helminth.* An elongated invertebrate belonging to one of the following phyla: Platyhelminthes (flatworms); Nemathelminthes or Aschelminthes, round- or threadworms; Acanthocephala, spiny-headed worms; and Annelida (Annulata), segmented worms. 2. Any small, limbless, creeping animal. 3. Median portion of the cerebellum. 4. Any wormlike structure.

For flatworm, hookworm, pinworm, etc., SEE UNDER: name of worm.

w. abscess. A. resulting from lodgment of a worm in the body.

w. fever. Fever due to irritation caused by worms in the intestinal canal.

wormian bones (wur'mĭ-ăn). Small, irregular bones in the course of the cranial sutures.

worsted test (wus'tĕd). Matching of the differently colored skeins of worsted yarn to detect color blindness. SYN: *Holmgren's test.*

wound (woond) [A.S. *wund*]. Break in the continuity of soft parts from violence or trauma to tissues.

In treating any wound, the patient should be given a tetanus toxoid "booster" injection if he has been immunized previously. If not, he must be given human tetanus antitoxin. If human tetanus antitoxin is not available, the equine form may be used but the patient must be tested for hypersensitivity prior to administering the full dose.

w., abdominal. Frequently sustained; ordinarily involves structure of abdominal wall.

In such instances, it may be treated as ordinary wounds. Where a cavity has been opened, and esp. if viscera have been exposed, they should be kept sterile and moist with a sterile normal salt solution prepared by dissolving a teaspoonful of salt in pint of warm water, or use the clearest water at hand, because allowing viscera to dry encourages the development of gangrene.

w., bullet. A puncture wound from a bullet. Usually there is a small point of entrance; if the bullet left the body, a larger point of exit; it is associated with injuries of bone, tendon, blood vessels, etc.

SYM: Depend on site, speed, and character of bullet.

F. A. TREATMENT: Antitetanic serum. Antiseptic to wound and dressing. Treat complications and shock.

w., cellulitis of. When wounds have been closed without drainage, esp. in such cases as appendicitis, local inflammation of the wound may occur.

SYM: Elevation of temperature from 4th to 7th day with tenderness. Inspect dressing and chart findings.

TREATMENT: Evacuation of the abscess; hot wet dressings.

w., contused. A bruise. It may be caused by a blunt instrument.

The skin need not necessarily be broken, but injury of the tissues under skin, leaving skin unbroken, causes more or less change in the normal musculature. The blood vessels underneath skin being ruptured cause discoloration. If extravasated blood becomes encapsulated it is termed *hematoma**; if it is diffused, an *ecchymosis.** More or less shock depending on the extent of the contusion.

TREATMENT: Cold compresses, pressure, and rest of part with elevation. When acute stage is over (24 to 48 hours), continued rest, heat, and elevation are prescribed. Aseptic drainage may be indicated.

w., crushing. If bleeding, apply cold cloths; if not, gently mold to proper shape, apply cloth dipped in warm water, and keep warm. If bone is fractured, apply splint.

w., fish-hook. Embedded fish hooks are notably difficult to remove. Push the hook through, then cut off barb with an instrument. These injuries frequently become infected, so carefully saturate with an antiseptic and cover with a dressing, and observe for several days.

w., gunshot. Penetrating or perforating wound which may contain a foreign body, as a bullet.

F. A. TREATMENT: Should be conservative. Apply antiseptic, sterile dressing; treat hemorrhage. If large vessels are torn, antitetanic serum to prevent lockjaw. *Do not probe.*

w., incised. A clean-cut wound.

Caused by a keen cutting instrument. There are no jagged edges. Any sharp cut in which the tissues are not severed is an incised wound. It may be either an aseptic or infected w., depending on circumstances which caused it.

An *aseptic* wound, or one occurring under surgical conditions, should heal if conditions are favorable and no contaminations due to pathogenic organisms or foreign material enter into it. During healing process, area of the wound must be kept aseptic. The skin must be cleansed with plain soap and water, and rinsed thoroughly, and covered securely with sterile dressings, preventing external contact with microorganisms. A clean wound should be left alone. The dressings should be changed only often enough to keep wound clean. There should be no squeezing or pulling of its edges.

w., lacerated. A torn wound.

It provides many avenues for infection. It is *not* a clean wound. The edges are ragged. May be caused by many kinds of implements, and the implement may be covered with any kind of pathogenic bacteria. These may be of a violent nature causing tetanus, or only a slight abscess. The infiltration of bacteria may cause any stage of a septic condition. In dealing with such wounds, all possibilities should be taken into consideration.

TREATMENT: The wound should be cleansed with antiseptic solution and ragged edges trimmed off, if too ragged. Some doctors advise that wet dressings be applied The patient should be given tetanus antitoxin. The wound should never be sealed. It is well to hold it open with some form of drain from a piece of sterile silkworm gut or a rubber drain.

w., nonpenetrating. One in which the surface of skin remains intact.

w., open. Contusion where skin is also broken, such as a gunshot w., incised w., or lacerated w.

w., penetrating. One in which the skin is broken and the agent causing the wound enters subcutaneous tissue or a deep-lying structure or cavity.

w., perforating. One in which the vulnerating body both enters and emerges from the cavity.

w., poisoned. This may be classed as a lacerated wound, or a punctured wound, depending on tearing of tissue.

The poisoned wound may be caused by a diseased animal, as a snake or a dog, or some of the wild animals, such as the coon or the squirrel.

TREATMENT: A poisoned wound should be treated the same as a punctured wound. Cauterize with silver nitrate; wet dressings should be applied. The animal, if possible, should be put under observation for rabies.

w., punctured. One made by sharp-pointed instrument, such as a dagger, an ice pick, or needle. The chief danger is from thrombosis and possible release of emboli. A puncture wound never gives access to int. of wound. Tetanus germs thrive in such a wound, as they live in darkness and progress rapidly without air. Inspect instrument that caused the wound.

TREATMENT: Tetanus antitoxin at once and apply moist dressings. If the patient does not respond, the punctured wound should be incised.

w., subcutaneous. Include all which are unaccompanied by break in skin. As contusions.

w. tearing off parts. If completely severed, treat same as lacerated wound. A few drops of carbolic acid should be used in water for washing wounds. Watch for shock. If parts are not completely severed, gently bring into position, apply splints where necessary, and bandage until surgical aid is obtainable. Watch for shock.

w., tunnel. One having a small entrance and exit and of uniform diameter.

W.R. Abbr. for *Wassermann reaction.*

wrinkle. 1. A crevice, furrow or ridge in the skin. 2. To make creases or furrows as in the skin by habitual frowning.

Wrisberg's cardiac ganglion (vrĭz'berg). A small ganglion sometimes found in cardiac plexus to the right of the ligamentum arteriosus.

W.'s cartilages. The cuneiform cartilages of the larynx.

W.'s nerve. The medial brachial cutaneous nerve, a branch of the medial cord of the brachial plexus. 2. The *nervus intermedius (pars intermedia),* a branch of the facial nerve lying between the motor root and the acoustic nerve.

wrist (rĭst) [A.S.]. The joint, or region, lying between the hand and the forearm.

w. bones. The carpus consisting of eight bones. For names SEE: *ossa carpi* under *skeleton.*

w. clonus. Irregular convulsive movements of the hand due to inability to control the muscles that bend the wrist backward.

w. clonus reflex. Lateral clonic movements of hand occurring when hand is held down at arm's length in extreme extension.

w. drop. Condition in which hand is flexed at wrist and cannot be extended; due to injury of radial nerve or paralysis of extensor muscles of wrist and hand.

w. joint. Joint formed by the radius and the first row of carpal bones.

wri'ter's cramp. An occupational disability due to excessive writing.

writing. The act of placing characters, letters, or words on a surface, usually paper, for the purpose of communicating ideas.

w., defects of. SEE: *agraphia.*

w., dextrad. Writing that progresses from left to right.

w., mirror. Writing so that letters and words are reversed and appear as in a mirror.

writing hand. Position seen in paralysis agitans marked by contraction of muscle of the hand. The fingers assume the position similar to holding a pen.

wryneck (rī'nĕk). Contracted state of 1 or more muscles of the neck, producing an abnormal position of the head. SYN: *loxia, torticollis.*

It is occasionally acute, due to cold or trauma; more commonly chronic and is then spastic in character and dependent upon nerve irritation. Has been produced by habitual malposition of the head assumed because of existing ocular defect. May be congenital.

When acute, generally passes away under influence of rest, heat, and time. Chronic may require friction, electricity, or stretching, section or removal of a portion of spinal accessory nerve. May be little benefit from any treatment.

w.s. Abbr. for *water soluble.*

wt. Abbr. for *weight.*

Wuchereria (vōō"kĕr-ē'rĭ-ă). A genus of filarial worms belonging to the superfamily Filarioidea, Class Nematoda. Common in warm regions of the world.

W. bancrofti. SYN: *Filaria bancrofti.* The causative agent of elephantiasis. Adults of the species live in lymph nodes and ducts of man. Females give birth to sheathed microfilariae which remain in internal organs during the day but at night are in circulating blood where they are sucked up by night-biting mosquitoes in which they continue their development, becoming infective larvae in about two weeks.

W. malayi. Species occurring in SE Asia and largely responsible for lymphangitis and elephantiasis in that region. Closely resembles *W. bancrofti.*

wuchereriasis (vōō"kĕr-ĕ-rī'ă-sĭs) SYN: *filariasis, elephantiasis, q.v.* Infestation with filaria worms of the genus *Wuchereria.*

Wunderlich's curve (voon'dĕr-lĭk). The fever curve typical of typhoid fever.

w/v. Abbr. for *weight in volume.* It indicates the amount (by weight) of a solid substance dissolved in a measured quantity of liquid. Per cent "weight in volume" expresses number of grams of an active constituent in 100 ml. of solution.

w/w. Abbr. for *weight in weight.* It indicates the amount (by weight) of a solid substance dissolved in a known amount (by weight) of liquid. Per cent "weight in weight" expresses the number of grams of an active constituent in 100 grams of solution.

Notes

Notes

X

X. 1. Abbr. of *Kienböck's unit.* 2. Roman numeral 10. 3. Symb. of *reactance.*

Xe. Chemical symbol for *xenon.*

xanthelasma (zăn-thĕl-ăz′mă) [G. *xanthos,* yellow, + *elasma,* plate]. 1. Yellow. 2. Flat or slightly raised yellowish tumor occurring in elderly persons, found most frequently on the upper and lower lids, esp. near the inner canthus. SYN: *xanthoma.*

xanthelasmoidea (zăn-thel-ăz-moy′dē-ă) [" + " + *eidos,* resemblance]. Chronic disease of childhood marked by wheals and followed by brownish-yellow patches. SYN: *urticaria pigmentosa.*

xanthellin (zăn-thĕl′ĭn). An antibiotic isolated from Bacillus subtilis in 1951.

xanthematin (zăn-thĕm′ă-tĭn) [" + *haima, haimat-,* blood]. A yellow substance derivable from hematin when treated with nitric acid.

xanthemia (zăn-thē′mĭ-ă) [" + *haima,* blood]. Yellow pigment in the blood. SYN: *carotenemia.*

xanthic (zăn′thĭk) [G. *xanthos,* yellow]. 1. Yellow. 2. Pert. to xanthine.

x. calculus. A urinary concretion containing xanthine.

xanthinuria (zăn′thĭn, -thēn) [G. *xanthos,* yellow]. A nitrogenous extractive contained in muscle tissue, liver, spleen, pancreas, and other organs, and in the urine, formed during the metabolism of nucleoproteins.

x. bases. Nitrogenous substances resulting from splitting up of nucleins. SEE: *purine bases.*

xanthinuria (zăn″thĭn-ū′rĭ-ă) [G. *xanthos,* yellow, + *ouron,* urine]. Excretion of large amounts of xanthine in the urine.

xanthochroia (zăn″thō-krō′ĭ-ă). Yellowish discoloration of the skin.

xanthochromia (zăn″thō-krō′mĭ-ă) [" + *chrōma,* color]. Yellow discoloration, as of the skin in patches or of the cerebrospinal fluid, resembling jaundice.

xanthochroous (zăn-thok′rō-ŭs) [" + *chroa,* color]. Having a yellowish or light complexion.

xanthocyanopia, xanthocyanopsia (zăn″-thō-sĭ-ăn-ō′pĭ-ă, -ŏp′sĭ-ă) [" + *kyanos,* blue, + *opsis,* sight]. A form of color blindness in which yellow and blue are distinguishable, but not red and green.

xanthocyte (zăn″thō′sīt). A cell containing yellow pigment.

xanthoderma (zăn″thō-der′mă) [" + *derma,* skin]. Yellowness of the skin. SYN: *xanthoplasty.*

xanthodont, xanthodontous (zăn′thō-dōnt, zăn-thō-dŏn′tŭs) [" + *odous, odont-,* tooth]. Having yellow teeth.

xanthogranulomatosis (zăn″thō-grăn-ū-lō″mă-tō′sĭs). SYN: *Hand-Schuller-Christian disease.* A disease characterized by exophthalmos, diabetes insipidus, and defects in membranous bones in which granulation tissue with cells containing cholesterol and its esters appear. It is related to eosinophilic granuloma and Letterer-Siwe disease. All three diseases are characterized by a histiocytic proliferation of unknown etiology.

xanthokyanopy (zăn″thō-kī-ăn′ō-pĭ) [" + *kyanos,* blue, + *opsis,* sight]. Partial blindness for color, yellow and blue only being discerned. SYN: *xanthocyanopia.*

xanthoma (zăn″thō′mă) [G. *xanthos,* yellow, + *-ōma,* tumor]. Flat, slightly elevated, soft, rounded plaque or nodule, usually on the eyelids.

They may occur in patches of yellowish macule on orbital regions, confined to middle life or later, and to the female sex, consisting of a degenerative process involving fibers of the orbicularis muscle.

x. diabeticorum. Cutaneous disease associated with diabetes mellitus.

x. dissemination. Condition characterized by presence of xanthoma throughout body especially on face, in tendon sheaths, and in mucous membranes.

x. mul′tiplex. Xanthomas all over the body.

x. palpebra′rum. X. affecting the eyelids.

x. tuberosum. A form which may appear on the neck, shoulders, trunk, or extremities, consisting of small, elastic, and yellowish-colored nodules.

xanthomatosis (zăn″thō-mă-tō′sĭs) [G. *xanthos,* yellow, + *ōma,* tumor]. Condition in which there is a deposition of lipid in tissues usually accompanied by hyperlipemia. Cholesterol may accumulate in tumor nodules (xanthoma) or in individual cells, especially histiocytes and reticuloendothelial cells. Also called *cholesterol lipidosis.*

xanthomelanous (zăn″thō-mĕl′ăn-ŭs) [" + *melas, melan-,* black]. Having black hair and an olive skin.

xanthopathy (zăn″thŏp′ă-thĭ) [" +*pathos,* disease]. Yellowish pigmentation of the skin. SYN: *xanthochromia, xanthoderma.*

xanthophane (zăn′thō-phān) [" + *phanein,,* to appear]. A yellow pigment in the retinal cones.

xanthoplasty (zăn″thō-plăs′tĭ) [" + *plassein,* to form]. Yellow color of the skin. SYN: *xanthoderma.*

xanthoproteic (zăn″thō-prō-te′ĭk) [" + *prōtos,* first]. Derived from or pertaining to xanthoprotein.

xanthoprotein (zăn″thō-prō′tē-ĭn) [" + *prōtos,* first]. Yellowish substance produced by heating proteids with nitric acid.

xanthopsia (zăn-thŏp′sĭ-ă) [G. *xanthos,* yellow, + *opsis,* sight]. Condition in which objects appear yellow.

xanthopsin (zăn-thŏp′sĭn) [" + *opsis,* sight]. Visual yellow, the visual purple produced by light acting on rhodopsin.

xanthopsis (zăn-thŏp′sĭs) [" + *opsis,* appearance]. Yellow pigmentation seen in cancers.

xanthopsydracia (zăn″thŏp-sĭ-drā′shĭ-ă) [" +*psydrax,* pustule]. Skin disease marked by the formation of yellow pustules or pimples on the skin.

xanthorrhea. Discharge of a yellow, purulent substance from the vagina.

xanthosis (zăn″thō′sĭs) [G. *xanthos,* yellow, + *ōsis,* condition]. A yellowing of the skin seen in carotenemia resulting from ingestion of excessive quantities of carrots, squash, egg yolk and other foods containing carotenoids. Condition usually harmless but it may indicate increase of lipochromes in blood due to other conditions such as hypothyroidism or diabetes.

xanthous (zăn′thŭs) [G. *xanthos,* yellow]. Yellow.

xanthuria (zăn″thū′rĭ-ă) [" + *ouron,*

urine]. Excretion of an excess of xanthine in the urine. SYN: *xanthinuria.*

X-chromosome. The sex chromosome, of importance in the determination of sex. SEE: *chromosome, X.*

Xe. Chemical symbol for *xenon.*

xeno-. Combining form meaning *strange, foreign.*

xenogenous (zĕn-ŏj'ĕn-ŭs) [G. *xenos,* strange, host, + *gennan,* to produce]. 1. Caused by a foreign body. 2. Originating in the host, as a toxin resulting from stimuli applied to cells of the host.

xenology (zē-nŏl'ō-gĭ). The study of parasites and their hosts and their relationships to each other.

xenomenia (zĕn-ō-mē'nĭ-ă) [G. *xenos,* strange, + *mēniaia,* menses]. Menstruation from a part of the body other than the normal one. SYN: *vicarious menstruation.*

xenon (zē'non) [G. *xenos,* strange]. A gaseous element in the atmosphere. At. wt. 131.30. At. no. 54. SYMB: Xe.

xenophobia (zĕn"ō-fō'bĭ-ă) [G. *xenos,* stranger, + *phobos,* fear]. Abnormal reluctance to meeting strangers.

xenophonia (zĕn"ō-fō'nĭ-ă) [G. *xenos,* strange, + *phōnē,* voice]. Alteration in accent and intonation of a person's voice due to defect of speech.

xenophthalmia (zĕn-ŏf-thăl'mĭ-ă) [" + *ophthalmia,* inflammation of the eye]. Inflammation of the eye caused by a foreign body.

Xenopsylla (zĕn-ō-sĭl'lă). A genus of fleas belonging to the family Pulicidae, order Siphonaptera.

X. cheopis. The rat flea, but other hosts include man and other animals. It is a vector and transmitter of a number of pathogens including *Hymenolepis nana,* the dwarf tapeworm, *Salmonella,* and causative organisms of bubonic and sylvatic plague, and endemic typhus.

xeransis (zē-răn'sĭs) [G. *xēros,* dry]. Loss of moisture in tissues or drugs brought about gradually. SYN: *siccation.*

xerantic (zē-răn'tĭk). Causing dryness. SYN: *siccant, siccative.*

xerasia (zē-rā'sĭ-ă) [G. *xēros,* dry]. Disease of the hair in which there is abnormal dryness, followed by brittleness, and eventually loss.

xero- (zē"rō-) [G.]. Prefix meaning *dry.*

xerocheilia (zē"rō-kī'lĭ-ă) [G. *xeros,* dry, + *cheilos,* lip]. Dryness of the lips; a type of cheilitis.

xeroderma (zē-rō-der'mă) [G. *xēros,* dry, + *derma,* skin]. Roughness and dryness of the skin; mild ichthyosis.

x. pigmento'sum. A rare disease of the skin starting in childhood marked by disseminated pigment discolorations, ulcers, cutaneous and muscular atrophy and death. SYN: *Kaposi's disease.*

xeroma (zē-rō'mă) [" + *-ōma,* mass]. An abnormally dry state of the conjunctiva. SYN: *xerophthalmia.*

xeromenia (zē-rō-mē'nĭ-ă) [" + *mēniaia,* menses]. The occurrence of the usual disturbances during menses without menstrual flow.

xeromycteria (zē-rō-mĭk-tē'rĭ-ă) [" + *myktēr,* nose]. Dryness of the nasal passages.

xeronosus (zē-rŏn'ō-sŭs) [" + *nosos,* disease]. Dryness of the skin.

xerophagia (zē-rō-fā'jĭ-ă) [" + *phagein,* to eat]. The eating of dry food only.

xerophthalmia (zē-rŏf-thăl'mĭ-ă) [G. *xēros,* dry, + *ophthalmos,* eye]. Conjunctival dryness with keratinization of epithelium following chronic conjunctivitis and in disease due to deficiency of vitamin A.

xerosis (zē-rō'sĭs) [G. *xēros,* dry, + *-ōsis,* condition]. 1. Abnormal dryness of skin, mucous membranes, or of the conjunctiva. 2. Normal sclerosis of tissues in the aged. SYN: *asteatosis.*

xerostomia (zē-rō-stō'mĭ-ă) [" + *stoma,* mouth]. Dryness of the mouth.

It occurs in diabetes, hysteria, paralysis of facial nerve involving chorda tympani, acute infections, some types of neuroses, and is induced by certain drugs such as nicotine and atropine; all arresting salivary secretion. SEE: *ptyalism.*

xerotes (zē'rō-tēz) [G. *xērotēs,* dryness]. Dryness of the body; dryness.

xerotocia (zē-rō-tō'shĭ-ă) [G. *xēros,* dry, + *tokos,* birth]. Dry labor.

xerotic (zē-rŏt'ĭk) [G. *xēros,* dry]. Dry; characterized by dryness.

xerotripsis (zē"rō-trĭp'sĭs) [" + *tripsis,* a rubbing]. Dry friction.

xiphi-, xipho- (zĭf-ĭ-, -o-) [G.]. Prefixes pert. to the *xiphoid cartilage.*

xiphisternum (zĭf-ĭ-ster'nŭm) [G. *xiphos,* sword, + *sternon,* chest]. The pointed process of the lower end of the sternum. SYN: *xiphoid cartilage.*

xiphocostal (zĭf"ō-kŏs'tăl) [" + L. *costa,* rib]. Relating to the xiphoid cartilage and the ribs.

x. ligament. One connecting the xiphoid cartilage to the cartilage of the 8th rib.

xiphodynia (zĭf-ō-dĭn'ĭ-ă) [" + *odynē,* pain]. Pain in the ensiform cartilage.

xiphoid (zĭf'oyd) [G. *xiphos,* sword, + *eidos,* process]. Sword-shaped, ensiform.

x. process. The lowest portion of the sternum, a sword-shaped cartilaginous process supported by bone.

It has no ribs attached to it, but some of the abdominal muscles are attached to it. It ossifies in the aged.

xiphoiditis (zĭf-oyd-ī'tĭs) [" + " + *-itis,* inflammation]. Inflammation of the ensiform or xiphoid cartilage.

x-ray. 1. Any of the radiations of an extremely short wave length, less than 5 Angstrom units, emitted primarily as result of sudden change in velocity of a moving electric charge and as the result of atomic changes of target due to this impact. Produced in vacuum tubes. Because of their penetrating ability and action on photographic film they are used in radiography. SYN: *roentgen ray.* 2. A photograph obtained by use of x-rays.

x. dermatitis. Cutaneous inflammation due to exposure to x-rays.

x. unit. Unit of x-ray dosage equal to 1/10 the erythema dose.

X-substances. Nonspecific, mildly toxic substances extracted from cultures of certain bacteria.

xylenin (zī'lē-nĭn) [G. *xylon,* wood]. A toxic substance extracted by xylene from tubercle bacilli.

xylo- (zī-lō-) [G.]. Prefix *pert. to or derived from wood.*

xylose (zī'lōs) [G. *xylon,* wood]. Wood sugar, a crystalline, nonfermentable pentose.

xyrospasm (zī'rō-spăzm) [G. *xyron,* razor, + *spasmos,* spasm]. Occupational neurosis of the fingers seen in barbers.

xysma (zĭz'mă) [G. *zysma,* filings]. Shreds of tissue sometimes seen in diarrhea stools.

xyster (zĭs'ter) [G. scraper]. File or rasp used in surgery.

Notes

Notes

Y

Y. Symb. of element *yttrium.*

yaghourt (yah-ghoort'). Yoghurt; yogurt,

yard [A.S. *gyrd,* a rod]. A measure of 3 feet or 36 inches. Equal to 0.9144 meter.

yava skin (yah'va skĭn). A form of elephantiasis due to the excessive use of kava. SEE: *elephantiasis.*

yaw. SYN: *maman pian.* The primary lesion of yaws.

y., mother. The primary lesion of yaws occurring at site of inoculation 3-4 weeks after infection.

yawn [A.S. *gānian,* to yawn]. 1. To open the mouth involuntarily, as in drowsiness or fatigue. 2. Involuntary act of gaping, accompanied by attempts at inspiration, excited by drowsiness.

yawning (yawn'ĭng) [A.S. *gānian,* to yawn]. Deep inspiration, gaping induced by drowsiness or fatigue. SYN: *oscitation.*

yaws (yawz) [Cariban]. An infectious tropical disease caused by a spirochete, *Treponema pertenue.* SYN: *frambesia.*

SYM: Febrile disturbances, rheumatism, eruption of tubercles with a caseous crust on hands, feet, face, and external genitals.

TREATMENT: Penicillin.

Yb. The symb. for *ytterbium.*

Y bacillus. A dysentery bacillus (*Shigella flexneri,* Hiss and Russell's Y bacillus).

Y car'tilage. The cartilage uniting the 3 pelvic bones at bottom of the acetabulum early in life.

Y-chromosome. One of a pair of sex chromosomes (X and Y) which play a role in the determination of sex. SEE: *chromosome,* Y.

yeast (yēst) [A.S. *gist*]. 1. A substance composed of aggregated cells (*Ascomycetes*) of minute unicellular sac fungi. 2. A commercial product composed of meal impregnated with living yeast.

yelk (yelk). Variant of yolk.

yellow (yĕl'ō) [A.S. *geolu*]. 1. One of the primary colors resembling that of a ripe lemon. 2. Colored yellow, as the skin in disease.

y. body. The corpus luteum, *q.v.*

y. enzyme. SEE: *enzyme, Warburg's yellow.*

y. fever. An acute infectious disease characterized by jaundice,. epigastric tenderness, vomiting, hemorrhages, and a febrile course consisting of 2 paroxysms.

ETIOL: A filtrable virus transmitted by the bite of a female mosquito, *Aedes aegypti.*

PERIOD OF INCUBATION: 3 to 6 days.

TREATMENT: Water and electrolyte balance should be carefully watched and in cases of persistent vomiting, parenteral fluids containing dextrose and saline should be given.

PROPHYLAXIS: Preventive measures include mosquito control by screening, spraying with DDT, etc. and destruction of breeding areas. Preventive vaccines are available for those who plan to travel, or live in areas where the disease is endemic.

SYM: *First Stage*: Disease begins with sudden onset of fever sometimes accompanied by a chill followed by pain in head, back, and limbs. Temperature rises rapidly till it reaches its maximum, 103° to 105° F. Face flushed, conjunctivae injected, pupils small, tongue coated, epigastrium tender, stomach irritable and unretentive, bowels constipated, urine scanty and albuminous. This stage lasts from a few hours to several days.

It is followed by a marked fall in temperature and an improvement in general symptoms. At this time convalescence may begin or patient may pass into second febrile paroxysm. Jaundice rarely appears before the third day.

Second Stage, Period of Intoxication: Three to nine days. Fever rises to its original height, skin becomes yellow, vomiting persistent, and ejected matter may contain dark blood (black vomit). Hemorrhages sometimes occur from other mucous membranes. Pulse rapid, but not proportionate to the fever. Urine becomes very scanty and contains albumin and casts. Death frequently results from exhaustion or uremia, though recovery may follow the gravest symptoms.

PROG: Always grave. Mortality 5% for natives of an area where the disease is endemic. In severe epidemics, 30 to 40%.

TREATMENT: There is no specific therapy. Absolute rest; cool, well-ventilated room; liquid diet. Vitamin K and calcium gluconate for hemorrhagic tendency. Dehydration and electrolyte balance must be controlled by appropriate fluid replacement therapy. Transfusion may be required. Control fever by cool applications. Analgesics for pain.

y. softening. A stage of softening of the brain marked by fatty degeneration and yellow discoloration.

y. spot. 1. SYN: *macula flava.* Yellowish nodule of ant. end of vocal cord. 2. Center of the retina, the point of clearest vision. SYN: *macula lutea.*

y. vision. Condition in which objects seem yellow in color. SYN: *xanthopsia.*

yerba (yer'ba) [Sp.]. An herb.

y. maté (mah'tā). Paraguay tea.

Yersin's serum (yer'sĭn). An antitoxic serum for the plague.

-yl [G.]. Suffix signifying, in chemistry, *a radical.*

-ylene [G.]. Suffix denoting, in chemistry, *a bivalent hydrocarbon radical.*

Y ligament. A y-shaped band covering the upper and front portions of the hip joint. SYN: *ligament, iliofemoral, q.v.*

yoghurt, yogurt (yōg'hert). A form of curdled milk, curdling being due to the action of *Lactobacillus bulgaricus.* Extensive claims have been made concerning the therapeutic value of yoghurt for various ailments. These have not been substantiated. SEE: *milk.*

yolk (yōk) [M.E. *yolke,* from A.S. *geolca*]. The contents of the ovum; sometimes only the nutritive portion. SYN: *vitellus.** SEE: *zona pellucida*

y. sac. Membranous sac surrounding food yolk in the embryo.

y. stalk. The umbilical duct connecting the yolk sac with the embryo.

Young-Helmholtz theory (yŭng-hĕlm'hōlts). Belief that color vision depends on 3 different sets of retinal fibers responsible for perception of red, green, and violet.

The loss of either red, green, or violet as color perceptive elements in the retina causes an inability to perceive a primary color or any color of which it forms a part.

Young's rule (yŭng). A rule for calculating the dose of medicine a child should receive. Divide the age by the age plus 12. The result represents the fraction of the adult dose suitable for the child. For example: a child of 4 years of age would require $\frac{4}{4+12} = \frac{1}{4}$ of the adult dose.

youth (yûth) [A.S. *geoguth*]. Period bet. childhood and maturity.

ypsiliform. Y-shaped.

y. s. Abbr. for *yellow spot* of the retina.

ytterbium (ĭ-tur'bĭ-ŭm). A rare metallic element. SYMB: Yb. At. wt. 173.04, at. no. 70.

yttrium (ĭt'rĭ-ŭm). A metallic element. SYMB: Y. At. wt. 88.905; at. no. 39.

Yvon's coefficient (ē'vŏn). The ratio bet. the amount of urea and phosphates in the urine.

Y's. tests. One for presence of acetanilide and the other for alkaloids in urine.

Z

Z. Abbr. for *Zuckung,* (Ger. *contraction*), *standard score* (statistics), *zero, zone.* 2. Symbol for *atomic number.*

Z disk. Intermediate (Ger. Zwischenscheibe) disk. SEE: *disk.*

Zaglas' ligament (zah'glahz). The part of the post. sacroiliac ligament from post. sup. spinous process of ilium to side of sacrum.

Zahn's lines or **ribs** (zahn). Transverse whitish marks on the free surface of a thrombus made by the edges of the lamellae of blood platelets.

Zander apparatus (zan'der). Mechanical means for massage and exercise designed by Zander about 1857.

Zang's space (zang). One bet. the 2 lower tendons of the sternomastoid muscle in the supraclavicular fossa.

zaranthan (zar-an'than) [Hebrew]. Scirrhous hardening of the breast.

zein (zē'ĭn) [G. *zeia,* a kind of grain]. A protein obtained from maize. It is deficient in tryptophan and lysine.

Zeiss' gland (zīs). One of the sebaceous glands at free edges of eyelids.

zelotypia (zē-lō-tĭp'ĭ-ă) [G. *zēlos,* zeal, + *typtein,* to strike]. 1. Morbid or monomaniacal zeal in the interest of any project or cause. 2. Insane jealousy.

Zenker's degeneration, zenkerism (zĕng'-kĕr, -ĭzm). A glassy or waxy, hyaline degeneration of skeletal muscles in acute infectious diseases, esp. in typhoid.

zeoscope (zē'ō-skōp) [G. *zein,* to boil, + *skopein,* to view]. Device for determining the alcoholic content of a liquid by means of its boiling point.

zephiran (zef'ĭ-ran). Proprietary name for refined benzalkonium chloride.

zero (zē'rō) [Italian *zero,* from Arabic *sifr,* a cipher]. 1. Figure corresponding to nothing. SYN: *cipher.* 2. The point from which the graduation of a scale commences.

On the centigrade and Réaumur scales the zero (0°) is the temperature of melting ice. On the Fahrenheit it is 32°. To obtain this fixed point the thermometer is immersed in melting ice, and when the mercury column ceases to fall, the level at which it remains is fixed as 0° on the C. and R. scales, and as 32° on the F. scale. SEE: *thermometer.*

z., absolute. The temperature at which all atoms and molecules cease movement, or at which all gases liquify. Approx. 273.2° C. or 459.8° F.

z., limes. SYMB: Lo. The greatest amount of toxin which, when mixed with one unit of antitoxin and injected into a guinea pig weighing 250 gm., will cause no local edema.

zestocausis (zĕs"tō-kaw'sĭs) [G. *zestos,* boiling hot, + *kausis,* a burning]. Cauterization with a tube containing heated steam.

Ziehl-Neelsen method. One for staining *Mycobacterium tuberculosis.*

zinc (zĭnk) [L. *zincum*]. A bluish-white, crystalline, metallic element. SYMB: Zn. At. wt. 65.37; at. no. 30. Sp. gr. 7.14. It boils at 906° C. It is found as a carbonate and silicate, known as *calamine,* and as a sulfide (blende).

z. ac'etate. USP. White, pearly crystals.

ACTION AND USES: Astringent and antiseptic. Used chiefly in eye solutions, in 1/10 to 5/10%.

z. chlo'ride. USP. White granular powder.

ACTION AND USES: Antiseptic, astringent, and escharotic.

z. ointment. An ointment consisting of 20% of zinc oxide mixed with petrolatum and white ointment, used in treating skin diseases.

z. ox'ide. USP. Very fine white powder.

ACTION AND USES: Slightly antiseptic and astringent. Used chiefly in the form of ointment, 20%.

z. salts. A bluish-white metal used to make various containers and also to "galvanize" iron to prevent rust. The most commonly used compounds are zinc oxide as a pigment for paints, in ointments, and in chloride and sulfate which resemble Epsom salts and have thus been accidentally administered. The salts are used also as a wood preservative, in soldering, and in medicine to neutralize tissue, and in dilute solutions as an astringent and emetic.

POISONING: SYM: Metallic taste with prompt burning of mouth, throat, esophagus, and stomach; violent vomiting, often bloody; increased salivation; painful diarrhea, and coma. If patient recovers, nervous complications are frequent.

F. A. TREATMENT: Wash out stomach and treat as for sulfuric acid.

z. stearate. USP. Very fine, smooth powder.

USES: A nonirritating antiseptic and astringent for burns, scalds, abrasions.

z. sul'fate. USP. White, transparent crystals.

ACTION AND USES: Externally, astringent and styptic. Internally, as an emetic.

Zinn's ligament (zĭn). Connective tissue giving attachment to the rectus muscles of the eyeball.

Z., zonule of. Suspensory ligament of lens of the eye. SYN: *zonula ciliaris.*

zirconium (zĭr-kō'nĭ-ŭm). A metallic element found only in combination. SYMB: Zr. At. wt. 91.22; at. no. 40.

Zn. Chemical symb. for *zinc.*

zoanthropy (zō-ăn'thrō-pĭ) [G. *zōon,* animal, + *anthropos,* man]. Delusion that one is an animal.

zoetic (zō-ĕt'ĭk) [G. *zōē,* life]. Pert. to life. SYN: *vital.*

zona (zō'nă) [L. *zona,* a girdle]. 1. A band or girdle. 2. An acute inflammatory disease, characterized by groups of small vesicles mounted on inflammatory bases, associated with neuralgic pain and following the distribution of certain nerve trunks. SYN: *herpes zoster.*

z. ciliaris. Ciliary processes taken together. SYN: *corona ciliaris.*

z. facia'lis. Herpes zoster of the face.

z. pellucida. Inner, thick, solid, membranous envelope of the ovum. It is pierced by many radiating canals, giving it a striated appearance.

z. radiata. SEE: *zona pellucida.*

zonal (zō'năl) [L. *zona*, girdle]. Pert. to a zone.

zonary (zō'nar-ĭ) [L. *zona*, a girdle]. Pert. to or shaped like a zone.

z. placenta. One arranged in the form of a broad ring around the chorion.

Zondek-Aschheim test (zŏn'dĕk ahsh'hīm). A test for pregnancy. SEE: *test, Aschheim-Zondek.*

zone (zōn) [L. *zona*, a girdle]. A small zone or belt.

z's., erotogenic. Areas of the body which when stimulated produce erotic desires. These areas include the *breasts, lips, genital* and *anal regions,* the *buttocks,* and sometimes the special senses which excite the libido, such as the smell of certain perfumes.

zonesthesia (zōn-ĕs-thē'zĭ-ă) [G. *zōnē*, girdle, + *aisthēsis*, sensation]. A sensation, as of a cord constricting the body. SYN: *cincture sensation.*

zonifugal (zō-nĭf'ū-găl) [L. *zona*, a band, + *fugere*, to flee]. Passing outward from within any zone or area.

zoning (zō'nĭng) [L. *zona*, a band]. The occurrence of a stronger fixation of complement in a lesser amount of suspected serum; a phenomenon occasionally observed in diagnosing syphilis by complement fixation method.

zonipetal (zō-nĭp'ĕt-ăl) [L. *zona*, a band, + *petere*, to seek]. Passing from without into a zone or area of the body.

zonula (zōn'ū-lă) [L. *zonula*, a tiny zone]. A small zone. SYN: *zonule.*

z. ciliaris. NA. Suspensory ligament of the crystalline lens.

zonular (zōn'ū-lar) [L. *zonula*, a tiny band]. Pert. to a zonula.

z. cataract. One with opacity limited to certain layers of the lens.

z. fibers. Interlacing ones of the zonula ciliaris.

z. spaces. Those bet. fibers of ligament of the lens.

zonule (zōn'ūl) [L. *zonula*, a tiny band]. A small band or area. SYN: *zonula.*

z. of Zinn. Suspensory ligament of the crystalline lens. SYN: *zonula ciliaris.*

zonulitis (zōn-ū-lī'tĭs) [" + G. *-itis*, inflammation]. Inflammation of Zinn's zonule.

zoodermic (zō"ō-der'mik) [G. *zōon*, animal, + *derma*, skin]. Performed with the skin of an animal, said of a method of skin grafting.

zoogenous (zō-ŏj'ĕn-ŭs) [" + *gennan*, to produce]. Derived or acquired from animals.

zooglea (zō"ō-glē'ă) [" + *gloios*, sticky]. A stage in development of certain organisms in which colonies of microbes are embedded in a gelatinous matrix.

zoograft (zō'ō-grăft) [G. *zōon*, animal, + L. *graphium*, a grafting knife]. A graft of tissue obtained from an animal.

zoografting (zō"ō-grăft'ĭng) [" + L. *graphium*, a grafting knife]. Use of animal tissue in grafting on a human body.

zooid (zō'oyd) [" + *eidos*, resemblance]. 1. Resembling an animal. 2. A form resembling an animal; an organism produced by fission. 3. An animal cell which can move or exist independently.

zoolagnia (zo"o-lag'nĭ-ă) [" + G. *lagein*, lust]. Sexual desire for animals.

zoologist (zō-ŏl'ō-jĭst). A person who specializes in the study of animal life.

zoology (zō-ŏl'ō-jĭ) [" + *logos*, a study]. The science of animal life.

zoomania (zo"o-ma'nĭ-ă) [" + G. *mania*, madness]. A morbid and excessive affection for animals.

zoonoses (zo-o-no'sēz). Diseases communicable from animals to man under natural conditions.

zooparasite (zō"ō-par'ă-sīt) [" + *parasitos*, parasite]. An animal parasite.

zoopathology (zō"ō-păth-ŏl'ō-jĭ) [G. *zōon*, animal, + *pathos*, disease, + *logos*, a study]. Science of the diseases of animals.

zoophagous (zō-ŏf'ăg-ŭs) [" + *phagein*, to eat]. Living upon animal food.

zoophilism (zō-ŏf'ĭl-ĭzm) [" + *philein*, to love, + *-ismos*, condition]. Abnormal love of animals.

zoophobia (zō"o-fō'bĭ-ă) [" + *phobos*, fear]. Abnormal fear of animals.

zoophyte (zō'ō-fīt) [" + *phyton*, plant]. A plantlike animal; any of numerous invertebrate animals resembling plants in appearance or mode of growth.

zooplasty (zō'ō-plăs-tĭ) [" + *plassein*, to form]. Transplantation of animal tissue to man.

zoopsia (zo-op'sĭ-ă) [" + G. *opsis*, vision]. Hallucinations involving animals.

zoosmosis (zō"ŏz-mō'sĭs) [" + *ōsmos*, impulsion]. Process of passage of living protoplasm into the tissues from blood vessels.

zoospore (zō'ō-spōr) [" + *sporos*, seed]. Any spore moving by means of flagella.

zootoxin (zō"ō-tŏks'ĭn) [" + *toxikon*, poison]. Any toxin or poison produced by an animal, as *snake venom.*

zoster (zŏs'ter) [G. *zōstēr*, girdle]. Acute inflammatory disease with vesicles grouped in the course of cutaneous nerves. SYN: *herpes zoster, zona.*

z. auricula'ris. Herpes zoster of the ear.

z. ophthal'micus. Herpes affecting the ophthalmic nerve.

zosteriform (zŏs-ter'ĭ-form) [" + L. *forma*, shape]. Resembling herpes zoster. SYN: *zosteroid.*

zosteroid (zŏs'ter-oyd) [" + *eidos*, form]. Resembling herpes zoster. SYN: *zosteriform.*

Z-plasty. A technique used in plastic surgery to relieve tension or scar tissue.

Zr. Chemical symbol for *zirconium.*

zweiback (swī'băk). A kind of bread, baked, then sliced and toasted. SERVING: 100 gm. Calories: 423. Other values: 10.7 gm. protein; 8,8 gm. fat; 74.3 gm. carbohydrate; 40 I.U. vitamin A.

zygapophysis (zī-găp-ŏf'ĭs-ĭs) [" + *apo*, from, + *physis*, growth]. One of the articular processes of the neural arch of a vertebra.

zygion (zĭj'ĭ-ŏn) [G. *zygon*, yoke]. Craniometrical point on the zygoma at either end of bizygomatic diameter.

zygodactyly (zī"gō-dăk'tĭl-ĭ) [" + *daktylos*, digit]. Fusion of 2 or more fingers or toes. SYN: *syndactylism.*

zygoma (zī-gō'mă) [G. *zygōma*, cheekbone]. 1. The long arch that joins zygomatic processes of the temporal and malar bones on the sides of the skull. SYN: *arcus zygomaticus* [NA]. 2. The malar bone. SYN: *os zygomaticum* [NA].

zygomatic (zī"gō-măt'ĭk) [G. *zygōma*, cheekbone]. Pert. to the zygoma.

z. arch. The formation on each side of the cheeks of the zygomatic process of each malar bone articulating with the zygomatic process of the temporal bone. SYN: *arcus zygomaticus* [NA].

z. bone. Bone on either side of the face below the eye. SYN: *malar bone; os zygomaticum* [NA].

z. process. 1. A thin projection from the temporal bone bounding its squamous portion. 2. A part of the malar bone helping to form the zygoma.

z. reflex. Movement of lower jaw toward percussed side when zygoma is percussed.

zygomaticoauricularis (zī"gō-măt"ĭk-ō-awrĭk"ū-lā'rĭs) [L.]. Muscle which draws the pinna of the ear forward. SEE: *Table of Muscles in Appendix.*

zygomaticum (zī"gō-măt'ĭk-ŭm) [L.]. The zygomatic bone.

zygomaticus (zī-gō-mat'ĭk-ŭs) [L.]. A muscle which draws the upper lip upward and outward. SEE: *Table of Muscles in Appendix.*

zygomaxillary (zī"gō-măks'ĭl-ar-ī) [G. *zygoma,* cheekbone, + L. *maxilla,* jaw] Pert. to the cheekbone and upper jaw.

z. point. A craniometrical point marked at the lower end of the zygomatic suture.

zygote (zī'gōt) [G. *zygōtos,* yoked]. Cell produced by union of two gametes. The fertilized ovum. SYN: *zygocyte.*

zymase (zī'mās) [G. *zymē,* leaven, + *ase,* enzyme]. Any of a group of enzymes* which, in the presence of oxygen, convert certain carbohydrates into carbon dioxide and water or, in absence of oxygen, into alcohol and carbon dioxide or lactic acid.

They are found in yeast, bacteria, and higher plants and animals. SEE: *ferment.*

zyme (zīm) [G. *zymē,* leaven]. A ferment; a disease-producing ferment, as the morbific principle of a zymotic disease.

zymogen (zī'mō-jĕn) [" + *gennan,* to produce]. A substance that develops into a chemical ferment or enzyme. It exists in an inactive form antecedent to the active enzyme. SYN: *proenzyme.* SEE: *pepsinogen, trypsinogen.*

zymogene (zī'mō-gēn) [" + *gennan,* to produce]. Microbe causing fermentation.

zymogenic (zī-mō-jĕn'ĭk) [" + *gennan,* to produce]. 1. Causing a fermentation. 2. Pert. to or producing a zymogen.

zymohydrolysis (zī"mō-hī-drŏl'ĭ-sĭs) [" + *hydōr,* water, + *lysis,* dissolution]. Decomposition brought about by a ferment. SYN: *zymosis, q.v.*

zymologic (zī-mō-lŏj'ĭk) [G. *zymē,* leaven, + *logos,* a study]. Relating to zymology.

zymologist (zī-mŏl'ō-jĭst) [" + *logos,* a study]. One who specializes in study of ferments.

zymology (zī-mŏl'ō-jī) [" + *logos,* a study]. The science of fermentation.

zymolysis (zī-mŏl'ĭ-sĭs) [" + *lysis,* a dissolution]. Changes produced by an enzyme; action of enzymes. SYN: *fermentation, zymosis, q.v.*

zymolyte (zī'mō-līt) [" + *lysis,* dissolution]. Substance upon which a ferment acts. SYN: *substrate.*

zymolytic (zī-mō-lĭt'ĭk) [" + *lytikos,* dissolved]. Causing fermentation; fermentative.

zymometer (zī-mŏm'et-er) [G. *zymē,* leaven, + *metron,* a measure]. Device for measuring fermentation. SYN: *zymosimeter.*

Zymonema (zī-mō-nē'mă) [" + *nēma,* thread]. A genus of fungi.

zymonematosis (zī"mō-nē-măt-ō'sĭs) [" + " + *-ōsis,* condition]. Infestation with Zymonema.

zymophore (zī'mō-fōr) [" + *phoros,* a bearer]. Noting the atomic group bearing the ferment.

zymophoric, zymophorous (zī-mō-for'ĭk, -mŏf'or-ŭs) [" + *phoros,* bearing]. Having fermentative properties.

zymophyte (zī'mō-fīt) [" + *phyton,* growth]. A microorganism causing fermentation.

zymoplastic (zī-mō-plăs'tĭk) [G. *zymē,* leaven, + *plassein,* to form]. Producing a ferment.

zymoscope (zī'mō-skōp) [" + *skopein,* to examine]. Device for determining zymotic power of yeast.

zymose (zī'mōs) [" + *ose,* sugar]. An enzyme that changes a disaccharide into a monosaccharide, such as cane sugar into invert sugar. SYN: *invertin.*

zymosimeter (zī-mōs-ĭm'ĕt-ĕr) [" + *metron,* a measure]. Device for determining amount of fermentation.

zymosis (zī-mō'sĭs) [G. *zymōsis,* fermentation]. 1. Fermentation. 2. Process by which an infectious disease is supposed to develop. 3. An infectious disease.

z. gas'trica. Organic acid in the stomach.

zymosthenic (zī-mōs-thĕn'ĭk) [G. *zymē,* leaven, + *sthenos,* strength]. Increasing the power and activity of an enzyme.

zymotic (zī-mŏt'ĭk) [G. *zymē,* leaven], Relating to or produced by fermentation.

Z., Z.', Z." Symbol for increasing strengths of contraction.

Notes

Appendix

Index to Appendix

Units of Measurement

Metric System

WEIGHTS

Scale	Table		Grams		Grains
Kilo	1 Kilogram	=	1,000.	=	15,432.35
Hecto	1 Hectogram	=	100.	=	1,543.23
Deca	1 Decagram	=	10.	=	154.323
Unit	1 Gram	=	1.	=	15.432
Deci	1 Decigram	=	.1	=	1.5432
Centi	1 Centigram	=	.01	=	.15432
Milli	1 Milligram	=	.001	=	.01543

Arabic numbers are used with weights and measures, as 10 Gm., or 3 ml., etc. Portions of weights and measures are usually expressed decimally. Grams should always be abbreviated with a capital initial, as Gm. A drop (gtt) of water is sometimes considered equivalent to a minim (m) but this is inaccurate.

CONVERSION TABLES FOR MEASURES MOST COMMONLY USED IN THE UNITED STATES*

Lengths	Cm.	Inches	Feet	Yards	Meters
1 centimeter	1.000	0.394	0.0328	0.01094	0.0100
1 inch	2.54	1.000	0.0833	0.0278	0.0254
1 foot	30.48	12.00	1.000	0.333	0.305
1 yard	91.4	36.00	3.000	1.000	0.914
1 meter	100.0	39.4	3.28	1.094	1.000
1 kilometer	100000.	39400.	3280.	1094.	1000.
1 mile	160903.	63360.	5280.	1760.	1609.

Volumes	Cc.	Fl. drams	Cu. in.	Fl. oz.	Quarts	Liters
1 cubic centimeter	1.000	0.270	0.0610	0.0338	0.001057	0.001000
1 fluid dram	3.70	1.000	0.226	0.1250	0.00391	0.00370
1 cubic inch	16.39	4.43	1.000	0.554	0.0173	0.01639
1 fluid ounce	29.6	8.00	1.804	1.000	0.03125	0.0296
1 quart	946.	255.	57.75	32.0	1.000	0.946
1 liter	1000.	270.	61.0	33.8	1.056	1.000

Weights	Gr.	Gm.	Ap. oz.	Lb.	Kilos
1 grain (gr.)	1.000	0.0648	0.00208	0.0001429	0.0000648
1 gram (Gm.)	15.43	1.000	0.03215	0.002205	0.001000
1 apothecary ounce	480.	31.1	1.000	0.06855	0.0311
1 avoirdupois pound	7000.	454.	14.58	1.000	0.454
1 kilogram	15432.	1000.	32.15	2.205	1.000

* RULES FOR CONVERTING ONE SYSTEM TO ANOTHER:

To Convert Grains, Drams, and Ounces into Grams or ml.:

Divide the number of grains by 15.
Multiply the number of drams by 4.
Multiply the number of ounces by 30.
The result = the number of grams or cc.

To Convert from the Metric System

Milligrams to grains: Multiply by 0.0154.
Grams to grains: Multiply by 15.
Grams to drams: Multiply by 0.257;
Grams to ounces: Multiply by 0.0311.

To Convert into Metric Fluid Measures

Minims to cubic millimeters: Multiply by 63.
Minims to cubic centimeters: Multiply by 0.06.

To Convert Metric Fluid Measures

Cubic millimeters to minims: Divide by 63 (or multiply by 0.016).
Cubic centimeters to minims: Multiply by 16.
Cubic centimeters to fluid ounces: Divide by 30 (or multiply by 0.033).
Liters to pints (U.S.): Multiply by 2.1.
Liters to pints (Imperial): Multiply by 1.76.

To Convert Centigrade Degrees to Fahrenheit Degrees

Multiply the number of centigrade degrees by 9/5 and add 32 to the result.
Example: 55°C. × 9/5 = 99 + 32 = 131° F.

To convert Fahrenheit degrees to centigrade degrees: Subtract 32 from the number of Fahrenheit degrees and multiply the difference by 5/9.
Example: 243° F. − 32 = 211 × 5/9 = 117.2° C.

Note: For practical purposes one cubic centimeter is equivalent to one milliliter. Technically one cc. is equal to 0.999972 ml.

TABLES OF DATA

Arabic numbers are used with weights and measures, as 10 Gm., or 3 ml., etc. Portions of weights and measures are usually expressed decimally. Grams should always be abbreviated with a capital initial, as Gm. A drop (gtt) of water is sometimes considered equivalent to a minim (m) but this is inaccurate.

UNITS OF LENGTH

Millimeters	Centimeters	Inches	Feet	Yards	Meters
1 mm. = 1.00	0.100	0.0394	0.00328	0.0011	0.0010
1 cm. = 10.0	1.00	0.394	0.0328	0.0109	0.0100
1 in. = 25.4	2.54	1.00	0.0833	0.0278	0.0254
1 ft. = 304.8	30.48	12.00	1.00	0.333	0.305
1 yd. = 914.	91.4	36.0	3.00	1.000	0.914
1 m. = 1000.	100.	39.4	3.28	1.094	1.00

1 μ = 1 mu = 1 micron = 0.001 millimeter. One mm. = 1000 μ.
1 km. = 1 kilometer = 1000 meters = 0.6215 mile.
1 mile = 5280 feet = 1.609 kilometers.

UNITS OF VOLUME

Cubic Centimeters*	Fluid Drams	Cubic Inches	Fluid Ounces	Quarts	Liters
1 cc. = 1.00	0.270	0.0610	0.0338	0.00106	0.00100
1 fl. ʒ = 3.70	1.000	0.226	0.1250	0.00391	0.00370
1 cu. in. = 16.39	4.43	1.000	0.554	0.0173	0.01639
1 fl. ℥ = 29.6	8.00	1.804	1.000	0.03125	0.0296
1 qt. = 946.	255.	57.75	32.00	1.000	0.946
1 L. = 1000.	270.	61.0	33.8	1.056	1.000

*See footnote, Appendix 4.
1 cubic millimeter = 0.001 cubic centimeter; 1 cc. = 1000 cu. mm.
1 gallon = 4 quarts = 8 pints = 3.78 liters.
1 pint = 473 ml.

UNITS OF WEIGHT

Grains	Grams	Apothecary Ounces	Pounds Avoirdupois	Kilograms
1 gr. = 1.000	0.0648	0.00208	0.0001429	0.000065
1 Gm. = 15.43	1.000	0.03215	0.002205	0.001000
1 ℥ = 480.	31.1	1.000	0.06855	0.0311
1 lb. = 7000.	454.	14.58	1.000	0.454
1 Kg. = 15432.	1000.	32.15	2.205	1.000

1 γ = 1 gamma = 1 microgram = 0.001 milligram; 1000 γ = 1 mg.
1 mg. = 1 milligram = 0.001 Gm.; 1000 mg. = 1 Gm.
1 grain = 64.8 mg.; 1 mg. = 0.0154 grain.

Weights and Measures

APOTHECARIES' WEIGHT

20 grains = 1 scruple
3 scruples = 1 dram
8 drams = 1 ounce
12 ounces = 1 pound

The ounce and pound in this are the same as in Troy Weight.

For abbreviations and symbols of these weights, see Appendix 12 through 15.

AVOIRDUPOIS WEIGHT

27$^{11}/_{32}$ grains = 1 dram
16 drams = 1 ounce
16 ounces = 1 pound
100 pounds = 1 cwt.
2000 pounds = 1 short ton
2240 pounds = 1 long ton
1 oz. Troy = 480 gr.
1 oz. Avoirdupois = 437½ grains
1 lb. Troy = 5760 grains
1 lb. Avoirdupois = 7000 grains

CIRCULAR MEASURE

60 seconds = 1 minute
60 minutes = 1 degree
90 degrees = 1 quadrant
4 quadrants = 360 degrees = circle

CUBIC MEASURE

1728 cubic inches = 1 cubic foot
27 cubic feet = 1 cubic yard
2150.42 cubic inches = 1 standard bushel
268.8 cubic inches = 1 dry (U.S.) gallon
1 cubic foot = about four-fifths of a bushel
128 cubic feet = 1 cord (wood)
40 cubic feet = 1 ton

DRY MEASURE

2 pints = 1 quart
8 quarts = 1 peck
4 pecks = 1 bushel

LIQUID MEASURE

4 gills = 1 pint
2 pints = 1 quart
4 quarts = 1 gallon
31½ gallons = 1 barrel
2 barrels = 1 hogshead

Barrels and hogsheads vary in size.

NOTE: A gallon (U.S.) is equal to 0.8327 British gallon. Therefore a British gallon is equal to 1.201 U.S. gallons.

LINEAR MEASURE

12 inches = 1 foot
3 feet = 1 yard
5½ yards = 1 rod
40 rods = 1 furlong
8 furlongs = 1 stat. mile
3 miles = 1 league

TROY WEIGHT

24 grains = 1 pwt.
20 pwts. = 1 ounce
12 ounces = 1 pound

Used for weighing gold, silver, and jewels.

MEASURES AND WEIGHTS EQUIVALENTS

General Measures: Approximate Equivalents: 60 gtt. = 1 teaspoonful. = 4 cc. or ml. = 60 minims = 60 grains. = 1 dram. = 1/8 ounce.

RS: avoirdupois m., apothecaries m., bushel, metric m., Troy weight, unit of measures.

HOUSEHOLD MEASURES AND WEIGHTS

	Equivalents
1 teaspoon*	1/8 fl. oz.; 1 dram
4 teaspoons	1 tablespoon
1 tablespoon	1/2 fl. oz.; 4 drams
16 tablespoons (liquid)	1 cup
12 tablespoons (dry)	1 cup
1 cup (ordinary)	8 fl. oz.
1 tumbler or glass	8 fl. oz.; 1/2 pint
16 fl. oz.	1 lb.
1 pint	1 lb.

*In this table, one teaspoonful will be assumed to be given as above. Some household teaspoons will hold 5 ml. of liquid substances.

ARTICLES

	Amount	Equivalents
Butter	1 pint, packed	1 lb.
	2 cups, packed	1 lb.
	1 tablespoon	1/2 oz.
Chocolate	1 square, baking	1 oz.
Coffee	4 1/3 cups	1 lb.
Cornmeal	2 2/3 cups	1 lb.
Eggs	9 large	1 lb.
Flour	1 quart	1 lb.
	4 cups	1 lb.; 1 qt.
	4 tablespoons	1 oz.
	Graham, 4 1/2 cups	1 lb.
	entire wheat, 3 7/8 cups	1 lb.
	pastry, 4 cups	1 lb.
Meat	2 cups, fine chopped	1 lb.
Oatmeal	2 2/3 cups	1 lb.
Oats	4 3/4 cups, rolled	1 lb.
Rice	1 7/8 cups	1 lb.
Rye	4 1/3 cups, meal	1 lb.
Sugar	brown, 2 2/3 cups	1 lb.
	confectioner's, 3 1/2 cups	1 lb.
	granulated, 2 cups	1 lb.
	powdered, 2 2/3 cups	1 lb.
Water	1 pint	1 lb.
	1 cup	8 oz.

Miscellaneous

UNITS OF TIME

1 millisecond = one thousandth (0.001) of a second

1 second = 1/60 of a minute

1 minute = 1/60 of an hour

1 hour = 1/24 of a day

UNITS OF TEMPERATURE

Given a temperature on the Fahrenheit scale; to convert it to Centigrade, subtract 32 and multiply by 5/9 Given a temperature on the Centigrade scale :to convert it to Fahrenheit, multiply by 9/5 and add 32.

UNITS OF ENERGY

1 gram/centimeter = 980.665 dynes/centimeter

1 foot-pound = 13,600,000 ergs = 13,825.5 gram-centimeters.

1 Calorie = 4.26649 × 10^7 gram-centimeters = 3085.46 foot-pounds

1 Calorie, *kg.* = 1 calorie, *gm.*

A large Calorie, or *kilocalorie*, is always written with a capital C.

TABLE OF pH

In trying to understand the following pH table, one need not be concerned about the intricate mathematical *theory* implied in the symbol "pH." If one concerns oneself with the *facts* one will find them simple and satisfying. One need only imagine oneself confronted with three beakers containing (*a*) a weakly acid solution, (*b*) pure water, (*c*) a weakly alkaline solution. If one is given a fourth, unknown, solution and tests it with litmus paper, phenolphthalein, and other indicators, one finds it possible to place the unknown in one of four places in the series, thus:

(1)	Un	Ac		W	—	Al	
(2)		Ac	Un	W	—	Al	
(3)		Ac	—	W	Un	Al	
(4)		Ac	—	W	—	Al	Un

Its position will depend on whether it is (1) strongly acid, (2) weakly acid, (3) weakly alkaline, or (4) strongly alkaline.

The pH scale is simply a series of numbers by which one states where a given solution would stand in a series of solutions arranged according to acidity or alkalinity. At one extreme (i.e., high pH) lies an alkaline solution made by dissolving 4 Gm. of sodium hydroxide in water to make a liter of solution; at the other is a solution containing 3.65 Gm. of hydrogen chloride per liter. Half-way between lies pure water, which is neutral. All other solutions can be arranged on this scale, and their acidity or alkalinity can be stated by giving the numbers that indicate their relative positions.

Tenth-normal HCl	1.00	Litmus is red in this range.
Gastric juice	*1.4	
Urine	*6.0	
Water	7.00	
Blood	7.45	Litmus is blue in this range.
Bile	7.5	
Pancreatic juice	8.5	
Tenth-normal NaOH	13.00	

Thus if one is told that the pH of a certain solution is 5.3, one can tell at once that it falls between gastric juice and urine on the above scale, is moderately acid, and will turn litmus red. The body fluids marked by asterisks above vary rather widely in pH, and typical figures have been used for the sake of definiteness. Urine samples obtained from normal people may have pH's anywhere between 4.7 and 8.0.

PREPARATION OF PERCENTAGE SOLUTIONS

When the metric system is used the preparation of percentage solutions is simple: a 1 per cent solution contains 1 Gm. in 100 ml.; a 0.1 per cent solution contains 0.1 Gm. (or 100 milligrams) per 100 ml.

When the apothecaries' system is used the following are helpful:

4.55 grains to the ounce, or 2.5 drams to 32 ounces; or 3.25 drams to 40 ounces, all make a 1 per cent solution.

To Prepare a Dilute Solution From One Which Is Stronger:

For example, to make 80 per cent alcohol from 95 per cent: Dilute 80 cc. of the 95 per cent alcohol to 95 cc. with distilled water.

Rule: Dilute a volume equal to the per cent desired to a volume equal to the per cent used.

See: *Dosage*, page D-43.

Table of Physical Constants of the Elements

Element*	Symbol	Valence	Atomic Number	Atomic Weight†	Density (g/ml)	Melting Point °C	Boiling Point °C
Actinium	Ac	3	89	(227)		1050.0	
Aluminum	Al	3	13	26.9815	2.70	660.0	2450.0
Americium	Am	3, 4, 5, 6	95	(243)	11.7		
Antimony	Sb	3, 5	51	121.75	6.62	630.5	1380.0
Argon	Ar	0	18	39.948	1.40	−189.4	−185.8
Arsenic	As	3, 5	33	74.9216	5.72	817.0	613.0‡
Astatine	At	1, 3, 5, 7	85	(210)		(302)	
Barium	Ba	2	56	137.34	3.5	714.0	1640.0
Berkelium	Bk	3, 4	97	(247)			
Beryllium	Be	2	4	9.0122	1.85	1277.0	2770.0
Bismuth	Bi	3, 5	83	208.980	9.8	271.3	1560.0
Boron	B	3	5	10.811	2.34	(2030)	
Bromine	Br	1, 3, 5, 7	35	79.904	3.12	−7.2	58.0
Cadmium	Cd	2	48	112.40	8.65	320.9	765.0
Calcium	Ca	2	20	40.08	1.55	838.0	1440.0
Californium	Cf	3	98	(251)			
Carbon	C	2, 4	6	12.0115	2.26	3727.0‡	4830.0
Cerium	Ce	3, 4	58	140.12	6.67	795.0	3468.0
Cesium	Cs	1	55	132.905	1.90	28.7	690.0
Chlorine	Cl	1, 3, 5, 7	17	35.453	1.56	−101.0	−34.7
Chromium	Cr	2, 3, 6	24	51.996	7.19	1875.0	2665.0
Cobalt	Co	2, 3	27	58.9332	8.9	1495.0	2900.0
Columbium	SEE: *Niobium*						
Copper	Cu	1, 2	29	63.546	8.96	1083.0	2595.0
Curium	Cm	3	96	(247)			
Dysprosium	Dy	3	66	162.50	8.54	1407.0	2600.0
Einsteinium	Es		99	(254)			
Erbium	Er	3	68	167.26	9.05	1497.0	2900.0
Europium	Eu	2, 3	63	151.96	5.26	826.0	1439.0
Fermium	Fm		100	(253)			
Fluorine	F	1	9	18.9984	1.11	−219.6	−188.2
Francium	Fr	1	87	(223)		(27)	
Gadolinium	Gd	3	64	157.25	7.87	1312.0	3000.0
Gallium	Ga	2, 3	31	69.72	5.91	29.8	2237.0
Germanium	Ge	4	32	72.59	5.32	937.4	2830.0
Glucinum	SEE: *Beryllium*						
Gold	Au	1, 3	79	196.967	19.3	1063.0	2970.0
Hafnium	Hf	4	72	178.49	13.1	2222.0	5400.0
Helium	He	0	2	4.0026	0.126	−269.7	−268.9
Holmium	Ho	3	67	164.930	8.80	1461.0	2600.0
Hydrogen	H	1	1	1.00797	0.071	−259.2	−252.7
Indium	In	3	49	114.82	7.31	156.2	2000.0
Iodine	I	1, 3, 5, 7	53	126.904	4.94	113.7	183.0
Iridium	Ir	3, 4	77	192.2	22.5	2454.0	5300.0
Iron	Fe	2, 3	26	55.847	7.86	1536.0	3000.0
Krypton	Kr	0	36	83.80	2.6	−157.3	−152.0
Lanthanum	La	3	57	138.91	6.17	920.0	3470.0
Lawrencium	Lw		103	(257)			
Lead	Pb	2, 4	82	207.19	11.4	327.4	1725.0
Lithium	Li	1	3	6.939	0.53	108.5	1330.0
Lutecium	Lu	3	71	174.97	9.85	1652.0	3327.0
Magnesium	Mg	2	12	24.312	1.74	650.0	1107.0
Manganese	Mn	2, 3, 4, 6, 7	25	54.938	7.43	1245.0	2150.0
Mendelevium	Md		101	(256)			
Mercury	Hg	1, 2	80	200.59	13.6	−38.4	357.0
Molybdenum	Mo	3, 4, 6	42	95.94	10.2	2610.0	5560.0
Neodymium	Nd	3	60	144.24	7.00	1024.0	3027.0
Neon	Ne	0	10	20.183	1.20	−248.6	−246.0
Neptunium	Np	4, 5, 6	93	(237)	19.5	637.0	
Nickel	Ni	2, 3	28	58.71	8.9	1453.0	2730.0
Niobium	Nb	3, 5	41	92.906	8.4	2415.0	3300.0
Nitrogen	N	3, 5	7	14.0067	0.81	−210.0	−195.8
Nobelium	No		102	(254)			
Osmium	Os	2, 3, 4, 8	76	190.2	22.6	2700.0	5500.0
Oxygen	O	2	8	15.9994	1.14	−218.8	−183.0
Palladium	Pd	2, 4, 6	46	106.4	12.0	1552.0	3980.0

*The 103 chemical elements known at the present time are included in this table. Some of those recently discovered have been obtained only as unstable isotopes.

†Based on Carbon-12. Figures enclosed in parentheses represent the mass number of the most stable isotope.

‡Element sublimes unless under pressure.

Element*	Symbol	Valence	Atomic Number	Atomic Weight†	Density (g/ml)	Melting Point °C	Boiling Point °C
Phosphorus	P	3, 5	15	30.9738	1.82	44.2	280.0
Platinum	Pt	2, 4	78	195.09	21.4	1769.0	4530.0
Plutonium	Pu	3, 4, 5, 6	94	(242)		640.0	3235.0
Polonium	Po	2, 4	84	(209)	(9.2)	254.0	
Potassium	K	1	19	39.102	0.86	63.7	760.0
Praseodymium	Pr	3	59	140.907	6.67	935.0	3127.0
Promethium	Pm	3	61	(145)		(1027)	
Protactinium	Pa		91	(231)	15.4	(1230)	
Radium	Ra	2	88	(226)	5.0	700.0	
Radon	Rn	0	86	(222)		(−71)	(−61.8)
Rhenium	Re		75	186.2	21.0	3180.0	5900.0
Rhodium	Rh	3	45	102.905	12.4	1966.0	4500.0
Rubidium	Rb	1	37	85.47	1.53	38.9	688.0
Ruthenium	Ru	3, 4, 6, 8	44	101.07	12.2	2500.0	4900.0
Samarium	Sm	2, 3	62	150.35	7.54	1072.0	1900.0
Scandium	Sc	3	21	44.956	3.0	1539.0	2730.0
Selenium	Se	2, 4, 6	34	78.96	4.79	217.0	685.0
Silicon	Si	4	14	28.086	2.33	1410.0	2680.0
Silver	Ag	1	47	107.868	10.5	960.8	2210.0
Sodium	Na	1	11	22.9898	0.97	97.8	892.0
Strontium	Sr	2	38	87.62	2.6	768.0	1380.0
Sulfur	S	2, 4, 6	16	32.064	2.07	119.0	444.6
Tantalum	Ta	5	73	180.948	16.6	2996.0	5425.0
Technetium	Tc	6, 7	43	(97)	11.5	2200.0	
Tellurium	Te	2, 4, 6	52	127.60	6.24	449.5	989.8
Terbium	Tb	3	65	158.924	8.27	1356.0	2800.0
Thallium	Tl	1, 3	81	204.37	11.85	303.0	1457.0
Thorium	Th	4	90	232.038	11.7	1750.0	3850.0
Thulium	Tm	3	69	168.934	9.33	1545.0	1727.0
Tin	Sn	2, 4	50	118.69	7.30	231.9	2270.0
Titanium	Ti	3, 4	22	47.90	4.51	1668.0	3260.0
Tungsten	W	6	74	183.85	19.3	3410.0	5930.0
Uranium	U	4, 6	92	238.03	19.07	1132.0	3818.0
Vanadium	V	3, 5	23	50.942	6.1	1900.0	3450.0
Xenon	Xe	0	54	131.30	3.06	−111.9	−108.0
Ytterbium	Yb	2, 3	70	173.04	6.98	824.0	1427.0
Yttrium	Y	3	39	88.905	4.47	1509.0	3030.0
Zinc	Zn	2	30	65.37	7.14	419.5	906.0
Zirconium	Zr	4	40	91.22	6.49	1852.0	3580.0

*The 103 chemical elements known at the present time are included in this table. Some of those recently discovered have been obtained only as unstable isotopes.

†Based on Carbon-12. Figures enclosed in parentheses represent the mass number of the most stable isotope.

Physiological Standards, Average Normal

Blood

(Expressed per 100 ml. (cc.) of whole blood unless otherwise stated)

Albumin (serum)	4–5 gm.
Ammonia (blood)	40–70 micrograms
Amylase	4–25 Russell units
Ascorbic acid	0.4–1.5 mg.
Bilirubin, total (indirect)	0.3 mg.
Bleeding time	1–5 min.
Calcium, total (serum)	8.5–10.5 mg.
Carbon dioxide content (serum)	26–28 mEq./L.
Chlorides (as chloride) (serum)	100–106 mEq./L.
Cholesterol, total (serum)	150–280 mg.
Clotting time (Lee-White method)	Below 20 min. 4th tube
Creatinine	0.7–1.5 mg.
Fibrinogen (plasma)	0.15–0.30 gm.
Glucose, fasting level	100 mg.
Hematocrit	42–50 mm. (males) 40–48 mm. (females)
Hemoglobin	13–16 gm. (males) 12–14 gm. (females)
Iodine, protein bound (serum)	3.5–8.0 micrograms
Iron, inorganic (plasma)	50–150 micrograms
Lactic acid	6–16 mg.
Lipids, total fatty acids	190–420 mg.
Magnesium (serum)	1.5–2.5 mEq./L.
Oxygen partial pressure	75–100 mm. of mercury
pH (serum)	7.35–7.45
Phosphorus, inorganic (serum)	3.0–4.5 mg.
Platelets	200,000–350,000/cu.mm.
Potassium (serum)	3.5–5.0 mEq./L.
Red Blood cells (Erythrocytes)	4,000,000–5,000,000/cu.mm.
Diameter	5.5–8.8 microns
Reticulocytes	0.5–1.5% of red cells
Sodium (serum)	136–145 mEq./L.
Sulfates, inorganic (serum)	0.5–1.5 mg.
Urea nitrogen (BUN)	8–25 mg.
Uric acid	3–7 mg.
Water	78%
White blood cells (Leukocytes)	5000–10,000/cu.mm.
Neutrophils (segmented)	54–62%
Lymphocytes	25–33%
Monocytes	3–7%
Eosinophils	1–3%
Basophils	0–0.75%

Cerebrospinal Fluid

Character	Clear; colorless; no coagulum
Pressure	70–180 mm. of water
Specific gravity	1.006–1.008
Total protein (Lumbar)	15–45 mg./100 ml.
Glucose	50–75 mg./100 ml.
Nonprotein nitrogen	12–30 mg./100 ml.
Chlorides	120–130 mEq./L.
Cells	0–5 mononuclear cells/cu.mm.
Colloidal gold reaction	Negative

Symbols

℞. Minim.
℈. Scruple.
ʒ. Dram.
f ʒ. Fluid dram.
℥. Ounce.
f ℥. Fluid ounce.
O. Pint.
℔. Pound.
℞. Recipe; take.
M. Misce; mix.
āā, āa. Of each.
A, Å. Angstrom unit.
C′. Complement.
c̄, c. [*L. cum.*]. With
E_0. Electroaffinity.
F_1. First filial generation.
F_2. Second filial generation.
mμ. Millimicron, micromillimeter.
μg. Microgram.
mEq. Milliequivalent.
mg. Milligram.
mg.%. Milligrams per cent; milligrams per 100 ml.
Qo_2. Oxygen consumption.
m-. Meta-.
o-. Ortho-.
p-. Para-.
s̄s̄, ss. [*L. semis*]. One-half.
′. Foot; minute; primary accent; univalent.
″. Inch; second; secondary accent; bivalent.
μ. Micron.
μμ. Micromicron.
+. Plus; excess; acid reaction; positive.
—. Minus; deficiency; alkaline reaction; negative.
±. Plus or minus; either positive or negative; indefinite.
#. Number; following a number; pounds
÷. Divided by.
×. Multiplied by; magnification.
=. Equals.
>. Greater than; from which is derived
<. Less than; derived from.
√. Root; square root; radical.
$\sqrt[2]{}$. Square root.
$\sqrt[3]{}$. Cube root.
∞. Infinity.
:. Ratio; "is to."
::. Equality between ratios; "as."
•. Birth.
†. Death.
°. Degree.
%. Per cent.
π. 3.1416—ratio of circumference of a circle to its diameter.
□, ♂. Male.
○, ♀. Female.
⇌. Denotes a reversible reaction.

Abbreviations, Prefixes, Suffixes

and

Latin and Greek Nomenclature

Principal Medical Abbreviations

Abbreviation	Latin	English Definition
a or āā	ana (Greek)	of each
a. c.	ante cibos	before meals
ad.	ad	to; up to
ad lib.	ad libitum	as desired
alt. dieb.	alternis diebus	every other day
alt. hor.	alternis horis	every other hour
alt. noc.	alternis noctus	every other night
aq.	aqua	water
aq. com.	aqua communis	common water
aq. dest.	aqua destillata	distilled water
aq. tep.	aqua tepida	tepid water
arg.	argentum	silver
av.	(French)	avoirdupois
bib.	bibe	drink
b. i. d.	bis in die	twice a day
b. i. n.	bis in noctus	twice a night
c̄	cum	with
C.	Centrigradus	centigrade
C.	congius	gallon
cap.	capsula	capsule
cc.	(French)	cubic centimeter
cg.	(French)	centigram
cm.	(French)	centimeter
comp.	compositus	compound
cong.	congius	gallon
def.	defaecatio	defecation
Dil., dil.	dilue	dilute
dr.	drachma	dram or drams
elix.	(Arabic)	elixir
emp.	emplastrum	a plaster
et	et	and
ext.	extractum	extract
F.		Fahrenheit (proper name)
Fld.	fluidus	fluid
fl. dr.	fluidrachma	fluid dram
fl. oz.	fluidus uncia	fluid ounce
Ft., ft.	fiat	let there be made
Gm.; gm.	gramme (French)	gram
gr.	granum	grain
Gtt., gtt.	guttae	drops
H.	hora	hour
h.n.	hac nocte	tonight
hor. interm.	horis intermediis	at intermediate hours
h.s.	hora somni	at bedtime or hour of sleep
hypo	Greek: under	hypodermically
inf.	infusum	infusion
L.		liter
lb.	libra	pound
liq.	liquor	liquid; fluid
M.	(French)	meter
m.	minimum	minim
mEq.		milliequivalent
mg.		milligram
mist.	mistura	mixture
ml.		milliliter
mm.	(French)	millimeter
n.b.	nota bene	note well
no.	numero	number
non rep.	non repetatur	don't repeat
noxt.	nocte; noxte	at night
O.	octarius	pint
ol.	oleum	oil
omn. hor.	omni hora	every hour
omn. noct.	omni nocte	every night
os.	os; ora	mouth
oz.	uncia	ounce
p.c.	post cibum	after food; after meals
per.		through or by
pil.	pilula	pill
p.o.	per os	by mouth
p.r.n.	pro re nata	as needed; as desired
pt.	(French; pinte)	pint
pulv.	pulvis	powder
Q.h.	quaque hora	every hour
Q. 2h.		every two hours

Abbreviation	Latin	English Definition
Q. 3h.		every three hours
q.i.d.	quater in die	four times a day
Q.s.	quantum sufficiat	a sufficient quantity
qt.	quartina	quart
quotid.	quotidie	every day
Q.v.	quantum vis	as much as you will
℞	recipe	take
rep.	repatatur	let it be repeated
s	sans	without
S.	signa	mark
S.c.	sub cutis	subcutaneously
Sig.	signetur	let it be marked
Sol.	solutio	solution
solv.	solve	dissolve
s.o.s.	si opus sit	if occasion require, if necessary
spt.	spiritus	spirit
sp. gr.	gravitus-heavy	specific gravity
ss.	semis	half
stat.	statim	immediately
syr.	syrupus	syrup
T.	temperatura	temperature
tab.	tabella	tablet
t.i.d.	ter in die	three times a day
t.i.n.	ter in nocte	three times a night
tr., tinct.	tinctura	tincture
ung.	unguentum	ointment
Ur.	urina	urine
vin	vinum	wine
vol. %.		volume per cent
Wt.		weight
w/v.		weight by volume

SEE: *Symbols*, p. App. 12.

A Glossary of Latin Medical Words

NOTE: Latin words which have become a part of the general medical vocabulary are listed in alphabetical order in the text.

abacus, -ī. *m.* Shelf.
abdōminālis, -e. Abdominal.
abdūcēns, -ntis. Leading or drawing from (the median line); applied, also, to 6th pair of cranial nerves.
aberrāns, -ntis. Wandering.
abstractum, -ī. *n.* Abstract.
accessōrius, -a, -um. Accessory.
accidō, -ere, -cidī. Occur; happen.
ācer, ācris, ācre. Sharp; severe.
acervulus, -ī. *m.* (Lit., little heap), acervulus.
acētābulum, -ī. *n.* (Lit., vinegar cup), the bony, cuplike, cavity of the hip joint; acetabulum.
acētās, -ātis. *m.* Acetate.
acētum, -ī. *n.* Vinegar.
acidum, -ī. *n.* Acid.
acinus, -ī. *m.* A terminal compartment or secreting portion of a gland; acinus.
acusticus, -a, -um. Auditory.
acūtus, -a, -um. Acute.
adeps, adipis. *m.* and *f.* Fat; lard.
adjūtor, -ōris. *m.* Helper; assistant.
adjuvō, -āre, -jūvī, -jūtus. Aid; assist.
adsum, -esse, -fuī. Be present.
aeger, -gra, -grum. Sick.
aegrōtus, -a, -um. Sick.
āēr, āēris. *m.* Air.
aeternus, -a, -um. Eternal.
aether, -is. *m.* Ether.
āla, -ae. *f.* Wing.
ālāris, -e. Winglike; alar.
albicāns, -ntis. Whitening; white.
albūgineus, -a, -um. White.
albulus, -a, -um. Whitish.
albus, -a, -um. White.
alcoholicus, -a, -um. Alcoholic.
aliquandō. Sometimes.
alius, -a, -ud. Other.
aloina, -ae. *f.* Aloin.
alter, -tera, -terum. Other.
altus, -a, -um. High.
alūmen, -inis. *n.* Alum.
alvus, -ī. *f.* Belly, or its contents.
amārus, -a, -um. Bitter.
amīcus, -ī. *m.* Friend.
āmissiō, -ōnis. *f.* Loss.
āmissus, -ūs. *m.* Loss.
ammōnium, -ī. *n.* Ammonium
amygdala, -ae. *f.* Almond.
anaestheticus, -a, -um. Producing insensibility; anesthetic.
anastomoticus, -a, -um. Anastomosing.
ānellus, -ī. *m.* Ring.
angulus, -ī. *m.* Angle.
anima, -ae. *f.* Breath; life.
anīsum, -ī. *n.* Anise.
ānnulāris, -e. Ringlike; annular.
ānnulus, -ī. *m.* Ring.
anterius, -a, -um. Anterior.
anticus, -a, -um. Foremost.
antidōtum, -ī. *n.* Antidote.
antimōnium, -ī. *n.* Antimony.
antimōniālis, -e. Of antimony; antimonial.
antipyreticus, -a, -um. Reducing the temperature; antipyretic.
antisepticus, -a, -um. Destroying germ life; antiseptic.
antitrāgus, -ī. *m.* A conical eminence opposite the tragus, *q.v.;* antitragus.
antīquus, -a, -um. Ancient.
aperiēns, -ntis. Laying open; laxative: aperient.
appellō, -āre, -āvī, -ātus. Call.
aptē. Aptly.
apud. Near.
aqua, -ae. *f.* Water.
aqueductus, -ūs. *m.* A canal; aqueduct.
aquōsus, -a, -um. Watery.
arbor, -oris. *f.* Tree.
arceō, -ēre, -uī, -tus. Ward off.
arcuātus, -a, -um (arcus, a bow). Curved like a bow.
arcus, -ūs. *m.* A bow; arch.
āreola, -ae. *f.* Small area (especially around the nipple).
argentum, -ī. *n.* Silver.
arōmaticus, -a, -um. Aromatic.
arsenicum, -ī. *n.* Arsenic.
arsenis, -itis. *m.* Arsenite.
artēria, -ae. *f.* Artery.
articulāris, -e. Articular.
articulō, -āre, -āvī, -ātus. Articulate.
artus, -ūs. *m.* Joint.
ascendēns, -ntis. Ascending.
asepticus, -a, -um. Free from putrefactive matter; aseptic.
asper, -a, -um. Rough.
astrictus, -a, -um. Bound up.
astūtus, -a, -um. Shrewd; artful.
atropīna, -ae. *f.* Active principle of belladonna; atropine.
attollēns, -ntis. Raising up; elevating.
attrāhēns, -ntis. Drawing to or towards.
audītōrius, -a, -um. Auditory.
aurantium, -ī. *n.* Orange.
auricula, -ae. *f.* (dim., **auris**). Auricle.
auris, -is. *f.* Ear.
axis, -is. *m.* (Lit., that about which a body turns), 2nd cervical vertebra; axis.
azygos. (Gr.) Without a fellow.
balneum, -ī. *n.* Bath.
basīlāris, -e. Basilar.
basis, -is. *f.* Base.
bene. Well.
benignus, -a, -um. Mild; benign; not malignant.
berberis, -idis. *f.* Barberry.
bibō, -ere, bibī. Drink.
bicarbonās, -ātis. *m.* Bicarbonate.
biceps, -cipitis. Two-headed.
bifidus, -a, -um. Cleft.
biliaris, -e. Pert. to or conveying bile; biliary.
bīnī, -ae, -a. Two each.
bismuthum, -ī. *n.* Bismuth.
bitartrās, -ātis. *m.* Bitartrate.
bonus, -a, -um. Good.
borās, -ātis. *m.* Borate.
brachiālis, -e. Of the arm; brachial.
brāchium, -ī. *n.* Arm.
brevis, -e. Short.
brōmidum, -ī. *n.* Bromide.
būbula, -ae. *f.* Beef.
būccinātor, -ōris. *m.* The trumpeter muscle; buccinator.
bulbus, -ī. *m.* Bulb.
caecus, -a, -um. Blind.
calamus, -ī. *m.* Reed.
calcaneum, -ī. *n.* The heelbone (os calcis)
calcium, -ī. *n.* Calcium.
calidus, -a, -um. Hot.
callōsus, -a, -um. Hard, tough.
calor, -ōris. *m.* Heat.
calumba, -ae. *f.* Calumba.
calvārium, -ī. *n.* The skullcap.
calx, -cis. *f.* Lime.
calyx, -icis. *f.* Cup; calyx.
camphora, -ae. *f.* Camphor.
camphorātus, -a, -um. Camphorated.
canāliculus, -ī. *m.* Small duct or canal.

canālis, -is. *m.* Canal.
canīnus, -a, -um. Of a dog, canine.
canis, -is. *m.* and *f.* Dog.
cānitiēs, -ēī. *f.* A gray color, hoariness.
cannabis, -is. *f.* Hemp.
cantharis, -idis. *f.* Spanish fly.
canthus, -ī. *m.* The corner or angle of the eye.
capiō, -ere, cēpī, captus. Take.
capitulum, -ī. *n.* Dim. (caput), **a knob or** protuberance of bone received into a concavity of another bone.
capsicum, -ī. *n.* Cayenne pepper; capsicum.
capsula, -ae. *f.* A small box; capsule.
carbō, -ōnis. *m.* Carbon; coal; charcoal.
carbolicus, -a, -um. Carbolic.
carbonās, -ātis. *m.* Carbonate.
cardamōmum, -ī. *n.* Cardamom.
careō, -ēre, -uī, -itus. Need; want.
carneus, -a, -um. Fleshy.
carpus, -ī. *m.* Wrist.
cartilāginōsus, -a, -um. Cartilaginous.
cartilāgo, -inis. *f.* Cartilage.
caruncula, -ae. *f.* (Dim., **carō,** flesh), a little piece of flesh; caruncle.
cataplasma, -atis. *n.* Poultice; cataplasm.
catharticus, -a, -um. Cathartic.
cauda, -ae. *f.* Tail.
caudātus, -a, -um. Having a tail; caudate.
causa, -ae. *f.* Cause.
causō, -āre, -āvī, -ātus. Cause.
cavernōsus, -a, -um. Hollow; cavernous.
cavitās, -ātis. *f.* Cavity.
cavus, -a, -um. Hollow.
celeriter. Quickly.
centrālis, -e. Central.
centrum, -ī. *n.* Center.
cephalalgia, -ae. *f.* Headache.
cērātum, -ī. *n.* Waxed dressing; cerate.
cerātus, -a, -um. Waxed.
cerevisa, -ae. *f.* Beer.
certus, -a, -um. Sure; certain.
cēterus, -a, -um. Other.
charta, -ae. *f.* Medicated paper.
chartula, -ae. *f.* Small paper (powder).
chirāta, -ae. *f.* Chirata.
chīrurgia, -ae. *f.* Surgery.
chīrurgus, -ī. *m.* Surgeon.
chlōral. *n.* Chloral.
chlōrās, -ātis. *m.* Chlorate.
chlōridum, -ī. *n.* Chloride.
chlōrōformum, -ī. *n.* Chloroform.
choledochus, -ī. *m.* Holding or receiving bile.
chorda, -ae. *f.* Cord.
chronicus, -a, -um. Chronic.
chylum, -ī. *n.* Chyle.
cibus, -ī. *m.* Food.
cicātrōsus, -a, -um. Full of scars, scarred.
ciliāris, -e. Ciliary.
cinchōna, -ae. *f.* Cinchona.
cinchonīna, -ae. *f.* Cinchonine.
cinereus, -a, -um. Ash-colored.
cinnamōmum, -ī. *n.* Cinnamon.
circulāris, -e. Circular.
circulatiō, -ōnis. *f.* Circulation.
circulus, -ī. *m.* Circle.
circum. Around.
circumdō, -dare, -dedī, -datus. Surround.
citō. Promptly; quickly.
citrās, -ātis. *m.* Citrate.
clārus, -a, -um. Clear, distinguished.
claudus, -a, -um. Lame.
clāvus, -ī. *m.* A corn, usually on the toes.
cludō, -ere, -sī, -sus. Shut; close.
cochlea, -ae. *f.* (Lit., snail shell), spiral cavity of the internal ear; cochlea.
cochleāre, -is. *n.* Spoon.
codeina, -ae. *f.* An alkaloid of opium; codeine.
coeliacus -a, -um. Relating to the stomach; celiac.
colicus, -a, -um. Of or pert. to the colon.
collateriālis, -e. Collateral.
collum, -ī. *n.* Neck.
colocynthis, -idis. *f.* Colocynth.
color, -ōris. *m.* Color.
cōlum, -ī. *n.* Large intestine; colon.
columna, -ae. *f.* Column.
comes, -itis. *m.* Companion.
commissūra, -as. *f.* A joining; commissure.
communicāns, -ntis. Communicating.
commūnis, -e. Common.
compōnō, -ere, -posuī, -positus. Compound.
conarium, -ī. *n.* (From Gr. κῶνος, a cone), a synonym for the pineal gland; conarium.
concha, -ae. *f.* (Lit., a shell), hollow part of the external ear; concha.
confectiō, -ōnis. *f.* Confection.
conium, -ī. *n.* Poison hemlock; conium.
conīveō, -āre, -nīvī. Blink; half close.
conjectūra, -ae. *f.* Guess.
contineō, -ēre, -tinuī, -tentus. Contain.
contrāhō, -ere, -xī, -ctus. Draw together; contract.
contusiō, -ōnis. *f.* Bruise.
cōnus, -ūs. *m.* Cone.
convalescō, -ere, -valuī. Recover health.
cor, cordis. *n.* Heart.
cornicula, -ae. *f.* Dim. (**cornus**), little horn
cornu, -ūs. *n.* Horn; horn-shaped process.
corōna, -ae. *f.* Crown.
coronārius, -a, -um. Encircling like a crown; coronary.
corpus, -oris. *n.* Body.
corrōsīvus, -a, -um. Corrosive.
corrugātor, -ōris. *m.* A muscle which wrinkles; corrugator.
cortex, -icis. *m.* and *f.* Bark; rind; external layer; cortex.
costa, -ae. *f.* Rib.
craniālis, -e. Cranial.
crās. *adv.* Tomorrow.
crassus, -a, -um. Gross; large.
creasōtum, -ī. *n.* Creasote.
crēber, -bra, -brum. Frequent.
crēdō, -ere, -credidī, -creditus. Trust; believe.
crēta, -ae. *f.* Chalk.
cribriformis, -e. Sievelike; cribriform.
cribrōsus, -a, -um. Having holes like a sieve.
crista, -ae. *f.* Crest; comb of a cock (gallus).
crūrālis, -e. Of the leg; crural.
crūreus, -a, -um. Of the leg.
crūs, crūris. *n.* The leg.
crusta, -ae. *f.* Crust.
cubēba, -ae. *f.* Cubeb.
cubitum, -ī. *n.* Elbow.
cuboideus, -a, -um. Cubelike; cuboid.
cum. With.
cuneiformis, -e. Wedge-shaped; cuneiform
cūra, -ae. *f.* Care.
cūrō, -āre, -āvī, -ātus. Treat; cure.
cutis, -is. *f.* Skin.
decem. Ten.
deciduus, -a, -um. That falls off.
decoctum, -ī. *n.* Decoction.
deferēns, -ntis. Bearing away.
defessus, -a, -um. Tired; wearied.
deformāns, -ntis. Deforming.
deformitās, -ātis. *f.* Deformity.
demonstrō, -āre, -āvī, -ātus. Show; prove.
dēns, dentis. *m.* Tooth.
dentātus, -a, -um. Toothed; dentate.
depressor, -ōris. *m.* That which depresses; depressor.
descendēns, -ntis. Descending.
dexter, -tra, -trum. Right.
diabeticus, -a, -um. Diabetic (*subst.*, one having diabetes).
diabolus, -ī. *m.* Devil.
dīcō, -ere, -dixī, dictus. Say.
diēs, -ēī. *m.* Day.
difficilis, -e. Difficult.
digitus, -ī. *m.* Finger (**digitus pedis,** a toe).
dilātor, -ōris. *m.* That which dilates: dilator.

dilūtus, -a, -um. Dilute.
dimidius, -a, -um. Half.
discipulus, -ī. *m.* A learner; pupil; student.
diū. For a long time.
diureticus, -a, -um. Diuretic.
dividō, -ere, -vīsī, -vīsus. Divide.
dō, dare, dedī, datus. Give.
doctus, -a, -um. Learned.
dolōr, -ōris. *m.* Pain.
dolōrōsus, -a, -um. Painful.
domicilium, -ī. *n.* Abode.
dorsālis, -e. Of the back; dorsal.
dorsum, -ī. *n.* Back.
dosis, -is. *f.* Dose.
drachma, -ae. *f.* Dram.
ductus, -ūs. *m.* Duct.
dulcis, -e. Sweet.
duo, duae, du. Two.
dūrus, -a, -um. Hard.
dyspepticus, -a, -um. Dyspeptic (*subst.*, a dyspeptic).
edō, -ere, -ēdi, -ēsus. Eat.
efferēns, -ntis. Bearing out or away; efferent.
effervescēns, -ntis. Boiling up.
elegāns, -ntis. Elegant.
ēluviēs, -ēī. *f.* Discharge.
emeticus, -a, -um. Causing vomiting; emetic.
ēminentia, -ae. *f.* Eminence.
emō, -ere, -ēmī, emptus. Buy.
empiricus, -ī. *n.* Quack; empiric.
emplastrum, -ī. *n.* Plaster.
ensiformis, -e. Sword-shaped; ensiform.
eō, īre, īvī, itus. Go.
epilepsia, -ae. *f.* Epilepsy.
epiploicus, -a, -um. Relating to the epiploön (omentum).
equīnus, -a, -um. Of a horse; equine.
ergota, -ae. *f.* Ergot.
errō, -āre, -āvī, -ātus. Wander; err.
ērudītus, -a, -um. Learned; educated; erudite.
et. And.
et-et. Both-and.
ethmoidālis, -e. (ἠθμός, a sieve), ethmoid
etiam. Even.
euonymus, -ī. *m.* Wahoo; Euonymus.
eupatōrium, -ī. *n.* Boneset; eupatorium.
excessus, -ūs. *m.* Departure.
excīdō, -ere, -īdī, -īsus. Cut out; excise.
excitō, -āre, -āvī, -ātus. Excite.
expectatiō, -ōnis. *f.* Expectation.
experimentum, -ī. *n.* Experiment.
expressiō, -ōnis. *f.* Expression.
exsiccātus, -a, -um. Dried out.
exsudō, -āre, -āvī, -ātus. Sweat out; exude.
externus, -a, -um. External.
extractum, -ī. *n.* Extract.
faciēs, -ēī. *f.* Face; countenance.
faciō, -ere, fēcī, factus. Make.
falx, -cis. *f.* Sickle (a sickle-shaped process).
familia, -ae (or -as). *f.* Family.
fasciculus, -ī. *m.* A small bundle of fibers.
febrifuga, -ae. *f.* Agent that reduces fever; febrifuge.
febris, -is. *f.* Fever.
fēmina, -ae. *f.* Woman.
femorālis, -e. Of the thigh; femoral.
fenestra, -ae. *f.* Window; an opening in the wall of the tympanum.
ferē. Almost.
ferrum, -ī. *n.* Iron.
fibrilla, -ae. *f.* Filament; fibril.
fibrōsus, -a, -um. Fibrous.
fides, -eī. *f.* Faith; trustworthiness.
fīdus, -a, -um. Faithful; trustworthy.
filia, -ae. *f.* Daughter.
filius, -ī. *m.* Son.
filix, -icis. *f.* Fern.
fimbria, -ae. *f.* Fringe.
fimbriātus, -a, -um. Fringed; fimbriated.
finiō, -īre, -īvī, -ītus. End; finish.
fiō, fierī, factus. Be made.
fissūra, -ae. *f.* Cleft; fissure.
flavus, -a, -um. Yellow.
flexilis, -e. Flexible.
flōs, flōris. *m.* Flower.
fluidus, -a, -um. Fluid.
flūmen, -inis. *n.* River.
fluō, -ere, fluxī, fluxus. Flow.
fluor, -ōris. *m.* Flux; flow.
foetidus, -a, -um. Offensive; fetid.
folium, -ī. *n.* Leaf.
folliculus, -ī. *m.* A small secretory sac; follicle.
fons, -ntis. *m.* Fountain; spring.
formō, -āre, -āvī, -ātus. Form.
fornicātus, -a, -um. Arched.
fornix, -icis. *m.* Arch; vault; fornix.
fortis, -e. Strong; brave.
fossa, -ae. *f.* Ditch; depression; fossa.
fovea, -ae. *f.* Small pit; depression.
fractus, -a, -um. Broken.
fragilitās, -ātis. *f.* Brittleness.
frēnum, -ī. *n.* A bridle; a membranous fold; frenum.
frigidus, -a, -um. Cold.
fructus, -ūs. *m.* Fruit.
frumentum, -ī. *n.* Corn; grain.
frustum, -ī. *n.* Piece; bit.
functiō, -ōnis. *f.* Execution; normal action; function.
fuscus, -a, -um. Brown.
fūsiformis, -e. Spindle-shaped; fusiform.
gallus, -ī. *m.* Cock.
ganglioniformis, -e. Ganglionlike.
gelsemium, -ī. *n.* Gelsemium; yellow jasmine (root).
gemellus, -a, -um. Paired; twin.
gena, -ae. *f.* The cheek.
geniōhyoglossus, -ī. *m.* Muscle attached to chin, hyoid bone and tongue.
gentiāna, -ae. *f.* Gentian.
genu, -ūs. *n.* Knee.
genus, generis. *n.* Kind.
germinātīvus, -a, -um. Germinative; germinal.
glabrus, -a, -um. Smooth.
glaciēs, -ēī. *f.* Ice.
globus, -ī. *m.* Globe.
glomerulus, -ī. *m.* Small ball, or tuft of vessels; glomerule.
glūteus, -a, -um (γογλστό, the buttock), of the buttock; gluteal.
glycerīnum, -ī. *n.* Glycerin.
glycerītum, -ī. *m.* Glycerite.
glycyrrhiza, -ae. *f.* Licorice.
gracilis, -e. Slender; graceful.
granulōsus, -a, -um. Granular.
granum, -ī. *n.* Grain.
gratus, -a, -um. Agreeable; pleasing.
gubernāculum, -ī. *n.* (Lit., a helm), applied to fetal cord directing descent of testes; gubernaculum.
gummi. Gum.
gustō, -āre, -āvī, -ātus. Taste.
gutta, -ae. *f.* Drop.
gyrus, -ī. *m.* Circle; ring; convolution (of the brain).
habeō, -ēre, -uī, -itus. Have.
habitō, -āre, -āvī, -ātus. Inhabit.
hallex, -icis, or hallux, -ucis. *f.* The great toe.
harmonia, -ae. *f.* Harmony, "suture of harmony."
helix, -icis. *f.* (ξυἕι , a tendril), outer ring of the external ear; helix.
hemisphericus, -a, -um. Hemispherical.
hēpar, hepatis. *n.* (Gr. Liver.
herba, -ae. *f.* Herb.
herī. Yesterday.
hiātus, -ūs. *m.* Opening; aperture.
hīc, haec, hoc. This.
hilāris, -e. Cheerful.
hīlus, -ī. *m.* Small fissure or depression.

hippocampus, -ī. *m.* (Lit., sea horse), applied to 2 convolutions of brain (major and minor); hippocampus.
homo, -inis. *m.* Man.
horribilis, -e. Horrible.
humānus, -a, -um. Human.
hūmor, -ōris. *m.* Fluid; humor.
hydrargyrum, -ī. *n.* Mercury.
hydrastis, -is. *f.* Golden seal **(root)**; hydrastis.
hyoideus, -a, -um. Hyoid.
Hyoscyamus, -ī. *m.* Henbane; Hyoscyamus.
īdem, eadem, idem. Same.
ignārus, -a, -um. Ignorant.
iliacus, -a, -um. Of or pert. to the flanks or ilium; iliac.
ille, illa, illud. He; she; it.
immōbilis, -e. Immovable.
immōbilitas, -ātis. *f.* Immobility.
impar, -is. Without a mate or fellow.
impediō, -īre, -īvī, -ītus. Hinder; check; prevent.
imperītus, -a, -um. Unskilled.
impūrus, -a, -um. Impure.
īmus, -a, -um. Lowest.
incisūra, -ae. *f.* Groove or notch.
Indicus, -a, -um. Indian.
infans, -ntis. *m.* and *f.* Infant.
inflammatiō, -ōnis. *f.* Inflammation.
infraspinātus, -a, -um. Beneath the spine (of the scapula); infraspinate.
infūsum, -ī. *m.* Infusion.
ingressus, -ūs. *m.* Entrance.
innominātus, -a, -um. Unnamed; innominate.
intermittō, -ere, -mīsī, -missus. Intermit.
internōdium, -ī. *n.* Space between 2 joints; internode.
internus, -a, -um. Inner.
interpositus, -a, -um. Placed between.
intertragicus, -a, -um. Between the tragus and antitragus.
intestīnum, -ī. *n.* Intestine.
intumescentia, -ae. *f.* An enlargement; intumescence.
inveniō, -īre, -vēnī, -ventus. Find; discover.
inversiō, -ōnis. *f.* Inversion.
iodidum, -ī. *n.* Iodide.
ipecacuanha, -ae. *f.* Ipecac.
ipse, ipsa, ipsum. Himself; herself; itself.
iris, iridis. *f.* Iris.
is, ea, id. He; she; it.
iter, itineris. *n.* Way; passageway.
jecur, jecinoris. *n.* Liver.
jūcundē. *adv.* Happily; pleasantly.
jūglans, juglandis. *f.* Walnut.
juguläris, -e. Jugular.
jūniperus, -ī. *f.* Juniper tree.
juvenis, -is. *m.* and *f.*, *adj.* and *subst.* Young; a youth.
labium, -ī. *n.* Lip.
lacer, -a, -um. Lacerated; mutilated.
lacrima, -ae. *f.* Tear.
lacrimālis, -e. Pert. to tears; lacrimal.
lactās, -ātis. *m.* A salt of lactic acid; lactate.
lactiferus, -a, -um. Milk-bearing; lactiferous.
lacus, -ūs. *m.* Lake; basin; reservoir.
lamella, -ae. *f.* Dim. **(lamina)**, layer.
lamina, -ae. *f.* Thin plate; layer.
lāna, -ae. *f*, Wool.
lassus, -a, -um. Weary.
laterālis, -e. Lateral.
lātus, -a, -um. Broad.
laudō, -āre, -āvī, -ātus. Praise.
lavandula, -ae. *f.* Lavender.
lavō, -āre, -āvī, -ātus or **lavi, lautus.** Wash.
laxātor, -ōris. *m.* A muscle that loosens; relaxer.
legō, -ere, -lēgī, lectus. Bring together; collect.
leniō, -īre, -īvī, -ītus. Calm; soothe; assuage.
lenticulāris, -e. Lentil-shaped (double-convex); lenticular.
lentus, -a, -um. Sticky.
letifer, -a, -um. Deadly.
levis, -e. Light.
lienālis, -e. Of the spleen.
ligamentōsus, -a, -um. Ligamentous.
ligamentum, -ī. *n.* Ligament.
lignum, -ī. *n.* Wood.
limbus, -ī. *n.* Border; band; **fringe.**
līmitāns, -ntis. Limiting.
limon, -ōnis. *f.* Lemon.
linea, -ae. *f.* Line.
lingua, -ae. *f.* Tongue.
linguālis, -e. Of the tongue; **lingual.**
linimentum, -ī. *n.* Liniment.
linum, -ī. *n.* Flax.
liquidus, -a, -um. Liquid.
lobulus, -ī. *m.* Lobule.
lobus, -ī. *m.* Lobe.
longitudinālis, -e. Longitudinal.
longus, -a, -um. Long.
lotiō, -ōnis. *f.* Wash; lotion.
lucidus, -a, -um. Clear; **transparent.**
lumbālis, -e. Of the loins; **lumbar.**
lumbus, -ī. *m.* Loin.
lūnula, -ae. *f.* Small crescent; **lunula.**
lupulīna, -ae. *f.* Yellow powder **from the** scales of the hop; lupulin.
luteus, -a, -um. Yellow.
luxatiō, -ōnis. *f.* Dislocation.
lympha, -ae. *f.* Chyle; lymph.
mācerō, -āre, -āvī, ātus. Soak; **macerate**
magister, -trī. *m.* Teacher; master.
magnus, -a, -um. Large; great.
māla, -ae. *f.* The cheekbone.
malignus, -a, -um. Malignant.
malus, -a, -um. Bad.
mandibulum, -ī. *n.* A jaw.
māne. *n.* Morning.
manūbrium, -ī. *n.* **(Lit., a handle, hilt)**; upper part of sternum; **manubrium.**
manus, -ūs. *f.* Hand.
massa, -ae. *f.* Mass.
masticō, -āre, -āvī, -ātus. Chew.
mastoideus, -a, -um. Nipplelike; **mastoid.**
mater, -tris. *f.* Mother.
māteria, -ae. *f.* Materials.
māternus, -a, -um. Maternal.
matrix, -īcis. *f.* Source; origin.
maxilla, -ae. *f.* Jawbone; jaw.
meātus, -ūs. *m.* Opening; **passage.**
mediānus, -a, -um. Middle; **median.**
medicāmen, -inis. *n.* Drug.
medicāmentārius, -a, -um. Medicated.
medicāmentum, -ī. *n.* Drug.
medicātus, -a, -um. Medicated.
medicīna, -ae. *f.* Medicine.
medicus, -ī. *m.* Physician; **doctor.**
medius, -a, -um. Middle.
membrāna, -ae. *f.* Membrane.
membrum, -ī. *n.* Member.
memoria, -ae. *f.* Memory.
mentha, -ae. *f.* Mint.
mentum, -ī. *n.* Chin.
mesentericus, -a, -um. Of the mesentery; mesenteric.
metus, -ūs. *m.* Fear.
mīles, -itis. *m.* Soldier.
minerālis, -e. Mineral.
misceō, -ēre, miscuī, mixtus. Mix.
miser, -a, -um. Poor; wretched.
mistūra, -ae. *f.* Mixture.
mītis, -e. Mild.
mitto, -ere, mīsī, missus. Send.
mobilis, -e. Movable.
mobilitās, -ātis. *f.* Mobility.
modiolus, -ī. *m.* (Lit., a small measure), hollow cone in the cochlea of the ear; modiolus.
molāris, -e (mola, mill), a term applied to the grinder teeth; molar.
molliō, -īre, -īvī, -ītus. Soften; mitigate.

mollis, -e. Soft.
molitiēs, -ēī. *f.* Softness.
mons, -ntis. *m.* Mountain.
montānus, -a, -um. Of a mountain; mountain (*adj.*).
monticulus, -ī. *m.* Dim. **(mons)**, small eminence.
morbus, -ī. *m.* Disease.
mordeō, --ēre, momordī, morsus. Bite.
moritūrus, -a, -um. About to die.
morphīna, -ae. *f.* Morphine.
morrhua, -ae. *f.* A genus of fishes, including the cod; cod.
mors, mortis. *f.* Death.
morsus, -ūs. *m.* Bite.
mortarium, -ī. *n.* Mortar.
mōtor, -ōris. *m.* That which moves; mover.
moveō, -ēre, mōvī, mōtus. Move.
mox. Presently; soon; directly.
mucilāgō, -inis. *f.* Mucilage.
mucōsus, -a, -um. Mucous.
mulceō, -ere, mulsi, mulsus. Soothe; allay.
multifidus, -a, -um. Many-clefted.
multus, -a, -um. Much; many.
muriāticus, -a, um. Muriatic.
musculus, -ī. *m.* Muscle.
mūtātiō, -ōnis. *f.* Change.
myristica, -ae. *f.* Nutmeg.
myrtiformis, -e. Shaped like the myrtle-leaf or berry; myrtiform.
nāris, -is. *f.* Nostril.
nāsus, -ī. *m.* Nose.
natō, -āre, -āvī, -ātus. Swim; float.
natūra, -ae. *f.* Nature.
nauta, -ae. *m.* Sailor.
naviculāris, -e. Boat-shaped; navicular.
neglectus, -a, -um. Neglected.
nēmō, -inis. *m.* and *f.* No one.
nervus, -ī. *m.* Nerve.
nescio, -īre, -īvi, -ītus. Not know; be ignorant of.
neurilemma, -atis. *n.* Nerve sheath.
nictitāns, -ntis. Winking.
nil. Nothing.
nimium. Too often.
nisi. Unless.
nitrās, -ātis. *m.* Nitrate.
nitricus, -a, -um. Nitric.
nitrōsus, -a, -um. Nitrous.
nōmen, -inis. *m.* Name.
nōminō, -āre, -āvī, -ātus. Name.
nōn. Not.
nondum. Not yet.
nōnus, -a, -um. Ninth.
nosco, -ere, nōvī, nōtus. Learn; know.
novem. Nine.
novus, -a, -um. New.
nox, noctis. *f.* Night.
nucha, -ae. *f.* Nape of neck.
nullus, -a, -um. No; none.
numerus, -ī. *m.* Number.
nunc. Now.
oblīquus, -a, -um. Oblique.
oblongātus, -a, -um. Oblong.
octō. Eight.
oculus, -ī. *m.* Eye.
officīna, -ae. *f.* Office.
officinālis ,-e. Officinal.
oleorēsīna, -ae. *f.* Oleoresin.
oleum, -ī. *n.* Oil.
olfactōrius, -a, -um. Olfactory.
omentum, -ī. *n.* Epiploön; omentum.
omnis, -e. Every; all.
operculum, -ī. *n.* (Lit., a cover or lid), applied to a group of convolutions in the cerebrum, between the 2 divisions of the fissure of Sylvius.
ophthalmicus, -a, -um. Of the eye; ophthalmic.
oppōnēns, -ntis. Opposing.
opticus, -a, -um. Optic.
opus, operis. *n.* Work.
orbita, -ae. *f.* **(orbis,** a circle), the cavity which lodges the eye; orbit.
ordō, -inis. *m.* Row.
orificium, -ī. *n.* Opening.
orior, -īrī, ortus. Arise.
ōs, ōris. *n.* Mouth.
os, ossis. *n.* Bone.
ossiculum, -ī. *n.* Small bone.
ostium, -ī. *n.* An opening.
ovālis, -e. Egg-shaped; oval.
oxalās, -ātis. *m.* A salt of oxalic acid, oxalate.
oxidum, -ī. *n.* Oxide.
palātum, -ī. *n.* Palate.
palpēbra, -ae. *f.* Eyelid.
pālus, -ūdis. *f.* Marsh; swamp.
pancreāticus, -a, -um. Pancreatic.
papillāris, -e. Resembling or covered with papillae; papillary.
pār, paris. *n.* A pair.
parasiticus, -a, -um. Parasitic.
paries, -iētis. *m.* Wall.
parō, -āre, -āvī, -ātus. Prepare.
pars, partis. *f.* Part.
partus, -ūs. *m.* Parturition; childbirth.
parvus, -a, -um. Small.
pater, -tris. *m.* Father.
patheticus, -a, -um. That which moves the passions; a name given to the 4th pair of nerves.
patria, -as. *f.* Fatherland; country.
paucus, -a, -um. Few.
pectinātus, -a, -um. Resembling the teeth of a comb; pectinate.
pectineus, -a, -um. Comblike.
pectiniformis, -e. Comblike.
pectus, pectoris. *n.* Breast; bosom.
pellūcidus, -a, -um. Transparent.
pensō, -āre, -āvī, -ātus. Weigh.
pepsīnum, -ī. *n.* Pepsin.
percolō, -āre, -āvī, -ātus. Filter; strain.
perforō, -āre, -āvī, -ātus. Bore through; perforate.
periculōsus, -a, -um. Dangerous.
perītus, -a, -um. Skilled.
peronēus, -a, -um. (*κερόνη* , fibula), relating to the fibula; peroneal.
persōna, -ae. *f.* Person.
perspiratōrius, -a, -um. Relating to perspiration; perspiratory.
pēs, pedis. *m.* Foot.
petō, -ere, -īvī, -ītus. Seek.
petrolātum, -ī. *n.* Petrolatum; vaseline.
petrōsus, -a, -um. Rocklike; petrous.
pharmacopoeia, -a. *f.* Pharmacopoeia.
phiala, -ae. *f.* Vial.
philosophus, -ī. *m.* Philosopher.
phosphās, -ātis. *m.* A salt of phosphoric acid; phosphate.
phrenicus, -a, -um. Of the diaphragm; phrenic.
physostigma, -atis. *n.* Calabar bean; physostigma.
piger, -gra, -grum. Lazy.
pigmentum, -ī. *n.* Pigment.
pilula, -ae. *f.* Pill.
pilus, -ī. *m.* Hair.
pineālis, -e. Resembling a pine cone; pineal.
pinna, -ae. *f.* (Lit., feather), pavilion of the ear; pinna.
piper, piperis. *n.* Pepper.
piperītus, -a, -um. Pepper, peppery.
pistillum, -ī. *n.* Pestle.
pituitārius, -a, -um. (pituita, phlegm or mucus), pituitary (applied to a reddish-gray body occupying the *sella Turcica* of the sphenoid bone, from a former erroneous belief that it discharged mucus into the nostrils).
pius, -a, -um. Tender.
pix, picis. *f.* Pitch.
plantāris, -e. Relating to the sole of the foot; plantar.
plānus, -a, -um. Flat; level; smooth.
plexus, -a, -um. Network; plexus.
plica, -ae. *f.* Fold.

plumbum, -ī. *n.* Lead.
poculum, -ī. *n.* Cup.
pollex, -icis. *f.* The thumb.
pomum, -ī. *n.* Apple.
pons, pontis. *m.* Bridge.
poples, poplitis. *m.* Ham of the knee; popliteal space.
poplitēus, -a, -um. Relating to the ham; popliteal.
populus, -ī. *m.* People.
portō, -āre, -āvī, -ātus. Carry.
portiō, -ōnis. *f.* Portion.
porus, -ī. *m.* Channel; canal.
post. Behind; after
posteā. Afterward
posticus, -a, -um. Hindmost.
potēns, -ntis. Powerful.
potiō, -ōnis. A drink; draught.
potō, -āre, -āvī, -ātus. Drink.
potus, -ūs. *m.* Drink.
praeparō, -āre, -āvī, -ātus. Prepare.
praeparatiō, -ōnis. *f.* Preparation.
praeputium, -ī. *n.* Foreskin; prepuce.
praescribō, -ere, -scripsī, -scriptus. Prescribe.
praescriptum, -ī. *n.* Prescription.
praesēns, -ntis. Present.
praestāns, -ntis. Excellent.
pressiō, -ōnis. *f.* Pressure.
primus, -a, -um. First.
princeps, -ipis. The first; chief; principal.
privō, -āre, -āvī, -ātus. Deprive.
prō. For; in behalf of.
processus, -ūs. *m.* A prominence; process.
profundus, -a, -um. Deep.
pronātor, -ōris. *m.* A muscle which turns the palm of the hand downward; pronator.
properō, -āre, -āvī, -ātus. Hasten.
proprius, -a, -um. One's own; special; proper.
prudēns, -ntis. Prudent.
pterygium, -ī. *n.* An eye disease; pterygium.
publicus, -a, -um. Public.
puella, -ae. *f.* Girl.
pugnō, -āre, -āvī, -ātus. Fight.
pulcher, -chra, -chrum. Beautiful.
pulmo, -ōnis. *m.* Lung.
pulmonālis, -e. Of the lungs; pulmonary.
pulverō, -āre, -āvī, -ātus. Powder; pulverize.
pulvis, pulveris. *m.* Powder.
punctum, -ī. *n.* Point.
puniō, -īre, -īvī, -ītus. Punish.
pūpilla, -ae. *f.* Pupil (of eye).
pupillāris, -e. Pupillary; applied to a delicate membrane which covers the pupil of the eye in the fetus.
purgātīvus, -a, -um. Purgative.
purificātus, -a, -um. Purified.
pūrus, -a, -um. Pure.
pyramidālis, -e. Pyramidal.
pyramis, -idis. *f.* Pyramid.
pyriformis, -e. Pear-shaped; pyriform.
quadrātus, -a, -um. Four-sided; square.
quadriceps, -cipitis. Four-headed.
quadrigeminus, -a, -um. Fourfold; four.
quaestiō, -ōnis. *f.* Question.
quam. Than.
quartus, -a, -um. Fourth.
quatuor. Four.
quatuordecim. Fourteen.
que. And.
quinīna, -ae. *f.* Quinine.
quis, quae, quid. Who; which; what.
quondam. Formerly.
quoque. Also.
quot. How many.
radiālis, -e. Of the radius; radial.
radiātus, -a, -um. Radiated.
rādix, -īcis. *f.* Root.
ramus, -ī. *m.* Branch.
rārō. Rarely.
rārus, -a, -um. Rare.
recens. Recently.
recipiō, -ere, -cēpī, -ceptus. Take.
recreō, -āre, -āvī, -ātus. Refresh.
rectus, -a, -um. Straight.
reductio, -ōnis. *f.* A bringing back.
reflexus, -a, -um. Turned back; reflected.
relevō, -āre, -āvī, -ātus. Relieve.
remedium, -ī. *n.* Remedy.
removeō, -ēre, -mōvī, -mōtus. Remove.
remittō, -ere, -mīsī, -missus. Send back; remit.
rēn, rēnis. *m.* (usually pl.), kidney.
rēnalis, -e. Of the kidney; renal.
reperiō, -īre, -perī, -pertus. Find.
reprimō, -ēre, -pressī, -pressus. Check repress.
requiesco, -ēre, -ēvī, -ētus. Rest.
rēs, reī. *f.* Thing.
rēsīna, -ae. *f.* Resin.
rēspīrātiō, -ōnis. *f.* Respiration.
rēte, -is. *n.* Net.
reticulāris, -e. Like a net; reticular.
retrāhēns, -ntis. Drawing back; retracting.
rheumatismus, -ī. *m.* Rheumatism.
ricinus, -ī. *m.* (Lit., a tick, which the seeds resemble), the castor oil plant (**Ricinus communis**).
rima, -ae. *f.* Slit; cleft.
rogō, -āre, -āvī, -ātus. Ask.
rosa, -ae. *f.* Rose.
rostrum, -ī. *n.* Beak.
rotundus, -a, -um. Round.
ruber, -bra, -brum. Red.
rubor, -ōris. *m.* Redness.
rūga, -ae. *f.* A wrinkle; fold.
rumex, -icis. *m.* and *f.* Sorrel.
sabulum, -ī. *n.* Sand.
saccharātus, -a, -um. Saccharated.
saccharum, -ī. *n.* Sugar.
sacciformis, -e. Saclike.
saccus, -ī. *m.* A sack or bag.
saepe. Often.
sal, -is. *m.* and *f.* Salt.
salicīnum, -ī. *n.* Salicin.
salicylās, -ātis. *m.* Salicylate.
salix, -īcis. *f.* Willow.
sānābilis, -e. Curable.
sanguis, -guinis. *m.* Blood.
sānitās, -ātis. *f.* Healing.
sānō, -āre, -āvī, -ātus. Heal; cure.
sapientia, -ae. *f.* Wisdom.
sapō, -ōnis. *m.* Soap.
sartōrius, -ī. *m.* The tailor's muscle; sartorius.
scāla, -ae. *f.* Ladder.
scalēnus, -a, -um. Of unequal sides.
scaphoideus, -a, -um. Boat-shaped; scaphoid.
schola, -ae. *f.* (Lit., leisure given to learning), school.
scientia, -ae. *f.* Knowledge; science.
scilla, -ae. *f.* Squill.
sciō, -īre, -īvī, -ītus. Know.
scrībō, -ēre, scripsī, scrīptus. Write.
scriptōrius, -a, -um. Of a writer; writer's
secundus, -a, -um. Second.
sed. But.
sēdes, -is. *f.* Seat.
segmentum, -ī. *n.* Segment.
sella, -ae. *f.* Saddle.
sēmicirculāris, -e. Semicircular.
sēmiellipticus, -a, -um. Semielliptical.
sēmilunāris, -e. Semilunar.
sēmimembranōsus, -a, -um. Semimembranous.
seminālis, -e. Seminal.
sēmis, sēmissis. *m.* Half.
sēmitendinōsus, -a, -um. Semitendinous
senectus, -tūtis. *f.* Old age.
senex, senis. *m.* Old man.
senilitās, -ātis. The feebleness of old age. senility.
sentiō, -īre, -sī, -sus. Feel

septem. Seven.
sequestrum, -ī. *n.* A portion of dead bone; sequestrum.
sermō, -ōnis. *m.* Conversation.
serrātus, -a, -um. Notched like a saw; serrated.
servus, -ī. *m.* Servant; assistant.
sesamoideus, -a, -um. Like a sesame seed; sesamoid (applied to a bone developed in a tendon).
seu. Whether.
signō, -āre, -āvī, -ātus. Write; direct.
simplex, -icis. Simple.
similō, -āre, -āvī, -ātus. Simulate.
sināpis, -is. *f.* Mustard.
sitis, -is. *f.* Thirst.
solitārius, -a, -um. Solitary.
somnificus, -a, -um. Sleep-producing.
somnus, -ī. *m.* Sleep.
sopor, -ōris. *m.* Deep sleep.
spectrum, -ī. *n.* Image.
spēs, speī. *f.* Hope.
sphenoideus, -a, -um. Wedge-shaped; sphenoid.
spīna, -ae. *f.* (A thorn), a process on the surface of a bone; the backbone.
spinālis, -e. Spinal.
spinōsus, -a, -um. Spiny.
spirālis, -e. Spiral.
spiritus, -ūs. *m.* Spirit.
splēnius, -a, -um. Resembling the spleen; applied to a muscle of the back and neck.
spongiōsus, -a, -um. Spongy.
squamōsus, -a, -um. Scaly; squamous.
stapēdius, -ī. *m.* A muscle acting upon the stapes; stapedius.
stertor, -ōris. *m.* Snoring.
stomachālis, -e. Stomachic.
stomachus, -ī. *m.* Stomach.
stramōnium, -ī. *n.* Jamestown weed; stramonium.
stria, -ae. *f.* Stripe; stria.
striātus, -a, -um. Striped; striated.
struō, -ēre, -xī, -ctus. Arrange.
strychnīna, -ae. *f.* Strychnine.
subacetās, -ātis. *m.* Subacetate.
subanconeus, -a, -um. Under the elbow.
subitō. Suddenly.
subitus, -a, -um. Sudden.
sublīmis, -e. Deep.
submuriās, -ātis. *m.* Submuriate.
subnitras, -ātis. *m.* Subnitrate.
subscapulāris, -e. Under the scapula; subscapular.
substantia, -ae. *f.* Substance.
subsultus, -ūs. *m.* A jumping; a twitching.
succus, -ī. *m.* Juice.
sudor, -ōris. *m.* Sweat.
sulcus, -ī. *m.* Furrow.
sulphonal. Sulfonal.
sulphās, -ātis. *m.* Sulfate.
sulphuricus, -a, -um. Sulfuric.
sum, esse, fui. Be.
sūmō, -ēre, -psi, -ptus. Take.
supercilium, -ī. *n.* Eyebrow.
superficialis, -e. Superficial.
superficiēs, -ēī. *f.* Surface.
supraspinātus, -a, -um. Above the spine (of scapula); supraspinate.
suppositōrium, -ī. *n.* Suppository.
suspensōrium, -ī. *n.* That which suspends.
suspensōrius, -a, -um. Suspensory.
sustentaculum, -ī. *n.* A prop; support.
sutūra, -ae. *f.* Seam; suture.
sympatheticus, -a, -um. Sympathetic.
symptōma, -atis. *n.* Symptom.
synoviālis, -e. Synovial.
tabacum, -ī. *n.* Tobacco.
taenia, -ae. *f.* A band. **t. semicirculāris.** A layer in the cerebrum; also, a genus of intestinal worms; the tapeworm.
talus, -ī. *m.* The heel.
tam. So.
tapētum, -ī. *n* (**tapēte,** carpet, tapestry), a lining membrane; also, the radiating fibers of the *corpus callōsum.*
taraxacum, -ī. *n.* Dandelion (root); taraxacum.
tarsus, -ī. *m.* Ankle.
tartaricus, -a, -um. Tartaric.
tartrās, -ātis. *m.* Tartrate.
tegō, -ēre, -xī, -ctum. Cover; protect.
tectōrium, -ī. *n.* A covering.
tectōrius, -a, -um. Protecting; covering.
temporālis, -e. Temporal.
tempus, -oris. *n.* Time.
tenax, -ācis. Holding fast; tenacious.
tendineus, -a, -um. Tendinous.
tendō, -ēre, tetendī, tentus. Stretch; reach.
tendō, -dinis. *m.* Tendon.
teneō, -ēre, -uī, -tus. Keep; hold.
tener, -a, -um. Delicate; tender.
tensor, -ōris. *m.* Stretcher; tensor.
tentō, -āre, -āvī, -ātus. Test; try.
tentōrium, -ī. *n.* A tent; covering.
tenuis, -e. Thin; small.
tepidus, -a, -um. Lukewarm.
terebinthina, -ae. *f.* Turpentine.
teres, -etis. Rounded; smooth.
tergum, -ī. *n.* Back.
terminus, -ī. *m.* End.
tertius, -a, -um. Third.
theobrōma, -ātis. *n.* Cacao (food of the gods).
thoracicus, -a, -um. Thoracic.
thyroideus, -a, -um. Having the shape of an oblong shield; thyroid.
tiglium, -ī. *n.* The specific name of the croton oil plant.
tinctūra, -ae. *f.* Tincture.
tonicus, -a, -um. Tonic.
tonsilla, -ae. *f.* Tonsil.
torcular, -āris. *n.* A wine press.
tracheālis, -e. Tracheal.
tractō, -āre, -āvī, -ātus. Handle.
tragus, -ī. *m.* (τράγος, a goat), small nipple in front of external auditory meatus; so called because sometimes covered with hair; tragus.
transversālis, -e. Transverse.
transversus, -a, -um. Transverse.
trapezoideus, -a, -um. Like a trapezium; trapezoid.
trauma, -atis. *n.* Injury; wound.
trēs, tria. Three.
triangulāris, -e. Triangular.
triceps, -ipitis. Three-headed.
trigeminus, -a, -um. Three-fold.
trigīnta. Thirty.
trigōnum, -ī. *n.* Triangle.
triquetrus, -a, -um. Three-cornered; triangular.
trochiscus, -ī. *m.* Troche.
tuba, -ae. *f.* (Trumpet), tube.
tuber, -eris. *n.* Swelling; protuberance.
tuberculum, -ī. *n.* A protuberance; tubercle.
tubulus, -ī. *m.* Small tube.
tubus, -ī. *m.* Tube.
tunica, -ae. *f.* Coat; covering.
tussiō, -īre, -īvī, -ītus. Cough.
tūtāmen, -minis. *n.* Means of defense; a protection.
tūtō. Safely.
tympanicus, -a, -um. Of the tympanum; tympanic.
ubi. Where.
ulna, -ae. *f.* Larger bone of forearm; ulna.
ulnāris, -e. Of the ulna; ulnar.
uncia, -ae. *f.* Ounce.
unciformis, -e. Hooked.
uncinātus, -a. -um. Hooked; uncinate.
unguentum, -ī. *n.* Ointment.
unguis, -is. *m.* Nail.
ūnus, -a, -um. One.
urbānus, -a, -um. Of the city; urbane.
urīna, -ae. *f.* Urine.

uriniferus, -a, -um. Urine-bearing; uriniferous.
usque. Continuously; constantly.
uterīnus, -a, -um. Of the uterus; uterine.
ūtilis, -e. Useful.
uvula, -ae. *f.* Dim. (**uva,** bunch of grapes), a small appendix or tubercle; uvula.
uxor, -ōris. *f.* Wife.
vaginālis, -e. Sheathlike; vaginal.
valeriānās, -ātis. *m.* Valerianate.
valetūdō, -inis. *f.* Health.
validus, -a, -um. Strong; sturdy; healthy.
valvula, -ae. *f.* Valve.
vās, vāsis. *n.* Vessel.
vasculōsus, -a, -um. Vascular.
vasculum, -ī. *n.* Small vessel.
vastus, -a, -um. Extensive; large.
vegetābilis, -e. Vegetable.
vehiculum, -ī. *n.* Vehicle.
vel. Either.
vēlum, -ī. *n.* Veil.
vēna, -ae. *f.* Vein.
vendō, -ēre, vendidī. Sell.
veneficus, -ī. *m.* Poisoner.
venēnum, -ī. *n.* Poison.
venōsus, -a, -um. Venous.
venter, -tris. *m.* Belly.
ventriculus, -ī. *m.* Dim. (**venter**), ventricle.
vērātrum, -ī. *n.* Hellebore; veratrum.
vermiformis, -e. Wormlike.
veru, -ūs. *n.* A spit (for roasting upon); used only in the term **verumontanum,** a longitudinal ridge in the floor of the male urethra.
verus, -a, -um. True.
vesica, -ae. *f.* Urinary bladder.
vesicatōrium, -ī. *n.* Blister.
vesicula, -ae. *f.* Vesicle.
vesiculāris, -e. Full of vesicles or cells; vesicular.
vestibulāris, -e. Relating to the vestibule of the ear; vestibular.
vetus, veteris. Old.
vigilō, -āre, -āvī, -ātus. Watch.
vīgintī. Twenty.
villus, -ī. *m.* Tuft of hair; villus.
vinculum, -ī. *n.* Link; chain.
vinum, -ī. *n.* Wine.
vir, virī. *m.* Man.
viridis, -e. Green.
vīs, vīs, pl. **vires, -ium.** *f.* Force; power.
viscus, -eris. *n.* Any internal organ of the body.
visiō, -ōnis. *f.* Vision.
vīsus, -ūs. *m.* Vision.
vīta, -ae. *f.* Life.
vitellus, -ī. *m.* Yolk.
vitreus, -a, -um. Resembling glass; vitreous.
vocālis, -e. Vocal.
vocō, -āre, -āvī, -ātus. Call.
vola, -ae. *f.* Palm of the hand (sole of the foot).
vorticōsus, -a, -um. Resembling an eddy or whirlpool.
vulnerō, -āre, -āvī, -ātus. Wound.
vulnus, vulneris. *n.* A wound.
vultus, -ūs. *m.* Countenance.
zincum, -ī. *n.* Zinc.
zingiber, -eris. *n.* Ginger.
zōna, -ae. *f.* Zone; belt.
zōnula, -ae. *f.* Little zone, or belt; zonule.

(*See also prescriptions*)

English, Latin and Greek Equivalents

acid. Acidum.
ague. Febris.
and. Et.
arm. Brachium. Gr., **brachion.**
artery. Arteria.
attachment. Adhaesio.
back. Tergum; dorsum.
backbone. Spina.
backward. Retro.
bath. Balneum.
beef. Bubula.
belly. Venter; abdomen.
bend. Flexus.
bile. Bilis. Gr., **chole.**
bladder. Vesica.
bleed. Fluere.
blind. Obscurus.
blister. Pustulo; vesicatorium.
bloat. Tumeo.
blood. Sanguis. Gr., **haima, aima.**
blood vessel. Vena.
body. Corpus. Gr., soma.
boiling (up). Effervescens.
bone. Os. Gr., osteon.
bony. Osseus.
bowels. Intestina; viscera.
bow-legged. Valgus.
brain. Cerebrum. Gr., egkephalon.
breach. Ruptura.
breast. Mamma. Gr., mastos.
breath. Halitus.
bubble. Pustula.
bulb. Bulbus.
buttock. Clunis. Gr., gloutos.
calcareous. Calci similis.
canal. Canalis.
cartilage. Cartilago. Gr., chondros.
catarrh. Coryza.
cavity. Caverna.
change. Mutatio.
chest. Thorax. Gr., thorax.
chin. Mentum. Gr., geneion.
choke. Strangulo.
clavicle. Clavicula.
confinement. Puerperium.
congestion. Conglobatio.
consumption. Phthisis, pulmonaria.
convulsion. Convulsio.
cord. Corda.
corn. Callus-clavus.
cornea. Cornu. Gr., keras.
costive. Astrictus.
cough. Tussio.
countenance. Vultus.
cramp. Spasmus.
crisis. Dies crisimus.
cup. Poculum.
cure. Sano.
curvature. Curvatura.
cuticle. Cuticula.
daily. Diurnus.
dandruff. Furfures capitas.
day. Dies.
dead. Mortuus; defunctus.
deadly. Lethalis.
deafness. Surditas.
decompose. Dissolvo.
dental. Dentalis.
depression. Depressio.
digestive. Digestorius; pepticus.
dilute. Dilutus.
discharge. Eluvies; effluens.
disease. Morbus.
dorsal. Dorsalis.
dose. Potio.
dram. Drachma.
drink. Bibo; potis.
dropsy. Hydrops; opis.
drug. Medicamentum.
duct. Ductus.
dysentery. Dysenteria.
ear. Auris. Gr., ous.
eat. Edo.
egg. Ovum.
elbow. Cubitum. Gr., agkon.
embryo. Partus immaturus.
emission. Emissio.
entrails. Viscera.
epidemic. Epidemus.
epilepsy. Morbus comitalis; epilepsia.
epileptic. Epilepticus.
erection. Erectio.
erotic. Amatorius.
eunuch. Eunuchus.
every. Omnis.
excrement. Excrementum.
excretion. Excrementum; excretio.
exhalation. Exhalatio.
exhale. Exhalo.
expel. Expello.
expire. Expiro.
external. Externus.
extract. Extractum.
eye. Oculus. Gr., ophthalmos.
eyeball. Pupula.
eyebrow. Supercilium.
eyelid. Palpebra.
eyetooth. Dens caninus.
face. Facies.
faculty. Facultas.
faint. Collabor.
fat. Adeps. Gr., lipos.
feature. Lineomentum.
febrile. Febriculosus.
fecundity. Fecunditas.
feel. Tactus.
fever. Febris.
film. Membranula.
filter. Percolo.
finger. Digitus. Gr., dactylos.
fistula. Fistula putris.
fit. Accessus.
flesh. Carnis. Gr., sarx.
fluid. Fluidus.
food. Cibus.
foot. Pes, pedis. Gr., pous.
forearm. Brachium.
forehead. Frons.
freckle. Lentigo.
gall. Bilis.
gangrene. Gangraena.
gargle. Gargarizo.
gland. Glandula.
gleet. Ichor.
gout. Morbus articularis; (in feet), podagra.
grain. Granum.
gravel. Calculus.
grinder tooth. Dens maxillaris.
gullet. Gula.
gum. Gingiva (of mouth).
gut. Intestinum.
hair. Capillus. Gr., thrix.
half. Dimidius.
hand. Manus. Gr., cheir.
harelip. Labrum fissum.
haunch. Clunis.
head. Caput. Gr., kephale.
heal. Sano.
healer. Medicus.
healing. Salutaris.
health. Sanitas.
healthful. Salutaris; saluber.
healthy. Sanus.
hear. Audio.
hearing. Auditio; (sense of) auditus.

heart. Cor. Gr., kardia.
heart burning. Redundatio **stomachi.**
heat. Calor; v. a. calefacio.
hectic. Hecticus.
heel. Calx, talus.
hirsute. Hirsutus.
homeopathic. Homeopathicus.
hysterics. Hysteria.
illness. Morbus.
incisor. Dens acutus.
infant. Infans; puerilis.
infect. Inficio.
infectious. Contagiosus.
infirm. Infirmus; debilis.
inflammation. Inflammatio; **(of lungs) in**flammatio pulmonaria.
injection. Injectio.
insane. Insanus.
intellect. Intellectus.
intercourse. Congressus.
internal. Intestinus.
intestine. Intestinum. **Gr., enteron.**
itch. Scabies.
itching. Pruritus.
jaw. Maxilla.
joint. Artus. Gr., **arthron.**
jugular vein. Vena **jugularis.**
kidney. Ren. Gr., nephros.
knee. Genu. Gr., **gonu.**
kneepan. Patella.
knuckle. Condylus.
labor. Partus.
labyrinth. Labyrinthus.
lacerate. Lacero.
larynx. Guttur.
lateral. Lateralis.
leech. Sanguisuga.
leg. Tibia.
leprosy. Leprosus.
ligament. Ligamentum. **Gr., syndesmos.**
ligature. Ligatura.
limb. Membrum.
lime. Calx.
listen. Ausculto.
liver. Jecur. Gr., **hepar, epar.**
livid. Lividus.
loin. Lumbus. Gr., **lapara.**
looseness. Laxitas.
lotion. Lotio.
lukewarm. Tepidus.
lung. Pulmo. Gr., **pneumon.**
lymph. Lympha.
mad. Insanus.
malady. Morbus.
male. Masculinus.
malignant. Malignus.
maternity. Conditio **matris.**
medicine. (Remedy) **Medicamentum.**
medicated. Medicatus.
milk. Lac.
mind. Animus.
mix. Misceo.
mixture. Mistura.
moist. Humidus.
molar. Dens **molaris.**
month. Mensis.
monthly. Menstruus.
morbid. Morbidus.
mouth. Os. Gr., **stoma.**
mucous. Mucosus.
muscle. Musculus. Gr., **mys.**
mustard. Sinapis.
nail. Unguis.
navel. Umbilicus. Gr., **omphalos.**
neck. Cervix; collum. Gr., **trachelos.**
nerve. Nervus. Gr., **neuron.**
nipple. Papilla.
no, none. Nullus.
normal. Normalis.
nose. Nasus. Gr., **rhis, ris.**
nostril. Naris.
not. Non.
nourish. Nutrio.
nourishment. Alimentus.
now. Nunc.
nudity. Nudatio.
nurse. Nutrix.
obesity. Obesitas.
ocular. Ocularis.
oculist. Ocularis **medicus.**
oil. Oleum.
ointment. Unguentum.
operator. Manus curatio.
opiate. Medicamentum **somnificum.**
optics. Optice.
orifice. Foramen.
pain. Dolor.
palate. Palatum.
palm. Palma.
parasite. Parasitus.
part. Pars.
patient. Patiens.
pectoral. Pectoralis.
pedal. Pedale.
phlegm. Pituita.
pill. Pilus.
pimple. Pustula.
plaster. Emplastrum.
poison. Venenum.
poultice. Cataplasma.
powder. Pulvis.
pregnant. Gravida.
prepare. Paro.
prescribe. Praescribo.
prescription. Praescriptum.
puberty. Pubertas.
pubic bone. Os pubis. **Gr., pecten.**
pulverize. Pulvero.
pupil. Pupilla.
purgative. Purgativus.
putrid. Putris.
quinsy. Cynanche; **angina.**
rash. Exanthema.
recover. Convalesco.
recumbent. Recubans.
recur. Recurro.
redness. Rubor.
remedy. Remedium.
respiration. Respiratio.
rheum. Fluxio.
rib. Costa.
rigid. Rigidus.
ringing. Tinnitus.
rupture. Hernia.
saliva. Sputum.
sallow. Salix.
salt. Sal.
salve. Unguentum.
sane. Sanus.
scab. Scabies.
scalp. Pericranium.
scaly. Squamosus.
scar. Cicatrix.
sciatica. Ischias.
scruple. Scrupulum.
seed. Semen.
senile. Senilis.
serum. Sanguinis **pars equosa.**
sheath. Vagina.
shin. Tibia.
shock. Concussio; **(of electricity), ictus** electricus.
short. Brevis.
shoulder. Humerus. Gr., **omos.**
shoulder blade. Scapula.
shudder. Tremor.
sick. Aegrotus.
side. Latus.
sinew. Nervus.
skeleton. Sceletos.
skin. Cutis. Gr., **derma.**
skull. Cranium. Gr., **kranion.**
sleep. Somnus.
smallpox. Variola.
smell. Odoratus.
soap. Sapo.
socket. Cavum.
soft. Mollis.
solid. Solidus.
solution. Dilutum.

soporific. Soporus.
sore. Ulcus.
spasm. Spasmus.
spinal. Dorsalis; spinalis.
spine. Spina.
spirit. Spiritus.
spittle. Sputum.
spleen. Lien.
spoon. Cochleare.
sprain. Luxatio.
stomach. Stomachus. Gr., gaster.
stone. Calculus.
stricture. Strictura.
sugar. Saccharum.
suture. Sutura.
swallow. Glutio.
sweat. Sudor. Gr., idros.
symptom. Symptoma.
system. Systema.
tail. Cauda.
take. Sumo.
tapeworm. Taenia.
taste. Gustatus.
tear. Lacrima.
teeth. Dentes.
tendon. Tendo. Gr., tenon.
testicle. Testis. Gr., orchis.
thigh. Femur.
throat. Fauces. Gr., pharygx.
throb. Palpito.
thumb. Pollex.
tongue. Lingua. Gr., glossa.
tonsil. Tonsilla.
tooth. Dens. Gr., odous.
troche. Trochiscus.
tube. Tuba.
twin. Geminus.
twitching. Subsultus.
ulcer. Ulcus.
unless. Nisi.
urine. Urina.
uterine. Uterinus.
vaccine. Vaccinum.
vagina. Vagina. Gr., kolpos.
valve. Valvula.
vein. Vena. Gr., phleps.
vertebra. Vertebra. Gr., spondylos.
vessel. Vas.
wash. Lavo.
water. Aqua.
wax. Cera.
waxed dressing. Ceratum.
weary. Lassus.
wet. Humidus.
windpipe. Arteria aspera.
wine. Vinum.
woman. Femina.
womb. Uterus. Gr., hystera; ystera.
worm. Vermis.
wound. Vulnus.
wrist. Carpus. Gr., karpos.
yolk. Luteum.

Latin and Greek Medical Words

LATIN EQUIVALENTS

COLORS

blue. Caeruleus; cyaneus; lividus.
black. Niger; nigra; nigrum.
brown. Fulvus.
crimson. Coccum; coccineus.
green. Viridis.
gray. Cinereus.
lemon. Citreum.
pink. Rosaceus.
purple. Purpura; purpureus.
red. Ruber.
scarlet. Coccineus.
violet. Violaceus.
white. Albus.
yellow. Flavus; luteus; croceus.

QUALITIES

bitter. Acerbus.
chill. Friguscolum.
cold. Frigidus.
dry. Aridus.
dull. Stupidus; hebes.
faintness. Languor.
fat. obesus; pinguis.
heat. Calor; ardor; fervor.
short. Brevis.
sour. Acidus.
sweet. Dulcis.
tall. Longus; celsus; procerus.
thick. Densus.
heavy. Gravis; ponderosus.
hot. Calidus; fervens; candens.
light. Levis.
liquid. Liquidus.
moist. Humidus; uvidus.
sharp. Acutus.
thin. Tenuis; macer.
warm. Calidus.
warmth. Calor.
weary. Lassus; languidus; fatigatus.
wet. Humidus.

METALS

gold. Aurum; aureus.
silver. Argentum; argenteus.
copper. Cuprum; cuprinus.
iron. Ferrum; ferreus.
tin. Stannum; plumbum album.

TIME

Words expressing periods of time.
afternoon. Post-meridiem.
age. Aetas; maturas; adultus; impubis.
autumn. Autumnus.
birth. Partus; natales.
breakfast. Prandium.
child. Infans; puer, filius.
day. Dies.
daily. Diurnus.
date. Status dies.
dawn. Prima lux.
death. Mors.
dinner. Cena.
evening. Vesper.
hour. Hora.
infant. Infans.
maturity. Maturitas; aetas matura.
meal. Epulae.
midnight. Media nox.
midsummer. Media aestas.
moment. Punctum.
month. Mens.
monthly. Menstruus.
morning. Matutinum.
night. Nox, noctis.
noon. Meridies.
old. Antiquus.
puberty. Pubertas.
second. Secundum.
spring. Ver; veris.
summer. Aestas.
sunrise. Solis ortus.
sunset. Solis occasus.
supper. Cena.
time. Tempus.
winter. Hiems, hiemis.
year. Annus.
young. Parvus; infans.
youth. Adolescentia.

RELATIONSHIP

aunt. Amita; matertera.
brother. Frater.
child. Infans.
cousin. Consobrinus.
father. Pater; paterfamilias.
husband. Maritus.
infant. Infans.
grandfather. Avus.
grandmother. Avia.
granddaughter. Neptis.
grandson. Nepos.
mother. Mater.
nephew. Fratris or sororis filius or sororis nepos.
niece. Fratris or sororis filia.
sister. Soror.
uncle. Patruus; avunculus.
widow. Vidua.
widower. Viduus.
wife. Uxor.

NUMERALS

SEE: Latin Numerals, in Appendix (Roman Numerals.)

Greek and Latin Singulars and Plurals

Singular	*Plural*
addendum	addenda
aden	adena
adenoma	adenomata
ala	alae
albacans	albacantes
amygdala	amygdalae
antenna	antennae
antiad	antiades
antrum	antra
apertura	aperturae
apex	apices
aponeurosis	aponeuroses
appendix	appendices
aqua	aquae
arcus	arcus
ascaris	ascarides
ascus	asci
atrium	atria
axis	axes
bacillus	bacilli
bacterium	bacteria
bronchus	bronchi
bulla	bullae
bursa	bursae
cactus	cacti
cadaver	cadavera
calcaneum	calcanea
calculus	calculi
calix	calices
cantharis	cantharides
canthus	canthi
cornu	cornua
corpus	corpora
crisis	crises
cuniculus	cuniculi
dens	dentes
diagnosis	diagnoses
diaphoreticus	diaphoretici
diastema	diastemata
digitus	digiti
dorsum	dorsi
echolatus	echolati
enema	enemata
ensis	enses
epididymis	epididymides
esthesis	estheses
fibroma	fibromata
filix	filices
filum	fila
flagellum	flagella
focus	foci
fornix	fornices
fossa	fossae
glans	glandes
gonad	gonades
gonococcus	gonococci
gyrus	gyri
ilium	ilia
keratosis	keratoses
labium	labia
lamina	laminae
loculus	loculi
locus	loci
medium	media
mucosa	mucosae
naevus	naevi
nodus	nodi
nox	noxa
os	ora
ovum	ova
papilla	papillae
pathema	pathemata
pes	pedes
petechia	petechiae
pilula	pilulae
polypus	polypi
ramus	rami
septum	septa
sequestrum	sequestra
serosa	serosae
spasmus	spasmi
spectrum	spectra
speculum	specula
sperma	spermata
stoma	stomata
sudamen	sudamina
sulcus	sulci
tarsus	tarsi
tela	telae
tinctura	tincturae
toxicosis	toxicoses
typha	typhae
ulcus	ulcera
varix	varices
vas	vasa
vesicula	vesiculae
vis	vires
viscus	viscera
vomica	vomicae
zygoma	zygomata

Numerals, Latin

Cardinals		Ordinals	
1.	unus	1st.	primus
2.	duo	2nd.	secundus
3.	tres	3rd.	tertius
4.	quattuor	4th.	quartus
5.	quinque	5th.	quintus
6.	sex	6th.	sextus
7.	septem	7th.	septimus
8.	octō	8th.	octāvus
9.	novem	9th.	nōnus
10.	decem	10th.	decimus
11.	ūndecim	11th.	ūndecimus
12.	duodecim	12th.	duodecimus
13.	tredecim	13th.	tertius decimus
14.	quattuordecim	14th	quartus decimus
15.	quīndecim	15th.	quīntus decimus
16.	sēdecim	16th.	septus decimus
17.	septendecim	17th.	septimus decimus
18.	duodēvīgintī	18th.	duodēvīcēsimus
19.	ūndēvīgintī	19th.	ūndēvīcēsimus
20.	vīgintī	20th.	vīcēsimus
21.	vīgintī ūnus, *or* ūnus et vīgintī	21st.	vīcēsimus primus, *or* prīmus et vīcēsimus
22.	vīgintī duo, *or* duo et vīgintī	22nd.	vīcēsimus secundus, *or* duo et vīcēsimus
28.	duodētrīgintā	28th.	duodētrīcēsimus
29.	ūndētrīgintā	29th.	ūndētrīcēsimus
30.	trīgintā	30th.	trīcēsimus
40.	quadrāgintā	40th.	quadrāgēsimus
50.	quīnquāgintā	50th.	quīnquāgēsimus
60.	sexāgintā	60th.	sexāgēsimus
70.	septuāgintā	70th.	septuāgēsimus
80.	octōgintā	80th.	octōgēsimus
90.	nōnāgintā	90th.	nōnāgēsimus
100.	centum	100th.	centēsimus
101.	centum ūnus, *or* centum et ūnus	101st.	centēsimus prīmus, centēsimus et prīmus
102.	centum duo, *or* centum et duo	102nd.	centēsimus secundus, centēsimus et secundus
200.	ducentī	200th.	ducentēsimus
300.	trecentī	300th.	trecentēsimus
400.	quadringentī	400th.	quadringentēsimus
500.	quīngentī	500th.	quīngentēsimus
600.	sēscentī, *or* sexcenti	600th.	sēscentēsimus
700.	septingentī	700th.	septimgentēsimus
800.	octingentī	800th.	octingentēsimus
900.	nōngentī	900th.	nōngentēsimus
1,000.	mīlle	1,000th.	mīllēsimus
2,000.	duo mīllia	2,000th.	bis mīllēsimus
10,000.	decem mīllia	10,000th.	decies mīllēsimus
100,000.	centum mīllia	100,000th.	centiēs mīllēsimus

Numerals, Roman

1	I	30	XXX	400	CD
2	II	40	XL	500	D
3	III	50	L	600	DC
4	IV	60	LX	700	DCC
5	V	70	LXX	800	DCCC
6	VI	80	LXXX	900	CM
7	VII	90	XC	1000	M
8	VIII	100	C	2000	MM
9	IX	101	CI	5000	$\overline{V}$
10	X	102	CII	10,000	$\overline{X}$
15	XV	200	CC	100,000	$\overline{C}$
20	XX	300	CCC	1,000,000	$\overline{M}$

Prefixes and Suffixes

a-, an. Negative.
a-, ab-, abs-. Away from.
ad-, -ad. Toward.
-aemia. Blood.
aer-. Air.
-aesthesia. Sensation.
-algesia, algia. Suffering; pain.
algi-. Pain.
all-. Other.
amb-. Both; on both sides.
amph-. Around; on both sides.
ana-, an-. Up.
angio-. Relating to blood or lymph vessels.
ante-. Before.
anti-. Against.
apo-. From; opposed.
-ase. Enzyme.
aut-, auto-. Self.
bi, bis-. Twice; double.
brachy-. Short.
brady-. Slow.
cac-, caco-. Bad; evil.
cat, cata, cath-. Down.
-cele. A tumor; a cyst; a hernia.
cent-. Hundred.
cephal-. Relating to a head.
chrom-, chromo-. Color.
-cide. Causing death.
circum-. Around.
co, com, con-. Together.
contra-. Against.
cyst-, -cyst. Bag; bladder.
-cyte. A cell.
dacry-. Tears.
dactyl-. Fingers.
de-. From; not.
deca-. Ten.
deci-. Tenth.
demi-. Half.
dent-. Relating to the teeth.
derma-. The skin.
di-. Double; apart from.
dia-. Through; between; asunder.
dipla, diplo-. Double.
dis-. Negative; double; apart; absence of.
-dynia. Pain.
dys-. Difficult; bad.
ec, ecto-. Out; on the outside.
-ectomy. A cutting out.
ef, es, ex, exo-. Out
-emesis. Vomiting.
-emia. Blood.
en-. In, into.
endo-. Within.
entero-. Relating to the intestine.
ento-. Within.
epi-. Upon.
-esthesia. Sensation.
eu-. Well.
ex-, exo-. Out.
extra-. On the outside; beyond.
fore-. Before; in front of.
-form. Form.
-fuge. To drive away.
galact, galacto-. Milk.
gaster, gastro-. The stomach; the belly.
-gene, -genesis, -genetic, -genic. Production; origin; formation.
glosso-. Relating to the tongue.
-gog, gogue. To make flow.
-gram. A tracing; a mark.
-graphy. A writing; a record.
hem, hemato-. Relating to the blood.
hemi-. Half.
hepa-, hepar-, hepato-. Liver.
hetero-. Other; indicating dissimilarity.
holo-. All.
homo, homeo-. Same; similar.
hydra, hydro-. Relating to water.
hyp, hyph, hypo-. Under.
hyper-. Over; above; beyond.
hypo-. Under.
-iasis. Condition; pathological state.
idio-. Peculiar to the individual or organ
ileo-. Relating to the ileum.
in-. In; into; not.
infra-. Beneath.
inter-. Between.
intra, intro-. Within.
-ism. Condition; theory.
iso-. Equal.
-itis. Inflammation.
-ize. To treat by special method.
juxta-. Near.
karyo-. Nucleus; nut.
kata-, kath-. Down.
kera-. Horn; indicates hardness.
kinesi-. Movement.
-kinesis. Motion.
lact-. Milk.
laparo-. The loin; relating to the loin or abdomen.
laryng, laryngo-. The larynx.
latero-. Side.
lepto-. Small; soft.
leuco, leuko-. White.
-lite, -lith. A stone; a calculus.
lith-. A stone.
-logia, -logy. Science of; study of.
-lysis. Setting free; disintegration.
macro-. Large; long; big.
mal-. Bad; poor; evil.
med-, medi-. Middle.
mega, megal-. Large; great.
-megalia or megaly. Large; great; extreme.
melan-, melano-. Black.
mes-, meso-. Middle.
meta-. Beyond; over; between; change, or transposition.
-meter. Measure.
metra, metro-. The uterus.
micro-. Small.
mio-. Less; smaller.
mono-. Single.
multi-. Many.
my, myo-. Muscle.
myel, myelo-. Marrow.
myxa, myxo-. Mucus.
neo-. New.
nephr, nephra, nephro-. Kidney.
neu, neuro-. Nerve.
niter, nitro-. Nitrogen.
non-, not-. No.
nucleo-. A nucleus.
ob-. Against.
oculo-. The eye.
-ode, oid. Form; shape; resemblance.
odont-. A tooth.
-oid. Form; shape; resemblance.
oligo-. Few.
-oma. A tumor.
omo-. Shoulder.
o-. An egg; ovum.
oophoron-. Ovary.
opisth-. Backward.
orchid-. Testicle.
ortho-. Straight; normal.
os-. A mouth; a bone.
-osis. Condition; disease; intensive.
oste, osteo-. A bone.
-ostomosis, ostomy. To furnish with a mouth or an outlet.
-otomy. Cutting.
oxy-. Sharp; acid.

pachy-. Thick.
pan-. All; entire.
para-. Alongside of.
path-, -path, -pathy. Disease; suffering.
-penia. Lack.
per-. Excessive; through.
peri-. Around.
-phobia. Fear.
-phylaxis. Protection.
-plasm. To mold.
-plastic. Molded; indicates restoration of lost or badly formed features.
-plegia. A stroke.
plur-. More.
pneu-. Relating to the air or lungs.
poly-. Much; many.
post-. After.
pre-. Before.
pro-. Before; in behalf of.
proto-. First.
pseud, pseudo-. False.
psych-. The soul; the mind.
py-, pyo-. Pus.
re-. Back; again.
retro-. Backward.
-rhage, -rhagia. Hemorrhage; flow.
-rhaphy. A suturing or stitching.
-rhea. To flow; indicates discharge.
sacchar-. Sugar.
sacro-. Sacrum.
salping, salpingo-. A tube; relating to a fallopian tube.
sarco-. Flesh.
sclero-. Hard; relating to the sclera.
-sclerosis. Dryness; hardness.
-scopy. To see.
semi-. Half.
-stomosis, stomy. To furnish with a mouth or outlet.
sub-. Under.
super, supra-. Above.
syn-. With; together.
tele-. Distant; far.
tetra-. Four.
thio-. Sulfur.
thyro-. Thyroid gland.
-tomy. Cutting.
trans-. Across.
tri-. Three.
-trophic. Relating to nourishment.
tropho-. Relating to nutrition.
uni-. One.
-uria. Relating to the urine.
urino, uro-. Relating to the urine or urinary organs.
vaso-. A vessel.
venter, ventro-. The abdomen.
xanth-. Yellow.

Anatomy and Physiology

Muscles of the Body with Their Action, Origin, Insertion and Innervation

The muscles in the body number over 650, the totals varying according to the authority, as some list as separate muscles what others regard as portions of adjacent muscles. Most of the muscles occur in pairs; 5 are single muscles.

HEAD AND FACE

attolens aurem (at-ōl'ĕnz aw'rĕm). SAME AS: *auricularis superior.*

attrahens aurem (ăt'ră-hĕnz aw'rĕm). SAME AS: *auricularis anterior.*

auricularis anterior (aw-rĭk"ū-lā'rĭs an-tē'rĭ-or). ACTION: Draws pinna of ear forward. ORIGIN: Superficial temporal fascia. INSERTION: Helix of ear anteriorly. INNERVATION: Facial. SYN: *atrahens aurem.*

auricularis posterior (aw-rĭk"ū-lā'rĭs pŏs-tē'rĭ-or). ACTION: Draws pinna of ear backward. ORIGIN: Mastoid process. INSERTION: Root of auricle. INNERVATION: Facial. SYN: *retrahens aurem.*

auricularis superior (aw-rĭk"ū-lā'rĭs sū-pē'rĭ-or). ACTION: Elevates pinna of ear. ORIGIN: Galea aponeurotica. INSERTION: Upper portion of pinna of ear. INNERVATION: Facial. SYN: *attolens aurem.*

buccinator (bŭk"sĭn-ā'tor). ACTION: Compresses cheek, retracts angle of mouth. ORIGIN: Alveolar process of maxilla, pterygomandibular ligament, buccinator ridge of mandible. INSERTION: Orbicularis oris. INNERVATION: Facial.

caninus (kā-nī'nŭs). SAME AS: *levator anguli oris.*

choroideus (kō-roy'dē-ŭs). SAME AS: *ciliaris.*

ciliaris (sĭl-ī-ā'rĭs). ACTION: Alters shape of crystalline lens in accommodation. ORIGIN: (1) Meridional: Junction of cornea and sclera. (2) Circular: Fibers forming a circle close to iris. INSERTION: (1) External layers of choroid. (2) Ciliary process. INNERVATION: Short ciliary.

compressor naris (kŏm-prĕs'or nā'rĭs). ACTION: Narrows nostril. ORIGIN: Nasal aponeurosis, superior maxilla above incisive fossa. INSERTION: Aponeurosis of bridge of nose. INNERVATION: Facial.

corrugator supercilii (kor'ū-gā-tor sū-pĕr-sĭl'ĭ-ī). ACTION: Draws eyebrows down and in. ORIGIN: Inner end of superciliary arch. INSERTION: Skin above orbital arch. INNERVATION: Facial.

depressor alae nasi (dē-prĕs'or ā'lē nā'sī). SAME AS: *depressor septi.*

depressor anguli oris (dē-prĕs'or ăng'-ū-lī ō'rĭs). ACTION: Depresses angle of mouth. ORIGIN: External oblique line of mandible. INSERTION: Angle of mouth. INNERVATION: Facial. SYN: *triangularis.*

depressor labii inferioris (dē-prĕs'or lā'-bĭ-ī ĭn-fē"rĭ-ō'rĭs). ACTION: Depresses lower lip. ORIGIN: External oblique line of the mandible. INSERTION: Lower lip and orbicularis oris. INNERVATION: Facial. SYN: *quadratus labii inferioris; quadratus menti.*

depressor septi (dē-prĕs'or sĕp'tī). ACTION: Draws outer wall of nostril downward. ORIGIN: Incisive fossa of superior maxillary bone. INSERTION: Septum and ala of nose. INNERVATION: Facial. SYN: *depressor alae nasi.*

dilatator naris anterior (dĭl'ă-tā-tor nā'-rĭs ăn-tē'rĭ-or). ACTION: Dilates apertures of nostril. ORIGIN: Cartilage of ala of nose. INSERTION: Border of ala. INNERVATION: Facial.

dilatator naris posterior (dĭl'ă-tā-tor nā'rĭs pŏs-tē'rĭ-or). ACTION: Dilates apertures of nostril. ORIGIN: Nasal notch of superior maxilla and the sesamoid cartilages. INSERTION: Integument of margin of nostril. INNERVATION: Facial.

epicranius (ĕp-ĭ-krā'nĭ-ŭs). Scalp muscles consisting of occipitofrontalis and temporoparietalis connected by galea aponeurotica.

frontalis (frŏn-tā'lĭs). SEE: *occipitofrontalis.*

levator anguli oris (lē-vā'tor ăng'ū-lī o'rĭs). ACTION: Elevates angle of mouth. ORIGIN: Canine fossa of maxilla. INSERTION: Angle of mouth and orbicularis oris. INNERVATION: Facial. SYN: *caninus.*

levator labii inferioris (lē-vā'tor lā'bĭ-ī ĭn-fē"rĭ-ō'rĭs). SAME AS: *mentalis.*

levator labii superioris (lē-vā'tor lā'bĭ-ī sū-pē"rĭ-ō'rĭs). ACTION: Elevates and extends upper lip. ORIGIN: Lower margin of orbit, malar bone. INSERTION: Upper lip. INNERVATION: Infraorbital branch of facial.

levator labii superioris alaeque nasi (lē-vā'tor lā'bĭ-ī sū-pē"rĭ-ō'rĭs ā-lē'kwĕ nā'sī). ACTION: Elevates upper lip, dilates nostril. ORIGIN: Nasal process of maxilla. INSERTION: Cartilage of ala of nose and upper lip. INNERVATION: Infraorbital branch of facial.

levator menti (lē-vā'tor mĕn'tī). SAME AS: *mentalis.*

levator palpebrae superioris (lē-vā'tor păl'pē-brē sū-pē"rĭ-ō'rĭs). ACTION: Raises upper eyelid. ORIGIN: Lesser wing of the sphenoid bone. INSERTION: Upper tarsal cartilage. INNERVATION: Oculomotor.

masseter (mă-sē'tĕr). ACTION: Mastication. ORIGIN: Zygomatic arch and malar process of superior maxilla. INSERTION: Angle, ramus, and coronoid process of mandible. INNERVATION: Mandibular division of trigeminal.

mentalis (mĕn-tā'lĭs). ACTION: Elevates and protrudes lower lip; wrinkles skin of chin. ORIGIN: Incisive fossa of mandible. INSERTION: Integument of chin. INNERVATION: Facial. SYN: *levator labii inferioris; levator menti.*

nasalis (nā-sā'lĭs). Consists of compressor naris and depressor septi.

obliquus oculi inferior (ŏb-lī′kwŭs ŏc′ū-lī ĭn-fē′rĭ-or). ACTION: Rotates eyeball up and out. ORIGIN: Orbital plate of superior maxillary bone. INSERTION: Sclerotic coat at right angles to insertion of rectus externus just below it. INNERVATION: Oculomotor.

obliquus oculi superior (ŏb-lī′kwŭs ŏc′ū-lī sū-pē′rĭ-or). ACTION: Rotates eyeball down and out. ORIGIN: Above optic foramen. INSERTION: By a tendon through trochlea to the sclerotic coat. INNERVATION: Trochlear.

occipitalis (ŏk-sĭp″ĭ-tā′lĭs)). SEE: *occipitofrontalis.*

occipitofrontalis (ŏk-sĭp″ĭ-tō-frŏn-tā′lĭs). Consists of (1) occipitalis and (2) frontalis bellies. ACTION: (1) Draws scalp back. (2) Draws scalp forward; raises eyebrows. ORIGIN: (1) Occipital and temporal bones. (2) Procerus, corrugator, and orbicularis oris muscles. INSERTION: Galea aponeurotica. INNERVATION: Facial.

orbicularis oculi (or-bĭk″ū-lă′rĭs ŏk′ū-lī). ACTION: Closes eyelid, wrinkles forehead vertically, compresses lacrimal sac. ORIGIN: (1) (*Pars lacrimalis*) Lacrimal bone. (2) (*Pars orbitalis*) Frontal processes of maxilla and frontal bone. (3) (*Pars palpebralis*) Inner canthus. INSERTION: (1) Joins palpebral portion. (2) Encircles orbit to orbit. (3) Outer canthus. INNERVATION: Facial.

orbicularis oris (or-bĭk″ū-lă′rĭs ō′rĭs). ACTION: Closes lips. ORIGIN: Nasal septum and canine fossa of mandible by accessory fibers. INSERTION: Buccinator and adjacent muscles surrounding mouth. INNERVATION: Facial.

orbicularis palpebrarum (or-bĭk″ū-lă′rĭs păl-pē-brā′rŭm). SAME AS: *orbicularis oculi (Pars palpebralis).*

orbitalis (or-bĭ-tā′lĭs). Circular division of ciliaris.

orbitopalpebralis (or″bĭ-tō-păl″pē-brā′lĭs). SAME AS: *levator palpebrae superioris.*

procerus (prō-sē′rŭs). ACTION: Draws skin of forehead down. ORIGIN: Bridge of nose. INSERTION: Skin over root of nose. INNERVATION: Facial. SYN: *pyramidalis nasi.*

pterygoideus lateralis (tĕr-ĭ-goyd′ē-ŭs lăt-ĕr-ăl′ĭs). ACTION: Brings jaw forward; moves jaw from side to side; opens jaws. ORIGIN: 1. Outer plate of pterygoid process. 2. Great wing of sphenoid and infratemporal ridge. INSERTION: Neck of condyle of mandible. INNERVATION: Lateral pterygoid from trigeminal n.

pterygoideus medialis (tĕr-ĭ-goyd′ē-ŭs mē-dĭ-ā′lĭs). ACTION: Closes jaw by raising and advancing it. ORIGIN: Pterygoid fossa of sphenoid bone. INSERTION: Inner surface of angle of mandible. INNERVATION: Medial pterygoid from trigeminal n.

pyramidalis nasi (pĭ-răm″ĭ-dā′lĭs nā′sī). SAME AS: *procerus.*

quadratus labii inferioris (kwăd-rā′tŭs lā′-bĭ-ī ĭn-fē″rĭ-ō′rĭs). SAME AS: *depressor labii inferioris.*

quadratus labii superioris (kwăd-rā-tŭs lā′bĭ-ī sū-pēr″ĭ-ō′rĭs). Composed of *levator labii superioris alaeque nasi, levator labii superioris, zygomaticus minor.*

quadratus menti (kwăd-rā′tŭs mĕn′tī). SAME AS: *depressor labii inferioris.*

rectus externus or **lateralis** (rĕk′tŭs ĕks-ter′nŭs, lăt-ĕr-ā′lĭs). ACTION: Rotates eyeball outward. ORIGIN: Margin of sphenoidal fissure and outer margin of optic foramen. INSERTION: Sclerotic coat. INNERVATION: Abducent.

rectus inferior (rĕk′tŭs ĭn-fē′rĭ-or). ACTION: Rotates eyeball downward. ORIGIN: Lower margin of optic foramen. INSERTION: Sclerotic coat. INNERVATION: Oculomotor.

rectus internus or **medialis** (rĕk′tŭs ĭnter′-nŭs, mē-dĭ-ā′lĭs). ACTION: Rotates eyeball inward. ORIGIN: Lower margin of optic foramen. INSERTION: Sclerotic coat. INNERVATION: Oculomotor.

rectus superior (rĕk′tŭs sū-pē′rĭ-or). ACTION: Rotates eyeball upward. ORIGIN: Upper margin of optic foramen. INSERTION: Sclerotic coat. INNERVATION: Oculomotor.

retrahens aurem (rĕt′ră-hĕns aw′rĕm). SAME AS: *auricularis posterior.*

risorius (rĭ-sō′rĭ-ŭs) (*laughing muscle*). ACTION: Draws angle of mouth outward and compresses cheek. ORIGIN: Fascia over masseter muscle. INSERTION: Angle of mouth. INNERVATION: Facial; buccal branch.

temporalis (tĕm-pō-rā′lĭs). ACTION: Closes jaws. ORIGIN: Temporal fossa and temporal fascia. INSERTION: Coronoid process of lower jaw. INNERVATION: Trigeminal; mandibular division. SYN: *temporal.*

tensor tarsi (tĕn′sor tar′sī). SAME AS: *Pars lacrimalis of orbicularis oculi muscle.*

triangularis (trī-ăng″gū-lā′rĭs). SAME AS: *depressor anguli oris.*

zygomaticus major (zī-gō-măt′ĭ-kŭs mā′-jor). ACTION: Draws upper lip backward, upward and outward. ORIGIN: Malar bone, zygomatic arch. INSERTION: Angle of mouth. INNERVATION: Facial.

zygomaticus minor (zī-gō-măt′ĭ-kŭs mī′-nor). ACTION: Draws the upper lip up and out. ORIGIN: Malar bone behind the maxillary arch. INSERTION: Angle of mouth, orbicularis oris. INNERVATION: Facial.

EAR

antitragicus (an-tĭ-tră′jĭ-kŭs). ORIGIN: Anterior part of antitragus. INSERTION: Opposite side at larger auricular fissure. INNERVATION: Posterior auricular branch of facial.

helicis major and **minor** (hĕl′ĭ-sĭs mā′jŏr, mī′nŏr). ACTION: Tighten the skin of auditory canal. ORIGIN: Tuberosity on helix. INSERTION: Rim of helix. INNERVATION: Auriculotemporal and posterior auricular.

obliquus auriculae (ŏb-lī′kwŭs aw-rĭk′ū-lē). ORIGIN: Conch of the ear. INSERTION: Fossa of antihelix. INNERVATION: Posterior auricular branch of facial.

stapedius (stă-pē′dĭ-ŭs). ACTION: Depress base of the stapes. ORIGIN: Interior of pyramid. INSERTION: Neck of stapes. INNERVATION: Tympanic branch of facial.

tensor tympani (tĕn′sor tĭm′păn-ī). ACTION: To draw the membrana tympani tense. ORIGIN: Temporal tube, eustachian tube and canal. INSERTION: Handle of malleus. INNERVATION: Branch of mandibular through otic ganglion.

tragicus (tră′jĭ-kŭs). ORIGIN and INSERTION: Outer part of tragus. INNERVATION: Temporal branch of facial.

transversus auriculae (trăns-vĕr′sŭs aw-rĭk′ū-lē). ACTION: Retracts helix. ORIGIN: Cranial surface of pinna. INSERTION: Circumference of pinna. INNER-

VATION: Posterior auricular branch of facial.

NECK

amygdaloglossus (ăm-ĭg″dă-lō-glŏs′ŭs). ACTION: Lifts edge of tongue. ORIGIN: Pharyngeal aponeurosis over tonsil. INSERTION: Continuous with palatoglossus.

azygos uvulae (ăz′ĭ-gōs ū′vū-lē). SAME AS: *uvulae.*

cephalopharyngeus (sĕf″ă-lō-făr-ĭn-jē′ŭs). SAME AS: *constrictor pharyngis superior.*

circumflexus palati (sĭr-kŭm-flĕks′ŭs păl-ă′tī). SAME AS: *tensor veli palatini.*

constrictor pharyngis inferior (kŏn-strĭk′-tor făr-ĭn′gĭs ĭn-fē′ĭ-ōr). ACTION: Narrows the pharynx, as in swallowing. ORIGIN: Sides of cricoid and thyroid cartilages. INSERTION: Posterior raphe of pharyngeal wall. INNERVATION: Pharyngeal plexus. SYN: *inferior constrictor; laryngopharyngeus.*

constrictor pharyngis medius (kŏn-strĭk′tor făr-ĭn′gĭs mē′dĭ-ŭs). ACTION: Narrows pharynx, as in swallowing. ORIGIN: Both cornua of hyoid bone and stylohyoid ligament. INSERTION: Middle of posterior pharyngeal wall. INNERVATION: Pharyngeal plexus. SYN: *middle constrictor; hyopharyngeus.*

constrictor pharyngis superior (kŏn-strĭk′-tor făr-ĭn′gĭs sū-pē′ĭ-ōr). ACTION: Narrows pharynx, as in swallowing. ORIGIN: Internal pterygoid plate, pterygomandibular ligament, jaw, side of tongue. INSERTION: Posterior pharyngeal wall. INNERVATION: Pharyngeal plexus. SYN: *superior constrictor; cephalopharyngeus.*

digastricus (dī-găs′trĭ-kŭs). Consists of (1) anterior and (2) posterior bellies. ACTION: (1) Draws hyoid bone forward. (2) Draws hyoid bone backward. ORIGIN: (1) Lower border of lower jaw. (2) Mastoid groove of temporal bone. INSERTION: Intermediate tendon between both bellies. INNERVATION: (1) Mylohyoid. (2) Facial.

genioglossus (jē-nī″ō-glŏs′ŭs). ACTION: Protrudes and retracts tongue, elevates hyoid. ORIGIN: Mental spine of inferior maxilla. INSERTION: Hyoid and bottom of tongue. INNERVATION: Hypoglossal.

geniohyoglossus (jē-nī″ō-hī″ō-glŏs′ŭs). SAME AS: *genioglossus.*

geniohyoideus (jē-nī″ō-hī-oyd′ē-ŭs). ACTION: Elevates and advances hyoid and helps to depress jaw. ORIGIN: Mental spine of inferior maxilla. INSERTION: Hyoid. INNERVATION: Hypoglossal. SYN: *geniohyoid muscle.*

glossopalatinus (glŏs″ō-păl-ă-tī′nŭs). ACTION: Elevates back of tongue and constricts fauces. ORIGIN: Undersurface of soft palate. INSERTION: Side of tongue. INNERVATION: Pharyngeal plexus. SYN: *palatoglossus.*

hyoglossus (hī″ō-glŏs′ŭs). ACTION: Depresses side of tongue and retracts tongue. ORIGIN: Cornua and body of hyoid. INSERTION: Side of tongue. INNERVATION: Hypoglossal.

hyopharyngeus (hī″ō-făr-ĭn-jē-ŭs). SAME AS: *constrictor pharyngis medius.*

laryngopharyngeus (lăr-ĭn″gō-făr-ĭn-jē′-ŭs). SAME AS: *constrictor pharyngis inferior.*

latissimus colli (lăt-ĭs′ĭ-mŭs kŏl′ī). SAME AS: *platysma.*

levator palati (lē-vā′tor păl′ă-tī). SAME AS: *levator veli palatini.*

levator veli palatini (lē-vā′tor vē′lī păl″ă-tī′nī). ACTION: Elevates soft palate. ORIGIN: Petrous portion of temporal bone and cartilaginous eustachian tube. INSERTION: Aponeurosis of soft palate. INNERVATION: Pharyngeal plexus.

lingualis (lĭng-gwā′lĭs). ACTION: Elevates sides and center of tongue. ORIGIN: Undersurface of tongue. INSERTION: Edge of tongue. INNERVATION: Hypoglossal.

longus capitis (lŏng′ŭs kăp′ĭ-tĭs). ACTION: Flexes head. ORIGIN: Transverse processes of 3rd to 6th cervical vertebrae. INSERTION: Occipital bone, basilar process. INNERVATION: Branches of 1st to 3rd cervical nerves. SYN: *rectus capitis anticus major.*

longus cervicis (lŏng′ŭs sĕr′vĭ-sĭs). SAME AS: *longus colli.*

longus colli (lŏng′ŭs kŏl′ī). Consists of three parts: (1) superior oblique, (2) inferior oblique, and (3) vertical. ACTION: Twists and bends neck forward. ORIGIN: (1) Transverse processes of 3rd to 5th cervical vertebrae. (2) Bodies of 1st to 3rd thoracic vertebrae. (3) Bodies of 3 upper thoracic and 3 lower cervical vertebrae. INSERTION: 1. Anterior tubercle of atlas. 2. Transverse processes of 5th and 6th cervical vertebrae. 3. Bodies of 2nd to 4th cervical vertebrae. INNERVATION: Branches of 2nd to 7th cervical nerves.

mylohyoideus (mī″lō-hī-oyd′ē-ŭs). ACTION: Elevates floor of mouth and hyoid, depresses jaw. ORIGIN: Mylohyoid line of mandible. INSERTION: Body of hyoid and median raphe. INNERVATION: Mylohyoid. SYN: *mylohyoid muscle.*

omohyoideus (ō″mō-hī-oyd′ē-ŭs). ACTION: Depresses hyoid. ORIGIN: Upper border of scapula. INSERTION: Hyoid bone. INNERVATION: Upper cervical through ansa hypoglossi. SYN: *omohyoid muscle.*

palatoglossus (păl″ă-tō-glŏs′ŭs). SAME AS: *glossopalatinus.*

palatopharyngeus (păl″ă-tō-făr-ĭn′jē-ŭs). SAME AS: *pharyngopalatinus.*

pharyngopalatinus (făr-ĭng″gō-păl-ă-tī′-nŭs). ACTION: Narrows fauces and shuts off nasopharynx. ORIGIN: Soft palate. INSERTION: Thyroid cartilage and aponeurosis of the pharynx. INNERVATION: Pharyngeal plexus.

platysma (plă-tĭz′mă). ACTION: Wrinkles skin of neck and chest; depresses jaw and lower lip. ORIGIN: Clavicle, acromion and fascia over deltoid, and pectoralis major. INSERTION: Lower border of mandible, risorius and opposite platysma. INNERVATION: Cervical branch of facial. SYN: *latissimus colli; tetragonus.*

rectus capitis anterior (rĕk′tŭs kăp′ĭ-tĭs ăn-tēr′ĭ-or). ACTION: Turns and inclines the head. ORIGIN: Base of atlas. INSERTION: Occipital bone, basilar process. INNERVATION: Between 1st and 2nd cervical.

rectus capitis anticus major (rĕk′tŭs kăp′ĭ-tĭs ăn-tī′kŭs mā′jor). SAME AS: *longus capitis.*

rectus capitis anticus minor (rĕk′tŭs kăp′ĭ-tĭs ăn-tī′kŭs mī′nor). SAME AS: *rectus capitis anterior.*

rectus capitis lateralis (rĕk′tŭs kăp′ĭ-tĭs lătĕr-ā′lĭs). ACTION: Inclines head laterally and supports it. ORIGIN: Transverse process of atlas. INSERTION: Jugular process of occipital bone. INNERVATION: Between 1st and 2nd cervical nerves.

salpingopharyngeus săl-pĭn″gō-făr-ĭn′jē-ŭs). ACTION: Elevates nasopharynx. ORIGIN: Eustachian tube close to nasopharynx. INSERTION: Posterior portion of the pharyngopalatinus. INNERVATION: Pharyngeal plexus.

scalenus anterior (skā-lē′nŭs ăn-tē′rĭ-or). ACTION: Elevates 1st rib and flexes neck. ORIGIN: Transverse processes of 3rd to 6th cervical vertebrae. INSERTION: Tubercle of 1st rib. INNERVATION: Cervical plexus. SYN: *scalenus anticus.*

scalenus medius (skā-lē′nŭs mē′dĭ-ŭs). ACTION: Elevates 1st rib and flexes neck. ORIGIN: Transverse processes of 2nd to 6th cervical vertebrae. INSERTION: First rib. INNERVATION: Cervical plexus.

scalenus posterior (skā-lē′nŭs pŏs-tēr′ĭ-ŏr). ACTION: Elevates 2nd rib and flexes neck. ORIGIN: Transverse processes of 4th to 6th cervical vertebrae. INSERTION: Second rib. INNERVATION: Cervical and brachial plexus. SYN: *scalenus posticus.*

sphenosalpingostaphylinus (sfē″nō-săl-pĭn″-gō-stăf-ĭ-lī′nŭs). SAME AS: *tensor veli palatini.*

sternocleidomastoideus (stĕr″nō-klī-dō-măs-toyd′ē-ŭs). ACTION: Rotates and depresses head. ORIGIN: By 2 heads, from sternum and clavicle. INSERTION: Mastoid process and outer part of superior curved line of occipital bone. INNERVATION: Spinal accessory. SYN: *sternomastoid muscle.*

sternohyoideus (stĕr″nō-hī-oyd′ē-ŭs). ACTION: Depresses hyoid bone. ORIGIN: Manubrium sterni and 1st costal cartilage. INSERTION: Body of hyoid bone. INNERVATION: Upper cervical through ansa hypoglossi. SYN: *sternohyoid muscle.*

sternothyreoideus (stĕr″nō-thī-rē-oyd′-ē-ŭs). ACTION: Depresses thyroid cartilage. ORIGIN: Sternum and 1st costal cartilage. INSERTION: Side of thyroid cartilage. INNERVATION: Upper cervical through ansa hypoglossi. SYN: *sternothyroid muscle.*

styloglossus (stī″lō-glŏs′ŭs). ACTION: Retracts and elevates tongue. ORIGIN: Styloid process. INSERTION: Side of tongue. INNERVATION: Hypoglossal.

stylohyoideus (stī″lō-hī-oyd′ē-ŭs). ACTION: Fixes hyoid, drawing it up and back. ORIGIN: Styloid process. INSERTION: Body of hyoid bone. INNERVATION: Facial. SYN: *stylohyoid muscle.*

stylopharyngeus (stī″lō-făr-ĭn′jē-ŭs). ACTION: Elevates and dilates pharynx. ORIGIN: Styloid process. INSERTION: Thyroid cartilage and side of pharynx. INNERVATION: Glossopharyngeal.

tensor palati (tĕn′sŏr păl-ă′tī). SAME AS: *tensor veli palatini.*

tensor veli palatini (tĕn′sŏr vē′lī păl″ă-tī′-nī). ACTION: Stretches soft palate. ORIGIN: Spine of sphenoid, scaphoid fossa of internal pterygoid process and eustachian tube. INSERTION: Posterior border of hard palate and aponeurosis of soft palate. INNERVATION: Otic ganglion, trigeminal nerve. SYN: *tensor palati; circumflexus palati; sphenosalpingostaphylinus.*

tetragonus (tĕt-ră-gō′nŭs). SAME AS: *platysma.*

thyreohyoideus (thī-rē-ō-hī-oyd′ē-ŭs). ACTION: Depresses hyoid bone; elevates thyroid cartilage if hyoid bone is fixed. ORIGIN: Side of thyroid cartilage. INSERTION: Cornu and body of hyoid bone. INNERVATION: Hypoglossal. SYN: *thyrohyoid muscle.*

uvulae (ū′vū-lē). ACTION: Elevates the uvula ORIGIN: Posterior nasal spine. INSERTION: Forms large part of uvula. INNERVATION: Pharyngeal plexus.

LARYNX AND EPIGLOTTIS

aryepiglotticus (ar-ĭ-ĕp-ĭ-glŏt′ĭk-ŭs). ACTION: Closes glottis opening. ORIGIN: Arytenoid cartilage. INSERTION: Epiglottis. INNERVATION: Laryngeal, recurrent.

arytenoideus (ăr-ĭ-tē-noyd′ē-ŭs). Consists of (1) arytenoideus obliquus and (2) arytenoideus transversus. ACTION: Closes glottis opening. ORIGIN: Arytenoid cartilage. INSERTION: (1) Aryepiglottic fold. (2) Crosses between the two cartilages of the obliquus portion. INNERVATION: Laryngeal, recurrent.

cricoarytenoideus lateralis (krī″kō-ăr-ĭ-tē-noyd′ē-ŭs lăt-ĕr-ă′lĭs). ACTION: Narrows glottis. ORIGIN: Upper border of arch of cricoid cartilage. INSERTION: Muscular process of arytenoid cartilage. INNERVATION: Laryngeal, recurrent.

cricoarytenoideus posterior (krī″kō-ăr-ĭ-tē-noyd′ē-ŭs pŏs-tē′rĭ-or). ACTION: Opens glottis. ORIGIN: Back of cricoid cartilage. INSERTION: Muscular process of arytenoid cartilage. INNERVATION: Laryngeal, recurrent.

cricothyroideus (krī″kō-thī-royd′ē-ŭs). ACTION: Tightens vocal cords. ORIGIN: Anterior surface of cricoid cartilage. INSERTION: Thyroid cartilage. INNERVATION:Laryngeal, superior. SYN: *cricothyroid.*

thyreoarytenoideus (thī″rē-ō-ăr-ĭ-tē-noyd′ē-ŭs). ACTION: Relaxes vocal cords. ORIGIN: Thyroid cartilage. INSERTION: Arytenoid cartilage. INNERVATION: Laryngeal, recurrent. SYN: *thyroarytenoid.*

thyreoepiglotticus (thī″rē-ō-ĕp-ĭ-glŏt′-ĭk-ŭs). ACTION: Depresses epiglottis. ORIGIN: Thyroid cartilage. INSERTION: Epiglottis and sacculus laryngis. INNERVATION: Laryngeal, recurrent. SYN: *thyroepiglotticus.*

BACK

accessorius (ăk″sĕs-sō′rĭ-ŭs). SAME AS: *iliocostalis thoracis.*

biventer cervicis (bī-vĕn′tĕr sĕr′vĭ-sĭs). SAME AS: *spinalis capitis.*

cervicalis ascendens (sĕr-vĭ-kă′lĭs ă-sĕn′-dĕns). SAME AS: *iliocostalis cervicis.*

complexus (kŏm-plĕks′ŭs). SAME AS: *semispinalis capitis.*

erector spinae (ē-rĕk′tor spī′nē). SAME AS: *sacrospinalis.*

iliocostalis cervicis (ĭl″ĭ-ō-kŏs-tā′lĭs sĕr′-vĭ-sĭs). ACTION: Extends cervical spine. ORIGIN: Angles of 3rd to 6th ribs. INSERTION: Transverse processes of 4th to 6th cervical vertebrae. INNERVATION: Branches of cervical. SYN: *cervicalis ascendens.*

iliocostalis dorsi (ĭl″ĭ-ō-kŏs-tā′lĭs dor′sī). SAME AS: *iliocostalis thoracis.*

iliocostalis lumborum (ĭl″ĭ-ō-kŏs-tā′lĭs lŭm-bō′rŭm). ACTION: Extends lumbar spine. ORIGIN: With sarcospinalis. INSERTION: In angles of 5th to 12th ribs. INNERVATION: Branches of dorsal and lumbar. SYN: *sacrolumbalis.*

iliocostalis thoracis (ĭl″ĭ-ō-kŏs-tā′lĭs thō-răs′ĭs). ACTION: Keeps dorsal spine erect. ORIGIN: Angles of 12th to 7th ribs. INSERTION: Sixth to 1st ribs and 7th cervical vertebra. INNERVATION:

Branches of dorsal. SYN: *iliocostalis dorsi; accessorius.*

interspinales (ĭn″tĕr-spī-nā′lēz). A series. ACTION: Support and extend vertebral column. ORIGIN: Undersurface of spine of one vertebra. INSERTION: Spine of vertebra above. INNERVATION: Branches of spinal.

intertransversales (ĭn-tĕr-trăns-vĕr-sā′-lēz). SAME AS: *intertransversarii.*

intertransversarii (ĭn″tĕr-trăns-vĕr-sā′-rĭ-ī). ACTION: Flex vertebral column. ORIGIN: Between transverse processes of contiguous vertebrae. INNERVATION: Branches of ventral and dorsal divisions of spinal. SYN: *intertransversales.*

latissimus dorsi (lăt-ĭs′ĭ-mŭs dŏr′sī). ACTION: Adducts, extends and rotates arm. ORIGIN: Lower thoracic and lumbar vertebrae, sacrum and tip of iliac crest. INSERTION: Intertubercular groove of humerus. INNERVATION: Brachial plexus.

levator scapulae (lē-vā′tor skăp′ū-lē). ACTION: Elevates posterior angle of scapula. ORIGIN: Transverse processes of four upper cervical vertebrae. INSERTION: Superior edge of scapula. INNERVATION: Dorsal scapular from 5th cervical, and branches of 3rd and 4th cervical. SYN: *levator anguli scapulae.*

longissimus capitis (lŏn-jĭs′ĭ-mŭs kăp′ĭ-tĭs). ACTION: Keeps head erect, draws it backward or to one side. ORIGIN: Upper thoracic and lower and middle cervical vertebrae. INSERTION: Mastoid process. INNERVATION: Branches of cervical. SYN: *trachelomastoid.*

longissimus cervicis (lŏn-jĭs′ĭ-mŭs sĕr′vĭ-sĭs). ACTION: Extends cervical spine. ORIGIN: Upper thoracic vertebrae. INSERTION: Ribs and upper lumbar and thoracic vertebrae. INNERVATION: Branches of dorsal divisions of spinal. SYN: *transversalis colli.*

longissimus dorsi (lŏn-jĭs′ĭ-mŭs dor′sī). SAME AS: *longissimus thoracis.*

longissimus thoracis (lŏn-jĭs′ĭ-mŭs thŏr-ā′sĭs). ACTION: Extends spinal column. ORIGIN: Transverse processes of lumbar and dorsal vertebrae. INSERTION: Lowest ribs and lumbar and dorsal vertebrae. INNERVATION: Lumbar and dorsal divisions of spinal. SYN: *longissimus dorsi.*

multifidus (mŭl-tĭf′ĭd-ŭs). ACTION: Rotates spinal column. ORIGIN: Sacrum, iliac spine, lumbar, cervical, and dorsal vertebrae. INSERTION: Laminae and spinous processes of next four vertebrae above. INNERVATION: Branches of dorsal divisions of spinal.

multifidus spinae (mŭl-tĭf′ĭd-ŭs spī′nē). SAME AS: *multifidus.*

obliquus capitis inferior (ŏb-lī′kwŭs kăp′ĭ-tĭs ĭn-fĕr′ĭ-or). ACTION: Rotates head. ORIGIN: Spine of axis. INSERTION: Transverse process of atlas. INNERVATION: Suboccipital.

obliquus capitis superior (ŏb-lī′kwŭs kăp′-ĭ-tĭs sū-pĕr′ĭ-or). ACTION: Rotates head. ORIGIN: Transverse process of atlas. INSERTION: Occipital bone. INNERVATION: Suboccipital.

rectus capitis posterior major (rĕk′tŭs kăp′ĭ′tĭs pŏs-tē′rĭ-or mā′jor). ACTION: Rotates and draws head backward. ORIGIN: Spine of axis. INSERTION: Inferior curved line of occipital bone. INNERVATION: Suboccipital. SYN: *rectus capitis posticus major.*

rectus capitis posterior minor (rĕk′tŭs kăp′ĭ-tĭs pŏs-tē′rĭ-or mī′nor). ACTION: Rotates and draws head backward. ORIGIN: Posterior tubercle of atlas. INSERTION: Inferior curved line of occipital bone. INNERVATION: Suboccipital. SYN: *rectus capitis posticus minor.*

rhomboideus major (rŏm-boy′dē-ŭs mā′jor). ACTION: Elevates scapula. ORIGIN: Spinous processes of 2nd to 5th thoracic vertebrae. INSERTION: Vertebral border of scapula below spine. INNERVATION: Dorsal scapular from brachial plexus.

rhomboideus minor (rŏm-boy′dē-ŭs mī′nor). ACTION: Retracts and elevates scapula. ORIGIN: Spinous processes of 7th cervical vertebra and 1st thoracic vertebra. INSERTION: Border of scapula above spine. INNERVATION: Dorsal scapular from brachial plexus.

rotatores (rō-tā-tō′rēz). ACTION: Extend and rotate the vertebral column. ORIGIN: Transverse processes of 2nd to 12th dorsal vertebrae. INSERTION: Lamina of next vertebra above. INNERVATION: Branches of dorsal divisions of spinal. SYN: *rotatores spinae.*

rotatores spinae (rō-tā-tō′rēz spī′nē). SAME AS: *rotatores.*

sacrolumbalis (sā″krō-lŭm-bā′lĭs). SAME AS: *iliocostalis lumborum.*

sacrospinalis (sā″krō-spī-nā′lĭs). ACTION: Extends vertebral column. ORIGIN: Sacrum, lumbar vertebrae, iliac crest. INSERTION: Iliocostalis and longissimus dorsi. INNERVATION: Posterior branches of spinal.

semispinalis capitis (sĕm″ĭ-spī-nā′lĭs kăp′ĭ-tĭs). ACTION: Rotates and draws head backward. ORIGIN: Transverse processes of upper six or seven thoracic and lower four cervical vertebrae. INSERTION: Occipital bone, between inferior and superior curved line. INNERVATION: Branches of dorsal divisions of cervical. SYN: *complexus.*

semispinalis cervicis (sĕm″ĭ-spī-nā′lĭs sĕr′vĭ-sĭs). ACTION: Erects cervical spine. ORIGIN: Transverse processes of upper five or six thoracic vertebrae. INSERTION: Spines from axis to 5th cervical vertebra. INNERVATION: Branches of dorsal divisions of spinal.

semispinalis colli (sĕm″ĭ-spī-nā′lĭs kŏl′ī). SAME AS: *semispinalis cervicis.*

semispinalis dorsi (sĕm″ĭ-spī-nā′lĭs dor′sī). SAME AS: *semispinalis thoracis.*

semispinalis thoracis (sĕm″ĭ-spī-nā′lĭs thō-rā′sĭs). ACTION: Erects vertebral column. ORIGIN: Transverse processes of 6th to 10th thoracic vertebrae. INSERTION: Spines of upper four thoracic and lower two cervical vertebrae. INNERVATION: Branches of dorsal divisions of spinal. SYN: *semispinalis dorsi.*

serratus posterior inferior (sĕr-ā′tŭs pŏs-tē′rĭ-or ĭn-fē′rĭ-or). ACTION: Draws ribs back and downward. ORIGIN: Spines of lower two thoracic and upper two lumbar vertebrae. INSERTION: Lower four ribs. INNERVATION: Branches of ventral divisions of 9th to 12th thoracic. SYN: *serratus posticus inferior.*

serratus posterior superior (sĕr-ā′tŭs pŏs-tē′rĭ-or sū-pē′rĭ-or). ACTION: Elevates the ribs. ORIGIN: Spines of 7th cervical and two upper thoracic vertebrae. INSERTION: Angles of 2nd to 5th ribs. INNERVATION: Branches of ventral divisions of thoracic. SYN: *serratus posticus superior.*

spinalis capitis (spī-nă'lĭs kăp'ĭ-tĭs). ORIGIN: Inconstant; from spines of upper dorsal and lower cervical vertebrae. INSERTION: Blends with the semispinalis capitis. SYN: *biventer capitis.*

spinalis cervicis (spī-nă'lĭs sĕr'vĭ-sĭs). ACTION: Extends cervical spine. ORIGIN: Spines of 5th, 6th, and 7th cervical vertebrae. INSERTION: Axis and, occasionally, the two vertebrae below. INNERVATION: Branches of cervical.

spinalis thoracis (spī-nă'lĭs thō-rā'sĭs). ACTION: Erects spinal column. ORIGIN: Spines of first two lumbar and last two thoracic vertebrae. INSERTION: Spines of middle and upper thoracic vertebrae. INNERVATION: Dorsal branches of spinal. SYN: *spinalis dorsi.*

splenius capitis (splē'nĭ-ŭs kăp'ĭ-tĭs). ACTION: Rotates and extends head. ORIGIN: Ligamentum nuchae, 7th cervical and first three thoracic vertebrae. INSERTION: Mastoid process and superior curved line of occiput. INNERVATION: Branches of dorsal divisions of cervical.

splenius cervicis (splē'nĭ-ŭs sĕr'vĭ-sĭs). ACTION: Rotates and flexes head and neck. ORIGIN: Spines of 3rd to 6th thoracic vertebrae. INSERTION: Transverse processes of 1st and 2nd cervical vertebrae. INNERVATION: Branches of dorsal divisions of cervical. SYN: *splenius colli.*

splenius colli (splē'nĭ-ŭs kŏl'ī). SAME AS: *splenius cervicis.*

supraspinatus (sū-pră-spī-nā'tŭs). ACTION: Abducts arm. ORIGIN: Supraspinatous fossa. INSERTION: Greater tuberosity of humerus. INNERVATION: Branches of suprascapular.

suspensorius duodeni (sŭs-pĕn-sō'rĭ-ŭs dū"ō-dē'nī). Wide, flat band of unstriped muscle attached to the left crus of diaphragm and continuous with the muscular coat of the duodenum at its line of junction with the jejunum.

trachelomastoid (trā"kē-lō-măs'toyd). SAME AS: *longissimus capitis.*

transversalis colli (trăns"vĕr-să'lĭs kŏl'ī) SAME AS: *longissimus cervicis.*

trapezius (tră-pē'zĭ-ŭs). ACTION: Draws head back and to the side, rotates scapula. ORIGIN: Superior curved line of occipital, spinous processes of 7th cervical and all thoracic vertebrae. INSERTION: Clavicle, acromion, base of spine of scapula. INNERVATION: Spinal accessory and cervical plexus.

ABDOMEN

cremaster (krē-măs'tĕr). ACTION: Raises testicle. ORIGIN: Midportion of inguinal ligament. INSERTION: Cremasteric fascia and pubic bone. INNERVATION: Genitofemoral.

obliquus externus abdominis (ŏb-lī'kwŭs ĕks-tĕr'nŭs ăb-dŏm'ĭ-nĭs). ACTION: Contracts abdomen and viscera. ORIGIN: Lower 8 ribs. INSERTION: Iliac crest, Poupart's ligament, linea alba, pubic crest. INNERVATION: Iliohypogastric, ilioinguinal, and branches of intercostal.

obliquus internus abdominis (ŏb-lī'kwŭs in-tĕr'nŭs ăb-dŏm'ĭ-nĭs). ACTION: Compresses viscera, flexes thorax forward. ORIGIN: Iliac crest, inguinal ligament, lumbar fascia. INSERTION: Few lowest ribs, linea alba, pubic crest. INNERVATION: Iliohypogastric, ilioinguinal, and branches of intercostal.

pyramidalis (pĭ-răm-ĭ-dă'lĭs). ACTION: Tightens linea alba. ORIGIN: Pubic crest. INSERTION: Linea alba. INNERVATION: Branch of 12th thoracic.

quadratus lumborum (kwăd-rā'tŭs lŭm-bō'rŭm). ACTION: Flexes trunk laterally and forward. ORIGIN: Iliac crest, iliolumbar ligament, lower lumbar vertebrae. INSERTION: Twelfth rib and the upper lumbar vertebrae. INNERVATION: Branches of 1st lumbar and 12th thoracic.

rectus abdominis (rĕk'tŭs ăb-dŏm'ĭ-nĭs). ACTION: Compresses abdomen. ORIGIN: Pubis. INSERTION: Cartilage of 5th to 7th ribs. INNERVATION: Branches of 7th to 12th intercostal.

sphincter pylori (sfĭnk'tĕr pī-lō'rī). A thickening of middle circular layer of the gastric musculature surrounding the pylorus.

transversalis abdominis (trăns"vĕr-să'lĭs ăb-dŏm'ĭ-nĭs). SAME AS: *transversus abdominis.*

transversus abdominis (trăns"vĕr'sŭs ăb-dŏm'ĭ-nĭs). ACTION: Compresses abdomen, flexes thorax. ORIGIN: Lumbar fascia, 7th to 12th costal cartilages, inguinal ligament, iliac crest. INSERTION: Xiphoid cartilage, linea alba, pubic crest and iliopectineal line. INNERVATION: Iliohypogastric, ilioinguinal, and branches of intercostal.

PERINEUM

accelerator urinae (ăk-sĕl-ĕ-rā'tōr ū-rī'nē). SAME AS: *bulbocavernosus.*

bulbocavernosus (bŭl-bō-kă-vĕr-nō'sŭs). ACTION: Constricts bulbous urethra in male; in female constricts urethra. ORIGIN: Central point of perineum and median raphe. INSERTION: Undersurface of bulb, spongy and cavernous part of penis; root of clitoris. INNERVATION: Perineal branch of pudendal.

coccygeus (kŏk-sĭj'ē-ŭs). ACTION: Supports coccyx, closes pelvic outlet. ORIGIN: Ischial spine and sarcospinous ligament. INSERTION: Coccyx and lowest portion of sacrum. INNERVATION: Third and 4th sacral.

compressor urethrae (kŏm-prĕs'ŏr ū-rē'thrē). SAME AS: *sphincter urethrae membranaceae.*

constrictor urethrae (kŏn-strĭk'tŏr ū-rē'thrē). SAME AS: *sphincter urethrae membranaceae.*

corrugator cutis ani (kor-ū-gā'tŏr kū'tĭs ā'nī). ACTION: Wrinkles skin of anus. ORIGIN: Submucous tissue, interior of anus. INSERTION: Subcutaneous tissue on opposite side of anus. INNERVATION: Sympathetic.

depressor urethrae (dē-prĕs'ŏr ū-rē'thrē). ACTION: Depresses urethra. ORIGIN: Ramus of ischium near the transversus perinei profundus. INSERTION: Fibers of constrictor vaginae.

erector clitoridis (ē-rĕk'tŏr klĭ-tŏr'ĭ-dĭs). SAME AS: *ischiocavernosus.*

erector penis (ĕ-rĕk'tŏr pē'nĭs). SAME AS: *ischiocavernosus.*

ischiocavernosus (ĭs"kĭ-ō-kă-vĕr-nō'sŭs). ACTION: Maintains erection of penis or clitoris. ORIGIN: Tuberosity of ischium and great sacrosciatic ligament. INSERTION: Corpus cavernosum of clitoris or penis. INNERVATION: Perineal branch of pudendal. SYN: *erector clitoridis* (in female); *erector penis* (in male).

ischiococcygeus (ĭs"kĭ-ō-kŏk-sĭj'ē-ŭs). SAME AS: *coccygeus.*

levator ani (lē-vā'tōr ā'nī). ACTION: Supports rectum and pelvic floor, aids in defecation. ORIGIN: Pubis, pelvic fascia, ischial spine. INSERTION: Rectum, coccyx and fibrous raphe of perineum. INNERVATION: Sacral and perineal.

sphincter ani externus (sfĭnk'tĕr ā'nī ĕks-tĕr'nŭs). ACTION: Closes anus. ORIGIN: Ring of fibers surrounding anus. INSERTION: Coccyx and central point of perineum. INNERVATION: Hemorrhoidal branch of pudendal.

sphincter ani internus (sfĭnk'tĕr ā'nī ĭn-tĕr'nŭs). ACTION: Contracts rectum and anus, but not voluntarily. ORIGIN: Muscular ring of rectal fibers above canal.

sphincter urethrae membranaceae (sfĭnk'-tĕr ū-rē'thrē mĕm-bră-nā'sē-ē). ACTION: Constricts membranous urethra. ORIGIN: Ramus of pubis. INSERTION: Behind and in front of urethra. INNERVATION: Perineal branch of pudendal. SYN: *compressor urethrae; constrictor urethrae.*

sphincter vaginae (sfĭnk'tĕr vă-jī'nē). SAME AS: *bulbocavernosus.*

sphincter vesicae (sfĭnk'tĕr vĕs'ĭ-kē). ACTION: Shuts off internal orifice of urethra. ORIGIN: Near urethra orifice of bladder. INNERVATION: Sacral and hypogastric.

transversus perinei profundus (trăns-vĕr'-sŭs pĕr-ĭ-nē'ī prō-fŭn'dŭs). ACTION: Assists compressor urethrae. ORIGIN: Ramus of ischium. INSERTION: Central tendon. INNERVATION: Perineal branch of pudendal.

transversus perinei superficialis (trăns-vĕr'sŭs pĕr-ĭ-nē'ī sū"pĕr-fĭsh-ĭ-ā'lĭs). ACTION: Tenses central tendon. ORIGIN: Ramus of ischium. INSERTION: Central point of perineum. INNERVATION: Perineal branch of pudendal.

THORAX

diaphragma (dī"ă-frăg'mă). ACTION: Increases chest capacity. ORIGIN: Ensiform cartilage, 7th to 12th ribs, arcuate ligaments and lumbar vertebrae. INSERTION: Central tendon. INNERVATION: Phrenic.

infracostales (ĭn"fră-kŏs-tā'lēz). SAME AS: *subcostales.*

intercostales externus (ĭn"tĕr-kŏs-tā'lēz ĕks-tĕr'nŭs). ACTION: Draw ribs together and raise ribs. ORIGIN: Lower border of rib. INSERTION: Upper border of rib below. INNERVATION: Intercostal.

intercostales internus (ĭn"tĕr-kŏs-tā'lēz ĭn-tĕr'nŭs). ACTION: Draw ribs together and lower ribs. ORIGIN: Lower border of rib. INSERTION: Upper border of rib below. INNERVATION: Intercostal.

levatores costarum (lē-vā-tō'rēz kŏs-tā'-rŭm). ACTION: Raise ribs; flex vertebral column. ORIGIN: Transverse processes of 7th cervical and upper eleven thoracic vertebrae. INSERTION: Rib next below. INNERVATION: Branches of intercostal.

subcostales (sŭb-kŏs-tā'lēz). ACTION: Draw ribs together and lower ribs. ORIGIN: Inconstant; inner surface of the ribs. INSERTION: Inner surface of one of ribs just below. INNERVATION: Intercostal.

transversus thoracis (trăns-vĕr'sŭs thōr-ā'-sĭs). ACTION: Narrows the chest. ORIGIN: Xiphoid cartilage and sternum. INSERTION: Costal cartilages, 2nd to 6th ribs. INNERVATION: Branches of intercostal.

triangularis sterni (trī"ăn-gū-lā'rĭs stĕr'-nī). SAME AS: *transversus thoracis.*

SHOULDER

deltoideus (dĕl-toy'dē-ŭs). ACTION: Raises arm and rotates it. ORIGIN: Clavicle, acromion process and spine of scapula. INSERTION: Shaft of humerus. INNERVATION: Axillary (circumflex) from brachial plexus. SYN: *deltoid.*

infraspinatus (ĭn"fră-spī-nā'tŭs). ACTION: Rotates arm back and out. ORIGIN: Infraspinous fossa of scapula. INSERTION: Great tuberosity of humerus. INNERVATION: Suprascapular from brachial plexus.

pectoralis major (pĕk-tō-rā'lĭs mā'jōr). ACTION: Flexes, adducts and rotates arm. ORIGIN: Sternum, clavicle, and cartilages of 1st to 6th ribs. INSERTION: Bicipital ridge of humerus. INNERVATION: Anterior thoracic from brachial plexus.

pectoralis minor (pĕk-tō-rā'lĭs mī'nōr). ACTION: Draws down scapula and point of shoulder, raises ribs. ORIGIN: Third to 5th ribs. INSERTION: Coracoid process of scapula. INNERVATION: Anterior thoracic from brachial plexus.

serratus anterior (sĕr-ā'-tŭs ăn-tēr'ĭ-ōr). ACTION: Elevates ribs, rotates scapula. ORIGIN: Upper 8 or 9 ribs. INSERTION: Angles and vertebral border of scapula. INNERVATION: Long thoracic from brachial plexus.

serratus magnus (sĕr-ā'tŭs măg'nŭs). SAME AS: *serratus anterior.*

subclavius (sŭb-klā'vĭ-ŭs). ACTION: Draws clavicle down and forward or elevates the 1st rib. ORIGIN: First rib and its cartilage. INSERTION: Undersurface of clavicle. INNERVATION: Special nerve with fibers from 5th and 6th cervical.

subscapularis (sŭb-skăp-ū-lā'rĭs). ACTION: Rotates humerus inward and lowers it. ORIGIN: Subscapular fossa. INSERTION: Lesser tubercle of humerus. INNERVATION: Subscapular.

supraspinatus (sūp-ră-spī-nā'tŭs). ACTION: Abducts and raises arm. ORIGIN: Supraspinous fossa of scapula. INSERTION: Greater tubercle of humerus. INNERVATION: Branches of suprascapular.

teres major (tē'rēz mā'jor). ACTION: Rotates arm inward, draws it down and back. ORIGIN: Axillary border of scapula. INSERTION: Lesser tubercle of humerus. INNERVATION: Branch of lower subscapular.

teres minor (tē'rēz mī'nor). ACTION: Rotates arm outward. ORIGIN: Axillary border of scapula. INSERTION: Greater tubercle of humerus. INNERVATION: Branch of axillary (circumflex).

ARM AND FOREARM

abductor pollicis longus (ăb-dŭk'tōr pŏl'ĭ-sĭs lŏn'gŭs). ACTION: Abducts thumb and wrist. ORIGIN: Dorsal surface of radius, ulna and interosseous membrane. INSERTION: Base of 1st metacarpal. INNERVATION: Branch of radial. SYN: *extensor ossis metacarpi pollicis.*

anconeus (ăn-kō'nē-ŭs). ACTION: Extends forearm. ORIGIN: Lateral epicondyle of humerus. INSERTION: Olecranon and posterior surface of ulna. INNERVATION: Branch of radial.

biceps brachii (bī'sĕps brā'kĭ-ī). ACTION: Flexes arm and forearm and supinates hand. ORIGIN: 1. Short head from coracoid process. 2. Long head from scapula above glenoid fossa. INSERTION:

Bicipital tuberosity of radius. INNERVATION: Musculocutaneous.

brachialis (brā″kĭ-ā′lĭs). ACTION: Flexes forearm. ORIGIN: Lower half of anterior surface of humerus. INSERTION: Coronoid process of ulna. INNERVATION: Musculocutaneous and radial.

brachioradialis (brā″kĭ-ō-rā″dĭ-ā′lĭs). ACTION: Flexes and supinates forearm. ORIGIN: Supracondylar ridge of humerus. INSERTION: Styloid process of radius. INNERVATION: Branch of radial. SYN: *supinator longus.*

coracobrachialis (kor-ă-kō-brā″kĭ-ā′lĭs). ACTION: Raises and adducts arm. ORIGIN: Coracoid process of scapula. INSERTION: Middle of inner border of humerus. INNERVATION: Musculocutaneous.

extensor carpi radialis brevis (ĕks-tĕn′-sŏr kar′pī rā″dĭ-ā′lĭs brē′vĭs). ACTION: Extends and abducts wrist. ORIGIN: External condyloid ridge of humerus. INSERTION: Base of 3rd metacarpal. INNERVATION: Branch of radial.

extensor carpi radialis longus (ĕks-tĕn′-sŏr kar′pī rā″dĭ-ā′lĭs lŏng′gŭs). ACTION: Extends and abducts wrist. ORIGIN: External condyloid ridge of humerus. INSERTION: Base of 2nd metacarpal. INNERVATION: Branch of radial.

extensor carpi ulnaris (ĕks-tĕn′sŏr kar′pī ŭl-nā′rĭs). ACTION: Extends and abducts wrist. ORIGIN: Lateral epicondyle of humerus. INSERTION: Base of 5th metacarpal. INNERVATION: Branch of radial.

extensor digiti quinti proprius (ĕks-tĕn′sŏr dĭj′ĭ-tī kwĭn′tī prō′prĭ-ŭs). SAME AS: *extensor digiti minimi.*

extensor digitorum communis (ĕks-tĕn′sŏr dĭj-ĭ-tō′rŭm kŏm-mū′nĭs). ACTION: Extends fingers and wrist. ORIGIN: External epicondyle of humerus. INSERTION: Second and 3rd phalanges. INNERVATION: Branch of radial.

extensor indicis (ĕks-tĕn′sŏr ĭn′dĭ-sĭs). ACTION: Extends index finger. ORIGIN: Dorsal surface of ulna and interosseous membrane. INSERTION: First tendon of extensor digitorum communis. INNERVATION: Branch of radial.

extensor ossis metacarpi pollicis (ĕks-tĕn′-sŏr ŏs′ĭs mĕt″ă-kar′pī pŏl′ĭ-sĭs). SAME AS: *abductor pollicis longus.*

extensor digiti minimi (ĕks-tĕn′sŏr dĭj′-ĭ-tī′ mĭn′ĭm-ī). ACTION: Extends little finger. ORIGIN: External epicondyle of humerus. INSERTION: Dorsum of 1st phalanx of little finger. INNERVATION: Branch of radial. SYN: *extensor digiti quinti proprius.*

extensor pollicis brevis (ĕks-tĕn′sŏr pŏl′ĭ-sĭs brē′vĭs). ACTION: Extends thumb and abducts 1st metacarpal. ORIGIN: Dorsal surface of radius. INSERTION: Base of 1st phalanx of thumb. INNERVATION: Branch of radial.

extensor pollicis longus (ĕks-tĕn′sŏr pŏl′ĭ-sĭs lŏng′gŭs). ACTION: Extends terminal phalanx of thumb and abducts hand. ORIGIN: Dorsal surface of ulna. INSERTION: Base of 2nd phalanx of thumb. INNERVATION: Branch of radial.

extensor primi internodii pollicis (ĕks-tĕn′sŏr prī′mī ĭn″tĕr-nō′dĭ-ī pŏl′ĭ-sĭs). SAME AS: *extensor pollicis brevis.*

extensor secundi internodii pollicis (ĕks-tĕn′sŏr sē-kŭn-dī ĭn″tĕr-nō′dĭ-ī pŏl′-ĭ-sĭs). SAME AS: *extensor pollicis longus.*

flexor carpi radialis (flĕks′or kăr′pī ra″-dĭ-ā′lĭs). ACTION: Flexes and abducts wrist. ORIGIN: Medial epicondyle of humerus. INSERTION: Base of 2nd metacarpal. INNERVATION: Branch of median. SYN: *radiocarpus.*

flexor carpi ulnaris (flĕks′or kăr′pī ŭl-nā′rĭs). Consists of (1) humeral head and (2) ulnar head. ACTION: Flexes and adducts wrist. ORIGIN: (1) Medial epicondyle of humerus. (2) Olecranon process and posterior border of ulna. INSERTION: Pisiform bone and 5th metacarpal. INNERVATION: Branch of ulnar.

flexor digitorum profundus (flĕks′or dĭj-ĭ-tō′rŭm prō-fŭn′dŭs). ACTION: Flexes the phalanges. ORIGIN: Upper three-fourths of shaft of ulna. INSERTION: Terminal phalanges of fingers. INNERVATION: Branch of ulnar and branch of median.

flexor digitorum sublimis (flĕks′or dĭj-ĭ-tō′rŭm sŭb-lī′mĭs). SAME AS: *flexor digitorum superficialis.*

flexor digitorum superficialis (flĕks′or dĭj-ĭ-tō′rŭm sū″pĕr-fĭsh-ē-ā′lĭs). Consists of three heads: (1) humeral, (2) ulnar and (3) radial. ACTION: Flexes middle phalanges and hand. ORIGIN: (1) Medial epicondyle of humerus. (2) Medial side of coronoid process. (3) Outer border of radius. INSERTION: Second phalanx of each finger. INNERVATION: Branches of median. SYN: *flexor digitorum sublimis.*

flexor pollicis longus (flĕks′or pŏl′ĭ-sĭs long′gŭs). ACTION: Flexes thumb. ORIGIN: Anterior surface of middle 3rd of radius. INSERTION: Terminal phalanx of thumb. INNERVATION: Branch of median.

palmaris longus (păl-mā′rĭs long′gŭs). ACTION: Tightens palmar fascia, flexes wrist. ORIGIN: Medial epicondyle of humerus. INSERTION: Transverse carpal ligament and palmar fascia. INNERVATION: Branch of median.

pronator quadratus (prō-nā′tor kwad-rā′tŭs). ACTION: Pronates forearm. ORIGIN: Lower 4th of ulna. INSERTION: Lower 4th of radius. INNERVATION: Volar interosseous.

pronator teres (prō-nā′tor tē′rēz). Consists of (1) humeral head and (2) ulnar head. ACTION: Pronates hand. ORIGIN: (1) Medial epicondyle of humerus. (2) Coronoid process of ulna. INSERTION: Lateral surface of shaft of radius. INNERVATION: Branch of median.

radiocarpus (rā″dĭ-ō-kăr′pŭs). SAME AS: *flexor carpi radialis.*

subanconeus (sŭb-ăn-kō′nē-ŭs). ACTION: Tightens posterior ligament of elbow. ORIGIN: Lower portion of humerus. INSERTION: Posterior ligament of elbow joint. INNERVATION: Radial.

supinator (sū″pĭ-nā′tor). ACTION: Supinates hand. ORIGIN: Lateral epicondyle of humerus; oblique line of ulna; elbow joint. INSERTION: Outer surface of radius. INNERVATION: Branch of radial. SYN: *supinator radii brevis.*

supinator longus (sū″pĭ-nā′tor long′gŭs). SAME AS: *brachioradialis.*

supinator radii brevis (sū″pĭ-nā′tor rā′-dĭ-ī brē′vĭs). SAME AS: *supinator.*

triceps brachii (trī′sĕps brā′kĭ-ī). Consists of three heads: (1) long, (2)

Table of Nerves

Name	BNA and NA Equivalents*	Origin	Function	Distribution
Abducent	N. abducens	Pons.	Motor	Lateral rectus muscle of eye.
Auditory	N. acusticus [BNA] N. vestibulocochlearis [NA]	Cochlea.	Special sense of hearing	Temporal lobes.
Auricular, great	N. auricularis magnus	Second and third cervical through cervical plexus.	Sensory	Side of neck; skin of ear and cheek.
Auricular, posterior	N. auricularis posterior	Facial.	Motor	Posterior auricular muscle.
Auriculotemporal	N. auriculotemporalis	Mandibular div. of trigeminal.	Sensory	Side of scalp.
Buccal	N. buccalis	Mandibular div. of trigeminal.	Sensory	Skin and mucous membrane of cheek.
Calcanean, internal	N. calcaneus medialis [BNA]	Posterior tibial.	Sensory	Sole of foot.
Cervical n., superficial (cutaneous cervical n.; transverse n. of neck)	N. cutaneus colli [BNA] N. transversus colli [NA]	Second and third cervical through cervical plexus.	Sensory	Skin of front of neck.
Chorda, tympani	N. chorda tympani	Facial.	Motor	Sublingual and submaxillary glands.
Ciliary, long	Nn. ciliares longi	Nasal.	Sensory and motor	Cornea, iris, and ciliary body.
Ciliary, short	Nn. ciliares breves	Ciliary ganglion.	Sensory and motor	Cornea, iris, and ciliary body.
Circumflex (Axillary)	N. axillaris	Posterior cord of brachial plexus.	Motor and sensory	Deltoid, teres minor, shoulder joint, and overlying skin.
Coccygeal	N. coccygeus	Spinal cord.	Motor and sensory	Coccygeus muscle and skin over coccyx.
Cochlear (See also Vestibulocochlear n.)	N. cochlearis	Auditory.	Special sense of hearing	Cochlea
Crural, anterior. See Femoral n.				
Cutaneous, internal	N. cutaneus antibrachii medialis [BNA] N. cutaneus antebrachii medialis [NA]	Inner cord of brachial plexus.	Sensory	Skin of inner aspect of forearm.
Cutaneous, lesser internal (n. of Wrisberg)	N. cutaneus brachii medialis	Inner cord of brachial plexus.	Sensory	Skin of inner aspect of upper arm.
Dental, inferior	N. alveolaris inferior	Mandibular div. of trigeminal.	Sensory and motor	Teeth of lower jaw, mylohyoid muscle, and skin of chin.
Dental, superior	N. alveolaris superior [BNA] Nn. alveolares superiores [NA]	Maxillary div. of trigeminal.	Sensory	Upper teeth and gums.
Digastric		Facial.	Motor	Stylohyoid and posterior belly of digastric muscle.

* Unless specifically designated, the nomenclature in this column is the same for BNA and NA.

Name	BNA and NA Equivalents	Origin	Function	Distribution
Facial (7th cranial n.)	N. facialis	Pons.	Motor	Muscles of expression.
Femoral (anterior crural n.)	N. femoralis	2nd, 3rd, and 4th lumbar.	Motor and sensory	Muscles and skin of thigh.
Frontal	N. frontalis	Ophthalmic div. of trigeminal.	Sensory	Skin of forehead.
Genitofemoral (genitocrural n.)	N. genitofemoralis	1st and 2nd lumbar.	Sensory and motor	Cremaster muscle and skin of groin and upper part of thigh.
Glossopharyngeal (9th cranial n.)	N. glossopharyngeus	Medulla oblongata.	Motor and sensory	Muscles and mucous membrane of pharynx, fauces, and posterior third of tongue.
Gluteal, inferior	N. gluteus inferior	5th lumber and 1st and 2nd sacral.	Motor	Gluteus maximus.
Gluteal, superior	N. gluteus superior	4th and 5th lumbar and 1st sacral.	Motor	Gluteus medius and minimus, tensor fasciae femoris.
Hypogastric	Ramus cutaneus anterior [BNA] N. hypogastricus [NA]	Iliohypogastric.	Motor and sensory	Muscles and skin of abdominal wall.
Hypoglossal (12th cranial n.)	N. hypoglossus	Hypoglossal nucleus in medulla oblongata.	Motor	Intrinsic muscles of tongue.
Iliac	Ramus cutaneus lateralis	Iliohypogastric.	Sensory	Skin of gluteal region.
Iliohypogastric	N. iliohypogastricus	1st lumbar.	Sensory and motor	Muscles and skin of hypogastrium.
Ilioinguinal	N. ilioinguinalis	1st lumbar.	Sensory and motor	Muscles of abdominal wall, skin of upper thigh, skin of root of penis and scrotum (in male), and skin of mons pubis and labium majus (in female).
Infraorbital	N. infraorbitalis	Maxillary div. of trigeminal.	Sensory	Skin of cheek and all upper teeth except molars.
Infratrochlear	N. infratrochlearis	Nasociliary.	Sensory	Skin of lower eyelid and root of nose, conjunctiva, and lacrimal sac and caruncle.
Intercostal	Nn. intercostales	Thoracic.	Sensory and motor	Muscles and skin of back, thorax, and upper abdomen.
Intercostobrachial	Nn. intercostobrachiales	2nd intercostal.	Sensory	Skin of axilla and medial side of arm.
Interosseous, anterior (volar interosseous n.)	N. interosseus volaris [BNA] N. interosseus anterior [NA]	Median.	Motor	Deep flexor and pronator muscles of forearm.

Name	BNA and NA Equivalents	Origin	Function	Distribution
Interosseous, posterior	N. interosseus dorsalis [BNA] N. interosseus posterior [NA]	Musculospiral (radial).	Motor and sensory	Muscles and skin of back of forearm and wrist.
Lacrimal	N. lacrimalis	Ophthalmic div. of trigeminal.	Sensory	Lacrimal gland, conjunctiva, and skin of upper eyelid.
Laryngeal, inferior	N. laryngeus inferior	Branch of recurrent laryngeal.	Motor	Muscles of larynx except cricothyroid.
Laryngeal, recurrent	N. recurrens	Vagus.	Motor	Muscles of larynx except cricothyroid.
Laryngeal, superior	N. laryngeus superior	Vagus.	Motor and sensory	Mucous membrane of larynx; arytenoid and cricothyroid muscles.
Lingual	N. lingualis	Mandibular div. of trigeminal.	Sensory	Mucous membrane of anterior two-thirds of tongue and floor and outer wall of mouth.
Lumbar	Nn. lumbales	Spinal cord.	Motor and sensory	Loins and front of lower abdomen and thigh to help in forming lumbar and sacral plexuses.
Mandibular	N. mandibularis	Trigeminal.	Motor and sensory	Teeth, gums, and skin of lower jaw and cheek; muscles of mastication; mucous membrane of anterior two-thirds of tongue.
Masseteric	N. massetericus	Mandibular div. of trigeminal..	Motor	Masseter muscle.
Maxillary	N. maxillaris	Trigeminal.	Sensory	Nasal pharynx, palate, teeth of upper jaw and skin of cheek.
Median	N. medianis	Internal and external cords of brachial plexus.	Motor and sensory	Pronators and flexors of forearm, two external lumbricales, thenar muscles, skin of palm of first four fingers.
Mental	N. mentalis	Inferior dental.	Sensory	Skin and mucous membrane of lower lip and chin.
Musculocutaneous	N. musculocutaneus	External cord of brachial plexus.	Motor and sensory	Flexors of upper arm and skin of external aspect of forearm.
Musculospiral. See Radial n.				

TABLE OF NERVES—*Continued*

Name	BNA and NA Equivalents	Origin	Function	Distribution
Mylohyoid	N. mylohyoideus	Inferior dental.	Motor	Mylohyoid muscle and anterior belly of digastric muscle.
Nasal (nasociliary n.)	N. nasociliaris	Ophthalmic div. of trigeminal.	Sensory	Ciliary ganglion, iris, conjunctiva, ethmoid cells, mucous membrane and skin of nose.
Nasopalatine	N. nasopalatinus	Meckel's ganglion (sphenopalatine ganglion).	Sensory	Mucous membrane of nose and palate.
Obturator	N. obturatorius	2nd, 3rd, and 4th lumbar through lumbar plexus.	Motor and sensory	Adductors of thigh, hip and knee joints; skin of inner aspect of thigh.
Occipital, greater	N. occipitalis major	2nd cervical.	Motor and sensory	Muscles of back of neck; skin over occiput.
Occipital, lesser	N. occipitalis minor	2nd and 3rd cervical.	Sensory	Skin behind ear and on back of scalp.
Occipital, third	N. occipitalis tertius	3rd cervical.	Sensory	Skin of back of head and nape of neck.
Oculomotor (3rd cranial n.)	N. oculomotorius	Floor of aqueduct of Sylvius.	Motor	All ocular muscles except lateral rectus and superior oblique.
Olfactory (1st cranial n.)	Nn. olfactorii	Olfactory lobe.	Special sense of smell	Nasal mucous membranes in olfactory region.
Ophthalmic	N. ophthalmicus	1st div. of trigeminal.	Sensory	Lacrimal gland, conjunctiva, skin of forehead, skin and mucous membrane of nose.
Optic (2nd cranial n.)	N. opticus	Corpora quadrigemina.	Special sense of sight	Retina.
Palatine, anterior, middle, and posterior	Nn. palatini	Meckel's ganglion.	Motor	Mucous membrane of palate.
Perineal	N. perinei	Pudendal.	Motor and sensory	Muscles and skin of perineum.
Peroneal, common (lateral popliteal n.)	N. peroneus communis	Sciatic.	Motor and sensory	Extensor muscles of lower leg and foot and overlying skin.
Phrenic	N. phrenicus	3rd, 4th, and 5th cervical.	Motor and sensory	Diaphragm.
Pneumogastric. See Vagus n.				
Popliteal, deep. See Tibial n.				
Popliteal, lateral. See Peroneal n., common.				
Pterygoid	N. pterygoideus	Mandibular div. of trigeminal.	Motor	Lateral and medial pterygoid muscles.
Pterygoid canal, n. of. See Vidian n.				

Name	BNA and NA Equivalents	Origin	Function	Distribution
Pudendal	N. pudendus	2nd, 3rd, and 4th sacral.	Sensory	Skin and muscles of perineum and genitalia.
Radial (musculospiral n.)	N. radialis	Brachial plexus.	Motor and sensory	Skin of back of entire arm and hand; extensor muscles of entire arm and hand.
Sacral	Nn. sacrales	Spinal cord.	Motor and sensory	Muscles and skin of loins and lower extremities.
Saphenous, external or short. See Sural n.				
Saphenous, internal or long	N. saphenus	Femoral.	Sensory	Skin of inner aspect of knee, leg, ankle and dorsum of foot.
Sciatic (great sciatic n.)	N. ischiadicus	Sacral plexus.	Motor and sensory	Muscles of calf and back of thigh; skin of lower calf and upper surface of foot.
Sphenopalatine	N. sphenopalatinus [BNA]	Maxillary div. of trigeminal.	Sensory	Meckel's ganglion.
Spinal accessory (accessory n.; 11th cranial n.)	N. accessorius	Floor of 4th ventricle and cervical cord.	Motor	Sternomastoid and trapezius muscles.
Stapedial	N. stapedius	Facial.	Motor	Stapedius muscle.
Stylohyoid		Facial.	Motor	Stylohyoid muscle.
Suboccipital	N. suboccipitalis	Posterior div. of 1st cervical.	Motor	Complexus oblique and rectus muscles of back of neck.
Subscapular	Nn. subscapulares	Posterior cord of brachial plexus.	Motor	Teres major and subscapularis muscles.
Supraclavicular, intermediate (supraclavicular n., middle; supraclavicular n.)	N. supraclavicularis medius [BNA] N. supraclavicularis medialis [NA]	3rd and 4th cervical.	Sensory	Skin of fossa below collar bone.
Supraclavicular, lateral (supraclavicular n., posterior; supra-acromial n.)	N. supraclavicularis posterior [BNA] N. supraclavicularis lateralis [NA]	3rd and 4th cervical.	Sensory	Skin of shoulder.
Supraclavicular, medial (supraclavicular n., anterior; suprasternal n.)	N. supraclavicularis anterior [BNA] N. supraclavicularis medialis [NA]	3rd and 4th cervical.	Sensory	Skin over upper part of thorax.
Supraorbital	N. supraorbitalis	Frontal.	Sensory	Forehead, upper eyelid, scalp, and frontal sinus.

TABLE OF NERVES—*Continued*

Name	BNA and NA Equivalents	Origin	Function	Distribution
Suprascapular	N. suprascapularis	5th and 6th cervical.	Motor	Supraspinatus and infraspinatus muscles and the shoulder joint.
Supratrochlear	N. supratrochlearis	Frontal.	Sensory	Skin of upper eyelid and root of nose.
Sural	N. suralis	Common peroneal and tibial n's.	Sensory	Skin of calf and medial side of foot to great toe.
Temporal, deep	N. temporalis profundus	Mandibular div. of trigeminal.	Motor	Temporal muscle.
Thoracic	Nn. thoracales [BNA] Nn. thoracici [NA]	Spinal cord.	Motor and sensory	Muscles and skin of thorax.
Thoracic, anterior	N. thoracalis anterior	Brachial plexus.	Motor	Pectoralis minor and major muscles.
Thoracic, long (posterior thoracic n.; external respiratory n. of Bell)	N. thoracalis longus [BNA] N. thoracicus longus [NA]	5th, 6th, and 7th cervical.	Motor	Serratus anterior muscle.
Tibial	N. tibialis	Sciatic.	Motor and sensory	Flexor muscles of back of knee joint and calf; skin of lower leg.
Trigeminal (5th cranial n.; trifacial n.)	N. trigeminus	Midbrain and pons.	Motor and sensory	Skin of face, tongue, teeth; muscles of mastication.
Trochlear (4th cranial n.; pathetic n.)	N. trochlearis	Floor of aqueduct of Sylvius.	Motor	Superior oblique muscle of eye.
Tympanic (Jacobson's n.)	N. tympanicus	Glossopharyngeal.	Sensory	Tympanum, eustachian tube, and structures of middle ear.
Ulnar	N. ulnaris	Medial cord of brachial plexus.	Motor and sensory	Muscles and skin of forearm and hand.
Vagus (10th cranial n.; pneumogastric n.)	N. vagus	Medulla oblongata.	Motor and sensory	Pharynx, larynx, heart, lungs, stomach.
Vestibulocochlear (8th cranial n.; acoustic n.; auditory n.)	N. vestibulocochlearis [NA]	Ganglion of Scarpa and ganglion of Corti.	Sense of hearing	Internal auditory meatus.
Vidian	N. canalis pterygoidei	Facial.	Sensory	Meckel's ganglion (sphenopalatine ganglion).
Zygomatic	N. zygomaticus	Maxillary div. of trigeminal.	Sensory	Skin of temple and cheek bone.

Nerve Plexuses of the Sympathetic and Cerebrospinal Systems

aortic (ā-or′tĭk) (*abdominal*). ORIGIN: Semilunar, lumbar ganglia, renal and solar plexuses. LOCATION: Sides and front of aorta. DISTRIBUTION: Inferior mesenteric, spermatic and hypogastric plexus. Filaments to inferior vena cava. (*thoracic*). ORIGIN: Thoracic ganglia of sympathetic nerve, cardiac plexus. LOCATION: Surrounding the thoracic aorta. DISTRIBUTION: Solar plexus, aorta.

***brachial** (brā′kĭ-ăl). ORIGIN: Anterior branches of 5th, 6th, 7th, 8th, cervical, and greater part of 1st dorsal nerves. LOCATION: Lower part of neck to axilla. DISTRIBUTION: Sixteen branches of suprascapular, subscapular, rhomboid, median, ulnar, musculospiral, posterior thoracic, musculothoracic, circumflex, musculocutaneous nerves.

cardiac (kar′dĭ-ăk) (*great or deep*). ORIGIN: Cardiac nerves of cervical ganglion of sympathetic and vagus. LOCATION: In front of bifurcation of trachea. DISTRIBUTION: Pulmonary, coronary and cardiac plexuses. (*superficial or anterior*). ORIGIN: Left superior cardiac nerve, branch of vagus and filaments of deep cardiac plexus. LOCATION: Beneath arch of aorta. Front of right pulmonary artery. DISTRIBUTION: Coronary and pulmonary plexuses.

carotid (kăr-ŏt′ĭd) (*external*). ORIGIN: Pharyngeal plexus, superior cardiac nerve and superior cervical ganglion. LOCATION: Around external carotid artery. DISTRIBUTION: External carotid artery and its branches. (*internal*). ORIGIN: Asympathetic plexus. LOCATION: Surrounding internal carotid artery. DISTRIBUTION: Tympanic plexus, sphenopalatine ganglion, abducens and oculomotor nerves, the cerebral vessels and the ciliary ganglion.

cavernous (kăv′ĕr-nŭs). ORIGIN: 3rd to 6th cranial nerves and ophthalmic ganglion. LOCATION: Cavernous sinus. DISTRIBUTION: Wall of internal carotid artery.

.eliac (sē′lĭ-ăk). ORIGIN: Solar plexus, branches from lesser splanchnic and vagus nerves. LOCATION: Behind stomach, in front of aorta at level of origin of celiac artery. DISTRIBUTION: Coronary, hepatic, pyloric, gastroduodenal, gastroepiploic and splenic plexuses. SYN: *solar plexus.*

***cervical** (ser′vĭ-kăl). ORIGIN: Anterior branches of first 4 cervical nerves. LOCATION: Beneath sternocleidomastoid muscle opposite first 4 cervical vertebrae. DISTRIBUTION: Cutaneous, muscular and communicating rami.

***coccygeal** (kŏk-sĭj′ē-ăl). ORIGIN: Fourth and 5th sacral and the coccygeal nerves. LOCATION: Dorsal surface of coccyx and caudal end of sacrum. DISTRIBUTION: Anococcygeal nerves.

cystic (sĭs′tĭk). ORIGIN: Hepatic plexus. LOCATION: At gallbladder. DISTRIBUTION: Gallbladder.

esophageal (ē-sō-făj′ē-ăl). ORIGIN: Vagus nerve, thoracic sympathetic ganglia. LOCATION: Around the esophagus. DISTRIBUTION: Esophagus.

gastric (găs′trĭk). ORIGIN: Celiac plexus and continuations of esophageal plexuses. LOCATION: Gastric artery. DISTRIBUTION: Abdominal viscera.

hemorrhoidal (hĕm″ō-roy′dăl). ORIGIN: Pelvic and inferior mesenteric plexuses. LOCATION: Rectum and sides of rectum. DISTRIBUTION: Rectum.

hepatic (hē-păt′ĭk). ORIGIN: Celiac plexus, left vagus, right phrenic. LOCATION: Accompanies hepatic artery. DISTRIBUTION: Liver.

hypogastric (hĭ″pō-găs′trĭk). ORIGIN: Aortic plexus and lumbar ganglia. LOCATION: Promontory of sacrum. DISTRIBUTION: Pelvic plexus.

***lumbar** (lŭm′bar). ORIGIN: First 4 lumbar nerves. LOCATION: Psoas muscle. DISTRIBUTION: Iliohypogastric, ilioinguinal, genitocrural, external cutaneous, obturator, accessory, and anterior crural nerves.

Meissner's (mĭs′nĕrs). ORIGIN: Superior mesenteric plexus (controls secretions of the bowels). LOCATION: Submucous coat of small intestines. DISTRIBUTION: Intestinal walls.

mesenteric (mĕs-ĕn-tĕr′ĭk). ORIGIN: Celiac plexus and left side of aortic plexus. LOCATION: Surrounding the inferior and superior mesenteric arteries. DISTRIBUTION: Descending colon, sigmoid, rectum, intestines.

myenteric (mĭ-ĕn-tĕr′ĭk). ORIGIN: Sympathetic system (controls peristalsis). LOCATION: Between the circular and longitudinal coats of small intestines. DISTRIBUTION: Intestinal walls.

ophthalmic (ŏf-thăl′mĭk). ORIGIN: Internal carotid plexus. LOCATION: Around ophthalmic artery and optic nerve. DISTRIBUTION: Optic region.

pancreatic (păn-krē-ăt′ĭk). ORIGIN: Splenic plexus. LOCATION: Near pancreas. DISTRIBUTION: Filaments to pancreas.

pancreaticoduodenal (păn-krē-ăt″ĭ-kō-dū″ō-dē′năl). ORIGIN: Hepatic plexus. LOCATION: Near head of pancreas. DISTRIBUTION: Filaments to pancreas and duodenum.

pelvic (pĕl′vĭk). ORIGIN: Hypogastric plexus, 2nd to 4th sacral nerves, 1st and 2nd sacral ganglia (pelvic brain). LOCATION: Side of rectum and bladder. DISTRIBUTION: Viscera of pelvis, pelvic plexus.

phrenic (frĕn′ĭk). ORIGIN: Solar plexus, semilunar ganglia. LOCATION: Accompanies phrenic artery to diaphragm. DISTRIBUTION: Diaphragm and suprarenal capsules.

prostatic (prŏs-tăt′ĭk). ORIGIN: Hypogastric plexus. LOCATION: Vesical arteries. DISTRIBUTION: Bladder.

pulmonary (pŭl′mō-nā″rĭ). ORIGIN: Anterior and posterior pulmonary branches of vagus and sympathetic nerves. LOCATION: Root of lungs, front and back. DISTRIBUTION: Root of lungs.

pyloric (pĭ-lor′ĭk). ORIGIN: Hepatic plexus.

* Plexuses of central nervous system.

LOCATION: Near pylorus. DISTRIBUTION: Filaments to pylorus.

renal (rē'năl). ORIGIN: Solar and aortic plexuses and semilunar ganglia. LOCATION: Renal artery. DISTRIBUTION: Kidneys, posterior vena cava, spermatic plexus.

***sacral** (sā'krăl). ORIGIN: Anterior branch of 4th and 5th lumbar and 1st, 2nd, 3rd, and 4th sacral nerves. LOCATION: Front of sacrum on piriformis muscle. DISTRIBUTION: Muscular, pudic, superior gluteal, great and small sciatic nerves.

solar (sō'lar) (*epigastric*). ORIGIN: Splanchnics and right vagus. LOCATION: Back of stomach. DISTRIBUTION: Semilunar ganglia, phrenic, suprarenal, renal, spermatic, celiac, superior mesenteric, and aortic plexuses. Called *abdominal brain*. SYN: *celiac plexus.*

spermatic (spĕr-măt'ĭk) (*ovarian*). ORIGIN: Aortic plexus. LOCATION: Accompanies spermatic vessels to testes or ovaries. DISTRIBUTION: Testes or ovaries.

splenic (splē'nĭk). ORIGIN: Celiac plexus, left semilunar ganglion, right vagus nerve. LOCATION: Accompanies splenic artery. DISTRIBUTION: Spleen, pancreatic plexus, left gastroepiploic plexus.

* Plexuses of central nervous system.

suprarenal (sū-pră-rē'năl). ORIGIN: Diaphragmatic, solar and renal plexuses. LOCATION: Around suprarenal capsules. DISTRIBUTION: Filaments to medulla of suprarenal capsules.

thyroid (thī'royd) (*inferior*). ORIGIN: Middle cervical ganglion. LOCATION: Around external carotid and inferior thyroid arteries. DISTRIBUTION: Larynx, pharynx, thyroid gland. (*superior*). ORIGIN: Superior laryngeal and cardiac nerves. LOCATION: Around the thyroid gland. DISTRIBUTION: Thyroid region.

uterine (ū'tĕr-ĭn). ORIGIN: Pelvic plexus. LOCATION: Accompanies uterine arteries. DISTRIBUTION: Cervix and lower part of uterus.

vaginal (văj'ĭ-năl). ORIGIN: Pelvic plexus. LOCATION: Vaginal walls. DISTRIBUTION: Vagina.

vertebral (vĕrt'ĕ-brăl). ORIGIN: First part thoracic ganglion, upper cervical nerves. LOCATION: Surrounding basilar and vertebral arteries. DISTRIBUTION: Vertebral and cerebellar regions.

vesical (vĕs'ĭ-kăl). ORIGIN: Pelvic plexus. LOCATION: Accompanies vesical arteries. DISTRIBUTION: Vesicula seminalis, vas deferens.

A. Cranial Nerves

Ref. Numbers Refer to Parts Supplied

Ref.	Cranial Nerve Supply to the	No.	Name of Nerve	Div. of Nerve
A	CHEEK—Tongue, teeth, ear and muscles of mastication	5th	Trigeminus or Trifacial	2nd
A 1			Great Sensory Nerve of head and face	3rd
B	EYE—Retina	2nd	Optic	
B 1	" Muscles of Orbit (rectus, *et al.*) and motor filaments to Iris	3rd	Oculomotor	
B 2	" " " (Supr. oblique)	4th	Trochlear or Patheticus	
B 3	" Conjunctiva, Lacrimal gland and eyelids	5th–7th	Trigeminus and Facial	1st div. of 5th
B 4	" Muscle of Orbit (external rectus)	6th	Abducent	
B 5	" Eyeball	3rd–5th	Oculomotor and Trigeminus	1st Div. Branches of
C	EAR—Tympanum	9th	Glossopharyngeal	
C 2	" External	5th	Trigeminus	3rd
C 1	" Muscles External, also Parotid Gland	7th	Facial	
C 3	" External	10th	Pneumogastric or Vagus	
C 4	" Middle	9th	Glossopharyngeal	
C 5	" Internal	8th	Auditory	
D	EXPRESSION—(Muscles of face, lips, etc.)	7th	Facial (Great Motor Nerve of Face Muscles)	
E	ESOPHAGUS	10th	Pneumogastric	
F	FOREHEAD—(Eyes and nose)	5th	Trigeminus	1st
G	FACE—Muscles of mastication, ear, cheek, tongue, teeth	5th	Trigeminus	2nd
G 1	" " " ear, cheek, tongue, taste, teeth	5th	Trigeminus	3rd
H	HEART	10th	Pneumogastric	
I	INTESTINES	10th	Pneumogastric	
J	LIVER	10th	Pneumogastric	Left Pneumogastric
K	LARYNX—Voice	10th	Pneumogastric	
K 1	" "	11th	Accessory Spinal	2nd
L	LUNGS	10th	Pneumogastric	
M	NOSE—Smell	1st	Olfactory	
M 1	" Mucous membrane	5th	Trigeminus	1st
M 2	" and lip	7th	Facial	
N	PALATE—Muscles	7th	Facial	
N 1	" Hard and soft (gums, tonsils and nose)	5th	Trigeminus	2. Meckel's Ganglion
O	PHARYNX	10th	Pneumogastric	
O 1	"	9th	Glossopharyngeal	also Meckel's Ganglion
O 2	"	11th	Accessory Spinal	2nd
P	STOMACH	10th	Pneumogastric	
Q	SPLEEN	10th	Pneumogastric	Right Pneumogastric
R	TEETH—Upper (4 incisors, 2 canine, 4 bicuspids, 6 molars)	5th	Trigeminus	2nd
R 1	" Lower (4 " 2 " 4 " 6 ")	5th	Trigeminus	3rd
S	TONSILS	9th	Glossopharyngeal	
S 1	"	5th	Trigeminus	2nd
T	TONGUE—(Papillae)	5th	Trigeminus	3rd
T 1	" Muscles	7th	Facial	
T 2	" Taste	9th	Glossopharyngeal	
T 3	" Muscles	12th	Hypoglossal	
T 4	" Circulation and secretion of Sub. Max. glands	7th	Facial	

A. CRANIAL NERVES *(Continued)*

Ref. Numbers Refer to Parts Supplied

Ref.	Name of Division	Function of Nerve	Principal Arteries
A	Superior Maxillary	Sensory[2]	Cheek—†Facial
A 1	Inferior	Sensory, Motor and Taste[2]	
B		Special Sense of Sight	Eye—13 brs. from Int. Carotid
B 1		Motor entirely	" ‡Infraorbital, from Ex. Carotid
B 2		Motor entirely	
B 3	Ophthalmic	5th Sensory[2] and 7th Motor[1]	
B 4		Motor entirely	
B 5	Also branches from Sympathetic	3rd Motor, 5th Sensory and Nutrition[3]	
C		Motor[4]	Ear—Post. †Auricular (Br. Ext. Car.)
C 2	Inferior Maxillary	Sensory[2]	" Ant. ‡Auricular (Br. Temporal)
C 1		Motor[1]	" ‡Auricular, †Posterior and ‡Ant.
C 3	Auricular branch	Sensory[3]	Deep Auricular, ‡Tympanic
C 4		Sensory[4]	‡Stylomastoid, Petrossal, ‡Vidian
C 5		Special Sense of Hearing	Int. Auditory
D		Motor	Face—†Facial
E	Esophageal branch	Motor and Sensory[3]	Esophagus—*Esophageal
F	Ophthalmic	Sensory[2]	(See Head)
G	Superior Maxillary	Sensory[2]	Face—†Facial
G 1	Inferior Maxillary	Sensory, Motor and Taste[2]	
H	Sup. Laryngeal branch	Motor and Sensory[3]	
I	Gastric branch	Motor and Sensory[3]	
J	Gastric branch	Motor and Sensory[3]	
K	Laryngeal branch	Motor and Sensory[3]	
K 1		Motor[5]	
L	Pulmonary branch	Motor and Sensory[3]	
M		Special Sense of Smell	Nose—‡Lateralis Nasi, ‡Nasal
M 1	Ophthalmic	Sensory[2]	Nasal Br. of Ophthalmic
M 2		Sensory and Motor[1]	
N		Motor[1]	Palāte—‡Dorsalis ‡Linguae (†lingual)
N 1	Superior Maxillary	Sensory[2]	
O	Pharyngeal branch	Sensory and Motor[3]	Pharynx—Asc'd †Pharyngeal
O 1		Sensory and Motor[4]	" "
O 2		Motor[5]	" "
P	Gastric branch	Motor and Sensory[3]	Stomach—*Gastric
Q	Gastric branch	Motor and Sensory[3]	Spleen—*Splenic
R	Superior Maxillary	Sensory[2]	Teeth—‡Inf. dental, ‖Sup. dental,
R 1	Inferior Maxillary	Sensory[2]	‡Alveolar
S		Sensory[4]	Tonsils—‡Dorsalis linguae, †asc'd Ph.
S 1	Meckel's Ganglion	Sensory[2]	" ‡Asc'd palat., ‡tonsilar, (†facial)
T	Inf. Maxillary (gustatory branch)	Sensory, Motor and Taste[2]	Tongue—‡Lingual (Ext .Carotid)
T 1		Motor[1]	" ‡Submental (†facial)
T 2	Lingual branch	Sensory, Motor and Spec. Nerve of Taste[4]	Asc'd †Pharyngeal (Ext. Carotid)
T 3		Motor entirely	
T 4	Chorda Tympani (§Br. of 7th)	Circulation and Secretion of Tongue	

B. The Twelve Pairs of Cranial Nerves

No.	Name	Div.	Branches	Function and Distribution*	Remarks
1	Olfactory		20	M	Its bulb is a lobe of the Cerebrum
2	Optic		None	B	
3	Oculomotor		Filaments	B1-B5	Great motor nerve of 5 of 7 muscles of eye
4	Trochlear or Patheticus		None	B2	Smallest cranial nerve
5	Trigeminus or Trifacial (Three Twins)	1st	Ophthalmic	B3-B5-F-M1	The great Sensory nerve of the head and face
	Trigeminus or Trifacial (Three Twins)	2nd	Superior Maxillary	A-G-N1-R-S1	
	Trigeminus or Trifacial (Three Twins)	3rd	Inferior Maxillary	A1-C2-G1-R1-T	
6	Abducent		Filaments	B4	(Leading from)
7	Facial or Portio Dura (Hard Portion)			C1-D-M2-N-F1-F4-B3	Great motor nerve of Facial Muscles
8	Auditory or Portio Mollis, of 7 (Soft Portion)			C5	
9	Glossopharyngeal			C-C4-O1-S-T2	Tongue and throat nerve
10	Pneumogastric (Vagus or Par Vagum)		12	C3-E-H-I-J-K-L-O-P-Q	Wandering nerve
11	Accessory Spinal	1 Ext.	Spinal portion		
		2 Int.	Accessory portion	K1-O2	Accessory to the Pneumogastric
12	Hypoglossal			T3	Hypoglossal (Under the tongue)

*To find the Function and Distribution of the Cranial Nerves, reference is given to Table "A" and "B."

B. CRANIAL NERVES *(Continued)*

No.	Function	Origin	Exit
1	Special Sense Smell	Frontal lobe, optic thalamus deeply and island of Reil, by three roots	Exit by 20 branches through the cribriform plate to the schneiderian membrane of nose
2	Special Sense Sight	Optic thalamus, corpora geniculata and corpora quadrigemina or optic lobes, which communicate with cerebrum and cerebellum	Through optic foramen to retina
3	Motor	Floor of aqueduct of Sylvius and inner surface of crus cerebri	Sphenoidal fissure to eye muscles
4	Motor of superior oblique mus. of eye	Valve of Vieussens, a thin plate of nervous matter above the fourth ventricle	Sphenoidal fissure to sup. oblique muscle of eye
5	Sensory	Superficial origin in, side of pons Varolii by two roots. Deep origin cerebellum and medulla oblongata and floor of fourth ventricle	1st Br. sphenoidal fissure and supraorbital foramen
	Sensory		2nd Br. foramen rotund and intraorbital foramen
	Sensory, Motor, Taste		3rd Br. foramen ovale and mental foramen
6	Motor of external rectus of eye	Fourth ventricle, deep origin posterior part of medulla oblongata	Sphenoidal fissure, between the two heads of the external rectus muscle
7	Motor	Floor of fourth ventricle	Internal auditory meatus through aqueductus Fallopii and stylomastoid foramen
8	Special Sense Hearing	Restiform body of 4th ventricle	Internal auditory meatus through the internal auditory canal
9	Mixed, Sensory, Motor, Taste	Medulla oblongata. Deeply from floor of fourth ventricle	Jugular foramen to back of tongue, middle ear, tonsils, pharynx and meninges
10	Mixed, Sensory and Motor	Medulla oblongata. Deeply from floor of fourth ventricle	Jugular foramen
11	Motor	Without cavity of cranium, lateral tract of spinal cord as low as the sixth cervical nerve	Enters cranium through the foramen magnum, uniting with the accessory portion which originates within the cranium and both make their exit through jugular foramen
	Motor	Within the cavity of the cranium, medulla oblongata deeply, near floor of 4th ventricle	
12	Motor	Medulla oblongata deeply from floor of 4th ventricle	Anterior condyloid foramen

EXPLANATION TABLES A AND B. CRANIAL NERVES

1st Pair—Olfactory, Special Sense of Smell.

2d " Optic, Special Sense of Sight.

3rd " Oculomotor, Great Motor of Eye, supplies five of the seven eye muscles.

4th " Trochlear or Patheticus, motor of superior oblique muscle of eye.

[2]5th " Trigeminus or Trifacial, great sensory nerve of head and face; divides into three portions, viz.: 1st Ophthalmic Sensory; 2nd Supr. Max. Sensory; 3rd Inf. Sensory, Max. Motor and a lingual nerve of the sense of taste.
Most difficult of all the cranial nerves to trace.

6th Pair—Abducent, Motor of External Rectus of Eye.

[1]7th " Facial or Portio Dura, great motor nerve of face muscles; exclusively motor at its origin, but it subsequently receives fibers from the (5th) Trigeminus, which give it some sensory function.

§Some anatomists claim that the Chorda Tympani nerve is a branch of the Sympathetic system.

8th Pair—Auditory, or Portio Mollis of 7th, Special Sense of Hearing.

[4]9th " Glossopharyngeal, in part a special nerve of taste, nerve of sensation, and also contains motor fibers.

[3]10th " Pneumogastric, Vagus of Par Vagum, (a mixed nerve) at its origin it is exclusively sensory, but lower down it is also motor and capable of providing both for sensation and motion in organs to which distributed.

[5]11th " Accessory Spinal, considered to be exclusively motor, but some authorities claim for it sensory fibers.
Accessory portion joins the vagus, to which it supplies its motor and some of its cardioinhibitory fibers.
Spinal portion supplies the trapezius and sternomastoid muscles.

12th " Hypoglossal, exclusively motor.

*Branches of the aorta. †Branches of branches of the aorta. ‡Branches of branches of branches of the aorta. ||Branches of branches of branches of branches of the aorta

Table of Arteries[1]

Name of Artery	Origin	Distribution	Branches
Acromial	Acromiothoracic.	Deltoid muscle.	
Acromiothoracic	Axillary.	Side of thorax and part of arm.	Acromial, clavicular, pectoral.
Adipose	Capsular arteries, small branches of thoracic aorta.	Adipose tissue of heart.	
Afferent	Interlobular of kidneys.	Glomeruli.	
Alar thoracic	Axillary.	Glands and tissue of the axilla.	
Alveolar	Internal maxillary.	Molar and bicuspid teeth.	
Anastomotic, of the arm	Brachial.	Elbow.	Anterior and posterior.
Anastomotic, of the sciatic	Sciatic.	External rotator muscles of thigh.	Branches of gluteal arterv
Anastomotic, of the thigh	Femoral.	Knee.	Superficial and deep.
Angular	Facial.	Lacrimal sac.	Infraorbital.
Aorta. SEE: *aorta,* in vocabulary.			
Appendicular	Ileocolic.	Mesentery of the vermiform appendix.	
Articular, middle, of knee	Popliteal.	Crucial ligaments and joint.	
Articular, superior, external of knee	Popliteal.	Femur and knee joint.	
Articular, superior, internal	Popliteal.	Knee joint. Vasti.	
Ascending	External circumflex.	Gluteal muscles and hip joint.	
Auditory, external	Internal maxillary.	Tympanum.	
Auditory, internal	Basilar.	Internal ear.	
Auricular	Occipital.	Auricle.	
Auricular, anterior, inferior	Temporal.	Auricle.	
Auricular, deep	Internal maxillary.	Tympanum and external auditory meatus.	
Auricular, left	Left coronary artery.	Left auricle; pulmonary artery.	
Auricular, posterior	Fifth branch of external carotid.	Back of auricle and part of neck.	Parotid, muscular, stylomastoid, auricular, and mastoid.
Auricular, right	Right coronary artery.	Right auricle, septum, and aorta.	
Axillary	Subclavian.	Brachial and seven branches.	Superior thoracic, acromiothoracic, long thoracic, alar thoracic, subscapular, ant. and post. circumflex.
Azygos (of knee)	Popliteal.	Crucial ligament, knee joint.	
Azygos	External plantar.	Articulations of tarsus.	
Azygos	Internal plantar.	Joints on inner side of foot.	Into branches of external plantar.
Azygos (of elbow)	Superior profunda.	Posterior part of elbow joint.	Anastomotica magna and interosseous recurrent.
Azygos (of shoulder)	Suprascapular.	Shoulder joint.	
Basilar	Right and left vertebral.	Brain.	Transverse, internal auditory, anterior cerebellar, superior cerebellar, posterior cerebral.

1 From *Appleton's Medical Dictionary,* Courtesy, Appleton Century Company.

TABLE OF ARTERIES—*Continued*

Name of Artery	Origin	Distribution	Branches
Bicipital	Anterior circumflex.	Long tendon of biceps and shoulder joint.	
Brachial	Axillary.	Arm and forearm.	Superior and inferior profunda, anastomotica magna, nutrient, muscular, radial, and ulnar.
Brachiocephalic	SEE: *Innominate a.*		
Bronchial, inferior	Thoracic aorta.	Bronchi and lungs.	
Bronchial, superior	Arch of aorta.	Bronchi.	
Buccal	Internal maxillary.	Muscles and integument of the cheek.	
Bulb, artery of	Internal pudic.	Erectile tissue of the corpus spongiosum.	
Calcanean, external	Posterior peroneal.	Outer side of foot and heel.	Anastomosing with external malleolar, external plantar and tarsal arteries.
Calcanean, inferior	External plantar.	External plantar muscles.	
Calcanean, internal	Posterior tibial and peroneal.	Inner side of heel and sole.	
Calcanean, middle	Posterior tibial.	Outer and back surface of os calcis.	
Capsular	SEE: *Suprarenal.*		
Carotid, common	Innominate (right); arch of aorta (left).	External and internal carotid.	
Carotid, external	Common carotid.	Front and back of neck, face, side of head, meninges, middle ear, thyroid, tongue, tonsils.	Internal maxillary, superior thyroid, lingual, facial, occipital, posterior auricular, superficial temporal.
Carotid, internal	Common carotid.	Brain, nose, orbit, internal ear, and forehead.	Anterior and middle cerebral, ophthalmic, tympanic, vidian, pituitary, gasserian, meningeal, communicating, anterior choroid.
Carpal	Radial.	Lower radius and wrist.	Anterior carpal rete.
Carpal	Ulnar.	Carpus.	Posterior carpal rete.
Cecal, anterior	Inferior mesenteric.	Front part of cecum.	
Cecal, posterior	Posterior mesenteric.	Back part of cecum.	
Celiac axis	Abdominal aorta.	Esophagus, stomach, duodenum, gallbladder, liver, pancreas, spleen.	Gastric, hepatic, splenic.
Cerebellar (three)	Basilar and vertebral.	Cerebellum.	Inferior and superior vermiform and hemispheral.
Cerebral, anterior and middle	Internal carotid.	Cerebrum.	
Cerebral, posterior	Basilar.	Cerebrum.	
Cervical, ascending	Inferior thyroid.	Neck.	Muscular, spinal.
Cervical, deep	Superior intercostal.	Neck.	Muscular, spinal.
Cervical, superficial	Transverse cervical.	Muscles of back of neck.	
Cervical, transverse	Thyroid axis.	Posterior cervical and scapular regions	

TABLE OF ARTERIES—*Continued*

Name of Artery	Origin	Distribution	Branches
Circumflex, anterior	Axillary.	Pectoralis major, biceps, shoulder joint.	Bicipital and pectoral.
Circumflex, posterior	Axillary.	Deltoid, teres minor, triceps, shoulder joint.	Acromial, articular, muscular, nutrient.
Coronary, left	Left anterior sinus of Valsalva.	Heart.	Left auricular, anterior interventricular, left marginal, terminal.
Coronary, right	Right anterior sinus of Valsalva.	Heart.	Right auricular, preventricular, right marginal, posterior interventricular, tranvserse.
Digital	External plantar.	Outer side second to fifth toes.	
Digital, palmar	Superficial palmar arch.	Sides of fingers.	
Dorsalis pedis	Anterior tibial.	Foot.	Tarsal, metatarsal, dorsalis hallucis, communicating.
Epigastric	External iliac.	Abdominal wall, femoral ring and cremaster.	Cremasteric, pubic, muscular, and terminal branches.
Facial	External carotid.	Pharynx and face.	Inferior palatine, tonsillar, glandular, muscular, submental, mesenteric, buccal, inferior labial, coronary of lips, lateralis nasi, angular.
Femoral	External iliac.	Lower part of abdominal wall, genitals, upper thigh.	
Gastric	Celiac axis.	Liver, esophagus, stomach.	Cardiac, esophageal, gastric and hepatic.
Gastroduodenal	Hepatic.		Gastroepiploic, pancreaticoduodenal, pyloric.
Gluteal	Internal iliac.	Gluteal muscles.	Deep and superficial gluteal.
Hepatic	Celiac axis.	Duodenum, liver, pancreas, stomach.	Gastroduodenal, pancreatic, subpyloric, terminal.
Iliac, common	Abdominal aorta.	Peritoneum.	Peritoneal, ureteric, external and internal iliac.
Iliac, external	Common iliac.	Lower limb.	Deep epigastric, circumflex, femoral.
Iliac, internal	Common iliac.	Pelvic and generative organs, inner thigh.	Anterior and posterior trunk.
Iliac, interior (anterior trunk)	Internal iliac.	Pelvic and generative organs and thigh.	Vesical, uterine, vaginal, obturator, sciatic, internal pudic, middle hemorrhoidal.
Iliac, interior (posterior trunk)	Internal iliac.	Muscles of hip and sacrum.	Gluteal, iliolumbar and lateral sacral.
Innominate	Arch of aorta.	Right side of head and right arm.	Right common carotid, right subclavian.
Intercostal, superior	Subclavian.	Neck and upper thorax.	Deep cervical, first intercostal, arteria aberrans.
Interosseous	Ulnar.	Deep muscles of the forearm.	Anterior and posterior interosseous.
Laryngeal, superior	Superior thyroid.	Muscles and mucous membrane of larynx.	
Lingual	External carotid.	Tongue.	Hyoid, dorsalis linguae, sublingual, ranine.
Mammary, internal	Subclavian.	Thorax.	Superior phrenic, mediastinal, pericardiac, sternal, anterior intercostal, perforating lateral intercostal, superior epigastric.

TABLE OF ARTERIES—*Continued*

Name of Artery	Origin	Distribution	Branches
Maxillary, internal	External carotid.	Structures indicated in names of branches.	Middle and small meningeal, inferior dental. deep temporal, tympanic, pterygoid, masseteric, buccal, posterior palatine, vidian. pterygopalatine, sphenopalatine, alveolar infraorbital.
Mediastinal, anterior	Internal mammary.	Superior and anterior mediastinums, thymus gland.	
Meningeal (four)	Ascending pharyngeal and posterior ethmoid.	Dura mater.	
Mesenteric, inferior	Abdominal aorta.	Descending colon, sigmoid flexure, rectum.	Colica sinistra, sigmoid, superior hemorrhoidal.
Mesenteric, superior	Abdominal aorta.	Small intestine, colon, cecum, ileum.	Inferior pancreaticoduodenal, colica media. colica dextra, ileocolic, vasa intestinae tenuis.
Musculophrenic	Internal mammary.	Diaphragm, 5th and 6th intercostal spaces, muscles of abdomen.	Phrenic, anterior intercostals, muscular.
Nasal	Ophthalmic.	Lacrimal sac, integuments of nose.	Lacrima :and transverse nasal.
Obturator	Internal iliac.	Pelvis and thigh.	Iliac, vesical, pubic, external and internal pelvic.
Occipital	External carotid.	Muscles of neck and scalp, meninges.	Muscular, auricular, meningeal, cranial branches, princeps cervicis.
Ophthalmic	Internal carotid.	Eye, adjacent structures, part of face.	Lacrimal, supraorbital, central of retina, ciliary, muscular, posterior and anterior ethmoid, palpebral, nasal, frontal.
Palmar arch (deep)	Radial.	Palm and fingers.	Perforating, palmar interosseous, recurrent.
Palmar arch (superficial)	Ulnar.	Palm and fingers.	Digital, cutaneous, muscular.
Pharyngeal, ascending	External carotid.	Pharynx soft palate, tympanum, meninges.	Meningeal, palatine, pharyngeal, prevertebral, tympanic.
Phrenic, superior	Internal mammary.	Diaphragm, pericardium pleura.	
Plantar arch	External plantar.	Anterior part of foot and toes.	
Plantar, external	Posterior tibial.	Sole and toes.	Anastomotic, calcaneal, cutaneous, posterior perforating, plantar arch.
Plantar, internal	Posterior tibial.	Inner side of foot.	Anastomotic, articular, cutaneous, muscular, superficial digital.
Popliteal	Femoral.	Knee and leg.	Cutaneous, superior and inferior muscular, superior external and internal articular, inferior external and interior articular, azygos articular, anterior and posterior tibial.
Profunda (deep femoral)	Femoral.	Thigh.	External and internal circumflex, three perforating.

TABLE OF ARTERIES—*Continued*

Name of Artery	Origin	Distribution	Branches
Profunda, inferior	Brachial.	Triceps, elbow joint.	
Profunda, superior	Brachial.	Humerus, muscles and skin of arm.	Articular, ascending, cutaneous, muscular, nutrient.
Pterygopalatine	Internal maxillary.	Pharynx, eustachian tubes, sphenoidal cells.	Eustachian, pharyngeal, sphenoid.
Pudic, external	Common femoral.	Skin and integument above pubes and external genitalia.	
Pudic, internal	Internal iliac, anterior trunk.	Generative organs.	Inferior hemorrhoidal, superficial and transverse perineal, muscular, artery of the bulb, of the corpus cavernosum, dorsalis penis.
Pulmonary	Right ventricle.	Lungs.	Right and left pulmonary.
Pyloric, superior	Hepatic.	Pyloric end of stomach.	
Radial	Brachial.	Forearm, wrist, hand.	Radial recurrent, muscular, anterior and posterior carpal, superficial volar, metacarpal, dorsalis pollicis, dorsalis indicis, deep palmar arch.
Renal	Abdominal aorta.	Kidney.	Inferior suprarenal, capsular, ureteral.
Scapular, dorsal	Subscapular.	Muscles of infraspinous fossa.	Infrascapular.
Scapular, posterior	Transverse cervical.	Muscles of scapular region.	Supraspinous and infraspinous, muscular, subscapular.
Sciatic	Internal iliac, anterior trunk.	Muscles and viscera of pelvis.	Coccygeal, inferior gluteal, muscular, anastomotic, articular cutaneous, vesical, rectal, etc.
Spermatic	Abdominal aorta.	Scrotum and testis.	Cremasteric, epididymal, testicular, ureteral.
Sphenopalatine	Internal maxillary.	Pharynx, nose and sphenoid cells.	Nasal, pharyngeal, ascending septal, sphenoid.
Spinal, anterior	Vertebral.	Spinal cord.	
Spinal, lateral	Vertebral.	Vertebrae and spinal canal.	
Spinal, posterior	Vertebral.	Spine.	
Splenic	Celiac axis.	Pancreas, great curvature of stomach, spleen.	Gastric, left gastroepiploic, splenic branches, small and large pancreatic.
Subclavian	Right—Innominate. Left—Arch of aorta.	Neck, thorax, arms, brain, meninges.	Vertebral, internal mammary, superior intercostal, thyroid axis.
Subscapular	Axillary.	Subscapularis, teres major, latissimus dorsi, serratus magnus, axillary glands.	Dorsal and infrascapular.
Suprarenal, inferior	Renal.	Suprarenal body.	
Suprarenal, middle	Aorta.	Suprarenal bodies.	
Suprarenal, superior	Phrenic.	Suprarenal bodies.	
Suprascapular	Thyroid axis.	Muscles of shoulder.	Inferior sternomastoid, nutrient, suprasternal, acromial, articular, supraspinous, and infraspinous.

TABLE OF ARTERIES—*Continued*

Name of Artery	Origin	Distribution	Branches
Temporal	External carotid.	Forehead, parotid gland, masseter muscle, ear.	Anterior auricular, middle, anterior and posterior temporal, transverse facial.
Thoracic, acromial	Axillary.	Muscles of shoulder, chest and arm.	Acromial, clavicular, humeral, pectoral.
Thoracic, alar	Axillary.	Axillary glands.	
Thoracic, long	Axillary.	Pectoral muscles, mammary and axillary glands.	
Thyroid axis	Subclavian.	Shoulder, neck, thorax, spine, cord.	Inferior thyroid, suprascapular, transverse cervical.
Thyroid, inferior	Thyroid axis.	Esophagus, larynx, muscles of neck.	Ascending cervical, esophageal, inferior laryngeal, muscular, tracheal.
Thyroid, superior	External carotid.	Omohyoid, sternohyoid, sternothyroid, thyroid gland.	Hyoid, sternomastoid, superior laryngeal, cricothyroid.
Tibial, anterior	Popliteal.	Leg.	Posterior and anterior tibial, recurrent, muscular, internal and external malleolar.
Tibial, posterior	Popliteal.	Leg, heel and foot.	Communicating, cutaneous, calcanean, internal and external plantar, malleolar, medullary, muscular, peroneal.
Ulnar	Brachial.	Forearm, wrist and hand.	Anterior and posterior ulnar, recurrent, common interosseous, muscular, nutrient, carpal, palmar arch.
Uterine	Branch of internal iliac.	Uterus.	Azygos, cervical, vaginal.
Vertebral	Subclavian.	Neck and cerebrum.	Anastomotic, lateral spinal, muscular, posterior cerebellar, posterior meningeal, posterior and anterior spinal.
Vesical, inferior	Internal iliac, anterior trunk.	Bladder, prostate, seminal vesicles, vagina.	
Vesical, superior	Internal iliac, anterior trunk.	Bladder.	Deferentia, ureteric.
Vidian	Internal maxillary.	Roof of pharynx, eustachian tube, tympanum.	Eustachian, pharyngeal, tympanic.

Table of Veins

Name	Description	Origin	Distribution
Alveolares superior and inferior (superior and inferior dental veins)	Veins supplying teeth and jaws. Anastomose with pterygoid plexuses.	Capillaries of teeth canals and gums.	Through jaws to structures of teeth. Between surfaces of maxillae below alveolar processes to v. facialis anterior at angle of jaw.
Angularis (angular vein)	Short superficial vein in nasal region.	Union of vv. nasofrontalis, frontalis, and supraorbitalis at root of nose.	From root of nose laterally to below eye.
Anonyma (innominate veins)	Paired veins without valves. Flow together to form vena cava superior.	Union of vv. jugularis interna and subclavia.	From sternoclavicular articulation to 1st right costal cartilage where they flow together to form vena cava superior.
Articulares genus (articular veins of knee)	Vein of knee.	Tissues of region of knee and m. articularis genu.	Tissues of region of knee to v. poplitea.
Articulares mandibulae (articular veins of mandible).	Deep veins of region of jaw; form large plexus lateral to ear. Anastomose with pterygoid plexus.	Plexus surrounding joint of jaw and tissues of external auditory canal region.	Region of jaw and adjacent structures diagonally downward to v. facialis posterior.
Auditivae internae (internal auditory)	Paired 2 from each ear. Arise in internal ear, pass through meatus acusticus internus. Drain blood from labyrinth.	From internal ear through meatus acusticus internus to sinus transversus or sinus petrosus inferior.	Empty into sinus transversus or sinus petrosus inferior.
Auriculares anteriores (anterior auricular veins)	Small veins of external ear structures.	Capillaries of tissues of external ear.	From tissues of external ear to v. facialis posterior in front of ear.
Auricularis posterior (posterior auricular vein)	Superficial vein of posterior skull region.	Capillaries of tissues of posterior portion of skull and mastoid emissarium.	From tissues of occipital region behind ear diagonally downward below ear to v. jugularis externa.
Axillaris (axillary vein)	Portion of large venous trunk from upper extremity in axillary region. Receives veins from arms and adjacent structures.	Union of deep brachial veins at lower margin of m. pectoralis major.	Region of axilla to clavicle.
Azygos (azygos vein)	Single vein draining blood from intercostal spaces, esophagus, bronchi, and mediastinal structures. Anastomoses freely with v. hemiazygos which flows into it.	Continuation of v. lumbalis ascendens dextra at diaphragm.	From level of diaphragm up posterior thoracic wall on right of vertebral bodies to v. cava superior.
Basilica (basilic vein)	Large superficial vein on medial and lateral aspect of arm and forearm. Anastomoses freely with v. cephalica.	Dorsum of hand at ulnar end of arcus venosus dorsalis.	Tissues of hand diagonally across back of hand to anterior surface of arm above elbow to upper 3rd of arm to flow into vv. brachiales.
Basivertebrales (basivertebral veins)	Veins of bodies of vertebrae.	Capillaries of vertebral bodies.	From body of each vertebra to venous plexuses of spinal column.
Brachiales (brachial veins)	Two large deep veins of upper arm.	Union of vv. ulnares and radialis at elbow.	From elbow on each side of forearm in deep tissues to unite to form v. axillaris.

Name	Description	Origin	Distribution
Bronchiales anteriores (anterior bronchiole veins)	Veins of bronchi.	Capillaries of bronchi.	From bronchi to anonyma separately or in common with other thoracic viscera.
Bronchiales posteriores (posterior bronchial veins)	Veins of posterior bronchial walls.	Capillaries of bronchial walls.	From tissues of bronchi to v. azygos at level of 4th to 6th thoracic vertebrae.
Bulbi urethrae (artery of bulb)	Corresponds to v. bulbi vestibuli in female.	Tissues of bulbus urethrae and muscles in region of trigone.	From tissues above rectum to trigone diagonally lateral to v. pudenda interna.
Canaliculi cochleae (vein of cochlear canal)	Vein of inner ear structures.	From capillaries of cochlea.	From cochlea through the canaliculus cochlea to bulbus v. jugularis superiores and jugularis interna.
Cava inferior (inferior vena cava)	Large venous trunk carrying blood from lower extremities, abdomen and trunk to right atrium. Branches from abdominal viscera flow into it.	Union of vv. iliacae communes in front of 4th or 5th lumbar vertebra.	Along posterior abdominal wall through liver and diaphragm diagonally upward in thorax to right atrium.
Cava superior (superior vena cava)	Large single venous trunk without valves, draining blood from upper part of body.	Union of two v. anonyma.	From first right costal cartilage downward to right atrium.
Cephalica (cephalic vein)	Superficial vein of arm and forearm. Anastomoses freely with v. basilica.	Dorsum of hand at radial end of arcus venosus dorsalis.	Tissues of hand, arm and forearm. Extends up lateral region of arm and forearm to v. axillaris at level of clavicle.
Cerebri externae and internae (superficial and inferior cerebral or Galen veins)	Have no valves. Collect blood from cerebral tissue.	From superficial tissues of cerebral surface and inferior substance of cerebrum.	From cerebrum through subarachnoid connective tissue of third ventricle to point where they flow together near the interventricular foramen.
Cerebri magna (magnus Galeni)	Large vein formed by union of vv. cerebri internae.	Capillaries of cerebrum.	From region of splenium corporis callosi forward to vena rectus.
Cervicalis profunda (deep cervical vein)	Deep vein of neck. Corresponds to arteria cervicalis profunda.	Plexus vertebralis posterior.	Posterior to v. jugularis interna to level of 7th cervical vertebra where it flows into vertebralis.
Circularis (circular sinus)	A blood channel in the region of the sella turcica.	Border of sella turcica.	Between 2 venae cavernosae.
Circumflexae femoris laterales (lateral circumflex femoral veins)	Veins of deep tissues of lateral aspect of thigh.	Capillaries of muscles in lateral region of thigh.	Laterally between m. rectus femoris and vastus intermedia diagonally upward to v. profunda femoris.
Circumflexae femoris mediales (internal circumflex veins)	Veins of medial and dorsal aspect of thigh and hip. Anastomose with v. glutaea.	Capillaries of tissues of knee joint and muscles of thigh.	From muscles of medial region of thigh upward beneath m. quadratus femoris to v. profunda femoris at its union with v. femoralis.
Circumflexa ilium profunda (deep circumflex iliac vein)	Vein of deep structures in iliac region.	Capillaries of deep muscles of upper portion of thigh and lower portion of abdomen.	From deep tissues from anterior superior spine of ileum along inner surface of pelvic brim to v. iliaca externa.
Circumflexa ilium superficialis (superficial circumflex iliac vein)	Superficial vein in lateral iliac region.	Capillaries of superficial tissues of lateral aspect of region of hip joint.	From superficial tissues from anterior iliac crest diagonally downward to flow into v. femoralis just before it enters external femoral ring.
Colica dextra (right colic vein)	Vein of ascending colon. Usually two.	Capillaries of walls of ascending colon.	From tissues of ascending colon through mesentery to v. mesenterica superior.

Name	Description	Origin	Distribution
Colica media (middle colic vein)	Vein of transverse colon.	Capillaries of walls of transverse colon.	From tissues of transverse colon through mesentery to v. mesenterica superior.
Colica sinistra (left colic vein)	Vein of descending colon. Anastomoses freely with vv. sigmoideae.	Capillaries of wall of descending colon.	From tissues of descending colon through mesentery laterally upward to v. mesenterica inferior.
Comitans lateralis	Vein of region of knee.	Capillaries of region of knee.	From tissues of leg and knee upward on either side of v. poplitea to flow into it.
Comitans medalis	Vein of region of knee.	Capillaries of region of knee.	From tissues of knee and leg upward to v. poplitea.
Cordis anteriores (anterior coronary veins)	Small veins of right ventricle.	Tissues of right ventricle.	From right ventricles near apex upward to flow directly into right atrium.
Cordis magna (coronary or great cardiac vein)	Large vein of anterior portion of ventricles.	Tissues of ventricles in region of apex.	From apex in anterior longitudinal sulcus upward to coronary sulcus left to right atrium through coronary sinus.
Cordis media (middle coronary vein)	Large vein of posterior portion of ventricles.	Capillaries of ventricles and ventricular septum.	From apex of heart along ventricles in longitudinal sulcus upward from apex to right atrium through coronary sinus.
Cordis parva (small or rt. cardiac vein)	Small vein of right atrium and ventricle.	Capillaries of right auricle and ventricle.	From branches in right auricle and ventricle along coronary sulcus to right atrium through coronary sinus.
Coronaria ventriculi (coronary vein of stomach)	Vein of stomach. Anastomoses with vv. gastroepiploica and pylorica.	Capillaries of upper portion of stomach.	From right or left along lesser curvature of stomach to vv. portae or lienalis near pylorus.
Costoaxillaris (costoaxillary vein)	Vein draining blood from middle portion of first 6th or 7th intercostal spaces.	Capillaries of upper intercostal spaces and veins.	From middle portion of upper 6 vv. intercostales to v. thoracoepigastrica.
Cutaneae abdominis et pectoris (subcutaneous abdominal and thoracic veins)	Veins in subcutaneous tissues of abdomen and thorax wall.	Capillaries of superficial tissues of body wall.	Throughout subcutaneous tissue of body wall by anastomoses to veins of neck, axilla and anterior abdominal wall.
Cystica (cystic vein)	Vein of gallbladder.	Capillaries of gallbladder.	From tissues of gallbladder downward to v. portae just below its entrance into liver.
Deferentiales	Veins of testes.	Capillaries of testes.	From testes along ductus deferens to plexus vesicalis.
Digitales communes pedis (common digital veins of foot)	Short veins on back of foot.	Union of vv. digitalis pedis dorsalis and intercapitulares.	From base of toes to venous arches of back of foot.
Digitales dorsales propriae (dorsal digital veins of hand)	Superficial veins of back of fingers. Anastomose freely with each other.	Capillaries of superficial tissues of fingers.	From tissues of fingers proximally along fingers dorsally to hand, uniting to form vv. digitales volares communes.
Digitales pedis dorsales (dorsal digital veins of foot)	Veins of toes on dorsal surface.	Capillaries of toes.	From tissues of toes to vv. digitales communes pedis at base of toes.
Digitales plantares (plantar digital veins)	Veins of toes on plantar surface.	From capillaries of toes.	Along plantar surface of toes to foot to become vv. metatarseae plantares.
Digitales volares communes (common digital vein of palm)	Superficial veins of palm of hand.	Capillaries of tissues of palm of hand.	From base of fingers to superficial venous arches of palm.

Name	Description	Origin	Distribution
Digitales volares propriae (palmar digital veins of hand)	Superficial veins of palmar surface of fingers. Anastomose freely with each other and dorsal veins.	Capillaries of superficial tissues of palmar surface of fingers.	Tissues of fingers along fingers to dorsal veins by vv. intercapitulares.
Diploicae (diploic veins)	Thin walled tubes in canals between the inner and outer skull surface. They have no valves except at mouth of vessels, form a network through the skull and are variable in distribution. Named from regions they drain.	Bony tissue between internal and external skull surfaces.	From bones of skull to venae durae matres and external veins of skull.
Dorsalis penis (dorsal vein of penis)	Large vein of penis along midline of dorsum.	Tissue of penis.	Along dorsum of penis upward to pelvis between symphysis pubes and urogenital trigon into plexus pudendalis in front of bladder.
Dorsales penis cutaneae (superficial veins of penis)	Small veins of skin of penis.	Capillaries of skin of penis.	From superficial tissues of penis laterally upward to v. pudendis externa.
Ductus venosus	Vein in liver functioning in fetal circulation, connecting v. umbilicalis and v. cava inferior.	V. umbilicalis.	From v. umbilicalis transversely through liver to v. cava inferior.
Duodenales (duodenal veins)	Veins of duodenum.	Walls of duodenum.	From duodenum by anastomoses to vv. iliocolica, colica media, and mesenterica superior.
Epigastricae superiores (superior epigastric veins)	Double veins of upper anterior abdominal wall. Anastomose freely with v. epigastrica inferior.	Capillaries of upper anterior abdominal wall.	From tissues of anterior abdominal wall along inner surface of m. rectus abdominis upward through diaphragm to form v. mammaria interna with v. musculophrenica.
Epigastrica inferior (inferior epigastric vein)	Vein of lower anterior abdominal wall. Tributaries drain blood from paraumbilical veins and superficial tissues of testes.	Capillaries of internal surface of lower anterior abdominal wall.	From internal surface of lower abdominal wall along m. rectus abdominus, diagonally across abdominal wall to flow into v. iliaca externa.
Epigastrica superficialis (superficial epigastric veins)	Veins draining blood from superficial regions of lower half of anterior abdominal wall.	Superficial tissues of lower portion of anterior abdominal wall.	From superficial tissues of abdominal wall, downward with many anastomoses diagonally to v. femoralis just outside entrance to external femoral ring.
Facialis anterior (anterior facial)	Superficial vein of face. Corresponds to arteria maxillaris externa. Drains blood from most of smaller superficial facial veins.	From union of vv. angularis and nasales externae at medial angle of eye.	Beneath superficial muscles of face. Diagonally across face from nose to angle to jaw where it flows into v. facialis communis.
Facialis communis (common facial vein)	Large vein of face beneath platysma.	Union of vv. facialis anterior and posterior.	From convergence of vv. faciales at angle of jaw to v. jugularis interna at level of hyoid bone.
Facialis posterior (posterior facial vein)	Deep vein of face. Branches drain deep structures of face.	Union of vv. temporalis superficialis and media.	From origin in front of ear downward through parotid gland behind ramus of mandible to angle of jaw where it forms v. jugularis interna.
Femoralis (femoral vein)	Large vein of thigh.	Continuation of v. poplitea.	From posterior region of knee through m. abductor magna upward beneath m. sartorius across thigh through femoral ring to become v. iliaca externa.

Name	Description	Origin	Distribution
Femoropoplitea (femoropopliteal vein)	Small superficial vein of dorsum of thigh and knee. Anastomoses with v. saphena magna.	Capillaries of superficial tissues in posterior region of knee.	From laterodorsal superficial tissues of knee transversely across and above knee through muscles to flow into v. poplitea.
Frontalis (frontal veins)	Superficial vein of skull, anastomosing with temporalis.	Capillaries of anterior region of scalp.	Anterior region of scalp down anterior midline diagonally across forehead to left of root of nose where it forms v. angularis.
Gastricae breves (short gastric veins)	Short veins of fundus of stomach, usually 3 to 5.	Capillaries of fundus of stomach.	From capillaries of fundus of stomach in gastrosplenic ligament to v. lienalis.
Gastroepiploica dextra (right gastroepiploic vein)	Vein of lower portion of stomach.	Capillaries of stomach.	Along lower portion of greater curvature of stomach to unite with v. gastroepiploica sinistra. Flows into v. mesenterica superior.
Gastroepiploica sinistra (left gastroepiploic vein)	Large vein of upper portion of stomach.	Capillaries of stomach.	Along greater curvature of stomach between it and spleen, unites with v. gastroepiploica dextra. Flows into v. lienalis.
Glutaea inferior (inferior gluteal vein)	Vein of lower region of hip. Anastomoses freely with v. glutaea superior.	Capillaries, gluteal and adjacent muscles.	From tissues of hip through pelvic wall to inner surface, to flow into v. hypogastrica.
Glutaea superior (superior gluteal vein)	Vein of upper region of hip. Anastomoses freely with v. glutaea inferior.	Capillaries of gluteal and adjacent muscles.	From tissues of hip through pelvic wall to inner surface to flow into v. hypogastrica.
Haemorrhoidales externae (external hemorrhoidal veins)	A plexus of veins on outer surface of rectum.	From internal plexus of rectum and veins of adjacent structures.	From outer surface of rectum to vv. pudendae internae, hypogastrica and mesenterica inferior by numerous branches.
Haemorrhoidales inferiores (inferior hemorrhoidal veins)	Veins of lower region of rectum and anus.	From plexus haemorrhoidalis externus of outer wall of rectum.	From region of anus diagonally lateral beneath m. glutaea to v. pudendae internae.
Haemorrhoidales internae (internal hemorrhoidal veins)	A plexus of veins in submucosa of rectum.	Tissues of rectum.	From inner wall of rectum through tissues of rectum by numerous branches to external plexus.
Haemorrhoidales mediae (middle hemorrhoidal veins)	Veins of middle region of plexus haemorrhoidalis externa.	Plexus haemorrhoidalis externa and tissues of bladder, prostate and seminal vesicles.	From plexus of outer rectal wall laterally to v. hypogastrica.
Haemorrhoidalis superior (superior hemorrhoidal vein)	Largest vein of region of rectum.	Capillaries of rectum and plexus on lower anterior lateral surface of rectum.	Posterior to rectum upward through mesorectum to flow into v. mesenterica inferior.
Hemiazygos (hemiazygos vein)	Single vein of lower left thoracic wall. Drains blood from intercostal veins. Anastomoses with v. azygos.	Continuation of v. lumbalis ascendens sinistra above diaphragm.	From diaphragm along left of vertebral bodies to v. azygos at 6th to 7th intercostal space.
Hemiazygos accessoria (accessory hemiazygos vein)	Drains blood from intercostal spaces above level of 6th to 7th intercostal space.	Capillaries of upper intercostal spaces.	From upper intercostal spaces along left margin of bodies of vertebrae to level of 6th to 7th intercostal space where it enters v. hemiazygos.
Hepaticae (hepatic veins)	Short, large veins from liver to v. cava inferior. Vary in number from 2 to 4.	Tissues of liver.	From lobes of liver to v. cava inferior, just below inferior surface of diaphragm.

Name	Description	Origin	Distribution
Hypogastrica (internal iliac or hypogastric vein)	Large, short vein draining blood from pelvis.	Convergence of veins of internal pelvic organs and structures.	From posterior pelvic wall upward and anterior to v. iliaca externa at brim of pelvis.
Ileocolica (ileocolic vein)	Vein of mesentery of ascending colon.	Capillaries of intestine in region of union of ileum and colon.	From region of lower portion of ascending colon and ileum through mesentery to unite with vv. colicae dextrae to flow into v. mesenterica superior.
Iliaca communis (common iliac vein	Large vein draining blood from pelvis and leg. Flow together to form v. cava inferior.	Union of vv. hypogastrica and iliaca externa.	Diagonally across pelvis from lateral region to meet in posterior midline.
Iliaca externa (external iliac vein)	Large vein from leg along anterior portion of rim of true pelvis. A continuation of v. femoralis.	V. femoralis, at its entrance into pelvis.	From v. femoralis behind inguinal ligament diagonally upward and backward to unite with v. hypogastrica to form v. iliaca communis.
Iliaca interna (see v. hypogastrica)			
Iliolumbalis (iliolumbar vein)	Vein of lower abdominal wall. Anastomoses to form collateral circulation with v. lumbalis ascendens.	Capillaries of tissues of body wall in lumbar regions.	From walls of false pelvis diagonally across inner surface of ilium to flow into v. hypogastrica or v. iliaca communis.
Intercapitulares (intercapitular veins)	Veins of hand in tissues between fingers.	Veins of fingers and tissues between fingers.	Connect between bases of fingers volar and dorsal veins of hand.
Intercavernous anterior and posterior (anterior and posterior intercavernous sinuses)	Unpaired blood channels connecting two cavernous sinuses, forming with them the circular sinus.	Layers of dura mater in region of hypophysis.	Anterior is in front and beneath hypophysis. Posterior is behind and beneath hypophysis.
Intercostales (intercostal veins)	Veins of intercostal spaces.	Capillaries of intercostal spaces.	From intercostal spaces to region along lower margin of ribs to vv. mammaria interna, azygos and costoaxillaris.
Intervertebrales (intervertebral veins)	Veins accompanying spinal nerves. Permit collateral circulation of venous plexuses of spinal cord.	From plexuses of spinal column.	Between vertebrae and between internal and external venous plexuses of spinal column.
Jugularis anterior (anterior jugular vein)	Superficial vein of anterior region of neck. Pair anastomose freely with other and adjacent veins.		From chin upon superficial muscles laterally downward across neck to v. jugularis externa or subclavia.
Jugularis externa (external jugular vein)	Large superficial vein in lateral region of neck. Main branches are vv. occipitalis and jugularis anterior.	From union of facialis posterior and auricularis posterior.	Below ear across sternocleidomastoid muscle beneath platysma down neck to v. subclavia.
Jugularis interna (internal jugular vein)	Largest vein of head and neck. Receives veins from face, neck, thyroid and larynx. With jugulares externa and anterior corresponds to arteria carotis communis.	Arises from capillaries of brain and regions of pharynx and neck, as direct continuation of v. transversus.	From foramen jugulare, where it connects with bulbus v. jugularis superioris downward on lateral wall of pharynx to junction with v. subclavia to form v. anonyma.
Labiales posteriores (labial veins)	Correspond to vv. scrotales posteriores.	Tissues of labia.	From labia to v. pudenda interna.

Name	Description	Origin	Distribution
Labiales (superior and inferior) (superior and inferior labial veins)	Superficial veins of the lips. Anastomose with each other	Capillaries of lips.	Tissues of lip to facialis anterior.
Lienalis (splenic vein)	Large vein draining blood from spleen and part of stomach.	Capillaries of spleen.	From spleen transversely across abdomen to head of pancreas where it forms v. portae with v. mesenterica.
Lingualis (lingual vein)	Vein of tongue corresponding to arteria lingualis. Anastomoses with vv. pharyngeae and thyreoidea superior.	From tongue along lower jaw to facialis. Capillaries of tongue and sublingual regions.	From tongue along lower jaw to vv. facialis or thyreoideae superiores.
Lumbales (lumbar veins)	Four or five veins of abdominal walls. Anastomose freely with each other.	Capillaries of walls of abdominal cavity.	From somatic tissues of abdomen posteriorly to v. cava inferior at various levels.
Lumbalis ascendens (ascending lumbar vein)	Vein parallel to v. cava inferior connecting lumbar veins.	Vv. Lumbales.	Along lateral border of spinal column through abdomen flowing into v. iliaca communis and continuing in thorax on right as v. azygos and on left as v. hemiazygos.
Mammaria interna (internal mammary)	Deep vein of chest draining blood from intercostal spaces. Double in the region m. transversus covered by m. transversus thoracis and single above it.	Union of vv. epigastricae superiores and musculophrenicae.	Between 7th and 10th ribs, lateral margin of inner aspect of sternum, beneath pleura, behind cartilages of the 1st to 7th rib to v. anonyma dextra at its junction with anonyma sinistra.
Mediana antebrachii (median antebrachial vein)	Superficial vein of forearm running between vv. cephalica and basilica. Anastomoses with them.	Tissues of hand and forearm.	From superficial veins of hand up forearm to v. basilica below elbow.
Mediana cubiti	Short vein of forearm for collateral circulation between vv. basilica and cephalica.	Tissues of forearm.	From v. cephalica below elbow diagonally across forearm to v. basilica at elbow.
Mediastinales anteriores (anterior mediastinal veins)	Veins of mediastinal region. May flow together or flow into veins of other viscera.	Capillaries of mediastinal viscera.	From mediastinal region to v. anonyma.
Mediastinales posteriores (posterior mediastinal veins)	Drain blood from posterior mediastinal structures.	Capillaries of mediastinal structures.	From posterior mediastinal structures to v. azygos at level of 9th to 11th thoracic vertebrae.
Meningeae (meningeal veins)	Multiple veins. Numerous in the dura mater of brain, anastomosing freely with each other. Usually accompany arteries with 2 veins for each artery.	Meninges of brain.	From meninges to sagittalis superior, sinus cavernosus and internal maxillary vein.
Mesenterica inferior (inferior mesenteric vein)	Large vein from mesentery of colon. Receives veins from region of rectum.	Capillaries of colon and rectum.	Through mesentery of colon upward to v. lienalis or v. mesenterica superior.
Mesenterica superior (superior mesenteric vein)	Large vein from small intestine which flows into v. portae.	Capillaries of mesentery of small intestines.	From mesentery of small intestines upward to head of pancreas to unite with v. lienalis to form v. portae.
Metacarpeae dorsales (dorsal metacarpal veins)	Superficial veins of back of hand. Anastomose freely with each other.	Capillaries of hand.	Superficial tissues of hand along metacarpal bones to venous arches of back of hand.

Name	Description	Origin	Distribution
Metacarpeae volares (palmar metacarpal veins)	Deep veins on both sides of hand. Anastomose with each other.	Capillaries of hand.	Deep tissues of palm of hand along metacarpal bone to palmar arches.
Metatarseae dorsales pedis (dorsal metatarsal veins)	Deep veins of back of foot.	Capillaries of deep structures of foot.	Along metatarsal bones toward ankle, uniting to form vv. tibiales anteriores.
Metatarseae plantares (plantar metatarsal veins)	Deep veins of solar aspect of foot.	Deep tissues of foot and vv. digitales plantares.	Along metatarsal bones to ankles and plantar venous arches.
Musculophrenicae (musculophrenic veins)	Veins of thoracic surface of diaphragm and lower thoracic wall.	Capillaries of thoracic surface of diaphragm and lower intercostal veins.	Along thoracic surface of diaphragm upward lateral to sternum to unite with vv. epigastricae superiores to form v. mammaria interna.
Nasales externae (external nasal veins)	Superficial veins of lower portion of nose.	Capillaries of lower portion of nose.	From tissue of nose to v. anterior facialis which they enter just below the eye.
Nasofrontalis (nasofrontal vein)	Short vein on each side of bridge of nose.	Capillaries in anterior of orbital cavity and region of frontal bone.	Between vv. supraorbitalis and angularis.
Obturatoria (obturator vein)	Vein draining blood from region of acetabulum and obturator foramen.	Capillaries of region of articulation of femur into pelvis.	Tissues of region of acetabulum and obturator foramen. Diagonally upward through tissues of region to enter pelvis on lateral aspect, diagonally backward and upward across pelvic wall to v. hypogastrica or iliaca externa.
Occipitalis (occipital vein)	Superficial vein of occipital region. Anastomoses with posterior vertebral plexus.	Capillaries of occipital region.	From superficial tissue of occipital region, and posterior vertebral plexus downward behind ear to v. jugularis externa below ear.
Oesophageae (esophageal veins)	Veins of esophagus.	Capillaries of esophagus.	From esophagus to v. azygos at level of 8th to 10th thoracic vertebrae.
Ophthalmica inferior (inferior ophthalmic vein)	Paired veins of floor of orbital cavity. Anastomose with superior ophthalmic veins.	Capillaries of lacrimal sac and eyelids.	From anterior of orbit between medial and interior wall of orbit to cavernous sinus.
Ophthalmica superior (superior ophthalmic vein)	Paired veins of orbital cavity. Have no valves. Anastomose with facial vein and inferior ophthalmic vein.	Capillaries of region of ethmoid and lacrimal bones, eyelids and ocular bulb.	From medial palpebral commissure of eye to cavernous sinus.
Ovarica (ovarian vein)	Vein of ovary.	Capillaries of ovaries and uterine tube and adjacent structures which form plexus around artery.	From plexus around artery upward from ovary across pelvic brim to become v. spermatica interna.
Palatina (palatine vein)	Deep vein of face corresponding to arteria palatina ascendens.	Capillaries of deep tissues of neck.	Deep tissues along ramus of jaw to v. facialis anterior at angle of jaw.
Palpebrales inferiores (inferior palpebral veins)	Veins of region of lower eyelid.	Capillaries of region of lower eyelid.	From region of lower eyelid to v. facialis anterior.
Palpebrales superiores (superior palpebral veins)	Veins of region of upper eyelid.	Capillaries of region of upper eyelid.	From region of upper eyelid to v. facialis anterior.
Pancreaticae (pancreatic veins)	Veins of pancreas.	Capillaries of pancreas.	From capillaries of tissues of pancreas by short veins which flow into v. lienalis at intervals.

Name	Description	Origin	Distribution
Pancreaticoduodenalis (pancreaticoduodenal vein)	Vein from duodenum and head of pancreas. Anastomoses freely with gastric veins.	Capillaries of duodenum and portions of pancreas.	Along duodenum between it and pancreas, upward to v. mesenterica superior just below its union with v. lienalis.
Parotidea anterior (anterior parotid vein)	Vein of parotid gland.	Capillaries of parotid gland.	From tissues of parotid gland to v. facialis anterior which it enters above angle of jaw.
Parotidea posterior (posterior parotid vein)	Vein of posterior portion of parotid gland.	Capillaries of posterior portion of parotid gland.	Posterior portion of parotid gland, interior to ear upward to union of v. temporalis superficialis with v. facialis posterior.
Parumbilicales (paraumbilical veins)	Small veins in region of umbilicus connecting superficial and deep veins.	Superficial tissues of region of umbilicus.	From superficial veins in umbilical region by anastomoses with vv. epigastricae to liver substance.
Pericardiacae (pericardial veins)	Veins of pericardium.	From capillaries of pericardium.	From pericardium to v. anonyma or to other veins of viscera which empty into it.
Peronaea (peroneal vein)	Deep vein of leg.	Veins of ankle and capillaries of tissues of leg.	From venous plexus in region of heel upward along lateral region of deep tissue to flow into v. tibialis posterior below knee.
Petrosus inferior (inferior petrosal sinus)	Paired blood channels in dura mater in temporal region.	Groove between petrous portion of temporal bone and basilar portion of occipital.	From petrous portion of temporal bone to superior jugular vein at its bulb.
Petrosus superior (superior petrosal sinus)	Paired blood channels in dura mater in temporal regions.	From region of petrous portion of temporal bone in the attached margin of tentorium cerebelli.	Between vena cavernosus and vena transversus.
Pharyngeae (pharyngeal veins)	Veins of pharyngeal region. Vary in number, from the plexus pharyngeus. Anastomose with veins of external ear, deep muscles of pharynx, palate and dura mater.	From plexus on outer pharyngeal surface.	From capillaries of pharyngeal region to v. jugularis interna or its adjacent branches at various levels.
Phrenica inferior (inferior phrenic)	Vein of abdominal surface of diaphragm.	Tissues of diaphragm.	Throughout abdominal surface of diaphragm to v. cava superior just below cava hiatus of diaphragm.
Phrenicae superiores (superior phrenic veins)	Paired veins of anterior wall of thorax, corresponding to arteriae pericardiacophrenicae.	Capillaries of pericardium.	From diaphragm through thoracic cavity in front of root of lung on pericardium to v. anonyma.
Plantares laterales (lateral plantar veins)	Veins of sole of foot.	Venous arches of sole of foot.	Along lateral margin of sole of foot upward to form vv. tibiales posteriores with vv. plantares mediales.
Plantares mediales (medial plantar veins)	Veins of sole of foot.	Venous arches of sole of foot.	Along medial aspect of sole of foot upward to form vv. tibiales posteriores with vv. plantares laterales.
Poplitea (popliteal vein)	Large vein in posterior region of knee. Has parallel median and lateral concomitants.	Union of vv. tibiales.	From vv. tibiales below knee in middorsal line upward to become femoral vein as it enters m. adductor.
Portae (portal vein)	Collects blood from digestive tract and conveys it to the liver. Terminates in capillary formation in liver	Union of vv. mesenterica superior and lienalis.	From head of pancreas upward posterior to bile ducts to hilum of liver to divide into right and left branch to liver.

Name	Description	Origin	Distribution
Profundae clitoridis (deep veins of clitoris)	Vein of clitoris.	Tissues of clitoris.	From clitoris to v. pudenda interna.
Profundae penis (deep veins of penis)	Vein of corpora cavernosa of penis. Branches anastomose freely with each other.	Capillaries of penis.	Above penis in crus penis. Flows into v. dorsalis penis at root of penis.
Profunda femoris (deep femoral vein)	Deep vein of thigh.	Capillaries of muscles of thigh.	From midregion of thigh upward beneath anterior muscles to v. femoralis.
Pudendae externae (external pudic veins)	Veins draining blood from superficial regions of medial aspect of upper thigh.	Capillaries of superficial tissues of lower abdomen, scrotum or labia.	Superficial tissues of lower abdomen and scrotum or labia, transversely across upper region of thigh to v. femoralis.
Pudenda interna (internal pudic vein)	Vein of pelvic floor draining blood from pelvic walls and penis or clitoris.	From anastomoses with v. dorsalis penis or clitoridis below symphysis pubis.	From trigonum urogenitale along pelvic wall backwards and upwards to flow into v. hypogastrica.
Pylorica (pyloric vein)	Small vein of pyloric region of stomach. Anastomoses with other gastric veins.	Capillaries of pyloric portion of stomach.	Along lesser curvature of stomach to v. portae near pylorus.
Radialis (radial vein)	Large deep vein on radial side of forearm.	Palmar arches of hand.	Palmar arches of hand along lateral side of forearm in deep tissues to unite with v. ulnaris at elbow to form vv. brachiales.
Rectus (straight sinus)	Single blood channel in layers of dura mater connecting superior and inferior sagittal sinuses.	At point of attachment of falx cerebri to tentorium cerebelli.	Between superior and inferior venous channel at base of skull.
Renales (renal veins)	Veins of kidney. Receive blood from veins of ureter. The v. spermatica interna flows into v. renalis on left.	From capillaries of kidneys by fusion of small vessels near hilum of kidney.	From hilus of kidney transversely across posterior abdominal wall to v. cava inferior.
Rete dorsale manus (dorsal venous rete of hand)	A network of veins on dorsal surface of hand at wrist.	Veins of dorsal surface of hands.	From vv. metacarpeae dorsales, flowing together and multiple anastomoses at wrist, becoming vv. basilica and cephalica.
Rete dorsale pedis (dorsal venous rete of foot)	A network of veins on back of foot at ankle.	Veins of dorsal surface of foot.	From vv. digitales pedis dorsales by multiple anastomoses to network of veins of ankle.
Sacralis lateralis (lateral sacral vein)	Vein of posterior pelvic wall. Forms plexus with v. sacralis media.	Capillaries of tissues of posterior pelvic wall.	From tissues of posterior wall upward laterally on pelvic surface of sacrum to flow into v. hypogastrica or iliaca communis.
Sacralis media (middle sacral vein)	Large vein of posterior pelvic wall. Forms plexus with v. sacralis lateralis.	Capillaries of tissues of posterior wall.	From tissues of pelvic wall in sacral region upward along sacrum in middle line to flow into v. hypogastrica or iliaca communis.
Sagittalis inferior (inferior longitudinal sinus)	Single blood channel between layers of dura mater at the base of the falx cerebri.	From regions of superior dura mater and skull.	Entire length of inferior free margin of falx cerebri.
Sagittalis superior (superior longitudinal sinus)	Single blood channel between layers of dura mater in sagittal plane. Triangular in shape.	Region of falx cerebri and anterior portion of skull cavity.	From crista galli of ethmoid bone along sagittal sulcus of frontal, parietal, and occipital bones into transverse sinus.

Name	Description	Origin	Distribution
Saphena magna	Large superficial vein of leg and thigh. Longest in body.	Capillaries of superficial tissues of leg and thigh and veins of foot.	Along medial aspect of leg from ankle upward across knee and thigh to enter femoral ring to flow into v. femoris.
Saphena parva (short saphenous vein)	Large superficial vein of back of leg.	Superficial veins of foot and capillaries of tissues of leg.	From ankle upward in middorsal line to above knee. Flows into v. saphena magna.
Scrotales anteriores (anterior scrotal veins)	Superficial veins of anterior region of scrotum.	Capillaries of superficial tissues of scrotum.	From anterior of scrotum transversely across thigh to v. pudenda externa.
Scrotales posteriores (posterior scrotal veins)	Veins of scrotum. Correspond to vv. labiales in female.	Capillaries of scrotum, posterior portion.	From scrotum upward laterally in perineum to pudenda interna in pelvic floor.
Sigmoideae (sigmoid veins)	Small veins of region of sigmoid flexure of colon.	Capillaries in region of sigmoid flexure.	Tissues of sigmoid colon through mesentery to v. mesenterica inferior.
Spermatica interna (spermatic vein)	Consists of 2 or 3 anastomosing vessels surrounding a. spermatica. Receives veins from ureters, peritoneum and kidney capsule.	From testicular vein in male and ovarian vein in female.	From brim of pelvis upward along posterior abdominal wall to v. cava inferior on right and v. renalis on left.
Sphenopalatina (sphenopalatine vein)	Vein draining deep structures of face and skull in nasal region.	Capillaries of deep nasal regions.	From nasal cavity through sphenopalatine foramen to pterygoid plexus in front of ear.
Sphenoparietalis (sphenoparietal sinus)	Paired blood channels of dura mater, from sphenoparietal region.	Capillaries of anterior temporal vein of diploe, middle meningeal and ophthalmomeningeal vein.	Each side of skull, behind coronal suture, to anterior end of sinus cavernosus.
Stylomastoidea (stylomastoid vein)	Corresponds to arteria stylomastoideus from middle and inner ear.	Capillaries of mastoid region and middle ear structures.	From mastoid and middle ear through stylomastoid foramen into facial canal behind ear to v. facialis posterior.
Subclavia (subclavian vein)	Large venous trunk to upper extremity. A continuation of v. axillaris in region of clavicle. Main tributaries are vv. transversa scapulae and coli.	V. axillaris and veins flowing into it from adjacent regions.	Beneath clavicle across first rib, to form v. anonyma with v. jugularis interna.
Submentalis (submental vein)	Superficial vein of under portion of chin. Anastomoses with v. lingualis and palatina.	Capillaries of region of chin.	From tissues of chin diagonally across chin to flow into v. facialis anterior or facialis communis below angle of jaw.
Supraorbitalis (supraorbital vein)	Vein of upper portion of orbital cavity.	Capillaries and superficial tissues in region of eye.	From superficial tissues of region of eye through supraorbital foramen along lateral wall of orbital cavity to nose where it joins v. nasofrontalis.
Suprarenalis (suprarenal vein.	Vein of adrenal glands.	Capillaries of adrenal glands.	·From tissues of adrenal glands to v. cava inferior on right and vv. renales on left.
Temporalis media (median temporal vein)	Superficial vein of lateral portion of skull. Anastomoses with vv. temporalis superficialis and supraorbitalis.	Lateral superficial plexus of skull.	From lateral superficial tissues of skull transversely downward from level of lateral canthus of eye through temporal muscle to join v. temporalis superficialis in front of ear.
Temporalis superficialis (superficial temporal vein)	Vein of superficial tissues of skull. Anastomoses freely with v. frontalis.	Superficial plexus of roof of skull.	Tissues of roof of skull diagonally downward to join vv. temporalis media in front of ear.

Name	Description	Origin	Distribution
Testicularis (testicular vein)	Vein of testes.	Capillaries of testes and epididymis which form close plexus around artery.	From tissues of testes and epididymis and plexus from veins of these organs through inguinal canal to become v. spermatica interna.
Thoracalis lateralis (long thoracic vein)	Long vein of lateral and anterior chest wall.	Capillaries of muscles in anterior chest and mammary glands.	Tissues of anterior chest muscles to v. axillaris with v. transversa colli.
Thoracoepigastrica (thoracoepigastric vein)	Superficial vein of trunk to permit collateral circulation between veins of arms and legs and trunk.	V. femoralis in inguinal region, and capillaries of superficial tissues of trunk.	Lateral wall of body from v. femoralis to v. thoracalis lateralis in axillary region below its union with v. axillaris.
Thymicae (veins of thymus)	Veins of thymus gland.	From capillaries of thymus gland.	From thymus gland to v. anonyma.
Thyreoidea ima (thyroid ima)	Large, short vein from plexus thyreoideus.	Plexus of thyroid.	From middle portion of plexus thyreoideus downward anterior to trachea to v. anonyma sinistra.
Thyreoideae inferiores (inferior thyroid veins)	Paired veins from plexus thyreoideus. Anastomose freely with thyreoideae superiores.	Plexus thyreoideus and regions of trachea, esophagus and larynx.	From thyroid plexus to v. jugularis interna at junction with subclavia.
Thyreoideae superiores (superior thyroid veins)	Two veins from superior portion of thyroid. Receive blood from vv. sternocleidomastoidea and laryngea.	Capillaries of thyroid.	From tissues of thyroid to v. jugularis interna at level of larynx, or to v. facialis communis.
Tibiales anteriores (anterior tibial veins)	Deep veins of anterior aspect of leg.	From union of vv. metatarseae dorsales pedis and capillaries of tissues of leg.	From dorsum of foot upward beneath m. tibialis anterior upward to knee, passing backward to flow into v. poplitea.
Tibiales posteriores (posterior tibial veins)	Deep veins of back of leg.	Union of vv. plantares and laterales and mediales in region of heel and capillaries of deep tissues of leg.	From ankle upward in median portion of deep tissues of posterior aspect of leg to flow into v. poplitea below knee.
Transversa colli (transverse cervical vein)	Drains blood from supraspinous region of scapula and neck.	Capillaries of supraspinous region of scapula and neck.	From supraspinous region of scapula diagonally across shoulder to v. axillaris with transversa scapulae.
Transversa faciei (transverse facial vein)	Superficial facial vein running directly upon masseter muscle and behind parotid gland.	Capillaries of middle portion of face.	From tissues of middle portion of face, transversely across face to v. facialis posterior in front of ear.
Transversa scapulae (transverse scapular vein)	Large vein of dorsal surface of scapula.	Capillaries of tissues of dorsal surface of scapula.	From tissues of dorsal scapular surface, two trunks on each side of scapular spine across shoulder to v. subclavia.
Transversus (lateral sinus)	Paired blood channels between layers of dura mater of base of skull. Cylindrical in shape.	Posterior region of skull cavity.	From internal occipital protuberance medially and inferiorly into internal jugular vein at jugular foramen.
Ulnaris (ulnar vein)	Large deep vein of medial side of forearm.	From palmar arches of hand.	From palmar arches of hand upward in deep tissues along ulnar side of forearm to form v. brachialis with v. radialis at elbow.
Umbilicalis (umbilical vein)	Vein carrying arterial blood from placenta to fetus.	Placental tissues.	Along umbilical cord through umbilicus to liver and ductus venosus.

Name	Description	Origin	Distribution
Urethrales (urethral veins)	Veins of corpus cavernosum urethrae.	Capillaries of urethra and adjacent regions.	From structures of urethra to plexus pudendalis behind symphysis pubis to v. pudenda interna.
Uterinae (uterine veins)	Veins carrying blood from uterus.	From tissues of uterus through plexus uterovaginalis.	From lateral margin of uterus in plexus uterovaginalis laterally to v. hypogastrica.
Uterovaginales (uterovaginal veins)	Plexus of veins around vagina at lateral margin of uterus.	Tissues of vagina and uterus.	From lower regions of uterus and vagina by multiple anastomoses to plexus pudendalis and v. ovarica.
Vertebrales externi anteriores and posteriores (anterior and posterior external vertebral plexuses)	Plexuses on external surfaces of spinal column.	From tissues of vertebrae from vv. intercostales and intervertebrales along anterior and posterior aspects of spinal column. Branches flow into vv. vertebrales interni.	From branches from tissues of spinal column and cord longitudinally in canal.
Vertebrales interni (internal vertebral veins)	Plexuses of veins running within spinal canal, the length of the canal.	Capillaries of vertebrae and tissues of spinal cord.	From foramen magnum. Empty into v. occipitalis and plexus basilaris superiorly and vv. sacrales inferiorly.
Vertebralis (vertebral vein)	Vein draining blood from plexus venosi vertebrales, v. occipitalis, deep muscles of neck and plexus vertebralis externi. Corresponds to cervical portion of arteria vertebralis.	From vena occipitalis and capillaries of veins of spinal canal and deep muscles of neck.	Foramen magnum downward lateral to arteria vertebralis through foramina transversaria of 1st, 6th or 7th cervical vertebra to external jugularis externa.
Vesicales (vesicular veins)	Veins of urinary bladder.	Tissues of bladder and plexus vesicalis.	From plexus vesicalis at base of bladder to v. pudenda interna.

Dietetics

Food Tables[1]

100 CALORIE PORTION TABLE

Foodstuffs	Weight		P., Gm.	F., Gm.	C., Gm.	Water, Gm.	P., Cal.	F., Cal.	C., Cal.	Vitamins			Minerals		
	Gm.	Oz.								A	B	C	Calcium (Ca), Gm.	Phosphorus (P), Gm.	Iron (Fe), Gm.
Breads, etc.:															
Rye, 1 thick slice	38.3	1.35	3.44	0.23	20.40	14.12	14.1	2.1	83.7	*	++	*	0.009	0.58	0.0006
White, 1 thick slice	37.1	1.31	3.37	0.59	19.75	13.10	13.8	5.6	81.0	+	+	— to +	0.010	0.035	0.00034
Whole wheat, 1 thick slice	39.7	1.40	3.85	0.36	19.83	15.25	15.8	3.4	81.2	+ to ++	++	— to +	0.020	0.072	0.00065
Zwieback, 3 pieces	23.2	0.82	2.27	2.30	17.09	1.34	9.3	21.4	70.0						
Flour, white, pastry, 3 tbs.	27.7	0.93	3.41	0.30	20.20	3.63	14.0	2.8	82.8	—	— to +	—	0.006	0.026	0.00023
Flour, whole wheat, 2¾ tbs.	27.1	0.95	3.74	0.52	19.50	3.10	15.3	4.1	80.0	+	++	—	0.009	0.025	0.0007
Cereals, dry:															
Cornflakes, 1⅓ cups	27.1	0.96	1.49	0.41	21.95		6.1	3.8	90.2						0.00055
Cornmeal, ⅓ cup	27.4	0.97	2.52	0.52	20.70	3.06	10.4	4.8	84.9	+	++	—	0.005	0.052	0.00025
Cornstarch, 3 tbs.	27.1	0.96	—	—	24.4		—	—	100	—	—	—			
Farina, 2 tbs.	26.9	0.97	2.86	0.37	20.50	2.72	11.7	3.4	84.0	—	— to +	—	0.006	0.035	0.00022
Grapenuts, 3 tbs.	26.3	0.95	3.03	0.26	20.20		12.0	2.0	85.4						
Macaroni. 1¼ cups	27.2	0.96	3.59	0.26	20.25	2.80	14.7	2.3	83.0	—	— to +	—	0.006	0.039	0.0003
Oatmeal, 2¼ tbs.	24.8	0.88	4.00	1.64	16.75	1.81	16.4	15.3	68.7	— to +	++	—	0.017	0.099	0.00096
Puffed rice, 1⅓ cups	26.2	0.93	2.16	0.07	21.9		8.9	0.6	90.0						
Rice, raw, 2 tbs.	27.8	0.97	2.22	0.08	22.0	3.42	9.1	0.7	90.2	—	—	—	0.003	0.027	0.00025
Shredded wheat, 1 biscuit	26.8	0.95	2.7	0.37	20.78	2.18	11.1	3.5	85.4	+	++	—	0.011	0.089	0.0012
Tapioca, pearl, 2½ tbs.	27.5	0.97	0.11	0.03	24.18	3.14	0.5	0.3	99.2	—	—	—	0.006	0.025	0.0004
Graham crackers, 6 or 7 small	23.3	0.82	2.33	2.19	17.18	1.26	9.6	20.4	70.4	+	++	—			
Soda crackers, 5	23.5	0.83	2.30	2.14	17.20	1.39	9.4	19.6	70.5	—	—	—	0.005	0.024	0.0004

+ indicates that the food contains the vitamin.
++ indicates that the food is a good source of the vitamin.
+++ indicates that the food is an excellent source of the vitamin.
— indicates that the food contains no appreciable amount of the vitamin.
* indicates that evidence is lacking or appears insufficient.
e.p. edible portion. a.p. as purchased.

[1]Boynton, *Cyclopedia of Medicine, Surgery, and Specialties,* F. A. Davis Company.

100 CALORIE PORTION TABLE—*Continued*

Foodstuffs	Weight		P., Gm.	F., Gm.	C., Gm.	Water, Gm.	P., Cal.	F., Cal.	C., Cal.	Vitamins			Minerals		
	Gm.	Oz.								A	B	C	Calcium (Ca), Gm.	Phosphorus (P), Gm.	Iron (Fe), Gm.
Dairy Products:															
Butter, 1 tbs.	12.6	0.45	0.13	10.70	—	1.38	0.5	99.5	—	+++	—	*	0.002	0.002	0.00003
Cheese, American, 1¼ in. cube	22.0	0.78	6.30	7.85	0.66	6.94	25.0	73.0	2.0	++	*	*	0.204	0.154	0.00028
Cheese, cottage, 5½ tbs.	89.0	3.12	18.50	0.89	3.80	64.10	76.0	8.3	15.6	+	*	*			
Cheese, full cream, 1½ in. cube	23.0	0.82	5.95	7.85	0.55	7.86	24.2	73.0	2.2	++	*	—			
Cream, "20 per cent," 4 tbs.	51.4	1.81	1.28	9.50	2.31	37.74	5.2	88.4	9.5	+++	++	— to +			
Cream, "40 per cent," 2 tbs.	25.3	0.90	0.57	10.12	0.76	12.28	2.3	94.2	3.1	+++	++	— to +	0.022	0.017	0.00008
Milk:															
Buttermilk, 1⅛ cups	275	9.70	8.30	1.29	13.20	250	34	12	54	+	++	— to +	0.289	0.266	0.0007
Condensed, sweetened, 1½ tbs.	30	1.06	2.4	2.5	16.2	8.1	10	23	67	+++	++	+	0.177	0.138	0.00036
Evaporated, unsweetened, 3¾ tbs.	59.0	2.08	5.8	5.4	6.3	40.25	24	50	26	+++	++	— to +			
Skim, 1⅛ cups	255	9.4	9.0	0.75	13.7	231	37	7	56	+	++	— to +	0.311	0.245	0.00064
Whole, scant ⅔ cup	140	4.9	4.6	5.6	7.0	122	18.9	51.7	28.6	+++	++	— to +	0.167	0.129	0.00033
Fats:															
Cottonseed oil, 1 tbs.	10.7	0.5	—	10.7	—	—	—	100	—	— to +	—	—			
Crisco, 1 tbs.	11.3	0.4	—	10.7	—	0.6	—	100	—	—	—	—			
Lard, 1 tbs.	11.3	0.4	—	10.7	—	0.6	—	100	—	— to +	—	—			
Oleo, 1 tbs.	12.9	0.42	0.15	10.6	—	0.7	0.6	99.5	—	— to +	—	—			
Fish:															
Haddock, e. p., generous serving	135.5	4.8	23.3	0.4	—	111	95.7	3.8	—	— to +	+	*	0.025	0.267	0.0013
Oysters, a. p., ⅜ cup	197	7	11.83	2.56	6.52	174	48.7	23.8	26.8	+ to ++	+ to ++	— to +	0.103	0.305	0.0087
Salmon, canned, ½ cup	49.7	1.76	10.82	6.02	—	31.6	44.3	56.0	—	+	*	*	0.011	0.124	0.0006

100 CALORIE PORTION TABLE—*Continued*

Foodstuffs	Weight		P., Gm.	F., Gm.	C., Gm.	Water, Gm.	P., Cal.	F., Cal.	C., Cal.	Vitamins			Minerals		
	Gm.	Oz.								A	B	C	Calcium (Ca), Gm.	Phosphorus (P), Gm.	Iron (Fe), Gm.
Fruits:															
Apples, fresh, 1 large......	157	5.6	0.63	0.78	22.1	132	2.6	7.3	90.5	+	+	++	0.011	0.019	0.0005
Apricots, dried, 7 halves...	35.1	1.24	1.65	0.35	21.9	10.3	6.8	3.3	90				0.023	0.041	0.0005
Banana, 1 small..........	99	3.5	1.28	0.6	21.7	74	5.3	5.5	89	+ to ++	+	++	0.009	0.031	0.0006
Blackberries, canned, 1 cup..................	168	6.0	2.2	1.7	18.3	145	9.0	15.6	75.2				0.029	0.057	0.001
Cantaloupe, e. p., average serving................	245	8.9	1.47	—	22.8	222	6.4	—	93.4	++	++	++	0.041	0.037	0.0007
Cherries, canned, ⅔ cup...	109	3.9	1.21	0.11	23.1	84	4.9	1.0	94.5	++	++	*	0.020	0.034	0.0004
Cranberries, a. p., 2 cups..	211	7.5	0.84	1.26	20.8	188	3.4	11.7	85.4	*	*	+	0.038	0.027	0.0012
Dates, dried, e. p., 4 or 5...	28.1	1.0	0.6	0.8	22.0	4.4	2.5	7.5	90.2	+	++	*	0.018	0.016	0.0008
Figs, dried, a. p., 1½ or 2..	30.8	1.1	1.32	0.1	22.8	5.8	5.4	0.8	93.6				0.050	0.035	0.0009
Grapes, e. p., 1 medium bunch................	100.5	3.6	1.3	1.6	19.3	77.7	5.4	15.0	79.3	+	+ to ++	+	0.019	0.031	0.0003
Grapefruit, ½...........	207	7.3	1.7	0.44	21.7	181	6.9	4.1	88.5	+	++	+++	0.043	0.041	0.0006
Lemons, e. p., 3 large.....	221	7.8	2.2	1.5	18.8	197	9.1	14.3	77.0	+	++	+++	0.080	0.049	0.0013
Oranges, e. p., 1 large.....	189	6.7	1.5	0.38	21.8	164	6.2	3.5	89.8	++	++	+++	0.085	0.040	0.0004
Peaches, canned, 3 halves..	206	7.3	1.4	0.21	22.25	182	5.9	2.0	91.5	+ to ++	+	+ to ++	0.033	0.049	0.0006
Peaches, fresh, e. p., 2 large..................	239	8.5	1.7	0.24	22.4	213	6.8	2.2	91.8	+ to ++	+	+	0.038	0.057	0.0007
Pears, canned, 3 halves....	128	4.5	0.38	0.38	23.1	104	1.6	3.5	94.5	*	*	— to +	0.019	0.033	0.0004
Pears, fresh, 1 large.......	154	5.4	0.92	0.77	21.7	129	3.8	7.2	89	*	+ to ++	+	0.023	0.040	0.0005
Pineapple, canned, 1 slice..	63.5	2.24	0.25	0.44	23.1	39.2	1.0	4.1	94.8	++	++	++			
Pineapple, fresh, 2 in. slice.	227	8.0	0.9	0.7	21.8	201	3.7	6.3	89.5	++	++	++	0.041	0.063	0.0011
Prunes, dried, e. p., 3 or 4..	32.4	1.14	0.7	—	23.7	7.2	2.8	—	97.2	++	++	—	0.017	0.034	0.001
Raisins, ¼ cup...........	31.4	1.1	0.72	0.94	21.5	4.6	3.0	8.7	88.1	—	+	—	0.020	0.041	0.0007

100 CALORIE PORTION TABLE—*Continued*

Foodstuffs	Weight		P., Gm.	F., Gm.	C., Gm.	Water, Gm.	P., Cal.	F., Cal.	C., Cal.	Vitamins			Minerals		
	Gm.	Oz.								A	B	C	Calcium (Ca), Gm.	Phosphorus (P), Gm.	Iron (Fe), Gm.
Fruits (continued):															
Raspberries, black, 1¼ cups	146	5.2	2.5	1.5	18.4	123	10.2	13.6	75.7	*	*	+++			
Rhubarb, e. p., 1 quart diced	423	15	2.5	3.0	15.3	399	10.4	27.5	62.7	*	*	+	0.190	.0131	0.004
Strawberries, e. p., 1½ cups	252	8.9	2.5	1.5	18.6	227	10.3	14.0	76.2	+	+	+++	0.103	0.070	0.002
Watermelon, e. p., large serving	324	11.4	1.3	0.65	21.7	300	5.3	6.0	89.0				0.035	0.010	
Grape juice, ½ cup	132	4.7	0.52	—	24.2	106	2.1	—	99.0	+	+ to ++	+	0.011	0.011	0.00030
Orange juice, 1 cup	233	8.2	—	—	24.4		—	—	100	++	++	+++	0.067	0.037	0.00046
Meat:															
Beef, liver, e. p., average serving	75.1	2.66	15.3	3.4	1.3	53.5	62.8	31.4	5.3	+ to +++	++	*	0.009	0.165	0.002
Loin medium fat, e. p., small serving	38.1	1.35	7.05	7.7	—	23.2	28.9	71.2	—	+	+	— to +	0.004	0.077	0.001
Round medium fat, e. p., small serving	47.8	1.7	9.7	6.5	—	31.2	39.7	60.4	—	+	+	— to +	0.006	0.104	0.0015
Lamb, leg, e. p., small serving	43	1.5	8.25	7.1	—	27.4	33.8	66	—	— to +	+	*	0.005	0.089	0.0012
Pork, bacon, medium fat, e. p., 2 or 3 slices cooked	15	0.53	1.48	10.1	—	3.0	6.1	93.7	—						
Ham, fresh, e. p., small serving	30.2	1.06	4.62	8.72	—	15.1	19.0	81.2	—	— to +	++	*	0.003	0.050	0.0007
Ham, smoked, e. p., boneless, small serving	30.6	1.08	4.56	8.73	—	12.2	18.7	81.2	—	— to +	++	—			
Sausage, a. p., 1 small	21.4	0.76	2.8	9.4	0.24	8.6	11.4	87.7	1.0	— to +	++	—			
Veal, cutlet, average serving	64.4	2.27	13.1	5.0	—	45.5	»3.3	46.1	—	— to +	+	—	0.008	0.141	0.0019

100 CALORIE PORTION TABLE—*Continued*

Foodstuffs	Weight		P., Gm.	F., Gm.	C., Gm.	Water, Gm.	P., Cal.	F., Cal.	C., Cal.	Vitamins			Minerals		
	Gm.	Oz.								A	B	C	Calcium (Ca), Gm.	Phosphorus (P), Gm.	Iron (Fe), Gm.
Miscellaneous:															
Eggs, whites	181	6.4	23.5	0.36	—	156	96.5	3.4	—	—	—	*	0.021	0.025	0.0002
Whole, e. p., 1¼	63	2.2	9.32	6.62	—	42.45	38.2	61.6	—	++	+ to ++	*	0.042	0.113	0.0019
Yolks, 1½	26.6	0.94	4.18	8.87	—	13.15	17.1	82.5	—	+++	++	*	0.036	0.139	0.0023
Gelatin, 3 tbs.	27.3	0.96	24.3	0.03	—		99.8	0.3	—						
Mayonnaise, 1 tbs.	11.3	0.40	0.14	10.7	0.03		0.6	99.5	0.1						
Soup, celery, canned, ¾ cup	182	6.4	3.8	5.1	9.1	161	15.6	47.2	32.3				0.065	0.054	
Soup, tomato, canned, 1 cup	245	8.7	4.4	2.2	13.7	220	18.1	25.1	56.3				0.088	0.073	
Nuts:															
Almonds, e. p., 10 to 15	14.9	0.53	3.14	8.21	2.58	0.72	12.9	77.1	10.5	+	++	*	0.036	0.070	0.0006
Peanuts, e. p., 20 to 25	17.7	0.63	4.57	6.85	4.33	1.63	18.8	63.6	17.7	+	++	*	0.013	0.071	0.0004
Peanut butter, a. p., 2 tbs.	15.9	0.56	4.66	7.40	2.70	1.09	19.1	68.8	11.1	+	++	*			
Walnuts, e. p., 10 to 15	13.8	0.45	2.30	8.77	2.23	0.35	9.4	81.6	9.1	+	++	*	0.012	0.050	0.0003
Poultry:															
Fowl, ½ serving	43.4	1.5	8.37	7.07	—	27.8	34.3	65.7	—	— to +	+	*	0.005	0.090	0.0012
Sugar:															
Granulated, 1⅜ tbs., 5 tps.	24.4	0.86	—	—	24.4	—	—	—	100	—	—	—			
Vegetables:															
Asparagus, fresh, 20 large stalks	435	15.4	7.85	0.87	14.4	410	32.2	8.1	59.1	++	+++	*	0.109	0.017	0.0044
Beans, baked, canned, 1⅓ cups	75	2.7	5.1	1.9	15.1	51.6	21	18	62	+	++	*			
Beans, dried, 2 tbs.	28.2	1.0	6.35	0.51	16.8	3.6	26.1	4.7	69.1	*	++	*	0.45	1.33	0.002

100 CALORIE PORTION TABLE—*Continued*

Foodstuffs	Weight		P., Gm.	F., Gm.	C., Gm.	Water, Gm.	P., Cal.	F., Cal.	C., Cal.	Vitamins			Minerals		
	Gm.	Oz.								A	B	C	Calcium (Ca), Gm.	Phosphorus (P), Gm.	Iron (Fe), Gm.
Vegetables (continued):															
Beans, fresh, string, 2¼ cups	232	8.1	5.4	0.70	17.4	207	22.1	6.5	71.4	++	++	++	0.107	0.121	0.0026
Beans, dried, lima, 2 tbs.	27.9	0.8	5.05	0.42	18.3	2.9	20.8	3.8	75.7				0.022	0.086	0.002
Beets, fresh, e. p., 3 to 5	211	7.4	3.4	0.21	20.5	185	13.8	2.0	84	— to +	+	+	0.556	0.075	0.0012
Cabbage, e. p., 1 small, 5 cups	313	11.2	5.0	0.94	17.4	284	20.4	8.8	71.5	+	++	+++	0.141	0.091	0.0034
Carrots, e. p., 5 medium	215	7.6	2.4	0.89	19.7	190	10	8	82	+++	++	++	0.120	0.099	0.0013
Cauliflower, a. p., 1 small	312	11	5.6	1.6	15.1	288	23	15	62	+	++	+	0.384	0.190	0.0019
Celery, e. p., 4 to 5 sma'l bunches	540	19	5.6	0.54	19.0	510	24	5	71	— to +	++	*	0.421	0.199	0.0027
Corn, green, e. p., ½ cup	100	3.54	2.8	1.2	19.0	75.4	11.5	11.2	78	+	++	+	0.006	0.103	0.0008
Eggplant, ¾	350	12	4.15	1.07	17.8	325	17	10	73	+	+	*	0.039	0.119	0.0018
Lentils, dried, 2½ tbs.	28	1.0	7.2	0.28	16.6	2.4	29.4	2.6	68	+	++	—	0.030	0.123	0.0002
Lettuce, e. p., 2 heads	505	18	6.1	1.5	14.7	479	24.9	14.2	60.3	+ to ++	++	+++	0.217	0.212	
Mushrooms, e. p., 20 to 25 small	216	7.5	7.6	0.9	14.7	190	31	8	60.2	— to +	+	—	0.037	0.231	
Onions, e. p., 5 medium	202	7.15	3.23	0.61	20.0	177	13.2	5.6	81.9	— to +	+	++	0.069	0.091	0.0012
Parsnips, e. p., 2 to 3	151	5.35	2.42	0.76	20.4	125	9.9	7	83.5	— to +	++	*	0.089	0.115	0.0009
Peas, green, ⅓ cup	97.6	3.45	6.85	0.5	16.5	73	28.2	4.5	67.5	++	— to ++	++	0.027	0.124	0.0017
Potato, boiled, 1 medium	103	3.4	2.6	0.10	21.4	78	10.5	0.93	87.8	+	++	+			
Potato, raw, 1 medium	118	4.16	2.6	0.12	21.7	92	10.6	1.1	89	+	++	++	0.017	0.058	0.0015
Potato, sweet, ½ medium	79.6	2.81	1.43	0.57	21.8	54.9	5.9	5.3	89	+ to ++	++	++	0.015	0.036	0.0004
Rutabagas	238	8.4	3.1	0.48	20.2	212	12.7	4.4	83	+		++	0.176	0.133	
Sauerkraut, 1¼ cups	363	12.8	6.15	1.83	13.8	322	25.2	17.2	56.6	+	+	+ to ++			
Spinach, cooked, 2 cups	174	6.15	3.7	7.1	4.5	156	15	66.3	18.5	+++	+	+ to ++			
Spinach, fresh, a. p.	412	14.6	8.7	1.24	13.4	380	35.4	11.5	54.8	+++	++	+++	0.276	0.280	0.0148

100 CALORIE PORTION TABLE—*Continued*

Foodstuffs	Weight		P., Gm.	F., Gm.	C., Gm.	Water, Gm.	P., Cal.	F., Cal.	C., Cal.	Vitamins			Minerals		
	Gm.	Oz.								A	B	C	Calcium (Ca), Gm.	Phosphorus (P), Gm.	Iron (Fe), Gm.
Vegetables (continued):															
Squash	211	7.5	3.0	1.1	19.3	186	12.3	9.8	79	++	*	*	0.038	0.061	0.0013
Tomato, canned, a. p., 1¾ cups	178	6.3	5.2	0.86	17.3	167	21.3	8	70.8	++	++	++ to +++			
Tomato, fresh, a. p., 5 small	433	15.3	3.9	1.73	16.9	408	16	16.1	69.1	++	++	+++	0.048	0.113	0.0017
Turnip, 2 cups, diced	245	8.65	3.2	0.48	19.9	220	13	4.5	81.5	− to +	++	++	0.157	0.118	0.0012

Recommended Daily Dietary Allowances, Revised 1968

(From Goldsmith, G. A.: The New Dietary Allowances. Nutrition Today 3: 16-19, Dec., 1968.)

								Fat Soluble Vitamins			Water Soluble Vitamins							Minerals				
	Age[1] Years from–to	Weight kg	lbs.	Height cm	in.	Kcalories*	Protein gm	Vitamin A Activity I.U.	Vitamin D I.U.	Vitamin E Activity I.U.	Ascorbic Acid mg	Folacin[3] mg	Niacin mg equiv.[4]	Riboflavin mg	Thiamine mg	Vitamin B_6 mg	Vitamin B_{12} μg	Calcium gm	Phosphorus gm	Iodine μg	Iron mg	Magnesium mg
Infants.....	0-1/6	4	9	55	22	kg x 120	kg x 2.2[2]	1500	400	5	35	0.05	5	0.4	0.2	0.2	1.0	0.4	0.2	25	6	40
	1/6-1/2	7	15	63	25	kg x 110	kg x 2.0[2]	1500	400	5	35	0.05	7	0.5	0.4	0.3	1.5	0.5	0.4	40	10	60
	1/2- 1	9	20	72	28	kg x 100	kg x 1.8[2]	1500	400	5	35	0.1	8	0.6	0.5	0.4	2.0	0.6	0.5	45	15	70
Children....	1- 2	12	26	81	32	1100	25	2000	400	10	40	0.1	8	0.6	0.6	0.5	2.0	0.7	0.7	55	15	100
	2- 3	14	31	91	36	1250	25	2000	400	10	40	0.2	8	0.7	0.6	0.6	2.5	0.8	0.8	60	15	150
	3- 4	16	35	100	39	1400	30	2500	400	10	40	0.2	9	0.8	0.7	0.7	3	0.8	0.8	70	10	200
	4- 6	19	42	110	43	1600	30	2500	400	10	40	0.2	11	0.9	0.8	0.9	4	0.8	0.8	80	10	200
	6- 8	23	51	121	48	2000	35	3500	400	15	40	0.2	13	1.1	1.0	1.0	4	0.9	0.9	100	10	250
	8-10	28	62	131	52	2200	40	3500	400	15	40	0.3	15	1.2	1.1	1.2	5	1.0	1.0	110	10	250
Males......	10-12	35	77	140	55	2500	45	4500	400	20	40	0.4	17	1.3	1.3	1.4	5	1.2	1.2	125	10	300
	12-14	43	95	151	59	2700	50	5000	400	20	45	0.4	18	1.4	1.4	1.6	5	1.4	1.4	135	18	350
	14-18	59	130	170	67	3000	60	5000	400	25	55	0.4	20	1.5	1.5	1.8	5	1.4	1.4	150	18	400
	18-22	67	147	175	69	2800	60	5000	400	30	60	0.4	18	1.6	1.4	2.0	5	0.8	0.8	140	10	400
	22-35	70	154	175	69	2800	65	5000	—	30	60	0.4	18	1.7	1.4	2.0	5	0.8	0.8	140	10	350
	35-55	70	154	173	68	2600	65	5000	—	30	60	0.4	17	1.7	1.3	2.0	5	0.8	0.8	125	10	350
	55-75+	70	154	171	67	2400	65	5000	—	30	60	0.4	14	1.7	1.2	2.0	6	0.8	0.8	110	10	350
Females....	10-12	35	77	142	56	2250	50	4500	400	20	40	0.4	15	1.3	1.1	1.4	5	1.2	1.2	110	18	300
	12-14	44	97	154	61	2300	50	5000	400	20	45	0.4	15	1.4	1.2	1.6	5	1.3	1.3	115	18	350
	14-16	52	114	157	62	2400	55	5000	400	25	50	0.4	16	1.4	1.2	1.8	5	1.3	1.3	120	18	350
	16-18	54	119	160	63	2300	55	5000	400	25	50	0.4	15	1.5	1.2	2.0	5	1.3	1.3	115	18	350
	18-22	58	128	163	64	2000	55	5000	400	25	55	0.4	13	1.5	1.0	2.0	5	0.8	0.8	100	18	350
	22-35	58	128	163	64	2000	55	5000	—	25	55	0.4	13	1.5	1.0	2.0	5	0.8	0.8	100	18	300
	35-55	58	128	160	63	1850	55	5000	—	25	55	0.4	13	1.5	1.0	2.0	5	0.8	0.8	90	18	300
	55-75+	58	128	157	62	1700	55	5000	—	25	55	0.4	12	1.5	1.0	2.0	6	0.8	0.8	80	10	300
Pregnancy..						+200	65	6000	400	30	60	0.8	15	1.8	+0.1	2.5	8	+0.4	+0.4	125	18	450
Lactation...						+1000	75	8000	400	30	60	0.5	20	2.0	+0.5	2.5	6	+0.5	+0.5	150	18	450

[1] Entries on lines for age range 22-35 years represent the reference man and woman at age 22. All other entries represent allowances for the midpoint of the specified age range.

[2] Assumes protein equivalent to human milk. For proteins not 100 percent utilized factors should be increased proportionately.

[3] The folacin allowances refer to dietary sources as determined by *Lactobacillus casei* assay. Pure forms of folacin may be effective in doses less than 1/4 of the RDA.

[4] Niacin equivalents include dietary sources of the vitamin itself plus 1 mg equivalent for each 60 mg of dietary tryptophan.

* One thousand calories (called a small calorie) equals one K calorie.

Vitamins

(Summary of Vitamins Significant in Human Diet)

Vitamin	Chief Functions	Results of Deficiency	Characteristics	Good Sources	Daily Allowances Recommended
VITAMIN A Provitamin, carotene	Essential for maintaining the integrity of epithelial membranes. Helps maintain resistance to infections. Necessary for the formation of rhodopsin and preventing night blindness.	*Mild:* Retarded growth. Increased susceptibility to infection. Abnormal function of gastrointestinal, genitourinary and respiratory tracts due to altered epithelial membranes. Skin dries, shrivels, thickens, sometimes pustule formation. Night blindness. *Severe:* Xerophthalmia, a characteristic eye disease, and other local infections.	Fat soluble. Not destroyed by ordinary cooking temperatures. Is destroyed by high temperatures when oxygen is present. Marked capacity for storage in the liver. NOTE: Excessive intake of carotene from which vitamin A is formed may produce yellow discoloration of the skin (carotenemia).	Animal fats butter cheese cream egg yolk whole milk. Fish liver oil. Liver Vegetable 1. green leafy, esp. escarole, kale, parsley 2. yellow esp. carrots. *Artificial:* Concentrates in several forms. Irradiated fish oils.	*Males (Ages 10-75$^+$ yrs.):* 4500 to 5000 I.U. *Females (Ages 10-75$^+$ yrs.):* 4500 to 5000 I.U. *In pregnancy:* 6000 I.U. *In lactation:* 8000 I.U. *Children:* 2000 to 3500 I.U. *Infants:* 1500 I.U.
THIAMINE Vitamin B_1	Important role in carbohydrate metabolism. Essential for maintenance of normal digestion and appetite. Essential for normal functioning of nervous tissue.	*Mild:* Loss of appetite. Impaired digestion of starches and sugars. Colitis, constipation or diarrhea. Emaciation. *Severe:* Nervous disorders of various types. Loss of coordinating power of muscles. Beriberi Paralysis in man.	Water soluble. Not readily destroyed by ordinary cooking temperature. Destroyed by exposure to heat, alkali or sulfites. Is not stored in body.	Widely distributed in plant and animal tissues but seldom occurs in high concentration, exception in brewer's yeast. Other good sources are: Whole grain cereals Peas, Beans Peanuts Oranges Glandular—heart, liver, kidney Many vegetables and fruits Nuts. *Artificial:* Concentrates from yeast. Rice polishings. Wheat germ.	*Males (10-75$^+$ yrs.):* 1.2 to 1.5 mg. *Females (10-75$^+$ yrs.):* 1.0 to 1.1 mg. *In pregnancy:* 1.1 to 1.2 mg. *In lactation:* 1.5 to 1.6 mg. *Children:* 0.6 to 1.1 mg. *Infants:* 0.2 to 0.5 mg.

Vitamin	Chief Functions	Results of Deficiency	Characteristics	Good Sources	Daily Allowances Recommended
RIBOFLAVIN Vitamin B_2	Important in formation of certain enzymes and in cellular oxidation. Normal growth. Prevention of cheilosis and glossitis. Participates in light adaption.	Impaired growth. Lassitude and weakness. Cheilosis. Glossitis. Atrophy of skin. Anemia. Photophobia. Cataracts.	Water soluble. Alcohol soluble. Not destroyed by heat in cooking unless with alkali. Unstable in light esp. in presence of alkali.	Eggs Green vegetables Liver Kidney Lean meat Milk Wheat germ Yeast, dried Enriched foods.	*Males (10-75⁺ yrs.):* 1.3-1.7 mg. *Females (10-75⁺ yrs.):* 1.3-1.5 mg. *In pregnancy:* 1.8 mg. *In lactation:* 2.0 mg. *Children:* 0.6 to 1.2 mg. *Infants:* 0.4 to 0.6 mg.
NIACIN Nicotinic acid Nicotinamide Antipellagra vitamin	As the component of two important enzymes, it is important in glycolysis, tissue respiration and fat synthesis. Nicotinic acid but not nicotinamide causes vasodilation and flushing. Prevents pellagra.	Pellagra. Gastro-intestinal disturbances. Mental disturbances.	Soluble in hot water and alcohol. Not destroyed by heat, light, air or alkali. Not destroyed in ordinary cooking.	Yeast Lean meat Fish Legumes Whole grain cereals and peanuts Enriched foods.	*Males (10-75⁺ yrs.):* 14 to 20 mg. *Females (10-75⁺ yrs.):* 12 to 16 mg. *In pregnancy:* 15 mg. *In lactation:* 20 mg. *Children:* 8 to 15 mg. *Infants:* 5 to 8 mg.
VITAMIN B_{12} Cyanocobalamin	Produces remission in pernicious anemia. Essential for normal development of red blood cells.	Pernicious anemia.	Soluble in water or alcohol. Unstable in hot alkaline or acid solutions.	Liver Kidney Dairy products. Most of vitamin required by humans is synthesized by intestinal bacteria.	*Males and Females (10-75⁺ yrs.):* 5 to 6 mcg. *In pregnancy:* 8 mcg. *In lactation:* 6 mcg. *Children:* 2 to 5 mcg. *Infants:* 1 to 2 mcg.
VITAMIN C Ascorbic acid	Essential to formation of intracellular cement substances in a variety of tissues including skin, dentine, cartilage and bone matrix. Important in healing of wounds and fractures of bones. Prevents scurvy. Facilitates absorption of iron.	*Mild:* Lowered resistance to infections. Joint tenderness. Susceptibility to dental caries, pyorrhea and bleeding gums. *Severe:* Hemorrhage. Anemia. Scurvy.	Soluble in water. Easily destroyed by oxidation, heat hastens the process. Lost in cooking particularly if water in which food was cooked is discarded. Also loss is greater if cooked in iron or copper utensils. Quick frozen foods lose little of their vitamin C. Stored in the body to a limited extent.	Abundant in most fresh fruits and vegetables, esp. citrus fruit and juices, tomato and orange. *Artificial:* Ascorbic acid. Cevitamic acid.	*Males (10-75⁺ yrs.):* 40 to 60 mg. *Females (10-75⁺ yrs.):* 40 to 55 mg. *In pregnancy:* 60 mg. *In lactation:* 60 mg. *Children:* 40 mg. *Infants:* 35 mg. The infant diet is likely to be deficient in vitamin C unless orange or tomato juice or other form is added.

Vitamin	Chief Functions	Results of Deficiency	Characteristics	Good Sources	Daily Allowances Recommended
VITAMIN D	Regulates absorption of calcium and phosphorus from the intestinal tract. Antirachitic.	*Mild:* Interferes with utilization of calcium and phosphorus in bone and teeth formation. Irritability. Weakness. *Severe:* Rickets, may be common in young children. Osteomalacia in adults.	Soluble in fats and organic solvents. Relatively stable under refrigeration. Stored in liver. Often assocated with vitamin A.	Butter Egg yolk Fish liver oils Fish having fat distributed through the flesh, salmon, tuna fish, herring, sardines Liver Oysters Yeast and foods irradiated with ultraviolet light. Formed in the skin by exposure to sunlight. Artificially prepared forms.	*Males and Females (10-22 yrs.):* 400 I.U. After age 22, none except during pregnancy or lactation. *In pregnancy:* 400 I.U. *In lactation:* 400 I.U. *Children:* 400 I.U. *Infants:* 400 I.U.
VITAMIN E Alpha tocopherol	Normal reproduction in rats. Prevention of muscular dystrophy in rats.	Red blood cell resistance to rupture is decreased.	Fat soluble. Stable to heat in absence of oxygen.	Lettuce and other green, leafy vegetables. Wheat germ oil Margarine Rice.	*Males* *(10-75⁺ yrs.):* 20 to 30 I.U. *Females* *(10-75⁺ yrs.):* 20 to 25 I.U. *In pregnancy:* 30 I.U. *In lactation:* 30 I.U. *Children:* 10 to 15 I.U. *Infants:* 5 I.U.
VITAMIN B_6 Pyridoxine	Essential for metabolism of tryptophan. Needed for utilization of certain other amino acids.	Dermatitis around eyes and mouth. Neuritis. Anorexia, nausea and vomiting.	Soluble in water and alcohol. Rapidly inactivated in presence of heat, sunlight or air.	Blackstrap molasses Meat Cereal grains Wheat germ.	*Males and Females (10-75⁺ yrs.):* 1.4 to 2.0 mg. *In pregnancy:* 2.5 mg. *In lactation:* 2.5 mg. *Children:* 0.5 to 1.2 mg. *Infants:* 0.2 to 0.4 mg.
FOLIC ACID Folacin	Essential for normal functioning of hematopoietic system.	Anemia.	Slightly soluble in water. Easily destroyed by heat in presence of acid. Decreases when food is stored at room temperature. NOTE: A large dose may prevent appearance of anemia in a case of pernicious anemia but still permit neurological symptoms to develop.	Glandular meats Yeast Green, leafy vegetables.	*Males and Females (10-75⁺ yrs.):* 0.4 mg. *In pregnancy:* 0.8 mg. *In lactation:* 0.5 mg. *Children:* 0.1 to 0.3 mg. *Infants:* 0.05 to 0.1 mg.

Medical Emergencies

Convulsions

Type	History	Clonic or Tonic	Pulse	Breathing	Color	Muscles	Pupils	Pathology	Treatment
1. Epilepsy. Grand mal type.	Previous history of "fits". Attack may be preceded by "aura". In some patients convulsions may occur only at night.	Generalized tonic, clonic type but may be focal.	Pulse is rapid.	Respirations are rapid, deep and stertorous.	Blue. Patient may become very cyanotic.	Rigid in tonic and in clonic origin.	Pupils may be contracted and occasionally of unequal size.	Abnormal electroencephalographic pattern.	Prevent the patient from injuring himself or from falling. Place on floor with pillow, etc. Use no stimulant. Do not place fingers in mouth but use a suitable padded gag to prevent patient's biting the tongue. Loosen clothing around neck.
2. Eclampsia.	Occurs in toxemia of pregnancy in antepartum and postpartum stages.	Prolonged tonic convulsions are characteristic with the whole body in a state of rigidity. Both tonic and clonic types may occur.	Pulse is rapid and becomes thready.	Respirations are irregular, shallow, and hissing. Breath-holding may occur.	Blue. Patient may become very cyanotic.	Rigidity of the body sets in. Extremities are flexed. General tonic spasm of body may be followed by clonic spasm.	Pupils may be dilated and may be of unequal size.	Hypertension. Pathologic changes in liver, kidney, brain and adrenals. Rapid gain of weight.	Control convulsions. Give proper antenatal care for toxemia of pregnancy. Control of diet, elimination and prevention of hypertension. Magnesium sulfate intramuscularly.
3. Apoplexy. Intracranial hemorrhage	Usually sequel to cerebral hemorrhage. May be result of vascular disease. Occurs usually after age of 40 years.	Usually tonic. May be limited to different areas, or to one side of the body.	Pulse is strong and of a bounding quality.	Respirations are deep and stertorous.	Red. Skin has a florid and flushed appearance.	Spastic in tonic usage with hemiplegia. One side of body shows paralysis. Other is normal.	Pupils may be unequal in size.	Arteriosclerosis. Intracranial hemorrhage.	Keep the patient absolutely quiet with an icecap to head. No stimulants. If vomiting, prevent aspiration of vomitus.
4. Hysteria.	Usually onset is not sudden. Is accompanied by laughter and crying. Seizure may be more prolonged than epilepsy.	May be of the stimulation types and take on those of epilepsy. Usually are of the tonic nature.	Pulse is normal. Shows no definite changes unless slightly rapid due to excitement.	Respirations may become rapid.	No change in color of skin.	Rigidity or relaxed as the victim wishes to demonstrate.	Pupils are normal and react to light. Muscles of eye resist when forced opening is attempted.	Patient seldom loses consciousness. May fall but not in an area where an injury may follow. Highly reactive to suggestion.	Inhalation of aromatic spirit of ammonia. Ice water dashed upon the face. Seizure is over usually when the audience disappears.

CONVULSIONS—*Continued*

Type	History	Clonic or Tonic	Pulse	Breathing	Color	Muscles	Pupils	Pathology	Treatment
5. Tetanus.	After injury—deep wound—and entrance of tetanus bacillus. Gunshot wound.	Tonic convulsions and tonic spasms of voluntary muscles.	Rapid pulse.	Rapid. Labored to irregular.	Cyanotic in convulsions.	Constant rigidity. Trismus may not appear for 24 hrs. after symptoms.	Normal.	Disease is due to the action of tetanus toxin, which is thought to act centrally rather than on the affected muscles.	Human tetanus immune globulin. Maintain airway. This may require tracheotomy. Oxygen therapy.
6. Uremic Convulsions.	Condition is usually accompanied by chronic or acute nephritis or chronic cardiac conditions. Marked edema noted.	Clonic (mild) to severe forms of muscle jerking.	Pulse rapid weak. Muscles are rigid (lends to imperceptibility).	Respirations are slow and stertorous.	Skin is pale, dry, scaly and has waxy appearance.	Tonic and clonic.	Pupils may be "pin point."	Arterial hypertension. Albuminuria. Suppression of urine. Visual disturbance.	Measures to reduce high blood pressure. Treatment by use of artificial kidney may be lifesaving.
7. Diabetic Convulsions.	Diabetes mellitus, hyperglycemia, acidosis.	Clonic and tonic.	Pulse rapid weak to irregular.	Deep breathing, rapid with extreme effort.	Dry skin. Very soft, cyanotic in convulsion.	Tonic and clonic.	Eye balls soft. Cataracts are frequent.	Generalized arteriosclerosis. Kidneys are enlarged. Degeneration in islets of Langerhans.	Use of insulin. Diabetic diet. Care of skin. Bed rest.

Dislocations

Type	History	Pathology	Muscles	Complications	Treatment	Strapping and Support	Differentiation
1. Neck.	Caused by violent twists or fall upon the head or diving into pool.	Bilateral dislocation. Severs spinal cord. Death follows. Nerve injury caused by tension or displacement. Permanent torticollis and limited neck motion.	Torticollis. Muscles spastic on uninjured side, relaxed on injured side.	Severance of cord. Pressure on cord causing predisposal to recurrence of dislocation, permanent torticollis, paralysis, death.	Keep patient in recumbent position in hyperextension of the neck. Reduction by leverage and not by manual traction. Keep traction by collar or plaster cast.	Reduction done by leverage. Application of plaster or rigid collar which must be worn until recovery of the ligaments to prevent recurrence.	Unilateral dislocation produces torticollis with head tilted on side and chin rotated away from displaced vertebrae. Reduction aids in complete disappearance of torticollis.
2. Back.	Sudden and violent twisting of the back.	Cervical dislocation—Paraplegia may occur. Respiratory failure or ascending myelitis. Dorsal dislocation. Urinary infection.	Affected side relaxed; uninjured side spastic. Muscle spasm holds back in rigidity with severe pain when any movement is made.	Damage to cord. Incomplete paraplegia. Failure to replace results in kyphosis deformity. Weakness and arthritis.	Do not allow patient to sit up or to be turned. Prepare patient for cast and brace. Control the pain. Watch for decubitus.	Treat as for fracture. Transport in prone position on rigid stretcher. Keep the body in hyperextension with cast or brace.	Compression fracture of first lumbar vertebrae is the most common injury of the spine. Decided excursion of the ilium (noted when the back is extended or flexed) is corrected. No crepitus. Discoloration, swelling, and persistent pain in muscle.
3. Shoulder.	ANTERIOR force was from behind—head of the humerus lies just below the coracoid process. POSTERIOR. Direct force upon the flexed elbow. Head of humerus is placed in front and lower than the axilla.	Rupture of tendon. Injury to circumflex nerve or brachial plexus. Disability. Injury to axillary vessels. Greater tuberosity (coracoid). Acromion processes fractured.	Muscle tension in the biceps muscle. Triceps muscle immobilized, may be slightly rigid.	Chronic arthritis. Cartilage displacement. Complete loss of function. Recurrences if a repeated injury or improper or inadequate mobilization after the first injury.	Kocher method of Replacement. Kept in sling. 1. Flex elbow to a right angle and place elbow against body. Rotate arm outward until forearm points away from body. 2. Keep elbow and arm (lower arm) flexed on upper. Raise elbow forward until it reaches a right angle position to the long axis (or horizontal) of the body. 3. Arm is directed obliquely inward and the hand placed on the opposite shoulder so that reduction or replacement is complete. Immobilize by sling. X-ray is necessary.		Dislocation of shoulder is corrected when the hand (unassisted) can be placed upon the opposite shoulder. Repeated recurrence of dislocation of the shoulder may be common.
4. Elbow.	In childhood between ages 8 to 12 years. Child falls upon the outstretched hand. Produces hyperextension of the elbow.	Elbow swollen. Held midway between flexion and extension. Head of radius is felt rotating behind humerus.	Tension in biceps muscle. Muscle ossification at the elbow.	Arthritis in joint. Muscle tissue ossification. Recurrence of dislocation.	Apply splint. Immobilize elbow until replacement can be made. Treat symptomatically.	Supinate the forearm. Make traction forward and downward on the forearm until radius and ulna slip back into position.	The ability to acutely flex the elbow when dislocation is satisfactorily reduced.

DISLOCATIONS—*Continued*

Type	History	Pathology	Muscles	Complications	Treatment	Strapping and Support	Differentiation
5. Wrist.	Caused by the hyperextended hand or by severe blows upon the dorsal portion of the wrist.	Dislocation of Semilunar bone. Flexion of the wrist is blocked by displaced bone. Usually results in a permanently weak wrist.	Muscles of back of hand tense. Usually marked swelling in area of the sprain.	Permanent pain, weakness and limitation of motion. Flexion limited. Displaced bones may have to be removed by surgical methods.	Surgical removal of displaced bone if unable to replace it. Support by splint or strapping. Cold applications for 24 to 48 hours.	Apply traction upon hand. Put firm pressure of the thumb upon the displaced bone.	Flexion of the wrist with slight limitations of motion and manifestation of weakness will indicate satisfactory reduction of the wrist.
6. Hand.	Most frequent in thumb due to forced hyperextension of the thumb or finger.	Head of metacarpal bone is wedged between flexor tendons (may necessitate an operation).	Marked muscle tension.	Deformity and permanent disability unless successful reduction is made.	Hyperextend the phalanx or thumb and then flex it. Use adhesive strapping. Cold applications for 24 to 48 hours.	Hyperextension of thumb as local pressure is made—thereby replacement is effected. Very early reduction is necessary.	Displacement of the thumb is the most frequent injury of the hand. Swelling, discoloration, and deformity (without point tenderness) are present.
7. Hip.	If posterior by indirect violence upon head of femur. If anterior by violent hyperabduction.	Injury to capsular and surrounding tissues of capsule of the acetabulum.	Posterior dislocation—hip is held rigidly flexed. Adduction, inward rotation and flexion of the thigh. Anterior dislocation—hip is immovable in abduction and external rotation. Knee flexed.	Torn tendons and ligaments. Fracture of the neck of femur.	1. Symptomatic for discomforts. 2. Splinting—since fracture is frequently a sequel. 3. Preparation for reduction of the dislocation.	Board or rigid splint. Keep limb in slight elevation unless fracture is imminent.	Reduction will be complete when flexion with extension and adduction of the thigh are possible.
8. Knee.	After violent fall or force upon knee.	Torn ligaments. Traumatized muscles of patellar and popliteal area. Loss of synovial fluid after rupture of bursa.	Rigid with pain. May include slight to marked swelling. Ecchymosis—slight or marked.	Disability and deformity. Permanently stiffened knee when synovial fluid is lost.	Splint as for fracture of femur and lower leg. Symptomatic (to relieve discomfort). Treat for shock.	Board or rigid splint. Keep knee and limb in slight elevation unless fracture is present.	The depression adjacent to the patella is diminished and complete flexion of the knee is restored.

DISLOCATIONS—*Continued*

Type	History	Pathology	Muscles	Complications	Treatment	Strapping and Support	Differentiation
9. Ankle.	From violence of undue weight or twisting upon the knee.	Production of scar tissue and contractures, which produce prolonged restriction of motion. Usually a short period of disability and then satisfactory recovery.	Rigid with pain. May include swelling and discoloration (May be delayed).	Fractures — Minor or Major as determined by accident. Temporary or permanent disability.	Continuous application of cold for 24 to 48 hours. Then heat, massage, and passive and active exercise.	Allow no use (fracture may be present). X-ray for fracture. Immobilize the foot and ankle on a pillow or a rigid splint.	Satisfactory reduction is made when the ankle can be dorsiflexed within a right angle.
10. Foot.	Force of violent nature upon plantar flexor of foot. Misstepping.	May include a compound dislocation of the ankle. Slight to increased amount of trauma and strain upon all soft tissue of foot.	Tense; and including marked swelling and discoloration.	Fracture of ankle. Weakness of muscles of plantar arch.	Continuous application of cold for 24 to 48 hours. Then heat, massage, and passive and active exercise.	Pillow splint or rigid splint as for fractures. Watch for swelling and cyanosis in part.	Satisfactory reduction is made when the displaced astragalus (projecting on the back of the foot) has been leveled.
11. Clavicle.	May be due to a heavy blow or fall upon the side of the shoulder.	Posterior dislocation causes pressure on structures at base of neck; rupture of sternoclavicular ligament.	Muscles are hyperextended. Fatigue results if prolonged.	Increased deformity and insecurity of movement of shoulder. Prolonged disability.	Symptomatic. Slight massage. Adhesive strapping. Sling for four weeks.	In recumbent position with small narrow sand bag between scapulae. Posterior Dislocation—press shoulders backward. Make traction on arm as it is held abducted at right angle—clavicle returns to position.	Complete reduction corrects the deformity at the sternoclavicular joint, no crepitus is present. Stretched ligaments and torn muscles are manifested by swelling, discoloration, and generalized pain. Shoulder has secure movement.
12. Jaw.	The too wide opening of the mouth, for example in yawning, laughing or eating.	Capsule of Glenoid fossa is too loose. Muscles are soft. Tissues aid in chronic displacement. Jaw becomes locked beneath maxillary prominence.	Muscles spastic. Later become fatigued.	Embarrassment in the unexpected recurrence. Trauma and fatigue in muscles. Predisposes infection.	Symptomatic treatment. Replacement by pressure of operator's thumbs upon molars until normal placement in the mandibular cavity.	Replacement. Jaw bandage (supporting).	Anterior dislocation manifests partly opened and locked jaws with the teeth projecting forward. Complete reduction will restore the jaw for normal occlusion.

Fractures

Type	History	Pathology	Complications	Hemorrhage	Color of Area	Treatment	Transportation
1. Simple	Fall or accident.	A complete fracture with no fragments compounding.	Pressure on the blood supply. Malunion. Osteomyelitis.	Subcutaneous or capillary.	Slight to marked increase in ecchymosis.	Splint before preparation for transportation. Reduction (depending upon skill of operator).	In splint.
2. Compound	Fall or accident.	Injury where either one or both fragments are through the skin.	Infection. Hemorrhage. Shock.	May or may not include hemorrhage.	Slight to marked increase in ecchymosis.	Immediate debridement in hospital. Further treatment elective.	Cover with sterile dressing. Maintain traction. For leg fracture use Thomas splint.
3. Greenstick	Fall or accident. (In children.)	Fracture is incomplete but there is bowing of the bone.	Complete fracture. Deformity.	Probably no hemorrhage will occur.	Discoloration may be slight. It may be marked.	Splint for preparation for transportation. Reduction of the curvature and place in cast.	Splint.
4. Comminuted	Injury due to crushing blow.	Bone is broken into two or more fragments.	Malunion. Unstableness. Infection.	Hemorrhage will occur in area of injury.	In area of deeper bones. Discoloration is delayed.	Splint before transportation. Replacement of fracture. Occasionally requires open reduction.	Splint and traction.
5. Impacted	Crushing force causing fracture. Fragments telescoped.	One fragment is jammed into another.	Deformity. Loss of function. Pain. Osteomyelitis.	Hemorrhage will occur in area of injury.	Discoloration according to extent of bone injury—it may be delayed.	Traction must be made while reduction and proper cast is fitted to hold extremity in place.	Splint and traction.
6. Transverse and 7. Spiral	Sudden twisting violence exerted upon extremity.	Fracture line across the bone. Fracture through the bone or around it.	Malfunction. Loss of function. Cuts off blood supply. Infection of bone.	Hemorrhage frequently occurs around area of fracture.	Same as compound fracture.	According to the site. Splint and traction.	Traction and immobilization.
a. Fracture of Skull	From a fall, or blow upon the skull.	In Vault with little or no intracranial trauma. Linear fracture may be overlooked. In Base serious compression in brain. Concussion injury to vital cranial nerves.	Concussion. Paralysis of limbs of the body. Infection of brain. Compression of brain.	Clots on the brain. Extent and nature determined by location of injury. Dangers of pressure upon the brain.	Linear fractures may be slight and overlooked. Bleeding (bright) from mouth and ears.	Place in dorsal recumbent position. Watch for infection. Allow skull base fractures to bleed. Limit fluids.	Place on rigid stretcher. Keep flat. Keep patient quiet.
b. Fracture of Neck	Diving into pools. Auto wrecks. Accidents.	Break extends through body of vertebrae or the laminae.	Death. Paralysis (total or partial).	No hemorrhage noted in the tissues.	No change in color of the skin.	Keep neck in hyperextension. Place rolled blanket under shoulders. Minor fracture needs traction for 5-6 weeks. Major (with cord injury) cast or collar for 10-12 months.	Patient must not move the neck under any consideration. Keep neck and head hyperextended. Restrain if necessary. Rigid stretcher or improvision for rigidity.

FRACTURES—*Continued*

Type	History	Pathology	Complications	Hemorrhage	Color of Area	Treatment	Transportation
c. Fracture of Back	Occurs after jack-knife fall and other accidents.	Usually crushing body of vertebrae.	Paralysis and Shock (depending upon the location of the fracture).	No hemorrhage in surrounding tissues.	Usually no change in color of the skin.	Extreme care in preparation and transportation. Rigid support. Place in hyperextension for 8 weeks. Body cast.	Place and secure in prone position. Keep patient in hyperextension. Restrain if necessary. Rigid stretcher or improvision.
d. Fracture of Coccyx	Falling into sitting position.	Fracture may be from sacral region or from tip of coccyx.	Constant pain. Abscesses. Osteomyelitis.	No hemorrhage in surrounding tissues.	No change in color of the skin.	Hot sitz bath after 24-48 hours of cold applications to area. Rest in bed. If not cured then operate (coccygectomy).	Carry patient on rigid stretcher. Keep in dorsal recumbent position.
e. Fracture of Pelvis	From a blow or crushing force.	Bone impairment. Involvement of sacral nerves. Paralysis, torn ligaments and lacerated muscles.	Rupture of bladder and rectum. Deformity and shortening of limb. Sprain of pelvic joints.	Same as in compound fracture. Discoloration may be delayed.	Same as in compound fracture if compound. Otherwise delayed.	Keep in dorsal recumbent position. After reduction keep prone. Reduction of fragments. Symptomatic treatment.	On rigid stretcher in dorsal recumbent position. Keep body extended.
f. Fracture of Femur or Thigh	Usually sudden and severe trauma to thigh.	Bone and nerve injury. Paralysis and permanent disability.	Deformity and shortening of the limb, where an endocrine disturbance is present. Severance of nerves and blood vessels. Paralysis and gangrene.	Same as in compound fracture. Discoloration may be delayed.	Same as in fracture of Pelvis.	Splint to leg and body. Keep patient flat. Provide and retain traction. Watch for shock.	Use rigid stretcher. Keep leg in traction until ready for reduction.
g. Fracture of Hip	Usually found in elderly people.	Fracture through neck or through trochanter or both.	Loss of function. Deformity shortening.	Hemorrhage but not in large amounts.	Ecchymosis but it may be delayed.	Traction. Smith Peterson Nail.	Place in Thomas Splint as improvised.
h. Fracture of Ankle (Potts Fracture)	From a sudden or forceful wrenching of the lower end of tibia and fibula.	Fracture of the lower ends of the fibula and tibia. Foot is displaced outward. Impairment of tissues, vessels, etc., from trauma.	Dislocation and sprains may occur simultaneously.	Same as in compound fracture. Discoloration.	Slight or marked areas of ecchymosis.	Immobilize immediately by pillow splint or rigid splint.	Keep limb well supported with slight elevation.
i. Fracture of Humerus	Result of a twisting force or blow upon upper arm.	Injury to the osseous structures. Trauma and lacerations of tissues, muscles, etc., if compound fracture.	Severance of nerves and blood vessels. Temporary deformity.	Slight—increased if compound fracture.	Slight or marked areas of discoloration.	Immobilize immediately by splint or sling (weight of forearm usually provides the necessary traction).	Keep arm in sling or splint.
j. Fracture of Forearm and Colles Fracture	Result of a twisting force upon the lower arm or wrist or from violence exerted upon the arm in preventing the body from falling.	Fracture and displacement of distal end of the radius. Tip of styloid process of ulna broken off. Backward displacement of radius.	Dislocations and sprains may be included. Trauma and swelling of tissues.	Slight—increased if fracture is not immediately immobilized.	Slight to marked.	Rigid splint, arm support with a sling.	Place in a sling after splinting.

Poisons and Poisoning

Toxic Substance	Probable Lethal Dose for Adult Humans (mg./kg. body wt.)*	Symptoms of Poisoning	Emergency Measures	Supportive and Follow up Treatment	Pathology
Acetophenetidin or Acetanilid	50 to 500 mg.	Sweating, nausea, vomiting, chills, ringing in ears, fall in blood pressure, circulatory collapse, cyanosis, coma, convulsions, death from respiratory failure.	Gastric lavage or induce emesis. Instill sodium bicarbonate into stomach. Whole blood or plasma. Artificial respiration or oxygen. Analeptics.	Keep patient warm and quiet. If cyanosis becomes severe, 1 to 2 mg./kg. of 1% methylene blue.	Methemoglobinemia, CNS stimulation, kidney and liver injury.
Acids (acetic, hydrochloric, nitric, phosphoric, sulfuric, etc.)	Variable	Immediate pain and corrosion of mucous membranes of mouth, throat and esophagus; difficulty in swallowing; stomach pain; nausea, coffee-ground vomitus; thirst; shock syndrome with death in circulatory collapse.	Give by mouth, magnesium oxide, milk of magnesia, lime water or aluminum hydroxide gel. Avoid carbonates as neutralizers. Give large amounts of water. Demulcents and morphine for pain.	Correct shock with fluids, plasma or whole blood. Tracheotomy or gastrectomy may become necessary.	Asphyxia from glottic edema, gastric and pyloric strictures and stenosis or perforation.
Amanita phalloides mushroom	Variable. May be only one mushroom.	After 6 to 15 hours, abdominal pain, nausea, vomiting, purging, weakness, thirst, shock syndrome, restlessness, delirium, hallucinations, coma, late jaundice, acute renal failure, death may be from cardiac, kidney, liver or CNS lesions.	Slurry of activated charcoal as lavage fluid, leaving some in stomach along with saline cathartic. Meperidine for pain.	Correct fluid and electrolyte balance. Prepare to treat renal or hepatic failure. Treatment with artificial kidney may be required.	Acute yellow atrophy of the liver, acute renal failure, cardiac damage
Aminophylline or Caffeine	50 to 500 mg.	Restlessness, excitement alternating with drowsiness, ringing in ears, fast pulse, nausea, vomiting, fever, diuresis, dehydration, thirst, tremor, delirium, convulsions, coma, death in cardiovascular and respiratory collapse.	Lavage, induce emesis and saline cathartic unless vomiting and purging have already begun. Treat CNS excitation with appropriate barbiturate therapy.	Oxygen and artificial respiration. Maintain fluid and electrolyte balance.	CNS stimulation and gastric ulceration.
Ammonia	Variable. Even a small amount may kill.	Irritation of eyes and respiratory tract (sometimes pulmonary edema, glottic spasm or laryngeal edema). Other symptoms are like Lye poisoning (See Lye in this table).	Give large amounts of water, dilute vinegar, lemon juice or orange juice. Demulcents and morphine for pain. Oxygen under pressure to help prevent pulmonary edema.	Treat for shock. Tracheotomy may be needed. NOTE: Do not give drugs such as narcotics which would depress respiration.	Corrosive esophagitis and gastritis, laryngeal edema, pulmonary edema.
d-Amphetamine	5 to 50 mg. but variable	Excitement, talkativeness, restlessness, tremors, dizziness, hyperactive reflexes, dry mouth, nausea, vomiting, diarrhea, palpitations, fever, dehydration, mydriasis, tachycardia, hallucinations, delirium, mania, convulsions, coma, death in circulatory collapse.	Gastric lavage with tap water or induce emesis. Treat symptoms of CNS with appropriate barbiturate therapy.	Isolate patient and avoid sensory stimuli. Ice packs and sponge baths for hyperpyrexia. Chlorpromazine may be required.	CNS and peripheral sympathetic stimulation; petechial hemorrhages in the brain.

*Most of these values from Gleason, M. N., Gosselin, R. E., Hodge, H. C. and Smith, R. P.: Clinical Toxicology of Commercial Products, 3rd ed. The Williams & Wilkins Co., Baltimore, 1969.

Toxic Substance	Probable Lethal Dose for Adult Humans (mg./kg. body wt.)*	Symptoms of Poisoning	Emergency Measures	Supportive and Follow up Treatment	Pathology
Aniline	50 to 500 mg.	Intense cyanosis, headache, nausea, dryness in throat, confusion, ataxia, vertigo, weakness, disorientation, drowsiness, heart block, death in cardiovascular collapse.	Lavage with 1:5000 potassium permanganate. Instill saline cathartic. Oxygen and artificial respiration. Give 1 to 2 mg./kg. of body weight of 1% methylene blue.	Whole blood transfusions if needed.	Intense methemoglobinemia; mild liver and kidney injury.
Antihistaminics, (for example: tripelennamine, diphenhydramine, Chlorpheniramine).	5 to 50 mg.	Drowsiness, lethargy, fatigue, ataxia, difficulty in vision, coma; however, sometimes only excitement is seen with tremors, anxiety, delirium, convulsions, hyperpyrexia, nausea, vomiting, diarrhea, death in cardiovascular collapse or respiratory arrest.	Lavage or induce emesis. Mild stimulants if depressed or cautious sedation if excited. Oxygen and artificial respiration.	Ice packs and alcohol sponges for hyperpyrexia.	Mechanism of death not precisely known. Cerebral edema is described.
Antabuse (disulfiran)	Unknown	Circulatory collapse.	Oxygen therapy, intravenous 5% flucose in water. Intravenous sodium ascorbate. In severe cases very slow injection of 5 ml. of a 2% solution of saccharated iron oxide may be of benefit.	Complete rest with postural drainage. Continue oxygen inhalation and maintain fluid balance.	Unknown.
Arsenic or Antimony	5 to 50 mg.	Symptoms may be delayed several hours. Metallic taste and odor of garlic on breath, burning pain throughout gastrointestinal tract, vomiting and purging, dehydration, shock syndrome, coma, convulsions, paralysis, and severe diarrhea which becomes bloody. Death may occur.	Gastric lavage. Administer dimercaprol (BAL) in accordance with supplier's dosage schedule.	Maintain fluid and electrolyte balance. Morphine for pain. Treat for shock. Treat anemia and renal failure if either is present.	Shock secondary to hemorrhagic gastroenteritis. Skin eruptions are of no toxicological significance.
Atropine	Less than 5 mg.	Dryness of mouth, burning pain in throat, thirst, mydriasis, skin is dry, hot and flushed, hyperpyrexia, tachycardia, palpitations, restlessness, excitement, confusion, mania, delirium. Death is rare.	Lavage with slurry of activated charcoal or 4% tannic acid. Pilocarpine will make patient more comfortable, but barbiturates must be used to control excitement. Do not use long-acting barbiturates. For depression use mild stimulants. If severe use oxygen and artificial respiration.	Oxygen and artificial respiration. Ice packs or alcohol sponges for hyperpyrexia. Catheterize if necessary. Ophthalmic pilocarpine.	Intense CNS excitation and parasympathetic paralysis.

POISONS AND POISONING—*Continued*

Toxic Substance	Probable Lethal Dose for Adult Humans (mg./kg. body wt.)*	Symptoms of Poisoning	Emergency Measures	Supportive and Follow up Treatment	Pathology
Barbiturates	50 to 500 mg.	Confusion, drowsiness, ataxia, vertigo, slurred speech, headache, stupor, coma, areflexia, cyanosis, hypotension, shallow pulse, cardiovascular collapse, death in respiratory arrest.	Establish airway, gastric lavage, artificial respiration, oxygen with CO_2 inhalation, maintain fluid and electrolyte balance. Use of artificial kidney to remove barbiturate has been helpful.	Record vital signs frequently. Correct airway obstruction. Oxygen and artificial respiration as needed. Antibiotic therapy if aspiration of vomitus has occurred.	CNS depression with respiratory arrest. Pulmonary edema occurs in prolonged coma.
Barium salts, Chloride and other soluble salts	Quite variable	Salivation, nausea, vomiting, abdominal cramps, violent and bloody diarrhea, slow and irregular pulse, ringing in ears, dizziness, twitching, convulsions or paralysis, death from respiratory failure and cardiac arrest.	Give rapidly by mouth, sodium magnesium or aluminum sulfate. Lavage or induce emesis, then leave more of the above in the stomach. Atropine or morphine may relieve abdominal pain. Quinidine or procainamide to prevent cardiac arrest.	Intravenous saline for dehydration. Treat for shock.	Violent peristalsis, atrial hypertension, cardiac disturbances, late kidney damage. Barium stimulates contraction of muscles.
Benzene or Xylene or Toluene	50 to 500 mg.	Burning sensation in mouth and stomach, nausea, vomiting, chest pains, cough, headache, giddiness, vertigo, ataxia, confusion, stupor, restless coma, death from respiratory failure or ventricular fibrillation. Late severe blood dyscrasias.	Lavage with tap water; leave mineral oil and saline cathartic in the stomach.	Oxygen, artificial respiration, parenteral fluids. Avoid fats, oils, alcohol and epinephrine.	Respiratory failure from CNS depression or ventricular fibrillation. Severe and possibly fatal bone marrow damage.
Benzene hexachloride	50 to 500 mg.	Irritability, vomiting, restlessness, ataxia, spasms, convulsions, coma, respiratory failure.	Lavage with tap water and instill saline cathartic into the stomach. Control convulsions by cautious use of barbiturates.	Rest and quiet. Avoid fats, oils, alcohol and epinephrine.	CNS depression, liver damage and hyaline changes in the renal tubules.
Boric acid and borate salts	50 to 500 mg.	Headache, nausea, vomiting, diarrhea, stomach pain, weakness, lethargy, restlessness, tremor, convulsions, coma. Distinctive, fine, bright red rash. Shock with death in vascular collapse.	Lavage stomach with 1% sodium bicarbonate solution and instill saline cathartic. Oxygen and plasma or whole blood transfusions as indicated.	Fluids and electrolytes for replacement therapy.	Cause of death not known. Both kidney and liver damage are occasionally reported.

Toxic Substance	Probable Lethal Dose for Adult Human (mg./kg. body wt.)*	Symptoms of Poisoning	Emergency Measures	Supportive and Follow up Treatment	Pathology
Botulinum toxin	Possibly most poisonous substance known to man. Microgram amounts are lethal.	After 12 to 36 hours: Nausea, vomiting, occasionally diarrhea, difficulties in vision and swallowing, weakness and paralysis of respiratory muscles. Profuse sweating and pulse is rapid and weak.	Lavage with tap water or a slurry of activated charcoal if within a few hours postingestion. Instill saline cathartic. Give specific or polyvalent botulinus antitoxin. NOTE: Call the U. S. Public Health Service, Atlanta, Georgia, telephone number 1-404-634-2561 for the location of nearest supply of antitoxin.	Oxygen and artificial respiration. Tracheotomy if needed.	Blocks transmission of nerve impulses at motor end plate. Congestion and hemorrhage in all organs, especially the CNS.
Bromides (sodium, potassium, ammonium, etc.)	500 to 5000 mg.	Prompt vomiting, drowsiness, irritability, ataxia, vertigo, confusion, mania, hallucinations, coma. Death is rare. Also seen are skin rashes, neurological signs, sensory disturbances, increased spinal fluid pressure.	Give sodium or ammonium chloride 2 to 4 Gm. daily in divided doses by any route. Give saline cathartic. If intoxication is severe enough use of artificial kidney to hasten removal of bromide may be indicated.	Maintain hydration and mild diuresis.	Acne-like skin eruption, inflammation of mucous membranes, CNS depression.
Cadmium Salts	Several hundred mg.	Nausea, vomiting, diarrhea, salivation, abdominal cramps, headache, vertigo, exhaustion, collapse, shock and immediate death or delayed from acute renal failure. Dusts and fumes are also very hazardous by inhalation producing pulmonary edema.	Demulcents; lavage with milk or water if vomiting is not prompt. Give saline cathartic. If pulmonary edema develops treat with positive pressure oxygen administration.	Maintain fluid and electrolyte balance. Prophylactic and supportive measures for liver injury or acute renal failure.	Severe gastroenteritis, mild liver damage, and acute renal failure. If inhaled as a dust or fume, produces pulmonary edema.
Camphor	50 to 500 mg.	Nausea, vomiting, feeling of warmth, headache, confusion, vertigo, excitement, restlessness, delirium, hallucinations, tremor, convulsions, depression, coma, death from respiratory failure.	Short-acting intravenous barbiturates to prevent or stop convulsions. Be very careful not to overdose. Gastric lavage with tap water.	Protect the patient from all possible sensory stimuli. Oxygen and artificial respiration as needed.	Intense CNS excitation.
Carbon disulfide	500 to 5000 mg.	Irritation of skin, eyes and mucous membranes, headache, nausea, vomiting, diarrhea, weak pulse, palpitations, fatigue, ataxia, vertigo, mania, hallucinations, CNS depression with respiratory paralysis.	Artificial respiration and oxygen. Lavage with tap water. Mild CNS stimulants.	Convulsions may be controlled by short-acting intravenous barbiturates.	CNS depression sometimes with permanent neurological sequelae.

Toxic Substance	Probable Lethal Dose for Adult Human (mg./kg. body wt.)*	Symptoms of Poisoning	Emergency Measures	Supportive and Follow up Treatment	Pathology
Carbon monoxide	1.5% concentration in the air will cause unconsciousness in a few minutes. Continued exposure to this concentration will cause death. Young children are more susceptible than adults.	Mild headache, breathlessness on moderate exertion, irritability, fatigue, nausea, vomiting, confusion, ataxia, syncope with periods of convulsions, incontinence of urine and feces, death from respiratory arrest.	Give oxygen with 5% CO_2 preferably with a face mask and artificial respiration if needed.	Keep patient warm. Use antibiotics at the first sign of infection. Give whole blood transfusions.	High concentrations of carboxyhemoglobin in circulating erythrocytes lead to an asphyxial death.
Carbon tetrachloride	5 to 10 ml. Total dose	Nausea, vomiting, intense abdominal pain, headache, confusion, drowsiness, CNS depression, coma, and death from respiratory arrest, circulatory collapse or ventricular fibrillation. Late kidney and/or liver injury with possible acute renal failure.	If swallowed: Gastric lavage or emetic. If inhaled: Artificial respiration, oxygen, stimulants but avoid alcohol.	No specific therapy but be prepared to treat renal and hepatic failure.	CNS depression, hepatic central lobular necrosis, necrosis of renal tubular epithelium.
Chloral hydrate	50 to 500 mg.	Symptoms much like those seen in barbiturate poisoning except that large doses produce vomiting from hemorrhagic gastritis and enteritis. Combinations of chloral hydrate and alcohol ("Mickey Finn") are no longer thought to exhibit more than simple additive depression.	See Barbiturates.	See Barbiturates.	CNS depression. May sensitize myocardium to endogenous epinephrine.
Chlorate salts or bromate salts	50 to 500 mg.	Vomiting, diarrhea, abdominal pain, methemoglobinemia, intravascular hemolysis, delirium, coma, convulsions, cyanosis, icterus, death in acute renal failure.	Gastric lavage. Demulcents and meperidine for pain. Oxygen and whole blood transfusions if needed.	Supportive treatment for acute renal failure.	Methemoglobinemia, intravascular hemolysis, acute renal failure.

Toxic Substance	Probable Lethal Dose for Adult Human (mg./kg. body wt.)*	Symptoms of Poisoning	Emergency Measures	Supportive and Follow up Treatment	Pathology
Chlordane or Heptachlor	50 to 500 mg.	Irritability, hyperexcitability, convulsions and tremors punctuated by periods of depression, late liver damage.	Gastric lavage with tap water, saline cathartic, ether or ultrashort-acting barbiturates for convulsions.	Oxygen and artificial respiration.	CNS excitement; severe gastroenteritis have been described.
Chlorpromazine or other phenothiazines	50 to 500 mg.	Drowsiness, somnolence, stupor, coma, areflexia, hypotension, tachycardia, hypothermia, restlessness, tremor, spasm, rigidity, convulsions, respiratory or vasomotor collapse.	Lavage with tap water. Levarternol for severe shock.	Fluids and electrolytes. Oxygen or artificial respiration. Blood transfusion may be required.	CNS depression, extrapyramidal seizures, liver damage.
Copper salts, sulfate	50 to 500 mg.	Prompt emesis, pain in mouth, esophagus and stomach, diarrhea with abdominal pain, metallic taste, shock, convulsions, paralysis, coma, death.	Lavage with milk or 1% potassium ferrocyanide, demulcents, morphine for pain.	Heat, artificial respiration.	Widespread capillary damage, kidney injury, liver damage.
Cyanide (sodium, potassium, hydrogen, etc.)	Less than 5 mg.	Large doses produce immediate death. In smaller doses an acrid taste is noted followed by numbness in the throat, anxiety, confusion, vertigo, hyperpnea then dyspnea, odor of bitter almonds on breath, unconsciousness followed by convulsions and death from respiratory arrest.	Start artificial respiration immediately, keeping airway clear. Give inhalations from amyl nitrite perles every 2 to 3 minutes for 15 to 20 seconds. Inject intravenously 10 ml. of freshly prepared 3% sodium nitrite over a 2- to 4-minute period. Do not remove needle. Urgency may necessitate use of nonsterile solutions. Through the same needle give 50 ml. of 25% sodium thiosulfate over a 10-minute period.	If symptoms recur, repeat injections at half doses at hourly intervals. Positive pressure oxygen. Gastric lavage may now be performed with 1:5000 potassium permanganate.	Cyanide combines with enzymes which are essential to transfer of oxygen to the cells. Death is due to tissue anoxia.
2,4-Dichlorophenoxyacetic acid (2,4-D)	50 to 500 mg.	Weakness, lethargy, diarrhea, spastic myotonia, ventricular fibrillation and cardiac arrest. Possibly hypermetabolism and hyperpyrexia with convulsions and coma.	Induce emesis or lavage with tap water. Quinidine may be of value for both cardiac symptoms and myotonia.	If fever occurs, treat vigorously with cold packs, alcohol sponges and other means for promoting heat loss.	Mechanism of death not known; abnormal EEG's have been recorded and severe protracted peripheral neuropathy has occurred.
DDT	50 to 500 mg.	Vomiting (may be delayed), numbness and tickling of lips, tongue and face, headache, sore throat, fatigue, tremors, ataxia, confusion, convulsions, coma, death from respiratory failure.	Lavage with tap water and instill saline cathartic. Phenobarbital may be given prophylactically or parenteral short-acting barbiturates to control convulsions once they have begun. O_2 plus 5% CO_2 inhalation.	Avoid fats, oils, alcohol, epinephrine, sensory stimuli. Calcium gluconate is said to be beneficial in controlling convulsions in addition to barbiturates.	No significant pathologic findings in animals except that from convulsions due to CNS excitation.

Toxic Substance	Probable Lethal Dose for Adult Human (mg./kg. body wt.)*	Symptoms of Poisoning	Emergency Measures	Supportive and Follow up Treatment	Pathology
Dieldrin or Aldrin	5 to 50 mg.	Headache, nausea, vomiting, dizziness, tremors, sudden convulsions alternating with periods of severe CNS depression and death from respiratory arrest.	Lavage with warm water unless convulsions have already begun. Instill saline cathartic. Control convulsions with appropriate barbiturate therapy.	Avoid sensory stimuli. Use oxygen and artificial respiration as needed.	Intense CNS stimulation; mild and transient kidney and liver injury.
Digitalis	50 to 500 mg.	Nausea, salivation, vomiting, headache, fatigue, weakness, drowsiness, confusion, disorientation, delirium, hallucinations, visual disturbances, death from ventricular fibrillation.	Slurry of activated charcoal followed by induced emesis or gastric lavage. Disturbances in cardiac rate and rhythm can be temporarily influenced by appropriate choices from atropine, potassium or salts, quinidine, procainamide or sodium EDTA.	Nitroglycerin for anginal pain. Preserve water and electrolyte balance.	Produces cardiac arrhythmia and all grades of impaired conduction. Striking lack of human pathologic changes in comparison with those seen in experimentally poisoned animals.
2,4 Dinitrophenol	5 to 50 mg.	Fatigue, insatiable thirst, sweating, flushing, nausea, vomiting, abdominal pain, restlessness, excitement, severe hyperpyrexia, tachycardia, hyperpnea, dyspnea, cyanosis, coma, death in respiratory or circulatory collapse.	Lavage with 5% bicarbonate solution and instill saline cathartic. Ice packs, alcohol sponges, cold water enemas to reduce body temperature.	Appropriate fluid therapy for dehydration or acidosis, mild stimulants, oxygen, artificial respiration.	Tremendously increased BMR through uncoupling of oxidative phosphorylation.
Ergot	5 to 50 mg.	Vomiting, diarrhea, dizziness, weak pulse, thirst, tingling in feet, numbness and coldness of extremities, variable effects on blood pressure, dyspnea, convulsions, loss of consciousness.	Slurry of activated charcoal by mouth followed by emesis or lavage. Instill saline cathartic.	Keep patient warm and quiet; massage extremities; treat for shock.	Congestion and inflammatory changes in gastrointestinal tract and kidneys. Gangrene of fingers and toes from persistent peripheral vasoconstriction.
Ethyl alcohol	Variable: one pint to more than one quart.	Emotional instability, mood depending on personality, circumstances and surroundings. Impaired motor coordination, slurred speech, ataxia, peripheral vasodilation with flushing, rapid pulse and sweating, nausea and vomiting, drowsiness, stupor and coma, peripheral vascular collapse, hypotension, tachycardia, hypothermia, death from respiratory or circulatory failure.	Lavage with tap water or 3% bicarbonate, mild stimulants, oxygen and artificial respiration.	Intravenous saline or lactate for circulatory collapse, dehydration or acidosis. Mild external heat. Avoid aspiration of vomitus. Watch for hypoglycemia in young children.	Irregularly descending CNS depression leading to respiratory or circulatory failure.

POISONS AND POISONING—*Continued*

Toxic Substance	Probable Lethal Dose for Adult Human (mg./kg. body wt.)*	Symptoms of Poisoning	Emergency Measures	Supportive and Follow up Treatment	Pathology
Ethylene glycol	Less than 5 mg.	Transient excitement, nausea, vomiting, abdomina cramps, weakness, muscle cramps, ataxia, vertigo, stupor, coma, death from respiratory paralysis or delayed acute renal failure with uremia.	Gastric lavage with 1:5000 potassium permanganate. Mild stimulants, oxygen and artificial respiration. Immediate treatment by use of artificial kidney is advisable.	Supportive measures for acute renal failure.	CNS depression and hydropic degeneration of renal tubular epithelium.
Ferrous or ferric salts	500 to 5000 mg.	Severe gastroenteritis; abdominal pain; vomiting and diarrhea both eventually becoming bloody; dehydration, pallor, cyanosis, shock leading to death in 3 to 4 hours.	Milk by mouth and induce vomiting if not already spontaneous. Gastric lavage with 5% sodium bicarbonate. The specific antidote desferroxamine should be given orally and intravenously in appropriate dose.	Intravenous fluids for dehydration and whole blood or plasma for shock.	Shock secondary to local tissue damage, mild hepatic cirrhosis and pyloric stenosis.
Fluoride (salts, sodium)	50 to 500 mg.	Peculiar taste, salivation, nausea, abdominal pain, vomiting, diarrhea, thirst, muscle weakness, tremors, central depression, death in shock.	Give 10 ml. of 10% calcium gluconate intravenously. Repeat at signs of tetany. Start drip of glucose in saline. Lavage with solution of lime water or calcium chloride, leaving some solution in the stomach.	Treat shock vigorously by keeping up blood volume and giving norepinephrine. Calcium gluconate intramuscularly to establish depots.	Hemorrhagic gastroenteritis, inhibition of cellular glycolysis, hypocalcemia.
Fluoroacetate (salts, sodium)	Less than 5 mg.	Vomiting; paresthesias of face; CNS excitation progressing to convulsions, punctuated by periods of severe CNS depression; disturbances in heart beat, ventricular fibrillation; death.	Induced vomiting or lavage. Leave 15 to 30 Gm. sodium or magnesium sulfate in stomach. Most effective antidote appears to be monoacetin which is not available in pharmaceutical form. Regardless of sterility considerations, inject this material in doses of 0.5 ml./kg. intramuscularly every half hour, or dilute 1 to 5 with sterile saline for intravenous use.	Oxygen, artificial respiration, short-acting barbiturates for convulsions.	Cardiac disturbances leading to fatal ventricular fibrillation.
Formaldehyde	500 to 5000 mg.	Pain in epigastrium; nausea, vomiting; anxiety; weak and rapid pulse; coma, collapse, death in respiratory failure.	Give 2 tablespoonfuls ammonium acetate solution, 1 teaspoonful of aromatic spirits of ammonia or 10 to 20 drops of household ammonia diluted with water.	Treat for shock; morphine for pain; antibiotics at the first signs of infection; bicarbonate or lactate for acidosis.	Inflammation and ulceration of gastrointestinal tract, acidosis, kidney damage, circulatory collapse.

POISONS AND POISONING—*Continued*

Toxic Substance	Probable Lethal Dose for Adult Human (mg./kg. body wt.)*	Symptoms of Poisoning	Emergency Measures	Supportive and Follow up Treatment	Pathology
Hydrogen sulfide or alkaline salts	Highly toxic 0.1 to 0.2% in air usually fatal.	Sudden collapse and unconsciousness in acute poisoning with death from respiratory paralysis. Subacutely, gas is an irritant to eyes, respiratory tract and skin.	Terminate exposure immediately; artificial respiration; oxygen with 5% CO_2; mild stimulants.	Antibiotics at first signs of infection.	No significant pathologic changes except in chronic poisoning in which pulmonary edema may be seen.
Hypochlorite salts or solutions (liquid household bleach)	Variable. Several ounces of usual household bleach (4 to 6% available chlorine)	Pain and inflammation of mouth, pharnyx, esophagus and stomach; coffee-ground vomitus; circulatory collapse; confusion; delirium; coma; edema of glottis. All systemic symptoms are secondary to local injury and shock.	Milk, egg whites, starch paste or milk of magnesia. Lavage with tap water or 2% sodium thiosulfate. Morphine for pain.	Treat shock with intravenous fluids. Tracheotomy or gastrectomy may be indicated.	Edema of pharynx, glottis or larynx. Perforation of stomach or esophagus. Fumes may produce pulmonary edema.
Iodine	5 to 50 mg.	Burning pain in mouth, throat and stomach; lips and mouth are stained brown; thirst; vomiting (blue vomitus if stomach contained starches), bloody diarrhea, anuria or strangury, urine containing albumin or blood. Death from circulatory collapse, asphyxia from glottic edema or aspiration pneumonia.	Give immediately by mouth starch solution, barley water or gruel. Lavage with starch solution or 2% sodium thiosulfate. Morphine for pain and mild stimulants as indicated.	Give fluids and electrolytes, supportive therapy for circulatory collapse, antibiotics for secondary infections, prepare for emergency tracheotomy.	Irritation and swelling within throat (glottic edema), esophagus and stomach. Shock secondary to fluid and electrolyte loss. More rarely, late esophageal stenosis.
Ipecac syrup or fluid-extract	Variable. 1 to 2 ounces of fluid-extract (14 times more concentrated than the syrup).	Nausea, vomiting, diarrhea, albuminuria, abdominal cramps, bloody vomitus and feces, dehydration, myocarditis, myocardial infarction, cardiac arrest or shock secondary to cardiac depression and fluid loss.	Lavage or induce emesis if spontaneous vomiting has not occurred. Do not give additional emetic agents. Saline cathartic if purging has not occurred. Once toxin has been removed. vomiting may respond to intravenous chlorpromazine.	General supportive and symptomatic measures for impending shock.	Intractable vomiting and diarrhea due to intense irritation of entire gastrointestinal tract leading to shock. Direct, specific cardiac damage.

POISONS AND POISONING—*Continued*

Toxic Substance	Probable Lethal Dose for Adult Human (mg./kg. body wt.)*	Symptoms of Poisoning	Emergency Measures	Supportive and Follow up Treatment	Pathology
Isopropyl alcohol	500 to 5000 mg.	Dizziness, incoordination, headache, confusion, stupor and coma. Symptoms closely resemble ethyl alcohol intoxication. Death from circulatory collapse or respiratory failure.	Lavage with tap water; oxygen and artificial respiration, mild stimulants.	Intravenous glucose and saline. Anticipate liver or kidney injury.	Acetonuria without glycosuria is pathognomonic. Severe CNS depression. Aspiration pneumonitis.
Kerosene (Coal Oil)	500 to 5000 mg. if retained in stomach, but a few ml. if aspirated can be lethal.	Burning sensation in mouth, throat and stomach; nausea, vomiting, diarrhea, drowsiness, restlessness, disorientation, coma. Signs of pulmonary involvement indicate grave prognosis of impending fulminating hemorrhagic bronchopneumonia.	If risks of lavage are undertaken, an endotracheal tube with inflatable cuff should be employed. Dilute bicarbonate is satisfactory lavage fluid; follow with the instillation of olive oil and saline cathartic.	Antibiotics for secondary infection and positive pressure oxygen	Severe chemical pneumonitis
Lead or its salts	30 Gm. (Chronic poisoning is much more common than acute.)	Dryness in mouth, burning pain in stomach and abdomen, constipation followed by diarrhea, muscular weakness, paralysis of extremities, skin cold and cyanotic, delayed severe anemia, death in peripheral vascular collapse or encephalopathy	Gastric lavage with magnesium or sodium sulfate. Morphine and atropine for pain. Milk or egg white as demulcent. Intravenous calcium salts may relieve colic. Intravenous calcium disodium edetate in accordance with supplier's directions.	Keep patient quiet. Maintain fluid and electrolyte balance.	Gastrointestinal inflammation, liver and kidney injury when sufficient lead has been absorbed. Precise mechanism of death is not known.
Lye, sodium and potassium hydroxides and carbonates	Total dose of 10 Gm. may be fatal.	Severe pain in mouth, difficulty in swallowing, gastrointestinal pain and purging, weak and rapid pulse, death in shock or asphyxia from glottic edema.	Large amounts of water by mouth; diluted vinegar or lemon juice; avoid emetics and lavage. Olive oil by mouth or milk and egg whites. Mild stimulants to prevent shock. Tracheotomy may be required.	Morphine for pain; fluids and electrolytes; cortisone. Use of bougies to prevent esophageal stricture.	Laryngeal or glottic edema; corrosion and possible perforation of upper gastrointestinal tract; late esophageal stenosis.
Meprobamate, Equanil or Miltown	500 to 5000 mg.	Drowsiness, relaxation, stupor, sleep, coma, areflexia, muscular flaccidity, severe and persistent hypotension.	Lavage or induce emesis; plasma or pressor agents for hypotension; mild stimulants.	Symptomatic and supportive care with frequent recording of vital signs.	No significant pathologic changes in tissues.

Toxic Substance	Probable Lethal Dose for Adult Human (mg./kg. body wt.)*	Symptoms of Poisoning	Emergency Measures	Supportive and Follow up Treatment	Pathology
Mercuric chloride or other soluble salts	5 to 50 mg.	Metallic taste and burning in mouth and throat; abdominal pain and cramps with nausea, vomiting; diarrhea and bloody stools; scanty urine containing albumin; collapse in shock with weak, rapid pulse, slow and shallow respirations, cold and clammy skin. If patient survives acute episode, he may die in renal failure after several days. Chronic mercury poisoning is also common with primarily neurological symptoms.	Egg white, milk or flour by mouth. Lavage with 3% sodium formaldehyde sulfoxylate. Dimercaprol (BAL) intramuscularly in accordance with supplier's directions.	Saline cathartic if purging has not already occurred. Demulcents and analgetics. Treat for shock. Prepare for management of acute renal failure.	Ulceration of gums and mouth, loosening of teeth, progressive peripheral neuritis are all seen in chronic poisonings or cases in which death is delayed. In acute cases, peripheral vascular collapse secondary to fluid or electrolyte loss, or acute renal failure is usual cause of death.
Methyl alcohol	500 to 5000 mg.	Exhilaration accompanied by headache, muscular weakness, nausea, vomiting and abdominal pain, delirium with visual disturbances which may progress to blindness, weak and rapid pulse, rapid and shallow respirations, cyanosis, coma, death from respiratory failure.	Gastric lavage with 5% sodium bicarbonate, leaving some solution in the stomach. Inject 3% sodium bicarbonate intravenously at the rate of 1000 ml. per hour but do not continue after acidosis is corrected.	Bed rest, treat for shock, mild external heat, stimulants as indicated, protect patient's eyes from light. Oxygen.	Intense metabolic acidosis. Partial to complete blindness due to atrophy of the ganglion cells of the retina if patient survives.
Morphine	5 to 50 mg.	Gross overdosages produce prompt depression, but smaller doses may cause transient period of excitement before drowsiness, weariness, loss of pain sensation, nausea, vomiting, pinpoint pupils, coma with muscular relaxation, slowing of respiratory rate, cyanosis, slow pulse, fall in blood pressure, death in respiratory arrest.	Gastric lavage, even if several hours after ingestion, with 1:10,000 potassium permanganate; saline cathartic left in stomach. Nalorphine is specific antagonist given intravenously in doses of 5 to 10 mg. Artificial respiration. Inhalation of oxygen with 5% CO_2.	Keep patient awake with mild stimulation. Correct airway obstruction. Maintain fluid and electrolyte balance. Keep patient warm.	Pulmonary congestion. Death is from respiratory failure due to central depression, but circulatory insufficiency may be contributory.
Muscaria mushrooms	Unknown but the ingestion of two or three *Amanita phalloides* type may be fatal.	Violent vomiting, diarrhea, apprehension, miosis, severe abdominal pain, irregular and slow pulse, slow and labored respirations, delirium, late stupor, death from cardiac arrest or circulatory collapse.	Slurry of activated charcoal by mouth. Lavage or induce emesis if not spontaneous. Saline cathartic. Atropine is specific antagonist, if the mushrooms contained muscarine. Artificial respiration.	Stimulants as indicated; external heat; oxygen inhalations; meperidine for pain; correct shock and dehydration by cautious fluid therapy.	Symptoms mimic intense parasympathetic stimulation. Severe hepatic, renal, and central nervous system damage.

POISONS AND POISONING—*Continued*

Toxic Substance	Probable Lethal Dose for Adult Human (mg./kg. body wt.)*	Symptoms of Poisoning	Emergency Measures	Supportive and Follow up Treatment	Pathology
Naphthalene (moth balls)	5 to 15 Gm.	Abdominal pain, nausea, vomiting, diarrhea, headache, diaphoresis, coma with or without convulsions. Certain individuals exhibit intense intravascular hemolysis accompanied by anemia, hematuria and renal insufficiency.	Induce emesis or lavage with tap water, saline cathartic, demulcents and mild stimulants.	Anemia from hemolysis may require whole blood transfusions. Supportive measures for acute renal failure.	Various states of central excitement or depression. Rarely, liver necrosis. Acute hemolytic anemia.
Nicotine	Less than 5 mg.	Burning sensation in mouth and throat, salivation, vomiting, diarrhea, headache, sweating, dizziness, weakness, pupils contracted at first then dilated, pulse slow at first then rapid, respirations deep and rapid at first then dyspneic, death from paralysis of respiratory musculature.	Slurry of activated charcoal as lavage fluid with additional portion left in stomach. Artificial respiration and oxygen.	Control convulsions with small doses of intravenous barbiturates. Relief for visceral symptoms is obtained with atropine and phenoxybenzamine (Dibenzyline).	Transient stimulation then depression of CNS, all autonomic ganglia and nerve endings in skeletal muscle.
Nitroglycerin	Less than 5 mg.	Prompt fall in blood pressure, intense throbbing in head, dizziness, faintness, excessive muscular relaxation, tremors, nausea, vomiting, skin flushed then cold and cyanotic, postural hypotension, paralysis, anoxic convulsions, death.	Gastric lavage or administer emetic. Mild stimulants as indicated. Oxygen and artificial respiration.	Keep patient in reclining position and comfortably warm. Transfusions, if needed, with whole blood or plasma.	Anoxia due to methemoglobinemia aggravated by stagnation of blood in capillaries, venules and veins from peripheral vasodilatation.
Nitrous fumes nitric oxide, nitrogen dioxide, sulfur dioxide, phosgene	Unknown	Only very high concentrations produce immediate pulmonary symptoms. After day or two, fatigue, restlessness, cough and other signs of developing pulmonary edema; increasing difficulty in breathing; cyanosis, coughing with frothy expectoration; lethargy, coma, circulatory collapse; death in asphyxia.	Enforce complete bed rest; positive pressure oxygen as needed. Antibiotics and steroids as indicated. Small doses of morphine.	Remove frothy exudates by suctioning. Good nursing care essential.	Asphyxial death due to blockage of gas exchange in lungs.
Oxalic acid and oxalate salts	50 to 500 mg.	Severe gastrointestinal irritation and intense pain in upper gastrointestinal tract; vomiting and intense thirst; pulse weak and thready; skin cold and cyanotic; twitching of facial musculature; convulsions, coma, collapse and death.	Give immediately by mouth large amounts of calcium lactate, lime water, magnesia or chalk or lavage cautiously with any of these. Intravenous calcium gluconate or chloride.	Keep patient quiet and in recumbent position. Morphine for pain; demulcents.	Severe gastroenteritis and secondary shock, hypocalcemia and kidney injury.

Toxic Substance	Probable Lethal Dose for Adult Human (mg./kg. body wt.)*	Symptoms of Poisoning	Emergency Measures	Supportive and Follow up Treatment	Pathology
Parathion, and other organo-phosphorus insecticides	Less than 5 mg.	Nausea, vomiting, diarrhea, abdominal cramps, salivation, headache, vertigo, runny nose, pinpoint pupils, generalized and profound muscular weakness, confusion, jerky movements, convulsions, coma, death in respiratory failure.	Give atropine 1 to 4 mg. intravenously immediately and repeat every 3 to 8 minutes until parasympathetic symptoms are controlled. Give oxygen and artificial respiration. If available, valuable adjunct is 2-PAM (pyridine aldoxime methiodide) in accordance with manufacturer's directions.	Endotracheal intubation or tracheotomy may be necessary. Keep patient under constant observation.	All signs and symptoms are referable to the inhibition of the enzyme, acetylcholinesterase, and consequent accumulation of acetylcholine at all nervous junctions where it is the chemical mediator.
Phenol	50 to 500 mg.	Corrosive burns in mouth, esophagus and stomach, abdominal pain, bloody diarrhea, pallor, sweating, weakness, headache, dizziness, ringing in ears, shock with weak pulse, fall in blood pressure and body temperature, shallow respiration, cyanosis, coma, death from respiratory failure. Skin contact produces pain followed by numbness and corrosive burn.	NOTE: If stomach wall is severely corroded passage of a tube into it may cause rupture of the stomach. Cautious lavage with olive oil. Avoid mineral oils and alcohol. As needed demulcents, morphine, mild respiratory stimulants. Wash skin areas with 50% alcohol or castor oil.	Moderate external heat. Treat shock conservatively and watch for signs of renal insufficiency. Systemic acidosis may require therapy with bicarbonate.	Corrosive burns of skin and mucous membranes, gastric perforation, more rarely esophageal stricture and kidney shutdown.
Phosphorus	Less than 5 mg.	Skin contact produces painful penetrating burns. Ingestion leads to burning pain in throat or abdomen with intense thirst followed by nausea, vomiting, diarrhea, odor of garlic on breath, luminescent vomitus and feces. Patient often appears to recover for several days then suddenly relapse with severe liver, kidney and cardiac damage.	Repeated washing of the stomach with 1% copper sulfate followed by 1:10,000 potassium permanganate. Leave liquid petrolatum in stomach. Give morphine for pain and vitamin K_1.	Intravenous saline and lactate for shock, dehydration and acidosis. Supportive therapy for delirium, hepatic insufficiency and renal failure. For several days avoid fats and oils in the diet because they promote absorption of phosphorus.	Fatty degeneration of liver, kidneys and heart.
Quaternary Ammonium Germicides	50 to 500 mg.	Burning pain in mouth and throat, restlessness, confusion, muscle weakness, CNS depression, labored breathing, cyanosis, asphyxial death.	Large quantities of milk or egg whites make good lavage fluids. No specific antidotes or antagonists are known.	Support respiration. If convulsions are persistent (rare), give intravenous short-acting barbiturates.	Nonspecific irritation, visceral congestion, cloudy swelling, mild pulmonary edema.

Toxic Substance	Probable Lethal Dose for Adult Human (mg./kg. body wt.)*	Symptoms of Poisoning	Emergency Measures	Supportive and Follow up Treatment	Pathology
Rotenone or Pyrethrum	Rotenone: 50 to 500 mg. Pyrethrum: from under 5 grams to more than 15 grams	Sensation of numbness in mouth; nausea, vomiting, gastrointestinal pain; tremors, convulsions, stupor; respiratory stimulation followed by depression; death from respiratory arrest.	Slurry of activated charcoal by mouth; induce vomiting or lavage with tap water, saline cathartic.	Support respiration, oxygen, mild sedation (avoid barbiturates), fluids. Glucose may be needed for hypoglycemia.	Severe hypoglycemia may be seen, otherwise the pathologic changes largely unknown.
Salicylate (sodium, methyl, acetylsalicylic acid)	50 to 500 mg.	Mild gastrointestinal pain, nausea, vomiting, deep and rapid breathing, headache, dizziness, ringing in ears, dimness of vision, irritability, nervousness, confusion, delirium, mania, convulsions, coma and death from respiratory failure with or without cardiovascular collapse.	Induce vomiting or lavage with 5% bicarbonate solution; saline cathartic.	Determine acid-base status and if acidosis is profound, institute sodium lactate therapy. Correct dehydration and hypoglycemia if present. Barbiturates, vitamin K, dialysis procedures or exchange transfusion as indicated.	Disturbed acid-base balance. Children often exhibit metabolic acidosis while adults more commonly show respiratory alkalosis. Intense CNS stimulation followed by depression.
Silver salts, nitrate, and other soluble salts	3.5 to 35 Gm. total dose.	Intense pain in mouth, throat and gastrointestinal tract; bloody stools; vertigo; coma, convulsions and death.	Gastric lavage with, or administration of, large quantities of table salt (sodium chloride) and water. Give saline cathartic.	Eggs and milk as demulcents, morphine for pain, stimulants as indicated; treat for shock; maintain fluid and electrolyte balance.	Severe corrosion of gastrointestinal tract. Deposits of metallic silver occur under skin in chronic poisoning, but these are of minor cosmetic concern.
Strychnine	Less than 5 mg.	Apprehension, stiffness of muscles, twitching of face and arms, sudden tetanic convulsions of entire body, cyanosis of face and lips, pulse slow and strong, death in 1 to 3 hours with face fixed in a grin and body arched in hyperextension.	Slurry of activated charcoal by mouth or gastric lavage with dilute permanganate or iodine; such procedures, however, are usually delayed until convulsions are controlled with chloroform, ether or intravenous barbiturates. NOTE: Do not give morphine.	Place patient in a quiet, dark room. Avoid drafts. Artificial respiration may be needed. Constant nursing care.	Stimulation of spinal cord leading to contraction of respiratory musculature and death from anoxia.
Thallium and salts, sulfate	5 to 50 mg.	Severe abdominal pain, vomiting, diarrhea, tremors, delirium, convulsions, paralysis, coma and death. Loss of hair is peculiar to chronic poisoning or cases of delayed death.	Induce emesis or lavage with 1% sodium or potassium iodide. Leave activated charcoal in stomach. Give saline cathartic and demulcents.	Treat for shock; maintain fluid and electrolyte balance; calcium salts or milk, symptomatic and supportive therapy for CNS disorders.	Hemorrhagic gastroenteritis and encephalopathy.

Toxic Substance	Probable Lethal Dose for Adult Human (mg./kg. body wt.)*	Symptoms of Poisoning	Emergency Measures	Supportive and Follow up Treatment	Pathology
Thiram or Disulfiram	50 to 500 mg.	Nausea, vomiting, diarrhea, ataxia, hyperexcitability, hypothermia, flaccid paralysis. If patient has also ingested ethyl alcohol in even trivial amounts, symptoms are quite different and include flushing, fall in blood pressure, palpitations, sweating, vertigo, confusion, circulatory collapse, coma and death.	Lavage with tap water. Strictly prohibit alcohol in all forms. Inhalations of oxygen.	Symptomatic and supportive care for gastrointestinal symptoms and neurological complications. In case complicated by alcohol, parenteral glucose, ascorbic acid, ephedrine and diphenhydramine may be beneficial.	Hyperemia, ulceration of gastrointestinal tract, renal and hepatic necrosis, demyelinization of cerebellum and medulla.
Turpentine	500 mg. to 5 Gm.	Sensation of warmth or pain in mouth, throat and stomach followed by abdominal pain, vomiting and diarrhea. Aspiration into lungs may cause pneumonitis. Excitement, ataxia, delirium and stupor, followed by convulsions, coma and death from respiratory failure.	Gastric lavage with weak bicarbonate solution, followed by demulcents and saline cathartic.	Morphine sulfate for intense pain and a short-acting barbiturate for excitement. Mild stimulation if indicated, e.g., caffiene sodium benzoate. Force fluids.	Irritation of kidneys; hematuria, albuminuria and sometimes complete urinary suppression. Kidney symptoms appear to be related to composition of the turpentine, and often never appear.
Warfarin	50 to 500 mg.	After few days of repeated ingestions: nosebleed; bleeding gums; pallor; hemorrhagic areas in skin, especially knees and buttocks; blood in urine or feces; death in hemorrhagic shock.	Gastric lavage with tap water in case of large single dose. Vitamin K is specific antidote and should be given until prothrombin levels return to normal. Whole blood transfusions may be necessary.	Replacement iron as ferrous sulfate.	Capillary dilatation and increased fragility with hypoprothrombinemia leading to internal hemorrhage.
Zinc salts, chloride, sulfate, acetate, etc.	50 to 500 mg.	Increased salivation, violent vomiting, purging, followed by prostration.	Lavage with milk or lime water. Follow with egg white and other demulcents. Morphine for pain.	Recumbent position, external heat to body, morphine for pain; treat for shock; maintain fluid and electrolyte balances.	Stricture of esophagus, pylorus, and destruction of glandular structure of stomach. Ulceration and/or perforation of the stomach.

*Most of these values from Gleason, M. N., Gosselin, R. E., Hodge, H. C., and Smith, R. P.: Clinical Toxicology of Commercial Products, 3rd ed. The Williams & Wilkins Co., Baltimore, 1969.

Dose Equivalent Expressed in Household Measures*

mg./kg.		mg./kg.	
Less than 5	A taste. Less than 7 drops	500 to 5000 (5 Gm.)	Between one ounce and one pint
5 to 50	Between 7 drops and one teaspoon	5000 to 15,000 (5 to 15 Gm.)	Between one pint and one quart
50 to 500	Between one teaspoon and one ounce	Greater than 15,000 mg. (15 Gm.)	Greater than one quart

*From Gleason, M. N., Gosselin, R. E., Hodge, H. C., and Smith, R. P.: Clinical Toxicology of Commercial Products, 3rd ed. The Williams & Wilkins Co., Baltimore, 1969.

Suffocation, Asphyxiation, Drowning

Type	History	Pathology	Symptoms and Color	Pulse	Breathing	Muscles	Pupils	Complications	Treatment
1. Drowning	Victim removed from body of water.	Waterlogging of lungs, and asphyxia are present.	Patient is unconscious. Color is gray and changing to blue (cyanosis).	When pulse is perceptible it is rapid and may be shallow.	If respirations are present the patient may gasp occasionally or very irregularly.	Muscles will be relaxed and body is very limp.	Pupils may be dilated.	Fracture of neck. Heart failure. Suffocation, shock and collapse.	Artificial respiration (mouth to mouth). External cardiac massage if needed. Oxygen—Treat for shock. Heart stimulants.
2. Gas Poisoning	Victim rescued from room with escaping gas from open jet or —victim overcome in closed garage.	Changes in the blood chemistry and then anemia is present. Respiratory paralysis which leads to death.	Patient unconscious. Color of the typical cherry red or pallor and cyanosis (carbon monoxide).	Pulse is rapid and may be irregular.	Respirations are usually slow but may be rapid and shallow very early after the exposure to gas.	Muscles are relaxed. Body is limp.	This varies with the type of gas poisoning.	Respiratory failure. Depletion of O_2 supply in the blood.	Artificial respiration. Oxygen. Shock treatment.
3. Choking	Edema of larynx. Diseases of the larynx. Foreign bodies are aspirated into the larynx.	Trauma of larynx.	Patient in a state of apprehension. Color—cyanotic.	Pulse is rapid due to exertion.	Respirations are very rapid or patient may gasp occasionally.	Muscles may be voluntarily contracted.	Pupils are dilated.	Pneumonia. Sinusitis. Complete obstruction of the bronchi. Lung abscess.	Manual removal or encourage coughing by slap on back. Tracheotomy may be required.
4. Strangulation and Hanging	Patient usually found during or after the act. Very definite signs of violence will be noted.	Fracture of cervical vertebrae. Suffocation. Trauma of Medulla by odontoid process of axis.	Unconscious or dead. Living patient is in a state of excitement or desperation. Color—cyanotic if body is long deceased.	Pulse may be perceptible. Pulse may be absent.	No respirations or respirations are very rapid or patient may gasp occasionally.	Muscles may be voluntarily contracted.	Pupils are dilated. Unequal if there is cerebral injury.	Fracture of neck. Suffocation. Contusions on neck.	Release pull of rope by placing chair under patient's feet, cut rope. Oxygen therapy. Artificial respiration. Treat for shock. Treat fractures.

Unconsciousness

Type	History	Color	Pupils	Muscles	Pulse	Breathing	Reflexes	Complications	Treatment
1. Shock	This condition is a result of a blow or damage to the central nervous system.	Skin cold, temperature subnormal. Skin is an ashen gray to cyanotic color.	Pupils are dilated.	Muscles are relaxed.	Pulse is rapid and becomes thready and feeble.	Respirations are rapid and shallow.	Reflexes diminished (not significant).	Respiratory and circulatory embarrassment to collapse and death.	Elevate foot of bed. Keep body warm. Transfusions usually indicated for depression of vascular system.
2. Bleeding	Victim of a trauma causing bright red spurting or welling bleeding. Bleeding after an operation.	Skin shows pallor which grows progressively worse to a yellow or greenish tinge.	Pupils are dilated.	Muscles are relaxed.	Pulse is rapid and becomes thready.	Respirations are rapid and shallow. Air hunger is evident.	Reflexes diminished.	Shock. Anemia. Heart failure. Death.	Digital pressure and tourniquet. Pad in joint. Keep patient quiet. Treat for shock. Transfusion if necessary.
3. Drowning	Victim is found unconscious in body of water. May have a fractured neck or skull.	Skin is cold and clammy and cyanotic.	Pupils are dilated.	Muscles are relaxed, unless death, then rigidity of rigor mortis.	If pulse is perceptible it will be rapid, weak or very irregular.	No respirations. Occasional gasp if alive.	Reflexes abolished.	Heart failure. Shock — Pneumonia — aspiration of foreign material.	Resuscitation (Mouth-to-mouth is most effective method if a manual positive pressure type of device is not available. Keep body warm but not hot. Stimulating drinks when conscious.
4. Gases	Victim rescued from a mine, a burning building, or room with open gas jet. Overcome in garage or car.	Skin is cyanotic and changing to the characteristic color, usually cherry red. (Carbon monoxide.)	Eyes fixed. Pupils are usually fully dilated. Varies with type of gas.	If alive, muscles are relaxed. If dead, rigor mortis.	Pulse is weak, slow and irregular.	Respirations irregular and jerky to only an occasional gasp.	Reflexes are abolished.	Respiratory failure. Asphyxia. Collapse.	Place the patient in the open air. Give oxygen and resuscitation (mouth-to-mouth). Treat for shock
5. Hanging	Victim is found hanging with constriction of the neck.	Skin is pale and face is cyanotic.	Pupils are dilatedand unequal if cerebral injury.	Muscles are relaxed. Varies with the level of tenure.	If strangulation is incomplete pulse is rapid, weak and irregular. If complete, pulse is absent.	Respirations have ceased or an occasional gasp is observed.	Reflexes are abolished.	Respiratory and circulatory failure. Fracture of neck.	Release the patient—cut the rope. Artificial respirations. Treat for shock and possible fracture of neck.

UNCONSCIOUSNESS—*Continued*

Type	History	Color	Pupils	Muscles	Pulse	Breathing	Reflexes	Complications	Treatment
6. Obstruction in throat	Victim has aspirated a foreign body or respiratory tract is obstructed by edema or disease.	Skin is cyanotic.	Pupils are dilated.	Sternal retraction. Muscles are tense with efforts in trying to breathe and to remove obstruction.	Pulse is rapid and very weak.	Respirations are deep and labored.	Reflexes are increased.	Asphyxia; pulmonary infection; shock.	Remove obstruction. Respiratory stimulant or give artificial respiration. Treat for shock. Tracheotomy if indicated.
7. Electric Shock	Victim is found after coming in contact with a "live wire."	Skin is pale, cold and clammy.	Pupils may be unequal.	Muscles are tense.	Weak and imperceptible pulse.	Respirations cease suddenly.	Deep tendon reflexes are usually increased.	Low voltage affects heart action, makes resuscitation impossible. High voltage affects the resp. center in medulla and patient may be resuscitated.	Release the patient from current with care. Artificial respiration by prone pressure. Electrical defibrillation may be required. If heart fails to resume contraction, use of an external cardiac pacemaker is indicated. Each moment of delay in using these techniques increases the chances of death.
8. Concussion	Head injury caused by fall or blow upon the head.	Skin pale, cold and clammy. Varies with degree of pathology.	Pupils are dilated. Varies with degree and area of injury.	Muscles may be spastic.	Pulse rate usually shows a slight increase. May be weak and rapid.	Respirations are usually deep.	Deep tendon reflexes may be increased.	Shock in severe cases. Paralysis of limbs may occur.	Bed rest. Keep patient flat and warm.
9. Epilepsy	History reveals the previous occurrence of "fits" or spells with or without aura.	Pallor to flush followed by cyanosis — may be slight and gradually increased to marked cyanosis.	Pupils are unequal. Eyes rolling.	Muscles may be spastic. Tonic type of convulsions is followed by the clonic type.	Pulse is usually rapid.	Respirations are deep and stertorous.	Reflexes may be increased.	Injuries in falling or biting the tongue. Patient may react violently (fighting others).	Bed rest. Prevent falling or biting tongue. Sedative—luminal.

UNCONSCIOUSNESS—*Continued*

Type	History	Color	Pupils	Muscles	Pulse	Breathing	Reflexes	Complications	Treatment
10. Drunkenness	History of fondness of alcohol; victim is unable to cope with the amount of intoxicants taken.	Color varies. Face may be flushed, skin is moist, relaxed and cool.	Pupils are usually dilated, but are equal.	Muscles are relaxed, body and limbs are limp.	Pulse is strong and slow.	Respirations are slow, deep, stertorous, accompanied by characteristic "lip blowing" and Cheyne-Stokes type of breathing.	Reflexes are usually increased.	Pneumonia.	Keep the body warm. If conscious give emetic. Gastric lavage. Give hot coffee or aromatic spirits of ammonia.
11. Stroke (Apoplectic)	Patient may have history of hypertension and arteriosclerosis. Usually past 40 years of age.	Skin is injected. May be cyanotic or ashen gray. Hot and dry to flushed (elevation of temperature).	Pupils vary, may be dilated, often unequal. In deep coma are inactive.	Muscles of the involved side (hemiplegia) are usually spastic with a facial palsy.	Pulse is slow, full with increased tension.	Respirations are slow, loud, usually deep.	Reflexes are diminished on one side. May be hyperactive on the other side.	Pneumonia—Injury from falling.	Rest and absolute quiet with head of bed elevated and feet lowered. Ice cap to head. No stimulants.
12. Narcotic Poisoning	History of addiction or idiosyncrasy for the drug.	Skin is ashen gray, cyanotic and cold.	Pupils are contracted to "pinpoint" if due to opiate derivative such as morphine or codeine.	Muscles are relaxed.	Pulse usually slow but varies with type of drug poisoning.	Respirations slow, irregular, stertorous.	Reflexes are diminished.	Addiction to drug or production of a marked sensitivity to a drug.	Removal of the drug by emetics or lavage. Use of antidotes. Specific counteractives.
13. Acid and Alkali Poisoning	History of accidental or intentional poisoning.	Clammy skin. Skin pale; face cyanotic.	Eyes sunken, staring. Pupils are dilated.	Tense. Patient in convulsion.	Rapid, feeble pulse.	Shallow, rapid, labored, irregular.	Reflexes are increased.	Corrosion of mucous membranes. Ulcers of stomach. Gastritis; jaundice.	For acids — Milk of magnesia, egg albumin, lime water, no chalk or alkaline carbonate. For Alkalies—Neutralize with acetic acid (vinegar). In both cases careful gastric lavage.
14. Mineral Poisoning	History of accidental or suicidal poisoning.	Skin is cold and clammy, pallor.	Eyes fixed, staring. Pupils are dilated.	Tense, convulsive to relaxed when in stupor.	Rapid, feeble to imperceptible.	Respirations are shallow, rapid, labored.	Reflexes are increased.	Nephritis. Liver degeneration. Colitis.	Gastric lavage—Emetics.

UNCONSCIOUSNESS—*Continued*

Type	History	Color	Pupils	Muscles	Pulse	Breathing	Reflexes	Complications	Treatment
15. Heat Exhaustion	Victim is overcome by the degree of heat in surrounding field of work and loss of sodium chloride through perspiration.	Skin may be pale and cool. Temperature is usually normal.	Pupils are moderately contracted.	Muscles are tense. Muscle cramps.	Pulse is rapid and may become weak.	Respirations shallow with rigidity of the chest muscles.	Reflexes are increased.	Shock.	Treat for shock (keep body warm). Give salt by mouth, and intravenous injections.
16. Heat Stroke (sun stroke or heat hyperpyrexia)	Victim has been exposed to intense degree or a prolonged period of heat from environment.	Skin is flushed (red) and hot when touched. Body temperature may be 106 or higher.	Pupils are dilated.	Muscles are relaxed.	Rapid and weak.	Respirations may be shallow and gasping or deep and slow.	Reflexes increased.	Suppressed sweating for prolonged period. Paralysis of vasomotor centers within medulla. Paralysis of heart, collapse and death.	Remove patient to cool area. Cold application to head and body. Rub body with ice or alcohol with ice in it. Fan body while this is being done to increase the rate of cooling. Keep in cold, wet sheet. Continue to lower body temperature. No stimulants or sedatives unless required to treat convulsions. Judge effectiveness of therapy by continual monitoring of rectal temperature.
17. Freezing	Victim is found after period of exposure to intense cold or prolonged period of exposure to the cold.	Frostbite—Skin is cold, pale and blanched. Frozen—skin is livid and later cyanotic, then turns to purplish or greenish black.	Pupils are dilated.	Muscles are tense and become very rigid.	Pulse is rapid and weak.	Breathing is slower and deeper. Patient falls into very deep slumber.	Reflexes are not discernible.	Pneumonia—certain damage due to mechanical destruction of the cells sloughing and gangrene of the part previously frozen.	Gradual warming of the parts. Slight massage of extremities for better circulation. Elevation of parts. Treatment of the dry gangrene.
18. Fainting	History of fatigue or shock or horrible sight or "light headedness."	Skin of face and the lips are blanched. Body is cold and clammy.	Pupils are normal.	Muscles are completely relaxed.	Pulse is rapid and thready.	Respirations are rapid and shallow.	Reflexes are slightly increased.	Shock is usually a serious complication. Body injury and fracture if patient falls.	Apply cold water to face, head and chest. Lower patient's head. Place head in low position. Give aromatic spirits of ammonia.

Wounds

Type	History	Pathology	Symptoms and Color	Complications	Treatment	Transportation	Points of Identification
1. Contusions.	History of blow or fall.	A bruise (hematoma) or petechial area with underlying injury.	Skin surface is rough, the area includes a large or small hematoma (depending upon the extent of injury).	Destruction of underlying tissue if hematoma is not aspirated early. Infection if skin is punctured or probed.	Alternate ice and warm applications to area of injury. Gentle massage of surrounding tissues not involved in injury.	Cover area with loose fitting bandage if skin is abraded. Keep the part well elevated if possible.	Skin is not broken. Tissues underlying skin may be slightly or very markedly crushed.
2. "Brush Burns" or Abrasions.	Area of injury has been subjected to rapid passing object or body thrown against rough surface. Ex:—skidding on wet grass.	Skin, mucous membranes show niches in skin. Top surface effaced with remaining surface dotted with small drops of blood.	Skin discolored. Top surface peeled off with fine bead-like dots of blood. Skin may also be impregnated with dirt and refuse.	Complications include infection developments. Recovery may show very rough unsightly scars.	Carefully brush away all loose dirt and debris. Cleanse the wound with soap and water. Use antiseptic solutions, ointment, and apply dressings. Tetanus toxoid or antitoxin as required.	Use loose applications of sterile dressings held in place by loose fitting triangle.	Top surface of the skin is brushed completely away, or remains very lightly attached to the area.
3. Lacerations.	History of an accident wherein sharp instruments have cut (lacerated) the area of the body.	Jagged or torn and roughened edges of tissues. May include evulsion of certain parts.	Injury has produced area of two raw or bleeding surfaces of the skin. Blood may be oozing or spurting from the wound.	Infection may develop. Septicemia may follow. Wound usually heals with very unsightly scar if not properly sutured.	Remove the large debris and dirt. Clean the wound by water dripping from sterile cloth or use soap and warm water, antiseptics and sterile dressings. Use mild antiseptics.	Cover the area of injury with loose application of dressings held by triangle or cravat bandage. Edges of wound may be united with flamed strip of adhesive tape. Tetanus toxoid or antitoxin as required.	Wound edges are jagged and irregular. Wound may contain amount of debris or dirt, and usually is infected.
4. Puncture.	Object may be still probing tissues, or patient may have been lifted from a rusty nail or thorn.	Tissues are pierced; small opening through the tissues (excellent course or inlet for infection).	Area usually manifests no bleeding. Trauma of tissues is usually evident.	Infection of the anaerobic type (Tetanus bacillus)—and septicemia.	Early indications of antitoxin. Probe the wound very carefully to enlarge bore for irrigation with antiseptic solutions. Tetanus toxoid or antitoxin as required. Treatment for prevention of gas gangrene may be required.	Cover the area with sterile dressings and triangle or cravat bandage.	Puncture site is very small. Object is usually withdrawn with fair amount of ease.

WOUNDS—Continued

Type	History	Pathology	Symptoms and Color	Complications	Treatment	Transportation	Points of Identification
5. Stab.	History of injury during a brawl or duel. Accident of fall or thrust upon blunt or heavy pointed object.	Size of hole in the tissues varies with the size of the instrument. Foreign material and pathogenic bacteria of anaerobic nature are usually introduced.	Evidence of the instrument that was used—such as knife, ice pick, etc. Victim shows pallor, syncope and later collapse.	Internal hemorrhage from or damage to organs underlying site of wound, such as puncture and collapse of lung, abdominal visceral injury or severance of a nerve. Pulmonary hemorrhage. Infection of body by anaerobic organisms—(Tetanus bacillus).	Cleanse and irrigate the wound when possible. Irrigation and inclusion of antiseptic drain or wet dressings. Early use of antitetanic sera. Tetanus toxoid or antitoxin as required.	Keep patient very quiet with head and chest slightly elevated. Treat for shock. If chest is involved then watch T.P.R. and blood pressure.	Large puncture site and very deep. Victim may still be pinned by the force of the blow.
6. Gun Shot.	History of an accident in care of a gun or pistol, etc. Victim of aimed shot or assailant.	Wound of single outer puncture site with deep injury (twisting and tearing of tissue) by buck shot, etc.	Aperture is small. Powder burns are occasionally found.	Shock, internal hemorrhage. Tetanus bacillus infection.	Early use of antitetanus sera. Cleanse and irrigate when possible. Wet antiseptic dressings. Debridement when necessary. Tetanus toxoid or antitoxin as required.	Keep patient very quiet. Head slightly lower than body. Treat for shock. Watch T.P.R. and blood pressure when hemorrhaging.	Puncture site. Deep wound shows characteristic twisting of the deeper tissues.
7. Bite: Human, animal, or insect.	History of bite of a rabid human, animal or reptile. Or the sting or bite of poisonous insect. Occasionally no history.	Tissue degeneration at site of wound. Muscular paralysis. Venom has a very drastic effect upon respiratory nerve centers.	Human—shape of denture. Dog—lacerated wound. Rabid disposition. Snake—two fang wound. Insect—elevated wheal with itching or burning sensation and pain or single or double red dot.	Infection introduced pathogenic organisms. Venom of toxic nature depresses victim. Death if too long delay in treatment.	1. Observe the victim. Enclose the dog. 2. Pasteur treatment if deemed necessary. 3. For snake bite apply tourniquet just tight enough to prevent venous return. Keep area cold with ice packs to prevent absorption of venom. Incision and suction as swelling rises. 4. Neutralize acid of "sting" with alkalies. 5. Treat for shock, respiratory stimulants for snake or insect venom. Specific antivenins are available for certain snake bites.	Avert apprehension. Keep patient quiet. Keep muscles of the area elevated and at rest.	1. Shape of denture. 2. Odor of colon bacillus about the wound (human bite). 3. Two fang puncture. Small red dot or presence of stinger.

The Interpreter

The Interpreter

OUTLINED IN FIVE LANGUAGES

Specially Arranged for Diagnosis

NOTE: The languages are listed as follows: *First:* English; *Second:* French; *Third:* German; *Fourth:* Italian; *Fifth:* Spanish.

INDEX

1. Good morning.
Bonjour.
Guten Morgen.
Buon giorno.
Buenos días.

2. How do you feel?
Comment vous sentez-vous?
Wie geht es Ihnen?
Come state?
¿Como se siente Vd.?*

3. Well?
Bien?
Gut?
Bene?
¿Bien?

4. Badly?
Mal?
Schlecht?
Male?
¿Mal?

5. Let me feel your pulse.
Laissez-moi tâter le pouls.
Lassen Sie mich Ihren Puls fühlen.
Lasciatemi sentire il polso.
Dejeme tomar el pulso.

6. Have you taken the medicine?
Avez-vous pris la médicine?
Haben Sie die Medizin genommen?
Avete preso la medicina?
¿Ha tomado Vd. la medecina?

7. Do you understand me?
Comprenez vous?
Verstehen Sie mich?
Mi capisce?
¿Me entiende Vd.?

8. Answer only. Yes or No.
Ne répondez que, Oui ou Non.
Antworten Sie nur Ja oder Nein.
Rispondete solamente, Si o No.
No me conteste Vd. más que si ó no.

9. Have you slept well?
Avez-vous bien dormi?
Haben Sie gut geschlafen?
Avete ben dormito?
¿Ha dormido Vd. bien?

10. Have you slept badly?
Avez-vous mal dormi?
Haben Sie schlecht geschlafen?
Avete mal dormito?
¿Ha dormido Vd. mal?

11. How does your head feel?
Comment va la tête?
Wie geht es Ihrem Kopf?
Come vi sentite il capo?
¿Como se siente la cabeza?

12. Does it still pain you?
Vous fait-elle encore mal?
Schmerzt er doch–
Fa male ancora?
¿Le duele todavia?

13. Can you eat?
Pouvez-vous manger?
Können Sie essen?
Potete mangiare?
¿Puede Vd. comer?

14. Not much?
Pas beaucoup?
Nicht viel?
Non molto?
¿No mucho?

15. Do you still feel very weak?
Vous sentez-vous encore très faible?
Fühlen Sie sich noch sehr schwach?
Vi sentite ancora molto débole?
¿Se siente Vd. muy débil todavía?

*Vd. = usted.

16. Yes?
Oui?
Ja?
Si?
¿Si?

17. No?
Non?
Nein?
No?
¿No?

18. What do you say?
Que dites vous?
Was sagen Sie?
Che cosa dite?
¿Qué dice Vd.?

19. Show me your tongue.
Montrez-moi votre langue.
Zeigen Sie mir Ihre Zunge.
Mostratemi la lingua.
Enseñeme Vd. la lengua.

20. Have you any pain?
Avez-vous des douleurs?
Haben Sie Schmerzen?
Avete dolore?
¿Tiene Vd. dolor?

21. Where have you pain?
Ou avez-vous des douleurs?
Wo haben Sie Schmerzen?
Dove avete dolore?
¿Dónde tiene Vd. dolor?

22. In the head?
A la tête?
Im Kopf?
Nella testa?
¿En la cabeza?

23. In the abdomen?
Au ventre?
Im Leib?
Nel ventre?
¿En el vientre?

24. In the chest?
A la poitrine?
In der Brust?
Nel petto?
¿En el pecho?

25. Show me where.
Montrez-moi où.
Zeigen Sie mir wo.
Mostratemi dove.
Enseñe me donde.

26. Did you take cold?
Avez-vous pris froid?
Haben Sie sich erkältet?
Avete preso un colpo d' aria?
¿Se ha resfriado Vd.?

27. Have you still that heavy pain?
Avez-vous encore cette douleur pesante?
Haben Sie noch den drückenden Schmerz?
Avete ancora quel dolore pesante?
¿Tiene Vd. todavía este dolor pesado?

28. Did you sleep a few hours?
Avez-vous dormi quelques heures?
Haben Sie einige Stunden geschlafen?
Avete dormito qualche ora?
¿Ha dormido Vd. algunas horas?

29. Say it once again.
Dites cela encore une fois.
Sagen Sie das wieder.
Ditelo ancora una volta.
Repitalo Vd. otra vez.

30. Are you hungry?
Avez-vous faim?
Haben Sie Hunger?
Avete fame?
¿Tiene Vd. hambre?

31. You may eat:—
Vous pouvez manger:—
Sie dürfen essen:—
Potete mangiare:—
Vd. puede comer.

32. Two eggs.
Quelques oeufs.
Ein paar Eier.
Un paio d' uova.
Dos huevos.

33. Toast.
Rôtie.
Geröstetes Brot.
Il pane abbrustolito.
Pan tostado.

34. Bread.
Du pain.
Brot.
Pane.
Pan.

35. Oysters.
Des huitres.
Austern.
Delle óstriche.
Ostras.

36. Chicken.
Du poulet.
Huhn.
Pollame.
Pollo.

37. Are you thirsty?
Avez-vous soif?
Haben Sie Durst?
Avete sete?
¿Tiene Vd. sed?

38. You may drink ice-water.
Vous pouvez boire de l'eau glaçée.
Sie dürfen Eiswasser trinken.
Potete bevere acqua ghiacciata.
Vd. puede beber agua con hielo.

39. Milk.
Du lait.
Milch.
Latte.
Leche.

40. Tea.
Du thé.
Tee.
Il té.
Té.

41. Coffee.
Du café.
Kaffee.
Il caffè.
Café.

42. Chocolate.
Du chocolat.
Schokolade.
La cioccolatta.
Chocolate.

43. Beef-tea.
Le bouillon.
Bouillon.
Brodo.
Caldo de carne.

44. Have you a good appetite?
Avez-vous bon appétit?
Haben Sie guten Appetit?
Avete buon appetito?
¿Tiene Vd. buen apetito?

45. You must be very careful.
Prenez bien des précautions.
Sie müssen sehr vorsichtig sein.
Dovete usare molte precauzioni.
Vd. debe tener mucho cuidado.

46. And remain on diet.
Et faites la diète.
Und Diät halten.
E rimanere a dieta.
Y quedarse en diéta.

47. In a few days you may eat food.
En quelques jours vous pourrez manger.
In einigen Tagen dürfen Sie essen.
In pochi giorni potrete mangiare.
En algunas dias podrá Vd. comer algo.

48. I will leave a prescription.
Je laisserai une ordonnance.
Ich werde Ihnen ein Rezept lassen.
Lascerò una ricetta.
Voy á dejarle una receta.

49. Don't be afraid.
N'ayez pas peur.
Sie brauchen Keine Angst haben.
Non abbiate paura.
No tenga Vd. miedo.

50. It is nothing serious.
Ce n'est rien de grave.
Es ist nichts ernstliches.
Non è nulla.
No es nada grave.

51. Speak slower.
Parlez plus lentement.
Sprechen Sie langsamer.
Parlate più adagio.
Hable Vd. mas despacio.

52. What is your name?
Quel est votre nom?
Wie heissen Sie?
Come vi chiamate?
¿Como se llama Vd.?

53. How old are you?
Quel âge avez-vous?
Wie alt sind Sie?
Che età avete?
¿Qué edad tiene Vd.?

54. Twenty.
Vingt.
Zwanzig.
Venti.
Veinte.

55. Twenty-three.
Vingt-trois.
Dreiundzwanzig.
Ventitre.
Veintitres.

56. Twenty-five.
Vingt-cinq.
Fünfundzwanzig.
Venticinque.
Veinticinco.

57. Thirty.
Trente.
Dreissig.
Trenta.
Treinta.

58. Thirty-five.
Trente-cinq.
Fünfunddreissig.
Trentacinque.
Treinta y cinco.

59. Forty.
Quarante.
Vierzig.
Quaranta.
Cuarenta.

60. Forty-two.
Quarante-deux.
Zweiundvierzig.
Quarantadue.
Cuarenta y dos.

61. Fifty.
Cinquante.
Fünfzig.
Cinquanta.
Cincuenta.

62. Sixty.
Soixante.
Sechzig.
Sessanta.
Sesenta.

63. An operation will be necessary.
Il sera nécessaire de faire une opération.
Eine Operation ist notwendig.
Una operazione è necessaria.
Habra que hacer una operacion.

64. Let the operation be made.
Laissez faire l'opération.
Lassen Sie die Operation machen.
Lasciate fare l'operazione.
Dejele Vd. hacer la operacion.

65. Do not be afraid.
N'ayez pas peur.
Haben Sie keine Angst.
Non abbiate paura.
No tenga Vd. miedo.

66. It is necessary.
Il le faut.
Es ist durchaus nöthig.
È necessario.
Es necesario.

67. You will not?
Vous ne voulez pas?
Sie wollen nicht?
Non volete?
¿Vd. no quiere?

68. To-morrow it will be too late.
Demain ce sera trop tard.
Morgen wird es zu spät sein.
Domani sarà troppo tardi.
Mañana será demasiado tarde.

69. You will?
Vous voulez bien?
Sie wollen?
Volete?
¿Vd. quiere?

70. That is right.
C'est bien.
Das ist recht.
Va bene.
Está bien.

71. Come to my office in the morning.
Venez à mon bureau le matin.
Kommen Sie vormittags in mein Büro.
Venite al mio ufficio nella matina.
Venga Vd. á mi oficina por la mañana.

72. At ten o'clock.
A dix heures.
Um zehn Uhr.
Alle dieci.
A las diez.

73. To-morrow afternoon.
Demain après-midi.
Morgen nachmittags.
Domani dopo il pranzo.
Mañana por la tarde.

74. At half-past two.
A deux heures et demi.
Um halb drei.
Alle due e mezzo.
A las dos y media.

75. At three o'clock.
A trois heures.
Um drei Uhr.
Alle tre.
A las tres.

76. At four o'clock.
A quatre heures.
Um vier Uhr.
Alle quattro.
A las cuatro.

77. At half-past four o'clock.
A quatre heures et demi.
Um halb fünf Uhr.
Alle quattro e mezzo.
A las cuatro y media.

78. Sunday.
Dimanche.
Sonntag.
Domenica.
Domingo.

79. Monday.
Lundi.
Montag.
Lunedi.
Lunes.

80. Tuesday.
Mardi.
Dienstag.
Martedi.
Martes.

81. Wednesday.
Mercredi.
Mittwoch.
Mercoledi.
Miercoles.

82. Thursday.
Jeudi.
Donnerstag.
Giovedi.
Jueves.

83. Friday.
Vendredi.
Freitag.
Venerdi.
Viernes.

84. Saturday.
Samedi.
Sonnabend.
Sabato.
Sábado.

85. Of what did your mother die?
De quoi est morte votre mère?
Woran ist Ihre Mutter gestorben?
Di che è morta vostra madre?
¿De qué murió su madre?

86. And your father?
Et votre père?
Und Ihr Vater?
E vostro padre?
¿Y su padre?

87. Your grandfather?
Votre grand-père?
Ihr Grossvater?
Il vostro nonno?
¿Y su abuelo?

88. Your grandmother?
Votre grand'mère?
Ihre Grossmutter?
La votra nonna?
¿Y su abuela?

89. Have you any sisters?
Avez-vous des sœurs?
Haben Sie Schwestern?
Avete sorelle?
¿Tiene Vd. hermanas?

90. Have you brothers?
Avez-vous des frères?
Haben Sie Brüder?
Avete fratelli?
¿Tiene Vd. hermanos?

91. Are you married?
Etes-vous marié?
Sind Sie verheiratet?
Siete sposato?
¿Está Vd. casado?

92. A widower?
Veuf?
Ein Witwer?
Siete vedovo?
¿Viudo?

93. A widow?
Veuve?
Eine Witwe?
Siete vedova?
¿Viuda?

94. Have you children?
Avez-vous des enfants?
Haben Sie Kinder?
Avete fanciulli?
¿Tiene Vd. hijos?

95. Are they yet living?
Vivent-ils encore?
Sind sie noch am Leben?
Vivono ancora?
¿Viven ellos todavía?

96. What have you been working at? Are you:—
A quoi avez-vous travaillé? Etes vous:—
Was haben Sie gearbeitet? Sind Sie:—
Che lavoro fate? Siete:—
¿Que oficio tiene Vd.?, es Vd.—

97. A laborer?
Un ouvrier?
Ein Arbeiter?
Un operajo?
¿Jornalero?

98. A baker?
Un boulanger?
Ein Bäcker?
Un fornajo?
¿Panadero?

99. A miller?
Un meunier?
Ein Müller?
Un mugnaio?
¿Molinero?

100. A butcher?
Un boucher?
Ein Fleischer?
Un macellajo?
¿Carnicero?

101. A tailor?
Un tailleur?
Ein Schneider?
Un sarto?
¿Sastre?

102. A shoemaker?
Un cordonnier?
Ein Schuhmacher?
Un calzolaio?
¿Zapatero?

103. A mason?
Un maçon?
Ein Maurer?
Un muratore?
¿Albañil?

104. What diseases have you had in your youth?
Quelles maladies avez-vous eu dans votre jeunesse?
Welche Krankheiten haben Sie in Ihrer Jugend gehabt?
Che malattie avete avuto nella vostra gioventù?
¿Qué enfermedades ha tenido Vd. cuando joven?

105. Have you had scarlet fever?
La fièvre scarlatine?
Haben Sie Scharlachfieber gehabt?
Avete avuto la febbre scarlatina?
¿Ha tenido Vd. Escarlatina?

106. Measles?
La rougeole?
Die Masern?
Morbillo?
¿Sarampion?

107. Typhoid fever?
La fièvre typhoïde?
Der Typhus?
La febbre tifoìde?
¿Tifoidea?

108. Rheumatism?
Le rhumatisme?
Rheumatismus?
Reumatismo?
¿Reumatismo?

109. Pneumonia?
Inflammation des poumons?
Lungenentzündung?
Polmonite?
¿Pulmonia?

110. The chills?
Les frissons?
Fieberfrösteln?
I brividi?
¿Escalofrio?

111. An attack of fever?
Une attaque de fièvre?
Einen Fieberanfall?
Un attacco di febbre?
¿Un ataque de calentura?

112. A venereal disease?
Une maladie vénérienne?
Eine Geschlechtskrankheit?
Malattie veneree?
¿Una enfermidad venerea?

113. The month.
Le mois.
Der Monat.
Il mese.
El mes.

114. The months.
Les mois.
Die Monate.
I mesi.
Los meses.

115. January.
Janvier.
Januar.
Gennaio.
Enero.

116. February.
Février.
Februar.
Febbraio.
Febrero.

117. March.
Mars.
März.
Marzo.
Marzo.

118. April.
Avril.
April.
Aprile.
Abril.

119. May.
Mai.
Mai.
Maggio.
Mayo.

120. June.
Juin.
Juni.
Giugno.
Junio.

121. July.
Juillet.
Juli.
Luglio.
Julio.

122. August.
Août.
August.
Agosto.
Agosto.

123. September.
Septembre.
September.
Settembre.
Septiembre.

124. October.
Octobre.
Oktober.
Ottobre.
Octubre.

125. November.
Novembre.
November.
Novembre.
Noviembre.

126. December.
Décembre.
Dezember.
Dicembre.
Diciembre.

127. In the spring.
Au printemps.
Im Frühjahr.
Nella primavera.
En la primavera.

128. In summer.
En été.
Im Sommer.
Nell' estate.
En el verano.

129. In autumn.
En automne.
Im Herbst.
Nell' autunno.
En el otoño.

130. In winter.
En hiver.
Im Winter.
Nell' inverno.
En el invierno.

131. Are you tired?
Etes-vous fatigué?
Sind Sie müde?
Vi sentite molto stanco?
¿Está Vd. cansado?

132. How are your stools?
Comment sont vos selles?
Wie ist der Stuhlgang?
Come andate del corpo?
Como son los evacuaciones de cuerpo?

133. Are they regular?
Sont-elles régulières?
Ist er regelmässig?
Andate regolarmente?
¿Son regulares?

134. Have you noticed their color?
Avez-vous remarqué la couleur de vos selles?
Haben Sie auf die Farbe geachtet?
Vi siete accorto di che colore?
¿Ha notado Vd. el color?

135. Are you constipated?
Etes-vous constipé?
Haben Sie Verstopfung?
Siete stitico?
¿Está Vd. estreñido?

136. Since when?
Depuis quand?
Seit wann?
Da quando?
¿Desde cuando?

137. Have you any diarrhea?
Avez-vous la diarrhée?
Haben Sie Durchfall?
Avete diarrea?
¿Tiene Vd. diarrea?

138. Do you pass any blood?
Y a-t-il du sang dans vos selles?
Ist Blut im Stuhl?
Fate del sangue?
¿Pasa Vd. sangre?

139. You don't perhaps know?
Vous ne vous en êtes pas aperçu?
Vielleicht wissen Sie es nicht?
Forse non vi siete accorto?
¿Quizas no se ha dado Vd. cuenta?

140. Have you vomited?
Avez-vous vomi?
Haben Sie erbrechen?
Avete vomitato?
¿Ha vomitado Vd.?

141. Do you still vomit?
Vomissez-vous encore?
Erbrechen Sie noch immer?
Vomitate ancora?
¿Vomita Vd. todavia?

142. Do you vomit blood?
Vomissez-vous du sang?
Erbrechen Sie hellrot?
Vomitate sangue?
¿Vomita Vd. sangre?

143. The blood.
Le sang.
Das Blut.
Il sangue.
La sangre.

144. Is it of a dark-or bright-red color?
Cela a-t-il une couleur fonçée ou claire?
Ist es dunkel oder hellroth?
E esso nero o pure rosso?
¿Es de color rojo oscuro ó claro?

145. Have you any pain?
Avez-vous des douleurs?
Haben Sie Schmerzen?
Avete dolori?
¿Tiene Vd. dolores?

146. In the abdomen?
Dans le ventre?
Im Leib?
Nel ventre?
¿En el vientre?

147. Here?
Ici?
Hier?
Qui?
¿Aquí?

148. There?
Là?
Da?
Qua?
¿Ahí?

149. Does it hurt?
Cela fait-il mal?
Schmerzt es?
Fa male?
¿Le duele?

150. Since when is your tongue that color?
Depuis quand votre langue a-t-elle cette couleur?
Seit wann hat Ihre Zunge jene Farbe?
De quanto tempo la vostra lingua è di questo colore?
¿Desde cuando tiene su lengua este color?

151. Are you warm?
Avez-vous chaud?
Ist Ihnen heiss?
Avete caldo?
¿Tiene Vd. calor?

152. Are you cold?
Avez-vous froid?
Ist Ihnen kalt?
Avete freddo?
¿Tiene Vd. frio?

153. Have you any nose-bleeding?
Saignez-vous du nez?
Haben Sie Nasenbluten?
Avete sangue dal naso?
¿Le sangra la nariz?

154. Have you had it?
Avez-vous saigné du nez?
Haben Sie Nasenbluten gehabt?
Lo avete avuto?
¿Le ha sangrado?

155. Have you no appetite?
N'avez-vous d'appétit?
Haben Sie keinen Appetit?
Non avete appetito?
¿No tiene Vd. apetito?

156. Since when?
Depuis quand?
Seit wann?
Da quando?
¿Desde cuando?

157. Try to recollect.
Cherchez à vous en rappeler.
Versuchen Sie sich zu erinnern.
Cercate di ricordarvi.
Trate Vd. de recordarse.

158. It is important to know how long you have felt this way.
Il est bien important de savoir depuis quand vous sentez ainsi.
Es ist von grosser Wichtigkeit zu wissen seit wann Sie sich so fühlen.
E necessario sapere de quando tempo vi sentite cosi.
Es necesario saber desde cuando se siente asi.

159. Have you any difficulty in passing your water?
Avez-vous de la difficulté à uriner?
Haben Sie Schwierigkeiten beim Wasserlassen?
Avete difficoltà nell' urinare?
¿Tiene Vd. dificultad en orinar?

160. Do you pass your water involuntarily?
Urinez-vous sans le vouloir?
Verlieren Sie Harn ohne es zu wollen?
Urinate involontariamente?
¿Orina Vd. sin querer?

161. Are any of your limbs swollen?
Avez-vous des membres gonflés?
Ist irgend eines Ihrer Glieder geschwollen?
Vi sentite gonflo in qualche parte?
¿Tiene Vd. alguna parte hinchada?

162. Let me see.
Laissez-moi voir.
Lassen Sie sehen.
Lasciatemi vedere.
Dejeme ver.

163. How long have they been swollen like this?
Depuis quand sont-ils gonflés ainsi?
Seit wann sind sie so angeschwollen?
Da quanto tempo che li avete cosí gonfi?
¿Desde cuando esta hinchado asi?

164. For how many days or weeks?
Depuis combien de jours ou de semaines?
Seit wievielen Tagen oder Wochen?
Da quanti giorni o settimane?
¿Desde cuantos dias ó semanas?

165. Were they ever swollen before?
Ont-ils jamais été ainsi gonflés?
Sind sie je früher so angeschwollen gewesen?
Li avete avuto mai gonfi prima?
¿Han estado hinchado antes?

166. Have you any difficulty in breathing?
Avez-vous de la difficulté à respirer?
Wird Ihnen das Atemholen schwer?
Avete nessuna difficoltà di respirare?
¿Tiene Vd. dificultad en respirar?

167. In getting on your feet?
A vous lever?
Beim Aufstehen?
Alzandovi?
¿En ponerse de pié?

168. Does it pain you?
Cela vous fait-il mal?
Schmerzt es?
Vi fa male?
¿Le duele a Vd.?

169. Whisper: One, two, three.
Dites à voix basse: un, deux, trois.
Flüstern Sie: eins, zwei, drei.
Dite piano: uno, due, tre.
Cuente Vd. a noz muy baya: uno, dos, tres.

170. Say it out loud.
A haute voix.
Sagen Sie es laut.
Ditelo ad alta voce.
A voz alta.

171. Cough.
Toussez.
Husten Sie.
Tossite.
Tosa Vd.

172. Cough again.
Toussez encore une fois.
Husten Sie noch einmal.
Tossite ancora.
Tosa Vd. otra vez.

173. That will do.
C'est bien.
Das ist genug.
Basta cosi.
Esta bastante.

174. Open your mouth.
Ouvrez la bouche.
Oeffnen Sie den Mund.
Aprite la bocca.
Abra Vd. la boca.

175. Since when do you cough?
Depuis quand avez-vous la toux?
Seit wann husten Sie?
Da quanto tempo avete la tosse?
¿Desde cuando tiene Vd. esta tos?

176. You cough a little?
Toussez-vous un peu?
Sie husten ein wenig?
Tossite solo poco?
¿Vd. tose poco?

177. Take a deep breath.
Prenez une respiration profonde.
Atmen Sie tief.
Prendete un gran respiro.
Tome Vd. una inspiración profunda.

178. Have you any pain in the shoulder-blades?
Avez-vous des douleurs dans les épaules?
Haben Sie Schmerzen in den Schulterblättern?
Avete dolori nelle spalle?
¿Tiene Vd. dolor en las hombros?

179. In the side?
Dans le côté?
In der Seite?
Nel fianco?
¿En el flanco?

180. In the back?
Dans le dos?
Im Rücken?
Nel dorso?
¿En la espalda?

181. Which side?
Quel côté?
Auf welcher Seite?
Quale lato?
¿En qué lado?

182. Right?
A droite?
Rechts?
A dritta?
¿Derecho?

183. Left?
A gauche?
Links?
A sinistra?
¿Izquierdo?

184. More at night?
Plus pendant la nuit?
Mehr bei Nacht?
Di più nella notte?
¿Mas durante la noche?

185. More in the daytime?
Plus pendant la journée?
Mehr bei Tag?
Pure nel giorno?
¿Mas durante el dia?

186. Do you expectorate much?
Expectorez-vous beaucoup?
Spucken Sie viel aus?
Sputate molto?
¿Expectora Vd. mucho?

187. About how much daily?
Combien à peu près par jour?
Ungefähr wie viel täglich?
Quanto al giorno in circa?
¿Mas ó menos que cantidad diaramente?

188. So much?
Autant?
So viel?
Tanto?
¿Tanto?

189. What is the color of your expectorations?
De quelle couleur est votre expectoration?
Welche Farbe hat der Speichel?
Che colore ha il vostro sputo?
¿Que color tiene la expectoración?

190. White?
Blanche?
Weiss?
Bianco?
¿Blanco?

191. Or yellow?
Jaune?
Gelb?
O gialliccio?
¿O amarillo?

192. Do you expectorate more?
Expectorez-vous plus?
Speien Sie mehr aus?
Sputate voi più?
¿Expectora Vd. mas?

193. Or less?
Ou moins?
Oder weniger?
O meno?
¿O menos?

194. Does it pain you to breathe?
Cela vous fait-il mal de respirer?
Spüren Sie Schmerzen beim Atmen?
Vi fa male di respirare?
¿Le duele al respirar?

195. Do you sweat much at night?
Transpirez-vous beaucoup la nuit?
Schwitzen Sie viel in der Nacht?
Sudate molto la notte?
¿Suda Vd. mucho de noche?

196. Have you lost flesh?
Avez-vous maigri?
Haben Sie abgenommen?
Siete dimagrito?
¿Ha perdido Vd. peso?

197. Sit down.
Asseyez-vous.
Setzen Sie sich.
Sedetevi.
Sientese Vd.

198. Stand up.
Levez-vous.
Stehen Sie auf.
Alzatevi.
Levantese Vd.

199. Walk a little way.
Allez quelques pas.
Gehen Sie einige Schritte.
Camminate un pò.
Ande Vd. algunos pasos.

200. Return; go backwards.
Revenez; allez en arrière.
Kommen Sie Aurück; gehen Sie rückwärts.
Ritornate; camminate all' indietro
Vuelva, ande Vd. para atras.

201. Do you feel like falling?
Vous semble-t-il que vous allez tomber?
Ist es Ihnen als ob Sie fallen müssten?
Vi sentite come se doveste cadere?
¿Le siente Vd. como que se caer?

202. Do you feel giddy?
Avez-vous le vertige?
Ist Ihnen schwindlig?
Avete delle vertigini?
¿Tiene Vd. vertigo?

203. Do you sometimes see things double?
Voyez-vous quelque-fois les choses en double?
Sehen Sie manchmal doppelt?
Vedete qualche volta le cose al doppio?
¿Vee Vd. algunas veces las cosas doble?

204. Let me see your eyes.
Montrez-moi vos yeux.
Lassen Sie mich Ihre Augen sehen
Fatemi vedere i vostri occhi.
Dejeme Vd. mirar sus ojos.

205. The eye.
L'œil.
Das Auge.
L' occhio.
El ojo.

206. The eyes.
Les yeux.
Die Augen.
Gli occhi.
Los ojos.

207. Look up.
Regardez en haut.
Schauen Sie hinauf.
Guardate sù.
Mire Vd. para arriba.

208. Look down.
Regardez en bas.
Schauen Sie hinunter.
Guardate abbasso.
Mire Vd. para abajo.

209. Look toward your nose.
Regardez vers votre nez.
Schauen Sie auf Ihre Nase.
Quardatevi il naso.
Mire Vd. á la nariz.

210. Look at me.
Regardez-moi.
Sehen Sie mich an.
Guardatemi.
Mireme Vd.

211. Did anything get into your eye?
Quelque chose vous est entrée dans l'oeil?
Ist Ihnen etwas ins Auge geflogen?
Vi è entrata qualche cosa nel l' occhio?
¿Le ha entrado algo en el ojo?

212. Did a stone hit you?
Vous a-t-on lançé une pierre?
Hat Sie ein Stein getroffen?
Vi hanno forse gettato una pietra?
¿Le han tirado una piedra?

213. Did you feel much pain at the time?
Avez-vous éprouvé beaucoup de douleurs alors?
Haben Sie gleich damals arge Schmerzen gespürt?
Avete sentito molto dolore allora?
¿Le ha dolido mucho entonces?

214. Is it worse now?
Est-ce pire maintenant?
Ist est jetzt schlimmer?
È peggio ora?
¿Está peor ahora?

215. Do your eyes water a good deal?
L'eau vous monte beaucoup aux yeux?
Tränen Ihre Augen stark?
Vi lacrimano gli occhi molto?
¿Le lagrimean mucho los ojos?

216. Can you not open your eye?
Ne pouvez-vous pas ouvrir l'œil?
Können Sie Ihr Auge nicht öffnen?
Non potete aprire il vostro occhio?
¿No puedę Vd. abrir el ojo?

217. Do not try to open it when you awaken.
N'essayez pas de l'ouvrir le matin en vous éveillant.
Versuchen Sie nicht, es beim Aufwachen zu öffnen.
Non forzate ad aprirlo nella mattina dopo il sonno.
No haga Vd. esfuerzos para abrirlo al dispertar.

218. I will give you something for that.
Je vous donnerai quelque chose pour cela.
Ich werde Ihnen etwas dafür geben.
Vi darò qualche cosa per questo.
Le daré algo para esto.

219. Use it regularly.
Servez-vous en régulièrement.
Gebrauchen Sie es regelmässig.
Usatelo regolarmente.
Tomale Vd. con regularidad.

220. Does the eyeball feel as if it were swollen?
L'œil vous semble-t-il gonflé?
Fühlt sich das Auge wie angeschwollen?
Vi pare come se il globo dell' occhio fosse gonfio?
¿El ojo le siente hinchado?

221. You must be careful not to go out yet.
Ayez soin de ne pas sortir.
Sie dürfen durchaus noch nicht ausgehen.
Dovete aver cura a non andar fuori.
Tenga Vd. cuidado de no salir todavía.

222. It would harm your eyes.
Cela nuirait à vos yeux.
Es würde Ihren Augen schaden.
Vi farà gran male ai vostri occhi.
Le haria daño á los ojos.

223. Since when has your eyesight failed you?
Depuis quand votre vue s'est elle diminuée?
Seit wann hat Ihre Sehkraft nachgelassen?
Da quando la vostra vista si è diminuita?
¿Desde cuando ha disminuido su vista?

224. Look here.
Regardez ici.
Schauen Sie hierher.
Guardate qui.
Mire Vd. para aca.

225. Can you see what this is on the wall?
Pouvez-vous voir ce que c'est sur le mur?
Können Sie sehen was hier an der Wand ist?
Potete vedere che cosa è questo nel muro?
¿Puede Vd. ver lo que esta en la pared?

226. You cannot?
Vous ne pouvez pas?
Sie können es nicht erkennen?
Non potete dire?
¿Vd. no puede?

227. Can you see it now?
Le voyez-vous maintenant?
Können Sie es jetzt sehen?
Potete vederlo adesso?
¿Le puede Vd. ver ahora?

228. And now?
Et maintenant?
Und nun?
Ed ora?
¿Y ahora?

229. What is it?
Qu'est-ce?
Was ist es?
Che cosa è?
¿Qué es esto?

230. Tell me what number it is.
Dites-moi quel est ce numéro.
Sagen Sie mir welche Nummer es ist.
Ditemi che numero è.
Digame Vd. que numero es este.

231. Tell me what letter it is.
Dites-moi quelle est cette lettre.
Nennen Sie mir diesen Buchstaben.
Ditemi che lettera è.
Digame Vd. que letra está.

232. Do you see things through a mist?
Voyez-vous tout á travers un brouillard?
Sehen Sie Alles durch einen Nebel?
Vedete cose come se fossero fra la nebbia?
¿Ve Vd. las cosas como en una niebla?

233. Can you see clearly?
Voyez-vous clairement?
Sehen Sie klar?
Potete vedere chiaro?
¿Puede Vd. ver claramente?

234. Better at a distance?
Mieux á une distance?
Besser aus einer Entfernung?
Meglio distanza?
¿Mejor á distancia?

235. Do exactly as I tell you.
Faites exactement ce que je vous dis.
Tun Sie genau wie ich Ihnen sage.
Fate esattamente ciò che io vi dico.
Haga Vd. exactamente como le digo.

236. It will get better.
Cela ira mieux.
Es wird besser werden.
Migliorerá.
Esto mejorará.

237. You must not lose courage.
Vous ne devez pas perdre courage.
Sie dürfen den Mut nicht verlieren.
Non dovete perdere corraggio.
No hay que perder el valor.

238. Let me see your hand.
Montrez-moi votre main.
Zeigen Sie mir Ihre Hand.
Fatemi vedere la vostra mano.
Enseñeme Vd. la mano.

239. Have you no power in it?
Est-elle complètement inerte?
Ist sie ganz kraftlos?
Non avete forza nella mano?
¿No tiene Vd. fuerza en la mano?

240. Grasp my hand.
Serrez-moi la main.
Drücken Sie mir die Hand.
Stringete la mia mano.
Apriete Vd. mi mano.

241. Can you not do it better than that?
Vous ne pouvez serrer plus fort que cela?
Können Sie nicht fester greifen?
Non potete farlo meglio?
¿No puede Vd. hacerlo mas fuerte?

242. Try again.
Essayez encore une fois.
Versuchen Sie es noch einmal.
Provateci di nuovo.
Prube Vd. otra vez.

243. The arm.
Le bras.
Der Arm.
Il braccio.
El brazo.

244. Since when is your arm so powerless?
Depuis quand votre bras a-t-il perdu la force?
Seit wann ist Ihr Arm so kraftlos?
Da quando il vostro braccio è senza forza?
¿Desde cuando no tiene Vd. fuerza en el brazo?

245. What did you feel in the beginning?
Qu'avez-vous senti au commencement?
Was haben Sie anfangs gespürt?
Che sentivate prima?
¿Qué ha sentido Vd. cuando esto empezó?

246. Shooting pains?
Des douleurs perçantes?
Stechende Schmerzen?
Dei dolori acuti?
¿Dolores agudos?

247. As if one were pricking you with pins?
Comme si on vous piquait avec des épingles?
Wie wenn man Sie mit Stecknadeln stäche?
Come se fossero delle spille?
¿Como si le estarian pieando con alfileres?

248. It came all of a sudden?
C'est venu tout d'un coup?
Ist es ganz plötzlich gekommen?
Venne tutto ad un tratto?
¿Ha venido de repente?

249. Early in the morning?
Le matin de bonne heure?
Frühmorgens?
Di buon mattino?
¿Temprano en la mañana?

250. Had you been drinking?
Vous-avez bu?
Waren Sie angetrunken?
Avevate bevuto?
¿Habia Vd. bebido?

251. Are you a drinking man?
Buvez-vous d'habitude?
Sind Sie Trinker?
Avete l' abito di bevere?
¿Tiene Vd. la costumbre de beber?

252. Had you been sleeping on your arm?
Vous êtes-vous endormi sur votre bras?
Sind Sie auf Ihrem Arm eingeschlafen?
Avete dormito col braccio sotto la testa?
¿Ha dormido Vd. encima del brazo?

253. You cannot remember?
Vous ne vous en souvenez pas?
Sie können sich nicht erinnern?
Non vi ricordate?
¿Vd. no puede recordarse?

254. Have you been much exposed to the wet weather?
Avez-vous été exposé au temps humide?
Sind Sie dem feuchten Wetter ausgesetzt gewesen?
Vi siete mai esposto alla umidità?
¿Ha estado Vd. mucho expuesto á la intemperie?

255. Raise your arm.
Levez le bras.
Heben Sie den Arm.
Alzate il vostro braccio.
Levante Vd. el brazo.

256. Raise it more.
Plus haut.
Höher.
Ancora di più.
Más alto.

257. Now the other one.
Maintenant l'autre.
Jetzt den andern
Adesso l'altro.
Ahora el otro.

258. Get up.
Levez-vous.
Stehen Sie auf.
Alzatevi.
Levantese Vd.

259. Can you not rise quicker?
Ne pouvez-vous pas vous lever plus vite?
Können Sie sich nicht schneller erheben?
Non vi potete alzare un po' più presto?
¿No puede Vd. levantarse más de prisa?

260. Is it impossible?
Est-ce impossible?
Ist es unmöglich?
È impossible?
¿Le es imposible?

261. That will do.
C'est assez.
Das ist genug.
Basta cosi.
Basta así.

262. Never mind.
N'importe.
Lassen Sie's gut sein.
Non importa.
No le hace.

263. Have you a pain in the pit of your stomach?
Avez-vous des douleurs dans le creux de l'estomac?
Haben Sie Schmerzen in der Magengrube?
Avete dolore nella bocca dello stomaco?
¿Tiene Vd. dolor en la boca del estomago?

264. Nausea.
La nausée.
Uebelkeit.
La nausea.
La nausea.

265. Does eating make you vomit?
Rendez-vous ce que vous mangez?
Erbrechen Sie nachdem Sie gegessen haben?
Mangiare vi fa vomitare?
¿El comer le hace vomitar?

266. When did your eyes begin to look yellow?
Quand vos yeux ont-ils commencé à prendre cette couleur jaune?
Wann begannen Ihre Augen so gelb auszusehen?
Da quando i vostri occhi son divenuti giallicci?
¿Cuando empezaban sus ojos a tener este color amarillo?

267. Have you stomach cramps?
Avez-vous des crampes d'estomac?
Haben Sie Magenkrämpfe?
Avete dolori acuti di stomaco?
¿Tiene Vd. calambre del estomago?

268. Since when is your tongue that color?
Depuis quand votre langue a-t-elle cette couleur?
Seit wann hat Ihre Zunge jene Farbe?
Da quando tempo la vostra lingua è di questo colore?
¿Desde cuando tiene su lengua este color?

269. Does your tongue feel swollen?
Est-ce que votre langue vous parait gonflée?
Fühlt sich Ihre Zunge wie angeschwollen?
Ve la sentite gonfia?
¿Le siente la lengua hinchada?

270. Have you ever had the chills?
Avez-vous jamais eu des frissons?
Haben Sie je Fieberfrösteln gehabt?
Avete mai avuto dei brividi di febbre?
¿Ha tenido Vd. escalofrios?

271. Do they come every day?
Les avez-vous tous les jours?
Kommt es jeden Tag?
Vi vengono tutti i giorni?
¿Les tiene Vd. cada dia?

272. At the same hour?
A la même heure?
Zur selben Stunde?
Alla stessa ora?
¿A la misma hora?

273. Have you any pain in the head?
Avez-vous des douleurs dans la tête?
Haben Sie Kopfschmerzen?
Avete dolori di testa?
¿Tiene Vd. dolor en la cabeza?

274. Did you fall, and how did you fall?
Etes-vous tombé? et comment êtes-vous tombé?
Sind Sie gefallen und wie sind Sie gefallen?
Siete caduto, e come siete caduto?
¿Ha caido Vd.? y como?

275. Did you faint?
Vous êtes-vous évanoui?
Sind Sie ohnmächtig geworden?
Siete svenuto?
¿Se ha desmayado Vd.?

276. Have you ever had fainting spells?
Avez-vous jamais eu des évanouissements?
Haben Sie je Ohnmachtsanfälle gehabt?
Siete mai svenuto regolarmente?
¿Ha tenido Vd. desmayos?

277. At intervals?
De temps à autre?
Dann und wann?
Ad intervalli?
¿De vez en cuando?

278. Are you subject to them?
Y êtes-vous sujet?
Haben Sie dieselben häufig?
Ne siete soggetto?
¿Se desmaya Vd. con frecuencia?

279. Had you them?
Les avez-vous eu?
Haben Sie dieselben gehabt?
Ne avete avuto?
¿Los ha tenido Vd.?

280. Never?
Jamais?
Niemals?
Mai?
¿Nunca?

281. How did this illness begin?
Comment cette maladie a-t-elle commencé?
Wie hat diese Krankheit begonnen?
Come ha incominciato questa malattia?
¿Como ha empezado este enfermedad?

282. When were you first taken sick?
Quand cette maladie a-t-elle commencé?
Wann hat diese Krankheit begonnen?
Quando vi siete ammalato la prima volta?
¿Cuando ha empezado este enfermedad?

283. Have you any pain in your bones?
Avez-vous des douleurs dans les os?
Haben Sie Schmerzen in den Knochen?
Vi sentite dei dolori nelle ossa?
¿Tiene Vd. dolor en los huesos?

284. The nerves?
Les nerfs?
Die Nerven?
I nervi?
¿Los nervios?

285. Are you nervous?
Etes-vous nerveux?
Sind Sie nervös?
Siete nervoso?
¿Esta Vd. nervioso?

286. The veins.
Les veines.
Die Adern.
Le vene.
Las venas.

287. The muscles.
Les muscles.
Die Muskeln.
I muscoli.
Los musculos.

288. The skull.
Le crâne.
Der Schädel.
El craneo.
El cerebro.

289. The temples.
Les tempes.
Die Schläfen.
Le tempia.
Las sienes.

290. The gums.
Les gencives.
Die Gaumen.
Le gengive.
Las encias.

291. The throat.
La gorge.
Der Hals.
La gola.
La garganta.

292. The neck.
Le cou.
Der Nacken.
Il collo.
El cuello.

293. The elbow.
Le coude.
Der Ellenbogen.
Il gomito.
El codo.

294. The thumb.
Le pouce.
Der Daumen.
Il police.
El dedo pulgar.

295. The foot.
Le pied.
Der Fuss.
Il piede.
El pié.

296. The leg.
La jambe.
Das Bein.
La gamba.
La pierna.

297. When did you sprain your foot?
Quand vous êtes-vous foulé le pied?
Wann haben Sie sich den Fuss verrenkt?
Quando vi siete dislocato il vostro piede?
¿Cuando se torcio Vd. el pié?

298. The stomach.
L'estomac.
Der Magen.
Lo stomaco.
El estomago.

299. The ribs.
Les côtes.
Die Rippen.
Le costole.
Las costillas.

300. The thigh.
La hanche.
Die Hüfte.
La coscia.
El muslo.

301. The heel.
Le talon.
Die Ferse.
Il calcagno.
El talon.

302. The lungs.
Les poumons.
Die Lungen.
I polmoni.
Los pulmones.

303. The liver.
Le foie.
Die Leber.
Il fegato.
El higado.

304. Did you ever have a liver disease?
Avez-vous jamais eu une maladie de foie?
Haben Sie je eine Leberkrankheit gehabt?
Avete mai avuto una malattia del fegato?
¿Ha tenido Vd. enfermedad del higado?

305. The hearing.
L'ouïe.
Das Gehör.
L' udito.
El oido.

306. Is it affected?
Est-elle affectée?
Ist es angegriffen?
È ammalato?
¿Está afectado?

307. Your memory.
Votre mémoire.
Ihr Gedächtniss.
La vuestra memoria.
Su memoria.

308. Is it good?
Est-elle bonne?
Ist es gut?
È essa buona?
¿Está buena?

309. Toothache.
Le mal aux dents.
Zahnschmerzen.
Dolor di denti.
Dolor de dientes.

310. Tuberculosis.
Tuberculose.
Tuberculose.
Tuberculosi.
Tuberculosis.

311. The skin.
La peau.
Die Haut.
La pelle.
El cutis.

312. A wound.
Une plaie.
Eine Wunde.
Una piaga.
Una llaga.

313. A corn.
Un cor.
Ein Hühnerauge.
Un callo.
El callo.

314. Did a dog bite you?
Un chien vous a-t-il mordu?
Hat Sie ein Hund gebissen?
Vi ha morsicato un cane?
¿Le ha mordido un perro?

315. Did a fly sting you?
Une mouche vous a-t-elle piqué?
Hat Sie eine Fliege gestochen?
Vi ha punto una mosca?
¿Le ha picado una mosca?

316. Did you prick yourself with a pin?
Vous êtes-vous piqué avec une épingle?
Haben Sie sich mit einer Stecknadel gestochen?
Vi siete punto con una spilla?
¿Se ha picado Vd. con un alfiler?

317. Since when have you this eruption?
Depuis quand avez-vous cette éruption?
Seit wann haben Sie dieser Ausschlag?
Da quanto tempo avete questa eruzione?
¿Desde cuando tiene Vd. esta erupcion?

318. Does it irritate much?
Cela irrite beaucoup?
Ist es sehr reizbar?
Vi irrita molto?
¿Le irrita mucho?

319. Did you take anything for it?
Avez-vous pris quelque chose pour cela?
Haben Sie etwas dafür genommen?
Avete preso qualche cosa per curarvi?
¿Ha tomado Vd. algo para curarlo?

320. Your arm feels paralyzed?
Votre bras vous parait être paralysé?
Ihr Arm erscheint Ihnen gelähmt?
Vi sentite il braccio paralizzato?
¿Su brazo se siente paralizado?

321. What have you worked at?
A quoi avez-vous travaillé?
Was haben Sie gearbeitet?
A che lavorate?
¿Que trabajo ha hecho Vd.?

322. This might be a case of lead poisoning.
Ceci pourrait être un cas d'empoisonnement causé par le plomb.
Dies ist möglicherweise eine Blutvergiftung durch Blei herbeigeführt.
Potrà essere un caso di avvelenamento da piombo.
Este podria ser envenenamiento por plomo.

323. I will use electricity.
Je me servirai de l'électricité.
Ich werde elektrischen Strom anwenden.
Userò dell' electricità.
Usaré electricidad.

324. You will get better.
Cela ira mieux.
Es wird besser werden.
Vi sentirete meglio.
Vd. mejorará.

325. Have you ever had hemorrhages?
Avez-vous jamais eu des hémorragies?
Haben Sie je Blutergüsse gehabt?
Avete avuto sbocco di sangue mai?
¿Ha tenido Vd. hemorragia?

326. You must not speak.
Vous ne devez pas parler.
Sie dürfen nicht sprechen.
Non dovete parlare.
No debe hablar.

327. Swallow small pieces of cracked ice.
Avalez des petits morceaux de glace.
Schlucken Kleine Eisstücke.
Ingoiate dei piccoli pezzettini di ghiaccio.
Trague Vd. pequeñas pieza de hielo.

328. Keep very quiet.
Restez bien tranquille.
Verhalten Sie sich sehr ruhig.
State tranquillo.
Quedese muy quieto.

329. Have you a pain in your side?
Avez-vous mal au côté?
Haben Sie Seitenschmerzen?
Avete dolori al fianco?
¿Tiene Vd. un dolor en el costado?

330. Did you burn yourself?
Vous êtes-vous brûlé?
Haben Sie sich verbrannt?
Vi siete bruciato?
¿Se ha quemado Vd.?

331. Did you sprain your foot?
Vous êtes-vous foulé le pied?
Haben Sie Ihren Fuss verstaucht?
Vi avete dislocato il piede?
¿Se torció Vd. el pie?

332. Hoarseness.
Enrouement.
Heiserkeit.
Raucedine.
Ronquera.

333. Have you a sore throat?
Avez-vous mal à la gorge?
Haben Sie Halsschmerzen?
Avete mal di gola?
¿Le duele la garganta?

334. Does it hurt you to swallow?
Avez-vous de la peine à avaler?
Spüren Sie Schmerzen beim Schlucken?
Vi fa male d'ingojare?
¿Le duele el tragar?

335. Does it hurt you to open your mouth?
Cela vous fait-il mal d'ouvrir la bouche?
Spüren Sie Schmerzen wenn Sie den Mund öffnen?
Vi fa male di aprire la bocca?
¿Le duele el abrir la boca?

336. The ear.
L'oreille.
Das Ohr.
L'orecchio.
El oido.

337. The ears.
Les oreilles.
Die Ohren.
Le orecchie.
Los oidos.

338. Have you ringing in the ears?
Avez-vous des bourdonnements d'oreilles?
Haben Sie Ohrenbrausen?
Vi tentennano le orecchie?
¿Tiene Vd. campaneo en los oidos?

339. Have you discharge from the ears?
La matière vous coule-t-elle des oreilles?
Eitern Ihre Ohren?
Vi sorte umore dalle orecchie?
¿Le sale material de los oidos?

340. Take one teaspoonful three times daily (in water).
Prenez-en une cuillerée à thé trois fois par jour (dans de l'eau).
Nehmen Sie einen Teelöffel voll dreimal täglich (in Wasser).
Bevetene un cucchiaio da tè tre volte al giorno (nell' acqua).
Toma Vd. una cucharadita de tè tres veces al dia (con agua).

341. Take two teaspoonfuls three times daily (in water).
Prenez-en deux cuillerées à thé trois fois par jour (dans de l'eau).
Nehmen Sie zwei Teelöffel voll dreimal täglich (in Wasser).
Bevetene due cucchiai da tè tre volte al giorno (nell' acqua).
Toma Vd. dos cucharaditas de té tres veces al dia (con agua).

342. Take three teaspoonfuls three times daily (in water).
Prenez-en trois cuillerées à thé trois fois par jour (dans de l'eau).
Nehmen Sie drei Teelöffel voll dreimal täglich (in Wasser).
Bevetene tre cucchiai da tè tre volte al giorno (nell' acqua).
Toma Vd. tres cucharaditas de té tres veces al dia (con agua).

343. Before meals.
Avant les repas.
Vor den Mahlzeiten.
Prima del pasto.
Antes de comer.

344. After meals.
Après les repas.
Nach den Mahlzeiten.
Dopo il pasto.
Despues de comer.

345. A pill.
Une pilule.
Eine Pille.
Una pillola.
Una pildora.

346. A powder.
Une poudre.
Ein Pulver.
Una polvere.
Un polvo.

347. Every hour.
Chaque heure.
Jede Stunde.
Ogni ora.
Cada hora.

348. Every two hours.
Toutes les deux heures.
Alle zwei Stunden.
Ogni due ore.
Cada dos horas.

349. Every three hours.
Toutes les trois heures.
Alle drei Stunden.
Ogni tre ore.
Cada tres horas.

350. Every four hours.
Toutes les quatre heures.
Alle vier Stunden.
Ogni quattro ore.
Cada cuatro horas.

351. Gargle.
Gargarisez.
Gurgeln Sie.
Gargarizzate.
Hacer gargaras.

352. Use injection.
Injectez.
Injizieren Sie.
Injettate.
Tomar una inyección.

353. Snuff.
Prisez.
Schnupfen Sie.
Annasate.
Aspirar (por la nariz).

354. Take a purgative.
Un purgatif.
Nehmen Sie ein Abführmittel.
Un purgativo.
Tome Vd. una purga.

355. Drop into one eye.
Laissez dégoutter dans un œil.
Träufeln Sie in das eine Auge.
Fate sgocciolare nell' occhio.
Vierta gotas en un ojo.

356. Drop into each eye.
Laissez dégoutter dans chaque œil.
Träufeln Sie in beide Augen.
Fate sgocciolare in ciascun occhio.
Vierta gotas en cada ojo.

357. Drop into right eye.
Laissez dégoutter dans l'œil droit.
Traüfeln Sie ins rechte Auge.
Fate sgocciolare nell' occhio.
Vierta gotas en el ojo derecho.

358. Drop into left eye.
Laissez dégoutter dans l'œil gauche.
Traüfeln Sie ins linke Auge.
Fate sgocciolare nell' occhio sinistro.
Vierta gotas en el ojo izquierdo.

359. Three times daily.
Trois fois par jour.
Dreimal täglich.
Tre volte al giorno.
Tres veces al dia.

360. In the morning.
Le matin.
Am Morgen.
Al mattino.
Por la mañano.

361. At noon.
A midi.
Mittags.
A mezzo giorno.
A mediodia.

362. At night.
Le soir.
Abends.
Alla sera.
Por la noche.

363. At bed-time.
A l'heure de se coucher.
Vor dem Schlafengehen.
All' ora di coricarsi.
Al acostarse.

364. Apply bandage to—.
Mettez un bandage à.
Nehmen Sie Bandagen.
Mettete una fasciatura.
Ponga Vd. un bendaje á—.

365. Apply ointment.
Appliquez un onguent.
Verwenden Sie Salbe.
Applicate un unguento.
Apliquese unguento.

366. Bathe with hot water.
Baignez avec de l'eau chaude.
Baden Sie mit heissem Wasser.
Bagnate con acqua calda.
Bañe con agua caliente.

367. Bathe with cold water.
Baignez avec de l'eau froide.
Baden Sie mit kaltem Wasser.
Bagnate con acqua fredda.
Bañe con agua fria.

368. Bathe with alcohol.
Baignez avec de l'alcool.
Baden Sie mit Alkohol.
Bagnate con lo spirito.
Bañe con alcohol.

369. Take a bath.
Prenez un bain.
Nehmen Sie ein Bad.
Prendete un bagno.
Tome Vd. un baño.

370. A sponge bath.
Un bain à l'éponge.
Ein Schwamm Bad.
Un bagno con la spugna.
Un baño con esponja.

371. A bran bath.
Un bain au son.
Ein Kleie Bad.
Un bagno con crusca.
Un baño con salvado.

372. A soda bath.
Un bain à la soude.
Ein Soda Bad.
Un bagno con soda.
Un baño con soda.

373. Paint the swelling with this.
Vous devez peindre l'enflure avec ceci.
Pinseln Sie die Geschwulst damit.
Dovete pitturare il gonfiore con questo.
Hay que pintar el hinchazon con esto.

Notes

Notes

Notes

Notes